W9-CYV-747

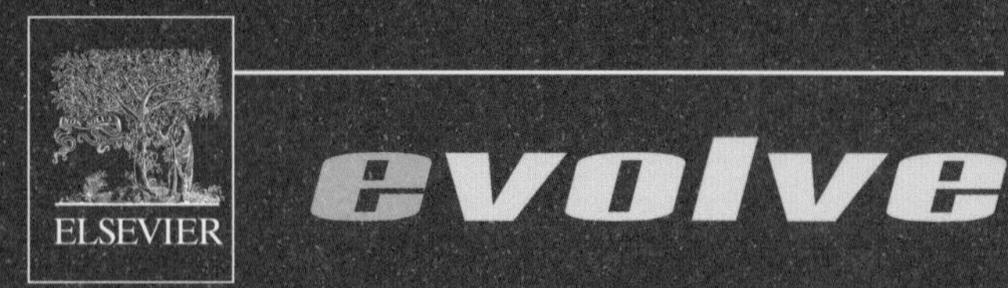

To access your Student Resources, visit the Web address below:

http://evolve.elsevier.com/Phipps

- **WebLinks**
  An exciting resource that lets you link to hundreds of websites carefully chosen to supplement the content of the textbook. The WebLinks are regularly updated, with new ones added as they develop.

Medical-Surgical Nursing

Health and Illness Perspectives

Medical-Surgical Nursing

Health and Illness Perspectives

Seventh Edition

Wilma J. Phipps, PhD, RN, FAAN
Professor Emeritus, Frances Payne Bolton School of Nursing
Case Western Reserve University
Cleveland, Ohio

Frances D. Monahan, PhD, RN
Professor and Director, Department of Nursing
Rockland Community College
State University of New York
Suffern, New York

Judith K. Sands, EdD, RN
Associate Professor, School of Nursing
University of Virginia
Charlottesville, Virginia

Jane F. Marek, MSN, RN, CS, CRNP
Adult Nurse Practitioner
Instructor, Frances Payne Bolton School of Nursing
Case Western Reserve University
Cleveland, Ohio

Marianne Neighbors, EdD, RN
Professor, School of Nursing
University of Arkansas
Fayetteville, Arkansas

ASSOCIATE EDITOR
Carol J. Green PhD, RN
Professor, Department of Nursing
Johnson County Community College
Overland Park, Kansas

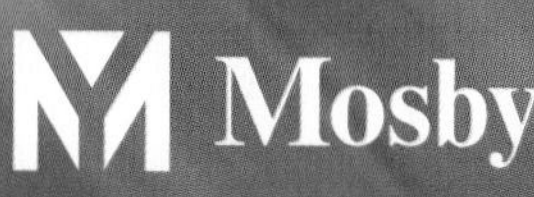

An Affiliate of Elsevier

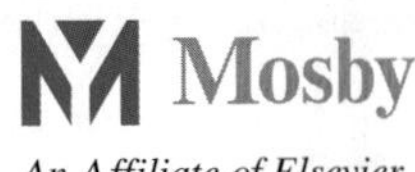

An Affiliate of Elsevier

11830 Westline Industrial Drive
St. Louis, Missouri 63146

MEDICAL-SURGICAL NURSING: HEALTH AND ILLNESS PERSPECTIVES,
SEVENTH EDITION

ISBN: 0-323-01804-1

NOTICE

Pharmacology is an ever-changing field. Standard safety precautions must be followed, but as new research and clinical experience broaden our knowledge, changes in treatment and drug therapy may become necessary or appropriate. Readers are advised to check the most current product information provided by the manufacturer of each drug to be administered to verify the recommended dose, the method and duration of administration, and contraindications. It is the responsibility of the licensed prescriber, relying on experience and knowledge of the patient, to determine dosages and the best treatment for each individual patient. Neither the publisher nor the author assumes any liability for any injury and/or damage to persons or property arising from this publication.

The Publisher

Library of Congress Cataloging-in-Publication Data

Medical-surgical nursing : health and illness perspectives / [edited by] Wilma J. Phipps ...[et al.].—7th ed.
p. ; cm.
Includes bibliographical references and index.
ISBN 0-323-01804-1
1. Nursing. 2. Surgical nursing. I. Phipps, Wilma J., 1925-
[DNLM: 1. Nursing Care. 2. Perioperative Nursing. 3. Nursing Process. WY 161 M4894 2003]
RT41 .M49 2003
610.73—dc21 2002029353

Vice President, Publishing Director: Sally Schrefer
Executive Editor: Michael S. Ledbetter
Senior Developmental Editor: Laurie K. Muench
Publishing Services Manager: Deborah Vogel
Project Manager: Mary E. Drone
Design Manager: Bill Drone

Chapter opening art created by: Julia E. Sokol, Philadelphia, PA

GW/QWK

Printed in China

Last digit is the print number: 9 8 7 6 5 4 3

We dedicate this book:

To my son, Charlie, for his encouragement during the completion of this manuscript

WJP

To the memory of my husband, William T. Monahan – the love and inspiration of my life

FDM

To the loving memory of my father, John C. Sarver, always my biggest fan

JKS

To Ian James Frank

JFM

To my husband and best friend, Larry Butler; my parents, Louis and Lillian Zadra; my sister, Marji Swickrath; and the rest of my family and friends who helped me get through this trying year with a smile

MN

Contributors

Sharon Aronovitch, PhD, RN, CETN
Assistant Professor, School of Nursing
Florida State University
Tallahassee, Florida

Kathleen Barta, MSN, RN, EdD
Associate Professor, Eleanor Mann School of Nursing
University of Arkansas
Fayetteville, Arkansas

Mary Jo Boehnlein, MSN, RN
Director of Perioperative Services
MetroHealth Medical Center
Cleveland, Ohio

Ellen K. Boyda, MS, RN, CRNP
Family Nurse Practitioner
Haverford College, Haverford, Pennsylvania;
Private Practice, Wilmington, Delaware

Sally Brozenec, PhD, RN
Assistant Professor, College of Nursing
Rush University
Chicago, Illinois

Bill Buron, MSN, RNC, FNP
Nursing Instructor
University of Arkansas
Fayetteville, Arkansas

Kim Bender Bushnell, MSN, RN
Interim Director, Nursing Program
Anne Arundel Community College
Arnold, Maryland

Pamela D. Dennison, MSN, RN
Clinician IV
University of Virginia Health System
Charlottesville, Virginia

Carolyn Eddins, MN, RN, CETN
Assistant Professor, School of Nursing
University of Virginia
Charlottesville, Virginia

Peggy Ellis, PhD, RN, FNP
Clinical Associate Professor
University of Missouri—St. Louis
St. Louis, Missouri

Jeanne M. Erickson, MSN, RN, AOCN
Clinical Instructor, School of Nursing
University of Virginia
Charlottesville, Virginia

Lisa Forsythe, MSN, RN
Clinician IV
University of Virginia Health System
Charlottesville, Virginia

Diane E. Fritsch, MSN, RN, CCRN, CS
Clinical Nurse Specialist
MetroHealth Medical Center
Cleveland, Ohio

Kathy Henley Haugh, MSN, RN
Assistant Professor, School of Nursing
University of Virginia
Charlottesville, Virginia

Cynthia Hollamon, MSN, RN, APN, CNP
Nurse Practitioner
University Hospitals of Cleveland
Cleveland, Ohio

Shelley Yerger Huffstutler, MSN, RN, DSN, FNP
Associate Professor, School of Nursing
University of Virginia
Charlottesville, Virginia

Carol Genet Kelley, PhD, RN, ANP, FNP, GNP
Project Director
Case Western Reserve University
Cleveland, Ohio

Arlene Keeling, PhD, RN
Associate Professor, School of Nursing
University of Virginia
Charlottesville, Virginia

Glenda Lawson, PhD, RN, APN
Associate Professor, Eleanor Mann School of Nursing
University of Arkansas
Fayetteville, Arkansas

Molly Loney, MSN, RN, AOCN
Education Nurse Specialist
Cleveland Clinic Foundation
Cleveland, Ohio

Carol Lynn Maxwell-Thompson, MSN, RN, FNP
Instructor, School of Nursing
University of Virginia
Charlottesville, Virginia

Joyce A. McConaughy, PhD, RN, CNS
Instructor, Eleanor Mann School of Nursing
University of Arkansas
Fayetteville, Arkansas

Michael McGillion, BScN, RN
Instructor, Department of Nursing
University of Toronto
Toronto, Ontario, Canada

Carol Meadows, MSNc, RNP, APN
Instructor, Eleanor Mann School of Nursing
University of Arkansas
Fayetteville, Arkansas

Gretchen G. Mettler, MS, RN, CNM
Instructor, Frances Payne Bolton School of Nursing
Case Western Reserve University
Cleveland, Ohio

Diana Lynn Morris, PhD, RN, FAAN
Associate Professor, Frances Payne Bolton School of Nursing
Associate Director for Programming
University Center on Aging and Health
Case Western Reserve University
Cleveland, Ohio

Lois Perry, MSN, RN, FNP
Clinician III, Outcomes Manager
University of Virginia Hospital
Charlottesville, Virginia

Kathryn B. Reid, MSN, RN, CCRN, FNP
Instructor, School of Nursing
University of Virginia
Charlottesville, Virginia

Katherine Russell, MSN, RN, ACNP
Adjunct Professor, School of Nursing
University of Virginia
Charlottesville, Virginia

Angela Sammarco, PhD, RN
Assistant Professor, Department of Nursing
College of Staten Island
City University of New York
Staten Island, New York

Lepaine Sharp-McHenry, MSN, RN, FACDONA
Consultant, Long-Term Care Nursing
Fayetteville, Arkansas

Sarah C. Smith, MA, RN, CRNO
Advanced Practice Nurse/Educational Associate
Department of Ophthalmology and Visual Sciences
University of Iowa Health Care
Iowa City, Iowa

Nan Smith-Blair, PhD, RN
Assistant Professor, Eleanor Mann School of Nursing
University of Arkansas
Fayetteville, Arkansas

Andreana Siu, DNSc, RN
Nurse Practitioner, Cardiology Division
VA Palo Alto Health Care System
Palo Alto, California

Audrey Snyder, MSN, RN, ACNP-CS
Instructor, School of Nursing
University of Virginia
Charlottesville, Virginia

Marianne C. Tawa, MSN, RN, ANP
Nurse Practitioner, Dermatology and Cutaneous Oncology
Dana Farber Cancer Institute
Boston, Massachusetts

Margaret M. Ulchaker, MSN, RN, CDE, NP-C
Adult Nurse Practitioner
Director of Patient Education/Research Coordinator
North Coast Institute of Diabetes and Endocrinology, Inc.
Westlake, Ohio

Judith H. Watt-Watson, PhD, RN
Graduate Coordinator, Associate Professor
University of Toronto
Toronto, Ontario, Canada

Kelly A. Weigel, MSN, RN, CNP
Instructor, School of Medicine
Case Western Reserve University
Cleveland, Ohio

Lynne C. Yurko, BSN, RN, CNA
Nurse Manager
MetroHealth Medical Center
Cleveland, Ohio

Reviewers

Deborah A. Bechtel-Blackwell, RNC, BSN, MS, PhD, WHCNP, ANP
Assistant Professor
University of South Carolina at Columbia
Columbia, South Carolina

Nancy Becker, RN, MS
Dean of Allied Health/Director of Nursing
Lehigh Carbon Community College
Schnecksville, Pennsylvania

Selma F. Brophy, RN, C, MSN, PhD
Associate Professor, College of Nursing
University of Wisconsin—Oshkosh
Oshkosh, Wisconsin

Teresa S. Burckhalter, RNC, MSN
ADN Faculty
Technical College of the Lowcountry
Beaufort, South Carolina

Joanne D. Cimorelli, RN, BS, CNOR, CRNFA
RN First Assistant
First Assistant Services
Havertown, Pennsylvania

Janet Coyne, RN, MSN
Instructor, School of Nursing
Crouse Hospital
Syracuse, New York

Mary E. Hanson-Zalot, RN, MSN, AOCN
Clinical Instructor, School of Nursing
Methodist Hospital
Philadelphia, Pennsylvania

Pameula S. Johnson, CCRN
Clinical Educator, Critical Care and Emergency Services
Nash HealthCare System
Wilson, North Carolina

Sharon Lambert, RN, DNS
Assistant Professor
McKendree College
Lebanon, Illinois

Holly Evans Madison, RN, MS
Chair, Nursing Department
Southern Vermont College
Bennington, Vermont

Deborah Marantides, RN, BSN, MSN, CS
Nurse Practitioner
VA Medical Center, University Hospitals of Cleveland
Cleveland, Ohio

Phyllis Peterson, RN, MN, AOCN
Assistant Professor
Our Lady of Holy Cross College
New Orleans, Louisiana

Anne R. Rentfro, RN, MSN, CS
Associate Professor
University of Texas at Brownsville
Brownsville, Texas

Bruce Austin Scott, RN, CS
Nursing Instructor, San Joaquin Delta College
Staff Nurse, Saint Joseph's Behavioral Health Center
Stockton, California

Louise A. Shirk, RN, BSN, MSN
Nursing Instructor
Midlands Technical College
Columbia, South Carolina

Thelma Allen Stich, RNC, CS, CDE
Assistant Professor, College of Nursing
Seton Hall University
South Orange, New Jersey

Margaret A. Tufts, RNC, BS, MS
Assistant Professor of Nursing
Quinnipiac University
Hamden, Connecticut

Linda Ulak, RN, EdD
Associate Professor, College of Nursing
Chair, Undergraduate Nursing
Seton Hall University
South Orange, New Jersey

Nancy C. Verdirame, RN, BSN, MSN
Instructor, Louise Obici School of Nursing
Suffolk, Virginia

Ann White, RN, PhD, MBA, CNA
Undergraduate Nursing Coordinator
University of Southern Indiana
Evansville, Indiana

Preface

The vision for this seventh edition of *Medical-Surgical Nursing* is of a text that presents the student with clear, comprehensive knowledge essential to practice. It uses a framework of supporting theory drawn from the health, natural, social and behavioral sciences, providing insight into the depth and breath of knowledge on which the discipline of nursing is based. Further, the text places knowledge within the context of current practice issues, models, and settings.

Chapters 1 through 18 address essential aspects of practice that cross the practice lines of specific areas of medical-surgical nursing. Included are chapters that focus on varied practice settings such as emergency, critical, acute, long-term, and home care; specific patient populations such as the older adult, the perioperative patient, and the dying patient; and nonspecific problems related to areas such as fluids and electrolytes, inflammation, and infection. A new chapter on Complementary and Alternative Therapies and new related boxes in various chapters orient the student not only to the use of these therapies as part of the patient's treatment plan but also to the need to assess for their use as part of ongoing self-care to develop an appropriate plan of care.

The focus of the balance of the chapters is on the management of specific medical-surgical problems grouped according to body system. An assessment chapter reviews anatomy and physiology, presents comprehensive directions for obtaining health history and physical assessment data, and discusses laboratory and other diagnostic studies, orienting the student to the care of patients with problems within each body system. One or more chapters discuss specific problems of the system. In these chapters specific disorders are discussed in terms of etiology, epidemiology, pathophysiology, and collaborative care. The collaborative care section includes diagnostic and management information, concisely presenting conditions and providing a comprehensive view of treatment, regardless of which professional member of the health care team is responsible for its direct implementation. Conditions that have a major independent nursing role are presented with a nursing care section developed around the Nursing Process steps of assessment, nursing diagnosis, planning, intervention, and evaluation and/or Patient Education.

Comprehensive knowledge essential to practice is highlighted in a variety of ways. Guidelines for Safe Practice boxes present the "how to's" of care in a detailed step-by-step format. Patient Teaching boxes present detailed patient teaching guidelines. Clinical Manifestations boxes for all major disease entities make information on signs and symptoms readily accessible. Nursing assessment sections in each Assessment chapter clearly direct the student how to perform an appropriate health assessment, and Geriatric Assessment boxes in these chapters reinforce the adaptations required to care effectively for this growing population.

The overall clarity of the presentation is enhanced by consistency from chapter to chapter. For example, all nursing diagnoses are from NANDA. Under Planning, all goals are in the future tense, and Evaluation statements are in the present tense. All Gerontologic Assessment boxes are found in the same location in each Assessment chapter and are organized in the same format. All Patient Teaching is presented in concise, easy-to-follow statements.

Nursing care plans are included throughout the text to reinforce the nursing role in the management of selected problems. These are consistent in format and use NANDA diagnoses, but they also identify NIC priority interventions and NOC suggested outcomes, placing the plans in the forefront of contemporary practice. Sample Clinical Pathways are included to reinforce current concepts of collaborative care. Healthy People 2010 boxes and Future Watch boxes further focus the student on the changing nature of professional practice and the need for continuing education. Research boxes are integrated throughout to provide applications to today's nursing practice, and Evidence-Based Practice boxes emphasize the importance of applying research to practice.

ANCILLARIES

Instructor's Resource, available on CD-ROM or online, includes chapter outlines, objectives, and overviews; teaching suggestions for classroom and practice applications; additional critical thinking questions; an updated 1500-question test bank in NCLEX format; and a collection of over 200 full-color images from the text.

CD-ROM Companion, packaged with the text, includes critical thinking case studies, review questions, and a vocabulary review with sound pronunciations.

Study Guide has been revised to include more activities, questions, and case studies designed to enhance student learning and stimulate critical thinking.

ACKNOWLEDGMENTS

A special thanks goes to the contributors of the sixth edition; their expertise and knowledge of current clinical practice added to the relevance and accuracy of the content and provided a strong base for this revision.

Wilma J. Phipps
Frances D. Monahan
Judith K. Sands
Jane F. Marek
Marianne Neighbors

Contents

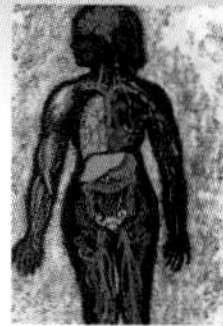

Unit I
PERSPECTIVES FOR NURSING PRACTICE

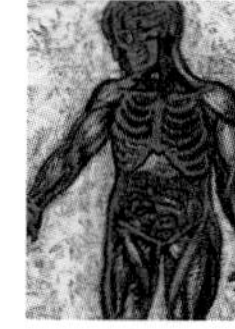

Unit II
CARE SETTINGS

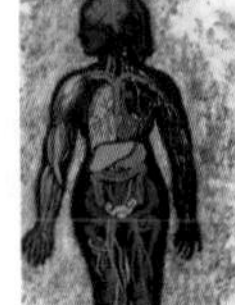

UNIT III COMMON PROBLEMS IN THE CARE OF ADULTS

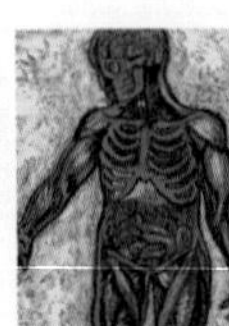

UNIT IV PERIOPERATIVE NURSING

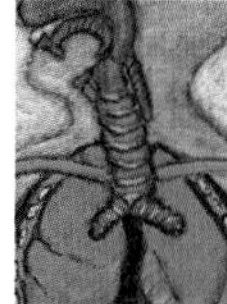

UNIT V
RESPIRATORY PROBLEMS

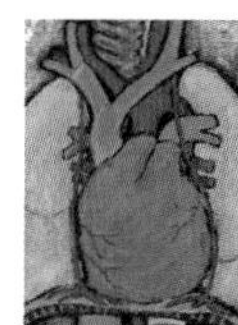

UNIT VI
CARDIOVASCULAR PROBLEMS

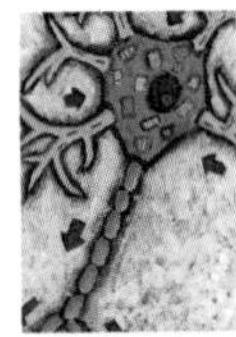

UNIT XII NEUROLOGIC PROBLEMS

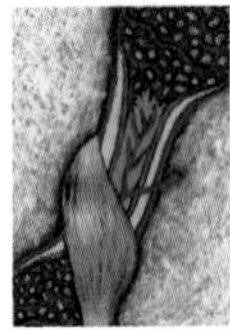

UNIT XIII MUSCULOSKELETAL PROBLEMS

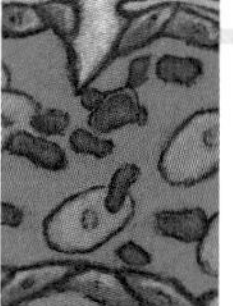

UNIT XIV Immunologic Problems

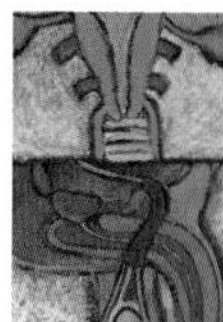

UNIT XV REPRODUCTIVE PROBLEMS

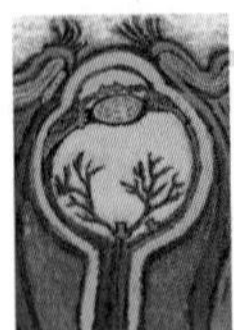

UNIT XVI EYE PROBLEMS

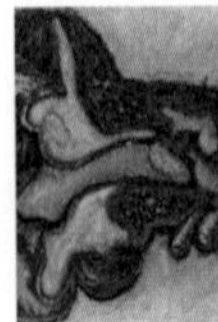

UNIT XVII EAR PROBLEMS

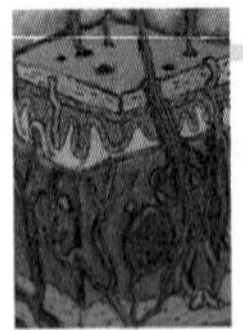

UNIT XVIII SKIN PROBLEMS

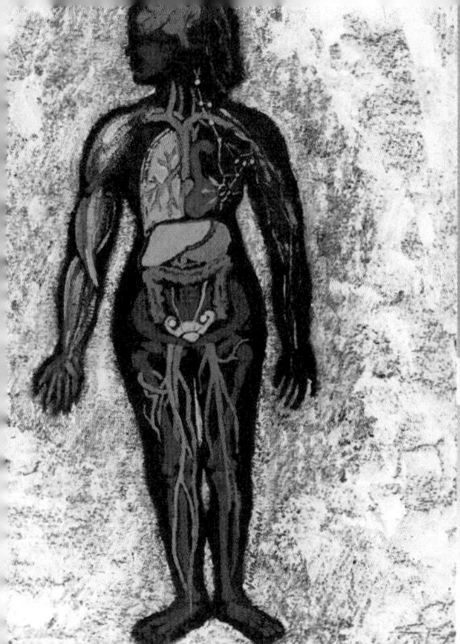

1 Medical-Surgical Nursing Today

Judith K. Sands

Objectives

After studying this chapter, the learner should be able to:

1. Discuss the major social and economic forces influencing the health care delivery system and the practice of professional medical-surgical nursing.
2. Describe the unique challenges confronting medical-surgical nursing practice in hospital settings.
3. Discuss how the future role of the medical-surgical nurse differs from the role practiced by most nurses today.
4. Outline the ways in which the nursing shortage of the early years of the twenty-first century is believed to be both different and more complex than nursing shortages of the past.
5. Identify the forces that have contributed to the expansion and acceptance of advanced practice nursing in the health care system.

The Chinese character for crisis, simultaneously representing both danger and opportunity, provides an appropriate background for any discussion of medical-surgical nursing practice in the early years of the twenty-first century. The danger is very real. The dramatic changes that have occurred in the last decade and a half have radically altered patient care. The hospital nursing workforce has been steadily eroded and replaced with a variety of minimally trained assistive personnel. Hospital stays continue to shorten while the patients in the beds become sicker and sicker. Technologic capabilities continue to expand at a furious pace and continuously raise the standards and expectations for bedside nursing practice. Overwhelming if not directly hostile work environments are driving increasing numbers of professional nurses away from acute care practice, and the next cycle of nursing shortage is clearly gaining strength nationwide. Nursing leaders and futurists alike suggest that this shortage may be different from those of the past in several significant ways. Widespread dissatisfaction about staffing levels and working conditions exist among professional nurses, and very real budgetary constraints negate the likelihood of an easy fix to these concerns. At the same time schools of nursing at all levels are reporting a steady erosion in enrollment levels while a relentless "graying" of the nursing workforce is occurring.

However, the picture is far from completely bleak. This is also a time of unprecedented opportunity for medical-surgical nurses, rich with both promise and excitement. Short hospital stays have greatly expanded the opportunities for nurses in home health, roles that are substantially different from those of the traditional public health nurse. Advanced practice roles of all types continue to evolve, and well-educated, experienced nurses are proving their worth in the system in a myriad of ways. Primary care nurse practitioners, nurse anesthetists, acute care nurse practitioners, clinical nurse specialists, care coordinators, and case managers are but a few of the many opportunities available to traditional medical-surgical nurses. The new focus on outcomes is allowing these practitioners to demonstrate their effectiveness in patient care management, patient satisfaction, and cost containment. The new millennium can clearly be characterized as both the "best of times and the worst of times" for medical-surgical nursing. Nurses are both blessed and cursed to live and practice in exciting times, depending on their perspective, and perhaps their greatest challenge as a profession is to stop being so highly reactive to change and instead to more proactively take responsibility for assertively and directly shaping their own futures. It is absolutely clear that the future of nursing as a profession will be directly affected by what nurses do or fail to do today.

THE CHANGING NATURE OF PRACTICE

The practice of medical-surgical nursing has traditionally been synonymous with acute care hospital nursing. Indeed, in the past virtually all medical-surgical nurses worked for hospitals and provided inpatient care, and few would argue with the assertion of the Academy of Medical-Surgical Nurses that the specialty is the backbone and foundation of virtually every health care organization.[1] Although most nurses are still employed in acute care settings, no trend in medical-surgical nursing practice is more pervasive than the reality of constant change. The health care industry in the United States has been and will continue to undergo rapid and profound change. There is no evidence of this pattern slowing or halting, and medical-surgical nursing practice must develop the ability to respond more quickly and effectively to these rapid shifts.

The most powerful impetus for change has been and continues to be the goal of reducing the cost of care. As a result, the focus of care delivery is increasingly shifting into the community in the attempt to contain or reduce costs, and futurists are clear that this trend will continue. Shortened hospital stays, increased acuity of inpatient care, rapid admission and discharge cycles, and the steady extension of services into the community have fundamentally changed the nature of medical-surgical practice. Today's medical-surgical nurses must manage much more than the traditional nursing skills and procedures. Contemporary nurses must have an understanding of the entire health care system, including its myriad complex mechanisms for distributing and reimbursing for services. Chronic illness management is increasingly recognized as the neglected aspect of care management, and medical-surgical nurses are logical resources for tackling this complex problem. However, as a result, the traditional scope of practice has expanded tremendously. No longer is it enough to provide excellent episodic acute nursing care. Quality care now encompasses and demands the full scope of nursing practice from health promotion, disease prevention, and early detection through acute care management and rehabilitation. Shifting most of these services into the community setting underscores the need for medical-surgical nurses to recognize and address the family and community as recipients of care as well as the patient. It also underscores the argument that medical-surgical nursing needs to rethink its mission to fully embrace the full spectrum of *adult health* nursing.

The various PEW commission reports of the early and mid 1990s clearly forecast these changes and outlined the responses that educational programs needed to make to adequately address the role changes that were forecast for professional nurses. A wide variety of specific competencies were addressed, but the dominant themes were the need for nurses to be[9]:

- Community-based
- Conversant in primary care strategies, health promotion and prevention
- Culturally competent
- Resource experts with an outcomes orientation
- Autonomous coordinators of care and effective collaborators
- Technologically competent in information management

This vastly expanded role underscores the expressed need for a much larger part of the practicing nurse population to be prepared at the BSN and MSN levels. These proportions have not changed substantially in recent years, and only one third of the current workforce is prepared at the baccalaureate level and just 10% hold master's degrees.[2]

SOCIAL CHANGES AND CHALLENGES

Aging

The percentage of U.S. citizens over 65 years of age has more than tripled since 1900. Persons over 65 are the fastest growing segment of our population, and persons over 85 years of age are the fastest growing proportion of the elderly population. It is estimated that the number of persons over 65 will exceed 50 million by the year 2020. Although the vast majority of older adults are healthy and continue to live independently in the community, the elderly consume over one third of health care services and comprise nearly half of all hospital admissions. Most older persons have at least one chronic medical condition and may experience multiple health problems. Their recovery process is typically slower, and many elders have compromised or scattered support systems that are severely stretched by the necessity to provide even short-term daily care. Common health problems include arthritis, hypertension, heart disease, cataracts, and hearing impairments. It is estimated that 23% of older adults living in the community experience difficulty with one or more activities of daily living.

The nursing home population is rising steadily, and about half of these patients are suffering from dementia. Long-term care costs are prohibitive and projected to rise at a rapid pace. With the Medicare program under constant threat of insolvency, it is unlikely that major new initiatives to support care of the elderly will emerge at the federal level. State initiatives are equally unlikely. There is tremendous opportunity for entrepreneurial nurses to find and implement methods of older adult care delivery that can continue to support the efforts of families to provide care in the home, as well as control costs and promote wellness in this frail population.

Poverty

The number of U.S. citizens living in poverty continues to defy both logic and intervention, but it is clear that the gap between the "haves" and the "have nots" in American society continues to widen. Women and children continue to be disproportionately affected by both poverty and homelessness and approximately half of the nation's poor are under the age of 18 or over the age of 65.

Medicaid is the most widespread form of health insurance for the poor, but it manages to cover less than half of those living in poverty. The remainder, greater than 40 million and growing slowly but steadily, are in the ranks of the working poor (i.e., persons who do not have health insurance, who cannot qualify for Medicaid, but who work part time or have low-paying full-time jobs that do not offer access to any health insurance). The relationship between poverty and health has been documented over and over again. The poor experience a higher prevalence of chronic disease and disability, frequently do not seek health care unless they are in pain or acutely ill, receive a disproportionate amount of their routine health care at urgent care facilities and emergency departments, and are often more preoccupied with obtaining food and shelter than in seeking preventive health services.

Cultural Diversity

The composition of American society is steadily changing from a Caucasian majority to an increasingly multicultural mix. The increase in persons of Latino or Hispanic heritage is particularly striking, and Latinos are rapidly becoming the dominant minority in the United States. Cultural diversity creates challenges to communication and understanding, as well as the potential for conflict between the patient and health care team concerning health beliefs, values, attitudes, and practices. This challenge is particularly important in the delivery of nursing care because nursing has been unsuccessful in recruiting significant numbers of students from any of the major minority populations to its ranks. The potential for misunderstanding and conflict is significant. Minority populations are one of the few remaining significant sources of new students to recruit into nursing, but the profession has been singularly unsuccessful to date in attracting minorities in any significant numbers.

Violence and Abuse

The United States is becoming a steadily more violent society, a trend that has profound implications for adult health nursing practice. Public health officials report a virtual epidemic of youth violence that consumes both the cities and the suburbs. Handgun violence is the second leading cause of death in the teenage population and the leading cause of death in young men ages 18 to 24 years of age.

Violence is frequently tied to conditions of poverty and hopelessness, disintegrating families, and substance abuse. Child abuse, domestic violence of all types, violence against women and elders, and violence against nurses are all causes for concerns and significant challenges to nursing practice. Nurses currently face a 16 times' greater risk of injury in the workplace than the national average. Violence is primarily concentrated in the acute care hospital and nursing home settings.

Spiraling Health Care Costs

Despite all of the aggressive downsizing, rightsizing, and reorganization efforts of the 1990s, the cost of health care continues to rise faster in the United States than in any other industrialized nation. Historically most health care in the United States has really been illness care, and it has proven to be exceedingly difficult to shift this orientation in a more balanced way toward prevention and health promotion. It has been shown over and over again that patients typically receive their health care from the most expensive professionals in the most expensive settings (acute care hospitals) and that much of that care is inefficiently or even wastefully used.

Our societal fascination with high technology has spurred tremendous medical advances, but it has also contributed to a voracious demand for services. Few patients or families are willing to forego an opportunity for improved health or extension of life if a diagnostic or treatment procedure exists that may improve their odds. Issues related to the prolongation of life challenge the system daily, but forums do not currently exist to rationally discuss the issues or begin to develop policy. Currently about 25% of all Medicare dollars are spent in the person's last year of life, with a huge proportion of this expenditure occurring in the last days or weeks. This occurs in the face of more than a decade of emphasis on advance directives and planning. Futile care remains a huge system issue. A mirror-image problem exists in neonatology where our ability to preserve life in grossly undersized preterm infants with widely variable and often questionable outcomes consumes astonishing sums of money daily.

Every industrialized country in the world today, except the United States, has some kind of national health system that guarantees a basic level of health care to all its citizens. Few Americans can afford to pay for health care out of their own pocket. It is estimated that the average individual may spend more than $5500 a year on insurance premiums, medications, physicians, and services. This figure is more than double that of 10 years ago and shows no sign of abating. Health care insurance is simply beyond the financial reach of most lower-income persons if it is not included in a job benefits program.

Nurses and the nursing profession must be alert to ways in which nurses can have the greatest impact on the changing health care delivery system. Nurses will have to become more comfortable with risk taking in identifying areas in which nursing can positively affect the health care system. Practicing nurses have been functioning in a defensive survival mode over the last decade. Too much of their conversation about practice has been directed to themselves, and they are not viewed as partners with the decision makers in service planning and provision. Medical-surgical nurses with advanced training and expertise can clearly be a significant part of any future solution to this enormous challenge, and every practicing nurse needs to be constantly thinking of how best to demonstrate the worth and cost-effectiveness of nursing care. Recent studies have clearly demonstrated that care by registered nurses promotes better patient outcomes, but an enormous amount of research is needed to clearly identify the patient outcomes that can be claimed as direct reflections of nursing care.[8] Entrepreneurship opportunities abound for those who can reach out and grab them, providing a variety of services cost-effectively in a variety of settings.

Genetics

Perhaps no contemporary trend has as much potential to revolutionize health care as the furious pace of knowledge development in the realm of genetics. The announcements of the initial successful mapping of the human genome have directed the spotlight of publicity and public attention to these accomplishments, but progress is startling and influential on a variety of fronts.

Society is close to being able to broadly identify an individual's predisposition to a given disease process and predict its onset, extent, and severity. Disease prevention and teaching strategies can then be tailored specifically to the person's own unique risk profile. These capabilities are already in our grasp with certain familial forms of bowel cancer, and carrier testing has been widely available for selected disease processes for years. Recombinant deoxyribonucleic acid (DNA) technology that joins parts of DNA, often from different species, already enables us to convert benign bacteria into factories for the production of insulin, cytokines, and growth factors. Potential applications are virtually limitless.

Mapping of the genome will be followed by an understanding of each gene's functions. This task is of particular importance as we attempt to harness or supplement the natural powers of the immune system. Pharmacogenics is exploring how genetics affects an individual's response to a

BOX 1-1 Nursing Roles and Responsibilities Related to Genetic Care

1. Collect and interpret genetic information from patient and family
2. Offer information and counseling to persons considering gene-based therapies
3. Facilitate decision making and informed consent related to gene-based therapies
4. Provide gene-based care
5. Monitor the effects of gene-based treatment
6. Advocate for patients on issues related to access to care, privacy, confidentiality, and the right not to participate in gene-based screening and care

particular disease or medication, and gene therapy is already being attempted to modify the course or nature of a disease process. Discovering the exact genetic nature and behavior of a tumor will allow us to tailor the chemotherapeutic plan to its unique characteristics.

The potential benefits of these discoveries are enormous, but so is the potential for abuse. Issues related to patient privacy and confidentiality are paramount, especially in relationship to workplace discrimination and access to health insurance. What will constitute a "preexisting condition" now if disease risk can be determined years in advance of its occurrence? Issues of autonomy are equally troublesome as society considers voluntary versus coercive testing procedures, and social justice issues are inevitable as issues of access to cutting edge gene therapy are discussed.

It is obvious that nurses will have to play a significant role in this uncharted world. Nurses are consistently named as the first providers that patients turn to with questions and concerns about their health care. Other roles for nurses in the future of genetics will vary by practice level and education but will certainly encompass all of those outlined in Box 1-1.[10]

Currently there are no avenues or mechanisms in place for addressing these very real concerns and protecting those most affected by them. The discussion has not even been initiated in any organized fashion at the state or national level. Once again it is likely that as a society individuals will be forced into addressing specific dilemmas and abuses as they arise rather than creating any comprehensive proactive policy.

THE REGISTERED NURSE IN MEDICAL-SURGICAL PRACTICE SETTINGS

The hospital has been the traditional practice site for most medical-surgical nurses for over 50 years and will continue to dominate the employment market into the foreseeable future despite all of the changes that have occurred in hospital care delivery in recent years. This is especially true for new graduate and inexperienced nurses. Contemporary hospital nursing evolved in the early 1940s as increasing technologic advances combined to bring more and more patient care into the institutional setting. Hospitals became the setting of first choice for care delivery and consumed increasing numbers of professional nurses. The advent of critical care units continued and greatly expanded this trend. The rise of critical care units also triggered a virtual explosion in expectations concerning the knowledge and skill base of medical-surgical nurses that has continued unabated into the present. Technology has triggered a constant expansion of expectations for practicing medical-surgical nurses.

Hospitals continue to employ most working registered nurses, although some shifts have occurred over the last decade and a half. Hospital employment of registered nurses peaked at about 65% of the workforce and still hovers around 60%. Labor department projections indicate a further decline in years to come, but it is not expected to fall below 53% of the workforce. Clearly hospital nursing will remain a dominant factor in medical-surgical practice in years to come, especially for entry-level nurses.

Current Challenges in Hospital Practice

Hospital-based nursing remains the most visible example of medical-surgical nursing practice and is clearly the most challenging for a variety of reasons. Although nurses are by far the largest single professional group in hospital care delivery, their overwhelming numbers have not translated into significant gains in either decision making or policy making concerning the redesign of patient care for the twenty-first century. Lip service is given to nursing's unique and essential role in coordinating the care patients receive in hospitals, but this unique role does not frequently get heard or addressed in the boardroom. Nursing care is universally recognized as the source of most of the "caring" that patients receive in the depersonalized hospital environment, and patients consistently express their faith and trust in nurses as caregivers, but again the centrality of this role has not translated into substantive power gains within the hospital hierarchy. The perceived erosion of the ability to consistently engage in this caring function is one of the most frequently expressed dissatisfactions in current hospital nursing practice.

Hospital downsizing in the 1990s provided a quick short-term solution to the acute financial woes experienced by hospitals in a radically changing world, but the replacement of registered nurses with increasing numbers of unlicensed assistive personnel has dramatically increased both the workload and the stress level of medical-surgical nurses. The predictable result has been a significant increase in worker burnout and a corresponding decline in both morale and nursing job satisfaction.[6]

The acuity and complexity of care demanded by patients in today's hospitals puts amazing demands on bedside nurses at a time when the pool of experienced clinicians continues to decline. The lack of adequate role models then predictably leads to early disillusionment and burnout of the newest and least experienced members of the profession. The hospital has reverted to being the care setting of last resort rather than the preferred site for care delivery, a status it had enjoyed for the last 50 years. The complexity and acuity of the care environment put extraordinary demands on nurses, and it is clear that new kinds of professionals are needed. Nurses are frequently undereducated at entry into practice for the complexities that they face. An ever-expanding knowledge base is an absolute of

BOX 1-2 Expectations for Nurses Working With Adult Populations

Expert nurses caring for adult populations must:

1. Be on the "cutting edge" of practice through continuous professional development.
2. Provide quality patient care that is sensitive to the physical, psychologic, cultural, and socioeconomic needs of individuals, families, groups, and communities.
3. Participate in outcomes measurement and program evaluation to ensure quality care.
4. Be politically active regarding issues that affect the health and well-being of the American public.
5. Use their knowledge of health economics to influence health resource allocations for the good of the American public.
6. Test interventions that support healthier lifestyles for U.S. citizens.
7. Demonstrate proficiency at patient care management through coordination of care, referrals, and resource utilization.
8. Demonstrate expert communication skills with consumers, patients, families, professional colleagues, and the media.

From Academy of Medical-Surgical Nursing: *Project tomorrow,* Pitman, NJ, 2000, AMSN.

BOX 1-3 Expectations for Nursing Programs Preparing Nurses for Acute Care Adult Health Practice

Nursing education programs must:

1. Provide a strong clinical foundation that students can apply to the care of adults and their families across settings.
2. Implement strategies that foster clinical decision making and critical thinking.
3. Strengthen content in organization and systems, cultural diversity, health care economics, political activism, and computer competency.
4. Focus research content on research utilization, outcomes measurement, and program evaluation.
5. Provide students with real work experience before employment in health care agencies.

Adapted from American Association of Colleges of Nursing: *Executive summary: a vision of baccalaureate and graduate nursing education,* Washington, DC, 1997, AACN; and American Organization of Nurse Executives: *Executive summary: nursing staffing survey,* Chicago, Ill, 1999, AONE.

daily practice, as is the need for highly skilled technologic care. But these are just the beginning. Patients are rapidly shuttled between home and hospital and back to the community setting. Hospital medical-surgical nurses must therefore also be highly skilled in health promotion and prevention strategies and play a substantive role in ensuring that patients receive needed services and supports after discharge.

The Academy of Medical-Surgical Nursing has outlined the skills and abilities needed by medical-surgical nurses today, and the scope is daunting. Even beginning nurses must have the leadership and management skills to direct teams and supervise unlicensed assistive personnel effectively. Delegation skills are critical. Nurses must have sufficient working knowledge of the financial and economic aspects of health care to manage resources effectively and articulate resource needs to administration. Nurses must understand and participate in quality assurance and improvement efforts and manage the increasing and often conflicting demands of multiple regulatory agencies. Computer competencies, data management, and outcomes measurement must become the daily language of every bedside nurse. The full list is presented in Box 1-2.

Nursing schools are obviously challenged to effectively prepare new graduates for this enormously complex practice world. The challenge comes at a time when schools are scrambling to find adequate numbers of well-prepared faculty and struggling with the dual challenges of declining availability of traditional inpatient education sites and the relative scarcity of rich learning opportunities for students in the community setting. The challenges to nursing education developed by major nursing organizations are summarized in Box 1-3.

The Shortage

Nursing shortage cycles have been chronic and recurring problems since the 1940s, but there are indications that this most

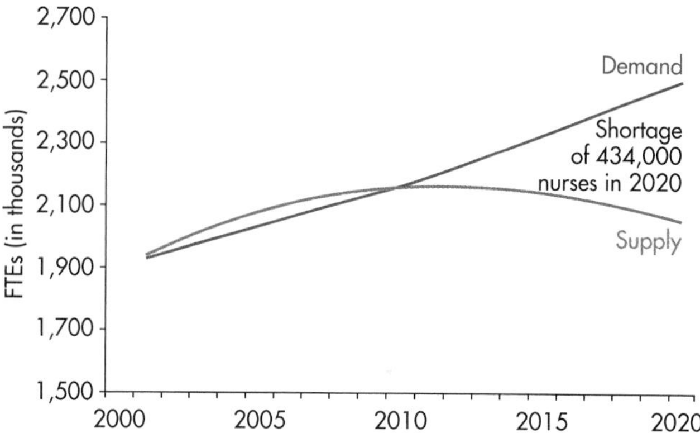

Figure 1-1 Forecast of total RN FTEs versus requirements estimated by the U.S. government, 2001-2020.

recent shortage may be both more severe and more difficult to resolve. A 1998 study reported that over 85% of hospitals were already experiencing a shortage and that conditions have steadily deteriorated in the intervening years.[7] Nursing demand is projected to continue to increase steadily throughout the first quarter of the twenty-first century, but federal predictions show a sharp decline in supply emerging by 2010 and continuing to worsen in the next decades toward a deficit of nearly a half million nurses (Figure 1-1). It is clearly already past time for creative action on this important issue.

Nursing remains a female-dominated profession, and few inroads have been made into enticing significant numbers of men into the profession. Men now represent just 7% of all nurses, a figure that is not substantially higher than the 5% that has been reported for years. The profession has also been uniformly unsuccessful in its effort to diversify racially and culturally, and only about 10% of nurses come from minority backgrounds (Figure 1-2). With all of the new

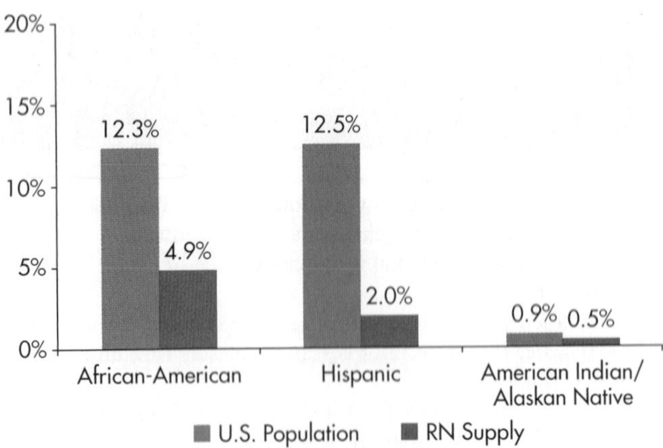

Figure 1-2 Racial composition of the U.S. population and RNs, 2000.

opportunities available to bright, ambitious women today, the failure to attract large numbers of men and minorities into nursing means that it is unlikely that the profession will be able to tap significant new sources of nurses to help meet the shortage. And, despite the widespread defections from traditional hospital employment, it is estimated that as many as 85% of the 2½ million licensed nurses in the United States are currently employed. There is not a huge inactive pool of clinically competent nurses to entice back into practice.[4] Finally, in the past it has been possible to successfully recruit both nationwide and abroad in a time of shortage, but the shortage of nurses is at present a worldwide phenomenon, and international recruitment is no longer a viable option for solving the problem.

The Graying of Nursing

Aging in the current nursing workforce is another factor that has the potential to make this current shortage both more severe and more prolonged (Figure 1-3). The average age of employed nurses is reported as 44 years of age, and the average nursing faculty member is over 50 years of age. The retirement of a large part of the nursing workforce in the not-too-distant future will play a significant role in this particular nursing shortage for the first time. Hospital nursing, which has traditionally employed younger nurses, will be hit particularly hard. Schools of nursing have been reporting small but steady declines in applications, enrollments, and graduations over the last 5 to 7 years; this decline is now reflected in the number of newly licensed nurses available for practice (Figure 1-4).

The age of newly licensed nurses is also continuing to rise and was reported by the American Nurses Association to be over 30 years in 2000.[3] The number of registered nurses under 30 years of age was 25% of the workforce in 1996 but had dropped to 9% by the year 2000.[5] Increasingly nursing is becoming a second career choice for individuals who are frequently drawn to its caring, interpersonal ethic. These individuals are often outstanding additions to the profession, but rising age at entry significantly compresses the years a nurse can commit to active professional participation, especially at the advanced practice and faculty level.

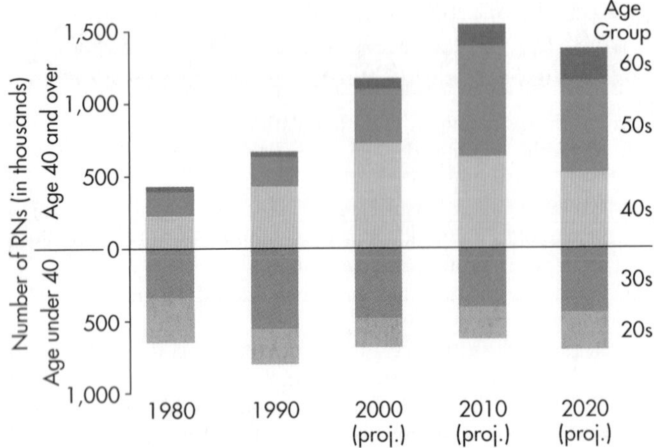

Figure 1-3 The aging RN workforce—number and distribution of RNs by age-group, 1980-2020 (projected).

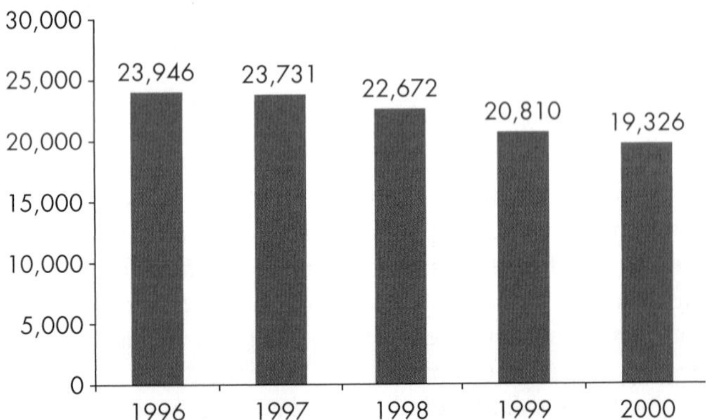

Figure 1-4 Graduates of generic (entry level) baccalaureate programs in nursing, 1996-2000.

OPPORTUNITIES IN MEDICAL-SURGICAL NURSING PRACTICE

The serious challenges that confront contemporary medical-surgical nursing practice are both complex and daunting. Hospital-based practice is clearly in crisis, and the economic environment in health care diminishes the likelihood of easy fixes for these complex and difficult issues. The future for general acute care nurses is uncertain at best and may not develop in the patient-centered ways that represent nursing's preferred future. However, at the same time that basic level practice is experiencing unparalleled challenges, advanced practice nursing is in the midst of an era of seemingly unlimited growth and opportunity.

Advanced Practice

All advanced practice roles are built on a solid foundation of advanced knowledge and skill. The possession of expert knowledge allows these nurses to earn the respect of their system colleagues and secure the increased scope of power and influence that nursing has pursued so unsuccessfully. The future for advanced practice nursing is very bright.

Advanced practice roles in nursing have traditionally emerged from unmet needs in the health care system. The clinical nurse specialist (CNS) role grew out of the clear need to improve the quality of patient care and the clinical practice of professional nursing in the decades following World War II. The technologic advances and explosion of knowledge that characterized these years demanded a new level of competence from clinical nursing leaders. The CNS role blossomed initially but lost substantial ground during the early years of downsizing and restructuring of the nursing workforce, with its clear preoccupation with trimming the workforce and reducing labor costs. The CNS role has been redesigned in recent years to better meet the needs of the health care system for skilled care management and coordination, especially the more effective management of specific populations in both the acute care and community settings. The role is proving to be both cost-effective and a source of increased patient satisfaction with care, and the need for nurses educated to provide these holistic sophisticated services continues to expand.

Nurse midwives have also experienced an unparalleled period of growth in use and acceptance. Standardization of the educational preparation has allowed midwifery to be accepted under the umbrella of advanced practice nursing, and obstetricians have slowly recognized midwives as an excellent means to expand their practices in a cost-effective way. Pregnant women are universally pleased with the holistic care that is at the center of midwifery practice and have contributed to their gradual acceptance by the larger health care system. Achieving hospital delivery privileges has been a long and difficult battle, but these privileges are becoming increasingly common as cost-conscious health maintenance organizations have added their support to the debate.

Nurse anesthesia is one of the oldest advanced practice roles and continues to demonstrate both its cost-effectiveness and safety for the management of routine procedures. The continuous focus on costs in the health care environment helps to ensure that the niche of nurse anesthetists in service delivery remains unchallenged.

The nurse practitioner role emerged in the 1960s in response to serious needs for primary care providers, especially in underserved areas. Family nurse practitioners dominate the practice environment today; but specialists in pediatrics, women's health, adult care, geriatrics, emergency care, and psychiatry are all well represented. The role has been heavily researched and has consistently demonstrated its general efficacy, patient satisfaction, and cost-effectiveness. Although independent practice remains a politically charged topic among physicians, there has been a slow but steady expansion of prescriptive authority and reimbursement for services by major insurance carriers.

The same unclear educational credentials that continue to plague basic nursing practice characterized the early years of the nurse practitioner movement. Finally, however, all advanced practice roles have been united under a framework of master's degree education and national certification that provides a sustainable foundation for expert knowledge and practice. There are some indications that the marketplace for nurse practitioner practice is reaching saturation in some areas, but most authorities agree that the pressure to control health care costs will continue to create new practice arenas for highly educated nurse practitioners. Long-term care provides an excellent example of a fertile area for nurse practitioners to successfully and positively influence both the quality of care and its cost.

The acute care nurse practitioner (ACNP) is the newest advanced practice role to develop, and once again it has been in response to system needs. ACNPs are demonstrating their ability to care for selected populations in the acute care setting in highly effective ways, releasing residents, fellows, and attending physicians to use their energy and time elsewhere. The potential for ACNPs to contribute to the acute care setting is enormous, and most health systems have just begun to explore the potential inherent in the role.

Technology

Any discussion of future influences and opportunities in medical-surgical nursing practice would be remiss not to include the rapid expansion of knowledge and growth of technology. This knowledge explosion requires a lifetime commitment to learning and adds credence to the concept of nurses as being primarily knowledge workers who need advanced education that includes both high-tech skills and basic research skills and the ability to assess outcomes. The classic example of these constantly increasing demands is the contemporary critical care nurse, whose job responsibilities seem to expand daily.

Technology is also opening uncharted areas for nursing care delivery. It allows the delivery of nursing care to patients in far-reaching locations by means of the telephone, facsimile, computer, or tele/videoconferencing. Triage, case management, and patient education are just a few of the natural pathways for nursing to explore using the technologic capabilities of the present and the future. They represent exciting opportunities for both institutional and entrepreneurial nursing service delivery.

As medical-surgical nurses we are certainly both blessed and cursed to practice in such challenging and interesting times. The early years of the twenty-first century challenge us to address the problems and concerns of hospital nurses and to strive to resolve the anti-intellectualism that has prevented nursing from taking its rightful place among the health care professions with a stronger educational base to support practice. These years also challenge us to ensure that the promise and potential of advanced practice works to the benefit of patients and nurses alike.

Critical Thinking Questions

1. Research the nature and scope of advanced practice in your local hospitals and community. Which advanced practice specialties are used? What is their scope of service and their degree of acceptance by physicians and consumers?
2. What strategies can you develop to communicate a more positive message about nursing as a career to: (a) elementary school

students, (b) middle school students, (c) high school students, and (d) college student peers?
3. What is the ethnic/racial composition of your nursing class? How well does it mirror the composition of the larger community? What suggestions do minority students have for making nursing more attractive to minority populations?
4. Explore some of the bills related to nursing education and practice before your state legislature and the U.S. Congress. Draft a letter to your state or federal representatives expressing the need to either support or reject these bills.

References

1. Academy of Medical-Surgical Nursing: *Project tomorrow,* Pitman, NJ, 2000, AMSN.
2. American Association of Colleges of Nursing: *The baccalaureate degree in nursing as minimal preparation for professional practice,* Washington, DC, 2000, AACN.
3. American Nurses Association: *Nursing facts: from the American Nurses Association,* 2000, website: http://www.nursingworld.org/readroom/fsdmogr.htm.
4. American Organization of Nurse Executives: *Perspectives on the nursing shortage: a blueprint for action,* Washington, DC, 2000, AONE.
5. Buerhaus, PI: Is another RN shortage looming? *Nurs Outlook* 46:103-108, 1998.
6. Gothberg, S: In pursuit of safe staffing, *Med-Surg Nurs: J Adult Health* 8:329-344, 1999.
7. Hay Group, Inc: *1998 nursing shortage study: preliminary report,* Philadelphia, 1998, Author.
8. Health Resources and Financing Administration: *Nurse staffing and patient outcomes in hospitals, executive summary,* 2001, Internet document: http://bhpr.hrsa.gov/dn/staff study.htm.
9. PEW Health Professions Commission: *Critical challenges: revitalizing the health professions for the twenty-first century,* San Francisco, 1995, Author.
10. Rieger PT: The gene genies, *Am J Nurs* 100(10):87-90, 2000.

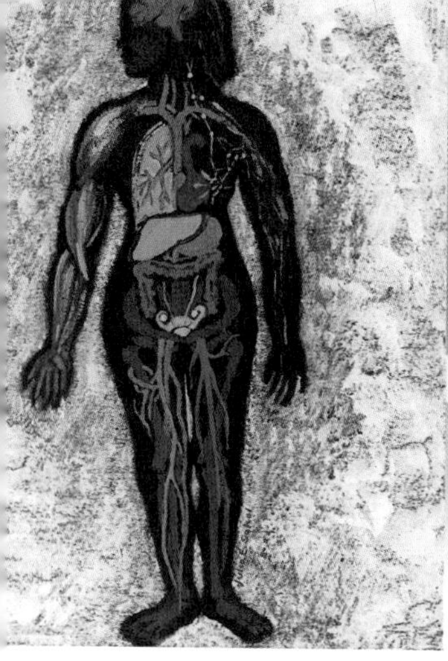

http://www.mosby.com/MERLIN/medsurg_phipps

Complementary and Alternative Therapies 2

Audrey Snyder

Objectives

After studying this chapter, the learner should be able to:

1. Contrast allopathic and homeopathic philosophies.
2. Define complementary and alternative therapies.
3. Describe the theory, practice, and patterns of use associated with commonly used complementary and alternative therapies.
4. Discuss the nurse's role in advising persons about complementary and alternative therapies.

Recovery from illness is one of life's most incredible phenomena. In today's society, the physician is typically viewed as the "healer," with other members of the health care team playing complementary roles in the prevention, detection, and treatment of disease. Yet human beings have existed for more than 2 million years, and for most of that long history people recovered from many illnesses without the assistance or intervention of high-technology scientific medicine. A vast array of healing practices clearly existed long before the advent of modern technology and scientific medicine.

In the natural course of any illness a person becomes ill, either acutely with symptoms such as pain, fever, nausea, or bleeding or insidiously with a gradual progression of symptoms. If the illness is mild and transient, the symptoms disappear with self-treatment or even no treatment. If the illness is more severe, or of longer duration, the person may seek expert help from a "healer," who is usually but not always a physician or nurse practitioner. Other choices for help exist, and these choices are affected by economic, social, and cultural factors. These other care options include a wide range of alternative, complementary, and ethnocultural/traditional therapies. Many individuals use, and move easily between, more than one health care therapy.

The ill person usually recovers or expects to recover. Recovery is by and large a natural biologic phenomenon that occurs regardless of the nature and extent of treatment provided. This fascinating process of recovery from illness defies full understanding but has been documented throughout human history. It also has stimulated the development of numerous forms of healing that attempt to explain or augment the natural phenomenon. Over the centuries natural healing has been attributed to all sorts of rituals, including cupping, leeching, and bleeding. From medicine man to herbalist, the art of healing has been passed down through succeeding generations. Every culture has its own traditional therapies that have been passed down through the years.

THE ALLOPATHIC PHILOSOPHY

The dominant health care system in the United States is "allopathic" and is predicated on a dualistic philosophy that sees the person as "body and mind." Allopathic practices are derived from scientific models of inquiry and involve the extensive use of technology. Interestingly, the word *allopathy* has two quite divergent origins. One origin is from a Greek root word meaning "other than disease." This root origin reflects the use of drugs in a health care therapy that may have no consistent or logical relationship to a patient's symptoms. The second origin of allopathy is from German roots that mean "all therapies." In this context allopathy is a "system of medicine that embraces all methods of proven value in the treatment of diseases." The American Medical Association adopted the second definition of allopathy in 1855 and has subsequently exclusively determined who can practice medicine in the United States. For example, in the 1860s the American Medical Association refused to admit women doctors to medical societies, practiced segregation, and demanded the purging of homeopaths from the practice of medicine.

Today allopathic physicians are becoming more accepting of other providers of health care such as homeopaths, osteopaths, and chiropractors, and even such traditional healers as lay midwives, and herbalists. Nursing education in the United States has also been firmly rooted in the domain of allopathic medicine because traditional physicians designed the original curricula and provided most of the instruction. However, nursing's "caring" ethic has always given professional nurses a more holistic view of patients and illness. This innate holism has made it easier for most nurses to accept the value and relevance of less traditional approaches. Today most nursing programs are incorporating education about complementary and alternative therapies into their curriculums.

THE HOMEOPATHIC PHILOSOPHY

The homeopathic health care philosophy is also practiced in the United States today, although it is less well known. Samuel C. Hahnemann developed homeopathic medicine in Germany between 1790 and 1810. Homeopathy, or homoeopathy, is derived from the Greek words *homoios* ("similar") and *pathos* ("suffering"). In the practice of homeopathy, the person, not the disease, is treated. Homeopathy has not been validated or endorsed by the dominant allopathic system, yet countless people use it. Homeopathy treats illness by giving very dilute medications that are derived from plant, animal, and mineral sources. Homeopathy espouses a holistic philosophy that sees health as a "balance of the physical, mental, and spiritual whole" and encompasses a wide range of health care practices that are often referred to as "complementary" or "alternative."[14] Complementary and alternative therapies include a range of philosophies, approaches, and therapies that conventional medicine does not commonly use, accept, study, understand, or make available. Yet, many of these therapies fit comfortably into nursing's holistic philosophies.

HISTORY OF COMPLEMENTARY AND ALTERNATIVE THERAPIES

The terms *alternative* and *complementary* therapy are often used interchangeably; but there are differences in their definitions and applications. Alternative therapies are used in place of traditional allopathic therapies, whereas complementary therapies are used in conjunction with traditional allopathic therapies.[14] The use of complementary and alternative therapies has grown steadily, particularly since the 1970s when the holistic health care movement blossomed in the United States. With the growing interest in these health care options, debate has also emerged concerning their usefulness and the role that they can play in a patient's health care. The growing body of knowledge, funded research, and an increase in communication between conventional and alternative practitioners, particularly since the early 1990s, has helped bridge some of the differences and quieted the debate; but there is more left to be done. The use of the term *integrative therapies* signals this more collaborative approach to patient care. It encompasses the treatment of patients with both traditional allopathic and alternative therapies concurrently. Throughout this chapter the abbreviation *CAT* is used to indicate the broad range of complementary and alternative therapies.

The concept of wellness means more than being momentarily healthy or without disease. Likewise, no illness is purely physical. Humans are complex, multidimensional beings with subtle interactions between body, mind, emotion, and spirit that serve to connect individuals to the environment and other people. The effects of illness manifest themselves physically, mentally, socially, and spiritually. Complete physical, mental, social, and spiritual well-being is the state often thought of as optimal health.

Some CATs are holistic and treat the whole person. Individuals use these holistic CATs because they foster an overall sense of well-being, offer the person a sense of control, and focus on healing the person rather than curing the disease. The use of holistic CATs establishes a partnership in which the patient is an active participant in both diagnosis and treatment.[2] Other CATs are more preventive in nature and seek to preserve or enhance the person's optimal health and thereby increase the person's resistance to disease.

Although many CATs have been in use for centuries in other countries, these therapies are just now achieving recognition and popularity in the United States. Advances in technology and communications, and the growing ability for our world to be a "global village" have broken down some of the barriers between CATs and conventional medicine. As more research is completed and the use of specific therapies accepted, some therapies will move from the CAT category to accepted practice.

Research on many CATs did not take place in the past because of a lack of research funds. In 1992 Congress established the Office of Alternative Medicine within the National Institutes of Health with a budget of $2 million to evaluate complementary and alternative medicine and to provide that information to the public. In 1998 the office was expanded to become the National Center for Complementary and Alternative Medicine (NCCAM) with a $50 million budget designed to stimulate, develop, and support research on complementary and alternative medicine (Table 2-1). It is no longer unrealistic to believe that the ability of consumers to access CATs may be a factor in an institution's ability to compete for and attract patients within a competitive health care environment.

A 1995 consensus conference group was called to evaluate the available research on CATs related to pain management, and the conference concluded that there is ample evidence that a number of well-defined complementary and alternative interventions exist that decrease pain and increase comfort. The preponderance of the evidence supports the efficacy of cognitive-behavioral applications. At present there is insufficient data to conclude that one intervention is inherently better than another for a given condition, yet evidence does support the conclusion that one approach may clearly be better than another for a given individual. Individual differences in response to treatment modalities have always been readily apparent in the practice literature.

The ability to successfully integrate CATs and traditional allopathic treatment is dependent on the creation of an environment of openness between health care providers and patients about the use of CATs. The use of CATs among Americans grew from 33% to 42% of the population between 1990 and 1997.[5] Yet most patients still report a reluctance to discuss their use of CATs with their primary care provider. Professional education is needed to improve patient-provider communication about CATs. One study reported that the use of unconventional therapies was associated with an increased use of physician services; this indicates a beginning trend in the use of practitioner-prescribed unconventional therapies as a complement to, rather than an alternative to, conventional

TABLE 2-1 National Center for Complementary and Alternative Medicine Funded Research Centers

Specialty	Center	Address
Addictions	Center for Addiction and Alternative Medicine Research Principal Investigator: Thomas J. Kiresuk, PhD	Center for Addiction and Alternative Medicine Research (CAAMR) Minneapolis Medical Research Foundation 914 South Eighth Street, Suite D917 Minneapolis, MN 55404 URL: http://www.mmrfweb.org/research/addicton&alt_med/index.html
Aging and women's health	Center for CAM Research in Aging and Women's Health Principal Investigator: Fredi Kronenberg, PhD	Center for CAM Research in Aging and Women's Health Columbia University College of Physicians and Surgeons 630 West 168th Street New York, NY 10032 URL: http://cpmcnet.columbia.edu/dept/rosenthal/
Arthritis	Center for Alternative Medicine Research on Arthritis Principal Investigator: Brian M. Berman, MD	Center for Alternative Medicine Research on Arthritis University of Maryland School of Medicine Division of Complementary Medicine 2200 Kernan Drive Baltimore, MD 21207-6693 URL: http://www.compmed.ummc.umaryland.edu/
Botanicals	Botanical Center for Age-Related Diseases Principal Investigator: Connie M. Weaver, PhD	Botanical Center for Age-Related Diseases Purdue University West Lafayette Division of Sponsored Programs West Lafayette, IN 47907-1021
Botanicals	Botanical Dietary Supplements for Women's Health Principal Investigator: Norman R. Farnsworth, PhD	Botanical Dietary Supplements for Women's Health University of Illinois at Chicago 809 S. Marshfield Avenue Chicago, IL 60612-7205
Botanicals	Center for Dietary Supplements Research Principal Investigator: David Heber, MD, PhD	UCLA Center for Dietary Supplements Research University of California at Los Angeles 10945 Le Conte Avenue, Suite 1401 Box 951406 Los Angeles, CA 90095-1406
Botanicals	Center for Phytomedicine Research Principal Investigator: Barbara N. Timmermann, PhD	Arizona Center for Phytomedicine Research University of Arizona College of Pharmacy 1703 E. Mabel P.O. Box 210207 Tucson, AZ 85721-0207
Cancer	Center for Cancer Complementary Medicine Principal Investigator: Adrian S. Dobs, MD	Johns Hopkins Center for Cancer Complementary Medicine Johns Hopkins University 720 Rutland Avenue Baltimore, MD 21205
Hyperbaric	Specialized Center of Research in Hyperbaric Oxygen Therapy Principal Investigator: Stephen R. Thom, MD, PhD	Specialized Center of Research in Hyperbaric Oxygen Therapy University of Pennsylvania 133 South 36th Street (6463801) Research Services, Mezzanine Philadelphia, PA 19104-3246
Cardiovascular diseases	Center for Complementary and Alternative Medicine Research in CVD Principal Investigator: Steven F. Bolling, MD	Center for Complementary and Alternative Medicine Adult Cardiac Surgery/Thoracic Transplantation The University of Michigan Taubman Health Care Center 2120, Box 0344 Ann Arbor, MI 48109 URL: http://www.med.umich.edu/camrc/index.html
Cardiovascular disease and aging in African-Americans	Center for Natural Medicine and Prevention Principal Investigator: Robert H. Schneider, MD	Center for Natural Medicine and Prevention Maharishi University of Management 1000 North 4th Street Fairfield, IA 52557
Chiropractic	Consortial Center for Chiropractic Research Principal Investigator: William C. Meeker, DC, MPH	Consortial Center for Chiropractic Research Palmer Center for Chiropractic Research 741 Brady Street Davenport, IA 52803 URL: http://www.palmer.edu

Continued

TABLE 2-1 National Center for Complementary and Alternative Medicine Funded Research Centers—cont'd

Specialty	Center	Address
Craniofacial disorders	Oregon Center for Complementary and Alternative Medicine Principal Investigator: B. Alexander White, DDS	Center for Health Research Kaiser Foundation Hospitals 3800 N. Interstate Avenue Portland, OR 97227-1110
Neurologic disorders	Oregon Center for Complementary and Alternative Medicine in Neurological Disorders Principal Investigator: Barry S. Oken, MD	Oregon Center for Complementary and Alternative Medicine in Neurological Disorders Oregon Health Sciences University 3181 SW Sam Jackson Park Road Portland, OR 97201
Neurodegenerative diseases	Center for CAM in Neurodegenerative Diseases Principal Investigator: Mahlon R. Delong, MD	Center for CAM in Neurodegenerative Diseases Department of Neurology Emory University School of Medicine 1639 Pierce Drive Atlanta, GA 30322
Pediatrics	Pediatric Center for Complementary and Alternative Medicine Principal Investigator: Fayez K. Ghishan, MD, DCH	University of Arizona Health Sciences Center Department of Pediatrics 1501 N. Campbell Avenue P.O. Box 245073 Tucson, AZ 85724-5073

medicine.[4] Insurance companies are also increasing their coverage for certain complementary and alternative therapies in an attempt to reduce the overall cost of health care and respond to consumer demand for services.

DEFINITION OF CATs

CATs are interventions for improving, maintaining, and promoting health and well-being; preventing disease; or treating illness that are not a part of the standard North American system of health care or disease prevention. A more definitive definition is still being developed.

Many CATs alleviate symptoms, but do not cure a disease process. CATs can decrease the symptoms associated with certain chronic conditions (e.g., cancer, heart disease, diabetes, arthritis, and chronic pain syndromes). CATs have been used to treat back pain, allergies, fatigue, arthritis, headache, neck problems, hypertension, sprain and strains, and insomnia. Most CATs incorporate the importance of mindfulness and attitude to healing. They also integrate the person's cultural background and personal beliefs into the treatment process. CATs are based on paradigms of the person as a whole, and this holism frequently complicates efforts to research the efficacy of CATs using a traditional scientific paradigm that looks at the impact of a therapy from just one perspective.

It continues to be extremely difficult to evaluate CATs in a familiar, scientific manner. The "gold standard" for clinical research involves the use of randomized controlled trials; but such trials cannot be used as the only method of evaluating safety, outcomes, effectiveness, and cost-effectiveness of CATs. New research strategies are needed. Nonspecific effects and placebo responses cannot be ignored. Research strategies must be capable of considering individual differences in response to therapies.

CLASSIFICATIONS OF CATs

The National Center for Complementary and Alternative Medicine has grouped complementary and alternative practices and therapies into five major domains: alternative medical systems, mind-body interventions, biologically based treatments, manipulative and body-based methods, and energy therapies.[12] Alternative medical systems are practiced by many cultures throughout the world. Examples include ayurvedic medicine, homeopathic or naturopathic medicine, and traditional Oriental medicine, which encompasses acupuncture, herbal medicine, Oriental massage, and *qi gong*.[13] Mind-body therapies enhance the mind's ability to affect bodily function. Meditation; hypnosis; dance, music, and art therapy; and prayer are included in this domain.

Biologically based therapies include natural products such as herbal products, special diets, orthomolecular therapies, and biologic therapies. Manipulative and body-based therapies include chiropractic and massage therapy. Energy therapies focus on biofield therapies (energy originating within the body) such as *qi gong, reiki,* and therapeutic touch; and electromagnetic field therapies (energy from other sources) such as pulsed fields or magnetic fields.[13]

Many therapies cross the boundaries of the domain classifications or may be used in combinations. For example, massage therapy is a body-based method but Oriental massage is a part of traditional Oriental medicine. *Qi gong* is an energy therapy but is also a part of traditional Oriental medicine. *Reiki* is an energy therapy and acupressure is a component of Oriental medicine. Both may be included in a massage session, which is a body-based therapy.

The following descriptions are not intended to be all inclusive but are meant to increase awareness of some common CATs. Additional information about particular therapies can be obtained from texts in the bibliography and organizations and web sites listed at the end of the chapter.

ALTERNATIVE MEDICAL SYSTEMS

Chinese Medicine

Chinese medicine is based on the belief that the body is pervaded with energy or *Qi,* which is produced from the air and food and travels throughout the body providing nourishment and engendering movement for the healthy and normal functioning of the body. There are extensive pathways or channels along which both *Qi* and blood travel that connect the surface of the body and the internal organs. The balance of yin and yang influences *Qi.* When yin and yang are balanced they work with the natural flow of *Qi* to help the body achieve and maintain health.

Traditional Chinese medicine includes a variety of therapies such as acupuncture, acupressure, auriculotherapy, moxibustion, and *qi gong.* Each of these is briefly described.

Acupuncture

Acupuncture has been in use for more than 23 centuries. Its use dates back to the Han Dynasty in the second century BC, and it has been known in the Western world since the seventeenth century.[9] Most states require a license, registration, and/or certification to practice as an acupuncturist (Box 2-1).

Acupuncture involves stimulating specific anatomic points in the body for therapeutic purposes such as pain reduction, healing, or physiologic changes. There are more than 2000 acupuncture points on the body that connect 12 main and 8 secondary pathways or meridians.[16] These points are most often stimulated using a thin, hair-sized needle, but practitioners may also use heat, pressure, friction, suction, laser light, or impulses of electromagnetic energy to stimulate the points. Basic science research suggests that neurologic pathways are the mechanism by which acupuncture relieves pain. High threshold sensory nerves at the acupuncture points are stimulated and send messages to the spinal cord, midbrain, and pituitary to release endorphins and block pain. Cortisol levels are also elevated, which may explain the prolonged pain relief achieved by patients with arthritis.

Acupuncture is believed to balance the body's *Qi* that flows through the 12 major meridians or energy pathways of the body. Each pathway and anatomic point is linked to internal organs and specific problems and pathologies can be accurately targeted. Illness is diagnosed by assessing the quantity and quality of *Qi* flowing through the channels and determining the individual's balance. After the assessment, points to stimulate are selected based on the theory that when *Qi* is blocked, it causes pain and dysfunction, and that restoration of flow is critical to the health of the body and mind.

Treatment focuses on removing the pathogenic agents that have invaded the channels, thus relieving the stagnation of *Qi* and blood that resulted from the presence of these agents. Chronic conditions generally require more acupuncture sessions than acute problems. Although our understanding of the action of acupuncture is fairly simplistic, its effects can be profound. Acupuncture is quite safe and is associated with a much lower incidence of complications than invasive surgical procedures. Possible adverse effects include infection and organ puncture (Box 2-2), and are a clear reminder that CATs as well as conventional therapies can produce adverse effects.

Acupuncture is among the most researched and documented of CAT practices. Randomized clinical trials provide evidence of its efficacy in treating osteoarthritis, back pain, painful menstrual cycles, and migraine headaches.[16] Because of the pervasive skepticism in conventional medicine regarding acupuncture and the fact that it requires individualized protocols, acupuncture is being clinically studied only with a limited number of conditions. At the National Institutes of Health consensus conference held in November 1997, a panel of experts scrutinized the research and literature on acupuncture to determine which conditions, based on published evidence, were best suited to acupuncture treatment.[11] Acupuncture was found to be effective in treating the nausea caused by surgical anesthesia and cancer chemotherapy as well as the pain experienced after dental surgery. Acupuncture was found to be useful by itself or combined with conventional therapies to treat addiction, headaches, menstrual cramps, tennis elbow, fibromyalgia, myofascial pain, ostoarthritis, lower back pain, carpel tunnel syndrome, and asthma.[11] It was also shown to assist in stroke rehabilitation. Third-party insurance carriers were then asked to reimburse for the use of acupuncture for these conditions.

Acupressure

Acupressure is a combination of acupuncture and massage in which the thumbs and fingertips apply pressure to stimulate pressure points along the acupuncture meridians. Acupressure may be incorporated into a massage therapy session.

Auricular Therapy

Auricular therapy is the diagnosis and treatment of pain and disease using the auricle or pinna of the ear. Points on

BOX 2-1 Choosing a Safe Acupuncture Practitioner

Check state laws regarding practitioner certification, licensure, and registration requirements.
Explore a potential practitioner's training, and experience, licensure, certification or registration.
Obtain a referral if possible.
Ensure that the practitioner uses new, sterile needles for each acupuncture session.

BOX 2-2 Contraindications to Acupuncture

Phobias to needles
Clotting disorders such as hemophilia
Pregnancy
Age less than 7 years
The influence of alcohol or narcotic medications
Dementia

the ear, which represent different parts of the body and its structure, are stimulated with needles, magnets, lasers, massage, or electricity. The technique has been useful in smoking cessation and addiction control therapy.

Moxibustion

Moxibustion uses the powdered leaves of moxa herb or mugwort *(Arthemisia vulgaris)*. The herb is burned above the skin or on an already inserted needle at the acupuncture points to apply heat and alleviate symptoms.

Qi Gong, Chi Kung, *and* T'ai Chi'

Qi gong, chi kung, and *t'ai chi'* all have their roots in Chinese martial arts training. *T'ai chi'* means "meditation in motion." Practice may involve vigorous exercise or slow movements and postures that focus on *Qi* in the body. The movements and postures are performed so that a continuous chain of movement occurs. The technique demands mindfulness of movement and breathing and can increase circulation. The routine is usually practiced daily as a part of an overall health maintenance program.

Homeopathy

Homeopathy was documented and systematized by Dr. Samuel Hahnemann, a German physician. It is based on the law of similiars—like cures like. The similia principle "suggests that any state of disturbance that is not corrected spontaneously (and leads to a state of 'disease') can be corrected by minute doses of a compound which at a higher dose can produce effects closely resembling the symptoms of the disease being treated; or by minute amounts of the compound actually causing the disease."[21,22] This theory was the basis for early vaccine development and current allergy treatment. The immune system is strengthened when it is exposed to a small amount of a disease component. The component is too weak to cause the disease but allows the body to fight off the related disease. Allergies can be treated in the same manner with the introduction of the allergen in small doses. The dose is progressively increased and an antibody response or resistance to the allergen develops.

Small doses of a compound, derived from plant, animal, or mineral sources, are given, which in large doses may produce symptoms of a disease in a healthy person. Frequently homeopathic remedies are prepared with tinctures of plants in ethyl alcohol or water. The mixture is shaken and strained over a 2- to 4-week period. Potentization is the combination of diluting and shaking of a substance. The higher potencies (meaning more dilute) are more powerful than lower potencies. Homeopathic medicines may be so dilute that there are no molecules of the original substance remaining, but it is believed that a pattern remains. Preparations may be given in tablet, granule, ointment, liquid, or suppository form. More than one remedy can be used to treat the same problem. Determination of a specific remedy is based on a person's unique pattern of symptoms. Homeopathy is one of the most difficult forms of CAT for persons to accept. Individuals simply do not expect it to work. Clinical trials have been positive; however, more research is needed (see Research box). There are very few documented adverse effects of homeopathy.

Research

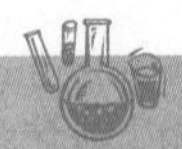

Reference: Linde K et al: Are the clinical effects of homeopathy placebo effects? A meta-analysis of placebo-controlled trials, *Lancet* 350:834, 1997.

In a review of 186 studies of homeopathy treatment, 89 of which fit predefined criteria for meta-analysis double blind or randomized placebo-controlled clinical trials, the clinical effects of homeopathy could not be explained solely by the placebo effect. Homeopathic medicine treatment was found to have a 2.24 times greater positive effect on patients than placebo alone.

Reference: Barnes J, Resch KL, Ernst E: Homeopathy for post-operative ileus: a meta-analysis, *J Clin Gastroenterol* 25(4):628, 1997.

Homeopathic remedies are advocated for the treatment of postoperative ileus, but data supporting their effectiveness based on clinical trials have been lacking. This study performed a meta-analysis of existing clinical trials to determine whether homeopathic treatment has any greater effect than placebo administration on the restoration of peristalsis after abdominal or gynecologic surgery. The analysis indicated a statistically significant ($p < 0.05$) weighted mean difference in the favor of homeopathic remedies of ≥12 C potency versus placebo. The evidence clearly suggests that homeopathic treatment can reduce the duration of postoperative ileus.

The American Institute of Homeopathy was founded in the United States in 1845 and was the first national medical society. Two years later the American Medical Association was founded, which slowed the growth of homeopathy. Homeopathy use experienced resurgence in the 1970s with the growth of the holistic health movement. Many current homeopathy practitioners have also been educated as allopathic medical doctors.

Homeopathic remedies can be purchased over the counter without a prescription, and health food stores may stock homeopathic preparations that are a combination of remedies. They contain minute amounts of several substances that have been found to be beneficial in treating the symptoms indicated on the label. The use of multiple substances is based on the premise that each substance has been beneficial in some patients; therefore one of the substances should work to correct the imbalance in an individual's body.

MIND-BODY AND SPIRITUAL THERAPIES

Mind-body and spiritual therapies include art therapy, biofeedback, color therapy, hypnosis, imagery, prayer and spiritual healing, relaxation techniques, and sound therapy including binaural beat technology. Mind-body medicine involves psychologic, social, and spiritual approaches (Box 2-3).

Hypnosis

Hypnosis is a state of attentive, focused concentration with suspension of some peripheral awareness. There are four components of a hypnotic state: absorption or deep contemplation of a theme or focus, controlled alteration of attention, dissociation or compartmentalization of one's experience, and

BOX 2-3 Four Categories of Mind-Body Therapies

Complementary and Alternative Medicine

Yoga
Qi gong
T'ai chi'

Behavioral Medicine

Psychotherapy
Meditation
Imagery
Hypnosis
Biofeedback
Support groups

Spirituality

Prayer and mental healing
Cross-cultural aspects

Overlapping

Art therapy
Music therapy
Dance therapy
Journaling
Humor
Body psychology

suggestibility or capacity for heightened responsiveness to instructions. Hypnosis has been used to treat pain, duodenal ulcers, irritable bowel syndrome, and nausea, as well as for smoking cessation. Some people are more susceptible than others to hypnosis.

Imagery

Imagery is an ancient healing technique that opens communication among perception, emotion, and bodily changes. It uses pictures and symbols and is a universal form of human thought. Guided imagery can be used to reduce pain, alter the course of a disease, and improve a patient's outlook concerning illness. Imagery can help the person feel more in control of their health or recovery process. Imagery may be used to treat anxiety, enhance the immune response, help children cope with the stress of illness, help cancer patients cope with pain, support the dying process, and provide support during stressful procedures[10] (Box 2-4). It can be used in conjunction with music to enhance healing, support coping, promote relaxation, and enhance postoperative recovery. Imagery has been used in psychotherapeutic settings to deepen patients' ability to reach therapeutic levels of insight and growth. Imagery is a strategy that can be easily integrated into the clinical practice of the bedside nurse, and nurses should familiarize themselves with the technique both didactically and experientially.

Imagery involves mental processes (as in imagining) that encourage attitude, behavior, or physiologic reactions. It attempts to cause an internal representation of events that involve the senses (vision, smell, touch, hearing, taste, and proprioception). It is believed to be the natural language of the unconscious mind and involves "thinking with one's senses," a lived experience. Physiologically, imagery communicates information between the mind, the senses, and the emotions so that psychologic insight and/or bodily responses can be used as agents of therapeutic change. The technique has been effectively adapted to help highly trained athletes prepare for competitive events.

Guided imagery uses cognitive techniques: simple visualization or direct suggestions, metaphor and storytelling, dream interpretation, drawing, and/or active imagination. The clinician actively engages the patient's capacity for imagery to influence or affect a specific outcome (Box 2-5). Imagery is a factor in the biofeedback process that allows subjects to learn how to alter their physiologic responses. The practice of imagery can contribute to insight and understanding into current concerns (i.e., imagery allows a patient to access inner wisdom), support symptom management (pain, depression, difficulty breathing), and improve the functional status of the patient.

Training in imagery facilitates its use. Interested clinicians can educate themselves, pursue personal growth work through imagery, practice on themselves, practice with colleagues, and take training programs (see Guidelines for Safe Practice box). Empiric research on the effectiveness of imagery is difficult to conduct but is sorely needed (see Research box). There is also a dearth of well-qualified practitioners.

BOX 2-4 Clinical Applications of Imagery

Perioperative pain and anxiety
Control of nausea and vomiting in chemotherapy
Pain management in cancer
Psychotherapy and depression
Restoration of physical function
Enhancement of the immune system
Wound healing
Control of HIV/AIDS anxiety and pain
Asthma management
Stress management
Control of burnout
Bulimia nervosa treatment

BOX 2-5 Types of Imagery

Diagnostic imagery: patients describe how they feel in sensory and emotional terms to guide the therapist in designing interventions.
Mental rehearsal imagery: prepares patients for medical procedures by teaching a relaxation strategy and guiding them through the procedure.
End-stage imagery: used to produce a specific physiologic or biologic change in the body such as enhancing immunity.

Guidelines for Safe Practice

The Use of Imagery

- Imagery techniques can alter blood glucose levels. Blood glucose should be monitored with the use of imagery in diabetic patients. Imagery may be contraindicated in unstable diabetic patients.
- Imagery can induce seizures in susceptible patients as it alters brain wave activity.
- It is inadvisable to use imagery for patients with a history of psychosis. Imagery is generally a safe technique, but it can evoke intense latent feelings and inner conflicts, and caution is necessary.
- Imagery should not produce harmful physical or psychologic effects in patients. Imagery is an adjunct, a support system, and not a replacement for clinical care.

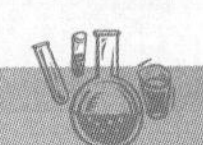

Research

Reference: Esplen, MJ: Guided imagery treatment to promote self-soothing in bulimia nervosa, *J Psychother Pract Res* 7:102, 1998.

This study explored the use of guided imagery therapy with a group of 50 subjects diagnosed with bulimia nervosa. Twenty-five of the subjects received 6 weeks of individual guided imagery therapy, which included weekly sessions of imagery and journaling. The other 25 subjects were assigned to a control group, which did journaling only. The frequency of bingeing and vomiting was determined, and measures of impulsivity, soothing, receptivity and aloneness were obtained. The imagery group had a mean reduction of binges of 74% ($p < 0.0001$) and a mean vomiting reduction of 73% ($p < 0.0001$). The guided imagery subjects also showed improvement on the psychologic measures of aloneness and the ability for self-comforting.

Spirituality

Spirituality is one's inward sense of something greater than the individual self, a personal awareness of dimensions of existence that extend beyond the physical domain. Spirituality encompasses a variety of perspectives, and personal biases and terminology can be confusing. Spirituality frequently involves but is different from religion. Religion is the outward, concrete experience of believing that there is something greater than the individual self. Religious care involves helping people maintain their belief systems and worship practices. Spiritual care on the other hand involves helping people maintain their personal relationship to a higher authority as defined by that person, and to identify meaning and purpose in life.

Spirituality is reported in all cultures. Concepts from the world of linear, material reality are inadequate to describe spirituality, which often is depicted through metaphors or poetry. In much of today's Western culture, material pursuits are valued more highly than spiritual ones. Material things can be quantified, analyzed, and manipulated. Spiritual understanding depends on a basic faith, and there is no tangible or physical benefit or value. Many people in today's more material world have a dismissive attitude toward spiritual therapies; if something is not physical and verifiable through the five senses, it is seen as nonsense or immaterial.

There is therapeutic potential in both spirituality and religion. The healing definition of spirituality is the intentional influence of one or more persons on a living system without using known physical means of interaction. Quieting the mind is usually a prelude to spiritual healing, which is predominately an activity of the mind as it impinges on matter. The planned use of spirituality includes the laying on of hands, intent, prayer, psychic healing, spiritual healing, faith healing, mental healing, and transpersonal healing. It can also involve the energy of heat, tingling, vibration, and color. It is unclear if there is an unidentified energy exchange or exchange of energy fields during the healing interaction.

There are two main types of spiritual healing. In the first the healer enters a prayerful altered state of consciousness and views the patient and self as one single entity. Prayer is a spiritual practice, and seeking medical care and using prayer are not mutually exclusive. There is no physical contact and no attempt to do anything or give anything. The only goal is to become one with the person and his or her god. In the second type, the spiritual healer touches the person and energy flows through the hand of the healer to the patient's area of pathology. The laying on of hands has been accepted by many cultures as a powerful means of healing. There are published reports of healers being able to influence a variety of cellular and other biologic systems through mental means. Physiologic function can be affected from a distance.

Spirituality positively correlates with physical and mental health, decreasing a variety of diseases. Positive effects have been shown in patients with cardiovascular disease, hypertension, cancer, and colitis. Spirituality also can affect how patients deal with aging and impending death.

Nurses need to explore spiritual and religious issues with patients as thoroughly as they do physical ones. Reports of spontaneous healing indicate that patients may occasionally heal themselves. The belief that life-threatening diseases such as cancer can disappear suddenly and completely is almost universal and is a more common belief than is generally acknowledged. This belief is usually coupled with the conviction that radical healing is somehow connected with one's state of mind. The belief that "miracles do happen" may help to restore hope and instill a fighting spirit, which are important to recovery from illness.

The experience of illness has the potential to transform a person. Illness can be a time of great personal growth. People may reexamine goals and values, clarify priorities, mend broken relationships, and discover inner resources. Spiritual experiences are individual, unique, and personal.

Prayer

Prayer is universal, a conscious relationship with the force of the universe, or God. It may take the form of intercessory prayer, confession, gratitude, or silent communion (see Research box).

Meditation

Meditation is a state of being in one's own essential nature. It refines consciousness so that thought and being are in tune

Research

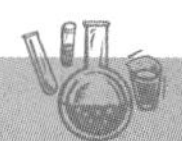

Reference: Harris WS et al: A randomized controlled trial of the effects of intercessory prayer on outcomes in patients admitted to the coronary care unit, *Arch Intern Med* 159(19):2273, 1999.

This study attempted to determine whether remote, intercessory prayer on behalf of hospitalized cardiac patients would reduce the incidence of adverse events and length of stay. A double-blind, controlled environment study was conducted involving 990 patients over 50 weeks. Patients were randomly assigned at admission to receive remote intercessory prayer from a prayer group or to receive simply the standard care. Patient names were given to teams in the prayer group who prayed for them daily for 4 weeks. The prayer group did not know and never met the patients. On retrospective chart review it was found that the prayer group showed a statistically significant beneficial effect in their coronary care unit course scores that reflect adverse events during hospitalization. No differences in length of stay were found.

with the universal plan. Quiet centering or meditation for just 20 minutes each day can redirect energies for healing and decrease stress. Meditation decreases oxygen consumption and cardiac and respiratory rates and is a component of some types of yoga. Meditation is contraindicated for persons who fear loss of control such as those with a history of schizophrenia or psychosis.

Yoga

Yoga is a philosophy that integrates the spiritual, mental, emotional, and physical aspects of life. The word *yoga* means the union of different aspects of the individual. There are several different types of yoga, but they all involve self-improvement through focused breathing, stretching, and meditation. Yoga emphasizes breath as the link connecting mind, body, spirit, and emotions. *Prana* or life force energy is taken in through the nose with breathing. Principles of the Alexander technique are derived from yoga. Yoga techniques have been used to improve blood pressure and treat depression, osteoporosis, and the discomforts associated with menopause.

Group Therapy

Group therapy provides mutual support, encouragement, and socialization. It can be used for psychologic therapy, to work through grief and loss, to lose weight, or to work on self-improvement. Group therapy usually centers around a common theme, for example, a breast cancer survivors support group.

Art and Color Therapy

Art, light, color, and environment affect mood and attitude. Art and color allow a person to express inner needs and desires, and record dreams and meditations. Art and color therapy may be used along with other mind-body therapies.

Music Therapy

Music is part of everyday life. Different parts of the body resonate to different sounds and pitches. Music therapy involves the use of sound to promote health. The controlled use of music can influence a person during illness or injury treatment. Some music is specifically recorded at 60 beats/min, the rate of the resting heart beat, to promote relaxation and a decrease in heart rate. This music has been used effectively in coronary care units, neonatal nurseries, and in cancer units. Music therapy is also used to decrease stress and anxiety. Binaural beat tapes use a combination of rhythm and beat, delivering it asynchronously and separately to each ear through headphones. Voice-guided imagery with voice over music or music over voice can also be used. Music chosen for relaxation must be selected to meet the individual's needs and preferences. Individual responses can be very different.

Biofeedback

Biofeedback involves the self-regulation or voluntary control of an internal state. Patients learn to regulate their physiologic functions in subtle ways through the use of noninvasive electronic monitoring equipment. The technique allows patients to participate in their own healing. It has been particularly helpful in treating hypertension, Raynaud's disease, migraines, and low back pain. Blood pressure, heart rate, skin temperature, electroencephalogram and electromyogram recordings have all been used with biofeedback to help patients learn a conditioned response.

RELAXATION THERAPY

Stress erodes health and well-being. It affects the nervous and immune systems, emotions, and how we relate to others. Stress management techniques may reverse disease and lower blood pressure and heart rate. Virtually all of the strategies described under mind-body therapies can also be effectively used as part of a stress management program.

Relaxation therapy can be somatic or cognitive. Somatic relaxation therapy uses observation to purposefully relax muscles, whereas cognitive relaxation therapy uses a mental device such as a word, sound, or breathing to relax the body and mind. Relaxation techniques are effective in reducing chronic pain such as headache, back pain, menstrual pain, orthopedic postoperative pain, and rheumatic pain. They are easy to teach and learn and can be used effectively by any nurse at the bedside. Relaxation is the foundation of techniques for prepared childbirth such as Lamaze, and is widely used in that setting.

Psychoneuroimmunology

Psychoneuroimmunology is the study of mechanisms that turn thoughts and feelings into chemical and neurologic sequelae. It explores the interaction between behavior, neural and endocrine activity, and the immune process. Psychological distress can suppress the immune system and increase the risk of illness. At the same time a person can work with mind and emotions to increase resistance to disease or to influence recovery. It has been used effectively to treat headaches; moderate blood pressure, heart rate, and rhythm; heal ulcers and irritable bowel syndrome; manage pain, anger, anxiety, and panic; and reduce muscle spasms.

BIOLOGICALLY BASED THERAPIES

Biologically based therapies include the use of natural products, both botanical and herbal, as well as nutritional supplements. This section discusses some commonly used nutritional supplements and herbal therapies (Table 2-2, see Future Watch box). Natural products represent one of the fastest growing consumer markets in the United States.

Herbal Medicine

Phytomedicine is the use of plant material for medicinal purposes. Every known culture has used healing plants as a basis for medicine (Box 2-6). Herbal and dietary supplements are not regulated like pharmaceuticals and lack the quality standards of pharmaceuticals. Different parts of plants yield different things. Herbal elements and content vary depending on the part of the plant harvested, time of year harvested, and soil content (Box 2-7). It also may take a period of time to build up blood levels of the active ingredient. Herbal products often are not as potent as commercially prepared medicines and may take several weeks to produce their effects. Herbal products are often assumed to be safe because they are natural, but natural does not always guarantee safety. There are potential adverse interactions between herbal products and prescribed drugs and foods, and they are not inherently a better option (see Patient Teaching box on p. 20). Patients are often not fully aware of the risks involved with the self-prescription of herbal products.

A new drug goes through a lengthy clinical trials process and then is patent protected to ensure that companies can earn back their investment. Herbal or natural products cannot be patented and are regulated as foods rather than drugs. All of the chemical ingredients of an herb may not be known. Plant-derived drugs are the chemically isolated constituents of plants (e.g., aspirin, digitoxin, atropine, and morphine). Prescribed drugs are purified, standardized, and thoroughly researched; and their pharmacodynamics are well known. This is not the case with herbal products and the presence of multiple ingredients may create unplanned synergistic effects.

Most available information on natural products and drug interactions is based on case reports rather than on clinical trials. Knowledge concerning drug-herbal interactions is limited by the lack of herbal product standardization, variations in purity and potency, the presence of multiple ingredients in products, product adulteration, misidentification of ingredients, and batch-to-batch and manufacturer variations related to crop conditions and yield.[20,21] The pharmacokinetics (absorption, distribution, metabolism, and elimination) and physiologic effects of most herbal products are poorly or in-

TABLE 2-2 Accessory Nutrients

Accessory Nutrient	Effect	Uses and Considerations
Alpha lipoic acid	Naturally occurring in the body, taken for its additional antioxidant effect; regenerates glutethione, vitamin E, vitamin C and other antioxidants in the body	Diabetes and HIV
Chromium	A necessary nutrient; deficiency contributes to adult diabetes and atherosclerosis. Chromium levels decrease with age.	Chromium picolate, the only active form, improves glucose transport across cells, lowers cholesterol and improves lipid profiles.
Cretine	Body enhancer, energy enhancer	Athletes use it to increase energy and endurance.
DHEA	Precursor to testosterone in males and progesterone in females. Builds muscle mass.	Should first have laboratory work to see if DHEA level is low. DHEA enhances mood and memory, improves immune system and can aid in the prevention of heart disease. *Caution: hormone precursors are as potent as hormones bought by prescription.*
Glucosamine	A key component in the synthesis of proteins found in joint cartilage. These proteins are negatively charged and attract water for the production of synovial fluid in the joints. It is theorized that when used as supplement, the body replenishes the synovial fluid and produces new cartilage.	Frequently recommended in the treatment of osteoarthritis, rheumatoid arthritis, tendonitis, gout, and bursitis. In Europe, nonsteroidals are used less, and glucosamine is used more. Used frequently in combination with chondrotin.
Melatonin	A hormone that regulates the body's circadian rhythms and sleep patterns	Useful for jet lag, helps to reset body clock with changing time zones if taken in new time zone at bedtime
NADH	Involved in the Krebs' cycle and production of energy	May play a role in the treatment of Parkinson's, depression and dementia and chronic fatigue syndrome; expensive
SAMe	Found in all living cells, a naturally occurring molecule, and a precursor to certain essential amino acids.	Used in the treatment of depressive disorders, osteoarthritis, migraine headaches, fibromyalgia, liver disease, and sleep disorders.

HIV, Human immunodeficiency virus; *DHEA,* dehydroergotamine mesylate; *NADH,* reduced form of nicotinamide-adenine dinucleotide; *SAMe,* S-adenosylmethionine.

completely understood, and caution must guide the use of any herbal product or nutritional supplement, especially during pregnancy and lactation (Boxes 2-8 and 2-9).

The 1994 United States Dietary Supplement Health and Education Act (DSHEA) regulates herbs as dietary supplements. Herbal products must now be labeled with side effects, contraindications, potential safety problems, and special warnings.

Future Watch
Two Accessory Nutrients

Superoxide dismutase (SOD) is an antioxidant that occurs naturally in the body. It is useful for treating soft tissue inflammation, inflammatory disease, and chronic bladder irritation. It is at present only available as an intramuscular injection because it is rapidly inactivated by the bowel when taken orally. Pain at the injection site is an unpleasant side effect. It has not yet been accepted for use in the United States, but it is currently being used on animals.

Coenzyme Q-10 (Ubiquinone) is used by cells to produce the energy needed for cell growth and maintenance. It is also used as an antioxidant or substance that protects cells from free radicals. It may function in tissues as a free radical scavenger, membrane stabilizer, or both. Oxygen atoms in the body contain pairs of electrons. During metabolism a single electron may be lost creating a free radical with a strong desire to replace its missing electron. It scavenges by taking an electron from a neighboring molecule, which sets up a chain of reactions that are destructive to body tissues. This process is a feature of most diseases, including cardiovascular disease and cancer. Antioxidants protect the cells against free radical damage. Coenzyme Q-10 is natural, but tissue levels decrease with age. Coenzyme Q-10 has been used to stabilize blood pressure, reduce shortness of breath and palpitations, and lessen heart muscle hypertrophy. It may have uses in treating ischemic heart disease, in heart failure, and in protecting the ischemic myocardium during surgery. In the United States Q-10 is sold as a dietary supplement, but recommended daily allowances (RDA) and treatment doses have not been established. It is not to be used during pregnancy or lactation.

Reference: National Institutes of Health: *Cancer Facts CAM, questions and answers about coenzyme Q-10, 2001,* website: http://cis.nci.nih.gov/fact/9-16.htm; Facts and Comparisons: *The review of natural products, potential herb-drug interactions,* Monograph, 1998.

BOX 2-6 General Principles Concerning Herbal Products

Herbal products are relatively safe due to the lower concentration of active ingredients.
A desired therapeutic effect takes time to develop.
Pharmacologic actions of herbal products are not well understood.
Herbal products are not usually appropriate in emergency or acute care situations.
Most often herbal products are used in patients with chronic illness with mild ambiguous symptoms.
Herbal products have the potential for drug interactions with prescribed drugs and each other, and there are contraindications to use.
Herbal products have the potential for multiple effects.

BOX 2-7 Preparations of Herbal Products

Infusions (tea): steeping herb is added to hot water.
Decoctions: decoctions are made from bark and roots
Juicing: parts are chopped and pressed to get the water-soluble parts.
Powder: dried plant is ground.
Syrup: herb is added to honey and brown sugar in water, then boiled and strained.
Tincture: herb is added to 5% alcohol. It stands 2 weeks, is shaken daily, and then strained and bottled.
Ointment: herb is added to hot petroleum jelly.
Poultice: crushed plant is mixed with hot moist flour or corn meal to make a warm paste and is applied to the skin.
Cold compresses: a cloth is soaked in a cooled infusion and applied to the affected part
Herb baths: herbs are crushed, and bath water is run over the crushed herbs.

BOX 2-8 Herbs Contraindicated During Pregnancy

Aloe
Autumn crocus
Black cohosh root
Buckthorn and berry
Cascara sagrada bark
Chaste tree fruit
Cinchona bark
Cinnamon bark
Coltsfoot leaf
Echinacea purpurea herb
Fennel oil
Combinations of licorice, peppermint, and chamomile
Combinations of licorice, primrose, marshmallow, and anise
Combinations of senna, peppermint oil, and caraway oil
Ginger root
Indian snakeroot
Juniper berry
Kava kava root
Licorice root
Marsh tea
Mayapple root
Petasite
Rhubarb root
Sage leaf
Senna

BOX 2-9 Herbs Contraindicated During Lactation

Aloe
Basil
Buckthorn bark and berry
Cascara sagrada
Coltsfoot leaf
Combinations of senna, peppermint oil, and caraway oil
Kava kava root
Indian snakeroot
Petasite
Rhubarb root
Senna

Patient Teaching
Using Herbal Products

- Discuss herbal products with your health care practitioner.
- Evaluate the available research on the use of the product.
- Research effective herbal dosages.
- Take note of all cautions listed.
- Consider herb-drug interactions.
- Investigate companies that market the herb. What are their quality standards?
- Choose a name brand company with quality control.
- Purchase the same brand each time.
- Take herbal products at the same time each day.
- Follow the manufacturers recommendations; for example, "drink with 8 oz. of water."
- Keep a log of any potential adverse reactions and report these to the health care practitioner.

The Food and Drug Administration (FDA) allows manufacturers to make certain health, nutrient content and structure/function claims on the labels, but the FDA must review the claims before marketing.[17] For example, companies can make limited structure or function claims such as: "promotes healthy prostate." One may also see statements on products such as "This statement has not been evaluated by the Food and Drug Administration. This product is not intended to diagnose, treat, cure or prevent disease." Therapeutic or drug effect claims are not allowed. Manufacturers of herbal products and dietary supplements are expected to voluntarily comply with good manufacturing practices. The 1997 Federal Commission on Dietary Supplements recommended that manufacturers provide science-based evidence about their products to consumers.

Licensed health care practitioners cannot prescribe natural substances to treat disease, although glucosamine handouts in orthopedic offices have somewhat changed this standard of practice. Many orthopedic physicians routinely recommend the use of glucosamine for joint cartilage regeneration. At present there is no official mechanism for the licensing or certification of herbalists in the United States.

In Germany herbs are available on the open market, but are carefully and thoroughly evaluated. The Institute for Drugs and Medical Devices, which is part of the Federal Health Agency in Germany and analogous to the Food and Drug Administration in the United States, reviews available information about a herbal product with an expert panel of pharmacists, physicians, toxicologists, epidemiologists, and other professionals.[1] The panel submits a summary report to the German Commission E, which acts as a separate regulatory body and provides information on herbal substances. Prepared monographs may include historical use and anecdotal evidence. The assessment of efficacy does not necessarily require new studies. The rapid globalization of markets for all products underscores the importance of achieving some degree of standardization and uniformity in product preparation around the world.

Commonly Used Herbal Products

A multitude of herbal preparations currently are on the market. The following section provides an overview of several commonly used herbal products. See the Research box for studies that have validated the usefulness of certain herbal products in patient care.

Ginkgo *(Kew tree, Maidenhair tree)*. Ginkgo is the oldest living plant on earth. In China it is a sacred tree, and Buddhists use it as a temple decoration. It increases general circulation, improves microcirculation, inhibits platelet aggregation, and inactivates oxygen free radicals. It is therefore useful for intermittent claudication as well as dementia syndromes such as Parkinson's disease. It does not appear to improve memory in healthy people but is effective with age-related changes. Ginkgo may slow the progress of Alzheimer's disease, but it is not a cure. Because gingko inhibits platelet aggregation, it should be used with caution after trauma or surgery. Bleeding is a potential side effect of use (see Guidelines for Safe Practice box). Ginkgo must be commercially prepared to decrease its toxin content.

Research

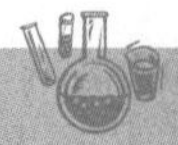

Reference: Ramesh PR: Managing morphine-induced constipation: a controlled comparison of an ayurvedic formulation and senna, *J Pain Symptom Manage* 16:240, 1998.

Researchers in a palliative care unit in India conducted a controlled trial comparing misrakasnejam (a liquid ayurvedic herbal preparation) with a conventional laxative tablet in the management of opioid-induced constipation in patients with advanced cancer. The results indicated that there was no statistically significant difference in the degree of laxative action; but the small volume of drug required, once a day dosing, and acceptable side effects made the misrakasnejam a good choice for the management of opioid-induced constipation.

Guidelines for Safe Practice
Cautions for the Use of Herbal Products

- Herbs that should be used cautiously with concurrent anticoagulant use: dong quai *(angelica sinensis)*, feverfew *(Tanacetum parthenium)*, garlic *(allium sativum)*, gingseng, ginger *(Zingiber officinale)*, and ginko *(ginko biloba)*. A general rule is that patients on anticoagulants should not use natural products.
- Milk vitch (loco weed, *astragulas*) is an immune system enhancer. Its use is contraindicated with autoimmune diseases.
- Chamomile may display a cross-sensitivity in persons allergic to ragweed, asters, and chrysanthemums.
- When using stinging nettles for allergy treatment, the freeze-dried preparation is needed.
- Ephedra is now being marketed in weight loss products and sports drinks. It has both bronchodilator and stimulant effects and can produce adverse cardiovascular side effects. It interacts with caffeine, decongestants, and stimulants. Deaths have been reported with its use in large quantities.
- Senna, when used for colonic stimulation, can potentiate cardiac glycosides, possibly by increasing the loss of potassium.
- Any patient who experiences an adverse reaction to a medication should be questioned about the use of herbal products. Potential herb-drug interactions should be reported by institution policy or directly to the Food and Drug Administration at MedWatch by phone 1-800-FDA-1088 or via the Internet at www.accessdata.fda.gov/scripts/medwatch.

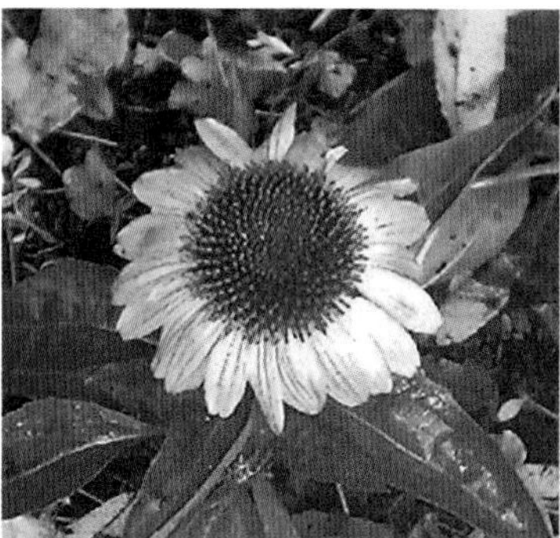

Figure 2-1 Echinacea, a member of the daisy family, bears a single flower with a cone-shaped center and purple rays. It is commonly seen in gardens in the United States.

Future Watch

St. John's Wort and Clinical Depression

The National Institutes of Health National Center for Complementary and Alternative Medicine has funded a study of St. John's wort for treating patients with clinical depression. Duke University Medical Center is coordinating a 3-year study in conjunction with 13 other clinical sites around the country. Patients are being enrolled in one of three treatment groups: one group will receive St. John's wort, a second group will receive a placebo, and the third will receive the antidepressant medication setraline (Zoloft).

Reference: National Center for Complementary and Alternative Medicine, St. John's Wort, 2001, website: http://nccam.nih.gov/fcp/factsheets/stjohnswort/stjohnswort.htm

Patient Teaching

Safe and Effective Use of Echinacea

- Echinacea is contraindicated with immunosuppressive therapy.
- It is often recommended that a person use echinacea for 10 days and then discontinue use because long-term use could cause harm. It should definitely not be used for longer than 8 consecutive weeks without a break.
- Echinacea should be taken at onset of cold symptoms and not used as a preventive therapy.

Gingseng. Gingseng has been used since colonial days. Gingseng increases resistance to stress and excessive activity and allows a person to endure adverse situations longer. Americans tend to use gingseng out of its proper context. The Chinese have a saying that "if you can feel your gingseng you've used too much." It is properly used to adapt to stress and has an invigorating and fortifying effect in times of fatigue or disability. However, ginseng can interact with anticoagulants and potentiate bleeding.

Echinacea (American Coneflower, Purple Cone Flower). Echinacea is an immune system enhancer. It has antiseptic, antiviral, and peripheral vasodilatory properties and can be used as supportive therapy for colds and flu. Many persons use it as a preventive, which is inappropriate use. It is most effective when used at the onset of cold symptoms to reduce the duration and severity of upper respiratory infections, both viral and bacterial (Figure 2-1; see Patient Teaching box).

Feverfew. Feverfew is a member of the sunflower family. It has antipyretic properties and acts like nonsteroidal antiinflammatory medications. It has been used to treat migraine headaches and arthritis and to reduce fever and inflammation. It also inhibits platelets, and caution should be used with anticoagulants. Feverfew can be effective in preventing migraine headaches, but it must be taken continually. It is not useful once a headache has started.

Garlic. Garlic has been valued throughout history. At times it was used as currency. It is often thought of as a cure all with antioxidant properties. It has a cholesterol-lowering effect (lowers low-density lipoprotein [LDL] cholesterol and triglycerides and raises high-density lipoprotein [HDL] cholesterol), regulates blood sugar, decreases blood pressure and platelet adhesiveness, prevents age-dependent vascular changes, and has antibacterial properties. It is often a major part of a Mediterranean diet and is believed to be helpful in avoiding heart disease, although its cholesterol-lowering and hypotensive effects may take months of use before positive effects are seen. It is not used with anticoagulants because it can prolong bleeding.

Ginger. Ginger root historically was chewed by sailors to decrease seasickness. Today it is used to prevent the nausea and vomiting associated with motion sickness, as a digestive aid and a peripheral circulatory stimulant. It is used cautiously with anticoagulants as it can potentiate bleeding.

Horse Chestnut. Horse chestnut decreases capillary permeability. It has been used to treat symptoms of venous insufficiency and to prevent varicose veins, but it cannot reverse them. Its effects seem to be equivalent to the use of compression stockings.

Kava Kava (*Piper methystium*). Kava kava acts as a sedative and sleep enhancer. It has been used for conditions of nervous anxiety, stress, and restlessness. It should not be combined with alcohol or central nervous system depressants (e.g., antipsychotics, sedatives, sleeping pills). The skin can turn yellow with excessive use and the preparation should not be used for more than 3 months. In some countries kava kava is used as a recreational drug.

St. John's Wort (*Hypericum perforatum*). St. John's wort has been used since medieval times as a treatment for mild to moderate depression. It is thought to work like a monoamine oxidase (MAO) inhibitor, and concurrent use with MAO inhibitors should be avoided.[15] There is increased evidence that St. John's wort interacts with many medications. Reported side effects include hypertension, headache, insomnia, arrhythmias, nervousness, tremors, seizures, stroke, and myocardial infarction (see Future Watch box).

Saw Palmetto (*Sabal serrulata*). Saw palmetto has both antiinflammatory and antiedema effects. It is used to treat the urination problems associated with stage 1 and 2 benign

Research

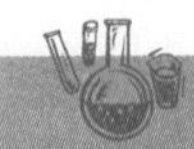

Reference: Marks LS, Hess DL, Dore FJ: Tissue effects of saw palmetto and finasteride: use of biopsy cores for in situ quantification of prostatic androgens, *Urology* 57:999, 2001.

A study supported by the Urological Sciences Research Foundation found that patients with benign prostatic hyperplasia (BPH) treated with saw palmetto for 6 months experienced a 32% decrease in dihydrotestosterone (DHT) levels in their prostate tissue. DHT is a hormone believed to be responsible for some of the prostate tissue enlargement associated with BPH. No statistically significant changes in DHT levels were noted in placebo-controlled patients. This study adds support to the anecdotal benefits of saw palmetto that patients and physicians have reported in the past.

prostatic hyperplasia. It may produce fewer side effects than common related pharmaceuticals (see Research box).

Tea Tree Oil. Tea tree oil has been used for centuries as a topical antiseptic. It has also been used for a multitude of skin conditions (e.g., athlete's foot and acne).

Valerian Root *(Valeriana officinalis)*. Valerian root works on GABA receptors, acting like the benzodiazepines. It has been used for restlessness, sleeping disorders based on nervous conditions, and insomnia. Its effects are immediate, but it does not work for everybody and is not recommended for chronic use.

NUTRITION

Nutrition is the science that studies the use of food to promote health and avoid disease, and nutrition is one of the most commonly used CATs. Patients recovering from trauma or major illness benefit from nutritional support, but nutrition also plays a major role in the prevention and treatment of chronic disease. Maintaining good nutrition in the face of chronic illness is challenging. Certain foods are associated with improvement of certain symptoms, and laboratory findings can guide nutritional supplementation. For example, instead of using hormone replacements to control menopausal symptoms, a patient may choose to supplement the diet with whole grain cereals, vitamin E, vitamin C, beta-carotene, fish oil, calcium, folate, vitamin B_6; and to use soy products because of their phytoestrogen content.

AROMATHERAPY

Aromatherapy involves the use of essential oils and hydrosols to promote personal health and beautify, balance, and heal the mind, body, and spirit. The use of aromatherapy dates back 5000 years. Distillation devices to extract oils were found in the ruins of Mesopotamia. Ancient cultures used plant oils for a variety of purposes. Egyptians embalmed with oil from frankincense and myrrh. More recently, soldiers in World Wars I and II carried lavender oil with them on the battlefield to disinfect wounds. In the 1930s Dr. René-Maurice Gattefosse coined the term *aromatherapy* and published a book that earned him the title of "father of modern aromatherapy." Chemically produced medications began to replace essential oils and herbs in medical treatment during the nineteenth century.

Aromatherapy oils are frequently used with massage. Oils are absorbed through the skin into the circulatory system and may be used in massage or baths; they can also be inhaled. Odors are transmitted to the brain via the olfactory nerve and stimulate the limbic system of the brain, which controls primitive needs such as hunger, thirst, and emotion. Odors also act on the hypothalamus, which controls the secretion of hormones in the endocrine system. Smells can affect intuition, emotion, and creativity. A person's reaction to an odor occurs on an emotional and largely subconscious level. Smell is connected with memory and some smells can evoke happy memories like a loved one's perfume or home-baked bread. Other smells are unpleasant (e.g., antiseptic smells of hospitals) and may even be painful if the memories are associated with a loved one who has died. Aromatherapy may be used with or without touch therapies.

Oils contain hormones, vitamins, natural antibiotics, and antiseptics. Oils are obtained by the process of distillation, where plant materials (roots, leaves, flowers, seeds, resins, and gums) from plants, flowers, shrubs, or trees are heated with water to release oils from the plant in a vaporized form. The steam and vapor are then condensed to a liquid state and the essential oil floats to the top of the water. The remaining water and micromolecules of essential oil are termed the hydrosol.

Essential oils are applied or inhaled to achieve physical, emotional, and spiritual balance and harmony. Aromatherapy hydrosols are mixed with a base oil of lotion and applied to the skin. They can be used in massage lotions, baths, compresses, steam inhalation, and hair and skin care products. They also may be used in aroma lamps or rings on light bulbs. Small quantities are therapeutic, but larger quantities could be toxic. Internal use is rarely recommended (Table 2-3; see Guidelines for Safe Practice box).

BACH FLOWER REMEDIES

Bach flower remedies are combinations of flower essences discovered by Edward Bach, a British physician. The combinations are selected from among 38 common, nontoxic flowers. The book, *The Twelve Healers,* is a reference guide used to help select the appropriate remedy for an individual state of mind. Rescue remedy is a combination of five flowers used to deal with everyday emergencies and is well known (Box 2-10). It is benign and produces no unpleasant reaction. It is preserved using brandy, which can be omitted, but the essence will not stay preserved as long. Two to four drops of an essence are placed under the tongue or in a glass of water and sipped throughout the day. Patients using Bach flower remedies may have a faint odor of alcohol on their breath. Hydrotherapy baths, douches, and packs can also be made with Bach flower remedies.

TABLE 2-3 Essential Oils and Reported Effects

Essential Oil	Reported Effect	Medicinal Uses
Cinnamon	Increases appetite	Promotes oral intake
Lavender	A natural antibacterial, antiseptic, and antiinflammatory agent	Headaches, muscular aches, insomnia, hypertension, heart palpitations
Clary sage	Muscle relaxant and digestive stimulant	Respiratory distress, premenstrual syndrome (PMS), and headaches *(contraindicated in pregnancy)*
Rosemary	Antiseptic, antidepressant, lowers blood pressure, and lowers blood glucose	Hypertension, hyperglycemia, colds, flu, asthma, and rheumatism
Geranium	Stimulates the adrenal cortex; functions as a diuretic, astringent, and antiseptic	Balances hormones; menopause, PMS, diabetes, kidney stones, sore throats; and skin problems
Peppermint	Stimulates digestion and settles the stomach	Used as an aid in quitting smoking; may relieve nausea and headaches; topically used as an insect repellent and antiseptic. *(Caution: it is too strong for use with infants.)*
Eucalyptus	Promotes respiration and open bronchioles; functions as an antiseptic, fever-reducer, pain reliever, and diuretic	Used for asthma, bronchitis, sinus infections, sore throat, kidney infections, and rheumatism
Chamomile	Antiinflammatory, pain reliever, fever reducer, and wound healer	Fever, wounds, pain
Rose	Antiseptic, relieves cramps, promotes menstruation	Fever, migraines, and PMS
Sandalwood	Antiseptic, diuretic, and expectorant	Fertility problems, and imbalances in urinary and reproductive systems
Myrrh	Soothes inflammation, clears congestion and secretions, antiseptic properties, and fungicidal agent	Wound healing and ulcers
Frankincense	Antiseptic, disinfectant, astringent, and wound healer	Bronchitis, colds, sinusitis, stomach and intestinal discomfort, and wound healing
Vanilla	Increases appetite	Promotes oral intake

Guidelines for Safe Practice

Cautions With the Use of Aromatherapy

- Many people are allergic to certain fragrances. Never suggest or use an aromatherapy with a patient without inquiring into allergies and the patient's preferences.
- Oils to avoid due to risk of toxicity or skin irritation: bitter almond, boldo leaf, calamus, jaborandi leaf, mugwort, mustard, pennyroyal, rue, sage, sassafras, savun, southernwood, tansy, thuja, wintergreen, wormseed, and yellow camphor.
- Oils to avoid during pregnancy: all of the above plus basil, clary sage, cypress, fennel, jasmine, juniper, marjoram, myrrh, peppermint, rose, rosemary, and thyme.
- Before using aromatherapy clinically, a health professional should complete a course in the medicinal uses of oils.

MANIPULATIVE AND BODY-BASED THERAPIES

Manipulative and body-based therapies focus on the integration of the structural and functional integrity of the body using manual methods. They may involve reeducation about movement as well as structured exercise. Bodywork and manipulative therapies with a structural focus include chiropractic, craniosacral, Trager, and Alexander technique. Neuromuscular therapies include reflexology and Trager. Structural and postural reintegration therapies include Rolfing and Alexander technique.

BOX 2-10 Rescue Remedy Ingredients

Star of Bethlehem
Rock rose
Impatiens
Cherry plum
Clematis

Massage

Massage therapy is perhaps the best known of the manipulative therapies and involves the manipulation of tissues to enhance healing and health. Massage manipulates the soft tissues (skin, muscles, tendons, ligaments, fascia) and structures within the soft tissue of the body for the purpose of normalizing these tissues.[8] Massage therapists may use their hands, forearms, or elbows to apply pressure and move the tissues of the body. Techniques include touch, stroking (effleurage), friction, vibration, percussion (tapotement), kneading (petrissage), stretching, compression, or passive and active joint movements.[8] Massage modalities include European massage, Swedish massage, deep tissue therapy, sports massage, manual lymph draining, and Esalen massage. The origins of massage can be found in Chinese folk medicine, the India yoga cult, and in Egyptian, Persian, and Japanese literature. The use of massage in the West disappeared during the Middle Ages and was relegated to an obscure place in folk culture. It has only recently reemerged as a major CAT therapy.

In 1900 Albert Hoffa published Technik Der Massage, which became the basis for all modern massage techniques. The polio epidemic of 1918 triggered a resurgence of interest in massage therapy in the United States and Europe, but its use again waned until the 1970s holistic health movement rekindled its popularity. Massage therapy is now reported to be the third most commonly used alternative therapy after relaxation techniques and chiropractic care.[6] A large study of emergency room staff found that massage was their most commonly used complementary therapy and the one they recommended most frequently to patients.[19]

Massage integrates mechanical, physiologic, reflexive, mind body, and energetic mechanisms. Massage affects the musculoskeletal, circulatory, lymphatic, nervous, and other body systems. It can reduce muscle tension and improve circulation; and slow stroke back massage has been shown to decrease heart rate, increase skin temperature, and decrease both systolic and diastolic blood pressure.[18] Massage has been reported to reduce acute and chronic pain and increase mobility and range of motion in the joints. It increases oxygen delivery to the tissues and improves the removal of lactic acid and other waste products from the cells. The levels of beta-endorphins have been shown to increase moderately after connective tissue massage, which decreases pain perception.

Massage also creates a state of relaxation that relieves anxiety and enhances the individual's sense of well-being. Mental centering can also occur. Deep massage can create a meditative state that recharges energy and activates the parasympathetic nervous system for restoration and rejuvenation.[8]

Touch is the fundamental medium of massage therapy. A therapist works with the patient to determine sensitivity to touch and the optimal pressure to use. Massage establishes a mind body connection between the therapist and patient in a safe and nonsexual environment. Used correctly touch conveys caring as well.

Many hospitals now use massage therapists to provide massage therapy for patients; examples of settings include cancer clinics, obstetrics and gynecology, postsurgical units, and rehabilitation units. Massage therapies may also be helpful in hospice settings or nursing homes. Massage therapies may also be offered to members of patient's families and to the staff to aid in stress reduction (Figure 2-2).[7] Treatment may also include other body-work and touch therapies. Massage therapists have frequently received additional training in medical massage to understand disease processes and indications and contraindications to therapy, and to be able to work in and around the medical environment.

Historically, nursing programs taught back massage as a part of nighttime care. Nurses massaged patients to help them relax. It is unfortunate that the move to highly technologic care erased this therapy from common use in nursing just as massage was achieving prominence as an alternative therapy. See the Research Boxes for current research concerning massage therapy.

Chiropractic

Chiropractic means hand work and refers to manual therapy that focuses on the spine and its effect on the nervous system.

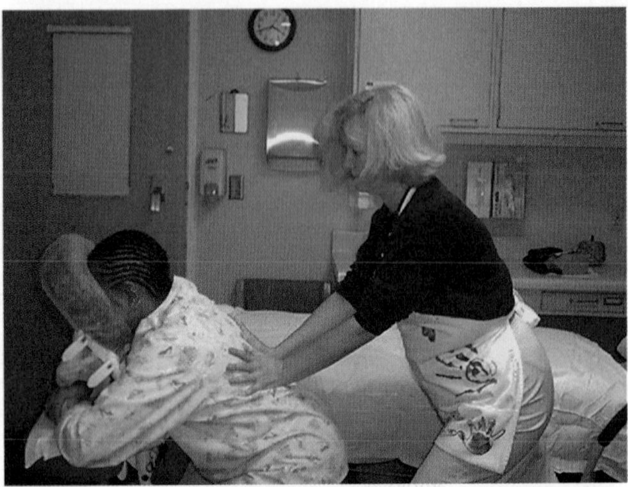

Figure 2-2 Many hospitals now use massage therapists to work along service lines providing massage therapy for specific types of patients. The massage therapist may also provide seated massage for hospital staff and family members.

Structural relationships are analyzed by the practitioner and manipulated to restore proper alignment and function. Chiropractic practitioners are the third largest medical specialty after medicine and dentistry, and practitioners are licensed in all 50 states. Chiropractic is an ancient healing art, but the position of chiropractic practitioners in health care has been rather contradictory. Chiropractic care is really more a mainstream than alternative therapy. Chiropractors use the patient history, physical examination, neuromuscular examination, radiographic examination, and laboratory or special studies to determine the appropriateness of chiropractic care for the individual patient.

Chiropractic care has been used to treat shoulder pain, low back pain, and temporomandibular joint disorders. Chiropractors use mobilization and manipulation as a treatment modality for spinal disorders, pain, altered musculoskeletal function, altered flexibility, and disturbed physical performance. Many studies have shown that chiropractic care for low back pain is more effective and less costly than conventional medical care. The 1994 AHCPR guidelines clearly state that spinal manipulation can alleviate low back pain, a condition that 70% to 80% of Americans experience at some time in their lives.[3]

Chiropractic care focuses on a strong patient-practitioner relationship that has demonstrated effectiveness in the treatment of headaches and neck pain, although more research is needed. Chiropractic treatment is not without risk; there is the potential for adverse outcomes such as brainstem or cerebellar infarction, spinal cord injury, vertebral fracture, tracheal rupture, diaphragm paralysis, and even death. Case reports are published in the literature, but hard data about complication rates are unavailable.

Craniosacral Therapy

Craniosacral therapy focuses on normalization of the craniosacral system. Dr. John Upledger, an osteopathic physician, developed craniosacral therapy in the 1970s. The therapy is based on the theory that there is a craniosacral rhythm or

Research

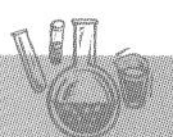

Reference: Field T et al: Massage reduces anxiety in child and adolescent psychiatric patients, *J Am Acad Child Adolesc Psychiatry* 31:25,1997.

Field and colleagues evaluated the effects of massage on cortisol levels in adolescent and younger psychiatric clients. Clients were found to be less depressed, less anxious, and had lower salivary cortisol levels after daily 30-minute massage sessions. Depressed subjects also had decreased urinary cortisol and epinephrine levels.

Reference: Field T et al: Job stress reduction therapies, *Altern Ther Health Med* 3:54, 1997.

Brief massage therapy sessions, music relaxation with visual imagery, muscle relaxation, and social support group sessions all were shown to have demonstrated effectiveness in reducing stress in hospital employees.

Reference: Cady SH, Jones GE: Massage therapy as a workplace intervention for stress reduction, *Percept Motor Skills* 84:157, 1997.

This study also demonstrated that massage therapy could effectively reduce stress in the workplace. In addition the participants systolic and diastolic blood pressures decreased after a 15-minute therapeutic massage administered in the work environment.

Research

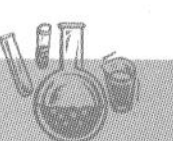

Reference: Richards KC: Effect of a back massage and relaxation intervention on sleep in critically ill patients, *Am J Crit Care* 7:288, 1998.

This study explored the effects of nighttime massage in the form of back rubs on the sleep quality of critically ill older men in an intensive care unit (ICU) setting. It found that a 6-minute nighttime massage incorporated into the evening routine by ICU nurses significantly improved the quality of the sleep of the critically ill subjects.

Reference: Smith MC et al: Benefits of massage therapy for hospitalized patients: descriptive and qualitative evaluation, *Altern Ther Health Med* 5:64, 1999.

This study explored the benefits of massage therapy for hospitalized clients. Clients experienced an increase in relaxation (98%), a sense of well-being (93%), and positive mood change (88%) after massage. More than two thirds of clients attributed enhanced mobility, greater energy, increased participation in treatment, and faster recovery to the massage therapy.

pulse motion that reflects the rise and fall of the cerebrospinal fluid within the dura mater compartment and occurs 6 to 12 times per minute in a healthy person. Dr. Upledger believed that the sutures of the skull are not entirely fused, as is commonly believed, but can be used to access the flow of cerebrospinal fluid through the dural membranes. The therapist works with the patient to identify where this pulsing rhythm is obstructed. The rhythm is monitored using light, gentle touch no heavier than 5 g (weight of a nickel). Once an obstruction is identified the practitioner assists the natural flow of fluid to help the body self-correct. Work in this area can increase energy flow and break up restrictions. Uses of craniosacral therapy include management of chronic fatigue syndrome, chronic headaches, joint problems, head injury, and stroke rehabilitation.

BOX 2-11 Principles of Trager

Finding elongation: length creates freedom of movement, which takes less effort.
Finding width: taking up our full space gives way to feeling.
Presence in relationships does matter.
Giving up weight makes one feel lighter.
Movements increase sensation.
Repetition is the way we learn and we learn our entire lives.
Assessment is treatment.

Trager

Trager uses gentle rhythmic movements or rocking to give the mind sensory information about where body parts are, and how they feel and move. The technique was developed by Milton Trager in the 1920s (Box 2-11). Trager connects a person to his or her body, stimulates deep relaxation, and focuses on quality of being from a model of optimal functioning. This approach provides a background for physical therapy, occupational therapy, massage therapy, chiropractic care, physical rehabilitation, and psychotherapy. Movement education can also involve Mentastics, a program of do-it-yourself exercises, to release psychophysiologic areas of holding in the mind and body.

Alexander Technique

Alexander technique is a system of posture and movement that uses the natural grace and poise of the body. It is a technique that focuses on postural reflexes or antigravity reflexes, "the use of ourselves." The technique was developed at the end of the nineteenth century by an Australian, Frederick Mathius Alexander, a Shakespearean reciter who consistently lost his voice after performances. He developed the Alexander technique and permanently cured his vocal problems. Since then his technique has been used for two main purposes, performing arts and physical therapy.

Alexander technique involves kinesthetic reeducation. Children have excellent use of their body from birth. A young child walks with an erect spine, free joints, and a large head that is balanced easily on the neck. Over time through environmental socialization, this poise is lost; with the Alexander technique it is retaught. The head needs to be floating forward and upward for optimal functioning. Alexander technique is a learned method to improve posture and movement dysfunction. Through one-on-one lessons with a teacher, a person learns how to move the body with minimal strain and maximum balance for optimal functional mobility and decreased pain. Over time a person acquires a sense of postural awareness enabling the person to automatically modify muscular responses to stress. Alexander technique has been clinically beneficial to persons with chronic pain conditions; traumatic injuries; back, hip, and neck dysfunction; repetitive stress injuries; neurologic dysfunctions; respiratory dysfunction; and posture or balance disorders.

Reflexology

Reflexology involves the use of the thumb and fingers to apply specific pressures to stimulate the reflex areas in the feet and hands that correspond to all the glands, organs, and parts of the body. It can improve the function of the whole body or a specific targeted area that may be distant from the area being stimulated. Energy flow is encouraged and impurities are removed to promote healing. Some form of reflexology has been practiced by many cultures throughout the ages, but its roots are in the ancient art of Oriental pressure therapy or acupuncture. All of these approaches are based on the theory that energy pathways exist throughout the body and that blockages of these pathways can lead to energy loss, discomfort, and illness. Reflexologists work each reflex, triggering release of stress and tension in the corresponding area or body zone and promoting an overall relaxation response. Patients express relief from tension and pain, a greater feeling of well-being, and increased energy.

Exercise

Exercise is movement that promotes health and fitness including cardiovascular endurance, muscle strength, and body flexibility. Appropriate physical activity and exercise conditions the heart and other muscles, and provides a sense of well-being. Stretching relaxes and loosens muscles, releases toxins, and increases blood flow. Lymph movement in the body is dependent on stretching and breathing. Exercise decreases stress hormones, improves relaxation, and helps the body deal with stress more effectively. Exercise can improve cardiovascular and pulmonary function, hypertension, diabetes, osteoporosis, and depression. Exercise has achieved such a prominent place in health and wellness programs in the United States that it is difficult for most people to consider it as a CAT.

ENERGY THERAPIES

All living systems are based on energy and vibration and all forms of "bodywork" interact with this energy in some way. Energy therapies include therapeutic touch, *reiki,* physioacoustics, and bioelectromagnetics.

Therapeutic Touch

Therapeutic touch was developed in 1972 by Dr. Delores Kreiger, a nurse and professor at New York University, and Dora Kunz, a natural healer. Contrary to what the name implies, the therapeutic touch practitioner focuses on modulating the patient's energy field rather than physically touching the patient. The technique is based on Rogers' theory of the unitary human being, which theorizes that the body is an open energy field that interacts with the environment. The practitioner consciously directs and sensitively modulates human energies. The therapist *centers* and then assesses the energy fields, *unruffles* or clears and immobilizes the energy field, directs energy and balances the energy field. Therapeutic touch has been used to decrease pain perception and anxiety, to improve wound healing, and to promote relaxation. Many nurses learn therapeutic touch techniques and use it in conjunction with nursing practice with consenting patients. It is one of the more controversial of the CATs among nurses.

Reiki

Reiki involves the use of intentional touch with a receptive patient to promote healing. The term *reiki* means "universal life force energy" and *reiki* practitioners draw energy into their bodies through the crown of their head. This energy then passes through the body and out of their hands to the patient. Specific hand placements are used during a session to cover the major human organs, focusing on the seven major energy charkas in the body. Healing can occur as energy passes to the patient (Box 2-12). *Reiki* practitioners may also perform self-healing techniques.

Vibrational Medicine

Vibrational medicine uses the fluctuating energy fields from electronic devices, the human voice, or musical instruments to promote health. Music, sound, and vibration can produce changes in heart rate, blood pressure, brain waves, and muscle contractions. For years low-frequency sound has been used in various forms to cause physiologic and psychologic effects.

Physioacoustics

Physioacoustics is the science of applying low frequency stimulation to the human body to obtain desired effects. It uses sine waves in the range of 20 to 120 Hz. The subject may sit in a special chair or lie on a special mattress. Preselected frequencies or sounds are played through simple speakers and are more felt than heard. A contraindication for vibrational therapy is an acutely herniated disk. Potential uses include stress, anxiety, and pain reduction.

Bioelectromagnetics

Bioelectromagnetics explores the interactions of electromagnetic fields and radiation with living tissues. Everything in our world is magnetic at some level and all physical bodies have magnetic fields. The earth itself has a geomagnetic field of 0.5 gaass. Exogenous static and electromagnetic fields influence and moderate the properties of biologic systems, yet there is no consensus about how they operate.

In Western culture magnetic fields are usually thought of as manufactured (e.g., the current in an electric outlet), even though the use of electromagnetic fields in health care is well known. Electrocardiograms and electroencephalograms have been used to measure electrical activity in the heart and brain for many years. Electricity and magnetism are frequently used in diagnosis (e.g., magnetic resonance imaging). Eye magnets have been used to remove shrapnel and a magnetic technique is used to treat retinal tears. External cardiac defibrillators and pacemakers are other common examples.

The use of magnets is currently being researched for a variety of purposes, although there is no proven protocol that sets out

BOX 2-12 Principles of Reiki

Just for today I will live the attitude of gratitude.
Just for today I will not worry.
Just for today I will not anger.
Just for today I will do my work honestly.
Just for today I will show love and respect for everyone.

the optimum dosage for therapeutic effects, maximum magnetic flux density, frequency of change in density, duration of exposure, or frequency of exposure. Magnets are currently being evaluated in wound healing, with the use of magnets that have less magnetism than the earth's magnetic surface. Magnetic support wraps are also being studied, although their therapeutic mechanism remains unclear. Theories include gene expression and an increase in blood flow. Dose, field strength, and duration must all be considered as variables in any study. One of the difficulties with blinded research in this area is how to effectively use magnetized versus sham magnets. It is important to consider competing effects, side effects, and cultural influences when evaluating any magnet research. Researchers are also continuing to evaluate the potential dangers of low-frequency fields. Individual case reports continue to speculate about the potential adverse effects of weak magnetic energies from cellular phones, high-tension power lines, and household appliances on the development of cancer, birth defects, and other health problems (see Chapter 15). Chairs with pulsed magnetic fields are being used with females with bladder incontinence and males after prostatectomy. Questions about the effectiveness of these interventions will gradually be resolved through clinical trials. Nurses will encounter persons using magnetic therapy in a variety of settings.

NURSING MANAGEMENT

The United States is undergoing rapid and profound changes in its demographic composition, and it is not unusual for nurses to come from different social, ethnic, cultural, and religious backgrounds than their patients. The provision of nursing care to persons using alternative and complementary therapies mandates that the nurse have an awareness of and sensitivity to the patient's unique sociocultural background and health promotion and disease prevention traditions.

Nurses must understand that patients may have differing world views and interpretations of health and illness that are based on their own unique life experiences and beliefs. Nowhere is this awareness and sensitivity more important than in dealing with complementary and alternative therapies. Patients from different cultures may have been using alternative therapies as their primary approach to health and illness care, and they may be extremely uncomfortable with and suspicious of mainstream Western medicine. Nurses need to be culturally aware of and sensitive to, as well as knowledgeable about, cultural beliefs and alternative practices. Some nurses believe that they should treat all patients the same. This attitude conveys a sense of equality but fails to acknowledge that very real cultural differences exist between people. It is not possible to act in exactly the same manner with all patients and still hope to deliver effective, individualized holistic care. Health beliefs and practices must be recognized and respected, not challenged or disparaged. Blending divergent viewpoints is difficult but not impossible, and nurses are important advocates for patients within the health care system.

Nursing was one of the first health professions to facilitate the use of CATs. Nursing deals with individuals as whole persons and CATs complement this philosophy. Many nursing programs have formally incorporated complementary health practices into the nursing curriculum. This formal knowledge allows the nurse to select interventions that can be easily integrated into the patient's belief system and lifestyle. It is not important to consumers of CATs that the nurse believe that a therapy is effective. Patients will still use them. Nurses need to increase their awareness of CATs health practices to be able to speak knowledgeably about their application, contraindications, and potential beneficial and adverse effects.

A variety of tools are available to assist the nurse to assess the patient and family from a CATs perspective. However, it is equally important for the nurse to carefully assess his or her own sociocultural heritage and health and illness beliefs. We are each the product of our own unique heritage and upbringing, and nurses are affected by this process as strongly as patients. The nurse cannot expect to enter any situation value free, but it is reasonable to expect the nurse to have a clear view of his or her own belief system and how it may affect a patient's care. Nurses are also representatives of the dominant allopathic health care philosophy and need to work carefully to communicate an openness to CATs as well as traditional practices of health and healing. Important assessment considerations related to CATs are summarized in Box 2-13.

The patient or family members are asked about the cause of the illness or problem in a manner that suggests a familiarity with traditional health beliefs as well as mainstream medical care. The patient and family may not believe in the epidemiologic or medical model of disease causation. Therefore they may not understand the rationale for modern treatment modalities and may choose not to follow the recommended treatment regimen. When health beliefs are acknowledged and respected, an impending cultural collision can be prevented. A compromise solution that recognizes the values of both sides is usually possible. One approach is to assume that all patients are using some type of traditional

BOX 2-13 Assessment Considerations Related to CATs

Native Language

Patient and family skills in English
    Speaking, understanding, reading, and writing
Availability of family, friends, or others to interpret
Availability of institutional interpreters

Cultural Heritage

Patient and family's cultural background
Health beliefs
Use of traditional health practices

Use of and Knowledge About CATs

Beliefs about CATs and their role in managing disease or supporting health
Experience with CATs
Use of traditional healers
CAT therapies in current use
    Effectiveness

therapy or CAT and state "tell me about the complementary or alternative treatments or products you are using." Conflicts between the patient's health beliefs and practices and the medical plan of care may be reflected in nursing diagnoses such as:

Ineffective therapeutic regimen management
Ineffective health maintenance
Deficient knowledge
Ineffective coping

Specific nursing interventions are directed toward the unique problems of each patient, but a few broad areas of intervention would be used by any nurse seeking to practice in a holistic and culturally competent way. Perhaps the most important nursing intervention is for the nurse to show respect for the patient's unique heritage and health care beliefs and to honestly attempt to blend those beliefs with the essential aspects of the patient's medical plan of care.

The nurse may be acting as a broker between the patient's traditional practices and the allopathic health care system, or may be attempting to introduce a CAT therapy to a patient who has never considered their use. Both roles require sensitivity and excellent communication skills. Successes may be small, such as facilitating patient access to unique cultural food items, or convincing an anxious patient to participate in a relaxation exercise, but their cumulative effect can be very powerful. As the care coordinator, the nurse is invaluable in interpreting the patient's beliefs and needs to the entire multidisciplinary care team. Health beliefs and practices, such as the use of special prayers and amulets, special foods, and traditional remedies, are integrated into the plan of care if possible.

It is especially important to consider the patient's heritage, educational level, and language skills when planning patient education. The assistance of a qualified interpreter may be appropriate. When patients are not comfortable speaking English, it is also important to plan additional time to orient the patient to the routines and equipment in use in the hospital setting. The nurse anticipates that the patient will be unfamiliar with most of the hospital environment, which can easily become overwhelming when language barriers make it difficult to ask needed questions.

CATs are used as interventions for a variety of nursing diagnoses (Box 2-14). Whenever CATs are introduced, the patient should receive information on the indications, contraindications, potential benefits, and any adverse side effects of the therapy (Box 2-15). The nurse may suggest that the patient keep a daily log of therapies used and document symptom improvement and any side effects experienced. Nurses assist patients to explore CAT therapies that are suitable for them and play an important role in helping patients to locate appropriate CAT practitioners to facilitate ongoing care after discharge (Boxes 2-16 and 2-17).

BOX 2-14 Nursing Diagnoses That May Incorporate CATs Into the Plan of Care

Constipation
Disturbed energy field
Ineffective health maintenance
Health-seeking behaviors
Risk for infection
Risk for injury
Deficient knowledge
Impaired memory
Acute pain
Chronic pain
Spiritual distress
Risk for spiritual distress
Readiness for enhanced spiritual well-being

BOX 2-15 Strategies for Introducing CATs to Clients

Identify the patient's goals for treatment (e.g., symptom management).
Assess the patient's knowledge, beliefs and interest in CATs.
Educate the patient on CAT options.
Offer options that may be beneficial to the patient.
Share current research outcomes.
Discuss expected outcomes of therapy.
Obtain clinical informed consent.
Ask the patient to evaluate the therapy following treatment.

Critical Thinking Questions

1. An elderly African-American man is dying of liver cancer. You've cared for him for several days and believe that you have established a rapport. As you enter his room tonight he tells you that he thinks the end is near and asks if you would spend a few minutes and pray with him.
   a. *How would you respond to his request?*
   b. *Would it matter if you were not religious yourself? Why or why not?*
   c. *If you do decide to pray with him, would this represent a "boundary violation" in your professional relationship?*
2. A 40-year-old woman who lives in a commune settlement has been suffering from severe low back pain and was admitted for a disk procedure. After visits from friends she tells you that she's thinking that a *reiki* practitioner might be able to help her and she asks you to help her discuss this with her physician.
   a. *How would you proceed?*
   b. *What would change, if anything, if you knew her physician considered CATs to be "completely worthless?"*
3. You are attending a dinner party and are introduced to some guests as a nurse and a graduate of the local university's School of Nursing. One man explodes, "Isn't that where that crackpot works who talks about therapeutic touch or some such nonsense?! How can any intelligent person get involved with something so ridiculous?" Respond.
4. Interview a senior member of your family about what traditional remedies or treatments they or their parents may have used for health maintenance or treatment. What CATs are currently practiced in your family?
5. Explore the community where you practice nursing and locate the CATs providers who are available to patients.

BOX 2-16 Evaluating CAT Therapies and Practitioners

Locate a CAT Practitioner

Recommendations from friends
Doctor's office or health center
Natural health center
Health food store
Internet
National organization referral programs

Assess the Safety and Effectiveness of a Therapy

Do the benefits outweigh the risks of treatment? Is there a benefit likely for the typical patient from the average practitioner? Discuss the therapy with the health care provider. Tell the practitioner of all conventional and alternative therapies currently being used.

Examine the Practitioner's Expertise and Credentials

Talk to state or local regulatory agencies with authority over practitioners who practice the therapy you seek. Does the practitioner meet their qualifications? Ask for references and talk with people who have experience with this practitioner. How was their experience? Talk with the practitioner in person to find out about education, additional training, licenses, and certifications. Is there a code of ethics for the professional organization?

Consider Service Delivery

How is the therapy given and under what conditions? Visit the practice setting. Are the conditions of the office or clinic acceptable? Does the service delivery adhere to regulated standards for medical safety and care?

Consider Costs

What therapies will your health insurance carrier cover or reimburse? Compare cost among several practitioners.

Consult Your Health Care Provider

Discuss all issues of treatment and therapies with your health care provider.

Adapted from National Center for Complementary and Alternative Medicine. Considering Complementary and Alternative Medicine, 2001, http://nccam.nih.gov/fcp/faq/considercam.html.

BOX 2-17 CAT Resources

American Academy of Medical Acupuncture
5820 Wilshire Blvd., Suite 500
Los Angeles, CA 90036
1-800-521-2262 or 323-937-5514
Fax 323-937-0959
http://www.medicalacupuncture.org

American Association of Oriental Medicine
433 Front St.
Catasauqua, PA 18032
Phone: (610) 266-1433
Toll Free:888-500-7999
Fax: (610) 264-2768
http://aaom.org E-mail:aaom1@aol.com

American Botanical Council
P.O. Box 144345
Austin, TX 78714-4345
Phone: (512) 926-4900
Fax: (512) 926-2345
www.herbalgram.org

American Holistic Medical Association
4101 Lake Boone Trail, Suite 201
Raleigh, NC 27607
(703) 556-9245
http://www.4woman.org/nwhic/references/mdreferrals/ahma.htm

American Holistic Nurses Association
PO Box 2130
Flagstaff, AZ 86003-2130
800-278-2462 (AHNA)
Fax 520-526-2752
www.ahna.org

American Massage Therapy Association
820 Davis Street, Suite 100
Evanston, IL 60201
847-864-0123
Fax: 847-864-1178
http://www.amtamassage.org

American Yoga Association
P.O. Box 19986
Sarasota, FL 34276
914-927-4977
Fax (941) 921-9844
http://www.americanyogaassociation.org

Association for Applied Physiotherapy and Biofeedback
10200 West 44th Avenue, Suite 304
Wheat Ridge, CO 80033-2840
800-477-8892, 303-422-8436
http://www.aapb.org

Center for Food Safety and Applied Nutrition
http://vm.cfsan.fda.gov

Food and Drug Administration
http://www.fda.gov

Homeopathic Educational Services
2124 Kittredge St.
Berkeley, CA 94704
800-359-9051
510-649-0294
Fax: 510-649-1955
http://www.homeopathic.com

Continued

BOX 2-17 CAT Resources—cont'd

National Center for Homeopathy
801 N. Fairfax St No. 306
Alexandria, VA 22314
877-624-0613
703-548-7790
Fax: 703-548-7792
http://www.healthy.net/nch/

National Certification Commission for Acupuncture and Oriental Medicine
11 Canal Center Plaza, Suite 300
Alexandria, VA 22314
703-548-9004
Fax: 703-548-9079
www.nccaom.org

National Certification for Therapeutic Massage and Bodywork
http://www.nctmb.com

National Institutes of Health
6120 Executive Boulevard
Rockville, MD 20092-9904
301-402-2466

NIH's National Center for Complementary and Alternative Medicine (NCCAM)
NCCAM Clearinghouse
P.O. Box 8218
Silver Spring, MD 20907-8218
Toll Free: 1-888-644-6226
Outside the U.S.: 301-231-7537, ext. 5
TTY: 1-888-644-6226
FAX: 301-495-4957
http://NCCAM.nih.gov

American Society for the Alexander Technique
P.O. Box 60008
Florence, MA 01062
Phone: 800.473.0620 or 413.584.2359
Fax: 413.584.3097
www.alexandertech.com

The Trager Institute
33 Millwood
Mill Valley, CA 94941-2091
415-388-2688
Fax 415-388-2710
http:www.trager.com

Craniosacral Therapy
The Upledger Institute
11211 Prosperity Farms Road, Suite D-325
Palm Beach Gardens, FL 33410
1-800-233-5880, ext.92012
561-622-4334
Fax: 561-622-4771
http://upledger.com
E-mail: upledger@upledger.com

References

1. American Botanical Council: *Popular herbs in the US market: therapeutic monographs,* Austin, TX, 1997, American Botanical Council.
2. Astin JA: Why patients use alternative medicine: results of a national study, *JAMA* 279:1548, 1998.
3. US Department of Health and Human Services: *Acute low back problems in adults,* Clinical Practice guideline No 14, AHCPR publication 95-0642, Rockville, MD, 1994, US Department of Health and Human Services, Public Health Service, Agency for Health Care Policy and Research.
4. Druss B, Rosenheck R: Association between use of unconventional therapies and conventional medical services, *JAMA* 282:651, 1999.
5. Eisenberg DD et al: Trends in alternative medicine use in the United States, 1990-1997: results of a follow-up national survey, *JAMA* 280:1569, 1998.
6. Eisenberg DD et al: Unconventional medicine in the United States, *N Engl J Med* 328(4):246, 1993.
7. Field T et al: Job stress reduction therapies, *Altern Ther Health Med* 3:54, 1997.
8. Fritz S: *Mosby's fundamentals of therapeutic massage,* St Louis, 1995, Mosby Lifeline.
9. Helms J: An overview of medical acupuncture, *Altern Ther Health Med* 4:35, 1998.
10. Menzies V: Guided imagery as a clinical intervention. Paper presented at the Graduate Nursing Seminar in Complementary and Alternative Therapies, University of Virginia, Charlottesville, Va, April 2001.
11. National Institutes of Health, Cancer Facts CAM, Questions and answers about coenzyme Q 10, 2001, website: http://cis.nci.nih.gov/fact/9-16.htm.
12. National Institute of Health Consensus Panel: Acupuncture, *National Institutes of Health Consensus Development Statement.* Sponsors: Office of Alternative Medicine and Office of Medical Applications of Research, Bethesda, Md, 1997, National Institutes of Health.
13. National Center for Complementary and Alternative Medicine, Major domains of complementary and alternative medicine, 2001, website: http://nccam.nih.gov/fcp/classify.
14. National Center for Complementary and Alternative Medicine, Considering Complementary and Alternative Medicine, 2001, http://nccam.nih.gov/fcp/faq/considercam.html.
15. National Center for Complementary and Alternative Medicine, St. John's Wort, 2001, website: http://nccam.nih.gov/fcp/factsheets/stjohnswort/stjohnswort.htm.
16. *NIH Consensus Statement on Acupuncture,* Bethesda, MD, 1997, National Institutes of Health.
17. *Popular herbs in the US market,* Therapeutic Monographs, 1997 American Botanical Council.
18. Smith MC et al: Benefits of massage therapy for hospitalized patients: descriptive and qualitative evaluation, *Altern Ther Health Med* 5:64, 1999.
19. Taylor AG et al: ED staff members' personal use of complementary therapies and their recommendations to ED patients: a southeastern US regional survey, *J Emerg Nurs* 24:495, 1998.
20. *The review of natural products: potential herb-drug interactions,* St Louis, 2000, Facts and Comparisons.
21. *The review of natural products: Ubiquinone,* St Louis, 1998, Facts and Comparisons.
22. Van Wijk R et al: The similia principle as a therapeutic strategy: a research program on stimulation of self-defense in disordered mammalian cells, *Altern Ther Health Med* 3:33, 1997.

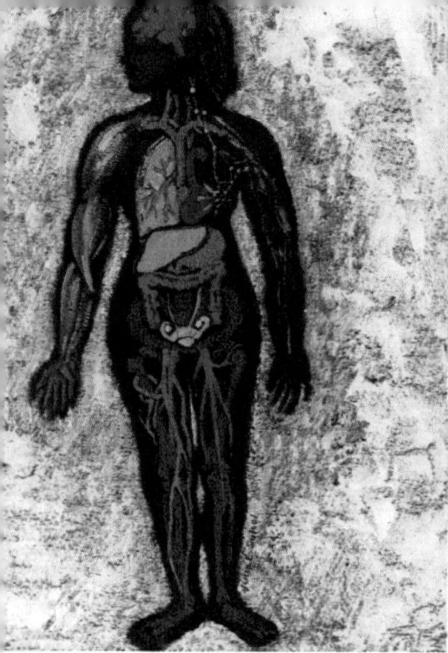

Promoting Healthy Lifestyles 3

Marianne Neighbors

Objectives

After studying this chapter, the learner should be able to:

1. Discuss the development of an agenda for health promotion in the United States.
2. Define terminology related to health promotion, risk reduction, and disease prevention.
3. Compare primary, secondary, and tertiary prevention.
4. Explain the role of physical activity, nutrition, tobacco use, substance abuse, responsible sexual behavior, injury and violence, self-responsibility, and regimen adherence in maintaining or interfering with healthy lifestyles.
5. Describe common tools that can be used to assess the elements of a healthy lifestyle.
6. Develop strategies to assist individuals to adhere to a health-promoting lifestyle.

Healthy lifestyles are increasingly recognized as a key component of optimal wellness in young adults, an essential tool for minimizing the incidence and severity of chronic illnesses and their complications, and an effective strategy for gaining control of the steadily rising costs of health care. Healthy lifestyles are the vehicle by which most of the goals of health promotion and disease prevention are implemented. Professional nursing has a natural connection with the promotion of healthy lifestyles. Nursing has been a strong voice for health promotion and disease prevention since Florence Nightingale first used the principles of hygiene and environmental management in care of the sick and wounded during the Crimean War. Her writings speak of providing the individual with such amenities as ventilation, clean air and water, clean linen, and warmth. She also promoted low noise levels, natural light, and safety in the workplace. Many other cultures, especially the primitive ones, have practiced health-promoting behaviors consistently. It was often the "civilized man" who brought disease and destruction to a once healthy population.

Although research showed the benefits of health promotion decades ago, it has received little support within a care system dominated almost exclusively by attention to disease and illness management. Today, after years of minimal attention in our society, health promotion programs are finally receiving due credit. Employers are starting to recognize the importance of long-term worksite health promotion programs because keeping employees healthy is an asset to the corporation. People are living longer, and the desire to maximize that increasing life span is strong. Our knowledge about the etiology of major causes of morbidity and mortality continues to unfold, and many of these diseases are at least partially related to lifestyle choices, especially in the areas of nutrition, exercise, risky sexual behavior, and alcohol and tobacco use. It is estimated that preventable illness accounts for 70% of the health care spending and that 50% of mortality is linked to lifestyle behaviors.[7] Nurses today have an unprecedented opportunity to make a significant impact on individual lives and positively affect the health of society by assisting people to make informed and healthful lifestyle choices.

Public health initiatives in the twentieth century began with an emphasis on halting the spread of infectious disease. Sanitation, immunization, and the development of antibiotics all combined to achieve tremendous successes. Diseases such as typhoid and smallpox have been virtually eliminated; while most childhood diseases have been brought under control with routine immunization, and epidemics such as polio have been almost totally eradicated. Equally impressive gains have been made through the development of sophisticated technology that can be used for mass population screening (e.g., mammography and Pap smears). A seemingly endless array of pharmacologic agents and high-tech interventions have perpetuated the widely held belief that all diseases and conditions would eventually be effectively controlled or eliminated.

The goal of disease eradication may still lie in the future, but now we are to some degree victims of our partial successes. Life spans continue to increase, and the elderly represent a steadily increasing proportion of the population. Chronic diseases are now the major challenges in health care, and the twofold goals of prevention and control have replaced cure. Aging is accompanied by a steadily increasing incidence of chronic illnesses. The challenge is to postpone or prevent these diseases as long as possible. The relationship between lifestyle choices and the incidence and severity of chronic illnesses is clear and indisputable. Genetics continues to play a crucial role in selected situations, but it is apparent that an individual's health status is, to at least some degree, a reflection of his or her style of living. This chapter addresses the major components of healthy lifestyles and nursing interventions to assist individuals to make health-promoting choices.

A NATIONAL AGENDA FOR HEALTH PROMOTION

The field of health promotion evolved together with the holism and wellness movement of the 1970s. Dunn's concept of "high-level wellness" epitomized this movement with its focus on a continual process of physical and psychoemotional self-actualization. When health promotion finally emerged on the national scene, however, its focus had been expanded to incorporate the fields of disease prevention and the maximization of health within the context of chronic illness. The first public health agenda for the United States was entitled Healthy People: *The Surgeon's Report on Health Promotion and Disease Prevention* and released in 1979.[12] In 1980 another document was released, *Promoting Health/Preventing Disease: Objectives for the Nation,* which specifically targeted areas of needed improvement for the nation in several areas: health status, increasing public awareness, decreasing risks, increasing services, and providing environmental protective measures.[13] For the first time the Surgeon General's office addressed the importance of the environment in influencing health and outlined the importance of government intervention and oversight to ensure these health objectives. The importance of clean air and water, food safety, and occupational safety were all included. Smoking was targeted as a national health hazard.

Healthy People 2000

National Health Promotion and Disease Prevention Objectives, released in 1989, was the next report of national health goals.[11] This document was produced as part of the contribution of the United States to the World Health Organization's (WHO) international project of "health for all by the year 2000." It was also a response to evaluation data indicating that many of the health objectives articulated for 1990 were not being met. Since the 2000 document release, progress has been made in a variety of areas of health concerns. However, continued progress is still imperative to build a healthy nation.[2]

Healthy People 2010

Understanding and Improving Health is the latest document presenting a vision for healthy people and public health opportunities that challenge health providers and planners to achieve new national health goals. The document attempts to reflect changes in demographics, advances in medicine interventions, pharmacotherapeutics and technology, and the impact of global interactions on the health of society. It includes 10 leading health indicators identified as key objectives, that highlight behavioral, physical and environmental factors that are important to the health of people (see Healthy People 2010 box). It also identifies goals by which to measure progress made relative to each health indicator (see Healthy People 2010 box), as well as 467 health-related objectives in 28 focus areas (see Healthy People 2010 box on p. 33).[10] Two of the major changes in demographics are addressed in Healthy People 2010 by a major goal relating to our aging nation and one relating to the diversity of our population. The underlying premise of the document is that the health of individuals is an integral component of the health of the community. Although our nation has seen a decline in childhood morbidity

Healthy People 2010

The Leading Health Indicators According to Healthy People 2010

- Physical activity
- Overweight/obesity
- Tobacco use
- Substance abuse
- Responsible sexual behavior
- Mental health
- Injury and violence
- Environmental quality
- Immunization
- Access to health care

From US Department of Health and Human Services: *Healthy People 2010: understanding and improving health,* Washington, DC, 2000, USDHHS.

Healthy People 2010

Goals for the Leading Health Indicators

- Improve health, fitness, and quality of life through daily physical activity.
- Promote health and reduce chronic disease associated with diet and weight.
- Reduce illness, disability, and death related to tobacco use and exposure to second-hand smoke.
- Reduce substance abuse to protect the health, safety, and quality of life for all, especially children.
- Promote responsible sexual behaviors, strengthen community capacity, and increase access to quality services to prevent sexually transmitted diseases (STDs) and their complications.
- Improve mental health and ensure access to appropriate, quality mental health services.
- Reduce disabilities, injuries, and deaths resulting from unintentional injuries and violence.
- Promote health for all through a healthy environment.
- Prevent disease, disability, and death from infectious diseases including vaccine-preventable diseases.
- Improve access to comprehensive, high-quality health care services.

From US Department of Health and Human Services: *Healthy People 2010: understanding and improving health,* Washington, DC, 2000, USDHHS.

and mortality, mortality from heart disease and stroke, and an increase in longevity, there needs to be an increased focus on promoting healthy behaviors, reduction of diseases, and promotion of healthy communities. Our health expenditures exceed most other countries, yet that has not improved our health record as compared to other developed countries.[9] The Healthy People 2010 objectives related to lifestyles and health promotion are presented in this chapter, and objectives related to specific diseases and conditions are included in chapters throughout this text.

Role of Professional Nursing

The central role of professional nursing in actualizing the commitment to health promotion and prevention is readily apparent. Nursing concepts and theories have focused on self-care, efficacy, and adaptation for decades. Nurses are acknowledged experts in health education and patient teaching and are well prepared to assume a leadership role in this area. In 1992 the American Nurses' Association (ANA) published *Nursing's Agenda for Health Care Reform,* which boldly called for a shift in the health care system from the predominant focus on illness and cure to a focus on wellness and care.[1] Nurses employed in community-based settings such as schools, industry, and clinics have found themselves on the cutting edge of the future in health care as potent social and economic forces have joined to catapult health promotion into national prominence. The cost of chronic illness management continues to drive the cost of health care steadily upward, and predictions for the future indicate more of the same. Effective self-care management within the context of a health-promoting lifestyle has been shown to decrease the need for office visits and hospitalization and therefore the cost to insurers.[6,9] Insurers, primarily in health maintenance organizations (HMOs), are acknowledging that it is cost-effective to invest in health promotion and prevention activities for their subscribers to delay or minimize disease management expenditures in the future. Nurses are quickly selected as the best-prepared health professionals to design and implement these activities.

Business and industry increasingly recognize that a healthy workforce decreases lost days from absenteeism and limits expenditures in copayments for health care. Screening services, diet teaching, and exercise facilities are now common benefits in the workplace as companies attempt to positively influence the health of their workers and minimize costs. Incentives for healthy lifestyles are provided in the form of discounts on insurance for nonsmokers or nondrinkers and for maintaining a healthy body weight. Occupational health nurses are at the center of these efforts and programs.

Education for effective self-care is a cornerstone of management in the acute care setting as well and is again the primary domain of nursing. Changes in acute care settings in an attempt to cut costs have made it extremely difficult for nurses to continue to effectively fulfill this vital role. The "baby-boom" generation, now part of our aging population, is a knowledgeable consumer and has high expectations of health care.[8] They have broad access to health information via the media and Internet. Many are profoundly active in self-care interventions and lifestyle changes to preserve good health. Nurses must continue to be committed to patient education for health promotion, a critical independent function, and claim it as an integral part of their practice in every setting. Professional nurses must also use opportunities to heighten the public's awareness of this important nursing function.

Healthy People 2010

Focus Areas

1. Access to quality health services
2. Arthritis, osteoporosis, and chronic back conditions
3. Cancer
4. Chronic kidney disease
5. Diabetes
6. Disability and secondary conditions
7. Education and community-based programs
8. Environmental health
9. Family planning
10. Food safety
11. Health communication
12. Heart disease and stroke
13. Human immunodeficiency disease
14. Immunization and infectious diseases
15. Injury and violence prevention
16. Maternal, infant, and child health
17. Medical product safety
18. Mental health and mental disorders
19. Nutrition and overweight
20. Occupational safety and health
21. Oral health
22. Physical activity and fitness
23. Public health infrastructure
24. Respiratory diseases
25. Sexually transmitted diseases
26. Substance abuse
27. Tobacco use
28. Vision and hearing

From US Department of Health and Human Services: *Healthy People 2010: understanding and improving health,* Washington, DC, 2000, USDHHS.

OVERVIEW OF HEALTH PROMOTION, RISK REDUCTION, AND PREVENTION

Health promotion, risk reduction, and prevention are broadly overlapping concepts, and healthy lifestyles play an essential role in all of them. Health promotion is the process of increasing awareness through health education about life activities such as eating, exercise, smoking, substance abuse, safety, and pollution. Risk reduction is the process of attempting to reduce one's risk, over time, of morbidity or mortality from chronic disease or acute events. Prevention is the broadest in scope and encompasses primary, secondary, and tertiary prevention.

Health Promotion

Health promotion can be broadly described as a process of fostering awareness, influencing attitudes, and identifying alternatives so that an individual can make informed lifestyle choices that help him or her achieve or maintain optimal levels of physical, mental, and emotional well-being. Health promotion targets personal habits, lifestyle patterns, and the environment to reduce risks and enhance health and well-being, thus strengthening the person's capacity to withstand physical and emotional stress. The concept of health promotion has expanded steadily over the last several decades. Originally directed primarily at young healthy adults seeking optimal wellness, health promotion is now acknowledged as an important goal for people of all ages and health status.

Risk Reduction

Although some would assume that health promotion activity automatically reduces risk, the term *risk reduction* is often separated to make note that using risk reduction strategies for chronic diseases and acute events (such as some accidents and other safety-related issues) is an integral component of healthy behavior. Because many people do not integrate healthy choices into their lifestyle behaviors until diagnosed with a chronic disease, it is important for nurses to educate patients who have been assessed and determined to be at high risk for morbidity or mortality about risk reduction strategies.

Primary Prevention

Most of the activities considered to be components of health promotion can be included within the parameters of primary prevention. Health promotion involves activities that help individuals achieve their maximal health potential. Activities include those designed to prevent the actual occurrence of specific diseases. For example, immunizations and chemoprophylaxis with drugs and other agents are administered to asymptomatic persons in an attempt to decrease their risk of developing disease. Healthy diet and exercise are also partially directed at prevention of diseases such as hypertension, cancer, and coronary artery disease. Societal initiatives as diverse as water fluoridation, nutrient enrichment in foods, clean air and water, the use of seat belts, and the elimination of domestic violence are all strategies for primary prevention. The scope of primary prevention is nearly limitless and is directly influenced by the economic and political climate of the society.

Secondary Prevention

Secondary prevention focuses on the early detection of diseases and their prompt and effective treatment, thereby limiting their seriousness and associated disability. Secondary prevention has expanded extensively over the last 30 years and includes many societal interventions. Examples include mammography; blood pressure, cholesterol, glaucoma, tuberculosis, and fecal occult blood screening; and prostate-specific antigen testing. Many other easier, low-cost screenings are being developed to diagnose morbidity sooner so that early interventions can be initiated. Major screening guidelines developed by eminent research and service groups, such as the American Heart Association and American Cancer Society, and the U.S. Preventive Services Task Force are presented throughout the text in conjunction with their associated disease processes. Treatment modalities are included in the area of secondary prevention and have traditionally received a majority of the health care expenditures.

Tertiary Prevention

Tertiary prevention is directed toward rehabilitation of the individual after an episode of disease or trauma. Tertiary prevention has gradually become the most significant target of health promotion activities. People rarely die today when diagnosed with diabetes, chronic obstructive pulmonary disease, coronary artery disease, hypertension, arthritis, or human immunodeficiency virus. Instead, they can be expected to live for many years, facing the challenges of optimal and effective disease management and pursuing wellness within the context of chronic disease. Chronic illness management is estimated to consume the major proportion of annual health care expenditures. The diagnosis or exacerbation of a chronic disease often creates a readiness point for the individual to be open to education concerning risk reduction and healthier living. Individuals who have never seriously considered changing their behavior and lifestyle may be prompted by the implications of their illness experience to make significant adjustments in their lifestyle. These readiness points are fertile areas for intervention by professional nurses engaged in illness care and management. The nurse's interventions are focused not only on the disease but on ways in which the patient can limit the seriousness and progression of the disease process and simultaneously improve quality of life.

Healthy Lifestyles

A healthy lifestyle is the way of living that includes all the behaviors that enhance the individual's health and reduces the risk of morbidity and mortality. These behaviors act in a cumulative manner to increase one's level of health and well-being. A healthy lifestyle is the result of choices that a person makes over the course of a lifetime. Lifestyles and health behaviors have their foundation within the family unit and reflect the family's unique cultural, ethnic, religious, and socioeconomic heritage and beliefs. These behaviors are powerfully reinforced each day as a child is growing up.[5] Outside influences such as peers, the media, and other life events greatly affect one's choices related to a healthy lifestyle.

Healthy lifestyles are practiced without the supervision of a health care provider, but they can be powerfully influenced by the attitudes and interventions of health professionals. Routine screenings, prenatal and well-child visits, school health education, and public information campaigns all provide opportunities to positively influence lifestyle choices. The patient contacts that occur during the treatment of episodic illnesses are also potential windows of opportunity for primary health promotion and prevention education by health professionals. It is particularly important for health professionals to use episodic illness contacts for health promotion education with young adults who visit a health professional infrequently and are usually in the process of establishing the lifestyle patterns that will carry them through their working years (see Evidence-Based Practice box.)

A FRAMEWORK FOR STUDYING HEALTHY LIFESTYLES

The *Healthy People 2010* document, with its 10 leading health indicators and related measurable goals, provides a current, useful framework for studying healthy lifestyles. Many of the

Evidence-Based Practice

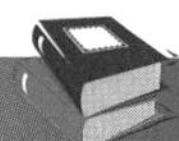

Reference: Sheahan SL: Documentation of health risks and health promotion counseling by emergency department nurse practitioners and physicians, *J Nurs Scholarship* 32(3):245, 2000.

The purpose of the study was to review the documentation of health risk factors and the health promotion counseling that occurred before discharge. Emergency department professionals such as nurse practitioners or physicians did the counseling. The emergency department is not usually regarded as an area where health promotion counseling occurs, but since patients who are at risk for health problems use them frequently, it is an area where identification of risk and counseling should be done. In this two-group comparative study investigators examined medical records of 305 nonacute ambulatory patients. The records sample was stratified and included 151 documented by nurse practitioners and 154 documented by physicians. They looked for specific risk factors, including alcohol use, dental caries, high blood pressure, obesity and tobacco use, and then documentation for counseling for the identified risk factors.

The sample reviewed was relatively young (mean age of 33), and over half of the individuals had at least one identified risk factor. However, only 22% received any counseling about health promotion strategies to reduce risk. Nurse practitioners were more likely to provide counseling about smoking cessation than were the physicians. The investigators concluded that there are many opportunities for identifying risk factors and counseling patients about reducing modifiable risk factors during emergency room visits. They recommended that all health care providers be aware of the goals in *Healthy People 2010* and begin identifying risk factors and documenting counseling completed at all patient encounters in the future.

Healthy People 2010

Goal and Objectives Related to Physical Activity

GOAL

Improve health, fitness, and quality of life through daily physical activity

OBJECTIVES

Increase the proportion of persons appropriately counseled about health behaviors.

Increase the proportion of adults with high blood pressure who are taking action (e.g., losing weight, increasing physical activity, and reducing sodium intake) to help control their blood pressure.

Reduce the proportion of adults who engage in no leisure-time physical activity.

Increase the proportion of adults who engage regularly, preferably daily, in moderate physical activity for at least 30 minutes per day.

Increase the proportion of adults who engage in vigorous physical activity that promotes the development and maintenance of cardiorespiratory fitness 3 or more days per week for 20 or more minutes per occasion.

Increase the proportion of adults who perform physical activities that enhance and maintain muscular strength and endurance.

Increase the proportion of adults who perform physical activities that enhance and maintain flexibility.

Increase the proportion of trips made by walking.

Increase the number of trips made by bicycling.

From US Department of Health and Human Services: *Healthy People 2010: understanding and improving health,* Washington, DC, 2000, USDHHS.

identified health indicators are associated with personal behaviors that can significantly decrease morbidity and mortality among individuals especially (1) physical activity, (2) overweight/ obesity, (3) tobacco use, (4) substance abuse, (5) responsible sexual behavior, (6) injury and violence, and (7) environmental quality. These indicators also line up fairly well with the major categories of risk factors for the primary causes of morbidity and mortality in the United States. Major categories of risk factors usually include age, hereditary factors, lifestyle factors (e.g., diet, exercise, stress, smoking, alcohol use), environmental factors (e.g., pollution, occupational exposure, poverty), and miscellaneous personal choice elements such as unprotected sex, failure to use seat belts, and drunk driving. The discussion in this chapter is limited to six major categories: (1) physical activity and rest, (2) diet and nutrition, (3) tobacco use and substance abuse, (4) sexual behavior, (5) injury and violence, and (6) self-responsibility and adherence to regimen. Risk factors and lifestyle choices associated with specific diseases and disorders are discussed throughout the text.

Physical Activity and Rest

The importance of exercise in a healthy lifestyle has been clearly demonstrated. Active adults live longer and are less likely to experience hypertension, coronary artery disease, diabetes, osteoporosis, selected cancers, and depression. Regular exercise increases physiologic health by improving circulation, increasing cardiovascular fitness and stamina, increasing or maintaining strength and flexibility, maintaining bone mass, increasing glucose tolerance, increasing the proportion of high-density lipoproteins, lowering declines in oxygen use and muscle mass related to aging, and reducing the risk of coronary artery disease.[3,4] Few interventions have such proven benefits supported by major, well-constructed research studies. The benefits of exercise are particularly well established for elders, who typically achieve sustained independence when they integrate active exercise into their lifestyle. The importance of exercise in weight control and in the prevention or delay of osteoporosis is also clearly established. Yet, research clearly indicates that American society is increasingly sedentary. This apparent dichotomy underscores the essential role that personal choice plays in lifestyle patterns. Why people initiate programs of exercise but often do not continue is being reviewed continually by researchers. Many personal characteristics are associated with physical activity such as motivation, self-efficacy, health risk, family orientation, and others that seem to affect one's choices about continued participation in moderate physical activity regimens. Some of the same characteristics affect one's choices about other health risks such as obesity and substance abuse (see Healthy People 2010 box).

Exercise is generally classified as either aerobic or anaerobic. Aerobic exercise is characterized by activities that involve the large muscle groups and that are performed in a rhythmic and continuous nature, usually for at least 15 minutes at a time. Examples include walking, bicycling, swimming, and dancing. Anaerobic exercise is characterized by bursts of energy expended in short time intervals. These activities include weight lifting, baseball, and wrestling. Although aerobic exercise contributes more directly to the development of cardiovascular fitness and endurance, moderate strength training also plays an important role in supporting muscle mass and strength, particularly for women and elders.

Sleep and rest are often grouped together and share many purposes. The precise function of sleep is still uncertain. It is known that the amount of sleep one requires varies with age, activity, and health status. Many adults report they do not get enough sleep. Modern lifestyles seem to contribute to our general "lack of sleep." The effects of stress are difficult to predict for each person, but the hectic pace of the average adult reduces the time available for restorative rest and sleep.

Our understanding of the more subjective area of rest is extremely limited. Physical rest plays an important role in healthy functioning. Adenosine triphosphate (ATP), which is necessary for all types of activities, is not actively stored by the body and must be continuously produced. Physical activity decreases the available pool of ATP, and rest is needed to replenish the supply. Rest also contributes to mental health through effective stress management. The activities that contribute to mental rest and relaxation vary tremendously among individuals and incorporate such diverse strategies as sports, reading, listening to music, and meditation.

DIET AND NUTRITION

The relationship between diet, overall health, and the development of a wide variety of disease processes receives constant attention in both the professional and popular literature today. New studies are reported daily that show a relationship between a dietary element and a disease process. Researchers suggest that dietary practices may be the single most important "choice" factor in determining health and longevity. New information is released daily. However, many of the reports are of preliminary work involving limited samples and draw conclusions from studies with less than rigorous designs. Quality diet research is difficult to perform and requires longitudinal approaches to yield data meaningful in affecting long-term health and well-being. Many of the study results appear to be contradictory and do not provide sufficient guidance to make lifestyle choices. Health care professionals need to remain current and informed about the scope of diet research to help consumers appropriately interpret and apply what they read and hear.

Diet has been found to directly affect the development of major disease processes. Media attention escalated in the 1970s and 1980s as dietary practices were clearly linked to the development of heart disease, diabetes, and selected cancers. Research exploded as the contributions and effects of specific elements were identified and described. Vitamins A, C, and E; beta carotene, fiber, cholesterol, and saturated fats; nitrates and nitrites; food additives and chemicals; and even water have all been spotlighted. Now other elements such as zinc and antioxidants are highlighted in the news as they are linked to positive health results.

The nutritional pyramid developed by the United States Department of Agriculture serves as the broad outline for information and teaching about nutrition (Figure 3-1). The pyramid contains five food groups instead of the four food

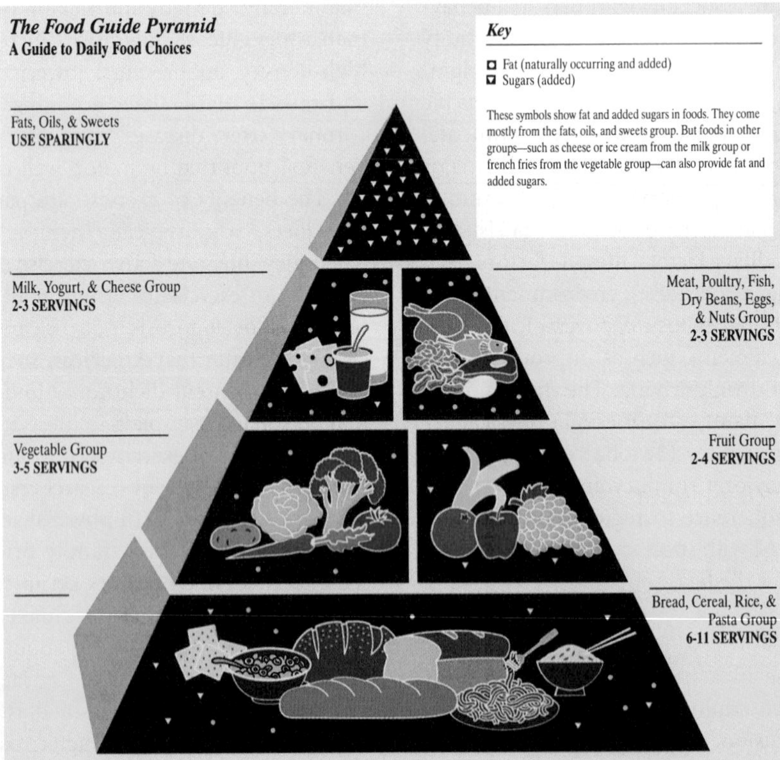

Figure 3-1 Food guide pyramid: a guide to daily food choices and numbers of servings.

groups previously described and is based on extensive research, which indicates that a decreased daily fat intake combined with five daily servings of fruits and vegetables significantly decreases the risk of coronary artery disease, diabetes, and cancer. Americans are increasingly aware of the importance of diet choices but have not been able to make significant changes in daily diet patterns. The "average" American diet still contains too much fat and is heavily skewed toward convenience and prepared foods (see Healthy People 2010 box below).

Current Issues in Diet and Nutrition

Nutrient research has become increasingly sophisticated, and the next decade will contribute much to our understanding of the effects of specific nutrients on such factors as immune system functioning, aging, and the development of chronic diseases. However broad social issues relating to diet and nutrition remain important concerns.

Obesity. Obesity is found in every age group and has gradually become a national health problem of significant proportions. Obesity affects about 50 million persons in the United States. This represents one in four European American adults and one in three African American and Hispanic adults. The links between obesity and numerous chronic diseases have been well established. Obesity is a major risk factor in coronary artery disease, hypertension, cerebrovascular accident, diabetes, arthritis, and some cancers. Some authorities consider obesity the second leading cause of preventable death in the United States after cigarette smoking. There is evidence that complex behavioral, genetic, and environmental factors result in obesity.

Obesity is a chronic disease requiring long-term management, and at present our knowledge base does not contain many effective treatment options. Persons of the same gender and body composition have similar basal energy requirements that can be predicted from their proportion of muscle tissue and body fat. However, these data represent only a beginning understanding of how various bodies metabolize nutrients and respond to increased and decreased demands. The futility of most standard treatment approaches reinforces these principles and has been amply demonstrated. However, weight control remains an important goal because even small percentages of weight loss are associated with significant declines in risks (see Healthy People 2010 box below).

Malnutrition. Malnutrition is still a problem in the United States despite a variety of social policy safety nets and interventions. The culture of poverty continues to steadily expand, and poor children are extremely unlikely to eat a diet that contains rich amounts of fruits and vegetables. Malnutrition is endemic in the homeless and in alcohol and drug abusers and is a growing concern in the rapidly increasing population of elders. The elderly experience steady declines in taste and smell, commonly lose their natural teeth, and increasingly live alone on fixed incomes. Protein calorie malnutrition is present in a significant minority of homebound elders and those in long-term care facilities. Inadequate protein intake is theorized to contribute to the loss of muscle tissue, which both increases the risk of falls in this population and leads to a steady decline in the ability to pursue or maintain an active, independent lifestyle.

Healthy People 2010
Goal and Objectives Related to Nutrition

GOAL

Promote health and reduce chronic disease associated with diet and weight.

OBJECTIVES

Increase the proportion of persons appropriately counseled about health behaviors.

Increase the proportion of persons who consume at least two daily servings of fruit.

Increase the proportion of persons who consume at least three daily servings of vegetables, with one-third being dark green or orange vegetables.

Increase the proportion of persons who consume at least six daily servings of grain products, with at least three being whole grains.

Increase the proportion of persons who consume less than 10% of calories from saturated fat.

Increase the proportion of persons who consume no more than 30% of calories from total fat.

Increase the proportion of persons who consume 2400 mg or less of sodium.

Increase the proportion of persons who meet dietary recommendations for calcium.

Increase the proportion of adults with high blood pressure who are taking action (for example losing weight, increasing physical activity, and reducing sodium intake) to help control their blood pressure.

From US Department of Health and Human Services: *Healthy People 2010: understanding and improving health,* Washington, DC, 2000, USDHHS.

Healthy People 2010
Goal and Objectives Related to Obesity

GOAL

Promote health and reduce chronic disease associated with diet and weight.

OBJECTIVES

Increase the proportion of persons appropriately counseled about health behaviors.

Reduce the proportion of adults who are obese.

Increase the proportion of adults who are at a healthy weight.

Increase the proportion of adults with high blood pressure who are taking action (e.g., losing weight, increasing physical activity, and reducing sodium intake) to help control their blood pressure.

Reduce the proportion of adults who engage in no leisure-time physical activity.

Increase the proportion of adults who engage regularly, preferably daily, in moderate physical activity for at least 30 minutes per day.

From US Department of Health and Human Services: *Healthy People 2010: understanding and improving health,* Washington, DC, 2000, USDHHS.

Osteoporosis

Osteoporosis is a disease characterized by low bone mass and structural deterioration of bone tissue. It affects about 24 million Americans, 15 to 20 million of whom are over 45 years old. About 40% of women who reach age 50 are expected to suffer from osteoporosis during their remaining life. It primarily affects the bones of the spine, hip, and wrists, resulting in 1.3 million fractures annually. Risk factors are many but include a diet low in calcium. The other factors related to osteoporosis are covered in Chapter 47, but the link between calcium content in the diet and the development or prevention of osteoporosis warrants inclusion among the issues related to nutrition and healthy lifestyles. The current recommended daily calcium intake of 1500 mg requires either extremely careful diet planning or appropriate supplementation.

Tobacco Use and Substance Abuse

Smoking has been a front-page story for many years now as the Surgeon General's office, numerous citizens' advocacy groups, some states, as well as individuals, have battled the powerful tobacco industry over the addictive qualities and health risks associated with the use of tobacco. The proposed settlement of $368.5 billion to states over the next 25 years still does not cover the past, present, and future health care expenditures related to tobacco use. The health risks of smoking have been clearly and specifically identified over the last 25 years, but progress related to smoking cessation has been slow, and tobacco use remains a major social concern.

The health consequences of tobacco use continue to be impressive. Smoking tobacco products is the main cause of preventable death in the United States. Approximately 400,000 Americans die each year of smoking-related illnesses. Secondhand smoke accounts for approximately 3000 deaths from lung cancer each year and has multiple adverse effects on the developing fetus (see Research box). From 20% to 30% of low-birth-weight infants can be attributed to maternal smoking during pregnancy, and 10% of the infant mortality rate is also attributed to maternal smoking. Lung cancer mortality rates are about 23 times higher for males who smoke than for nonsmokers. Although most Americans are aware that smoking is directly associated with the incidence and mortality of lung cancer and chronic obstructive pulmonary disease, many are unaware of its contribution to cancers of the bladder, kidney, pancreas, and female reproductive organs. Smoking, combined with heavy alcohol use, dramatically increases the incidence of many gastrointestinal tract cancers. Smoking also contributes to the incidence of coronary artery disease, hypertension, peripheral vascular disease, and cerebrovascular disease.

As nicotine is inhaled into the lungs it is absorbed into the bloodstream. Approximately 15% of the nicotine travels to the brain, where it is absorbed within 7 seconds of inhalation. Nicotine stimulates the release of catecholamines, particularly epinephrine. This release of epinephrine causes tachycardia, constricts the peripheral vessels, raises the blood pressure, and produces a feeling of euphoria. The effects of the nicotine on the blood vessels persist well after the cigarette has been smoked. Over time many smokers are able to regulate their intake of nicotine to produce and sustain the feeling of euphoria without the negative side effects of either over dosage or withdrawal. Nicotine is also one of the most powerful known addictions, which is why efforts directed at preventing smoking are so essential.

Cigarette smoke also contains carbon monoxide, which binds to the hemoglobin in the blood and has a binding capacity 200 times stronger than that of oxygen. The oxygen-carrying capacity of the red blood cells is significantly decreased. In high-risk individuals a decreased oxygen-carrying capacity results in hypoxia, impairs vision and thinking, and increases the incidence of atherosclerosis. Cigarette smoking is not the only problem. Tobacco may also be chewed (snuff) or smoked in cigars and pipes. Many individuals believe that these methods are "safe" because the nicotine and tar contaminants are not inhaled, but these forms of tobacco use cause their own health-related problems. Smoking cigars and pipes and chewing tobacco are among the leading causes of cancers of the lips, tongue, mouth, larynx, and esophagus.

Eliminating a smoking habit is extremely difficult and requires a significant commitment, but its importance to any discussion of healthy lifestyles is readily apparent (see Healthy People 2010 box on p. 39, top left).

In addition to tobacco use, substance abuse is a lifestyle behavior that has incredible consequences on the health of the individual. Substance abuse is a significant problem throughout society. It is estimated that substance abuse-related illnesses and treatments cost more than $90 billion a year. Substance related mental disorder is the diagnosis often used rather than drug addiction. Substances abused include alcohol, amphetamines, caffeine, cocaine, depressants, hallucinogens, inhalants, marijuana, nicotine, narcotics, and sedatives.

Research

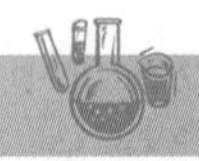

Reference: Martinelli AM: Testing a model of avoiding environmental tobacco smoke in young adults, *J Nurs Scholarship* 31(3):237, 1999.

Environmental tobacco smoke has been shown to be detrimental to an individual's health. The exposure is common among young adults but is preventable.

The purpose of the study was to test a model of avoiding environmental tobacco smoke in 18- to 25-year-old young adults. The explanatory model, consisting of gender, self-efficacy, situational influences and other health promotion behaviors, was based on Pender's health promotion model. Previous studies indicated that young adults who live or associate with smokers are more likely to smoke. Those at lower risk for smoking are ones who report valuing health and participating in healthy behaviors.

A convenience sample of 136 undergraduate students was used in the study. Instruments used included self-reported data on an individual characteristic questionnaire, the General Self-Efficacy Scale, the Health Promotion Lifestyle Profile, and the ETS Avoidance Scale. Results indicated that some of the tendency to avoid environmental tobacco smoke was accounted for by gender, self-efficacy not living with smokers, and using other health promotion strategies. The investigators concluded the model could provide useful information for developing prevention programs for young adults.

The Center for Substance Abuse Treatment (under the U.S. Department of Health and Human Services) has developed a National Treatment Plan Initiative that plans to coordinate research evaluating programs with curative measures in communities, establish standards of care, make effective drug treatment available, and improve public awareness and acceptance of substance abuse rehabilitation (see Healthy People 2010 box).

Healthy People 2010

Goal and Objectives Related to Tobacco Use

GOAL

Reduce illness, disability, and death related to tobacco use and exposure to secondhand smoke

OBJECTIVES

Increase the proportion of persons appropriately counseled about health behaviors.
Reduce tobacco use by adults.
Increase smoking cessation attempts by adult smokers
Increase abstinence from alcohol, cigarettes, and illicit drugs among pregnant women.
Reduce the proportion of nonsmokers exposed to environmental tobacco smoke.

From US Department of Health and Human Services: *Healthy People 2010: understanding and improving health,* Washington, DC, 2000, USDHHS.

Healthy People 2010

Goal and Objectives Related to Substance Abuse

GOAL

Reduce substance abuse to protect the health, safety, and quality of life for all, especially children.

OBJECTIVES

Increase the proportion of persons appropriately counseled about health behaviors.
Reduce past month use of illicit substances.
Reduce the proportion of persons engaging in binge drinking of alcoholic beverages.
Reduce the proportion of adults who exceed guidelines for low-risk drinking.
Reduce the treatment gap for alcohol problems.
Reduce the treatment gap of illicit drugs in the general population.
Increase the number of admissions to substance abuse treatment for injection drug use.
Reduce drug-related hospital emergency department visits.
Increase abstinence from alcohol, cigarettes, and illicit drugs among pregnant women.
Increase the number of communities using partnerships or coalition models to conduct comprehensive substance abuse prevention efforts.

From US Department of Health and Human Services: *Healthy People 2010: understanding and improving health,* Washington, DC, 2000, USDHHS.

Responsible Sexual Behavior

Responsible sexual behavior can prevent sexually transmitted disease as well as unwanted pregnancies. Both of these can contribute to morbidity and even mortality among individuals, especially young adults. Sexually transmitted diseases (STDs) are among the most common and most serious diseases in the public health arena in the United States. Approximately 15 million new cases occur annually. More than 20 types of STDs have been identified. They are epidemic in young adults and even teenagers. According to the Centers for Disease Control and Prevention, STDs cost the health care system more than $10 billion per year (not including treatments for human immunodeficiency virus [HIV] infection). STDs affect men and women of all backgrounds, ethnic groups, and economic status. The incidence is rising partly owing to our changing sexual practices, sexual activity beginning in earlier ages, and young people marrying later.

Health problems caused by STDs tend to be more serious in women because they often have more subtle symptoms and seek treatment only after serious problems develop. STDs in pregnant women are associated with spontaneous abortion, prematurity, low-birth-weight infants, and congenital infections. Chlamydial infections are the most common of all bacterial STDs, with about 4 to 8 million occurring each year. Genital herpes, genital warts, and gonorrhea are also extremely common and on the rise. The incidence of syphilis has decreased dramatically over the last 25 years, but cases are still diagnosed each year, and it may be on the rise again.

Although the onset of acquired immunodeficiency syndrome (AIDS) seemed to alert the public to the devastation of STDs, sexual responsibility is still a significant lifestyle behavior that has not been adopted by a large proportion of the population. Significant progress has been made in terms of public education, but prevention efforts still lag behind the goals set (see Healthy People 2010 box on p. 40).

Injury and Violence

The nation's morbidity and mortality rate from injury and violence is excessive. Motor vehicle accidents, shootings, falls, fires, poisonings, and drowning account for most deaths in this category. Motor vehicle accidents cause most of the serious and chronic injuries. Nurses in acute care settings will take care of many patients hospitalized for injuries, some of them permanent, from automobile accidents. Although death rates are highest in teenagers and young adults, they are common in all age groups. Alcohol-related crashes account for almost half of the deaths from automobile accidents. Reducing the numbers of impaired drivers and increasing the use of safety equipment (e.g., seat belts, infant car seats) is imperative. Safety education programs for young adults are ongoing but keeping alcohol out of the hands of drivers is the real key.

Violence in the nation is an increasing problem. Homicide is one of the leading causes of death in children. Young adult males, especially African-Americans, are at high risk for being victims of homicide. Causes of violence such as stress, poverty, inadequate education, media influences, and others are documented in the literature. The effects of stress have been

Healthy People 2010

Goal and Objectives Related to Sexually Transmitted Diseases

GOAL

Promote responsible sexual behaviors, strengthen community capacity, and increase access to quality services to prevent sexually transmitted diseases (STDs) and their complications.

OBJECTIVES

Increase the proportion of persons appropriately counseled about health behaviors.
Increase the proportion of adults in publicly funded HIV counseling and testing sites who are screened for common bacterial sexually transmitted diseases(STDs) (chlamydia, gonorrhea, and syphilis) and are immunized against hepatitis B virus.
Reduce the proportion of adults with genital herpes infection.
Reduce AIDS among adolescents and adults.
Reduce the number of new cases of AIDS among adolescents and adult men who have sex with men.
Reduce the number of new cases of AIDS among adolescents and adult men who have sex with men and inject drugs.
Increase the proportion of adults with TB who have been tested for HIV.
Increase the proportion of HIV-infected adolescents and adults who receive testing, treatment, and prophylaxis consistent with current Public Health Service treatment guidelines.

From US Department of Health and Human Services: *Healthy People 2010: understanding and improving health,* Washington, DC, 2000, USDHHS.

extensively studied from both physiologic and psychological perspectives, and the negative effects of chronic and excessive stress are well delineated. Chronic stress negatively affects health and is associated with an increased incidence of injury and vulnerability to infection. Over half of the adult population consistently reports that they have experienced at least moderate stress in the previous 2 weeks. The incidence of chronic stress rises sharply among well-educated and highly paid individuals. Role stress in particular has received a lot of attention in the last 20 years. Modern lifestyles force many women to experience career versus family conflicts and challenge increasing numbers of women and men to address the multiple demands of single parenthood. The effects of stress are difficult to predict for any individual, but the hectic pace of many contemporary lifestyles significantly reduces the time available for restorative rest and sleep. The number of adults who report that they are "not getting enough sleep" continues to rise and that increases the stress level. The nurse assists individuals and families to anticipate and recognize stress, prevent it from developing into violence, and develop coping strategies to manage stress (see Healthy People 2010 boxes related to Injury and Violence Prevention in Chapter 7).

Self-Responsibility and Regimen Adherence

Healthy lifestyles do not just happen. They are the result of conscious and unconscious choices and of commitments to specific, daily behaviors. Therefore the area of self-responsibility is the sixth major and perhaps the single most important element of a healthy lifestyle. Any professional involved in health promotion must understand and respect the complex personal, social, political, and economic factors that shape individual lives. It is a fact of the human experience that most people make the easiest choices available to them. The list of self-responsibility issues is almost endless. Most of our current social ills are tied at least in part to individual choices that reflect neither a pattern of health promotion nor self-responsibility. Health care professionals must be aware that they cannot make anyone choose a healthy lifestyle, and adhering to a healthy lifestyle regimen can be a complex challenge.

Regimen adherence is one of the most complex and frustrating phenomena facing health care professionals involved in health promotion and patient teaching. Multiple studies have validated the fact that up to 50% of study populations do not adhere to professional recommendations concerning either disease management or health promotion activities. This fact is reflected in the slow progress and steady resistance associated with even "simple" regimens such as seat belt use, regular daily flossing, and weekly exercise. Dietary changes have proven to be particularly resistant to change because they involve choices that must be made several times every day. People cannot simply abstain from food as they can from tobacco or alcohol use. There are multiple behavior determinants that affect one's capacity to choose and stay with healthy lifestyle behaviors. Such determinants include motivation, socialization, self-efficacy, stress, environment, and other factors. Education and awareness are, of course, important elements of lifestyle choices, but they are not the sole factors. People can commonly state the rationale for lifestyle changes and practices but may still be unable to implement this knowledge in their everyday lives, a fact that is clearly demonstrated in smoking cessation.

Pender's model of health promotion continues to be an effective way to illustrate the forces involved in influencing behavior and lifestyle change (Figure 3-2). Pender identified factors that affect the person's perceptions of the problem, factors that modify behaviors, and factors that influence the likelihood of health-promoting actions. Motivation to participate in health-promoting behaviors is influenced by the individual's perceptions about health in general and perceptions of self, including self-concept and perceived control of the environment. Persons who do not value health, who do not see a need to improve their health status, or who are not self-motivated are less likely to engage in health-promoting activities. The person's age, sex, and ethnicity are among the many potential modifying factors that may be active in any given situation. Identifying an individual's unique and specific modifying factors requires careful and sensitive assessment. The influence of family and friends can also be powerful factors. Research indicates that family support for health-promoting activities enhances a person's successful adaptation to a health promotion regimen.

Perceived barriers to health promotion and regimen adherence include concrete factors such as cost and availability, as well as highly personal and unique factors such as the reactions of significant others. Major factors that have been iden-

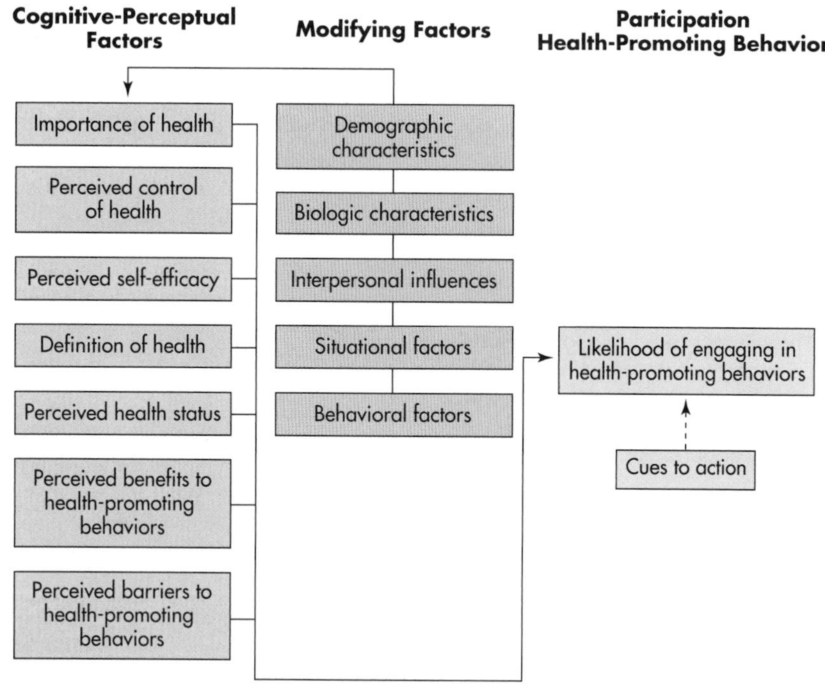

Figure 3-2 Pender's health promotion model.

> **BOX 3-1 Major Factors Affecting Regimen Adherence**
>
> Amount of time the regimen requires
> Visibility of the regimen to others
> Amount of energy required to complete the regimen
> Difficulty of the regimen
> Amount of discomfort associated with the regimen
> Frequency of action required
> Expense of the regimen
> Duration of need for the regimen
> Amount of disruption to "normal" activities
> Perceived effectiveness of regimen in controlling or preventing the disease or condition

tified as barriers to regimen adherence are summarized in Box 3-1. The complexity of the regimen appears to be particularly important. Simpler lifestyle changes are typically easier to make. The degree of behavior change required and the duration of need for the regimen are also critical variables. Changes that must be implemented "for life" are particularly difficult for individuals to sustain over time.

NURSING MANAGEMENT

ASSESSMENT

Assessment is perhaps the most critical phase of the nursing process when working with individuals and families to promote healthy lifestyles. A great deal of time and money have been expended in this country on public information campaigns and education materials designed to positively affect lifestyle choices. The public education approach is grounded in the belief that when people understand the importance of making recommended lifestyle changes, they will be able to incorporate those changes into their daily lives. The fallacies of this approach are apparent in our own lives. Most of us can clearly state the health advantages of selected lifestyle changes, but few of us are able to easily make those changes. Most of us want "easy" answers to difficult issues with minimum disruption of our daily habits. Broad-based educational approaches commonly fail to adequately consider individual value systems and are insensitive to differences in various cultural groups.

The assessment challenge of the professional nurse is to understand the lived experience of the patient and family—their values, priorities, life circumstances, interests, intellect, situational constraints, and support network. Valid and reliable assessment tools can gather pieces of information, but an in-depth understanding of the person's life circumstances emerges from skilled interviewing. This assessment and interviewing process can also be used to establish a working relationship or partnership with the person and family (see Research box on p. 42).

A wide variety of assessment and screening tools exist for evaluating components of the healthy lifestyle. A full presentation of the range of tools is beyond the scope of this chapter. A well-developed functional health pattern assessment tool will provide preliminary data concerning areas such as health beliefs and values, sleep and rest, and exercise. A basic tool can be used to reveal the areas needing in-depth assessment. Examples of the types of tools or questions that can be used in the initial assessment of the components of the healthy lifestyle are displayed in Boxes 3-2 through 3-4.

Research

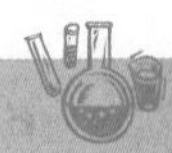

Reference: Kavanagh T et al: Risk profile and health awareness in male offspring of parents with premature coronary heart disease, *J Cardiopulm Rehabil* 20:172, 2000.

The purpose of the study was to assess risk and determine the health awareness of males whose parents had premature coronary heart disease. The premise was that a genetic predisposition combined with environmental or lifestyle risk factors increased ones risk. Increasing awareness and early detection of risk in these individuals would be appropriate public health intervention to protect this population. The sample was a group of 571 sons of parents with premature coronary heart disease. A risk assessment, measurement of body dimensions, blood values, and cardiopulmonary exercise testing was completed on the subjects. A follow-up questionnaire was sent out 2 years after the evaluation.

Although subjects were concerned about the family history, 23% were smokers and 75% were inactive. The 2-year follow-up data showed the subjects reported increased awareness of risk, with more subjects participating in exercise and weight reduction programs. The study showed that sons of parents with premature coronary heart disease exhibit modifiable risk factors. These may be reduced through appropriate screening, education, and counseling sessions.

BOX 3-2 Subjective Assessment Categories for Health Risk Appraisal

General background information, including family history
Preventive measures practiced
Gender specific questions
Diet
Exercise patterns
Safety measures
Use of over-the-counter drugs, complementary, and alternative therapies
Stress and coping patterns
Rest and sleep patterns
Alcohol or other substance use and abuse
Tobacco use

Objective assessment is also included in the data-gathering process related to healthy lifestyles. The components vary substantially according to the setting and purpose of the nurse's interactions. Common objective areas for assessment include:

General appearance
Height and weight compared with standard reference tools
Body mass index (BMI) calculated by dividing the weight in kilograms by the height in meters squared (20 to 25 kg/m^2 is a healthy range for adults)
Skinfold measurements
Range of motion of joints
Treadmill exercise tolerance assessment
Laboratory tests (e.g., cholesterol, lipids, hemoglobin, hematocrit)
Vital signs (respirations, pulse, blood pressure)

BOX 3-3 Sample Assessment Questions for Health Beliefs

Health Perception– Health Management Pattern

1. How has your general health been?
2. Have you had any colds in the past year? Have you had any absences from work/school?
3. What are the most important things done to keep healthy? Do you think these things make a difference to health?
4. Do you use any "home remedies" to cure ailments or ease pain?
5. Have you had any accidents (home, work, driving)?
6. In the past, has it been easy to find ways to follow suggestions of doctors or nurses?
7. If appropriate: What do you think caused this illness? Action taken when symptoms perceived? Results of action?
8. If appropriate: What is important to you while you are here? How can we be most helpful?

BOX 3-4 Sample Brief Dietary/Nutritional Assessment Form

Name _______ Age _______ Health History ___________
Ht _____ Wt _____ BMI ____ Recent change in weight
(if yes, note cause)___________
Food Allergies _________ Food Type Preferences _________
Cultural or Religious Dietary Influences___________
Medications, including nutritional supplements ___________
Usually daily nutritional intake ___________
Patterns of eating (e.g., time, size of meals, snacks) _________
Difficulty with meals (e.g., preparing, shopping problems) ____
Difficulty eating (e.g., chewing, swallowing, digesting) _______
Food safety practices ___________
Usual meal preparer ___________
Other problems with diet or nutrition ___________

NURSING DIAGNOSES

A wide variety of nursing diagnoses may be applicable in any specific patient situation. Promotion of healthy lifestyles will be a goal in working with adults of all ages, regardless of their baseline health status. Efforts can be directed at improving the health status of individuals who are basically healthy, decreasing risk factors in individuals who are asymptomatic but at risk for particular disease processes, and improving the health of individuals already experiencing chronic diseases who need to adhere to a health regimen. The following diagnoses can serve as broad umbrellas for these unique situations. (NOTE: The diagnosis of health-seeking behaviors does not use the standard *related to* etiology and simply states the desired area for knowledge or change.)

Diagnostic Title	Possible Etiologic Factors
1. Health-seeking behaviors	Exercise plan to improve fitness and minimize the effects of osteoporosis
2. Ineffective health maintenance	Oral intake in excess of metabolic requirements; eating in response to stressors
3. Potential for effective therapeutic regimen management	Desire to quit smoking

EXPECTED PATIENT OUTCOMES

The appropriate outcomes will vary greatly, reflecting the unique personal and etiologic factors of the diagnosis. Sample outcomes for the situations reflected in the diagnoses identified above might include:

1. Will participate in a regular physical exercise program that includes weight-bearing exercise of at least 30 minutes' duration a minimum of three times per week

2a. Will verbalize an intent to modify the diet in ways that conform to the recommended food pyramid

2b. Will balance food intake and energy expenditure to support a 1 pound per week weight loss

2c. Will identify alternative coping mechanisms for dealing with life stress without excess food intake

3a. Will describe the short- and long-term health effects of tobacco use

3b. Will verbalize the desire to eliminate tobacco use

3c. Will significantly reduce the amount of tobacco used daily or quits

INTERVENTIONS

1. Promoting an Optimal Body Weight

The complexity of weight loss has been addressed earlier in the chapter. All weight management approaches focus on establishing a lifelong balance between food intake and energy expenditure that supports gradual weight loss if needed. Diet has always received the most attention in weight loss efforts and diet changes remain appropriate, but most exotic and highly restrictive plans have proven to be ineffective for long-term weight control.

Diets are individualized with the caloric intake planned at a level below the person's maintenance needs. Although there are "ideal" weight charts available, the Body Mass Index (BMI) is a better measurement of overweight because it applies to both men and women regardless of their frame size or muscle mass (Figure 3-3). It does not work for pregnant women, competitive athletes, or frail elders. The loss of 1 pound of fat per week requires a calorie deficit of 500 calories per day. Weight loss for some persons may be achieved by eating three average balanced meals a day. Other persons are more successful with frequent small meals. When caloric intake is severely reduced there is often a large initial weight loss through water loss. A plateau is then reached, which lasts 7 to 10 days and may be very discouraging to the dieter. Weight loss then continues at a slower rate as the body adapts to the decreased caloric intake by decreasing the metabolic rate. Weight loss programs should be integrated with moderate exercise programs for the most effective results. Exercise promotes the loss of fat rather than lean body tissue and positively affects serum insulin and lipid levels. Adding regular exercise also improves general health and well-being and allows the individual increased flexibility in daily dietary intake. Support from others appears to be critical. Having a weight-loss/exercise partner is usually beneficial. Positive results are often obtained in the context of weight loss groups such as Weight Watchers.

The use of appetite suppressants is controversial because of long-term inefficiency and associated health risks. Most over-the-counter diet aids contain phenylpropanolamine and bulk-producing agents. Phenylpropanolamine is a sympathomimetic with mild anorectic action but no adverse central nervous system effects. Its effectiveness as a weight loss drug in humans remains questionable. Bulk-producing agents such as methylcellulose expand the stomach and provide a sense of fullness, but the same effect can be achieved by drinking two or three glasses of water before each meal.

Prescription drugs such as sibutramine (Meridia) suppress the appetite but should be used in conjunction with other treatments such as exercise and nutritional alterations. Previously approved drugs such as fenfluramine (Redux) and phentermine for appetite suppression in severe obesity were very promising, but a surprising incidence of heart valve problems and cases of pulmonary hypertension have resulted in the withdrawal of these drugs from the American market. The future of pharmacologic support for weight loss therefore remains unclear. The surgical management of severe obesity is discussed in Chapter 33.

Limiting Acohol Use

Alcohol use must be included in any discussion of a healthy diet. Alcohol use is pervasive in American society, and the potential for abuse and addiction is tremendous. Although high in calories, alcohol has no nutrient benefits and contributes to a wide variety of medical disorders, including alcoholic cirrhosis. The nurse carefully explores the individual's use of alcohol and its meaning in his or her life. If a person does not currently use alcohol, there is no reason to begin. However, if alcohol use is important the individual can safely and appropriately incorporate it into the lifestyle. Some modest health benefits have even been attributed to the occasional use of alcohol in the form of red wine. Daily alcohol intake should be limited to no more than two cans of beer, two small glasses of wine, or two drinks containing no more than 1½ ounces of alcohol each.

1. Promoting Exercise

The nurse attempts to assist the person to establish and maintain a program of regular moderate exercise to enhance physical and emotional health. A variety of exercise plans can be used to achieve this goal, but any exercise program should have moderate weight-bearing exercise as its foundation. The recommendations for amount, intensity, and duration of exercise have varied somewhat over the last decade. It is generally agreed that moderate intensity exercise that involves the large muscles and takes place at least three times per week for 30 to 60 minutes can achieve reduction in risk for cardiovascular disease and stroke, in addition to assisting in maintaining a healthy weight.[4] Higher levels of frequency, intensity, and duration can be established for individuals as appropriate. Regular exercise increases the person's energy and feeling of well-being; the individual should feel replenished, not depleted. Moderate-intensity exercise, with brisk walking as the classic example, carries a very low risk of injury and is achievable for adults of all ages.

Body Mass Index Chart

BMI ▶	18	19	20	21	22	23	24	25	26	27	28	29	30	31	32	33	34	35	36	37	38	39	40	41
Height ▼	Weight in Pounds ▼																							
60 ins	96	97	102	107	112	118	123	128	133	138	143	148	153	158	163	168	174	179	184	189	194	199	204	209
61 ins	98	100	106	111	116	122	127	132	137	143	148	153	158	164	169	174	180	185	190	195	201	206	211	217
62 ins	101	104	109	115	120	126	131	136	142	147	153	158	164	169	175	180	186	191	196	202	207	213	218	224
63 ins	105	107	113	118	124	130	135	141	146	152	158	163	169	175	180	186	191	197	203	208	214	220	225	231
64 ins	108	110	116	122	128	134	140	145	151	157	163	169	174	180	186	192	197	204	209	215	221	227	232	238
65 ins	110	114	120	126	132	138	144	150	156	162	168	174	180	186	192	198	204	210	216	222	228	234	240	246
66 ins	115	118	124	130	136	142	148	155	161	167	173	179	186	192	198	204	210	216	223	229	235	241	247	253
67 ins	120	121	127	134	140	146	153	159	166	172	178	185	191	198	204	211	217	223	230	236	242	249	255	261
68 ins	122	125	131	138	144	151	158	164	171	177	184	190	197	203	210	216	223	230	236	243	249	256	262	269
69 ins	125	128	135	142	149	155	162	169	176	182	189	196	203	209	216	223	230	236	243	250	257	263	270	277
70 ins	130	132	139	146	153	160	167	174	181	188	195	202	209	216	222	229	236	243	250	257	264	271	278	285
71 ins	134	136	143	150	157	165	172	179	186	193	200	208	215	222	229	236	243	250	257	265	272	279	286	293
72 ins	137	140	147	154	162	169	177	184	191	199	206	213	221	228	235	242	250	258	265	272	279	287	294	302
73 ins	140	144	151	159	166	174	182	189	197	204	212	219	227	235	242	250	257	265	272	280	288	295	302	310
74 ins	145	148	155	163	171	179	186	194	202	210	218	225	233	241	249	256	264	272	280	287	295	303	311	319
75 ins	148	152	160	168	176	184	192	200	208	216	224	232	240	248	256	264	272	279	287	295	303	311	319	327
76 ins	152	156	164	172	180	189	197	205	213	221	230	238	246	254	263	271	279	287	295	304	312	320	328	336

BMI less than 18.5, underweight; BMI 18.5-24.9, healthy weight; BMI 25-29.9, overweight; BMI 30-39.9, obese; BMI 40 and above, extremely obese.

Figure 3-3 Healthy body mass index ranges for Americans. (Adapted from NHLBI Obesity Education Initiative, NIH, www.nhlbi.nih.gov.)

Consensus is lacking about who needs a physical examination or cardiac screening before beginning an exercise plan. Adults under 45 years of age who do not have significant cardiac risk factors can usually safely begin an exercise program without preliminary screening. The nurse encourages these individuals to begin slowly, increase intensity progressively, and report the occurrence of any unusual or unexplainable symptom promptly. Adults over age 45 or at known risk of cardiovascular problems should consult with their physician before beginning an exercise program.

An exercise prescription specifically delineates the type, frequency, intensity, and duration of exercise. Intensity and duration can steadily increase as the person's conditioning improves. In addition to this basic aerobic plan, the individual may also be counseled to include some strength training. Strength training has proven to be very effective for women seeking to minimize the progression of osteoporosis and for elders who need to maintain muscle mass, strength, balance, and flexibility.

The nurse instructs the person about the importance of both range of motion and stretching exercises before the aerobic phase of exercise, and the importance of a slow cool down period at the conclusion of exercise so the heart rate can gradually return to its resting level. These precautions help protect the muscles and joints from injury and prevent the incidence of post-exercise hypotension and syncope.

Exercise is also commonly prescribed as part of tertiary prevention for persons with chronic illnesses. Exercise has been shown to increase tolerance for activities of daily living (ADL), increase appetite, decrease anxiety and depression, and promote adjustment. The exercise program is specifically tailored to the person's unique needs and abilities. Exercise is begun at a low intensity, and both frequency and duration are modified as needed. Walking, cycling, and swimming are often well tolerated. When specific exercise prescriptions are indicated (e.g., after myocardial infarction or with chronic obstructive pulmonary disease), an exercise physiologist will typically perform the assessment and set the program parameters.

The nurse uses in-depth assessment to determine the patient's perceived barriers and supports for exercise. Getting started is typically the biggest barrier to the establishment of a regular exercise plan. Both home-based and workplace programs are effective for various groups of people. The nurse reminds the individual that expensive equipment and health club memberships are not necessary for a successful exercise plan. A partner to share the exercise is a strongly positive motivator for most people. Walking remains an ideal choice for many people because the risk of injury is low, the intensity and duration are easily controlled, and the exercise requires no special training. Adherence to the plan remains a challenge, however, and an exercise plan can easily fall into disuse. Some strategies that can be used to foster adherence to an exercise regimen are included in the Patient Teaching box.

Patient Teaching

Strategies for Establishing a Successful Exercise Plan

1. Exercise should be fun or at least pleasurable. Find an activity that you can enjoy.
2. Establish specific time periods for exercise and plan them into your week. You are more likely to exercise if it is a scheduled event.
3. Start in small increments and progress slowly. Monitor your body's response to increases in intensity or duration.
4. Set small, attainable goals and reward yourself as you achieve each goal.
5. Wear proper clothing and use exercise equipment correctly.
6. Be sure to warm up and cool down thoroughly before and after exercise.
7. Avoid exercising in extremes of heat, cold, or humidity.
8. Avoid exercising for about 2 hours after a heavy meal. Do not eat for about 1 hour after active exercise.
9. Share the activity with a friend, or consider joining a structured exercise class. Many community agencies sponsor exercise groups such as swimming, low impact aerobics, and mall walking.

BOX 3-5 Dietary Guidelines for Americans

Aim for Fitness

Aim for a healthy weight.
Be physically active each day.

Build a Healthy Base

Let the pyramid guide your food choices.
Choose a variety of grains daily, especially whole grains.
Choose a variety of fruits and vegetables daily.
Keep food safe to eat.

Choose Sensibly

Choose a diet low in saturated fat and cholesterol and moderate in total fat.
Choose beverages and foods to moderate your intake of sugars.
Choose and prepare foods with less salt.
If you drink alcoholic beverages, do so in moderation.

Source: Dietary Guidelines for Americans 2000, USDA.

2a. Promoting a Healthy Diet

The guidelines for healthy eating for adults of average risk, presented in Box 3-5, are fairly straightforward, and are built on the food guide pyramid. The guidelines emphasize distribution and variety and reflect current knowledge that good nutrition involves a balance of nutrients, fiber, fluids, vitamins, and minerals. The diet stresses the importance of vegetables, fruits, and grains in the daily diet and encourages individuals to decrease their intake of saturated fats and cholesterol. Individuals who are already experiencing chronic illnesses or who are assessed as being at higher risk may need more specific guidelines concerning the balance and distribution of foods. A more detailed description of the principles of healthy eating is provided in the Patient Teaching box on p. 46.

The nurse assists the person to use the food guide pyramid for effective daily meal planning. Using initial assessment

Patient Teaching
Guidelines for Healthy Eating

1. Always eat breakfast.
   a. Drink 100% fruit juice with breakfast or later in the day.
   b. Eat some fruit with the breakfast or take some to work with you.
2. Reduce your daily fat intake to no more than 30% of your total calories (no more than 10% should be from saturated fats) and reduce your cholesterol intake to less than 300 mg/day.
   a. Use "lite" or low-fat dairy products.
   b. Use only a tablespoon of salad dressing.
   c. Choose lean cuts of meat, trim the fat, and drain the grease.
   d. Use reduced-fat margarine or spreads.
   e. Substitute low-fat or fat-free baked goods, cookies, and ice cream.
   f. Leave the cheese off foods unless low fat type.
3. Maintain a reasonable protein intake within the stated fat restriction.
   a. Choose lean roast beef or grilled chicken.
   b. Keep portions to regular and small; do not "double or super size" portions.
4. Eat five or more servings of vegetables and fruits daily. Be sure to include green and yellow vegetables and citrus fruits.
   a. Use ready-to-eat vegetables for snacks.
   b. Use fresh fruit for snacks.
5. Increase your intake of complex carbohydrates by eating six or more servings of breads, cereals, and legumes.
   a. Choose oatmeal for breakfast and whole grain cereals.
   b. Eat beans and soy products more frequently.
6. Increase the fiber in your diet to 20 to 30 g/day. Add small amounts of fiber daily, and be sure to maintain a liberal intake of water.
   a. Choose more cruciferous vegetables for salads and side vegetables.
   b. Add fiber supplements to foods.
7. Drink five to eight 8-ounce glasses of water each day.
   a. Substitute water for sodas, tea, and coffee at least two to three times a day.
8. Limit the amount of salt you consume each day to 6 g (slightly more than 1 tsp).
   a. Refrain from adding it during cooking and avoid adding salt at the table.
   b. Eat salty foods sparingly, especially salty snacks that are also usually high in fat.
9. Refrain from alcohol intake.
   a. Consume no more than 12 ounces of beer, 4 ounces of wine, or 2 to 3 ounces of liquor a day.

findings to identify needed dietary changes. Second, the nurse integrates the patient's dietary restrictions, likes and dislikes, and cultural factors to assist in meal planning. Most sedentary women and older adults need about 1600 total calories per day; this represents the lower end of the serving range on the pyramid. Men usually need about 2200 calories per day, which reflects the upper end of the serving range. Box 3-6 gives examples of standard servings for meal planning purposes. Individuals need to pay particular attention to the serving size for meat because 2 to 3 ounces is a much smaller amount than most people would usually regard as a serving. The individual

BOX 3-6 The Food Guide Pyramid: Standard Foods—What Counts as 1 Serving?

Bread Group

1 slice of bread
½ English muffin or bagel
1 cup ready-to-eat cereal
½ cup cooked cereal or pasta

Fruit Group

1 medium apple, banana, or orange
¾ cup cooked or canned fruit
¾ cup fruit juice

Vegetable Group

1 cup raw leafy vegetables
½ cup cooked or chopped raw vegetables
¾ cup vegetable juice

Meat Group

2-3 ounces* cooked meat, fish, or poultry
1 cup cooked dry beans or peas
2 eggs or 4 tbsp peanut butter

Milk Group

1 cup milk, yogurt, or ice cream
1-2 ounces cheese
½ cup cottage cheese

*1 ounce of meat or cheese is the size of a matchbox; 3 ounces are the size of a deck of cards; 8 ounces are the size of a paperback book.
Source: US Department of Agriculture and the US Department of Health and Human Services.

can use a blank pyramid to adapt the general guidelines to his or her own unique food likes and dislikes. A blank pyramid also facilitates incorporation of cultural or religious food practices into the meal planning process. These can be listed under the appropriate food group on the pyramid.

The average American diet is at least 10% to 15% higher in total fats than is recommended. Fats should be used only sparingly as illustrated in the pyramid. This point becomes even more important for persons who have multiple risk factors or who already have heart or vascular disease. This emphasis on reducing dietary fat is reflected in the *Healthy People 2010* nutrition goal and objectives.

The nurse encourages individuals to have their baseline cholesterol level determined and provides some simple strategies for reducing dietary fat and cholesterol (see Patient Teaching box on p. 47). Reducing fat and cholesterol is often an extremely difficult change because it targets foods popular in American culture such as high fat cheeses, red meat, and cold cuts. The nurse may also need to teach about the major sources of fat and cholesterol in the average diet.

Permanent diet changes are difficult to sustain and are more likely to be successful when modifications are made gradually. For example, the change to skim milk can be made gradually by first switching to 2% milk and then decreasing the milk fat content again several weeks later. Altering the entire diet is rarely successful, so the nurse encourages the per-

Patient Teaching
Reducing Fat Content in the Diet

1. Eat fish or shellfish at least twice a week. Clams, scallops, and oysters contain less cholesterol than crab, shrimp, and lobster.
2. Eat lean, well-trimmed meat. Trim loose fat.
3. Use skinless chicken and trim loose fat. Light meat has less cholesterol than dark meat.
4. Prepare foods by broiling, roasting, or baking. Avoid frying.
5. Use low-fat or nonfat dairy products.
6. Use tub margarine rather than stick. Stick margarine has more saturated fat, particularly the trans-fatty acids.
7. Use low-fat or nonfat salad dressings. Read labels carefully.
8. Use low-saturated-fat oils such as canola or safflower.
9. Consider the use of substitutes, such as egg substitutes, cooking sprays, cream and butter powders, and products using fat substitutes.

son to select one or two important changes on which to focus his or her efforts. These changes can then be supported through printed materials, written or pictorial, prepared at a reading level that is appropriate and acceptable to the person. Whenever possible diet discussion and teaching should incorporate the whole family or social unit. Success is rarely possible when the family does not endorse the needed changes. This is especially true when the patient is not the primary food preparer. The messages given to the patient must be practical and consider financial resources and other environmental constraints such as access to food and equipment for food preparation. When the desired changes are complex, consultation with a dietitian is usually appropriate. The dietitian initiates the teaching, and the nurse reinforces the learning by providing additional explanations about the diet and helping the patient adapt current dietary patterns to meet the new diet prescription.

Older adults and others living alone may face additional challenges in eating a healthy diet. The strong social role of food in our society is commonly lacking for persons living alone. Food preparation and consumption can become haphazard and erratic. Small, frequent meals and supplements can be helpful when people have difficulty sustaining an adequate intake. Meals-on-wheels programs and senior center services can be viable alternatives for homebound elders or those with limited mobility.

Food Labels

Food labels can be an important source of information, and the nurse teaches the individual to interpret labels accurately. There has been much legislation lately regarding labeling of foods including what dietary supplements are added and amounts, how to label juice products, clarifying the meaning of terms such as *low*, *reduced*, and *lean*, noting trans-fatty acids and nutrient content claims. The legislation attempts to facilitate consumer decision making about foods and their contents and additives; however, labels are still difficult to understand and tedious to read. The nurse attempts to ensure that individuals understand and use the information that is provided on labels to make appropriate diet choices.

Supplements

Complementary and alternative therapies have become very popular in recent years, and dietary supplements are a major part of this booming industry. Many individuals are routinely exposed to "the benefits" of dietary supplements in the media. It is estimated that the majority of adults in the United States take one or more dietary supplements daily. The nurse determines the person's current use of vitamins, minerals, and other supplements. The need for routine, broad-spectrum supplementation is established after carefully assessing the person's daily intake.

Specific supplementation of vitamins A, B, C, or E may be used as chemoprophylaxis to reduce the risk of certain cancers or to bolster immune function. The need for calcium supplementation is explored with women and all elders. If an individual does not consume dairy products, the average diet provides only about 300 mg of calcium per day, which is far below the recommended level of 1500 mg. Each milk product serving provides another 300 mg. A combined calcium and vitamin D supplement is recommended for adults who are not routinely meeting their daily calcium needs through food.

2b. Promoting Rest and Sleep

The nurse will help the person plan for adequate daily rest and sleep. It is easy to allow lifestyle issues to interfere with sleep patterns. Most people experience sleep difficulties at some time, but these problems are usually amenable to correction by simple measures such as avoiding caffeine, making the environment conducive for sleep, avoiding late naps, and engaging in relaxation activities. Exercise can also be used to increase well-being and promote sleep, and the nurse encourages the patient to engage in regular exercise for its multiple positive health benefits. People experiencing actual sleep disorders face more complex challenges. Stress also negatively affects the individual's ability to achieve adequate rest and sleep. The nurse helps patients improve their overall coping abilities.

2c. Promoting Adherence to a Healthy Lifestyle

The many benefits of healthy lifestyles are well documented. Most of the components of a healthy lifestyle are low tech, low cost, and seemingly simple. Yet the vast majority of adults do not integrate these components into their daily lives. Simply educating people about health risks and benefits does not significantly change behavior. This calls into question the cost-effectiveness of the time and money expended on outreach education for the public.

The challenges related to regimen adherence are very real and frustrating for health care professionals. The difficulties inherent in making lifestyle changes need to be acknowledged in interactions with patients and families. Regimen adherence is a classic example of personal choice and personal control. The nurse needs to be aware of and respect the person's right to make personal choices that conflict with recommended behaviors. The nurse must also realize that professionals are limited in their ability to "force" positive changes. This does not mean, however, that intervention and teaching are either inappropriate or a waste of time. Successful health promotion outreach acknowledges that the individual retains control over his or her own life choices, but nurses commonly encounter people at moments of readiness when life events have conspired to make health status improvement a priority in the person's life (see Evidence-Based Practice box on p. 35). These opportunities to effect positive change must not be squandered.

The nurse begins by assisting the individual to identify supports and barriers to change and to differentiate between actual and perceived barriers. Teaching and health education remain important parts of the overall intervention plan, but the nurse recognizes that they represent the beginning of intervention and not the end. The nurse is responsible for providing the patient with adequate information to make choices; the nurse is not responsible for the choices that are made. Successful change reflects the person's inner drives and goals. Values clarification can help the person recognize and articulate his or her values related to health and personal responsibility. The nurse directly addresses the issue of self-responsibility and personal choice and helps the person recognize how his or her lifestyle behavior is either congruent or incongruent with the person's core values. The nurse then assists the person to address areas of values conflict. This may provide sufficient impetus for the person to initiate needed behavior change.

The person is next assisted to set goals for health promotion and lifestyle change. The nurse needs to be positive and supportive of the patient's goals. Even seemingly minor changes are positive steps and can reduce health risks and improve overall health. The critical starting point is the person's commitment to take responsibility for his or her health.

The nurse then assists the individual to develop and implement a plan that addresses the targeted lifestyle changes. Appropriate family and community resources and supports are identified. The nurse helps the person explore acceptable alternatives for overcoming actual barriers to adherence. The person must believe that the problem is solvable and that he or she is competent to solve it. The nurse needs to be enthusiastic about the person's ability to make needed changes and provide the individual with positive reinforcement for his or her efforts and accomplishments. Behavior modification principles state that positive reinforcement of desired behaviors increases the likelihood that the behavior will be repeated.

Numerous other practical strategies can be effective in promoting adherence to a health promotion regimen. These include keeping the regimen as simple as possible and allowing the person to adapt it as needed to his or her lifestyle. Formal contracting can occasionally be a powerful tool and underscores the importance of working collaboratively with the patient and family. The family plays a critical role in determining successful outcomes. The nurse needs to be thoroughly familiar with the community resources that are available to help the person integrate the regimen into his or her lifestyle. Printed materials, phone calls, and direct referrals to community support groups can help the person take that important first step. Other strategies that can be effective in promoting adherence to a health promotion regimen are in the Guidelines for Safe Practice box.

3. Promoting Smoking Cessation

The hazards of smoking are well known and widely accepted in American society, but more than 46 million persons continue to smoke. Nicotine has been identified as the primary addictive component of cigarettes, and the power of nicotine addiction is now well recognized. Becoming nicotine free is an enormous challenge that has a high risk of failure. The American Cancer Society estimates that more than 70% of smokers would like to quit smoking but have either failed in their efforts to quit or fear making the attempt. This number is expected to rise as society continues to make it more difficult and unacceptable to smoke in public settings. The discouraging success rates of smoking cessation efforts reinforce the fears and hesitancies of current smokers. Almost 17 million smokers attempt to quit smoking each year, but only 1 million actually succeed in becoming and remaining smoke free.

There are clearly no magic programs that can create successful nonsmokers. A variety of approaches exist to assist smokers in their efforts to quit, and each has had some degree of success. Hypnosis, acupuncture, aversion therapy, 12-step support programs, psychotherapy, and various forms of nicotine replacement in gums, patches, nasal sprays, and pills are all in use. The programs with the greatest success appear to be those that combine a behavior modification approach with some form of nicotine pharmacologic support. It is important to remember, however, that a significant portion of successful "quitters" use no formal program and simply decide to quit

Guidelines for Safe Practice

Strategies to Increase Patient Adherence to a Therapeutic Regimen

1. Plan collaboratively with the patient. Remember, the regimen belongs to the individual and not to the nurse.
2. Include the family in all planning and teaching if this involvement is acceptable to the patient.
3. Support the person's overall coping abilities.
4. Simplify the needed regimen as much as possible.
5. Assist the person to incorporate the regimen into his or her preferred pattern of daily activities as much as possible. Encourage the person to tailor the regimen as needed to make it "fit."
6. Be sure that the patient and family understand the rationale for all activities. Provide appropriately written materials for them to keep as references.
7. Explore the idea of contracting with the person for needed behavior change.
8. Provide lots of positive feedback for efforts.
9. Initiate the process of referral to appropriate community self-help and support groups as appropriate. Provide the person with contact phone numbers and addresses and written materials about services. Make the initial telephone contact, if appropriate.

"cold turkey." Each smoker clearly has unique needs for support through this process. The American Cancer Society and the American Lung Association are excellent sources of information about specific smoking cessation resources that are available in any local community.

The nurse must remain aware that no one can make someone else quit smoking, no matter how important this action may be from a health perspective. Ultimately, the motivation and effort must come from the individual. However, every health care professional needs to use every opportunity to reinforce education about the hazards of smoking and provide encouragement to persons who are interested in or willing to try smoking cessation. Patients commonly report that no health care professional has ever directly addressed the need for them to stop smoking or encouraged them to try. Approaching patients about the need to quit is clearly the most significant nursing intervention. Nurses commonly interact with patients at times when life and health circumstances have combined to create a readiness point for life changes, and these opportunities need to be promptly and enthusiastically used.

A basic approach to smoking cessation that can be used with any smoker includes the four *A*'s: ask, advise, assist, and arrange. The nurse *asks* the patient about the nature of the patient's smoking habit and *advises* smoking cessation. If acceptable to the patient, the nurse *assists* the patient to develop a specific plan for smoking cessation and then *arranges* appropriate follow-up monitoring and support. Self-help materials such as brochures, pamphlets, and tapes may prove helpful and should be available in any health care setting. Family involvement and support are critical and can be a defining variable for long-term success. Some type of planned social support during the transition process is helpful for most people. This may involve the family or finding a "buddy" to make smoking cessation a joint effort. Other general behavioral strategies to support smoking cessation are in the Guidelines for Safe Practice box.

Nicotine replacement therapy (NRT) preparations were developed to minimize withdrawal symptoms while the smoker learns to live without his or her accustomed smoking-related habits. The power of these habits is reflected in the common yearning for a cigarette after meals, or the expression of not knowing what to do with one's hands without a cigarette. Nicotine gum was the first major cessation-assistant. Nicotine patches were developed next and offered first by prescription and then for over-the-counter purchase. The principle of each product is to slowly release sufficient nicotine into the bloodstream to minimize cravings. These products are helpful for many people but are no panacea for withdrawal control; however, they can be a useful adjunct to a more holistic plan to stop smoking. The use of nicotine replacement therapies and the antidepressant bupropion helps some people stop smoking. Studies have shown higher long-term rates of smoking cessation using either bupropion alone or in combination with a nicotine patch.

The patches release nicotine through the skin, and skin irritation is the most common side effect. Patients are strongly cautioned not to smoke while using the patch because the risk of nicotine overdose exists, particularly for patients with preexisting cardiac disease. Overdose symptoms include headache, abdominal pain, nausea, and vomiting and can progress to severe hypotension and prostration. Patients should also be aware of the predictable symptoms associated with nicotine withdrawal. These symptoms range in severity and duration for any individual but can be extremely severe at times of intense cravings. Classic withdrawal symptoms include irritability, anger, anxiety, restlessness, hunger, decreased concentration, and cravings. Nicotine gum must be used correctly to be effective. It is not a traditional gum and cannot be used in that way appropriately. Principles of safe use are summarized in the Guidelines for Safe Practice box on p. 50. Nicotine is now also available in nasal sprays and inhalers (Table 3-1).

Guidelines for Safe Practice

Assisting a Patient to Stop Smoking

1. Assist individual to set a firm "quit" date.
2. Inform individual about available choices for nicotine replacement (e.g., gum, patches of varying concentrations, nasal sprays, pills). Teach about safe and correct use.
3. Explore the advantages of a smoking cessation contract.
4. Encourage the person to use a buddy system or designate a support person to call when he or she experiences cravings.
5. Explore effectiveness of regular gum, hard candy, and so on for use during cravings.
6. Avoid social activities and situations where people smoke during the first weeks of abstinence.
7. Restrict the intake of caffeine if restlessness and anxiety are pronounced symptoms.
8. Incorporate daily exercise into the cessation plan.
9. Use relaxation strategies and imagery to control cravings. Help the person to construct an image of himself or herself as a nonsmoker.
10. Provide regular and enthusiastic support and encouragement for efforts. Openly express confidence that the person can be successful in quitting.
11. Encourage the person to set aside his or her "cigarette money" and spend it on another form of reward for nonsmoking.
12. Encourage involvement with community supports for quitting as available. Remind the family to be enthusiastic and supportive of the person's efforts.

EVALUATION

Evaluation is specifically targeted to the outcomes that were developed to address the person's unique situation. The range of potential evaluation activities is broad. Successful achievement of the sample outcomes related to a healthy lifestyle would be indicated if the patient:

1. Participates consistently in a program of aerobic and strength-building exercise for 30 minutes three times each week.

2a. Plans meals that incorporate the recommendations from the food pyramid.

TABLE 3-1 Common Medications for Smoking Cessation Programs

Medication/ Delivery Method	Action	Intervention
Bupropion (Wellbutrin, Zyban)	Inhibits the reuptake of dopamine, norepinephrine, and serotonin	Assess for therapeutic effect—smoking cessation after 7 weeks; risk of seizures; withdrawal symptoms such as headache, nausea, vomiting. Teach patient to use caution when driving, to avoid alcohol ingestion, to notify provider if pregnant, and that effects may take 2-4 weeks and treatment lasts 7-12 weeks.
Nicotine gum (Nicorette, Nicorette DS)	Acts as an antagonist at the nicotinic receptors in the central and peripheral nervous systems	Assess for adverse side effects such as irritation of the buccal membranes or patient misuse. Teach patient to chew slowly and not to chew over 45 minutes.
Nicotine patch (Habitrol, Nicoderm, Nicotrol)	Acts as an antagonist at the nicotinic receptors in the central and peripheral nervous systems	Assess for therapeutic effects. Teach patient how to use properly, to cease smoking immediately when using the patch treatment, to keep out of reach of children, and not to use if pregnant.
Nicotine nasal spray (Nicotrol NS)	Acts as an antagonist at the nicotinic receptors in the central and peripheral nervous systems	Assess for therapeutic effects. Teach patient proper use of spray.
Nicotine inhaler (Nicotrol Inhaler)	Acts as an antagonist at the nicotinic receptors in the central and peripheral nervous systems	Assess for therapeutic effects. Teach patient proper use of inhaler.

Guidelines for Safe Practice

Safe Use of Nicotine Gum

- Remember that nicotine gum is not standard gum.
- Take a piece of nicotine gum and chew it a few times to break it down. Chewing will release a "peppery" taste. When this occurs, the gum is parked between the gum and cheek. Do not continue to chew it.
- The nicotine takes several minutes to reach the brain, so the effects are less intense than those achieved with smoke inhalation.
- Repeat at intervals, continuing the chew-and-park strategy for about 30 total minutes.
- Excessive chewing can release the nicotine too quickly. The nicotine mixes with the saliva and may cause dizziness, nausea, and soreness in the mouth and throat. It is not effectively absorbed into the bloodstream and does not reduce cravings.
- Do not smoke while chewing the nicotine gum.

2b. Maintains target goal weight.
2c. Uses exercise and progressive relaxation to deal effectively with stress.
3a. Correctly describes the adverse health consequences of smoking.
3b. Expresses desire to remain a nonsmoker.
3c. Has not smoked cigarettes for 6 months and no longer uses patches or nicotine gum.

Critical Thinking Questions

1. A 38-year-old single mother with four children between the ages of 8 and 16 works full time and finds it difficult to find time to exercise. She has been slowly gaining weight and is dissatisfied with both her appearance and fitness. Her father died in his forties of a heart attack, and she expresses concern that she is following in his footsteps.

   She has actual barriers to establishing an exercise program. She has minimal disposable income, the children get home from school at different times and are all involved in school or community activities, and she is the only driver in the family. She states that she is always tired. What approach would you take to help her achieve her stated goal of improving her fitness, considering the constraints of her lifestyle?
2. A single college student in her twenties is basically healthy but is concerned that she spends so much time studying that her exercise regimen has really become lax. She has not gained any significant weight but no longer feels "toned." She states she does not sleep well and often studies all night. She has a significant family history of coronary artery disease, osteoporosis, and skin cancer. She is asking for your guidance to help her establish a healthier lifestyle.

   Where should you start in counseling and helping her make appropriate changes in her lifestyle? What areas seem most important right now? What other health areas of concern should you talk to her about? How important is her family history?
3. A successful executive is recovering from a mild heart attack. He is about 35 lb overweight and admits to an erratic meal pattern. He skips meals, eats a lot of junk food, travels a great deal, and eats heavily when he is entertaining clients. His wife is of Italian background and is an excellent cook. He acknowledges that he needs to make some changes in his diet to decrease the risk of

another heart attack and says that he is willing to listen as long as you do not start advocating "the nuts and berries stuff."

Establish your priorities. What areas will you target and how will you begin to assist him in making changes in his diet?

4. A 55-year-old woman has a history of heart disease and takes medication for hypertension, arthritis, and insulin-dependent diabetes. She has smoked cigarettes for more than 30 years and admits to daily alcohol use. She is disabled from her job, lives alone, and is a recent widow. She is quite overweight but states that "all the women in my family are fat and we all live to be 80." She needs to make numerous changes in her lifestyle. The physician wants her to lose weight, bring down her lipid and cholesterol levels, begin exercising, and gain better control of her diabetes. She has confided in you that she thinks it is all "much ado over nothing," and she is satisfied with things as they are. "After all," she says, "I'm not in the market for another husband."

   The goal for this woman is clearly to establish a healthier lifestyle. Where will you begin? Establish goals and priorities and explain your rationale.

References

1. American Nurses' Association: *Nursing's agenda for health care reform,* Kansas City, Mo, 1992, American Nurses' Association.
2. Andersen RE: Healthy people 2010 steps in the right direction, *Physician Sports Med* 28(10):7, 2000.
3. DiPietro L, Dziura J: Exercise: a prescription to delay the effects of aging, *Physician Sports Med* 28(10):77, 2000.
4. Franklin BA, Sanders W: Reducing the risk of heart disease and stroke, *Physician Sports Med* 28(10):19, 2000.
5. Kavanaugh T et al: Risk profile and health awareness in male offspring of parents with premature coronary health disease, *J Cardiopulm Rehabil* 20(3):172, 2000.
6. Nisbeth O, Klausen K, Andersen LB: Effectiveness of counseling over 1 year on changes in lifestyle and coronary heart disease risk factors, *Patient Educ Counsel* 40:121, 2000.
7. Orleans CT et al: Rating our progress in population health promotion: report card on six behaviors, *Sci Health Promotion* 14(2):75, 1999.
8. Reynolds C: The future of health care: implications for health promotion, *Art Health Promotion* 3(6):1, 1999.
9. Richmond JB: Building the next generation of healthy people, *Public Health Rep* 6(114):212, 1999.
10. US Department of Health and Human Services: *Healthy People 2010: understanding and improving health,* Washington, DC, 2000, USDHHS.
11. US Department of Health and Human Services, Public Health Service: *Healthy People 2000: national health promotion and disease prevention objectives,* Pub No PHS 91-50212, Washington, DC, 1990, US Government Printing Office.
12. US Surgeon General: *Healthy People: the Surgeon General 's report on health promotion and disease prevention,* Washington, DC, 1979, Department of Health, Education and Welfare.
13. US Surgeon General: *Health promotion/disease prevention: objectives for the nation,* Washington, DC, 1980, USDHHS.

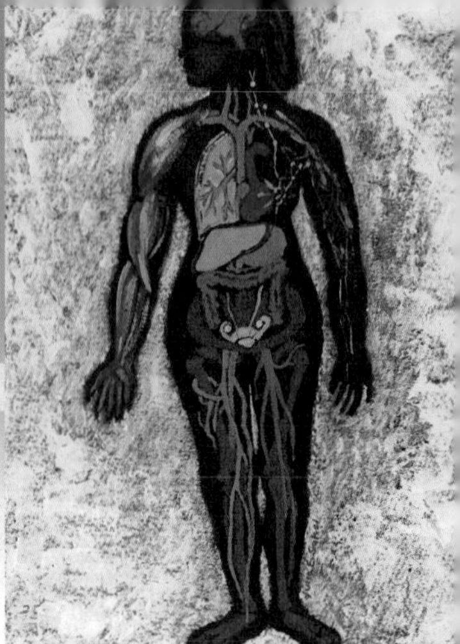

4 Nursing Care of Older Adults

Diana Lynn Morris

Objectives

After studying this chapter, the learner should be able to:

1. Discuss the focus of assessment in older patients.
2. Distinguish between primary and secondary changes of aging.
3. Describe unique patterns of illness in older adults.
4. Explain domains of functional assessment to be addressed in all older patients.

HISTORICAL PERSPECTIVES

Human beings have the longest life span of any animal species, with the potential to live 125 years. For centuries mystery and myth have surrounded the phenomenon of aging. Aristotle believed later life to be period of disengagement while Plato described the development of wisdom in old age. Further, the ancient Greeks believed that life force heat was gradually used up in the normal process of aging. They observed then, as has been confirmed today, that old people are subject to a host of health problems, including dyspnea, joint pains, dizzy spells, insomnia, and visual and hearing losses.

The teachings of Sir Francis Bacon (1561 to 1626) marked the beginning of the scientific approach to aging. Bacon believed that the effects of aging accounted for the physical decline of joints and vision. According to Bacon, factors slowing or accelerating the effects of aging included physical stature, temperament, environment, diet, and heredity. These factors remain important correlates that affect health even today. Metchnikoff (1845 to 1916) regarded aging as a natural physiologic process beginning at the moment of conception, and Nasher (1863 to 1944) argued that age-related diseases were distinct from aging as a normal process. Today, we continue to emphasize the need to distinguish between normal aging changes and secondary aging changes (diseases). In 1909, Nasher used the word *geriatrics* to refer to diseases of old age. In 1927 Rybrikov, a Russian psychologist, referred to the aging process as the study of *gerontology.* Over time, the following five basic characteristic patterns of aging have been identified:

1. Increased mortality with age
2. Changes in the chemical composition of the body, including a decrease in lean body mass, an increase in fats and lipofuscins, and cross-linking of collagen tissues
3. Progressive deteriorative changes
4. Reduced ability to adapt to environmental changes
5. Increased vulnerability to multiple diseases

Nurses have cared for older adults and their family members throughout history. In 1904 the *American Journal of Nursing* published an article on old age and disease. The American Nurses Association (ANA), guided by an understanding of normal aging, the unique needs of older adults, and a commitment to scientific care, established a division of geriatric nursing in 1966 to develop standards of nursing care for older adults. In 1995 the ANA revised the 1981 standards of care to guide generalist and advanced practice nurses caring for older adults. These standards, which serve as a model for practice, apply to all settings and can be used to evaluate care. Seven factors have been identified as basic considerations in providing gerontologic nursing care (Box 4-1). The focus of care is on determining the strengths of older adults and then promoting their use to maximize independence.[5] Three groups constitute those collectively referred to as older adults: the young-old (ages 64 to 74 years); the middle-old (ages 75 to 84 years); and the old-old (ages 85 and older).

Demographic Trends

America is a nation of aging people. In colonial times, half the population was younger than 16 years old. In 1900 life expectancy at birth was 49 years. From 1980 to 1990, a period described as "the graying of America," the American population of old-old—those 85 years and older—increased by 38%, whereas the numbers of persons ages 65 to 84 years increased only 20% and those younger than 65 years of age increased by only 8%. By 1990 the so-called "baby boomers" constituted one third of the population of the United States, and the number of older adults reached 30 million. It is predicted that by 2010 the number of older adults will reach 39 million and by 2030, 70 million. This age-group, which composed 4% of the population in 1900, will increase 20% by the year 2030, with the largest growth occurring among members of ethnic minorities and those older than 85 years. Hispanic-American older adults will increase by 328%, Asian/Pacific Islanders by 285%, American Indians/Eskimos/Aleuts by 147%, and white Americans by only 81%.[2] Americans indeed reflect an aging population, with four- and five-generational

BOX 4-1 Factors Specific to Gerontologic Nursing

Nurses caring for older adults need to consider the following:
1. The ramifications of the aging process
2. The differing rates at which people age
3. The cumulative effect of the aging person's loss(es)
4. The interrelationship between social, economic, psychologic, and biologic factors
5. The frequently atypical response of the elderly to disease and its treatment
6. The accumulated disabling effects of multiple chronic illnesses or degenerative processes
7. The cultural values associated with aging and social attitudes toward aging

Source: American Nurses Association: *Scope and standards of gerontological nursing practice,* Washington, DC, 1995, The Association.

families becoming common as more and more American live into their 100s.

Other dramatic demographic trends include the lower rates of life expectancy for nonwhite persons compared with white persons and the higher number of older women than men. In 1991 life expectancy was 72.5 years for African-American women and 79.3 years for Caucasian women. In 1986 African-American men had a life expectancy of 66 years compared with 72.6 years for Caucasian men. Although the proportions of both men and women in the older than 65 age groups will increase over the next decade, the population of women older than age 65 outnumbers that of men by about 6.1 million. The majority of noninstitutionalized older adults live with families; however, this trend is reversed for those 85 years of age and older. About 50% of persons 65 and older live in suburbs, 27% live in central cities, and 23% live in non-metropolitan areas.[2]

These demographic trends have had a significant impact not only on families and the labor force but also on the health care system. More and more older adults are living longer with chronic illnesses and functional disability and surviving catastrophic acute illnesses. The health care needs of these persons will continue to increase. Those caring for this aging population will need increased knowledge and skills to help this group maintain health and function and avoid complications—all of which will affect the quality and cost of care for older adults.

Improving the quality of life, rather than searching for means to increase longevity, is of utmost importance. According to *Healthy People 2010,* the major goal is to increase the quality and length of healthy life for all Americans. For older Americans in particular, the focus is on maintaining functional health, preventing disability, and reducing disparities in care and treatment.

Significance for Nursing

The U.S. Public Health Service report *Healthy People 2010* is a guide for health professionals and the citizen-consumer.[44] The document provides guidelines for nurses in their daily practice as they provide care to patients. Nurses can anticipate that this report will be used to provide direction for national health policies and future health care priorities and reimbursement. The publication provides a common ground for collaboration with other health care professionals and health service agencies.

The strength of *Healthy People 2010* is that it focuses on increasing the quality and years of healthy life. Thus health promotion and disease prevention strategies, traditionally emphasized in nursing practice, are incorporated into interventions to achieve health objectives. The second goal is particularly important for aging cohorts that have increasing numbers of ethnic minorities. Many minority older adults have experienced a lack of access to health services and differential treatment by providers over their lifetimes. All nurses can use this document to support the care and education of patients in all types of settings, no matter what disease process is being treated. The report also provides information about the health promotion and disease prevention needs of specific groups according to characteristics such as age, race and ethnicity, and economic status.

ASSESSMENT OF OLDER ADULTS

General Issues

Skillful, knowledge-based assessment is the foundation for providing quality nursing care to older adults. In gerontologic and geriatric care, the focus of assessment is the older adult's level of function. A basic premise is that function is multidimensional and includes physical, mental, and social function. Further, the position taken in this chapter is that an elder's functional health is influenced by spiritual well-being.

There is a great deal of heterogeneity in the way that people age. Health concerns for aging persons are multidimensional, requiring critical evaluation of what is normative and what is the result of disease. In ethnic minority groups, secondary aging changes and chronic illnesses may present in the late middle years, resulting in earlier functional decline and disability. In addition, illnesses in older adults can present differently than in younger persons. Nurses may need to use geriatric assessment guidelines with middle-aged adults.

Older adults who are hospitalized are at increased risk for institutionalization. Often such institutionalization is a result of the loss of the ability to carry out activities of daily living (ADLs) and instrumental activities of daily living (IADLs). Thus time spent on a thorough baseline assessment of an elder's health status with emphasis on functional abilities and periodic follow-up assessment can potentially prevent disability and additional health care cost.

In the 1990s geriatric research has focused on failure to thrive in older adults, a phenomenon first addressed in children.[28,31,45] Failure to thrive in older persons leads to catastrophic disability and preventable deaths. This syndrome can be observed in hospitalized older adults and could be seen on admission or be noted for the first time during hospitalization. Failure to thrive in older adults may be multifaceted and result from factors other than disease processes, such as poor nutrition, medications, alcohol use, social isolation, losses, and depression.[32] Nurses in acute and long-term care settings, therefore, can prevent and assess for failure to thrive in older adults.

Institutionalization and failure to thrive are extreme examples of negative health outcomes for hospitalized older adults. However, any loss of functional abilities can dramatically affect the quality of life and well-being of older adults.[24,34] A holistic nursing assessment is the necessary foundation for the care of each older adult patient and collaboration with other health care providers. The focus of geriatric assessment is function, and the goal is to enhance or maintain function while preventing loss of function and subsequent disability. Health care providers should assist persons to maintain functional health and sustain active life expectancy for as long as possible. Thus, the emphasis for gerontologic care in the new millennium is to decrease the disability curve for aging persons. Nurses will play a key role in meeting this challenge through health assessment that directs primary, secondary, and tertiary intervention. Older adults and their family members will be the focus in this endeavor.

The following sections present critical areas of nursing assessment to be addressed when caring for older adults no matter what the clinical setting or the acute and chronic diseases being treated. Topics include primary and secondary aging changes, differences in illness presentation, ADLs/IADLs, falls, spirituality, sexuality, family, nutrition, cognition and sensory perception, depression and suicide, alcohol and medication use, and sleep. The order of presentation of these topics is not meant to imply a hierarchical structure. Although the concepts are presented separately, an elder's functional health status is often affected by the interaction of factors in the physical, mental, social, and spiritual domains. For example, if one has decreased physical function, one can become depressed; if one is depressed, there is a decrease in physical function.

Primary and Secondary Aging

Critical to any approach to an integrated, functional assessment of older adults is understanding of and the ability to differentiate between primary (normative) aging changes and secondary changes (disease related). Normal aging changes are called *primary changes.* Such effects of aging—for example, thinning hair and decreased pulmonary capacity—have been demonstrated through research to occur universally. Increasing knowledge provides evidence that many changes once thought to be associated with aging, such as arthritis and dementia, are actually *secondary changes* and do not occur universally as part of aging. Also the muscle atrophy and weakened joints seen in many older adults have been discovered to be related more to a sedentary lifestyle than to a primary change of aging. Primary changes of aging are summarized in Table 4-1 and Figure 4-1.

In addition to the primary changes of aging listed in Table 4-1 and Figure 4-1, some other variations in organ function bear mentioning. First, the variation in organ function among individuals is much greater in older adults than in younger persons.

Second, the rate of decline from one function to another varies. Basal metabolic rate and total body water of older adults decrease only minimally to about 80% of that of young adults.[14] On the other hand, renal blood flow and maximum breathing capacity show a significant decline in most older persons.

A third major change related to the aging process occurs in response to stress. Although an older person may have adequate cardiac output at rest, stress in the form of an infection, exertion, or emotional shock will decrease cardiac output, and it will take much longer for it to return to the person's baseline level. In addition, there is a loss of reserve capacity related to a decline in coordination of brain interactions. This decline causes a slowing of reaction time and a greater susceptibility to infection and accidents.

Unique Patterns of Illness Among Older Adults

A hallmark of gerontology is that disease may have atypical presentations in older adults (Table 4-2). Often acute illnesses are superimposed on several chronic illnesses complicated by the effects of primary aging. A careful history, as well as knowledge about the unique clinical presentation in older adults, aids the nurse in assessment, establishing nursing diagnoses, and intervening effectively. In assessing the health and illness of older adults, some general patterns must be recognized. First, an age-related decline in immune function results in a less rapid and less effective response to infections and in an increased incidence of autoimmune and malignant disease. Second, stress situations (either physiologic or psychosocial) may produce more pronounced reactions in older persons and may require a longer time for readjustment. Third, complex functions that require multisystem coordination show the most obvious decline and require the greatest compensation and support. Fourth, older adults frequently have atypical manifestations of an illness. Confusion, restlessness, or other altered mentation is a common occurrence in the presence of illness, including psychiatric disorders such as depression. Obscure or unexplained deterioration of health or function should not be accepted as normal aging and must be evaluated carefully. Multiplicity and chronicity of disease are common among older adults, and many have several chronic ailments.

FUNCTIONAL ASSESSMENT OF OLDER ADULTS—COMMON CONCERNS

Activities of Daily Living and Instrumental Activities of Daily Living

Assessment is a critical step in effective nursing care for older adults. The global aspects of health in older adults can be separated into three major concepts: absence of disease, performance of basic self-care activities, termed *activities of daily living (ADLs),* and performance of more complex activities, called *instrumental activities of daily living (IADLs).*

As early as the late 1800s, information on functional health as an estimate of morbidity was obtained in Europe and the United States. During the 1940s classifications of disability included self-care activities of dressing, toileting, and

TABLE 4-1 Primary Changes of Aging

Body System	Change
Skin	Loss of subcutaneous supportive tissue
	Decreased sebaceous secretions
	Thinning and graying hair
Muscular	Increased fat substitution for muscle
	Muscle atrophy
Skeletal	Loss of calcium from bones
	Shrinkage of vertebral disks
	Deterioration of cartilage
Pulmonary	Reduced chest wall compliance
	Decreased breathing capacity
	Decreased vital capacity
	Increased residual volume
	Reduced cough reflex
	Reduced ciliary activity
Cardiac	Endocardial thickening
	Thickened heart valves
	Decreased cardiac output (under stress)
Vascular	Progressive stiffening of arteries
	Artherosclerotic plaques
Renal	Decreased blood flow
	Decreased glomerular filtration rate
	Reduced nephrons
	Decreased creatinine clearance
Liver	Minimal change
Bowel	Minimal change
Gastrointestinal	Minimal loss of digestive enzymes
	Decreased absorption
Endocrine	Decreased utilization of insulin
	Cessation of progesterone
	Decline, then plateau of estrogen
	Gradual decline in testosterone
Vision	Deterioration in ability of lens to focus
	Loss of color sensitivity
	Decreased dark adaptation
	Decreased peripheral vision
	Decreased sensitivity to glare
Hearing	Increased threshold for high frequencies
	Difficulty in speech discrimination
	Degeneration of cochlea and auditory pathways
Sexual	Minimal change in amount of sexual response
	Increase in time for full sexual response
	Decreased vaginal lubrication
	Increased refractory period for men

From Rossman I: *Clinical geriatrics,* ed 3, Philadelphia, 1986, JB Lippincott.

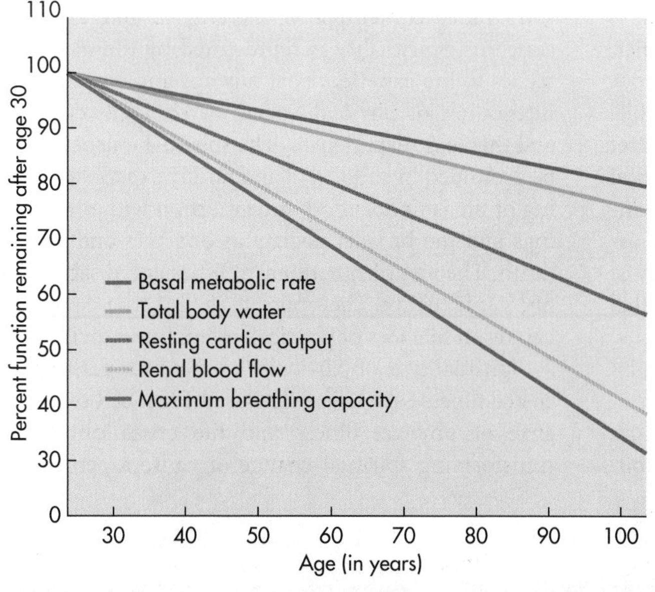

Figure 4-1 Changes in biologic function with aging.

TABLE 4-2 How Illness Changes With Age

Problem	Classic Presentation in Young Adults	Presentation in Older Adults
Urinary tract infection	Dysuria, frequency, urgency, nocturia	Dysuria is often absent; frequency, urgency, nocturia are sometimes present. Incontinence, confusion, anorexia are other signs
Myocardial infarction	Severe substernal chest pain, diaphoresis, nausea, shortness of breath	Sometimes no chest pain or atypical pain location such as in jaw, neck, shoulder may be present. Shortness of breath may be present. Other signs are tachypnea, arrhythmia, hypotension, restlessness, syncope
Pneumonia (bacterial)	Cough producing purulent sputum, absent; chills and fever and/or elevated white blood cell count	Cough may be productive, dry, or chills and fever, pleuritic chest pain, elevated white count also may be absent. Tachypnea, slight cyanosis, confusion, anorexia, nausea and vomiting, tachycardia may be present
Congestive heart failure	Increased dyspnea (orthopnea, paroxysmal nocturnal dyspnea), fatigue, weight gain, pedal edema, night cough and nocturia, bilateral basilar rales	All of the manifestations of young adult and/or anorexia are seen: restlessness, confusion, cyanosis, falls
Hyperthyroidism	Heat intolerance, fast pace, exophthalmos, increased pulse, hyperreflexia, tremor	Slowing down (apathetic hyperthyroidism), hyperreflexia, lethargy, weakness, depression, atrial fibrillation, and congestive heart failure may be seen
Depression	Sad mood and thoughts, withdrawal, crying, weight loss, constipation, insomnia	Any of classic signs, plus memory and concentration problems, weight gain, increased sleep may be present

Modified from Henderson ML: Assessing the elderly: altered presentation, *Am J Nurs* 85(10):110, 1985

ambulation. Since that time, three self-maintenance components have consistently been identified: basic ADLs (bathing, eating, and toileting), more complex social activities of living (shopping, managing finances, cooking, housekeeping, transportation, and managing medications), and the ability to use a telephone and cope with other aspects of one's environment—that is, IADLs.

Functional disability has been shown to correlate with physical illness, self-care ability, complications during hospitalization, rehabilitation potential, and even mortality. Therefore the concept of functional ability in older adults has become a valuable health indicator. Measures of functional status that examine the ability to function independently despite disease are the most useful clinical and research indicators of older adults with multiple chronic and acute illnesses. The Administration on Aging reports that 52.5% of older adults have at least one disability[2]; 14% have difficulty with ADLs, and 21% have some problem with IADLs.

In addition to assessing the respiratory, cardiovascular, digestive, neurologic, and other body systems of the older patient, the nurse must carefully assess functional self-care ability. Subtle changes in appetite or ambulation or even the onset of urinary incontinence may be the initial and only clinical indicator of infections such as pneumonia, urinary tract infections, or even myocardial infarctions. Several functional assessment tools and scales have been widely used in a variety of clinical settings, including the Katz ADL scale and the Barthel index.

Risk of Falls

A major health concern that threatens the function of older adults is the risk of falls that can result in injury and disability.[47] Even falls that do not result in serious injury may affect an elder's function and quality of life. Concern about the risk of falls is heightened when an older adult is admitted to a hospital or long-term care facility. Fortunately, assessment tools (Box 4-2) and protocols are available to assist clinicians in identifying older patients who are at risk. All older patients should be assessed on admission for risk of falling, and then a protocol to prevent a fall from occurring should be instituted.

Spiritual Well-Being

Spirituality focuses on the meanings one attaches to life, particularly one's own life experience. For some individuals, spirituality includes a connection with and commitment to a particular religious orientation and religious institution. However, belief in specific religious dogma or belonging to a church may not be part of a person's spirituality. Bianchi[7] describes aging as a "spiritual journey" that synthesizes a person's inner contemplative experience and external human concerns. Spirituality is represented by the meaning one attaches to life experiences at any age and represents a holistic integration of physical, social, psychologic, cultural, sexual, and theologic experiences. The spiritual journey of aging may be grounded in childhood and family experiences. The meaning of life is understood in connection with other human beings and the broader society as one ages and moves toward death. The loss of functional abilities and disability can affect one's spirituality. The opposite is also true. Spiritual distress can result in a loss of physical, mental, and social function.[27,32]

Spirituality is of particular concern for persons who experience illness (see Evidence-Based Practice box). The experience of physical illness and life crises can precipitate a transforming spiritual change or cause a person to become

BOX 4-2 Risk of Falls Assessment Tool

Fall Assessment Scoring System — POINTS

I. AGE

65-79 Years	1	
80 & Above	2	I. ☐

II. MENTAL STATUS

A. Oriented at all times or comatose	0	
Confusion at all times	2	II.A ☐
Intermittent confusion	4	
B. Agitated/uncooperative/anxious-moderate	2	
Agitated/uncooperative/anxious-severe	4	II.B ☐

III. ELIMINATION

Independent and continent	0	
Catheter and/or ostomy	1	
Elimination with assistance	3	
Ambulatory with urge incontinency or episodes of incontinence	5	III. ☐

IV. HISTORY OF FALLING WITHIN SIX MONTHS

No history	0	
Has fallen one or two times	2	
Multiple history of falling	5	IV. ☐

V. SENSORY IMPAIRMENT

Sensory impairment (blind, deaf, cataracts, not using corrective device)	1	V. ☐

VI. ACTIVITY

Ambulation / transfer without assistance	0	
Ambulation / transfer with assist of one or assistive device	2	VI. ☐
Ambulation / transfer with assist of two	1	

VII. MEDICATIONS

- ☐ Narcotics ☐ Tranquilizers ☐ Sleeping aids
- ☐ Diuretics ☐ Chemotherapy ☐ Antiseizure / antiepileptic

For the above medications, check how many the patient is taking currently at home or that the patient will be taking in the hospital

No medications	0	
1 medication	1	
2 or more medications	2	VII. ☐

Add one more point if there has been a change in these medications or dosages in the past 5 days

A score of 10 or more indicates a high risk for falling. TOTAL ☐

Indicate high risk and care plan. SCORE ☐

If the patient does not meet a score of 10, but in the nurse's judgment is at risk to fall, initiate the high-risk fall protocol.

From MacAvoy S, Skinner T, Hines M: Clinical methods: fall risk assessment tool, *Appl Nurs Res* 9(4):213, 218, 1996.

Evidence-Based Practice

Reference: Fehring RJ, Miller JF, Shaw C: Spiritual well-being, religiosity, hope, depression, and other mood states in older people coping with cancer, *Oncol Nurs Forum* 24(4):663, 1997.

One hundred older patients whose average age was 73 years from two acute care units were interviewed. There were 33 men and 67 women with lung, breast, or colon cancer. A positive relationship was found between intrinsic religiosity, hope, and positive mood states. Thus older adults with higher religiosity and hope scores had less depression. Older patients with lower levels of intrinsic religiosity and hope were more likely to be depressed and have negative mood states. The implications are that nurses need to assess the religiosity and spiritual well-being of older cancer patients. Further, nurses can implement care plans with older patients that support the patient's search for a sense of meaning and hope as a means of coping with illness.

more introspective and contemplative.[17] The nurse can help a patient explore the meaning of a particular physical or life crisis. This process helps patients find meaning in their lives through definitions of self and personhood that go beyond physical abilities.

The nurse can be instrumental in helping patients express themselves and find meaning in the illness experience. The nurse can provide nonjudgmental support and advocacy for patients and their families as they seek meaning within the illness experience.

To support older adults' spiritual well-being, nurses need to include an assessment of older adults' spirituality that goes beyond questions about religious affiliation. Older adults should still be asked basic questions about religious practices that comfort them, help them cope, and provide a sense of security. However, spiritual well-being has dimensions beyond religious practices that represent only one aspect of older adults' self-care. The JAREL Spiritual Well-Being Scale has been developed for use with older adults.[30] The JAREL scale includes 21 questions for the older patient to answer that the nurse then scores to identify areas of spiritual concern (Box 4-3). Also, a clinical assessment and intervention protocol has been developed for spiritual well-being that can be used to assess a person's spiritual experience during an illness episode.

Sexuality

Both men and women maintain interest in sexual activity into the late adulthood years. More women cease having sexual activity after age 65 than do men. The primary reasons for the cessation are lack of an acceptable sexual partner for widows or an ailing husband for married women (rather than lack of interest).

Cultural attitudes toward older adults influence both genders. Older men and women frequently are thought of as sexually unattractive and lacking in ability to engage in sex. However, Masters and Johnson found that although sexual responses are slower, older adults still have the same phases of excitement, plateau, orgasm, and resolution as younger persons.[35]

However, sexual problems occur more frequently for older adults. Women may have dyspareunia as a result of vaginal thinning and decreased lubrication. These factors are caused by postmenopausal steroid starvation. Men tend to be affected by secondary impotence related to performance anxiety and low self-esteem. Diabetes, alcohol, and medications for hypertension are other prominent causes of impotence.

Masters and Johnson report a condition known as "widowers' syndrome."[35] After an extended period of sexual inactivity, a man cannot achieve or maintain an erection. An equivalent condition occurs in women: the vagina constricts and undergoes atrophic changes. The conclusion is that those who do not engage in sexual activity lose the ability to do so.

Sexuality is more than the physical act of intercourse. Older persons continue to need human companionship and love and affection.[21,37,41] Nurses need to be aware of components of sexuality and how older adults may be affected by chronic illness, loss of a partner, and the need for touch. It is imperative that nurses become more aware of and knowledgeable about the specific needs of gay and lesbian older adults,[11] groups who are overlooked and often stigmatized. Being sensitive to family dynamics is just as important for a newly married couple in their seventies as for a young couple. Through counseling the nurse can explain aging changes and suggest vaginal lubrication for women and extra physical stimulation for men. Changes in sexual position and styles of lovemaking are appropriate for those with disabling disease.

Older adults are susceptible to sexually transmitted disease, although not in the same numbers as younger adults.[20,38] Acquired immunodeficiency syndrome (AIDS) is becoming increasingly prevalent in older adults as the epidemic spreads among all age groups. The "at risk" categories differ for older adults (e.g., not as many are intravenous drug abusers), and the disease trajectory may progress differently.[48] However, other risk factors are present (e.g., the decline in the ability of the immune system to ward off infections makes older adults more susceptible to organisms of sexually transmitted diseases). Women in particular are more vulnerable because of the friable vaginal lining that occurs with aging. A final, and often difficult issue for the nurse, is the need to determine if older adults are or have been the victims of sexual abuse and violence. Sexual violence against older women is believed to be a growing problem and should be determined as a component of geriatric assessment.

Family

Although the institutions of marriage and the family are still viewed as the most acceptable in the media and much of society, there is increasing tolerance for diversity in living patterns. Alternatives to traditional family life that are increasingly common include cohabiting with members of the same or opposite sex, living alone, becoming a single parent, remaining a childless couple, and living communally. Other alternative family structures include homosexual couples who

BOX 4-3 JAREL Spiritual Well-Being Scale

Directions: Please circle the choice that **best** describes how much you agree with each statement. Circle only **one** answer for each statement. There is no right or wrong answer.

	Strongly Agree	Moderately Agree	Agree	Disagree	Moderately Disagree	Strongly Disagree
1. Prayer is an important part of my life.	SA	MA	A	D	MD	SD
2. I believe I have spiritual well-being.	SA	MA	A	D	MD	SD
3. As I grow older, I find myself more tolerant of others' beliefs.	SA	MA	A	D	MD	SD
4. I find meaning and purpose in my life.	SA	MA	A	D	MD	SD
5. I feel there is a close relationship between my spiritual beliefs and what I do.	SA	MA	A	D	MD	SD
6. I believe in an afterlife.	SA	MA	A	D	MD	SD
7. When I am sick I have less spiritual well-being.	SA	MA	A	D	MD	SD
8. I believe in a supreme power.	SA	MA	A	D	MD	SD
9. I am able to receive and give love to others.	SA	MA	A	D	MD	SD
10. I am satisfied with my life.	SA	MA	A	D	MD	SD
11. I set goals for myself.	SA	MA	A	D	MD	SD
12. God has little meaning in my life.	SA	MA	A	D	MD	SD
13. I am satisfied with the way I am using my abilities.	SA	MA	A	D	MD	SD
14. Prayer does not help me in making decisions.	SA	MA	A	D	MD	SD
15. I am able to appreciate differences in others.	SA	MA	A	D	MD	SD
16. I am pretty well put together.	SA	MA	A	D	MD	SD
17. I prefer that others make decisions for me.	SA	MA	A	D	MD	SD
18. I find it hard to forgive others.	SA	MA	A	D	MD	SD
19. I accept my life situations.	SA	MA	A	D	MD	SD
20. Belief in a supreme being has no part in my life.	SA	MA	A	D	MD	SD
21. I cannot accept change in my life.	SA	MA	A	D	MD	SD

 From Hungelmann J et al: Focus on spiritual well-being: harmonious interconnectness of mind-body-spirit—use of the JAREL spiritual well-being scale, *Geriatr Nurs* 17(6):262-266, 1996.

make a lifelong commitment and choose to raise a family. Divorce, a common occurrence today, is a highly stressful event that often creates a crisis. Most adults who are divorced, however, go on to marry again. In fact, in more than 45% of all marriages, one or both partners were married previously, with either or both spouses having children from previous marriages, resulting in what is called a *blended family*.[9] Families of older adults also reflect this diversity in family structure. Family, however defined, provides intimacy, affection, and instrumental support to older adults. Also, older adults may be part of multigenerational families and households. Sometimes four or five generations live together and share resources and family tasks. For some older adults, family intimacy and support take place in unrelated (by blood) groups who may or may not live in the same household.

Issues of divorce and alternative lifestyles are often thought of as applying only to the younger generation. However, older adults are part of diverse family configurations and partnerships. Thus assessment of the older adult's family as a means of social support is essential, particularly in supporting the functional health and well-being of the older adult. The nurse also needs to assess the role of the older patient in providing support to the family. Questions can easily be asked about who older adults get help from when they need it for specific activities, in whom they confide, whether the support is adequate, and most important whom that they could really count on if they needed something. Many instruments that measure what support is needed are lengthy, but a short form is available. The Caregiver Well-Being Scale developed by Tebb[39] includes 45 questions about caregivers' satisfaction with basic human needs and ADLs. In addition, older patients should be asked about what type of support they provide to their family network. In fact many older adults, particularly women, are family caregivers.

We have moved beyond the simpler caregiving model of the sandwich-generation woman who is caring for children and aging parents. Today an older female caregiver who is 70 years old and admitted for knee replacement could be caring for a 90-year-old mother, a husband, and a grandchild. A 66-year-old male patient could be giving care to a 44-year-old mentally disabled daughter. The literature abounds with evidence of the physical, psychologic, and financial stress caregivers experience. Of particular concern are the negative health sequelae of caregiving, particularly depression.[36,40,48] Caregivers may ignore their own health and symptoms because of the demands of caregiving. Also, many caregivers experience changes in dietary habits and sleep, have an increased use of psychotropic medications, and are unable to carry out their normal self-care activities. Several research instruments are available to assess caregiver stress and burden as well as caregiver reward. The nurse needs to determine if older patients are caregivers, to whom they are providing care, whether they have assistance with their caregiving, and if they have special concerns while they are in the hospital. When concerns are identified, the older adult can be referred to a clinical nurse specialist or social worker for further evaluation and follow-up monitoring.

Finally an essential component of family assessment is screening for family violence. Older adults are not exempt from being victims or perpetrators.[6,49] For some older persons, family violence has been an established family pattern. Fulmer and O'Malley also address assessment of elder neglect that results in impaired function.[18] There may be an increased risk for older adults being cared for by a family caregiver owing to the stress of caregiving. The risk for violence by a family caregiver is greater when there are decreases in the care recipient's function and a lack of adequate formal and informal support for the caregiver. Thus nurses who care for older adults need to determine if older patients are being exposed to violence and neglect in the home. The nurse needs to be aware that in some states mandatory reporting of elder abuse and neglect is required.

Nutrition

Nutritional requirements of older adults are essentially the same as for other adults, except that calorie needs diminish because of a decrease in lean body mass relative to fat (which burns fewer calories).[14] Fiber (i.e., fruits, vegetables, whole-grain bread, and cereals), although undigestible, is an important constituent in the diet. Fiber holds water in the fecal mass, which softens the stools and enhances regular evacuation. The incidence of diverticulitis, colon cancer, or gallstones is thought to be influenced by diets chronically low in fiber. Persons at or near age 65 may still have a life expectancy of 15 or more years during which dietary fiber deficiencies might play a role in development of colon cancer, diverticulitis, or gallstones. Because the latter disorders and constipation are common problems in older adults, moderate amounts of fiber become regularly included in the diet.

Water is vital for function and temperature regulation. A number of situations may predispose older adults to a deficiency in body water. Approximately 50% of the body's water supply is obtained from solid foods; therefore a reduction in calorie intake may mean that water intake from food sources is not adequate. Some older adults, especially those who are chronically ill, may have a defective thirst sensation mechanism, resulting in a diminished awareness of the body's signal to increase fluid intake. Finally, the older person may lose water from commonly occurring conditions such as diarrhea, excessive perspiration, or polyuria or from the use of diuretics. In the event of a water deficit, older people should be encouraged to consume more fluids, particularly water (minimum of 1500 to 2000 ml/day unless contraindicated by conditions such as congestive heart failure).

Many older adults, especially those who are ill, frequently are malnourished and have inadequate levels of energy expenditure through regular activity or exercise. A state of malnutrition can have a marked detrimental affect on an older adults quality of life.[46] Diets often are deficient in calcium, vitamins A and C, iron, and zinc. A vitamin-mineral supplement may be indicated. Other than acute and chronic illnesses, possible causes of malnutrition are changes in taste, vision, smell, or dentition; limited financial resources; psychologic factors such as boredom and lack of companionship when eating; edentia;

BOX 4-4 The Mini Nutritional Assessment Tool

Last Name: ______________ First Name: ______________ M.I. ______ Sex: ______ Date: ______

Age: ______ Weight, kg: ______ Height, cm: ______ Knee Height, cm: ______

Complete the form by writing the numbers in the boxes. Add the numbers in the boxes and compare the total assessment to the Malnutrition Indicator Score.

Anthropometric Assessment

	Points
1. Body mass index (BMI) (weight in kg)/(height in m)^2 a. BMI < 19 = 0 points b. BMI 19 to < 21 = 1 point c. BMI 21 to < 23 = 2 points d. BMI ≥ 23 = 3 points	❑
2. Mid-arm circumference (MAC) in cm a. MAC < 21 = 0.0 points b. MAC 21 ≤ 22 = 0.5 points c. MAC > 22 = 1.0 points	❑ ❑
3. Calf circumference (CC) in cm a. CC < 31 = 0 points b. CC ≥ 31 = 1 point	❑
4. Weight loss during last 3 months a. weight loss greater than 3 kg (6.6 lbs) = 0 points b. does not know = 1 point c. weight loss between 1 and 3 kg (2.2 and 6.6 lbs) = 2 points d. no weight loss = 3 points	❑

General Assessment

	Points
5. Lives independently (not in a nursing home or hospital) a. no = 0 points b. yes = 1 point	❑
6. Takes makes more than 3 prescription drugs per day a. yes = 0 points b. no = 1 point	❑
7. Has suffered psychological stress or acute disease in the past 3 months a. yes = 0 points b. no = 2 points	❑
8. Mobility a. bed or chair bound = 0 points b. able to get out of bed/chair but does not go out = 1 point c. goes out = 2 points	❑
9. Neuropsychological problems a. severe dementia or depression = 0 points b. mild dementia = 1 point c. no psychological problems = 2 points	❑
10. Pressure sores or skin ulcers a. yes = 0 points b. no = 1 point	❑

Dietary Assessment

	Points
11. How many full meals does the patient eat daily? a. 1 meal = 0 points b. 2 meals = 1 point c. 3 meals = 2 points	
12. Selected consumption markers for protein intake • At least one serving of dairy products (milk, cheese, yogurt) per day? yes ❑ no ❑ • Two or more servings of legumes or eggs per week? yes ❑ no ❑ • Meat, fish or poultry every day? yes ❑ no ❑ a. if 0 or 1 yes = 0.0 points b. if 2 yes = 0.5 points c. if 3 yes = 1.0 points	❑ ❑
13. Consumes two or more servings of fruits or vegetables per day? a. no = 0 points b. yes = 1 point	❑
14. Has food intake declined over the past 3 months due to loss of appetite, digestive problems, chewing or swallowing difficulties? a. severe loss of appetite = 0 points b. moderate loss of appetite = 1 point c. no loss of appetite = 2 points	❑
15. How much fluid (water, juice, coffee, tea, milk, . . .) is consumed per day? (1 cup = 8 oz.) a. less than 3 cups = 0.0 points b. 3 to 5 cups = 0.5 points c. more than 5 cups = 1.0 points	❑ ❑
16. Mode of feeding a. unable to eat without assistance = 0 points b. self-fed with some difficulty = 1 point c. self-fed without any problem = 2 points	❑

Self-Assessment

	Points
17. Do they view themselves as having nutritional problems? a. major malnutrition = 0 points b. does not know or moderate malnutrition = 1 point c. no nutritional problem = 2 points	❑
18. In comparison with other people of the same age, how do they consider their health status? a. not as good = 0.0 points b. does not know = 0.5 points c. as good = 1.0 points d. better = 2.0 points	❑ ❑

Assessment Total (max. 30 points) ❑❑❑

Malnutrition Indicator Score		
≥ 24 points	well-nourished	❑
17 to 23.5 points	at risk of malnutrition	❑
< 17 points	malnourished	❑

From Guigoz Y, Vellas B, Garry PJ: Assessing the nutritional status of the elderly: the Mini Nutritional Assessment as part of geriatric assessment, *Nutr Rev* 54(1):S59-S65, 1996.

lifelong faulty eating patterns; fads and misconceptions regarding certain foods; lack of energy to prepare food; inability to feed oneself; and lack of sufficient knowledge of the essentials of a well-balanced diet. Living arrangements may affect dietary patterns; older men who live alone were found to have less adequate diets than older women living alone.

Older persons often enter the hospital in a poorly nourished state because of chronic illness or other factors previously described. Trauma, surgery, or sepsis may increase nutritional demands and cause further nutritional deficiencies, particularly in protein and calories, to develop rapidly. Often, a poor state of nutrition on admission, increased nutritional needs, and decreased appetite coexist in hospitalized older adults. A nutritional assessment, including a record of food intake over several days and weight on admission with regular weight checks thereafter, should be a priority in nursing to detect deficiencies early.

It has been suggested that nutritional status be considered a "vital sign."[12] This is particularly true for older adults in acute care. Poor nutrition can lead to functional losses, and functional losses can lead to poor nutrition. For example, in a study of older nuns a 3% weight loss over 1 year increased the risk of an individual becoming dependent in ADLs.[42] Other researchers have reported that protein-energy undernourishment in older middle-aged patients (55 to 64 years) and older patients is a strong risk factor for mortality 1 year after discharge from a hospital. Therefore one dimension of a geriatric assessment should be nutritional screening. The Mini Nutritional Assessment (MNA) is a relatively simple screening instrument that can be used with older adults in acute care settings (Box 4-4).[22] Some of the areas included in the MNA are dietary habits, medication use, and functional items such as ADLs, dental health, and depression. A simple method to monitor nutritional status used in long-term care is monthly weighing of all older adults.

Cognition and Sensory Perception

Older adults differ from their younger counterparts in several aspects of cognitive and perceptual function. Changes occur in the central nervous system, but the function of the peripheral motor neurons and the autonomic nervous system remains relatively constant throughout the life span.

Cognitive Function

Cross-sectional studies have shown that the highest overall intelligence test performance occurs at some time between the late teens and late twenties. People in their thirties, forties, and fifties tend to score somewhat lower. However, longitudinal evidence has shown that general intelligence either remains the same or increases slightly during the adult years. Certain factors such as education and other sociocultural advantages may influence intellectual development and performance.

The measure of one's intelligence is more than a score on a standardized examination. Intelligence can include a person's capacity for creativity and understanding of how systems work. Creativity and productivity are possible in old age. Older adults do not lose the capacity for creativity as they age. Some, for the first time, have the time to pursue artistic talents that had not been fully developed because of work and family obligations. Active use of mental capacity throughout life contributes to mental productivity in old age.

Aging changes listed in Box 4-5 affect complex processes such as learning, memory, language, and mentation. Although loss of memory is not considered a primary aging change, many older persons have progressively increasing problems with short-term memory. Older persons may need more time to take in information and can experience some problems with retrieval of stored information (memory). Although persons of advancing age perform less well on neuropsychologic tests, this performance is not necessarily associated with impaired function. Therefore any change in cognitive function in the older adult must be taken seriously, and the etiology of the change explored. A change in cognitive function is often the first indication that an elder's health status has changed. Older adults with cognitive changes may be misdiagnosed with irreversible organic brain disease (e.g., Alzheimer's disease). This results in an increased risk of institutionalization. The cause of the cognitive changes may be an undiagnosed medical condition that is reversible with treatment. Reversible cognitive changes may actually be symptoms of disease, depression, and delirium owing to toxic effects of drugs, dehydration, fecal impaction, infection, and overstimulation to name only a few causes. Changes in cognitive function should then trigger aggressive global assessment of the elder's health status starting with evaluation of the presence of disease or adverse drug effects.

The following is an example of what can happen to an older adult who experiences cognitive changes and the underlying cause is misdiagnosed.

> A 72-year-old woman had a heart attack while on her way to another town to visit her ill husband. She was hospitalized and, when her husband died unexpectedly 24 hours later after elective surgery, was unable to attend the funeral. Despite continued complications, she is now being prepared for discharge. The physician has asked her daughter to meet him to discuss the need to place her mother in a nursing home. The physician says this is necessary because the patient can no longer care for herself, is unable to remember things, and is becoming senile. The daughter places her mother, who does not seem to be the person she once knew, in a nursing home. However, she does seek another opinion to be sure the physician was right. Severe depression is subsequently diagnosed, and her mother is treated. The mother is now back living in her own home, driving her car, participating actively in church, and traveling to visit the grandchildren.

BOX 4-5 Aging Changes Affecting Cognition and Perception

- Decreased brain weight
- Diminished enzyme activity
- Slowed reflexes
- Decreased sensory receptors for temperature, pain, and tactile discrimination
- Weakening of interneuron connections
- Increased response time
- Chronic hypoxia

BOX 4-6 NEECHAM Confusion Scale

NAME/ID: ______________________ DATE: ________ TIME: ________
SCORED BY: ________________

Level 1: Processing

Processing–Attention: (Attention-Alertness-Responsiveness)

_4 *Full attentiveness/alertness:* responds immediately and appropriately to calling of name or touch—eyes, head turn; fully aware of surroundings, attends to environmental events appropriately
_3 *Short or hyper attention/alertness:* either shortened attention to calling, touch, or environmental events or hyperalert, overattentive to cues/objects in environment
_2 *Attention/alertness inconsistent or inappropriate:* slow in responding, repeated calling or touch required to elicit/maintain eye contact/attention; able to recognize objects/stimuli, although may drop into sleep between stimuli
_1 *Attention/alertness disturbed:* eyes open to sound or touch; may appear fearful, unable to attend/recognize contact, or may show withdrawal/combative behavior
_0 *Arousal/responsiveness depressed:* eyes may/may not open; only minimal arousal possible with repeated stimuli; unable to recognize contact

Processing–Command: (Recognition-Interpretation-Action)

_5 *Able to follow a complex command:* "Turn on nurse's call light" (must search for object, recognize object, perform command)
_4 *Slowed complex command response:* requires prompting or repeated directions to follow/complete a complex command; performs complex command in "slow"/overattending manner
_3 *Able to follow a simple command:* "Lift your hand or foot Mr. ________" (only use 1 objective)
_2 *Unable to follow direct command:* follows command prompted by touch or visual cue—drinks from glass placed near mouth; responds with calming affect to nursing contact and reassurance or hand holding
_1 *Unable to follow visually guided command:* responds with dazed or frightened facial features, and/or withdrawal resistive response to stimuli, hyper/hypoactive behavior; does not respond to nurse gripping hand lightly
_0 *Hypoactive, lethargic:* minimal motor/responses to environmental stimuli

Processing–Orientation: (Orientation, Short-Term Memory, Thought/Speech Content)

_5 *Oriented to time, place, and person:* thought processes, content of conversation or questions appropriate; short-term memory intact
_4 *Oriented to person and place:* minimal memory/recall disturbance, content and response to questions generally appropriate; may be repetitive, requires prompting to continue contact; generally cooperates with requests
_3 *Orientation inconsistent:* oriented to self, recognizes family but time and place orientation fluctuates; uses visual cues to orient; thought/memory disturbance common, may have hallucinations or illusions; passive cooperation with requests (cooperative cognitive protecting behaviors)
_2 *Disoriented and memory/recall disturbed:* oriented to self/recognizes family; may question actions of nurse or refuse requests, procedures (resistive cognitive protecting behaviors); conversation content/thought disturbed; illusions and/or hallucinations common
_1 *Disoriented, disturbed recognition:* inconsistently recognizes familiar people, family, objects; inappropriate speech/sounds
_0 *Processing of stimuli depressed:* minimal response to verbal stimuli

Level 2: Behavior

Behavior–Appearance:

_2 *Controls posture, maintains appearance, hygiene:* appropriately gowned or dressed, personally tidy, clean; posture in bed/chair normal
_1 *Either posture or appearance disturbed:* some disarray of clothing/bed or personal appearance or some loss of control of posture, position
_0 *Both posture and appearance abnormal:* disarrayed, poor hygiene, unable to maintain posture in bed

 From Miller J et al: The assessment of acute confusion as part of nursing care, *Appl Nurs Res* 10(3):143, 1997.

Continued

The focus of assessment for the nurse then is the level of cognitive function in older patients, and cognitive screening is done first. If impairment is present, then information about the person's level of function before hospitalization is obtained from a family member. For those who have impaired function on admission, cognitive screening should continue throughout the hospital stay. A variety of cognitive screening instruments is available. The two most commonly used are the Short Portable Mental Status Questionnaire (SPMSQ), which is quick and easy to administer; and the Mini-Mental Status Examination (MMSE), which includes questions that require some level of reading and writing literacy and motor function. The SPMSQ and MMSE should be used as screening tools only. If a patient's score is indicative of cognitive impairment, the nurse should refer the elder for further evaluation.

During hospitalization, the older patient's cognitive function needs to be assessed on an ongoing basis. This is necessary because older patients are at risk for developing acute confusional states. Researchers have found that nurses are able to clinically assess marked cognitive impairment but may miss some of the subtle signs of cognitive changes that put the patient at risk for decreased function. The NEECHAM Confusion Scale provides nurses with an instrument for systematic, clinical evaluation of acute confusion (Box 4-6).

BOX 4-6 NEECHAM Confusion Scale—cont'd

Behavior–Motor:

4 *Normal motor behavior:* appropriate movement, coordination and activity, able to rest quietly in bed; normal hand movement
3 *Motor behavior slowed or hyperactive:* overly quiet or little spontaneous movement (hands/arms across chest or at sides) or hyperactive (up/down, "jumpy"); may show hand tremor
2 *Motor movement disturbed:* restless or quick movements; hand movements appear abnormal—picking at bed objects or bed covers, etc.; may require assistance with purposeful movements
1 *Inappropriate, disruptive movements:* pulling at tubes, trying to climb over rails, frequent purposeless actions
0 *Motor movement depressed:* limited movement unless stimulated; resistive movements

Behavior–Verbal:

4 *Initiates speech appropriately:* able to converse, can initiate and maintain conversation; normal speech for diagnostic condition, normal tone
3 *Limited speech initiation:* responses to verbal stimuli are brief and uncomplex; speech clear for diagnostic condition, tone may be abnormal, rate may be slow
2 *Inappropriate speech:* may talk to self or not make sense; speech not clear for diagnostic condition
1 *Speech/sound disturbed:* altered sound/tone; mumbles, yells, swears or is inappropriately silent
0 *Abnormal sounds:* groaning or other disturbed sounds; no clear speech

Level 3: Physiologic Control

Physiologic Measurements:

Recorded Values:	*Normal Values:*	
Temperature	(36°-37°)	______Periods of apnea/hypopnea present? 1 yes, 0 no
Systolic blood pressure (BP)	(100-160)	______Oxygen therapy prescribed? 0 no, 0 yes, but not on, 2 = yes, on now.
Diastolic BP	(50-90)	
Heart rate (HR):	(60-100)	
Regular/irregular	(circle one)	
Respirations	(14-22) (count for 1 full minute)	
O_2 saturation	(93 or above)	

Vital Function Stability: (Count abnormal systolic BP and/or diastolic BP as one value; count abnormal and/or irregular HR as one; count apnea and/or abnormal respirations as one; and abnormal temperature as one.)

2 BP, HR, temperature, respiration within normal range with regular pulse
1 Any one of the above in abnormal range
0 Two or more in abnormal range

Oxygen Saturation Stability:

2 O_2 saturation in normal range (93 or above)
1 O_2 saturation 90 to 92 or is *receiving oxygen*
0 O_2 saturation below 90

Urinary Continence Control:

2 Maintains bladder control
1 Incontinent of urine in last 24 hours or has condom catheter
0 Incontinent now or has indwelling or intermittent catheter or is anuric

	Total Score of:	Indicates:
______ Level 1 Score: Processing (0-14 points)	0-19	Moderate to severe confusion
______ Level 2 Score: Behavior (0-10 points)	20-24	Mild or early development of confusion
	25-26	"Not confused," but at high risk for confusion
______ Level 3 Score: Integrative Physiologic Control (0-6 points)	27-30	"Not confused," or normal function
______ Total NEECHAM (0-30 points)		

Sensory-Perceptual Function

Pain, temperature, taste, and touch are all dulled to some extent as one ages. Hearing and vision also become less acute, and the older adult experiences presbyopia and presbycusis. Long-distance vision, night vision, and tolerance for glare decrease; and the older person has more difficulty hearing high tones and discriminating speech in noisy situations. These changes in hearing and vision[23] are of particular concern when assessing the older adult because these sensory losses affect the older person's ability to communicate with significant others and the outside world. Older adults' ability to receive information can become compromised. For example, what appears to be recent memory loss may actually be the result of being unable to take written or spoken information. Specifically, hearing impairment can result in social isolation and depression in the older adult. In persons 70 years of age and older, 33% report hearing problems, 18% report visual impairments, and 8.6% report that they have both hearing and vision impairment.[8] Assessment of hearing and vision should begin by asking the patients to describe (1) what problems they may be having, (2) when they were first aware of the problems, (3) whether there have been recent changes, and (4) what they are doing to accommodate losses, including assistive devices. Ebersole and Hess describe basic, clinical observations of the older patient's behavior that can be performed by the nurse to assess hearing.[14] They include, but are not limited to, speech quality and loudness, turning head toward speaker, asking that things be repeated, not being able to follow clear directions, not responding to environmental sounds, and thinking that people are talking about him or her. The nurse should also assess the patient for inappropriate anger or irritation when spoken to by staff. In addition, anytime an older adult (or the family) complains of hearing difficulties, the inner ear should be visually inspected to assess for cerumen impaction. Vision can be easily assessed by using a pocket-sized Snellen chart.

Depression and Suicide

Depression remains the major mental health problem in older adults and can lead to disability and premature death.[3,43] However, this treatable disorder goes largely unrecognized, undiagnosed, or misdiagnosed; therefore it remains untreated. Acute and primary health care providers are in the best position to assess the presence of depression in older patients. Depression and depressive symptoms are found in 8% to 20% of community dwelling older adults[4,13,19] and 17% to 35% of older adults seen in primary care.[25] It has been suggested that late-life depression is a geriatric syndrome with multiple etiologies that requires interdisciplinary, multidimensional geriatric assessment. Depression in older adults results in decreased functional health in multiple domains and can lead to suicide (see Evidence-Based Practice box).

Evidence continues to show that people become more suicidal as they age, with older white men committing suicide at a rate six times higher than the general population.[29] It is important for nurses to know that 75% of older adults who commit suicide have visited a primary care physician in the month before the suicide.[10] Of great concern is a 16% increase in suicide in 80- to 84-year-olds from 1980 to 1996.[43] Suicidal behaviors may be aggressive and highly lethal or more covert such as refusal to eat and not taking necessary medication. Some older men who commit suicide commit homicide first by killing their spouses. Even if the older adult is not clinically depressed, the person may be experiencing a level of depressive symptoms that result in functional impairment and poor health. The good news is that depression is treatable in older adults, and timely appropriate care can prevent suicidal behaviors.

Evidence-Based Practice

Reference: Moore SL: A phenomenological study of the meaning of life in suicidal older adults, *Arch Psychiatr Nurs* 11(1):29, 1997.

Eleven older adults ages 64 to 92 were interviewed about their suicidal feelings. The main theme that described the older adults' experience was one of alienation. Suicidal older adults talked about broken connections with significant people and a loss of meaningful activities. Respondents spoke of despair, pain, and suffering (Psychache); the feeling that family and others no longer cared about them (No One Cares); and feeling loss of control, loss of independence, and disappointed (Powerlessness). The implications are that assessment should be focused not only on feelings of hopelessness, but also on older persons' sense of connectedness to family, friends, and meaningful activities. Further, the nurse can help the older adult develop a self-care plan that includes continued involvement with people and life-enhancing activities.

Depression presents differently in older adults than in younger persons. Older persons may find it less acceptable to acknowledge depression. Therefore structured instruments are helpful in screening. The nurse can easily screen for depression using the Center of Epidemiological Studies Depression Scale (CES-D) or Geriatric Depression Scale (GDS) (Box 4-7). These instruments can be included in the nursing assessment form or used as an addition to it. The questions can be asked of the older patient or read by the older patient and easily scored by the nurse. The CES-D and GDS measure the presence of depressive symptoms but are not used for differential diagnosis of major depression. Standard questions for suicide assessment can be used to assess whether suicidal thoughts are present. If depressive symptoms and suicidal ideas or behaviors are observed, the older person should be referred for more complete psychiatric evaluation.

Alcohol and Medication Use and Misuse

Assessment of alcohol, medication, and drug use and abuse is an essential component of geriatric assessment. Although data about illicit drug use in older adults are minimal and the types and amount of actual use are uncertain, assessment of illicit drug use is important and may become more so, given younger cohorts' patterns of multiple substance use. Reasons for the importance of this aspect of assessment are many. First, alcohol, medication, or drug misuse, abuse, or addiction can result in a variety of functional deficits and have negative

BOX 4-7 Geriatric Depression Scale (Short Form)

Choose the best answer for how you felt over the past week.

	Please circle	
1. Are you basically satisfied with your life?	yes	no
2. Have you dropped many of your activities and interests?	yes	no
3. Do you feel that your life is empty?	yes	no
4. Do you often get bored?	yes	no
5. Are you in good spirits most of the time?	yes	no
6. Are you afraid that something bad is going to happen to you?	yes	no
7. Do you feel happy most of the time?	yes	no
8. Do you often feel helpless?	yes	no
9. Do you prefer to stay at home, rather than going out and doing new things?	yes	no
10. Do you feel you have more problems with memory than most?	yes	no
11. Do you think it is wonderful to be alive now?	yes	no
12. Do you feel pretty worthless the way you are now?	yes	no
13. Do you feel full of energy?	yes	no
14. Do you feel that your situation is hopeless?	yes	no
15. Do you think that most people are better off than you are?	yes	no

The following count as one point. Scores >5 indicate probable depression.

1. No	6. Yes	11. No
2. Yes	7. No	12. Yes
3. Yes	8. Yes	13. No
4. Yes	9. Yes	14. Yes
5. No	10. Yes	15. Yes

effects on body systems. Second, even nonproblematic use of alcohol in young and middle adulthood may result in functional losses and organ damage because of normal aging changes. Third, alcohol and medications can have a variety of interactive effects that are detrimental and even life threatening. Finally, the clinical presentation of substance (alcohol, prescribed, and over-the-counter medications) interaction, misuse, and abuse is frequently mistaken by clinicians for irreversible dementia.[26]

Alcohol and the Older Adult

Although alcohol use and misuse decrease with age, 4% of older adults abuse or are dependent on alcohol, and 10% are considered problem drinkers.[1] Currently, African-American men and women have the highest rates in persons 65 years of age and older, followed by Hispanic men, and then Caucasians.[41]

Two patterns of alcoholism have been identified in older adults. Some older alcoholics began drinking at an early age and have survived into their elder years. Other older adults are late-onset drinkers who began abusing alcohol in their later years. The abuse often begins in the fifth decade, but alcoholism and related health problems may not be detected until the sixth decade. Of course the abuse of alcohol can occur at any time during the aging process and may actually be a symptom of other functional health problems such as depression and social isolation or may be a self-care behavior to manage insomnia or pain.

Because of the social stigma and cultural values related to alcohol use, it is important that nurses be aware of their personal beliefs about alcohol and experiences with those that use

BOX 4-8 The CAGE Assessment: Four Questions About Drinking

The following answers count as one point. Scores >5 indicate probable depression.

C Have you ever felt you should **c**ut down on your drinking?
A Have people **a**nnoyed you by criticizing your drinking?
G Have you ever felt bad or **g**uilty about your drinking?
E Have you ever taken a drink first thing in the morning (**e**ye opener) to steady your nerves or get rid of a hangover?

Positive answers to two or more questions suggest that you may have a problem with drinking.

One or more responses from an elder are significant and deserves follow-up.

or abuse it. An additional area to address is the attitudes of professionals toward older adults who drink, including differences in attitudes related to the gender of the elder. The beliefs, values, and attitudes of professionals can be barriers to accurate assessment. Nurses also need to recognize that older adults may present barriers to assessment because of their own beliefs and attitudes about alcohol use and abuse. Several screening instruments are now available and are easily integrated into multidimensional geriatric assessment such as the CAGE Assessment (Box 4-8) and the Older Alcohol Screening Test (EAST) (Box 4-9).[16] One does not have to be an expert in substance abuse to effectively use alcohol-screening instruments. The role of the clinical nurse is to assess an older adult's pattern of alcohol use and screen for abuse so that appropriate referral and management can be implemented. Screening can identify the potential for problems with drug

BOX 4-9 Elderly Alcohol Screening Test (EAST)

Directions: If a statement says something true about you, put a check in the "Yes" box. If a statement says something not true about you, put a check in the "No" box. Please answer all questions.

1. Have you ever drunk alcohol? ❑ Yes ❑ No
2. Do you feel that you are a normal drinker? ❑ Yes ❑ No
3. Have you ever awakened the morning after drinking the night before and found that you could not remember a part of the evening? ❑ Yes ❑ No
4. Does your spouse, the people you live with, or your children ever worry or complain about your drinking? ❑ Yes ❑ No
5. Can you stop drinking without a struggle after 1 or 2 drinks? ❑ Yes ❑ No
6. Do you ever feel bad about your drinking? ❑ Yes ❑ No
7. Do friends, your children, or other relatives think you are a normal drinker? ❑ Yes ❑ No
8. Have you ever used alcohol instead of prescribed medications from your doctor to treat your health problems? ❑ Yes ❑ No
9. Do you try to limit your drinking to certain prescribed times of the day or to certain places? ❑ Yes ❑ No
10. Are you always able to stop drinking when you want to? ❑ Yes ❑ No
11. Have you ever been evicted, asked to move, or been denied access to any older living accommodations or recreational facilities because of your drinking? ❑ Yes ❑ No
12. Have you ever attended a meeting of Alcoholics Anonymous (AA)? ❑ Yes ❑ No
13. Have you gotten physically or verbally aggressive when drinking? ❑ Yes ❑ No
14. Has drinking ever created problems between you and your spouse, your children, or other family members? ❑ Yes ❑ No
15. Have your children ever avoided contact with you, or not allowed you to see or visit your grandchildren because of your drinking? ❑ Yes ❑ No
16. Has your spouse (or any other family member) ever gone to anyone for help about your drinking? ❑ Yes ❑ No
17. Have you ever lost any friends or had disagreements with neighbors because of your drinking? ❑ Yes ❑ No
18. Have you ever neglected eating, your own daily health maintenance, or your family for 2 or more days in a row because of your drinking? ❑ Yes ❑ No
19. Have you ever drunk to relieve the pain and sorrow due to the loss of or death of your spouse or other loved ones? ❑ Yes ❑ No
20. Do you drink before noon? ❑ Yes ❑ No
21. Have you ever been told by your doctor that you have liver trouble? ❑ Yes ❑ No
22. Have you ever had severe shakes, heard voices, or seen things that were not there after heavy drinking? ❑ Yes ❑ No
23. Have you ever gone to anyone for help about your drinking? ❑ Yes ❑ No
24. Have you ever been hospitalized because of your drinking? ❑ Yes ❑ No
25. Have you ever been a patient in a psychiatric hospital or on a psychiatric ward of a general hospital where drinking was part of the problem? ❑ Yes ❑ No
26. Have you ever been at a psychiatric or mental health clinic or gone to a doctor, a social worker, clergyman, or counselor for help with an emotional problem in which drinking played a part? ❑ Yes ❑ No

Elderly Alcohol Screening Testing Scoring

	YES	NO		YES	NO		YES	NO		YES	NO
1.	0	0	8.	2	0	15.	2	0	22.	5	0
2.	0	2	9.	0	0	16.	2	0	23.	5	0
3.	1	0	10.	0	2	17.	3	0	24.	5	0
4.	1	0	11.	2	0	18.	3	0	25.	5	0
5.	0	2	12.	2	0	19.	1	0	26.	5	0
6.	1	0	13.	2	0	20.	1	0			
7.	0	2	14.	2	0	21.	2	0			

Total possible score: 50
0-3 points: Probably not alcoholic
4-9 points: 80% diagnostic of alcoholism
10 points: Virtually 100% diagnostic of alcoholism

and alcohol interactions and identify those at risk for symptoms of alcohol withdrawal.

Medication and the Older Adult

The use of both prescribed and nonprescribed medications increases with age. Older adults consume disproportionately more of all kinds of drugs than do middle adults, partly because they experience more chronic illness. Medications provide tremendous benefits to older adults, but they also can create problems for the patient, family, and health care provider. Management may be further complicated by a lack of knowledge regarding ethnopharmacology. The medication regimen may be complex and troublesome for the patient or family to administer, and as a result drug misuse can easily occur. Misuse is defined as overmedication, undermedication, inappropriate prescription by the professional, or errors in amount and administration. Some misuse can result in drug dependency. Medications may be difficult to tolerate and can cause unpleasant side effects, and negative interactions with foods may occur. Other medications may cause adverse reactions and interactions or unpredictable responses in older adults. Misuse, dependency, and drug interactions often result in loss of physical, mental, and social function.[15]

Drug Absorption. Numerous age-related physical changes in older adults affect the response to medications. The absorption of drugs may be influenced by the presence or absence of nutrients or by the decrease of hydrochloric acid that normally occurs with aging; drugs that depend on an acid medium may be absorbed less efficiently. Absorption also may be altered because the rate of transit through the gastrointestinal system tends to slow with age.

Drug Distribution. Distribution of drugs within the body is affected by the loss of lean body mass and the increased proportion of body fat. Fat-soluble drugs tend to be stored in fat, thereby decreasing the intensity of the reaction while increasing the duration. Within the bloodstream the distribution of drugs is affected by the amount of serum protein, specifically albumin, available as binding sites for drugs. In aging persons, the serum albumin levels tend to be lower, resulting in altered concentrations of bound (inactive) and unbound (active) drugs. Unbound drugs in the circulation are active in producing the effects of the drug. The unbound drug can be excreted by the kidneys or metabolized by the liver. A principal mechanism of drug interaction seems to be the displacement of one drug by another from these protein-binding sites. For example, warfarin may be displaced by aspirin, indomethacin, and other drugs, causing increased anticoagulation activity.

Drug Metabolism. The metabolism of drugs in older adults may be altered by lower levels of enzyme activity in the liver. The result of prolonged or incomplete metabolism is an increase in the half-life of some drugs that allows the drug to exert its effect for a longer period.

Drug Excretion. The kidney is the primary route of excretion of drugs. Changes with aging such as decreased renal plasma flow to the kidney, decreased glomerular filtration rate, and decreased number of functional tubules combine to result in inefficient excretion of active drug. This increases the risk of accumulation of drugs to potentially toxic levels because of decreased renal clearance. The decreased rate of excretion and the changes in binding sites in the blood unite to prolong the elevated blood level and activity of many drugs. Digoxin has a narrow margin of safety and is an example of a drug that is critically affected by the change in renal excretion.

Medications have a definite place in the therapeutic regimen for the older adult, but they must be handled carefully (see Evidence-Based Practice box). One general principle in medication therapy is that the drug level should be built up gradually, and the lowest dose and the fewest possible number of drugs should be used. Nurses should check for untoward reactions to medications and report them to the health care provider. The basis for ongoing assessment of an older adult's response to medication is a thorough medication history (Box 4-10). Information from the nutritional assessment of the elder can be used to identify possible food interactions.

Evidence-Based Practice

Reference: Sarah Cole Hirsch Institute, *Helping older adults manage their medication*, Cleveland, OH, 2000, Frances Payne Bolton School of Nursing, Case Western Reserve University.

This State of the Science review addresses research findings regarding medication management and adherence in older adults. Recommendations address assessment of factors that influence adherence and nursing interventions to promote adherence. It is reported that adherence is affected by impaired cognition; use of psychoactive drugs; patients' lack of confidence in their memory; impaired vision and small motor skills; complexity of medication regimen; use of over-the-counter drugs; financial constraints; and problems with access to home care. Several interventions are delineated: initiate self-administration of medication while an inpatient; provide multidisciplinary medication education with repeated oral and written instruction; create individualized medication (written) schedules based on older adult's daily schedule at home; simplify regimens; modify labeling and use color coding on labels and written schedules; modify containers; develop a plan for refilling medication once home; use postdischarge multidisciplinary monitoring and follow-up; and, include technologic aids such as voice mail reminders, interactive computers and medication organizers.

Sleep-Wake Patterns

Sleep is a basic requirement for all human beings. Sufficient sleep is needed to maintain energy levels, physical appearance, and well-being. Certain changes in sleep and sleep patterns seem to occur as part of normal aging.[33] These include a prolonged sleep latency (time it takes to fall asleep), an increase in the number of awakenings during the sleep period, a decrease in slow-wave sleep (thought to be associated with physical restoration), and a decrease in rapid eye movement sleep that occurs in advanced old age (thought to be associated with mental restoration). These changes often result in more fragmented sleep than that experienced in earlier years. Although many older adults adapt to these normal sleep changes, others experience acute or chronic insomnia. Physical problems that cause shortness of breath, frequency of urination, incontinence, impairment of mobility, or confusion may disrupt sleep. Other contributing factors include certain drugs (e.g., some antihypersensitive drugs) and environmental factors such as temperature, light, noise, and type of bed and location.

Because quality of sleep can have far-reaching effects on the individual's general well-being, an essential component of the nurse's health assessment of older adults must include an evaluation of sleep. A sleep problem that is identified should be analyzed to determine its onset, subjective complaint (how the problem is described by the patient), previous treatments and effectiveness, and sleep patterns before the onset of the problem. Sleep problems are of particular concern during hospitalization when the normal daily routines of older adults are disrupted and they are exposed to new environmental stimuli. Promotion of adequate sleep is based on assessment of an individual's sleep-wake pattern on admission. The

BOX 4-10 Patient Medication History*

General Considerations: What is the client/patient's:

1. Cognitive level ______
2. Visual acuity and ability to read labels ______
3. Hand/muscle coordination (to pour, uncap/cap bottle) ______
4. Ability to swallow without difficulty ______
5. Level of ADL: independent [ ] needs help [ ] ______
6. Lifestyle patterns (alcohol, smoking, activity) ______
7. Beliefs and attitudes toward:
   Self ______
   Illness ______
   Treatments ______
   Prescribing physician or nurse ______
8. Living conditions: alone [ ], with others [ ] ______
   Relationship with others ______
9. Ability to afford cost of medication ______

Specific Medication History:

10. Medications currently taking (ALL prescribed by ALL physicians and nurses providing care):
    Prescribed: ______
    Over-the-counter:
    for pain ______
    constipation ______
    sleep ______
    vitamins ______
    health food products ______
11. Knowledge (reason for taking drug): ______
    Times and frequency of self-medication: ______
12. Are medications shared with: family [ ], friends [ ]
    If so who ______
13. ADR (adverse drug reaction[s]):
    Has experienced ADR(s): yes [ ] no [ ]
    If yes, how was it handled ______
14. Incidence of overuse or underuse of medication:
    yes [ ] no [ ] Describe ______
15. Storage:
    How is medication stored ______
    Where stored ______
    Reason kept that way ______
16. Disposition of old drugs (how handled): ______

From Ebersole P, Hess P: *Toward healthy aging: human needs and nursing response,* ed 5, St Louis, 1998, Mosby.
*If medications administered by spouse or other, the assessment should be done to ascertain caregiver's ability.

nurse's assessment includes a description of the elder's sleep patterns and activities during waking periods, including periods of rest, exercise, and "naps." The elder should be asked about usual bedtime routines as well as what factors disturb and enhance sleep. Some older adults are still working, some are retired from evening or night jobs, or some are caregivers and may have a sleep-wake pattern that differs from the hospital routine. These data are then used to accommodate the older adult's normal sleep-wake cycle as closely as possible.

Critical Thinking Questions

1. You are chairing a committee to revise the preadmission assessment for 1-day surgery patients. Sixty percent of the patients admitted are 65 years of age and older. What specific assessment items will you suggest be included for all older adult patients?
2. An 83-year-old woman is recovering from hip replacement surgery. She is refusing to eat or take part in therapy. She complains that something is wrong with her head and she has a disease that is "rotting" her brain. She is suspicious about what her roommate is saying to the nurses about her. At times she is confused and does not remember what he has been told from shift to shift. What areas of function do you need to assess to determine what is affecting her status?
3. A 69-year-old man has been hospitalized for 10 days after complications following a myocardial infarction. Three days ago it seemed that he would be discharged soon. However, he has now become lethargic and has been sleeping frequently throughout the day. What information from the chart may be helpful in determining what has caused the changes in his condition?
4. You are assigned to a recuperative care unit of the hospital. Most of the patients are older adults with complications from chronic illnesses that exacerbated their present problems. What should you be noting in the review of the charts before assessing your patients? What assessment data are important to ascertain on all patients on this unit because of their older adult status?

References

1. Adams WL, Cox NS: Epidemiology of problem drinking among the older, *Int J Addict* 30(13):1469, 1995.
2. Administration on Aging (AoA), *A profile of older Americans: 2000,* Washington, DC, 2000, US Department of Health and Human Services.

3. Administration on Aging (AoA), *Older adults and mental health: issues and opportunities,* Washington, DC, 2001, US Department of health and Human Services.
4. Alexopoulos GS et al: "Vascular depression" hypothesis, *Archiv Gen Psychiatr* 54:915, 1997.
5. American Nurses Association (ANA): *Scope and standards of gerontological nursing practice,* Washington, DC, 1995, ANA.
6. Ayres MM, Woodtli A: Concept analysis: abuse of ageing caregivers by older care recipients, *J Adv Nurs* 35(3):326, 2001.
7. Bianchi EC: *Aging as a spiritual journey,* New York, 1990, Crossroad.
8. Campbell VA et al: Surveillance for sensory impairment, activity limitation, and health related quality of life among older adults—United States, 1993-1997, *Morb Mortal Wkly Rep CDC Surveill Summ* 48(8):131, 1999.
9. Carter B, McGoldrick M, editors: *The changing family life cycle,* Boston, 1989, Allyn & Bacon.
10. Center for Mental Health Services: *National strategy for suicide prevention,* Rockville, MD, 2000, US Department of Health and Human Services.
11. Claes JA, Moore W: Issues confronting lesbian and gay older adults: the challenges for health services and human service providers, *ZZJ Health Hum Serv Adm* 23(2):181, 2000.
12. Cope KA: Nutritional status: a basic "vital sign," *Home Health Nurs* 12(2):29, 1994.
13. Devon CAJ: Suicide in the older: how to identify and treat patients at risk, *Geriatrics* 51(3):67, 1996.
14. Ebersole P, Hess P: *Toward healthy aging: human needs and nursing response,* ed 5, St Louis, 1998, Mosby.
15. Finlayson RE: Misuse of prescription drugs in the older adult, *Int J Addict* 30(13):1647, 1995.
16. Fioritto P, editor: *Alcoholism and aging: a matter of substance,* ed 2, Cleveland, 1997, School of Medicine, Case Western Reserve University.
17. Fry PS: The unique contribution of key existential factors to the prediction of psychological well-being of older adults following spousal loss, *Gerontologist* 41(1):69, 2001.
18. Fulmer TT, O'Malley TA: *Inadequate care of the older: a health care perspective on abuse and neglect,* New York, 1987, Springer.
19. Gallo JJ, Lebowitz BD: The epidemiology of common late-life mental disorders in the community: themes for the new century, *Psychiatr Serv* 50:1158, 1999.
20. Genke J: HIV/AIDS and older adults: the invisible ten percent, *Care Manag J* 2(3):196, 2000.
21. Grigg E: Sexuality and older people, *Elder Care* 11(7):12, 1999.
22. Guigoz Y, Vellas B, Garry PJ: Assessing the nutritional status of the older: the Mini Nutritional Assessment as part of geriatric evaluation, *Nutr Rev* 54(1):S59, 1996.
23. Guralnik JM: The impact of vision and hearing impairments on health in old age, *J Am Geriatr Soc* 47(8):1029, 1999.
24. Guralnik JM et al.: The impact of disability in older women, *J Am Med Womens Assoc* 52:113, 1997.
25. Gurland BJ, Cross PS, Katz S: Epidemiological perspectives on opportunities for treatment of depression, *Am J Geriatr Psychiatr* 4(suppl 1):S 7, 1996.
26. Gurnak AM, editor: Introduction: special issue on drugs and the older, *Int J Addict* 30(13):1461, 1995.
27. Herriot CS: Spirituality and aging, *Holis Nurs Pract* 21(8):60, 1996.
28. Hollinger-Smith L, Buschmann MB: Failure to thrive: predicting older nursing home residents at risk, *Clin Gerontol* 20(4):65, 1999.
29. Hoyert DL, Kochanke KD, Murphy SL: Deaths: final data for 1997, *National Vital Statistics Reports* 47(9), 1999. Hyattsville, MD, National Center for Health Statistics.
30. Hungelmann J et al: Focus on spiritual well-being: harmonious interconnectedness of mind-body–spirit—use of the JAREL Spiritual Well-Being Scale, *Geriatr Nurs* 17(6):262, 1996.
31. Jamison MST: Failure to thrive in older adults, *J Geront Nurs* 23(2):8, 1997.
32. Katz IR, DiFilippo S: Neuropsychiatric aspects of failure to thrive in late life, *Clin Geriatr Med* 13(4):623, 1997.
33. Kramer CJ, Kerkhof GA, Hofman WF: Age differences in sleep-wake behavior under natural conditions, *Personality Individ Dif* 27(5):853, 1999.
34. Leveille SG et al: Aging successfully until death in old age: opportunities for increasing active life expectancy. *Am J Epidemiol* 149(7):654, 1999.
35. Masters W, Johnson V: *Human sexual response,* Boston, 1966, Little, Brown & Co.
36. Musil C: Health of grandmothers as caregivers: a ten month follow-up, *J Women Aging* 12(1-2):129, 2000.
37. Pangman VC, Sequiure M: Sexuality and the chronically ill older adult: a social justice issue, *Sexuality and Disability* 18(1):49, 2000.
38. Szirony TA: Infection with HIV in the older population, *J Geront Nurs* 25(10):25, 1999.
39. Tebb S: An aid to empowerment: a caregiver well-being scale, *Health Soc Work* 20(2):87, 1995.
40. Teel CS, Press AN: Fatigue among older adults in caregiving and noncaregiving roles, *West J Nurs Res* 21(4):498, 1999.
41. Trudel G, Turgeon L, Pichi L: Marital and sexual aspects of old age, *Sexual and Relationship Therapy* 15(4):381, 2000.
42. Tully CL, Snowdon DA: Weight change and physical function in older women: findings from the nun study, *J Am Geriatr Soc* 43:1394, 1995.
43. US Department of Health and Human Services (USDHHS): *Mental health: a report of the surgeon general,* Rockville, MD, 1999, USDHHS, SAMSHA, CMHS, NIH, NIMH.
44. US Department of Health and Human Services, Public Health Services: *Healthy people 2010: national health promotion and disease prevention objectives,* Washington, DC, 2000, US Government Printing Office.
45. Verdery RB: Failure to thrive in older people, *J Nutr Health Aging* 2(2):69, 1998.
46. Vetta F: The impact of malnutrition on the quality of life in the older, *Clin Nutr* 18(5):259, 1999.
47. Wallman HW: Comparison of older nonfallers and fallers on performance measures of functional reach, sensory organization, and limits of stability, *J Gerontol A Biol Sci Med Sci* 56(9):M580, 2001.
48. Whitlatch CJ et al: The stress process of family caregiving in institutional settings, *Gerontologist* 41(4):462, 2001.
49. Windham DA: The millennial challenge: elder abuse, *J Emerg Nurs* 26(5):444, 2000.

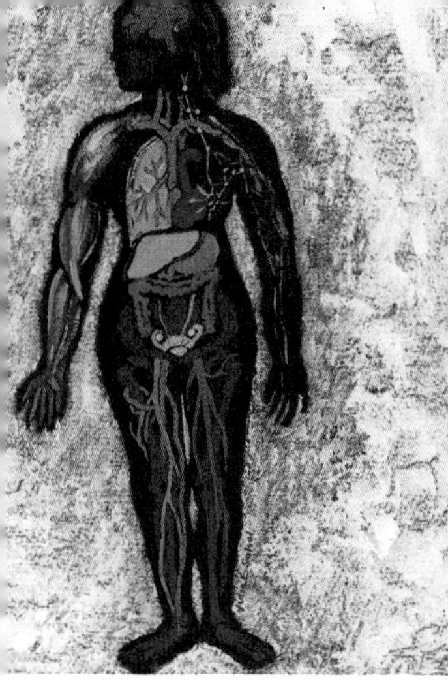

http://www.mosby.com/MERLIN/medsurg_phipps

Chronic Illness 5

Wilma J. Phipps

Objectives

After studying this chapter, the learner should be able to:

1. Differentiate between acute and chronic illness.
2. Describe factors that influence chronic illness.
3. Identify areas of assessment for the chronically ill person.
4. Describe psychosocial interventions for the person with a chronic illness.
5. Describe provisions of the Americans With Disabilities Act.

The prevention and management of chronic disease is one of the major challenges facing the health care system today. Awareness of unmet needs among persons with long-term health problems is increasing, and it is recognized that individuals have needs that extend beyond the strictly medical. Their problems demand the use of multiple sources of help and care, especially since the coping abilities of chronically ill persons often are reduced because of advancing age; serious functional impairment and disability; and limited personal, social, and financial resources.

Chronic disease is not an entity in itself but an umbrella term that encompasses long-lasting diseases, which often are associated with some degree of disability. Although each chronic illness is unique and has a different impact on the individual, family, and community, there is a common core of problems and complications that the nurse must understand to competently care for any person with a long-term illness.

INCIDENCE AND PREVALENCE OF CHRONIC DISEASE

The incidence and prevalence of chronic diseases have increased since the beginning of the twentieth century. Incidence refers to the number of cases of illness that had their onset during a specified period of time. Health statistics commonly report the number of new cases for a calendar year. Prevalence refers to the total number of cases at a given point in time. Thus prevalence rates are higher than incidence rates because they include all persons (cases) with a specified condition (old cases) and those who acquired the condition during a specified period of time (new cases).

The reason for the increase in both the incidence and prevalence of chronic diseases is that fewer persons are dying from acute diseases. Mortality from infectious diseases such as whooping cough and chickenpox in children and pneumonia in persons of all ages has decreased. Improved sanitation, the introduction of effective vaccines and mass immunizations, and the discovery of antibiotics have all contributed to this decrease in deaths from infectious diseases.

According to recent surveys, an estimated 99 million Americans have one or more chronic conditions, and the number is expected to increase annually. By the year 2010, 120 million persons will be affected (Figure 5-1).

Disability

Disability refers to any long- or short-term reduction of activity as the result of an acute or a chronic condition. Limitation of activity is used to describe a long-term reduction in a person's ability to perform the kind or amount of activity associated with a particular age-group. Restriction of activity is generally used to refer to a relatively short-term reduction in a person's activity below his or her normal capacity.

The latest available figures from the U.S. Bureau of the Census show that the number of persons with some limitation in activity has been increasing each year. In 1994, 54 million people in the United States, or roughly 21% of the population, had some level of disability. Although the rates of disability are relatively stable or declining slightly for those 45 years and older, rates are on the rise among younger people. A related finding is that the number of persons with limited activity decreased as family income increased. This seems to indicate that persons from higher income levels may be better educated about preventive health measures and that they are able to afford better diet, better housing, and better medical care.

ACUTE VERSUS CHRONIC ILLNESS

An acute illness is one caused by a disease that produces symptoms and signs soon after exposure to the cause, that runs a short course, and from which there is usually a full recovery or an abrupt termination in death. An acute illness may become chronic. For example, a common cold may develop into chronic sinusitis. A chronic illness is one caused by disease that produces symptoms and signs within a variable period of time, that runs a long course, and from which there is

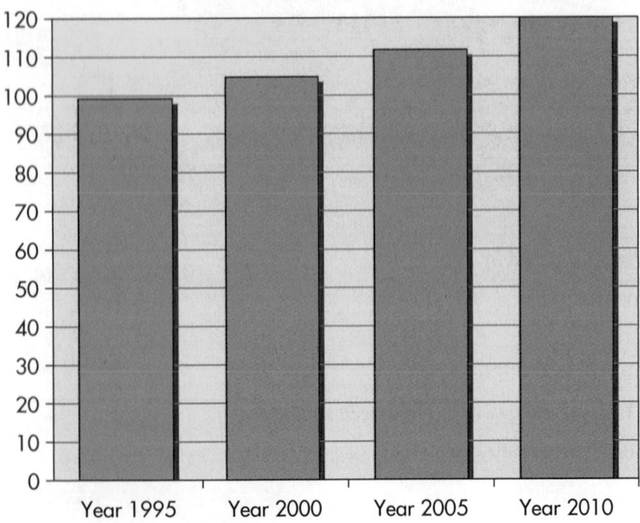

Figure 5-1 Estimated number of people with chronic conditions (in millions).

only partial recovery. Criteria used to define chronic conditions on the National Health Survey are as follows: (1) the conditions were first noticed 3 months or more before the date of the interview, or (2) they belong to a group of conditions (including heart disease and diabetes) that are considered chronic, regardless of when they began. These criteria are in accordance with the definition of the Commission on Chronic Illness, which states that chronic illness is any impairment or deviation from normal that has one or more of the following characteristics:

1. The illness or impairment is permanent.
2. The illness or impairment leaves residual disability.
3. The illness or impairment is caused by nonreversible pathologic alteration.
4. The illness or impairment requires a long period of supervision, observation, or care.

The symptoms and general reactions caused by chronic disease may subside with proper treatment and care. The period during which the disease is controlled and symptoms are not obvious is known as remission. However, at a future time the disease may become active again with recurrence of pronounced symptoms. This is known as an exacerbation of the disease.

Exacerbations of chronic disease often cause the patient to seek medical attention and may lead to hospitalization. The needs of a patient who has an acute illness can be very different from those of the patient with an acute exacerbation of a chronic disease. For example, a young person may enter the hospital with complaints of fever, chest pain, shortness of breath, fatigue, and a productive cough. If the diagnosis is pneumonia, the patient usually can be assured of recovery after a period of rest and a course of antibiotic treatment. If, however, the diagnosis is rheumatic heart disease and the patient is being admitted to the hospital for the third, fourth, or fifth time, reassurance is not so definite, clear-cut, or easy to give. In such a case it is necessary to begin planning care that will extend beyond the period of hospitalization, taking into consideration many aspects of the patient's total life situation. The concerns of the patient who has repeated attacks of illness are very different from those of one who has a short-term illness.

Further, the needs of patients who are admitted to the hospital with an acute illness but who also have an underlying chronic condition must not be overlooked. For example, elderly patients who enter the hospital with pneumonia may receive treatment for the pneumonia and recover from this illness. However, they may still be hampered by the arteriosclerotic heart disease and arthritis that they have had for years. Also, these two chronic conditions may have been aggravated by the acute infection, or the return to former activity may be hindered by joint stiffness resulting from bed rest and inactivity. Consideration of a patient's multiple diagnoses is essential if new problems associated with the chronic illness are to be prevented.

The National Health Survey classifies chronic physical conditions into the following categories: (1) selected skin and musculoskeletal conditions, (2) impairments (visual, hearing, speech, paralysis, deformity, or orthopedic impairment), (3) selected digestive conditions, (4) selected conditions of the genitourinary, nervous, endocrine, metabolic, and blood and blood-forming systems, (5) selected circulatory conditions, and (6) selected respiratory conditions.

Many chronic conditions cause a limitation of activity, which affects the lifestyle of those affected. Studies document that, although the impact of acute illness has diminished, the burden of chronic health problems and related disability has increased.

Approximately 14% of the population experiences some activity limitations, whereas almost half of the persons over 65 years of age are limited in their activities by one or more chronic conditions. Some activity limitations are associated with mental disabilities, but most are the result of physical handicaps caused by heart conditions and arthritis. Because chronic disability increases in direct proportion to age, persons older than 65 years of age are most prone to severe chronic disability.

The inability to work or to move about greatly influences the kind of medical treatment and health supervision needed by persons who have a chronic illness. Some persons need only periodic medical examination and perhaps continuing treatment with medications; others may require complete physical care. Some have a disease that progresses very slowly without remissions, whereas others may have episodes of acute illness and then seem comparatively well for a time. Each person requires a thorough assessment to determine the stage of the illness, the course the illness is likely to take, the type of care needed, and the method by which that care will be delivered if the individual is to be helped appropriately.

FINANCING CHRONIC ILLNESS CARE

As the number of persons with chronic conditions increases, so do the direct medical costs. Figure 5-2 shows the estimated medical costs for 1995, 2000, 2005, and 2010.[13] The cost of the care of persons with chronic conditions includes hospital care, physician care, other costs, and nursing home care. The "other" category includes the cost of prescriptions, dental care, nonphysician practitioners, home health care, medical equipment for use in the home, and emergency care.[13] The allocation of these costs is shown in Figure 5-3. Because there is no organized federal system of care for those with chronic conditions, individual states are evaluating models for delivering cost-effective care to this population. Also, the Robert Wood Johnson Foundation has a national program, "Building Health Systems for People With Chronic Illness," that is examining various ways to organize and pay for care for this population.[28] Some of the approaches being considered by individual states are managed care models. There is also a teamwork approach being studied by the Wisconsin Department of Health and Human Services. In this model the patient can choose a physician, and then community-based organizations

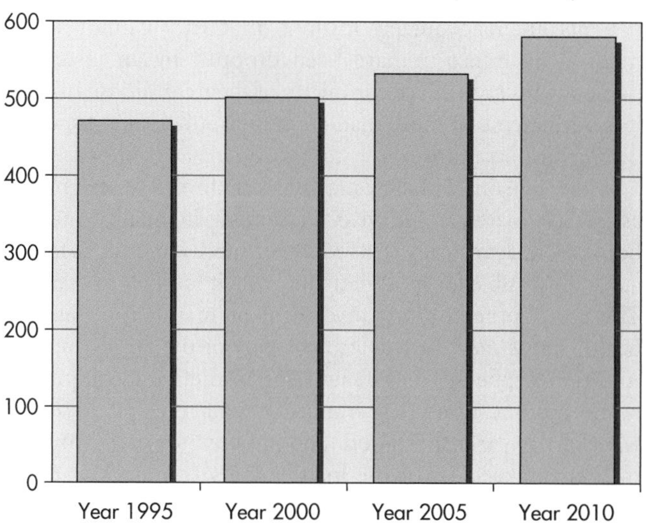

Figure 5-2 Estimated direct medical costs (in millions).

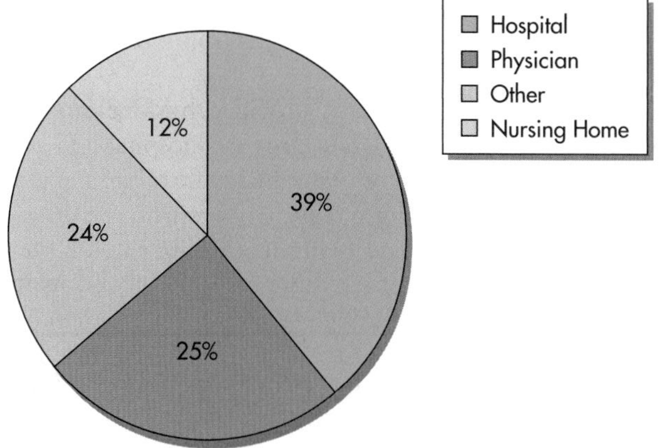

Figure 5-3 Direct medical costs for persons with chronic conditions.

put together a caregiving team that works with the physician to develop a comprehensive care plan. The plan is developed with the participant in his or her own home, if possible. This approach helps to identify the individual's strengths, disabilities, and lifestyle preferences, as well as the capabilities of his or her informal support network. In the Wisconsin plan the patients are called "participants" to indicate that they are part of the planning process.

The goal in most programs for persons with chronic conditions is to keep them at home, if possible. This is less costly, and most persons prefer to stay in their own homes as long as necessary services are available to them.

A related issue under study is that of long-term care insurance. Although long-term care insurance is available in most states, sales have been slow. There is a particular concern because of the number of "baby boomers" who will be retiring in the next 15 to 20 years. More of these persons will need to have private insurance because public financing mechanisms will be inadequate to cover their needs. However, it is almost impossible for persons with chronic conditions to obtain private insurance. Therefore it is important that they obtain insurance before they become chronically ill. The "Program to Promote Long-Term Care Insurance for the Elderly," sponsored by the Robert Wood Johnson Foundation, is designed to promote this goal.

FACTORS INFLUENCING THE OCCURRENCE AND MANAGEMENT OF CHRONIC ILLNESS

Age

Different age-groups have different kinds of experiences with acute and chronic diseases. The young are more likely to experience short, intense, acute conditions that are quickly over. Elderly persons are more likely to have long, drawn-out chronic diseases; nevertheless, it is true that anyone can have either an acute or a chronic disease at any age. Chronic illness and disability may date from birth (e.g., spina bifida with neurologic damage); or they may originate in childhood, adolescence, or early adult life (e.g., multiple sclerosis or rheumatoid arthritis). The major chronic illnesses among those 65 years and older identified in the National Health Survey are arthritis, diabetes, heart disease, and hypertension.

Because of strides made in pediatric medicine, children who 30 years ago would have died of diseases such as cystic fibrosis are living longer. The reduction in death rates among the younger age-groups has allowed a higher percentage of the population to reach the age of greatest risk for chronic diseases. Cancer develops far more frequently in older than in younger persons. Because the average age of our population continues to rise, about 30% of persons now alive will eventually develop cancer.[1]

A commonly asked question is, "When does aging end and illness begin?" Differences found in age-groups or changes found in individuals as they age represent normal aging (i.e., a universal, intrinsic process of growth and development that is inevitable, irreversible, and not preventable). Remissions and exacerbations are possibilities with chronic illness; they are not with aging. Even though aging, a normal process, is distinct from chronic disease, a pathologic process, chronic illness often accompanies aging. The problems of aging and chronic disease are influenced in major ways by each other (e.g., the social problems confronting older adults are strongly influenced by the presence and severity of chronic disabilities).

Race and Ethnicity

Some chronic diseases are more prevalent among members of particular racial or ethnic groups than among others. For example, diabetes among African-Americans is about 70% more prevalent than among Caucasian Americans, and among Hispanics it is nearly double that for Caucasian Americans. The prevalence of diabetes among American Indian and Alaska Natives is more than twice that for the total population.

Other examples include hypertension, which occurs more often among African-Americans and Hispanics than among Caucasians; tuberculosis, new cases of which develop in disproportionately high numbers among Hispanics and Asian and Pacific Islanders in the United States; and cervical cancer, which occurs in women of Vietnamese origin five times more often than in Caucasian women.

Biologic and genetic characteristics of African-Americans, Hispanics, American Indians, Alaska Natives, Asians, Native Hawaiians and/or Pacific Islanders do not explain these disparities in chronic illness. They are most likely the result of complex interactions among genetic variations; environmental factors; and specific health behaviors such as smoking, diet, and exercise.

Geographic Location

Twenty-five percent of Americans live in rural areas defined as places with fewer than 2500 residents. In rural areas the rates of heart disease, cancer, and diabetes exceed those for urban areas. This may reflect the fact that people living in rural areas are less likely to use preventive screening services or exercise regularly and have less timely access to emergency services and specialty care. In 1996 20% of the rural population was uninsured, compared with 16% of the urban population.

Cultural Values

Western culture tends to be cure oriented. Therefore health care for acute conditions is often more valued than health care for the chronically ill. In contrast with working with the exciting aspects of sophisticated and mechanical technology, caring for chronically ill persons is often considered boring. The continual struggle to cope with day-to-day living soon becomes tedious for chronically ill persons, their families, and health professionals. The rewards of treating chronic illness cannot be measured by a cure but by the degree to which complications are prevented and persons are helped to function at their optimal level.

The cultural context has many symbolic meanings, beliefs, and values that health professionals need to understand to meet individual health needs. Some persons may view their chronic disease as a form of punishment from God. Thus they may experience a sense of guilt. Those who view their chronic disease as a "leper phenomenon" may experience a sense of social rejection. Others may see their chronic illness as a destructive force without meaning or simply as a physical response of the body. Appreciation of the person's beliefs and behavior in the context of his or her cultural heritage rather than denial of the cultural influence increases understanding between the health professional and the chronically ill person. Differences do not imply deviance. It is possible to introduce health practices in a manner congruent with an individual's cultural values.

Personal Cost of Disability

Chronically ill persons and their families are subjected to great personal and emotional losses that must be dealt with—loss of self-esteem, loss of status within the family, loss of independence, feelings of rejection, and feelings of helplessness are only a few. These can be more devastating than economic deprivation, which is a constant problem for many.

The economic cost to the patient and family is considerable. The cost of hospitalization rises yearly. Frequent or extended hospitalization and medical expenses can be ruinous if patients are inadequately insured or if they cannot afford medical insurance or have been dropped by an insurance company because of the chronicity of their condition. In 2002 it is estimated that more than 40 million Americans are without medical insurance.

Many persons with chronic illness are forced to seek public assistance merely to survive. Placement in quality nursing homes, which typically costs $3000 or more a month, is financially impossible for most patients or their families to manage. The cost of medications to control or maintain a patient's health status may deplete a major part of the family budget. Additional expenses may include special diets and equipment, home modifications (e.g., ramps or widening of doors for wheelchairs), transportation, and support services provided by homemakers, day or live-in attendants, or nurses.

The ability of the individual family to pay its own way is determined in part by which member of the family becomes disabled. Older studies showed that the family suffered less economic deprivation if the wife was disabled. In those studies three fourths of the chronically ill persons unable to carry out their jobs were men. Today, however, more and more households are headed by women who are single parents and are the only wage earners for the family. Women who head households need additional help and support, and nurses should be sensitive to their needs.

Some financial assistance is provided by Medicare. This federally administered program provides hospital and medical insurance protection for persons 65 years of age and older, as well as for those younger than 65 years who are disabled and eligible for Social Security benefits. Persons under age 65 who are medically indigent because of health problems may be eligible for assistance through the Medicaid program.

Medicare primarily pays for acute care services. According to the Health Care Finance Agency (HCFA), 58% of Medicare costs covers payments to hospitals, 24% covers physician costs, 14% covers "other" services, and only 5% goes to nursing homes.

Recent changes in federal funding have altered Medicare and Medicaid programs. Persons ages 65 years and older receiving Social Security benefits have a higher fee deducted from their monthly payments to pay for their Medicare premiums. Medicare Part A pays for hospitalization; Medicare Part B covers medical expenses and physician care. Since January 1, 1998, Medicare Part A pays all but $764 for the first 60 days of hospitalization and Medicare Part B covers physician bills, physical therapy treatments, rental of wheelchairs, and other equipment.

As of January 2002, each beneficiary pays a quarterly premium of $150.00 for Part B coverage. The premium is deducted from the beneficiary's social security check. Persons not receiving social security are billed for the monthly premiums quarterly. The monthly premium usually increases yearly. Part B does not cover the cost of medicine, eyeglasses, hearing aids, or dentures. Medicare reimbursement is commonly 80% of the amount billed. Most persons covered by Medicare purchase supplemental health insurance (co-insurance or "gap" insurance) to cover the expenses not reimbursed by Medicare.

There have been severe cutbacks in Medicaid, which is administered by state governments. For example, persons seeking Medicaid assistance in Ohio are not eligible if they have assets of more than $1500. Until recently a person was allowed to keep his or her home if a spouse was living in it. However, some persons who were financially well off were advised by lawyers to "spend down their assets" to become eligible for Medicaid. That is, they were advised to transfer their assets to children or other relatives so that it appeared they were unable to pay for nursing home care. Because Medicaid was intended to be a program for the indigent, several governors proposed more stringent eligibility standards, and some states have passed laws that make it impossible for well-to-do persons to receive Medicaid after they have "spent down their assets." In some states a person is allowed to keep his or her home if a spouse is still living in it; however, the house will be sold by the state after the death of the spouse to recover the amount of Medicaid assistance received by one or both spouses. Because of large state budget deficits beginning in the 1990s, several governors are proposing even more stringent eligibility standards for Medicaid.

Thus persons with chronic illnesses may have considerable difficulty paying for prescribed therapy. For example, antiinflammatory agents used to treat arthritis are very expensive. Many of these medications cost between $0.75 and $1.35 each, and the usual dose is three times daily. Persons with other chronic conditions such as Parkinson's disease may be taking even more expensive drugs (costing as much as $1200/month). It is not uncommon for persons with limited resources to have to decide whether to purchase medications or food because there is not enough money for both.

EPIDEMIOLOGY OF CHRONIC DISEASE

Epidemiology examines the distribution of chronic disease, as well as the measurement of health status in the general population. It is both a body of knowledge and a method for obtaining knowledge. As a methodology, epidemiology can be used to assist in explaining the multifactorial causal patterns of chronic diseases.

Problems in Determining Causality of Chronic Diseases

Some of the factors that contribute to the difficulty of studying the cause of chronic disease are:

1. *Multifactorial nature of etiologic factors.* The operation of multiple factors is particularly important in chronic diseases. The interaction of factors may be purely additive or synergistic (i.e., the combined potential for harm of many risk factors is more than the sum of the individual factors). They interact, reinforce, and even multiply each other. Asbestos workers, for example, have increased lung cancer risk. Asbestos workers who smoke have 30 times more risk than co-workers who do not smoke and 90 times more risk than persons who neither smoke nor work with asbestos.
2. *Absence of a known agent.* Because no specific diagnostic test exists for many chronic diseases, the distinction between persons with a disease and those free of disease may be more difficult to establish than with most infectious diseases.
3. *Long latent period.* Many chronic diseases have a long latent period. The latent period is the equivalent of the incubation period in infectious disease, except that it is generally longer. Because of the extended latency, it is often difficult to link antecedent events with outcomes. However, increasing evidence shows that onset of ill health is strongly linked to influences of physical, social, economic, and family environments. It is easy to identify the common exposure to chickenpox in a school setting, but it is much more difficult to identify the impact of drastic alterations in family circumstances caused by mental disorders or slow-onset physical illnesses.
4. *Indefinite onset.* The problem of pinpointing the initial occurrence of the disease exists with many chronic conditions such as degenerative diseases and mental illnesses. The vague onset of chronic illnesses makes it is difficult to collect statistics on the number of new cases in any given year.
5. *Differential effect of factors on incidence and course of disease.* Factors in the socioeconomic environment that affect health include income level, housing, employment status, culture, and lifestyle. For example, Mormons who abstain from smoking and alcohol have lower cancer rates than the general population as a whole.
6. *Disease-specific mortality rates.* These rates are difficult to determine with chronic illness because death may result from factors other than the chronic disease itself.

One approach for studying chronic illness from an epidemiologic viewpoint is to emphasize that interrelated factors determine illness (i.e., disease is a process that results from the breakdown of many factors: biologic, cultural, economic, emotional, and social). The multiple interactions involving the host, the environment, and the agent sometimes are described as the "web of causation." With this approach an attempt is made to identify the multiple related factors that lead to the disease process. Until a disease can be understood as a web of causation, it is difficult to make rational decisions regarding therapeutic interventions, and it is even more difficult to identify early preventive actions. To develop a chain of causation, one must identify first the natural history of disease by systematic studies of groups of people.

Natural History of Chronic Disease

All diseases have a natural history. For example, chronic diseases extend over time and develop through a sequence of stages. When people speak of the epidemiology of a disease, they are referring to its natural history (i.e., the outcomes of a particular disease are observed over time, and the numbers of the affected persons developing each outcome are measured). This information is used to predict an individual's possible future health. Knowledge of the natural history of disease allows intervention to prevent or limit the effects of diseases. The stages involved in the natural history of a disease are:

1. *Stage of susceptibility.* The disease has not yet developed, but the groundwork has been laid by the presence of factors that favor its occurrence. These may be referred to as risk factors. The need to identify risk factors is becoming more apparent because chronic diseases are a greater health challenge than ever before. Some major risk factors are environmental and behavioral and therefore are amenable to change (e.g., smokers can be persuaded to give up smoking).
2. *Stage of presymptomatic disease.* No manifestation of disease is present, but pathologic changes have begun. An example of presymptomatic disease is atherosclerotic changes in coronary vessels before any overt signs or symptoms of illness appear.
3. *Stage of clinical disease.* By this stage sufficient anatomic or functional changes have occurred so that recognizable signs of disease exist. At present the natural history of many diseases is not completely understood. For example, it is not known why some individuals with several risk factors do not develop clinical disease, whereas others with fewer risk factors do.
4. *Stage of disability.* Disability, which can result from an acute or a chronic condition, reduces a person's activity. The extent of protracted disability resulting from chronic disease is very significant to the person and society because of the person's reduced income, the impact on his or her psychosocial roles, and the burden on community resources.

The subtlety of the natural history of chronic diseases often leaves the person unaware of a disease process for an extended period. Recently, predisposing characteristics or habits that help identify the person at risk to develop a particular chronic disease have been studied extensively. By altering habits of eating, rest, activity, or smoking, the course of certain chronic illnesses such as emphysema, hypertension, diabetes, or heart disease may be changed. Unfortunately, many chronic conditions begin without the individual's awareness of significant physiologic changes. An important step in prevention is early detection of these changes.

PREVENTION OF CHRONIC DISEASE

Because chronic disease evolves over time and pathologic changes may become irreversible, the goal is to detect risk factors as early as possible. Although these diseases differ from their infectious disease predecessors, it is now clear that many are preventable.

CHRONICALLY ILL PERSONS AND THEIR FAMILIES

The effects of chronic illness on the affected person and family members are numerous and varied. The first impact of the disability may nearly immobilize them. Time must be provided for them to talk through their concerns and fears before they can be expected to begin coping with their new situation.

Marked changes are often required in family living as a result of chronic illness. Some families may find themselves drawn closer together. Other families may drift apart, the individual members being incapable of helping one another. At times, chronic illness may threaten a person's basic emotional stability, and the whole situation may be unbearable to others. Sometimes the person's emotional needs may not have been apparent to family members early in the illness, but when such needs grow obvious, relatives feel inadequate to cope with the situation. The length of illness, periodic hospitalizations, and increased financial, emotional, and social burdens are stressors that threaten the family's integrity.

Chronic illness imposes additional problems of learning how to cope with restrictions on activities of daily living, how to prevent or identify medical crises that occur, and how to carry out treatment regimens as delineated by the health care provider. Family members also need to learn about the restrictions, not only to be of assistance to the chronically ill person but also to adjust to resultant disruptions in their own activity patterns.

Because chronic illness may have periods of exacerbation when symptoms become more acute and medical crises may occur, patients and family members need to know which symptoms must be reported to the health care provider, as well as the time interval for reporting these symptoms. They also need to know how to contact the provider and what measures to take if a medical crisis occurs. For example, if a person has a history of myocardial infarction, family members must know what to do if the person experiences severe chest pain. Should they call 911? Should the person be taken immediately to a hospital emergency department? Should the physician be contacted first? Patient and family members should plan in advance the sequence of actions to take during a medical crisis, depending on the nature and extent of the presenting symptoms.

Family Influences on Illness

Definition of Family

The definition of family has changed over time. In the past the concept of family as extended family was considered the societal norm. With the advent of urbanization, the norm became the nuclear family (mother, father, and children). Today the concept of family includes the single-parent family, the reconstituted family, and the gay or lesbian couple, among others. Family may be defined according to geographic proximity, as in shared households or residential retirement homes. Family also may be defined by shared emotional bonds between individuals or by one's support network. For this reason, in this discussion family is regarded as those people whom the ill individual or spokesperson identifies as family. A flexible definition of the family is especially important among ethnic families such as African-Americans and Mexican-Americans. African-American elders often consider blood, marriage, or friendship relationships as equivalent; and caregivers treat personal care aides of the same cultural background as kin.[4] These nonblood relationships are referred to as fictive kin. In addition, Mexican-Americans use a "compadre" system or coparent who assumes the parenting role should anything happen to the natural parents.[4]

Models of Family Functioning

Models of family functioning provide ways of thinking about the family that allow one to understand and predict behavior. Models are useful because they suggest ways that families may be helped. The two models described here are useful to nurses when they think about how families cope with illness. When selecting a theoretic framework of family functioning to address an ethnically diverse population, the nurse needs to determine if the definition of the family addresses changes in today's family compositions. For example, family systems theory assumes that family members must be together to have relationships. However, family members who live at a distance may be just as intimate as those who live together. Anthropologic and developmental perspectives suggest that family must be legally sanctioned or that all families go through the same stages at the same time. Because these two perspectives fail to address nonblood relationships or the earlier ages at which many minority families go through some of the developmental stages, they provide less guidance to the nurse for planning interventions. However, despite its limitations, family systems theory is still one of the most frequently used family theories because of its focus on the interaction of the family members with the external environment.

Family Systems Theory

The family systems perspectives is derived from general systems theory, as described in the work of Ludwig von Bertalanffy.[32] Family systems theory conceptualizes the family as an open system that functions within the broader context of the environment. The more open the family system, the greater is the exchange of information with the environment. Within the boundary of the family, dynamic interactions between the members or subsystems (such as the subsystem of parents or children) are governed by the family's organization. The organization of the family system is characterized by roles, relationships, expectations, and rules.

The terms *roles, relationships, expectations,* and *rules* are used to define organization in the family systems literature. Family members occupy and function in roles in relationship to one another. They seem to function in these roles according to the expectations of the whole family. Thus one family member may take on the role of breadwinner, whereas another may take on the role of homemaker. One family member may be the decision maker, another may be the primary caregiver for the small children, and another may be the caregiver for the chronically ill adult.

The term *rules* applies to the family expectations about how each person in his or her role relates to other family members; this becomes a standard for behavior over time. Whether spoken or implicit, these rules result in patterns of relating that characterize the family's interpersonal relationships and their attempts to maintain equilibrium.

The dynamic interactions that take place within the family are governed by the family's organization. According to family systems theory, the interactions are directed toward achieving and maintaining equilibrium within the system. Homeostasis reflects the family's striving to maintain equilibrium in the face of internal or external changes. Other family theorists refined the thinking on homeostasis with development of the concepts of morphogenesis and morphostasis. Morphostasis describes maintenance of the status quo within the family system, and morphogenesis reflects the ability of the family to change its basic structure and organization to survive and remain viable. Morphogenesis and morphostasis describe the family system as existing in a dynamic balance between change and stability in response to the environment.

Certain principles describe the characteristics of a system. The principle of circular causality describes family as a group of individuals who are interrelated such that changes in one member evoke changes in another, which in turn affect the first individual. That is to say, individuals living in a family do not exist in a vacuum. They are constantly affected by the behavior of others in the family, which in turn affects their own behavior.

The principle of nonsummativity holds that the family as a whole is more than the sum of the individuals who make up that family. A family cannot be described by the characteristics of its individuals alone because this does not allow for the interaction among them. Thus one cannot look at each member of a family individually and have an appreciation of the characteristics of the family as a whole.

Understood within the framework of family systems theory is the idea that the organism of the family is constantly moving toward goals. The principle of equifinality states that different outcomes may have the same beginnings and that different beginnings may lead to the same outcomes. Because families are open systems, they are constantly exchanging information with the larger environment. Thus the outcome of the system is affected by more than just its initial conditions.

The family systems framework suggests several key assessment areas for the nurse (Box 5-1).

Family Stress Theory

Family stress theory stems from the work of Hill,[11,12] who described families' responses to dealing with the loss of the

BOX 5-1 Family Systems Theory—Key Assessment Areas

1. What are the family rules related to the patient, caregiver, and all other identified family member roles?
2. How flexible is each family member in creating and adapting roles to accommodate changes in the patient's health?
3. What are the patient and family goals related to the illness?
4. What environmental sources of information and support are known and unknown to the family?

father-husband after he was drafted into the armed services. Hill's ABC=X conceptualization of the family's response to stress serves as the foundation for investigation and theory building in the area of family stress research. Although researchers have made some modifications over the years to provide clarity and empiric support to the framework, it has remained essentially unchanged. This family crisis framework can be stated as follows:

A (the event) + Interacting with B (the family's crisis-meeting resources) + Interacting with C (how the family defines the event) = 5X (the crisis)

The A factor represents the stressor event, which can be either external or internal to the family. It can result from normative changes or catastrophic events. In this chapter the chronic illness itself is the stressor event to the family.

The B factor represents family resources, which may be of two types. Resources may be (1) those already available to the family, or (2) coping resources strengthened or developed in response to the crisis event. Resources already available to the family might include a family member who is a health care professional or who has had previous experience in caring for an ill person. The B factor represents the area of the family stress framework that has received the most attention by researchers. Two of the most important internal resources are the adaptability and cohesion of the family unit.

The C factor represents the family's perception of the crisis. This is related to the family's view of the seriousness of the event, as well as what the event means to the family. If a family has experienced the death of a member from a stroke, the family might view a stroke in a second family member more seriously than would another family.

The X factor represents the crisis as experienced by the family. It is the outcome of the stressor event for the family after it is interacted on by family resources and perceptions.

Adaptability and Cohesion

Family adaptability is the family's ability to reorganize and change roles, rules, and patterns of interaction in response to either situational or developmental stress. Adaptability refers to how flexible family members are in changing roles to accommodate changes in the family. To the extent that family members can be flexible in their roles, rules, and patterns of interaction, the family can successfully manage changes brought about by having a chronically ill member. Families who cannot make the necessary changes in their role structure and who have difficulty changing family rules are described as being rigid. Families at the opposite end of the adaptability continuum are described as being chaotic; they experience such dramatic role shifts and changes in rules that family members often do not know what rules apply.

Family cohesion describes the extent to which family members feel bonded to each other and concerned and committed to the family. Cohesion is conceptualized as being on a continuum. Extreme cases of cohesion are (1) enmeshment, an overinvolvement of family members in each other's lives and, at the other end, (2) disengagement, in which family members are detached from the family and have little commitment to it. Healthy families lie somewhere between these two extremes. A sense of commitment in family members is vital if the ill member is to be cared for and the family is to continue.

Characteristics of Families

Particular qualities either increase the family's resources or add to the "pileup," a term used to describe the family experience of having additional stressors at the time of a stressor event. The nurse's awareness of a family's characteristics can give insight into the amount of burden families experience and the resources families have in caring for an ill member. These characteristics include but are not limited to the ones discussed in the following paragraphs.

Familial Relation to the Patient

Spouses and adult children experience caregiving in different ways. Spouses are more concerned about their health and see their physicians more often, rate their own health as poorer, report more stress symptoms, and use more psychotropic medications than do adult children. The negative effects on the spouse caregiver's health may be related to the spouse's hesitancy to make use of respite services. Respite services are designed to give a few hours to several days of relief from caregiving activities. Thus the nurse must assess the caregiver's awareness of services and the cultural acceptability of these services and encourage the use or creation of respite by the caregiver. To minimize potential guilt feelings, the nurse should stress the importance of respite for the caregiver's health and continued quality of patient care.

In contrast, adult children are more concerned about family, time, and emotional conflicts. Consequently, adult children often express more burden and place their parents in nursing homes more readily than do spouse caregivers. The fact that adult children perceive more burden may be related to the infrequent visits of family and friends and time spent relaxing.[16] Nevertheless, adult children use respite services more readily and report more benefits than do spouses. Finally, wives are more bothered by their cognitively impaired husband's frequent dangerous behaviors and embarrassing acts, and adult children are more stressed by a parent's inability to bathe himself or herself or stay alone.

Gender

Just as differences exist between spouses and adult children, so do differences exist between the genders. Wives tend to be more distressed/burdened during the initial stages of their caregiving role than are husbands, and some women throughout the experience describe the situation as more confining and oppressive than do men. Nevertheless, with the passage of time, some wives perceive less burden and reflect attitudes comparable with those of husband caregivers.[36]

Sons perform and experience the caregiving role differently and do not sense any major caregiving problems.[14] This low perception of problems probably is related to the fact that sons often delegate the physically intimate caregiving activities to their wives (i.e., the daughter-in-law) and focus on managing their parents' financial concerns. Daughters usually do not have the opportunity to delegate these activities. Therefore daughters may sense more caregiving problems.

The family life cycle also affects family responses. The family may have the burden of caring for both young children and elderly parents, although sometimes older children or young adults can share in the caregiving. Middle-aged daughters are more likely than older wives to have parental, employment, and marital obligations competing with caregiving. As the patient's level of impairment increases and the need for the daughter's assistance increases, so does the daughter's sense of burden[9] and rewards.[20] Older husbands are more likely than sons to experience burden as caregivers because older men are likely to be full-time caregivers and sons are more likely to be part-time caregivers. Determining where the family is in its life cycle can assist the nurse in identifying potential areas of needed support.

Ethnicity

When focusing on diseases such as Alzheimer's, the nurse needs to consider the patient's and family's ethnic heritage.[31] The patient's ethnic heritage may produce different human responses to the same phenomenon. Individual responses to catastrophic illness are filtered through differing belief systems and practices. Consequently nurses need to consider the influence of family culture on the selection of coping strategies. Caucasian caregivers are more burdened when the patient has dementia and is unable to perform[22] daily living tasks such as preparing meals, laundering clothes, shopping, and paying one's bills. In contrast, African-American caregivers are less burdened by the amount of supervision needed by Alzheimer's patients than are Caucasian caregivers, but they are more burdened by a variety of physical disabilities that require more physical labor. The higher level of burden from physical disabilities among African-American caregivers may reflect their overall poorer health status compared with that of Caucasian caregivers. Nevertheless, Caucasian caregivers are more likely to institutionalize persons with a dementia than are African-American caregivers.

Family composition also affects the family response. The family may be large, with several persons who can share in the caregiving, or it may be a single-parent household already pressed to care for its members. The nurse must assess not only the actual participation of household members in caregiving activities but also the caregiver's perceived helpfulness of these acts of caregiver support. A large household does not always mean shared caregiving, and a small household does not always mean more limited support.

Socioeconomic Status

Socioeconomic status determines whether a family can afford to hire extra help to compensate for the activities usually performed by the patient and whether the cost of the illness places an added financial strain on the family.

Employment Status

The employment situation of the caregiver is also important. The female caregiver may have been forced to quit her job or decrease her hours of work because of caregiving demands. Women who continue to work experience absences, work interruptions, loss of pay, decreased energy to do their jobs well, limited job choices, and a desire to not work.[3] Often women who are forced to quit their jobs score the lowest on mental health measures, which suggests that work may provide some respite for caregivers. Obviously, as the caregiving family's income decreases, the ability to purchase services to support the caregiver will decrease. A nurse referral of the family to a social worker may be helpful to the family at this point.

Problem Solving

Family members may or may not have the knowledge and ability to do the problem solving required to care for an ill member and also meet the family's demands. The perceived caregiver costs and rewards and the helpfulness of available social support are majors factors in the ability to cope.

Family Health

Family health is also important. The caregiver may have a chronic illness as well as the patient, a situation that often occurs in a family of elderly persons. African-American caregivers often have as many as four chronic illnesses.[18]

Support Network

A support network composed of persons external to the family who can help the members carry out their tasks and give them emotional support is important for coping. African-American older adults living in the South have larger, more diverse support networks composed of family, relatives, friends, and fictive kin than do African-American elders living in the North.[5] Fictive kin or "para-kin" are unrelated individuals with whom interpersonal relationships are so close that they [the fictive kin] are viewed as family members.[10] In addition, fictive kin have the same familial obligations as "blood" relatives. Living in the South tends to increase the actual frequency of support. Not only does the region of the country affect the family's caregiver activity, it also affects the type of services used. African-American urban older adults use more health services than do rural African-American elders.[4] Rural older adults turn first to their families in the case of illness, but urban elders turn to the hospital. The generally higher incomes of urban elders make services more affordable for them than for rural elders. Furthermore, African-Americans, Native Americans, poor Caucasian persons, and others living in small towns and rural areas are far more dependent on unpaid family members and friends than on public and private service agencies for meeting their everyday needs in life. Also, there are fewer of these services available.

Social Support

It is important to determine whether the family is receiving help with the care needs of the patient, with the family's emotional needs, and with activities outside of the household. Can the family identify persons who visit them, call them, provide respite to them, and/or assist them with decision making? The caregiver's perception of social support decreases the feelings of burden and social isolation.

Religion

The nurse should never overlook the role of the patient's and family's religion during an illness and particularly a hospitalization. Religion can affect the patient's practices, acceptable treatments, and attire.[14] Prayer is especially important in the lives of African-Americans and Muslims. For many African-Americans, frequent prayer demonstrates their belief in the power of God to cure any disease in a faithful person. If the person is not cured, the person failed to demonstrate sufficient faith. Similarly, devout Muslims must pray to Allah, their supreme being, five times a day. The Muslim patient may be found kneeling on a prayer rug facing Mecca, the Holy Land, during these times. It is important for nursing staff members to assess and arrange for the times the patient will need privacy for prayer. Failure to integrate prayer times into the patient's treatment plan may result in tension between the family and health care professionals. Sometimes the patient's faith that God will provide a cure may interfere with the patient's ability to realize that God sends cure through the hands of health care professionals. Health care professionals may need to employ the assistance of a local religious leader to stress this point.

At other times a patient's religion may forbid the acceptance of a treatment. For example, Jehovah's Witnesses refuse blood transfusions, and Orthodox Jews refuse the use of anything electrical on the Sabbath. For Jehovah's Witnesses to accept a blood transfusion means choosing to give up eternity with Jehovah. Although the health care professional may disagree with the Jehovah's Witness patient's beliefs, he or she must still respect and support the patient. For the Orthodox Jew, the Sabbath begins at sundown Friday and ends at sundown Saturday. During the Sabbath, work of any kind is prohibited, including driving, using the telephone, handling money, and even pushing an elevator button. While caring for one Orthodox Jewish woman with renal failure, the nurses on her medical floor rearranged the time of her hemodialysis on Friday from afternoon to the morning hours. Consequently, when the Sabbath began, this patient already had returned to her room and was not in need of the electric elevator for transportation. Furthermore, the patient used battery-powered candles so that she did not have to operate the electric lights. Finally, when the patient needed the head of her bed raised, although she was capable of operating the bedside switches, the nurse brought the patient a bedside bell so that she could call for assistance.

Observance of the Sabbath has ramifications for discharge planning. Because of the prohibition against operating a vehicle on the Sabbath, it is important to plan discharge of the Orthodox Jewish patient before or after the Sabbath. Otherwise the patient's family has to find a non-Orthodox Jew to pick up the patient from the hospital. The only exception to strict adherence to these practices is in a situation of life or death. For example, a young Jewish boy was severely injured one Saturday afternoon while playing football. He needed to go to the hospital immediately. The only person available to take him was his Orthodox Jewish grandfather, who drove him the 25 miles to the hospital. Once the boy was safely admitted, his grandfather walked home.

Sometimes patients wear religious symbols, which the nurse must treat respectfully. These religious symbols include rosaries for Catholics, sacred threads around necks or arms of Hindus, medicine bundles for Native Americans, red ribbons for Mexican children, and mustard seeds, which are worn by some Mediterranean people to ward off the evil eye. When a medical procedure needs to be performed, removal of these religious symbols may be a problem. After explaining the rationale for removing the symbol in a calm, soothing tone, the nurse should gently place the symbol in close contact with or at least within eyesight of the patient.

These are just a few cultural characteristics of families that can affect the family's experience with chronic illness. As positive attributes, they can be indicators of family resources. As negative attributes, they may be predictors of deficits in family coping.

The family stress theory suggests several key assessment areas for the nurse (Box 5-2).

Compliance

Persons with chronic illness often are labeled as "compliant" or "noncompliant" in carrying out regimens prescribed for them. There are many factors that influence the person's ability or motivation to carry out the prescribed regimen. If the

BOX 5-2 Family Stress Theory—Key Assessment Areas

1. What does the illness mean to the family? Are there different meanings among family members?
2. What family characteristics serve as indicators of possible coping resources?
3. What family characteristics suggest possible deficits in family coping?
4. Has the illness increased or decreased the family's cohesion?
5. Which religious beliefs and practices must be integrated into the plan of care?

person does not carry out the regimen (noncompliant), it does not necessarily mean that he or she is refusing to do so deliberately, although this may sometimes occur.

The nurse needs to assess the situation, including the patient's value system (health beliefs, cultural influence, spiritual values),[19] to determine the reasons that the patient is not complying with therapeutic recommendations. The following are some possible reasons for nonadherence to a prescribed therapy[19]:

- Failure to understand or internalize the reason for the recommendations
- Procedures that are difficult to learn and carry out
- Time required to carry out therapy
- Inability to pay for prescribed therapy
- Side effects of therapy (e.g., medications or exercises)
- Embarrassment about carrying out the regimen in front of others
- Social isolation and lack of support and positive reinforcement

Conflicts occur within the family structure when one family member recognizes the importance of carrying out the prescribed regimen but another does not. For example, a wife may see the need for continuing check-ups and medication for her husband's hypertension, whereas he may perceive this as a needless expense because he feels well and has no symptoms. Persons vary from time to time in the extent of compliance. Those who are not hospitalized are their own health care agents, and they (or their significant others) determine the actions that are taken.

Coping mechanisms that have been developed should not be tampered with unless, based on a thorough understanding of the situation, viable and more appropriate alternatives can be proposed. If the goal of maintaining the chronically ill person in the optimal state of health is being interfered with by the individual's or the family's attitudes or capacities, a change in those attitudes or capacities is necessary, but it must be a change that is mutually acceptable. In preparation for giving the highest level of care to persons with a chronic illness, the nurse may find it helpful to review research in this area.

ASSESSMENT OF THE PERSON WITH A CHRONIC ILLNESS

Before a plan of care can be devised for the chronically ill person, a thorough assessment of needs and capabilities is carried out. Included in such an assessment are the individual's physical, psychologic, social, and financial status.

Physical Status

Because medical diagnoses do not accurately reflect the physical status and functioning of the chronically ill person, the use of a profile system or assessment tool may be instituted as a guide for those working with the patient. Assessment is made in six different categories: (1) physical condition, including cardiovascular, pulmonary, gastrointestinal, genitourinary, endocrine, and cerebrovascular disorders; (2) upper extremities—structure and function—including the shoulder girdle and cervical and upper dorsal spine; (3) lower extremities—structure and function—including the pelvis and lower dorsal and lumbar sacral spine; (4) sensory components relating to speech, vision, and hearing; (5) excretory function, including the bowels and bladder; and (6) mental and emotional status. The ability of the person to carry out activities of daily living (e.g., dressing, feeding, bathing, brushing teeth, combing hair, using the toilet, and moving from place to place) specifically needs to be assessed. The completed assessment should indicate in what areas the patient has difficulty and the extent of that difficulty. Such a guide can be used in planning goals for care, both immediate and long term, and is useful in assisting the individual and the family to make realistic plans for care. Because a chronic condition is not static, reassessment is carried out at regular intervals to identify improvement or regression.

The impact of chronic illness on the person's desire for or ability to participate in sexual activities also should be assessed. Changes in body appearance, shortness of breath, and musculoskeletal or neurologic impairments cause some persons to think that they can no longer be sexually active. In addition, the side effects of certain medications tend to decrease sexual desire or cause impotence. The nurse should determine if concern about sexual ability is a problem for the person, and, if it is, appropriate action, including referral, should be taken. (See Chapter 52 for more information about sexuality in health and illness.)

Psychologic Status

Assessment of the person's psychologic needs and capabilities includes determining attitudes and stage of adaptation to the illness, feelings concerning how the illness affects the family or significant others, and the person's own goals in regard to living with an illness. For example, those who are almost totally helpless as a result of a long-term chronic condition may seem to have no interest in learning ways to help themselves. Family members may react in the same manner and be of little help to them. Both the affected person and family need interest and support from nurses and other professionals as they learn to cope with the change in their life situations.

Feelings of anxiety, frustration, irritability, bitterness, and guilt may be expressed by some chronically ill persons who face unending pain and loss of economic and social security. Some persons become obsessed with their health problems and spend much of each day thinking about what will happen and what to do. Guilt may result from being unable to work and support oneself or from the belief, as a result of a search for some purpose or reason for the affliction, that one must deserve the suffering. Depression is common among chronically ill persons, especially those who feel powerless. Powerlessness can be the result of feeling unable to control or overcome what has happened to one. Patients who are depressed may be suicidal, and the nurse should be alert to cues that the patient may be contemplating suicide.

Coping skills may be challenged by persistent, ongoing problems such as chronic pain, recurring medical expenses, or continuing difficulties in carrying out activities of daily living. Usual coping methods may become impossible (e.g., a person who usually copes by expending energy in physical activity may become unable to do so). The person who usually copes by discussing problems with family members will need to find an alternative method if family communication patterns break down. The person can be helped to identify usual coping methods and to explore alternative approaches when necessary.

It is important to recognize that chronically ill persons or their families may suffer from unresolved sadness known as chronic grief. Chronic grief may be defined as accumulated or prolonged grief. It extends over long periods, with permanent characteristics developing in many persons, and carries with it a potential for decreased functioning. The causes are varied, and new waves of grief are constantly triggered. One example is grief caused by the losses associated with aging: youth, dreams, jobs, hair, friends, family, health, visual acuity, social role, money, body parts, and mobility. Each loss is accompanied by grief, which builds on previous grief, just as individual bricks create a wall. In chronic grief the person may be faced with repeated acute episodes. These episodes may coincide with exacerbation of the condition, facing a new limitation, or meeting new indignities. Each new episode requires a renewed struggle back and forth through the various stages of grief.

The nurse can assist by listening and helping the person explore feelings and the content related to these feelings. Because the grief is ongoing, family members also can be helped to identify their feelings and strengthen the communication patterns within the family structure for normal support of its members.

Social and Financial Status

Social and financial status must be considered because both relate specifically to the kind of support and resources available to meet the person's goals. For example, it would be unrealistic to plan for a hydraulic bathtub chair if the patient cannot afford it, if family members are unavailable to help operate it, or if the patient's apartment manager will not permit it to be installed. Alternative methods of helping the patient to take a tub bath would have to be explored.

The social assessment includes living arrangements, family roles, support of significant others, cultural and social group memberships, education, and vocational and avocational activities. The data collected through the performance of this kind of thorough assessment should make it possible to devise a plan of care directed toward the accomplishment of attainable goals that are mutually acceptable to the patient, the family, and the caregivers.

ROLE OF THE NURSE IN CHRONIC ILLNESS

Clarifying Nurse-Patient Values

Before nurses can work effectively with chronically ill persons, they need to be able to distinguish between their own values, standards, and goals and those of the patient. In day-to-day contact with individuals who are making little or no progress, it is tempting to make plans for their future because of a sincere interest in helping them. This is particularly true when the patient's age is similar to one's own. There may be a feeling that something must be done to speed progress. The nurse may become frustrated by the feeling of wanting to do something or wanting to see some marked change. However, he or she must recognize that management of the care of the chronically ill person requires a slow-moving, persistent pace with possibly little or no change for a long time. The person's physical and mental condition must be maintained at its present level or improved, and efforts must be made to progress and encourage the family's adaptation to the patient's condition. Eagerness and readiness to progress are determining factors for the future. The "doing" in the care of the chronically ill person is not always a physical action with the hands. Often the maintenance of a positive approach and attitude and a demonstration of real interest are the greatest help to the patient. Teaching patients to perform activities related to their own care independently rather than performing those activities for them also may lead to progress.

Promoting Self-Care

Asking the person to identify what is meaningful is a primary step toward helping develop self-care. Physical needs are of paramount importance for chronically ill persons. Meeting these physical needs provides a way to convey to such individuals an interest in their progress and welfare. Chronically ill persons who are hospitalized should be allowed to perform as much of their own care as possible. Persons who have been independent in self-care before hospitalization should not be allowed to regress in these abilities if at all possible. Helping patients to take their own baths or showers, attend to toilet needs, and groom themselves can give some sense of accomplishment and help them maintain their self-respect. Helping them to be dressed appropriately promotes a sense of wellness. Success in performing parts of their own self-care may be stimulating enough to strengthen ill persons' motivation; they and their families then may make amazing strides in thinking through and working out future problems themselves. For their planning to be realistic and ultimately functional, all health care personnel must teach chronically ill persons the total physiologic ramifications of their disability, as well as methods of coping with those ramifications.

Persons who are in their homes or in substitute homes should be encouraged to dress in regular, comfortable street clothing rather than pajamas or gowns. Visitors to the home and family members who constantly see such individuals dressed in bedclothes think of them as sick and are reminded of their illness. Seeing them dressed as usual helps to maintain normal attitudes, relationships, and expectations.

Promoting Self-Esteem

The care of chronically ill persons requires alertness in feeling, seeing, and hearing. Continued warmth and interest are necessary to the self-esteem of any chronically ill person. Very often a relationship based on an understanding of these requirements promotes self-esteem and helps the individual to become highly motivated. It may be taxing to listen to the same questions and say the same things day after day, but the nature of chronic illness may require this attention, and the manner in which responses are given will convey warmth and interest. The world of chronically ill persons, whether they are in the hospital or elsewhere, becomes narrowed and circumscribed. They treasure and are interested in those things and those people who are close to them. Their conversations may be largely about themselves, their immediate environment, a few close objects, and the persons who are close to them. Although they may be confined to bed and to their room, others can keep them up-to-date on outside news. Depending on their level of adaptation to their illness, they may welcome hearing about outside events, or they may not be able to think beyond themselves. When they reach the stage of being able to look beyond themselves, newspapers, magazines, radio, or television or creating something with their own hands may help to keep up their interest in others and in outside events.

Supporting the Person with a Progressive Disability

Health care personnel must be prepared to provide care for patients whose disease will follow a course of progressive disability, as with multiple sclerosis, rheumatoid arthritis, or Alzheimer's disease. In these instances goals of care must be modified to retard the downhill progression of disability rather than to achieve maintenance or improvement of physical status. Helping the patient and family cope with progressive deterioration and in some cases eventual death is a demanding task.

Providing Community Resources

There has been increasing interest in providing programs for chronically ill persons and in assisting them and disabled persons to assume a more active role in their communities. Volunteer workers may act as readers both in hospitals and in homes or may assist with other diversional activities. Institutions receiving federal funds are required to make aids such as ramps available to persons who are unable to climb stairs or who are in wheelchairs. With the development of structural changes that facilitate mobility, some persons with physical limitations are more involved in local activities and associations. Nurses can assist by supporting the further development of these structural changes in all community buildings and by encouraging the participation of chronically ill persons in community activities of interest. Various information sources may be obtained from national organizations involved with chronic illness and disability. Many of these agencies have services available in the community (Box 5-3). Programs,

BOX 5-3 Community Resources Involved in Chronic Health Problems

GENERAL

Alzheimer's Disease and Related Disorders Association
Suite 1015
Skokie, IL 60076
(847) 933-2413

American Association of Diabetes Educators
100 West Monroe St., Suite 400
Chicago, IL 60603
(800) 338-3633

American Association of Retired Persons
601 E St. NW
Washington, DC 20049
(202) 434-2277
e-mail: www.aarp.org

American Cancer Society
1599 Clifton Rd., N.E.
Atlanta, GA 30329
(404) 486-0100
(800) ACS-2345
e-mail: www.cancer.org

American Diabetes Association
National Center
1701 N. Beauregard St.
1660 Duke St.
Alexandria, VA 22311
(703) 549-1500
(800) DIABETES
e-mail: www.diabetes.org

American Heart Association
7272 Greenville Ave.
Dallas, TX 75231
(214) 373-6300
(800) 242-8721
e-mail: www.americanheart.org

American Lung Association
1740 Broadway
New York, NY 10019
(212) 315-8700
e-mail: www.lungusa.org

American Parkinson Disease Association
1250 Hylan Blvd., Suite 4B
Staten Island, NY 10305-1946
(718) 981-8001
(800) 223-2732
e-mail: www.apdaparkinson.com

Arthritis Foundation
1330 W. Peachtree St.
Atlanta, GA 30309
(404) 872-7100
(800) 283-7800
e-mail: www.arthritis.org

Association of Retarded Citizens (ARC-U.S.)
1010 Wayne Ave., Suite 650
Silver Spring, MD 20910
(301) 565-3842

Brain Injury Association (NHIF)
105 N. Alfred St.
Alexandria, VA 22314
(703) 236-6000
(800) 444-6443

Continued

BOX 5-3 Community Resources Involved in Chronic Health Problems—cont'd

Cystic Fibrosis Foundation
6931 Arlington Rd.
Bethesda, MD 20814
(301) 951-4422
(800) 344-4823

Epilepsy Foundation of America (EFA)
4351 Garden City Dr.
Landover, MD 20785-7223
(301) 459-3700
(800) EFA-1000

International Life Sciences Institute–North America (ILSINA)
One Thomas Circle, NW
Ninth Floor
Washington, DC 20005
(202) 659-0074

Juvenile Diabetes Foundation
120 Wall St.
New York, NY 10005-4001
(212) 785-9500
(800) JDF-CURE
e-mail: www.jdf.org

Leukemia and Lymphoma Society
1311 Mamaroneck Ave.
White Plains, NY 10605
(914) 949-5213
(800) 955-4LSA
e-mail: www.leukemia.org

March of Dimes Birth Defects Foundation (MDBDF)
1275 Mamaroneck Ave.
White Plains, NY 10605
(914) 428-7100

Muscular Dystrophy Association, Inc.
3300 E. Sunrise Dr.
Tucson, AZ 85718
(520) 529-2000
e-mail: www.mdausa.org

National Association for Down's Syndrome
P.O. Box 4542
Oak Brook, IL 60522
(630) 325-9112

National Association for Visually Handicapped
22 W. 21st St.
New York, NY 10010
(212) 889-3141
e-mail: www.staff@navh.org

National Council on the Aging
409 3rd St. SW, Suite 200
Washington, DC 20024
(202) 479-1200
e-mail: www.ncoa.org

National Easter Seal Society (NESS)
230 W. Monroe St., Suite 1800
Chicago, IL 60606
(312) 726-6200
(800) 221-6827
e-mail: www.sealsnepa.com

National Hemophilia Foundation
116 W. 32nd St., 11th Floor
New York, NY 10001
(212) 328-3700
e-mail: www.hemophilia.com

National Jewish Medical & Research Center
1400 Jackson St.
Denver, CO 80206
(303) 388-4461

National Kidney Foundation
30 E. 33rd St., Suite 1100
New York, NY 10016
(212) 889-2210
e-mail: www.kidney.org

National Mental Health Association
1021 Prince St.
Alexandria, VA 22314-2971
(703) 684-7722
(800) 969-NMHA

National Multiple Sclerosis Society
733 3rd Ave.
New York, NY 10017
(212) 986-3240
(800) FIGHT-MS
e-mail: www.nmss.org

Parents of Children with Down Syndrome (PODS)
P.O. Box 10416
11600 Nebel St.
Rockville, MD 20849
(301) 916-4985

Shriners Hospitals for Crippled Children
2900 Rocky Point Dr.
Tampa, FL 33607
(813) 281-0300
(800) 237-5055
e-mail: www.shrinershq.org

Sickle Cell Disease Association of America (SCDAA)
200 Corporate Pointe, Suite 495
Culver City, CA 90230-8727
(310) 216-6363
(800) 421-8453

United Cerebral Palsy Associations
1660 L St. NW, Suite 700
Washington, DC 20036-5602
(202) 776-0406
(800) USA-5UCP
e-mail: www.ucpa.org

United Ostomy Association
11772 MacArthur Blvd., Suite 200
Irvine, CA 92612-2405
(949) 660-8624
(800) 826-0826

BOX 5-3 Community Resources Involved in Chronic Health Problems—cont'd

REHABILITATION

Architectural and Transportation Barriers Compliance Board
1331 F St. NW, Suite 1000
Washington, DC 20004
(202) 272-0080

Mainstream, Inc.
6930 Carroll Ave., Suite 240
Takoma Park, MD 20912
(301) 891-8777
(800) 661-8239
e-mail: www.mainstream.org

National Information Center for Children and Youth with Disabilities (NICHCY)
Box 1492
Washington, DC 20013-1492
(202) 884-8200
800-695-0285
e-mail: nichcy@aed.org

National Spinal Cord Injury Association (NSCIA)
6701 Democracy Blvd., Suite 300
Bethesda, MD 20817
(301) 588-6959

Paralyzed Veterans of America
801 18th St. NW
Washington, DC 20006
(800) 424-8200

Various types of information may be obtained by contacting these national organizations. In addition, services of the various agencies usually are available at the local level.

BOX 5-4 Provisions of Americans with Disabilities Act

1. Employers may not discriminate against a qualified person with a disability in hiring or promotion.
2. Employers can ask about the person's ability to perform a job but may not ask if someone has a disability or use tests that tend to screen out persons with disabilities.
3. Employers need to provide "reasonable accommodation" to individuals with disabilities, including job restructuring and modification of equipment.
4. Employers do not need to provide accommodations that impose an "undue hardship" on business operations.
5. Employers with 25 or more employees were to comply by July 1992.
6. Employers with 15 to 24 employees were to comply by July 1994.

Transportation

1. New public transit buses must be accessible to persons with disabilities.
2. Transit authorities must provide comparable paratransit or other special transportation services to persons with disabilities who cannot use fixed route bus service, unless an undue burden would result.
3. Existing rail systems were required to have an accessible car per train by July 1995.
4. New rail cars must be accessible.
5. New bus and train stations must be accessible.
6. Key stations in rapid, light, and commuter rail systems had to be made accessible by July 1993, with extensions up to 20 years for commuter rail (30 years for rapid and light rail).
7. All existing Amtrak stations must be accessible by July 2010.

Public Accommodations

1. Restaurants, hotels, and retail stores may not discriminate against persons with disabilities.
2. Auxiliary aids and services must be provided to persons with hearing or vision impairments or other persons with disabilities, unless an undue burden would result.
3. Physical barriers in existing facilities must be removed, if removal is readily achievable. If not, alternative methods of providing the service must be offered, if they are readily achievable.
4. All new construction and alterations of facilities must be accessible.

Telecommunications

Companies offering telephone service must offer telephone relay services to persons who use telecommunication devices for the deaf (TTDs) or similar devices.

State and Local Governments

State and local governments may not discriminate against qualified persons with disabilities.

facilities, and legislation of this nature reflect the public's increasing awareness of the difficulties faced by chronically ill and disabled persons.

Advocating for the Chronically Ill

Nurses have a responsibility to inform the disabled about their rights under the law. Therefore nurses should be aware of provisions of the Americans With Disabilities Act, which was passed by Congress in 1990 and is called by some the Civil Rights Act for the disabled. It provides protection to the estimated 48 million Americans with disabilities. Its four main components address employment, public services, public accommodations and services operated by private entities, and telecommunication services (Box 5-4). A copy of the Americans With Disabilities Act, Public Law 101-239, can be obtained free from the U.S. Government Documents Office in Washington, DC, or from one's congressional representative.

As citizens all nurses can advocate for the disabled and chronically ill by helping to articulate their needs to the general public. Nurses can be active in their own communities to ensure that the public accommodations and public service provisions are carried out.

CONCEPTUAL FRAMEWORKS FOR CHRONIC ILLNESS

Trajectory of Chronic Illness

Beginning in the 1960s social scientists began to develop a conceptual framework for examining chronic illness. Anselm Strauss, a sociologist, was responsible for some of the earliest work. He and fellow sociologist, Barney Glazer, developed A Chronic Illness Trajectory Framework with the term *trajectory* being borrowed from the physical sciences. A trajectory is defined as a course of illness over time plus the actions taken by patients, families, and health professionals to manage or shape the course. When nurses and nurse researchers began to use the trajectory, they adapted it to fit their understanding of the trajectory of chronic illness based on their experiences with persons who were chronically ill. Over time the dynamic and changing character of chronic illnesses resulted in nine phases being delineated in the framework. These phases are pretrajectory, trajectory onset, stable, unstable, acute, crisis, comeback, downward, and dying phases of chronic illness. Table 5-1 defines these phases and identifies appropriate management goals for each. Selected aspects of the trajectory and its phases are discussed in the following paragraphs.

Comeback refers to returning to a satisfactory way of life following a crisis of a chronic condition within any physical or psychosocial limits imposed by the condition. The work of comeback is threefold: physical recovery, limitations stretching, and psychosocial reintegration.[15] Physical recovery refers to the healing process that occurs after major body trauma. Limitations stretching refers to the formal rehabilitation process and to what the person discovers about his or her body once at home and on his or her own. Some patients discover that they can stretch their limitation through repeated attempts and reach higher levels of activity than originally expected. However, there are limits to how far one can stretch, and the remaining disabilities must be accepted.

Psychosocial reintegration refers to the psychologic and social aspects of learning to live with the disabilities that remain, plus the identity reconstitution that occurs as an illness and the ramifications are incorporated into the framework of the

TABLE 5-1 Trajectory Phases

Phase	Definition	Goal of Management
Pretrajectory	Genetic factors or lifestyle behaviors that place an individual or community at risk for the development of a chronic condition	Prevent onset of chronic illness
Trajectory onset	Appearance of noticeable symptoms; includes period of diagnostic workup and announcement by biographic limbo as person begins to discover and cope with implications of diagnosis	Form appropriate trajectory projection and scheme
Stable	Illness course and symptoms under control; biography and everyday life activities being managed within limitations of illness; illness management centers in the home	Maintain stability of illness, biography, and everyday life activities
Unstable	Period of inability to keep symptoms under control or reactivation of illness; biographic disruption and difficulty in carrying out everyday life activities; adjustments being made in regimen, with care usually taking place at home	Return to stable
Acute	Severe and unrelieved symptoms or the development of illness complications necessitating hospitalization or bed rest to bring illness course under control; biography and everyday life activities temporarily placed on hold or drastically cut back	Bring illness under control and resume normal biography and everyday life activities
Crisis	Critical or life-threatening situation requiring emergency treatment or care; biography and everyday life activities suspended until crisis passes	Remove life threat
Comeback	A gradual return to an acceptable way of life within limits imposed by disability or illness; involves physical healing, limitations stretching through rehabilitative procedures, psychosocial coming to terms, and biographic reengagement with adjustments in everyday life activities	Set in motion and continue to move the trajectory projection and scheme forward
Downward	Illness course characterized by rapid or gradual physical decline accompanied by increasing disability or difficulty in controlling symptoms; requires biographic adjustment and alterations in everyday life activity with each major downward step	To adapt to increasing disability with each major downward turn
Dying	Final days or weeks before death. Characterized by gradual or rapid shutting down of body processes, biographic disengagement and closure, and relinquishment of everyday life interests and activities	To bring closure, let go, and die peacefully

From Hyman RB, Corbin JM: *Chronic illness: research and theory for nursing practice,* New York, 2001, Springer.
Biography, Life course made up of the many aspects of the self. It is the temporal dimension of identity. Together biography and the self constitute identity. Biographic impact refers to the manner in which these many aspects of self-care can be affected by illness or its management.[34] *Everyday life activities,* Actions of daily living through which persons live out the many aspects of their selves.[34] *Coming to terms,* The process of making the identity adaptations that are necessary to live with chronic conditions.[34] *Limitations management,* The alterations and adaptations by which persons carry out these activities.[34]

person's life. Comeback is a gradual process, and it is difficult to say whether it is ever fully achieved.[15]

Promoting comeback is complicated. It involves locating individuals and their families within the total framework of their lives, including their physical condition and psychologic and social contexts, and using this information to help patients embark and remain on the comeback trail until they reach their potential. Nurses by virtue of being there are the ones to guide this practice.[9]

Stable Phase

In the stable phase symptoms are under control. In some chronic diseases such as multiple sclerosis, when symptoms are under control, the disease is considered to be in remission. Maintaining health-promoting behaviors that often conflict with activities of daily living may be tiresome and demanding. When health-promoting behaviors are not maintained, the possibility of complications and destabilization are probable.

One study reinforces how difficult it is to carry out health-promoting activities on a daily basis when one has a chronic condition. Fatigue, inconvenience, disabilities, lack of time and money, and conflicting role responsibilities were the reasons given for not exercising regularly. For these reasons contact with nurses who provide ongoing monitoring and reinforcement of healthy lifestyle is essential, even during stable periods, to minimize relapses and complications.[15]

Unstable Phase

An unstable trajectory denotes a period in the chronic illness when the person is not considered "acutely ill" and yet symptoms are not under control and direct medical intervention is indicated to stabilize the condition. This period is marked by uncertainty and the patient's questions such as, "Is it possible to bring the symptoms under control? Will the disabilities increase? Was the condition discovered early enough?" With diseases such as cancer the uncertainty is even greater, because one can never be sure what the outcome will be.[15] Because medical management is frequently on an outpatient basis, patients and families often have to cope on their own when the support of nurses could be very helpful.[15] By reaching out into the community and maintaining contact with persons during unstable periods, nurses can help persons to develop strategies for managing the uncertainties that illness brings into their lives.[15]

Downward Phase

In this phase there is progressive bodily deterioration. Symptoms of disabilities intensify despite efforts to contain them. The patient may deteriorate until death occurs, or the disease can be arrested for a period of time. Chronic sorrow may develop as patients experience symptoms and disability. The nursing goal is to stay on top of the chronic disease and slow the rate of decline.[15]

Dying Phase

In this phase there are profound physiologic and psychosocial changes. The need for a nursing presence during the difficult weeks or months of dying cannot be overemphasized.[15] This period may be even more difficult for patient and family if the patient is dying from acquired immune deficiency syndrome and the family has been unaware that the patient is human immunodeficiency virus–positive.

•••

The trajectory framework is a dynamic one because the trajectory changes as the person's condition changes. This framework offers nursing a foundation for developing a model of nursing care that: (1) is specifically geared toward the problems of the chronically ill, (2) is comprehensive in scope, and (3) gives directions to practice teaching, research, and policy.[34]

Shifting Perspective Model of Chronic Illness

A second model of chronic illness is the shifting perspective model. This was derived from a metasynthesis of 292 qualitative research studies about the reported experiences of adults with chronic illness and was published in 2000 (see Research box). The persons involved in the metastudy reviewed research from nursing, medicine, and allied health reported from January 1986 to January 1996. These reports appeared in referenced journals, research-based books, or theses that investigated the experience of the person living with a chronic illness.

Research

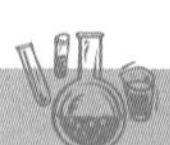

Reference: Paterson BL: The shifting perspectives model of chronic illness, *J Nursing Scholarship* 33:21-26, 2001.

The purpose of this study, a metasynthesis, was to analyze and synthesize 292 qualitative research reports that investigated the experience of living with a chronic illness from the perspective of the person with the disease. "Perspectives of chronic illness determine how people respond to the disease, themselves, caregivers, and situations that are affected by the illness such as employment" (p. 23). Two perspectives emerged in this analysis. The "illness in the foreground" perspective is characterized by a focus on sickness, suffering, loss, and burden associated with a chronic illness. This perspective is commonly seen in persons newly diagnosed with chronic illness, but it also may reappear in response to new symptoms. The "wellness in the foreground" perspective is characterized by seeing the chronic illness as an opportunity for change in several life realms. This perspective is gained by learning about the disease, creating supportive environments, developing personal skills needed to manage the disease, and sharing knowledge of the disease with others. It allows the person to focus on other aspects of life. Perceived threats to control may initiate a shift from a wellness to an illness perspective, and processes involved in moving back to a wellness perspective have also been identified. Health care professionals can assist persons with chronic illness to identify and understand their perspectives and the fluctuations that may be expected. Some evidence exists to support the notion that health care professionals can assist with shifts to wellness perspectives. Changes in approach to the care of a person with a chronic illness to fit the perspective at hand may also be necessary.

In contrast with the trajectory model phases, the shifting perspective model of chronic illness acknowledges that the chronically ill live in the dual kingdoms of well and sick.[23] Sometimes the person's illness is in the foreground and at other times wellness is in the foreground (Figure 5-4).

Illness in the Foreground

In this stage the focus is on the sickness, loss, and burden associated with living with a chronic illness; "the chronic illness is viewed as destructive to self and others."[23] People in this phase are self-absorbed in their illness perspective and often have difficulty attending to the needs of significant others. This phase occurs most often in the newly diagnosed individual who is overwhelmed by the disease.[23] It can be protective, allowing time for the person to deal with changes in the body caused by the chronic illness. It also can be used to develop coping behaviors such as conserving energy by limiting what the sick person can do.

Wellness in the Foreground

In the wellness in the foreground perspective, the self, not the diseased body, becomes the source of identity. The body becomes something to which things are done, not what controls the person.[23]

People gain this perspective in several ways:

- Learning as much as they can about their disease
- Creating supportive environments
- Developing personal skills such as negotiating
- Identifying their body's unique patterns of response
- Sharing knowledge with others

They shift from being a victim of circumstances to a creator of circumstances.

Distancing from the illness allows for focus on the emotional, spiritual, and social aspects of life rather than on the diseased body. Persons reporting this change have a greater appreciation of life and loved ones and give greater attention to others, often acting as an advocate for people with the disease.[23]

Shifting From Wellness to Illness in the Foreground

The major factor that causes a shift from wellness to illness in the foreground is the perception of threat to control. These threats are personally defined and may not be seen as threats by observers. Any threat to control that exceeds the person's threshold of tolerance will cause a shift in perspective from wellness to illness in the foreground.[23]

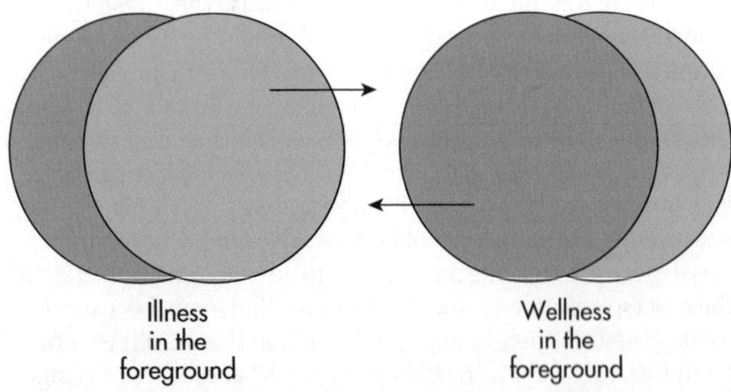

Figure 5-4 The shifting perspectives model of chronic illness.

Persons with chronic illness select people with whom they can share their experiences in ways that will not be detrimental to their preferred perspective. Those with illness in the foreground perspective may choose practitioners who emphasize symptoms of the disease. Those with a wellness in the foreground perspective may search for practitioners who assume a holistic stand.[23]

Many health care professionals are caught in a tradition of rehabilitating people with chronic illness by assisting them to accept limitations imposed by their disease. This approach can be contraproductive. For example, losses and limitations may not be viewed negatively by a person with chronic illness but rather as opportunities for transformation.[23]

SUMMARY

The ultimate goal of nursing in chronicity is to help patients to shape the illness course while maintaining quality of life. This dual goal is achieved through a type of nursing care termed *supportive assistance.*[34] Targets of nursing care are individual, family, community, and society. Specific nursing actions include direct care, teaching, counseling, making referrals, making arrangements, and monitoring. The center of care for the chronically ill is the home where the day-to-day activities of prevention and management of the chronic disease take place. Institutions such as hospitals and rehabilitation centers are backup resources. Because focus of care in chronicity is not cure but prevention, interventions are aimed at fostering prevention or helping the person to live with illnesses should they occur. "Of all the health professions, only nurses have the skills, knowledge, and vision to organize and provide the comprehensive and technologically complex care that chronically ill patients require."[34]

Critical Thinking Questions

1. You are caring for two patients, both of whom have advanced, progressive multiple sclerosis. One family adapts well to the debilitated state of their family member, whereas the other family members drift and are unable to offer their support to the patient. Offer an explanation for this difference in family reaction.
2. How may the care of one person with a chronic illness be generalized to the care of other persons with chronic illnesses?
3. On admission to the hospital of a patient with a chronic illness, the nurse performs a thorough physical assessment but makes no mention of psychologic assessment of the patient. Should this oversight be called to her attention, or is the physiologic assessment more important?
4. What resources are available in your community for the care of the chronically ill? Are the facilities adequate for the number of persons needing care? How are these facilities supported financially?

References

1. American Cancer Society: *2001 cancer facts and figures,* Atlanta, 2001, The Society.
2. Reference deleted in proofs.
3. Brody E et al: Work status and parent care: a comparison of four groups of women, *Gerontologist* 27(2):201-208, 1987.
4. Capitman JA: *Long-term care use by minority elderly: an eldercare information packet,* Waltham, Mass, 1992, Brandeis University.
5. Coontz S, Parson M Raley G, editors: *American families: a multicultural reader,* New York, 1999, Routledge.
6. Reference deleted in proofs.
7. Reference deleted in proofs.
8. Reference deleted in proofs.
9. George L, Gwyther I: Caregiver well-being: a multidimensional examination of family caregivers of demented adults, *Gerontologist* 26(3):253-259, 1986.
10. George L: Social participation in later life: black-white differences. In Jackson JS, editor: *The black American elderly: research on physical and psychosocial health,* New York, 1988, Springer.
11. Hill R: *Families under stress,* New York, 1949, Harper & Brothers.
12. Hill R: Generic features of families under stress, *Soc Casework,* 1958, pp 139-150.
13. Hoffman C, Rice D, Sung H: Persons with chronic conditions: their prevalence and costs, *JAMA* 276(18):1473-1479, 1996.
14. Horowitz A: Sons and daughters as caregivers to older parent: differences in role performance and consequences, *Gerontologist* 25(6):612-617, 1985.
15. Hyman RB, Corbin JM, editors: *Chronic illness research and theory for nursing practice,* New York, 2001, Springer.
16. Johnson C, Catalano D: A longitudinal study of family supports to impaired elderly, *Gerontologist* 6:612-615, 1983.
17. Reference deleted in proofs.
18. Kauffman C et al: *Characteristics and needs of black caregivers and their elderly clients in personal care homes,* Washington, DC, 1987, American Red Cross.
19. Kim MJ, McFarland GK, McLane AM: *Pocket guide to nursing diagnoses,* ed 5, St Louis, 1995, Mosby.
20. Kinney J, Stephens M: Hassles and uplifts of giving care to a family member with dementia, *Psychol Aging* 4(4):402-408, 1989.
21. Reference deleted in proofs.
22. Morycz R et al: Racial differences in family burden: clinical implications for social work, *J Gerontol Soc Work* 10(1/2):133-154, 1987.
23. Paterson BL: The shifting perspectives model of chronic illness, *J Nurs Scholarship* 33(1):21-26, 2001.
24. Reference deleted in proofs.
25. Reference deleted in proofs.
26. Reference deleted in proofs.
27. Reference deleted in proofs.
28. The Robert Wood Johnson Foundation: Chronic Care in America: the system that isn't, *Adv Issue* 4:1, 9-10, 1996.
29. Reference deleted in proofs.
30. Reference deleted in proofs.
31. Valle R: Cultural and ethnic issues in Alzheimer's disease family research. In Light E, Lebowitz B, editors: *Alzheimer's disease treatment and family stress directions for research,* Rockville, Md, 1989, National Institute of Mental Health.
32. von Bertalanffy L: General systems theory and psychiatry. In Ariti S, editor: *American handbook of psychiatry,* ed 2, New York, 1974, Basic Books.
33. Reference deleted in proofs.
34. Woog P, editor: *The chronic illness trajectory framework—the Corbin and Strauss nursing model,* New York, 1992, Springer.
35. Reference deleted in proofs.
36. Zarit S, Reever K, Bah-Peterson J: Relatives of the impaired elderly: correlates of feelings of burden, *Gerontologist* 20(6):649-655, 1980.
37. Reference deleted in proofs.

http://www.mosby.com/MERLIN/medsurg_phipps

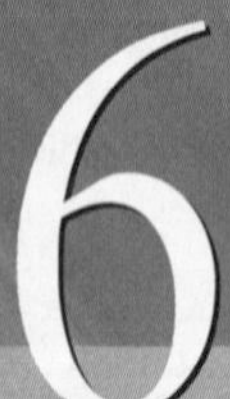

Loss, Grief, Dying, and End-of-Life Care

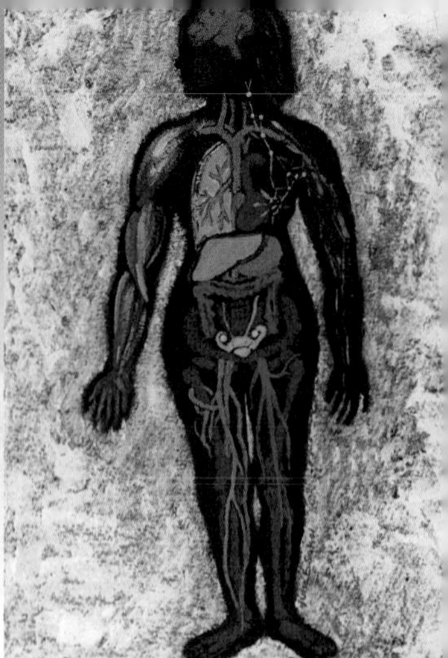

Molly Loney

Objectives

After studying this chapter, the learner should be able to:

1. Recognize how loss affects the individual, family, and community during life changes and the dying process.
2. Identify death as a significant loss and transition in human development.
3. Describe the process of normal grieving and the range of its manifestations.
4. Compare bereavement theories in terms of key tasks for the individual and the family in their grief work.
5. Identify behaviors that place the dying person and family at risk for poor bereavement outcomes.
6. Identify current societal attitudes that influence how nurses, patients, and families respond to situations in which someone is dying or has died.
7. Describe nursing strategies useful in assessing and meeting the needs of the dying individual and family through palliative care.
8. Discuss factors that affect quality of life for the individual and family during the dying process.
9. Describe self-care strategies for nurses in managing the demands of caring for a dying patient and a grieving family.

When we think of loss, we think of the loss through death of people we love. But loss is a far more encompassing theme in our lives. For we lose not only through death, but also by leaving and letting go and moving on. And our losses include not only our separations and departures from those we love, but our conscious and unconscious losses of romantic dreams, impossible expectations, illusions of freedom and power, illusions of safety—and the loss of our own younger self . . . the self that thought it always would be unwrinkled and invulnerable and immortal.

These losses are a part of life—universal, unavoidable, inexorable. And these losses are necessary because we grow by losing and leaving and letting go.[67]

INTRODUCTION

Throughout time, society has been preoccupied with questions regarding living and dying, while searching for immortality. Despite modern technology and increasing efforts to control the inevitable, death remains a part of life, and end-of-life care remains an important part of nursing practice.

Facing the end of life is one of the most difficult losses humans may experience.[7] Although loss and grief are common to any developmental stage or transition, death in all cultures is finite. Losses surrounding dying can be overwhelming and deplete coping resources, as well as the integrity of the individual, family, and community.

The thoughts people have about death affect their lives in many ways. Some are peaceful and inspiring, whereas others generate anxiety and fear. Living in the shadow of death can motivate further growth[29] and allow the dying person to transcend suffering, or it can create a crisis for the dying individual and his or her family.[4] In any culture, how people respond to dying is dependent on the meaning that death has in the life cycle of the dying person, the family, and the community.[26,58,64] Ferrell summarized the many ways that death can positively affect our view of life[17]:

Death helps one savor life.
It provides an opposing standard against which to judge being alive.
It gives a sense of individual existence.
It helps give life meaning.
It allows one to evaluate personal achievements.
It allows retrospective analysis of one's life.
It gives one strength to express convictions.
It reveals the importance of intimacy.

Reactions of family and the community can provide needed support or lead to isolation for the dying person.[23,61,65] Reactions of health care professionals can either enhance or disrupt the quality of care they offer the dying person.[25,27,44] In learning ways to enhance quality of life and guide the patient and family through the dying process, it becomes important for nurses to understand their own experience with loss, grief, and dying.

This chapter offers an understanding of loss, the experience of grief in anticipating or surviving death, factors influencing grieving, societal and ethical issues surrounding death and dying, and nursing strategies for providing end-of-life care that meet the changing needs of the dying person, family, and self. Perhaps the most beneficial way to learn to effectively care for dying persons and their families is to understand our own perspectives and those of others on loss, grief, and death.

THE LOSS EXPERIENCE

Loss is a natural part of human existence. It is a universal experience that is interwoven into daily life. Loss is a pattern that is repeated as one faces change or developmental challenge.[19] As a child learns to become progressively independent in terms of feeding, going to school, making friends, surviving puberty, driving, and earning wages, a loss occurs for both the parents and the child.

Loss is an important force in a person's life because it implies the removal of someone or something that had meaning to the individual.[25] It has been defined as any change that reduces the probability of reaching some desired goal or that deprives a person suddenly of a valued possession or relationship.[7] Although it can be caused by a negative change or a positive developmental event, loss always represents some form of deprivation.[51] According to Viorst,[67] persons grow by having to give up some deep attachment or cherished part of themselves to gain a new level of autonomy and mastery.

Bowlby[7] views loss within a framework of early childhood attachment. During periods of high vulnerability and uncertainty, as in childhood, persons develop strong bonds of affection with significant others who meet their basic needs. These significant others offer safety and security beyond simply meeting physical needs for food and shelter. If attachment bonds are threatened or broken, as with the death of a mother, separation anxiety ensues.[25] The ways in which the person learns to cope with this loss of attachment and need gratification in childhood can be a predictor of later coping with adult loss.[72]

Whether a person faces separation or some other significant life changes, experience with loss can result in a crisis. A crisis occurs whenever a person is unable to manage stress and meet basic needs in the usual way. If past coping skills become ineffective or the stress becomes overwhelming, the individual perceives a threat to self-integrity and a loss of control. Feelings of vulnerability and anxiety trigger an adaptive response, and the person tries to resolve the stress by avoidance, finding support, or becoming immobilized.[4] The tension and uncertainty that accompany crisis and loss can motivate regression or growth, depending on the presence of key balancing factors.[39] Mastery of this tension and uncertainty involves balancing the stressors with realistic perceptions, using available supports, and regaining some control by tapping constructive coping skills.[4,39] Growth results when a person develops more resilience in managing life changes in the face of the loss.[29]

TYPES OF LOSS

As a component of crisis, loss can be categorized as developmental or situational. Developmental loss involves any predictable change in status, roles, relationships, or bodily function that normally occurs in life. Although developmental losses require adaptation, we are socially and culturally prepared for making social and biologic transitions in reaching a new level of growth and maturity.[4] Situational loss involves an unanticipated change in roles, relationships, or function. The person lacks preparation or role modeling in terms of effective adaptation, except through experience with previous situational losses. Natural disasters, accidents, unemployment, and illnesses are situations that challenge the person's usual adaptive response and may precipitate life crises.[73] Any illness represents several losses occurring simultaneously in all areas of one's life. Situational losses can overwhelm the individual, with each component involving a "small death" and bringing the inevitable reality of one's own mortality into closer focus.[19]

Loss can also be conceptualized as simple, symbolic, or compound. A simple loss involves the loss of a familiar object, such as misplacing a favorite pair of earrings. The loss carries little attachment value and can easily be replaced. If, however, the earrings were a gift from a grandmother, the loss becomes symbolic and carries with it special meaning. Symbolic losses are secondary losses to simple loss and signify cherished roles, relationships, or identities.[50] Compound loss involves several symbolic losses occurring together. If the earrings were a gift from a deceased grandmother with whom the person had a special relationship, then the loss becomes compound.[72] Examples of compound loss in this situation include loss of history, support, friendship, maternal figure, self-image, and childhood innocence. Although initially difficult to identify, symbolic losses are important to recognize because they offer insight into possible meanings behind a loss.[53]

Loss can be experienced even when it is not observed. Depending on the degree of threat to self or others, anticipation of loss can trigger an adaptive response similar to that experienced with an actual loss.[27] Anticipatory loss experienced during a progressive and terminal illness can be as challenging and painful as the death of a loved one as the dying person and family confront uncertainty over an inevitably tragic future.[56] Although uncertainty can serve as a motivating force, it can also overwhelm and deplete the adaptive reservoir for coping with loss.[56]

LOSS WITHIN THE FAMILY

Loss does not occur in a vacuum.[26] An individual's perception of loss is often magnified as each family member and the family as a whole struggle to make sense out of the experience.[12] Because a family is an interactive and functional network of significant relationships, any change in one member affects others.[23] Callanan and Kelley[10] described the family as a mobile, whose balance and structure are disrupted by loss.

Families try to adapt to change or loss by holding onto the way things were to preserve the family's integrity and identity as a unit. The family of the dying person faces unyielding demands not only in meeting the needs of the dying person, but also in meeting the daily needs of all the family members.[25,65] Uncertainty and confusion can develop over roles, relationships, rules, and responsibilities.

A teenage son may assume head-of-the-household responsibilities to support his mother and younger siblings when his father is given a prognosis of 3 months or less for end-stage cancer. Although the son may be seeking independence, his added responsibilities prevent him from playing on the basketball team, excelling in school, and getting together with his friends. He is faced with loss of a father figure, normalcy, social support, sources of recognition/achievement, and a somewhat predictable future.

Conflicts may arise between the older son and siblings who do not recognize his authority. The son and his mother may also be challenged in maintaining their parent-child relationship because of the mother's need for love and intimacy from a male figure. The father may experience loss in feeling inadequate to maintain his role as father and head of the household. The family faces tremendous losses: loss of normalcy; loss of an authority figure and role model; loss of predictability, security, and rules; and loss of relationships with the father.

BOX 6-1 Factors Influencing Loss

Individual	Family
Age	Individual factors
Personality	*plus*
Developmental level	Family's stage of development
Past experience	Family rules and roles
Role modeling	Belief system and culture
Perception of intensity of loss	Patterns of communication
Meaning of attachment	Perception of threat to family integrity
Types of loss	Flexibility in roles
Replaceability	Repertoire of coping skills
Timing of experience	Relationship to community
Disruption from loss	Use of community supports
Threat to self and significant other(s)	
Coping skills	
Availability of supports	

FACTORS INFLUENCING LOSS

Individuals differ in their perceptions of loss and their abilities to adapt to loss in growth-producing ways. When the loss represents a major life change, adaptation is challenged. Each person interprets the meaning and extent of loss on the basis of many factors, such as personality, cultural and religious background, and coping resources. The extent to which a loss is intensified depends on the importance of the attachment, the possibility of replacing the object or relationship, the person's age and developmental stage, the amount of personal and social disruption caused by the loss, and the availability of a supportive environment (Box 6-1).[19,51,72] The more cumulative and meaningful a loss is, the greater are its threat and its intensity. Aging, terminal illness, and death represent multiple and often overwhelming losses for any person or family, regardless of adaptive resources.[13,56]

In addition to intensity and meaning, timing is an important factor in determining how loss is perceived. If a person is preoccupied with mastering a developmental task, such as accepting retirement, his or her ability to deal with other life changes may be reduced. If the same person is also confronted with the sudden death of a spouse, he or she may experience greater difficulty in adaptation. Each loss requires time and effective coping skills for successful integration. Loss cannot be viewed globally. Each person and family will define loss differently. The loss experience is analogous to an onion, with multiple interfacing layers. To understand the experience, each layer needs to be peeled away and examined from an inside view, even if the process is painful.

Each loss in life is experienced uniquely in terms of the involved person's or family's developmental stage (Table 6-1), as well as the experience's meaning, relationship to other losses, intensity, and timing.[51,53,72] Individuals also vary in the length of time needed to adapt to or recover from the loss experience. Although a year has been used in the past as a time frame for measuring recovery from a significant loss, current research suggests that true recovery may take years, depending on influencing factors.[72]

DEATH AND LOSS

Although death can be defined as a normal life crisis and a fact of life,[4] it is the most significant loss experienced by an individual or family in today's society.[70] It represents not only separation from an important relationship, but also an inevitability that we all face. Despite awareness of our own mortality, death in our culture usually is perceived as untimely and incongruent with the laws of nature, especially when the death is caused by an illness or an accident.[19] Death challenges individuals and families to search for "reasons why" in their belief systems and lifestyles. Because of such searching, death always implies several interfacing losses that serve only to remind the survivor(s) of the loved one's death.[25,53] Concomitant losses of role relationships, normalcy, a shared future, identity as a unit (as with a couple or family), a sense of control over life events, intimacy, social support, a role model, and social approval can be symbolic aspects of a loved one's death.[51] As a point of transition and potential for growth, the intensity and complexity of death challenge the individual's and the family's coping skills. Supportive nursing interventions often are needed to promote the transition from crisis to growth.[4,56]

How successful a family is in adapting to loss depends on the family's developmental stage, rules, belief system, cultural ties, communication patterns, role flexibility, perceptions of threat from the loss, coping skills, and social supports (see Box 6-1).[25,61] When a family faces a loss due to death during a period of high stress or major transition, adaptation is difficult and the family is at risk for ongoing crises.[4,12,13]

LOSS WITHIN THE COMMUNITY

Loss also has an impact on the community and its members, especially when the loss is finite, as with death. All cultures and religions acknowledge death openly or indirectly as a significant loss, both to the family and to the community as a whole. What dying and death mean to the individual and fam-

TABLE 6-1 Developmental Impact of Loss and Death

Age	Concept of Death	Potential Impact
Younger than 2 years	Self-centered	Death as need deprivation
2-5 years	Temporary and concrete	Death as separation, with no distress or fear
5-9 years	Concrete and logical; unable to link cause/effect; magical thinking	Death as punishment, with anxiety or fear of bodily harm
9-12 years	Realistic; able to see as inevitable and finite	Death as separation, with fear of leaving home and family; may have daydreams and poor grades
12-18 years	Abstract and realistic; able to anticipate and predict	Death as threat to independence, with fear of being different from peers; may act out with drugs, alcohol, anger, or aggression
18-25 years	Abstract and realistic	Death as disruption of lifestyle and separation from peers
25-45 years	Abstract and realistic	Death as disruption of family unit/roles and threat to history/future
45-65 years	Abstract and realistic	Death as disruption in productivity in family/work
65 years-death	Philosophic	Death as series of chronologic losses, with separation from support net works

Adapted from Silverman PR, Nickman SL, Worden IW: Detachment revisited: the child's reconstruction of a dead parent, *Am J Orthopsychiatry* 62(4):494-503, 1992; Tipton K: How to discuss death with patients and families, *Nursing 99* 29(9):10-12, 1999.

ily, as well as how they try to adapt to the loss, comes from their culture. It is critical to recognize that[8,28,58]:

- Culture is not stagnant and can change daily.
- Members of the same family or community may interpret and practice their identified cultural beliefs differently.
- Each person and family facing death can experience compounded loss if their cultural patterns of responding to loss are not acknowledged or respected.
- Persons who are dying and their families have much to teach health care professionals about their preferences in how they face a major loss, such as death.

LOSS AND THE NURSE

Occupational stress involving loss is part of the daily experience of nurses, especially those who work with patients facing terminal illnesses and death.[66] By remaining caring and empathic, nurses become vulnerable to identifying with their patients' and families' losses.[32] The observable loss of a patient's independence after cancer has caused irreversible spinal cord compression can symbolize personal losses in the nurse's own family history, as well as professional helplessness.[27,38] A conflict may arise if a nurse perceives his or her role as primarily curing. With the current emphasis in medical care on using technology for cure, nurses are at risk for loss of control, fear of failure, and loss of professional satisfaction when their patients are beyond cure.[66]

Because loss is a universal phenomenon that is experienced by patients, their families and communities, and the nurses who support them, it becomes important to understand the process of adaptation.

GRIEF: AN ADAPTIVE RESPONSE TO LOSS

Grief and bereavement are companions of adulthood as loss is faced with increasing frequency in the life cycle. Each loss affects the individual and the family by prompting an adaptive response.[4,7,25] Figure 6-1 is an illustrative diagram of adaptation to the loss experience. Separation from something or

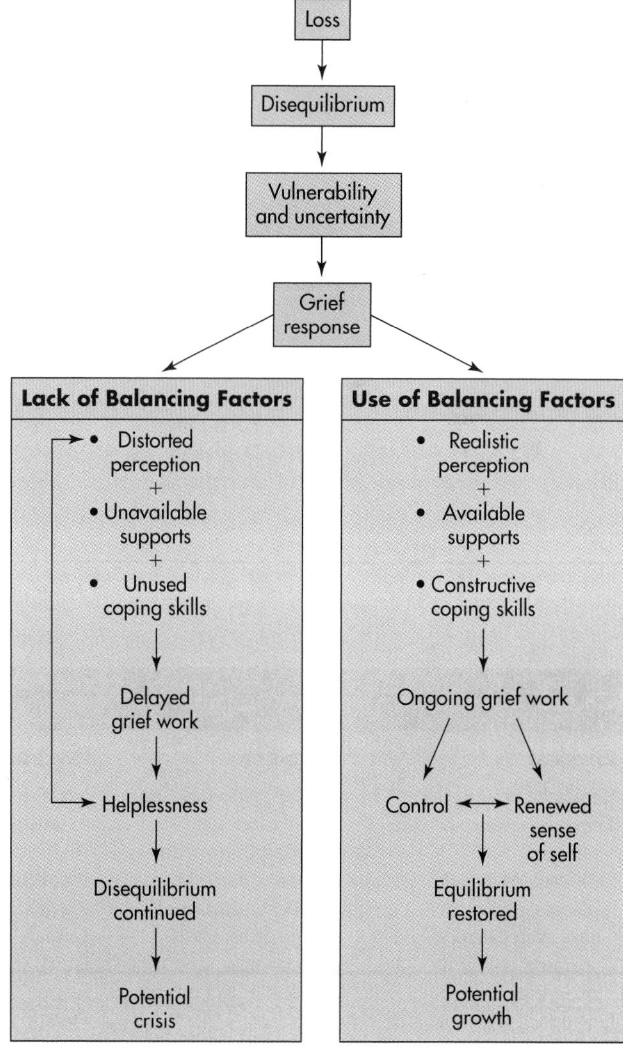

Figure 6-1 Adaptation to the loss experience.

someone of value triggers certain instinctive behaviors through which the person tries to hold onto what is being lost. Such behaviors are the basis for grieving.[7,51,72]

Grief refers to the subjective state of anticipating or suffering the loss of a person or object with whom a significant relationship existed. Although used interchangeably with *bereavement,* the term *grief* refers to the normal, expected process of adapting to any loss. It is the total response to the separation caused by the loss, which involves psychologic, spiritual, cognitive, social, and somatic dimensions.[43,45]

What makes grief difficult to conceptualize is its universal nature and individual expression. Grief is a lived experience and depends on each person's or family's perceptions of what is lost and what the loss means at a given point in time.[46] Not only can grief manifest differently from one individual to another, but the individual's and family's expressions of grief can change over time. Because loss is a component of human development, grieving can help a person to adapt to a loss, as well as grow from the experience.[4,19,29]

Mourning refers to the cultural and social response to loss, which includes any manifestation of grief. It is learned through role modeling and socialization during childhood. The term *mourning* is an important one because it often implies how grief is expressed by the individual and family within their cultural norms.[8,53,58,72]

HISTORICAL PERSPECTIVE: THE GRIEF PROCESS

In 1915 Freud described grief as a process of gradual withdrawal of the energy that ties the bereaved person to the lost object or person who died. Freud also described grief as a reaction to loss that triggered ego defenses to reduce anxiety and discomfort. The reaction involved a gradual withdrawal of the energy that tied the grieving person to the person who died.[19] In studying victims of fire and war, Lindemann[34] expanded on the definition by identifying both psychologic and physical responses to acute loss. Engel[14] legitimized grief as a discrete syndrome with common causative factors and universal manifestations.

Several later theorists have attempted to aid our understanding of grief by defining specific behaviors associated with grief and the sequence in which they occur (Table 6-2). Most agree that grief is an ongoing process of adaptation involving movement through stages or phases of (1) shock and disbelief, (2) awareness and acceptance of the reality of the loss, (3) intense experience of pain and disorganization over the loss, and (4) recovery or reestablishment of homeostasis.

In working to identify the unique needs of dying patients, Kübler-Ross[28] described five sequential stages of grief, from an initial period of shock and emotional numbness through eventual acceptance of the impending or past loss. Although

TABLE 6-2 Comparison of Grief Theories

Stage	Lindemann	Kübler-Ross	Bowlby	Worden	Rando
Initial	Shock and disbelief	Shock and denial	Numbing	Accepting reality	Recognizing loss
Acute grief	Acute mourning	Anger Bargaining Depression	Yearning and searching Disorganization	Experiencing the pain Withdrawing	Reacting to separation Recollecting and reexperiencing
Recovery	Resolution	Acceptance	Reorganization	Reinvesting	Relinquishing old bonds Readjusting Reinvesting

BOX 6-2 Common Manifestations of Grief

Physical	Cognitive	Psychologic	Social	Spiritual
Headache, dizziness Tightness in throat or chest Shortness of breath, deep sighing Changes in eating, elimination, and sleeping Feeling empty, exhausted Restlessness Malaise Sexual arousal changes	Lack of concentration Foggy thoughts Preoccupation with loss Hallucinations (auditory and visual) Bargaining Searching for reason for loss	Numbness, dulled senses Anxiety Preoccupation with fears Denial Guilt Anger Hostility, resentfulness Ambivalence Crying Sadness, depression	Withdrawal, isolation Dependency Helplessness Busy with tasks, chores Takes on traits of dying person Holds onto possessions of dying person Performance difficulties in work and family roles Loneliness	Doubting past beliefs, faith Hopelessness Searching for meaning of loss Changes in religious practices

her conceptualization offered an intimate view of grieving, her stages have been misinterpreted as a series of steps that occur in a neat, chronologic order. This misinterpretation, which implies that grief is one-dimensional, does not account for individual differences in mourning or adaptation.

Bowlby[7] offered a similar stepwise model of the grief process as a developmental stage for coping with separation from a significant love object or source of need fulfillment. Worden[72] helped redefine grief from a holistic perspective and identified four tasks of grieving in the Harvard Bereavement Study of elderly widows. A key component is the need to experience the pain of loss in all its dimensions, including physical, cognitive, psychologic, social, and spiritual distress (Box 6-2).

Worden[72,73] offered further insight into the complex grief process, including:

- Grief does not follow any order or sequence.
- Grief is an individual process through which individuals and families progress at their own rate and in their own ways.
- Although painful, grief is the only way to adapt to loss.
- Grief may be so painful for some that the process is denied or delayed, leading to physical complaints and psychologic illness.
- Losses such as death require grief work to reconcile the loss. With each new developmental stage and anniversary of the loss, individuals and families try to make sense of past losses in light of their current situation, roles, and relationships.
- Unresolved grief may resurface and compound current losses.
- Even with support, some people never work through their grief.

Rando[50] described grief experienced in times of overwhelming stress or severe trauma as *complicated mourning,* defined as abnormal or unresolved grief that persists over time, disrupts one's lifestyle, and interferes with a six-phase process of mourning. Clark[11] elaborated on the definition of *posttraumatic stress* as exposure to a traumatic event that leads to the survivor's reexperiencing the event in repeated intrusive images that impair the survivor's daily functioning. Although initially associated with war and disasters, such an extreme reaction can result from suffering multiple losses during the dying process, as well as bearing witness to the suffering of others.[3] Solari-Twadell and colleagues[59] added a dynamic, multidimensional structure to the grief process by comparing grief to a pinwheel. "Winds of loss" within the context of an individual's or family's history drive the ongoing cycle of grieving until emotional surrender and acceptance occur.

Grieving has been described as a three-dimensional roller coaster with unpredictable ups and downs. The person and family experiencing grief feel "off balance," with no idea of what to expect or of how to return to what used to be a normal course. Ups and downs occur without warning as one emotion comes after another, with forward-and-backward movement. The difficulty lies in regaining some sense of control and realizing that finding a way back to a pregrief lifestyle may mean having to ride the roller coaster's entire course.

DEATH AND GRIEF

Grief is a period of adjustment that requires making a transition in the way one thinks and interacts with the world.[45] Working through grief over dying involves changes in roles, relationships, and identities. As a turning point, death can be a time of immobilization and crisis or potential for growth. Successfully negotiating and making the transition between living and dying can build communication and coping skills in a family, as well as strengthen the family members' ability to face future losses in life.[4,12,27,72]

Responses by Survivors

Understanding the grieving process and recognizing the behavioral manifestations that usually occur can assist the nurse in preparing survivors for what to expect or to help them make sense of their feelings and somatic symptoms. The age of the survivor can impact the experience of loss (see Evidence-Based Practice box). Timing of the sharing of information, as well as the type and amount of information given at any one session, is important. Understanding the various processes and behaviors, both anticipated and unexpected, of bereaved persons may help to avert misunderstandings and help to strengthen the survivors and enable them to grow during the period of grieving. Sharing experiences helps grieving persons. Recognizing the "normal" nature of the experiences, even those that seem somewhat bizarre, opens the way for working through the experience.[51,53,62,72]

Evidence-Based Practice

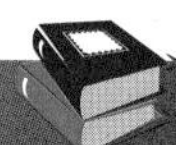

Reference: Hegge M, Fischer C: Grief responses of senior and elderly widows: practice implications, *J Gerontol Nurs* 26(2):35-43, 2000.

The purpose of this study was to describe how the death of a life partner compounded the simultaneous and cumulative losses associated with aging. Interviews were conducted with 22 senior widows (ages 60 to 74) and 17 elderly widows (ages 75 to 90), using an open-ended tool and convenience sample. Interviews were audiotaped, transcribed, and analyzed for patterns. Responses of each group were coded for recurrent themes, similarities, and differences.

Findings reinforced previous grief literature in describing grief as an erratic cycle with peaks and valleys of reactions, but the widows' grief was not experienced in orderly or predictable stages. Both groups identified loneliness as a major problem, but financial issues were more troubling for senior widows. Disruptions in sleeping, eating, and activities of daily living were more troubling for elderly widows. Senior widows described more intense reactions than elderly widows, who described their losses as expected.

Both groups used religion and reminiscing to cope. Senior widows relied more on friends, whereas elderly widows relied primarily on family for support. Senior widows described a gradual renewal of interest in pursuing their personal goals, whereas elderly widows revised their goals to prepare for their own death, with hopes of rejoining the deceased spouse. Knowledge about how age can affect grief can be useful in assessing and supporting both senior and elderly widows.

Shock and Disbelief

The initial response may begin when a terminal prognosis is made and usually lasts for several weeks beyond the funeral.[25] Regardless of whether or not the death was anticipated, the immediate response is shock, numbness, and disbelief. The survivors may feel a sense of unreality, and as a consequence they may appear to be "taking the death well." After the funeral this feeling of unreality or numbness changes to feelings of pain and separation. Survivors may experience somatic symptoms, including muscular weakness, tremors, and tightness of the throat. They may experience diaphoresis, sigh deeply, have cold or clammy sensations, become anorexic, or feel exhausted. Bereaved persons exhibit extremes of behavior. They may become sedentary and do little or nothing except nap. On the other hand, they may be so hyperactive that they are unable to sit quietly or sleep. They may experience extremes of mood, such as profound sadness, anger, depression, or guilt, or find themselves laughing without an explanation. They may have difficulty concentrating. Coupled with these extremes in mood and behavior may be a continuance of disbelief, although the death is comprehended intellectually. "Searching behaviors," which include dreams in which the deceased is alive and experiences of "seeing" the deceased or "feeling" the deceased's touch are common. During this phase, offers of comfort are often rejected because the bereaved is focusing on the deceased.[51,53,70]

Yearning and Protest

For several weeks the bereaved have feelings of yearning and protest. They may feel anger toward the deceased for leaving them, toward God for allowing the death to occur, or toward the caregivers for not returning the deceased to health. They may be jealous of others who still have their loved ones. The survivors may wish they had been the ones to die. During this period the bereaved may find it difficult to share their feelings or thoughts because they question their own sanity. Knowing that others have had similar thoughts and feelings sometimes helps to normalize the experience.[38,51,72]

Anguish, Disorganization, and Despair

As the bereaved begin to focus more on themselves and the numbness and rage begin to fade, they begin to recognize the reality and finality of the loss. New feelings and accompanying behaviors emerge. The bereaved may experience a sense of confusion, aimlessness, inability to make decisions, apathy, or a loss of confidence. During this period they may also experience loneliness and depression.

The bereaved experience mood extremes and intense feelings, which are often frightening to them. They fear they will lose emotional control and, as a defense mechanism, become self-centered. Family members and friends may interpret this behavior as selfish and either reprimand them or withdraw. Neither behavior is helpful to the bereaved.[51,53,59,72]

The experience of anguish leads to a new awareness of the preciousness of life. Life appears fragile. The bereaved may display intense fear of being hurt or worry over the welfare of family members. At the same time, they may smoke or resort to alcohol or chemical abuse. Other health-risking behaviors, such as lack of rest, may occur.

The wish and need to cry fulfill an important function in acknowledging the loss and in receiving support from others. Memories and mental images of the deceased are void of negative characteristics. Feelings of guilt, remorse, fear, and regret may surface. Opportunities to reminisce and to share feelings with others are helpful.[38,52,72]

Identification

The bereaved may adopt the behavior, admired qualities, and mannerisms of their lost beloved ones. Some may take on the symptoms of the last illness of the lost loved one. Care must be taken to distinguish symptoms associated with physical illness from those associated with loss. Symptoms associated with loss will abate as the loss is resolved.[22,51,72]

Reorganization and Restitution

The feelings and symptoms of grieving gradually subside; they do not suddenly disappear. Bereaved persons tell us they have periods of depression, as well as periods of well-being as life begins to make sense once again. Reorganization and restitution generally begin approximately 6 months after the loss and last for a few years. The process may be considerably longer or shorter and still be within normal range. Contrary to old popular beliefs, although life stabilizes, the pain of loss may remain for a lifetime. Reactions to loss recur around circumstances that are poignant reminders of the deceased—birthdays, anniversaries, and holidays.[38,51,53,65,72]

FACTORS AFFECTING THE GRIEF RESPONSE

Many factors combine to affect the degree of stress felt and the particular response of survivors to a death. The major factors include (1) the type of relationship lost, (2) the nature of the death, (3) the characteristics of the survivor, (4) the cultural background, and (5) the nature and use of the support network.[35,58,63]

Type of Relationships and Roles

Feelings of helplessness and emptiness may result after the death of someone such as a parent, spouse, or significant other, on whom one has been dependent. Perhaps more significant is the intense void that accompanies the loss of the survivor's role as a caring family member. This sense of loss is intensified in proportion to the survivor's reliance on the deceased for self-validation, identity, and linkage to social and friendship networks.[51,58,63,65]

Identities and roles are related. A survivor—widow, widower, daughter, or son—is left with incomplete skills because the usual division of labor in everyday life is lost. Loss of children creates its own special problems. The normal course of life events is disrupted when the young die before the old. Feelings of guilt and self-blame may be more pronounced.[51,72]

Nature of the Death

The nature of the death and the circumstances after a death affect the grieving process. The closer the circumstances are to what the survivors perceive as a "good" death, the more comforting it will be. If survivors' perceptions of the death include intense suffering, confusion over treatment goals, or untimely death (either premature or prolonged), the death may become more difficult to reconcile.[17]

Anticipatory grieving or grieving that began before the loss may ease the transition once a loss is complete. However, excessive anticipation and repeated cycles of anticipatory grief may deplete a survivor's energy to complete the grieving process when the death finally occurs.[27,44,51,63]

Social and Cultural Background

One's cultural background has a profound influence over how illness and death are experienced, as well as how health care professionals are viewed.[26] Cultures all over the world recognize grief and death, but each culture is unique in how it defines what are acceptable expressions of grief.[25,58] Although it is difficult to categorize grief responses from all cultures, some general guidelines can be a useful frame of reference (Table 6-3). Encouraging feedback and validating cultural patterns with survivors in dealing with death can acknowledge and honor their beliefs and promote grieving without compounding loss.[8,58]

Social Support

Social support is critical to promoting grieving in survivors. Grieving means expressing the multidimensional pain of the loss with others who both listen and acknowledge what has happened. Such acknowledgment gives survivors opportunities to[23,27,61]:

- Release feelings.
- Begin to find some meaning out of the dying experience.
- Share unresolved concerns.
- Validate information about what happened.
- Remember involvement in trying to support the dying person.
- Find some beginning closure.

Supportive networks are available but may not be used by survivors in an effort to remain composed or protective. Survivors may need to look outside their immediate circle of support when all are involved in sharing the grieving. The shared experience of grieving may prevent members of the family or network from supporting the most immediate family member(s).[23]

Because inadequate social support for grieving is associated with intense emotions and delayed grief, it becomes important to help survivors share their perceptions of available supports they can use.[3,13,23,60]

GRIEF RESOLUTION

Debate continues over whether one can ever recover from the experience of loss.[51,70] Lindemann[34] suggested that grief resolution could occur within a few weeks of the loss. Other findings recognize that grief is more appropriately measured in years.[70]

Because grieving is such an individual process, with a wide range of possible manifestations, how can we assess if and when an individual has successfully completed grief work? Engel[15] defined successful mourning as the ability to remember comfortably and realistically both the pleasures and disappointments of the lost relationship. A change in perspective is the key to grief recovery. This change in perspective occurs when the person can rise above the emotions of the loss and view the situation more objectively, while finding some meaning in the loss experience.[22,64] This change in perspective occurs when the person can rise above the emotions of the loss and view the situation more objectively, while finding some meaning in the loss experience.

Worden[73] further clarified what is meant by grief recovery. Recovery is not simply letting go of the lost object or person. Instead, it is the negotiating and renegotiating of the meaning of the loss over time. Their view reinforces the thought that loss may be permanent and unchanging, but like development, the grief process is ongoing.

Wolfelt[71] offered *reconciliation* as the term that best describes how acute grief is processed or worked through. Reconciliation means moving on with life even without the presence of the lost object. In reconciliation there is a renewed energy and a sense of confidence, an ability to fully acknowledge the loss, and a capacity to become reinvolved in normal activities of daily living. Reconciliation involves acknowledging that loss is a difficult yet necessary or growth-facilitating part of life. Wolfelt's view focuses on reconciliation as a process, not as an event or outcome. As human beings, we never get over grief; rather, we become reconciled to it.

A person's success in grieving at a given point in time will affect future experiences of loss and adaptation. With any loss comes the reliving or resurfacing of old issues involving separation and helplessness. If these issues are not acknowledged in some way and their associated feelings worked through, the griever may carry the pain of the experience into the future.[9,51,70,72] Cumulative, unresolved loss has been identified as a significant risk factor for morbidity after bereavement.[45,47,51,73] It not only can change perception but also can confront the person with overwhelming feelings of grief at some future time. When needs for grief work are ignored or denied, even a minor change in the person's routine can serve as a catalyst to resurrect the intensity and burden of past losses.[50,72] Unresolved loss or grief that is ignored becomes a crisis for the affected individual and family and causes impairment of the usual activities of daily living (Box 6-3).

NURSING MANAGEMENT OF GRIEVING PERSON

According to Worden,[72] the role of the caregiver is to assist the griever in releasing emotional ties to the deceased despite the discomfort and sorrow it causes and in subsequently replacing the type of interaction lost. The griever must be persuaded to participate in grief work that entails accepting the pain of facing and experiencing the loss. A number of strategies are available to assist grievers. Worden has grouped these into broad phases that roughly correspond to the process of grief—from

TABLE 6-3 Views of Death Among Major Cultures

Cultural Group	Meaning	Life After Death	Grief Expression	Values
African-American	Natural process Associated with hospitalization	Part of God's plan Eternal life means heaven or oneness with God	Very open in sharing mourning in funeral rituals and church Physical and emotional	Respect aged persons Large extended family and community support Appearance/dress brings social recognition Food as social bond
Native American	Natural and celebrated process Harmony with nature and gods	Cycle of rebirth in different life forms Spirit lives in oneness with nature/gods	Composed and stoic Search for chance to meet death	Honor aged persons Actively prepare for death with rituals Multigenerational family (including ancestors) over individual Food and herbs for healing
Asian	Natural process Expect to suffer	Cycle of rebirth until reach eternal freedom of spirit	Stoic Somatic complaints	Honor aged and dying persons Maintain status quo and save face Family over individual Formal relationships
East African	Natural and celebrated process Never random event	Transition time between life and death when dead are present Cause as honor or punishment	Very open in sharing mourning with music and dance	Honor aged and dying persons Multigenerational family and community over individual
Hispanic	Natural process Dying as suffering	Life created by death of the gods Reach spiritual state based on how died and family	Men are stoic; women are vocal Somatic complaints	Do not see consequences for health behaviors Extended family and community over individual Open with affection Food for healing
Islam	Natural process At peace with Allah and man	Phases of afterlife depending on faith/loyalty (believers find beauty; nonbelievers find ugliness) Day of judgment expected	Stoic with outsiders, especially women Open crying after funeral	Honor men and aged persons Family and Koran rule Standards for social conduct Relative obliged to stay with dying persons to pray for atonement After-death care and funeral rituals to prepare for judgment
Judaism	Expected but feared process Dying as suffering	Through memories of loved ones and Israeli heritage Hope for new world with coming of prophets	Open in sharing suffering and loss with times of mourning (first week/month, anniversary)	Respect aged persons in maintaining history Dying persons are never left alone until burial After-death and funeral rituals Religious community over individual
Western	Natural process in Europe Feared process to be controlled in United States	Purgatory as transition until released by prayer for Catholicism Heaven as eternal life for faithful versus hell	Open mourning in Europe Denial and time-limited mourning in United States	Respect aging in Europe Deny and fear aging in United States Individual autonomy in United States Family and church support during funeral ritual

Modified from Irish D, Lundquist K, Nelsen K: *Ethnic variations in death, dying, and grief,* Washington, DC, 1993, Taylor & Francis; Kemp C: *Terminal illness: a guide to nursing care,* Philadelphia, 1995, JB Lippincott.

BOX 6-3 Signs of Poor Bereavement Outcomes

Overactivity without a sense of loss
Taking on symptoms belonging to the deceased
Development of psychosomatic illness
Withdrawal from relationships with close friends and family members
Hostility and rage against persons associated with the death or loss
Wooden and formal conduct that masks rage and hostility
Lasting loss of social interaction skills
Destructive behavior (e.g., giving away one's belongings, substance abuse)
Prolonged and agitated depression, with risk of suicide
Feelings of worthlessness, self-blame, and need for punishment
Intense feeling that death or loss occurred yesterday
Inability to talk about the deceased without emotional distress a year after the loss
Intense grief triggered by a relatively minor event
False euphoria after the loss
Overidentification with the deceased
Phobias about illness or death
History of prolonged grieving
Inability to carry out usual activities of daily living

Data from Kübler-Ross E: *On death and dying,* New York, 1969, Macmillan; Worden W: *Grief counseling and grief therapy,* ed 3, New York, 1995, Springer; Rando T: *Treatment of complicated mourning,* Champaign, Ill, 1993, Research Press.

shock to reintegration. These activities are useful to health care professionals in helping the bereaved.

ASSESSMENT

Health History

Planning interventions for helping grieving persons help themselves must be preceded by accurate assessment of where persons are in their grief, as well as what factors are influencing their grief.[35] Encouraging the grieving individual and family to tell their own stories and describe their lived experiences can provide insight into their grieving and help promote grief expression. Assessment cues indicating active grieving are:

- Perception of loss(es) shared in conversation
- Preoccupation with fears (suffering, abandonment, loss of control, or helplessness)
- Asking "Why me?" and "Why us?" questions
- Preoccupation with or avoidance of discussing loss(es)
- Verbalizing feelings of "going crazy," "being numb," "loneliness," or "life is empty"
- Reviewing what he or she did or did not do to help the dying person or the family (e.g., comments with the theme of guilt or blame)
- Somatic complaints
- Talking about suicide
- Verbalizing doubts in past religious belief/faith and fairness in the world
- Report of change in eating, sleeping, and/or elimination

Physical Examination

Objective assessment of the grieving person are likely to include:

- Deep sighing, changes in breathing patterns
- Restlessness, agitation
- Shortened attention span
- Apathy
- Inability to express feelings without intense emotions (e.g., crying, anxiety, sadness, or anger)
- Lack of emotional expression when talking about loss(es)
- Dependent behavior
- Withdrawal from family and friends
- Keeping very busy with chores
- Changes in performing daily roles in family and at work
- Taking on behaviors characteristic of the dying person

Trying to interpret the importance of any of these cues without having a perception of loss can make assessment difficult. Any assessment needs to be validated and updated on an ongoing basis. Reassessment may address such major topics as:

- Acceptance of the reality of the loss
- Evaluation for need for medical attention and treatment
- Identification of unresolved grief
- Detection of illogical thoughts

Instruments have been developed to identify persons at risk for difficulty in the grieving process or to identify the problems of persons who experience prolonged bereavement-related distress in widowhood. Behaviors suggestive of the inability to resolve grief include:

- Searching
- Yearning
- Preoccupation with the deceased
- Crying
- Disbelief about the loss
- Feeling stunned by the loss
- Lack of acceptance of loss of spouse

NURSING DIAGNOSES

Human responses to the loss of a loved one are varied. Although other nursing diagnoses may be applicable, the one most commonly recognized among persons who experience loss is grieving. Grieving is an appropriate diagnostic category for those seeking to promote wellness and to facilitate healing associated with significant loss. At the same time, normal grieving may be associated with dysfunctional or distorted behaviors[3,50] that can be recognized in a variety of secondary diagnoses.

Grieving is the ultimate price of loving, of attachment, and of a meaningful relationship.[7,72] In some instances the person is unable to mourn in a manner that allows for resolution of the grief and reinvestment in life.[45,51,73]

The North American Nursing Diagnosis Association (NANDA) recognizes two independent nursing diagnostic categories in relationship to grieving: (1) anticipatory grieving and (2) dysfunctional grieving. *Anticipatory grieving* is defined as "the state in which an individual or group experiences reactions in response to an expected significant loss,"[20,64] and *dysfunctional grieving* is defined as "the state in which an individual or group experiences prolonged unresolved grief and engages in detrimental activities."[3,15]

Diagnostic Title	Possible Etiologic Factors
1a. Anticipatory grieving	Perceived loss of a significant other, physiologic or psychosocial well-being, or personal possessions
1b. Dysfunctional grieving	Actual or perceived object loss; thwarted grieving response to loss; absence of anticipatory grieving; multiple losses; chronic fatal illness; loss of others; loss of physiologic/psychosocial well-being; prolonged denial; intense pining and yearning; ambivalent relationship with the deceased; severe self-reproach; multiple crises; lack of support from family; history of ineffective coping

Other secondary diagnoses relevant to persons experiencing loss include anxiety, spiritual distress, hopelessness, impaired thought processes, self-esteem disturbance, and ineffective coping. Etiologic factors for these diagnoses include loneliness, social isolation, financial difficulties, hostility, substance abuse, hallucinations, fear, anger, inability to understand or find meaning in the loss, sorrow, guilt, and anger toward God. The bereaved may exhibit somatic symptoms while grieving; relevant nursing diagnoses include self-care deficit, altered nutrition, and sleep pattern disturbance.

EXPECTED PATIENT OUTCOMES

The expected outcomes associated with grief and the work that is entailed in the grieving process include remembering the loved one without emotional pain and reinvesting emotional energy in life so that the capacity to love is not lost.[19]

Expected patient outcomes for the grieving person may include but are not limited to:[70,72]

1a,b. Will face the pain
Will experience the pain in all its dimensions
Will withdraw from ties to the deceased
Will adjust to an altered environment without the deceased
Will renew or form new relationships
Will recall memories without intense grief

INTERVENTIONS

1a,b. Facilitating Resolution of Grief

Understanding the grieving process as a normal part of living provides the basis for nursing assessments and interventions. Nursing actions in response to the bereaved call for a delicate blending of being present, listening, expressing honest feelings, and inviting the bereaved to share their experiences and emotions.[35,37,48,66,68]

After the death, appropriate nursing interventions begin with making contact and assessing the bereaved in his or her grief to plan appropriate future interventions. A relationship must be established, and the nurse must be present physically and emotionally to offer security and support.

When working with the bereaved, the nurse needs to take the initiative and reach out in a concrete way. The nurse should not say, "Call me if you need me," but should be specific in how he or she can assist or get others to assist. For example, the nurse might say, "How about if I call your sister to accompany you to select the casket?" or "Suppose I arrange for you to attend a widow-to-widow meeting?" The nurse should not take refusals personally or give up. Offers of assistance should be repeated because grievers initially may be unable to respond to and appreciate offers of help but will benefit over time. Physical contact, hugging, touching, and hand-holding are used as appropriate. These actions are important early in the process to convey that the griever is not alone. If the griever is a person who does not like to be touched, simply sitting nearby is more comforting. Regular expression of feelings should be encouraged to help prevent the grieving person from becoming overwhelmed and unable to function. Security should be provided through direction concerning meals, rest, and priorities of activities for the day or week. Others should be encouraged to take charge of routine functions and responsibilities of the bereaved (e.g., running errands or preparing meals). Family members should be helped to focus on one problem at a time, addressing problems to which practical solutions can be found before addressing more complicated problems. Most important, the nurse must also give people "permission" to grieve by displaying neutral (i.e., nonjudgmental) attitudes and behaviors. Verbal and nonverbal behavior should communicate compassionate support. For example, when the griever's voice cracks, facial muscles quiver, and eyes water, and the bereaved turns to the nurse, the nurse should lean forward, relax, and not turn away or offer a tissue, but allow the griever to cry. The nurse's comfort and approval is displayed through body language, and actions speak louder than words.

Grieving persons should not be allowed to remain isolated. Family members should be encouraged to be present after all the intensity of the funeral has subsided, because social supports generally decrease weeks or months after a death, when the bereaved is forced to resume life without the loved one. Self-help groups can be suggested, and the grievers assisted to attend. A family perspective must be maintained, and the nurse must remember that the family is changed.

Patient/Family Education

Nursing interventions and guidelines for teaching the patient and family facing death are found in the Guidelines for Safe Practice box.

EVALUATION

Progress in grieving is difficult to measure because of its ongoing nature and wide range of manifestations.[51,66,72] Assessment

Guidelines for Safe Practice

Grief Support

NURSING INTERVENTIONS

A. Establish therapeutic nurse-patient relationship.
B. Encourage patient/family to talk about the loss and express feelings.
C. Acknowledge feelings and the stress involved in dealing with the anticipated or actual losses.
D. Use self and caring presence to help grieving persons feel connected to someone who cares.[11,18,39]
E. Encourage patient/family to discuss what the loss means to them.
F. Introduce and encourage use of health care supports.
G. Encourage patient and family to share their thoughts about impending death and grieving with each other.
H. Guide patient/family in problem solving to deal with the loss.
   1. Examine ways they have dealt positively with past losses.
   2. Identify changes needed to adjust now within family or work roles, relationships, responsibilities, and expectations.
   3. Discuss realistic and available resources to use in making needed changes.

PATIENT/FAMILY TEACHING

A. Review the normal grief process and its nature.
B. Reinforce that everyone deals with grief in his or her own way.
C. Explain that feelings over loss are natural and necessary for recovery, even if they are uncomfortable.
D. Reinforce the importance of expressing feelings, even negative ones, with someone supportive.
E. Emphasize the need to maintain positive habits of self-care when grieving (e.g., eating, sleeping, and elimination).
F. Reinforce patient's need for normalcy, support, control, and self-esteem when faced with impending death.
G. As questions are raised, briefly review with the dying person and family:
   1. What to expect in the dying process
   2. Choices about the quality of life left that the dying person can make
   3. Consequences of those choices (e.g., electing no resuscitation does not mean hastening death)
   4. Measures being taken to offer comfort and some control

Specific Grief Behaviors

A. Denial
   1. Encourage patient/family to describe their loss and their perception of the experience.
   2. Avoid confronting.
   3. Help discuss changes that have occurred in life since the anticipated or actual loss.
   4. Give opportunities every shift to share feelings.
   5. Acknowledge patient/family perceptions and feelings.

A. Review normalcy of the grief process.
B. Briefly explain denial as a protective mechanism, and the need to give time for each person to work through awareness in his or her own way.
C. Review ways to support a grieving loved one who is in denial.
D. Explain to family how the dying person may continue denial until the moment of death to maintain hope.

B. Bargaining
   1. Encourage patient/family to ask questions as they arise.
   2. Acknowledge patient/family's wish that everything was "back to normal."
   3. Encourage patient/family to express underlying feelings.
   4. Help patient/family identify realistic versus possibly unrealistic hopes.

A. Offer consistent information.
B. Encourage everyday communication of questions with patient's physician.
C. Anticipate patient/family needs by explaining briefly all tests, procedures, and care.
D. Help patient/family discuss changing goals (from aggressive treatment to palliative care).

C. Guilt
   1. Encourage patient/family to express negative or ambivalent feelings constructively.
   2. Help patient/family to examine what they do versus do not have direct control over.
   3. Acknowledge patient/family's wanting to resolve losses.
   4. Help define what is realistic control (e.g., maintaining independence with activities of daily living [ADLs]).

A. Reinforce normalcy of the grief process.
B. Review concrete ways to maintain some sense of control.
C. Review with dying patient ways to remain helpful, if desired, to family.
D. Review with family specific ways members can help support and care for their dying loved one.
E. Reinforce what care they are giving that is helping.
F. Help redefine goals of treatment to palliative care.

D. Anger
   1. Encourage patient/family to express negative feelings in constructive ways.
   2. Acknowledge anger as a legitimate feeling in grief.
   3. Redirect inappropriate expression of anger toward self or others.

A. Reinforce normalcy of the grief process and importance of expressing all feelings, even if negative.
B. Review available and constructive outlets for expressing anger.
C. Review self-care strategies to prevent anger from building up without some release.

E. Depression
   1. Encourage patient/family to maintain their ADLs and routine as physically able.
   2. Help patient/family express sadness over loss (e.g., in talking about lifestyle changes in present and future).
   3. Provide privacy when crying.

A. Reinforce normalcy of the grief process versus prolonged depression.

Continued

Guidelines for Safe Practice

Grief Support—cont'd

E. Depression—cont'd
   4. Help patient/family:
      a. Find some positive aspect or characteristic of present situation.
      b. Find ways to maximize any positive features.
      c. Identify specific hope(s) for the future.
   5. Refer to appropriate health care support for suicidal thoughts that include an intent and plan.
   6. Encourage patient to participate in activities that increase his or her self-esteem.
   7. Encourage patient/family to still celebrate moments of joy in everyday life, despite facing death (e.g., sitting in garden for 30 minutes, watching a family video).

B. Reinforce depression as a protective mechanism and the need to give each person the time to work through this stage. Explain available resources on the health care team.
C. Reinforce important ways to build up the dying person's self-esteem (e.g., reminiscing, telling the loved one how much he or she did in the past for the family, grace in facing death).

tools can help identify individual manifestations in the bereaved over time, but fluctuations in the grieving experience are to be expected. Any assessment needs to be ongoing to reflect movement through the experience of loss and the process of grief.[33] Interventions that are appropriate for one person may not be useful and may even be harmful to another person.

The grief experience can present an overwhelming challenge to the grieving person, family, and nurse. To face the challenge, measurable outcomes need to be established for each person on the basis of the individual's sociocultural situation. The outcomes serve as a yardstick of progress and offer hope that the intensity of grieving will not last forever.

Resolution of the grieving process is successful if the grieving person[51,53,73]:

1a,b. Acknowledges the loss and its impact on changing roles and/or relationships

Talks about the reality of the loss (e.g., son's deceased father will not be taking him to the park to play ball anymore).

Begins to incorporate the reality of the loss (e.g., wife no longer sets place at table for deceased husband).

Displays some sign(s) of grieving (e.g., cognitive, social, physical, and/or psychologic)

Indicates an absence of:

- Destructive behavior (e.g., suicidal thoughts, alcohol, or drug abuse).
- Signs of poor bereavement outcomes.

Uses some constructive means to express feelings with a significant other or health care professional about the loss.

Establishes and maintains activities of daily life routine in meeting own needs (e.g., rest, nutrition, fluids, elimination).

Identifies at least one grief support in significant other or health care professional.

Begins to set some goals for own future and has decreasing preoccupation with the loss.

Evaluation methods that can be useful in measuring grief recovery include the following:

- Perceptions of the grieving person and family about the experience
- Observations of responses to nursing interventions
- Comparisons of current grief behavior with baseline behavior
- Functional status of the grieving person and family in maintaining usual lifestyle
- Mutual discussion of goals and ways to work toward goal achievement
- Perceptions of the nurse about own grief history

When complicated grief is evident, psychiatric intervention may be required. Parkes and Weiss[45] identified persons exhibiting the following behaviors as requiring psychiatric care:

- An extreme depressive reaction manifested by persistent sadness with no shifts to a normal state; an unresponsiveness to warmth; extreme expressions of guilt and identification symptoms
- Psychotic break with reality (neurotic anxiety; obsessions; phobic, hysteria, or schizophrenic reactions; acting and speaking as though the deceased were still present)
- Suicidal tendencies (self-punitive acts, often to expiate guilt)
- Excessive drinking, drug abuse, or promiscuity (as substitutes for the deceased)

Although the discussion in this section focuses primarily on the survivors, all involved are experiencing loss. The dying person, perhaps, is facing the greatest loss of all.[9] Everyone involved is grieving. The principles apply to all from different perspectives. Nursing care of dying persons includes multiple processes.

Dying persons and their families and friends may or may not experience the grieving process in the same way. Dying persons may grieve over the loss of physical function, the loss of past abilities, the ultimate loss of life, and separation from all they know and love. At the same time, significant others may grieve over the potential loss of the loved one, the hurt they feel, and the emptiness they anticipate.[51,64,65,72]

FACING DEATH: THE FINAL LOSS

Despite the amazing advances of science, technology, nursing, and medical knowledge, dying continues to be a part of living. The fact is that at some future time we will cease "to be." In a sense, we are dying even as we are living. To conceptualize living and dying as the opposite ends of a continuum creates a false dichotomy. Living and dying are not opposite ends of a continuum: they are the continuum.[29,38] Recent attention to quality of life in persons who are dying has focused on advocating for integration of palliative care into the entire course of the illness so that death is a natural transition instead of a crisis.[4,9,10] When we interact with persons who are known to have a life-threatening illness, we are more directly confronted with their dying and our own vulnerability. This confrontation evokes anxiety, and thus we become more aware of the dying component of living. Although we may identify with the suffering and sorrow of persons as they live their dying, we interact with living persons. To appreciate our own and others' responses to loss, dying, and death, we need an understanding of the context in which they occur and of our own views and reactions within varying contexts.[38]

SOCIETAL, CULTURAL, AND SOCIAL PERSPECTIVES

Dying and Death: The Differences

Dying is different from death. Dying, a part of living, is a process—the process of coming to an end. Death, the permanent cessation of all vital functions—the end of human life—is an event and a state. The event is the moment of death; the state is that of being dead.[9,38]

Both dying and death have unique aspects that evoke fears, anxieties, and uncertainties.[53,59,72] Some aspects of dying, such as physical and emotional pain, the loss of others, and the inability to function in familiar ways, may also occur under other circumstances (e.g., illness, retirement, or relocation) and therefore are not unique to dying. The unique aspect of dying is that it ends in death. People have no prior experiences to help them understand what it means to be dead. Questions surface: Can dead persons think? Do they have feelings? What is it like to be dead? Is there another life? Where will they go?

At the same time that death is a unique event, it is universal. Because it is universal, each society has had to develop its own beliefs, norms, mores, restrictions, and standards related to loss, dying, and after-death practices. Appropriate ways to respond in one societal or cultural group may be inappropriate in another. Each society dictates the standards and practices that it will support. Thus members of a society have a prescribed set of behaviors from which to choose.[43,58]

In general, the dominant view of dying, death, and loss of members of any one society is a function of how death fits into the teleologic view of life. Individual responses reflect the dominant societal view. However, the repertoire of responses of dying persons or of the survivors is also determined by personal beliefs and one's subcultural group (e.g., social, cultural, religious) affiliations. For instance, Americans may view dying similarly, but their responses may be influenced by their religious beliefs, their views on life after death, their social class, and their occupations.[38,43]

Prevailing Societal Attitudes

Death denial, death defiance, death acceptance, and desire for death are four prevailing societal attitudes toward death. As these general attitudes are discussed, it is important to remember that they may vary in different situations, depending on whose death is involved.

Recognition of the prevailing attitudes and their differences helps health care professionals to understand the process of dying, guides them when interacting with others, helps them avoid conflicts among themselves, and, most important, enhances their communication abilities and thus their patient care. Quality care for dying persons and family members must remain the constant goal of health care professionals.[18,66]

No attitude is good or bad; attitudes are merely different. Our behavior reflects our attitudes. If we recognize our own attitudes toward dying and death in a particular situation, as well as those of other persons involved, we may better understand why all of us feel the way we do and why we are acting the way we are. This recognition and understanding may not always lead to agreement, but it can contribute to modifications of behavior and to decreased conflict in decision making. These attitudes are explored briefly in the following sections.

Death Denial. Western society has been described as a death-denying society.[43,69,73] Many people avoid the subject of dying and death. Health care professionals, particularly physicians, have been described as being unwilling to talk with patients about their dying.[9,19,44] Both health care professionals and family members often justify their stance by expressing the belief that they are "protecting" the dying person.

The question is, whom are they really protecting? In most situations they are protecting themselves; that is, consciously or unconsciously, they weigh the impact on themselves and decide—or choose—not to act because of fear of the reaction or response. The following questions often arise: What will happen to me? Will I lose emotional control? Will the other person shout, cry, or become angry? Will family members become angry? Will the physician become angry? Will I know what to do or say? What if they do not react at all?

In nursing, a death-denying attitude has taken on a negative connotation. This attitude is neither good nor bad; however, the actions and consequences of an attitude can be evaluated as good or bad. For example, a death-denying attitude may contribute to a lack of open communication about dying, but it also may contribute to continuing to give care in bleak situations. On the other hand, a behavior or action such as continuation of care may reflect more than one attitude; for example, it may reflect both death denial and death defiance.[38,51]

Death Defiance. Death defiance is a part of the Judeo-Christian heritage. Throughout the ages people have fought for causes or ideologies, even though they knew that they might die in the attempt. This attitude is reflected in hospitals, especially in critical care units or during emergency situations. The cause is saving a life; the battle is with death. Although staff members do not die in the battle, they are open to loss. If the patient dies, staff members live with the sense of a battle lost. Moreover, they face again the inevitability of death, despite modern technology.[66] Death defiance is helpful as we fight for life. It is not helpful when we do not also attend to the realities of the situation.

Death Acceptance. Death acceptance is viewing death as a normal, natural, and integral part of living. Becker, a prominent philosopher, defined the resignation to and acceptance of our limited existence as the central task for achieving maturity. With this acceptance, death becomes the conclusion of life's plan. It sounds so simple. Intellectually it calms the fear and pain of dying and of facing our own mortality. Like other attitudes toward death, however, this attitude is not a panacea.[38]

For some, death acceptance is the ultimate achievement of maturation, a form of self-actualization. The dying person must achieve this attitude alone; it cannot be forced on the dying person by others. The value of the death acceptance attitude can be judged by actions and behaviors of the dying person only. An adaptable sense of hope may be needed for the dying to accept death.[16,72]

Desire for Death. The fourth attitude, the desire for death, is more common in our society than people generally like to admit.[9] People may desire their own death or the death of others.

Many circumstances give rise to the desire to die or for someone else to die. One major reason is the search for relief from suffering. Suffering takes many forms, including pain, loneliness, disability, fear, uncertainty, and economic and emotional crises. If fear and suffering were prevented with compassionate symptom management, physician-assisted suicide would not exist.[9,17,43]

Other reasons that contribute to the desire to die may be associated with a relief from suffering, but are expressed in a different way. Some persons search for reunion with loved ones. Still others look forward to death as a last phase in the fulfillment of life.

Recognition of how people express their desire to die is important. In many instances the expression of the desire to die is the dying person's or family member's way of confirming his or her recognition that death is inevitable within a predictable period of time in the near future.[10,62]

Meaning of Death

The knowledge that death is imminent within a predicted period of time adds reality to feelings of fear, anxiety, and uncertainty.[27,38,44] As a result, persons facing imminent death experience these emotions differently than do healthy persons who are speculating about what it is like to be dying. Healthy persons speak of death in the abstract; they talk about the death of another or project it into the distant future. Casual comments such as "We all have to die someday," "We are all dying from the time we are born," or "Everyone has to die of something," reflect what Freud called "unconscious immortality."[19] The fact that people can continue to think about others who have died causes them to unconsciously believe in their own immortality. Hearing of someone else's dying or death, however, forces them to face their own finiteness.

Neither the casual comments nor unconscious beliefs are inherently good or bad. However, such comments offer little in the way of understanding or support when they are made to a dying person or to his or her family. Such statements usually are in response to the discomfort we feel when someone tells us that death is imminent. A more understanding response might be, "I'm sorry to hear that."[38,52]

Views toward dying and death vary considerably. Even when we are discussing hypothetical situations, our closeness to dying or to a dying person can influence our views and our responses.[63,64] The same data are seen differently from different perspectives. It is important to identify the referent under discussion whether we are talking in theoretic terms or about practical situations. In other words, from whose perspective are we evaluating the situation: my perspective, your perspective, the patient's perspective, or a family member's perspective? Lack of recognition of different perspectives can lead to poor communication, faulty nursing judgments, and inappropriate nursing interventions.[38]

Quality of Life

What constitutes quality of life? Who can predict what the quality of life will be during the dying process? Can one person judge the quality of life of another, especially if the other is dying?

Much has been written about what constitutes quality of life from the research perspective, but there is little information on what constitutes quality of life for the dying person. It has been suggested that if the known instruments were used to measure quality of life, most dying persons would receive low scores, because most instruments focus on objective physical, behavioral, psychologic, and economic results of disease and treatment and less on measures of a general sense of well-being, happiness, or satisfaction.[9,17,18] Dying persons may perceive quality of life differently than those who are living with an acute or chronic illness or who are well.[25,46,58] McMillan[42] studied perceptions of quality of life in cancer patients receiving hospice care. The findings reinforce that social and spiritual aspects of quality of life are enhanced with hospice care (see Research box). What constitutes quality of life differs from person to person and for any one person during the various stages of life.

In considering the dying person, what contributes to the meaningfulness of life may be a more cogent question than what constitutes quality of life.[18] For example, depression can be expected, but how much and for how long? A person can live with pain, anxiety, and fear, but how much and for how long? How much control does the person have over the situation? Can we increase the control he or she can have in the situation, although the person has lost control over dying? Do the symptoms detract from the meaning of life from the perspective of the dying person? Sometimes trials and tribulations contribute to a person's growth.[4,29]

Dying persons must have freedom to choose a style of dying and then be assisted in that choice. Patients' preferences are important because they make explicit the values of personal autonomy and self-determination.[9,18,31,43,54]

Informed consent, then, becomes an important factor in supporting meaningfulness of life. It includes giving people at the end of life sufficient information about their diagnoses, prognoses, and possible therapies so that they can make informed choices about how they will live or die and about who will help them and in what ways. Informed consent is a person's agreement to allow something to happen on the basis of a full disclosure of facts needed to make an intelligent decision.[19,31,54] To give informed consent, the individual must be competent to make decisions regarding medical treatment. A guardian may be assigned to persons deemed incompetent to make their own decisions.[31,49] Dying persons have the right to refuse treatment or to request it. The nurse has the responsibility to provide information regarding treatment and to respect the patient's decisions. Nursing can also provide a safe environment for patients as they deal with uncertainty.[35,49,54]

QUALITY OF DEATH

Rights of Dying Persons

The rights of dying persons have been recognized by both the American Nurses Association and the American Medical Association.[1,,2,43] Both organizations have standards for meeting these rights (Boxes 6-4 and 6-5). One right of dying persons is the right to know that they are seriously ill and that they may die. The assumption is that such information ensures that they will have more control over what happens to them. As a result, they can participate more fully in decisions about their care and will have the opportunity to complete unfinished business.

Research

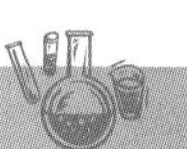

Reference: McMillan S: The quality of life of patients with cancer receiving hospice care, *Oncol Nurs Forum* 23(8):1221-1228, 1996.

This descriptive study evaluated the impact of hospice services on quality of life for cancer patients and their families. Using the Hospice Quality of Life Index, 118 cancer patients receiving hospice care at home and their primary caregivers were surveyed using a convenience sample. Sampling was done within 48 hours of hospice admission and after 3 weeks of hospice service. Results with factor analysis showed high mean scores of quality of life involving social and spiritual issues, with low mean scores involving physical needs and functional issues.

BOX 6-4 Elements of Quality Care for Patients in the Last Phase of Life

Preamble

In the last phase of life, people seek peace and dignity. To help realize this, every person should be able to fairly expect the following elements of care from physicians, health care institutions, and the community.

Elements

1. The opportunity to discuss and plan for end-of-life care
2. Trustworthy assurance that physical and mental suffering will be carefully attended to and comfort measures intently secured
3. Trustworthy assurance that preferences for withholding or withdrawing life-sustaining intervention will be honored
4. Trustworthy assurance that there will be no abandonment by the physician
5. Trustworthy assurance that dignity will be a priority
6. Trustworthy assurance that burden to family and others will be minimized
7. Attention to the personal goals of the dying person
8. Trustworthy assurance that care providers will assist the bereaved through early stages of mourning and adjustment

From American Medical Association: *Elements of quality care for patients in the last phase of life,* Chicago, 1997, AMA.

BOX 6-5 Position Statement on the Nurse's Role in End-of-Life Decisions

Nursing and the Patient Self-Determination Act

Summary: The American Nurses Association (ANA) believes that nurses should play a primary role in implementation of the Patient Self-Determination Act, passed as part of the Omnibus Budget Reconciliation Act of 1990. It is the responsibility of nurses to facilitate informed decision making for patients making choices, particularly at the end of life. The nurse's role in education, research, patient care, and advocacy is critical to the ongoing implementation of the Patient Self-Determination Act within all health care settings.

Nursing Care and Do-Not-Resuscitate Decisions

Summary: The American Nurses Association (ANA) believes that nurses bear a large responsibility at the time a patient experiences cardiac arrest for either initiating resuscitation or ensuring that unwanted attempts to resuscitate do not occur. Nurses face ethical dilemmas concerning confusing or conflicting do-not-resuscitate (DNR) orders.

Forgoing Medically Provided Nutrition and Hydration

Summary: The American Nurses Association (ANA) believes that the decision to withhold medically provided nutrition and hydration should be made by the patient or surrogate with the health care team. The nurse continues to provide expert and compassionate care to patients who are no longer receiving medically provided nutrition and hydration.

Promotion of Comfort and Relief of Pain in Dying Patients

Summary: The American Nurses Association (ANA) believes that the promotion of comfort and aggressive efforts to relieve pain and other symptoms in dying patients are obligations of the nurse.

Nurses should not hesitate to use full and effective doses of pain medication for the proper management of pain and the dying patient. The increasing titration of medication to achieve adequate symptom control, even at the expense of life, thus hastening death secondarily, is ethically justified.

From American Nurses Association: *Position statement on the nurse's role in end-of-life decisions,* Washington, DC, 1997, ANA.

Another right is the right to die in an atmosphere of hopefulness.[16] Persons have a right to die in peace and dignity, surrounded by loved ones and unencumbered by tubes and machines. They have a right to privacy. Dying persons are entitled to be cared for by sensitive, caring, knowledgeable people who attempt to understand them and their loved ones. They are entitled to die as free from pain or other discomforts as is possible.[57,64] Comfort contributes to peaceful dying and alleviates fears of suffering.[18]

Advance Directives

The Patient Self-Determination Act (1991) mandates that the rights of persons who are dying are upheld. The law advocates death with dignity when terminal illness precludes treatment and maintains the right of all patients to make health care decisions and to refuse lifesaving treatment, even if they are unable to communicate.[18,31,54,64] Advance directives ensure that the patient's treatment preferences are upheld.

Hospitals, nursing homes, and hospices are responsible for informing patients about advance directives and treatment decisions. Responsibilities of the health care agency include:

1. On admission, advising patients of their rights
    a. To accept or refuse medical care in the event that they become terminally ill
    b. To make advance directive decisions
2. Documenting the process and the patient's decision
3. Implementing advance directive policies within the institution or agency
4. Providing ongoing staff education about rights and policies regarding advance directives

Each state has detailed laws that define the types of advance directives that are legally binding. The state statute should be consulted before advising patients. In all states, making an advance directive decision includes designing a living will and/or designating a durable power of attorney for health care.[31,49,54]

Living wills direct decisions for withholding or withdrawing of life-sustaining treatment when the patient is in a terminal condition and death is imminent. Traditionally, life-sustaining treatment has included cardiopulmonary resuscitation and mechanical ventilation. However, with the growing number of court cases, questions have arisen about inclusion of nutrition and hydration, as well as specific conditions for offering life support measures.[49,54] These documents outline the person's health care preferences and offer directives to physicians in the event that the person becomes unresponsive from accidental trauma or end-stage disease.[31,49]

A durable power of attorney for health care is another type of advance directive that authorizes a designated party to make health care decisions in the event that the authorizing person becomes unresponsive or unable to make his or her own decisions. Included are special directions for life-sustaining treatments and hydration/nutrition issues, but not authorization to make financial decisions.[31,49,54]

Copies of advance directives should be given to family members, physicians, the person's attorney, and the person's religious advisor. Individuals are advised to sign and date them at least yearly. An open discussion with significant others about one's philosophy of life and desires related to the process of dying is perhaps the most effective way of ensuring a meaningful death—or what has been referred to as a "good" death.[9,10,31,62]

Despite legislation, many individuals remain unaware of their rights in preparing an advance directive (see Research box). Nurses are instrumental in ensuring that advance directives are incorporated into admission assessments and ongoing education for the patient and family. Patients may need guidance in initiating discussion about end-of-life decisions with their family members and physicians, especially when facing cumulative loss and grief. Patients have the right to decline preparing an advance directive, but nurses need to use sensitive communication techniques in following up on such choices.[31,62] Such a decline may represent the patient's attempt to protect family members from added grief or meet their unrealistic expectations about "beating" a terminal prognosis. Choosing an advance directive can help patients and their families speak the unspeakable, acknowledge their shared grief, gain a sense of control in facing an uncertain future, and prevent potential conflicts at the end of life.[50,53]

Good Death/Bad Death

Many nurses, and in fact people in general, express concern over dying with dignity or dying a good death. Is there such a thing as a good death? There is no one good death; rather, there are many. There is no one right way to die, just as there is no one right way to live. Dying with dignity, or a good death, is really an ideal. The terms offer little in the way of guiding care. There are many views about what constitutes a good death: to die as one lived, to die without pain, or to die in the company of loved ones are all answers. A good death involves individual perceptions of the living-dying process, as well as shared observations of the death event. A death is more likely to be labeled as good when dying is viewed as a part of living and not as a separate phenomenon. A good death is also associated with the way all persons involved interact with each other preceding and during the event—that is, if there is harmony rather than conflict.[9,38,43]

Research

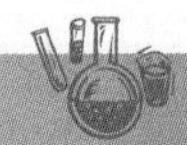

Reference: Gilbert M et al: Determining the relationship between end-of-life decisions expressed in advance directives and resuscitation efforts during cardiopulmonary resuscitation, *Outcomes Manage Nurs Pract* 5(2):87-92, 2001.

The purpose of this study was to determine how useful patients' advance directives are to health care team members in making end-of-life treatment decisions. Medical records of 135 adult patients who had undergone cardiopulmonary resuscitation in the past year were reviewed. Only 35 of the patients had an advance directive, and only 36% outlined specific guidelines for directing end-of-life care. The remaining patients had a vague or nondirective document. The study reinforces the need for members of the health care team to provide patients with information and resources to document their specific wishes for end-of-life care.

Sometimes nurses refer to deaths as normal or abnormal. Deaths are perceived as normal or good when most or all persons involved perceive that all was done that could be done or the wishes of the patient are respected and accepted by most persons involved. In these instances there is a sense of loss, but the loss is accompanied by a sense of fulfillment and closure. Nurses may label deaths as bad or abnormal when there is conflict over the type or length of treatment, the wishes of the patient are ignored, or there are bad feelings about a lack of honesty, especially with family members.

The dying experience can leave a lasting impression on survivors. Depending on their perceptions, family members may retain images of pain, depression, and helplessness.[9,18,23] People's attitudes toward dying and when people should die, as well as the characteristics of the dying person, will also influence how they interpret the experience.

Age and Premature Death

There was a time when people did not make a connection between aging, loss of body function, and general progressive debilitation and dying. The expectations of living have changed as life expectancies have changed. During the Roman period, life expectancy was 20 years; it increased to 35 years during the Middle Ages. By the late 1800s Americans could anticipate living 50 years, but few persons lived past the age of 60 or 70 years. In contemporary American life, people not only anticipate living more than 70 years, they expect to do so as active, functioning individuals.[43]

Many people believe that any age is too young to die. Some perceive that people do not die of natural causes or of old age, but as a result of accidents, homicides, or suicides, or while receiving treatment for a recognized, diagnosed clinical problem such as heart disease, stroke, disseminated intravascular coagulation, or total body failure. According to this perception, most deaths can be interpreted as being avoidable, unnecessary, and premature. If death always is interpreted as being avoidable, unnecessary, or premature, it follows that someone must be blamed. Who can be blamed? The physician? The hospital? Society? Perhaps it is the fault of the person who died for not seeking help sooner. This interpretation of death as always being avoidable contributes to conflict and guilt.[18,43]

Prolonged Dying

Just as there is concern over premature death, there is concern over prolonged dying.[9,50] Through modern technology and therapy we have become adept at maintaining life in the desperately ill person. Unfortunately, at times the same techniques used to maintain life during temporary crises create dilemmas related to what constitutes life. When are we prolonging dying rather than life? Our ability to prolong dying leads to many moral and ethical issues related to life and death.[27,55]

Dying: An Achievement or a Failure?

Although most dying people express resentment, fear, or sorrow over the major changes that are forced on their lives by progressive debilitation, some view dying as an achievement.[19] Some persons, especially those with a prolonged course of living with dying, focus on living their dying so as to die well. People who believe that dying well is an achievement sometimes are described by health care professionals as denying or defying death. These people recognize their dying but choose therapy or choose to go home and participate in their customary activities. They live their dying the way they wish, and thus from their own perspective they die well. These persons seem to do more than adjust or accommodate. They rise to an unseen challenge and in so doing expand their living rather than extend their dying. They transcend what their illness presents as limitations and find strength in facing uncertainty.[18,64]

A small number of persons may perceive dying as a personal failure or may attribute it to external forces. Some dwell on all they could have accomplished were it not for their illness. They usually exude a sense of powerlessness and futility and express overt anger. Others appear depressed, helpless, and resigned to their situation.[9,38,53]

How people perceive their dying may change throughout the course of their dying. Attitudes, like physical capabilities, do not remain static. Dying encompasses the whole person; it is an emotional, behavioral, and physical process.[25,29]

FUNERALS AND AFTER-DEATH RITUALS

All societies have funeral practices associated with care and disposal of the body and with the expected behavior of the bereaved. Funerals and after-death rituals serve many positive functions for the bereaved.[8,58] They include:

- A gathering of friends and family offers sympathy, a recognition of the loss, communication of caring—in short, social support. Wakes, viewings, and visitations are forms of gatherings for family and friends. Nurses and other health care professionals accomplish similar tasks by reviewing together what occurred and sharing past experiences about the person who died or others who have died.
- The use of ritual, which is often religious in nature, offers some reason for or lends some meaning to death.
- Visual display of the dead body assists survivors with reaching closure or accepting the finality of death.
- There is an opportunity to display grief publicly in a procession that ends at the place of final disposition.
- Burial, entombment, or cremation of the body reinforces the idea of preservation of life on earth and, for some, provides a place to return for prayer or reminiscence.
- Material expenditure for funerals is one way to communicate "the loss of the bereaved to society."

All major changes in life have rituals to help individuals and society adapt to the changed state and cope with the disequilibrium that occurs during the transition from one state to another (e.g., birth, marriage, and death). Funerals serve as a rite of passage from life to death, validate the life of the deceased, and act as a testimony that a life has been lived.*

*References 13, 19, 50, 51, 56, 58, 72.

Funerals meet the needs of mourners and society by offering spiritual, psychologic, and social benefits to the survivors.[38]

THE END-OF-LIFE TRAJECTORY

Chronicity of Dying

The nature of dying has changed. Because of modern therapies and technology, patterns of illness have shifted from acute infectious diseases to chronic conditions; as a result, dying has become a chronic process. With the exception of some acute problems such as myocardial infarction, severe infections, or trauma, most dying persons experience chronic problems with multiple pathophysiologic alterations. These alterations usually are permanent and result in disability, with a need to adjust to loss and to accommodate to change. Multiple series of losses can affect a person's behavioral responses and ability to cope.[43,50,64]

Dying takes on many characteristics of chronic illness. Like other chronically ill persons, those who are dying express feelings of being socially displaced or isolated. They grieve over the loss of former activities and abilities. They express sorrow over the continued loss of friends, business associates, and acquaintances. They talk of being alive and yet not able to live. They are expected to be present oriented rather than future oriented.[13,25]

Whenever the anticipated life span is perceived as shortened, persons may be viewed as chronically ill or dying and treated differently. The chronicity of their dying may force them into experiencing a social death while they are functionally and biologically very much alive. Many factors contribute to promoting social dying long before the event of death; these factors are discussed in the next section.[19,25,43]

The Living-Dying Interval

The theoretic stages and phases of dying help in assessing and understanding a situation. The ultimate goal is quality care for dying persons and their families. Nursing interventions help the patient and family achieve that goal. An awareness of patterns of living and dying assists in understanding the nature of grief and dying. The four major patterns and their various combinations are based on the clinical courses of dying patients (Figure 6-2). These patterns are descriptive, not predictive, and are useful for understanding the variations of behavior among dying persons. They also demonstrate the futility of expecting persons to pass through a series of stages of behavior in any fixed sequence.[38]

Peaks and Valleys

The pattern of peaks and valleys is characterized by periods of greater health (peaks) and periods of crises (valleys). Dying persons refer to the peaks as "hopeful highs" and the valleys as "terrible or depressing lows." Although there are times of greater health, the overall course is downward to the event of death. Many hospitalizations and many moments of increased expectation and dashed hopes are associated with the experience of dying in this pattern. The uncertainties are great; fluctuations in behavior and difficulties in planning and adjustment are to be expected as goals and plans change.[38,52]

Descending Plateaus

The pattern of descending plateaus is characterized by an unpredictable number of progressive degenerative steps, with plateaus (periods of stable health) lasting an indeterminate period of time. Again, the overall general course is downward. People do not return to their former level of health or functioning after each crisis. Like the pattern of peaks and valleys, the course is fraught with uncertainty and anxiety about whether another crisis will occur and cause more debilitation. This pattern is associated with expressions of futility and anger. Dying persons and their families grieve over the fact that functional ability is lost despite concerted rehabilitative efforts.[38]

Downward Slopes

The pattern of downward slopes is characterized by a consistent, persistent, easily discernible downward course. Unlike the other patterns, death is expected within a predictable period of time measured in hours or days. In most instances the dying person loses consciousness, and there is little time to prepare family members for the death of their loved one. These deaths usually occur in critical care units.[38]

Gradual Slants

The fourth pattern of living-dying, the pattern of gradual slants, is characterized by a low ebb of life, gradually and almost imperceptibly culminating in death. Generally, these persons experience a debilitating bodily insult from which there is little recovery. In many instances the person is no longer conscious and life is maintained by life support systems. This pattern is associated with many of the following questions:

- When should life support systems be discontinued?
- Where should these persons be cared for?
- Who should be responsible for their care?

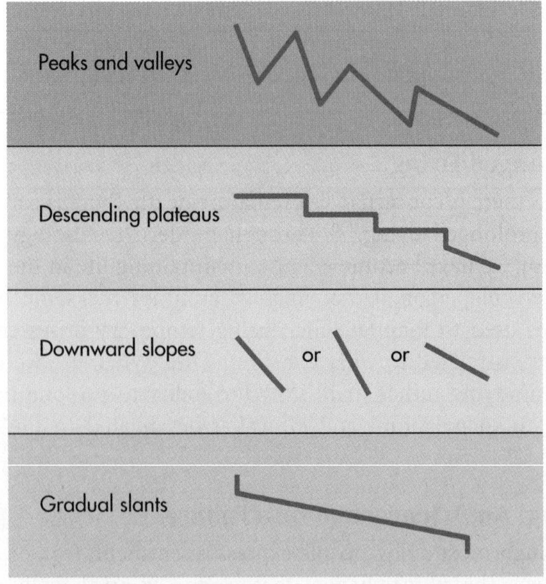

Figure 6-2 Martocchio's patterns of living-dying.

In reality, many combinations of the four patterns may occur in one person's experience of living-dying. For example, a person's pattern may change from peaks and valleys to a downward slope or from a downward slope to a gradual slant.[38]

Choice: A Need and a Right

Dying persons should be free to choose how and when they are told of their prognosis.[9,18,25,66] Some have recently advocated an individual's choice for deciding how and when he or she will die.[9,31,49]

Dying persons describe a system of filtering out or listening only to what they want to know or to realize. They tell us about how they listen to the facts initially but do not hear them until later. Dying persons, as well as other persons facing an extreme crisis, describe reaching an emotional readiness when they are ready to process information. Sometimes patients look for confirmation of what they think they heard.[10,32,65,74] The person who recognizes that death is imminent should be allowed to talk about his or her concerns and seek the support of family and friends.[10,38,62]

Other patients choose not to see or to hear—choose not to know. If that is their informed choice, then it is inappropriate to push them to know that which they do not want to see or hear. The refusal of the patient to know or to discuss the facts creates a challenge for caregivers and family, primarily in communication.[27,38,49]

Role of Confidant

Nurses can introduce the element of choice by fulfilling the patient's need for a confidant who will initiate and allow honest talk. The role of confidant is a necessary but difficult one. Talking about dying is not easy, and periods of awkwardness and expressions of fear are inevitable.[10,62]

Dying persons look to the confidant for honesty and acceptance as they search for understanding of their state. The length of time that relationships exist with patients who have long-term chronic illnesses provides both the opportunity and the obligation for nurses to establish authentic relationships with dying patients, relationships in which nurses can be viewed as confidants.*

The role of the confidant is primarily to be present, to listen, and to guide as the dying person grapples with the experience of dying. The confidant can help make the period of transition from living to dying a time for a deepening feeling of closeness and a time for reinforcing family relationships.[35,48,68,74] An atmosphere of emotional closeness is a significant part of the confidant relationship. Within this context patients can develop and share their agendas for the future, for quality of life, and for what they truly want without the need to protect the nurse from difficult truths.[10,41] Challenging communication issues confront the nurse confidant and require sensitivity in supporting the patient and family during the dying experience. Callanan and Kelley[10] have described nursing interventions that help operationalize the confidant role (Box 6-6).

*References 10, 27, 35, 37, 62, 65.

Impact on the Family

Thus far we have focused on the dying person, but the impact of the knowledge that death is imminent extends beyond the dying person to his or her family, social groups, and the society in which he or she lives.

Cohesive or Disruptive Force

The experience of dying may serve as a cohesive force in some families and a disruptive force in others. In general, families who have responded to stressors or crises as a unified force in the past will offer each other strength and support. For families who have strained relationships, the dying experience may promote further strain.[23,65]

Family members generally express remorse over the fact that a family member had to come face-to-face with death before they realized how much they needed each other or cared for each other. But unless this recognition is coupled with assistance in learning how to make the relationship grow, it will not necessarily lead to greater social and emotional solidarity.[23,65]

Family Control

Dying persons at times use their dying to control the behaviors of family members. When dying persons use dying as a means of control for self-gain or as a weapon, the result is

BOX 6-6 Communicating With the Dying Patient and Family

1. Listen to everything the dying patient says for important cues of near-death awareness or messages for the family.
   a. Talking about travel, anticipated change, or going home can symbolize approaching death.
2. Help the dying patient describe and share the meaning behind what he or she says, even if it is confusing.
3. Help the family interpret the dying patient's messages and behavior.
   a. Hallucinations can represent the dying patient's sensing the presence of family members who have previously died.
   b. Reinforce subtle signs of recognition and comfort when family members visit.
   c. Inform the family when the patient shows signs of imminent death.
4. Encourage and guide family communication with the dying patient, whether verbally or through touch.
5. Gently ask about anything not understood.
6. Accept without judgment what the dying patient says.
7. Validate the normalcy of grieving and uniqueness of the patient's own experience.
8. Allow the dying patient to control the conversation. If periods of silence occur, stay with the patient quietly.
9. If silence lasts for more than 10 minutes, acknowledge the patient's efforts in trying to communicate.
10. Let the patient know when leaving the room.
11. Encourage the patient to reminisce when able.
12. Encourage the dying patient and family to put into words any unfinished business.

Adapted from Callanan M, Kelley P: *Final gifts,* New York, 1997, Bantam; Zerwekh J: The truth-tellers: how hospice nurses help patients confront death, *Am J Nurs* 94(2):30-34, 1994.

anger, resentment, and perhaps retaliation by family members. Retaliation usually takes the form of not visiting, not phoning, or visiting for only short periods. It is an attempt by family members to protect themselves from the control of the dying person even while they wish to be close and loving.

The problem becomes more serious for the family members and the dying person alike if the dying person is being cared for at home. The dying person usually recognizes the antagonism of family members but may interpret it as withdrawal or isolation.[38] Often the dying person may feel rejected and unloved and may not understand that the family loves him or her but not the behavior.

Dying at Home

Although biomedical technologic advances continue to encourage that the locus of dying be the hospital, hospice care provides another alternative. Hospice nursing is coordinated with the multidisciplinary team to help the terminally ill patient maintain physical, psychosocial, and spiritual well-being in whatever life is remaining. Managing symptoms, building family support, and linking the family to community support are central goals.[57,64]

With the increased emphasis on hospice and palliative care and the pressures by Medicare and other insurers to discharge patients as soon as aggressive treatment is discontinued, more persons may choose to die in the privacy of their own homes surrounded by family. *Palliative care,* as defined by the World Health Organization, is the active and total care of people whose disease is not responding to curative treatment. The philosophy of hospice care is based on palliative care. The goals of palliative care are comfort, control, and quality of living until death.[9,57,64]

To have those we love die at home, cared for by family, may fulfill the romantic ideas we may have surrounding dying. However, it takes proper, careful, and advance planning. Two major factors usually are considered: the economic situation and the dying person's wishes. Other important factors to be considered pertain to environmental and caregiver resources. Unless all factors are discussed in advance, family members may be ill prepared to deal with the simplest tasks. They may not know how to change an occupied bed. They may be concerned about how, what, or even whether to feed the dying person. Family members are suddenly expected to assume nursing responsibilities that they may not desire or feel prepared to do, such as changing dressings, irrigating wounds, and administering medications.[8,23,25,65]

Family members need guidance and accessible resources to meet their own needs, as well as the needs of their loved one, as they face the end of life. Nurses can help reinforce the importance of self-care for family health and stability.[30] Family members who wish to care for their loved one at home need information about what to expect and help in mobilizing resources. Anticipating ways to meet the needs of the dying person can offer the family some sense of control. Planning backup relief for grocery shopping, running errands, and taking a break from caregiving 24 hours a day can help family members attend to the family and the dying person. Neighbors and friends can often be recruited to support the family, especially the family caregiver. By focusing on self-care, nurses can help family members strengthen and develop coping skills and use resources within the community.[64]

NURSING MANAGEMENT OF DYING PERSON AND FAMILY

ASSESSMENT

Health History

Nursing assessment is an ongoing process throughout end-of-life care. It is part of the dying person–family–nurse relationship and continues through the family-nurse relationship at the death of the patient. A thorough initial assessment with subjective input from the dying person and family provides the basis for relationships. Assessment criteria are listed in Box 6-7.

Physical Examination

The ultimate cause of death depends on the specific disease process, but certain physiologic changes occur to all persons as they approach death. Irreversible failure of the vital organs precedes death. The nurse should recognize the clinical manifestations of death and prepare the family and patient for the impending death. Being present for the death of a loved one may assist the survivors in resolving their loss.

Failure of the respiratory system is characterized by Cheyne-Stokes breathing, which results from alterations in blood P_{CO_2} levels. The hyperpneic and apneic cycles associ-

BOX 6-7 Nursing Assessment of the Dying Person and Family

Dying Person and Family Perceptions

General Perceptions of Each Individual

Awareness of clinical diagnosis and prognosis
Philosophy of living while dying and views regarding dying
Perceptions of self and effect of the dying process on self
Expected physiologic and behavioral changes
Past experiences with major illnesses or crises
Shared experiences with major illnesses or crises

Perceived Strengths, Desires, and Hopes

Personal abilities and coping techniques
Personal support systems
Availability of resources
Beliefs; religious convictions; cultural views of dying, death, and bereavement
Past experiences with death
Expectations about care and dying, use of life supports (present and future)

Input From Nurse

Beliefs, values, attitudes, responses
Support systems: personal and professional
Expertise, including incorporating others in care

ated with Cheyne-Stokes breathing continue until asphyxia and respiratory failure occur. Heart failure may occur as a result of the increased load on the heart and increased ventricular filling during the hyperpneic phase. The results of heart failure include decreased perfusion, ischemia, and eventually cell death. Eventually, compensation is no longer effective, and myocardial ischemia, liver congestion, and pulmonary congestion result.

Physical changes associated with failing respiratory and cardiac systems include cool skin; skin color changes such as pallor, jaundice, or mottling; weak, thready pulse; respiratory stridor (due to accumulated secretions in the larynx or trachea—sometimes termed *death rattle*); decreased urine output; reduced gastrointestinal motility resulting in impaction; and incontinence as the sphincter muscles relax. Decreased oral intake and a decreased or absent swallow reflex are also present. As the patient approaches death, the peripheral pulses may not be palpable, and it may be necessary to palpate the carotid or auscultate the apical pulse. The extremities feel cool and appear cyanotic as a result of decreased peripheral circulation. The mucous membranes may be dry as a result of decreased fluid intake and, in the case of the oral mucosa, mouth breathing.

Although some patients remain alert to the end, inadequate cerebral perfusion generally leads to decreased neurologic functioning, manifested as confusion, disorientation, delirium, lethargy, and/or apathy. Surges of energy may also occur. Severe neurologic deterioration is characterized by stupor, absence of reaction to painful stimuli, and coma. The pupils react to light sluggishly and, as the person experiences neurologic failure, become nonreactive. A wide range of emotional responses also can be expected. Anxiety, fear, restlessness, agitation, or withdrawal are not uncommon. Some dying persons may exhibit unusual or inappropriate behavior, perhaps as a result of anxiety. The nurse may observe the dying person speaking to someone when there is no one in the room. Speaking to a deceased loved one in the hours preceding death has been reported around the world and is recognized as part of the dying process.

Signs of imminent death include respiratory congestion, including respiratory bubbling and Cheyne-Stokes respirations that become progressively more shallow until they cease; fixed and dilated pupils with a glassy stare; damp, cold, and mottled skin, especially in the extremities; decreased sensorium, with talk about leaving on a trip or seeing deceased significant others; bowel and bladder incontinence; weak and irregular pulse; and progressive hypotension.[6,27,66]

NURSING DIAGNOSES

As one reviews the various nursing assessment criteria in caring for dying persons and their significant others, it becomes clear that analyses of the data may lead to identification of nearly all the NANDA nursing diagnoses over the course of the dying process. The complex physiologic, psychologic, social, and spiritual dynamics that accompany dying help explain the presence of the multiple primary and secondary nursing diagnoses. Perhaps the greatest challenge to nurses is prioritizing—which nursing diagnoses should be addressed and in which order?

Among the most important diagnoses to address are those related to symptom management and grieving. The physical symptoms that accompany the dying process depend on the particular pathophysiology of the disease responsible for the life-threatening state and other preexisting health problems. Assessing and understanding the cause of the symptoms is central to determining appropriate interventions. Following is a brief outline of some of the most common nursing diagnoses associated with care of dying persons as they relate to major symptoms or problems. Nursing interventions for these diagnoses are found in the section related to the presenting problem.

In addition to the nursing diagnoses associated with physical symptoms, other applicable nursing diagnoses relate to psychosocial and spiritual dimensions. The following are examples that may be relevant: fear, compromised coping, ineffective family coping, interrupted family processes, powerlessness, social isolation, and spiritual distress.

Because the needs of the dying person and family are complex, it has been suggested that nursing diagnoses and interventions be combined under one heading entitled "terminal care syndrome."[38] As in nursing management of the grieving person, the primary nursing diagnosis for care of the dying person and family is anticipatory grieving.

Diagnostic Title	Possible Etiologic Factors
1. Anticipatory grieving	Loss of significant other, changes in family unit and roles

EXPECTED PATIENT OUTCOMES

Expected patient outcomes for the dying person and his or her family may include [23,35,38,53] but are not limited to:

1. Will meet psychologic needs and resolve feelings regarding imminent death
   Family will identify resources (external and internal) to deal with the patient's eventual death
   Will accept imminent death, will verbalize feelings, will accept support from family, friends, and nursing staff
   Patient and family will express their feelings and acknowledge the impact of the grieving process
   Will identify factors that can be controlled, will participate in care and decision making as possible
   Will experience a dignified death, congruent with his or her personal philosophy, culture, and advance directive decisions

INTERVENTIONS

1. Facilitating Resolution of Grief

To be of most assistance to dying persons and their families, nurses must be realistic about how much they can relieve suffering. Nurses cannot stop the dying process, nor can they take away the pain of loss. A realistic perspective helps make the experience better and facilitates grief. Nurses can intervene more effectively if they accept the fact that fear of pain and suffering is a natural part of facing death.[17,66]

The nursing needs of dying persons are the nursing needs of living persons. The range of activities is as broad as for any diverse population of patients, family, and significant others. Nursing interventions may occur either at home or in various institutional settings. Attention to physical care is a major part of caring for dying persons. Maintenance of comfort, both physical and emotional, is of primary importance to the dying patient. Teaching family members how to maintain the patient's comfort allows their participation and promotes their feelings of competence and well-being.[23,64] Family members may need help in recognizing how small gestures, such as gently rubbing lubricant on the dying person's lips or rinsing the person's face with a cool washcloth, can offer comfort. The patient's culture determines what suggestions the family will accept and what comforting interventions family members offer the dying patient.[8,58]

Nurses can also assist patients and families in maintaining control over their individual lives as much as possible to ensure dignity and self-esteem through the end of life.[35,64,66] Expert nursing behaviors have been identified that sensitively address the dying patient's and family's need for control in providing symptom relief, interpreting signs of dying, sharing control, and providing information (Table 6-4).[6,41,66]

Patient/Family Education

The family should be taught in simple terms the physiology of death. Explaining that the gradual slowing of body systems includes the gastrointestinal system may help the family accept the patient's refusal of foods or fluids. As death approaches, nausea, vomiting, and pain may result from overloading the gastrointestinal tract. Gurgling respirations, shortness of breath, and generalized body edema may result from trying to "push" fluids when body systems are slowing down.

The patient and family need information about what is being done to relieve pain and other distressing end-of-life symptoms, like terminal restlessness. Dispelling fears of addiction may help the dying person and family accept medication for pain or agitation when offered. The family can be encouraged to use nonpharmacologic methods of pain control, such as reading a favorite story to the patient or bringing in favorite music, when appropriate, to help the patient relax.[21,36]

The nurse also serves as a resource for reexamining treatment decisions and answering difficult questions regarding issues such as organ donation and autopsy. Listening to what the patient or family is asking is the key to knowing what information or support is needed. Even after advance directive choices are made, the dying patient or family may need to repeatedly talk through the decision and what it will mean.[6,23,65,66] Helping the family focus on respecting the patient's preferences can help clarify goals of care.

Nursing responsibilities include being knowledgeable about organized support systems, agencies, and independent resources within the community. Nurses in any health care setting need to be prepared to assist patients and their families in contacting and using these resources. Inquiries related to the many alternative modes of care for dying persons, such as hospice, home care, nursing home care, and other forms of institutional care, should be answered openly and honestly. If the nurse cannot answer the patient's or family's questions, they should be referred to those who can supply the answers.[35,58,64]

EVALUATION

To evaluate the effectiveness of nursing interventions, patient behaviors should be compared with those stated in the expected patient outcomes. Successful achievement of patient outcomes is indicated if:

1. Patient and family members share feelings regarding imminent death.
   Family members acknowledge their losses, and the impact of loss on the family.
   Patient receives support from family and friends.
   Patient and family begin to use coping skills and resources.
   Patient and family make decisions regarding end-of-life treatment and activities.
   Patient experiences a dignified natural death according to his or her wishes.

TABLE 6-4 Guidelines for Supportive Nursing Behaviors in Terminal Care

Key Areas	Positive Behaviors
Providing comfort	Reducing physical and psychologic pain
Responding to family	Meeting family's ongoing need for information Facilitating transition from focus on cure to palliation Helping members find something to do and reducing potential for future regret
Responding after death	Creating a peaceful scene for survivors Supporting realization by family that death has occurred Demonstrating respect during postmortem care
Responding to anger	Communicating with empathy and respect even when anger is directed at nurse Offering acknowledgment and redirecting to constructive outlets
Responding to colleagues	Providing emotional support and feedback
Finding personal growth	Defining a professional and personal commitment in caring for dying person Reflecting on stories of sharing the dying process with patients and their families

Adapted from McClement S, Degner L: Expert nursing behaviors in care of the dying adult in the intensive care unit, *Heart Lung* 24(5):408-419, 1995; Steeves R: Loss, grief, and the search for meaning, *Oncol Nurs Forum* 23(6):897-903, 1996.

Goals that are mutually set with the dying patient and family will be more achievable. Although accepting losses and death may be encouraged, helping the dying patient and family find some peace in the dying experience is a more realistic outcome.[6,10,35,72]

NURSES' GRIEF

Nurses also experience loss when a nurse-patient relationship ends with the death of the patient. It is important for nurses to recognize the universal experience, as well as signs of their own grieving. Losing a patient can remind nurses of other losses of patients, family, or friends. Nurses may view a patient's death as a personal failure, with a corresponding loss of control and self-esteem. If the nurse is unable to help prevent suffering or resolve a family conflict before a patient's death, the nurse may feel inadequate. It is crucial for nurses to evaluate the differences they have made for their patients and their families, even in the face of death. Recognition of specific successes and contributions leads to feelings of achievement and helps nurses cope with the loss. Cumulative loss over time can challenge nurses' well-being and professional satisfaction.[50,66]

Like patients and their families, nurses need a supportive environment in which to express their grief. Many institutions have established bereavement resources for health care workers, ranging from on-call employee assistance programs to walk-in pastoral care to group debriefing sessions with a trained facilitator. Peer support is an important source of validation and grief support. Peer support can be accomplished through formal or informal sharing of common experiences in a group setting. One-to-one interactions with a trusted peer or significant other may alleviate some of the stress related to working with dying persons.[35,66] Although potentially stressful, caring for patients and their families at the end of life offers nurses countless opportunities to make a difference in promoting quality of living and dying.

SPECIAL ISSUES IN BEREAVEMENT

Ethical Perspectives

To help a person die well is to support that person's sense of self-respect, dignity, and choice until the last moment of life. Achievement of this goal entails skilled and compassionate nursing care to maximize comfort and minimize suffering. The goal is to provide calm, sensitive, individualized nursing care to each person so that dying, the final human experience, is as free of pain and anxiety as possible.[2,9,18]

Historically the profession and activities of nursing have been concerned with life and based on two fundamental principles: (1) all people should live as whole persons and (2) all people should live long and healthful lives. The expectation has been that nurses and physicians will help to fulfill these principles.[38,68]

In the past, nurses and physicians fulfilled their obligations by striving to save lives. Death often was caused by infection and communicable disease. Many people died at young ages.[19,25] With advances in pharmaceuticals, anesthesia, surgical techniques, and life-sustaining technologies, persons who would have succumbed to life-threatening illnesses now seek treatment to restore health and function. The capacity to prolong life and to ease the pain and suffering of seriously ill persons has improved to a great extent. The improvement has been accompanied by some difficult consequences. Increasingly, deaths occur in institutions. In many instances, deaths occur in critical care units to the sound of monitors. More and more often, death is caused by someone's decision rather than by the failure of the body systems.[9]

Death becomes impersonal when the body and the tubes and machines become one and when there is only a deteriorating organ system present. The situation becomes so confusing that those involved have conferences to determine whether life or death is being prolonged.[43] Family members long to return to normal living. They search for help in making life-and-death decisions for loved ones who are no longer able to contribute to decision making. Staff members search for relief from a situation fraught with dilemmas.[9,23]

Discussions of issues such as "quality of life," "right to die," "death with dignity," "living wills," and "informed consent" in lay and professional literature demonstrate the extent and awareness of the conflicts associated with modern therapies that extend life, but at great cost.[9,55] Concern over decisions regarding life-and-death issues has led to the development of organizations that represent differing views. The Hemlock Society, the Society for the Right to Die, and the Americans United for Life[19] are examples of a few of these organizations.[49,54,57]

The question of who should decide under what circumstances is important. Other important questions include the following: What is death? What constitutes informed consent? When are therapies ordinary, and when are they extraordinary? Should all life be preserved, regardless of quality? Should pain be treated, even though the medication may shorten the life span? What constitutes euthanasia? Is there a distinction between active and passive euthanasia? Is suicide a person's right? All these questions create ethical issues that can make coping with death and dying overwhelming for patients, family members, and the health care team.[38]

Ethical Issues

Many ethical issues evolve around indications for medical and nursing interventions. These issues arise from questions such as the following: When should medical therapies be started or stopped? When should life supports be discontinued? What constitutes death?

Withholding or Withdrawing Treatment

Appropriate consideration of withholding or withdrawing specific therapy occurs when (1) the therapy offers no reasonable expectation of the patient's attaining any human awareness, (2) the therapy is proving medically ineffective and useless after sufficient trial, or (3) the therapy is perceived from the expressed point of view of the patient (or the decision-making representative) as cumulatively a greater burden than a benefit.[54,55,57]

When decisions are made to withhold or withdraw life-sustaining treatment, the goal of medical and nursing care focuses on keeping the patient comfortable, avoiding suffering and pain, and providing support, comfort, and care on a physical, emotional, and spiritual level. Identifying those procedures not directed to supportive care becomes more difficult once medical procedures designed to prolong life are withheld or withdrawn. Perhaps the most controversial area is that of determining the proportionate benefit and burden of medical (artificial) nutrition and hydration.[16,25,27] The issue of withdrawing treatment, once it is started, is also present.

Euthanasia

The term *euthanasia* comes from the Greek words meaning "good or pleasant death." It implies that under some circumstances a person may prefer death to life. Euthanasia, or "mercy killing," is a topic surrounded by controversy. At the present time, there is no agreement on whether death is ever preferable to life or on what constitutes euthanasia.[25,55]

The more common distinctions made when discussing euthanasia are those of active and passive and voluntary and involuntary. *Active euthanasia* refers to an act that directly and intentionally shortens a person's life. It is an act of commission. *Passive euthanasia* usually refers to an act of omission—letting death occur by either withholding or withdrawing treatment that might prolong a person's life.[54,55] When considering questions related to euthanasia, there is a continuum ranging from a strict belief in the sanctity of life (antieuthanasia, treating at all costs) to passive euthanasia (letting die) to active euthanasia (ending life, killing).

A persistent moral issue is the question of whether letting death occur is morally equivalent to killing, or whether omission is equivalent to commission. No action is an action. Both active and passive euthanasia are intentional choices. The distinction seems to be that of the intent of the action. The 1986 statement by the American Medical Association Council on Ethical and Judicial Affairs[1,19] holds that the patient and/or immediate family can decide to "discontinue all means of life-prolonging medical treatment" even "if death is not imminent but a patient's coma is beyond doubt irreversible." The New Jersey Supreme Court implicitly invoked this distinction when it held that judgments about therapy should be made in terms of the degree of invasiveness of the treatment and its chance of success.[55] Ethicists have distinguished ordinary treatment from extraordinary treatment by stating that ordinary treatment offers a reasonable prospect of benefit for the patient without excessive pain, expense, or inconvenience.[27,55]

In more direct terms, killing is wrong, but letting someone die in the sense of not instituting extraordinary efforts or by discontinuing extraordinary treatments is morally permissible. In fact, most physicians accept that killing a patient is morally wrong and thus not permissible, but in some circumstances it may become morally required to let a patient die.[9] Nurses generally accept the same view.

Suicide

Quality of living and quality of dying may be closely associated. A person with a terminal illness may assess the situation and decide that living with pain, disability, or despair is not living.[9,17,18] He or she may ask the question, Is it better to take measures to bring about a peaceful death than to continue in such a state?

Suicide, or voluntary euthanasia carried out by the individual on his or her own behalf, has been seen variously as an affirmation of life, a denial of life, and a questioning of life. The traditional religious teaching of the Western world since St. Augustine has condemned all forms of self-destruction. Suicide was and still is considered by some to be a sin and an interference with God's will.[40,55] Many assert that human beings do not have the power of disposal of their bodies. They can only treat their bodies as they choose in relation to self-preservation. These views are being challenged in society today as they have been in the past.[15] Some physicians suggest that under some circumstances, when death is imminent, persons who are severely ill should be helped by their physicians to commit suicide. They distinguish this element of the population from the lonely, elderly, and physically handicapped, for whom they do not advocate assisted euthanasia. They point out that although few laws exist in the United States to cover physician participation, they do exist in Uruguay, Switzerland, Peru, Japan, and Germany. Some cultures, such as the Japanese, and some individuals favor suicide over other negative values such as dishonor.[8,58]

Individual and societal views regarding suicide run the gamut from opposition to suicide under all conditions and at all costs, to suicide as justifiable under some conditions, to suicide as a person's right. The question of an individual's right to autonomy or self-determination is a basic consideration in discussing suicide. Those who oppose suicide under all conditions usually use some form of the argument that "life is a gift, and no one has the right to take a life." Those at the opposite end of the continuum argue that a person has the right to determine his or her own fate, even if it means destroying his or her own life. Other considerations in arguments opposing suicide include viewing suicide as cowardly, a crime against society, an insult against humanity, and an act that brings great pain to the survivors.[9,55]

Suicide is of particular concern to health care professionals who may be in a position to offer other alternatives and thus prevent it. It is difficult to evaluate what constitutes suicide. Is refusal to eat or to continue with prescribed therapies a form of suicide, or must there be an overt act, such as an overdose of medications? Is suicide always a voluntary act, or is a person driven to suicide by rejection of others or by pain that might have been controlled?[9,25,40] When is suicide justifiable in the person known to be dying? What do you do when a patient who is dying slowly and painfully asks for your assistance in ending it all?

Nurses and physicians are committed to another imperative—to never abandon care.[10,55,66] Never abandoning care includes ensuring that a dying person is not alone, that others are aware of his or her dying, and that he or she is free of pain and anxiety. It is not an obligation to assist in ending life. In fact, the ethical basis for suicide prevention is the psychologic thesis that a suicide attempt is often a cry for help rather than a firm decision to end one's life.[15,34,50] Thus nurses and physicians have a legal and ethical obligation to assess and recognize suicidal risk and depression in patients and to make efforts to assist them in receiving counseling.[40,55]

The impact of pain is really a quality-of-life question that can best be evaluated by the dying individual experiencing the pain.[17,18] If quality of life is determined by the person living the life, is suicide a purely personal decision? It seems that the quality of life of survivors also should be considered. When the survivors have had no prior warning or part in the decision, and when the suicide is not perceived as an action to achieve comfort, the anguish to the survivors is great. For some the anguish never ends; grief is compounded by guilt, shame, and even anger.[50,72]

Suicide may be a form of control by the dying person, or it may be a form of escape. Some dying people seek an escape from loss of control over the event of dying; others seek an end to suffering.[17,40,50] Nurses can be influential in providing dying persons and their families with a sense of control by assisting with problems such as pain control, bowel and bladder control, and depression. They can decrease the uncertainty of the situation by explaining what the dying person and family can anticipate over the coming days. Nurses can involve other members of the interdisciplinary team in offering the dying patient and/or family tangible support through referrals.[27,35] Music, art therapy, and imagery can be used to help patients and their family members express and work through the process of grieving, as well as provide relaxation and diversion from symptom distress[5,21,36] (see Complementary & Alternative Therapies box). Pastoral care can offer opportunities for dying patients and their families to make sense of their experience in terms of their religious beliefs.[55] Social workers can help facilitate family communication and end-of-life planning when conflicts are present.[66] By coordinating involvement of the interdisciplinary team, nurses can further enhance quality of life.[10,52,66]

Definitions of Death

Much controversy surrounds the question, "What is death?" Is death the irreversible cessation of respiration and circulation, or is death the irreversible cessation of all functions of the brain, including the brainstem? In addition, different cultures have different definitions of death.[8,58]

The term *brain dead,* in use for some time, still causes much confusion. Originally it referred to a person whose lungs were activated by a ventilator but whose centers in the brainstem were destroyed. Removal from the support system would result in death as a result of the inability of the person to resume spontaneous breathing. *Brain dead* is also used to mean that the person is dead in the sense that a functioning brain is the seat of identity. What decision can be made about persons in a "persistent vegetative state"? They show no evidence of cortical functioning but continue to have sustained capacity for spontaneous breathing and heartbeat.[6,9,19,55]

Advocates use definitions that reflect their values and provide them with a rationale to act. Each appeal or action has its own consequences. For example, some definitions of brain death provide more latitude for organ transplantation and experimentation. The rationale for this latitude is that the removal of organs from the person who is brain dead aids the living. This is a worthy endeavor, but does retrieving organs lead to violation of the dead? What are the constraints? Who gives consent for donation?

There are no clear rules that dictate decisions in these matters. Decisions are accompanied by conflict, insecurity, and discomfort. The conflict and emotions that accompany decisions about the life or death of another are entirely appropriate because they are irreversible.[27,55]

The important factor in any ethical issue, regardless of whether it is dealing with euthanasia, suicide, or treatment decisions, is to be aware of the values or forces that lead us to make the decisions we do. An understanding of our own values and perspectives, as well as of formal ethical systems, does not give explicit answers to dilemmas. However, it does help us to be consistent and communicate with others in a way that is understandable. This does not ensure agreement, but it does facilitate discussion and attention to different perspectives and to the consequences of actions.

Complementary & Alternative Therapies

Potential Evidence-Based Benefit(s) of Music, Art Therapy, and Imagery

- Increased self-awareness
- Decreased perception of stress
- Increased endorphins and sense of well-being
- Increased lymphocytes and immune response
- Decreased anxiety and fear
- Decreased perception of pain
- Decreased nausea and vomiting
- Increased communication with significant others
- Increased sense of hope
- Increased peacefulness over anticipated loss

Source: Bartrop R et al: Depressed lymphocyte function after bereavement, *Lancet* 16:834, 1997; Mariano C: Holistic integrative therapies in palliative care. In Matzo M, Sherman D, editors: *Palliative care nursing: quality care to the end of life,* New York, 2001, Springer.

Critical Thinking Questions

1. A 60-year-old woman is admitted for evaluation of progressive back pain, weakness, and weight loss. She is scheduled for magnetic resonance imaging (MRI) to rule out a possible spinal cord tumor. The nurse is preparing the patient for the MRI scan when the patient remarks, "Why bother? I am going to die like my father no matter what." How should the nurse respond?
2. A 45-year-old man with advanced lung cancer and multiple metastases is admitted to the hospital with a do-not-resuscitate (DNR) order. Since requesting DNR status, he has become unresponsive. The patient's wife wants the physician to reverse her husband's DNR order and asks the nurse for help. How should the nurse respond?
3. A 24-year-old woman who suffered severe head injuries following a motor vehicle accident is near death. Her family is at the bedside around the clock and asks the nurse if they can be involved in her physical care. Develop a plan to enable the family to care for their loved one and assist them in the grieving process.

References

1. American Medical Association: *Elements of quality care for patients in the last phase of life,* Chicago, 1997, AMA.
2. American Nurses Association: *Position statement on the nurse's role in end-of-life decisions,* Washington, DC, 1997, ANA.
3. American Psychiatric Association: *Diagnostic and statistical manual of mental disorders: DSM-IV-TR,* ed 4, Washington, DC, 2000, APA.
4. Aquilera D, Messick J: *Crisis intervention: theory and methodology,* St Louis, 1994, Mosby.
5. Bartrop R et al: Depressed lymphocyte function after bereavement, *Lancet* 16:834, 1997.
6. Berry P, Griffie J: Planning the actual death. In Ferrell B, Coyle N, editors: *Palliative nursing,* New York, 2001, Oxford University Press.
7. Bowlby J: Attachment and loss: retrospect and prospect, *Am J Orthopsychiatry* 52(4):644-677, 1972.
8. Brown-Saltzman K: Multicultural perspectives in palliative care, *Oncol Nurs Forum* 3:41-47, 1994.
9. Byock I: *Dying well: the prospect for growth at the end of life,* Evanston, Ill, 1997, Riverhead.
10. Callanan M, Kelley P: *Final gifts,* New York, 1997, Bantam.
11. Clark C: Posttraumatic stress disorder: how to support healing, *Am J Nurs* 97(8):27-32, 1997.
12. Davies B: *Fading away: the experience of transition in families with terminal illness,* Amityville, NY, 1995, Baywood.
13. Ebersole P: *Toward healthy aging: human needs and nursing response,* ed 5, St Louis, 1998, Mosby.
14. Engel G: Is grief a disease? *Psychosom Med* 3(1):18-22, 1961.
15. Engel G: A life setting conducive to illness: the giving-up–given-up complex, *Ann Intern Med* 69(2):293-300, 1968.
16. Farnslow-Brunjes C: Hope: offering comfort and support for dying patients, *Nursing 97* 27:54-57, 1997.
17. Ferrell B: *Suffering,* Boston, 1997, Jones & Bartlett.
18. Ferrell B et al: Dignity in dying, *Nurs Manage* 31(9):52-57, 2000.
19. Freud S: *Instincts and their vicissitudes: collected papers,* New York, 1915, Basic Books.
20. Gilbert M et al: Determining the relationship between end of life expressed in advance directives and resuscitation efforts during cardiopulmonary resuscitation, *Outcomes Manage Nurs Pract* 5(2):87-92, 2001.
21. Ginnette C et al: Transformation through grieving: art and the bereaved, *Holist Nurs Pract* 13(1):68-69, 1998.
22. Glick I, Weiss RS, Parkes CM: *The first year of bereavement,* New York, 1974, John Wiley & Sons.
23. Goetschius S: Caring for families: the other patient in palliative care. In Matzo M, Sherman D, editors: *Palliative care nursing: quality care to the end of life,* New York, 2001, Springer.
24. Hegge M, Fischer C: Grief responses of senior and elderly widows: practice implications, *J Gerontol Nurs* 26(2):35-43, 2000.
25. Kemp C: *Terminal illness: a guide to nursing care,* ed 2, Philadelphia, 1999, JB Lippincott.
26. Koenig BA, Gates-Williams J: Understanding cultural differences in caring for dying patients. In Caring for patients at the end of life (special issue), *West J Med* 163:244-249, 1997.
27. Kramer L et al: The nurse's role in interdisciplinary and palliative care. In Ferrell B, Coyle N, editors: *Palliative nursing,* New York, 2001, Springer.
28. Kübler-Ross E: *On death and dying,* New York, 1969, Macmillan.
29. Kübler-Ross E: *Living with death and dying,* New York, 1997, Touchstone.
30. Laferriere R: Orem's theory of practice: hospice nursing care, *Home Healthc Nurse* 13(5):50-54, 1995.
31. Lark J, Gatti C: Compliance with advance directives: nurses' view, *Crit Care Nurs Q* 22(3):65-71, 1999.
32. Larson D: *The helper's journey,* Champaign, Ill, 1993, Research.
33. Lev E, Munroe B, McCorkle R: A shortened version of an instrument measuring bereavement, *J Nurs Stud* 30(3):213-226, 1993.
34. Lindemann E: Symptomatology and management of acute grief, *Am J Psychiatry* 151(6 suppl):155-160, 1944.
35. Loney M: Death, dying, and grief in the face of cancer. In Burke C, editor: *Psychosocial dimensions of oncology nursing care,* Pittsburgh, 1998, Oncology Nursing Society.
36. Mariano C: Holistic integrative therapies in palliative care. In Matzo M, Sherman D, editors: *Palliative care nursing: quality care to the end of life,* New York, 2001, Springer.
37. Martocchio B: Authenticity, belonging, emotional closeness, and self-representation, *Oncol Nurs Forum* 14(4):23-27, 1985.
38. Martocchio BC: Grief and bereavement: healing through hurt, *Nurs Clin North Am* 20(2):327-341, 1985.
39. Maslow A: *Motivation and personality,* New York, 1954, Harper & Brothers.
40. Massie MJ, Gagnon P, Holland JC: Depression and suicide in patients with cancer, *J Pain Symptom Manage* 9(5):325-338, 1994.
41. McClement S, Degner L: Expert nursing behaviors in care of the dying adult in the intensive care unit, *Heart Lung* 24(5):408-419, 1995.
42. McMillan S: The quality of life of patients with cancer receiving hospice care, *Oncol Nurs Forum* 23(8):1221-1228, 1996.
43. Metzger M, Kaplan K: *Transforming death in America: a state of the nation report,* Washington, DC, 2001, Last Acts.
44. Oaks J, Ezell G: *Dying and death: coping, caring, understanding,* Scottsdale, Ariz, 1993, Goruch.
45. Parkes CM, Weiss RS: *Recovery from bereavement,* New York, 1983, Basic Books.
46. Pilkington F: The lived experience of grieving the loss of an important other, *Nurs Sci Q* 6(3):130-138, 1993.
47. Prigerson H et al: Complicated grief and bereavement-related depression as distinct disorders: preliminary empirical validation in elderly bereaved spouses, *Am J Psychiatry* 152(1):22-30, 1995.
48. Radziewicz R: Go light your world, *Oncol Nurs Forum* 24(10):1689-1694, 1997.
49. Ramsey C: Legal aspects of palliative care. In Matzo M, Sherman D, editors: *Palliative care nursing: quality care to the end of life,* New York, 2001, Springer.
50. Rando T: *Treatment of complicated mourning,* Champaign, Ill, 1993, Research Press.
51. Rando T, editor: *Clinical dimensions of anticipatory mourning: theory and practice in working with the dying, their loved ones, and their caregivers,* Champaign, Ill, 2000, Research Press.
52. Ray C: Seven ways to empower dying patients, *Am J Nurs* (5):56-57, 1996.
53. Sanders C: *Grief: the mourning after—dealing with adult bereavement,* ed 2, New York, 1999, John Wiley & Sons.
54. Scanlon C: Public policy and end-of-life care: the nurse's role. In Ferrell B, Coyle N, editors: *Palliative nursing,* New York, 2001, Oxford University Press.
55. Schwarz J: Ethical aspects of palliative care. In Matzo M, Sherman D, editors: *Palliative care nursing: quality care to the end of life,* New York, 2001, Springer.
56. Selder F: Life transition theory: the resolution of uncertainty, *Nurs Health Care* 10(8):437-451, 1992.
57. Sheehan D, Foreman W: *Hospice and palliative care: concepts and practice,* Sudbury, Mass, 1996, Jones & Bartlett.
58. Sherman D: Spirituality and culturally competent palliative care. In Matzo M, Sherman D, editors: *Palliative care nursing: quality care to the end of life,* New York, 2001, Springer.
59. Solari-Twadell P et al: The pinwheel model of bereavement, *Image J Nurs Sch* 27(4):323-326, 1995.
60. Spiegel D: *Living beyond limits: new hope and help for facing life-threatening illness,* New York, 1993, Times Books.
61. Spitzer A, Bar-Tal Y, Golander H: Social support: how does it really work? *J Adv Nurs* 22:850-854, 1995.
62. Stanley K: Silence is not golden: conversations with the dying, *Clin J Oncol Nurs* 4(1):34-40, 2000.

63. Steele L: The death surround: factors influencing the grief experience of survivors, *Oncol Nurs Forum* 15(5):575-581, 1990.
64. Super A: The context of palliative care in progressive illness. In Ferrell B, Coyle N, editors: *Palliative nursing,* New York, 2001, Oxford University Press.
65. Tipton K: How to discuss death with patients and families, *Nursing 99* 29(9):10-12, 1999.
66. Vachon M: The nurse's role: the world of palliative care nursing. In Ferrell B, Coyle N, editors: *Palliative nursing,* New York, 2001, Oxford University Press.
67. Viorst J: *Necessary losses,* New York, 1986, Simon & Schuster.
68. Watson J: *Human science and human care,* New York, 1988, National League for Nursing.
69. Weisman A: *On dying and denying: a psychiatric study of terminality,* New York, 1972, Behavior.
70. Wolfelt A: *The journey through grief: reflections on healing,* Fort Collins, Col, 1997, Companion.
71. Wolfelt A: A systems approach to healing the bereaved child, *Bereavement,* 10:8-11, 1997.
72. Worden W: *Grief counseling and grief therapy,* ed 3, New York, 1995, Springer.
73. Worden W: *Children and grief: when a parent dies,* New York, 1996, Guilford.
74. Zerwekh J: The truth-tellers: how hospice nurses help patients confront death, *Am J Nurs* 94(2):30-34, 1994.

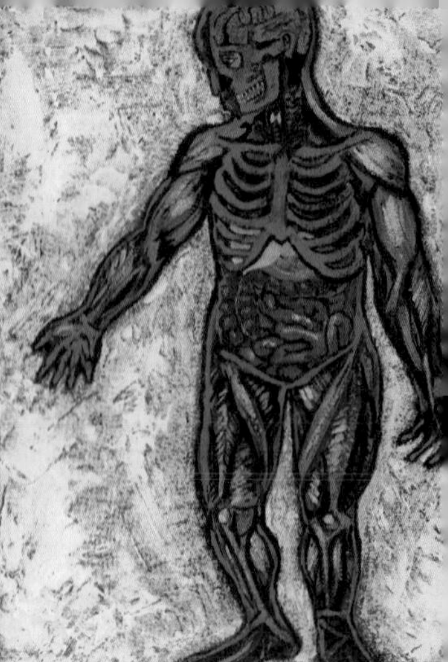

7 Emergency Care

Kim Bender Bushnell

Objectives

After studying this chapter, the learner should be able to:

1. Discuss the unique challenges of nursing practice in an emergency care setting.
2. List nursing interventions that increase patient and staff safety in the emergency department.
3. Identify the components of an initial trauma assessment.
4. Describe the principles of collaborative management of the trauma patient.
5. Discuss the role of the emergency department nurse in caring for a person who was sexually assaulted.
6. Outline the guidelines for care of victims of intimate partner violence.

Emergency nursing is a diverse and multidimensional specialty area of professional nursing. It crosses all age groups and includes care that ranges from disease management and injury prevention to lifesaving resuscitative measures. Astute decision-making abilities, analytic and scientific inquiry, and critical thinking skills are very much a part of the practice of the emergency department (ED) nurse.

The demands on emergency nursing continue to grow and become more challenging as health care changes. A continued increase in the incidence of violence and the numbers of uninsured, and the advent of managed care provide for a challenging practice arena. Managed care, one of the primary financing mechanisms for health care, is of great importance in current ED practice as insurance programs increasingly dictate who receives care, what care can be provided, and which care settings may be used. The challenge of providing health care to the large numbers of uninsured and underinsured individuals and families falls heavily on departments of emergency services, which are commonly used in lieu of a primary care provider. Combined market forces and legislation seem to indicate that managed care payment mechanisms will continue to be a major force in health care for the foreseeable future.

This chapter on emergency care provides an overview of the unique environment of emergency nursing, triage practice, trauma assessment, and the impact of violence on emergency nursing practice.

SCOPE OF PRACTICE FOR EMERGENCY NURSING

The scope of emergency nursing practice encompasses assessment, analysis, nursing diagnosis, outcome identification, planning, implementation of interventions and evaluation of human responses to perceived, actual, or potential; sudden or urgent; and physical or psychosocial problems that are primarily episodic or acute, and that occur in a variety of settings.[3] Treatment of these problems may require minimal care or lifesaving measures, patient and family education, appropriate referral, and discharge planning. The quality of practice depends on the nurse's psychomotor, interpersonal, and decision-making skills. Care is delivered in a variety of settings, including the acute care facility, the prehospital and military settings; clinics and health maintenance organizations; ambulatory care centers; and business, educational, industrial, and correctional institutions. Some of the many characteristics unique to emergency nursing practice are listed in Box 7-1.

Emergency nursing activities occur in a sequential arrangement or flow pattern based on the acuity of the person's condition. Emergency nursing includes provision of care to persons whose problems range from nonacute to life threatening. In fact, most persons who request ED service are ambulatory and have nonacute conditions; therefore many EDs have developed a specific care area for these individuals. Some hospitals use the terms *fast track* or *urgent care* to identify a designated area in or near the ED for persons with nonacute conditions. These areas may be open only after physicians' offices have closed, or they may provide quick service 12 to 24 hours a day. Fast-track or urgent care areas have been developed because these care environments are less expensive treatment areas. Persons treated in these areas require less time with the health care staff because of the nature of their signs and symptoms. Regardless of whether EDs are designed to separate the nonacute from the acutely ill person, and regardless of ability to pay, every person requesting care must be evaluated on arrival.

BOX 7-1 Characteristics Unique to Emergency Nursing Practice

1. Assessment, analysis, nursing diagnosis, planning, implementation of interventions and treatment of emergent, urgent, and nonurgent individuals of all ages
2. Triage and prioritization
3. Emergency operations preparedness
4. Stabilization and resuscitation
5. Crisis intervention for unique patient populations, such as sexual assault survivors
6. Provision of care in uncontrolled or unpredictable environments
7. Consistency as much as possible across the continuum of care

Modified from Emergency Nurses Association: *Standards of emergency nursing practice,* ed 4, St Louis, 1999, Mosby.

BOX 7-2 Four-Color–Coded Disaster Triage System

0–Black: Dead

1–Red: Critical or Life-Threatening

These victims have a reasonable chance of survival only if they receive immediate treatment. Emergency treatment is initiated immediately and continued during transportation. This category includes victims with respiratory insufficiency, cardiac arrest, hemorrhage, and severe abdominal injury.

2–Yellow: Serious

These victims can wait for transportation after they receive initial emergency treatment. They include victims with immobilized closed fractures, soft-tissue injuries without hemorrhage, and burns on less than 40% of the body.

3–Green: Minimal

Victims in this category are ambulatory, have minor tissue injuries, and may be dazed. They can be treated by nonprofessionals and held for observation if necessary.

Triage

Triage is a vital function in all EDs. More than 100 million people seek ED care in the United States each year.[10] All patients presenting to the ED need to be accurately triaged. A registered nurse fulfills the role of triage nurse. The word *triage* is derived from the French word *trier,* meaning "to pick out or sift."[12] The triage system is used to identify those patients whose condition is most seriously compromised so that they are the first to receive medical intervention. The choosing, sorting out, and placing of priorities on care have been practiced since patient care began and have been used extensively in disasters and wars. A standardized four-color-coded triage system (used during disasters) quietly communicates to all health care providers the priority of treatment (Box 7-2). However, triage as a systematic method to be used by health care personnel in both prehospital situations and EDs has come into its own.

The most important function of triage is to provide an initial assessment of patients so that the right person is directed to the right place at the right time. This assessment is the basis for the assigning of a triage urgency category (see Complementary & Alternative Therapies box).

Persons who need to be seen immediately have an emergent or life-threatening situation; persons who need to be seen as soon as possible have an urgent condition that has the potential of becoming a life-threatening situation; and persons

Complementary & Alternative Therapies

Assessment Question

The topic of alternative and complementary therapies is important for emergency nurses. Many patients are using unconventional treatments but not informing members of the health care team. It is imperative that both emergency nurses and physicians ask about the patient's use of these therapies, including herbal preparations.

Some therapies can have side effects and/or potentiate the effects of some medications. Many people have a false sense of security when a product is declared "natural." Garlic is a natural product and has an antihypertensive effect but may also increase bleeding times unbeknown to the patient.

Some common therapies include:

Acupuncture	Naturopathic medicine
Herbal preparations	Nutrition and nutritional supplements
Homeopathy	Reflexology
Imagery	Spirituality
Music therapy	Therapeutic touch

Obtaining correct information regarding use of alternative and complementary therapies during the triage or assessment process is imperative.

Source: Milton D: Using alternative and complementary therapies in the emergency setting, *J Emerg Nurs* 24(6):500-508, 1998.

Research

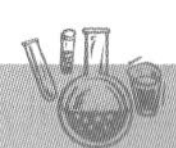

Reference: Fry M: Triage nurses order x-rays for patients with isolated distal limb injuries: a 12-month ED study, *J Emerg Nurs* 71(16):17, 2001.

The objective of this study was to determine whether triage nurses could safely, accurately, and appropriately order x-ray studies for patients with distal limb injuries. Lengthy waiting times tend to increase anxiety for both patients and personnel. The nursing staff at the study institution decided to investigate ways to improve service delivery, such as expediting triage care by extending their triage role to include ordering distal limb x-rays. All adult patients presenting to the emergency department (ED) of a tertiary teaching hospital for 12 months with distal limb injuries were eligible for the study. Excluded were those with severe pain or evidence of neurovascular compromise. All ED distal limb x-ray studies ordered during the study period were analyzed for type, frequency, and abnormality. The conclusion was that with structured education, triage nurses safely assessed patients and ordered appropriate x-ray studies before physician assessment. Data indicated that all staff believed that this new triage practice had increased patient satisfaction and improved patient flow and waiting times.

who can be seen as time allows have nonurgent conditions, with no life-threatening symptoms at the time of presentation and no symptoms that typically become life threatening. This system of prioritization of patients is used by the Emergency Medical Service (EMS) system. The use of these common terms provides for understanding of the situation and more uniform prehospital and in-hospital communication and care. Fast track or urgent care areas treat patients with urgent or nonurgent conditions. Persons with emergent conditions are seen in the main ED area (see Research box).

To increase efficiency and best outcome for patients, many EDs have developed a chest pain center (CPC) within their department. The goal of the CPC is the immediate diagnosis and treatment of acute myocardial infarction. Patients are triaged directly into the CPC with a triage category of emergent. Box 7-3 presents a listing of the typical emergent, urgent, and nonurgent complaints of persons seeking care at a level I trauma center over a 24-hour period. Level I trauma centers are usually based in large metropolitan teaching hospitals. The levels of trauma care are covered later in this chapter.

Triage and Managed Care

All ED health care providers must be well informed about the provisions of the Consolidated Omnibus Reconciliation Acts (COBRA) and the Emergency Medical Treatment and Active Labor Act (EMTALA), which outline guidelines for service provision and reimbursement in EDs. The EMTALA provisions require that each patient who comes to the ED must receive a screening examination to determine whether an emergency condition exists. Many patients come to the ED without preauthorization from their managed care organization. The responsibility for providing a medical screening examination and securing preauthorization falls on the ED staff.

Triage and Computerized Tracking

A universal concern in all EDs is patient flow. Computerized tracking provides clinicians with an automated patient locator board. Patient name, arrival time, chief complaint, and caregiver names are available on the screen. Registration and triage personnel are always aware of open beds and the location of patients via the patient tracking systems.

BOX 7-3 Presenting Complaints of Persons Seeking Emergent, Urgent, or Nonurgent Care at a University Teaching Hospital Over a 24-Hour Period

- Abdominal pain
- Abdominal problem
- Alcohol intoxication
- Assault
- Asthma
- Back pain
- Behavioral problem
- Broken tooth
- Cardiopulmonary arrest
- Cardiovascular problem (chest pain)
- Cough
- Depression
- Diarrhea
- Difficulty breathing
- Dizziness
- Earache
- Electrical shock
- Environmental injury (heat stroke)
- Eye injury
- Eye problem (blurred vision)
- Eye problem (infection)
- Eye problem (conjunctivitis/pink eye)
- Fever
- Foreign body removal
- Genital problem (sore and discharge)
- GI bleeding (black stools)
- GI bleeding (bloody stools)
- GI bleeding (vomiting blood)
- Head injury
- Head wound (cut/scrape)
- Headache
- Head/neck problem (stiff neck)
- Hernia
- Insect bite
- Joint pain
- Lower extremity injury (sprain/strain)
- Lower extremity problem (swelling, no history of injury)
- Lower extremity wound (cut)
- Meningitis
- Multiple injuries (auto accident)
- Multiple problems (achy, dizzy, tired)
- Multiple trauma
- Multiple wounds (cuts, scrapes from fall)
- Nausea/vomiting
- Neck injury
- Neck wound
- Neurologic problem (confusion)
- Neurologic problem (weak one side, unable to walk)
- Nosebleed
- Overdose
- Palpitations (heart racing, skipping beats)
- Pregnancy problem (abdominal pain)
- Pregnancy problem (bleeding)
- Rash
- Respiratory problem (drowning)
- Seizures
- Shortness of breath
- Sick (feel bad, tired, irritable)
- Trunk injury
- Trunk wound
- Unresponsive
- Upper extremity injury
- Upper extremity problem (swelling, inflammation)
- Upper extremity wound (cut)
- Urinary problem (burning, pain, frequency, blood in urine)
- Vaginal bleeding (nonpregnant)
- Vomiting
- Weakness
- Wheezing

Tracking systems take advantage of abbreviations, symbols, color codes, and icons to note current patient status. Many systems also use color codes to identify which caregivers have already seen a patient, as well as admission or discharge pending information. The tracking system can also be used to improve efficiency in gathering triage information during initial patient assessment and is an excellent tool for research and analysis of department utilization. Computerized tracking also improves communication among department personnel.

Critical Pathways in Emergency Departments

Time tracking of patients in the ED is essential for many reasons, such as to ensure quality of care practice, to track and trend workload activity, and to have appropriate staffing to match workload. Many hospitals are using critical (clinical) pathways to achieve these goals. Use of critical pathways in the ED increases the consistency and rapidity of diagnosis and treatment, with earlier initiation of intervention being key to effectiveness.[8] For example, a person with an arm injury and signs of a fracture will have an x-ray examination to determine the type of fracture. A critical pathway for this type of patient identifies the x-ray examination as the major diagnostic activity to be accomplished and a time frame for completion, such as 20 minutes after the assessment and evaluation by the ED physician and the ED nurse. Once mutually identified interventions, outcomes, and times are determined for a particular patient population or diagnosis, the nurse can assume that the interventions and outcomes should be completed within the time period. Critical pathways are tools and guidelines that provide standardization of care, consistency with interventions, and a means to evaluate effectiveness of care. Thus critical pathways promote quality of care, increase effectiveness of care, increase staff communication, and increase staff and patient satisfaction.

Communication

Maintaining effective communication in any clinical setting is a challenge; however, in the ED the challenge is compounded because of the number of health care personnel involved in the care of the patient and because of the emergent situation. All health care providers should keep in mind that communication is the process through which the patient-clinician relationship develops. The patient may base his or her perception of care provided on the communication and interpersonal skills demonstrated by the nurse, as well as the level of the nurse's competence.

Regardless of the type or location of the emergent incident, one extremely important communication need is the ability to access emergency help. All agencies and communities that provide health care have a code or system that activates a call for help within an extremely short period. Most communities in the United States (but not all) have a 911 access number for activating the EMS system. The chain of survival following emergent injuries requires excellent communication skills to access care and initiate appropriate emergency services.

Managing violent situations in the ED also requires the nurse to use excellent communication skills. Nurses need to be able to deescalate a pattern of violent behavior before it is out of control. Appropriate techniques to deescalate such a situation include a calm and interested demeanor, a lowered and controlled voice, and a willingness to avoid interrupting the verbal responses of those involved. If a nurse finds it impossible to apply these communication skills in a particular situation, another nurse may be asked to take over or assist.

Environment

The nurse working in the emergency arena focuses on controlling environmental factors that can infringe on quality care. Noise is a major environmental factor and a significant stressor in the ED. Nurses must make an effort to work quietly and to identify this approach (quiet work) as a standard for the ED. As new EDs are being constructed, soundproofing is being included whenever possible. However, many other noise-controlling behaviors can be implemented, including:

- Setting all telephones on soft ring
- Equipping all dispatch radios with telecommunication devices that limit the broadcast to one person (e.g., earphones, telephones)
- Setting alarms on monitors as low as safely possible
- Closing doors quietly and as appropriate
- Use of pagers (on vibrate mode) to locate staff, rather than overhead paging
- Implementation of these guidelines greatly enhances the quality of the caregiving environment.

Emergency Environment and Violence

Treating critically ill and injured patients is stressful enough without the addition of violent acts. It is estimated that between 1 and 2 million workplace assaults occur annually and almost half of these occur in health care institutions. Nurses are more likely to suffer nonfatal injuries while at work than any other professional.[2]

Violence is often triggered by stressors that patients and families are unable to cope with effectively. Stress, pain, fear, long waits, and noxious stimuli are environmental variables that may trigger a violent act.[7] Other environmental triggers are unpleasant waiting areas, lack of access to refreshments, insufficient and uncomfortable seating, and lack of feedback to patients and significant others about a patient's condition or progress. Attention to these details deescalates the potential for violent behavior and provides a safer working environment.

External violence in the ED setting has increased in association with the continued increase in street violence, family violence, and drug and alcohol use. Nurses are often called on to manage both the victim and the victimizer in the health care setting. Health care providers always need to be extremely aware of their environment and its potential for violence. Triage nurses and registration staff are at greater risk because they are often situated at the entrance of the ED and in a more isolated location. Steps to increase security within the ED are reviewed in Box 7-4.

BOX 7-4 Measures to Increase Security in the Emergency Department

1. Limited access (should be as few entrances to the ED treatment area as possible)
2. Metal detectors
3. Security personnel at entrances
4. Secure triage areas
5. Placement of panic buttons
6. Video cameras
7. Enforce visitor control measures
8. Protective glass

Legal and Forensic Considerations

Nurses must be aware of state and local regulations that require mandatory reporting of cases of suspected child and elder abuse, accidental deaths, and suicides. Each ED has written policies and procedures to assist nurses and other health care providers in making appropriate reports.

Physical evidence is real, tangible, or latent matter that can be visualized, measured, or analyzed. ED nurses are often called on to collect evidence, and all hospitals should have policies governing the collection of forensic evidence. It is of utmost importance that the chain of custody be followed to ensure the integrity and credibility of the evidence. The chain of custody is the pathway that evidence follows from the time it is collected until it has served its purpose in the legal investigation of an incident.

TOPICS OF CONCERN IN EMERGENCY CARE

Trauma

Trauma is the most common cause of death in persons younger than 44 years old and is the fifth leading cause of death in persons of all age groups. More than 400 Americans die each day from injuries resulting primarily from motor vehicle crashes, firearms, poisonings, suffocation, falls, fires, and drowning. Unintentional injuries are a major source of morbidity and mortality in the United States; therefore accident prevention is a major public health goal.[13] The U.S. Public Health Service and the American Public Health Association actively promote accident prevention. National health care objectives for the year 2010 related to accidents, derived under the direction of the Department of Health and Human Services, are listed in the Healthy People 2010 box. Suggestions for achieving these goals include:

- Enacting laws
- Requiring use of vehicle safety belts, motorcycle helmets, child restraints, and bicycle helmets
- Requiring that handguns be designed to minimize the likelihood of accidental discharge, especially by children
- Requiring adoption of a graduated driver licensing model law
- Increasing functional smoke detectors to at least on every floor
- Teaching injury prevention and control in all schools

Healthy People 2010
Objectives Related to Unintentional Injury Prevention

1. Reduce deaths caused by unintentional injuries.
2. Reduce nonfatal unintentional injuries.
3. Reduce deaths caused by motor vehicle crashes.
4. Reduce pedestrian deaths on public roads.
5. Increase use of safety belts.
6. Increase use of child restraints.
7. Increase the proportion of motorcyclists using helmets.
8. Increase the number of states and the District of Columbia that have adopted a graduated driver licensing model law.
9. Increase the number of states and the District of Columbia with laws requiring bicycle helmets for bicycle riders.
10. Reduce residential fire deaths to no more than 1.2 per 100,000 people.
11. Reduce deaths from falls.
12. Reduce drowning.
13. Reduce hospital emergency department visits for nonfatal dog bite injuries.
14. Increase functioning residential smoke alarms.
15. Reduce deaths by poisonings.

Modified from US Department of Health and Human Services: *Healthy people 2010: understanding and improving health,* Washington, DC, 2000, USDHHS.

- Requiring use of effective head, face, eye, and mouth protection for sports that pose risk of injury

Prevention of Trauma

Accidents are the underlying cause of trauma. Although accidents have no single cause, human error is a predominant factor. Onset of illness such as a cerebrovascular accident or myocardial infarction accounts for only a small percentage of accidents. More than one half of all accidents involving motor vehicles are the result of improper driving practices or human error. A much smaller percentage of accidents are caused by vehicle defects or poor road conditions. Alcohol is a factor in approximately 50% to 75% of all fatal motor vehicle crashes. Young drivers are significantly overrepresented in alcohol- and drug-related crashes. Illegal drugs, as well as many legally prescribed medications, can slow reaction time and contribute to the occurrence of accidents.

The home is a dangerous place. Falls account for about half the deaths that result from trauma in the home, and they are usually preventable. Falls commonly occur as persons, particularly the elderly, walk from room to room. Some falls are caused by heavily waxed floors, loose rugs, poor lighting, scattered toys, and other preventable conditions (Box 7-5). People fall from roofs, windows, high ladders, and steps, often because they have not used proper equipment or taken appropriate precautions.

Burns and other injuries result from improper use of solvents and cleaning agents. The number of electrical appliances used in the home has increased the danger of electrical shock and fire from overloaded circuits. Many persons die in fires caused by cigarette ashes dropped on furniture or rugs or dis-

BOX 7-5 Measures to Increase Home Safety

Floors

Anchor large rugs and carpets.
Use nonskid backing on small rugs.
Avoid floor wax unless nonskid.

Stairs

Ensure uniform height.
Use nonskid treads.
Mark risers with contrasting color.
Have strong hand rails at appropriate heights.
Have adequate lighting.

Bathroom

Have hand rails in tub or shower and by toilet.
Use skid proof bath mats.
Apply treads in tub or shower floor.
Have shower seat for elderly or unstable persons.

Other

Have smoke alarms on every level.
Have working fire extinguisher in kitchen.
Have escape ladder if home is more than 1 story.
Secure all medications and cleaning products out of reach of children.

carded in waste containers, and by cigarettes that are dropped when the smoker falls asleep. Homeowners with older heating systems need to be encouraged to have these systems checked for gas leaks or other unsafe features. Members of a household should hold fire drills and know what to do if a fire occurs. Smoke alarms in kitchens, bedrooms, hallways, and basements should be considered essential.

Children are the victims of most accidental poisonings, although adults also are at risk. All poisonous substances should be kept in original containers, tightly capped, and *never* placed in containers such as soft-drink containers, drinking glasses, or cups. Medications should never be removed from the source bottle and placed in an unmarked bottle. Likewise, medications should never be taken from unmarked or poorly marked containers.

Head injuries are the most serious type of injury sustained by pedal cyclists of all ages. Almost one third (30%) of the pedal cyclists killed in traffic crashes in 1998 were between 5 and 15 years old.[13] Bicycle helmets are effective in decreasing bicycle-related head injuries. Emergency nurses are in a unique position to teach children proper bicycle safety.

As scooter sales have increased so have injuries. The Consumer Product Safety Commission recently reported that ED-treated injuries related to lightweight scooters have increased 700% since May 2000. Children younger than 15 years sustain 90% of the injuries. Fractures and dislocations accounted for 29% of the injuries. Proper safety gear, such as, helmets, wrist guards, and knee and elbow pads are effective in decreasing scooter injuries.[4]

Nurses should also alert the public to the importance of accident prevention. As participants in legislative activities, community committees, and community education, nurses must continually emphasize the role of human error and violence in trauma. Legislative initiatives focus on prevention as the primary method for decreasing the incidence, effects, and related costs of trauma to society.

Good Samaritan Statute

Nurses may encounter trauma situations as bystanders or because of trauma to family members. When an off-duty nurse happens on an accident, an ethical and moral, if not a legal duty, to stop and render assistance exists. To encourage professionals to help accident victims, the legislatures of all states have passed statutes that grant health care professionals immunity from liability for negligent acts. These statutes, named after the biblical "Good Samaritan," state that a health care professional who stops and aids accident victims without compensation will not be liable for untoward results related to his or her acts.

There is an exception to the Good Samaritan statute. The law does not exempt a nurse from acts that constitute gross negligence. The statute states that if care was rendered in good faith and an emergency existed, the nurse will be free from liability. However, if the nurse acts willfully, with gross negligence, a judgment of liability is possible.

Trauma Centers

Trauma centers are classified according to national designations that are implemented by state rules and regulations. Facilities are classified as level I, level II, or level III trauma centers. Level I–designated facilities are usually tertiary referral centers located in large metropolitan areas and have a strong commitment to manage all types of trauma and emergencies. To offset the cost of the trauma service, as well as to ensure that clinical skills are maintained at a high level, at least 1000 trauma patients per year are treated. A level I trauma center must have clinicians and specialists immediately available 24 hours a day. Level II trauma facilities have similar characteristics, with the exception of in-house availability of specialists. Specialists are on call and must be available within an established time frame, usually 20 to 30 minutes.[1] Level III facilities are most often located in smaller institutions in communities in which a level I or II facility is unavailable. Level III centers have a responsibility to adequately stabilize trauma patients and follow clear and concise protocols for transfer to level I or II facilities. Facilities may also elect to have a nontrauma ED. This designation needs to be clearly communicated to the local community and EMS systems.

Collaborative Care Management of Trauma

Emergency nurses and trauma systems can have an impact on patient outcomes by understanding the trimodal distribution of trauma deaths. The trimodal distribution illustrates the time frame in which the highest incidences of death occur after injury. The first peak occurs within minutes of injury, and death usually results from severe injury to the brain, upper spinal cord, heart, aorta, and other major blood vessels. The second peak occurs within 2 hours of injury and death is related to subdural or epidural hematomas, hemopneumothorax, ruptured spleen, lacerated liver, fractured femurs, or other injuries causing major blood loss. The third peak occurs days to weeks after the injury, and death usually results from complications such as sepsis and multiple organ failure.[11]

In the prehospital care setting nurses and paramedics (e.g., flight crews, rescue squad) can possibly reduce the first death peak with rapid and accurate lifesaving interventions. The second death peak is of importance to all ED nurses because it usually occurs in EDs.

Trauma is a "team sport." All members of the trauma team must work together efficiently and effectively to deliver optimal and comprehensive trauma care. The emergency nurse is an important member of the trauma team, and although he or she may provide trauma care in a variety of settings, certain nursing functions are common to trauma patient care, regardless of the setting (Box 7-6).

Assessment

In trauma care a systematic process for initial assessment of the trauma patient is crucial for recognizing life-threatening conditions and initiation of appropriate interventions. This process is summarized in Box 7-7 in order of priority.

The initial assessment of all trauma patients (prehospital or ED) is based on specific priorities of care. The initial assessment is divided into primary and secondary surveys and should be completed within minutes unless resuscitative measures are needed. If life-threatening conditions exist, the assessment should not proceed until appropriate interventions are instituted to manage these problems.

The primary survey is an assessment of airway, breathing, and circulation. Disability (brief neurologic assessment) is also part of the primary survey, as is exposing the patient to ensure assessment of all body areas. The secondary survey is a systematic head-to-toe assessment, with the objective of recognizing all injuries. It is also important to check cervical stability, especially before moving the patient. If possible, additional information is gathered at this time, such as mechanism of injury, patient information, past medical history, allergies, tetanus status, and current medications. Figure 7-1 presents information on complete primary and secondary surveys.

The primary and secondary surveys begin the initial cycle of trauma care[1]:

1. Cycle I: field stabilization and resuscitation
2. Cycle II: in-house resuscitation and operative phase
3. Cycle III: critical care
4. Cycle IV: intermediate care
5. Cycle V: rehabilitation

Assessment, analysis, and action are ongoing in the trauma situation. Figure 7-2 depicts another part of a trauma flow record, which reveals ongoing data that are recorded and demonstrates how some of the data from the primary and secondary surveys are combined to identify a trauma score. Other information being collected and recorded includes fluids; medications; blood, or blood components administered and the response of the patient; urine, blood, nasogastric, and other secretion loss; and cardiac rate and rhythm strips.

Analysis of data occurs concurrently with data collection. Some of the major judgments demanded of the nurse caring for the patient who has experienced trauma are presented next.

Multiple Trauma. Many trauma patients sustain *multiple trauma,* or injury to two or more body systems (Box 7-8). Motor vehicle crashes and falls, two major causes of trauma, may involve injury to the head or neck, an extremity, or the chest or abdominal area. Penetrating wounds to the chest wall may also affect the abdomen.

Persons with severe injuries require administration of intravenous fluids as soon as possible to prevent or control shock. In the field or ED, two or three large-bore intravenous catheters are placed to administer fluids and drugs. A central line may be inserted. An indwelling bladder catheter is inserted to monitor urinary output, as well as core body temperature.

In multiple trauma the trauma team first focuses on the highest priority problem of the particular patient and then moves to the next highest priority problem. Some problems

Text continued on p. 129.

BOX 7-6 Nursing Trauma Care Activities

1. Perform a rapid, initial assessment of the trauma patient to identify injuries.
2. Institute appropriate lifesaving interventions.
3. Monitor patient responses to resuscitative efforts.
4. Communicate with other team members.
5. Perform as a patient advocate.
6. Document care of the trauma patient.

Source: Rea R: *Trauma nursing core course provider manual,* ed 5, Chicago, 2000, Emergency Nurses Association.

BOX 7-7 Trauma Assessment

Primary Survey

Airway
Breathing
Circulation
Disability
Expose

Secondary Survey

Rapid head-to-toe assessment to determine all injuries

BOX 7-8 Severe Injuries Often Seen in Multiple Trauma

Crushing and penetrating chest injuries
Crushing pelvic injuries
Spinal cord injuries
Multiple bone or soft-tissue injuries
Injuries causing hemorrhage with shock
Head injuries with decreasing level of consciousness

TRAUMA FLOW SHEET

University of Virginia Medical Center
Emergency Medical Services
Trauma Flow Sheet

Patient Name Label

Date: ____________________

Arrival time: ___:___ Injury time ___:___ Transferred from: ____________________

Arrived by: Helicopter: ____________________ Squad: ____________________ ALS/BLS

Documentation received: ER Record X-Rays CT Scan

Mechanism: **MVA:** Driver/Passenger Location in vehicle: ____________________ Carseat Y/N

Restraint: Type: ____________________ Vehicle damage: ____________________

Vehicle speed: High/Low Rollover Ejected Head-on T-Bone Rear-end

Pedestrian struck/Fall: Speed of vehicle/Height of fall: ____________________

GSW/stab: Caliber/Size of weapon: ______________ Distance: ______________

Other: ____________________

Past Medical HX: Cardiac Renal Respiratory HTN Diabetic Other: ____________________

Medications: ____________________

Allergies: ____________________ **Approx. wt:** ______________ **kg**

Last menses: ____________________ **Last tetanus:** ____________________

HPI: ____________________

____

____

Family Notification: Notified/Enroute Phone consent Y/N Unable to notify Present

Contact person: ____________________ Phone: ____________________

Prehospital Intervention

Airway: Oral/Nasal Combi Intubated

O_2: High flow Cannula None BVM

IV Access: GA _____ Total fluid _______

IV Access: GA _____ Total fluid _______

Immobilized: Y/N

CPR: Y/N Time begun: __:__

Procedure: ____________________

Procedure: ____________________

Response

Service	Time	PTA	Name
Trauma res	__:__	___	____________
Trauma chief	__:__	___	____________
Neurosurgery	__:__	___	____________
Anesthesia	__:__	___	____________
Radiology	__:__	___	____________
E.R. Attending	__:__	___	____________
Surg. Attending	__:__	___	____________

Primary Survey

Airway: Patent Obstructed

Intervention: Oral/Nasal Airway size _____ MM

Intubated: Oral/Nasal size _____ MM Depth _____ CM

Procedure: Cric size _____ MM Depth _____ CM

Breathing: No Distress Distressed <10 >26 Assisted BVM/Vent

Expansion: Symmetrical/Asymmetrical Flail R/L Tracheal Deviation R/L

Intervention: O_2-high flow Assisted – BVM

Chest tube R/L Size _____ FR Amt out _____ CC

Chest tube R/L Size _____ FR Amt out _____ CC

Circulation: Skin – Warm Dry Moist Cool Pink Pale Cyanotic

Cap refill – Brisk Delayed None

Pulses Present: All present Deficit ____________________

Obvious Bleeding site ____________________

Intervention: Bleeding control

IV Access: Cent/Periph site ______________ GA _____ NS/LR by ______________

IV Access: Cent/Periph site ______________ GA _____ NS/LR by ______________

Procedure: Thoracotomy ACLS Protocol ATLS Protocol

Other: ____________________

Disability: Awake Responds to verbal Responds to pain Unresponsive

Figure 7-1 Trauma flow sheet–primary and secondary surveys.

Continued

Secondary Survey

Time:___:___

Date:__________

Neuro:
Mental status: A V P U   GCS: E__V__M__
Pupils: R __ L __ EOM: Intact Deficit ________
Drainage: Nasal Ears R/L Clear/Bloody None
Motor and sensory: Grossly intact Deficits ________
Other: ________

Respiratory:
Trachea: Midline Deviated R/L
Chest expansion: Symmetrical/Asymmetrical Flail R/L
Resp effort: Unlabored 12-18/min Distressed <10 >26 Absent
Breath sounds: R ______ L ______
Other: ________

Cardiovascular:
Skin: Warm/Dry Other ________
Cap refill: Normal Delayed
Pulses: All present Deficit ________
Heart sounds: S1, S2 Rub Murmur Other ________
Other: ________

GI/GU:
Abd: Soft/Nontender Flat Firm Rigid Distended Tender ________
Pelvis: Stable Unstable
Bowel sounds: Y/N Other ________
Rectal: Heme: +/− Tone: NL Flaccid
Blood at urinary meatus: Y/N
Other: ________
Skeletal: ________

Interventions

Time

___:___ Cardiac monitor
___:___ NIPB
___:___ Pulse oximeter
___:___ 12 LD EKG
___:___ Foley size ___ Heme +/−
___:___ NG/OG size ___ Heme +/−
___:___ ICP bolt
___:___ A-line- Rad R/L Fem R/L
___:___ DPL
___:___ Warming ________

Radiology

Time in Time out

___:___ ___:___ Portable C-spine, Pelvis, Chest
___:___ ___:___ Plain films
___:___ ___:___ CT ________
___:___ ___:___ A-Gram ________
___:___ ___:___ Repeat ________
___:___ ___:___ Repeat ________

___:___ C:spine cleared by: ________
___:___ C-collar removed by: ________
___:___ Backboard removed by: ________

Musculoskeletal

A	= Abrasion	H	= Hematoma
B	= Burn	L	= Laceration
D	= Deformity	M	= Amputation
E	= Ecchymosis	P	= Penetrating
F	= Foreign body	T	= Tenderness
		Av	= Avulsion

Rule of Nines

Burns

2 3 4 5 6 7 8 9

Pupil Gauge
Diameter by millimeter

Glasgow Coma Score

Eyes	Open spontaneously	4
	To verbal command	3
	To painful stimuli	2
	No response	1
Verbal	Oriented and converses	5
	Disoriented and converses	4
	Inappropriate words	3
	Incomprehensible sounds	2
	No response	1
Motor	Obeys command	6
	Localizes pain	5
	Flexion/Withdrawal	4
	Flexion/Abnormal	3
	Extension	2
	No response	1

Pediatric Coma Scale

Eye Opening	
Spontaneous	4
To verbal command or shout	3
To pain	2
No response	1
Best Verbal Response	
> 5 years	
Oriented and converses	5
Disoriented and converses	5
Inappropriate words	3
Incomprehensible sounds/garbled	2
No response	1
2-5 years	
Appropriate words and phrases	5
Inappropriate words	4
Cries, screams	3
Moans, grunts	2
No response	1
0-23 months	
Smiles, coos, cries appropriately	5
Cries	4
Inappropriate crying, screaming	3
Moans, grunts	2
No response	1
Best Motor Response	
Obeys commands	6
Localizes pain	5
Withdraws (normal flexion)	4
Abnormal flexion (decorticate)	3
Extension (decerebrate)	2
No response	1

Figure 7-1, cont'd Trauma flow sheet–primary and secondary surveys.

Intake

IV #	Time	Solution	Amt.	Amt. Inf.	PO

Total infused ☐

Blood Products

Bag #	Time	Product	Amt.	Site	Amt. Inf.

Total infused ☐

Output

Time	Urine	NGT	CT-RT	CT LT
Totals				

Total output ☐

Arterial Blood Gases

Time	PH	PC02	P02	HC03	BE	Fi02

Labs **Date:** ______

Sent	**Time**
Type and cross X ___	___ : ___
Trauma bloods	___ : ___
UA/C&S	___ : ___
Beta HCG	___ : ___
Spun HCT	___ : ___
Repeat HCT: ______	___ : ___
Other: ______	___ : ___

Urine dip : Heme +/−

DPL : In ______ Out ______ Heme +/−

Other: ______

Results

WBC	___	GLUC	___	CA	___
HGB	___	NA	___	MG	___
HCT	___	K	___	PHOS	___
PLT	___	CL	___	AMY	___
PT	___	C02	___	BILI	___
PTT	___	BUN	___	BETA	___
Lactic acid	___	CR	___	ETOH	___

Belongings

Clothes - Cut off	Necklace
Shirt/Sweater	Hearing aid
Pants	Glasses
Dress/Skirt	Contacts
Shoes/Socks	Denture
Underwear	Upper
Coat/Jacket	Lower
Wallet/Purse	
Money $ ______	
Watch	
Ring	Other ______
Earring	Other ______
Bracelet	Other ______

Disposition: With patient / To family / Police / Morgue

Safe/Security Envelope # ______

Figure 7-2 Trauma flow sheet.

Continued

Time	BP	HR	RR	SA 02	T	GCS					Meds	Notes Date: ______
						E	V	M				

Time	MD Order	Time	MD Order
	DT .5 ml IM X 1 if >5 years since previous		
	Gastrografen 1/4 oz in 240 cc H20 PO/NG q20′ until CT (or 10cc/kg - Peds) prn / as possible		
	Ancef 1 gram IV now		
	Foley to straight drainage		
	Gastric tube to suction		
	O_2 ______________________		
	Fentanyl 50-100 mcg IV PRN pain with SBP >100 and RR > 16		
	Versed 1 - 2 mg IV PRN sedation with SBP > 100 and RR > 16		

Primary RN signature ________________ Procedure RN ____________ Recording RN ____________

Disposition: Unit/Room ______________________ Home time: ___ : ___

Report given to: ______________________________ RN. By: ______________________________ RN.

UPJ-960798/1074 Revised 12/95

Figure 7-2, cont'd Trauma flow sheet.

such as penetrating wounds of the heart and aorta require immediate surgery. In other types of injury, if bleeding is controlled, surgery can be delayed while the team focuses on other problems. Although the trauma team has priorities, the needs of the total patient must be kept in focus.

The trauma team must always consider that treatment of one system may add to the problems of another injured system. For example, large amounts of fluid given to prevent or alter renal problems may compromise an inadequate ventilatory system, leading to failure of both systems. Assessment, analysis, and action in trauma require focusing on these multiple-system problems.

Airway and Breathing. The rate, depth, and character of respirations provide clues to the presence of ventilatory, central nervous system (CNS), or metabolic problems. Most trauma victims breathe a little faster than normal (18 to 24 respirations per minute). In the presence of abnormal respiratory effort (nasal flaring; suprasternal, intercostal, or substernal retractions), the airway may be partially obstructed. The following respiratory findings suggest specific emergency care problems:

1. Rate
    a. Slow (below 10 respirations per minute): ventilatory or CNS problems
    b. Rapid (above 26 respirations per minute): hypoxia, acidosis, and shock
2. Depth
    a. Shallow: shock, chest pain, and chest injuries
    b. Deep: hypoxia, hypoglycemia, and metabolic acidosis
3. Sounds
    a. Inspiratory stridor: upper airway obstruction (above tracheal bifurcation)
    b. Expiratory wheezes or stridor: lower airway obstruction
4. Frothy, blood-tinged sputum: lung injury, pulmonary edema, and pulmonary embolus

Circulation. Pulse quality, locations, and rate are assessed. Skin color and any obvious sources of bleeding are assessed. Life-threatening conditions that may be found when assessing circulation include uncontrolled external bleeding, shock, and pericardial tamponade.

Persons who sustain major trauma or a major stressor to the body usually develop shock (hypovolemic, neurogenic, multisystem failure shock). Signs of shock vary depending on the type and severity of the shock (see Chapter 14).

Disability–Neurologic Assessment. After the primary survey is completed, a neurologic assessment is performed. Level of consciousness may be altered in trauma, and such alterations have many causes (Box 7-9). Refer to Unit 12 for further information regarding neurologic assessment and injury.

General Trauma Interventions

Some general principles of management for accidental injuries or sudden illnesses serve as guidelines in giving first aid at a scene.

BOX 7-9 Possible Causes of Changes in Level of Consciousness

1. Hypoxia (decreased oxygen to brain)
    a. Respiratory insufficiency
        (1) Airway obstruction from foreign body, secretions
        (2) Pneumothorax
        (3) Spinal cord injury
    b. Shock
        (1) Cardiogenic cardiac arrest
        (2) Hypovolemic hemorrhage
        (3) Multisystem failure shock
2. Metabolic (chemical brain depressants)
    a. Extrinsic
        (1) Drugs: alcohol, narcotics, barbiturates, antihistamines, tranquilizers
        (2) Poisons: carbon monoxide, carbon tetrachloride, hydrocarbons, methane gas
    b. Intrinsic
        (1) Ketones: diabetic ketoacidosis, starvation
        (2) Glucose: hypoglycemia, hyperglycemia
        (3) Ammonia: liver failure
        (4) Urea: kidney failure
        (5) Hormonal hypofunction: hypothyroidism, adrenocortical insufficiency
        (6) Electrolyte imbalance: sodium, potassium, calcium, hydrogen ions
3. Brain pathologic conditions
    a. Trauma: concussion, brainstem contusion, intracranial hematoma
    b. Seizures: epilepsy, tumors, idiopathology
    c. Cerebrovascular accident: cerebral hemorrhage, thrombosis
    d. Tumors: benign, malignant
    e. Infections: meningitis, encephalitis

- Remain calm and think before acting.
- Summon assistance or be sure that emergency services has been contacted.
- Identify yourself as a nurse to victim and bystanders.
- Do a primary survey for *priority* data (cessation of breathing or heartbeat, interference with breathing, hemorrhage, coma).
- Carry out measures as indicated by the primary survey (see Box 7-7).
- Do a secondary survey.
- Keep the victim lying down or in the position in which he or she is found (unless cardiopulmonary resuscitation [CPR] is necessary), protected from dampness or cold. Position the person to support airway management and some degree of comfort.
- Avoid unnecessary handling or moving of the victim; move the victim only if danger is present.
- If the victim is conscious, explain what is occurring and provide assurance that help is on the way.
- Do not give oral fluids if there is a possibility of abdominal injury or if anesthesia will be necessary within a short time.

Lifesaving measures are implemented when the primary survey indicates the presence of breathing or circulatory difficulties. After breathing has been reestablished and excessive bleeding controlled, other interventions are carried out when the secondary survey is completed.

Rescue squad and ED personnel are trained to detect and respond to the patient's physical life-threatening needs. Because these needs assume priority, it is easy to overlook the psychologic needs of the patient and significant others. The impact of severe trauma or critical illness can be devastating not only for the patient but for the patient's family and significant others. Care of the emergency patient always extends beyond the patient to the psychosocial care of the patient's family and friends. In times of crisis families need support but may not be able to provide it for each other. Emergency nurses must be there to help provide empathy, support, and direction, as well as act as resource persons. A calm, interested approach that conveys concern for the victim as a person is helpful.

Giving information frequently during all phases of emergency care to both patient and significant others helps them understand what is occurring, thereby decreasing some of the anxiety. During resuscitation attempts, it is imperative that contact be made with the family. The family needs clear information regarding their family member's prognosis and condition. The nurse contacts chaplains, social workers, or family friends who can stay with the family. Some hospitals have volunteers who can stay with patients or families during crisis periods. The nurse is honest and does not offer false hope about the patient's condition or expected outcome.

The nurse offers family and friends the option of seeing the patient, even if only for a fleeting moment before the patient is rushed to surgery or an intensive care unit. This contact is crucial for the family. If the patient has injuries or multiple tubes, the nurse prepares the family members for what they will see before taking them into the room.

Sexual Assault: Rape

Sexual assault is a horrifying, even life-threatening, experience. The number of reported rapes has been steadily increasing, but it is still estimated that two to three times that number of rapes go unreported. It is estimated that 17% of rape victims are between 13 and 16 years old.[14]

Accurate statistics about rape, rapists, and victims of rape are difficult to compile because of the large number of unreported cases. There are also many misconceptions concerning rape. Some facts include:

1. Rape occurs among persons of all social classes.
2. Rape occurs mostly between persons of the same race.
3. Most rapes are committed by someone the victim knows.
4. Males, especially young boys, may be rape victims; the attacker usually is a heterosexual male.
5. During the rape the victim may be unable to resist the attack.

Sexual Assault Resource Agencies

Sexual assault resource agencies are available in many cities. The services of these centers differ but usually include one or more of the following:

1. Direct service and counseling to the survivor
2. Service to professional agencies (health, law)
3. Community education

Service to health professionals and community education are efforts to help change the system for the rape victim.

Many victim services agencies are staffed by volunteers who serve as victim advocates throughout the medical examination and police interview. Some form of follow-up service, such as counseling, may be available. Some resource agencies also have attorney volunteers who offer the victim legal advice or representation.

Rape Trauma Syndrome

Rape is a traumatic event for the victim physically, psychologically, and socially. *Rape trauma syndrome* refers to the emotional state of discomfort and stress resulting from memories of an extraordinarily catastrophic experience. Patients show a wide range of emotions as well as various physical responses, including gastrointestinal irritability; genitourinary disturbance; and sleeping, eating, and sexual disruption.[5]

Rape is an act of physical violence, and force often is used. A weapon may be used either to threaten or injure the victim, or the hands or fists may be used to beat or choke the victim. Injury also can occur if the victim struggles or attempts to defend herself. The vagina and perineum may be injured by the force of the sexual attack, and the rectum also may be lacerated if anal sex has been attempted. Sexually transmitted diseases, including human immunodeficiency virus (HIV), may be contracted.

The psychologic trauma of rape usually is severe; the rape victim is in a state of crisis. Fear is an overwhelming emotion because the victim perceives the rape as life threatening. Other feelings expressed by victims are depersonalization, shame, degradation, defilement, violation, guilt, humiliation, and anger. The victim not only has been harmed or threatened with harm but also may have been subjected to multiple sexual assaults by one or more persons. Fellatio (oral sex) commonly is demanded, and some rapists will urinate on the victim before leaving. There is also the fear of pregnancy or contracting a sexually transmitted disease.

The person who has been raped goes through the same phases as any person facing a crisis situation. The initial phase is one of shock, disbelief, and disorganization. After the initial acute phase, there is a period of pseudoequilibrium when the victim rationalizes the event or attempts to suppress thoughts concerning the rape. Later, as the survivor tries to reorganize her life, there may be periods of depression, phobic reactions, and nightmares.

The rape victim also experiences sociologic crisis. If the victim is married, the marital relationship may be affected. If she is single, she often fears repeated occurrences and may feel the need to relocate, especially if the attack occurred in her home or apartment. The victim needs to make decisions about the incident, because loss of needed support from family and friends may occur. Job security or relationships with co-workers may be threatened. Sociologic problems may emerge during the initial emergency period and may take considerable time to resolve. The social importance of rape in the overall context of violence is reflected in its inclusion in the Healthy People 2010 objectives presented in the Healthy People 2010 box.

Prevention

All individuals need to know basic rape prevention measures to help prevent rape from occurring (Box 7-10). Some communities include issues of rape and self-defense in secondary school curricula. Classes in self-defense are available in most communities. Sexual assault agencies and police stations may provide information about classes in the local community.

Persons who are raped may seek medical help directly or call the police, who will then take the person to the appropriate facility for medical examination. Some survivors fear reprisal by the rapist or are unwilling to let others know about the rape and therefore do not seek medical attention. Rape survivors need to be encouraged to report the incident.

Most hospitals have developed protocols for care of the rape survivor in the ED, including the following measures:

1. High priority in triage
2. Provision for privacy without leaving the victim alone
3. Provision of a victim advocate (such as a worker from the sexual assault resource agency)
4. Development of sexual assault nurse examiner (SANE) programs
5. Routines to ensure protection and comfort of the victim (if the hospital does not have a SANE program)
   a. Person(s) designated to have primary contact with the victim
   b. Authority of the primary contact person to make the decision about the victim's readiness for medical examination or police interview (if no life-threatening injury is present)
   c. Ensure "chain of evidence" for specimens is maintained (i.e., clear documentation of injuries and collection and storage of specimens according to protocols)

Sexual Assault Nurse Examiners

Providing care to survivors of sexual assault involves unique challenges. The victim requires skilled and empathetic care to begin the process of emotional recovery; but professional, thorough, and accurate examination is essential to gather the evidence needed for successful prosecution of the rapist. The sexual assault nurse examiner role was developed to respond to the multiple challenges of caring for survivors of sexual assault. The first SANE program was developed in Memphis, Tennessee, in 1976, and the role has rapidly spread throughout the country.[6] The SANE is able to provide a more time-efficient evidentiary examination process by shortening the time a victim may have to wait for a physician or resident to be available to complete the examination. The forensic quality of the examination is improved as well, because the SANE knows exactly what forensic evidence to collect and how to meet the crisis intervention needs of the survivor.

NURSING MANAGEMENT

ASSESSMENT

The victim is asked many questions by the SANE to determine the details of the assault and the nature and extent of all

Healthy People 2010

Objectives Related to Violence

1. Reduce homicides.
2. Reduce maltreatment and maltreatment fatalities of children.
3. Reduce the rate of physical assault by current or former intimate partners.
4. Reduce the annual rate of rape or attempted rape.
5. Reduce sexual assault other than rape.
6. Reduce physical assaults.
7. Reduce physical fighting among adolescents.
8. Reduce weapon carrying by adolescents on school campuses.
9. Reduce firearm-related deaths.
10. Reduce the proportion of persons living in homes with firearms that are loaded and unlocked.
11. Reduce nonfatal firearm-related injuries.
12. Increase the number of states and the District of Columbia with statewide ED surveillance systems that collect data on external causes of injury.

Modified from US Department of Health and Human Services: *Healthy people 2010: understanding and improving health,* Washington, DC, 2000, USDHHS.

BOX 7-10 Rape Prevention Measures

Prevention of Attack

Set house lights to go on and off by timer.
Keep light on at all entrances.
Install safety locks on windows and doors.
Have key ready before reaching door of house or car.
Look in car before entering.
Never let strangers enter the house; insist on identification from all service personnel; check identity with agency if suspicious.
Do not list first name on mailbox or in telephone directory.
Be alert when walking; stay in lighted areas.
Walk down center of street if possible.
Avoid lonely or enclosed areas.

If Attacked

Run toward a lighted house; yell "Fire!"
Spit in rapist's face; act bizarre; vomit.
Rip off rapist's glasses.
Step hard on rapist's foot (instep).
Aim at eyes; try to gouge eyes, scrape face.
Hit throat at Adam's apple (larynx).
Use fighting and screaming with caution; this may scare some rapists, encourage others.
Try talking to avoid rape.
Make close observations about rapist, car, location.

injuries. The victim's general demeanor and emotional state are assessed. The victim may express feelings of degradation, shame, guilt, and feeling "dirty" and may express anger toward the assailant or project the anger toward health care personnel. The SANE also collects data related to pain or discomfort (localized, generalized, or diffuse). The victim may complain of a sore throat if choking occurred or if oral sex was forced. Nausea may also be present. Some victims respond emotionally and cry, shake, laugh inappropriately, or are extremely restless. Other victims appear outwardly calm and subdued.

The expertise of the SANE is particularly important in the assessment of objective signs of the rape. A head-to-toe assessment is conducted for signs of physical trauma. Any serious physical trauma is treated before collection of evidence. Data regarding the victim's last menstrual period, medical history, history of the assault, and vital signs are obtained.

Evidence Collection

After the SANE explains the procedure to the survivor and obtains her permission, the collection of evidence begins. This process is both time consuming and difficult for the survivor. Most states have standardized kits for evidence collection and storage. The SANE collects scrapings from beneath the victim's fingernails, pulls head and pubic hairs, obtains saliva samples, swabs the genitalia and vagina, and conducts a vaginal examination. Some SANE protocols also include colposcopy to obtain photographic evidence of all injuries. A colposcope is a movable microscope that is positioned outside an inserted speculum, and it can provide significant magnification of microtrauma and internal injuries. Used to assess trauma that is difficult to visualize without magnification, the colposcope also has a camera attached to take photographs of the injuries.

A pregnancy test is done, and tests for HIV antibody are performed. Tests for other sexually transmitted diseases may be conducted and repeated at appropriate intervals.

NURSING DIAGNOSES

Diagnostic Title	Possible Etiologic Factors
1. Rape-trauma syndrome	No etiology is necessary with acute phase of this diagnosis

EXPECTED PATIENT OUTCOMES

Expected patient outcomes for the victim experiencing rape trauma syndrome may include but are not limited to:

- **1a.** Will acknowledge the traumatic effect of the rape
- **1b.** Will begin to express feelings and responses to the rape
- **1c.** Will identify available rape counseling and support resources in the community
- **1d.** Will understand rationale for treatment and evidence collection procedures

INTERVENTIONS

1. Providing Emotional Support

Most victims need to talk with someone who cares about what is happening to them and who is nonjudgmental. The nurse uses crisis intervention theory to decide how best to help the survivor. Many hospitals have contacts with sexual assault agencies, and the victim is given the choice of having a victim advocate from the center be present during the entire examination period, both medical and legal. Interviews by the police are often done as a team interview with the SANE.

Preparation for the physical examination is carried out in advance. Having a pelvic examination after a sexual assault can be a traumatic experience, especially if the survivor has never had a pelvic examination.

1. Addressing Sexual Concerns

The survivor often has concerns related to sexuality. Time is needed to work through these concerns, and long-term counseling is helpful for many victims.

Concern about possible pregnancy depends on the circumstances—whether the woman is in the childbearing years, whether birth control was used during the assault, and at what point in the menstrual period the rape occurred. If pregnancy is a possibility, postcoital hormone contraceptive therapy usually is offered.

Concern about sexually transmitted diseases is common. Antibiotic therapy is given after the initial examination as a preventive measure. The victim needs to know that medical follow-up assessment is important and that she should be retested for sexually transmitted diseases and screened for HIV infection at appropriate intervals. In addition, the woman may experience vaginal discharge, itching, and a burning sensation caused by an acute vaginal infection (vaginitis).

1. Planning for Discharge

Clean clothes need to be provided, and no survivor of sexual assault should ever be sent home alone. Every ED should maintain a current list of battered women's shelters. Social workers may be called on to help the victim secure a safe place to stay. The survivor needs to know about the availability of follow-up medical and counseling services. Some medical centers have psychiatrists who are especially expert in counseling rape survivors. The survivor may go to the police station to follow up with the police report after medical care is completed (see Guidelines for Safe Practice box).

EVALUATION

To evaluate effectiveness of nursing interventions, compare patient behaviors with those stated in the expected patient outcomes. Successful achievement of patient outcomes for the survivor of rape experiencing rape trauma syndrome, acute phase, is indicated by the victim's ability to:

- **1a.** Express the understanding that she is a victim in the assault, and not to blame herself.
- **1b.** Express her feelings about the rape.
- **1c.** Identify community resources available for support and counseling and express a commitment to seek follow-up support.

Intimate Partner Violence

Research suggests that 10% to 15% of all women who come to the ED are victims of intimate partner violence (IPV).

Guidelines for Safe Practice

Care Provided to the Sexual Assault Survivor

1. Assess severity of all injuries and treat accordingly.
2. Provide a safe environment.
3. Obtain consent for evidence collection.
4. Document chief complaint and history of assault.
5. Complete vital signs, history of medications, allergies, and pertinent health history.
6. Observe and document emotional status.
7. Observe and document physical injuries (written, diagrams, and photographs).
8. Observe and document genital injuries (using toluidine blue dye, Wood's light, and colposcopy).
9. Complete evidence collection.
10. Order laboratory studies per protocol.
11. Order additional testing based on the results of the examination.
12. Plan for the patient's discharge, including referrals, prescriptions, and follow-up care.

Evidence-Based Practice

Reference: Glass N, Dearwater S, Campbell J: Intimate partner violence screening and intervention: Data from eleven Pennsylvania and California community hospital emergency departments, *J Emerg Nurs* 27(2):141, 2001.

Routine screening for intimate partner violence (IPV) should be done during all assessments of emergency department (ED) patients. The ED is often the only contact the abused women may have with health care providers.

The objective of this study was to provide clinical practice recommendations for screening and interventions for IPV in EDs. Eleven mid-sized community level EDs in Pennsylvania and California were used as the setting for the study. An anonymous survey inquiring about physical, sexual, and emotional IPV was conducted over 2 years. The majority of both abused and nonabused women supported routine screening for IPV. Fewer than 25% of women stated they were asked about IPV by ED staff. This study provides evidence supporting standard protocols for routine screening for IPV. This information is important for health care providers who are seeking to improve their identification and care for abused women.

The link between IPV and sexual assault is striking, as many as 33% to 46% of women who have been physically abused by their partner were also sexually assaulted. Absenteeism from work as a result of abuse costs businesses $3 billion to $5 billion and another $100 million in medical costs each year. Battering is the largest single cause of injury to women today.[9]

For many of the 4 to 8 million women who are abused each year, the ED is their primary source of medical care after abusive episodes. Although the battered woman may come to the ED, opportunities for IPV intervention are often lost because health care providers do not ask the right questions (see Evidence-Based Practice box). Physicians and nurses should directly ask all injured women if they are in an abusive relationship. Battered women cannot be predicted based on socioeconomic status, race, profession, or educational level. Battering is an equal-opportunity problem.

ED staff follows several principles in caring for patients suspected of sustaining physical abuse. First, nurses incorporate questions and observations into the initial patient assessment. Historical questions and examination techniques may elicit information or evidence about IPV. Victims may not readily share this information if it is not solicited; however, if given the opportunity, the victim often shares the information. Second, nurses must know the resources available for victims of IPV. Financial help and "safe housing" are often priority concerns. Victims, once placed in safe environments, can be helped to use the legal system to maintain their safety. Long-term counseling, vocational rehabilitation, and other support are necessary to promote total health. Last, the ED staff must have clear procedures on how to handle victims of IPV and must define the process used to notify local authorities.

Critical Thinking Questions

1. While skating on her new in-line skates, a young woman was hit by a bicyclist. You are the first to arrive at the scene of the accident. The woman is sitting up, crying, alert, but anxious. What should you do?
2. During a triage assessment a patient reports she was just raped. What is her triage category? Describe the various procedural steps that will be taken during her examination.
3. A 28-year-old man fell off a roof while working. He has a wrist fracture, several small lacerations, and a swollen ankle. You are the triage nurse in a busy ED. To what category will you assign him when presented for care? Provide rationales for your decision.
4. While working in the ED, you receive a call stating that paramedics will be bringing in at least 15 victims from a motor vehicle accident. Some are listed in critical condition. How will you prepare for this event? What type of triage will be necessary? How will you ensure that there is effective and appropriate communication among the personnel in the ED, the patient, families, paramedics, and media?

References

1. Cardona V et al: *Trauma nursing from resuscitation through rehabilitation,* Philadelphia, 1995, WB Saunders.
2. Erickson L, Williams-Evans A: Attitudes of emergency nurse regarding patient assaults, *J Emerg Nurs* 26(3):210, 2000.
3. Emergency Nurses Association: *Standards of emergency nursing practice,* ed 4, St Louis, 1999, Mosby.
4. Flaherty L: From the feds, *J Emerg Nurs* 27(1):59, 2001.
5. Girardin B: Care of the sexually assaulted patient. In Girardin B et al, editors: *Color atlas of sexual assault,* St Louis, 1998, Mosby.
6. Ledray L, Simmelink K: Efficacy of SANE evidence collection: a Minnesota study, *J Emerg Nurs* 23(1):75, 1997.

7. Mayer BW, Smith FB, King CA: Factors associated with victimization of personnel in emergency departments, *J Emerg Nurs* 25(5):361, 1999.
8. Mayer T, Augustine J: Managed care and triage, *Top Emerg Med* 19(2):12, 1997.
9. Nelms ST: An educational program to examine emergency nurses' attitudes and enhance caring interventions with battered women, *J Emerg Nurs:* 25(4):290, 1999.
10. Nourjah P: *National ambulatory medical care survey: 1997 ED summary (vital and health statistics),* Atlanta, 1999, Centers for Disease Control and Prevention.
11. Rea R: *Trauma nursing core course provider manual,* ed 5, Chicago, 2000, Emergency Nurses Association.
12. Somerson SW, Markovchick AB: Development of the triage system. In Salluzo R et al, editors: *Emergency department management: principles and applications,* St Louis, 1997, Mosby.
13. US Department of Health and Human Services: *Healthy People 2010: Understanding and improving health,* Washington, DC, 2000, USDHHS.
14. Virginians Aligned Against Sexual Assault: *Virginia statewide public awareness campaign against violence information packet,* Richmond, 1998, Virginians.

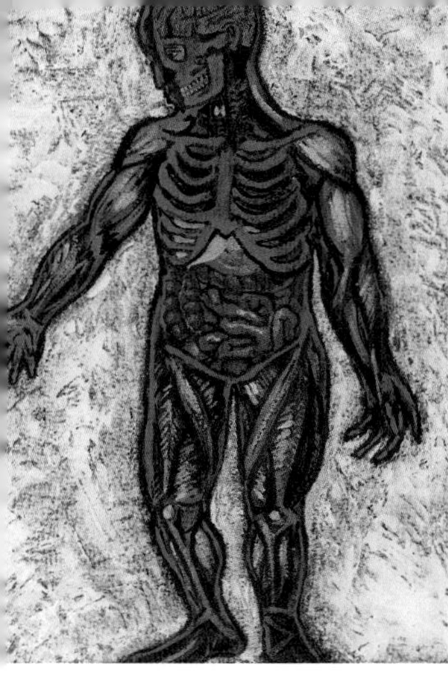

http://www.mosby.com/MERLIN/medsurg_phipps

Critical Care 8

Nan Smith-Blair

Objectives

After studying this chapter, the learner should be able to:

1. Describe the role of the critical care nurse.
2. Describe how the Standards for Nursing Care of the Critically Ill, the Principles of Critical Care Nursing Practice, and the Scope of Critical Care Nursing Practice impact the quality of care patients and families receive.
3. Describe the physical and psychologic environment of critical care units.
4. Identify the types of data needed for the care of critically ill patients.
5. Identify essential assessment parameters required in the care of critically ill patients.
6. Develop interventions to alleviate physiologic stressors that are specific to the critical care setting.
7. Explain the rationale for interventions to prevent and alleviate physiologic, psychologic, and social stressors for the critically ill patient and family.

The delivery of critical care as we know it today originated from the need to centralize specially trained personnel and equipment in a separate area of the hospital to optimize the care of critically ill and injured patients. The concept of gathering patients together for care can be traced back to Florence Nightingale, who wrote[24]:

> It is not uncommon, in small country hospitals, to have a recess or small room leading from the operating theatre in which the patients remain until they have recovered, or at least recovered from the immediate effects of the operation. (p. 89)

Nurses began to group their most unstable patients closer to the nurses' station so they could provide "watchful vigilance" or intensive observation. As Louisa May Alcott noted[2]:

> I had managed to sort out the patients in such a way that I had what I called "my duty room, my pleasure room, and my pathetic room," and worked for each in a different way. One, I visited, armed with a dressing tray, full of rollers, plasters, and pin; another, with books, flowers, games, and gossip; a third, with teapots, lullabies, consolation, and, sometimes, a shroud. (p. 41)

Since the earliest days of nursing, the sickest patients have been placed near the nurses' station, underlining the importance of frequent assessment and rapid intervention. From the development of postoperative wards and polio centers to triage centers during various wars, to the evolution of the coronary care unit, this concentration of highly specialized caregivers with access to unique technology has remained the guiding principle for the evolution of critical care environments.

Today's critical care unit continues to be a unique, high-paced environment in which the most sophisticated medical, nursing, and technical interventions are integrated to combat life-threatening illness. These units are referred to as intensive care units (ICUs), critical care units, coronary care units (CCU), and other names that identify the type and intensity of patient care. The one constant in all the various units is that nursing has always played a unique role. The role of the nurse in the care of the critically ill patient remains the key to the success of the critical care unit. Through the vigilant observation of a patient's ever-changing condition, the critical care nurse is able to monitor the complex treatment regimen, quickly identify problems and initiate appropriate therapies, and intervene to prevent or correct life-threatening situations. However, the focus of critical care nursing practice no longer only focuses on the patient's critical illness/injury. Critical care nurses have broadened their focus to include preventive care and risk modification to decrease future patient hospitalizations.

This chapter provides an overview of some common aspects of critical care nursing and the critical care environment. Effects of the critical care environment on patient, family, and staff are discussed. Assessment of the critically ill patient is described, followed by selected interventions designed to alleviate physiologic, psychologic, and social stressors experienced by critically ill patients, families, and clinicians who staff the units.

CRITICAL CARE NURSING PRACTICE

Critical care nursing is concerned with human responses to life-threatening problems, such as major surgery, trauma, infection, and shock, as well as prevention of potential life-threatening conditions. The critical care nurse is responsible for ensuring that all critically ill patients and families receive optimal care through a process of establishing goals for patient care and providing mechanisms for nurses to assess the achievement of the patient's progress toward the goals[5] (Box 8-1). The American Association of Critical Care Nurses (AACN), established in 1969, is the largest nursing specialty organization in the world. It is committed to providing resources to maximize nurses' contributions to the care of critically ill patients and families through stressing the values of accountability, advocacy, integrity, collaboration, leadership, lifelong learning, quality innovation, and commitment.[4] Clinical competencies for nurses practicing in critical care have been established by AACN and include clinical judgment and reasoning skills with the ability to make decisions and critically think. The critical care nurse must provide clinical practices tailored to the needs of each individual patient and family through collaboration with the health care team members to meet desired patient outcomes. The AACN vision statement reflects a guide for critical care nursing practice that includes a "healthcare system driven by the needs of the critically ill patients where critical care nurses make their optimal contributions."[4] Critical care nurses have long been recognized for the patient advocacy role as listed in Box 8-2.

BOX 8-1 Principles of Critical Care Nursing Practice

- The critical care nurse maintains the established standards of critical care nursing practice.
- The critical care nurse continually updates knowledge necessary for competence.
- The critical care nurse, as an integral part of the multidisciplinary health care team, coordinates care delivered to patients and supports families within the critical care environment.
- The critical care nurse recognizes the stresses involved in the critical care environment, and creates a compassionate and humanistic climate by providing support to patients, families, and colleagues. The critical care nurse must also identify psychologic and physiologic limitations when providing care.
- The critical care nurse respects the rights of patients, families, and colleagues in the promotion or prolongation of life by individualizing each patient situation.
- The critical care nurse identifies the values of patients, families, colleagues, and self, and incorporates those beliefs and attitudes into situations of ethical dilemmas.
- The critical care nurse adheres to the Code of Ethics of the American Nurses Association.

Source: American Association of Critical Care Nurses: *Conceptual model of critical care nursing* (position statement), Aliso Viejo, Calif, 1981, AACN.

THE CRITICAL CARE UNIT ENVIRONMENT

Physical Environment

Many of the early critical care units were originally small spaces carved out of existing recovery rooms or other areas in the hospital. Soon, however, the ICU emerged as a distinct area for care of complex patients, different from the recovery room in that patients were also admitted from outside the hospital and from other units. The units were also staffed 24 hours a day, 7 days a week. Today's CCU is designed, equipped, and staffed to meet the anticipated needs of patients in life-threatening situations. The physical layout is frequently a modified circle that allows for direct visualization of all patients at all times. Patients may be separated into individual cubicles with glass windows for visualization or situated in a large open area with curtains for partitions. The advantage of direct nurse-patient visualization is accompanied by the disadvantages of limited privacy and patient exposure to frequent crisis interventions.

Although direct visualization of patients facilitates patient monitoring, maximizes the use of available staff, and is required by some hospital accrediting organizations, the cost to the patient in terms of sensory overload and loss of control can be significant. Optimal patient care requires that a careful and sensitive balance be maintained between the needs of patients and those of caregivers.[8,23]

The central nurse's station contains sophisticated monitoring and even video equipment that enables nurses to continuously monitor vital data for each patient. Supplies and equipment in critical care areas are highly sophisticated and must be readily accessible. Certain technologies are available for constant use at each bedside (e.g., cardiac monitor, oxygen, hemodynamic monitoring equipment, and suction equipment), whereas others must be available within seconds (defibrillator, ventilator, 12-lead electrocardiogram [ECG] machine, emergency medications). Still other technologies must be available for constant or intermittent use with certain patient populations (e.g., intraaortic balloon pumps, con-

BOX 8-2 Role of the Critical Care Nurse as Patient Advocate

- Support the right of the patient or surrogate to informed decision making
- Intervene when the best interest of the patient is in question
- Help the patient obtain necessary care
- Respect the values, beliefs, and rights of the patient
- Provide education and support to help the patient or the patient's designated surrogate make decisions
- Represent the patient in accordance with the patient's choices
- Support the decisions of the patient or the patient's designated surrogate or transfer care to an equally qualified critical care nurse
- Intercede for patients who cannot speak for themselves in situations that require immediate action
- Monitor and safeguard the quality of care the patient receives
- Act as liaison between the patient, the patient's family, and health care professions.

tinuous venovenous hemofiltration or hemodialysis, extracorporeal membrane oxygenator, temporary or permanent pacemakers, ventricular assist devices, intermittent conventional hemodialysis, and a variety of pumps for infusion of intravenous fluids or enteral feedings).

The concentration of complex technologic equipment also combines to create a unique hazard in the critical care environment—the risk of electrical microshock. The invasive monitoring and therapeutic interventions used with critically ill patients often create a direct pathway to the heart (e.g., central venous pressure lines, pulmonary artery catheters, and temporary pacemakers). Direct contact with stray or leaked current could prove fatal, particularly to critically ill patients whose resistance may be further decreased through other breaks in skin integrity or through electrolyte imbalances. Critical care nurses are responsible for the safe and proper use of electrical equipment, as well as for the implementation of appropriate electrical safety precautions.[7]

As the need for more specialized and sophisticated critical care equipment grows, the critical care patient often becomes surrounded by a sea of machinery. As the patient increases in complexity, additional technology may be required for comprehensive care resulting in the available space becoming quickly overwhelmed with monitoring and other care-delivery equipment. The use of centralized or headwall power columns, which are designed to support the complex power needs for monitoring equipment, oxygen, suction equipment, and electrical outlets; to store equipment; and to provide a workspace at each patient's bedside, has become popular in newer or remodeled critical care environments. With the advent of microprocessing and digital processing, continued research and development of critical care equipment focuses on how to provide the most service in the smallest available space. Figure 8-1 illustrates a typical high-technology critical care environment.

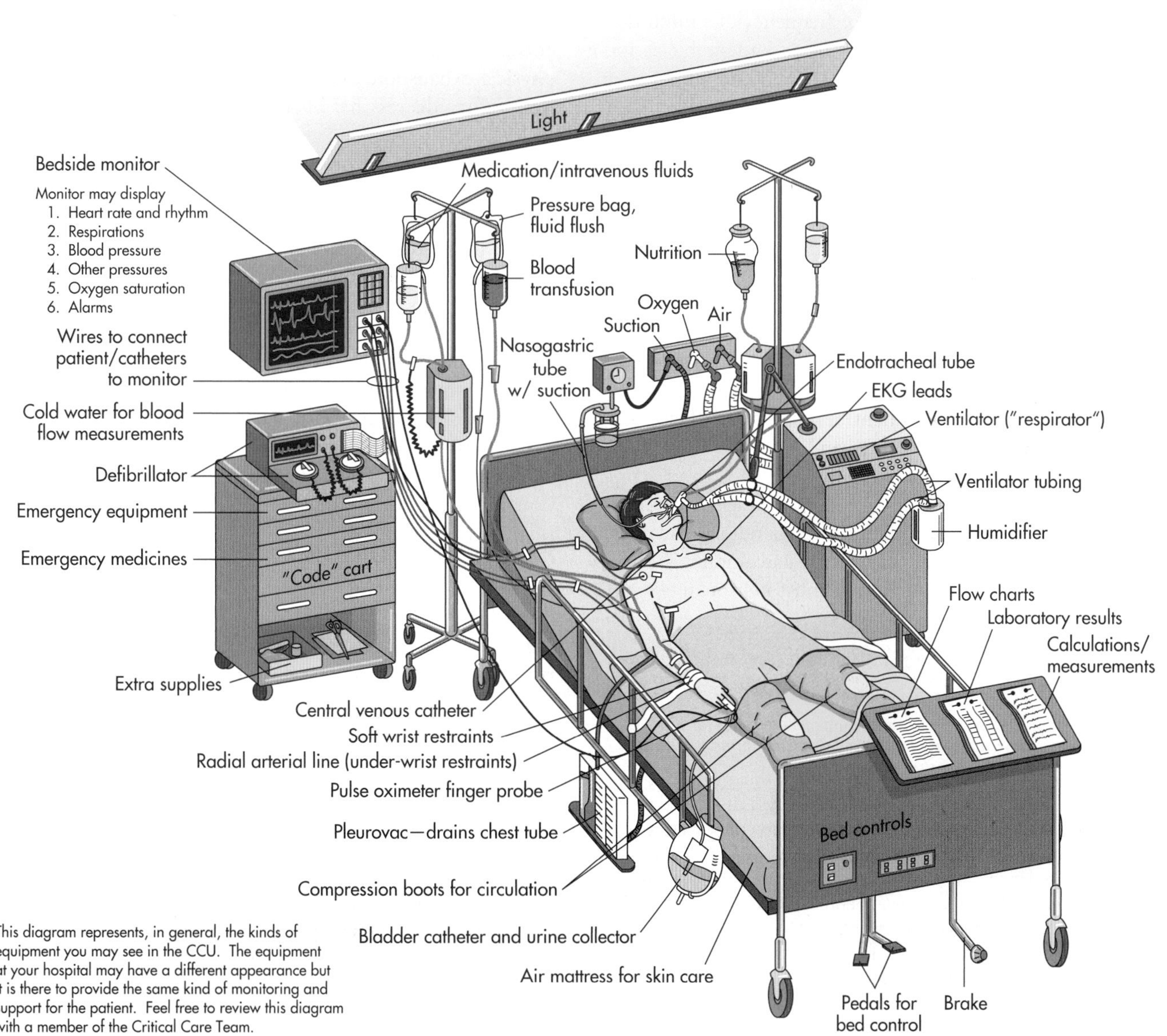

Figure 8-1 A look at a critical care unit room and equipment.

Psychologic Environment

The critical care environment confronts patients with advanced forms of medical and nursing therapies. Although the patient and family are partially aware of the dynamics of critical care, their attention primarily focuses on the appearance of this confusing and frightening environment: flashing lights; buzzing machines; painful procedures; and a noisy, brightly lit, crowded, hyperactive environment. The stressors on the patient and family are immense. The recovery period from psychologic stressors experienced in critical care may extend well past discharge from the hospital.[21] Some factors that precipitate stress, especially in the ICU environment, are sensory deprivation and overload, sleep deprivation, and acute confusion.

Sensory Deprivation and Overload

The level and variety of sensory stimulation that allow an individual to interact optimally with the environment involves the stimulation of all five senses. The optimal level varies significantly among individuals. Patients in a CCU have little or no control over the amount and/or frequency of stimuli that they receive. Too many stimuli can be as undesirable as too few stimuli. Critical care environments rarely contain the type of sensory stimuli that are familiar or understandable to patients. Instead, the majority of the sounds, sights, and smells are unique to the CCU. Unfamiliar voices, equipment noise, continuous bright lights, and frequent assessment interventions all add to the patient's stress level. This level of stimulation also does not disappear during the night and is in fact minimally diminished.[29]

Patient stimulation in the critical care environment is continuous, 24 hours a day, 7 days a week. Staff members may not realize the impact of this level of stimuli and frequently perpetuate it. Staff, of course, are also able to leave the high-energy critical care environment at the end of their shift, whereas the patient is unable to escape it.

Years of research indicate that sensory overload and deprivation in the critical care environment frequently result in perceptual distortion, hallucinations, and paranoia. The nurse needs to be constantly aware of the type and amount of stimuli directed toward the patient and must help maintain the level of stimulation within tolerable limits.[15,32] Research has found that a concentrated effort by staff to reduce environmental stimuli increases the likelihood of patients being able to sleep (see Research box). Every effort should be made to reduce noise and other controllable variables and assist the patient to understand this complex environment, thereby reducing the stress of the unknown.

Research

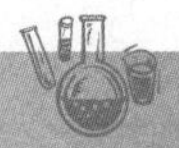

Reference: Olson DM et al: Quiet time: a nursing intervention to promote sleep in neurocritical care units, *Am J Crit Care* 10:74-78, 2001.

This study examined whether implementing a "quiet time" protocol to reduce external environmental stimuli was associated with in increase in sleep among patients in a neurocritical care unit. Patients whose Glasgow Coma Scale score was 10 or greater were observed eight times a day from 2 to 4 AM and from 2 to 4 PM, during which time the environmental sounds and lights were decreased. The percentage of patients observed asleep was significantly higher during the time the "quiet-time" period was implemented than during a control period. The researchers concluded that efforts by staff to reduce environmental stimuli during descrete time periods increases the likelihood of sleep in patients in the neurocritical care unit.

SLEEP DEPRIVATION

An essential part of the 24-hour cycle, sleep accounts for approximately one third of a person's life. An adequate amount of uninterrupted sleep is essential to prevent exhaustion or illness and maintain physiologic and psychologic well-being. Rapid eye movement (REM) sleep, an important component for mental restoration, occurs primarily in the last cycles of uninterrupted sleep and is the most likely form of sleep to be affected by sleep deprivation in the ICU.[20,31]

Hourly intervention is frequently necessary in the CCU to maintain physiologic homeostasis. This recurrent disruption in the sleep cycle quickly leads to a lack of REM sleep. Adverse effects of REM sleep deprivation include irritability, anxiety, physical exhaustion, and disruption of metabolic functions. Respiratory distress has also been associated with a lack of REM sleep.[14]

The bedside nurse must assess the patient and determine if adequate periods of uninterrupted time have been provided to promote all stages of sleep. Sleep periods should be included in the plan of care and adhered to as much as possible.[25] Consideration must be given to the importance of interventions vs. the necessity of uninterrupted sleep periods. Patients should not be subjected to activity or stressful procedures during the early morning hours unless they are imperative to maintain homeostasis. Visiting times should also be tailored to balance the needs of the patient and family while supporting adequate rest. Recent studies suggest that longer but less frequent visits may be more desirable than the traditional plan of a few minutes each hour.

ACUTE CONFUSION

The risk of developing acute confusion is high in the critical care setting. The high-technology environment is overwhelming and can be frightening for the patient. The presence of serious or traumatic illness adds additional psychologic and physiologic stress. Confusion is common among all patients in ICUs but especially older patients. It has a rapid onset and is generally reversible but can be very distressing for both patient and family.[13] Symptoms of acute confusion include hallucinations (both visual and auditory), restlessness, memory impairment, and fluctuations in the patient's level of awareness.[17]

Initial patient assessment should include information about the patient's mental status before admission. If the patient was able to adequately perform activities of daily living, it is reasonable to expect that the patient can return to that level of functioning once the acute confusion resolves.

Overwhelming stress is a frequent contributor to acute confusion, and the nurse must make every effort to make the critical care environment therapeutic rather than stressful. In the recent past, patients were physically restrained to protect them from harm. This type of intervention controls the patient's behavior but frequently increases the patient's confusion and causes a level of struggle or combativeness that may necessitate chemical sedation. Interventions ideally focus on removing stressors rather than adding to the problem. Current thinking focuses on alternatives to physical restraints. Fostering reality orientation by spending time with the patient and encouraging interaction with family and significant others should be a priority with the confused patient.[27]

Reality orientation is an ongoing, repetitive regimen of providing information to the patient at regular intervals and again as needed. This intervention is initiated immediately after admission to the ICU and is maintained until the patient can repeat the information on request.[27]

THE CRITICAL CARE NURSE

The critical care environment is also an exceptionally stressful environment for the nursing staff. The stress on the nursing staff stems partially from very high expectations: advanced knowledge of physiology related to all body systems, astute observational and physical assessment skills, ability to quickly prioritize and make decisions regarding patient care, and technical proficiency in operating the highly sophisticated equipment.[11] Nurses are also increasingly faced with complex ethical issues that consume their time and emotional energy. In addition, the constant vigilance and emergency-ready atmosphere may promote an uneasy sense of impending crisis. Critical care nurses must be able to remain calm in stressful circumstances and communicate effectively with the patient and family during crisis situations.

Most critical care nurses select this area of practice at least in part because they feel stimulated by a fast-paced environment where they are expected to effectively integrate a detailed knowledge base, excellent assessment skills, and significant technologic proficiency. Manageable stress levels can promote creativity and productivity. However, continuous high-level stress can be as detrimental to the nurse as to the patient. Box 8-3 summarizes some of the multiple stressors that can be present in the critical care environment.

Critical care nurses must understand how stressors affect the patient and family, but they must also be aware of the presence and effects of their own stressors. Critical care nurses must guard their own physical and psychologic health and recognize how insufficient or ineffective coping mechanisms can lead to burnout.

All critical care clinicians should be aware of the symptoms of stress and develop strategies for recognizing and decreasing their own stress levels. Most young professionals graduate from nursing school with skill and commitment toward meeting the needs of patients and families. It is essential that these clinicians also develop an ability to understand and respond appropriately to their own needs for support in the daily work environment as well as the needs of their colleagues. Failure to develop self-care strategies may decrease the nurse's ability to respond appropriately to patient needs and ultimately leads to nurse burnout and exit from the health care field.

Long-term involvement with patients in a critical care environment is a relatively new phenomenon and is accompanied by significant new stressors. Technology currently enables medical science to extend the life of some critically ill patients for significant periods of time. Patient populations, such as those awaiting organ transplantation, may have critical care hospitalizations that extend over weeks to months. Consistent nurse caregivers are clearly helpful to the patient and family in coping with the stressors of the critical care environment, and these nurses are more likely to develop a strong therapeutic relationship with the patient and family. They may even be able to more quickly assess and respond to

BOX 8-3 Stressors on Patients, Families, and Staff in the Critical Care Environment

Patient/Family	Staff
Unfamiliar environment, new faces	Expectations of self
Noise, light levels	Expectations of peer, clinical supervisors, other health care team members, hospital administrators
Sensory deprivation/ overload	Intricate machinery and techniques
Interruption of sleep/ wake cycles	Closed, crowed work area
Inaccessibility of family, friends	Constant contact with seriously ill, dying patients
Lack of privacy	Continual vigilance over multiple patients
Lack of information/understanding of prognosis, care plan	Constant emergency readiness
Lack of information/ understanding of policies, procedures	Sustained high activity level
Anticipation of painful interventions	Limited breaks away from high-stress unit
Confusion/disorientation related to physiologic factors	Limited communication with many patients related to intubation or altered level of consciousness
Impaired communication related to intubation	Limited opportunity to communicate with families
Observation of crisis interventions in other patients	Isolation from other nurses in hospital
Fear related to diagnosis	Ethical conflicts related to issues of resuscitation and use of life-support equipment
Fear of death	Legal issues
Conflict between patient/family goals and staff goals	Exposure to infectious diseases
Pain	

changes in the patient's condition. However, nurses caring for patients on an ongoing basis may also find themselves becoming so close to the circumstances of the patient's illness that their own psychologic health suffers. It is important for the clinician to be able to recognize when caring for a patient on an ongoing basis results in undue stress and to develop strategies for protecting his or her mental health. Strategies include:

- Development of support networks among nursing peers.
- Use of employee assistance personnel (counselors, social services personnel, and chaplains; critical stress debriefing) to cope with stressful circumstances.
- Development of interests outside of the critical care environment to help keep personal and professional worlds separate.
- Careful self-evaluation of the values, beliefs, and feelings associated with the critical care milieu.
- Use of a multidisciplinary team approach to nursing care. Multiple resources are available to the critical care clinician to accomplish the work of patient care. The nurse collaborates with direct caregivers such as physicians; respiratory, speech, and physical therapists; and other care providers such as nutritionists, pharmacists, venipuncture teams, chaplains, social workers, radiology technicians, clerical assistants, and hospital volunteers.
- Acknowledgment of the need to occasionally change assignments to provide respite care for the clinician.
- Scheduling of regular clinical care conferences with the patient, significant others, and other multidisciplinary team members to help the patient feel less dependent on the nursing staff. The use of conferences allows the patient and family to provide important input into the overall plan of care and feel the tangible involvement of various members of the multidisciplinary team. This approach is particularly important for the long-term critical care patient. Care goals can be reevaluated, modifications agreed on, or new goals established.

Experience has demonstrated that new graduate nurses can succeed in a critical care environment, but the hiring of novice nurses requires careful attention to both their orientation and mentoring.[26] Particular emphasis needs to be focused on the need for novices to develop both expertise in clinical skills and the emotional maturity needed for handling the stresses of the critical care environment. The experienced clinician more quickly identifies the subtle changes in the condition of a critical care patient. If adequate time, support, and supervision are not provided to the new graduate clinician, the presence of a novice simply escalates the stress experienced by other critical care clinicians. Ultimately patient care can suffer.

CARING FOR A DYING PATIENT IN CRITICAL CARE

The death of a critically ill patient can be the source of tremendous emotional stress to the nurse. To help protect self against overwhelming stress caused by a patient's death, when caring for a dying patient the nurse should:

- Examine his or her own feelings about death.
- Listen attentively to the expressed needs of the patient and family.
- Remain available to the patient and family both physically and emotionally.
- Use touch, if culturally acceptable, in caring for the patient and family.
- Reassure the patient and family that the patient will continue to receive skilled and compassionate care even if a "do not resuscitate" decision has been made.
- Attempt to remain nonjudgmental about family or hospital issues.
- Respect the strengths and limitations of the patient/family relationship, which existed long before the patient-hospital relationship.
- Include the family in care.
- Provide for patient and family privacy.
- Provide the opportunity for the family to exercise religious or cultural traditions.

Providing comprehensive care to critically ill patients and their families is a challenging opportunity. The critical care nurse combines the technologic sophistication of this unique setting with a personal, individualized care approach to maximize the potential outcomes for the patient.

ETHICAL DECISION MAKING IN CRITICAL CARE

In many ways technologic advances in health care have evolved faster than society's ability to understand and keep pace with the associated ethical dilemmas. Life can be prolonged in ways that were previously impossible. Not infrequently life can be maintained past all known hope of recovery. Tremendous emotional, financial, legal, and social ramifications exist as patients are stabilized into conditions for which long-term health care options are limited. For example, few families and even fewer skilled care facilities have the resources to care for a patient who requires continuous mechanical ventilation.

With the advent of advance directives, nurses frequently assume responsibility for gathering information about the patients' wishes concerning the extent of their care or treatment. Patients frequently have not prepared advance directives or are incompetent to render such a decision, leaving the family and significant others to determine the type and extent of medical care the patient would or would not want in this situation. Critical care nurses frequently assist families with highly emotional decisions such as foregoing resuscitation or withdrawing life support systems. Assisting families with these decisions is painfully complex.

All health care professionals must examine their own beliefs about life and death, termination of life, organ/tissue donation, and use of limited resources. Education and support for the nurse are available from formal classes, support groups, peers, and hospital ethics committees. Ethics committees are also available to patients, families, and staff members who wish consultation and support in difficult or divisive situations.

Biomedical advances at times seem to challenge the compassionate aspects of care giving. The critical care nurse is the professional caregiver best qualified to play a pivotal role in identifying and supporting the patient's wishes.

NURSING MANAGEMENT

The nursing process is the same in critical care situations as it is in any other patient setting. Management of critically ill patients requires establishment of a database, identification of actual and potential nursing diagnoses and collaborative problems, delineation of priorities, definition of outcome criteria, execution of the planned interventions, and modification of future interventions and plans on the basis of current outcomes. Management of critically ill patients differs from management of other patients because of an ever-changing database, a larger number of complex and interrelated problems, frequent priority reorganization, a greater variety of equipment and methods for measuring changes in patient status, and time limitations imposed by the patient's rapidly changing condition.[6]

ASSESSMENT

The assessment process for the critically ill patient differs from the assessment of other patients only in terms of the technologies used to assist in data collection. The cardiac monitor, hemodynamic monitoring lines, and laboratory analyses provide data that must be incorporated into the total patient assessment. Technologies are adjuncts to the data the nurse gathers through observation, history taking, and physical examination. Monitored data are useless unless correlated with physical findings and integrated into meaningful analysis by the critical care nurse.

The complete history and physical examination provide the necessary foundation for further ongoing data collection in the critical care setting, and the importance of accurate and thorough initial information cannot be overemphasized. However, the multiple sources of data and the continually fluctuating condition of critically ill patients make constant priority reorganization a necessity. The critical care nurse continually updates the database to reformulate short-term goals and interventions.

Patient assessment must be thorough, yet rapid. The physical and psychologic reactions of an entire organism under stress must be considered and not limited by the usual or the expected. Patient assessment also must be organized and repetitive so that small alterations or deviations from previous findings will be apparent. Finally, the assessment must be individualized, with time and attention given to particularly significant aspects.

Health History

The patient may be admitted to critical care as either a direct admission (usually through the emergency department), as a transfer from another patient care division in the same or a different hospital, or as a postoperative admission after certain operations. Data from the patient and family, written history, and the transfer report of other nurses are all integrated into the patient's initial treatment plan. Consultation between transferring and receiving nursing unit staffs is essential to accomplish this process effectively. These data sources help ensure continuity of care and communication of all issues important to the patient or family. The nurse carefully explores the patient's and family's response to the need for critical care placement. A full patient profile may be deferred until later in the hospitalization, as hemodynamic stabilization is always the first priority of care. The initial contact with the critical care personnel sets the tone for all future interactions and is an invaluable opportunity for the nurse to demonstrate competence and caring and begin to establish the essential foundation of trust.

Physical Examination

The physical assessment of the patient, while augmented by the technology of the ICU, still uses the skills of inspection, palpation, percussion, and auscultation to determine the patient's care needs and evaluate responses to interventions. The critical care nurse combines these physical assessment skills with information received from the patient and appropriate monitoring data to establish an initial plan of care and set priorities. In the critical care setting physical assessment may take place hourly or even more frequently as patient status dictates. All disciplines involved in the patient's care participate in the ongoing assessment process from their own perspective. The ongoing dynamic and collaborative nature of critical care assessment allows for rapid responses to be made to any changes in patient status but may also contribute significantly to the patient's sensory overload. The need to evaluate status changes frequently may leave the patient with little time for rest and privacy. Significant nursing skill is required to balance the need for information gathering with the need for patient rest. It may take years of experience for the nurse to gather and synthesize several pieces of data simultaneously, thoroughly, and rapidly, with the least disruption to the patient.

Monitored Data

Nurses in all clinical settings use tools such as stethoscopes, sphygmomanometers, thermometers, and scales to collect patient data. Critical care nurses also have access to tools such as cardiac monitors, hemodynamic pressure lines, intracranial pressure monitoring devices, and airway pressure monitoring devices that are capable of continuous data collection. The explosion in critical care technology since the 1970s provides the critical care nurse with amazing quantities of objective data. Digital computerized monitoring systems that occupy less space and provide more capabilities than ever before are widely available. The most sophisticated patient data management systems take information from all the monitored parameters (ECG, respirations, intraarterial pressure, pulmonary artery pressure, venous oxygen saturation [SvO_2], central venous pressure, intracranial pressure, and body temperature), combine it with manually entered data (such as body weight, height, intake and output, and times of drug administration), and produce a wide array of hemodynamic and pulmonary calculations and patient response trends for analysis by critical care practitioners.

Technologic adjuncts to critical care assessment are continuously undergoing change, combining older and well-tested monitoring systems with newer advances. Certain types of monitoring equipment are in use in all critical care environments. Waveforms and other data produced by these devices may be viewed continuously on a video screen or be graphed for a permanent record. Many monitoring systems involve use of fluid, tubing, and transducer equipment, which act as portals of entry for microorganisms. Strict aseptic technique is essential to prevent complications associated with nosocomial infections.

Cardiac Monitoring. Cardiac monitoring is a noninvasive procedure that poses minimal risk to the patient. It consists of placing conductive electrodes on the patient's chest that recognize the electrical activity of the heart and relay it to a video display screen. Depending on the sophistication of the monitoring equipment, the clinician may be able to view the patient's ECG and heart rate at the bedside and at remote locations in the critical care unit, monitor changes during activity (with mobile equipment), and set flexible monitoring parameters as changes in cardiac status occur. Parameters may include changes in heart rate and rhythm, respiratory rate and rhythm, analysis of dysrhythmias, and even changes in specific ECG segments, such as the ST segment for ischemia recognition. Alarms notify the clinician when preset limits have been reached. Most monitors default to preset limits if the clinician does not set specific alarm parameters and only allow clinicians to silence the alarms for limited periods of time.[12,18]

Hemodynamic Monitoring. Hemodynamic monitoring refers to invasive monitoring of the arterial or venous system. Monitoring is accomplished through catheters that measure changes in air and fluid pressures and can also be used to administer intravenous fluids and obtain arterial or venous blood for laboratory analysis. The air and fluid pressure readings are interpreted by transducers connected to the system and display the results as waveforms on cardiac monitoring equipment (Figure 8-2). The two most commonly used hemodynamic monitoring systems are intraarterial monitoring and pulmonary artery monitoring.

It is important for the nurse to verify the digital display of waveform values with a manual sphygmomanometer, regularly calibrate the transducer equipment with the transducer positioned at specific landmarks on the patient's body, and assess the entire system for patency and accuracy.[9] Research has demonstrated that in patients with a stable hemodynamic status, measurements obtained in a 30-degree lateral and in a supine position are essentially the same (see Research box). A thorough knowledge of waveform interpretation is required

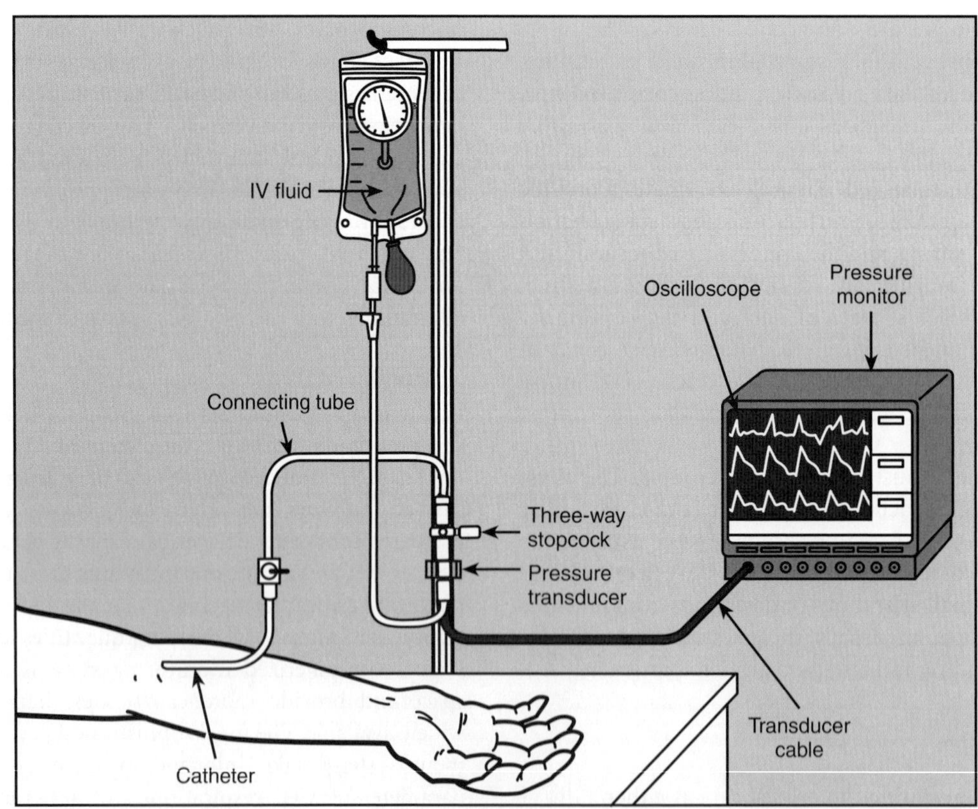

Figure 8-2 Components of a pressure monitoring system. The cannula, shown entering the brachial artery, is connected via pressure tubing to the transducer. The transducer converts the pressure wave into an electronic signal. The transducer is wired to the electric monitoring system, which amplifies, conditions, displays, and records the signal.

to appropriately interpret and respond to the values displayed on the screen or on a manual printout. Even minor errors in reading and interpreting values or small problems in the patency of the system, such as a tiny air bubble in the transducer system, can result in inaccurate data and may cause profound complications for the patient. Aseptic technique is critical to the maintenance of these systems with the least possible risk to the patient. Ongoing assessment of the patient's response to the equipment is also critical to avoid dangerous complications such as air emboli, bleeding, malposition of catheters, tissue damage, or hemodynamic compromise as a result of foreign body insertion or malposition.

Intraarterial Monitoring. Intraarterial monitoring involves inserting a catheter into an artery, usually through the radial or femoral artery, and connecting the catheter to a high-pressure flush system filled with either a heparinized or nonheparinized saline solution. The high-pressure flush counterbalances arterial resistance to maintain patency of the system. Intraarterial systems display a continuous reading of the patient's blood pressure and provide ready access to obtain arterial blood gas or other laboratory specimens.[1]

Pulmonary Artery Monitoring. Pulmonary artery monitoring involves inserting a catheter through the subclavian or internal jugular vein and advancing it into the pulmonary artery, usually under fluoroscopic guidance to ensure accurate placement. These catheters have several lumens encased within a larger lumen, and each opens at a different point along the length of the catheter. Each lumen may be used for fluid administration, and specific lumens may be used to attach monitoring and transducer equipment. The large bore of the lumens and placement of the catheter in large arteries permit administration of caustic intravenous solutions that could damage peripheral veins. A balloon at the distal tip of the catheter is filled with approximately 1 ml of air when the natural flow of blood through the patient's heart pulls the balloon into place in the pulmonary artery.[28]

When the catheter is correctly placed, the balloon is deflated. Monitoring and transducer equipment is attached to the catheter. The catheter and monitoring equipment are used to obtain significant data about the patient's hemodynamic and cardiac function. Available data include pulmonary artery and central venous pressure recordings and cardiac output measurements. Combining these values with parameters such as blood pressure and body surface area make it possible to calculate additional information that is not directly available from catheter readings. Newer monitoring equipment calculates these values automatically when data are entered into the database, decreasing the chance for error from manual calculation. The pulmonary artery catheter rapidly provides valuable information to evaluate the patient's response to vasoactive drugs by providing data about left and right heart function. It is also a significant tool for managing severe cardiac failure and cardiogenic shock.

Central Venous Pressure Monitoring. A central venous pressure (CVP) catheter may be used in lieu of a pulmonary artery catheter when evaluation of pulmonary artery pressure and left heart function are not required. CVP catheters may be connected to a transducer and used to measure right heart pressures and deliver intravenous fluids, but they are more limited in the scope of data they provide than are pulmonary artery catheters. A newer type of central line is called a peripherally inserted central venous catheter (PICC). The external portion of the PICC is assessed and maintained by nurses, and patients and families may be instructed in these techniques for home use. PICC lines are long-dwell catheters that require the same aseptic care as other central lines. They can be used to administer long-term intravenous fluid therapy but at present have no monitoring capabilities. PICC lines are more commonly used for long-term fluid and medication administration.[16,30]

Intracranial Pressure Monitoring. Monitoring intracranial pressure (ICP) involves placement of a catheter through the skull into either the subarachnoid space or the cerebral ventricle to monitor changes in pressure within the cranial cavity. A transducer and tubing system gather the data that are displayed on the monitoring screens. Newer monitoring systems have the capacity to sense changes in intracranial pressure and display pressure readings on a bedside monitor without the use of fluid-filled pressure tubing and transducer systems. Although insertion through the skull into the cranial cavity is still required, these newer systems reduce the risk of contamination by microorganisms. Patients with unstable intracranial pressure may be quite sensitive to routine nursing interventions such as turning, suctioning, and changes in bed position.[33] Continuous display of ICP readings allows the nurse to constantly evaluate the patient's responses to all interventions and take prompt action if the patient's pressure reaches unsafe levels. The catheter also can be used to aspirate

Research

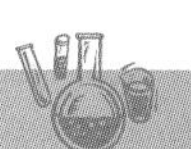

Reference: Bridges EJ et al: Effect of the 30° lateral recumbent position on pulmonary artery and pulmonary artery wedge pressures in critically ill adult cardiac surgery patients, *Am J Crit Care* 9(4):262-275, 2000.

This study sought to determine and compare the effect of 30-degree right and left lateral and supine positions on pulmonary artery and pulmonary artery wedge pressures after cardiac surgery in adult patients. Despite the beneficial effects of lateral positioning, many patients are positioned supine for prolonged periods to obtain hemodynamic information. The study used an experimental repeated-measures design with 35 patients deemed stable hemodynamically 12 to 24 hours after cardiac surgery. Subjects were randomly assigned to one of two position sequences with pulmonary artery and pulmonary artery wedge pressures measured in each position. A significant difference in pulmonary artery systolic, end-diastolic, and mean pressures were noted between patients positioned in the 30-degree lateral position and the supine position, although mean differences were small. No significant differences were noted in pulmonary artery wedge pressures between the two positions. The authors concluded that pulmonary artery and pulmonary artery wedge pressure values obtained with the patient in a 30-degree lateral position could be used interchangeably with values obtained with the patient in the supine position during the first 12 to 24 hours after cardiac surgery if the patient is hemodynamically stable.

cerebrospinal fluid for analysis or culture and to relieve elevated ICP. The nurse is also responsible for identifying changes in pressure readings, analyzing trends, evaluating patient responses to interventions or therapies, and preventing complications.

Continuous Airway Pressure Monitoring. Continuous airway pressure monitoring (CAPM) is a simple noninvasive technique that uses a transducer cable, high-pressure tubing (as used for measuring pulmonary and arterial pressures), and a display monitor. The monitoring equipment is connected to a ventilator circuit at the Y connector near the airway. Standard calibration procedures are used, but the monitoring tubing is filled with air, not fluid, and the transducer can be at any level while calibration is performed. The absence of fluid in the transducer system minimizes the risk of infection. The waveforms produced by CAPM may be continuously displayed, graphed, and compared with hemodynamic waveforms. The waveforms produced by the system enable the clinician to continuously monitor the patient's response to various modes of mechanical ventilation or to mechanical ventilation itself, and assess the patient's response to therapeutic interventions.[3]

CAPM is also useful in identifying one of the most common complications of mechanical ventilation—patient-ventilator asynchrony or intolerance. Asynchrony can result from mechanical malfunction, inappropriate ventilator mode selection and inadequate inspiratory flow rate, airway obstruction from excessive secretions, or patient anxiety or agitation. Asynchrony increases the work of breathing and can result in inadequate gas exchange. When a patient experiences asynchrony, the CAPM waveforms deviate from the expected patterns, alerting the nurse to the need for prompt intervention. CAPM can be especially helpful in monitoring sedated, very ill, or chemically relaxed patients who may be unable to subjectively communicate patient-ventilator intolerance. CAPM provides the bedside nurse with continuous visual assurance that the patient is receiving adequate ventilation and that chemical relaxation is being delivered at an appropriate dose. Any interruption of ventilation is immediately apparent by waveform absence.[10]

Analysis of the patient's waveforms and comparison with expected waveforms allow the care team to evaluate the patient's response to mechanical ventilation and modify the plan if necessary. Hemodynamic pressure data frequently serve as the foundation of treatment for critically ill patients. However, both real and artificial changes in the hemodynamic waveforms occur in response to pressure gradients produced by the pulmonary and systemic circulation. True pressures can be further obscured by tachypnea and underlying cardiac pathologic conditions. CAPM may be used in these situations to help standardize measurements. Simultaneous graphing of CAPM and pulmonary artery pressures provides a clear visual picture of end expiration. CAPM has thus been shown to be a simple, cost-efficient, and effective adjunct to critical care monitoring.

Summary of Monitoring. The preceding discussion presents a few of the invasive and noninvasive monitoring tools available to critical care clinicians. In all cases the nurse must be knowledgeable about the proper use and maintenance of the equipment including the normal appearance of the waveform associated with each line, standard interventions used to prevent complications, signs and symptoms of actual complications, and techniques used to troubleshoot the monitoring systems when problems develop. The patient risk associated with invasive monitoring lines is significantly reduced when knowledgeable personnel manage the lines. In addition to the various invasive lines used for monitoring, critical care nurses also must be skillful in using central lines for medication, fluid, and nutrition administration.

As monitoring techniques become increasingly sophisticated, it is tempting to treat the patient solely based on the numbers and waveforms produced by the equipment. It is essential for the clinician to remember that these data must always be combined with data obtained from routine physical assessment that include the patient's general appearance and subjective response to all therapeutic measures. A flat line on a waveform may be the result of a disconnected wire or tubing rather than a change in the patient's condition. The nurse must remain vigilant and keep one eye on the monitor and one eye on the patient to avoid treating the equipment instead of the patient. The nurse must also individualize the use of each monitoring technique to the uniqueness of each patient situation.

NURSING DIAGNOSES

The range of nursing diagnoses that can be appropriate in any specific critical care patient situation is virtually limitless. The discussion of nursing interventions that follows addresses broad categories of interventions that are applicable in a wide variety of situations. Similarly, commonly encountered nursing diagnoses might include but are certainly not limited to:

Diagnostic Title	Possible Etiologic Factors
1. Decreased cardiac output	Alterations in preload or after load, disturbances in cardiac rate/rhythm
2. Impaired gas exchange	Altered oxygen supply, changes in the alveolar capillary membrane
3. Ineffective tissue perfusion	Interruption of blood flow, (cerebral, cardio-exchange problems pulmonary)
4. Anxiety	Situational crisis, threat of death or disability
5. Acute confusion	Sensory deprivation/overload, lack of sleep, pain, hypoxia
6. Deficient knowledge: critical care environment and routines	Lack of exposure
7. Interrupted family processes	Temporary family disorganization and role changes
8. Deficient knowledge: discharge	Fear of the unknown and lack of previous experience from ICU and future care needs

EXPECTED PATIENT OUTCOMES

Expected patient outcomes are tailored to the unique needs of each individual patient. Broad outcomes that commonly apply to the identified nursing diagnoses include:

1. Will maintain systolic blood pressure above 100 mm Hg, urine output greater than 30 ml/hr, and cardiac rate and rhythm within acceptable limits
2. Will demonstrate satisfactory pulmonary function (adequate blood oxygenation, hemoglobin saturation, and forced expiratory volume in 1 second [FEV_1]) and exhibit a satisfactory respiratory rate and pattern.
3. Will exhibit stable vital signs and intracranial pressure no greater than 15 mm Hg
4. Will report an increase in psychologic comfort and an absence of restlessness or other behavioral manifestations of anxiety
5. Will experience fewer episodes of confusion
6. Will expresse understanding of routines and environment of the critical care unit
7. Will identify stress of critical care admission on the family unit and personal and community resources available to assist with coping
8. Will express understanding of changing care needs and or the transfer to another setting

INTERVENTIONS

1, 2, 3. Maintaining Cardiac Output, Gas Exchange, and Tissue Perfusion

The ultimate goal of nursing intervention for any patient is to promote, sustain, and restore optimal levels of physiologic, psychologic, and social functioning. However, in a critical care setting, the immediate goal of ensuring a patient's survival determines the priorities for intervention; physiologic problems must be addressed first. Once life-threatening stressors have been alleviated, priorities can be reevaluated, and other problems addressed.

Physiologic priorities are determined by the degree of threat to the person's survival. Certain body systems are more prone to disorders requiring intensive therapeutic interventions and are frequently encountered in the critical care unit. At the most basic level, these priorities can be organized in the same "ABC" framework as basic cardiac life support. Establishment of airway, breathing, and circulation remains the foundation for therapeutic management of the critical care patient. When the ABCs of basic life support are applied, the critical care nurse is able to move from the most pressing to least pressing patient problems. When a critical care nurse determines that a patient's physiologic status has begun to deteriorate, actions are immediately taken to reverse the problem. Correct positioning of the endotracheal tube with suctioning as needed to ensure an unobstructed airway ensures airway patency. The nurse then assesses the patient's ability to breathe and the effect of physical restraints or physiologic conditions such as acute respiratory failure. Circulatory needs, such as the establishment of normal cardiac rhythm, intravenous access for administration of medications, and adequate cardiopulmonary perfusion of vital organs, are addressed next. The critical care clinician may continue to use this basic ABC principle in ongoing assessments to ensure that problems are recognized before complications develop.

4,5. Reducing Anxiety and Confusion

In addition to continuous assessment for physiologic derangements, the nurse also must focus attention on recognizing the psychologic stressors that confront the patient and family. The emotional discomfort and distress that the patient and family endure not only affect the patient's psychologic health but also have a direct impact on physical recovery.

The initial step in preventing or alleviating psychologic stress is to identify the patient and family's perception of the critical event. Their perceptions will be affected by their individual personalities, current psychologic health, general understanding of the present situation and its projected outcome, tolerance for ambiguity, and normal patterns of coping. Initial perceptions are often significantly affected by previous exposure to similar events, either positive or negative, and general level of familiarity with medical interventions and the hospital environment. Specific interventions nurses can use in any setting to reduce the psychologic stress of illness are described next.

Because the critically ill person is separated from familiar surroundings and is dependent on others to meet the most basic needs, the patient becomes partially or totally isolated from usual support systems. Feelings of helplessness, powerlessness, loneliness, and depersonalization, as well as disturbances in body image, are common. Modes of expressing and therefore relieving the frustration, anger, hostility, fear, and depression generated by these feelings are limited by the physical constraints of the critical care environment. Consistently assigned caregivers can be an effective way to establish a therapeutic relationship with the patient and family.

An atmosphere of openness and acceptance that encourages expression of feelings can help provide patients with a means of coping. The nurse talks openly and honestly with patients and attempts to decrease the patient's feelings of depersonalization, isolation, and alienation. Anger and hostility are often indications of fear and anxiety. Depression and withdrawal may be signs of hopelessness, loneliness, powerlessness, or loss and are normal and expected. The nurse encourages the patient and family to express their feelings and assists the patient to identify the fears and concerns that may be causing unusual or inappropriate behavior. The nurse is nonjudgmental and avoids communicating a message that the patient's behavior is "wrong" or unacceptable.

Nurses or other health care team members who help patients talk about feelings must be ready to accept whatever emotionally laden information might be expressed. Nonjudgmental recognition and acceptance of the patient's feelings help reinforce the patient's right to the feelings.

Intubated patients are unable to express their feelings freely even when alert and oriented and are therefore particularly vulnerable to psychologic stressors. It is natural to communicate less with persons who cannot talk easily, and the nurse must guard against this. Strategies such as keeping a letterboard, paper and pencil, or a "magic slate" within the patient's reach and providing assistance to the patient help reduce the sense of isolation. However, such methods do not allow the patient to truly express feelings and concerns. The nurse carefully assesses the patient for cues concerning his or her emotional state and anticipates common concerns among critically ill patients. The nurse can verbalize the potential concerns, allowing the patient to validate them as appropriate. The direct expression of empathy for the patient and family conveys acceptance and understanding.

6. Providing Information

The patient's perception of stressors and not the stressor itself determines the patient's reaction to the illness and the critical care environment. It is essential that the patient and family receive adequate information and simple explanations. Without explanations the critical care environment presents a mysterious and threatening array of noxious stimuli, which may be perceived as extremely unnatural and even magical. The highly sophisticated equipment increases the patient's feelings of vulnerability, and the patient may worry that the cardiac monitor is actually keeping the heart beating, that a blood transfusion indicates hemorrhaging, or that chest physiotherapy signifies pneumonia. A common misconception of patients after coronary artery bypass surgery is that "open heart" surgery involved cutting the heart wide open and sewing it back together again. Such a perception can lead to a drastic alteration in body image.

The nurse is an important source of information for the patient and family and he or she usually leads the patient education effort. Patient teaching in critical care has a short-term focus. Pain, discomfort, weakness, anxiety, and transient confusion are some of the obstacles to learning that critical care patients experience. The nurse provides simple repetitive explanations of all interventions and their purposes and introduces the patient and family to the overall plan for ongoing care. Patients may not understand or believe what they are told the first time, and anxiety and denial may prevent accurate retention. The nurse may need to reinterpret and reiterate the diagnosis, prognosis, goals of treatment, types of interventions, and expectations of the patient and family during the entire critical care stay. Primary caregivers ideally provide explanations to encourage continuity of care and minimize the confusion of differing approaches and wording. If the patient and family are apprised of the patient's current status, as well as all changes in plans, the situation can be perceived accurately, and they are able to plan realistically for the future and participate fully as members of the health care team.

7. Supporting Family Involvement and Expression of Feelings and Needs

The essence of crisis intervention is helping persons cope with a major life crisis that a critical illness may precipitate. Critical care nursing is far broader in scope and more future oriented than crisis intervention alone, but specific situations frequently require the immediacy and limited focus of crisis intervention. At the time of crisis the nurse assists the patient and family to establish short-term goals and minimizes the number and scope of decisions they must make. As the crisis situation stabilizes, the nurse provides the patient and family with more information and assists them to accept additional responsibility for decision making and goal setting.

When the patient and family are knowledgeable about the goals of therapy and understand the patient's diagnosis, current status, and prognosis, they can be involved in many aspects of care planning and make decisions consistent with the treatment regimen.

Involvement of significant others decreases the patient's feelings of powerlessness, frustration, and anxiety. The family is likely to be needed in a direct caregiver role at some point in the patient's recovery, and it is important for the multidisciplinary team to begin including them in care planning as soon as possible. The patient is reassured by having a loving advocate represent his or her wishes and concerns. Even when a patient is unconscious, visits by key support figures who talk to and touch the patient may have positive, if immeasurable, effects on the patient while helping to decrease the family's feelings of helplessness.[22]

The nurse actively involves all alert patients in goal setting and care planning. The nurse seeks to increase the patient's feeling of personal control in structuring the daily schedule of activities. The knowledge that the preferences of the patient are important to the nursing staff and that the patient is viewed as capable of making decisions reinforces the importance of the patient's role in recovery.

The environment of the CCU presents multiple stresses to both the patient and family. Narcotics and sedatives, anxiety, hypoxia, sleep deprivation, and multiple metabolic derangements all combine to create acute confusion, disturbed thought processes, and perceptual distortions. The nurse uses reality orientation on an ongoing basis to assist patients to regain their mental stability. Although some environmental factors cannot be altered, the nurse can use a variety of strategies to control the sensory level of the critical care unit.

Critical care units are increasingly recognizing the importance of visits by the patient's significant others in minimizing the psychologic stressors of the environment. The practice of restrictive and minimal visitation is increasingly being replaced by varying degrees of open visitation. Open visitation policies range in scope from longer and more frequent visitation hours to the practice of true open visitation where the patient and family participate fully in care activities and care team rounds. Although these policies appear to improve the ability of the patient and family to develop trust and a therapeutic relationship with the care team, the nurse must be careful to avoid overwhelming the family with the daily stress and sensory overload of the critical care unit. With more open visiting in place it is frequently important for the nurse to encourage significant others to meet their own needs for rest, nutrition, psychosocial support, relaxation, and spiritual renewal. Many significant others need to be supported in their decision to leave the critical care environment at regular intervals even when visitation policies would allow them to remain.[19]

In the critical care setting the patient's physiologic needs often assume priority over psychologic needs, and the patient's needs as a social being may be virtually ignored. Limited visiting hours, the strange technical environment, and the aura of danger in the critical care unit isolate patients from their supportive family and friends and prevent them from participating in their usual social roles. For the most part, staff members view a person who is critically ill primarily in the patient role. The more significant roles of spouse, parent, child, lover, sibling, friend, or provider may go virtually unrecognized unless staff members initiate interventions to provide continuity in these relationships.

Continuity in social roles is fostered through some of the same types of interventions used to reduce psychologic stress: increasing visiting between patient and family; including the family in discussions of disease process, prognosis, and plans of care; and reporting by family of events and activities occurring in the other significant spheres of the patient's life. Relaying telephone messages between the patient and distant friends is one way the nurse can help the patient maintain contact with his or her broader external world.

One of the most effective and important ways to prevent disruption in relationships is for the nurse to carefully prepare family or friends for their first visit with the patient in the critical care unit. The patient's physical appearance and the critical care environment are explained thoroughly before the visitor enters. Visitors need to understand the patient's level of consciousness, as well as ability to communicate and comprehend communication. They need to understand the importance of their presence to the patient and the patient's need for their support. When visitors approach the bedside, the nurse remains with them if possible to facilitate their initial interaction with the patient. Family frequently needs to be encouraged to touch the patient and offer other physical expressions of their love and support. Fear of hurting the patient or disrupting the multiple monitoring devices can virtually immobilize the family member. The nurse can help family members find safe places to stand and explain the basic purpose of the various lines and tubes. The nurse also encourages the family to speak with the patient, especially unconscious or intubated patients. At each subsequent visit the nurse caring for the patient meets with the family to answer questions and apprise them of the patient's progress.

In addition to supporting the maintenance of the patient's current roles and relationships, the critical care nurse also recognizes the inevitability of actual role change for some patients and families during a critical illness. Roles of provider, decision maker, employer, and employee may be altered, reversed, or eliminated. Family and friends may need to assume some or all of the responsibilities of the patient at this time.

During the critical phase of illness the family members are trying to cope with significant role changes and may need help in working through problems that arise as family members and friends assume or fail to assume these additional responsibilities. The nurse needs to be sensitive to these challenging problems and provide the family with professional guidance, such as from a social worker, to assist in reorganizing themselves and their resources. The nurse may help the family appoint a temporary family representative, someone who knows and is able to represent the wishes of the family as a whole and who can be contacted in the event of emergency. The nurse also may help the family to plan visiting schedules that meet the patient's needs without preventing family members from fulfilling their own responsibilities. This is a period of great emotional stress for both patient and family.

8. Patient/Family Education: Preparing for Transfer

Transfer from the CCU to another setting can cause significant stress for patients and their families. The critical care area represents security and protection with its sophisticated electronic equipment and attentive, highly skilled staff members. Patients know that transfer means moving to an area where there are fewer nursing personnel per patient, less direct contact with nursing personnel, no automatic or obvious monitoring devices, and no direct observation of the patient from the nurses' station. Greater independence and higher levels of activity will be expected of patients on the transfer unit, and the support of familiar nursing staff members will be lost. Patients may experience ambivalent feelings about the transfer, particularly if they do not feel as well or as independent as anticipated at the time of transfer.

The anxiety precipitated by the transfer can be prevented or reduced if the patient and family are taught to interpret the meaning of particular signs and symptoms and are helped to understand the true purpose of equipment and routines. The nurse continuously points out the signs that indicate patient progress. The nurse begins to include transfer plans in discussions with the family as soon as the patient's condition begins to stabilize. This helps the family to adjust and prepare for the relocation. Along with the projected date of transfer, the patient and family need to know what to expect on the new unit and what will be expected of them. Ideally a nurse from the receiving unit meets the patient and family before transfer. After transfer, visits from the critical care staff are helpful in conveying ongoing concern for the patient's welfare, as well as in providing objective validation of continued progress. With careful planning and execution, transfer from the critical care unit can be a triumphant rather than a traumatic event.

With the increasing trend toward managed care insurance plans and decreased scope of third-party reimbursement for hospitalization, patients are increasingly discharged directly from the critical care environment to the home. These patients may require a wide variety of care regimens that their significant others need to manage effectively. Families are also frequently required to perform various nursing therapies. A family member may need to learn to manage sophisticated machinery such as home ventilators or oxygen equipment and understand how to safely troubleshoot routine problems with machinery. Critical care clinicians need to begin working with the patient's family early in the hospitalization to establish a good therapeutic relationship and ensure that home issues are resolved before the day of discharge. Family caregivers must be both technically proficient and confident that they can effectively manage the patient's care. The nurse can instill that confidence in a family caregiver, and confidence is an essential component of successful home management. Planning for respite care for a family caregiver is also important to ensure that the caregiver does not become overwhelmed with the multiple responsibilities of home care. Early referral to community-based home care agencies is also essential to provide the patient and family with the needed physical and psychologic resources to manage the transition to home. Discharge is otherwise a lonely and overwhelming experience.

EVALUATION

To evaluate the effectiveness of nursing interventions. the patient's behaviors are compared with those stated in the expected patient outcomes. Achievement of outcomes is successful if the critically ill patient (and in the case of outcomes 7 and 8, the family):

1. Maintains all monitored parameters within specified limits.
2. Demonstrates satisfactory gas exchange and pulmonary function.
3. Has stable vital signs and ICP level within accepted limits.
4. Reports increased psychologic comfort and is free of behaviors indicative of anxiety.
5. Remains oriented to self and surroundings.
6. Expresses understanding of the nature and scope of critical care monitoring and interventions.
7. Functions successfully with the assistance of personal and community resources.
8. Expresses understanding of changing care needs and transfer to another setting.

COLLABORATIVE CARE

The care of critically ill patients and their families involves members of a multidisciplinary team that includes numerous disciplines (e.g., nursing, medicine, respiratory, occupational, social services, pharmacy, rehabilitation). It is the nurse's responsibility to coordinate patient care, which is best served by a collaborative approach. When a collaborative environment is fostered, the focus is on finding the best solution to patient care issues based on the unique talents and contributions of all concerned parties. The patient's interests remain the highest primary concern among members of the multidisciplinary team.

COLLABORATIVE PROBLEMS

Many patient care problems with which critical care nurses must deal are physiologic complications that nurses manage using both nurse and physician driven interventions and protocols. Such collaborative problems should be labeled *Potential Complication*. This label alerts the nurse that the nursing focus for the identified collaborative problem is to prevent or reduce the severity of the physiologic event. For example, a collaborative problem critical care nurses may encounter frequently is *Potential Complication: Arrhythmias.* Nurses monitor for the development of arrhythmias and, when they occur, implement a protocol of treatment that has been previously established and approved by the medical staff. This allows appropriate use of the critical care nurse's assessment skills, critical thinking, and timely implementation of prescriptive orders from medicine to quickly alleviate the problem.

Critical Thinking Questions

1. Discuss how critical care nursing has evolved over the century, including the contributions of the professional organization to critical care nursing practice.
2. What are some of the common stressors critical care nurses face and how can nurses reduce the stress associated with each stressor?
3. How does the use of critical care monitoring technology affect the delivery of patient care in the critical care environment?
4. How does the critical care nurse use a multidisciplinary approach to optimize patient care planning?

References

1. Ahrens T: Hemodynamic monitoring, *Crit Care Nurs Clin North Am* 11:19, 1999.
2. Alcott LM: *Hospital sketches,* Boston, 1863, James Redpath,.
3. Aloi A, Burns SM: Continuous airway pressure monitoring in the critical care setting, *Crit Care Nurse* 15:66, 1995.
4. American Association of Critical Care Nurses. Mission, vision, and values (position statement). Aliso Viejo, CA, 1999b, Internet document: http://www.aacn.org.
5. American Association of Critical Care Nurses. Role of the critical care nurse (position statement). Aliso Viejo, CA, 1999a, Internet document: http://www.aacn.org.
6. American Association of Critical Care Nurses. Standards for acute and critical care practice. Aliso Viejo, CA, 1999c, Internet document: //http:www.aacn.org.
7. Baas LS, Beery TA, Hickey CS: Care and safety of pacemaker electrodes in intensive care and telemetry nursing units, *Am J Crit Care* 6:302, 1997.
8. Bray KA, Hearn K: Critical care unit design: establishing operations, Part 3, *Nurs Manage* 24(3):64A-C, 64F, 64H, 1993.
9. Bridges EJ et al: Effect of 30° lateral recumbent position on pulmonary artery and pulmonary artery wedge pressures in critically ill adult cardiac surgery patients, *Am J Crit Care* 9:262, 2000.
10. Burns SM: Protocols for practice: applying research at the bedside. Continuous airway pressure monitoring, *Crit Care Nurse* 21:66, 2001.
11. Currey J, Worrall CL: Making decisions: nursing practices in critical care, *Aust Crit Care* 14:127, 2001.
12. Drew BJ, Krucoff MW: Multilead ST-segment monitoring in patients with acute coronary syndromes: a consensus statement for healthcare professionals. ST-Segment Monitoring Practice Guideline International Working Group, *Am J Crit Care* 8:372, 1999.
13. Foreman MD et al: Delirium in elderly patients: an overview of the state of the science, *J Gerontol Nurs* 27:12, 2001.
14. Freedman NS et al: Abnormal sleep/wake cycles and the effect of environmental noise on sleep disruption in the intensive care unit, *Am J Respir Crit Care Med* 163:451, 2001.
15. Gammon J: The psychological consequences of source isolation: a review of the literature, *J Clin Nurs* 8:13, 1999.
16. Goh RH: Team approach to vascular access: CINA conference '99, *CINA-J*, Sept 15:53-55, 1999.
17. Granberg-Axell A, Bergbom I, Lundberg D: Clinical signs of ICU syndrome/delirium: an observational study, *Intensive Crit Care Nurs* 17:72, 2001.
18. Jacobson C: Bedside cardiac monitoring, *Crit Care Nurse* 18:82, 1998.

19. Krapohl GL: Visiting hours in the adult intensive care unit: using research to develop a system that works, *Dimens Crit Care Nurs* 14:245, 1995.
20. Lee KA: Sleep and fatigue, *Annu Rev Nurs Res* 19:249, 2001.
21. Maddox M, Dunn SV, Pretty LE: Psychosocial recovery following ICU: experiences and influences upon discharge to the community, *Intensive Crit Care Nurs* 17:6, 2001.
22. Mendonca D, Warren NA: Perceived and unmet needs of critical care family members, *Crit Care Nurs Q* 21:58, 1998.
23. Moore K: Critical care unit design: a collaborative approach, *Crit Care Nurs Q* 16:15, 1993.
24. Nightingale F: *Notes on hospitals,* ed 3, London, 1863, Longman, Green, Longman, Roberts and Green.
25. Olson DM et al: Quiet time: a nursing intervention to promote sleep in neurocritical care units, *Am J Crit Care* 10:74, 2001.
26. Porte-Gendron RW et al: Baccalaureate nurse educators' and critical care nurse managers' perceptions of clinical competencies necessary for new graduate baccalaureate critical care nurses, *Am J Crit Care* 6:147, 1997.
27. Rapp CG: Acute confusion/delirium protocol, *J Gerontol Nurs* 27:21, 2001.
28. Shaffer RB: Arterial catheter insertion(assist), care, and removal. In Lynn-McHale DJ, Carlson KK, editors: *AACN procedure manual for critical care,* ed 4, Philadelphia, 2001, WB Saunders.
29. Solsona JF et al: Are auditory warnings in the intensive care unit properly adjusted? *J Adv Nurs* 35:402, 2001.
30. Todd J: Clinical. Peripherally inserted central catheters and their use in IV therapy, *Br J Nurs* 8:140, 142, 144, 1999.
31. Topf M, Thompson S: Interactive relationships between hospital patients' noise-induced stress and other stress with sleep, *Heart Lung J Acute Crit Care* 30:237, 2001.
32. West S: How do nurses prevent sensory imbalance occurring in the intensive care unit? *Nurs Crit Care* 1:79, 1996.
33. Winkelman C: Effect of backrest position on intracranial and cerebral perfusion pressure in traumatically brain-injured adults, *Am J Crit Care* 9:373, 2000.

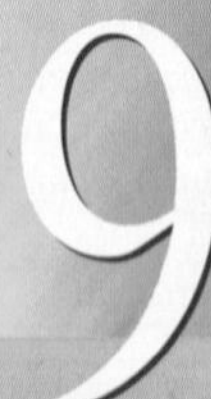

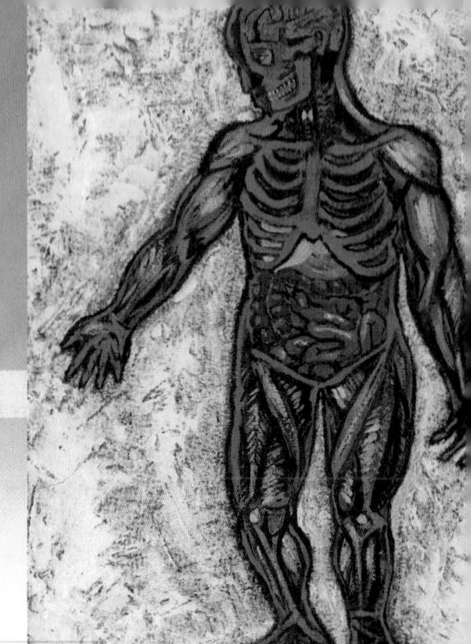

9 Community-Based Care

Marianne Neighbors

Objectives

After studying this chapter, the learner should be able to:

1. Describe the trends in community-based care for medical-surgical clients.
2. Describe the agencies delivering care in the community for medical-surgical clients.
3. Discuss the nursing responsibilities related to managing the transition from acute care to community-based care.
4. Apply the nursing process in planning care for clients and their families in community settings.
5. Discuss the unique challenges of the community as an environment for providing nursing care.
6. Identify current social, ethical, and economic issues related to community-based care.
7. Describe the unique factors related to nursing care of clients in the home.

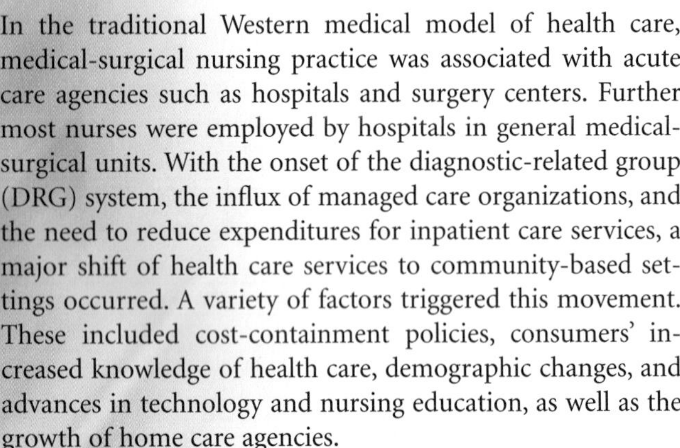

In the traditional Western medical model of health care, medical-surgical nursing practice was associated with acute care agencies such as hospitals and surgery centers. Further most nurses were employed by hospitals in general medical-surgical units. With the onset of the diagnostic-related group (DRG) system, the influx of managed care organizations, and the need to reduce expenditures for inpatient care services, a major shift of health care services to community-based settings occurred. A variety of factors triggered this movement. These included cost-containment policies, consumers' increased knowledge of health care, demographic changes, and advances in technology and nursing education, as well as the growth of home care agencies.

Community-based medical-surgical care is defined as the delivery of health services to clients and families where they live, work, or go to school. The focus of the care is on acute and chronic conditions that require interventions and, at times, continuous services and follow-up. The nurse's role in the delivery of care in these settings is diverse.[15]

TRENDS IN COMMUNITY-BASED CARE

As the cost for in-hospital care increases, as technology becomes more sophisticated, and as the health care consumer becomes more knowledgeable and takes on a greater responsibility for self-care, health care services will continue to move to the community as the base for the delivery of care. An increasing number of surgeries that previously required hospitalization are now routinely performed in outpatient settings. More care is being delivered in the home, in schools, and at the worksite. With the resources given to health promotion and risk reduction, an even greater number of services will be offered in community-based settings than ever before. Some experts have predicted that 75% of all health care will be delivered in community settings by the year 2025. This opens a multitude of opportunities for nurses to focus their care giving and teaching in a variety of new settings.[16]

PRACTICE ROLES AND SETTINGS INCLUDED IN COMMUNITY-BASED CARE

Health care in community-based settings is often managed by a team of multidisciplinary professionals including the physician, registered nurse, dietitian, social worker, physical or occupational therapist, respiratory therapist, clergy, nursing care assistants, and others. The medical-surgical nurse of today must be knowledgeable, highly skilled, and increasingly independent to handle the health care needs of clients in community-based settings. Care delivered by medical-surgical nurses in nonhospital settings is based on the nursing process. Assessment skills are crucial in defining the nature of clients' needs. Setting goals for the client and determining appropriate interventions that can be delivered in the community setting may require the expertise and ingenuity of the health care team. Services may be delivered by the nurse or may be delegated to other appropriate health care personnel. Evaluation of the client's status and continued need for care is an ongoing process.

The setting for delivery of health care in the community may be an ambulatory clinic, outpatient surgery center, adult day care center, school health office, nurse-managed center, long-term care facility, rehabilitation center, hospice care facility, public health unit, occupational health office, correctional facility, or the home. Practice roles vary among these community settings. Nurses may find themselves with many colleagues to support and assist them in an ambulatory surgery or clinic setting, but are usually independent in industrial, school, or home environments. Components of the nursing roles include providing care to clients at various points on the wellness-illness continuum, working with multidisciplinary teams of health care professionals, and meeting the needs of diverse populations in the community. Specific responsibilities of the nurse vary with the setting and particular agency.

Ambulatory Clinic

Medical-surgical care in the community is commonly provided in an ambulatory clinic. Clients are familiar with visiting the physician's office or other clinic for many of their acute health care needs. Nurses employed in these clinics may be working with physicians or may be nurse practitioners who retain autonomy in their practice. This is common in "free clinics," community support clinics, and in some government-run clinics in indigent areas.

Outpatient Surgery Center

Free-standing outpatient surgical centers have become quite commonplace in the past few years. With the advent of improved surgical techniques and advanced technology, many surgeries that previously needed to be performed in a hospital setting are now done in these centers. A variety of surgical procedures can be performed safely and the client discharged after a short recovery period. Medical-surgical nurses in these centers usually do preoperative assessments and education for clients, assist with the surgical procedures in the operating suite, and also care for clients after the surgery. In some cases they may also be responsible for postoperative teaching and even follow-up at home.

Adult Day Care Center

Adult day care centers provide supervision, meals, and some health care for elderly clients during the daytime. Nurses in these settings may be doing assessments and care planning, providing treatments and health education, and supervising other assistive personnel at the center. They work with families and the multidisciplinary health care team to develop and implement the care plans for the clients served by the day care center.

School Health Office

School health offices are established to provide services for students. In kindergarten through grade 12 (k-12) school systems, school nurses are expected to assess and treat acute conditions, respond to emergencies, administer medications, maintain health records, and deliver ongoing care for students with chronic health problems. The school nurse monitors the school environment for health and safety issues and engages in health education for students, staff, and parents. An in-depth knowledge of state mandates for school health, growth and development, health promotion and education, first-aid, and usual childhood problems and diseases is necessary for nurses in this setting. The school nurse has become an integral component of the k-12 school environment.

In addition to school nursing at this level, school nurses are employed at the university/community college level to care for the health needs of the student population. Nurses in this setting are often focused on common recurring medical surgical problems such as respiratory diseases, nutritional disorders, and acute emergency problems. Health centers on college campuses may be nurse-managed centers or ambulatory clinics with physicians, nurses, laboratory, and pharmacy services. One of the major roles of the nurse in this setting is health promotion and education.

Nurse-Managed Center

Nurse-managed health centers are facilities that are controlled by nurses. Care is usually provided by nurse practitioners and other nurses and health service personnel. Physicians are usually not employed by the centers but may be on advisory boards. Nurse-managed clinics are especially common on university campuses. The nurse practitioner is the primary care provider at the center. Health promotion and health education are usually integral components of the practice at nurse-managed health centers.

Long-Term Care Facility

Long-term care facilities in the community provide services to elderly and medically frail clients who cannot be cared for at home. The nurse's role in long-term care is usually focused on medical-surgical care needed to preserve functioning, restore health, and treat chronic disease, and support clients and families during the dying process. See Chapter 10 for information on the long-term care setting.

Rehabilitation Center

Rehabilitation centers provide special services to clients with complex problems that require extensive professional intervention. Subacute rehabilitation centers deliver care to clients who require some medical monitoring during the rehabilitation period. Nurses in these facilities may be performing interventions just as in hospitals during the client's stay, or they may be more directed toward the care and treatment of the client with disabilities. The most frequent medical-surgical problems seen in rehabilitation nursing include cerebrovascular accident (CVA or stroke), amputation, paralysis from back injuries or brain injuries, and postsurgical cases such as total hip or knee replacements. The nurse in this setting must be familiar with the pathophysiology, prognosis, and recovery period of these disorders. Because some clients in rehabilitation settings have minimal recovery ability, the nurse should also be adept at psychologic interventions. Good communication is a major priority. Progress for some clients may be extremely slow, and both the client and family can easily become frustrated. The nurse also works with families or other care providers to assist them in learning to care for the client at home.

Hospice Care Center

The hospice care center is a facility that cares for terminally-ill clients. The medical-surgical nurse working in a hospice care center is usually delivering palliative care to clients. Care is focused on preservation of dignity, comfort, and emotional and spiritual support. In addition, ongoing consultation with the hospice team and support for family and significant others are components of the nurse's role in this setting. Hospice care may also be delivered in the home or in long-term care facilities. See Chapter 6 for additional information on end of life care.

Public Health Unit

The county public health unit is the facility with the responsibility for the health of the community as a whole. The nurse in this facility provides a variety of services to clients such as immunizations, maternity services, assessment of children, treatments for communicable diseases, birth control, and interventions for other acute and chronic medical problems. The most common adult medical-surgical problems seen at the health unit are chronic respiratory disorders such as asthma, tuberculosis and emphysema, diabetes, cardiovascular diseases, sexually transmitted diseases, and nutritional disorders such as iron deficiency anemia. The public heath nurse is instrumental in education programs for these clients to help them understand their disease processes, medications and treatments, and to prevent complications. The nurse may be actively involved in case-finding (tracking contacts) when a person is diagnosed with tuberculosis, hepatitis, or any other communicable disease; distributing medications to the client and contacts for prevention; monitoring adherence to the prescribed regimen; and follow-up testing and education. Because sexually transmitted diseases continue to plague society, public health nurses play an important role in prevention, counseling, and treatment of these diseases. The nurses are also involved with epidemiology, education, and environmental safety.

Occupational Health Office

Occupational health is concerned with preserving and protecting the health of employees. The nurse in an occupational health office is usually involved with employee physical examinations, environmental health and safety, workplace initiatives, acute assessment and intervention, and health promotion (Figure 9-1). The Occupational Safety and Health Administration (OSHA) has standards for workplace health and safety that the nurse implements in cooperation with other assigned personnel. The Healthy People 2010 document has a goal and objectives specifically addressing occupation health issues (see Healthy People 2010 box).

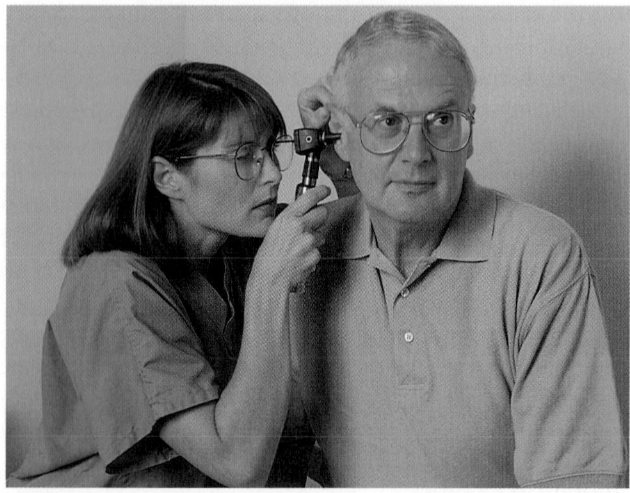

Figure 9-1 An occupational health nurse checks the ears of an industrial employee. Hearing loss can be a significant problem in industrial plants if preventive measures are not in place.

Healthy People 2010

Goal and Objectives Related to Occupational Health

GOAL

Promote the health and safety of people at work through prevention and early detection.

OBJECTIVES

- Reduce deaths from work-related injuries.
- Reduce work-related injuries resulting in medical treatment, lost time from work, or restricted work activity.
- Reduce the rate of injury and illness cases involving days away from work due to overexertion or repetitive motion.
- Reduce pneumoconiosis deaths.
- Reduce deaths from work-related homicides.
- Reduce work-related assaults.
- Reduce elevated blood lead levels from work exposure.
- Reduce occupational skin diseases or disorders among full-time workers.
- Increase the proportion of worksites employing 50 or more persons that provide programs to prevent or reduce employee stress.
- Reduce occupational needle stick injuries among health care workers.
- Reduce new cases of work-related, noise-induced hearing loss.

From US Department of Health and Human Services: *Healthy People 2010: understanding and improving health,* Washington, DC, 2000, USDHHS.

Correctional Facility

Nursing in a correctional facility focuses health care efforts on primary and secondary preventive services as well as some treatment interventions. The facility may be a local jail, a youth detention center, or a state or federal prison. The medical-surgical nurse in this community-based setting is involved with assessments, triage, counseling, and common recurring illness treatments. Health promotion and health education may also be a major focus of the nurse's role.

The Home

Home care for clients has become an increasingly important part of the health care system because clients are being discharged from acute care hospitals while still in need of nursing services. The ongoing changes in managed care organizations and Medicare have lessened hospital admissions and increased early discharges. As a result, admissions to home health services have increased. Home health nursing is recognized as a specialty in nursing[2] and has Standards of Practice. The American Nurses Association has also published a "Scope of Practice" guide for home health nursing.[1] Home health nursing practice requires the competencies of the acute medical-surgical nurse with enhanced proficiency in case finding, screening, assessment, critical thinking, teaching, collaboration, and health promotion. In addition, home health nurses often work with children, families, and older adults, so knowledge of health care needs and interventions across the lifespan is necessary.

TRANSITION FROM ACUTE CARE TO COMMUNITY-BASED SETTINGS

The transition from acute care to community-based settings can be made smoother and easier for clients and families through efficient discharge planning. Whether the client is being discharged to a long-term care facility, to the home, or to another community-based care agency, discharge planning includes assessing client needs at discharge, making arrangements and referrals for follow-up care and assistance, and coordinating the various professional and volunteer services in the community. Hospital discharge planning takes a wide variety of forms, from a cursory assessment of needs by an assigned staff nurse on the day of discharge to a multidisciplinary planning process conducted under the guidance of an institution-wide or unit-based discharge planner.[8] This individual is usually a professional nurse, but social workers also fulfill this responsibility in some institutions. Effective discharge planning is by nature a multidisciplinary group process that should begin with admission and be on-going throughout the hospital stay. Planning complex discharges usually necessitates a team conference in which professionals from a variety of disciplines discuss the client's discharge needs and plans with the client, if possible, and the family. However, the luxury of team conferences for discharge planning is not readily available to support the discharge of most clients, and the nurse planner often must work individually with each discipline to determine the full extent of the client's needs for service and support after discharge. Keeping the client and family fully involved in the planning process is challenging but essential.

Nurses working in discharge planning may be expected to serve as case managers in a managed care environment. This role can take a variety of forms. Case-managed care is supported by private industries and the federal government as a means of reducing insurance costs and making early hospital discharge to a community setting such as the home safe and less expensive. The nurse case manager can be employed by a home health agency, a hospital, a health maintenance organization (HMO) discharge program, or an insurance company. Some nurse entrepreneurs have established their own companies that provide case-managed services for major insurance carriers or the employees of large corporations. Their responsibility is to meet the client needs in the best manner while maintaining cost-effective care delivery (see Research box).

The nurse case manager may provide direct care to clients or coordinate the efforts of other personnel involved in the client's care. In either role the case manager conducts a detailed assessment of the client's needs, discusses options with the client and family, arranges for selected services to be coordinated with the home care agency staff, and ensures quality care by evaluating client outcomes on a regular basis. Open communication among the client, family, and nurse case manager is essential for successful transition to the home or other community-based care service.

HOME HEALTH CARE

Since a major area for delivery of medical-surgical nursing care in the community is in the home, the unique aspects of home health care are presented here. Home health nursing focuses on acute and chronic problems and delivers specific care to the client in the home. Services provided in the home include skilled nursing care, ventilator care, pediatric or newborn care, psychiatric care, parenteral nutrition, and chemotherapy (Box 9-1). Home care agencies may also offer services such as personal care, homemaker assistance, light

Research

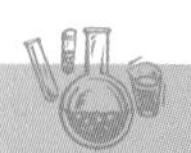

Reference: Hays BJ, Sather L, Peters DA: Quantifying client need for care in the community: a strategy for managed care, *Public Health Nurs* 16(4):246, 1999.

The study looked at the validity and reliability of a modified version of the Community Health Rating Scale (CHRIS), which is used to measure clients' need for care. It was used to determine an intensity measure, referring to the extent to which the client will benefit from the delivery of health care services. Intensity of need for care was defined as the quantification of need for the services. The CHRIS is a tool that focuses on four domains. It uses clients in its analysis in the domains of physiologic, environmental, psychosocial, and health behaviors, and families in all but the physiologic domain.

Historically nurses have been involved in assessing and reporting clients' needs. The recent trend of managed care has initiated the need for quantifying these needs. The collection of data related to this is important for the measurement and analysis of outcome achievement and to determine the cost of care delivery. Gathering comprehensive data in the community is difficult but necessary to future efficient practice.

Researchers refined the tool that was first developed by Peters to make it simpler and more effective for the purpose of providing an index of need for care. Case studies were used to present data to two panels of nurse raters. They validated the appropriateness of the tool. Because managed care requires nurses to present information about a client's health and illness patterns and needs over a period of time, nurses need a tool that can collect the necessary data. The modification of the CHRIS has provided a tool that could be useful for rating intensity of need for care. The study showed the refined CHRIS tool was reliable and valid for this purpose. The modified tool is more practical and user friendly than the original CHRIS. It provides opportunity for nurses to quantify need for care data on clients in the community.

TABLE 9-1 Number of Home Health Care Workers (1998) and Certified Agency Full-Time Employees (1999)

Type of Employee	Number of Employees	Number of Medicare Full Time Equivalents (FTEs)
Registered Nurse	129,304	100,696
Licensed Practical Nurse	40, 849	25,032
Physical Therapy Staff	14,849	14,032
Home Care Aides	326,633	82,069
Occupational Therapists	4348	3548
Social Workers	9379	5012
Other	146,989	41,562
Totals	672,351	271,951

From National Association for Home Care, from 2000 Basic statistics about home care.

BOX 9-1 Common Home Care Service Lines

- Intermittent skilled services
- Hospice services
- Home medical equipment—beds, wheelchairs, ventilators
- Psychiatric program
- Early obstetrics discharge
- Parenteral therapy program—hydration, antibiotics, total parenteral nutrition, chemotherapy
- Respite program
- Rehabilitation program—occupational therapy, physical therapy, speech therapy
- Personal care services—activities of daily living
- Supplies
- Private duty
- Pediatric home care
- Ventilator care
- Newborn home care
- Oncology program
- Prenatal monitoring

housekeeping, yard work, pick-up and delivery of goods/supplies, respite care, and personal home management.

Agencies providing home care services may be private for-profit or not-for-profit, or public, associated with the county heath department, or associated with hospitals. Some of the private agencies are also associated with larger institutions or health care corporations or they may be free-standing, independent agencies in the community. Freestanding proprietary agencies account for about 41% and hospital agencies about 30% of the total Medicare-certified agencies.[5]

Trends in Home Health Care

The number of home-bound clients with complex medical needs is rising rapidly owing to economic trends in health care, technologic innovations, and population demographics. Simultaneously giant mergers in health care agencies, budget constraints, advancing technology, and the Outcomes Assessment Information Set (OASIS) are significantly affecting home health care agencies and home health nursing practice.[11] More than 7700 Medicare-certified agencies currently provide home care services.[5] Noncertified home care agencies and hospices are also numerous but remain outside Medicare for several reasons. Many of them do not provide the kinds of services that Medicare covers, or they do not provide skilled nursing care and are not eligible to participate in Medicare. The number of registered nurses practicing in the home care setting has steadily increased as has the overall number of employees providing home health services (Table 9-1). Expenditures for home care in 1998 were in excess of $36 billion. This figure, though impressive, still represents only 3% of the total national expenditure on health care. However, hospital-based home care is included with hospital expenditures, and private pay to independent providers is not included in this data so the figures do not truly represent the dollars spent on home health services.[4] The home health payments accounted for about 4% of Medicare benefits payments in 2000. The Medicare expenditures from 1990 to 1996 increased rapidly but have declined since. Changes in the Medicare benefit system account for the dramatic decrease in spending for home health during the past few years.[3] This issue certainly places pressure on agencies to maximize services without increasing costs.

Home care has been documented as cost-effective, and cost considerations were clearly some of the driving forces behind the dramatic growth of home care in the past, but with the result of changes imposed by the Balanced Budget Act of 1997, the benefits in the home health area of Medicare were reduced significantly.[6] It seems to be well accepted by health personnel and by consumers that the privacy and safety of the home environment are clear preferences as the site of care for most clients and families. Other advantages of home care over institutional care include decreased nosocomial infection and improved nutritional status. Home care allows for the resumption of more normal interactions and routines. Care can be more easily personalized to the unique needs of the client and family, and clients experience a greater sense of control and higher morale when they are cared for in their home environments.

Technologic progress has influenced home care greatly. Clients can now be monitored at home through computer linkages to sophisticated diagnostic systems. Technologic innovations such as small, easily programmed intravenous infusion pumps have made parenteral home therapies safe and

Research

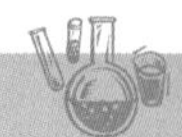

Reference: Anderson AA et al: Unplanned hospital readmissions: a home care perspective, *Nurs Res* 48(6):299, 1999.

The purpose of the study was to describe clients who had unplanned readmissions to an acute care (hospital) setting during the first 100 days of receiving home care services. Because many clients are now being cared for in the home after hospitalization, investigators found a need for more data about when and why clients had readmissions to the acute care setting during this care delivery time. To determine which clients had unplanned readmissions, the Hospital Readmission Inventory (HRI) was used to review records of 916 patients from 11 midwestern home care agencies. The HRI is an audit tool with established validity and reliability.

The study found that most clients were referred to a home care agency after a 9-day hospital stay for either cardiovascular, respiratory or neoplastic disorder. The greatest percentage of readmissions was due to new problems developed because of the already diagnosed chronic disease problem. Clients with chronic diseases were most susceptible to infections after discharge and complications of the already existing disease. Most of the readmissions occurred after an average of 18 days at home. The most common symptoms experienced included gastrointestinal distress and respiratory and cardiac problems. The study concluded that chronic illness was the best predictor for hospital readmission after discharge and ongoing home care. The complexity and multisystem problems associated with chronic disease puts clients at high risk for readmission.

affordable. A variety of respiratory therapies, ranging from oxygen compression tanks to mechanical ventilators, are widely used today with elders or clients with multiple chronic illnesses. Infusion of blood, home defibrillators, and home monitoring of clients at risk for cardiac dysrhythmias are common today. The changing demographics of our population also have influenced the need for more home health care. The numbers of elders will more than double by the year 2030, whereas the younger generation is decreasing in numbers. Home care is delivered to clients of all ages, but increasing age and functional disability are two major predictors of the need for home care. Elders represent more than 50% of the home care population.[9]

Home care is clearly successful in meeting the complex care needs of many clients in their preferred setting. However, maintaining health in the home setting after an acute illness that required hospitalization of a person with a chronic disease is difficult. Hospital readmissions of this type of client with problems such as pneumonia are common (see Research box).

Family involvement is integral to the success of home care, and the direct or unspoken message to families is an expectation that they assume this care giving role regardless of the cost. The interest or willingness of the family is rarely seriously considered. The burden of care giving can be extensive yet difficult to formally quantify. Not all homes are suitable for care giving, especially when high-technology care is required, and the demands of monitoring and implementing high-technology care can overwhelm the caregiver.

The needs of home care clients vary significantly. Needs range from assistance with personal care and activities of daily

BOX 9-2 Medical-Surgical Problems Commonly Managed by Home Health Nurses and Home Service Agencies

- Neoplasms and palliative care for terminal cancer clients
- Chronic pain
- Peripheral vascular disorders
- Metabolic/endocrine disorders especially diabetes mellitus
- Chronic obstructive pulmonary disorders
- Nutritional and digestive disorders
- Musculoskeletal and neurologic disorders
- Acute injuries and infections
- Genitourinary disorders
- Chronic pediatric disorders
- Hematologic disorders

living (ADLs), to long-term technology support, to short-term skilled interventions after surgery. One or two home visits or around-the-clock nursing care may be required. Clients diagnosed with cancer make up the largest group of clients treated in the home environment. Clients with peripheral vascular disorders and diabetes are the second and third most frequently seen clients by home health care agencies. Other major types of disorders that are treated in the home are listed in Box 9-2.

The home as the environment for nursing care offers a particular challenge to the nurse. Working in home care is an autonomous practice. Over time, nurses delivering care in the home must adapt to each client's individual needs, resources, and health beliefs. It is a challenging practice that requires organizational skills, good communication, and flexibility.[12] Nurses use many standard medical-surgical nursing skills to provide care to their clients, but they also need to develop special skills to work effectively with clients in their homes. The home care nurse's caseload routinely includes clients with diverse illnesses such as cardiac disease, respiratory disease, diabetes, cancer, and neurologic problems. The home care nurse may provide or direct nursing services to assist with ADLs, manage wound care and high-technology interventions, and teach families self-management skills. The home health nurse works with clients and families to promote self-care and independence and to improve the quality of life for the client.[12]

Discharge Planning in Home Health

Discharge planning truly needs to be initiated at admission and then continued as an ongoing process throughout the hospitalization. Short hospital stays necessitate prompt initiation of the planning process if a serious gap in services is to be successfully avoided. It is not uncommon for clients with complex needs to be discharged and then wait for 24 to 48 hours before they are first contacted by the home care agency. Families are left alone to cope with the client's needs during the most vulnerable portion of the transition home and may not have the necessary skills, equipment, or support to provide needed care. This service gap can have serious consequences for both the client's care and the family members' confidence in their ability to successfully manage care at home. The arrival of the home care nurse becomes not support but family rescue. Ideally, the home health nurse who is responsible for planning the client's care at home should visit the client before discharge to the home and assess the medical needs, special equipment requirements, physical and financial restrictions, and ability of the family to provide care and emotional support. Unfortunately this first contact is usually viewed more as a luxury than a necessity, and families take clients home with little knowledge of who will be providing needed care and support.

The goal of effective discharge planning is to provide the client and family with the following: (1) information about what to expect after discharge, (2) instruction in appropriate self-care, (3) identification of family and community resources, (4) awareness of procedures to follow for emergencies, (5) knowledge of follow-up care, (6) family teaching specific to the client's concerns, and (7) explanation of home care services, telephone numbers, and, when possible, introductions to home care personnel.

The plan for discharge from home care services begins with the initial visit to the client (in hospital or in the home) and focuses on setting realistic outcomes that can be achieved. The home health nurse in the discharge planning role follows up with an evaluation visit and completes the discharge summary for the home health agency.[10]

Determining Discharge Planning Needs

Discharge planning for home care includes a careful assessment of the client's home environment. The unique demands of the client's physical care are compared with the resources available in the home (e.g., running water, refrigeration, and dry storage space). The nurse also assesses the client and family's resources and support systems, including the immediate and extended family, neighbors, friends, and religious supports. A basic discharge planning assessment is presented in Box 9-3.

The nurse needs to determine whether the client and family have adequate coping mechanisms to manage the illness and the common stressors of home care. The client's attitude toward discharge to home, family members' reactions to the caregiver role, and the family's ability to accept help from the home care team all influence the outcome of care. Before discharge to home care, the client and family's attitudes toward home care are determined. The client's motivation to return home and the family's willingness to provide and accept home care are important determinants of successful home management. The client and family's perceptions and concerns about recovery will influence acceptance of home care.

BOX 9-3 Discharge Planning Needs Assessment

Home Environment

Living arrangements
House or apartment
One floor or multilevel
Stairs—how many to reach bedrooms, bathrooms, kitchen
Adequacy of heating, cooling, electricity, plumbing, telephone service, etc.

Care Needs

Equipment and supplies
Adequacy of storage facilities

Support Systems

Who is present in the home, family roles?
Extended family, kinship network
Family coping strategies
Knowledge of and willingness to use external supports from community
Friendship, neighborhood, community, and church supports available

Learning Needs

Knowledge base
Skill acquisition
Comfort with caregiver role

Emotional Responses

Feelings about diagnosis, discharge, and home care expectations
Potential role conflicts and burdens for caregivers

Financial Assessment

Family resources
Insurance coverage
Supplemental care expenses

Financial Assessment

Financial assessment must be undertaken before discharge because home care can be a significant financial burden for families. Home health care can be expensive and is usually not completely reimbursable. Client and family self-payments are the second-largest source of payments for home care services. Cost analyses indicate that home care expenses vary in relation to the type, intensity, and length of services needed. Medicare, Blue Cross-Blue Shield, and an increasing number of private insurance companies pay for acute, posthospital home care services to reduce the length of hospital stay. For such coverage, however, the care required must be defined as intermittent rather than ongoing. Medicaid and a few insurers will pay for longer-term home care services for those whose condition is chronic. Supplemental coverage can be obtained in some cases from agencies that provide old-age assistance, workers' compensation, disability, Medicaid, or other financial aid programs.

Even when care is reimbursable, the family must usually pay deductibles, and only a percentage of the total cost is reimbursable. There may also be extra expenses associated with home care that are not covered by any insurance or government program, and these can become significant out-of-pocket expenses. For example, utility bills may increase because of equipment necessary for care. Special services from a pharmacist or supplies such as enteral feeding products may be costly yet are reimbursable only on a limited basis. Caring for the client in the home also may have caused a family member to quit work or reduce employment hours, thus reducing income.

BOX 9-4 Financial Resources Screening Checklist

1. Check the governmental or private resources available to the client (benefits vary with each plan):

_________ Medicaid	_________ Financial help (family)
_________ Medicare A (home care services)	_________ Disability payments
_________ Medicare B (home care equipment)	_________ Retirement pensions
_________ Health insurance including HMOs and PPOs	_________ Welfare programs
_________ Employer insurance	_________ Meals-on-Wheels
_________ Social Security	_________ United Way agencies
_________ American Cancer Society (free equipment, bandages)	_________ Private insurance
_________ Multiple Sclerosis Society (wheelchair loans)	_________ Savings accounts
_________ Volunteer or charitable organization resources	_________ Veterans Administration
_________ Old-age assistance	_________ Military retirement
_________ Supplemental Security Income	

2. Do you think that your total income for this year was enough to meet your (the client and other family members) usual monthly expenses and bills?
   _________ Yes _________ No
3. In the past 6 months, has money been spent on the client's physician, hospital, nursing home, or medication bills that have not been reimbursed by insurance?
   _________ Yes _________ No

Each of the major reimbursement sources varies in the requirements the client must meet, the lengths of time benefits are allowed, and the types of equipment or supplies provided. Typically the complete descriptions of the therapies, equipment, and services covered are included in the manuals available from each insurer.

Financial assessment is often difficult for nurses to undertake, and in larger hospitals this aspect of discharge planning is usually the responsibility of a social worker. However, nurses need access to financial data to ensure that clients receive the full benefits for which they are eligible under government or private insurance. Nurses need to understand the services that are reimbursed by different insurers. In today's economic climate, with the high costs of health care, even middle-income families may need assistance because they may be ineligible for governmental programs or other assistance. Box 9-4 lists financial resources that may be available to clients requiring home care. The involvement of a social worker or financial discharge planner who is aware of the current eligibility and reimbursement criteria is essential, especially for elders.

Case Management in Home Health

The unique charge of the nurse case manager in home health includes early identification of high-risk clients and clients with high-cost service needs. The nurse case manager organizes the treatments, choosing treatment alternatives that control the overall cost to the health care provider agency and/or third-party payer. The case manager performs ongoing assessments of the needs of the clients and finds resources to meet the identified needs. The nurse also identifies expected outcomes for the services delivered and time frames for completion of the goals and evaluation of the outcomes.[10] The use of nurse case managers in home health has proven to be cost-effective and successful over time.

Reimbursement Issues for Home Health Services

Medicare is the single largest reimbursement source for home care services. The serious concern over Medicare's level of reimbursement for home care is reflected in the fact that there has been a 26% decline in Medicare-certified home health agencies since 1997.[9] Medicare's service and reimbursement guidelines are used as models for most other insurers. Home care cannot be initiated without a physician order, and it cannot proceed without a physician-approved plan of care (Box 9-5).[10] The basic requirements for service and scope of reimbursable services for Medicare and Medicaid are summarized in Box 9-6.

Home care reimbursement may also come from the Veteran's Administration, CHAMPUS, the Older American Act, and Title XX Social Services Block Grant. Most insurers cover skilled care, assessment and monitoring of unstable conditions, and initial teaching for self-care.[10] The home health nurse should have knowledge of the reimbursement methods and eligibility requirements and review them frequently, as the guidelines change frequently. The continued medical dominance of the health care system and its persistent focus on illness are reflected in the fact that general health maintenance, health promotion, and interventions such as psychoemotional support are not covered services, despite the complexities of most home care situations. Covered services do not consider the full range of nursing practice or the

BOX 9-5 Medicare's Required Data for the Plan of Care

1. All pertinent diagnoses
2. A notation of the beneficiary's mental status
3. Types of services, supplies, and equipment ordered
4. Frequency of visits to be made
5. Client's prognosis
6. Client's rehabilitation potential
7. Client's functional limitations
8. Activities permitted
9. Client's nutritional requirements
10. Client's medications and treatments
11. Safety measures to protect against injuries
12. Discharge plans
13. Any other items the home health agency or physician wishes to include

realities of the lives of most clients and caregivers. This often creates dilemmas for the nurse who may identify a need for services that cannot be delivered owing to reimbursement constraints.[13]

Cultural Issues in Home Health Care

Effective home care acknowledges and incorporates the client's cultural background and religious beliefs. The plurality of American society necessitates that the nurse have knowledge of the client's cultural beliefs and respect for the client's unique cultural orientation. There may be cultural or religious conflicts between the client, family, and health care professional's approaches to the client's care. The nurse should remember that this is the client's home and the client is in control. The home health nurse is a guest in this setting.[10] Clients and families may ignore the advice and teachings offered by the health care team and elect not to follow the prescribed regimen. Control over the client's care is clearly in the hands of the client and family.

Family Issues in Home Health Care

The dynamics of the extended family may also need to be explored and used. The promotion of client and family involvement in care is fundamental, as the home care nurse recognizes that self-care may be the only option when insurance and other benefits are depleted.

Families can easily become overwhelmed with the burdens of caregiving. To manage home care, family members must acquire new knowledge and skills, be motivated to help the client, and adapt to the changes in role expectations of family members. The home health nurse needs to empower the client and family to participate more fully in the decision making and the care needed.[2]

The problems typically reported by families who provide home care include the burden of providing daily physical care, steady financial drain, and lack of support or resources. Many family members are employed full-time and cannot arrange their schedules to meet the care needs of the client. Other problems include the stress of learning the skills needed to

BOX 9-6 Eligibility Requirements for Medicare and Medicaid Home Care Services

Medicare

Covers skilled nursing, physical therapy (PT), occupational therapy (OT), and speech therapy; medical supplies and equipment; and home health aide or social services if delivered in conjunction with skilled service. Persons covered:

1. 65 years or older and entitled to Social Security benefits
2. Under 65 years if qualifies for Social Security disability benefits
3. End-stage renal disease clients

Requirements:

1. Must be homebound
2. Services must be "medically necessary" and be prescribed in a physician plan of care
3. Must require skilled nursing, PT, or speech/language therapy

NOTE: The skilled provider is authorized to (a) assess an acute process or change in condition, (b) teach about a new or acute situation, and (c) perform a skilled procedure or hands-on service that requires the skill, knowledge, and judgment of a registered nurse.

Medicaid

Must cover intermittent nursing service, a home health aide, and medical supplies and equipment. May cover PT, OT, speech/language therapy, private duty nursing, or personal care services. Persons covered:

1. Recipients of Aid to Families with Dependent Children (AFDC)
2. Recipients of Aid to the Aged, Blind, and Disabled (AABD) with income criteria
3. Others who meet federal or state income guidelines

NOTE: States have some discretion in determining which groups their Medicaid programs will cover and the financial criteria for Medicaid eligibility. To be eligible for federal funds, states are required to provide Medicaid coverage for most individuals who receive federally assisted income maintenance payments, as well as for related groups not receiving cash payments. States also have the option to provide Medicaid coverage for other "categorically needy" groups. These optional groups share characteristics of the mandatory groups, but the eligibility criteria are somewhat more liberally defined.

Requirements:

1. Must be homebound
2. Services must be "medically necessary" and be prescribed by a physician
3. Additional requirements vary by state; participation in case management may be required

perform the care or to handle the necessary equipment and facing ethical dilemmas such as end-of-life issues with the client and family members.[10,13] Long-term caregiving may also require structural remodeling of the home and result in social isolation for the caregivers. The greatest challenge for the home care nurse is assisting families to find solutions that work within the context of their own unique lifestyle.

The need for custodial or respite care also may be apparent. Care of dying clients in the home has increased significantly with the success of the hospice movement.[7] Home care nurses must be open to discussion of spiritual concerns, life review, and reconciliation. Families may also wrestle with decisions about long-term care placement for the home client and seek the nurse's advice. The home health nurse may refer the family to a social worker or directly to a long-term care facility for information.[13]

NURSING MANAGEMENT

The family home is a unique environment for providing care to the adult client and must be taken into account in the development of the client's plan of care. The combined influences of the physical and psychologic environments of the home continuously affect the outcomes of care provided. The physical environment of the home and the psychologic factors affecting home care are assessed and evaluated by the nurse in light of the effects on the client and family.

The concept of self-care is extremely important in home care. It does not mean the client or family can take care of all the client's needs; rather it reflects the type of complex interaction between the home health nurse and the household members. As explained by Rice, the self-care model is used as a means to promote independent living and increase quality of life for the client.[14] This model incorporates a group of subconcepts such as self-efficacy, self-determination, health beliefs, locus of control, and mutual participation of the client and family in the home plan of care, all of which are important to the individual receiving care in the home. This self-care model enhances the competence, independence, and decision making of the household and sustains and improves life and health for the client.[14]

Growing numbers of clients and their families successfully manage home care with mechanical ventilators, parenteral nutrition infusions, home hemodialysis, intravenous antibiotics or chemotherapy, and other life-sustaining interventions. Home care, even in the face of technologic dependency, allows families to exert control over their lives and maintain their highest level of functioning.

ASSESSMENT

The home care nurse must be skillful in conducting client and environmental assessment. Careful assessment of the client's needs should have been completed as part of the discharge planning process, but the home care nurse needs to promptly and efficiently verify the accuracy of the predischarge assessment and determine any additional or unique needs for equipment, care, or support.

Assessment of Expectations

Both the client and family's willingness and motivation for home care must be assessed in light of their expectations. Their knowledge of the treatment plan, equipment management, and client's needs should also be assessed. The roles and responsibilities of the family caregiver(s) versus the nurse or home health aide may need to be clarified. It is important to ensure that family caregivers have thoughtfully considered the changes in their daily lives and schedules that will result from the assumption of the challenges of caregiving.

BOX 9-7 Caregiver Role Assessment

1. How have the responsibilities of family members changed since the client has been at home?
2. How do you and other family members feel about these changes in responsibility?
3. Has your health changed since you have been caring for the client at home? If so, describe how.
4. Family members tell us they have emotional reactions to the changes in the person they are caring for. What has your experience been with these emotional reactions?
5. Family members often state that responsibilities of home care can be overwhelming and difficult. Do you find this true or not true?
6. Family members also have found they have gained strengths or a sense that they are successful in caring for the client at home. Do you find this to be true or not true?
   Tell me the successes you have experienced.
   Tell me about when you have not felt successful.

Cultural values may make it extremely difficult for some families to accept the prescribed treatment regimen. Fear of exposing personal lifestyles and information might affect the acceptance of having the nurse in the client's home. Sensitivity to cultural beliefs and family values is important to the success of the overall treatment plan. Cultural network resources can also be explored as an additional source of potential support for the family. The success of home care depends to a large extent on the ability and willingness of family members or significant others to draw on and use internal and external resources. Internal resources include the family's or individual's positive attitudes toward home care, ability to problem solve or seek advice, and willingness to accept help or assistance from external resources. Accepting help from friends, neighbors, and church or community groups often is difficult for families. The home health care nurse can determine the availability of these and other external resources and then assess the family's willingness to accept such help.

Each family member's reactions to the role he or she carries out in relation to home care influences the family's internal resources. The home care nurse may need to periodically assess family members' role responsibilities in home care inasmuch as these change over time. Also, individual reactions to responsibilities and the energy required to carry them out vary with the length of time that caregiving continues. Situational depression in both clients and caregivers is not uncommon. Families also react to changes, whether improvement, decline, or stabilization, in the client's condition during home care. Interview questions that can be used to assess caregiver roles and reactions are listed in Box 9-7.

When family responses are regularly assessed and evaluated, the nurse may be able to promptly intervene with assistance in obtaining occasional or regular respite care so that the caregivers can spend some worry-free time away from the caregiving situation. The nurse must realize that as home care continues, the resources, motivation, and emotional reactions of the family and client will change and must be taken into account in revising the home care plan.

Assessment of the Home

The home is the physical environment for delivery of nursing care. Criteria used to assess the safety of the home depend to some extent on the client's abilities and needs. The home of a client who is discharged with special equipment may require alterations to provide a safe environment for care. Modifications in the home environment for safety also may be based on the client's disabilities or physical condition, such as the need for high-rise toilet seats, grab bars in the bathroom, or changing a living room into a bedroom. Throw rugs may need to be removed, a ramp added, or a doorway widened to accommodate a client using a walker or wheelchair and to promote safety in the home.[10]

Guidelines for assessing the physical environment should always include basic information about the home within that community. The location of the residence in relation to necessary home care services, durable medical equipment companies, and care sites for emergencies is important. Another factor is the availability of transportation to and from needed resources such as a pharmacy or physician's office.

The physical environment of the home should always be assessed for basic factors that affect the client's health and adjustment to home care. Adequacy of heating, cooling, electrical outlets, plumbing, and refrigeration, as well as access to a telephone, should be determined. Lack of these basic resources does not preclude home care, however, unless they are necessary for safety.

Infestation by insects or rodents can also compromise the safety of the client and ability to maintain cleanliness for needed care supplies. Plumbing and toilet facilities are also assessed in light of the client's care needs. The actual physical layout of the home, particularly in relation to the client's bedroom, also is assessed. The client may be bedridden, unable to climb stairs, or restricted to one area because of medical equipment. Creative problem solving may be necessary to ensure that family members can use the space in their home in the way they desire and that medical equipment does not cause too much noise or interference. Physical modifications are often necessary to support long-term care provision.

The family and client should also be assessed for knowledge of emergency procedures. Each family should know how to use the community's emergency telephone system and how to contact the home health care nurse for less serious situations. Family members can be taught cardiopulmonary resuscitation. An exit plan should be made in case of fire, especially when the client is unable to walk or has difficulty with mobility. Equipment checks are a specific and important part of home care assessment. Typically, each piece of equipment comes with written materials that outline the safety checks, cleaning procedures, and routine maintenance. The family must understand the manuals and incorporate safety checks into everyday schedules.

Assessment of the Client

Assessment of the adult client in the home environment encompasses many of the same data collection procedures used in the acute care setting, but the client and family caregivers are the major data collectors. The client and family caregivers are asked to describe the client's condition and discuss any concerns. The nurse may never have seen the client before the initial home visit and may have only the limited data provided on the home care referral form. The nurse depends on the family's observations and monitoring for ongoing specific data.

Assessment proceeds in an orderly fashion. The nurse asks the client and family members about their concerns and gathers specific data about each identified medical problem, nursing diagnosis, or symptom that the client is experiencing. Because an interval of several days or more may occur between visits, detailed assessment is necessary to provide a solid basis for comparison on follow-up visits.

Assessment also includes the client and primary caregiver's responses to home management. The primary caregiver is the person who provides most of the physical or daily care for the client. This may be a spouse, parent, sibling, significant other, grown child, or friend. Multiple persons may be involved in the client's home care. The responsibility of providing care can be both physically and psychologically demanding, and the nurse needs to openly assess the severity of the burden being experienced by the caregivers.

Assessment of the Treatment Plan

The treatment plan outlines the general care the client needs and any special skills the client and family must master. General areas for assessment include basic care needs, medications, nutrition, home environment, emergency procedures, specific client needs, and equipment checks. General care assessment includes needs for assistance with hygiene, elimination, communication, rest and activity schedules, transportation, socialization, and continued contact with health care professionals.

The treatment plan includes prescriptions for medication, diet, exercise, and physical or psychologic care. The nurse discusses with the client the specific therapy he or she was given and exactly how it is being carried out. In addition, the nurse asks the client and family about any difficulties with treatments, obtains their opinions about the benefits or drawbacks of the therapy, and discusses these issues with them.

The nurse also identifies all prescription and over-the-counter medications in use and the client and caregivers' knowledge of their purpose, desired effects, proper administration, and possible side effects. Careful consideration is given to the possibility of adverse drug interactions among the medications. Written client education materials about all medications should be available as resources for the client and family to refer to, and the nurse reviews these carefully with the client and caregiver to ensure understanding.

Confusion over multiple medications is a common problem. Clients may resume taking medications they took before hospitalization but that no longer are prescribed. The nurse asks about what is taken daily and when it is taken and requests the client to count the remaining number of pills in the prescription to determine how many were taken. Assessing actual dose taken versus prescribed dose is critical because there may be various reasons why clients and families change the dosage, including finances or forgetfulness.

Drug boxes can be another useful way to assist the family in medication administration and allow the nurse to more accurately monitor the client's adherence to the medication regimen. Regular assessment of the supply of medications also helps ensure that necessary prescriptions are refilled before they run out.

The nurse also regularly assesses the client's nutritional status. The ability to follow through on diet prescriptions is affected by food costs, accessibility, and lifelong eating patterns. Objective data about nutritional status obtained through interval measurements of body weight, intake and output, or calorie counts can be useful.

Assessment of Learning Needs

To promote quality, cost-effective care, education of clients and families is extremely important. The nurse must be skillful in assessing readiness to learn, providing information, and evaluating outcomes of teaching. The nurse should be familiar with the general principles of teaching/learning and adult learning theory. The education process begins with assessment and diagnosis of learning needs. Assessing the client and family's understanding of the illness and its treatment establishes a baseline for teaching.[10] The nurse also must assess the family members desire for information. In addition to information about the client's biologic condition, family members have personal knowledge and skills needs.

Any barriers to learning that the client and family may have need to be assessed. Learning is influenced by attitudes, beliefs, and values and varies for each person through the various stages of home health care. The nurse should reinforce positive behavior changes. Clients and families learn best when they believe the information is relevant to their situation and important to them.[10] Clients and families who are in a stage of denial will have difficulty learning.

NURSING DIAGNOSES

Nursing diagnoses are based on the assessment data collected in the home and on the data gathered through discharge planning. The nursing diagnoses should reflect each family's actual and potential strengths as well as problems and responses to the condition, treatment plan, and rigors of home care. By diagnosing strengths, the nurse identifies abilities family members can use in dealing with the actual and potential problems they face. The nurse also analyzes the data to determine the coping skills, external resources, and other family strengths essential for managing the home care alone.

A wide variety of diagnoses may be applicable in any particular situation. These include all of the specific disorder-related diagnoses identified throughout the text. A few diagnoses are more specifically applicable to the uniqueness of the home care situation. One example relates to the problem of *relocation stress syndrome* in which clients and family members experience stress and anxiety when they leave the acute care setting. This problem needs to be acknowledged and planned for before the client's discharge from the acute care setting. Extensive preparation, through teaching and involvement of the client and family in coordinating resources that are readily accessible and economically feasible, lessens relocation stress.

Other commonly encountered diagnoses in home care are presented in the following chart:

Diagnostic Title	Possible Etiologic Factors
1. Risk for impaired home maintenance	Lack of knowledge of home care and community resources
2. Risk for caregiver role strain	Unrealistic expectations or demands, insufficient opportunities for respite
3. Risk for loneliness	Time demands of caregiving, inability to participate in family and social activities
4. Decisional conflict	Uncertainty about choices for meeting long-term needs

EXPECTED CLIENT OUTCOMES

The ultimate goal of home care is to assist the client and family to their maximal level of functioning. In some cases this may be the client's complete recovery and return to work. In other situations, maximal function may be the family's ability to manage the client's care in the home without professional assistance.

Specific client outcomes will again reflect the unique aspects of each client and family situation and their identified needs. The following are broad outcomes that would be applicable for the home care-related diagnoses addressed previously.

Client and caregivers:

- **1a.** Will demonstrate the ability to perform necessary client care skills
- **1b.** Will identify needs for further skills or knowledge to effectively manage the client's home care regimen
- **1c.** Will adapt the home environment successfully to ensure client safety
- **2a.** Will successfully balance care giving demands with other components of lifestyle
- **2b.** Will obtain routine respite services to ensure time away from caregiving
- **3.** Will identify ways to increase meaningful social interactions and relationships
- **4a.** Will discuss advantages and disadvantages of options for long-term care management
- **4b.** Will share fears and concerns regarding choices for long-term care and reactions of others

INTERVENTIONS

1. Gaining Access to the Home

Home care services may be crucial to the client's successful discharge and home maintenance, but clients and families may still view the process as an invasion of their privacy. Providing nursing care in a person's home cannot be undertaken without developing a successful approach to home care services. Preferably, the nurse and other professionals in the acute care setting initiate discharge planning, and family members accept the need for the home care nurse and possibly other professionals in their home.

Ideally the first visit with the client and family should be conducted in the hospital before discharge, but often the first visit is to the home. Therefore the initial contact with the client is almost always by telephone. The nurse clearly identifies herself or himself and the home care agency and makes arrangements for the initial home visit, which should take place as soon as possible to confirm the client's specific care needs. A specific appointment is set up, and the nurse clarifies with the family members how they prefer the nurse to enter the home. An agency contact telephone number is provided to the family for use in making changes in the appointment schedule or to access assistance in case of an abrupt change in the client's status. This initial phone contact sets the tone for the nurse's working relationship with the client and family and begins the process of rapport and trust building. When timely and appropriate discharge planning has been performed, the transition to home care can be smooth.

Safety concerns for the nurse working in the community setting are always important, especially on the first home visit. The nurse always needs to be aware of the environment and sensitive to environmental cues that would indicate an unsafe situation. Family members can be approached with questions about safe places to park, walk, and use phones in their neighborhood (see Guidelines for Safe Practice box).

Families are often unsure of the nurse's exact role in the home and need to clearly understand the scope and boundaries of the nurse's practice. At the first visit the client's needs are assessed and available home care options are discussed. Control of the home care situation clearly rests with the client and family, and this fact must be recognized and respected. The nurse is often welcomed to the home in a social manner on the first home visit and may be offered refreshment. The nurse should remember that she (he) is a guest in the home and any personal beliefs or feelings about the client's lifestyle should not be addressed. The nurse uses this visit to establish trust, rapport, and a working relationship with the client and the primary caregiver. The nurse emphasizes the collaborative nature of their partnership in the client's care. Clear expectations should be set about the time limits for the initial visit and future ones. The nurse explains the steps of the assessment process and the services that will be provided.[10]

Clear information is also provided to the client and family about the costs of home care services, insurance reimbursement, and other economic details that the family will need. Options to reduce home care expenditures safely, such as family members providing wound dressing changes 3 days a week or the nurse reducing visits to twice weekly, should be explored. The nurse should note that most insurers have restrictions on the lifetime number of visits that the client can receive. Insurers also have limits on how much they will pay for selected client conditions. Discussing the economics of the health care situation with families can be difficult, but helping them understand that cost-effective use of their insurance will maintain coverage for them at a later date is essential (see Evidence-Based Practice box). The initial visit concludes with mutual understanding and agreement about the client's care needs, the distribution of care responsibilities between the family and home care agency, and the frequency and nature of future visits.

Guidelines for Safe Practice

Safety Precautions for Home Visiting

1. Let the agency know your planned schedule in advance and phone numbers of the clients to be visited.
2. Have accurate information about the exact location of the client's home and parking availability. Always carry a detailed street map.
3. Park in a well-lighted, busy area near the client's home. If possible, schedule visits only during daylight hours.
4. Reconfirm appointments with the family before arrival.
5. Maintain your car in good working order. Keep the car free of personal belongings. Keep any needed supplies in the trunk, and always keep the car locked.
6. Avoid carrying a purse or wearing jewelry.
7. Be alert at all times. If you do not feel safe, leave the area. Visit high-crime areas only with a second nurse, never alone.
8. If a client, family member, or visitor is drunk or hostile, leave the home and then reschedule the visit.
9. If a serious argument, fight, or abuse is occurring in or around the home, leave and then report the incident to the proper authorities.
10. Always carry agency identification and emergency phone numbers. A cellular phone provides added security.

Evidence-Based Practice

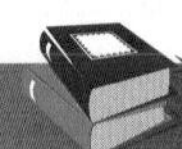

Reference: Madigan EA, Fortinsky RH: Alternative measures of resource consumption in home care episodes, *Public Health Nurs* 16(3):198, 1999.

In the past, the resources allotment for home health care has been designated by number of visits. Recent research into the economics of home care services shows that resource consumption should be reviewed by alternative measures. Measures such as cost-based episodes of care and cost per discipline or per intervention should be assessed. This may be a more reliable benchmark for planning for resources needed for care delivery in the home.

The purpose of this study was to provide data on measures of resource consumption in home care episodes. Alternative measures include both time and costs as the two major dimensions. The investigators studied 102 home health clients from 10 agencies in Ohio. Each client had an episode of care while remaining in the home. The mean time per visit was 46 to 55 minutes, but there were differences in the number of visits provided by various disciplines. The mean cost per day was about $43, and the mean cost per episode was $1160. The investigators found that there were no observable differences between disciplines in the time spent with the client per visit. The investigators also found that the discipline-specific costs per day were significantly different. These findings can give home care agencies information on costs that can be used to review their present fee for specific services.

1,2,3. Implementing Family Education

The knowledge and skills that the client and family must have to manage the client's care safely and effectively are specifically related to the client's unique diagnosis and treatment plan. Client/family teaching is directed at (1) understanding the illness and treatment plan, (2) competence in managing the client's care, and (3) fostering effective coping with the lifestyle implications of home care. Understanding the client's and family's lifestyle helps the nurse to plan with them about how to make necessary changes with the least disruption. When a care regimen causes minimal disruptions in lifestyle, the client is more likely to comply with it. Teaching is more effective when it includes not only knowledge of treatment but also assistance in tailoring the needed care regimen to meet the unique lifestyle circumstances and preferences of the family. Flexibility and creative problem solving are essential.

Implementation of teaching plans can take many forms in home health care. The use of computer-assisted instruction and videotapes in the home has been successful. Demonstrating a technique and having the caregiver or client "return demonstrate" the technique is a way to ensure the individual understands the correct way to perform the procedure. Methods of teaching that incorporate the whole family and emphasize the need to change behavior are most likely to have positive results. Using praise and reinforcement and providing an opportunity to ask questions and to evaluate learning effectiveness are important parts of implementation.

Research on home-based client/family education indicates that behaviorally oriented programs that emphasize changing the environment in which clients care for themselves are the most successful in improving the clinical course of chronic diseases. An example of environmental modification would include rearranging furniture so that it is in the field of vision of the client who is rehabilitating from a CVA and has residual hemianopsia. Modification of the environment actively enlists the client in changing behavior to meet desired objectives.

Establishing cues as reminders for new behaviors increases adjustment to home care. For example, encouraging clients with many treatments to try to schedule these with meals or other regular activities helps them remember to perform the activities.

The nurse must remember to bring teaching materials for the home visit even if the client has received handouts before discharge. Duplication of materials and information reinforces previous teaching. The nurse builds on teaching materials already given to the client so that it does not appear that only new content is being taught. Also, duplication of teaching efforts must be avoided. For example, the nurse and physical therapist should decide who will be responsible for teaching range-of-motion exercises, thus reducing duplication of effort.

The nurse should be aware of the client and family member's ability to read and/or understand the material. If English is a second language in the household, it is imperative that the nurse determine if caregivers understand the material. Sometimes using fewer written words and more descriptive pictures is helpful in households where the literacy is poor or English is not the primary language. Not only should the printed word be at an appropriate level for the client but also the vocabulary used by the nurse. Results of client education studies indicate that common "medical words" are not understood by clients. Using the client's own terms is usually most effective. Even for functionally literate clients, the stress associated with illness may reduce their comprehension of spoken words, written materials, and even visual teaching resources.

Cultural factors such as beliefs related to health practices also affect the client's response to teaching. The nurse should adapt to the cultural practices of the client and caregivers if the particular practice is not harmful to the client.

Documentation of specific teaching activities is also crucial. Although client education is clearly one of the most essential professional interventions in home care, it remains a struggle to secure reimbursement for education services. Reteaching clients is usually not reimbursable, regardless of learning or need, and thus must be included in other reimbursable care or charged directly to the family. Medicare considers teaching a skilled care activity and reimburses for it if there is justification for the need. Box 9-8 summarizes the guidelines for teaching activities for home health services. Clients and families often state that carrying out procedures they were taught or observed in the hospital seems more complicated at home. Adaptations in procedures are often necessary in the home, and health care personnel are not immediately available to provide assistance. The caregivers' confidence in their ability to successfully and safely manage care may falter. The complexity of scheduling the total care, including bathing, feeding, and technical treatments, may be difficult. The varied aspects of transferring learning into the home situation ideally need to be discussed with the family before the client's discharge. An emphasis on problem solving that incorporates the client and family environment, including daily routines, is helpful. The nurse reassures family

BOX 9-8 Medicare Guidelines for Teaching

The activities that require the skills of a licensed nurse and are reimbursable by Medicare include (but are not limited to) teaching:

- Self-administration of injectable medications
- Bowel or bladder training if dysfunction exists
- Maintenance of peripheral and central venous lines
- Administration of intravenous medications
- Diabetic management
- Wound care if complex
- Self-catheterization
- Gastrostomy/enteral feedings
- Ostomy care
- Application of specialized dressings
- Ambulation with assistive devices
- Use of prosthesis, braces, crutches, walker, cane
- Preparation of a therapeutic diet
- Performance of activities of daily living if special equipment is necessary

members that they can contact the home health agency if they have questions at any time.

Physical problems of the client and caregiver may make learning the self-care regimen more difficult, especially for older adults. Pain, electrolyte imbalances, or the primary disease process can alter the client's cognitive functioning and prevent the client from being an active partner in the learning process. The client may also simply lack sufficient mental or physical energy for learning. Arthritic problems may compromise an elderly caregiver's ability to master psychomotor tasks. The effort to manipulate small objects such as needles and syringes can be frustrating. Nurses must determine any physical changes that might hamper learning and take steps to alleviate these barriers when teaching clients and families.

Another personal factor that can make a difference in the client and family's learning is mental or psychologic state. Much has been written about how anxiety affects perceptions and behavior. It generally is accepted that persons who have moderate to severe anxiety may be able to focus only on their immediate concerns. Consequently, the information given during hospitalization, when the client and family are experiencing moderate to severe anxiety, may be so distorted that the person does not learn what is intended. Nurses may need to use methods to reduce anxiety so that the client and family can attend to learning. For some clients, complex equipment may be overwhelming and create increased anxiety. The nurse initially may need to perform the technical care and gradually teach self-care as the client or family is able to manage it.

2, 3. Reducing Caregiver Role Strain

It is stressful on families and other caregivers when changes occur in their schedules owing to a client's health care needs. Home care management requires adaptations to new routines, responsibilities, and learning requirements. The work can be mentally and physically taxing for the caregivers. This may result in family members feeling overwhelmed and even angry with the client. The changes tax the family's resources in terms of both money and time.

Home care alters communication patterns and generally disorganizes a family, at least temporarily. The length of home care affects coping within the family. The longer that home care is required, the more the family's coping skills can become depleted. More situational crises arise during prolonged home care, thus further challenging the family's coping abilities. Other contributing factors include past experiences and realistic expectations of home care. Families with positive past experiences who can accurately predict the length of home care and who have realistic expectations about the daily schedule are better able to cope with prolonged home care.

Family members' fatigue and stress are problems the home care nurse must assess and address. The nurse can assist family members to adjust to the disruptions that have been created and support them in adjusting to these disruptions. Although the family may be reluctant to accept help from outside the family, the nurse should provide information and strategies to find outside assistance with the care needed and for financial support when necessary. Social support in the form of helping with everyday care, contacts with a network of peers, acceptance of caregiving by family members, and provision of emotional concern or praise seems to ease the perception of burden in a caregiver.

The nurse also ensures that the family is aware of and appropriately accessing all support systems available in the community. Volunteer organizations may be available to assist with transportation for physician or clinic appointments, and charitable organizations such as the American Cancer Society can be a source of supplies and equipment that can decrease the costs of care. Local communities typically have a variety of specific social support resources that can be mobilized to assist the family.

Religious denominations, neighborhood associations, community centers, voluntary service groups, and professionally led support groups can all be sources of social support. These groups can be used so that the client or family caregiver does not become isolated and overburdened with care. In addition, if the family has an adequate financial resource base, the part-time involvement of a compatible home health aide to assist with daily care demands can release the primary caregiver to devote some time and attention to his or her own needs.

Caring for a family member in the home may alter individual members' everyday activities, interactions, and pattern of social contacts. Participation in religious, leisure, and school activities may be affected. Caregivers may lose familiar and meaningful family interactions such as intimate talks, humorous exchanges, the comfort of physical contact through hugs, and the joy of intimate sexual contact. The caregiver can feel increasingly isolated from normal social contact. The possibility of acute loneliness in both client and caregiver in the context of overwhelming daily care demands is a real concern.

Friends may fear that activities are too much of a physical strain for the client with a chronic illness and quit visiting or offering to take the client out to church or to the store. Extended family members and friends may believe that visiting the home causes the family more grief over the client's disability. The nurse can assist the family to explore how home care has changed family function. Family members' own descriptions will help clarify the alterations in communications and personal exchanges they are experiencing. The client and family need assistance to anticipate these problems and suggestions on how to deal with such reactions. Respite care can be an essential strategy for addressing the problems associated with both caregiver burden and its risk of associated loneliness.

4. Assisting With Decision Making

Dealing with a client's chronic disability and its home care management creates constraints on family members' daily schedules and use of the home for activities. The family must make many decisions each day about the client's home care. These decisions may result in conflicts between family members. The client and family members have direct responsibility for managing such conflicts. Clients and families experiencing chronic illness must live with the constraints imposed by the disease and the home care.

Insufficient financial resources are a common problem reported by families at home. Reimbursements from insurance companies or Medicare vary widely and are constantly changing. The home care nurse must be skilled in understanding governmental regulations and advocating for the client's eligibility for coverage. The nurse may enlist the help of a social worker familiar with home care coverage regulations to ensure that information on the costs of home care covered by insurers is made available to the family. In addition, the nurse (with the assistance of the social worker) needs to identify any voluntary sources of financial support for families.

The nurse also must be concerned about specialty services available to the family. In some instances, the technical support services needed by the client may be at such a distance that safety is a concern. When this occurs, the nurse must ensure that the family recognizes and can readily manage emergencies such as equipment failure or lack of supplies.

The physical and financial burdens of caregiving may eventually overwhelm the family's coping abilities and necessitate a decision about placement of the client for long-term care. This is usually an exceedingly stressful decision for everyone concerned. The home care nurse can assist caregivers to realistically evaluate their situation, explore alternatives, and achieve a degree of comfort related to their ultimate decision. The collaborative involvement of a social worker to explore realistic placement options and associated costs can be helpful.

EVALUATION

1,2,3,4. Evaluation consists of making a judgment as to whether home care has been successful. This judgment depends on comparison of the client and family's status with the expected outcomes of home care.

If the client's physical function falls short of the expected outcomes, the nurse must identify factors contributing to this problem. The nurse may see signs that the client's pathophysiologic condition is worsening. Referral to the physician or arrangements for transportation to a medical facility may be necessary. Evaluation might reveal that the expected outcomes have not been achieved. The client may have misunderstood what he or she was taught, the resources arranged at discharge may not have been obtained, or the family members may have found home care overwhelming. Expected outcomes may have been unrealistic in terms of the allotted time. The nurse reassesses the situation and establishes new outcomes in conjunction with the client and family.

Evaluation also reveals many instances in which clients have achieved their expected outcomes. The nurse should acknowledge this with the client and family. When families are given recognition for their achievements, they feel supported in their efforts. All evaluation data, whether indicative of outcome achievement or not, must be documented. Evaluation data may be used for justification for reimbursement of extended home care or for the involvement of other home care resources. For the client to continue to receive Medicare home health care benefits beyond the 2 to 3 weeks of intermittent care allowable, "exceptional circumstances" must be proved. Clients may qualify for up to 2 months of home care reimbursement when the nurse provides data that document the need for continued home care.

Outcomes assessment data from an individual client may be blended with data from clients with similar needs to project future trends and needs in home care. These data are used to refine the clinical pathways used for effective case management. Outcome data can also be used to evaluate the quality of nursing care, to determine whether specific nursing interventions were successful, and to determine whether resource allocation was appropriate within the specific situation. The need for predictable, cost-effective nursing interventions is great, and data from home care are an important source of client data.

DOCUMENTATION

Documentation plays an essential role in nursing practice in any setting, and home care is no exception. The client's home health service record establishes a legal record of the care provided, demonstrates that established standards of care have been met, and serves as the basis for cost reimbursement. Agencies are becoming increasingly dependent on third-party reimbursement, and appropriate documentation is the key to cost recovery. Documentation takes an increasing amount of time for the home health nurse, as Medicare and Medicaid reimbursement guidelines dictate the exact and narrow nature of reimbursable services These elements must be clearly reflected in the documentation of each home visit. Standardized forms are usually used for documentation, especially if reimbursement is from Medicare. The client should understand the need for the detailed documentation and that confidentiality is maintained.[10] The nurse may use a combination of written notes, tape-recorded notes, or a laptop or hand-held computer, and the use of these tools should be shared with the family.

As is true with hospital-based care, each agency uses its own unique documentation forms and procedures, but common elements characterize effective documentation. Documentation is completed as soon as possible after care is provided, and time should be scheduled into the visit parameters to allow for this task to be accomplished. Laptop computers enable the nurse to promptly record data and transmit it to the agency in a timely way. Details of assessment, care delivered, and health teaching are recorded, as well as all attempted or completed telephone contacts with the client and family.[10] Box 9-9 contains some tips for accurate and appropriate home care documentation.

The Omaha System of documentation is becoming increasing popular in home health agencies. It is a standardized language for documentation and care planning that is coded for ease of reimbursement.[3] Clinical pathways are also being used in the home setting to establish the nature and goals of nursing interventions. They provide a solid framework from which to construct accurate documentation.

BOX 9-9 Home Care Documentation

Whatever form the documentation takes, it should clearly indicate:
1. Why the service was initiated
2. What skilled interventions are needed and why
3. Where the plan of care is going
4. What plans exist for preparing the client to manage without home visits

Unique Elements in Home Care Documentation
1. The client's basic homebound state needs to be regularly reaffirmed because this is the primary criterion for care. The limitations that keep the client homebound need to be reiterated (e.g., fracture, paralysis, shortness of breath, pain).
2. Documentation needs to reflect the client's ongoing need for care. Entries focus on the client's limitations rather than strengths and progress.
3. Entries should provide specific factual information about the exact services provided.
4. Each reimbursable service needs to be reflected in the documentation. The need for every visit must be clearly indicated.
5. The entry should clearly indicate in what way the care has been tailored to meet the unique needs of the client or home situation.

Critical Thinking Questions

1. A 59-year-old woman was recently discharged from the acute care hospital, after having bilateral total knee surgery, to a community-based rehabilitation center for continued physical therapy. She will be returning home after a week in the center. You are her case manager and will be finding resources in the community for her ongoing care needs, implementing the treatment plan, and monitoring the outcomes of the interventions for her HMO. While hospitalized, she was also diagnosed with type 2 diabetes mellitus. Develop a plan of care for her ongoing care needs. What referrals will need to be made? How will you evaluate her progress? How can you monitor the costs of her care and institute cost-saving strategies?
2. A 75-year-old man has severe coronary artery disease, a history of myocardial infarction, and hypertension. He is on multiple medications and frequently forgets to take them. What strategies would you use to assist him to improve his adherence to the medication regimen?
3. A 36-year-old ex-school teacher is quadriplegic as a result of a motor vehicle accident. She has pressure wounds on her coccyx. She lives alone but has friends and family who visit her frequently. She also has a home health aide who comes in twice a day to prepare meals and assist with bathing. You are visiting her daily to treat and dress the pressure wounds. She states she is losing weight but does not care because she is tired of living this way. How should you respond to her? What resources are available in your community to assist her? What ethical dilemmas are present here?
4. A 62-year-old woman has metastatic breast cancer and is now homebound. Her health insurance was cancelled when she had to quit her job. Her husband is 75 years old and unable to meet her daily care needs. The couple lives on his Social Security benefits and his small pension. What resources will you explore to meet the couple's needs for care and support?

References

1. American Nurses Association: *A statement on the scope of home health nursing practice,* 1992, American Nurses Publishing.
2. American Nurses Association: *Standards of Practice for home health nursing,* 1986, American Nurses Publishing.
3. Bowles KH: The Omaha System as a potential bridge between hospital and home care, *Online J Nurs Inf,* vol 3, no 1, 1999.
4. Clarke C: *Home care compliance manual,* Gaithersburg, 1999, Aspen.
5. Demel B, Baker JR: Effects of the home care interim payment system on access to home care for people on Medicare, *Care Manage* 2(2):108, 2000.
6. Holland DE: Determining the relevance of a certification exam to home health care nursing practice, *Care Manage J* 1(3):197, 1999.
7. Ladd RE et al: What to do when the end is near: ethical issues in home health care nursing, *Public Health Nurs* 17(2):103, 2000.
8. Naylor MD et al: Client problems and advanced practice nurse interventions during transitional care, *Public Health Nurs* 17(2):94, 2000.
9. National Association for Home Care: *Basic statistics about home care,* Washington, DC, 2000, http://www.nahc.org.
10. Neighbors M, Monahan FD: *A practical guide to medical-surgical nursing in the home,* Philadelphia, 1998, WB Saunders.
11. Neal LJ: Research supporting the congruence between rehabilitation principles and home health nursing practice, *Rehab Nurs* 24(3):115, 1999.
12. Neal LJ: Neal theory of home health nursing practice, *Image* 31(3):251, 1999.
13. Rantz MJ et al: The future of long-term care for the chronically ill, *Nurs Adm Q* 25(1):51, 2000.
14. Rice R: Key concepts of self-care in the home: implications for home care nurses, *Geriatr Nurs* 19(1):52, 1998.
15. Stanhope M, Lancaster J: *Community health nursing,* ed 5, St Louis, 2000, Mosby.
16. Van-Ort S, Townsend J: Community-based nursing education and nursing accreditation by the Commission on Collegiate Nursing Education, *J Prof Nurs* 16(6):330, 2000.

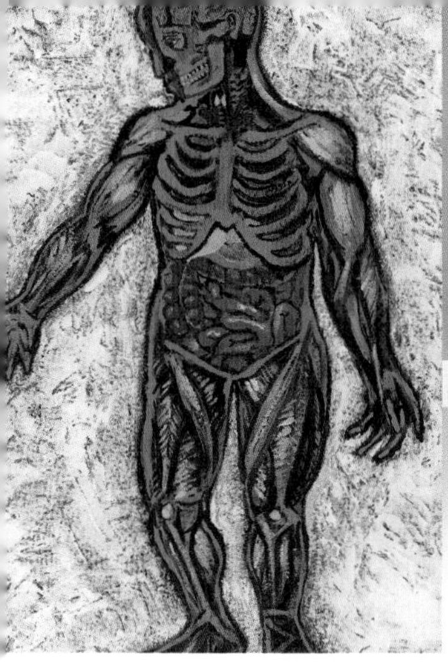

Long-Term Care 10

Lepaine Sharp-McHenry

Objectives

After studying this chapter, the learner should be able to:

1. Describe the trends of health care needs in the long-term care setting.
2. Discuss the regulatory process and its impact on care provided in nursing facilities.
3. Identify current challenges facing long-term care that threaten the delivery of quality care.
4. Apply the nursing process in using the Resident Assessment Instrument.
5. Analyze factors essential to effective delivery of care in the long-term care setting.

Before the mid-1960s long-term care (LTC) was provided mostly by families (as it is today), sometimes with hired help, and sometimes by purchasing care in private institutions. Unfortunately, very dependent people with no family care options or financial resources had little choice among charity sponsored or county homes (occasionally called almshouses and poor farms) where they might get housing and meals. States also established chronic illness hospitals for people with mental illness, dementia, developmental disability and severe physical disabilities; but public funding and standards of care suffered from little public visibility and little accountability for the use of funds. Exposure of adverse conditions might prompt temporary public attention, but problems would often recur. When the most vulnerable citizens are out of sight and dependent on the kindness of others, they can be at risk.

Today LTC refers to services provided to individuals who need ongoing health care or assistance with activities of daily living. It includes subacute, rehabilitative, medical, skilled nursing, and supportive social services for those with functional limitations or chronic health conditions. The nurse's role in LTC is multifaceted, but depends heavily on knowledge of medical-surgical conditions, nutrition, pathophysiology, pharmacology, growth and development, and psychoemotional needs of individuals with chronic disorders. Although LTC primarily meets the needs of the elderly, other population groups, such as individuals with disabilities or AIDS, also benefit from it. During the mid 1990s, the American Nurses Association reframed its definition of LTC to reflect a broader scope, encompassing all population groups and allowing for more varied care settings. In years past LTC often referred only to nursing homes; however, this trend is changing. To meet the increasing needs of an aging population, the LTC continuum has greatly expanded. LTC services are now provided in nursing facilities, skilled nursing facilities (SNFs), residential care and assisted living facilities, congregate day care, home, and other community-based settings. (See Box 10-1 for definitions and abbreviations of common terminology relating to LTC.)

There are approximately 1.5 million people who live in the 17,023 nursing facilities in this country. There are 1.8 million nursing facility beds. Of this number in 1999 and 2000, 122,732 were special-care beds. Alzheimer's disease special-care beds accounted for 71% of the total beds in special-care units.[3] People age 85 and older are the most common users of LTC. Nearly one in four (24.5%) lived in a nursing home in 1990. Between 1884 and 2020, America's 85 and older population is projected to double to 7 million and swell to between 19 and 27 million by 2050, making these seniors the fastest

BOX 10-1 Common Terminology Used in Long-Term Care

ICF (Medicaid): Intermediate Care Facility, Medicaid certified facility
SNF (Medicare): Skilled Nursing Facility, Medicare skilled unit that cares for clients with skilled needs as determined by Medicare
PPS (Medicare): Prospective Payment System, predetermined rate of reimbursement for Medicare long-term care services
ICF/MR: Intermediate Care Facility for Mentally Retarded
IPS (Medicare): Interim Payment System
RAI: Resident Assessment Instrument
RAP: Resident Assessment Protocols
MDS: Minimum Data Set: Federally mandated standardized assessment tool used in nursing facility that participates in the Medicare and Medicaid Programs.
Provider: The facility or owner of the facility who provides long-term care services
NF: Nursing Facility, nursing homes that provide either Medicare and/or Medicaid services.

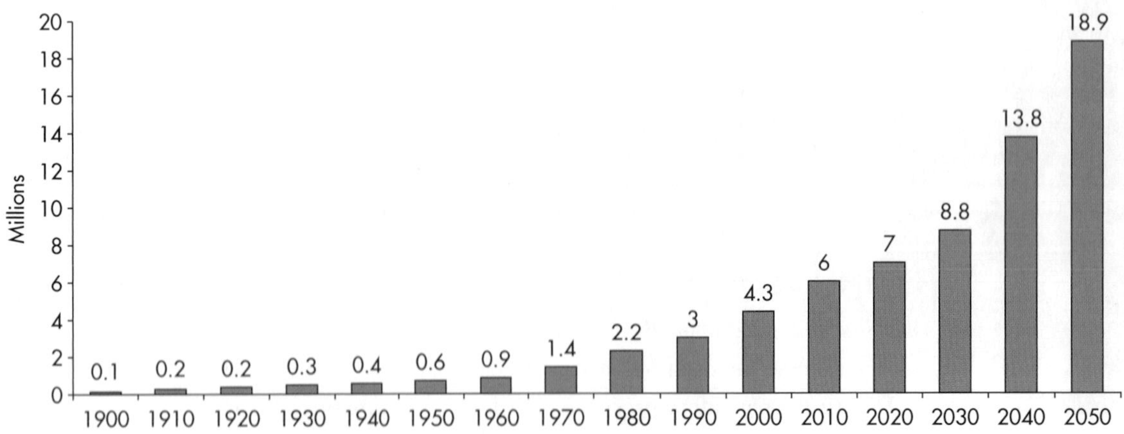

Figure 10-1 Population 85 years and over: 1900 to 2050.

growing segment of the population. Figure 10-1 illustrates the dramatic upsurge in the 85+ population. From 2010 to 2030, the number of baby boomers age 65 to 84 will grow by an estimated 80% while the population age 85 and older will grow 48%.[10]

Despite the development of noninstitutional LTC services, the need and demand for nursing home care will continue to increase over the next several decades. The major factors contributing to this growth are the expanding population of the frail older adults with significant functional disabilities, fewer available and qualified caregivers, and a lack of regular and consistent access to community services.[1] The increasing need for LTC will not only affect how services will be delivered but also their financial feasibility on the current system.

REIMBURSEMENT

In the 1940s and 1950s health insurance emerged as an employment benefit for large companies. Pricing and cost of health services rose along with insurance coverage, and the problem of insuring those with the greatest risk of needing care became increasingly apparent. For older individuals and those with disabilities or chronic illness, commercial insurance was generally unavailable or unaffordable. As families felt the effects of the high cost of caring for elderly and disabled people without insurance, pressure grew for establishing a public system of health care financing to cover "uninsurable" people. The situation was made more pressing by closure of mental hospitals when new medications made it possible to stabilize mental illness. Many frail individuals of all ages with profound disabilities and no financial resources still needed residential care. Reimbursement concerns became a major issue in health care nationally.

Medicare and Medicaid

After years of debate Medicare was enacted in 1965, establishing the federal system of financing acute care and posthospital care for seniors on a short-term basis (100 institutional days or 100 home visits). Later it was expanded to cover people with disabilities and end-stage renal disease, and home care benefits were liberalized.

Medicaid was enacted in 1966, making both acute care and institutional LTC available to people who were financially destitute, through combined state and federal funding. This is a "safety net" for those least able to purchase health care. Together Medicare and Medicaid brought substantial funds to the LTC marketplace. Access to care was extended to millions who previously had little or none. The programs also helped finance construction of buildings and the purchase of medical equipment. A boom in construction of nursing facilities and establishment of home health agencies followed enactment of these programs.

Medicare and Medicaid operated heavily on trust, reimbursing providers of services without effective mechanisms to control how the funds were used. Basic essentials such as nursing services and food services (counted as "routine services") could be manipulated to cut costs, while funds were diverted to other uses such as transportation, administrative salaries, marketing, interior design, and profits. Ancillary service charges, paid on the basis of "allowable cost" without limit or much challenge, grew in size and number. Some corporations that own nursing facilities acquired ancillary service companies, many of which have been quite profitable.

By 1980 Medicare expenditures in "cost-based" reimbursement to hospitals were escalating. Congress reacted by instituting a prospective payment system (PPS) whereby rates of payment for care were established in advance according to the diagnosis or procedure that brought the client to the hospital. More than 400 diagnosis-related groups (DRGs) were identified with a payment rate assigned to each. Hospitals now had the incentive to treat and discharge a client as soon as possible so the cost of care did not exceed the fixed payment.

By 1984 clients were being diverted in greater numbers to home health agencies (HHAs), SNFs, rehabilitation hospitals, and LTC hospitals after short hospital stays. Many were in unstable condition needing skilled services with rehabilitation. Facilities and agencies needed more personnel, more equipment, and more specialized skills. A boom in Medicare spending for postacute care services ensued but did not necessarily relieve the stress on facility staff. Staff was not necessarily increased in proportion to the responsibilities in many extended

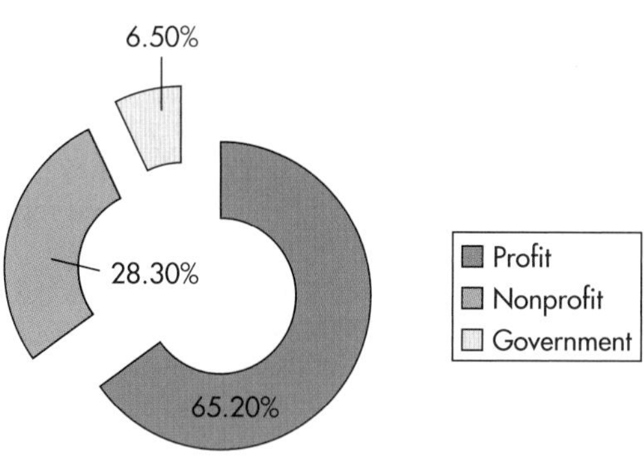

Figure 10-2 Nursing facility ownership.

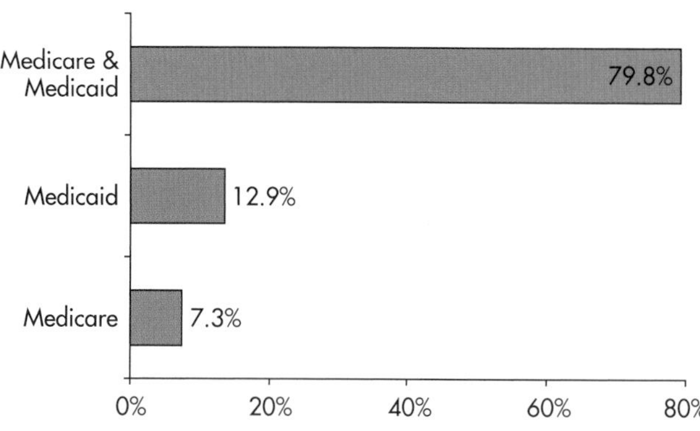

Figure 10-3 Nursing facility certification.

care facilities with SNFs units. Medicaid and private pay residents who also required a great deal of personal and skilled care primarily populated many of these facilities.

With generous public funding, LTC became "big business" after the mid-1960s. For-profit companies dominate the nursing home industry (> 65.2% in 2000) and set standards that affect competing not-for-profit companies (28.3% in 2000).[3] (See Figure 10-2 for nursing facility ownership in the United States.)

In many cases, larger multifacility companies have acquired individually owned facilities and small group chains. Less than 7% of certified facilities are government owned. Beyond maintaining financial viability of an agency or institution, a provider company has the responsibility to deliver the care that has been purchased by the resident /his family or the government program paying for the care. Companies also want to produce earnings for owners. Nurse employees are key players in assessments that determine payment for care and in delivering the care. The quality of nursing care enhances a company's reputation and attracts new business where competition exists in the market. However, the nurse's role as company "team player" in meeting financial goals must be continually consistent with professional commitment to serve clients' best interests.

Long-Term Care Reform

Most Americans thought little about the cost of health care for a long time. However, in the 1960s when Medicare was passed, government became a major purchaser of health care services for one segment of the American people—the elderly. As this group grew in size, the amount of money paid out by the government increased. At the same time, federal and state governments were paying for additional health care services for the poor through the Medicaid program. The number of people served by Medicaid had also grown, adding to the percentage of federal dollars purchasing health care for certain groups of Americans.

Growth of managed care plans throughout the 1990s has exacerbated the trend of early hospital discharges to SNFs and HHAs, rehabilitation hospitals and LTC hospitals. Insurers (including Medicare and HMOs) limit their costs in hospital contracts, and the hospitals in turn limit client days in the hospital. More clients requiring technical support (e.g., intravenous lines, respirators) have been transferred to SNFs and HHAs. In 1998 total expenditures for nursing facility care accounted for 7.6% of total health spending. However, Medicaid spending on nursing facility care was nearly one fourth (23.8%) of the nation's total expenditures for all Medicaid programs. Nursing facility Medicare expenditures were 4.8% of total Medicare spending. The number of facilities duly certified by Medicaid and Medicare continues to increase. According to the latest data, 79.8% are duly certified, 12.9% Medicaid only, and 7.3% Medicare only (Figure 10-3).[3]

The 1997 Balanced Budget Act mandated significant cuts in anticipated Medicare spending by instituting PPS in home health agencies and SNFs. Early anecdotal reports indicated a negative impact on nursing services staffing. Within a year HHA closures and reduction in nursing staff were being attributed to sharp revenue cuts under Medicare's Interim Payment System.

In some SNFs, despite greater responsibilities, nursing staff was reported to have been reduced. The PPS for SNFs phase-in began July 1, 1998. This resulted in Medicare reimbursement for skilled nursing care in LTC facilities to be based on clinical needs of residents and the nursing resources necessary to meet those needs. Medicare residents of LTC facilities are classified into a case mix group associated with the Resource Utilization Group Version III (RUG-III) case mix classification system to determine the payment the nursing home will receive for providing care.[13] The classification is based on a nationally mandated standardized assessment instrument called the Resident Assessment Instrument (RAI), which identifies functional deficits and care needs by reference to Resident Assessment Protocols (RAPs) and documents them in a Minimum Data Set (MDS). These instruments are discussed in more detail later in the chapter.

Computerized analysis of the MDS classifies each resident into one of the 44 homogeneous case mix groups in the RUG-III system, which is the basis for reimbursement. This system is also used for Medicaid reimbursement in some states. Registered nurses coordinate frequent assessments and related care plans during a resident's Medicare SNF benefit stay. These assessments determine the classification of residents for reimbursement purposes, and preliminary assessments can also be used to assist in selecting new admissions.

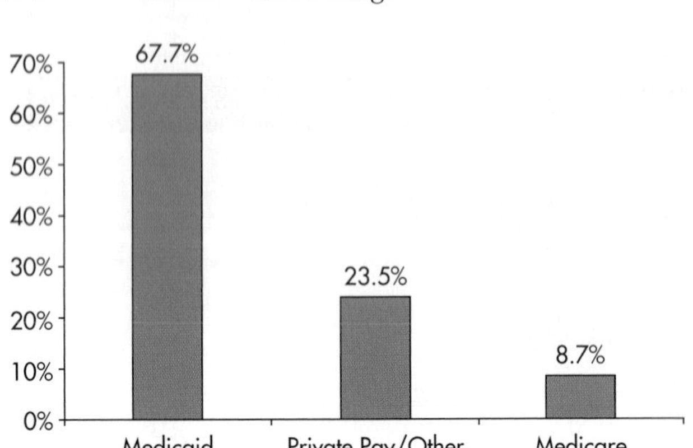

Figure 10-4 Nursing facility residents by payer source.

The primary payer source for nursing facility residents in our country comes from Medicaid at 67.7%, followed by Private Pay/Other at 23.5%, and the remaining 8.7% from Medicare (Figure10-4).[3] According to the American Health Care Association, our nation's LTC financing system steers people toward impoverishment and reliance on Medicaid, a government welfare program. However, Medicaid will not withstand the demographic tidal wave of aging baby boomers. Proposed cuts in Medicaid will present tremendous problems for the nation unless there is a fundamental shift to a system that relies more heavily on private LTC insurance. It can help protect Americans from financial ruin as they grow older and ease the fiscal burden on state and federal governments. By the end of 1994 more than 3.8 million people had purchased LTC insurance policies, compared with 815,000 by December 1987. LTC insurance sales continue to grow at an annual average rate of about 25%. LTC insurance is becoming a more viable option to the American people as policy rates and benefits become more attractive and economical.[2]

As the population ages, more resources are needed to cover the rising cost of LTC. Numerous federal efforts have been attempted to reduce the Medicare budget with much opposition from consumers. As federal and state tax dollars continue to be the primary source of funding for LTC services, regulatory accountability becomes essential to ensure that high standards of care are maintained.

REGULATIONS

Along with the implementation of Medicare and Medicaid in the mid 1960s, federal nursing home regulations were introduced. Before 1965 most nursing home regulation was the responsibility of the state; however, with enactment of Medicare and Medicaid in 1965, federal involvement in payment for nursing home services increased substantially, as did involvement in regulating services provided with federal funds. Nursing homes that provide services to Medicare and Medicaid beneficiaries enter into provider agreements with the Centers for Medicare and Medicaid Services (CMS) (formerly the Health Care Financing Administration [HCFA]) for Medicare and the individual state Medicaid agencies for Medicaid. To obtain and sustain the agreements (and thereby establish eligibility to receive payment for services rendered to beneficiaries), nursing homes must meet certain requirements set forth in the Social Security Act and implementing regulations in the Code of Federal Regulations (CFR) 483, Subpart B. Nursing homes have the option of participating in either the Medicare or Medicaid program, both, or neither. Unless they participate in neither program, they are subject to the federal regulations that govern the Medicare and Medicaid programs.

In the 1970s investigations conducted by the U.S. Public Health Service's Division of Nursing, state legislative commissions and congressional committees revealed widespread poor care and deplorable conditions of harmful neglect in nursing homes. Inadequate staffing for good care was repeatedly cited. Ineffective regulation by state and federal government was seen as part of the problem. These revelations led to temporary tightening of enforcement but not enough systemic improvement to stop repeated cases of failure to provide sufficient nursing services. No substantial staffing requirements were enacted because of industry opposition and government reluctance to commit to paying the cost of good staffing.

In 1982 the HCFA proposed changes in regulation of SNFs and ICFs that would have reduced government oversight of nursing homes. This was countered by Congress for the HCFA to fund a study of nursing home regulation by the Institute of Medicine (IOM) at the National Academy of Sciences.

Recommendations of the IOM's Committee on Nursing Home Regulation issued a report "Improving the Quality of Care in Nursing Homes." This report was based on both objective information and a consensus of professional opinions.[11] This led to enactment of the 1987 Nursing Home Reform Act by HCFA commonly referred to as Omnibus Budget Reconciliation Act (OBRA '87) within the nursing home industry.[20]

Nursing Home Reform Act

The Nursing Home Reform Act discontinued the Medicaid ICF authorization except for ICFs caring for people with "mentally retardation" (ICF/MRs). It replaced ICF authorization with Nursing Facility (NF) authorizations, and extended SNF licensed nurse-staffing requirements to Medicaid NFs. It did not establish staffing requirements for direct caregivers and licensed nurses in proportion to number of residents.

This law set new requirements for resident assessments, resident rights, nurse aide training, monitoring psychiatric medications and restraints, and medical direction. These new regulations dramatically changed the delivery of LTC. As a result, the LTC industry became one of the most regulated industries in the country. Resident rights were a significant aspect of OBRA '87. Residents were guaranteed the right to a dignified existence, self-determination, and communication with and access to persons and services inside and outside the facility (see Patient Teaching box).

It is clearly understood that OBRA '87 instituted minimum quality of care standards that established the least acceptable care that can be provided to residents in LTC facilities. Failures to meet these minimum standards indicate the delivery of substandard care. These standards are free of geographic

Patient Teaching
Resident Rights

Nursing Facilities must guarantee that each resident:
Is informed of all rules and regulations before or at the time of admission.
Is told of all services available and the cost.
Is informed of the right to complete an advance directive.
Is fully informed of his or her condition and is given opportunity to help plan the medical treatment.
If transferred or discharged only for medical reasons, nonpayment, or the welfare of other clients; must be given notice and may appeal.
Is encouraged to exercise his or her right as a client and citizen.
May manage his or her personal affairs.
May not be mentally or physically abused.
Be free from restraints unless used as directed by a physician only as necessary to protect from self-harm.
Is assured of confidentiality of all his or her personal and medical records.
Is treated with dignity and respect by the staff, including having privacy for certain types of treatment and for personal needs.
May not be forced to perform services for the home.
May visit and talk privately with anyone he or she chooses, and can send and receive mail unopened.
May participate in social, religious, and community activities at his or her discretion.
If married, is given private facilities in which to meet his or her spouse, and if a married couple is together in a home, they must be allowed to share a room.
May retain and use personal clothing and possessions as space permits, unless to do so would infringe on the rights of other clients.

boundaries and apply to every SNF and nursing facility in the United States that participate in the Medicare and Medicaid reimbursement programs. States may have additional regulations, but they must meet the minimum requirements set forth by HCFA. HCFA guidelines are organized into 15 categories (Box 10-2).

Standard Survey

Each state is required to have a plan for survey and certification of LTC facilities. This plan must comply with federal guidelines mandated by HCFA to determine whether LTC facilities meet requirements for participation in the Medicare and Medicaid programs. State survey agencies are required to conduct unannounced annual surveys. The survey must be conducted by a multidisciplinary team of professionals and must include a registered nurse. Other professionals that may be included in the survey are physician, physical therapist, speech therapist, occupational therapist, dietitian, sanitarian, engineer, licensed practical nurse, or social worker.

A standard survey must include (1) a case mix stratified sample; (2) a survey of the quality of care furnished, as measured by indicators of medical, nursing, rehabilitative care, dietary and nutrition services, activities and social participation, sanitation, infection control, and the physical environment; (3) an audit of written plans of care and residents' assessments to determine accuracy of such assessments and the adequacy of such plans of care; and (4) a review of compliance with residents' rights requirements.

When an SNF or NF is found to be not in compliance with requirements for participation in the Medicare and Medicaid programs, remedies may be imposed to ensure prompt compliance with program requirements. There are numerous remedies that may be imposed in addition to termination of the provider agreement. See Box 10-3 for remedies imposed for failure to meet requirements for participation in Medicare and Medicaid programs.

Enforcement Initiatives

In July 1998, March 1999, and July 1999, reports by the U.S. General Accounting Office note that enforcement of Medicare and Medicaid regulations by both federal and state authorities had been ineffective.[17-19] This was acknowledged by President Clinton's simultaneous initiative on improved enforcement.

BOX 10-2 Long-Term Care Regulatory Categories

Resident Rights
Admission, Transfer, and Discharge Rights
Behavior and Facility Practices
Quality of Life
Resident Assessment
Quality of Care
Nursing Services
Dietary Services
Physician Services
Special Rehabilitative Services
Dental Services
Pharmacy Services
Infection Control
Physical Environment
Administration

Source: *Federal Register* Vol. 56, No. 187, Rules and Regulations 48867-48878.

BOX 10-3 Remedies for Failure to Comply with Medicaid and Medicare Requirements

- Termination of agreement
- Temporary management
- Denial of payment, including:
  1. Denial of payment for all individuals, imposed by HCFA, to a
     a. Skilled nursing facility, for Medicare
     b. State, for Medicaid or
  2. Denial of payment for all new admissions
- Civil money penalties
- State monitoring
- Transfer of residents
- Closure of the facility and transfer of residents
- Directed plan of correction
- Directed in-service training
- Alternative or additional state remedies approved by HCFA

Source: Health Care Financing Administration, HHS 488.406 42 CFR Ch IV (10-1-99)

Insufficient staffing was repeatedly cited by witnesses at hearings convened by the U.S. Senate Special Committee on Aging, echoing a theme heard in state and congressional hearings since the 1970s. As a result, investigations of nursing home care and more stringent enforcement procedures were imposed on LTC facilities.

In early 1999 steps to address this problem as legislators in as many as 21 states drafted bills to improve staffing in nursing homes across the country. A number of these bills were based on the Consumers Minimum Staffing Standard for Nursing Homes developed by experienced LTC nurses and recommended by the National Citizens Coalition For Nursing Home Reform (website: www.nccnhr.org).

NURSE STAFFING

Medicare SNF staffing requirements were exceedingly minimal. The law required that SNF services be authorized by a licensed physician and that a licensed nurse (registered nurse [RN] or licensed practical or vocational nurse [LPN/LVN]) be on duty at all times, including an RN for 8 consecutive hours of each day. Implementing this regulation required that each SNF employ a full-time RN Director of Nursing. Medicaid nursing homes, called Intermediate Care Facilities (ICFs), were required to have a licensed nurse (RN or LPN/LVN) on duty on the day shift 7 days a week as charge nurse. If the charge nurse was not a RN, at least 3 hours of weekly consultation with a RN was required.

On the federal level, neither Medicare nor Medicaid set a standard for the number of nursing personnel in proportion to the number of beneficiaries being cared for in the nursing home. Neither program set standards for nurse aide training. States often set additional staffing requirements for facility licensure, but these were still too minimal, and in many cases were more protective of state funds than of beneficiaries.

The IOM report "Improving the Quality of Care in Nursing Homes" released in 1986 cited widespread inadequate care in U.S. nursing homes and related this to too few professional nurses, inadequate training and supervision of nursing assistants, excessive workloads for these direct caregivers, and inadequate government oversight of the care. The report called for more professional nurse staffing, required assessment and documentation of each resident's care needs, required nurse aide training, and improved regulation, oversight, and enforcement.[13] The IOM report was the impetus for the implementation of the Omnibus Budget Reconciliation Act (OBRA '87); however, it did not establish staffing requirements for direct caregivers and licensed nurses in proportion to number of residents.

OBRA '87 required that facilities certified by Medicare and Medicaid must have a nursing services department headed by a registered nurse (RN) Director of Nursing (DON), who is a full-time employee. Except in facilities of 60 or fewer beds, the DON may not be counted as direct care staff. A staff RN must be on duty 8 consecutive hours of each day, and a licensed nurse (RN or LPN/LVN) must be on duty at all other times. Waivers of these requirements are allowed in certain situations. For Medicare SNFs, 2 days a week of the 8-hour RN requirement can be waived by the U.S. Secretary of Health and Human Services if diligent effort by the facility to obtain the nurses at prevailing nursing home compensation was unsuccessful, a physician ensures it will not harm residents, and a physician or RN is on call. This is noted in the Social Security Act sec.1819 (b)(4)(C)(ii). For Medicaid nursing facilities, any of the licensed nurse requirements can be waived by the state if diligent effort by the facility to obtain the nurses at prevailing nursing home compensation was unsuccessful, a physician ensures it will not harm residents, and a physician or RN is on call. This is noted in the Social Security Act sec.1919 (b)(4)(C)(ii).

Vacancy rates for nursing personnel began to soar in the late 1980s. Hospitals across the country reported persistent vacancies and nursing school enrollments dropped. A devastating nursing shortage then developed quickly. Positions were going unfilled for more than a year in many rural facilities. Home care agencies had growing caseloads while LTC facilities were full and needed RNs. States across the country set up commissions to study the nursing shortage to identify ways in which to address and resolve the issue. The American Medical Association proposed the use of a registered care technologist, or RCT. This was supported by many health care administrators to alleviate the shortage of licensed nurses, but it sent shock waves through the nursing profession. The RCT would not be part of the nursing care delivery team, but rather supervised by the local Medical Boards; however, this proposal did not come to fruition.

Today a critical concern is still the growing demand for qualified nurses in LTC. Another important challenge facing LTC is the recruitment and retention of staff that provide direct care for the elderly. Certified nursing assistants (CNAs) and LPNs make up the majority of direct care staff in LTC settings with NAs making up approximately 43% of LTC staff while providing 90% of direct care.[14] Experts anticipate that the need for qualified caregivers in nursing homes will increase. According to estimates by the U.S. Department of Labor's Bureau of Labor Statistics, nursing homes will need 600,000 new CNAs by early next decade, when the first wave of baby boomers begins to need LTC.

The nursing shortage in LTC has become a serious social issue that may adversely affect the provision of effective resident care. Studies conducted in the early 1990s indicated that the nurse vacancy rates were considerably higher in nursing homes compared with other practice settings. A national survey conducted by the American Nurses Association showed that 66% of nursing homes reported increased nurse workloads, and a majority of these homes reported an increase in nurse hours worked.

In 1996 the IOM was again charged with studying the Adequacy of Nurse Staffing in Hospitals and Nursing Homes: Is It Adequate? This Committee concluded that there was a need for increased funding of research related to staffing levels, skill mix, and studies focused on quality of care and outcomes in nursing homes. The Committee recommended "Congress require a 24-hour presence of registered nurse coverage by the year 2000 in nursing facilities as an enhancement of the current 8-hour requirement specified under OBRA '87." The use of geriatric nurse specialist and geriatric nurse practitioners was recommended, as was increased emphasis on the educational preparation of directors of nursing.[12]

Since 1997 nurse-staffing levels have not improved. The average U.S. nursing facility has provided a total of 3.5 hours per resident day of RNs, LVN/LPNs, NAs, and DON time. Of the 3.5 hours, 60% or 2.1 hours are given by NAs and that figure has remained constant since 1994.[9] These figures reflect only averages. In fact, half of US nursing facilities provides fewer than 3.5 total and 2 nursing assistant hours per resident day.[21] Studies have shown that inadequate nurse staffing and poorly trained staff contribute to negative resident outcomes. For example, inadequate staffing and lack of professional supervision has been reported to contribute to dehydration in nursing homes[13] (see Evidence-Based Practice box).

In 1999 The U.S. Office of the Inspector General confirmed the many chronic and recurring quality problems in nursing homes. State surveyors reported that nursing home staffing shortages and inadequate staff expertise were major factors in poor quality. In an effort to explore the need for a national minimum staffing standard for nursing facilities, an expert panel of leading nurse researchers, educators, and administrators in LTC, consumer advocates, health economists, and health services researchers convened at the John A. Hartford Institute for Geriatric Nursing Division of Nursing at New York University. The expert panel on nursing home care found that the average nursing staff level in some nursing homes is too low to ensure high quality care. The panel recommended 24-hour RN supervision, additional education and training, and minimum staffing standards for nursing administration. It was also recommended that minimum ratios of caregivers and licensed nurses to clients be established, depending on the time of day and client needs, and recommended that residents received at least 4.5 hours of direct care each day[8] (see Future Watch box).

Evidence-Based Practice

Reference: Kayser-Jones J et al: Factors contributing to dehydration in nursing homes: inadequate staffing and lack of professional supervision, *J Am Geriatr Soc* 47:1187, 1999.

The purpose of the study was to investigate the factors that influenced fluid intake among nursing home residents who were not eating well. The study design used was prospective, descriptive, and anthropologic. Two proprietary nursing homes with 105 and 138 beds, respectively, were study sites. Forty nursing home residents participated. Data were collected by participant observation, event analysis, bedside dysphagia screening, mental and functional status evaluation, assessment of level of family/advocate involvement, and chart review. Data were gathered on the amount of liquid served and consumed over a 3-day period. Daily fluid intake was compared with three established standards: Standard 1 (30 ml/kg body weight), Standard 2 (1 ml/kcal/energy consumed), and Standard 3 (100 ml/kg for the first 10 kg, 50 ml/kg for the next 10 kg, 15 ml/kg for the remaining kg).

The residents' mean fluid intake was inadequate; 39 of the 40 residents consumed less than 1500 ml/day. By using three established standards, we found that the fluid intake was inadequate for nearly all the residents. The amount of fluid consumed with and between meals was low. Some residents took no fluids for extended periods, which resulted in their fluid intake being erratic and inadequate even when it was resumed. During the data collection, 25 of the 40 residents had illnesses/conditions that may have been related to dehydration.

When staff is inadequate and supervision is poor, residents with moderate to severe dysphagia, severe cognitive and functional impairment, aphasia or inability to speak English, and a lack of family or friends to assist them at mealtime are at great risk for dehydration. Adequate fluid intake can be achieved by simple interventions such as offering residents preferred liquids systematically and by having an adequate number of supervised staff help them to drink while properly positioned.

Future Watch

Proposed Minimum Staffing Standards for Nursing Homes in United States

ADMINISTRATION STANDARD

Full-time RN with a bachelor's degree as director of nursing (a provision for grandfathering current RN directors would be allowed for a specified time period)

Part-time RN assistant director of nursing (full-time in facilities of 100 beds or more; this person may also be the MDS coordinator)

Part-time RN director of in-service education (preferably with gerontology training; full-time in facilities of 100 or more)

Full-time RN nursing facility supervisor on duty at all times, 24 hr/day, 7 days/week

DIRECT CARE STAFFING STANDARD

The minimum number of direct care staff must be distributed as follows:

Minimum level direct care staff (RN, LVN/LPN, or CNA):

Day shift	1 FTE for each 5 residents	(1.6 hr. per resident day)
Evening shift	1 FTE for each 10 residents	(0.8 hr per resident day)
Night shift	1 FTE for each 15 residents	(0.53 hr per resident day)

Minimum licensed nurses (RN and LVN/LPN) providing direct care, treatments and medications, planning, coordination, and supervision at the unit level:

Day shift	1 FTE for each 15 residents	(0.53 hr/resident day)
Evening shift	1 FTE for each 20 residents	(0.40 hr/resident day)
Night shift	1 FTE for each 30 residents	(0.27 hr/resident day)

Minimum total number of direct nursing care staff is 4.13 hr/resident day. Total administrative and direct and indirect nursing hours is 4.55 hr/resident day. Staffing must be ADJUSTED UPWARD for residents with higher nursing care needs.

Source: Harrington C et al: Experts recommend minimum nurse staffing standards for nursing facilities in the United States, *Gerontologist* 40(1):5, 2000.

RN, Registered nurse; *MDS*, minimum data set; *LVN/LPN*, licensed vocational/licensed practical nurse; *CAN*, certified nurse assistant; *FTE*, full-time employee; *NA*, nursing assistant. This builds on the Nurse Staffing Standards accepted by the National Citizen's Coalition for Nursing Home Reform (1995).

Continued

Future Watch—cont'd

Proposed Minimum Staffing Standards for Nursing Homes in United States

MEALTIME NURSING STAFF

Direct care staff standards will take into account specific needs of residents at mealtimes. At all mealtimes there will be:

- 1 nursing FTE for each two to three residents who are entirely dependent on assistance
- 1 nursing FTE for each two to four residents who are partially dependent on assistance

Nursing staff that assist with feeding should be CNAs who are adequately trained in feeding procedures and they should be supervised by licensed nurses.

EDUCATION AND TRAINING

All licensed nurses in nursing homes must have continuing education in care of the chronically ill and disabled and/or gerontologic nursing (at least 30 hours every 2 years).

NAs should have a minimum of 160 hr of training, including training in appropriate feeding techniques.

NURSE PRACTITIONERS

Each nursing home is strongly urged (but not required) to have a part-time geriatric or adult nurse practitioner and/or a geriatric clinical nurse specialist on staff (full-time for 100 beds or more).

In 1998 a new method to monitor staffing levels in nursing facilities materialized as a result of consumer advocates who were able to persuade President Clinton and the HCFA to develop a consumer information system to inform the public about current staffing levels in each nursing facility. This consumer information system was established for all 16,000 certified nursing facilities by the HCFA using the Internet. In 1999, nurse-staffing information was added to the information system. This website, www.Medicare/Nursing HomeCompare.htm, allows the public to compare up to three nursing facilities in the United States at one time. Another attempt to increase monitoring of staffing levels in nursing facilities across the country came through new legislation passed in the federal budget act (Benefits Improvement and Protection Act of 2000). This regulation requires nursing facilities that receive Medicare or Medicaid funding to post daily "the number of licensed and unlicensed nursing staff directly responsible for resident care in the facility. This information shall be displayed in a uniform manner (as specified by the Secretary) and in a clearly visible place."[4]

At the beginning of the twenty-first century, when nursing facility care should have improved, many nursing facility residents have experienced worsening outcomes.[6] As the older population grows, as well as a continued trend toward nursing homes caring for more cognitively impaired, frail elderly with chronic conditions continues, the failure to increase nursing facility staffing will have a negative impact on the health and well-being of these individuals. Unless federal and state regulatory agencies are willing to establish mandated staffing levels and provide the resources to support it, adding more professional nurse staffing will continue to be a challenge.

LONG-TERM CARE FACILITY

The nursing facility is a fascinating, complex microcosm. It is a temporary place of recovery and rehabilitation for posthospital short-term residents. It is respite and support for families and is the home and community for the residents. This is the reason individuals who live in LTC facilities are called residents rather than clients. The LTC facility is an employer and place of career development for health care personnel. It is also a business, competing with others for customers. One LTC facility may be part of a larger business, or a group of facilities, that may own other companies supplying medical equipment and services.

The nursing facility is a system of interacting departments that offers all basic services for supporting and sustaining life for very dependent people. By law and regulation it must provide a safe environment for residents and staff. To function well it must have clear lines of responsibility and authority. Each facility is unique because of its location, the residents who live there, and the people who manage and work in the home. However, there are probably many similarities, especially among the more than 17,000 facilities that are certified for Medicare and or Medicaid participation.

HFCA requires the LTC facilities to have a governing body. The Board has fiduciary responsibility for financial viability of the company. It approves operating and capital expenditure budgets. The Board is accountable for conforming with all relevant laws and regulations. It initiates and/or has oversight of mission, goals, objectives, and policies. The Board selects and delegates responsibility to an Administrator and/or a management company, who reports back to the Board. Although each LTC facility is different, the following discussion outlines elements of facility organization that are common to many (Figure 10-5).

All departments are essential to the organization, although some have only a few employees. The Nursing Services Department has by far the most employees, making up 60% of all nursing home personnel. It is responsible for ensuring that direct and individualized personal care is available to each resident 24 hours a day.

The Administrator is chief executive of the facility, with authority delegated from the Board or CEO of the corporation. He or she must be licensed as a nursing home administrator in the state where the facility is located. The Administrator is responsible for compliance with all local, state, and federal law and regulation, keeping the facility ready for inspection at all times. He or she must ensure that the facility obtains required licenses, permits, and approvals in a timely manner and maintains Medicare and Medicaid certification (if the facility participates in these programs). Business and financial management is a primary responsibility.

Each facility participating in Medicare and Medicaid must have a licensed physician as Medical Director, who is responsible for implementation of resident care policies and the delivery of medical care. State law for nursing facilities serving

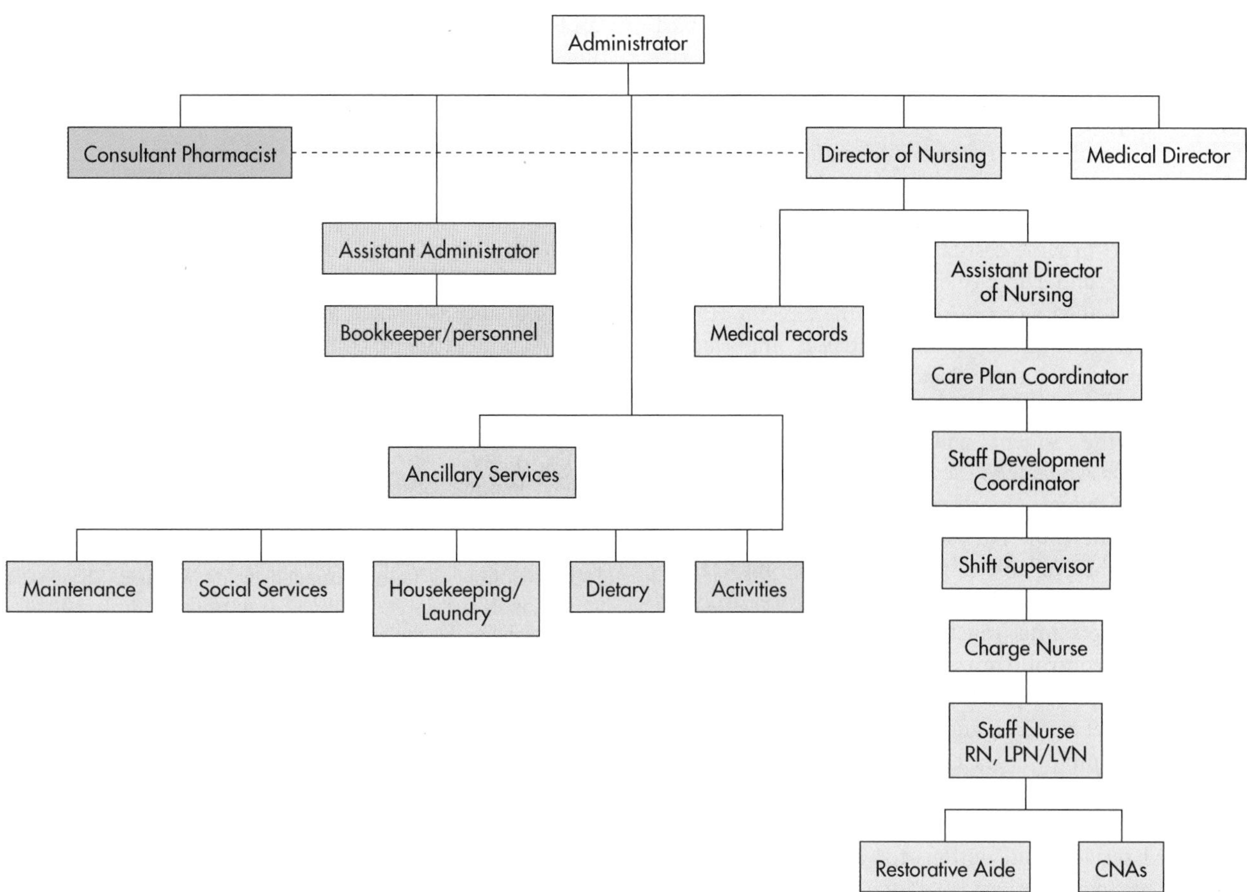

Figure 10-5 Nursing facility organizational chart.

only private pay residents may also require this. The Medical Director may be on staff part-time or full-time. The Medical Director must ensure that each Medicare and Medicaid resident has an admitting order from a physician and is seen by a physician whenever needed and at least every 30 days for 3 months after admission and every 60 days thereafter. Physicians may delegate routine medical visits and orders to a clinical nurse specialist, nurse practitioner, or physician assistant if this is permitted under state law. The Medical Director also conducts Medicare utilization review in coordination with the nursing department and rehabilitation professionals—a process of considering the progress of posthospital residents every few days to certify and recertify their eligibility for the Medicare SNF benefit.

The Medical Director participates in or ensures physician approval of an interdisciplinary care plan for each resident. He or she reviews and makes decisions concerning medical records problems, incident reports, infection reports, and consultant pharmacy reports. He or she participates in the Quality Assessment and Infection Control Committee meetings at least quarterly to track quality issues with the DON and others.

Nursing services must be sufficient to provide supportive restorative care that allows each resident to attain and maintain the highest practicable physical, mental, and psychosocial well-being. The Nursing Services department must have the capacity to meet special needs of residents for medication and treatments, including injections, ostomy care, urinary catheter care, enteral and parenteral feeding, respiratory care (including tracheotomy care, suction, and oxygen administration), foot care and assistance with use of prostheses, hearing aids, glasses, and dentures. Basic nursing care must ensure that the resident has adequate nutrition, hydration, and assistance as needed with activities of daily living: eating, bathing, dressing, grooming, personal hygiene, toileting, transferring from bed to chair, and mobility. Restorative care to help residents regain lost function, recover strength, and heal wounds is integral to good nursing care. To avoid complications in very dependent residents, there must be particular emphasis on preventive care such as ensuring adequate nourishment and liquid intake, range of motion, frequent turning and supportive positioning to relieve pressure and stasis, mouth care, and cleansing and lubrication of skin. The continuing challenge for nursing services is to organize the care so that all elements are provided consistently. In addition to direct care staff, many nursing facilities employ a Care Plan Coordinator who frequently may also serve as the assistant DON. This person's primary responsibility is to coordinate the interdisciplinary care plan process. A Staff Development Coordinator may also be employed to coordinate in-service education and orientation training.

The facility must employ a qualified dietitian at least part time. The dietitian makes an assessment of each resident's nutritional needs, participates in interdisciplinary care planning, and plans therapeutic diets. The dietitian must interact with the nursing department to obtain information about residents' acceptance of meals and preferences in foods, ability to chew and swallow foods, need to alter consistency or content of foods, need to provide assistance with meals, amount of nutritional intake, and evidence of retention and assimilation of food (e.g., weight gain or loss). A full-time director of food service must also be employed if the dietitian is employed on a part-time basis. The dietary department is responsible for planning, preparation, and delivery of regular meals and therapeutic diets to the residents and must make between-meal nourishing snacks available to the residents. Breakfast must be served no more than 14 hours after the evening meal was served. A substitute choice of foods with comparable nutritious value must be available to residents at each meal. Handling, storage, and preparation of foods must meet accepted state standards. Personnel must meet health standards and observe infection control requirements in handling foods.

All Medicare- and Medicaid-certified facilities must provide medical social services, and in facilities of 120 beds or more, they must employ at least one full-time qualified social worker. The social services department assesses psychologic and social needs of residents and their families and helps them locate needed services and options for assistance with payment if needed. Social workers collaborate with nursing in interdisciplinary care planning and work closely with families in planning admissions, discharges, and transfers. Some social workers are qualified to provide individual counseling or therapy for a resident. Social workers often play a key role in interviewing families of prospective residents and making preliminary determinations of care needs and sources of payment. A social worker may help plan and convene Resident Council and Family Council meetings.

Federal law requires an activities program to enhance the quality of life for each resident. The facility must employ an activities professional or recreational therapist. Ideally the program involves a plan for individualized activity of interest for each resident, whether bed-bound, chair-bound, or ambulatory. There may be only one professional and an activities aide to help carry out the program, so a great deal of collaboration with nursing is needed. Cooperative planning between nursing and the activities department can do much to ensure that the program reaches all residents, even if some stay in their rooms. Nursing personnel need to schedule resident care to allow time for, and transport to, activities each day. Unit conferences and care planning in collaboration with families allow staff to identify diversions and activities related to each resident's individual interests and tastes, and plan for these to be incorporated into the resident's day.

In recent years the development of new approaches has brought more interest, sense of community participation, and personal autonomy to the lives of nursing home residents. William Thomas, MD, has pioneered a concept called The Eden Alternative, which allows live animals, growing plants, and visiting children to be a regular part of daily life in nursing facilities (Box 10-4).

His newest concept, The Green House Project, is founded on the idea that the physical and social environments in which LTC is delivered should be warm, smart, and green. The concept comes from the Eden Alternative method of empowering staff by making the resident the center of the community and enlivening the nursing home environment with plants, animals, and children (Box 10-5).

For quality assurance, a medical records specialist may routinely audit resident clinical records for consistency, com-

BOX 10-4 The Eden Alternative

The Eden Alternative has become the most famous of the "alternative methods of organizing care and staff management" in the nation's nursing homes founded by Dr. William Thomas. The mission of the Eden Alternative is to improve the quality of life for individuals who live in long-term care (LTC) facilities. The core vision for this organization is to teach the concept that LTC facilities are not institutions for the frail and elderly but rather habitats for human beings that can be both vibrant and vigorous and be inclusive of Mother Nature. The long-term goal of the Eden organization is to build a coalition of successful Eden facilities that will remake the way people think about LTC. They want to eliminate the loneliness, helplessness, and boredom of institutional care. They believe bringing in other living creatures, revitalizing the surrounding environment, and providing daily spontaneity will accomplish this. The Eden Alternative is based on 10 principles:

1. The three plagues of loneliness, helplessness, and boredom account for the bulk of suffering in a human community.
2. Life in a truly human community revolves around close and continuing contact with children, plants, and animals. These ancient relationships provide young and old alike with a pathway to a life worth living.
3. Loving companionship is the antidote to loneliness. In a human community, we must provide easy access to human and animal companionship.
4. To give care to another makes us stronger. To receive care gracefully is a pleasure and an art. A healthy human community promotes both of these virtues in its daily life, seeking always to balance one with the other.
5. Trust in each other allows us the pleasure of answering the needs of the moment. When we fill our lives with variety and spontaneity, we honor the world and our place in it.
6. Meaning is the food and water that nourishes the human spirit. It strengthens us. The counterfeits of meaning tempt us with hollow promises. In the end they always leave us empty and alone.
7. Medical treatment should be the servant of genuine human caring, never its master.
8. In a human community, the wisdom of the elders grows in direct proportion to the honor and respect accorded to them.
9. Human growth must never be separated from human life.
10. Wise leadership is the lifeblood of any struggle against the three plagues. For it, there can be no substitute.

Source: The Eden Alternative Homepage, website: www.edenalt.com, 2001.

pleteness, and accuracy and collaborate with the Medical Director, attending physicians, and Nursing Service personnel to promote compliance with standards. The medical records department may be given the responsibility of transmitting MDS data for each Medicare and Medicaid resident to the state, on admission and periodically as required thereafter. These assessments must be retained in the resident's record as well. Closed records must be maintained in conformance with state law and in an orderly manner in a secure place for at least 5 years from discharge (adults).

A housekeeping supervisor trains personnel and oversees their work in a schedule of daily and periodic cleaning of furniture surfaces, rooms, halls, bathrooms, and utility rooms to maintain a clean, comfortable environment for residents and staff. Infection control and safety practices must be followed in the collection and disposal of trash, handling and storage of cleansers, insecticides, and cleaning materials. Maintenance of every aspect of buildings, grounds, and equipment in the facility, auxiliary power, and conformity to the fire safety code is also an administrative responsibility. Nursing personnel must be instructed to contact the engineer or other maintenance personnel to report any aspect of the equipment, building, and grounds that needs repair.

Laundry services are essential to nursing services to ensure that clean linens for beds, bathing, and clean clothes for residents are available at all times. Some facilities contract with outside laundries. Whatever the arrangement, auxiliary clean linen supplies should be available in the facility at all hours. Nursing service must ensure safe handling of soiled linens to protect laundry workers. There must be close coordination between nursing and laundry services for timely receipt and storage of clean linens and transport of soiled linens to the laundry. Although some families launder clothes at home for a resident, the facility often is responsible for laundering residents' personal clothing.

Nursing works closely with ancillary service providers, transmitting physician orders, arranging schedules to coordinate with their services, ensuring appropriate documentation in the residents' clinical records, and ordering necessary supplies. A Licensed Consultant Pharmacist must review the medication regimen for each Medicare and Medicaid resident at least once a month to confirm the appropriateness of prescriptions, doses, and combinations of drugs. The pharmacist also inspects the labeling, expiration dates, and storage conditions of medications and biologicals, as well as records of receipts and disposition of all controlled substances.

Nursing facilities are also required to have the following services available to its residents:

- Physical therapy, occupational therapy, and speech/language therapy professionals retained on staff or their services obtained by contract with outside providers
- Respiratory therapy services (may be arranged through hospitals with which the facility has a transfer agreement)
- Laboratory, radiology, and other diagnostic services provided by agreement with providers of these services if they are not available at the facility
- Transportation provided in insured company cars with approved drivers, and/or by contract with outside taxi and ambulance services
- Agreements to provide services retained with one or more licensed dentists and providers of foot care (licensed podiatrist or physician)
- Provision for resident access to religious services and spiritual counseling

BOX 10-5 The Green House Project

Green House Project, founded by Dr. William Thomas, is an attempt to design, build, and test a radically new approach to residential long-term care (LTC) for the elderly. It is founded on the idea that the physical and social environment in which we deliver LTC can and should be warm, smart, and green. The Green Houses themselves will be small (6 to 8 person) community homes where people requiring skilled nursing services can live and receive the care they need. They will be linked with a sophisticated health care delivery network that can ensure quality, provide expertise, organize back up staffing, and deliver back office support.

The houses will fit the character of the neighborhoods in which they are built. Inside, warmth will be created through the floor plan, furnishings, décor, and, most important, the people. A small number of caregivers will share ongoing responsibilities for the elders and the house. Developing intimate relationships will be made easier by the fact that each Green House will provide a minimum of 36 hours of staffing a day, 6 hours per elder per day, a standard above that provided in conventional, facility-based LTC. The house will be filled with useful but unobtrusive technology that ensures safety and promotes quality of care, rigor in record keeping, and community and family involvement. It will be the Einstein of smart houses. Finally, we recognize that people find great pleasure in the company of animals, the laughter of children, and the growth of green plants. Past experience with the Eden Alternative has shown, time and again, that contact with the living world is a major factor in both quality of life and improved clinical outcomes. The Green Houses must indeed be green.

The fundamental principals of the Green House Project are:

- Creating warmth
- New logic of smallness
- Rethinking hierarchy
- The power of informality
- Using smart technology
- The power of green

The ultimate idea is to create a place that is full of hope, life, and vitality.

The Faxton-St Luke's Healthcare System of Utica, NY, was the first to pilot the Green House Project. Residents moved into the first four of seven planned Green Houses starting Spring 2001. These first Green Houses are small community homes for six to eight residents, purposely located within a 15-minute radius of the health care system's central campus. The 3500- to 4000-square foot homes are built from scratch, are designed to integrate into the surrounding community, and contain four or five private and semiprivate (for couples) bedrooms.

Source: The Green House Project www.thegreenhouseproject.com, 2001.

In the facility, many departments must function as one unit to meet the needs of its residents. Admission to a nursing facility is often a difficult decision affecting numerous aspects of a person's life. Ensuring that the facility functions properly and according to mandated standards is essential to the physical, emotional, social, psychologic, and spiritual well-being of each resident. When all requirements are met, the objective is to enhance the quality of life for each resident who lives in the facility.

NURSING HOME ADMISSION

The goal of nursing home care is to provide necessary care and services that will attain or maintain the highest practicable physical, mental, and psychosocial well-being as determined by the comprehensive assessment and plan of care. The facility must ensure that the resident obtains optimal improvement or does not deteriorate within the limits of the resident's right to refuse treatment, or within the limits of recognized pathology, or the normal aging process.

As individuals age, the likelihood of using a nursing facility increases. In a study conducted in 1997 on expected lifetime use of nursing facility services, 20% of all men can expect to be admitted to a nursing facility at least once. Of the total female population, 34% can anticipate at least one admission to a nursing facility.[3] The Census Bureau estimates that as the elderly population in the United States increases, the number of nursing facility residents will increase to 2.9 million by the year 2020.[15]

Of the 1.8 million nursing facility beds, 1.5 million are occupied. As women's life spans continue to exceed their male counterparts, one can expect to see women being the largest users of LTC services. The typical nursing facility resident is a white female. Women have historically accounted for 75% of residents in nursing homes. In 1997 women accounted for 72% of the total.[16]

Many factors affect family members' decision to place a loved one in a nursing facility. Although care-receiver attributes can be useful in predicting nursing home placement, it is believed that caregiver characteristics appear to be more important predictors of placement[5] (see Research box).

Family involvement is essential to foster a smooth transition from home to a nursing facility. They are consumers, as is the resident. It is important to understand their role in this process. Many have been primary caregivers for extended periods and will find it difficult to shift roles over night. There are many things that the facility staff can do to develop a close collaborative relationship with family members (Box 10-6).

An admission to a nursing facility can be as short as 3 months for some and as a long as years for others. The length of stay depends on the health needs of the individual. It has been noted that widows, divorcees, or never married individuals are more likely to spend more days in a nursing facility than those who are married. The National Center for Health Statistics indicates that the most frequently cited admission diagnoses in 1997 for males and females were related to diseases of the circulatory system.

Research

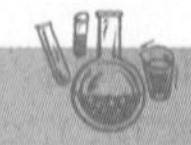

Reference: Hagen B: Nursing home placement: Factors affecting caregivers' decisions to place family members with dementia, *J Gerontol Nurs* 27(2):44, 2001.

The purpose of this study was to explore factors influencing caregivers' decision-making process related to placing an elderly family member with dementia in a nursing home. The exploratory, descriptive study used qualitative methodology to examine the decision-making process of caregivers considering nursing home placement of their family member suffering from dementia. The purposive sample consisted of five individuals caring for a family member with dementia at home. Recruitment of participants occurred through a geriatric outreach program in a large, urban Canadian hospital. Selection criteria for inclusion in the study were:

- Caregivers must be caring for an older family member (older than age 65) with dementia.
- Caregivers must be living in the same residence as the family member with dementia.
- Caregivers must be the primary source of care and decision making for the family member.
- Caregivers must be considering nursing home placement of their family member, but have not yet made a formal application for placement.

Recruitment and data collection took place over 2 months. Data collection ended after repeated in-depth interviews with five participants, when the point of data saturation was reached. Of the sample, four participants were female and one was male. They ranged from 34 years to 72 years old. The sample included two daughters, two wives, and one son. Data were analyzed concurrently with data collection, using the constant comparative method.

The study found a number of factors that influenced placement-related decision making, including independence, perceived presence of others, fear of loneliness, negative nursing home attitudes, sense of existential self, and guilt. The study suggested that the decision to place a family member in a nursing home is complex, and it may be necessary to address deeper issues with clients who are unable to make a decision about nursing home care.

BOX 10-6 Keys to Resident/Family Satisfaction

The keys to resident and family satisfaction include:

- Keeping open communication (keep the family informed of the resident's health status and changes)
- Viewing the family as an ally
- Encouraging family involvement in the care (clarifying the scope of participation through the facility policies)
- Encouraging participation in the care planning process and care meetings
- Promoting and supporting an active Resident Council
- Promoting and supporting an active Family Council
- Encouraging the staff to understand and respect the residents' rights

In all 42% of nursing facility clients suffers from some level of dementia and 33% have documented symptoms of depression. The percentage of clients receiving preventive skin care has risen noticeably since 1994, from 28% to 60% of the total

MDS + TRIGGERS + RAPS ⟶ COMPREHENSIVE ASSESSMENT
UTILIZATION
GUIDELINES

Figure 10-6 RAI framework.

Assessment (MDS/Other) ⟶ Decision Making (RAPs/Other) ⟶ Care Plan Development ⟶ Care Plan Implementation ⟶ Evaluation

Figure 10-7 Problem identification process.

client population in 1999 and 2000. Just over 16% of the clients received rehabilitative therapy at the facility. A total of 50% of nursing home residents were receiving psychoactive drugs in 1999 and 2000. Just over 2% of clients do not speak English as their dominant language.[3]

Nationally in 1999 and 2000, nursing facilities reporting information about their residents in their most recent standard survey indicated that their residents on average require assistance with or are dependent on nursing staff for 3.75 activities of daily living (ADLs). The five ADLs are eating, bathing, dressing, toileting, and transferring. ADL dependence is a measure of resident acuity that helps facilities gauge the needs of their resident population. The area of greatest dependency was identified as bathing; 94% of all nursing facility residents were dependent on staff or required assistance with bathing. Nearly 86% are either dependent or require assistance to dress; 20% require some assistance with eating and 19% are dependent on staff for eating; 79% require assistance from or are dependent on staff for toileting.[3]

Despite unprecedented treatments and technology available to health care professionals, residents in nursing facilities have experienced an increase in negative outcomes. During the last 8 years, there has been an increase in resident contractures, the number of residents in bed all or most of the times, the use of psychotropic drugs, and incontinence.[7,9] Improving the outcomes and quality of life for nursing facility residents is a primary concern for consumers, nursing, administrators, and regulatory agencies. Proper nurse staffing is paramount to ensure accurate and thorough assessment of each resident to prevent deterioration and promote his or her highest practicable level of physical, mental, and psychosocial well-being.

NURSING MANAGEMENT

Resident Assessment Instrument

The Nursing Home Case-Mix and Quality Demonstration is the official title for the project where case mix methodology for nursing homes was refined. This project can trace its origins to the Institute of Medicine study, "Improving the Quality of Care in Nursing Homes," and from there to the nursing home reforms of 1987, which were convenient amendments to the Budget Reconciliation Act. This legislation mandated a resident specific MDS. After several generations of revision, this data set has become the primary source of information for both monitoring quality and establishing payment. Data collected in this standardized assessment tool are electronically transmitted to the HCFA to establish an information database. A second source of data on nursing facilities is from OSCAR, the federal On-Line Survey Certification and Reporting System. This information is used to identify care trends, resident profiles, reimbursement, staffing, admissions, discharges, etc. The data allow HCFA to compare LTC facilities within each state, regionally, and nationally.

Nurses were given significant mandated responsibility in the Nursing Home Reform Act commonly referred to as Omnibus Budget Reconciliation Act (OBRA '87) within the nursing home industry. A registered nurse must coordinate the interdisciplinary assessment of each resident's care needs at least four times a year and with each significant change in health status and functional capacity. The plan of care for each resident must reflect the care needs identified in the assessment. The RAI is a powerful tool for clinicians and provides a regulatory framework that supports and promotes good clinical practice. Federal requirements state that facilities must use a RAI that has been specified by the state. This assessment system provides a comprehensive, accurate, standardized, reproducible assessment of each LTC facility resident's functional capabilities and helps staff to identify health problems. See Figure 10-6 for a schematic of the overall RAI framework.

There are four types of federally mandated assessments:

1. Admission (Initial) Assessment must be completed by the 14th day of the resident's stay in the facility (42 CFR 483.20 (b)(4)(I)/F 273).
2. Annual reassessment must be completed within 12 months of most recent full assessment (42 CFR 483.20 (b)(4)(v)/F 275).
3. Significant change in status reassessment must be completed by the end of the 14th calendar day following determination that a significant change has occurred (42 CFR 483.20 (b)(4)(9iv)/F 274).
4. Quarterly Assessment is a set of MDS items, mandated by State (contains at least HCFA established subset of MDS item). Must be completed no less frequently than once every 3 months (42 CFR 483.20 (b)(5)F 276).

The nursing profession's problem identification model is called the nursing process. The RAI provides a structured, standardized approach for applying a problem identification process in LTC facilities. Figure 10-7 depicts how the problem identification process would look as a pathway.

Minimum Data Set, Resident Assessment Protocols, and Utilization Guidelines

The RAI consists of three basic components: the MDS, RAPS, and Utilization Guidelines specified in state operations manuals. Use of the three components of the RAI yields information about a resident's functional status, strengths, weaknesses, and preferences and offers guidance on further assessment after problems have been identified. Each component flows naturally into the next as follows:

- MDS: A core of screening, clinical, and functional status elements including common definitions and coding categories, that forms the foundation of the comprehensive assessment for all residents of LTC facilities certified to participate in Medicare or Medicaid. The items in the MDS standardize communication about resident problems and conditions within facilities, between facilities, and between facilities and outside agencies. The triggers are specific resident responses for one or a combination of MDS elements. The triggers identify residents who either have or are at risk for developing specific functional problems and require further evaluation using RAPs designated within the State-specified RAI. Currently, the MDS is in its second version. Because it is a lengthy assessment and care screening tool, it is not reprinted here but can be accessed on the Internet at www.hcfa.gov/medicaid/mds20/mds20.pdf.
- RAPs: A component of the utilization guidelines, the RAPs are structured, problem-oriented frameworks for organizing MDS information and examining additional clinically relevant information about an individual. RAPs help identify social, medical, and psychologic problems and form the basis for individualized care planning. There are 18 problem-oriented RAPs, each of which includes MDS-based "trigger" conditions that signal the need for additional assessment and review (Box 10-7). The legend summarizes which MDS item responses trigger individual RAPs and has been designed as a helpful tool for facilities if they chose to use it. It is a worksheet, not a required form. The triggered conditions are indicated in the appropriate column on the RAP Summary Form. Based on the review of assessment information, the interdisciplinary team decides whether the triggered condition affects the resident's functional status or well-being and warrants a care plan intervention. The decision to proceed to care planning should be indicated on the RAP Summary Form.
- Utilization Guidelines: Provides instructions concerning when and how to use the RAI.
- Because RNs have the primary responsibility for completing this assessment tool, it behooves nursing facilities to ensure that RNs in nursing home practice not only possess the skills to accurately complete the assessment but also are knowledgeable of its purpose and key role in the LTC setting.

BOX 10-7 RAP Problem Areas

- Delirium
- Cognitive loss
- Visual function
- Communication
- ADL functional/rehabilitation potential
- Urinary incontinence and indwelling catheter
- Psychosocial well-being
- Mood state
- Behavioral symptoms
- Activities
- Falls
- Nutritional status
- Feeding tubes
- Dehydration/fluid maintenance
- Dental care
- Pressure ulcers
- Psychotropic use
- Physical restraints

Source: Long-Term Care Facility Resident Assessment Instrument (RAI) User manual, HCFA, October 1995.

Interdisciplinary Care Plan

Once the comprehensive assessment is completed, it provides the foundation on which the care plan is formulated. The care plan is a roadmap that provides a guide for all staff to ensure that decline of the resident's condition is avoided, if possible. The focus should be not only resolution of clinical problems but also prevention of further decline. Facilities are mandated to develop a comprehensive care plan for each resident that includes measurable objectives and timetables to meet a resident's medical, nursing, mental, and psychosocial needs that are identified in the comprehensive assessment.

The care plan must describe:

- The services that are to be furnished to attain or maintain the resident's highest practicable physical, mental, and psychosocial well-being.
- Any services that would otherwise be required under 42 CFR 483.25 but are not provided because of the resident's rights under 483.10, including the right to refuse treatment.

The comprehensive care plan must be developed within 7 days after completion of the comprehensive assessment. It must be prepared by an interdisciplinary team that includes the attending physician, a registered nurse with responsibility for the resident, other appropriate staff in disciplines as determined by the resident's needs, and to the extent practicable, the resident, the resident's family, or the resident's legal representative. The care plan must be periodically reviewed and revised by a team of qualified individuals after each assessment. The services provided or arranged by the facility must meet professional standards of quality and be provided by qualified persons in accordance with each resident's written plan of care.

Most nursing facilities use a computer program for analyzing the MDS, which then produces a standardized care plan. The facility is then responsible to individualize the care plan to meet the needs of each resident. The care plan should address the needs, strengths, and preferences of the resident as reflected in the comprehensive assessment. It should be prevention focused and address a plan for managing risk factors. Objectives should reflect realistic measurable outcomes with time frames. Interventions must be appropriate for the identified needs of the resident and may involve other disciplines outside nursing. A clear mechanism should be in place to ensure that all disciplines complete and document their intervention and its effect and results. Progress notes are often used to accomplish this.

Care plans are not static documents and should reflect changes in the resident's condition. The care plans must be translated into instructions or checklists for the caregivers of each resident. Unit charge nurses (LPNs or RNs) assign resident care responsibilities to direct care staff. Direct care staff should be able to describe the care, services, and expected outcomes of the care they provide. Also, they should possess a general knowledge of the care plan and services being provided by other therapists and understand the expected outcomes of this care and the relationship of these expected outcomes to the care they provide. Once this process is complete, the objective is to improve the quality of life for each resident in the facility.

Documentation

Federal guidelines require that clinical records on each resident be maintained in accordance with professional standards and practices. They must be complete, accurately documented, readily accessible, and systemically organized. The clinical record must include sufficient information to identify the resident, a record of the assessments, the plan of care, services provided, results of preadmission screening conducted by the state, and progress notes.[1] Medicare requires documentation, which includes a nursing assessment, to be completed each shift for residents who are receiving skilled services. Medicaid documentation frequency and content requirements vary from state to state. In addition to Medicare and Medicaid requirements, nursing facilities may have additional facility specific documentation requirements.

A complete clinical record contains an accurate chronologic representation of the actual experiences of the resident in the facility. Documentation should include sufficient information that indicates that the facility is aware of the status of the resident. The documentation should also show that the effects of care provided and response to treatments are being assessed and addressed. Effective documentation portrays a picture of the resident's progress, change in condition, and changes in treatment. Good documentation practice should show progress toward achieving care plan goals. This allows clinicians access to accurate information that aids in making good clinical judgments for treatment interventions. Failure to maintain and record accurate objective and subjective data obtained from assessments, residents, family, or caregivers can result in negative outcomes, inappropriate treatment, or no treatment at all. As in all clinical settings, proper documentation is key to effective communication between and among disciplines and staff.

Critical Thinking Questions

1. An elderly woman was admitted to an LTC facility 10 days ago. She knows that it is winter and even comments on the frost outside her window but thinks that she is living in a hotel. She gets lost getting from her room to the dining room and back again. She recognizes most of the staff members' faces but can remember only a few names. The CNAs must assist her with dressing or she will put items on backwards or in the wrong order. Her glasses are often left in the last place she visited. The staff must remind her to finish her meals or she will wander from the table. Her weight is stable. Her table is by the window and she often locates it without help, except at supper. When she is at the table, she will rock back and forth and tear her napkin into little pieces. She cannot remember if she has eaten her meals after only a few minutes. Her family says she has been confused like this for the past year, but agrees that it did get worse about a month ago. She was started on Elavil for depression 6 weeks ago and takes Tylenol as needed for arthritis pain. How can the use of the RAI assist you to define her needs? What strategies would you use to address her confusion?
2. An 87-year-old woman is admitted to an LTC facility with arthritis and chronic obstructive pulmonary disease. She weighs 65 lbs. She is malnourished, frail, and very weak. Her skin is in good condition except for two small skin tears on her right lower leg. She has an advance directive that indicates she wants all measures taken except the use of tube feedings. Discuss alternatives to improve her nutritional status and prevent further decline.
3. A 72-year-old man was admitted to the Medicare unit for rehabilitation after sustaining a fall at home and having an open reduction internal fixation of the left hip. He is alert and oriented to time, place, and person. He is very resistant to care and does not want to be in the facility. He tries to get up without assistance. He nearly suffered another fall on his second night in the facility trying to climb over the side rails. What interventions would be most effective in ensuring his safety? What is the nursing facility's responsibility in terms of maintaining a safe environment for this resident?
4. A woman diagnosed with Alzheimer's dementia-type has been a resident in an LTC facility for 2 months. She is confused and disoriented most of the time. She constantly wanders in and out of other residents' rooms. She paces the halls constantly until she is exhausted. She has attempted to exit the building on numerous occasions but has never gotten further than the front entryway of the facility. She is a very fast walker and can be combative at times. What alternatives are available to prevent her from escaping and injuring herself? How might improved staffing patterns assist with this issue?

References

1. American Geriatrics Society, Regulation and quality of care standards in nursing facilities, *J Am Geriatr Soc* 48:1519, 2000.
2. American Health Care Association (AHCA), Long term-care insurance: debunking the myths, 2001, website: http://www.ahca.org/brief/bg-ltc.htm.
3. American Health Care Association Health Services Research and Evaluation Group: *Facts and trends: the nursing facility sourcebook*, Washington, DC, 2001, American Health Care Association.
4. Benefits Improvement and Protection Act of 2000, 42 U.S.C. 139995I-3(b)§1919(b), 2000.
5. Hagen B: Nursing home placement: factors affecting caregivers' decisions to place family members with dementia, *J Gerontol Nurs* 27(2):44, 2000.
6. Harrington C: Nursing home staffing: a need for humane policy, nursing facility staffing policy: a case study for political change, *Policy Politics Nurs Practices* 2:2, 2001.

7. Harrington C, Carrillo H: The regulation and enforcement of federal nursing home standards, *Med Care Res Rev* 56(4):471, 1999.
8. Harrington C et al: Experts recommend minimum nurse staffing standards for nursing facilities in the United States, *Gerontologist* 40:1, 2000.
9. Harrington C et al: Nursing facilities staffing, residents, and facility deficiencies, 1991-1999, Reports prepared for Health Care Financing Administration, University of California, 2000, website: www.hcfa.gov/medicaid/ltcomep.
10. Hobbs FB, Damon BC: 65+ in the United States, U.S. Bureau of the Census, 1996, *Current Population Reports Special Studies,* pp 23-190, Washington, DC, 1996, US Government Printing Office.
11. Institute of Medicine: *Improving the quality of care in nursing homes,* Washington, DC, 1986, National Academy Press.
12. Institute of Medicine: *Nursing staff in hospitals and nursing homes: Is it adequate?* Washington, DC, 1996, National Academy Press.
13. Kayser-Jones J et al: Factors contributing to dehydration in nursing homes: inadequate staffing and lack of professional supervision, *J Am Geriatr Soc* 47:1187, 1999.
14. Forum For State Health Policy Leadership: Severe shortage of nursing aides puts quality of long-term care in jeopardy, *State Health Notes* 21:322, 2000.
15. US Bureau of the Census: *Statistical Abstract of the United States:* 1998, We the American Elderly, Washington, DC, 1998, US Government Printing Office.
16. US Department of Health and Human Services: *An overview of nursing home facilities: Data from 1997 national nursing home survey,* Publication No. DHHS (PHS) 2000-1250 0-0169 (2/00), Hyattsville, MD, 2000, US Department of Health and Human Services, Center for Disease Control and Prevention, National Center for Health Statistics.
17. US General Accounting Office, *California nursing homes: care problems persist despite federal and state oversight:* Report to the Special Committee on Aging, US Senate, (GAO/HEHS 98-202), Washington, DC, 1998.
18. US General Accounting Office, *Nursing homes: additional steps needed to strengthen enforcement of federal quality standards,* Report to Special Committee on Aging, US Senate, (GAO/HEHS 99-46), Washington, DC, 1999.
19. US General Accounting Office, *Nursing homes: complaints investigation processes often inadequate to protect residents,* Report to Special Committee on Aging, US Senate, Washington, DC, 1999.
20. US General Accounting Office, *Nursing home care: the unfinished agenda, 1987 Omnibus Budget Reconciliation Act (OBRA '87),* Report to Special Committee on Aging, US Senate, Washington, DC, 1986.
21. Wunderlich, GS, Kohler P, editors: *Institute of Medicine, Improving quality of long-term care,* Washington, DC, 2000, National Academy of Sciences.

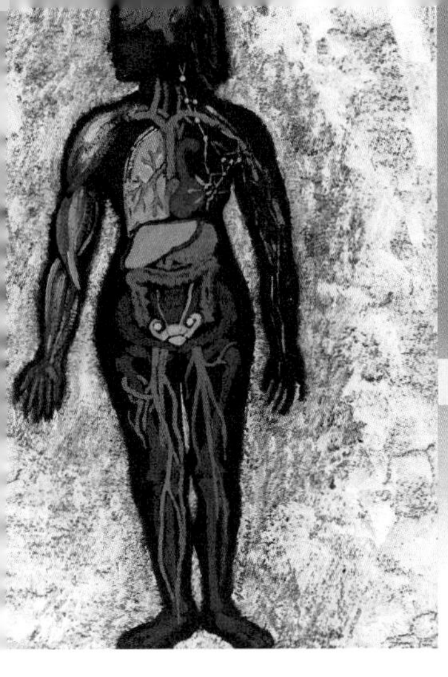

Inflammation and Infection

11

Bill Buron, Frances D. Monahan

Objectives

After studying this chapter, the learner should be able to:

1. Differentiate between inflammation and infection.
2. Describe the inflammatory process and the biologic basis of related signs and symptoms.
3. Explain the chain of infection.
4. Identify risk factors for infection.
5. Differentiate between passive and active immunization using examples of each.
6. Identify common child and adult immunizations by name and recommended use.
7. Describe measures to prevent and control nosocomial infections.
8. Cite the major components of the CDC guidelines for Standard and Transmission-Based Precautions used in hospitals.
9. Explain the nursing care required of patients experiencing inflammation and/or infection using the steps of the nursing process.

Inflammation and infection commonly occur simultaneously in the body; however, they are two separate processes. Inflammation is always present with infection, but infection is not always present with inflammation.

Inflammation is a complex reaction to injury or death of cells or tissues. Inflammation is a defense mechanism initiated to control and/or eliminate the offending agent and prepare an environment conducive to healing and repair. The inflammatory process is initiated by any type of injury: microbial, mechanical, or thermal. Hence it follows a bee sting, a burn, or a deep vein thrombosis. It may also occur after more serious events such as myocardial infarction. The inflammatory process takes place in the healthy tissue adjacent to dead or injured cells. The infectious process is one type of injury that initiates the inflammatory process. An example is cellulitis, which is an acute, diffuse, spreading, suppurative inflammation of the deep subcutaneous tissues usually caused by bacterial infection of a cutaneous wound or lesion.[1]

Infection follows the invasion of cells and/or tissues by living microorganisms such as bacteria, viruses, or fungi. Although nonliving objects may place an individual at risk for infection (as in the case of a splinter leading to infection in a finger), it is the actual invasion of the microorganisms that causes the infection.

The body has a complex array of defenses designed to prevent and combat infection-causing microorganisms and other injurious agents. These defenses are both nonspecific and specific.

Nonspecific defenses, which are the external and internal mechanisms that do not require exposure to a specific antigen for their development, constitute natural immunity. These defenses include the barrier protection of the skin and mucous membranes, the action of chemical substances such as lysozyme (an enzyme that can break down cell walls of bacteria), phagocytosis (ingestion of particles such as microorganisms or cell fragments by a phagocytic cell where they are ultimately killed and digested), and the action of protein substances such as interferon, which among other things enhances phagocytosis. The inflammatory response as a whole is a nonspecific internal defense that occurs if the nonspecific external responses are breached.

The body's specific defenses consist of specific immunity against particular microorganisms or molecular entities. This acquired immunity results from exposure to antigens or transfer of antibodies from one individual to another.

The anatomy and physiology involved in both natural and acquired immunity are discussed in detail in Chapter 48. The inflammatory response as a clinical phenomenon and clinical concepts of infection and infection control are discussed in the following paragraphs.

INFLAMMATORY RESPONSE

When injury occurs in the body, all the nonspecific and, to some degree, the specific defense mechanisms are directed toward localizing the effects of the injury, protecting against microbial invasion at the site, and preparing the site for repair. This process is called *inflammation.*

Any type of exogenous (outside the body) or endogenous (inside the body) injury can initiate the inflammatory response: heat, cold, irradiation, chemical (toxin or poison), trauma including surgery, infection, immunologic injury (hypersensitivity reaction), ischemic damage, or neoplasia. Whatever the stimulus, the response itself is the same, but the degree of response varies with the degree and severity of the injury.

Inflammations can be classified as acute or chronic. Acute inflammations are characterized by a sudden onset, a marked fluid exudative response, and a duration of 1 to 2 weeks. After the injurious agent is removed, the inflammation resolves, and healing with return of normal function ensues. Chronic inflammations have a slower, more insidious onset (over weeks, months, or years) and are characterized by increased cellular exudation. Scarring and loss of functional tissue may occur. Chronic inflammation can occur when acute inflammation is unsuccessful in resolving the injury or when persistent irritation exists. A granuloma is a lesion composed of modified macrophages surrounded by a rim of mononuclear leukocytes that may result from chronic inflammation. Granulomas can effectively wall off infectious organisms.

Knowledge of the physiologic changes that occur during the inflammatory process is essential to understanding the pathophysiology and clinical manifestations of a variety of diseases. For example, the death of heart muscle that occurs with myocardial infarction causes an inflammatory response. Fat deposits (atheromas) on blood vessel walls that injure the lining of the vessel wall also initiate an inflammatory response. Similarly, irritation of the peritoneum by trauma or bacterial invasion can cause inflammation of the peritoneum (peritonitis).

Steps in the Inflammatory Response

Three major physiologic events occur during the inflammatory process: the vascular response, fluid exudation, and cellular exudation (Table 11-1). The vascular response consists of a transitory vasoconstriction (stress response) followed immediately by vasodilation. This occurs as a result of vasoactive chemical substances such as histamine, serotonin, or kinins being released at the site of injury or invasion.[7] The amount of blood flow to the area is thus increased (hyperemia), causing redness and heat. Chemical mediators also cause increased permeability of the capillary walls. This, along with the increased hydrostatic pressure in the injured area secondary to the increased blood flow, results in the exudation of fluid out of the capillaries and into the interstitial spaces. This extra fluid in the interstitial spaces of the tissues acts to dilute toxins and microorganisms that are in the area and serves as the vehicle by which phagocytes and nutrients needed for healing reach the injured site.[31]

Fluid exudation from the capillaries into the interstitial spaces begins immediately and is most active during the first 24 hours after injury or invasion. Initially the fluid exudate is primarily serous fluid, but as the capillary wall becomes more permeable, protein (albumin) is lost into the interstitial spaces. This increases the colloid osmotic pressure in these spaces, which encourages more fluid exudation. The swelling of the tissue from the fluid in the interstitial spaces is called edema.

Cellular exudation refers to the migration of white blood cells (WBCs) (leukocytes) through the capillary walls into the affected tissue. An increased number of WBCs are attracted to the vessels in the affected area as a result of chemotactic substances being released from the tissues by cell injury and complement activation. The WBCs adhere to the capillary wall and then pass through the widened endothelial junctions of the capillary wall. Neutrophils (polymorphonuclear leukocytes, PMNs), which make up about 60% of the circulating WBCs, are the first leukocytes to respond, usually within the first few hours. The neutrophils ingest the bacteria and dead tissue cells (Figure 48-3); and then die, releasing proteolytic enzymes that liquefy the dead neutrophils, dead bacteria, and other dead cells (pus). Monocytes, which continue the phago-

TABLE 11-1 Summary of the Steps in the Inflammatory Response

Steps	Mediators	Outcome
1. Injury	Physical, chemical, biologic, immunologic stimulus	Cell and tissue injury
2. Vascular response		
a. Vascular dilation	Histamine, plasmin, serotonin, kinins, prostaglandins released or activated by injury	Dilation of vessels, causing stasis of blood and margination of leukocytes
b. Fibrin clot formation	Activation of clotting mechanism	Containment of irritants
3. Fluid exudation	Histamine, kinins, prostaglandins cause opening of venule-endothelial cell junction	Fluid exudation into tissues
4. Cellular exudation		
a. Leukocyte exudation	Chemotactic substances released by complement activation, clot formation, injured cells	Passage of leukocytes from blood to site of injury and accumulation there
b. Attack and engulfment of foreign materials	Neutrophils, macrophages	Removal and digestion of bacteria, foreign particles, damaged tissues
5. Healing	Fibroblasts produce collagen fibers, tissue regeneration	Resolution of inflammation, formation of scar tissue

cytosis, and lymphocytes, which play a role in the antigen-antibody response at the site, appear later (see Chapter 48).

The inflammatory response prepares the tissue for healing and contains the spread of bacterial invasion. To prevent the spread of bacteria, fibroblasts are attracted to the area and secrete fibrin, a threadlike substance that encircles the affected area to wall it off from healthy tissue. If interference occurs with this walling-off process, bacteria can spread into the surrounding tissue. Thus abscesses should not be incised and drained until they have "come to a head," which indicates the walling-off process is completed.

Local Manifestations of Inflammation

The five cardinal symptoms of inflammation were identified many centuries ago: (1) redness (rubor) and (2) heat (calor) caused by the hyperemia, (3) swelling (tumor) caused by the fluid exudate, (4) pain (dolor) caused by the pressure of the fluid exudate and by chemical (bradykinin and prostaglandins) irritation of the nerve endings, and (5) loss of function of the affected part caused by the swelling and pain. The amount of pain and related loss of function depend on the location and extent of injury.

Regional Lymph Node Manifestations

If bacteria cannot be contained locally, they may spread to other parts of the body by means of the lymph system or bloodstream. If picked up by the lymph stream, the bacteria are carried to the nearest lymph node where they can be ingested and destroyed. If the bacteria are virulent enough to resist the action of the lymph nodes, leukocytes are brought in by the bloodstream to attack and engulf the bacteria in the node. The node then becomes swollen and tender because of the accumulation of phagocytes, bacteria, and destroyed lymphoid tissue. This process is known as lymphadenitis. Swollen lymph nodes can be palpated primarily in the neck, axilla, and groin.

Systemic Manifestations

Moderate-to-severe inflammatory responses can produce systemic manifestations. The three major systemic manifestations are (1) increase in body temperature (fever), (2) increase in WBCs in peripheral circulation (leukocytosis), and (3) increased erythrocyte sedimentation rate (ESR).

Generalized fever is produced by the release of substances known as endogenous pyrogens at the inflammatory site.[12] These pyrogens consist of substances from injured cells, materials released by WBCs that accumulate at the site, and components of the cell wall of invading bacteria. The pyrogens include prostaglandins, leukotrienes, bacterial endotoxins, and interleukin-1. These substances are carried to the temperature-regulating center in the hypothalamic region of the brain, where they signal a resetting of the body temperature set-point. The body responds by increasing heat production and decreasing heat loss. As long as the pyrogens remain in circulation, the set-point stays elevated. The fever response is part of the defense mechanism and helps increase production of antimicrobial agents such as interferon. It also tends to support increased phagocytic activity of some cells, including macrophages.

Leukocytosis develops when leukopoietins, agents released from damaged cells and from WBCs accumulating at the inflammatory site, are carried by the circulation to the bone marrow, where WBCs are produced. When leukopoietins reach the bone marrow, they signal the release of mature neutrophils held in reserve there. This leads to an immediate increase in the WBC count in the peripheral circulation to more than 10,000 mm^3. Chemotactic agents then draw these cells to the inflammatory site. Leukopoietins also increase the production of WBCs in the bone marrow. With prolonged inflammation the bone marrow stores of WBCs are depleted, and the synthesis of mature WBCs may not be able to keep pace with the needs of the inflammatory site; thus the marrow releases more immature neutrophils as the inflammation continues. These less mature cells, known as bands, become more prevalent in the peripheral circulation and indicate a significant ongoing inflammation. The condition sometimes is referred to as a "shift to the left." This clinical phrase was derived from the past clinical laboratory method of counting the less mature cells and tabulating them in the left-hand columns of differential count forms.

With inflammation an increased ESR also occurs; that is, when an anticoagulant is added to the blood in the laboratory, the red blood cells (RBCs) (erythrocytes) settle to the bottom of a test tube more rapidly than normal. This increase in the ESR is believed to be caused by an increase in fibrinogen, a blood protein essential to the healing process. The ESR is elevated during the acute inflammatory stage of infection, which indicates that the body's defense mechanisms for the repair of damaged tissue are operating.

Repair and Healing

Inflammation prepares the injured area for healing and hence is sometimes referred to as the first stage of the healing process. For healing to proceed, inflammation must have subsided and pus and dead tissue must have been removed. Pus is a local accumulation of dead phagocytes, dead bacteria, and dead tissue. The bacteria most frequently causing this reaction are staphylococci, streptococci, *Neisseria* organisms, and *Pseudomonas aeruginosa (Pseudomonas pyocyanea)*. A collection of pus that is localized by a zone of inflamed tissue is called an abscess (Figure 11-1). When pus collects in a preexisting cavity such as the pleura or gallbladder it is called empyema. If an abscess within the body develops a suppurating channel and ruptures onto the surface or into a body cavity, it is called a sinus. If a tubelike passage forms from an epithelium-lined organ or normal body cavity to the surface or to another organ or cavity, it is called a fistula.

Once the inflamed area is clean or debrided, the phase of healing called *reconstruction* begins. New cells are produced to fill in the space left by the injury. These cells may be normal, functional (parenchymal) cells regenerated by the affected tissue, or they may be fibrotic cells known as scar tissue, which serve only to fill in the injured area. When *regeneration* occurs and the structure and function of damaged tissue are restored, *resolution* is said to have occurred. Some body tissues readily regenerate; others do not. Tissues such as the bone marrow, the epithelial layer of the skin, and the mucous membrane of the respiratory, gastrointestinal (GI), and genitourinary tracts

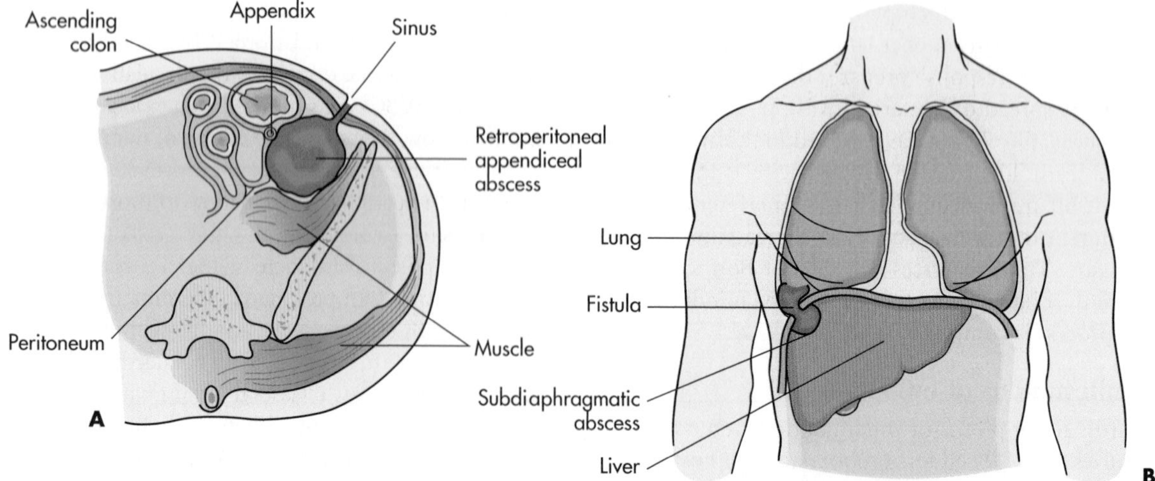

Figure 11-1 **A,** Cross section of torso showing appendiceal abscess with sinus that has developed through abdominal wall. **B,** Subdiaphragmatic abscess that has developed fistula opening into pleural cavity.

consist of labile cells that continually regenerate over the life span. Hence regeneration in response to injury is rapid and effective. Tissues such as bone, liver, pancreas, and kidney have parenchyma composed of stable cells that normally stop regenerating when full growth is attained but are capable of regeneration when injury occurs. Regeneration of these tissues occurs over a longer period than tissues composed of labile cells. Nerve cells, skeletal muscle cells, and cardiac muscle cells are permanent or fixed cells and are unable to regenerate. These are always replaced with fibrous tissue. If a large amount of tissue is destroyed, replacement with parenchymal cells may not be possible, regardless of the type of tissue, and abnormalities of healing such as keloids or adhesions may form. See Chapters 18 and 61 for further discussion.

Instead of healing, necrosis (death of the tissue) may occur. Bacteria, both pathogens and nonpathogens, often invade the necrotic tissue and cause decomposition, which is called gangrene. The body defenses are useless in preventing or curing gangrene because little or no blood can reach the area. Gangrenous tissue must be completely removed before healing can occur.

INFECTIOUS DISEASE PROCESS

Infection is the presence in the body of a pathogen that multiplies and produces effects that are injurious to the host. Pathogens include bacteria, viruses, mycoplasma, chlamydia, fungi, and parasites (worms, protozoa, and arthropods such as the scabies mite). Injury may result from the presence and spread of the pathogen through the body tissues or from the effects on the body of toxins produced by the pathogen. Exotoxins are soluble protein substances secreted by the pathogen that destroy cells in the surrounding tissue. Endotoxins are substances present in the cell walls of gram-negative bacteria. They are released when the cell wall is disrupted and cause nonspecific effects such as fever and inflammation. In large amounts they can also cause abnormal bleeding or clotting and hypotension.

Pathogens differ in both invasiveness and toxigenicity. Some organisms, such as pneumococci, are highly invasive and virtually nontoxigenic. Others, such as *Clostridium tetani,* have high toxicity but low invasiveness. An infection is symptomatic if it causes clinical signs and symptoms and asymptomatic if no perceivable clinical or subclinical signs or symptoms are present.

Pathogenic organisms that are present in the body but do not produce injury or incite an injurious body response are said to be colonizing the body. Colonization with microorganisms often occurs in patients who have an endotracheal or tracheostomy tube in place. Colonization of nasal passages or skin surfaces with *Staphylococcus aureus* is also common. It is often unclear whether a person has an infection or colonization, but either one can be a source of infection to self and others.

Chain of Infection

A common sequence of events known as the chain of infection underlies development of all infectious diseases. The links in this chain are a *causative agent, reservoir, portal of exit* from the reservoir, *mode of transmission, portal of entry* to a susceptible host, and a *susceptible host* (Figure 11-2).

First, a causative agent, or pathogen, must exist. This can be a bacterium, virus, fungus, rickettsial organism, protozoa, or helminth (worm). Second, there must be a reservoir where the agent can be found, that is, a place where it lives and multiplies. The reservoir can be animate (human or animal) or inanimate (e.g., soil, water, intravenous solutions, equipment). Human reservoirs can be asymptomatic carriers, colonized individuals, or persons with an acute clinical infection. Carriers can (1) be incubating the agent before the onset of signs and symptoms, (2) have a subclinical infection, (3) be in the convalescent stage of an infection, or (4) be chronic carriers of the agent. Viral hepatitis B is an example of an infectious disease that can be transmitted by human carriers in all these stages. If the organisms normally live on the skin or mu-

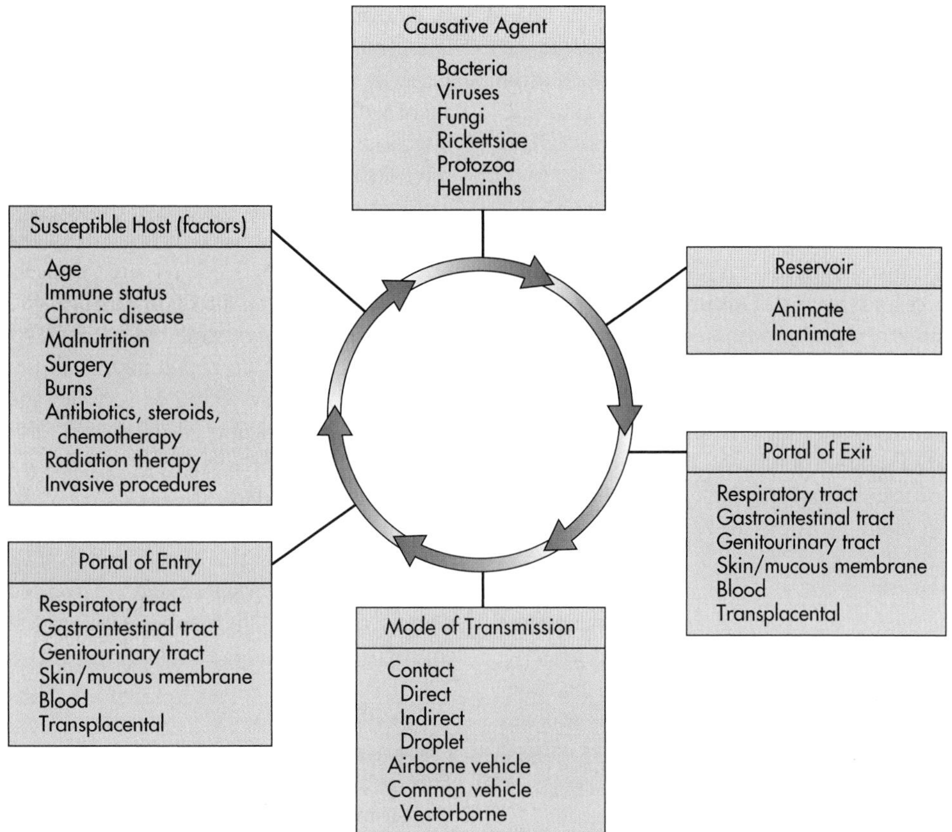

Figure 11-2 The infectious disease process.

TABLE 11-2 Distribution of Normal Microbial Flora

Region of Body	Sterile Areas	Nonsterile Areas	Microorganisms
Skin	None	All skin	*Staphylococcus, Bacillus, Corynebacterium, Mycobacterium, Streptococcus,* transient environmental organisms
Respiratory tract	Larynx, trachea, bronchi, bronchioles, alveoli, sinuses	Nose, throat, mouth	*Staphylococcus, Candida, Streptococcus, Neisseria, Pneumococcus,* oral organisms
Gastrointestinal tract	Esophagus, stomach, upper small intestine	Esophagus and stomach (transiently), large intestine	Gram-negative rods, *Streptococcus, Bacteroides, Proteus, Clostridium, Lactobacillus*
Genitourinary tract	Cervix, uterus, fallopian tubes, ovaries, prostate gland, epididymides, testes, bladder, kidneys	External genitalia, anterior urethra, vagina	Skin organisms, *Lactobacillus, Bacteroides*
Body fluids and cavities	Blood, pleural fluid, synovial fluid, spinal fluid, lymph, etc.	None	

cous membranes of the host, the reservoir is said to be endogenous (Table 11-2). All other reservoirs are exogenous sources of infection. Often the reservoir of an agent responsible for an outbreak of an infection is not readily apparent and may never be identified. If the process of infection is well understood, however, appropriate and effective control measures can be instituted, even though the original reservoir of the causative agent is not known.

The agent must have a portal of exit from the reservoir. If the reservoir is human, the portal of exit can be (1) the respiratory tract, (2) the GI tract, (3) the genitourinary tract, (4) open lesions on the skin, or (5) across the placenta.

Once the agent has left the reservoir, it needs a mode of transmission to a host. Transmission can be by contact, air, common vehicle, or vector. *Contact transmission* includes direct, indirect, or droplet contact.

Direct Contact Transmission

This type of transmission occurs when there is spread of infection from the source to the host without the presence of an intermediate object. This happens when there is physical contact with or skin shedding onto the host. Gonorrhea is an example of a disease transmitted by direct contact.

Indirect Contact Transmission

With this type of transmission there is an intermediate object between the source and the host. This intermediary can be the contaminated hands of a person who has had contact with an infected source and then touches a susceptible host without washing the hands. An inanimate object that has been contaminated by an infectious source is known as a fomite. Bed linen, respiratory therapy equipment, tissues, and silverware are examples of fomites that can be responsible for the indirect transmission of an infectious agent.

Droplet Transmission

This type of transmission occurs when the infectious agent is expelled from the reservoir in the form of droplets, as happens with a sneeze or cough. These droplets do not become airborne but settle on surfaces 3 to 4 feet from their source. Meningococcal meningitis and influenza are examples of diseases transmitted in this manner.

Airborne Transmission

Airborne transmission occurs when the infectious agent expelled from the source remains suspended in the form of droplet nuclei or dust in the air. A host then inhales the agent. These droplet nuclei measure 1 to 5 mm and are smaller than the droplets in droplet transmission, and thus air currents can carry them. Chickenpox (varicella zoster) and tuberculosis are diseases that can be spread by this route.

Common Vehicle Transmission

Common vehicle transmission occurs when a contaminated inanimate vehicle acts as the intermediary for the infectious agent from the source to multiple hosts. Contaminated water, food, and intravenous fluids are common vehicles. Salmonellosis and hepatitis A are examples of diseases that can be transmitted in this way.

Vector-Borne Transmission

Vector-borne transmission occurs when there is an animate intermediary from the source to the recipient. For example, mosquitoes are the intermediaries in the transmission of malaria, and ticks serve as the intermediary in the spread of Rocky Mountain spotted fever and Lyme disease.

Once the infectious agent has been transmitted to a host, it must gain entry into the host. The portals of entry are similar to the portals of exit from the human reservoir and include the respiratory tract, the GI tract, the genitourinary tract, breaks in the skin or mucous membranes, and across the placenta. These portals of entry are usually the first areas colonized by infecting microorganisms.

The final step in the process after the inoculation of the host is the maturation and multiplication of the infectious agent. Entry of an infectious agent into a host does not mean that the agent will proliferate and cause infection. Whether or not an infection occurs depends on the dose of the infecting agent received, the organism's virulence, and the host's susceptibility. The healthy human body is extremely resistant to infection; however, when the basic biologic defense mechanisms of the body are compromised, an organism has a much greater chance of causing an infection. Chapter 48 deals with many biologic defense factors exhibited by the host to prevent infection and injury. Some factors that increase host susceptibility to infection are (1) very young or very old age; (2) impaired immune status as occurs with certain disease states such as human immunodeficiency virus (HIV) infection, diabetes, cancer, and other chronic disease; (3) therapeutic treatments such as radiation and certain drugs, especially antibiotics, steroids, and chemotherapeutic agents; (4) surgery; (5) burns; (6) poor nutritional status; and (7) invasive procedures (intravenous catheters, chest tubes, urinary catheters) that break through the normal external defense barriers.

Pathophysiology

Once a pathogen gains access to a susceptible host, a time known as the incubation period passes before the clinical symptoms of infection appear. During this period the organism is establishing itself, spreading to target organs or tissues, and proliferating within various areas of the body. The incubation period varies, depending on the organism and the condition of the host. The incubation period can last from a few hours to years but is often predictable and diagnostically significant. The prodromal period follows the incubation period. This second period is characterized by the onset of symptoms, which are usually nonspecific. Common prodromal symptoms are malaise, anorexia, headache, muscle aches, and joint pain. As the pathogen begins to rapidly multiply and spread, the acute period ensues. The acute period is characterized by local manifestations of infection, which are due to the inflammatory response. Hence these are the classic signs and symptoms of inflammation: redness, heat, swelling, pain, and limitation of use.

Systemic manifestations of the acute period include fever and chills, along with tachycardia and tachypnea resulting from increased metabolic demand. Other specific symptoms depend on the type of injury elicited by the virulent pathogen and its site within the body. The final phase of the infectious process is the convalescent period. During this stage healing occurs and symptoms disappear.

Infection may be localized (having a focal point of symptoms or injury) or generalized (having systemic involvement), and its course may be acute or chronic. An acute infection often incites an immediate violent host response. The outcome of the infection (pathogen over host or host over pathogen) is determined within a relatively short time, as seen in mumps, plague, or smallpox. In a chronic infection the pathogen establishes itself more insidiously within the host, does not cause immediate damage, and tends to provoke less of a host response, as in tuberculosis and aspergillosis. Many acute infections become chronic and vice versa.

COLLABORATIVE CARE MANAGEMENT

Infection Control

Historical Perspective

Infection control has become a recognized discipline only in the past 25 years, although the principles governing it have been in existence for some time. In the middle of the nineteenth century Semmelweiss, an obstetrician in Vienna, demonstrated the significance of hand washing in combating the transmission of infection. He observed that the incidence of puerperal fever, a major cause of postpartum mortality, was much higher on the ward where the medical students trained than on the ward attended by the midwives. Although the role of microorganisms in causing infection was not yet realized, Semmelweiss believed that somehow the medical students could be transmitting disease from the autopsy suite to maternity patients. He showed that when the students and physicians were required to wash their hands and rinse them in a chlorinated lime solution before a delivery, the incidence of puerperal fever decreased greatly. The idea that hand washing alone could prevent the spread of disease met with much opposition by his colleagues. Better acceptance came after Pasteur, Lister, and Koch developed the germ theory of disease and related asepsis to the prevention of the spread of disease. At about the same time, Nightingale made significant contributions to sanitation and isolation practices. From this evolved an era in which medical asepsis was practiced more by ritual than with true understanding of the specific principles on which it was based.

During World War II, with the successful use of sulfonamides and penicillin to treat infection and the development of new antibiotics, a false sense of security developed about infection control. It soon became apparent, however, that antibiotics were not the sole answer to infection control. Organisms once well controlled by antibiotics demonstrated the ability to develop resistant strains. In the late 1950s and the 1960s, outbreaks of penicillin-resistant *S. aureus* infections were common, and gram-negative organisms such as *Pseudomonas,* which were previously considered nonpathogenic, were suddenly implicated as the cause of infections acquired in the hospital. Along with drug resistance and the emergence of newly recognized pathogens, the number of persons at risk for secondary infections increased owing to longer life expectancy, the use of immunosuppressive agents, and an increase in the use of invasive procedures to diagnose and treat disease.

The rise in hospital infections made it necessary to examine preventive and control measures and to reemphasize the use of aseptic techniques. In 1970 an international conference to address the problem of hospital-acquired (nosocomial) infections was held in Atlanta. As a result, the Centers for Disease Control and Prevention (CDC) in Atlanta set forth guidelines for prevention and control of infections in hospitals. The CDC is constantly updating and revising its recommendations based on epidemiologic studies and research findings. The American Hospital Association (AHA) and the Joint Commission on Accreditation of Healthcare Organizations (JCAHO), a major private accrediting agency, looked at the ethical and economic issues relating to nosocomial infections and established standards for programs in infection control. The purpose of these programs is to decrease morbidity and mortality from infections, as well as to reduce the cost of infections that could have been prevented. Consumer awareness of the problem also contributed to the attention given the issue of infection control. In the early 1970s only 10% of hospitals in the United States had infection surveillance and control programs; by the end of the decade nearly all had them. The field of infection control is constantly evolving, with the identification of new pathogens and advances in research uncovering new information that impacts current thinking and practices.

In the late 1980s and early 1990s, antimicrobial-resistant organisms became more prevalent in both the developing world and in hospitals in the United States.[8,30] Examples of such organisms include vancomycin-resistant enterococci and multidrug-resistant tuberculosis. Indiscriminate use of antibiotics and noncompliance with prescribed therapy are largely responsible for this situation.[29]

Today all health care facilities should have infection control practitioners (ICPs) and policies that address the issues of employee health and safety and patient care practices. Incorporated in these policies are Occupational Safety and Health Administration (OSHA) guidelines to protect health caregivers from exposure to bloodborne pathogens such as hepatitis B, hepatitis C, and HIV.[2] Discovery of HIV as the pathogen responsible for the current epidemic of acquired immunodeficiency syndrome (AIDS) has provided the incentive to develop safer practices to protect health caregivers from all bloodborne pathogens. Determining the modes of transmission of HIV has helped the CDC and ICPs to develop new systems (Standard Precautions) for personnel to use when caring for all patients. ICPs are a valuable resource, as they interact with hospital departments, surveying for infections and teaching prevention and control. When a question or problem about infection control arises, the ICP should be contacted without hesitation. Questions may arise that deal with clinical procedures, products for cleaning and disinfection, waste disposal, isolation systems, or personnel health issues.

Hospital personnel are most at risk for infection with HIV from needlestick injuries (see Evidenced-Based Practice box).[16] Programs to prevent needlestick injuries and to present factual information are essential. The most recent revision to OSHA's bloodborne pathogens standard deals with needlestick safety. The Needlestick Safety and Prevention Act, enacted in 2001, requires employers to adopt safer needle devices and maintain a log of contaminated needlestick injuries.[19]

Evidence-Based Practice

Reference: Jagger J, Perry J: Exposure safety: safeguarding sharps disposal, *Nurs 2000* 30:10, 2000.

This study examined contributing factors related to 3666 percutaneous sharps injuries to health care workers employed by nine hospitals. The researchers divided the timing of the injuries into two different categories. The authors defined "disposal failures" as those injuries that occurred after needle use, but before needle disposal. Examples included injuries from sharps left on bedside tables or floors. The second injury category consisted of injuries that occurred during the process of disposal or were caused by a previously disposed-of device. Included in this category were injuries that occurred as health care workers were stuck by a sharp as they tried to place it in the disposal container. Many of these injuries were related to overflowing disposal containers, or from sharps placed in inappropriate containers (such as the trash can). In all 68% of the injuries occurred before the sharp device reached the disposal container; 32% of the injuries occurred at the time of the disposal or were caused by a previously disposed-of device. The study did not include injuries that occurred from recapping or disassembly of a sharps device.

After examining the events associated with percutaneous injuries, the authors listed important points to consider when handling sharps. They recommended that health care workers consistently replace disposal containers before they are full. Health care workers should be educated that discarding sharps in standard trash containers or leaving them on beds or floors can seriously harm others. Whenever possible, health care workers should use devices with safety features that shield or blunt needles or blades during and after use. Finally, disposal containers should be within easy reach before using a sharp. The authors concluded that following these simple rules will significantly reduce percutaneous sharps injuries.

INFECTION CONTROL IN THE COMMUNITY

A *communicable disease* is any disease that is highly transmissible to other persons. Efforts to recognize and control communicable diseases are the responsibility of national, state, and local agencies. On the national level, the CDC is responsible for programs aimed at the prevention and control of communicable and other preventable disease in the United States. The CDC provides epidemiologic and laboratory services to state health facilities on request. It enforces quarantine regulations and conducts foreign quarantine activities; administers international programs for the control of malaria, smallpox, and measles; and provides consultation to other nations on the control of preventable diseases. It also collects, tabulates, and assesses data on reportable diseases from state health departments and publishes the findings in the *Morbidity and Mortality Weekly Report (MMWR)*. Through its continuous surveillance, the CDC is able to detect new cases of disease and intervene to control disease outbreaks. In addition, the CDC is instrumental in providing guidelines and recommendations for infection control.

Control of infectious diseases in the United States is the responsibility of each state. State health officers usually delegate this responsibility to a division of communicable diseases in which a staff of physicians, nurses, veterinarians, and sanitary engineers works closely with a state epidemiologist in the detection, assessment, and control of specific reportable diseases.

Local public health departments work in conjunction with state health departments in this effort. Physicians and health care facilities have a responsibility to report communicable diseases promptly to the health department. Health agencies in the community then use the reported data to determine potential or real problems, identify the causative agent and if possible its source, and identify the population at risk. A plan to control the problem, care for those exposed, and protect the population at risk is then devised and implemented.

Prevention and Control Measures

Prevention and control measures are many and varied in that they address each of the different links in the chain of infection. Environmental measures are used to eliminate or reduce the number of infectious agents directly or by elimination or reduction of reservoirs, vectors, fomites, and common vehicle transmitters. Thus the prevention and control of disease in the community involves control measures such as proper sanitation to ensure a pure water supply and proper disposal of sewage and other potentially infectious materials. These measures have been legislated into building codes, state laws, and federal regulations. Regulations also address health practices in institutions that handle, package, and prepare foods. Another example of an environmental control measure is spraying a designated area to kill mosquitoes, which are implicated in the spread of viral encephalitis. Spraying usually is done only after an outbreak has been identified.

Other prevention and control measures are designed to prevent infection by focusing on increasing the resistance of potential hosts and controlling transmission via the portals of exit and entrance. Depending on the communicable disease, care of exposed persons and protection of the population at risk for contracting the disease may entail prophylaxis, immunization, or only careful monitoring of new cases. Often, simple adherence to basic principles of hygiene is sufficient. The local or state health department determines the need for additional measures. Attempts are made to reach those at risk and to inform them of the preventive measures. Education of the public is a key component of these efforts.

Immunization Programs

The goal of immunization programs is to prevent infectious disease by inducing a specific immune response resulting in acquired immunity for immunized individuals. Acquired immunity is specific immunity. It protects against a single, unique agent through development of specific antibodies or responsive cells in the body. It is acquired from contact with the agent (antigen) or through the introduction of specifically protective antibodies or cells into the body. Refer to Chapter 48 for a detailed discussion of the immune response and acquired immunity.

Acquired immunity may result from a natural or artificial encounter. Immunity acquired naturally results from natural conditions such as recovery from a disease. In artificially acquired immunity the antigen or protective antibodies were

TABLE 11-3 Types of Acquired Specific Immunity

Type of Immunity	Acquisition of Immunity	Protection	Examples
Active			
Antibodies synthesized by body in response to antigenic stimulation	*Natural:* natural contact with antigen through clinical or subclinical case	*Development:* develops slowly; protective levels reached in a few weeks *Duration:* long-term; often lifetime *Spectrum:* specific to antigen contacted	Recovery from childhood diseases (e.g., chickenpox, measles, mumps)
	Artificial: immunization with antigen	*Development:* develops slowly; protective levels reached in a few weeks *Duration:* several years; extended protection with "booster" doses *Spectrum:* specific to antigen immunized against	Immunization with live or killed vaccines; toxoid immunization
Passive			
Antibodies produced in one individual transferred to another	*Natural:* transplacental and colostrum transfer from mother to child	*Development:* immediate *Duration:* temporary; several months *Spectrum:* all antigens that mother has immunity to	Maternal immunoglobulins in neonate
	Artificial: injection of serum from immune human or animal	*Development:* immediate *Duration:* temporary; several weeks *Spectrum:* all antigens that source has immunity to	Injection of pooled human gamma-globulin; injection of animal hyperimmune sera

purposely introduced into the body by vaccination. The immunity also may be active or passive. When an individual produces the antibodies within the body, the immunity is termed *active.* When an individual receives the protective antibodies from some other source, the immunity is termed *passive.* Thus, when antibodies are transferred from the mother across the placenta, the child is said to have a natural passive immunity. When a vaccine is given so that antibodies are produced within the body, the immunized person is characterized as having an artificial active immunity. Table 11-3 summarizes the different types of acquired specific immunities.

Immunity to harmful agents is a relative state. The effects of different dosages of an infectious organism or the toxic products of such organisms in experimental studies clearly show that administration of sufficiently large numbers of an organism or high dosages of a toxin can overwhelm even the most highly immunized animal. Further, when the normal mechanisms of defense are breached, even in the highly resistant host, disease can result. Thus acquired immunity to infection is not always an absolute condition but depends on many complex variables. These include not only the defense mechanisms of the host but also the dosage, route of contact, and virulence of the harmful agent.

If 90% of the population is protected against organisms that require continued passage through humans to reproduce and live, the disease caused by the organism can be virtually eliminated because there are too few susceptible hosts to allow the organism to spread. This type of group protection is called herd immunity. It is ineffectual, however, against organisms such as tetanus bacilli that can exist indefinitely in the soil. Thus for protection against this type of organism, each person must be immunized. If like diphtheria in the United States, the disease is not prevalent in the environment, or, like tetanus, is not spread from person to person by direct contact, the inoculation must be repeated at regular intervals to maintain protection. This inoculation is called a *booster dose,* and usually consists of one-tenth the original inoculating dose.

An inoculation often causes a local tissue response. Symptoms of inflammation and sometimes ulcerations appear at the site of the injection, and symptoms of widespread tissue involvement such as slight febrile reactions, general malaise, and muscle aching are common for 1 or 2 days. Delayed symptoms follow the initial inoculation because the immune response system must become sensitized to the antigen. The systemic reaction to subsequent inoculations usually occurs sooner and is less severe because the immune response is stimulated at once. The local reaction also is less severe than that after the initial inoculation because the organisms have less opportunity to produce inflammation.

Primary Immunization Schedules

Recommendations concerning current immunization schedules are found in *Morbidity and Mortality Weekly Reports,* which presents recommendations of the U.S. Public Health Service's Advisory Committee on Immunization Practices (ACIP). The reader should refer to this resource when questions arise about proper immunization practices, prophylaxis, interruption in immunization schedules, or adverse reactions and side effects. Individuals may refer to the National Immunization Program Home Page at http://www.cdc.gov/nip/ for up-to-date immunization recommendations (Table 11-4).[14]

The immunization schedule for diphtheria, pertussis, tetanus (DPT) begins with one dose of combined toxoid and vaccine when an infant is 2 months old. The next two doses

TABLE 11-4 Recommended Childhood Immunization Schedule United States, January-December 2001

Vaccines[1] are listed under routinely recommended ages. Bars indicate range of recommended ages for immunization. Any dose not given at the recommended age should be given as a "catch-up" immunization at any subsequent visit when indicated and feasible. Ovals indicate vaccines to be given if previously recommended doses were missed or given earlier than the recommended minimum age.

Age / Vaccine	Birth	1 mo	2 mos	4 mos	6 mos	12 mos	15 mos	18 mos	24 mos	4-6 yrs	11-12 yrs	14-18 yrs
Hepatitis B[2]		Hep B #1										
			Hep B #2				Hep B #3				Hep B[2]	
Diphtheria, tetanus, pertussis[3]			DTaP	DTaP	DTaP		DTaP[3]			DTaP	Td	
H. influenzae type b[4]			Hib	Hib	Hib	Hib						
Inactivated polio[5]			IPV	IPV		IPV[5]				IPV[5]		
Pneumococcal conjugate[6]			PCV	PCV	PCV	PCV						
Measles, mumps, rubella[7]						MMR				MMR[7]	MMR[7]	
Varicella[8]							Var				Var[8]	
Hepatitis A[9]										Hep A—in selected areas[9]		

Approved by the Advisory Committee on Immunization Practices (ACIP), the American Academy of Pediatrics (AAP), and the American Academy of Family Physicians (AAFP).

1. This schedule indicates the recommended ages for routine administration of currently licensed childhood vaccines, as of 11/1/00, for children through 18 years of age. Additional vaccines may be licensed and recommended during the year. Licensed combination vaccines may be used whenever any components of the combination are indicated and its other components are not contraindicated. Providers should consult the manufacturers' package inserts for detailed recommendations.
2. **Infants born to HBsAg-negative mothers** should receive the first dose of hepatitis B (Hep B) vaccine by age 2 months. The second dose should be at least one month after the first dose. The third dose should be administered at least 4 months after the first dose and at least 2 months after the second dose, but not before 6 months of age for infants.
   Infants born to HBsAg-positive mothers should receive hepatitis B vaccine and 0.5 ml hepatitis B immune globulin (HBIG) within 12 hours of birth at separate sites. The second dose is recommended at 1-2 months of age and the third dose at 6 months of age.
   Infants born to mothers whose HBsAg status is unknown should receive hepatitis B vaccine within 12 hours of birth. Maternal blood should be drawn at the time of delivery to determine the mother's HBsAg status; if the HBsAg test is positive, the infant should receive HBIG as soon as possible (no later than 1 week of age).
   All children and adolescents who have not been immunized against hepatitis B should begin the series during any visit. Special efforts should be made to immunize children who were born in or whose parents were born in areas of the world with moderate or high endemicity of hepatitis B virus infection.
3. The fourth dose of DTaP (diphtheria and tetanus toxoids and acellular pertussis vaccine) may be administered as early as 12 months of age, provided 6 months have elapsed since the third dose and the child is unlikely to return at age 15-18 months. Td (tetanus and diphtheria toxoids) is recommended at 11-12 years of age if at least 5 years have elapsed since the last dose of DTP, DTaP, or DT. Subsequent routine Td boosters are recommended every 10 years.
4. Three *Haemophilus influenzae* type b (Hib) conjugate vaccines are licensed for infant use. If PRP-OMP (PedvaxHIB® or ComVax® [Merck]) is administered at 2 and 4 months of age, a dose at 6 months is not required. Because clinical studies in infants have demonstrated that using some combination products may induce a lower immune response to the Hib vaccine component, DTaP/Hib combination products should not be used for primary immunization in infants at 2, 4, or 6 months of age, unless FDA-approved for these ages.
5. An all-IPV schedule is recommended for routine childhood polio vaccination in the United States. All children should receive four doses of IPV at 2 months, 4 months, 6-18 months, and 4-6 years of age. Oral polio vaccine (OPV) should be used only in selected circumstances. (See *MMWR* May 19, 2000/49(RR-5); 1-22).
6. The heptavalent conjugate pneumococcal vaccine (PCV) is recommended for all children 2-23 months of age. It also is recommended for certain children 24-59 months of age. (See *MMWR* Oct. 6, 2000/49(RR-9); 1-35).
7. The second dose of measles, mumps, and rubella (MMR) vaccine is recommended routinely at 4-6 years of age but may be administered during any visit, provided at least 4 weeks have elapsed since receipt of the first dose and that both doses are administered beginning at or after 12 months of age. Those who have not previously received the second dose should complete the schedule by the 11- 12-year-old visit.
8. Varicella (Var) vaccine is recommended at any visit on or after the first birthday for susceptible children (i.e., those who lack a reliable history of chickenpox as judged by a health care provider and who have not been immunized. Susceptible persons 13 years of age or older should receive 2 doses, given at least 4 weeks apart.
9. Hepatitis A (Hep A) is shaded to indicate its recommended use in selected states and/or regions, and for certain high risk groups; consult your local public health authority. (See *MMWR* Oct. 1, 1999/48(RR-12); 1-37).

For additional information about the vaccines listed above, please visit the National Immunization Program Home Page at http://www.cdc.gov/nip/ or call the National Immunization Hotline at 800-232-2522 (English) or 800-232-0233 (Spanish).

are given at 2-month intervals. The fourth dose is given between 15 and 18 months. This schedule maintains adequate antibody levels until the child enters kindergarten, when the final immunization is given. Booster doses of tetanus and diphtheria are started between the ages of 11 and 12 years and are recommended every 10 years thereafter.

In 1997 the American Academy of Pediatrics (AAP) recommended more frequent use of inactivated poliovirus vaccination (IPV), instead of oral poliovirus vaccine (OPV) for routine immunization against poliovirus. Since then, the occurrence of vaccine-associated paralytic poliomyelitis (VAPP) has decreased.[9] Because of this correlation and the serious risks associated with poliovirus, beginning in early 2000, the AAP recommended that IPV be administered for the entire series of routine childhood vaccination. The vaccine should be administered at 2 months, 4 months, 6 to 18 months, and 4 to 6 years. Oral poliovirus vaccine (OPV) should be used only in selected circumstances.[9]

A single dose of measles, mumps, rubella (MMR) virus vaccine, live, is given when the child is 12 to 15 months old. A second dose of MMR is given at age 4 to 6 years or 11 to 12 years. Children who have not been vaccinated as infants can be vaccinated at any age.

Mumps vaccine, live attenuated, should not be administered before 12 months of age because of the persistence of maternal antibodies, which may interfere with seroconversion.

Most cases of measles are now seen in young adults, whereas before the vaccine became available in 1969, most cases occurred in school-age children. Women in childbearing years should be tested for rubella antibodies if they cannot document immunization, because rubella infection in the first trimester of pregnancy is associated with neonatal morbidity and mortality (congenital rubella syndrome). If antibodies are not present, vaccination is recommended. Because of the theoretic risk to the fetus, women of childbearing age are vaccinated only if they are not pregnant, and they are counseled not to become pregnant for 3 months after vaccination.

Administration of *Haemophilus influenzae* b (Hib) vaccine conjugate is recommended at 2, 4, and 6 months of age. A booster dose is recommended at 12 to 15 months.

Varicella is considered to be a self-limiting disease of childhood; however, the virus is likely to inflict serious harm if contracted by infants, adults, adolescents, and immunocompromised individuals.[6] Varicella vaccine was first introduced in 1995. Since then it has become more widely used. The CDC now recommends routine administration one time between the ages of 12 and 18 months for those who lack a reliable history of chickenpox. They also recommend one-time administration for all children under 13 years old who lack a reliable history. For children and adults over the age of 13, who lack a reliable history, the CDC recommends two doses given at least 4 weeks apart.[6]

It is important for the nurse to recognize and differentiate between common and serious immunization reactions. Nurses should take a proactive role in educating patients on the importance of monitoring for these reactions so that early treatment can be initiated when warranted. Common and serious immunization reactions are presented in Table 11-5.[28]

Adult Vaccination

Proper protection against certain diseases is as important for adults as it is for children. If not already protected, all adults should be vaccinated against measles, mumps, rubella, and varicella. They should also receive a booster immunization against tetanus and diphtheria every 10 years after the primary series is completed. All adults over the age of 65 and those under age 65 with serious, long-term illnesses should be vaccinated with influenza yearly.[11] Protection is obtained by giving an injection of influenza vaccine in October. Infants and children up to 9 years old who are at risk are given a subvirion (split-virus) vaccine in two doses 4 weeks apart. A yearly booster dose is needed to maintain and update immunity. Persons who are allergic to eggs or egg products should not be immunized because of the danger of hypersensitivity reactions.

The pneumococcal vaccine should be given at least once to immunocompromised adults and all adults over the age of 65.[11]

Hepatitis A vaccine was introduced in 1995. It should be administered on a selective basis; that is, only groups at a high risk are immunized. For example, the CDC recommends that hepatitis A vaccine be administered to individuals in communities with a high rate of hepatitis A, and travelers to developing countries.[5] It is also recommended for intravenous drug users, persons with multiple sexual partners or homosexual men, and day care workers.

Table 11-6 summarizes important information about commonly used vaccines. In the United States a marked reduction has occurred in the incidence of infectious diseases that can be prevented by immunization; however, there has been a decline in the number of children being immunized because of inaccessibility and cost. Free immunizations are no longer equally available in all 50 states because of the reduction in federal money used to support local immunization efforts. Infections formerly seen only in children are now occurring more frequently in adults because of lack of immunizations and resulting failure of the population to develop acquired immunity during early childhood.

Air travel has further heightened concern about the spread of infectious disease because of its elimination of the barriers of time and distance. A person with an infectious disease can easily come from a remote area of the world to a major population center where the disease can be readily spread to a susceptible public.

Passive Immunization

Antibodies produced by other persons or by animals such as the horse, cow, and rabbit can be introduced into a person's bloodstream for protection against attack by a pathogen. This protection is temporary, usually lasting only a few weeks, and stimulates no production of antibodies by the recipient. It is called artificial passive immunity. Artificial passive immunization is given to a person who has been exposed to a disease and has no natural or artificial active immunity. It usually is administered before the disease develops but may be given to modify disease symptoms. To be effective after the disease has developed, however, it must be administered early, before extensive damage to body tissue occurs.

TABLE 11-5 Common and Serious Immunization Reactions

Immunization	Common, Harmless Reactions	Serious Reactions
DTaP	Pain, tenderness, swelling, or redness at the injection site for 24-48 hours (51%). Fever for 24-48 hours (47%). Painless lump (or nodule) at the injection site 1 or 2 weeks later. Mild drowsiness (32%), Fretfulness (53%), or poor Appetite (21%) for 24-48 hours.	Fever over 105° F, or 40.5° C (0.3%). Crying for more than 3 hours (1%). High-pitched, unusual cry (0.1%). Convulsions (0.06%). Collapse with shocklike state (0.06%). Any other unusual reaction.
MMR	Fever of 101° to 103° F (38.3° to 39.5° C) for 2 or 3 days. Measles vaccine rash: a mild pink rash, mainly on the trunk; nonpruritic, lasting less than 3 days (5%).	Anaphylactic reaction (to the egg in the vaccine). Hives, shock, wheezing, stridor, and swelling of the mouth or throat beginning within 2 hours of the time the child received the vaccine.
Polio	None.	Paralytic polio (symptoms include a stiff neck, muscle tenderness, and weakness). This is very rare and occurs mainly in immunocompromised children or the adults who care for them, usually within 30 days of when the vaccine was given.
HIB	Sore injection site or mild fever (1.5%).	None reported.
Hep B	Sore injection site (30%) or mild fever (3%).	None reported.
Influenza	Pain, tenderness, or swelling at the injection site within 6 to 8 hours (10%). Fever of 101° to 103° F, or 38.3° to 39.5° C (18%). Fevers mainly occur in young children.	Anaphylactic reaction if allergic to the egg in the vaccine. Common symptoms of a severe allergic reaction are hives, shock, wheezing, stridor, and swelling of the mouth or throat beginning within 2 hours of the time the vaccine was administered.
Chickenpox (Varicella)	Pain or swelling at the injection site for 1 to 2 days. Fever than begins 2 to 4 weeks after the vaccination and lasts 1 to 3 days. (NOTE: Never give aspirin for any symptom within 6 weeks of receiving a vaccine [Reye's syndrome has been linked with the use of aspirin to treat fever or pain caused by a virus]). For a fever or pain, give acetaminophen. Mild rash at the injection site or elsewhere on the body. The rash begins 5 to 26 days after the vaccine, looks like a few chickenpox lesions, and usually lasts a few days.	None reported.

From Schmitt BD: Immunization Reactions, Clinical Reference Systems Annual, 2000.

Passive immunization usually is reserved for persons to whom the disease would be detrimental. For example, it rarely is given to prevent a disease such as chickenpox or mumps in healthy children because they are at an optimal age for the body to respond immunologically with minimal adverse effects. Passive immunization is given to all age groups exposed to pathogens that cause serious diseases, such as hepatitis A or B, diphtheria, tetanus, or rabies. Antivenins, which are given to persons bitten by poisonous snakes or black widow spiders, are other examples of passive immunologic products.

Products used for passive immunization may be specific to the disease. Antitoxins and immune animal and human sera are examples. These materials contain elevated levels of immune globulins, which can specifically detoxify the toxin, neutralize the virus, or inactivate the bacterium. The whole blood of a patient who has recently recovered from a disease against which antibodies are produced also may be used. Antitoxins are available for diphtheria, tetanus, botulism, gas gangrene, and the venom of snakes. Human immune serum is available for measles, tetanus, and rabies.

Immune serum globulin (ISG), or gamma-globulin, is an antibody-rich fraction of pooled plasma from normal donors. The rationale for pooling plasma is that someone among the donors will have had the diseases and will have developed antibodies against them. The globulin fraction of the plasma carries the antibodies, and because it is known not to transmit the hepatitis virus, it is considered safe to use. Because of occasional side effects, it is now recommended that the use of ISG be limited to those disorders in which its efficacy has been definitely established. These are measles prophylaxis or modification, viral hepatitis type A prophylaxis or modification, and immunodeficiency diseases.

Special human ISGs are derived from the sera of persons previously immunized or convalescing from specific diseases. Tetanus immune globulin (human) is of value in prophylaxis and treatment of tetanus in persons who have not received

TABLE 11-6 Description of Selected Vaccines

Vaccine	Description	Comments
DPT		
Diphtheria	Toxoid Inactivated Diphtheria toxin	Booster dose every 10 years
Tetanus	Inactivated Tetanus toxoid	Booster dose every 10 years For contaminated wound management, additional booster given if more than 5 years since last booster dose
Pertussis	Killed whole *Bordetella pertussis*	Not recommended for persons older than 7 years of age because risk of pertussis low and reaction possibly severe
Measles	Live attenuated virus vaccine	Contraindications: pregnancy, immunocompromised state, history of anaphylactic reaction to eggs
Mumps	Live attenuated virus vaccine	Contraindications: pregnancy, immunocompromised state, history of anaphylactic reaction to eggs
Rubella	Live attenuated rubella virus grown in human diploid cells	Contraindications: pregnancy, immunocompromised state
Polio		
OPV	Live attenuated oral poliovirus vaccine	Contraindications: pregnancy, immunocompromised state
IPV	Inactivated poliovirus vaccine	Administered by subcutaneous injection, contraindicated in pregnancy
Influenza	Inactivated whole or disrupted (split) influenza viruses	Antigenic content annually changed to reflect influenza A and B virus strains in circulation; administered annually; contraindication: history of anaphylactic hypersensitivity to eggs
Pneumococcal	Purified preparation of 23 different types of pneumococcal capsular polysaccharide	Should be given to persons 2 years and older who have chronic illnesses specifically associated with increased risk for pneumococcal disease and to all healthy adults over 65 years
Hepatitis A	Killed whole virus grown in human diploid cells	Administered by intramuscular injection with booster in 6 to 12 months
Hepatitis B		
Recombinant deoxyribonucleic acid (DNA)	Purified surface antigen of virus produced by recombinant yeast cells	Given in series of three injections, first followed by other two, 1 and 6 months later; indicated for persons who have routine or frequent contact with blood and body fluids; contraindicated for persons allergic to yeast
Human serum	Purified, inactivated surface antigen of virus from plasma of human carriers	Administration schedule same as for recombinant DNA form; recommended for hemodialysis patients
Haemophilus influenzae b (Hib)	Bacterial polysaccharide conjugated to protein	Administration schedule may vary depending on brand of vaccine used
Varicella	Live attenuated virus vaccine	Administered by intramuscular injection; transmission of virus to susceptible persons can occur; contraindications: pregnancy, immunocompromised state

prior immunization. Hepatitis B immune globulin (human) is available for prophylaxis after exposure to hepatitis B. Zoster immune globulin (human) is available for restricted use for prophylaxis against chickenpox.

NURSING MANAGEMENT IN IMMUNIZATION

Ensuring proper storage and handling of vaccines is basic to an immunization program. A refrigerator with freezer, used only for vaccines and medication with daily monitoring of temperatures, contributes to vaccine efficacy (Box 11-1).

The nurse is responsible for assessing persons before immunization for any contraindication to the vaccine being used. Vaccines prepared in chicken or duck embryos may

BOX 11-1 Vaccine Handling and Storage

Read storage requirements for all vaccines.
Monitor expiration dates monthly.
Date open vials and use within specified time.
Monitor refrigerator and freezer temperatures daily and log.
Store OPV and varicella vaccine frozen (freezer at 7° F [−14° C]).
Refrigerate DPT, diphtheria toxoid, tetanus-diphtheria, IPV, Hib, hepatitis B, pneumococcal, influenza (35°-46° F [2°-8° C]; do not freeze).
Protect MMR from light and excessive heat at all times.
Use small cooler with ice packs for high-use times.
Dedicate refrigerator for storage of vaccine and medication only.

BOX 11-2 Additional Considerations for Vaccine Administration

In general, inactivated vaccines and live vaccines (except cholera and yellow fever) can be administered simultaneously in separate sites.
Whenever possible, live vaccines should be administered on the same day or at least 30 days apart.
Purified protein derivative (PPD) testing for tuberculosis can be done on the same day as live virus vaccines are given or 4 to 6 weeks later.
Live attenuated vaccines should not be given at the same time as passive immunization because passively acquired antibodies can interfere with the response to live attenuated virus vaccines.
Pregnant women should not receive live attenuated vaccines because of the theoretic risk to the fetus.
If a person has a febrile illness, it is usually best to wait until recovery before vaccination.

cause an allergic reaction in persons allergic to eggs. Substances containing horse serum, such as tetanus antitoxin, should never be given unless a small amount of the substance has been injected intradermally (a sensitivity test) and no "hive" reaction about the injection site has been produced after 20 minutes because many people are allergic to horse serum. Active immunologic products should not be given while a person has a cold or other infection because the inflammatory reaction from the immunization will be greater than usual.

Children with histories of allergy often are not given routine immunization against diseases for which there is herd immunity because the danger of severe allergic response to the immunization is greater than the danger of contracting the disease. These children should be immunized against diseases such as tetanus, however, and immunization is achieved by giving the vaccine or toxoid in small doses over several weeks or months. The package inserts accompanying the immunologic product should always be read carefully to determine the indications, precautions, and side effects.

Live attenuated virus vaccines should not be given to persons with immunodeficiency, because virus replication after administration may be unchecked in these individuals. As noted earlier, OPV viruses are excreted by the recipient of the vaccine and are communicable to other persons. For this reason, IPV has recently replaced the previously recommended series of OPV. Other factors to be considered in the administration of vaccines are listed in Box 11-2.

Before leaving the clinic, the person or family members should be instructed about the expected effects of an inoculation and told to contact the physician or to report to a hospital emergency room if any other symptoms develop. The person is cautioned not to scratch any lesion produced by an inoculation. If a severe local reaction with redness, swelling, and tenderness occurs, the physician may order the application of hot, wet dressings. If the lesion is open, these dressings should be sterile.

When antitoxins, antisera, or antivenins are given, the patient is kept under observation for 20 to 30 minutes. Symptoms of severe allergic response usually appear within that time. Epinephrine 1:1000 should be available for immediate administration if an allergic response occurs.

PATIENT/FAMILY EDUCATION

Probably the greatest responsibility of the nurse relative to immunization programs is to teach the public the advantages of immunization and encourage widespread participation in programs recommended by the local public health officer. It is advisable to provide the public with the following information: disease protection given, why immunization is desirable, and when booster doses should be obtained. The relative safety of the immunization and the advantages of immunization early in life also should be stressed.

HEALTH CARE WORKERS

Persons employed in health care facilities should be evaluated for immunity against chickenpox, rubella, measles, polio, diphtheria, tetanus, and hepatitis B. Persons at risk for occupational hepatitis B infection or chickenpox should be offered vaccine at the time of employment. Persons with negative tuberculin skin tests should be retested every 6 to 12 months, depending on the prevalence of tuberculosis in the area. Yearly chest roentgenograms are no longer recommended for the routine management of persons with positive tuberculin test reactions. After the initial roentgenogram following a skin test conversion, annual films have not been shown to be of significant clinical value and are not cost-effective in monitoring persons for early disease. If occupational exposure to infectious disease occurs, Personnel Health should be consulted for prophylaxis and follow up monitoring.

INFECTION CONTROL IN THE HOSPITAL

A nosocomial infection is not present or incubating when a person is admitted to the hospital but develops after admission as opposed to a community-acquired infection, which is present or incubating at the time of admission to the hospital. Nosocomial infections are a major problem in that they increase patient morbidity, mortality, and hospital costs.

Approximately 2 million patients in acute care facilities in the United States develop nosocomial infections. The direct annual patient care cost associated with these infections is approximately $3.5 billion.[15]

The incidence of nosocomial infection varies with the type of hospital. This can be attributed to differences in the size of hospitals, the severity of illness in the patient population, susceptibility of the patient population, and the number of staff members who have hands-on contact with the patients. The patient with the greatest risk of developing a nosocomial infection has a chronic illness, a prolonged hospital stay, and the most direct contact with various hospital personnel (e.g., physicians, students, nurses, therapists). These factors hold true for variations in infection rates not only between institutions but also within an institution. Certain patient care areas are considered to be high-risk areas for the development of

TABLE 11-7 Modes of Transmission of Some Common Pathogens

Pathogen	Common Reservoir
Gram-positive cocci	
Staphylococcus aureus	Contaminated objects, hands, and nasal tracts of health care workers, air, self
Group A streptococci	Direct contact, air, hands, rarely objects
Enterococcus group	Self, hands of health care workers, environmental surfaces
Gram-negative rods	
Escherichia, Klebsiella, Enterobacter	Self, hands of health care workers, contaminated solutions
Proteus, Salmonella, Providencia, Serratia, Citrobacter	Contaminated food and water, hands of health care workers, self
Pseudomonas	Contaminated environment, hands, self
Anaerobic bacteria	
Clostridium, Bacteroides	Self, contaminated environment, hands
Fungal organisms	
Yeasts	Self, hands of health care workers
Fungi	Air, contaminated environment
Viruses	
Varicella	Air, direct contact
Herpes	Self, direct contact, air
Rubella	Direct contact, air
Hepatitis B and C	Contaminated instruments, sharps, direct contact

nosocomial infections. Hospital units housing patients with altered host defenses or who experience invasive procedures and/or devices are high-risk areas.

Persons at Risk

Factors that predispose a person to nosocomial infection include (1) age, with the very young and the very old being the most susceptible; (2) impairment of normal immune defenses because of an underlying disease process such as cancer, chronic renal disease, chronic lung disease, diabetes, or AIDS; (3) impairment of the normal immune defenses because of the therapy being given, such as radiation, steroids, or chemotherapy; (4) use of antibiotics, which can eliminate the patient's normal flora, providing opportunity for colonization with pathogenic and drug-resistant organisms that may then cause infection; (5) use of invasive diagnostic and therapeutic procedures and devices, which bypass the patient's normal defense barriers and thus provide a portal of entry into the body (e.g., indwelling urinary catheters, monitoring devices, intravenous catheters, and respiratory assistive devices); (6) surgery; (7) burns; (8) lengthy hospitalization; and (9) severity of the underlying disease, which is probably the most important factor predisposing to nosocomial infection.

A patient admitted to the hospital with a community-acquired infection may develop a superinfection with another organism during the hospitalization. Often this superinfection is with a more virulent or drug-resistant organism. For example, a patient admitted with a leg ulcer infected with *S. aureus* may develop further infection (not colonization) with *P. aeruginosa.* If this infection progresses to involve the bloodstream, a secondary bacteremia has occurred.

The most common site for a nosocomial infection is the urinary tract; 75% of these infections are related to instrumentation, including indwelling urinary catheters, catheterizations, and urologic procedures. Infected surgical wounds, followed by lower respiratory tract infections, cutaneous infections, and bloodstream infections (some associated with the use of intravascular lines), are the next most frequently encountered types of nosocomial infections. Together these sites account for about 35% of all nosocomial infections.

Pathogens Causing Nosocomial Infections

The pathogens typically responsible for nosocomial infections and their usual reservoirs are listed in Table 11-7.

Escherichia coli continues to account for most reported nosocomial urinary tract infections. *S. aureus* and coagulase-negative staphylococci, part of the patient's own flora, are the main organisms causing nosocomial surgical wound infections. *P. aeruginosa* and *S. aureus* are the most common pathogens causing nosocomial pneumonia. Coagulase-negative staphylococci and *S. aureus* are the pathogens most frequently causing nosocomial primary bacteremia.[23]

The reservoirs for *S. aureus* are the respiratory tract and skin. From 10% to 15% of the general population can be persistent carriers of this organism, which is harbored in the anterior nares. Among persons working in hospitals, the carrier rate may be as high as 25% to 30%. Nasal carriers, especially those with respiratory tract infections, are potential sources of environmental and human contact contamination. Methicillin-resistant *S. aureus* (MRSA) is of special concern. Methicillin is one of the penicillins specifically developed to treat *S. aureus,* infections which are common in surgical wounds and on the skin. Although MRSA is no more virulent than methicillin-sensitive *S. aureus* (MSSA), it is more difficult and expensive to treat. The antibiotic of choice for treating MRSA infection is vancomycin. Institutions have used various strategies in an attempt to eradicate MRSA colonization in their patient populations. These include cultures on admission, periodic surveillance cultures, isolation, and various antibiotic protocols. All have proved to be largely ineffective.

Enterococci resistant to vancomycin (VRE) have emerged as a significant pathogen within the last 5 to 10 years. Enterococci are normally found in the GI tract and in the female genital tract, but can be important nosocomial pathogens. Resistance to vancomycin has developed as a result of indiscriminate use of antibiotics. Limited treatment options are a serious concern with VRE. Because of the progressive antibiotic resistant nature of VRE, no single antibiotic is currently available that can eradicate it. In fact, many primary care providers are actually beginning to treat VRE by stopping all antibiotics and simply waiting for normal flora (bacteria) to repopulate and replace the VRE strain. Alternatively a combination of several drugs is prescribed. Transmission-Based as well as Standard Precautions should be implemented as soon as VRE is suspected.[29]

Group A streptococci *(Streptococcus pyogenes)* are gram-positive organisms, strains of which cause streptococcal sore throat, scarlet fever, and streptococcal skin infections. A particularly virulent strain of this organism is responsible for necrotizing fasciitis. Streptococci are found in animate reservoirs, particularly the pharynx and nares, of personnel and patients.

Other organisms involved in nosocomial infections include gram-negative coliform bacteria, *Escherichia, Klebsiella,* and *Enterobacter,* all of which live in the human intestinal tract. Although these organisms usually are susceptible to antibiotics, they have the capacity to develop antibiotic resistance. The large reservoir of coliform organisms within the general population can be a source of self-infection or cross-infection from the hands of hospital personnel through the ingestion of foods or through the contamination of other materials. Some strains of these organisms are more likely than others to produce infection. The more pathogenic strains seem to gain ascendency in patients who are receiving antibiotic therapy; immunodeficient patients are particularly susceptible to infection by coliform bacteria.

Although *Salmonella* organisms usually are acquired outside the hospital, the organism is readily transmissible and can be the cause of nosocomial infection. It is transmitted by direct or indirect contact with an infected person or through food (especially raw eggs), dairy products, or water contaminated with the organism. The CDC recommends that no one eat raw or partially cooked eggs. Patients with sickle cell disease, HIV, or malignancies are more vulnerable to infection from these organisms.

P. aeruginosa, a gram-negative organism, is present throughout the hospital environment in areas such as sinks and nebulizers where water is always present. It is a frequent cause of infection in patients with leukopenia secondary to burns, leukemia, cystic fibrosis, and various immunodeficiency syndromes. It also is known to be a significant cause of infection in patients receiving prolonged courses of antibiotics, immunosuppressive drugs, and inhalation therapy. *P. aeruginosa* can be a threat to patients undergoing instrumentation (tracheostomy and urinary tract catheterization) and receiving renal transplants. Neonates, particularly premature infants, as well as elderly and debilitated persons, are the most vulnerable.

Serratia marcescens and *Serratia liquefaciens* are gram-negative organisms, the reservoirs for which are soil and water. They are found in the same hospital locations as *Pseudomonas. S. marcescens,* previously thought to be nonpathogenic, was used because of its red pigmentation to mark airflow and settling patterns of bacteria. It is now recognized as a pathogen that can cause severe infection in a susceptible host. The *Serratia* organisms develop resistance to antibiotics rapidly and can be devastating if an outbreak occurs in an intensive care or burn unit. Because the mode of transmission is through direct or indirect contact on the hands of personnel or on contaminated articles, good hand washing and aseptic techniques are the most effective measures to prevent such outbreaks.

Candida albicans is a yeastlike fungus that can cause infection, especially in immunocompromised patients or those receiving antibiotics. These patients have a decrease in normal flora, which provides a niche for the *Candida* organisms to settle in and proliferate. Antibiotics suppress bacterial growth but do not affect fungal growth; special antifungal agents are necessary to control these infections unless the normal flora returns after discontinuance of the antibiotics.

Prevention and Control Measures for Nosocomial Infections

In the hospital many potential sources of infection exist including patients, personnel, visitors, equipment, and linens. Patients may become infected with organisms either from the external environment (exogenous) or, as is often seen in the severely immunocompromised host, from their own internal organisms (endogenous). Virtually any microorganism can be a potential pathogen to the immunocompromised patient. Most of the causative organisms are present in the patient's external environment and are introduced to the body through direct contact or contaminated materials. Discussion of specific control measures follows, but it must be remembered that in many instances nosocomial infections could be prevented simply by the use of strict aseptic technique when giving care and by greater restraint in the use of invasive procedures and antibiotics.

Control of External Environment

Health care providers should be in good health and keep their immunization status up to date. They should report to the employee health service when they feel ill. Visitors also should be in good health, and their number should be limited to prevent overcrowding in the patient's room. Staff members should wear clean clothing and observe good personal hygiene practices, especially thorough hand washing, which decreases transient and resident flora on the hands and thus acts as a deterrent to cross-infection by the hands. Friction and rinsing are the two most important components of good hand washing (Box 11-3). Ample hand washing facilities are necessary throughout the hospital and should be used by all personnel before and after patient contact; after contact with excretions, secretions, wound drainage, or any contaminated articles; and before any clean or sterile procedure or contact with clean or

BOX 11-3 Guidelines for Proper Hand Washing

1. Wet hands.
2. Apply cleansing agent.
3. Apply friction and scrub hands together on front, back, between fingers, and all surfaces.
4. Scrub for a minimum of 10 seconds.
5. Rinse thoroughly to remove all lather and debris.
6. Dry thoroughly.
7. Discard paper towels used for drying.
8. Use second towel to turn off water faucets and avoid recontamination.

Reference: Mayone-Ziomek JM: Handwashing in healthcare, *Dermatol Nurs* 10:1, 1998.

sterile equipment. Hand washing is the most effective method for preventing nosocomial infection.[3,21,30,33] Although this has been a classic concept stemming from before the years of Florence Nightingale, there is growing concern among the CDC about compliance with "proper" hand washing.[22]

The problem of hand washing compliance is becoming an even greater issue with the increasing presence and associated mortality of antibiotic resistance.[20] On observation, a study found that of 2834 opportunities for hand washing, health care personnel washed their hands only 48% of the time.[26] As a way to increase compliance, new hand washing products are becoming available that may offer promising alternatives to the traditional "soap and water" method (see Future Watch box).[34] Many pathogens have the ability to live outside the human body for extended periods. Recent research found that 3 of 10 chair seat cushions contained VRE on the surface. After contamination experiments, all samples were positive at 72 hours and 1 week after inoculation. Thus it is recommended that in addition to frequent hand washing, a sheet folded four times or a bath blanket folded in half be placed on seat cushions to prevent transmission of infection.[24]

It is important that dermatologic conditions of the hands be corrected, because dry, cracked skin can more readily become colonized with pathogens, and broken skin is more difficult to rid of transient and resident flora. The person with a skin problem on the hands also tends to avoid proper hand washing, because it can further increase dryness and irritation. The person with active herpes simplex infection of the hand (herpetic whitlow) should not give direct patient care until the lesion has healed. Staff members also should develop the habit of working from clean procedures to dirty procedures when delivering patient care. For example, the nurse should adjust the intravenous infusion rate and check the intravenous site before changing the bed of an incontinent patient.

Housekeeping and sanitation practices should be strictly observed to reduce dust and environmental reservoirs of organisms, especially in high-risk areas such as nurseries, operating rooms, and intensive care units. Spills of blood or other body fluids should be cleaned up promptly with an approved hospital disinfectant or a 1:10 dilution of 5.25% sodium hypochlorite (household bleach and water). Linens should be changed with as little contact with the nurse's uniform as possible. Linen should not be thrown on the floor or shaken in the air, because this not only further contaminates the linen but also stirs up dust particles and creates air currents that can transmit pathogens. Waste products should be disposed of in the appropriate receptacle. State and federal laws regulate the disposal of infectious waste from health care institutions. Items such as needles and syringes, laboratory cultures and tissue specimens, and other disposable items that are saturated with blood or body substances are considered regulated infectious waste. Regulated infectious waste must be incinerated or treated to render it noninfectious before disposal. Other waste materials from patient rooms may be disposed of as regular trash. Proper cleaning and sterilization of contaminated reusable articles and equipment are essential.

An often forgotten, reusable item that is a common source of infection in the health care setting is the stethoscope (see Research box). To decrease the risk of transmitting infection with stethoscopes, several simple guidelines should be followed (Box 11-4).[17]

Air is generally not considered an important factor in nosocomial cross-infection. However, in the case of *Aspergillus* spores and *Mycobacterium tuberculosis,* adequate air exchanges are necessary to reduce the number of organisms. Minimal standards for air exchanges in patient care areas are published by the Department of Health and Human Services. Minimal air changes of outdoor air per hour range from 2 in patient rooms to 15 in operating rooms.

Future Watch
Alcoholic Solutions Replacing Soap and Water?

From Zaragoza M et al: Handwashing with soap or alcoholic solutions? A randomized clinical trial of its effectiveness, *Am J Infect Control* 27:258, 1999.

A recent prospective, randomized, clinical trial studied the effectiveness of an alcoholic solution hand washing compared with the "gold standard" soap and water hand washing during regular work hours on clinical wards of a large public university hospital. The subjects, 47 health care workers, were randomly assigned to regular hand washing (with liquid soap and water) or hand washing with an alcoholic solution. The number of colony-forming units (CFUs) on agar plates (after hand printing) in three different samples was counted before and after hand washing.

Results showed a 49.6% decrease in the number of CFUs for soap and water, and a 88.2% decrease in CFUs for the alcoholic solution. When the average number of CFUs recovered after the procedure of both methods were compared, a statistically significant difference in favor of the alcoholic solution hand washing ($P<0.001$) was discovered.

In 9.3% of the subjects studied, the alcoholic solution method of hand washing worsened minor preexisting skin conditions. However, for most people, the alcoholic solutions were effective and safe and, with future research, may prove to be an effective alternative to the traditional soap and water method in health care environments where compliance rate is poor due to lack of sinks and/or work overload.

Research

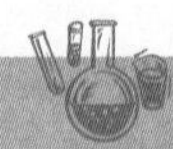

Reference: Marinella M et al: The stethoscope: a potential source of nosocomial infection? *Arch Intern Med* 157:786, 1997.

The purpose of this study was to assess bacterial contamination on the stethoscope diaphragm and under the plastic rim that secures the diaphragm of a variety of health care personnel on two different units in a large university hospital. The study also compared the effectiveness of different cleaning agents and assessed the transmissibility of bacteria on the stethoscopes to human skin.

A total of 11 genera and species of organisms were isolated. The most prominent organism isolated, recovered from 87.5% of stethoscope diaphragms and 100% of rim areas, was coagulase-negative staphylococcus. Another prominent bacterium isolated was *Staphylococcus aureus* (27.5% of diaphragms and 25% of rim areas). The mean number of total colony forming units (CFUs) was approximately 158 per diaphragm and approximately 289 per rim.

Of the cleaning agents studied, the most effective was isopropyl alcohol. After cleaning with alcohol, the diaphragms contained approximately 0.2 CFUs, and the rims contained approximately 2.2 CFUs ($P=0.01$). Cleaning with soap and water did not significantly reduce bacterial levels on either the diaphragm or rim areas.

Finally, the study revealed that *M. luteus* could be transferred from a stethoscope to human skin, making it likely that other bacteria could also be transferred.

BOX 11-4 Stethoscope Safety Tips

If possible, use a hospital-issued stethoscope that is kept in a single designated area. This prevents the use of stethoscopes throughout the facility and traveling outside the facility.

Disinfect stethoscopes regularly. Use isopropyl alcohol, which is not only readily available, but also less corrosive to metal and rubber than other germicides. Alternatively, 70% ethyl alcohol can be used.

Before and after every shift, wipe down the stethoscope, starting at the earpieces (which helps prevent the spread of ear infections among the staff), continuing down the tubing, and ending around the bell and diaphragm. Take the diaphragm apart to remove dust, lint, or debris and clean it well before reassembling it.

Wipe the bell and diaphragm with alcohol between each use. Also be sure to clean the entire stethoscope after using it on a patient with a known infection.

Use disposable covers. Available in various styles, the most useful covers are designed for single use. They are made of thin plastic, which prevents crackling sounds. Most covers protect the bell and diaphragm and the tubing leading to the stethoscope's bifurcation. Ask the infection control coordinator about these covers. Their cost may be offset by fewer nosocomial infections and, therefore, fewer unpaid hospital days.

Some clinicians use nondisposable covers that fit over the stethoscope tubing. These can also be a source of infection. If you use one, be sure to wash the nondisposable cover every day to decrease the chances of transmitting microbes.

Encourage the physician to use your stethoscope when he/she assesses one of your patients. That way, he/she can avoid contaminating his/her own stethoscope and perhaps exposing the next patient to infection.

For some patients, such as those with an antibiotic-resistant infection, you may want to leave a stethoscope in the patient's room for use on that patient only. Check with the infection control coordinator for guidelines.

Reference: Lambright Eckler JA: Stethoscope safety tips, *Nurs* 27:10, 20, 1997.

Control of Internal Environment

Reducing the endogenous sources of infection is more difficult than control of the external environment because the source is often the patient's normal flora. Preventive measures aim to decrease the risk of the infection by increasing the patient's defense mechanisms. Teaching the patient about good nutrition and personal hygiene is a practical measure that is part of nursing care. Maintaining the patient's normal flora and preventing colonization with pathogens that can serve as a source of infection are other effective measures, but these are not always possible when patients are receiving antibiotics or undergoing chemotherapy, which disrupt the normal flora and promote colonization. Appropriate use of antibiotics for prophylaxis and treatment helps prevent colonization with pathogens and decreases the incidence of infection with drug-resistant organisms. A summary of major prevention and control measures is provided in the Guidelines for Safe Practice box.

Prevention of Urinary Tract Infections

As mentioned previously, urinary tract infections (UTIs) are the most common nosocomial infections seen in the hospital. Most of these infections are associated with catheterization and instrumentation of the urinary tract. Urinary catheters should be used only when absolutely necessary. If a catheter must be used, it should be removed as soon as medically feasible, because the longer the catheter is in place, the greater the risk of infection. To prevent transmission of bacteria into the bladder, strict aseptic technique is necessary during insertion of the catheter. Bacteria that are present around the catheter-meatal junction also can be transmitted on the tip of the catheter into the bladder along the thin layer of mucus that surrounds the catheter in the urethra. For this reason the catheter should be securely anchored to prevent it from moving in and out of the urethra. Movement of the catheter can track bacteria into the urethra and up into the bladder along the mucous sheath. Furthermore, the catheter-meatal junction should be kept clean; the patient incontinent of stool can pose a challenge in this regard. In some institutions, antiseptic agents are used to cleanse the meatus, and antimicrobial agents are applied around the catheter-meatal junction. Both of these practices are considered controversial. Good hand washing techniques by personnel, cleansing of the patient's meatal area with soap and water, and proper anchoring of the catheter are considered effective ways to reduce the incidence of UTIs in patients with indwelling catheters.

Another portal of entry for bacteria is through the distal catheter-proximal drainage tube junction. Every time the system is disconnected, the risk of introducing bacteria into the

Guidelines for Safe Practice

Prevention and Control of Nosocomial Infections

CONTROL OF EXTERNAL ENVIRONMENT (EXOGENOUS SOURCES OF INFECTION)

Health Care Providers

1. In good health—do not care for patients when ill
2. Keep immunizations current
3. Practice effective hand washing between each patient
   If skin dry, rough, or broken, seek appropriate attention
   If active herpes simplex infection of hand (herpetic whitlow), do not give direct patient care until lesion healed
4. Appropriate use of personal protective equipment, based on degree of risk of exposure (e.g., gloves, mask, apron, face shield, shoe covers, air respirator)

Housekeeping and Sanitation

1. Bed linens not shaken in air or thrown on floor
2. Proper disposal of wastes—solid and liquid
3. Proper cleaning and sterilization of contaminated articles
4. Proper ventilation for adequate air exchanges
   Modern hospitals-patients' room air is under negative pressure
   Negative pressure keeps air from patients' rooms from moving into hallways
5. Proper mopping and damp dusting to remove dust and other environmental reservoirs of infection

CONTROL OF INTERNAL ENVIRONMENT (ENDOGENOUS SOURCES OF INFECTION)

1. Preventive measures aimed at increasing patient's defense mechanisms and thus reducing risk of infection
   Teach patient about good nutrition
   Teach patient about personal hygiene, especially hand washing
2. Be aware that normal flora of patient can be disrupted when patient is receiving antibiotics or chemotherapy and colonization may occur
   Give antibiotics on time as scheduled
   Teach patient about appropriate use of antibiotics and dangers of taking them when not prescribed by physician

system increases; thus a closed drainage system should be maintained. Bladder irrigations should not be a routine practice. If irrigation is necessary, a sterile disposable syringe and sterile solution should be used. If frequent irrigations are necessary, as with transurethral prostatectomy in which blood clots are common, a three-way catheter drainage system with continuous bladder irrigation is recommended. In this way a closed system is maintained. Urine specimens should be obtained from the rubber portal on the drainage tubing. The portal should be cleansed with an antiseptic before insertion of the needle into the portal.

Another portal of entry of bacteria into the system is through the collection bag. The bag should be kept below the bladder level at all times to prevent reflux of urine into the bladder. In addition, the bag should be kept off the floor, and the emptying spout should be cleansed with an antiseptic after the urine is emptied. The container used to collect the urine from the bag must be used for only one patient; it should not be shared among patients.

A final control measure in preventing nosocomial UTIs is to place patients with urinary catheters in separate rooms. This is helpful in preventing cross-infection among patients.

Prevention of Respiratory Tract Infections

After urinary tract infections, pneumonia is the second most common nosocomial infection; however, pneumonia is by far the most deadly nosocomial infection.[4] A major risk factor is respiratory intubation because endotracheal, nasotracheal, and tracheostomy tubes bypass the patient's defense mechanisms of the upper respiratory tract. The importance of proper maintenance and decontamination of respiratory therapy equipment in preventing nosocomial pneumonias is well established. Hand washing is essential before and after contact with patients and respiratory assist devices, which contain moisture and are ideal reservoirs for organisms, especially gram-negative species such as *Pseudomonas* and *Serratia.* Suctioning is a sterile procedure necessitating the use of sterile equipment and irrigants (see Chapter 21). Surgical procedures that lead to impaired coughing also are an increased risk. Preoperative patient teaching that stresses the importance and proper technique of coughing and deep breathing is essential to the success of reducing postoperative pulmonary infection. Inappropriate use of antibiotics should be avoided to minimize oropharyngeal colonization with gram-negative bacteria, which, if aspirated, may lead to serious pneumonia. Debilitated patients should be protected from the hazards of aspiration, especially while eating.

Prevention of Bacteremias

Many blood infections (bacteremias) occur secondary to infections at another site; thus prevention may depend greatly on control of the underlying infection. Some bacteremias result from the use of intravascular devices and systems. The sources of infection in these instances are the hands of staff members, the patient's skin, or infusions contaminated either from mishandling by hospital personnel or, less often, at the time of manufacture. Intravenous and intraarterial catheters should be inserted under aseptic conditions, and catheter insertion sites should be cared for aseptically. The insertion site is treated as an open wound and is assessed frequently for any sign of infection, such as redness, swelling, exudate, purulence, warmth, or pain.

Central lines should have a sterile dressing to prevent contamination of the insertion site. Peripheral catheters should be changed every 72 hours or more often if a complication such as infiltration or phlebitis occurs. The catheter is secured to prevent in-and-out movement and tracking of bacteria into the cannula site. Aseptic technique should be followed during the mixing and adding of drugs, changing the infusion, or manipulating connections or stopcocks. The tubing should be changed every 72 hours.[25] Before beginning infusion of a solution, the nurse should check it for turbidity, particulate matter, and leaks in the system. Hyperalimentation solutions require special adherence to these practices because they are composed of nutrients that provide an excellent culture medium for organisms. *Candida* infections occur frequently in patients receiving hyperalimentation, particularly those who are immunocompromised.

Protection by Isolation

The purpose of isolation is to protect both the caregiver from exposure to infectious agents and the patient from cross-infection.

Some general principles apply regardless of the type of isolation. Barriers such as gowns, gloves, and masks should be used only once and then discarded in an appropriate receptacle before leaving the patient's room. These barriers should be conveniently available for each patient room. Hands must be washed before and after each patient contact even when gloves are worn.

In 1996 the CDC and HICPAC published revised guidelines for isolation precautions in hospitals.[10,27] These new guidelines incorporate the major tenets of what was previously known as universal precautions (UP) and body substance isolation (BSI). Neither UP nor BSI addressed prevention of airborne, droplet, and direct contact modes of transmission. In the early 1990s concern with preventing transmission of tuberculosis including multidrug-resistant tuberculosis required additional precautions. At the same time, the prevalence of multidrug-resistant organisms was increasing, and hospitals needed new ways to deal with this problem. The new CDC/HICPAC guidelines for isolation precautions in hospitals were developed to address these concerns.

The precautions are described as two tiered. The first tier, Standard Precautions, combines UP and BSI techniques and is to be used with all patients regardless of whether the diagnosis is known. These precautions apply to (1) blood, (2) all other body fluids and secretions except sweat, regardless of whether they contain visible blood, (3) nonintact skin, and (4) mucous membranes. Table 11-8 lists the techniques used for Standard Precautions.

The second tier, Transmission-Based Precautions, is designed to reduce the risk of airborne, droplet, and contact transmission. It is used when caring for patients with documented or suspected infection with highly transmissible or epidemiologically important pathogens for which Standard Precautions may be insufficient. The three types of transmission-based precautions are (1) airborne precautions, (2) droplet precautions, and (3) contact precautions. Standard Precautions are used in combination with one or more of the Transmission-Based Precautions, depending on the disease identified.

Airborne Precautions are to be used to prevent airborne transmission of organisms contained in dust particles or the droplet nuclei of evaporated droplets (5 μm or less). Special air handling, which may include negative pressure, frequent air exchanges, direct-to-the-outside exhaust, high efficiency particulate air (HEPA) filters, or ultraviolet light, is necessary to prevent airborne transmission. Placing the patient with suspected or diagnosed tuberculosis in a private room with negative pressure room air and 12 air exchanges per hour and having the staff entering the room use HEPA filter respirators is an example of Airborne Precautions. The patient should stay in the room with the door closed until sputum smears indicate that he or she is no longer infectious.

Droplet Precautions are used to prevent contact between the conjunctiva or mucous membrane of the nose or mouth with large-size (larger than 5 μm) particle droplets containing microorganisms generated by cough, sneeze, or talking or by a procedure such as suctioning or bronchoscopy. Generally these droplets are a risk only to persons within a 3-foot radius of the source. They quickly settle onto surfaces and can no longer be inhaled. Placing the patient with suspected *Neisseria meningitidis* pneumonia in a private room and wearing a mask while working within 3 feet of the patient is an example of Droplet Precautions.

Contact Precautions are used to interrupt transmission of epidemiologically important organisms by direct (skin to skin) or indirect (skin to contaminated item) contact. Placing the patient with *Clostridium difficile* diarrhea in a private room with single-use or dedicated-to-the-patient equipment and donning a gown and gloves to enter the room to perform any patient care procedure is an example of Contact Precautions.

TABLE 11-8 Standard Precautions Techniques

Item	Precautions
Hand washing	After touching blood, body fluids, secretions, excretions, contaminated items, whether or not gloves are worn
Gloves	When touching blood, body fluids, secretions, excretions, and contaminated items and when performing invasive procedures; remove gloves promptly after use and wash hands
Mask, eye protection, face shield	To protect mucous membranes of the eyes, nose, and mouth during activities that are likely to generate splashes or sprays of blood, body fluids, secretions, and excretions
Private room	Indicated if personal hygiene is poor or if body substances contaminate the environment
Needles	Dispose of uncapped and unbent needles at point of use in puncture-resistant container: one-handed or device-assisted recapping if necessary
Soiled linen	Placed in leak-proof bags: gown and gloves worn by laundry workers sorting all soiled linen
Reusable equipment	Bagged for transport to decontamination area: gowns, gloves, masks, and eye protection worn by decontamination personnel

Modified from Garner JS and the Hospital Infection Control Practices Advisory Committee: Guidelines for isolation precautions in hospitals. Part II. Recommendations for isolation precautions in hospital, *Am J Infect Control* 22:24-52, 1996.

Because of the special considerations for preventing the spread of VRE, HICPAC developed separate recommendations outlining the additional precautions needed.[13] Contact isolation is used in conjunction with Standard Precautions, with each institution adapting the HICPAC recommendations based on their particular circumstances and endemic rate.

Table 11-9 is a synopsis of types of precautions and patients requiring the precautions. Table 11-10 is a list of clinical syndromes or conditions warranting additional empiric precautions to prevent transmission of epidemiologically important pathogens pending confirmation of diagnosis. Table 11-11 is a list of type and duration of precautions needed for selected infections.

TABLE 11-9 Types of Precautions

Standard Precautions

Use Standard Precautions for the care of all patients

Airborne Precautions

In addition to Standard Precautions, use Airborne Precautions for patients known or suspected to have serious illnesses transmitted by airborne droplet nuclei. Examples of such illnesses include:

(1) Measles
(2) Varicella (including disseminated zoster)*
(3) Tuberculosis

Droplet Precautions

In addition to Standard Precautions, use Droplet Precautions for patients known or suspected to have serious illnesses transmitted by large particle droplets. Examples of such illnesses include:

(1) Invasive *Haemophilus influenzae* type b disease, including meningitis, pneumonia, epiglottitis, and sepsis
(2) Invasive *Neisseria meningitidis* disease, including meningitis, pneumonia, and sepsis
(3) Other serious bacterial respiratory infections spread by droplet transmission, including:
- (a) Diphtheria (pharyngeal)
- (b) Mycoplasma pneumonia
- (c) Pertussis
- (d) Pneumonic plague
- (e) Streptococcal pharyngitis, pneumonia, or scarlet fever in infants and young children

(4) Serious viral infections spread by droplet transmission, including:
- (a) Adenovirus*
- (b) Influenza
- (c) Mumps
- (d) Parvovirus B19
- (e) Rubella

Contact Precautions

In addition to Standard Precautions, use Contact Precautions for patients known or suspected to have serious illnesses easily transmitted by direct patient contact or by contact with items in the patient's environment. Examples of such illnesses include:

(1) Gastrointestinal, respiratory, skin, or wound infections or colonization with multidrug-resistant bacteria judged by the infection control program, based on current state, regional, or national recommendations, to be of special clinical and epidemiological significance
(2) Enteric infections with a low infectious dose or prolonged environmental survival, including:
- (a) *Clostridium difficile*
- (b) For diapered or incontinent patients: enterohemorrhagic *Escherichia coli* 0157: H7, *Shigella,* hepatitis A, or rotavirus

(3) Respiratory syncytial virus, parainfluenza virus, or enteroviral infections in infants and young children
(4) Skin infections that are highly contagious or that may occur on dry skin, including:
- (a) Diphtheria (cutaneous)
- (b) Herpes simplex virus (neonatal or mucocutaneous)
- (c) Impetigo
- (d) Major (noncontained) abscesses, cellulitis, or decubiti
- (e) Pediculosis
- (f) Scabies
- (g) Staphylococcal furunculosis in infants and young children
- (h) Zoster (disseminated or in the immunocompromised host)*

(5) Viral/hemorrhagic conjunctivitis
(6) Viral hemorrhagic infections (Ebola, Lassa, or Marburg)

From Garner JS and the Hospital Infection Control Practices Advisory Committee: Guidelines for isolation precautions in hospitals. Part II. Recommendations for isolation precautions in hospitals, *Am J Infect Control* 22:24-52, 1996.
*Certain infections require more than one type of precaution.

TABLE 11-10 Clinical Syndromes or Conditions Warranting Additional Empiric Precautions to Prevent Transmission of Epidemiologically Important Pathogens Pending Confirmation of Diagnosis

Clinical Syndrome or Condition	Potential Pathogens	Empiric Precautions
Diarrhea		
Acute diarrhea with a likely infectious cause in an incontinent or diapered patient	Enteric pathogens	Contact
Diarrhea in an adult with a history of recent antibiotic use	*Clostridium difficile*	Contact
Meningitis	*Neisseria meningitidis*	Droplet
Rash or exanthems, generalized, cause unknown		
Petechial/ecchymotic with fever	*N. meningitidis*	Droplet
Vesicular	Varicella	Airborne and Contact
Maculopapular with coryza and fever	Rubeola (measles)	Airborne
Respiratory infections		
Cough/fever/upper lobe pulmonary infiltrate in an HIV-seronegative patient and/or a patient at low risk for HIV infection	*Mycobacterium tuberculosis*	Airborne
Cough/fever/pulmonary infiltrate in any lung location in an HIV-infected patient and/or a patient at high risk for HIV infection	*M. tuberculosis*	Airborne
Paroxysmal or severe persistent cough during periods of pertussis activity	*Bordetella pertussis*	Droplet
Respiratory infections, particularly bronchiolitis and croup, in infants and young children	Respiratory syncytial or parainfluenza virus	Contact
Risk of multidrug-resistant microorganisms		
History of infection or colonization with multidrug-resistant organisms	Resistant bacteria	Contact
Skin, wound, or urinary tract infection in a patient with a recent hospital or nursing home stay in a facility where multidrug-resistant organisms are prevalent	Resistant bacteria	Contact
Skin or wound infection		
Abscess or draining wound that cannot be covered	*Staphylococcus aureus,* group A streptococcus	Contact

From Garner JS and the Hospital Infection Control Practices Advisory Committee: Guidelines for isolation precautions in hospitals. Part II. Recommendations for isolation precautions in hospitals, *Am J Infect Control* 22:24-52, 1996.
HIV, Human immunodeficiency virus.

Diagnostic Tests

Diagnostic tests are an important adjunct in the diagnosis of an infection. The complete blood count is simple but important because a systemic response to infection is the variation in number and type of leukocytes (WBCs) in the peripheral circulation. The normal WBC count in blood is 5000 to 10,000 WBCs/mm^3. With the presence of a serious infection the number of WBCs rises above 10,000/mm^3. Leukocyte values between 10,000 and 20,000 are considered slightly elevated, 20,000 to 40,000 moderately elevated, and more than 40,000 greatly elevated. In a few infectious diseases the number of WBCs in circulation actually drops, which is also significant.

Five types of mature WBCs are found in circulation: neutrophils, eosinophils, basophils, lymphocytes, and monocytes. Each type plays a more or less specific role in body defense (see Chapter 48); therefore different diseases produce different reactions among the WBC populations in the blood. These changes in patterns of distribution are detected not only by counting the total number of WBCs in a stained blood smear, but also by classifying them according to morphology and calculating the relative percentage of each cell type present. This type of count is known as a differential count. As described earlier, an increase in the number of immature neutrophils is commonly referred to as a "shift to the left" and may indicate an acute infection. The differential count may provide information that can be correlated with other clinical data to help diagnose an infection. Table 11-12 provides some general correlations between leukocyte response and infectious diseases.

Other tests used to assess for infection include skin tests, radiologic tests, gallium and indium scans, ultrasound, computed tomography and magnetic resonance imaging scans, microbiologic cultures, and serologic antibody titers. Examples of data obtainable from such tests include an increase in ESR; the appearance of C-reactive protein; the presence of proteinemia; positive bacterial, viral, and fungal cultures; and positive radiologic findings, all of which may indicate the presence of an infection.

Proper collection and handling of laboratory specimens are essential to ensure accurate laboratory results. Inappropriate collection or handling of specimens may lead to unnecessary delays in test results or inaccurate results, thus affecting the

TABLE 11-11 Type and Duration of Precautions Needed for Selected Infections and Conditions

Infection/Condition	Precautions	
	Type*	Duration†
Abscess		
Draining, major[a]	C	DI
Draining, minor or limited	S	
Acquired immunodeficiency syndrome	S	
Anthrax		
Cutaneous	S	
Pulmonary	S	
Creutzfeldt-Jakob disease	S	
Gastroenteritis		
Campylobacter species	S	
Clostridium difficile	C	DI
Cryptosporidium species	S	
Escherichia coli		
Enterohemorrhagic O157:H7	S	
Diapered or incontinent	C	DI
Giardia lamblia	S	
Salmonella species (including *S typhi*)	S	
Gonorrhea	S	
Hepatitis, viral		
Type A	S	
Diapered or incontinent patients	C	F[a]
Type B-HBsAg positive	S	
Type C and other unspecified non-A, non-B	S	
Type E	S	
Herpes simplex (*Herpesvirus hominis*)		
Mucocutaneous, disseminated or primary, severe	C	DI
Mucocutaneous, recurrent (skin, oral, genital)	S	
Herpes zoster (varicella-zoster)		
Localized in immunocompromised patient, or disseminated	A,C	DI
Localized in normal patient	S	
Hookworm disease (ancylostomiasis, uncinariasis)	S	
Human immunodeficiency virus (HIV) infection[c]	S	
Influenza	D	DI
Meningitis		
Aseptic (nonbacterial or viral meningitis; also see enteroviral infections)	S	
Fungal	S	
Haemophilus influenzae, known or suspected	D	U(24 hrs)
Neisseria meningitides (meningococcal) known or suspected	D	U(24 hrs)
Pneumococcal	S	
Multidrug-resistant organisms, infection or colonization		
Gastrointestinal	C	CN
Respiratory	C	CN
Pneumococcal	S	
Skin, wound, or burn	C	CN
Parvovirus B19	D	F[b]

Adapted from Centers for Disease Control and Prevention: Type and duration of precautions needed for selected infections and conditions, Washington, DC, 1997, website: www.CDC.gov.

*Type of Precautions: A, Airborne; C, Contact; D, Droplet; S, Standard; when A, C, and D are specified, also use S.

†Duration of precautions: CN, until off antibiotics and culture-negative; DI, duration of illness (with wound lesions, DI means until they stop draining); U, until time specified in hours (hrs) after initiation of effective therapy; F, see footnote.

[a]Maintain precautions in infants and children <3 years of age for duration of hospitalization; in children 3 to 14 years of age, until 2 weeks after onset of symptoms; and in others, until 1 week after onset of symptoms.

[b]Maintain precautions for duration of hospitalization when chronic disease occurs in an immunodeficient patient. For patients with transient aplastic crisis or red-cell crisis, maintain precautions for 7 days.

[c]Discontinue precautions *only* when TB patient is on effective therapy, is improving clinically, and has three consecutive negative sputum smears collected on different days, or TB is ruled out. Also see CDC "Guidelines for Preventing the Transmission of Tuberculosis in Health-Care Facilities."(23)

Continued

TABLE 11-11 Type and Duration of Precautions Needed for Selected Infections and Conditions—cont'd

Infection/Condition	Precautions	
	Type*	Duration†
Pneumonia		
Adenovirus	D, C	DI
Bacterial not listed elsewhere (including gram-negative bacterial)	S	
Burkholderia cepacia in cystic fibrosis (CF) patients, including respiratory tract colonization	S	
Chlamydia	S	
Fungal	S	
Haemophilus influenzae		
Adults	S	
Infants and children (any age)	D	U(24 hrs)
Legionella	S	
Meningococcal	D	U(24 hrs)
Multidrug-resistant bacterial (see multidrug-resistant organisms)		
Mycoplasma (primary atypical pneumonia)	D	DI
Pneumococcal	S	
Multidrug-resistant (see multidrug-resistant organisms)		
Pneumocystis carinii	S	
Pseudomonas cepacia (see *Burkholderia cepacia*)	S	
Staphylococcus aureus	S	
Streptococcus, group A		
Adults	S	
Infants and young children	D	U(24 hrs)
Viral		
Adults	S	
Infants and young children (see respiratory infectious disease, acute)		
Staphylococcal disease (*S aureus*)		
Skin, wound, or burn		
Major	C	DI
Minor or limited	S	
Enterocolitis	S	
Multidrug-resistant (see multidrug-resistant organisms)		
Pneumonia	S	
Scalded skin syndrome	S	
Toxic shock syndrome	S	
Streptococcal disease (group A streptococcus)		
Skin, wound, or burn		
Major	C	U(24 hrs)
Minor or limited	S	
Streptococcal disease (group B streptococcus), neonatal	S	
Streptococcal disease (not group A or B) unless covered elsewhere	S	
Multidrug-resistant (see multidrug-resistant organisms)		
Syphilis		
Skin and mucous membrane, including congenital, primary, secondary	S	
Latent (tertiary) and seropositivity without lesions	S	
Tinea (fungus infection dermatophytosis, dermatomycosis, ringworm)	S	
Toxoplasmosis	S	
Tuberculosis		
Extrapulmonary, draining lesion (including scrofula)	S	
Extrapulmonary, meningitis	S	
Pulmonary, confirmed or suspected or laryngeal disease	A	F[c]
Skin-test positive with no evidence of current pulmonary disease	S	
Urinary tract infection (including pyelonephritis), with or without urinary catheter	S	
Wound infections		
Major[a]	C	DI
Minor or limited[b]	S	
Zoster (varicella-zoster)		
Localized in immunocompromised patient, disseminated	A, C	DI
Localized in normal patient	S	

TABLE 11-12 White Blood Cell Response to Infections

Leukocyte Response	Associated Infectious Process
Increase in neutrophils (neutrophilia)	Typical in many acute local and systemic infections caused by bacteria (especially pyogenic bacteria), rickettsia, some viruses, and a few protozoa
Decrease in neutrophils (neutropenia)	Frequent in salmonellosis, brucellosis, whooping cough, overwhelming bacterial infections, influenza, infectious mononucleosis, hepatitis A infection, mumps, rubella, rubeola, and some rickettsial and protozoan diseases
Increase in eosinophils (eosinophilia)	Frequent in allergic reactions, chronic skin disease, helminthic infections, and scarlet fever
Increase in lymphocytes (lymphocytosis)	Frequent in chickenpox, mumps, measles, infectious mononucleosis, influenza, whooping cough, syphilis, tuberculosis, salmonellosis, viral hepatitis, and viral pneumonia; sometimes in convalescent phase of acute bacterial infection
Increase in monocytes (monocytosis)	Common in tuberculosis, chickenpox, brucellosis, mumps, syphilis, and certain rickettsial diseases; may occur in certain viral and protozoan diseases and in convalescent phase of acute bacterial infections
Decrease in lymphocytes (lymphocytopenia)	Human immunodeficiency virus

patient's therapy. When an infection is suspected, culture specimens are obtained from the suspected site. In the patient with a fever of unknown origin, culture specimens typically are obtained from the blood, urine, sputum, and other possible sources of infection such as aspirates of body fluid, or intravenous catheter tips. It is imperative that these cultures be obtained before the initiation of antibiotic therapy because antibiotics can suppress any bacteria present causing inaccurate or false-negative culture results.

Cultures should be obtained in a manner that avoids contamination. Aseptic preparation of the culture site, observance of aseptic technique, and placement of specimens in an appropriate container are crucial factors to be observed in ensuring the best sample. Once obtained, the specimen must be properly stored and transported promptly to the laboratory. Each institution should have guidelines for the proper method of collecting and handling specimens for the laboratory. All specimens must be accompanied by the correct requisition and include the following information: (1) patient's name, (2) date and time of collection, (3) test requested, (4) type of specimen, (5) how the specimen was obtained (e.g., clean void or catheter urine, expectorated sputum, or tracheal aspirate), and (6) where the results are to be sent. A record of all tests is kept to avoid unnecessary duplication of tests.

Interpretation of laboratory results is sometimes difficult because of normal flora, which reside in a commensal (intimate) relationship with the host. The skin, upper respiratory tract, vagina, urethra, and bowel are examples of body sites in which normal bacterial flora can be found. The bacteria found vary from site to site, and knowledge of the normal flora is helpful in discerning the significance of laboratory culture results. It must be emphasized that laboratory results alone cannot be used to make diagnostic and therapeutic decisions. Rather, they are used in conjunction with the patient's clinical status to make appropriate diagnostic and therapeutic decisions.

Selection of an antibiotic on the basis of culture and sensitivity least disrupts the normal flora while providing effective control of the infecting organism. For an immediate response to a serious infection, a broad-spectrum antibiotic is chosen with activity against types of organisms identified in a Gram stain. Once the culture has grown, the organism has been identified and sensitivities have been determined, the spectrum of the antibiotic can be safely narrowed.

NURSING MANAGEMENT

ASSESSMENT

Health History and Physical Examination

Signs and symptoms of infection can be both local and systemic and vary with the phase of the infection (see p. 188), the agent responsible for the infection, and the site of the infection. (For details on host response to specific infectious disease, see the particular chapter that discusses the disease site.) Examples of signs and symptoms of infection in specific areas of the body that should be assessed for as part of the history and physical examination are listed in Box 11-5. Systemic signs and symptoms that should be assessed for include prodromal symptoms of weakness, headache, light-headedness, congestion, muscle aches, joint pain, decreased appetite, or malaise, as well as later signs such as fever, increased pulse rate, hypotension, altered mental status, or even jaundice, shock, confusion, and convulsions.

Of all the clinical symptoms mentioned, fever (pyrexia) is one of the most valuable diagnostic indicators of infection. Although not all fevers are the result of an infectious process, most persons with an infectious disease develop fever as a systemic response to the infectious agent.

None of the signs and symptoms present in localized or generalized infections is diagnostic by itself, as other disease processes can produce the same signs and symptoms; however, they are helpful clues in the diagnosis of a suspected infectious process.

BOX 11-5 Subjective and Objective Data Suggesting Infection

Localized Infection

Subjective	*Objective*
Pain	Inflammation
Tenderness	Edema
Warmth	Redness
Swelling	Warmth
Itching	Exudate or drainage
	Amount
	Color
	Consistency
	Odor

Respiratory Tract Infection

Subjective	*Objective*
Sore throat	Redness of throat
Congestion	Rales
Cough	Rhonchi
Sputum production	Cough
Chest pain	Type
Stuffy nose	Frequency
Runny nose	Sputum
	Amount
	Color
	Consistency
	Odor

Gastrointestinal Tract Infection

Subjective	*Objective*
Anorexia	Vomitus
Nausea	Frequency
Vomiting	Amount
Diarrhea	Color
	Consistency
	Odor

Gastrointestinal Tract Infection—cont'd

Subjective	*Objective*
	Diarrhea
	Frequency
	Amount
	Color
	Consistency
	Odor

Genitourinary Tract Infection

Subjective	*Objective*
Urgency	Frequency
Frequency	Amount
Burning or painful urination	Color
	Odor
Change in color or smell of urine	Purulent, foul discharge
	Presence of WBCs and bacteria
Flank or pelvic pain	Urinalysis
Discharge	Culture
Itching	

Generalized Infection

Subjective	*Objective*
Malaise	Fever
Muscle aches	Elevated WBC count
Headache	Hypotension
Weakness	Altered mental status
Joint pain	Confusion
Anorexia	Convulsions
	Shock
	Tachycardia

WBC, White blood cell.

NURSING DIAGNOSES

Nursing diagnoses are determined from analysis of patient data. Nursing diagnoses for the patient with an infection include:

Diagnostic Title	Possible Etiologic Factors
1. Acute or chronic pain	Inflammation, edema, circulating bacterial toxins
2. Hyperthermia	Release of endogenous pyrogens in response to an infectious agent
3. Fluid volume	Altered temperature regulation
4. Fatigue	Increased metabolic energy production
5. Knowledge: infection, treatment, and health-promotion techniques	Lack of exposure, lack of recall, or information misrepresentation

Other diagnoses are applicable, depending on the type and location of infection. Examples include a patient with osteomyelitis who would be at risk for altered mobility or a patient with meningitis who would be at risk for altered cerebral tissue perfusion. The patient is always at risk for developing a systemic infection.

EXPECTED PATIENT OUTCOMES

Expected patient outcomes for the patient with an infection may include but are not limited to:

1. Will report relief of discomforts of malaise, mylagia, and fever
2. Will return to normal temperature after defervescence
3. Will maintain adequate fluid volume for proper functioning
4. Will report decreased level of fatigue
5. Will verbalize understanding of rationale for diagnosis (e.g., radiologic examinations, cultures, and CBC) and treatment regimen

On the national level, the U.S. Department of Health and Human Services publishes an ongoing document that includes a list of goals for all Americans designed to improve the health of the nation as a whole. Goals related to this chapter from the most recent document, *Healthy People 2010,* may be found in the Healthy People 2010 box.[32]

Healthy People 2010

Goals Related To Infection Control

Although the last 100 years have seen a reduction in the incidence of infectious diseases (e.g., control of smallpox, diphtheria and polio) through development of vaccines, underimmunized groups still exist. The persistence of many vaccine-preventable infections remains a threat to public health. Without prevention of disease and the promotion of a healthy lifestyle, many consumers demand antibiotics for a cure. This leads to the increasing problem of antibiotic resistance. "Healthy People 2010" goals related to control of infection are:

- Reduce or eliminate indigenous cases of vaccine-preventable disease.
- Increase the proportion of providers who have measured the vaccination coverage levels among children in their practice population within the past 2 years.
- Increase the proportion of children who participate in fully operational population-based immunization registries.
- Reduce chronic hepatitis B virus infections in infants and young children (perinatal infections).
- Achieve and maintain effective vaccination coverage levels for universally recommended vaccines among young children.
- Maintain vaccination coverage levels for children in licensed day care facilities and children in kindergarten through first grade.
- Increase the proportion of young children and adolescents who receive all vaccines that have been recommended for universal administration for at least 5 years.
- Increase routine vaccination coverage levels for adolescents.
- Increase hepatitis B vaccine coverage among high-risk groups.
- Reduce hepatitis A.
- Reduce hepatitis C.
- Increase the proportion of persons with chronic hepatitis C infection identified by state and local health departments.
- Reduce hospitalization rates for immunization-preventable pneumonia and influenza.
- Increase the proportion of international travelers who receive recommended preventive services when traveling in areas of risk for select infectious diseases: hepatitis A, malaria, and typhoid.
- Increase the proportion of local health departments that have established culturally appropriate and linguistically competent community health promotion and disease prevention programs.
- Reduce invasive early onset group B streptococcal disease.
- Reduce the number of courses of antibiotics for ear infections for young children.
- Reduce the number of courses of antibiotics prescribed for the sole diagnosis of the common cold.
- Reduce hospital-acquired infections in patients in intensive care units.
- Reduce vaccine-associated adverse events.

By attaining these goals, the American public should be able to make significant progress in meeting the two overarching goals (increase quality and years of healthy life, and eliminate health disparities) by the year 2010.

From US Department of Health and Human Services: *Healthy People 2010: understanding and improving health,* Washington, DC, 2000, USDHHS.

INTERVENTIONS

1. Promoting Comfort

Both pharmacologic and nonpharmacologic methods of pain relief are indicated (see Chapter 12). Analgesics such as acetaminophen or nonsteroidal antiinflammatory agents (NSAIDs) are effective in reducing discomfort related to fever. NSAIDs decrease the inflammatory response. Both acetaminophen and NSAIDs may be used as antipyretics.

2. Promoting Normothermia

Fever is a protective response to pathogens. Treatment is focused on eradicating the causative organism from the body. Nursing interventions include administration of antipyretics and antibiotics to treat the underlying cause of infection. The patient should be monitored for therapeutic and adverse effects of the antibiotic. The nurse should make sure the causative organism is sensitive to the prescribed antibiotic. Superinfection is a side effect of antibiotic therapy and may occur with extended use of certain antibiotics.

Additional methods of reducing fever include use of hypothermia blankets, ice packs, and tepid water baths. The nurse should be careful not to cool the patient too quickly, as this can produce shivering. Shivering causes increased heat production and oxygen consumption. The use of hypothermia blankets should be discontinued when the patient's temperature is within 1 to 3 degrees of the desired temperature.

Vital signs should be monitored including an accurate assessment of core temperature. Seizures and a decreased level of consciousness are potential complications of fever. Dysrhythmias can be caused by dehydration. The patient should be bathed and given dry linen after defervescence.

3. Promoting Adequate Fluid Volume

Fever causes fluid loss from evaporation of body fluids and increased perspiration. Signs of dehydration include increased thirst, dry mucous membranes, and decreased skin turgor. Encouraging intake of oral fluids and possibly administering intravenous fluids are necessary to support circulating volume and tissue perfusion. The nurse should assess the degree of diaphoresis as the body attempts to increase heat loss by evaporation, conduction, and diffusion. Accurate record of intake and output is necessary to assess all sources of fluid loss.

4. Promoting Rest

The nurse should encourage adequate rest during the acute phase of infection. The patient should be encouraged to be as independent as possible. Together the nurse and patient should plan for increased levels of activity. Scheduling tests and activities when the patient is fully rested is beneficial.

5. Patient/Family Education

The patient and family should be informed of the purpose of treatment modalities. Education regarding medication is essential to prevent recurrence of infection and drug resistance. The importance of completing the entire course of antibiotic therapy to prevent reinfection should be stressed. Health promotion techniques such as hand washing and avoiding sources of infection should be included in the teaching plan.

Persons with infections frequently are cared for at home. The community health nurse often is asked to teach family members how to care for the patient and how to protect family members, friends, and neighbors. Many of the same principles of infection control apply in the home as in the hospital. Nurses should incorporate the information included in the Patient Teaching box into daily educational plans as an effort to reduce infection. Additional general principles for home care of persons with an infection are discussed here.

Hand washing is considered the most effective measure in preventing the spread of infection in the home. Hands should be washed before care and after contact with body substances (blood, urine, feces, sputum, vomitus, or wound drainage). Caregivers should wear a smock or coverall to protect their clothes. Gloves should be worn when handling body substances. Soiled dressings, used disposable gloves, and other disposable items that contain body substances should be put in plastic bags before being discarded in the trash. All liquid waste can be flushed down the toilet. Used needles and syringes should be put in a puncture-resistant plastic container or can, which is tightly closed before discarding in the trash. Disposable dishes are not required. Dishes and linen should be washed in hot soapy water. A cup of bleach should be added to the detergent to disinfect laundry soiled with blood. Blood and body substance spills should be cleaned up using an effective household disinfectant. If gloves are not available, plastic bags can be worn to protect the caregiver's hands. All persons should be taught to cover the nose and mouth when coughing. In general, it is not considered necessary for the caregiver to wear a mask in the home.

EVALUATION

To evaluate effectiveness of nursing interventions, compare patient behaviors with those stated in the expected patient outcomes. Achievement of outcomes is successful if the patient with infection:

1. States discomfort is relieved.
2. Maintains core temperature within normal range for 24 hours.

Patient Teaching

Information To Be Included in Public Education Programs To Reduce Infection

1. Vaccines that are available to prevent infection
2. Need to report symptoms of generalized infections that persist more than 24 hours (see Table 11-9)
3. Rationale for completion of entire course of prescribed antibiotics; concept of developing resistance
4. Need to report signs of antibiotic allergy immediately: itching, rash, and respiratory swelling
5. Rationale for reserving antibiotic use for severe infections; avoid disrupting normal body flora

3. Maintains adequate fluid volume.
4. Participates in usual levels of activity.

5a. Describes rationale for diagnostic examinations.
5b. Completes prescribed course of antibiotics.
5c. Verbalizes understanding of treatment regimen.

Critical Thinking Questions

1. A 65-year-old patient with type 2 diabetes is admitted for a femoral popliteal bypass graft for impaired circulation to his left lower extremity. Two months before this admission, he was discharged after treatment for an infected left foot ulcer, which grew MRSA and was colonized with VRE. What precautions would you take in planning care for this patient?
2. A patient is admitted with a persistent lung lesion in the left upper lobe. Lung cancer is suspected. A bronchoscopy is performed and acid-fast bacillus cultures subsequently grow *Mycobacterium tuberculosis.* The patient had not been in isolation before these results. What action would you take regarding possible exposure of other patients and personnel?
3. A patient is admitted for chemotherapy for treatment of acute myelocytic leukemia. He has a right subclavian catheter triple lumen catheter for infusion of his chemotherapy and total parenteral nutrition. The site is inspected daily. The nurse tells the patient the line must be changed because of induration at the site. Explain why this may have occurred and possible consequences.
4. A patient brings her 5-year-old child in for a routine examination. When completing the health history, the nurse finds that the child has never received any immunizations. The patient states, "My mom told me those shots don't work; they just hurt the kids." How would you respond to this? What would be included in your plan of care based on this information?

References

1. Abbas A, Lichtman A, Pober J: *Cellular and molecular immunology,* Philadelphia, 1994, WB Saunders.
2. American Hospital Association: *OSHA's final bloodborne pathogen standard: a special briefing,* Chicago, 1992, The Association.
3. Bennett JV, Brachman PS, editors: *Hospital infections,* Boston, 1992, Little, Brown.
4. Carroll P: Preventing nosocomial pneumonia, *RN* 61:6, 1998.
5. Centers for Disease Control and Prevention: Hepatitis A: new focus for immunization guidelines, *Consultant* 40:1, 2000.
6. Centers for Disease Control and Prevention: Protecting more patients from varicella: updated guidelines, *Consultant* 39:8, 1999.
7. Clerici M et al: Cytokine production patterns in cervical intraepithelial neoplasia: association with papillomavirus infection, *J Natl Cancer Inst* 89:3, 1997.
8. Cohen ML: Epidemiology of drug resistance: implications for a post-antimicrobial era, *Science* 257:1050, 1992.
9. Committee on Infectious Diseases: Prevention of poliomyelitis: recommendations for use of only inactivated poliovirus vaccine for routine immunization, *Pediatrics* 104:6, 1999.
10. Garner JS, Hospital Infection Control Practices Advisory Committee: Guidelines for isolation precautions in hospitals. Part I. Evolution of isolation practices. Part II. 11.11. Recommendations for isolation precautions in hospitals, *Am J Infect Control* 22:24, 1996.
11. Gindler J et al: Successful immunization for children and adults, *Patient Care* 31:9, 1997.

12. Goldman L, Bennett JC: *Cecil textbook of medicine,* ed 21, Philadelphia, 2000, WB Saunders.
13. Hospital Infection Control Practices Advisory Committee: Recommendations for preventing the spread of vancomycin resistance, *Infect Control Hosp Epidemiol* 16:105, 1995.
14. http://www.cdc.gov/nip/
15. http://www.nursingmanagement.com
16. Jagger J, Perry J: Safeguarding sharps disposal, *Nurs 2000* 30:10, 2000.
17. Lambright Eckler JA: Stethoscope safety tips, *Nurs* 27:10, 1997.
18. Marinella MA et al: The stethoscope: a potential source of nosocomial infection?, *Arch Intern Med* 157:7, 1997.
19. Martin M: Bloodborne pathogens, *Occup Hazards* 63:4, 2001.
20. Massey S: Influencing handwashing behavior, *Nurse Pract* 25:2, 2000.
21. Mayhall CG, editor: *Hospital epidemiology and infection control,* Baltimore, 1996, Williams & Wilkins.
22. Mayone-Ziomek JM: Handwashing in healthcare, *Dermatol Nurs* 10:3, 1998.
23. McMillan G: Minimizing the threat of nosocomial infection, *J Am Acad Physicians Assistants* 14:1, 2001.
24. Noskin GA et al: Persistent contamination of fabric-covered furniture by vancomycin-resistant enterococci: implications for upholstery selection in hospitals, *Am J Infect Control* 28:4, 2000.
25. Pearson ML, Hospital Infection Control Practices Advisory Committee: Guideline for prevention of intravascular device-related infections, *Infect Control Hosp Epidemiol* 17:438, 1996.
26. Pittet D et al: Compliance with handwashing in a teaching hospital, *Ann Intern Med* 130:2, 1999.
27. Pugliese G: Medical news: infection control indicators in 1996, *Infect Control Hosp Epidemiol* 17(1):81, 1996.
28. Schmitt BD: Immunization reactions, *McKesson clinical reference systems:* pediatric advisor 2001.2.
29. Sheff B: VRE & MRSA: putting bad bugs out of business, *Nurs Manage* 30:6, 1999.
30. Soule BM, Larson EL, Preston GA: *Infections and nursing practice: prevention and control,* St Louis, 1995, Mosby.
31. Tenover FC, Hughes JM: The challenges of emerging infectious diseases: development and spread of multiply-resistant bacterial pathogens, *JAMA* 275:300, 1996.
32. U.S. Department of Health and Human Services: *Healthy People 2010: understanding and improving health,* Washington, DC, 2000, USDHHS.
33. Wenzel RP, editor: *Prevention and control of nosocomial infections,* Baltimore, 1993, Williams & Wilkins.
34. Zaragoza M et al: Handwashing with soap or alcoholic solutions? A randomized clinical trial of its effectiveness, *Am J Infect Control* 27:3, 1999.

12 Pain

Judith H. Watt-Watson, Michael McGillion

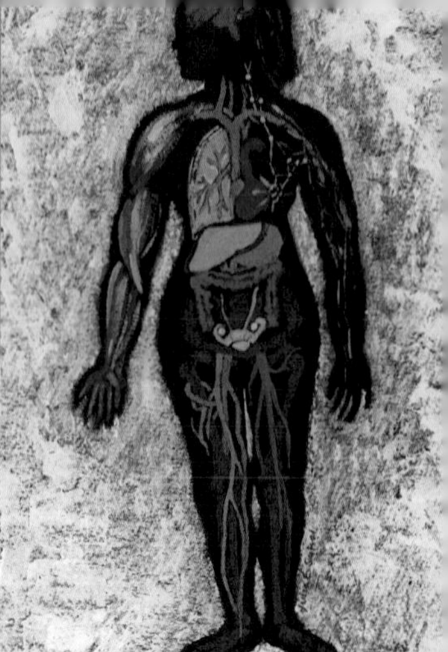

Objectives

After studying this chapter, the learner should be able to:

1. Describe some common misbeliefs about pain management.
2. Describe the physiology of pain and related theories of pain transmission.
3. Compare factors that influence perception of and response to pain.
4. Differentiate between acute and chronic pain.
5. Compare pain assessment tools used in clinical practice.
6. Describe pharmacologic and nonpharmacologic approaches to pain management.
7. Identify five nursing interventions for pain management.
8. Explain the purpose and methods of the team approach for chronic pain management.

NATURE OF THE PROBLEM

Pain relief is a management problem for many patients, their families, and the health professionals caring for them. Although pain is experienced by everyone to some degree, responses to it are unique for each person. Difficulties in recognizing and understanding someone else's pain are clinically well known. The International Association for the Study of Pain[31] has defined pain as an unpleasant sensory and emotional experience associated with actual or potential tissue damage or described in terms of such damage. Pain therefore is multidimensional and entirely subjective. With verbal children or adults, only the person experiencing the pain can describe or evaluate it. Pain can be evoked by a multiplicity of stimuli, but the reaction to it cannot be measured objectively. Pain is a learned experience that is influenced by the entire life situation of each person.

McCaffery and Pasero's definition[28] that pain is "whatever and whenever the person says it is," has changed practice by focusing health professionals' attention on the subjectivity of pain. Patients' self-reports about their pain are the key to effective management. However, we now realize that interpreting this definition at the simplest level may cause problems. Patients do not always admit to pain. They do not necessarily know how and when to tell us that they are hurting and/or they expect to have severe pain, so they are not going to complain. Patients may also not differentiate between pain and what the pain means to them, that is, suffering. Therefore the focus on the individuality of pain in both of these definitions underlines the importance of careful listening and valuing of patient information to understand the patient's pain experience as completely as possible.

Pain accompanies many disorders, as well as some therapies. It is a sensation that is frequently feared by persons undergoing surgery. Although some persons with cancer do not experience pain, it is one of the major concerns people have about cancer.

Relief of pain and discomfort is a major nursing objective and one that requires skill in both the art and science of nursing. Knowledge about concepts related to pain, data collection, and useful therapies is essential. Sensitivity and empathy, trying to understand what the person is experiencing, are important components of a systematic approach to the patient in pain. Too often management decisions are made without valid assessment and evaluation, including sufficient input from patients. Consequently, pain management is ineffective.

Pain is now referred to as the fifth vital sign. The new pain management standards from the Joint Commission on Accreditation of Healthcare Organizations[20] (JCAHO) (http://www.jcaho.org) and the Canadian Pain Society (CPS) Position Statement on Pain Relief[50] both emphasize that patients have a right to the best pain relief possible and that measures to prevent or reduce acute pain are a priority. The JCAHO Statement on Pain Management[20] includes the following directives:

1. Inform patients at the time of their initial evaluation that relief of pain is an important part of their care and that health providers need to respond quickly to reports of pain.
2. Ask patients on initial evaluation and as part of regular assessments about presence, quality, and intensity of pain and use the patient's self-report as the primary indicator of pain.

3. Work together with the patient and other health care providers to establish a goal for pain relief and develop and implement a plan to achieve that goal.
4. Review and modify the plan of care for patients who have unrelieved pain.

The Canadian Pain Society's management principles in its Position Paper[50] are similar:

1. Unrelieved acute pain complicates recovery.

   Unrelieved pain after surgery or injury results in more complications, longer hospital stay, greater disability, and potentially long-term pain.
2. Routine assessment is essential for effective management, including patient's self-report where possible, to minimize or prevent pain.

   Pain is a subjective and highly variable experience. Therefore patients' self-report of pain should be used whenever possible. For patients unable to report pain, a nonverbal assessment method must be used. Health professionals have a responsibility to assess pain routinely, to believe patients' pain reports, to document pain reports, and to intervene to prevent pain.
3. The best pain management involves patients, families, and health professionals, where patient-families are encouraged to communicate the severity of pain and health professionals are knowledgeable about pain relief options.

   Patients and families must be informed that they have a right to the best pain relief possible and are encouraged to communicate the severity of their pain.

   Patients, families, and health professionals need to understand pain management strategies, including nonpharmacologic techniques and the appropriate use of opioids.

ETIOLOGY

Pain results from a variety of causes, and its trajectories have different patterns. Some patients may experience both acute and persistent pain depending on the complexity of the problem. Acute pain is usually short-lived with a known cause or pathologic process. Trauma, infection, inflammation, diagnostic tests, surgeries, and treatments are common sources of acute pain. Recurrent acute pain can occur in people who experience headaches, dysmenorrhea, arthritis, sickle cell anemia, cancer, or inflammatory bowel disease. Chronic pain is defined as pain that persists beyond the usual time for healing to occur.[31] The term is usually used to describe pain that has been present for more than 3 months. Chronic pain may occur with progressive diseases such as cancer, acquired immunodeficiency syndrome (AIDS), sickle cell anemia, and multiple sclerosis and with neuropathic pain syndromes such as postherpetic neuralgia. Some patients have idiopathic chronic pain for which the cause is not known.

Unnecessary pain can result from incomplete pain assessments or treatments based on assumptions rather than on patient data. Regardless of the etiology of pain, the foundation for effective pain management is to believe that all pain is real and that malingerers (people who deliberately lie about their pain) are rare (fewer than 2%). Patients' self-reports of their pain are critical to the choice of strategies and the evaluation of the effectiveness of interventions. It is important to recognize that patients in pain will not necessarily ask for help until they are in severe pain,[52] and they may use words such as "pressure" or "soreness" instead of "pain."

Both children and elderly adults frequently experience unrelieved pain because health professionals incorrectly assume that their age minimizes the pain experience.[49] Careful observation, especially of facial expressions at rest and during movement, is particularly important with infants and with cognitively impaired elders. Instruments that are clinically easy to use are now available to help assess pain in vulnerable populations unable to verbally communicate pain.[18,33]

Unrelieved acute pain has numerous negative consequences. Postoperative pain can cause cardiovascular, pulmonary, and gastrointestinal (GI) complications.[4,23,25,36] Atelectasis after surgery has been found to be greater in patients with higher pain intensity.[40] Moreover, early unrelieved postoperative pain for thoracotomy patients was the only factor that significantly predicted pain 18 months later in a major study.[22] Both the CPS and JCAHO have emphasized the importance of effective pain management to meet managed care demands for earlier patient mobilization, reduced hospital stays, and reduced costs. Most important of all is research that suggests that early treatment of acute pain before it begins, when possible, may prevent future long-term pain.[21]

EPIDEMIOLOGY

Pain is a common reason for seeking help from health care professionals. Millions of patients have surgery every year, and unrelieved pain continues to be reported for the majority of patients after surgery. Although 90% of cancer pain can be controlled, about 40% to 80% of cancer patients report moderate to severe pain.[38] Unfortunately, people in a variety of settings continue to experience considerable pain in spite of effective treatment options.

From Marks and Sachar's[27] findings to the present,[52] research repeatedly has demonstrated that significant numbers of hospitalized patients experience moderate to severe pain unrelieved by treatment.[31] Contributing factors include inadequate knowledge and problematic attitudes of physicians and nurses, which have been well documented.[7,8,10] Although health professionals more recently have supported the principle of pain relief, this goal does not appear to have significantly altered practice. Health professionals either have not recognized unrelieved pain or have tolerated poor pain relief as the norm. Many patients have not been asked by health professionals about their pain, or discrepancies have been documented between patients' pain ratings and ratings by health professionals.[10,29,52] This problematic communication is compounded if patients expect to have pain while hospitalized or are reluctant to ask staff members for help.[52] Some commonly held misbeliefs influence our practice and may contribute to this ineffective pain management (Box 12-1).[49] These misbeliefs are crucial to recognize and correct because they influence our approaches to both the assessment and management of pain.

Minimal or no pain should be the goal of pain management. A hospital admission should not automatically mean a pain experience for any patient, including older adults, children, and infants. Patterns of pain intensity vary, and the diagnosis and/or type of surgery is not an effective basis for determining the amount of pain the person is experiencing or the analgesic required. Although not all pain can be eliminated, the use of multiple modalities usually can decrease the intensity to at least the minimal range.

Pain is a complex experience, and multiple strategies are more effective than single-modality treatment in alleviating pain. Incorrect beliefs about analgesic administration, particularly opioids, frequently result in the undermedication of patients.[52,53]

It is difficult to understand and recognize another person's pain. Therefore it is crucial to gain as much information about the patient as possible rather than making assumptions about what may be happening.[45] The nurse must be vigilant about personal expectations, biases, and factors that may interfere with the ability to deliver individualized nursing care. One study found that among 180 patients who underwent an appendectomy, patients who were older and of an ethnic minority (Asian, African-American, or Hispanic) received significantly smaller doses of opioids postoperatively than did Caucasian patients.[29]

PHYSIOLOGY

Theories of Pain

Various theorists through the centuries have tried to explain pain[30] (Box 12-2). Aristotle's perception of pain as an emotion or "passion of the soul" was rejected by specificity theorists who accepted Descartes' separation of the body from the mind. Specificity theorists believed that pain messages were carried in a specific straight-line transmission from receptors in the periphery to a central pain center; therefore, pain was considered to equal the degree of injury. Pattern theorists questioned this premise because it was evident that people responded differently to the same stimulus. Instead, they proposed that patterns of impulses were more important than specificity in explaining pain. Although these theories contributed to understanding pain mechanisms, all had major

BOX 12-1 Misbeliefs About Pain

Misbeliefs are incorrect beliefs that are accepted as truths and frequently used to guide practice.

Misbeliefs About the Pain Experience

1. Patients should expect to have pain in the hospital.
2. Obvious pathologic conditions, test results, and type of surgery determine the existence and intensity of pain.
3. People who are in pain always have observable signs.
4. Chronic pain is not as serious a problem for people as acute pain.
5. Patient self-reports of pain are not accurate.
6. All patients will tell us when they are in pain and will use the term *pain.*

Misbeliefs About Pain Management

1. One pain treatment or strategy is all that is needed.
2. Addiction is a major problem with people taking opioids for pain.
3. Patient-controlled analgesia is not appropriate for oral analgesia.
4. Patients must demonstrate pain before receiving analgesic medication.
5. People who respond to placebos do not have real pain.
6. Injectable opioids are the most effective.
7. Respiratory depression is a common and severe side effect of opioids in all patients.

Misbeliefs About Pain and Age

Children, Including Infants

1. Children do not experience pain.
2. Children cannot accurately describe their pain.
3. Children should not be given opioids for pain.
4. Opioids are best given by the intramuscular route.
5. Children forget painful experiences.
6. Children who are playing or sleeping do not have pain.
7. Parents should not stay with children during painful procedures.

The Older Adult

1. Pain is a normal part of getting older; pain sensation decreases with age and therefore can never be very intense.
2. Opioids are too potent for elderly patients.
3. Pain cannot be assessed with elderly patients who are cognitively impaired.

From Watt-Watson J: Misbeliefs about pain. In Watt-Watson J, Donovan M, editors: *Pain management: nursing perspective,* St Louis, 1992, Mosby, pp 36-58.

BOX 12-2 Theories of Pain Transmission

Affect Theory

Pain is an emotion and its intensity depends on the meaning of the part involved.
Limitations: Does not include physiologic aspects.

Specific Theory

Specific pain receptors project impulses over neural pain pathways to the brain.
Limitations: Does not account for psychologic aspects of pain perception and variability of response.

Pattern Theory

Pain results from combined effects of stimulus intensity and summations of impulse in the dorsal horn of the spinal cord.
Limitations: Does not account for psychologic aspects.

Gate Control Theory

Pain impulses can be controlled by a gating mechanism in the substantia gelatinosa of the dorsal horn of the spinal cord to permit or inhibit transmission. Gating factors include effect of impulses transmitted over fast or slow conducting nerve fibers and effects of descending impulses from the brainstem and cortex.

limitations. Melzack and Wall built on the relationships between these theories in proposing their gate control theory (GCT) in 1965. The GCT contributed considerably to our current understanding of the transduction, transmission, modulation, and perception of the pain process.[16]

According to the GCT,[29,44] pain is not a simple, sensory experience but a complex integration of sensory, affective, and cognitive dimensions. Pain involves dynamic interactions between ascending and descending neural systems along with ongoing balancing of inhibitory-excitatory mechanisms. Pain perception and responses to pain are not predictable but vary with each person and experience. This variability results from the modulation of noxious (painful) input at several levels of the central nervous system.

Excitatory stimuli, both painful and innocuous, are converted into an action potential that stimulates the primary afferent neurons in the periphery. The message is then transmitted by these neurons to converge onto common second-order neurons in the dorsal horn of the spinal cord. The substantia gelatinosa (SG) in the dorsal horn is the major site where modulation of painful stimuli results from complex excitatory and inhibitory processes acting as a "gate." The GCT postulates that increased activity in the large, non-nociceptive primary afferent neurons (A-beta), such as that produced with massage or transcutaneous electrical nerve stimulation, can reduce pain messages carried by the small, nociceptive afferent neurons (A-delta and C) to cells in the SG.[44,54] As a result, further transmission of the pain message is inhibited. However, if pain impulses reach a critical level without being blocked, they will be transmitted to second-order neurons in the SG. Pain impulses then are transmitted by nociceptive pathways, which ascend from the second-order neurons to the thalamus and cerebral cortex. These ascending tracts transmit sensory-discriminative data about the quality and intensity of pain, contribute to the motivational-affective dimension about the meaning of pain, and activate descending inhibitory systems. Pain transmission can be blocked by descending inhibition involving neurotransmitters such as enkephalin, serotonin, and norepinephrine.

Impulses sent to the brainstem, the center for motivational-affective and sensory-discriminative actions, can influence cognition or evaluation in the cortex. Impulses are then sent from the cortex back to the SG via corticospinal pathways to inhibit or permit passage of pain impulses. Note in Table 12-1 the various factors that can open or close the gate.

Melzack and Wall[30] emphasized that noxious stimuli enter an already active nervous system that is a compilation of past experience, culture, anticipation, and emotion. Cognitive processes related to the meaning of the pain act selectively on sensory input and motivation to influence pain transmission via the descending tracts to the dorsal horn. As a result, the amount and quality of pain are determined by individual factors such as previous pain experiences and one's concept of the cause of pain and its consequences. Cultural values can influence how one feels and responds to pain. Therefore pain is a highly personal experience and more than just a painful stimulus. For example, there is no one standard response to surgery, and the same pain-relieving intervention may not be effective for all patients.

The Pain Process

The process by which a painful stimulus is perceived involves the four steps of transduction, transmission, modulation, and perception.[16] Transduction and transmission involve processing the pain message from the nociceptors to the spinal cord. Modulation in the spinal cord will determine whether the stimuli will be perceived as pain.

Transduction

Transduction, or receptor activation, involves converting the painful stimulus into an impulse that is carried from the periphery to the central nervous system (CNS). The pain receptors, or nociceptors, are free nerve endings of unmyelinated or lightly myelinated afferent neurons. Nociceptors are located extensively in the skin and mucosa and less frequently in selected deeper structures, such as viscera, joints, arterial walls, and bile ducts. Nociceptors respond to harmful or potentially harmful stimuli that may be chemical, thermal, or mechanical.

The noxious stimulus creates an action potential that activates the nerve fiber to send the impulse to the CNS. Chemical stimuli for pain include histamines, bradykinin, prostaglandins, and acids, some of which are released by damaged tissues. Anoxic tissue also releases chemicals that lead to pain. Tissue

TABLE 12-1 Factors Affecting Pain Transmission Based on the Gate Control Theory

Site	Close Gate (Block Transmission)	Open Gate (Permit Transmission)
Fibers	Impulses transmitted by large, fast, myelinated A-beta and A-alpha fibers	Impulses transmitted by slow, small, A-delta and C fibers
	Stimulation of unaffected skin areas (e.g., massage)	Stimulation of affected skin areas (e.g., sun-burned skin)
Brainstem (descending pathway)	Endorphin effect	No endorphin effect
	Sufficient or maximum sensory input (e.g., distraction)	Insufficient sensory input (e.g., monotony)
Cortex	Past experiences	Past experiences
	Feelings of pain control	Anxiety

swelling may cause pain by creating pressure (mechanical stimulation) on nociceptors in adjoining tissues.

Transmission

Pain impulses are transmitted to the spinal cord by two types of fibers: thinly myelinated faster-conducting A-delta fibers and slower-conducting unmyelinated C fibers. Easily localized pain that may be described as "sharp" or "pricking" is transmitted by the A-delta fibers. An example of this type of pain is that felt by a needle prick. More diffuse pain that may be described as "burning," "dull," or "aching" results from impulses transmitted by the C fibers. Impulses transmitted on the larger diameter myelinated A-beta and A-alpha fibers have an inhibitory effect on those transmitted over A-delta and C fibers.

The primary afferent nerve fibers enter the spinal cord through the dorsal root and synapse onto second-order neurons within six interconnected levels or laminae in the dorsal horn (Figure 12-1).

Lamina II comprises an area called the substantia gelatinosa, which is the major site for modulation of nociceptive input. Substance P is released at synapses in the SG and is thought to be a major neurotransmitter of pain impulses.

Secondary neurons synapse with projection neurons in the spinal cord. The pain impulses then cross the spinal cord over interneurons and connect with ascending spinal pathways. The most important ascending pathways for nociceptive impulses located in the ventral half of the spinal cord are the spinothalamic tract (STT) and the spinoreticular tract (SRT). The STT is a discriminative system and conveys information about the nature and location of the stimulus to the thalamus and then to the cortex for interpretation. Impulses transmitted over the SRT, which goes to the brainstem and part of the thalamus, activate the autonomic and limbic (motivational-affective) responses. The ultimate perception of pain is dependent on modulation of neuronal impulses in ascending pathways in relation to the activation of descending inhibitory systems.

Modulation

Discovery of receptors in the brain to which opiate compounds bind led to the discovery of two naturally occurring endogenous morphine-like pentapeptides (5-amino acid compounds), met-enkephalin and leu-enkephalin. These enkephalins are classified as endorphins (from the terms endogenous and morphine). Other endorphins, such as beta-endorphin, also have been identified. The endorphins are thought to suppress pain by (1) acting presynaptically to inhibit release of the neurotransmitter substance P or (2) acting postsynaptically to inhibit conduction of pain impulses.[30] The endorphins are found in high concentration in the basal ganglia of the brain, thalamus, midbrain, and dorsal horn of the spinal cord.

Descending spinal pathways, from the thalamus through the midbrain and medulla to the dorsal horns of the spinal cord, conduct nociceptive inhibitory impulses. Serotonin, norepinephrine, and endorphins are released by descending fibers and inhibit the release of neurotransmitters. Therefore

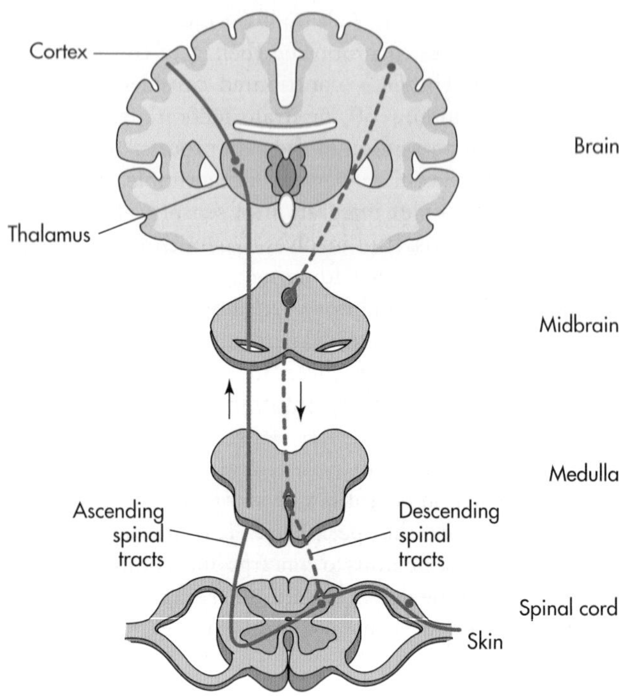

Figure 12-1 Pathways of pain transmission to and from cortex.

nociceptive stimuli will not be transmitted to second-order neurons. Treatment modalities such as electrical stimulation by means of transcutaneous electrical nerve stimulators can activate opiate analgesia. Acupuncture is also thought to use the opiate pathways.

Perception

Pain is multidimensional and highly variable. Pain is a subjective, very personal experience that can be influenced by factors such as the meaning of the situation that is unique to each person. Tolerance to pain varies within and between individuals experiencing the same noxious stimulus. Responses to pain are influenced by individuals' interpretation of pain and its meaning to them.

Pain Tolerance. Across cultures there is great uniformity in the minimum level of noxious stimulus that people report as pain.[9] This level is called the pain detection threshold.[30] It is primarily biologic in nature and is relatively consistent within an individual, relative to the location and type of stimulus. In contrast, pain tolerance involves the cognitive-affective dimension of pain, is very subjective, and varies widely within and between individuals and cultures.

Pain tolerance is the maximum degree of pain intensity a person is willing to experience and can be increased or decreased by numerous factors (Box 12-3). Tolerance can vary between different individuals in the same situation and in the same individual in differing situations. For example, a woman with a tender breast lump may complain of more pain if her mother died of breast cancer. Individual persons can respond in many ways to any level of pain intensity, and pain tolerance is influenced by the meaning of the pain to the individual. It is important to remember that there is no right or wrong way

BOX 12-3 Factors That Influence Pain Tolerance

Increase Tolerance	Decrease Tolerance
Alcohol	Fatigue
Drugs	Anger
Hypnosis	Boredom
Warmth	Anxiety
Rubbing	Persistent pain
Distraction	Stress
Faith	Depression
Strong beliefs	

to experience pain, and the pain experience is subjective and unique to each person.

The Meaning of Pain. Pain has different meanings for each person and may differ for the same person at different times. Pain initially has an important protective function by warning the person of impending tissue damage. However, with persistent pain, meanings can change. Some examples of the meanings of pain include:

- Harm or damage
- Complication, such as infection
- New illness
- Recurrence of illness
- Fatal disease
- Increasing disability
- Loss of mobility
- Aging
- Healing
- Necessary for cure
- Punishment for sins
- Challenge
- Appreciation for suffering of others
- Something to be tolerated

Numerous factors influence the meaning of pain for an individual, including age, gender, sociocultural background, environment, and past or present experiences.[35] For example, two women may be experiencing pain from a fractured leg. To the 75-year-old woman living alone with few social contacts, pain may be interpreted on the basis of fear of aging and inability to maintain her independent living status. The 28-year-old lawyer might interpret the pain as an expected nuisance, with the realization that healing will occur and she can get back to work soon.

Response to Pain. People respond to pain in different ways, depending on their perception of the pain, including what it means to them. Some may be fearful, apprehensive, and anxious, whereas others are tolerant and optimistic. Some weep, moan, scream, beg for relief or help, threaten to destroy themselves, thrash about in bed, or move about aimlessly when in severe pain; others lie quietly in bed and may only close their eyes, grit their teeth, bite their lips, clench their hands, or perspire profusely when experiencing pain.

On the basis of their cultural beliefs some persons have been taught to endure severe pain without reacting outwardly, whereas others are taught to be very expressive when experiencing any degree of pain. People whose health beliefs and education emphasize prevention tend to accept pain as a warning to seek help, expecting that the cause of pain will be found and cured.

BOX 12-4 Factors That Influence Responses to Pain

- Meaning of pain to individual person
- Degree of pain perception
- Past experience
- Cultural values
- Social expectations
- Physical and mental health
- Parental attitudes toward pain
- Setting in which pain occurs
- Fear, anxiety
- Usual way of responding to stressors
- Age
- Preparation for pain context
- Health professionals' responses

Researchers for many years have attempted to examine how ethnicity influences patients' pain behavior. Research has been inconclusive because of methodology issues as to what differences exist and how they impact pain perception and response.[22,33] Cleeland[9] examined the relationship between standardized self-report numerical scales of pain intensity and pain interference with cancer patients from several countries. His findings indicated cross-cultural similarity in the self-report ratings. All samples used activity and affect to report how patients reacted to pain. What differed was the focus of interference (e.g., work and activities versus mood and relationships). Therefore it is important to recognize that ethnic groups may differ in their perception and response to pain, including whether they will approach the caregiver for help. However, there are also many variations within groups, and it is important not to stereotype any group.

Numerous factors influence individuals' responses to pain (Box 12-4). One cannot predict how any given person will respond, and value judgments should not be made concerning how a patient responds. It is important for health professionals to recognize misbeliefs about expected pain responses that prevent effective pain management.

PATHOPHYSIOLOGY

The pathophysiology of pain includes the processes that are thought to contribute to pathophysiologic or persistent pain, i.e., how the nervous system is changed with repeated noxious stimuli. The duration and site of pain determine its clinical manifestations.

Prolonged Pain

Acute pain results when the sensory endings of primary afferent nerve fibers are activated by strong noxious stimuli, and the brain interprets the input carried by them as painful. This pain is called *nociceptive* as it results from the activity of healthy, intact nociceptive afferent fibers that are aroused only by intense stimuli. Prolonged pain that is evoked by repeated or sustained noxious stimuli that sensitize and change the nervous system is called *neuropathic* pain.[11] Three key processes help to explain prolonged or chronic pain problems.[11]

Peripheral sensitization occurs when tissue trauma or infection causes sensitization of peripheral nociceptors so that weak, nonpainful stimuli cause pain. An example is sunburn. This process is thought to be mediated by inflammatory mediators such as bradykinins and prostaglandins. Intervention strategies to decrease the inflammatory response, such as ice, nonsteroidal antiinflammatory drugs (NSAIDs), and sometimes immobilization of the area using a splint or cast, are essential. Peripheral neuropathic pain can arise when otherwise intact sensory neurons become hyperexcitable and begin to discharge at abnormal (ectopic) locations along their course. The most important locations of this discharge are at the sites of nerve injury and the associated dorsal root ganglion. Postherpetic neuralgia after shingles is an example. Prevention using early diagnosis of acute herpes zoster, vaccination to prevent chickenpox, and antiviral therapy for acute zoster have become current practices. Central sensitization involves a progressively increased response to repeated noxious stimuli and hyperexcitability in the dorsal horn (windup). As a result, weak, nonpainful stimuli can cause pain by central amplification (allodynia). For example, surgery can cause central sensitization that increases postoperative pain intensity and the need for analgesia. Therefore perioperative analgesic strategies, including opioids, regional anesthesia, and preemptive analgesia (see Chapter 18) are thought to reduce this sensitization.[43] Patient-controlled analgesia after surgery helps patients prevent or maintain minimal pain levels and also prevents this sensitization. Central amplification is thought to involve *N*-methyl-daspartate (NMDA) receptors, and NMDA antagonist drugs such as ketamine and dextromethorphan may help to reduce this.[5]

Longevity of Pain

There are two types of pain syndromes that may occur separately or together: acute and chronic. Unfortunately, many health care professionals do not make this differentiation and provide care for the person experiencing chronic pain as though it were acute pain. There are differences between acute and chronic pain (Table 12-2), and the approaches to pain relief are usually different, although some of the same techniques may be used.

Acute Pain

Acute pain is essentially a transient episode and informs the person that something is wrong. The onset is usually sudden from a perceived cause, and the painful areas can generally be well identified.

Sudden severe pain activates the autonomic nervous system, which may produce signs of sympathetic overactivity. These signs include tachycardia, increased blood pressure, pupillary dilation, diaphoresis, and stimulation of adrenal medullary secretion. In some situations, such as with severe visceral pain of sudden onset, vasodilation may occur with a subsequent fall in blood pressure and shock. Continuous painful stimulation can also produce a steadily maintained reflex contraction of adjacent or distant muscles, such as abdominal rigidity in persons with intraabdominal pain.

Acute pain is commonly accompanied by increased muscle tension and anxiety, both of which may contribute to increased perception of pain (Figure 12-2). If the pain is moderate or severe, overt physiologic and behavioral signs facilitate assessment of the pain. The person usually seeks pain relief.

Chronic Pain

Chronic pain persists beyond the usual time for healing and is often present clinically beyond 4 weeks. Chronic pain may begin as acute pain but then persists (e.g., full-thickness burns), or the onset may be so insidious that the person cannot state specifically when it was first experienced. The source of the pain may be unknown or impossible to determine, such as intractable pain associated with some cancers. The pain sensation can be more diffuse than acute pain so the person is unable to identify a specific pain site. Chronic pain is a major health problem with economic and social implications for

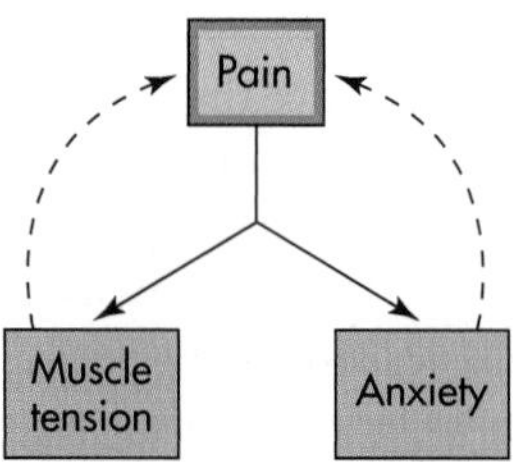

Figure 12-2 Acute pain.

TABLE 12-2 Comparison of Acute and Chronic Pain

Characteristic	Acute Pain	Chronic Pain
Onset	Usually sudden	May be sudden or develop insidiously
Duration	Transient (up to 3 months)	Prolonged (months to years)
Pain localization	Pain vs. nonpain areas generally well identified	Pain vs. nonpain areas less well identified; intensity becomes more difficult to evaluate (change in sensation)
Clinical signs	Signs of sympathetic overactivity (such as increased blood pressure)	Usually no change in vital signs (adaptation)
Purpose	Warning that something is wrong	Meaningless; no purpose
Pattern	Self-limiting or readily corrected	Continuous or intermittent; intensity may vary or remain constant
Prognosis	Likelihood of eventual complete relief	Complete relief usually not possible

both society and the approximately 25% to 30% of the population who suffer from it.[6]

Chronic pain is characterized by irritability (often compounded by insomnia), which leads to decreasing interests and isolation from friends and family.[51] Added to this is the centering of the person's life on the pain experience, with increasing feelings of helplessness and hopelessness as the pain persists. Ultimately the person may withdraw from social interactions (Figure 12-3). Responses to chronic pain can vary, and the unique pattern for each person and family needs to be considered.

The patient's world centers on ways to modify the pain experience. These patients undergo tremendous disruptions in many aspects of their usual activities, including work, family roles, socialization, sleep, and leisure.[51] Some patients go from one physician to another seeking pain relief, which takes time, effort, and money. Even as they seek relief, they often lose faith in the ability of anyone to help them. The lack of continuity of care augments the problem. Physicians often feel helpless when the patient continues to report pain. The development of pain clinics and inpatient pain teams has led to successful control of chronic pain for some (but not all) persons. Information about pain centers in the United States and Canada is presented in Box 12-5.

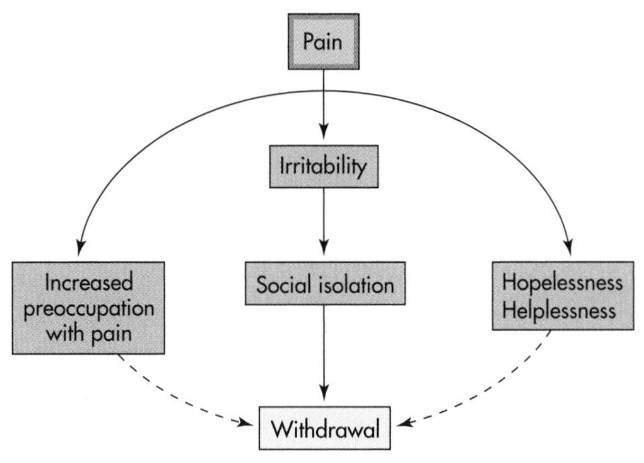

Figure 12-3 Chronic pain.

Specific Types of Pain

Somatic versus Visceral Pain

Pain may originate in the skin and subcutaneous tissue (superficial pain), in the muscles and bones (deep somatic pain), or in the body organs (visceral pain). Somatic and visceral pain differ in their characteristics, particularly in the quality of pain, localization, causes, and accompanying symptoms (Table 12-3).

Referred Pain

Referred pain is felt in areas other than those stimulated by injury or disease. For example, the person having a heart attack may only report pain radiating down the left arm, when in fact the tissue damage is occurring in the myocardium.

BOX 12-5 Organizations Providing Information About Pain-Relief Centers in the United States and Canada

American Chronic Pain Association, Box 850, Rockland, CA 95677; (916)632-0922; fax: (916)632-3208; website: www.members.tripod.com/,widdy/ACPA.html

National Chronic Pain Outreach Association, 7979 Old Georgetown Rd., Suite 100, Bethesda, MD 20814; (540)997-5004; fax: (540)997-1305; E-mail: ncpoa1@aol.com

Canadian Pain Society, (613)234-0812; fax: (613)234-9894; website: www.canadianpainsociety.ca

North American Chronic Pain Association of Canada (NAC-PAC), 6 Handel Court, Brampton, Ontario, Canada L6S 14; (905)793-5230; fax: (905)793-8781; E-mail: nacpac@sympatico.ca

International Association for the Study of Pain, 909 N.E. 43rd St.; Suite 306, Seattle, WA 98105; (206)547-6409; fax (206)547-1703; E-mail: IASP@locke.hs.washington.edu

American Council for Headache Education, 875 Kings Highway, Suite 200, West Deptford, NJ 08096; (800)255-2243

The Migraine Association of Canada, Suite 1912, 365 Bloor St., E., Toronto, Ontario M4W 3L4, Canada; (416)920-4916; fax: (416)920-3677; www.migrane.ca; to order information: (800)663-3557; 24-hour information line: (416)920-4917

Commission for the Accreditation of Rehabilitative Facilities, 101 N. Wilmot Rd., Suite 500, Tucson, AZ 85711; written inquiries preferred

TABLE 12-3 Comparison of Superficial, Somatic, and Visceral Pain

	Type of Pain		
	Superficial	Somatic	Visceral
Characteristic	Skin and Subcutaneous Tissue	Deep Muscles and Bones	Internal Organs
Quality	Sharp, pricking, burning	Sharp or dull and aching	Sharp or dull and aching, cramping
Localization	Good	Poor	Poor
Referred pain	No	No	Yes
Provoking stimuli	Cut, abrasion, excessive heat or cold, chemicals	Cut, pressure, heat, ischemia, displacement (bone)	Distention, ischemia, spasms, chemical irritants (no cutting)
Autonomic reactions	No	Yes	Yes
Reflex muscle contractions	No	Yes	Yes

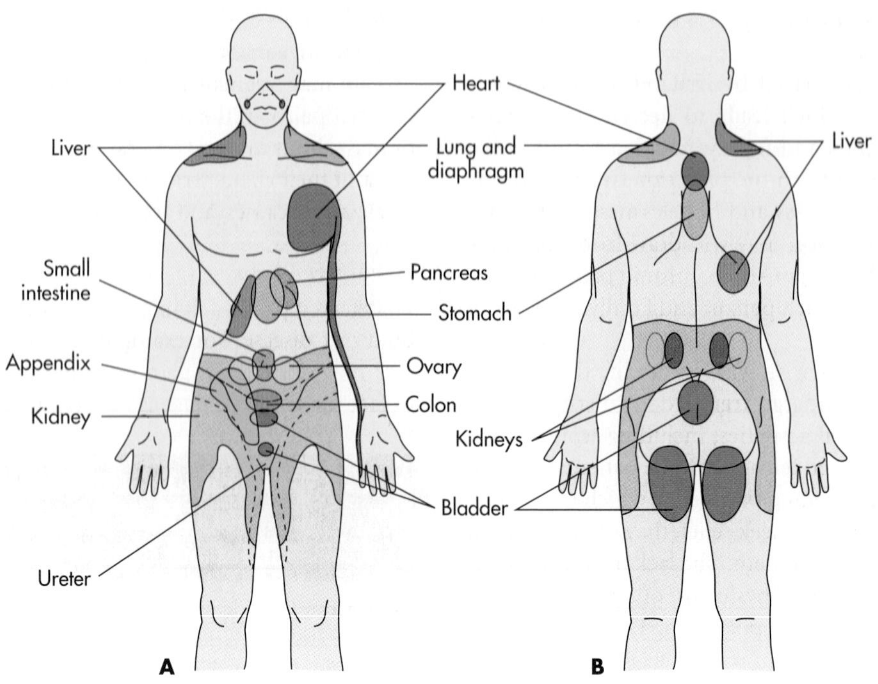

Figure 12-4 Usual sites of referred pain. **A**, Front. **B**, Back.

Referred pain occurs most often with damage or injury to the visceral organs, and the pain is referred to cutaneous surfaces (Figure 12-4). The origin of referred pain is complex and not clearly understood and may relate to one or more of the following[30]:

1. Referred pain usually occurs in structures that developed from the same embryonic dermatome.
2. Visceral and somatic nerves enter the nervous system at the same spinal level and share the same spinothalamic tracts.
3. Somatic pain is more common, and the person has "learned" to interpret signals conducted on certain pathways as being somatic in origin.

The cutaneous pattern of various types of referred pain is fairly constant and frequently seen in practice. The nurse should be able to recognize the possibility of visceral organ disease in patients who report cutaneous pain.

Psychogenic Pain

The term *psychogenic pain* has been used to describe pain for which no pathologic condition has been found or in which the pain appears to have a greater psychologic basis than a physical one.[31] It is important to remember that diagnostic tests are not definitive measures and may not be sophisticated enough to detect all pathophysiologic changes. Distinguishing between physical and emotional components of pain is difficult, and it is important to remember that all pain is real.

Neuropathic Pain

Neuropathic pain arises from injury to the nervous system and can occur in different forms. Sharp, spasmlike pain can occur along the course of one or more nerves, such as the trigeminal nerve in the face (trigeminal neuralgia or tic douloureaux) and the sciatic nerve (sciatica) in the lower back and extremity. Severe burning pain can be associated with injury to a peripheral nerve in the extremities. As a result, the patient may go to great lengths to protect against irritating stimuli, which may be something as simple as the noise of a plane overhead.

Phantom limb pain is pain experienced in a surgically removed extremity. This problem is more likely to develop in those who had significant pain before amputation, and it may persist long after healing has occurred. This phenomenon has only recently been successfully prevented in the postoperative period by the administration of effective preemptive analgesia before surgery. Refer to Chapter 25 for a discussion of the management of amputation.

COLLABORATIVE CARE MANAGEMENT

Pharmacologic Approaches

Analgesics

Two groups of analgesics, as well as adjuvant medications, are important components of effective pain management. Opioid analgesics, such as morphine, act mainly on the CNS to alter the perception of pain. Nonopioid analgesics, such as aspirin, block impulses mainly in the periphery and decrease inflammation-related pain by inhibiting the synthesis of prostaglandins. For some types of pain, such as pain with bone cancer, analgesics from both groups are necessary. Adjuvant medications such as amitriptyline (Elavil) help relieve some types of neuropathic pain such as that with postherpetic neuralgia (shingles).[48]

Standard doses are helpful guidelines for analgesic prescription and administration, but dosages need to be evaluated for each individual patient. Although most nurses do not prescribe analgesics, they do make administration choices about the type, dose, and frequency when drug options are given. Nurses are also responsible for evaluating the effectiveness of the medication, monitoring for side effects, and advocating change when needed. It is important to understand the concept of an equianalgesic dose. An equianalgesic dose is the dose of one analgesic that has the same pain-relieving effect as another drug. This concept makes it possible to change one analgesic for another, or to change the route of administration, for example from parenteral to oral opioid doses. Equianalgesic dosing also allows comparisons to be made between weak analgesics such as codeine for mild pain, versus stronger analgesics such as morphine for moderate to severe pain. Equianalgesic doses of common opioids are presented in Table 12-4.

Opioid Analgesics. Opioid analgesics can be classified according to the strength of their effect; for example codeine is a weak opioid and morphine is a strong opioid. Opioids are also classified as agonist, antagonist, or mixed agonist-antagonist opioids, depending on their effect at mu, delta, and kappa receptor sites. For example, morphine is an agonist as it binds to and activates the receptors, mainly mu, to produce analgesia. Antagonist opioids, such as naloxone, bind to a receptor without activating it; they also block and displace agonist opioids such as morphine and prevent their analgesic effect. Butorphanol (Stadol) is an example of a mixed agonist-antagonist that acts like naloxone when given to someone who is taking an agonist such as morphine on a regular basis. Therefore, people receiving agonist opioids should not be given concurrent agonist-antagonist opioids or a state of withdrawal will result.

Opioids are the most effective analgesic for the relief of moderate to severe pain and must be given on a regular basis to prevent pain from recurring. Side effects of opioids vary with the physiologic state of the patient. Constipation is the most common side effect. Naloxone (Narcan) will reverse any depressive effect.

When opioids are administered, it is important to distinguish between the effects of tolerance, dependence, and addiction as noted here:

Tolerance: Larger doses needed to produce the same analgesic effects

Dependence: Need to continue use of drug to prevent symptoms of withdrawal

Addiction: Behavioral pattern of compulsive drug use; drug used for psychologic effect

Drug tolerance occurs with some patients and with some conditions, usually when the patient's pain is first being controlled and/or when the pain increases. This is a physiologic response and requires increasing the dose until pain relief is attained. The dose can be steadily increased because there is no ceiling or maximum amount of opioid that can be given. Physical dependence and drug tolerance are involuntary behaviors and are the physiologic result of frequent ongoing opioid administration. Although physical dependence and tolerance develop, symptoms of withdrawal rarely occur because, as pain decreases, the dosage is gradually tapered and no symptoms are experienced. Physical dependence and drug tolerance do not represent addiction, and the fear of addiction should not prevent opioid administration, because addiction in hospitalized patients rarely occurs.

Administration Routes. Opioids can be administered by a variety of routes. The oral route is preferred unless the patient is vomiting, is unable or not permitted to swallow, or is in acute pain. Slow-release preparations, such as MS Contin, are given every 8 to 12 hours, allowing less focus on the pain and better control with fewer side effects. In addition to intramuscular and subcutaneous injection, opioids can also be administered rectally, transdermally, sublingually, epidurally, and intravenously.[1,19,28] When intravenous access is not possible, sublingual and rectal routes should be considered as alternatives to injections.

Epidural infusions of opioids such as morphine or fentanyl can be administered through a catheter placed in the epidural or intrathecal space by the physician (Figure 12-5). An infusion device attached to the line provides a continuous supply of the opioid. This method relieves pain without diminishing CNS function. Patients with intractable pain can be well managed at home using this route.[1,19,28]

Epidural administration is extremely effective, but patients still experience the common related side effects of opioid administration. See the Guidelines for Safe Practice box for a summary of side effect management. In addition, patients frequently complain of pruritis (itching), which can be severe. Antihistamines and comfort measures are effective for many patients, but it is occasionally necessary to reduce the opioid dosage or administer low-dose naloxone (Narcan), which generally controls the itching without reversing the analgesic effect.

Patient-controlled analgesia (PCA) is a method that allows patients to administer their own opioids whenever they feel it is necessary. PCA may involve oral medications or an infusion system with a pump. With a PCA pump, the patient pushes a button to release a set amount of opioid by bolus intravenously, subcutaneously, or epidurally. A basal rate of infusion may be ordered in addition to the on-demand dosage. A refractory period prevents delivery of another bolus before a preset time interval. The device also records the patient's attempts to receive the opioid in a given time period. A suggested protocol[1,19,28] for intravenous PCA includes loading doses such as 3 to 5 mg of morphine, repeated every 5 minutes until the pain is decreased.[13] On-demand doses are usually 0.5 to 1.5 mg of morphine every 6 minutes to a maximum of 10 mg/hr. With shorter hospital stays, patients need to be given oral analgesics as soon as possible and have their pain well managed before discharge. Equianalgesic oral opioids can be started before or when the last PCA dose is given.

People using PCA tend to take less total analgesia than those receiving intermittent injections.[15,28] PCA is used for the management of postoperative pain, other types of acute pain such as sickle cell crisis, and for cancer pain.[13,15]

Sedation and Analgesia. Sedation and analgesia (previously known as conscious sedation) involves the administration of drugs to produce a state of sedation and analgesia (see Chapter 17 for additional discussion). This medically controlled state of depressed consciousness allows the patient to (1) maintain protective reflexes, (2) maintain a patent airway

TABLE 12-4 Equianalgesic Doses of Opioids Commonly Used for Severe Pain

Name	Equianalgesic Dose (mg) Oral	Parenteral*	Comments
Morphinelike agonists			
Morphine	30†	10	Standard of comparison for opioid analgesics; sustained-release preparations (MS Contin, Oramorph-SR) release drug over 3-12 hours
Hydromorphone (Dilaudid)	7.5	1.5	Slightly shorter duration than morphine
Oxycodone	30	—	
Methadone (Dolophine)	20	10	Good oral potency; long plasma half-life (24-36 hours) Accumulates with repetitive dosing, causing excessive sedation (on days 2-5)
Levorphanol (Levo-Dromoran)	4	2	Long plasma half-life (12-16 hours) Accumulates on days 2-3
Fentanyl	—	0.1	Transdermal fentanyl (Duragesic) 25-50 μg/hour roughly equivalent to 30 mg sustained-release morphine q8hr Because of skin reservoir of drug, 12-hour delay in onset and offset of transdermal patch; fever increases dose rate
Oxymorphone (Numorphan)	—	1	5 mg rectal suppository = 5 mg morphine intramuscularly
Meperidine (Demerol)	300	75	Slightly shorter acting than morphine Normeperidine (toxic metabolite) accumulates with repetitive dosing, causing central nervous system excitation; avoid in patients with impaired renal function or who are receiving monoamine oxidase inhibitors
Mixed agonist-antagonists			
Nalbuphine (Nubain)	—	10	Not available orally; not scheduled under Controlled Substances Act Incidence of psychotomimetic effects lower than with pentazocine; may precipitate withdrawal in opioid-dependent patients
Butorphanol (Stadol)	—	2	Like nalbuphine
Dezocine (Dalgan)	—	10	Like nalbuphine May precipitate withdrawal in opioid-dependent patients; subcutaneous injection irritating
Partial agonists			
Buprenorphine (Buprenex)	0.4		Not available orally; sublingual preparation not yet in United States; less abuse potential than morphine; does not produce psychotomimetic effects May precipitate withdrawal in opioid-dependent patients; not readily reversed by naloxone; avoid in labor

Adapted from American Pain Society Quality of Care Committee.[3]

*These are standard intramuscular (IM) doses for acute pain in adults and also may be used to convert doses for intravenous (IV) infusions and repeated small IV boluses. For single IV boluses, use half the IM dose.

†Some experts argue that 60 mg of oral morphine is the more accurate equivalent dose and suggest caution in converting patients from high doses of oral morphine to other drugs if the 30-mg equivalent is used.

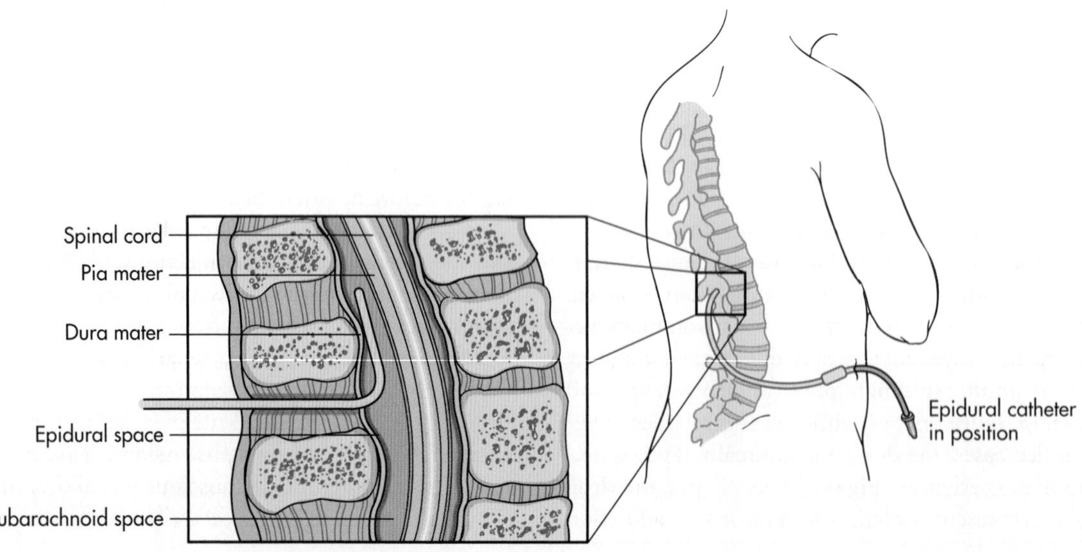

Figure 12-5 Site of epidural catheter placement.

Guidelines for Safe Practice

Managing Opioid Side Effects

OPIOID SIDE EFFECTS

Hypotension (particularly postural hypotension)
Decreased respirations and decreased cough
Dizziness and sedation
Constipation
Nausea

PREVENTING CONSTIPATION

Opioids bind to receptor sites in the gastrointestinal (GI) tract and slow GI motility. The resultant constipation is best managed by administering a stool softener or stimulant as soon as the opioid is started. Monitor the patient's bowel pattern carefully and ensure adequate fluids.

MANAGING SEDATION

The sedative effects of opioids on the central nervous system last from 1 to 3 days and then tolerance is built up. Initially it may be beneficial to allow the patient to catch up on needed sleep. If problematic:

- Reduce the opioid dose, add a nonsteroidal antiinflammatory drug if possible, or administer more frequently.
- Change the opioid and evaluate the patient's response.
- Monitor respiratory rate and track the patient's sedation level using a sedation scale.
- Have a reversal agent available for use if needed (e.g., Naloxone [Narcan]).

MANAGING NAUSEA

Nausea is believed to result from stimulation of the chemoreceptor trigger zone in the brain and decreased GI motility. Tolerance to the effects usually develops within a few days. If problematic:

- Administer an antiemetic such as prochlorperazine (Compazine). Administer on a scheduled basis and not as needed.
- Add metoclopramide (Reglan) if antiemetics are initially ineffective.
- Change the opioid if nausea persists.

PREVENTING RESPIRATORY DEPRESSION

Effective pain relief allows the patient to be more active in self-care, get out of bed, and ambulate more freely, which counter the effects of respiratory depression. In addition:

- Encourage deep breathing and the use of incentive spirometry.
- Monitor the patient's sedation level. Respiratory depression is usually only a problem when sedation becomes excessive.

ENSURING SAFETY

Orthostatic hypotension and dizziness cause an increased risk for injury. Patients are taught to change positions slowly and should be monitored in their early attempts to be out of bed.

independently and continuously, and (3) respond to physical stimulation or verbal command (e.g., "open your eyes"). There is a sedation continuum that nurses involved in the administration of these drugs must understand. Under the direction of a physician, the nurse may be responsible for the medication and monitoring of people receiving conscious sedation. Policies or guidelines, appropriately trained personnel, and necessary equipment are prerequisites to safely administer sedation.

Nursing care of the patient under conscious sedation requires expert knowledge of the agents being used and continuous 1:1 monitoring because of the risk of respiratory depression. As such, special training within the clinical setting is required. This training usually involves learning institution-specific protocols for preparing and administering the sedative agents, continuous assessment, and maintaining/supporting the patient's airway until recovery.

Nonopioid Analgesics. Mild to moderate pain generally can be controlled by nonopioid analgesics, most commonly NSAIDs such as aspirin, and by acetaminophen. Acetaminophen (Tylenol, Datril) is comparable to aspirin in analgesic effect, but unlike aspirin, lacks any antiinflammatory action. Although acetaminophen does not alter the prothrombin level and has fewer side effects, overdoses can cause severe liver damage. This analgesic is useful for persons who are allergic to aspirin and for whom aspirin is contraindicated, such as persons with peptic ulcers.

The NSAIDs are the most widely used analgesics because of their general lack of serious side effects and their effectiveness in pain relief.[1,19,28] These drugs act primarily by inhibiting the synthesis of prostaglandins, which "sensitize" nerve endings and trigger pain. In lower doses, NSAIDs have analgesic properties; in higher doses there is antiinflammatory action in addition to analgesia. NSAIDs are used to control the moderate pain of dysmenorrhea, arthritis and other musculoskeletal disorders (see Chapter 47), postoperative pain, and migraine headaches. Other indications include analgesia for patients with bone cancer. NSAIDs commonly used for pain management are listed in Table 12-5.

NSAIDs and particularly acetylsalicylic acid (aspirin) inhibit platelet aggregation and increase bleeding time. Common side effects include GI disturbances, dizziness, tinnitus, and headache. Persons who are hypersensitive to aspirin also may be hypersensitive to other NSAIDs. In addition to blocking prostaglandin synthesis, salicylates also produce analgesia by blocking pain impulses peripherally or centrally, possibly in the hypothalamus. Aspirin is also a weak vitamin K antagonist and prolongs prothrombin time when given in large doses. Therefore, aspirin is contraindicated for persons receiving anticoagulants or other NSAIDs. Aspirin should be avoided by persons with a history of bleeding disorders or peptic ulcer and by children and teenagers because of the risk of Reye's syndrome.

Two classifications of NSAIDs are now available: the traditional COX-1 inhibitory agents that block prostaglandins in gastric mucosa and hemostasis and the new COX-2 inhibitory agents that are thought to be selective to pain, inflammation, and fever.[42] Irritation of the gastric mucosa is a common side effect of COX-1 NSAIDs, and dyspepsia can occur with COX-2. Therefore these drugs should be taken with meals or with a snack such as a glass of milk.

Adjuvant Medications. Adjuvant drugs may be given with analgesics to augment pain relief.[1,19,28] They also may be an option for pain relief when other analgesics are not effective.

Sedatives and antianxiety agents sometimes are prescribed for persons with pain. These drugs do not have any analgesic effects, but may permit relaxation and sleep, decrease anxiety, prevent an increase in pain, or enable the person to cope more effectively with the pain.

TABLE 12-5 Common Medications for Mild-to-Moderate Pain

Drug	Action	Intervention
Acetylsalicylic acid (aspirin)	Inhibits formation of prostaglandins, which are involved in the production of pain and inflammation Blocks pain impulses peripherally and/or centrally, possibly in the hypothalamus Is a weak vitamin K antagonist and prolongs prothrombin time Powerfully inhibits platelet aggregation	Teach patient to: Minimize gastric irritation by taking with food, full glass of liquid, or antacid Consider enteric coated preparations if gastrointestinal (GI) upset persists Immediately report the incidence of any bleeding (e.g., bruising, gums, nose bleed, urine, stool)
Ibuprofen (Advil, Motrin) Naproxen, naproxen sodium (Anaprox, Naprosyn, Aleve) Ketoprofen (Orudis) Fenoprofen (Nalfon) Mefenamic acid (Ponstel)	As above, inhibits prostaglandin synthesis Inhibits platelet aggregation	Teach patient to: Take on an empty stomach with a full glass of water unless GI upset occurs As above, report any incidence of bleeding
Ketorolac tromethamine (Toradol)		When given intramuscularly, the drug must be administered deeply into a large muscle

Phenothiazines such as promethazine (Phenergan) do not potentiate the analgesic effect of opioids. However they do increase opioid-related sedation, hypertension, and respiratory depression and should not be used for pain relief.[19] In some persons sedatives and antianxiety agents may lead to disorientation and agitation, which can increase the pain and decrease the person's ability to cope. Treating pain with analgesics is the more effective and preferred method.

Tricyclic antidepressants such as amitriptyline (Elavil) produce analgesia at doses lower than those used for depression. These drugs are useful in nerve injury pain, such as with postherpetic neuralgia (shingles). They are believed to prevent the uptake of serotonin and norepinephrine in the descending inhibitory modulation in the spinal cord and reduce sensitization mechanisms. Low doses are used for analgesia (an average of 570 mg daily).[48]

A variety of other medications may be used as adjuvants for pain relief. Anticonvulsants such as phenytoin (Dilantin) and carbamazepine (Tegretol) are used to suppress abnormal (ectopic) nerve discharges that occur in nerve injury pain such as trigeminal neuralgia.[19] Dexamethasone (Decadron), a corticosteroid, is helpful in relieving pain from increased intracranial pressure, nerve compression, spinal cord compression, bowel obstruction, and bone metastases. Corticosteroids block the production of arachidonic acid, which is necessary for the synthesis of prostaglandins and other inflammatory chemicals that cause pain.[19] These drugs also stimulate appetite and may elevate mood. Counterirritants are over-the-counter drugs that relieve local pain by producing counterirritation (stimulation of the large A-beta fibers). Examples of counterirritants include ointments containing methylsalicylate (oil of wintergreen) or ethyl aminobenzoate and oil of cloves (for toothaches).

Nonpharmacologic Approaches

Nonpharmacologic approaches can be used with analgesics for effective pain management.[1,19,28] This type of intervention can alter pain transmission, modify the response to pain, and modify the pain stimulus. Physical strategies that are invasive and/or non-nursing acts will be discussed in this section. Nursing measures will be discussed under Nursing Management.

Altering Pain Transmission

Electrical Stimulators. The purpose of electrical stimulators is to modify the pain stimulus by blocking or changing the painful stimulus with stimulation perceived as less painful. The gate control theory suggests that stimulating large myelinated A-beta fibers closes the "gate" to pain stimuli.[30] Selected forms of electrical stimulation may activate the descending inhibitory system.

Transcutaneous electrical nerve stimulation (TENS) uses a battery-powered stimulator worn externally. This convenient, nonintrusive, nonaddictive type of pain therapy can be learned easily by the patient. Success is variable, and the device is usually used with other pain therapies.

A number of TENS devices are available; all consist of a battery-powered portable pulse generator about the size of a pocket pager. Control knobs on the generator permit adjustment of the impulse. The generator is connected by a pair of cables to electrically conductive adhesive electrodes placed at appropriate sites on the skin. TENS delivers a balanced biphasic potential in a waveform.

TENS appears to be most useful for postoperative pain, posttraumatic pain, phantom limb pain, peripheral neuralgias, low back pain, and muscle pain. Although it can be effective with mild or moderate pain, it is less effective for severe pain.[46] Nurses are responsible for monitoring the effectiveness of treatments and for patient teaching concerning the safe use of TENS (see Patient Teaching box).

TENS electrodes should not be placed over hair, irritated or open skin, sutures, the carotid sinus (may produce bradycardia), laryngeal or pharyngeal muscles (may trigger spasms), or the uterus of a pregnant woman. A cardiac pacemaker may interfere with TENS effects. Suggested electrode

Patient Teaching
The Use of TENS

Teach patients to:
1. Remove and clean electrodes daily.
2. Wash skin with soap and water.
3. Allow skin to air dry.
4. Wipe skin with a prep pad before reapplying the conductor pad.
5. Check the battery if numbness or tingling is not felt during treatments.
6. Report if sensation is either absent or uncomfortable.

BOX 12-6 Neurosurgical Procedures for Pain Control

Neurectomy: severing of nerve fibers from the cell body
Rhizotomy: resection of posterior nerve root before it enters spinal cord
Cordotomy: severing of ascending anterolateral pain-conducting pathways of spinal cord
Sympathectomy: excision or destruction of one or more sympathetic ganglia or nerves

placement may include (1) directly over the painful area, (2) at trigger points along the nerve pathways, or (3) at trigger points in the same dermatome as the pain. Spinal cord stimulators are similar to TENS except that they are intrusive procedures. Instead of electrode placement on the skin, the electrodes are placed on or near the spinal cord. This is achieved either surgically over the ventral surface of the spinal cord or percutaneously through the back into the epidural space. Because the percutaneously inserted spinal cord electrical stimulator can be inserted under local anesthesia, it is preferred over surgical placement of dorsal column stimulator electrodes. Postoperative care after dorsal column stimulator implantation includes the same care that follows laminectomy (see Chapter 47), with monitoring for infection and leakage of cerebrospinal fluid.

Nerve Block. A nerve block involves the injection of substances such as local anesthetics or neurolytic agents (e.g., alcohol or phenol) near the nerve(s) to block the conduction of impulses and for the symptomatic relief of pain. Nerve blocks are used to treat chronic pain associated with peripheral vascular disease, trigeminal neuralgia, causalgia, and cancer.

Acupuncture. Acupuncture is an ancient form of disease treatment that can be used for pain relief. Developed in Asia, this method has become more popular in Western countries. Small needles are skillfully inserted and manipulated at specific body points, depending on the type and location of pain. The gate control theory provides the best explanation for the effectiveness of acupuncture. The local stimulation of large-diameter fibers by the needles "closes the gate" to pain. It is not known to what extent the psyche and the power of suggestion contribute to the effectiveness of this therapy.

Neurosurgical Procedures. Neurosurgical procedures do not play a major role in management of chronic pain.[18] Major limitations include short duration of relief, occurrence of dysesthesia (pain induced by gentle touch of the skin), central pain syndrome (burning sensations in skin areas lacking sensation from surgical afferent interruptions), and possible further neurologic dysfunction.[28] However, for constant, relentless chronic pain that cannot be controlled by analgesics (intractable pain), various neurosurgical procedures may be used to reduce or eliminate the pain (Box 12-6). Other forms of pain control usually are attempted before neurosurgical intervention.

Modifying Pain Response

A wide range of strategies are available for modifying the pain response. Many of these strategies are within the realm of independent nursing practice and are discussed in the next section. Others may be used by nurses with special training but frequently are interventions used by other members of the collaborative care team.

Behavior Modification. Behavior modification consists of a planned change in the way a person behaves by means of rewarding desired behavior and ignoring undesirable behavior. Forms of behavior modification are used unconsciously all the time: a young child "throwing a tantrum" may be ignored, but as his behavior becomes more appropriate, his mother may reward him with her time and attention.

Behavior modification may be useful for persons with chronic pain. For example, one protocol for patients with chronic low back pain is to set a limit of 10 minutes daily for discussion of their pain experiences (with the exception of data-gathering interviews). Pain medications are prescribed on a regular schedule to dissociate the feelings of pain with inappropriate use (reward) of analgesics or other unhealthy behaviors.

In using behavioral methods to alter pain-associated behavior or to encourage patient activities, success will occur only with a consistent approach on the part of the health care team. Although patients should always be praised for their efforts to comply or assist with treatment regimens, a true behavior modification program requires careful analysis of patient behavior and the development of a specific and comprehensive treatment plan.

Biofeedback and Autogenic Training. Some persons are able to alter their body functions through mental concentration. In biofeedback training a machine that monitors brain wave activity (electroencephalograph) is used. The individual concentrates on slowing his or her brain wave activity to rates at which pain and distress are unlikely to cause discomfort (i.e., complete relaxation). It may take many months of regular practice to achieve the desired level of control. The nurse should encourage and praise the person's efforts.

In autogenic training the same type of self-regulation is used to alter various autonomic nervous system functions, such as pulse, blood pressure, and muscle tension. The use of transcendental meditation and other methods of concentration and self-control may achieve the same degree of autoregulation without the use of sophisticated physiologic monitoring equipment.

Hypnosis. Hypnosis may be used in the treatment of various conditions, particularly when these conditions are aggravated by tension and stress. Patients are helped to alter their perception of pain through the acceptance of positive suggestions made to the subconscious. Many persons are able to learn self-hypnosis. Individuals vary widely in their suggestibility and readiness to try this approach. The nurse's most helpful role may be to support the patient's desire to make hypnosis work.

NURSING MANAGEMENT

ASSESSMENT

Effective pain management can occur only when systematic and regular assessments take place. An important nursing intervention is assessing subjective and objective data at least once a shift and often more frequently when pain is anticipated.[24] Patient input is important, and it is unfortunate that research has shown that health professionals and patients assess pain differently.[9,52] It is crucial to gather as much information as possible from the patient to avoid making incorrect assumptions about pain. To aid in data collection and to evaluate the effectiveness of interventions, a variety of pain assessment tools are available.[12,28]

Although many patients continue to experience postoperative pain, many will not ask for help[47,52] (see Research box). For this reason it is best to use a numeric rating scale (e.g., 0 to 10 scale, where 0 is no pain and 10 is the worst possible pain) to validate the pain the patient is experiencing. The Wong Baker Faces Scale has been translated into several languages and is an alternative for both children and adults. The numeric rating scale is valid and easy to use. The frequency of assessment will vary depending on the intensity of the patient's pain and the pharmacokinetics of the analgesic given. If the pain intensity does not decrease after analgesic administration, further assessment is indicated, including drug choice and dosage.

Health History

Before pain occurs, it is useful to obtain data concerning the patient's expectation for pain relief. Many persons are unaware that they are expected to speak out when they have pain or discomfort. Some patients think they will be considered "complainers" or "bad patients" if they state that they are in pain.[45]

It is distressing to note that most patients have previously experienced severe pain and continue to expect severe pain after surgery.[52] Patients need to be asked on admission about their expectations, knowledge, and concerns about pain. They should then be taught how and when to verbalize their discomfort and the various methods available for pain relief. As already mentioned, the best assessment of pain is the patient's own evaluation.

Data to be collected by the nurse include the location, intensity, quality, timing (onset, duration, frequency, cause), and aggravating and relieving factors. One approach for evaluating these characteristics is the use of the mnemonic PQRST:

Research

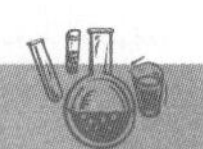

Reference: Watt-Watson J et al: The impact of nurses' empathic responses on patients' pain management in acute care, *Nurs Res* 49:4, 2000.

In this study 225 patients were interviewed on their third day after coronary bypass graft surgery, along with their assigned nurses (n = 94) to examine the relationship between nurses' empathic responses and their patients' pain intensity and analgesic administration after surgery. Most patients reported moderate to severe pain, yet received only 47% of their prescribed analgesia. Two thirds of patients did not see their nurse as a resource for their pain management. Although most patients said they would not ask for help with pain, their nurses expected them to. Nurses' responses to pain intensity were moderately empathic and did not influence their patients' pain intensity or analgesic use. Deficits in knowledge and misbeliefs about pain management, which would have limited empathic responses, were evident.

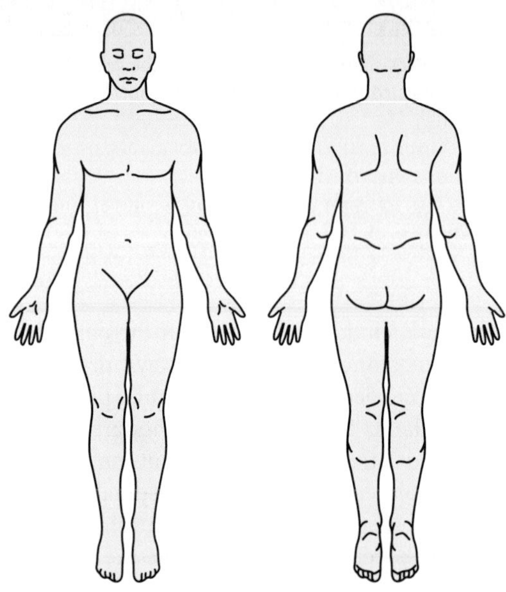

Figure 12-6 Body diagrams for pointing out sites of pain.

BOX 12-7 Examples of Pain Intensity Rating Scales

Categoric scale
0—No pain
1—Mild pain
2—Discomforting pain
3—Distressing pain
4—Horrible pain
5—Excruciating pain

Numeric scale*

0—1—2—3—4—5—6—7—8—9—10
No pain ... Worst pain imaginable

Visual analog scale (VAS)*

No pain ... Worst possible pain

*A 10-cm baseline is recommended for the numeric scale and visual analog scale.

FLOW SHEET — PAIN

Patient ______________________________ Date ______________

*Pain rating scale used ______________________________

Purpose: To evaluate the safety and effectiveness of the analgesic(s).

Analgesic(s) ordered: ______________________________

Time	Pain rating*	Analgesic	R	P	BP	Level of arousal†	Other‡	Plan and comments

* Pain rating: A number of different scales may be used. Indicate which scale is used and use the same one each time. Two common examples:
- 0 to 10 with 0 being no pain and 10 being as bad as it can be.
- Melzack's scale:
0 = no pain; 1 = mild; 2 = discomforting; 3 = distressing; 4 = horrible; 5 = excruciating

† Possible arousal scale: 1 = wide awake; 2 = drowsy; 3 = sleeping; 4 = difficult to arouse

‡ Possibilities for other columns: bowel function, activities, nausea and vomiting, other pain relief measures. Identify the side effects of greatest concern to patient, family, physician, nurses, etc.

Figure 12-7 Flow sheet for monitoring patient's response to pain.

P: *Provoking factors: what makes the pain worse or relieves it*
Q: *Quality: dull, sharp, crushing*
R: *Region or radiation: site and radiation to other areas*
S: *Severity or intensity*
T: *Time: onset, duration, frequency, cause*

Diagrams of the body can help patients point out the sites of their pain (Figure 12-6). Pain intensity can be assessed using several measures as outlined in Box 12-7. An efficient, reliable, and valid approach is to ask the patient to use a numerical rating to describe the pain or discomfort: 0 (no pain) to 10 (worst pain possible). Ratings need to be documented and intervention options discussed for ratings greater than 3. Ratings can be recorded on a vital sign sheet similar to temperature and blood pressure data. More detailed flow sheets are also helpful to provide ongoing assessment of progression of the pain and the response to various interventions (Figure 12-7). Pain intensity should be assessed at least once a shift or more often if the patient rated his or her pain at 4 or greater (0 to 10) and is receiving interventions for pain (such as analgesics, relaxation exercises, or TENS). When acute pain has subsided, further data can be collected about the meaning of pain for the person. Long-term pain requires a much more in-depth assessment. Hospitals or pain clinics using a team approach in providing care to the person with chronic pain often develop their own pain history form or questionnaire. This history may be collected by one or more health team members. Types of data collected to assess a patient experiencing chronic pain include:

- Demographic data
- Sociocultural data
- History of the pain pattern from time of onset
- Factors perceived to increase or decrease the pain
- Effects of the pain on the person's lifestyle including work, family responsibilities, sexuality, leisure, sleep, nutrition, and activity
- Meaning of the pain for the person
- Effects of the patient's pain on other family members or friends
- Measures used in the past and present for relief of pain and their effectiveness

Physical and Behavioral Examination

Physiologic and behavioral data help the nurse identify possible pain or discomfort in a person who has not reported pain or is unable to do so (see Clinical Manifestations box). Physiologic signs of pain result from activation of the sympathetic nervous system. With very severe pain, neurogenic shock may result from the stress to the system. The behavioral signs are not specific to pain; therefore, if the observable data suggest that pain may be present, subjective data must be elicited to validate the assumption where possible.

Specific physical and behavioral data required to assess the patient's pain include:

- Appearance (grimacing, gritting teeth, clenching fists, lying rigidly as if afraid to move)
- Motor behavior
- Affective and verbal responses
- Vital signs
- Skin moisture and color
- Inspection and gentle palpation of painful area; identify trigger points that initiate pain, if present

Sometimes the patient's behavior does not seem to match his or her verbalization of pain. For example, the patient may request an analgesic, a back rub, or other measure to relieve pain; but when the nurse arrives to carry out the request, the patient is asleep. It must be emphasized here that the patient who is sleeping or lying quietly is not necessarily pain-free. The patient may be exhausted from the pain, and sleeping is a coping mechanism. Patients may also use distraction such as talking and joking with visitors to manage unrelieved pain. The person's self-report of pain is the key to effective management.

Physiologic signs of pain can disappear quickly for the person with acute pain and are typically not present with chronic pain because of the body's compensatory mechanisms. Although there is adaptation to the pain stimuli, the pain persists. The absence of physiologic signs, therefore, does not indicate absence of pain. Prolonged pain, however, may create changes in the person's appearance over time, perhaps as a result of decreased activity, decreased appetite, lack of sleep, or lack of interest in appearance because of fatigue or depression.

Behavioral responses to chronic pain are varied and unique to the individual person. Here, also, there may be few overt signs to indicate the presence of pain. Changes usually occur in daily patterns related to sleeping, eating, socialization, and libido. If the person is extremely depressed because of the ongoing pain, withdrawal behaviors may be noted.

Pain assessment is particularly complex when the person is unable to describe what he or she is experiencing, for example, patients with developmental issues or cognitive impairment. Older people with normal to moderately impaired cognitive functioning, as well as some severely impaired elderly, have been found capable of rating their pain using self-report scales.[26] Research is ongoing to develop valid behavioral measures to help assess pain more accurately in this population (see Research Box).

Clinical Manifestations

Acute Pain

PHYSIOLOGIC SIGNS

Pulse: increased rate
Respirations: increased depth and frequency
Blood pressure: increased systolic and diastolic
Diaphoresis, pallor
Dilated pupils
Muscle tension (face, body)
Nausea and vomiting (if pain is severe)

BEHAVIORAL SIGNS

Rigid body position
Restlessness
Frowning
Clenched teeth
Clenched fists
Crying
Moaning

Research

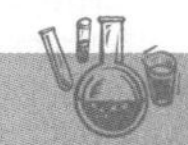

Reference: Feldt, K.: The checklist of nonverbal pain indicators (CNPI), *Pain Management Nurs* 1:1, 2000.

The CNPI was designed to measure pain behaviors in cognitively impaired elders. Pilot testing of the instrument with people over 65 years ($X = 83$ years) with hip fractures demonstrated that pain was poorly tolerated in older patients, particularly those who were very elderly and those who were cognitively impaired. Nurses in both acute and long-term care settings have indicated a need for a measure to assess pain in cognitively impaired elders. The CNPI is a simple dichotomous measure of six observed pain behaviors and includes verbal and nonverbal vocalizations, grimacing, bracing, rubbing, and restlessness. The CNPI has preliminary reliability and validity and further testing is in progress.

NURSING DIAGNOSES

Nursing diagnoses are determined from analysis of patient data. Nursing diagnoses for the patient with pain include the following nursing diagnoses but can also include a wide variety of associated diagnoses that reflect the patient's unique experience and response to the pain.

Diagnostic Title	Possible Etiologic Factors
1. Acute pain	Tissue pressure, inflammation, trauma or effects of surgery and other treatments
2. Chronic pain	Nervous system sensitization from factors listed for pain; actual etiology unclear
3. Deficient knowledge	Lack of previous instruction, misunderstanding pain, management strategies

Examples of other pain-related diagnostic titles that may be appropriate after health history and physical examination analyses include:

Activity intolerance
Anxiety
Breathing pattern, ineffective
Constipation
Fatigue
Hopelessness
Powerlessness
Self-care deficit
Sexual dysfunction
Sleep pattern disturbance
Social isolation

EXPECTED PATIENT OUTCOMES

Expected outcomes for the person experiencing acute pain may include but are not limited to:

1a. Will state that pain is decreased to a low rating (e.g., 4) on a scale of 0 to 10 (0, no pain; 10, most severe pain imaginable)
1b. Will demonstrate relaxed facial expression and body position and participates in activities
1c. Will discuss concern about asking for help and taking analgesics

Expected outcomes for the person experiencing chronic pain may include but are not limited to:

2a. Will state plans to participate in ongoing therapies
2b. Will state plans for increasing independence in activities in daily living
2c. Will identify supports for encouragement and help

Outcomes for the person with acute and/or chronic pain include but are not limited to:

3a. Will verbalize factors that alter the pain and effective control measures
3b. If future pain is a possibility after being discharged, the person or significant other will:
Explain how, when, and for how long to apply heat or ice or to exercise to relieve pain
Explain prescribed medications (actions, dosages, frequency, side effects
Describe when to seek medical assistance if pain is not relieved as expected
Express comfort after using previously effective modalities

INTERVENTIONS

Pain is a complex experience involving sensory, affective, and behavioral components that requires a multimodal treatment approach. Pain such as muscle spasms in the lower back may be relieved more effectively by heat and ultrasound than by medications. Strategies such as breathing exercises, muscle relaxation, imagery, and distraction do not replace analgesics for patients who need pharmacologic management, but can be useful adjuncts in treatment. Nonpharmacologic interventions can be effective in reducing the dose of medication required and in decreasing the pain while the patient waits for pain medication to work. Because pain is multidimensional, encouraging patients to use a broad range of pain relief methods results in more effective pain management. Patients may bring their own previously successful strategies that need to be encouraged, for example, the use of music, humor, or Tai Chi.

Planning for Pain Management

The nurse's role in planning and monitoring outcomes of care is critical to effective pain management. The initial thorough assessment serves as the foundation on which priorities are established and treatment strategies are devised. The Guidelines for Safe Practice box contains some basic principles of pain management to guide the planning period.[1] The patient's ability and desire to play an active or passive role in using pain relief measures need to be considered. Decreased ability results from severe pain, fatigue, sedation, depression, or unconsciousness. Decreased desire or will occurs in some persons with chronic pain who have experienced numerous failures in pain relief. The nurse is able to function independently with many interventions, but careful planning with other members of the health care team is necessary to ensure that all have the same patient outcomes or goals in mind. The patient and family are included in all planning activities if possible.

One aspect of the treatment plan that often is forgotten or omitted is incorporating measures the *patient* thinks may help relieve the pain, even if these measures differ from those usually carried out in that institution. Without encouragement, the patient may hesitate to mention these remedies (e.g., nonprescription liniments, special applications of heat and cold,

Guidelines for Safe Practice

ABC Principles of Pain Assessment and Planning

A Ask about pain regularly.
Assess pain systematically.
B Believe the patient and family in their reports of pain and what relieves it.
C Choose pain control options appropriate for the patient, family, and setting.
D Deliver interventions in a timely, logical, and coordinated fashion.
E Empower patients and their families.
Enable them to control their course to the greatest extent possible.

unusual positioning, or favorite homemade foods or drinks). If there are no contraindications to the remedy the patient wishes to try, the health care team may consider using it before trying other relief measures.

Time constraints can make planning difficult. However, planning for the same group of health care providers to care for the patient would help ensure a more consistent approach and plan of care. The small group of health care team members and the patient can develop a plan of care in which the patient's decisions are honored, and a daily routine can be developed that reduces anxiety and frustration. The plan should include, if appropriate, premedication before uncomfortable procedures, specified blocks of time for rest or napping, and coordination between various departments such as physical therapy and occupational therapy. For some patients fatigue is a significant problem and regular visits to off-unit departments should be interspersed with rest periods; for other patients the most beneficial plan includes ensuring that they go directly from one department to the next so that time is not wasted getting in and out of bed or performing other painful maneuvers.

1. Managing Acute Pain

Using Physical Noninvasive Measures

Cutaneous (dermal) stimulation. Cutaneous stimulation is thought to innervate the large A-beta fibers, closing the gate to impulses from the periphery.[54] TENS is a previously discussed example that may be ordered by the physician. Strategies that can be used by nurses include massage, light rubbing of the area involved or of a contralateral site, whirlpool baths, heat, or cold. These interventions are effective, simple, low risk, and not time consuming and do not require expensive equipment. Patients may need to try several to find which ones have the best effects. Box 12-8 lists various alternatives for the application of heat. The Guidelines for Safe Practice box at right reviews the basic principles for the safe use of these interventions.

Positioning

Patients who are immobilized or who splint (guard) a body part to minimize pain need to be encouraged to perform passive and/or active exercises when possible to prevent complications. Premedication may be necessary to prevent or reduce pain. For example, when the body or an extremity is moved, supporting the trunk or extremity prevents an increase in pain by unilateral pulling on muscles, joints, and ligaments. Interventions for nurses and home caregivers to reduce the pain associated with positioning are summarized in the Guidelines for Safe Practice box at bottom of column.

Modifying the Environment

The patient's physical environment can create sensory overload and potentiate the pain stimuli. If nurses would stand still for 5 minutes in the patient's environment and watch and listen, they might understand that some patients

BOX 12-8 Alternatives for Heat Application

1. Superficial heat
   a. Dry heat: heating pad, hot-water bottle, lamp, sun
   b. Moist heat: whirlpool baths, soaks, hydrocollator packs
2. Deep heat
   a. Short-wave diathermy
   b. Ultrasound vibration
   c. Microwave diathermy (contraindicated if implanted cardiac pacemaker)

Guidelines for Safe Practice

Using Heat and Cold Effectively

1. Explain the options available and involve the patient in choosing which options to use. Ice is rarely the patient's first choice, but it probably has a better chance than heat of being an effective pain reliever.
2. Apply heat and cold directly to the site of pain, but if this is not possible they can also be used:
   a. around the painful site.
   b. between the pain and the brain.
   c. beyond the pain.
   d. on the opposite side of the body from the pain site.
   e. over acupuncture or trigger point sites.
3. Use heat and cold at a comfortable intensity. They should not cause pain.
4. Apply heat and cold for 20 to 30 minutes at a time. The minimum effective time is about 10 minutes. Ice should not be applied for longer than 10 minutes to minimize the chance of tissue damage.
5. Encourage the patient to explore options for frequency of application. Alternating heat and cold can be effective in some situations.
6. Protect the skin with the use of either heat or cold and assess the skin after every application.
7. Use heat and cold before pain becomes severe whenever possible.

Adapted from McCaffery M, Pasero C: *Pain: clinical manual*, ed 2, St Louis, 1999, Mosby.

Guidelines for Safe Practice

Reducing Pain With Positioning

1. Give analgesics to prevent or minimize pain before care is given if pain is anticipated.
2. Use a turning sheet for patients with severe neck, back, or general trunk pain.
3. Place a pillow under a painful joint when helping a patient change position.
4. Support limbs at the joints rather than the muscle bellies when handling an extremity.
5. Use special beds (Rotorest, water bed) for patients with severe general or trunk pain.
6. Avoid bumping the bed or moving it suddenly.
7. Use bed cradles to support linens off painful extremities.
8. Assist with range of motion and evaluate joint flexibility.

are almost continuously bombarded with noise and visual stimulation. Modifying the environment may be helpful, but not all patients respond positively to the same environment. Some patients may benefit from a quiet room with minimal lighting, whereas others prefer a bright environment with sources of distraction such as television or music. The nurse can explore possible changes with the patient and implement any acceptable suggestions. Potential environmental modifications are listed in the Guidelines for Safe Practice box.

Administering Analgesics

The American Pain Society (APS) quality improvement guidelines[2,3] identify the two most important components of care for patients with acute pain or cancer pain as being assessment and treatment with analgesic medication. Monitoring outcomes is an important component of their guidelines (Box 12-9). When health professionals are more knowledgeable about pain assessment and management, they are better prepared to clarify patient concerns and help them with management. Patients may have concerns about being a "good" patient or fears about analgesics that interfere with their reporting pain[45] (see Research box; Box 12-10). Nurses need to ask patients about these concerns. Nonpharmacologic methods are required as well as medications for therapy to be effective.

Addiction from taking opioids continues to be a concern for both health professionals and patients. Persons receiving opioids for pain relief very rarely develop addiction. The incidence of opioid addiction in hospitalized patients is less than 1%.[39] Patients are taking opioids for pain relief and not for the psychologic effect. Patients who are concerned about becoming addicted can be asked, "Would you take this medication if you were not in pain?" Unfortunately, health professionals are also overly concerned about addiction, and opioids are underprescribed by physicians and underadministrated by nurses.[52]

Patients can also refuse to take opioid analgesics because of side effects such as constipation and nausea. Laxatives and stool softeners should be given to any patient receiving opioids on a regular basis. Nausea and vomiting are experienced by some; these patients usually respond well to antiemetics. Sedation and drowsiness may occur for the first 48 to 72 hours, but one needs to consider that the patient may be catching up on sleep lost because of the pain. A sedation scale may be used to monitor level of arousal (Box 12-11). Respiratory depression is rarely a problem with standardized doses and careful titration. Strategies for managing opioid side effects are summarized in the Guidelines for Safe Practice box on p. 223.

Guidelines for Safe Practice

Modifying the Environment

1. Move the patient to a quieter room away from the center of activity.
2. Dim bright lights; pull shades if sunlight is intense.
3. Keep verbal interactions at a minimum when pain is severe.
4. Encourage other patients to use headphones or keep television or radio at a reasonable level.
5. Control the number of persons entering the patient's room according to patient's wishes.
6. Explore the effect of soft music or nature sound tapes.

BOX 12-9 American Pain Society Guidelines for Managing Acute Pain

1. Recognize and treat pain promptly.
   a. Chart and display patients' self-report of pain.
   b. Commit to continuous improvement of one or several outcome variables.
   c. Document outcomes based on data and provide prompt feedback.
2. Make information about analgesics readily available.
3. Promise patients attentive analgesic care.
4. Define explicit policies for use of advanced analgesic technologies.
5. Examine the process and outcomes of pain management with the goal of continuous improvement.

BOX 12-10 Patient Concerns about Reporting Pain and Using Analgesics

Addiction: believe it occurs if they take frequent medication
Tolerance: believe they need to "save" medication for later pain
Side effects: fear constipation, nausea, mental confusion
Fatalism: expect pain to be inevitable and not treatable
Being a good patient: means not complaining
Distract physician: pain management wastes time that could be spent on treatment
Progress: reporting pain means acknowledging disease progression
Injections: believe major route is by injection which is not wanted

From Ward S et al: Patient-related barriers to management of cancer pain, *Pain* 52:319, 1993.

Research

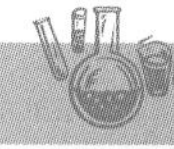

Reference: Ward S et al: Patient-related barriers to management of cancer pain, *Pain* 52:319, 1993.

In this study 207 patients with cancer attending six outpatient oncology clinics were asked to identify their concerns about reporting pain and using pain medication. Between 37% and 85% of patients reported concerns, particularly about addiction, side effects, and interpersonal communication issues with health professionals. "Good patients" were thought to avoid talking about pain by 45% of this sample. Women were more concerned about side effects than men. Patients who were older, were less educated, or had lower incomes were more likely to have concerns. Patients with more concerns had higher pain levels and were undermedicated. Health professionals need to assess and address patients' concerns about reporting pain and using analgesics, particularly if they are older and less educated.

BOX 12-11 Sample Sedation Scale for Monitoring Opioid Side Effects

S = Sleep, easy to arouse
1 = Awake and Alert
2 = Slightly drowsy, easily aroused
3 = Frequently drowsy, arousable, drifts off to sleep during conversation
4 = Somnolent, minimal or no response to physical stimulation

From McCaffery M, Pasero C: *Pain: clinical manual*, ed 2, St Louis, 1999, Mosby.

Guidelines for Safe Practice

Using Opioid Analgesics Effectively

1. Base all analgesic decisions on thorough and ongoing patient assessment.
2. Individualize the route, dosage, and schedule using the oral route wherever possible.
3. Administer opioid analgesics regularly around the clock if pain is present most of the day. Give analgesics to prevent or minimize pain.
   a. PRN dosing may be used late in the postoperative course when continuous pain is no longer present or expected. Ask the patient regularly for pain ratings to ensure adequate control.
4. Become familiar with the dose and duration of the major strong opioids such as morphine, hydromorphone, oxycontin, and fentanyl.
   a. Morphine is the standard strong opioid. However, individuals respond differently and other opioid analgesics maybe be necessary because of idiosyncratic side effects.
   b. Several types of analgesics may be used together to maximize effects (e.g., adding NSAIDs).
   c. Titrate the dose and administration interval to ensure adequate analgesia and minimize side effects.
   d. Meperidine (Demerol) should be reserved for very brief courses in patients who have allergies or intolerance to morphine and morphine derivatives.
5. Monitor patients closely for pain relief, particularly when beginning or changing analgesic regimens. Change the regimen as needed.
6. Recognize and treat side effects as soon as possible.
7. Use cognitive/behavioral and nonpharmacologic interventions appropriately to augment analgesic pain management.

Adapted from American Pain Society (APS): *Principles of analgesic use in the treatment of acute pain and cancer pain*, ed 4, Glenview, Ill, 1999, The Society.

Nursing activities related to PCA include maintaining the system, assessing the effectiveness of and the patient's response to analgesia, monitoring for side effects, and recording the number of times the patient activates the system. The patient and family members need to know how to monitor the patient's response to the medication and how to care for the PCA system if the patient is at home. Patients need to understand how and when to push the button to get a medication dose. They need to be encouraged to take the next dose when pain increases above mild intensity or above the desired level identified by the patient. In the hospital, the medication button should be clearly differentiated from the call button for help, such as by color or shape. No one but the patient should press the PCA button.

Patients and families as well as health professionals need to understand how to assess pain and the importance of giving analgesic medication regularly to prevent or reduce pain to a mild level when possible. The importance of preventing or minimizing acute pain needs to be stressed. Patients should be provided education to manage their pain. They have the right to determine their analgesic intake, but it is important to make sure they have adequate knowledge with which to make this decision. Refer to the Guidelines for Safe Practice box at left for a summary of basic principles of effective opioid analgesic administration.

The *placebo response* occurs when people experience pain relief from an intervention that may not be directly related to the applied pain relief method. Health professionals can cause a positive placebo response by the ways they interact with patients. If a person expects relief from pain, anxiety and muscle tension decrease, and less pain is experienced. The nurse's empathic approach toward the patient such as listening without judgment, giving ways to express pain and the right to do so, and recognizing the person's unique responses help to facilitate pain relief indirectly. Medication placebos such as giving saline injections instead of an opioid or giving oral doses of inappropriate drugs such as meperedine, 50 mg PO, are unethical.

There are some special considerations for analgesic use with elderly patients. Unrelieved pain in this population has been shown to result in problems after surgery such as confusion. Opioids usually are well tolerated by elders as long as the person is closely monitored for response to the analgesic prescribed.[19,37] Guidelines to help minimize the risk of side effects from the use of opioids and NSAIDs in the elderly patient are found in the Guidelines for Safe Practice boxes on p. 233.

2. Managing Chronic Pain

In recent years knowledge of the nature of chronic pain and the need for coordinated efforts of different health care professionals have resulted in the establishment of pain clinics and inpatient pain teams for control of chronic pain.

Persons with chronic persistent pain sometimes are admitted to a hospital for evaluation or initiation of treatment by a multidisciplinary health care team. One example is a team for evaluation and treatment of chronic back pain or substance abuse. Each team member evaluates the patient separately and shares his or her assessment in a team conference during which a specific treatment plan is developed. Protocols are developed for the approach to be used for control of the chronic pain; all persons providing patient care during the hospitalization need to become familiar with the protocols so that a consistent approach is used.

Nursing responsibilities include patient assessment, documenting observations, carrying out phase-related activities, and patient teaching. The culmination of the hospitalization is a discharge conference with the patient and family members in which future treatment plans and recommendations are presented and discussed.

Guidelines for Safe Practice

Use of Opioids With Elderly Patients

1. Height, weight, and body surface are not accurate measures for determining drug dosages in elders.
2. Analgesics usually last longer in elders because their renal and hepatic clearance rates are slower.
3. Age is not significant in determining dose, but it is important in determining frequency of dose.
4. Dose is based on the therapeutic response and undesirable side effects (confusion, untoward central nervous system effects, respiratory depression).
5. Elders may be hesitant to ask for pain relief. Monitor patients closely for nonverbal signs of pain. The stress of unrelieved pain leads to fatigue, anxiety, and confusion, which are physically and psychologically debilitating.
6. Review other medications the patient is taking to avoid drugs that may interact unfavorably with the analgesic.

Guidelines for Safe Practice

Use of Nonsteroidal Antiinflammatory Drugs (NSAIDs) With Elderly Patients

Precautions to be observed with the use of NSAIDs in older adults include:

1. NSAIDs cause more ulcers and bleeding episodes in elders than they do in younger adults.
2. Elders with renal impairment are at increased risk for liver and renal toxicity and need to be monitored closely for signs of toxicity, including serum levels of the NSAID.
3. GI disturbances from decreased prostaglandin production can be reduced by the administration of misoprostol (see Chapter 33). The NSAIDs should also be buffered by food and liquid.

Most patients with chronic pain profit from an ongoing association with a multidisciplinary pain clinic. Most pain clinics use a team approach that includes physicians (internists, anesthesiologists, surgeons, and psychiatrists), nurses, physical and occupational therapists, social workers, psychologists, vocational rehabilitation counselors, and appropriate others. Each pain clinic is organized differently and emphasizes different aspects of pain relief. Common approaches to the holistic management of chronic pain include:

Behavior modification (with patient's approval)
Medications: NSAIDs, tricyclic antidepressant, and opioids
Exercise and activity prescriptions
Hypnosis, acupuncture, or other cognitive/behavioral strategies
Family education to support planned goals/activities

The responsibility of the nurse varies depending on the available team members and may include patient assessment, documentation of observations, creating and maintaining a therapeutic milieu, providing emotional support for patient and family, and patient teaching. Nurses who work in pain clinics must be skilled in nurse-patient interactions, be knowledgeable about the mechanisms of pain and the effectiveness of various treatment modalities, and possess patience and understanding as they assist patients in reaching their goals.

BOX 12-12 Common Simple Modes of Distraction

1. Playing games, watching television
2. Talking with someone
3. Listening to favorite music
4. Rhythmic breathing.
5. Focusing on an object

Guidelines for Safe Practice

Modifying the Environment To Reduce Anxiety

1. Help the patient explore concerns related to the pain (meaning of pain for the patient).
2. Emphasize the importance of the patients' role in communicating their pain to the nurse (e.g., 0 to 10 pain intensity).
3. Respect the patient's response to pain, even if it differs considerably from what the nurse expects.
4. Teach the family and close friends ways in which they can help the patient, such as massage, encouraging the patient to use distraction or relaxation techniques, or supporting painful parts when moving or changing the patient's position. People often feel helpless when observing a loved one in pain and may need help themselves to cope.
5. Arrange for someone to be with the patient if the person fears being alone.
6. Talk with family or close friends and help them to allay their anxieties so that these are not transmitted to the patient.
7. Use gentle touch in patient interactions if it is acceptable to the patient.

3. Patient/Family Education

Teaching distraction and relaxation strategies. Patients can be taught to modify their sensory input to control pain by activities that promote distraction or relaxation.[1] Because anxiety increases pain, measures taken to decrease anxiety may help to decrease pain. Distraction interferes with the pain stimulus, thereby modifying the patient's awareness of the pain. Mild or moderate pain can be modified by focusing on activity in the environment. A quiet environment providing little or no sensory input actually can intensify the pain experience because the person has nothing to focus on but the painful stimulus.

Distraction requires the active participation of the individual in an effort to block out the painful stimulus. This can be enhanced by involving two or more sensory modalities, such as vision, hearing, touch, or movement. The distractors must be powerful enough to involve the person's total interest without resulting in fatigue. Pain of long duration requires a variety of meaningful distractions. Examples of common easily used distractors are listed in Box 12-12. Strategies for modifying the environment to reduce anxiety are found in the Guidelines for Safe Practice box above.

Full relaxation decreases the muscle tension and fatigue that usually accompany pain; it also helps to decrease anxiety, thereby preventing augmentation of the pain stimulus. In addition, relaxation techniques can be an effective form of distraction. The use of relaxation techniques has been shown to be effective in treating chronic pain and insomnia.[28] Relaxation exercises may be especially beneficial for persons with chronic pain to help reduce stress that may exacerbate the pain and to help the person achieve a sense of control—and more effectively cope with the pain. There is less evidence validating relaxation as an effective intervention for reducing acute pain.[28] There are numerous forms of relaxation techniques; most tend to focus on the repetition of a word, sound, or phrase or repetition of an activity, such as deep breathing, jaw relaxation, or yawning. Success with a relaxation technique requires active patient involvement and practice and encouragement.

Using Guided Imagery

Guided imagery is a term that describes the use of images to improve physiologic status, mental state, self-image, or behavior.[1,29] Progressive muscle relaxation exercises before the use of this approach facilitate the imaging process. Imagery techniques require practice to be effective and the level of concentration required may be unattainable for patients who are fatigued from acute or chronic pain. Imagery can be used simply to support mental relaxation by visualizing oneself in a favorite setting such as a quiet beach, or it can be a more active part of the pain management plan. Patients can use complex images of their pain such as fire that is gradually extinguished to add a level of conscious control to the pain experience. The technique works best when the patient selects the image and decides how it is to be used.

Complementary and Alternative Therapies

The use of complementary and alternative therapies are well suited as adjuncts to the management of acute and chronic pain. Relaxation techniques and massage are commonly used for the treatment of back and chronic pain.[28] Another modality, the use of music, has been successful in decreasing postoperative pain levels. The use of companion animals may also be an effective method of relaxation for some patients.[28] For patients who are unable to actively engage in relaxation techniques, superficial massage can be an effective option for reducing muscle tension and anxiety.[28] By providing muscle relaxation, pain may also be reduced. The most easily accessible areas of the body to massage are the back and shoulders, but the hands and feet may also be used. Therapeutic touch may be helpful to patients in pain[28,41] (see Complementary & Alternative Therapies box).

EVALUATION

Achievement of outcomes is successful if the patient with pain:

1a. Assesses pain intensity as 4 or less on a 0 to 10 scale.
1b. States that he or she does not have pain before the next analgesic dose or that mild pain is acceptable.
1c. Mobilizes and participates in usual activities easily and comfortably.
1d. Is free of side effects such as constipation or nausea.
1e. Asks for help with pain relief when needed.
2a. Participates in holistic chronic pain program.
2b. Is independent in usual activities of daily living, work, family activities, and leisure.
2c. Accurately evaluates the need for additional programs and support.
3a. Patient and family: Know how to use several nonpharmacologic pain relief measures such as heat or cold at home.
3b. Accurately describe action, side effects, dose, and frequency of all medications.
3c. State when and from whom they will seek help if pain is not relieved as expected.

Complementary & Alternative Therapies

Therapeutic Touch

The rationale for the success of therapeutic touch is not clearly understood and related research is limited. Therapeutic touch is rejected outright by many health care professionals, but it has been shown to be helpful for some patients and some types of pain. Before implementing this technique, the nurse would require special education and training. The nurse undergoes a brief period of meditation before deliberately moving his or her hands over the patient's body to assess, direct, or modulate body energy patterns. The nurse does not touch the patient's skin. In theory, the nurse is focusing his or her own internal energy and then transmitting this healing energy to the patient.

Critical Thinking Questions

1. If you were a scientist who wanted to develop an ideal analgesic, what properties would you borrow from the opioids and the NSAIDs if you could select only two properties from each? What side effects would you eliminate if you could eliminate one from each group? Why did you make the choices you made?
2. How does the assessment of acute pain differ from the assessment of chronic pain? Think about two patients for whom you have provided care—one with acute pain and one with chronic pain. In what ways did their responses to pain differ, and how did these responses influence different management approaches?
3. Compare the equianalgesic doses and the duration of action for analgesics ordered for patients you are caring for during a 24-hour period.
4. Your 45-year-old male patient says he can be strong and stand his pain, which he rates as 8 (0 to 10). From your understanding of pain pathophysiology and analgesics, how would you respond?
5. Interview three or four patients who are using a nonpharmacologic pain intervention. Compare and contrast the method, frequency of use, patient satisfaction, and effectiveness for pain relief. Were several modalities used, and was the combination of approaches successful?

References

1. Agency for Health Care Policy and Research (AHCPR): *Management of cancer pain*, Rockville, Md, 1994, US Department of Health and Human Services.

2. American Pain Society (APS): *Principles of analgesic use in the treatment of acute pain and cancer pain,* ed 4, Glenview, Ill, 1999, The Society.
3. American Pain Society (APS) Quality of Care Committee: Quality improvement guidelines for the treatment of acute and cancer pain, *JAMA* 274:1874, 1995.
4. Benedetti C, Bonica J, Belluci G: Pathophysiology and therapy of postoperative pain: a review. In Benedetti C, Chapman C, Moricca G, editors: *Recent advances in the management of pain,* New York, 1984, Raven Press.
5. Bennett G: Update on the neurophysiology of pain transmission and modulation: focus on the NMDA-receptor, *J Pain Symptom Manage* 19(1)(Suppl):2-6, 2000.
6. Bonica I, editor: *The management of pain,* ed 2, Philadelphia, 1990, Lea & Febiger.
7. Brunier G, Carson G, Harrison D: What do nurses know and believe about patients in pain? Results of a hospital survey, *J Pain Symptom Manage* 10:436, 1995.
8. Clarke E et al: Pain management knowledge, attitudes and clinical practice: the impact of nurses' characteristics and education, *J Pain Symptom Manage* 11(1):18, 1996.
9. Cleeland C et al: Effects of culture and language on ratings of cancer pain and patterns of functional interference. In Jensen T, Turner J, Wiesenfeld-Hallin, Z, editors: *Proceedings of the 8th World Congress on Pain,* vol 8, Seattle, 1997, IASP Press.
10. Cleeland C et al: Pain and its treatment in outpatients with metastatic cancer, *N Engl J Med* 330(9):592, 1994.
11. Devor M: Pain mechanisms and pain syndromes. In Campbell J, editor: Pain 1996—an updated review, *IASP Refresher Course Syllabus,* Seattle, 1996, IASP Press.
12. Donovan MI: A practical approach to pain assessment. In Watt-Watson JH, Donovan MI, editors: *Pain management: nursing perspective,* St Louis, 1992, Mosby.
13. Dunbar P, Chapman R, Buckley P, Gavrin J: Clinical analgesic equivalence for morphine and hydromorphone with prolonged PCA, *Pain* 68:265, 1996.
14. Ferrell B, McCaffery M, Grant M: Clinical decision making and pain, *Cancer Nurs* 14:289, 1991.
15. Ferrell B, Nash C, Warfield C: The role of patient-controlled analgesia in the management of cancer pain, *J Pain Symptom Manage* 7:149, 1992.
16. Fields H: *Pain,* Toronto, 1987, McGraw-Hill.
17. Feldt K: The Checklist of Nonverbal Pain Indicators (CNPI), *Pain Manage Nurs* 1(1):13, 2000.
18. Gylbels J, Tasker R: Central neurosurgery. In Wall P, Melzack R, editors: *Textbook of pain,* London, 1999, Churchill Livingstone.
19. Hardman J, Limbird L: *Goodman and Gilman's the pharmacological basis of therapeutics,* ed 9, New York, 1996, McGraw-Hill.
20. Joint Commission on Accreditation of Healthcare Organizations (JCAHO), website: http://www.jcaho.org.
21. Kalso E: Prevention of chronicity. In Jensen T, Turner J, Wiesenfeld-Hallin Z, editors: *Proceedings of the 8th World Congress on Pain,* vol 8, Seattle, 1997, IASP Press.
22. Katz J: Perioperative predictors of long-term pain following surgery. In Jensen T, Turner J, Wiesenfeld-Hallin, Z, editors: *Proceedings of the 8th World Congress on Pain,* vol 8, Seattle, 1997, IASP Press.
23. Kehlet H: Pain relief and modification of the stress response. In Cousins M, Phillips G, editors: *Acute pain management,* New York, 1986, Churchill Livingstone.
24. Kessenich K: Cyclo-oxygenase 2 inhibitors: an important new drug classification, *Pain Manage Nurs* 2(1):13, 2001.
25. Kollef M: Trapped-lung syndrome after cardiac surgery: a potentially preventable complication of pleural injury, *Heart Lung* 19(6):671, 1990.
26. Manz B et al: Pain assessment in the cognitively impaired and unimpaired elderly, *Pain Manage Nurs* 1(4):106, 2000.
27. Marks RM, Sachar EJ: Undertreatment of medical inpatients with narcotic analgesics, *Ann Intern Med* 78:173, 1973.
28. McCaffery M, Pasero C: *Pain: clinical manual,* ed 2, St Louis, 1999, Mosby.
29. McDonald D: Gender and ethnic stereotyping and narcotic analgesic administration, *Res Nurs Health* 17:45, 1994.
30. Melzack R, Wall PD: *The challenge of pain,* New York, 1996, Penguin Books.
31. Merskey H, Bogduk N: *Classification of chronic pain: descriptions of chronic pain syndromes and definitions of pain terms,* ed 2, Seattle, 1994, IASP Press.
32. Miaskowski C et al: Assessment of patient satisfaction utilizing the American Pain Society's quality assurance standards on acute and cancer-related pain, *J Pain Symptom Manage* 9(1):5, 1994.
33. Mitchell A, Brooks S, Roane D: The premature infant and painful procedures, *Pain Manage Nurs* 1(2):58, 2000.
34. Neill K: Ethnic pain styles in acute myocardial infarction, *West J Nurs Res* 15(2):531, 1993.
35. Oberle K: Pain, anxiety and analgesics: a comparative study of elderly and younger surgical patients, *Can J Aging* 9(1):13, 1990.
36. O'Gara P: The hemodynamic consequences of pain and its management, *J Intensive Care Med* 3:3, 1988.
37. Pasero C, McCaffery M: Postoperative pain management in the elderly. In Ferrell B, Ferrell B, editors: *Pain in the elderly,* Seattle, 1996, IASP Press.
38. Payne R, Paice J: Cancer pain clinical practice guidelines for clinicians and patients: rationale, barriers to implementation, and future directions. In Payne R, Pratt R, Hil C, editors: *Assessment and treatment of cancer pain,* vol 12, Seattle, 1998, IASP Press.
39. Porter J, Jick H: Addiction rare in patients treated with narcotics, *N Engl J Med* 303(2):123, 1980.
40. Puntillo K, Weiss S: Pain: its mediators and associated morbidity in critically ill cardiovascular surgical patients, *Nurs Res* 43(1):31, 1994.
41. Spross J, Burke M: Nonpharmacological management of cancer pain. In McGuire D, Yarbro C, Ferrell B, editors: *Cancer pain management,* Boston, 1995, Jones & Bartlett Publishers.
42. Sunshine A: A comparison of the newer COX-2 drugs and older nonopioid oral analgesics, *J Pain* 1(3)(Supp 1):10, 2000.
43. Taylor B, Brennan T: Preemptive analgesia: moving beyond conventional strategies and confusing terminology, *J Pain* 1(2):77, 2000.
44. Wall P: Comments after 30 years of the gate control theory, *Pain Forum* 1:12-22, 1996.
45. Ward S et al: Patient-related barriers to management of cancer pain, *Pain* 52:319, 1993.
46. Ward S, Gordon D: Application of the American Pain Society quality assurance standards. *Pain* 56:266, 1994.
47. Ward S, Gordon D: Patient satisfaction and pain severity as outcomes in pain management: a longitudinal view of one setting's experience, *J Pain Symptom Manage* 11(4):242, 1996.
48. Watson CPN, Watt-Watson J: Treatment of neuropathic pain: antidepressants and opioids, *Pain Res Manage* 4:168:2000.
49. Watt-Watson J: Misbeliefs. In Watt-Watson J, Donovan M, editors, *Pain management: nursing perspective,* St Louis, 1992, Mosby.
50. Watt-Watson J et al: Canadian Pain Society Position Statement on Pain Relief, *Pain Res Manage* 4(2):75, 1999.
51. Watt-Watson J, Evans R, Watson CP: Relationships among coping responses and perceptions of pain intensity, depression and family functioning, *Clin J Pain* 4(2):101, 1988.
52. Watt-Watson J et al: The impact of nurses' empathic responses on patients' pain management in acute care, *Nurs Res* 49:4, 2000.
53. Watt-Watson J, Graydon J: Impact of surgery on head and neck cancer patients and their caregivers, *Nurs Clin North Am* 30:659, 1995.
54. Woolf C, Thompson J: Stimulation-induced analgesia: transcutaneous electrical nerve stimulation (TENS) and vibration. In Wall P, Melzack R, editors: *Textbook of pain,* London, 1994, Churchill Livingstone.

13 Fluid, Electrolyte, and Acid-Base Imbalance

Andreana Siu, Ellen K. Boyda

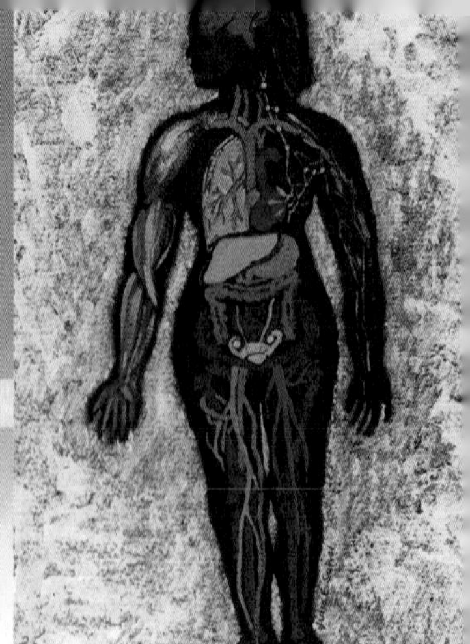

Objectives

After studying this chapter, the learner should be able to:

1. Describe the mechanisms that maintain fluid, electrolyte, and acid-base balance.
2. Compare the mechanisms and effects of fluid deficit and excess.
3. Discuss the mechanisms and effects of deficits and excesses of sodium, potassium, calcium, and magnesium.
4. Describe the mechanisms that maintain acid-base balance.
5. Differentiate between metabolic and respiratory acidosis and alkalosis.
6. Apply the pathophysiologic principles of acid-base balance to the interpretation of arterial blood gas (ABG) measurements.
7. Analyze components of ABGs to identify the type of acid-base disturbance.
8. Describe the causes and effects of each type of acid-base imbalance.
9. Use ABG findings in formulating the care of the patient with an acid-base imbalance.
10. Describe the management of patients with a fluid, electrolyte, or acid-base imbalance.

INTRODUCTION

Fluid, electrolyte, and acid-base balance is fundamental to the process of life. In the presence of a severe imbalance, the most perfectly conditioned heart cannot beat; neurons either cannot transmit or fire uncontrollably; digestion cannot take place; skeletal muscle cannot contract. At the cellular level, operations and exchanges that are essential to the life of the cell cannot take place.

Although medical therapy to prevent and treat fluid, electrolyte, or acid-base disturbances is the responsibility of the physician, nurses play a major role in all aspects of patient care for those at risk for developing a disturbance or those with a disturbance. Nursing responsibilities include:

- Recognizing situations likely to cause imbalances
- Intervening to prevent imbalances
- Carrying out preventive and therapeutic measures prescribed by the physician and monitoring patients' responses to these measures
- Recognizing signs and symptoms of fluid, electrolyte, or acid-base disturbances
- Monitoring patients to prevent and/or identify onset of imbalances related to their specific conditions or treatments
- Alleviating the effects of disturbances on the comfort and safety of patients.
- Educating patients, where appropriate, to manage their underlying condition in order to prevent an acid-base imbalance.

This chapter presents an overview of normal fluid, electrolyte, and acid-base balance. The prevention, causes, assessment, and nursing management of the most commonly encountered fluid, electrolyte, and acid-base imbalances are reviewed. Each imbalance is discussed separately, although in most instances a disturbance in the balance of one is accompanied by a resultant disturbance in one or several of the others. Nursing interventions are listed where applicable throughout the text, but are reviewed in more detail in the Nursing Management section.

Etiology

Fluid and electrolyte imbalances are common problems of patients in all clinical settings. Physiologic homeostasis is closely related to fluid and electrolyte balance, and alterations in fluid balance usually are accompanied by electrolyte abnormalities. Any disease process can potentially affect the fluid and electrolyte balance. The causes of deficits or excesses are varied and are discussed separately in each section.

Physiology: Maintenance Of Fluid And Electrolyte Balance

This section briefly reviews basic principles from chemistry and physiology that govern homeostasis. Major electrolytes are presented, but the pathophysiologic states that result from their imbalance are more thoroughly dealt with in subsequent sections.

BODY FLUID AND ELECTROLYTE COMPARTMENTS, DISTRIBUTION, AND FUNCTION

Fluid and electrolytes are found within the body either in the cell (intracellular) or outside the cell (extracellular). The *extracellular fluid* (ECF) compartment is further subdivided into the *interstitial fluid* (fluid between the cells) and *intravascular fluid* (fluid in the blood vessels) compartments. A third type of fluid, *transcellular fluid*, denotes fluid separated by a layer of epithelial cells from other ECF.[17] Transcellular fluid includes digestive juices, fluid in the pleural cavity, synovial fluid, lymphatic fluid, intraocular fluid, and cerebrospinal fluid. Some authorities consider this to be a part of the extracellular compartment, and others consider it a separate compartment. Transcellular fluid makes up 1% to 3% of body weight. Under normal circumstances, the amount of transcellular fluid does not fluctuate much during the day and therefore has little impact on fluid balance.

Water is the largest single constituent of the body, accounting for 45% to 75% of body weight. The volume and distribution of body water vary with age and gender (Figure 13-1). In the newborn, almost 75% of the body weight is water, with the greatest percentage found in the extracellular compartment. The volume and distribution change over time. In the young adult man, 60% of the body weight is water, with two thirds of this being in the intracellular compartment. In the average young woman, approximately 50% of body weight is water. The difference between men and women is predominantly the result of the difference in water content of muscle and fat tissues. Skeletal muscle cells holds more water than fat cells. Women in general have a higher ratio of fat to skeletal muscle than men.

Body water has multiple functions. Intracellular fluid (ICF) provides the internal aqueous medium for cellular chemical function. The extracellular water maintains blood volume and serves as the body's transport system to and from cells. Body water cushions and lubricates, helps give the body its structure, hydrolyzes food in the digestive system, and acts as a reactant and medium for the chemical reactions that occur within the cell. Adequate body water balance is necessary for (1) the maintenance of normal body temperature, which is achieved by distributing heat and by cooling the body via evaporation from the skin; (2) the elimination of waste products; and (3) all transportation within the body.

Electrolytes are chemical compounds that develop an ionic charge when dissolved in water. The most prominent of these are the positively charged ions *(cations)*—hydrogen, sodium, potassium, magnesium, and calcium—and the negatively charged ions *(anions)*—chloride, bicarbonate, sulfate, and phosphate. The precise concentrations of the electrolytes are vital to body functions that require particular ions or pH. Electrolytes also serve to maintain fluid osmolarity and volume within the intracellular and extracellular compartments. All body fluids contain electrolytes (Table 13-1).

Nurses practicing in acute and critical care areas handle solutions containing multiple electrolytes. These solutions can

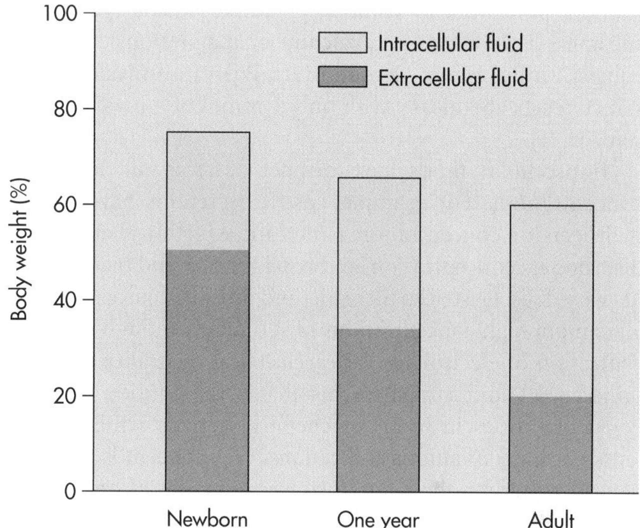

Figure 13-1 In the newborn infant more than half of total body fluid is extracellular. As the child grows, proportions gradually approximate adult levels.

TABLE 13-1 Normal Electrolyte Content of Body Fluids

Electrolytes* (Anions and Cations)	Extracellular: Intravascular (mEq/L)	Extracellular: Interstitial (mEq/L)	Intracellular (mEq/L)
Sodium (Na^+)	142	146	15
Potassium (K^+)	5	5	150
Calcium (Ca^{++})	5	3	2
Magnesium (Mg^{++})	2	1	27
Chloride (Cl^-)	102	114	1
Bicarbonate (HCO_3^-)	27	30	10
Protein ($Prot^-$)	16	1	63
Phosphate (HPO_4^{-2})	2	2	100
Sulfate (SO_4^{-2})	1	1	20
Organic Acid	5	8	0

*Note that the electrolyte level of the intravascular and interstitial fluids (extracellular fluids) is approximately the same and that sodium and chloride contents are markedly higher in these fluids, whereas potassium, phosphate, and protein contents are markedly higher in intracellular fluid.

be as diverse as dialysate and hyperalimentation solution. Although the concentration of these solutions is calculated by teams of medical, nursing, and pharmacy specialists, it is useful for nurses who are handling these solutions to have a general understanding of the systems of measurements used.

One system involves measurement of the number of electrically charged particles per liter of fluid. The unit of measurement can be in milliequivalents (mEq) per liter or in millimoles (mmol) per liter. To understand the difference between milliequivalents and millimoles, it is necessary to first understand the concept of valence. Valence reflects the number of hydrogen atoms that can be held in combination or displaced in a reaction by one atom of an element. Examples of a univalent substance are sodium (Na^+), potassium (K^+), and chloride (CL^-). Examples of a bivalent substance are calcium (Ca^{++}) and magnesium (Mg^{++}). To convert from millimoles to milliequivalents, the millimole value is multiplied by the valence of the substance. If a substance is *univalent* (e.g., sodium, potassium or chloride), 1 mmol equals 1mEq. If a substance is *bivalent* (e.g., calcium or magnesium), 1 mmol equals 2 mEq. Hence, 2 mmol (2 mEq) of a univalent substance reacts chemically with only 1 mmol of a bivalent substance.

Transcellular fluids have distinct patterns of electrolyte concentrations. For example, gastric secretions have a high hydrogen ion concentration, pancreatic secretions have a high bicarbonate concentration, and renal tubular and bladder fluids vary daily. Gastric, pancreatic, and intestinal juices and bile all contain high concentrations of sodium. Although the concentration of electrolytes varies, electrical neutrality is maintained in all fluid compartments; that is, the solution contains equal quantities in terms of chemical activity (milliequivalents per liter) of anions and cations. This concept is essential to understanding the laboratory measurement of anion gap, which is discussed later in the chapter.

Each electrolyte has specific functions. The general functions of all electrolytes are to (1) promote neuromuscular irritability, (2) maintain body fluid volume and osmolarity, (3) distribute body water between fluid compartments, and (4) regulate acid-base balance.

In addition to the milliequivalent values, it is also important to take into account the concentration of electrolytes in solution. The terms *osmolality* and *osmolarity* refer to concentration. Technically, these two terms mean slightly different things. Osmolality refers to the number of dissolved particles (or solute) in 1000 g (or 1 kg) of distilled water. Osmolarity, on the other hand, is most accurately used when referring to the concentration of particles in 1000 ml of solution or osmoles per liter of solution. In the clinical setting, the concentrations dealt with are much smaller so osmolality or osmolarity is reported in milliosmoles (thousandth of an osmole).[21] Thus, osmolality is measured in milliosmoles per kilogram of water, and osmolarity is measured in milliosmoles per liter of water[24]; 1kg of water is equivalent to 1 L in volume. Therefore, since the dissolved particles occupy a certain volume in the solution, the total volume in 1 kg of water will be 1 L of water plus the relatively small volume occupied by the solutes. The difference in the terms osmolality and osmolarity is of practical interest to a research chemist who may be using electrolytes dissolved in different types of solutions. In clinical practice the difference in these terms is negligible because of the low solute concentrations in the body fluids, all of which are basically water. Throughout this chapter the term *osmolarity* is used.

The significance of plasma osmolarity is that it is the main regulator of the release of antidiuretic hormone (ADH). In the state of dehydration osmolarity rises, stimulating the release of ADH, which signals the kidneys to conserve water and produce concentrated urine.

Measuring plasma and urine osmolarity is useful in several circumstances. Plasma osmolarity averages 290 ± 5 mOsm/kg and is relatively constant from day to day. Symptoms resulting from increased osmolarity usually occur at levels greater than 350 mOsm. Coma occurs at approximately 400 mOsm or greater. An osmolar gap exists when the measured and calculated (or expected) values differ by more than 15 mOsm/kg. This signifies the presence of substances in the plasma or urine that are not normally found in homeostasis (i.e., toxins or poisons).

NORMAL EXCHANGE OF FLUID AND ELECTROLYTES

In the healthy human being, body fluids (water and electrolytes) are constantly being lost and replaced. The fluid that is lost is not pure water but contains some electrolytes; thus both water and electrolytes must be replaced daily. Knowing the approximate concentrations of fluid and electrolytes in the various compartments enables the nurse to anticipate which imbalance will occur with abnormal losses from any particular site.

Body fluids are lost daily from the kidneys, respiratory tract, gastrointestinal tract, and skin. Negligible amounts are also lost in saliva and tears. Two processes demand continual expenditure of water: control of body heat and excretion of metabolic waste products. The volume of fluids used in these processes depends on factors such as external temperature, humidity, metabolic rate, and physical activity. In normal fluid balance, output equals intake. A balanced diet provides excess amounts of electrolytes and they are excreted. The result is that balance is maintained. This balance is regulated primarily by the function of the kidney tubules.

Table 13-2 summarizes the normal routes of gains and losses of fluid in an adult consuming approximately 2500 calories/day. Note that approximately two fifths of the normal fluid intake is obtained from water in food, or "preformed water." Solid foods such as meat and vegetables are 60% to 90% water. The fact that a large quantity of water is obtained from food has important implications if a person's food intake decreases substantially.

The insensible route (skin, respiratory tract, and gastrointestinal tract) accounts for approximately two fifths of fluid lost daily. These losses are not perceptible. Insensible loss through the skin refers to invisible perspiration, not visible sweat. When visible perspiration occurs, the loss of

TABLE 13-2 Normal Fluid Intake and Loss in Adult Consuming 2500 Calories/Day (Approximate Values)

Intake Route	Amount of Gain (ml)	Output Route	Amount of Loss (ml)
Water in food:	1000	Skin:	500
Water from oxidation:	300	Lungs:	350
Water as liquid:	1200	Feces:	150
		Kidneys:	1500
TOTAL	2500	TOTAL	2500

water through the skin is greater than the normal 500 ml/day. Fecal loss is proportionately larger in the presence of diarrheal or loose stools. Certain pulmonary conditions cause a loss greater than the normal 350 ml/day from the lungs. It is important to note that increased fluid loss through the insensible routes also results in the loss of electrolytes.

INTERNAL REGULATION OF BODY WATER AND ELECTROLYTES

The human body uses a number of remarkable operations to closely regulate both the volume and composition of body fluids. Fluid and electrolyte balance depends on an adequate intake and output. This means that the intake must equal the output.

The control of intake and output is regulated by various internal mechanisms. In this section the regulation of body water and major electrolytes is summarized. See standard physiology texts for a more in-depth review.

Thirst

The major control of fluid intake is thirst. The thirst center is located in the ventromedial nucleus of the hypothalamus. Impulses from this center can stimulate the cerebral cortex, which interprets this stimulation as the perception of thirst. The thirst center itself is stimulated by hypertonic body fluid, isoosmotic contraction, decreased blood pressure, decreased cardiac output, dryness of the mouth, and angiotensin. How these factors generate the stimulus to the thirst center is not fully understood. The dehydration of cells in the thirst center is thought to stimulate the neurons, which transmit an impulse to the cerebral cortex, which in turn translates the sensation to that of thirst. Most of the time thirst is not consciously thought of as a control of water intake. Social and cultural habits exert an important influence on the quantity and type of liquid that human beings drink. This may be an important consideration in some plans of care. Some evidence suggests that human beings also have a salt appetite. This may be important during periods of extreme sodium depletion, such as with prolonged heat exposure and perspiration.

Kidney

The major organ controlling ECF and electrolyte balance is the kidney. In addition to its commonly portrayed function as the organ of excretion of some metabolites and drugs, the kidney plays a powerful role in maintaining a vital balance of substances such as sodium, potassium, bicarbonate, chloride, H^+, glucose, and others. When the kidney properly regulates the balance of water and ions, homeostasis is achieved. This is accomplished through filtration, resorption, secretion, and synthesis.

Filtration occurs through the glomerular membrane. This membrane contains three layers: the capillary endothelium, the inner wall of Bowman's capsule, and the basement membrane. By design, the outer and inner layers of the glomerular membrane leak. The cells do not adhere to each other and have spaces between them to permit the passage of small molecules. The larger molecules, particularly proteins, are constrained by these small spaces. The large negatively charged molecules have more difficulty passing through the basement membrane owing to the ionic charge relationships within the membrane itself.[13]

Glomerular filtration in the kidney is determined by three factors: glomerular capillary blood pressure, the hydrostatic pressure of Bowman's capsule, and plasma protein concentration (see Chapter 38). Many factors and pathophysiologic states can affect these three factors and thus change glomerular filtration. Conditions such as shock and hypertension change glomerular capillary blood pressure. Changes in the pressure of Bowman's capsule can be caused by urinary obstruction. A decrease in plasma protein concentration can occur with increased loss, decreased intake, or decreased production of proteins. Damage to the basement membrane of the capsule, as with glomerular nephritis, decreases filtration from the glomeruli.

Within the renal lumen the dynamics of resorption and excretion are driven by molecular polarity. Nonpolar molecules are reabsorbed more easily than polar ones and can be affected by introducing drugs that specifically block transport through the tubular epithelium. An example of these is the thiazide diuretics, which block the resorption of sodium in the distal tubule. Because the sodium is then excreted, for osmotic reasons water follows. There is a subsequent volume loss in ECF. Resorption of sodium in the renal tubule involves active transport throughout its length. This is not true of other organic molecules, which depend on carrier proteins that are specific to certain areas of the tubule.

Molecules that do not filter through the glomerulus pass into the efferent renal arteriole to the peritubular capillaries, where they are secreted into the tubular lumen. Some molecules are neither filtered nor secreted significantly (albumin).

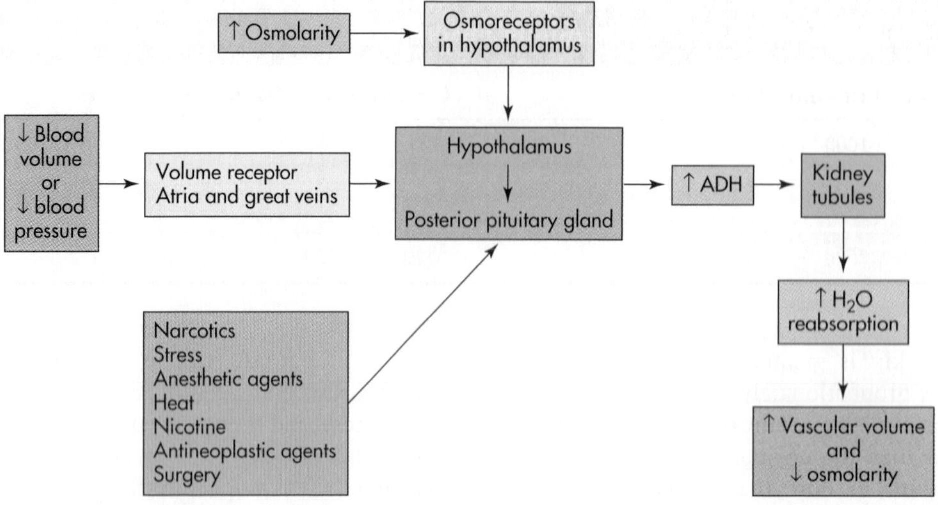

Figure 13-2 Factors and mechanisms involved in antidiuretic hormone (ADH) production and effect of ADH.

However, some are both filtered and secreted (potassium). Finally, the kidney synthesizes certain molecules such as bicarbonate, which affect osmolarity and acid-base balance.[13]

Antidiuretic Hormone

ADH is a hormone produced by the supraoptic and paraventricular nuclei of the hypothalamus and released from the posterior pituitary gland. The neurons in the hypothalamus receive input from volume receptors in the left atrium and great veins and from osmoreceptors in the hypothalamus. Volume receptors are stimulated by changes in atrial blood volume or blood pressure. Impulses from the volume receptors are transmitted by afferent nerve fibers to the hypothalamus. Increased blood volume or blood pressure augments the firing of the volume receptors, stimulates the hypothalamus, and inhibits ADH production. Conversely, decreased blood volume or blood pressure dampens the firing of the volume receptors and stimulates the production of ADH.

Osmoreceptors are stimulated by changes in cell size. The addition of water to the body fluids increases the size of the cells in the osmoreceptor and leads to a decrease of ADH production. A loss of water causes the cells to shrink and stimulates the secretion of ADH. Angiotensin, narcotics, stress, heat, nicotine, antineoplastic agents, and anesthetic agents also stimulate the secretion of ADH. Figure 13-2 depicts the factors and mechanisms involved and the results of ADH production.

ADH acts on the kidney cells by stimulating 39′,5′-cyclic adenosine monophosphate (AMP) release, which regulates cellular metabolism. In the kidney, ADH causes increased water resorption in the distal convoluted tubules and collecting ducts. Additionally, it stimulates the sodium pump in the loop of Henle and regulates the rate of blood perfusion, both of which lead to water resorption. Under the influence of ADH, the kidney can concentrate urine to 1200 mOsm/kg H_2O. The conservation of water increases blood volume and pressure and decreases osmolarity. Because ADH can be secreted in response to factors other than a deficit of water (narcotics, anesthetic agents, and stressors), fluid overload can occur.

Inappropriate ADH secretion can be a life-threatening event. This condition is known as the *syndrome of inappropriate secretion of ADH (SIADH).* The features of this phenomenon are plasma hyponatremia and hypotonicity. Simultaneously, the urine is itself hypertonic and contains appreciable amounts of sodium. In this syndrome there is an absence of hypokalemia and edema. Cardiac, renal, and adrenal functions are normal. Despite the decreased urine output there is no evidence of dehydration or hypovolemia. The presence of low serum blood urea nitrogen and uric acid levels assists in confirming the diagnosis. The secretion of ADH is "inappropriate" in that it continues despite the decreased osmolarity of the plasma. The serum sodium concentration and serum osmolarity are the most easily available indices of this process. The treatment consists of restriction of fluid intake and, when applicable, therapy for the underlying disorders (e.g., administration of cortisone for Addison's disease or discontinuation of causative medications). Administration of salt (sodium chloride solutions) is usually of transient benefit, but is useful in patients in whom water intoxication is severe.[18]

Aldosterone-Renin-Angiotensin System

Aldosterone is a hormone produced by the zona glomerulosa of the adrenal cortex. It increases the kidney's resorption of sodium and thus water in the proximal tubules and the distal convoluted tubules. In the complete absence of aldosterone, a person may excrete 25 g of sodium per day, whereas if large quantities of aldosterone are present no sodium is excreted.

The major stimulus for aldosterone production is a reflex initiated by the kidney. Cells in the kidney monitor sodium levels and blood volume. When the serum sodium level or the blood volume decreases, the juxtaglomerular cells in the kidney secrete a protein, *renin.* Renin acts on *angiotensinogen,* a plasma protein formed in the liver to produce *angiotensin I.* This, in turn is converted to *angiotensin II* by yet another en-

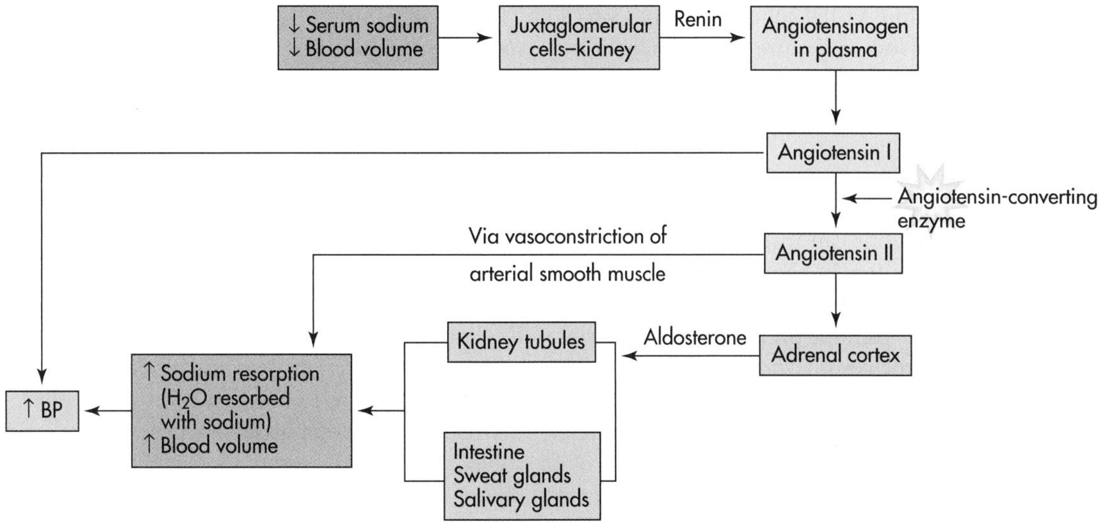

Figure 13-3 Factors and mechanisms involved in aldosterone production and effects of aldosterone production.

zyme called angiotensin-converting enzyme. Angiotensin II stimulates the adrenal cortex to secrete aldosterone. Aldosterone causes the retention of sodium by the kidneys, intestines, and sweat and salivary glands. In addition, angiotensin II causes vasoconstriction of arterial smooth muscle, which results in a decrease in glomerular filtration rate and the occurrence of systemic hypertension.

Some aldosterone may be secreted in response to adrenocorticotropic hormone. Sodium and water retention may be precipitated by liver failure because aldosterone is catabolized by a normally functioning liver. Figure 13-3 depicts the factors and mechanisms involved as well as the effects of aldosterone production.

Atrial Natriuretic Peptide

Atrial natriuretic peptide (ANP), also called atrial natriuretic factor, is a hormone produced from specialized cells in the atrial muscle of the heart. This substance is a 28-amino acid peptide released in response to stretching during periods of volume overload, such as congestive heart failure, renal failure, hypertension, and certain dysrhythmias. ANP may also be secreted in direct response to a number of vasopressor substances, including vasopressin and epinephrine.[12] The main effects of ANP are direct arterial vasodilation, increased glomerular filtration rate, and diuresis (due to the increased renal blood flow).[28] It is speculated that ANP may be the primary counteractant of the plasma renin-angiotensin-aldosterone system.[14]

Sodium

Sodium, the most abundant extracellular cation, influences the degree of water retention. Deficiency may result in neuromuscular dysfunction. Excess may result in hypertension. Ingestion and excretion control the total volume of plasma sodium, while the degree of its dilution in water determines the concentration, or osmolarity, of plasma sodium. Factors affecting the volume and osmolarity of plasma sodium include (1) ingestion of sodium, (2) excretion of sodium, (3) ADH, (4) aldosterone-renin-angiotensin system, and (5) ANP.[18]

Regulation of sodium balance is accomplished by the same mechanisms that regulate fluid balance. An increase in serum sodium level causes an increase in plasma osmolarity. This in turns stimulates the thirst center to increase water intake and the posterior pituitary to release more ADH. ADH causes the kidney to retain water and as a result normalizes the serum osmolarity. When serum sodium level drops, the reverse happens. The sensation of thirst diminishes leading to a decrease in water intake. The release of ADH is also suppressed, which leads to increased water excretion. Aldosterone is also secreted by the adrenal cortex to increase sodium resorption in the renal tubules.

Potassium

Potassium (K^+) is the major intracellular cation and regulates intracellular osmolarity. Not only is potassium an important participant in the control of acid-base balance, it is also important in the conduction of nerve impulses and promotion of proper skeletal and cardiac muscle activity. Because of potassium's role in the excitability of nerves and muscles, it is important that the extracellular concentration of potassium be maintained within the narrow, normal range. Potassium values are shown in Table 13-1.

The major excretion site of excess potassium is the kidney. Most excess potassium (80% to 90%) is excreted in the urine, and the remainder is excreted by the gastrointestinal tract. Potassium is completely filtered by the kidney, but most of the filtered potassium is reabsorbed in the proximal tubules and the loop of Henle. Glomerular filtration of potassium plays only a minimal role in normal potassium excretion. The control of renal excretion of potassium resides in the ability of the distal tubular cells to secrete potassium into tubular fluid. As extracellular potassium levels rise, more potassium moves into the cells, including the distal tubular cells. The higher concentration in the cells facilitates potassium secretion into tubular fluid because of the gradient difference between the distal tubular cells and the fluid in the tubular lumen. Conversely, if potassium intake is low or if more potassium is lost through the gastrointestinal tract, the potassium level in the distal tubules is decreased. This causes a decrease in the gradient, and less potassium is secreted.

Even though glomerular filtration plays only a minimal role in the amount of potassium excreted in the urine, it is important because certain situations can interfere with the resorption of the filtered potassium in the proximal tubules, leading to an increased loss of potassium. Osmotic diuretics and disease states that produce osmotic diuresis are examples. Tubular diuretics, such as hydrochlorothiazide and furosemide, also enhance the loss of potassium.

When potassium level increases in the ECF, two additional mechanisms to maintain serum potassium level come into play: secretion of aldosterone and the hydrogen-potassium exchange. Aldosterone increases the amount of potassium secreted by the distal tubules. The aldosterone-secreting cells of the adrenal cortex are sensitive to the extracellular concentration of potassium. If the extracellular concentration of potassium increases, aldosterone is secreted and stimulates the distal tubular cells to secrete more potassium. The renin-angiotensin system is not involved in this stimulation of aldosterone.

The hydrogen-potassium exchange mechanism also contributes to the maintenance of potassium balance. In the case of hyperkalemia (high potassium level in the serum or ECF), potassium moves into the cell in an attempt to lower the serum potassium level. To maintain electrical neutrality, hydrogen ions move out of the cell and this can lead to acidosis. The opposite is also true for hypokalemia. Potassium moves from the cell into the ECF in an attempt to raise the serum potassium level. In exchange, hydrogen ions move into the cell and this can lead to alkalosis.

The same hydrogen-potassium exchange mechanism is also responsible for the maintenance of acid-base balance. An abnormal hydrogen ion concentration in the arterial blood, as in the case of acidosis or alkalosis, can cause a transcellular shift in potassium. The existence of a low hydrogen ion concentration (alkalosis) causes hydrogen ions to move from the cells into the ECF compartment. To maintain electrical neutrality, potassium moves into the cell causing a relative hypokalemia. Conversely, a high hydrogen concentration (acidosis) causes hydrogen to move into the cells and potassium to move from the ICF compartment to the ECF compartment causing a relative hyperkalemia.

Calcium

Factors Affecting Distribution

Calcium (Ca^{++}) plays a major role in the promotion of neuromuscular irritability and muscular contractions. Calcium and phosphorus are found primarily in the bones and teeth (99%), with a very small amount dissolved in the blood (1%). The amounts of dissolved calcium and phosphorus are in inverse relationship. As one increases, the other decreases. This inverse relationship must be maintained; if both are elevated at the same time, they form an insoluble precipitate. The dissolved part of calcium is carried in the blood in two forms: bound to protein, particularly albumin, and ionized. The serum levels that usually are reported are measures of total dissolved calcium (both bound and ionized). The ionized fraction can be measured separately, but this is a more expensive test and is not routinely performed. Only the ionized fraction is involved in the promotion of neuromuscular activity.

The ionized portion must be maintained within fine limits because a decrease in ionized calcium has profound effects on the body, one example of which is tetany. In a person with normal serum protein and albumin levels and a normal calcium level, the ionized fraction is usually a little more than 50% of the total dissolved level. Because part of the dissolved calcium is bound to protein, the concentration of serum calcium varies as the protein level varies. If the total protein and albumin levels fall, the total serum calcium level falls. Patients with serum calcium levels below normal resulting from a decrease in protein or albumin may exhibit no symptoms of hypocalcemia because, although their total calcium level is low, the ionized fraction may still be within normal limits.

The ratio between the dissolved calcium that is bound and the ionized fraction is affected by acid-base status. Acidosis causes more calcium to be ionized, whereas alkalosis causes more of the ionized fraction to become bound to protein. These changes are probably not detrimental to people with a normal serum calcium level. However, alkalosis in a person who already has a low serum calcium level can lead to tetany. Calcium also binds to other agents such as citrate, which normally is metabolized by the liver. Because citrate is commonly used as an anticoagulant in stored blood, patients receiving a large number of transfusions rapidly should be watched carefully for signs of hypocalcemia. Some authorities recommend that for every 3 to 4 U of blood given rapidly, the patient should receive 10 ml of calcium gluconate.[6]

Control of Calcium Levels

The serum level of calcium depends on three hormones: parathyroid hormone, vitamin D, and calcitonin. *Parathyroid hormone* is produced by the parathyroid gland in response to decreased serum calcium levels. It causes increased movement of calcium from the bone, increased absorption of calcium from the gastrointestinal tract, and increased resorption of calcium from the renal tubules. These activities result in increased serum calcium levels. Parathyroid hormone also increases the excretion of phosphorus by the kidneys.

Vitamin D is formed by the action of sunlight on a provitamin present in the skin and can be obtained in its completed form from dietary sources. The liver and kidney hydroxylate vitamin D to its active form, which is essential for the absorption of calcium from the gastrointestinal tract. Parathyroid hormone cannot increase the absorption of calcium from the gastrointestinal tract unless activated vitamin D is present. In addition, vitamin D significantly increases the effectiveness of parathyroid hormone in bone resorption (demineralization). The major control point for the blood concentration of vitamin D is the hydroxylation step in the kidney, which is stimulated by parathyroid hormone. The feedback mechanism begins with a low calcium level stimulating the secretion of parathyroid hormone, which then activates vitamin D; both then increase the absorption of calcium from the gastrointestinal tract and the resorption (demineralization) of calcium from the bone.

Calcitonin, a hormone produced by the thyroid gland, decreases calcium levels by preventing bone resorption (demineralization) of calcium. It opposes the effects of parathyroid hormone and vitamin D on bones. High calcium levels stimulate the thyroid gland to release calcitonin, which inhibits the release of calcium from the bone, thus lowering serum calcium levels.

Magnesium

Magnesium is one of the major intracellular cations. It is responsible for many of the intracellular enzyme reactions, including carbohydrate metabolism and protein synthesis. It also plays a role in sodium and potassium transport, neuromuscular excitability, as well as in calcium absorption through its effect on the parathyroid hormone.

Both the gastrointestinal system and the kidneys are responsible for the regulation of magnesium balance. When the serum magnesium level falls, the gastrointestinal tract absorbs more magnesium and excretes less in the feces. Similarly, the kidney conserves magnesium by increasing its resorption at the proximal tubule and the loop of Henle. When the serum magnesium level rises, the kidney excretes the excess in the urine.

MOVEMENT OF FLUID AND SOLUTES BETWEEN COMPARTMENTS

The components previously discussed are not static, nor are the different compartments of fluid closed to each other. Instead, there is a constant dynamic interchange between compartments. Materials are carried to and waste products removed from the cells via the movement of solutes and water.

Solute and Fluid Transport Between Extracellular and Intracellular Compartments

Solutes, including electrolytes, flow across cell membranes by passive or active processes. Passive transport of solute across a membrane is called *diffusion.* Solutes move from a more concentrated solution to a less concentrated solution until both are equal. If a higher concentration of a substance exists outside the cell, it will diffuse into the cell if the cell membrane is permeable. Cell membranes are largely lipid; hence lipid-soluble molecules enter easily. Certain water-soluble molecules can diffuse into cells with the assistance of proteins in the cell membrane by the process of *facilitated diffusion.*

Some electrolytes and other solutes flow from lower to greater concentrations or against the concentration gradient by active transport. An example is the sodium-potassium pump. To accomplish this uphill feat requires the help of carrier ions and energy. The energy source is in the form of adenosine triphosphate (ATP). It has been shown that with the expenditure of one high-energy phosphate bond from ATP, three sodium ions move out of the cell, and two potassium ions move into the cell. Active transport uses a large percentage of the energy formed each day, because sodium and potassium are constantly diffusing into and out of the cell. Active transport is required to keep the proper concentrations of the two electrolytes within the cell.

Water, like solutes, moves between the extracellular and intracellular compartment. The movement of water is controlled by the osmolarity of the two compartments. Sodium is the main regulator of extracellular osmolarity, and potassium is the main regulator of intracellular osmolarity. Unaided, water moves in a predictable direction from high concentration to low concentration. The movement of water from an area of low osmolarity (high water concentration) to an area of high osmolarity (low water concentration) is called *osmosis* and continues until the osmolarity between the two compartments is equal. For example, if the water content increases or the solute content decreases in the extracellular compartment, water moves into the cells to equalize osmolarity. Should the reverse conditions prevail and the solute concentration increase extracellularly beyond the intracellular concentration, the flow of water also reverses until osmolarity is equalized. Solutes also move back and forth between the two compartments, but the cell membrane is more permeable to water than it is to solutes. For this reason, fluid movement between the extracellular compartment and the intracellular compartment is primarily regulated by osmosis.

The mechanisms controlling water and sodium levels also control osmolarity and thus the movement of fluid between the extracellular and intracellular compartment. Various pathologic states including disease and trauma can affect osmolarity and cell membrane permeability. These in turn are the causes of cellular edema or cellular dehydration, the signs and symptoms of which are discussed later in the chapter.

Fluid Transport Between Vascular and Interstitial Spaces

The control of fluid movement between the vascular and interstitial spaces is defined by Starling's law of the capillaries. Two different types of pressure influence the flow of fluid between the vascular space and the interstitial space. These are hydrostatic pressure and colloid osmotic pressure (oncotic pressure). *Hydrostatic pressure* is the pressure caused by blood pressing against the walls of the blood vessels. Hydrostatic pressure also exists in the tissue but is minimal (5 mm Hg or less), and some authorities believe that the hydrostatic pressure in the tissue is actually a negative pressure.[27] Hydrostatic pressure effectively pushes fluid out of the vascular bed into the interstitial space.

Colloid osmotic pressure is the pressure needed to overcome the pull of proteins (colloids), especially albumin, in the blood. The proteins do not pass freely through the walls of the capillaries because of their size. A few proteins are present in the interstitial space, but a much larger concentration is in the intravascular space. The colloid osmotic pressure within the vascular space serves to *pull* or *absorb* fluid from the interstitial space.

The difference between hydrostatic pressure and colloid osmotic pressure in the vascular space determines the movement of fluid between the vascular and interstitial spaces. For example, in Figure 13-4 the hydrostatic and the colloid osmotic pressures in the tissue would be zero. The hydrostatic pressure at the arteriole end of the capillary (approximately 40 mm Hg) is greater than the hydrostatic pressure at the venule end of the capillary (approximately 10 mm Hg). The colloid osmotic pressure stays approximately the same throughout the vascular bed and equals about 25 mm Hg.

The difference between the hydrostatic pressure and the colloid osmotic pressure at the arteriole end of the capillary is +15 mm Hg (40 mm Hg −25 mm Hg = 15 mm Hg) and favors the movement of fluid out of the vascular compartment. The difference between the hydrostatic pressure and the colloid osmotic pressure at the venule end of the capillary is −15 mm Hg (10 mm Hg − 25 mm Hg = −15 mm Hg) and favors the movement of fluid into the vascular compartment (see Figure 13-4).

Hydrostatic pressure can be conceived of as "push," and colloid osmotic pressure as "pull." These forces are constantly opposing each other in the movement of solutions and substances. The competing forces fall into four categories.

1. *Vascular hydrostatic pressure* is the blood pressure at the capillary level, which is related to the pressure wave each time the heart contracts.
2. *Vascular colloid osmotic pressure* is the pull exerted by the plasma proteins in the blood, which normally remains fairly constant. However, if a large amount of protein leaves the capillary, vascular osmotic pressure drops, further reducing the vascular spaces' ability to retain fluid.
3. *Interstitial fluid hydrostatic pressure* is the push exerted by interstitial fluid against tissues and individual cells, especially those making up the capillary membrane.
4. *Interstitial fluid colloid osmotic pressure* is the pull exerted by the protein in the interstitial fluid.[7]

Overall this system allows fluids high in nutrients and oxygen to diffuse out of the vascular bed at the arteriole end of the capillary and fluids containing waste products to move back into the vascular bed at the venule end of the capillaries. The system is not perfect, however, and some fluid is left in the interstitial space. In addition, some protein may escape from the vascular bed and, if allowed to accumulate, acts as a force to pull even more fluid from the vascular space. The lymphatic system picks up the excess fluid and the escaped proteins and returns them to the vascular space.

Many factors affect hydrostatic pressure. At the arteriole end of the capillary, the hydrostatic pressure depends on the volume and viscosity of blood, force of the heartbeat, and resistance of the blood vessels. Hydrostatic pressure at the venous end depends on the venous pressure. In turn, the venous pressure depends on the structural integrity of the veins, respiration, and skeletal muscle contractions. The colloid osmotic pressure depends on the protein level. The protein level itself is dependent on dietary intake, the liver's ability to produce proteins, and the body's ability to retain, not lose, protein. Various pathologic states can interfere with any of these mechanisms and result in edema.

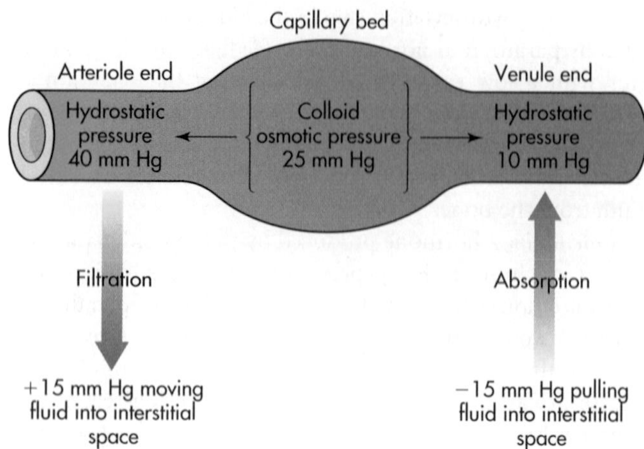

Figure 13-4 Pressure difference across capillary provides for movement of fluid, nutrients, and waste between interstitial and vascular spaces.

FLUID IMBALANCE

Sodium is the most prevalent electrolyte in the ECF. Therefore changes in ECF volume are often associated with alterations in sodium balance and may be described in the context of that abnormality. As a result of fluid and electrolyte imbalance, patients may experience severe, potentially life-threatening pathologic changes.

When a change occurs in the sodium/water ratio, a disturbance in osmolarity results; that is, the ECF becomes hypoosmolar or hyperosmolar. When the change in ECF volume occurs with a proportionate change in extracellular solutes (particles dissolved in solution, i.e., electrolytes, urea, or glucose), the ECF remains isotonic. Loss of fluid balance may occur as a result of fluid excess or deficit. The fluid disruption may be associated with hypoosmolarity or hyperosmolarity, or the fluid may remain isotonic (Table 13-3).

As with all clinical problems, the same pathophysiologic change is not of equal significance to all people. For instance, consider a 24-hour viral syndrome with associated nausea and diarrhea. In one individual, this may result in some extracellular volume depletion, but not significant electrolyte disturbance. On the other hand, the same viral syndrome in someone without the ability to concentrate urine (due to hormonal or renal factors) may cause severe, even life-threatening fluid and electrolyte imbalance. Therefore it is essential to evaluate each episode of real or potential fluid imbalance in the specific physiologic context in which it occurs. That is, consider the patient from a holistic perspective.

FLUID DEFICIT

An ECF deficit may occur as a result of (1) reduced fluid intake, (2) loss of body fluids, or (3) sequestration (compartmentalizing) of body fluids.

Etiology

Decreased Intake. Anyone without fluids available to drink, who is unable to take fluids independently, or who does

TABLE 13-3 Water and Sodium Imbalances

Type of Imbalance	Water Imbalance	Sodium Imbalance
Hyperosmolar	Water ↓ in relation to sodium and other solutes	Sodium or other solutes ↑ in relation to water
Hypoosmolar	Water ↑ in relation to sodium and other solutes	Sodium ↓ in relation to water
Isotonic volume excess	Water ↑ proportionally with sodium	Sodium ↑ proportionally with water
Isotonic volume deficit	Water ↓ proportionally with sodium	Sodium ↓ proportionally with water

not respond to thirst appropriately may develop a fluid deficit. Patients who are unable to ask for fluids, identify their need for fluid, or swallow easily may develop a fluid deficit. Thus someone with a cerebrovascular accident and aphasia may be unable to communicate a desire for fluids or may have difficulty swallowing fluids that are offered. A confused or disoriented patient may be unaware of thirst. Patients who are comatose, weak, or catatonic may develop fluid deficits because of the inability to ask for fluids, swallow, or respond to thirst. People with oropharyngeal discomfort may avoid oral fluid intake in an effort to avoid worsening the pain. In a disaster such as a flood or an earthquake, a supply of potable water or fluids may be unavailable, and people may suffer dehydration as a result.

Fluid Loss. Excessive fluid loss is common and occurs for a variety of reasons. Most of the fluid in the gastrointestinal tract is absorbed in the small intestine and proximal colon, leaving only small amounts to be excreted with the feces. In disease states with severe diarrhea, however, liters of fluid can be lost via the gastrointestinal tract resulting in severe volume deficits in a short period. Other losses from the gastrointestinal tract, such as vomiting, gastrointestinal suctioning, and bleeding, may also result in significant fluid loss. Table 13-4 shows ECF volumes.

Polyuria can be associated with a fluid deficit. For instance, diabetes insipidus is a clinical syndrome that results in excessive loss of urine. The etiology may be central or nephrogenic, acquired or congenital. Diabetes insipidus may occur as a result of another disease or be provoked by a variety of drugs. It is characterized by polyuria and polydipsia. If a patient with diabetes insipidus is able to maintain adequate intake, severe fluid shifts are avoided. However, anything that interferes with fluid intake quickly results in severe volume depletion.[24]

Fluid loss may be provoked by changes in the osmolarity of ECF. For example, in diabetes mellitus, large amounts of glucose can accumulate in the blood. If diabetic ketoacidosis develops, ketone bodies collect as well. In response to these increased solute levels, a hyperosmolar state occurs, which leads to an osmotic diuresis and concomitant fluid loss.[21]

Many other problems may result in significant fluid loss. Hyperventilation, marked perspiration, bleeding, diaphoresis, and excessive tracheostomy secretions are examples of other potential causes of fluid deficit.

Sequestration of Body Fluids. Occasionally ECF can be sequestered in areas that do not normally contain a large volume of fluid. The pleural, peritoneal, and pericardial cavities are potential spaces that generally contain only a small amount of fluid. Table 13-5 shows fluid collection in potential spaces.

TABLE 13-4 Extracellular Fluid Volume*

	Approximate ml of Fluid (Daily)
Saliva	1500
Gastric juice	2500
Intestinal juice	2000
Pancreatic juice	1500
Bile	500
TOTAL	8000 ml/24 hr

*Note that approximately 8 L of fluid are used daily for digestive purposes. Normally most of this fluid is resorbed. Some of each of the ions found in blood plasma is present in each of the fluids listed, but the individual concentration varies with each fluid.

In some clinical problems one or more of these potential spaces may contain a large volume of fluid that has been lost from the vascular space.[9] This sequestration of body fluids in a potential space is called *third-spacing* and is associated with an intravascular volume deficit. Although not lost from the body, the fluid is unavailable for use. Therefore, symptoms consistent with volume deficit may develop. Eventually, when the fluid begins to return to the vascular space, symptoms of volume overload may be evident. Third-spacing may occur in the context of several clinical problems, for example, during the postoperative period after major abdominal surgery, with pancreatitis, and with hepatic failure.[13]

Pathophysiology

How the body reacts to a fluid deficit depends on whether it is due to an isotonic, hyperosmolar, or hypoosmolar imbalance. As mentioned earlier, isotonic imbalance occurs when the change in ECF volume occurs with a proportionate change in extracellular solutes. The water/sodium ratio remains unchanged. An example of fluid deficit related to isotonic imbalance is hemorrhage. When fluid volume deficit occurs as a result of isotonic imbalance, the thirst center is stimulated to increase water consumption, ADH secretion is increased to increase water resorption from the renal tubule, and the renin-angiotensin-aldosterone system is also stimulated to increase sodium and water resorption. Since the imbalance is isotonic, the osmolarity between the extracellular and intracellular compartments are the same, and there is no water

TABLE 13-5 Fluid Collection in Potential Fluid Spaces

Potential Fluid Space	Location	Fluid
Intrapleural	Between lung and chest wall	Pleural effusion
Pericardial	Between heart and pericardial sac	Pericardial effusion
Peritoneal	Between intestines and abdominal wall	Ascites

movement by osmosis between the two compartments. The cells neither swell nor shrink as a result of the isotonic fluid volume deficit.

A fluid volume deficit may also occur with sodium loss or sodium excess. When the extracellular sodium content is low, renal absorption of water is diminished in an attempt to restore normal proportions of sodium to water in the ECF. The resulting fluid deficit occurs as a result of the hypoosmolar state. Fluids lost through vomiting, diarrhea, and sweating have a high sodium content, which may precipitate hyponatremia. Diuretics (thiazides, loop, and potassium-conserving) may also contribute to sodium loss. In a hypoosmolar state, the osmolarity in the ECF compartment is lower than that in the ICF compartment. As a result, water moves by osmosis from the ECF compartment to the ICF compartment resulting in cellular swelling.

Fluid deficit may occur in hypernatremia as well. For example, in diabetes insipidus large amounts of urine are excreted, and the sodium content of the ECF becomes more concentrated. Hyperosmotic dehydration occurs. When an ECF deficit occurs as a result of hyperosmotic state, ADH secretion is increased in an attempt to maintain an adequate circulating blood volume. Water also moves out of the cell to replace water lost from the extracellular compartment resulting in cellular shrinkage. If the water deficit is not corrected, the cells eventually become unable to compensate for extracellular losses and cellular dehydration ensues. When cells are unable to continue providing water to replace the ECF, signs of circulatory collapse appear. As both intracellular and ECF volumes decrease, cell function is impaired as a result of inadequate diffusion of food, oxygen, and waste products. Because brain cells are particularly sensitive to these metabolic alterations, mental changes occur.

Thirst and weight loss are early symptoms of water deficit and become more pronounced as the deficit increases.[5] It should be noted that weight loss is not present with third-spacing phenomena, as fluid has not been lost from the body, just to a nonfunctional compartment. Signs of ECF depletion are listed in the Clinical Manifestations box.

As a fluid deficit evolves, body temperature begins to rise, and fever may develop. A dry mouth and throat may cause difficulty with speech. When cells are unable to continue providing water to replace the ECF losses, signs of circulatory collapse ensue: blood pressure drops, tachycardia occurs, and the respiratory rate increases. Signs and symptoms of moderate and severe water deficits are presented in Table 13-6.

Clinical Manifestations
Extracellular Fluid Depletion

Skin: poor turgor
Mouth: dry mucous membranes
Cardiovascular: postural hypotension (early), low blood pressure, tachycardia, increased respiration, decreased vein filling
Weight: loss
Urine: low output, increased specific gravity

Collaborative Care Management

Nurses are instrumental in preventing fluid volume deficit. Identification of vulnerable patients is essential. Included are those with (1) a compromised mental state who may not recognize or respond appropriately to thirst; (2) physical limitations that impair the ability to obtain adequate fluids and nutrition; (3) disease states that may alter fluid and electrolyte balance; or (4) limited access to adequate food and fluids due to social, environmental, recreational, or occupational circumstances.

When a patient at risk for fluid and/or electrolyte imbalance is identified, a plan of care is developed. The patient and family members should be educated about the importance of adequate fluid and nutrition intake. Collaboration among the nurse, patient, family members, and other health care providers results in an ongoing plan for the continued assessment and treatment of problems. An evaluation of serum electrolytes is essential for the recognition of specific problems. An accurate record of intake and output is maintained. A detailed action plan to replete fluid and restore electrolyte balance is initiated. Factors that may alter fluid and/or electrolyte states, such as certain medications (particularly diuretics), hyperventilation, fever, burns, diarrhea, and diabetes, must be noted and appropriate interventions undertaken.

A fluid volume deficit may be mild to severe. People who are mildly dehydrated may notice only symptoms of increased thirst or dry mouth. On the other hand, the fluid deficit may be so profound as to be associated with circulatory collapse and eventually death. Obviously, severe fluid depletion is a clinical emergency requiring rapid but thoughtful fluid repletion, restoration of electrolyte balance, and perhaps circulatory support. While hemodynamic stability is being established, efforts are directed toward identification and treatment of the underlying cause. Once the etiology and pre-

TABLE 13-6 Water Deficit

	Moderate Deficit	Severe Deficit
Skin	Flushed, dry	Cold, clammy
Mouth	Dry mucous membranes	Dry, cracked tongue
Eyes	—	Soft, sunken eyeballs
Cardiovascular system	—	Tachycardia, low blood pressure, rapid respirations
Central nervous system	Apprehension, restlessness	Lethargy, coma
Blood	—	Hemoconcentration, increase in hematocrit, BUN, electrolytes
Urine	High specific gravity, scant amount (except with osmotic diuresis)	Oliguria, concentrated urine
Other	Thirst, weight loss	Thirst, weight loss, fever

BUN, Blood urea nitrogen.

cise nature of the deficit are established, interventions specific to the pathophysiologic mechanisms can be initiated, and plans to prevent future compromise developed.

Fluid replacement needs are often calculated according to weight. Because 1 L weighs 1 kg, the amount of weight (in kilograms) lost during the period of fluid depletion approximates the volume of water deficit. That is, if 2 kg were lost, the approximate fluid loss is 2 L. Repletion requires intake of the volume lost plus an additional 1.5 L to fulfill the current daily needs.[13] Fluid replacement may require several days of therapy to avoid the complications of rapid volume infusion such as intercompartmental fluid shifts and pulmonary edema.

Oral fluid resuscitation is preferable, but if the patient is unable to tolerate oral fluids, intravenous therapy may be ordered. The type of intravenous solution is based on the patient's fluid and electrolyte status as well as volume needs and is discussed in greater detail later in the chapter.

Vital signs should be assessed regularly. Postural (orthostatic) hypotension is common in persons with a fluid volume deficit. To assess for postural blood pressure changes, the blood pressure is taken with the patient supine. It is then taken with the patient sitting and again with the patient standing. A drop in the systolic blood pressure of more than 15 mm Hg or a heart rate increase of more than 15 beats/min is consistent with intravascular volume depletion.[13] The patients should be observed closely during evaluation for postural hypotension. Marked reductions in standing blood pressure can result in dizziness and, if severe, in syncope. The patient should not be left unattended. If significant symptoms occur, the patient should be quickly assisted to a sitting or supine position. Daily weighing is useful to monitor fluid balance as well. Laboratory results should be reviewed for serum and urine electrolytes and abnormalities reported so that appropriate adjustments in therapy can be initiated.

FLUID EXCESS

Etiology

Fluid excess may occur as a result of (1) overhydration, (2) excessive sodium intake, or (3) failure of renal or hormonal regulatory functions.

Overhydration

Polydipsia may occur in the setting of psychiatric (often psychotic) disorders, SIADH, and certain head injuries involving the hypothalamus. Under normal circumstances, the renal response to increased fluid intake causes the excretion of large volumes of urine to maintain fluid balance. However, when regulatory pathophysiologic conditions such as renal dysfunction exist, intake may substantially exceed output, and ECF overload may occur.

An iatrogenic fluid excess may occur as a result of intravenous or nasogastric fluid administration. Intravenous fluids such as 0.9% sodium chloride and lactated Ringer's solution contain significant amounts of sodium and may not be tolerated well in large volumes, particularly in compromised patients.

Excessive Sodium Intake

Dietary sodium indiscretion may result in hyperosmolarity of the ECF, which promotes renal conservation of fluid. As the ECF volume expands to restore normal osmolarity, signs of extracellular volume excess develop.

Failure of Regulatory Mechanisms

As mentioned earlier, excess or inappropriate secretion of ADH occurs in response to stressors, drugs, and anesthetics. SIADH may also accompany inflammatory conditions of the lung (tuberculosis, pneumonia, and abscesses) and brain (encephalitis and meningitis), endocrine disturbances, certain infections in the lungs, and some malignancies. ECF volume increases in response to the increased ADH. Other endocrine problems, such as hyperfunction of the adrenal glands and adrenal adenomas, may result in aldosterone excess. Aldosterone promotes sodium retention which, in turn, results in mild volume expansion.

Pathophysiology

ECF excess can be evident in a hypoosmolar or hyperosmolar milieu. SIADH illustrates hypoosmolar overhydration. Initially ADH stimulates the renal tubules to absorb water. As the extracellular volume expands and the sodium remains static, the fluid becomes progressively hyponatremic. When the ECF is hypoosmolar, fluid moves into the cells to equalize the concentration on both sides of the cell membrane, resulting in cellular swelling. Because brain cells are particularly sensitive to the increase in intracellular water, the most common signs of hypoosmolar overhydration are changes in mental status. Confusion, ataxia, and convulsions may also occur (see Clinical Manifestations box).

In hypernatremic states, as may occur with increased sodium intake, increased aldosterone secretion, or Cushing's syndrome (see Chapter 29), extra body water is retained in an attempt to restore a normal proportion of ECF and sodium. The fluid volume excess occurs in response to a hyperosmolar state.

Fluid volume excess is associated with a weight gain that may develop over a short time (e.g., several pounds in a 24-hour period). Peripheral edema may occur, particularly in hyperosmolar overhydration. Signs of circulatory overload include neck vein distention, crackles in the lungs, and bounding pulse. If fluid excess is severe or cardiac function is compromised, pulmonary edema and respiratory failure can occur. Assessment techniques are covered in greater detail later in the chapter.

Collaborative Care Management

The goals of treatment are to restore normal fluid balance, provide symptomatic care until balance is achieved, and prevent future fluid volume excess. Identification of patients vulnerable to fluid overload is essential. Patients with altered renal, cardiac, hypothalamic, and adrenal function are at risk for fluid imbalance.

Pharmacologic therapy includes the administration of diuretics, as long as renal failure is not the cause of the excess fluid. Thiazide diuretics are used initially. If these are not effective, loop diuretics (furosemide) are prescribed. Accurate monitoring of intake and output, weight, and electrolytes are important nursing responsibilities.

Patients on a low-sodium diet need to know foods to avoid. Education is imperative if sodium restriction is indicated. Long-term dietary modifications may be necessary to control fluid volume. Many processed foods contain large amounts of sodium; patients should be taught to read product labeling so that high-sodium foods can be avoided. Patients and family members should be educated about food preparation techniques and seasoning options that minimize sodium use. Assistance with meal planning may be necessary. Sometimes it is necessary to limit fluid intake to avoid overhydration. This may be particularly difficult in the setting of psychogenic polydipsia.

As with fluid deficits, fluid volume excess ranges from mild to severe. Mild volume overload may be associated with transient polyuria. On the other hand, severe volume overload, particularly in persons with compromised renal or cardiac function, may be associated with pulmonary edema, a potentially life-threatening emergency. Once again, if the patient's condition is stable, the primary goal of therapy is identification of the etiology of fluid imbalance and institution of the appropriate therapy.

Clinical Manifestations

Overhydration

Changes in behavior: confusion, incoordination, convulsions
Hyperventilation
Sudden weight gain
Warm, moist skin
Increased intracranial pressure: slow bounding pulse with an increase in systolic and decrease in diastolic blood pressures
Peripheral edema, usually not marked

Excess fluid in the tissues results in poor cellular nutrition as cells are pushed farther apart and away from capillaries. Normal exchange of nutrients and wastes is interrupted. Edematous tissues are therefore poorly nourished, susceptible to trauma and infection, and heal poorly. Caution must be taken to protect edematous parts of the body from prolonged pressure, injury, and temperature extremes. Skin over these parts should be kept well lubricated to prevent dryness. If edematous areas are exposed to extensive moisture from incontinence or perspiration, they should be cleansed and dried frequently to prevent maceration.

EDEMA

Edema is a collection of excess fluid in body tissue. Usually, edema is extracellular, but it may be intracellular as well. Although edematous states may exist in the setting of overhydration, edema is not the same as overhydration. The distinction is important. Do not assume that edema indicates fluid volume overload. Whenever edema is noted, the nurse assesses the patient for potential etiologies such as inflammation, vascular impairment, tissue injury, and volume excess.

Etiology

Intracellular Edema. Cellular membrane permeability may be altered when the cell is severely deprived of nutrients or when cell metabolism is so profoundly altered that normal movement of electrolytes across the cell membranes fails. Thus intracellular edema may occur as a result of reduced tissue metabolism and severely impaired cellular nutrition.

When impaired tissue blood flow deprives cells of nutrition, the transmembrane electrolyte movement that maintains intracellular osmotic neutrality becomes dysfunctional. Normally, sodium ions leak into the intracellular space and are removed by active transport mechanisms. In patients with severe cellular malnutrition, ionic pump integrity is compromised, and the sodium cannot be removed from the cell. The relative hypertonicity of the intracellular space results in the osmotic intrusion of water and causes cellular swelling.[16] This usually heralds tissue death and may be seen in severe peripheral vascular disease or hypothermic injury.

Cellular swelling may also develop as a result of the enhanced cellular membrane permeability that occurs in inflammation. Sodium and other ions leak into the cell interior and osmotically attract fluid, resulting in cellular edema. In-

TABLE 13-7 Causes of Edema According to Underlying Physiologic Mechanism

Fluid Pressure	Oncotic Pressure
Increased capillary fluid pressure	Decreased capillary oncotic pressure
Increased venous pressure	Loss of serum protein
Vein obstruction	Burns, draining wounds, fistulas
Varicose veins	Hemorrhage
Thrombophlebitis	Nephrotic syndrome
Pressure on veins from casts, tight bandages, or clothing	Chronic diarrhea
Increased total volume with decreased cardiac output	Decreased intake of protein
Congestive heart failure	Malnutrition
Fluid overloading	Kwashiorkor
Sodium and water retention, increased aldosterone	Decreased production of albumin
Decreased renal blood flow	Liver disease
Congestive heart failure	**Increased Interstitial Oncotic Pressure**
Renal failure	Increased capillary permeability to protein
Increased production of aldosterone	Burns
Cushing's syndrome	Inflammatory reactions
Aldosterone added to system	Trauma
Corticosteroid therapy	Infections
Inability to destroy aldosterone	Allergic reactions (hives)
Cirrhosis of liver	Blocked lymphatics: decreased removal of tissue fluid and protein
	Malignant diseases
	Surgical removal of lymph nodes
	Elephantiasis

tracellular edema is part of the complex response to endotoxins seen in septic shock.[16]

Extracellular Edema. Extracellular edema is much more common than intracellular edema. The two general causes of ECF accumulation are (1) leakage of plasma fluid across a capillary membrane into an interstitial space (as occurs in pulmonary edema) and (2) collection of fluid in interstitial spaces resulting from compromised lymphatic function.

Pathophysiology

Leakage of plasma into an interstitial space may occur as a result of (1) increased capillary fluid (hydrostatic) pressure, (2) decreased plasma colloid osmotic pressure, and/or (3) increased capillary permeability (Table 13-7).

Increased Capillary Fluid Pressure. An increase in capillary fluid pressure results from vascular compartment overload. The high pressure pushes fluid out of the vessels into the surrounding interstitial tissues. If there is increased hydrostatic pressure in the pulmonary vasculature, fluid is pushed across the alveolar-capillary membrane into the interstitial spaces of the lung. If the fluid accumulation is sufficient, pulmonary edema occurs.[16]

Increased capillary filtration pressure may be caused by giving too much fluid within a short period of time to a person who, because of advanced age (reduced vessel elasticity) or circulatory or renal disease, cannot dispose of the surplus. As the pressure gradient increases, fluid moves into the interstitium.

Decreased Plasma Colloid Osmotic Pressure. Proteins in the blood (particularly albumin) are necessary to create the oncotic pressure that holds fluids in the vessels. When the colloid osmotic pressure is decreased, fluid moves out of the vascular compartment into the interstitial space. When serum proteins are low because of inadequate intake (severe malnutrition), loss through denuded skin (burns and wounds), renal disease, or decreased production in the liver, edema results.[16]

Increased Capillary Permeability. An increase in capillary permeability allows plasma protein to leak into the interstitual space. This results in the movement of fluid into the interstitial space, an increase in the interstitual colloid osmotic pressure and in edema.[16] This process is operative in many infectious states, in burns, and with histamine release. Increased capillary permeability contributes to the profound pulmonary compromise in adult respiratory distress syndrome (see Chapter 21).

Compromised Lymphatic Function. Blockage of lymphatic flow can quickly result in significant fluid accumulation. When lymphatic flow is blocked, proteins that have leaked into the interstitial space have no route of escape. As protein accretion occurs, the colloid osmotic pressure rises, and fluid moves into the interstitium.[16] Lymphatic blockage may occur in infections, as a result of an occlusive tumor, or as a result of surgical node excision.

Collaborative Care Management

Treatment is dependent on the cause of the edema. Nursing management of persons with edema is discussed in the section on Interventions.

ELECTROLYTE IMBALANCE

As noted earlier, sodium, potassium, calcium, and magnesium are the principal cations in the body. Chloride and bicarbonate are the principal anions. Life cannot be sustained unless body fluids contain exactly the right amount of each in the right concentration within each of the fluid compartments. In addition, no single electrolyte can be out of balance without causing other electrolytes to be out of balance also.

SODIUM

Sodium is the predominant electrolyte in ECF. The normal concentration of sodium in the blood is 135 to 145 mEq/L. Its concentration is the major determinant of ECF volume. Sodium is essential for many physiologic activities, including maintenance of acid-base balance, cellular membrane active and passive transport mechanisms, and intracellular metabolism. Disorders of sodium balance are commonly seen in clinical practice and generally occur in association with fluid imbalance.

Hyponatremia

Hyponatremia refers to a serum sodium concentration less than 135 mEq/L.

Etiology

Hyponatremia is common with thiazide diuretic use, but it may be seen with loop and potassium-sparing diuretics as well. Although diuretic-provoked hyponatremia is generally mild, it can become severe if confounded by other factors that cause sodium wasting or if sodium intake is markedly restricted, as may be the case in patients with severe congestive heart failure.

Hyponatremia occurs frequently in patients with acquired immunodeficiency syndrome (AIDS), and in patients with midspectrum human immunodeficiency virus (HIV) infection. The etiology may be multifactorial: vomiting and diarrhea, SIADH, adrenal insufficiency, and salt-wasting syndrome.[3]

Postoperative hyponatremia is common and may be related to several factors, including temporary alteration in hypothalamic function, loss of gastrointestinal fluids by vomiting or suction, or hydration with nonelectrolyte solutions. Although equally common in men and women, postoperative hyponatremia is a much more serious complication in premenopausal women. The etiology of this gender/age-related aberrance is unknown. Nevertheless the effects of hyponatremia may clearly be more devastating and potentially fatal in premenopausal women.[21] Judicious monitoring of serum sodium levels and careful assessment for symptoms of hyponatremia are critical for all postoperative patients.

Sodium depletion may also occur as a result of profuse sweating, gastrointestinal or biliary drainage, and draining fistulas. Recall that there are numerous etiologies for SIADH; each also represents a potential cause of hyponatremia.

Pathophysiology

Sodium loss from the intravascular compartment causes fluid from the water to diffuse into the interstitial spaces. As a result, sodium in the interstitial fluid is diluted. The decreased osmolarity of ECF that exists with sodium loss creates a condition similar to water excess; that is, water moves into the cells by osmosis and leaves the extracellular compartment depleted. This differs from water intoxication because there is not an excess of total body water, but an intercompartmental movement of water that depletes the extracellular compartment.

The laboratory test for plasma sodium does not always give an accurate indication of total body sodium. Some clinical conditions in which the level of serum sodium is not an accurate indicator of total body sodium are listed in Table 13-8. Sodium readily combines with bicarbonate and chloride to help maintain acid-base balance. Signs and symptoms of hyponatremia are presented in the Clinical Manifestations box on p. 251.

Collaborative Care Management

Recognition of people at risk for hyponatremia is essential to its prevention. Athletes and persons working in hot environments are encouraged to hydrate with fluid and electrolytes. If salt is not replaced along with water, hyponatremia can occur. Management includes educating vulnerable people to recognize signs of sodium depletion and maintaining sufficient sodium and water intake to replace skin and insensible fluid loss. Generally an increased dietary intake of sodium and fluid provides adequate treatment.

People with adrenal insufficiency require special instructions to manage their disease safely. Education about the im-

TABLE 13-8 Comparison of Serum Sodium Levels with Total Body Sodium*

Condition	Serum Sodium	Total Body Sodium
Prolonged sweating	Low (hyponatremia)	Low
Diuretics and low-sodium diets	Low	Low
Addison's disease	Low	Low
Edema (cardiac, renal hepatic disease)	Low or normal	High
Excretion of dilute urine, early stages of gastrointestinal sodium loss	Normal	Low
Excess oral or IV sodium intake	High (hypernatremia)	High
Water and sodium loss with water loss	High	Low

*Note that a low or high serum level does not necessarily correspond with total body sodium.

portance of sodium and fluid balance and the rationale for prescription medications is important. Daily weighing and intake and output monitoring are useful.

The general goal of treatment for hyponatremia is to correct sodium imbalance and restore normal fluid and electrolyte homeostasis. However, specific interventions are guided by the severity of the hyponatremia and the clinical presentation. In the presence of severe hyponatremia and marked symptoms (seizures, coma, and respiratory arrest), aggressive intervention is required. In mild hyponatremia, simply increasing dietary sodium or restricting the pure water intake may be sufficient to correct the imbalance.

As sodium replacement is undertaken, monitoring of serum sodium values is continued to assess the effectiveness of therapy, and the patient is evaluated for signs of worsening hyponatremia. Patients receiving vigorous repletion therapy should be monitored for further deterioration of mental status that may occur with too rapid replacement.[21]

If sodium cannot be given orally or by gastric feeding, intravenous fluids are necessary. Generally 0.9% sodium chloride or lactated Ringer's solution is prescribed. Hypertonic sodium solutions are given only in emergency situations and with judicious monitoring to avoid dangerous complications.

Too rapid restoration of sodium balance may provoke brain injury owing to rapid fluid shifts. The recommended rate of repletion is controversial. It has been suggested that maximum sodium replacement for asymptomatic individuals is 0.5 mEq/L/hr or 12 mEq/L/day. However, 1.5 to 2 mEq/L/hr for 3 to 4 hours is appropriate for severely hyponatremic patients showing significant neurologic deficits.[24]

Monitoring of fluid balance is always important when intravenous fluids are given. Patients with compromised cardiac or renal function are particularly vulnerable to fluid overload. Patients should be assessed regularly for the signs of fluid accumulation previously described.

Hypernatremia

A serum sodium level above 145 mEq/L is termed hypernatremia. Hypernatremia may occur as a result of fluid deficit or sodium excess.

Etiology

Because sodium is inextricably linked to fluid regulation, hypernatremia frequently occurs with fluid imbalance. Hypernatremia develops when an excess of sodium occurs without a proportional increase in body fluid or when water loss occurs without proportional loss of sodium.

Excess dietary or parenteral sodium intake, watery diarrhea, and diabetes insipidus increase the risk of hypernatremia. Thirst is the normal defense mechanism against hypernatremia. People with a preserved thirst mechanism, who have the cognitive ability to process that desire, have unlimited access to fluids, and retain the motor ability to drink those fluids are probably able to avoid hypernatremia. People most vulnerable to hypernatremia are infants, the elderly, those with physical or mental status compromise, and people with hypothalamic dysfunction.

Pathophysiology

If sodium becomes concentrated in the ECF, osmolarity rises, water leaves the cell by osmosis and enters the extracellular compartment to dilute fluids there, and the cells are water depleted. The presence of hypernatremia suppresses aldosterone secretion, and sodium is excreted in the urine. Signs and symptoms of hypernatremia are listed in the Clinical Manifestations box below.

Collaborative Care Management

Preventive measures include the recognition of persons at risk for the development of hypernatremia. Bedridden patients should have water readily available. Those who are unable to access water at will should be offered fluids at least every 2 hours. A patient with diabetes insipidus and fluid deprivation requires diligent attention to fluid replacement. An accurate record of intake and output permits quick recognition of a negative fluid balance.

The elderly, the very young, and debilitated patients require careful monitoring to avoid electrolyte imbalance. People with kidney failure, congestive heart failure, or increased aldosterone production may require dietary sodium restriction.

Usually osmolar balance can be restored with oral fluids. If not, the parenteral route may be necessary. Correction of chronic hypernatremia should not exceed a rate of 0.7

Clinical Manifestations

Hyponatremia

Headache
Muscle weakness
Fatigue and apathy
Postural hypotension
Anorexia, nausea, and vomiting
Abdominal cramps
Weight loss

SEVERE

Mental confusion
Delirium
Shock
Coma

Clinical Manifestations

Hypernatremia

Thirst
Dry, sticky mucous membranes
Low urinary output
Firm, rubbery tissue turgor

SEVERE

Manic excitement
Tachycardia
Death

mEq/L/hr. In acute, symptomatic states, more rapid correction is indicated: 6 to 8 mEq/L/hr in the first 3 to 4 hours, followed by a rate not to exceed 1 mEq/L/hr.[21]

Fluid resuscitation must be undertaken with particular caution in patients with compromised cardiac or renal function. The nurse should closely monitor the patient's response to fluids and be alert to symptoms of fluid overload.

POTASSIUM

The normal concentration of potassium in the blood is 3.5 to 5.5 mEq/L. Because most of the potassium in the body is intracellular, the serum potassium level does not necessarily indicate the total body potassium content. Maintenance of serum potassium concentration within the normal range, however, is vital to normal body functions.

Potassium has a direct effect on the excitability of nerves and muscles, contributes most to the intracellular osmotic pressure, and helps maintain acid-base balance and normal kidney function. A potassium deficit is associated with excess alkalinity (alkalosis) of the body fluids, and a potassium excess accompanies an excess of acid (acidosis). These conditions are discussed in more detail in the acid-base section of this chapter.

Potassium is the major cation of the cells. During the formation of new tissues (anabolism) or when glucose is converted to glycogen, potassium enters the cell. With tissue breakdown (catabolism), such as that occurring with trauma, dehydration, or starvation, potassium leaves the cell. The body conserves potassium less effectively then, even when the body needs it. Normally about 5% of the total body potassium is excreted each day.

Hypokalemia

A low level of serum potassium, less than 3.5 mEq/L, is known as *hypokalemia.*

Etiology

The patient who has food withheld for several days, is dehydrated, or is given large amounts of parenteral fluids with no replacement of potassium develops potassium depletion. The parenteral administration of 5% dextrose in water without the addition of potassium tends to dilute the potassium in the ECFs. This dilution, in addition to the lack of a balanced diet and to potassium loss caused by catabolism of body proteins, accounts for many instances of electrolyte imbalance in the postoperative patient. People who eat an inadequate diet, who take no food for an extended period, or who are losing large amounts of fluid from the gastrointestinal tract through vomiting, diarrhea, or a draining fistula usually are given intravenous solutions that contain potassium.

Severe hypokalemia may be seen in patients with purging eating disorders who induce vomiting or abuse laxatives. Chronic hypokalemia may provoke some adaptive response, as even the severely depleted person may not demonstrate symptoms usually seen with marked hypokalemia.[4] Medications such as diuretics, amphotericin B, some penicillins, and gentamycin may precipitate hypokalemia as a result of renal potassium loss.[21] Aldosterone promotes potassium excretion by the kidneys. Therefore primary or secondary hyperaldosteronism provokes hypokalemia.[24] Figure 13-5 summarizes the causes and effects of hypokalemia.

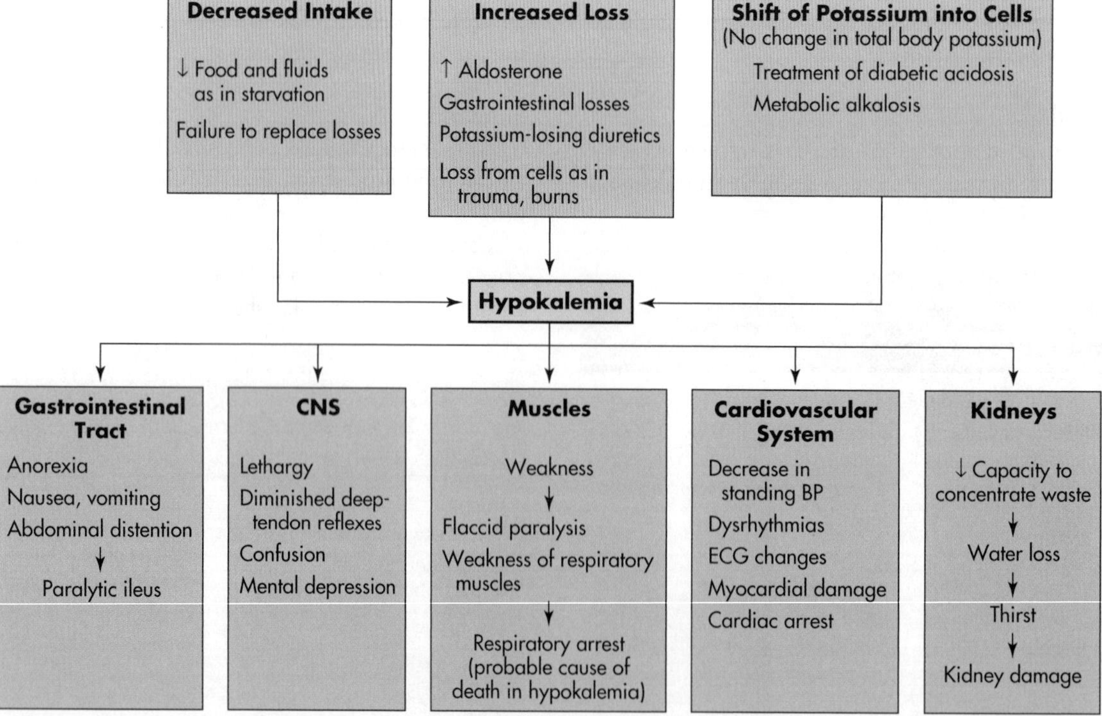

Figure 13-5 Causes and effects of hypokalemia.

Pathophysiology

Movement of sodium (inward) and potassium (outward) across the cell membrane causes depolarization of the membrane and initiates an action potential, which creates nerve and muscle activity. When extracellular potassium concentration is low, the resting membrane potential increases (hyperpolarization), and the cell becomes less excitable. For this reason, the major symptoms of hypokalemia are muscle weakness and atony.

Recall that potassium moves out of the cells when hydrogen ions move into the intracellular compartment in acidosis. Therefore hyperkalemia accompanies acidosis. As the acidosis is treated, potassium moves back into the cells, and hypokalemia may develop. In alkalosis the potassium concentration is lowered because of (1) movement of potassium into cells and (2) potassium excretion by the kidneys as hydrogen ions are being retained.

Whenever sodium is retained in the body through resorption by the kidney tubules, potassium is excreted. Thus whenever aldosterone secretion is increased, such as during the stress response, potassium is excreted. Potassium also may be lost in the urine when there is considerable urinary output and as a result of therapy with certain diuretics (the thiazides and furosemide) and the corticosteroids.

Potassium balance is critical for the maintenance of normal cellular metabolism and excitation. Potentially life-threatening cardiac dysrhythmias may occur in the setting of potassium imbalance. Hypokalemia potentiates the action of digitalis preparations; hence patients receiving these drugs are at particular risk for cardiac rhythm disturbance.

Collaborative Care Management

Hypokalemia can be prevented by being alert to the conditions that cause potassium depletion (vomiting, diarrhea, and diuretics) and by monitoring the patient for early warning signs. If there is an order for enemas until results are clear, the nurse should not give more than three enemas to a patient without consulting the physician.

Patients receiving potassium-wasting diuretics should be educated about their effects and taught the importance of adequate dietary intake of potassium. They should be cautioned that in the presence of other problems provoking potassium loss, their health care provider should be contacted.

With severe hypokalemia the patient may die unless potassium is administered promptly. The safest way to administer potassium is orally. When potassium is given intravenously, the rate of flow must be monitored closely to prevent hyperkalemia and a host of cardiac dysrhythmias. Because it is very irritating to the vein, potassium must be diluted before intravenous administration. The usual rate of infusion generally does not exceed 20 mEq/hr. As cardiac dysrhythmias may be provoked by both hypokalemia and hyperkalemia, cardiac monitoring is useful; it is essential for those with marked disturbance.

In some instances of severe depletion, potassium may be given in a concentrated solution (40 mEq/100 ml) over 4 hours. When it is delivered in this concentrated manner, an intravenous infusion pump is essential to safely control the flow rate. If possible, a central line is desirable for the concentrated infusion, owing to the irritating nature of the solution.

Persons who are receiving potassium-wasting diuretics should be instructed to include foods high in potassium in their diet (Table 13-9). If low serum potassium levels are shown to result from diuretic therapy, a potassium supplement may be prescribed, usually in the form of potassium chloride (elixir of potassium chloride), or a potassium-sparing diuretic such as triamterene (as found in Dyazide) may be used. People taking diuretics at home should be taught to recognize symptoms of potassium depletion, such as muscle weakness, anorexia, nausea, and vomiting, and to report these symptoms to the health care provider. Because potassium supplements are irritating to the gastrointestinal tract, they should be taken with at least one-half glass of water.

Hyperkalemia

A serum potassium level greater than 5.5 mEq/L is termed *hyperkalemia.* This condition does not occur as frequently as hypokalemia, especially if renal function is normal.

Etiology

Hyperkalemia is caused by the movement of potassium out of the cells, increased intake of potassium, and decreased excretion of potassium. Movement of potassium out of the cells occurs with severe tissue damage in sepsis, fever, trauma, or surgery. This movement also occurs in metabolic acidosis and insulin deficiency/hyperglycemia.

The kidney's efficient excretion of potassium is a safety factor that guards against hyperkalemia. However, people with impaired renal function are at risk for hyperkalemia. This is a particularly important consideration when medications (angiotensin-converting enzyme inhibitors, beta-blockers, cyclosporine, nonsteroidal antiinflammatory drugs, lithium, heparin, and others) that also promote potassium retention are prescribed for persons with renal dysfunction.[28] Potassium supplements are generally avoided for people with aldosterone deficiency, as these individuals have a tendency for developing hyperkalemia.

Spurious hyperkalemia may result from drawing a test blood sample from a site proximal to the site of an infusion containing potassium, by using a needle for blood collection that is of so small a bore that cell lysis occurs (21 gauge or smaller), or by drawing the sample after prolonged tourniquet application particularly in combination with isometric hand grip.[21] Spurious potassium elevation must be ruled out before treatment is instituted, or iatrogenic hypokalemia may be provoked. See Figure 13-6 for causes and effects of hyperkalemia.

Pathophysiology

Time is an important factor in the development of hyperkalemia. A rapid increase in serum potassium of only 1 to 3 mEq/L can be lethal. On the other hand, some persons with renal failure develop severe hyperkalemia slowly and seem to be able to adjust to the potassium excess with few symptoms.

TABLE 13-9 Foods High in Potassium

Food Source	Amount	mEq
Fruits		
Apricots		
Canned	½ c	6.0
Dried	4 halves	5.0
Fresh	3 small	8.0
Banana	1 small	9.6
Strawberries	1 c	6.3
Grapefruit sections	¾ c	5.1
Melon		
Cantaloupe	½ small	13.0
Honeydew	¼ medium	13.0
Watermelon	½ slice	5.0
Nectarine	1 medium	6.0
Orange	1 medium	5.1
Orange juice	½ c	5.7
Peach		
Dried	2 halves	5.0
Fresh	1 medium	6.2
Protein foods		
Beef	3 oz	8.4
Chicken	3 oz	9.0
Frankfurters	1	3.0
Liver	3 oz	9.6
Pork	3 oz	9.0
Veal	3 oz	11.4
Scallops	1 large	6.0
Turkey	3 oz	8.4
Milk		
Whole	1 c	8.8
Powdered, whole	¼ c	10.0
Buttermilk	1 c	8.5
Skim	1 c	8.8
Powdered, skim	¼ c	13.5
Vegetables*		
Asparagus		
Fresh	½ c	4.7
Frozen	½ c	5.5
Beans		
Dried, cooked	½ c	10.0
Lima	½ c	9.5
Beet greens	½ c	8.5
Broccoli	½ c	7.0
Cabbage, raw	1 c	6.0
Carrots, raw	1 large	8.8
Celery, raw	1 c	9.0
Collards	½ c	6.0
Mushrooms, raw	4 large	10.6
Mustard greens	½ c	5.5
Peas, dried	½ c	6.8
Potato		
Baked, white	½ c	13.0
Boiled, white	½ c	7.3
Baked, sweet	½ c	8.0
Spinach	½ c	8.5
Tomatoes	½ c	6.5
Brussels sprouts	2/3 c	7.6
Squash, winter, baked	½ c	12.0
Miscellaneous		
Peanut butter	2 tbsp	5.0
Nuts, unsalted	25	4.5
Beverages that contain large amounts of cocoa, cola drinks, and dry, instant coffee and tea		

*Most raw vegetables contain potassium, much of which is lost during cooking.

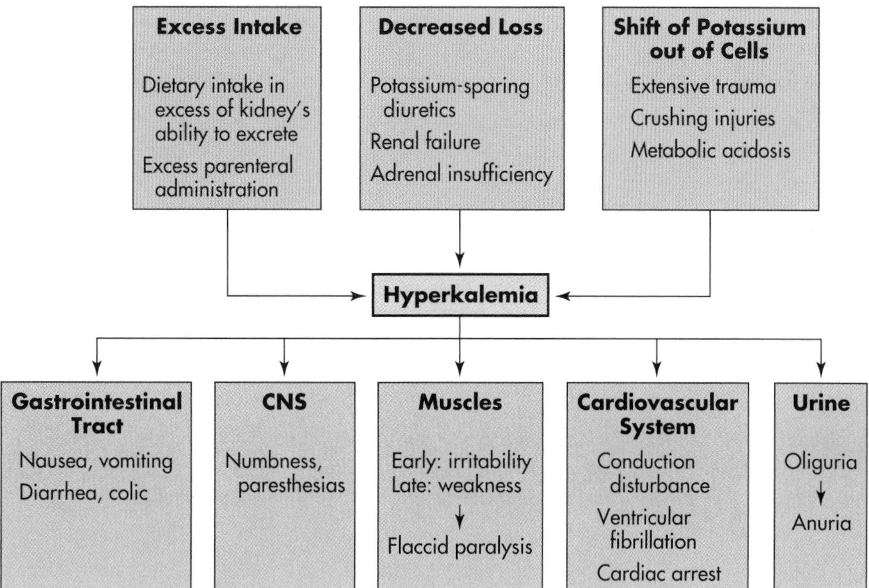

Figure 13-6 Causes and effects of hyperkalemia.

Alterations in the stimulation properties of muscle may result in weakness, even paralysis, in patients with severe hyperkalemia. Generally, these problems do not occur until the serum potassium exceeds 8 mEq/L.[21] Nausea, diarrhea, and intestinal colic may also occur in hyperkalemia. Alterations in cardiac muscle stimulation (depolarization) and relaxation (repolarization) occur as well. These changes in the myocardial action potential result in changes in the surface electrocardiogram, such as wide QRS complexes and tall, peaked T waves. Ventricular dysrhythmias and cardiac arrest may occur.

Collaborative Care Management

Patients at risk for hyperkalemia should be identified. People with impaired renal function should be cautioned about the possibility of hyperkalemia and advised to avoid over-the-counter medications (such as nonsteroidal antiinflammatory drugs) that may provoke hyperkalemia and salt substitutes that are high in potassium. Intravenous potassium repletion should be monitored carefully to avoid iatrogenic hyperkalemia.

The severity of the hyperkalemia guides therapy. Mild hyperkalemia may be relieved by simply withholding the provoking agent (i.e., potassium supplement or medication). With more severe hyperkalemia, a cation-exchange resin, such as polystyrene sulfonate (Kayexalate) may be ordered. Exchange resins act by exchanging the cations in the resin for the potassium in the intestine. The potassium is then excreted in the stool. Bowel function must be maintained if this therapy is to be effective. Potassium-wasting diuretics may be prescribed to promote further loss. If the patient is in acute renal failure, dialysis will be necessary to eliminate the excess potassium.

Severe hyperkalemia (generally greater than 6 mEq/L) is a medical emergency and requires prompt intervention. These patients should be in a unit where continuous cardiac monitoring may be done. Aggressive treatment is indicated if tall, peaked T waves, wide QRS complexes, or ventricular dysrhythmias are present on 12-lead electrocardiogram. Intravenous calcium gluconate may be prescribed to counteract the cardiac effects of hyperkalemia; insulin infusions and intravenous sodium bicarbonate may be used to promote intracellular uptake of potassium.

CALCIUM

Calcium is necessary for many physiologic activities: nerve transmission, cardiac excitability, muscular contraction, blood clotting, and hormone regulation. The normal total serum calcium level is 8.5 to 10 mg/dl. This includes the nonionized (bound to albumin and in combination with citrate or phosphate) and ionized (metabolically active) calcium.[21]

Both vitamin D and parathyroid hormone must be present for calcium to be absorbed from the gastrointestinal tract. As you recall, parathyroid hormone maintains the serum calcium level within normal limits by mobilizing calcium from bone. Calcium is excreted principally through the gastrointestinal tract, with normally only very small amounts being lost in the urine.

Hypocalcemia

Hypocalcemia is defined as a total serum calcium concentration of less than 8.5 mg/dl or an ionized calcium concentration of less than 4 mg/dl.

Etiology

Calcium deficit results from inadequate intake, vitamin D deficiency, hypoparathyroidism, interruption of normal calcium absorption from the gastrointestinal tract, excess loss of calcium through the kidneys, and kidney disease leading to the inability of the kidney to change provitamin D to functional vitamin D. People with pancreatic disease or disease of

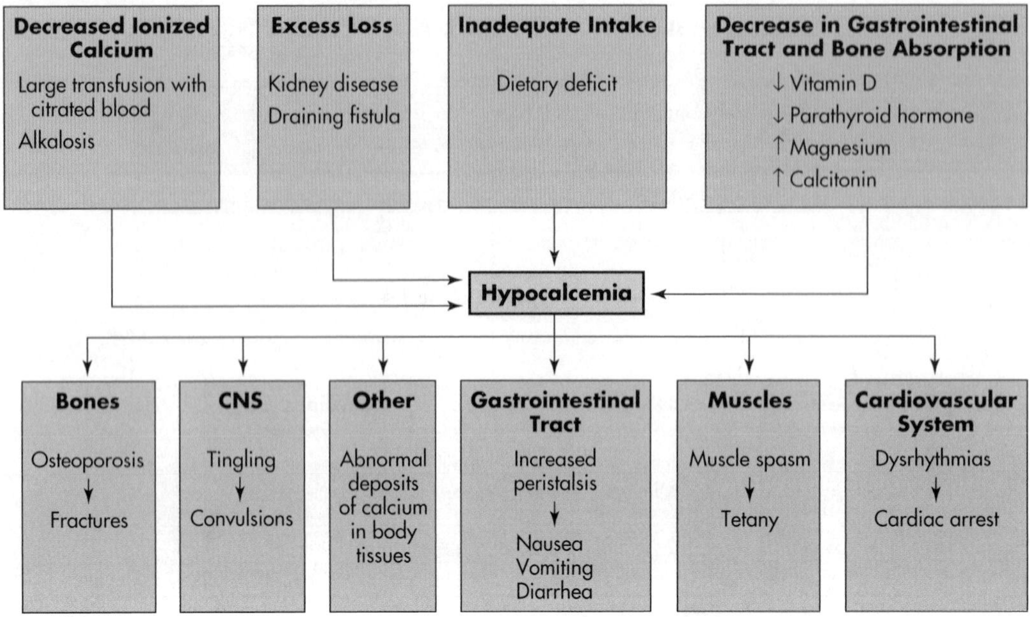

Figure 13-7 Causes and effects of hypocalcemia.

the small intestine may fail to absorb calcium normally from the gastrointestinal tract and may excrete large amounts of calcium in the feces. Persons with chronic pancreatitis have chronic hypocalcemia related to vitamin D deficiency. Draining intestinal fistulas also cause excess calcium loss.

The hypocalcemia seen with chronic alcoholism is probably multifactorial. Decreased calcium intake, malnutrition, acid-base disturbance, associated pancreatitis, hepatic dysfunction, and gastrointestinal loss are all potential contributors. The causes and effects of hypocalcemia are shown in Figure 13-7.

Pathophysiology

Calcium ions are thought to line the pores of cell membranes. Because both calcium and sodium ions carry a positive charge, they tend to repel each other. The presence of calcium in the pores of cells (especially neurons) has a blocking effect on permeability to sodium. When serum calcium levels are low, this blocking effect is minimized; sodium then moves more easily into the cell, and depolarization takes place more readily.16 This results in increased excitability of the nervous system, leading to muscle spasm, tingling sensations, and, if severe, convulsions and tetany. Skeletal, smooth, and cardiac muscle functions are all affected by overstimulation.

Tetany is the most characteristic sign of severe hypocalcemia. The patient who has calcium deficiency usually complains first of numbness and tingling of the nose, ears, fingertips, or toes. If calcium is not given at this time, painful muscular spasms (tetany), especially of the feet and hands (carpopedal spasms), muscle twitching, and convulsions may follow.

Two tests are used to elicit signs of calcium deficiency. *Trousseau's sign* is elicited by grasping the patient's wrist or inflating a blood pressure cuff on the upper arm to constrict the circulation for a few minutes. Palmar flexion, a positive response, may be present in hypocalcemia. *Chvostek's sign* is elicited by tapping the patient's face lightly over the facial nerve (just below the temple). Facial muscle twitching indicates a positive Chvostek's sign. Although positive Trousseau's and Chvostek's signs may be present in hypocalcemia, neither is very sensitive nor specific. That is, a person may have hypocalcemia in the absence of these signs or not have hypocalcemia in the presence of these signs.

Calcium is important for normal cardiac muscle function as well as normal impulse propagation. Hypocalcemia may be associated with myocardial pump dysfunction, hypotension, and a host of potentially life-threatening cardiac dysrhythmias.

As almost half of the total serum calcium is bound to albumin, the report of serum calcium must be evaluated with consideration of the total albumin. In the presence of a normal serum albumin concentration, ionized calcium constitutes 47% of the total serum calcium. However, in the case of hypoalbuminemia, ionized serum calcium may be easily underestimated. On the other hand, in the presence of alkalosis, an ionized serum calcium deficit may be unrecognized. Alkalosis promotes the binding of calcium to protein; hence less calcium is available for physiologic activities. Therefore, with alkalosis (pH 7.4), the patient may be hypocalcemic as a result of a low level of ionized calcium, despite a normal total serum calcium level.[21]

Hypocalcemia often coexists with hypomagnesemia. Magnesium affects the availability and action of parathyroid hormone. When hypocalcemia occurs as a result of hypomagnesemic hypoparathyroidism, the treatment of choice is magnesium replacement.[21]

Collaborative Care Management

Inadequate calcium intake, excess calcium loss, and vitamin D deficiency place persons at risk for developing hypocal-

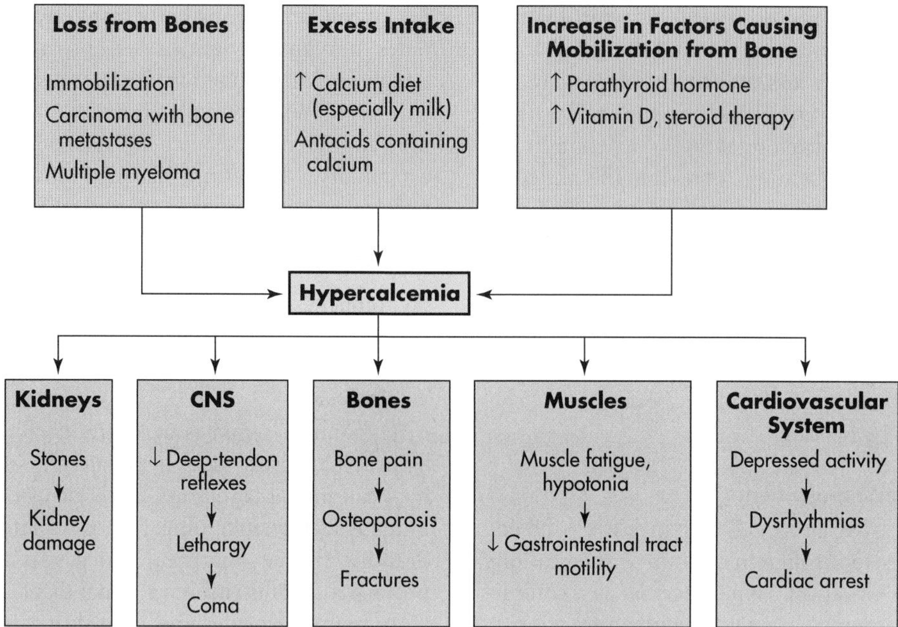

Figure 13-8 Causes and effects of hypercalcemia.

cemia. Patients who have extremely poor diets or who have calcium-depleting conditions should be monitored for signs of hypocalcemia. Patients should be educated about the importance of adequate calcium and vitamin D intake.

Patients undergoing thyroid, parathyroid, and radical neck surgery are particularly vulnerable to hypocalcemia secondary to parathyroid hormone deficit. Monitoring of serum calcium levels and correction of deficits are important for these patients.

As discussed earlier, patients receiving transfusions of large amounts of whole blood are at risk for hypocalcemia. Citrate is added to stored blood to prevent coagulation. When the blood is transfused, the citrate binds with circulating calcium. Usually, this does not present a problem, because the citrate is quickly metabolized by the liver. However, if the patient has a preexisting calcium deficit, has a hepatic dysfunction that impairs metabolism, or is receiving large amounts of whole blood very rapidly, hypocalcemia may occur. Vulnerable patients should have serum calcium levels checked during and/or after transfusions.[21]

For persons with acute hypocalcemia, 10 to 20 ml of a 10% intravenous solution of calcium gluconate given slowly may be prescribed. Although calcium chloride provides more readily available ionized calcium, it is so irritating to the vein that it is generally not used. Patients receiving intravenous calcium replacement should have continuous cardiac monitoring.

For patients with mild hypocalcemia, a high-calcium diet or oral calcium salts may be sufficient. When decreased parathyroid hormone or vitamin D is the causative factor, these substances must be supplied. When the serum phosphorus level rises, the calcium level falls. Hence aluminum hydroxide gel can be given to lower a high serum phosphorus concentration (via phosphorus binding of calcium).

After thyroid, parathyroid, or radical neck surgery, patients must be watched closely for symptoms of calcium deficiency because of the possibility that the parathyroid glands may have been inadvertently removed or are temporarily suppressed by local edema. Intravenous calcium gluconate should always be available for emergency use during the postoperative period.

Bone demineralization may occur with prolonged hypocalcemia. Therefore, although patients should ambulate cautiously, they should be encouraged and assisted to do so to minimize bone resorption.

Hypercalcemia

Hypercalcemia refers to a total serum calcium concentration greater than 10 mg/dl.

Etiology

Hypercalcemia can result from excessive intake of calcium, especially in milk and absorbable calcium-containing antacids (milk-alkali syndrome), from excessive vitamin D intake, and from conditions that promote release of calcium from the bones into ECF. These causes and their effects are shown in Figure 13-8.

The most common causes of hypercalcemia, however, are malignancy and hyperparathyroidism (see Chapters 15 and 29). An elevated serum calcium level may occur in malignancy as a result of tumor secretion of parathyroid hormone or alteration of bone metabolism.[21]

Pathophysiology

Hypercalcemia acts like a cellular sedative, depressing nerve and muscle activity. Generalized muscle weakness may be noted. Deep tendon reflexes may be decreased or absent. Myocardial function is altered, and cardiac dysrhythmias may occur. Gastrointestinal motility decreases and constipation, nausea, and vomiting may occur. Mental status changes (lethargy, confusion, memory loss, and coma) may occur.

With immobilization calcium leaves the bone and becomes concentrated in the ECF. Normal retention of calcium in the bones is caused by weight-bearing forces on the skeleton. When a large amount of calcium accumulates in the ECF and passes through the kidneys, calcium can precipitate and form stones (calculi), a relatively common complication of immobility.

Calcium precipitates more readily in alkaline solution. This can be a problem in a person with a urinary tract infection, which increases the alkalinity of the urine, because renal calculi are more likely to be formed.

Collaborative Care Management

Mild hypercalcemia may be treated with hydration and education about avoiding foods high in calcium or medications that promote calcium elevation. Hypercalcemia as a complication of immobilization may be avoided with ambulation as appropriate when the person is able, and the use of active weight-bearing exercises as appropriate. Appliances such as a trapeze or resistance devices may be applied to a hospital bed to provide opportunities for exercise. When a patient cannot ambulate or do active exercises, a tilt table may be used for weight-bearing exercise.

People with marked hypercalcemia have often lost calcium from their bones or have malignant involvement of bone; therefore special care should be taken to prevent pathologic fractures. Although exercising is important to minimize further demineralization, consideration must be given to the danger of fractures, and an individualized plan of care developed.

Careful attention must be directed to the prevention of renal calculi. Encouraging oral fluids can help prevent concentrated urine. Unless contraindicated, 3000 to 4000 ml of fluid per day is desirable. Acid-ash fruit juices, cranberry juice, and prune juice are particularly useful, as they promote a more acid urine, thus discouraging stone formation.

Severe hypercalcemia is a medical emergency. Continuous cardiac monitoring is necessary and emergency equipment should be readily available. Initial treatment for severe hypercalcemia is hydration. As the hydration regimen may be vigorous (possibly several hundred ml/hr for several hours, cardiac and renal status must be assessed before the fluids are begun and reassessed at least every 2 hours during fluid therapy. Intravenous furosemide may be given to promote diuresis. If additional treatment is required, calcitonin and/or plicamycin (Mithramycin) may be given to prevent bone resorption. Serum and urinary electrolytes should be checked every 2 hours during treatment of severe hypercalcemia.[28] An example of a Clinical Pathway for the patient with hypercalcemia is found on pp. 259 and 260.

MAGNESIUM

The normal serum magnesium level is 1.5 to 2.5 mEq/L. Most is found in bone, 30% to 35% in the ICF, and only a small amount in the ECF. Therefore serum magnesium levels do not necessarily reflect total body magnesium. Magnesium participates in many enzymatic reactions, especially those involving energy use or production. It also affects the release of acetylcholine at neuromuscular junctions and is therefore important in the maintenance of normal neural and muscular excitability. Magnesium has a sedative effect on the central nervous system similar to that of calcium.

Hypomagnesemia

Hypomagnesemia is a serum magnesium level of less than 1.5 mEq/L.

Etiology

Hypomagnesemia is a common clinical problem. It frequently coexists with hypokalemia and less often with hypocalcemia. Magnesium levels may be decreased as a result of many factors, including: (1) loss of intestinal fluids through draining fistulas, diarrhea, and gastrointestinal suction; (2) prolonged malnutrition; (3) renal disorders; (4) drug therapy with aminoglycosides and loop diuretics; and (5) endocrine disorders, such as increased secretion of ADH, aldosterone, and thyroid hormone, and diabetes mellitus. The hypomagnesemia often seen in chronic alcoholism is multifactorial and related to decreased dietary intake of magnesium, increased gastrointestinal losses, and intestinal malabsorption.[21] Causes and effects of hypomagnesemia are shown in Figure 13-9.

Cardiac patients may be at particular risk for hypomagnesemia for several reasons. Renal conservation of magnesium occurs at the loop of Henle. Loop diuretics, commonly prescribed for cardiac patients, enhance magnesium loss. Gastrointestinal edema, common in patients with congestive heart failure, diminishes intestinal resorption of magnesium and provokes gastrointestinal symptoms that promote magnesium loss. The effects of digitalis preparations are potentiated by a low magnesium level. Therefore when hypomagnesemia occurs, the patient is at risk for digitalis toxicity. In some cases, hypomagnesemia may contribute to the development of atherosclerosis, coronary artery spasm, and cardiomyopathy. Hypomagnesemia also increases urinary loss of potassium. For this reason, patients who are hypomagnesemic are also often hypokalemic. Magnesium deficit in that situation may precipitate life-threatening cardiac dysrhythmias.

Pathophysiology

A low serum magnesium level leads to increased neuromuscular irritability by increasing acetylcholine release, increasing the sensitivity of the myoneural junction to acetylcholine, diminishing the threshold of excitation of the motor nerve, and enhancing the force of myofibril contraction.[24] Magnesium is excreted by the gastrointestinal tract when a large amount of calcium is present, as the calcium is preferentially absorbed. The kidneys effectively conserve magnesium when intake is low.

Metabolically, magnesium is closely interrelated with both calcium and potassium. Hypomagnesemia is suspected when hypocalcemia and hypokalemia are refractory to treatment. Magnesium inhibits transport of parathyroid hormone from

clinical pathway *The Patient With Hypercalcemia*

Directions:
1. Review coordinated care track (CCT) approximately every 8°.
2. Appropriate and completed interventions need no additional documentation.
3. Cross through any interventions that are not applicable.
4. Circle any intervention not completed.
5. The plan of care—nursing interventions and outcome evaluation statements—may be added to the CCT as necessary.

DRG 239 Expected LOS 5 days
Physician(s) ______________________
____
Admit Date ______________________
Discharge Date ______________________
Primary Diagnosis
____
____
Date of last Chemo ______________________
Date of last Radiation ______________________
____

Comorbid Conditions:
☐ CHF ☐ COPD
☐ IDDM
☐ Angina
☐ Dehydration
☐ Malnutrition

Imprint/Label

Complications during this admission:
☐ Pulmonary embolus ☐
☐ Deep vein thrombosis ☐
☐ ☐
☐ ☐

Risk Factors:
☐ Obesity ☐ ETOH/Substance Abuse ☐ Smoking ☐

DATE	PROBLEM LIST	DISCHARGE CRITERIA	DATE INITIALLY MET	MET ON DISCHARGE	
				YES	NO
	1. Confusion 2. Safety 3. Constipation 4. Dehydration 5. Renal failure	1. Normal calcium level 2. Patient/caregiver has knowledge, resources, and ability to provide care outside of the hospital environment. 3. Able to consume 1000 cc fluid/day. 4. Renal function returns to prehypercalcemic level.			
		Explain any discharge criteria not met:			

Courtesy The Cleveland Clinic Foundation, Department of Advanced Practice Nursing, Cleveland, Ohio, 1996.
ADL, activities of daily living; *CHF,* congestive heart failure; *COPD,* chronic obstructive pulmonary disorder; *IDDM,* insulin-dependent diabetes mellitus (type 2).

Continued

clinical pathway *The Patient With Hypercalcemia—cont'd*

TIME FRAME LOCATION	HOSPITAL DAY 1 DATE UNIT	HOSPITAL DAY 2 DATE UNIT	HOSPITAL DAY 3 DATE UNIT	HOSPITAL DAY 4 DATE UNIT	HOSPITAL DAY 5 DATE UNIT
PATIENT SATISFACTION	"HOW CAN WE ENHANCE YOUR STAY AT THE CCF?"	"HOW CAN WE ENHANCE YOUR STAY AT THE CCF?"	"HOW CAN WE ENHANCE YOUR STAY AT THE CCF?"	"HOW CAN WE ENHANCE YOUR STAY AT THE CCF?"	"HOW CAN WE ENHANCE YOUR STAY AT THE CCF?"
DISCHARGE PLANNING PATIENT EDUCATION	Identify primary caregiver ______ Identify learning needs	Team conference Consult Social Worker, Chaplain Teach signs/symptoms of hypercalcemia Teach aspiration precautions	Team & family conference Consult Hospice Consult ASC Evaluate need for SQ injection teaching if pt. to be discharged on calcitonin	Confirm discharge disposition SQ injection teaching if pt. to be discharged on calcitonin	Give RTC appts.
TESTS/ PROCEDURES/ CONSULTS	CBC, SMA 17 Weigh patient Monitor I & O IV hydration and diuresis	Calcium level Weigh patient Monitor I & O IV hydration and diuresis	Calcium level Weigh patient Monitor I & O Decrease IV hydration	Calcium level Weigh patient Monitor I & O Consider discontinuing the IV hydration	Calcium level Weigh patient Monitor I & O
ALLIED HEALTH	Nutrition Services ☐ Palliative Care Consult ☐				
NURSING INTERVENTIONS	Initiate calcitonin per doctor's order Establish usual bowel pattern ______ Institute bowel regimen for constipation (i.e., stool softeners, laxatives, enemas) Aspiration precautions Assess swallowing before giving fluids/food Review meds pt taking prior to admission Exclude meds contributing to confusion or hypercalcemia (i.e., Vit D, antacids, etc.)	Continue calcitonin per doctor's order Continue bowel regimen for constipation (i.e., stool softeners, laxatives, enemas) Assess for bowel movement Aspiration precautions Assist patient with ADL	Evaluate need for further calcitonin Continue bowel regimen for constipation (i.e., stool softeners, laxatives, enemas) Assess for bowel movement Aspiration precautions Assist patient with ADL	Evaluate need for further calcitonin Continue bowel regimen for constipation (i.e., stool softeners, laxatives, enemas) Aspiration precautions Assist patient with ADL	Aspiration precautions Assist patient with ADL Continue bowel regimen for constipation (i.e., stool softeners, laxatives, enemas)
OUTCOME CRITERIA	Vital signs stable Weight stable or ↓ from admission Drug therapy initiated Patient satisfaction addressed	Free from injury No aspiration Calcium level decreased from admission Patient satisfaction addressed	Calcium level decreased from previous day Patient satisfaction addressed Free from injury No aspiration	Free from injury No aspiration Calcium level decreased from admission Patient satisfaction addressed	Able to verbalize s/s of high calcium Free from injury No aspiration Normal calcium level Patient satisfaction addressed

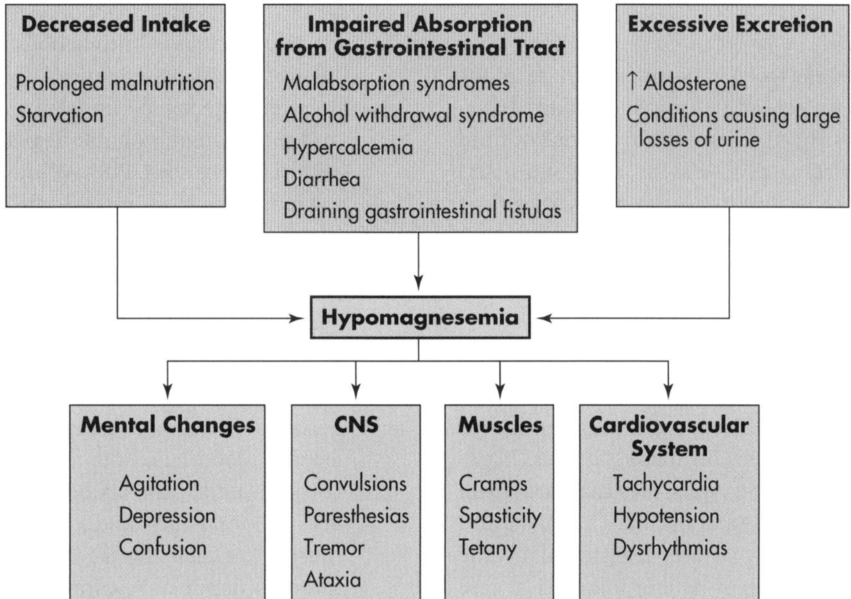

Figure 13-9 Causes and effects of hypomagnesemia.

the glands, causing a decrease in the amount of calcium being released from bone that results in a calcium deficit. Hypomagnesemia usually manifests with behavioral and neurologic symptoms such as confusion, increased reflexes, tremors, muscle spasms, arrhythmias, and paresthesias.[21]

Collaborative Care Management

Recognition of patients at risk for hypomagnesemia is important. People taking loop diuretics and digoxin should be encouraged to consume foods rich in magnesium, such as fruits, vegetables, cereals, and milk.[8] As magnesium is primarily an intracellular electrolyte, serum magnesium levels may be normal, despite total body magnesium depletion. Recognition of signs and symptoms of magnesium deficiency should not be ignored. Magnesium is essential for potassium resorption, so if hypokalemia does not respond to potassium replacement, hypomagnesemia should be suspected.[21]

Treatment of the underlying cause is the first consideration in hypomagnesemia. If the deficit is severe, parenteral magnesium replacement is indicated. When intravenous administration of magnesium is necessary, continuous cardiac monitoring is advisable. The infusion should be given via an infusion pump so that accurate dosing is assured. Patients experiencing mental status changes as a result of the hypomagnesemia require special attention be given to safety measures.

Hypermagnesemia

Hypermagnesemia is a serum magnesium level greater than 2.5 mEq/L.

Etiology

Hypermagnesemia seldom develops in the presence of normal renal function. However, magnesium excess may inadvertently occur as a result of magnesium replacement or when magnesium sulfate is administered to prevent seizures resulting from eclampsia. Therefore careful assessment of patients receiving magnesium therapy is essential.

Pathophysiology

Magnesium has what might be loosely described as a sedative effect: As the magnesium level rises, the patient becomes drowsy and lethargic and reflexes diminish. Respirations may become so severely depressed that respiratory arrest occurs. Because a loss of deep tendon reflexes occurs before severe respiratory problems occur, periodic assessment of reflexes during magnesium administration is essential. Cardiac effects of hypermagnesemia include slow heart rate and atrioventricular conduction block. As peripheral vasodilation occurs, hypotension, flushing, and increased skin warmth may be noted.[21]

Collaborative Care Management

Patients with impaired renal function are at risk of hypermagnesemia and should be cautioned to avoid over-the-counter medications that contain magnesium (e.g., Milk of Magnesia and Mylanta). Any patient receiving parenteral magnesium therapy should be assessed frequently for signs of hypermagnesemia.

Withholding magnesium-containing medications may correct mild hypermagnesemia. For renal failure, dialysis may be required for adequate treatment. Severe hypermagnesemia may require treatment with intravenous calcium gluconate (10 to 20 ml of 10% calcium gluconate administered over 10 minutes). If cardiorespiratory collapse is imminent, the patient may require temporary pacemaker and ventilator support.[21]

NURSING MANAGEMENT OF PATIENT WITH FLUID AND ELECTROLYTE IMBALANCES

Nursing management of persons with alterations in fluid and electrolyte imbalances is discussed in the following section.

ASSESSMENT

Health History

Imbalances in fluid and electrolytes occur as part of many clinical conditions. They also can be caused by many treatment regimens. The nurse needs to be alert to the risk of fluid and electrolyte imbalances and assess for their signs and symptoms (Table 13-10). The health history needs to explore existence of risk factors as well as the occurrence of these clinical manifestations. Information as to time of onset, extent, and aggravating and relieving factors needs to be obtained.

Data of particular importance in assessing fluid and electrolyte imbalance are the comparison of intake to output and changes in the patient's weight. These are nursing measures that can be instituted independent of doctors' orders. If patients and families are given explanations, they can participate in measuring and recording intake and output. The intake and output are totaled at intervals that are determined by the severity of the patient's condition. A patient in a critical care unit may have hourly measurements, whereas a patient in a step-down unit or on a medical floor may have them totaled once per shift.

Physical Examination

Because symptoms of fluid and electrolyte imbalance are frequently not specific, a good rule is to be alert for changes in behavior, level of consciousness, vital signs, skin, turgor, muscle strength, and condition of mucous membranes. Baseline observations made during the first encounter with a patient are essential for comparison with subsequent observations to detect changes. Specific physical examination findings and their meaning in terms of fluid and electrolyte balance are:

Body temperature can both indicate fluid and electrolyte imbalance or can cause the imbalance. Dehydration (with resultant increased serum sodium) causes temperature elevations. Fluid volume excess unrelated to infection can cause a decrease in body temperature. A profound decrease in circulating blood volume results in extremities that are cool to the touch. With fever, because of increases in metabolism and respiration, fluid loss is increased.

Pulse rate is affected by imbalances in potassium, sodium, and magnesium; volume depletion; and plasma to interstitial space shift. Pulse volume is affected by circulating blood volume. Dysrhythmias can indicate imbalances in potassium and magnesium.[16]

Respiration is a sensitive indicator of body pH. An example of this is the respiratory pattern in metabolic alkalosis, which is evidenced by decreased rate and depth and periods of apnea. Slow, shallow respirations favor carbon dioxide retention and hence carbonic acid and hydrogen ions. The changes caused by the alkalotic state of the arterial blood gases depress the respiratory centers to compensate for the alkalosis. Hypoventilation also occurs in potassium and calcium imbalances owing to muscle weakness. Metabolic acidosis increases both the rate and depth of respirations as the lungs attempt to blow off the carbon dioxide. During periods of abnormalities, respirations should be counted for a full 2 minutes.

Blood pressure variations are useful in evaluating fluid disturbances. In circulatory volume loss, the systolic pressure falls faster than the diastolic, resulting in diminished pulse pressure.

Jugular neck veins provide a built-in manometer for central venous pressure, providing the patient is not in congestive heart failure. Flat neck veins in a supine patient indicate decreased plasma volume. Normal jugular vein distention at a 45-degree angle is no higher than 2 cm above the sternal angle. Jugular neck veins distended from the manubrium to the angle of the jaw indicate high venous pressure.[18]

Hand veins are another useful measure of plasma volume. Normally, hand veins empty in 3 to 5 seconds when elevated. Conversely, they fill in 3 to 5 seconds when placed in a dependent position. Decreased plasma vol-

TABLE 13-10 Assessment of Fluid and Electrolyte Imbalance

Parameter	Fluid Excess	Fluid Loss/Electrolyte Imbalance
Behavior	Tires easily; change in behavior, confusion, apathy	Change in behavior, confusion, apathy
Head, neck	Facial edema, distended neck veins	Headache, thirst, dry mucous membranes
Upper gastrointestinal tract	Anorexia, nausea, vomiting	Anorexia, nausea, vomiting
Skin	Warm, moist, taut, cool feeling where edematous	Dry, decreased turgor
Respiration	Dyspnea, orthopnea, productive cough, moist breath sounds	Changes in rate and depth of breathing
Circulation	Loss of sensation in edematous areas, pallor,* bounding pulse, ↑ blood pressure	Pulse rate changes, dysrhythmias, postural hypotension
Abdomen	Increased girth, fluid wave	Distention, abdominal cramps
Elimination	Constipation	Diarrhea, constipation
Extremities	Dependent edema, "pitting," discomfort from weight of bedclothes	Muscle weakness, tingling, tetany

*Pallor: edema decreases the intensity of skin color by increasing the distance between the skin surface and the pigmented or vascular areas. In the dark-skinned person, pallor is observed by absence of underlying red tones that give brown and black skin "glow." The brown skin appears more yellow-brown, and the black skin appears more ashen gray.

ume causes the hand veins not to show or to fill more slowly. Increased plasma volume causes the hand veins to empty more slowly.

Assessments of skin turgor and mucous membranes are commonly used in detection of fluid volume. In normal skin turgor, gently pinched skin should fall back to its normal position when released. Because of decreased elasticity, evaluating skin turgor is not useful in the elderly. Mucous membranes in mouth breathers can be dry from evaporative processes rather than a fluid volume deficit. However, the area where the cheek and gum meet should be moist even in mouth breathers as long as they have no fluid volume deficit.

The type of edema that represents excess interstitial fluid (pitting edema, dependent edema, or refractory edema) is an obvious indication of increased total body sodium. As has been explained previously, edema is not produced by retention of water alone. In assessing the patient, it is important to differentiate between pitting edema and lymphedema. Pitting edema is an excessive accumulation of interstitial fluid and is either generalized or localized. When the amount of generalized edema is great, it is termed *anasarca.* To demonstrate the presence of edema, the thumb is pressed into the skin against a bony surface. When the thumb is withdrawn, an indentation persists for a short period of time. The depth of the indentation should be estimated and recorded in millimeters. Terms such as "3+" are meaningless and should not be used. The distribution should also be noted. Obstruction of lymphatic channels produces *lymphedema.* Lymphedema is differentiated by its woody or brawny feel, as opposed to the more pliant feel of interstitial edema.

Episodes of muscular weakness, fatiguability, and decreased activity tolerance may be descriptive of potassium deficit.

Severe ECF deficit produces sunken eyes, whereas excess ECF produces periorbital edema.

Behavior, while not diagnostic, can augment other observations. Sharp decreases in plasma pH cause disorientation and finally coma. With alkalosis, one of the symptoms is overexcitability, such as unexplained anxiety or nervousness. The extreme of this spectrum can be convulsions.[18]

Laboratory Values

Laboratory determinations of serum levels of the specific electrolytes also help in making decisions concerning electrolyte excesses or deficits. When there is water excess, hemodilution occurs and the hematocrit, blood urea nitrogen (BUN), and electrolyte levels are decreased. With excessive fluid loss hemoconcentration occurs, and the hematocrit, BUN, and electrolyte levels are increased. Urine specific gravity and anion gap are also useful measurements of fluid and electrolyte balance.

NURSING DIAGNOSES

Nursing diagnoses are determined from analysis of patient data. Nursing diagnoses for the patient experiencing fluid and electrolyte imbalances include, but are not limited to:

Diagnostic Title	Possible Etiologic Factors
1. Deficient fluid volume	Active fluid volume loss (hemorrhage, diarrhea, gastric intubation, wounds, diaphoresis), inadequate fluid intake, failure of regulatory mechanisms, sequestration of body fluids
2. Excess fluid volume	Excess fluid intake, excess sodium intake, compromised regulatory mechanisms

EXPECTED PATIENT OUTCOMES

Expected outcomes for patients with fluid and electrolyte imbalances may include but are not limited to:

1,2. Will maintain functional fluid volume as evidenced by adequate urinary output, stable weight, normal vital signs, normal urine specific gravity, moist mucous membranes, balanced intake and output, elastic skin turgor, prompt capillary refill, and absence of edema

2. Will verbalize understanding of treatment plan and causative factors that led to the imbalance

INTERVENTIONS

1,2. Intake and Output Monitoring

Intake and output monitoring is essential to determine the degree of fluid deficit or excess. The intake record should show the type and amount of all fluids the patient has received and the route by which they were administered. This includes fluids taken orally, parenterally, rectally, or by tubes (e.g., percutaneous esophageal gastrostomy [PEG], nasogastric). A record of solid food intake is sometimes necessary, especially with very young children. Foods that are eaten in a semisolid state but which are basically water based such as gelatin or Popsicles are recorded as fluids. In a strict sense, milk-based fluids are considered solids and as such are not totaled in with fluids. Ice chips are recorded by dividing the amount of chips by one half (60 ml of chips would equal 30 ml of water). Patients may receive a considerable amount of fluid intake through the frequent sucking of ice chips.

The output record is equally important. Vomitus, gastrointestinal drainage, and liquid stools are measured as accurately as possible and are described by color, content, and odor. Gastric secretions are normally watery and pale yellow-green; they usually have a sour odor. However, if the acid-base balance has been upset, gastric secretions may have a fruity odor because of the presence of ketone bodies (acetone). Bile is somewhat thicker than gastric juice and may vary in color from dark green to brown. It has an acrid odor, and patients may report a bitter taste if vomiting bile. Intestinal contents vary from dark green to brown, are likely to be quite thick, and have a fecal odor. The amount of fluid used in irrigating nasogastric tubes is added to "intake" and needs to be subtracted from total drainage before it is recorded. It is difficult to determine accurately the amount of water lost in the stools; but a record of the consistency, color, and number of stools and the approximate amount of each provides a reasonable estimate.

Disease states that cause increased vascular hydrostatic pressure and/or interstitial fluid colloid osmotic pressure result in fluid loss to the interstitial spaces, or third spacing. Examples of this are pleural or peritoneal effusions and ascites from hepatic or renal disease. Drainage of peritoneal or pleural fluid during the active disease state can exacerbate intravascular losses caused by continued shifts from the vascular compartment. Peritoneal or pleural fluid drainage is also noted as output, with the amount and color (clarity) recorded. Body weights are used to track fluid shifts and retention such as is found in third spacing. Body weight is discussed in more detail later in this chapter.

Noting the character and volume of urine is essential to evaluating fluid and electrolyte status. Urinary output is documented by recording the time and amount of each voiding. If renal function is a major concern, as in a severely burned patient, an indwelling catheter is inserted to measure the amount of urinary output hourly. The fluid intake is then regulated with respect to the output. Obviously, accuracy is critical. A frequent complaint is that nothing is more difficult to obtain in a modern hospital than an accurate record of urinary output. The patient and family should be instructed to save all urine. Measuring devices can be placed under the toilet seat to collect urine. Signs posted on the patient's chart and in the utility room and bathroom help to prevent discarding urine before it is measured.

Another parameter of importance in evaluating fluid and electrolyte status is the specific gravity of the urine. Specific gravity indicates the kidney's ability to dilute or concentrate urine. It is the weight of a specified amount of urine compared with the weight of an equal amount of distilled water. The specific gravity of water is 1.000. The specific gravity of urine in healthy persons ranges from 1.003 to 1.030. A highly concentrated specimen implies a state of dehydration; a dilute sample in a person with healthy kidneys indicates adequate hydration or possibly overhydration. As a matter of interest, a more accurate way of ascertaining renal concentrating ability is the simultaneous measurement of serum and urine osmolarity. The normal serum osmolarity is 290 (5 mOsm/kg) and the range of urine osmolarity is 40 to 1600 mOsm/L.[13]

As previously stated, to maintain chemical neutrality the total concentration of cations and anions must be equivalent in all body fluids in terms of milliequivalents per liter. However, because there are a number of anions and cations present in the blood that are not routinely measured, a "gap" exists between the total concentration of anions and cations and the concentration normally measured in the serum. This gap is composed primarily of unmeasured anions and is calculated by the formula Na $(Cl + HCO_3^-)$. The mean is approximately 12 mEq/L (range 8 to 16 mEq/L). The anion gap has important diagnostic significance in acid-base disorders, particularly metabolic acidosis. An increased anion gap may indicate endogenous metabolic acidosis, anion ingestion (ethylene, methanol, paraldehyde, and salicylates), acidosis secondary to therapeutic agents (paraldehyde, penicillin, and carbenicillin), and increased plasma proteins. A decreased anion gap may indicate increased unmeasured cations (hypercalcemia, hyperkalemia, and hypermagnesemia) or increased globulins (found in myeloma or lithium toxicity). Four commonly occurring clinical conditions associated with a high anion gap include (1) renal failure, (2) ketoacidosis, (3) reactions to drugs or toxins, and (4) lactic acidosis. In the absence of renal failure or intoxication with drugs and toxins, an increase in anion gap is assumed to be due to ketoacids or lactate accumulation.

All drainage from body orifices or artificial openings should be measured. This would include drainage from an ileostomy or a T tube after exploration of the common bile duct or from any catheter draining a surgical area. If there is excessive drainage from a wound, it may be necessary to weigh the dressings. Fluid loss is the difference between the wet dressings and the dry weight of the dressing.

Fluid aspirated from any body cavity such as the abdomen (paracentesis) or pleural space (thoracentesis) must be measured. The fluid contains not only electrolytes and water but also proteins. Blood loss from any part of the body is measured carefully. Diaphoresis is difficult to measure without special laboratory equipment. In some patients, however, it may be important to estimate the loss of fluid by this route. A careful note of excessive perspiration and its duration is made. If the clothing and bed linen become saturated, wet and dry weights may be taken. Accurate recording of body temperature helps the physician determine how much fluid should be replaced. Fluid loss through the skin and lungs increases as the body temperature rises. A patient who has a high fever and is breathing rapidly can lose as much as 2500 ml of fluid per day through the lungs.

1,2. Daily Weight

Trends in weight are often the best way to determine the onset of dehydration or the accumulation of fluid, either as generalized edema or as "hidden" fluid in body cavities. An increase of 1 kg in weight is equal to the retention of 1 L (1000 ml) of fluid in the edematous patient. If the weight record is to be accurate, the patient must be weighed on the same scale at the same hour each day and be wearing the same amount of clothing. Circumstances that may affect the weight should be kept as nearly identical as possible from day to day. Usually weights are taken early in the morning after the patient had voided for the first time, but before he or she has eaten or defecated. When precise weights are needed, all clothing and even wound dressings are removed. A person maintained on intravenous fluids other than those specifically designed for parenteral nutrition can be expected to lose approximately 0.2 to 0.5 kg/day.

1. Replacement of Fluid and Electrolytes

General Principles

Replacement of fluid and electrolyte losses is accomplished by one of the following: (1) oral intake, (2) tube feeding, (3) intravenous infusion, and/or (4) total parenteral nutrition.

The healthiest method of fluid and electrolyte replacement is by oral intake because it is believed to maintain motility and integrity of the gastrointestinal system.

When fluids can be metabolized by the gastrointestinal system but cannot be swallowed, interventions are used to bypass the esophagus. Examples are the use of nasogastric tubes, PEG tubes, and gastrostomy tubes (see Chapter 33). Normal saline solution and plain water should also be given by slow drip to replace daily fluid loss. When it is not possible for a patient to take food or fluid through the alimentary tract, the most common method of replacement is by intravenous infusion. Usually a vein in an extremity is used; however, when these are unavailable, a vein in the neck or groin is used. The intravenous infusion may be given by threading a needle or an intracatheter into a vein and securing it by taping it in place at the insertion site. An alternate method of access is to make an incision (cutdown) and thread a polyethylene catheter (intracatheter) into the vein. A peripheral inserted central catheter (PICC) is such an intravenous device. The insertion site is usually the brachial vein, and the catheter tip lies in the superior vena cava, providing a peripheral access to the central circulatory system. This access device permits use of more concentrated and/or irritating solutions than can be safely or comfortably administered with peripheral access devices. PICC lines also allow long-term administration of antibiotics, chemotherapeutic agents, parenteral nutrition, or hydrating fluids. RNs certified in the procedure may insert PICC lines.

Fluids administered by any route are most effective when apportioned over a 24-hour period, which helps maintain normal body fluid levels and provides better regulation of the electrolyte balance. This in turn prevents end metabolic products from being excreted in concentrated form, which reduces the potential of formation of calculi and renal damage. In addition, fluid spacing prevents circulatory overload, which may result in fluid and electrolyte shifts. Side effects from rapid fluid and electrolyte shifts include diarrhea and pulmonary edema. Side effects such as these can precipitate significant morbidity, and in some cases can contribute to mortality in severely ill patients.

Concentrated solutions of sodium, glucose, or protein should always be given slowly because they require body fluids for dilution. Hypertonic solutions cause fluid to diffuse from the tissues to equalize concentrations in the vascular compartment. The rapid dilution by the volume of blood in the superior vena cava makes it the preferred site for infusions of hypertonic solutions. An example of a hypertonic solution is the solution used for total parenteral nutrition (see Chapter 34).

Administering large amounts of a hypertonic solution into the alimentary tract causes a rapid shift of fluid from the vascular compartment into the intestinal lumen with a resultant decrease of blood volume. This process can lead to shock. "Dumping syndrome," which sometimes occurs after a gastric resection, is caused by this abnormal shift of fluid (see Chapter 33). In older therapies to reduce cerebral edema an attempt would be made to shift the edema through administration of hypertonic solutions. Newer pharmacologic therapies for cerebral edema are more precise and safer. It is important to remember that unless in the tightly controlled situation of a "fluid challenge," administration of a large amount of fluid is potentially dangerous, even in an apparently healthy person. Under most circumstances, fluids of any kind should be replaced at the speed with which they are lost.

The size of the patient is another important consideration in fluid administration. The small adult has less fluid in each compartment, especially in the intravascular system. Hence, a small person becomes seriously dehydrated more quickly than a larger adult but needs fluid replacement at a lesser volume than a larger person. Also, persons with small or inelastic vasculature become overhydrated easily.

Promoting Oral Intake

Adults who have no circulatory or renal malfunction usually are given between 2500 and 3000 ml of fluids per day. Precautions should be taken so that the overzealous patient does not drink too much fluid in a day or does not take in too much (three to four glasses) at one time. Excessive water intake may cause water intoxication.

When they are ill, many people find it difficult to eat or drink despite the need to do so. Nurses have a responsibility to encourage adequate food and fluids, thereby avoiding the need for parenteral hydration or nutrition. Water-based fluids such as fruit drinks, lemonade, punch, and noncarbonated beverages may be considered within the water requirement. Juicy fruits and Popsicles are yet another way of offering fluids. Despite being water-based, coffee, tea, and some colas have a diuretic effect; caution should be exercised when using them to meet a fluid requirement. Carbonated beverages also have a high sodium content. In a strict sense, milk, eggnog, ice cream, frozen yogurt, cocoa, and nutritional supplements such as Ensure or Sustacal are actually considered solids because they are either protein-, lipid-, or milk-based. Soup and bouillon can provide both fluid and electrolytes. Sport drinks that are high in electrolytes are another way of replacing fluid and electrolytes. It is important to remember the bolus concept when using sport drinks for replacement. Sometimes it is necessary to dilute the sport drink with water to avoid diarrhea. Be sure that the replacement modality is permitted in the patient's diet. For example, regular soda or sport drinks would be poor choices for fluid replacement in the diet of a person with diabetes because both contain large amounts of glucose.

The methods used in presenting food and fluid to patients may influence their consumption; often a small amount of either offered at frequent intervals is more useful than a large amount presented less often. Serving foods the patient is familiar with and likes helps to stimulate appetite. For example, familiar carbonated beverages are helpful to a nauseated patient. Consideration should always be given to the cultural and aesthetic aspects of eating.

Mouth care should be given to a dehydrated patient before and after meals and before bedtime. Dry oral mucous membranes (xerostomia) may lead to disruptions in the tissues of the oral cavity. Care should be taken to avoid irritating foods (spicy foods or those with high acidic content or fluids with temperature extremes). Stimulation of saliva may be aided by hard candy or chewing gum. Alternatively, an order for carboxymethylcellulose (artificial saliva) may be obtained. Lips should be kept moist and well lubricated.

Vomiting and diarrhea are common symptoms of many illnesses, and most people suffer from them from time to time. Sodium and potassium are lost in vomiting and diarrhea, whereas chloride is lost only in vomitus. Replacement fluids include salty broth (for sodium replacement) and tea (for potassium replacement). Sport drinks are another electrolyte replacement option discussed earlier. Orange juice is an old standard for replacing potassium. Soda crackers are a sodium replacement option if fluids are not well tolerated.

A patient with a draining fistula from any portion of the gastrointestinal tract loses sodium, calcium, and potassium and requires dietary supplementation. Milk will replace all the losses, and the patient who is lactose tolerant should be instructed to increase milk intake over normal levels. Medications are available for those with lactose intolerance. Lactase enzyme preparations, available over the counter, enhance the digestion of milk in those who are unable to do so. Consultation with a knowledgeable dietitian can yield a wealth of information concerning milk substitutes used for specific replacement needs. Patients with a permanent fistula or ostomy need to be especially careful to supplement sodium and potassium if vomiting, diarrhea, or fever occurs, which adds to their high electrolyte loss.

It is helpful to know the relative amount of various essential nutrients contained in the most commonly used foods. When losses must be restored, the patient needs to consume more than the usual daily requirement. Bananas, citrus fruits, all fruit juices, some fresh vegetables, coffee, and tea are relatively high in potassium and low in sodium. Salty broth and tomato juice provide extra sodium in addition to potassium. Milk, meat, eggs, and nuts are high in protein, sodium, and potassium. Current nutrition literature and the dietitian or nutritionist should be consulted liberally.

The nurse may encounter an order to "force" or "encourage" fluids. The amount required depends on the size of the patient, the amount of fluid loss, and the patient's circulatory and renal status. Taking these factors into account, the nurse is required to make an informed judgment to determine the amount. This information is then relayed to the rest of the nursing care team, including involved family members, or other caretakers.

If an elderly person living at home complains of pronounced weakness without apparent cause, the nurse should ask if cathartics or enemas have been used. If so, stopping this practice, replacing the sodium and potassium loss, and increasing fluid may reverse this symptom. Then the nurse may address the issue of proper bowel care.

Any patient with renal or circulatory impairment (shock, cardiac decompensation, or constriction of blood vessels resulting from disease) may develop electrolyte imbalances. Sodium and water may be held in the tissues, the potassium level of the blood may increase, acidosis may develop from inadequate tissue oxygenation, or the kidneys may be unable to excrete waste products properly. Patients with cardiac and renal impairments are instructed to avoid foods containing high levels of sodium, potassium, or bicarbonate.

Tube Feeding

Either water, a physiologic solution of sodium chloride, high protein liquids, or a regular diet can be blended, diluted, and given by gavage (see Chapter 33). As previously mentioned, high-protein tube feeding can cause water deficit through osmotic diuresis. The water content in the tube feeding needs to be increased when (1) the patient complains of thirst, (2) the protein or electrolyte content of the tube feeding is high, (3) the patient has a fever or a disease causing an increased metabolic rate, (4) the urinary output is concentrated, or (5) signs of water deficit develop.

Parenteral Fluids

Types of Solutions. The nurse needs to be familiar with the commonly used parenteral solutions (Table 13-11). The physician's order will include the type and amount of solution and the rate of administration. A hypotonic solution of 5% dextrose in distilled water is often given for short-term use in patients with hypernatremia. It is also used as a vehicle for drug administration via minibag. Dextrose 5% in saline solution may be given depending on the serum levels of sodium and vascular volume; potassium chloride is frequently added to meet normal intake needs and replace losses. Dextrose 5% in 0.2% normal saline is generally used as a maintenance fluid.

TABLE 13-11 Solutions for Intravenous Use

Contents of Solutions	Cations (mEq/L)		Anions (mEq/L)				HCO$_3^-$		Glucose
Type of Solution	Na^+	K^+	Ca^{++}	Mg^{++}	NH_4^-	Cl^-	Lactate	PO_4^-	(g/L)
5% dextrose in water									50
10% dextrose in water									100
Normal saline (0.9%)	154					154			
Ringer's solution	147	4	4			155			
5% dextrose in Ringer's lactate	130	4	3			109	28		50
Ringer's lactate	130	4	3			109	28		
5% dextrose in 0.2% saline	34					34			50
5% dextrose in 0.45% saline	77					77			50

With the addition of 20 mEq/L of potassium chloride, it provides the electrolytes at the maintenance requirement. Dextrose 5% in $^1/_2$ normal saline is generally used as a replacement solution for losses caused by gastrointestinal drainage. A physiologic solution of sodium chloride (0.9% normal saline) is given primarily when sodium chloride has been lost in large amounts and to patients with hyponatremia. Sodium and chloride deficit occurs with loss of gastrointestinal fluids, with burns, and with vascular volume deficits. Because it is isotonic, the normal saline solution remains in the extracellular space. For this reason, it is often given for fluid challenges and during resuscitation. Balanced solutions that contain several electrolytes may be used to replace fluid loss in surgical patients. Ringer's solution and lactated Ringer's solution are examples.[20]

Body needs for carbohydrates may be partially met by giving fructose or 10% to 20% glucose in distilled water. These solutions are hypertonic and therefore require additional water for excretion.

Amino acid preparations (Aminosol) are generally given into the central vasculature rather than peripherally. They are generally components of total parenteral nutrition solutions. Whole blood or packed red cells are used to replace blood loss; but plasma, 25% salt-poor albumin, or plasma expanders can be given to substitute for blood protein loss and are used to reestablish normal volume and prevent shock. Dextran, the most commonly used plasma volume expander, increases the oncotic pressure of the blood, thus increasing the resorption of fluid from interstitial spaces and increasing plasma volume. Low-molecular-weight dextran decreases the blood viscosity and allows greater flow of blood through the capillaries. Thus it is useful in treating cardiogenic, hemorrhagic, or septic shock (see Chapter 14). Dextran may cause a prolonged bleeding time and is contraindicated in patients with renal failure, severe bleeding disorders, and severe congestive heart failure.[21]

Administration. The speed at which intravenous solutions containing electrolytes are infused should be regulated according to the patient's condition and electrolyte concentration. The patient is watched carefully for untoward signs, which would include those of excess fluids or electrolytes. Hyperkalemia can be particularly dangerous because it may cause cardiac arrest. When solutions containing electrolytes are administered, the nurse monitors the urinary output carefully. Marked decreases are reported immediately to the physician. Because the kidneys select the ions needed and excrete the surplus, a normal output is essential. If the nurse is planning the sequence of intravenous fluids, hydrating fluids such as half-strength physiologic solution of sodium chloride or glucose in water should be given first for the patient with a primary water deficit. Renal failure and untreated adrenal insufficiency are contraindications for the use of potassium. If these conditions are known or suspected, the nurse should verify orders for potassium administration. Physicians usually write the daily intravenous fluid orders after reviewing the most recent blood chemistry results.

The rate of administration of fluids is ordered by the physician and depends on the patient's illness, the fluids to be administered, and the patient's basic state of health. An infusion is rarely run at a rate faster than 4 ml/min. If the infusion is given continuously or in the presence of impaired cardiac or renal function, the rate of administration is rarely faster than 2 ml/min. The usual rate for fluid loss replacement is 3 ml/min. This rate allows time for the fluid to diffuse into ECF compartments and avoids circulatory overload or increases in the blood volume to the point of producing a diuretic effect. It is important to note that when administering an intravenous infusion by gravity, different brands of administration equipment vary in drops per milliliter. To determine the rate of delivery, the nurse must check the packaging of the equipment used. The most important factor in determining the rate of delivery is the millimeters per minute, not drops per minute. The correct number of drops per minute is dependent on the millimeters per minute to be administered.

For reasons cited earlier in the text, nurses should question the practice of increasing the rate of flow of intravenous solutions to complete the infusion at a specified time. The rate of flow should never be increased when administering parenteral nutrition. Nurses should recognize the signs of pulmonary edema (bounding pulse, engorged peripheral veins, hoarseness, dyspnea, cough, and rales) and monitor patients for signs of fluid overload (see Chapter 21). Persons at risk include those receiving concentrated solutions or rapid infusions, and those whose age or physical condition places them at special risk. At the first sign of increased blood volume, the rate of flow should be reduced to "keep vein open" rate (20 to 30 ml/hr depending on institution policy), and the physician should be notified. Particular care needs to be taken when delivering fluids to infants, elderly patients with circulatory or renal impairments, patients with cardiac disease, those who have had plasma shifts such as burn patients, and those with extensive tissue trauma from other causes. Patients whose plasma has shifted need to be watched carefully because the shift reverses itself after a few days, flowing from the interstitial spaces to the vascular space. This may potentiate an increase in blood volume with resulting pulmonary edema.

It is imperative that the nurse check the labels of fluid containers carefully for correct content and accurately record the fluids given. Expiration dates are also an important feature of the container label. Patients receiving fluids intravenously are monitored for symptoms of hypervolemia or hypovolemia so that rates can be adjusted accordingly (Table 13-12). The insertion site is checked regularly, several times per shift, for signs of infiltration or inflammation. If infiltration occurs, the infusion should be stopped immediately and relocated. Peripheral intravenous sites are generally rotated every 72 hours. Dressing changes over peripheral intravenous sites are also changed every 3 days; institutional policy may vary. Electrolyte solutions that contain potassium are irritating. Extravasation of these solutions may cause tissue necrosis. Infiltration of these solutions require a physician's attention. When dextran and other plasma expanders or other protein solutions are being given, the patient is observed for anaphylactic reaction (apprehension, dyspnea, wheezing, tightness of chest, angioedema, itching, hives, and hypotension) (see Chapter 49).

TABLE 13-12 Complications of Intravenous Fluid Therapy

Observations	Nursing Actions
Circulatory Overload	
Bounding pulse, venous distention, hoarseness, dyspnea, cough, pulmonary rales, restlessness	Notify physician Reduce flow to "keep open" rate Raise head of bed to facilitate breathing
Local Infiltration	
Decreased rate or cessation of fluid flow Tissue around needle or catheter site cold, pale, swollen, hard Complaint of local pain	Stop infusion Arrange to restart infusion at another site Apply moist heat Elevate lower arm
Thrombophlebitis	
Pain, redness, warmth, edema along vein	Same as for local infiltration Cold compresses may be applied initially
Pyrogenic Reaction	
Fever, chills, general malaise, nausea, and vomiting 30 min after infusion started Hypotension (if severe)	Switch to another infusion solution and run at "keep open" rate Notify physician Monitor vital signs Save infusion fluid for culture
Anaphylactic Reaction (With Proteins)	
Apprehension, dyspnea, wheezing, tightness of chest, itching, hypotension	Switch infusion to nonprotein solution and run at "keep open" rate Notify physician Monitor vital signs

Pronounced and continued thirst despite the administration of fluids is not normal and should be reported to the physician. In the immediate postoperative period, this kind of thirst suggests internal hemorrhage, temperature elevation, or some other untoward development. In the chronically ill patient, thirst may indicate the onset of a disease such as diabetes mellitus in which extra water is used by the kidneys to eliminate glucose. Thirst is also a symptom of hypercalcemia.

Patient/Family Education

Education of the patient and family is important in the prevention and early detection of future fluid and electrolyte imbalances. Many of the principles discussed in the Interventions section have relevance as home-going instructions. Patients at particular risk for developing imbalances include those with chronic diseases, especially renal insufficiency, congestive heart failure, diabetes, and cancer. The teaching plan should include the signs and symptoms of deficit or excess, causative factors, and measures to prevent alterations in homeostasis. If drug therapy is included in the treatment plan, the patient and family should be instructed regarding the correct method of administrating the medication, correct dose, and therapeutic and adverse effects.

Depending on the type of deficit or excess, certain food or fluids may be encouraged or restricted. The patient and family should be provided with a list of foods that are permissible, as well as those to be avoided. The nurse should instruct the patient to discriminate between fresh and prepared foods and read the package labels to determine the nutritional content of prepared foods. For example, the patient needing restrictions in potassium should be instructed to avoid organ meats, fresh and dried fruits, and salt substitutes. The patient should also be provided with a list of foods and their fluid content. Obviously it is important to include the caretaker in the teaching. The patient and caretaker should be informed of the need for periodic reassessment. Teaching should also include measures to prevent complications such as alterations in skin integrity or oral mucosa and infection. Skin assessment and care are important points to include in teaching. Persons with fluid excess and deficits are at risk for breaks in skin integrity. Caregivers should be taught positioning techniques for patients with mobility restrictions. Bony prominences and edematous skin are prone to breakdown. Healing is especially difficult in persons with edema.

■ EVALUATION

To evaluate the effectiveness of the nursing interventions, compare patient behaviors with those stated in the expected patient outcomes. Achievement of outcomes is successful if the patient with disturbances in fluid and electrolyte imbalance:

1. Maintains functional fluid volume level with adequate urinary output, vital signs within patient's normal limits, specific gravity of urine within 1.003 and 1.035,

moist mucous membranes, stable weight, intake equal to output, elastic skin turgor, and no edema.

2. States possible causes of imbalance and plan to prevent recurrence of imbalances.
3. Reports a decrease or absence of symptoms causing discomfort.

ACID-BASE BALANCE

Etiology

Before discussing the etiology of acid-base disturbances, it is essential to review the normal values of the acid-base system. If information about acid-base balance is to be useful, it is important to know how to interpret arterial blood gases (ABGs) so intervention can take place when the body is unable to restore a normal acid-base balance in the face of a disturbance.[9] An ABG measurement gives the information needed to determine if the primary disturbance of acid-base balance is respiratory or metabolic in nature. Analysis of the patient's arterial blood gases requires an arterial puncture, which must be obtained with utmost care and caution to both the technician and patient (see Guidelines for Safe Practice box).

Arterial blood gases give information about a patient's oxygenation, ventilation, and acid-base status. See Table 13-13 for the parameters, normal values, definitions, and implications. It is important to note the patient's temperature on the requisition when the blood sample is drawn, as the ABGs must be corrected for temperature, especially fever, which increases oxygen consumption and metabolic rate.[9]

The information ABG measurements provide reflects the functional status of alveolar and capillary diffusion, alveolar ventilation, pulmonary circulation, and pulmonary gas exchange. The partial pressure of oxygen in arterial blood ($Pa{O_2}$) is a measurement of the pressure oxygen exerts in its free form when dissolved in the plasma.[2] Normal $Pa{O_2}$ values range from 80 to 100 mm Hg. The partial pressure of carbon dioxide in arterial blood ($Pa{CO_2}$) reflects the measurement of the pressure of CO_2 dissolved in the plasma., which reflects the pulmonary component of the ABGs.[2] Normal $Pa{CO_2}$ values are 35 to 45 mm Hg. The level of the buffer bicarbonate is measured by the HCO_3, which reflects the renal component of the ABGs.[2] The normal value is 22 to 26 mEq/L. Base excess is a calculated measurement that indicates the number of buffering ions in the blood. Base excess normal ranges are −2 to +2 (mmol/L). The anion gap reflects the difference between the unmeasured cations (K^+, Mg^{++}, and Ca^{++}) and unmeasured anions (albumin, organic anions, HPO_4^-, and SO_4^- and is useful in identifying types of metabolic acidosis. For example, an anion gap of 16 to 20 indicates acidosis caused by retention of organic acids as in diabetic ketoacidosis. A normal range for anion gap is 12 (±4) mEq/L.[22]

Physiology: Regulation of Acid-Base Balance

Acids, Bases, and pH. Acids are substances having one or more hydrogen ions ($[H^+]$) that can be liberated into a solution. Bases are substances that can accept or bind H+ ions in a solution. Acid-base balance is actually homeostasis of the hydrogen ion concentration in body fluids.[1] The need for multiple mechanisms to maintain acid-base balance arises from the importance of the H^+ ion concentration on the operation of cellular enzymes and function of vital organs (especially the brain and heart).[1] The body produces large amounts of acids from normal metabolism every day, yet despite this large addition of acids to the body fluids, the H^+ ion concentration remains low.

> ## *Guidelines for Safe Practice*
> **Drawing Arterial Blood Gases**
>
> Performing an arterial puncture requires knowledge of the anatomy and physiology of the arterial system as well as skill in the technique of arterial puncture. For patient well-being and safety, an Allen's test should be performed on the artery from which the blood is to be drawn (usually the radial artery). If a blockage is found in the ulnar artery, another site should be chosen.[14] Once the puncture is complete, the radial artery (or whichever artery is used) must be compressed by the practitioner's fingers for a minimum of 5 minutes to ensure that bleeding has stopped and to avoid the risk of hemorrhage from the site. The most common problems in taking an arterial blood sample include bleeding, vessel obstruction, and infection.[14] In addition, as in all situations where blood is handled, strict Standard Precautions must be adhered to for protection of all involved (see Chapter 11 for Standard Precautions).
>
> Reference: Williams AJ: Assessing and interpreting arterial blood gases and acid-base balance, *BMJ* 317:1213, 1998.

Hydrogen ion concentration is represented by the pH. This pH scale was devised by chemists to express the small quantity of H+ ions in blood or body fluids.[22] The pH is the negative logarithm of the concentration of H^+ ions; therefore, as H^+ ion concentration increases, the pH decreases and vice versa. A low pH, therefore, indicates an acidic solution, while a high pH indicates a basic or alkaline solution.[1] A change in pH by 1 unit results in a 10-fold change in H^+ concentration.[15] Even minute changes (e.g., a change from 7.4 to 7.3) result in a major increase in H^+ ion concentration in the solution.

Normal arterial blood pH is 7.35 to 7.45. When the pH is in this range, the ratio of base ions to acid ions is 20:1. If there is an increase of H^+ ions, the pH decreases ($<$7.35), and the patient is said to have acidemia. The process of becoming acidemic is called *acidosis*. Alternately, if the ratio of bases to acids is increased (i.e., if there is an excess of bases), the pH increases ($>$7.45), and the patient is said to have alkalemia. The process of becoming alkalemic is called alkalosis.

Hydrogen ions circulate throughout the body fluids in two forms: the volatile hydrogen of carbonic acid and the nonvolatile form of hydrogen in organic acids, such as sulfuric, hydrochloric, pyruvic, phosphoric, and lactic acids. In a day's time many acids are produced as the end products of metabolism. In the normal person, the lungs excrete 13,000 to 30,000 mEq/day of the volatile hydrogen in carbonic acid

(H_2CO_3) as CO_2, and the kidneys excrete approximately 50 mEq/day of nonvolatile acids. Mechanisms that regulate acid-base balance include chemical buffer systems, the respiratory system, and the kidneys (Table 13-14).[22]

Chemical Buffer Systems. The body cells are very sensitive to changes in pH; hence the pH must be kept relatively constant within the narrow range of normal. The chemical buffer systems, with their almost instantaneous effect, serve this function.

A buffer is a substance that can act as a chemical sponge, by either soaking up or releasing hydrogen ions so that the pH value remains stable. The main buffer systems of the body are the carbonic acid–bicarbonate system, the phosphate system, and protein buffer system. The carbonic acid–bicarbonate buffer system is the system that is monitored clinically. If this buffer system is stable, the other buffer systems are stable.[1]

Carbonic Acid-Bicarbonate Buffer System. The carbonic acid–bicarbonate system is present in ECF (ECF). Carbonic acid is formed by the combination of carbon dioxide and water: $CO_2 + H_2O \rightleftarrows H_2CO_3$. When a strong base is added to the body fluids, it is buffered by carbonic acid to a bicarbonate salt and water: $H_2CO_3 + NaOH \rightarrow NaHCO_3 + H_2O$. When a strong acid is added to the system, the bicarbonate buffer changes it to a salt and carbonic acid: $HCl + NaHCO_3 \rightarrow NaCl + H_2CO_3$. This carbonic acid then dissociates into carbon dioxide and water that can be excreted by the lungs and kidneys.

The ability to maintain a stable pH depends essentially on maintenance of the normal ratio of 20 parts bicarbonate to 1 part carbonic acid (Figure 13-10). The body strives to maintain this ratio at all times. This is done by retaining or blow-

TABLE 13-13 Arterial Blood Parameters Used for the Analysis of Acid-Base Status

Parameter	Normal Value	Definition and Implications
PaO_2	80-100 mm Hg	Partial pressure of oxygen in arterial blood (decreases with age) In adults <60 years: 60-80 mm Hg = mild hypoxemia 40-60 mm Hg = moderate hypoxemia <40 mm Hg = severe hypoxemia
pH	7.40 (±0.05 [2 SD]) 7.40 (±0.02 [1 SD])	Identifies whether there is academia or alkalemia; the value using 2 standard deviations (SD) from the mean is the common clinical value. PH <7.35 = acidosis; pH >7.45 = alkalosis
$[H^+]$	40 (±2) nmol/L or nEq/L	The hydrogen ion concentration may be used instead of the pH
$PaCO_2$	40 (±5.0) mm Hg	Partial pressure of CO_2 in the arterial blood PCO_2 <35 mm Hg = respiratory alkalosis PCO_2 >45 mm Hg = respiratory acidosis
CO_2 content	25.5 (±4.5) mEq/L	Classic method of estimating $[HCO_3^-]$; measures HCO_3^- + dissolved CO_2 (latter is generally quite small except in respiratory acidosis)
Standard HCO_3^-	24 (±2) mEq/L	Estimated HCO_3^- concentration after fully oxygenated arterial blood has been equilibrated with CO_2 at a PCO_2 of 40 mm Hg at 38° C; eliminates the influence of respiration on the plasma HCO_3^- concentration.
Base excess	0 (±2) mEq/L	Reflects pure metabolic component Base excess = 1.2 × deviation from 0 Negative in metabolic acidosis Positive in metabolic alkalosis Misleading in respiratory and mixed acid-base disturbances Not essential for interpretation of acid-base disturbances
Anion gap	12 (±4) mEq/L	Anion gap (or delta) reflects the difference between the unmeasured cations (K^+, Mg^{++}, Ca^{++}) and unmeasured anions (albumin, organic anions, HPO_4^-, $SO_4^=$); useful in identifying types of metabolic acidosis; value >16-20 indicates acidosis is caused by retention of organic acids (for example, diabetic ketoacidosis)

Useful Formulas

Plasma anion gap = $[Na^+] - ([HCO_3^-] + [Cl^-])$

Calculation of third acid-base parameter when two are known:

$$[H^+] = 24 \times \frac{PaCO_2}{[HCO_3^-]}$$

Conversion of pH into $[H^+]$ (use formulas below):

pH of 7.4 5 $[H^+]$ of 40 mEq/L

For every 0.1 increase in pH above 7.4, multiply 40 × 0.8

For every 0.1 decrease in pH below 7.4, multiply 40 × 1.25

For example, pH of 7.60 = 40 × 0.8 × 0.8 = $[H^+]$ of 26 mEq/L

From Price SA, Wilson LM: *Pathophysiology: clinical concepts of disease processes,* ed 6, St Louis, 2003, Mosby.

ing off CO_2 by the lungs or by retaining or excreting HCO_3^- by the kidneys. This relationship is expressed in Figure 13-11.

Phosphate Buffer System. The phosphate buffer system is most active in the ICF; it is especially active in the kidneys. Like bicarbonate, phosphate can accept spare hydrogen ions. Conversely, one molecule of phosphoric acid can donate up to three hydrogen ions to make up for any hydrogen ion deficits. Phosphate groups may occur free in plasma or bound to certain organic compounds.

The phosphate system is composed of sodium and other cations in combination with $H_2PO_4^-$ ion and HPO_4^- ion. Because phosphate is excreted by the kidneys, this system is helpful in buffering fluids in the renal tubules.

Protein Buffer System. The protein buffer system is located in the plasma and inside the cells; the protein hemoglobin in red blood cells is one of the proteins involved. Although most protein buffers are intracellular, they assist in buffering ECF. The protein buffer system is found throughout the body and is therefore the most plentiful chemical buffer system in the body.[22]

Respiratory Control of pH. The respiratory control center in the brain responds to increases of carbon dioxide and hydrogen ions in body fluids. Rate and depth of respiration are in turn controlled by the respiratory control of pH as follows: (1) when the pH value decreases (more acidic), respiratory rate and depth are increased, and there is greater excretion of carbon dioxide through the lungs; thus less carbon dioxide is present to produce carbonic acid by the reaction, $CO_2 + H_2O \rightleftarrows H_2CO_3$, and the pH increases toward alkalinity; and (2) when the pH value rises above the normal range (more alkaline), the respiratory center is depressed, rate and depth of respiration decrease, carbon dioxide is retained, and more carbonic acid is formed, moving the pH toward acidity. The respiratory system is extremely efficient and reacts within minutes to changes in acid-base balance.

Because carbon dioxide is constantly being formed as a product of metabolism, the concentration of carbon dioxide in ECFs must be continuously balanced between the rate of metabolism and the rate of pulmonary excretion. The buffering capacity of the respiratory system is more than double that of all the chemical buffers combined.

TABLE 13-14 Mechanisms Regulating Acid-Base Balance

Action Time	Effect
Chemical Buffers in Cells and Extracellular Fluid	
Instantaneous	Combine with acids or bases added to the system to prevent marked changes in pH
Respiratory System	
Minutes to hours	Controls CO_2 concentration in ECF by changes in rate and depth of respiration
Kidneys	
Hours to days	Increases or decreases quantity of $NaHCO_3$ in ECF Combines HCO_3^- or H^+ with other substances and excretes them in urine

ECF, Extracellular fluid.

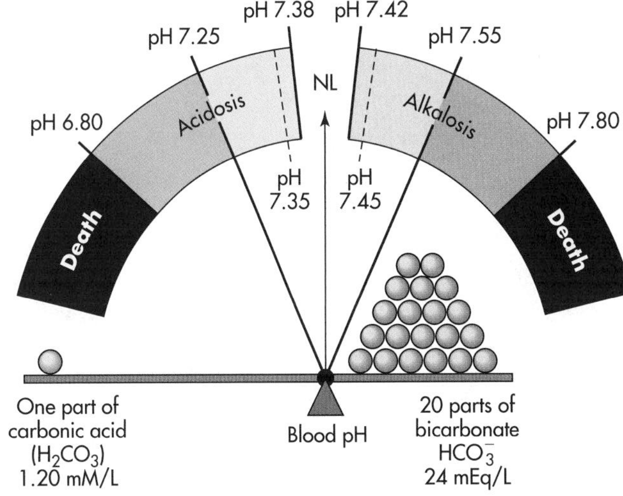

Figure 13-10 Note that the relationship of 1 part carbonic acid to 20 parts bicarbonate maintains hydrogen ion concentration (pH) within normal limits. Increase in H_2CO_3 or decrease in HCO_3^- causes alkalosis.

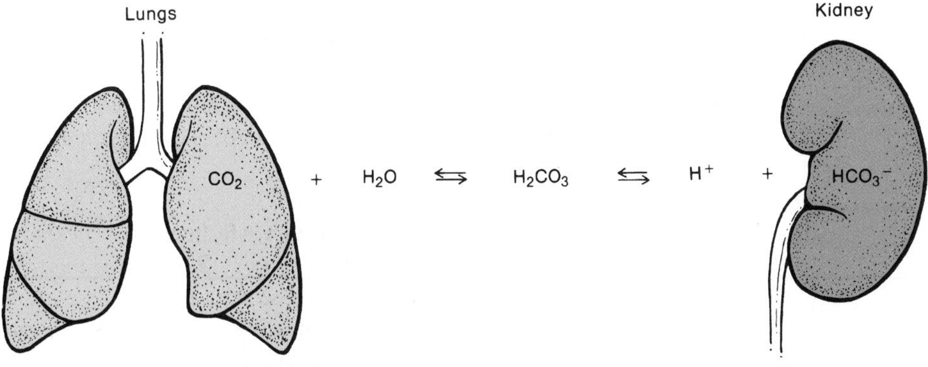

Figure 13-11 The lungs help control acid-base balance by blowing off or retaining CO_2. The kidneys help regulate acid-base balance by excreting or retaining HCO_3^-.

TABLE 13-15 Expected Directional Changes with Acid-Base Imbalances

	pH	HCO_3^-	Pco_2
Respiratory Acidosis			
Uncompensated	↓	Normal	↑
Partly compensated	↓	↑	↑
Compensated	Normal	↑	↑
Respiratory Alkalosis			
Uncompensated	↑	Normal	↓
Partly compensated	↑	↓	↓
Compensated	Normal	↓	↓
Metabolic Acidosis			
Uncompensated	↓	↓	Normal
Partly compensated	↓	↓	↓
Compensated	Normal	↓	↓
Metabolic Alkalosis			
Uncompensated	↑	↑	Normal
Partly compensated	↑	↑	↑
Compensated	Normal	↑	↑

From Sands JK, Dennison PE: *Clinical manual of medical-surgical nursing concepts and clinical practice,* ed 3, St Louis, 1995, Mosby.

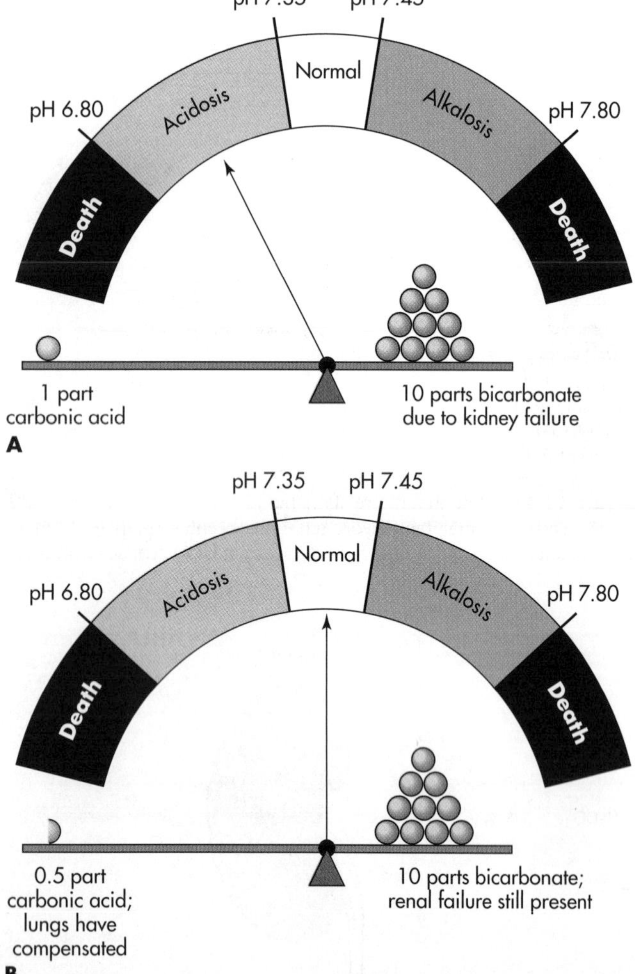

Figure 13-12 **A,** Example of metabolic acidosis. Bicarbonate is decreased because of renal failure. Carbonic acid to bicarbonate ratio is 10:1; acid is present. **B,** Example of compensation. Note that acid is also decreased. Ratio returned to 20:1; pH level is normal.

Renal Regulation of pH. Although chemical buffers and respiratory regulation have limited ability to make complete adjustments in the pH level, renal regulation is powerful and complete in its adjustments in the pH level of body fluids. However, this response takes hours to days to accomplish. The renal regulation of pH is affected by control of the retention or excretion of bicarbonate and hydrogen ions. The kidneys usually excrete an acid urine because of the excess of acid metabolic products (nonvolatile acids), which must be eliminated by the renal route. Normally almost all of the bicarbonate formed by the kidneys is retained.

Hydrogen ions secreted by kidney tubule cells and bicarbonate filtered into the glomerular filtrate combine in the kidney tubules to form carbon dioxide and water, which is excreted through exhalation (CO_2) and in urine (H_2O). In acidosis, excess hydrogen ions are secreted into the kidney tubules, where they combine with buffers and are excreted in the urine. In alkalosis, bicarbonate ions enter the tubules, which, lacking hydrogen ions that they normally combine with to form carbonic acid, combine instead with sodium or other cations and are excreted in the urine. Hydrogen ions can be exchanged for sodium and potassium ions in the kidney tubules; therefore excretion or conservation of hydrogen ions can result in imbalances of sodium and potassium.

Pathophysiology

Compensatory Mechanisms. The kidneys and lungs also have a compensatory function in maintaining acid-base balance. In a disease state that leads to an acid-base imbalance, the normal bicarbonate-carbonic acid ratio of 20:1 is lost. In response, the kidneys attempt to compensate for changes in blood CO_2 by making a corresponding change in blood bicarbonate, and the lungs attempt to compensate for abnormal changes in blood bicarbonate by making corresponding

TABLE 13-16 Types of Acid-Base Disturbances and Compensatory Mechanisms

Physiologic Causes	Expected Response	Method of Compensation
Respiratory Acidosis		
Carbonic acid excess: lungs not removing sufficient CO_2 (hypoventilation)	Acute: For every 10 mm Hg increase in $Paco_2$, 1 mEq/L increase in HCO_3^- Chronic: For every 10 mm Hg increase in $Paco_2$, 3.5 mEq/L increase in HCO_3^-	Bicarbonate production by kidneys increased; bicarbonate retained and chloride excreted instead by kidneys; secretion and excretion by hydrogen ions in urine increased
Respiratory Alkalosis		
Carbonic acid deficit: lungs removing too much CO_2 (hyperventilation)	Acute: For every 10 mm Hg decrease in $Paco_2$, 2 mEq/L increase in HCO_3^- Chronic: For every 10 mm Hg decrease in $Paco_2$, 5 mEq/L increase in HCO_3^-	Kidneys increase excretion of bicarbonate ions
Metabolic Acidosis		
Bicarbonate deficit: retention of acid metabolites, diabetic ketoacidosis, excess acid intake (salicylate poisoning), hyperkalemia, or loss of bicarbonate	For every 1 mEq decrease in HCO_3^-, 1.2 mm Hg decrease in $Paco_2$	Increased rate and depth of respiration cause increased excretion of CO_2 by lungs; formation of bicarbonate ions in the kidneys increased
Metabolic Alkalosis		
Bicarbonate excess: excess intake (sodium bicarbonate, carbonated drinks) or retention of bicarbonate, potassium depletion, loss of acid	For every 1 mEq increase in HCO_3^-, 0.7 mm Hg increase in $Paco_2$	Rate and depth of respiration decreased; lungs retain more CO_2; kidneys excrete bicarbonate

Adapted from Price SA, Wilson LM: *Pathophysiology: clinical concepts of disease processes,* ed 6, St Louis, 2003, Mosby.

changes in blood CO_2 (Table 13-15). Compensation is an effort to maintain the normal 20:1 ratio. Figure 13-12 is an example of what happens in metabolic acidosis and the compensatory mechanism of the lungs that occurs to correct the imbalance. See Table 13-16 for types of acid-base imbalances and the expected compensatory responses.

Another compensatory mechanism that can be used by the body in the presence of acid-base problems is shifting of hydrogen ions from the extracellular to the intracellular compartment or vice versa. With an increased level of hydrogen ions (metabolic acidosis), these ions can be shifted into the intracellular compartment in exchange for potassium. This shift alone increases the pH level of the blood. In addition, because the hydrogen ion concentration is now higher in the renal tubule cells, hydrogen is excreted in exchange for the reabsorbed sodium. In metabolic alkalosis, hydrogen ions are pulled from the intracellular compartment, and potassium ions are shifted into the intracellular compartment. Again, this shift alone helps to lower the pH level. Also, because potassium ion concentration is now higher in the renal tubule cells, potassium is excreted for the conserved sodium, and hydrogen ions are also conserved. These compensatory mechanisms can lead to hyperkalemia when acidosis is present and hypokalemia when alkalosis is present.

It must be remembered that the buffer systems and the compensatory mechanisms provide for only temporary adjustment, and the underlying cause of the disturbance must be ultimately identified and corrected. However, the kidneys can make permanent adjustments, as seen in persons who have respiratory acidosis as a result of chronic obstructive pulmonary disease (COPD) (see Chapter 21). It should be noted that the body's own compensatory mechanism will never overcompensate for a primary imbalance.

Types of Acid-Base Disturbances. The two types of acidosis and alkalosis are respiratory and metabolic. The major effect of acidosis is depression of the central nervous system, as evidenced by disorientation followed by coma. Alkalosis is characterized by overexcitability of the nervous system, and the muscles may go into a state of tetany and convulsions. Acid-base imbalance always produces an imbalance of the body's other cations as well; thus symptoms of these imbalances can also occur. Therefore, using a systematic approach to assessment of acid-base disturbances is imperative (Box 13-1). An alternative method to assessing an acid- base disturbance can be approached by looking at the H model (see Future Watch box).

Respiratory Acidosis: Carbonic Acid Excess. Any factor that decreases the rate of pulmonary ventilation increases the concentration of dissolved carbon dioxide, carbonic acid, and hydrogen ions and results in respiratory acidosis. An excess of carbon dioxide (hypercapnia) over a period of time can cause carbon dioxide narcosis. In this condition, carbon dioxide levels are so high that they no longer stimulate respirations but depress them. Associated with the decreased respiratory rate are lack of oxygen and hypoxia. CO_2 narcosis can occur in chronic obstructive pulmonary disease. During respiratory acidosis, potassium moves out of the cells, producing hyperkalemia. Ventricular fibrillation may then occur if the blood potassium level is greatly increased.

BOX 13-1 A Systematic Approach to the Assessment of Acid-Base Disturbances

Begin With a High Degree of Clinical Suspicion

1. Examine the clinical history for disease processes that may lead to simple acid-base disorders.
   a. This requires knowledge of the pathogenesis of the various acid-base disorders.
   b. For example, one might expect a person with advanced chronic obstructive pulmonary disease to develop respiratory acidosis.
2. Note clinical signs and symptoms that suggest an acid-base disorder.
   a. Unfortunately, many of the signs and symptoms of an acid-base disorder are subtle or nonspecific.
   b. For example, Kussmaul respirations in a diabetic patient may represent respiratory compensation for metabolic acidosis.
3. Examine laboratory reports of the electrolytes and other data that suggest disease processes associated with acid-base disorders.
   a. For example, hypokalemia is often associated with metabolic alkalosis.
   b. For example, an elevated serum creatinine level indicates renal insufficiency, and renal insufficiency and failure are usually associated with metabolic acidosis.

Evaluate Acid-Base Variables to Identify The Type of Disorder

1. First, examine the arterial blood pH to determine the direction and magnitude of the acid-base disturbance.
   a. If decreased, the patient has acidemia with two potential causes: metabolic acidosis or respiratory acidosis.
   b. If increased, the patient has alkalemia with two potential causes: metabolic alkalosis or respiratory alkalosis.
   c. It is helpful to note that the renal and respiratory compensations rarely return the pH to normal so that a normal pH in the presence of changes in the $PaCO_2$ and HCO_3^- suggests a mixed disorder; for example, a person with a combined respiratory acidosis and metabolic alkalosis might have a normal pH.
2. Examine the respiratory ($PaCO_2$) and metabolic (HCO_3^-) variables in relation to the pH to tentatively characterize the primary disturbance as a respiratory, metabolic, or mixed disorder.
   a. Is the $PaCO_2$ normal (40 mm Hg), increased, or decreased?
   b. Is the HCO_3 normal (24 mEq/L), increased, or decreased?
      (1) Optional: Is there a base excess or deficit?
   c. In a simple acid-base disorder, the $PaCO_2$ and HCO_3^- are always altered in the same direction.
   d. Deviation of the $PaCO_2$ and HCO_3^- in opposite directions indicates the presence of a mixed acid-base disorder.
   e. Make a tentative decision about the primary disturbance by correlating the findings with the clinical situation.
3. Estimate the expected compensatory response to the primary acid-base disorder.
   a. If the compensatory response is greater or less than expected, a mixed acid-base disorder is suggested (an acid-base nomogram may also be used to help identify a mixed acid-base disorder).
   b. Calculate the plasma anion gap.
      (1) If increased (0.16 mEq/L), metabolic acidosis is most likely.
   c. Compare the magnitude of fall in plasma [HCO_3^-] with the increase in the anion gap; these should be similar in magnitude.
      (1) If the anion gap has risen more than in [HCO_3^-], this suggests that a component of the metabolic acidosis is due to HCO_3^- loss.
      (2) If the increase in anion gap is much greater than the fall in [HCO_3^-], there is a coexistent metabolic alkalosis.
4. Make the final interpretation.
   a. Simple acid-base disorder
      (1) Acute (uncompensated) or
      (2) Chronic (partially or fully compensated)
   b. Mixed acid-base disorder
   c. Normal or wide anion gap: metabolic acidosis

From Price SA, Wilson LM: *Pathophysiology: clinical concepts of disease processes,* ed 6, St Louis, 2001, Mosby.

Future Watch

Using the H Model To Identify an Acid-Base Disorder

Interpreting the results of arterial blood gas analyses is made easy by the use of a simple strategy called the H model. The H model uses the values of the patient's pH, $PaCO_2$, and HCO_3^- level. The left axis of the H model is $PaCO_2$, which represents the respiratory system. The right axis of the model is HCO_3^- level, which represents the metabolic system. The mean values of these two parameters (PaCO2 of 40 mm Hg. and HCO_3^- of 24 mEq/L) are connected to form the center line, which is referred to as "baseline." When a deviation from the baseline occurs, an acid-base disturbance is present. When the patient's actual values are plotted on this chart, it is easy to visualize where the abnormality is in relation to normal, or "baseline."

This method may be an easier way to determine the acid-base disturbance for those practitioners less familiar with acid-base balance. Look for more information on this method in the future.

Reference: Kirksey KM, Holt-Ashley M, Goodroad BK: An easy method for interpreting the results of arterial blood gas analysis, *Crit Care Nurse* 21(5):49, 2001.

Respiratory acidosis can result from a number of pathologic conditions that cause hypoventilation and CO_2 retention: (1) damage to the respiratory center in the medulla; (2) obstruction of respiratory passages, for example, pneumonia or chronic bronchitis; (3) loss of lung surface for ventilation, for example, atelectasis, pneumothorax, emphysema, or pulmonary fibrosis; (4) weakness of respiratory muscles, for example, poliomyelitis or hypokalemia; and (5) severe depression of respirations, for example, as a result of an overdose of respiratory depressant drugs. COPD is the most common cause of chronic respiratory acidosis.[10] Causes of respiratory acidosis are summarized in Box 13-2.

Respiratory Alkalosis: Carbonic Acid Deficit. Excessive pulmonary ventilation decreases hydrogen ion concentration and thus causes respiratory alkalosis. A common cause of respiratory alkalosis is hyperventilation. A person who hyperventilates blows off large amounts of carbon dioxide. Hyperventilation may be caused by anxiety, pain, hypoxia, or lesions affecting the respiratory center in the medulla (brain tumor or

BOX 13-2 Causes of Respiratory Acidosis

Damage to respiratory center in medulla (head injury)
Depression of respiratory center by drugs (narcotics, ethanol, barbiturates, anesthetics)
Obstruction of respiratory passages: pneumonia, chronic bronchitis, emphysema, pulmonary edema
Loss of lung surface for ventilation
Atelectasis
Pneumothorax
Emphysema
Pulmonary fibrosis
Kyphoscoliosis
Weakness of respiratory muscles
Poliomyelitis
Hypokalemia
Guillain-Barré syndrome
Amyotrophic lateral sclerosis (ALS)
Increased carbohydrate intake from tube feedings in patients being mechanically ventilated

BOX 13-3 Causes of Respiratory Alkalosis

Hyperventilation syndrome (caused by anxiety, hysteria)
Hyperventilation caused by:
- Fever
- Hypoxia
- Pain
- Pulmonary disorders (pulmonary emboli, asthma, pneumonia)
- Lesions affecting the respiratory center in the medulla
- Brain tumor
- Encephalitis, meningitis
- Excess assisted ventilation
- Hyperthyroidism
- Gram-negative sepsis

encephalitis). Other causes of respiratory alkalosis are conditions that greatly increase metabolism (hyperthyroidism) and the overventilation of patients with mechanical ventilators.[11] Causes of respiratory alkalosis are summarized in Box 13-3.

Metabolic Acidosis: Bicarbonate Deficit. When excess organic acids are added to the body fluids or when bicarbonate is lost, a metabolic acidosis results.

In conditions such as uncontrolled diabetes mellitus or starvation, glucose either cannot be used or is unavailable for oxidation. The body compensates for this by using body fat for energy, producing abnormal amounts of ketone bodies in the process. In an effort to neutralize the ketones and maintain the acid-base balance of the body, plasma bicarbonate is exhausted. The resultant acid-base imbalance is called metabolic acidosis, or *ketoacidosis.* This condition can develop in anyone who does not eat an adequate diet and whose body fat must be burned for energy. The reason that nutrition experts criticize extremely low-carbohydrate or high-protein-no carbohydrate reduction diets is the resulting ketoacidosis.[23] Metabolic acidosis can also develop whenever excessive amounts of lactic acid are produced, such as in prolonged strenuous muscle exercise or when oxidation takes place in cells without adequate oxygen, which may occur in heart failure or shock. Loss of large amounts of alkaline intestinal secretions, such as in severe diarrhea or through fistulas, can also create a bicarbonate deficit.

BOX 13-4 Causes of Metabolic Acidosis

Increased acid production
Ketoacidosis (uncontrolled diabetes mellitus, alcoholism, starvation)
Uremic acidosis (renal failure)
Lactic acidosis (shock, respiratory or cardiac arrest)
Increased acid ingestion
Salicylates, ethanol, ethylene glycol
Loss of bicarbonate
Severe diarrhea
Intestinal fistulas
Adrenal insufficiency
Hypothyroidism

BOX 13-5 Causes of Metabolic Alkalosis

Loss of stomach acid
Gastric suctioning
Persistent vomiting
Excess alkali intake (e.g., overuse of antacids, Milk of Magnesia, or $NaHCO_3^-$; citrate in blood) transfusions
Intestinal fistulas
Hypokalemia
Cushing's syndrome or aldosteronism
Potassium-depleting diuretic therapy

The normal functioning kidney excretes an excess of hydrogen ions in conditions of acidosis and, in so doing, retains potassium so that hyperkalemia, as well as acidosis, is present. In kidney failure, metabolic acids accumulate in the bloodstream.[26] Causes of metabolic acidosis are listed in Box 13-4.

Metabolic Alkalosis: Bicarbonate Excess. When excessive amounts of acid substance and hydrogen ions are lost from the body or when large amounts of bicarbonate or lactate are added orally or intravenously, the result is an imbalance in which there is an excess of base elements. This imbalance, called *metabolic alkalosis,* does not occur as often as metabolic acidosis. In alkalosis, potassium enters the cells and hypokalemia results. An excess of bicarbonate in distal tubular fluid causes obligatory potassium loss.

Metabolic alkalosis can occur in the following conditions: (1) loss of hydrochloric acid from the stomach caused by vomiting or gastric drainage from a nasogastric tube (loss of chloride leaves more sodium to combine with and retain bicarbonate in the kidneys); (2) loss of potassium ions through intestinal fistulas, diarrhea, or in the urine; (3) ingestion of large amounts of sodium bicarbonate or other systemic antacids to treat indigestion or ulcers; (4) infusion of excessive amounts of bicarbonate or lactate intravenously; (5) diuretic therapy; and (6) excessive mineralocorticoids.[19] Causes of metabolic alkalosis are listed in Box 13-5.

Collaborative Care Management

Respiratory Acidosis. Treatment is aimed at enhancing alveolar ventilation to improve the exchange of carbon dioxide and oxygen. This objective is accomplished by identifying and treating the cause of the inadequate ventilation. Bronchodilators may be used to reduce bronchial spasm. Respiratory infections may be treated with antibiotics. Postural drainage and chest clapping are necessary for persons with airway obstruction. Adequate hydration is also important to assist in removal of secretions. Supplemental oxygen and assisted ventilation may be used as necessary.

Because the respiratory center is narcotized by the increased amounts of carbon dioxide, a lowered oxygen tension in the blood (or hypoxemia) then becomes the stimulus for respiration. If a patient whose respiratory drive is dependent on a low PO_2 level is given large amounts of oxygen, the stimulus for breathing is removed, and respirations cease. For this reason, uncontrolled oxygen delivery is never used with patients with carbon dioxide narcosis.

Low-flow oxygen (1 to 3 L/min) is given to a patient with COPD who maintains a chronically high PCO_2 level. Respiratory treatments are usually given using compressed air or room air instead of oxygen in these situations. If signs of ventilatory failure are present, the PCO_2 level is greater than 50 to 60 mm Hg, and the PO_2 level is less than 50 mm Hg, the patient may require intubation and mechanical ventilation.[10]

The major nursing responsibility is to recognize patients who have the potential for developing respiratory acidosis because of conditions that interfere with normal respiratory gas exchange. A patient whose airway is compromised by the presence of secretions must be encouraged to cough frequently or may need to undergo nasopharyngeal or tracheal suctioning. Pulmonary hygiene measures may be used to promote removal of secretions.

Respiratory Alkalosis. Treating the underlying condition usually resolves the respiratory alkalosis. Respiratory alkalosis becomes especially dangerous when it leads to cardiac dysrhythmias caused partly by a decreased serum potassium level. If a patient who is receiving assisted ventilation complains of dizziness or shows any signs of muscle irritability, it is likely that the depth of respiration is too great, and the respiratory rate or volume of the machine should be decreased. If tetany is present, calcium gluconate is given intravenously. Renal function must be maintained to promote renal compensation of the disturbance.

Metabolic Acidosis. Treatment of acidosis is directed primarily toward the underlying cause and the restoration of electrolyte balance. If the acidosis is severe, intravenous sodium bicarbonate is sometimes given. Bicarbonate preparations must be administered with caution, because they can induce a metabolic alkalosis and lead to tetany and convulsions. When acidosis is caused by renal failure, renal dialysis is necessary.

As the acidosis is corrected, potassium moves back into cells, and hypokalemia develops. If a patient being treated for acidosis needs to receive potassium, it is given after the

TABLE 13-17 Major Signs and Symptoms and Therapy for Acid-Base Imbalances

Signs and Symptoms	Therapy
Respiratory Acidosis	
Hyperpnea	Bronchodilators
Visual disturbances	Postural drainage
Headache	Chest clapping
Late: confusion, drowsiness, coma	Mechanical ventilation
Potassium excess	
Respiratory Alkalosis	
Lightheadednes	Treatment of underlying condition
Numbness or tingling of fingers or toes	
Late: tetani, convulsions	
Potassium deficit	
Metabolic Acidosis	
Headache and mental dullness	Treatment of underlying condition
Kussmaul's respirations	Sodium bicarbonate (IV)
Late: disorientation, coma	Fluid and electrolyte replacement
Potassium excess	
Metabolic Alkalosis	
Confusion, dizziness	Treatment of underlying condition
Numbness or tingling of fingers or toes	Diuretic: acetazolamide (Diamox)
Late: tetani, convulsions	
Potassium deficit	Fluid and electrolyte replacement

acidosis has been partially corrected and as the pH level is returning to normal. It is important to bear in mind that even though acidosis is accompanied by hyperkalemia, the patient may be potassium depleted. The potassium leaves the cells in exchange for the hydrogen ions, and much of it is excreted.

Maintenance of adequate respiratory function in a patient with metabolic acidosis facilitates the excretion of carbon dioxide. If the kidneys are functioning well, they can help correct the acidosis by producing more bicarbonate. Because some conditions that lead to metabolic acidosis cause a hyperosmolar state as well, osmotic diuresis will take place, and the patient needs fluid replacement along with careful monitoring of intake and output. If changes in the sensorium have resulted, safety precautions are instituted.

Metabolic Alkalosis. Treatment is aimed at correcting the cause of the metabolic alkalosis. It may be as simple as cessation of excessive antacid ingestion or discontinuing a nasogastric tube. Sodium chloride or ammonium chloride may be given orally or intravenously if the alkalosis is severe. If the condition is associated with loss of sodium chloride, then potassium, given as potassium chloride, must be restored because it is lost with the sodium. A diuretic that acts as a carbonic anhydrase inhibitor (Diamox) may help relieve the alkalosis by increasing the excretion of bicarbonate in the kidneys.

The nurse assists in the maintenance of optimal respiratory function so that compensation can take place through this mechanism. Careful monitoring of the patient for adequate renal function and safety precautions are important in the nursing care of patients with metabolic alkalosis. Because convulsions may occur, precautions are taken for the patient's protection.

It is important to treat the underlying cause of the acid-base imbalance (Table 13-17). In mixed acid-base imbalances, signs and symptoms as well as management vary.

NURSING MANAGEMENT OF PATIENT WITH RESPIRATORY ACIDOSIS

ASSESSMENT

Health History

Data to be collected include complaints of headache, confusion, lethargy, nausea, irritability, anxiety, dyspnea, and blurred vision.[10] Whenever possible, always ask the patient or family if there is any preexisting disease or illness which will help in making the diagnosis.

Physical Examination

Physical assessment should include assessing for changes in mental status from confusion to lethargy, to stupor, and then to coma. Tachycardia and hypertension may be present as well as cardiac dysrhythmias. Respirations should be assessed for quality, rate, and depth. Adequacy of airway patency must also be determined.[10] Hyperkalemia results from movement of potassium out of cells as the hydrogen ions move in.

NURSING DIAGNOSES

Nursing diagnoses for the patient with respiratory acidosis are determined from analysis of patient data and may include but are not limited to:

Diagnostic Title	Possible Etiologic Factors
1. Impaired gas exchange	Hypoventilation
2. Disturbed thought processes	Central nervous system (CNS) depression
3. Anxiety	Hypoxia, hospitalization
4. Risk for ineffective family coping	Illness of family member
5. Ineffective airway clearance	Hypoventilation, secretions
6. Ineffective breathing pattern	Hypoventilation, dyspnea

EXPECTED PATIENT OUTCOMES

Expected patient outcomes for a patient with respiratory acidosis include but are not limited to:

1. Will maintain patent airway and adequate breathing rate and rhythm with return of ABGs to patient's normal level
2. Will be alert and oriented to person, place, and time or to his or her normal baseline level of consciousness (LOC)
3. Will cope with anxiety
4. Will exhibit effective coping and awareness of effective support systems
5. Will have secretions that are normal for self in amount and can be raised
6. Will maintain adequate rate and depth of respirations, using pursed lip and other breathing techniques when necessary (as in the patient with COPD)

INTERVENTIONS

1. Supporting Effective Gas Exchange

The patient with respiratory acidosis requires thorough and frequent assessment of breath sounds, respiratory rate and rhythm, and maintenance of a patent airway. The nurse needs to be prepared for the use of artificial airways. Providing a position of comfort (which is usually sitting upright) for the patient allows for ease of respirations. Obtaining and monitoring ABG results and vital signs and reporting changes in the patient's condition are crucial to patient care. The nurse provides and monitors supplemental oxygen as ordered. Turning the patient every 2 hours and as needed (PRN), providing pulmonary hygiene as ordered and PRN, adequate hydration, comfort measures such as mouth care, and assisting with activities of daily living are all part of nursing care for this patient. The patient should be instructed regarding coughing and deep breathing techniques and management of disease condition, especially COPD.

2. Coping With Disturbed Thought Processes

The patient with respiratory acidosis requires frequent neurologic assessment. The person's baseline LOC should be documented and monitored frequently. Reorientation to reality is done as necessary by providing calendars, clocks, familiar objects, and frequent family visits.

3. Relieving Anxiety

Assess the patient for visible signs of anxiety. Provide a calm, relaxed environment. Give clear, concise explanations of treatment plans. Encourage the patient to express feelings. Provide comfort measures. In addition to orienting the patient to reality frequently, providing support and information to the patient and family helps allay anxiety and fears. Relaxation techniques may be useful in reducing anxiety. The patient must be monitored for signs of respiratory depression, which is an adverse effect if narcotic analgesics are given. Assist the patient to identify coping mechanisms to deal with anxiety and stress.

4. Enhancing Coping Mechanisms

Patients in respiratory acidosis are frequently confused, anxious, and often belligerent (from high PCO_2 levels). The patient's family often feels anxious and has difficulty coping. The nurse provides support and information to family members about the patient's ongoing condition and reassures them that there is a physiologic cause for the patient's behavior. The nurse encourages questions and open communication with all involved and facilitates family and physician communication.

5. Promoting Airway Clearance

Meticulous care to airway patency is important for the patient's recovery. Regular breathing and coughing exercises should be implemented as well as nasopharyngeal suctioning when necessary. Good hydration is important to keep the secretions thin and moist. Chest physiotherapy may be helpful in raising secretions deep within the lungs.

6. Promoting an Effective Breathing Pattern

Adequate alveolar ventilation must be maintained. This may necessitate mechanical ventilation. Teaching the patient proper breathing techniques as well as panic control breathing will aid in providing and maintaining an effective breathing pattern.

Patient/Family Education

The nurse develops an individualized teaching plan based on patient and family learning needs. Diet, medications, breathing techniques, as well as signs and symptoms of respiratory acidosis are some potential learning needs. Patients with COPD are at high risk for this acid-base disorder and may require further pulmonary rehabilitation.[10]

EVALUATION

To evaluate the effectiveness of the nursing interventions, compare patient behaviors with those stated in the expected outcomes. Achievement of outcomes is successful if the patient with respiratory acidosis:

- **1a.** Demonstrates improved ventilation and oxygenation.
- **1b.** Has vital signs, ABGs, and cardiac rhythm within own normal range
- **2.** Returns to baseline LOC.
- **3.** Reports reduced anxiety.
- **4.** Family uses adequate coping mechanisms.
- **5.** Is able to raise secretions on own.
- **6.** Demonstrates effective breathing techniques.

NURSING MANAGEMENT OF PATIENT WITH RESPIRATORY ALKALOSIS

ASSESSMENT

Health History

Any reports of anxiety (most common cause of hyperventilation), shortness of breath, muscle cramps or weakness, perioral tingling, palpitations, panic, and dyspnea must be fully explored.[6]

Physical Examination

Light-headedness and confusion occur as a result of cerebral hypoxia. The person with respiratory alkalosis may exhibit hyperventilation, tachycardia or arrhythmia, muscle weakness, and a positive Chvostek's sign or Trousseau's sign indicating a low ionized serum calcium level secondary to hyperventilation and alkalosis.[25] Deep tendon reflexes may be hyperactive, the patient's gait may be unsteady, and muscle spasms or tetany may be present.[11] The patient may be agitated, irrational, belligerent, or psychotic. Seizures may occur in extreme cases. Serum potassium levels will be decreased. Any patient who is on mechanical ventilation should be monitored regularly because of the risk of hyperventilation, which will cause respiratory alkalosis.

NURSING DIAGNOSES

Nursing diagnoses for the patient with respiratory alkalosis are determined from analysis of patient data and may include but are not limited to:

Diagnostic Title	Possible Etiologic Factors
1. Anxiety	Stress, fear
2. Ineffective breathing pattern	Hyperventilation, anxiety
3. Disturbed thought processes	CNS excitability, irritability
4. Risk for injury	Change in LOC and potential for seizures

EXPECTED PATIENT OUTCOMES

Ascertaining and treating the cause or causes of the patient's anxiety and hyperventilation are the goal. Expected outcomes for the patient with respiratory alkalosis may include but are not limited to:

1. Will report decreased anxiety; verbalizes methods to cope with anxiety
2. Will return to normal respiratory rate and rhythm or at least decreased hyperventilation, with return to baseline ABGs
3. Will exhibit reorientation to person, place, and time as per patient's baseline
4. Will be free from injury

INTERVENTIONS

1. Allaying Anxiety

The patient with respiratory alkalosis usually hyperventilates because of anxiety. The nurse helps to allay the anxiety and gives antianxiety medications as ordered. Sometimes the intervention may be having the patient breathe into a paper bag. This will trap CO_2, allowing the patient to rebreathe and thus increase the CO_2 level and slow the respiratory rate. Relaxation techniques may be useful adjuncts to allay anxiety.

2. Promoting an Effective Breathing Pattern

A thorough frequent assessment of respiratory rate and rhythm is essential, in addition to encouraging the patient to slow his or her respiratory rate. Maintain a calm, comforting attitude when dealing with the patient and family. Position the patient to promote maximal ease of inspiration. Assist the patient with relaxation techniques.

3. Coping With Disturbed Thought Processes

The patient may need frequent reorientation. If possible, ask the family to bring in familiar objects from home, such as calendars, clocks, or photographs. Encourage the family to assist in reorientation. Reading the paper aloud or watching the news may be helpful to review current events. When giving instructions, use simple direct statements and allow the patient adequate time to respond.

4. Preventing Injuries

The patient should be frequently assessed for potential injuries. A neurologic assessment should be performed and documented. Any changes in neurologic functioning should be reported. Use the agency's fall prevention program and/or family members to prevent falls or injuries. Institute seizure precautions as needed. Assess the environment for potential hazards. Assess the patient's muscle strength in addition to gross and fine motor coordination.

Patient/Family Education

The nurse develops an individualized teaching plan based on the etiology of the patient's respiratory alkalosis, for example, a stress reduction class to learn other strategies to decrease stress as a cause of hyperventilation. The patient and family should be taught how to prevent, recognize, and treat hyperventilation. The patient and family should be taught safety precautions for medications, especially those containing aspirin.

Health Promotion and Prevention

Referrals for psychiatric counseling may be necessary to relieve the patient's anxieties. Other strategies may include teaching the patient muscle relaxation techniques, controlled therapeutic breathing, and visualization techniques.

EVALUATION

To evaluate the effectiveness of nursing interventions for the patient experiencing respiratory alkalosis, compare the patient's condition with the stated expected outcomes. Achievement of outcomes is successful if the patient with respiratory alkalosis:

1. Reports reduction in anxiety levels.
2a. Demonstrates effective normal breathing pattern.
2b. Has ABG results within patient's normal baseline.
3. Returns to baseline LOC and orientation level.
4. Remains free from injury; no seizure activity.

NURSING MANAGEMENT OF PATIENT WITH METABOLIC ACIDOSIS

ASSESSMENT

Health History

Any reports of anorexia, nausea, vomiting, abdominal pain, headache, and thirst if the patient is dehydrated must be fully explored.

Physical Examination

On physical examination findings indicative of metabolic acidosis may include confusion; hyperventilation; warm, flushed skin; bradycardia and other dysrhythmias; decreasing LOC[22]; nausea, vomiting, or diarrhea; Kussmaul respirations, and acetone breath, especially if acidosis is due to ketoacidosis. Symptoms may progress to coma if untreated.

NURSING DIAGNOSES

Nursing diagnoses for the patient with metabolic acidosis are determined from analysis of patient data and include but are not limited to:

Diagnostic Title	Possible Etiologic Factors
1. Disturbed thought processes	Secondary to CNS depression
2. Decreased cardiac output	Dysrhythmias
3. Risk for injury	Secondary to altered mental state
4. Risk for imbalanced fluid volume	Diarrhea, renal failure

EXPECTED PATIENT OUTCOMES

Once the underlying cause is detected and treated, expected outcomes for the patient with metabolic acidosis include but are not limited to:

1. Will return to usual baseline LOC
2. Will return to normal baseline parameters for vital signs with improved cardiac output and decreased or resolved dysrhythmias
3. Will remain in a safe, secure environment without injury
4. Will maintain fluid and electrolyte balance and stabile renal status

INTERVENTIONS

1. Coping With Disturbed Thought Processes

The nurse monitors the patient's LOC frequently and reorients as necessary. Other interventions include monitoring vital signs, especially respiratory rate and rhythm; blood pressure to assess cardiac output; temperature to assess for fever; and ABGs to assess the effects of treatment. Cardiac monitoring may be indicated to detect any dysrhythmias. Correcting the underlying cause is essential (e.g., diabetic ketoacidosis, renal failure, electrolyte imbalance).

2. Supporting Cardiac Output

Monitoring vital signs, intake and output, and fluid and electrolyte balance will be important to restore adequate cardiac output as well as to assess the effectiveness of treatment. Cardiac monitoring may be indicated to detect any dysrhythmias as well as evaluate cardiac status.

3. Promoting Safety

The nurse provides a safe, secure, monitored environment for the patient. Safety precautions are especially important for a confused patient.

4. Promoting Return of Fluid and Electrolyte Balance

The nurse monitors the patient's intake and output to restore adequate fluid balance. The nurse also administers the treatment prescribed to correct the cause of the metabolic acidosis per medical order.

Patient/Family Education.

An individualized teaching plan is formulated by the nurse to meet patient and family needs. If ketoacidosis is the cause, teaching about diabetes may be instituted to prevent recurrence of symptoms.

EVALUATION

To evaluate effectiveness of nursing interventions, compare patient behaviors with those stated in the expected patient outcomes. Achievement of outcomes is successful if the patient with metabolic acidosis:

1. Exhibits baseline-level of consciousness and orientation.
2. Returns to normal baseline parameters for vital signs and cardiac output with cardiac dysrhythmias resolved.
3. Remains free from injury.
4. Maintains fluid and electrolyte balance and stabile renal function.

NURSING MANAGEMENT OF PATIENT WITH METABOLIC ALKALOSIS

ASSESSMENT

Health History

The health history may include reports of prolonged vomiting or nasogastric suctioning; frequent self-induced vomiting; muscle weakness; light-headedness; ingestion of large amounts of licorice or antacids; use of diuretics; muscle cramping, twitching, or tingling; and circumoral tingling.[25]

Physical Examination

The patient may exhibit mental confusion, dizziness, and changes in LOC. Other data may include hyperreflexia, tetany, dysrhythmias, seizures, respiratory failure, a positive Chvostek's or Trousseau's sign if the patient has a low ionized serum calcium level, decreased hand grasps secondary to muscle weakness, and generalized muscle weakness. A decreased calcium and/or potassium level may be present. There may be impaired concentration and potentially seizures. Electrocardiographic changes consistent with hypokalemia may be present.[19]

NURSING DIAGNOSES

Nursing diagnoses for the patient with metabolic alkalosis are determined from analysis of patient data and include but are not limited to:

Diagnostic Title	Possible Etiologic Factors
1. Disturbed thought processes	CNS excitation
2. Decreased cardiac output	Dysrhythmias and electrolyte imbalances
3. Risk for injury	Muscle weakness, tetany, confusion, and possible seizures
4. Risk for imbalanced fluid volume	Nasogastric drainage, diuretic therapy, fistula

EXPECTED PATIENT OUTCOMES

Expected outcomes for the patient with metabolic alkalosis may include but are not limited to:

1. Will be oriented to time, place, and person as per baseline status
2. Will return to normal baseline range for cardiac output with resolution of electrolyte imbalances and cardiac dysrhythmias
3. Will maintain a safe, secure environment
4. Will maintain normal fluid volume

INTERVENTIONS

1. Coping With Disturbed Thought Processes

The nurse monitors the patient's LOC and reorients the patient frequently. The use of familiar objects with frequent visits of significant others aids in reorienting the patient.

2. Supporting Cardiac Output

Monitoring vital signs, intake and output, and fluid and electrolyte balance will be important to restore adequate cardiac output as well as to assess the effectiveness of treatment. Cardiac monitoring may be indicated to detect any dysrhythmias as well as evaluate cardiac status.

3. Promoting Safety

The nurse maintains a safe, secure environment for the patient. The nurse institutes seizure precautions and falls prevention as necessary.

4. Promoting Return of Fluid and Electrolyte Balance

The nurse monitors serum electrolytes and ABGs and administers replacement therapy such as potassium and chloride as ordered. The nurse observes the patient for any signs or symptoms of electrolyte deficiencies. Antiemetics may be administered to relieve vomiting. Diuretic therapy should be stopped or reduced as ordered by the physician. An accurate record of intake and output should be kept.

Patient/Family Education

The type of teaching depends on the etiology of the alkalosis. The goal of patient and family education is to prevent recurrence of the imbalance. The patient and family should be taught signs and symptoms of metabolic alkalosis to detect the onset of any recurrence. If the cause of alkalosis was related to diuretic therapy, reinforcement regarding correct medication use is warranted. Information should be given regarding excessive use of antacids. Teaching the patient how to manage persistent vomiting may prevent future episodes of metabolic alkalosis. If an eating disorder is suspected, a referral to a psychologist and nutritionist is indicated.

EVALUATION

To evaluate the effectiveness of nursing interventions, compare patient behaviors with those stated in the expected patient outcomes. Achievement of outcomes is successful if the patient with metabolic alkalosis:

1. Manifests mental status that has returned to baseline.
2. Is free of cardiac dysrhythmias.
3. Remains free from injury.
4. Maintains fluid balance at baseline level.

GERONTOLOGIC CONSIDERATIONS

Older adults, particularly those with COPD, are at risk of developing acid-base disorders that can lead to respiratory depression. Older patients are also at risk of developing any acid-base imbalance as a result of susceptibility to pH disturbances caused by normal physiologic aging. In addition, several medications may alter the activity of normal pH compensating mechanisms. Preexisting or underlying conditions such as renal, cardiac, pulmonary, and endocrine disorders increase the risk of an elderly person developing an acid-base disturbance. Once an acid-base disorder develops, the older patient is less able to compensate for imbalances because of age-related changes in the kidneys.

Critical Thinking Questions

1. A patient on your unit has a diagnosis of dehydration. The physician has ordered "force fluids." You must make a judgment as to type and amount since these were not specified in the order. Identify the additional patient data needed to make an appropriate nursing decision.
2. A patient with advanced cancer of the lung has been nauseated for several weeks after chemotherapy and has become malnourished. A serum chemistry profile indicates a serum albumin level of 2.2 mg/dl. Identify the data relevant for assessing calcium balance/imbalance and data needed to confirm your conclusions about the patient's electrolyte status.
3. A patient has end-stage AIDS and an opportunistic infection of the small intestine, which at this stage of his HIV infection can be treated but not cured. The opportunistic infection gives him copious amounts of diarrheal stools. Identify the foods and fluids and the information needed to approximate amounts needed to maintain fluid and electrolyte balance.
4. An 83-year-old patient with cardiomegaly and periodic episodes of atrial fibrillation insists on taking laxatives several times per week. Evaluate the risk this situation presents to fluid and electrolyte balance, and list the possible consequences. Describe a detailed teaching plan to correct this.
5. A well-toned 30-year-old engineer has volunteered to ride his bicycle in a 150-mile ride for charity that will take place over 2 days. This event is planned for early August, when the ambient temperature averages 85° to 90° F. As the nursing consultant helping to plan this event, list the fluid and electrolyte considerations for riders such as this patient.
6. A 32-year-old administrative assistant comes to the urgent care center with a 72-hour history of vomiting secondary to influenza. She is lethargic and states, "My muscles are twitching." Her respirations are 18/min and heart rate is 110 beats/min, and she has a fever of 100.4° F (orally). Her blood pressure is 110/68 which she states "is about normal for me." Her ABG values are as follows:
   pH: 7.57
   Pa_{O_2}: 92
   Pa_{CO_2}: 41
   HCO_3:36
   Describe her acid-base status, probable cause for the imbalance, and treatment.
7. A 55-year-old man, whose wife died unexpectedly last week, is found by his daughter to be unconscious on the sofa. On the coffee table is an empty bottle labeled Seconal. He is rushed to the emergency room. Objective data include:

ABGs	Vital Signs
pH: 7.13	BP: 104/68
Pa_{O_2}: 53	Respirations: 7/min and shallow
Pa_{CO_2}: 70	Heart rate: 82/min
HCO_3: 23	Temperature: 99.6° F (rectally)

   What is your analysis of the situation? What treatment is indicated?

References

1. Adrogue HE, Adrogue HJ: Acid-base physiology, *Respir Care* 46(4):328, 2001.
2. Blood gas analysis, supplement to *Crit Care Nurse* 20:6, 2000.
3. Bevilacquq J: Hyponatremia in AIDS, *Bailliere's Clin Endocrinol Metab* 8(4):837, 1994.
4. Bonne O et al: Adaptation to severe chronic hypokalemia in anorexia nervosa: a plea for conservative management, *Int J Eating Disord* 13(1):125, 1993.
5. Boyda EK, Kee J: Knowledge base for patients with fluid, electrolyte and acid-base imbalances. In Monahan FD, Neighbors M, editors: *Medical-surgical nursing: foundations for clinical practice,* ed 2, Philadelphia, 1998, WB Saunders.
6. Brensilver J, Goldberger E: *A primer of water, electrolyte and acid-base syndromes,* ed 8, Philadelphia, 1996, Oxford University Press.
7. Cirolia B: Understanding edema, *Nursing* 96 26(2):68, 1996.
8. Cohn JN et al: New guidelines for potassium replacement in clinical practice: a contemporary review by the National Council on potassium in clinical practice, *Arch Intern Med* 160(16):2429, 2000.
9. Coleman NJ: Evaluating arterial blood gas results, *Aust Nurs J* 6(11):1, 1999.

10. Epstein KE, Nirupam S: Respiratory acidosis, *Resp Care* 46(4):366, 2001.
11. Foster GT, Vaziri ND, Sassoon CSH: Respiratory alkalosis, *Resp Care* 46(4):37, 2001.
12. Giles T et al: Prolonged hemodynamic benefits from a high-dose bolus injection of human atrial natriuretic factor in congestive heart failure, *Clin Pharmacol Ther* 50:557, 1991.
13. Goldberg S: *Clinical physiology made ridiculously simple,* Miami, 1997, MedMaster Inc.
14. Gottlieb SS et al: Prognostic importance of atrial natriuretic peptide in patients with chronic heart failure, *Am Coll Cardiol* 13:1534, 1989.
15. Gould BE: *Pathophysiology for the health-related professions,* Philadelphia, 1997, WB Saunders.
16. Guyton AC, Hall JE: *Textbook of medical physiology,* ed 10, Philadelphia, 2000, WB Saunders.
17. Heitz UE, Horne MM: *Pocket guide to fluid, electrolyte, and acid-base balance,* ed 4, St Louis, 2001, Mosby.
18. Hudak C et al: *Critical care nursing: a holistic approach,* ed 7, Philadelphia, 1997, JB Lippincott.
19. Khanna A, Kurtzman NA: Metabolic alkalosis, *Resp Care* 46(4):354, 2001.
20. Klotz, RS: The effects of intravenous solution on fluid and electrolyte balance, *J IV Nursing* 21(1):20, 1998.
21. Metheny NM: *Fluid and electrolyte balance nursing considerations,* ed 4, Philadelphia, 2000, JB Lippincott.
22. Price SA, Wilson LM: *Pathophysiology: clinical concepts of disease processes,* ed 6, St Louis, 2001, Mosby.
23. Remer T: Influence of diet on acid-base balance, *Semin Dial* 13(4):221, 2000.
24. Rose BD: *Clinical physiology of acid-base and electrolyte disorders,* ed 5, New York, 2000, McGraw-Hill.
25. Sommers MS, Johnson SA: *Davis's manual of nursing therapeutics for diseases and disorders,* Philadelphia, 1997, FA Davis.
26. Swenson ER: Metabolic acidosis, *Resp Care* 46(4):342, 2001.
27. Tallis, RC, Fillit, SH, Brocklehurst TJ: *Brocklehurst's textbook of geriatric medicine and gerontology,* ed 5, New York, 1998, Churchill Livingstone.
28. Young L, Koda-Kimble M: *Applied therapeutics: the clinical use of drugs,* ed 7, Philadelphia, 2001, JB Lippincott.

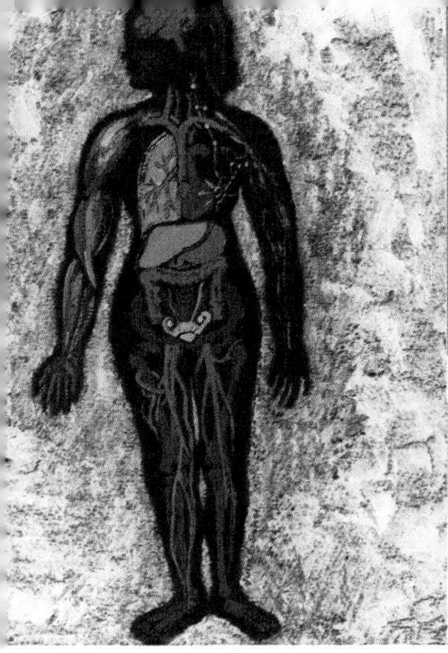

Shock 14

Nan Smith-Blair

Objectives

After studying this chapter, the learner should be able to:

1. Define physiologic shock.
2. Correlate the four classifications of shock with their pathophysiology.
3. Discuss the progression of clinical manifestations through the three stages of shock.
4. Identify assessment findings related to each type of shock.
5. Identify medical and nursing management strategies in the treatment of shock.
6. Describe methods of fluid replacement during shock.
7. Correlate effects of pharmacologic agents used to treat shock with nursing measures for patients receiving drug therapy.

NATURE OF THE PROBLEM

Shock is a complex physiologic entity representing a diverse group of life-threatening circulatory conditions. Mortality rates from uncomplicated hemorrhagic shock are low provided adequate replacement of blood volume is instituted early. Despite advances in the assessment and treatment of this complex physiologic syndrome, however, mortality rates from other forms of shock continue to range from 65% to 80%. Shock may develop in any patient, in any setting. Mortality rates from shock depend on the patient's physiologic state before the initial incident, the duration of the shock state, and response to therapy. Early recognition of clinical manifestations and initiation of therapeutic measures may halt the progression of shock and prevent mortality.

PHYSIOLOGY

Every cell in the body needs adequate tissue perfusion to provide the necessary supply of oxygen and nutrients and to remove metabolic by-products. In shock, blood flow to vital organs becomes inadequate and/or the cells become unable to extract and use oxygen and substrates. If left untreated, this functional impairment of cells, tissues, organs, and body systems progresses to multiple organ dysfunction and death.

HEMODYNAMIC PRINCIPLES

The circulatory system is composed of the heart, large blood vessels, and microcirculation (also called the peripheral or capillary circulation). These three components function interdependently to maintain an adequate cardiac output and tissue perfusion. Adequate blood flow depends on:

- Adequate amounts of blood for the heart to pump
- Effective pumping by the heart
- Constriction and dilation of blood vessels to maintain normal blood pressure

Shock results when one or more of these functions is disrupted.

Patients in shock may require placement of an arterial catheter and an indwelling balloon-flotation pulmonary artery catheter and use of sophisticated bedside monitors to evaluate cardiac function, circulating blood volume, and physiologic response to treatment (Figure 14-1). From these measured pressures, various hemodynamic parameters can be obtained and used to assess the mechanisms that support normal cardiovascular function: cardiac output, preload, afterload, and systemic and pulmonary vascular resistance (Table 14-1).

Cardiac Output

Cardiac output reflects the amount of blood the heart pumps from the ventricles in 1 minute. Determinants of cardiac output include heart rate and stroke volume. Stroke volume is defined as the amount of blood ejected by the ventricle with each heartbeat. It is influenced by three factors: preload, afterload, and contractility. Changes in either heart rate or stroke volume can change cardiac output. As metabolic needs of the body change, the heart adjusts cardiac output by altering either heart rate or stroke volume.

Heart Rate

Heart rate is influenced by the autonomic nervous system. Sympathetic innervation results in an increase in heart rate, whereas parasympathetic innervation results in a decrease in heart rate. Healthy individuals can increase cardiac output up to three times normal for short periods by increasing the heart rate. Increases in heart rate decrease diastolic filling time, allowing less time for the coronary arteries to be perfused. In individuals with reduced cardiac reserve, as in ischemic heart disease, increasing heart rate may actually decrease cardiac output as myocardial oxygen demand becomes greater than myocardial oxygen supply.

Preload

Preload is defined as the amount of stretch in the ventricle at the end of diastole. As blood returns to the ventricle, the ventricle distends, myocardial fibers stretch, and the force of contraction increases. The amount of ventricular stretch at end of

TABLE 14-1 Hemodynamic Terms and Normal Values

Pressure	Acronym	Normal Range	Definition
Cardiac output	CO	4-6 L/ min	Volume of blood pumped by each ventricle each minute;
Cardiac index	CI	2.4-4.0 L/min/m^2	CO divided by body surface area; indexed to body surface area to adjust for differences in body size
Central venous pressure	CVP	2-4 mm Hg	Pressure created by volume in the right side of the heart
Stroke volume	SV	60-70 ml	Amount of blood ejected by the ventricle with each heartbeat
Systemic vascular resistance	SVR	900-1400 dynes/sec/cm^{-5}	Resistance to blood flow created by systemic vasculature (arteries and arterioles) against which the left ventricle must pump to eject its volume; as SVR increases, CO decreases
Pulmonary vascular resistance	PVR	30-100 dynes/sec/cm^{-5}	Resistance to blood flow created by the pulmonary arteries and arterioles against which the right ventricle must pump to eject its volume

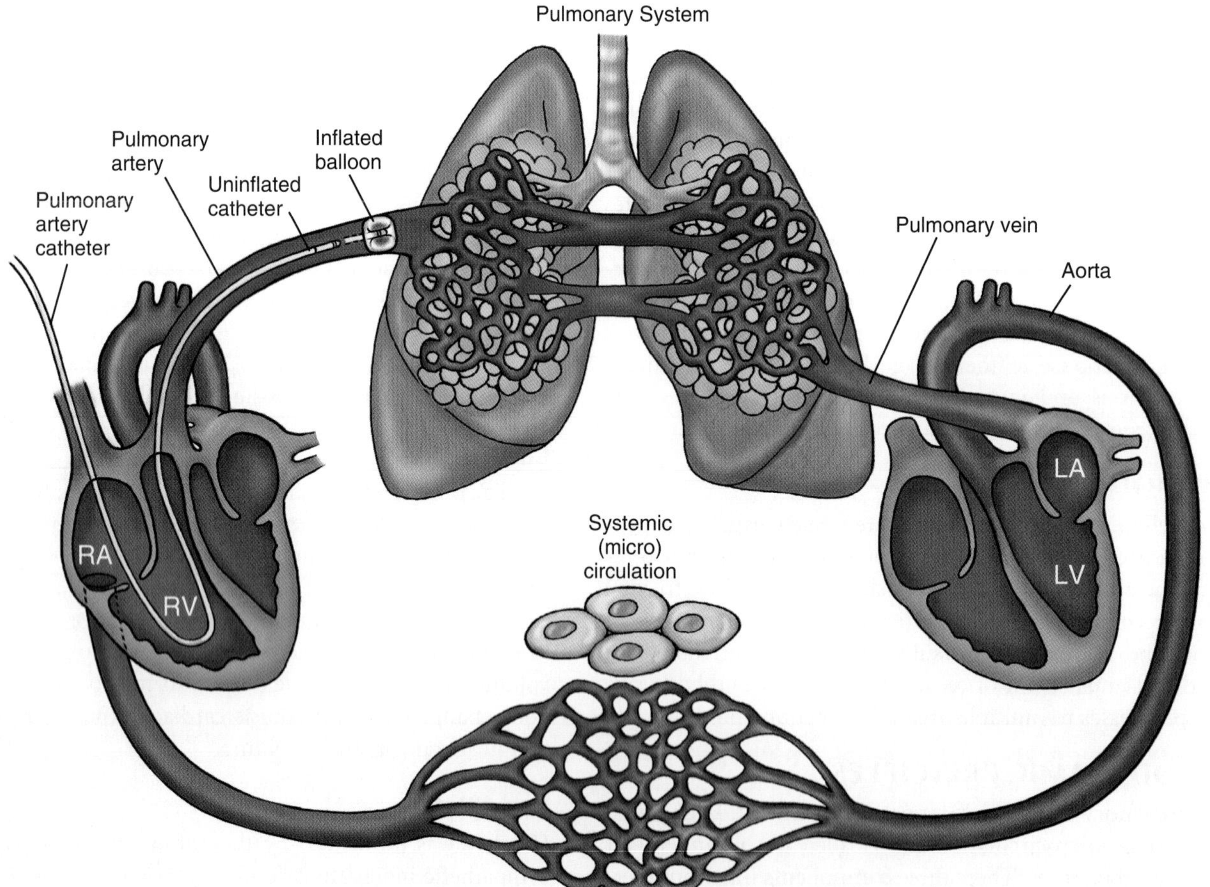

Figure 14-1 Pulmonary artery catheter position. When the balloon is deflated, pressures in the pulmonary artery can be measured. When the balloon is inflated, blood flow propels the catheter until the tip "wedges" in a small arterial branch. Pressure is normally transmitted from the left side of the heart through the pulmonary artery wedge pressure. *LA,* left atrium; *LV,* left ventricle; *RA,* right atrium, *RV,* right ventricle.

diastole determines the pressure on the walls of the ventricle. End-diastolic pressure refers to the amount of pressure in the ventricle. The fundamental control mechanism, the Frank-Starling law of the heart, states that as the normal left ventricle accepts increases in volume, it distends and cardiac output is increased until a critical point is reached. After that critical point, further increases in filling volume beyond the maximum length-tension relationship will result in a decrease in stroke volume and cardiac output. Thus preload is a function of the volume of blood presented to the ventricle and compliance (ability of the ventricle to stretch) of the ventricle at the end of diastole. Factors affecting volume include changes in venous return, total blood volume, and atrial kick. Factors affecting ventricular compliance include the "stiffness" and thickness of the muscular wall.

Afterload

Afterload is defined as ventricular wall tension or stress during systolic ejection. Systemic vascular resistance influences left ventricular afterload. Pulmonary vascular resistance affects right ventricular afterload. Increased afterload usually results in an increase in the work of the heart. Factors that oppose ejection of blood from the ventricle increase afterload. Afterload may be increased in conditions that impede aortic or pulmonary outflow (aortic stenosis or pulmonary stenosis), obstruction in the outflow tract (septal hypertrophy), increased systemic or pulmonary vascular resistance (vasoconstriction), or an increased blood volume or viscosity. As resistance to left ventricular ejection increases, stroke volume decreases. Conversely, as systemic resistance falls, stroke volume from the left ventricle increases. The ability of the heart to contract and respond to alterations in preload and afterload significantly affects cardiac output.

Contractility

Contractility refers to the heart's contractile force or inotropy (*ino*, strength; *tropy*, enhancing). Inotropy can be either positive (stronger contraction) or negative (weaker contraction). Contractility is negatively influenced by myocardial ischemia and underlying heart disease. Contractility can also be altered by a variety of pharmacologic agents, especially those mimicking the sympathetic nervous system (sympathomimetic, adrenergics).

Control of Peripheral Circulation

Intrinsic control mechanisms of blood flow to individual vascular beds are through response of arteriolar smooth muscle to products of metabolism causing either vasodilation or vasoconstriction. Other factors influencing this balance include local release of catecholamines, histamine, acetylcholine, serotonin, angiotensin, adenosin, and prostaglandins. These factors are released in response to tissue injury, hypoxemia, or hormones. Local circulation is also influenced by temperature and carbon dioxide.

Extrinsic control of peripheral blood flow is mediated by the central nervous system. The autonomic nervous system exerts dual antagonistic control over organ systems via sympathetic and parasympathetic fibers. Stimulation of the vasoconstrictor region in the medulla causes an increase in mean arterial pressure and heart rate by enhancing sympathetic nervous system outflow and inhibiting parasympathetic nervous system outflow. Sympathetic outflow targets resistance vessels causing vasoconstriction. Inhibition of these areas causes the opposite effect, vasodilation. Sympathetic fibers causing vasoconstriction supply arteries, arterioles, and veins. Capacitance vessels (veins) are also responsive to sympathetic stimulation, but the effects are not as easily seen as on the arterial side.

OXYGEN TRANSPORT PRINCIPLES

All forms of shock involve impaired delivery of oxygen to the tissues. Variables that influence oxygen transport include the amount of oxygen delivered to the tissues, oxygen consumption by the tissues, and the oxygen extraction ratio (Table 14-2).

Oxygen delivery depends on blood flow (cardiac output), the amount of hemoglobin available to carry oxygen, and the percentage of arterial oxygen hemoglobin saturation. The body normally delivers three to four times more oxygen to the tissues than they need for normal metabolism. Any condition that reduces cardiac output, hemoglobin availability, or hemoglobin saturation has an impact on the amount of oxygen delivered to tissues.

Oxygen consumption represents the body's demand for oxygen and is a reflection of tissue metabolism. Reduced oxygen consumption is common in all forms of shock and may be due to a reduction in blood flow (delivery) as in hypovolemic or cardiogenic shock due to an uneven distribution of blood as occurs in septic shock. The magnitude of the oxygen consumption deficit in patients experiencing shock has been correlated with mortality rates.

Oxygen consumption and delivery can be measured using a specialized pulmonary artery catheter. The oxygen extraction ratio (VO_2/DO_2) provides an estimate of the balance between tissue oxygen demand (consumption) and oxygen supply (delivery). It also provides an indication of the ability of the tissues to extract and use the oxygen delivered.

TABLE 14-2 Oxygen Transport Terms

Term	Acronym	Definition
Oxygen delivery	DO_2	Amount of oxygen delivered to the tissues each minute; reflects the ability of the circulatory system to supply oxygen to the tissues
Oxygen consumption	VO_2	Amount of oxygen used by the tissues each minute; reflects the body's total metabolism
Oxygen extraction ratio	VO_2/DO_2	Ratio of oxygen consumption to oxygen delivery; indicates the ability of the tissues to extract and use oxygen delivered

ETIOLOGY

Shock may be classified as hypovolemic, cardiogenic, or distributive.

Hypovolemic Shock

Hypovolemic shock is the most common type of shock. It is caused by a loss of whole blood, plasma, or interstitial fluid in quantities such that the body's metabolic needs can no longer be met. The etiologic factors in hypovolemic shock are listed in Box 14-1.

Hypovolemic shock develops from an absolute or relative hypovolemia. Absolute hypovolemia results from an external loss of fluid from the body, as in hemorrhage. Relative hypovolemia results from an internal shift of fluid from the intravascular space to the extravascular space. It may occur as the result of an increased capillary permeability, decreased colloidal osmotic pressure, or loss of intravascular integrity. Reduced intravascular blood volume leads to a decrease in the amount of blood returning to the heart (venous return). This, in turn, decreases the amount of blood received by the ventricles during diastolic filling (preload) and a decrease in the amount of blood available for ejection from the ventricle (stroke volume). As compensatory mechanisms begin to fail and can no longer maintain cardiac output, tissue perfusion to organ systems significantly decreases (Figure 14-2).

Clinical manifestations of hypovolemic shock depend on the severity of fluid loss and the person's ability to compensate for the loss. Disease processes, age, amount of blood loss, rate of loss, and length of time over which the loss occurs all affect how quickly clinical manifestations of hypovolemic shock occur. Hemorrhagic shock is divided into four classes: early, moderate, progressing, and profound. Assessment findings for each of these classes are listed in Table 14-3. The clinical presentations of the various types of hypovolemic shock are all similar to the presentation of hemorrhagic shock.

Class I hemorrhagic shock represents a fluid loss of up to 15% and may be tolerated without any symptoms if compensatory mechanisms are effective in maintaining cardiac output.

Class II hemorrhagic shock represents more significant volume losses of 15% to 30%. The body tries to initiate compensatory mechanisms to return to homeostasis. The heart rate increases to between 100 and 120 beats/min in response to sympathetic nervous system stimulation. The patient's blood pressure remains normal, but the pulse pressure is narrowed. Urinary output ranges from 20 to 30 ml/hr. Capillary refill time is prolonged.

Class III hemorrhage shock occurs with major blood losses of 30% to 40% of total volume. The patient becomes increasingly anxious and progressively confused. Systolic blood pressure drops below 80 mm Hg and pulse pressure is narrowed. Respirations increase in rate and depth. Urine output falls to 5 to 15 ml/hr. Capillary refill continues to be prolonged.

Class IV hemorrhagic shock represents a severe blood loss of greater than 40% of the total volume. The patient develops severe hypotension. Heart rate may exceed 140 beats/min, and respirations may exceed 35 per minute. Urine output decreases to only negligible amounts. Peripheral capillary refill time is significantly longer than 3 seconds.

BOX 14-1 Etiology of Hypovolemic Shock

Loss of Blood Volume

External

Trauma
Gastrointestinal bleeding
Surgery

Internal

Hemothorax
Ruptured aortic aneurysm
Hemoperitoneum
Retroperitoneal hemorrhage
Loss of plasma volume
Burns
Desquamated-exudated lesions
Loss of other body fluids

Gastrointestional

Severe vomiting
Severe diarrhea

Renal

Diabetic ketoacidosis
Hyperosmolar nonketotic diabetes
Diabetes insipidus
High output renal failure
Adrenal insufficiency
Diuretic therapy

Cardiogenic Shock

Cardiogenic shock refers to a shock response generated when the heart's ability to pump blood becomes impaired. This impairment decreases cardiac output. If peripheral vascular resistance is not adequate to compensate for a decrease in tissue perfusion, shock may develop. Cardiogenic shock can be caused by dysfunction of the left ventricle, right ventricle, or both. It may result from primary ventricular ischemia, structural problems, or dysrhythmias. Etiologic factors in cardiogenic shock are listed in Box 14-2.

The most common cause of cardiogenic shock is a loss of contractile elements of the myocardial muscle owing to ischemia. This usually results from ischemia related to acute myocardial infarction. Cardiogenic shock develops when 40% or more of the functional myocardium has been damaged after either a massive acute myocardial infarction (AMI), or the cumulative results of several smaller AMIs. Massive damage usually occurs in the anterior wall of the left ventricle.

Structural problems may cause cardiogenic shock if forward motion of blood is disrupted. Causes include papillary muscle rupture and septal rupture. Regurgitant or stenotic valve lesions also interrupt forward flow of blood through the heart and may result in abrupt onset of congestive heart failure progressing to shock.

Dysrhythmias affecting heart rate can disrupt pump function and cause cardiogenic shock. Bradydysrhythmias can

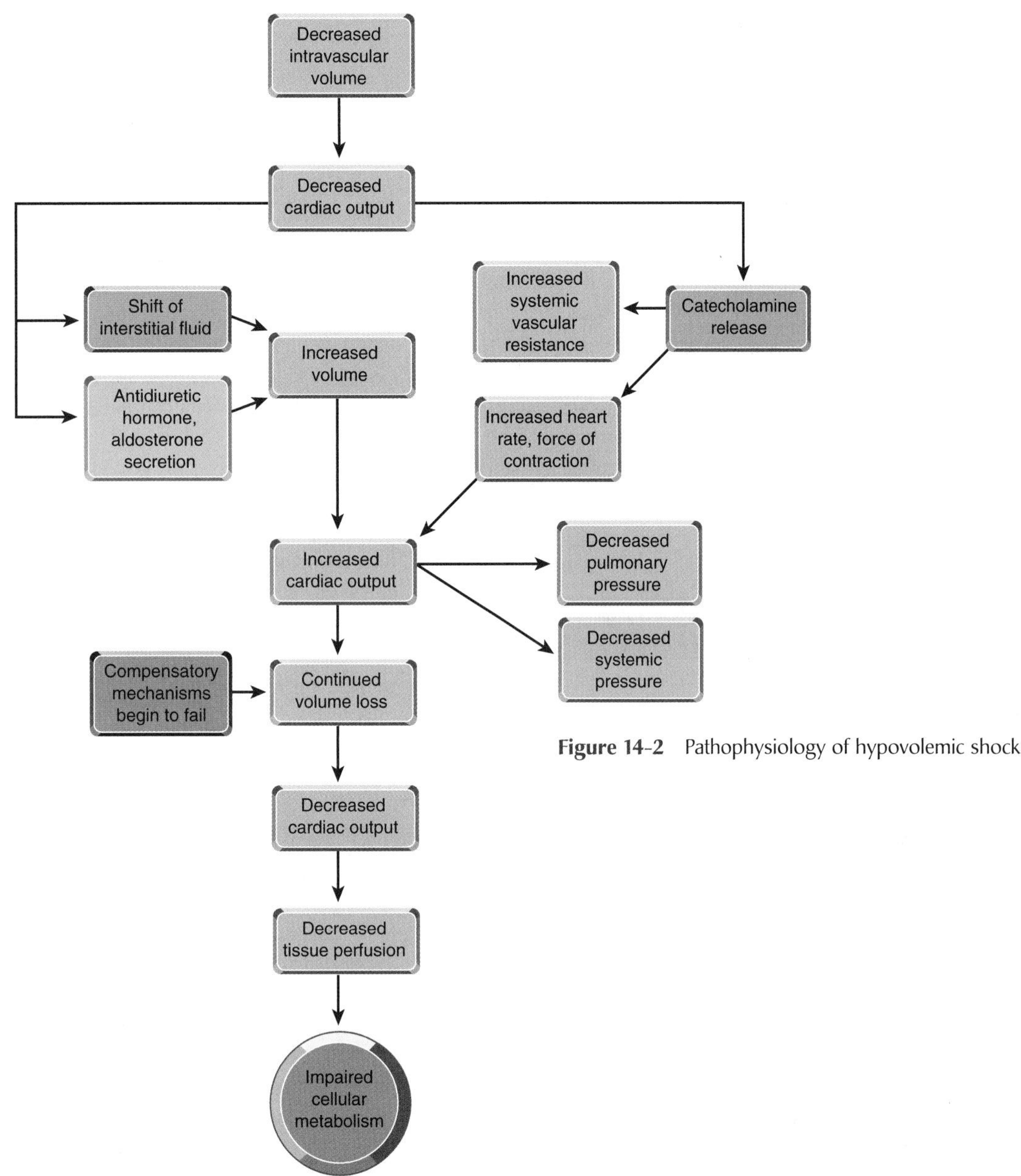

Figure 14-2 Pathophysiology of hypovolemic shock.

TABLE 14-3 Clinical Manifestations of Hypovolemic Shock

Parameter (For a 70-kg man)	Class I (Early)	Class II (Moderate)	Class III (Major or Progressive)	Class IV (Severe or Profound)
Approximate blood volume loss (ml)	Up to 750	750-1500	1500-2000	2000 or more
% of blood volume	Up to 15%	15%-30%	30%-40%	40% or more
Neurologic/behavioral status	Slightly anxious/ anxious	Mildly anxious, restless; muscle fatigue and weakness evident	Agitated, confused, progressive decrease in activity; progressive thirst evident	Stuporous, lethargic, unresponsive; dilated pupils may be evident
Heart rate	<100	>100 Mild tachycardia	>120 Tachycardia	140 or higher; irregular pulse; decreased pulse, amplitude
Blood pressure	Normal	Normal/decreased	Decreased	Severe hypotension
Pulse pressure (mm Hg)	Normal/increased	Decreased	Decreased	Decreased
Respirations	14-20, normal	20-30, normal	30-40, hyperpnea	>35, shallow, irregular
Urine output (ml/hr)	30 or more	20-30	5-15	Negligible
Capillary blanch best	Normal	Slight delay	Defined delay	No refilling observed
Skin	Pale, flushed, slightly cool	Slightly cold, pale	Cold and moist	Cold and cyanotic, mottled

From McQuillian KA, Wiles CE: Initial management of traumatic shock. In Cardona DV et al: *Trauma nursing from resuscitation through rehabilitation,* Philadelphia, 1988, WB Saunders.

lower cardiac output, especially in patients unable to compensate by increasing their stroke volumes. Conversely, in tachydysrhythmias, as the heart rate increases, diastolic filling time decreases, reducing stroke volume because the filling time is too short.

When the left ventricle is unable to pump blood forward adequately, three primary problems result. First, the amount of blood ejected from the ventricle with each heart beat (stroke volume) decreases. This subsequently decreases cardiac output, blood pressure, and tissue perfusion. Second, as blood pressure falls, coronary artery perfusion decreases, which in turn decreases myocardial muscle perfusion. The increased workload and oxygen demand of the myocardium exacerbates myocardial ischemia and predisposes the patient to further muscle damage creating a viscious cycle. Third, the amount of blood remaining in the left ventricle at the end of systole increases. If the primary problem involves the left ventricle, this increased end-systolic volume eventually leads to increased ventricular filling pressure. Increased filling pressures are transmitted back to the left atrium and then to the pulmonary circulation. This increases pulmonary vascular pressure, causing fluid to move into the interstitial space and intraalveolar spaces, resulting in pulmonary congestion, hypoxia, and deteriorating blood gases. Increased pulmonary pressures are eventually reflected backward to the right ventricle, causing both left and right ventricular failure. As the ventricular pressures remain elevated, systemic manifestations of right-sided heart failure become evident (Figure 14-3).

Compensatory mechanisms initially may be able to maintain blood pressure and adequate tissue perfusion to vital organs. However, as the left ventricle fails to effectively pump blood out to the circulatory system, compensatory mechanisms begin to fail and clinical manifestations develop. The patient shows a decrease in sensorium, systolic blood pressure falls to less than 90 mm Hg, and diastolic pressure increases, narrowing the pulse pressure. Heart rate increases above 100 beats/min. A weak, thready pulse develops and heart sounds reveal a diminished S1 and S2 caused by decreased contractility. A summation gallop may be audible over the left apex from increased pressure in the left ventricle and decreased compliance. Skin becomes pale, cool, and moist from peripheral vasoconstriction. A variety of dysrhythmias may occur, depending on the underlying problem.

Urinary output progressively decreases to less than 30 ml/hr, and the urine becomes concentrated. Urinalysis shows increased osmolarity and specific gravity and decreased urine sodium. Blood urea nitrogen and serum creatinine levels rise as waste products are no longer excreted effectively.

BOX 14-2 Etiologic Factors in Cardiogenic Shock

Ventricular Ischemia

Myocardial infarction
Open heart surgery
Cardiac arrest

Structural Problems

Valvular dysfunction
Septal rupture
Papillary muscle rupture
Ventricular aneurysm
Cardiomyopathies
Intracardiac tumors

Dysrhythmias

Bradydysrhythmias
Tachydysrhythmias

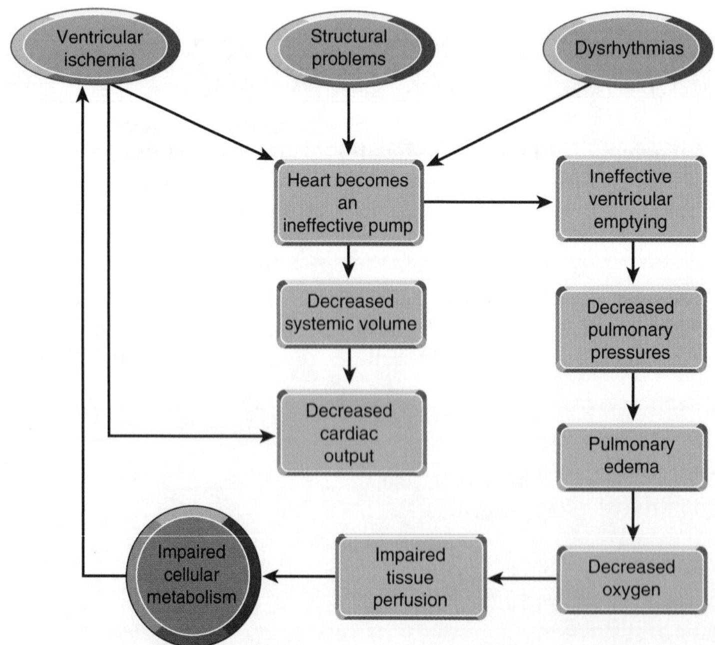

Figure 14-3 Pathophysiology of cardiogenic shock.

Respiratory rate and depth increase in an attempt to improve oxygenation. Arterial blood gases initially demonstrate respiratory alkalosis, but this progresses quickly to respiratory and metabolic acidosis with hypoxemia from alveolar hypoventilation. Auscultation of the lungs reveals crackles and wheezes.

Distributive Shock

Distributive shock results from inadequate vascular tone that leads to massive vasodilation. Although vascular volume remains normal during distributive shock and the heart pumps blood adequately, the size of the vascular space increases. The result is a maldistribution of blood within the circulatory system. This disproportion between blood volume and capillary vessel size effectively decreases blood pressure. Distributive shock is frequently subdivided into three types: (1) septic, (2) neurogenic, and (3) anaphylactic.

Septic Shock

Septic shock is a multisystem response to infection in which, unlike other forms of shock, the fall in blood pressure and resultant insufficient perfusion of vital organs does not respond to fluid administration. In reporting nations worldwide, the incidence of sepsis has increased to an estimated 400,000 cases per year, of which approximately 100,000 episodes of septic shock are treated in the United States. Mortality from septic shock remains between 50% and 60%, with patients usually succumbing to refractory hypotension or progressive multiple organ failure.[3]

Septic shock generally occurs in immunocompromised patients, infants, the elderly, or patients undergoing procedures in which the risk of significant bacterial contamination may occur. Microorganisms implicated in sepsis and septic shock are listed in Box 14-3. The initial infection produces an overwhelming systemic inflammatory response triggered by release of endotoxins, formyl peptides, exotoxins, and proteases from gram-negative organisms; or exotoxins, enterotoxins, hemolysins, peptidoglycans, and lipoteichoic acid from gram-positive organisms. These substances exert a harmful effect on the vascular, coagulation, and immune systems. Bacterial toxins stimulate release of macrophage-derived cytokines that intensify the inflammatory response. Nitric oxide is released from endothelial cells, vascular smooth-muscle cells, and macrophages and is postulated to be a major mediator of vasodilation, hypotension, and myocardial depression seen in septic shock. The immune system becomes so overwhelmed that the system designed initially to protect the body now works against it. The antiinflammatory substances released to modulate the inflammatory response produce a period of immune depression after the initial shock episode, placing the patient at an additional risk of a nosocomial infection and death.

Four primary pathophysiologic changes occur in septic shock. They include myocardial depression, massive vasodilation, maldistribution of the intravascular volume, and formation of microemboli. Myocardial depression occurs when the ventricular force of contraction decreases from biochemical mediators, including myocardial depressant factor, endotoxins, tumor necrosis factor, endorphins, complement products, and leukotrienes. Massive vasodilation and increased capillary permeability reduce the amount of blood returning to the heart (decreased preload). Afterload decreases as well, from massive vasodilation that occurs secondary to the release of such mediators as bradykinin, endorphins, complement products, histamine, and prostaglandins. Although plasma volume is normal in the early phases of septic shock, it becomes maldistributed as shock progresses because of increased capillary permeability, selective vasoconstriction, and vascular occlusion. Increased capillary permeability allows protein and fluid to shift to the interstitial and intracellular compartments. However, not all vascular beds vasodilate. Stimulation of the sympathetic nervous system and prostaglandin and other biochemical mediators cause selective vasoconstriction in the pulmonary, renal, and splanchnic circulations.

Activation of the clotting system and aggregation of neutrophils cause formation of microemboli that become lodged in the small blood vessels, causing some vascular beds to receive more blood than they need, whereas others receive too little. This maldistribution of blood leads to hypoxia and a lack of nutritional support to some areas, causing cellular dysfunction that ultimately ends in cell death.

The early stage of septic shock is characterized by a hyperdynamic or warm phase as compensatory mechanisms are activated (Table 14-4). During this phase, massive vasodilation occurs in venous and arterial beds causing a decrease in systemic vascular resistance. Venous dilation decreases venous return to the heart and decreases preload. Dilation of the arterial beds decreases afterload. The patient's blood pressure declines in response to reduced preload and afterload. Blood pressure is decreased with a widened pulse pressure because of the vasodilation. The skin becomes warm and flushed in appearance as a result of the massive vasodilation. The heart rate increases

BOX 14-3 Causative Microorganisms Implicated in Septic Shock

Gram-negative bacteria
- *Bacteroides*
- *Escherichia coli*
- *Enterobacter* spp.
- *Klebsiella pneumoniae*
- *Pseudomonas aeruginosa*
- *Serratia marcescens*
- *Haemophilus influenzae*

Gram-positive bacteria
- *Staphylococcus aureus*
- *Staphylococcus epidermidis*
- *Streptococcus pneumoniae*
- *Clostridium* spp.

Fungi
Protozoa
Parasites
Rickettsiae
Spirochaeta
Viruses

TABLE 14-4 Clinical Manifestations of Septic Shock

	Hyperdynamic Phase	Hypodynamic Phase
Cardiac output/cardiac index (CO/CI)	Increased	Decreased
Systemic vascular resistance (SVR)	Decreased	Increased
Right atrial pressure (RAP)	Decreased	Increased
Pulmonary capillary wedge pressure (PCWP)	Decreased	Increased
Heart rate	Increased	Increased
Respiratory rate	Increased	Decreased
Blood pressure	Decreased	Decreased
Pulse pressure	Wide	Narrow
Skin	Warm, pink, flushed	Cool, pale, clammy
Level of consciousness	Decreased	No response to painful stimuli
Urinary output	Decreased	Anuria
Temperature	Increased	Increased/decreased

to compensate for the hypotension and increased metabolic acidosis and sympathetic nervous system stimulation and adrenal stimulation. A ventilation/perfusion mismatch occurs in the lungs as a result of pulmonary vasoconstriction. The respiratory rate increases to compensate for the hypoxemia. Crackles develop as increased pulmonary capillary membrane permeability leads to pulmonary edema. Arterial blood gases values reveal respiratory alkalosis, metabolic acidosis, and hypoxemia. Level of consciousness is altered and the patient becomes disoriented, confused, combative, or lethargic. The patient's temperature rises in response to the pyrogens released from invading microorganisms.

As septic shock progresses, the patient's condition deteriorates to a hypodynamic phase, with a fall in cardiac output and profound hypotension developing. This phase results from ventricular failure caused by myocardial hypoxemia, release of myocardial depressant factor, and acidosis, producing an increase in afterload. Tachycardia occurs as the body attempts to compensate for the decline in cardiac output and hypotension. Peripheral vasoconstriction causes increased systemic vascular resistance to compensate for the falling blood pressure. The patient's skin now is pale, cold, and clammy (see Future Watch box).

Future Watch

New Treatment in Septic Shock on the Horizon?

Nitric oxide synthase (NOS) of the inducible subtype (iNOS) may play a pivotal role in vasodilation associated with septic shock. A number of biochemical pathways are involved. Current research has focused on inhibition through L-arginine analogs, depletion of arginine, inhibition of cofactors, modulating gene transcription, and scavaging nitric oxide to prevent the detrimental effects of iNOS. The focus of future clinical trials may identify iNOS-specific agents that are clinically useful to combat the effects of vasodilation seen in septic shock.

Reference: Schoonover LL, Stewart AS, Clifton GD: Hemodynamic and cardiovascular effects of nitric oxide modulation in the therapy of septic shock, *Pharmacotherapy* 20(10):1184-1197, 2000.

Neurogenic Shock

Neurogenic shock is characterized by massive vasodilation from loss or suppression of sympathetic tone. It is a temporary condition associated with injury or disease of the upper spinal cord or brainstem or developing after administration of general or spinal anesthesia. Neurogenic shock can be caused by any condition that interrupts sympathetic nerve impulse transmission or blocks sympathetic outflow form the vasomotor center in the brain. Interruption of sympathetic activity occurs with trauma to the spinal cord or medulla, conditions that disrupt the supply of oxygen to the medulla, or conditions that deprive the medulla of glucose (such as an insulin reaction). Other causes of neurogenic shock include high-level spinal anesthesia, ganglionic- and adrenergic-blocking drugs, severe emotional stress, pain, depressive drugs, and drug overdoses.

The onset of neurogenic shock may occur within minutes of the injury, and the condition may last for days, weeks, or months depending on the precipitating cause. Lack of sympathetic tone leaves a dominant parasympathetic nervous system, which results in massive vasodilation. Neurogenic shock creates a relative hypovolemia in which the blood volume is distributed inappropriately. Vasodilation decreases venous return and cardiac output, resulting in hypotension. Inhibition of the baroreceptor response results in the loss of compensatory reflex tachycardia so that the heart rate cannot increase in response to the reduction in blood pressure. Loss of vasomotor tone in cutaneous blood vessels disrupts thermoregulation, so the patient must depend on the environment for temperature regulation.

Anaphylactic Shock

Anaphylaxis is a sudden, life-threatening hypersensitivity reaction to an antigen. It is characterized by massive vasodilation and increased capillary permeability. Unless treatment begins immediately, the patient quickly develops shock.

TABLE 14-5 Manifestations of Shock

Parameter	Compensatory Shock	Progressive Shock	Refractory
Heart rate	Increased	>150 /min; often irregular	>150 /min; irregular
Blood pressure	Adequate to perfuse vital organs Low normal to normal blood pressure	No longer able to perfuse vital organs Blood pressure <80-90 mm Hg	<80 mm Hg; may not be audible
Arterial Pulses	Rapid, weak, thready	Thready, weak, rapid; may not be palpable	Weak, thready, or non-palpable
Skin	Cool, moist, pale	Cold, cyanotic, mottled	Cyanotic, mottled
Respirations	Increased rate and depth	Rapid, shallow, rales	Respiratory failure
Arterial blood gases			
PaO_2	Decreased	Decreased	Severely decreased
$PaCO_2$	Decreased	Increased	Increased
pH	Increased	Decreased	Severely decreased
Level of consciousness	Restlessness, agitation, lethargy, mental cloudiness, confusion; responds to verbal stimuli and follows simple commands	No longer responds to verbal stimuli; response to painful stimuli deteriorates from flexion, extension to flaccid	Flaccid
Pupils	Dilated; reactive to light	Dilated, response to light may deteriorate from sluggish to absent	May be fixed, dilated
Urinary output	<0.5 ml/kg/hr	<0.5 ml/kg/hr	Anuria or neglible

Anaphylaxis is mediated by immunoglobulin E (IgE) antibody. IgE is produced after the first exposure to an antigen. It binds to the surface of mast cells and basophils. During subsequent exposures, the antigen binds to and cross-links antigen-specific IgE molecules on the surface of tissue mast cells, initiating mast cell degranulation and release of vasoactive, chemotactic, and enzymatic mediators, including histamine, eosinophilic chemotactic factor of anaphylaxis (ECF-A), neutrophilic chemotatic factor of anaphylaxis (NCF-A), proteinases, heparin, serotonin, leukotrienes, prostaglandins, and platelet-activating factor.[11]

These chemical mediators cause vasodilation, increased capillary membrane permeability, bronchoconstriction, and coronary capillary permeability. Shock develops as a consequence of hypotension from profound vasodilation and low cardiac output. Increased capillary permeability and peripheral pooling of blood cause the relative fluid volume deficit. As a result of the rapid and profound development of shock, normal compensatory mechanisms are unable to reverse or retard the development of this process. Death can result because of severe hypoxemia secondary to bronchoconstriction or cardiovascular collapse.

Early recognition of anaphylaxis is crucial because, within minutes, it can progress to shock, respiratory arrest, and cardiovascular collapse. The earliest signs of systemic anaphylaxis include feelings of anxiety and uneasiness, flushing, diaphoresis, sneezing, and weakness. These are quickly followed by nausea, dizziness, itching, and sometimes edema; and severe hypotension from vasodilation and increased capillary permeability quickly follow.

PATHOPHYSIOLOGY

The clinical syndrome of shock results from sustained, inadequate tissue perfusion leading to alterations in tissue metabolism and function at the cellular and organ system level. Untreated, the patient progresses through a continuum of shock stages manifested by specific signs and symptoms that vary according to the patient's individual response and ability to compensate. Shock stages are compensatory, progressive, and irreversible (also called refractory). Manifestations of the shock stages are summarized in Table 14-5.

Compensatory Stage

The compensatory stage of shock is characterized by an initial decrease in cardiac output and tissue perfusion. The resulting reduction in delivery of oxygen and nutrients at the cellular level decreases aerobic metabolism and increases anaerobic metabolism, resulting in the production of lactic acid. Compensatory mechanisms begin and, at least initially, maintain adequate cardiac output and tissue perfusion. No clinical manifestations are evident during this early stage of shock.

Initial compensatory mechanisms are complex, widespread, and aimed largely at maintaining blood pressure within a low normal to normal range with adequate perfusion to vital organs. The sympathetic nervous system is quickly activated when arterial blood pressure falls. Pressoreceptors in the arterial walls of the aorta and carotid sinuses sense a decrease in pressure and transmit signals to the vasomotor center in the medulla. The autonomic nervous system signals sympathetic nerve fibers throughout the body to discharge norepinephrine. This release causes arterioles to constrict, which assists in increasing arterial pressure. The adrenal medulla is stimulated to release the catecholamines epinephrine and norepinephrine into the bloodstream. Stimulation of $beta_1$-adrenergic receptors in the heart increases the rate and force of contraction. Stimulation of $beta_2$-adrenergic receptors causes coronary artery vasodilation and increased blood flow to the myocardium to meet the increased oxygen demand of the heart. Alpha-adrenergic receptor stimulation causes vasoconstriction. This results in blood being shunted away from organs, including skeletal muscles, fat, and skin. Arterioles in vital organs, such as the heart and brain, remain open and continue to receive blood flow.

Chemoreceptors in the aorta and carotid arteries respond to decreased arterial oxygen tension by sending signals to the respiratory center in the brain. The respiratory center responds by increasing the rate and depth of respirations, which results in a respiratory alkalosis.

Decreased cardiac output and vasoconstriction in the kidneys result in decreased renal perfusion. Resultant renal ischemia stimulates the release of renin by the juxtaglomerular apparatus. Circulating renin reacts with angiotensinogen produced in the liver, resulting in production of angiotensin I. A converting enzyme in the lungs converts angiotensin I to angiotensin II. Angiotensin II, a potent vasoconstrictor, helps to increase blood pressure and venous return. It also stimulates release of aldosterone from the adrenal cortex, causing reabsorption of sodium and water and increased venous return to the heart. Reduced renal perfusion results in oliguria, with urinary output falling below 0.5 ml/kg/hr. Further reductions in cardiac output result in additional decreases in urinary output.

Catecholamine stimulation also causes contraction of the radial muscle of the iris, causing pupillary dilation. Vasoconstriction of the vessels in the skin and stimulation of the sweat glands cause the skin to be cool, pale, and moist. Decreased tissue perfusion in the liver stimulates breakdown of glycogen stores to increase availability of glucose for energy production. This results in increased blood glucose levels.

How long the body can maintain tissue perfusion and homeostasis depends on the patient's general health and reserves. Compensatory mechanisms may be able to maintain arterial blood pressure and tissue perfusion only briefly. If the underlying cause of shock is not managed, the patient progresses to the next stage of shock.

Many of the clinical manifestations of compensated shock result from an excess of catecholamines and other vasoconstricting hormones and from increased sympathetic neural activity to the heart and vasculature. Sinus tachycardia is present, with heart rates exceeding 100 beats/min. Respirations become deep and rapid. Blood gas analysis reveals respiratory alkalosis and hypoxemia. In most forms of shock the skin is cool, moist, and clammy, especially in the extremities. However, in patients with distributive forms of shock (septic, neurogenic, and anaphylactic), inappropriate peripheral vasodilation occurs and the extremities may remain warm. Urine volume is reduced. An altered sensorium may be characterized by restlessness and agitation. The pupils are dilated, and blood glucose levels increase. The nurse must be aware that underlying disease states, such as diabetes, or the effects of such drugs as beta-blockers or vasodilators may mask the compensatory responses of tachycardia and vasoconstriction.

Progressive Stage

As shock progresses, compensatory mechanisms can no longer compensate for decreased cardiac output and fail to maintain blood pressure sufficient to perfuse vital organs. Physiologic changes that initially helped shunt blood to vital organs become ineffective and organs begin to malfunction. The primary cause of the shock disorder must be corrected quickly, or severe hypoperfusion of organs will lead to multisystem organ failure.

As cellular metabolism shifts from aerobic to anaerobic as a result of prolonged cellular hypoxia, production of adenosine triphosphate decreases, reducing metabolic cellular processes. The net result is decreased oxygen consumption. Glycolysis results in conversion of pyruvate to lactate. Increased lactate levels cause metabolic acidemia and promote cardiac dysrhythmias. The decrease in adenosine triphosphate availability also causes the sodium-potassium pump to malfunction. Active transport of sodium and potassium across the cell membrane diminishes. Sodium ions accumulate inside the cell causing intracellular swelling. As organelles inside the cell begin to swell, their function deteriorates. Potassium collects outside the cell. Changes in the sodium-potassium ion concentration cause the resting membrane potential to become more positive, leading to development of dysrhythmias.[9]

Bradykinin and myocardial depressant factor are important vasoactive polypeptides that appear to play a significant role in shock. Bradykinin produces vasodilation, increased capillary permeability, smooth muscle relaxation, and infiltration of an area with leukocytes. Bradykinin is thought to have a major impact in later stages of shock and may be a factor in the development of associated pulmonary insufficiency. Myocardial depressant factor is released in response to splanchnic ischemia and appears to depress cardiac muscle contraction, further contributing to a decreased cardiac output.

Metabolic acidosis worsens and causes precapillary sphincters to relax. Postcapillary vasoconstriction continues, creating increased resistance and decreased capillary flow rates. Capillary hydrostatic pressure increases, causing fluid to move out of the capillary beds into the interstitial space. Interstitial edema further decreases blood return to the heart. As capillary flow rates decrease, microemboli can form, placing the patient at risk of developing disseminated intravascular coagulation.

As pulmonary capillary bed hypoperfusion persists, alveolar cells become ischemic and unable to produce surfactant. This causes alveoli to collapse, producing massive microatelectasis and reduced pulmonary compliance. Ischemia also increases pulmonary capillary permeability, allowing fluid to leave pulmonary capillaries producing interstitial and intraalveolar edema. Pulmonary edema drastically reduces diffusion of oxygen and intensifies hypoxemia. Respiratory insufficiency and failure commonly occur with persistent shock states.

Prolonged kidney hypoperfusion potentiates development of acute tubular necrosis, progressing to renal insufficiency and acute renal failure. Toxic waste products cannot be excreted, resulting in an increase in blood urea nitrogen and serum creatinine levels.

Prolonged hypoperfusion of the liver reduces the organs ability to perform important functions adequately. The impaired functions include metabolism of drugs and hormones and the conjugation of bilirubin. As a result of the latter, bilirubin accumulates in the blood and causes jaundice. The liver loses its ability to metabolize waste products such as ammonia and lactic acid. As cellular damage occurs and death approaches, intracellular enzymes are released into the blood and can be observed as increases in serum glutamic-oxaloacetic transaminase, serum glutamic-puruvic transaminase, and lactic dehydrogenase. Pancreatic hypoperfusion and ischemia result in release of pancreatic enzymes amylase and lipase.[9]

Clinical manifestations associated with the progressive stage of shock include decreased blood pressure with a narrow pulse pressure, decreased heart rate, decreased urine production, increased urine specific gravity, decreased creatinine clearance, increased serum creatinine, and blood urea nitrogen. Peripheral edema develops from altered capillary fluid dynamics.

Decreased cerebral blood flow causes further decreases in the level of consciousness. As the persistent hypoperfusion state continues, more stimulation is required to elicit a response from the patient. Response to painful stimuli progressively decreases until the patient becomes flaccid (no response to painful stimuli).

Respiratory rate increases and the patient develops audible crackles as a result of interstitial pulmonary edema. Arterial blood gases show metabolic and respiratory acidosis with hypoxemia.

Refractory Stage

Irreversible or refractory shock is the final stage of shock. The body becomes refractory to all therapeutic measures attempted. Multiple organ failure develops and produces signs and symptoms of cardiac, respiratory, neurologic, hepatic, gastrointestinal, pancreatic, and hematologic failure. Intractable circulatory failure develops as blood pressure and heart rate continue to decrease. The shock state is so profound and degree of cellular destruction so severe that death is imminent.

COLLABORATIVE CARE MANAGEMENT

Therapeutic management of the patient in shock is determined by the stage of shock and the patient's signs and symptoms. Collaborative care in the management of patients in shock is essential to improve the patient's chances of survival. Therapy to maintain tissue perfusion in the shock patient may be simple, involving only volume replacement, or complex, involving volume replacement, pharmacologic manipulation, and mechanical support. The role of the nurse is vital in identifying subtle parameters of inadequate perfusion and the effectiveness of medical interventions. The nurse plans, implements, and evaluates appropriate nursing interventions to limit effects of inadequate perfusion while concurrently collaborating with the physician and other health care professionals to implement medical therapies to reverse the shock state. Details of treatment are included under the intervention section later in this chapter.

NURSING MANAGEMENT

ASSESSMENT

Nursing management of a patient in shock is both complex and challenging. By remaining aware of the risk of shock in susceptible patients, the nurse may be able to recognize signs and symptoms that signal the onset of shock and correct them before they can progress. Assessment must be accomplished quickly, almost simultaneously with initiation of treatment. Assessment steps include watching for changes in clinical manifestations and monitoring hemodynamic parameters and laboratory values to detect subtle changes warning of progression of the shock state. Frequent nursing assessments are required, because the patient's condition can change significantly in minutes. Concise documentation should reflect the patient's condition and response to therapeutic interventions.

Health History

The nurse must rapidly collect a pertinent history from the patient or family, focusing on risk and causative factors that may explain signs/symptoms of the evolving shock disorder. Questions should relate to recent illnesses, infections, trauma, surgery, and medication use. When obtaining this information from the patient, the nurse should note how the patient responds to the questions as well as the patient's attention span, general mood, and behavior. Some of the early manifestations of shock may include difficulty in maintaining focus on the question being asked; expressing a sense of restlessness; and changes in mood, mental status, or behavior. If possible, the nurse should validate suspected mood and behavior changes with family members or the patient's significant other.

Physical Examination

Hypovolemic Shock

It is essential to identify the sources of fluid loss and estimate the amount lost. Assess quickly for abnormalities in gastrointestinal, skin, and renal losses; plasma-to-interstitial fluid shifts (third-spacing); or hemorrhage. If possible, correct this fluid loss immediately. Also perform a quick overview assessment to identify and treat any life-threatening problems. Monitor blood pressure, heart rate, and respiratory rate and depth closely. Assess the skin for color and temperature. Check the patient's level of consciousness. Watch the patient's hydration and perfusion status by monitoring urine output, peripheral pulses, capillary refill time, condition of the mucous membranes, and presence of pallor or cyanosis.

Cardiogenic Shock

Rapidly assess the patient's level of consciousness and cardiopulmonary status. Check for blood pressure less than 90 mm Hg, decreased sensorium, and reduced skin temperature. Monitor the patient for chest pain, dysrhythmias, a heart rate over 100 beats/min, weak and thready pulse, and diminished heart sounds. As soon as the patient is stabilized, obtain a medical history and current data needed to detect diseases or medications that could cause or aggravate the shock syndrome. Observe for dyspnea, cyanosis, crackles or wheezes, rapid and shallow breathing, and chest expansion. Evaluate blood gas values for development of metabolic acidosis and hypoxemia. As the left ventricle fails and fluid backs up into the pulmonary system and the right side of the heart, signs and symptoms may include neck vein distention, positive hepatojugular reflux, and increased central venous pressure values. Monitor hemodynamic status via pulmonary artery catheter for a cardiac index of less than 2.2 L/min/m^2, increased pulmonary artery wedge pressures, and increased systemic vascular resistance. Observe for a urinary output of less than 30 ml/hr.

Distributive Shock

Suspect anaphylactic shock if the patient has cutaneous effects (pruritus, generalized erythema, urticaria, and angioedema) or difficulty breathing, especially if you find inspiratory stridor or hoarseness or if the patient reports a sensation of fullness or a lump in the throat or dysphagia. Tachypnea is present in all early stages of distributive shock. As the shock state continues, however, and respiratory muscles tire, the respiratory rate declines. Other assessment findings may include vomiting, diarrhea, cramping, abdominal pain, urinary incontinence, and vaginal bleeding. Assess for severe hypotension, but remember that pulse pressure is widened in the hyperdynamic stages of septic shock, and narrowed in the later stages of septic, neurogenic, and anaphylactic shock. Assess the patient's heart rate for tachycardia (bradycardia is a common finding in neurogenic shock). Examine the skin. In neurogenic shock, the skin may be warm and dry from pooling of blood in the extremities and loss of vasomotor control in surface vessels that normally control heat loss. Warm, flushed skin may also occur in the hyperdynamic stage of septic shock; however, as shock progresses, the skin becomes pale, cool, and clammy.

Because changes in level of consciousness represent decreased cerebral perfusion, assess frequently for such changes. Assessment of hemodynamic parameters in anaphylactic and neurogenic shock reveals:

- Decreased cardiac output and cardiac index.
- Decreased central venous pressure and pulmonary capillary wedge pressures (from venous vasodilation).
- Decreased systemic vascular resistance (from arterial vasodilation).

Changes in hemodynamic parameters in the hyperdynamic phase of septic shock include increased cardiac output and cardiac index, decreased central venous pressure and pulmonary capillary wedge pressures, and decreased systemic vascular resistance. As the shock state progresses to the hypodynamic phase, cardiac output and cardiac index fall, central venous pressure and capillary wedge pressures increase, and systemic vascular pressure increases.

NURSING DIAGNOSES

Nursing diagnoses and their prioritization are determined from analysis of patient data. Because of the complex nature of shock, it is essential that all nursing diagnoses be managed simultaneously. Nursing diagnoses for the person with shock may include but are not limited to the following:

Diagnostic Title	Possible Etiologic Factors
1. Impaired gas exchange	Decreased lung compliance, interstitial edema, changes in alveolar capillary membrane permeability
2. Decreased cardiac output	Changes in myocardial contractility, preload, and afterload; inadequate distribution of blood volume; or loss of systemic vasomotor tone
3. Ineffective tissue perfusion	Impaired myocardial contractility, reduced circulating blood volume, or deficient fluid volume
4. Deficient or excess fluid volume	Hemorrhage or fluid shifts associated with loss of plasma proteins (hypovolemic shock); increased levels of aldosterone and antidiuretic hormone secondary to reduced renal perfusion, and sodium retention (cardiogenic shock); distributional volume loss with fluid shifts to the interstitial space (distributive shock)

EXPECTED PATIENT OUTCOMES

Expected patient outcomes for the person with shock may include but are not limited to:

1. Will have improved gas exchange in the lungs with resultant adequate oxygenation of all body tissues
2. Will have adequate cardiac output with perfusion to all body tissues
3. Will maintain a cardiac output adequate to circulate blood to the body's tissues
4. Will maintain adequate fluid volume

INTERVENTIONS

Treatment of shock varies depending on the cause of the shock, the organ systems affected, and the preexisting condition of the patient. As with all life-threatening conditions, care priorities follow the basic principles of Airway, Breathing, and Circulation. However, shock is treated most effectively if the underlying cause can be determined quickly and treated.

1,2,3,4. Collaborative Medical/Nursing Interventions

Current medical interventions for treating shock are aimed at increasing oxygen delivery to cells and include increasing cardiac output and index, increasing hemoglobin value, and increasing oxygen saturation. Interventions include a combination of fluid, pharmacologic, and mechanical therapies to reverse the altered circulatory component and improve clinical symptoms. Successful management relies on accurate nursing assessments, data analysis, implementation of medical therapies, and evaluation of the patient's response to treatment. A multidisciplinary approach to the management of these complex patients will assist the patient in reaching a positive outcome.

1. Improving Oxygenation

Most patients in shock have some degree of hypoxemia. Oxygen is usually administered because tissues are already suffering from oxygen deprivation caused by decreased blood flow. Because the energy system of the body is impaired, muscles used in ventilation may not function adequately, and breathing may have to be assisted. The major complication is acute respiratory distress syndrome (ARDS), which occurs secondary to reduced pulmonary blood flow and increased pulmonary vascular resistance. Pulmonary capillary permeability increases leading to noncardiogenic pulmonary edema. Surfactant production is reduced, resulting in decreased pulmonary compliance and hypoxemia that becomes refractory to oxygen therapy. If symptoms of ARDS develop, the patient may require intubation and mechanical ventilation using positive end-expiratory pressure. Positive pressure at the end of expiration prevents surfactant-deficient alveoli from collapsing, resulting in atelectasis.[8] Nursing actions include implementing measures to optimize oxygenation and ventilation including positioning, effective secretion removal, and preventing desaturation of oxygen during nursing care.

2, 3. Improving Cardiac Output and Tissue Perfusion

When the left ventricle becomes severely impaired, as in cardiogenic shock or in the late stages of any type of shock, the patient may require pharmacologic, mechanical, and surgical interventions to improve myocardial performance.

Pharmacologic Management

The major treatment goals are to enhance the effectiveness of the heart's pumping action and to improve tissue perfusion. Pharmacologic management of shock is based on manipulation of contractility, preload, afterload, and heart rate. A list of commonly used drugs is found in Box 14-4.

BOX 14-4 Drugs Use to Improve Cardiac Output

Drugs That Increase Cardiac Contractility

Inotropic Agents

Dopamine (Intropin)—beta-dosing range
Dobuatmine (Dobutrex)
Amrinone (Inocor)
Epinephrine (Adrenalin)
Isoproterenol (Isuprel)
Norepinephrine (Levophed)
Digoxin (Lanoxin)

Drugs That Alter Preload/Afterload

Vasoconstrictor Agents

Epinephrine (Adrenalin)
Norepinephrine (Levophed)
Dopamine (Intropin)-alpha-dosage range
Metaraminol (Aramine)
Phenlyephrine (Neo-Synephrine)
Ephedrine

Vasodilator Agents

Nitroprusside (Nipride, Nitropress)
Nitroglycerin (Nitrol, Tridil)
Hydralazine (Apresoline)
Labetalol (Normodyne, Trandate)

Improving Contractility. Positive inotropic drugs are used to increase contractility, cardiac output, and tissue perfusion. They are used in the treatment of cardiogenic and distributive shock. They also increase myocardial oxygen demand by increasing the workload of the heart. Therefore these agents must be used with caution in patients with ischemic heart disease or cardiogenic shock.

Drugs such as dopamine, dobutamine, and low doses of epinephrine stimulate beta-receptor sites in the heart causing improved myocardial contractility and improved cardiac output.

Altering Preload. The primary treatment to improve preload is the administration of fluids. Pharmacologic agents may also be given to improve preload in the treatment of hypovolemic and in distributive shock. Vasopressors, such as epinephrine and norepinephrine, cause vasoconstriction and increase venous return to the heart. Vasopressors should be used with caution in hypovolemic shock patients, as the primary need of these patients is fluid replacement. In patients in cardiogenic shock, preload reduction may be required to decrease the workload on the heart. Vasodilators are used to decrease the heart's workload by reducing peripheral vascular resistance. Commonly used vasodilators include nitroglycerin and nitroprusside. Continuous blood pressure monitoring during administration of nitroglycerin or nitroprusside is essential, as either drug can cause hypotension.

Altering Afterload. Afterload reflects the force the heart must overcome to eject blood. In distributive shock, systemic vascular resistance is low. To increase vascular tone and improve venous return to the heart (preload), drugs that increase afterload such as norepinephrine, phenlyephrine, or high doses of dopamine may be required. In patients in cardiogenic shock, reducing afterload may be necessary to reduce the workload of the heart. Because of their vasodilation actions, nitroglycerin and nitroprusside are commonly used afterload reducing agents.

Other Drugs. Early coverage with appropriate intravenous antibiotics is an important factor in successful treatment of septic shock. Broad-spectrum antibiotics to cover gram-positive, gram-negative, and anaerobic organisms are ordered until culture and sensitivity reports are obtained. Once the organism is identified, coverage should be tailored according to which antibiotic the organism is most susceptible.

Mechanical Management

Intraaortic balloon counterpulsation (IABP) may be indicated for temporary circulatory assistance to restore hemodynamic stability in patients in cardiogenic shock. A polyurethane balloon is inserted percutaneously through the femoral artery and positioned just distal to the left subclavian artery (Figure 14-4). The balloon is inflated during diastole and deflated in systole. The overall effects of counterpulsation are to increase coronary perfusion and cardiac output, and decrease preload and afterload. Intraaortic balloon pump counterpulsation is an effective means of decreasing the work of the myocardium and decreasing oxygen consumption.[5] Patients who require IABP therapy need to monitored closely for development of complications including emboli formation,

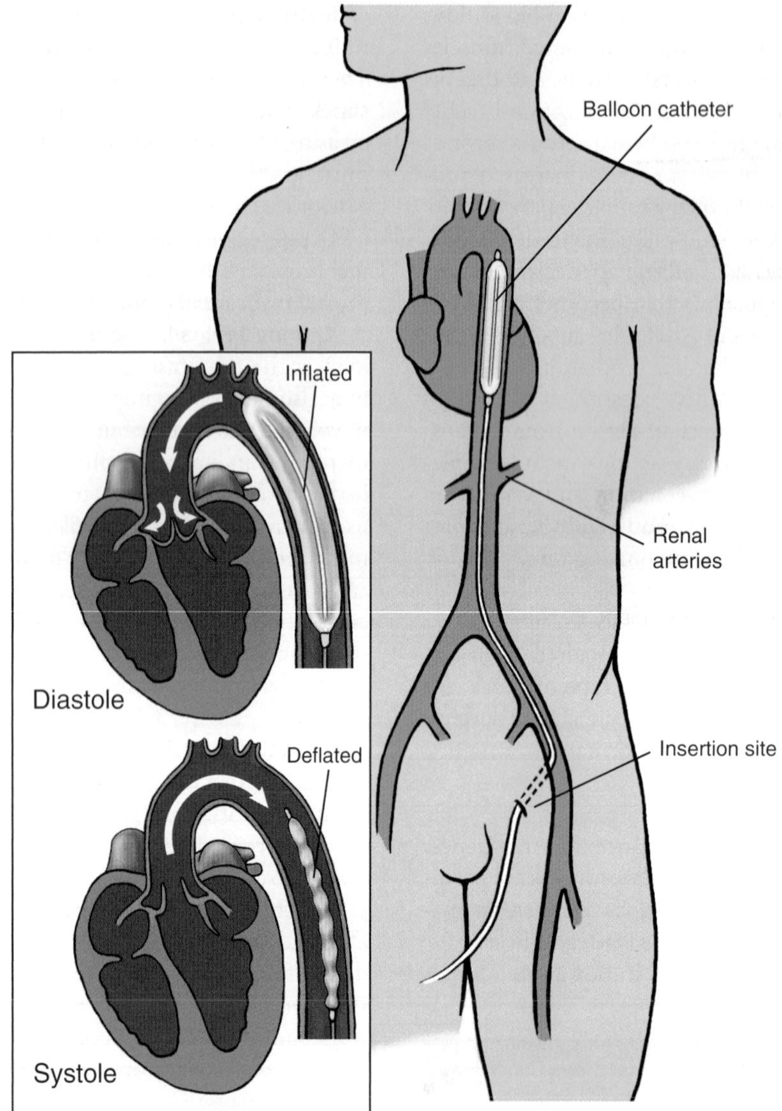

Figure 14-4 Placement of intraaortic balloon pump catheter.

thrombocytopenia, improper balloon placement, bleeding, balloon rupture, and circulatory compromise of the cannulated extremity.

Ventricular assist device is used to temporarily support the failing ventricle not responding to intraaortic balloon pump and pharmacologic therapy.[9] These devices can support the function of a single ventricle or the whole heart. They divert blood from the failing ventricle or ventricles and pump it back into the aorta (left ventricular assist device), the pulmonary artery (right ventricular assist device), or both arteries. Heart transplantation may be an option for a small percentage of patients with severe myocardial damage and cardiogenic shock.

The *pneumatic antishock garment (PASG),* also known as military antishock trousers, external counter-pressure devices, and G suits raise blood pressure by increasing systemic peripheral resistance and possibly cardiac output[4] (Figure 14-5). These inflatable garments also put direct pressure on bleeding sites helping to control bleeding in pelvic and long-bone fractures, and abdominal and extremity vascular injuries. The PASG is usually instituted in emergency situations in the field. However current guidelines suggest that, in addition to use for prehospital stabilization, PASG may be beneficial in hypotension resulting from ruptured abdominal aortic aneurysm, suspected pelvic fracture, anaphylactic shock unresponsive to standard therapy, uncontrollable lower extremity hemorrhage, and severe traumatic hypotension (a palpable pulse is present, blood pressure is nonobtainable). Contraindications for use of PASG include patients with pulmonary edema, pregnancy, impaled objects, evisceration of the abdomen, and thoracic and diaphragmatic trauma.[6]

If a patient is admitted with a PASG in place, the nurse monitors the circulatory status of the lower extremities and assesses for the reappearance of shock symptoms. As the patient stabilizes, the PASG is removed by gradual reduction in the pressure in the garment compartments. The abdominal

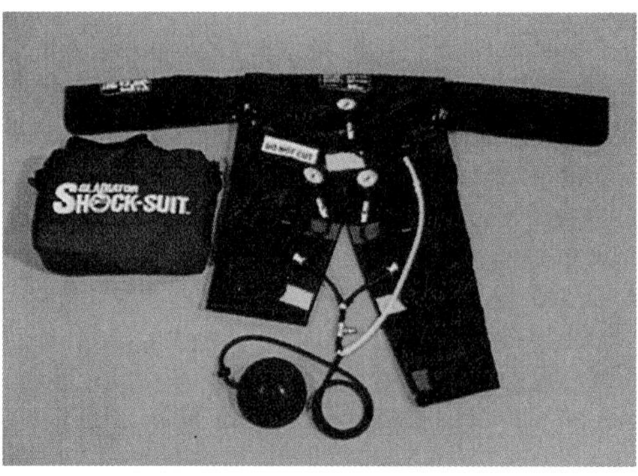

Figure 14-5 Pneumatic antishock garment with abdominal and leg compartments, valves, and foot pump.

section is deflated first, allowing gradual redistribution of blood volume followed by deflation of the lower extremities. The patient's vital signs are monitored closely and pressure reapplied if shock symptoms appear until other stabilization measures can be implemented.

Surgical/Invasive Interventions

Invasive cardiac procedures, such as percutaneous transluminal coronary angioplasty, thrombolytic therapy, stent placement, rotoblade therapy, and laser therapy are used to attempt early revascularization of an occluded coronary artery following an acute myocardial infarction complicated with cardiogenic shock. Early use of these procedures has resulted in greater survival rates in patients less than 75 years old.[7]

Patient Positioning

Traditionally the patient in shock has been placed in the Trendelenburg position. This position should be avoided if possible in shock states because it causes fluid to rapidly shift to the upper thorax, activating baroreceptors in the aortic arch and carotid arteries. Activation of these receptors sends misleading signals that blood pressure is elevated, shutting off the body's sympathetic nervous system response to the shock state. Instead, placing the patient in a supine position with the legs slightly elevated promotes venous return from the legs to the heart, and improves cardiac output and organ perfusion. If this type of position impairs the patient's ventilation, elevation of the patient's head 30 to 45 degrees should aid breathing.

4. Fluid Therapy

Fluid resuscitation has been a mainstay in the management of patients in shock. Benefits of fluid administration include increasing intravascular volume, increasing venous return to the heart (preload), improved cardiac contractility, and increased cardiac output. The goal of fluid therapy is to improve tissue perfusion. The nurse should collaborate with the physician regarding the administration of fluid and accurately monitor intake and output and daily weights of the patient. Nursing intervention also includes minimizing fluid through limiting blood sampling and applying pressure to bleeding sites.

Patients in severe shock may require immediate and rapid volume replacement. A minimum of two large-bore intravenous catheters (No. 14 or 16) should be inserted into the patient to provide routes for immediate and rapid administration of large volumes of fluids and medications. The large peripheral veins in the antecubital fossa are recommended. Severe vasoconstriction and venous collapse may dictate the physician performing a venous cut-down for vascular access. A multilumen central venous catheter or pulmonary arterial catheter can also be used to administer large fluid volumes and to measure hemodynamic status. In patients not responding to fluid infusion or who have underlying cardiac or renal disease, the insertion of a pulmonary-artery catheter should be considered.[3]

The major goals in treating hypovolemic shock are to find and aggressively control the source of blood loss and to reverse that loss with administration of appropriate fluids to restore tissue perfusion. At times, fluid replacement is the only therapy needed in this type of shock. Distributive and septic shock are accompanied by hypovolemia because fluid is leaking out of the capillaries and because the vascular space has increased with vasodilation. Patients with cardiogenic shock may also require fluid therapy, although many may require fluid restriction or removal of fluid. Fluid administration in these patients must be monitored closely. Before institution of fluid therapy, a pulmonary artery catheter is inserted, and the pulmonary end-diastolic pressure is measured. If the pressure is less than 18 mm Hg and the cardiac index is less than 2.2 L/min, volume replacement should be given.

Fluid Challenge

Once intravenous access has been established, a fluid challenge of 200 ml to 2 L of crystalloid solution is infused intravenously to see if fluid administration improves circulation and therefore oxygen delivery. Nursing responsibilities include obtaining baseline hemodynamic measurements, administering the fluid challenge, and assessing the patient response. The patient's hemodynamic status should be carefully monitored during such fluid challenges especially in patients suspected of having impaired left ventricular function. Patient response to this initial bolus of fluid determines further treatment with additional fluids, or the addition of other therapeutic modalities.[10]

Fluid Selection

The selection of resuscitation fluid remains controversial. The physician's choice of fluid or fluids is determined by the cause of the volume deficit and the patient's clinical status. The goal of fluid therapy is to return laboratory and hemodynamic values to the patient's normal baseline levels. The nurse should carefully monitor the patient's response to fluid therapy. Fluids are generally classified as either crystalloid or colloid solutions (Table 14-6).

Crystalloids are inexpensive and readily available solutions. These fluids move freely from the intravascular space into the tissues. Lactated Ringer's solution closely resembles plasma and is commonly used to expand intravascular volume and is

TABLE 14-6 Fluids Used for Replacement Therapy in Shock

Type	Uses/Indication	Special Considerations
Crystalloid Solutions		
Isotonic		
Normal saline	Increase plasma volume Replace body fluid	Improves plasma volume without changing normal sodium concentration or serum osmolality Red blood cell (RBC) mass should be adequate if large volumes are being infused to prevent decrease in oxygen carrying capacity. Potential fluid overload due to sodium content. Does not improve oncotic pressure
Lactated Ringer's solution	Increase body fluid Buffer acidosis	Lactate is converted to bicarbonate in liver and buffers acidosis Increased lactic acidosis in shock conditions caused by lactate Potential fluid overload due to sodium content Added K^+ may cause problems in renal failure or adrenal insufficiency patients Use with caution in patients in shock or with hypoperfusion as lactate conversion requires aerobic metabolism
Ringer's solution	Replace body fluid Provide additional K^+ and Ca^{++}	Does not contain lactate so may be used in treatment of shock Potential fluid overload due to sodium content High chloride concentration may cause hyperchloremic metabolic acidosis
Hypotonic		
½ Normal saline	Raise total body fluid volume	Potential for interstitial and intracellular edema due to rapid movement of this fluid from vascular space. Dilution of plasma proteins and electrolytes
5% dextrose in water (D_5W)	Raises total fluid volume Provides 0.2 kcal/ml	Acts as free water and is distributed throughout all body compartments Prevents hyperosmolar states Dilution of plasma proteins and electrolytes can occur due to rapid metabolism of glucose and free water
Colloid Solutions		
Plasma protein fraction	Expands plasma volume Increases serum colloid osmotic pressure	Prepared from pooled plasma Reduced risk of hepatitis due to processing procedure Osmotically equivalent to plasma Low risk of hepatitis Deficient in clotting factors Can cause hypotension with rapid infusion (>10 ml/min) Does not protect against human immunodeficiency virus (HIV) contamination risk Use with caution in patients with congestive heart failure (CHF) and renal failure
5% or 25% (salt poor) albumin	Increases plasma colloid osmotic pressure Expands plasma volume 25% albumin used in patients with pulmonary edema, peripheral edema, and hypoproteinemia	Administration rate <2-4 ml/min with 5%; <1 ml/min with 25% Diuretic may be administered with 25% albumin to ensure diuresis May precipitate CHF after rapid infusion in patients with circulatory overload and compromised cardiovascular function Rare transmission of hepatitis virus Albumin is an important protein for drug and ion transport
Plasma Expanders		
Hetastarch (Hespan)	Expands plasma volume	Similar volume expansion characteristics as 5% albumin but effects last up to 36 hours; maximum infusion rate 20 ml/kg/hr Low risk of allergic and anaphylactic reactions Cost is ~½ albumin or plasma protein fraction No danger of hepatitis transmission Possible dilution of clotting factors (monitor clotting and platelet counts), plasma proteins and decreased osmotic pressure Causes a rise in serum amylase level (>200 ml/100 ml) persisting up to 4 days due to action of amylase in hetastarch degradation Infuse through separate line if possible

TABLE 14-6 Fluids Used for Replacement Therapy in Shock—cont'd

Type	Uses/Indication	Special Considerations
Blood and Blood Products		
Whole blood	Replaces blood volume Provides intravascular volume	Increases oxygen carrying capacity of blood Potential risk of hepatitis, HIV transmission; allergic reactions Requires type and cross-matching Should be stored at 1°-6° but must be warmed 20-30 minutes before use or use approved blood warmer device Administered via Y–connector tubing with normal saline; must use blood filter
Packed red blood cells Packed concentrate Fresh frozen (leukocyte poor)	Increases hematocrit Improves oxygen-carrying capacity of blood	Used to prevent excess fluid administration in patients with cardiogenic shock Fewer risks of metabolic complications than stored bank whole blood Risk of hepatitis, HIV transmission, and allergic reactions Type and cross-matching required Does not provide adequate volume alone for volume replacement in hypovolemic shock Monitor for clotting derangements when more than 20 U are administered; give 1 U fresh frozen plasma/each 4 U of RBCs to replenish clotting factors
Human plasma Fresh frozen Dried	Increases osmotic pressure to improve circulating volume Restored plasma volume Restores clotting factors (except platelets)	Effective for rapid volume replacement Contains clotting factors Potential risk for hepatitis and HIV transmission, and allergic reactions Administer as soon as possible after thawing to prevent deterioration of clotting factors V and VIII

HIV, Human immunodeficiency virus; *RBCs,* red blood cells.

usually infused at an amount of 3 ml for each 1 ml of blood loss. If large volumes of crystalloids are required, the potential for development of hemodilution of red blood cells (RBCs) and plasma proteins may be of concern. Hemodilution of RBCs may impair delivery of oxygen to tissues. Hemodilution of plasma proteins decreases colloidal osmotic pressure and places the patient at risk for pulmonary edema.

Colloids contain proteins that increase osmotic pressure and remain in the vascular system longer than crystalloids. The improved osmotic pressure holds and attracts fluid into vascular compartment. The patient may require smaller volumes of colloids infused.

Use of colloids has been recommended in a number of resuscitation guidelines and intensive care management algorithms.[2,13] The U.S. Hospital Consortium Guidelines recommend colloid administration in hemorrhagic shock until blood products are available and in nonhemorrhagic shock following an initial crystalloid infusion.[15] More recently, a review of research findings indicates that resuscitation with colloids did not reduce the risk of death compared to crystalloids in patients with trauma, burns, and after surgery. Fluid resuscitation with colloid solutions is considerably more expensive than with crystalloids and therefore should be used only if their effect can be shown to be clearly superior to that of crystalloids[1] (see Research box).

Blood Administration. Whole blood, packed red blood cells, washed red blood cells, fresh frozen plasma, and platelets

Research

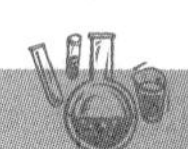

Reference: Alderson P et al.: Colloids versus crystalloids for fluid resuscitation in critically ill patients (Cochrane Review), *The Cochrane Library,* Issue 2, Oxford, 2001, Update Software.

A meta-analysis was used to synthesize the evidence of the effects on mortality from randomized or quasirandomized controlled trials comparing colloid and crystalloid fluid resuscitation in critically ill patients. Thirty-six studies were reviewed in which participants were randomized or quasirandomized to treatment groups (receiving colloids of either Dextran 70, hydroxyethal starches, modified gelatins, albumin or plasma protein fraction) or a control group (receiving either isotonic or hypertonic crystalloids). All participants were adult patients who were critically ill as a result of conditions such as trauma, burns, or surgery, or had other critical conditions such as complications of sepsis. A pooled relative risk factor was used to examine the risk of death. Results of albumin or plasma protein fraction (18 trials with a total of 641 patients) demonstrated a pooled relative risk factor (RRF) of 1.34, hydroxyethylstarch (7 trials with a total of 197 patients) a RRF of 1.16; modified gelatin (4 trials with 95 patients) a RRF of 0.50; dextran (8 trials with 668 patients) a RRF of 1.24; and dextran in hypertonic crystalloid with isotonic crystalloid (8 trials with 1283 patients) and RRF of 0.88. The researchers concluded there was no evidence that resuscitation with colloids reduces risk of death compared to crystalloids in patients with trauma, burns, and after surgery.

Implication for practice: Crystalloid solutions, which are less expensive than colloid solutions, are as effective as colloid solutions in the fluid resuscitation of patients.

are administered for the treatment of major blood loss. Patients are typed and cross-matched to identify their blood type, to determine presence of the Rh factor, and to ensure compatibility with the donor blood to prevent blood transfusion reactions. In extreme emergencies, the patient may be transfused with O-negative blood (universal donor blood type).

Blood and blood products are given until the hemoglobin is 10g/dl or greater.[8] Packed red blood cells increase blood volume and oxygen-carrying capacity without placing the patient at risk of volume overload associated with whole blood. One unit of packed RBCs increases the hematocrit by 3% and the hemoglobin value by 1g/dl.[12]

Administration of blood products in the treatment of shock is not free of risks especially when massive transfusions are required. Because blood for transfusion contains an anticoagulant to prevent clotting while the blood is being stored, the patient who receives large amounts of blood may develop clotting defects. Stored blood is also deficient in platelets and other clotting factors. When massive transfusions are required, fresh frozen plasma, which contains all clotting factors except platelets, is administered to restore coagulation factors. One unit of fresh frozen plasma is given for every 4 to 5 U of blood transfused.

Massive transfusion of cold blood can result in hypothermia, which can cause cardiac dysrhythmias. If blood is to be rapidly infused, it should be warmed before administration using approved blood warmer devices (see Guidelines for Safe Practice box).

Although all blood is transfused through a standard blood filter, when several units are administered, some debris resulting from aggregation of platelets, leukocytes, and fibrin can pass through the filter. This debris is eventually filtered out of the blood by the pulmonary capillaries, and causes little difficulty in patients who receive only a few units of blood. Nonetheless, it is recommended that microfilters be used when massive transfusions (10 U of whole blood or packed cells in less than 24 hours) are given.

Guidelines for Safe Practice

Safe Administration of Multiple Units of Blood

1. Ensure typing and cross-matching for blood type, Rh factor, and compatibility with donor blood is performed before administration of each unit.
2. Administer blood products through at least a 20-gauge, preferably an 18-gauge or larger catheter.
3. Do no infuse intravenous medications into the same port with blood.
4. Administer all transfusions with a blood filter to trap debris and tiny clots.
5. Use approved blood warmers when massive transfusions are required to prevent hypothermia.
6. Monitor closely for signs of transfusion reaction, fluid overload, acidosis, hyperkalemia, and coagulation disorders.

The pH value of stored blood is lower than that of normal blood. The added anticoagulant makes the blood more acidic. In addition, because blood is stored in an airtight bag, the metabolism that continues is anaerobic, and the end products are lactic and pyruvic acids.

Blood Substitutes. Currently three types of red cell substitutes under investigation are not yet part of conventional volume replacement therapy. These agents are perfluorocarbon emulsions, cell-free hemoglobin, and liposome encapsulated hemoglobin.[14] Red cell substitutes do not require type and cross-matching, can act as potent plasma volume expanders, and have significant capacity for carrying oxygen. Because these substances do not transmit viral or bacterial infection and do not cause immunosuppression, they offer considerable promise and advantages for the future.

EVALUATION

To evaluate the effectiveness of nursing and medical interventions, compare patient responses with those stated in the expected outcomes. Achievement of outcomes is successful if the patient in shock:

1. Has improved gas exchange and adequate oxygenation as evidenced by: an airway that is patent and clear of secretions; arterial blood gas values within normal limits: pH 7.35 to 7.45, $PaO_2 \geq 80$ mm Hg, $PaCO_2$ 35 to 45 mm Hg, $SaO_2 \geq 95\%$; respiratory rate 12 to 20 beats/min, breath sounds clear to auscultation; absence of cyanosis; capillary refill $\leq$3 seconds.
2. Demonstrates signs of hemodynamic stability as evidenced by: heart rate <100 beats/min; systolic blood pressure >110 mm Hg or within 10 mm Hg of baseline; cardiac output 4 to 8 L/min and/or cardiac index >2 L/min/m^2; central venous pressure 0 to 8 mm Hg; pulmonary capillary wedge pressure 8 to 12 mm Hg; systemic vascular resistance 800 to 1400 dynes/sec/cm^{-5}; warm extremities with capillary refill time <3 seconds; absence of dysrhythmias or presence of hemodynamically stable dysrhythmias; normal sensorium.
3. Has increased tissue perfusion as evidenced by signs of: hemodynamic stability as listed previously; being alert and oriented to time, place, and person; adequate peripheral tissue perfusion (skin warm and dry, absence of cyanosis, capillary refill <3 seconds); urine output >30 ml/hr; no dysrhythmias present; arterial blood gases within normal limits.
4. Has intravascular volume within normal limits as evidenced by: stable hemodynamic variables as listed previously; body weight within 5% of baseline; balanced fluid intake and output; urine output >30 ml/hr; fluid and electrolyte balance as demonstrated by laboratory data within normal limits (electrolytes, hematocrit, hemoglobin, blood urea nitrogen, and serum creatinine); normal body temperature; demonstrates adequate peripheral perfusion (skin warm and dry; absence of cyanosis).

Critical Thinking Questions

1. During report the nurse from the previous shift tells you that your patient, admitted with the diagnosis of cardiogenic shock, is to receive a fluid challenge. What special considerations should be taken when administering fluids to this patient?
2. While assessing the 48-hour IV flow rates on a patient receiving a vasoactive drug, you note that each shift has been infusing the drug at a different rate. What are some of the possible explanations for the variation in the flow rates?
3. Compare and contrast assessment findings of a patient in cardiogenic shock and a patient in hypovolemic shock.
4. Discuss the rationale for *not* using the Trendelenburg position to increase a patient's blood pressure.

References

1. Alderson P et al: Colloids versus crystalloids for fluid resuscitation in critically ill patients (Cochrane Review), *The Cochrane Library,* Issue 2, Oxford, 2001, Update software.
2. Armstrong RF et al: *Critical care algorithms,* Oxford, 1994, Oxford University Press.
3. Astiz ME, Rackow EC: Septic shock, *Lancet* 351:1501, 1998.
4. Domeier RM et al: Use of pneumatic antishock garment (PASG), *Prehosp Emerg Care* 1:32, 1997.
5. Fink M: Shock: an overview. In Rippe R et al, editors: *Intensive care medicine,* ed 3, Boston, 1996, Little, Brown.
6. Hankins D, Freeman S: Prehospital devices. In Tintinalli J, Ruiz E, Krome R, editors: *Emergency medicine: a comprehensive study guide,* ed 4, New York, 1996, McGraw-Hill.
7. Hochman JS et al: One-year survival following early revascularization for cardiogenic shock, *JAMA* 285(2):190, 2001.
8. Hollenberg S, Parillo J: Shock. In Fauci AS et al, editors: *Harrison's principles of internal medicine,* New York, 1998, McGraw-Hill.
9. Jimenez E: Shock. In Civetta R, Taylor R, Kirby R, editors: *Critical care,* Philadelphia, 1997, Lippincott-Raven.
10. Leier CV: Approach to the patient with hypotension and shock. In Kelley WN, editor: *Texbook of internal medicine,* ed 3, Philadelphia, 1997, Lippincott-Raven.
11. Marquardt DL: Anaphylaxis. In Stein JH: *Internal medicine,* ed 5, St Louis, 1998, Mosby.
12. Tierney L, Messina L: Blood vessels and lymphatics. In Tierney L, McPhee S, Papadakis M, editors: *Current medical diagnosis and treatment,* Stamford, Conn, 1999, Appleton & Lange.
13. Venmeulen LC et al: A paradigm for consensus: the university hospital consortium guidelines for the use of albumin, nonprotein colloid, and crystalloid solutions, *Arch Intern Med* 155(4):373, 1995.
14. Winslow R: New transfusion strategies: red cell substitutes, *Ann Rev Med* 50:337, 1999.
15. Yim JM et al: Fluid resuscitation with colloids or crystalloid solutions in critically ill patients: a systematic review of randomized controlled trials, *BMJ* 155(22):2450, 1998.

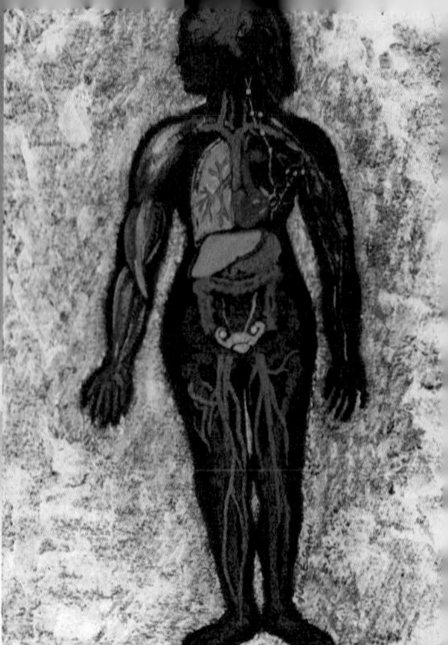

15 Cancer

Jeanne M. Erickson

Objectives

After studying this chapter, the learner should be able to:

1. Describe epidemiologic trends in the incidence of cancer.
2. Identify the factors related to carcinogenesis.
3. Describe the pathophysiology of cancer, including the characteristics of malignant cells, growth of neoplasms, and nature of metastases.
4. Relate the pathophysiologic changes of cancer to common clinical manifestations.
5. Identify the nurse's role in the prevention and early detection of cancer.
6. Apply the nursing process to care of the patient in the diagnostic and treatment phases of cancer.
7. Explain the rationale for the major types of cancer therapy.
8. Discuss the major nursing care concerns for patients undergoing surgery, radiotherapy, chemotherapy, or biotherapy for treatment of cancer.

NATURE OF THE PROBLEM

Cancer was recognized in ancient times by skilled observers who gave it the name "cancer" (*L. cancri*, crab) because it stretched out in many directions like the legs of a crab. The term cancer is an "umbrella" word used to describe a group of more than 100 diseases in which cells multiply and spread without restraint, destroying healthy tissue and endangering life.

Few diseases cause greater feelings of anxiety and apprehension than cancer. Its physiologic and psychologic impact on patients and their families causes profound changes in their lifestyles. Cancer treatments may last a lifetime and too often do not result in the cure that patients hope for. Many myths surround malignant disease, often focusing on its incurability and fostering feelings of hopelessness and dread. Yet much progress has been made in the prevention, early detection, and treatment of cancer to improve survival rates and the quality of life for those undergoing treatment.

Cancer nursing has been recognized as a subspecialty in the nursing profession since 1975. Today, the Oncology Nursing Society has more than 25,000 members and is the largest organization of oncology professionals in the world. Oncology nurses care for patients of all ages and both genders in a variety of settings that range from the acute care hospital to ambulatory care clinics, home care agencies, and hospices. Oncology nurses fill the roles of care provider, case manager, genetic counselor, researcher, educator, and consultant. Outside of the clinical setting, oncology nurses provide important cancer education to the public in industry, schools, and community forums. Oncology nursing care requires a broad base of knowledge in both pathophysiology and psychosocial areas and frequently involves complex technical and psychomotor skills. Patients and their families look to oncology nurses for assistance and guidance in all phases of the illness, during prevention and screening programs, from diagnosis, throughout therapy, to terminal care.

To be an effective support to the patient with cancer, the nurse must be aware of the emotional impact that a cancer diagnosis has on the patient and family because this emotional response affects every aspect of nursing care. In addition, nurses need to identify their own feelings about cancer and their responses to their role in cancer care. Nurses may share the same fearful attitudes about cancer that exist in society. For this reason it is important that all nurses examine their own feelings about cancer and try to work through them, both by increasing their knowledge of the disease and its treatment and by discussing feelings openly with members of the health care team. Nurses who have resolved their own feelings are more able to help patients and their families during the cancer experience and more likely to feel satisfied with their work. Cancer nursing challenges the creativity, skill, and commitment of the nurse.

ETIOLOGY

Multistep Process of Carcinogenesis

Carcinogenesis is a dynamic and multistep process that is influenced by many independent variables. Cellular, genetic, immunologic, and environmental factors interact to cause the

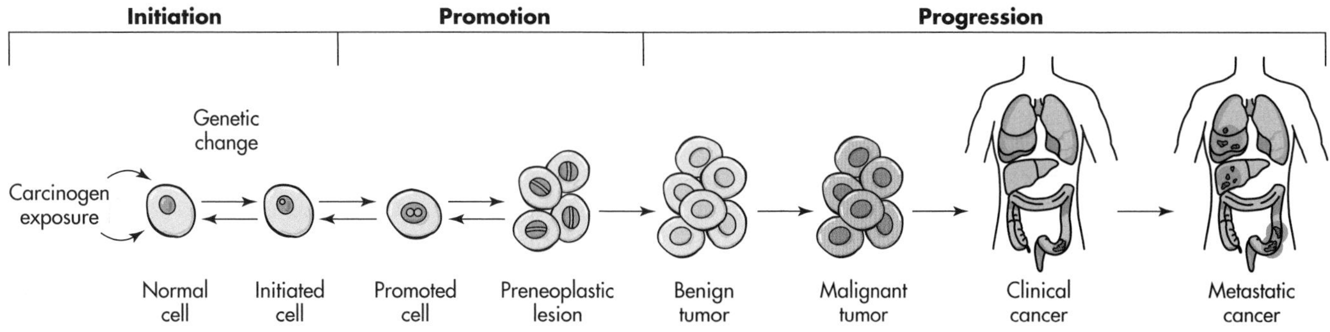

Figure 15-1 Multistage process of carcinogenesis.

abnormalities that result in the malignant process. A series of genetic mutations are core to the development of cancer, and a number of endogenous and exogenous factors can be involved in these mutations. Endogenous factors include age; specific genetic abnormalities, either spontaneous or inherited; and immunologic deficiencies. Exogenous factors include such factors as radiation, tobacco, and chemicals known to cause cellular damage.

The complex process of carcinogenesis, or the development of cancer, involves three overlapping and multistep stages: initiation, promotion, and progression (Figure 15-1). In initiation, a single genetic change occurs in a normal cell, altering cellular growth and/or function. During promotion, the altered cell continues to undergo additional malignant changes. Progression involves the continued growth of the cell population containing the malignant phenotype. In both the initiation and promotion stages, the carcinogenic process can be stabilized or reversed if the cell has the ability to repair or control the genetic alteration. In the final stage of progression, however, reversal of carcinogenesis is no longer possible.[10]

Specific genes regulate cellular proliferation through the production of various proteins and enzymes.[26,32] Proto-oncogenes are the normal genes that regulate cell growth. When mutations occur in proto-oncogenes, they become oncogenes and can allow uncontrolled cell growth to occur. Tumor suppressor genes inhibit cellular growth and program cellular death, or apoptosis. For example, the p53 tumor suppressor gene on chromosome 17 prevents cells with DNA damage from replicating, and mutations to the p53 gene are found in half of all human cancers. A third type of gene is the DNA mismatch or repair gene, which functions to identify a mismatched nucleotide in DNA and orchestrate the necessary repairs. A mutation to this gene prevents recognition and repair of such errors.

A number of growth factors, growth factor receptors, and activating factors have been identified as components of the intracellular communication network. These substances regulate growth signals between the cell and its nucleus. Several growth factors are used as tumor markers and give prognostic information. Overexpression of the growth factor receptor HER-2/neu, for example, is linked to a more aggressive breast cancer in younger women.

Risk Factors
Cancer

ENDOGENOUS

Age
- Cancer incidence increases with age.

Genetic heritage
- Some cancers exhibit a clear inheritance pattern.

Hormonal factors
- Do not act as primary carcinogens, but appear to influence the process of carcinogenesis.

Immunologic factors
- Malignant cells are antigenically different and should be recognized and destroyed by an intact immune system.

EXTERNAL

Drugs and chemicals
- Multiple drugs and chemicals are proven carcinogens.

Radiation
- Both ionizing and ultraviolet radiation can cause cancer.

Tobacco
- Tobacco is the single most lethal known carcinogen.

Nutrition
- Diets high in fat and calories are associated with an increased risk of cancer.

Sexual practices
- Early onset sex and multiple partners are associated with cancer in females.
- Breast cancer incidence is higher in women who marry and get pregnant at an older age.

Viruses
- Several viruses have been shown to cause cancer.

Psychosocial factors
- Life stressors are unproven but suggested causes of cancer.

Risk Factors

Carcinogens can be endogenous or exogenous factors, and common factors are listed in the Risk Factors box. They cause cancer either by damaging the genes that regulate normal cellular growth or by enhancing the growth of abnormal cells already present (e.g., by accelerating cell division). Major endogenous factors associated with cancer growth include age, genetic heritage, and immune competence. The primary external or exogenous factors include tobacco, radiation, diet, chemicals, and certain infections.

Age

Age is a major risk factor associated with cancer development. The probability of developing an invasive cancer is between 1% and 2% from birth to age 39, about 8% to 9% from ages 40 to 59, and rises to 22% for women and 33% for men between the ages of 60 and 79.[12] Several theories have been proposed to explain this increase in cancer that accompanies aging. First, older people have been exposed to a greater cumulative number of carcinogens over a longer period of time, increasing the chances for malignant transformations. Second, older cells may be less capable of repairing the genetic abnormalities that result in cancer. And finally, a weakened immune system in older persons may play a role in allowing the abnormal cellular growth of cancer.

Genetic Heritage

Most cancers are not inherited, but occur as random events in people with little or no relevant family history. Nevertheless, some tumors appear to occur in an inherited form. The two major patterns of transmission are dominant inheritance, which requires inheritance of only one altered copy of a gene to produce cancer susceptibility, and recessive inheritance, which requires two altered copies of a gene (one from each parent) to cause cancer susceptibility.

Approximately 10% of all cancers are inherited.[19] Three main categories of familial cancers are inherited cancer syndromes, genetic disorders, and familial clusters of cancer. Inherited cancer syndromes tend to be autosomal dominant and involve many different genes that regulate cell growth or DNA repair. These syndromes are usually diagnosed at an early age and may be associated with multiple primary tumors. The Li-Fraumeni syndrome is an example of such a disorder and is characterized by an increased risk of soft tissue sarcoma, breast cancer, and other cancers. This syndrome is associated with inheritance of an altered p53 tumor suppressor gene. A second example is the breast/ovarian cancer syndrome, linked with the BRCA1 gene, a mutated tumor suppressor gene, on chromosome 17. Female carriers of BRCA1 have a substantially higher risk of developing breast and ovarian cancers. Other examples are hereditary nonpolyposis colon cancer and xeroderma pigmentosum, which creates an increased risk for skin cancers.

A group of genetic disorders that have primarily nonmalignant manifestations are also associated with a predisposition to malignant disease. Ataxia-telangiectasia is a genetic syndrome associated with breast cancer and leukemia. Muir-Torre syndrome is associated with basal and squamous cell carcinomas as well as multiple internal malignancies.

Finally, cancer seems to "cluster" in some families at a higher than statistically expected incidence, but the associated genetic factors have not yet been clearly identified. Breast cancer is a common example of a cancer that clusters in families. A second breast cancer susceptibility gene, located on chromosome 13, appears to be present in some familial clusters of breast cancer. Table 15-1 lists cancers with a known hereditary link.

Hormonal Factors

Evidence suggests that hormones may be connected with the development of certain cancers. In addition, some metabolites of cancers may act as antihormones or have new physiologic effects. Hormones do not appear to be primary carcinogens but seem to influence carcinogenesis in three ways: (1) through a preparatory action on the target tissues, making them susceptible to the carcinogenic agent; (2) through a "permissive" influence on carcinogenesis, allowing the process to progress; and (3) by a conditioning effect on the tumor. Hormones can either inhibit or enhance tumor growth. Hormone therapy and some surgical therapies (hypophysectomy and oophorectomy) are based on this principle. There is evidence that tissues that are endocrine responsive (e.g., breast, endometrium, prostate) do not develop cancer unless stimulated by their growth-promoting hormones. Estrogens have been associated with adenocarcinomas of the vagina, hepatic tumors, breast tumors, and uterine cancer.

In addition to tissue stimulation by the hormone, carcinogenesis may be influenced by the duration of the hormonal effect. The longer the preparative influence of the hormone, the greater the chance of cancer development.

Precancerous Lesions

Certain benign lesions and tumors have a tendency toward malignant change. The cancers may be preventable if minor precursor conditions can be located and treated early. Precancerous lesions belong to a large and heterogeneous group; in some cancer is inevitable, whereas in others the risk is so low that medical intervention is unnecessary. Precancerous conditions include polyps of the colon and rectum, certain pigmented moles, dysplasias of the cervical epithelium, Paget's disease of the bone, senile keratoses, and leukoplakias of the oral mucous membranes.

Immunologic Factors

Scientists have become increasingly aware of the role of the immune system in the natural history of malignant disease. Mutated cells that become malignant are antigenically different from normal cells and should be recognized as foreign by the body's cell-mediated immune system. When the immune response is initiated, the malignant cell should be destroyed. The function of an immune surveillance system against cancer is suggested by the following points: (1) the high incidence of cancers during early childhood and older age—periods when the immune system is weak, (2) an increased tumor incidence in persons who have immunodeficiency diseases associated with a defect in cellular immunity, and (3) the increased incidence of neoplasia (e.g., non-Hodgkins lymphoma) in persons who receive immunosuppressive drugs such as cyclosporine or azathioprine to prevent organ transplant rejection.

Research continues to investigate why the initial tumor cells are able to progress to clinical cancer when an intact im-

TABLE 15-1 Common Hereditary Cancer Syndromes and Associated Cancer Susceptibility Genes

Syndrome/Condition	Associated Cancer	Gene
Ataxia-telangiectasia	Leukemia, lymphoma, breast cancer, and other solid tumors	ATM
Beckwith-Wiedemann syndrome	Wilms' tumor, adrenal carcinomas, hepatoblastomas	Linked to chromosome 11p
Breast/ovarian cancer syndrome	Breast cancer, ovarian cancer, prostate cancer, colon cancer	BRCA1
	Breast cancer (male and female), ovarian cancer	BRCA2
Cowden's disease	Breast cancer, thyroid cancer, colonic neoplasms	Linked to chromosome 10q22-33
Familial adenomatous polyposis (Gardner syndrome)	Colon polyposis (adenomas), desmoid tumors, osteomas, thyroid cancer, hepatoblastoma	APC
Fanconi anemia	Leukemia, esophageal cancer, hepatoma	FACC
Gorlin syndrome	Basal cell carcinoma, brain tumors, ovarian cancer	Linked to chromosome 9q
Hereditary nonpolyposis colorectal cancer (Lynch syndromes)	Gastrointestinal (GI) cancers, endometrial cancer, ovarian cancer, ureteral cancer	hMSH2, hMLH1, hPMS1, hPMS2
Li-Fraumeni syndrome	Breast cancer, sarcoma, brain tumors, leukemia, adrenocortical carcinoma	p53
		p16
Muir-Torre syndrome	GI and genitourinary cancers, skin cancer, breast cancer, benign breast tumors	hMSH2, hMLH1
Multiple endocrine neoplasia type I	Pancreatic cancer, pituitary adenomas	Linked to chromosome 11q
Multiple endocrine neoplasia type II	Thyroid cancer, pheochromocytomas	RET
Neurofibromatosis	Pheochromocytomas, optic gliomas	NF1
Peutz-Jeghers syndrome	GI cancer, breast cancer, uterine cancer, ovarian cancer, testicular cancer	Linked to chromosome 19p
		Linked to chromosome 1
		RB1
Von Hippel-Lindau syndrome	Hemangioblastoma, renal cell cancer, pheochromocytomas	VHL
		WT1
Xeroderma pigmentosum	Skin cancer, melanoma, leukemia	RAD2

Adapted from Calzone KA: Genetic predisposition testing, *Oncol Nurs Forum* 24:713, 1997.

mune surveillance system exists. Some tumors arise in areas that are poorly served by the immune system, such as the central nervous system or the retrobulbar aspect of the eye. Some tumors fail to stimulate antibody formation because they are so similar to normal cells. The normal control system for the immune response may become overactive and suppress the immune system. Finally, some persons may lack the genetic ability to mount an effective immune response.

The normal immune system is capable of detecting and destroying as many as 10 million cancer cells at a time. However, when a tumor grows at a rate faster than the normal immunologic response can effectively handle, the tumor will continue to grow unchecked. Typically, a tumor must measure at least 1 cm in diameter before it can be detected by conventional diagnostic methods. Unfortunately a tumor 1 cm in diameter already contains more than 1 billion cells. The role of the immune system is discussed further in Chapter 49.

Drugs and Chemicals

Many chemicals, drugs, and products in the environment are known to be carcinogenic; hundreds more are suspected to be associated with the development of cancer. As long ago as 1775, an increased incidence of scrotal cancer was recognized in men employed as chimney sweeps in English homes where coal was burned as fuel. Coal tar, an end product of coal combustion, is now acknowledged as the first occupational chemical carcinogen. Important links between cancer and the environment have been identified from studying patterns of incidence and mortality. As people move from place to place throughout the world, however, the baseline incidence and mortality rates for each type of cancer change. It is theorized that up to two thirds of all cancers may be related to environmental factors.

The Occupational Safety and Health Act of 1970 authorized the Occupational Safety and Health Administration to enforce maximal allowable concentrations of exposure to known carcinogens (threshold limit values [TLVs]), but the task is difficult because the identification of potential human carcinogens in the environment and workplace is a lengthy and time-consuming process. The Department of Health and Human Services publishes a biennial report listing proven carcinogens, including the risk of exposure and exposure standards. The Ninth Report was published in 2000, and the carcinogens included in the report are listed in Box 15-1.

Certain drugs have also been shown to be carcinogenic. Oral contraceptives were first recognized as having carcinogenic potential for breast cancer, but are now known to also exhibit a protective effect against ovarian and endometrial cancers. In 1971 a rare form of vaginal cancer in women was linked to the ingestion by their mothers of diethylstilbestrol (DES), which was prescribed to prevent spontaneous abortion.

Cancer therapy itself may increase the risk for other cancers. Alkylating agent chemotherapy, such as chorambucil, cyclophosphamide, and thiotepa is accompanied by significant subsequent risk of acute leukemia and other malignancies. Consequently use of these drugs is limited to those cases for which no comparable alternative therapy exists.

BOX 15-1 Substances Known to be Carcinogens in Humans

Aflatoxins
Alcoholic beverage consumption
Analgesic mixtures containing phenacetin
Arsenic compounds
Asbestos
Azathioprine
Benzene
Benzidine
Bis (Chloromethyl) ether
Busulfan
1,3-Butadiene
Cadmium and cadmium compounds
Chlorambucil
Methyl CCNU
Chloromethyl methyl ether
Coal tar
Coke oven emissions
Creosote (coal and wood)
Cristobalite
Cyclophosphamide
Cyclosporin A
Diethylstilbestrol
Direct Black 38
Direct Blue 6
Dyes that metabolize to benzidine
Environmental tobacco smoke
Erionite
Ethylene oxide
Lead chromate
Melphalan
Methoxsale with ultraviolet A therapy
Mineral oils
Mustard gas
Myleran
2-Naphthylamine
Piperazine estrone sulfate
Quartz
Radon
Silica
Smokeless tobacco
Sodium equilin sulfate
Sodium estone sulfate
Solar radiation and exposure to sunlamps and sunbeds
Soots
Strong inorganic acid mists containing sulfuric acid
Strontium chromate
Tamoxifen
Tars
Thiotepa
Thorium dioxide
Tobacco smoking
Tridymite
Vinyl chloride
Zinc chromate

Radiation

Various forms of radiation, both waves and particles of energy, can cause cancer. Ionizing radiation consists of electromagnetic waves or material particles that have sufficient energy to ionize atoms or molecules (i.e., remove electrons from them) and thereby alter their biochemical behavior. Large amounts of radiation can be lethal to living cells. Ultraviolet radiation is composed of lower energy electromagnetic waves, but is still capable of causing carcinogenic changes.

Ionizing Radiation. Every living thing is exposed to small amounts of radiation from natural elements in the earth, such as uranium. This is known as natural background radiation. Other sources of exposure include diagnostic or therapeutic x-rays, manufactured radioisotopes, and other industrial sources. Problems with radiation did not appear until after 1895, when the roentgen-ray (x-ray) machine was developed and became widely used in the diagnosis of disease. The development of this machine was followed by the discovery of radium, used for the treatment of cancer.

Radiologists working with the early equipment showed a higher than normal incidence of skin cancer. Workers employed in painting radium on watch dials had high rates of oral and sinus carcinomas and osteosarcomas. Survivors of the atomic bombs dropped on the Japanese cities of Hiroshima and Nagasaki during World War II were exposed to high doses of radiation. Within 10 years, a variety of cancers were diagnosed in this population at higher than normal incidence rates.

Radiation exposure results in breakage of either a single or double strand of the DNA helix. The damage is permanent and cumulative after each additional radiation exposure. Exposure of the entire body significantly increases the amount of radiation received. For this reason all of the body except the part being treated is protected from exposure when radiation is administered for therapeutic purposes.

The amount of exposure a patient receives from a series of radiographs taken for diagnostic purposes depends both on the machine used and the skill of the technician. A fluoroscopic examination usually entails more exposure than the use of radiography. The exposure of the average nurse working in a hospital and occasionally assisting a patient while a radiograph is taken is almost negligible.

High-dose radiation exposure can cause leukopenia, leukemia, bone cancer, and sterility or damage to the reproductive cells. Because of this risk, persons whose daily work exposes them to radiation wear film badges. The badge, which contains photographic film capable of absorbing radiation, is developed each month to measure cumulative radiation exposure. Personnel who are becoming overexposed are temporarily reassigned.

Because radiation poses a danger to a fetus, particularly between the second and sixth weeks of gestation, pregnant women usually are not employed in radiology departments or in caring for patients receiving radioactive materials.

Ultraviolet Radiation. Many Americans eagerly seek a tanned skin despite proof that sun exposure can cause cancer. Ultraviolet radiation from the sun or from a tanning bed can act as an initiator, a promoter, a cocarcinogen, and an immunosuppressive agent. Wavelengths that range from 200 to 400 nm, which include both ultraviolet A and B waves, can cause skin damage. In particular, wavelengths from 290 to 310 nm produce severe erythema of the skin and cause the maximum number of carcinogenic changes.[10] Skin cancer occurs most commonly in persons who work in the open air, such as sailors, construction workers, and farmers, and on areas of the body most exposed to sunlight. Light-complexioned individuals seem to be the most susceptible to the carcinogenic effects of the sun.

Radon and Electromagnetic Field Effects. Radon is a colorless, odorless gas that results from the decay of uranium. It emanates from soil and rocks, and can be found in underground mines as well as underground basements. Prolonged breathing of radon gas at high levels has been linked to an increased incidence of lung cancer. Radon levels can be lowered by improving ventilation of the building or mine. Home monitoring kits are available, and the Environmental Protection Agency has established guidelines for controlling radon levels.

The effect of living or working near electromagnetic fields (EMFs) is a recent environmental concern. EMFs are extremely low frequency energy fields, and exposure can come from household appliances, electrical power lines, and electricity-generating facilities. Electrical power lines generate both electric and magnetic fields that can easily pass through body tissue and most materials. The intensity of the EMF is in proportion to the electrical energy running through the lines. The nearer one is to the source (within 50 m), the greater the exposure. Whether EMFs are carcinogenic remains unclear, but a weak association in leukemia incidence has been shown in children who live near high-voltage electric lines. Occupational exposure has been linked to an increased incidence of leukemia and brain tumors. Cellular telephones are also being studied as a source (and thus a risk) of EMF exposure.[30]

Lifestyle Practices

Smoking and Tobacco Use. Tobacco smoke is the single most lethal known carcinogen, responsible for up to 30% of all cancer deaths in the United States.[30] Cigarette smoking is the most important risk factor for lung cancer, and lung cancer is the most common cause of cancer death among both women and men in America. Cigarettes are also linked to cancers of the mouth, pharynx, larynx, esophagus, pancreas, kidney, bladder, and colorectum. Passive smoking, or the inhalation of tobacco smoke in the environment (ETS), also causes several thousand cancer deaths each year. Nevertheless, about one in four adults still smokes cigarettes, and more than 3000 children and adolescents begin smoking each day.[9]

Tobacco contains a number of different agents that initiate and/or promote malignant transformation over time. Correlation exists between cancer mortality and the number of cigarettes smoked daily, the number of years a person has smoked, and the age at which the person began to smoke. Smokers have a lung cancer risk 10 to 25 times greater than that of a nonsmoker.[17] There are immediate as well as long-term benefits of stopping smoking. People who stop smoking live longer and can cut their risk of dying from lung cancer by at least 50%. They also reduce their risk of heart disease and pregnancy-associated problems.

Many smokers have changed to filtered cigarettes, pipe smoking, or the use of smokeless tobacco (plug, leaf, snuff) in the misguided belief that their cancer risk will be lessened or eliminated. Evidence is abundant that there is no "safe" cigarette and that smokeless tobacco is equally unsafe because it places the user at higher risk for head and neck cancers.

The carcinogenic effects of tobacco smoke are also released into the environment and research indicates that ETS contains most of the same carcinogenic compounds that have been identified in mainstream smoke. Consequently, nonsmokers inhaling the ambient air near a cigarette smoker are exposed to the same carcinogens as the smoker; and their risk for lung cancer, cardiovascular disease, and other respiratory conditions also increases.

Since 1971 cigarette advertising has been banned on television and radio. At the same time, the warning on cigarette packages was changed from "Caution: cigarette smoking may be hazardous to your health" to either "Warning: the surgeon general has determined that cigarette smoking is dangerous to your health" or a more definitive statement asserting that smoking may cause cancer, heart disease, and emphysema. In 1990 federal law prohibited the sale of tobacco products to minors. Legislation limiting public smoking and the sale of tobacco products will continue to be important interventions in the effort to reduce smoking-related diseases and cancers.

Nutrition. Diet is the second most significant lifestyle factor contributing to cancer. Nutrition research has increased steadily over the past decade, and a variety of studies indicate a relationship between dietary components and the development of cancer.

The consumption of a diet high in fat and calories has been associated with an increased risk for colon, breast, prostate, pancreatic, and endometrial cancer.[30] These cancers are more prevalent in the United States and Europe and may in part be related to the consumption of red meat and other foods that are high in fat content. Large-scale, long-term studies of the effect of dietary fat on the incidence of breast and uterine cancer are needed to confirm or rule out the risk.

Diets high in fiber content appear to offer some protection against colon cancer. Fiber is believed to reduce cancer risk by diluting colon contents, decreasing colon transit time, and thus limiting contact with carcinogens. Fruits, vegetables, and whole grain foods, which are good sources of vitamins C and D, beta-carotene, and selenium, appear to have a cancer-deterrent effect. These vitamins and minerals, known as antioxidants, assist in the repair of cellular damage caused by free radicals. Free radicals damage the genetic makeup of the cell and its natural ability to resist cancer.

A significant association exists between high alcohol intake and cancer of the mouth, pharynx, larynx, and esophagus. Alcoholism is also associated with smoking and a variety of vitamin and dietary deficiencies. It is speculated that alcohol consumption and nutritional deficiencies may enhance carcinogenesis by increasing the metabolic activity of specific tobacco carcinogens. These tumors occur with greater frequency in men, African-Americans, older adults, and persons from lower socioeconomic groups and urban settings.

Sexual/Reproductive Factors

Sexual practices play a role in the incidence of several cancers. Carcinoma of the uterine cervix is less common in virgins than in sexually active women. The incidence is higher in those who have first coitus at an early age, who have an early first marriage, and who have had multiple sex partners. Teenage women are at greater risk for cervical dysplasia, a precursor stage in the development of cancer of the squamocolumnar junction, possibly because of greater exposure to as yet unidentified carcinogenic viruses.

Carcinoma of the penis is virtually unknown among circumcised men. The means by which circumcision provides protection is not clear but may be related to better hygiene.

The correlation between sexual activity and breast cancer is the reverse of that for the cancer of the uterine cervix. Women who develop breast cancer tend to marry and become pregnant later in life. A woman's age at the birth of her first child and ages at menarche and menopause are also relevant factors in the subsequent development of breast cancer. Women who give birth to their first child before age 20 have only one third the risk of women older than age 35 who deliver a first child. This fact is not used to advocate for pregnancy at an early age but to help women make informed decisions on when to begin a family. The physiologic rationale for these phenomena may be related to the length of time in which a woman is exposed to her own endogenous sex hormones.

Viruses and Other Microorganisms

Several viruses have been identified as causes of cancer.[30] The prevalence and spread of these viruses are of most concern in developing countries, where communicable disease rates are highest. More than 30 different types of the human papilloma virus are involved in cancers of the genitals and anus, especially affecting women. Cervical cancer, for example, may result from transmission of the virus during sexual intercourse. Hepatitis B and C can cause liver cancer. The Epstein-Barr virus, which causes mononucleosis, is also associated with cancer of the upper pharynx, Hodgkin's lymphoma, and non-Hodgkin's lymphoma. The human immunodeficiency virus can cause Kaposi's sarcoma and lymphoma. *Helicobacter pylori,* a bacterium, causes stomach ulcers and is also associated with stomach cancer. Studies are focusing on how and why these microorganisms produce carcinogenic changes in humans.

Psychosocial Factors

Stressors such as life changes, loss of a significant other, and personality variables have been suggested as etiologic factors in the development of cancer. Determination of how a person's state of mind affects the immune and hormonal systems is not easily explained. Research with persons with acquired immunodeficiency syndrome has indicated that a positive state of mind can influence survival with the disease. Most reports are anecdotal in nature, however, and further studies in psychoneuroimmunology will be needed to determine the mechanism for these complex interactions.

Social support in the form of institutions, family, and friends also may be an important variable. The person with minimal social support and maximal need may be at a higher risk for developing cancer. In addition, lack of social support may adversely affect coping responses to therapy and to the illness. At present, however, how one defines the nature of social support and the degree to which it is present or lacking are unclear.

EPIDEMIOLOGY

The study of epidemiology is essential to identify patterns of cancer occurrence and help determine prevention and early detection strategies, treatment, and research priorities in cancer care. Cancer affects human beings wherever they live and whatever their race, color, cultural background, or economic status.

Overall cancer incidence declined between 1992 and 1998 after two decades of increasing cancer rates.[16] Decreased incidence rates have occurred for the leading cancers, including prostate, colorectal, and lung; breast cancer incidence, which has been stable during the 1990s, may be decreasing in younger women. However, more than 1,250,000 new cases of cancer are diagnosed annually; thus cancer remains a major health problem. According to population figures, approximately 44% of men and 38% of women now alive in the United States will develop some form of cancer in their lifetime.[12]

The death rate from cancer has also shown a steady decline in the last decade. One notable exception is the continuing increase in lung cancer deaths in women, but even this increase has recently slowed. Although the incidence of breast cancer has increased, death rates continue to decline. These improvements in survival can be attributed to (1) diagnosis of more cancers in the early localized stage, (2) early treatment of more patients, and (3) development of new diagnostic, treatment, and support modalities. Improved survival rates are seen for many cancers, including cancers of the cervix, uterus, thyroid, kidney, and bladder, as well as for melanoma, Hodgkin's disease, and leukemia. Other diverse and relatively uncommon cancers, however, show an increase in incidence. This group of cancers includes melanoma, acute myeloid leukemia, soft tissue cancers, and non-Hodgkin's lymphoma.

Despite numerous advances an estimated 553,400 Americans will still die from cancer each year—more than 1500 people a day. The actual number of cancer deaths continues to increase because of an aging and expanding population. Unfortunately, large disparities in cancer incidence and mortality occur across racial and ethnic groups. African-American men and women experience higher incidences of cancer and poorer survival than Caucasian men and women, although these differences may be lessening. The disparity in survival reflects both diagnosis of cancer at later disease stages, and poorer survival within each stage of diagnosis. Table 15-2 lists estimates of the number of new cases of cancer and deaths from cancer in 2001.

More than 8 million Americans are living today who have had a diagnosis of cancer and received treatment.[4] The overall 5-year survival rate for cancer is approximately 60%, and many will be cured of their cancer. "Cure" refers to those persons who have no evidence of active disease and have a life expectancy comparable to that of a person who has never had cancer.

Gender and Site

Basal and squamous cell skin cancers are the most prevalent cancers, with over a million cases diagnosed each year. Luckily these skin cancers are highly curable and not included in the

TABLE 15-2 Estimated Numbers of New Cancers and Cancer Deaths in 2001*

	New Cancers	Cancer Deaths†
All Sites	1,268,000	553,400
Oral cavity and pharynx	30,100	7,800
Digestive system	235,700	131,300
Respiratory system	184,600	162,500
Bones and joints	2900	1,400
Soft tissue (including heart)	8700	4,400
Skin (excluding basal and squamous)	56,400	9,800
Breast	193,700	40,600
Genital system	286,800	58,500
Urinary system	87,500	25,000
Eye and orbit	2100	200
Brain and other nervous system	17,200	13,100
Endocrine system	21,400	2,300
Lymphoma	63,600	27,600
Multiple myeloma	14,400	11,200
Leukemia	31,500	21,500
Other and unspecified primary sites	31,400	36,200

Adapted from Greenlee R et al: Cancer Statistics, 2001, *CA Cancer J Clin* 51:15, 2001.
*Most recent available statistics.
†Rounded to the nearest 100; excludes in situ carcinomas except urinary bladder.

analysis of the more invasive cancers. For men the most common sites of cancer are the prostate, lung, and colon/rectum. Prostate cancer accounts for about for 31% of new cancers each year. For women the top three cancer sites are the breast, lung, and colon/rectum. Breast cancer accounts for 31% of new cancers in women.

Deaths from lung, prostate, and colorectal cancers cause 52% of deaths in men. In women, lung, breast, and colorectal cancer cause 51% of deaths. Lung cancer has been the leading cause of death in women since 1987 and now accounts for 25% of all cancer deaths in women. The death rate from lung cancer in women continues to increase, although the rate of increase has slowed in recent years.

The average cancer mortality in developed countries is higher for men than for women. During the last 40 years a decrease in mortality from cancer among American women is the result of a sharp reduction in the number of deaths caused from uterine cancer. The death rate from cancer involving the female genital tract has dropped to one third to one half the rate of 25 years ago. There is ample evidence that the increased use of the Pap test to detect lesions of the cervix has resulted in earlier treatment and a higher rate of cure. Figure 15-2 compares cancer incidence and deaths in 2001* by site and gender.

Age

Cancer has been called a disease of aging. Some researchers believe that if people live long enough, they will eventually develop a malignancy. Although cancer is the leading cause of death in women 35 to 74 years old, the three most prevalent malignancies (lung, breast, colorectal) peak between ages 55 and 74 years. In men, this same age span reflects the years in which the most deaths occur from lung, colorectal, and prostate cancer.

Today the average life expectancy is 76.7 years. The population over age 65 has been steadily growing and now makes up about 13% of the population. By 2030, this population will represent 20% of the U.S. population.[1] In addition, Hispanic, African-American, Native-American, and Asian-Pacific ethnicities make up a growing percentage of the older population. This "graying of America" has an immense impact on the health care system and health care policies (see Chapter 4).

Access to health care for many elders is influenced by a variety of factors. The older population may be limited by the financial constraints of a fixed income and inadequate health insurance; limited transportation; and cultural, ethnic, or religious practices that may not be part of mainstream medical care. These factors may help to explain why elderly persons typically are diagnosed with advanced cancers and do not participate in prevention and screening programs. In addition, elders tend to have more chronic disease states, with signs and symptoms that can mask a malignancy, thereby preventing early detection. The ability of older adults to withstand the rigors of treatment is also questioned because of physical conditions that may affect their nutrition, memory, and mobility. Because of these concerns, older patients may not be offered the same treatment options as younger patients, and they may not be represented adequately in clinical trials.

Race

With the exception of breast cancer, the incidence and mortality rates for the most common cancers are higher in African-Americans than in Caucasian Americans.[12] The 5-year survival rate for African-Americans diagnosed with cancer is only 49% compared with 62% for Caucasian Americans. Lower survival rates result from diagnosis at later stages of the disease, as well as lower survival at each stage, suggesting possible differences in treatment, tumor characteristics, or other factors.

Hispanic-Americans, Asian-Americans/Pacific Islanders, and Native-Americans have lower incidence and mortality rates for cancers than do either African-Americans or Caucasian Americans. Yet an American Cancer Society survey showed that Hispanic-Americans are not adequately aware of cancer warning signs and ways to reduce cancer risk, and they tend not to seek screening or treatment.

Cultural and ethnic behaviors and beliefs, as well as socioeconomic factors such as poverty and access to health care, play important roles in how quickly a person will seek health care and treatment. Health care insurance is often unavailable or too expensive for certain minority groups.

Geographic Factors

There are differences in the worldwide distribution of cancer. For example, primary cancer of the liver is common in

*Most recent available statistics.

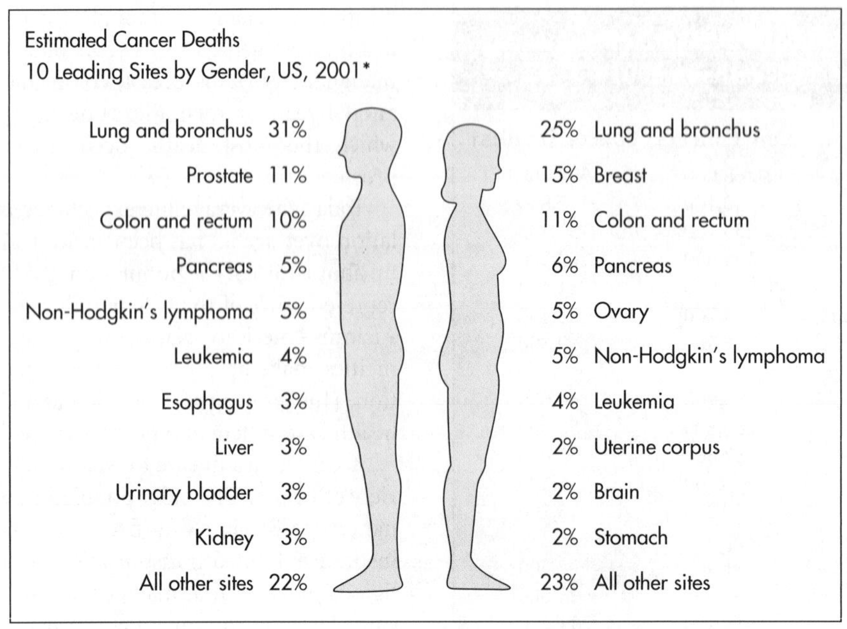

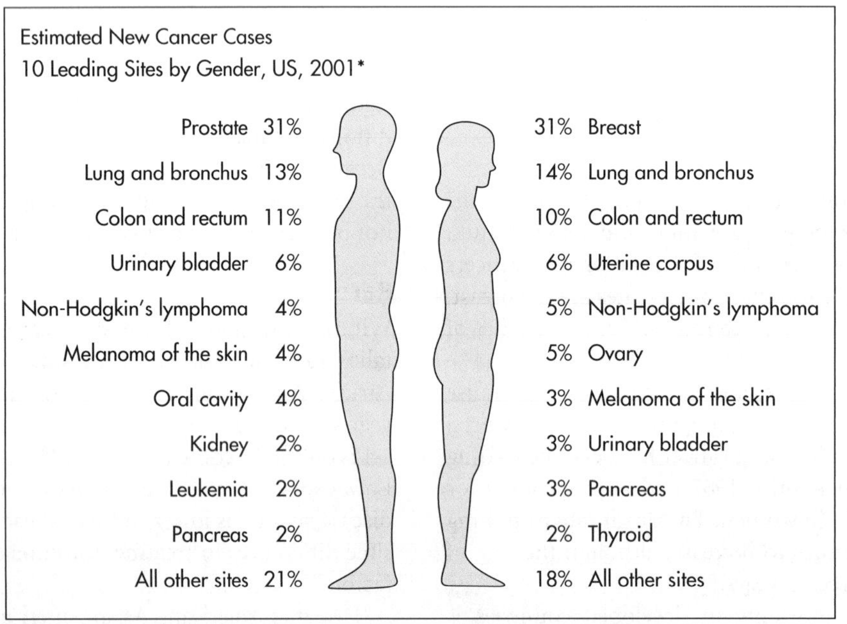

Figure 15-2 Estimated U.S. cancer deaths by gender, 2001. *Most recent available statistics.

Indonesia and parts of Africa and Asia but rare in other regions. Cancer of the breast is more common in the United States and Western Europe than it is in Japan. Ugandans, Nigerians, and South African blacks are at lowest risk for cancer of the lung, stomach, large intestine, uterus, and kidney. Genetic differences among populations may contribute to international variations but are unlikely to explain all variations, because migration from one country to another results in major changes in the cancer incidence pattern.

Factors Affecting Prognosis

Trends in cancer epidemiology are evaluated to determine why the incidence of certain cancers has decreased, increased, or remained the same. There is reason to believe that the cure rate and prognosis of cancer would improve substantially with earlier recognition and more complete reporting of early signs. Delay may be related to the patient's perception of (1) the chance of having cancer, (2) the possibility of early detection and treatment, (3) the inconvenience of examination, (4) the need for relief of symptoms, (5) the need for reassurance, and (6) the ability to pay for health care.

Success in treating many cancers awaits better and more sensitive diagnostic aids to detect lesions in their early stages. In parts of the body that are easily examined, such as the skin and cervix, early recognition and prompt treatment often result in cure.

Prognosis also is affected by the intrinsic characteristics of the tumor, such as histologic type and grade, size, and rate of growth. Other important factors are age and the general condition of the patient. The presence of debilitating conditions, such as infection, chronic obstructive pulmonary disease, or malnutrition, may adversely affect the outcome.

PHYSIOLOGY

The knowledge of cell kinetics, or how cells grow and divide, is necessary to understand the process of cancer development and the principles of cancer treatment. Much of what is now known about cancer cells is the result of research in which normal cells were transformed into malignant cells in a controlled laboratory setting. Transformation to a malignant cell is recognized as a multistep process that originates in a single proliferating cell. The transformed cell then has an altered ability to differentiate and proliferate.

Normal Cellular Proliferation

Characteristics of Normal Cells

Normal tissue contains large numbers of mature cells of uniform size and shape, each containing a nucleus of uniform size. Within each nucleus are the chromosomes, and within each chromosome is deoxyribonucleic acid (DNA), the giant molecule whose chemical composition controls the characteristics of ribonucleic acid (RNA), found in the nucleoli and cytoplasm of the cell. RNA regulates cell growth and function. When the ovum and sperm unite, the DNA and RNA within the chromosomes of each govern the differentiation and future course of the trillions of cells that finally develop to form the adult organism. In the development of various organs and parts of the body, cells undergo differentiation in size, appearance, and arrangement. Under the microscope, the pathologist can examine tissue and determine its origin in the body.

Normal Cell Growth

In normal tissue cellular growth takes place by an orderly process in response to a need such as trauma, surgery, or an inflammatory event. Once the need is met, cell multiplication stops. Normal cells recognize the presence of other cells near them by means of the process of contact inhibition. When cells are in close contact with other cells, they normally adhere closely together. This contact is responsible for inhibiting overlap of cells and disorganized growth. With normal cells, these restraints on growth are maintained until the need for new cells arises because of cell death. Some cell turnover rates are rapid, as in the bone marrow, skin, and gastrointestinal tract, because the need for cell replacement in these areas is greater than in slower-growing tissue. Finally, normal cells do not migrate but have a designated location, with the exception of certain blood cells.

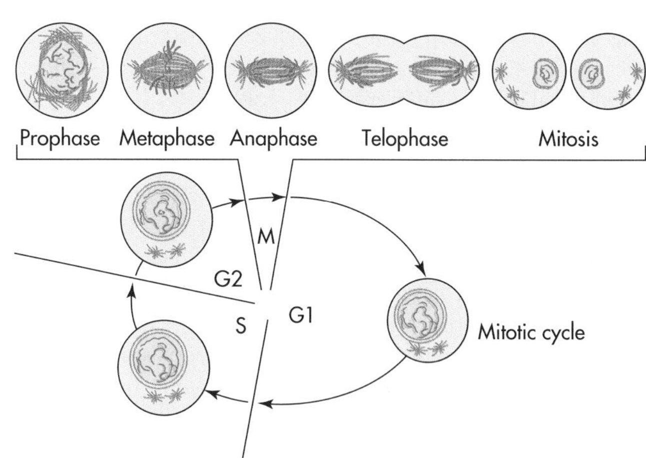

Figure 15-3 Cell cycle. *G1,* RNA/protein synthesis; *S,* DNA synthesis; *G2,* RNA/protein synthesis and interphase; *M,* mitosis.

Cell Cycle

Mitosis refers to the splitting of one cell into two cells during the cell cycle. The concept of cell cycle time is pertinent to understanding normal cell replication and has implications for drug use in cancer therapy. Cell cycle time may be described as the interval from mitosis of a cell to its mitosis into daughter cells. There is a stationary period (G0) of apparent rest after mitosis takes place. The cells are not in the cycle but are viable and capable of undergoing mitosis if necessary. The cell cycle is divided into four phases (Figure 15-3): (1) a quiescent phase consisting of G1 (G denotes a gap) in which RNA and protein synthesis begins; (2) S, a period of DNA synthesis; (3) G2, further RNA and protein synthesis and the development of the mitotic spindle; and (4) mitosis (M). The cell cycle is controlled by the cell nucleus, which receives signals from growth-regulating proteins that stimulate or suppress cell division. As described earlier, certain genes, including proto-oncogenes and tumor suppressor genes, code for these proteins.

Differentiation

All body tissue is derived from stem cells, which are immature cells with no specific cell lineage. These cells have the ability to proliferate rapidly and renew themselves as needed and to develop specialized functions as they grow and mature. The process of cellular differentiation causes the cells to resemble their normal forebears and have fully mature, specialized function and morphology. For example, all kidney cells are similar but are different from muscle cells, and each type has its specialized function.

The method by which differentiation takes place is unknown. One theory is that all cells carry the same genetic material but that selective repression of different genetic characteristics occurs because of buildup of different repressor substances in the cytoplasm. Different cells repress different genetic characteristics. Cell differentiation, once begun, proceeds along a path toward specialized function that cannot then revert to a previous immature state. Figure 15-4 shows the normal cellular differentiation process.

PATHOPHYSIOLOGY

Alterations in Cell Growth

Malignant or cancerous growths represent one form of abnormal cell growth. Other types of cellular growths are benign and include hyperplasia and hypertrophy. Hyperplasia is an increase in cell number, whereas hypertrophy is an increase in cell size but not number. Although many neoplasms are characterized by hyperplasia, normal tissues also may undergo hyperplasia. Wound healing, callus formation, and growth in embryonic tissue are all normal forms of hyperplasia.

Metaplasia is a reversible process in which one adult cell type in an organ is replaced by another adult cell type. The new cell type usually is not one normally seen in the area in which metaplasia occurs. The change of columnar or pseudostratified columnar epithelium of the respiratory tract to squamous epithelium or squamous metaplasia represents the most common type of metaplasia. Dysplasia is an alteration in adult cells characterized by changes in their size, shape, and organization. Neoplasia is abnormal cellular division not necessary for normal cell growth and development. These terms are summarized in Table 15-3.

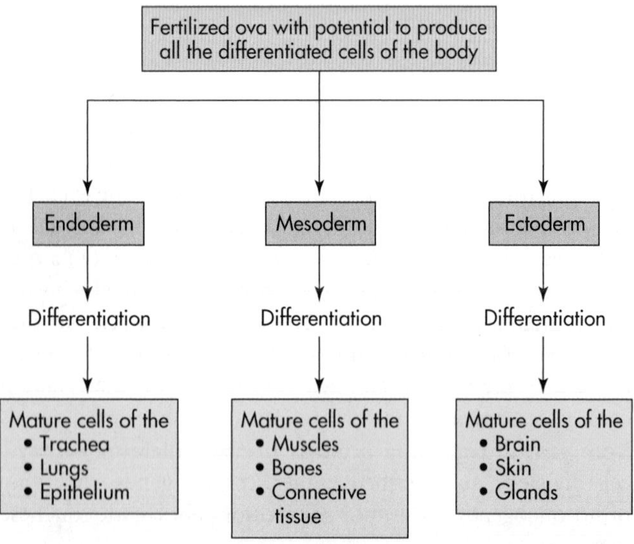

Figure 15-4 Normal cellular differentiation.

Benign tumors show normal cell growth patterns, even though the new tissue growth is not needed. Benign tumors closely resemble the tissue from which they arose and often perform the same function, such as moles on the skin. Benign tissues usually bind closely together and do not invade other tissues. Once removed, benign tumors usually do not recur.

Malignant cells, by contrast, do not show normal growth patterns, dividing almost continuously. Cancer cells gradually lose the appearance of the cells from which they arose, often becoming smaller and rounder with a larger nucleus. The grading system for cancer reflects how much the cancer cells resemble the tissue of origin. Generally a cancer with more poorly differentiated cells has a poorer prognosis because of a higher degree of malignancy. The total loss of differentiation is termed anaplasia. Cancer cells do not serve any useful function, do not exhibit contact inhibition, and migrate through blood vessels and tissues, spreading to and growing in other body locations, a process called metastasis. The differences between benign and malignant tissue growth are summarized in Table 15-4.

Metastasis

Metastasis is the major cause of cancer death.[14] The presence of metastases is an important prognostic factor for many cancers, and research continues to uncover important details of this malignant process. Mechanisms that contribute to metastasis include angiogenesis, or formation of a new blood supply; motility, alterations in cell adhesion, and mechanisms to escape immune detection.

Angiogenesis involves the migration and proliferation of endothelial cells from existing blood vessels near the tumor. Both positive and negative regulators of angiogenesis influence the formation of a new blood supply to nourish the metastatic tumor. Tumor cells produce motility factors, which enable them to circulate through blood vessels and lymphatics. Cell adhesion molecules on the cell surface are important mediators that allow detachment of tumor cells from the pri-

TABLE 15-3 Terms Denoting Cellular Changes

Type of Cellular Change	Definition	Example
Mitosis	Formation of new cell by cell division	Normal cell growth
Hyperplasia	Increase in cell number	Breast epithelium in pregnancy
Hypertrophy	Increase in cell size	Increase in muscle cell size with exercise
Atrophy	Decrease in cell size	Decrease in muscle cell size with disuse
Metaplasia	Replacement of one adult cell type by a different adult cell type	Replacement of columnar epithelium of respiratory tract by squamous epithelium
Dysplasia	Changes in cell size, shape, and organization	Changes in cervical epithelium in long-standing cervicitis
Anaplasia	Reverse cellular development to a more primitive cell type	Irreversible change accompanying cancer
Neoplasia	Abnormal cellular changes and growth of new tissues	Malignancies

mary tumor site. Finally, tumor cells escape the immune system in a variety of ways, including secretion of immunosuppressive factors and cellular proteins that have no antigenic structure. With better understanding of the metastatic cascade, a greater potential exists for development of therapies that can interrupt this invasive process (see Future Watch box).

Cancer spreads in several different ways (Figure 15-5). Cancer cells differ from normal cells in their unique ability to move without restraint into surrounding tissue. Tumor cells lack adhesiveness (the ability to stay in contact with other cells), so they can easily break away from the tumor mass of which they are a part and directly invade surrounding tissues. This is referred to as local invasion. Local spread may involve hemorrhage, necrosis, ulceration, and fibrous replacement of the involved tissues. This produces the typical local effects of ulcerating, bulky, hemorrhagic masses; or indurative, fibrosing lesions with tissue fixation, distortion of the structure, and the dimpling of the skin that may be seen in some breast cancers.

TABLE 15-4 Differences between Benign and Malignant Neoplasms

Benign	Malignant
Limited growth potential	May proliferate rapidly or grow slowly
Localized	Spread (metastasize) throughout the body
Fibrous capsule	No enclosing capsule
Rarely recur after removal	May recur even after treatment
Usually regular in shape	Irregular shape with poorly defined border
Cells similar to cell of parent tissue (well differentiated)	Cells much different from parent cells (poorly differentiated)
Expansive growth	Infiltrative growth

Future Watch

Inhalation Therapy With an Angiogenesis Inhibitor Drug for Kaposi's Sarcoma

Angiogenesis inhibitors prevent a tumor from establishing its own blood supply. These agents also stop tumors from disrupting normal tissue structures that allows tumor invasion and metastasis. One agent, IM862, is a protein that inhibits production of two angiogenesis growth factors. Since the drug can be absorbed through mucous membranes, it is administered with nose drops. In one clinical trial, patients with Kaposi's sarcoma were randomized to receive one of two administration schedules of IM862. Nearly half of the 44 patients had more than 50 lesions at the start of the trial. Thirty six percent had either complete or partial remissions, with a median duration of 8 months. Adverse effects were mild and temporary. Larger randomized trials with IM862 are currently underway.

Reference: Tulpule A et al: Results of a randomized study of IM862 nasal solution in the treatment of AIDS-related Kaposi's sarcoma, *J Clin Oncol* 18:716, 2000.

Infection may accompany the local infiltration. The cancer cells tend to spread along the path of least resistance, such as in tissue clefts, along blood vessels, or along the perineural spaces. The fibrous capsule that covers some organs may limit tumor growth. For example, primary tumors of the kidney, liver, or testes may increase the size of the organ without destroying the capsule. Local spread is not an orderly process but one that occurs unequally and haphazardly. Because of local spread, any surgical attempt to remove the cancer must include a margin of surrounding tissues to ensure removal of all malignant cells.

Cancer also spreads by lymphatic permeation and embolization. Once cells have invaded the lymph vessels, they may detach and become emboli, which lodge in the lymph nodes, forming a metastatic lesion. Spread then continues to

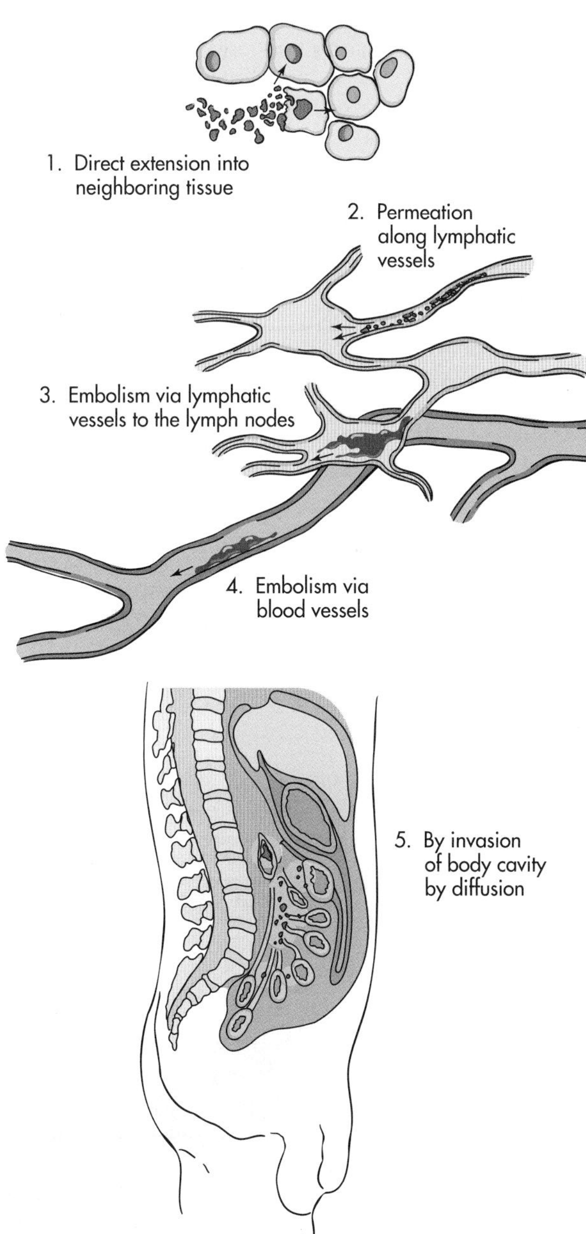

Figure 15-5 Modes of dissemination of cancer.

the next group of nodes and into other organs. The presence of cancer in the lymph nodes is certain evidence of spread, but even if lymph node metastasis does not occur, there still may be dissemination of malignant cells through the blood (see Evidence-Based Practice box). Lymphatic and vascular dissemination may take place concurrently. Vascular spread can result in more widely disseminated disease because of the ability of tumor cells to move freely through both the lymphatic and venous systems. Blood-borne cancer cells escape from the bloodstream by a process of attachment and invasion through endothelial cells lining the blood vessel (Figure 15-6).

Evidence-Based Practice

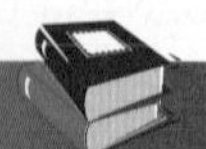

Reference: Bass SS et al: Effects of postinjection massage on the sensitivity of lymphatic mapping in breast cancer, *J Am Col Surg* 192:9, 2001.

Researchers investigated the effectiveness of massage following injections of blue-dye and a radiocolloid for sentinel lymph node (SLN) identification in patients with breast cancer. The first study group of 134 patients received a 5-minute massage after injection of the blue dye, and the second group of 230 patients received a 5-minute massage after injection of a radiocolloid. The control group was 230 patients who received no massage. SLN was identified in 88% of blue-dye patients who received massage, versus 73% of blue-dye patients who were not massaged. In the radiocolloid group, SLN identification was 91.3% in the massaged group and 81.7% in women who were not massaged. Based on these results, the researchers recommend that injections of the blue-dye and radiocolloid should be followed by a 5- to 6-minute massage before axillary exploration. This practice can maximize SLN identification to detect the early spread of breast cancer.

Finally, cancer can spread by diffusion, the spread of clumps of cancer cells from the surface of the tumor by mechanical means. This type of spread is particularly prevalent in serous cavities such as the abdominal or pleural cavity. In the peritoneal cavity, cells tend to gravitate to the pelvis. Cancer cells also can be implanted, or "seeded," during a surgical procedure, causing metastatic lesions. Metastasis may regress or disappear without apparent cause and remain dormant for many years, only to resume growth years later.

Sites of Metastases. The site of metastatic spread depends on the venous or lymphatic drainage of the organ involved, type of cancer, and tissue factors in potential metastatic sites. Various body tissues seem to have different attractions for metastases, common sites being, in order, the liver, lungs, bone, brain, and adrenal glands. The spleen, muscle, and skin are rarely involved. Table 15-5 shows the pattern of metastasis of some common primary tumors.

Classifying and Naming Neoplasms

Tumors derive their names from the type of tissue involved (Table 15-6), but classification of malignant tumors is difficult because many cancers contain several types of cells, including

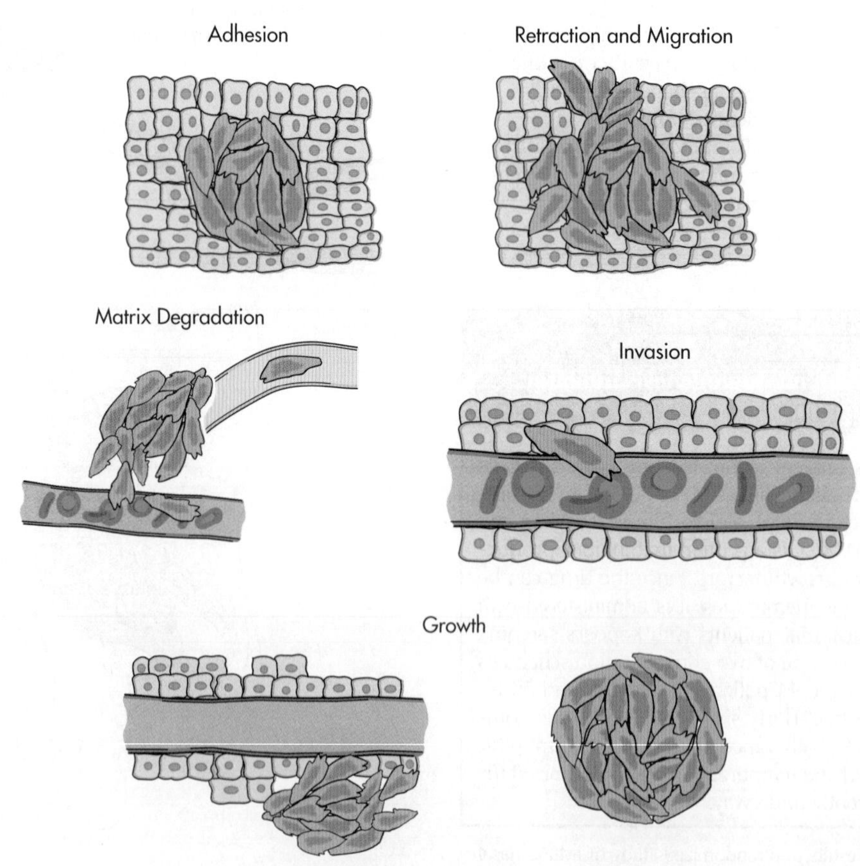

Figure 15-6 Process of dissemination of cancer cells from the bloodstream.

benign tissue. In general, the names of benign tumors carry the suffix *oma* after the name of the parent tissue, for example, neuroma or fibroma; but there are exceptions.

Cancers may be classified according to the cell type of origin. Two main cell types are epithelial and mesenchymal (connective tissue). The term *carcinoma* denotes a malignant tumor of epithelial cells, and the term *sarcoma* denotes a malignant tumor of connective tissue cells. Carcinomas may be further classified as arising from glandular epithelium with the prefix *adeno* or arising from the squamous epithelium with the word *squamous.* When a malignant tumor contains all three types of embryonal tissue, it is termed a *teratoma.* Tumors that originate during the primitive blastula embryonic phase have the suffix *blastoma.* Other terms may be added to describe the histology, or tissue structure, within the tumor, such as follicular or cystic.

Tumors also are classified according to cellular maturity. When there is complete loss of identity with the tissue of origin, the tumor is called undifferentiated (anaplastic). Some tumors are known by the names of the scientists who first described them, for example, Hodgkin's disease and Wilms' tumor. Other tumors are named after the organ from which they arise, for example, hepatoma and thymoma. In a small percentage of cases, the tissue of origin may never be identified, despite aggressive investigation including postmortem examination. Such cases, termed cancer of unknown primary, are

TABLE 15-5 Sites of Metastasis in Common Cancers

Cancer	Sites of Metastasis
Bladder	Bone Bone marrow Brain Liver Lung Skin
Breast	Adrenal glands Bone Brain Liver Lung Lymph nodes • Axillary • Internal mammary • Supraclavicular Skin
Lung	Adrenal glands Bone Brain Liver Lung (ipsilateral) Lymph nodes • Hilar • Mediastinal
Prostate	Bone Kidney Liver Lung Lymph nodes • Perineural • Sacral • External iliac • Lumbar • Pelvic Seminal vesicles
Cervical	Bone Liver Lung Lymph nodes • Femoral • Iliac • Hypogastric
Endometrial	Lymph nodes • Femoral • Iliac • Hypogastric
Ovarian	Lymph nodes • Iliac • Inguinal • Paraaortic • Retroperitoneal Peritoneal surfaces • Bladder • Diaphragm • Intestines • Liver
Testicular	Bone Brain Liver Lymph nodes • Pelvis • Paraaortic • Supraclavicular
Colorectal	Adrenal glands Bone Brain Liver Lung Lymph nodes • Inguinal • Perineal
Leukemia	Central nervous system (CNS) Skin Testes
Melanoma	Liver Lung Lymph nodes: Regional
Head and neck	Bone Liver Lung Lymph nodes: Regional
CNS tumors	Rarely metastasize Seeding to distant CNS structure (e.g., spinal cord)

From Hawkins R: Mastering the maze of metastasis, *Oncol Nurs Forum* 28:959, 2001.

TABLE 15-6 Classification of Neoplasms

Parent Tissue	Benign Tumor	Malignant Tumor
Epithelium		
Skin and mucous membrane	Papilloma Polyp	Squamous cell carcinoma Basal cell carcinoma Transitional cell carcinoma
Glands	Adenoma Cystadenoma	Adenocarcinoma
Endothelium		
Blood vessels	Hemangioma	Hemangiosarcoma Angiosarcoma
Lymph vessels	Lymphangioma	Lymphangiosarcoma
Bone marrow		Multiple myeloma Ewing's sarcoma Leukemia Lymphosarcoma Lymphangioendothelioma
Lymphoid tissue		Reticular cell sarcoma (difficult to classify because of cell embryology) Lymphatic leukemia Malignant lymphoma
Connective Tissue		
Embryonic fibrous tissue	Myxoma	Myxosarcoma
Fibrous tissue	Fibroma	Fibrosarcoma
Adipose tissue	Lipoma	Liposarcoma
Cartilage	Chondroma	Chondrosarcoma
Bone	Osteoma	Osteogenic sarcoma
Synovial membrane	Synovioma	Synovial sarcoma
Muscle Tissue		
Smooth muscle	Leiomyoma	Leiomyosarcoma
Striated muscle	Rhabdomyoma	Rhabdomyosarcoma
Nerve Tissue		
Nerve fibers and sheaths	Neuroma Neurinoma (neurilemoma)	Neurogenic sarcoma Neurofibrosarcoma
Ganglion cells	Neurofibroma	Neuroblastoma
Glial cells	Ganglioneuroma Glioma	Glioblastoma Spongioblastoma
Meninges	Meningioma	
Pigmented Neoplasms		
Melanoblasts	Pigmented nevus	Malignant melanoma Melanocarcinoma
Miscellaneous		
Placenta	Hydatidiform mole Dermoid cyst	Chorion-epithelioma (choriocarcinoma) Embryonal carcinoma Embryonal sarcoma Teratocarcinoma

frequently adenocarcinoma by histologic classification, metastatic at the time of diagnosis, and have a poor prognosis.

Methods of Classifying Degree of Malignancy

The degree of malignancy, or grade, is based on microscopic examination of the tissue. Tumors are graded by Arabic numerals into four grades. A higher grade means the tissue appears more abnormal and generally is more aggressive. A grade 1 tumor is the most differentiated (most like the tissue of origin) and therefore the least malignant, whereas a grade 4 is the least differentiated (unlike the tissue of origin) and has a high degree of malignancy. The grade of a tumor can guide decisions about treatment and provide prognostic information, although tissue differentiation may vary within a tumor

BOX 15-2 Classification of Malignant Lesions by Grade and Stage

Grade*	Stage*
Grade 0	*Stage 0*
Normal tissue	Cancer in situ
Grade 1	*Stage I*
Well differentiated, with minimal deviation from tissue of origin	Tumor limited to tissue of origin
Grade 2	*Stage II*
Moderately well differentiated, with evidence of structural changes from normal tissue of origin	Limited local spread
Grade 3	*Stage III*
Poorly differentiated, with extensive structural changes from normal tissue of origin	Extensive local and regional spread
Grade 4	*Stage IV*
Very anaplastic, with no resemblance to tissue of origin	Widespread metastasis

*Not all malignant lesions will have a direct correlation between grade and stage. The pathologist will make the final determination.

BOX 15-3 TNM Staging Classification System

Tumor	
T0	No evidence of primary tumor
T1S	Carcinoma in situ
T1, T2, T3, T4	Ascending degrees of tumor size and involvement
Nodes	
N0	No evidence of disease in lymph nodes
N1a, N2a	Disease found in regional lymph nodes; metastasis not suspected
N1b, N2b, N3	Disease found in regional lymph nodes; metastasis suspected
Nx	Regional nodes cannot be assessed clinically
Metastasis	
M0	No evidence of distant metastasis
M1, M2, M3	Ascending degrees of metastatic involvement of the host, including distant nodes

BOX 15-4 Seven Warning Signs of Cancer

1. **C**hange in bowel and bladder habits
2. **A** sore that does not heal
3. **U**nusual bleeding or discharge
4. **T**hickening or a lump in the breast or elsewhere
5. **I**ndigestion or difficulty in swallowing
6. **O**bvious change in a wart or mole
7. **N**agging cough or hoarseness

and change over time. Staging is a form of classification that describes the gross extent of the tumor and its spread (metastasis) throughout the body. This classification is critical to the physician in planning the appropriate treatment and giving prognostic information (Box 15-2).

Determination of the cancer stage and the site of the original tumor are vital for planning therapy. The International Union Against Cancer (UICC) and the American Joint Committee on Cancer (AJCC) have devised the TNM system of classification: T, primary tumor; N, regional lymph nodes; M, metastases. The TNM system is a uniform system used worldwide for describing the anatomic extent of most solid cancers (Box 15-3). The system provides a type of "shorthand" notation to describe the particular tumor. The purpose of the TNM system is to create categories that can be used to describe all cases and also allow subsequent and more detailed information to be added as it becomes known. Accurate classification is important for treatment planning, end results reporting, communication, and clinical trials research.

Clinical Manifestations of Cancer

The clinical manifestations of cancer may be diverse and affect multiple systems, depending on the site and size of the tumor. Nurses need to be aware of the more common signs and symptoms of cancer to aid in the early detection of cancer. Box 15-4 lists seven warning signs of cancer. In addition, any unexplained weight loss or pain, fatigue, night sweats, or irregularities in the genital or neurologic system should be investigated as possible symptoms of cancer.

Tumors can cause serious problems if they obstruct the lumen of tubular structures such as the ureter, trachea, or intestinal tract. Intraspinal and intracranial tumors cause symptoms because of the pressure they exert within a closed space. Tumors also may degenerate or cause atrophy and ulceration of overlying epithelium. Hemorrhage and infection may also develop at the site. In addition, many cancers cause a variety of systemic effects that may occur either early or late in the disease course and depend on the location and activity of the tumor. Hematologic and immunologic abnormalities such as infection and bleeding, hormonal and endocrine changes, and neuromuscular disorders may result from a malignant process.

COLLABORATIVE CARE MANAGEMENT

Prevention and Health Promotion

Nurses play a major role in educating the public about primary and secondary cancer prevention. The government's health initiative, Healthy People 2010, outlines multiple objectives related to cancer prevention and control[31] (see Healthy People 2010 box). Nurses have many opportunities to promote these initiatives through public education.

Even though the public has a greater knowledge of cancer than ever before, positive attitudes about cancer and the

Healthy People 2010

Objectives Related to Cancer

1. Reduce the overall cancer death rate to 159.9 deaths per 100,000 population or by 21%.
2. Reduce the lung cancer death rate to 44.9 deaths per 100,000 population or by 22%.
   a. Target risk factors of cigarette smoking, occupational exposures, and air pollution.
3. Reduce the breast cancer death rate to 27.9 deaths per 100,000 population or by 20%.
   a. Encourage mammography screening.
   b. Target risk factor of obesity.
4. Reduce the death rate from cancer of the uterine cervix to 2.0 deaths per 100,000 females.
   a. Encourage screening with a Pap test.
   b. Encourage protection against sexually transmitted diseases.
5. Reduce the colorectal cancer death rate to 13.9 deaths per 100,000 population or by 34%.
   a. Target risk factors of obesity, diet, and alcohol intake.
   b. Encourage screening and early detection tests.
6. Reduce the oropharyngeal cancer death rate to 2.7 deaths per 100,000 population or by 10%.
   a. Target risk factors of alcohol and tobacco use.
7. Reduce the prostate cancer death rate to 28.8 deaths per 100,000 males or by 10%.
   a. Encourage participation in trials to identify benefits of screening and treatments.
8. Reduce the rate of melanoma cancer deaths to 2.5 deaths per 100,000 population or by 11%.
   a. Target risk factor of sun exposure.
9. Increase to 75% the proportion of persons who limit sun exposure, use sunscreens and protective clothing when exposed to sunlight, and avoid artificial sources of ultraviolet light.
10. Increase to 85% the proportion of physicians and dentists who counsel their at-risk patients about tobacco use cessation, physical activity, and cancer screening.
11. Increase to 97% of women aged 18 years and older who have ever received a Pap test, and to 90% of women aged 18 years and older who received a Pap test within the preceding 3 years.
12. Increase to 50% the proportion of adults who receive a colorectal cancer screening examination.
13. Increase to 67% the proportion of women aged 40 years and older who have received a mammogram within the preceding 2 years.
14. Increase the number of states to 45 that have a statewide population-based cancer registry that captures case information on at least 95% of the expected number of reported cancers.
15. Increase to 70% the proportion of cancer survivors who are living 5 years or longer after diagnosis.

From US Department of Health and Human Services: *Healthy People 2010: understanding and improving health,* Washington, DC, 2000, USDHHS.

health care system are essential if persons are to adhere to good health practices. Many factors play a role in whether a person will change an unhealthy or undesirable behavior after receiving health teaching. What individuals believe about their susceptibility, the costs of changing the behavior, and the health message are examples of influential factors. In addition, many barriers have been identified that prevent optimal success of cancer screening programs.[23] Barriers associated with health care providers include lack of time and expertise to integrate comprehensive cancer screening. Patient barriers include lack of funds, transportation, or support to access the screening program. Finally, the health care system may have inadequate resources to offer comprehensive screening. A population with increasing cultural diversity also presents challenges to effective screening. For example, certain minority groups, the poor, and the less educated are less likely to access screening programs. Nurses need to consider a wide range of issues when designing and participating in cancer prevention and screening activities.

Anxiety and fear about cancer may also immobilize the individual. A cancer diagnosis, aspects of treatment, and uncertainty about prognosis can be frightening. People may view cancer as the inevitable loss of a job, income, and an enjoyable lifestyle, as well as premature death. All nurses can emphasize the positive aspects of the early diagnosis of cancer and how early diagnosis can mean a greater chance for cure and a normal lifestyle. An estimated one third of persons for whom a cancer diagnosis is made are cured by medical treatment. Another one third could perhaps be cured by medical treatment if the cancer were diagnosed early enough. The 5-year survival rate for all cancers is 60% and continues to increase with continuous discoveries that improve diagnosis and treatment methods.

Primary Prevention

A cancer risk factor may be defined as something specific to an individual that increases the possibility of developing a malignancy. Risk factors are identified and reduced whenever possible. Three types of risk factors for cancer have been identified. Lifestyle factors are those over which the person has some control, especially tobacco use, diet, alcohol use, sunlight exposure, and sexual practices. Environmental factors include exposure to carcinogens and are at times beyond the individual's control. Genetic factors—conditions inherited at conception—are not usually controllable, but genetic counseling may provide guidance about risk reduction and early detection strategies.

Primary prevention attempts to reduce a person's exposure to any known risk factors that might lead to disease.[22] This is an insurmountable task in cancer prevention, inasmuch as all risk factors are not known or have not been proved as factors in specific cancer development. However, substantial evidence demonstrates a direct link between certain environmental and lifestyle factors and cancer development. Examples include smoking and lung cancer, excessive sun exposure and skin cancer, and low dietary fiber content and colon cancer.

Nurses must have knowledge of these cancer risk factors and be active in educating the public. Nurses can teach in both the hospital and clinic settings, where health promotion and counseling are routine components of everyday practice. Participation in community health fairs as well as conducting

BOX 15-5 Treating Tobacco Use and Dependence: a Guide for All Clinicians

1. Identify tobacco use and assess willingness to quit.
2. For tobacco users willing to quit, implement the "5 As":
   a. *Ask* about tobacco use.
   b. *Advise* all users to quit.
   c. *Assess* willingness to make a quit attempt.
   d. *Assist* the patient with a plan to quit.
      Set a date.
      Give practical counseling.
      Identify social supports.
      Recommend the use of approved pharmacotherapy.
      Provide supplementary materials.
   e. *Arrange* scheduled follow-up.
3. For tobacco users unwilling to quit, implement the "5 Rs":
   a. Explain why quitting is personally *relevant.*
   b. Highlight the *risks* of tobacco use.
   c. Identify the potential *rewards* of stopping.
   d. Identify the *roadblocks* to quitting.
   e. *Repeat* at every opportunity.
4. For former smokers, implement relapse prevention strategies.
   a. Discuss benefits from cessation.
   b. Emphasize the success in quitting.
   c. Discuss any problems or threats encountered.

Adapted from Fiore MC et al:. *Treating tobacco use and dependence: quick reference guide for clinicians,* Rockville, Md, October 2000, US Department of Health and Human Services, Public Health Service.

public education in schools and places of business are also roles where nurses can educate the public about cancer prevention.

Every nurse has the responsibility to promote a tobacco-free and smoke-free lifestyle. Tobacco is the leading cause of disease and death in the United States, and effective treatments for tobacco dependence are available. In 2000 the Public Health Service, in collaboration with a multidisciplinary panel of consultants, published a reference guide for clinicians, "Treating Tobacco Use and Dependence," to assist all clinicians in incorporating tobacco dependence interventions into their practice.[9] The interventions include identifying and assessing tobacco use in every patient, providing patients who are willing to quit with the appropriate interventions, treating patients who are not willing to quit at this time with motivational interventions, and, finally, providing relapse prevention treatment to patients who have recently quit using tobacco. The plan is summarized in Box 15-5.

Primary prevention for skin cancer involves avoiding excessive and prolonged exposure to the sun and other sources of ultraviolet radiation, such as tanning beds. These practices are especially important for persons with light-complexioned skin. Nurses remind patients that skin damage from the sun occurs even without sunburns, and that regular use of a sunscreen with a sun protection factor of 15% or higher can significantly reduce the lifetime incidence of skin cancer.

Strategies to prevent colon cancer include nutritional interventions as well as the removal of precancerous adenomatous polyps. The dietary risk factors for colon cancer include a diet high in animal fat, low in fiber, and high in alcohol consumption. Nurses counsel patients to limit the amount of fat and alcohol in their diet and include sources of fiber (Box 15-6). Because it is known that colorectal cancers arise from precursor adenomatous polyps, removing such polyps can reduce the risk of subsequent colon cancer.

BOX 15-6 Nutritional Recommendations to Reduce Cancer Risk

Choose Most of the Foods You Eat From Plant Sources.

Eat five or more servings of fruits and vegetables each day. Include other foods from plant sources, such as whole grain breads and cereals, rice, and beans.

Limit Your Intake of High-Fat Foods, Particularly From Animal Sources.

Choose foods low in fat and limit consumption of meats, especially high-fat and red meats.

Be Physically Active: Achieve and Maintain a Healthy Weight.

Be at least moderately active for 30 minutes on most days of the week. Stay within your healthy weight range.

Limit Consumption of Alcoholic Beverages, If You Drink At All.

Modified from American Cancer Society: *Cancer prevention & early detection: facts & figures—2001,* Atlanta, 2001, The Society.

Chemoprevention involves the use of chemical agents to reverse or suppress the malignant process. A number of chemoprevention trials have been instituted, and many agents have been identified as having potential benefit for use with individuals with an increased risk for certain cancers. In 1998, the drug tamoxifen was shown to reduce the chance of developing breast cancer by 49% in premenopausal and postmenopausal women at increased risk.[10] Another drug, raloxifene, was also shown to reduce the incidence of breast cancer. The STAR trial is currently evaluating whether raloxifene is as effective as tamoxifen in reducing breast cancer risk. Additional chemoprevention trials are underway.

The importance of identifying cancer risk through genetic counseling is growing as more information about genetic mutations are linked to cancer development. Patients with and without family histories of cancer seek information about their unique cancer risks, and new methods to answer these questions are becoming more widely available. Patients whose test results indicate a genetic predisposition to cancer may be referred for additional surveillance, prophylactic surgery, chemoprevention, or risk avoidance. Nurses in many settings are likely to encounter patients who seek information about their genetic risk, and nurses need to know how and when to refer patients for genetic counseling. Oncology nurses also have the opportunity to specialize in cancer genetics. Cancer genetics nursing roles include performing risk assessments, educating about risk and risk-reduction options, as well as coordinating individualized cancer surveillance plans.[23] Nurses who practice in this arena must also be sensitive to the ethical issues associated with identifying individuals at high risk for cancer.

Secondary Prevention

Secondary prevention efforts are aimed at early diagnosis and prompt effective treatment for persons without clinical signs or symptoms of cancer. Once the diagnosis is known, definitive treatment is begun. For successful secondary prevention, there must be a means to detect and cure the cancer at an early stage. Most cancer screening programs are examples of secondary prevention activities.

At present, early detection methods are not available for all cancers. Screening tools that have enabled the detection of early asymptomatic cancers and are known to reduce cancer mortality include mammograms and Pap smears. Use of the prostate-specific antigen (PSA) to detect early stage prostate cancer has also caused dramatic declines in the mortality rates for prostate cancer. The use of chest x-ray films to screen for lung cancer has been largely unsuccessful because of their low sensitivity in detecting early lesions. Clinical trials are investigating the feasibility of low radiation dose computed tomography (CT) as a screening tool for lung cancer. The American Cancer Society (ACS) has developed guidelines for early detection of common cancers for average-risk individuals with no symptoms (Table 15 -7). In addition, the ACS recommends that individuals with higher risks for particular cancers have more frequent and/or additional examinations. Health care professionals together with the patient can choose the most appropriate early-detection protocol that meets the individual's risk potential. The goal is to discover early cancer in persons who have no symptoms.

The nurse's role in screening and early detection begins with a sound knowledge of cancer, known risk factors, and the treatment modalities available.[18] Cancer risk assessment must be an integral part of every interaction the nurse has with the public. Data obtained from interviews, the nursing history, physical examinations, social and family histories, health surveys and questionnaires, and employment records help the nurse determine the person's individual cancer risk factors.

Nurses can teach women that the breast, lung, gastrointestinal tract, and uterus are the most common sites of cancer in women. Women are taught to examine their breasts each

TABLE 15-7 American Cancer Society Recommendations for the Early Detection of Cancer in Average Risk, Asymptomatic People

Cancer Site	Population	Test or Procedure	Frequency
Breast	Women, age 20+	Breast self-examination	Monthly, starting at age 20
		Clinical breast examination	Every 3 years, ages 20-39 Annual, starting at age 40*
		Mammography	Annual, starting at age 40
Colorectal	Men and women, age 50+	Fecal occult blood test (FOBT) and flexible sigmoidoscopy†	Annual FOBT and flexible sigmoidoscopy every 5 years, starting at age 50
		-or-	
		Flexible sigmoidoscopy	Every 5 years, starting at age 50
		-or-	
		FOBT	Annual, starting at age 50
		-or-	
		Colonoscopy	Colonoscopy every 10 years, starting at age 50
		-or-	
		Double contrast barium enema (DCBE)†	DCBE every 5 years, starting at age 50
Prostate	Men, age 50+	Digital rectal examination and prostate specific antigen test	The PSA test and the DRE should be offered annually, starting at age 50, for men who have a life expectancy of at least 10 years‡
Cervix	Women, age 18+	Pap test and pelvic examination	All women who are, or have been, sexually active, or have reached age 18 should have an annual Pap test and pelvic examination; after a woman has had 3 or more consecutive satisfactory normal annual examinations, the Pap test may be performed less frequently at the discretion of the physician
Cancer-related check-up	Men and women, age 20+	Examinations every 3 years from ages 20 to 39 years and annually after age 40; the cancer-related check-up should include examination for cancers of the thyroid, testicles, ovaries, lymph nodes, oral cavity, and skin, as well as health counseling about tobacco, sun exposure, diet and nutrition, risk factors, sexual practices, and environmental and occupational exposures	

From Smith R et al: American Cancer Society Guidelines for the early detection of cancer: update of early detection guidelines for prostate, colorectal, and endometrial cancer, *CA: Cancer J Clin* 51:38, 2001.

*Beginning at age 40, annual clinical breast examination should be performed before mammography.

†Flexible sigmoidoscopy together with FOBT is preferred compared with flexible sigmoidoscopy alone.

‡Information should be provided to men about the benefits and limitations of testing.

month immediately after the menstrual period or, after menopause, on a designated day each month and to have mammography at regular intervals. Even though the value of breast self-evaluation (BSE) in early detection has been questioned in recent research, nurses should still encourage BSE until conclusive evidence is found. Women of all ages should know the importance of reporting any abnormal vaginal bleeding or discharge that occurs between menstrual periods or after menopause. Women are encouraged to have routine gastrointestinal screening and gynecologic examinations and to take precautions against sexually transmitted diseases. (See Chapter 53 for details of early symptoms of cancer of the female reproductive system.)

Men should be made aware that their risk is greatest for cancers of the prostate, lung, and gastrointestinal tract. Men can be screened for colorectal cancer with routine fecal occult blood testing and sigmoidoscopy, and they can be screened for prostate cancer with the digital rectal examination and PSA test. The incidence of testicular cancer overall is small; however, it is most prevalent in young men between the ages of 15 and 40 years. Regular testicular self-examination, like BSE in women, is important for this age group.

Older adults as a group require more individualized health teaching about cancer risk and detection methods. This population may already have other chronic illnesses and take several medications. New symptoms, therefore, may be difficult to recognize as early warning signs of cancer. The elderly may be reluctant to undergo routine screening or to report new physical complaints because of their fears of cancer, a tenuous financial state, or feelings of hopelessness if a diagnosis of cancer is made. Health care professionals need to encourage elders to participate in health education and screening programs and tailor these programs for the unique needs of this population. Nurses in all settings need to incorporate cancer assessment as well as teaching about early detection into the care of elders.

Diagnostic Tests

Laboratory Tests

Many laboratory tests are pertinent to the diagnosis of cancer. Laboratory tests can be used to diagnose a specific organ malfunction or metabolic aberration that may reveal a benign or malignant condition. Some common tests used in cancer detection include a complete blood count, a serum chemistry profile (sodium, potassium, chloride, carbon dioxide, bicarbonate, glucose, blood urea nitrogen), and examination of body fluids, such as sputum and urine, for blood. More specific tests measure the presence of tumor markers, or proteins associated with specific cancers, in serum or body fluids. For example, a serum PSA test may be done if prostate cancer is suspected, or a carcinoembryonic antigen test may be performed for follow-up testing of suspicious lesions of the gastrointestinal tract or to monitor for disease progression after treatment. Tumor markers can also monitor the patient's response to cancer therapy (Table 15-8). Newer laboratory techniques used in the diagnosis of cancer include radioimmunoassays and flow cytometry. Radioimmunoassay techniques measure tumor antigen in the serum using radiolabeled antigens. Flow cytometry identifies cellular and DNA characteristics of the tissue that may yield important diagnostic and prognostic information (e.g., to differentiate the types of leukemia).

Cytology

In 1942 Dr. George Papanicolaou showed that the diagnosis of cancer could be made from the study of cells that have sloughed or exfoliated from a tumor. These cells are found in body secretions such as cervical discharges, sputum, gastric washings, pleural fluid, and urinary washings. The secretion is spread on a slide, stained, and examined by a pathologist, who can classify the tissue as benign, dysplastic ("suspicious"), or malignant. The main use of the Pap smear, as it is often called, is to diagnose cancer in an asymptomatic person and to identify precancerous lesions or noninvasive cancer. If suspicious cells are found, a biopsy must be performed to confirm the diagnosis of cancer. The Pap smear is most widely used for examining cervical washings.

Tumor Imaging

Radiographs, or x-ray studies, are commonly obtained to provide two-dimensional views of organs. Because air, bone, and soft tissue absorb x-rays differently, their structure and function can be distinguished on the film. Chest x-ray studies and mammograms are common radiographic examinations used in the diagnosis of cancer.

CT provides three-dimensional views of internal structures. CT scans are some of the most useful and most used tests in the diagnosis of cancer because they can detect smaller lesions than x-rays.

TABLE 15-8 Markers Used to Detect and Monitor Cancer

Markers	Associated Tumor
Human chorionic gonadotropin, beta subunit (B-HCG)	Testicular cancer, choriocarcinoma
Bence Jones protein	Multiple myeloma
Alpha-fetoprotein (AFP)	Testicular, choriocarcinoma, pancreas, colon, lung, stomach, liver
Carcinoembryonic antigen (CEA)	Lung, gastrointestinal, breast, pancreas
Prostate specific antigen (PSA)	Prostate
CA-125	Ovarian, pancreas, breast, colon, lung, liver
CA-19-9	Ovarian, pancreas
CA-15-3	Breast

Other radiographic tests use contrast media to better outline and distinguish structures. The barium enema and the intravenous pyelogram, which studies the genitourinary tract, are common examples of contrast studies. Nuclear medicine procedures involve scanning organs after the ingestion or instillation of a radiolabeled material. Diseased organs often show increased or abnormal uptake of the radioisotope. Such scans may be used to study the bones, liver, and thyroid.

Positron emission tomography (PET) studies glucose metabolism in body tissues and is proving useful in differentiating varying rates of tissue metabolism. Because tumors have a high rate of glycolysis, malignant tissues accumulate higher concentrations of radioactive glucose compounds, which are detected with gamma camera tomography. PET scans can accurately map organ structures and define malignant masses.

Ultrasound probing, or echography, is performed by means of an electronic instrument that detects and records echoes of sound when they are reflected at the junction of tissue with different densities. The procedure is helpful in differentiating between cystic and solid tumors.

Magnetic resonance imaging (MRI) uses a magnetic field and radiofrequency waves to align hydrogen nuclei in tissues. A computer then analyzes the tissues for abnormalities. The results can be enhanced with the use of contrast agents. MRIs are contraindicated for persons with any implanted metallic device that is susceptible to the magnetic pull of the MRI machine. Table 15-9 lists some common scanning procedures used to diagnose cancer

Invasive Diagnostic Techniques

Biopsy. A biopsy is the only definitive way to diagnose cancer. It is essential to obtain and accurately identify an adequate tissue sample before any cancer therapy is prescribed. An incisional biopsy involves the surgical removal of a section of the neoplasm. If the tumor is small and can be removed in its entirety an excisional biopsy is performed. When possible, an aspiration biopsy (needle biopsy), which removes a small plug of tumor by a needle or syringe, is used to avoid the larger incisional or excisional biopsy. Needle biopsy, although inexpensive and relatively simple to perform in an outpatient setting, has the potential of missing the malignant focus and "seeding" tumor cells along the needle track as it is inserted and withdrawn.

The biopsy specimen is examined to establish a histologic diagnosis and identify important cytologic features of the tumor. A growing number of cancers are now associated with cytogenetic abnormalities, such as chromosomal translocations and deletions. Chronic myelogenous leukemia (CML) has long been associated with the Philadelphia chromosome that features a translocation between chromosomes 9 and 22, forming the BCR-ABL oncogenic protein that has high tyrosine kinase activity. This oncogene is now the target of a new genetic therapy, Gleevec. Other cytogenetic changes can be used as tumor markers and yield prognostic information. In acute myelogenous leukemia the presence of chromosomal translocations such as t(15;17) and t(8;21) indicates a good prognosis. The HER/2neu growth factor receptor is an important marker in breast cancer.

Endoscopy. Hollow metal tubes equipped with a light are used to illuminate various body cavities, permitting visual inspection of the interior of the cavity being examined. These instruments are commonly referred to as scopes and are named for the organs they visualize. A bronchoscope is used to examine the bronchus; a gastroscope is used to visualize the stomach; and a proctoscope is used to visualize the anus and sigmoid colon. Many abdominal structures can be examined by laparoscopy or by the insertion of the instrument into the abdominal space. The laparoscope can be used to inspect the liver, diaphragm, and peritoneum as well as gastrointestinal, gynecologic, and genitourinary structures, thus avoiding a

TABLE 15-9 X-ray and Scanning Procedures Used in Cancer Diagnosis

Study	Procedure	Comment
Lymphangiography	Oil-based blue dye and procaine (Novocain) injected in skin of web between first and second toes or index and second fingers to show lymphatic drainage of extremities	Used in diagnosing lymph and metastatic cancer. Lymphomatous nodes have "foamy" or "lacy" structure. Metastatic nodes have "moth-eaten" appearance. Bluish-green skin discoloration from dye may last 1 week
Xeroradiography	X-ray image on plate of selenium-coated metal	Provides picture of soft tissue
Tomography	X-ray image with ability to penetrate dense shadows	Provides picture of soft tissue
Thermography	Constructs photographic images of surface temperature	Identifies skin temperature elevations over inflammatory or malignant lesions
Computed tomography (CT) scan	X-ray beam and use of computer	Produces images of plane sections of body; identifies size and location of tumors
Magnetic resonance imaging (MRI)	Magnetic fields	Produces a cross-sectional image of the body; spares patient from x-ray exposure
Positron-emission tomography (PET)	Scanners that rotate around patient; image formed by positrons emitted by isotope injected into or inhaled by patient	Allows viewing of brain and body processes in three dimensions; gives a picture of biochemical and metabolic processes

major surgical procedure. A biopsy specimen of a mass or secretions in the organ can be obtained during any of these endoscopic procedures.

Diagnostic tests provide critical information about the primary tumor, extent of the disease, and its stage. The natural course of each specific cancer and its pattern of spread are considered when looking for evidence of the tumor throughout the body. Table 15-10 outlines some common malignancies and diagnostic tests used in their evaluation.

Nursing Management During the Diagnostic Phase

The nurse's role during the phase of diagnostic testing for cancer is to prepare the patient for each test and procedure, explain the rationale for the test, and inform the patient of where and when the test will take place. Nurses may also be involved in obtaining laboratory specimens, assisting with radiology procedures, and interpreting test results. Tests and procedures often require the patient to go without food, and tests can disrupt normal activity and sleep patterns. Some tests cause discomfort, including being immobilized in uncomfortable positions for lengthy intervals, placement of catheters or needles, or use of distasteful or uncomfortable contrast materials. Nursing interventions emphasize the patient's physical and emotional comfort. Premedication with analgesics, antiemetics, or sedatives may be necessary to ensure the patient's physical comfort during the procedure.

Patients and families often experience a great deal of anxiety about the possibility of a cancer diagnosis. Although the word cancer may not be mentioned, it is usually an overriding fear for both patients and their families. Diagnostic tests and procedures can cause anxiety and apprehension even when the rationale for their use is clearly explained. Nurses offer support to the patient and the entire family at this critical time.

Hospitalization of a family member and the fear of a cancer diagnosis can lead to changes in family roles that cause some members to assume responsibilities and tasks that are new and uncomfortable to them. The spouse or adult children may need to take on the role of decision maker and caretaker

TABLE 15-10 Common Malignant Conditions and Commonly Used Diagnostic Tests and Procedures*

Malignancy	Laboratory Tests and Procedures Used
Breast cancer	Breast physical examination Ultrasound Mammography Tissue and lymph node biopsy
Lung cancer	Chest x-ray Computed tomography (CT) scan Sputum cytology Fiberoptic bronchoscopy with biopsy and bronchial washings Medastinography (endoscopic examination of mediastinum and nodes)
Gastrointestinal cancers	
Esophagus	Chest x-ray CT scan Magnetic resonance imaging (MRI) Esophagoscopy and biopsy Barium contrast studies (barium swallow)
Stomach	As above Gastric secretion analysis Carcinoembryonic antigen (CEA)
Colorectal	As above Stool guaiac Barium enema Proctosigmoidoscopy and biopsy
Liver	As above Liver biopsy Liver enzyme studies
Genitourinary cancers	
Prostate	Digital rectal examination Bone scan Biopsy Urinalysis Laboratory: prostatic-specific antigen, serum acid phosphatase
Bladder	Cytology Cystoscopy (internal examination of bladder) Intravenous pyelogram (IVP) (examination of calyx, pelvis, and lower part of urinary tract using contrast medium) Urinalysis
Kidney	CT scan Renal angiogram, sonogram X-ray studies of kidney, ureters, and bladder Urinalysis IVP
Gynecologic cancers	
Cervix	Colposcopy (examination of the vagina and cervix by means of a magnifying lens) Biopsy Papanicolaou (Pap) test (smear)
Ovary	Pelvic physical examination Pap test IVP Barium enema Urinalysis
Uterus	Endometrial biopsy and aspiration

*The diagnostic tests cited are not a comprehensive list of tests and procedures used to detect specific cancers, but are only a representative sample of diagnostic aids used.

and possibly provide financial assistance. Families and significant others have the same information needs as the patient, including knowledge of the test results, information about the diagnosis and prognosis, and options for treatment. Nurses assist the patient and family to gain a sense of control and hope when the diagnosis of cancer is first made.

Treatment of Cancer

Once a diagnosis of cancer is confirmed and the extent of disease is defined, the patient and health care team begin the complex process of determining the most effective and appropriate therapy. The choice of treatment is based on characteristics of the patient, information about the specific cancer, and choices related to both quantity and quality of life. Cancers can be treated with surgery, radiation therapy, chemotherapy, and biologic therapy. Today most patients with cancer are treated with a combination of therapies referred to as multimodality therapy.

Surgical Management

Of the four major forms of cancer therapy (chemotherapy, radiation therapy, biotherapy, and surgery), surgery is the oldest and most widely used option. Surgery may be used for cancer diagnosis and staging, cure, adjuvant treatment, control of oncologic emergencies, or palliation of symptoms. Trends in cancer surgery include the use of more ambulatory procedures, minimally invasive approaches, and multimodality treatment plans.

The initial role of surgery in cancer therapy is diagnosis and staging of disease. Most cancers require tissue samples to confirm the diagnosis. Surgery is often the best way to obtain these samples. The type of surgical biopsy and its extent depend on the site and characteristics of the tumor.

When surgery is used for cure, the malignant lesion must be small, localized, and amenable to complete surgical removal. It is standard procedure to remove a wide margin of tissue surrounding the involved organ and to dissect the regional lymph nodes at the time of surgery. This technique can greatly reduce the incidence of local recurrence and increase survival rates, especially in tumors that disseminate through the lymphatics. However, the benefits of extensive surgery must be weighed against the prolonged recovery period and the disfigurement caused by more radical resections. Since the advent of newer and more potent cytotoxic agents and improved radiotherapy techniques, more conservative surgery is the accepted norm so that the patient has a better cosmetic outcome and more normal body function. Adjuvant, meaning aiding or assisting, chemotherapy or radiotherapy can be given before or after surgery to eliminate any microscopic cancer not removed by the surgery.

Surgical approaches for early stage breast cancer illustrate the trend toward less invasive therapy. Breast conservation techniques, such as lumpectomy followed by radiation therapy, have replaced the radical mastectomy. Lymphatic mapping and sentinel node biopsy are now performed rather than full axillary node dissections in some patients with early breast cancer. In this approach, a radiocolloid dye is injected into the tumor site and scanned with a gamma probe. The primary lymph node drainage site, or sentinel node, is identified, excised, and examined. If the sentinel node has no evidence of tumor, theoretically the cancer has not spread further down the lymph node chain and a full axillary dissection is not performed. The patient can be spared the additional surgery as well as the potential pain, immobility, and lymphedema associated with axillary node dissections.[13]

Surgery as a palliative procedure is a useful intervention for patients with more advanced disease. Palliative surgery may be used to reduce the bulk of an unresectable tumor or to stabilize a pathologic fracture. Examples of other palliative procedures include a jejunostomy tube for nutritional support or a tracheostomy to relieve tracheal obstruction. The formation of a colostomy to relieve colon obstruction and a laminectomy for spinal cord decompression are surgical procedures that improve the patient's quality of life but do not affect the cancer itself. Surgery can also provide pain control through a variety of surgical blocks.

Surgical interventions can also be used to support other treatment modalities such as radiation and chemotherapy. Surgical placement of a vascular access device enables safer chemotherapy administration. Applicators, which hold internal sources of radiation therapy, are commonly placed in the operating room with the patient under general anesthesia. Finally, reconstructive surgical procedures play an important role in improving body function and appearance for the patient with cancer. Breast reconstruction after mastectomy and facial reconstruction after head and neck surgery are commonly performed. Table 15-11 provides examples of surgical interventions currently used in the treatment of

TABLE 15-11 Surgical Approaches to Cancer Care

Intervention	Example
Diagnosis	Breast biopsy
Staging	Staging laparotomy Second-look laparotomy
Treatment of primary tumor	Curative resection (abdominal perineal resection)
Reconstruction, rehabilitation	Breast reconstruction Continent urostomy or ileostomy
Palliative	Endocrine ablation Pericardial window
Adjuvant	Paraaortic node dissection Hickman line insertion
Complications of other methods	Excision of bowel stricture Excision of radionecrotic tissue
Resection of metastases	Partial hepatectomy Pulmonary resection
Cytoreductive	Abdominal soft tissue sarcomas Ovarian peritoneal carcinoma
Emergencies	Obstruction Hemorrhage
Cancer prevention	Colectomy (familial polyposis) Orchidopexy (testicular tumors)

From McCorkle R et al: *Cancer nursing,* ed 2, Philadelphia, 1996, WB Saunders.

cancer. The operative procedures used to treat various types of cancer are discussed in later chapters under the specific organ systems.

NURSING MANAGEMENT OF PATIENT UNDERGOING CANCER SURGERY

PREOPERATIVE CARE

Before surgery the health care team assesses the patient's physical and emotional status to predict how well the patient can withstand the proposed surgical procedure and rehabilitation. Important factors to consider include age, nutritional status, and performance status, as well as the presence of any comorbid medical problems and the results of laboratory and diagnostic tests. Several performance scales are used to evaluate the patient's functional status, such as the Karnofsky Scale, outlined in Box 15-7. Other scales include the Eastern Cooperative Oncology Group (ECOG) scale, and the World Health Organization scale, which give the patient a score of 0 (bedridden or totally disabled) to 4 (asymptomatic and independent).

The presence of other physical problems, such as diabetes, arthritis, or heart disease, can complicate recovery from surgery. The patient may already have compromised respiratory function or limited mobility. The nurse notes these preexisting conditions before surgery and individualizes the patient's postoperative plan of care as necessary.

Patients need to be informed about postoperative care routines. Specific questions and concerns should be answered as honestly and promptly as possible. Discussion of the immediate postoperative period should occur, including any special equipment that may be needed, such as catheters, monitors, infusion lines, or chest tubes.

BOX 15-7 Karnofsky Performance Scale

A Subjective Assessment Tool to Assess and Compare the Patient's Activity and Performance Ability

Description	Score
Normal; no complaints; no evidence of disease	100
Able to carry on normal activity; minor signs or symptoms of disease	90
Normal activity with effort; some signs or symptoms of disease	80
Cares for self; unable to carry on normal activity or to do active work	70
Requires occasional assistance but is able to care for most needs	60
Requires considerable assistance and frequent medical care	50
Disabled; requires special care and assistance	40
Severely disabled; hospitalization is indicated, although death is not imminent	30
Hospitalization is necessary; very sick; active supportive treatment necessary	20
Moribund; fatal processes progressing rapidly	10
Dead	0

Relieving Anxiety

During the preoperative phase of care, the nurse develops a therapeutic relationship with the patient and family. Open and honest communication can assist the patient to maintain a realistic sense of hope. Explanations of the various tests and test results, as well as the goal of surgery (cure, palliation, or supportive treatment), help both patient and family be more active and informed in treatment decisions.

The age and physical status of the patient have considerable impact on acceptance of a cancer diagnosis, as well as on postoperative recovery and rehabilitation. Elderly persons may fear dying or becoming a burden to their families, both physically and financially. Patients in early adulthood to middle age have more physical stamina but may also have many emotional concerns. These patients are in their most productive years in relation to careers, educational opportunities, and sexual activity. They may fear loss of job security, financial independence, disfigurement, role adjustments within the family and community, and loss of reproductive capacity. Nurses need to discuss specific concerns with the patient and provide support with information and necessary resources.

Supporting Optimal Physical Status

The nutritional status of the patient requires careful assessment and intervention before surgery. Signs of poor nutrition or cachexia may develop before medical intervention is sought and before a definitive cancer diagnosis is confirmed. Patients may need nutritional support before surgery. Oral supplements, high in protein and calories, or total parenteral nutrition (TPN) if the patient cannot take and retain oral feedings, may need to begin in the preoperative period. The nurse emphasizes the importance of good nutrition with the patient and family. Sound nutrition helps the patient heal more quickly and have more strength and energy and usually means a shortened recovery time. Blood or blood products may need to be administered to patients with anemia. Autologous blood donations can be scheduled if the patient is healthy and the surgery is not imminent. The nurse assesses and documents the patient's response to these preoperative interventions and establishes priorities for high-risk areas that will need special interventions after surgery.

Postoperative Care

Preventing Infection and Bleeding

Meticulous postoperative care is especially important for patients with cancer because many patients are already physically compromised or immunodeficient before surgery as a consequence of the disease process and diagnostic testing. Patients are at increased risk for infection because of the presence of invasive devices, such as drains, indwelling catheters, and intravenous lines. The nurse carefully monitors each potential source for infection, documents findings, arranges for culture of any suspicious drainage, and notifies the physician immediately. Maintenance of strict asepsis is critical in the care of immunocompromised patients. The nurse teaches the patient and other caregivers the signs of infection and how to prevent, detect, and manage infectious complications. Visitors with an infectious process are advised to refrain from physical contact with the patient during this critical period. Antibiotic therapy to cover a wide range of organisms may be prescribed. (See Chapter 18 for a more detailed discussion of postoperative care and Chapter 11 for information about inflammation and infection control.)

Many patients with cancer are at risk for bleeding, and nurses carefully monitor for signs of postoperative bleeding. Bedside assessment includes clinical signs of bleeding at incision sites as well as results of laboratory tests.

Promoting Comfort

Comfort measures to alleviate and control pain are priority interventions for all postoperative patients. The patient following cancer surgery has the same type of analgesic needs as other surgical patients; however, the cancer patient may require larger and more frequent doses of analgesics to achieve adequate pain control. (See Chapter 12 for an in-depth discussion of pain control.)

Nurses ensure that the patient receives sufficient analgesia to relieve postoperative pain. Nursing interventions include prompt administration of pain medication as well as ongoing assessment to ensure effective relief and minimize side effects. Nurses are important advocates for needed changes in drug selection, dose, or administration schedule to achieve optimal pain relief. PCA pumps are popular options to manage postoperative pain because the pumps provide prompt medication administration, resulting in greater patient satisfaction. Relaxation, deep breathing, and imagery may also be components of the pain management plan. Sufficient pain relief ensures that optimal ambulation, nutrition, and participation in self-care (bathing, dressing, elimination) can be achieved.

Maintaining Functional Status

Because many cancer patients are elderly and physically debilitated before surgery, nursing interventions strive to increase and restore the patient's physical stamina as quickly as possible. The nurse capitalizes on all opportunities to enhance the patient's physical strength by active and passive exercises and the use of assistive devices such as canes or walkers. The nurse can enlist the aid of physical and occupational therapists to help achieve this goal. Early ambulation and activity after surgery are important to prevent deep vein thromboses.

Promoting Nutrition

Many factors influence the postoperative nutritional status of the patient with cancer. The catabolic state that exists during the perioperative period requires high caloric and protein replacement. The patient may have already been in a malnourished state before surgery, showing moderate to severe weight loss, decreased muscle mass, loss of adipose tissue, and an impaired immune response. The surgical procedure itself may necessitate anatomic alterations that interfere with normal ingestion, digestion, and absorption of nutrients. The nurse and dietitian are challenged to devise a plan for nutritional support that the patient can accept and follow. Strategies vary with each individual patient but include daily weights, daily calorie counts, offering food preferences when possible, teaching the importance of compliance with the prescribed diet; and providing oral, enteral, or parenteral supplements. Good oral hygiene and dentition help facilitate oral intake. Encouraging ambulation, diversional activities, and family visits during mealtimes may add to the patient's enjoyment and compliance with the nutrition regimen. The nurse needs to carefully evaluate how well the nutritional plan is working for the patient and family.

Providing Emotional Support

One of the first questions the patient may ask when awakening from anesthesia after surgery is "Was it cancer?" or "Did they get it all?" The family often asks the same questions. Fear that the tumor was malignant or unresectable is normal. The nurse anticipates these questions and is prepared to respond appropriately. Dealing honestly with the patient is essential to maintaining therapeutic communication and credibility. The nurse needs to be cognizant of what the surgeon has communicated to the patient so that the information conveyed is clear and consistent. For those patients who desire spiritual comfort, a minister, rabbi, or the hospital chaplain is contacted to provide strength and support.

After cancer surgery the patient faces the prospect of changes in lifestyle, role, and self-concept. Nurses need to be able to identify patients who are facing a critical loss or change. Patients who have had a mastectomy, colostomy, or gynecologic surgery may be especially troubled by body changes that make them feel less attractive and less functional. Patients may need encouragement to verbalize and discuss these reactions. Depression may manifest as mood disturbances, changes in activity, appetite, sleep, or sexual dysfunction many months after surgery. Nurses have a responsibility to explore the patient's feelings and concerns about changes in body image. The nurse encourages the inclusion of the partner in any discussion or information-sharing session related to family relationships or the patient's sexuality. The patient and the patient's partner need to be aware of the patient's decreased energy level during the postoperative and rehabilitation stage. Sexual desire or the ability to perform sexually may diminish. Alternative methods of sexual expression (e.g., hugging, caressing, alternative positioning) are suggested, and information is provided on alternatives such as breast reconstructive surgery or sexual stimulants and prostheses. Patients need to know that grieving a lost body part or function is natural, and the nurse actively supports the patient during this time. Support groups are helpful to many people, and the nurse ensures that the patient receives the name and phone number of appropriate groups in the local community, or initiates contact directly with patient's permission.

Biotherapy

Principles Underlying Biotherapy. The immune system and the immune response to cancer have been studied for many years. Studies of cancer in both animals and humans show that when the normal cell becomes malignant, it often undergoes biochemical changes that result in the formation of new cellular antigens that may trigger the immune response. A normally functioning immunosurveillance mechanism should recognize and eliminate these cancer cells, thus preventing uncontrolled cancer growth and spread within the body; but tumor cells can escape immune detection, either by an ineffective or altered antigen on the tumor cell, a suppressed immune response, or an overwhelming number of tumor cells that the immune system is incapable of controlling.

The link between cancer and the immune system is also illustrated when (1) some tumors spontaneously regress, (2) cancer incidence increases in persons who are immunosuppressed (posttransplant patients, the elderly), (3) metastatic tumor size decreases after surgical removal of the primary tumor, and (4) metastatic disease becomes dormant after successful local treatment of a tumor. These observations have stimulated continuing research on the role of the immune system and how the immune response can be enhanced to fight cancer growth.

The focus of biotherapy, or immunotherapy, is manipulation of the immune system through the use of naturally occurring biologic substances (cells, cell products) or genetically engineered agents and drugs that modify the body's immune response to cancer or cancer therapy. Biotherapy is now established as a major category of cancer therapy and is effective alone or in conjunction with surgery, chemotherapy, and radiation therapy. A number of biologic agents have been developed to function as regulators and messengers of immune function.

Types of Biotherapy. Biotherapy agents can be classified into five major categories: cytokines, monoclonal antibodies (MABs), cellular therapies, and immunostimulants.[25] Cytokines are proteins that mediate and regulate various immune functions. The most common cytokines are the interferons (IFNs), interleukins (ILs), and hematopoietic growth factors (HGFs). The next class of biologic agents is MABs, which are antibodies produced by hybridoma techniques for specific antigens on tumor cell surfaces. Cellular therapy uses activated immune cells such as lymphokine-activated killer cells and tumor-infiltrating lymphocytes. Immunostimulant therapy includes vaccine therapy, where the patient is vaccinated with a variety of antigens to stimulate a nonspecific immune response or a tumor-specific immune response. Finally, retinoids are natural derivatives of retinol, or vitamin A, and stimulate cellular differentiation. Table 15-12 presents the common biotherapy agents and their clinical applications.

Interferons. IFNs are a group of glycoproteins (alpha, beta, gamma) produced by T lymphocytes in response to viral infections or other stimuli. IFNs bind to receptors on nearly all the cells in the body. All nucleated cells are capable of IFN production, which can be induced by natural or synthetic agents. IFNs are synthetically produced by recombinant DNA technology by the insertion of genes for an IFN of each category into *Escherichia coli.*

IFNs have the ability to alter cellular metabolism in both normal and cancer cells. IFNs produce changes in viral RNA and protein synthesis, and inhibit the function of several oncogenes. IFNs also can activate natural killer cells, mediators that can identify and destroy some tumor cells. IFNs can be used alone or in combination with other chemotherapy agents.

Three types of IFNs are manufactured: alpha, beta, and gamma. Each type is distinct and has unique dosing parameters, administration guidelines, and side effects. Interferon-alpha first received Federal Drug Administration approval for the treatment of hairy cell leukemia and has since been approved for the treatment of chronic myelogenous leukemia and Kaposi's sarcoma and as adjuvant therapy for melanoma. It is manufactured under the trade names of Intron-a and Roferon-a. IFNs are administered in a variety of regimens, by subcutaneous and intravenous routes, bolus and infusion methods, and high and low doses. The most common side effects of interferons are the flulike symptoms of fatigue, fever, chills, myalgias, and headache. Mild to moderate myelosuppression and alterations in mood and cognition may also occur with interferon therapy.[6]

Interleukins. Interleukins are a group of biologic factors that stimulate and increase a number of other immune cells and other cytokines, including lymphocytes, macrophages, complement factors, and monocytes. They are produced by thymus cells and are involved in cell-mediated immunity. Of the 17 interleukins identified, IL-2 has been most thoroughly studied. IL-2 is produced by recombinant technology and is used in the treatment of renal cell cancer and melanoma. IL-2 can be administered subcutaneously or as a continuous or bolus intravenous infusion. IL-2 is being studied using both low-dose outpatient regimens and high-dose schedules requiring critical care monitoring. Side effects of IL-2 can affect every major organ system. In addition to flulike symptoms, IL-2 can cause a vascular leak syndrome, which causes tachycardia, hypotension, edema, and pulmonary side effects such as dyspnea and pulmonary edema. Neurologic toxicity, nephrotoxicity, and hepatotoxicity as well as skin changes and gastrointestinal upset can also occur.[11]

Growth Factors. HGFs are glycoproteins that stimulate the development of hematopoietic cell lines. The proteins attach to the surface of a stem cell and stimulate the cell to proliferate, differentiate, and mature. Some HGFs stimulate a single cell type, whereas others stimulate multiple cell lines. Granulocyte colony–stimulating factor (G-CSF) stimulates the growth and activation of neutrophils. Granulocyte-macrophage colony–stimulating factor (GM-CSF) stimulates the production of neutrophils, eosinophils, and macrophages. Both G-CSF and GM-CSF have shown the ability to accelerate bone marrow recovery of neutrophil counts after myelosuppressive therapy. The use of these factors has dramatically decreased the sepsis-related morbidity and mortality caused by the prolonged bone marrow suppression that follows chemotherapy and bone marrow transplant. With decreased bone marrow suppression, patients can receive their full course of chemotherapy without delays or toxicity. G-CSF and GM-CSF are usually given as subcutaneous injections, but may also be given by the intravenous route.

Erythropoietin (EPO) is recombinant growth factor approved for the treatment of anemia associated with end-stage

TABLE 15-12 Selected Biotherapy Agents With FDA-Approved Applications

Agent	Category	Definition and Biologic Actions	Approved Indications
Interferons	Cytokine	Family of glycoprotein hormones with antiviral, immunomodulatory, and antiproliferative effects	
Interferon-alpha		Derived primarily from leukocytes	Hairy cell leukemia Kaposi's sarcoma Condyloma acuminata Chronic hepatitis B Chronic hepatitis C Chronic myelogenous leukemia Adjuvant therapy for melanoma
Interferon-beta		Derived primarily from fibroblasts	Multiple sclerosis
Interferon-gamma		Derived from activated T lymphocytes	Chronic granulomatous disease
Interleukins IL-2	Cytokine	Molecular messengers between cells of the immune system; they activate cells of the immune system and stimulate the production of other cytokines; 17 interleukins have currently been identified	Melanoma, renal cell carcinoma
Monoclonal antibodies	Antibodies	Pure immunoglobulins derived from a single cell (hybridoma); they bind to target antigens on tumor cells and signal other cells of the immune system to destroy the tumor through phagocytosis or by complement-mediated lysis	
Satumomab pendetide			Detection of colon and ovarian cancer
Capromab pendetide			Detection of prostate cancer
Rituximab (Rituxan)			CD 20^+ B-cell non-Hodgkin's lymphoma
Trastuzumab (Herceptin)			Breast cancer with HER2 protein overexpression
Gemtuzumab (Mylotarg)			CD 33^+ AML
Growth factors			
GM-CSF	Hematopoietic growth factor	Natural hormonelike protein produced by a variety of immune cells that stimulates the maturation, differentiation, and proliferation of granulocytes and monocytes/macrophages	Accelerate myeloid recovery in lymphoid malignancies and post-BMT; mobilize stem cells for transplantation
C-CSF	Hematopoietic growth factor	Natural hormonelike protein produced by a variety of cells, mainly monocytes and macrophages, as well as endothelial cells, fibroblasts, and stromal cells that stimulates the growth and activation of granulocyte precursor cells	Reduce the severity, duration, and sequelae of neutropenia; mobilize stem cells for transplantation
Erythropoietin	Hematopoietic growth factor	Natural hormone produced by the kidney that regulates and controls red blood cell production and maturation	Chemotherapy-related anemia Anemia related to chronic renal failure and zidovudine administration in patients with HIV
Retinoids	Vitamin A derivatives	Class of agents that perform a significant role in vision, growth, reproduction, epithelial cell differentiation, and immune function	All-*trans*-retinoic acid in the treatment of acute promyelocytic leukemia Bexarotene for cutaneous T-cell lymphoma

Adapted from Rieger PT: Biotherapy: an overview. In Rieger PT, editor, *Biotherapy: a comprehensive review,* Boston, 2001, Jones and Bartlett.
GM-CSF, Granulocyte-macrophage colony-stimulating factor; *G-CSF,* granulocyte colony–stimulating factor; *HIV,* human immunodeficiency virus.

renal disease and myelosuppressive cancer therapy. EPO can effectively decrease the transfusion requirements for anemic patients and improve their quality of life. EPO is most commonly given as subcutaneous injections but may also be given as an intravenous infusion.

IL-11 is the newest HGF and is used to stimulate platelet production in patients who are at high risk for severe thrombocytopenia. Although the other HGFs have generally mild side effects, IL-11 is associated with mild to moderate toxicity, especially fluid imbalance and cardiac arrhythmias, and its use must be carefully evaluated in the clinical setting. IL-11 is administered as subcutaneous injections.

Monoclonal Antibodies. MABs are produced by hybridoma techniques that involve immunizing animals (usually mice) with antigen, and then fusing B cells from the mouse's spleen with tumor cells to make hybrid cells. MABs can be produced to bind with almost any antigen. They are effective in the serologic detection of tumors because malignant cells often express antigens that are not usually found on the surfaces of normal cells. These markers may be sensitive enough to detect early cancer and can be used to monitor the progress of disease in patients undergoing therapy.

Rituximab is a MAB used in the treatment of B-cell lymphomas whose cells express the CD20 surface antigen. Rituximab binds with the CD20 antigen on the malignant B cells, causing cell-mediated cytotoxicity. Herceptin is another MAB used in the treatment of breast cancers that express the HER2 antigen on its cells. Herceptin binds to the HER2 antigen and causes cell death. MABS are usually administered as intravenous infusions and can be used alone or in combination with chemotherapy. The most common adverse effect of MAB use is an infusion-related symptom complex in which patients experience fever, chills, and rigors during administration of the drug. This syndrome usually occurs with the initial but not with subsequent treatments and is usually not serious enough to discontinue treatment.[7]

Ongoing research efforts with cellular therapies and vaccines will no doubt provide new applications for biologic agents in cancer diagnosis and therapy. The use of biotherapy is expensive because of the complex technology required to produce these products. Continued research to attach anticancer drugs and radioisotopes to tumor-specific immune cells may provide therapies that are able to seek out and destroy only cancer cells, thus protecting normal cells and decreasing side effects.

Collaborative Care Management. Flulike side effects are associated with several biotherapy agents, including interferon and interleukin. These side effects include fever, chills, rigors, headache, and malaise. Fevers and myalgias can be prevented and alleviated by the use of acetaminophen as a premedication or around the clock to promote comfort. Nonsteroidal antiinflammatory drugs (NSAIDs) may also be used, but aspirin and aspirin-containing products should be avoided because of the risk of bleeding in myelosuppressed patients. Nurses use comfort measures to keep the patient warm and well hydrated. Meperidine administration may be used to relieve chills and rigors. Rest, relaxation, and diversional activities are encouraged.[27] Flulike symptoms are generally worse with initial doses of the biotherapy agents and diminish over time. This adaptation is called tachyphylaxis.

Fatigue is reported by almost all patients receiving biotherapy and is a common cause for reducing dosage or discontinuing therapy because the effects are cumulative. Many other factors may contribute to fatigue, including anemia, poor nutrition, and disease status; and these causes are also addressed. Nurses help patients identify strategies to conserve energy and establish priorities for activities that require energy. Nurses counsel patients to seek a balance between rest and activity. Rest periods in a calm, stress-free environment are incorporated into each day's activities. An exercise plan individualized to the patient's tolerance is also recommended. Nurses also encourage the use of relaxation and stress reducing activities such as listening to music or reading.

Neurologic toxicities include somnolence, anxiety, depression, and mental status changes. Nurses must be skilled in mental status examination and complete baseline as well as ongoing assessments. Antidepressants and behavioral therapy are prescribed, but in severe cases, doses of the MAB may need to be reduced or discontinued to relieve these side effects.

Cardiovascular and pulmonary toxicities are most commonly associated with high-dose IL-2 therapy. Potential cardiotoxicities include arrhythmias and hypotension. Fluid retention can result in weight gain, as well as periperhal and pulmonary edema from vascular leak syndrome. IL-2 increases capillary permeability and allows fluid to leak from the vessels to interstitial spaces. Nurses carefully monitor fluid balance and are prepared to manage severe fluid imbalance and hypovolemic shock if necessary.

Severe gastrointestinal toxicity from biotherapy is not common, but patients may experience anorexia, nausea, and diarrhea. Nurses offer these patients strategies to optimize nutritional intake and use appropriate antiemetic and antidiarrheal medications.

An infusion-related complex of symptoms can also occur, especially during the initial administration of an MAB. This symptom complex includes fever, chills, and urticaria, and can, in rare cases, progress to bronchospasm, hypotension, and angioedema. Nurses prevent and manage this syndrome by using premedications (acetaminophen and diphenhydramine), gradually increasing the rate of the MAB infusion, and closely monitoring the patient during the initial MAB infusion.[20] Skin rashes and local injection site reactions may also occur. Hematologic effects are usually mild and reversible.

Many biotherapy agents must be reconstituted or diluted and should be prepared immediately before administration. Biotherapy agents are generally unstable at room temperature and must be transported in a cooler to maintain stability.

Patient/Family Education. Patients receiving biotherapy need a basic understanding of their cancer, how the immune system functions in relation to cancer, and why biotherapy is being prescribed. Biotherapy agents have a number of side effects, including flulike symptoms, fatigue, hypersensitivity reactions, and various organ toxicities (Table 15-13). The intensity and duration of toxicity depend on the agent used; its dose, route, and schedule; and any other concurrent therapy. Most side effects occur shortly after administration and are reversible when the drug is discontinued. Agents given continuously for long periods may lead to chronic and cumulative toxicity, such as fatigue. Each symptom can create significant discomfort when experienced alone, but when the patient must deal with the combined effects, care needs are significantly increased.

Nurses who care for patients receiving biotherapy need to educate patients and families about the type of biotherapy they are receiving, provide for safe administration of the agents, and assess for and manage side effects. Although side effects vary, the patient and caregiver are made aware of the most common ones. A printed instruction sheet that addresses prevention,

TABLE 15-13 Common Side Effects of Biotherapy Agents

Biotherapy Agent	Common Side Effects	Occasional
Interferon	Myelosuppression Anorexia Fever and chills Fatigue Headache and myalgias Hepatotoxicity	Mental status changes Bone pain Diarrhea Flushing Nausea Skin rash
Granylocyte colony–stimulating factor (GCSF)	Increased WBC count	Bone pain Injection site reactions Headache
Erythropoietin	Increased RBC count	Headache
Interleukin–11 (Oprelvekin)	Increased platelet count	Fluid retention Peripheral edema Tachycardia
Monoclonal antibodies	Fever and chills Flushing Fatigue	Anorexia Bronchospasm Diarrhea Headache Hypotension Hepatotoxicity Mucositis Myalgias Myelosuppression Nausea Skin rashes
Interleukin-2	Anorexia Capillary leak syndrome Fever, chills, flushing Fluid retention and peripheral edema Fatigue Headache and myalgias Diarrhea Hypersensitivity Hepatotoxicity	Mental status changes Skin rash Pulmonary edema Mucositis

Adapted from Rieger PT: Patient management. In Rieger PT, editor: *Biotherapy: a comprehensive overview,* ed 2, Boston, 2001, Jones and Bartlett.
WBC, White blood cell; *RBC,* red blood cell.

management, and reporting of side effects lends the patient support and helps facilitate compliance with therapy. Patients need to understand the level of monitoring that is required during therapy, whether in the intensive care unit or in the home environment. If the patient will be self-administering the biotherapy agent, the nurse teaches the patient proper drug preparation and storage, techniques for subcutaneous injections, and safe handling and disposal of all equipment and drug materials.

Radiotherapy

Radiotherapy, or the use of radiation in the treatment of disease, has been used since the discovery of x-rays in 1895 and radium in 1898. Today, radiotherapy is included in the therapy of more than half the patients with cancer at some point. Radiotherapy can be prescribed as a single, curative modality or used as a palliative measure to relieve symptoms of metastatic disease. Radiotherapy can also be combined in a multitude of ways with chemotherapy and surgery.

Radiation Physics. Ionizing radiation, either natural or manufactured, contains energy that is capable of breaking the chemical bonds in molecules, which can lead to cellular damage or cell death. Therapeutic ionizing radiation is classified into two types: electromagnetic and particulate. Electromagnetic radiation includes x-rays and gamma rays—energy rays that have no mass. Special machines produce x-rays, and radioactive materials emit gamma rays. Both x-rays and gamma rays penetrate deep into tissue before releasing their energy and causing cellular changes. Particulate radiation has mass and includes particles of radiation such as electrons, neutrons, alpha particles, and others. Because of their mass, these particles cannot penetrate deeply into tissues and instead release their energy into cells close to the surface (Figure 15-7).

Radiotherapy can be delivered to the patient in one of three ways. External radiation, or teletherapy, directs radiation from an external source toward the body. External sources of radiotherapy are usually megavoltage machines, such as the linear accelerator, which produce gamma and electron radiation.

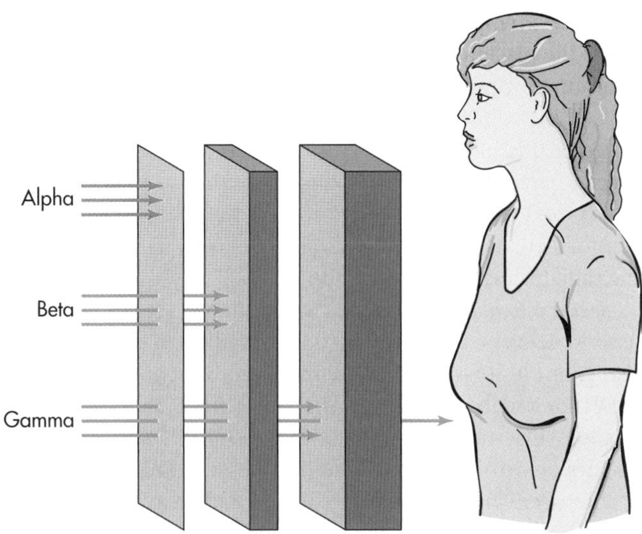

Figure 15-7 Relative penetrating power of three types of radiation.

TABLE 15-14 Radiosensitivity of Selected Body Organs

Organ	Radiosensitivity
Bone marrow	High
Ovaries	
Testes	
Intestine	
Skin	Medium high
Oral cavity and esophagus	
Vagina, cervix	
Growing bone and cartilage	Medium
Fine vasculature	
Mature bone and cartilage	Medium low
Kidney	
Liver	
Thyroid	
Muscle	Low
Brain and spinal cord	

Machines that produce higher energy particles with varying biologic effects are currently being researched and are in limited use around the world.

Radiation therapy is prescribed in units called grays (Gy) or in centigrays (cGy). In the past the dosage was measured by the amount of radiant energy absorbed by tissues and expressed in the unit rad. An external radiation treatment can range from 1 minute to a few minutes. The exact duration depends on the dose to be delivered, the energy, type of radiation beam, and depth of the tumor.

Brachytherapy, or internal radiation, places a radioactive source directly inside the body. The radioactive source may be sealed in a needle, seed, or wire, and temporarily implanted in the tumor. The radioactive source may also be unsealed, in the form of a systemic intravenous or oral preparation.

Radiation Biology. Ionizing radiation causes cell death either through direct damage to the double strands of DNA or as a consequence of biochemical changes that interfere with cellular repair and reproduction.[15] Before radiation therapy is prescribed, the radiosensitivity of the target tissue is determined. Radiosensitivity is a measure of the potential susceptibility of cells to injury from ionizing radiation and the speed at which damage will occur. All body tissue has a known degree of radiosensitivity (Table 15-14). The radiation oncologist must calculate the maximal treatment dosage that can be administered without compromising the normal tissues surrounding the tumor. Other considerations include the patient's age, tumor size and stage, degree of spread, and overall prognosis if radiation is used to treat the tumor.

Cells that are in the mitosis (M) phase of the cell cycle are the most sensitive to the effects of radiation; however, damage also may occur during DNA synthesis (S phase). Tissues that have high proliferative rates, such as the bone marrow, skin, and gastrointestinal tract, are most affected by radiation. Tumor resistance to radiation can be a major problem that is usually related to tissue hypoxia. Hypoxic cells are known to be radioresistant and require about three times as much radiation as a well-oxygenated cell requires to achieve the same degree of cell kill. Cell kill refers to the number of tumor cells expected to be destroyed after a radiation treatment. Tumor cells become hypoxic when they outgrow the nearest capillary blood supply during their growth. The mechanism of how hypoxia makes a cell radioresistant is not fully understood.

Although the goal of radiotherapy is to achieve maximum tumor cell kill while sparing normal tissue, it is impossible to completely avoid injury. The total dose of radiation is divided into multiple small doses and typically delivered daily over a period of weeks. This theoretically allows the normal cells time to repair themselves. Cancer cells do not have the same ability to repair and reverse the changes caused by radiation as do normal cells and are more likely to die. With external radiation, fractionization divides the total dose of radiation into a small number of equal fractions, which are usually delivered once daily over a period of weeks. Hyper or accelerated fractionization, two or more treatments per day, may be used in selected cases. Radiotherapy may also be delivered as a "split course" of therapy, where the patient receives part of the total dose followed by a rest of 1 to 2 weeks until the final cumulative dose is achieved. This plan is advantageous for several reasons. Normal cells that received a sublethal dose of radiation have time to repair the damage. Tumor cells that were in a nonsensitive cycle phase may progress to a more radiosensitive phase; therefore a larger cell kill will be attained when treatment is resumed.

Types of Radiotherapy

External Radiotherapy. External radiation may be used alone or in conjunction with surgery. Used alone radiation therapy can cure cancer of the skin, oral cavity, larynx, uterine cervix, prostate, pelvis, and early stages of Hodgkin's disease. When radiation is used in conjunction with surgery, it is used either for cure or palliation of symptoms. Cancers of the head and neck, lung, breast, uterus, bladder, bone, and testes can be cured with combined surgery and radiation.

When cure is the anticipated outcome, the radiation may be administered before or after surgery. The rationale for preoperative treatment is to decrease tumor size, increase the potential for removal of the entire tumor during surgery, eradicate subclinical disease that might be present beyond the intended surgical field, and eradicate lymph nodes where disease could form or support metastasis. The disadvantage of preoperative radiation is a delay in wound healing in normal tissues that were within the treatment field.

Postoperative radiation therapy usually is performed to eradicate any residual tumor and subclinical disease. Higher doses can be administered than could have been used before surgery. The most cited disadvantage of postoperative radiotherapy is the need to delay the treatment until postoperative wound healing is complete.

Radiation therapy can also be combined with chemotherapy. A number of medications, called radiosensitizers, can be used to enhance the effect of radiation therapy. These drugs act in a variety of ways (e.g., changing the oxygenation of the tissue). Other medications are radioprotectors, which help to protect tissue against the damage caused by radiation therapy.

Stereotactic radiosurgery is a specialized technique that delivers a single dose of radiation directly to a small tumor, such as an intracranial lesion. Also known as the gamma knife, this procedure requires rigid head immobilization, occasional sedation or analgesia, tumor localization with CT or MRI scans, and sophisticated computer imaging.

Before any treatment is initiated, the patient is thoroughly examined by the radiation oncologist and undergoes a simulation, or planning, phase. The precise target area where the tumor is located is defined, and the anatomic area to receive the radiation, called a port, is outlined with either ink markings or small permanent tattoo markings. These outlines are essential so that only the small, defined area or port receives the radiation. The simulation phase may take several hours for planning and positioning.

Different ports may be used on different days, or the port position may be changed at intervals so that an optimal yet safe dose of radiation is given through each port. The patient may need to assume difficult or uncomfortable positions during the treatment, and immobilization is critical for accurate delivery of the radiation. Specific immobilizing or positioning devices may be necessary to help maintain proper positioning during the treatment, and these are made specifically for the patient. Pediatric and elderly patients often require casts or molds, special boards, or safety belts to help them maintain the correct position. The need for organ-shielding devices also is determined during simulation.

The pretreatment phase may require several sessions in the radiation oncology department. A picture of the patient in the exact desired position, with immobilizing devices and shields in place, is kept in the patient's treatment file. The photograph helps technicians responsible for administering the radiation to correctly position the patient for each treatment. The technician documents the treatment number, cumulative dose, patient position and immobilizing devices used, and any specific patient concerns or problems encountered.

Brachytherapy (Internal Radiation Therapy). Brachytherapy is the placement of radioactive sources on or directly into a tumor. A number of cancers can be treated with brachytherapy (Table 15-15). Internal radiation may be delivered by sealed or unsealed techniques. In either type of brachytherapy, special precautions are necessary because care providers can be exposed to the radioactive source. Radiation safety interventions are based on the radioisotope used, its location, and the radiation emitted.

Sealed Internal Radiotherapy. Sealed internal radiotherapy is used to deliver a concentrated dose of radiation directly to the malignant lesion or tumor area and can be at a low-dose rate (LDR) or a high-dose rate (HDR). LDR brachytherapy usually involves insertion of radioactive substances within hollow cavities or within tissues. Table 15-16 lists radioisotopes commonly used in brachytherapy. These radioactive substances may be placed in molds, plaques, needles, wires, special applicators, or ribbons.

Placement of the sealed container is carried out in the operating room, radiation department, or a treatment room. Exact positioning of the container is essential so the tumor receives the maximum dose of radiation while exposure of normal tissues and organs is minimized. X-ray films are taken to verify appropriate placement. The patient then returns to a

TABLE 15-15 Cancers Treated with Brachytherapy

Cancer	Technique	Radioactive Source
Endometrial	Intracavitary	Radium, cesium
Cervical	Intracavitary	Radium, cesium
Prostate	Interstitial	Iodine, gold
Breast	Interstitial	Iridium
Ocular melanoma	Plaque therapy	Cobalt, iodine
Head and neck	Interstitial thermal	Iridium, cesium
Rectal	Interstitial	Cesium
Esophageal	Intraluminal	Cesium
Bronchogenic	Endobronchial	Iridium, iodine

From Dow KH et al: *Nursing care in radiation oncology,* ed 2, Philadelphia, 1997, WB Saunders.

TABLE 15-16 Radioisotopes and Their Properties

Radioisotope	Symbols	Half-Life	Type
Cesium-137	^{137}Cs	30 years	Beta, gamma
Gold-198	^{198}Au	2.7 days	Beta, gamma
Iodine-125	^{125}I	60 days	Beta, gamma
Iodine-131	^{131}I	8 days	Beta, gamma
Iridium-192	^{192}Ir	74.4 days	Beta, gamma
Phosphorus-32	^{32}P	14.3 days	Beta
Radium-226	^{226}Ra	1620 years	Alpha, gamma
Strontium-90	^{90}Sr	28.1 years	Beta

From Dow KH et al: *Nursing care in radiation oncology,* ed 2, Philadelphia, 1997, WB Saunders.

private hospital room where the radioactive substance is inserted. This is called afterloading and is a technique used to prevent unnecessary exposure of staff members in various departments to the radiation source. The length of time the radiation material is left in place depends on the element used and the dose that has been prescribed. Time ranges from a few hours to several days, and the patient remains hospitalized for this period. HDR brachytherapy is a second technique for positioning an applicator into the tumor cavity. The radiation source, in the form of pellets or tubes, is loaded into the applicator through wires by remote control and then unloaded at the end of the treatment, which lasts several minutes. HDR treatments may be scheduled weekly for several weeks. HDR brachytherapy can be completed in an outpatient setting and does not require hospitalization.[8]

Unsealed Internal Radiotherapy. Unsealed internal radiation is delivered to the patient by mouth or as an intravenous solution. One example is the radioisotope, iodine-131, which is used to treat thyroid cancer. Because the isotope is excreted in all body fluids, persons caring for the patient can be exposed to the radiation from the patient (external exposure) or from contact with the patient's discharges that contain the radioactive substance (internal exposure). It may be inhaled, ingested, or absorbed through the skin. The exposure risk varies with each of the substances used, and safety for the staff members caring for the patient depends on a thorough knowledge of the substance used and its action within the body. Special precautions are not needed with the tracer doses used for diagnostic procedures.

Other radioisotopes commonly used for unsealed brachytherapy include radioactive phosphorus (^{32}P) and gold (^{198}Au). These substances may be administered orally, intravenously, or by direct instillation into a body cavity. Each isotope is a potential source of radiation exposure for health care personnel. The mode of elimination from the body varies with the specific isotope; but generally traces are found in urine, feces, emesis, sputum, wound drainage, and perspiration. Caregivers need to follow specific instructions from radiation oncology personnel to minimize radiation exposure when working with these patients.

Protection of Health Care Professionals From Radiation Hazards. Radiotherapy can be a source of occupational radiation exposure to caregivers, and radiation safety guidelines must be carefully followed to minimize the risk. Radiation therapy rooms are shielded with concrete and lead walls, and no one enters the room during the treatment. Patients with internal radiation sources that emit gamma rays expose caregivers to radiation for varying periods of time, and the length of time that a staff member can be safely exposed is important in planning care. The time interval required for the radioactive substance to be half dissipated is called its half-life. This period varies widely, but as the end of the half-life is reached, danger from exposure decreases.

Exposure to radiation can be controlled in three ways: time, distance, and shielding. Caregivers should minimize time spent with the patient and maximize their distance from the patient. Radiation is subject to the inverse-square law. A person who stands 2 m away from the source of radiation receives only one fourth as much exposure as when standing only 1 m away. At 4 m only one sixteenth of the exposure is received (Figure 15-8). Lead gloves and aprons are used during x-ray and fluoroscopy procedures, but lead is insufficient to

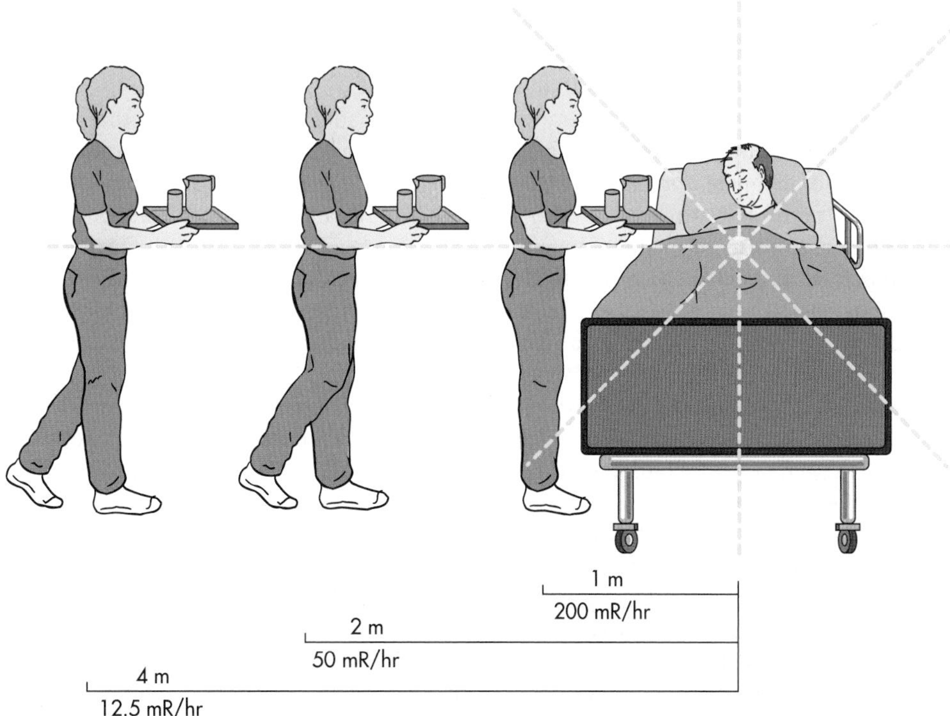

Figure 15-8 Nurse nearest source of radioactivity (patient) is exposed to more radioactivity.

TABLE 15-17 Possible Sequelae of Radiation Therapy

Anatomic Site	Acute Sequelae (Early)	Late Sequelae
Brain	Earache, headache, dizziness, hair loss, erythema	Hearing loss, damage to middle or inner ear, pituitary gland dysfunction, cataracts, and brain necrosis
Head and neck	Odynophagia, dysphagia, hoarseness, xerostomia, dysgeusia, weight loss	Subcutaneous fibrosis, skin ulceration, necrosis, thyroid dysfunction, dental decay, osteoradionecrosis of mandible, delayed wound healing, damage to middle and inner ear
Lung and mediastinum or esophagus	Odynophagia, dysphagia, cough, hoarseness pneumonitis, carditis	Progressive fibrosis of lung, dyspnea, chronic cough; esophageal stricture Rare: chronic pericarditis, myelopathy
Breast or chest wall	Odynophagia, dysphagia, hoarseness, cough; pneumonitis (asymptomatic); carditis; cytopenia	Fibrosis, retraction of breast; lung fibrosis; arm edema; chronic endocarditis, myocardial infarction Rare: osteonecrosis of ribs
Abdomen or pelvis	Nausea, vomiting, abdominal pain, diarrhea; urinary frequency, dysuria, nocturia; cytopenia	Proctitis, sigmoiditis; rectal or sigmoid stricture; colonic perforation or obstruction; contracted bladder, urinary incontinence, hematuria, vesicovaginal fistula; rectovaginal fistula; leg edema; scrotal edema, sexual impotency; vaginal retraction or scarring; sterilization Rare: damage to liver or kidneys
Extremities	Erythema, dry/moist desquamation	Subcutaneous fibrosis: ankylosis, edema; bone/soft tissue necrosis

From Perez CA, Brady LW: *Principles and practices of radiation oncology,* ed 3, Philadelphia, 1998, JB Lippincott.

stop gamma rays during brachytherapy. Shields, however, may be effective reminders to caregivers to more safely manage the time spent with the patient. Some hospitals have single, lead-lined rooms designated for implant patients. Radiation safety guidelines require that personnel who deliver radiotherapy or care for brachytherapy patients wear dosimetry badges to measure their radiation exposure. Care for brachytherapy patients is rotated among a team of nurses, and no pregnant caregiver is assigned to deliver care.

Staff education is important to ensure compliance with the safety and monitoring procedures involved with radiotherapy. Hospitals in which therapeutic doses of radioactive isotopes are administered are required to designate a radiation safety officer. The radiation safety officer, often a physicist, determines the precautions to be observed in each situation, and nurses consult the safety officer as needed to address questions and concerns. Most hospitals post printed instruction sheets detailing the precautions to be followed and warning all staff of the radiation risk. Health care givers should be fully acquainted with all precautions and meticulous in carrying them out.

Side Effects of Radiation Therapy. Because radiotherapy is a local treatment, most side effects are site-specific, depending on which organs and tissues are within or close to the treatment field. Side effects can be classified as acute or late. Acute toxicities occur within days and affect tissues with a rapid renewal rate, such as the skin, bone marrow, and mucosal lining of the gastrointestinal tract and vagina. Late toxicities occur months or years after treatment, and may be due to injury to the blood vessels and connective tissue that surround the treatment field. Late effects include cataracts, pulmonary fibrosis, and strictures. Table 15-17 indicates the early and late local toxicities of radiation therapy to various anatomic sites.

Radiation therapy also has carcinogenic potential. It is known that secondary malignancies develop in patients previously treated with radiation therapy. Skin cancer, leukemia, non-Hodgkin's lymphoma, and sarcoma are all associated with radiation exposure. Although these cases are rare and multiple factors are probably involved in radiation carcinogenesis, nurses may need to address this concern with patients.

Most patients receiving radiotherapy experience skin reactions in the treatment port. Slight initial erythema, from the effect of radiation on capillary blood flow, progresses to pronounced erythema in 2 to 3 weeks and then begins to fade. The skin reaction may progress further to dry desquamation and then moist desquamation. Skin folds, such as the axilla and groin, are at higher risk for skin reactions. Temporary hair loss, or alopecia, in the treatment area also occurs in about 3 weeks. Figure 15-9 illustrates typical radiotherapy skin reactions of erythema and dry desquamation. Long-term effects, including ulceration, fibrosis, and atrophy, may occur months after irradiation is completed and are attributed to changes in endothelial permeability, edema, and increased skin temperature. Scoring systems to evaluate skin toxicity have been developed, and an example is displayed in Table 15-18.

Nearly all patients receiving radiation therapy experience fatigue. Complicated by other disease and treatment factors, the loss of energy and feeling of tiredness may be cumulative and have profound effects on the patient's quality of life. Bone marrow suppression is also a common side effect, because bone marrow is extremely radiosensitive and likely to be af-

TABLE 15-18 Acute Radiation Morbidity Scoring Criteria (RTOG) and Late Radiation Morbidity Scoring Scheme (RTOG, EORTC) for Skin

0	Grade 1	Grade 2	Grade 3	Grade 4	Grade 5
Acute Morbidity					
No change over baseline	Follicular, faint or dull erythema, epilation, dry desquamation, decreased sweating	Tender or bright erythema, patchy moist desquamation, moderate edema	Confluent, moist desquamation, other than skin folds, pitting edema	Ulceration, hemorrhage, necrosis	
Late Morbidity					
None	Slight atrophy, pigmentation change, some hair loss	Patchy atrophy, moderate telangiectasia, total hair loss	Marked atrophy, gross telangiectasia	Ulceration	Death directly related to radiation late effect

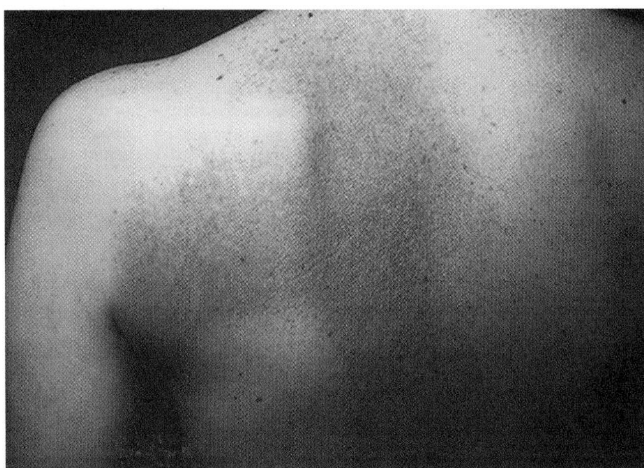

Figure 15-9 Erythema and dry desquamation of the skin in response to external radiotherapy.

fected in almost every treatment port. Recovery of the bone marrow depends on the dose used and the tumor volume treated.

NURSING MANAGEMENT OF PATIENT RECEIVING RADIOTHERAPY

Before planning care for the patient receiving radiotherapy, the nurse must have an in-depth understanding of the treatment plan. The goal of therapy should be specifically identified and details about the type of radiation, frequency of treatments, and treatment ports must be obtained. Effective interdisciplinary communication is essential.

ASSESSMENT

Health History

Aspects of the health history of particular importance when caring for a patient receiving radiotherapy are:

- Age
- Medical history
- Medications
- Allergies
- Social support
- Learning ability
- Financial status
- Knowledge of planned treatment
- Concerns related to radiation treatment

Physical Examination

Physical examination of the patient receiving radiotherapy should focus on:

- Performance status
- Nutritional status
- Elimination pattern
- Mobility
- Skin and mucous membrane integrity

The nursing assessment is the initial step in ascertaining the patient's overall physical and emotional state, including the patient's perception of the effects of radiotherapy on well-being and lifestyle. The patient may have many fears and concerns about radiation and may also be facing the fears of a new diagnosis of cancer. Nurses effectively address these fears with information, support, and counseling.

The nurse assesses the patient's understanding of the cancer and the use and goals of radiation therapy. Does the patient know the number of treatments to be administered, the daily schedule, the area of the body to be irradiated, and the radiotherapy procedures?

The nursing assessment also includes the patient's health history and current physical status. The presence of chronic conditions and symptoms is noted because they may present problems during therapy. Immobility or pain from arthritis or recent surgery, for example, may prevent the patient from assuming necessary positions.

The nutritional state of the patient is evaluated and interventions are planned if the patient is malnourished or at high risk for nutritional complications. Poor nutrition and a history of recent weight loss affect the ability of the patient to withstand a long course of treatment.

The condition of the patient's skin, especially skin that lies within the treatment field, is evaluated before the start of therapy. Because skin is always undergoing cellular renewal, it is extremely vulnerable to the effects of radiation. Skin that has been damaged from cancer or surgery or irritated from a dermatologic condition is noted. The effects of radiation on the body are cumulative. Thus if an area requires treatment in the future, the skin will be even more vulnerable to damage.

The age of the patient may also influence the outcome of treatment. Immune system function declines with age, regeneration of the bone marrow takes longer in elderly persons, and the effects of fatigue are more pronounced. The skin and mucosa are less elastic and take longer to repair after injury. Consequently, older adults have less tolerance to radiation than a younger person with the same cancer. Finally, older persons may be more fearful and anxious about therapy, especially if they recall experiences with the early days of radiotherapy or have confusion or memory loss related to other illnesses.

NURSING DIAGNOSES

Diagnostic Title	Possible Etiologic Factors
1. Deficient knowledge	Unfamiliar with treatment plans, procedures, and side effects
2. Risk for impaired skin integrity	Dry or wet desquamation in radiation port
3. Fatigue	Poor nutrition, pain, immobility, other treatments
4. Imbalanced nutrition: less than body requirements	Nausea, stomatitis, diarrhea, anorexia
5. Risk for infection	Decreased white blood cell count, impaired skin integrity, stomatitis, iatrogenic factors
6. Impaired oral mucous membranes	Radiation port in head/neck area
7. Diarrhea	Radiation port in lower abdomen

EXPECTED PATIENT OUTCOMES

Expected patient outcomes for the patient undergoing radiotherapy for cancer may include but are not limited to:

1. Will be able to describe goal of treatment, planned schedule for treatment, and anticipated side effects
2. Will maintain intact skin in radiation port without signs of infection
3. Will maintain self-care activities without significant fatigue
4. Will maintain adequate nutritional intake and desired weight
5. Will maintain a normal temperature and has no signs of infection
6. Will have moist, intact oral mucous membranes
7. Will experience normal bowel elimination pattern

NURSING INTERVENTIONS

1. Providing Patient/Family Education

The nurse plays a vital role in dispelling patient and family fears and teaching about radiation therapy. The nurse clarifies and reinforces information about the number of treatments planned, the body area to be irradiated, and the nature of the preliminary planning and treatment sessions. During the initial phases of treatment, the patient needs the nurse's support to adjust to the reality of a new diagnosis of cancer, accept prognostic information, and understand therapy goals. When outpatient radiotherapy is planned, the nurse assesses the type and availability of the patient's support system, financial concerns, and transportation issues. The nurse arranges additional support for any area of need.

Some patients fear that they will be "radioactive" after treatment and a danger to others around them. Others are anxious that radiation will be painful. Both are misconceptions. No sensation is felt during treatment. The patient is informed that he or she will be alone in the treatment room but continuously monitored on television and able to talk to the radiation technician at all times. Immobilizing devices, such as special molds or casts, may be used to maintain proper body position during treatment. Treatments are generally completed in minutes. Patients who are highly anxious or unable to lie still during the treatment period may require sedation. Visiting the radiation therapy facility may allay some common fears.

The nurse teaches the patient about common side effects that may be anticipated with radiotherapy. Because many patients receive radiotherapy on an outpatient basis, teaching about self-care measures to prevent and manage side effects is critical.

2. Maintaining Skin Integrity

Skin care measures vary among institutions, but generally include measures to keep the skin clean, dry, and protected from irritants.[28] Examples of suggested skin care measures for the radiation treatment field are addressed in the Guidelines for Safe Practice box. The nurse provides the patient with written

> ***Guidelines for Safe Practice***
>
> **Preventing Skin Irritation During Radiation Therapy**
>
> 1. Cleanse radiation field (area within ink markings or inside tattoo outline) daily with mild soap and water. *Do not* erase ink markings if present.
> 2. Clean and keep dry skin folds that overlap and places where moisture collects (abdominal skin folds, under and between pendulous breasts, between buttocks or perineum).
> 3. Avoid use of perfumed soaps, lotions, or deodorant on involved skin surface.
> 4. Guard against irritation from belts, bras, rough clothing on treatment field. Cotton clothing is least irritating.
> 5. Do not use heating pads, hot water bottles, or ice packs on treated field.
> 6. Avoid exposure to sunlight. If unavoidable, use sunscreen for protection.
> 7. Use an electric razor only to shave within treatment area.
> 8. Avoid scratching, vigorous rubbing, or massage of the treatment field.
> 9. Do not apply any lotions, powders, or ointments to treated area unless advised to do so by radiologist.

instructions about skin care and verifies the patient's understanding. The nurse also provides support and interventions for patients who have lost scalp hair, as this side effect may be particularly distressing. Specific skin care measures are warranted if moist desquamation occurs. Various ointments and dressings may be prescribed for skin protection and comfort.

3. Managing Fatigue

Decreased energy levels and fatigue are common symptoms during radiotherapy, especially when daily treatments are taken over several months. Concurrent problems such as anemia, malnutrition, and recovery from surgery may worsen the fatigue from radiotherapy. The nurse assesses for the severity and impact of fatigue on the patient's quality of life. Factors that contribute to fatigue are addressed, such as therapy for anemia and effective pain management. The nurse encourages patients to incorporate rest periods throughout the day and ensure adequate sleep at night. The nurse may need to counsel patients about reducing activities that demand too much energy, incorporating a mild exercise/activity plan into their daily routine, and the use of distraction or relaxation. These strategies are all known to help with fatigue.[5]

4. Promoting Nutrition

Maintaining good nutrition with a diet high in carbohydrates, protein, and calories supplies the necessary energy for daily activities. The nurse incorporates nutritional assessment into routine care. Weight is checked at least weekly to determine if the patient's dietary intake is sufficient or if additional supplements are needed. The nurse assesses for symptoms such as anorexia, nausea, mucositis, dysphagia, and diarrhea, which compromise intake, and plans strategies to manage these symptoms. Antiemetics and antidiarrheal agents can be used as well as local measures and analgesics to manage mouth or throat pain with eating. Patients receiving therapy through head and neck ports may require aggressive nutritional support (e.g., placement of a percutaneous feeding tube and the use of enteral feedings). The nurse plays an integral role in evaluating the appropriateness and effectiveness of nutritional interventions throughout the course of radiotherapy.

5. Monitoring Myelosuppression

Laboratory studies are monitored at intervals during treatment to determine the effects of therapy on bone marrow production of white blood cells (WBCs), red blood cells (RBCs), and platelets. The nurse also assesses patients for early signs of infection, anemia, and bleeding, which can result from bone marrow suppression, especially in patients receiving concurrent chemotherapy. Interventions to manage these serious complications, such as antibiotic therapy, blood transfusions, and growth factor support may be necessary to complete the course of radiotherapy. Myelosuppression is discussed in more detail on p. 340.

6. Managing Mucositis

Mucositis, or inflammation of the mucosal membranes of the gastrointestinal or genitourinary tract, occurs when this tissue is included in the radiation port. The inflammation can be severe, causing pain, ulceration, and bleeding. When mucositis occurs in the mouth and throat, the nurse implements measures to keep the mouth and throat clean. Mouth rinses, such as salt and peroxide solutions, are usually recommended for cleansing. Patients should avoid spicy and acidic foods, alcohol, and tobacco. Patients may have difficulty swallowing and complain of heartburnlike pain. Local anesthetics as well as systemic analgesics may be necessary to relieve pain. Radiotherapy to mouth and throat ports causes a severe dry mouth, called xerostomia, as well as taste changes, called dysguesia. The nurse educates patients about dietary strategies to deal with these symptoms (e.g., the use of artifical saliva solutions) and stresses the importance of mouth care measures (see p. 353). Cystitis, urethritis, and vaginitis may occur when radiotherapy is given through a pelvic port. The nurse needs to encourage specific hygiene measures and high fluid intake to relieve discomfort and assess for and institute treatment for any local infections.

7. Controlling Diarrhea

Patients receiving radiotherapy to abdominal ports are at risk for both nausea and diarrhea. Nausea can usually be controlled with the regular use of an antiemetic. The nurse encourages the patient to consume a low-residue diet and use antidiarrheal agents as needed to control diarrhea. Assessment of fluid and electrolyte status is imperative when these side effects are severe to prevent dehydration and electrolyte abnormalities.

EVALUATION

To evaluate the effectiveness of nursing interventions, compare patient behaviors with those stated in the expected patient outcomes. Achievement of outcomes is successful if the patient undergoing radiotherapy for cancer:

1. Is knowledgeable about the planned radiation treatment and incorporates measures to prevent side effects into the daily routine.
2. Is free of signs of skin inflammation, breakdown, or infection.
3. Maintains independence in all self-care activities.
4. Consumes a balanced diet and maintains a stable weight.
5. Is normothermic and exhibits no signs of infection.
6. Has intact oral mucous membranes without evidence of inflammation, breakdown, or infection.
7. Passes soft stool daily.

Chemotherapy

Advances in knowledge concerning cancer growth and the development of a vast array of chemotherapeutic agents have led to concomitant advances in cancer treatment. Improvement in overall survival and longer disease-free intervals can be directly attributed to the use of chemotherapeutic agents, particularly in combination chemotherapy regimens and as adjuvant therapy. The last 50 years, and particularly the last decade, have brought rapid change and excitement into clinical practice.

Chemotherapy like other treatment modalities may be used for cure, as a means to achieve long-term control of cancer growth, or as palliation to temporarily shrink a tumor mass. When chemotherapy is used at a time when the malignant cell population is small and likely to be susceptible, complete tumor cell eradication is possible. Table 15-19 shows the responsiveness of various neoplastic diseases to chemotherapy.

Adjuvant chemotherapy refers to chemotherapy administered in conjunction with either surgery or radiation therapy. It is aimed at the destruction of micrometastases believed to be present but too small to be detected by current diagnostic techniques. Left untreated, micrometastases have a high potential for tumor growth and cancer recurrence.

Clinical Trials. Chemotherapeutic drugs are carefully tested before being approved for use as cancer treatment. The National Cancer Institute coordinates a rigorous drug-screening process for potential new agents. This process identifies compounds with antitumor activity, shows the activity in animal studies and establishes the pharmacologic aspects of the drug (kinetics, absorption, dose, metabolism, and excretion), and defines toxicity. Drugs then go through the four phases of clinical trials outlined in Table 15-20. Participation in various phases of clinical trials is available at cancer treatment centers across the country. Nurses need to be informed about the clinical trials process and assist patients to evaluate the risks and benefits of participation. Patients receiving cutting edge treatments need extensive support and education throughout the treatment period.

Principles of Chemotherapy. Normal and malignant cells progress through various phases in the cell cycle as they replicate. Most chemotherapy agents cause cell death by interrupting cell growth and replication at some point in the cell cycle (Figure 15-10). Drugs are classified by their mechanism of action. Drugs that act during a particular point of the cell cycle are termed cell cycle phase-specific drugs, whereas drugs that are active throughout the cell cycle are called phase-nonspecific drugs (Figure 15-11). Chemotherapy drugs are selected for use with a particular tumor based on tumor characteristics, such as the fraction of tumor cells in replication at a given time, tumor size, and location.

Cell Population Growth. Chemotherapy is most effective when the tumor is small and growing rapidly, a time when a relatively high proportion of cells are undergoing division. At this time, tumor cells are more sensitive to drugs that are toxic to dividing cells (phase-specific drugs). Larger, slower-growing tumors respond better to drugs that act regardless of whether a cell is dividing (phase-nonspecific drugs).

Cell-Kill Hypothesis. Chemotherapy is thought to kill a fixed percentage of the total number of cancer cells. Theoretically, if a drug had a 90% cell-kill rate and 1 million cells were present, the first treatment course would kill 900,000 cancer cells, leaving 100,000. The second treatment would again destroy 90% of the cells, leaving 10,000. Again, theoretically, after a number of chemotherapy treatments, only one cell would remain and that would be killed by the body's immune system (Figure 15-12). The cell-kill hypothesis explains why chemotherapy is scheduled in multiple courses over time.

Combination Chemotherapy. Most chemotherapy agents are given as a combination regimen. Combination chemotherapy has a therapeutic effect superior to single-agent therapy for many cancers, because drugs that attack the tumor cells in various ways can produce maximal tumor kill. The use of multiple drugs also decreases the likelihood of the tumor becoming resistant to a specific therapy, a process similar to

TABLE 15-19 Neoplastic Disease Response to Chemotherapy

Response	Neoplastic Disease
Cures in advanced cancer	Gestational trophoblastic tumor Acute lymphoblastic leukemia Acute myeloblastic leukemia Hodgkin's disease Non-Hodgkin's lymphoma (children) Diffuse histiocytic lymphoma Burkitt's lymphoma Testicular tumors
Cures with adjuvant chemotherapy	Wilms' tumor Osteogenic sarcoma Rhabdomyosarcoma
Minor responses with chemotherapy/adjuvant chemotherapy; no demonstrable prolongation of life	Non–small cell lung carcinoma Head and neck cancer Stomach cancer Cervical cancer Melanoma Cancer of the adrenal cortex Soft tissue sarcoma
Complete and partial remissions with uncertain prolongation of survival with chemotherapy/adjuvant chemotherapy	Multiple myeloma Ovarian cancer Endometrial cancer Neuroblastoma Colorectal cancer Liver cancer
Complete remissions and increased survival with chemotherapy/adjuvant chemotherapy	Breast cancer Small cell lung carcinoma Acute myeloblastic leukemia Non-Hodgkin's lymphoma Prostate cancer Chronic granulocytic leukemia Hairy cell leukemia

TABLE 15-20 Phases of Clinical Trials for Chemotherapeutic Drugs

Phase	Purpose
I	Identify toxic reactions; determine optimal dose within safe limits and set schedule
II	Determine extent of antineoplastic activity
III	Compare action of new drug with standard antineoplastic drugs
IV	Determine effect on advanced cancer, effect of combined therapy with other antineoplastic drugs, and effect with adjuvant therapy

antibiotic resistance. Drugs included in combination chemotherapy protocols have the following characteristics:

- Are active when used alone
- Have different mechanisms of action
- Have a biochemical basis for possible synergism
- Do not produce toxicity in the same organs
- Produce toxicity at different times after administration

Dose Intensity. Chemotherapy is most effective when sufficient doses of the drugs are delivered within a specified period of time to achieve maximal tumor kill. Many factors, however, can disrupt the treatment plan, particularly toxicity, which may necessitate dose reductions or delays. Dose reductions often translate into a significant reduction in clinical response when highly active cancers are treated. Many options are now available to ensure the dose intensity of curative regimens, including the use of hematopoietic growth factor support.

Tumor Resistance to Chemotherapy. Malignant neoplasms can become resistant to both single and multiple chemotherapeutic agents. This resistance may be present before any treatment has begun, termed primary resistance, as a result of a specific genetic trait. Secondary resistance may be acquired during treatment, probably as a result of spontaneous genetic alterations such as mutations, translocations, and deletions, which occur as the cell divides. These genetic alterations then change the drug's mechanism of action or metabolism within the cell. A tumor that initially responded to chemotherapy with shrinkage or decreased growth begins to increase in size and/or metastasize. Multiple-drug resistance (MDR) can occur when several agents are used in combination, and acquired MDR is documented for many chemotherapy drugs. Research into MDR is aimed at identifying and interfering with the molecular and biochemical changes that lead to resistance.

Chemotherapeutic Agents. Drugs may be classified as alkylating agents, antimetabolites, plant (vinca) alkaloids, antitumor antibiotics, and steroids. Table 15-21 lists chemotherapeutic agents by classification, action, toxicities, and nursing interventions.

Common Side Effects of Chemotherapy. Chemotherapy causes injury to normal cells as well as cancer cells. The bone marrow, gastrointestinal epithelium, and hair follicles are the most sensitive to chemotherapy because of their high rate of growth. Other side effects include fatigue and specific organ toxicities, such as pulmonary fibrosis, cardiotoxicity (congestive heart failure), genitourinary effects (cystitis, renal damage, sterility), hepatic toxicity, and neurotoxicity (numbness and tingling of the hands and feet, motor weakness). Nurses

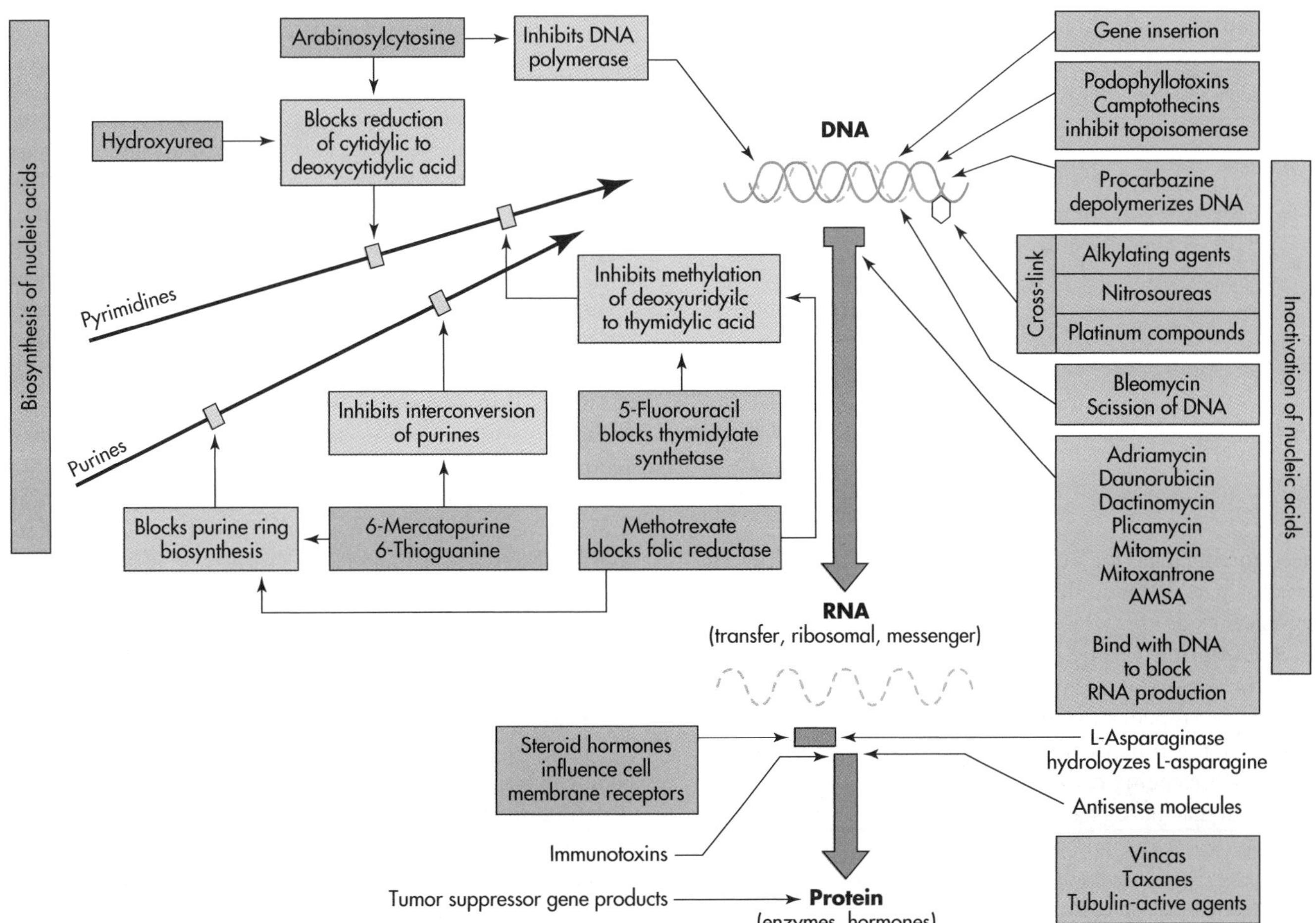

Figure 15-10 Mechanism of action for chemotherapeutic and biologic agents.

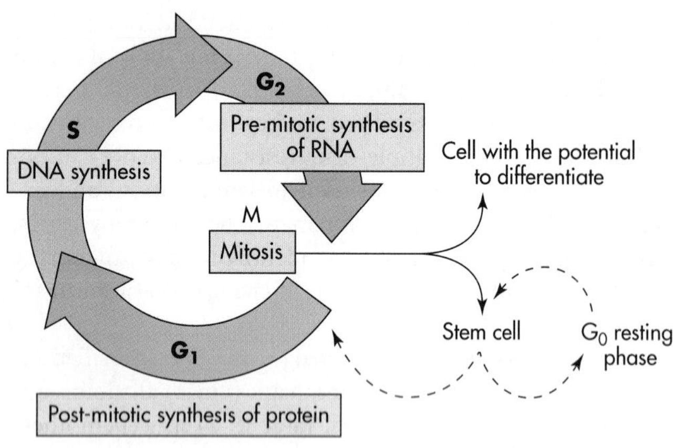

Cell Cycle Phase-Specific Agents

G_1 Phase
Asparaginase
Prednisone

S Phase
Antimetabolites
Cytarabine
5-fluorouracil
Hydroxyurea
Methotrexate
Thioguanine

G_2 Phase
Antibiotic
Bleomycin
Podophyllotoxin
Etoposide

Mitosis
Vinca alkaloids
Vinblastine
Vincristine
Vindesine
Paclitaxel

Cell Cycle Phase-Nonspecific Agents

Alkylating Agents
Busulfan
Carboplatin
Chlorambucil
Cisplatin
Cyclophosphamide
Dacarbazine
Ifosfamide
Mechlorethamine
Melphalan
Thiotepa

Antibiotics
Bleomycin
Dactinomycin
Daunorubicin
Doxorubicin
Mitomycin

Nitrosoureas
Carmustine (BCNU)
Lomustine (CCNU)
Semustine (MeCCNU)

Miscellaneous
Mitoxantrone
Navelbine
Procarbazine

Figure 15-11 Common cancer chemotherapeutic agents and their activity within the cell cycle.

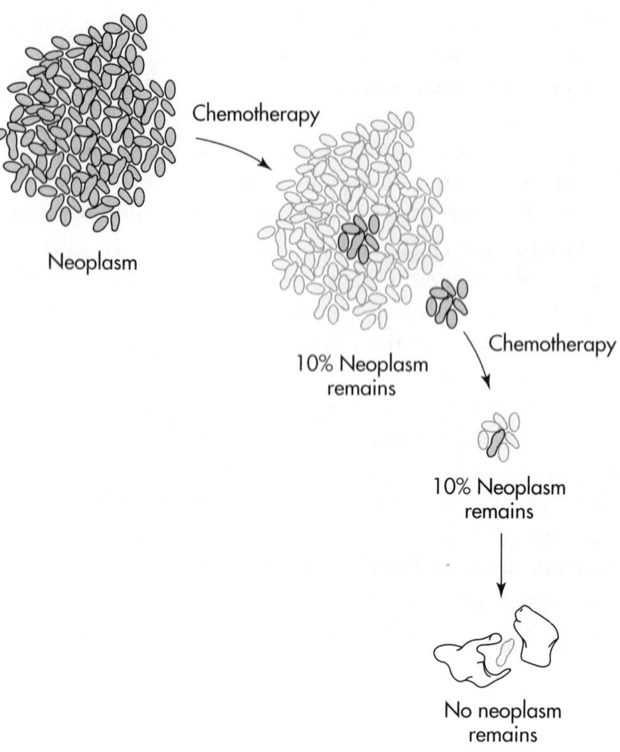

Figure 15-12 Cell-kill theory. Chemotherapy destroys 90% of neoplasm; repeated chemotherapy repeats process until the last neoplastic cell is killed by the body's immune response.

need to anticipate the possible side effects of each drug and work as part of the health care team to prevent and manage significant side effects.

Bone Marrow Effects. Many chemotherapy agents are toxic to the bone marrow and produce myelosuppression, which results in neutropenia, thrombocytopenia, and anemia. Myelosuppression can be the dose-limiting factor for many drugs, and life-threatening complications of infection and bleeding can result. Each drug has a predictable nadir, or point in time when WBCs, RBCs, and platelets will be at their lowest point. For many drugs, the nadir occurs 7 to 10 days after drug administration. Blood counts are obtained before chemotherapy administration and at regular intervals to identify the nadir and monitor the bone marrow recovery.

The most serious complication of myelosuppression is infection, which is the leading cause of morbidity and mortality in patients with cancer. Neutropenia, or neutrophils less than 1000 mm^3, is a critical risk factor for infection, as neutrophils form the primary defense against bacterial invasion. A minor infection in a person with neutropenia can result in septic shock within a few hours. Intact skin and mucous membranes are also important defenses against infection. Common sites for infections in myelosuppressed persons are the oropharynx, lungs, urinary tract, and skin.

Signs of early infection may be absent or diminished in neutropenic patients. Without neutrophils, patients do not develop the classic and common signs of infection such as redness, swelling, and pus formation. Mild localized tenderness and fever, defined as a temperature over 38.5° C, may be the only indications of a potentially dangerous infection.

The patient is at a significant risk for bleeding when the platelet count is $<50,000/mm^3$. The occurrence of bleeding may be minor, such as bruising or a nosebleed, or can be serious hemorrhage in the brain or gastrointestinal tract.

Patients with anemia exhibit signs of altered tissue perfusion, which can affect every organ system and cause a variety of symptoms. These patients may complain of symptoms that range from fatigue, decreased endurance, and headache to tachycardia, angina, dizziness, and dyspnea at rest.

Gastrointestinal Effects. Patients receiving chemotherapy commonly experience constipation and diarrhea. These symptoms may be a direct side effect of a particular chemotherapy

TABLE 15-21 Chemotherapy Agents Commonly Used to Treat Cancer

Drug	Action	Nursing Intervention
Alkylating Agents*		
Busulfan (Myleran) Cyclophosphamide (Cytoxan) Chlorambucil (Leukeran) DTIC Ifosfamide (Ifex) Melphalan (Alkeran) Nitrogen mustard (mechlorethamine) Thiotepa (Thioplex)	Alkylating agents are cell cycle non-specific and act against already formed nucleic acids by cross-linking DNA strands, thereby preventing DNA replication and transcription of RNA	Monitor for major toxicities Hematopoietic Anemia Leukopenia Thrombocytopenia Gastrointestinal Nausea and vomiting Diarrhea Reproductive Infertility Change in libido Ovarian and sperm suppression Genitourinary Cystitis and renal toxicity
Nitrosureas		
Carmustine (BCNU) Lomustine (CCNU) Streptozocin (Zanosar) Platinum-containing compounds Carboplatin (Paraplatin) Cisplatin (Platinol)	Alkylating agents that cross the blood-brain barrier Also alter functions of cell membrane and mitochondria	Drug specific Hemorrhagic cystitis (cyclophosphamide and ifosfamide) SIADH (cyclophosphamide) Nephrotoxicity (cisplatin) Ototoxicity (cisplatin)
Antimetabolites		
Capecitabine (Xeloda) Cytosine arabinoside (ARA-C) (Cytosar-U) Deoxycoformycin (pentostatin) Floxuridine (FUDR) Fludarabine phosphate Gemcitabine (Gemzar) Methotrexate 6-Mercaptopurine (6-MP) 6-Thioguanine (6-TG) 5-Fluorouracil (5-FU)	Act by interfering with synthesis of chromosomal nucleic acid; antimetabolites are analogs of normal metabolites and block the enzyme necessary for synthesis of essential factors or are incorporated into the DNA or RNA and thus prevent replication; are cycle specific	Monitor for major toxicities (depend on specific drug) Hematopoietic Bone marrow suppression Anemia Leukopenia Thrombocytopenia Gastrointestinal Mucositis/stomatitis Diarrhea Nausea and vomiting Alopecia Photosensitivity (5-FU, FUDR, methotrexate)
Antitumor Antibiotics		
Bleomycin (Blenoxane) Dactinomycin or actinomycin D (Cosmegen) Daunorubicin (Daunamycin) Doxorubicin (Adriamycin) Idarubicin (Idamycin) Mitomycin (Mutamycin) Mitoxantrone (Novantrone) Plicamycin (Mithramycin, Mithracin)	Interfere with synthesis and function of nucleic acids and inhibit RNA and DNA synthesis Agents are cycle nonspecific	Monitor for major toxicities Hematopoietic Bone marrow suppression Gastrointestinal Mucositis/stomatitis Anorexia, nausea, vomiting Integumentary Alopecia Tissue necrosis if extravasation of vesicant drugs Cardiac and pulmonary toxicity (doxorubicin, daunorubicin, idarubicin) Pulmonary fibrosis (bleomycin) Radiation recall (dactinomycin, daunorubicin, doxorubicin)

*Be aware of potential to develop second malignancy later in life (e.g., leukemia) when on alkylating agents.
RBC, Red blood cell; *SIADH,* syndrome of inappropriate antidiuretic hormone; *WBC,* white blood cell.

Continued

TABLE 15-21 Chemotherapy Agents Commonly Used to Treat Cancer—cont'd

Drug	Action	Nursing Intervention
Hormonal Agents		
Androgens Testosterone propionate Fluoxymesterone (Halotestin)	Alter pituitary function and directly affect the malignant cell	Monitor for major toxicities Fluid retention Masculinization
Corticosteroids Dexamethasone (Decadron) Hydrocortisone sodium succinate (Solu-Cortef) Methylprednisolone sodium (Solu-Medrol) Prednisone (Meticorten)	Lyse lymphoid malignancies and have indirect effects on malignant cells	Monitor for major toxicities Fluid retention Hypertension Diabetes Increased susceptibility to infection
Estrogens Diethylstilbestrol Estradiol	Suppress testosterone production in males and alter the response of breast cancers to prolactin	Monitor for major toxicities Fluid retention Feminization Uterine bleeding
Progestins Estramustine (Emcyt) Megestrol (Megace) Medroxyprogesterone (Provera)	Promote differentiation of malignant cells	
Estrogen antagonists Leuprolide (Lupron) Tamoxifen (Nolvadex)	Compete with estrogens for binding with estrogen receptor sites on malignant cells	Monitor for side effects Minimal with occasional headache Hot flashes
Antiadrenal Aminoglutethimide	Produces the equivalent of a medical adrenalectomy, thereby inhibiting the formation of estrogens and androgenesis and function of nucleic acids and inhibit RNA and DNA synthesis Agents are cycle nonspecific	Monitor for side effects Adrenal insufficiency
Vinca Alkaloids		
Vinblastine (Velban) Vincristine (Oncovin) Vindesine sulfate Vinorelbine (Navelbine)	Bind to proteins within the cells, causing metaphase arrest thus inhibiting RNA and protein synthesis Act in M phase	Monitor for major toxicities Myelosuppression (except vincristine) Peripheral neuropathy Constipation Extravasation Alopecia
Epipodophyllotoxins		
Etoposide (VP-16) Teniposide (VM-26)	Act in late G2 and S phase; cause breaks in DNA strands; interfere with topoisomerase II enzyme reaction	Monitor for major toxicities Myelosuppression Nausea and vomiting Alopecia Hypotension
Taxanes		
Paclitaxel (Taxol) Docetaxel (Taxotere)	Act in G2 and M phase; stabilize microtubule to inhibit cell division	Monitor for major toxicities Myelosuppression Hypersensitivity Alopecia Peripheral neuropathy (paclitaxel) Fluid retention (docetaxel)

TABLE 15-21 Chemotherapy Agents Commonly Used to Treat Cancer—cont'd

Drug	Action	Nursing Intervention
Camptothecins		
Irinotecan (Camptosar) Topotecan (Hycamtin)	Act in S phase; inhibit topoisomerase I enzyme reaction	Monitor for major toxicities Myelosuppression Diarrhea Alopecia Flulike syndrome (topotecan)
Other		
Hydroxyurea (Hydrea)	S-phase antimetabolite	Monitor for major toxicities Myelosuppression Nausea and vomiting Stomatitis
L-Asparaginase (Elspar)	Inhibits protein synthesis	Monitor for major toxicities Nausea and vomiting Hypersensitivity
Thalidomide	Inhibits angiogenesis	Monitor for major toxicities Sedation, peripheral neuropathy, constipation, skin rash

drug and can be worsened by factors such as altered dietary intake and activity, other medications such as opiods, or surgical procedures. The gastrointestinal tract is also susceptible to complications of infection and bleeding.

Stomatitis. Stomatitis, an inflammation of the oral mucous membranes, is a common side effect of many chemotherapy drugs (Box 15-8). Effects range from mild erythema to severe and painful ulcerations on the lips and in the mouth and throat. The peak effect of chemotherapy on the mucosal cells occurs 7 to 10 days after treatment and typically parallels the myelosuppressive effects of the drug.

Nausea and Vomiting. Patients with cancer have often identified nausea and vomiting as the most uncomfortable and distressing side effects of chemotherapy. Much progress has been made in understanding how chemotherapy causes nausea and vomiting, and new treatments have dramatically improved the management of these symptoms. In addition to the many chemotherapy drugs that can cause severe nausea and vomiting, other physical and emotional factors may also complicate the problem.

Chemical, visceral, central nervous system, and vestibular input can initiate the physiologic processes that cause nausea and vomiting (Figure 15-13). The vomiting center (VC) and the chemoreceptor trigger zone (CTZ) on the floor of the fourth ventricle coordinate the nausea and vomiting response. Chemical triggers include chemotherapy, which may directly stimulate the CTZ or cause secretion of serotonin antagonists (5-HT3) by the gastrointestinal tract, which in turn stimulate the VC. Visceral triggers of nausea occur when physical or emotional factors stimulate the vagus nerve. Central nervous system factors, such as psychologic distress, and vestibular mechanisms, which cause vertigo or imbalance, may also play a role. Chemotherapy agents vary greatly in their potential to cause nausea (Table 15-22). Chemotherapy typically causes a pattern of nausea that peaks within the first 12 hours and may be followed by delayed nausea that lasts 2 to 5 days. Patients may also experience anticipatory nausea, which is a conditioned response that develops after initial courses of chemotherapy.

BOX 15-8 Drugs Causing Stomatitis

Bleomycin (Blenoxane)
Doxorubicin (Adriamycin)
Cytosine arabinoside (Ara-C)
Cyclophosphamide (Cytoxan)
Daunorubicin (Cerubidine)
Methotrexate
5-Fluorouracil (5-FU)

For the outpatient nausea may interfere with the ability to continue work. Persistent vomiting can result in fluid and electrolyte imbalance, general weakness, and weight loss. A decline in nutritional status makes the person more susceptible to infection and less able to tolerate therapy. The onset and duration of both nausea and vomiting vary greatly from patient to patient and with the drugs given.

Alopecia. The alopecia that results from cancer therapy is one of the most traumatic psychologic side effects patients with cancer experience. Hair loss is a constant reminder of cancer, makes the illness visible to others, and causes significant changes in body image.

Not all chemotherapy drugs cause alopecia, and the degree of hair loss depends on the dose of the drug and method of administration. When it does occur, hair loss ranges from mild scalp thinning to complete loss of all body hair. Hair loss

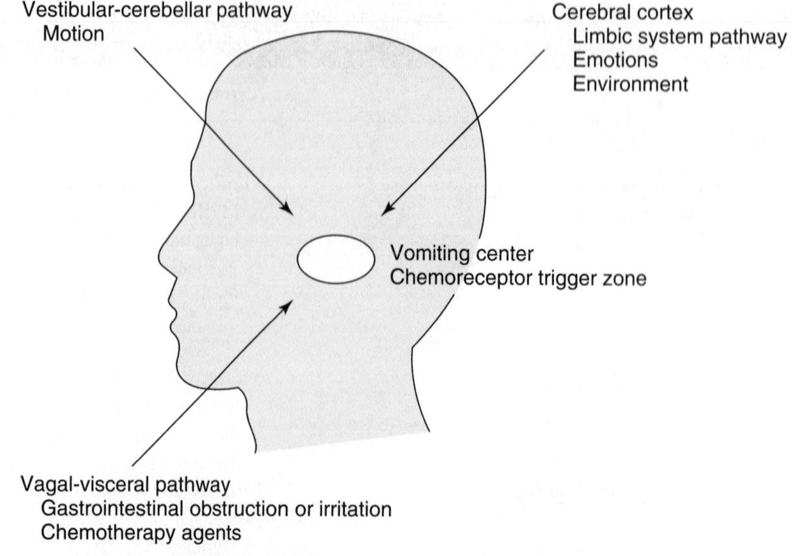

Figure 15-13 Pathways of nausea and vomiting.

TABLE 15-22 Emetogenic Potential of Common Chemotherapy Agents

Incidence	Agent	Onset (hours)	Duration (hours)
High	Cisplatin	1-6	24-48$^+$
	Dacarbazine	1-3	1-12
	Cyclophosphamide	4-12	12-24$^+$
	Cytarabine (high dose)	1-4	12-48$^+$
	Etoposide (high dose)	4-6	24$^+$
	Methotrexate (high dose)	1-12	24-72
Moderate	Doxorubicin	4-6	6$^+$
	5-Fluorouracil	3-6	24$^+$
	Carboplatin	4-6	12-24
	Daunorubicin	2-6	24
	Topotecan	6-12	24-72
	Ifosfamide	3-6	24-72
	Irinotecan	6-12	24$^+$
Low	Bleomycin	3-6	—
	Cytarabine	6-12	3-12
	Etoposide	3-8	—
	Methotrexate	4-12	3-12
	Vinblastine	4-8	—
	Gemcitabine	—	—
	Vinorelbine	—	—
	Fludarabine	—	—
	Vincristine	4-8	—
	Paclitaxel	4-8	—
	Docetaxel	—	—
	Hydroxyurea	—	—

Adapted from Camp-Sorrell D: Chemotherapy: toxicity management. In Yarbro CH et al, editors, *Cancer nursing: principles and practice,* ed 5, Boston, 2000, Jones and Bartlett.

usually begins 2 to 3 weeks after the start of therapy and is reversible, with regrowth usually occurring 1 to 2 months after treatment. New hair growth may take up to a year to occur and may have a different thickness and texture.

Sexual Dysfunction. Cancer chemotherapy affects the germinal epithelium of the ovary and testes, and many patients experience reproductive dysfunction during and after chemotherapy. Cycle-nonspecific agents such as the alkylating agents are most commonly associated with altered fertility. For female patients, age is an important predictor of whether these changes will be permanent. Women less than 30 years old are more likely to regain ovarian function because they have more oocytes that are not undergoing constant mitosis. Women may become amenorrheic during chemotherapy followed by a period of irregular menstrual cycles. Perimenopausal women receiving chemotherapy are likely to become menopausal and develop the short- and long-term symptoms and complications of estrogen depletion. The testes are more susceptible to the effects of chemotherapy because of the constant mitosis necessary for sperm production. Testicular damage results in decreased sperm production and sperm and semen abnormalities. The incidence and length of time for recovery depend on the particular drug and dose the patient has received. Both men and women have regained the ability to conceive children after chemotherapy.

Fatigue. Fatigue is a common side effect for many patients receiving chemotherapy and may seriously compromise the patient's quality of life. Many factors play a role in causing fatigue, including the physical, psychologic, and social changes that result from cancer and cancer therapy. Chemotherapy causes fatigue when cellular metabolism is altered and the end products of cellular destruction accumulate in the body. Fatigue is a subjective experience but does have objective consequences. Fatigued patients complain of feeling weak and having no energy, feelings which are not relieved with adequate rest. They may be unable to complete normal activities of daily living without feeling exhausted.

Specific Organ Toxicities. Certain chemotherapy agents cause specific organ toxicity, affecting the heart, lung, liver, kidney, and bladder. The organ damage may be permanent. The anthracycline agents directly damage the cardiac cells. Short-term side effects include electrocardiogram changes and heart failure may develop over time. Pulmonary fibrosis may develop with the use of bleomycin and other lung toxicities may occur with cytarabine, cyclosphosphamide, and a number of other drugs. Liver toxicity can develop, especially with the use of higher doses of drugs. Nephrotoxicity is a dose-limiting side effect of cisplatin and is also associated with high-dose methotrexate. Hemorrhagic cystitis is a bladder complication seen with cyclophosphamide and ifosfamide use. Drugs that are known to cause irreversible organ damage are administered within cumulative lifetime dose limits. Nurses are frequently responsible for monitoring total doses for those drugs that have cumulative lifetime limits.

Cryoprotective Agents. Some organ toxicity may be prevented or minimized with the use of medications that protect normal tissue called cryoprotectants. Three cryoprotectant agents are currently available for use, but others are under investigation. Dexrazoxane (Zinecard) is used to decrease the cardiotoxicity associated with doxorubicin, and mesna (Mesnex) is used to decrease the hemorrhagic cystitis caused by ifosfamide. The third agent, amifostine (Ethyol), may protect a broad range of normal tissues, including the kidney, gastrointestinal tract, lung, and nerves, from the effects of many chemotherapy agents. Because cryoprotective agents have a side-effect profile of their own, the risks and benefits of their use must be considered in the treatment plan.

Hypersensitivity Reactions. A number of chemotherapy drugs are associated with hypersensitivity reactions, and nurses administering or caring for patients receiving these drugs must institute specific precautions. Box 15-9 lists drugs that have a significant risk of hypersensitivity reactions. Nursing protocols outline specific interventions related to the administration of these medications (e.g., the use of premedication, frequent monitoring, and standing orders for emergency care).

BOX 15-9 Immediate Hypersensitivity Reactions: Predicted Risk of Chemotherapy

High Risk

L-asparaginase*
Paclitaxel

Low-to-Moderate Risk

Anthracyclines
Bleomycin
Carboplatin
Cisplatin
Cyclosporine
Docetaxel
Etoposide
Melphalan*
Methotrexate
Procarbazine
Teniposide

Rare Risk

Cytosine arabinoside
Cyclophosphamide
Chlorambucil
Dacarbazine
5-Fluorouracil
Ifosfamide
Mitoxantrone

From Oncology Nursing Society: *Cancer chemotherapy guidelines and recommendations for practice,* Pittsburgh, 1999, Oncology Nursing Press.
*Significantly increased risk with IV route.

BOX 15-10 Vesicant Chemotherapy Agents

Dactinomycin
Daunorubicin
Doxorubicin
Epirubicin
Idarubicin
Mechlorethamine
Mitomycin
Vinblastine
Vincristine
Vindesine
Vinorelbine

Chemotherapy Administration. Chemotherapy administration is primarily the responsibility of a registered nurse who must be knowledgeable about the pharmacology and dosing of the drug, as well as competent in drug preparation, administration, and management of toxicity. The Oncology Nursing Society recommends, and various state boards of nursing and many health care institutions require, that nurses who administer chemotherapy complete formal chemotherapy education programs to ensure competent practice.

Preventing Extravasation. A number of chemotherapy agents cause tissue damage if they extravasate or leak out of the vein and infiltrate soft tissue. These drugs, termed vesicants, cause severe tissue ulceration and necrosis when extravasated in a significant amount (Box 15-10). Nurses who administer chemotherapy institute specific safety protocols for vesicant administration. The nurse monitors for possible intravenous infiltrations and immediately institutes appropriate treatment to minimize tissue damage, including the application of heat and cold and the administration of specific antidotes. Although infrequent, extravasation injuries do occur with central venous access devices (VADs).

Special Handling of Chemotherapy. Chemotherapy drugs are associated with serious side effects, including carcinogenicity and teratogenicity. Health care workers who handle antineoplastic drugs can be exposed to low doses of the drug by direct contact, inhalation, and injection and can be at risk for some of the same side effects associated with therapeutic use. Because the long-term effects of chronic exposure are not completely known, guidelines for safe handling of these agents have been established. The Occupational Safety and Health Administration (OSHA) of the U.S. Department of Labor and other health care institutions have developed the guidelines summarized in the Guidelines for Safe Practice box. It is essential that any health care provider working with cytotoxic drugs follow these guidelines to prevent injury to self and others.

Routes for Chemotherapy Administration. The method of administration for each drug is based on its pharmacokinetic properties as well as characteristics of the patient and cancer. The route of choice is one that delivers the optimal amount of drug to the tumor. Chemotherapeutic agents can be given orally, subcutaneously, intramuscularly, intravenously, and topically. Chemotherapy drugs can also be directly instilled into the bladder, peritoneum, or cerebrospinal fluid. These latter routes allow high-dose concentrations of the drug to the tumor site without undue systemic effects and may be used when a malignant organ or tissue cannot be treated surgically. Administration of chemotherapy into the cerebrospinal fluid, called the intrathecal route, can be done either by a lumbar

Guidelines for Safe Practice

Safety in Handling Chemotherapeutic Agents

A. Prevention of inhalation of aerosols
   1. Mix all drugs in an approved class II or III vertical airflow biologic safety cabinet (BSC), wearing gloves made of latex or nitrile at all times. Surgical masks do not prevent aerosol inhalation and should not be used. Eye and face barriers should be worn if splashes are likely to occur or sprays or aerosols are used.
   2. Prime all IV bags within the BSC before adding the drug. Use a maintenance bag of normal saline or D_5W to prime the tubing and all the chemotherapy bags afterward.
   3. Break ampules by wrapping a sterile gauze pad or alcohol wipe around the neck (decreases chance of droplet contamination).
   4. Vent vials with only enough air to allow the drug to be aspirated easily using a hydrophobic filter needle.
   5. Syringes and needles used in cytotoxic drug preparation should not be crushed, clipped, or recapped. They should immediately be placed in a sharps container labeled "cytotoxic waste" for disposal.
   6. Use a gauze pad when removing syringes and needles from IV injection ports or spikes from IV bags.

B. Prevention of drug absorption through the skin
   1. Wear latex or nitrile gloves and a gown made of nonpermeable fabric with a closed front and cuffed long sleeves.
   2. Change gloves every 60 minutes.
   3. Remove gloves immediately after spilling drug solution on them or puncturing or tearing them.
   4. Wash hands before putting on gloves and after removing them.
   5. Cover the work surface with a plastic-backed absorbent pad; change pad when cabinet is cleaned or after a spill.
   6. Clean all surfaces or the BSC before and after drug preparation in accordance with manufacturer's instructions. Discard equipment used in a leakproof, puncture-proof, chemical-waste container.
   7. Use syringes and IV sets with Luer-Lok fittings.
   8. Place an absorbent pad under injection sites to catch accidental spillage.
   9. Label all antineoplastic drugs with a chemotherapy warning label.
   10. Wash skin areas thoroughly with soap and water as soon as possible in the event of skin contact with drugs.
   11. Flush eyes with eye solution or clean water in the event of eye contact; seek medical attention.

C. Prevention of ingestion
   1. Do not eat, drink, chew gum, apply cosmetics, store food or smoke in drug preparation areas.
   2. Wash hands before and after preparing or giving drugs.
   3. Avoid hand-to-mouth or hand-to-eye contact when handling the drugs.

D. Safe disposal
   1. Discard nonsharp cytotoxic waste products in a leakproof, puncture-proof sealable plastic bag of a different color than regular trash bags. Label as "cytotoxic waste."
   2. Use a leakproof, puncture-proof container labeled as "cytotoxic waste" for needles and sharp, breakable items.
   3. Keep waste containers in labeled, covered waste containers for disposal.
   4. Housekeeping personnel should be instructed in safe procedures and should wear latex or nitrile gloves and gowns of nonpermeable fabric.
   5. All waste produced by cytotoxic drug administration in the home should be placed in a sealed receptacle and transported in the nonpassenger area of a vehicle to the home agency for disposal.

E. Prevention of contamination by body fluids
   1. Wear latex or nitrile gloves and disposable, nonpermeable fabric when handing any body fluids.
   2. Empty waste products into the toilet by pouring close to the water to avoid splashing. Close the lid and flush two to three times (in the home).
   3. Wear gloves and gown when handling linen soiled with body fluids; place in isolation linen bag for separate laundry.
   4. Place soiled linens in separate, washable pillow cases and wash twice, separately from other household linens (in the home).
   5. A standard duration of 48 hours is accepted as the time after which most cytotoxic drugs will have been metabolized or excreted. For most cytotoxic agents, urine excretion is complete within 48 hours after administration (range of 1-6 days) and stool excretion is complete within 7 days (range of 5-7 days).

puncture or by using a cerebrospinal (Ommaya) reservoir (Figure 15-14).

Intravenous Drug Administration. The intravenous route is the most common route for chemotherapy administration. Chemotherapy can be administered through standard peripheral intravenous lines, but patients who require long-term repeated venous access, receive intensive chemotherapy regimens, or have poor peripheral vein access will usually receive chemotherapy through a centrally placed VAD. A central VAD is an intravenous catheter located in a central vessel, usually positioned in the superior vena cava, with its tip at the entrance to the right atrium. The type of VAD depends on treatment variables and the patient's general condition and preference. Centrally located catheters allow for intermittent or continuous administration of chemotherapy agents, blood and blood products, other medications, and TPN. These catheters may have single, double, or triple lumens for multidrug administration. Central VADs can be short term, such as percutaneous subclavian catheters, which are nontunneled, sutured catheters, usually used when immediate central access is needed (Figure 15-15). Long-term VADs are tunneled and cuffed and made out of softer silicone, so that they may stay in place for years. The technique of "tunneling" the catheter beneath the skin helps to prevent bacterial entry and growth along the catheter tract. All tunneled catheters have a small "cuff" around which fibroblasts form and help secure the catheter in place. Figure 15-16 shows positioning of a tunneled and cuffed central VAD. The exit site of central catheters requires a sterile dressing change, and each catheter lumen must be flushed to maintain patency when it is not being used. Protocols for dressing changes and flushing vary among institutions.

Implanted VADs, or ports, are tunneled and cuffed catheters attached to a reservoir made out of titanium or steel with a self-sealing septum (Figure 15-17). The port is placed in a subcutaneous pocket in the upper chest, and the catheter does not have an external segment. The catheter is accessed by inserting a noncoring needle through the skin and into the reservoir. When the catheter is not in use, no external dressing is used and flushing is required only once a month.

Peripherally inserted central catheters (PICCs) are catheters that are inserted into a peripheral vein and advanced into a central vein. Access is usually obtained via the cephalic or basilic vein in the upper arm. This technique allows for easier insertion. External dressing and daily flushing procedures are necessary to maintain the patency of the catheter.

Complications with all VADs include local and systemic infection, thrombosis, occlusion, and air embolism.[21] Local infection can occur at the exit site of the catheter, along the

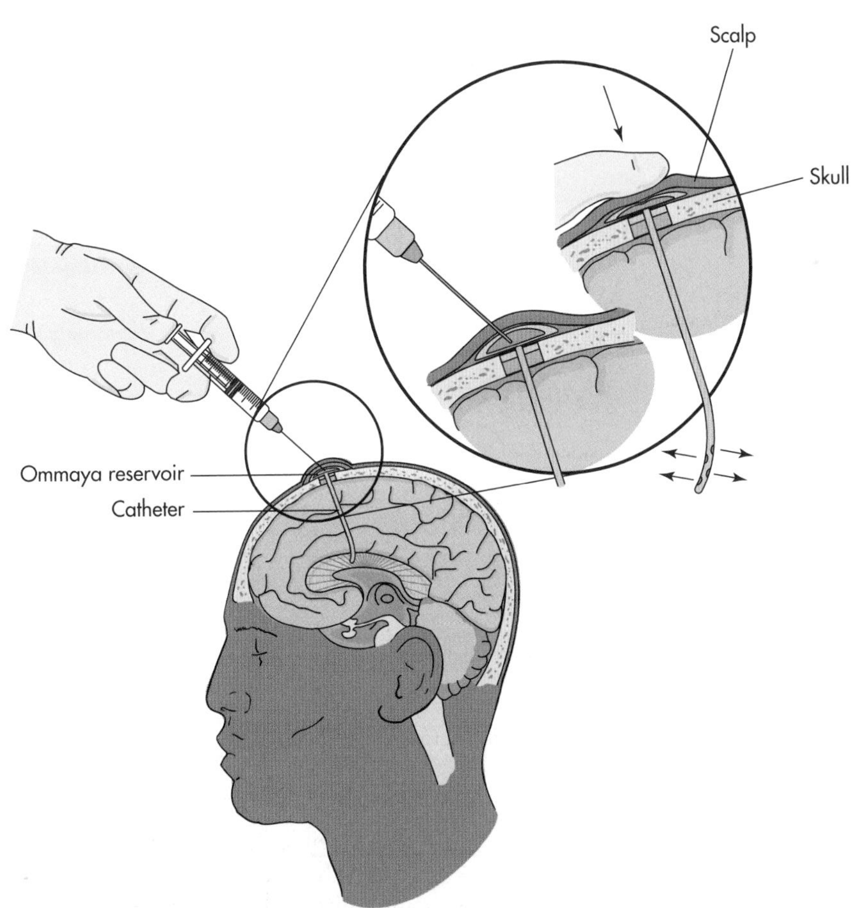

Figure 15-14 Ommaya reservoir for administration of chemotherapeutic agents directly into the central nervous system. NOTE: Medication is administered into reservoir and moves through a catheter into the lateral ventricle.

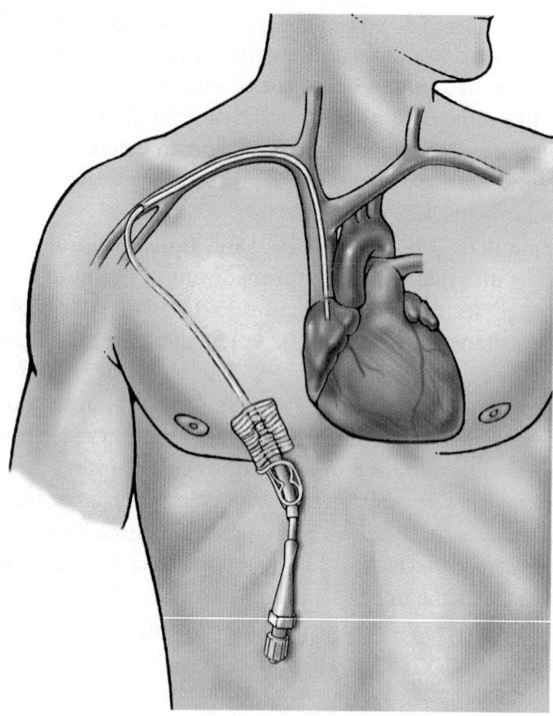

Figure 15-15 Central venous catheter in place.

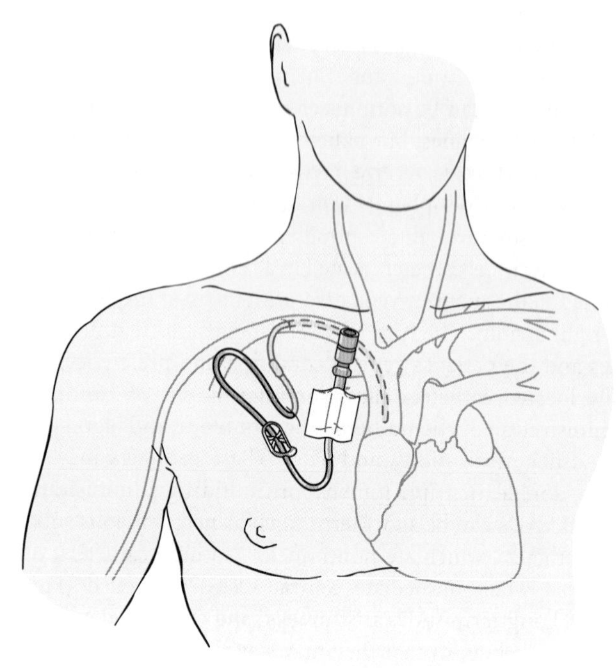

Figure 15-16 Tunneled catheter.

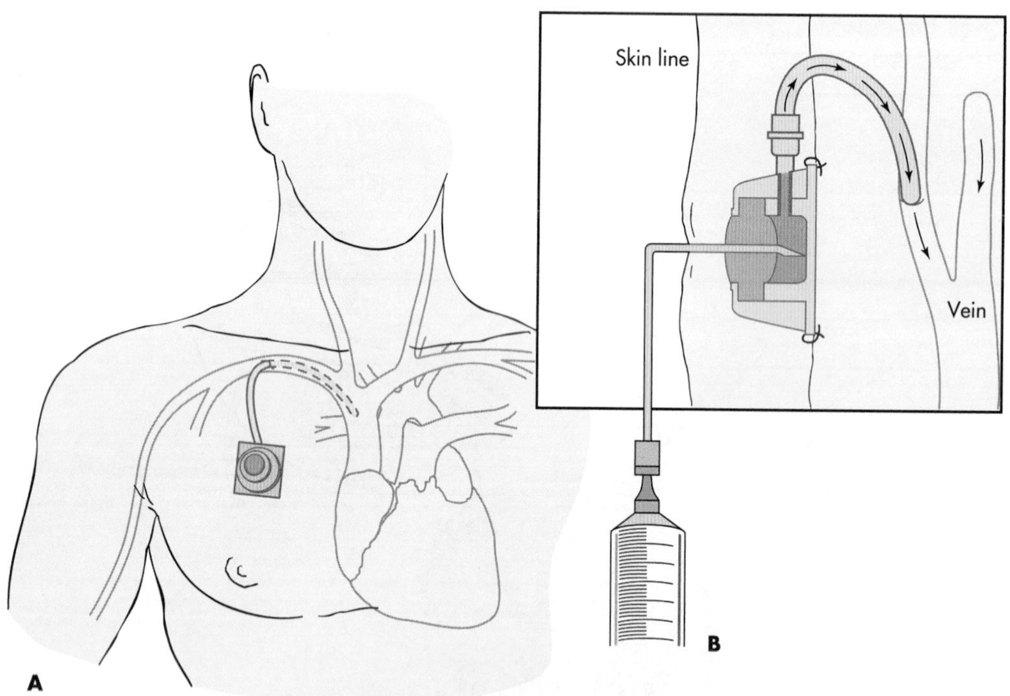

Figure 15-17 **A**, Implanted port. **B**, Cross section of port with needle access.

tunnel, or at the pocket of a port. Thromboses can occur around and along the catheter, preventing blood flow in the vessel around the catheter. Compromised circulation can affect the extremity as well as the face and neck. Thromboses can also occur within the catheter, causing difficulty with infusion of fluids and withdrawal of blood. A comparison of VADs is presented in Table 15-23.

Delivery of chemotherapy in the home is possible with the use of either external or implantable pump systems. The pumps have electronic internal power sources so that either intermittent or continuous drug administration is possible. The external pumps are small and lightweight and attach to either a belt or shoulder strap, so that the patient can maintain normal activities. External pumps require a competent patient

TABLE 15-23 Comparison of Venous Access Devices

Type of Device	Advantage	Disadvantage
Peripheral catheter	Easy and quick to insert at the bedside No major complications No self-care	Short life span (3 days) Discomfort and difficult insertion for some Not safe for certain drugs and infusions
Non-tunneled central venous catheter	Inserted at the bedside Safe for all fluids and blood drawing	Short-term Not for outpatient use
Peripherally inserted central catheter (PICC)	Can remain for 6 months or longer Easier to insert and less expensive than other central catheters Safe for all fluids and blood drawing	Inserted in angiography May limit arm mobility and activities Requires self-care for dressing changes and flushes Blood drawing may be difficult
Tunneled central venous catheter	Can remain for years Good for long-term, intense, frequent IV therapy Safe for all fluids and blood drawing	Inserted in angiography Causes minor insertion discomfort Requires self-care for dressing changes and flushes Higher risk of infection
Implanted port	Can remain for years Requires no self-care Maintains body image and mobility Low infection rate Safe for all fluids and blood drawing	More difficult and expensive insertion in angiography Causes minor insertion discomfort More difficult removal Minor discomfort with needle access

and/or caregiver to receive instruction in the care and maintenance of the delivery system.

Implantable pumps are inserted with a technique similar to implanted ports. The catheters are placed into the selected vein or artery, and a subcutaneous pocket for the pump is created near the site. The chemotherapy drug is injected into the chamber of the pump with a needle inserted through the skin. The most common complication of implantable pumps is the development of a seroma over the pump pocket. This accumulation of sterile fluid may require aspiration

Dose Calculation and Drug Preparation. Chemotherapy doses are usually based on the individual's body surface area (BSA). BSA is calculated using the patient's height and weight. Both high-dose and low-dose regimens can be prescribed for many commonly used drugs. It is critical that the drug prescription be accurate and complete to avoid dosing or administration errors. Many institutions have strict guidelines concerning who can prescribe chemotherapy and how the orders are processed. Because of the hazards of handling chemotherapy, special procedures for both drug preparation and transportation are necessary.

NURSING MANAGEMENT OF PATIENT RECEIVING CHEMOTHERAPY

ASSESSMENT

Chemotherapy, with its many side effects, can adversely affect the patient in a variety of ways. The nurse is constantly alert for signs and symptoms that could indicate the presence of chemotherapy side effects.

Health History

Aspects of the health history of particular importance when caring for a patient undergoing chemotherapy are:

- Age
- Comorbid health problems, current treatment
- Medical history, family history
- Medications in use, prescribed and over the counter
- Allergies to food, drugs
- Social support, family composition
- Learning ability, education level, occupation
- Financial status, insurance coverage
- Understanding of chemotherapy and its use in cancer treatment
- Knowledge of planned treatment and expected side effects.

Physical Examination

Physical examination of the patient receiving chemotherapy should focus on:

- Performance status
- Body surface area (height and weight)
- Venous access
- Nutritional status, recent weight gain/loss
- Elimination patterns, current problems with constipation/diarrhea
- Mobility, activities of daily living
- Skin and oral mucous membrane integrity
- Neurologic status
- Cardiovascular status
- Pulmonary status

NURSING DIAGNOSES

Diagnostic Title	Possible Etiologic Factors
1. Deficient knowledge	Unfamiliarity with chemotherapy regimen, schedule, side effects
2. Risk for infection	Neutropenia
3. Risk for injury: bleeding	Thrombocytopenia
4. Impaired gas exchange	Anemia

5. Nausea	Effects of chemotherapy
6. Imbalanced nutrition: less than body requirements	Nausea, anorexia, early satiety, stomatitis
7. Disturbed body image	Alopecia, weight loss, alterations in sexual function
8. Impaired oral mucous membranes	Stomatitis, esophagitis

EXPECTED PATIENT OUTCOMES

Expected patient outcomes for the patient receiving chemotherapy may include but are not limited to:

1. Will describe the goal of chemotherapy, the chemotherapy schedule, and the potential side effects
2. Will have no evidence of fever or any untreated signs of infection
3. Will not experience episodes of uncontrolled bleeding
4. Will not complain of dyspnea, chest pain, dizziness, or weakness related to anemia
5. Will not experience nausea or have uncontrolled episodes of vomiting
6. Will maintain desired weight and have adequate nutritional intake
7. Will acknowledge changes in body image and demonstrate positive coping strategies
8. Will maintain intact oral mucous membranes and will not complain of pain related to stomatitis

NURSING INTERVENTIONS

1. Providing Patient/Family Education

The nurse first clarifies the goal of chemotherapy for the patient, whether chemotherapy is to be used for cure, palliation of symptoms, or as adjuvant therapy. The nurse needs accurate and detailed information about the patient's cancer, its stage and extent, and the proposed chemotherapy regimen and may play a role in any interdisciplinary team conference to plan the most appropriate treatment regimen.

Knowledge of the planned chemotherapy protocol provides information about the major side effects to be expected and what supportive interventions are indicated. The nurse then develops an individualized patient teaching and care plan.

The assessment interview clarifies the patient's expectations of therapy and explores the patient's fears or anxieties about the treatment. Patients facing chemotherapy for the first time usually know of someone who has been treated with chemotherapy and can often recite its many associated negative aspects. They wonder if they will face the same discomforts, such as nausea and vomiting, weight loss, and hair loss. Patients who have previously undergone chemotherapy may fear resumption of therapy and express doubts regarding its effectiveness. They doubt the wisdom of subjecting themselves once again to the adverse side effects that go along with therapy. It is important for the nurse to respect and support the unique response of each patient. Each patient is reassured that every effort will be made to prevent and control undesirable side effects. The nurse provides honest, detailed, and realistic information at a level that meets the patient's needs.

Patients commonly express concern related to the cost of a lengthy course of chemotherapy, especially if they have inadequate health insurance. They may fear becoming a financial drain on family resources, since most treatment regimens require frequent clinic visits and repeated hospitalizations. Transportation, child care, and work responsibilities are also possible areas of concern. The nurse attempts to understand each patient's unique situation and plan collaboratively to address individual concerns.

2. Preventing and Managing Infections

Nursing interventions to prevent infection include measures to maximize the patient's own defenses against infection, minimize sources of infection, and aggressively identify and treat infection. The nurse teaches the patient about the risk for infection, specific signs and symptoms of infection, and how infections can be prevented and treated. Patients who will be at home need to have a thermometer and know how to use it. Patients are taught to report a fever as well as any new sign of infection and need specific instructions about whom to notify and when.

The patient needs to maintain good personal hygiene, particularly skin and mouth care. Protocols for specific VAD, wound, or tube care are emphasized. The patient should avoid contact with family, staff, or visitors who have an infection. Caregivers should practice thorough hand washing before any patient contact. The frequency of patient assessments depends on the degree of myelosuppression expected with the regimen. Patients undergoing induction chemotherapy for leukemia, for example, may require assessment and measurement of vital signs every 4 hours with daily monitoring of blood counts. The patient receiving a monthly outpatient regimen may have blood counts checked weekly with a physical assessment before each treatment.

Any sign of infection in a neutropenic patient is considered to be a medical emergency that requires immediate treatment. Physical and laboratory examinations are performed to determine the site of infection, and aggressive antimicrobial therapy is instituted to control the infection. Colony-stimulating factors (CSFs) are increasingly being used to reduce the severity and duration of neutropenia following chemotherapy. G-CSF and GM-CSF are WBC growth factors given as subcutaneous injections for several days after chemotherapy administration (see p. 327). Many patients are taught to self-administer this medication and need to be taught about drug preparation and subcutaneous injection technique. Infection precautions are summarized in the Guidelines for Safe Practice box on p. 351, left.

3. Preventing and Managing Bleeding Episodes

The myelosuppressed patient is at risk for bleeding because of an inadequate number of platelets. Bleeding precautions are instituted to maintain the integrity of the skin and mucous membranes. The patient is assessed for signs and symptoms of bleeding, including occult blood in body fluids. The platelet count is monitored as indicated by the degree of bleeding risk. A platelet count below 10,000/mm^3 or the presence of active

Guidelines for Safe Practice

The Patient With Neutropenia

1. Maximize the patient's own defenses against infection.
   a. Implement skin care regimen to maintain skin integrity.
   b. Implement oral hygiene regimen to maintain integrity of the mouth.
   c. Avoid intramuscular and subcutaneous injections, rectal temperatures, and rectal medication administration.
   d. Avoid invasive procedures, such as urinary catheterizations.
   e. Avoid medications likely to mask a fever, such as aspirin, acetaminophen, and steroids.
2. Minimize the patient's exposure to sources of infection.
   a. Emphasize the need for thorough hand washing for all persons who have physical contact with the patient.
   b. Restrict persons with colds and infections from physical contact with the patient.
   c. Limit dietary intake of fresh fruits and vegetables, or wash them thoroughly.
   d. Limit patient contact with obviously infected items, such as cat litter and bird cages.
3. Assess for signs and symptoms of infection.
   a. Monitor vital signs as indicated.
   b. Monitor total white blood count and neutrophil count as indicated.
   c. Examine potential sites of infection, including lungs, skin, intravenous sites, mouth, and perirectum.
4. Implement a plan for aggressive antimicrobial therapy.
   a. Immediately report temperature greater than 101° F or any new sign of infection.
   b. Obtain bacterial and fungal cultures of body fluids before starting initial antibiotic therapy.
   c. Administer broad-spectrum antimicrobial therapy as soon as possible and adjust coverage as necessary. Check drug allergies and monitor for side effects.
5. Administer G-CSF or GM-CSF therapy as prescribed.
   a. Teach patient self-administration technique if necessary.
6. Educate patient and family about the risk of infection.
   a. Inform the patient about the relative risk of infection.
   b. Implement a teaching plan that includes:
      (1) Symptoms of infection
      (2) Self-care measures to prevent infection
      (3) When and how to report symptoms of infection
      (4) How potential infections will be treated

bleeding in a thrombocytopenic patient indicates the need for platelet transfusion. Nurses need to be knowledgeable about the safe administration of platelet transfusions, including how to prevent and control transfusion reactions. The Guidelines for Safe Practice box at right outlines nursing interventions to prevent bleeding in thrombocytopenic patients.

4. Supporting Tissue Perfusion

The patient with anemia experiences multiple symptoms related to poor tissue perfusion, such as fatigue, dyspnea, and headaches. Patients who are symptomatic or who experience severe anemia may require RBC transfusions to temporarily restore RBC levels during treatment. Nurses are responsible for the safe administration of blood products and the identification and management of RBC transfusion reactions. Therapy with EPO, an RBC growth factor, can prevent severe anemia related to chemotherapy, reducing the need for transfusions and preventing the common symptoms. EPO is given as a subcutaneous injection, usually on a weekly schedule.

Guidelines for Safe Practice

The Patient With Thrombocytopenia

1. Minimize source of trauma as cause of bleeding.
   a. Avoid intramuscular and subcutaneous injections, rectal temperatures, and rectal medication administration.
   b. Avoid aspirin, aspirin-containing products, and nonsteroidal antiinflammatory drugs, which may increase bleeding.
   c. Minimize venipunctures and other invasive procedures, such as urinary catheterization.
   d. Apply pressure to venipuncture sites for 5 minutes.
   e. Implement mouth care regimen with soft toothbrushing. Avoid flossing and other dental procedures.
   f. Use only electric shavers for hair removal.
   g. Provide assistance with activity as necessary to prevent falls.
   h. Limit activities likely to cause trauma, such as contact sports.
2. Assess for signs and symptoms of bleeding.
   a. Inspect potential sites of bleeding, such as skin, nose, and mouth.
   b. Check sputum, urine, stool, emesis, and other body fluids for occult blood.
   c. Monitor platelet count as indicated.
3. Administer platelet transfusions when platelet count is $<10,000/mm^3$, when there is active bleeding, or before an invasive procedure.
4. Educate patient and family about the risk of bleeding.
   a. Inform the patient about the relative risk of bleeding.
   b. Implement a teaching plan that includes:
      (1) Symptoms of bleeding, such as bruises, petechiae, nose bleeds, blood in urine, stool, sputum, or emesis
      (2) Self-care measures to prevent bleeding
      (3) When and how to report symptoms of bleeding
      (4) How potential episodes of bleeding would be treated

5. Preventing and Managing Nausea and Vomiting

The gastrointestinal tract is highly sensitive to the effects of chemotherapy. Anorexia, nausea, and vomiting are common problems. Diarrhea or constipation can also occur. The outcome can be weight loss and fluid volume deficit, which can lead to serious malnutrition and dehydration. Nausea and vomiting are two of the more dreaded side effects of chemotherapy. Although nausea and vomiting are expected with many chemotherapy agents, advances in the use of antiemetics have successfully reduced their incidence and severity. A variety of antiemetic agents with different mechanisms of action are available, and agents are prescribed based on the severity of the problem (Table 15-24). Both premedication with antiemetics before treatment and scheduled coverage during chemotherapy are essential. Antiemetics should also be available in case patients experience delayed nausea for several days after therapy. The nurse evaluates the effectiveness of the antiemetic regimen and makes adjustments as needed for subsequent courses of treatment. If diarrhea or constipation

TABLE 15-24 Examples of Antiemetic Regimens for Chemotherapy-Related Nausea

Type of Nausea	Examples of Regimen
Low	No antiemetic premedication or Prochlorperazine 10-20 mg PO premedication then qid prn or Metoclopramide 10-20 mg PO premedication then qid prn
Moderate	Ondansetron 8-16 mg PO 1 hour before chemotherapy then 8 mg bid or Granisetron 1 mg PO 1 hour before Chemotherapy then 1 mg bid
Severe	Ondansetron 8-16 mg PO 1 hour before Chemotherapy then 8 mg q8h bid or Granisetron 1 mg PO 1 hour before Chemotherapy then 1 mg bid and Dexamethasone 10-20 mg PO 1 hour before chemotherapy
Delayed	Prochloperazine 10 mg PO q6h × 2 days or Prochlorperazine spansule 15 mg PO q12h × 2 days and Dexamethasone 4 mg PO q6h × 2 days
Anticipatory	Lorazepam 1-2 mg PO

occurs, the nurse uses dietary strategies in addition to the use of pharmacologic agents to promote regular bowel function. When fluid losses are moderate, the nurse encourages a higher fluid intake and monitors fluid balance. Intravenous rehydration may be necessary when fluid losses are severe.

6. Promoting Nutrition

Anorexia, nausea, vomiting, and stomatitis can also put the patient at risk for altered nutrition. The nurse emphasizes that eating a nourishing diet helps to maintain energy and meet body nutrient and repair needs. A comprehensive care plan needs to address all the contributing factors that may compromise dietary intake. Nausea needs to be controlled, as noted previously. Oral care that relieves mouth and throat dryness or discomfort is instituted. The patient may need to rest before meals to help conserve energy for eating. Patients with anorexia often are more hungry at breakfast than other meals, especially when they have had an uninterrupted night of sleep. The nurse encourages a diet high in calories and proteins, and suggests the consumption of multiple small meals and snacks throughout the day. Creative strategies to make mealtimes more pleasant may also enhance intake, such as the company of others, a comfortable position, and an environment free of noxious stimuli. The nurse monitors body weight frequently to evaluate the effectiveness of nutritional interventions. Additional interventions include a diet history, anthropometric measurements, and laboratory data evaluation. Oral supplements or enteral feedings may be ordered if the patient has a severely limited intake but maintains a functional gastrointestinal tract. TPN is used with patients who are at severe risk of malnutrition and unable to tolerate gastrointestinal feedings. Certain chemotherapy protocols can also result in weight gain as described in the Evidence-Based Practice box.

Evidence-Based Practice

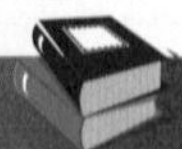

Reference: McInnes JA, Knobf MT: Weight gain and quality of life in women treated with adjuvant chemotherapy for early-stage breast cancer, *Oncol Nurs Forum* 28:675, 2001.

Weight gain is a documented side effect for women receiving adjuvant chemotherapy for breast cancer. This study documented the weight changes of 50 women with breast cancer who were receiving adjuvant chemotherapy. The researchers monitored the women for 36 months and identified factors associated with weight changes, as well as the effect of weight changes on quality of life. One year after treatment began, 62% of women experienced a weight gain that ranged from 5 to 27 pounds. After 2 and 3 years, respectively, 68% and 40% of women maintained significant weight gains. Premenopausal women gained more weight over time than postmenopausal women. Tamoxifen administration was not a significant factor associated with weight gain. Although weight gain was distressing to these women, it did not significantly affect quality of life as measured by several quality of life instruments. Nurses need to teach this patient population about weight gain as a side effect and develop strategies to prevent and manage this problem, which can lead to other health problems as well as disturbances in body image.

7. Promoting a Positive Body Image

Alopecia, weight loss, changes in body function and appearance, and altered social roles can all affect the patient's body image, or feelings about oneself. Chemotherapy treatments can cause all of these changes, and the nurse needs to assess their impact on each individual.

Patients scheduled for chemotherapy that causes hair loss are informed of this likelihood early in the course of therapy so they can be prepared when hair loss occurs. Some patients shave their heads or cut their hair very short in preparation for hair loss. Others choose to use wigs, head scarves, or caps to compensate for hair loss, and the nurse provides counseling and information about these resources early in the therapy. At present, there is no intervention available that prevents hair loss, although basic research is showing promise in this area (see Future Watch box). Hair dyes, permanents, and vigorous hair brushing are avoided to minimize thinning. The patient is reassured that hair loss is temporary and hair will regrow after chemotherapy is discontinued, perhaps with a different shade and texture.

Patients who experience alterations in sexuality or sexual function also need specific counseling and interventions. The nurse provides information on the expected side effects of chemotherapy related to sexual function, such as amenorrhea, decreased sperm function, infertility, and risk to a fetus. Patients of reproductive age are advised to use birth control

Future Watch
An End to Chemotherapy-Related Hair Loss?

Cyclin-dependent kinase 2 (CDK2) is an enzyme involved in cell division, and inhibition of CDK2 has been shown to prevent chemotherapy-induced alopecia. Researchers developed a synthetic compound, GW8510, and used topical applications on newborn rats who were then administered chemotherapy. GW8510 was 100% effective in preventing hair loss in half of the animals, and substantially reduced hair loss in others. No side effects were reported, and the treatment did not appear to interfere with the anticancer effect of the chemotherapy.

Reference: Davis S et al: Prevention of chemotherapy-induced alopecia in rats by CDK inhibitor, *Science* 291(5501):134, 2001.

measures during the treatment period to avoid conception. Treatment side effects such as nausea, fatigue, and anxiety may also affect sexual desire. The nurse addresses these side effects and answers general and specific questions about sexual concerns. The nurse can make appropriate referrals when more intensive counseling and interventions are necessary.

8. Managing Stomatitis

Chemotherapy agents disrupt the integrity of mucous membranes, causing dryness, painful ulcerations, and infections. Although this inflammation can affect mucosal cells throughout the gastrointestinal, genitourinary, and respiratory tracts, oral problems are the most common (also see p. 337). The nurse closely inspects the patient's mouth, including the lips, teeth, gum, tongue, palates, and throat to identify any lesions or abnormalities. Patients may report the early signs of mouth dryness and increased sensitivity. A cleansing and hydrating mouth care regimen started at the beginning of chemotherapy can reduce the severity of mucositis.[33] The Guidelines for Safe Practice box outlines a mouth care program for chemotherapy patients. Patients may develop infections, such as the raised blisters of herpes and the white patchy lesions of candida, and antibiotics may be prescribed. Analgesics are prescribed to treat the pain that accompanies severe mucositis. Nutritional therapy may be prescribed when mucositis significantly limits oral intake.

EVALUATION

To evaluate the effectiveness of nursing interventions compare patient behaviors with those stated in the expected outcomes. Achievement of outcomes is successful if the patient receiving chemotherapy:

1. Accurately describes the purpose of the treatment plan and side effects that can be expected.
2. Remains free of infection and has an intact skin.
3. Does not experience bleeding and protects self from injury and bruising.
4. Is free of dyspnea, chest pain, and dizziness.
5. Reports occurrences of nausea and vomiting are mild and well controlled by prescribed medications.
6. Consumes a well-balanced diet and maintains desired body weight.
7. Discusses changes in body image and speaks positively of self.
8. Remains free of oral inflammation, ulcers, and infection.

Guidelines for Safe Practice
Mouth Care for the Patient Receiving Chemotherapy

Brush teeth with a soft toothbrush after meals, snacks, and at bedtime.

1. Rinse mouth after brushing with salt solution (half teaspoon of salt in 8 ounces of water) or with mouthwash containing less than 6% alcohol.
2. Remove and clean dentures after meals, snacks, and at bedtime.
   a. Do not wear dentures that do not fit well or when the mouth is sore.
3. Floss teeth at least daily.
   a. Omit flossing if it causes pain or if at high risk for infection or bleeding.
4. Apply protective lubrication to lips.
5. Avoid irritants, such as tobacco and alcohol.
6. If mouth dryness occurs:
   a. Increase mouth rinses to every 2 to 4 hours.
   b. Increase fluid intake.
   c. Consider use of artificial saliva.
7. If mouth soreness develops:
   a. Use topical anesthetics.
   b. Implement dietary strategies to avoid foods that are spicy, hard, coarse, and acidic.
   c. Consider use of systemic analgesics.
8. If infection develops, use local or systemic antimicrobial medications.
9. Consult with health care providers before having any dental procedures.

Other Cancer Treatment Modalities

Bone Marrow Transplantation. The goals of bone marrow transplantation are to replace diseased bone marrow with healthy bone marrow or to rescue health bone marrow from dose-intensive therapy for a solid tumor. Malignant conditions treated with bone marrow transplantation include acute and chronic leukemias, preleukemic states, lymphoma, multiple myeloma, neuroblastoma, and breast cancer. There are three types of bone marrow transplants: syngeneic, in which the bone marrow donor is an identical twin and tissue is a perfect human leukocyte antigen (HLA) match; allogeneic, in which bone marrow comes from a related or unrelated donor and may or may not be HLA-matched; and autologous, in which the patient's own bone marrow cells are used. Bone marrow stem cells can be harvested from the posterior iliac crests during a surgical procedure, or blood stem cells designated to become bone marrow cells can be harvested from the patient's peripheral blood using plasmapheresis. Collection of stem cells in the peripheral blood through plasmapheresis is much easier than harvesting marrow cells and stem cells also engraft more rapidly than transplanted marrow cells.[24] Chemotherapy and the administration of growth factors "mobilize" the patient's stem cells, and they can then be collected with less possibility of tumor cell contamination. Bone marrow transplant is discussed in more detail in Chapter 51.

Autologous peripheral stem cell transplantation has become the most common type of marrow transplant because most patients do not have a donor for HLA-matched bone marrow. The Evidence-Based Practice box compares patient outcomes with these procedures.

In every marrow transplant regimen the patient is treated with high doses of chemotherapy, radiotherapy, or a combination of both. The therapies carry significant toxicity, and the patient requires intensive support with blood products, antibiotics, and growth factors during the period of engraftment, which may last several weeks. In addition to mucositis, myelosuppression, and various organ toxicities, allogeneic transplants also have the risk of acute and chronic graft-versus-host disease, which causes skin, liver, and gastrointestinal abnormalities. The transplant process is complex and requires interdisciplinary coordination of care during every phase.

Gene Therapy. Advances in the understanding of cancer as a genetic disease have led to new therapies that are directed toward the genetic mutation of cancer itself. Gene therapy involves the identification and treatment of the defective gene function underlying the patient's cancer. Treatment may involve the transfer of a new gene that compensates for the genetic alteration in the cancer cells.

Evidence-Based Practice

Reference: Lee SJ et al: Recovery after stem-cell transplantation for hematologic diseases, *J Clin Oncol* 19:242, 2001.

Patients need information about long-term morbidity after transplantation to make informed decisions about the treatment. This study surveyed 320 autologous and allogeneic transplant recipients at 6, 12, and 24 months after transplant. Three types of information were obtained from patients: (1) objective measures of health status, such as event-free survival and need for medications and rehospitalization; (2) qualitative assessment of quality of life; and (3) identification of bothersome symptoms. Results showed that autologous patients had better objective recovery and quality of life measures than allogeneic patients at 6 months. At years 1 and 2, however, the groups were roughly equal in these recovery parameters, with 60% agreeing to statements of recovery at 1 year, and increasing to 80% percent at 2 years. Fewer than one third of patients in both groups reported being extremely bothered or bothered a lot by symptoms at any of these time intervals. Patients in both groups were bothered the most by persistent fatigue, financial problems, and sexual difficulties after their transplants. In addition, the mortality in the allogeneic group was higher than in the autologous group over 2 years (overall survival of 78% versus 48%); thus the actual probability of these outcomes would be lower for the allogeneic group. When counseling patients about transplantation treatment options, health care providers need to give information about long-term survival, in terms of both mortality and specific morbidity concerns.

Two examples of gene therapy already in use are the biotherapy agent all-transretinoic acid (ATRA), used for the treatment of acute promyelocytic leukemia (APL), and STI 571 (Gleevec) for chronic myelogenous leukemia (CML) and gastrointestinal stromal tumor. In APL, a chromosomal translocation, t(15;17), results in production of a protein responsible for abnormal myeloid differentiation. ATRA binds to altered retinoic acid receptors on the abnormal gene and halts production of the carcinogenic protein. In CML, the target for gene therapy is the Philadelphia chromosome, t(9;22), a reciprocal translocation that occurs between chromosome 9 and 22 in the bone marrow. The result of this chromosomal abnormality is production of an abnormal enzyme that instructs cells to reproduce uncontrollably. Gleevec inhibits the activity of the mutant enzyme.

As more specific cancer genes and gene products are identified, further therapies will be developed that can halt abnormal cell growth at the molecular level. Nurses are challenged to become educated in the area of cancer genetics to be prepared to administer gene therapy in the clinical setting. New treatments might include therapies that restore normal p53 function and cellular death, inhibit DNA and RNA coding for abnormal proteins, or interfere with cellular signals that allow uncontrolled cellular growth. Because these therapies are directed specifically toward the growth of cancer cells, their effects on normal cells and subsequent toxicities should be minimal.

Complementary and Alternative Therapies for Cancer. Complementary therapies are therapies used in addition to the conventional cancer treatments of surgery, radiation, and chemotherapy. These therapies often improve the patient's functional status and sense of well-being. Examples of complementary therapies include massage, aromatherapy, relaxation therapy, meditation, and yoga. Alternative therapies also include practices that were once considered outside of American biomedicine, such as acupuncture, herbal remedies, and homeopathy. These therapies are currently being researched for their proven positive effects on patients. The National Institutes of Health and the National Center for Complementary and Alternative Medicine conducts and coordinates research efforts that examine these types of therapies.

Nurses need to know what complementary and alternative health care therapies their patients may be using, and this question should be included in initial patient assessments. The popularity of many of these therapies continues to grow, and more than half of patients with cancer may be using these therapies in addition to their prescribed treatments.[29] Some of these therapies are recognized as helpful approaches, and it is often possible to incorporate them into the patient's treatment regimen. Other therapies may add undesirable or harmful effects to the patient's regimen. For example, some herbs can increase the patient's risk of bleeding or increase sedation (Box 15-11). Other patients may reveal that they are pursuing the use of unconventional or unproven therapies instead of standard treatment. This may be especially true for patients with limited options for treatment who continue to look for a cure or for patients with unrealistic fears about the side effects of radiation or chemotherapy. Nurses need to answer questions and provide information about alternative and complementary therapies in a nonjudgmental way to help patients make informed decisions about their therapy and support the patient's right to make informed choices that deviate from mainstream approaches.

Oncologic Emergencies

Oncologic emergencies include a variety of complications associated with cancer or its treatment. These syndromes may signal a new diagnosis of cancer or occur as the cancer progresses. Emergencies include obstructions such as spinal cord compression, superior vena cava syndrome, and tracheal or bowel obstruction; or increased intracranial pressure, caused by tumor growth in and around major organs. Metabolic crises include hypercalcemia, tumor lysis syndrome, syndrome of inappropriate antidiuretic hormone secretion (SIADH), hyperviscosity, and disseminated intravascular coagulation. In some cases, such as siadh, the cancer cells secrete a hormonelike substance that causes abnormal chemical and metabolic processes. In other cases, cancer treatment can precipitate the crisis, as in tumor lysis syndrome. Some common oncologic emergencies are listed in Table 15-25.

Nurses need to be alert to patient populations at risk for oncologic emergencies. Nursing assessments often detect signs and symptoms that indicate an impending crisis. Early diagnosis and immediate treatment of these life-threatening conditions are critical. During these crises, the patient may require transfer to an intensive care unit for hemodynamic monitoring and cardiopulmonary support. Continuity of care and emotional support for the patient and family are essential. In most cases successful treatment of the emergency requires control of the underlying cancer process in addition to supportive therapy.

BOX 15-11 Herbs That Increase Risk of Bleeding or Sedation

Increase Sedation	Increase Risk of Bleeding
Calamus	Alfalfa
Calendula	Angelica
California poppy	Anise
Capsicum	Arnica
Catnip	Asa foetida
Celery	Bogbean
Couch grass	Boldo
Elecampane	Capsicum
German chamomile	Celery
Goldenseal	Chamomile
Gotukola	Clove
Hops	Danshen
Jamaican dogwood	Fenugreek
Kava	Feverfew
Lemon balm	Garlic
Sage	Ginger
St. John's wort	Gingko
Sassafras	Horse chestnut
Siberian ginseng	Horseradish
Skullcap	Licorice
Shepherd's purse	Meadowsweet
Stinging nettle	Onion
Valerian	Papain
Wild carrot	Passionflower
Wild lettuce	Poplar
Withania root	Prickly ash
Yerba mansa	Quassia
	Red clover
	Tumeric
	Wild carrot
	Wild lettuce
	Willow

From Decker GM, Myers J: Commonly used herbs: implications for practice, *Clin J Oncol Nurs,* vol 5(suppl), 2001.

Cancer Pain

Pain is one of the most feared effects of cancer, although contrary to popular belief, it is usually one of the last symptoms to appear. Pain is generally not a problem in the early, localized stage of disease. About 30% of patients with cancer experience pain while undergoing treatment. As the cancer progresses and metastasizes, more than 90% of patients experience pain.[2]

Alleviation of pain is the responsibility and obligation of health care professionals. The Oncology Nursing Society (ONS) developed a position paper on cancer pain in part because pain management is a significant clinical problem faced by the nurse caring for cancer patients and because cancer pain has been poorly managed. The ONS statement makes the nurse responsible for the coordination of pain management, including effective assessment, intervention, and evaluation of the pain.

Patients with cancer experience pain from three sources. First, tumors directly cause pain of three types: somatic, visceral, or neuropathic. Somatic pain is caused by tumors that infiltrate cutaneous or connective tissue, such as muscle, bone, and blood vessels. One common example is the pain from bone metastases. Visceral pain results from organ involvement, such as pancreatic cancer. Neuropathic pain results from involved nerve fibers or central nervous system tissue, such as a peripheral neuropathy. These pain syndromes have distinct characteristics (Table 15-26). Patients can also experience pain from cancer therapy. Examples include acute pain related to diagnostic procedures, postoperative pain, or pain that results from mucositis caused by chemotherapy. Finally, as many as 10% of patients experience significant pain from a condition or disease unrelated to their cancer, such as migraine headaches or arthritis.

Each type of pain may be further classified as acute or chronic. Acute pain is caused by reversible tissue damage and resolves in the time frame of tissue healing. Chronic pain persists longer than 3 months and may be related to tissue damage. Chronic pain does not resolve within a specific time frame. Patients with cancer commonly have pain of several etiologies and durations.

A commonly used conceptual framework suggests that cancer pain is multidimensional, consisting of physiologic, sensory, affective, cognitive, behavioral, and sociocultural

TABLE 15-25 Oncologic Emergencies

Type	Pathophysiology	Clinical Manifestations
Obstructive		
Increased intracranial pressure	Increased brain mass from tumor, hemorrhage, or edema; alteration in internal jugular vein flow caused by head/neck tumor or by surgical resection—results in alteration in function	Change in mental status, vomiting, headache, dizziness, seizures (see Chapter 42)
Spinal cord compression	Primary or metastatic lesions causing disruption of reflexes and motor function because of neuron impairment and interruption of motor or sensory nerve fibers; symptoms depend on location.	Flaccid paralysis, paresthesias, locomotion difficulties, respiratory impairment at C5 level (see Chapter 44)
Superior vena cava (SVC) syndrome	Obstruction of the SVC caused by primary (usually lung cancer) or metastatic tumors in the mediastinal or paratracheal nodes	Dyspnea, facial and neck swelling, chest pain, cough, dysphagia, ruddy edematous face
Tracheal obstruction	Reduction in lumen from tracheal stenosis, extrinsic compression, or mass in lumen	Signs and symptoms of inadequate gas exchange and respiratory function (see Chapter 21)
Metabolic		
Hypercalcemia	Bone disease or metastasis increases bone resorption with bone destruction and release of calcium in the extracellular fluid; it is believed the tumor may produce (1) a substance that enables bone resorption of calcium or (2) ectopic parathyroid hormone that increases serum calcium levels	Nausea and vomiting, constipation, muscle weakness, coma, dysrhythmias, polyuria, nephrolithiasis (see Chapter 13)
Tumor lysis syndrome	Rapid tumor cell destruction after cytotoxic chemotherapy may result in release of intracellular electrolytes; may occur in cancers characterized by rapid cell growth (leukemia and lymphomas)	Hyperphosphatemia (oliguria, azotemia), hyperkalemia, hyperuricemia (nausea and vomiting, lethargy, anuria, azotemia), hypocalcemia (see Chapter 13)
Syndrome of inappropriate antidiuretic hormone secretion	Increase in antidiuretic hormone seen in cancers such as lung carcinoma (especially small cell), duodenal and pancreatic carcinoma, thymoma, lymphomas, uterine carcinoma, and central nervous system tumors; may also occur with some chemotherapeutic agents (cyclophosphamide)	Fluid and electrolyte and neurologic changes (see Chapter 42)
Hyperviscosity	Increased blood viscosity from increase in cell number, loss of flexibility of cells, or overproduction of serum proteins; this causes increased resistance to blood flow	Bleeding from gastrointestinal or urinary tracts or puncture sites; visual disturbance, headache, dizziness, weakness, dyspnea, distended neck veins
Anaphylaxis	Hypersensitivity responses (I, II, III, IV) caused by chemotherapeutic agents (asparaginase, cisplatin, etoposide, paclitaxel, docetaxel, bleomycin, melphalan)	Signs of anaphylactic reactions (see Chapter 49
Septic shock	Increased susceptibility to infection from impaired immune system or effect of immunosuppressive agents, leading to bacterial septicemia	Signs and symptoms of septic shock (see Chapter 14)
Disseminated intravascular coagulation	Chronic bleeding consumes all clotting factors; may also result from sepsis	Thrombocytopenia, bleeding of mucous membranes and tissues (see Chapter 27)
Cardiac Toxicities		
Cardiac tamponade	Intrapericardial pressure increases from accumulation of fluid from direct tumor invasion, metastatic lesion, or infection or from pericardial thickening after radiation; results in decreased diastolic ventricular filling, decreased stroke volume and cardiac output	Dyspnea, cough, chest pain, muffled heart sounds, cyanosis, edema, decreased systolic pressure, decreased central venous pressure (see Chapter 24)
Cardiomyopathy with congestive heart failure	Chemotherapeutic drugs (such as anthracyclines, mithramycin, mitomycin, and cyclophosphamide) appear to damage cardiac myofibrils, causing sarcoplasmic reticular swelling that leads to destruction of the myofibril; hypertrophy of the heart muscle ensues with decreased function	Acute: tachycardia, dysrhythmias Chronic: signs of congestive heart failure (see Chapter 24)

TABLE 15-26 Pathophysiology of Cancer Pain

Cause	Type of Pain
Bone destruction with infraction (fracture without displacement)	Increased sensitivity over area or sharp continuous pain
Obstruction of a viscus (gastrointestinal or genitourinary tract)	Severe, colicky, crampy type of pain; may be dull, diffuse, poorly localized
Obstruction of an artery, vein, or lymphatic	Dull, diffuse, aching (caused by arterial ischemia, venous engorgement, edema)
Infiltration, compression of peripheral nerves or nerve plexus	Continuous, sharp, or stabbing pain; sometimes hyperesthesia or paresthesia
Infiltration or distention of integument, fascia, or tissue (e.g., ascites)	Localized, dull aching pain
Inflammation, infection, and necrosis of tissue	Varied pain caused by pressure or ischemia

TABLE 15-27 Roles of the Primary Therapies in the Management of Cancer Pain

Primary Therapy	Major Pain Indications
Radiation therapy	Painful bony metastases Epidural spinal cord compression Cerebral metastases Tumor-related compression or infiltration of peripheral neural structures
Chemotherapy	Nociceptive or neuropathic pain syndromes caused by tumors likely to respond to chemotherapy
Surgery	Stabilization of pathological fractures Spinal cord decompression Relief of remediable bowel obstructions Drainage of symptomatic ascites
Antibiotic therapy	Overt infections (e.g., pelvic abscess or pyonephrosis) Occult infections (e.g., in head and neck tumors or ulcerating tumors)

Source: Cherny NJ, Portenoy RK: The management of cancer pain, *CA Cancer J Clin* 44(5):272, 1994.

dimensions.[34] The physiologic dimension includes the physical and anatomic details of pain. The sensory dimension is the patient's description of the pain, including its location, intensity, and quality. The affective dimension consists of psychologic or personality traits associated with the pain, such as depression or anxiety. The cognitive dimension is the meaning that the patient assigns to the pain. For example, a patient may feel that the onset of a new pain indicates tumor recurrence. Behavioral dimensions include the patient's behaviors related to the pain, such as mood, activity, and expression. Finally, the sociocultural dimension addresses how the patient's specific age, culture, religion, and roles influence the patient's experience of pain. These dimensions are complex and intertwined, with various cause-and-effect relationships. Nurses need to identify and understand the importance of these dimensions in the patient's pain experience.

Collaborative Care Management. The goal of pain management is to provide pain relief that enables the patient to carry on with normal activities of daily living without symptoms of discomfort. The multidimensional character of pain requires an integrated, multidisciplinary approach, often consisting of several interventions. Recently, the Joint Commission on Accreditation of Healthcare Organizations revised its pain management standards to emphasize the importance of pain assessment and management for every patient. The presence of pain is to be documented as a fifth vital sign, and patients in pain are to be comprehensively assessed. The use of a standard pain assessment tool can facilitate a comprehensive examination.[3]

Pain management for patients with cancer includes the use of appropriate therapies to control the cancer, pharmacologic measures to manage the patient's perception of pain, and a variety of nonpharmacologic measures to provide additional relief. Surgery, chemotherapy, and radiation therapy may all be appropriate treatments for pain; and examples of their use in pain management are listed in Table 15-27. Pharmacologic therapy with several classes of drugs is the foundation of pain control. Patients may be prescribed nonopioid analgesics, opioids, or other agents that contribute to pain relief, such as antidepressants or anticonvulsants. Principles of pain management include using the least invasive route possible and ensuring around-the-clock administration to maintain therapeutic blood levels. The World Health Organization offers guidelines for the use of analgesics (Figure 15-18). Mild pain is treated with nonopioid medications, such as NSAIDs or adjuvant drugs. As pain increases, opioids are used, increasing in potency and dose as necessary. Opioids can also be combined with nonopioids and adjuvant drugs for improved pain relief. Nonpharmacologic measures for pain include behavioral techniques, such as relaxation or diversional activities; meditation, hypnosis, or imagery; and the use of heat and cold, cutaneous stimulation, and massage. See Chapter 12 for a discussion of pain assessment and management.

Patient/Family Education. Pain may not be effectively managed for a variety of reasons, including caregiver's lack of knowledge about pain management principles, inadequate assessment, and inadequate use of available analgesics. In addition, patients may not follow through with self-care measures for pain control out of fear of addiction, inadequate understanding of the regimen, a belief that nothing can be done to relieve their pain, or lack of financial and supportive resources to obtain analgesics. The nurse discusses pain management with the patient and family and emphasizes the importance of promptly reporting the presence of pain, using adequate doses of analgesics to gain control of the pain, and regular dosing to sustain effective analgesic blood levels. The nurse also teaches

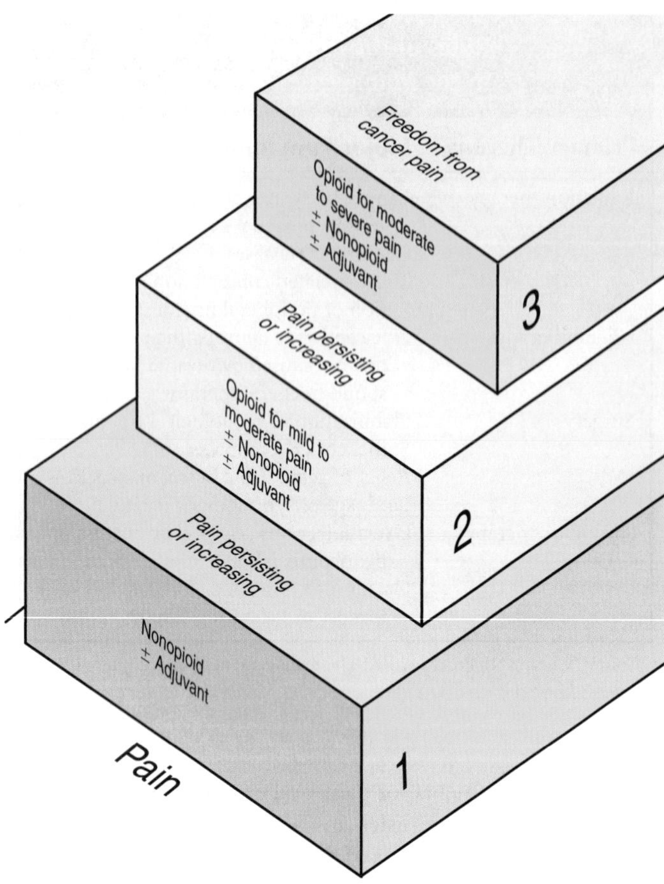

Figure 15-18 World Health Organization three-step analgesic ladder.

the patient about the physiologic phenomena of tolerance and dependence and reassures the patient that regular use of an opioid is both safe and appropriate and does not constitute addiction.

Certain populations of patients present unique challenges to effective pain management. Older adults and former substance abuse patients need careful planning to effectively manage pain and control side effects. In hospice or palliative care settings issues related to euthanasia and assisted suicide may enter into discussions about pain management, necessitating careful ethical reasoning, education, and interventions.

Ensuring patient comfort is a priority for nurses who care for patients in pain. Until the patient receives adequate pain relief, it is difficult to achieve any other patient outcome. Although complete absence of pain can be a difficult goal to achieve, especially in patients with advanced cancer, the nurse reassures patients that every effort will be made to find the most effective pain regimen. The nurse needs to intervene promptly when pain crises occur or when ongoing assessments reveal that the patient's pain is not well controlled. The nurse must advocate for patients when adjustments in pain regimens need to be made. Nursing strategies for dealing with the cancer patient's pain are listed in the Guidelines for Safe Practice box.

Guidelines for Safe Practice

Dealing Effectively With Cancer Pain

Know the patient and the pattern of pain experienced. Document findings.
Use an organized pain assessment method that is easy to use and that provides sufficient data to assist in selecting the most appropriate intervention for relief.
Understand the pharmacology of the drugs being used, including classification, probable side effects, route of administration, expected outcomes in terms of when to expect pain relief to occur.
Understand the difference between addiction, dependence, and tolerance.
Use appropriate drug combinations.
Advocate for effective analgesic regimens.
Become familiar with equianalgesic doses of common analgesics.
Provide patient and family teaching related to pain control.

RESOURCES FOR CANCER EDUCATION, DETECTION, AND TREATMENT

Federal recognition of the need to give intensive assistance to cancer educational programs began in 1926 when Congress proclaimed April of each year as National Cancer Control Month. In 1937 the National Cancer Institute was created within the National Institutes of Health to coordinate an extensive program of research in the field of cancer. With the passage of the National Cancer Act in 1971, cancer clinical research centers were developed across the country to translate research results into medical practice so that the most up-to-date professional cancer care would be widely available to cancer patients.

Today a variety of oncology-related organizations provide free information about cancer care to consumers. This information is available in print and on websites. With rapid advances in informatics, consumers and health professionals have immediate access to the most current information about even the rarest medical conditions. As a result, consumers of cancer care today are more educated than ever before. Nurses are challenged to know and use the same technology to be able to answer the questions of well-informed patients. Box 15-12 provides a list of organizations that may be used as resources by patients with cancer as well as cancer care providers.

Critical Thinking Questions

1. You are speaking to a group of senior citizens at a local retirement center about the three most common cancers for men and women. What are the three most common cancers? What information would you give this audience about risk factors, prevention and early detection strategies for these cancers?
2. Your son is doing a school project on dangerous chemicals that are present in our environment. He asks you what substances are known to cause cancer. What are some substances that are known to cause cancer? What references can you recommend?

BOX 15-12 Oncology-Related Organizations

Alliance for Lung Cancer Advocacy, Support, and Education
1601 Lincoln Avenue
Vancouver, WA 98660
www.alcase.org

American Brain Tumor Association
2720 River Road
Des Plaines, IL 60018
www.ABTA.org

American Cancer Society
1599 Clifton Road NE
Atlanta, GA 30329-4251
www.cancer.org

American Lung Association
1740 Broadway
New York, NY 10019-4374
www.lungusa.org

American Society of Clinical Oncology
225 Reinekers Lane, Suite 650
Alexandria, VA 22314
www.asco.org

Cancer Information Service
National Cancer Institute
Building 31, Room 10A 03
Bethesda, MD 20892
www.nci.nih.gov

Leukemia and Lymphoma Society
600 Third Avenue
New York, NY 10016
www.leukemialymphoma.org

National Alliance of Breast Cancer Organizations
9 E. 37th Street, 10th Floor
New York, NY 10016
www.nabco.org

National Coalition for Cancer Survivorship
1010 Wayne Avenue, Suite 505
Silver Spring, MD 20910
www.cansearch.org

National Marrow Donor Program Coordinating Center
3433 Broadway Street, NE, Suite 500
Minneapolis, MN 55413
www.marrow.org

National Ovarian Cancer Coalition
2335 East Atlantic Boulevard, Suite 401
Pompano Beach, FL 33062
www.ovarian.org

National Prostate Cancer Coalition
1158 15th St. NW
Washington, DC 20005
www.4npcc.org

Oncology Nursing Society
501 Holiday Drive
Pittsburgh, PA 15220
www.ons.org

Susan G. Komen Breast Cancer Foundation
5005 LBJ Freeway
Suite 370
Dallas, TX 75224
www.komen.org

United Ostomy Association
19772 MacArthur Blvd. Suite 200
Irvine, CA 92612-2405
www.uoa.org

3. A 48-year-old woman recently diagnosed with breast cancer with axillary lymph node involvement is in the clinic to receive her first chemotherapy treatment with doxorubicin (Adriamycin) and cyclophosphamide (Cytoxan). What side effects will you teach her to expect? What self-care measures will you teach her to prevent and manage these side effects?
4. A 69-year-old retired man with squamous cell carcinoma of the tonsil will begin a 6-week course of radiation therapy to ports that include the primary tumor site and lymph nodes in the neck. What side effects will you expect with this radiation therapy plan? What assessments and interventions will be important for you to include in his care?
5. A 60-year-old man with multiple myeloma was admitted to your unit in a pain crisis. Until last night, his pain had previously been controlled with oxycodone, 10 mg every 6 hours as needed. What criteria will you include in your pain assessment? What principles of pain management will you consider when implementing new analgesics?

References

1. Administration on Aging (AOA)/Department of Health and Human Services, 2001, website: http://aoa.dhhs.gov.
2. Ashby T, Dalton J: Pain assessment and management in people with cancer. In Nevidjon BM, Sowers KW, editors: *A nurse's guide to cancer care,* Philadelphia, 2000, JB Lippincott.
3. Berry PH: Getting ready for JCAHO: just meeting the standards of really improving pain management? *Clin J Oncol Nurs* 5:110, 2001.
4. Bradley CJ et al: Physical, economic, and social issues confronting patients and families. In Yarbro CH et al, editors: *Cancer nursing: principles and practice,* ed 5, Boston, 2000, Jones and Bartlett.
5. Clark PM, Lacasse C: Cancer-related fatigue: clinical practice issues, *Clin J Oncol Nurs* 2:45, 1998.
6. Cuaron L, Thompson J: The interferons. In Rieger PT, editor: *Biotherapy: a comprehensive overview,* ed 2, Boston, 2001, Jones and Bartlett.
7. DeJulio JE: Monoclonal antibodies: overview and use in hematologic malignancies. In Rieger PT, editor: *Biotherapy: a comprehensive overview,* ed 2, Boston, 2001, Jones and Bartlett.

8. Dunne-Daly C: Principles of brachytherapy. In Dow KH et al, editors: *Nursing care in radiation oncology,* ed 2, Philadelphia, 1997, WB Saunders.
9. Fiore MC et al: *Treating tobacco use and dependence: quick reference guide for clinicians,* Rockville, Md, 2000, US Department of Health and Human Services, Public Health Service.
10. Foltz AT, Mahon SM: Application of carcinogenesis theory to primary prevention, *Oncol Nurs Forum* 27(suppl):5, 2000.
11. Gale DM, Sorokin P: The interleukins. In Rieger PT, editor: *Biotherapy: a comprehensive overview,* ed 2, Boston, 2001, Jones and Bartlett.
12. Greenlee RT et al: Cancer statistics, 2001: *CA Cancer J Clinicians* 51:15, 2001.
13. Gross RE: Current issues in the surgical treatment of early stage breast cancer, *Clin J Oncol Nurs* 2:55, 1998.
14. Hawkins R: Mastering the intricate maze of metastasis, *Oncol Nurs Forum* 28:959, 2001.
15. Hilderley LJ: Principles of teletherapy. In Dow KH et al, editors: *Nursing care in radiation oncology,* ed 2, Philadelphia, 1997, WB Saunders.
16. Howe HL et al: Annual report to the nation on the status of cancer, 1973-1998, *J Natl Cancer Inst* 93:824, 2001.
17. Ingle RJ: Lung cancer. In Yarbro CH et al, editors: *Cancer nursing: principles and practice,* ed 5, Boston, 2000, Jones and Bartlett.
18. Jennings-Dozier K, Mahon SM: Cancer prevention and early detection: from thought to revolution, *Oncol Nurs Forum* 27(suppl):3, 2000.
19. Knudson A: Hereditary cancer: theme and variations, *J Clin Oncol* 15:280, 1997.
20. Kosits C, Callaghan M: Rituximab: a new monoclonal antibody therapy for non-Hodgkin's lymphoma, *Oncol Nurs Forum* 27:51, 2000.
21. Lin EM: Venous access devices. In Nevidjon BM, Sowers KW, editors: *A nurse's guide to cancer care,* Philadelphia, 2000, JBLippincott.
22. Mahon SM: Principles of cancer prevention and early detection, *Clin J Oncol Nurs* 4:169, 2000.
23. Mahon SM: The role of the nurse in developing cancer screening programs, *Oncol Nurs Forum* 27(suppl):19, 2000.
24. McCarthy PL et al: Stem cell transplantation: past, present, and future. In Buchsel PC, Kapustay PM, editors: *Stem cell transplantation: a clinical textbook,* Pittsburgh, 2000, Oncology Nursing Press.
25. Rieger PT: Biotherapy: an overview. In Rieger PT, editor: *Biotherapy: a comprehensive overview,* ed 2, Boston, 2001, Jones and Bartlett.
26. Rieger PT: Emerging strategies in the management of cancer, *Oncol Nurs Forum* 24:728, 1997.
27. Shelton BK: Flu-like syndrome. In Rieger PT, editor: *Biotherapy: a comprehensive overview,* ed 2, Boston, 2001, Jones and Bartlett.
28. Sitton E: Managing side effects of skin changes and fatigue. In Dow KH et al, editors: *Nursing care in radiation oncology,* ed 2, Philadelphia, 1997, WB Saunders.
29. Sparber A et al: Use of complementary medicine by adult patients participating in cancer clinical trials, *Oncol Nurs Forum* 27:623, 2000.
30. Trichopoulos D, Li FP, Hunter DJ: What causes cancer? *Sci Am* 275:80, 1996.
31. U.S. Department of Health and Human Services: *Healthy People 2010: understanding and improving health,* Washington, DC, 2000, USDHHS.
32. Williams JK: Principles of genetics and cancer, *Semin Oncol Nurs* 13:68, 1997.
33. Wojtaszek C: Management of chemotherapy-induced stomatitis, *Clin J Oncol Nurs* 4:263, 2000.
34. Yeager KA, McGuire DB, Sheidler VR: Assessment of cancer pain. In Yarbro CH et al, editors: *Cancer nursing: principles and practice,* ed 5, Boston, 2000, Jones and Bartlett.

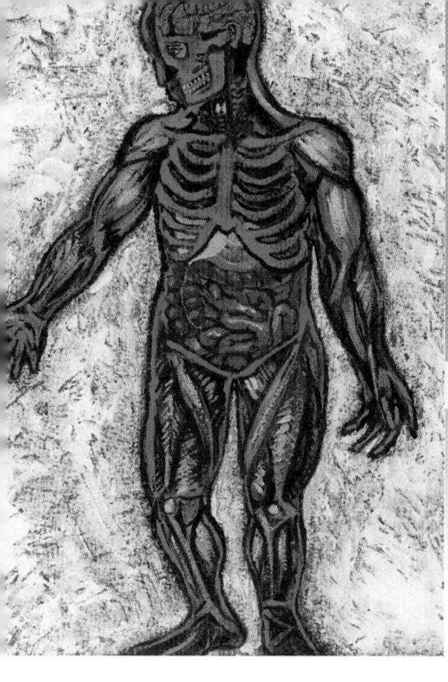

http://www.mosby.com/MERLIN/medsurg_phipps

Preoperative Nursing 16

Jane F. Marek, Mary Jo Boehnlein

Objectives

After studying this chapter, the learner should be able to:

1. Identify the major influences on the emergence of perioperative nursing.
2. Describe the preoperative phase as a component of the surgical experience.
3. Identify different classifications of surgeries.
4. Identify the biopsychosocial responses of patients to surgery.
5. Discuss the components and significance of the preoperative patient assessment.
6. Explain the potential for postoperative complications.
7. Identify nursing diagnoses for the preoperative patient.
8. Discuss expected patient outcomes for the preoperative phase.
9. Discuss nursing interventions in the preoperative phase.
10. Discuss final preparations for the preoperative patient.

HISTORICAL PERSPECTIVE

History of Surgery

Surgery is defined as "the branch of medicine dealing with manual and operative procedures for correction of deformities and defects, repair of injuries, and diagnosis and cure of certain diseases."[28] The word *surgery* comes from the Greek *kheirurgos,* which means working by hand. Hippocrates, the father of surgery, reportedly used wine or boiled water for wound irrigations as early as 450 BC. By AD 130 to 200 surgery became a specific medical discipline. At that time, the Greek physician Galen was said to have boiled his instruments before use. A variety of surgical techniques were practiced throughout the following years. During the 1500s ligatures were used to control bleeding. Morton's use of ether at Massachusetts General Hospital in 1846 heralded the advent of anesthesia as an adjunct to surgery. Use of anesthesia permitted the physician to perform slower, more precise, and pain-free procedures. Despite these advances, wound infection and mortality rates were high. In the mid to late 1800s, the mortality rate for patients undergoing amputation reportedly was as high as 40%.[24]

Not until the middle of the nineteenth century did surgery emerge as a true medical specialty. Ignaz Semmelweiss's work in 1847 showed the importance of hand washing between procedures and patients in decreasing the incidence of puerperal fever after childbirth. In 1867 Joseph Lister published his work on antisepsis in which he advocated the use of antiseptics such as carbolic acid sprays during surgery to kill microorganisms. However, Semmelweiss and Lister's methods were not adopted until the 1880s and were then followed by the introduction of the principles of aseptic technique. The late 1890s brought forth improvements in diagnostic tools, including the discovery of x-rays in 1895 and advancements in the development of surgical instrumentation. At the turn of the century most surgical procedures were limited to the abdomen. William and Charles Mayo, who had performed only 54 abdominal surgeries between 1889 and 1892, published an article in 1904 describing the results of 1000 abdominal procedures.[24] Surgical techniques continued to develop as thoracic, neurologic, and cardiovascular procedures were introduced. Throughout the twentieth century advances in anesthesia, the surgical environment, and technology have allowed more predictable and safer outcomes for patients.

Perioperative Nursing: Past and Present

In the early 1900s many surgical procedures were performed in the patient's home. Nursing's role focused on preparing the environment and supporting the patient. Increasingly complex procedures and greater demands on the physician's time made performing surgery in the home inconvenient for the surgeon, patient, and family. To accommodate these needs, physicians began performing surgery in private medical boarding houses, which provided both hotel and nursing services.[24] By the 1920s and 1930s most physicians were affiliated with hospitals. Nursing's primary role was providing technical assistance to the surgeon.

Perioperative nursing is an outgrowth of operating room (OR) nursing as it was practiced in its early years. Contemporary perioperative nursing practice is patient-centered rather than task-oriented.

The role of the registered nurse in the operating room has been expanded, defined, and standardized through the efforts of the members of the perioperative nurses' professional organization, the Association of Operating Room Nurses (AORN). The AORN defines the perioperative nurse as follows:

> The registered nurse who, using the nursing process, designs, coordinates, and delivers care to meet the identified needs of patients whose protective reflexes or self-care abilities are potentially compromised because they are having operative or other invasive procedures. Perioperative nurses possess and apply knowledge of the procedure and the patient's intraoperative experience throughout the patient's care continuum. The perioperative nurse assesses, diagnoses, plans, intervenes, and evaluates the outcome of interventions based on criteria that support a standard of care targeted toward this specific population. The perioperative nurse addresses the physiological, psychological, socio-cultural, and spiritual responses of the individual that have been caused by the prospect or performance of the invasive procedure.[2]

Using the American Nurses' Association (ANA) Code for Nurses with Interpretive Statements, AORN developed perioperative nursing explications of the Code for Nurses. The explications provide perioperative nurses with a framework to relate the ANA code to their own practice.

The preoperative phase begins when the decision for surgical intervention is made. The scope of nursing activities includes, but is not limited to, preoperative assessment of the patient's physical, psychologic, and social states; the planning of nursing care that is required to prepare the patient for surgery; and the implementation of nursing interventions. This phase ends when the patient is safely transported to the OR and transferred to the OR nurse for care.

Movement of the patient onto the OR bed begins the intraoperative phase; this period lasts until the patient is admitted to the postanesthesia care unit. During this phase nursing responsibilities focus on the continuing assessment of the patient's physiologic and psychologic status and the planning and implementation of effective nursing interventions to promote safety and privacy and to prevent wound infection and promote healing. Specific nursing activities include providing emotional support to the patient during induction of anesthesia and throughout the procedure, establishing and maintaining functional positioning, maintaining asepsis, protecting the patient from electrical hazards, assisting in fluid balance, ensuring accurate sponge and instrument counts, assisting the surgeon, and communicating with both the patient's family and other health care team members. Other nursing roles include the RN first assistant (RNFA) and certified registered nurse anesthetist (CRNA) (see Chapter 17).

The postoperative phase "begins with admission to the postanesthesia care area and ends with a resolution of surgical sequelae."[2] Nursing activities include ongoing assessment of changes in the physical and psychologic status of the patient, along with appropriate planning, implementation, and evaluation of care. Nursing interventions include frequent monitoring of airway patency, vital signs, and neurologic status, as well as assessing and maintaining fluid and electrolyte balance, pain management, management of the surgical site, and providing a thorough summary report of the patient's status to the nurse receiving the patient on the unit and to the patient's family or friends.

SURGICAL PROCEDURES

Types of Surgery

Most surgical procedures are given names that describe the site of the surgery and the type of surgery performed. For example, appendectomy refers to removal (-ectomy) of the appendix. Common surgical suffixes are listed in Box 16-1. Some surgeries carry the name of the surgeon who developed the technique, such as the Billroth procedures (partial gastrectomies). Surgeries may be classified according to the degree of risk, extent, purpose, anatomic site, timing, or physical setting.

Degree of Risk

The degree of risk involved in the surgical procedure is classified as either minor or major. *Minor surgery* is simple surgery that presents little risk to life. Many minor surgeries are performed with the use of local anesthesia, although general anesthesia may be used (see Chapter 17). *Major surgery* is more extensive than minor surgery and may involve risk to life. Major surgery usually is performed with use of general or regional anesthesia.

Extent

The extent of the surgical procedure can be classified as minimally invasive, open, simple, or radical. *Minimally invasive procedures* are usually performed with the use of fiberoptic endoscopes and do not require traditional or extensive incisions. Endoscopes may be introduced through natural openings in the body or through porthole incisions, which also permit passage of surgical instruments. Endoscopic procedures have both diagnostic and therapeutic purposes and can be used alone or in conjunction with open techniques. Endoscopic procedures can be performed on a variety of anatomic sites. Examples of endoscopic and endoscopically assisted procedures are found in Table 16-1. Minimally invasive procedures usually result in improved patient outcomes including fewer postoperative complications, decreased length of hospital stay, reduced postoperative pain, and earlier resumption of normal activities.

Open procedures involve the traditional opening of the body cavity or body part to perform the surgery. Because of the more extensive surgical approach, the patient may experi-

BOX 16-1 Common Surgical Suffixes

-ectomy: removal of an organ or gland
-rrhaphy: repairing
-ostomy: providing an opening (stoma)
-otomy: cutting into
-plasty: formation or plastic repair
-scopy: looking into

ence more postoperative pain and a longer recovery period. The extent of the procedure may also influence postoperative infection rates. Infection rates increase with the length of procedure; it is estimated that the infection rate doubles for every hour the surgical procedure continues.[4,14]

Simple procedures are generally limited to a defined anatomic location and do not require extensive exposure and dissection of adjacent tissue. In contrast, *radical procedures,* which are usually associated with malignancies, involve dissection of tissue and structures beyond the immediate operative site. In most cases, adjacent lymph nodes, muscle, and fascia that have been invaded by tumor are excised.

Purpose

Surgical procedures may be classified according to their indications. Breast biopsy is an example of a *diagnostic* procedure performed to determine the cause of symptoms or origin of the problem. The goal of *curative* surgery, for example an appendectomy, is to resolve a health problem or disease state by removing the involved tissue. *Restorative* or *reconstructive* surgical procedures are performed to correct deformity, repair injury, or improve the functional status of the individual. Procedures done to relieve symptoms without the intent to cure are termed *palliative. Ablative* surgery is performed to excise tissue that may contribute to or worsen the patient's existing medical condition (e.g., an orchiectomy performed for a patient with prostatic cancer). *Cosmetic* surgery is preformed for aesthetic purposes.

TABLE 16-1 Types of Endoscopic/Endoscope-Assisted Surgical Procedures

Surgical Specialty	Possible Procedures Performed
General	Cholecystectomy Colectomy Appendectomy Herniorrhaphy Modified Whipple procedure Nissen fundoplication
Orthopedic	Anterior cruciate ligament repair Carpal tunnel release Acromioplasty Diskectomy
Gynecologic	Tubal ligation Laparoscopic assisted vaginal hysterectomy Hysteroscopy
Ear, nose, throat	Temporal mandibular joint repair Nasal polypectomy Ethmoidectomy Frontal antrostomy
Urology	Prostatectomy Nephrectomy Bladder neck suspension
Cardiothoracic	Mediastinoscopy Lymph node dissection Coronary artery bypass

Anatomic Site

Another way of classifying surgical procedures is by location of body parts or systems, such as cardiovascular surgery, chest surgery, intestinal surgery, or neurologic surgery. Information specific to these types of surgery can be found in appropriate chapters elsewhere in the text.

Timing or Physical Setting

The timing of surgical intervention may be classified as *elective, urgent,* or *emergent.* Planned, nonessential surgical procedures are classified as elective. Urgent procedures are unplanned and require timely intervention but do not pose an immediate threat to life. Emergent procedures must be performed immediately to preserve life and limb. The same principles related to preoperative care apply to all types of surgery, although modifications must be made for emergent surgical intervention because of the limited preoperative time.

Ambulatory surgery does not require inpatient admission and may be performed under general, local, or regional anesthesia. The patient is admitted to the facility on the day of surgery, remains for postoperative care, and is discharged within 23 hours. Origins of ambulatory surgery can be traced to Egypt as early as 3000 BC. Rapid-acting anesthetic agents, minimally invasive surgical techniques, technologic advances, and changes in reimbursement policies by the federal government and third-party payers all contributed to the emergence of ambulatory surgery as a safe and cost-effective method of providing surgical services. Ambulatory surgical care facilities include hospital-based centers, hospital-affiliated satellite centers, free-standing facilities, and physicians' offices.

In the past all patients were admitted to the hospital for preparation 1 or more days before surgery. Same-day surgery is the response to the national mandate to reduce health care costs. The patient is admitted to the hospital on the day of the procedure and remains hospitalized after surgery. Patient assessment and preoperative teaching are conducted on an outpatient basis before admission.

SPECIAL CONSIDERATIONS FOR THE PATIENT IN THE SURGICAL SETTING

Surgery is a unique experience for each patient, depending on the individual's underlying psychosocial and physiologic factors. Although hospital personnel consider some operations minor procedures, surgery is always a major experience for the patient and family. Surgery is a stressor that produces both physiologic stress reactions (neuroendocrine responses) and psychologic stress reactions (anxiety, fear). Surgery is also a social stressor, requiring family adaptation to temporary or permanent role changes.

Neuroendocrine Response to Surgery

Impending surgery evokes the physiologic stress response. The body's response to impending stress is coordinated by the central nervous system. The central nervous system activates the hypothalamus, the sympathetic nervous system, the anterior and posterior pituitary glands, and the adrenal medulla and cortex. This activation results in the release of catecholamines and hormones, which are responsible for the physiologic events that occur in response to stress.

Systemic effects of the neuroendocrine response are manifested by many complex changes in the body. Some of these changes include increased heart rate and blood pressure, increased blood flow to the brain and vital organs, decreased motility and blood flow to the gastrointestinal tract, increased gastric acid production, elevated blood glucose, increased respiratory rate, increased perspiration and piloerection, dilation of pupils, and platelet aggregation. The nurse's knowledge of the patient's physiologic response to stress is vital for planning and implementing care throughout the perioperative experience.

The Psychologic Response

Anxiety is a normal adaptive response to the stress of surgery and can occur at any time throughout the perioperative period. Potential sources of anxiety include anticipation of impending surgery, pain and discomfort, changes in body image or function, role changes, loss of control, family concerns, or potential alterations in lifestyle. Previous surgical experiences may positively or negatively affect the patient's level of anxiety. Anxiety may be decreased if the patient views the surgery as having positive results, such as curing disease, relieving discomfort, or creating a more attractive physical appearance. In contrast, anxiety usually is increased when the underlying pathologic condition is, or is perceived to be, life-threatening.

Physiologic manifestations of anxiety include increased pulse and respiratory rate, increased blood pressure, abdominal distress, and increased urinary frequency. Mild levels of anxiety are known to enhance learning and performance; however, moderate to high levels of anxiety may interfere with the individual's ability to make informed decisions and decrease effective coping mechanisms.[7] In the surgical patient, extended or excessive periods of anxiety or stress can lead to increased protein breakdown, decreased wound healing, altered immune response, increased risk of infection, and fluid and electrolyte imbalance.

Fear is another emotional response that can result from a perceived impending threat such as surgery. Fear of the unknown and loss of control are the most common responses to facing surgery. Other fears are more specific and related to the type, extent, and purpose of surgery (Box 16-2). Fears concerning pain, disfigurement, disability, or death may be realistic or may be influenced by lack of information or the personal experiences of others. The patient with incapacitating fear or anxiety warrants intervention before proceeding with surgical intervention.

BOX 16-2 Fears Related to Surgery

General

Fear of unknown
Loss of control
Threat to sexuality

Specific

Diagnosis
Anesthesia
Pain
Disfigurement
Loss of function
Death

The Sociologic Response

The usual role of a person hospitalized even for 1 day is disrupted. This disruption inevitably causes role adaptation on the part of other family members and friends as they help with transporting the patient to and from the hospital, psychologic support of the patient, child care, and other family responsibilities. Inability to work also may be a problem to both the patient and family. Job security may be threatened and financial stress may result.

Family members often experience more anxiety than the patient because of their own feelings of helplessness concerning the surgery. Family and friends may be anxious for a variety of reasons, including concern about prognosis and potential changes in lifestyle or routines. The stress of providing emotional support for the patient may also place an added burden on the family or caregiver. Personal experiences with surgery and anesthesia may influence the family's perception of the current situation.

LEGAL AND ETHICAL ISSUES

Informed Consent

The informed consent process protects a patient's right to self-determination and autonomy regarding surgical intervention. Before surgery the patient is asked to a sign a statement consenting to the operative procedure. The consent implies that the patient has been given the information necessary to understand the nature of the procedure, as well as the known and possible consequences. The physician is responsible for providing the patient with sufficient information to weigh the risks and benefits of the proposed surgery (disclosure duty). This information usually includes the nature of the surgery with its benefits, risks, prognosis if treatment is withheld, and alternative treatment modalities. Legal responsibility for obtaining informed consent from the patient resides with the physician. Failure of the surgeon to provide the patient or legal guardian with full disclosure can result in litigation for negligence. Although nurses may be named in litigation, there is legal precedence that the sole responsibility for obtaining informed consent lies with the physician. At least 23 states have ruled that neither nurses nor institutions have the independent duty to obtain a patient's informed consent for surgical or invasive procedures.[16] In some instances, however, nurses and institutions may have a legal duty to ensure that informed consent has been obtained.[17] AORN's explications of the ANA Code of Ethics ensure the nurse's ethical obligation to confirm that appropriate consent for surgery has been obtained.[2] In addition to the surgeon, the anesthesia provider also has the legal responsibility to provide the patient or legal guardian full disclosure regarding the risks and benefits of any anesthetic agents or medications that may be administered during the procedure. The Joint Commission on Accreditation of Health Care Organizations (JCAHO) requires the anesthesia provider to attest that informed consent regarding the risks of anesthesia has been obtained.

The necessary components of the consent document include the patient's full legal name; surgeon's name; specific procedure(s) to be performed; signature of the patient, next of kin, or legal guardian; witness(es); and date. Witnessing the informed consent does not ensure that the patient has a complete understanding of the surgical procedure and its consequences. By signing the consent form, the witness validates *only* identification of the patient or legal substitute, mental status of the patient at time of signature (alert and competent and not under the effects of mind-altering substances), and voluntary signature.

Signing of the official consent form primarily provides evidence that the consent process has occurred and that the patient is aware of the concept of informed consent. The role of the nurse in this process is one of patient advocate. The nurse should verify that the patient has discussed with the physician and the anesthesia provider the risks and benefits of the surgery and alternatives to surgical intervention. If this discussion has not taken place, the nurse should consult with the physician. To facilitate the decision-making process, the nurse should also assess the patient's understanding of what is to occur during and after surgery and clarify any misconceptions. It is imperative that this process occurs before the patient receives any sedation. If an adult is incapable of giving informed consent, consent must be obtained from the next of kin. The order of kin relationship for an adult, as determined from legal interstate succession, is usually spouse, adult child, parent, and sibling. A parent or legal guardian usually provides consent for a minor child. Emancipated minors, that is, minors who are married or earning their own livelihood and retaining the earnings, can sign their own consent forms. The signature of the husband or wife of a married minor is also acceptable. In an emergency, the surgeon may operate without written permission of the patient or family, although every effort is made to contact a family member or guardian if time permits. Consent in the form of a telephone call is permissible in this situation. Two persons must witness the call. If no family member or legal guardian can be contacted, two physicians who are not associated with the procedure may make the decision for surgical intervention. In this circumstance, a relative must sign an operative consent as soon as possible. Patients who are illiterate must understand the verbal explanation of the consent process and may sign the form with an *X*. This process must be witnessed by two persons. Translators must be provided for patients with language barriers. The legal guardian may sign the consent form for mentally incompetent persons; in the guardian's absence, a court of competent jurisdiction may legalize the procedure.

It should also be noted that the patient has the right to refuse surgical intervention. A patient has the right to withdraw informed consent at any time before the procedure if that decision is reached voluntarily and rationally. The nurse's responsibility is to support the patient's decision.

Advance Directives

Patients' rights of autonomy and self-determination are protected by The Patient Self-Determination Act of 1991 (PSDA). By law patients are required to be informed of their rights in decision making regarding health care choices. *Advance directives* are developed by state law and allow an individual to indicate his or her preferences for treatment if he or she is unable to make independent health care decisions. A *living will* and *durable power of attorney for health care* are common examples of advance directives. The patient completes both documents while still competent. A living will outlines the patient's wishes regarding medical care, artificially supplied nourishment, life support, and resuscitation measures. The durable power of attorney identifies the person who is authorized to make decisions on the patient's behalf if the patient becomes incapacitated. The PSDA does not apply to all health care settings. Any institution receiving Medicare or Medicaid funds is required by the PSDA to inform patients about their states' advance directives and whether such documents have been executed. The perioperative nurse must be aware of a patient's decisions regarding advance directives.

Do-Not-Resuscitate Orders

As discussed in the preceding paragraphs, advance directives concern decisions regarding end-of-life treatments. The decision not to initiate cardiopulmonary resuscitation is written as a specific directive by a physician, which is termed a *do-not-resuscitate (DNR) order.* Perioperative nurses may encounter patients with DNR orders who are undergoing surgical procedures to improve the quality of life or for palliative care. DNR orders are not automatically suspended when the patient enters the operating room. The AORN's position statement on perioperative care of patients with DNR orders is supported by the PSDA, JCAHO, the ANA Code for Nurses, and "A Patient's Bill of Rights." The AORN position statement asserts the following: "Required reconsideration of DNR decisions with patients is an integral component of the care of patients undergoing surgery."[2] Reviewing the DNR status ensures that the risks and benefits of anesthesia and surgery are discussed with the patient or family before surgery. Discussion should include goals of surgical treatment, potential for and nature of resuscitative measures, and possible outcomes with and without resuscitative efforts. The patient or the individual with durable power of attorney will decide whether to maintain, suspend, or modify the DNR orders during anesthesia and surgery. If the DNR order is suspended during the intraoperative period, there must be documentation indicating when it is to be reinstated. The perioperative nurse has the responsibility to support the patient's decisions regarding end-of-life treatment choices and the patient's right to refuse treatment.

NURSING MANAGEMENT

ASSESSMENT

Health History

Assessment of the patient during the preoperative phase begins with the initial contact between patient and nurse and is ongoing throughout the perioperative period. Assessment should be holistic, reflecting the physiologic, psychologic, spiritual, and social needs of the patient and the family or significant others (Box 16-3).

BOX 16-3 Preoperative Subjective Data Collection

Reason for Seeking Care/History of Present Illness

Demographic data
Allergies
- Iodine
- Medications
- Latex
- Cleansing solutions
- Adhesive tape

Medications and substance use
- Smoking
- Recreational drugs
- Alcohol
- Prescription medication
- Over-the-counter medications

Herbal and nutritional supplements
Cultural and religious background
Psychosocial status
Functional assessment
Level of anxiety
Medical history
Review of systems
Surgical and anesthetic history
Perception of surgical procedure
Perception of pain
Assessment of surgical risk

BOX 16-4 CAGE Questionnaire

CAGE Questionnaire

C: Have you felt a need to *cut down* on your drinking?
A: Have you ever felt *annoyed by criticism* of your drinking?
G: Have you ever felt *guilty* about your drinking?
E: Have you ever felt the need for an *eye-opener* drink?

Patient assessment occurs in a variety of settings. The nurse's initial contact with the patient may be in the physician's office, preadmission testing area, inpatient hospital unit, ambulatory surgery facility, or over the telephone. A complete health history is compiled to identify factors that may increase surgical risk or contribute to the development of postoperative complications. The goal of preoperative assessment is to identify individuals at risk for intraoperative and postoperative complications and implement interventions to decrease risk and improve surgical outcomes. In the following sections not every component of the health history is addressed, only data that have a particular relevance for the preoperative patient are discussed. It is important, however, to elicit a complete health history from the patient and/or family. For a complete discussion of obtaining the health history refer to a text on physical examination.

Allergies

The patient should be assessed for allergies to iodine, medications, latex, cleansing solutions, and adhesive tape. The type of reaction should be documented in the patient's record. This information is needed because many of these products are used throughout the surgical procedure. Povidone-iodine is commonly used during surgery for cleansing the patient's skin. If the patient is unsure whether he or she has an allergy to iodine, the nurse should question the patient regarding allergies to shellfish because of the high iodine content. Iodine is also a component of many contrast media that may be used during surgery. Patients with latex allergies require special latex-free supplies and equipment. Latex allergy is discussed in Chapter 17.

Medications and Substance Abuse

Data regarding history of smoking, substance abuse, and prescribed and over-the-counter medications are collected. These data are important because of the potential adverse interactions of these substances with some anesthetic agents and increased risk for perioperative complications.

Smoking, first identified as a risk factor for postoperative pulmonary complications in 1944, increases postoperative risk even in individuals without chronic lung disease. Patients who smoke are at an increased risk for postoperative atelectasis. Eight weeks of abstinence from smoking before surgery is necessary to decrease the risks of postoperative pulmonary complications.[22,23] Although patients who stop smoking 8 weeks before surgery have better postoperative outcomes, some sources show decreased mortality and morbidity in patients who stop smoking only 24 hours before surgery.[19] During the preadmission interview, patients should be provided with the benefits of smoking cessation and offered information regarding smoking cessation techniques.

Drug and alcohol use can alter the effects of anesthetic and analgesic agents, and patients who use these substances may require adjustments of the recommended dosages of these agents. In addition to an accurate history of recreational drug use, it is important to elicit an accurate history of alcohol consumption. Unidentified alcohol use may result in withdrawal symptoms in the surgical patient whose regular alcohol intake is decreased or discontinued. An accepted screening tool for potentially problematic alcohol consumption is the CAGE questionnaire (Box 16-4) developed by Ewing in 1984.[21]

A thorough history of medication use is essential. Many types of prescription and over-the-counter (OTC) medications may affect reactions to anesthetics or surgery (Table 16-2). Medication history is of particular importance in the preoperative assessment of the older adult; data reveal an estimated 75% of community dwelling elders take at least one prescription medication per day. Concurrent use of multiple medications presents a challenge in the assessment of the older adult, as the typical older adult receives between 12 and 17 prescriptions annually and may take up to four to five medications at one time.[13,25] The use of multiple medications significantly increases the elderly patient's potential for drug interactions, adverse side effects, and interactions with anesthetic agents.

TABLE 16-2 Common Prescription and Over-the-Counter Medications and Their Effects on Anesthesia and Surgery

Medications	Effect	Potential Interaction and Nursing Implication
Anticoagulants		
Aspirin	Inhibit platelet aggregation	Aspirin should be discontinued 7 days before surgery
Heparin	Inhibit action of antithrombin	Monitor for bleeding May be discontinued before surgery
Low-molecular-weight heparins	Inhibit factor Xa	Monitor for bleeding Increased bleeding risks with other anticoagulants May be given before surgery for prophylaxis for deep vein thrombosis
Warfarin	Interfere with vitamin K-dependent coagulation factors	Monitor coagulation studies, International Normalized Ratio, prothrombin time Usually discontinued 2-4 days before elective surgery Highly protein bound; drug interactions may potentiate anticoagulant effects
Nonsteroidal anti-inflammatory drugs	Block prostaglandin synthesis Inhibit platelet aggregation Prolong bleeding time Significant analgesic and antipyretic properties	Cautious use in patients with impaired renal and hepatic function Monitor for bleeding Increased risk of bleeding with concomitant use of anticoagulants May increase blood pressure in normotensive and hypertensive individuals Decreases hypotensive response to thiazides, beta-blockers, and vasodilators
Steroids	Decrease neuroendocrine response, antiinflammatory and immunosuppressive action, delayed wound healing	Maintain drug therapy perioperatively (dosages may need to be temporarily increased), may be given IV intraoperatively Monitor for bleeding Monitor closely for signs and symptoms of infection
Antihypertensives	Possible perioperative cardiac complications, including myocardial infarction and congestive heart failure	Maintenance of antihypertensive therapy before and day of surgery Perioperative monitoring of blood pressure and pulse
Diuretics	Lower blood pressure, treatment of edema	Fluid and electrolyte imbalance
Insulin	Lower blood sugar	Stress response will increase dosage requirements NPO status and decreased intake will decrease dosage requirements IV fluids containing glucose can increase dosage requirements
Analgesics (opiate agonists)	Central nervous system depressant	Monitor for respiratory depression and suppression of cough reflex Drug tolerance Synergistic effects with other central nervous system depressants
Antihistamines	H_1 receptor antagonist Anticholinergic properties	Potentiates central nervous system depressant effects of benzodiazepines, barbiturates, phenothiazines, and opioids Monitor for tachycardia Cautious use for patients with hypertension
Decongestants	Sympathomimetic	Cautious use in patients with hypertension and cardiac disease Increased pressor effects and toxicity with other sympathomimetics (epinephrine)

IV, Intravenously.

In addition to prescribed medications, the patient must also be assessed for use of OTC medications. More than 600 medications previously requiring a prescription are now available over the counter. An estimated 30% of North Americans use at least one OTC preparation in a 2-day period.[12] The use of self-administered OTC drugs and the use of prescribed medications compound the elderly patient's risk for drug interactions and reactions to anesthesia.

Herbs and Nutritional Supplements

Complementary and alternative therapies encompass practices and beliefs outside of the dominant health system that are used to prevent or treat illness or to promote health.[27] Refer to Chapter 2 for further discussion of complementary and alternative therapies.

Although used extensively in Europe and Asia for years, dietary supplements, vitamins, minerals, and homeopathic and herbal products are examples of nontraditional therapies that are becoming increasingly popular in the United States, where sales of these products exceeded $13 billion in 1999. An estimated 70 million Americans and 80% of persons in developing countries use herbal remedies and these numbers are expected to continue to increase.[5]

The terminology for these products is often confusing; herbs also known as botanicals, nutraceuticals, or phytomedicines are medicinal plants and possess pharmacologic properties. Although 25% of traditional medications are derived from plants, in the United States herbs are classified as dietary supplements, not medications, and hence are under control of the Federal Trade Commission rather than the U.S. Food and Drug Administration (FDA).[5] In 1994 the Dietary Supplement Health and Education Act (DSHEA) was passed and established regulations for dietary supplements. The significance to health care providers and consumers is that herbal products lack the rigorous control and approval process required by the FDA for medications. Under DSHEA regulations, the FDA can restrict use of a dietary supplement only if proven unsafe. Currently there are no regulations regarding purity, identification of ingredients, or manufacturing processes for herbals and dietary supplements[8]; however, the FDA does issue warnings and responds to medical complaints regarding dietary supplements.

Media exposure, marketing, and accessibility of herbal products contribute to the increased use of these products among Americans. Many consumers mistakenly assume that all herbal products are safe and do not realize the implications of their use, including side effects and potential drug-herb interactions. Studies estimate that one of every five persons taking prescription medications also takes herbal products, and 15 million adults may be at risk for potential drug-herb interactions.[11] Of particular interest to the perioperative nurse is that 40% to 70% of patients taking herbal products do not disclose the use of these products to the health care provider.[5,6,27] Compounding this is the fact that many providers do not specifically question patients regarding the use of alternative therapies during the assessment interview. Therefore it is essential that the preoperative assessment includes specific questions regarding the use of herbal products and other complementary and alternative therapies.

There is a paucity of data regarding the use of herbal products and anesthetic interactions and the benefit of discontinuing these products before surgery. Currently the American Society of Anesthesiologists (ASA) has no formal standard of care specific to phytomedicines. Information released by the ASA, however, advises clinicians that patients discontinue herbal medications at least 2 to 3 weeks before surgery.[1] In practice, this may be impossible, as most patients are not seen that far in advance for elective surgery. The perioperative nurse may see many patients who are still taking herbal medications at the time of surgery; therefore it is the responsibility of the perioperative nurse to be aware of the common names, actions, side effects, drug-herb interactions, and perioperative implications of commonly used herbal products (Table 16-3). Until standards are established by the ASA, the perioperative nurse needs to know the institutional policies regarding discontinuation of these products before surgery.

TABLE 16-3 Commonly Used Herbs and Perioperative Implications

Herb	Common Name	Common Uses	Perioperative Implications
Echinacea augustifolia	Purple coneflower	Immune stimulant Antiinfective	Possible allergic reactions Risk of hepatotoxicity with other hepatotoxic drugs or long-term use May decrease effectiveness of corticosteroids Contraindicated in patients with immune disorders
Ephedra sinica	Ma-Haung Ephedrine Natural ecstasy	Appetite suppressant Bronchodilator Antitussive Athletic performance enhancement	Sympathomimetic effects include increased heart rate and blood pressure Risk of arrhythmias with cardiac glycosides or halothane Potential complications include hypertension, myocardial ischemia and infarction, cardiac arrest, seizures, respiratory depression, bronchodilation, stroke, and urinary retention Enhanced sympathomimetic effects with methyldopa Potential life-threatening interactions with monoamine oxidase inhibitors
Tanacetum parthenium	Feverfew Midsummer daisy	Migraine prophylaxis Antipyretic Antiarthritic Menstrual irregularity	May inhibit platelet activity and increased bleeding time Avoid concomitant use with aspirin, warfarin and other anticoagulants, and thrombolytics

TABLE 16-3 Commonly Used Herbs and Perioperative Implications—cont'd

Herb	Common Name	Common Uses	Perioperative Implications
Allilum sativum	Garlic	Hyperlipidemic Antibiotic Antihypertensive Antiplatelet and antithrombolytic Antioxidant	Inhibits platelet aggregation May potentiate warfarin May increase International Normalized Ratio (INR) and prothrombin time May cause gastrointestinal upset May decrease blood glucose levels
Zingiber officinale	Ginger	Prevention of motion sickness Analgesic and antiinflammatory particularly for treatment of rheumatoid arthritis and osteoarthritis	Anticoagulant action In large doses increases risk of bleeding and dysrhythmias
Panax ginseng *P. quinquefolius*	Ginseng root	Decreases fatigue and stress Enhances well-being and energy level	May cause tachycardia and hypertension especially with use of cardiac stimulants Inhibits platelet aggregation May decrease effectiveness of warfarin May decrease INR and PT Lowers blood glucose May potentiate effects of digoxin May cause electrocardiogram changes Assess for ginseng abuse syndrome (insomnia, hypotonia, and edema)
Ginkgo biloba	Ginkgo	Increases cerebral blood flow Improves memory and mental functioning Antioxidant Decreases symptoms of peripheral vascular disease, vertigo, and tinnitis	Inhibits platelet-activating factor, increases risk of bleeding Prolongs bleeding time Increases effects of anticoagulants Side effects include subconjuctival hemorrhage and spontaneous subdural hematoma
Piper methysticum	Kava-kava Kawa	Anxiolytic	Potentiates effects of central nervous system depressants, anesthetics, and alcohol
Glycyrrhiza glabra	Licorice	Antiulcer agent (gastric and duodenal ulcers) Expectorant	Contraindicated in chronic hepatic disease, renal disease, and hypokalemia May increase hypertension and edema May cause electrolyte imbalance (particularly hypokalemia) Neutralizes antibiotics May potentiate corticosteroids
Hypericum perforatum	St. John's wort	Antidepressant Anxiolytic	May prolong sedative effects of anesthesia and opioids Contraindicated with use of selective-seratonin reuptake inhibitors and ephedra Possible interactions with warfarin, steroids, benzodiazepines, calcium channel blockers, and protease inhibitors
Valeriana officinalis	Valerian	Mild sedative Hypnotic Anxiolytic Muscle relaxant	Risk of hepatotoxicty with other herbs (particularly skullcap and mistletoe) Long-term users may require increased dosage of anesthetics Prolongs sedative effects of anesthesia Potentiates action of barbiturates and alcohol Avoid concomitant use with sedatives and anxiolytics

Cultural and Religious Background

Cultural and ethnic background influences an individual's response to health, illness, surgery, and death. An awareness of cultural differences may enhance the nurse's knowledge of how the surgical experience may be perceived by the patient and family. In addition, responses to pain may be influenced by cultural and ethnic background. If a patient's cultural background includes a language barrier, arrangements should be made for an interpreter to be present throughout the perioperative process.

Like cultural beliefs, religious beliefs also influence individual and family responses to health, illness, pain, surgery, and death. Religion can be a source of support and comfort for the patient. Some religions allow for little individual control over the environment and therefore may dictate the degree or level of medical interventions a patient chooses. Awareness of a patient's individual religious beliefs enables the nurse to appropriately support the patient's decisions regarding care throughout the perioperative period. For example, the nurse would be supportive of a Jehovah's Witness's refusal to receive blood transfusions.

Psychosocial Status

Assessment of the social situation of the patient, the patient's family, and significant others is necessary to coordinate postoperative care, discharge needs, and follow-up care. The patient's role in the family and social support network should be evaluated during the preoperative interview. The primary source of psychologic support for the patient is usually the family or significant others. Knowledge of the patient and family's coping mechanisms enables the nurse to assist them in coping effectively with the impending events. The patient's financial status and insurance coverage should also be assessed, as these factors may have considerable implications for the immediate surgical intervention, hospitalization, and follow-up care.

Functional Assessment

The patient should be assessed for his or her ability to perform activities of daily living (ADLs). Functional status can be assessed by interviewing the patient or by using a standardized tool such as the Sickness Impact Profile. The patient's preoperative level of functioning provides a baseline and can be used in projecting the person's ability for postoperative self-care. An important consideration is whether the proposed surgery will result in a decline in the person's functional status. Potential discharge needs should be assessed during the preoperative evaluation. If it is anticipated that the patient will need assistance with ADLs, a caregiver(s) should be identified. If the patient is expected to experience a significant change in role or loss of independence, both the patient and family may need counseling and support. Social service referrals can be initiated at this time. The case manager or discharge coordinator is the primary facilitator for discharge needs including medical equipment and supplies, home care, and therapy requirements.

Level of Anxiety

Anxiety is a common response to the stressors of surgical intervention. Signs of anxiety in the presurgical patient are no different from those in other persons and can be observed in a number of ways. Highly anxious persons may talk rapidly, ask many questions without waiting for answers, repeat the same questions, or change topics frequently during the interaction. They may deny that they have any worries or fears, but their actions are contrary to this denial. Some patients will not talk about the forthcoming surgery, responding only in monosyllables, whereas others may cry and display anger; both behaviors are overt signs of anxiety. In some instances, patients may not be able to identify specific concerns, and further exploration may be indicated.

Anxiety results in elevated levels of cortisol and adrenaline, which are normal physiologic responses to stress. If unmanaged or prolonged, anxiety may lead to increased protein breakdown, decreased wound healing, increased risk of infection, altered immune response, and fluid and electrolyte imbalances. Changes in sleep patterns also provide clues about increased anxiety. Major causes of insomnia are worry, fear, and concerns about the future.

The effect of family members or significant others on the patient's level of anxiety needs to be determined. Some family members or significant others may increase the patient's anxiety by hovering over the patient, displaying anxious behaviors, or offering false reassurances. Others are calm, and it is observed that the patient's anxiety is reduced when they are present. Before surgery and throughout the perioperative experience, family members are often more anxious than the patient, perhaps because of feelings of powerlessness and helplessness.

Medical History

The medical history should focus on preexisting medical conditions and a family history of medical conditions that may increase operative risk, such as myocardial infarction and diabetes mellitus. A thorough review of systems is taken to collect data on all body systems. The nurse should inquire about any past hospitalizations and illnesses and collect data to determine the presence of systemic or chronic disease. The presence of chronic disease may place the patient at higher risk for developing surgical or anesthetic complications. However, the mere presence of chronic disease does not always increase surgical risk. The nature and extent of the disease or diseases and the degree to which they are under control are important variables. Nursing assessment and documentation of these factors are critical in the preoperative period.

Surgical and Anesthetic History

The nurse assesses the patient's previous experiences with surgery and anesthesia. These data provide the surgical team with information regarding any reactions or complications to surgical procedures or anesthetics. The patient's and family's previous surgical experiences can affect the upcoming event and influence physical and psychologic responses to the procedure.

To determine potential problems with airway maintenance and endotracheal intubation, the patient should be questioned regarding any problems with cervical mobility, mouth opening, dentures or loose teeth, and problems with the temporal mandibular joint. In addition, the patient should be assessed for a history of adverse reactions to anesthetic agents or medications used perioperatively. Nausea and vomiting are common side effects of many medications used perioperatively. Knowledge of the patient's previous problems with postoperative nausea and vomiting can influence the choice of medications used for anesthesia and analgesia.

Another indication for assessing the patient's anesthetic history is to determine the risk for serious complications such as malignant hyperthermia. A family history of anesthetic complications should also be elicited, as malignant hyperthermia is an autosomal-dominant inherited syndrome. A positive family history for malignant hyperthermia may include a sudden or unexplained death while the patient is under anesthesia (see Chapter 17).

The patient should be questioned for any problems with incisions or wound healing. African-Americans and persons with darkly pigmented skin are prone to keloid formation. Keloids are an increased growth of collagen fibers and fiberblasts that form at the site of tissue injury, including surgical incisions. If the patient is prone to keloid formation, the surgeon may inject a corticosteroid during the surgical procedure to reduce scar tissue formation.

Perception of Surgical Procedure

The patient's level of understanding of the proposed surgical procedure and postoperative routine is determined. It is important for the nurse to explore the patient's understanding and expectations of treatment. The patient should be assessed for informed consent and an accurate understanding of the procedure and its proposed outcomes. Knowing the level of the patient's understanding of the surgical event is required before any teaching can take place. It is important to find out exactly how the surgery is perceived because persons respond on the basis of their perceptions. If possible, the nurse should clarify any misunderstandings or misconceptions; however, the patient may need to be referred to the surgeon for further information, particularly regarding informed consent.

Perception of Pain

In 2000 JCAHO established a standard requiring that all patients have their pain assessed and appropriately managed. The latter includes the provision of postoperative discharge pain management instructions. This standard applies to patients in hospitals, outpatient surgery centers, and other health care institutions accredited by JCAHO.[20]

Preoperative assessment of the patient's perception of pain is necessary for effective postoperative pain management. A complete pain assessment (see Chapter 12) and an assessment of the patient's expectations for pain management after surgery should be performed. It is important to include the family in the assessment and pain management plan. A preoperative pain assessment provides a baseline and allows for comparison of the patient's level of postoperative pain.

Assessment of Surgical Risk

Every person responds to the surgical experience in a unique way. A number of variables influence psychologic and physiologic responses throughout the entire surgical experience. Some of these include age, the presence of chronic disease or disabilities, impaired nutritional status, and type of surgical procedure. The type of procedure performed influences the degree of risk involved. Surgical mortality is higher in thoracic and abdominal procedures. Regardless of the type of procedure being performed, it is important to consider the individual's preoperative health status.

> **_Future Watch_**
>
> **Prediction of Surgical Risk**
>
> A new rating system developed in England may help is assessing the biologic age of older adults, and thus predict their surgical risk. The star rating is a simple assessment tool that grades patients' performance and lifestyles and provides a rough estimate of their biologic age. No physiologic measurements or questionnaires are necessary; the assessment criteria can be determined during the initial health history.
>
> The rating system is as follows:
>
> - Five star: physically and mentally intact
> - Four star: physical deterioration requiring adaptation of lifestyle and mental deterioration to level of forgetfulness and intellectual blunting
> - Three star: physical or mental frailty that threatens independent living, which is maintained only by the input of others
> - Two star: independent existence no longer possible
> - One star: bed or chair bound; requires help with feeding, washing, and toilet needs; has advanced dementia with the inability to recognize family members
>
> If further research supports the validity of this system as a reliable predictor of surgical risk, it is an easy tool to implement in clinical practice. Reliable prediction of surgical risk may influence elderly patients' decisions regarding treatment and surgical intervention.
>
> Reference: Farquharson SM et al: Surgical decisions in the elderly: the importance of biological age, *J R Soc Med* 94:232, 2001.

Age

Although other demographic data are collected, age is particularly relevant in the assessment of the patient. Age affects surgical and postoperative outcomes (see Future Watch box). Between the ages of 30 and 40 the functional capacity of each organ system decreases by approximately 1% annually.[7] The age of the surgical patient identifies those individuals at increased risk for surgical and postoperative complications. Refer to the section on gerontologic considerations for further discussion.

American Society of Anesthesiologists Status

Surgical risk can be assessed by different methods. An objective method of determining the degree of risk for a particular patient has been developed by the ASA. The scale is based on the number and severity of preexisting medical conditions independent of the proposed surgical procedure. Higher ASA scores indicate a greater risk of perioperative complications and death. The anesthesiologist or anesthetist performs the patient assessment and classification before surgery. Table 16-4 contains the classification status.

Cardiac Status

Intraoperative cardiac events including myocardial infarction, unstable angina, congestive heart failure, dysrhythmias, and

TABLE 16-4 Physical (P) Status Classification of the American Society of Anesthesiologists

Status*†	Definition	Description and Examples
P1	A normal healthy patient	No physiologic, psychologic, biochemical, or organic disturbance
P2	A patient with a mild systemic disease	Cardiovascular disease with minimal restriction on activity; hypertension, asthma, chronic bronchitis, obesity, or diabetes mellitus
P3	A patient with a severe systemic disease that limits activity, but is not incapacitating	Cardiovascular or pulmonary disease that limits activity; severe diabetes with systemic complications; history of myocardial infarction, angina pectoris, or poorly controlled hypertension
P4	A patient with severe systemic disease that is a constant threat to life	Severe cardiac, pulmonary, renal, hepatic, or endocrine dysfunction
P5	A moribund patient who is not expected to survive 24 hours with or without the operation	Surgery done as last recourse or resuscitative effort; major multisystem or cerebral trauma, ruptured aneurysm, or large pulmonary embolus
P6	A patient declared brain dead whose organs are being removed for donor purposes	

Modified from the American Society of Anesthesiologists, ASA, 520 N. Northwest Highway, Park Ridge, IL 60068.
*In status P2, P3, and P4 the systemic disease may or may not be related to the cause for surgery.
†For any patient (P1 through P5) requiring emergency surgery, an E is added to the physical status (e.g., P1E, P2E). ASA 1 through ASA 6 is often used for physical status.

sudden cardiac death are the leading cause of mortality and morbidity in the operative patient.[22] After surgery cardiac complications continue to be a leading cause of morbidity and mortality. The patient is at highest risk for myocardial infarction 3 to 6 days after the surgical procedure.[19] Patients with a questionable or positive history of cardiac disease may need a cardiac consultation before undergoing elective surgery.

The patient with coronary artery disease is at a significantly higher risk for development of perioperative complications. The presence and severity of angina should be assessed. A standardized tool such as the Canadian Cardiovascular Society (CSS) Angina Classification System or the Goldman Index (identifies clinical risk factors for adverse cardiac outcomes after noncardiac surgery) can be used for preoperative assessment. The health history should include questions regarding the presence of chest pain at rest, during physical activity, and with exercise. Patients with unstable angina should be referred for cardiac clearance before surgery.

Persons with congestive heart failure (CHF) are at increased risk for perioperative pulmonary and cardiac arrest. If digoxin is used to manage left ventricular dysfunction, these patients may also be at risk for perioperative dysrhythmias. Patients with known arrhythmias should be stabilized and controlled before surgery to reduce the risk for perioperative complications.

Hypertension is a common comorbid condition among preoperative patients. Perioperative complications of hypertension include myocardial infarction, CHF, cerebrovascular accident, and death. Elective surgery should be delayed until severe hypertension is under control. Patients with mild to moderate hypertension controlled with medication are usually maintained on their antihypertensive regimen before and including the day of surgery.[22]

Certain types of surgical procedures are associated with a higher risk of postoperative cardiac complications. Procedures associated with a higher risk include major vascular, thoracic, major abdominal, and emergency surgery.

Pulmonary Status

Identification of patients at risk for pulmonary complications is an important component of the preoperative assessment. Postoperative pulmonary complications occur almost as frequently as postoperative cardiac complications and may prolong the patient's hospital stay by 1 to 2 weeks.[23]

Perioperative pulmonary complications include pneumonia, respiratory failure, bronchospasm, atelectasis, hypoxemia, and exacerbation of chronic lung disease. Risk factors known to contribute to the development of postoperative pulmonary complications include smoking, advanced age, chronic obstructive pulmonary disease (COPD), asthma, morbid obesity, and type of surgery (thoracic, cardiac, and upper abdominal procedures). Persons receiving inhalant anesthetics are also at risk for the development of pulmonary complications, particularly atelectasis and pneumonia. Table 16-5 summarizes the major risk factors for postoperative pulmonary complications.

Any condition that restricts movement of the chest wall places the person at risk for perioperative respiratory complications. Persons with morbid obesity may have difficulty with chest wall expansion owing to excessive weight on the thoracic cavity. Obese persons may also be dyspneic when lying supine.

TABLE 16-5 Risk Factors for the Development of Postoperative Pulmonary Complications

Risk Factor	Effect
Smoking	Irritation of lining of bronchial passages
Chronic obstructive lung disease	Airway obstruction, increased mucus, decreased ciliary action to remove secretions, bronchoconstriction, bronchospasm, decreased ventilatory capacity, hypoxemia
Respiratory infection	Increased secretions, blockage of bronchial passages and alveoli
Skeletal deformities	Impaired ventilation, susceptibility to infection (kyphoscoliosis, rheumatoid arthritis of the spine)

The patient should be questioned for a history of neuromuscular disease including muscular dystrophy, myasthenia gravis, and polio. Neuromuscular disease impairs respiratory muscle function and may result in hypoventilation, decreased ability to remove secretions, and hypoxemia.

Length of surgery has also been identified as a risk factor for the development of pulmonary complications. Procedures lasting longer than 3 hours are associated with a higher risk of pulmonary complications. The type of anesthesia also influences development of pulmonary complications. Research indicates a lower risk of pulmonary complications in persons who have received epidural or spinal anesthesia than those receiving general anesthetics.[23]

Smoking causes blood vessel constriction and increased secretions. The carbon monoxide in smoke binds with hemoglobin, decreasing tissue oxygenation. The increased lung compliance, increased airway resistance, and chronic mucus hypersecretion found in COPD may lead to inadequate ventilation, severe hypoxemia, dysrhythmias, and respiratory failure. Patients with asthma are at an increased risk for bronchospasm during intubation, extubation, and postoperatively.

Assessment of the patient's respiratory status should include questions regarding exercise intolerance, dypsnea on exertion, unexplained dyspnea, the presence of a cough, and increased sputum production. The patient should be asked specifically about his or her ability to climb stairs and the number of stairs that cause dypsnea. The preoperative interview should also include questioning the patient regarding a history of sleep apnea, which has been linked to near fatal respiratory complications (see Research box).

To reduce the risk and severity of perioperative pulmonary complications, the patient's pulmonary status should be optimized before surgery. The presence of respiratory infection may delay elective surgery.

Renal Status

Decreased renal function is another factor associated with increased surgical risk. A decline in kidney function can impair the body's ability to excrete waste products, medications, and anesthetic agents. It is important to consider that elderly patients over age 70 have some impairment in renal function as a result of the aging process. Persons with chronic renal insufficiency are at risk for adverse events in the perioperative period owing to alterations in electrolyte balance, acid-base balance, platelet function, fluid balance, and immune function. It is important to realize that a number of patients with renal disease have concomitant diabetes and hypertension and thus are at increased risk for developing complications from

Research

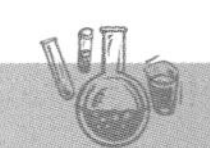

Reference: Jarrell L: Preoperative diagnosis and postoperative management of adult patient with obstructive sleep apnea syndrome: a review of the literature, *J Perianesthesia Nurs* 14(4):193, 1999.

Patients with a history of obstructive sleep apnea syndrome (OSAS) are at risk for developing postoperative respiratory complications. Individuals with OSAS can experience near fatal postoperative respiratory complications after administration of general anesthesia.

General anesthesia causes a decrease in the neural stimulation of the upper airway musculature; this, in conjunction with an OSAS patient's narrowed upper airway, puts the patient at risk for prolonged apneic events, hypoxia, hypercapnia, and cardiac dysrhythmias in the postoperative period. Many persons are unaware they have OSAS; therefore it is crucial to identify these individuals during the preoperative evaluation to ensure appropriate perioperative care.

Extensive review of current research reveals that there is no standard method to diagnose OSAS. Laboratory tests are available to diagnose this syndrome, but because of inconvenience and cost they are not frequently used.

Although questionnaires have been designed to classify the various symptoms of OSAS, health care providers have no validated, reliable, predictive tool to diagnose OSAS. Symptoms such as unacceptable habitual snoring, apneic periods reported by others, and daytime somnolence can be predictors for the diagnosis. Research indicates that using these identified symptomatic data in conjunction with risk factors, including gender (males have a greater propensity towards OSAS) and obesity as indicated with the body mass index (BMI), enhances the practitioner's ability to identify patients with OSAS.

Because of lingering sedative and respiratory depressant effects of general anesthesia, patients with OSAS are at a high risk for hypoxemia in the postoperative period. Research indicates that treatment with nasal continuous positive airway pressure (N-CPAP) both before surgery and immediately after extubation may permit unlimited usage of sedatives, anesthetics, and analgesics throughout the perioperative period.

There is a paucity of nursing research that addresses the needs of the OSAS patient in the perioperative period. Additional nursing research is needed to provide validated methods to provide quality perioperative nursing care to patients with or suspected of having OSAS.

coexisting illness. During the perioperative period, acute kidney failure (AKF) can develop in the patient with preexisting renal insufficiency and also in the patient without renal disease. Factors contributing to the development of AKF include intraoperative hypotension, sepsis, and type of surgical procedure. The incidence of AKF in the person without preexisting renal disease is 1.5% to 2.5% for cardiac surgical procedures and more than 10% in patients undergoing supraceliac abdominal aortic aneurysms.[15] It is important to remember that administration of nephrotoxic drugs and administration of contrast media can also result in postoperative AKF.

Hepatic Function

Because of the metabolic functions of the liver, assessment of hepatic functioning is an important component of the patient's preoperative evaluation. Patients with liver dysfunction are at risk for perioperative complications including hemorrhage, altered pharmacokinetics, hepatic and kidney failure, encephalopathy, hepatitis, and infection.

The patient with liver disease who receives general anesthetic agents, mechanical ventilation, or spinal or epidural anesthesia experiences a decrease in hepatic blood flow during surgery, which may lead to ischemic injury. Volatile anesthetic agents such as halothane and enflurane depress cardiac output and systemic pressure, resulting in decreased hepatic blood flow. If assessment reveals the presence of acute, viral, or alcoholic hepatitis or cirrhosis, elective surgery may need to be postponed.

Neurologic Status

Assessment of neurologic status establishes baseline function and identifies patients at risk for perioperative neurologic complications. Perioperative stroke and acute delirium are the most common neurologic complications.

Patients at risk for perioperative stroke include the elderly, smokers, and individuals with hypertension, coronary artery disease, and diabetes. The incidence of perioperative stroke is 2% to 5% in patients undergoing cardiac procedures and less than 1% in patients undergoing noncardiac procedures[15]; however, more than 80% of perioperative strokes occur in the postoperative period, usually as a result of atrial fibrillation and carotid stenosis.

Patients with a history of recent transient ischemic attacks are also at increased risk for perioperative stroke and should be referred for further evaluation before surgery. Persons with a history of a recent stroke should have elective procedures delayed for at least 2 weeks, depending on the severity of the neurologic insult.[15]

Delirium is an acute, reversible state of agitated confusion characterized by hallucinations; disorientation; distractibility; insomnia; and emotional, physical, and autonomic overactivity. Risk factors identified for the development of delirium include advanced age, drug and alcohol withdrawal, medication side effects, sepsis, pain, electrolyte and acid-base imbalance, sensory deprivation and sensory overload, cardiac dysrhythmias, myocardial infarction, and stroke. Persons undergoing surgery for aortic aneurysm and noncardiac thoracic surgery are also at an increased risk for developing delirium.[22] If preoperative assessment reveals the presence of risk factors, medications such as meperidine and benzodiazepene should be avoided, as they increase the risk of developing postoperative delirium.[22] Early identification of patients at risk enables the nurse to be alert for signs of emerging delirium in the postoperative period. Refer to Chapter 18 for further discussion of delirium.

Hematologic Status

Hematologic assessment of the patient is essential, especially in procedures with an expected blood loss. Patients should be questioned regarding a history of anemia, bleeding disorders, and hematologic malignancies. A history of blood transfusions and any adverse reactions to blood or blood products should be elicited. It is also important to ask if the patient has donated his or her own blood (autologous donation) for the surgical procedure. A thorough medication history is important, paying particular attention to medications that inhibit platelet functioning. Common medications that impair platelet functioning include anticoagulants, nonsteroidal anti-inflammatory drugs (NSAIDs), aspirin, tricyclic antidepressants, alcohol, and beta-blockers. The nurse should consult with the anesthesiologist or surgeon to determine when and if these medications need to be discontinued before surgery.

Persons with a history of atrial fibrillation, venous thromboses, and mechanical heart valves are often treated with the oral anticoagulant warfarin. Warfarin therapy increases the patient's risk for bleeding and hemorrhage. Preoperative management of these patients is a challenge, as discontinuing anticoagulant therapy increases the risk for thromboembolism. However, there is no evidence in the literature to support the best practice for managing patients on long-term anticoagulant therapy. The nurse needs to consult with the surgeon and anesthesiologist regarding perioperative management of anticoagulation therapy.

Another cornerstone of the preoperative assessment is questioning the patient about a history of deep venous thrombosis (DVT) and pulmonary embolism. Risk factors for the development of DVT include age over 40 years, prior history of DVT, decreased mobility, pelvic or cardiovascular surgery, total hip and total knee surgery, fracture or trauma, history of smoking, use of estrogen, and obesity. Refer to Chapter 25 for a full discussion of DVT.

Endocrine Function

Diabetes mellitus is a common condition, and perioperative management of the patient with diabetes depends on the type of diabetes and treatment modality. Patients with diabetes mellitus are at risk for delayed wound healing and infection. The presence of obesity, advanced age, and complications resulting from diabetes place the patient at additional risk. Many patients with diabetes also have cardiovascular and renal disease and are at an increased risk for negative perioperative outcomes.

The goal of managing patients with diabetes in the perioperative period is stabilization of blood glucose levels. The trauma of surgery and accompanying factors such as stress, nothing-by-mouth (NPO) status, anesthesia, tissue trauma, and reduced postoperative activity all affect the regulation of blood glucose levels. Refer to Chapter 30 for further discussion of diabetes.

Thyroid disorders are common conditions that affect the outcomes of surgical patients. Hypothyroidism commonly occurs in elderly patients and is often undiagnosed. The signs and symptoms of decreased thyroid function may be confused with normal signs of aging. Myxedema coma, an extreme form of hypothyroidism, may occur perioperatively as a result of the stress of the surgery itself. Severe hypofunction of the thyroid gland places the patient at risk for developing intraoperative hypotension, CHF, cardiac arrest, and death. Persons with mild to moderate hypothyroidism experience few perioperative complications.[15]

Persons with increased thyroid function are also at risk for development of perioperative complications. Patients with hyperthyroidism are at risk for perioperative cardiac dysrhythmias, ischemia, and the development of thyroid storm. Thyroid storm may also be precipitated by the stress of surgery or severe illness. The nurse should consult with the anesthesiologist regarding perioperative pharmacologic management of the patient with thyroid dysfunction.

Immunologic Status

Assessment of the immunologic status of the surgical patient is important because of the immune system's role in the body's physiologic response to stress and trauma. A decrease in immune functioning can lead to impaired wound healing and infection. As a result of the normal aging process, the elderly patient has decreased immune functioning. The patient should be questioned about any history of risk factors for immunosuppression such as cancer, diabetes mellitus, chemotherapy, radiation therapy, and long-term steroid use.

Oral steroids are commonly prescribed to treat a variety of conditions. Persons on exogenous steroids will continue to require steroids throughout the perioperative period. The perioperative nurse should consult with the anesthesiologist for dosage recommendations during the perioperative period. Patients on long-term steroid therapy are at risk for the development of adrenal insufficiency. Refer to Chapter 29 for further discussion of adrenal insufficiency.

Nutritional Status

Patients with impaired nutritional status are at high risk for developing complications from surgery or anesthesia. An estimated 50% of hospitalized patients have some degree of malnutrition, which can adversely affect postoperative outcomes.[9] Patients most likely to have nutritional deficiencies are the elderly and those who are chronically ill, particularly persons with gastrointestinal tract conditions or malignant tumors. As a result of malnutrition, the patient may experience negative nitrogen balance, failure of blood clotting mechanisms, alterations in wound healing, increased risk of infection, electrolyte imbalance, and increased risk of morbidity and mortality.

The patient's nutritional status should be assessed. Data gathered should include any changes in appetite, fluctuations in weight (intentional and unexplained weight loss or gain), and special dietary requirements. These data are relevant in predicting postoperative outcomes and determining nutritional requirements in the postoperative period. A nutritional consult may be indicated at the time of the preoperative evaluation.

The person who is emaciated or cachectic or who has lost weight below an acceptable level usually has a prolonged postoperative recovery. The malnourished person already has diminished reserves of carbohydrates and fats, so body proteins are used to provide the necessary energy requirements to maintain metabolic functioning of cells. Nitrogen imbalances are greater than normal and less protein is available for healing. Collagen, the connective tissue that is the substance of scar tissue, is a protein. Wound healing therefore becomes considerably delayed, and wound separation and infection may occur.

If the surgery is not emergent and can be delayed for several weeks, the malnourished patient is placed on a high-protein, high-carbohydrate diet before surgery. In the preoperative or postoperative period, total parenteral nutrition may be given until the patient is able to tolerate a high-protein, high-carbohydrate diet by mouth. High protein intake does not result in increased body protein unless there is sufficient carbohydrate to provide the necessary energy. Activity or exercise also is required for protein synthesis.

Nutritionally depleted patients usually have a deficiency of vitamins. Vitamins B_1, C, and K are necessary for wound healing and clot formation; and supplemental vitamins may be prescribed for malnourished patients. Box 16-5 identifies common causes of malnutrition that may affect perioperative outcomes and delay postoperative recovery.

Patients who are 10% over their ideal weight are considered obese and are at risk for increased morbidity and mortality from concomitant systemic disease. The obese patient is often malnourished from lack of appropriate nutrient intake. Obesity is known as a risk factor for a number of chronic diseases and also presents a risk factor for surgery, including enlarged organs such as heart, kidneys, and liver.

Anesthesia poses additional risks for the obese patient. During induction, intubation, and maintenance of anesthesia,

BOX 16-5 Common Causes of Malnutrition

Chronic infection
Inflammatory bowel disease
Immune disorders
Chronic pancreatitis
Carcinoma (increased with stomach or colon)
Liver disease
Renal disease
Congestive heart failure
Weight loss (10% of body weight in 3 months before surgery)
Abdominal trauma
Severe multiple trauma (especially pelvic, hip, and leg fracture)
Major burns
Wound sepsis
Acute pancreatitis
Small bowel fistulas
Severe peritonitis

there are additional concerns while caring for the obese patient. Increased abdominal pressure while in the supine position may reduce ventilation capacity, and inefficient ventilation may prolong induction time. Higher doses of anesthetic agents are required for maintenance of anesthesia because of continuous uptake by adipose tissue. After surgery the adipose tissue retains fat-soluble anesthetic agents that are slowly eliminated, prolonging the recovery period.

During surgery fluctuations of vital signs are more common in the obese person, resulting from the excessive demands on the cardiovascular system. Operating time may be increased because of difficulties in exposing the surgical site. The surgeon incising through layers of fatty tissue has to exert more traction on the tissues to expose the surgical site, which increases trauma to the tissues. Incisional hernias may occur at a later date.

During the immediate postoperative period obese patients often require more assistance with turning, coughing, and deep breathing. Excess fat deposits often limit movement of the diaphragm, thereby decreasing ventilation. It is also more difficult for obese persons to move about, and they may require additional assistance. Both decreased activity and decreased diaphragmatic expansion are contributing factors to development of postoperative pulmonary complications. In addition, obesity and decreased activity increase the risk for thrombophlebitis.

Although weight reduction usually cannot be accomplished before surgery, it is important for the nurse to identify obesity as a risk factor and make appropriate plans for perioperative management. In the preoperative evaluation the patient can be offered information on the benefits of maintaining an ideal body weight, nutritional guidelines, and methods of weight reduction.

GERONTOLOGIC CONSIDERATIONS

There are approximately 35 million persons aged 65 years and older in the United States, composing approximately 13% of the total population.[18] The number of older persons continues to increase; individuals 85 years and older are the fastest growing segment of the elderly population. It is estimated that the average 65-year-old person is expected to live another 17.5 years.[3]

The perioperative nurse must be aware of the special considerations required for assessment of the elderly patient. Regardless of the setting, the perioperative nurse will encounter elderly patients. A total of 20% of all surgical procedures are performed on the elderly, and one third of patients in ambulatory surgical centers are 65 years or older.[3,26] The elderly patient is at high risk for developing perioperative complications regardless of the presence of concomitant disease. Compounding this fact, it is estimated that 80% of older adults have multiple health problems. The presence of comorbid conditions and emergency procedures increase morbidity and mortality.[3,26] The increased incidence of mortality and postoperative complications are associated with cardiac disease, pulmonary complications, sepsis, and kidney failure.

The ability of the elderly patient to tolerate surgery depends on the extent of the physiologic changes that have occurred with the aging process, the duration of the surgical procedure, and the presence of chronic illness. Surgical procedures that present an increased risk for elderly patients include abdominal, thoracic, neurosurgical, and emergency procedures. The normal aging process produces a general decline in organ function, alterations in pharmocokinetics, and alterations in thermoregulatory ability. The nurse's knowledge of the normal aging process is essential for planning perioperative interventions for the geriatric patient. A summary of physiologic changes associated with aging that may affect care of the patient in the perioperative setting is presented in Table 16-6.

In addition to the physiologic alterations in the geriatric patient, the nurse also needs to be aware that physiologic and psychologic stressors may cause confusion. It is important to determine the reason for confusion. Common causes of confusion include hypoxia, electrolyte imbalance, cerebral hemorrhage, diabetes, infection, dehydration, medications, Alzheimer's disease, and unfamiliar surroundings.

Depression and alcohol abuse are common in the elderly and are often undiagnosed. Both can affect postoperative patient outcomes and therefore need to be assessed in the preoperative period.

While performing the preoperative assessment, it is important to remember that elderly persons vary in the extent to which the physiologic changes associated with aging occur. The greater the number of physiologic changes, the greater the potential for the patient to develop perioperative complications.

Physical Examination

The nurse performs a complete head-to-toe physical assessment. Objective data are collected and recorded in the preoperative phase for two reasons: (1) to obtain baseline data for comparison during the intraoperative and postoperative phases and (2) to identify potential problems that may require preventive nursing interventions before surgery. If the

TABLE 16-6 Age-Related Physiologic Changes and Associated Perioperative Complications

Physiologic Changes	Potential Perioperative Complications
Cardiovascular ↓ Elasticity of blood vessels ↓ Cardiac output ↓ Stroke volume ↑ Peripheral vascular resistance Fibrosis of electrical conduction system ↓ Sensitivity to baroreceptors	Shock (hypotension), fluctuations in blood pressure, dysrhythmias, thrombosis with pulmonary emboli, delayed wound healing, postoperative confusion, hypervolemia, decreased response to stress

TABLE 16-6 Age-Related Physiologic Changes and Associated Perioperative Complications—cont'd

Physiologic Changes	Potential Perioperative Complications
Respiratory	
↓ Elasticity of lungs	Loss of laryngeal reflexes, aspiration, atelectasis, pneumonia, postoperative confusion
Chest wall rigidity	↓ Gas exchange
↑ Residual lung volume	Ineffective cough
↓ Forced expiratory volume	Difficulty maintaining airway
↓ Vital capacity	Difficult intubation
↓ Alveolar volume	
↓ Ciliary action	
Thoracic kyphosis	
Arthritic changes of cervical spine	
Costochondral calcification	
Tenacious sputum	
Renal	
↓ Renal blood flow	Prolonged response to anesthesia and drugs, overhydration with IV fluids, hyperkalemia
↓ Glomerular filtration rate	Delirium
↓ Muscle tone in ureters, bladder, urethra	Drug toxicity
	Electrolyte and acid-base imbalance
	Edema
↓ Bladder tone	Incomplete bladder emptying, urinary tract infection, urinary incontinence, urinary retention, urinary frequency
↓ Bladder capacity	
Benign prostatic hypertrophy	
Gastrointestinal	
↓ Intestinal motility	Aspiration, paralytic ileus
Delayed gastric emptying	Constipation, fecal impaction
↓ Liver mass	
↓ Hepatic blood flow	Altered drug metabolism
Neurologic	
↓ Number of brain cells	Cognitive deficits, confusion, delirium
↓ Neurons	Misinterpretation of stimuli
↓ Cerebral blood flow	Injury
Presbycusis	Falls
Presbyopia	↑ Anxiety
↓ Proprioception	
Changes in sleep patternsn	
Musculoskeletal	
↓ Muscle mass, tone, and strength	Immobililty, deep vein thrombosis, atelectasis, pulmonary embolism, pneumonia
Loss of bone mass	Positioning difficulty, pathologic fracture
↓ Bone density	Falls
Degenerative joint disease	
Integumentary	
↓ Elasticity	Pressure ulcers, bruising
Small vessel fragility	Delayed wound healing
↓ Lean body mass, ↑ in overall body fat	Delayed recovery from anesthetics because of storage in adipose tissue
↓ Subcutaneous fat	Hypothermia
Immunologic	
Fewer killer T cells	↓ Ability to protect against invasion by pathogenic microorganisms
↓ Response to foreign antigens	Delayed wound healing, wound infection
Metabolic	
↓ Gamma-globulin level	↓ Inflammatory response
↓ Plasma proteins	Delayed wound healing, wound dehiscence or evisceration
↓ Serum albumin	Altered fluid dynamics, edema
	↓ Binding capacity with potential for ineffective drug dosing
Benign hypothermia (temperature < 98.6° F)	↑ Cardiac workload, hypoxia, intraoperative and postoperative hypothermia
↓ Basal metabolic rate	Delayed shivering, delayed recovery from anesthetics
Impaired thermoregulatory ability	

patient has been hospitalized, the admission history and physical assessment should contain much of the pertinent data that can serve as baseline data before surgery. Preoperative vital signs are assessed and documented. Any abnormalities in the patient's physical assessment are documented and reported to the attending surgeon and anesthesiologist for further evaluation. The surgical procedure may be canceled based on the severity of the abnormal findings. Refer to individual assessment chapters for a complete discussion of each body system.

Much information can be obtained from the initial contact with the patient. The patient may have special needs such as visual impairment, hearing deficit, cognitive impairment, or language barrier.

The general survey should include an assessment of the patient's mood, affect, and level of anxiety. During the interview the patient may manifest anxiety by changing the subject frequently, repeating, avoiding certain topics, and increasing or decreasing interaction. Objective signs of anxiety include increased pulse and respiratory rate, moist palms, frequent hand movements, increased urination, and restlessness.

A general overview of the patient's functional status can be obtained by observing the individual's gait, ability to transfer, and performance of ADLs. The patient should also be assessed for any prostheses such as artificial limbs or eyes, dentures, or hearing aids.

Preoperative assessment of cardiovascular status is essential to identify patients at risk for perioperative cardiac complications. Vital signs are obtained. The nurse screens the patient for undiagnosed hypertension. Heart sounds are auscultated, and the presence of extra sounds, irregular rate and rhythm, or murmurs are noted. The nurse evaluates the extremities for the presence and quality of peripheral pulses, capillary refill, warmth, color, and edema.

A preoperative baseline assessment of respiratory status is important for early identification of patients at high risk for developing postoperative respiratory complications. Respiratory assessment should include respiratory rate, effort, and rhythm; chest excursion; use of accessory muscles; auscultation of breath sounds; and pulse oximetry.

Adequate renal function is necessary to maintain fluid and electrolyte balance during the perioperative period. The nurse observes the patient's urine for color, clarity, quality, amount, and odor. Urinary tract infection, if present, is treated with antibiotics before surgery.

The patient's neurologic status, including level of consciousness, orientation, and motor and sensory function, is evaluated. This information is necessary to detect any abnormalities from baseline functioning that may occur during the perioperative period. The patient is also evaluated for sensory deficits such as problems with vision, hearing, and sensation.

The patient's musculoskeletal status is assessed for abnormalities in joint structure and function. Limitation in range of motion or arthritis may interfere with intraoperative patient positioning. It is important to assess range of motion of the cervical spine because of the positioning required for endotracheal intubation. Persons with alterations in musculoskeletal function may be predisposed to postoperative complications associated with immobility.

The patient's integumentary system is assessed for integrity and areas prone to the development of pressure ulcers. Breaks in the skin, decreased subcutaneous tissue, and other pathologic changes in the skin will affect intraoperative patient positioning and placement of monitoring devices, skin preparation, and placement of surgical drapes and other surgical equipment.

An assessment of the hydration status of the patient is important because of potential alterations in fluid volume balance resulting from NPO status, administration of intravenous fluids, intraoperative and postoperative hemorrhage, and excessive wound drainage. Physical examination findings that suggest alterations in hydration status may include weight outside of ideal range, decreased muscle tone, lack of subcutaneous tissue, dry and flaky skin, brittle nails, decreased skin turgor, dry mucous membranes, edema, and adventitious breath sounds.

An assessment of the patient's nutritional status should include height, weight, and body mass index (BMI). BMI is an important prognostic indicator for the development of chronic disease. Obesity is defined as a BMI of 30 kg/m^2 and overweight as a BMI of 25 kg/m^2. Other factors affecting nutritional status include the presence of loose teeth, improperly fitting dentures, and poor dentition. Persons weighing more than 300 pounds require a special operating room bed and other equipment both intraoperatively and postoperatively. The operating room personnel need to be notified of these special patient care requirements.

Diagnostics

Laboratory and diagnostic testing are performed before the patient is cleared for surgery. Patient age and physical condition, type of procedure and anesthetic, and institutional requirements determine the extent of laboratory testing. Laboratory and diagnostic testing may take place in a variety of settings and at varying times before the procedure depending on institutional protocol and reimbursement regulations. Admission panel testing protocols are based on patient history and age and type of procedure. Because of the high incidence of coronary artery disease, male patients over 40 years old and female patients over 50 years old generally require an electrocardiogram (ECG). Chest radiography is not relevant as a routine preoperative screening test but may be indicated for patients at high risk for pulmonary complications. Other tests may be indicated according to the patient's medical history, risk factors, and the proposed surgical procedure. Refer to Table 16-7 for examples of common preoperative tests.

If surgical blood loss is anticipated, a blood sample is sent for type and screen or type and cross-matching so that packed RBCs are available for transfusion during and after surgery. Ideally the patient should have a preoperative hematocrit of at least 30% to 45% and hemoglobin of at least 10 g/dl. Patients undergoing procedures in which the anticipated blood loss is greater than 500 ml should have a higher preoperative hemoglobin and hematocrit than patients undergoing procedures without significant blood loss.[19] In the case of elective surgery,

TABLE 16-7 Common Preoperative Diagnostic Tests

Test	Indication	Possible Findings
Complete blood count with differential	Procedures with anticipated significant blood loss Chronic illness or disease History of infection	Baseline hematologic function Anemia Infection Blood dyscrasias
Serum electrolytes (blood urea nitrogen, creatinine)	Age over 60 years (age may vary with institutional protocol) Chronic disease Renal disease Liver disease Use of diuretics	Electrolyte imbalance Acid-base imbalance Hydration status Renal functioning Hepatic function Hypoglycemia Hyperglycemia (with fasting glucose)
Coagulation studies (prothrombin time, partial thromboplastin time, international normalized ratio)	Bleeding disorders Anticoagulant use Procedures with anticipated significant blood loss Liver disease	Baseline coagulation status Predict risk of perioperative bleeding Response to anticoagulant therapy Liver disease
Liver enzymes	History of liver disease History of/or current alcohol abuse	Hepatic functioning
Beta-human chorionic gonadatropin	Women of childbearing years	Pregnancy status
12-Lead electrocardiogram	Males over 40 years old Females over 50 years old History of cardiac disease	Cardiac rhythm Dysrhythmias Ischemia Infarct
Chest radiograph	History of pulmonary disease Thoracic surgical procedures Significant smoking history (per institutional protocol)	Heart size Chronic obstructive pulmonary disease Pneumonia Structural abnormalities Heart failure
Pulmonary function tests	Establish baseline pulmonary functioning Evaluate/predict risk for perioperative complications History of pulmonary disease Significant smoking history (per institutional policy)	Obstructive or restrictive lung disease
Urinalysis	Procedures involving instrumentation of urinary tract Urologic symptoms	Urinary tract infection Kidney disease

the patient may choose to do autologous donation. Use of the patient's blood eliminates the risk of contracting hepatitis or human immunodeficiency virus from blood transfusions. According to the guidelines of the American Association of Blood Banks, the patient's hematocrit must be at least 34%, and the white blood cell count must be below 12,000/mm^3 for autologous donation. Donations must be completed at least 72 hours before surgery, and the blood may be used up to 36 days after donation. The patient may be advised to take an iron supplement after donation, depending on the number of units donated and baseline hematocrit. The patient should be informed about autologous donation at the time the decision is made for surgical intervention to allow sufficient time for donation.

NURSING DIAGNOSES

Nursing diagnoses are determined from analysis of patient data. Nursing diagnoses for the preoperative patient may include but are not limited to:

Diagnostic Title	Possible Etiologic Factors
1. Deficient knowledge	Lack of familiarity with perioperative routines
2. Anxiety	Fear of the unknown Fear of pain Cost of care, lack of insurance Body image changes Change in health status

3. Risk for ineffective airway clearance	Anesthesia, sedation, pooled secretions, surgical procedure, immobility, decreased cough
4. Risk for ineffective peripheral tissue perfusion	Venous stasis, increased coagulability of blood, immobility

EXPECTED PATIENT OUTCOMES

Expected patient outcomes for the patient during the preoperative phase may include but are not limited to:

1. Will verbalize an understanding of perioperative routines; will demonstrate satisfactory performance of postoperative exercises
2. Will describe techniques to control anxiety; will attest to an increase in psychologic and physiologic comfort
3. Will demonstrate effective coughing, clear breath sounds, adequate air exchange, and patent airway
4. Will demonstrate adequate peripheral tissue perfusion as evidenced by palpable, symmetric, peripheral pulses; warm, dry skin; absence of edema, erythema, and calf tenderness; will verbalize knowledge of treatment regimen

INTERVENTIONS

Having identified the patient's specific needs and formulated nursing diagnoses, the nurse must collaborate with other health care professionals to implement the plan for treatment, teaching, and emotional support for the patient. A major focus of nursing intervention during the preoperative period is teaching and psychologic preparation of the patient and family.

1. Patient/Family Education: Preoperative Patient Education

The purpose of preoperative teaching is to provide information that addresses individual learning needs, promotes safety, promotes psychologic comfort, promotes patient and family involvement in care, and promotes compliance with instructions. Changes in health care challenge the perioperative nurse in implementing preoperative patient education programs in shortened time frames and in alternative settings. Research indicates that effective preoperative teaching has been associated with reduced anxiety levels, earlier ambulation, and increased involvement in postdischarge self-care activities.[7] The preoperative information helpful to most patients relates to preoperative tests and activities, events related to the surgery, and expectations about what will happen postoperatively. Most patients are less anxious and participate more effectively if they know the reasons for tests and perioperative activities. There is inconclusive evidence regarding the most effective time frame for implementing preoperative teaching. The teaching can be done in the physician's office, via the telephone, or in a preadmission testing area before the scheduled surgery date. When preparing the teaching plan, it is important to consider how much time the nurse will have to teach the patient and what information is vitally necessary for the patient to know. The length of the teaching session influences the effectiveness of the teaching. Several shorter periods of instruction, 20 minutes or less, are more effective than longer periods.[10] It is important to make sure to allow time to answer questions and address patient and family concerns. The nurse must assess how much information the patient wants to gain. Giving the patient or family more information than they want may result in increased anxiety and stress.

It is also important to remember that most patients will only retain less than 50% of what is taught immediately after the teaching session.[10] Nursing interventions to increase patient and family retention include repetition and review of content using multisensory channels including printed materials, videos, and demonstrations. The nurse should select the most effective method of patient instruction based on the patient's learning preferences and resources available. Written materials that can be kept for future reference, video and audiotapes, anatomic models, and examples of equipment or prostheses can all be used for teaching. A teaching plan using diverse methods can be most effective for patients who learn more readily by using a combined approach.[10] It is important to remember that some adults in the United States are functionally illiterate and will not benefit from printed materials with reading levels above the fourth- or fifth-grade levels. With this information in mind, the nurse needs to assess the appropriateness of printed materials when using them for patient education.

The preoperative education plan should begin with an assessment, including baseline knowledge of the patient and family, readiness to learn, barriers to learning, patient and family concerns, and learning styles and preferences. Another important intervention is to ensure the patient's physical comfort before initiating teaching. For an in-depth discussion of the principles of teaching and learning refer to a fundamentals of nursing textbook.

The content of preoperative teaching focuses on information that will increase patients' familiarity with procedural events, thus decreasing anxiety; information regarding activities to enhance physiologic healing; and information on prevention of postoperative complications. Content should include information about events that will occur during the surgical experience (procedural), what the patient may experience during the perioperative period (sensory), and what actions may help decrease anxiety (behavioral) (Box 16-6).

2. Anxiety Reduction

Impending surgery may result in anxiety because it is associated with fear of the unknown, pain, waiting for surgery, body image changes, treatments, fear of not being asleep during the surgical procedure, altered functioning, loss of control, and death. It is the responsibility of the registered nurse to assist the patient and his or her family and significant others in identifying sources of anxiety and implementing effective coping mechanisms.

The level of the patient's anxiety affects the receptiveness and ability to comprehend preoperative instructions. Giving someone information does not necessarily mean that the person understood the information. Mild anxiety enhances learning. However, moderate levels of anxiety are characterized by selective inattention, and severe levels of anxiety may completely impede the individual's ability to comprehend information, thus making learning impossible. When the level

BOX 16-6 Preoperative Teaching Content

Procedural

Informed consent
Preoperative screening (laboratory, diagnostic tests, history, physical assessment)
Arrival time
Preoperative routines (bowel prep, antimicrobial shower, skin prep, vital signs, clothing, personal belongings)
NPO status (see Evidence-Based Practice box)
Preoperative medication
Transfer to surgical suite (timing, holding area, surgical waiting room, visiting hours, duration of procedure)
Postanesthesia care unit routines
Presence of intravenous lines, surgical drains, surgical incision, catheters
Pain control methods (preemptive analgesia, oral, intravenous, epidural, patient controlled analgesia)
Postoperative routines (coughing and deep breathing exercises, leg exercises, antiembolism stockings, pneumatic compression devices, ambulation, diet advancement, expected discharge date, home care needs)

Sensory

Needle insertion
Medication effects (drowsiness, dry mouth, amnesia)
Operating room environment (cold, monochromatic, surgical attire, warm blankets, hard narrow bed, bright lights, noise, face mask for gaseous inhalation)
Pain (incisional, muscular, sore throat)
Dizziness when standing or ambulating for the first time
Sensations associated with invasive devices (e.g., Foley catheter, nasogastric tube), postoperative equipment (e.g., pneumatic compression devices, antiembolism hose)

Behavioral

Demonstration and explanation of exercise routines (coughing, deep breathing, incentive spirometry, leg exercises)
Transfer techniques, splinting of incision, progressive ambulation

of anxiety has decreased sufficiently for learning to take place, the nurse should assist the patient in methods to facilitate learning and enhance problem solving. The nurse can help the patient recall effective coping mechanisms or explore alternative methods of coping with the current situation.

Empowering patients by increasing their sense of control before surgery is essential for decreasing patient anxiety. Loss of control is one of the fears associated with surgery. Allowing patients to participate in decisions concerning their care allows them to maintain some control over events. Patients also may be taught activities that help decrease anxiety and gain a sense of control. The most common interventions to decrease anxiety are deep breathing, relaxation exercises, music therapy, and guided imagery. More recent interventions incorporating holistic nursing include humor, touch therapy, aromatherapy, acupressure, massage, and animal-assisted therapy (see Research box).

The nurse must consider the patient's family and friends when planning psychologic support. The patient's family members or close friends are usually as anxious as the patient. This anxiety can be transmitted to patients, increasing their anxiety levels. The same principles described in exploring concerns and giving information to the patient hold true for significant others. Family involvement in preoperative education decreases the anxiety of both the patient and family, with resultant increased satisfaction with care and increased patient cooperation with routines.

An important source of anxiety for the presurgical patient is fear of pain. The topic of postoperative pain control should be initiated at the preoperative interview. Understanding that pain will be present but controlled may help relieve this common source of anxiety and also add to the patient's sense of control. Dispelling myths about pain and pain management can allay fears and decrease anxiety. Common myths include the following: (1) pain is necessary, (2) taking pain medication will cause addiction, and (3) women experience less pain than men. Education regarding pain management should include medications used, potential side effects, alternative pain relief measures, methods to assess pain, expected course of pain, and most important the patient's role in the pain management plan. A more recent method of controlling postoperative pain, as well as the anticipatory anxiety associated with the pain experience, is preemptive analgesia (see Chapter 17).

Use of Medications

The anxious preoperative patient may require medication to relieve anxiety and promote comfort during this stressful time. If the nurse's assessment reveals the need for medication to reduce anxiety, the anesthesiologist should be consulted.

3. Minimizing the Potential for Respiratory Complications

Teaching the patient about the necessity of deep breathing and coughing after surgery is a common component of preoperative education. Deep breathing facilitates oxygenation and removal of residual inhalant anesthetics and also prevents alveolar collapse, which may lead to atelectasis. Effective coughing removes secretions that may block the airways. All patients potentially at risk for postoperative pulmonary complications are taught deep breathing and coughing exercises before surgery to enhance performance and increase patient participation in postoperative recovery routines.

All patients need to know how to correctly perform diaphragmatic breathing because it increases lung expansion by permitting the diaphragm to descend fully. Although many men normally breathe diaphragmatically, few women do so. With diaphragmatic breathing, the abdomen rises with inspiration and falls with expiration. The nurse assesses the patient's normal breathing pattern by placing a hand lightly on the patient's abdomen and asking the patient to take a deep breath. If diaphragmatic breathing does not occur naturally, the patient can be taught to inspire deeply while pushing the abdomen up against the hand.

Deep breathing and coughing exercises are performed with the patient in a sitting position. The nurse instructs the patient to take a breath through the nose and exhale through the mouth. The patient is then instructed to take a deep breath

Evidence-Based Practice

Reference: Madsen M, Brosnan J, Nagy VT: Perioperative thirst: a patient perspective, *J Perioperative Nurs* 13(4):225, 1998.

A long established protocol for presurgical patients is restricting food and fluids after midnight before surgery. This practice is based on Mendelson's classic study done in 1946, which recommended food and fluid restrictions as a measure to decrease gastric acid aspiration and resultant pneumonitis in obstetric patients receiving anesthesia. Recent research has refuted Mendelson's findings and evidence indicates that healthy patients should be allowed to consume unrestricted clear fluids up to 2 to 3 hours before elective surgery. Contrary to Mendelson's findings, there is a low incidence of pulmonary aspiration and death resulting from aspiration during surgery. In fact, recent studies show that prolonged fluid restriction may actually increase the volume of gastric secretions and decrease the pH, both increasing the risk of aspiration.

Despite evidence to the contrary, many institutions still adhere to the NPO after midnight guidelines. A 1996 survey of university anesthesiology programs and ambulatory surgical centers indicated that 43% of the respondents had not revised their fasting guidelines, despite recommendations from current literature. Another survey of anesthesiologists and nurses showed the length of preoperative fasting ranged from 3.75 to 29 hours, with a mean fasting of 11 hours. The length of fasting was primarily determined by the time of the surgical procedure, rather than individual patient need. Midnight seems to be the universal time from which to begin fluid and food restriction.

Although there is little evidence documenting the amount of discomfort caused by prolonged preoperative fasting, there is concern that this practice is particularly difficult for children and the elderly, who are vulnerable to dehydration. Preoperative fasting has also been linked to headache, especially in persons with a history of chronic headache.

The purpose of this study was to determine the amount of discomfort experienced by patients undergoing elective surgery in a hospital that practices traditional NPO after midnight fasting guidelines. The convenience sample consisted of 50 adults, mostly male, undergoing elective surgery in a metropolitan acute care medical center. Types of surgeries included cardiothoracic, orthopedic, neurosurgical, urologic, vascular, and general procedures. Persons undergoing emergency procedures or those with recent nausea and vomiting, gastrointestinal pathology, pregnancy, and conditions causing delayed gastric emptying were excluded from the study. Participants were interviewed 48 hours after recovering from the effects of anesthesia and given a structured questionnaire developed with input from surgical nurses. Patients were asked to rate their discomfort levels using a 5-point Likert scale on not being able to drink after midnight, not being able to eat after midnight, the ability to sleep after surgery, and worry after surgery. Additional data were collected regarding the number of hours of fasting, medications taken by mouth the morning of surgery, the amount of fluid taken with the medication, and any other concerns regarding the surgical experience.

Results showed thirst caused the most discomfort and hunger caused the least discomfort. Patients reported more discomfort caused by thirst than discomfort caused by worrying about the surgery. An overwhelming majority of participants reported discomfort from thirst before surgery; they further elaborated on the discomfort caused by thirst in a final open-ended question during the interview. Descriptors included comments such as, "horrible dry mouth, cotton balls, sore and dry, mouth stuck together, couldn't swallow, so thirsty I almost went crazy."

Limitations of this study include the small sample size and the majority of male participants. However, the results clearly indicate thirst is a significant source of discomfort in surgical patients who have excessive fluid restrictions before surgery. Other studies have shown that hospital convenience is often the primary reason for adhering to traditional presurgical fluid restrictions, despite evidence that supports more liberal fluid restriction. Patient care guidelines for fasting should be based on evidence, rather than hospital convenience. As patient advocates nurses are in a prime position to promote practices that decrease patient suffering. Changing practices regarding fasting routines requires the cooperation of the surgical staff, anesthesiologists, and nursing working together to provide the best individualized patient care.

Research

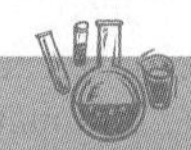

Reference: Norred CL: Minimizing preoperative anxiety with alternative caring-healing therapies, *AORN J* 72(5):838, 2000.

This review of the use of alternative therapies to minimize preoperative anxiety is based on Dr Jean Watson's philosophy and science of caring. Watson, well known for her caring theory, brings together the caring and compassion of nursing with traditional medical therapy in a holistic approach to nursing practice. Central to Watson's theory of nursing is caring and the therapeutic relationship between patient and nurse.

This holistic approach to patient-nurse interactions can be particularly beneficial to the perioperative nurse. It is well known that surgical patients experience stress and anxiety. Research indicates the most common concerns of surgical patients are fear of death and the need for caring during the operative experience. One of the key nursing interventions during the perioperative experience is to assist patients to reduce and manage anxiety and stress. The therapeutic relationship is the cornerstone of developing a trusting relationship with the patient, which can then be enhanced by the use of caring-healing therapies of holistic nursing.

One therapy that may be an effective intervention to decrease anxiety during induction of anesthesia or sedation is hypnosis. In a randomized, controlled study of 60 patients undergoing plastic surgery, hypnosis was effective in decreasing analgesic requirements and anxiety during conscious sedation. Hypnosis has been an effective intervention to decrease acute and chronic pain.

Guided imagery is another effective intervention for perioperative patients. In a study of patients undergoing elective colorectal surgery, those who used guided imagery perioperatively experienced less preoperative and postoperative pain and required 50% fewer narcotics than the control group. Guided imagery has also been effective in facilitating the healing process, to control both acute and chronic pain, and to decrease anxiety and fear.

Aromatherapy is another intervention that may be an effective measure to allay anxiety. Initial studies indicate that lavender has a therapeutic effect on brain waves and may encourage healing; however, further research is needed to validate the effectiveness of aromatherapy in reducing anxiety in perioperative patients. Watson suggests a drop of lavender on a surgical mask may help alleviate the patient's anxiety and decrease unpleasant odors that may be encountered in the operating room.

Music therapy has been shown to be an effective tool in decreasing anxiety and analgesic requirement. Tactile therapy, including touch and massage, may also be effective interventions in the perioperative setting.

Although further research is needed to validate the effectiveness of alternative therapies in caring for perioperative patients, these therapies can be adjuncts to traditional approaches to patient care. Anxiety is a common problem in surgical patients, and combining holistic therapies with a caring, therapeutic relationship may be effective in reducing anxiety and improving patient well-being.

through the nose and mouth, hold the breath for 3 to 5 seconds, and then exhale completely through the mouth. Deep breathing exercises are repeated three times; the patient is then instructed to cough (Box 16-7).

It is important for the patient to hold the breath for 3 seconds to promote alveolar expansion. If there is difficulty with a deep cough, encourage the patient to do a "huff" cough. Repeated huff coughs often stimulate a deep cough. The patient also is shown how to splint an incision with a pillow, a towel, or his or her hands to help decrease pain while coughing.

An additional method of promoting lung expansion is with the use of an incentive spirometry device. Various models are commercially available. The patient is taught to seal the lips around the mouthpiece and inhale. Once maximal inhalation is achieved, the patient should hold his or her breath for 3 seconds and then exhale slowly. The patient should not exceed 10 to 12 breaths per minute. The device can be set to a predetermined volume to achieve maximum lung expansion (Figure 16-1).

4. Promoting Peripheral Tissue Perfusion

A variety of nursing interventions are directed toward promoting adequate peripheral circulation. Measures used to decrease venous stasis include antiembolism hose, pneumatic compression devices, leg exercises, early ambulation, adequate hydration, and deep breathing. Venous stasis in the postoperative period may lead to DVT, thrombophlebitis, and the potential formation of pulmonary embolus.

Antiembolism stockings, alone or in combination with pneumatic compression devices (also known as intermittent pulsatile compression devices or sequential compression devices), are often used perioperatively to enhance venous return in the lower extremities. The pneumatic compression device provides intermittent periods of compression starting from the ankle and progressing proximally to promote venous return. The nurse must measure the patient's lower extremities to obtain the appropriate size of sleeves and stockings. These devices are applied in the operating room and are continued until the patient is ambulatory (Figure 16-2).

BOX 16-7 Deep Breathing and Coughing Exercise

Deep Breathing

- Lie in semi-Fowler's or high Fowler's position with knees flexed to relax abdomen and allow full chest expansion.
- Place a hand lightly on the abdomen.
- Breathe in slowly through nose, letting chest expand and feeling abdomen rise against hand.
- Hold breath for 3 seconds.
- Exhale slowly through pursed lips (abdomen contracts).
- Repeat deep breathing three times, then cough (see next).

Coughing

- Breathe in as described previously.
- Count to 3.
- On "3," cough *deeply* three times.
- If unable to cough deeply, do repeated "huff" coughs (forced expiration with glottis open).

Respirex® 2

To prevent problems with breathing after surgery, it is important to inflate your lungs and keep them clear of secretions. Respirex 2 will help you do this.

To use your Respirex, follow these steps:

1. Place yourself in a sitting position or as upright as you can.
2. Put the mouthpiece in your mouth and make a tight seal with your lips.
3. Take in a slow, deep breath to raise and keep the ball between the 600 and 900 mark. When your lungs are completely full, hold your breath.
4. As soon as you stop inhaling, the ball will fall. Continue to hold your breath for 5 secs before breathing out. This forces air down into your lungs.
5. Repeat this process 10 times, slowly, every hour while you are awake. Pause briefly between breaths.

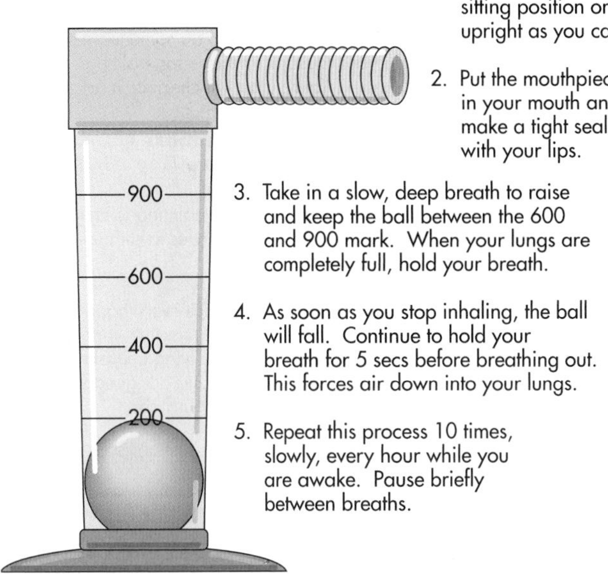

Figure 16-1 Patient instructions for using incentive spirometer.

Intermittent Pulsatile Compression Device (IPC)

The intermittent pulsatile compression device (IPC) gives a regular, gentle massage (or compression) to both legs. This action helps you avoid complications brought about by being less active after surgery.

The IPC is a pair of plastic wrap-around stockings or sleeves. They are put on both legs before surgery. Each sleeve is connected to a small compressor which inflates the sleeves and applies pressure to the calves of your legs. You will feel the pressure as a "milking" action or gentle massage. The pressure lasts for about 10 seconds of each minute. The sleeves then deflate and the process is repeated in a minute.

The sleeves will be removed once you are more active and recovering from surgery. Your nurses will help you with this device and answer any questions you may have after surgery.

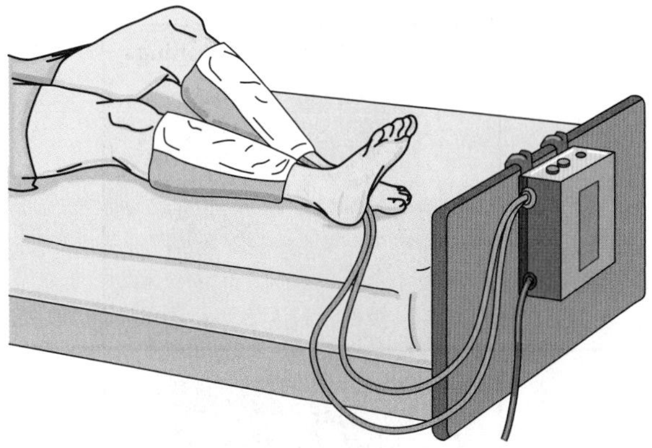

Figure 16-2 Patient instructions for intermittent pulsatile compression device.

Leg exercises help prevent venous congestion and promote peripheral tissue perfusion. The nurse teaches the patient leg exercises before surgery and has the patient perform a return demonstration using proper technique. Refer to Figure 16-3 for an example of teaching material pertaining to postoperative leg exercises.

Additional interventions to decrease venous stasis include early ambulation, frequent turning, and active or passive

Postoperative Leg Exercises

After surgery you will need to do some leg exercises. These exercises will help the blood circulation in your legs and keep your muscles in shape for walking. Before surgery, your nurse will help you practice the exercises you need to know. Your nurse will check or mark the exercises below that you need to practice.

☐ **Ankle Pumps**
(See Figure 1)

- Move both ankles by pointing toes up, then down, then in circles to stimulate circulation.
- Repeat at least 10 times every hour.
- You may do this while lying on your back or when sitting and dangling your feet over the side of your bed.

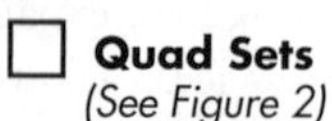

Quad Sets
(See Figure 2)

- Lying on your back with both legs straight, tighten your thigh muscles so that the backs of your knees press down into the bed.
- Hold your muscles tight for 5 seconds.
- Exhale slowly while holding your muscles tight. Relax.
- Repeat at least 5 times every hour.

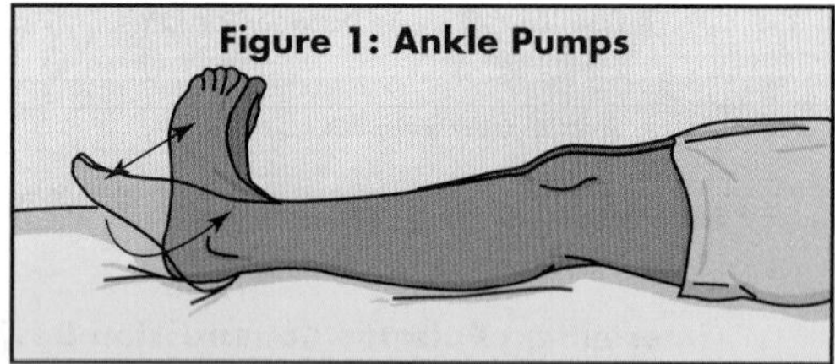

Figure 1: Ankle Pumps

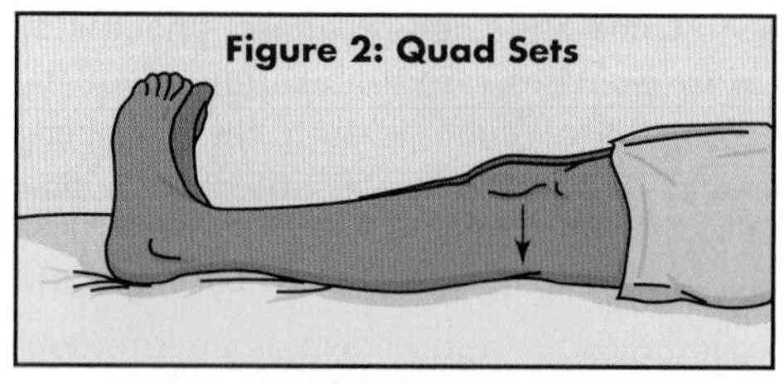

Figure 2: Quad Sets

☐ **Gluteal Tightenings**
(See Figure 3)

- Lying on your back, tense your buttocks muscles tightly as if holding back a bowel movement.
- Hold these muscles tight for 5 seconds.
- Exhale slowly while holding your buttocks tight. Relax.
- Repeat at least 5 times every hour.

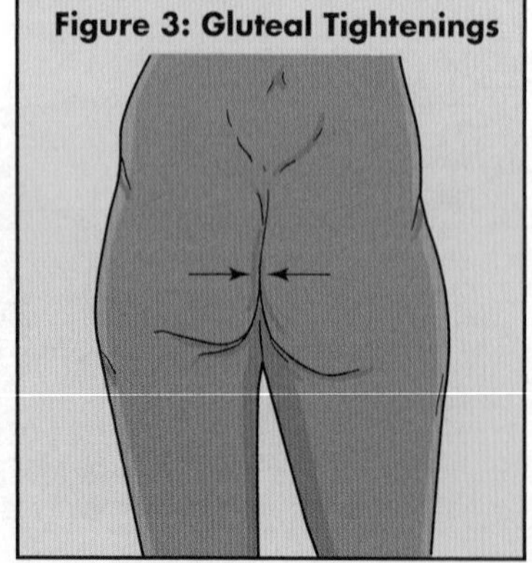

Figure 3: Gluteal Tightenings

☐ **Straight Leg Raises***
(See Figure 4)

- Lying on your back, bend your right hip and knee so your foot rests flat on the bed. This helps to take the strain off your lower back.
- Keeping your left knee straight, point your toes toward the ceiling and lift the leg a few inches off the bed. Exhale slowly while lifting your leg.
- Slowly lower your leg to the bed. Rest.
- Repeat at least 5 times. Then do the same exercise 5 times with your right leg. Do straight leg raises 4 times a day.

** DO NOT do this exercise if you are having abdominal surgery, or if you have back problems.*

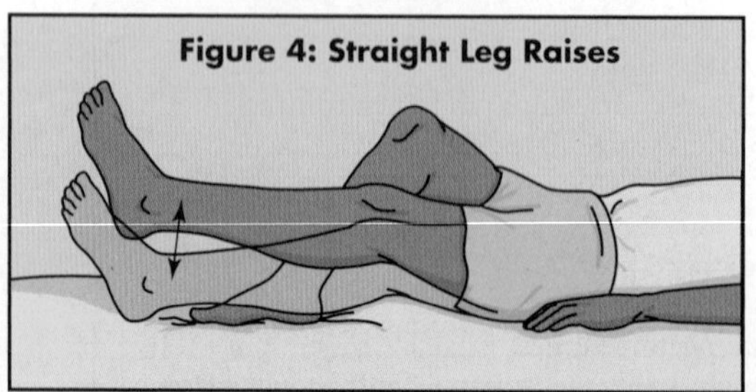

Figure 4: Straight Leg Raises

Figure 16-3 Patient instructions for postoperative leg exercises.

range-of-motion exercises. Early mobilization prevents pulmonary and circulatory complications, prevents pressure ulcers, stimulates intestinal motility, and decreases pain.

Final Preparations for Surgery

In the final phase of preoperative nursing care the nurse is responsible for ensuring that the patient is ready to be safely transferred to the surgical suite. All of the patient's personal belongings are identified and secured. The patient dons a hospital gown and removes all personal clothing. If the patient is wearing nail polish or artificial nails, one or more fingernails/toenails are exposed to allow for accurate assessment of capillary refill and pulse oximetry. Jewelry is usually removed; however, rings may be taped according to institutional policy. Objects such as eyeglasses or prostheses sent to the operating room with the patient may become lost or damaged. For this reason, prostheses such as dentures and prosthetic limbs or eyes are usually removed, labeled, and placed in safekeeping. Dentures are removed, labeled, and placed in a denture cup. If dentures are not removed the patient's airway may be compromised with induction of anesthesia. The presence of dental caps is documented, and this information is also relayed to the anesthesiologist. Patients are usually allowed to wear hearing aids to the surgical suite. This allows the patient to communicate with the surgical team throughout the perioperative period. The presence of the hearing aid must be documented to prevent loss or damage. Patients who want to take religious items or jewelry to the operating room are usually permitted to do so. To prevent loss of the item, a paper emblem obtained from a religious representative is sometimes substituted.

To ensure patient safety, it is necessary to verify the surgical site, particularly in the circumstance where laterality is involved (e.g., right or left eye for cataract extraction). The nurse must thoroughly review the medical record and operative consent to validate the type of surgical procedure and the surgical site. The patient's role is to verbally confirm the surgical procedure and to mark the operative site if applicable. Some institutions have the patient mark the appropriate extremity or site with a sticker or skin marking pen. This verification process is documented in the medical record on the preoperative checklist.

In addition to the surgical consent form, the nurse is responsible to verify the need for any special consent forms. A special consent form would be indicated for a patient's refusal of blood transfusions or blood products, patients undergoing an amputation, and in some circumstances sterilization procedures.

Premedication

Before any premedication is given, it is imperative to ascertain that the consent form has been completed, signed, and placed in the chart. The purposes of premedication are to decrease anxiety and provide sedation, to decrease secretion of saliva and gastric juices, to prevent or decrease nausea and vomiting, and to relieve pain and discomfort (Table 16-8). These med-

TABLE 16-8 Common Premedications

Drug	Action	Nursing Intervention/Implication
Midazolam (Versed)	Short-acting parenteral benzodiazepene Central nervous system (CNS) depressant Muscle relaxant Anxiolytic Anticonvulsant Anterograde amnesic effects (will impair memory of perioperative events) Used in conscious sedation and short surgical procedures	Monitor for CNS depression; effects potentiated with other CNS depressants Monitor respiratory status and vital signs closely Avoid rapid injection which increases risk of respiratory depression Hypotension may occur if used with opoid agonist analgesic Prolonged half-life in obese patients Inform patient of amnesic effects
Diazepam (Valium)	Anxiolytic Anticonvulsant Transient analgesia with intravenous administration	Monitor for CNS depression; effects potentiated with other CNS depressants Monitor respiratory status and vital signs closely Monitor patient for hypotension, muscular weakness, tachycardia, and respiratory depression when administered parenterally Monitor patients for adverse reactions including drowsiness, ataxia, and urinary retention (more common in the elderly)
Lorazepam (Ativan)	Most potent benzodiazepine Skeletal muscle relaxant Anxiolytic Sedative Hypnotic Impairs memory of perioperative events	Monitor for CNS depression; effects potentiated with other CNS depressants Monitor respiratory status and vital signs closely Monitor patient for drowsiness and sedation Inform patient of amnesic effects Additive effects with other CNS depressants

Continued

TABLE 16-8 Common Premedications—cont'd

Meperedine hydrochloride (Demerol)	CNS agent Opiate agonist analgesic	Monitor respiratory status and vital signs closely; tachycardia, hypotension, and respiratory depression may occur Sedation and dizziness are common side effects; ensure patient safety after administration
Morphine sulfate	Opium alkaloid Opiate agonist Produces analgesia, sedation, euphoria, and miosis	Monitor for CNS depression; effects potentiated with other CNS depressants Monitor respiratory status and vital signs closely, respirations ≤ 12/min may indicate toxicity Sedation and dizziness are common side effects; ensure patient safety after administration Nausea and puritis are common side effects Promote coughing and deep breathing postoperatively, as cough and sigh reflexes are depressed with opiate analgesics
Fentanyl citrate (Sublimaze, Duragesic)	CNS depressant Opiate agonist Sedative Analgesic Supplement to general and regional anesthesia	Monitor for CNS depression; effects potentiated with other CNS depressants Monitor respiratory status and vital signs closely Respiratory depressant effect may persist longer than analgesic effect; have opioid antagonist (naloxone) and resuscitative equipment available
Atropine sulfate	Autonomic nervous system agent Anticholinergic Antimuscarinic Sympatholytic Mydriatic and cyclopegic Antisecretory and vagolytic effects (suppresses salivation, perspiration, and respiratory tract secretions) Used before surgery to reduce incidence of laryngospasm, reflex bradycardia, and hypotension during general anesthesia	Monitor vital signs closely, especially pulse May cause urinary retention Smaller doses usually required in elderly patients Elderly patients may exhibit CNS stimulation or drowsiness; ensure patient safety after administration
Glycopyrrolate (Robinul)	Effects similar to atropine	Monitor vital signs closely Monitor for urinary retention, particularly in elderly patients Dizziness and blurred vision may occur; ensure patient safety after administration
Scopolamine hydrobromide (Hyoscine)	Autonomic nervous system agent Anticholinergic Parasympatholytic Antimuscarinic Produces amnesia and sedation	Monitor respiratory status and vital signs closely Monitor for excitement and disorientation shortly after administration; ensure patient safety after administration
Promethazine hydrochloride (Phenergan)	Long-acting phenothiazine derivative Produces sedative, amnesic, and antiemetic effects Adjunct to analgesics for pain control	Monitor for CNS depression; effects potentiated with other CNS depressants Monitor respiratory status and vital signs closely Depressed cough reflex and xerostomia may occur Sedation and dizziness are common side effects; ensure patient safety after administration
Hydroxyzine hydrochloride (Vistaril, Atarax)	CNS depressant Anticholinergic Antihistamine Bronchodilator Relieves anxiety May be given to reduce analgesic requirements before or after surgery	Monitor for CNS depression; effects potentiated with other CNS depressants Drowsiness and dizziness are common side effects; ensure patient safety after administration

ications commonly are given "on call to the OR" but also may be given just before anesthesia induction in the operating room suite. Premedications may be omitted altogether, depending on the preference of the anesthesiologist. Once premedications have been administered, it is essential that the patient be kept in bed with the side rails up to ensure safety.

Preoperative Checklist

A preoperative checklist is a method of summarizing patient data and the final preparations for surgery (Figure 16-4). The patient is transferred to a stretcher and transported to the operating room. The patient's chart and archival records, if any, accompany the patient.

Preoperative Checklist

	Yes	No	N/A
ID Band			
Allergies (if Yes, band applied and chart labeled) • Type __________ • Reaction __________			
Surgical site verified with patient/significant other			
Surgical site is marked by patient/significant other			
Surgical consent signed, dated, and witnessed			
Special consents signed, dated, and witnessed (if Yes, identify specific consents(s) • Special consent(s) __________			
Advanced directives			
History and physical examination completed			
Surgical prep completed • Voided • Catheterized			
I & O flowsheet on chart			
Vital signs flowsheet on chart			
Medication record on chart			

Valuables

Circle if applicable:	**Disposition**
Dentures/partial plates	
Hearing aid	
Wigs/hairpins/hairpieces	
Jewelry	
Glasses/contact lenses	
Prosthesis	
Acrylic nails/nailpolish removed	
Other __________	

Figure 16-4 Preoperative checklist.

Continued

Level of Consciousness

	Yes	No	N/A
Alert and oriented × 3			
Confused			
Lethargic			
Awake			
Unresponsive			
Other • Comments ______			

Functional Status

ROM or physical limitations (specify) ______

Sensory function

- Visual ______
- Auditory ______
- Tactile ______

Language barrier ______

Comments ______

Diagnostic

	On Chart WNL	ABNL: Physician Notified	N/A
CBC			
K			
Glucose			
bHcg			
Sickle prep			
ECG			
Blood products T&S ___ # of units ______ T&C ___ # of units ______ autologous donation ___ # of units ______			
Other ______			

Figure 16-4, cont'd Preoperative checklist.

Ht. ______________ Wt. ______________

Vital signs: T ___ P ___ R ___ BP ___ Pulse oximetry ______________

Pain rating (0-10) ______________

NPO status ______________

IV Fluids:

IV Site ______________ Catheter size ______________

Solution ______________

Rate ______________

Premedications:

Drug: ______	Dosage: ______	Route: ______	Time Given: ______
Drug: ______	Dosage: ______	Route: ______	Time Given: ______

Other medications taken by patient day of surgery:

Drug: ______	Dosage: ______	Route: ______	Time Taken: ______
Drug: ______	Dosage: ______	Route: ______	Time Taken: ______

Preoperative teaching completed: Yes ____ No ____

Patient accompanied by: ______________

Comments: ______________

Signature: ______________ Date: ______ Time: ______

Review of preoperative checklist by operating room nurse:

Signature: ______________ Date: ______ Time: ______

Figure 16-4, cont'd Preoperative checklist.

EVALUATION

To evaluate the effectiveness of nursing interventions, compare patient behaviors with those stated in the expected patient outcomes. Achievement of outcomes is successful if the patient undergoing surgical intervention:

1. Participates in and complies with perioperative instructions, exercises, and routines and verbalizes an understanding of rationales for care.
2. States psychologic and physiologic comfort is increased and describes own anxiety and uses effective coping mechanisms.
3. Demonstrates effective coughing and deep breathing exercises and adequate air exchange.

3a. Demonstrates correct use of incentive spirometer.

4. Identifies factors to improve peripheral circulation.

4a. Demonstrates correct performance of leg exercises.

DOCUMENTATION

The nursing report serves as a concise evaluation of the care given during the preoperative phase. Biopsychosocial assessment data are recorded and all pertinent data communicated to the operating room nurse. Preoperative teaching content and the patient and family's responses should be recorded. In addition, any relevant social factors that need to be considered while the patient is in surgery should be reported. Vital signs, preoperative medications, and laboratory and diagnostic results are recorded on the patient's medical record.

Critical Thinking Questions

1. A 45-year-old man is scheduled for a gastric stapling surgery for morbid obesity. He is seen in the preadmission testing for preoperative evaluation. The history reveals the patient is single and lives alone; his elderly parents live nearby and are supportive; he has a history of smoking, sedentary lifestyle, and is employed as a computer programmer. Physical assessment data include weight of 177 kg (390 pounds), BMI 52, BP 188/100, P 96, R 18.
   What other assessment data are needed to complete the patient's preoperative evaluation?
   What possible psychosocial needs should be addressed?
   What laboratory and diagnostic tests are indicated for this patient?
   What pertinent data and special care needs should be communicated to the operating room nurse?
   Describe the content of preoperative teaching for the patient and his family.
2. An 85-year-old widow residing in an assistive living facility is admitted for repair of a pathologic hip fracture. Past medical history includes breast cancer and degenerative joint disease. She has a daughter who lives out of state and a few friends at her residence. Her advance directive includes a durable power of attorney for health care and a wish for no life-sustaining treatment and resuscitation measures. During the preoperative interview she displays anxiety and expresses concerns about not waking up after surgery.
   Describe the plan of care for this patient.
   Describe interventions to help manage her anxiety and address her concerns.
   What needs to be addressed with the patient, surgeon, anesthesiologist, and operating room staff concerning her advance directive while in the operating room?

References

1. Ang-Lee MK, Moss J, Chun-Su Y: Herbal medicines and perioperative care, *JAMA* 286(2):208, 2001.
2. Association of Operating Room Nurses, Inc: *2001 Standards and recommended practices,* Denver, Colo, 2001, AORN Publications.
3. Bailes BK: Perioperative care of the elderly surgical patient, *AORN J* 72(2):86, 2000.
4. Bond G: Infection control assessment in the perioperative setting, *Semin Perioperative Nurs* 8(1):24, 1999.
5. Brumley C: Herbs and the perioperative patient, *AORN J* 72(5):783, 2000.
6. Cott J et al: Drug-herb interactions: how vigilant should you be? *Patient Care Nurse Pract* 3(10):17, 2000.
7. Dunn D: Preoperative assessment criteria and patient teaching for ambulatory surgery patients, *J Perianesthesia Nurs* 13(5):274, 1988.
8. Flanagan K: Perioperative assessment: safety considerations for patients taking herbal products, *J Perianesthesia Nurs*16(1):19, 2001.
9. Fortunato NH: *Berry & Kohn's operating room technique,* ed 9, St Louis, 2000, Mosby.
10. Geier KA: A practical guide to improving patient outcomes, *Orthop Nurs* 19:(May/June Suppl):22, 2000.
11. Hatcher T: The proverbial herb, *Am J Nurs* 101(2):36, 2001.
12. Lowe NK, Ryan-Wenger NM: Over-the-counter medications and self-care, *Nurse Pract* 24(12):34, 1999.
13. Mahoney D, Zhan L, Eckler M: Preventing drug-drug interactions among older adults: guidelines and clinical application, *Am J Nurse Pract* 3(1):7, 1999.
14. Mangram AJ et al: Guideline for prevention of surgical site infection, 1999, *Infect Control Hosp Epidemiol* 20(4):247, 1999.
15. Mason JE, Freeman B: Perioperative medical care. In Doherty GM et al, editors: *The Washington manual of surgery,* ed 2, Philadelphia, 1999, Lippincott Williams & Wilkins
16. Murphy EK: Continuing developments in informed consents, *AORN J* 72(4):717, 2000.
17. Murphy EK: Preparation of the patient for the procedure: legal and ethical considerations. In Phippen ML, Wells MP, editors: *Patient care during operative and invasive procedures,* Philadephia, 2000, WB Saunders.
18. Older Americans 2000: Key Indicators of Well-Being/Federal Interagency Forum on Aging-Related Statistics, 2000, Internet document: http://www.agingstats.gov/chartbook2000/population.html
19. Patton CM: Preoperative assessment of the adult patient, *Semin Perioperative Nurs* 8(1):42, 1999.
20. Petersen C: Clinical issues, *AORN J* 73(3):701, 2001.
21. Seidel HM et al: *Mosby's guide to physical examination,* ed 4, St Louis, 1999, Mosby.
22. Shurpin K, DeSimone ME: Preoperative evaluation, *Am J Nurse Pract* 12(2):7, 1998.
23. Smitana GW: Preoperative pulmonary evaluation, *N Engl J Med* 340(12):937, 1999.
24. Starr P: *The social transformation of American medicine,* New York, 1982, Basic Books.
25. Stupay S, Siversten L: Herbal and nutritional supplement use in the elderly, *Nurse Pract* 25(9):56, 2000.
26. Tappen RM, Muzic J, Kennedy P: Preoperative assessment and discharge planning for older adults undergoing ambulatory surgery, *AORN J* 73(2):464, 2001.
27. Tsen LC et al: Alternative medicine use in presurgical patients, *Anesthesiology* 93(1):148, 2000.
28. Venes, D, editor: *Taber's cyclopedic medical dictionary,* ed 19, Philadelphia, 2001, FA Davis.

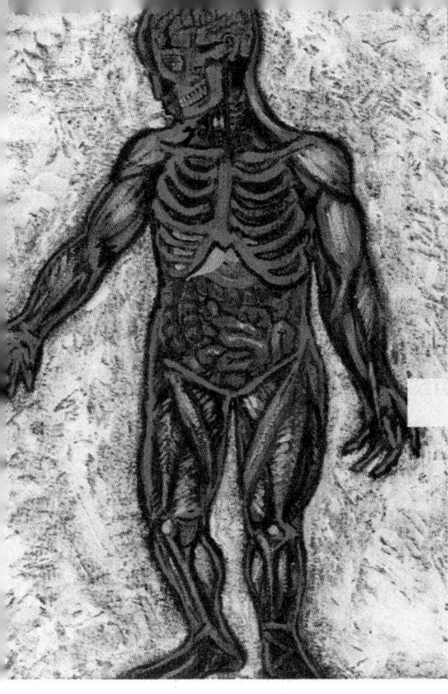

Intraoperative Nursing

17

Mary Jo Boehnlein, Jane F. Marek

Objectives

After studying this chapter, the learner should be able to:

1. Describe the intraoperative phase as a component of the surgical experience.
2. Identify the subspecialties in surgery.
3. Describe the roles of each member of the surgical health care team.
4. Discuss the significance of aseptic technique maintenance.
5. Explain the purpose of appropriate attire in the surgical suite.
6. Compare and contrast the different types of anesthesia.
7. Describe the physiologic stress responses to anesthesia and surgery.
8. Describe the components of the intraoperative patient assessment.
9. Formulate appropriate nursing diagnoses for the intraoperative patient.
10. Explain the potential for the development of intraoperative complications.
11. Identify desired patient outcomes for the intraoperative phase.
12. Discuss nursing interventions to minimize intraoperative risks.
13. Explain the basis for evaluation of nursing interventions during the intraoperative period.

INTRAOPERATIVE PHASE

The intraoperative phase begins with the transfer of the patient onto the operating room (OR) bed and continues until the patient is admitted to the postanesthesia care unit (PACU). Assessment of the patient's physiologic and psychosocial needs provides the nurse with information to determine the nursing diagnoses that are congruent with intraoperative nursing interventions. The intraoperative nursing care plan is developed from assessment data, nursing diagnoses, and identification of expected patient outcomes. The plan is designed to address individual patient needs and safely facilitate the surgical procedure. Throughout the entire intraoperative period, the nurse functions as an active team member who is able to quickly alter the plan in response to changes in the patient's condition.

SURGICAL SPECIALTIES

Surgery emerged as a true medical specialty in the mid-nineteenth century. The work of Ignaz Semmelweiss, Louis Pasteur, and Joseph Lister became the basis for the current aseptic practices used in the OR.

General surgery is the basis for all surgical specialties. Surgical specialties emerged as a result of understanding the etiology of various disease processes and using specific treatments for various parts of the body. Each specialty involves surgical procedures performed on a specific system or anatomic region (Box 17-1).

INTRAOPERATIVE PATIENT CARE TEAM

The coordinated efforts of the surgical team are required to deliver safe and effective intraoperative patient care. To accomplish this goal, team members must work as a coordinated unit. Each member of the surgical team must be familiar with the specific surgical procedure, adhere to policies and procedures, and be able to adjust quickly to alterations in the patient's condition and the surgical procedure.

The OR team is divided into categories based on the responsibilities of its members. Members of the scrubbed sterile team scrub their hands and arms, don sterile gowns and gloves, maintain sterility, and work in the sterile field. Members of this team consist of the primary or operating surgeon, assistants to the surgeon, and the scrub nurse.

Members of the nonscrubbed, nonsterile surgical team function outside the sterile field. Team members are responsible for ensuring patient safety, positioning the patient, monitoring the patient, maintaining sterile technique, handling nonsterile supplies and equipment, and providing items for the sterile team. Members of the nonsterile team include the

BOX 17-1 Procedures of Surgical Subspecialties

General Surgery

Digestive system structures, abdominal wall, thyroid, and breast—e.g., mastectomy, bowel resection, ventral herniorrhaphy

Gynecology and Obstetrics

Female reproductive system—e.g., hysterectomy, cesarean section

Genitourinary Surgery

Male reproductive system, male and female renal system—e.g., prostatectomy, cystoscopy

Orthopedic Surgery

Musculoskeletal system—e.g., knee reconstruction, fracture repair, spinal fusion, total joint arthroplasty

Neurosurgery

Brain, spinal cord, and nerves—e.g., cerebral aneurysm clipping, laminectomy

Thoracic and Cardiovascular Surgery

Pulmonary structures, heart, great vessels, and peripheral vascular system—e.g., lung resection, femoral-popliteal vein bypass graft, mitral or aortic valve repair

Ophthalmic Surgery

Eye structures—e.g., corneal transplantation, vitrectomy, cataract removal

Otorhinolaryngology, Head and Neck Surgery

Ear, nose, throat, trachea, and esophagus—e.g., stapedectomy, laryngectomy, tracheostomy

Plastic and Reconstructive Surgery

Congenital or trauma-induced abnormalities or disfigurement, cosmetic corrections (e.g., skin grafting, cleft palate repair, face lift)

circulating nurse, anesthesiologist and anesthetists, and other allied personnel.

Primary Surgeon and Assistants

The primary or operating surgeon has the knowledge, skill, and expertise to successfully perform the identified surgical procedure. The surgeon is responsible for determining the preoperative diagnosis, the choice and execution of the surgical procedure, the explanation of the risks and benefits of the surgical procedure to the patient, obtaining informed patient consent for the surgical procedure, and the postoperative management of the patient's care.

Under the direction of the operating surgeon, the surgeon's assistant is responsible for exposing the surgical site, providing hemostasis to prevent blood from obscuring the anatomy, and assisting with suturing throughout the operative procedure. The first assistant may be a surgeon, resident, registered nurse first assistant (RNFA), advanced practice nurse, surgical assistant, or physician's assistant.

The Association of Operating Room Nurses (AORN) acknowledged the role of the RN as a first assistant to the surgeon and adopted an official statement recognizing the RNFA in 1984. The association defined the scope of practice, requirements, education, and clinical privileges that are required for the RNFA. On the basis of the AORN statement, many state boards of nursing have accepted the AORN statement and have incorporated RNFA functions into the scope of nursing practice.[3]

Scrub Nurse

The scrub nurse role may be performed by an RN or an OR scrub technologist. The scrub nurse must have an understanding of the specific surgical procedure and the anatomy and physiology of the involved system. Some of the scrub nurse's responsibilities include the preparation of supplies and equipment on the sterile field; maintenance of patient safety and integrity of the sterile field; observation of the scrubbed team members for breaks in sterile technique; provision of appropriate sterile instrumentation, sutures, and supplies to the operating surgeon; and adherence to established policies and procedures for sponge, instrument, and sharps counts.

To perform this role effectively, the scrub nurse must possess manual skills and dexterity and strictly adhere to the principles of aseptic technique. All duties need to be consistently performed with precision and accuracy to ensure the patient's safety throughout the surgical procedure.

Circulating Nurse

The circulating nurse is an RN whose responsibility is to serve as the patient advocate while coordinating events before, during, and after the surgical procedure. The circulating nurse is responsible for creating a safe environment for the patient, managing the activities outside the sterile field, and providing nursing care to the patient.

Before and during administration of the anesthetic, the circulating nurse provides emotional support to the patient and assists the anesthesia team during the induction period. Throughout the surgical procedure, the circulating nurse implements measures to ensure patient safety, obtains supplies and equipment for the sterile team members, and enforces policies and procedures. The circulating nurse is also responsible for documenting intraoperative nursing care and ensuring that surgical specimens are identified and placed in the appropriate media. Some of the other responsibilities of the circulating nurse include enforcing the principles of aseptic technique; recognizing and implementing actions to resolve possible environmental hazards that involve the patient or surgical team members; ensuring that sponge, instrument, and sharps counts are completed and appropriately documented; and communicating relevant information to individuals outside of the OR, such as family members and other health care workers.

Anesthesiologist and Anesthetist

An anesthesiologist is a physician who specializes in administering anesthetic agents and monitoring the patient's response to the agents. An anesthetist is an individual who administers anesthetics under the direct supervision of an anesthesiologist or surgeon. Anesthetists may be resident physicians or a certified registered nurse anesthetist.

In the preoperative period, the anesthesiologist and anesthetist evaluate the patient and determine the appropriate anesthetic to be administered. Intraoperative responsibilities include anesthetizing the patient, providing appropriate levels of pain relief for the patient, monitoring the patient's physiologic status, and providing the best operative conditions for the surgeon. In the immediate postoperative period, the anesthesiologist assumes medical responsibility for the patient.

Other Personnel

A number of allied personnel also contribute to meeting the needs of the surgical patient. Pathologists, radiologists, radiology technicians, perfusionists, environmental services personnel, and clerical staff are a few of the many individuals whose skills and expertise are necessary to provide assistance to the surgical team and ultimately to the patient.

THE SURGICAL ENVIRONMENT

Design of the Surgical Suite

A surgical suite is designed to provide a safe therapeutic environment for the patient. The design of the suite addresses issues of traffic patterns, infection control, safety, and efficiency.

Traffic Control

Traffic in and out of the operating suite is kept to a minimum. Only essential personnel are allowed inside the operating room. As the number of persons increases, potential contamination from bacterial shedding and air turbulence increases.

Traffic control patterns are designed to address activity and movement into and out of the surgical suite, as well as within the suite. The floor plan of a surgical suite is divided into three zones. The three-zone concept was developed to define the areas within the surgical suite by the types of activities that occur within each area. The three zones are known as the unrestricted area, the semirestricted area, and the restricted area.

The unrestricted area provides an entrance to and exit from the surgical suite. The holding area, PACU, lounges, dressing rooms, and offices are located in the unrestricted area. In this area street clothes may be worn and traffic is not restricted. The semirestricted area provides access to restricted zones and peripheral support areas within the surgical suite. Peripheral support areas consist of storage for clean and sterile supplies, work areas for processing supplies and equipment, and corridors to the individual ORs. Scrub attire and hair covering must be worn in the semirestricted area. The restricted area includes the individual operating rooms, scrub areas, substerile rooms, and clean core areas. In this area scrub attire, hair covering, and masks must be worn.

Infection Control

The design of the OR and the materials used within it are chosen to address issues of infection control and safety. Materials used in the interior of the OR address issues of environmental control.

Ceiling and walls are constructed of nonporous, smooth, fire-resistant materials that are easy to clean with microbial agents. Tile wall covering is not advocated because of the potential for microorganisms to grow in porous grout lines.

Materials used for floor coverings have the same specifications as the walls and ceiling. The floors need to be highly wear resistant with slip-proof surfaces to prevent personnel injury.

Sliding doors are used to prevent air turbulence in the OR. Fire regulations dictate that doors should be able to swing open if needed.

Environmental Conditions

Temperature and humidity are environmental conditions that need to be controlled to reduce the incidence of infection. Temperature within an OR is maintained between 20° and 22° C (68° and 75° F). Most pathogenic bacteria metabolize and reproduce at or near normal body temperature. Bacterial growth may be inhibited by keeping room temperature below body temperature. The lower room temperature also helps decrease the surgical patient's metabolic demands. The relative humidity in the OR is maintained within the range of 40% to 60%. This level of humidity diminishes bacterial growth and restricts static electricity.

Many ORs have high-efficiency particulate air filters in the air systems to assist with infection control. Inlet air is dispersed from vents in the ceiling and exhausted through vents at the floor level. Slightly less air is exhausted than is introduced, creating a positive pressure gradient within the room. The positive pressure prevents potentially contaminated air from entering the room. This is why all doors to individual ORs remain closed except for patient and team members' entry and exit. There should be at least 15 room air exchanges per hour in each operating room. Three of the exchanges should be fresh air exchanges.[22,23]

INFECTION CONTROL

Surgical wound infections account for 25% of nosocomial infections and 38% of all postoperative infections.[4] They rank as the second most common nosocomial infection and occur in 2% to 5% of patients that undergo surgical procedures each year. An estimated 500,000 infections occur annually, prolonging the hospital stay by 7.4 days with total costs exceeding $10 billion annually. Surgical wound infections are the most common cause of morbidity and mortality for the surgical patient.[9] Additional sources of nosocomial infection for the surgical patient include postoperative pneumonia and pneumonia related to ventilator use and bacteremia related to the surgical procedure and/or intravenous catheter insertion.[9]

Asepsis is defined as the absence of microorganisms that cause disease. Surgical asepsis promotes tissue healing by deterring pathogens from coming into contact with the surgical wound. Practices that suppress, reduce, and inhibit infectious processes are known as aseptic technique.

Infection control policies and procedures guide the practice of aseptic technique in the operating room. The policies and procedures are based on principles of microbiology and bacteriology. Infection control policies are guided by

AORN-recommended practices for perioperative nursing. The AORN has developed recommended practices for aseptic technique, surgical attire, environmental services activities, sterilization of supplies and equipment, surgical hand scrub, and cleansing of skin.

All members of the OR team are responsible for strict adherence to aseptic technique. It is essential that OR nurses acquire a surgical conscience. *Surgical conscience* is defined as vigilant adherence to aseptic technique throughout the entire perioperative period. This involves constant examination and observation of the patient, OR environment, and personnel. A surgical conscience is completely developed when the nurse automatically attends to sterile technique. To develop a surgical conscience, the nurse must understand the principles of asepsis and sterile technique, acquire self-discipline in managing nursing practice, and develop good communication and assertiveness skills to identify patient needs and communicate breaks in sterile technique.

Basic Rules of Surgical Asepsis

Strict adherence to aseptic technique minimizes the potential for contamination of the sterile field and wound infection. Protocols for creating and maintaining a sterile field have been developed from the seven AORN-recommended practices for maintaining a sterile field. Six of the practices address practice issues and are briefly discussed. The seventh practice addresses the administrative function of establishing and reviewing policies and procedures related to the practice of aseptic technique.

Recommended practice I states that "scrubbed persons function within a sterile field."[2,3] Scrubbed personnel wear sterile gowns and gloves at the surgical field. Gowns and gloves provide a barrier to restrict the transfer of microorganisms from the scrubbed person's hands and clothing to the surgical wound. The gown of a scrubbed team member is considered sterile in front from the chest to the level of the sterile field, and the sleeves are sterile from 2 inches above the elbow to the stockinette cuff. The stockinette cuff portion of the gown is unsterile and needs to be completely covered by a sterile glove. The unsterile areas of the surgical gown include the neckline, shoulder, axillary region, and back. Articles dropped below the waist or table level are considered contaminated.

The second recommended practice states that sterile drapes are used to create a sterile field.[2,3] Surgical drapes provide a barrier that impedes the movement of microorganisms from a nonsterile area to a sterile area. Sterile drapes are placed on the patient, equipment, and furniture used within the sterile field. Draped tables are sterile only at the table level; items extending over the table edge are contaminated. Handling of drapes should be kept to a minimum. When placing sterile drapes, gloved hands are protected by a cuff of the drape (Figure 17-1).

Practice III states that all items used in the sterile field are sterile.[2,3] If there is a question about the sterility of an item, it must be considered unsterile. Packaging materials must guarantee that items will remain sterile until removed. Before opening a sterile package it must be inspected for seal integrity, tears, pinholes, the presence of a sterilization indicator, and the expiration date as indicated.

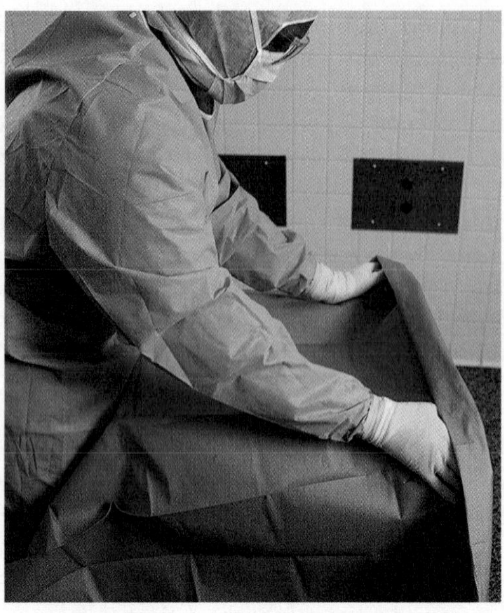

Figure 17-1 Scrub nurse protects gloves with cuff of drape when opening inner wrapper of pack, which will serve as sterile table cover.

The fourth practice addresses the introduction of supplies into the sterile field. Supplies that are introduced into the sterile field are to be delivered in a manner that ensures the sterility of the item and maintains the integrity of the sterile field.[2,3] A sterile package is opened from the far side first and the near side last; wrapper tails are held when the item is presented to the sterile field (Figure 17-2). Solutions are poured to prevent splashing of liquids onto the field. After a bottle of sterile solution is opened the entire contents must be presented to the sterile field or discarded. The edges of a bottle cap are considered nonsterile after the cap is removed. If the cap is replaced, the sterility of the bottle contents cannot be ensured; therefore the remaining contents must be discarded.

Recommended practice V addresses maintenance and monitoring of the sterile field. The possibility for contamination increases with time; therefore the sterile field should be established as close to the time of use as possible. Unattended sterile fields are considered contaminated.[2,3]

Movement within or around the sterile field by personnel is addressed in recommended practice VI.[2,3] The integrity of the sterile field must be maintained by individuals moving within or around the sterile field. Only scrubbed personnel touch and reach over sterile areas. Sterile persons remain close to the sterile field and never turn their backs to the field. Sterile individuals change positions by passing back-to-back or face-to-face. Unscrubbed personnel only touch and reach over nonsterile areas. Unscrubbed team members must not walk between sterile fields and must approach sterile fields by facing them.

Infection Control Practices for Operating Room Personnel

All individuals working in the operating room serve as a major source of microbial contamination to the environment because of the large quantities of bacteria that are present in the respiratory tract and on the skin, hair, and attire of all persons. To re-

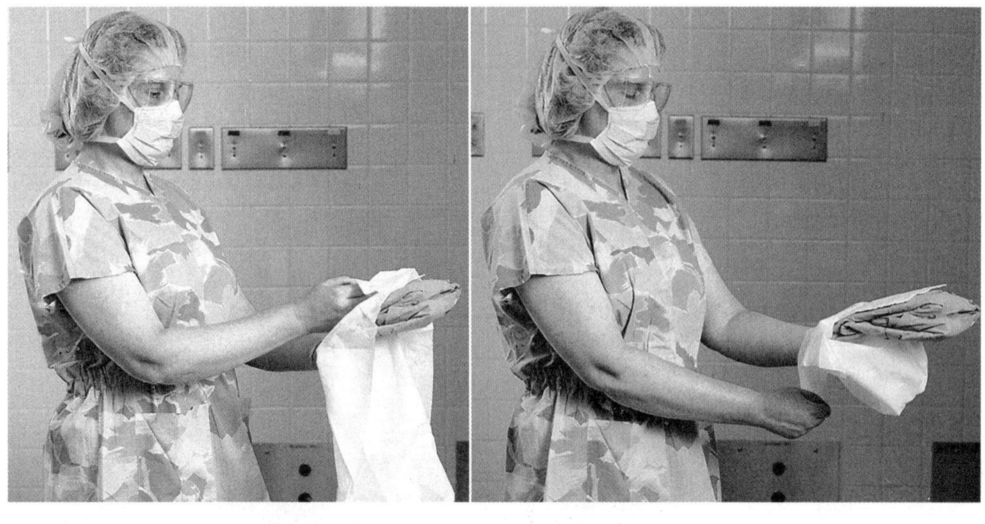

Figure 17-2 A, When opening sterile package, scrub nurse opens corner nearest body last to avoid potential contamination of inner pack. B, To prevent nonsterile corners of outer wrapper from touching scrub nurse or sterile field, scrub nurse draws back corners of opened wrapper when presenting inner package.

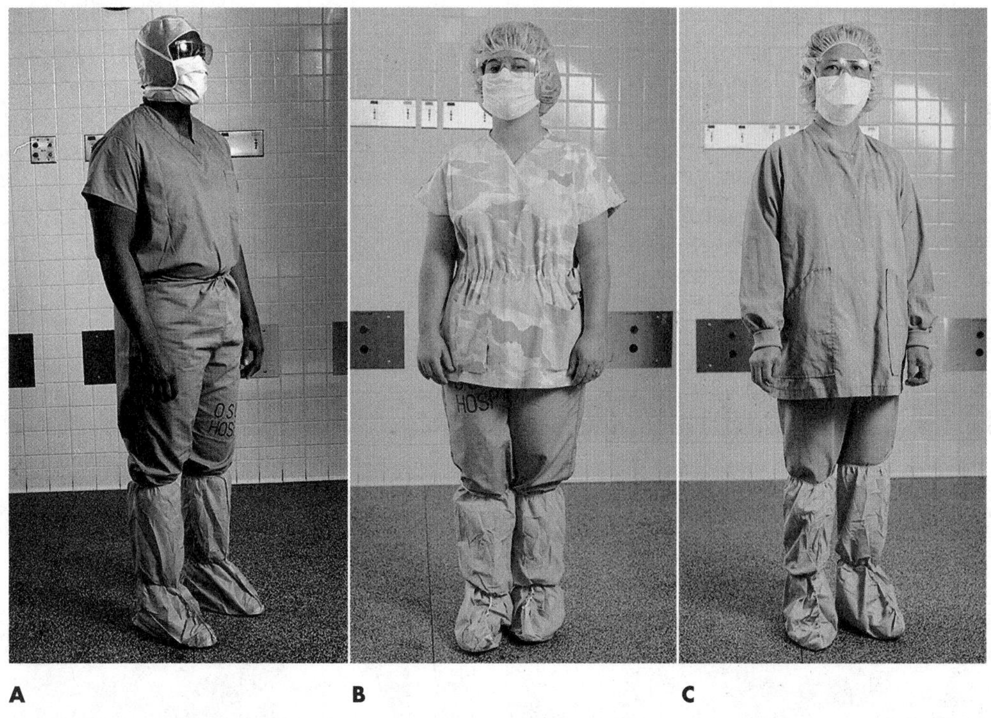

Figure 17-3 Proper surgical attire. A, Two-piece scrub suit with shirt tucked in. B, Tunic top. C, Non-scrubbed personnel with long-sleeved jacket.

duce the risks of OR personnel serving as sources of infection for the patient, it is necessary for everyone to wear surgical attire in the semirestricted and restricted areas of the OR. Surgical attire also provides personnel protection from exposure to infectious microorganisms and hazardous substances. Surgical attire includes a scrub suit, hat or hood, and face mask or shield.

Surgical Attire

Dressing in OR attire proceeds from head to toe. The surgical hat is put on first to prevent contamination of the scrub clothes with hair or dandruff. The hat must be clean and free of lint, and must completely cover all head and facial hair. If the hat does not provide sufficient coverage of facial hair, a hood should be worn.

Scrub suits are put on after the hair is covered. The suits, which are laundered daily, should be made of material that meet the requirements of the National Fire Protection Agency and should be closely woven to minimize bacterial shedding. Scrub shirts are either tied at the waist or tucked into the scrub pants to decrease bacterial shedding and to prevent contamination of the sterile field by a loose shirt. Unscrubbed personnel should wear long-sleeved warm-up jackets to prevent possible shedding of microorganisms from bare arms (Figure 17-3).

Footwear should be comfortable. In the interest of safety, clogs, open-toe, and cloth athletic shoes are not recommended. Literature suggests that the use of shoe covers in the OR does not affect the incidence of postoperative wound infection.[22] Shoe covers are a part of personal protective equipment and are to be worn whenever it is expected that splashes or spills will happen. If worn, they should be changed when torn, soiled, or wet and removed when leaving the surgical suite.

Masks are necessary to prevent contamination of the surgical environment by respiratory droplets. A mask is to be worn where sterile supplies are open and in areas where scrubbed persons are present. The mask must totally cover the nose and mouth and must be secured to prevent ventilation from the sides of the face. It is either on or off; it should not be saved by being hung around the neck, placed on the forehead, or placed in a pocket. When removing a mask, care should be taken to prevent contamination of the hands. The filter portion of the mask should not be touched. The mask should be removed only by touching its strings; once removed, it should be immediately discarded (Figure 17-4).

Face shields and protective eyewear are also part of surgical attire. These items are protective barriers used to decrease the risk of splash or spraying of fluids into the mucous membranes of the mouth, nose, and eyes. All personnel who are in close proximity to the operative site should wear protective eyewear.

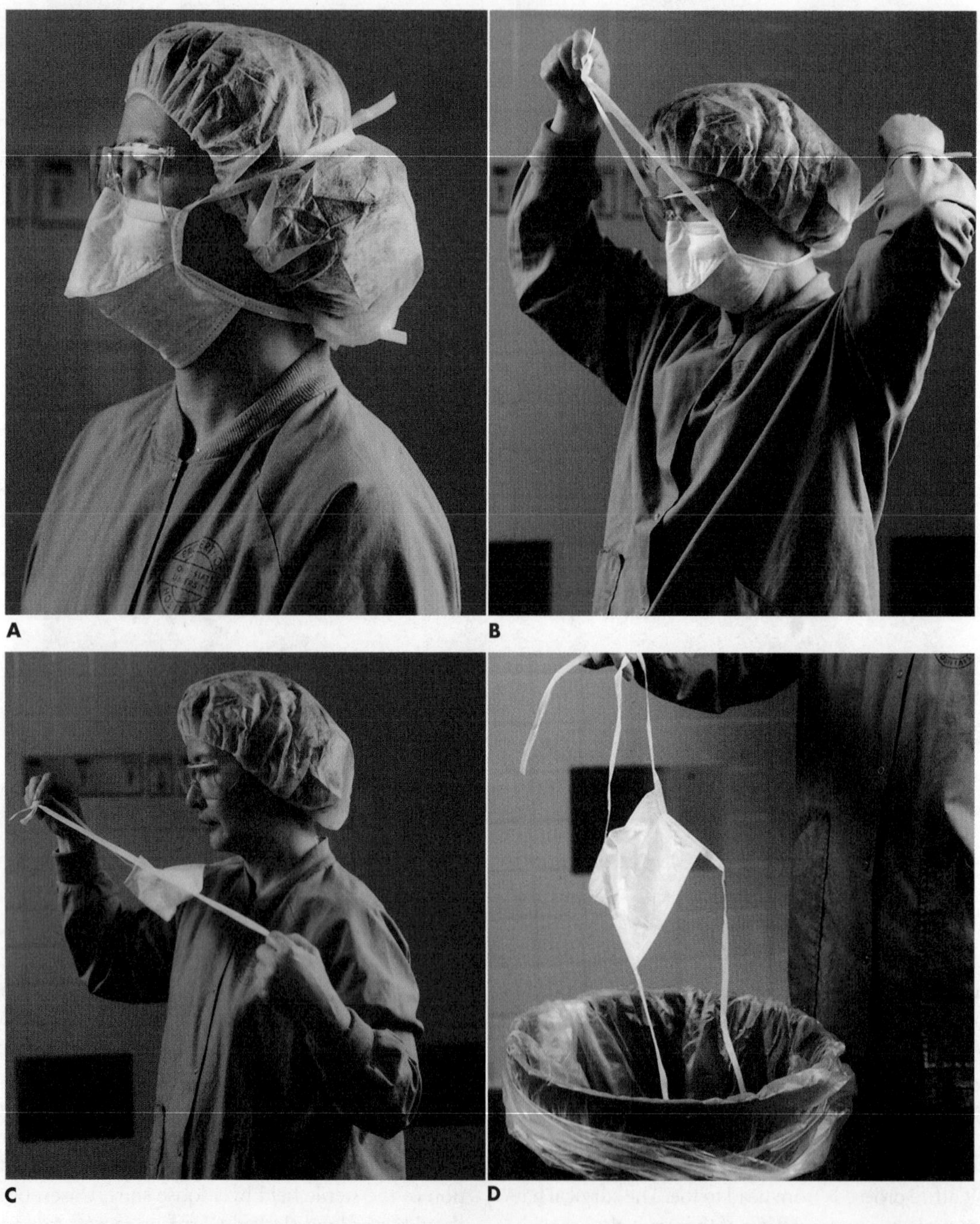

Figure 17-4 Proper handling of mask. **A,** Edges of properly worn mask conform to facial contours when mask is applied and tied correctly. **B** and **C,** Personnel should avoid touching filter portion of mask when removing it. **D,** Masks should be discarded on removal.

Lead aprons and thyroid shields are protective attire worn to protect OR personnel from radiologic exposure. These items are worn when personnel must be present during fluoroscopic procedures or when x-rays are used intraoperatively.

Ideally OR attire should never be worn outside of the surgical suite because this creates a two-way hazard. Any contaminants that come in contact with the OR team members can become airborne and find susceptible hosts outside of the surgical suite. Conversely, bacteria present outside the OR may be carried back to the surgical suite. If changing scrub attire is not feasible, head and shoe coverings are removed and the scrub clothes are covered. The preferred method is to use a clean cover gown that closes in the back. If a lab coat is worn, it must be completely buttoned to protect the front of the scrub suit. On return to the department, clean scrub attire should be put on because cover gowns and lab coats are ineffective barriers to potential external contaminants.

Standard Precautions

A discussion of aseptic technique maintenance is not complete without mention of Standard Precautions. Uncontained blood and body fluids—an inevitable part of surgery—present a great hazard to operating room personnel. Because routine medical history and examination cannot identify all patients with human immunodeficiency virus, hepatitis, or other blood-borne pathogens, Standard Precautions are used for all patients. Table 17-1 provides some examples of intraoperative applications of Standard Precautions.

The proper handling and disposition of needles, knife blades, and sharp instruments, along with strict compliance with the Centers for Disease Control and Prevention's (CDC) practices of Standard Precautions protects OR personnel. Other protective mechanisms for health care workers are the Occupational Safety and Health Association's (OSHA) revised blood-borne pathogens standard for 2001 and federal legislation. These revised standards and the federal Needlestick Safety and Prevention Act have mandated changes for the protection of health care workers who are exposed to blood from needles and other sharps. Provisions require the use of engineering controls, including safer medical devices such as needleless systems and sharps with built-in injury protectors. Other requirements include an exposure control plan and sharps injury log for documenting and tracking exposure.[13,25,28] Adherence to these practices, along with strict maintenance of aseptic technique, minimizes the chance of transmission of pathogens between patients and personnel.

Sterilization of Supplies

Microorganisms that do not normally invade healthy tissue are capable of causing infection if introduced directly into the body. For this reason all supplies and instruments used for the surgical procedure must be properly sterilized. Sterilization renders items safe for contact with tissue without transmission of infection as long as their sterility is maintained.

Sterilization processes for instruments and products used in the surgical suite must be performed according to guidelines established by the regulatory agencies that conduct research and set guidelines for the methods, products, and equipment used in sterilization processes. These agencies include the CDC, OSHA, AORN, Food and Drug Administration (FDA), and American Association for Medical Instrumentation (AAMI). Table 17-2 summarizes methods of sterilization.

Although the sterilization process prevents the potential spread of disease via surgical instruments and other supplies used during the surgery, data indicate that some pathogens are not susceptible to the normal sterilization processes. *Prions,* abnormal isoforms of cellular proteins, are unlike all other known pathogens and do not contain genetic material. Prions are responsible for the transmission of Creutzfeldt-Jakob disease and other encephalopathies including "mad cow" disease (bovine spongiform encephalopathy). These highly resistant pathogens can survive routine sterilization and disinfection processes, including steam sterilization, dry heat, ethylene

TABLE 17-1 Intraoperative Applications of Standard Precautions

Nursing Action	Potential Contaminant	Precautions
Changing the blood-filled suction liner at the end of the procedure	Blood splashing out of suction liner	Goggles or face shield, nonsterile gloves
Transferring an actively bleeding trauma patient to the operating room bed	Direct contact with blood	Goggles or face shield, nonsterile gloves, fluid-resistant apron or gown
Organizing blood-filled sponges for the sponge count	Direct contact with blood-contaminated items	Goggles or face shield, nonsterile gloves
Removing or changing the surgical knife blade	Cuts and direct contact with blood	Manufacturer's safety device, instrument, or surgical clamp to disassemble knife blade and handle
Sharps handling and disposal	Needlestick injury, contaminated sharps	Needleless systems; hands-free technique for passing sutures, knife blades, and other sharp instruments; one-handed recapping technique; blunt suture needles; resheathing needle; written exposure control plan and sharps injury log

TABLE 17-2 Major Methods of Sterilization

Method	Manner of Sterilization	Advantages	Disadvantages
Steam	Steam under pressure infiltrates permeable materials with moist heat, causing the denaturation and coagulation of the cellular protein system → death of microbe or spore.	Safe Easy Economic Permeates porous substances Leaves no film on items	Items cannot be sensitive to heat Steam and moisture may corrode items Ineffective against prions
Chemical (ethylene oxide gas)	Chemical disrupts cellular protein metabolism and reproduction → death of microbe or spore.	Effective for heat-sensitive items Noncorrosive Permeates dry substances Leaves no film on items	Time consuming Expensive Toxic by-products can formulate
Plasma	Low-temperature hydrogen peroxide creates a gas plasma. The gas plasma consists of ions, electrons, and neutral atomic particles. Free radicals in gas interact with cellular membranes, enzymes, or nucleic acids → death of microbe or spore.	Faster than ethylene oxide gas Dry nontoxic method By-products (water and oxygen) are environmentally safe No aeration Safe for heat-sensitive items Noncorrosive to metal	Ineffective against prions Incompatible with cotton-woven fabric and paper Ineffective on small-diameter cannulae Ineffective against prions

oxide, and plasma sterilization.[26] The CDC and World Health Organization, AORN, and Joint Commission of Accredited Healthcare Organizations (JCAHO) are all working to develop protocols for sterilization processes that will ensure sterilization of instruments and supplies that come in contact with prions and thus prevent transmission of these virulent pathogens.

Surgical Scrub

The purpose of a surgical scrub is to remove dirt and microorganisms from the hands, fingernails, and forearms; decrease the resident microbial count to minimum levels; and retard the regrowth of microorganisms. This is accomplished by a mechanical washing of the fingernails, hands, and arms with an antimicrobial soap.

The microbial flora of the skin are classified as transient and resident bacteria. Transient flora are acquired by contact and loosely adhere to the skin. The majority of transient microorganisms are removed by chemical and mechanical methods.

Resident flora are found deep in the skin in hair follicles and sebaceous glands. These microorganisms are shed from the body as old cells move from the dermal to the epidermal layer of the skin with perspiration and other skin secretions. Because of these actions, resident flora are potential sources of contamination. Resident bacteria are decreased but not completely removed during the surgical scrub.

The skin cannot be sterilized; however, it can be made surgically clean. Obtaining surgically clean skin involves a mechanical process that removes transient flora with friction along with a chemical process that decreases the number of flora on the epidermis with the use of an antimicrobial detergent.

Various antimicrobial detergents meet the criteria for effectiveness. The effective agent must be a broad-spectrum antimicrobial, fast-acting in decreasing the microbial count, able to leave a residue on the skin to reduce regrowth of bacteria, and nonirritating and nonsensitizing. The most commonly used agents are povidone-iodine and chlorhexidine gluconate products. The gold standard for surgical hand preparation in Europe has been agents containing alcohol because of its high degree of antimicrobial activity. Alcohol is rapid acting and provides the greatest reduction in the number of skin microbes. Using a combination of alcohol and chlorhexidene gluconate is more effective than an alcohol product alone in reducing the numbers of colonizing flora and promoting residual antibacterial properties on the skin.[21]

The procedure and types of material used for the surgical scrub vary among institutions. Regardless of the procedure, certain criteria must be met by all personnel before beginning the surgical scrub.

Only individuals who are free of skin problems and upper respiratory infections should scrub. Skin cuts and abrasions can discharge serum, which can provide an environment for microbial growth and therefore increase the potential for infection. Fingernails must be kept short to prevent tearing of surgical gloves and clean to prevent harboring of microorganisms. Nail polish that is chipped or worn for more than 4 days appears to foster larger amounts of bacteria. It is recommended that if nail polish is worn it should be freshly applied and free of chips. Artificial nails prevent effective hand washing by harboring gram-negative microorganisms and should not be worn.[3]

There are two accepted methods for performing a surgical hand scrub: the timed scrub procedure and the brush-stroke procedure. Both are effective and follow an anatomic pattern of scrub, beginning at the fingertips and ending with the elbows. New evidence may support a brushless technique. There is inconclusive evidence to support the best practice for length of scrub time (see Research box).

In the timed scrub each anatomic area of the hands and forearms is scrubbed for an identified length of time with special attention given to the fingers and hands. At the conclusion of the timed scrub, the hands and arms are rinsed.

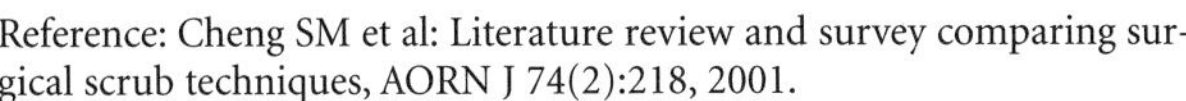

Research

Reference: Cheng SM et al: Literature review and survey comparing surgical scrub techniques, AORN J 74(2):218, 2001.

Reference: Gruendemann BJ, Bjerke NB: Is it time for scrubbing with an alcohol-based agent? AORN J 74(6): 859, 2001.

Reference: Larson E et al: Comparison of different regimes for surgical hand preparation, AORN J 73(2):412, 2001.

Reference: Association of Operating Room Nurses: 2001 Standards and recommended practices, Denver, 2001, AORN publications.

The surgical hand scrub has been a cornerstone of aseptic practices in the operating room since the 1800s. A number of research studies address the best practices for performing the surgical hand scrub. Currently differences exist regarding the agents used and the time and method for performing the scrub. There are no North American guidelines for the duration of scrubbing time or method of scrub technique.

Times for performing the scrub vary from 2 to 6 minutes. European and Australian studies have concluded that 3 to 4-minute scrubs are as effective as 5-minute scrubs with the use of specific agents. However, recommendations in the United States are conflicting and vary from 2 to 5 minutes.

Methods vary, including a brush or sponge or a hand scrub with an alcohol rub to follow. The European standard is a minimum of a 2-minute hand scrub followed by an alcohol rub.

Chlorhexidine gluconate, iodophors, and triclosan are all proven antimicrobial agents. There are no data to support the efficacy of foam surgical scrubs as an appropriate scrubbing agent.

Alcohol is an effective agent due to its rapid action and ability to decrease the number of skin microbes. In addition, alcohols are nontoxic and nonallergenic. The use of alcohol has not been widely adopted in the United States, largely because of concern over skin drying and flammability. Adding emollients or rehydrating agents and the use of enclosed dispensing systems are effective measures to address these concerns. The use of alcohol-based solutions may also decrease the amount of scrub time.

Long considered the best practice, mechanical scrubbing using a brush has been shown to actually increase skin shedding, skin damage, and the microbial skin counts of health care workers. With repeated brushing, the outer layers of the epidermis may be damaged or removed, exposing the flora of deeper layers. The damage to skin as a result of repeated brushing may actually increase the risk and rate of transmission of infection from health care workers to patients.

On the basis of an extensive literature review, a change in practice is recommended. The new procedure consists of a prewash and scrub with or without water, performed by rubbing an alchohol-based antimicrobial agent on the hands and arms.

Before implementing a change in practice, several areas of concern need to be addressed. These include length of scrub time, the use of artificial nails and nail polish, nail length, and the use of hand lotions. The new method must meet FDA requirements and AORN standards. An effective way to implement and evaluate the change in practice must also be accomplished.

TABLE 17-3 Surgical Scrub Guidelines

Action	Comments
1. Don surgical attire, making sure all hair and jewelry are covered and mask is properly secured.	Surgical attire decreases possible contamination from the operating room to the patient.
2. Remove all jewelry from hands and arms.	Jewelry harbors microorganisms that may not be removed during hand washing.
3. Moisten hands and arms and wash to 2 inches above the elbows with an antiseptic agent.	A prescrub loosens surface debris.
4. Clean nails and subungual areas with nail cleaner under running water.	Improperly cleaned fingernails and subungual areas can harbor microorganisms.
5. Rinse hands and arms. Allow water to flow from fingertips to elbows, taking care not to splash surgical attire.	Elevating hands higher than the elbows facilitates water flowing from the cleanest area down the arm. Moisture on scrub attire contaminates the sterile gown.
6. Moisten scrub brush, create lather, and begin the surgical scrub at the fingertips, progressing to the digits, palm, and the back of the hand.	The scrubbing is done vigorously with the scrub brush held perpendicularly to the digit. All sides of the digit and web spaces are scrubbed. Depending on institutional policy, this step initiates either the timed scrub or the scrub-count process.
7. Scrub forearms to 2 inches above the elbow.	Each side of the arm is scrubbed in a circular motion to 2 inches above the elbow.
8. Discard the scrub brush into the appropriate container. Rinse hands and arms thoroughly. Keep hands elevated and proceed into the operating room.	Same comments as for No. 5.

The brush stroke scrub differs from the timed scrub method only in that there is a defined number of brush strokes used for each area of the fingers, hands, and arms. Methods of rinsing and entering the operating room are the same as for the timed scrub process. See Table 17-3 for surgical scrub guidelines.

Patient Skin Preparation

The recommended practices developed by AORN provide a guideline for preoperative skin preparation of the operative site. The goal of skin preparation is to reduce the risk of postoperative wound infection by (1) removing soil and transient microbes from the skin, (2) reducing the resident microbial count to subpathogenic amounts in a short period of time and with the least amount of tissue irritation, and (3) inhibiting rapid rebound growth of microbes.

Skin preparation can be performed before the induction of anesthesia. If the preparation is done when the patient is awake, the circulating nurse needs to explain the purpose of the procedure, attend to the patient's privacy by avoiding unnecessary exposure, and provide for the patient's comfort and safety.

Hair is removed from the surgical site only when necessary. Methods for hair removal include wet shaving, use of clippers, and use of a depilatory. There is a greater incidence of wound infection in patients who are shaved before surgery than for patients who have not had a shave preparation, who have a smaller amount of hair clipped, or on whom a depilatory is used.[3,30] When performing a shave preparation, care should be taken to prevent nicks, scratches, or cuts because any breaks in the skin surface provide a medium for the growth of microorganisms and a resultant infection.

The preparation begins with a mechanical scrubbing at the incision site and is extended in a circular fashion away from the site to the periphery. At the periphery the preparation sponge is considered contaminated and is discarded. The soiled sponge is never brought back over the area previously scrubbed. Each time the area is scrubbed a new sponge is used.

When it is necessary to prepare an area that includes an open draining wound or a body orifice, the practice of cleansing from the incision site to the periphery is modified. The alterations of the preparation are based on the principle that the cleaning proceeds from clean to dirty areas. The most contaminated area is scrubbed last, even if it is the site of the surgical incision.

ANESTHESIA

The field of anesthesiology is acknowledged as a major contributor to medicine and has enabled the growth and scientific development of modern surgery. The term *anesthesia* is derived from the Greek word *anaisthesis* meaning "no sensation."[23]

In the early nineteenth century alcohol or opium was given to patients for pain relief or for muscle relaxation during surgical procedures. Surgeons had to work rapidly to complete the surgical procedure because these drugs were unable to provide sufficient pain relief or relaxation. In 1842 the surgeon Crawford Long began using ether as an anesthetic for surgical patients, but he did not publish his work until 1849. In 1846 dentists Horace Wells and William Morton used nitrous oxide for dental extractions. Later that year William Morton demonstrated the use of ether as an effective method for rendering a surgical patient unconscious. Morton's work provided the foundation for the modern practice of anesthesia.[15]

Anesthesia is the limited or total loss of feeling with or without loss of consciousness. The two broad classifications of anesthesia are general and local. General anesthesia produces unconsciousness; local anesthesia creates a loss of sensation in a particular area. The method of administering the anesthesia and the choice of anesthetic agent for a particular patient are determined by the anesthesiologist (Table 17-4). Factors that influence the decision include the patient's preference; the patient's age, physical status, and emotional status; presence of coexisting disease; type and length of the surgical procedure; patient's position during the surgical procedure; postoperative recovery from specific anesthetic agents; and any requirements of the surgeon. The American Society of Anesthesiologists developed a classification system to identify risk factors based on the patient's health status (see Chapter 16). As part of the preoperative evaluation the anesthesiologist classifies the patient according to the physical status.

Operating room nurses do not administer anesthetic agents, but they must have an understanding of the various anesthetics used in surgery, the methods of administration, and the potential side effects and complications. This knowledge enables the nurse to plan intraoperative nursing care and to assist the anesthesia team.

Types of Anesthesia

General Anesthesia

General anesthesia is the depression of the central nervous system by administration of drugs or inhalation agents. The exact methods by which general anesthetic agents produce unconsciousness, analgesia, and muscle relaxation are unknown. It is thought that each anesthetic affects the central nervous and musculoskeletal systems in unique ways and works with multiple sites and areas to create these effects.[18,23]

Depth of Aesthesia. For anesthesia to be safe, the anesthesiologist must monitor its depth or level. Guidelines to estimate the depth or level of anesthesia used to be based on clearly delineated physiologic changes and reflex responses that were seen with the administration of ether (Box 17-2). Because ether is no longer used, physiologic responses may vary with the variety of agents and techniques used today. However, these guidelines can still be used to estimate the depth of anesthesia.

A more recent method of monitoring the depth of anesthesia and sedation is the Bispectral Index (BIS). The BIS is a simple monitoring device that provides a number representing the depth of anesthesia. The number ranges from 100 (fully conscious) to 0 (absence of brain activity); 40 represents profound coma. Although sources vary, research indicates that patients with the depth of anesthesia maintained at a BIS of 45 to 65 allows less anesthetic, no intraoperative awareness, faster recovery, and reduced postoperative complications.[27] Although BIS seems to be a consistent marker for the depth of anesthesia, one disadvantage is that BIS values vary depending on the combination of anesthetic agents used.[12,34]

Phases of General Anesthesia. The three phases of general anesthesia are the induction phase, maintenance phase, and emergence phase. *Induction* begins with the administration of intravenous agents or with the inhalation of a combination of anesthetic gases and oxygen. Endotracheal intubation is performed during this phase. This phase is completed when the patient is ready for positioning, skin preparation, or the incision.

Once it is safe for any of these activities to commence, the patient has entered the *maintenance* phase of anesthesia. During this phase the anesthesiologist maintains the appropriate levels of anesthesia with inhalation agents and intravenous medications. The anesthesiologist pays close attention to the surgical field and anticipates the surgeon's actions in order to alter the depth of anesthesia whenever necessary.

TABLE 17-4 Comparison of Types of Anesthesia

Type	Expected Result	Method of Administration	Risks
General	Reversible unconsciousness Analgesia Anesthesia Amnesia Muscle relaxation (immobility) Depression of reflexes	Inhalation Intravenous injection	Oral or dental injury Cardiac or respiratory arrest Residual muscle paralysis Hypertension Hypotension Hypothermia Hyperthermia Renal dysfunction Neurologic dysfunction
Regional			
Spinal	Analgesia Anesthesia Muscle relaxation	Anesthetic agent injected into the cerebrospinal fluid (CSF) in the subarachnoid space	Hypotension Total spinal anesthesia (inadvertent high level of spinal anesthesia, causing respiratory arrest and complete paralysis) Neurologic complications (tinnitis, arachnoiditis, meningitis, paresthesias, bowel/bladder dysfunction, paralysis) Headache Infection
Epidural	Analgesia Anesthesia Muscle relaxation	Anesthetic agent injected into epidural space and CSF	Dural puncture Intravascular injection with possible convulsions, hypotension, cardiac arrest Hypotension Total spinal anesthesia Neurologic complications Hematoma Infection
Nerve block	Anesthesia of selected nerve	Local anesthetic injected around peripheral nerve	Inadvertent intravascular injection Nerve damage
Intravenous (Bier block)	Anesthesia of extremity (usually used on upper extremity)	Anesthetic agent injected into veins of arm or leg while using a pneumatic tourniquet	Infection Pain from tourniquet Overdose or toxicity of anesthetic agent Infection
Monitored anesthesia care	Analgesia Anesthesia Amnesia Decreased level of consciousness with ability for purposeful responses to verbal and tactile stimuli Ability to independently maintain airway Safe monitoring of patient Anxiety relief	Anesthesia provider present to monitor patient May supplement local or regional anesthetic with analgesics, sedatives, or amnestics	Same as for local or regional Respiratory depression with use of adjuvant drugs
Sedation and analgesia (conscious sedation)	Ability to maintain independent cardiorespiratory function Decreased level of consciousness with ability for purposeful responses to verbal and tactile stimuli Sedation Analgesia Amnesia Anxiety relief Rapid safe return to activities of daily living	Intravenous injection May or may not have anesthesia provider in attendance; RN may have responsibility for patient monitoring	Oversedation Respiratory depression, apnea Airway obstruction Hypotension Aspiration
Local	Depresses peripheral nerves and blocks conduction of pain impulses	Administration of anesthetic agent by surgeon to a specific area of the body by topical application or local infiltration	Allergic reaction Toxicity Cardiac or respiratory arrest Anxiety due to "awake" state of patient Infection

BOX 17-2 Stages of General Anesthesia

Stage I begins with the administration of anesthetic agents and ends with the loss of consciousness. This is also known as the relaxation stage.

Stage II begins with the loss of consciousness and ends with the onset of regular breathing and loss of eyelid reflexes. This stage is referred to as the excitement or delirium phase because it is often accompanied by involuntary motor activity. The patient must not receive any auditory or physical stimulation during this period.

Stage III begins with the onset of regular breathing and ends with the cessation of respirations. This stage is known as the operative or surgical phase.

Stage IV begins with the cessation of respiration and leads to death.

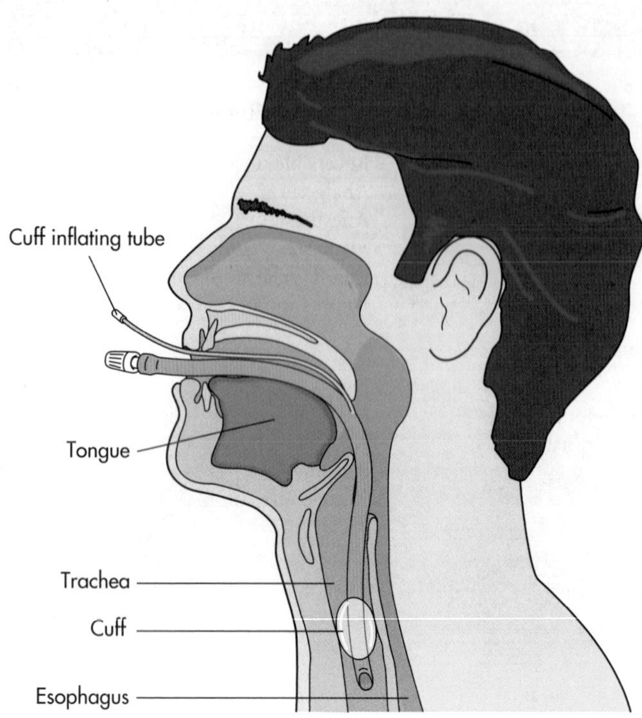

Figure 17-5 Endotracheal tube in position.

The *emergence* period begins when the anesthesiologist decreases the anesthetic agents and the patient begins to awaken. Extubation usually occurs during this period. Potential complications during this period include laryngospasm, vomiting, slow spontaneous respirations, and uncontrolled reflex movement.

Balanced Anesthesia. Balanced anesthesia is one of the most commonly used methods of administering general anesthesia. This method combines various agents to produce hypnosis, analgesia, and muscle relaxation with a minimum of physiologic disturbances. Each agent is administered for a specific purpose. Intravenous barbiturates are used for induction, regional anesthetics are used for muscle relaxation and analgesia, and inhalation agents are used for maintenance. Variations of this technique are used depending on the patient's physical status and the requirements of the surgical procedure.

Inhalation Anesthesia. Inhalation anesthesia is produced by administering a mixture of anesthetic gases and oxygen directly to the lungs. The gases are passed into pulmonary circulation, delivered to the brain and other body tissues, and are readily eliminated through the respiratory system. These agents are administered to the patient by a face mask or directly into the lungs through an endotracheal tube (Figure 17-5).

The endotracheal tube may have a balloon that is inflated after insertion; the balloon fills the tracheal space, lessening the chance of aspiration of gastric contents. Regardless of the skill of the anesthesiologist, an endotracheal tube may cause some irritation to the trachea and subsequent edema. After surgery it is not uncommon for the patient to report a sore, irritated throat. Some of the more common inhalation anesthetics in use are described in Table 17-5.

Several measures are used during inhalation anesthesia to promote the safety of both patient and health care workers. Oxygen is administered by mask or endotracheal tube throughout the procedure. The percentage of oxygen saturation in the blood is measured by pulse oximetry or in some cases by arterial monitoring. A scavenging method for waste anesthetics (carbon dioxide absorber) must be used to avoid unnecessary exposure to health care personnel. In addition, breathing circuits, masks, endotracheal tubes, and reservoir bags are all disposable, providing a clean circuit for each patient, thus avoiding potential cross-contamination.

Intravenous Anesthetic Agents. Intravenous drugs are also used to achieve a safe, reversible state of anesthesia. Patients may prefer an intravenous anesthesia induction because it is rapid and generally pleasant. Because of patient satisfaction it has become a routine practice to induce general anesthesia with intravenous agents regardless of the agent used for maintenance.

Intravenous anesthetic agents can be used alone or as supplements to inhalation agents (Table 17-6). Intravenous agents provide hypnosis, sedation, amnesia, and/or analgesia and are injected into a peripheral vein. Unlike inhalation agents, which are reversed by discontinuing the drug and ventilating the lungs with 100% oxygen, intravenous drugs must be metabolized by the liver and excreted by the kidneys.

Opioid Analgesics. Opioids provide analgesia and sedation and can be used in high doses as anesthetics for short surgical procedures (Table 17-7). These drugs are administered either in bolus doses or by continuous intravenous infusion. The opioids do not produce muscle relaxation; in fact they may cause an increase in muscle tone. Neuromuscular blocking agents are used during surgery to counteract this action.

After surgery patients who receive high-dose opioid anesthesia are susceptible to respiratory depression. Patients may hypoventilate and become hypoxic; therefore careful monitoring of vital signs is necessary in the postoperative period. Opioid-induced respiratory depression can be reversed with the administration of an opioid antagonist such as naloxone (Narcan).

Neuromuscular Blocking Agents. Neuromuscular blocking agents are used as adjuncts to anesthetic agents. The major action of the neuromuscular blocking agents is the relaxation of voluntary muscles. These agents are used to facilitate the

TABLE 17-5 Commonly Used Inhalation Agents

Agent	Indication	Advantages	Disadvantages
Nitrous oxide (N_2O)	Maintenance; sometimes for induction	Rapid induction and emergence; additive effects to other anesthetics	Poor muscle relaxation; can depress myocardium; risk of hypoxia with high does or faulty anesthesia machine
Desflurane (Suprane)	Induction; used in ambulatory surgery and shorter procedures	Rapid induction and emergence; low lipid-solubility, good choice for obese patients	Can cause coughing with induction; causes ↑ heart rate and ↓ blood pressure
Enflurane (Ethrane)	Maintenance; sometimes for induction	Good relaxation; permits larger amounts of epinephrine to be used than with halothane	Can cause ↑ heart rate and ↓ blood pressure; risk of nephrotoxicity; slightly irritating odor
Halothane (Fluothane)	Maintenance; sometimes for induction	Rapid induction and emergence; pleasant, nonirritating odor	Sensitizes myocardium to epinephrine; ↓ heart rate and arterial blood pressure; risk for arrhythmias; risk of hepatoxicity; delayed emergence in obese patients
Isoflurane (Forane)	Maintenance; sometimes for induction	Good relaxation; rapid induction and emergence; little myocardial depression; safe for patients with hepatic and renal disease	↑ Heart rate; slightly irritating odor
Sevoflurane (Ultane)	Induction (often with mask); maintenance	Rapid induction and emergence; pleasant odor	Risk of nephrotoxicity; costly

TABLE 17-6 Commonly Used Intravenous Agents

Agent	Indication	Advantages	Disadvantages
Diazepam (Valium)	Amnesia; hypnotic; sedation; analgesia	Good sedation	Prolonged duration; irritating to vein
Etomidate (Amidate)	Induction	Rapid induction and emergence; fewer cardiovascular and respiratory effects than thiopental	Pain with injection; may cause spontaneous muscle movements; ↑ incidence of nausea and vomiting after induction; costly
Ketamine (Ketalar)	Induction; occasional maintenance; good for dressing changes, wound debridement, and short diagnostic procedures; may be administered intravenously, intramuscularly, orally, or rectally	Short acting; patient maintains airway; produces amnesia; good choice for patients with reactive airway disease	May cause emergence reactions including confusion, hallucinations, euphoria; may cause ↑ heart rate and blood pressure; ↑ intracranial pressure;no muscle relaxation
Methohexital sodium (Brevitol)	Induction	Rapid onset and very short duration of action	May cause hiccups; respiratory depression, apnea; laryngosapasm; hypotension; pain with injection
Midazolam (Versed)	Hypnotic; sedation; analgesia; amnesic; anxiolytic	Rapid onset and short duration; no pain with injection	Respiratory depressant; prolonged effect with obese patients
Propofol (Diprivan)	Induction; maintenance; good choice for short procedures and ambulatory surgery	Rapid onset and short duration; other properties include antiemetic, antipruritic, anxiolytic	Respiratory depression, may cause apnea after induction; bradycardia; ↓ blood pressure; may cause tremors, dystonia, and spontaneous muscle movement during induction and emergence; pain at injection site
Thiopental sodium (Pentothal)	Induction; brief anesthesia without analgesia	Rapid induction and emergence; anticonvulsant	Respiratory depression, apnea; laryngospasm; hypotension

TABLE 17-7 Commonly Used Opioid Analgesics

Agent	Indication	Advantages	Disadvantages
Alfentanil (Alfenta)	Induction; balanced anesthesia	Rapid onset and short duration	Respiratory depression, apnea; half-life prolonged in patients with cirrhosis; nausea
Fentanyl (Sublimase, Duragesic)	Surgical analgesia; supplement to other anesthetic agents	Rapid onset and short duration	Circulatory and respiratory depression
Remifentanil (Ultiva)	Induction and maintenance; surgical analgesia	Rapid action; easily titrated	Respiratory depression; nausea; costly
Sufentanil (Sufenta)	Balanced anesthesia; surgical analgesia; supplement to other anesthetic agents	Rapid onset and recovery; seven times more potent than fentanyl	Respiratory depression, apnea; skeletal muscle rigidity; pruritis

TABLE 17-8 Commonly Used Neuromuscular Blocking Agents

Agent	Indication	Advantages	Disadvantages
Depolarizing Muscle Relaxant			
Succinylcholine (Anectine)	Intubation; short procedures	Rapid onset; short duration	Bradycardia; respiratory depression; increased intracranial pressure; causes muscle fasciculation and release of potassium; avoid in patients with renal failure, burns, neuromuscular disease; causes ↑ intracranial pressure (ICP); postoperative dysrhythmias
Nondepolarizing muscle relaxants			
Atracurium (Tracrium)	Intubation; maintenance	Good choice for patients with renal and hepatic disease; minimal cardiovascular effects	Respiratory depression; cautious use in patients with cardiovascular disease and asthma due to histamine release
d-tubocurarine chloride (Curare)	Maintenance; may be given before depolarizing agent (succinylcholine)	No effect on intellectual functions or consciousness	↓ Blood pressure, circulatory collapse; respiratory depression, apnea, bronchospasm; may cause histamine release; no anesthetic or analgesic properties
Pancuronimum (Pavulon)	Maintenance	Rapid action; five times as potent as tubocurarine with less histamine release	May ↑ heart rate and blood pressure in high doses; respiratory depression
Rocuronium (Zemuron)	Intubation; maintenance	Rapid onset	↑ Heart rate; prolonged effects in patients with renal or hepatic dysfunction
Vecuronium (Noruron)	Intubation; maintenance	Minimal cardiovascular effects; little histamine release	Prolonged effects in patients with renal or hepatic dysfunction

passage of endotracheal tubes, prevent laryngospasm, control muscle tone throughout the surgical procedure, and decrease the amount of general anesthesia used. Neuromuscular blocking agents interfere with the transfer of impulses from the motor nerves to the voluntary muscle cells.

The two categories of neuromuscular blocking agents are depolarizing and nondepolarizing agents (Table 17-8). Depolarizing agents react with receptors at the end plate region of the muscle and begin depolarization of the muscle membrane, which causes muscle contraction. The muscle contraction is uncoordinated and is referred to as muscle fasciculation. After surgery patients may complain of muscle stiffness and soreness resulting from muscle fasciculation.

Nondepolarizing agents cause paralysis of the voluntary muscles, are slower acting, and have a longer duration than depolarizing agents. These agents vary with rate of onset and duration and may interact with other drugs such as antibiotics and lead to prolonged muscle relaxation.

Regional Anesthesia

Regional anesthesia causes a temporary loss of sensation in a particular portion of the body by the use of local anesthet-

TABLE 17-9 Commonly Used Local Anesthetic Agents

Agent	Indication	Advantages	Disadvantages
Bupivacaine (Marcaine, Sensoracaine)	Epidural, spinal, peripheral nerve block, local	Minimal cardiovascular effects; addition of epinephrine to ↓ rate of absorption also ↓ risk of systemic toxic reaction; prolongs anesthetic effects	Elderly more at risk for systemic toxic reaction; overdose can cause cardiac arrest
Lidocaine (Xylocaine)	Epidural, spinal, peripheral, intravenous blocks, local	Short acting; low toxicity	Overdose can lead to cardiac and respiratory arrest and convulsions; cautious use in patients with family history of malignant hyperthermia
Procaine hydrochloride (Novocain)	Spinal, peripheral nerve block, local	Rapidly absorbed from injection site; low toxicity; no local irritation	Low potency; possible anaphylaxis
Tetracaine (Pontocaine)	Spinal; topical	Long duration; 10 times more potent than procaine	Slow onset; possible anaphylaxis; 10 times more toxic than procaine; higher risk of systemic toxicity

TABLE 17-10 Advantages and Disadvantages of Regional Anesthesia

Advantages	Disadvantages
Simplicity	Lack of patient acceptance—patient's fear of being awake during the surgical procedure
Reasonable cost	Impracticality of anesthetizing certain areas of the body
Easily induced	Insufficient duration of anesthesia—patient's fear anesthetic will wear off prematurely
Minimum equipment required	Rapid absorption of agent into circulation can lead to cardiac arrest
↓Postoperative care requirements	
Fewer systemic effects on body functions	
Avoidance of adverse effects of general anesthesia	
↓ Nausea and vomiting	
Can be used for a variety of patients in circumstances where general anesthesia is contraindicated	

ics. Local anesthetics temporarily prevent generation and conduction of nerve impulses and may or may not affect motor functions (Table 17-9).

Regional anesthetics are used with patients in whom general anesthesia is contraindicated. The advantages and disadvantages of its use are outlined in Table 17-10. The types of regional anesthesia are spinal, epidural, nerve block, and intravenous or Bier block.

Spinal Anesthesia. Spinal anesthesia is usually administered for surgical procedures performed on the lower abdomen, inguinal region, perineum, or lower extremities. With the patient lying on one side curled into a fetal position or in a sitting position, a local anesthetic agent is injected into the cerebrospinal fluid in the subarachnoid space (Figure 17-6). After injection of the local anesthetic, there is an almost immediate onset of anesthesia at the site.

The duration and level of spinal anesthesia are determined by the site and speed of injection, body height or length of the vertebral column, specific gravity of the anesthetic agent, intraabdominal pressure, and position of the patient immediately after injection. Patient position is extremely important when using hyperbaric agents (agents with a specific gravity heavier than that of the spinal fluid), because gravity moves the anesthetic agents to the lowest point of the vertebral column. Altering the position of the patient causes the hyperbaric agent to be directed up, down, or to a particular side of the spinal cord.

One of the most common postoperative complaints of patients who have spinal anesthesia is headache. The headache occurs because cerebrospinal fluid leaks out of the dura from the opening made by the spinal needle. This leads to a decreased pressure within the spinal cord, which causes the headache when the patient assumes an upright position. Treatment modalities include strict bed rest in the supine position for 24 to 48 hours, hydration, analgesia, epidural blood patch (5 to 20 ml of the patient's blood is injected at the puncture site), and application of an abdominal binder to increase pressure. The severity and occurrence of postspinal headaches have been reduced by using a needle that separates the dural fibers instead of cutting them with a blunt-bevel needle.[23]

Epidural Anesthesia. Epidural anesthesia is achieved when a local anesthetic agent is injected through the intervertebral space into the space surrounding the dura mater in the spinal column (see Figure 17-6). The anesthesia is administered either through a single dose or intermittently through an epidural catheter. This type of anesthesia is used in abdominal,

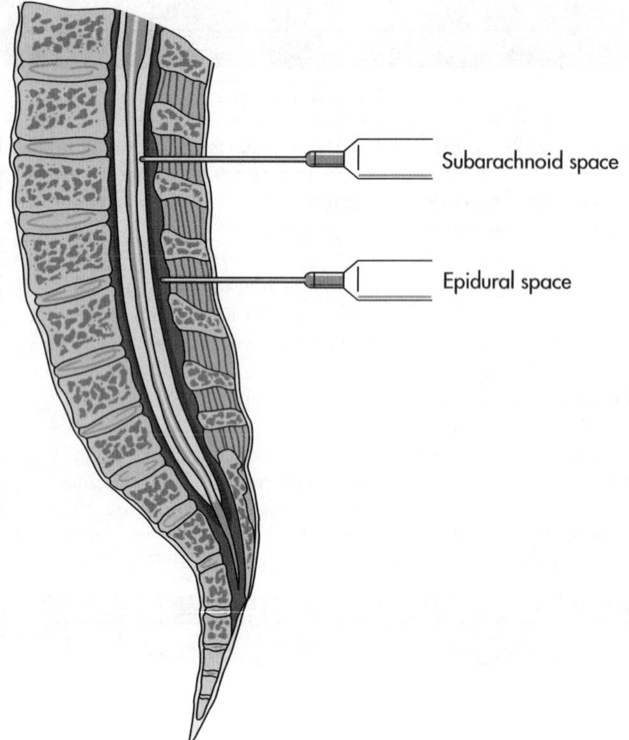

Figure 17-6 Agent is injected into subarachnoid space for spinal anesthesia or into epidural space for epidural anesthesia.

genitourinary, and lower extremity procedures. In contrast to spinal anesthesia, epidural anesthesia requires greater doses of local anesthetics, has a slower onset of anesthesia, and is not dependent on the patient's position for the level of anesthesia. Advantages include the ability to titrate dosing throughout the procedure and decreased incidence of postoperative headache and neurologic complications.

Nerve Block. A nerve block is achieved with the injection of a local anesthetic into or around a nerve or group of nerves that innervates the operative site. Examples include intercostal, axillary, and digital blocks. Nerve blocks are used to interfere with sensory, motor, or sympathetic transmissions. Onset and length of the block depend on the amount and concentration of the anesthetic. Besides intraoperative use, nerve blocks are also used to relieve chronic pain.

Intravenous Regional Anesthesia. Intravenous regional anesthesia or Bier block is achieved by administering local anesthetic agents into the venous system of an exsanguinated extremity. A tourniquet is used to prevent the agent from entering the systemic circulation. When the tourniquet is deflated at the end of the procedure, the patient is monitored for systemic effects of the local anesthetic, which may cause cardiovascular or central nervous system complications. Advantages of this technique are a quick onset of anesthesia and a short recovery time. The major disadvantage of this technique is that it is limited to procedures lasting 2 hours or less. If the tourniquet is inflated longer than 2 hours, tissue damage can occur.

Monitored Anesthesia Care

Monitored anesthesia care, like general anesthesia, uses sedatives and other anesthetic agents but in lower dosages that allow the patient to remain responsive and breathe independently. Indications are for minor surgeries or as a supplement to local or regional anesthesia. Advantages for the patient include anxiety relief, amnesia, analgesia, comfort, and safety. A member of the anesthesia team is present to monitor the patient's vital signs, respiratory status, and cardiac status and administer oxygen as needed. In addition to monitoring the patient's physical status, the anesthesia provider can administer intravenous analgesics, sedatives, or amnestic agents as necessary for patient comfort.

Sedation and Analgesia

The American Society of Anesthesiologists (ASA) in conjunction with JCAHO has developed standards and definitions for levels of sedation and anesthesia. Moderate sedation and analgesia, formerly known as conscious sedation (see also Chapter 12), is a drug-induced depression of consciousness in which the patient is able to respond purposefully to verbal commands and tactile stimulation. Cardiovascular function is usually maintained, and the patient is able to independently maintain an airway and spontaneous ventilation.[19] Moderate sedation and analgesia is commonly administered to patients undergoing ambulatory surgical procedures and short surgical or diagnostic procedures that require sedation and amnesia. Advantages for the patient include relief of fear and anxiety, elevation of pain threshold, maintenance of consciousness and protective reflexes, amnesia, and a quick return to normal activities.

Orders for medications used during sedation and analgesia must be written by the physician performing the procedure or anesthesia provider. The American Nurses Association and AORN have determined that registered nurses may administer these medications, assess patient's responses, and monitor the patient during the procedure.[24] Qualifications of nurses administering medications and protocols for patient care during sedation and analgesia vary by state and institution.

Local Anesthesia

Local anesthetic agents can be used alone or in conjunction with other types of anesthesia including inhalation and intravenous agents. The patient's condition, the procedure performed, and the use of other agents determine whether an anesthesia provider will be present to monitor the patient. In some instances the registered nurse is responsible for patient monitoring. To ensure patient safety and quality of care the AORN has developed recommended practices for nurses who monitor patients receiving local anesthetics.

Local anesthesia interferes with the initiation and transmission of nerve impulses by the use of mediations administered topically or injected by local infiltration, regional block, or field block (anesthetic agent is injected into a wide area surrounding the surgical site). Motor and sensory nerves are affected, resulting in paralysis of both voluntary and involuntary muscles. The action of the local anesthetic and systemic

TABLE 17-11 Patient Monitoring Methods during Anesthesia

Parameter	Methods
Arterial blood pressure	Auscultation method using blood pressure cuff and stethoscope
	Direct measurement with arterial cannulation and connection to pressure transducer (arterial line)
	Automatic device that measures systolic, diastolic, and mean blood pressure and heart rate
Heart rate	Palpation of superficial artery
	Auscultation of the heart with a precordial or esophageal stethoscope
	Doppler monitoring probe applied to radial pulse
	Electrocardiogram with continual display
Respiratory status	Direct observation of chest movements
	Auscultation of the chest with a stethoscope or esophageal stethoscope
Body temperature	Skin surface probes or strips applied to body to monitor surface temperature
	Core temperature probe inserted into nasophyarynx, esophagus, bladder, or rectum*
Urinary output	Indwelling urinary catheter
Pulse oximetry	Noninvasive measurement of arterial oxyhemoglobin saturation (Sao_2)
Capnography—end-tidal carbon dioxide ($EtCO_2$)	Noninvasive measurement of end-tidal concentration of carbon dioxide
	Detects changes in respiratory, circulatory, or metabolic status
	Useful to detect onset of inadvertent hypothermia, malignant hyperthermia, and anesthesia equipment problems
BIS Monitor	Using electroencephalogram technology to monitor depth of anesthesia

*Note that core temperature is best measured via esophageal or pulmonary artery probes. Bladder and rectal temperatures are not universally accepted as a true measurement of core temperature.

absorption are affected by local blood flow and vascular supply to the region. Medications may be given to either increase or decrease the rate of absorption; for instance epinephrine can be added to the local agent causing vasoconstriction and increased anesthesia time. Another advantage of adding epinephrine to the local anesthetic is decreased bleeding at the surgical site.

The patient may experience a burning and stinging sensation with injection of the local agent. Side effects include allergic and toxic reactions. Although the physician is administering the local anesthetic, it is important to monitor the amount of medication the patient is receiving, as toxic reactions are dose-related. Another factor that may lead to toxic reactions is the addition of epinephrine owing to increased catecholamine response.[33] Signs of toxicity may include tachypnea, bradycardia or tachycardia, perioral numbness, tinnitus, drowsiness, metallic taste, paresthesias, tremors, seizures, and coma.

Other Types of Anesthesia

Induced hypothermia may be used as an adjunct to other anesthetic agents. Hypothermia refers to the reduction of body temperature below normal to reduce oxygen and metabolic requirements. Extracorporeal cooling, a method of bloodstream cooling, consists of removing the blood from a major vessel, circulating it through coils immersed in a refrigerant, and returning it to the body through another vessel. Bloodstream cooling is the fastest method for producing hypothermia and is used primarily for patients undergoing open-heart surgery and brain surgery.

Monitoring the Patient

During any surgical procedure the patient is subjected to many stressors. Potent anesthetic agents, tissue trauma, blood loss, and positioning are all stressors that can interfere with and alter the patient's respiratory and cardiovascular status. Continuous monitoring and assessment are necessary to detect changes in the patient's physiologic status and to initiate necessary treatment in a timely manner.

Basic intraoperative monitoring standards have been developed by the ASA. The AORN has developed Standards of Care to guide the practice of nurses working in the perioperative setting. Both organizations have determined that the basic standards include performing electrocardiograms (ECGs); monitoring blood pressure, heart rate, and temperature; and continuous monitoring of ventilation, circulation, and level of consciousness. Both invasive and noninvasive methods are used for monitoring the patient. Automatic devices are also used to assist in the monitoring processes (Table 17-11). It is imperative that the anesthesiologist and nurse be familiar with the functions and uses of the specialized equipment and ensure that it is in proper working order. Even with the availability of automatic monitoring equipment, it is necessary for the anesthesiologist or nurse to remain in close contact with the patient to immediately observe any significant physiologic changes.

During the procedure, monitoring of the anesthetized patient's vital functions is primarily the responsibility of the anesthesiologist. Throughout the surgical procedure the circulating nurse assists in patient monitoring by estimating and reporting blood loss, measuring urine output, and assessing the patient's overall status. In emergent situations, the circulating nurse provides assistance to the anesthesia team.

Nurse's Role During Induction and Emergence

The induction of and emergence from general anesthesia are critical points in the intraoperative care of the patient. During induction the circulating nurse should remain at the bedside to provide the patient with physical and psychologic support and to assist the anesthesia provider. The circulating nurse should ensure a quiet calm atmosphere; excessive noise and movement of the patient should be avoided at this time. The circulating nurse may be asked to assist the anesthesia provider by providing pressure to the cricoid cartilage before intubation. This technique, known as Sellick's maneuver, prevents aspiration and regurgitation of stomach contents by obstructing the esophagus and is commonly performed for patients at risk for pulmonary aspiration (see Research box).

There are similar concerns for patient care during emergence from general anesthesia. To ensure safety the circulating nurse should remain at the patient's side to ensure safety and provide assistance to the anesthesia provider. Maintenance of a patent airway and ventilation are the primary responsibility of the anesthesia provider; however, the nurse needs to be available to assist as necessary. Safety and comfort are primary nursing concerns as the patient may exhibit retching, vomiting, shivering, or restlessness during emergence.

Anesthesia Complications

Anesthetic-related operative mortality rate is relatively low. For a healthy person the risk is about 0.01%. Some of the more common complications of anesthesia are related to untoward reactions to the anesthetic agent. The major complication is cardiac arrest. Laryngospasm and inhalation of gastric contents are serious potential complications that may occur during the emergence or induction phase of general anesthesia.

As discussed in Chapter 16, evidence does not support the traditional NPO past midnight fasting guidelines. The ASA revised guidelines for healthy patients undergoing elective procedures recommend the following minimal fasting periods: clear liquids 2 to 4 hours, a light meal 6 hours, and meat and fatty foods 8 hours.[36] It is important to remember that these are recommendations only and clinical practice may vary.

Both general and regional anesthesia cause a dilation of peripheral blood vessels and a drop in blood pressure. Venous blood pools in dependent areas, reducing blood return to the heart and lungs for oxygenation and redistribution. General anesthesia depresses the medulla, which maintains cardiac

Research

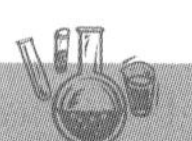

Reference: Koziol CA, Cuddeford JD, Moos DD: Assessing the force generated with application of cricoid pressure, *AORN J* 72(6):1018, 2000.

Pulmonary aspiration of gastroesophageal contents during induction is a serious complication of general anesthesia. The application of cricoid pressure, or Sellick's maneuver, is a standard of care for patients at risk for pulmonary aspiration. However, the effectiveness in preventing aspiration depends on the technique of the person performing the maneuver. Nurses at the patient's side during induction are in a key position to perform this maneuver.

Applying pressure to the cricoid cartilage as a means to avoid airway obstruction was described as early as the 1770s. In 1961 Sellick described this technique for induction of patients undergoing emergency and obstetrical anesthesia.

Cricoid pressure is most often applied to patients at risk for pulmonary aspiration. Patients at risk include those with increased gastric volume, elevated gastric pressure, or impaired laryngeal-pharyngeal function, usually as a result of decreased level of consciousness. Nonfasting patients and those with prolonged periods of fasting are both at risk for aspiration as a result of increased gastric volume. Other causes of increased gastric volume include delayed gastric emptying, diabetic neuropathy, bowel obstruction, and opioid administration. Common causes of elevated gastric pressure include nausea, vomiting, ascites, obesity, and pregnancy.

Cricoid pressure is performed by compressing the cricoid cartilage against the body of the sixth cervical vertebra, thus obstructing the esophagus. Cricoid pressure is applied when laryngeal reflexes are lost as a result of administration of anesthetic agents and is continued until a cuffed endotracheal tube is correctly placed. When the maneuver is correctly performed, cricoid pressure provides better visualization with the laryngoscope and allows for smooth intubation. Improperly applied cricoid pressure may allow aspiration and distort or obstruct the airway.

Although widely accepted as an effective method, both nursing and medical literature before the mid-1990s contained ambiguous information regarding correct performance of the application of cricoid pressure, particularly regarding the amount of force necessary. Recent research has shown that 3 to 4 kg of force is necessary to achieve obstruction of the esophagus, effectively preventing aspiration of gastroesophageal contents into the airway. Research has also shown there is a wide variation of cricoid force applied by anesthesia care providers, nurses, and paramedical personnel in the clinical setting.

The primary purpose of this study was to assess perioperative nurses' knowledge regarding the recommended amount of cricoid pressure. Researchers also studied the amount of cricoid force applied to a model of the cricoid cartilage.

This study was conducted in a community hospital, veterans hospital, and an AORN professional meeting. The convenience sample consisted of 102 perioperative nurses. Participants were given a questionnaire designed to measure their knowledge regarding cricoid pressure. The nurses were also given a model to demonstrate the amount of force they typically apply to a patient in the OR.

On the questionnaire only 5% of the participants identified the correct amount of cricoid pressure, 78.5% under estimated, and 16.5% over estimated the correct amount. Only 13% of the participants applied the correct amount of pressure on the model. Again the majority (69.5%) applied less than the recommended force.

Clearly results indicate a startling lack of knowledge and skill regarding cricoid pressure among perioperative nurses. Education and training to provide the cognitive knowledge and skill to effectively perform the application of cricoid force should be included in the orientation program of all persons who may perform this technique. Following the orientation performance could be measured by annual clinical competency testing. Further research could replicate this study using a larger random sample of perioperative nurses as well as including anesthesia care providers.

output and peripheral vascular constriction. Muscle relaxants reduce the milking action of normal muscles that assists in venous return. The anesthesiologist constantly monitors the patient and is prepared to compensate for complications of these changes when they occur. The circulating nurse, knowledgeable about anesthesia methods, patient risk factors, complications, and preventive interventions, is able to provide efficient and appropriate assistance to the anesthesia team members. Common postoperative complications and interventions used to prevent or treat them are discussed in Chapter 18.

Malignant Hyperthermia

Malignant hyperthermia (MH), first identified in the 1960s, is a serious and potentially fatal complication of general anesthesia. Even though MH occurs most commonly during induction or during the surgical procedure, it can occur in the PACU or on the nursing unit 24 to 72 hours after surgery. Malignant hyperthermia can also recur 24 to 72 hours after surgery. Malignant hyperthermia reportedly occurs in 1 in 50,000 adults and 3 in 15,000 children.[20,35] This hypermetabolic syndrome is more common in children with a mean age of 18.3 years.[20] With prompt recognition and treatment, the mortality rate is less than 10%.[35]

Malignant hyperthermia is a genetic autosomal dominant defect that results in a disorder of muscle metabolism. It is triggered by certain anesthetic agents (Box 17-3) and extreme physiologic and emotional stress. A genetic defect in the muscle cell membrane permits anesthetic agents to trigger a sudden increase of calcium ions within the muscle cells. The rapid increase of calcium starts a series of biochemical reactions that elevate the metabolic rate, causing hyperthermia (with temperatures rising to 43° C), muscle rigidity, respiratory and metabolic acidosis, and cell breakdown. Muscle rigidity occurs in 75% of patients with MH.[20] Diagnostic findings include hypercalcemia, metabolic and respiratory acidosis, hyperkalemia, hypermagnesemia, and elevated serum creatine phosphokinase (CPK).

Jaw spasms or fasciculations after administration of succinylcholine during induction should alert the anesthesiologist to the potential for an MH episode. The earliest and most consistent clinical sign of MH is unexplained ventricular dysrhythmia, specifically tachycardia or premature ventricular contractions, which is associated with an increase in end-tidal carbon dioxide. Other clinical symptoms include tachypnea, cyanosis, dysrhythmias, skin mottling, unstable blood pressure, elevated levels of CPK, and elevated levels of myoglobin. As a result of desaturation, blood at the surgical field may appear dark. The patient's temperature may rise 1° C to 2° C every 5 minutes and may exceed 43° C. Because it occurs in the late stages, an elevated temperature is not a reliable indicator of MH. The patient's urine may appear dark due to rhabdomyolysis (breakdown of striated muscle with excretion of myoglobin in urine). Other late clinical manifestations of MH include hyperkalemia, acute renal failure, left-sided heart failure, disseminated intravascular coagulation (DIC), pulmonary embolus, and neurologic deficits.

Treatment of the patient experiencing MH includes immediate cessation of the inhalation agent or muscle relaxant, administration of 100% oxygen, cooling with ice packs or cooling blankets, lavaging body cavities with iced saline, restoration of acid-base balance, treatment of hyperkalemia, and rapid intravenous infusion of dantrolene. Cooling measures should be discontinued when the patient's temperature reaches 38° C.

Dantrolene is the only known treatment able to stop an MH crisis. Dantrolene provides skeletal muscle relaxation and retards the biochemical actions that cause muscle contractions. Dosage recommendations by the Malignant Hyperthermia Association of the United States include an initial bolus of 2 to 3 mg/kg with subsequent dosing of up to10 mg/kg.[35]

Identification of patients at risk is the primary method for prevention of MH. The preoperative history should include an assessment of the patient's previous experience with surgery, unexplained complications or death of family members associated with anesthesia, or known muscular abnormalities. The CPK level may also be elevated, but this is not specific to MH because elevations may also occur as a result of alcoholism or muscle disease. A history of heatstroke in the patient or family may be significant. The key assessment finding in identifying those at risk for MH is unexplained death under general anesthesia. For persons with suspected MH, diagnosis is confirmed by preoperative muscle biopsy. Patients identified at risk for developing MH may be given dantrolene preoperatively as prophylaxis. Anesthetic agents known to trigger MH should not be administered. Family members of individuals with known MH should undergo diagnostic testing as a prophylactic measure.

Inadvertent Hypothermia

Hypothermia is a more common complication than hyperthermia. Inadvertent hypothermia should not be confused with induced hypothermia, a special anesthetic technique used during cardiac, neurosurgical, and transplant surgery.

Inadvertent hypothermia, a drop in core temperature to 35° C or below, is classified as mild, moderate, or severe. Untreated or severe hypothermia can lead to coma and death; below 20° C brain activity ceases. Inadvertent hypothermia

BOX 17-3 Anesthetic Agents Triggering Malignant Hyperthermia

Inhalation Agents

Halothane
Enflurane
Isoflurane
Desflurane
Sevoflurane

Neuromuscular Blocking Agent

Succinylcholine

Nondepolarizing Muscle Relaxant

Tubocurarine chloride

occurs in 60% to 90% of surgical patients and is associated with such adverse effects as shivering, patient discomfort, decreased drug metabolism, coagulopathy, increased catecholamine production, and postoperative myocardial infarction.[14] Because of decreased metabolism, the patient may have delayed recovery from anesthesia and increased postoperative morbidity and mortality.[11]

Anesthesia inhibits the reflexes that generate heat and decreases the thermoregulatory center in the hypothalamus, decreases the basal metabolic rate, and increases vasodilation. Anesthesia also causes normal protective reflexes such as shivering to be lost. In the OR the body may lose core heat by exposure to a cool environment, infusion of intravenous fluids, skin preparation with cool solutions, cold dry anesthetic gases, and via the surgical incision. Patients receiving general anesthesia commonly experience a 1° (−17.2° to −17.5° C) to 1.5° F loss in core temperature during the first hour of anesthesia.[15] Preoperative sedation, the length of the procedure, and blood and fluid losses add to the heat loss. Inadvertent hypothermia may result in cardiac dysrhythmias, metabolic acidosis, hyperglycemia, coagulopathy, decreased platelet aggregation, and coma. The usual signs of hypothermia are often masked by administration of anesthetic agents, and symptoms may not be evident until the postoperative period. Symptoms include shivering, speech impairment, cyanosis, decreased blood pressure, weak pulse, and dilated pupils. Shivering occurs as a hypothalamic response to a drop in core temperature and as result of some anesthetic agents. Untreated shivering can lead to increased O_2 consumption (as much as 400%), increased cardiac workload, cardiac ischemia, decreased cerebral blood flow, and hypoxia.[7,23]

Hypothermia also decreases the body's immunologic functioning. The incidence of surgical wound infection is increased in hypothermic patients.[7,11]

Intraoperative interventions to prevent and treat heat loss include humidification and warming of anesthetic gases; warming of blood products, IV fluids, and irrigation fluids; and various warming devices.

PHYSIOLOGIC STRESS RESPONSES TO SURGERY AND ANESTHESIA

Surgery affects all body systems and stimulates the physiologic response to stress. The physiologic components involved in the stress response include the central nervous system, hypothalamus, sympathetic nervous system, anterior and posterior pituitary glands, adrenal medulla, and adrenal cortex. Not all of these components are necessarily involved in the response to surgery. Refer to a physiology text for a thorough discussion of the stress response.

Neuroendocrine Responses

Neuroendocrine responses play a major role in the patient's reaction to the stress of surgery. Responses include stimulation of the autonomic nervous system (primarily the sympathetic nervous system) and stimulation of selected hormones (primarily aldosterone and glucocorticoid hormones from the adrenal cortex and antidiuretic hormone from the posterior pituitary). Table 17-12 summarizes the endocrine stress responses to surgery.

Stimulation of the sympathetic nervous system serves to protect the body from further damage. Vasoconstriction of peripheral blood vessels enables the body to compensate for blood loss and redirect blood flow to critical areas such as the heart and brain. Increased cardiac output also helps maintain blood flow. Severe trauma or excessive blood loss, however, will overwhelm the compensatory mechanisms, and blood pressure will fall. Certain types of anesthetics or high spinal

TABLE 17-12 Endocrine Stress Responses

Physiologic Changes	Results	Effect
↑ Norepinephrine secretion	Peripheral vasoconstriction ↓ Gastrointestinal activity	Helps maintain blood pressure when circulating volume is decreased May lead to anorexia or constipation
↑ Aldosterone secretion	Sodium retention	Maintains circulating blood volume Increases susceptibility to fluid overload Decreases urinary output
↑ Glucocorticoid secretion	Gluconeogenesis ↑ Protein catabolism Ketogenic effect Antiinflammatory effect ↑ Platelet production Increased gastric acid secretion	Provides energy to meet stress of surgery Provides an additional energy source Provides amino acids for cell synthesis after tissue destruction Provides fat as an energy source Increases susceptibility to infection Promotes clotting to prevent bleeding Contributes to development of thrombophlebitis
↑ Antidiuretic hormone (ADH) secretion	Sodium and water reabsorption in the kidney tubules	Maintains circulating blood volume Increases susceptibility to fluid overload Decreases urinary output Potential for hypokalemia

anesthesia also may interfere with the compensatory vasoconstriction, producing hypotension.

Another sympathetic response is decreased gastrointestinal activity, which may have an adverse effect on the patient. Before surgery psychologic stress may result in anorexia and constipation and postoperatively, the patient may experience anorexia, gas pains, and constipation from decreased peristalsis in the gastrointestinal tract.

Adrenocortical activity is increased in response to the trauma of surgery, producing greater amounts of aldosterone and cortisol. Aldosterone is released primarily from the adrenal cortex in response to activation of the renin-angiotensin system. Aldosterone acts on the distal kidney tubule cells causing sodium and water resorption and excretion of potassium and hydrogen ions. Aldosterone helps maintain vascular volume and blood pressure, which may compensate for blood and fluid loss during surgery.

During the first 24 to 48 hours after surgery increased aldosterone secretion is accompanied by an increase in antidiuretic hormone (ADH) secretion by the posterior pituitary gland. Water is resorbed by the kidney resulting in decreased urine output. Spontaneous diuresis occurs as the amount of ADH is decreased, usually in about 2 to 4 days.

Cortisol is released from the adrenal cortex and has major effects on glucose, protein, fat metabolism, and fluid and electrolyte balance; it also has antiinflammatory and immunosuppressant effects. Glucocorticoids also play a major role in the maintenance of blood pressure and cardiac output. Increased levels of cortisol in response to stress may stimulate gastric acid secretion, possibly resulting in ulceration of the gastric mucosa. Excessive cortisol may also result in poor wound healing, increased risk of infection, and decreased inflammatory response.

The stress response to surgery varies in intensity depending on the type and duration of surgery, the health of the individual patient, and the body's ability to adapt and respond to the stressor. Understanding the body's physiologic response to stress is critical to understanding the effects of prolonged or unresolved stress and the impact of surgical intervention on the patient's overall health and well-being.

Metabolic Responses

After surgery the patient is in a relative state of starvation; metabolism is increased and fluid and nutrient intake is decreased. Carbohydrate metabolism increases as a result of the increased production of glucocorticoid hormones. Usually there are periods when the patient is not permitted to eat and receives only intravenous fluids. The patient without oral intake experiences a daily fluid loss of more than 1200 ml/day. Maintenance fluids should be administered on the basis of body weight and at a rate sufficient to maintain urine output. Additional fluids may be needed to replace intraoperative blood or other fluid loss.

Anorexia also may occur as part of the stress response, thus adding to the problem of inadequate carbohydrate intake even if food is permitted by mouth. The body must meet its glucose needs by the breakdown of stored liver glycogen or by the synthesis of glucose from noncarbohydrate sources.

Fat metabolism increases to allow mobilization of fat from the cells as an energy source. With the decreased intake of carbohydrates and fats after surgery, body fats are metabolized for energy and the patient may lose weight. Protein metabolism is increased after surgery to supply essential amino acids necessary for tissue healing. The net effect of these metabolic processes depends on the patient's preoperative nutritional state.

OTHER CONSIDERATIONS

Bloodless Surgery

Bloodless surgery avoids the use of allogenic blood products. It is an alternative for patients with objections to receiving blood and blood products. Bloodless surgery reduces or eliminates the need for transfusions. Initially intended for Jehovah's Witnesses and patients with objections to receiving blood products, bloodless surgery can be used for any surgical patient. The concern regarding the risks of allogenic transfusion and blood shortages have resulted in more widespread application of bloodless techniques.

Techniques to decrease the need for blood transfusion include preoperative autologous blood donation, intraoperative techniques to improve hemostasis, minimally invasive procedures, and the use of regional versus general anesthesia. Medications such as erythropoieton and iron can be given before surgery to increase preoperative hemoglobin levels.

Surgical techniques to improve hemostasis include the use of gamma-knife radiosurgery, electrocautery, radiofrequency ablation, and laser beam coagulation. Intraoperative methods to conserve blood include hypotensive anesthesia, which lowers the mean arterial blood pressure and decreases the risk for bleeding; moderate levels of hypothermia; hemodilution; cell salvage; and the use of volume expanders and topical and systemic hemostatic agents.

Latex Allergy

Allergic reactions to latex were reported as early as the 1930s; however, the number of reported cases has increased since the introduction of Universal Precautions in the 1980s. Among health care workers the incidence of latex allergy may be as high as 17% in contrast to the estimated 1% incidence in the general population.[17]

Latex allergy is an immune reaction to one or more proteins in natural rubber latex. Surgical gloves and many of the supplies used in the perioperative area contain latex, which can cause an allergic response in latex-sensitive individuals (Box 17-4). The allergic response can be life threatening; therefore it is essential for perioperative nurses to be able to deal with patients and other health care workers who develop a reaction to latex.

Natural Rubber Latex

Natural rubber latex originates from the white milky sap of the *hevea brasilinesis* plant, more commonly known as the

BOX 17-4 Examples of Medical Supplies Containing Latex

- Adhesive tape
- Airways
  - Nasal
  - Oral
- Breathing bags
- Breathing circuits
- Bulb syringes
- Catheters
  - Foley
  - Straight
  - Central venous
  - Pulmonary artery
- Elastic bandages
- Electrode pads
- Fluid-warming blankets
- Gloves
- Intravenous ports
- Rubber stoppers on multidose vials
- Stethoscope tubing
- Ventilator bags
- Syringe plungers
- Wound drains

rubber tree. During the refinement process many accelerators, antioxidants, emulsifiers, stabilizers, extenders, colorants, retardants, ultraviolet light absorbers, and fragrances are added to the sap. The resulting product contains 2% to 3% latex protein.[16]

Reactions to Latex

There are two types of reactions to latex products. Type I sensitivity produces an immediate reaction and is the most serious form of hypersensitivity. Type IV sensitivity or contact dermatitis produces a delayed response and is the most common form of hypersensitivity (Table 17-13). It is thought that a type IV reaction may potentially progress to a type I reaction.[16]

Type I reactions are systemic in nature. Immunoglobulin E (IgE) antibodies are produced in response to the latex allergen. The IgE binds onto receptors on mast cells and basophils. Subsequent exposure to the latex protein causes mast cell proliferation, the release of basophil histamine, and subsequent anaphylaxis. The reactions occur suddenly and range from a skin flare response to wheezing and bronchospasm.

In contrast, there is no antibody formation with a type IV or cell-mediated reaction. Macrophages and T lymphocytes are activated in response to the allergen. Activation of the T lymphocytes and macrophages causes tissue inflammation and contact dermatitis. The onset of the reaction is slow and usually requires hours of contact before the appearance of symptoms. The reaction is localized to the area of contact. Type IV reactions are responses to substances used in the manufacturing process and are associated with wearing latex gloves and are therefore not considered true latex allergies.[16]

Routes of Exposure

Five routes of exposure to the latex protein can cause severe reactions in latex-sensitized individuals. Cutaneous exposure to medical supplies such as anesthesia masks, tourniquets, ECG electrodes, adhesive tape, fluid warming blankets, and elastic bandages can trigger reactions in susceptible patients.

Many of the severe reactions to latex have occurred as a result of the latex protein coming in contact with the mucous membranes of the mouth, vagina, urethra, or rectum. Oral mucosal reactions have occurred in response to the products used in dentistry, as well as to other medical products such as nasogastric tubes. Serious reactions have also been reported as a result of exposure of the vaginal mucosa to latex during examinations, sexual intercourse, deliveries, and abortions. Although contact of examination gloves, enema kits, and rectal pressure catheters with the rectal mucosa has precipitated reactions, the most severe mucous membrane reactions have occurred as a result of contact of the rectal mucosa with catheters used during barium enemas.

Inhalation of the latex proteins also causes severe reactions. Inhalation reactions have been most commonly associated with anesthesia equipment and endotracheal tubes; however, exposure to the latex protein through the aerosolization of glove powder has also been reported. In this circumstance the latex protein binds to the powder used in the gloves. When the gloves are removed from the box or from the hands, the powder is aerosolized and the particles dissipate onto surgical drapes and sponges. The aerosolization increases the risk of exposure for all sensitized individuals.

During the surgical procedure internal tissue absorbs the latex protein. A reaction is triggered when internal organs come in contact with surgical gloves and other products such as irrigation syringes, instruments, and catheters used throughout the surgical procedure.

The intravascular administration of latex proteins is not well understood. It is postulated that reactions occur from the use of disposable syringes, medications stored in vials with latex plugs, and intravenous tubing with latex ports.

Individuals at Risk for Developing Latex Allergy

A number of groups of individuals are at risk for developing a latex allergy. Individuals at greatest risk are those with neural tube defects. This patient population undergoes multiple surgeries, uses rubber catheters for urinary or bowel programs, and has multiple exposures to latex gloves in daily care. Other at-risk populations include individuals who have urinary conditions requiring continuous or intermittent catheterization; a history of allergies and asthma; a history of reactions to latex products; a history of multiple surgical procedures, especially bowel procedures; food allergies to bananas, avocados, tropical fruits, kiwis, potatoes, and chestnuts (possible cross-reaction between the food and the latex allergens); and health care workers with daily exposure to latex products. It is estimated that health care workers may use as many as 40 to 50 pairs of gloves per day.[10] Because of the increased incidence of latex allergy among perioperative staff, nonlatex surgical gloves are being used in many settings (see Research box).

TABLE 17-13 Reactions to Latex Products

Type I Reactions	Type IV Reactions
IgE activated (antibody formation)	T cell activated (no antibody formation)
Systemic responses	Localized responses
Cutaneous→flushing, diaphoresis, pruritus	Symptoms resolve in 72 to 96 hours
Gastrointestinal→nausea, vomiting, cramping, diarrhea	Individual remains sensitized and will react with every contact
Cardiovascular→hypotension, tachycardia, dysrhythmias	
Respiratory→dyspnea, bronchospasm, laryngeal edema	
Rapid onset of reactions	Delayed onset of reactions
Immediate response	Primary reaction occurs within 18 to 24 hours
	Subsequent reactions can develop sooner
Can be life threatening	Causes discomfort but is not life-threatening

Intraoperative Patient Management

A thorough history must be obtained after surgery to provide safe intraoperative patient care for individuals who are identified as at high risk for a systemic reaction to latex. Once the patient has been identified as having a latex allergy, the information must be documented and relayed to all other health care workers who provide care. The patient and patient's family should be assured that the team is aware of the latex allergy. The perioperative plan of care that addresses protective measures needs to be explained to the patient and the patient's family members. Patient and family education should include instructions regarding management of symptoms and prevention of further allergic reactions.

During the surgical procedure the circulating nurse ensures that only latex-free products are used. The anesthesia team ensures that the breathing circuit, face mask, and ventilator bag are latex-free. Rubber stoppers are removed from vials, and medications are drawn directly from multidose vials. Glass syringes are used to draw medications. Medications are injected through three-way stopcocks instead of through rubber ports. Latex-free tape is used when applying the dressing.

Education and Prevention

Because of the prevalence of latex allergy, education and prevention concern health care workers. Because the natural latex protein attaches to the powder used on gloves, the FDA has mandated that powder levels on all surgical and examination should be decreased. By 2002 the powder levels on surgical gloves must be 15 mg/dm^2 and those on examination gloves to 10 mg/dm^2. Standards are already in place to limit the amount of residual powder by 50% on powder-free latex and latex-free gloves.[17]

Latex products have been the gold standard for protection because of the excellent barrier protection. Barrier protection has been shown to vary among different brands of latex gloves. Although more research is indicated, nonlatex gloves may be a more effective barrier against small pathogens than latex gloves.[29]

Because of the prevalence of latex allergy among health care workers, prevention is an initiative of Healthy People

Research

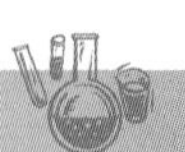

Research: Korniewicz DM et al: Implementing a nonlatex surgical glove study in the OR, *AORN J* 73(2):435, 2001.

Because of increased incidence of latex allergies among health care workers nonlatex surgical gloves are being used in the operating room. Despite their increased use, there is little known about the performance of nonlatex gloves. This federally funded study is being performed in a 23-room OR at a university hospital in Baltimore. The purpose of the study is to evaluate patterns of use and the number of leaks in sterile nonlatex surgical gloves used during surgical procedures. The study is also evaluating health care workers' satisfaction with nonlatex gloves. Specific questions include: Do nonlatex surgical gloves provide the same barrier protection and protection against needlestick injuries as latex gloves?

Two brands of latex and five brands of nonlatex gloves are evaluated monthly in the 23 operating rooms. To date more than 12,000 surgical procedures have been performed among all surgical services; 12,703 (6,366 latex and 6,337 nonlatex) gloves have been collected and analyzed. Data are collected from all health care workers involved in the surgical procedure, including surgeons, first assistants, surgical residents, and the scrub team.

After the surgical procedure the used gloves are collected and are inspected for barrier protection and leaks using the recommended standards of the U.S. Food and Drug Administration. Data are collected from the health care workers regarding their role during the procedure, dominant hand, length of time working in the OR, allergies, and perception of needlestick injuries. Monthly data are collected from all involved staff to evaluate satisfaction with the specific glove.

A total of 800 health care workers have participated in the study. Currently 60% to 80% of the staff are completing the user satisfaction forms weekly. After the first month of study, participation declined to 80 to 100 staff members per week.

Although data collection for this study is ongoing, participation trends among staff are declining. To obtain relevant data for any study, consistent ongoing participation is essential. To encourage staff's full participation in a research study, the authors recommend the following: consistent communication among staff regarding the purpose and progress of the study, feedback regarding status of the study, and sufficient orientation for staff regarding the study design and data collection methods. Finally, they recommend a pilot test allowing suggestions from participants.

2010, the National Occupational Research Agenda, and the National Institute for Occupational Safety and Health (NIOSH). OSHA has mandated that powder-free and nonlatex gloves be provided to employees who are allergic to latex. The FDA has required that manufacturers of medical devices clearly label items containing latex. NIOSH also recommends environmental measures to decrease the number of latex dust particles through cleaning of furniture, carpeting, and ventilation systems. When latex gloves are necessary, it is recommended to use powder-free gloves, and to avoid wearing oil-based lotions.

The national objective of Healthy People 2010 is to increase the number of health care facilities that use prevention strategies to protect employees from latex allergies. Education of employees should include strategies to decrease exposure in high-risk and sensitive individuals, alternatives to natural latex products, management of symptoms and treatment of latex allergy, and finally mandatory annual review of latex allergy protocols.

Gerontologic Considerations

As discussed in Chapter 16, many elderly patients have multiple chronic health problems that affect recovery from surgical intervention. Morbidity associated with geriatric surgical patients is usually due to preexisting medical problems. Morbidity and mortality rates for patients 65 years of age and over with comorbid conditions undergoing elective surgical procedures is 4 times higher and 20 times higher for emergent procedures.[8]

The perioperative nurse needs to understand the effects of aging and chronic disease on the outcome of surgery for the elderly patient. This knowledge allows the nurse to use the nursing process to ensure safe patient care throughout the perioperative experience. Although many of the intraoperative interventions are the same for any patient undergoing anesthesia and surgery, to meet the special care needs of the geriatric patient, the circulating nurse recognizes the patient's increased risk for inadvertent hypothermia, the risk for cardiovascular complications, and the potential complications related to intraoperative positioning.

Inadvertent Hypothermia

Body temperature is regulated in the anterior hypothalamus. Cutaneous thermoreceptors detect alterations in ambient temperatures and signal the anterior hypothalamus. The sensors in the anterior hypothalamus monitor the temperature of cerebral blood flow. The difference between those temperatures and a set point determined by the hypothalamus triggers the heat-generating response. This response is influenced by age, exercise, medications, and anesthetics.[7]

The body's normal response to heat loss and cold is shivering to generate heat. Because of impaired thermoregulatory ability, the shivering response to cold is less sensitive in older adults than in younger patients. A slower metabolic rate, decreased cardiovascular reserve, thinning of skin, loss of subcutaneous tissue, and diminished muscle mass affect the geriatric patient's ability to produce and conserve body heat. The stress of surgery and anesthesia also suppresses the heat-producing responses in elderly patients. Intraoperative routines, environmental factors, and anesthesia-related factors can also affect perioperative thermoregulation in the geriatric patient (Box 17-5).

The patient is assessed for the risk of hypothermia. This includes assessment of physiologic status and body size. Knowledge of the extent of the surgical procedure along with the type of anesthesia planned assists the circulating nurse to formulate a plan of patient care that will decrease intraoperative body heat loss. Increasing the temperature in the OR; covering the patient with warm blankets; warming anesthetic gases, intravenous fluids, and irrigation solutions; warming skin preparation fluids; covering the patient's head; and limiting exposure of body surface are measures that can be taken to prevent inadvertent hypothermia in the elderly patient.

Positioning

The potential for postoperative skin problems presents a significant risk for the geriatric patient. Decreased adipose tissue, poor skin turgor, decreased peripheral circulation, and tissue fragility can cause postoperative skin problems. Arthritis, deceased range of motion, and skin fragility make patient positioning one of the most important aspects of intraoperative patient care. In addition to the threat of skin problems, improper positioning can also cause joint pain unrelated to the surgical procedure.

Anesthesia Considerations

Geriatric patients require special consideration when undergoing anesthesia. The normal aging process causes a variety of physiologic changes that affect the geriatric patient's response to anesthesia. The patient's response to anesthesia may be unpredictable and significant. Diminished physiologic reserves, preexisting medical conditions, and the physical stress caused by anesthesia and surgical intervention pose increased risk. Thorough preoperative assessment and careful anesthesia management can improve patient outcomes.

The geriatric patient is more susceptible to the action of medications. Decreased liver and kidney function and re-

BOX 17-5 Factors Affecting Perioperative Thermoregulation in Geriatric Patients

Procedural

- Intravenous infusion of cool solutions
- Irrigation of incision sites with cool solutions
- Lengthy surgical procedures
- Surgical procedures involving large body surfaces or open cavities

Environmental

- Cool air temperature in the operating room
- Air currents related to air exchanges within the operating room

Anesthetic

- Inhalation of cool nonhumidified gaseous agents

duced cardiac output affect the metabolism and excretion of drugs from the body. Therefore geriatric patients generally require lower doses of anesthetic agents and take longer to eliminate them.

The presence of pulmonary disease or pulmonary insufficiency may pose ventilatory difficulties. Alterations in the airway of elderly patients also cause ventilatory difficulties. Loss of teeth and alterations in jaw contours can cause an inadequate fit of the anesthesia mask. Decreased range of motion in the jaw, head, and neck presents difficulties for intubation.

NURSING MANAGEMENT

The unique nature of the intraoperative environment creates an inevitable focus on the many technical activities required to facilitate the surgical procedure and maintain patient safety. However, the perioperative nurse is also responsible for meeting the patient's psychosocial needs.

Several factors have an impact when considering the nurse-patient relationship during the operative phase. The operative phase of the perioperative experience is short, and the patient may be sedated or unconscious most of the time. However, the nurse has a great deal of impact on the patient in a short period of time. The experience is almost universally stressful for all patients. Allowing patients to participate as much as possible in their perioperative care may improve the quality of care. Explanations of procedures and events are critical, because patients may not know what questions to ask. These types of interventions may allow a sense of security and effective coping, thereby making the operative experience a positive one.

ASSESSMENT

When patients are admitted to the OR suite, the perioperative nurse must assess the patient's physical and emotional status, paying particular attention to any factors that would increase surgical risk. A preoperative interview should take place on the patient's arrival to the OR admission suite. Astute interviewing skills and communication of a caring attitude are important for a thorough assessment of both physical and emotional status of the patient.

Health History and Physical Examination

Preoperative data should include an assessment of the physiologic and psychosocial health status. Psychosocial assessment should include the patient's family or significant other. The patient is typically brought to the holding area by transport personnel. The circulating nurse reviews the health history and physical examination that was completed preoperatively, validates the data, and assesses the patient for any changes. During this interview the circulating nurse reviews the chart and preoperative checklist and assesses and verifies the patient's physical and psychologic readiness for surgery (Box 17-6).

After a review of the information accumulated during the immediate preoperative assessment, the nurse formulates nursing diagnoses, expected patient outcomes, and an intraoperative plan of care. Assessment continues during the patient's transfer to the OR, positioning on the OR bed, induction of anesthesia, and during and immediately after the surgical procedure.

NURSING DIAGNOSES

The nursing diagnoses discussed in this chapter focus on high-incidence problem areas for patients during a surgical intervention. The North American Nursing Diagnosis Association (NANDA) does not recommend the routine use of Risk for Infection for patients undergoing surgery. The use of this diagnosis should be limited to high-risk patients. We have included this diagnosis to enable the learner to become familiar with routine standards of care and aseptic practices used in the operating room. Note that the nursing diagnoses Risk for Latex Allergy Response and Latex Allergy Response can be used to guide nursing care for patients with latex allergy.

Nursing diagnoses for the patient in the intraoperative phase of surgery may include but are not limited to:

Diagnostic Title	Possible Etiologic Factors
1. Anxiety	Unfamiliar environment; fear of impending surgery/anesthesia, intraoperative diagnosis; loss of control; role change
2. Risk for perioperative-positioning injury	Immobility, decreased range of motion, contractures, altered nutritional status, elderly, edema, surgical procedure longer than 2 hours, loss of sensory protective responses related to anesthesia, chronic disease, venous stasis
3. Risk for trauma injury	Burns from chemical or electrical hazards, physical hazards, retention of foreign objects
4. Risk for postoperative wound infection	Excessive body cavity exposure, decreased body defense mechanisms, preoperative health status of patient

BOX 17-6 Perioperative Assessment Data

- Identification of patient, presence of identification bracelet
- Verification of procedure, surgical site, and surgeon by patient; consent form
- Preprocedural vital signs and pain rating
- NPO status
- Review allergy and medication history
- Mobility, functional status
- Presence of prostheses, implants
- Mental and sensory status
- Pulmonary status
- Cardiovascular status
- Renal and hydration status
- Skin integrity
- Nutritional status
- Religious, cultural, and philosophic beliefs
- Expectations of treatment
- Review laboratory and diagnostic findings
- Anticipated need for blood products

5. Risk for imbalanced body temperature	Cool operative environment, inhaled anesthetics, prolonged exposure, cool solutions, elderly, malignant hyperthermia
6. Risk for imbalanced fluid volume	Major invasive procedures, rapid loss of blood/body fluid during the surgical procedure, stress of surgical intervention, anticoagulant therapy, trauma, preexisting disorders (e.g., bleeding disorders), elderly
	Rapid intake of excessive fluid or sodium, stress of surgical intervention, corticosteroid therapy, preexisting conditions (e.g., Cushing's syndrome, congestive heart failure), elderly

EXPECTED PATIENT OUTCOMES

Expected patient outcomes for the patient in the intraoperative phase of surgery may include but are not limited to:

1. Will demonstrate little or no subjective or objective evidence of anxiety
2a. Will remain free from neuromuscular and neurovascular deficits or injury related to surgical positioning
2b. Will remain free from injury and signs of skin and tissue injury beyond 24 to 48 hours after the procedure
3. Will remain free from injury or trauma related to electrical, chemical, and physical factors
4. Will remain free of postoperative wound infection
5a. Will maintain desired intraoperative body temperature
5b. Will maintain body temperature within normal range in the immediate postoperative period
6. Will demonstrate fluid balance

INTERVENTIONS

Having identified the patient's specific needs and formulated nursing diagnoses, the nurse must collaborate with other members of the health care team to implement the plan for patient care during the intraoperative phase of the surgical experience. As discussed previously, anesthesia and all the components of the surgical experience place great stress on the body and may result in postoperative complications. The major focus of intraoperative nursing interventions during this period is maintenance of patient safety and prevention of postoperative complications. The nurse is responsible for documentation of all nursing interventions and the patient's response to care. At the completion of the surgical procedure the circulating nurse gives a report to the nurse in the receiving unit.

2. Minimizing Anxiety

Most patients experience some anxiety when facing a surgical intervention. As discussed in Chapter 16, an important part of preoperative nursing intervention is helping the patient cope with anxiety. Anxiety may be due to preconceived ideas and fears related to the surgical experience, illness, and hospitalization. Perioperative events such as the disclosure of possible complications, anesthesia, intraoperative diagnosis, or postoperative pain may trigger an increase in anxiety level immediately before surgery.

Interventions at this time focus on providing support by gentle physical contact, maintaining personal dignity, ensuring a quiet and unhurried surgical environment, attending to the needs of the patient, and providing comfort measures such as a warm blanket or pillow. In addition, providing information about the environment and explaining the rationale for nursing interventions decreases the patient's fear of the unfamiliar environment. Soothing words and an empathic attitude help promote a nurturing atmosphere in the OR's high-technology environment. Patient-centered care remains the focus of the perioperative nurse. By communicating an overall attitude of caring and providing physiologic and emotional support, nurses can make a noticeable difference in a patient's preoperative emotional state. The successful use of anxiety-reducing interventions may reduce or eliminate the need for anxiolytic medications. During induction of anesthesia, the nurse's close proximity to the patient and provision of comfort and support help minimize the patient's fears and facilitate induction.

2. Minimizing Risks for Injury to Skin and Tissues Due to Positioning

The patient may be placed in a variety of positions for the surgical procedure. A thorough knowledge of the physiologic effects of pressure is necessary to keep the patient free from injury and trauma resulting from complications of positioning.

Injury may occur to tissues and neurovascular structures as a result of positioning required for the surgical procedure. Positioning affects the cardiovascular, respiratory, neurologic, and integumentary systems. Prolonged pressure on the bony prominences, pressure on the peripheral nervous or vascular systems, or the shearing force of sheets and drapes during patient movement may be responsible for pressure ulcers.

A pressure ulcer as defined by the Agency for Healthcare Research and Quality (AHRQ) is a lesion caused by unrelieved pressure that results in damage to the underlying tissues.[6] In the acute care patient population the incidence of pressure ulcers ranges from 2.7% to 29% and dramatically increases to 12% to 66% in surgical patients.[6,31]

Tissue perfusion is a critical factor in the development of pressure sores. Normal capillary interface pressure is 23 to 32 mm Hg. Pressures in excess of normal can alter tissue perfusion and cause ischemia.[1] However, pressures as low as 11 to 20 mm Hg may occlude blood flow in elderly patients and those with hemiplegia and peripheral vascular disease.[31] Gravity forces patients against the hard surface of the OR bed and compresses skin, muscle, and bone and increases capillary interface pressures. Compression of vessels, external pressure, uneven body weight distribution, and constant pressure on bony prominences can result in pressure sores. Compounding this, anesthetic agents lower blood pressure and alter tissue perfusion, which may also result in tissue damage.[6]

Tissue damage resulting from prolonged pressure on the OR bed may not be visible for several days. Pressure ulcers that originate in the operating room develop outwardly from the muscle and subcutaneous tissue and progress to the dermis and epidermis.[6,31] Reddened skin areas that appear 1 to 2 days after surgery are commonly mistaken for burns. These incorrectly diagnosed reddened areas may then progress to stage III or stage IV pressure ulcers within 6 days.[31]

Pressure injuries commonly occur over bony prominences, such as the occiput, spine, scapulae, coccyx, sacrum, or calcaneous. Figure 17-7 illustrates common surgical positions and indicates the associated pressure points. Commonly used operative patient positions are described in Table 17-14.

Several risk factors have been identified as contributing to the development of pressure ulcers in the surgical patient (see Risk Factors box). The circulating nurse should assess the patient for risk factors during the preoperative interview. A common complication of anesthetized patients is associated with vasoconstriction and decreased subcutaneous oxygen tension, resulting in increased surgical wound infections. Because of the correlation of hypothermia and tissue viability the relationship between hypothermia and the development of pressure ulcers has been explored (see Research box).

The respiratory system is influenced greatly by positioning. The thoracic cage normally expands in all directions except posteriorly. The respiratory system is most vulnerable in the prone and the lithotomy positions owing to the mechanical restriction of lung expansion at the ribs or sternum. The diaphragm is unable to fully descend against the abdominal musculature and respiratory function is impaired.

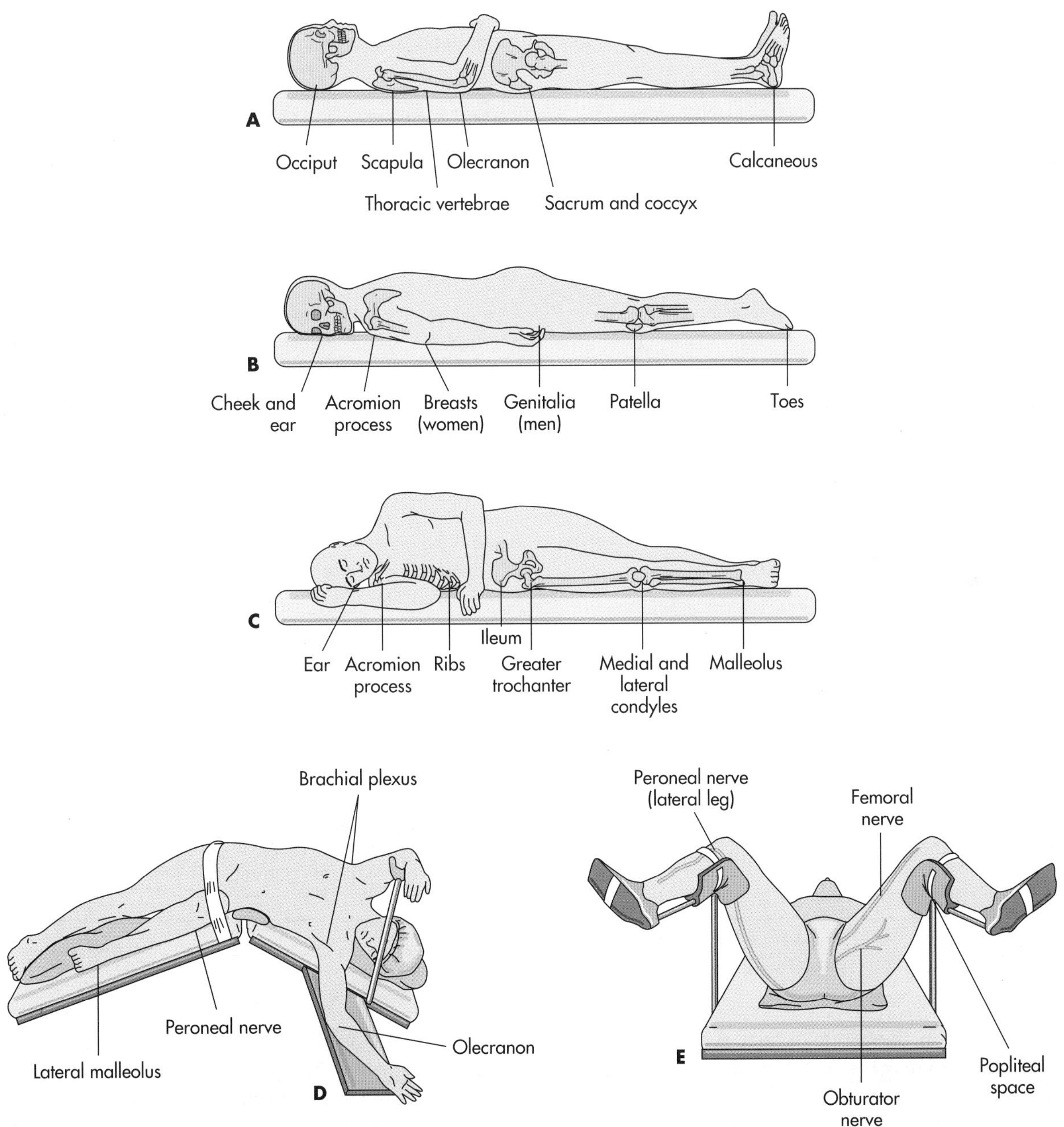

Figure 17-7 Examples of common surgical positions and their associated potential pressure points. **A**, Supine (dorsal recumbent) position. **B**, Prone position. **C**, Lateral position. **D**, Lateral (kidney) position. **E**, Lithotomy position.

TABLE 17-14 Commonly Used Operative Patient Positions

Description	Comments
Supine	
Flat on back with arms at side, palms down, legs straight with feet slightly separated	Most commonly used position; venous pooling in the legs may result from a reduction of venous pressure
Prone	
Patient lies on abdomen with face turned to one side, arms at sides with palms pronated, elbows slightly flexed; feet elevated to prevent plantar flexion	Patient is anesthetized in supine position and then placed prone; chest rolls or frame used for support; respiratory excursion is decreased; risk for injury to head, eyes, nose, facial nerve, genitalia, and breasts
Trendelenburg	
Patient supine; head and body are lowered into a head-down position; knees are flexed by "breaking" table	Respiratory excursion is decreased from upward movement of abdominal viscera; cerebral edema or venous thrombosis may occur because of congestion of the cerebral vessels
Lithotomy	
Patient lies on back with buttocks to edge of table; thighs and legs are placed in stirrups simultaneously to prevent muscle injury; head and arms are secured to prevent injury	Elastic wraps or antiembolic stockings may be used on legs to prevent thrombus formation; risk for vein compression in legs, increased intraabdominal pressure, injury to obturator and femoral nerves because of flexion of thighs; injury to common peroneal nerve caused by fibular neck resting against stirrups; risk for acute hypotension when legs are lowered; avoid abduction greater than 90 degrees of arms
Lateral	
Patient lies on side; table may be bent in middle	Risk for injury to dependent brachial plexus and dependent common peroneal nerve, pressure sore development over the dependent greater trochanter of femur; potential interference with cardiac action because of possible shift in heart position

Risk Factors

Development of Pressure Ulcers in Surgical Patients

SITUATIONAL (RELATED TO OPERATING ROOM (OR) ENVIRONMENT)

- Type of surgery (vascular, cardiac, and orthopedic)
- Surgical position
- Type of surgical exposure and method of retracting tissues
- Length of procedure (over $2\frac{1}{2}$ to 3 hours)
- Standard OR mattress
- Positioning devices
- Warming blankets
- Anesthetic agents
- Vasoactive drugs
- Shearing forces
- Friction
- Moisture from preparation and irrigating solutions

PATIENT-RELATED

- Advanced age
- Body weight (obesity and malnourished)
- Cormobid disease (diabetes, cardiovascular disease, peripheral vascular disease, pulmonary disease, paralysis)
- Decreased immune functioning
- Compromised tissue perfusion
- Decreased range of motion
- Immobility
- Compromised skin condition preoperatively
- Low preoperative albumin level
- Low score on Braden scale
- Evidence of preoperative anxiety or fear

Reference: Armstrong D, Bortz P: An integrative review of pressure relief in surgical patients, *AORN J* 73(3):645, 2001; Schultz A et al: Etiology and incidence of pressure ulcers in surgical patients, *AORN J* 70(3):434, 1999.

Several changes in the cardiovascular system that occur with positioning also may result in complications. A tight restraint, crossed legs, or limb hyperextension can compromise blood flow by compression of a vessel against a bony structure and may result in venous stasis or ischemia. Rapid changes of position may cause sudden hypotension. An example of this occurs when legs are lowered quickly from the lithotomy position. The lithotomy position also may lead to circulatory pooling in the lumbar region and compression of abdominal contents on the inferior vena cava and abdominal aorta. In both situations, there is a decrease in venous return, which affects cardiac output.

Most of the problems associated with the neurologic system are not discovered until recovery from anesthesia is com-

Research

Reference: Scott EM et al: Effects of warming therapy on pressure ulcers—a randomized trial, *AORN J* 73(5):921, 2001.

Pressure ulcers in the surgical patient is a common and expensive problem with an estimated annual cost in the United States of $3.6 billion. The incidence of pressure ulcers in surgical patients is as high as 66% for older patients undergoing orthopedic procedures; for other surgical patients the incidence ranges from 8.5% to 35%. Risk factors for the development of pressure ulcers in surgical patients include immobility; circulatory and metabolic changes as a result of anesthesia and surgical trauma; operating room bed mattress pressure; diabetes; albumin levels; and patients undergoing reconstructive surgery for existing pressure ulcers, vascular, cardiac and orthopedic procedures. Length of surgical procedure as a risk factor has not been supported in all studies.

Intraoperative hypothermia is a common problem among surgical patients and may influence tissue viability. Hypothermia is associated with longer hospital stays, variations in serum potassium level, increased risk of myocardial ischemia and cardiovascular complications, increased arterial blood pressure, impaired coagulation, and decreased subcutaneous oxygen tension through vasoconstriction. The reduced oxygen tension has been correlated with an increased incidence of surgical wound infections of patients undergoing colorectal surgery.

The relationship between intraoperative hypothermia, tissue viability, and wound infection has been established. This study explores the possible relationship between core temperature, peripheral circulation, and oxygen delivery to the skin and deeper tissues. The researchers hypothesized that control of intraoperative hypothermia would reduce the incidence of postoperative pressure ulcers. They also sought to identify other contributing factors to the development of pressure ulcers and to explore the relationship between the patient's intraoperative core temperature and tissue viability.

This was a prospective randomized clinical trial conducted on patients in the English National Health Service. Inclusion criteria included age 40 years and older, absence of existing sacral pressure ulcers, and patients scheduled for major surgery with an expected length of stay of 5 days. The following surgical specialties were included: orthopedic, colorectal, gastrointestinal, urology, and vascular.

A total of 324 patients were included in the study—161 in the treatment group and 163 in the control group. Patients in the control group received standard care that consisted of automatic regulation of ambient temperature, minimal patient exposure, and use of warm blankets immediately after surgery. Treatment group patients received standard care plus the use of a forced-air warming blanket and an intravenous fluid warmer. Data were also collected regarding comorbid conditions affecting peripheral circulation, smoking history, steroid use, and American Society of Anesthesiologist status. Core temperature was measured via tympanic thermometers. The dependent variable was the development of a pressure ulcer defined as nonblanchable hyperemia persisting longer than 24 hours or break in the skin.

Results indicated a 46% relative risk reduction and a 4.8% absolute risk reduction of pressure ulcers in patients receiving the warming therapy. In all, 26 patients developed pressure ulcers at three sites (sacrum, heel, and buttock).

As expected, core temperatures of patients undergoing general anesthesia were significantly lower than those with regional anesthetics. A statistically significant greater number of patients with general anesthesia developed pressure ulcers compared with those receiving regional anesthesia. Although in general, older patients developed pressure ulcers, patients who received the standard care and developed pressure ulcers were younger. Patients who developed pressure ulcers had lower body mass indices (BMIs) than those who did not. ASA status, although not statistically significant, seemed to be an indicator of pressure ulcer risk. More than 90% of patients were ASA status II or III.

Although not statistically significant, results are of clinical significance. Although hypothermia may occur in patients receiving regional or general anesthesia, body temperatures tended to be lower in patients receiving general anesthesia. General anesthesia was also associated with a higher incidence of pressure ulcer development. Both these results support the research hypothesis.

Forced air warming blankets are safe and easy to use and are not associated with thermal injury. The cost of the use of the warming blanket is low compared with the cost associated with treatment of pressure ulcers. Although further research is needed, forced-air therapy may be an effective intervention to treat hypothermia and to reduce the incidence of pressure ulcer development in the surgical patient. Other areas needing further research include BMI and ASA status and relationship to the development of pressure ulcers.

plete. Postoperative sedation may mask symptoms of peripheral nerve damage. Most postoperative peripheral neuropathies result from an inappropriate positioning on the operating bed, usually as the result of direct mechanical pressure. Ischemia and insufficient blood supply caused by stretching or compression are chief factors in nerve injuries. The lithotomy position is especially likely to cause injury to the saphenous and common peroneal nerves. These injuries result from either misplaced stirrups or acute flexion of the thighs. In all positions in which the arms are extended on armboards, hyperextension of the arms may cause damage to the brachial plexus.

The circulating nurse assists the surgeon and the anesthesia care provider in safely positioning the patient for the surgical procedure. Ensuring the patient's comfort and safety and proper positioning with the appropriate devices can minimize complications associated with positioning (see Table 17-14). Distribution of body weight should be as even as possible, and the patient should be maintained in correct alignment.

The type of positioning device used depends on the individual patient, type of procedure, and the surgeon's preference. Positioning devices come in a wide variety of shapes, styles, and materials. Some examples include foam pads and mattresses, face guards, sand bags, bean bags, air mattresses, gel pads, frames, and rolls. The device chosen should maintain the desired intraoperative position and minimize the potential for injury by redistributing pressure and preventing excessive stretching. To reduce pressure, the device must have the documented ability to reduce capillary interface pressure to 32 mm Hg or less. Ideally, the device should be durable, nonallergenic, radiolucent, easily stored, resistant to moisture and microorganisms, able to be disinfected or disposed of;

and cost-effective. The standard OR mattress is less effective than foam and gel mattresses in reducing pressure, although none have been shown to be effective in reducing pressure below 32 mm Hg. Bath blankets, turn sheets, and heating blankets all commonly used in positioning increase pressure up to 44 mm Hg.[31]

To avoid stretching and compression of nerve and muscle tissue, positioning of extremities must not exceed a 90-degree angle to the body. Bony prominences such as heels, elbows, and sacrum are vulnerable pressure points and should be well padded. The safety strap should be applied 2 inches above the knees to avoid pressure on the popliteal nerve. Compression of the popliteal nerve from stirrups or knee braces also should be avoided.

Surgical equipment, such as pneumatic saws and drills and retractors, placed directly on the patient may lead to pressure injuries. The circulating nurse monitors members of the team at the field to ensure that they do not lean on the patient during the procedure. Antiembolic stockings or intermittent pneumatic compression devices may be used to decrease venous pooling in the lower extremities.

Changing positions gradually is important to prevent drastic shifts in blood volume from one area of the body to another. Foam-filled cushions can be used to maintain adequate respiratory excursion and to prevent pressure on the chest, breasts, genitalia, and abdominal structures. Refer to the Guidelines for Safe Practice box for nursing interventions associated with intraoperative patient positioning.

Guidelines for Safe Practice

Preventing Complications of Surgical Positioning

- Maintain patient in correct alignment, and distribute body weight equally.
- Any positioning devices should maintain normal intracapillary pressure of 32 mm Hg or less.
- If foam overlays are used, they should be constructed of thick dense foam that resists compression.
- Towels, blanket rolls, and pillows are not effective in reducing pressure and may cause injury due to friction.[3]
- Gel pads are effective in reducing overall pressure in a large surface area.
- Pad all bony prominences.
- Use antiembolic hose and intermittent pneumatic compression devices to decrease venous pooling as indicated.
- Change patient positions gradually to avoid drastic shifts in blood volume.
- Avoid local compression from safety straps, knee braces, stirrups, equipment, or personnel.
- Avoid stretching and compression of neuromuscular and vascular structures.
- Position extremities at no more than a 90-degree angle to the body.
- After positioning the patient's body alignment and tissue integrity should be reassessed.
- Documentation of positioning should include preoperative assessment; position, type, and location of devices; names and titles of personnel; and postoperative assessment.

A detailed procedure for each surgical position should be written and available for OR personnel who are responsible for or assist with positioning of patients. Detailed documentation by the circulating nurse should include the preoperative skin condition, type of position, any intraoperative changes in positioning, placement of extremities, type and placement of positioning aids and supplemental padding, and the site of placement of the electrosurgical conduction pad.

3. Reducing Injury from Electrical, Chemical, and Physical Hazards

The OR is an area containing many potentially life-threatening and mechanically injurious situations related to electrical shock, burn, fire, and explosions. Many nursing activities are focused on the protection of the patient from electrical, chemical, and physical hazards. It is imperative that all members of the surgical health care team have current knowledge of the equipment and supplies most often involved in such incidents. The most significant hazards are inadequately trained personnel, malfunctioning equipment as a result of improper maintenance, inappropriate design of OR suites, and inappropriate surveillance by team members.

Federal regulations mandate the marketing and safety standards of electronic devices used in the operating room. When electrical equipment is in use, hazards can be minimized or prevented by the following nursing interventions:

Use only electrical equipment designed for OR use
Use cords of adequate length
Ground the patient correctly
Test equipment before use
Establish and follow sound clinical engineering testing and maintenance programs
Participate in in-service sessions for new equipment, and maintain an adequate knowledge base for correct use of all electrical equipment
Verify that correct attachments for a piece of equipment are being used
Report faulty equipment immediately
Maintain humidity levels at 50% or higher to minimize static electricity
Prevent the pooling of fluids under the patient

The use of electricity introduces hazards of electric shock, power failure, and fire to patients. If a voltage exists between any two electrical conductors touching the patient, the flow of current can result in electric shock or electrocution. If the voltage is high enough, ventricular fibrillation and sudden death may result.

Laser (light amplification by stimulated emission of radiation) technology is an effective treatment modality; however, it presents hazards for patients and members of the surgical team. As the high-powered beams of light are directed into tissue, the resultant intense heat vaporizes the tissue and causes a rapid coagulation of blood vessels. When lasers are used, special equipment is necessary to protect both the patient and surgical team members. Eye protection specific to the type of laser (e.g., argon, carbon dioxide) is used to prevent retinal damage from misdirected beams of light. If aberrant light beams land on surgical drapes, they can cause fire. Improperly functioning surgical instruments can deflect light to other tissue. Measures such as the use of coated instruments, wet towels on the field, smoke evacuation methods, and warning signs on the door of the operative suite are routinely taken to protect the patient and OR team members.

Chemical hazards in the operating room include exposure to solutions used for cleaning, cementing bone, gas sterilization of instruments, and skin preparation. Iodine and iodophors are two of the most effective bactericidal agents used for preoperative skin scrubbing but are irritants to the skin if the concentration is too high. Alcohol, which sometimes is used in incision site preparation, is flammable. Precautions necessary for prevention of injury from any hazardous chemicals are many. All personnel must be aware of and follow safe chemical usage recommendations set by the hospital's safety department and the manufacturing company. It is imperative that the circulating nurse determine or verify any patient allergies that may increase risk of injury from certain solutions intended for use during the surgical procedure. To prevent skin irritation and electrical shock or burn, solutions used for skin preparation should not be allowed to pool under the patient.

It is the responsibility of the circulating nurse to protect the patient from injury from physical hazards. Prevention of injury includes careful movement during positioning, use of appropriate positioning methods, and use of protective devices such as side rails and safety straps. Safe transfer of the patient to or from the operating room bed is accomplished with lift devices or a minimum of four people. Safety can be promoted by ensuring that sufficient support help is obtained for the transfer, that all tubes are visible and protected from inadvertent removal, and that the movement is coordinated among all team members.

To ensure that injury does not occur from misidentification of the patient or the correct operative site, it is mandatory that the circulating nurse verify the patient's identity and operative site. The circulating nurse must bring any discrepancy or concerns to the attention of the surgeon, anesthesiologist, patient, and when necessary, the hospital administrator.

Prevention of Foreign Object Retention

Because of the high level of risk to the patient related to foreign object retention in the surgical wound, counting materials used during a surgical procedure is an important intraoperative nursing intervention. Sponges, sharps, and instruments are counted before the procedure, as additional items are added, at initial closure, and finally at skin closure. An additional count is necessary when either the scrub or circulating nurse leaves the case. Policies and procedures must be written with specific guidelines to be followed for the counting of items during each surgical procedure. The surgical count should be performed by both the circulating and scrub nurse.

The AORN recommended practices state that sharps should be counted on all procedures. Sponges and instruments should be counted on procedures in which there is a possibility that such items could be retained.[3] For example, procedures in which a major body cavity is opened or a deep incision is made would necessitate both a sponge and an instrument count.

Sponges and other products have radiopaque markings and in the event of an incorrect count, an x-ray film can be obtained to determine the presence of the missing item in the patient. All counts performed are documented and placed in the patient's record. Any corrective action taken in the event of a discrepancy and the resultant outcome are also recorded.

3. Minimizing Risks for Postoperative Wound Infection

All patients who undergo surgery have the potential to acquire an infection. Surgical intervention breaks down some of the body's primary defenses against infection. Infection can prolong hospital stay and can even endanger the life of a patient. Protecting the patient from infection is a major goal of intraoperative nursing interventions. The goal of nursing interventions is to control the number and types of microorganisms present during surgery. Many of the activities that are directed toward achieving this goal are related to monitoring and controlling the environment. The most important measure in preventing postoperative wound infection is adherence to meticulous aseptic technique principles and to transmission-based precautions. The entire surgical team has a responsibility to uphold principles of aseptic technique and follow the policies and procedures established to ensure that the surgical suite is protected from unnecessary risks resulting from increases in microbial population.

Creating and maintaining the sterile field is the responsibility of both the circulating and scrub nurses. The standards and recommended practices for perioperative nursing provide guidelines in areas related to the maintenance of a sterile field. These areas include basic aseptic technique, traffic patterns in the surgical suite, environmental controls, OR attire, sterilization, barrier materials, surgical hand scrub, and preoperative skin preparation of patients. Throughout the surgical procedure, the circulating nurse monitors adherence to aseptic technique principles by all surgical team members and ensures that breaks in technique are corrected.

The CDC recommends the classification of surgical wounds to predict the probability of postoperative infection. The circulating nurse is responsible for assigning and documenting the classification. Wounds are classified as clean, clean contaminated, contaminated, or dirty (Table 17-15). Documentation of the appropriate wound classification assists the infection control nurse with follow-up planning and nosocomial wound infection reporting.

Surgical site infections account for 38% of postoperative infections and are the most common nosocomial infection for surgical patients.[4] Research has shown that despite strict aseptic technique, *Staphylococcus aureus* has been found at clean surgical sites.[9] Most surgical incisions are sufficiently sutured together and covered with an occlusive dressing making them resistant to infection for the first 24 hours after surgery.[9] Exceptions to this are wounds with a drain in place or those left open to heal by secondary intention (see Chapter18). Surgical

TABLE 17-15 CDC Surgical Wound Classification

Classification	Definition	Examples
Clean wound	Uninfected, primary closure Closed wound drainage system No inflammation present	Total knee arthroplasty Mitral valve replacement Breast biopsy
Clean contaminated wound	Respiratory, alimentary, or genitourinary tract entered without spillage No sign of infection, minor break in sterile technique	Total abdominal hysterectomy Radical prostatectomy Pneumonectomy
Contaminated wound	Major break in aseptic technique Signs of infection Contamination from gastrointestinal tract Open fresh traumatic wound	Appendectomy for ruptured appendix Laparotomy for perforated bowel
Dirty wound	Old trauma with necrotic tissue Preexisting infection Perforated viscera Acute inflammation	Incision and drainage of abscess

site infections are the result of pathogens acquired exogenously from personnel or the environment or from the patient's own organisms. The patient's own organisms are responsible for most surgical site infections and are thought to be implanted at the time of surgery.[9] Of particular concern is the emergence of antibiotic-resistant strains of both gram-negative and gram-positive organisms including methicillin-resitant strains of *S. aureus* (MRSA) and vancomycin-resistant strains of *enterococcus* (VRE).

Because of antibiotic resistance, surgical antimicrobial prophylaxis should be used judiciously. Surgical prophylaxis refers to a brief course of antibiotic therapy administered just before an operation begins.[22] Intravenous infusion is the most common route of antibiotic administration. The goal of surgical antimicrobial prophylaxis is to reduce the number of pathogens resulting from intraoperative contamination and is not intended to prevent postoperative contamination.[22] Antibiotics are chosen based on which microorganisms are most likely to be found at the surgical site. The surgical wound classification described earlier can be helpful in estimating postoperative infection rates and the need for antibiotic therapy.

Cefazolin, a first-generation cephalosporin, is effective against many gram-positive and gram-negative organisms and is generally regarded as the antimicrobial agent of choice for surgical prophylaxis in clean operations. If the patient has a penicillin allergy, alternatives are clindamycin and vancomycin. It is important to remember that vancomycin should not be used routinely for antimicrobial prophylaxis. To achieve maximum effectiveness, 1 to 2 g of cefazolin should be administered to patients at least 30 minutes before incision time.[22] Antibiotics are most effective when they are present in tissues before bacteria enter the surgical site. A single dose of antibiotics is sufficient for most surgical procedures. However, more research is needed to determine the needs of patients undergoing lengthy surgical procedures. Nursing responsibilities include assessing the patient for drug allergies, administering the correct drug at the correct time, and monitoring the patient for therapeutic and adverse effects of the drug. Maintaining sterile technique during venipuncture and fluid administration is also essential to prevent any further sources of infection.

Promoting Wound Healing

The etiology of wound infection is diverse and may be related to the environment, host, or pathogen (wound healing is discussed in Chapter 18). Appropriate closure and drainage of dead space facilitate wound healing.

Wound healing by *primary intention* occurs in most surgical incisions. After the operation is completed, the wound edges are closed. Primary closure is indicated for clean straight incision lines with all layers of the wound able to be well approximated.

Closure of an incision with minimal trauma is facilitated by placing sutures or other materials (Table 17-16) in close approximation to achieve an anatomically secure wound. Sutures, staples, drains, or any foreign body at the surgical site may promote inflammation and increase the risk of a surgical site infection.[22] Monofilament sutures have been shown to produce the least amount of inflammation.[22] Surgical stapling is believed to cause less reaction than suturing. Wound edges will not heal readily if not in close contact. A dead space may occur from separation of wound edges or from air trapped between layers of tissue. Serum, blood, or other fluid may accumulate in a dead space and prevent healing.

If it is anticipated that fluid may collect in a body area near the wound after surgery, the surgeon usually inserts a tube or drain to permit the fluid to escape. Drains are usually made of latex or silicone. One end of the tube or drain is placed in or near the organ or cavity to be drained, and the other end is passed through the body wall, usually through a separate small incision near the operative site. A closed suction drain placed through a separate incision distant from the operative incision reduces the risk of infection. Suction drains create a negative pressure in a reservoir. The negative pressure gently suctions fluid from the wound into the attached reservoir. The Hemovac and Jackson-Pratt drains (Figs. 17-8 and 17-9) are

TABLE 17-16 New Options in Wound Closure

Material	Uses	Advantages
2-Octyl cyanoacrylate (Dermabond)	Surgical topical adhesive used as alternative to skin sutures For primary skin closure and simple lacerations Falls off naturally in 5 – 10 days Applied by single-use applicator Not suitable for areas under tension, movement, or below the skin	Superior cosmetic results Forms firm bond Faster application time, rapid setting Reduces risk of needlestick injuries
Adhesive strips (Suture strip)	Indicated for primary wound closure of skin incisions and skin tears or lacerations as an alternative to sutures	Latex-free Water-resistant Improved cosmetic results Reduces risk of needlestick injuries
Zippers (Medi-Zip)	Zipper adheres to skin by two adhesive strips; wound edges are sealed as zipper is closed Primary wound closure	Reduces tissue inflammation, risk of infection, and postoperative scarring Quick application (faster than suturing) Reduces risk of needlestick injuries

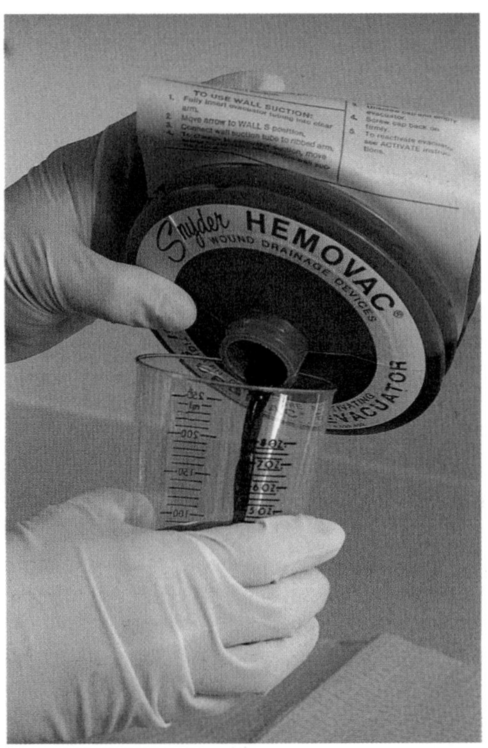

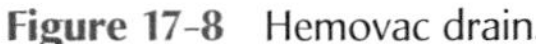
Figure 17-8 Hemovac drain.

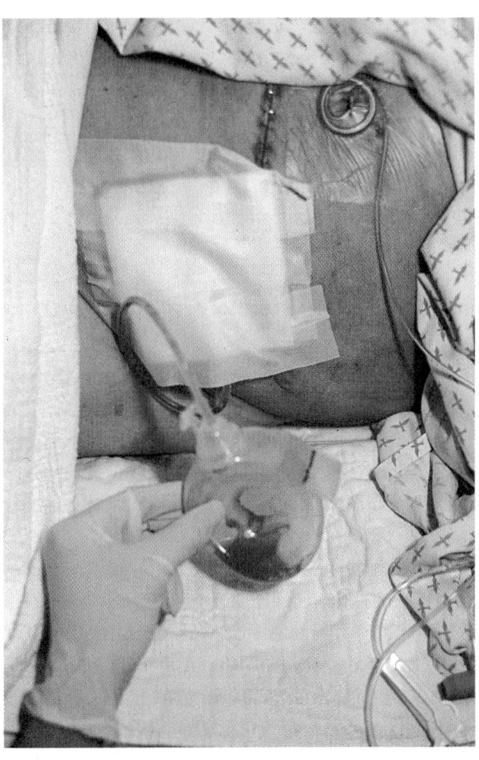
Figure 17-9 Jackson-Pratt drain.

examples of closed-suction drainage systems. Closed drains also may be attached to wall or portable suction devices for a greater range of suction capacity. The level of suction is based on the amount and area to be evacuated. Some suction drains contain filters and have the capacity for reinfusion of blood products, for example, Gish and Solcotrans drains. In some cases, drainage is by gravity through a tube, such as a T tube (Figure 17-10) or Penrose drain. Colonization of drain tracts increases with time; therefore drains should be left in place the shortest amount of time to accomplish the evacuation of hematomas or seromas.

Nursing interventions related to drains focus on the preparation of the drainage system components, assessment of patency and drainage, and accurate documentation. After the surgeon places the tubing, the drain is assembled using sterile technique. Patency of the system and the amount, type, color, and consistency of the drainage is assessed. The type and location of drainage and the drainage assessment

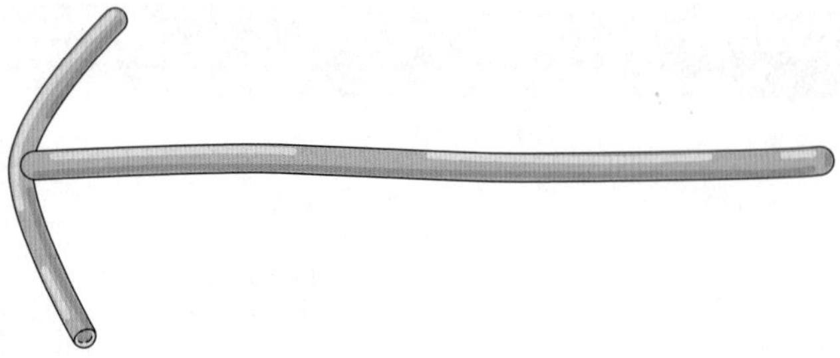

Figure 17-10 T tube drain.

are recorded and reported to the nurse in the postoperative receiving unit.

Dressings

Protecting the incision site from contamination is a means of minimizing risk for postoperative wound infection. Most surgical wounds are closed by primary intention. After the wound is closed, a sterile dressing is applied and maintained for 24 to 48 hours.[5] There are inconclusive data to support maintaining a dressing beyond 48 hours as a method to prevent infection and promote healing.[5] Dressings also absorb drainage, protect the incision from trauma, and give support to the incision and surrounding skin. The circulating nurse is responsible for ensuring dressing security and documenting the condition of the dressing before the patients is transferred to the postoperative unit.

5. Minimizing Risk for Alteration in Normothermia

Hypothermia

Factors that put patients at risk for alterations in body temperature are trauma, advanced age, malnutrition, prolonged preoperative inactivity, and sedation. The greatest heat loss occurs in the first hour of surgery; therefore heat conservation methods should be initiated early by the perioperative nurse.

Prevention is the best treatment of hypothermia. An intervention that can be initiated immediately after admission to the OR is the application of warm blankets. Before surgery begins, the patient should remain covered as much as possible. This necessitates that an ample supply of blankets be available in warming cabinets at all times. Blankets should be warmed to 105° F (40.5° C) and changed every 15 minutes. Another intervention that is used successfully during preoperative preparations is a radiant lamp. The application of thermal coverings, especially a covering for the head, is recommended to reduce radiant heat loss. During surgery an automatic thermal blanket is often placed under the patient.

The temperature and humidity of the room should be controlled. The nurse should ensure that the patient's skin is exposed as little as possible during positioning, prepping, and draping. Skin prep solutions can be warmed before use. The nurse should ensure that the sheets and drapes on and under the patient are dry, both to prevent heat loss and skin irritation and to maintain asepsis. A forced-air warming device (Bair Hugger) is commonly used during surgery to conserve body temperature.

Core body temperature should be monitored throughout the procedure. Sites for measurement of body temperature are chosen based on accessibility, comfort, and safety. Pulmonary artery monitoring provides the most accurate measurement but is an invasive technique. Tympanic membrane measurement correlates closely to core temperature because of the proximity of the carotid arteries that supply blood both to the tympanic membrane and the hypothalamus.[32] Body temperature can also be measured by probes inserted into the esophagus, rectum, or urinary bladder, although rectal and bladder readings may overestimate core temperature.[32] If the patient is intubated, an esophageal probe may be inserted for continuous temperature monitoring. Temperature probes placed in the distal third of the esophagus are closely correlated with core temperature. Temperatures measured in the mid or proximal esophagus are affected by inhaled gases and are not reliable.

During most surgical procedures a large amount of fluid is administered intravenously and topically for wound irrigation. The circulating nurse ensures that all fluids presented to the anesthesiologist or added to the surgical field are warm. In the immediate postoperative period, warm blankets are applied as soon as surgical patient drapes are removed.

Hyperthermia

Hyperthermia occurs less frequently than hypothermia in the surgical patient. Malignant hyperthermia generally occurs in response to certain anesthetics. Other risk factors for hyperthermia include dehydration, fever, vasoconstriction from medication, endocrine disorders such as thyroid disease, and intracranial infection or injury to the hypothalamus.

During surgery nursing interventions for cooling include removing excessive drapes, applying alcohol or cool water to the patient's skin, assisting with the monitoring of vital signs, using an automatic cooling blanket, and assisting with the preparation and administration of cool intravenous fluids and emergency medications. A preoperative baseline temperature should be recorded for all patients. Core body temperature should be monitored throughout the procedure.

As with all nursing interventions, documentation should include all measures taken, equipment used (including serial numbers and temperature settings), and patient responses to treatment. Communication with the postoperative receiving unit is imperative for the continuity of patient care. This is especially important in cases in which an alteration in normothermia resulted in an emergent situation.

6. Promoting Fluid Balance

Intraoperative monitoring of fluid loss and adequate replacement is a high priority throughout the procedure for both anesthesiologist and circulating nurse. The nurse assists the anesthesiologist in monitoring the patient during surgery.

In the surgical patient alterations in fluid balance include the risk for both hypovolemia and hypervolemia. Hypovolemia can be defined as isotonic fluid loss from the extracellular space. An excess of isotonic fluid in the extracellular (interstitial or intravascular) compartment results in hypervolemia. Untreated hypovolemia (loss of 40% or more of intravascular volume) can lead to hypovolemic shock. Hypervolemia may result from excessive isotonic fluid replacement or excessive blood or plasma replacement. Fluid shifts into the intravascular space may be caused by administration of albumin and hypertonic IV fluids. Hypervolemia, if not corrected, can result in pulmonary edema and congestive heart failure. Electrolyte imbalance may also occur as a result of preexisting disease, surgical stress, preoperative steroid or diuretic use, preoperative regimens such as enemas or laxatives, and gastric suction and lavage.

Nursing interventions to promote fluid volume balance include monitoring of vital signs, particularly pulse and blood pressure, and accurate monitoring of intake and output of all fluids, including irrigation and blood loss. An indwelling urethral catheter is inserted before the start of surgery if the patient is at risk for fluid volume imbalance, for the critically ill patient if the surgery is expected to be lengthy, or if significant blood loss is anticipated. Urine output is recorded hourly. Blood loss is monitored by keeping an accurate record of the fluids administered into the wound, the amount of fluid suctioned from the operative site, and the amount of saturation of all sponges (sponges may be weighed for a more accurate estimation).

Common causes of fluid volume deficit include bleeding, decreased intake due to NPO status, inadequate IV fluid replacement, excessive gastrointestinal losses, evaporation of fluid from exposed cavities during surgery, inhalation of dry anesthetic gases, and third-spacing of fluid. Third-spacing occurs when fluid moves out of the intravascular space, but not into the intracellular space, as a result of increased capillary membrane permeability or decrease in plasma colloid osmotic pressure. The fluid may shift into the surgical site such as the abdominal or pleural cavity. Third-space fluid losses may be significant after extensive tissue dissection; other causes include peritonitis, bowel obstruction, ascites, and hypoalbuminemia.

Treatment goals related to hypovolemia include replacement of lost fluids, maintenance of normal blood pressure, and restoration of blood volume. To increase blood volume isotonic fluids such as normal saline or lactated Ringer's solution are administered. Blood replacement may be necessary if blood loss exceeds 1200 ml or the hematocrit drops below 30%. Blood or blood products may be transfused to compensate for the loss or to prevent shock. Transfusions may be homologous or autologous. Blood products include whole blood, packed red cells, fresh frozen plasma, platelets, serum albumin, and blood substitutes. Assessment of the available blood and ordering of additional blood must be performed continuously to remain ahead of anticipated needs. Before administration of any blood product the necessary identification and safety precautions must be followed.

During the procedure blood may be recovered from the field for autotransfusion. Blood can be suctioned from the wound, body cavity, or drapes and sponges. All blood recovery devices must be approved by the FDA. If a microfibrillar collagen has been used for hemostasis, blood may not be salvaged because of the risk of DIC or adult respiratory distress syndrome. Persons with known systemic infections or open trauma are not candidates for autotransfusion.

If intraoperative cell salvage is used, the nurse must be familiar with the use of autotransfusion devices. Three basic systems available for autotransfusions are cell salvage processors, canister collection systems, and salvage collection bags. All components of the system are sterile and disposable. If not used intraoperatively, the blood collected may be processed and bagged for transfusion postoperatively. Alternative methods include salvaging blood from reinfusion drains. The blood is anticoagulated and may be collected for a maximum of 6 hours; the red cells are reinfused intravenously. The anesthesiologist records all blood products given, the amount of solutions used by the surgeon, the estimated blood loss, and all intraoperative events concerning fluid imbalances.

Patient/Family Education

The patient and family should be instructed about perioperative routines on arrival in the OR suite. Although this information was covered in a teaching session (location will vary depending on circumstances), reinforcement is beneficial because of the anxiety the patient may be experiencing. Anticipating both the patient and family's questions helps allay their concerns. The family should be told where to wait and the anticipated length of events. During the procedure and recovery period, the nurse can communicate the patient's status to the family.

EVALUATION

Evaluation of intraoperative patient care is achieved by comparing the patient's responses to interventions with the expected outcomes. Achievement of outcomes is successful if the intraoperative patient:

- **1.** Shows little subjective or objective evidence of anxiety.
- **2a.** Is free from neurovascular and neuromuscular injuries related to surgical positioning.
- **2b.** Exhibits intact skin with no evidence of pressure beyond 24 to 48 hours.
- **3.** Shows no signs of injury or trauma from electrical, chemical, or physical factors.
- **4.** Exhibits no swelling or redness at the incision site.
- **5a.** Has body temperature at desired intraoperative level.
- **5b.** Is at or near normothermia.
- **6.** Maintains stable vital signs without evidence of hypovolemia or cardiac overload.

Feedback about postoperative findings from nursing peers on patient care units can supply valuable information for evaluation and should be encouraged. In ambulatory surgery settings, a follow-up telephone call to the patient at home should be made by nursing personnel. This can be useful in obtaining feedback about the nursing care received during the surgical intervention.

Critical Thinking Questions

1. An 80-year-old woman is scheduled for a hemiarthroplasty for a fractured left hip. On arrival in the holding room her oral temperature is 36.1° C. She is oriented to person only. Her past history includes hypertension, congestive heart failure, and type 2 diabetes. What elements of her history will influence her intraoperative management? What nursing interventions should be included in her plan of care to prevent complications?
2. A 46-year-old woman is scheduled for a right breast biopsy. During the immediate preoperative interview the circulating nurse notes that the patient's perception of the procedure is not congruent with the scheduled surgical procedure and informed consent. What actions by the circulating nurse are appropriate?
3. A 28-year-old man with paraplegia is scheduled for a skin graft for a stage IV pressure ulcer. He has a documented history of type I allergic response to latex. Devise an intraoperative plan of care for the patient.
4. A 35-year-old woman involved in a motor vehicle accident is brought to the OR for an emergent abdominal exploration. Preoperative assessment reveals a hematocrit of 32% and hemoglobin of 10 g/dl. The patient is also a Jehovah's Witness and refuses receipt of any blood products. What intraoperative techniques may be used to reduce this patient's risk for bleeding?
5. A patient is scheduled for cosmetic surgery with sedation and analgesia. As the nurse assigned to monitor this patient, develop the intraoperative plan of care.

References

1. AORN recommended practices for positioning the patient in the perioperative practice setting, *AORN J* 73(1):231, 2001.
2. AORN recommended practices for maintaining a sterile field, *AORN J* 73(2):477, 2001.
3. Association of Operating Room Nurses: *2001 Standards and recommended practices,* Denver, Colo, 2001, AORN Publications.
4. Adams A: Surgical site infections: another look at banishing bugs, *Nurs 2000* 30(6):50, 2000.
5. Adams A: Preventing surgical site infection (SSI): guidelines at a glance, *Nurs Manage* 32(8):46, 2001.
6. Armstrong D, Bortz P: An integrative review of pressure relief in surgical patients, *AORN J* 73(3):645, 2001.
7. Arndt K: Inadvertent hypothermia in the OR, *AORN J* 70(2):203, 1999.
8. Bailes BK:Perioperative care of the elderly surgical patients, *AORN J* 72(2):186, 2000.
9. Bond G:Infection control assessment in the periopertive setting, *Semin Periop Nurs* 8(1):24, 1999.
10. Davis BR: Perioperative care of patients with latex allergy, *AORN J* 72(1):47, 2000.
11. Defina GA, Lincoln J: Prevalence of inadvertent hypothermia during the periopertaive period: a quality assurance and performance improvement study, *J Perianesthesia Nurs* 13(4):229, 1998.
12. Drummond JC: Monitoring depth of anesthesia, *Anesthesiology* 93(3):876, 2000.
13. Eck E, DeBaun B, Pugliese G: OSHA compliance: needlestick prevention requires planning, products, and people, *Infect Control Today* 5(8):32, 2001.
14. Ensminger J, Rose M: Preventing inadvertnent hypothermia-a success story, *AORN J* 70(2):298, 1999.
15. Fortunato NH: *Berry and Kohn's operating room technique,* ed 9, St Louis, 2000, Mosby.
16. Gritter M: The latex threat, *AJN* 98(9):26, 1998.
17. Hamann CP, Rodgers PA, Sullivan K: Latex allergy update, *Infect Control Today* 5(3):34, 2001.
18. Hemmings HC, HopkinsPM: *Foundations of anesthesia: basic and clinical sciences,* St Louis, 2000, Mosby.
19. Joint Commission for Accreditation of HealthCare Organizations: Standards and intents for sedation and anesthesia care, *Comprehensive Accreditation Manual for Hospitals,* 2001, website: http://www.jcaho.org/standard/aneshap.html.
20. Karlet MC: Malignant hyperthermia: considerations for ambulatory surgery, *J Perianesthesia Nurs* 13(5):304, 1998.
21. Larson RN et al: Comparison of different regimens for surgical hand preparation, *AORN J* 73(2):412, 2001.
22. Mangram AJ et al: Guideline for prevention of surgical site infection, 1999, *Infect Control Hosp Epidemiol* 20(4):247, 1999.
23. Meeker MH, Rothrock JC: *Alexander's care of the patient in surgery,* ed 11, St Louis, 1999, Mosby.
24. Messinger JA et al: Getting conscious sedation right, *AJN* 99(12):44, 1999.
25. Murphy EK: Needlestick safety and prevention act, *AORN J* 73(2):458, 2001.
26. Muscarella LW: Assessing the risk of Creutzfeldt-Jakob disease, *Infect Control Today* 5(8):28, 2001.
27. Pandit SK: Ambulatory anesthesia and surgery in America: a historical background and recent innovations, *J Perianesthesia Nurs* 14(5):270, 1999.
28. Perry J: The blood-borne pathogens standard, 2001, *Nursing 2001* 31(6):32, 2001.
29. Peters S: Held hostage breaking free from latex allergy, *Adv Nurse Pract* 7(6):53, 1999.
30. Ramsey CA: Preoperative measures to prevent surgical site infections, *Infect Control Today* 4(5):54, 2001.
31. Schultz A et al: Etiology and incidence of pressure ulcers in surgical patients, *AORN J* 70(3):434, 1999.
32. Scott EM et al: Effects of warming therapy on pressure ulcers-a randomized trial, *AORN J* 73(5):921, 2001.
33. Singer EA: Local anesthesia: principles and techniques for the primary care nurse practitioner, *Am J Nurse Pract* 4(10):27, 2000.
34. Sleigh JW et al: The bispectral index: a measure of depth of sleep? *Anesthesia Analg* 88:659, 1999.
35. Stolworthy C, Haas RE: Malignant hyperthermia: a potential fatal complication of anesthesia, *Semin Periop Nurs* 1(1):58, 1998.
36. Warner MA et al: Practice guidelines for preoperative fasting and the use of pharmacologic agents to reduce the risk of pulmonary aspiration: application to healthy patients undergoing elective procedures, *A Report by the American Society of Anesthesiologists,* October 21, 1998.

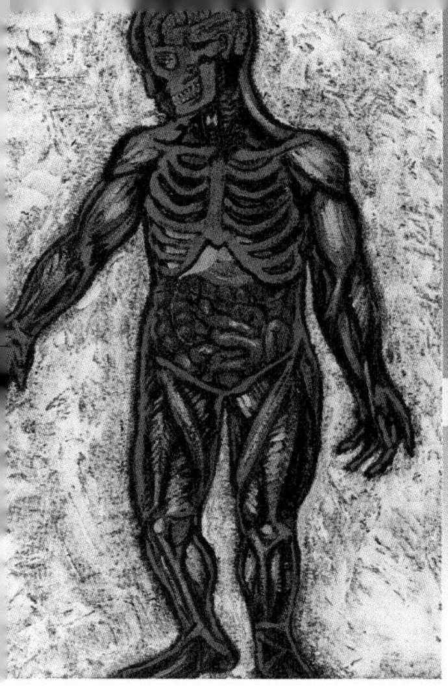

http://www.mosby.com/MERLIN/medsurg_phipps

18 Postoperative Nursing

Mary Jo Boehnlein, Jane F. Marek

Objectives

After studying this chapter, the learner should be able to:

1. Describe the postoperative phase as a component of the surgical experience.
2. Identify postoperative complications that may compromise a patient's safety and stability after anesthesia and surgical intervention.
3. Discuss patient risk factors for potential postoperative complications.
4. Discuss postoperative patient assessment.
5. Formulate relevant postoperative nursing diagnoses.
6. Identify desired patient outcomes for the postoperative phase.
7. Describe nursing interventions to prevent or treat postoperative complications.
8. Describe the interventions to minimize anxiety in patients and their families during the postoperative course.
9. Discuss the relevance of evaluation and documentation of nursing care interventions.
10. Identify the benefits of follow-up communication and referrals for the patient's later postoperative recovery.

The postoperative phase begins with the transfer of the patient from the operating room to the appropriate postoperative unit and ends with the discharge of the patient from the surgical facility or the hospital. The focus of nursing care in the postoperative phase is the patient's return, as quickly as possible, to an optimal level of functioning.

The primary focus of this chapter is the nursing care of the patient in the postanesthesia care unit (PACU). The postoperative nursing care on the patient care unit is reviewed in lesser detail. The nursing diagnoses and interventions address the postoperative patient care needs in both the PACU and the patient care unit.

The immediate postanesthesia phase presents multifaceted challenges in patient care. Anesthesia and surgical interventions place great stress on all body systems (see Chapter 17). The postanesthesia nurse must understand the patient's risks for postoperative complications and be prepared to quickly implement appropriate interventions should an acute change in the patient's status occur.

To meet the criteria for transfer from the PACU to the clinical unit or to the home, the patient must be stable and free from symptoms of complications. The potential for the development of postoperative complications continues beyond the immediate postoperative phase. Ongoing nursing assessment is essential to providing care after the patient is transferred to a specific clinical unit. Nursing interventions focus on minimizing the potential for postoperative complications and planning for recovery and discharge. Effective preoperative patient teaching (see Chapter 16) prepares the patient for a role in facilitating the recovery course; this information is reinforced in the postoperative period.

It is common practice to be discharged the day of surgery or after a short stay in the hospital. In addition to economic incentives, improvements in surgical and anesthetic techniques have made ambulatory and short-stay surgery both safe and efficient. As a result, the patient and family have an increased responsibility for self-care and have more complex teaching and discharge needs. For this reason, assessing the patient's needs and providing relevant information are crucial responsibilities for nurses who care for patients in the early postoperative period.

HISTORICAL BACKGROUND

General anesthesia has been used since the late 1890s and surgical procedures date back to the Egyptian age. In contrast, a specially designated area for the recovery of postsurgical patients is comparatively new, dating to the 1860s. Florence Nightingale described the use of a small room adjacent to the operating theater where the patient remained until he or she recovered from the immediate effects of the operation.[9] Even though Nightingale described this concept in the nineteenth century, it was World War II that had the greatest impact on the development of the modern-day PACU. Because of the shortage of nurses there was a need to centralize patients and equipment to efficiently deliver care.

Many PACUs opened in the 1940s after it was discovered that a specialized unit decreased patient morbidity and mortality and shortened length of stay.[19] Postoperative mortality within the first 24 hours after administration of anesthesia and surgical intervention was caused by airway obstruction, laryngospasm, hemorrhage, cardiac arrest, or medication error. Other factors that contributed to mortality included a lack of standardized patient care and an absence of medical and nursing supervision.[9] As a result of these findings, many hospitals opened these units staffed with specially trained nurses for the care of patients recovering from anesthesia. Today, most patients recovering from general or regional anesthesia are transferred from the operating room (OR) to the PACU before discharge or transfer to a nursing division. Critically ill patients may be directly transferred from the OR to an intensive care unit (ICU).

IMMEDIATE POSTANESTHESIA CARE

The PACU is usually located adjacent to the operating rooms. The basic design consists of a large open room divided into individual patient care spaces. The number of spaces depends on the number of individual operating rooms in the surgical suite. In general, there are 1 to 1.5 PACU patient care spaces per OR. Each individual patient care space is supplied with a cardiac monitor, blood pressure monitoring device, pulse oximeter, airway management equipment, suction, and oxygen. Emergency medications and equipment are centrally located. Isolation rooms are available if needed. The length of stay in the PACU is generally less than 24 hours.

Personnel

Registered nurses in the PACU have an in-depth knowledge of anesthetic agents and patient responses to these agents, pain management techniques, surgical procedures, and potential complications. The PACU nurse demonstrates competence in physical assessment and managing emergency situations.

In 1986 the American Society of Post Anesthesia Nurses (ASPAN) developed specialty certification for registered nurses working in the PACU. Certification in ambulatory postanesthesia is available for nurses working in ambulatory surgical settings.[9] Other staff assisting the nurse in the PACU includes licensed practical nurses and unlicensed assistive personnel.

Phases of Postanesthesia Care

The ASPAN has identified three distinct phases of care: the preanesthesia phase, postanesthesia phase I, and postanesthesia phase II. The focus of the preanesthesia phase is the patient's emotional and physical preparation before surgery. Postanesthesia phase I encompasses the care of the patient emerging from anesthesia through until the patient is physiologically stable and does not require one-to-one care. During this phase the PACU nurse makes a preliminary assessment of breath sounds, respiratory effort, oxygen saturation, blood pressure, cardiac rhythm, level of consciousness, and muscle strength. Postanesthesia phase II begins when the patient's level of consciousness returns to baseline and the patient has a patent airway, intact upper airway reflexes, manageable pain, and stable pulmonary, cardiac, and renal functioning. During this phase the patient is transferred to the nursing division or short-stay unit.

NURSING MANAGEMENT

NURSING CARE CONSIDERATIONS IN THE POSTANESTHESIA CARE UNIT

The PACU nurse cares for a diverse patient population ranging from the ambulatory surgical patient to the individual requiring continuous invasive monitoring and mechanical ventilation. The diversity of operative procedures and anesthetic techniques presents a challenge to PACU nurses.

Transfer to the Postanesthesia Care Unit

The circulating nurse informs the PACU of the patient's estimated time of arrival in the unit and also of any special care needs or equipment required. A detailed report is given when the patient is admitted to the unit.

Physical Assessment

The nurse/patient ratio on admission to the PACU is 1:1. While connecting the monitoring equipment, applying oxygen, and making an immediate physiologic assessment, the PACU nurse receives reports from the anesthesiologist, surgeon, and circulating nurse. The verbal report includes data regarding the surgical procedure and intraoperative patient responses. Data in the report are based on recommendations made by the ASPAN in 1992 (Box 18-1).[19] The anesthesiologist is in attendance until the PACU nurse accepts responsibility for the patient. The American Society of Anesthesiologists Standards mandates the anesthesiologist's presence for Postanesthesia Care.[19]

After the verbal reports and immediate assessment of the patient's airway, respiratory, and circulatory status, the PACU nurse performs a more thorough patient assessment. The ASPAN has also made recommendations for the components of the initial PACU assessment (Box 18-2). Nursing units differ in the method of organizing patient assessment data. Some use a head-to-toe approach; others use a major body systems approach (Figure 18-1).

Nursing care in the immediate postoperative phase focuses on maintaining ventilation and circulation, monitoring oxygenation, monitoring level of consciousness, preventing shock, and managing pain. Assessments of respiratory, circulatory, and neurologic functions are performed and documented at frequent intervals. Neurologic status is ascertained by observing the patient's level of consciousness. Response to verbal or noxious stimuli is noted. Pupils are assessed for responsiveness to light and accommodation. Equality and

BOX 18-1 Patient Status Report on Admission to the Postanesthesia Care Unit

Patient demographics
Need for life-support equipment
Allergies
Pertinent medical history
ASA status
Baseline vital signs
Surgical procedure performed
Intraoperative positioning
Type and length of anesthetic
Time and type of reversal agents given
Estimated blood loss
Amount of intraoperative fluid replacement
Urine output
Intravenous and invasive lines
Medications administered
Laboratory data
Vital signs
Intraoperative procedure performed
Presence of implants
Dressings
Drainage tubes and locations with recorded output
Patient skin condition
Orders to be initiated in postanesthesia care unit
Presence of family in waiting area
Preoperative anxiety level

ASA, American Society of Anesthesiologists.

BOX 18-2 Nursing Assessment in the Postanesthesia Care Unit

- Vital signs
  - Presence of artificial airway
  - Ventilator settings as needed
  - Oxygen saturations
  - Respiratory assessment
  - Blood pressure (cuff or arterial line)
  - Pulse (apical, peripheral)
  - Monitored cardiac rhythm
  - Temperature (include method of measurement)
- Level of consciousness
  - Ability to follow commands
  - Pupillary response
- Urinary output
- Skin integrity
- Neurovascular assessment of extremities (as appropriate)
- Motor assessment
- Pain
  - Location
  - Presence
  - Severity
  - Character
  - Pain scale rating
- Patient-controlled analgesia
- Dressings
- Condition of surgical wound
- Drainage tubes
  - Type
  - Location
  - Amount and character of drainage
  - Patency
- Presence of intravenous lines
  - Type and location of site
  - Type, amount, and rate of solution infusing
- Additional monitoring parameters (as appropriate)
  - Intracranial
  - Central venous
  - Arterial line
  - Pulmonary artery
- Position of patient
- Patient safety needs
  - Side rails
- Level of psychosocial support
- Anxiety
- Numeric score (as applicable)

Adapted from Meeker MH, Rothrock JC: *Alexander's care of the patient in surgery,* ed 11, St Louis, 1999, Mosby.

strength of handgrip also are assessed. A handgrip sustained for 5 seconds is an indication that neuromuscular function is returning. The ability to move all extremities is also assessed and noted.

Many institutions use clinical pathways to deliver safe, efficient, and cost-effective patient care. An example of a Clinical Pathway (coordinated care track) for use in the PACU can be found on p. 431.

Laboratory and diagnostic data are also used for patient assessment in the PACU. Objective assessment of the patient's respiratory status may include pulse oximetry, arterial blood gases, and chest x-ray. The patient's heart rate and rhythm are continuously monitored via electrocardiogram. Frequent assessment of the patient's hematologic and renal status may be indicated, especially if there were significant intraoperative blood and fluid losses.

Pain

Pain (see Chapter 12) is a common occurrence after nearly all types of surgical procedures. Postoperative pain is most severe after intrathoracic, intraabdominal, and major orthopedic surgeries. Surgical pain is usually acute and is classified as nociceptive pain. Nociceptive pain results from tissue trauma during surgery, that is, from cutting, pulling, and manipulating tissues and organs and positioning and pressure areas during surgery. Stimulation of nerve endings by chemical substances released at the time of surgery or from tissue ischemia caused by interference of blood supply to tissues also contribute to pain. Reduced blood supply may be caused by pressure, muscle spasm, or edema. Somatic pain occurs as a result of trauma to bone, joint, muscle, connective tissue, or skin. Pain can be further classified as either somatic or visceral. The quality of somatic pain is usually aching or throbbing and localized. Extensive tissue dissection and prolonged retraction of muscle and fascia contribute to the development of somatic pain.

Visceral pain occurs as a result of trauma to the visceral organs. Visceral pain occurring as a result of tumor involvement is usually described as localized and aching. Obstruction of

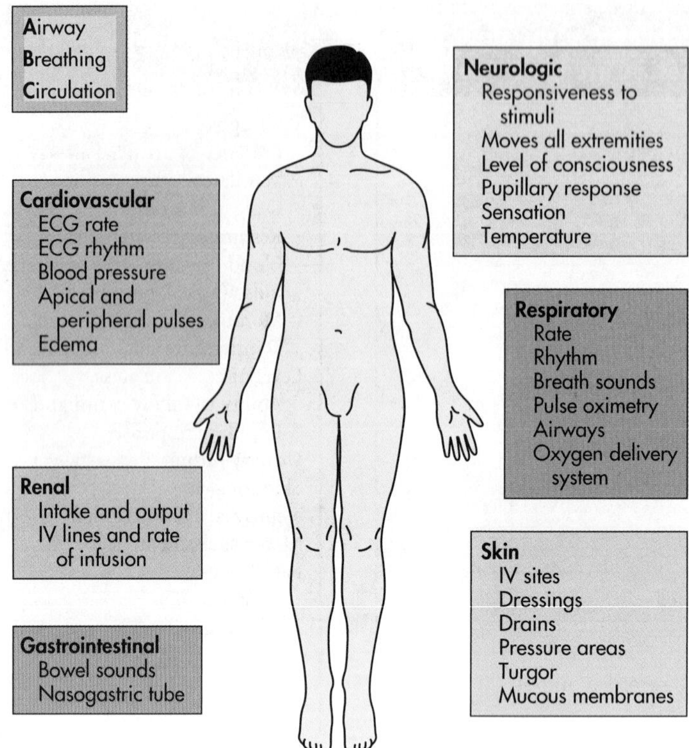

Figure 18-1 Body system approach to assessment.

hollow visceral organs usually results in intermittent cramping and poorly localized pain.

After surgery other factors can contribute to the pain sensation: distended bladder, gas used for insufflation during endoscopic procedures, infection, distention, muscle spasms surrounding the incisional area, tight dressings or casts, and the patient's pain threshold and response to pain. The presence of pain can prolong recovery because it can interfere with return to activity.

Anxiety in the PACU Environment

The environment of a postanesthesia unit is sometimes noisy and hectic. Florence Nightingale first noted that unnecessary noise is detrimental to patients.[9] Patient care needs change swiftly and sometimes dramatically. A balance of caring and technologic skills provides a safe and supportive approach to patient care that can help to relieve patient anxiety.

On awakening from anesthesia, the patient needs frequent reorientation and reassurance of not being alone. The patient also needs to know that the operation is over and that recovery from anesthesia is satisfactory. Careful explanations of procedures should be given even when it appears that the patient is not alert. The patient who has had regional anesthesia should be reassured that sensation and movement in the extremities will return.

Reassurance should be offered that family or significant others have been notified of the patient's safe arrival in the recovery room. Research has shown that family visitation in the PACU benefits both patients and family and may be a simple intervention to relieve anxiety.[27] PACU traditionally has not been an area where visitation has been allowed, but evidence supporting this practice may influence change in visitation policies.

Most surgeons discuss the results of the operation with the patient and family immediately after the surgery. Family members commonly are highly anxious about the patient's condition and may not perceive or understand all that the surgeon tells them. Patients often experience periods of amnesia during the hours when they first regain consciousness and may not remember what they have been told. To provide satisfactory answers to the patient's and family members' questions, the nurse needs to know what information was given. The family also needs to know what to expect when the patient returns to the unit and when the patient is ready for discharge.

Some of the concerns that were present in the preoperative period (see Chapter 16) may continue into the postoperative period. These concerns generally focus on the performed surgery, the results of the surgery, and the temporary or permanent effects that may change a patient's lifestyle. The patient may have concerns about changes in roles, body image, return to work, lifestyle, emotional status, economic implications of the surgery, or prognosis.

Assessment for Complications

Respiratory. Assessing respiratory status is of primary importance during the immediate postoperative period. Both a patent airway and adequate respiratory function should be ascertained. Immediate respiratory complications that may occur include airway obstruction, hypoxemia, hypoventilation, aspiration, and laryngospasm.

clinical pathway *Postanesthesia Care Unit Coordinated Care Track*

Patient Classification: III
DATE:

PATIENT IMPRINT

TIME FRAME	TIME OF ADMISSION: 0-30 MIN	30-90 MIN	90-180 MIN	TIME OF TRANSFER: 3-6 HR
Patient Satisfaction	Pediatric support person at bedside		What can we do to enhance your stay with us?	
Discharge Planning	Identify risk factors for prolonged recovery		Plan for bed availability	Discharge to Regular Nursing Floor (RNF) or extended recovery/ICU
Airway Management	Airway Assessment Ventilator settings as ordered/O_2 as ordered Monitor O_2 Saturation Vital signs per protocol	Assess for readiness to wean	Wean ventilatory support/O_2 per protocol	Wean to room air Incentive spirometry q2h after extubation
Hemodynamic Management	Hemodynamic monitoring Hemodynamic support as necessary	Monitor need for hemodynamic support	Wean from hemodynamic support as tolerated	
Nursing and Medical Interventions	Identify patient by name and arm band Identify allergies Level of consciousness assessment Dressing assessment Systems assessment Dermatome assessment Report from anesthesia Initiate surgical-specific protocols Pain management—provide pharmacological therapies Rewarming initiated IV and arterial line management Initiate stir-up regimen (wake up) Place necessary consults Admission documentation	Review chart for patient information Pain management—provide pharmacological and nonpharmacological therapies Review orders Implement physician orders Continue stir-up regimen Emotional support Treat nausea/vomiting if necessary Monitor for potential surgical complications	Labs, x-rays complete Consults complete Wean from rewarming devices Patient repositioned Mouth care given Monitor for potential surgical complications Assess need for extended observation	Monitor for potential surgical complications Assess need for extended observation or ICU care
Patient Education	Family notified patient in PACU Orient to person, place, and time Explain activities of care while providing care	Answer patient questions Reinforce pain scale	Family called for update on patient's condition Orient to expectations of PACU discharge	Family visit for 15 minutes Instruct on postop pain management Instruct on importance of coughing, deep breathing, and exercising limbs
Outcome Criteria	Vital signs within normal parameters Oxygenation within normal range Dressing and drains intact	Vital signs within normal parameters Dressing and drains intact No excessive bleeding Pain minimized	Oriented to person and place/returned to baseline mentation Hemodynamically stable	Postanesthesia Score >8 Temp 35.5°-38.4° C Coughing and deep breathing Pain < 4 Minimal nausea/vomiting No evidence of surgical complications All appropriate physician orders initiated

Courtesy Cleveland Clinic Foundation, Department of Advanced Practice Nursing, Cleveland, Ohio.

Respiratory complications are the leading cause of morbidity and mortality in the immediate postoperative period.[25,26] Although respiratory complications are more common in patients with known respiratory disease or other risk factors, the potential for complications exists for all patients (see Chapter 16).

Airway Obstruction. The amount of airway support required depends on the individual patient, anesthetic technique, and type of surgery. Patients may be admitted to the PACU with an endotracheal tube or laryngeal mask airway in place. However, anesthesia techniques often allow extubation or airway removal in the operating room as the patient emerges from general anesthesia, recovers reflexes, and is able to respond to verbal stimuli. A serious complication for patients recovering from general anesthesia is airway obstruction.

Airway obstruction is commonly thought to occur as a result of movement of the tongue (relaxed from anesthesia) into the posterior pharynx (Figure 18-2), anesthetic-induced changes in pharyngeal and laryngeal muscle tone; laryngospasm; edema; and secretions or other fluid collecting in the pharynx, bronchial tree, or trachea. Clinical manifestations include gurgling, wheezing, stridor, sternal and intercostal retractions, hypoxemia, and hypercarbia. Initial treatment consists of administration of 100% oxygen, physical maneuvers to maintain airway (jaw-thrust maneuver), suctioning of secretions, and insertion of an oral or nasal airway. Insertion of an oral airway must be accompanied by the jaw-thrust maneuver. If these interventions are unsuccessful, endotracheal intubation, cricothyroidotomy, or tracheostomy may be necessary.

Another population at risk for the development of airway obstruction are patients with a history of obstructive sleep apnea syndrome (OSAS). OSAS is caused by complete or partial collapse of the pharynx during inspiration resulting in airway obstruction and is associated with hypoxemia, apnea, and interrupted sleep. The effects of anesthesia increase the risk for airway obstruction. Airway obstruction is most likely to occur in the recovery phase of general anesthesia in patients with OSAS.[12] Patients with OSAS are also at risk for hypoxemia because of the residual effects of anesthetic agents. The patient should be monitored for periods of apnea and arrhythmias; oxygen saturation should be continuously monitored.

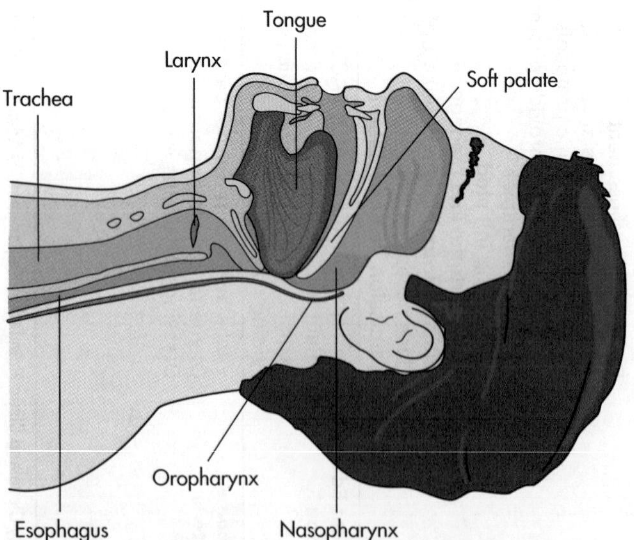

Figure 18-2 Obstruction of airway by tongue blocking oropharynx in unconscious person lying supine.

Hypoxemia. Hypoxemia is a common complication that occurs in the immediate postoperative period. Hypoxemia may occur as a result of hypoventilation, which diminishes the exchange of oxygen between the alveoli and the atmosphere. The following factors contribute to the risk for hypoventilation and hypoxemia:

- Opioids (respiratory center depression)
- Insufficient reversal of neuromuscular blocking agents (residual muscle paralysis)
- Increased tissue resistance (emphysema, infections)
- Decreased lung and chest wall compliance (pneumonia, restrictive diseases)
- Obesity, gastric and abdominal distention
- Constrictive dressings
- Incision site close to the diaphragm
- General anesthesia
- Postoperative pain

Aspiration. Aspiration is the inhalation of gastric contents or blood into the tracheobronchial system. Aspiration usually is caused by regurgitation; however, aspiration of blood may result from trauma or surgical manipulation (e.g., after tonsillectomy). Aspiration of gastric contents can cause chemical irritation, pneumonitis, destruction of tracheobronchial mucosa, and an increased risk of secondary infection. Risk factors for aspiration include decreased level of consciousness, dysphagia, delayed gastric emptying, head and neck surgery, history of hiatal hernia, and emergent intubation of a patient with a full stomach.

Laryngospasm. Laryngospasm is a spasm of laryngeal muscle tissue and may manifest as complete or partial closure of the vocal cords, resulting in airway obstruction. Untreated, laryngospasm can cause hypoxia, cerebral damage, and death. Airway irritation is a major causative factor for the development of laryngospasm. Certain anesthetic agents, laryngoscope blades used in intubation, endotracheal tube placement, or surgical stimulation (e.g., bronchoscope passage) can cause irritation. In the PACU, repeated suctioning and irritation by the endotracheal tube or artificial airway can cause laryngospasm after extubation. Symptoms of laryngospasm include dyspnea, crowing sounds, hypoxemia, and hypercapnia.

Cardiovascular. Assessing the patient's status for postoperative complications is a priority for nursing care. Hypotension, hypertension, and cardiac dysrhythmias occurring as a result of the influence of anesthetic agents on the central nervous system (CNS), myocardium, and peripheral vascular system are the most commonly encountered cardiovascular complications in the immediate postanesthesia period.

Hypotension. Hypotension is generally defined as a systolic pressure of 90 mm Hg or below or as a 20% decrease from the patient's baseline measurement.[19] The most common cause of hypotension is a decreased preload secondary to hypovolemia;

other causes include failure of the heart muscle to pump adequately and reduced peripheral vascular resistance.[19] Hemorrhage, inadequate fluid replacement, pneumothorax, vasodilation caused by drugs or anesthetic agents, or pulmonary embolus can contribute to hypovolemia. A common cause of postoperative hypotension is blood loss or inadequate fluid replacement. Other causes of hypotension include shock, ischemia, hypoxia, myocardial infarction, dysrhythmias, third-space fluid loss, and congestive heart failure. Clinical manifestations of hypotension and hypovolemia include increased heart rate, decreased urinary output, pallor of extremities, confusion, and restlessness.

Hypertension. Hypertension can be defined as a 20% to 30% increase from the patient's preoperative or baseline level. Common causes of hypertension include pain; reflex vasoconstriction in response to hypoxia, hypercarbia, or hyperthermia; preexisting hypertension; sympathetic stimulation; bladder distention; and anxiety. Persons with known hypertension or a history of cardiac disease are at increased risk for postoperative complications. Treatment of hypertension depends on the etiology. Untreated hypertension may lead to cardiac dysrhythmias, myocardial ischemia and infarction, left ventricular failure, pulmonary edema, and cerebrovascular accident.

Cardiac Dysrhythmias. Common dysrhythmias occurring in the immediate postoperative period include sinus tachycardia, sinus bradycardia, and supraventricular and ventricular dysrhythmias. Causes include preexisting cardiac disease, hypoxia, hypercarbia, respiratory acidosis, fluid and electrolyte imbalance, hypothermia, and pain. Determination of etiology is essential before initiating treatment. Initial treatment includes assessment of airway patency, adequate ventilation, medications, and supplemental oxygen.

Thermoregulation. Premedication, anesthesia, and the stress of surgery interact in a complex fashion to disrupt normal thermoregulation (see Chapter 17). Both hypothermia and hyperthermia are associated with physiologic alterations that may interfere with recovery. Patients at the age extremes and those who are extremely debilitated are at even greater risk for the development of postoperative temperature abnormalities.

Hypothermia. Prevention of abnormalities in thermoregulatory responses begins preoperatively with the nursing admission history (see Chapter 16). As many as 90% of surgical patients and 60% to 90% of those admitted to the PACU experience some degree of hypothermia.[6,7] After surgery hypothermia can extend recovery and increase postoperative morbidity. Delayed recovery time results from prolonged elimination of muscle relaxants and delayed drug metabolism by the liver and kidneys.

Anesthetic gases trigger heat loss by causing peripheral vasodilation. After induction of anesthesia, the body's homeostatic mechanisms in response to cold are decreased and the core temperature drops lower than normal before the body is able to begin adaptive responses. Some inhalation agents and muscle relaxants given during surgery decrease heat production and impede the shivering response.

Shivering, an involuntary skeletal muscular activity initiated by the hypothalamus to produce heat, is a compensatory mechanism in response to hypothermia and normally occurs with a 1° C drop in temperature. As the body temperature decreases, the basal metabolic rate drops 5% to 7% per degree Celsius of heat loss.[1] Shivering, the normal response to cold, increases oxygen demands by 300% to 400% and increases the metabolic rate 50% to 100%, resulting in increased myocardial workload.[1] For the patient without cardiac disease there are usually no significant sequelae; however, the patient with coronary artery disease or cardiac myopathy may decompensate.

Hypothermia also affects coagulation. Fibrinolysis increases and platelet activity decreases as the body temperature drops. Thus the risk of bleeding is increased. However, lengthy surgical procedures and venous stasis still can lead to the development of deep vein thrombosis (DVT) in hypothermic patients.

Hypothermia also causes decreased cerebral blood flow, resulting in CNS depression. The hypothermic patient may exhibit dilated pupils, slowed reactions and thought processes, and decreased coordination.[1]

Vasoconstriction occurs as a result of hypothermia. Vasoconstriction probably causes a fluid shift from the extracellular space, resulting in intravascular volume loss. Vasodilation occurs as the patient rewarms and approaches normothermia. To avoid hypovolemia during rewarming, the patient may require large amounts of intravenous fluids.

Objective signs of hypothermia include tachypnea, shivering, and tachycardia, but may be difficult to detect in the anesthetized patient as a result of the effects of anesthetics. Inadvertent hypothermia is often not detected until the immediate postoperative period when the effects of anesthesia are wearing off.

Rewarming is essential in the immediate postoperative care of the patient in the PACU. Unrecognized or untreated periods of hypothermia can pose a significant risk for patients during this period.

Hyperthermia. Hyperthermia is defined as core temperature above 39° C. In the early postoperative period hyperthermia may be caused by an infectious process, sepsis, or malignant hyperthermia. Although malignant hyperthermia is most often associated with the intraoperative period, it may occur or recur 24 to 72 hours after surgery. If unrecognized or untreated malignant hyperthermia will result in death (see Chapter 17).

Fluid Volume. Fluids are lost during surgery through blood loss and increased insensible fluid loss as a result of hyperventilation and exposed skin surfaces. Because of fluid retention at the surgical site, fluids also may be "lost" to the circulation after major surgery in which tissue dissection was extensive.

Excessive blood volume lost during surgery requires intraoperative and postoperative replacement therapy. Blood, blood products, colloids, and crystalloids may need to be replaced. In addition, volume may be replaced with intravenous fluids such as normal saline or lactated Ringer's solutions. Postoperative parenteral fluid requirements vary with the patient's preoperative status and the surgical procedure.

The normal body response to the stress of surgery is renal retention of water and sodium. For at least 24 to 48 hours after surgery, fluids are retained by the body because of the stimulation of antidiuretic hormone as part of the stress response to trauma and the effect of anesthesia. During surgery renal vasoconstriction and increased aldosterone activity also occur, leading to increased sodium retention with subsequent water retention. Overhydration can occur with vigorous fluid replacement, especially in the small older patient. Both water intoxication and pulmonary edema can occur, depending on the type and amount of fluids given.

Electrolyte disturbances also may be seen in the postoperative period. Although these disturbances are more common in patients with diabetes and kidney failure, they also may occur in the young, the elderly, and the debilitated patient. Such electrolyte disturbances should be treated promptly (see Chapter 13).

The patient receiving fluids intravenously is monitored for signs of pulmonary edema (dyspnea, cough, adventitious lung sounds, bounding pulse, jugular vein distention) or water intoxication (change in behavior, confusion, warm moist skin, sodium deficit). The patient also is monitored for fluid and electrolyte imbalances. Extra potassium may be necessary to replace losses from gastric suctioning.

If hydration is adequate, a patient usually voids within 6 to 8 hours after surgery. Fluid intake will exceed fluid output during the first 24 to 48 hours. Although 2000 to 3000 ml of intravenous fluid usually are given on the operative day, the first voiding may not be more than 200 ml, and the total urine output for the operative day may be less than 1500 ml. As body functions stabilize, fluid and electrolyte balance returns to normal within 48 hours.

Gastrointestinal. Nausea and vomiting are common postoperative problems affecting many patients in the PACU. These disturbing occurrences are often associated with general anesthesia, obesity (caused by decreased elimination of anesthetic agents), abdominal surgery, the use of opiate analgesics, history of motion sickness, and psychologic factors. Postoperative vomiting can lead to fluid and electrolyte imbalance, dehydration, stress on abdominal incisions, aspiration, and increased intracranial pressure. Vomiting, diarrhea, and prolonged nasogastric intubation may result in the loss of gastrointestinal secretions high in sodium and potassium (see Chapter 13).

Anesthetic Complications

Complications of General Anesthesia. Prolonged somnolence and muscle weakness are major nervous system complications that may occur immediately after general anesthesia has been achieved. Failure to awaken promptly or completely is usually the result of the anesthetic's residual effect. Other causes of stupor include severe hypoxia, hypothermia, metabolic imbalances, hyponatremia, hyperglycemia, and severe hypercapnia. Muscle weakness usually results from prolonged effects of muscle relaxants. Kidney failure and electrolyte imbalances can delay recovery from muscle relaxants. Emergence delirium is another alteration in level of consciousness that may occur during the immediate postanesthesia phase. In this short-lived state, the patient exhibits increased motor activity, disorientation, and vocalizations.

Complications of Regional Anesthesia. Complications, although rare, can occur if a patient has received spinal or epidural anesthesia. These complications are the result of neurologic injury caused by local anesthetic toxicity, needle trauma, or cord ischemia. Symptoms can include hypoxia, agitation, hypotension, nausea, and motor or sensory loss.

ONGOING POSTOPERATIVE NURSING CARE CONSIDERATIONS

Discharge From the Postanesthesia Care Unit

The PACU nurse documents all assessments and interventions for the duration of the patient's stay in the unit (Figure 18-3). Patients usually remain in the PACU until their vital signs are stable and they are capable of reasonable self-care. Discharge from the PACU is determined by physician order or a numeric scoring system (postanesthesia recovery [PAR] score) approved by the department of anesthesia. The Aldrete score is the most common tool in use. There are two Aldrete recovery scores, one for phase I recovery and one for phase II. The phase I Aldrete score (Table 18-1) measures respiration, activity, circulation, consciousness, and oxygen saturation (or color). Each criterion is scored from 0 to 2, with a total score of 9 or 10 warranting discharge from the PACU. The phase II Aldrete score (Table 18-2) is used for patients who have progressed from phase I and are now conscious or those who have received local or regional anesthesia.

Depending on admission status, the patient may be discharged to a short-stay unit, home, or an inpatient unit. If the patient remains hospitalized, the PACU nurse telephones the report to a nurse on the inpatient unit who will assume responsibility for care. The report includes information regarding the patient's preoperative history, surgical procedure and recovery, type of anesthetic and medications administered, and physician orders.

Admission to the Surgical Unit

If the patient is to remain hospitalized, he or she is transferred from the PACU to the surgical division. The patient is oriented to the room, call light is within reach, and side rails are up until the patient is completely oriented. The nurse on the surgical division completes a head-to-toe patient assessment and reviews all perioperative documentation.

Assessment for Complications

Respiratory

Risk factors for the development of respiratory complications include chronic obstructive pulmonary disease, smoking, advanced age, thoracic and upper abdominal surgical procedures, marked obesity, and the presence of acute respiratory infections (see Chapter 16).[3,16] Only 2% to 5% of patients without significant risk factors experience significant pulmonary complications.[16] The most common respiratory complications are atelectasis, pneumonia, and pulmonary embolus. The majority of postoperative respiratory complications are the result of anesthesia and poor postoperative pain control.

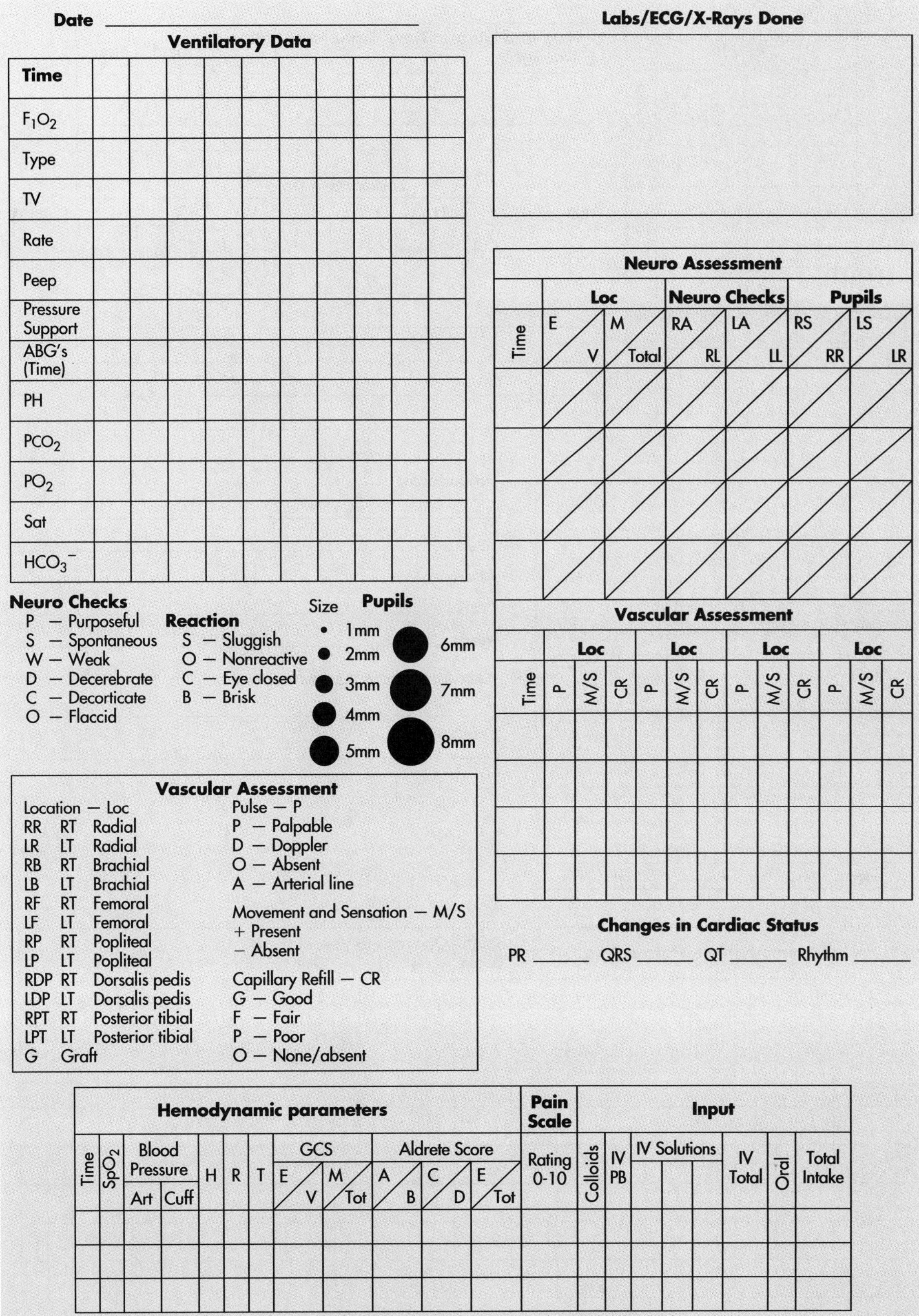

Date ______________________________

Ventilatory Data

Time										
F_1O_2										
Type										
TV										
Rate										
Peep										
Pressure Support										
ABG's (Time)										
PH										
PCO_2										
PO_2										
Sat										
HCO_3^-										

Labs/ECG/X-Rays Done

Neuro Assessment

Time	Loc		Neuro Checks		Pupils	
	E / V	M / Total	RA / RL	LA / LL	RS / RR	LS / LR

Neuro Checks
P — Purposeful
S — Spontaneous
W — Weak
D — Decerebrate
C — Decorticate
O — Flaccid

Reaction
S — Sluggish
O — Nonreactive
C — Eye closed
B — Brisk

Pupils
Size
1mm
2mm
3mm
4mm
5mm
6mm
7mm
8mm

Vascular Assessment

Time	Loc			Loc			Loc			Loc		
	P	M/S	CR	P	M/S	CR	P	M/S	CR	P	M/S	CR

Vascular Assessment

Location — Loc
RR RT Radial
LR LT Radial
RB RT Brachial
LB LT Brachial
RF RT Femoral
LF LT Femoral
RP RT Popliteal
LP LT Popliteal
RDP RT Dorsalis pedis
LDP LT Dorsalis pedis
RPT RT Posterior tibial
LPT LT Posterior tibial
G Graft

Pulse — P
P — Palpable
D — Doppler
O — Absent
A — Arterial line

Movement and Sensation — M/S
+ Present
– Absent

Capillary Refill — CR
G — Good
F — Fair
P — Poor
O — None/absent

Changes in Cardiac Status

PR ______ QRS ______ QT ______ Rhythm ______

Hemodynamic parameters													Pain Scale	Input							
Time	SpO_2	Blood Pressure		H	R	T	GCS			Aldrete Score			Rating 0-10	Colloids	IV PB	IV Solutions			IV Total	Oral	Total Intake
		Art	Cuff				E / V	M / Tot		A / B	C / D	E / Tot									

Figure 18-3 Postanesthesia care unit record.

Continued

Output					
Total Output	Emesis	NG	Urine Foley	Urine Void	Irrigation

Drug and Dosage	**Route**	**Time**	**Signature**

Blood Sugar	**Insul**	**Time**

Laboratory Data							
Na / K	Cl / CO_2	Glu / BUN	Cr / WBC	RBC / Hgb	Hct / Plat	PT / pt. cont.	PTT / pt. cont.

Procedures:

____

____

Allergies ____________________

PMH ____________________

Meds __________ **EBL/IVF** __________

Post Anesthesia Assessment

____

Anesthesiologist

____

Surgeon

____ General ____ Spinal ____ Epidural

____ AMC ____ Local ____ Other

Drug & Dosage	Route	Time	Signature

Hemodynamic Parameters															**Pain Scale**	**Operative Site(s)**	**Ventilatory Data**			**Input**							
Time	SpO_2	Blood Pressure		H	R	T	GCS			Aldrete Score					Rating 0-10		Airway	O_2 Percent		Colloids	IV PB	IV Solutions			IV Total	Oral	Total Intake
		Art	Cuff				E / V	M / Tot		A / B	C / D	E / Tot															

Figure 18-3, cont'd Postanesthesia care unit record.

Glasgow Coma Scale (GCS)

	≥ 2 yrs.	≤ 2 yrs.
E — Eyes		
4	Open spontaneously	Open spontaneously
3	Open to speech	Open to speech
2	Opens to pain	Opens to pain
1	No response	No response
V — Verbal		
5	Oriented	Coos and babbles
4	Confused	Irritable cry
3	Inappropriate words	Cries to pain
2	Incomprehensible words	Moans to pain
1	No response	No response
T	Intubated or TRACH	
M — Motor		
6	Obeys commands	Spontaneous movements
5	Localizes pain	Withdraws to touch
4	Withdraws to pain	Withdraws to pain
3	Flexion	Flexion (decorticate)
2	Extension	Extension (decerebrate)
1	No response	No response

Activity (A)
2 — Able to move 4 extremities voluntarily
1 — Able to move 2 extremities voluntarily
0 — Unable to move any extremities

Discharge summary ______ Time ______
Level of consciousness ______
BP: ___ P: ___ R: ___ T: ___
Breath sounds: ______
Bowel sounds: ______
Dressings: ______
______
Neurovascular checks: ______
______
Pt. belongings: ______
PO intake ______ Urine: ______
IV intake: ______ Emesis/NG ______
Other: ______ Drains: ______
Total in: ______ Total out: ______
Discharge IV and site: ______
Other: ______

Plan of Care

Standard Care Statement Initiated:

____ Post/Anesthesia Patient ____ Other ______

Additional Protocols Initiated

Evaluation of Goals: By discharge patient will: ______

Met	Not Met	N/A		
____	____	____	1. Achieve/Maintain pre-anesthetic and optimal level of respiratory function.	______
____	____	____	2. Achieve (pre-anesthetic) normal fluid and electrolyte balance.	______
____	____	____	3. Express a decrease or improvement in discomfort as evidence by verbal/non-verbal communication.	______
____	____	____	4. Acknowledge understanding of recovery procedures.	______

Output								Progress Notes
Total Output	Emesis	NG	Urine Foley	Urine Void	Irrigation			**Admission Assessment** IV Site ______ Breath Sounds ______ Drains ______ Bowel Sounds ______

The patient has met the criteria for discharge:

Anesthesiologist signature: ______

Recovery RN ______ Transferred to: ______

Transported by: ______ Report given to: ______

Written discharge instruction given ______
Title

Figure 18-3, cont'd Postanesthesia care unit record.

TABLE 18-1 Aldrete's Modified Phase I Postanesthetic Recovery Score

Patient Sign	Criterion	Score
Activity	Able to move 4 extremities*	2
	Able to move 2 extremities*	1
	Able to move 0 extremities*	0
Respiration	Able to deep-breathe and cough	2
	Dyspnea or limited breathing	1
	Apneic, obstructed airway	0
Circulation	BP ± 20% of preanesthesia value	2
	BP ± 20–49% of preanesthesia value	1
	BP ± 50% of preanesthesia value	0
Consciousness	Fully awake	2
	Arousable (by name)	1
	Nonresponsive	0
Oxygen saturation	Spo_2 >92% on room air	2
	Requires supplemental O_2 to maintain Spo_2 >90%	1
	Spo_2 <90% even with O_2 supplement	0
Color	Pink or normal	2
	Pale or dusky, mottled, or flushed	1
	Cyanotic	0

From Aldrete JA: Discharge criteria. In Thomson D, Frost E, editors: *Baillière's Clinical anesthesiology: postanaesthesia care,* London, 1994, Baillière-Tindall.
*Voluntarily or on command.
BP, Blood pressure; *Spo_2*, oxyhemoglobin saturation determination via pulse oximetry.

TABLE 18-2 Aldrete's Phase II Postanesthetic Recovery Score

Patient Sign	Criterion	Score
Activity	Able to move 4 extremities*	2
	Able to move 2 extremities*	1
	Able to move 0 extremities*	0
Respiration	Able to deep-breathe and cough	2
	Dyspnea, limited breathing, or tachypnea	1
	Apneic or on mechanical ventilator	0
Circulation	BP ± 20% of preanesthesia level	2
	BP ± 20–49% of preanesthesia level	1
	BP ± 50% of preanesthesia level	0
Consciousness	Fully awake	2
	Arousable on calling	1
	Not responding	0
Oxygen saturation	SPo_2 >92% on room air	2
	Requires supplemental O_2 to maintain Spo_2 >90%	1
	Spo_2 <90% even with O_2 supplement	0
Dressing	Dry and clean	2
	Wet but stationary or marked	1
	Growing area of wetness	0
Pain	Pain-free	2
	Mild pain handled by oral meds	1
	Severe pain requiring IV or IM meds	0
Ambulation	Can stand up and walk straight†	2
	Vertigo when erect	1
	Dizziness when supine	0
Fasting-feeding	Able to drink fluids	2
	Nauseated	1
	Nauseated and vomiting	0
Urine output	Has voided	2
	Unable to void but comfortable	1
	Unable to void and uncomfortable	0

From Aldrete JA: Discharge criteria. In Thomson D, Frost E, editors: *Baillière's Clinical anaesthesiology: postanaesthesia care,* London, 1994, Baillière-Tindall.
*Voluntarily or on command.
†May be substituted by Romberg's test, or picking up 12 clips in one hand.
NOTE: The total possible score is 20. A score of 18 or more is required before patient discharge.
BP, Blood pressure; *IV,* intravenous; *IM,* intramuscular; *Spo_2*, oxyhemoglobin saturation determination via pulse oximetry.

Atelectasis. Atelectasis is the collapse or incomplete expansion of the lung and usually occurs within 36 hours after surgery. Common presenting symptoms are dyspnea and hypoxia, which may be accompanied by fever, crackles, or diminished or absent breath sounds. Inadequate lung expansion is a primary cause of postoperative atelectasis. The effects of anesthesia, reluctance to cough and deep breathe resulting from inadequate pain control or location of the surgical incision, and immobility contribute to inadequate lung expansion.

Pneumonia. Pneumonia is an inflammation of the lung resulting from infection and may affect one or more lobes of the lung. In the surgical patient pneumonia often develops in the dependent lower lobes as a result of inadequate lung expansion and retained secretions. Postoperative pneumonia generally occurs after the third postoperative day. Common presenting symptoms are dypsnea, fever, chills, productive cough, and pleuritic chest pain.

Pulmonary Embolism. A clot or part of a clot may break away and flow through the heart into the pulmonary circulation until it occludes a pulmonary vessel (pulmonary embolism). Emboli alter the pulmonary circulation and decrease the function of the right and left sides of the heart. Pulmonary embolism (PE) is a complication of DVT; more than 80% of the clots originate in the lower extremities.[3] PE is a serious postoperative complication; 10% to 15% of patients with PE will die. Assessment for PE is challenging; symptoms are often vague and nonspecific. Common signs and symptoms are tachypnea, anxiety, tachycardia, dyspnea, pleuritic chest pain, cyanosis, and hypoxia. Signs of a pulmonary embolism de-

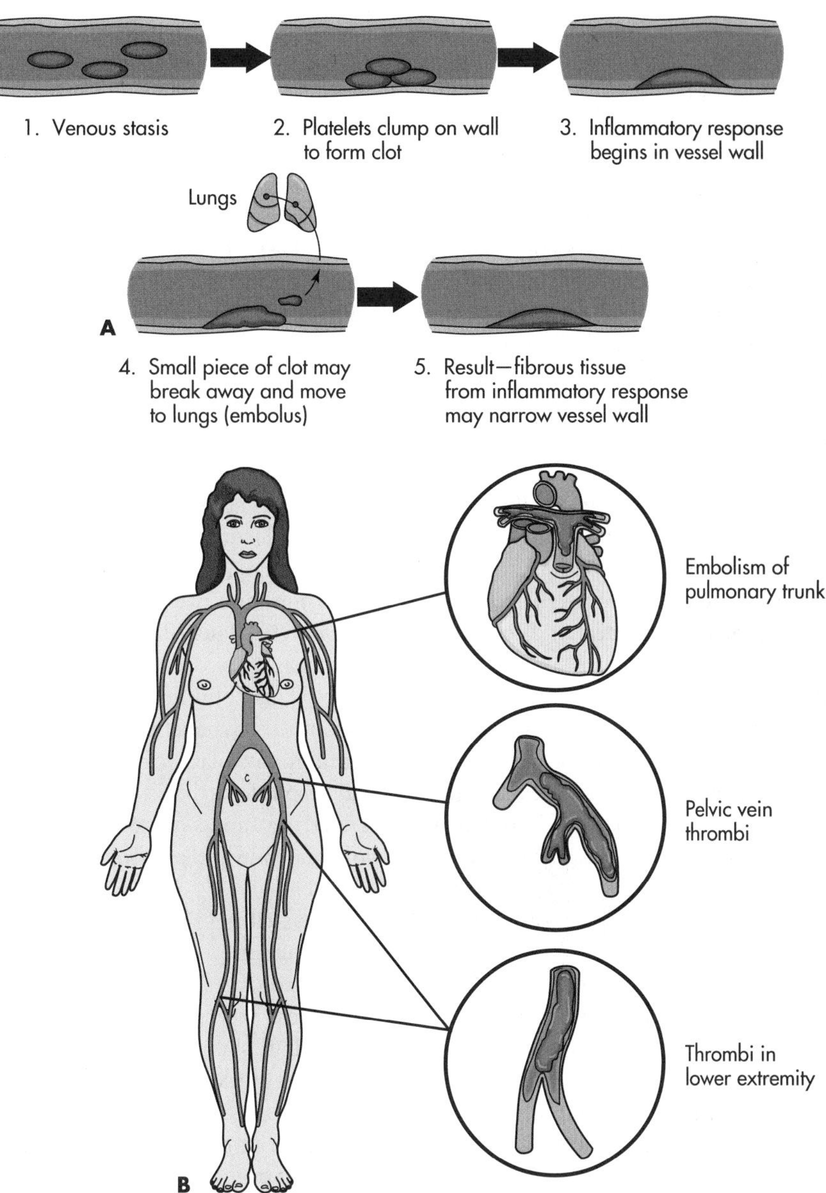

Figure 18-4 **A,** Formation of thrombus on wall of vein after venous stasis, resulting in narrowing of blood vessels. **B,** Common locations of venous thrombi.

pend on the size of the blood vessel that has been occluded. In some patients, pulmonary embolism causes sudden death. Any complaints of sudden sharp thoracic or upper abdominal pain or dyspnea, as well as any signs of shock, should be reported immediately to the physician (see Chapter 21).

Cardiovascular

Immediate complications of hypotension and dysrhythmias were previously discussed. Later complications include venous thrombosis and pulmonary embolism. Early recognition and management of cardiovascular complications before they become serious are critical.

Venous Thrombosis. The formation of clots (DVT) in the veins of the pelvis and the lower extremities impairs circulation and is a potentially serious postoperative complication. DVT may also develop into PE.

Three factors (Virchow's triad) contribute to the formation of DVT: damage to the endothelial lining of the vein, venous stasis (slowing of blood flow), and hypercoagulability. Platelets adhere to the vessel wall, with the resulting inflammatory response stimulating blood coagulation and fibrin development, resulting in a blood clot on the vessel wall (thrombophlebitis). Postoperative clots often form in a vein of the foot, calf, thigh, or pelvis. The clot grows, usually in the direction of the slow-moving blood. Clots can occur in either a deep or superficial vein (Figure 18-4).

Postoperative venous stasis occurs for a number of reasons. A major contribution to venous stasis is immobility. Every time the leg is moved, the muscle compresses the vein, pushing the blood toward the heart (venous pump); valves prevent the blood from moving backward. Ambulation and mobility promote return of venous blood to the heart and prevention of venous stasis.

Risk factors include a history of DVT, clotting abnormalities, immobility, obesity, type of surgery (lower extremity, pelvic, and abdominal), trauma, malignancy, and oral contraceptive use. Other factors include prolonged sitting with the legs dependent, decreased mobility, intestinal distention, pressure on the popliteal area, anesthetic effects, and tight dressings or casts on lower extremities. Typical signs and symptoms of DVT include pain, edema, erythema, local tenderness, palpable cord, and calf circumference inequality. A positive Homans' sign (calf pain on dorsiflexion of the foot) is often associated with DVT but is not a reliable indicator. See Chapter 25 for further discussion of DVT.

Gastrointestinal

Postoperative gastrointestinal complications include hiccoughs, nausea and vomiting, abdominal distention, paralytic ileus, and abdominal compartment syndrome. These gastrointestinal disturbances can cause a great deal of discomfort for the patient.

Hiccoughs. Hiccoughs (singultus) are produced by involuntary contraction of the diaphragm and rapid closure of the glottis. This annoying postoperative complication interferes with eating and sleeping, and is among the most exhausting postoperative complications. The exact cause of hiccoughs is unknown, but postoperative hiccoughs are associated with abdominal distention, irritation of the diaphragm or phrenic nerve, and peritonitis. Fortunately, hiccoughs usually resolve within a few hours.

Nausea and Vomiting. Postoperative nausea and vomiting (PONV) is one of the most common complications after general anesthesia and occurs in 25% to 30% of surgical patients.[29] Particularly distressing to the patient, nausea and vomiting prolongs recovery time, increases length of stay and hospital costs, and increases postoperative morbidity. Research identified nausea as the cause for 25% of same-day surgery patients' admissions to inpatient units and as a contributor to longer lengths of stay than for patients who did not experience nausea.[11] Other studies reveal that as many as 71% of patients cite nausea and vomiting as the reason for their negative postoperative experience.[20]

Factors associated with PONV include the use of inhalation agents particularly nitrous oxide, opioid use before or during anesthesia, type of surgical procedure (abdominal, gynecologic, and eye and ear), duration of surgical procedure, dehydration, obesity, history of motion sickness, history of PONV, paralytic ileus, pain, and anxiety. Isoflurane, enflurane, and halothane are less emetogenic than older agents and nitrous oxide but are still associated with significant PONV. Propofol (Diprivan), a newer intravenous agent, is associated with a lower incidence of PONV. PONV occurs three times more frequently in adult females than males; there is also a higher incidence in children.[10,29]

Nausea and vomiting may result in fluid and electrolyte imbalance and increased risk of aspiration, and may produce tension on the incision. In addition to these deleterious effects, patients have identified nausea and vomiting as more distressing than pain or the surgery itself.[20]

Abdominal Distention. Postoperative abdominal distention is a result of an accumulation of nonabsorbable gas in the intestines caused by manipulating the bowel during surgery, swallowing of air during recovery from anesthesia, and passing of gases from the bloodstream to the atonic portion of the bowel. Distention persists until normal bowel tone and peristalsis resumes, usually within 24 hours. Most patients experience distention to some degree after abdominal and renal surgery.

Patients with abdominal distention may report diffuse abdominal pain. Gas pains in the intestinal tract, which usually occur as peristalsis returns, can be extremely painful. Distention may cause dyspnea by pressure on the diaphragm and may lead to atelectasis. Abdominal girth is increased because of the collection of gas. Acute gastric dilation may produce signs of shock (restlessness; rapid, weak thready pulse; hypotension) and overflow vomiting.

Paralytic Ileus. Paralytic ileus, a decrease or absence of peristalsis, may occur after abdominal surgery or peritoneal injury. This condition is characterized by diffuse abdominal discomfort, hypoactive or absent bowel sounds, distention, vomiting, and lack of flatus. Fever, decreased urine output, and respiratory distress may accompany this condition. Untreated or unrecognized paralytic ileus may lead to hypovolemia, fluid and electrolyte imbalance, shock, and death (see Chapter 34).

Stress Ulcer. Erosion of the gastric or duodenal mucosa that occurs in previously unaffected individuals as a result of the physiologic and psychologic stressors of surgery is known as a stress ulcer. Epigastric pain and bleeding are common presenting symptoms. Histamine-2 receptor antagonistic agents (famotidine) and proton pump inhibitors (omeprazole) are effective in reducing gastric acidity and volume during the perioperative period. Antacids (sodium bicarbonate or sodium citrate) are also effective in reducing gastric acidity, but not gastric volume. These agents may be prescribed as prophylaxis for the development of stress ulcers.

Abdominal Compartment Syndrome. A compartment is an anatomic space consisting of muscles, nerves, and blood vessels surrounded by a nonelastic covering. Compartment syndrome occurs when increased pressure causes ischemia and compromises the viability of the tissues within the space. Although compartment syndrome most often occurs in the extremities, abdominal compartment syndrome (ACS) occurs in association with abdominal surgery or trauma.

ACS occurs as a result of increased intraabdominal pressure and intraabdominal hypertension, which may be caused by an accumulation of fluid or gas, trauma, coagulopathy, abdominal packing after emergency laparotomy, hemorrhage, intestinal obstruction, ascites, severe intraabdominal infection, and liver transplantation. Increased pressure within the compartment causes decreased tissue perfusion, acidosis, and eventually tissue necrosis. Signs and symptoms include abdominal distention, decreased urinary output, decreased cardiac output, tachycardia, hypercapnia, and tachypnea.

Normal intraabdominal pressure is 0 mm Hg. After abdominal surgery or trauma, pressure may increase to 15 mm Hg.[21] It has not been determined at what level of pressure ACS develops, and symptoms occur with varying levels of pressure. Cardiac output decreases with pressures of 10 mm Hg, hypotension and oliguria occur at pressures of 15 to 20 mm Hg, and anuria occurs at pressures in excess of 40 mm Hg.[21] Although intraperitoneal monitoring is the most accurate method of measuring intraabdominal pressure, this method requires placement of a tube in the abdomen, which increases the patient's risk for infection or bowel injury. A more commonly used method of measuring intraabdominal pressure is by monitoring bladder pressure via a Foley catheter. Changes in intraabdominal pressure are reflected by changes in bladder pressure.

Elevated intraabdominal pressure can result in respiratory, cardiovascular, and renal dysfunction, as well as increased intracranial pressure. Treatment goals are immediate release of intraabdominal pressure and preservation of cardiac, respiratory, neurologic, and renal function. The type of treatment depends on the cause of the increased pressure.

Urinary

Urine retention is characterized by the inability to void over a 6- to 8-hour period. Urine retention may occur after spinal anesthesia or surgery of the rectum, colon, or gynecologic structures as a result of local edema or temporary disturbance of the innervation of the bladder musculature. Postoperative urine retention usually resolves within 48 hours. Box 18-3 summarizes common causes of postoperative urine retention.

With urine retention, light palpation of the bladder (over the lower part of the abdomen just above the symphysis pubis) usually elicits discomfort, and distention may be present. In some cases, the patient voids frequently in small amounts, but without discomfort, to relieve pressure in the overdistended bladder. This pattern is called retention with overflow.

If the patient is unable to void after 6 to 8 hours, straight catheterization may be necessary until bladder tone returns. An indwelling Foley catheter is not recommended.

Another postoperative complication is urinary tract infection. Causes include urine retention and catheterization. Prolonged immobility leading to urinary stasis may also be a contributing factor. Signs of urinary tract infection include frequency, dysuria, hematuria, and fever. These symptoms usually are observed 24 to 48 hours after surgery.

BOX 18-3 Causes of Postoperative Urine Retention

- Effects of anesthetics that interfere with bladder sensation and the ability to void
- Epidural analgesia
- Medications (opioids and anticholinergics)
- Recumbent position
- Pelvic, perineal, bowel surgery
- Prolonged immobility
- Sympathetic nervous stimulation resulting from pain, fear, or anxiety

Wound Status

Types of Healing. Tissues may heal by one of three ways: primary, secondary, or tertiary intention (Figure 18-5). Wound healing by *primary intention* occurs in most surgical incisions. The incision is a clean straight line with all layers of the wound (muscle, fascia, subcutaneous tissue, and epithelial tissue) well approximated by suturing. If these wounds remain free of infection and do not separate, healing occurs rapidly with minimal scarring.

Wound healing by *secondary intention* occurs when the edges of the wound cannot be approximated, such as with ulcers or contaminated or infected wounds whose management requires they be left open. Healing by secondary intention occurs from the inside out by a filling in of the wound with granulation tissue. There is usually extensive scar tissue formation. Healing time is longer than by primary intention and these wounds have a greater possibility for infection.

Tertiary intention, or delayed primary closure, occurs when there is a delay of 3 to 5 days or more between injury and suturing. These wounds are initially left open because of possible contamination, allowing the inflammatory process in the wound bed to decrease the bacterial count and risk of infection. Tissue edges are approximated as well as possible after the wound is clean. The amount of scarring depends on the type of wound.

Influencing Factors. Major factors that can delay wound healing include advanced age, nutritional status (malnutrition or obesity), vascular disease, decreased immune status, diabetes, corticosteroid use (suppresses inflammation), presence of foreign bodies, infection, dead space, irradiation (affects fibroblastic activity), and local wound factors (vascular supply to the wound, wound temperature, and type and method of

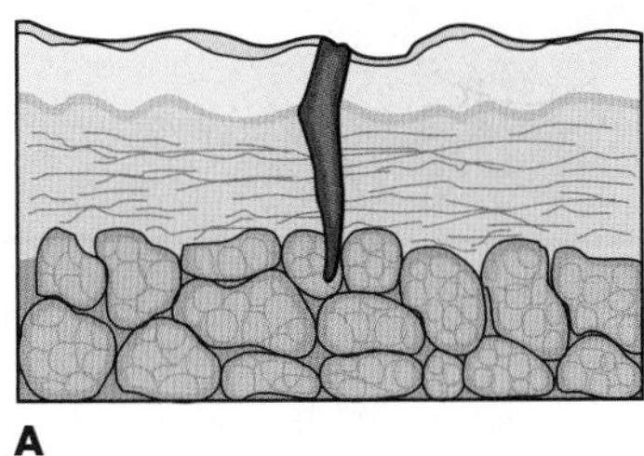
A

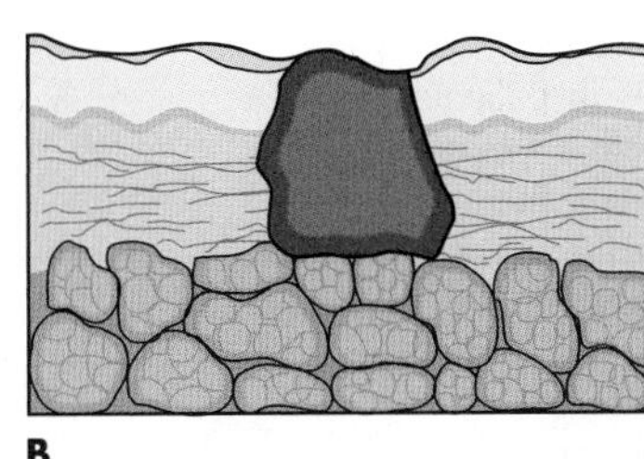
B

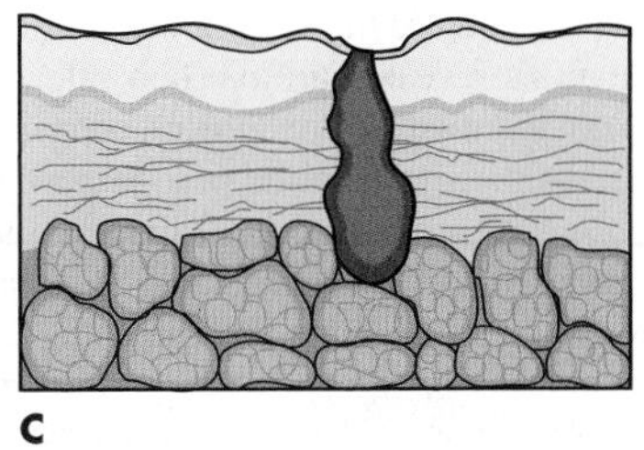
C

Figure 18-5 Types of wound healing. **A,** Primary. **B,** Secondary. **C,** Tertiary.

closure). Enzymatic activity in wounds is highest during the early stages of wound healing; therefore new wounds are more sensitive to factors that delay healing.

Hemorrhage. Hemorrhage is most likely to occur within 48 hours after surgery. The slipping of a ligature (suture) or the dislodging of a clot may cause hemorrhage. During surgery bleeding from small vessels may go unnoticed because of decreased blood pressure or use of a tourniquet. Hemorrhage may occur with the reestablishment of blood flow. Careful assessment of wound dressings, drainage systems, and blood counts (hemoglobin and hematocrit) is required.

Wound Infection. After surgery the patient remains at risk for wound infection, a major nosocomial infection. Excessive body cavity exposure and decreased body defense mechanisms are among the contributing factors to postoperative wound infection. A wound may become infected as a result of factors intrinsic to the patient, factors that delay healing, or the effectiveness of aseptic technique used by health care personnel. Hypothermia is also associated with an increased risk of surgical site infection.[14] Mild hypothermia increases the risk of surgical site infection by causing vasoconstriction and decreased oxygenation to the wound space, impairing the action of local phagocytes (neutrophils) (see Future Watch box). Experimental methods to combat the detrimental effects of hypothermia include administration of supplemental oxygen and local heating of incisions with an electrically powered bandage.[14]

Objective signs of infection include pain, fever, edema, erythema, purulent discharge, and leukocytosis. Understanding the principles of Standard Precautions, wound healing, and wound care is imperative when caring for the surgical patient.

Wound Dehiscence and Evisceration. *Wound dehiscence* is a partial to complete separation of the surgical incision. *Wound evisceration* is protrusion of an internal organ through the incision and onto the skin. Both wound dehiscence and evisceration typically occur in the abdomen (Figure 18-6). Dehiscence most commonly occurs 3 to 10 days after surgery, before the formation of collagen.

Wound separation that occurs during the first 3 postoperative days usually is related to technical factors, such as suturing technique. Dehiscence usually is associated with obesity, abdominal distention, vomiting, coughing, or infection. Factors such as cachexia, hypoproteinemia, avitaminosis, increased age, decreased resistance to infection, malignant tumor, multiple trauma, chronic steroid use, and hypothermia can also contribute to separation. Many of these complications can be prevented by identification of persons at risk and preventive nursing interventions (patient instruction regarding respiratory exercises, early ambulation, splinting the incision, and aseptic technique).

On a subjective level, the patient may report a "giving" sensation at the incision or a feeling of wetness. If evisceration

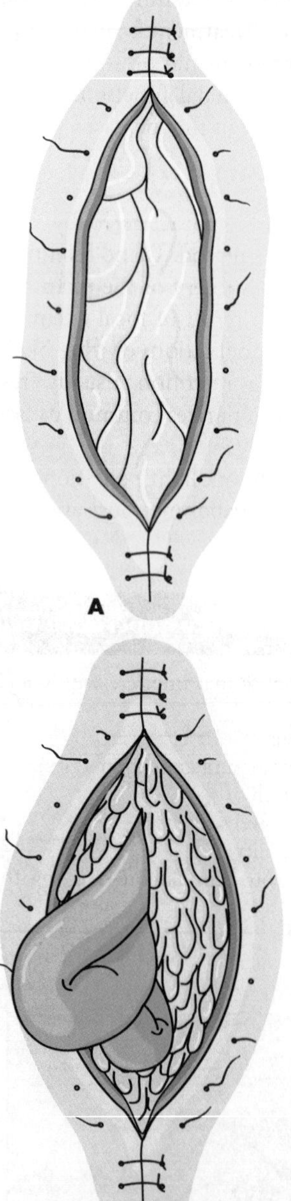

Figure 18-6 **A,** Wound dehiscence. **B,** Wound evisceration.

Future Watch
Preoperative Warming

The purpose of the study was to determine if preoperative warming of patients who were undergoing short (less than 1 hour) clean procedures would decrease postoperative infection rates. A total of 521 patients were randomly assigned to a standard or experimental group. The patients assigned to the standard group were not warmed before surgery; those in the experimental group received local and systemic warming for at least 30 minutes before the start of the surgical procedure.

Data analysis revealed an infection rate of 14% in patients who were not warmed before surgery, compared with a 4% rate for those patients who received preoperative warming therapy. Data suggest that preoperative warming assists in the prevention of postoperative wound infection. The authors recommend further studies to support the findings.

Reference: Melling AC et al: Effects of preoperative warming on the incidence of wound infection after clean surgery: a randomized controlled trial, *Lancet* 358(9285):876-880, 2001.

has occurred and a loop of bowel is obstructed, the patient will report severe localized pain at the incision. The dressing will be saturated with clear pink drainage. The wound edges may be partially or entirely separated, and loops of intestine may be lying on the abdominal wall. Signs of shock may occur. Both dehiscence and evisceration are surgical emergencies and require immediate repair.

GERONTOLOGIC CONSIDERATIONS

Because of the changes associated with the aging process, the prevalence of chronic diseases, alteration in fluid and nutrition status, and the increased use of medications, the older patient has special care requirements in the postoperative period. Older patients commonly have a slower recovery from anesthesia because of the increased time required to eliminate sedatives and anesthetic agents.

Respiratory complications in the older patient are increased with a history of pulmonary disease and with abdominal procedures because of the proximity of the surgical site to the diaphragm. The older patient is at a higher risk for aspiration, postoperative atelectasis, and pneumonia because of diminished airway reflexes and less efficient coughing. The physiologic changes in the pulmonary system alter lung function, which causes a reduced partial pressure of arterial oxygen tension (PaO_2). The physiologic changes in conjunction with the effects of opioids, muscle relaxants, and the presence of residual anesthetic agents increase older patients' risks for developing hypoxia. Hypoxia in the older adult may be exhibited as combativeness or restlessness.

Older patients are also at risk for hypertension, myocardial ischemia, and the development of congestive heart failure, which can occur as a result of fluid overload. As discussed in Chapter 17, the older patient is also susceptible to inadvertent hypothermia. This risk continues in the postoperative period, particularly in the PACU.

Pain

A common misconception is that pain perception or sensitivity decreases with age. Pain management in the older adult should be based on the assumption that the neurophysiologic processes involved in nociception are not affected by age.[18] Acute pain in the older patient may be inadequately treated, perhaps as a result of underreporting the presence or level of pain. However, the older adult is more likely to have atypical acute pain.[18] Older patients are frequently given lesser dosages of opioids than those given to younger patients. Research indicates that older postoperative patients received only 24% to 27% of prescribed analgesics.[18] Untreated pain can negatively affect patient outcomes and result in depression, anxiety, falls, sleep disruption, increased length of stay, and increased health care costs.[10,13,18]

Obstacles to assessment of pain in older adults include hearing and vision impairment, cognitive impairment, and the patient's reaction to and report of pain. Although cognitive impairment may be present in some older patients, in a study of nursing home residents with mild cognitive impairment, 83% were able to use at least one pain intensity scale to describe their pain.[10] Although pain is known to be a multidimensional concept, pain intensity is thought to be the most important component of pain assessment in the postoperative period.[10]

Mental Status

Older patients often experience changes in mental status in the perioperative period. Changes in mental status may be attributed to medications, pain, anxiety, depression, or confusion. Although the severity of symptoms may vary, depression, delirium, and dementia often have similar symptoms. Patients may also be affected by a combination of these disorders, which poses a challenge in identifying the cause of the patient's change in mental status.

Confusion is commonly categorized as acute or chronic. Acute confusion is also known as *delirium.* Chronic confusion or *dementia* is a long-term progressive process characterized by memory and cognitive impairment.

Delirium

Delirium is a temporary, usually reversible, altered state of consciousness with a change in cognition that is not explained by a known dementia.[15,24] An estimated 30% to 60% of all older inpatients may experience delirium.[2] Risk factors for developing delirium in the postoperative period include age greater than 80 years, transfer to unfamiliar surroundings, disruption in lifestyle, pain, and age-related changes that decrease the brain's ability to adapt to change.[24] Common causes for delirium include infection, malignancy, fractures, trauma, acute myocardial infarction, congestive heart failure, stroke, metabolic disorders, hypothermia or hyperthermia, blood loss, dehydration, urine retention, and opioid use. Symptoms are vague and vary with the individual; however, common symptoms may include disorientation, difficulties with social interactions, restlessness, agitation, disrupted sleep-wake cycles, lethargy, or memory loss.

In most cases acute confusion can be resolved by treating the underlying physiologic cause. However, 25% persons with persistent delirium experience irreversible brain damage and or death.[15]

Assessment of the patient's baseline mental status and close monitoring for early alterations and changes in cognition are important nursing interventions. A mental status instrument such as the Mini-Mental State Examination is an easy reliable method of monitoring changes in cognition and mental status and can alert caregivers to potential problems.

Dementia

The incidence of dementia increases with age; 10% of persons 65 years and older and 40% of persons 85 years and older have symptoms of dementia.[2] Alzheimer's type is the most common form of dementia, accounting for 60% to 70% of cases.[8] Other disorders that cause dementia include Parkinson's disease, multiple sclerosis, stroke, drug or alcohol toxicity, acquired immunodeficiency syndrome, and hydrocephalus.

Dementia is caused by destruction of brain tissue and is usually not reversible. In general, the onset is insidious and symptoms are progressive. It is important to note that a patient with chronic dementia may experience delirium as a result of hospitalization, medications, or acute illness.

Dementia is characterized by memory and cognitive impairment including language disturbance, changes in behavior and personality, decreased ability to perform activities of daily living (ADLs), and memory loss. Older hospitalized patients may exhibit symptoms of increased agitation and confusion in the late afternoon, a phenomenon known as *sundowning.* Sundowning may occur in patients with or without dementia. Factors thought to contribute to sundowning include sleep disturbances, sleep apnea, decreased functioning of the hypothalamus, decreased visual acuity, and lack of structure in the afternoon or early evening.[24]

NURSING DIAGNOSES

Nursing diagnoses are determined from postoperative analysis of patient assessment data. Not all relevant nursing diagnoses are addressed. Others include:

Surgical recovery, delayed
Oral mucous membrane, altered
Nutrition, altered: less than body requirements
Constipation
Sleep pattern disturbance
Skin integrity, impaired, risk for
Body image disturbance
Anxiety

Nursing diagnoses for the postanesthesia patient may include, but are not limited to:

Diagnostic Title	Possible Etiologic Factors
1. Ineffective airway clearance	Increased secretions secondary to anesthesia, ineffective cough, airway obstruction, pain, improper positioning
2. Ineffective breathing pattern	Anesthetic and drug effects, incisional pain, recumbent position, constrictive dressings
3. Risk for activity intolerance	Bed rest, deconditioning, increased metabolic demands of surgery
4. Acute pain	Surgical procedure, intraoperative positioning
5. Risk for imbalanced fluid volume	Excess/insufficient intravenous fluids, stress on renal/endocrine systems
6. Nausea	Effects of anesthetic agents, pain, abdominal distention, medications, stress, movement in the immediate postoperative period
7. Risk for ineffective tissue perfusion (peripheral)	Venous stasis, deep vein thrombosis
8. Urinary retention	Surgery, anesthesia, and drug effects
9. Risk for injury (trauma)	Residual anesthesia effects, delirium, dementia, disorientation
10. Risk for infection	Surgical procedure, iatrogenic factors, intrinsic factors
11. Deficient knowledge	Lack of exposure, discharge needs

EXPECTED PATIENT OUTCOMES

Expected patient outcomes for the postanesthesia patient may include but are not limited to:

1. Will maintain a patent airway with lungs clear to auscultation
1a. Will remain free of aspiration of secretions, fluids, or vomitus
1b. Will demonstrate effective coughing and deep breathing techniques
1c. Will demonstrate correct use of incentive spirometer
2. Will maintain effective breathing pattern, with easy respirations of normal rate and depth
3. Will ambulate and perform activity without dyspnea, fatigue, or significant change in vital signs
3a. Will display pulse and blood pressure at or near preoperative baseline
4. Will demonstrate decreased pain by absence of facial grimacing, guarding, or diaphoresis
4a. Will report pain intensity at 4 or less on a scale of 0 to 10
5. Will demonstrate fluid balance as evidenced by balanced intake and output, elastic skin turgor, moist mucous membranes, and vital signs within baseline range
6. Will report relief from nausea and vomiting and abdominal distention
7. Will demonstrate adequate peripheral tissue perfusion
7a. Will experience adequate venous return and absence of deep vein thrombosis and pulmonary embolism
8. Will empty the bladder within 6 to 8 hours after surgery
9. Will remain free of injury-related to falls or confusion
10. Will display timely healing of surgical wound without signs of infection
11. Will verbalize understanding of postoperative routines and discharge plan

INTERVENTIONS

1. Promoting Optimal Respiratory Function

Promotion of optimal respiratory function begins in the PACU and continues throughout the patient's hospital stay. The effects of neuromuscular blocking agents used in general anesthesia to facilitate endotracheal intubation and relaxation during the surgical procedure may need to be reversed. Barbiturates, opioids, muscle relaxants, and inhalation anesthetic agents depress respirations; naloxone (Narcan) may be used for reversal of postoperative opioid depression. Nondepolarizing muscle relaxants may be reversed with antagonists such as anticholinesterases. The anesthesiologist determines if it is necessary to administer drugs to reverse anesthetic effects.

The goals of respiratory care for the postanesthesia patient are to maintain airway patency and to promote adequate ventilation, thereby preventing hypoxemia and hypercapnia. Nursing management plays a critical role in the prevention of respiratory complications.

1a. Maintaining Airway Patency

The patient may arrive in the PACU with an oral, nasal, or pharyngeal airway or an endotracheal tube. The airway or endotracheal tube remains in place until the patient is able to breathe independently and maintain his or her own airway.

If airway obstruction occurs, it may be necessary to insert an airway or intubate the patient. The insertion of an oral airway alone may be insufficient to relieve airway obstruction caused by anesthetic-induced changes in the pharynx and larynx and may need to be accompanied by the jaw-thrust maneuver and positive-pressure ventilation.

The pharyngeal airway is most commonly used (Figure 18-7) and keeps the air passage open and the tongue forward until the pharyngeal reflexes have returned. The airway should be removed as soon as the patient begins to awaken and has regained cough and gag reflexes. After this time, the presence of an airway can be irritating and can stimulate gagging, vomiting, or laryngospasm.

An endotracheal tube allows mechanical ventilation, prevents the tongue from falling back, and prevents airway obstruction resulting from laryngospasm. A cuffed endotracheal tube also prevents aspiration. The tube should be left in place until spontaneous and adequate respirations are ensured. The patient is extubated when he or she is awake, maintains the airway, and maintains spontaneous and adequate respirations, as evidenced by the patient's ability to raise the head and grip a hand, as well as by normal blood gas or oxygen saturation levels.

Excessive secretions from the nasopharynx or tracheobronchial mucosa can lead to partial or complete airway obstruction (Figure 18-8). Pooled secretions in the lower airways as a result of inadequate inspiration and immobility after surgery may result in hypostatic pneumonia. Removal of these secretions in the early postoperative period can prevent airway obstruction and infection. If the patient is unable to effectively clear secretions, the secrections must be removed by suctioning. Often pharyngeal suctioning is all that is required. If endotracheal suctioning (see Chapter 21) is necessary, the patient should be hyperventilated with 100% oxygen before and after each introduction of the catheter into the trachea. When thick secretions are a problem, humidification is increased to keep secretions as thin as possible and to prevent dry air from further irritating the respiratory passages.

Airway obstruction may also occur as a result of aspiration. Secretions aspirated into the tracheobronchial tree can cause pneumonia. The patient may require suctioning until the cough and gag reflexes are present. The patient is at risk for aspiration until protective reflexes are regained. Until protective reflexes have returned, side lying is the best position to prevent aspiration.

1b, 1c. Promoting Coughing

Patients should have received preoperative instructions regarding deep breathing, cough (huff coughing), and the use of incentive spirometry (see Chapter 16). The patient should perform deep breathing, coughing, and incentive spirometry every hour while awake. The patient should also be encouraged to turn and move about in bed if able, or be repositioned at least every 2 hours if unable. The patient should be encouraged to sit in a chair if permitted because maintaining an upright position promotes optimal lung expansion. If fluids are not contraindicated, an intake of at least 2500 ml should be encouraged to thin secretions and reduce drying of mucous membranes.

The postsurgical patient may be reluctant to cough and deep breathe because of pain, particularly after thoracic or abdominal procedures. The nurse ensures the patient's pain is adequately controlled before beginning respiratory exercises; however, it is important to remember that opioids depress respirations and the cough reflex.

Teaching the patient to splint the incision may help promote coughing. The patient can be taught to splint the incision with a folded sheet or small pillow. Splinting prevents excessive muscular strain around the incision and reduces acute pain. Family members should be included in the

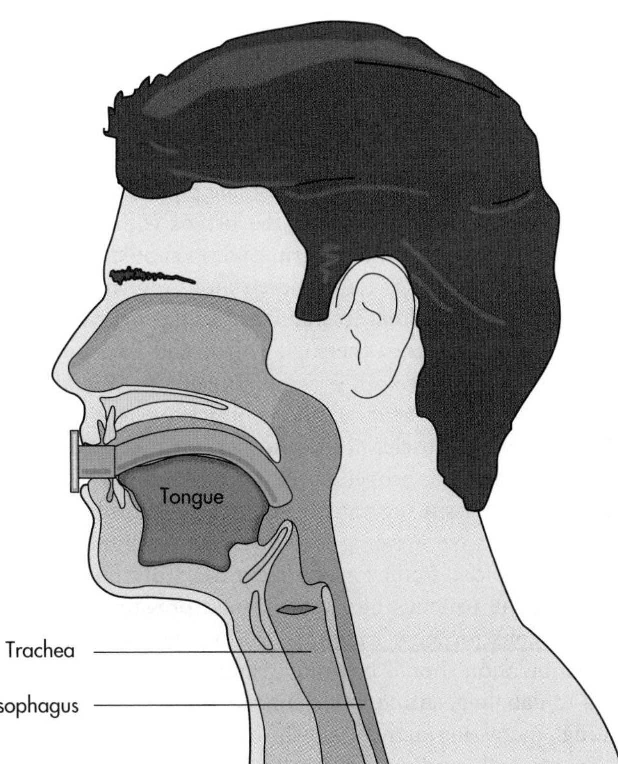

Figure 18-7 Pharyngeal airway in place to prevent tongue from blocking oropharynx.

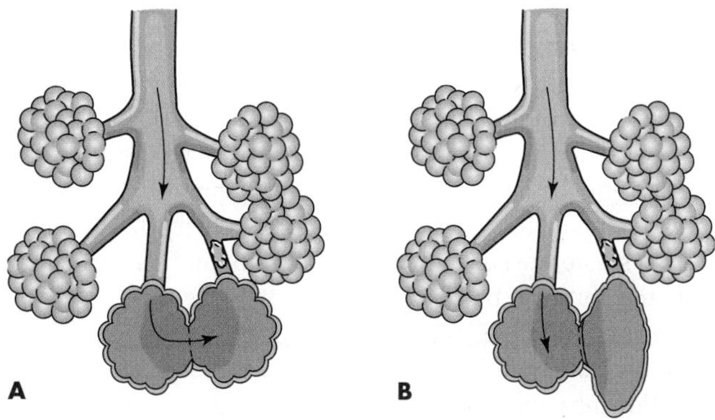

Figure 18-8 Mucous plug blocking alveolar duct in obstructive atelectasis. **A,** Aeration of blocked alveolus through intraalveolar duct with deep inspiration. **B,** Collapse of blocked alveolus with shallow inspiration.

demonstration and teaching. They can be instructed to remind the patient to perform breathing exercises and coughing at regular intervals.

The lungs are auscultated before and after ventilatory measures to determine effectiveness. If the patient is unable to effectively clear secretions, respiratory tract suctioning may be required. Patients with a history of respiratory disease may also require nebulizer treatments or bronchodilators. Postoperative nursing interventions to facilitate adequate ventilation are continued throughout the postoperative course, as the effects of anesthesia may persist for days, particularly in older and obese patients.

2. Promoting Effective Breathing

Oxygen therapy, coughing and deep breathing, and proper positioning can promote an effective breathing pattern. Almost all patients receive oxygen in the postoperative period because anesthesia decreases pulmonary expansion and can lead to hypoxemia or atelectasis. Oxygen can be administered by nasal cannula, facemask, or endotracheal tube.

The duration of postoperative oxygen therapy depends on the individual patient. As a general rule, all patients should receive oxygen at least until they are conscious and able to take deep breaths on command. Prolonged use of oxygen therapy is guided by oxygen saturations and/or arterial blood gas determinations. Patients with thoracic or upper abdominal incisions or preexisting pulmonary disease may require a longer length of oxygen therapy.

Continuous monitoring of oxygen saturation (Sao_2) level is a necessary postoperative intervention. Respiratory assessment should include the respiratory rate and depth, chest excursion, the use of accessory muscles, and the presence of tachypnea or dyspnea. Symptoms of hypoxemia include restlessness, anxiety, change of mental status, and a decrease in Sao_2.

Pain management and positioning are important interventions to promote effective breathing patterns and optimal respiratory function. Anxiety may affect respiratory function, causing the patient to hyperventilate or take shallow breaths. Nursing interventions to decrease anxiety may help promote effective breathing.

3. Promoting Activity

Encouraging early activity and mobility in the postoperative period can reduce the risk and severity of cardiovascular, pulmonary, gastrointestinal, and urinary complications. The patient's ability to tolerate activity should be assessed by monitoring the patient's vital signs and respiratory and circulatory status before and after initiating activity. In addition, the nurse should assess the patient's motor and sensory function and ability to perform ADLs.

Early ambulation is especially important in the older postoperative patient. Cardiovascular deconditioning can manifest as fluid imbalance, decreased cardiac output, and increased resting heart rate. Signs of cardiac decompensation may occur in response to activity; these include fatigue, confusion, dizziness, nausea, pallor, palpitations, angina, bradycardia (decrease in heart rate greater than 10 beats per minute), decreased systolic blood pressure, and increased diastolic blood pressure. If these symptoms occur, the activity should be stopped immediately. Other signs of activity intolerance include excessive dyspnea or tachypnea after activity or failure to return to the resting pulse rate within 3 to 4 minutes.[4]

The effects of cardiovascular deconditioning can be minimized by having patients sitting or in an upright position as soon as possible several times a day. The patient should be taught to change positions slowly, gradually increase activity, and allow for adequate rest periods. Range of motion activities should be encouraged at least once a shift for patients who are unable to ambulate or tolerate activity. If the patient is unable to perform active range of motion, the nurse should perform passive range of motion exercises. A physical therapy referral may be needed for muscle strengthening activities and progressive ambulation.

To avoid the multisystemic complications of immobility, patients are ambulated as soon as permitted by the surgeon. Most patients are dangled the evening of surgery or the next day. After the patient demonstrates the ability to assume the upright position without orthostatic changes or syncope, activity is advanced as tolerated. Before surgery the patient should have been instructed regarding the proper technique of isometric leg exercises (see Chapter 16). Until the patient is fully ambulatory, these exercises should be performed at least every 2 hours.

Before getting out of bed for the first time, the patient is dangled. Dangling is done to assess the patient's activity tolerance and ability to withstand progressive ambulation. When a patient stands, blood shifts from the thorax to the pelvis and lower extremities because of the effects of gravity. This redistribution of blood is accompanied by a drop in arterial pressure, which then activates compensatory mechanisms to maintain blood pressure.

Several interventions can be used to prevent orthostatic changes in blood pressure when dangling or ambulating for the first time. Isometric leg exercises help prevent muscle deconditioning; these along with the use of with antiembolic hose help promote venous return. Patients should be taught to take slow, deep breaths to promote venous return and to prevent vagal stimulation. To maintain spatial orientation, remind patients to keep their eyes open and look ahead. To maintain venous flow while standing, patients should be instructed to wiggle their feet and contract the leg muscles. By contracting the muscles of the lower extremities, a 90 mm Hg force is generated, propelling blood back to the heart. The nurse should assist the patient to change positions gradually and avoid passive standing for more than 3 minutes to avoid pooling of blood in the lower extremities. Continuous assessment of the patient's heart rate, blood pressure, color, and level of consciousness is essential throughout the procedure.

Ambulation should be gradual and progressive: sitting in bed to dangling, sitting in a chair, standing, and then ambulating. Increasing activity slowly helps to maintain muscle tone, strength, and endurance. To increase patient cooperation in postoperative ambulation, the nurse should ensure that the patient's pain is under control before ambulation. Uncontrolled pain can limit transfer ability and tolerance of ambulation.

4. Promoting Comfort

Pain is a complex process that involves sensory stimuli, neural processes, individual experiences, cultural background, and anxiety. Pain results in the stress response with accompanying changes in the cardiovascular system, hormonal release, anxiety, tension, and muscle contraction. From the patient's point of view the distress of postoperative pain is probably the most significant postoperative problem. In the United States, 75% of surgical patients report inadequate relief of acute postoperative pain.[17] Adequate and prompt pain relief is a critical nursing intervention. Effective management of pain (see Chapter 12) begins with a trusting nurse-patient relationship. Involving patients in their pain management program is essential. Active participation and empowerment can increase the effectiveness of a pain management program.

In the immediate postanesthesia period it is important to remember that opioid analgesics may produce respiratory depression and nausea and vomiting. It is a challenge to find the proper medication, dosage, and timing of administration that produces the least amount of adverse side effects. The goal is to keep the patient comfortable without overmedication. The nurse should adjust the dose and interval of medication until satisfactory pain relief is achieved. It is usually necessary to administer opioids during the first 12 hours after major surgery. If severe pain is expected, medication should be offered to the patient at regular intervals around the clock to maintain effective blood levels.

Two goals of effective pain management are preventing pain and maintaining a pain intensity rating that is tolerable for the patient. Methods to provide effective postoperative pain relief include preemptive analgesia, around-the-clock administration of analgesics, patient-controlled analgesia (PCA), as needed or PRN dosing, management of breakthrough pain, and nonpharmacologic interventions. Nonopioids, opioids, and adjuvant medications can be used to manage postoperative pain (see Evidence-Based Practice box). Balanced or multimodal analgesia, which combines opioid, nonsteroidal antiinflammatory, and local anesthetics, has been shown to be an effective technique to manage postoperative pain.[18,28]

Routes of administration include intravenous, epidural, spinal, and oral. Other techniques more commonly used in ambulatory surgery include wound infiltration or instillation and the use of intraarticular anesthetics or opioids following general anesthesia. Anesthetic techniques such as the addition of morphine to the local anesthetic in nerve blocks and ketorolac to intravenous regional anesthesia have been shown to provide prolonged postoperative analgesia for ambulatory surgery patients.[28] Because of shortened lengths of hospital stay and the volume of ambulatory surgery patients, oral routes may become more common choices for treatment of acute postoperative pain. The goal of these new delivery systems is to provide portable, safe analgesia with lower doses and fewer adverse side effects (see Future Watch box).

Evidence-Based Practice

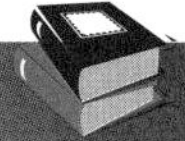

Reference: Summers S: Evidence-based practice part 3: acute pain management of the perianesthesia patient, *J Perianethesia Nurs* 16(2):112-120, 2001.

Evidence supports that postoperative patients do not receive adequate postoperative pain relief. More than 30 million surgical procedures are performed annually in the United States, and most patients require postoperative pain management. Research indicates that up to 75% of postoperative patients do not receive adequate pain control because of myths and misconceptions of health care providers about opioid abuse, addiction, and dependence. Although it is also known that postanesthesia care unit (PACU) patients often do not receive the prescribed dose of opioids, little is known regarding the treatment of pain by PACU nurses. Pain management protocols have been developed by the American Pain Society and the Agency for Health Care Policy and Research to guide clinical practice. The 1999 Joint Commission on Accreditation of Healthcare Organizations (JCAHO) guidelines mandated evaluation of the effectiveness of pain management for all patients.

The three classes of drugs used to manage postoperative pain are opioids, nonopioids, and adjuvants.

1. Opioids: morphone, hydromorphone, oxycodone, fentanyl, meperidine, pentazocine, dezocine
2. Nonopioids: acetaminophen, nonsteroidal antiinflammatory drugs (NSAIDs)
3. Adjuvants: anticonvulsants, tricyclic antidepressants, benzodiazepines, corticosteroids, phenothiazines, antihistamines, dextroamphetamine, alpha-receptor blocker, caffeine (Although adjuvant drugs are more commonly used to treat chronic pain, they may be used to manage acute postoperative pain.)

It is well established that the patient's report of pain is the best measure for nurses to assess and treat pain. Research supports that when a 0 to10 pain scale is used, 0 to 3 rating reflects mild pain, 4 to 6 moderate, and 7 to 10 severe pain. Research also indicates which medications are most effective in treating different levels of pain.

- Moderate pain: adjuvant drugs and NSAIDs combined with a short-acting opioid (codeine, oxycodone, hydrocodone, tramadol, and propoxyphene)
- Severe pain: opioids combined with NSAIDs and adjuvants

Evidence regarding inadequate pain relief in surgical patients, reliability of pain scales, and data supporting medication choice based on pain level all provide a sound basis to guide clinical practice. More research is needed regarding treatment of pain by PACU nurses. Evidence supports implementation of a pain management protocol for patients in the PACU to increase patient satisfaction and meet JCAHO standards.

Preemptive analgesia, first described in1986, blocks the painful (nociceptive) stimuli from entering the CNS before the surgical procedure. This method results in less pain and lower pain intensity in the postoperative period. There is controversy regarding when this intervention should be implemented, before the surgical incision, before the onset of pain, or during the postoperative period. Some clinicians recommend that preemptive analgesia include preoperative, intraoperative, and postoperative administration of analgesics such as nonsteroidal antiinflammatory drugs (NSAIDs) to reduce

Future Watch

Opioid Delivery Systems

New methods of opioid administration deliver analgesia on demand or in continuous dosing. These new delivery systems include subcutaneous patient-controlled analgesia (PCA); iontophoresis (transfer of the ions of soluble salts into the tissues by direct current); and fentanyl given transdermally, intranasally, and via the oral mucosa. Currently, transdermal fentanyl is usually not recommended for managing acute or postoperative pain because of respiratory depression and other side effects. Subcutaneous PCA has been studied using oxymorphone, hydromorphone, and morphine. Initial studies show the subcutaneous route as effective as intravenous PCA, although higher doses of the subcutaneous medication were required. The use of disposable pumps may allow subcutaneous PCA to be prescribed for patients having ambulatory surgery. Although still being researched, iontophoresis may provide an alternative to transdermal delivery of opioids. Similar to the transdermal route, iontophoresis has a more rapid onset and offers the option of on-demand dosing. Following orthopedic surgery, intranasal on-demand fentanyl was found to be as effective as intravenous PCA fentanyl in relieving postoperative pain. Following total hip or knee replacement surgery, oral transmucosal fentanyl provided a rapid onset of analgesia, few side effects, and lower dosages than required for intravenous PCA fentanyl.

Reference: Tong D, Chung F: Pain control in the perioperative period, *Surg Clin North Am* 79(2):401-430, 1999.

nociceptive input, local anesthetics to block sensory input, and opioid administration.[18]

Analgesics have greater effect if they are administered before pain becomes severe. Assessment of the patient's pain is the first priority. The patient's report is the most reliable indicator of pain intensity (see Evidence-Based Practice box). The visual analog scale or numerical rating scales are reliable valid tools to measure pain intensity. The faces rating scale can be used for nonverbal patients or those with language barriers.

Around-the-clock dosing provides stable serum levels of analgesics. Another advantage is the assurance that analgesia is provided to patients who may be hesitant to ask for pain medication or to report their pain. Around-the-clock dosing may be given by the oral or intravenous route. A provision for treating breakthrough pain (see Chapter 12) should accompany around-the-clock dosing.

PCA (see Chapter 12) involves the participation of patients in their pain management and avoids delay between the patient's request for and administration of analgesia. The effective use of PCA is based on the assumption that patients can best evaluate and manage their own pain. The patient must be evaluated before surgery to determine whether PCA is an appropriate choice for postoperative pain management.

PCA may be administered by the oral, subcutaneous, intravenous, or epidural route. Although intravenous or epidural routes are more commonly used, oral PCA involves the use of a wrist pouch and pain diary.[22] Subcutaneous, intravenous, and epidural routes use an infusion control device for medication delivery. The infusion control device can be set to administer a basal rate of medication, and/or the patient can receive a predetermined bolus of opioid by activating a hand control when pain relief is desired. It is important to remember that no one but the patient may push the PCA button! Assessing and documenting the patient's response to the PCA therapy are nursing responsibilities. Other nursing interventions include assessing for side effects such as respiratory depression, excessive sedation, nausea, vomiting, and pruritis.

Epidural analgesia usually combines the use of opioids and local anesthetics. Drugs most commonly used include morphine, fentanyl, hydromorphone, and bupivacaine. Using both an opioid and local anesthetic reduces side effects and may help prevent paralytic ileus and reduce respiratory and cardiovascular complications.[23] Epidural catheters should be well secured with tape, and great care must be taken to prevent displacement of the catheter. The catheter site should be assessed for signs of infection. In addition to the assessment associated with intravenous PCA, the patient should be assessed for hypotension, headache, motor and sensory deficits, urine retention, and local anesthetic toxicity (tinnitus, metallic taste, irritability, dysrhythmias, and seizures). A pain management team or anesthesiologist usually coordinates management of patients with PCA.

The amount of analgesic medication required by patients varies according to the patient's age and type of surgery. Numerous individual variables relate to pain perception and reaction. In general, after the first 48 to 72 postoperative hours, pain usually decreases in severity and may be controlled by a less potent analgesic. Physicians commonly write PRN orders for different analgesics and doses, thus permitting the nurse to select the combination that best meets the patient's immediate needs.

Pain is often accompanied by anxiety. The PACU environment, which is usually very busy and sometimes noisy, may contribute to anxiety and pain. Dimming the lights, providing privacy, playing soothing music, and involving family when feasible may alleviate some stress associated with the environment (see Research box).

Nonpharmacologic methods for managing pain and anxiety are helpful adjuncts to traditional methods of pain management (see Complementary & Alternative Therapies box). Comfort measures such as positioning or the use of heat or cold may help alleviate the patient's pain. Relaxation techniques are another strategy to control stress, anxiety, and the muscle tension associated with pain. To promote the effectiveness of relaxation techniques, the patient should be in a quiet environment, have an object to contemplate, and assume a comfortable position. The Agency for Health Care Policy and Research guidelines for managing pain, which use a holistic and interdisciplinary approach, is a useful reference for clinicians. Inadequate pain management can lead to prolonged healing time, increased length of stay, and patient dissatisfaction.[23]

Pain may also influence other aspects of the patient's recovery. To increase patient cooperation in postoperative ambulation, the nurse should ensure that the patient's pain is under control before ambulation. Uncontrolled pain can limit

Research

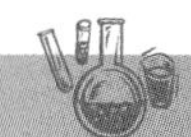

Reference: Shertzer KE, Keck JF: Music and the PACU environment, *J Perianesthesia Nurs* 16(2):90-102, 2001.

Pain is a common problem in the postanesthesia care unit (PACU) and unrelieved pain is a common cause of increased length of stay in the PACU. In addition to increased cost, unrelieved pain results in multisystem complications. It is well known that a combination of pharmacologic and nonpharmacologic interventions provides the most effective pain relief. However, medications traditionally have been the primary method of pain relief in the PACU. Noise has been identified as contributing to patient's discomfort in the PACU, primarily as a result of hormone release in response to stress. A significant source of noise in the PACU is staff members' conversation and the ringing of telephones. Studies have shown that patients require higher doses of analgesia when noise levels in the PACU are high. Music has been established as an effective intervention for managing postoperative pain.

This study was conducted at a large Veterans Administration hospital and investigated the effects of soothing music and decreased noise on the pain of patients in the PACU. The sample consisted of 97 patients who underwent same-day surgery. Pain intensity was measured using a numeric rating scale. Patients in the experimental group experienced a reduction in pain during their PACU stay and also viewed their PACU stay as more positive than those in the control group. This study supports the use of nonpharmacologic methods in the PACU as an effective method to decrease patients' pain and improve their perioperative experience.

Complementary & Alternative Therapies

Pain Management

Nonpharmacologic nursing interventions in addition to analgesics can be effective in reducing patients' postoperative pain. Nonpharmacologic methods of pain management may enhance the effect of medications. Relaxation and music have been found to be effective in reducing pain after major abdominal surgery. Acupuncture, massage, and guided imagery have been effective in reducing pain associated with cardiac bypass surgery. Other complementary therapies effective in managing pain include hypnotherapy, prayer, T'ai chi, and aromatherapy using touch. All of these therapies involve relaxation. Relaxation may be effective in reducing the fear and anxiety associated with pain.

Aromatherapy may enhance immune function, promote relaxation, and may even have analgesic effects. The use of these nonpharmacologic therapies may be effective interventions for a holistic approach to managing patients' postoperative pain.

Reference: Buckle J: Aromatherapy in perianesthesia nursing, *J Perianesthesia Nurs* 14(6):336-344, 1999; VanKooten ME: Non-pharmacologic pain management for postoperative coronary artery bypass graft surgery patients, *Image* 31(2):157, 1999.

transfer ability and tolerance of ambulation. Pain can also cause rapid, shallow breathing and a hesitancy to cough, which may lead to stasis of pulmonary secretions, atelectasis, and pneumonia.

Postoperative Pain Management for the Older Adult

The principles of pain management that apply to the younger population are also appropriate for older adults. Analgesics with the fewest side effects and shortest half-lives should be used. The first-line treatment is morphine; hydromorphone, fentanyl, and controlled-release oxycodone are also effective.[18]

Although opioids have no analgesic ceiling, dosages should be reduced for older patients. Because older adults experience a higher peak effect and longer duration of analgesia, they may be more sensitive to the analgesic effects of opioids.[18] The initial dose of an opioid should be 25% to 50% of the suggested adult dosage and should be slowly increased to achieve satisfactory pain control.[18] Because of altered distribution and excretion of drugs, the potential for side effects is greater for the older population. For patients with adequate pain control, reducing the dose of the opioid by 25% to 50% may be an effective method to manage side effects. For patients without adequate pain control, decreasing the opioid dose and adding an NSAID may both reduce the incidence of side effects and provide adequate pain control. Nonpharmacologic methods also may be effective adjuncts.

Patients generally develop tolerance to the respiratory depressant effects of opioids 72 hours after administration. It should be noted that tolerance to most opioid side effects, except constipation, develops over time.[18] Because of the increased incidence of constipation in older adults, preventing opioid-related constipation is an important intervention. A laxative or stool softener should be prescribed while the patient is receiving opioids and until regular bowel habits resume.

Because of the quick onset and ease of titration, the intravenous route of opioid administration is the best route for severe pain control for older postoperative patients. Intramuscular injections should be avoided because of the decreased muscle mass in older persons. Hypothermia often occurs in older patients recovering from anesthesia and until the patient is normothermic, drug absorption may be delayed because of injection into a cold muscle.

Although clinicians may be reluctant to prescribe intravenous PCA for older patients, this is an effective method of pain control as long as the patient has been screened for the cognitive and physical ability to use the PCA. It may be possible to modify the PCA equipment for patients who are physically unable to use the equipment. During the preoperative interview the nurse should spend time explaining the use of the PCA, and this information should be reinforced in the postoperative period. Monitoring of sedation and respiratory status is an important assessment for older patients with PCAs.

For older patients unable to tolerate PCA, lower doses of pain medications administered on a routine basis rather than PRN provides more effective pain control. Other options include short-term use of NSAIDs for management of postoperative pain. Although NSAIDs are effective in managing moderate levels of pain and avoid opioid-induced side effects, the risk of gastrointestinal irritation, renal insufficiency, and platelet dysfunction may outweigh their benefits. These medications must be used with caution and only on a short-term basis. Intravenous ketorolac is an option for the older patient; contraindications include renal disease, cirrhosis, heart failure, or dehydration. For patients older than 65 years, the usual dose must be decreased by 50% and the daily dose should not exceed 60mg.[18] Use of ketorolac should not exceed 5 days.

5. Maintaining Fluid and Electrolyte Balance

Fluid volume deficits require fluid replacement after major surgery. The nurse should expect the patient's urinary output to be less than intake for the first 48 hours after surgery because of increased secretion of antidiuretic hormone and intraoperative blood loss. Intake and output should be balanced after 48 hours.

Most patients receive intravenous fluids to maintain fluid and electrolyte balance. The exact amount and type of fluid administered depend on the surgical procedure, estimated intraoperative blood loss, as well as the patient's age, weight, body surface area, preoperative status, intraoperative course, and individual response to stress. A solution of 5% dextrose in 0.9% sodium chloride commonly is given, or lactated Ringer's solution may be given for prolonged periods to supply the necessary electrolytes. Potassium may be added to an intravenous solution to prevent hypokalemia. Careful monitoring of the patient's intravenous fluid administration is essential to ensure adequacy of replacement and prevention of fluid overload. In some instances intravenous replacement therapy may be ordered for excessive gastrointestinal fluid losses.

Nursing interventions associated with intravenous therapy include assessing the site for correct placement and signs of infection, assuring patency of the lines, assessing the patient's fluid balance, and monitoring the flow rate, at least hourly. Infusion rates vary, but the average for an adult patient in the PACU ranges from 80 to 150 ml/hr. An infusion control device is usually used.

Evaluation of hydration status includes assessing the patient's intake and output, skin turgor, mucous membranes, weight, level of consciousness, and vital signs. Output including urine and that from nasogastric tubes and drainage devices should be carefully monitored.

The patient should also be assessed for the presence of edema. Adventitious lung sounds, dyspnea, orthopnea, and jugular vein distention are signs of fluid overload and should be reported to the physician. Laboratory values also reflect the patient's fluid balance; these include serum electrolytes, albumin, complete blood count, creatine, and blood urea nitrogen.

Oral administration of fluids is begun as soon as bowel sounds are positive and the cough and gag reflexes are present. Ice chips or sips of water are offered first. Oral care should be offered frequently for patients recovering from general anesthesia and those who cannot take food or liquids by mouth.

6. Relieving Nausea and Vomiting

PONV is a distressing complication for patients. The etiology of PONV includes anesthetic agents, paralytic ileus, and opioid use. Traditional methods of treating PONV include using anesthetic agents with fewer emetogenic properties (propofol) and postoperative antiemetics. Nontraditional methods such as acupressure may complement traditional approaches of treating PONV (see Complementary & Alternative Therapies box). Antiemetics such as ondansetron (Zofran), trimethobenzamide hydrochloride (Tigan), or prochlorperazine maleate (Compazine) may be administered. If vomiting is caused by gastric distention, a nasogastric tube may be passed to drain stomach contents.

Vomiting can result in aspiration of stomach contents. To prevent possible aspiration, the patient should be placed in a side-lying position. Frequent oral care is provided. Removing offensive odors from the environment and providing distraction with music or relaxation techniques may be effective interventions. When vomiting has subsided, and unless contraindicated, ice chips, sips of clear liquids, or small amounts of dry solid food may relieve the patient's nausea. Excessive vomiting may result in fluid and electrolyte imbalance, particularly hypokalemia. Accurate recording of intake and output and monitoring of serum electrolytes and chemistry results are important interventions.

6. Relieving Abdominal Distention

Abdominal distention may lead to nausea and vomiting. Ambulation is one of the most effective means for stimulating peristalsis and expelling flatus. Ambulation usually is begun and encouraged as early as permissible. Dilation of the stomach can be relieved by aspiration of fluid or gas with a nasogastric tube. It is important to assess bowel function before resuming oral

Complementary & Alternative Therapies

Effects of Acupressure on the Incidence of Postoperative Nausea and Vomiting (PONV)

Despite the use of anesthetic agents with less emetogenic properties, PONV continues to be a common postoperative complication. Opioid use before or during anesthesia increases the incidence of PONV. This study examined the use of acupressure, a traditional form of Chinese medicine, as a complement to traditional treatment of PONV.

Acupressure is a form of acupuncture that places constant pressure on acupuncture points without puncturing the skin. The researchers used elastic wristbands (Sea-Bands) that exert pressure on the anterior surface of the wrist. Other studies have shown these bands to be effective in controlling nausea and vomiting in pregnancy, motion sickness, and surgical patients.

This study evaluated the effectiveness of the wristbands on ambulatory surgery patients and patients in the postanesthesia care unit who were at high risk for PONV. Although the results were inconclusive, earlier research outside the United States indicates the effectiveness of wristbands as an adjunct to control PONV. Recommendations for further research include a larger scale study with larger sample size.

Reference: Windle PE et al: The effects of acupressure on the incidence of postoperative nausea and vomiting in postsurgical patients, *J Perianesthesia Nurs* 16(3):158-162, 2001.

intake. The abdomen should be assessed for the presence of bowel sounds. When appropriate, the diet should be resumed gradually and advanced as tolerated. Hot or cold liquids and carbonated beverages tend to cause excess gas and should be avoided when peristalsis is sluggish; ice chips do not have the same effect because the water warms before it reaches the stomach. The patient should be encouraged not to use a straw to sip fluids to avoid excess intake of air into the stomach.

7. Promoting Tissue Perfusion

Adequate tissue perfusion is important in the postoperative period to provide oxygenation to all tissues, especially to the traumatized tissue to aid in wound healing. Pallor in light-skinned patients and a dullness or decrease in red tones in dark-skinned patients indicates decreased circulation. In dark-skinned persons, examining the oral mucous membranes is another way to assess for pallor. Vasoconstriction may result from cold temperatures or a decrease in the amount of circulating blood as a result of blood loss or from the neuroendocrine response to stress. The nail beds are assessed for prompt capillary refill.

Significant changes from baseline vital signs or output from drains should be reported to the physician. A weak, thready pulse with a significant drop in blood pressure may indicate hemorrhage or circulatory failure. The surgeon, anesthesiologist, or both are notified at once if any of these signs occur, especially if signs of shock are present. Oxygen therapy is initiated to increase the oxygen saturation of the circulating blood. Treatment for shock may be necessary (see Chapter 14).

Trauma to vein walls during surgery, hypercoagulability as a result of surgical trauma, and venous stasis associated with decreased activity or positioning during surgery all contribute to the potential for development of thromboembolism in the postoperative patient. Nursing management often can prevent postoperative thrombophlebitis and pulmonary embolism.

Nursing interventions begin with assessment of peripheral pulses; skin integrity, temperature, color, and texture; capillary refill; presence of edema; presence of pain; and motor and sensory function of the lower extremities. The nurse should also assess the calves for symmetry, pain, tenderness, redness, and a palpable venous cord. Homans' sign is not a reliable indicator for presence of DVT. Only 10% of patients with DVT will exhibit a positive Homans' sign; false-positive results are also common.[5] Calf circumference should be monitored and recorded in patients at risk for DVT; differences greater than 2 cm should be reported to the physician.[4] Isometric leg exercises should be initiated as soon as the patient is able. Leg exercises increase venous return, strengthen calf muscles, and encourage collateral circulation. These exercises should be performed hourly while awake and should be continued until the patient is ambulatory.

Antiembolic stockings may be applied during the preoperative period to facilitate blood return from the lower extremities to the heart and remain in place until the patient is ambulatory. Positioning should not compromise circulation; no pressure should be permitted on the popliteal area. Restrictive dressings should be avoided. Elevating the legs increases venous return and decreases edema. If legs are supported on pillows, pressure should be equally distributed along the entire leg. When sitting, the patient should be encouraged to cross legs only at the ankles. Intermittent external pneumatic compression devices may be used, either alone or in combination with antiembolic hose on the lower extremities. They should also remain in place continuously until the patient is ambulatory.

Pharmacologic therapy may also be indicated to prevent thrombus formation. Unfractionated heparin and low-molecular-weight heparin (LMWH) both inhibit platelet function and are options for prophylaxis for DVT in postoperative patients. The risks of heparin therapy in the surgical patient include bleeding, wound disruption, and thrombocytopenia. The usual prophylactic dose of unfractionated heparin is 5000 units subcutaneous every 8 to 12 hours; the first dose should be administered within 6 to 12 hours after surgery. Enoxaparin, a LMWH, is usually given in 30- to 40-mg doses every 12 hours for DVT prophylaxis after abdominal or orthopedic surgery. For patients receiving LMWH and epidural analgesia, there is an increased risk of epidural hematoma. After epidural catheter removal, the dose of LMWH should be held for at least 2 hours; the patient should be assessed for neurologic function and bleeding.

Before therapy is initiated, the patient should be assessed for bleeding disorders, pregnancy, peptic ulcer disease, and use of aspirin or other anticoagulants. During anticoagulation therapy, laboratory data to be assessed include complete blood count and clotting studies. Bleeding precautions should be maintained while the patient is receiving anticoagulants.

8. Promoting Urinary Elimination

Urine output is closely monitored after surgery until normal urinary tract function is reestablished. A urine output of at least 30 ml/hour is required to maintain adequate kidney function. Urine output typically is less than fluid intake during the first 24 to 48 hours because of the fluid shifts that occur in response to the stress of surgery. In addition, the specific gravity of the urine will be elevated. The bladder is palpated for distention when output is low to identify possible urinary retention. Urine retention may occur as a result of sympathetic stimulation associated with pain, anxiety, or the depressant effects of anesthesia or opioid analgesics. Signs of urine retention include a report of bladder fullness; frequent voiding of small amounts (25 to 60 ml), bladder distention, and dribbling of urine.

An indwelling urinary catheter is inserted during surgery before major surgical procedures and is removed after surgery as soon as possible. Patients receiving epidural anesthesia will have an indwelling urinary catheter while the epidural catheter is in place. Meticulous catheter care is imperative. Fluids by mouth are encouraged as soon as they can be tolerated. Increasing the patient's fluid volume aids in flushing the bladder. The nurse should ensure patency of the catheter; catheter irrigation should be performed as ordered. Patients with indwelling catheters should also be monitored for signs of infection.

Initial postoperative voiding may be facilitated by measures such as offering fluids, getting the patient up to the bathroom or commode as permitted, providing interventions to stimulate the micturation reflex (running water in the bathroom and pouring water over the perineum), and ensuring adequate time and privacy. Measures to decrease pain and anxiety may help by blocking stimulation of the sympathetic nervous system. To avoid adverse side effects of opioid use, once the patient's severe pain is controlled, nonopioids should be given for reports of pain.

If the patient is unable to void within 6 to 8 hours after surgery, straight catheterization may be ordered. The catheter may be left in for continuous drainage, depending on the volume of urine obtained. If signs of urine retention are present, the physician may order the residual volume to be checked postvoiding. Urinary residuals greater than 100 ml or 25% of the bladder capacity may require an indwelling catheter and further evaluation.

9. Preventing Injury

The nurse who provides postanesthesia care must place great emphasis on patient safety until the patient is fully awake or has complete return of sensation after regional blocks. The unconscious patient must be protected from falling and injury as a result of improper positioning. Side rails should be maintained in the upright position. The patient's call light should be within close reach and interventions to prevent falls should be implemented.

Interventions to reduce delirium, particularly in older adults, include frequent orientation, use of familiar items, relaxation tapes, massage, prevention of dehydration, and ensuring a quiet, restful environment. Hypnotics may be used to treat delirium. If the patient is agitated and poses a threat to self, an order for restraints may be necessary. However, every alternative should be exhausted before initiating restraints! The patient must be reevaluated frequently for the need to continue restraints. Each institution should have a protocol for the use of restraints based on federal guidelines. While restraints are in use, the nurse must ensure that safety and patient care needs are met. It is important to note that use of restraints may increase agitation in the older patient. Emotional support and explanations to the family regarding the use of restraints are important interventions to reduce stress and anxiety.

10. Preventing Wound Infection

Adherence to standard precautions and meticulous wound care are major components of nursing interventions to prevent infection. Interventions to prevent wound infection are necessary throughout the postoperative course. Frequent assessment of the surgical site and accurate recording of findings are vital in the immediate postoperative period. Laboratory data to be assessed include the complete blood count for an elevation in white blood cell count and wound culture results for the growth of organisms. The surgeon should be notified if signs of infection or complications are noted. Adequate nutrition is an essential component for the healing process. The patient should be encouraged to consume adequate calories, protein, and vitamin C to aid in wound healing. Diet instructions are included in the discharge teaching as well.

Wound Care

Meticulous care of the surgical incision is an important nursing measure to promote wound healing. When a surgical wound site is redressed or treated, strict aseptic technique must be followed. Wounds treated with primary closure should be covered with a sterile dressing for 24 to 48 hours. There is inconclusive evidence to support the use of dressings beyond 48 hours.[14] Wounds healing by secondary intention or delayed primary closure are usually packed and covered with a sterile dressing.

If drains are present, the insertion sites should be assessed for signs of infection. A closed drainage system should be maintained and tubing should be secured to avoid displacement of the drain. Accurate recording regarding the amount and character of output from drains is critical. Excessive or abnormal drainage should be reported immediately to the surgeon. Commonly used drains are discussed in Chapter 17.

Antibiotics may be ordered as prophylaxis against infection (see Chapter 17). Administration of antibiotics must take place at the scheduled times to maintain adequate blood levels.

Hemorrhage can interfere with wound healing. When bloody drainage is noted on a dressing, the amount can be outlined with a pen and reassessed at 10- to 15-minute intervals. If necessary, a pressure dressing can be applied over an existing dressing. Constant monitoring of vital signs is required. It may be necessary for the patient to return to surgery for ligation of the bleeding vessel.

Wound Dehiscence and Evisceration

If wound dehiscence or evisceration occurs, the surgeon is notified immediately. The patient is placed in a low Fowler's position, kept quiet, instructed not to cough, and provided with emotional support. Protruding viscera are covered with a warm, sterile saline dressing. Interventions to treat shock are initiated if signs and symptoms of shock are present (see Chapter 14). A minor wound dehiscence may be either resutured or allowed to remain open and heal by secondary intention. In the presence of infection or drainage, the wound usually is left open. The treatment for evisceration is immediate closure of the wound under local or general anesthesia.

11. Patient/Family Education

Patient and family education in the postoperative period begins with what was taught in the preoperative period (see Chapter 16). Explanations regarding rationales for treatment may increase patient cooperation and compliance with postoperative routines. Planning for discharge requires additional teaching. The nurse will have to instruct the patient regarding postoperative medications (dose, frequency, administration techniques, adverse effects), wound care, diet, signs and symptoms of infection and complications; activity restrictions; and the plan for follow-up care. The patient will need clarification regarding when to resume showering or bathing; there is inconclusive evidence of when to resume these activities.[14] The patient may also need supplies for wound care. A family member or significant other should be included in the teaching, especially if the patient will require assistance at home. Written materials are helpful to reinforce what was covered in the teaching session. It is important to assess the patient's and family's literacy level when providing written materials. The average adult in the United States cannot read above the eighth grade level; it is recommended that patient education materials be written at the fourth to sixth grade level.[30]

It is important for the nurse to recognize that the patient who is discharged directly to home after surgery may be unable to absorb a great deal of information. Therefore a follow-up telephone call should be made by nursing personnel to complete both the education and evaluation. The nurse also can provide emotional support and referral if necessary. Referrals to home health nurses, rehabilitation programs, support groups, and other health professionals also should be made based on individual patient needs.

EVALUATION

To evaluate the effectiveness of nursing interventions, compare patient behaviors with those stated in the expected patient outcomes. Achievement of patient outcomes is successful if the surgical patient in the postoperative phase:

1. Maintains a patent airway, with lungs clear to auscultation.
1a. Is free from aspiration of secretions, fluids, or vomitus.
1b. Demonstrates effective coughing and deep breathing techniques.
1c. Demonstrates correct use of incentive spirometer.
2. Maintains effective breathing pattern, with easy respirations of normal rate and depth.
3. Tolerates activities and ambulates without dyspnea, fatigue, or significant change in vital signs.
3a. Displays pulse and blood pressure at or near preoperative baseline.
4. Demonstrates decreased pain and absence of facial grimacing, guarding, or diaphoresis.
4a. Reports pain intensity at 4 or less on a scale of 0 to 10.
5. Demonstrates fluid balance as evidenced by balanced intake and output, elastic skin turgor, moist mucous membranes, and vital signs within baseline range.
6. Reports relief from nausea, vomiting, and abdominal distention.
7. Demonstrates adequate peripheral tissue perfusion as evidenced by adequate venous return and absence of DVT and PE.
8. Voids within 6 to 8 hours after surgery, continues with normal pattern, urine output of at least 30 ml/hr.
9. Is free from injury related to falls or confusion.
10. Displays timely healing of surgical wound free from infection.
11. Verbalizes understanding of postoperative routines and discharge plan.

Many institutions have developed surveys that ask patients to evaluate the care and attention received while hospitalized. These postoperative surveys can be a valuable quality improvement tool. Feedback obtained from the surveys has been used to modify standards of patient care.

The postanesthesia patient care record is a legal document and should be clear and concise. Standards of care or clinical pathways for care should be used. Evaluations of care and variations from the standard of care should be thoroughly documented.

Critical Thinking Questions

1. An 81-year-old woman has been transferred to your unit from the PACU. She has undergone an exploratory laparotomy for bowel obstruction. She received general anesthesia and 1 U of packed red blood cells during the operation. She has a history of congestive heart failure and hypertension. She has a Jackson-Pratt drain to self-suction and a nasogastric tube to continuous suction. Five percent dextrose in 0.45% saline is infusing via a central venous catheter at 100 ml/hr. Medication history includes digoxin 0.125 mg PO qd, Lasix 40 mg PO qd, and lisinopril 20 mg PO qd. Describe the assessments you would make in priority order and the rationale for each. What laboratory tests would you expect to be ordered for the next few days? Provide the rationale for each. What complications is this patient most at risk of developing and why? Develop a postoperative plan of care for this patient.
2. A 25-year-old woman is being discharged after major abdominal surgery. Her postoperative course has been complicated by wound dehiscence and infection. She is scheduled for delayed closure after resolution of the infection. Discuss the discharge needs of this patient.
3. A 54-year-old man is being discharged after a split-thickness skin graft to a sacral pressure ulcer. Past medical history includes paraplegia resulting from a motor vehicle accident. He is married with 2 teenage boys and is employed as a sales manager and will have to be off work for at least 2 months. How might his medical condition and prolonged recovery time affect his role performance within his family and job? Describe how normal wound healing might be altered for this patient. What assessments must be made before his discharge? What information would you give him as home-going instructions?
4. Describe components of a pain management protocol that can be used for patients in the PACU.
5. You are caring for a 45-year-old woman who has undergone a total abdominal hysterectomy. She is obese and smokes 1½ packs of cigarettes a day. She has an intravenous PCA and rates her pain at an 8. You observe her repeatedly pressing the button of the PCA device, and she is reluctant to perform respiratory exercises or get out of bed because of her severe pain. Describe appropriate nursing interventions and rationales for this patient.

References

1. Arndt K: Inadvertent hypothermia in the OR, *AORN J* 70(2):203, 1999.
2. Bailes BK: Perioperative care of the elderly surgical patient, *AORN J* 72(2):186, 2000.
3. Bryan CL, Homma A: The respiratory system. In Rakel RE, Bope ET, editors: *Conn's current therapy,* Philadelphia, 2001, WB Saunders.
4. Carpenito LJ: *Nursing diagnosis application to clinical practice,* ed 8, Philadelphia, 2000, JB Lippincott.
5. Church V: Staying on guard for DVT & PE, *Nursing 2000* 30(2):35, 2000.
6. Defina J, Lincoln J: Prevalence of inadvertent hypothermia during the perioperative period: a quality assurance and performance improvement study, *J Perianesthesia Nurs* 13(4):229, 1998.
7. Ensminger J, Moss R: Preventing inadvertent hypothermia—a success story, *AORN J* 70(2):298, 1999.
8. Fetzer SJ: Dementia: a complex symptom, *J Perianesthesia Nurs* 14(4):228, 1999.
9. Fortunato NM: *Berry & Kohn's operating room technique,* ed 9, St Louis, 2000, Mosby.
10. Gordon DB: Pain management in the elderly, *J Perianesthesia Nurs* 14(6):367, 1999.
11. Gunta K, Lewis C, Nuccio S: Prevention and management of postoperative nausea and vomiting, *Orthop Nurs* 19(2):39, 2000.
12. Jarrell L: Preoperative diagnosis and postoperative management of adult patients with obstructive sleep apnea syndrome: a review of the literature, *J Perianesthesia Nurs* 14(4):193, 1999.
13. Larsen PD: Effective pain management in older patients, *AORN J* 71(1):205, 2000.
14. Mangram AJ et al: Guideline for prevention of surgical site infection, 1999, *Infect Control Hosp Epidemiol* 20(4):247, 1999.
15. Martin JH, Haynes LCH: Depression, delirium, and dementia in the elderly patient, *AORN J* 72(2):209, 2000.
16. Mason JE, Freeman B: Perioperative medical care. In Dorherty GM et al, editors: *The Washington manual of surgery,* ed 2, Philadelphia, 1999, Lippincott Williams & Wilkins.
17. Mayer DM et al: Speaking the language of pain, *AJN* 101(2):44, 2001.
18. McCaffery M, Pasero C: *Pain clinical manual,* ed 2, St Louis, 1999, Mosby.
19. Meeker MH, Rothrock JC: *Alexander's care of the patient in surgery,* ed 11, St Louis, 1999, Mosby.
20. Monti S, Pokorny M: Preop fluid bolus reduces risk of post op nausea and vomiting: a pilot study, *Internet J Adv Nurs Pract* 2000 4(2): website: http://www.icaap.org/iuicode?88.4.2.3.
21. Nebelkopf H: Abdominal compartment syndrome, *AJN* 99(11):53, 1999.
22. Pasero C: Oral patient-controlled analgesia, *AJN* 100(3):24, 2000.
23. Pasero C, McCaffery M: Providing epidural analgesia, *Nursing 9* 29(8):34, 1999.
24. Ratchford J: Confusion in the elderly. In Ratchford J, editor: *Continuing education for nurses 2001,* Lakeway, Texas, 2001, National Center for Continuing Education.
25. Shurpin K, DeSimone ME: Preoperative evaluation, *Am J Nurse Pract* 2(2):7, 1998.
26. Smetana GW: Preoperative pulmonary evaluation, *N Engl J Med* 340(12):937, 1999.
27. Sullivan EE: Family visitation in PACU, *J Perianesthesia Nurs* 16(1):29, 2001.
28. Tong D, Chung F: Pain control in the perioperative period, *Surg Clin North Am* 79(2):401, 1999.
29. Windle PE et al: The effects of acupressure on the incidence of postoperative nausea and vomiting in postsurgical patients, *J Perianesthesia Nurs* 16(3):158, 2001.
30. Winslow EH: Patient education materials, *AJN* 101(10):33, 2001.

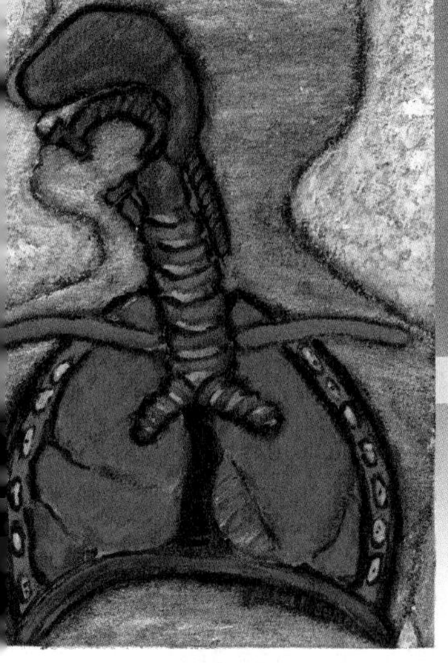

Assessment of the Respiratory System 19

Shelley Yerger Huffstutler

Objectives

After studying this chapter, the learner should be able to:

1. Identify the structural components of the respiratory system.
2. Differentiate ventilation from respiration.
3. Explain the respiratory system's primary function of gas exchange.
4. Describe the mechanisms that control ventilation.
5. Discuss the defense mechanisms of the lungs.
6. Explain age-related changes in the respiratory system.
7. Identify subjective and objective data needed to obtain a complete respiratory assessment.
8. Describe diagnostic tests and related nursing care commonly used to evaluate respiratory conditions.

An activity that most of us rarely think about in our daily lives is breathing air in and out of our lungs. However, the ease or discomfort of breathing has a major impact on the quality of our daily activities. The act of breathing involves two interrelated processes, ventilation and respiration. Ventilation is the movement of air into and out of the lungs. Respiration refers to the exchange of oxygen and carbon dioxide across cell membranes.

This chapter initially provides a review of the anatomy and physiology of the respiratory system. This is followed by a discussion of the subjective and objective data essential to the health assessment of a patient experiencing a respiratory problem. Tests commonly used to diagnose and monitor patients with respiratory dysfunction are then described.

ANATOMY AND PHYSIOLOGY

Upper Airway

Nose and Sinuses

The nose functions primarily as the organ of smell and as a passage through which air travels on its way in and out of the lungs. The upper part of the nose is supported by bone, and the lower part is supported by cartilage. The external openings to the nose are the nostrils or nares. These lead into the two nasal cavities, which are separated by the nasal septum.

Mucus-lined curved bony projections, called turbinates, form the lateral walls of the nasal cavities (Figure 19-1) and provide a large surface area for warming, humidifying, and filtering the inspired air. Because the turbinates have a rich blood supply, air that is inhaled is heated almost to body temperature by the time it reaches the posterior nasopharynx. The inspired air is also humidified by the nose and is 100% saturated with water vapor by the time the air reaches the alveoli. This humidification results in an insensible fluid loss of 250 ml/day. Filtration of large particles of dust and other matter is accomplished by trapping of the particulates by the nasal hairs. These irritants can trigger the sneeze reflex to remove the foreign particles. In addition, the mucous membrane of the turbinate bones entraps small particles where they are propelled by cilia (hairlike projections that beat in a wavelike motion) to the pharynx for swallowing or expectoration.

Each turbinate has an opening for draining the nasolacrimal ducts and four paranasal sinuses (Figure 19-2). The sinuses are air-filled spaces lined with mucous membrane that is continuous with that of the nose. Their primary purpose is to produce mucus for the nasal cavity and promote vocal resonance and timber.

Pharynx

The pharynx, or throat, is divided into the nasopharynx, oropharynx, and laryngopharynx (Figure 19-3). Because it is the only opening between the nose and mouth and the lungs, any obstruction of the pharynx (e.g., tissue swelling, presence of a foreign body, or the tongue falling back into the pharynx) can lead to cessation of ventilation. The nasopharynx is posterior to the nose and above the soft palate and contains the adenoids and openings of the eustachian tubes. The oropharynx is located in the posterior portion of the mouth and contains the tonsils. The adenoids and tonsils are made up of lymphoid tissue that helps to filter bacteria or other foreign matter that enters the nose and throat. The laryngopharynx opens into the larynx and esophagus.

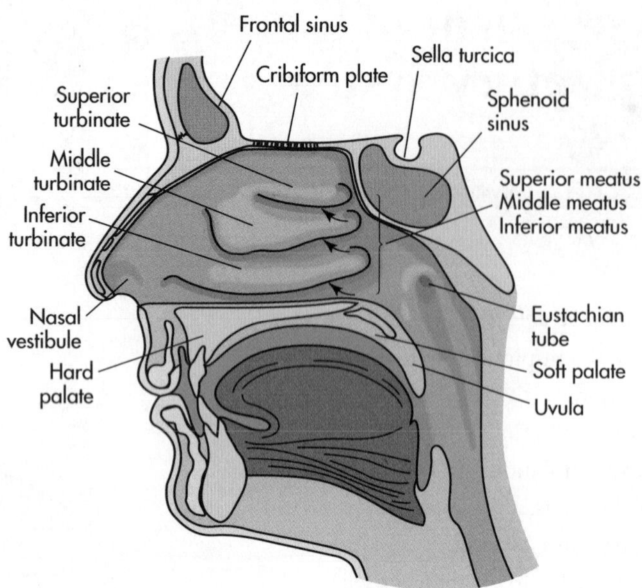

Figure 19-1 Lateral wall of nose, showing superior, middle, and inferior turbinates.

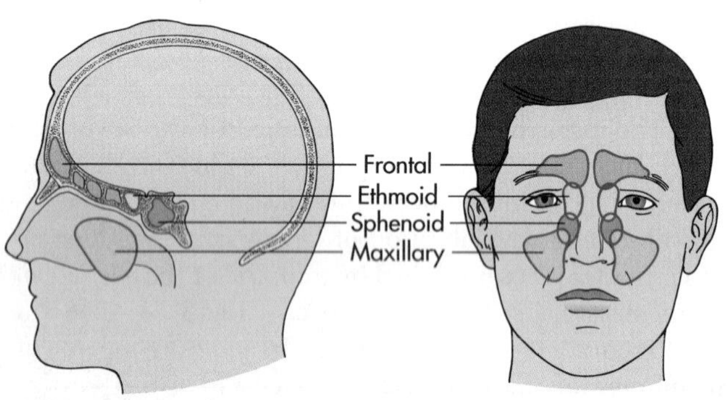

Figure 19-2 Location of sinuses.

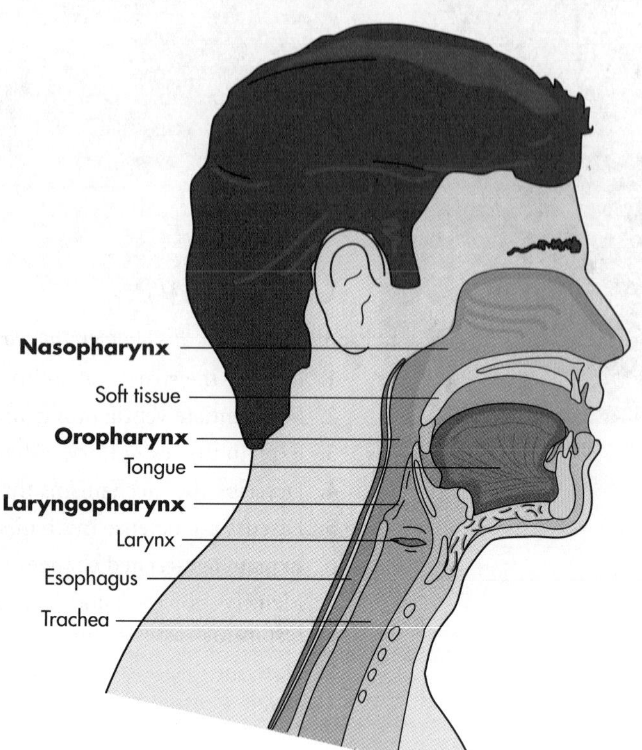

Figure 19-3 Sagittal section of head showing pharynx and larynx.

Larynx

The larynx, also known as the *voice box,* connects the pharynx to the trachea. It is made up of cartilage, muscle, and ligaments (Figure 19-4) and houses the vocal cords, which form the V-shaped opening of the glottis or entrance to the larynx. Sound is produced as exhaled air is forced through a closed glottis causing the vocal cords to vibrate. The closing of the glottis also allows for an increase in intrathoracic pressure that is needed when a person is coughing or lifting. The entrance to the larynx is protected by the epiglottis. This leaf-shaped lid of fibrocartilage covers the glottis during swallowing to prevent aspiration of food or fluids into the lungs. The larynx is innervated by the laryngeal nerve, which initiates the cough reflex in response to stimulation by foreign particles, dry mucous membranes, and other irritants. Damage to the laryngeal nerve results in paralysis of the laryngeal muscles and allows foreign materials to enter the lungs.

Lower Airway

Trachea, Bronchi, and Bronchioles

As inhaled air passes through the larynx, it enters the lower airway, which consists of the trachea, bronchi, bronchioles, and terminal respiratory units (Figure 19-5). The trachea, commonly known as the windpipe, connects the larynx to the right and left mainstem bronchi. The point at which the trachea bifurcates into the right and left bronchi is called the carina. The carina contains cough receptors that can be easily stimulated, for example, by tubes such as suction catheters or endotracheal tubes. The landmark used to locate the carina is the manubriosternal junction, often called the angle of Louis.

The trachea and bronchi are supported by incomplete cartilaginous rings that prevent airway collapse when the pressure in the thorax becomes negative. The trachea shares a small muscle with the esophagus at the point where the cartilaginous rings do not meet. This is a potential site for a tracheoesophageal (T-E) fistula. Cuffed tubes, such as endotracheal or tracheostomy tubes, may lead to T-E fistulas as a result of high pressures within the cuffs.

These lower airways are lined with goblet cells that produce mucus, which traps debris and ciliated epithelium that propels foreign particles toward the pharynx for removal. Mucus and particles are removed from the airway by swallowing, coughing, or sneezing. See Chapters 20 and 21 for a complete discussion of pulmonary defense mechanisms.

The bronchi enter the lungs through an opening called the hilus. The right bronchus is wider and shorter than the left bronchus, extending nearly vertically from the trachea. Aspiration or misplaced intubation is more likely to occur with the right lung due to this anatomic feature. Thus it is important to secure an endotracheal tube so that proper ventilation can be maintained. If the tube is misplaced or slips into the right bronchus, air will not be able to enter the left lung. The left bronchus is narrower and extends at more of an acute angle

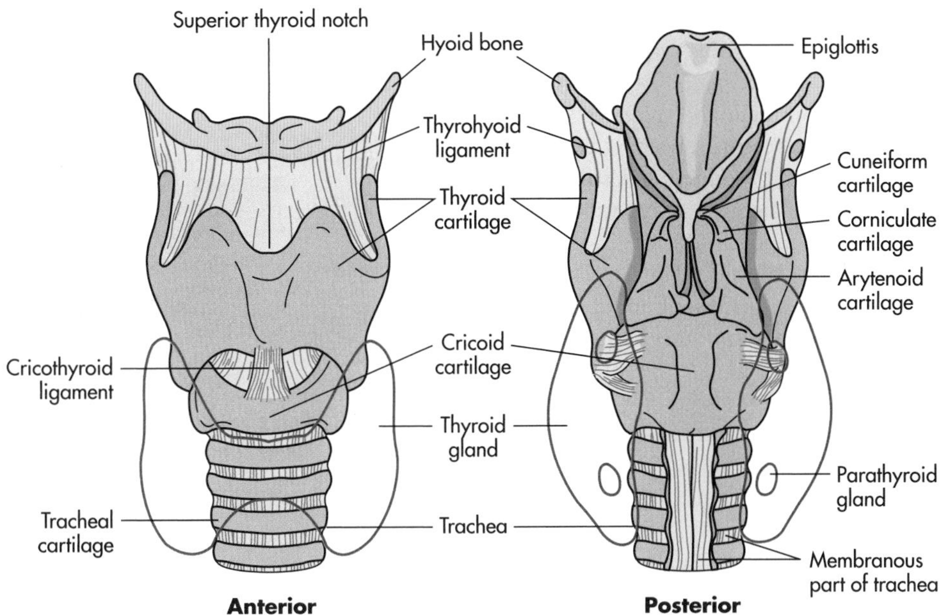

Figure 19-4 Larynx.

off the trachea, making it more difficult to pass a catheter into it for removal of secretions from the left lung.

The right and left mainstem bronchi divide into smaller branches: the left bronchus divides into two lobar branches, and the right bronchus divides into three lobar branches. The lobar branches divide into segments that further subdivide into subsegmental bronchi, terminal bronchi, bronchioles, terminal bronchioles, and respiratory bronchioles. Respiratory bronchioles divide further into respiratory terminal bronchioles, alveolar ducts, alveolar sacs, and alveoli.

The bronchioles contain no cartilage for support. The patency of these airways is determined by smooth muscle, which relaxes or contracts, thus affecting their diameter. The diameter of the airway determines the amount of airway resistance. For example, if the radius of the airway was cut in half, the resistance would increase by 16 times. Mucous plugs, bronchoconstriction, airway edema, and external compression of the airway are conditions that increase airway resistance and impair airflow into the lungs. Cilia and secretory gland cells that aid in the removal of dust and particles are absent at the level of the terminal bronchioles (see Figure 19-5, *B*).

Terminal Respiratory Unit

The structures distal to the terminal bronchioles are collectively referred to as *acini* or terminal respiratory units (see Figure 19-5, *A*). The acini include the respiratory bronchioles, alveolar ducts, alveolar sacs, and alveoli.

The adult lung contains approximately 300 million alveoli or a surface area equivalent to the size of a tennis court. The alveoli are interconnected by tiny openings, called pores of Kohn, which are present in the alveolar epithelium. The pores allow air movement between alveoli that promotes even distribution of air and collateral ventilation if a small airway becomes obstructed; however, they also allow bacteria to move from alveolus to alveolus.

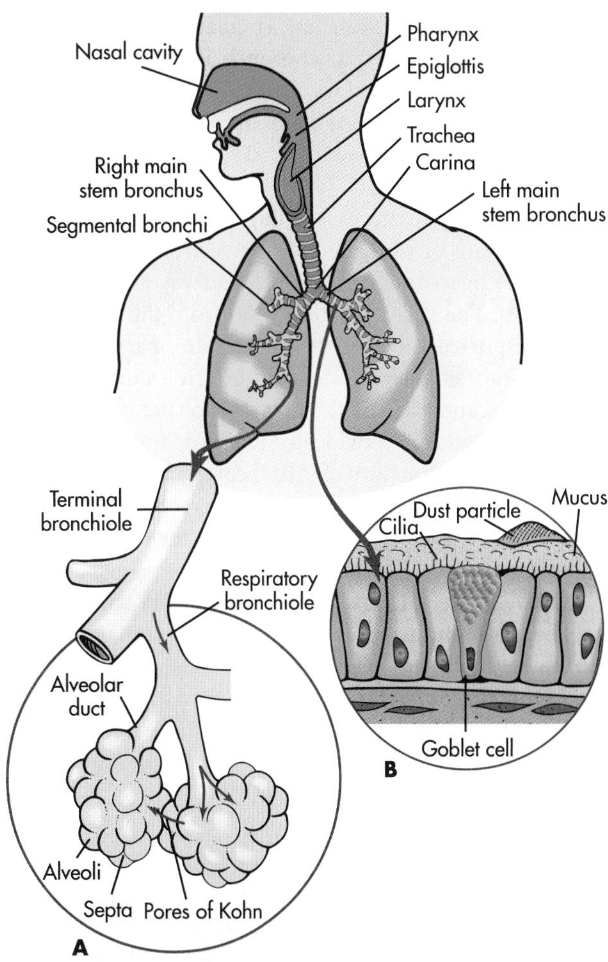

Figure 19-5 Respiratory system. **Inset A**, Acinus, or pulmonary functional unit. **Inset B**, Ciliated mucous membrane.

The alveolar sacs contain three types of cells. Type I alveolar cells are flat squamous cells. These cells form the alveolar epithelium, which is the site of gas exchange. Type II alveolar cells produce surfactant, a lipoprotein that reduces surface tension within the alveolus and contributes to the elastic properties of lung tissue. Surfactant production is stimulated when alveoli are stretched. Thus sighing, active ventilation, and adequate tidal volumes are important factors in the production and release of surfactant. Alveoli collapse, a condition called *atelectasis,* without adequate surfactant and a number of lung diseases, including acute respiratory distress syndrome, can result. Alveolar macrophages are the third type of cell found in the alveolar sacs. Macrophages are phagocytic cells that are responsible for ingesting and removing bacteria and other foreign particles from the alveolar surface. The macrophages transport the microorganisms to the lymphatics or bronchioles for removal via the mucociliary escalator. The alveolar macrophage is one of the most important defense mechanisms against lung infection.

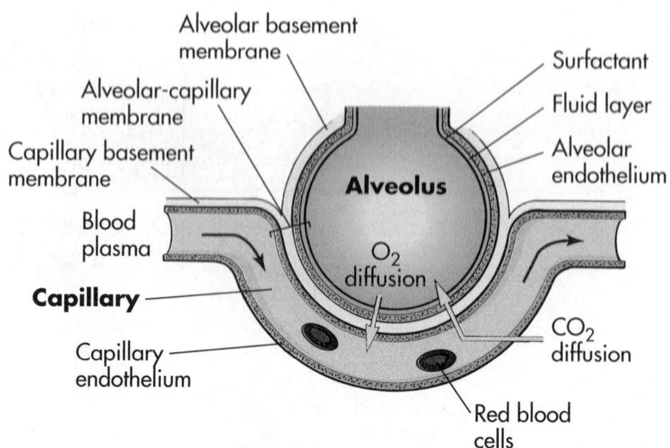

Figure 19-6 Blood transport of oxygen.

Lung Circulation

Pulmonary and Bronchial Blood Supply

The lungs receive blood from both pulmonary and bronchial circulation. Bronchial circulation provides nutrients to the tissues of the tracheobronchial tree and warms and moistens inspired air but does not participate in gas exchange. The bronchial arteries originate from the thoracic aorta. Blood is returned from the bronchial system to the left atrium by the azygos vein.

Pulmonary circulation is a high-volume, low-pressure circuit by means of which blood received from the right ventricle of the heart interacts with the airway at the terminal bronchioles. The deoxygenated blood from the right ventricle is transported through the main pulmonary artery that branches into smaller arteries and arterioles and finally to the alveolar capillaries of the acini. Once the blood is oxygenated and carbon dioxide is removed, the blood is returned to the left atrium of the heart via the pulmonary veins. The oxygenated blood then enters the left ventricle where it is pumped out of the aorta into the systemic circulation.

The alveoli are surrounded by a pulmonary capillary network. Each alveolus is separated from the pulmonary capillary by an interstitial space (Figure 19-6), a distance of less than 1 mm. At this site, oxygen travels from the alveolus into the capillary blood for distribution to the cells of the body and carbon dioxide passes out of the blood into the alveolus for passage to the external environment.[2]

Lungs and Thoracic Cage

Thoracic Cage

The thoracic cage is composed of the ribs, sternum, scapulae, and vertebral column. The thoracic cage houses the lungs, heart, great vessels, lymph nodes, thymus gland, and esophagus. Intercostal muscles lie between the ribs, and the diaphragm forms the floor of the thoracic cage. See Figure 19-7 for the anatomy of the thorax and lungs.

Lungs

The lungs are conical-shaped structures that extend from just above the clavicles to the eleventh or twelfth rib. Although their primary function is gas exchange, the lungs also serve as a reservoir for blood, for inactivation of vasoactive substances such as bradykinin, and for conversion of angiotensin I into angiotensin II. The right lung has three lobes (upper, middle, and lower); the left lung has two lobes (upper and lower). A serous membrane called the parietal pleura lines the inside of the thoracic cavity. It is continuous with the visceral pleura that covers the surface of the lungs.[4] The area between these two closely opposed pleurae forms a potential space known as the pleural space. It contains a few milliliters of serous fluid that facilitates pleural surface adhesion and allows the pleural surfaces to slide over each other without friction during inhalation and exhalation. An abnormal accumulation of fluid or exudate in this potential space is called pleural effusion.

Ventilation

Air moves in and out of the lungs as a result of changes in the pressure gradient between the atmosphere and alveoli caused by inspiratory and expiratory muscular mechanics. The movement of air is from an area of greater pressure to an area of lesser pressure. The pressure gradient between the atmosphere and the thoracic cavity is established by changes in the size of the thoracic cavity.

Inspiratory Muscles

Inhalation is an active process that requires contraction of the inspiratory muscles, including the diaphragm, external intercostal muscles, and scalene muscles. The diaphragm is a large dome-shaped muscle that flattens during contraction, initiating inspiration. It is the primary muscle of breathing and is innervated by the right and left phrenic nerves. Injury or damage to the phrenic nerves causes paralysis of the diaphragm, adversely affecting lung movement on the affected side. The chest will move up instead of downward on the side of the paralysis during inspiration. This is known as paradoxic movement. Contraction of the external intercostal and scalene muscles causes the anterior part of the thoracic cage to rise during inspiration, increasing the chest dimensions. During

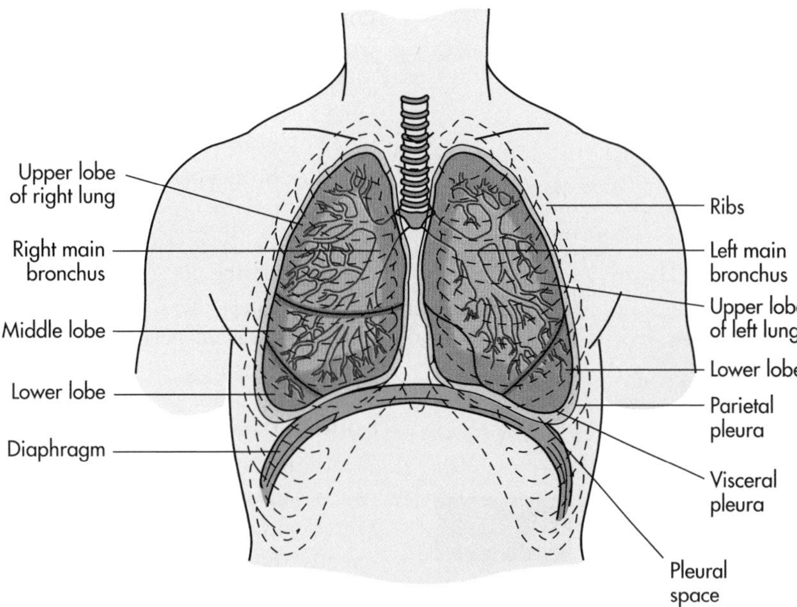

Figure 19-7 Anatomy of thorax and lungs.

exercise or in diseased states the sternocleidomastoid muscles, accessory muscles used to assist in inhalation, raise the sternum resulting in an increased diameter of the thoracic cage. Because of the change in the size of the thorax, the resultant increase in volume causes a change in pressure such that the intrapleural pressure, as well as the intrapulmonary pressure or airway pressure, decreases in relation to atmospheric pressure. This pressure gradient causes air to move into the lungs.

Expiratory Muscles

Exhalation is normally a passive process produced by elastic recoil of the chest wall and the lungs. Relaxation of the diaphragm and intercostal muscles decreases the size of the thoracic cage. Active exhalation that results from disease, exercise, or coughing causes the internal intercostal and abdominal muscles to contract. Contraction of these accessory muscles causes the ribs to move upward, abdominal contents to rise, and diaphragm to move upward. The resultant decrease in volume leads to an increase in the intrapulmonary and intrapleural pressures. The pressure gradient that is created between the atmosphere and the airways causes the air to flow out of the lungs.

Compliance and Elasticity

Two properties that permit the lungs to expand and return to their resting state are compliance and elasticity. Compliance is a quality of yielding to pressure and represents the ease with which the lungs can be stretched while consuming a volume of air. Determinants of compliance include the elastic recoil of the lung and chest wall, along with the alveolar surface tension. An increase in compliance means that the lungs are abnormally easy to inflate; a decrease in compliance indicates stiffness or difficulty in inflating the lungs.

Elasticity of the chest wall is determined by the musculature and bones of the thoracic cage and is reduced in patients with bony deformities, abdominal distention, and obesity. Elastic recoil of the lungs is the tendency of the lungs to return to the resting state. The elasticity of the lungs is determined by the elastic and collagen fibers of the lungs. The fibers are stretched out when the lungs are inflated and contract when the lungs are deflated. Conditions in which lung tissue stiffens, such as pulmonary fibrosis or interstitial lung disease, result in a decrease in compliance.

Gas Exchange

Diffusion

Gas movement across the alveolar-capillary membrane occurs by the process of diffusion. Once the inspired oxygen reaches the alveoli, oxygen diffusion occurs into the pulmonary capillary due to the greater partial pressure of oxygen of alveolar air in contrast to the partial pressure of oxygen in venous blood. Carbon dioxide diffuses in the opposite direction because the partial pressure of carbon dioxide of venous blood is greater than the partial pressure of carbon dioxide of alveolar air (Figure 19-8). Diffusion of oxygen is decreased by the following four factors: (1) a decrease in atmospheric oxygen, (2) a decrease in alveolar ventilation, (3) a decrease in alveolar-capillary surface area, and (4) an increase in thickness of the alveolar capillary membrane.

Ventilation-Perfusion

Ventilation-Perfusion Ratio

Efficient gas exchange is dependent on a balance between ventilation or air flow (V) and perfusion or blood flow (Q). In other words, areas that receive ventilation should be well perfused with blood, and areas that receive blood flow should be capable of ventilation.

In the normal lung alveolar ventilation is about 4 L/min and pulmonary capillary blood flow is about 5 L/min. Gravity causes greater blood flow to the lower portion of the lungs.

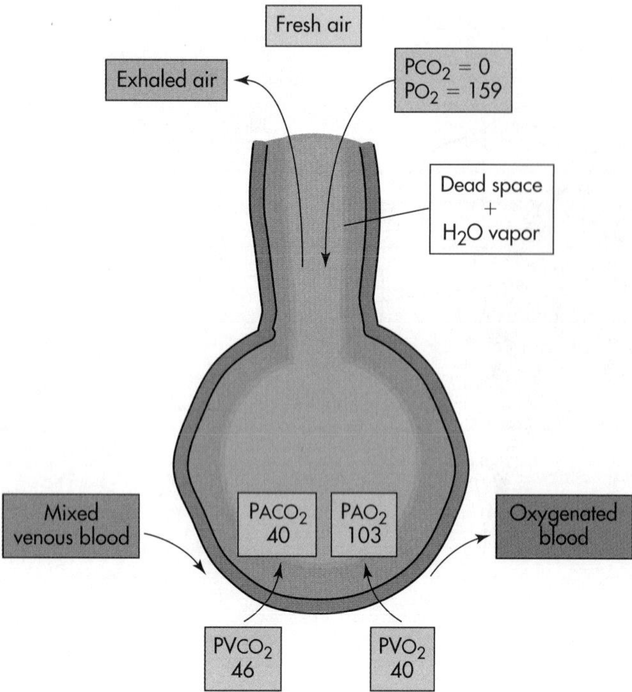

Figure 19-8 Diffusion of gases across the alveolocapillary membrane. PCO_2 and PO_2, partial pressure of carbon dioxide and oxygen; $PACO_2$ and PAO_2, alveolar PCO_2 and PO_2; $PVCO_2$ and PVO_2, mixed venous PCO_2, and PO_2.

Thus, in an upright person the bases of the lungs receive a greater volume of blood than the apices. If a patient is in the supine position, the dependent portions of the lungs receive more blood flow than the upper parts. Similarly, ventilation is not uniformly distributed. In an upright person, the upper parts of the lungs contain a greater residual volume of gas and the alveoli are less compliant than in the lower parts of the lungs; thus, more gas is distributed to the bases of the lungs. These slight imbalances in ventilation and perfusion have little effect on overall gas exchange in normal lungs. The overall V/Q ratio of normal lungs is 0.8.

Mismatched ventilation and perfusion may occur as a result of dead air space and shunting of blood. Dead air space refers to those areas of the respiratory tract that are ventilated but not perfused by the pulmonary circulation and therefore do not allow gas exchange. There are two types of dead space: anatomic and alveolar. Anatomic dead space consists of the conducting airways above the level of the alveolus. Alveolar dead space consists of alveoli that are not perfused. Alveolar air space may be the result of normal factors such as gravity or may be due to disease. Impaired blood flow in relation to the amount of ventilation to the alveoli or excessive ventilation relative to blood flow results in mismatch. For example, blood flow (perfusion) to the alveoli may be blocked by a pulmonary embolus, yet the alveoli may be well ventilated. Perfusion also may be blocked when gas pressure within the alveolus is greater than within the capillary, causing the capillary to collapse. These are both examples of high V/Q ratios resulting in dead-space ventilation or "wasted" ventilation. The air does not participate in gas exchange but does contribute to the work of breathing.

Low V/Q ratios indicate that the lungs are poorly ventilated in relation to the amount of blood flow. For example, blood flow to the alveolus may be normal but fluid in the alveolus, bronchospasm, or mucus plugs increase airway resistance and may prevent adequate ventilation. As a result V/Q inequality, or shunting, now exists. The blood perfuses the area of the lung that is not ventilated; thus, blood is "shunted" past the area and no gas exchange occurs. This is known as wasted perfusion. Figure 19-9 shows examples of V/Q relationships.

Control of Respiration

Breathing can be viewed as an automatic loop process in which sensors (chemoreceptors) continually feed data to a central processor (medulla oblongata and pons). Subsequently, the respiratory muscles are directed to adjust ventilation to meet the needs of the body (Figure 19-10). In addition, an override feature (cerebral cortex) exists, so that ventilation can be consciously altered. The major sensors are the central and peripheral chemoreceptors. Other receptors that affect ventilation include the neural receptors (stretch receptors and J receptors).

Central Chemoreceptors

Central chemoreceptors, located near the medulla, are sensitive to hydrogen ion concentration (pH) in the spinal fluid. Carbon dioxide readily crosses the blood-brain barrier and combines with water to form carbonic acid, which dissociates into hydrogen ions. A change in arterial carbon dioxide levels affects the pH of the cerebrospinal fluid, which in turn stimulates the chemoreceptors. There is an increase in the depth and rate of ventilation when carbon dioxide levels increase and a decrease in the depth and rate of ventilation when the carbon dioxide levels decrease.

Ventilation is regulated primarily by the central chemoreceptor response to changes in arterial carbon dioxide levels and its effect on the pH of the cerebrospinal fluid. However, the central chemoreceptors become less sensitive in patients with chronically high carbon dioxide levels and low oxygen levels. In these patients, the peripheral chemoreceptors are the primary stimuli for ventilation.

Peripheral Chemoreceptors

Peripheral chemoreceptors, located in the carotid bodies and aortic arch, primarily respond to low arterial blood oxygen levels (PaO_2, 60 mm Hg) and signal the respiratory center in the medulla. Efferent signals are then sent to the respiratory muscles to increase the ventilatory rate. Patients who rely on their hypoxic drive for breathing (e.g., those with chronic obstructive pulmonary disease [COPD]) depend on the peripheral chemoreceptors for control of ventilation. Administration of an uncontrolled amount of oxygen or failure to monitor arterial PaO_2 levels with oxygen administration in these patients can depress or abolish their hypoxic ventilatory drive, and death may result.

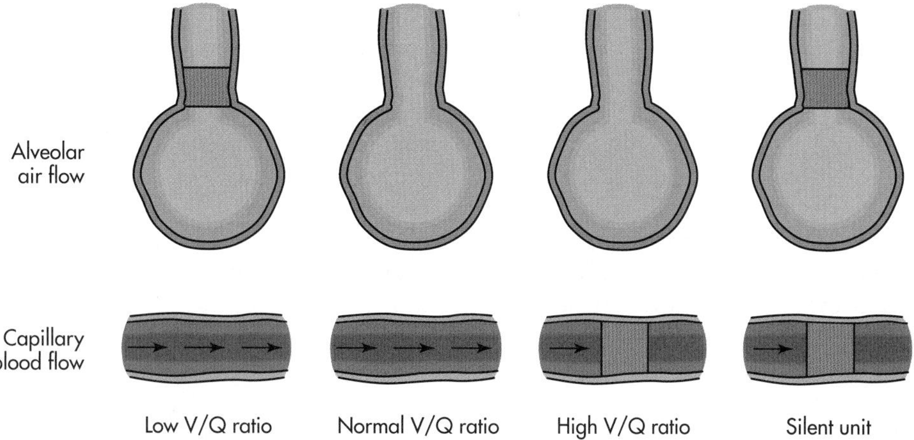

Figure 19-9 Range of ventilation to perfusion ratios from zero to infinity.

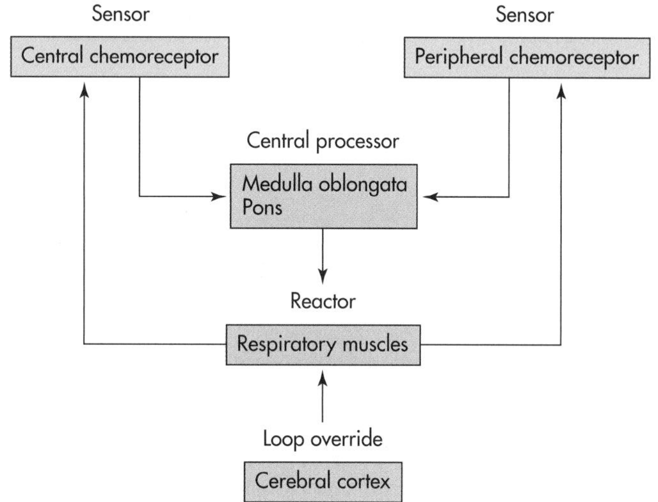

Figure 19-10 Respiratory control loop.

Neural Receptors

The stretch receptors located in the conducting airways respond to changes in the pressure within the airways. Inspiration is inhibited once the lungs are inflated, an effect known as the Hering-Breuer inflation reflex, which acts to prevent overinflation of the lungs. J receptors, located in the alveolar walls, respond with rapid shallow breathing in conditions associated with an increase in interstitial fluid volume such as pulmonary edema and pneumonia.[3]

Physiologic Changes With Aging

Changes in respiratory anatomy and physiology that occur with aging can produce variations in clinical findings. The thoracic cage becomes rigid from cartilage calcification, osteoporosis of the ribs, and arthritic changes in the joints of the ribs. Kyphosis, or accentuated dorsal curvature of the thoracic spine (hunch back), may also occur with aging. An increase in the anteroposterior diameter of the chest occurs in older adults.

Chest wall compliance is reduced because of stiffening of the chest wall and a loss in elastic recoil of the lungs associated with advanced age. This results in increased work of breathing. Muscle strength also decreases with aging affecting lung volumes and pressures; however, respiratory muscle strength may be enhanced with exercise. Structural changes within the lungs include calcification of bronchial cartilages, increased anatomic dead space, decreased diameter of noncartilaginous bronchioles, increased size of the pores of Kohn, and enlarged alveolar ducts. Pulmonary diffusion capacity decreases because of a loss in the surface area of the alveolar-capillary membrane and inequalities in the distribution of air or blood. The room air alveolar-arterial oxygen gradient (PAO_2-PaO_2) increases with aging. Arterial oxygen pressure (PaO_2) levels are lower, but carbon dioxide levels and pH are not affected by age. Ventilatory and heart rate responses to brief periods of hypoxia or hypercarbia are blunted. Sleep apnea may be observed in older adults but has not been reported to be clinically significant. Although total lung capacity is relatively unchanged, the effects of aging on lung volumes and spirometry include an increase in residual volume, a decrease in forced vital capacity, a decrease in forced expiratory volume, a decrease in maximum voluntary ventilation, and a decrease peak expiratory airflow.

Any or all of these changes may be noted by the nurse assessing the older adult patient.

HEALTH HISTORY

Respiratory assessment should be tailored to the patient's health status. If the patient exhibits signs of respiratory distress such as increased restlessness, paradoxic breathing pattern, increased ventilatory rate, complaints of dyspnea and/or use of accessory muscles, the subjective information should be deferred and an abbreviated physical assessment performed. Once the patient is physiologically stable, data collection can resume. Information can also be obtained from a significant other, if available.

Common Symptoms

The most common pulmonary symptoms for which persons seek health care include dyspnea, cough, increased sputum production, hemoptysis, wheezing, and chest pain. Upper airway symptoms include nasal obstruction, nasal discharge, sinus pain, sore throat, and hoarseness.

Dyspnea

Dyspnea, which is defined as difficult breathing, is one of the most common clinical manifestations of respiratory disease. The term is used to describe both difficult or labored breathing observed by another and a patient's subjective experience of breathlessness or breathing discomfort. A defining attribute of dyspnea is that it is a distinctly distressful sensation. Terms used to describe the sensation include chest tightness, suffocation, not getting enough air, choking, and smothering.[7] Dyspnea is distinct from tachypnea (an increased respiratory rate) or hyperpnea (an increased depth of respiration) because of the associated discomfort. As for any symptom, comprehensive data about the timing and characteristics of dyspnea needs to be collected as part of the assessment. Pertinent data related to timing include whether the problem is acute or chronic (persisting over time with only the intensity of the symptom changing), whether it is episodic or paroxysmal, the date and type (sudden or gradual) of onset, duration, and frequency. Characteristics to be explored include perceived severity, phase of the respiratory cycle affected (inspiratory, expiratory, or both), associated factors such as time of day, seasonal or weather changes, exposure to environmental irritants, anxiety, activity, and body position. Relationship to body position is important, as two distinct types of dyspnea are orthopnea, which is breathlessness on assuming the recumbent position, and paroxysmal nocturnal dyspnea (PND), which is the sudden onset of difficult breathing while sleeping in the recumbent position. Symptoms such as use of respiratory accessory muscles, dilated nostrils, tachycardia, and cyanosis, which are commonly associated with dyspnea also need to be identified. Some studies reveal that the qualitative characteristics vary by disease category. Persons with asthma report severe but episodic dyspnea and may report complete resolution of symptoms between episodes. Persons with emphysema, chronic bronchitis, and pulmonary vascular disease report constant dyspnea.[7] Additional studies have tried unsuccessfully to link the worsening of dyspnea with the degree of deterioration of lung function.[5]

Assessing the severity of dyspnea, particularly when referencing the subjective experience of breathlessness, is particularly challenging but critical for patient evaluation and management decisions. One method used to objectify and quantify the subjective sense of breathlessness is described in the Evidence-Based Practice box. A second is use of the self report visual analog scale illustrated in Figure 19-11. This scale can be used to evaluate the effectiveness of interventions and to monitor the patient's response to therapy. A third approach to assessing dyspnea is by determining its effect on activities of daily living (ADLs). This approach is valuable because chronic dyspnea has been shown to result in the reduction of physical activity and may affect the person's ability to work, socialize, and perform usual ADLs. Consequences of chronic dyspnea affect all aspect of a person's life. Fatigue frequently accompanies dyspnea. Dyspnea during moderate exertion causes the reduction of physical activities resulting in physical deconditioning. Physical deconditioning then results in dyspnea with only mild exertion and eventually with ADLs.[6] To determine the effect of dyspnea on ADLs, the patient is asked, "How does your breathing difficulty affect your ability to bathe, dress, and groom yourself; walk or exercise; prepare meals and eat; get about your home; climb stairs; sleep; perform chores and hobbies; get to the bathroom; maintain family and social relationships; maintain employment; perform sexually; and attend activities away from home?"

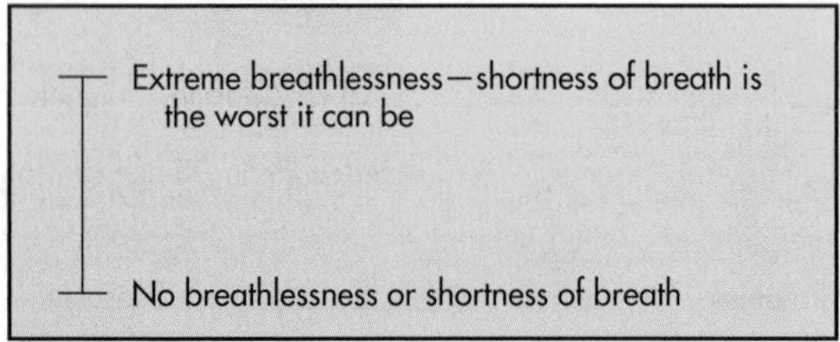

Figure 19-11 Breathlessness visual analog scale. The patient is asked to place a mark on the line between no breathlessness and extreme breathlessness at the place that corresponds with his or her severity of breathlessness.

Evidence-Based Practice

Reference: Kendrick KR, Baxi SC, Smith RM: Usefulness of the modified 0-10 Borg scale in assessing the degree of dyspnea in patients with COPD and asthma, *J Emerg Nurs* 26(3):216, 2000.

This study focused on routine and triage assessment of subjective dyspnea using the modified Borg scale (MBS) in a hospital emergency department serving adult veterans. A total of 400 male veterans aged 24 to 87 years presented with a chief complaint of dyspnea. The assessing physician identified 102 of these patients as having acute bronchospasm; 42 were diagnosed with asthma, and 60 were diagnosed with chronic obstructive pulmonary disease (COPD). All study patients with acute bronchospasm were able to use the MBS to rate their perception of severity of dyspnea before the treatment modality (metered dose inhaler or nebulizer) and after treatment. As the peak expiratory flow rates (PEFRs) and SaO_2 percentages increased, the MBS scores of difficulty breathing decreased. For the asthma groups the mean MBS score decreased from 5.1 at triage baseline to 2.4 after treatment. Likewise, COPD patients experienced a decrease in their MBS scores from 6.0 at triage baseline to 3.0 after treatment. The researchers concluded that the MBS is a valid and reliable assessment tool for dyspnea. The MBS correlated well with other clinical parameters and could be useful when assessing and monitoring outcomes in patients with acute bronchospasm. Patients who used the MBS rated the tool with a high degree of satisfaction on ease of use and found the language scale adequately expressed their dyspnea. The emergency department triage and primary care nursing staff rated the MBS as highly satisfactory, stating the tool was quick and easy to use. Respiratory assessment in the triage notes and nursing notes were streamlined to consistently include three respiratory measures: MBS, SaO_2, and PEFR. Long respiratory narratives were found unnecessary in many cases. In addition, the MBS provided an important element of subjective assessment when evaluating the severity of dyspnea.

Chronic dyspnea, chronic fatigue, and the reduction of physical activities lead to loss of previous role identification, inability to earn a living, social isolation, and, often, depression.[7] People with chronic dyspnea need preventive and therapeutic plans for dealing with both acute and chronic distress. It is essential that nurses assess the level of dyspnea experienced by the individual, understand its effects on health, and offer tools to help with its management. One research study looked at the nurse's intervention for patients with breathlessness (see Research box).

Cough

Coughing has two main functions. It protects the lungs from aspiration, and it helps propel foreign matter and excess mucus up through the airways. Receptors for the cough reflex are located in the tracheal and bronchial mucosa, with the largest concentration found in the larynx, carina, and bifurcations of the large and medium-sized bronchi. When these receptors are stimulated, impulses are transmitted primarily via the afferent nervous pathways (vagus, phrenic, and spinal motor nerves) to expiratory musculature (larynx, tracheobronchial tree, diaphragm, and abdominal wall). Cough is a common symptom of airway disease.

Cough is described as acute, chronic, or paroxysmal (periodic forceful episodes that are difficult to control), and as productive, nonproductive, or dry progressing to productive. Productive refers to the production of sputum. Not all patients with a productive cough expectorate sputum; sometimes, the sputum is swallowed. However, the term *productive cough* is used when sputum is produced regardless of the patient's ability to expectorate it. Coughs can also be described as barking, hoarse, or hacking.

Cough must be analyzed in terms of its onset (gradual or sudden), duration and frequency, pattern (occasional, on arising, with activity), perceived severity (effect on activities of daily living, e.g., inability to eat, talk, or sleep), aggravating factors (hot or cold weather or exercise), associated symptoms (e.g., sputum production, chest tightness, fever, or choking), and alleviating factors (medications, treatments, and folk remedies). Even though cough is an important defense mechanism, cough lasting longer than 2 to 3 weeks may indicate serious respiratory dysfunction and should be evaluated.

Sputum Production

As described previously, a mucus blanket lines the epithelial layer of the tracheobronchial tree and cleanses it of inhaled particles and debris. The goblet cells and submucosal glands produce mucus. The cilia propel the mucus (which contains foreign particles, pus, blood, and debris) upward toward the pharynx where it is coughed up, suctioned, or swallowed. Normal sputum is clear and thin and averages 100 ml/day. With pulmonary disease sputum can change in amount and/or characteristics, and the type of change can be reflective of the specific type of pathology present. Thus it is important to assess baseline sputum characteristics. Sputum is described in terms of color, consistency, and amount. Color varies widely. It can be clear as with noninfectious processes, creamy yellow as seen in staphylococcal pneumonia, green as seen in *Pseudomonas* pneumonia, "currant jelly" as seen in *Klebsiella* pneumonia, rusty as seen in pneumococcal pneumonia, or pink and frothy as seen with pulmonary edema. Consistency may be thick, viscous (gelatinous), or watery. Sputum may also be described as mucoid or mucopurulent. Amount of sputum is assessed using objective measurements such as teaspoons, tablespoons, or cups rather than subjective terms such as "scant" or "moderate." Sputum is most accurately assessed by seeing it as opposed to accepting the patient's description.

Hemoptysis

Hemoptysis is the coughing up of blood or blood-tinged sputum. Hemoptysis is usually frothy with air bubbles, alkaline in pH, and bright red. The source of bleeding may be from anywhere in the upper or lower airways, or from the lung parenchyma. Hemoptysis must be distinguished from hemetemesis, which is vomiting blood that originates in the gastrointestinal tract. Hemetemesis is never frothy, has an acid pH, and may be mixed with food particles. If it has been in the stomach long enough to be acted on by the digestive enzymes, it is dark red or coffee grounds–like in appearance. Epistaxis must be considered as a potential cause of hemoptysis. The amount of hemoptysis should be quantified in teaspoons, tablespoons, or cups. The coughing up of 400 to 600 ml of blood in a 24-hour period is considered to be a massive amount and requires immediate evaluation.[9]

Wheezing

Wheezing is a continuous, high-pitched, whistling sound produced when air passes through narrowed or obstructed airways. It generally occurs during expiration but can be heard throughout the respiratory cycle. Wheezing is usually heard with a stethoscope; however, it may be audible to the patient or heard by others in close proximity to the patient. Information to be collected related to wheezing includes presence of

Research

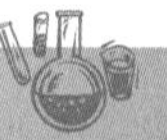

Reference: Bredin M et al: Multicentre randomized controlled trial of nursing intervention for breathlessness in patients with lung cancer, *Br Med J* 318:2000.

Studies demonstrating effective nursing interventions to assist patients with dyspnea are limited. Positive results were demonstrated in a study with lung cancer patients cared for in a nurse-led clinic. The interventions included:

- A detailed assessment of patient's dyspnea and factors that improved or exacerbated it
- Advice and support for patients and families on ways of managing dyspnea
- Training in breathing control techniques, activity pacing, progressive muscle relaxation, and psychosocial support

The interventions group reported significant improvement in dyspnea, levels of depression and physical symptoms, improved ability to perform activities of daily living, and reduced levels of anxiety and distress secondary to dyspneic episodes.

factors that can cause bronchospasm and produce wheezing, such as asthma, exposure to physiologic irritants, stress, or anxiety. Snoring may be reported because if airway obstruction is present, "stridor" or loud snoring may be experienced. Patients who awake frequently because of loud snoring may be experiencing sleep apnea syndrome.

Chest Pain

Chest pain can result from several conditions. A detailed investigation is required to differentiate chest pain of cardiac origin from that of other causes. Chest pain of cardiac origin is described in Chapter 23. Chest pain of pulmonary origin can originate from the chest wall, parietal pleura, or lung parenchyma. Table 19-1 summarizes the characteristics of pulmonary chest pain.

Upper Airway Symptoms

Symptoms to be explored related to the upper airway include difficulty breathing through the nose, nasal discharge, sinus pain, or vocal change. Changes in voice can be caused by obstruction or congestion of nasal passages as well as inflammation of the vocal cords (hoarseness). Hoarseness may be associated with tumors, recurrent laryngeal nerve damage, or laryngitis. Patients may experience hoarseness after removal of an endotracheal tube.[4]

Respiratory Risk Factors

In addition to a review of the symptom(s) or reason(s) the patient is seeking health care, the patient should be interviewed about risk factors associated with respiratory dysfunction. The most important risk factors to explore include smoking, past pulmonary illnesses, or exposure to respiratory infections, predisposition to genetic disorders, and exposure to environmental irritants. The psychosocial effects of any respiratory disorder also need to be explored with the patient.

Smoking

Smoking has been implicated as a major cause of lung disease. There is a strong relationship between smoking and the development or exacerbation of chronic bronchitis, emphysema, asthma, lung cancer, and respiratory infections. Passive smoke has also been implicated in increasing the risk for nonsmokers. The *Healthy People 2010* document has a goal and objectives for smoking reduction and cessation. (See Chapter 3 for a list of the objectives related to tobacco use.) The patient's current and past history of tobacco use must be assessed. Patients should be questioned about the type of tobacco (cigars, cigarettes, or pipe) as well as the number of packs and number of years smoked. Pack-years (for cigarette use) can be determined with the following equation: Pack-year = number of years smoked × number of packs smoked per day (e.g., 20 years of 2 packs/day = 540 pack-years). Questions regarding any attempts to quit smoking and exposure to second-hand smoking (in the home or at work) should also be asked. If the patient has quit smoking, pack-years are still determined in addition to the length of time the patient has stopped smoking. The use of cigars, pipes, marijuana, and smokeless tobacco is measured as amount used per day.

Respiratory Disorders

A history of respiratory illnesses and hospitalizations for lung diseases or disorders should be obtained (e.g., childhood allergies, frequent respiratory infections, influenza, frequent colds, pneumonia, pleurisy, emphysema, asthma, chronic sinusitis, chest surgery or trauma, tuberculosis, and adult-onset allergies). Any exposure to tuberculosis, other respiratory infections, or travel to areas with risk for respiratory infections such as histoplasmosis (Southwest United States) or coccidioidomycosis (Southwest United States, Central America, or Mexico) should be explored.

Family History

Some respiratory diseases have a genetic component, so the patient must be asked if there is a family history of allergy, asthma, atopic dermatitis, or lung cancer. Also obtain a family history of documented α_1-protease inhibitor deficiency or cystic fibrosis. A strong family history of emphysema or the development of respiratory symptoms at an early age could prove helpful in identifying patients who are candidates for genetic testing and counseling. Panlobular emphysema is a disease that usually affects young adults and is caused by an α_1-protease inhibitor deficiency. Cystic fibrosis is a disease that involves mucus-secreting and eccrine sweat glands. The overproduction of secretions affects the lungs by obstructing respiratory passages, impairing oxygenation, and impairing mucociliary clearance.

TABLE 19-1 Characteristics of Pulmonary Chest Pain

Origin	Characteristics	Possible Cause
Chest wall	Well-localized, constant ache increasing with movement	Trauma, cough, herpes zoster
Pleura	Sharp, abrupt onset, increasing with inspiration or with sudden ventilatory effort (cough, sneeze), unilateral	Pleural inflammation (pleurisy) Autoimmune and connective tissue disease
Lung parenchyma	Dull, constant ache, poorly localized	Benign pulmonary tumors Carcinoma
	Well-localized, sharp, sudden onset	Pneumothorax
	Sudden onset, increasing stabbing pain on inspiration, may radiate	Pulmonary embolus and infarction

Environmental Irritants

Assess the patient's exposure to pollutants and irritants such as dust, fumes, gases, coal dust, and other allergens. Inquire about the workplace and type of work the patient does as well as the home environment and adjacent area to determine potential exposure to irritants. Inquire about hobbies to check for exposure to allergens or pollutants such as pets, glues, and paints. Also, gather information about family member's occupations because this may be helpful in determining the source of the patient's respiratory complaint.

Psychosocial History

Respiratory problems can affect a patient's functional status; therefore it is important to obtain a history of the patient's perception of the situation as well as coping skills and resources. The quality of life may be perceived as diminished by patients with respiratory disorders.

Need satisfaction is important to understanding the patient's functional performance. Assess the patient's sense of self, sense of control, and satisfaction with family life, safety-security needs, leisure activities, financial resources, and social support. Although symptoms may affect psychosocial functioning, psychosocial effects of a respiratory disorder may also impair cognitive functioning and adaptation to the disorder. This may be manifested as sleeping difficulties, irritability, helplessness-hopelessness, tension-anxiety, depression, and isolation.

An assessment of emotional responses that occur with dyspnea and other respiratory symptoms is important to understanding the patient's experiences. Anxiety is frequently experienced as are depression and hostility. Assessing emotional responses such as anxiety, fear, or panic may assist the health care provider in selecting interventions that are more likely to be successful. Inquiring about the degree of emotional response and the extent of physical and/or psychologic impairment yields a more complete assessment of the patient. These data are relevant for the health care provider to incorporate in the plan of care.

Review of Other Systems

Ask the patient about problems with swallowing and ambulating, as well as any history of neurologic or muscular disease. Factors that may adversely affect respiratory function include immobility, dysphagia, and diseases affecting muscular strength (e.g., amyotrophic lateral sclerosis, myasthenia gravis, stroke). It is helpful to perform a general review of other body systems to assist the patient in recalling all signs and symptoms.

PHYSICAL EXAMINATION

The nurse collects objective data on the patient during the physical examination. The vital signs and upper and lower airways are assessed for deviations from the normal for the patient's age and health problems.

Respiratory Vital Signs

Respiratory Rate and Ventilation

The respiratory rate should be counted and the depth and rhythm of the breathing pattern assessed. The expansion of the chest should be bilaterally symmetric. See Figure 19-12 and Table 19-2 for normal and abnormal breathing patterns.

Pulse Oximetry

Pulse oximetry, referred to as Spo_2, is a painless, noninvasive procedure used to assess oxygenation. The normal Spo_2 value is greater than 95%. An arterial blood gas analysis can provide a Sao_2 measurement that can be compared with the

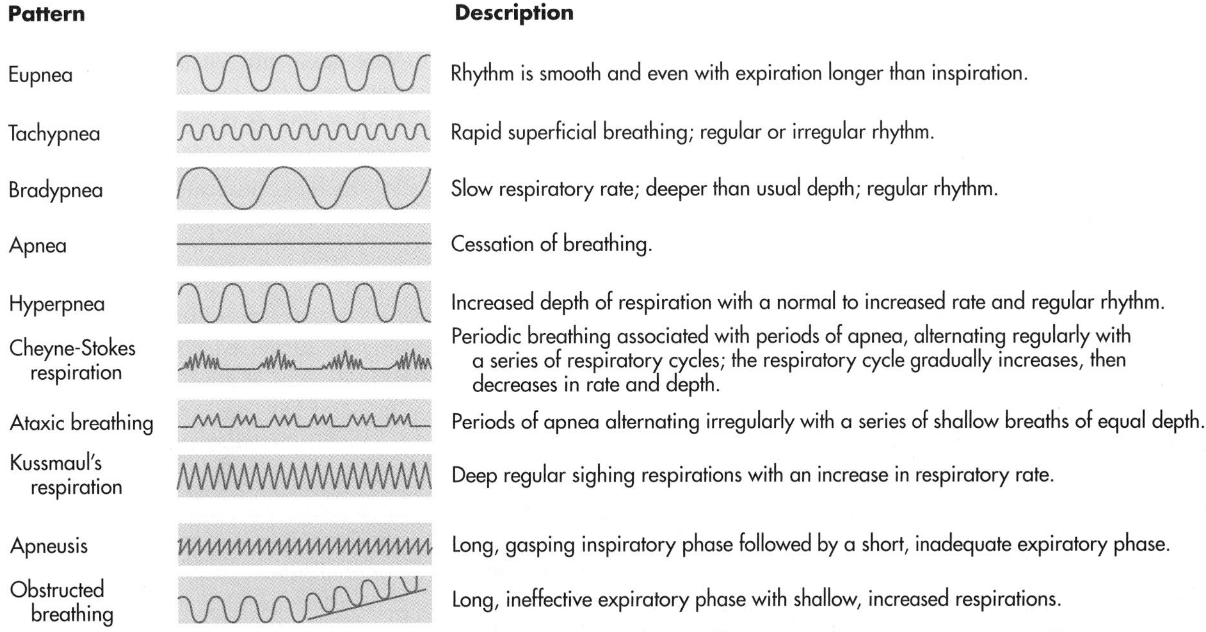

Figure 19-12 Respiratory patterns.

TABLE 19-2 Possible Findings by Inspection in a Pulmonary Examination

Observe	Normal	Abnormal
General appearance	Quiet respiration Sitting or reclining without difficulty Skin translucent, appears dry Nail beds pink Mucous membranes pink and moist*	Lips puckered when exhaling (pursed-lip breathing) Nasal flaring Audible wheezing Restless and apprehensive Leans forward with hands or elbows on knees (tripod position) Skin: diaphoretic, dull pale, or ruddy Cyanosis: skin or mucous membranes have bluish cast Central cyanosis: results from decreased oxygenation of blood† Peripheral cyanosis: result of local vasoconstriction or decreased cardiac output Digital clubbing: painless enlargement of terminal phalanges related to chronic tissue hypoxia
Trachea	Midline in neck	Tracheal deviation; displacement either lateral, anterior, or posterior Jugular venous distention Cough: strong or weak, dry or wet, productive or nonproductive Sputum production: amount, color, odor, and consistency
Rate	Eupnea: 12 to 20	Tachypnea: rate >20 breaths/min Bradypnea: rate <10 breaths/min
Breathing pattern	Minimal effort with inspiration: passive, quiet expiration Inspiration/expiration ratio: 1:2 Male: diaphragmatic breathing Female: thoracic breathing	Accessory muscle breathing Paradoxic: part of chest wall moves in during inhalation and out during exhalation Stridorous: audible, loud, low-pitched sound with inhalation and exhalation
Thoracic configuration	Symmetric appearance Anteroposterior (AP) diameter less than transverse diameter Spine straight Scapulae on same horizontal plane	Chest expands unevenly Muscular development asymmetric Barrel chest: AP diameter increased in relation to transverse diameter Kyphosis: increased thoracic curvature Scoliosis: increased lateral curvature Scapular placement asymmetric

*Dark-skinned people might have normal bluish-pigmented mucous membranes.
†Central cyanosis is relevant to respiratory status. Observe nail beds, mucous membrane, and lips.

Spo_2 value when pulse oximetry is initiated to establish reliability; therefore the need for blood gas analysis is decreased.

Mixed Venous Oxygen Saturation (Svo_2)

Svo_2 measurement is a valuable tool used to assess oxygenation status in the critically ill person. It can be measured continuously or periodically with a specialized pulmonary artery catheter (see Chapter 22). Svo_2 provides information about the amount of oxygen that is supplied to the tissues relative to the oxygen demand at the tissue level. Oxygen demand reflects the amount of oxygen extracted for use at the tissue level. Normal Svo_2 is 60% to 80% and indicates adequate tissue perfusion. A decrease in Svo_2 (<60%) signifies that the oxygen demand is greater than the supply. An increase in Svo_2 (>80%) signifies that the oxygen supply is greater than the oxygen demand. A value of <60%, or a change of +10% from the patient's baseline, is significant.

Upper Airway

Examination of the upper airway includes inspection of the nose and nasal septum for deformities and asymmetry. Some septal deviation is common in adults and is usually asymptomatic (Figure 19-13). Pressing each naris closed while asking the person to sniff inward through the other naris assesses the patency of each. The nasal mucosa and turbinates are observed for color, edema, exudate, or polyps. Excessive redness, edema, exudate, or bleeding is an abnormal finding. Red, swollen nasal mucous membranes accompanied by watery to mucopurulent nasal discharge indicates acute rhinitis. Nasal mucosa that is swollen, pale, boggy, and usually gray to dull red indicates allergic rhinitis.

The sinuses are palpated for signs of tenderness over the frontal and maxillary areas. Transillumination can be performed if infection is suspected. Normally, the sinuses demonstrate differing degrees of a red glow. When disease is present, however, the light will not penetrate the sinuses and the red glow will not be seen through the hard palate or above the eyebrow.

The oropharynx is examined with a tongue blade and a light source. The anterior and posterior tonsillar pillars, uvula, tonsils, and posterior pharynx are inspected for color, symmetry, evidence of exudate, edema, ulcerations, and tonsillar enlargement. Some tonsils are enlarged without being infected, especially in the younger population. The uvula should be

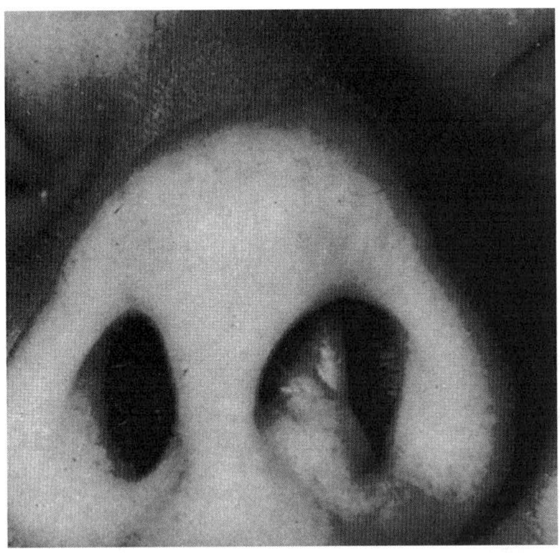

Figure 19-13 Septal deviation. Anterior end of septal cartilage is dislocated and projects into nasal vestibule.

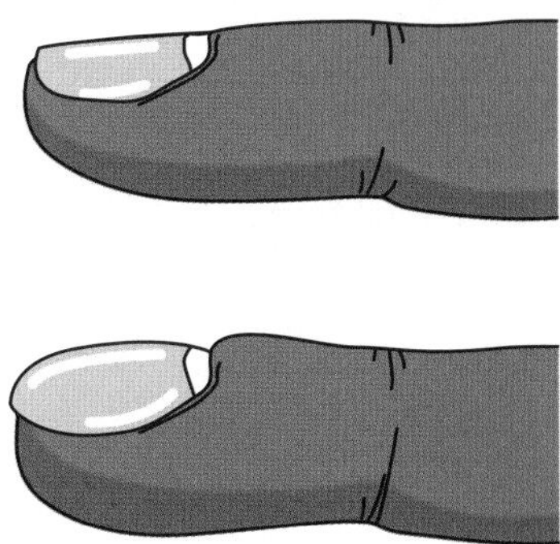

Figure 19-14 Comparison of normal nail *(top)* and digital clubbing *(bottom)*.

TABLE 19-3 Possible Findings by Palpation in a Pulmonary Examination

Palpate	Normal	Abnormal
Skin and chest wall	Skin nontender, smooth, warm, and dry	Skin moist or exceedingly dry Crepitation—"crackling" when skin palpated-caused by air leak from lung into subcutaneous tissue
Fremitus*	Spine and ribs nontender Symmetrical, mild vibrations felt on chest wall during vocalization	Localized tenderness Increased fremitus—a result of vibration through more solid medium, such as lung tumors; pneumonia Decreased fremitus—a result of vibration through increased space (excess air) in the chest, such as pneumothorax or chronic obstructive pulmonary disease Asymmetric fremitus is always abnormal
Lateral chest expansion	Symmetric 3-8 cm expansion†	Expansion less than 3 cm, painful or asymmetric†

*Normal fremitus varies from person to person. A patient's baseline must be established.
†Reduced expansion can result from either an overexpanded chest (barrel chest) or from a restricted chest.

midline and rise with phonation. The gag reflex is also tested. Absence of a gag reflex affects the patient's ability to manage the airway.

Chest and Lungs

Inspection

Note the patient's thorax for shape and symmetry. The anteroposterior diameter should be less than the transverse diameter (1:2 to 5:7). Observe the color of the lips, skin, and nail beds. Assess for indicators of respiratory distress such as nasal flaring or use of accessory muscles. Inspect the fingers for clubbing (Figure 19-14). Table 19-2 indicates possible findings.

Palpation

The chest and spinal column are palpated for tenderness, bulges, and abnormalities; the trachea is palpated for position; and the chest is palpated for symmetry of expansion. All areas of the chest should be palpated for fremitus. To do this, the patient is asked to repeat a phrase (e.g., "99") while the examiner places the palms of the hands against the patient's chest. Fremitus increases with lung consolidation since sound is conducted better through a dense structure than through a porous one. Normal and abnormal findings are presented in Table 19-3.

Percussion

Percussion is used to assess lung fields and diaphragmatic excursion (Figure 19-15). Percussion tones are produced from vibration created by tapping the chest wall. The type of percussion note depends on the density of the underlying tissue and the amount of air through which the vibration travels. A resonant percussion note predominates in healthy, adult lung tissue. Hyperresonant sounds are produced over areas of trapped gas, such as emphysema. Dull percussion sounds are produced in conditions such as atelectasis, pneumonia, and pleural effusion. Table 19-4 identifies normal and abnormal percussion findings.

Auscultation

Auscultation of breath sounds and voice sounds provides valuable information about the lungs and pleura. The patient

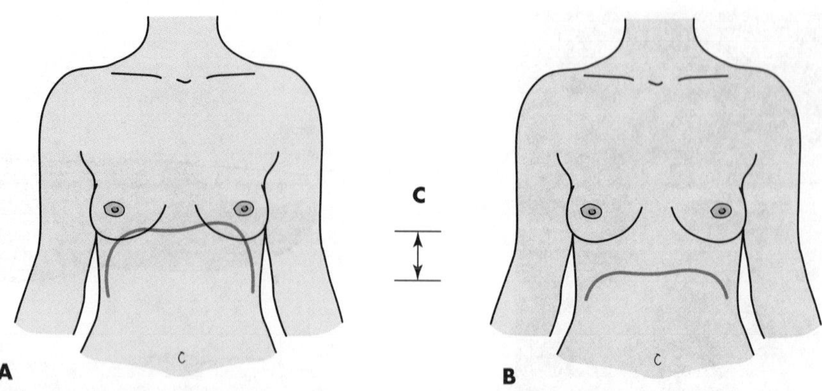

Figure 19-15 Diaphragmatic excursion. **A**, Position of diaphragm at full-end expiration. **B**, Position of diaphragm at full-end inspiration. **C**, Range of diaphragmatic movement–distance from expiration to inspiration.

TABLE 19-4 Possible Findings by Percussion in a Pulmonary Examination

Percussion	Normal	Abnormal
Lung fields	Resonance: low-pitched, hollow, easily heard sounds; equal quality bilaterally	Hyperresonant: heard with air trapping (emphysema or pneumothorax) Dull or flat: results from decreased air in lungs (tumor, atelectasis, fluid)
Diaphragm position and movement	Resting diaphragm at 10th thoracic vertebra Each hemidiaphragm moves 3-6 cm	High position-stomach distention or phrenic nerve damage Decreased or no movement in either hemidiaphragm*

*Decreased excursion can result from hyperinflated lungs pushing down on diaphragm, diaphragmatic disorders, or loss of diaphragmatic innervation.

is instructed to take slow, deep breaths through the mouth during the examination. Using the diaphragm of the stethoscope, the examiner listens systematically to all lung fields and compares breath sounds of the right and left sides during inspiration and expiration (Figure 19-16). Three normal and distinct breath sounds are produced based on the specific area of the respiratory tract. Characteristics of breath sounds can be found in Table 19-5.

Adventitious breath sounds (Table 19-6) are caused by moving air colliding with secretions in the tracheobronchial passageways, or by the inflation of previously deflated airways. They can be caused by any pathologic condition that is associated with excess mucus or fluid, tissue inflammation, bronchospasm, or airway obstruction. These are "added" sounds that are not normally auscultated in the lungs. Another abnormal auscultatory finding is diminished or absent breath sounds. This finding indicates either obstruction or changes in the elasticity of lung fibers. Conditions that lead to alveolar hypoventilation include COPD, pleurisy, and pneumothorax.

Normal voice sounds are usually muffled and indistinct while listening with the stethoscope. Pathology that increases lung density enhances transmission of voice sounds (Table 19-7). Assessment of voice sounds is not part of the routine examination; it is done when pathology is suspected.[1]

Assessment measures and variations in normal findings relevant to the care of older adults are presented in the Gerontologic Assessment box. Also identified are disorders common in older adults, which may be responsible for abnormal assessment findings.

Gerontologic Assessment

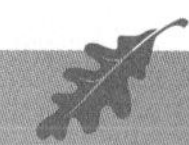

Inspect the chest.
- Increased chest diameter and kyphosis occur with aging and result in decreased chest expansion.

Check ability to breathe deeply and cough forcefully.
- Decreased muscular strength and reduced chest wall compliance with decreased chest expansion impair the ability to deep breathe and cough, increasing the risk of low arterial oxygen levels and atelectasis. Decreased ability to handle secretions increases the risk of aspiration.

Auscultate breath sounds.
- Crackles may be heard and breath sounds decreased due to shallow breathing and/or atelectasis related to the factors cited above.

Observe carefully for signs of respiratory infection.
- Overall, respiratory defenses function less effectively with age, increasing the risk of infection.

When reviewing the results of pulmonary function tests, expect the following:
- Increased residual volume
- Decreased forced vital capacity
- Decreased forced expiratory volume
- Decreased maximum voluntary ventilation

COMMON DISORDERS IN OLDER ADULTS

Emphysema
Chronic bronchitis
Asthma
Pneumonia

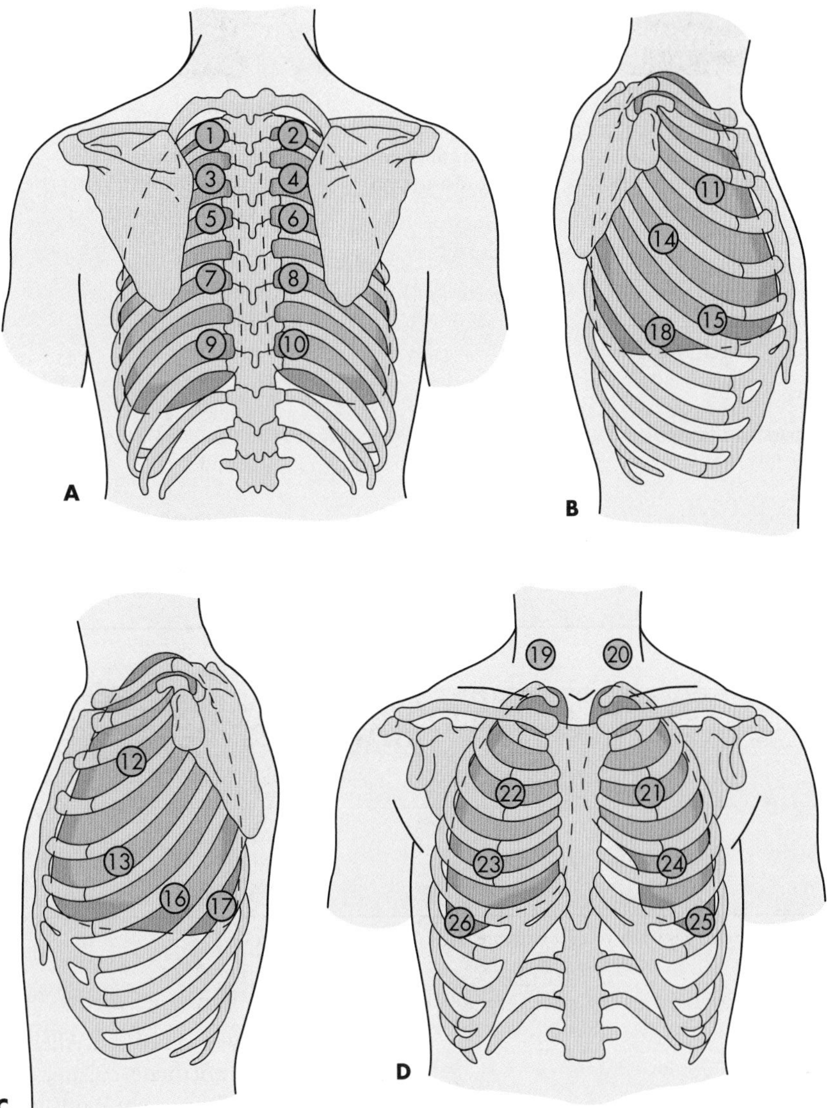

Figure 19-16 Numbers indicate a recommended sequence for percussion and auscultation during a routine screening examination. **A**, Posterior thorax. **B**, Right lateral thorax. **C**, Left lateral thorax. **D**, Anterior thorax.

TABLE 19-5 Characteristics of Breath Sounds

Sound	Duration of Inspiration and Expiration	Diagram of Sound	Pitch	Intensity	Normal Location	Abnormal Location
Vesicular	Inspiration>expiration 5:2		Low	Soft	Peripheral lung	Not applicable
Bronchovesicular	Inspiration = expiration 1:1		Medium	Medium	First and second intercostals spaces at the sternal border anteriorly; posteriorly at T4 medial to scapulae	Peripheral lung
Bronchial (tubular)	Inspiration<expiration 1:2		High	Loud	Over trachea	Lung area

From Malasanos L et al: *Health assessment,* ed 4, St Louis, 1990, Mosby.

TABLE 19-6 Abnormal (Adventitious) Lung Sounds

Type	Physiology	Auscultation	Sound	Possible Condition
Crackles	Air passing through fluid in small airways, or sudden opening of deflated weakened airways	More commonly heard during inspiration	Fine high-pitched or coarse low-pitched popping sounds that are short and discontinuous	Pneumonia, heart failure, atelectasis, emphysema
Rhonchi	Large airway obstructed by fluid	Heard commonly during expiration	Low-pitched continuous snoring sound	Chronic obstructive pulmonary disease (COPD), bronchospasm, pneumonia
Wheezes	Air passing through narrowed airways	Can be heard throughout inspiration and expiration	High-pitched whistling sound	Airway obstruction, bronchospasm as in asthma, COPD
Pleural friction rub	Rubbing of inflamed pleura	May occur throughout respiratory cycle, heard best at base of lung at end of expiration	Scratching, grating, rubbing, creaking	Inflamed pleura, pulmonary infarction

TABLE 19-7 Voice Sounds*

Type	Instruction to Patient	Sound	Abnormal
Egophony	Say prolonged "e"	Muffled "e"	"a"
Whisphered pectoriloguy	Whisper "1, 2, 3"	Muffled "1, 2, 3"	Loud, clear "1, 2, 3"
Bronchophony	Say "1, 2, 3"	Muffled "1, 2, 3"	Loud, clear "1, 2, 3"

*Examiner auscultates for characteristic changes when voice sounds are transmitted through chest wall.

DIAGNOSTIC TESTS

Laboratory Tests

Complete Blood Count

The complete blood count provides information about red blood cells (RBCs), hemoglobin, hematocrit, and white blood cells (WBCs). The RBC count is valuable in assessing overall oxygen-carrying capacity. Normally there are 4 million (female) to 5 million (male) RBCs in each cubic millimeter of blood, and each RBC contains an estimated 280 million hemoglobin molecules. Oxygen that diffuses into the pulmonary capillary chemically attaches to the hemoglobin for transport to the tissues. An abnormally low hemoglobin level can adversely affect the body's ability to carry oxygen to the cells to meet the metabolic needs of the body. Hemoglobin is the iron-containing pigment of the RBCs, and hematocrit is the volume of RBCs within a given volume of blood. The WBC count provides information regarding infection or immune system dysfunction.

Arterial Blood Gases and Acid-Base Balance

Arterial blood gas analysis provides information about oxygenation, ventilation, and acid-base balance. It is valuable in assessing the efficiency of pulmonary gas exchange and the presence of an acid-base disorder.[8] The arterial blood gas parameters are shown in Table 19-8. A blood sample is obtained by direct puncture of a radial, brachial, or femoral artery. If the radial artery is to be used, Allen's test is performed first to ensure there is adequate collateral blood flow to the hand (Figure 19-17). To prevent clotting of the sample, a preheparinized syringe is used to collect the blood. Once the 2 ml of blood is obtained, air bubbles are expelled, and the syringe is sealed with an impermeable cap to prevent contact with room air. The blood sample is placed on ice until analyzed. Arterial punctures are contraindicated in patients receiving thrombolytic agents.

An indwelling arterial catheter is commonly used to obtain blood samples in the critically ill; the catheter should be flushed per hospital protocol to prevent clotting. Continuous arterial blood gas monitoring is also performed in certain instances.

Nursing Care. The purpose of the test and its procedure is explained to the patient. If the patient is receiving supplemental oxygen, the amount of oxygen should be noted. The oxygen should not be changed or removed (unless ordered) before the test. Other interventions in the plan of care should be withheld for 20 minutes before the test. No other preparation is necessary. After the arterial puncture is made, constant, firm, direct pressure is applied to the puncture site for 5 minutes, or longer for patients with blood-clotting abnormalities. Subsequently, the site is observed for bleeding and hematoma formation. The involved extremity is also monitored for cir-

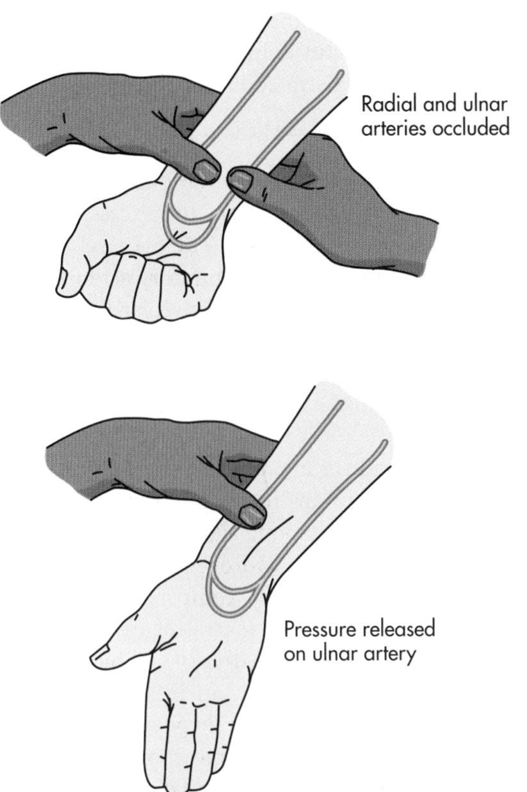

Figure 19-17 Allen's test. Hold patient's hand with palm up. Have patient clench and unclench hand while occluding the radial and ulnar arteries. The hand will become pale. Lower the hand and have the patient relax the hand. While continuing to hold the radial artery, release pressure on the ulnar artery. Brisk return of color (5 to 7 seconds) demonstrates adequate ulnar blood flow. If pallor persists for more than 15 seconds, ulnar flow is inadequate and radial artery cannulation should not be attempted.

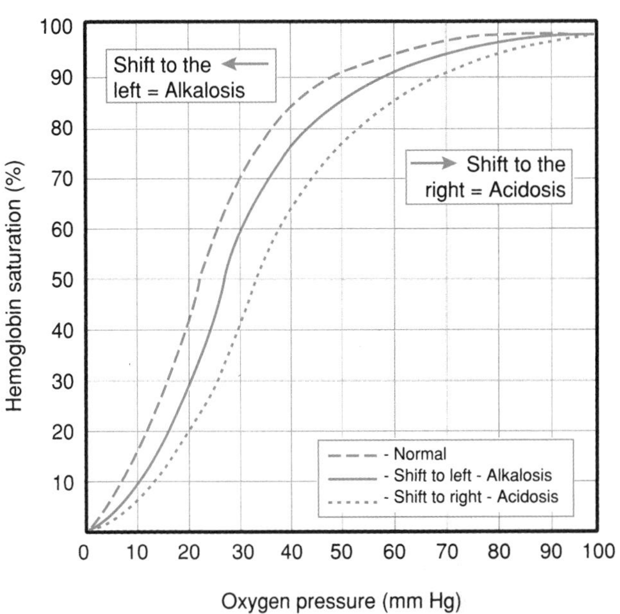

Figure 19-18 Oxyhemoglobin dissociation curve.

TABLE 19-8 Arterial Blood Gases

Parameter	Measurement	Value
Acid-base-balance	pH: hydrogen ion concentration	Normal: 7.35-7.45 Alkalemia: ↑7.45 Acidemia: ↓7.35
Oxygenation	PaO_2: partial pressure of dissolved O_2 in blood	Normal: 80-100 mm Hg Hyperoxemia: ↑100 mm Hg Hypoxemia: ↓80 mm Hg 95%-98%
Ventilation	SaO_2: percentage of O_2 bound to hemoglobin $PaCO_2$: partial pressure of CO_2 dissolved in blood	Normal: 35-45 mm Hg Hypercapnia: ↑45 mm Hg Hypocapnia: ↓35 mm Hg

culatory impairment, which if it occurs, must be reported immediately.

Oxygenation. Both partial pressure of oxygen (PaO_2) and oxygen saturation (SaO_2) levels are measured to determine the adequacy of arterial blood oxygenation. PaO_2 is oxygen dissolved in arterial blood. The PaO_2 can be used to assess the need for oxygen therapy or a change in it. SaO_2 measures the percentage of the hemoglobin that is combined with oxygen. About 98% of the oxygen-carrying capacity of blood is accounted for by oxyhemoglobin, with the partial pressure of oxygen acting as the driving force for this chemical combination.

Oxyhemoglobin Dissociation Curve. The relationship of PaO_2 to SaO_2 is demonstrated in the oxyhemoglobin dissociation curve. Although the percentage of hemoglobin that is bound with oxygen increases as the PaO_2 increases, this relationship is not directly linear. Many factors affect the affinity of the heme molecule for oxygen. The sigmoid curve represents the saturation percentages that occur at various PaO_2 levels (Figure 19-18). In the upper portion of the curve, hemoglobin has an increased affinity for oxygen, so that large changes in PO_2 levels can be tolerated without significantly changing the saturation. For example, at a PO_2 of 100 mm Hg, hemoglobin saturation is 97%; even if the PO_2 level should decrease to 70 mm Hg, the saturation would only decrease to 94%. This serves as a protective mechanism that ensures adequate tissue oxygenation despite mild hypoxemia. However, once the PO_2 level falls below 60 mm Hg, oxygen saturation drops sharply and reduces the ability of the hemoglobin to transport oxygen.

The affinity of hemoglobin for oxygen is influenced by several factors. For example, hypothermia, alkalosis, and hypocapnia are associated with reduced tissue metabolism. These conditions cause the oxyhemoglobin dissociation curve to shift to the left. This shift results in an increased affinity of hemoglobin for oxygen resulting in less oxygen being released to the tissues. Thus, a patient who has an alteration in pH (alkalosis) will have more oxygen-bound hemoglobin (i.e., a higher SaO_2, than an patient who has the same PaO_2 but with a pH in the normal range).

A shift in the oxyhemoglobin dissociation curve to the right means there is decreased affinity of the hemoglobin for oxygen; thus, oxygen is easily released from the hemoglobin. Fever, acidosis, and hypercapnia are conditions that shift the curve to the right. These conditions produce an increased need for oxygen because of the associated increase in tissue metabolism. A patient with a lowered pH (acidosis) will have a lower SaO_2 than a patient who has the same PaO_2 with a pH in the normal range. Another condition that causes a shift to the right is an increase in 2,3-diphosphoglycerate.

The amount of oxygen that is delivered to the tissues depends on oxygen saturation, hemoglobin, and cardiac output. PaO_2 and SaO_2 levels may be normal; however, if the patient is anemic or has inadequate cardiac output tissue oxygenation may be inadequate. Thus arterial blood gas results should not be used in isolation in planning care.[10]

Ventilation. $PaCO_2$ is the partial pressure of carbon dioxide in the blood and is a parameter that measures the adequacy of ventilation. $PaCO_2$ levels depend on the amount of carbon dioxide produced by the body and the ability of the lungs to eliminate it. A decrease in the ventilatory rate, or alveolar hypoventilation, causes the lungs to retain carbon dioxide. This results in an elevated $PaCO_2$ level (hypercapnia). An increase in the ventilatory rate, or alveolar hyperventilation, causes carbon dioxide to be blown off, resulting in a decrease in $PaCO_2$ level (hypocapnia). $PaCO_2$ levels are used to assess the need for or change in mechanical ventilatory support.

Acid-Base Balance. Arterial blood pH is a measurement of hydrogen ion concentration and reflects the acidity or alkalinity of the blood. As the hydrogen ion concentration increases, the blood becomes more acidic and the pH value falls. When the hydrogen ion concentration decreases, the blood becomes more alkaline, and the pH value rises. Excess acid can be the result of a respiratory or metabolic disorder, or a mixed respiratory and metabolic disorder.

Carbon dioxide combines with water to form carbonic acid. Carbonic acid, in turn, dissociates to form hydrogen and bicarbonate ions, as illustrated in this equation:

$$CO_2 + H_2O \longleftrightarrow H_2CO_3 \longleftrightarrow HCO_3 + H$$

When there is an excess of carbon dioxide in the blood, a result of alveolar hypoventilation, the excess carbonic acid and H ions produce an acidemia. The pH level is below 7.35 and the patient is in a state of respiratory acidosis. When the $PaCO_2$ level decreases as a result of alveolar hyperventilation, too much carbon dioxide is blown off. The decrease in carbonic acid and H ions produces an alkalemia. The pH level is greater than 7.45 and the patient is in a state of respiratory alkalosis.

In metabolic acidosis an accumulation of metabolic acids causes the increase in hydrogen ion concentration of the blood; conversely, in metabolic alkalosis the excessive loss of acids causes the decrease in hydrogen ion concentration. The respiratory system can rapidly compensate for a metabolic acid-base imbalance by either increasing or decreasing ventilation. If a metabolic acidosis (decrease in bicarbonate level) develops, the lungs respond by increasing ventilation and blowing off excess carbon dioxide (hypocapnia). Conversely, if a metabolic alkalosis (increase in bicarbonate level) develops, the lungs respond by decreasing ventilation and retaining carbon dioxide (hypercapnia). The kidneys also respond to acid-base imbalances by excreting bicarbonate or resorbing bicarbonate ions and secreting hydrogen ions. However, this compensatory mechanism occurs over several days, whereas the respiratory system changes occur within minutes.

An imbalance in acid-base balance may be a result of a respiratory disorder, a metabolic disorder, or a combination of both. Thus, an acid-base assessment requires an evaluation of all three parameters: $PaCO_2$, pH, and bicarbonate levels. See Chapter 13 for more information.

α_1-Antitrypsin Assay

α_1-Antitrypsin is a globulin that inhibits certain enzymes from destroying the alveolar walls. α_1-Antitrypsin deficiencies are inherited; patients with this deficiency are highly susceptible to lung tissue destruction at an early age. This blood test is valuable in the identification of patients with the genetic abnormality that greatly increases their risk for development of emphysema without the usual predisposing factors.[10]

Sputum Analysis

A sputum sample may be ordered for microbiologic and cytologic testing. Sputum examination may be helpful in evaluating patients in whom tuberculosis, pneumonia, and lung cancer are suspected. Gram stains and cultures define a causative organism. Sensitivity is a test ordered in conjunction with the culture that identifies antibiotics to which the organisms present in the sputum are sensitive and prevent further growth. An acid-fast bacilli stain is used to diagnose tuberculosis. Cytologic examination identifies cell types to aid in diagnoses, such as in lung cancer. However, an absence of malignant cells in the specimen cannot be interpreted as an absence of cancer. Sputum examination may also reveal the presence of parasites, macrophages, or other cells that aid in the evaluation of lung disease.

To collect a sputum sample, have the patient rinse the mouth with water, take a series of deep breaths, and then cough to raise sputum and expectorate it into a sterile container. To do this correctly, the patient needs to understand the difference between saliva and sputum, and may need to practice deep breathing and coughing. Patients need to be instructed to notify the staff as soon as a specimen is collected.

Sputum specimens are best collected as the patient awakens in the morning. A bronchodilator or inhalation of a hypertonic solution may be ordered for patients who have difficulty raising secretions. Patients who are intubated, or have a tracheostomy placed, will require suctioning via the artificial airway with a catheter and special collection container. Sputum specimens can also be obtained by invasive methods such as transtracheal aspiration or fiberoptic bronchoscopy.

Throat Culture

A throat culture is performed to help identify microorganisms so that appropriate treatment can be initiated. To obtain the throat culture, ask the patient to tilt the head back and open the mouth. A tongue depressor is used so that the swab is less likely to come in contact with the normal flora of the mouth. Both tonsillar pillars and the posterior pharynx should be swabbed. The swab is placed in the culture tube, labeled, and transported to the laboratory.

Radiologic Tests

Chest Roentgenograms

Chest radiographs are obtained to diagnose disorders of the lung, to evaluate effectiveness of treatment, to determine the extent and location of disease, and to assess the progression of lung disease. In addition, chest radiographs can be used to evaluate proper placement of catheters and tubes. Chest radiographs are usually performed in the radiology department where the patient stands in an upright position with the anterior chest pressed against the film cassette holder. This produces a posteroanterior (PA) radiograph in which the x-ray beam travels through the patient's posterior chest to the x-ray film. However, if the patient is acutely ill, the x-ray can be taken at the bedside with a portable x-ray machine. If the patient can sit up, the radiograph is taken with the x-ray camera positioned toward the patient's anterior chest, and the x-ray beam travels through the anterior chest to the x-ray film that is placed behind the patient's back. This is referred to as an anteroposterior view. A lateral radiograph is generally taken along with a PA radiograph. Generally the left side of the chest is pressed against the film cassette, and the x-ray beam travels through the side of the body. Figure 19-19 shows PA and lateral chest radiographs. Special views such as the oblique, lordotic, or decubitus may be obtained to visualize specific parts of the chest. In preparation for the radiograph all metal objects above the waist are removed. During the test the patient is asked to take a deep breath and hold it. There is no discomfort, although the temperature of the room and film cassette holder may be cool. Personnel may be positioned behind a lead wall or wear lead aprons while the radiograph is taken. Possible radiographic findings are listed in Table 19-9.

Computed Tomography

Computed tomography (CT) scanning, with or without the use of radiopaque contrast media, uses computer programming to permit visualization of multiple cross-sectional "slices" of the lung. Each tomogram represents a specific part of the lung. Lesions that are not clearly visualized on chest radiography can be evaluated more clearly with CT. For this test the patient must remove all metal articles and lie still on an examination table while the x-ray machine rotates to take

TABLE 19-9 Radiographic Findings

Trachea	Midline, translucent, tubelike structure found in the anterior mediastinal cavity
Clavicles	Equally distant from the sternum
Ribs	Thoracic cavity encasement
Mediastinum	Shadowy-appearing space between the lungs that widens at the hilum
Heart	Solid-appearing structure with clear edges visible in the left anterior mediastinal cavity; cardiothoracic ratio should be less than half the width of the chest wall on a posteroanterior (PA) film; cardiac shadow appears larger on an anteroposterior (AP) film
Carina	Lowest tracheal cartilage at the bifurcation
Mainstem bronchus	Translucent, tubelike structure visible approximately 2.5 cm from the hilum
Hilum	Small, white, bilateral densities present where the bronchi join the lungs; left bronchus should be 2 to 3 cm higher than the right
Bronchi	Not usually visible
Lung fields	Usually not completely visible except for "lung markings" at periphery Blackened area without tissue markings suggests pneumothorax Patchy infiltrates suggest pneumonia, atelectasis
Diaphragm	Rounded structures visible at bottom of the lung fields; right side is 1 to 2 cm higher than the left; costophrenic angles should be clear and sharp Loss of costophrenic angle sharpness suggests pleural effusion Flattened diaphragm suggests emphysema

films. If a contrast medium is to be used, the patient must be questioned about iodine sensitivity before the test and informed that a warm, flushed feeling and a salty taste in the mouth may be experienced.

Fluoroscopy

Dynamic information about the chest, such as diaphragmatic movement or lung expansion and contraction, can be evaluated with fluoroscopy. Fluoroscopy is a technique used to observe movement in the area being filmed while the specific study is in progress. It can also be used in conjunction with other procedures, such as bronchoscopy, when a biopsy of the lung is obtained. This technique exposes the patient to greater doses of radiation than the standard chest radiograph and is reserved for select patients.

Magnetic Resonance Imaging

Magnetic resonance imaging (MRI) is able to produce cross-sectional images of the body that are helpful in detecting subtle lesions. It is superior to CT scanning in detecting lesions of the chest wall and congenital heart disease. However, CT scanning is better for most thoracic abnormalities. The test takes about an hour and all metal objects must be removed before it is performed. Any patient who has an implant made of ferromagnetic material cannot undergo MRI since the device (e.g., prosthetic valve) could shift. The imager may also interfere with the functioning of a cardiac pacemaker.

Ventilation/Perfusion Lung Scan

Lung scan procedures involve the use of a scanning device that records the pattern of pulmonary radioactivity after the inhalation (ventilation lung scan) or intravenous injection (perfusion lung scan) of gamma ray-emitting radionucleotides. These scans provide the clinician with a visual image of the distribution of ventilation and perfusion in the lungs. Valuable information about ventilation-perfusion patterns can aid in the diagnosis of parenchymal lung disease and vascular disorders, such as pulmonary embolism. For the ventilation scan the patient is required to breathe a small amount of radioactive gas through a ventilation system. During the

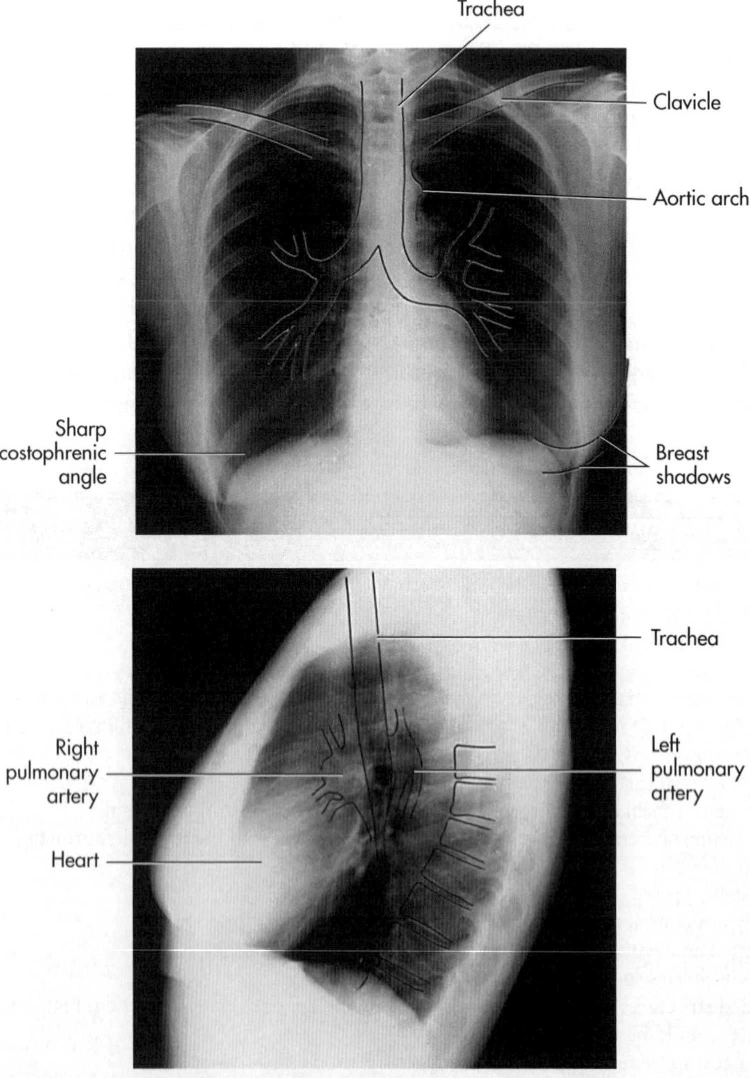

Figure 19-19 Location of structures on a chest radiograph.

procedure the patient must be able to take a breath and hold it. If a perfusion lung scan is to be performed, the patient receives an injection of a radioactive agent and the camera takes a series of images. For this, an accurate preprocedure weight is needed so that the dosage of radioactive agent can be calculated and the patient must be assessed for allergies. No special care is needed after the test.

Pulmonary Angiography

Pulmonary angiography visualizes the pulmonary vascular system and is used to detect pulmonary emboli and a variety of congenital and acquired lesions of the pulmonary vessels. Additional data obtained in conjunction with this test include measures of pulmonary pressures, cardiac output, and pulmonary vascular resistance. A radiopaque material is injected into a catheter that has been introduced into a peripheral vein and advanced through the right side of the heart to the pulmonary artery. A series of radiographic films are then taken to follow the distribution of the contrast material throughout the pulmonary vascular system. The catheter is removed at the completion of the test and a pressure dressing applied (see Guidelines for Safe Practice box).[9]

Special Tests

Pulmonary Function Tests

Pulmonary function testing is a noninvasive method of assessing the functional capacity of the lungs. These tests cannot be used in isolation to diagnose specific disease but are integral to the diagnostic process. Pulmonary function tests (PFTs) are used to evaluate pulmonary disability, to evaluate pulmonary function in patients before surgery, to evaluate the patient's disease progression and response to therapy, and to differentiate obstructive lung disease from restrictive lung disease. The patient is asked to breathe into a mouthpiece that is connected to a spirometer. Nose clips are applied to permit mouth breathing only; the patient is required to inhale deeply, hold his or her breath, and then quickly and forcefully exhale. It may take several attempts on behalf of the patient to perform successfully. Shortness of breath or light-headedness may be experienced.

Nursing Care. The purpose of the test and its procedure is explained to the patient. Food and fluids are not restricted; however, the test should not be scheduled after a meal since the diaphragm will be exerted during the test. Medications that may affect respiration are omitted before the PFTs, unless specifically ordered to be given. Height and weight are obtained measurements before the test. After the PFTs, the patient's respiratory status is assessed.

Spirometry. Spirometry is the most common pulmonary function test conducted. It is a test in which lung capacities (the sum of two or more lung volumes), lung volumes, and flow rates are determined. The patient breathes through a mouthpiece connected to a spirometer that measures the air moving through the apparatus. A graphic tracing of the lung volumes and capacities is recorded (Figure 19-20).

Tidal volume periodically increases in spontaneously breathing healthy patients. This is referred to as sighing. Patients whose breathing pattern is shallow without sighing are at risk for atelectasis and pneumonia. Tidal volume is monitored closely in critically ill patients who are mechanically ventilated.

Vital capacity (VC) reflects the muscle strength and volume capacity of the lung. It is important to maintain an effective cough, to take a deep breath, and to clear the airways of secretions. In addition to evaluating respiratory function before surgery, vital capacity is used to monitor and diagnose pulmonary disorders. VC provides information about airway resistance when measured as forced vital capacity. One of the most meaningful clinical measurements is the forced expiratory volume (FEV). The FEV measures the amount of air in liters that is forcefully expired over a specified amount of time, generally 1, 2, or 3 seconds. When compared with the forced vital capacity (FVC), the FEV can identify the pulmonary impairment as restrictive or obstructive. In obstructive disease

Guidelines for Safe Practice

The Patient Undergoing Pulmonary Angiography

PREANGIOGRAPHY

- Explain the purpose of the test and its procedure.
- Give the patient nothing by mouth for 4 to 6 hours before the test.
- Check for the signed consent form.
- Check laboratory data: electrolytes, complete blood count, blood urea nitrogen, creatinine, and clotting studies should be within normal limits.
- Assess the patient for allergies to contrast media.
- Obtain baseline vital signs before the procedure.
- Inform the patient that the dye may cause flushing, coughing, and a warm sensation.

IMMEDIATELY AFTER ANGIOGRAPHY

- Monitor vital signs every 15 minutes.
- Observe dressing and site for bleeding or hematoma development every 15 minutes.
- Assess site for infection or thrombophlebitis (swelling, warmth, redness, or pain).
- Maintain bed rest for 4 to 6 hours.

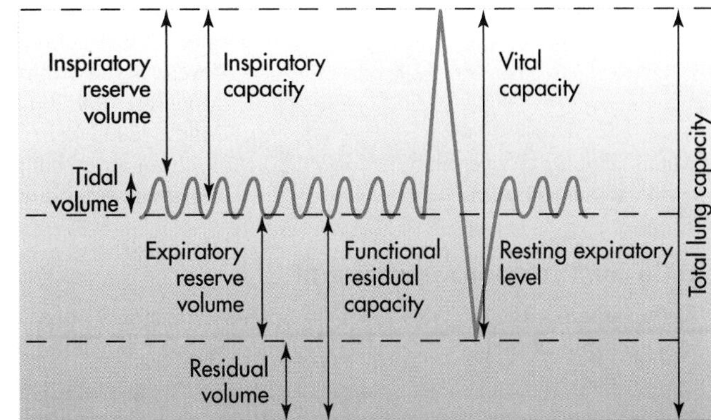

Figure 19-20 Lung volumes and capacities illustrated by spirography tracing.

TABLE 19-10 Definitions and Implications of Pulmonary Function Tests

	Definitions	Implications
Lung Volume (Nonoverlapping Measures)		
Tidal volume (V_T) ~500 ml	Volume of gas inspired and expired with a normal breath	Decrease in V_T without an increase in respiratory rate can lead to hypoventilation and respiratory acidosis
Inspiratory reserve volume (IRV) ~3000 ml	Maximal volume that can be inspired from the end of a normal inspiration	Not widely used clinically
Expiratory reserve volume (ERV) ~1000 ml	Maximal volume that can be exhaled by forced expiration after a normal expiration	Limited use clinically
Residual volume (RV) ~1500 ml	Volume of gas left in lung after maximal expiration	Expressed as a ratio >33% of VC suggests presence of chronic obstructive pulmonary disease Normal in restrictive disease
Lung Capacities (Combinations of Various Volumes)		
Inspiratory capacity (IC): IC = V_T + IRV = 3500 ml	Maximal amount of air that can be inspired after a normal expiration	Not widely used clinically
Functional residual capacity (FRC): FRC = ERV + RV = 2500 ml	Amount of air left in lungs after a normal expiration	Reflects expanding forces of chest wall and recoiling forces of lungs When lung tissue is lost, the chest wall forces have less opposition, thus increasing FRC
Vital capacity (VC): VC = V_T + IRV+ ERV = 4500 ml	Maximal amount of air that can be expired after a maximal inspiration	Reflects ability to deep breathe, cough, and clear the airways
Forced vital capacity (FVC)	Maximal amount of air that can be expelled with a maximal effort after a maximal inspiration	VC that is forcefully exhaled Important index to evaluate patients before surgery for postoperative respiratory complications: 20 ml/kg of ideal body weight indicates that the patient is at risk for complications
Total lung capacity (TLC): TLC = V_T + IRV + ERV + RV = 6000 ml	Total amount of air in lungs after maximal inspiration	Determined by size, age, and sex Increased in obstructive disease and decreased in restrictive disease
Volume/Time Relationships		
Minute volume (VE): VE = 4-12 L/min	Volume inspired and expired in 1 min of normal breathing	Index of ventilation Should increase with fever, pain, exercise, and acidosis
Forced expiratory volume in 1 sec (FEV_1): FEV_1/FVC = 75% of VC in 1 sec FEV_3/FV = 95%	Amount of air expelled in the first second of forced vital capacity maneuver	Reflects airflow characteristics; expressed as a percentage of FVC Severe decline in FEV_1 results in hypercapnia and respiratory acidosis Forced expiratory flow (FEF 25-75) is an early indicator of obstructive disorders and reflects degree of airway patency
Peak expiratory flow (PEF)	Maximum flow rate achieved during FVC Degree of obstruction: Severe: <100 L/min Moderate: 100-200 L/min Mild: >200 L/min	Correlates with FEV_1 Useful to assess response to treatment
Maximal voluntary ventilation (MVV): MVV = 170 L/min	Amount of air exchanged per minute with maximal rate and depth of respiration	Quick assessment of lungs Reflects compliance, airway resistance, and respiratory muscle status
Diffusion/Perfusion Measurement		
Diffusing capacity (D_{LCO}) = 25 ml/min/mm Hg	Assesses ability of gas molecules to cross alveolar-capillary membrane	Reported as raw number and percentage of predicted value
Nitrogen washout	Determines maldistribution of ventilation	Displayed on a tracing showing a curved pattern If slope of the pattern is uneven, uneven ventilation is suspected

blocked airways interfere with expiration more than inspiration. When airway obstruction (resistance) increases, airflow rates decrease. The amount of time necessary to forcefully exhale an amount of air after full inspiration is increased in obstructive disease. The FEV/FVC ratio is low. In restrictive disease air can be expelled rapidly, and the FEV/FVC ratio is usually high. Most patients should be able to exhale approximately 75% of their VC in 1 second.[9]

Functional residual capacity (FRC) reflects the volume of gas remaining in the lungs at the end of a normal passive exhalation and is in continuous contact with pulmonary capillary blood. If FRC is decreased, alveoli collapse, and gas exchange is adversely affected.

Lung volumes and capacities are defined, and clinical implications of each measurement are provided in Table 19-10. Normal values for PFTs are expressed in milliliters, liters, liters per second, or liters per minute or as a percentage of predicted normal depending on the test performed.

Pulmonary function testing can also be performed during bronchial provocation and while a patient is exercising to identify triggers to bronchospasm, to determine if the obstruction (bronchospasm) is reversible with bronchodilator therapy, and to determine the extent of exercise limitation. Bronchodilators are generally withheld before the bronchial provocation test.

Flow-Volume Loops. Flow-volume loops aid in distinguishing obstructive from restrictive lung disorders and intrathoracic from extrathoracic disorders. Inspiratory and expiratory volumes are plotted against flow rates to produce a flow-volume loop. Figure 19-21 presents a comparison of various flow-volume loops. Typically a patient with obstructive airway disease has a "scooped out" appearance in the expiratory flow curve. In restrictive disease there is a symmetric reduction in volume and flow; it appears as a smaller version of a normal flow-volume loop.

Pulmonary Diffusion Capacity. The ability of gas to diffuse across the alveolar-capillary membrane is measured by a test called diffusing capacity of the lung for carbon monoxide (D_{LCO}). One method involves the patient breathing in a known amount of carbon monoxide and exhaling it after 10 seconds of breath holding (to allow the gas to diffuse across the alveolar-capillary membrane). The carbon monoxide concentration in the blood is estimated by the amount of carbon monoxide exhaled. A normal value is approximately 25 ml/min/mm Hg; however, predicted values are based on age, height, and gender. The D_{LCO} is decreased in patients with lung disorders that involve the alveolar-capillary membrane such as emphysema and interstitial lung disease.

Thoracentesis

Thoracentesis involves the insertion of a needle into the pleural space to instill medications into the pleural space, biopsy the pleura, or remove pleural fluid (Figure 19-22). Aspiration of pleural fluid may be done for gross or microscopic examination and/or to relieve respiratory distress. Therefore, thoracentesis may be performed for diagnostic or therapeutic

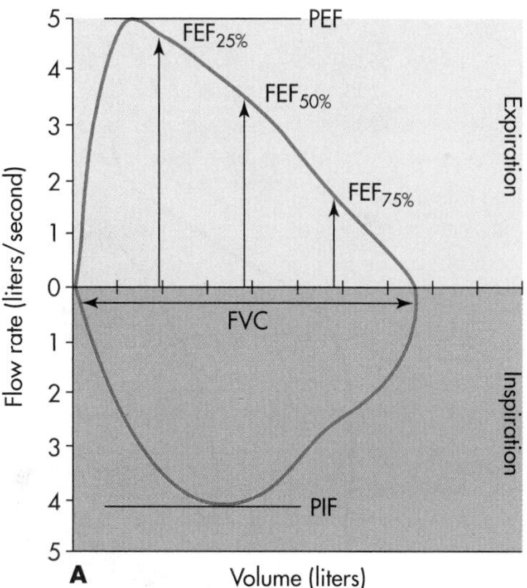

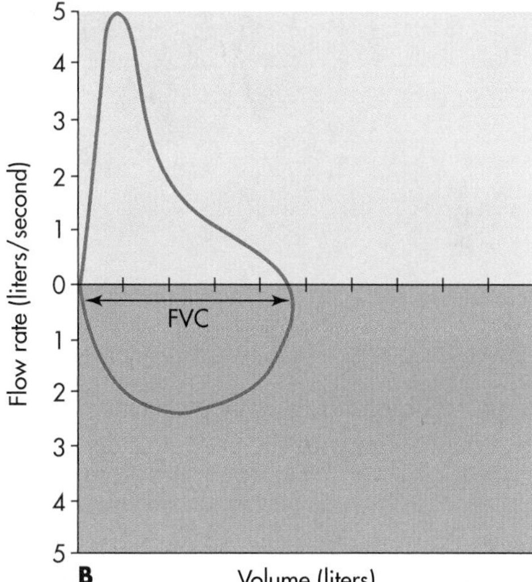

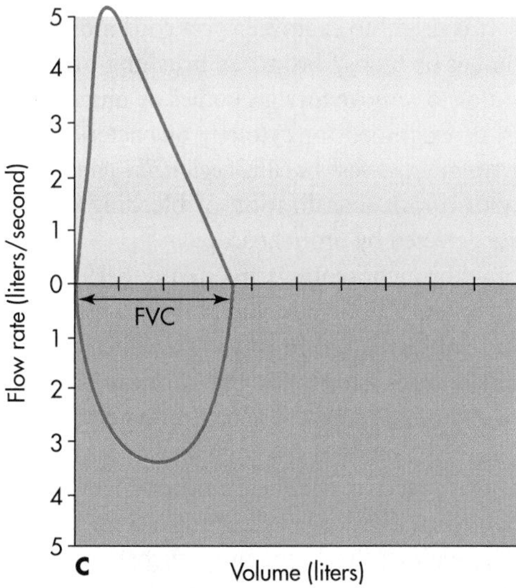

Figure 19-21 Flow volume loops. **A,** Peak expiratory flow (PEF); peak inspiratory flow (PIF); forced expiratory flow at X% of FVC (FEF%), and forced vital capacity (FVC); **B,** Obstructive disorder. **C,** Restrictive disorder.

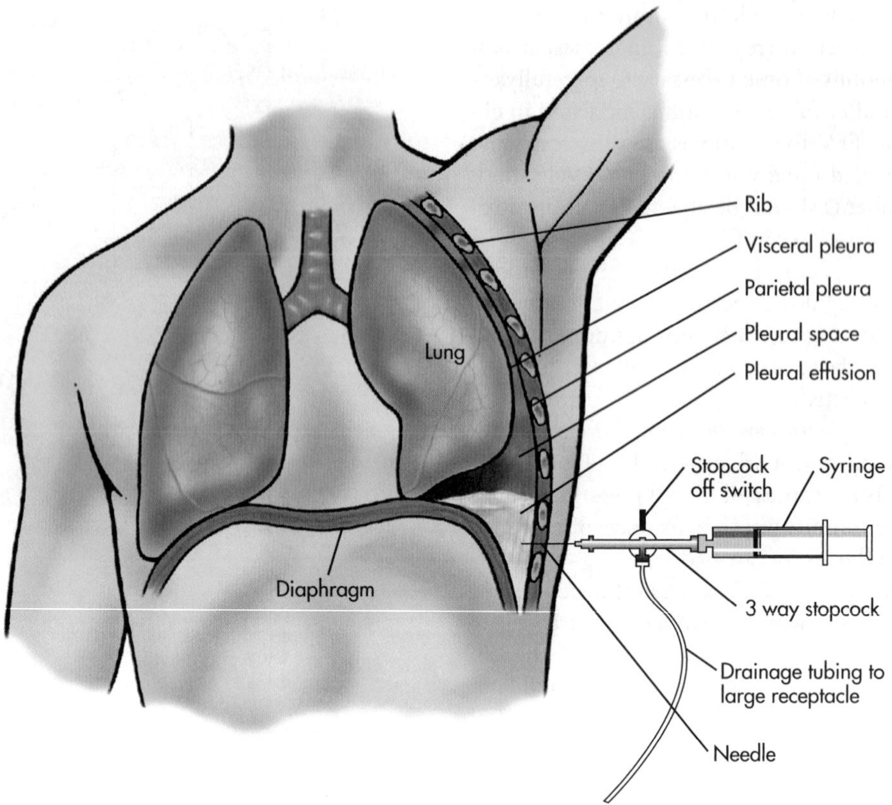

Figure 19-22 Thoracentesis.

purposes. The procedure is usually performed at the bedside or in a treatment room with the patient under local anesthesia (see Guidelines for Safe Practice box, p. 479, top left).

Endoscopy

Bronchoscopy

Bronchoscopy is used to diagnose and treat airway and lung disorders. It is useful to examine vocal cord movement, to obtain specimens by biopsy-bronchial brushing-bronchoalveolar lavage, and/or to remove foreign bodies or mucus plugs. Specimens can be examined for cytology or bacteriology and cultured for fungi, acid-fast bacilli, *Legionella pneumophila,* and *Pneumocystis carinii.* Localization of bleeding or tumor sites can also be detected by bronchoscopy.

Fiberoptic bronchoscopy is frequently performed because of the instrument's small size and ability to visualize the segmental and subsegmental bronchi. The fiberoptic scope has two channels: one channel for the clinician to visualize the structures and one channel to accommodate equipment such as biopsy forceps, suction, cytology brush, or oxygen. A local anesthetic is sprayed or swabbed on the tongue and oropharynx; subsequently the scope is introduced into the nose (the mouth or an endotracheal tube or tracheostomy tube can also be used). The anesthetic is also applied to the scope; additional anesthetic may be applied through the scope as advancement occurs toward the vocal cords and carina.

Bronchoscopy with the rigid bronchoscope is generally performed in the operating room because general anesthesia is required. It is usually reserved for removing foreign objects, controlling massive hemoptysis, placing airway stents, and dilating tracheobronchial strictures. If bronchoscopy is performed under general anesthesia, the care is similar to that for any patient undergoing general anesthesia. Prebronchoscopy and postbronchoscopy care can be found in the Guidelines for Safe Practice box, p. 479, top right.

Laryngoscopy

Indirect laryngoscopy involves the placement and rotation of a laryngeal mirror in the back of the mouth to visualize the larynx. It is used for examination and removal of tissue or foreign objects. Direct laryngoscopy is performed under local or general anesthesia and involves the insertion of a laryngoscope through the mouth into the larynx for examination. Biopsy of a tumor or removal of a foreign object can be accomplished. Postlaryngoscopy care is similar to postbronchoscopy care. Preprocedural and postprocedural care are similar to that for any patient undergoing general anesthesia.

Mediastinoscopy

Mediastinoscopy is an operative procedure that allows visualization and biopsy of lymph nodes. The procedure is helpful in diagnosing cancer, tuberculosis, histoplasmosis, and other diseases. A mediastinoscope is an instrument similar to a bronchoscope; however, it is inserted through a small incision in the suprasternal notch. The scope is advanced into the mediastinum where lymph nodes can be inspected and biopsied. The proce-

Guidelines for Safe Practice
The Patient Undergoing Thoracentesis

1. The procedure is explained, and a signed consent form is obtained. Emphasize the importance of not moving, breathing quietly, and not coughing during the procedure to avoid damage to the pleura and lung. Explain that the local anesthetic may cause a slight burning sensation and pressure may be felt when the needle is inserted.
2. Assess the patient's respiratory status and vital signs before the procedure. Pulse oximetry may be monitored. Supplemental oxygen should not be discontinued.
3. If possible, the patient should sit on the edge of the bed with the affected side closest to the foot of the bed. Support the patient's feet with a footstool. Raise the bedside table and put pillows on the table so that the patient can lean forward and rest his or her head and crossed arms comfortably on the pillows. If the patient is unable to sit up, place him or her in the position indicated by physician.
4. Reassure the patient and provide physical support, such as holding the patient's hand, as needed.
5. Monitor vital signs, general appearance, and respiratory status throughout the procedure. Up to 1 L of fluid may be removed at one time. If the patient develops pernicious coughing, reexpansion pulmonary edema should be suspected and the procedure terminated. Other signs and symptoms to monitor include hypotension, increased shortness of breath, bloody sputum, tracheal deviation, vasovagal reflex, and hypoxemia.
6. After the needle is withdrawn, a sterile occlusive dressing is applied, and the patient can assume a position of comfort.
7. A postprocedural chest radiograph is taken to check for a possible pneumothorax.
8. Manage postprocedural pain.

dure is generally performed in the operating room with the patient under general anesthesia. A small incision is made to allow entrance of the scope. After the procedure, the incision is sutured and the patient is taken to the postanesthesia care unit to recover. Preprocedural and postprocedural care is similar to that for any patient undergoing general anesthesia and surgery. Pneumothorax, hemoptysis, subcutaneous crepitus of neck or face, and laryngeal nerve damage (hoarseness, changes in vocal patterns, and difficulty in swallowing) are potential complications.

Thoracoscopy

Thoracoscopy is an operative procedure that allows visualization of the contents of the thoracic cavity. It can be used to obtain biopsies, resect tumors, perform esophageal operations, resect pericardium, and perform many other thoracic surgical procedures. A simple fiberoptic mediastinoscope, a rigid bronchoscope, a flexible bronchoscope, or a video-assisted laparoscopic instrumentation may be used to perform thoracoscopy. A general or local anesthetic may be administered, depending on the extent of the procedure. Two to four small chest incisions are made to insert the instrument. The lung on the operative side is allowed to collapse to permit a more panoramic view of the intrathoracic structures and keep the lung immobile while the surgeon performs the desired procedures. A chest tube is inserted and connected to a closed drainage system at the completion of the procedure. Preprocedure and postprocedure care is similar to that for any patient undergoing general anesthesia and surgery.[9] Care of the patient with a chest tube can be found in Chapter 21.

Guidelines for Safe Practice
The Patient Undergoing Flexible Bronchoscopy

- Respiratory rate and pattern are monitored and lungs are auscultated. Observe for changes in breathing pattern and breath sounds.
- Oxygen saturation may be monitored with pulse oximetry.
- Patient is given nothing by mouth until cough and gag reflexes return.
- Patient is positioned in a semi-Fowler's or side-lying position.
- Patient is monitored for bleeding, laryngeal edema, or laryngospasm (stridor) and increasing shortness of breath.
- If a biopsy was performed, explain to the patient that sputum may be blood streaked.
- Manage throat discomfort with warm saline gargles or throat lozenges.

References

1. Estes ME: *Health assessment and physical examination,* Albany, NY, 1998, Delmar Publishers.
2. http://www-medlib.med.utah.edu/WebPath/LUNGHTML/LUNGIDX.html.
3. Hansen M: *Pathophysiology: foundations of disease and clinical interventions,* Philadelphia, 1998, WB Saunders.
4. Jarvis C: *Physical examination and health assessment,* ed 3, Philadelphia, 2000, WB Saunders.
5. Lareau S et al: Dyspnea in patients with chronic obstructive pulmonary disease: Does dyspnea worsen longitudinally in the presence of declining lung function? *Heart Lung* 28:1, 1999.
6. Luce JM, Luce JA: Management of dyspnea in patients with far-advancing lung disease, *JAMA* 285:10, 2001.
7. McCarley C: A model of chronic dyspnea, *J Nurs Scholarship* 31:3, 1999.
8. Metules TJ: Use ABGs when precision counts, *RN* 63:10, 2000.
9. Nettina SM: *The Lippincott manual of nursing practice,* ed 7, Philadelphia, 2001, JB Lippincott.
10. Sacher RA, McPherson RA: *Widman's clinical interpretation of laboratory tests,* ed 11, Philadelphia, 2000, FA Davis.

20 Upper Airway Problems

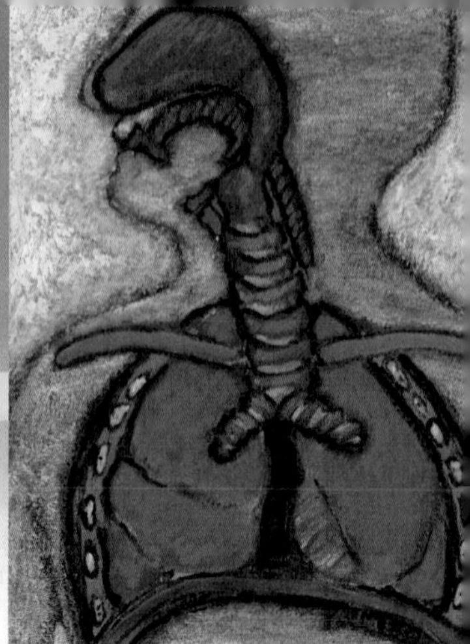

Glenda Lawson

Objectives

After studying this chapter, the learner should be able to:

1. Compare the etiology, pathophysiology, clinical manifestations, and management of infections of the nose and sinuses.
2. Compare acute pharyngitis with acute follicular tonsillitis in relation to etiology, clinical manifestations, and management.
3. Describe the nursing care of the patient after nasal surgery.
4. Identify conditions that cause obstructions of the upper airway and their management.
5. Describe clinical manifestations and management of the patient experiencing epistaxis.
6. Identify the special needs of the patient diagnosed with carcinoma of the upper airway structures.
7. Contrast the nursing care of the patient after a partial laryngectomy with that of the patient after a total laryngectomy with radical neck dissection.
8. Differentiate among the three speech methods that can be used by patients after a total laryngectomy.
9. Outline the nursing care for the patient who has an endotracheal tube or tracheostomy.
10. Describe the home care interventions and patient teaching necessary for the patient with a permanent tracheostomy tube.

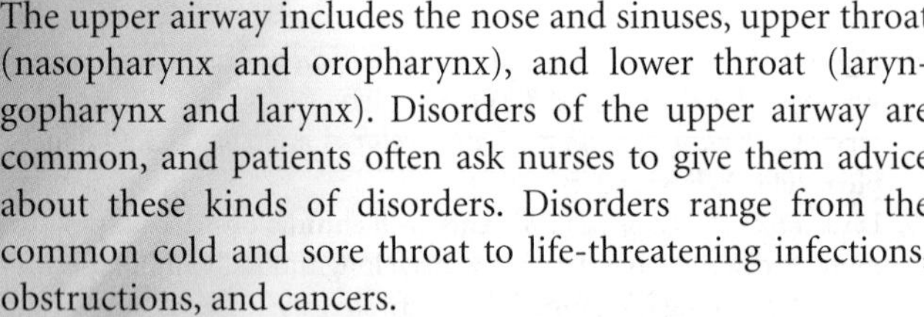

The upper airway includes the nose and sinuses, upper throat (nasopharynx and oropharynx), and lower throat (laryngopharynx and larynx). Disorders of the upper airway are common, and patients often ask nurses to give them advice about these kinds of disorders. Disorders range from the common cold and sore throat to life-threatening infections, obstructions, and cancers.

Disorders that affect the nose or olfactory nerve may lead to anosmia, or loss of the sense of smell. Anosmia may result from (1) nasal obstruction, which prevents air currents from reaching the olfactory epithelium; (2) skull fracture across the cribriform plate at the roof of the nose where part of the olfactory nerve enters the nose; (3) viral infections, which affect the olfactory nerve; or (4) meningiomas, which form in the olfactory area. Parosmia, or a perverted sense of smell, may also be present during sinusitis or an upper respiratory tract infection.

INFECTIONS OF THE NOSE AND SINUSES

The skin around the external nose is easily irritated during acute attacks of rhinitis or sinusitis. Furunculosis (boils) and cellulitis occasionally develop. Infections around the nose are extremely dangerous because the venous blood supply from this area drains directly into the cerebral venous sinuses. Septicemia therefore can occur easily, so pimples or lesions in the area should not be squeezed. If any infection in or around the nose persists or shows even a slight tendency to spread or increase in severity, a physician should be consulted. Herpetic lesions, often referred to as fever blisters, may develop around the nose and mucous membranes. These lesions are commonly associated with viral infections. If scratched, they can spread to other areas of the body or to other persons. Other infections that involve the upper airway as a portal of entry and site of symptoms, and that were of little concern before the bioterrorism of the autumn of 2001, are anthrax, and smallpox (see Future Watch box).

RHINITIS

Etiology/Epidemiology

The term *rhinitis* refers to inflammation of the mucous membrane of the nose. Rhinitis may be acute or chronic.

Acute rhinitis, also known as coryza or the common cold, is an inflammatory condition of the mucous membranes of

Future Watch

Will Smallpox Resurface? Will Evidence of Anthrax Increase?

With the events of September 2001, the question of smallpox resurfacing and the incidence of anthrax increasing are, unfortunately, possible realities. As a result of such awareness, government officials are asking all health care workers to have a basic understanding of these diseases, including their presenting signs and symptoms and treatment/management options. Although a great deal of information on smallpox and anthrax is available, listed below are focus points for providing a basic foundation.

SMALLPOX

Forms of Disease

Variola minor: <1% mortality rate
Variola major: 30% mortality rate

Incubation Period

12 to 14 days with a range of 7 to 17; no evidence of viral shedding

Clinical Manifestations

There is a sudden onset of influenza-like symptoms, including fever, malaise, headache, prostration, severe back pain, and less often, abdominal pain and vomiting. Two to three days later, the temperature falls and the patient feels somewhat better, at which time the characteristic rash appears, first on the face, hands, and forearms and then, after a few days, on the trunk. Lesions also develop in the mucous membranes of the nose and mouth and ulcerate very soon after their formation, releasing large amounts of virus into the mouth and throat.

Infectivity

Persons carrying the virus during the incubation period cannot infect others. The frequency of infection is highest after face-to-face contact with a patient once fever has begun and during the first week of rash, when the virus is released via the respiratory tract. Although patients remain infectious until the last scabs fall off, the virus shed from the skin is not highly infectious.

Transmission

Smallpox is transmitted from person to person by infected aerosols and air droplets spread by face-to-face contact with an infected person after fever has begun, especially if symptoms include coughing. The disease can also be transmitted by contaminated clothes and bedding, although the risk of infection from this source is much lower.

Treatment

Vaccine administered up to 4 days after exposure to the virus provides protective immunity and can prevent infection or ameliorate the severity of the disease. Otherwise, no treatment, other than the management of symptoms, is currently available.

Infection Control in Health Care Facilities

Health care providers, attendants, and mortuary workers, even if vaccinated, should wear gloves, caps, gowns, and surgical masks.

All contaminated instruments, excretions, fluids, and other materials should be decontaminated chemically or by heat or incineration.

Contaminated clothing and bedding, if not incinerated, should be autoclaved or washed in hot water containing sodium hypochlorite.

Fumigation of the premises may be done with formaldehyde.

Cadavers should be cremated, in a properly designated facility, whenever possible, and all persons coming in contact with them should be vaccinated or at least placed on daily fever watch. Body bags treated with sodium hypochlorite may also be used.

Reference: World Health Organization: *Weekly Epidemiol Rec* 76(44):337-344, 2001.

ANTHRAX

Anthrax is an animal disease that has been around for thousands of years and rarely causes serious disease in humans. However, when anthrax spores get inside the body, they grow rapidly and produce "anthrax toxin," which is so deadly it can kill even after the infection has been controlled.

Forms of Disease

Skin: curable with antibiotics; 20% mortality without treatment
Inhalational: most deadly form of the disease
Gastrointestinal: high mortality

Incubation Period

Within 7 days

Clinical Manifestations

Skin anthrax starts with a papule at the site of inoculation. After several days it becomes a vesicle and then a painless ulcer with an area of black eschar in the middle. Antibiotic treatment cures this infection, but untreated, skin anthrax results in overwhelming septicemia and death. Inhalation anthrax begins with mild, nonspecific upper respiratory and flulike symptoms, including fever, muscle aches, and fatigue. As early as 1 day after these symptoms appear—but up to 2 weeks later—acute symptoms of respiratory distress and shock occur. This form of the disease is often fatal.

Infectivity

People can catch anthrax from infected animals or contaminated animal products. More uncommon but most deadly is anthrax caught by inhaling spores, thousands of which must be inhaled before infection develops.

Transmission

Skin infection is transmitted by direct contact with contaminated articles, soil, or infected tissue. Inhalation anthrax is transmitted by aspiration of spores. Gastrointestinal anthrax is transmitted via ingestion of undercooked contaminated meat. Spores remain infectious for years.

Treatment

Early treatment with antibiotics is essential. The two recommended antibiotics are doxycycline and ciprofloxacin (Cipro). Because anthrax spores can stay in the lungs for a long time, antibiotic treatment should continue for 60 days. Some forms of anthrax created as biologic weapons have been reported to be resistant to these drugs, but no hard evidence exists to support these reports. It is important to remember that no antibiotic treatment should be started unless the appropriate authorities have warned of an anthrax outbreak.

Infection Control in Health Care Facilities

- Patients are isolated until lesions are free of anthrax bacilli.
- Spores require steam sterilization or burning.

Reference: Smith M: Senior medical editor, *WebMD*, Oct 2001.

the nose and accessory sinuses caused by a filterable virus. It affects almost everyone at some time and occurs most often in the winter, with additional high incidences in early fall and spring. Some of the known causes of the common cold are 100 serotypes of rhinoviruses, coronoviruses, adenoviruses, echoviruses, influenza and parainfluenza viruses, and coxsackievirus. The common cold is spread by droplet nuclei from sneezing, and the condition is contagious for the first 2 to 3 days.

Colds may also be spread by the contaminated hands of persons who are frequently sneezing and blowing their noses or by fomites, such as a telephone used by these persons. Secondary invasion by bacteria may cause pneumonia, acute bronchitis, sinusitis, and otitis media.

Allergic rhinitis (hay fever) is a type I hypersensitivity reaction that develops as a result of inhaled allergens. More than 35 million Americans have allergic rhinitis.[10] Inhaled allergens are classified as outdoor (seasonal; also classified as acute) or indoor (perennial; also classified as chronic). The outdoor allergens are pollens of trees, grasses, or weeds. The indoor allergens are spores of molds, dust mites, and animal dander. Although some persons believe they are allergic to flowers, this is often not so, because many flowers, such as roses, are insect pollinated. Only flowers that are pollinated by pollen in the air can cause an allergic reaction. The medications commonly used to treat allergic rhinitis are listed in Table 20-1.

Chronic rhinitis is a chronic inflammation of the mucous membrane characterized by increased nasal mucus. Chronic rhinitis may be the result of repeated acute infection, allergy, or vasomotor rhinitis, which is thought to be associated with an instability of the autonomic nervous system caused by stress, tension, or some endocrine disorder. Often it presents as a nasal allergy, but an allergen cannot be identified. Rhinitis can also be caused by the overuse of nosedrops or medication via nasal sprays. This is a rebound phenomenon that usually disappears within 1 to 2 weeks after the nasal medication is discontinued.

Pathophysiology

All types of rhinitis cause sneezing, nasal discharge with nasal obstruction, and headache, but the pattern of these symptoms varies with each (Table 20-2). A sore throat often,

TABLE 20-1 Common Medications for Allergic Rhinitis

Drug	Action	Intervention
Nonsedating Antihistamines		
Fexofenadine (Allegra) Cetirizine (Zyrtec) Loratadine (Claritin) Desloratadine (Clarinex) Astemizole (Hismanal)	Prevents release of histamine and other substances causing symptoms	Evaluate effectiveness.
Low-Dose Steroid Nasal Sprays		
Beclomethasone (Vancenase, Beconase) Flunisolide (Nasalide) Fluticasone (Flonase) Triamcinolone (Nasacort) Budesonide (Rhinocort, Rhinocort Aqua) Mometasone (Nasonex) Dexamethasone (Dexacort, Decadron)	Depresses inflammatory reactions	Evaluate effectiveness. Ask patient to demonstrate use of nasal spray.
Other Nasal Sprays		
Cromolyn sodium (Nasalcrom)	Reduces mucus production and swelling	Evaluate effectiveness. Ask patient to demonstrate use of nasal spray.
Ipratopium (Atrovent)	Blocks ability of nervous system to stimulate nasal mucous glands	Assess for allergy to atropine; may cause sensitivity to the decongestant.

TABLE 20-2 Symptoms of Rhinitis

Symptom	Acute Rhinitis	Allergic Rhinitis	Chronic Rhinitis
Nasal discharge	Initially watery, then mucoid	Thin, watery	Serous, mucopurulent, or purulent
Eyes	Tearing during early phase	Tearing, itching	No tearing
Turbinates	Edematous	Pale, edematous, mucoid	Enlarged
Nasal polyps	No	Sometimes	Sometimes
Headache	Generalized	Generalized	Generalized

but not always, accompanies these symptoms because of early dryness followed by irritation from postnasal drainage. With acute rhinitis, signs of acute inflammation such as early chilliness followed by "feverishness" and malaise also are present. If uncomplicated, a cold is usually self-limiting and lasts for about 1 week.

In chronic rhinitis, acute symptoms are absent. The chief complaint is nasal obstruction accompanied by a feeling of stuffiness and pressure in the nose. Polyp formation may occur, and vertigo may be present.

Collaborative Care Management

No specific treatment exists for the common cold. The goals of treatment are to (1) relieve symptoms, (2) inhibit spread of the infection, and (3) reduce the risk of bacterial complications such as sinusitis and otitis media. Studies have indicated that oral antihistamines are not effective in treating viral upper respiratory tract infections. They are helpful, however, in treating allergic rhinitis. Decongestants (sympathomimetic amines) are the recommended treatment for relieving nasal congestion and enhancing eustachian tube function. Decongestants can be purchased over the counter (OTC) and are administered as nasal drops or sprays two or three times a day for no more than 3 days (see Guidelines for Safe Practice box). Topical decongestants include oxymetazoline (Afrin) and phenylephrine nasal sprays (Neo-Synephrine). In persons with severe congestion these medications facilitate the uptake of other topical drugs such as nasal cromolyn (Nasalcrom) and corticosteroid sprays.

The side effects of decongestants include rebound nasal congestion (with chronic use), nervousness, and transient increases in blood pressure. Decongestants are contraindicated in patients receiving tricyclic antidepressants or monoamine oxidase inhibitors. Room humidifiers are helpful in liquefying secretions and thus promoting draining and decreasing congestion.

For allergic rhinitis the treatment similarly consists of maintaining an allergen-free environment. Hyposensitization or desensitization (administering the allergen in gradually increasing doses to establish an "immunity") may be helpful. Antihistamines give relief to most persons, but their effectiveness often decreases as the "hay fever season" continues. In addition, side effects such as sleepiness or "dribbling" of urine, can sometimes affect activities of daily living.

For chronic rhinitis a careful medical follow-up is indicated. When nasal obstruction persists, surgery may be necessary to remove polyps (polypectomy) or to revise septal tissue (septoplasty).

If the nasal passages are dry, a nasal spray of normal saline can be purchased OTC, or it can be made by mixing 1 teaspoon of salt in 1 quart of water. The homemade solution should be made fresh daily. The solution is best administered from a spray bottle with both nostrils open.

Patient/Family Education. Guidelines for instructing the patient and family about rhinitis can be found in the Patient Teaching box.

SINUSITIS

The sinuses are air-filled cavities lined with mucous membranes. The term *sinusitis* refers to any inflammation of the mucous membranes. Sinusitis is a common disorder, although it has become less common since the advent of antibiotics. Often patients who complain of sinusitis do not have a sinus infection but some other disorder. Of all the patients who

Guidelines for Safe Practice
Self-Administration of Nosedrops

Instruct patient to:

1. Wash hands.
2. Assume a position that will facilitate the flow of medication, such as one of the following:
   a. Sit in chair and tip head well backward.
   b. Lie down with head extended over edge of bed.
   c. Lie down with pillow under shoulders and head tipped backward.
3. Turn head to the side that will receive the drops.
4. Place no more than 3 drops of solution into each nostril at one time (unless otherwise prescribed).
5. Remain in position with head tilted backward for 3 to 5 minutes to permit solution to reach posterior nares.
6. If marked congestion is still present 10 minutes after nosedrop insertion, another drop or two of solution may be administered (nasal constriction from first insertion may facilitate additional drops reaching posterior nares).

Patient Teaching
The Patient With Rhinitis

1. Obtain additional rest.
2. Drink at least 2 to 3 L of fluid daily.
3. Use nasal spray or nosedrops two or three times per day as ordered (see Guidelines for Safe Practice box).
4. Prevent further infection.
   a. Blow nose with both nostrils open to prevent infected matter from being forced into eustachian tube.
   b. Cover mouth with disposable tissues when coughing and sneezing to prevent droplet nuclei from contaminating the air.
   c. Dispose of used tissues carefully.
   d. Avoid exposure when possible (i.e., avoid crowds, people with colds, specific allergens). Older adults and those with chronic lung disease are particularly vulnerable and should have a flu shot yearly.
   e. Wash hands frequently and especially after coughing, blowing the nose, sneezing, and so on. Evidence suggests that many colds are transmitted from person to person by hand contact and from touching objects handled by a person with a cold.
   f. Seek medical attention for:
      (1) High fever, severe chest pain, earache
      (2) Symptoms lasting longer than 2 weeks
      (3) Recurrent colds

consult an otolaryngologist because of "sinus trouble," few actually have sinusitis.

Sinusitis may be acute or chronic.

Acute Bacterial Sinusitis

Etiology/Epidemiology

The most common types of acute sinusitis are allergic and viral. It is often difficult to distinguish between these two types, although the patient's history may be helpful. Allergic sinusitis is usually seasonal, and redness and itching of the eyes may be present. Viral sinusitis is usually accompanied by fever, malaise, and systemic symptoms such as achiness. There may also be a history of recent exposure to an infected person. Common viral causes of sinusitis are rhinovirus, influenza virus, adenovirus, and parainfluenza virus.[9] The next most common form of sinusitis is acute bacterial sinusitis. Pathogens most often causing acute bacterial sinusitis include *Streptococcus pneumoniae, Haemophilus influenzae,* beta-hemolytic streptococci, *Klebsiella pneumoniae,* and various anerobic organisms.

Pathophysiology

The first symptom of acute bacterial sinusitis is usually a stuffy nose followed by slowly developing pressure over the involved sinus. Other signs and symptoms include general malaise, persistent cough, postnasal drip, headache, slightly elevated or normal temperature, and mild leukopenia. Symptoms worsen over 48 to 72 hours, culminating in severe localized pain and tenderness over the involved sinus (Table 20-3 and Figures 20-1 and 20-2). The patient often believes that the pain is due to an infected tooth.

In acute frontal and maxillary sinusitis, pain usually does not appear until 1 to 2 hours after awakening. It increases for 3 to 4 hours and then becomes less severe in the afternoon and evening. Usually this is due to increased drainage as a result of gravity from standing during the day.

There may be bloody or blood-tinged discharge from the nose in the first 24 to 48 hours. The discharge rapidly becomes thick, green, and copious, blocking the nose. The throat may become inflamed and sore on one side because of the purulent discharge.

On examination the involved nasal mucosa is hyperemic and edematous, and the turbinates are enlarged. X-ray films show that the involved sinus is clouded, and a fluid level is visible (Figure 20-3).

TABLE 20-3 Location of Pain With Sinusitis

Sinus	Pain Location
Maxillary	Over cheek and upper teeth (Figure 20-1)
Frontal	Above eyebrow (Figure 20-1)
Ethmoid	Medial and deep in eye (Figure 20-2)
Sphenoid	Deep behind eye, over occiput, or top of head

Collaborative Care Management

Diagnostic tests include transillumination of the sinuses, conventional sinus x-ray films, computed tomography (CT), and magnetic resonance imaging (MRI). Fiberoptic examination of the nose (rhinoscopy) may also be used. For the majority of patients, however, a diagnosis of sinusitis is made without radiographic studies.

Management of acute bacterial sinusitis centers on relief of pain and shrinkage of the nasal mucosa. Ibuprofen (Advil) and an oral decongestant such as pseudoephedrine (Sudafed) are commonly prescribed. The decongestant is given orally or by nasal spray for 2 to 3 days. In some patients codeine (usually Tylenol No. 3) may be required for pain relief, and it may need to be taken for several days. Giving Tylenol No. 3 and ibuprofen at alternate times assists in managing fever.[11]

The antibiotic of choice is amoxicillin for 10 days. Failure of the infection to respond to amoxicillin is an indication for aspiration of the maxillary sinus to obtain a specimen for culture and sensitivity. A list of the antimicrobial agents used to treat acute sinusitis can be found in Box 20-1. If a patient does not improve after 5 days of amoxicillin, a change in antibiotics may be necessary. The antibiotics are usually taken for 10 to 14 days.

Patients may obtain relief from saline nasal sprays, steam from a shower, or a humidifier. Hot wet packs applied to the face over the infected sinus(es) either continuously or for 1 to 2 hours at a time four times a day may provide symptomatic

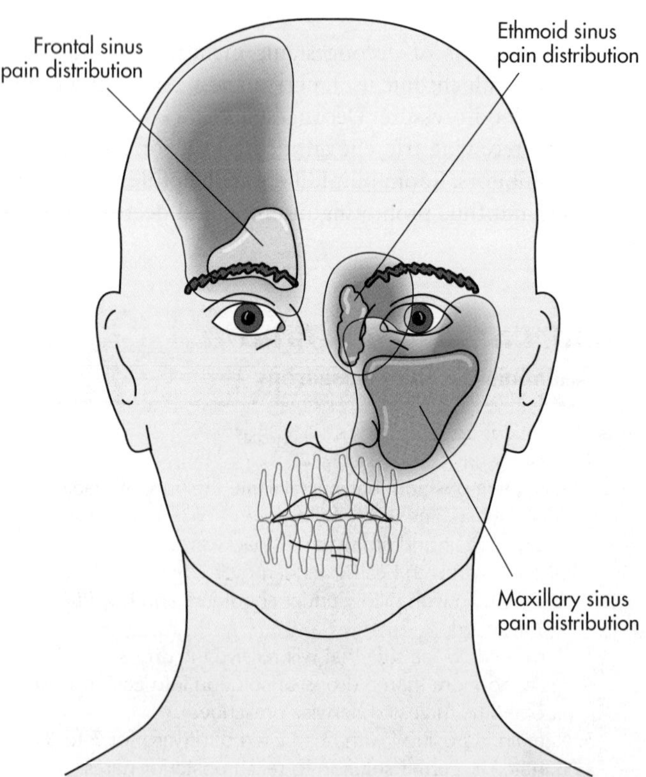

Figure 20-1 Sinus pain: area of local tenderness and pain referral. Maxillary sinus pain often is referred to the teeth. Frontal pain is generally localized to the supraorbital area. Ethmoid pain is generally deep to the eye.

relief. A washcloth wrung out in hot water is a convenient way to provide wet packs, as are wet cloth towels slightly warmed in a microwave.

Acute frontal sinusitis with pain, tenderness, and edema of the frontal or sphenoid sinus may require hospitalization because of the risk of intracranial complications or osteomyelitis. High-dose intravenous antibiotics and nasal decongestants orally or by spray are usually ordered. When the infection has subsided, an oral antibiotic is prescribed and the patient is discharged home. In some cases osteomyelitis of the frontal bone occurs with *Staphylococcus aureus,* the most common causative organism.

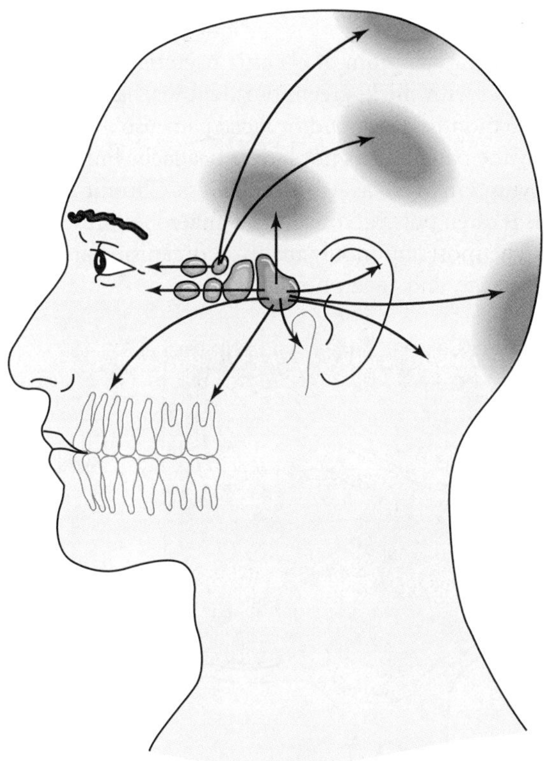

Figure 20-2 Pain from anterior ethmoid is deep to the eye. Pain from posterior ethmoid cells and sphenoid is referred to the eyes, teeth, ears, or temporal area of the occiput.

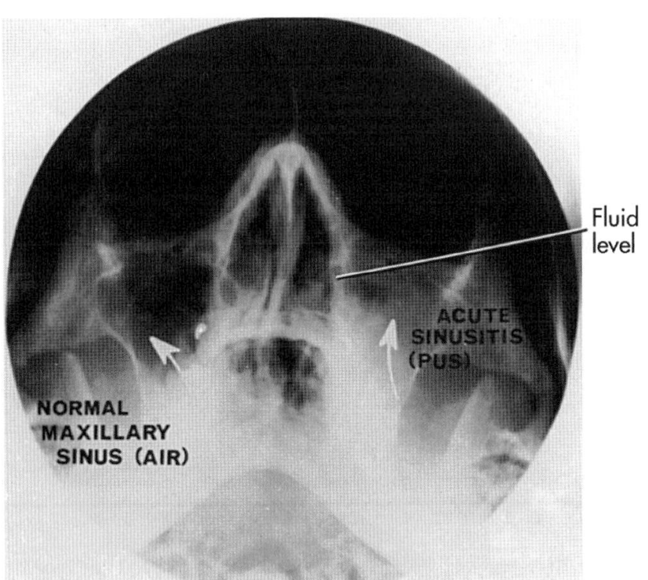

Figure 20-3 X-ray film of maxillary sinus showing normal sinus on left and acute sinusitis with clouding and visible fluid level on right.

Sinusitis of fungal origin ranges from a mild infection resembling chronic sinusitis to a severe, life-threatening invasive infection. Noninvasive fungal sinusitis caused by *Aspergillus* and *Candida* is often found in patients following other infections or prolonged administration of antibiotics. Treatment may require surgical drainage of the sinuses.

Invasive fungal sinusitis is most likely to occur in transplant patients, patients receiving chemotherapy, patients with acquired immunodeficiency syndrome (AIDS), or persons with poorly controlled diabetes. *Aspergillus* and *Mucor* are two types of fungi most prone to causing invasive disease. Symptoms include facial fullness, cranial neuropathies, and pain. Proptosis of the eye, facial swelling, and blood-tinged nasal discharge may be present. On examination the nasal mucosa appears gray or black. The diagnosis is confirmed by biopsy of the affected membranes. Treatment consists of hospitalization, intravenous amphotericin B, aggressive surgical management, and attempts to correct the underlying immunodeficiency.

Patient/Family Education. The patient is instructed to get plenty of rest and to increase fluid intake to 2 to 3 L per day. The medication regimen is explained, and the patient or family is given a written copy. For patients taking antibiotics, the importance of taking the antibiotics as prescribed is stressed and the patients are told to contact a health care provider if no change in symptoms occurs after 5 days of taking the medication. It is also stressed that ibuprofen and any decongestant need to be taken as prescribed. The patient is told to use a nasal spray or steam from the shower to keep nasal mucosa moist[11] and to seek medical attention if any of the following occur:

- Increase in bloody drainage from the nose
- Severe headache or increased pain in the face, teeth, or ears
- Elevation of temperature above 99° F (23° C) or persistent elevated temperature

BOX 20-1 Antimicrobial Therapy for Acute Bacterial Sinusitis

Amoxicillin (Amoxil, Trimox, Wymox)
Loracarbef (Lorabid)
Amoxicillin–clavulanate potassium (Augmentin)
Cefaclor (Ceclor)
Cefprozil (Cefzil)
Cefuroxime axetil (Zinacef IV, Ceftin PO)
Doxycycline (Vibramycin, Monodox)
Trimethoprim-sulfamethoxazole (Bactrim, Septra)
Clarithromycin (Biaxin)
Azithromycin (Zithromax)

- Increase in fatigue or general achiness
- Increased nasal stuffiness and inability to clear secretions from the nose
- Purulent or foul-smelling nasal discharge

Subacute Bacterial Sinusitis

Etiology/Epidemiology

The measures described previously cure a large majority of patients with acute bacterial sinusitis. A subacute infection persists in the remaining few.

Pathophysiology

Persistent purulent nasal discharge is the only constant symptom. A sinus x-ray film or CT scan determines whether one or more than one sinus is involved. Because it is uncommon for acute bacterial sinusitis to persist, when an infection lingers, an unusual causative organism must be suspected. Special culture and sensitivity techniques may be required to identify the particular organism to be treated, especially if it is an anaerobe. Antibiotic sensitivity studies are essential. The most commonly isolated organisms are *Haemophilus influenzae, Streptococcus pneumococcae,* and *Branhamella catarrhalis.*

Collaborative Care Management

Infections are treated with antibiotics to which the causative organisms are sensitive, usually penicillin or amoxicillin, unless the patient is allergic to them. Systemic sulfonamide therapy or erythromycin with a sulfonamide is used for infections caused by *B. catarrhalis,* which is resistant to penicillin and amoxicillin. Other treatment consists of nasal vasoconstriction, moist heat applied to the sinus(es), and irrigation of the involved sinus; no pain medication is required, since pain is not severe. An antral puncture, which can be repeated several times without causing permanent damage to the nose or maxillary sinus, is commonly used for irrigation of the maxillary sinus. Anesthesia is achieved by placing a cotton applicator moistened with 5% cocaine solution high under the inferior turbinate against the lateral wall of the nose. A second applicator is placed under the middle turbinate. After the anesthesia takes effect (in about 5 to 10 minutes), a 16- to 18-gauge needle is inserted under the turbinate until the needle pierces the medial wall of the antrum and enters the sinus cavity (Figure 20-4). A syringe is attached to the needle, and purulent material or air is aspirated from the cavity. The aspirated material is sent to the laboratory for culture and sensitivity testing. Saline solution is instilled to wash out the sinus. Antibiotic solutions may be used, but mechanical cleansing is more important than the solution used (Figure 20-5).

It is impossible to irrigate the ethmoid sinuses directly; thus ethmoiditis is treated systemically. Antibiotics are usually prescribed for 10 to 14 days.

Patient/Family Education. Treatment of subacute bacterial sinusitis is focused on preventing chronic bacterial sinusitis.

Chronic Bacterial Sinusitis

Etiology/Epidemiology

Chronic bacterial sinusitis develops when irreversible mucosal damage occurs. Damage can result from recurrent attacks of sinusitis or from suppurative sinusitis either being untreated or inadequately treated during the acute or subacute phase.

Pathophysiology

The major symptom of chronic bacterial sinusitis is nasal congestion with thick, green, purulent discharge, present for at least 3 months. Fever and/or facial pain also may be present. Usually the patient does not have a headache but may experience symptoms such as lightheadedness. Chronic bacterial sinusitis is often polymicrobial, with anaerobes present in most cases. The most commonly involved organisms are *S. aureus, H. influenzae,* and anaerobes.

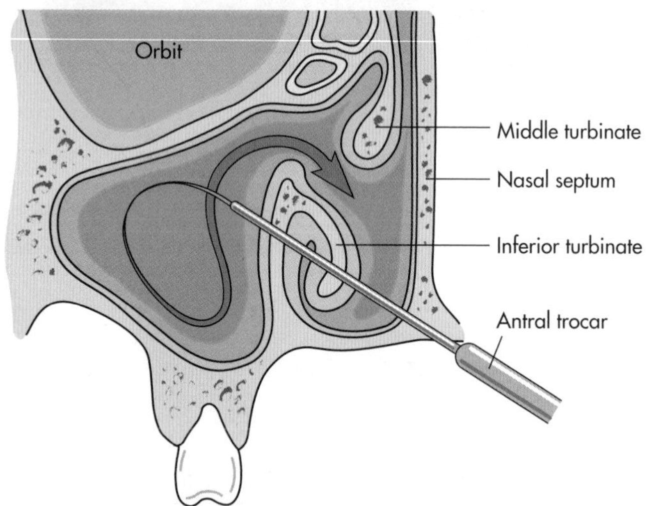

Figure 20-4 Antral puncture. Trocar inserted under inferior turbinate (through medial wall of antrum). Contents of the sinus are washed into the nose through the natural ostium.

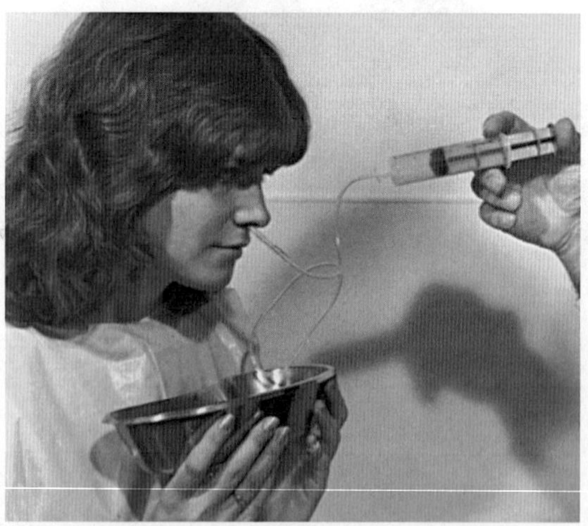

Figure 20-5 Irrigation of maxillary sinus. With the head tipped forward, solution returns via the natural ostium and out the anterior portion of the nose for examination and/or culture.

Collaborative Care Management

Diagnostic Tests. The sinuses can be aspirated to obtain organisms for culture and sensitivity. A CT scan of the sinuses is used to determine if there is blockage of the nasal sinus drainage system, polyps, mucus plugs, or other findings that would require endoscopic sinus surgery. Before endoscopic sinus surgery is used to treat chronic sinusitis, the patient is also evaluated with nasal endoscopy and coronal CT scans. The nasal endoscopy reveals subtle changes that cannot be seen in an anterior rhinoscopy using a nasal speculum, and the coronal CT scan determines the underlying cause of sinusitis. The coronal CT scan is best performed after acute inflammation has subsided and medical treatment has been attempted.

Medications. Decongestants are usually sufficient treatment. Patients who do not have fever, facial pain, or tenderness are not usually helped by antibiotics. When antibiotics are necessary, the results of the culture and sensitivity are used to determine the appropriate antibiotic. Antibiotics are usually prescribed for 2 to 3 weeks.

Treatments. Nasal saline irrigations and surgery are the major treatments.

Surgical Management. Treatment of chronic sinusitis involves surgery to remove all diseased soft tissue and bone, to provide adequate postoperative drainage, and to obliterate the sinus cavity when necessary. The goal of surgery is to eradicate infection and leave contiguous structures intact. Several types of surgical procedures are used to treat patients with chronic sinusitis.

Functional Endoscopic Sinus Surgery. In functional endoscopic sinus surgery (FESS), also known as endoscopic sinus surgery, a fiberoptic endoscope that illuminates and magnifies is used to enter the sinus. The underlying principle of this type of surgery is to focus on reestablishment of sinus ventilation and to identify the actual site of the pathology so that a more limited operation may be performed.[11] In FESS normal sinus bone is opened wide, ensuring adequate drainage from the sinuses and alleviating current infection.

FESS allows patients with sinus disease to be treated without hospitalization and prevents facial scarring and extended recovery periods. Although the main use of FESS is to treat recurrent or chronic sinus disease, it can be used for other purposes, including (1) the removal of polyps, foreign bodies, or other growths; (2) treatment of recurrent or chronic pain caused by nasal or sinus blockage; and (3) examination with the patient under anesthesia, usually with a biopsy.

The surgical goals of FESS include removing diseased tissue, promoting sinus drainage, improving sinus ventilation, removing objects or masses, and alleviating pain. The procedure can be performed with the patient under local or general anesthesia. If local anesthesia is used, the procedure is performed in an ambulatory surgery center, where the patient is kept for 2 to 3 hours postoperatively and then discharged.

In FESS, small nasal endoscopes are used to dissect the diseased tissue, which is located by CT scan. In early sinus disease the air cells are opened to allow for ventilation and drainage. In advanced disease the air cells may need to be removed. A major advantage of fiberoptic endoscopy is that all of the diseased tissue can be removed while preserving more healthy tissue, thus preserving more of the function of the sinus.

Diet. Patients may eat whatever they wish, but the nasal packing and postoperative swelling usually decrease appetite. Protein intake to aid healing is emphasized, and patients may be able to take milk-based drinks. Additional fluids are encouraged.

Activity. The patient is encouraged to take it easy and rest more than usual for the first week to allow the body to heal.

Referrals. Usually no referrals are necessary.

Caldwell-Luc Sinus Surgery. The Caldwell-Luc procedure, also known as a radical antrum operation, is the generally accepted operative procedure for chronic maxillary sinusitis that cannot be cured with antibiotics and other medical therapy. Local or general anesthesia may be used.

The procedure is performed through an incision under the upper lip (Figure 20-6). Part of the anterior bony wall of the antrum is removed, producing a permanent window (Figure 20-7). All of the diseased mucosa and periosteum is removed through the window. The bone of the lateral wall of the nose in the inferior meatus, which divides the nose from the antrum, is also removed. The mucous membrane and periosteum of the lateral wall of the nose are preserved and fashioned into a hinged flap.

The antrum may be packed to prevent bleeding. Packing is removed through the nose 24 to 48 hours after surgery. As the maxillary sinus heals, the exposed bone is covered by mucosa. Numbness of the upper lip and upper teeth may be present for several months after a Caldwell-Luc operation, because some nerves to these structures pass through the site of the incision.

Diet. Because of the oral incision, only fluids are given for at least 24 hours and then a soft diet is followed for several days. The need to increase protein intake to aid healing is emphasized.

Activity. The patient is encouraged to rest more than usual for the first 5 to 7 days to allow the body to heal. Raising the

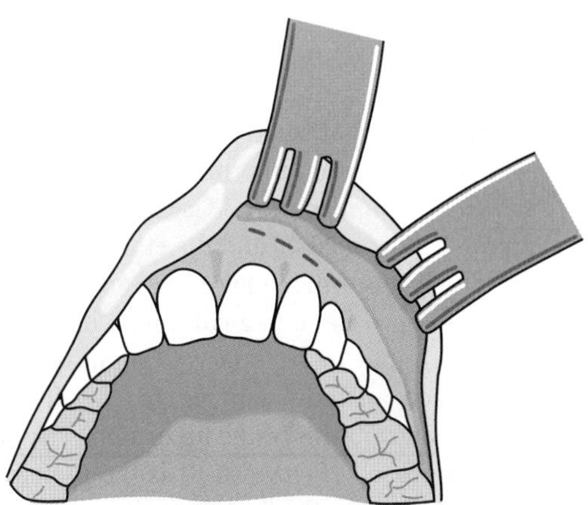

Figure 20-6 The incision into the maxillary sinus (Caldwell-Luc surgery) is made under the upper lip.

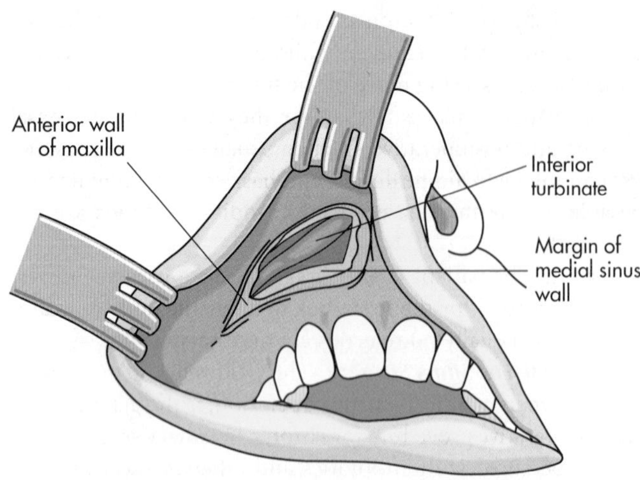

Figure 20-7 Caldwell-Luc surgery. After removal of the sinus mucosa or polypoid tissue, a window is made into the nose along its floor, allowing dependent drainage from the maxillary sinus. The incision is closed with absorbable sutures.

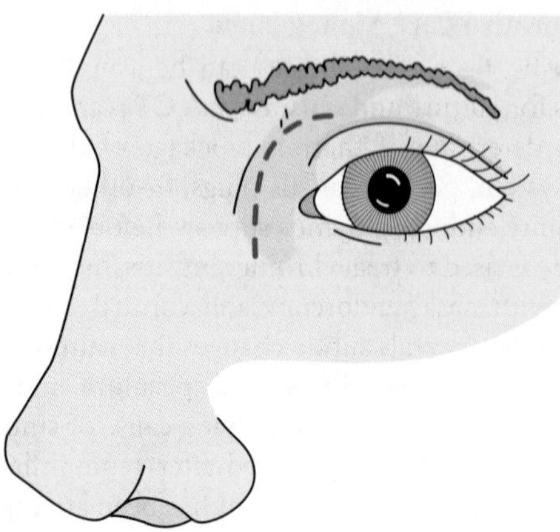

Figure 20-8 Medial canthal incision for external ethmoidectomy.

head of the bed 30 degrees facilitates drainage and decreases nasal edema.

Referrals. Usually no referrals are necessary.

Ethmoidectomy. An ethmoidectomy, which entails removal of ethmoid air cells, is performed to remove diseased mucosa, nasal polyps (which commonly originate in the ethmoid cells), or mucoceles from the ethmoid sinus. A mucocele is a mucous cyst that is a consequence of repeated infection. Repeated infection causes the sinus ostia from the ethmoid sinus to become blocked by thickened mucosa or scar tissue. Thus mucus cannot drain; it builds up, and a cyst forms. The mucocele continues to enlarge, resulting in pressure necrosis on surrounding bone. It can be seen as a mass at the medial canthus.

Three surgical approaches are used in performing an ethmoidectomy: transnasal, transantral, and external. General or local anesthesia with sedation may be used. Removal of ethmoid air cells creates a single large cavity that is packed for 24 to 48 hours.

In the transnasal approach, the surgery is performed using a headlight and operating microscope or endoscope. This approach is technically difficult, and complications involving the orbit can cause cerebrospinal fluid rhinorrhea.

In a transantral ethmoidectomy a Caldwell-Luc incision is used (see Figures 20-6 and 20-7) and the ethmoid air cells are removed from below. It is difficult to remove anterior ethmoid air cells using this approach, and a combined intranasal and transantral approach may be necessary. Complications of the transantral approach include damage to the infraorbital nerve, which causes numbness of the lip or upper teeth.

The external approach (Figure 20-8) is the preferred one for ethmoid surgery because it allows better visualization and reduces the risks of complications such as damage to the optic nerve and cerebrospinal fluid leak. A pressure dressing is usually applied over the operative eye to prevent postoperative edema.

Diet. Fluids are given freely for the first 24 hours, progressing to a soft diet. The need to increase protein intake to aid in healing is emphasized.

Activity. The patient is encouraged to rest more than usual for the first postoperative week.

Referrals. Usually no referrals are necessary.

Sphenoid Sinus Surgery. Surgery of the sphenoid sinus can be accomplished using an endoscopic technique, through an external or transantral ethmoidectomy approach, or through a transseptal approach. The ethmoid sinus is usually removed, and the anterior wall of the sphenoid sinus opened. Diseased tissue is removed, along with the mucous membrane lining the sinus. To facilitate drainage directly into the nasopharynx, the sinus ostium is opened wide.

Diet. Fluids are given freely for the first 24 hours, progressing to a soft diet. The need to increase protein intake to aid in healing is emphasized.

Activity. The patient is encouraged to rest more than usual for the first 5 to 7 days after the surgery.

Referrals. Usually no referrals are necessary.

Frontal Sinusectomy. The use of the osteoplastic flap operation makes frontal sinus surgery different from that performed on the other sinuses. Surgery of the other sinuses basically provides for an open, well-drained cavity, which in the past proved inadequate for the frontal sinuses because recurrence of disease was common. The osteoplastic flap operation allows for complete removal of diseased mucosa of the frontal sinus and for obliteration of the sinus so that it is no longer functional or continuous with the inner nose.

The osteoplastic flap procedure is performed through a "gull-wing" or "crossbow" incision. In men the incision extends along the eyebrows and connects along the bridge of the nose. In women, for whom baldness usually is not a problem in later life, the incision connects both temporal areas a few centimeters posterior to the hairline. Both incisions give excellent postoperative cosmesis and are extended to the periosteum of the bone overlying the frontal sinus.

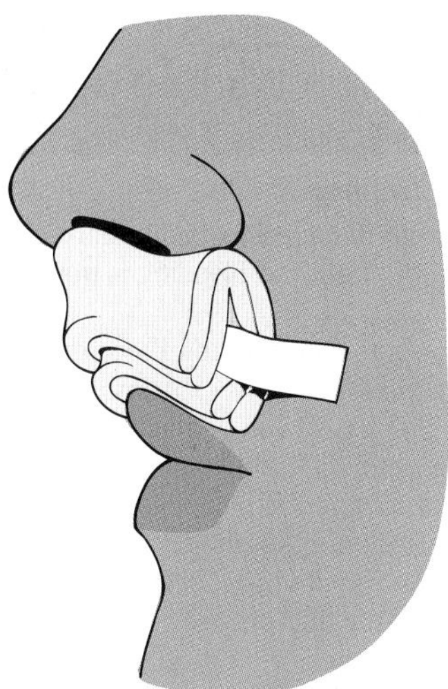

Figure 20-9 Dressing placed under nose to catch nasal drainage. Sometimes called a mustache dressing or a drip pad.

The skin overlying the sinus is reflected, and a radiograph of the frontal sinus (obtained before surgery) is used as a template for sawing the lateral and superior borders of the anterior frontal bone. The anterior bone is then reflected inferiorly, thus exposing the entire contents of the frontal sinus. The mucosa is removed under direct vision, and an operating microscope is used to ensure that all fragments of mucosa are removed. An incision is then made in the left lower abdominal quadrant, and subcutaneous fat is obtained for adipose obliteration of the sinus. The bony flap and skin are then repositioned, and a pressure dressing is applied to minimize postoperative swelling.

After surgery, pain in the frontal area is not significant after 24 hours. Pain in the abdominal area, however, often lasts several days, and serous drainage from this area is common after the drain is removed. Sutures are removed on about the fifth postoperative day. Because nasal packs are not used, special oral hygiene care is not needed. Preoperative and postoperative teaching for patients having sinus surgery can be found in the Guidelines for Safe Practice box.

Diet. Fluids are given freely for the first 24 hours, progressing to a soft diet. The need to increase protein intake to aid in healing is emphasized.

Activity. The patient is encouraged to rest more than usual for the first week after surgery.

Referrals. Usually no referrals are necessary.

NURSING MANAGEMENT OF PATIENT UNDERGOING FUNCTIONAL ENDOSCOPIC SINUS SURGERY

PREOPERATIVE CARE

Because FESS is an outpatient procedure, preadmission tests and preoperative teaching are scheduled a few days before surgery. The postoperative routine also is reviewed with the patient at this time so that the patient can determine in advance of surgery the preparations, if any, that will need to be made at home. All information that needs to be taught to the patient perioperatively for any sinus surgery is found in the Patient Teaching box.

POSTOPERATIVE CARE

If inflammation or infection is noted during the surgery, antibiotics are administered and continued for a total of 10 to 14 days. Some surgeons also order a steroid nasal spray for a few days. To keep the mucosa moist, all patients begin normal saline sprays after packing is removed. Saline irrigations may be necessary for those with considerable nasal crusting.

Self-care information is reinforced before discharge. The patient's progress is assessed via a phone call within 24 hours.

Guidelines for Safe Practice

Care of the Patient After Nasal Surgery

Nursing care after nasal surgery includes:

1. Assessment for signs of hemorrhage: excessive blood on nasal dressing, bright red vomitus, repeated swallowing (check back of throat with penlight for blood running down throat), rapid pulse, restlessness
2. Assessment for signs of infection: fever, elevated white blood cell (WBC) count
3. Measures to relieve discomfort and promote effective breathing
   a. Mid-Fowler's position to decrease local edema
   b. Cool mist via collar or face tent
   c. Ice compresses over nose for 24 hours as needed
   d. Psychologic support and sedation as needed
   e. Use of flashlight or penlight to examine back of throat to ensure that packing has not slipped to back of throat, where it could gag patient
   f. Frequent oral care
   g. Change of dressing under nose as needed (Figure 20-9)
4. Promotion of good nutrition
   a. Encourage food as tolerated.
   b. Encourage increased fluid intake.
5. Patient/family teaching
   a. Avoid blowing nose for 48 hours after packing has been removed.
   b. Avoid constipation and straining (Valsalva's maneuver) and vigorous coughing until healing occurs, because it can cause bleeding.
   c. Expect stools to be tarry for several days.
   d. Expect face to be discolored around eyes and nose for several days.
   e. Cosmetic effect from nasal surgery cannot be judged for 6 to 12 months (time required for tissue to return to normal and for scar resolution).

Patient Teaching
The Patient Undergoing Sinus Surgery

PREOPERATIVE TEACHING

Determine patient's understanding of the surgical procedure. Clarify misconceptions and answer patient's and family's questions. Explain that patient will:

1. Have nothing to eat or drink for 6 to 8 hours before surgery.
2. Receive a sedative before surgery.
3. Feel pressure, not pain, during surgery.
4. Have a nasal pack for 24 to 48 hours after surgery and may feel like he or she has a "head cold."
5. Have a mustache dressing after surgery (see Figure 20-9).
6. Have "black eyes" and swelling around the nose and eyes for 1 to 2 weeks after surgery.
7. Have a prescription for pain medication as needed.

POSTOPERATIVE TEACHING

Precautions for the First Week

1. Do not blow your nose until after your first office visit, usually 3 to 5 days after surgery. Blowing your nose puts too much pressure on the surgical site. Following Caldwell-Luc surgery, the nose should not be blown for 2 weeks.
2. If you feel fluid or congestion in your nose, gently sniff back the fluid and spit it into a tissue.
3. Try not to sneeze, because this will put too much pressure on the surgical site. If you must sneeze, keep your mouth open and sneeze through your mouth.
4. Do not bend over, and do not lift heavy objects; both put excessive pressure on the surgical site.
5. Avoid constipation (Valsalva's maneuver [straining] can cause bleeding).
6. Additional precautions for patients with Caldwell-Luc surgery include:
   a. Do not chew on affected side until incision heals.
   b. Use caution with oral hygiene to avoid injury to the incision.
   c. Avoid wearing dentures for about 10 days.

Managing Pain

1. The discomfort after surgery is more of an ache and pressure from the packing in the nose than actual pain.
2. The pain may increase during the week after surgery because of swelling and secretions in the sinus.
3. Most patients obtain relief by taking acetaminophen. If your physician expects you will have more pain, another medication will be prescribed.
4. Never take aspirin or any product containing aspirin, because aspirin can cause bleeding.

Taking Care of the Drainage

1. Expect the drainage to increase after surgery.
2. A small amount of bright red bleeding is normal and may continue for a week.
3. Old blood that accumulated during the surgery is reddish brown, and it will drain for a week or more. It is of no concern.
4. A small dressing (dry pad) will be placed beneath your nose to absorb any drainage.
5. You may need to change the pad several times each day, depending on the amount of drainage. The drainage pad can be discontinued when the drainage stops.
6. After drainage stops, a thicker, yellowish green drainage may continue for several weeks.

Breathing Difficulties

1. Your head may feel stuffy, and the mucous membranes of your nose may swell. This is nórmal and expected.
2. Stuffiness will increase during the first week after surgery and then decrease over the next couple of weeks, and breathing through your nose should improve.
3. Keeping your head elevated and sleeping with an extra pillow will help make you more comfortable. In this position there will be less swelling and better drainage of nasal secretions.
4. A cool mist humidifier at the bedside will help loosen secretions and prevent crusting of the nose. Be sure to follow the manufacturer's directions for cleaning the unit so that bacteria will not grow, be dispersed into the air, and infect you or others.
5. At the postoperative visit, the packing will be removed and you will be given instructions for cleaning your nose.

Rest and Activity

1. Since the body needs extra rest for at least a week to heal, take it easy the first week and then return to normal activities. The usual time to be off work or school is 5 to 7 days unless you work in a dusty or dirty environment.
2. After a week, swimming, jogging, or other such exercises are usually permitted. If bright red bleeding occurs, stop activity until bleeding stops, and then gradually resume activity.

Self-Monitoring

1. Report signs of infection (fever, purulent discharge) to surgeon.
2. Expect ecchymoses of the nose and eyes to begin to change color over the next 1 to 2 weeks.
3. Expect tarry stools from swallowed blood for a few days.
4. Take prophylactic antibiotics as prescribed; do not stop until all medication is taken.

NURSING MANAGEMENT OF PATIENT UNDERGOING CALDWELL-LUC SURGERY, ETHMOIDECTOMY, SPHENOIDECTOMY, OR FRONTAL SINUS SURGERY

■ PREOPERATIVE CARE

For the convenience of the patient, preadmission tests and preoperative teaching should be scheduled for the same day, usually a few days before surgery. The patient is admitted to the hospital the morning of surgery. As indicated in the section on FESS, all information that needs to be taught to the patient perioperatively for any sinus surgery is found in the Patient Teaching box.

■ POSTOPERATIVE CARE

Because general anesthesia is usual, the patient is positioned well onto the side to facilitate removal of secretions and to maintain the airway. This position also prevents swelling of the surgical site and aspiration of bloody drainage. Cool mist is administered by face tent or collar to prevent drying of secretions and to keep mucous membranes moist.

When the patient recovers from anesthesia, the head of the bed is elevated to a mid-Fowler's position to prevent edema and promote drainage. The patient is reminded to sniff secretions to the back of the mouth, where they can be expectorated. Ice compresses are applied over the nose or over the maxillary or frontal sinuses for a few hours after surgery to help reduce swelling in the operative area, constrict blood vessels, reduce bleeding, and relieve pain.

The patient is monitored for:

- Excessive bleeding from the nose (Frequent swallowing is a clue.)
- Decreased visual acuity, especially diplopia, which indicates damage to the optic nerve or muscles of the globe of the eye
- Pain over the involved sinus, which may indicate an infection or inadequate drainage
- Elevated temperature (The temperature must be taken rectally or aurally; it cannot be taken orally because of packing in the nose, which causes mouth breathing.)

Because of increased dryness of the lips, mouth care using a soft toothbrush is given frequently, and lubricant applied. Mouthwash can be used to manage halitosis. If there is an oral incision, mouth care is given before meals to improve appetite and after meals to remove food debris, which could lead to infection. A liberal fluid intake is urged to prevent drying of secretions. Also, the patient may be very thirsty because of dry mouth from mouth breathing.

GERONTOLOGIC CONSIDERATIONS

The care for an older adult having sinus surgery is the same as that already described. However, if the patient has coexisting disease, attention must be given to assessment of affected organs and functions. In addition, the patient may be hospitalized for a day or two to carefully monitor the status and prevent complications.

SPECIAL ENVIRONMENTS FOR CARE

Community-Based Care

Since sinus surgery is usually done on an outpatient basis, postoperative care is completed in the home after initial stabilization and discharge.

COMPLICATIONS

Complications of sinusitis usually are the result of either inadequate therapy during the acute stage or a delay in treatment. Signs and symptoms of complications include:

- Generalized persistent headache
- Vomiting
- Convulsions
- Chills or high fever
- Edema or increasing swelling of the forehead or eyelids
- Blurring of vision, diplopia, or persistent retroocular pain
- Signs of increased intracranial pressure
- Personality changes or dulling of the sensorium
- Increase in white blood cell count above 20,000 mm^3

Serious complications that may develop from untreated chronic sinusitis include cavernous sinus thrombosis, bacteremia or septicemia, and osteomyelitis.

Orbital Complications. Seventy five percent of orbital infections are caused by extension from paranasal sinusitis, usually involving the ethmoid sinuses. Orbital infection can cause inflammatory edema, orbital cellulitis, subperiosteal abscess, orbital abscess, and cavernous sinus thrombosis. Complications are treated vigorously with intravenous antibiotics and, in the case of abscess, incision and drainage.

Cavernous sinus thrombosis is a particularly serious complication that occurs when there is extension of infection through the venous pathways (usually the angular vein) to the cavernous sinus. The patient is very ill, with chills and a temperature as high as 41° C (106° F). There is pain deep behind the eye, and the patient becomes toxic and sometimes semicomatose. The primary treatment of cavernous sinus thrombosis is intravenous antibiotics, without which death can occur in 48 to 72 hours.

INFECTIONS OF THE PHARYNX AND LARYNX

ACUTE PHARYNGITIS

Etiology/Epidemiology

Acute pharyngitis is the most common throat inflammation. It may be caused by hemolytic streptococci, staphylococci, other bacteria, filterable viruses, or fungi. Group A beta-hemolytic streptococci (GABHS) are the cause of up to 30% of the cases of acute pharyngitis. The most common cause, however, is viruses, which account for 70% of the cases of acute pharyngitis. There is also increased evidence of gonococcal pharyngitis caused by the gram-negative diplococcus *Neisseria gonorrhoeae.* The disease is increasingly found in both men and women. When gonorrhea is suspected, a throat culture is indicated. A severe form of acute pharyngitis often is termed *strep throat* because of the frequency of streptococci as the causative organism.

Pathophysiology

Dryness of the throat is a common complaint associated with pharyngitis. The throat appears red, and soreness may range from slight scratchiness to severe pain with difficulty in swallowing. A hacking cough may be present. Children often develop a very high fever, whereas adults may have only a mild elevation of temperature. Symptoms usually precede or occur simultaneously with the onset of acute rhinitis or acute sinusitis. Pharyngitis is also a common manifestation of infectious mononucleosis. Signs and symptoms of the different types of pharyngitis are summarized in the Clinical Manifestations box.

Collaborative Care Management

Acute pharyngitis usually is relieved by hot saline throat gargles and mild OTC analgesics. An ice collar also may provide comfort. For adults, acetylsalicylic acid administered

Clinical Manifestations

Pharyngitis

GROUP A BETA-HEMOLYTIC STREPTOCOCCAL
Sore throat, slightly elevated temperature, malaise

GONOCOCCAL OR VIRAL
Minimal discomfort
Fever, diffuse sore throat

INFECTIOUS MONONUCLEOSIS (EPSTEIN-BARR VIRUS)
Sore throat, cervical lymphadenopathy, and fever

FUNGAL (ESPECIALLY CANDIDIASIS [THRUSH])
Pus, dysphagia, white plaques in mouth or on pharyngeal walls

Patient Teaching

The Patient With Pharyngitis or Tonsillitis

1. Use warm saline gargles, ice collars, moist inhalations, and frequent mouth care for comfort.
2. Drink at least 2 to 3 L of fluids daily.
3. Observe for symptoms of recurrence requiring medical attention: fever, excessive pain, pus, dysphagia.
4. Obtain prophylactic antibiotic therapy for pharyngitis in patients with a history of rheumatic fever or infective endocarditis to prevent reinfection.

orally as a gargle or in Aspergum may be prescribed. Lozenges containing a mild anesthetic may help relieve local soreness. Moist inhalations may help relieve throat dryness. A liquid diet usually is better tolerated than solid food, and fluids up to at least 2.5 L/day are encouraged. Oral hygiene may prevent drying and cracking of the lips and usually refreshes the mouth. The person should remain in bed if the temperature is elevated and should have extra rest if afebrile.

A throat culture is necessary to identify the infecting organism. If beta-hemolytic streptococci are identified, the drug of choice is penicillin. For the person allergic to penicillin, erythromycin or another antibiotic is prescribed. Persons with a history of bacterial endocarditis or rheumatic fever are usually given penicillin prophylactically if they are not allergic.

The prescribed course of antibiotic therapy varies from 7 to 12 days, depending on the organism and the severity of infection. Patients must understand that they should continue therapy for the prescribed number of days even if they are symptom free.

Patient/Family Education. The major role of the nurse is patient teaching, which is presented in the Patient Teaching box. It is important to stress the need for strict hand washing, use of separate eating utensils, and covering one's mouth when coughing and sneezing in order to reduce the spread of infection.

ACUTE FOLLICULAR TONSILLITIS

Etiology/Epidemiology

Acute follicular tonsillitis is an acute inflammation of the tonsils and their crypts. It is usually caused by a *Streptococcus* organism. It is more likely to occur when the person's resistance is low, and it is common in children and young adults, especially mouth breathers or those with a history of asthma and chronic upper respiratory tract infections.

Pathophysiology

The onset is almost always sudden, and symptoms include sore throat, pain on swallowing, fever, chills, general muscle aching, and malaise. These symptoms often last for 2 to 3 days. The pharynx and tonsils appear red, and the peritonsillar tissues are swollen. Sometimes a yellowish exudate drains from crypts in the tonsils. A throat culture usually is taken to identify the infecting organism.

Collaborative Care Management

The patient with acute tonsillitis is encouraged to rest and take generous amounts of fluids orally. Warm saline throat irrigations may be ordered, and antibiotics are given for streptococcal pharyngitis. Acetaminophen (Tylenol) and sometimes codeine sulfate may be ordered for pain and discomfort. An ice collar applied to the neck may relieve discomfort. Occasionally with extreme cases, physicians may prescribe intramuscular or oral steroids to reduce inflammation.

Patient/Family Education. Because the person with acute tonsillitis is usually cared for at home, the nurse should help in teaching the general public the care that is needed (see Patient Teaching box). Nurses working in clinics, industry, schools, physicians' offices, emergency departments, and the community have many opportunities to do this teaching. It is also important to teach the patient that untreated tonsillitis can adversely affect the heart and kidneys and can lead to chorea and pneumonia. The incidence of these complications is decreasing with early diagnosis and the widespread use of penicillin. Many physicians believe that persons who have recurrent attacks of tonsillitis should have a tonsillectomy. This procedure is usually performed 4 to 6 weeks after an acute attack has subsided.

A peritonsillar abscess is an uncommon local complication of acute follicular tonsillitis in which infection extends from the tonsil to form an abscess in the surrounding tissues. The presence of pus behind the tonsil causes difficulty in swallowing, talking, and opening the mouth; the difficulty in swallowing may be so great that the person is unable to swallow. Pain is severe and may extend to the ear on the affected side.

If antibiotics to which the infecting organism is sensitive are administered early, infection subsides. If the peritonsillar abscess is caused by anaerobic organisms, hydrogen peroxide (an oxidizing agent) in the form of a mouthwash may help relieve symptoms. Acute streptococcal or staphylococcal tonsillitis may also cause a peritonsillar abscess to form. If an abscess forms, it is incised and drained. During the procedure, the patient's head usually is lowered, and suction is applied as soon as the incision is made to prevent the patient from aspirating the purulent drainage. Warm saline irrigations, an ice collar, or narcotics may relieve discomfort. If acute follicular tonsillitis is treated adequately, peritonsillar abscess is not likely to occur.

ACUTE LARYNGITIS

Etiology/Epidemiology

Simple acute laryngitis is an inflammation of the mucous membrane lining the larynx accompanied by edema of the vocal cords. It may be caused by a cold, by sudden changes in temperature, or by irritating fumes.

Pathophysiology

Symptoms vary from a slight huskiness to complete loss of voice. The throat may be painful and feel scratchy, and a cough may be present.

Collaborative Care Management

Laryngitis in adults usually requires only symptomatic treatment. Individuals diagnosed with laryngitis are advised to remain indoors and to avoid using their voice for several days or weeks, depending on the severity of the inflammation. Steam inhalations may be soothing, and cough syrups or home remedies for coughs provide relief to some patients. Smoking or being near others who are smoking should be avoided. Additional fluids by mouth help prevent dehydration and drying of the throat. Chronic laryngitis occurs in people who use their voices excessively, who smoke a great deal, or who work continuously where there are irritating fumes. Hoarseness usually is worse in the early morning and in the evening. There may be a dry, harsh cough and a persistent need to clear the throat. All persons with persistent hoarseness should be examined by laryngoscopy to rule out cancer of the larynx. Treatment of chronic laryngitis consists of removal of irritants, voice rest, correction of faulty voice habits, steam inhalations, and cough medications. Additional fluids by mouth are encouraged to prevent dehydration and drying of the throat.

Patient/Family Education. The nursing role is mainly patient teaching, which focuses on:

- The need to take antibiotics as prescribed (to not stop antibiotics when feeling better)
- The need for an increase in fluid intake
- For smokers, the need to stop smoking and, for both smokers and nonsmokers, the need to avoid irritating fumes and secondhand smoke
- Precautions to be observed in using steam inhalations

CHRONIC ENLARGEMENT OF THE TONSILS AND ADENOIDS

Etiology/Epidemiology

Tonsils and adenoids are lymphoid structures located in the oropharynx and nasopharynx. They reach full size in childhood and then begin to atrophy during puberty. When adenoids enlarge, usually as a result of chronic infections but sometimes for no known reason, they cause nasal obstruction. The person breathes through the mouth, snores loudly, may have a dull facial expression, and may have reduced appetite because the blocked nasopharynx can interfere with swallowing. Hypertrophy of the tonsils does not usually block the oropharynx but may affect speech and swallowing and cause mouth breathing.

Approximately 30% of cases of tonsillitis are caused by group A beta-hemolytic streptococci or staphylococci. Another organism such as a pneumococcus, gram-negative organism, or a virus also can be the causative agent.

Pathophysiology

The tonsils are red and swollen with yellow or white exudate found mainly in the crypts of the tonsils. Signs and symptoms include fever, dry throat, malaise, dysphagia, otalgia, and a feeling of fullness in the throat. Occipital, tonsillar, submaxillary, submental, and cervical chain lymph nodes are often swollen and palpable.

Collaborative Care Management

The tonsils and adenoids are removed when they become enlarged and cause symptoms of obstruction, when they are chronically infected, when the person has repeated attacks of tonsillitis, or after repeated peritonsillar abscesses. No specific tests are used to determine whether or not surgery is indicated.

Chronic infections of these structures usually do not respond to antibiotics and may become foci of infection by spreading organisms to other parts of the body, such as the heart and the kidneys. However, if patients are not candidates for surgery, antibiotic therapy is usually continued throughout contamination. Antibiotic therapy coupled with surgery is the primary treatment.

Tonsillectomy in adults may be performed with either general or local anesthesia. After the tonsils are removed, pressure is applied to stop superficial bleeding. Bleeding vessels are tied off with sutures or by electrocoagulation. The person is monitored carefully for hemorrhage, especially when sleeping, because a large amount of blood may be lost without any external evidence of bleeding. The physician may be able to control minor postoperative bleeding by applying a sponge soaked in a solution of epinephrine to the site. The person who is bleeding excessively often is returned to the operating room for surgical treatment to stop the hemorrhage. Use of sutures causes more pain and discomfort than electrocoagulation, and the patient may be unable to take solid foods for several days. Most otolaryngologists prescribe acetaminophen instead of aspirin for pain after a tonsillectomy because aspirin increases the tendency for bleeding.

The tough, yellow, fibrous membrane that forms over the operative site begins to break away between the fourth and eighth postoperative days, and hemorrhage may occur. The separation of the membrane accounts for the throat being more painful at this time. Pink granulation tissue soon becomes apparent, and by the end of the third postoperative week the area is covered with normal mucous membrane.

Guidelines for Safe Practice

Care of the Patient After Tonsillectomy

1. Position patient on side until fully awake after general anesthesia or in mid-Fowler's position when awake.
2. Monitor for signs of hemorrhage: frequent swallowing (inspect throat), bright red vomitus, rapid pulse, restlessness.
3. Promote comfort.
   a. Give 30% cool mist via collar.
   b. Apply ice collar to neck (will also reduce bleeding by vasoconstriction).
   c. Use acetaminophen in place of aspirin.
4. Give appropriate food and fluids.
   a. Give ice-cold fluids and bland foods during initial period (e.g., ice chips, frozen juice bars, gelatin).
   b. Milk is usually not given because it may increase mucus and cause patient to clear throat.
   c. Advance to normal diet as soon as possible.
5. Instruct patient in self-care.
   a. Avoid attempting to clear throat immediately after surgery (may initiate bleeding).
   b. Avoid coughing, sneezing, vigorous nose blowing, and vigorous exercise for 1 to 2 weeks.
   c. Drink fluids (2 to 3 L/day) until mouth odor disappears.
   d. Avoid hard, scratchy foods, such as pretzels, popcorn, or toast, until throat is healed.
   e. Report signs of bleeding to physician immediately.
   f. Expect more throat discomfort between fourth and eighth postoperative days because of membrane separation.
   g. Expect stool to be black or dark for a few days because of swallowed blood.
   h. Resume normal activity immediately, as long as it is not stressful and does not require straining.

Before surgery, patients must be allowed nothing by mouth (remain NPO) after midnight, be infection free at the time of surgery, and meet criteria for the specific form of anesthesia to be used. Postoperative care is outlined in the Guidelines for Safe Practice box. Postoperative assessments focus primarily on identification of complications of tonsillectomy, namely, hemorrhage and respiratory obstruction related to edema of local tissue.[14]

Patient/Family Education. Providing the patient with information regarding the normal postoperative expectations will assist in reducing anxiety levels. See the patient teaching section in the Guidelines for Safe Practice box.

LARYNGEAL PARALYSIS AND EDEMA

LARYNGEAL PARALYSIS

Etiology/Epidemiology

Laryngeal paralysis may result from disease or injury of either the laryngeal nerves or the vagus nerve. Causes include aortic aneurysm, mitral stenosis, laryngeal cancer, subglottic or cervical esophageal tumors, bronchial carcinoma, neck injuries, severing or stretching of the recurrent laryngeal nerve during thyroidectomy, and prolonged intubation of patients in intensive care units.

Pathophysiology

One or both vocal cords may be paralyzed. If only one cord is involved, the airway is adequate and only the voice may be affected. Improvement of voice quality in persons with unilateral cord paralysis has been achieved by injecting a small quantity of Gelfoam or Teflon into the paralyzed cord. This swells the cord and pushes it toward the midline, where the other cord can approximate it better during phonation.

Bilateral paralysis impairs the airway and causes incapacitating dyspnea, stridor on exertion, and a weak voice. A sudden bilateral vocal cord paralysis is uncommon and usually results from a massive cerebrovascular accident or blunt trauma, both of which are usually incompatible with life. Treatment of bilateral cord paralysis is aimed at restoring the airway, not at improvement of the voice.

Collaborative Care Management

The primary diagnostic test is laryngoscopy. This and other tests used, along with their purposes, are listed in Table 20-4. Depending on the patient's symptoms, one or more of the following medications may be prescribed. If the patient is experiencing gastroesophageal reflux, antacids, which neutralize gastric acid, or H_2 inhibitors, which reduce the amount of gastric acid produced, may be ordered.

If the patient has signs and symptoms of an infection, appropriate antibiotics are prescribed. For patients with swelling of the vocal cords, systemic steroids are often ordered, and for those with spastic movements of the cords, botulinum may be injected.

Treatment of cord paralysis may involve excision of nodules or polyps, or a thyroplasty, in which a stent is inserted to reapproximate the vocal cords, may be performed. A tracheostomy may be necessary to maintain the airway.

Other possible procedures include an arytenoidectomy, in which a portion of one of the arytenoid cartilages is resected, thus increasing the diameter of the posterior portion of the glottis sufficiently to improve breathing.

Patient/Family Education. Patient/family education is directed at providing information specific to any of the treatments listed above and to prepare the patient for home care and any further follow-up that may be needed.

ACUTE LARYNGEAL EDEMA

Etiology/Epidemiology

Acute laryngeal edema is a medical emergency and not to be confused with laryngeal paralysis. Laryngeal edema may be caused by anaphylaxis, urticaria, acute laryngitis, serious inflammatory disease of the throat, or edema after intubation.[6]

Pathophysiology

Acute laryngeal edema narrows or closes the airway, which must be immediately restored if life is to be maintained.

TABLE 20-4 Diagnostic Tests and Purposes

Test	Purpose
Indirect laryngoscopy	To diagnose vocal cord abnormality
Videostroboscopy (observe vocal cord vibration during phonation): fiberoptic laryngoscope is attached to videotape to record actual cord motion	To diagnose abnormal vibrations of cord
Electromyography	To determine innervation and thus movement of vocal cord(s)
Computed tomography scan	To determine cause of vocal cord paresis or paralysis, such as tumor or aneurysm along course of recurrent laryngeal nerve

Adapted from Sigler BA, Schuring LT: *Ear, nose and throat disorders,* St Louis, 1993, Mosby.

Collaborative Care Management

Treatment of acute laryngeal edema consists of administration of an adrenal corticosteroid or epinephrine and intubation or tracheostomy if necessary. Edema of the larynx caused by irradiation of the larynx or tumors of the neck may be chronic and may also require tracheostomy.

Patient/Family Education. Patient/family education focuses on the necessity for proper medical evaluation by a physician or nurse practitioner. Also, information specific to any of the treatments listed in previous paragraphs is provided.

NASAL DEFORMITIES/OBSTRUCTIONS

RECONSTRUCTION OF THE NOSE

Etiology/Epidemiology

The nasal septum is made up of cartilage and bone joined by a fibrous attachment. The septum separates the nose into two cavities, provides support, and acts as a shock absorber for the floor of the frontal fossa. Normally the septum of the nose is straight and thin. As a person ages, the septum tends to become deviated to one side or the other, and an irregular projection may develop on it.

Deformities of the nose may be present from birth or develop as the result of trauma to the nose from sports injuries, automobile crashes, abnormal vasculature, nasal illicit drug use, and the like. Trauma can result in overgrowth of fibrous tissue that fills in the fracture and causes bowing of the septum. There can also be loss of nasal septal cartilage from trauma or infection, resulting in marked concavity, referred to as a saddle nose.

Although some deformities may seem minor to the casual observer, they may be considered major by the person who is not pleased by the appearance of his or her nose. The patient's desire for a change in the size or shape of the nose may be unrelated to function and be for cosmetic reasons.

Pathophysiology

The primary effect of a deviated septum or nasal fracture is obstruction to breathing through the nose. A deviated septum may also alter the velocity with which air passes through the nose and hence can interfere with filtering, warming, and humidifying inspired air. As a result, the nasal mucosa becomes dry and crusty, nasal bleeding increases, and changes in the lining of the nose develop. Patients may also experience difficulty in breathing through the nose or mouth, postnasal drip, nasal discharge, and/or loss of smell or taste.

Collaborative Care Management

The most common test used to confirm nasal fractures is x-ray examination. For cosmetic reasons, high-tech tests are usually performed in the surgeon's office that allow the patient to examine several methods of repair and reconstruction and provide the patient with an actual view of what the repair might look like when completed.

Cosmetic surgery on the nose is referred to as rhinoplasty, or as nasoseptoplasty when the septum is involved. Preparation of the patient is important so that the patient does not have unrealistic expectations about the surgery. Bone and cartilage may be removed from the nose if it is irregular, or they may be inserted if a defect such as a saddle nose is being corrected (Figure 20-10). Most rhinoplasties are performed with the patient under local anesthesia. The incision is usually made at the end of the nose inside the nostril so that it is not conspicuous.

Preoperative care is primarily focused on facilitating open communication with the patient so that the procedure and what it entails is understood. It is important that the patient be secure with the decision to have surgery and that he or she has a realistic expectation of the outcome. Depending on the extent of surgery needed, some surgeons prefer to revise the nose a little at a time in order to allow the patient some time to get used to his or her new look. Whereas some changes are subtle and take a while to be noticed, some changes are evident immediately. Also, subtle changes can sometimes turn to overt changes as a result of the development of scar tissue or keloids in the nasal cavity. Sometimes patients return to the clinic for several steroid injections in order to keep scarring minimal.

A nasoseptoplasty involves reconstruction of the nasal septum. In this procedure an incision is made through the mucosa at the caudal end of the septal cartilage. The septal mucous membranes are elevated, and the septal cartilage is separated from its bony attachments and straightened. The

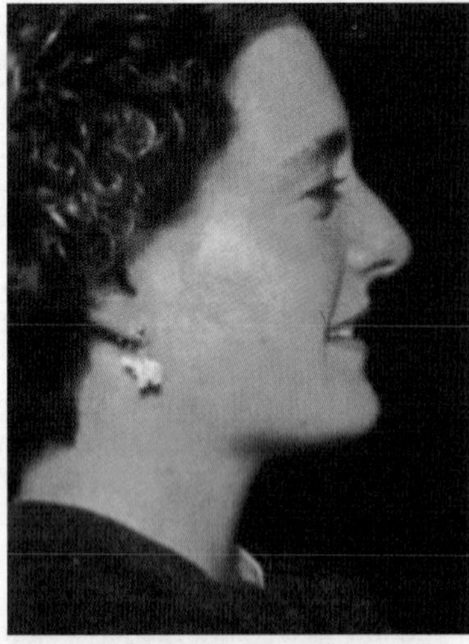
A

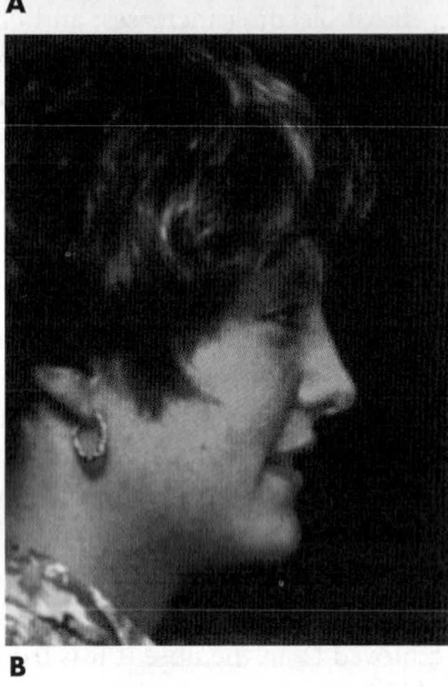
B

Figure 20-10 Rhinoplasty. **A**, Preoperative lateral view. **B**, Postoperative lateral view.

septal mucous membranes are then approximated to prevent bleeding.

Nasal septal splints made of plastic or Silastic are inserted into the nose to prevent synechiae (a type of scar tissue) and to keep the septum in place. The nose may be packed for several days to prevent a hematoma from forming between the septal flaps and to support the septum. The patient is usually given antibiotics until the packing is removed. The splints and nasal packing are removed by the surgeon. Reconstruction of the external nose (rhinoplasty) is often combined with septoplasty.

Following a rhinoplasty/nasoseptoplasty, the nose is usually protected with a plaster of paris splint, an adhesive tape dressing, or a plastic mold. Firm healing develops on about the tenth day. Ecchymosis and swelling are present around the eyes and nose for 10 to 14 days after surgery. It will be several weeks before the final results of the surgery are evident.

The patient is placed in mid-Fowler's position to decrease local edema, and cool mist is given via a collar or face tent. Iced compresses are usually applied to the nose to lessen the discoloration, bleeding, and discomfort, and to hasten fluid resorption from the surgical site. Patients can usually apply their own iced compresses.

The patient is monitored for signs of hemorrhage (see Guidelines for Safe Practice box for nasal surgery on p. 489). Some oozing on the dressing below the nose is expected, and this dressing may be changed as necessary (see Figure 20-9). If bleeding becomes pronounced, the surgeon is notified and equipment for repacking the nose is prepared. This equipment consists of a hemostat tray containing gauze packing, umbilical tape for posterior packing, a few small gauze sponges, a small catheter (used for inserting a postnasal plug), packing forceps, tongue blades, and scissors. The surgeon may require a head mirror, good light, epinephrine 1:1000 or other vasoconstrictor, 4% topical lidocaine (Xylocaine) or 4% cocaine solution, applicators, a nasal speculum, and suction.

Because packing blocks the passage of air through the nose, a partial vacuum is created during swallowing, and the person may complain of a sucking action when attempting to drink. Postnasal drainage, the presence of old blood in the mouth, dryness of the mouth from mouth breathing, and loss of the ability to smell often lead to anorexia. Frequent mouth care is important.

If the patient was given intravenous anesthesia, clear liquids are recommended until nausea subsides. Progression to a regular diet can then be implemented. Activity is limited for a minimum of 7 to 10 days to prevent injury.

Patient/Family Education. Patient/family education is described in the Guidelines for Safe Practice box. In addition, the patient is instructed to report signs of complications. Complications of nasal deformities are usually identified as being physical or psychosocial in nature. Physical complications prevent the normal exchange of air through the nasal pathway and can lead to chronic dryness and irritation of the nasal mucosa and decreased ability to breathe, especially at night when sleeping on the nonaffected side. Psychosocial complications include alterations in body image, self-concept, and shyness, often to the point of social isolation, depending on the degree of deformity or the patient's perception of the degree of deformity.

HYPERTROPHIED TURBINATES

Etiology/Epidemiology

Long-standing allergic rhinitis and low-grade inflammation may cause permanent enlargement of the turbinates, especially the inferior turbinate.

Pathophysiology

The turbinates lose most of their normal ability to expand and shrink. This results in continuous nasal obstruction (Figure 20-11).

Collaborative Care Management

Hypertrophied turbinates may be medically treated with aerosols containing corticosteroids such as beclomethasone dipropionate (Beconase, Vancenase) or dexamethasone (Decadron, Turbinaire). These aerosols are used for their antiinflammatory effect.

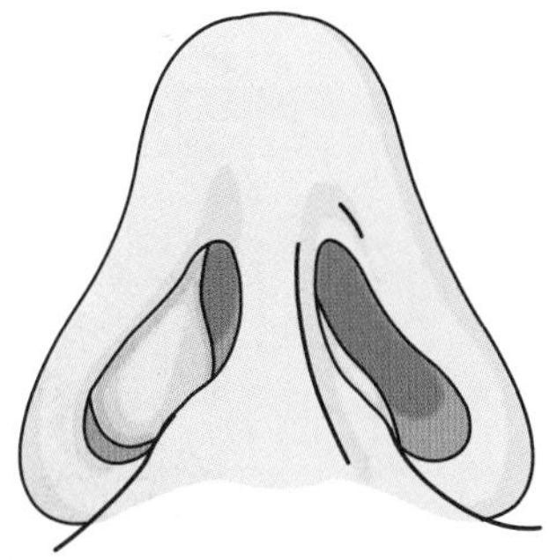

Figure 20-11 Hypertrophic turbinate.

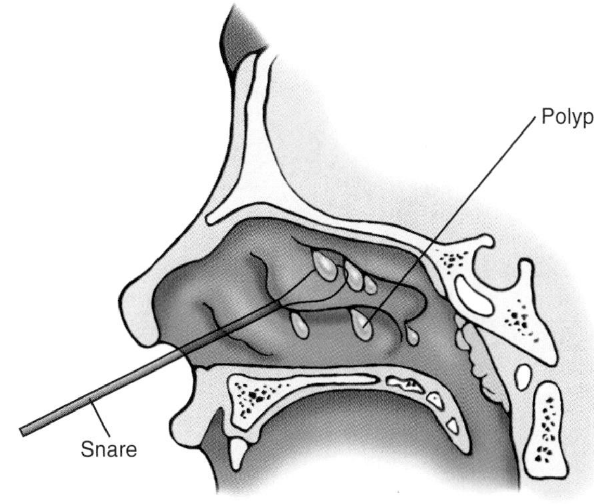

Figure 20-12 A nasal snare is used to remove nasal polyps. After the nose is anesthetized, the nasal snare is slipped around the polyp; it is transected, and forceps are used to remove the transected polyp.

Although not used as often since the advent of corticosteroid aerosols, laser surgery on the turbinates may still be used to restore the airway. Debulking (resection) of the hypertrophied mucosa may be necessary. When surgery is necessary, the care and teaching of the patient is the same as that for patients undergoing nasal surgery.

Patient/Family Education. Explanations of the problem and potential treatment pathways should be given to the patient and family. If surgery is necessary, the patient should be instructed before and after surgery about the procedure and care needs, as outlined in the Guidelines for Safe Practice box for nasal surgery.

NASAL POLYPS

Etiology/Epidemiology

Nasal polyps are grapelike growths of the sinus mucosa that project into the cavities of the nose and paranasal sinuses. The exact cause of nasal polyposis is unknown, but some believe it is related to the inflammatory response. Supporting this theory is the fact that persons with chronic viral or bacterial infections have a higher incidence of nasal polyps. Nasal polyps are common and affect men twice as often as women. They are typically associated with allergies, cystic fibrosis, asthma, disorders of ciliary motility, chronic rhinitis, and chronic sinusitis.

Patient Teaching
The Patient With Nasal Polyps

1. Elevate the head of the bed to decrease nasal edema and improve breathing through the nose.
2. Increase humidity to thin secretions and reduce dryness of the nose. Use a central humidifier on the furnace or use a room humidifier. Increase fluid intake and use a saline nasal spray.
3. Prevent respiratory infections by avoiding persons with upper respiratory tract infections and avoiding crowds. Notify the physician at the first sign of infection so that appropriate therapy can be started.
4. Take medications as ordered. Be aware of side effects such as drowsiness if antihistamines are prescribed.
5. Seek prompt medical attention if there are signs of recurrence of polyp(s).

Pathophysiology

Some of the patients with nasal polyps also have symptoms of asthma and intolerance to aspirin, indomethacin, and other nonsteroidal antiinflammatory drugs (NSAIDs). The cause of the triad of nasal polyps, asthma, and aspirin sensitivity is unknown, but the patient may have an acute asthmatic attack in response to infection, anesthesia, surgery, or the administration of aspirin, all of which could be considered stressors for the hyperresponsive airway of the person with asthma.

Collaborative Care Management

Nasal polyps can be treated with corticosteroid sprays or by local injection of a steroid into the polyp. Steroid sprays are used for long-term reduction of polyp size, to prevent recurrence, and to reduce the inflammatory response, thus reducing swelling.

Antibiotics such as amoxicillin or erythromycin are prescribed when infection is present. Persistent polyps may require nasal polypectomy (Figure 20-12) or removal of polyps via Caldwell-Luc surgery, in which the maxillary sinus is entered.

Patient/Family Education. The major role of the nurse is in patient teaching. The points to be emphasized are listed in the Patient Teaching box.

TRAUMA TO THE UPPER AIRWAY

FRACTURES OF THE NASAL BONES AND SEPTUM

Fractures of the nasal bones and septum commonly occur from relatively minor injuries, such as falls, or from more severe injuries, such as automobile accidents or fights. If there is no displacement of the bone, no obstruction to the airway, and no cosmetic deformity, treatment is not needed. When airway obstruction or bone displacement occurs, simple

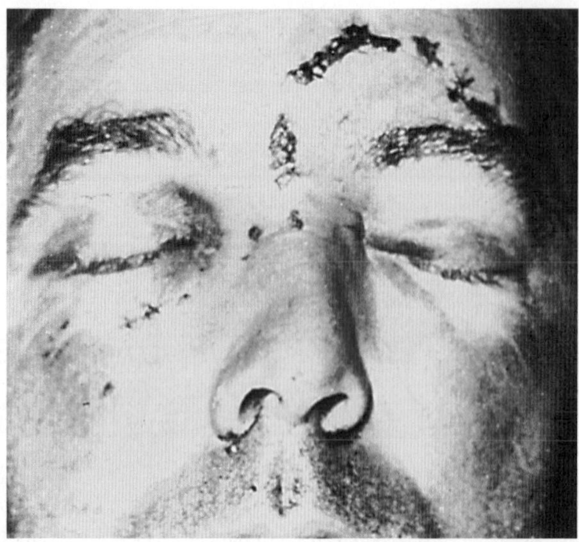

Figure 20-13 Laterally displaced fracture of nose secondary to trauma. Pressure on convex side will restore alignment.

reduction of the fracture is performed (Figure 20-13). Most simple nasal fractures can be reduced by applying firm pressure on the convex side of the nose. Nasal fractures should be reduced within the first 24 hours if at all possible. Local anesthesia is often used. After 24 hours the reduction becomes more difficult and may require general anesthesia.

FRACTURES OF THE MAXILLARY AND ZYGOMATIC BONES

Fractures of the maxillary and zygomatic bones are often seen after automobile accidents, fights, or severe falls in sporting events. These fractures are generally reduced with the patient under anesthesia. Patients may also require wiring of the teeth, with all the attendant problems of that procedure.

EPISTAXIS

Etiology/Epidemiology

Epistaxis (nosebleed) usually originates from the tiny blood vessels in the anterior part of the septum. Bleeding from the posterior part is more common in older adults and is more likely to be severe. Nosebleeds are more common in men than in women.

The most common cause of epistaxis is trauma to the nasal mucosa from damage by a foreign object. Other causes include picking the nose, local irritation of the mucous membrane from lack of humidity in the air, chronic infection, violent sneezing, or blowing the nose. Systemic causes include coagulation defects, such as hemophilia, leukemia, and purpura.

Pathophysiology

Although persons with hypertension do not have more nosebleeds than do normotensive persons, they tend to bleed more profusely when they do have a nosebleed. Nosebleed is usually unilateral, and some persons are more prone to nosebleed than are others. Persons with frequent nosebleeds should have a complete physical examination to determine the cause.

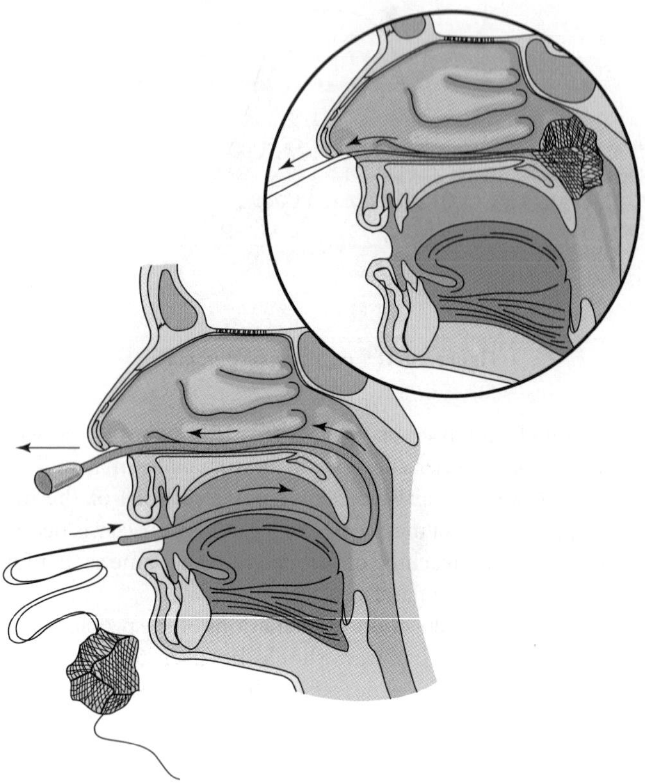

Figure 20-14 Postnasal packing. A pack is attached to the catheter and then pulled through the mouth to the posterior aspect of the nasopharynx.

Guidelines for Safe Practice

Initial Care of the Patient With Epistaxis

1. Have patient sit up leaning forward with head tipped downward to prevent swallowing or aspiration of blood.
2. Use fingers to compress soft tissues of nose against septum and maintain pressure for at least 5 minutes.
3. Apply ice or cold compress to nose to constrict blood vessels.
4. If bleeding does not stop with direct pressure, place a cotton ball soaked in a topical vasoconstrictor (e.g., phenylephrine [Neo-Synephrine]) into nose and apply pressure.
5. Instruct patient not to blow nose for several hours after a nosebleed.
6. Notify physician.

Collaborative Care Management

Most nosebleeds can be controlled with simple measures (see Guidelines for Safe Practice box). If these measures are ineffective, medical intervention is necessary. After identifying the site of the bleeding, the physician cauterizes the bleeding point with a silver nitrate stick or electrocautery. If the bleeding point cannot be seen, a postnasal pack may be inserted (Figure 20-14). Because this procedure is extremely painful and may cause complications, patients should be admitted to the hospital. For example, the pressure of the postnasal pack may stimulate the sinopulmonary reflex, causing the patient to

Research

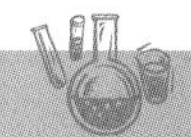

Reference: Holland NJ et al: The Foley catheter in the management of epistaxis, *Int J Clin Pract* 55(1):14-5, 2001.

Although the urinary Foley catheter has never been specifically designed or licensed for use in treating epistaxis, it has been used for that purpose for many years, and its use is again being revisited. Researchers in the United Kingdom collected data via telephone questionnaire using a sample of 90 ear, nose, and throat physicians in two countries within the United Kingdom. Their aim was to determine how many departments were using the Foley catheter for managing epistaxis, to determine whether licensed nasal balloon devices were available, and to determine if there had been any complications associated with the use of either of these devices. Results of the study found that 83 (92%) ear, nose, and throat departments used the Foley catheter for management of epistaxis and 44 (49%) departments had licensed balloon devices available. The researcher reported that although the majority of departments were using the catheter, only 22% of the physicians questioned were aware that the Foley catheter was not licensed for use in the nose. It is important to note that researchers also reported that most of the complications reported with using nasal balloon devices were complications associated with the foley catheter.

stop breathing. In this situation the pack must be removed immediately. If no problems occur, the pack is left in place for 48 to 72 hours and then gently removed.[8] Management includes adequate oxygenation, humidification, analgesia, bed rest, blood transfusions, intravenous fluids, systemic antibiotics, and sedation. If the posterior pack fails to control the bleeding, another pack may be placed and the patient may be taken to surgery for ligation of the internal maxillary artery or to the radiology department for embolization of the bleeding vessels.

Severe epistaxis causes apprehension because of the profuse bleeding from the nose and into the throat. The person is kept in mid-Fowler's position and is urged not to swallow blood because doing so may cause nausea and vomiting. The position of the postnasal pack must be checked frequently by viewing the posterior oropharynx for bleeding or slippage.[18] Nasal packs may slip out of place and cause airway obstruction. The patient is monitored for signs of complications (confusion, agitation, increased lethargy, and changes in vital signs, especially in respirations and pulse). Nasal packs also make eating and swallowing difficult; a liquid diet is usually better tolerated (see Research box).

Patient/Family Education. Patient education for epistaxis is focused on the proper treatment of nosebleeds and recognition of when medical care is needed. The proper method for stopping nosebleeds is presented in the Guidelines for Safe Practice box.

MALIGNANCIES OF THE UPPER AIRWAY: OVERVIEW

Malignancies involving the upper airway can occur in several sites, including (1) the lip and oral cavity; (2) the pharynx: nasopharynx, oropharynx, and laryngopharynx; (3) the larynx; (4) the paranasal sinuses; (5) the salivary gland; and (6) the thyroid gland. See Chapter 32 for cancer of the mouth and pharynx and Chapter 29 for cancer of the thyroid.

BOX 20-2 TNM System for Staging of Head and Neck Cancer

Stage I	T_1, N_0, M_0
Stage II	T_2, N_0, M_0
Stage III	T_3, N_0, M_0; T_1, T_2, or T_3, N_1, M_0
Stage IV	T_4, N_0 or N_1, M_0
	Any T, N_2 or N_3, M_0
	Any T, any N, M_1

T, Primary tumor extent or size; *N,* regional lymph node (number, size, and location); *M,* presence or absence of distant metastases.

Ninety percent of cancers of the head and neck are squamous cell carcinoma. Squamous cell carcinomas of the head and neck can metastasize to regional lymph nodes. Metastasis is greatest in those areas with rich lymphatic supply, such as the floor of the mouth, tongue, pharyngeal wall, nasopharynx, and supraglottic larynx. There is little correlation between cervical metastases and the size of the primary lesion, because even small lesions may have regional metastases.

The lung is the most common site of distant metastasis. Metastases to the liver and skeleton are less common, and metastasis to the brain is rare.

The diagnosis is confirmed by biopsy, CT scan, and MRI. The CT scan is used to differentiate between benign and malignant lesions, determine tumor extension, and identify the presence of bony destruction. The MRI scan with gadolinium enhances tumor imaging in soft tissues and shows tumor extension and tumor secretions. The radiolucency of the tumor and its secretions are different, which is why both can be identified on MRI with gadolinium.

Treatment of squamous cell carcinomas of the head and neck depends on the size of the primary tumor and the presence of nodal metastasis. The usual system for staging head and neck cancer is the TNM (tumor, node, metastasis) system, which is based on the number, size, and location of the metastases to either the same, the opposite, or both sides of the neck (Box 20-2).[15] Persons with stage III or IV disease are automatically placed in the advanced-stage category requiring combined therapy with radiotherapy, surgery, and chemotherapy.

Persons with stage I or II cancer of the head and neck can be treated with either primary radiotherapy or surgical intervention with equal success. Radiotherapy is given either preoperatively or postoperatively, depending on the experience and wishes of the surgeon. Chemotherapy may also be used, but it is considered experimental at this time. A chemotherapeutic regimen used alone or as an adjuvant to radiotherapy and resection for squamous cell carcinoma of the head and neck has yet to be standardized.

When cervical lymph node metastases are identified at the time of surgery, a neck dissection is performed. In the past a radical neck dissection involved removal of all affected nodes, lymphatic tissues with the submandibular gland, the sternocleidomastoid muscle, the internal jugular vein, and the spinal accessory nerve. Advances in surgical techniques have led to modified neck dissection, in which an attempt is made to preserve the sternocleidomastoid muscle, internal jugular vein, various chains or sections of lymph nodes, and spinal nerves by themselves or in combination. As previously stated, patients have radiation treatments before or after neck dissection, depending on surgeon preference, the condition of the patient, and the site of the tumor.

Persons at high risk for upper airway cancers are those who work in high-risk areas where toxic fumes are present, including tobacco or secondhand smoke; those who consume alcohol; those with a family history of these cancers; and those 50 years of age and older. Referral to an ear, nose, and throat (ENT) specialist for further evaluation is necessary for anyone who meets high-risk criteria or questions the character of a noted lesion or node.

CARCINOMA OF THE NASAL CAVITY AND PARANASAL SINUSES

Etiology/Epidemiology

Carcinoma of the nasal cavity has its highest incidence in men between 60 and 70 years of age. Exposure to certain substances has been implicated in some malignancies of the nasal cavity. These substances include wood dust and leather dust (inhaled by furniture workers) and exposure to nickel compounds, chromate compounds, hydrocarbons, nitrosamines, and dioxane. The risk is higher among those who dip snuff, work in the shoe industry, or are textile and asbestos workers.

> ***Clinical Manifestations***
>
> **Carcinoma of the Nasal Cavity and Paranasal Sinuses**
>
> MAXILLARY SINUS
>
> There may be a bump on the hard palate. Nasal obstruction and bleeding occur as the tumor breaks into the nasal cavity. Swelling of the cheek occurs with pain. Swelling of the gums may cause toothache or result in ill-fitting dentures. If the tumor impinges on the infraorbital nerve, there may be numbness of the cheek, increased lacrimation, exophthalmos, and diplopia. More advanced tumors may result in displacement of the eye, extraocular muscle palsy, hyperesthesia of the cheek, and inability to open the mouth.
>
> FRONTAL SINUS
>
> Patients commonly have swelling and frontal pain that mimics a sinus headache. Pain occurs when the tumor invades bone and causes bony destruction. If the tumor invades the ethmoids and orbit, the eye on that side will be displaced, resulting in double vision (diplopia).
>
> SPHENOID SINUS
>
> A major complaint is steady, deep-seated temporoparietal headaches. Because of its close proximity to the cavernous sinus, a tumor extending into this area causes compression of the third, fourth, and sixth cranial nerves, causing diplopia.
>
> ETHMOID SINUS
>
> These tumors cause medial orbital swelling, puffiness of the face, decreased vision, excessive tearing (epiphora), and olfactory complaints. Death is caused by direct extension of the tumor into the vital areas of the skull.

Pathophysiology

The majority of persons give no history of exposure to high-risk substances. Most, however, have signs and symptoms of a long-standing chronic sinusitis. Common complaints include a stuffy nose, sinus headache, and facial pain.

Signs and symptoms of malignancies of the nasal cavity and paranasal sinuses are listed in the Clinical Manifestations box.

Collaborative Care Management

Treatment consists of radiation therapy followed by complete surgical excision of the maxilla. This combination is more effective at eradication than either radiation or surgery alone. Some surgeons prefer that radiation be given 8 to 10 weeks before surgery; other surgeons prefer surgery followed by radiation therapy. Chemotherapy used in conjunction with surgical intervention and radiation may improve long-term survival.

Surgery for maxillary sinus and palate tumors consists of removal of the entire jaw (maxillectomy), removal of the entire palate (hard and soft), and when necessary, removal of one eye (orbital exenteration) (Figures 20-15 and 20-16). Split-thickness skin grafts are usually applied to the oral defect remaining after surgery. After healing, a dental prosthesis replaces the hard palate and floor of the nose. The patient then has nearly normal speech, swallowing, and appearance. Early diagnosis and treatment greatly affects the surgical outcome.

Radical surgery is required because of the danger of recurrence. Meningitis is a potential postoperative complication, and prophylactic antibiotics are usually prescribed.

Maintenance of an airway postoperatively is critical for these patients, and sometimes a tracheostomy is performed. A nasogastric tube is inserted to ensure adequate liquid and caloric intake, because eating is difficult until the prosthesis is fitted. Several different prostheses are usually needed before a final one fits, because the cavity shrinks as healing progresses. Often they need to be readjusted and sized weekly.

Postoperative care is summarized in the Guidelines for Safe Practice box. Persons who undergo radical surgery of this type have a number of emotional adjustments to make. Alteration in their physical appearance is readily visible; the person feels conspicuous and different. In addition to disfigurement, these patients have all the normal fears of surgery and of cancer. Fear, anger, and grief are normal reactions to the situation. Fear is focused on concerns about the future, the ability to live normally, and being rejected. Anger and grief are common responses to the loss and the helplessness to control the loss. Oral communication also may be a problem immediately after surgery, and every effort is made to allow the person to express needs and feelings by writing if necessary. Conveying compassion and concern to the person is important.

Guidelines for Safe Practice

Care of the Patient After Paranasal Surgery

Nursing care after paranasal surgery includes:

1. Routine tracheostomy care.
2. Administration of nasogastric tube feedings.
3. Monitoring for signs of meningitis: fever, headache, stiff neck, neck rigidity.
4. Mouth care. A gentle spray or oral irrigation may be used. Oral irrigating solutions include saline and hydrogen peroxide, weak sodium bicarbonate, or an antibiotic solution. It is important to know where the suture line is to prevent damage to it when irrigating the mouth. Because the patient may have difficulty in swallowing, it may be necessary to aspirate the irrigating solution from the mouth, and care must be taken to prevent trauma to the sutures by the suction. Management of saliva may also be a problem because of the swallowing difficulty.
5. Dressing care. The patient will have a bolster/bolus dressing or packing in the maxillary sinus cavity. Observe packing to ensure that it is intact and not hanging loose in the back of the throat, where it can cause gagging.
6. Assessing adjustment to the prosthesis. Adjustment may be a problem because of a poor fit. If the prosthesis creates pressure, it leads to pain. If eating causes nasal regurgitation, the prosthesis may need adjustment.
7. Providing information on long-term follow-up after discharge. The patient will be seen weekly for at least 6 weeks. If receiving radiation therapy postoperatively, he or she will be seen for several more weeks.
8. Eye prosthesis. Radiotherapy must be completed before the patient can be fitted for an ocular prosthesis, and it may take 4 to 6 months for healing to occur and the patient to be ready for the eye prosthesis.

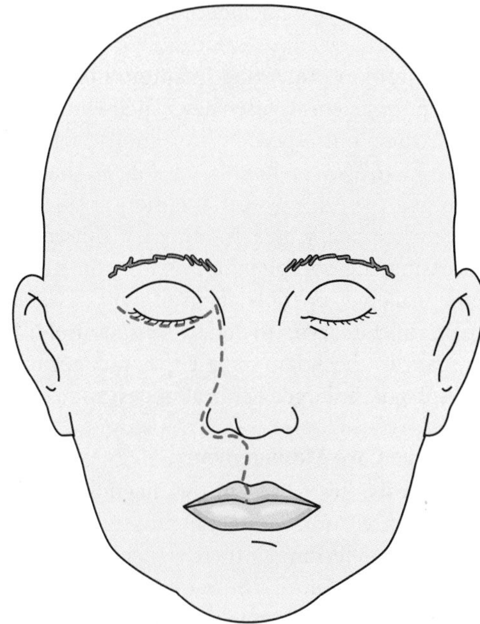

Figure 20-15 Weber-Fergusson incision for maxillectomy.

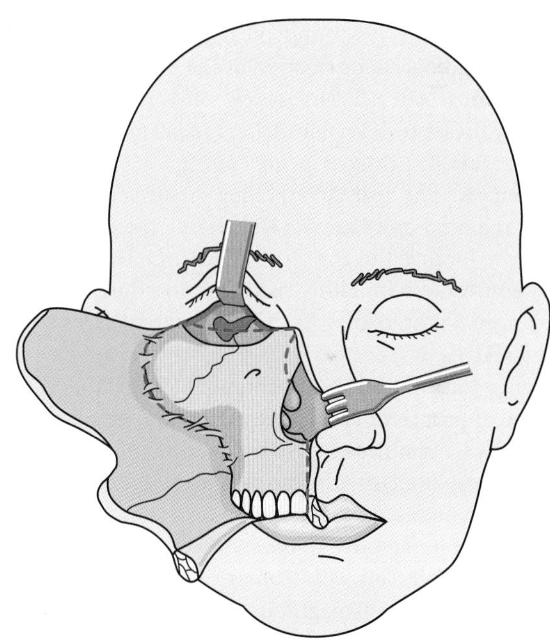

Figure 20-16 Demonstration of exposure and block removal of maxilla with eye preservation. If the tumor extends through the floor of the orbit, the eye must be removed with the maxilla.

Patient/Family Education. Patient education should be focused on "prevention" or early detection. Patients must be taught how to identify the risk factors. Referrals should be offered to those with further questions, a history of longstanding chronic sinusitis, concerns, or a need for follow-up on an already-identified lesion.

CARCINOMA OF THE LARYNX

Etiology/Epidemiology

Squamous cell carcinoma of the larynx is increasing in frequency. It is estimated that in the United States more than 12,600 new cases and more than 3800 deaths associated with carcinoma of the larynx occur every year.[3]

Epidemiology

Cancer of the larynx is five times more common in men than in women, and it occurs most often in persons over 60 years of age. There appears to be a relationship between cancer of the larynx and heavy smoking, heavy alcohol intake, chronic laryngitis, vocal abuse, and family predisposition to cancer. Because of an increase in the number of women who are heavy smokers, the incidence of carcinoma of the larynx among this group is increasing.[12]

Pathophysiology

Squamous cell carcinoma can arise from any part of the laryngeal mucous membrane. It is often preceded by leukoplakia. Cancer of the larynx limited to the true vocal cords rarely spreads to the cervical lymph nodes because of the limited lymphatic supply. Elsewhere in the larynx (epiglottis, false vocal cords, and pyriform sinuses), lymphatic vessels are abundant, and cancer of these tissues often spreads rapidly and metastasizes early to the deep lymph nodes of the neck. Tumors of the supraglottic and infraglottic portions of the larynx have a 35% to 40% incidence of metastasis to mid to low jugular nodes.

The most common presenting symptom of laryngeal cancer is persistent hoarseness, often associated with otalgia and dysphagia. Anyone, but especially any smoker, who becomes progressively hoarse or is hoarse for longer than 2 weeks should be urged to seek medical attention at once. If treatment is given when hoarseness first appears (caused by the tumor's preventing the complete approximation of the vocal cord), a cure usually is possible. Signs of metastases of cancer to other parts of the larynx include a sensation of a lump in the throat, pain in the Adam's apple that radiates to the ear, dyspnea, dysphagia, enlarged cervical nodes, and cough.

Collaborative Care Management

Diagnostic Tests. Tests used in the diagnosis of laryngeal cancers include direct and indirect fiberoptic laryngoscopy; a chest x-ray film to determine if there is metastasis to the lung, a second primary tumor, or chronic obstructive pulmonary disease; a barium swallow to rule out metastasis to the esophagus, determine the extent of the tumor, and evaluate swallowing ability; and a CT scan to determine if there is metastasis to lymph nodes or adjacent structures. If laryngeal ulceration or a mass is found on laryngoscopy, a biopsy is taken for pathologic confirmation of the diagnosis.

Medications. After laryngoscopy, only pain medications are usually prescribed. Preadmission medications such as digitalis preparations or diuretics are continued.

Treatments. The primary therapy is surgical excision or primary radiotherapy. Patients with early-stage lesions (T_1 or T_2) that are localized to the glottis have an 85% to 90% cure rate when treated with either of these procedures. Surgery is either an endoscopic laser excision or partial laryngectomy (Table 20-5).

Patients with more extensive tumors (T_3 or T_4) require a combined approach of surgical resection and preoperative or postoperative radiotherapy. Newer treatment regimens add chemotherapy with cisplatin and 5-fluorouracil along with radiotherapy in an attempt to preserve the larynx. Chemotherapy alone is never curative in these cancers.

If these therapies fail, if the tumor recurs, or if there are extensive tumors with cartilaginous invasion, a total laryngectomy is required. Some patients also require a modified neck dissection.

Surgical Management

Hemilaryngectomy. In hemilaryngectomy, or vertical partial laryngectomy, one half of the larynx is removed (Figure 20-17). This procedure is usually well tolerated. The patient is not allowed to swallow for 7 to 10 days postoperatively, but difficulty in swallowing is not a long-term problem. The quality of the voice is adequate for communication.

Removal of more than one half of the larynx or a portion of the second vocal cord is called a subtotal laryngectomy. Removal of more of the second cord causes more difficulty in swallowing. Thin liquids are the most difficult to swallow, and thickened liquids and soft foods are recommended. Speech pathologists are often consulted to assist patients with swallowing technique.

Supraglottic Laryngectomy. When the supraglottis is invaded by cancer, a supraglottic laryngectomy (horizontal partial laryngectomy) is performed (Figure 20-18). Because the true vocal cords are preserved, the patient's voice quality is excellent. The major postoperative problem is the danger of aspiration because of difficulty swallowing. Aspiration may occur because the major reflex arc that causes closure of the larynx is initiated by sensory receptors in the supraglottic larynx, which has been removed. These patients need special swallowing training postoperatively. Patients take variable amounts of time to learn to swallow safely, and it may be 2 to 3 weeks or longer before oral feedings are started. When aspiration is suspected, methylene blue dye, grape juice, or food coloring is added to drinks and swallowed, and the color is checked for in tracheal secretions.

After a partial laryngectomy a temporary tracheostomy tube is inserted. It is removed when edema in the surrounding tissues subsides. The person is not on absolute voice rest but is advised not to use the voice until the surgeon gives specific approval (usually 3 days after surgery). In the past, whispering was allowed, but it is now believed that whispering can further damage the voice. The person usually adjusts readily to the relatively minor limitations of speech.[23]

Total Laryngectomy. When cancer of the larynx is advanced, a total laryngectomy may be performed. This includes

TABLE 20-5 Laryngectomy Surgery for Cancer

Type	Description	Voice Result	Swallowing Ability
Partial Laryngectomy			
Hemilaryngectomy	Opening into larynx through thyroid cartilage with removal of diseased false cord, arytenoid, and one side of thyroid cartilage	Hoarse voice	Initially need swallowing therapy to learn how to swallow without aspirating
Supraglottic partial laryngectomy	Horizontal incision passes above true cords (leaving cords intact) with removal of epiglottis and diseased tissue	Normal voice	Same as above
Total laryngectomy	Removal of epiglottis, thyroid cartilage, and three or four tracheal rings; closure of pharynx with trachea; permanent tracheostomy	No voice	No swallowing problem

removal of the epiglottis, thyroid cartilage (larynx), hyoid bone, cricoid cartilage, and three or four rings of the trachea. The pharyngeal opening to the trachea is closed, and the remainder of the trachea is brought out to the neck wound and sutured to the skin to form a permanent tracheostomy through which the patient breathes (Figure 20-19). The patient loses the sense of smell because breathing through the nose is impossible. Initially the person has a runny nose because sniffing in and out is not possible. The person has no voice because of loss of the larynx. Nursing care of the patient

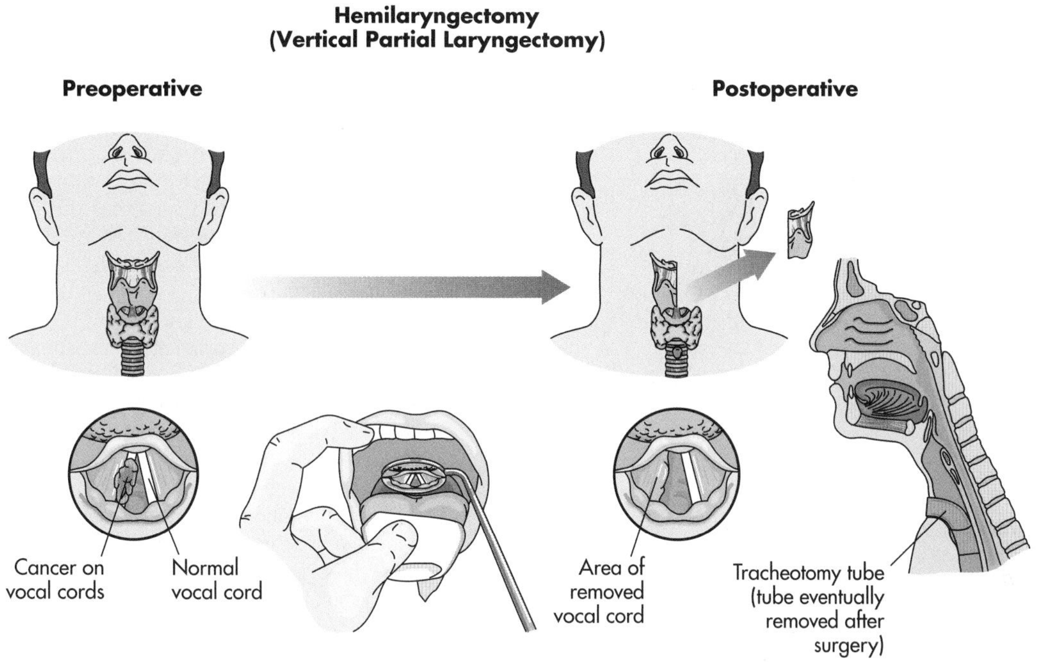

Hemilaryngectomy
(Vertical Partial Laryngectomy)
Preoperative
Postoperative
Cancer on vocal cords
Normal vocal cord
Area of removed vocal cord
Tracheotomy tube (tube eventually removed after surgery)

Figure 20-17 Technique of hemilaryngectomy (vertical partial laryngectomy).

Supraglottic Laryngectomy
(Horizontal Partial)
Planned tissue to be excised
Tracheotomy opening
Preop. Frontal View
Tongue
Trachea
Preop. Lateral View
Postop. Lateral View
Tracheotomy tube (tube eventually removed after surgery)

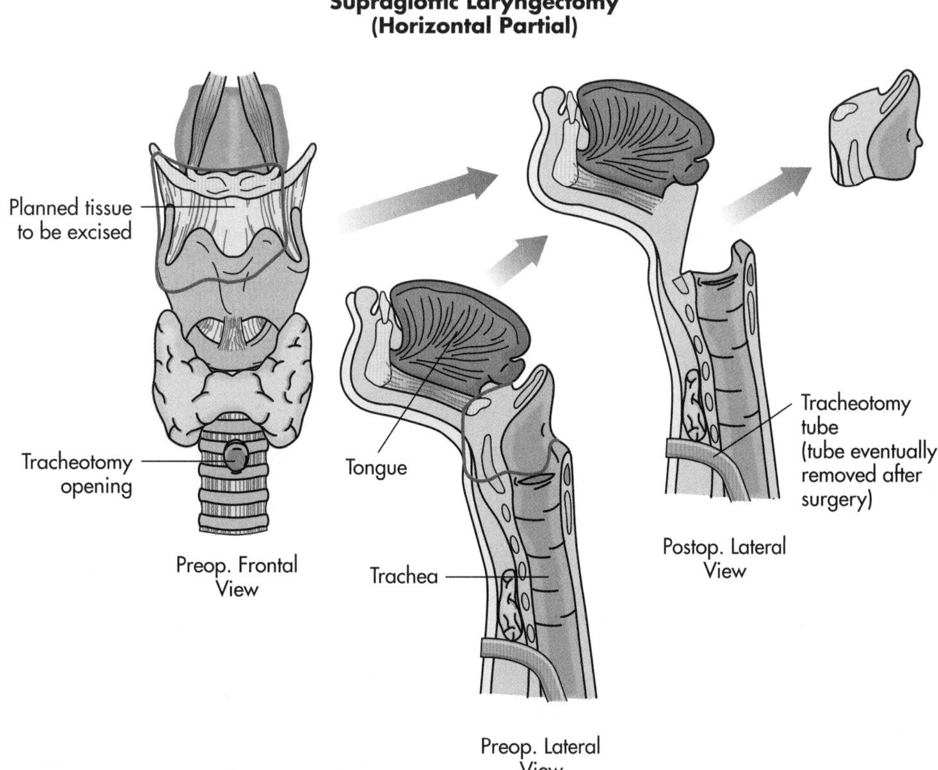

Figure 20-18 Technique of supraglottic laryngectomy. Removal of endolaryngeal structures from tip of epiglottis down to laryngeal vertical.

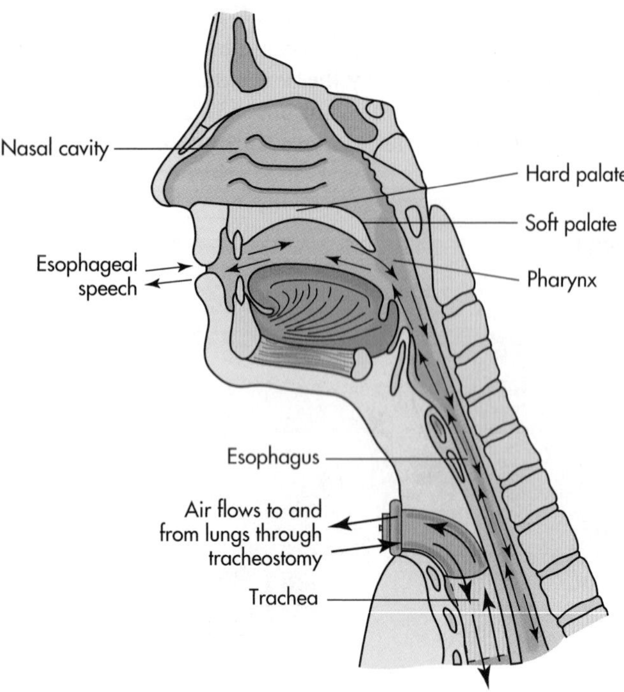

Figure 20-19 Permanent tracheostomy: no connection exists between trachea and esophagus.

after a total laryngectomy is outlined in the Guidelines for Safe Practice box and the Nursing Care Plan.

Radical Neck Dissection. A radical neck dissection may be performed along with the laryngectomy when risk of metastasis to the neck is high (i.e., when the size and location of the primary tumor are known to result in metastasis or when palpable cervical lymph nodes are found during surgery). In a radical neck dissection the submandibular salivary gland, sternocleidomastoid muscle, internal jugular vein, and spinal accessory nerves are removed. This extensive surgery is done to ensure complete removal of node-bearing tissue or to prevent nodal spread. In some patients modifications of a radical neck dissection are performed. These are referred to as selective, modified, conservative, or functional neck dissections and are used when the nodal metastatic disease is not far advanced. Radical neck dissection causes atrophy of the trapezius muscle, and the shoulder droops on the side of surgery.

Patients can be assisted by the physical therapist or nurse in range-of-motion exercises, which will gradually replace the function of the lost muscles with that of other muscles.[6] Initially the patient may have some difficulty lifting the head and must place the hands with fingers interlocked behind the head to lift it from the pillow.

The patient can breathe best in a mid-Fowler's position. This position helps reduce facial edema, improve circulation, and reduce or prevent headaches from lymphedema. Pressure dressings are not recommended in radical neck dissection, because they compromise the blood supply to the skin flaps protecting the vital neck structures.[7]

Guidelines for Safe Practice

Care of the Patient After Total Laryngectomy

Nursing care after a total laryngectomy includes:

1. Comfort and airway management
   a. Elevate head of bed 45 degrees.
   b. Encourage coughing, deep breathing every 4 hours.
   c. Maintain oxygen to tracheostomy collar.
   d. Assess airway patency every shift and as needed.
   e. Assess vital signs, quality and rate of respiration, and skin color (pallor, cyanosis).
   f. Auscultate lungs every shift and as needed.
2. Suture line and stoma care
   a. Assess suture line and stoma site every 4 hours.
   b. Report erythema, purulent drainage, hematoma.
   c. Care for suture line and stoma site as ordered by surgeon.
   d. Monitor drain function and output.
   e. Maintain suction to drain at level ordered.
   f. Milk tubing every 1 to 2 hours for 24 hours, and then every 4 hours and as needed.
   g. Report changes in amount and color of drainage or air leak.
3. Fluid/food and hygiene needs
   a. Monitor hydration and ensure adequate fluid intake to maintain healthy oral mucosa; provide mouth care at least three times daily.
   b. Record intake and output every shift.
   c. Weigh daily at the same time and in the same amount of clothing.
   d. Provide stoma and stoma vent care every shift and as needed.
   e. Administer enteral feedings per order.
   f. Assess patient's tolerance of feedings.
   g. Assess bowel sounds every shift and as needed.
   h. Report intolerance to feedings (nausea, fullness, inability to tolerate prescribed amount of feedings).
   i. Record amount, consistency, and frequency of stools.
   j. Assess swallowing ability and provide support when oral diet resumes.
4. Patient/family education and support
   a. Begin teaching laryngectomy care.
   b. Assess anxiety level and provide emotional support.
   c. Assist patient in communicating.
   d. Provide patient with writing materials, picture board.
   e. Use questions that can be answered "yes" or "no."
   f. Reinforce use of artificial speech device and encourage its use.
   g. Monitor patient's reaction to change in body image.
   h. Be sensitive to patient's reactions to changes in appearance.
   i. Provide time to listen to patient.
   j. Encourage use of Lost Chord or New Voice Club.
   k. Prepare patient for discharge.
   l. Monitor ability of patient or significant other to perform airway management care.
   m. Provide patient with a list of supplies necessary for home care.
   n. Provide information about soft diet.
   o. Review written instructions in home-going booklet with patient and family.
   p. Refer to home nursing staff to assess patient's ability to perform self-care at home.
   q. Refer to speech pathologist for voice/speech rehabilitation.

Nursing Care Plan *Patient Undergoing Total Laryngectomy*

DATA Mr. K., a 68-year-old man, had noted progressive hoarseness for several months. Indirect laryngoscopy and biopsy confirmed cancer of the larynx, and he was admitted for a total laryngectomy. His wife has been attentive and supportive.

On admission the nurse identified that the patient:

- Was visibly apprehensive (paced the floor, was restless, asked repeated questions)
- Had as a major concern the extent of his cancer and its effect on his speech postoperatively
- Is 175 cm (5 feet 10 inches) tall; weight on admission was 68 kg (150 pounds)
- Wears glasses for near vision, which is poor without glasses

During surgery the larynx was removed and a permanent tracheostomy was performed with insertion of a temporary laryngectomy tube. A nasogastric tube was inserted, which will be removed after Mr. K. is swallowing well.

Today (the first postoperative day) Mr. K. again appears apprehensive (restless, points frequently to his tracheostomy, pulls on his wife's hand, and points to the cord on the call light). Breath sounds are clear in the upper lobes but absent in the lower lobes. Codeine and acetaminophen have been prescribed for pain.

NURSING DIAGNOSIS **Ineffective airway clearance related to secretions in upper airway and laryngectomy tube**
GOALS/OUTCOMES Will remain free of airway obstruction

NOC Suggested Outcomes
- Respiratory Status: Airway Patency (0410)
- Respiratory Status: Gas Exchange (0402)
- Respiratory Status: Ventilation (0403)
- Aspiration Control (1918)

NIC Suggested Interventions
- Artificial Airway Management (3180)
- Airway Suctioning (3160)
- Respiratory Monitoring (3350)
- Aspiration Precautions (3200)

Nursing Interventions/Rationales
- Place patient in semi-Fowler's position. *This position uses gravity to help expand the thorax and decrease pressure on the lower lung lobes.*
- Suction laryngectomy tube as needed as evidenced by noisy respirations, increased pulse and respiratory rate, and restlessness (suction requirements vary between 2 and 4 hours). *Air blowing through secretions produces noisy respiration; pulse and respirations are increased when oxygen intake is decreased; restlessness may indicate decreased oxygenation.*
- Provide tracheostomy care. *Keeping the tracheostomy tube patent facilitates air exchange and decreases the risk for infection.*
- Provide humidification. *Humidity helps keep secretions liquid for easier removal and prevents the formation of mucus plugs.*
- Encourage deep breathing and coughing exercises. *Deep breathing helps aerate the lower lung lobes; coughing helps the patient expel secretions.*

Evaluation Parameters
1. Respirations effortless, quiet, and at baseline rate
2. Breath sounds clear at all lobes

NURSING DIAGNOSIS **Anxiety related to breathing difficulties and inability to communicate**
GOALS/OUTCOMES Will report reduction in level of experienced anxiety following use of coping mechanisms

NOC Suggested Outcomes
- Anxiety Control (1402)
- Coping (1302)
- Psychosocial Adjustment: Life Change (1305)

NIC Suggested Interventions
- Anxiety Reduction (5820)
- Calming Technique (5880)
- Coping Enhancement (5230)
- Presence (5340)
- Coping Enhancement: Speech Deficit (4976)

Nursing Interventions/Rationales
- Carry out regular suctioning of tracheostomy after explaining benefit to patient. *If the patient knows the tube will be suctioned frequently and that suctioning will keep his airway open, fear of possible asphyxiation may diminish.*
- Develop a means of communication (e.g., cards with needs printed clearly or paper for writing). Be sure patient wears his glasses. *When patients can communicate their needs, fear and resultant anxiety are often relieved.*
- After the initial postoperative time period and if patient's wife is willing and able, teach her how to suction the tracheostomy. *Participating in her husband's care may help the wife to feel that she is helping, thus reducing her anxiety. Anxiety can be transferred from wife to husband.*

Continued

Nursing Care Plan *Patient Undergoing Total Laryngectomy—cont'd*

- Encourage patient to care for his own tracheostomy when feasible. *Self-care increases self-confidence and enhances feelings of control over the situation, thus reducing anxiety.*

Evaluation Parameters

1. Accurately verbalizes signs of anxiety
2. Demonstrates use of anxiety-lowering strategies
3. Demonstrates use of positive coping mechanisms

NURSING DIAGNOSIS **Acute pain related to surgery**
GOALS/OUTCOMES Will achieve pain-free status

NOC Suggested Outcomes

- Pain Control (2120)
- Comfort Level (2100)
- Pain Level (2120)

NIC Suggested Interventions

- Analgesic Administration (2210)
- Pain Management (1400)
- Coping Enhancement (5230)
- Medication Management (2380)

Nursing Interventions/Rationales

- Administer prescribed analgesics to prevent pain from becoming severe. *Analgesics decrease the transmission and perception of pain stimuli.*
- Encourage nonpharmacologic measures to reduce pain, such as relaxation exercises or distraction. *Many nonpharmacologic measures minimize pain perception.*
- Provide nose and mouth care while nasogastric tube is in place. *The nasogastric tube may produce irritation of the nares. The mouth becomes dry and uncomfortable from open-mouth breathing and decreased lubrication. The tube makes swallowing fluids difficult and may cause an earache.*

Evaluation Parameters

1. Reports satisfaction with pain control methods
2. Reports feeling comfortable
3. No evidence of pain (grimace, withdrawn behavior, complaints of pain)

NURSING DIAGNOSIS **Risk for imbalanced nutrition: less than body requirements related to difficulty swallowing**
GOALS/OUTCOMES Weight will remain within 5 pounds of baseline weight

NOC Suggested Outcomes

- Nutritional Status (1004)
- Nutritional Status: Food and Fluid Intake (1008)
- Nutritional Status: Nutrient Intake ((1009)

NIC Suggested Interventions

- Nutrition Management (1100)
- Nutritional Monitoring (1160)
- Nutrition Therapy (1120)
- Enteral Tube Feeding (1056)

Nursing Interventions/Rationales

- Administer prescribed tube feeding via nasogastric tube until patient is able to swallow well. *Tube feedings provide greater adequacy of nutrients than intravenous fluids. Swallowing is impaired initially from postoperative edema of the lower pharynx.*
- Give only fluids until patient is swallowing well after removal of the nasogastric tube. *Initially fluids are easier to swallow past edematous areas of the throat than are solid foods.*
- Explain anatomic changes that have taken place in patient and that there is no connection between the esophagus and the tracheostomy. *An explanation regarding anatomic changes may reduce the patient's concern about choking.*
- Stay with patient during initial eating of semisolid and solid foods. *He may fear choking and not be willing to swallow initially. Encouragement by the nurse with the assurance of suctioning if necessary may give the patient more confidence regarding swallowing.*
- Use measures to encourage eating as necessary (e.g., tray for patient's wife so they can eat together, selection of desired foods). *Returning to usual eating patterns may encourage the patient to eat.*
- Encourage patient to monitor his own weight two to three times per week until baseline weight is regained. *Participating in own weight monitoring may encourage the patient to eat.*

Evaluation Parameters

1. Swallows without difficulty
2. Food intake is sufficient to maintain baseline weight

Nursing Care Plan *Patient Undergoing Total Laryngectomy—cont'd*

NURSING DIAGNOSIS **Impaired verbal communication related to laryngectomy**
GOALS/OUTCOMES Will resume communication with use of electronic larynx

NOC Suggested Outcomes
- Communication Ability (0902)
- Communication: Expressive Ability (0903)

NIC Suggested Interventions
- Communication Enhancement: Speech Deficit (4976)
- Anxiety Reduction (5820)
- Referral (8100)

Nursing Interventions/Rationales
- Encourage patient to communicate via an established system (e.g., electrolarynx, hand signals, writing) during the initial period following surgery. *After removal of the larynx, sounds cannot be made by pervious method of vibrating vocal cords. Alternative methods of communication allow the patient to make his needs and wishes known.*
- Support activities of speech therapist: (a) encourage practice with electronic device; (b) discuss availability of mechanical devices for speech or telephone use. *Until the patient has a tracheoesophageal puncture (TEP), an electronic larynx will help him communicate. Having the ability to communicate raises self-confidence and allows greater personal control.*

Evaluation Parameters
1. Begins to communicate with others
2. Participates in speech rehabilitation
3. Voices satisfaction with ability to communicate needs

NURSING DIAGNOSIS **Risk for impaired skin integrity related to surgical incision**
GOALS/OUTCOMES Will remain free of skin breakdown

NOC Suggested Outcomes
- Tissue Integrity: Skin and Mucous Membranes (1101)
- Wound Healing: Primary Intention (1102)

NIC Suggested Interventions
- Infection Protection (6550)
- Incision Site Care (3440)
- Skin Surveillance (3590)

Nursing Interventions/Rationales
- Maintain sterile technique when cleaning incision and changing dressings. *Keeping the incision clean promotes healing and prevents infection.*
- Monitor drainage device for patency. *Maintaining drain patency prevents the formation of a hematoma under tension. A hematoma places pressure on the suture line, interfering with approximation of wound edges and increases the risk for wound dehiscence, venous congestion, and possible necrosis of the flap.*
- Assess appearance of the wound and report changes promptly. *To detect changes in skin integrity early so that corrective measures can be taken quickly.*

Evaluation Parameters
1. Surgical incision shows evidence of healing
2. No evidence of hematoma or dehiscence

NURSING DIAGNOSIS **Risk for infection related to surgery and potentially altered nutritional status**
GOALS/OUTCOMES Will show no evidence of wound infection

NOC Suggested Outcomes
- Immune Status (0702)
- Nutritional Status (1004)
- Risk Control (1902)

NIC Suggested Interventions
- Infection Protection (6550)
- Skin Surveillance (3590)
- Wound Care (3660)
- Infection Control (6540)

Nursing Interventions/Rationales
- Clean suture line every 4 hours and as needed using sterile technique. *Keeping the suture line clean prevents infection and promotes healing.*
- Monitor negative drainage system for patency. *Prevents hematoma formation and reduces the opportunity for bacteria to grow in the hematoma, which is an excellent culture media.*
- Milk drainage tubing as necessary. *To prevent hematoma formation and resultant infection.*

Continued

Nursing Care Plan — Patient Undergoing Total Laryngectomy—cont'd

- Monitor for signs of localized infection (redness, warmth, tenderness, swelling) and systemic infection (elevated white blood cell [WBC] count, fever, lethargy). *Treatment for infection can be instituted more quickly when signs of infection are recognized early.*

Evaluation Parameters
1. Drainage flows from draining tubing
2. Suture line is free of redness, swelling, warmth, and tenderness
3. Temperature within normal limits
4. WBC count within normal limits

NURSING DIAGNOSIS **Deficient knowledge related to lack of previous experience**
GOALS/OUTCOMES Will accurately describe and participate in self-care

NOC Suggested Outcomes
- Knowledge: Health Resources (1806)
- Knowledge: Infection Control (1807)
- Knowledge: Treatment Procedures (1814)

NIC Suggested Interventions
- Teaching: Psychomotor Skill (5620)
- Teaching: Procedure/Treatment (5618)

Nursing Interventions/Rationales
- Teach patient (1) description of anatomic changes; (2) care of the stoma, including self-suctioning; (3) methods of protecting the stoma; and (4) availability of community resources. *When the patient learns how to provide his own care, it will give him self-confidence and control over his situation. Care is needed to keep the tracheostomy open for air exchange. Resources such as the Lost Cord Club are available to persons experiencing laryngectomy.*
- Repeat teaching frequently. *Stress interferes with learning. There is too much information to learn at one time. Therefore repetitive teaching enhances learning.*
- Encourage patient to maintain a soft diet for at least 2 weeks following discharge. *Soft foods are easier to swallow, allowing the patient to develop self-confidence with eating a variety of foods.*

Evaluation Parameters
1. Expresses interest in assuming self-care
2. Accurately demonstrates wound care
3. Accurately describes at-home care

NURSING DIAGNOSIS **Disturbed body image related to altered anatomic appearance and function**
GOALS/OUTCOMES Will accept body changes and integrate those changes into view of self

NOC Suggested Outcomes
- Body Image (1200)
- Psychosocial Adjustment: Life Change (1305)
- Acceptance: Health Status (1300)

NIC Suggested Interventions
- Body Image Enhancement (5220)
- Emotional Support (5270)
- Coping Enhancement (5230)

Nursing Interventions/Rationales
- Prepare patient and significant other preoperatively for changes in appearance and loss of voice. *Clarify their perception of information provided by the surgeon and speech pathologist to allow for corrections of misunderstandings.*
- Provide time to discuss with patient and family their feelings regarding expected changes preoperatively and actual changes postoperatively. *Allows the opportunity to ventilate feelings of anger and grief in a safe environment.*
- Refer patient and family to other services as needed (e.g., speech pathology, social work) and to community support groups for patients undergoing laryngectomy. *Supports multidisciplinary approach to patient care. Helps the patient understand the roles of others. Allows discussion with other patients who have had the same experiences.*

Evaluation Parameters
1. Begins to talk about bodily changes and their impact on his life
2. Asks for information about support groups and referrals
3. Participates in support group discussions

Often a Hemovac (Figure 20-20) or another suction device is attached to drains placed in the incision in the operating room. Its purpose is to maintain constant drainage from the neck wound and prevent pressure on the skin flaps. The drain is checked regularly to see that it is working properly and there is no edema, which might indicate that a hematoma is developing. The tubing is milked every 1 to 2 hours for the first 24 hours after surgery and then every 4 hours and as needed. Changes in the amount or color of drainage should be reported to the surgeon.

Radical neck dissection can be performed without laryngectomy for persons whose primary malignant lesion is in the oral cavity, oropharynx, or parasinuses. Often the procedure accompanies other procedures and is referred to as a composite resection. Composite resections may consist of radical neck dissection plus removal of the mandible; removal of the mandible with resection of the floor of the mouth; or removal of the mandible, the floor of the mouth, and the tongue. Patients who undergo a composite resection usually have a tracheostomy.

Emotional reactions to this type of radical surgery may be profound. Disfigurement is readily visible, and reactions to the change in body image are marked. In addition to the usual fears of surgery and cancer, the patient having a composite resection may have fears of rejection and fears concerning the future.[7]

Nursing care for patients after a radical neck dissection is outlined in the Guidelines for Safe Practice box.

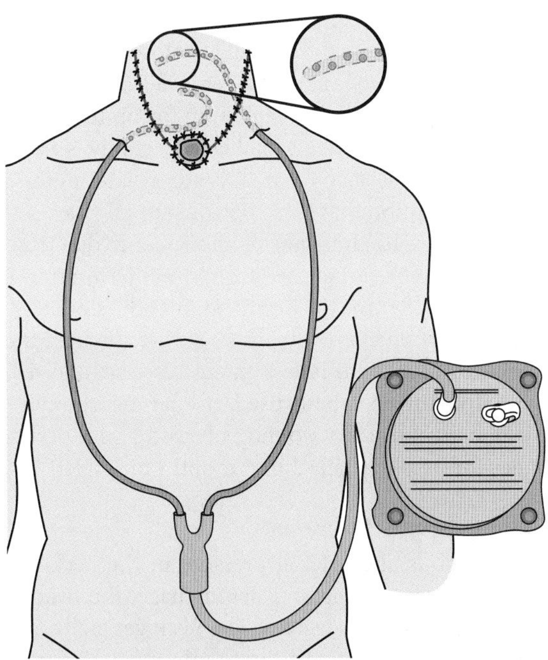

Figure 20-20 Hemovac apparatus for constant closed suction. In this system of wound drainage, suction is maintained by a plastic container with a spring inside that tries to force apart the lids and thereby produces suction that is transmitted through plastic tubing. Neck skin is pulled down tight, and no external dressing is required. The container serves as both a suction source and a receptacle for blood. It is emptied as required, and drainage tubes are left in the neck for 3 days.

Guidelines for Safe Practice

Care of the Patient After Radical Neck Dissection

Nursing care after radical neck dissection includes:

1. Comfort and airway management
   a. Elevate head of bed 30 degrees.
   b. Maintain oxygen mist therapy if ordered.
   c. Encourage coughing, deep breathing, and use of incentive spirometer.
   d. Assess airway for signs and symptoms of increasing airway obstruction (stridor, dyspnea, increased pulse and respiratory rate).
   e. Monitor vital signs every 4 hours.
2. Wound assessment and care
   a. Maintain venous access with large-bore needle.
   b. If hemorrhage occurs: stat-page physician, apply direct pressure, suction airway, and reassure patient.
   c. Care for suture line as ordered.
   d. Maintain drainage output, color, and consistency.
   e. Maintain suction to drain.
   f. Milk tubing every 1 to 2 hours for 24 hours; and then every 4 hours and as needed.
   g. Check for air leak in drain.
   h. Assess for signs and symptoms of infection of suture line (erythema, pus, elevated temperature).
   i. Assess skin flap every shift for signs and symptoms of poor drain patency or infection: swelling, bleeding, oozing of suture line, or dehiscence.
   j. Monitor intake and output and record every shift.
3. Prevention of complications
   a. Monitor shoulder droop secondary to loss of nerve supply to trapezius muscle and inability to raise hand over head.
   b. Reinforce need to do shoulder-strengthening exercise three times per day.
   c. Consult physical therapist with concerns about patient's exercises.
   d. Monitor for difficulty in swallowing related to postoperative swelling and xerostomia (dry mouth) from radiation therapy preoperatively.
4. Nutritional management
   a. Monitor patient's ability to ingest optimal caloric intake.
   b. Weigh daily at same time and with same amount of clothing.
   c. Consult with dietitian and physician if desired caloric intake cannot be met.
   d. Explain about role of diet in wound healing.
5. Patient/family teaching and support
   a. Provide emotional support.
   b. Monitor depression, which is not uncommon after disfiguring surgery.
   c. Identify members of patient support system and involve them and patient in planning and giving care.
   d. Plan for specific time to provide emotional support.
   e. Help patient verbalize feelings about having cancer, changes in body image, and changes in lifestyle.
   f. Refer to home care nursing staff to assess patient's ability to care for self at home.
   g. Teach suture line care for home going. Cleanse site with half-strength hydrogen peroxide followed by antibiotic ointment twice daily to keep incision line free of crusting.
   h. Provide optimal pain management.
   i. Encourage activity to prevent permanent disability.[5]

Diet. Diet includes tube feedings after surgery, progressing to a soft diet. Protein is encouraged for wound healing.

Activity. The patient is up in a chair on the first postoperative day and can walk in the hall beginning on the second postoperative day.

Referrals. Common referrals for patients who have undergone a laryngectomy include social services, speech pathology, respiratory therapy, and physical therapy.

NURSING MANAGEMENT OF PATIENT UNDERGOING LARYNGEAL SURGERY

PREOPERATIVE CARE

Before surgery the patient who is to undergo a total laryngectomy is told by the physician that breathing will occur through a permanent opening made in the neck and that normal speech will not be possible. This information is often depressing to the patient because it may threaten economic status, as well as quality of life. The patient meets with a speech pathologist before surgery to learn about options for postoperative rehabilitation and speech. In some instances a visit from another person who has made a good recovery from total laryngectomy and who has undergone rehabilitation successfully is helpful. In other instances the visit may depress the patient further. Careful assessment must be made to determine if the patient will benefit from such a visit and whether the visit should be made preoperatively, immediately after surgery, or later in the recovery period.

In some medical centers the visit is planned for 5 to 7 days after surgery. Even though the patient and significant other may be hesitant about the visit, they often indicate afterward that the visit was helpful and improved their outlook about the patient's future.

Many large cities have a Lost Chord Club or a New Voice Club, and the members are willing to visit hospitalized patients. Information regarding these clubs may be obtained by writing to the International Association of Laryngectomees.*[1] Local speech rehabilitation centers may supply instructive films and other resources. The local chapters of the American Cancer Society and the local health department also have information. If possible, the family should also learn about the method of esophageal speech that the person will be learning.

IMMEDIATE POSTOPERATIVE CARE

Like all patients who have had head and neck surgery, patients who have undergone a laryngectomy require hemodynamic monitoring, airway monitoring, and wound and flap monitoring after surgery.

Maintaining a Patent Airway

Some degree of airway obstruction is common in patients after a partial laryngectomy, from either preoperative radiotherapy or swelling from surgery close to the airway.

To prevent emergency airway situations, a tracheostomy is performed at the time of surgery.[16] A cuffed tracheostomy tube is generally inserted to (1) allow ventilation after surgery until the patient wakes from anesthesia, (2) prevent blood from the surgical site from entering the tracheobronchial tree, (3) prevent pharyngeal and gastric secretions from soiling the bronchial tree, and (4) maintain an adequate airway when edema from surgery or radiation is expected.

The tracheostomy cuff is kept inflated until the morning after surgery or until the patient can manage his or her secretions. The patient is suctioned every 2 to 4 hours to prevent the buildup of secretions in the tracheobronchial tree or in the tracheostomy tube. When the cuffed tracheostomy tube is being suctioned, the patient is suctioned orally before the cuff is deflated to prevent aspiration of secretions accumulated above the cuff. In some centers 3 to 5 ml of sterile saline may be instilled in the tube to soften and dislodge thickened secretions.

Patients receive cool mist therapy with a T tube. They also receive incentive spirometry and chest physiotherapy and, if necessary, aerosol and systemic bronchodilators.

When a cuffed tracheostomy tube is no longer necessary (not earlier than the third postoperative day), an uncuffed tube is inserted. Cuffless tubes are less harmful to the trachea, interfere less with swallowing, and minimize aspiration. Because there is no cuff, secretions cannot accumulate above it. Also, the cuffless tube allows the patient to occlude the tube with a finger and speak, which is a significant psychologic boost to the patient. Because the patient is able to expectorate secretions and has an adequate airway, the tracheostomy tube is plugged for increasing periods of time. The goal is to remove the tube and allow the opening to close by secondary intention. Some patients' tubes are removed 5 to 7 days after surgery; other patients' tubes remain in for up to 10 days.

Care for the person after a total laryngectomy is essentially the same as that described for tracheostomy later in the chapter with the exception that these persons usually have a laryngectomy tube in place. It is shorter and wider in diameter than a tracheostomy tube. Some patients may not have a tube in the laryngeal stoma after the operation because the stoma is a permanent one kept open initially by the sutures because the surgeon believes that there is less tissue reaction and a better laryngeal stoma if no tube is used. If a laryngectomy tube is used, it remains until the wound is healed and a permanent fistula has formed—usually 3 to 6 months or longer.

Maintaining Proper Positioning

To reduce venous and arterial pressure in the neck and decrease the risk of swelling and hemorrhage, the head of the bed is elevated 30 to 45 degrees. The neck generally is maintained in a slightly flexed position to minimize tension on the suture lines. However, some patients require greater neck flexion or rotation to minimize tension or flexion of the flaps used for reconstruction. If the procedure is uncomplicated, the patient is usually up in a chair on the first postoperative day and is able to walk in the hall with assistance on the second day.

*American Cancer Society, Inc., 1599 Clifton Road NE, Atlanta, GA 30329, (404) 320-3333 or (800) ALS-2345.

Managing the Wound

In head and neck surgery, complications are always a threat because of extensive undermining of subcutaneous tissues to elevate the skin flaps, contamination at the time of surgery when the upper aerodigestive tract is entered, and the poor quality of tissue in persons who receive preoperative radiotherapy.

The surgical site is closed either with interrupted or running sutures or staples, and the wound is left exposed (no dressing). Monitoring of the wound site is critical to safe patient care, and the persons caring for the patient need to be familiar with the initial appearance of the wound so that any changes are readily apparent. The viability of the skin flaps is assessed by noting the color, temperature, capillary refill, and induration. Slight erythema and induration of the skin flaps are normal in the early postoperative period. The incision should be kept free of crusting and exudates.

The suture line is assessed for signs of approximation, edema, color, and drainage. The incision is cleansed with half-strength hydrogen peroxide solution using clean technique. Cotton swabs are used to remove crusts. Antibiotic ointment is applied to the wound to seal the suture line. Drain exit sites and the tracheostomy incision receive the same care as the suture line. A minimal amount of bleeding from skin edges is normal in the immediate postoperative period. A more diffuse ooze of darker, red blood, along with swelling of the wound, indicates that a hematoma is developing, and the surgeon must be notified immediately. It is especially important to closely monitor the wounds of patients who received radiotherapy preoperatively because they are more prone to wound dehiscence or the development of a pharyngocutaneous fistula.

Maintaining the Closed Drainage System

A closed drainage system with continuous suction is used to eliminate dead space and prevent accumulation of blood, serum, and other secretions under the skin flaps. Many drainage systems are available (e.g., Davol, Hemovac, Jackson-Pratt), and all provide a continuous negative pressure of 80 to 120 mm Hg. They are monitored for function, the presence of air leaks, and the type and amount of drainage. If the drainage system is not functioning properly, a massive hematoma under tension can develop, which may require that the patient return to surgery for exploration, control of bleeding, and restoration of the drainage system.

If air continuously seeps into the drainage system, negative pressure will not be maintained. Air leaks should be corrected immediately. If the air leak is through the suture line, the problem can be solved by adding sutures or applying thick antibiotic ointment to the incision. In some situations a circular dressing is applied to the neck if no reconstruction flap is involved. If the air leak is minimal, the drain can be connected to wall suction. When a massive air leak occurs, the drain may need to be replaced and the leak obliterated. When the tubing is milked, the wound is examined to determine if fluid is accumulating under the flaps.

The type and amount of drainage are recorded every 8 hours. The amount of drainage in the first 16 hours can vary from less than 100 ml to as much as 300 ml. Initially the drainage is sanguineous to serosanguineous. The drains are removed when the drainage is less than 30 ml per 24-hour period. Purulent or granular serous drainage mixed with air (with an odor to it) is considered abnormal and indicates a probable pharyngocutaneous fistula.

ONGOING POSTOPERATIVE CARE

Nutrition

A nasogastric tube, inserted during the surgical procedure, is used for the instillation of food and fluids at regular intervals after both partial and total laryngectomy (Figure 20-21). The use of a nasogastric tube to give food is thought to minimize contamination of the pharyngeal and esophageal suture lines and to prevent fluid from leaking through the wound into the trachea before healing occurs. The nasogastric tube is removed as soon as the person can swallow safely. The person who has undergone a total laryngectomy requires careful attention during his or her first attempts to swallow, even though aspiration cannot occur because the trachea is no longer communicating with the esophagus. The person who has undergone a partial laryngectomy, especially a supraglottic laryngectomy, has to relearn swallowing and is at significant risk for aspiration. After tube feedings are discontinued, soft, formed foods, such as ice cream and mashed potatoes, are begun. The patient is instructed to hold the breath, flex the head, and tilt it toward the unaffected side; place a small amount of food on the back of the tongue; swallow; and then cough to expel any food that entered the trachea. Other foods and fluids are added to the diet as the patient masters the technique of swallowing.

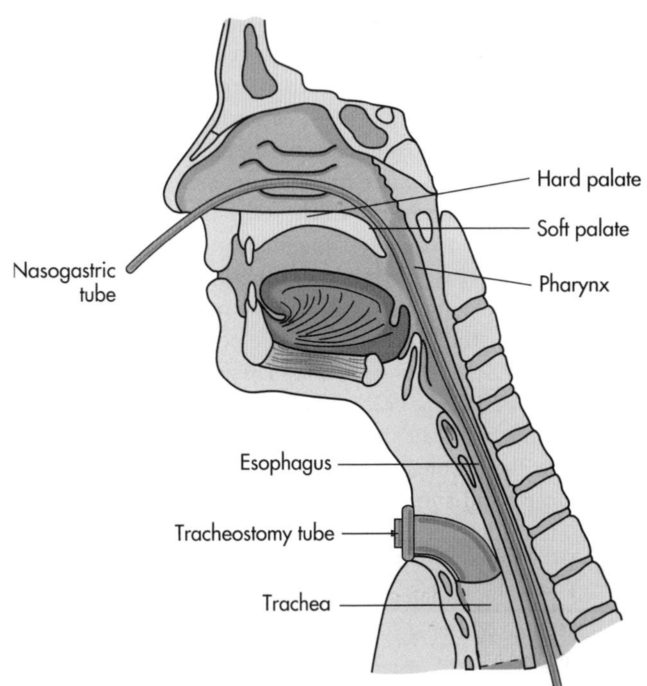

Figure 20-21 Position of tracheostomy tube and nasogastric tube after total laryngectomy.

The sense of smell is affected after a total laryngectomy because breathing through the nose is impossible; therefore the patient does not receive normal olfactory sensations. Some patients report that they are able to smell, and most have drainage from the nose for a period of time. See the Guidelines for Safe Practice boxes for a summary of postoperative care of the patient after a total laryngectomy and for postoperative care of the patient after neck dissection. Also see the Nursing Care Plan for the patient undergoing a total laryngectomy.

Body Image

Some alteration of appearance is readily visible, which may cause the person to feel somewhat conspicuous. Anger, grief, or denial may be part of the normal response to the change in body image.[23]

Speech Rehabilitation

There are three types of speech possible after a total laryngectomy: (1) speech via an artificial larynx, or electrolarynx, which is learned immediately after surgery; (2) esophageal speech; and (3) tracheoesophageal speech.[13]

Until recently, esophageal speech, which is speech produced by expelling swallowed air (burping) across constricted tissue in the pharyngoesophageal segment, was the primary speech method used after laryngectomy. Although this method of speech was successful for many laryngectomees, others could never learn to use it. In addition, the use of radiotherapy after a total laryngectomy, which is increasing, causes fibrous tissue to form, making esophageal speech difficult to master.

For tracheoesophageal speech, a tracheoesophageal puncture (TEP) is made to create a tracheoesophageal fistula large enough to permit the insertion of a valve prosthesis. Some surgeons create the tracheoesophageal fistula after the larynx has been resected and a frozen section reveals that all of the carcinoma has been removed. Other surgeons prefer to wait until the patient has completed postoperative radiotherapy. This may be as long as 3 to 6 months after surgery. The reason for deferring creation of the tracheoesophageal fistula is that this allows time for edema of the incision to abate. Also, radiotherapy may cause shrinking of the skin around the incision. The tracheoesophageal fistula may require an overnight hospital stay, or the procedure may be performed in an outpatient setting. In this procedure a small fistula is created from the superior wall of the tracheal stoma into the proximal wall of the esophagus. A red rubber catheter is pulled through the fistula into the esophagus at the 12 o'clock position of the laryngostoma and sutured into place (Figure 20-22, *A*). The end of the catheter is occluded with a plug or an umbilical clamp, or a knot is tied in the catheter. The patient is discharged with the catheter in place. The prosthesis is inserted 5 to 7 days later by the speech pathologist or the surgeon. The patient is taught how to speak with the TEP at this time. Figure 20-22, *B*, shows placement of the prosthesis.

The prosthesis is a hollow silicone tube with a one-way valve that is open at the tracheal end and closed with a horizontal slit at the laryngopharyngeal end. When the patient talks, air pressure opens the closed end, permitting air to enter the laryngopharynx. When the patient stops talking, the laryngopharyngeal end closes, preventing saliva from draining into the trachea. Because air is diverted from the trachea into the esophagus, this form of speech is referred to as tracheoesophageal speech.[13]

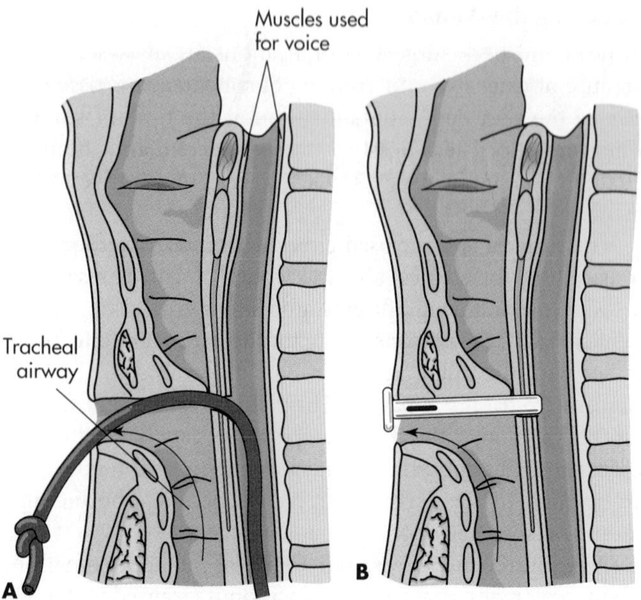

Figure 20-22 Tracheoesophageal puncture (TEP). **A,** Placement of red rubber catheter into TEP. Note knot in end of catheter to prevent passage of stomach contents. **B,** Placement of voice prosthesis into TEP.

The stoma must be occluded during speech, either by placing a finger over the opening of the valve or by using a special tracheostomal valve inserted after the patient has learned to use the prosthesis. The patient or family must be taught to remove, clean, and reinsert the voice prosthesis rapidly so that the fistula does not stenose.[22] Not all patients and families are comfortable with removing and cleaning the prosthesis, and considerable support by the speech pathologist may be necessary. The patient and family need to be taught how to place a rubber catheter into the fistula if the prosthesis comes out (see Figure 20-22, *A*). After placement, the catheter is knotted and taped to the chest. The patient should then see a physician.[22]

Advantages of tracheoesophageal speech include more rapid restoration of voice, speech that is closer to normal in rate and phrasing, and speech that is more pleasing than speech with an electrolarynx. Disadvantages include reliance on a prosthesis and the possibility that the tracheoesophageal fistula may stenose.[6] For these reasons, all three methods of speaking are still in use, and none are mutually exclusive. In fact, some patients find it useful to use more than one of the methods (Box 20-3).

Information about devices used to produce electronic speech can be obtained from the American Cancer Society or from the local telephone company.[1] Information about esophageal speech can be obtained from the American Speech

BOX 20-3 Speech Methods After Total Laryngectomy

Tracheoesophageal Prosthesis

Formation of a tracheoesophageal fistula with insertion of a silicone prosthesis that produces a sound in the esophagus (see Figure 20-22, *B*)

Esophageal Speech

Speech produced by expelling swallowed air (burping) across constricted tissue in the pharyngoesophageal segment

External Speech Aids

Mechanical devices such as a vibrator or electronic artificial larynx used externally

and Hearing Association,*[4] the International Association of Laryngectomees, and the American Cancer Society.

The speech pathologist teaches the patient to use esophageal speech after all therapy (including postoperative radiotherapy) is completed and swelling of the incision has abated.[23] This may not occur until 3 to 6 months after surgery. To learn esophageal speech, the patient must first practice burping. This provides the moving column of air needed for sound, and folds of tissue at the opening of the esophagus act as the vibrating surface. The patient must learn to coordinate articulation with esophageal vocalization made possible by aspirating air into the esophagus. The new voice sounds are natural, although somewhat hoarse. The qualities of speech provided by the use of the nasopharynx are still present. The patient may have digestive difficulty while learning to speak; this is caused by swallowing air during practice, by unusual strain on abdominal muscles, and by nervous tension. Digestive difficulties usually abate with proficiency in speaking.

Most patients learn esophageal speech best at a specialized speech clinic, and some individuals may need to go to a nearby city for this instruction. Motivation and persistent effort are essential in learning this kind of speech. Encouragement from the professional staff and from the patient's significant other is important to the patient's morale. Use of an electronic artificial larynx is taught by the speech pathologist 1 to 2 days postoperatively. Various mechanical devices are available, and newer ones permit a natural type of speech, providing pitch inflection and volume control. The patient's speech pathologist, the local chapter of the American Cancer Society, or the local telephone company can provide information about purchasing these devices.[1]

Reconstructive Surgery

Because of the extensive surgery required to treat malignancies of the head and neck, reconstructive surgery has become common practice. In the past, skin grafts and pedicle or rotation skin flaps were used for reconstruction. Today myocutaneous flaps and free flaps are the major reconstructive flaps used to reconstruct large deficits caused by extensive tumor resection and traumatic defects of the head and neck.[4]

Myocutaneous Flaps

Myocutaneous flaps use the axial blood supply that supplies muscle mass, as well as cutaneous and subcutaneous tissue. The inclusion of muscle with its blood supply when transferring the skin allows for a much greater range of rotation of the flap. The pectoralis major, the latissimus dorsi, the trapezius, and the sternocleidomastoid muscles can be used for myocutaneous flaps.

Free Flaps

Free flaps consist of harvested tissue separated from the donor site with the vein and artery. The vein and artery are anastomosed to recipient vessels close to the defect (microvascular anastomosis). It is also possible to harvest flaps containing soft tissue and bone to reconstruct the mandible after mandibulectomy.

Close postoperative monitoring of any type of skin flap is essential. Monitoring includes:

- Direct observation unless the wound is completely covered with a dressing. Some surgeons exteriorize (bring to the outside) a small segment of buried flaps for monitoring purposes.
- Use of Doppler to monitor patency of the anastomoses. The surgeon indicates the area where the Doppler is to be applied. Assessments are hourly for at least the first 24 hours.

To prevent clot formation in the recipient graft, the hematocrit is kept below 30 and sometimes as low as 25 before blood replacement is considered. Some surgeons order low-dose aspirin or even heparin to prevent clot formation. Persons with a below-normal hematocrit fatigue easily because the oxygen-carrying capacity of the blood is reduced.

GERONTOLOGIC CONSIDERATIONS

A total laryngectomy is very traumatic for the patient in many ways. Because the older adult is even more susceptible to complications, anxiety, and poor wound healing, caring for an elderly patient who has undergone a laryngectomy is a challenge. The nurse should be knowledgeable about the patient's history and the presence of complicating, preexisting conditions that require monitoring during the postoperative period. If the patient has preexisting communication difficulties, communication challenges are enhanced in the postoperative phase. The patient may be referred for additional nursing care on discharge to the home.

SPECIAL ENVIRONMENTS FOR CARE

Critical Care Management

Most patients undergoing major head and neck surgery are placed in an intensive care unit or a specialized ENT unit because of their need for invasive monitoring and intensive nursing care. Following a laryngectomy, most patients leave the intensive care unit and move to a step-down unit in 5 to 7 days.

*10801 Rockville Pike, Rockville, MD 20852.

Patient Teaching
Home Care of the Patient After Laryngectomy

Home care of the patient after a laryngectomy can be difficult. It is frightening for both the patient and the family until they become familiar with the equipment and care needed. The nurse should help them feel comfortable with the new responsibilities by reinforcing instructions, providing detailed written instructions, allowing them to demonstrate techniques with nursing supervision, and planning time for questions and concerns. The following additional information should be explained to the patient and family:

1. The nose normally filters and warms air that we breathe. This function is lost with a tracheostomy or stoma; therefore extra humidity is necessary to moisten the air. The following are measures that can increase humidity:
   a. Use a cool mist in the room where you spend most of your time. Also use it in your bedroom at night.
   b. Cover the stoma during the day with a dampened stoma cover and moisten it when it dries.
   c. Wash the stoma with a washcloth and warm water and soap daily to remove crusts of mucus that form inside and outside of the stoma. Do not use paper tissues to clean around the stoma because they may contain lint that may be inhaled into the stoma. Crusts that are difficult to remove can be softened with hydrogen peroxide or a few drops of saline solution.
   d. Use a syringe or eyedropper to instill 3 to 5 ml of normal saline into your laryngectomy vent or stoma. This loosens mucus plugs before suctioning. Normal saline can be made by boiling 1 teaspoon of table salt in 1 quart of tap water for 20 minutes, cooling the solution, and placing it in a clean bottle with a lid. Make new solution every 2 days, because it does not contain a preservative.*
   e. Keep the stoma covered when you go outside to prevent cold air, dust, or pollen from getting in the tube or stoma. Use a scarf, bib, crocheted cover, or shirt that buttons at the neck.
   f. If the skin around the stoma becomes irritated, apply a thin coat of plain petroleum jelly or zinc oxide. Take care not to place it too close to the stoma to avoid inhaling it.
2. The following are additional instructions or precautions:
   a. You can bathe in a tub or take a shower, being careful to keep soap and water from entering the tube or stoma. A stoma shower guard or a handheld shower can be used.
   b. You can shampoo as long as you keep shampoo and water out of the stoma. You may need someone to help you shampoo.
   c. Men can shave using an electric or a manual razor. Be sure to cover the stoma so that lather and particles do not fall into the opening.
   d. You may not swim because water would enter your lungs.
   e. Drink at least 8 to 10 glasses of fluid daily. More fluid is needed during hot weather or when home heating is in use.
   f. Avoid persons who have colds or the flu or are not feeling well.
   g. Call your physician immediately if you feel like you are getting a cold or other respiratory tract infection.
   h. You can use antihistamines or decongestants, but be aware that they dry secretions; drink extra fluids and increase humidity while taking them.
   i. Increasing your activity helps thin secretions and makes them easier to cough or suction up.
   j. Wear a medical identification bracelet or carry a card stating that you are a neck breather. Emergency cards stating, "I am a total neck breather" can be obtained from your local branch of the American Cancer Society.
   k. Persons who have undergone a total laryngectomy often have dry mouth and bad breath. Brush with fluoride toothpaste and floss your teeth at least after breakfast and at bedtime. Keep your mouth fresh and clean by using baking soda and salt gargle (1 teaspoon of salt, 1 teaspoon of baking soda, and 1 quart of water).
3. Observe for complications.
   a. Complications may include hematoma, wound dehiscence, tissue loss, pharyngocutaneous fistula, and carotid artery rupture.
   b. If these are present, a physician should be seen.

*This step may not be prescribed for all patients.

Home Care Management

Home care of the patient after a laryngectomy is outlined in the Patient Teaching box.

COMPLICATIONS

Complications related to the surgical wound include hematoma, wound dehiscence, tissue loss, pharyngocutaneous fistula, and carotid artery rupture. Complications of myocutaneous and free flaps include venous or arterial congestion, flap necrosis, and slough.

THE COMPROMISED AIRWAY

Etiology/Epidemiology

The airway can be partially or completely obstructed by many conditions, several of which are discussed earlier in this chapter. With partial airway obstruction the individual displays respiratory distress and produces sounds such as gurgling, snoring, or stridorous ventilations.

Pathophysiology

When the airway is completely obstructed, the conscious person has no breath sounds and displays signs of severe respiratory distress progressing to respiratory arrest. Airway obstruction is confirmed in the unconscious person when attempts to ventilate the person do not produce chest movement and no expiratory air passes from the individual's airway.

Collaborative Care Management

Airway Management. The type of intervention used to reestablish and maintain airway patency depends on the individual's level of consciousness, his or her respiratory status,

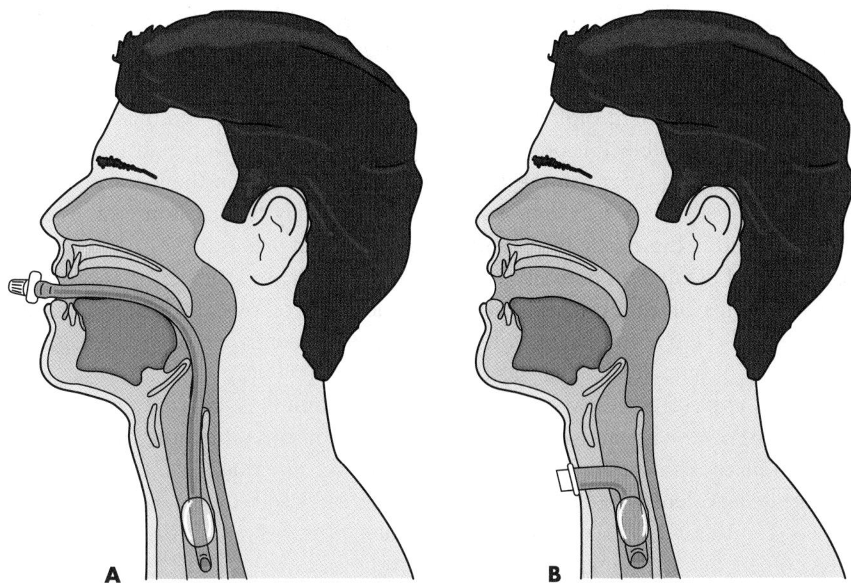

Figure 20-23 A, Position of endotracheal tube. B, Position of tracheostomy tube.

and the cause of airway obstruction. The conscious person with an obstructed airway must be assessed for adequacy of air exchange. If the individual can talk and cough, air exchange is adequate and interventions can be focused on the underlying cause. The conscious person with a completely obstructed airway is unable to speak or cough and soon loses consciousness if the obstruction is not relieved. Special maneuvers such as chest or abdominal thrusts and back blows are administered if the obstruction is caused by a foreign object blocking the airway. Organizations such as the American Heart Association and the American Red Cross offer training programs to certify proficiency in these basic lifesaving techniques.

In the unconscious individual the tongue falls back, covering the glottis. Lifting the chin moves the tongue forward, opening the airway. An alternative position to keep the tongue from obstructing the unconscious person's glottis is to place the individual in a side-lying position.

When a person has a mechanical obstruction of the airway and is expected to be unconscious for some time, it may be necessary to use an artificial airway.

Artificial Airways

Oral Airways. The simplest type of artificial airway is an oropharyngeal airway. The oropharyngeal airway keeps the tongue from falling back over the glottis. This type of airway is never used in a conscious individual, because it may cause vomiting or laryngospasm. An oropharyngeal airway must be inserted correctly to avoid pushing the tongue back against the glottis.

The esophageal gastric airway consists of a face mask with two ports. The lower port is for the esophageal tube, which is introduced into the esophagus to prevent reflux of gastric contents. The upper port is used for ventilation. The esophageal gastric tube airway is never inserted into a conscious person.

Endotracheal Tubes and Tracheostomy. When a person is no longer able to maintain his or her own airway, an endotracheal tube or a tracheostomy is necessary. An endotracheal tube is usually chosen initially as a means of providing the airway; a tracheostomy is performed only if airway maintenance is necessary for longer than 10 to 14 days or if trauma to the airway prevents the use of an endotracheal tube. Although a tracheostomy has the disadvantage of a higher risk of infection, it is much more comfortable than an endotracheal tube and allows the person to eat. It is also necessary when a patient requires prolonged mechanical ventilation.

In endotracheal intubation a tube is passed through either the nose or the mouth into the trachea (Figure 20-23, *A*), whereas in a tracheostomy an artificial opening is made in the trachea, into which a tracheostomy tube is inserted (Figure 20-23, *B*). These procedures are used to (1) establish and maintain a patent airway, (2) prevent aspiration by sealing off the trachea from the digestive tract in the unconscious or paralyzed person, (3) permit removal of tracheobronchial secretions in the person who cannot cough adequately, and (4) treat the patient who requires positive-pressure mechanical ventilation that cannot be given effectively by mask. Whether an intubation or a tracheostomy is performed initially depends on the facilities available and the wishes of the physician. Most physicians consider it safer to do an emergency endotracheal intubation and then perform a tracheostomy as a nonemergency procedure in the operating room if prolonged support of the airway is needed. The endotracheal tube is not removed until after the tracheostomy opening is made.

A tracheostomy is necessary when an endotracheal tube cannot be inserted or when it is contraindicated, as in severe burns or laryngeal obstruction caused by tumor, infection, or vocal cord paralysis. Once the airway is secured, either by intubation or tracheostomy, secretions are aspirated and well-humidified oxygen is usually given. If the patient is unable to sustain respiration, a mechanical ventilator is attached to either the endotracheal tube or the tracheostomy tube. When mechanical ventilation is required, a cuffed tube is used. Usually an endotracheal tube is not left in place longer than 10 to 14 days. If the patient is unable to maintain a patent airway after this period of time, a tracheostomy is performed.

The endotracheal tube is made of plastic with an inflatable cuff so that a closed system with the ventilator can be maintained (Figure 20-24). The tube is inserted via the mouth or nose through the larynx into the trachea. If an oral endotracheal tube is used, a rubber airway or bite block is often necessary to prevent the patient from biting down on the tube and obstructing the airway.

Two potentially fatal complications can occur in patients with endotracheal tubes: accidental extubation and displacement of the endotracheal tube. Tips of endotracheal tubes have been shown to shift as much as 2 cm in the trachea when patients flex or extend their necks or laterally tip their heads. Usually the endotracheal tube is affixed to the patient's face with waterproof tape above and below the lips and around the endotracheal tube to keep it in place. This method can cause facial skin breakdown, especially in patients with leukemia or who are immunosuppressed. For this reason, commercially available endotracheal tube holders that use no tape are available (Figure 20-25).

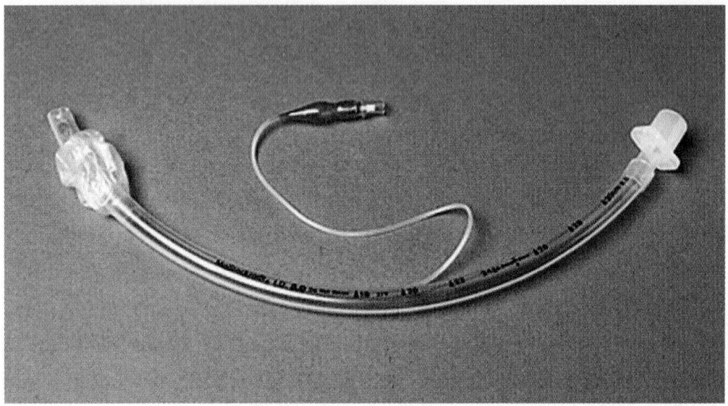

Figure 20-24 Endotracheal tube.

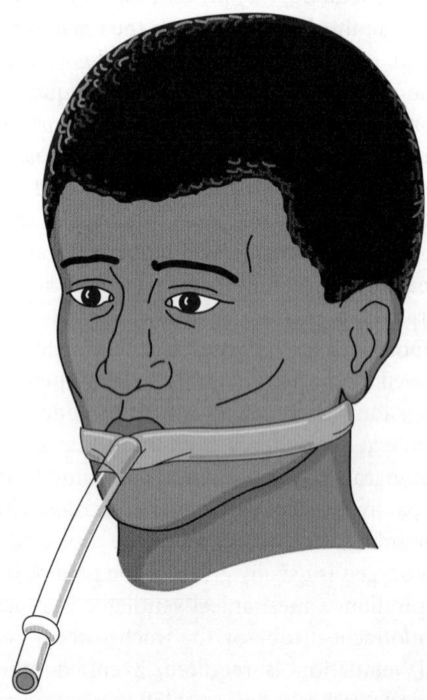

Figure 20-25 Comfit endotracheal tube holder.

Tracheostomy tubes are usually made of silicone, pliable plastic, or metal. Most adult-sized plastic tracheostomy tubes have a cuff that is inflated with air to fill the space between the outside of the tube and the trachea. The cuff provides a sealed airway for positive-pressure mechanical ventilation and prevents aspiration in the unconscious person during tube feedings. Usually tracheostomy tubes do not need to be changed more often than every 2 to 3 weeks. Low-pressure cuffs are less likely to cause damage to the trachea. When secretions are thick and copious, the tube may have to be changed weekly or more frequently. Some tracheostomy tubes have a single lumen; others have both an inner and an outer cannula. The outer cannula is changed only by the physician or a specially prepared nurse; the inner cannula is removed regularly by the nurse for cleaning. Twill tapes are attached to each side of the tube and tied securely on the side of the neck to prevent the tube from becoming dislodged when the patient coughs or moves. The tapes are not tied behind the patient's neck because lying on the knot may cause skin irritation and a pressure sore.

Should the tracheostomy tube be coughed out, the opening may close and the patient will be unable to breathe. Therefore a tracheal dilator or curved hemostat is kept at the bedside so that the opening can be held open until the physician arrives to insert a new tracheostomy tube. Some surgeons prefer to place a retention suture on each side of the tracheostomy opening and tape the end of the suture to the skin. If the opening shows signs of closing, tension can be placed on the sutures to widen the opening.

A small dressing may be placed under the tracheostomy tube. Although drainage should be minimal, the wound is inspected frequently for bleeding during the immediate postoperative period. The dressings are changed as they become soiled with mucous drainage.

Depending on the patient's condition, a tracheostomy can be either temporary or permanent; the person who has undergone a total laryngectomy has a permanent tracheostomy. The patient who has had a tracheostomy performed is apprehensive and is often fearful of choking. Thus when feasible, the procedure is thoroughly explained to the patient before surgery. Both the patient and the family need to understand that the patient will be unable to speak, that the nurses will be able to communicate with the patient, and that constant attendance will be provided until the patient can manage his or her own airway safely.

A fenestrated tracheostomy tube has an opening on the upper surface of the outer cannula that allows air inspired through the nose and mouth to pass through the tube. When the external opening is plugged, air can pass over the vocal cords, allowing the individual to talk. If ventilatory assistance is required, the inner cannula can be inserted so that the patient can be connected to a mechanical ventilator.

NURSING MANAGEMENT OF PATIENT WITH AN ENDOTRACHEAL OR TRACHEOSTOMY TUBE

Endotracheal airways irritate the trachea, resulting in increased mucus production, so the patient must be assessed regularly for excess secretions and suctioned as often as necessary to maintain a patent airway. Because endotracheal airways bypass the upper airway, which normally humidifies and warms inspired air, an external source of cool, humidified air also must be provided to avoid thickening and crusting of bronchial secretions.

Interventions to minimize the risk of infection are essential because an endotracheal or tracheostomy tube provides a direct route for introduction of pathogens into the lower airway, increasing the risk of infection. All respiratory therapy equipment should be changed every 24 hours, and any equipment that touches the floor must be replaced. Water that condenses in equipment tubing must be removed but never poured back into the humidifier reservoir because it may contain pathogens. Frequent mouth care must be provided because secretions tend to pool in the mouth and in the pharynx, particularly if the cuff of the tube is inflated. Mouth care is also important because an endotracheal tube or oral airway increases the risk of ulceration or abrasion of the lips and oropharynx.

The lips, tongue, and oral cavity must be inspected regularly, and the oral cavity cleaned with swabs soaked in saline. A moisturizing agent is applied to cracked lips. The oropharynx is gently suctioned as needed.

Adequate nutritional intake must be maintained. The person with an endotracheal tube is kept NPO, so nourishment is given parenterally or by gastrointestinal feedings. Gastrointestinal supplemental feedings are preferred because they maintain the function of the gut, provide more nutrition than intravenous feedings, pose less infection risk, and are more economical than intravenous feedings (Box 20-4).

The patient with a tracheostomy tube is usually able to swallow and have a normal oral intake. Some experts prefer that the cuff on the tracheostomy tube be inflated while the patient is eating to prevent aspiration. Others believe that the inflated cuff bulges into the esophagus and makes swallowing more difficult, and they therefore prefer that the cuff be deflated. Nursing assessment will determine which technique to use. Methylene blue dye can be swallowed before each feeding or mixed with the tube feeding. If the dye does not appear in tracheal secretions, it is safe to proceed with the meal.

BOX 20-4 Administering Gastrointestinal Feedings to the Intubated Patient

1. Assess for bowel sounds and tube placement.
2. Elevate the head of the bed at least 45 degrees.
3. Inflate the tracheostomy tube cuff. If using a Salem sump nasogastric tube, check the amount of residual feeding. If half the volume of the feeding to be given remains, the tube feeding is withheld.
4. Administer the tube feeding over 20 to 30 minutes. Keep the head of the bed elevated for 45 to 60 minutes after the feeding.
5. Assess at regular intervals for aspiration.
6. Assess regularly for tube placement and residual stomach contents.

Adequate ventilation and oxygenation must be ensured. Lung sounds must be assessed regularly. Unless the individual's underlying lung pathology alters lung ventilation, breath sounds should be heard bilaterally, and chest expansion should be symmetric. If an endotracheal tube is inserted too far, it will slip into one of the mainstem bronchi (usually the right) and occlude the opposite bronchus and lung, resulting in atelectasis on the obstructed side. Even if the endotracheal tube is still in the trachea, airway obstruction results if the end of the tube is located on the carina (the area at the lower end of the trachea at the point of bifurcation of the mainstem bronchi). This results in dry secretions that obstruct both bronchi. Although these complications are more common with the use of an endotracheal tube, they can occur with a tracheostomy tube, especially in a small person with a short neck. In either situation the tube is pulled back until it is positioned below the larynx and above the carina. The tube is then fastened securely in place.

For maximum ventilation and lung perfusion, the patient is turned and repositioned every 2 hours.

Respiratory frequency, tidal volume, and vital capacity are assessed, and postural drainage, percussion, and vibration performed as appropriate.

Tube placement must be maintained. The tube is kept secured around the neck with tape or specially designed ties, and placement is assessed at regular intervals. The endotracheal tube is marked to establish a landmark for position comparison and to measure and document the length of tube that extends beyond the patient's lips. A spare tube is always kept at the bedside. Tapes or ties are changed whenever soiled to decrease skin irritation.

Patients with endotracheal tubes or tracheostomy tubes with the cuff inflated cannot talk. Therefore the call light (or tap bell) should be kept within the patient's reach, the patient should be reoriented frequently, and an acceptable communication mode must be established. Questions should be asked so that the patient can indicate a simple "yes" or "no" response by nodding the head, using hand signals, or squeezing the nurse's hand. Some patients may be able to use an erasable board or notepad to communicate. It is also important to talk to the patient, explain all procedures, and reinforce that the ability to speak will return when the tube is removed. Family and friends should be encouraged to talk to the patient and offer support.

Although the low-pressure cuffs used today reduce the risk of tracheal wall damage, it is important to inflate the cuff with the correct amount of air (Box 20-5).

During the immediate extubation period, special precautions must be observed. The patient must be monitored for signs of upper airway obstruction secondary to laryngeal edema. These signs include increased respiratory distress, increased restlessness, hoarseness, and laryngeal stridor. The adequacy of the cough and gag reflexes also must be assessed. After removal of a tracheostomy tube, there is a temporary air leak at the incision site. Therefore the patient must be instructed to occlude the opening with a finger in order to speak. The tracheal stoma is suctioned if needed. However,

BOX 20-5 Inflating an Endotracheal or Tracheostomy Cuff

The cuff should be inflated to a volume that provides adequate occlusion around the tube without increasing the risk of tracheomalacia, tracheal stenosis, tracheoesophageal fistula, or erosion through a major blood vessel. Inflate the cuff as follows:

1. Using a 10- or 20-ml syringe, slowly inject air into the cuff.
2. As air is introduced, assess for air leak around the tube. This is determined by (a) the ability of the patient to talk or make sounds and (b) the ability of the nurse to feel air coming from the patient's nose or mouth.
3. When the airway is sealed and no passage of air around the tube can be detected, remove 0.5 ml of air. This creates a "minimal leak" and ensures that the lowest possible pressure is being exerted on the tracheal wall.
4. Auscultate over the trachea while ventilating the patient with either an Ambu bag or a mechanical ventilator. A small amount of air should be heard gurgling past the cuff.
5. If an adequate seal cannot be obtained with 25 ml of air, notify the physician.
6. The exact pressure in the cuff can be measured by connecting the pilot balloon to a handheld meter. To do this, the balloon is inflated with a syringe, in the normal fashion, until a seal is obtained. The syringe is removed, and the meter attached. The meter reading, in cm H_2O, is then recorded, and the pressure in the cuff is checked each shift to ensure consistency.

frequent use of the stoma for suctioning can delay closure and healing of the tracheostomy incision.

NURSING MANAGEMENT OF PATIENT WITH A TRACHEOSTOMY

Although nursing care of persons with either endotracheal or tracheostomy tubes is similar, patients with tracheostomies have additional nursing care needs (see Clinical Pathway). Analgesics and sedatives are given judiciously so as not to depress the respiratory center. The patient is suctioned as often as necessary. In some cases every 1 to 2 hours may be sufficient. Patients who are conscious can usually indicate when they need to be suctioned; however, the need for suctioning can be determined easily by the sound of the air coming from the tracheostomy tube, especially after the patient takes a deep breath. When respirations are noisy and pulse and respiratory rates are increased, the patient needs to be suctioned. The patient should also be suctioned if any other sign of respiratory distress occurs. If mucus is blocking the inner cannula of the tracheostomy tube and cannot be removed by suction, the inner cannula is removed to open the airway. When the mucus is thick, the inner cannula should be cleaned and replaced at once because the outer tube may also become blocked. If, despite these measures, the patient becomes cyanotic, the physician should be summoned immediately. A patient who is able to cough up his or her own secretions probably will require suctioning less frequently. The amount of mucus subsides gradually, and the patient eventually may go for several hours without being suctioned. However, even when secretions are minimal, the patient is apprehensive and needs constant attendance.[8,19]

Research has shown that using normal saline instillation as part of the suctioning procedure facilitates mobilization of mucous tracheal secretions and does not cause oxygen desaturation.[20] However, other research has found that the instillation of a 5-ml bolus of normal saline before suctioning of mechanically ventilated patients who were in the intensive care unit of an academic medical center had an adverse effect on oxygen saturation and that this adverse effect worsened over time. This study recommended that instillation of normal saline before suctioning should not be used routinely in patients receiving mechanical ventilation who have pulmonary infections.[1]

Maintaining Air Humidification

Because an endotracheal or tracheostomy tube bypasses the upper airway, the patient's ability to humidify and warm inspired air is lost. Therefore whether the patient is on or off the ventilator, the inspired air should be humidified to prevent mucosal irritation and drying of secretions. Large-bore tubing is needed to provide mist, because water particles condense in small-bore tubing. A noticeable difference in the viscosity of secretions is evident in patients who do not receive mist for even as short a period as 30 minutes. Other important nursing care measures and observations vary with the route of intubation—via the larynx or from below the larynx.[8] The patient who has an endotracheal tube in place usually has an increased volume of oropharyngeal secretions because of irritation from the tube. The patient also has great difficulty swallowing (especially if an oral tube is used), necessitating frequent oropharyngeal suctioning.

Providing Nourishment

The patient with an endotracheal tube is kept NPO. Nourishment is given intravenously or by nasogastric tube feedings. The patient with a tracheostomy tube in place is usually able to swallow and have a normal oral intake.

Weaning From the Tracheostomy Tube

Patients who have had tracheostomies for a period of time may require progressive weaning before the tracheostomy tube can be safely removed (decannulation). The cuff is deflated to determine the patient's ability to handle secretions without aspiration. If no aspiration occurs, a smaller, uncuffed tube is inserted to determine the patient's ability to breathe around the tube and through the nose and mouth. Next, the opening of the tracheostomy tube is occluded for 24 hours to ensure that the patient can breathe through the nose and mouth without difficulty. If the patient tolerates this procedure, the tracheostomy tube is removed and decannulation is accomplished. An occlusive dressing is applied to the stoma site to promote healing.[19]

For patients with a permanent tracheostomy, care continues in the home as presented in the following paragraphs.

clinical pathway *Tracheostomy*

TIME FRAME LOCATION	HOSPITAL DAY POD DAY OF SURGERY DATE UNIT	HOSPITAL DAY POD 1 DATE UNIT	HOSPITAL DAY POD 2 DATE UNIT
Discharge Planning	Identify caregiver and other support services: __________	Identify caregiver and other support services: __________	Identify caregiver and other support services: __________
Patient Education	Identify learning needs Assess knowledge of surgical procedure	Assess knowledge of surgical procedure and postop supports	Initiate patient education record Begin teaching trach/wound care
Adjunct Interventions	Respiratory therapy Consult Speech Pathology	Respiratory therapy	Speech pathology if patient has persistent aspiration Screen for physical therapy
Nursing/Medical Interventions	Monitor vital signs q4h, I&O, labs, IV fluids Airway: HOB elevated, oxygen via cool mist trach collar, I/S, trach care/suction qsh and prn Wound: wound/stoma care qsh, IV ATB Nutrition: NPO Provide emotional support and reassurance regarding trach	Monitor vital signs q4h, I&O, labs, IV fluids Airway: HOB elevated 45°, oxygen via cool mist trach collar, I/S, trach care/suction qsh and prn Deflate trach cuff Wound: wound/stoma care qsh, IV ATB Nutrition: clear liquids; advance as tolerated Provide emotional support and reassurance regarding trach Activity: up in chair	Monitor vital signs q4h, I&O, labs, IV fluids Airway: HOB elevated 45°, oxygen via cool mist trach collar, I/S, trach care/suction qsh and prn Wound: wound/stoma care qsh, IV ATB Nutrition: advance diet as tolerated; D/C IV with good PO intake Provide emotional support and reassurance regarding trach Activity: ambulate with assistance
Outcome Criteria	Vital signs stable Adequate urine output Patent airway Oxygen saturation >90% No wound complications Patient/family satisfaction addressed	Vital signs stable Voiding Mobilizing secretions effectively Oxygen saturation >90% No wound complications Increased PO intake without aspirating Receptive to teaching Patient/family satisfaction addressed	Vital signs stable Voiding Mobilizing secretions effectively Oxygen saturation >90% No wound complications Increased PO intake without aspirating Receptive to teaching Patient/family satisfaction addressed

TIME FRAME LOCATION	HOSPITAL DAY POD 3 DATE UNIT	HOSPITAL DAY POD 4 DATE UNIT	HOSPITAL DAY POD 5 DATE UNIT
Discharge Planning	Identify caregiver: __________	Identify caregiver: __________	Identify caregiver: __________
Patient Education	Continue teaching/return demonstration	Continue teaching/return demonstration	Continue teaching/return demonstration
Adjunct Interventions	Respiratory therapy Physical therapy (if needed)	Respiratory therapy Physical therapy (if needed)	Respiratory therapy Physical therapy (if needed)
Nursing/Medical Interventions	Monitor vital signs, I&O, labs, IV fluids Airway: HOB elevated 45°, oxygen via cool mist trach collar, I/S, trach care/suction qsh and prn Wound: wound/stoma care qsh, IV ATB Nutrition: diet as tolerated Activity: ambulate independently	Monitor vital signs, I&O, labs Airway: HOB elevated 45°, trach care/suction qsh and prn, change to button trach Wound: wound/stoma care qsh IV antibiotics Nutrition: diet as tolerated Anxiety: emotional support Activity: ambulating	Monitor vital signs, I&O, labs Airway: HOB elevated 45°, oxygen via cool mist trach collar, I/S, trach care/suction qsh and prn Wound: wound/stoma care qsh D/C antibiotics Nutrition: diet as tolerated Anxiety: emotional support Activity: ambulating
Outcome Criteria	Vital signs stable Voiding Mobilizing secretions effectively Oxygen saturation >90% Stable wound Adequate PO intake Receptive to teaching Patient/family satisfaction addressed	Vital signs stable Voiding Tolerates trach change Mobilizing secretions effectively Oxygen saturation >90% Stable wound Adequate PO intake Progressing with teaching Patient/family satisfaction addressed	Vital signs stable Voiding Mobilizing secretions effectively Patent airway Oxygen saturation >90% Stable wound Good PO intake Progressing with teaching Patient/family satisfaction addressed

Continued

clinical pathway *Tracheostomy—cont'd*

TIME FRAME LOCATION	HOSPITAL DAY POD 6 DATE UNIT	HOSPITAL DAY POD 7 DATE UNIT	HOSPITAL DAY POD 8 DATE UNIT
Discharge Planning	Identify caregiver: ______	Identify caregiver: ______	Identify caregiver: ______
Patient Education	Reinforce teaching/evaluation	Reinforce teaching/evaluation	Reinforce teaching/evaluation
Adjunct Interventions	Respiratory therapy Physical therapy (if needed)	Respiratory therapy Physical therapy (if needed)	Respiratory therapy
Nursing/Medical Interventions	Monitor: vital signs, I&O, labs Airway: trach care/suction qsh/prn Wound: wound/stoma care qsh Nutrition: diet as tolerated Activity: ambulating	Monitor: vital signs, I&O, labs Airway: trach care/suction qsh/prn Wound: wound/stoma care qsh Nutrition: diet as tolerated Activity: ambulating	Monitor: vital signs, I&O, labs Airway: trach care/suction qsh/prn Wound: wound/stoma care qsh Nutrition: diet as tolerated Activity: ambulating
Outcome Criteria	Vital signs stable Voiding Mobilizing secretions effectively Stable wound Oxygen saturation >90% Good PO intake Progressing with teaching Patient/family satisfaction addressed	Vital signs stable Voiding Mobilizing secretions effectively Oxygen saturation >90% Stable wound Good PO intake Progressing with teaching Patient/family satisfaction addressed	Vital 8signs stable Voiding Mobilizing secretions Oxygen saturation >90%, Stable wound Good PO intake Able to do trach/wound care D/C criteria met Patient/family satisfaction addressed

Patient Teaching

Home Care of the Patient With a Permanent Tracheostomy Tube

INCREASING ENVIRONMENTAL HUMIDITY

1. Use a cool mist humidifier in the room where you spend most of your time.
2. Use it in your bedroom when you are napping or sleeping.

SUCTIONING THE TRACHEOSTOMY TUBE

1. Gather the supplies you need.
   a. Suction machine
   b. Suction catheter (No. 14 French whistle-tip)
   c. Two nonsterile gloves
   d. A clean basin or sink
   e. Hydrogen peroxide
   f. Clean 4 × 4 fine-mesh gauze pads
   g. Jar of tap water or normal saline (Use distilled water if you have well water.)
   h. Clean cotton-tipped swabs
   i. Clean pipe cleaners or small brush
   j. Clean washcloth and towel
   k. Tracheostomy tube ties
   l. Clean scissors
   m. Plastic or paper bag for disposal of soiled materials
2. Wash hands thoroughly with soap and water.
3. Sit or stand in front of the mirror (can use the mirror over the sink in the bathroom).
4. Put on gloves.
5. Suction the tracheostomy tube.
6. If your tube has an inner cannula, remove it. (If your tube does not have an inner cannula, go to step 12.)
7. Clean the inner cannula in the basin. Pour hydrogen peroxide over it until it is clean.
8. Clean the inner cannula with pipe cleaners or a small brush. Discard used pipe cleaners in a disposable bag.
9. Rinse the cannula thoroughly with normal saline, tap water, or distilled water.
10. Dry inside and outside of the cannula with 4 × 4 fine-mesh gauze. Discard used gauze in a disposable bag.
11. Reinsert the inner cannula and lock it in place.
12. Remove the soiled gauze dressing from your neck and dispose of it in a disposable bag.
13. Inspect the skin around the stoma for any signs of irritation or infection, such as redness, hardness, tenderness, drainage, or a foul smell. If any of these are present, call your nurse or physician after you finish your tracheostomy tube care.
14. Soak cotton-tipped swabs in hydrogen peroxide. Use swabs to clean the exposed parts of the outer cannula and the skin around it. Discard in a disposable bag.
15. Wet the washcloth with tap water, normal saline, or distilled water. Wipe away hydrogen peroxide and clean the skin around the stoma.
16. Dry the area around the stoma with the clean towel.
17. Change the ties using twill tape recommended to you.
18. Do not completely remove the old tie until you have a new one in place.
19. Cut twill tape as you have been taught.
20. Place fine-mesh gauze under the tracheostomy tie and neckplate by folding it or cutting a slit.
21. Remove your gloves and discard them in the same bag used for soiled gauze.
22. Wash your hands with soap and warm water.
23. Wash the basin and small brush with soap and warm water.
24. Put the washcloth and towel in the laundry.
25. Wash your hands again.

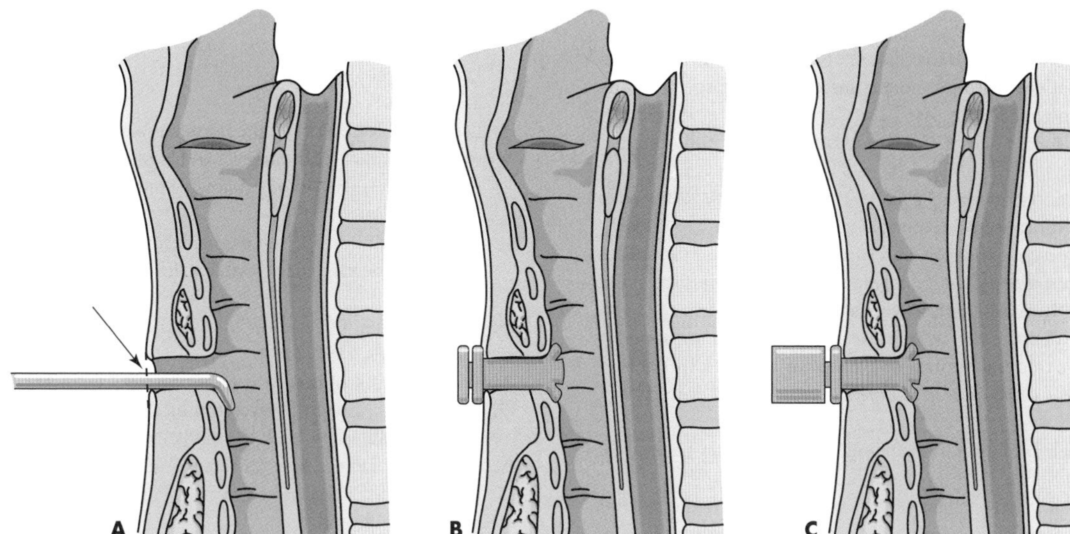

Figure 20-26 Tracheal button. **A,** A bent pipe cleaner is inserted into the stoma to measure the stoma depth. The pipe cleaner is gently pulled back to hook on the anterior tracheal wall. The distance from the pipe cleaner bend to the skin surface determines the length of the tracheostomy button. As an alternative, several different sizes of tracheal buttons are tried to determine which one is most comfortable for the patient. **B,** A solid plug inserted into the tracheostomy button prevents the button from being coughed out and allows the patient to breathe through the upper airway and vocalize. **C,** A hollow tube adaptor ("one-way" valve) replaces the stoma plug to allow for suctioning and inspiration through the button and expiration and vocalization through the upper airway.

Patient/Family Education

Persons to be discharged with a tube in place are taught to care for and change the tube while in the hospital. A mirror is necessary for this procedure, which the patient may begin a few days after surgery. The patient should also practice suctioning the tracheostomy tube before discharge.[17] Patients who go home with the tracheostomy tube in place must be provided with necessary supplies or with instructions as to where to get supplies. The patient will need suction equipment, which can be rented for home use or obtained in many communities through the local chapter of the American Cancer Society.[1]

The patient should be given written instructions about how to care for the tracheostomy tube, and the instructions should be reviewed with the patient and significant other before discharge. Points to be included in the written instructions are listed in the Patient Teaching box.[21]

Tracheal buttons are used in some patients with a permanent tracheal stoma. A tracheal button is a hollow Teflon tube with a serrated distal end that is inserted into the tracheal stoma, where the end fits against the anterior tracheal wall (Figure 20-26). When the button is in place, a solid plug is inserted to spread the distal end flanges, which secures the tube in place. The button keeps the stoma tract open and allows the patient to breathe, vocalize, and clear secretions through the upper airway.

If the patient has difficulty breathing, the solid plug can be removed and the patient can be ventilated with an Ambu bag fitted with an adaptor. Routine suctioning through the tracheal button is discouraged because the suction catheter tends to hit the posterior wall of the trachea, causing ulceration and bleeding. If the tracheostomy tube must be reinserted after several hours or days, it can be easily reinserted because the stoma has been kept open with the button.

Critical Thinking Questions

1. Compare and contrast the upper respiratory tract infections most commonly seen in adults. What variations in treatments and medications are used for the infections?
2. A patient you are caring for has had a temporary tracheostomy for approximately 8 hours. You notice that the patient's SaO_2 levels have dropped from 97% to 89% within the past hour. What mechanical problems will you look for? What parts of the physical examination will you use to further assess the situation? What immediate and long-term action will you implement?
3. What specific behavior might indicate that an individual who has undergone radical neck surgery or a permanent laryngectomy is not adjusting to his or her change in appearance? How can the nurse help the patient to cope effectively with this change?
4. What home care teaching tips would you give to a patient who had just been discharged with a tracheostomy tube in place? How can the nurse help alleviate the fears of the patient?
5. What special needs does the patient with a permanent tracheostomy have? Discuss the communication problems the patient might face. How does this situation differ from that of the patient who has undergone a laryngectomy?

References

1. Ackerman MH, Mick DJ: Instillation of normal saline before suctioning in patients with pulmonary infections: a prospective randomized controlled study, *Am J Crit Care* 7(4):261, 1998.
2. American Cancer Society: *Cancer facts and figures 1998,* Atlanta, 1998, ACS.
3. American Cancer Society: *Health information seekers,* 2001, website: http://americancancersociety.org/.
4. American Speech, Language, and Hearing Association: *Communication facts: special populations: augmentative and alternative communication,* 2001, website: http://www.asha.org/index.htm.
5. Byers RM, Roberts DB: The selective neck dissection for upper aerodigestive tract carcinoma: indications and results. In Robins KT, editor: *Advances in head and neck oncology,* San Diego, 1998, Singular.
6. Clark LC: Rehabilitation for the head and neck cancer patient, *Oncology* 12(1):81-94, 1998.
7. Cyr MH, Hickey MM, Higgins TS: Tracheal, esophageal conditions and care. In Harria LL, Huntoon MB, editors: *Core curriculum for otorhinolaryngology and head-neck nursing,* New Smyrna Beach, Fla, 1998, Society of Otorhinolaryngology and Head-Neck Nurses.
8. Harkin H, Russell C: Tracheostomy patient care, *Nurs Times* 97(25):34, 2001.
9. Higgins TS et al: Nasal cavity, paranasal sinuses, nasopharynx conditions and care. In Harria LL, Huntoon MB, editors: *Core curriculum for otorhinolaryngology and head-neck nursing,* New Smyrna Beach, Fla, 1998, Society of Otorhinolaryngology and Head-Neck Nurses.
10. Krouse JH: Introduction to sinus disease: anatomy and physiology, *ORL Head Neck Nurs* 17(3):6-16, 1999.
11. Krouse JH, Krouse HJ: Introduction to sinus disease: diagnosis and treatment, *ORL Head Neck Nurs* 17(2):7-12, 1999.
12. Landis SH et al: Cancer statistics, 1999, *CA Cancer J Clin* 49(1): 8-31, 1999.
13. Leder SB, Blom, ED: Tracheoesophageal voice prosthesis fitting and training. In Blom ED, Singer MI, Hamaker RC, editors: *Tracheoesophageal voice restoration following total laryngectomy,* San Diego, 1998, Singular.
14. McKenna M: Postoperative tonsillectomy/adenoidectomy hemorrhage: a respective chart review, *ORL Head Neck Nurs* 17(3):18-21, 1999.
15. Miaskowski C, Buchsel P: *Oncology nursing: assessment and clinical care,* St Louis, 1999, Mosby.
16. Reed V: Breath of life, *Nurs Stand* 14(50):22, 2000.
17. Rudy SF, McCullagh L: Overcoming the top 10 self-care learning barriers, *ORL Head Neck Nurs* 19(2):8, 2001.
18. Santos PM, Lepore ML: Epistaxis. In Baily BJ, Calhoun KH, editors: *Head and neck surgery—otolaryngology,* ed 2, Philadelphia, 1998, Lippincott-Raven.
19. Serra A: Tracheostomy care, *Nurs Stand* 14(42):45, 2000.
20. Schwenker D, Ferrin M, Gift AG: A survey of endotracheal suctioning with instillation of normal saline, *Am J Crit Care* 7(4):255, 1998.
21. Schreiber D: Trach care at home: a how-to guide, *RN* 64(7):43, 2001.
22. van-der-Torn M et al: Alternative voice after laryngectomy using a sound-producing voice prosthesis, *Laryngoscope* 111(2):336, 2001.
23. Zeine L, Larson M: Pre and post-op counseling for laryngectomees and their spouses: an update, *J Commun Disord* 32(1):51, 1999.

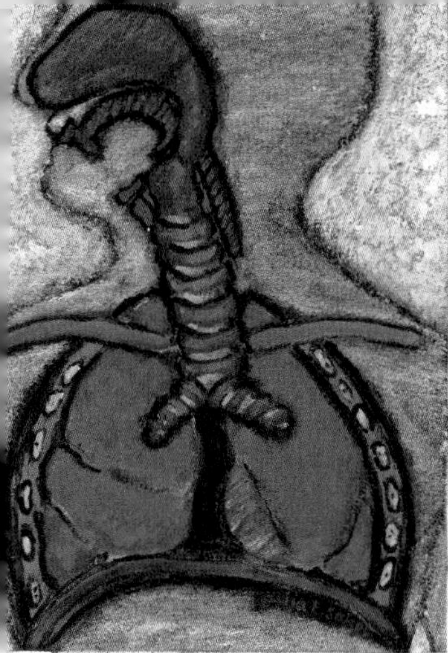

http://www.mosby.com/MERLIN/medsurg_phipps

Lower Airway Problems

21

Pamela D. Dennison

Objectives

After studying this chapter, the learner should be able to:

1. Differentiate between restrictive and obstructive pulmonary disorders.
2. Compare community-acquired and hospital-acquired pneumonia.
3. Describe incidence, preventive measures, and current challenges in the diagnosis and treatment of tuberculosis.
4. Compare fungal infections of the respiratory tract.
5. Describe incidence, prevention, and therapy for lung cancer.
6. Write a teaching plan for the patient who is to have resectional surgery of the lung.
7. List five precautions to be observed in the care of chest tubes and a closed drainage system, and give the rationale for each.
8. Explain the pathophysiology of acute lung injury and adult respiratory distress syndrome.
9. Explain the pathophysiology of and interventions for chronic bronchitis, pulmonary emphysema, and asthma.
10. Describe a method for teaching the patient with chronic obstructive pulmonary disease to use a metered-dose inhaler and an inhaler with a spacer.
11. Discuss the clinical manifestations of cystic fibrosis in adults.
12. Describe the nature of respiratory failure and the care of the patient with an endotracheal tube and mechanical ventilation.
13. Discuss the indications for and advantages of noninvasive methods of providing mechanical ventilation.
14. Differentiate among a closed, an open, and a tension pneumothorax in terms of signs and symptoms, treatment, and nursing management.

Many diseases, both acute and chronic, affect the respiratory system. Considerable change in the incidence of diseases affecting the respiratory system has occurred in recent decades. Although the incidence of some pulmonary diseases such as lung abscess and bronchiectasis has decreased, the incidence of other pulmonary diseases such as chronic bronchitis and emphysema has increased. In addition, the reduction in immunologic competence that occurs with cancer chemotherapy, immunosuppressant medications given after organ transplantation, or acquired immunodeficiency syndrome (AIDS) has resulted in an increase in opportunistic lung infections caused by microorganisms that were rarely pathogenic in the past.

The most significant pulmonary diseases are those that are chronic, and these have increased dramatically in recent years. Current statistics indicate that more than 17 million Americans have emphysema, asthma, or chronic bronchitis.[41] This number can be expected to increase yearly as the number of older adults in our society increases. Because most diseases of the respiratory tract are not reportable, the full extent of both acute and chronic illness is difficult to estimate. However, known facts about disability from chronic pulmonary diseases indicate that these diseases are a major health problem and that they cause tremendous losses in productivity in the United States. The Social Security Administration reports that disability payments to persons with chronic pulmonary problems are second only to payments to persons with heart problems.

Early symptoms of respiratory diseases are probably those most often ignored by the general population. With the exception of acute pulmonary disorders, the major factor preventing early diagnosis and treatment of pulmonary diseases is the insidious nature of their signs and symptoms. Medical attention is needed for cough, difficulty breathing, production of sputum, shortness of breath, and nose and throat irritations that do not subside within 2 weeks, since these symptoms suggest respiratory disease.

CLASSIFICATION OF PULMONARY DISORDERS

The classification of lung diseases used in this chapter differentiates the pulmonary disorders on the basis of etiology and how they affect ventilation. Lung diseases are divided into restrictive and obstructive ventilatory disorders. A third category, pulmonary vascular disorders, also alters the ability of the lung to carry out respiration effectively.

Restrictive Disorders

In restrictive lung disease, expansion of the lungs is limited. Static lung volumes are diminished as a result of decreased lung or thoracic compliance (Table 21-1). Patients with a restrictive disorder may demonstrate respiratory alkalosis caused by a compensatory increase in respiratory rate to offset diminished lung volumes. When the increased respiratory rate no longer adequately compensates for the diminished lung volumes, hypoxemia (low arterial blood oxygen) occurs. Clinically, persons with restrictive disorders exhibit some degree of dyspnea. Often they become dyspneic only on exertion. As the restrictive disease progresses, however, persons become dyspneic at rest. In addition, persons with restrictive disorders often have a dry, hacking cough. Table 21-2 lists major disorders that result in primarily restrictive ventilatory defects.

Obstructive Disorders

Obstructive lung disease includes any process that limits airflow on expiration. Both lung compliance (lung expansibility) and airway resistance are increased. These pathophysiologic changes alter the ability to move air out of the lungs, which results in characteristic changes in both static and dynamic lung volume measurement (see Table 21-1). Clinically, persons with obstructive lung disease may exhibit a prolonged expiration time, increased anteroposterior (AP) diameter of the thorax, and hyperresonance on percussion. Persons with pulmonary disorders characterized by the preceding description have been identified as having chronic obstructive pulmonary disease (COPD).

TABLE 21-1 Comparison of Pulmonary Function Test Results in Restrictive and Obstructive Disease

Test	Restrictive	Obstructive
FVC	Decreased	Decreased or normal
RV	Decreased	Increased
TLC	Decreased	Normal or increased
RV/TLC	Normal or increased	Significantly increased
FEV_1/ FVC	Normal or increased	Decreased
FEV_3/FVC	Normal or increased	Decreased

FVC, Forced vital capacity; *RV*, residual volume; *TLC*, total lung capacity; *FEV*, forced expiratory volume (in 1, 3 seconds).

Pulmonary Vascular Disorders

Pulmonary vascular disorders are the third category of pulmonary disorders considered in this chapter. Pulmonary vascular disorders include any process that results in the narrowing or occlusion of pulmonary blood vessels. In pulmonary vascular disease, efficiency of pulmonary respiration is compromised, usually resulting in hypoxemia. Clinically, patients have dyspnea, increased respiratory frequency, digital clubbing, atelectasis, and chest pain. Pulmonary vascular disease may result from primary pulmonary hypertension or as a result of either circulatory or lung disease. Only pulmonary vascular disease related to pulmonary emboli and pulmonary infarction is discussed here.

RESTRICTIVE LUNG DISORDERS

INFECTIOUS DISEASES

Acute Bronchitis

Acute inflammation of the conductive airways is common, especially among children and older adults.

Etiology/Epidemiology

Bronchitis can be acute or chronic. (Chronic bronchitis is discussed later in this chapter.) Acute bronchitis is an inflammation of the bronchi and usually the trachea; thus the more correct term for this illness is *tracheobronchitis.* Although acute bronchitis occurs most often in persons with chronic lung disease, it also occurs as an extension of an upper respiratory tract infection in persons without underlying lung disease and is therefore communicable. It may also be caused by physical or chemical agents such as dust, smoke, or volatile fumes. As air pollution increases, the incidence of acute bronchitis increases. There is a marked seasonal incidence that peaks in late winter or spring.[54] Acute bronchitis is typically viral, but bacterial pathogens such as *Streptococcus pneumoniae* and *Haemophilus influenzae* may also cause bronchitis either as a primary or a secondary infection (Box 21-1).

TABLE 21-2 Restrictive Pulmonary Diseases

Type of Disorder	Disease Example
Parenchymal inflammation	Pneumonia, adult respiratory distress syndrome
Space-occupying lesion	Benign or malignant tumor
Diffuse pulmonary disease	Silicosis, fibrosis
Pleural disease	Pleural effusion
Lung collapse	Pneumothorax, atelectasis
Resectional surgery	Pneumonectomy
Neuromuscular disorder	Poliomyelitis, Guillain-Barré syndrome
Central nervous system depression	Narcotic overdose, cerebral edema

Pathophysiology

In the healthy person the defense mechanisms of the respiratory tract usually destroy or remove inhaled microbes. However, when defenses are weakened, the potentially pathogenic bacteria that normally reside in the nose and pharynx may colonize the mucosa of the trachea and bronchi. As part of the inflammatory process, there is increased blood flow to the affected area, causing an increase in pulmonary secretions. A painful cough with sputum production, low-grade fever, and malaise are common symptoms. The patient may have pain beneath the sternum caused by inflammation of the tracheal wall. Symptoms usually last 1 to 2 weeks but may continue for 3 to 4 weeks. Rhonchi and wheezes are heard on chest examination. If symptoms worsen and there is a high fever, shortness of breath, pleuritic chest pain (pain on inspiration), rapid respirations, and rales (crackles) or signs of consolidation on physical examination of the chest, pneumonia is suspected.

Collaborative Care Management

Diagnosis is based on the history and symptoms. Respiratory viruses are the most common infectious agents. Bacterial cultures of sputum are of limited use, and viral cultures are unnecessary. Chest x-ray findings are usually normal.[54]

Treatment of acute bronchitis is mainly symptomatic and supportive. It depends on the patient's age and the presence of other complicating illnesses. Reassurance, increased fluid intake to 2 to 3 L/day to thin secretions, and mild analgesic-antipyretic therapy with aspirin, acetaminophen, or ibuprofen every 4 to 6 hours for comfort are frequently all that is needed. If nocturnal cough is preventing sleep, codeine or dextromethorphan may be prescribed. Over-the-counter cough and cold remedies are not recommended, since they may dehydrate bronchial secretions and make them more difficult to remove. For patients with wheeze or other respiratory discomfort, a bronchoactive medication such as an inhaled $beta_2$-agonist is often prescribed. Antibiotics are usually not prescribed unless there is evidence of bacterial infection or if symptoms last more than 2 weeks in elderly patients or in persons with chronic diseases such as diabetes mellitus, cirrhosis, congestive heart failure, or COPD, who are at high risk for pneumonia. During known epidemics of influenza A virus, amantadine or rimantadine may be given early in the course of the disease to minimize symptoms.[18] All patients are urged to avoid environmental tobacco smoke, which is further irritating to the respiratory tract, and those who smoke are urged to quit.

Patient/Family Education. Nursing care is supportive and is directed toward helping the patient with prescribed therapy and avoiding future infection. Teaching for effective coughing to expel airway mucus is particularly important.

To produce an effective cough, the patient is taught to inspire deeply, hold the breath a few seconds, and cough two or three times with the mouth open and without taking another breath. This sequence is repeated several times, and then the patient is told to rest. This technique is believed to work because the cleansing action of cough in the large airways takes place primarily during the first one or two coughs of the cough sequence. The sequential nature of the coughing promotes the movement of mucus along the pulmonary tree from the lower airways to the mouth for expectoration. This type of controlled cough and forced expiration technique is known as the huff cough technique.

If a bronchoactive medication is ordered, the patient is also taught how to use an inhaler with a spacer.

BOX 21-1 Infectious Causes of Acute Bronchitis

Viruses

Rhinovirus
Adenovirus
Influenza A and B
Parainfluenza virus
Respiratory syncytial virus (RSV)

Bacteria

Streptococcus pneumoniae
Haemophilus influenzae
Moraxella catarrhalis
Bordetella pertussis
Mycoplasma pneumoniae
Chlamydia pneumoniae (TWAR strain)

Bacterial Infections

Pneumonia

Etiology. Pneumonia is an acute inflammation of lung tissue. It can result from infectious agents being inhaled or transported to the lungs via the bloodstream. It can also be due to noxious fumes or radiation treatment.

Epidemiology. Pneumonia is the most common cause of death from infectious disease in the United States. More than 4 million cases of pneumonia occur in the United States yearly. Most types of pneumonia are communicable, with the mode of transmission depending on the infecting organism. In recent years there have been significant changes in pathogens causing bacterial pneumonia and dramatic shifts in antimicrobial resistance patterns. Many new antimicrobial agents have been developed in response to pathogen resistance. These include β-lactamase inhibitors, fluoroquinolones, macrolides, and azalides.[25]

Pneumonia is classified as community-acquired pneumonia (CAP) or hospital-acquired pneumonia (HAP), depending on where the infection was acquired. With the rise in the elderly population, an increasingly important form of CAP is nursing home–acquired pneumonia (NHAP). HAP, also referred to as nosocomial pneumonia, includes the subset of ventilator-associated pneumonia (VAP).

Pathophysiology. Pneumonia results in inflammation of lung tissue. Depending on the particular pathogen and the host's physical status, the inflammatory process may involve different anatomic areas of the lung parenchyma and the pleurae.

Community-Acquired Pneumonia. CAP is an acute infection of the pulmonary parenchyma that is associated with symptoms of lower respiratory tract disease and accompanied by new infiltrates on x-ray or auscultory findings consistent with pneumonia in a patient who is not hospitalized or residing in a long-term care facility for the 14 days before the onset of illness.[54]

CAP is responsible for 10 million physician visits, 500,000 hospitalizations, and 45,000 deaths annually in the United States.[54] It may affect healthy individuals, but more than 70% of the cases occur in persons with preexisting disease (e.g., COPD, coronary artery disease, diabetes mellitus, malignancy, and alcohol abuse) or impaired host defenses. The mortality rate for persons with CAP ranges from less than 1% among outpatients to 30% among those requiring hospitalization.[54] The incidence of specific pathogens varies among patient populations and is dictated by host and environmental factors. *Streptococcus pneumoniae* is the most common cause of CAP in all age-groups; *Mycoplasma pneumoniae* primarily affects adolescents and young adults, but it can cause severe pneumonia in older adults and debilitated persons. *Haemophilus influenzae* and aerobic gram-negative bacteria have increased as a cause and are responsible for 12% of cases of CAP. *Legionella pneumoniae* accounts for about 6% of cases of CAP but is associated with a disproportionately high rate of respiratory failure and death.[69]

CAP is heralded by the symptoms of fever, rigors, sweats, new cough with or without sputum, a change in the color of the sputum, chest discomfort, and the onset of dyspnea.

NHAP is a form of CAP. Pneumonia is a leading cause of morbidity, hospitalization, and death among older adults living in nursing homes. The annual Medicare expenditures for acute hospitalization exceed $3.5 billion, and as many as 28% of Medicare beneficiaries admitted with pneumonia come from skilled nursing facilities. NHAP is defined as a new radiologic pulmonary infiltrate not solely attributable to heart failure, cancer, or pulmonary embolus, with at least one of the following major criteria or two of the following minor criteria. Major criteria are cough, sputum production, and fever; minor criteria are dyspnea, pleuritic chest pain, altered mental status, pulmonary consolidation, and increased white blood cell (WBC) counts.

Hospital-Acquired Pneumonia. Pneumonia is the second most common nosocomial infection in the United States and the leading cause of death from nosocomial infections. Nearly 1% of patients admitted to the hospital develop pneumonia, and nearly one third die. Up to 60% of patients in intensive care units (ICUs) develop pneumonia. The mortality rate is high because of coexisting diseases and the prevalence of gram-negative bacteria that are resistant to many antibiotics. About 80% of cases of HAP are caused by gram-negative bacteria. The remaining cases result from gram-positive bacteria (*Staphylococcus aureus* and *Streptococcus* species). *Pseudomonas aeruginosa* causes 20% to 30% of cases of nosocomial pneumonia and is the most common pathogen found in these patients. The second most common pathogen responsible for nosocomial pneumonia is *S. aureus,* which occurs when there are impairments in host defenses or other risk factors (e.g., indwelling and central venous catheters, chronic renal failure, treatment in a neurosurgical ICU, coma, recent surgery, arteriovenous shunts or fistulas). *Enterobacter* species are the third most common cause of nosocomial pneumonia. Risk factors for HAP are summarized in the Risk Factors box.

HAP occurs with aspiration of endogenous oropharyngeal bacteria into the lower respiratory tract. Oropharyngeal and tracheal colonization with gram-negative bacteria often occurs when patients have impaired defenses or serious underlying disease. Colonization of the stomach may lead to subsequent colonization of the airway and lower respiratory tract. Agents that increase gastric pH (e.g., antacids, H_2 antagonists) are associated with higher rates of nosocomial pneumonia in critically ill patients being mechanically ventilated.

Intubation and mechanical ventilation greatly increase the risk of bacterial pneumonia. VAP is pneumonia that occurs in a patient treated with mechanical ventilation when pneumonia is neither present nor developing at the time of intubation. It is a serious problem with significant morbidity and mortality. The overall mortality rate for VAP ranges from 54% to 71%, and it adds an additional 5 to 7 days to the hospital stay of surviving patients and billions of dollars to the nation's health care costs.[28] Aspiration of bacteria from the oropharynx, leakage of contaminated secretions around the endotracheal tube, patient position, and cross-contamination from respiratory equipment and health care providers are important factors in the development of VAP. Environmental factors implicated in the transmission of bacteria are contaminated ventilator tubing and inadequate hand washing by medical staff. Studies on hand washing demonstrate consistent lack of compliance with recommendations for prevention of infection. Observational studies of nurses show 8-second handwashing technique rather than the recommended 10-second technique. These same observational studies also demonstrate only a 22% compliance by nurses with the recommendation for hand washing before and after patient contact.[28] Nosocomial pneumonia can also be spread hematogenously to the lung from infections in wounds, soft tissue, or the urinary tract.

Risk Factors

Hospital-Acquired Pneumonia

- Treatment in an intensive care unit (ICU)
- Mechanical ventilation (those requiring 48 hours or more of ventilation in an ICU have a 10% to 20% chance of developing pneumonia)
- Endotracheal intubation or tracheostomy
- Recent surgery
- Debilitation or malnutrition
- Invasive devices
- Neuromuscular disease
- Depressed level of alertness
- Aspiration
- Antacid use
- Age 60 or older
- Prolonged hospital stay
- Any serious underlying disease

Viral Pneumonia. Viruses cause approximately 8% of cases of pneumonia in hospitalized adults. The incidence of viral infection as a cause of pneumonia is underestimated because of the insensitivity of viral diagnostic methods. The importance of the different viruses as causes of pneumonia varies with the season and the age distribution of the population. Respiratory synctial virus (RSV) is an increasingly recognized cause of pneumonia, but during outbreaks, influenza virus accounts for over 50% of cases in adults. Some cases of viral pneumonia have a rapid, relentless, and fatal course with generalized alveolar and interstitial infiltrates, development of adult respiratory distress syndrome, and progressive respiratory failure.[54]

Collaborative Care Management. Not all patients with pneumonia have to be hospitalized. In general, persons ages 55 years and younger who are in good health and have no serious preexisting condition (e.g., COPD, ethanol abuse, congestive heart failure, renal failure, liver disease, cerebrovascular accident, malignancy, debilitation) can be treated on an outpatient basis as long as they respond well to oral therapy. Persons who develop systemic toxicity, debilitation, respiratory failure, or hypoxemia are usually hospitalized. Administration of parenteral antibiotics for 2 to 3 days often improves these patients' conditions sufficiently so that oral antibiotics can be substituted and treatment continued on an outpatient basis. Guidelines for the treatment of NHAP are being developed on the basis of initial studies. Initial indications are that a significant number of nursing home residents with pneumonia can be treated successfully with oral antibiotics in the nursing home.[55]

Diagnostic Tests. Chest x-ray films demonstrate consolidation of lung involvement and the distribution of involvement. Diffuse involvement is characteristic of atypical pneumonia, and lobar involvement is characteristic of typical pneumonia. Chest x-ray findings also document pleural effusion. Sputum studies for culture, sensitivity, and Gram stain are done to identify the causative organism. To be accurate, sputum must be obtained from a deep cough before the start of antibiotic therapy and must arrive in the laboratory for processing within 2 hours. If a sputum specimen is unable to be obtained by coughing, it may be obtained by transtracheal aspiration or by bronchoscopy with aspiration, biopsy, or bronchial brushing. An elevated WBC count (15,000 to 25,000/mm^3) is consistent with bacterial pneumonia, and positive blood cultures are found in 18% of patients hospitalized with CAP.[69] Cold agglutinins and complement fixation studies are done when a viral cause is suspected. Arterial blood gas (ABG) studies or pulse oximetry are used to monitor oxygenation status. Hypoxemia and respiratory alkalosis are common, although if underlying chronic respiratory disease is present, respiratory acidosis may occur.

Thoracentesis may be done to obtain a pleural fluid specimen for analysis if pleural effusion is present.

Medications. Unless the clinical findings and Gram stain are classic for a specific organism, initial treatment of CAP is with a broad-spectrum antimicrobial. Therapy is then modified when the results of culture and sensitivity are received.

HAP (including VAP), with its high mortality rate, requires aggressive therapy. Therapy is often empiric and uses combinations of broad-spectrum antibiotics. Many experts recommend treatment with a third-generation cephalosporin or an anti-*Pseudomonas* penicillin-β-lactamase inhibitor combined with an aminoglycoside. HAP caused by methicillin-resistant *S. aureus* is treated with vancomycin.

Bronchoactive medications delivered as inhaled aerosols directly to the respiratory tract may be ordered to decrease respiratory symptoms of rhonchi (gurgles) and wheezing. The success of this therapy, which minimizes systemic drug exposure and side effects,[61] depends on the effective use of aerosol delivery devices. The devices most commonly used to administer orally or nasally inhaled aerosols are the metered-dose inhaler (MDI) with or without a reservoir (holding chamber or spacer) device, the small-volume nebulizer, and the dry-powder inhaler (DPI).

With spontaneous breathing, an inhaled aerosol distributes to the lungs and to the stomach through swallowing of the oropharyngeally deposited drug. The therapeutic effect is achieved by absorption in the airway; the systemic effects are caused by absorption in the airways and gastrointestinal (GI) tract. Studies have repeatedly demonstrated that only about 15% of the dose is delivered by MDI, DPI, or nebulizer. Patient technique may significantly decrease the amount of delivered dose.[61] Nursing plays a major role in teaching and assessing the correct use of aerosol therapy devices.

A spacer is a molded plastic reservoir that can be fitted onto an inhaler to deliver medication more safely and effectively. This device makes it unnecessary to coordinate breathing as carefully as with the standard inhaler, and thus patients are medicated more effectively. With enhanced delivery of medication to the lungs, it may be possible to reduce the number and volume of puffs required, thereby reducing the cost of medication. Once the medication is in the spacer, the patient can take several breaths, inhaling each time from the spacer, to receive the entire dose. Inhalers with spacers can be used to deliver most bronchoactive medications. The correct use and care of an MDI and spacer is shown in Figure 21-1.

Pharmacologic management of viral pneumonia in the healthy host primarily consists of early antimicrobial therapy for secondary bacterial infections. Specific antiviral therapy may also be beneficial.

Treatments. Oxygen is given to maintain an adequate saturation level. Turning, coughing, and deep breathing to promote airway clearance and effective respiration are performed regularly.

Diet. A high-calorie, high-protein diet with frequent small feedings is usually prescribed.

Activity. Early mobilization and activity progression are encouraged with alternating periods of activity and rest. Initially, fatigue and other constitutional symptoms limit patient activity to the chair and bedside commode.

Referrals. Common referrals for the patient with CAP requiring hospitalization include a dietitian, physical therapist, respiratory therapist, and social worker.

How To Use Your Metered-Dose Inhaler the Right Way

Using an inhaler seems simple, but most patients do not use it the right way. When you use your inhaler the wrong way, less medicine gets to your lungs. (Your doctor may give you other types of inhalers.)

For the next 2 weeks, read these steps aloud as you do them or ask someone to read them to you. Ask your doctor or nurse to check how well you are using your inhaler.

Use your inhaler in one of the three ways pictured below (**A** or **B** are best, but **C** can be used if you have trouble with **A** and **B**).

Steps for Using Your Inhaler

Getting ready
1. Take off the cap and shake the inhaler.
2. Breathe out all the way.
3. Hold your inhaler the way your doctor said (A, B, or C below).

Breathe in slowly
4. As you start breathing in **slowly** through your mouth, press down on the inhaler **one** time. (If you use a holding chamber, first press down on the inhaler. Within 5 sec, begin to breathe in slowly.)
5. Keep breathing in **slowly**, as deeply as you can.

Hold your breath
6. Hold your breath as you count to 10 slowly, if you can.
7. For inhaled quick-relief medicine (β_2-agonists), wait about 1 min between puffs. There is no need to wait between puffs for other medicines.

A. Hold inhaler 1 to 2 in in front of your mouth (about the width of two fingers).

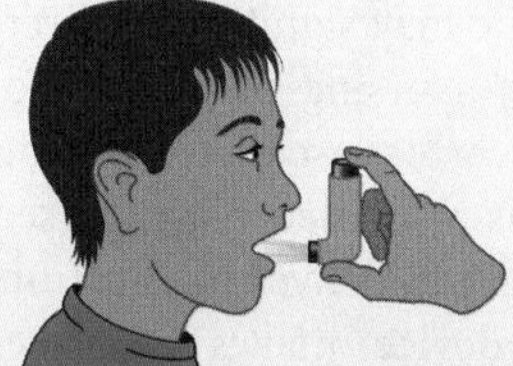

B. Use a spacer/holding chamber. These come in many shapes and can be useful to any patient.

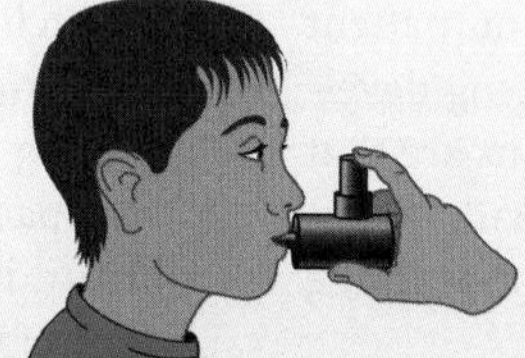

C. Put the inhaler in your mouth. Do not use for steroids.

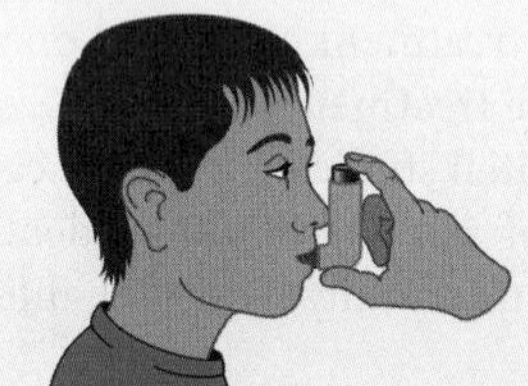

Clean Your Inhaler as Needed

Look at the hole where the medicine sprays out from your inhaler. If you see "powder" in or around the hole, clean the inhaler. Remove the metal canister from the L-shaped plastic mouthpiece. Rinse only the mouthpiece and cap in warm water. Let them dry overnight. In the morning, put the canister back inside. Put the cap on.

Know When to Replace Your Inhaler

For medicines you take each day (an example):
Say your new canister has 200 puffs (number of puffs is listed on canister) and you are told to take 8 puffs per day.

$$8 \text{ puffs per day} \overline{)\,200 \text{ puffs in canister}} = 25 \text{ days}$$

So this canister will last 25 days. If you started using this inhaler on May 1, replace it on or before May 25.

You can write the date on your canister.

For quick-relief medicine take as needed and count each puff.

Do not put your canister in water to see if it is empty. This does not work.

Figure 21-1 How to use a metered-dose inhaler.

NURSING MANAGEMENT OF PATIENT WITH PNEUMONIA

ASSESSMENT

Health History

Data to be collected to assess the patient with pneumonia include:

- History and character of onset and duration of cough, fever, shaking chills, chest pain, sputum production (amount, color, consistency)
- Self-care modalities used to treat symptoms
- History of exposure to persons with upper respiratory tract infection or pulmonary irritants
- History of recent antibiotic use (bacterial identification may be obscured by prior antibiotic use)
- Report of patient's ability to maintain activities of daily living (ADLs)

Physical Examination

Physical assessment of the patient with pneumonia includes:

- Vital signs

Check for elevated temperature. Elevation may be marked (39° C to 40° C [102.2° F to 104° F]) or low grade. Also check for tachycardia and tachypnea.

Pulmonary examination

Inspect for accessory muscle retraction, central cyanosis, respiratory grunting on expiration, and restricted chest movement. Palpate for decreased expansion on the affected side of the chest and for increased tactile fremitus. Percuss for dullness over areas of consolidation. Auscultate for bronchial breath sounds, inspiratory crackles (rales), decreased vocal fremitus due to pleural effusion, and egophony due to consolidation.

NURSING DIAGNOSES

Nursing diagnoses are determined from analysis of patient data. Nursing diagnoses for the person with pneumonia may include but are not limited to:

Diagnostic Title	Possible Etiologic Factors
1. Ineffective airway clearance	Increased sputum production, fatigue, tracheobronchial inflammation
2. Impaired gas exchange	Alveolocapillary membrane changes, inflammatory process, secretions impairing oxygen exchange across alveolocapillary membrane
3. Risk for spread of infection	Compromised lung defense system
4. Activity intolerance	Generalized weakness, imbalance between oxygen supply and demand
5. Acute pain	Pleural inflammation, coughing paroxysms
6. Imbalanced nutrition: less than body requirements	Infectious process, sputum production
7. Deficient knowledge: condition, treatment	Lack of exposure to or unfamiliarity with information

EXPECTED PATIENT OUTCOMES

Expected patient outcomes for the person with pneumonia may include but are not limited to:

1. Will demonstrate effective cough with expectoration (Both cough and sputum production should decrease within 72 hours of treatment initiation. Patients with chronic lung disease will return to prepneumonia status.)
2. Will demonstrate improved ventilation and adequate oxygenation of tissues, with return of ABG results to baseline
3. Will remain free of new infection
4. Will require minimal assistance with ADLs
5. Will report absence of chest pain
6. Will demonstrate improved appetite

7a. Will state when influenza and pneumonia vaccines should and should not be taken (not during acute illness)

7b. Will list signs and symptoms to be reported to the physician

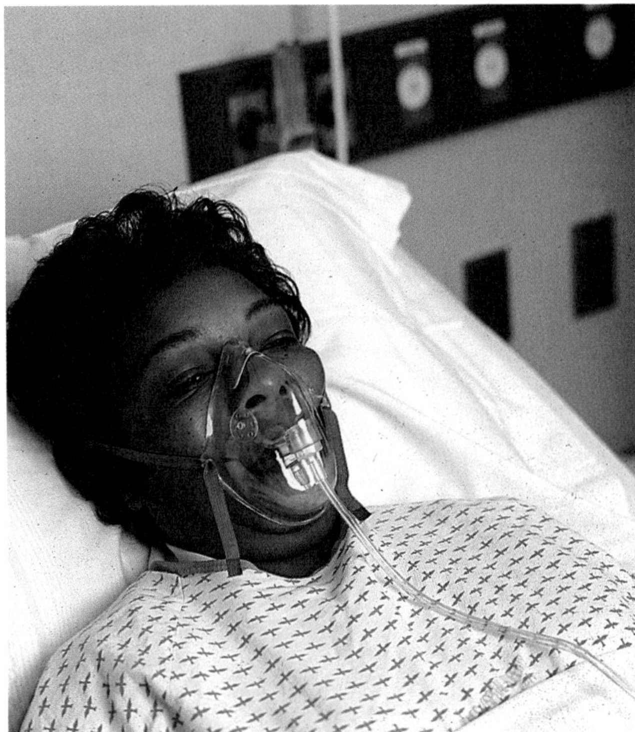

Figure 21-2 Simple oxygen mask.

7c. Will describe the cause and factors contributing to the occurrence of pneumonia

INTERVENTIONS

1. Maintaining Effective Airway Clearance

Dehydration results in thick, tenacious secretions, so fluid intake adequate to thin secretions and enable them to be expectorated easily must be ensured. If the patient does not have cardiovascular disease requiring fluid restriction, a fluid intake of 3 to 4 L/day should be provided. The best liquefying agent is water.

Changing the patient's position frequently will assist in mobilizing secretions. The nurse should also assist with nebulizer therapy and support effective coughing by teaching the proper technique and splinting the chest if needed because of muscle soreness. The patient who is unable to clear his or her own airway should be suctioned using sterile technique. Bronchoactive medications are administered as ordered, and the patient monitored for side effects and response to therapy.

2. Facilitating Breathing and Oxygenation

The patient is helped to breathe deeply and expand the chest to increase ventilation. The nurse places the patient in a position that facilitates breathing, typically an upright or semi-upright position. A pillow placed lengthwise at the patient's back provides support and thrusts the thorax slightly forward, allowing freer use of the diaphragm. The patient who must be upright to breathe may find it restful to put the head and arms on a pillow placed on an overbed table or to sit up in a big armchair with a footrest used to prevent dependent edema.

Oxygen by mask or cannula (Figures 21-2 and 21-3) is usually ordered when the partial pressure of oxygen (PaO_2) is less

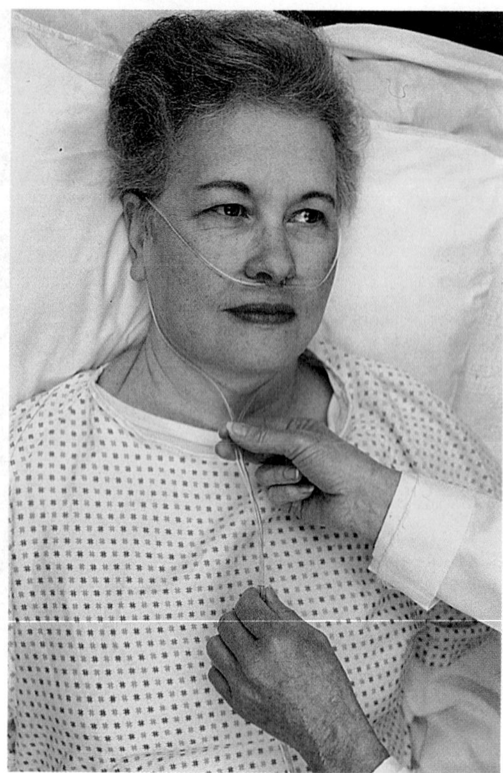

Figure 21-3 Nasal cannula.

than 60 mm Hg. When supplemental oxygen is necessary, it may be administered by nasal prongs or by mask. The method used depends on the patient's condition and the concentration of oxygen required. The nurse needs to be familiar with the various devices used to administer oxygen and, when oxygen is in use, must check the equipment frequently to ensure that it is working properly. Table 21-3 compares oxygen delivery systems.

The nurse monitors the patient for signs of hypoxemia. The patient with hypoxemia may not be breathless or cyanotic because cyanosis does not occur until there is 5 g or more of deoxygenated hemoglobin. In persons with anemia, all the available heme is completely saturated with oxygen, and thus these persons are never cyanotic, even though they may be hypoxemic. Thus an increase in the pulse rate or restlessness may be the first indication that the patient is experiencing hypoxemia. Patients receiving oxygen therapy are also monitored with ABG studies and pulse oximetry. Oxygen therapy is administered at the lowest concentration needed to achieve desired ABG values and/or pulse oximetry saturations.

3. Preventing Spread of Infection

When Standard Precautions are used, respiratory isolation is unnecessary. Hand washing is the most important way to prevent the spread of pneumonia from one patient to another via the hands of hospital personnel. Reducing the likelihood of gram-negative colonization of patients is also a primary consideration. For this reason, many hospitals have instituted tighter control policies on the use of antibiotics except in situations where a review panel of physicians approves their use. A reduction in the use of antibiotics also reduces the incidence of antibiotic-resistant hospital flora, which is the source of many nosocomial infections. Proper administration of medications and treatments is also important in preventing the spread of infection. Before administration of any prescribed antibiotic is begun, sputum for Gram stain and culture and blood for blood culture are collected. Antibiotic blood levels are maintained by giving antibiotics at scheduled times. Newer recommendations in the treatment of the hospitalized patient with uncomplicated CAP include a 2- to 3-day period of intravenous (IV) antibiotics followed by oral therapy. Patients may be discharged after they have demonstrated an ability to tolerate one dose of oral antibiotic.[18]

4. Assisting With Activities of Daily Living

Activities need to be spaced to prevent fatigue and respiratory distress. Response to physical activity must be monitored and activities adjusted to prevent overexertion. Activity levels are increased gradually on the basis of patient response. The need for supplemental oxygen with increased activity (based on oxygen saturation) must be carefully assessed. Methods to conserve energy should be included in patient teaching.

5. Promoting Comfort

The patient is monitored for chest pain, and character and location are noted. The patient is assisted to a position of comfort, usually with the head of the bed elevated 45 to 90 degrees. Analgesics (aspirin, acetaminophen, codeine) are administered as needed and prescribed. The hands are used to splint the chest when the patient coughs. Frequent mouth care is given, and the lips and nares are protected with a water-soluble lubricant. The patient is kept warm and dry to avoid chilling.

6. Promoting Adequate Nutrition and Hydration

Total daily intake is monitored. Oral fluids are encouraged as permitted. If the patient is receiving IV fluids, the rate is monitored. The patient is observed for signs of fluid volume deficit or excess. Meals that are appealing and appetizing to the patient are provided. Small, frequent feedings are offered. High-carbohydrate and high-protein foods are encouraged. Oral care is provided before and after meals.

7. Patient/Family Education

The major teaching emphasis is prevention. The nurse begins by assessing the patient's understanding of pneumonia by asking questions such as how is pneumonia transmitted and what are the risk factors for it. Proper handling of secretions is taught, including the importance of covering the nose and mouth with tissue when coughing or sneezing; discarding tissues in a paper or plastic bag for disposal; expectorating into an appropriate container; and washing the hands after coughing, sneezing, and expectorating. The importance of follow-up care and the need for vaccinations to prevent respiratory infections are reinforced. The nurse explains that persons at risk for developing complications of influenza should receive

TABLE 21-3 Comparison of Oxygen Delivery Systems

Delivery System	Indications	Concentration	Flow Rate	Considerations
Low Flow				
Nasal cannula	Patient with spontaneous respirations and oxygen requirements of less than 50%	32%-36%	2-6 L/min with no respiratory distress; 5-6 L/min with onset of respiratory distress	Oxygen concentration will increase about 4% for each increase of 1 L/min Questionable efficacy in patients who are mouth breathing
Simple face mask	Patient with spontaneous respirations	35%-60%	6-8 L/min	Liter-per-minute flow should be *at least* 6 to prevent accumulation and rebreathing of expired carbon dioxide May not be well tolerated by claustrophobic patient Effective for patients who are mouth breathing
Partial rebreather face mask	Patient with spontaneous respirations and oxygen requirements greater than 50%	65%-75%	6-10 L/min	Flow rates should be high enough to ensure that reservoir bag remains inflated during inspiration *and* expiration
Nonrebreather face mask	Spontaneously breathing patient with profound hypoxia or oxygen requirement	85%-95%	8-12 L/min	Flow rates should be high enough to ensure that reservoir bag remains inflated during inspiration *and* expiration
High Flow				
Venturi mask	Patient with spontaneous respirations	24%-50%	Varies (consult manufacturer's directions)	Good for use in patients who require delivery of precise oxygen concentrations Prescribed by concentration, not flow rate
Positive Pressure				
One-way valve pocket mask	Patient requiring assistance or control of ventilation	50%-55% (with oxygen supplement)	10-15 L/min	Prevents direct contact between health care provider and patient Easier to use and obtain adequate tidal volumes than bag-valve mask Should be used with oropharyngeal or nasopharyngeal airway in place to prevent gastric distention
Bag-valve mask	Patient requiring assistance or control of ventilation	Approaching 100% with reservoir; 45%-50% without reservoir	10-15 L/min	Prevents direct contact between health care provider and patient Should be used with oropharyngeal or nasopharyngeal airway in place to prevent gastric distention Difficult to use; inexperienced operators may not deliver adequate tidal volumes Short-term device of choice once endotracheal intubation achieved

From Somerson SJ et al: Mastering emergency airway management, *Am J Nurs* 96(5):25, 1996.

an annual influenza vaccine unless they are allergic to eggs or egg products or have had a previous reaction to vaccine.[18] Pneumonia polysaccharide vaccine is given only every 3 to 5 years. Booster vaccine is recommended 5 years after initial vaccination in all patients originally immunized before the age of 65.

EVALUATION

To evaluate the effectiveness of nursing interventions, compare patient behaviors with those stated in the expected patient outcomes. Achievement of patient outcomes is successful if the patient:

1. Has reduced cough and sputum and clear lung sounds.

2. Maintains PaO_2, $PaCO_2$, pH, and pulse oximetry within normal limits or at baseline level.
3. Is free of new infection.
4. Participates in ADLs.
5. Is free of chest pain.
6. Displays an improved appetite.
7. States the need for the influenza and pneumococcal vaccines, as well as for follow-up care (notifying physician) if cough persists, fever lasts for more than 48 hours, fatigue is overwhelming, or generalized achiness is present.

GERONTOLOGIC CONSIDERATIONS

Respiratory tract infections, and pneumonia specifically, are important causes of disease and death in older adults. In the United States 687,000 hospitalizations and 74,000 deaths caused by pneumonia occur annually among older adults. About 2% to 9% of these are caused by RSV.[29] Risk factors for pneumonia in older adults include alcoholism, asthma, immunosuppressive therapy, chronic lung disease, heart disease, institutionalization, and age greater than 70 years.[22] Nurses working with older persons need to be aware of their vulnerability to pneumonia, particularly because the presence and cause of pneumonia in older adults, whether community, nursing home, or hospital acquired, is not straightforward. The atypical presentation in elderly patients may delay diagnosis and treatment. In these patients the usual symptoms and signs (cough, crackles, rhonchi [gurgles], fever, chills, rigors, and chest pain) may be absent. Elderly patients with pneumonia may present with confusion, weakness, lethargy, failure to thrive, anorexia, abdominal pain, and episodes of falling, incontinence, delirium, and/or headache. Fever and chest consolidation may be absent. Tachypnea also has been shown to be a reliable indicator of lower respiratory tract infection in this population. Interventions are directed toward preventing pneumonia by teaching older adults to receive a vaccination for influenza yearly and pneumonia vaccination as indicated. Also, the importance of maintaining activity, good nutrition, and good health practices should be emphasized.

SPECIAL ENVIRONMENTS FOR CARE

Home Care Management

Persons discharged from the hospital after being admitted with CAP who are otherwise in fairly good health still require 4 to 6 weeks before they feel completely well. Recuperation requires extra rest and gradual resumption of activities, including return to work. Many people find it easier to resume work on a part-time basis until they have more energy. An adequate, balanced diet is essential, as are rest periods and adequate sleep at night. Generally the older the person, the longer the period of recovery, although many young people recovering from pneumonia remark, "I can't believe how tired I am."

Persons with HAP have an even more protracted period of recovery because their pneumonia may be superimposed on a chronic condition such as COPD. They are likely to be even more restricted in their activities because of chronic shortness of breath and resultant fatigue.

Persons living alone should have someone in the home at least part of each day to assist with ADLs such as bathing, dressing, and meal preparation. The nurse caring for the patient or a social worker should make a referral to a home health agency before the patient is discharged, unless the patient has a significant other to assist with these activities. These patients also need to be monitored closely by their health care provider and often need assistance in going to follow-up appointments.

COMPLICATIONS

With the advent of antibiotics and better diagnostic measures such as x-ray procedures, complications during or after pneumonia are rare in otherwise healthy persons. Atelectasis, delayed resolution, lung abscess, pleural effusion, empyema, pericarditis, meningitis, and relapse are complications that were common in the past. The patient must understand the importance of strict adherence to the prescribed medical treatment. Careful and accurate observation and sufficient time for convalescence also help ensure that the average patient has a smooth recovery. Older adults and those with a chronic illness are likely to have a relatively long course of convalescence from pneumonia and are at higher risk for complications.

Tuberculosis

In 1900 tuberculosis (TB) was the leading cause of death in the United States. It remained a major cause of death until the introduction of antituberculosis drug therapy in the late 1940s and early 1950s. Although TB is considered to be preventable and curable, it demands constant public health surveillance.

Etiology

TB is an infectious disease caused by the bacillus *Mycobacterium tuberculosis* or the tubercle bacillus, an acid-fast organism.

Epidemiology

TB is a global problem, and worldwide the number of cases of TB has continued to increase. The World Health Organization (WHO) estimates that approximately one third of the world's population is infected with *M. tuberculosis*.[54] TB is responsible for more deaths of young and middle-aged adults than any other disease except for AIDS. In 1997 there were approximately 8 million new TB cases and 2 million deaths due to TB. The highest rates occur in sub-Saharan Africa and south Asia. The lowest rates are reported in western Europe and North America. Targets for TB control established recently by the World Health Assembly include cure of 85% of the sputum smear-positive TB cases detected and detection of 70% of the estimated new sputum smear-positive TB cases.[81] In the United States and in developing countries, the epidemic of infection with the human immunodeficiency virus (HIV) has had a major impact on the incidence of TB. The United States experienced a resurgence of TB from 1986 to 1992 as a result of deteriorating public health services, increasing incidence of HIV, and development of disease among immigrants who arrived with latent disease. In response, TB control programs enhanced efforts to promptly identify persons with active TB and initiate and complete appropriate therapy. These efforts brought about a historically low case rate in 1998 of 18,361.[68]

TB continues to disproportionately affect poor, homeless, and HIV-infected persons. Cities with the highest number of persons positive for HIV, especially among drug abusers, also have the highest number of TB cases. These cities more likely have a large number of immigrants, many of whom come from countries in which TB is endemic. A major concern is that many persons with HIV are infected with TB organisms resistant to most chemotherapeutic agents used to treat TB. When this is true, infected persons pass their resistant organisms to those they infect, making treatment of newly infected persons particularly difficult. Because HIV infection is an important risk factor for developing TB among persons who have a positive tuberculin test, the Centers for Disease Control and Prevention (CDC) recommends that all HIV-infected persons be screened for active TB and, if infected, receive appropriate therapy. Also, persons with active TB and all tuberculin-positive persons should be evaluated for HIV infection.

Pathophysiology

When an individual with no previous exposure to TB (negative tuberculin reactor) inhales a sufficient number of tubercle bacilli into the alveoli, TB infection occurs. The body's reaction to the tubercle bacilli depends on the susceptibility of the individual, the size of the dose, and the virulence of the organisms. Inflammation occurs within the alveoli (parenchyma) of the lungs, and natural body defenses attempt to counteract the infection.

Macrophages ingest the organisms and present the mycobacterial antigens to the T cells. CD4 cells secrete lymphokines that enhance the capacity of the macrophages to ingest and kill bacteria. Lymph nodes in the hilar region of the lung become enlarged as they filter drainage from the infected site. The inflammatory process and cellular reaction produce a small, firm, white nodule called the primary tubercle. The center of the nodule contains tubercle bacilli. Cells gather around the center, and usually the outer portion becomes fibrosed. Thus blood vessels are compressed, nutrition of the tubercle is impaired, and necrosis occurs at the center. The area becomes walled off by fibrotic tissue, and the center gradually becomes soft and cheesy in consistency. This latter process is known as caseation necrosis. This material may become calcified (calcium deposits), or it may liquefy (liquefaction necrosis). The liquefied material may be coughed up, leaving a cavity, or hole, in the parenchyma of the lung. The cavity or cavities are visible on chest x-ray films and result in the diagnosis of cavitary disease.

Most individuals who are exposed to TB and develop a TB infection (confirmed by a positive tuberculin test) do not develop an active case of TB. The only x-ray evidence of their TB infection is a calcified nodule known as a Ghon tubercle. The evidence on x-ray films of enlarged hilar lymph nodes and the Ghon tubercle are referred to as the primary complex.

Persons who have the primary complex have become sensitized to the tubercle bacillus. This causes an antigen-antibody reaction when the person receives the antigen in the form of a purified protein derivative (PPD) or old tuberculin in a tuberculin test, and so the tuberculin test is said to be positive. This sensitization, once developed, usually remains throughout life unless something compromises the immune response. Evidence suggests that most persons who have a positive tuberculin reaction and take isoniazid (INH) prophylactically convert from a positive to a negative tuberculin test. This protection is believed to last for life. A positive tuberculin test does not mean that one has active TB, however, and nurses should explain this to persons undergoing the test.

TB is unlike other infections. Usually other infections disappear completely when overcome by the body's defenses and leave no living organisms and generally no signs of infection. *However, persons who have been infected with tubercle bacilli harbor the organism for the remainder of their lives unless they have received prophylactic INH.* Tubercle bacilli remain in the lungs in a dormant, walled-off, or so-called resting state. When a person is under physical or emotional stress, these bacilli may become active and begin to multiply. The development of active TB is believed to be caused by defects in T-cell function, macrophage function, or both. However, it is generally accepted that only 1 out of 10 persons with a positive tuberculin test ever develop active TB, and the incidence is expected to be much lower among those who receive preventive therapy with INH.

TB that occurs several years after the primary infection is known as reactivation TB.

TB is more likely to occur in persons with HIV infection because in HIV infection, progressive depletion and dysfunction of CD4 cells occur, along with defects in macrophage and monocyte function. Recent studies have estimated that patients who are co-infected with HIV and TB have higher rates of TB reactivation, higher rates of acute disease, higher rates of extrapulmonary disease, and malabsorption of anti-TB medications.[30] Two mycobacterial organisms are found in persons with AIDS. In developed countries the *Mycobacterium avium-intracellulare* complex (MAC) is the organism found in middle-class AIDS patients who have no history of IV drug use, whereas pulmonary TB caused by *M. tuberculosis* is more common in AIDS patients from developing countries and in persons from inner-city minority populations who have a history of IV drug use.

The WHO has revised the international definitions used in TB control in order to establish consistent, clear, and relevant definitions of the common basic terms for use by everyone involved in these efforts[81] (Table 21-4).

Extrapulmonary TB has taken on increased importance because of its extremely high rate of occurrence, usually along with pulmonary TB, in persons with HIV infection. TB is spread to other parts of the body via blood (hematogenously) or lymph (lymphogenously).

Mycobacteria other than tubercle bacilli (MOTT), formerly referred to as atypical acid-fast bacilli, include *Mycobacterium kansasii*, MAC, *Mycobacterium xenopi*, *Mycobacterium marinum*, *Mycobacterium fortuitum*, and *Mycobacterium chelonei*. These are strongly acid-fast organisms, but they differ from *M. tuberculosis* on culture. They are being

TABLE 21-4 Classifications of Tuberculosis

Tuberculosis suspect	Any person who presents with symptoms or signs suggestive of tuberculosis (TB)
Case of TB	Person in whom TB has been bacteriologically confirmed or diagnosed by a clinician
Definite case of TB	Person with culture positive for *Mycobacterium tuberculosis* complex
Pulmonary TB, sputum smear positive	Two or more sputum smear examinations positive for TB, or one sputum smear examination positive for acid-fast bacilli (AFB) plus x-ray abnormalities consistent with active pulmonary TB, or one sputum smear positive for AFB plus sputum culture positive for *M. tuberculosis*
Pulmonary TB, sputum smear negative	At least three sputum specimens negative for AFB, x-ray abnormalities consistent with active TB, no response to a course of broad-spectrum antibiotics, and decision by a clinician to treat with a full course of anti-TB chemotherapy
Extrapulmonary TB	TB of organs other than the lungs (e.g., pleurae, lymph nodes, abdomen, genitourinary tract, skin, joints and bones, meninges); diagnosis based on one culture-positive specimen or histologic or strong clinical evidence consistent with active extrapulmonary TB, followed by a decision by a clinician to treat with a full course of anti-TB chemotherapy
New patient	Person who has never had treatment for TB or who has taken anti-TB drugs for less than 1 month
Relapse	Patient previously treated for tuberculosis who has been declared cured or had treatment completed and is diagnosed with bacteriologically positive (smear or culture) TB
Failure	Patient who, while on treatment, is sputum smear positive at 5 months or later during the course of treatment
Chronic	A patient who is sputum positive at the end of a re-treatment regimen

Adapted from World Health Organization, Revised international definitions in TB control, *Int J Tuberc Lung Dis* 5(11):1071-1072, 2001.

isolated with increasing frequency from immunocompromised patients (persons with HIV infection or AIDS, transplant patients, and patients undergoing antineoplastic chemotherapy). MOTT have been found in soil and water and less commonly in foodstuffs and are considered to be opportunistic organisms. MOTT identified in sputum specimens may mean that the person is colonized and does not have invasive disease. MOTT are often isolated from the sputum of patients with pneumoconiosis, chronic bronchitis, COPD, a past history of TB, bronchiectasis, and chronic aspiration from esophageal disease. Table 21-5 summarizes these nontuberculosis organisms.

MAC is the most common bacterial infection in patients with AIDS. It occurs in 30% to 50% of AIDS patients. Patients with MAC have fever, night sweats, weight loss, diarrhea, lymphadenopathy, and anemia. The diagnosis is usually made from isolator blood cultures, bone marrow, lymph node, or liver biopsy. It is also diagnosed by acid-fast smear of stool in patients with disseminated infection.

Multidrug-resistant (MDR) TB has become a major problem in the United States. The emergence of MDR TB means that increased efforts are required to find every TB patient and to ensure that he or she is treated with multidrug therapy initially in an effort to prevent further drug resistance. It is also important to protect other patients and health care workers from becoming infected by patients with MDR TB. The problem is especially great in institutions caring for large numbers of patients with HIV, many of whom also have MDR TB.

TABLE 21-5 Mycobacteria Other Than Tubercle Bacilli Associated With Human Disease

Organism	Sites Typically Involved	Suggested Therapy
M. avium-intracellulare complex (MAC)	Lung, disseminated (AIDS)	Amikacin; clofazimine (Lamprene); RIF, EMB, and clarithromycin
M. kansasii	Lung	INH, RIF, and EMB for 12-24 months
M. xenopi	Lung	Amikacin, clofazimine, RIF, and EMB (perhaps clarithromycin and quinolone)
M. marinum	Skin, soft tissue	RIF, trimethoprim-sulfamethoxazole, or minocycline as single agents
M. fortuitum	Soft tissue Pulmonary Disseminated	Amikacin (parenteral) and cefoxitin or imipenem for 4-6 weeks
M. chelonei	Soft tissue	Often resistant to INH and PZA; may respond to four or more drugs; surgical excision of localized disease

AIDS, Acquired immunodeficiency syndrome; *EMB*, ethambutol; *INH*, isoniazid; *PZA*, pyrazinamide; *RIF*, rifampin.

Collaborative Care Management

The most critical issues in the management of TB involve the recognition of patients at risk and strategies to ensure completion of therapy. The increasing use of directly observed therapy (DOT) has been key to control efforts in developed, as well as developing, countries. The DOT strategy for TB control is based on five elements considered essential to a successful TB control program. These elements include:

1. Government commitment to make TB a priority program and to provide resources for nationwide coverage
2. Use of sputum smear microscopy for case detection among persons with persistent cough

3. An uninterrupted drug supply for treatment
4. Use of standardized chemotherapy, the patient's commitment to completing treatment, and the involvement of a health care worker to observe the patient taking each dose of medication
5. A recording and reporting system for monitoring treatment outcomes to reach targets of 85% cure, and training and supervision of health care workers and community volunteers[32]

Diagnostic Tests. Diagnostic testing for TB is slow and not ideally sensitive. Tests include the tuberculin skin test, sputum smear and culture, and chest x-ray examination.

Skin testing is performed to evaluate the body's cell-mediated immune function and to determine the body's sensitivity to infectious agents or allergens. A positive reaction is manifested by induration (thickening or hardening) at the site of the injection within a specified time period. Testing for *M. tuberculosis* with tuberculin-PPD is a common type of skin test. A positive reaction indicates that the individual has developed antibodies to the infectious agent, but it does not confirm active disease. A positive skin test reaction must be substantiated with other diagnostic evidence before active disease can be confirmed. Skin controls are sometimes administered to individuals along with the PPD skin test. If the reaction to the control is positive but the reaction is negative for PPD, it is unlikely that the individual has TB. If the reaction to the control is negative, the individual is "anergic" (i.e., has an altered cellular immunity system) and other tests must be performed to make the diagnosis of TB. The nurse should explain the purpose of the test and its procedure (see Guidelines for Safe Practice box).

Sputum smears and cultures are also used in the diagnosis of TB. If microscopic study of a slide prepared from the sputum of an individual reveals tubercle bacilli, the individual is said to have positive sputum, which confirms the diagnosis of TB. However, most persons with TB do not have positive sputum on smear, and a positive sputum culture is necessary to confirm the diagnosis.

Results of chest x-ray films and sputum examinations either rule out the possibility or confirm a diagnosis of TB. Because it is impossible to differentiate between typical bacilli and MOTT by a sputum smear, cultures are obtained on all persons. Cultures are also used for antimicrobial susceptibility (sensitivity) studies. Despite the introduction of improved culture media, the tubercle bacillus grows slowly on artificial media, and culture reports are not available for 3 to 6 weeks. Newer approaches to culturing the bacillus are under development.

Blood-streaked sputum in the absence of pronounced coughing may be the first indication to the person that something is wrong. Pathologic changes may have occurred in the lungs, but sputum examination may not show tubercle bacilli. However, if the nodules produced in the parenchyma of the lung become soft in the center and then caseated and liquefied, the liquefied material may break through and empty into the bronchi and be raised as sputum. Cavities in the lung may appear on x-ray films and may be present in more than one lobe of the lung.

Guidelines for Safe Practice

Administering the Mantoux Test

1. Draw up 0.1 ml (or amount specified by manufacturer) of purified protein derivative (PPD), using a tuberculin syringe and ½-inch, 25- to 27-gauge needle.
2. Cleanse the site (ventral forearm) with alcohol and let dry.
3. Keeping skin slightly taut, insert the needle (bevel upward) just beneath the skin surface.
4. Inject the solution, creating a 6- to 10-mm bleb. Do not massage the area after withdrawing the needle.
5. Read the test site with a millimeter ruler 48 to 72 hours after injection. The site should be lightly palpated to determine the presence or absence of induration. The largest diameter of induration should be measured and recorded in millimeters. Any erythema at the site should also be noted. Erythema alone does not indicate a positive result.
6. Interpretation of induration:
   a. 10 mm or more: highly significant for past or present infection
   b. 5 through 9 mm: doubtful reaction; however, retesting may be required
   c. 0 through 4 mm: little or no sensitivity; however, if individual's history indicates exposure, the test should be repeated in 4 to 6 weeks, since it may take this long for a tuberculin test to convert from negative to positive

Medications. Current TB treatment regimens are effective yet problematic, and there has been minimal research interest in the development of new tools to address this public health problem. When the ideal combination of available drugs is used, the duration of treatment requires a minimum of 6 months. Low-income countries aim for 8 months of therapy. Medical regimens for TB are associated with high levels of nonadherence.

Accomplishing the goals of therapy requires individualization, often with creative innovations to foster patient compliance. Because of the public health considerations related to TB, successful therapy needs to be viewed as the sole responsibility of those supervising the care of the patient.

To avoid the emergence of drug-resistant organisms, the Advisory Council for the Elimination of Tuberculosis recommends the following regimen for beginning therapy for TB.

Susceptibility Testing. All persons from whom *M. tuberculosis* is isolated should have drug susceptibility testing performed on the first isolate. Drug susceptibility testing should also be performed on additional isolates from patients whose cultures fail to convert to negative within 3 months of beginning therapy.

Initial Regimen. Initial treatment should be with four drugs (Table 21-6). During the first 2 months the patient should receive INH, rifampin (RIF), pyrazinamide (PZA), and either ethambutol (EMB), or streptomycin (SM), with daily dosing for at least 2 weeks. When drug susceptibility results are available, the regimen should be altered as needed. There are two models for dosing during the remaining period:

1. The initial daily dosing followed by 6 weeks of twice-weekly dosing of the same four drugs followed by 4 months of twice-weekly dosing of INH and RIF
   or
2. Daily dosing with INH, RIF, PZA, and EMB or SM until drug resistance is ruled out (8 weeks of dosing), followed by 4 months of INH and RIF

These first 2 months, when the bacterial burden is greatly reduced and patients become noninfectious, are called the "intensive" or "bactericidal" phase. The "continuation" or "sterilizing" phase of 4 to 6 months is required to eliminate persisting bacilli and minimize the risk of relapse.[57] Sputum cultures should be monitored monthly for patients with positive cultures. Conversion to negative should occur in 85% of patients.[18]

Health care and correctional facilities that are experiencing outbreaks of TB resistant to INH and RIF or that are resuming treatment of a patient who has been treated for TB in the past may need to begin patient treatment with five or six drugs as initial therapy. As global rates of MDR TB are rising, patients are being treated with a combination of second-line drugs that are more expensive, more toxic, and less effective. The most common second-line drugs include para-aminosalicylic acid (PAS), cycloserine, clofazimine, thiacetazone, and quinolones (see Future Watch box).

Immunosuppressed Patients. HIV infection and other factors that compromise the immune system make patients more susceptible to the development of resistant organisms. For this reason, it is recommended that patients with HIV and TB be treated for a total of 9 months and for at least 6 months after their sputum converts to negative. If drug susceptibility results are not available, EMB or SM should be considered for the entire course of therapy because of the rapid progression of TB while the patient is receiving inadequate therapy. TB therapy poses additional risk for HIV patients because the medication regimen has the potential to interact with other medications, especially antiretroviral agents.

Treatment of Extrapulmonary Tuberculosis. The regimen that is used for treating pulmonary disease is also used to treat extrapulmonary disease. Some experts believe that therapy should be for 9 months instead of 6 months for patients with disseminated TB, miliary disease, TB of bones and joints, and TB of the lymph glands.

Treatment of Tuberculosis During Pregnancy. Therapy is essential for pregnant women who have TB. SM is not used because it may cause congenital deafness. Routine use of PZA is not

TABLE 21-6 Common Medications for Tuberculosis

Drug	Classification	Common Side Effects	Tests	Remarks
Isoniazid (INH)	Bactericidal; penetrates all body tissues and fluids, including cerebrospinal fluid (CSF)	Peripheral neuritis, hepatitis, rash, fever	AST (formerly SGOT), ALT (formerly SGPT) (not as routine)	Daily alcohol intake interferes with metabolism of isoniazid and increases risk of hepatitis; antacids containing aluminum interfere with absorption of INH.
Rifampin (RIF)	Bactericidal; penetrates all body tissues, including CSF	Hepatitis, febrile reactions, thrombocytopenia (rare), hepatotoxicity increases when given with INH	AST, ALT, platelet count (not as routine)	Urine, sweat, tears may turn orange temporarily; decrease effectiveness of oral contraceptives, anticoagulants, corticosteroids, barbiturates, hypoglycemics, and digitalis.
Ethambutol (EMB)	Bacteriostatic; does not penetrate CSF; penetrates other body fluids	Optic neuritis (reversible with discontinuation of drug; very rare at 15 mg/kg skin rash)	Visual acuity; red-green color discrimination; GI irritation	No significant reaction with other drugs. Check vision monthly. Give with food.
Pyrazinamide (PZA)	Bacteriostatic or bactericidal depending on susceptibility of mycobacterium	Hyperuricemia, hepatitis, arthralgia, GI irritation	Uric acid, AST, ALT	Obtain baseline liver function tests and repeat regularly. Give with food; drink 2 L of fluid daily.
Streptomycin (SM)	Bactericidal, aminoglycoside; disrupts protein synthesis; poor penetration into body tissues and CSF	Eighth cranial nerve damage (vestibular or ocular); damage often irreversible; nephrotoxicity	Vestibular function; audiograms; creatinine level determined before therapy started	Monitor kidney function monthly. Monitor vestibular function with caloric stimulation test monthly. Monitor hearing with audiograms monthly. Meningitis is treated with intrathecal or subarachnoid instillation of SM.

ALT, Alanine transaminase; *AST,* aspartate transaminase; *GI,* gastrointestinal; *SGOT,* serum glutamic-oxaloacetic transaminase; *SGPT,* serum glutamate pyruvate transaminase.

recommended because the risk of birth defects in the fetus has not been determined. Nine months of therapy with INH, RIF, and EMB is recommended. Women may breastfeed while receiving TB therapy because the concentration of the drugs in breast milk is so low that drug toxicity does not develop in the newborn.

Control of Nosocomial Tuberculosis. The control of the spread of TB to hospital employees is based on three tenets: tuberculin skin testing and chest x-ray studies for new employees, isolation of clinical cases, and a high level of suspicion for TB among new admissions. Concern about occupational transmission is heightened by the increasing levels of TB incidence. Recent transmissions to health care workers have been due to failure to diagnose, delays in laboratory identification of TB, delays in recognition of drug resistance, and lapses in infection control practices. The prevention of nosocomial TB is supported by 1997 Occupational Safety and Health Administration (OSHA) standards that require (1) an active surveillance program using the tuberculin PPD test, (2) isolation of persons with suspected TB, (3) negative-pressure isolation rooms, and (4) the use of particulate respirators.

Diet. A well-balanced diet containing the essential food groups with a vitamin supplement is recommended. Persons who are homeless or have limited incomes may require food vouchers with which to obtain additional food. Those who are poorly nourished or underweight may benefit from six small feedings of high-calorie, high-protein foods daily rather than three large meals.

Activity. Patients with TB require increased periods of rest to promote healing and alleviate fatigue. Participation in ADLs is encouraged to increase activity tolerance and build muscle strength.

Referrals. The most common referrals are to social services, nutritionists, and community health nursing. Patients who are homeless or have limited incomes are referred to social services for assistance with food and shelter. To prevent infecting others, some patients should not return to their previous living conditions until their sputum cultures are negative for acid-fast bacilli. Environmental factors are of extreme importance in influencing the transmission of the disease. A nutritionist should meet with the patient and significant others to review the basic food groups and the amount of each nutrient required by the patient. Ways to provide extra calories in small, frequent meals is helpful information. A community health nurse should meet with the patient and significant other to develop a plan for follow-up care.

Future Watch
New Developments in Tuberculosis Drugs

There is encouraging news about the development of new drugs for tuberculosis (TB). Longer-acting rifamycins may provide for more widely spaced intermittent treatment and a reduction in the number of directly observed doses. Rifapentine was approved for treatment of TB in the United States in 1998, and rifabutin has been recommended for human immunodeficiency virus (HIV)–infected TB patients, who cannot receive rifampin because of interactions with antiretroviral agents. A significant advance in TB treatment has also come from the development of the broad-spectrum fluoroquinolone antibiotics (moxifloxacin, gatifloxacin). They have proven successful in the treatment of patients and are now among the preferred "second-line" drugs for multidrug-resistant TB. Two novel classes of compounds also are of interest. Oxazolidinones have been developed as broad-spectrum antimicrobials and seem to have substantial antimyocobacterial activity. The other class is the nitroimidazopyrans. These are drugs related to nitroimidazoles that have been studied in the past as possible anti-TB drugs. The most promising compound, PA-824, has an action against *Mycobacterium tuberculosis* comparable with that of isoniazid (INH). It also appears to have a sterilizing effect that could shorten TB treatment considerably.

Reference: O'Brien RJ, Nunn PP: The need for new drugs against tuberculosis, *Am J Respir Crit Care Med* 163(5):1055-10058, 2001.

NURSING MANAGEMENT OF PATIENT WITH TUBERCULOSIS

ASSESSMENT

Health History

Any history of signs and symptoms of TB is explored (see Clinical Manifestations box). It is also important to determine whether the patient has had a known exposure to a person with TB. Often the source of the infection is unknown and never determined. Close contacts of the patient need to be identified so that they may undergo examination to determine whether they are infected and have active disease or a positive tuberculin test.

Physical Examination

Physical assessment of the patient with TB focuses on the pulmonary examination and the general health status. Attention is directed to determining the presence of a productive cough, adventitious breath sounds, afternoon temperature elevation, tuberculin skin test reaction of 10 mm induration or more, and pulmonary infiltrates visible on a chest x-ray film.

Clinical Manifestations
Pulmonary Tuberculosis

CONSTITUTIONAL SYMPTOMS

Low-grade fever
Pallor
Chills
Night sweats
Easy fatigability
Anorexia
Weight loss

PULMONARY SYMPTOMS

Cough productive of a scant amount of mucoid sputum
Purulent, blood-stained sputum if cavitation has occurred
Dyspnea: late in the disease
Chest pain: late in the disease

NURSING DIAGNOSIS

Nursing diagnoses for the person with TB may include but are not limited to:

Diagnostic Title	Possible Etiologic Factors
1. Risk for spread/reactivation of infection	Inadequate defense mechanisms, environmental exposure, insufficient knowledge to avoid exposure, inadequate therapeutic interventions
2. Ineffective airway clearance	Increased sputum, decreased energy/fatigue
3. Ineffective therapeutic regimen management	Complicated and lengthy medical regimen, economic difficulty, lack of follow-up care, side effects of therapy
4. Activity intolerance	Unable to perform ADLs because of fatigue

EXPECTED PATIENT OUTCOMES

Expected patient outcomes for the person with TB may include but are not limited to:

1. Will explain measures such as compliance with chemotherapy regimen and measures to prevent spread of TB, such as covering the mouth and nose with tissues when coughing or sneezing and proper disposal of used tissues
1a. Will state name, dose, actions, and side effects of prescribed medications
1b. Will explain the rationale for two, three, or four chemotherapy agents taken together
1c. Will explain the relationship between drug-resistant organisms and the need to take chemotherapy agents as directed
1d. Will explain why the health care provider should be notified immediately if for any reason chemotherapy agents cannot be taken (e.g., side effects)
1e. Will state where to receive a new supply of chemotherapy agents and the date it is to be obtained
1f. Will state the need and plan for follow-up care
1f(1). Will list signs and symptoms that indicate the need for immediate medical care (increased cough, hemoptysis, unexplained weight loss, fever, night sweats)
1f(2). Will state when and where the next sputum test or x-ray film is to be taken
1f(3). Will identify the plan for accessing follow-up care
2. Breath sounds will be clear
2a. Will clear the airway by effective coughing
2b. Amount of sputum will be reduced
3. Will demonstrate behaviors necessary to maintain the therapeutic regimen
4. Will participate in ADLs

INTERVENTIONS

TB is a multifaceted problem that requires a multipronged approach. Nurses can be key to TB control by developing an individualized interventional strategy. Nurses can identify needed ancillary services, monitor the patient's progress, and change the strategy if it is not working.

1. Preventing Spread of Infection

The most important factor in the transmission of TB is overcrowded living conditions. To prevent the transmission of TB from person to person, it is necessary to prevent contamination of the air with *M. tuberculosis.* This is accomplished by treating the patient with antituberculosis drugs and teaching the patient to cover the nose and mouth with a tissue when coughing, sneezing, and laughing so that droplet nuclei are not discharged into the air. Most persons who adhere to the antiinfective prescribed therapy and do not have other mitigating factors such as immunosuppression convert their sputum from positive to negative in 2 to 3 weeks (see Patient Teaching box).

2. Improving Airway Clearance

To improve airway clearance, the patient is taught to sit upright in a chair or in bed. If the patient is confined to bed at home, he or she may find it helpful to sit on the side of the bed with the feet on a chair. The patient is taught to take two or three deep breaths, cover the mouth with tissues, and then cough. Using this method when coughing decreases fatigue because it requires less expenditure of energy. Many patients can cough most effectively when the mouth is moist, and sips of water or a warm beverage such as tea or coffee can be encouraged before coughing. For patients with thick, tenacious sputum, fluid intake is encouraged to thin the secretions and make them easier to expectorate. Water is considered by many experts to be the most effective sputum-liquefying agent.

3. Enhancing Management of Therapeutic Regimen

To encourage patient understanding of the complex therapeutic regimen in order to promote adherence, health care professionals must encourage open discussion and solicit questions and concerns from the patient and family. Also, patience is required, and the information may need to be repeated often for clarity and to promote understanding. It is best to strive for continuity of teaching by coordinating care that involves both acute care and home care or public health clinicians. All questions should be answered as completely as

Patient Teaching

Preventing the Transmission of Tuberculosis

Patient must take antituberculosis drugs as prescribed.
- Drugs are always taken as combination of at least four drugs initially.
- Drugs must be taken uninterruptedly.
- Both of the above are necessary to prevent development of resistant strains of *Mycobacterium tuberculosis.*

Prevent contamination of air with *M. tuberculosis.*
- Cover nose and mouth with disposable tissues when coughing, sneezing, or laughing.
- Place used tissues in paper or plastic bag for disposal.

possible, supplying information appropriate to the patient's educational level and ability to comprehend what is being taught. Written materials with diagrams and drawings that reinforce what is being taught are helpful. All written materials should be reviewed with the patient and, whenever possible, a family member before they are given to the patient. For patients who do not speak English, a translator and written materials in the patient's language are necessary. Concerns about interpersonal or financial problems indicate the need for a social services referral.

4. Increasing Activity Tolerance

During the acute phase of the illness, persons with TB experience fatigue and have difficulty completing ADLs. Increasing activity tolerance involves careful assessment of the physiologic response to activity and planning for progressive increases based on patient tolerance. In some settings activities may require measures to prevent exposure of susceptible individuals. Respiratory isolation may hinder patient interest in activity, especially when wearing a mask is required. The nurse needs to reinforce the need for isolation while also promoting a positive self-image and increasing activity.

Patient/Family Education

Health Promotion/Prevention. The major priority of TB prevention and control programs is that all persons with TB be promptly identified and treated with an adequate course of drug therapy. A special effort must be made to identify TB among foreign-born U.S. residents from countries with high TB rates. These high rates reflect the global nature of TB as a public health problem.

Primary and Secondary Prevention. For TB to be eliminated, the organism must be prevented from being transmitted from one person to another. Persons with latent TB (positive PPD test, no clinical signs of disease) who are at risk for progression to active TB are treated with INH 300 mg/day for 6 to 12 months (Box 21-2). Preventive INH therapy is more than 90% effective in patients who adhere to a 52-week regimen.[18] It is a common misconception that INH therapy for latent infection is contraindicated in patients over age 35. If INH-associated hepatitis occurs, the symptoms are mild, nonspecific, and similar to those of any viral illness. Contraindications to the use of INH preventive therapy are (1) previous INH-associated liver disease; (2) severe adverse reactions to INH, such as fever, chills, rash, and arthritis; and (3) acute liver disease of any etiology.[18] Persons receiving INH preventive chemotherapy may also receive pyridoxine concurrently to reduce the incidence of central nervous system (CNS) effects or peripheral neuropathies. They should be seen monthly by a health care provider to reinforce the importance of adhering to the regimen and to be monitored for any serious side effects. Because most cases of TB in patients with HIV infection occur in those with a history of a positive tuberculin test, all persons with HIV infection should be considered for preventive therapy with INH.

Vaccination. Efforts continue in search of a more satisfactory TB vaccine. Presently bacille Calmette-Guérin (BCG) is used worldwide except in the United States and the Netherlands. Vaccination is compulsory in many developing countries and officially recommended in others. The vaccine contains attenuated tubercle bacilli that have lost their ability to produce disease. It produces a subclinical infection that results in sensitization of T lymphocytes and cross-immunity. In most instances it produces a positive PPD reaction, so it is administered only to persons who have a negative reaction to the tuberculin test. The vaccine should be given intradermally only by persons who have had careful instruction in the proper technique. A multiple-puncture disk is used to give the vaccine. Possible complications of vaccination are local ulcers, which occur in a relatively high percentage of persons vaccinated, and abscesses or suppuration of lymph nodes, which occur in a small percentage of persons vaccinated.[18]

Protection of Health Care Workers. To protect nurses and other health care providers caring for patients who have a positive TB smear or culture, the following measures are indicated:

- First and foremost, emphasis is on preventing *M. tuberculosis* from being expelled into room air by the patient. Patients must be instructed to cover their noses and mouths with tissues when coughing and sneezing. Those who are too ill to do so or who are confused should have a surgical mask put over their nose and mouth.
- The patient should be placed in a private room, and the door to the hallway is kept closed.
- If the patient must leave the room for tests or procedures, he or she should wear a mask or particulate respirator with a one-way valve.
- The air pressure in the room should be negative. This allows air to flow into the room when the door is opened and prevents room air from moving out into the hallway.
- The air in the room is exchanged several times every hour, with two of the exchanges being with fresh air from the outside (the evidence is inconclusive as to the optimal number of air exchanges required). Air from the

BOX 21-2 Priorities for Preventive Therapy With Isoniazid Among Tuberculosis-Infected Persons

1. Persons with human immunodeficiency virus (HIV) infection
2. Recent contacts of persons with infectious tuberculosis (TB)
3. Persons with recent skin test conversions
4. Persons with recent TB disease who have been inadequately treated
5. Persons with negative sputum cultures and stable fibrotic lesions on chest radiographs consistent with inactive TB
6. Persons with medical conditions that increase the risk of TB
   Leukemia or lymphoma
   Silicosis
   Diabetes mellitus
   Gastrectomy
   End-stage renal disease
   Antibodies to HIV

patient's room should be directly vented to the outside and not recirculated within the hospital.

- High-energy particulate air (HEPA) filters should be installed in ventilation ducts.
- Ultraviolet lights high on walls or ceilings in patient rooms can be used to disinfect room air. They are placed so that they do not cause a risk to the patients or health care workers.
- Personnel caring for patients should wear a disposable particulate respirator. The respirator should fit snugly over the nose and mouth to prevent as much room air as possible from getting in around the edges. The particulate respirator filters out organisms as small as 1 m; *M. tuberculosis* organisms are 3 to 5 m. Compliance with the use of the particulate respirators has been a problem because of discomfort.
- All health care workers should know their tuberculin status. All workers who are tuberculin negative should be tested yearly with PPD. Those who have not had a recent test should receive a baseline tuberculin test on employment and then yearly. Workers who have inadvertently been exposed to a patient with TB (often before the diagnosis of TB is made) should have a tuberculin test 8 to 12 weeks after exposure. It takes this period for a test to convert from negative to positive. The CDC recommends that health care workers involved in the care of patients receiving cough-inducing procedures, such as bronchoscopy and tracheal suctioning, should be tested with tuberculin at least every 6 months.[68]
- Health care workers who convert from a negative to a positive tuberculin test should have an examination to rule out active TB. Those refusing therapy should have a yearly chest x-ray.

EVALUATION

To evaluate the effectiveness of nursing interventions, compare patient behaviors with those stated in the expected patient outcomes. Achievement of patient outcomes is successful if the patient:

1a-d. Explains the rationale for taking anti-TB drugs without interruption; demonstrates use of a pillbox or empty egg carton to distribute each day's supply of medications divided according to the number of times taken, along with a checklist to record each dose as it is taken; states the name, dose, actions, and side effects of the medications.

1e,f. States the date of the next sputum test and the date and time of the next chest x-ray examination; states the date and time of the next appointment with the medical provider; states signs and symptoms that indicate the need for immediate medical care (e.g., an increase in dyspnea or appearance of hemoptysis); states when and where to get medications.

2a,b. Has minimal cough; covers the nose and mouth with a tissue when coughing or sneezing and disposes of tissues as taught; has decreased sputum; has clear breath sounds.

3. Identifies and uses available resources for follow-up care, support with the medication regimen, and housing if needed.

4. Participates in ADLs; reports measurable increase in activity tolerance.

GERONTOLOGIC CONSIDERATIONS

Many older persons were exposed to TB when they were children and have a positive tuberculin test. This indicates that they have dormant tubercle bacilli walled off in their lungs. When these persons are subjected to physical or emotional stress, they may develop active TB. Also, with aging, the immune system may be less able to react to the tuberculin test or respond effectively to an infection. This increases the risk of undiagnosed infection, which can be transmitted to others. Thus it is recommended that older adults, including those in nursing homes, have a yearly chest x-ray examination. If an active case of TB is found in a nursing home resident, more frequent x-ray examinations of other residents are necessary.

Many older adults, especially those who are frail, have a poor appetite and need special attention to their nutritional needs. Other older persons with limited financial resources need help in obtaining an adequate diet. Asking the person to keep a daily food diary can help determine whether the person's diet is sufficient to support healing of the TB.

SPECIAL ENVIRONMENTS FOR CARE

Home Care Management

Following an initial acute care hospitalization, most persons with active TB can return home and periodically visit a TB clinic or other treatment facility. A community or public health nurse will assess the home environment and determine whether the patient can be relied on to take all medications as prescribed or whether there is another adult in the home who can be responsible for ensuring that the patient takes all medications as prescribed. If not, other provisions for DOT are necessary. The nurse is responsible for teaching the patient about medications, handling secretions, protecting others from infection, and eating an adequate diet. Generally, patients who take their medications as prescribed convert their sputum from positive to negative within 3 to 4 weeks. Faithful covering of the nose and mouth with tissues when coughing or sneezing prevents contamination of air in the home. Because the incidence of TB is high among persons who are HIV positive, the patient should be encouraged to have an HIV test.

It is also important that persons who have had sustained contact with someone who has TB have a tuberculin test and appropriate follow-up care. Contacts who have a positive tuberculin test are offered prophylactic treatment with INH and will need follow-up with periodic chest x-ray examinations.

COMPLICATIONS

The complication of greatest concern is the development of a resistant strain of TB that may be extremely difficult to treat and will require hospitalization while effective drug therapy is sought. HIV may also develop, and it may not be possible to determine which of the two diseases occurred first.

Rigorous treatment of both diseases is required, and hospitalization is often necessary.

Lung Abscess

Etiology/Epidemiology

A lung abscess is a pus-containing necrotic lesion of the lung parenchyma that often contains an air-fluid level. It may be associated with infections, pulmonary infarction, malignancy, and necrosis secondary to silicosis and coal miners' pneumoconiosis. Lung abscess secondary to aspiration is much less common since the introduction of antibiotic treatment, and the prognosis has improved, with a mortality rate of 15% to 20%. The prognosis is relatively poor, however, for elderly, debilitated, malnourished, and immunocompromised patients. Large abscesses and aerobic bacteria are associated with the worst outcomes.[36]

Pathophysiology

Infected material lodges in the small bronchi and produces inflammation. Partial obstruction of the bronchus results in retention of secretions beyond the obstruction and the eventual necrosis of tissue. The necrotic lung tissue is coughed up, and an air-filled cavity is left in the lung. Aspirated food particles and perigingival debris, which contains both aerobic and anaerobic organisms, are the most common causes of lung abscess secondary to aspirated substances. Laboratory cultures of sputum or transtracheal aspirates are necessary to identify the causative organism. Lung abscess may follow bronchial obstruction caused by a tumor, foreign body, or stenosis of the bronchus. Metastatic spread of cancer cells to the lung parenchyma may also cause an abscess, and occasionally the infection appears to have been borne by the bloodstream. Bronchoscopy may be used to identify the infected segment and to obtain specimens for culture. Signs and symptoms of an acute lung abscess are presented in the Clinical Manifestations box.

Collaborative Care Management

Most diagnoses of lung abscess are made from chest x-ray films. If blood and pleural fluid cultures are negative, the identification of the causative agent requires an invasive procedure, such as bronchial lavage or percutaneous lung aspiration.

The course of lung abscess is influenced by the cause of the abscess and by the type of drainage that can be established. If the purulent material drains easily, the patient may respond well to segmental postural drainage, antibiotic therapy, and good general supportive care.

Antibiotic therapy is based on the identified pathogen and may be continued for up to 8 weeks. Most cavities close within 6 weeks, but occasionally a cavity may persist for months. Foul-smelling sputum usually disappears within a few days, whereas cough and non–foul-smelling sputum may continue for a longer period. Usually the patient begins to feel better during the first week of therapy, but it may take up to 2 months for the temperature to return to normal. In some patients uninfected cavities or fibrosis may persist.

If the patient does not improve with the above therapy, bronchoscopy is performed to improve drainage and search for a possible obstruction to drainage, such as carcinoma or a foreign body. Rarely, surgical resection of the abscessed area is needed.

The person with a lung abscess is very ill and requires hospitalization. Care of the patient with a lung abscess is presented in the Guidelines for Safe Practice box. Of equal importance to caring for the patient with a lung abscess is the prevention of lung abscess in hospitalized patients. Nursing interventions that decrease the risk of lung abscess begin with monitoring patients who are at risk for aspiration (i.e., those with a reduced level of consciousness, depressed cough and/or gag reflexes, impaired swallowing, a tracheostomy, or an endotracheal tube). These patients should be elevated to the highest or best position for eating and drinking. Patients receiving enteral feedings should also be carefully positioned and closely monitored to ensure that the tube is in the stomach. Frequent mouth care should be provided to persons with diminished levels of consciousness. Patients who are vomiting should be placed on their side in postanesthesia position to reduce the risk for aspiration. For patients unable to expectorate secretions from the mouth and oropharynx, oral suctioning may be necessary.

Clinical Manifestations
Acute Lung Abscess

- High fever: 39° C (102° F)
- Chills and prostration
- Cough and sputum production common
- Night sweats, pleuritic chest pain, anemia, and occasionally hemoptysis
- Putrid sputum in about 50% of patients—foul odor evident in patient's room
- Weight loss in about 40% of patients (foul-smelling and foul-tasting sputum often causes anorexia)
- Mortality rate of primary abscess is 5%
- Up to one third of patients 45 years of age and older with a lung abscess also have carcinoma. A diagnostic bronchoscopy should be considered for all high-risk patients, even if they respond well to therapy.

Guidelines for Safe Practice
The Patient With Lung Abscess

- Monitor vital signs at least every 4 hours because temperature may spike in afternoon and may persist for as long as 2 weeks.
- Place patient in comfortable position. If patient is conscious, he or she usually is more comfortable with headrest at 45 to 90 degrees.
- Help patient cough up sputum. This helps drain abscess.
- Collect sputum for culture and sensitivity tests to determine organism and antibiotic therapy. This monitors effectiveness of therapy and whether resistant organisms are developing.
- Do postural drainage. This facilitates drainage from the abscess.

Empyema

Etiology/Epidemiology

Empyema is the presence of fluid containing pus within a body cavity, typically the pleural space. It usually occurs after pleural effusion secondary to other respiratory diseases, such as pneumonia, lung abscess, TB, and fungal infections of the lung, and also after thoracic surgery or chest trauma. It is reported in 1% to 2% of patients hospitalized with community-acquired pneumonia. Empyema can result from staphylococcal infection.

Pathophysiology

There are three stages of empyema:

Stage I: exudative phase	The fluid stage of empyema
Stage II: fibrinopurulent phase	The pleural effusion becomes infected with cellular debris
Stage III: organizing phase	The empyema is chronic and characterized by a thick, inelastic pleural peel that traps and compresses the lung

The signs and symptoms of empyema are presented in the Clinical Manifestations box.

Collaborative Care Management

Treatment of empyema requires vigorous pleural drainage and antimicrobial therapy. Initial treatment is often serial thoracentesis with aspiration of the cavity and instillation of antibiotics into the pleural space. Oral or IV antibiotics may also be given. An alternative method of drainage is closed-chest drainage, in which a trocar is inserted between the ribs at the base of the cavity, a chest catheter is inserted through the trocar, the trocar is removed, and the tube is connected to water-seal drainage. Pus then drains from the cavity into the collection chamber. For closed drainage to be successful, the pus must be thin enough to drain out of the pleural space, and the lung must be able to reexpand to fill the pleural space. When the fluid is loculated, the chest tube may require ultrasound or computed tomography (CT)–guided placement. In some cases fibrinolytic agents may be instilled via the chest tube to promote drainage. The agents most commonly used include streptokinase and urokinase. Urokinase has the advantage of being less allergenic. Both work by activating plasminogen, which is converted to plasmin, which then degrades fibrin and clots, helping to liquefy the drainage. In the event that none of these measures effectively drains the pleural space within a few days or if the lung fails to reexpand to obliterate the space, surgery is necessary.

For second-stage empyema, a newer procedure of video-assisted thoracostomy has demonstrated good success. In instances of chronic empyema in which a fibrinous peel has formed on the visceral pleura, preventing the lung from reexpanding and filling the space left after the empyema cavity was drained, decortication may be necessary. In decortication, the fibrinous peel is removed from the visceral pleura by blunt dissection, freeing the lung so that it can reexpand and fill the pleural space. With both of these procedures, two chest tubes are inserted into the pleural space and connected to water-seal drainage with additional suction. A repeat chest CT scan and assessment of the patient's clinical condition are important in evaluating response to therapy.[16]

Patient/Family Education. Nursing care depends on the type and effectiveness of the procedure and the patient's symptoms. Some patients require oxygen therapy. Antibiotics are given, and the response is monitored. Activity is reduced initially, on the basis of patient tolerance, but progressed gradually to prevent debilitation. Coughing and deep breathing exercises may be indicated to improve ventilation. In some cases the patient goes through several treatments before the empyema space is closed. This can be frustrating, and the patient can become very discouraged. A major nursing role is to support the patient and family during the various procedures. Keeping the patient and family apprised of progress and any treatments to be done is important.

> ***Clinical Manifestations***
> **Empyema**
>
> Fever
> Dyspnea
> Anorexia
> Pleuritic chest pain
> In addition to the above, the following may be found on examination:
> - Unequal chest expansion
> - Weight loss with malaise
> - Pleural friction rub
> - Foul-smelling sputum
> - Decreased lung sounds in area of empyema

Fungal Infections

North America is home to three major endemic mycoses that give rise to major fungal infections of the lungs: histoplasmosis, coccidioidomycosis, and blastomycosis. The causative agents are found in soil. They are classified as deep mycoses because there is involvement by the parasite of deeper tissues and internal organs. Most of the clinical presentations are mild and self-limiting, but each of these diseases can be problematic to certain populations and can become disseminated, requiring aggressive treatment.

Histoplasmosis

Etiology/Epidemiology. Inhalation of spores of *Histoplasma capsulatum* causes histoplasmosis. Spores are found in soil contaminated by the excrement of birds and bats, such as that around chicken coops, bird roosts, and in caves. The excrement enhances the growth of the organism in soil by accelerating sporulation.[78] Activities that disturb contaminated soil sites are associated with exposure to the spores, and air currents may carry them for miles. Extensive skin testing suggests that as many as 50 million people in the United States have been infected by *H. capsulatum,* and up to 500,000 new infections occur yearly. Most healthy people who are infected remain asymptomatic.

Pathophysiology. The inhaled spores are phagocytized by alveolar macrophages within which they germinate. The spores form yeast cells and multiply by budding. There is a primary infection with involvement of regional lymphatics and early dissemination to other organs via lymphatics and blood. Yeast cells spread to the liver, spleen, and bone marrow and are phagocytized by reticuloendothelial cells. The process in the lung involves necrosis and healing by fibrotic encapsulation, and eventually the original parenchymal foci and hylar lymph nodes show calcification.

The severity of illness after inhalation exposure to *H. capsulatum* varies and depends on the intensity of exposure and the immune state of the host. Some individuals are asymptomatic; others develop a flulike pulmonary illness with cough, chest pain, dyspnea, headache, fever, arthralgia, anorexia, erythema nodosum, hepatomegaly, and splenomegaly. Patchy infiltrates may be seen on chest x-ray films. In most individuals T-cell immunity develops in 10 to 14 days, and the initial infection is self-limiting and does not require antifungal chemotherapy. However, some immunocompromised persons may develop a rapidly progressive primary infection that is fatal without antifungal therapy.

Chronic histoplasmosis (CPH) develops almost exclusively in patients with underlying lung disease. There are recurrent episodes of necrotizing segmental or lobar granulomatous pneumonitis, which has a tendency toward cavity formation, contraction, fibrosis, and compensatory emphysema. Patients exhibit cough, dyspnea, fever, and weight loss.

Progressive disseminated histoplasmosis (PDH) occurs in 1 in 2000 exposed individuals with very low resistance to infection (infants, older adults, and immunocompromised persons). Rarely disseminated histoplasmosis occurs in adults of both genders and all ages with no known immune disorder. These persons have fever, weakness, weight loss, hepatosplenomegaly, leukopenia, and oropharyngeal ulceration. Adrenal insufficiency occurs in about 50% of these persons.

Collaborative Care Management. Skin testing for histoplasmosis is used only for screening purposes. In endemic areas, 90% to 95% of young adults have positive test results. The person should be tested with histoplasmin, tuberculin, blastomycin, and coccidioidin because of the likelihood of cross-reaction. The strongest skin reaction indicates the likely cause of the infection. Positive diagnosis of fungal disease may be based on direct demonstration of intracellular yeasts in smears of bone marrow; biopsy specimens of lymph nodes, liver, or spleen; or cultures of bone marrow, blood, or sputum. Agglutination, precipitation, and complement fixation tests also may be used to help establish the diagnosis of histoplasmosis. These serology tests become positive about 1 month after the primary infection. Titers of serial tests are used to determine activity of the infection. In histoplasmosis, chest films demonstrate a nodular infiltrate similar in appearance to TB. The WBC count is usually normal, although in acute cases it may increase to 13,000/mm^2. Leukopenia and anemia may be present in persons with disseminated disease.

In many cases the disease is self-limiting and no antifungal therapy is needed. When it is needed, administering and monitoring the effects of medications is the major focus of treatment. Antifungal therapy consists primarily of amphotericin B (Fungizone), itraconazole (Sporanox), or ketoconazone (Nizoral). The duration of therapy depends on the type of infection, the condition of the patient's immune system, and the agent used. Amphotericin B is given intravenously. The dose and length of therapy are determined by the difficulty in eradicating the infection and the likelihood of relapse. The therapy may last 2 to 3 weeks or 2 to 3 months. Amphotericin B has many toxic properties, including local phlebitis, systemic reactions, renal toxicity, hypokalemia, and anemia. In rare instances, anaphylaxis, bone marrow suppression, and cardiovascular and hepatic toxicity develop. Systemic toxicity (chills, fever, aching, nausea, and vomiting) can be lessened by premedication with acetaminophen along with 25 to 50 mg of diphenhydramine (Benadryl) orally. Heparin and hydrocortisone succinate (Solu-Cortef) are sometimes added to the infusions to minimize phlebitis. A bone scan should be performed before starting amphotericin B therapy.

A reversible azotemia occurs when amphotericin B is administered. The level of azotemia is monitored by biweekly blood urea nitrogen (BUN) or serum creatinine determinations. A BUN value of greater than 40 mg/dl or a creatinine level nearing 3 mg/dl indicates a need to reduce the drug or temporarily stop it. Therapy is not continued until the azotemia is improved. Serum potassium levels are checked biweekly, and hypokalemia is treated with oral potassium. Anemia is common, and the hematocrit usually stabilizes at 25% to 35%. Other antifungals that may be used are itraconazole and ketoconazole. Itraconazole is administered orally with food because food enhances its absorption. An initial loading dose is followed by lower maintenance doses. Treatment with itraconazole 200 mg once or twice per day for 12 to 24 months is indicated for all patients with CPH. Those patients requiring hospitalization for ventilatory insufficiency, general debilitation, or an inability to tolerate itraconazole are usually treated with amphotericin B.[78]

Itraconazole and amphotericin B are the treatment choices in PDH histoplasmosis. Persons with AIDS who develop PDH have a relapse rate of 80% after treatment. For this reason, the goal of therapy is lifelong suppression as opposed to cure. Amphotericin B, which is administered intravenously weekly or twice weekly, is highly effective but inconvenient and not well tolerated. Itraconazole 200 mg once or twice daily is the treatment of choice for those patients who have shown a positive response to a lengthy course of amphotericin B, usually for 12 weeks. Antigen levels may be monitored every 3 to 6 months to ensure that concentrations remain negative or low.[78]

Ketoconazole is also administered orally and is fairly well tolerated by patients. Toxicity appears to be minimal; pruritus, minor GI intolerance, and liver function abnormalities have been reported. However, most studies demonstrate that ketoconazole is less effective than itraconazole.

In the management of fungal disease, promoting comfort is also important. The patient should be positioned to facilitate breathing, and measures such as the use of antipyretics and cool sponge baths initiated to reduce fever (if present).

Patient/Family Education. Persons with mycotic diseases can be seriously ill and may require long-term therapy (as long as 2 to 3 months or more) with IV antifungal agents. Because these diseases are not well understood by the public, the patient and family need to feel comfortable in discussing concerns with the nurse. The nurse is responsible for providing factual information, clarifying misconceptions, and helping the patient and family understand the disease, its therapy, and the required follow-up. Patients require close medical follow-up for 1 year to prevent relapse. The patient and family must understand the need to avoid infected areas or to wear a protective mask if they have to be in an infected area.

Coccidioidomycosis

Etiology/Epidemiology. Coccidioidomycosis is caused by inhalation of spores of *Coccidioides immitis,* which are found in desert soil and dispersed in dust in the spring. The disease is endemic in the desert areas of the southwestern United States. Susceptibility to the infection is in part genetically determined. Coccidioidomycosis is 50 times more common in Filipino men and 10 times more common in African-American men than in Caucasian men. This increased susceptibility to progressive disease in these groups of men parallels their susceptibility to TB. The increased susceptibility of some races to diseases such as coccidioidomycosis and TB is believed to be the result of a genetically determined impairment of their capacity to develop cellular immunity to infection.

Pathophysiology

The pathophysiologic process that occurs after inhalation of spores is believed to be similar to that described under Histoplasmosis. Disseminated disease is marked by hilar adenopathy, and fungi can be isolated from lymph nodes. A pneumonic disease with necrosis and cavitation may occur after development of delayed hypersensitivity. The disease process is controlled and resolved in most persons as a result of cellular immunity mechanisms. Approximately 60% of infected persons are asymptomatic, with the remainder having symptoms that range from flulike to frank pneumonia. Progressive disseminated coccidioidomycosis or progressive pulmonary disease is found only in those persons whose ability to resist infection or develop immunity has been compromised in some way.[79]

X-ray films of the chest may show pneumonic infiltrate, hilar adenopathy, pleural effusion, or cavitary lesions 2 to 4 cm in size. These cavities usually close spontaneously within 2 years of detection. Approximately 5% of persons with primary pulmonary involvement have residual lung lesions such as cavities or nodules. Only about 0.5% of infected individuals go on to develop a severe, progressive mycosis.

Extrapulmonary dissemination of coccidioidomycosis can occur. One of the sites of dissemination is the meningeal surface of the brain. If there is any indication of CNS involvement, a lumbar puncture is performed. A positive complement fixation titer in the spinal fluid is diagnostic of meningitis. Dissemination can also occur to skin, soft tissue, liver, and bones; the patient is monitored by physical examination of the skin, gallium scanning of soft tissue, and bone scans.

Collaborative Care Management. Coccidioidin 1:10 or 1:100 is used to test for the disease. The test is read in 48 hours. It takes 3 to 6 weeks after exposure for the test to become positive. In severe disseminated disease the test may be negative, indicating that the patient's immune system is no longer able to respond.

As with histoplasmosis, agglutination, precipitation, and complement fixation tests may be used to help establish the diagnosis. These serology tests become positive about 1 month after the primary infection. Titers of serial tests are used to determine activity of the infection.

Surgical intervention for lesions that are localized may involve either excision or drainage to facilitate healing. Management of coccidiomycosis is otherwise similar to that of histoplasmosis.

Blastomycosis

Etiology/Epidemiology. Blastomycosis is caused by inhalation of *Blastomyces dermatitidis* spores, which are carried on air currents. The incidence of blastomycosis is difficult to specify because there is not a good skin test for it.[54]

Pathophysiology. Although skin lesions that appear as small, nonitchy papular or pustular lesions on exposed parts of the body, such as the hands and face, may be the first evidence of blastomycosis, the initial site of infection is in the lung. It is assumed that inhaled spores are phagocytized in the alveoli as part of the primary infection. Thus the pathogenesis of blastomycosis is similar to that of TB, histoplasmosis, and coccidioidomycosis. The infection spreads to other organs by lymph and blood. The skin, bones, and prostate are the most common sites of spread. Acute pulmonary blastomycosis in the form of a self-limiting pneumonia can occur. Otherwise, blastomycosis is a chronic progressive disease with a mortality rate of about 90% when untreated. For this reason, treatment is recommended for every person in whom the diagnosis is established.

Collaborative Care Management. Management of blastomycosis is similar to the management of histoplasmosis.

• • •

The clinical manifestations and medical therapy for the three major fungal lung infections are summarized in Table 21-7.

TABLE 21-7 Clinical Manifestations and Medical Therapy for Fungal Lung Infections

Type of Infection	Clinical Manifestations	Medical Therapy
Histoplasmosis	Severe infections; acute onset with fever, chest pain, dyspnea, prostration, weight loss, wide-spread pulmonary infiltrates, hepatomegaly, and splenomegaly; no symptoms in some persons, benign acute pneumonitis in others	Drug(s) of choice: amphotericin B (Fungizone IV); 75% of patients are cured. Ketoconazole (Nizoral) 400 mg orally daily at bedtime or with meals; without treatment, patient with disseminated disease will die.
Coccidioidomycosis (Valley fever, San Joaquin Valley fever)	Asymptomatic upper respiratory tract infection in about 60% of those who inhaled spores: 40% have symptoms ranging from flulike illness to frank pneumonia	Amphotericin B IV. Therapy required for only 10% of those with symptoms; remainder have spontaneous remission. Ketoconazole orally.
Blastomycosis	Skin lesions that appear as small papular or pustular lesions on exposed parts of the body, such as hands and face Peripheral development of lesions, may become raised but do not itch	Amphotericin B IV; mandatory in immunocompromised patients. Ketoconazole orally. Miconazole (only for patients who cannot tolerate amphotericin or ketoconazole).

IV, Intravenously.

OCCUPATIONAL LUNG DISEASES

Many pulmonary diseases are believed to be caused by substances inhaled in the workplace. Occupational lung diseases are more common in blue-collar workers than in white-collar workers, in industrialized areas than in rural areas, and in small and medium-sized businesses than in larger industrial plants.

In some instances it is debatable whether a person's lung disease is clearly occupation specific. This is especially true in cases of bronchitis, asthma, emphysema, or cancer, because all of these conditions can be caused or aggravated by several factors found in many different occupations and by nonoccupational factors such as smoking and air pollution.

Millions of Americans are believed to have job-related diseases. Because these diseases are not reportable, exact statistics do not exist. The U.S. Department of Health and Human Services has estimated that 400,000 persons develop job-related diseases each year and that there are 100,000 deaths each year from occupational diseases. The National Heart, Lung, and Blood Institute reports that lung diseases cause more than half of these deaths. More than 5 billion dollars per year is paid out in workers' compensation for job-related illnesses and injuries.

It is well documented that smokers develop occupational lung disease more often than nonsmokers and that smokers' lungs are more vulnerable to the effects of these diseases than are nonsmokers' lungs. The combined effects of cigarette smoke and industrial pollutants are great. The risk of developing chronic bronchitis, emphysema, lung cancer, and heart disease is much increased when the worker smokes. Some of these risks, such as lung cancer in persons who worked with asbestos and who also smoked, are becoming more widely known.

Occupational lung diseases can be divided into several categories. The major ones are (1) the pneumoconioses, including silicosis and coal worker's pneumoconiosis (black lung disease); (2) asbestos-related lung disease; and (3) hypersensitivity diseases, including occupational asthma, allergic alveolitis (farmer's lung), and byssinosis (brown lung disease). The etiology, epidemiology, pathophysiology, clinical manifestations, and prevention of the major occupational lung diseases are presented in Table 21-8.

Collaborative Care Management

Medical therapy for these patients depends on the patient's signs, symptoms, and complications.

The major role of nurses is to be knowledgeable about the cause and prevention of occupational lung diseases so that appropriate information and teaching can be presented to the public. The nurse may be key in identifying that the patient's presenting symptoms may be occupation related. A careful occupational history is essential. Questions such as "Do you see dust or mist in the air?" "Do you blow dust from your nose or cough it up at the end of the day?" and "Are your symptoms different on the first day of the work week?" may provide significant clues to occupational exposure and risk.

Patient/Family Education. Occupational lung diseases are preventable. However, concerted efforts by the public, government agencies, and industry are necessary if these diseases are to be prevented. Government action has been slow and in some instances has occurred only in response to public interest groups that have lobbied for stricter regulation of harmful substances. However, countervailing economic and political pressures have sometimes prevented laws from being passed or have resulted in less strict laws being passed because of the costs involved in meeting the strict standards required to control certain hazards. Measures recommended by the American Lung Association to reduce the incidence of occupation-related lung diseases include:

- Public education about the relationship between polluted air in the workplace and lung diseases

TABLE 21-8 Major Occupational Lung Diseases

Type	Etiology and Epidemiology	Pathophysiology	Clinical Manifestations and Prevention
Pneumoconioses*			
Simple (chronic) silicosis	Inhaled silica dust; most common form seen in miners, foundry workers, and others who inhaled relatively low concentrations of dust for 10-20 years	Dust accumulated in tissue → tissue reaction with whorl-shaped nodules throughout lungs	Breathlessness with exercise; 20%-30% progress to confluent silicosis
Complicated silicosis (also called confluent silicosis)	20%-30% of persons with chronic silicosis develop this form	Progressive massive fibrosis (PMF) throughout lungs → ↓ lung function and cor pulmonale	Breathlessness, weakness, chest pain, productive cough with sputum; dies of cor pulmonale and respiratory failure
Acute silicoproteinosis	Rapidly progressive disease, leading to severe disability and death within 5 years of diagnosis	Inflammatory reaction within alveoli, diffuse fibrosis Rapid progression to respiratory failure	Prevention: dust control and improved ventilation can reduce dust levels; sandblasters in enclosed spaces can use special suits and breathing apparatuses; some experts believe such protective measures are still inadequate
Complicated progressive massive fibrosis (PMF)	3% of persons with simple silicosis develop PMF; occurs in miners with heavy deposits of coal dust in lungs; *may appear suddenly years after miner has left the mines;* workers who smoke have 5-6 times more lung obstruction than nonsmoking workers; cigarette smoking causes chronic bronchitis and emphysema	Fibrosis develops in some of dust-laden areas; fibrosis spreads, and fibrotic areas coalesce; eventually most of lung is stiffened and useless	PMF shortens life span; may die of respiratory failure, cor pulmonale, or superimposed infection; most silicosis-associated deaths are in persons older than age 65 years; National Institute for Occupational Safety and Health (NIOSH) concerned about number of young persons dying from silicosis; occupations of these young persons include operators of machines used to crush, grind, mix, and blend materials; painters/paint spray operators; construction workers; and laborers More deaths occur in minorities; more women are developing silicosis Prevention: dust control; abrasive blasting with silica sand, to prepare surfaces for painting = exposure to 200 times NIOSH recommendations; workers need to be educated about NIOSH recommendations for avoiding prolonged overexposure to silica dust
Asbestos-Related Lung Disease			
	Asbestos causes lung cancer, malignant mesothelioma of pleura and periosteum, cancer of the larynx, and certain gastrointestinal cancers; also causes asbestosis, a progressive fibrotic lung disease; risk of these diseases increases with repeated exposure and length of time since first exposure; declared a human carcinogen by the Environmental Protection Agency (EPA) and International Agency for Research on Cancer of the World Health Organization (WHO) Total number of deaths in United States eventually caused by exposure to	Fibrosis caused by asbestos called asbestiosis; asbestos fibers accumulate around terminal bronchioles; the fibers surround iron-rich tissue, forming ferruginous bodies with characteristic picture on x-ray film; more asbestos bodies as more fibers are inhaled; after 20-30 years of exposure, fibrosis begins in lungs; if heavy exposure, appears in 4-5 years	After fibrosis begins, cough, sputum, weight loss, increasing breathlessness; most die within 1-5 years of first symptoms Treatment with radical pleurectomy and pneumonectomy; survival only 1-2 years Prevention: enforcement of regulations governing mining, milling, and use of asbestos; a guiding principle of AHERA is that asbestos in a building poses no hazard to health unless fibers become airborne and can be inhaled;

*Also known as "dust in the lungs."

TABLE 21-8 Major Occupational Lung Diseases—cont'd

Type	Etiology and Epidemiology	Pathophysiology	Clinical Manifestations and Prevention
Asbestos-Related Lung Disease–cont'd			
	asbestos is estimated to exceed 200,000; 20%-25% of deaths from workers with heavy exposure are from lung cancer; cancer related to degree of exposure and to cigarette smoking, which enhances carcinogenic properties of asbestos; *asbestos workers who smoke are 90 times more likely to develop lung cancer as smokers with no exposure to asbestos* Four commercially important forms of asbestos: chrystolite, crocidolite, amosite, and anthophylline; chrystolite accounts for 95% of current world production; nearly all asbestos used in North America is mined in Quebec, Canada; crocidolite is 2-4 times more potent than chrystolite or amosite in causing mesothelioma; all forms equally potent as cause of lung cancer; new use of asbestos almost completely ended in United States and other developed nations as a result of government bans and market pressures; asbestos extensively and aggressively marketed by Canada and other exporting nations in the developing world, where sales remain strong Asbestos Hazard Emergency Response Act (AHERA), passed in 1986, tightened controls on use of asbestos in the United States; mesothelioma accounts for 7%-10% of deaths in asbestos workers; inoperable and always fatal; can occur after very little exposure to crocidolite; has been reported in wives of asbestos workers and in persons living near asbestos plants; cigarette smoking not a contributing factor in these persons; inhalation of only a few fine, straight crocidolite factors are necessary; swallowing of asbestos-contaminated sputum responsible for cancer of larynx, esophagus, stomach, and intestines	Occurs in persons exposed to crocidolite fibers of a certain size; needlelike shape of crocidolite fibers enables them to pass through lung tissue to pleura	removal of asbestos required only when asbestos is visibly deteriorating or when renovation is imminent Protective masks must be used when working with asbestos
Hypersensitivity Diseases			
	Hypersensitivity diseases fall into occupational category when antigen is found primarily in workplace; lung hypersensitivity can occur in bronchi, bronchioles, or alveoli; coarse dust causes bronchial reactions; fine dust provokes small airway and alveolar reactions		
Occupational asthma	More common in 10% of population who are atopic (genetic tendency to develop an allergy); nonatopic persons can also become sensitized; substances with antigenic properties include detergent	Hypersensitivity reaction mediated by histamine → bronchoconstriction and ↑ mucus production; repeated attacks if cause	Wheezing is major symptom Prevention: total elimination of antigen; desensitization not successful

Continued

TABLE 21-8 Major Occupational Lung Diseases—cont'd

Type	Etiology and Epidemiology	Pathophysiology	Clinical Manifestations and Prevention
Hypersensitivity Diseases—con't			
	enzymes, platinum salts, cereals and grains, certain wood dusts, isocyanate chemicals used in polyurethane paints and other products, agents used in printing, and some pesticides	unrecognized and asthma is untreated; may lead to permanent obstructive lung disease; asthmatic response that is well established can be provoked by other factors (house dust, cigarette smoke) and by fatigue, breathing cold air, and coughing	
Hypersensitivity pneumonitis (allergic alveolitis [farmer's lung])	Hypersensitivity disease caused by fine organic dust inhaled into smallest airways; cause of farmer's lung is moldy hay; other dusts can cause allergic alveolitis—these include moldy sugar cane and barley, maple bark, cork, animal hair, bird feathers and droppings, mushroom compost, coffee beans, and paprika; often disease is named for cause (mushroom worker's lung, etc.); fungus spores growing in the apparent antigen are thought in many cases to be real cause of disease	Alveoli are inflamed, inundated by white blood cells, sometimes filled with fluid; if exposure infrequent or level of dust low, symptoms are mild, and treatment not sought, chronic form develops over time; eventually, fibrosis occurs, and fibrosis may be so well established that it cannot be arrested	Symptoms begin some hours after exposure to offending dust and include fatigue, shortness of breath, dry cough, fever, and chills; symptoms may be severe enough to require emergency treatment and hospitalization; acute attacks treated with steroids; recovery may take 6 weeks, and patient may have residual lung damage; real cure is permanent separation of patient and antigen Prevention: properly dried and stored farm products (hay, straw, sugar cane) do not cause allergic alveolitis; presumably fungi only grow in moist conditions
Byssinosis (brown lung)	Occupational disease occurs in textile workers; mainly in cotton workers but also afflicts workers in flax and hemp industries; cause is found in bales of raw cotton that contain not only cotton fibers but fragments of cotton plant; something in plant matter, rather than pure cotton, is cause	Chronic bronchitis and emphysema develop in time; constriction of bronchioles in response to something in crude cotton; symptoms of asthma and allergy persist as long as there is exposure to cotton antigen	Tightness in chest on returning to work after a weekend away (Monday fever); strong relationship between amount of dust inhaled and symptoms; persistent productive tight chest with chronic bronchitis and emphysema; person leaves industry as respiratory cripple Prevention: dust control measures; pretreating bales of cotton by washing with steam and other agents may inactivate causative agent; try to detect persons who are likely to become sensitized to cotton dust and keep them out of high-risk areas

- General commitment to reduce, eliminate, or avoid air pollution in the workplace
- Elimination of the most prevalent and notorious lung hazard—cigarette smoke

Education of the public includes not only employers and employees but also engineers and planners who design operations; buyers and purchasers who select ingredients, cleaning agents, and equipment; and physicians and nurses who care for persons with occupation-related diseases. Many times, workers who are instructed about the hazards involved in certain occupations and workplaces are helpful in deciding what preventive measures need to be taken to combat or minimize the effects of hazards. The commitment to reduce, eliminate, or avoid pollution of workplace air requires full consideration of possible health effects whenever operations are planned and improvement of conditions whenever possible.

SARCOIDOSIS

Etiology /Epidemiology

Sarcoidosis is a multisystem granulomatous disease that primarily affects the lungs and lymphatic systems of the body. The cause of sarcoidosis is unknown. However, there is a growing body of knowledge that indicates it may result from exposure of a genetically susceptible host to specific environmental agents. It is worldwide in distribution and is most common in young and middle-aged adults. In the United States it is most common in African-American women.

Pathophysiology

There is evidence of an antigen-antibody reaction manifested by a reticuloendothelial response in which both thymus-derived (T) cells and plasma (B) cells participate. It is believed that the antigen is airborne, because bilateral hilar lymphadenopathy is commonly present at the onset and bronchopulmonary macrophages are increased.

The central pathologic event involves the growth of noncaseating granulomas and proliferation of lymph tissue. The patient with sarcoidosis may initially complain only of vague symptoms of malaise, fever, aching in the joints, or weakness. In addition to mediastinal lymph node enlargement, ocular manifestations, such as uveitis and conjunctivitis, and dermatologic changes, such as erythema nodosum, are often found. Symptoms of pulmonary sarcoidosis are also nonspecific but may include a dry cough, dyspnea, chest pain, and in some cases, bronchial hyperreactivity.[46]

Diagnosis of sarcoidosis is based on x-ray film findings, transbronchial lung biopsy, and organ biopsy showing noncaseating granulomas. Chest x-ray findings are abnormal in more than 90% of patients, typically showing bilateral hilar lymph node enlargement. Organ biopsy yields the most conclusive evidence of sarcoidosis and is most helpful in differentiating it from Hodgkin's disease and TB.

Other tests useful in the diagnosis of pulmonary sarcoidosis include a gallium scan and bronchoalveolar lavage (BAL) with flexible fiberoptic bronchoscopy. The fluid obtained from BAL is examined to determine the degree of active inflammation in the lung and the need for therapy. Changes in pulmonary function tests (PFTs) are present in only 20% of patients with stage 1 sarcoidosis but are found in 40% to 70% of patients in the later stages. Gas exchange is preserved until late in the clinical course.[6]

Collaborative Care Management

In many patients sarcoidosis is a benign, self-limiting process that resolves within 2 years of diagnosis with no residual damage. Other patients have an acute or chronic form of the disease. The optimal treatment regimen for pulmonary sarcoidosis is still being determined. Recent studies indicate that early stages require no treatment, and systemic steroids have shown positive results for those patients with more involvement. Steroid therapy is initially started at high doses and tapered over a year. The patient is then followed medically for several years for signs of relapse. Relapse usually occurs within 3 to 6 months after the discontinuation of steroids. Several cytotoxic agents have been used to treat sarcoidosis. There is limited research indicating when they should be used. When used, methotrexate and azathioprine are the preferred agents.

About 10% of patients develop the chronic form of sarcoidosis. These patients are treated with low-dose steroids (5 to 10 mg every other day) for years. In this form the disease proceeds to nodular granulomatous depositions in lung tissue and eventual pulmonary fibrosis. In severe cases, pulmonary hypertension and cor pulmonale develop. Lung and other organ transplantations have been successfully performed in patients with end-stage sarcoidosis. However, posttransplantation recurrent sarcoid lesions have been seen. Posttransplantation immunosuppression helps to control these lesions.

Nursing care needs vary with the severity of the patient's signs and symptoms and medical therapy.

Patient/Family Education. Teaching the patient about the precautions and side effects of steroid therapy is a major nursing function when caring for the patient with sarcoidosis.

BOX 21-3 Effects of Smoking on Lung Cancer Risk

Smokers are 10 times more likely to develop lung cancer than those who never smoked.
Heavy smokers are more likely to die of lung cancer than light smokers, suggesting a dose-response effect.
Risk associated with smoking increases with the number of years a person smokes.
Risk decreases steadily after a person stops smoking.
Cigarette smokers have a higher death rate than pipe smokers.
Nonsmoking wives of smokers have a significantly higher risk of lung cancer than nonsmoking wives married to nonsmokers.

CANCER OF THE LUNG

Etiology

Cancer of the lung may be either metastatic or primary. Metastatic tumors may follow malignancy anywhere in the body. Metastasis from the colon and kidney is common. Metastasis to the lung may be discovered before the primary lesion is known, and sometimes the location of the primary lesion may be found only at autopsy.

Epidemiology

Lung cancer is the leading cause of cancer death in both men and women in the United States. Increases in its incidence closely coincide with increases in cigarette smoking (Box 21-3). It is estimated that 87% of lung cancers are attributable to smoking.[1] In 1999 in the United States there were an estimated 160,000 deaths from lung cancer and 172,000 new cases.[2]

The increase in death rates for both men and women is directly related to cigarette smoking. The cancer death rate for male cigarette smokers is more than double that for nonsmokers, and the rate for female smokers is 67% higher than that for nonsmokers. It is projected that mortality from lung cancer among women will continue to rise until 2010.

A history of smoking, especially for 20 years or more, is a prime risk factor. Other risk factors include exposure to certain industrial substances such as arsenic, specific organic chemicals, radon, and asbestos, particularly in those who smoke. It is estimated that asbestos workers who smoke have a 6 to 10 times greater incidence of lung cancer than the general population. Some evidence also suggests a genetic predisposition to lung cancer.[33]

Because no effective treatment exists for lung cancer, emphasis is on prevention. The cure rate for lung cancer is about 10%, and the 5-year survival rate is only slightly higher. The cure rate has not significantly improved since 1950 despite advances in surgery, chemotherapy, and radiation. Success with therapy could be enhanced with early diagnosis and treatment. Unfortunately, about one third of the persons with lung cancer have inoperable cancer when first seen by a physician.

Lung Cancer Screening. Although there are numerous recommendations for screening and early detection of breast, colorectal, and prostate cancers, there are currently no such recommendations for lung cancer. Because of the tremendous impact of lung cancer on individuals, families, and society, there is a growing interest in early detection and screening. The reluctance to recommend screening is due to limited data to support improved outcomes from screening. Newer studies are showing that when stage I cancer is resected, 5-year survival can be as high as 70%.[34] Recent and current studies are examining the beneficial effect of low-dose CT scanning in asymptomatic but at-risk populations. The populations identified as being at-risk and eligible for screening include smokers or former smokers who are (1) 60 years of age or older, (2) have at least a 10–pack-year smoking history, (3) have no known history of malignancy, and (4) are fit to undergo thoracic surgery. CT scanners are capable of detecting very small nodules and thus help to diagnose lung cancer earlier. There are also clinical trials seeking to identify biomarkers for lung cancer applied to sputum specimens.[15]

Pathophysiology

Four major histologic types account for more than 90% of all lung cancers. These include adenocarcinoma, large cell and squamous cell carcinoma, and small cell lung cancer (SCLC) (Figure 21-4). Small cell cancer grows the most rapidly and, in general, is the most responsive to cytotoxic chemotherapy.[18] As with other types of cancer, lung cancer is staged.

Staging for SCLC is a simple two-stage system.[38] This reflects the fact that more than 70% of SCLC cases are metastatic at the time of diagnosis and therefore inoperable for cure. The two stages are (1) limited (indicating that the tumor is confined) and (2) extensive (indicating metastasis). The TNM (tumor, node, metastasis) International Staging System for Lung Cancer is used for non–small cell lung cancer (NSCLC) and is presented in Box 21-4.

Cancer of the lung may metastasize to nearby structures, such as the prescalene lymph nodes, the walls of the esophagus, and the pericardium, or to distant areas, such as the brain, liver, kidneys, adrenal glands, or skeleton. In general, the overall cure rate for all types of lung cancer is only about 10%.[18] Survival rates of patients with NSCLC depend on the size of the tumor, nodal status, and degree of metastasis.

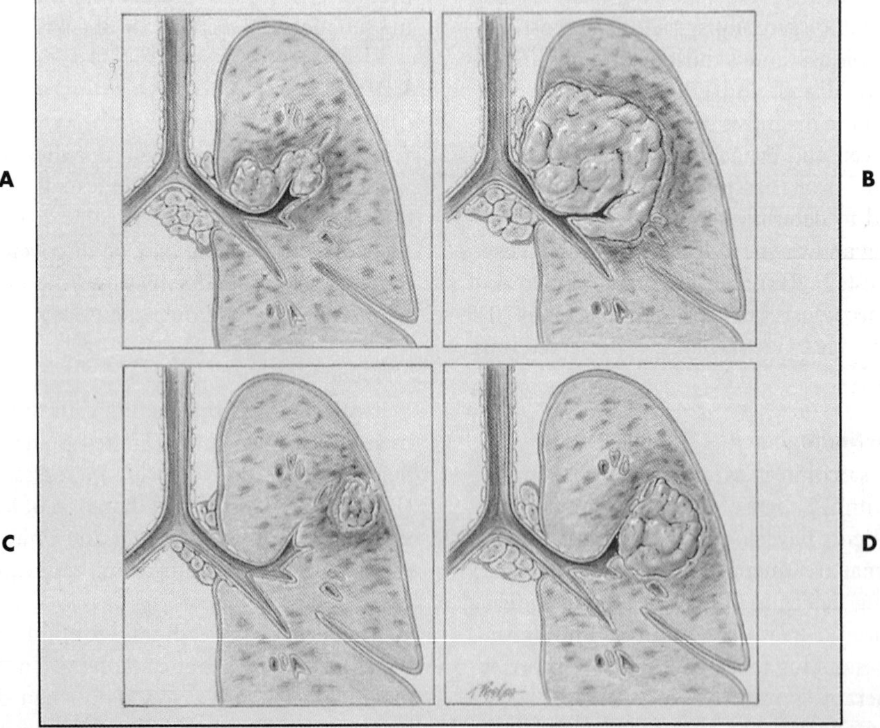

Figure 21-4 Cancer of the lung. **A**, Squamous (epidermoid) cell carcinoma. **B**, Small cell (oat cell) carcinoma. **C**, Adenocarcinoma. **D**, Large cell carcinoma.

A patient's signs and symptoms depend on several factors, including the location of the lesion. In approximately 10% of cases, patients are asymptomatic and the cancer is identified on a routine chest x-ray film. Of patients with cancer of the lung or bronchus who have symptoms, approximately 75% have a cough and approximately 50% have hemoptysis. Shortness of breath and a unilateral wheeze are also common. Extrapulmonary intrathoracic signs and symptoms occur with peripheral pulmonary lesions that perforate into the pleural space. These include pain on inspiration, friction rub, pleural effusion, edema of the face and neck when the superior vena cava is involved, fatigue, and clubbing of the fingers. In the latter stages of the disease, weight loss and debility usually indicate metastases, especially to the liver.

Collaborative Care Management

Diagnostic Tests. Confirmed diagnosis of lung cancer requires histologic examination of the tumor. Specimens for examination may be obtained by fiberoptic bronchoscopy, percutaneous transthoracic needle biopsy, endoscopic ultrasonography with fine-needle aspiration, sputum collection, or surgery. Fiberoptic bronchoscopy is the procedure of choice for obtaining tissue for diagnosis from centrally located lesions. Tissue samples can be removed from visible tumors, and brushing and washing of peripheral lesions can be performed. When hilar or mediastinal lymph nodes are involved, transbronchial needle biopsy via a bronchoscope is done to obtain nodal tissue for examination. Procedural risks include respiratory failure, pneumothorax, and bleeding. Percutaneous transthoracic needle biopsy is the procedure of choice for diagnosing malignancy in peripheral lung nodules. The procedure is performed using CT guidance or, less commonly, fluoroscopy or ultrasonography. Analysis of tissue samples can provide a specific diagnosis and sometimes the cell type. Complications include pneumothorax and hemoptysis. Endoscopic ultrasonography with fine-needle aspiration is becoming the accepted procedure for diagnosis and staging of lung cancer. In this procedure an echoendocoscope is used to obtain tissue specimens via fine-needle aspiration. There are no reported complications. Cytologic analysis of sputum is the safest and least expensive way to diagnose lung cancer. In this approach, a sample of sputum is examined for bacteria and cancer cells. For best results, a 3-day pooled sample is used. Diagnostic yield also has been shown to increase with induction of sputum rather than spontaneous expectoration. Finally, lesions may be excised through a small incision. Video-assisted thoracoscopy or thoracotomy is useful for performing small diagnostic wedge excisions.

Many other diagnostic tests are used in the diagnosis and staging of lung cancer. A lateral chest x-ray film is able to depict tumors, especially those on the periphery. A contrast-enhanced CT scan or magnetic resonance imaging (MRI) can differentiate an underlying mass from atelectasis or inflammation. A CT scan is also used to reveal malignant pleural effusions, which usually mean inoperability. MRI can be used to differentiate involvement of visceral pleura from involvement of parietal pleura, thus identifying chest wall invasion. CT of the chest is widely accepted as a tool for diagnosis and staging, but it has significant specificity limitations. It may best identify sites of metastasis.[4] Positron emission tomography (PET) is more sensitive than CT or MRI and aids in the diagnosis of both primary and metastatic sites. PET also has been found to

BOX 21-4 International Staging System for Lung Cancer: TNM Descriptors for Non–Small Cell Lung Cancer

Primary Tumor (T)

T_X	Primary tumor cannot be assessed or tumor proven by the presence of malignant cells in sputum or bronchial washings and not visualized by imaging or bronchoscopy
T_0	No evidence of primary tumor
T_{is}	Carcinoma in situ
T_1	Tumor ≤3 cm in dimension; surrounded by lung or visceral pleura
T_2	Tumor ≥3 cm in dimension; involves main bronchus; invades visceral pleura; associated with atelectasis
T_3	Tumor of any size that directly invades the chest wall, diaphragm, mediastinal pleura, or parietal pericardium
T_4	Tumor of any size that invades the heart, great vessels, trachea, esophagus, vertebral body, or carina; or tumor with pleural or pericardial effusion

Regional Lymph Nodes (N)

N_X	Regional lymph nodes cannot be assessed
N_0	No regional lymph node metastasis
N_1	Metastasis to ipsilateral hilar lymph nodes, intrapulmonary nodes
N_2	Metastasis to ipsilateral mediastinal or subcarinal lymph nodes
N_3	Metastasis to contralateral mediastinal, hilar, scalene. or supraclavicular lymph nodes

Distant Metastasis (M)

M_X	Presence of distant metastasis cannot be assessed
M_0	No distant metastasis
M_1	Distant metastasis present

Adapted from Hyer JD, Sivestri G: Diagnosis and staging of lung cancer, *Clin Chest Med* 21(1):95-106, 2000.

be effective in staging NSCLC. Thoracentesis is routinely performed if there is evidence of pleural effusion clinically or on a CT scan. Thoracoscopy is useful for evaluating pleural seeding and for examining mediastinal nodes. Mediastinoscopy is better than a CT scan or MRI for assessing mediastinal metastases and effectiveness of preoperative radiation therapy or chemotherapy.

Medications. Historically NSCLC has not been considered amenable to cytotoxic chemotherapy, but more recently developed regimens have improved response rates and survival. Combination therapy that includes cisplatin plus etoposide, vinorelbine, paclitaxel, docetaxel, or gemcitabine has demonstrated the best results. Patients who are most likely to benefit from chemotherapy include those with minimal weight loss, less extensive disease spread, and good functionality.[18] The most widely used chemotherapy regimens for SCLC, which is the most responsive type of lung cancer to cytotoxic agents, include cyclophosphamide, doxorubicin, and etoposide; cisplatin and etoposide; or ifosfamide, carboplatin, and etoposide.[18] Medications to control pain, hypertension, or other coexisting disease are also a part of the patient's treatment.

Treatments. Radiation therapy given concurrently or alternating with chemotherapy appears to improve survival, but it may also increase the risks for myelosuppression and esophagitis.

Surgical Management. Assessment of surgical risk for pulmonary resection considers age, pulmonary reserve, presence of cardiovascular disease, and presence of disease so extensive it would require a pneumonectomy. Mortality and morbidity related to pulmonary resection increase significantly in persons older than 70 years of age. Some studies suggest higher mortality and morbidity in those 60 to 65 years of age. ABG studies and PFTs are used to measure pulmonary reserve. A $PaCO_2$ greater than 45 mm Hg indicates inoperability, whereas a PaO_2 less than 60 mm Hg suggests that pulmonary resection would be risky. An exception is when the low PaO_2 is caused by complete airway obstruction that results from desaturated blood entering the pulmonary veins from a perfused but nonventilated lung (ventilation-perfusion [V/Q] mismatch). The PFTs are used to evaluate the risk for pulmonary resection. A predicted postoperative forced expiratory volume in 1 second (FEV_1) of more than 800 ml is required in most adults. Most patients with an FEV_1 less than 30% of predicted are usually unable to tolerate pneumonectomy.

Coronary artery disease is present in about 80 of every 1000 patients older than age 65. Previous myocardial infarction, especially when surgery would be necessary less than 6 months after infarction, increases the risk. Left ventricular dysfunction, including signs of heart failure, indicates high risk of death after pulmonary resection. Unstable angina must be controlled before resection. Hypertension has to be under control. Frequent premature ventricular contractions are signs of severe heart disease and are associated with increased perioperative complications and death. Pneumonectomy is associated with higher risk than lesser procedures, particularly for patients age 70 and over, and especially with surgery of the right lung.

Principles of Thoracic Surgery. Endotracheal anesthesia is used for surgery involving the lung in which the pleural space is entered. Endotracheal anesthesia makes it possible to keep the uninvolved ("good") lung expanded and functioning when the chest is opened and atmospheric pressure enters the pleural space.

The pressure in the pleural space (the space between the visceral and parietal pleura) is subatmospheric (less than 760 mm Hg) and is referred to as negative. When the pleura is entered surgically or with trauma to the chest wall, atmospheric (positive) pressure enters the pleural space, and the lung on that side collapses. After resectional surgery of the lung (except pneumonectomy), one or two drainage tubes are inserted into the pleural space. Each tube is connected to a negative-pressure closed drainage system. This system allows air and fluid to drain from the pleural space and prevents air or fluid from entering the pleural space. In all resectional surgery (except pneumonectomy) the remaining portions of the lung must overexpand and fill the space left by the resected portion. The removal of air and fluid from the pleural space aids in the expansion of the remaining portion of the lung and helps reestablish negative pressure in the pleural space.

Types of thoracic surgery along with indications for each type are presented in Box 21-5. An exploratory thoracotomy is performed to confirm a suspected diagnosis of lung or chest disease. The usual approach is by a posterolateral parascapular incision through the fourth, fifth, sixth, or seventh intercostal space. Occasionally an anterior approach is used. The ribs are spread to give the best possible exposure of the lung and hemithorax. The pleura is entered and the lung examined, a biopsy usually is taken, and the chest is closed. This procedure may also be used to detect bleeding in the chest or other injury after trauma to the chest. Because the pleural space was entered, a chest tube and closed drainage system are necessary (Figure 21-5).

A pneumonectomy (the removal of an entire lung) is most often performed to treat bronchogenic carcinoma (Figure 21-6, *B*). It may also be used to treat TB. However, a pneumonectomy is performed only in cases in which a lobectomy or segmental resection will not remove all of the diseased tissue. A thoracotomy incision is made in either the posterior or anterior chest. Before the lung can be removed, the pulmonary artery and vein are ligated and then cut. The mainstem bronchus leading to the lung is clamped, divided, and sutured or stapled. To ensure an airtight closure of the bronchus, a pleural flap may be placed over it and sutured into place. This is not necessary if staples are used. The phrenic nerve on the operative side is crushed, causing the diaphragm on that side to rise and reduce the size of the remaining space. Because there is no lung left to reexpand, drainage tubes are not usually used. Ideally, the pressure in the closed chest is slightly negative. The fluid left in the space consolidates in time, preventing the remaining lung and the heart from shifting toward the operative side (mediastinal shift).

In a lobectomy one lobe of the lung is removed (Figure 21-6, *C*). In addition to being a treatment of lung cancer, it is used to treat bronchiectasis, emphysematous blebs or bullae,

BOX 21-5 Types of Thoracic Surgery and Indications for Their Use

Exploratory Thoracotomy

To confirm suspected diagnosis of lung or chest disease, especially carcinoma; to obtain a biopsy; being replaced by noninvasive procedures (thoracoscopy)

Pneumonectomy

Removal of a lung: bronchogenic carcinoma when lobectomy will not remove all of lesion; tuberculosis when other surgery will not remove all of diseased lung

Pneumomectomy

Lung reduction surgery to reduce lung volume and decrease tension on respiratory muscles in persons with emphysema

Lobectomy

Removal of one lobe of lung: bronchogenic carcinoma confined to a lobe; bronchiectasis; emphysematous blebs or bullae; lung abscess; fungal infections; benign tumors; tuberculosis

Bilobectomy

Removal of two lobes from right lung: bronchogenic carcinoma when lobectomy will not remove all of disease

Sleeve Lobectomy

Resection of main bronchus or distal trachea with reanastomosis to a distal uninvolved bronchus: bronchogenic carcinoma to preserve functional parenchyma

Segmental Resection

Segmentectomy; removal of one or more lung segments: bronchiectasis; lung abscess or cyst; metastatic carcinoma; tuberculosis

Wedge Resection

Removal of pie-shaped section from surface of lung: well-circumscribed benign tumors; metastatic tumors; localized inflammatory disease, including TB

Decortication

Removal of a fibrinous peel from visceral pleura: chronic empyema

Thoracoplasty

Removal of ribs: residual air space after resectional surgery; chronic empyema space

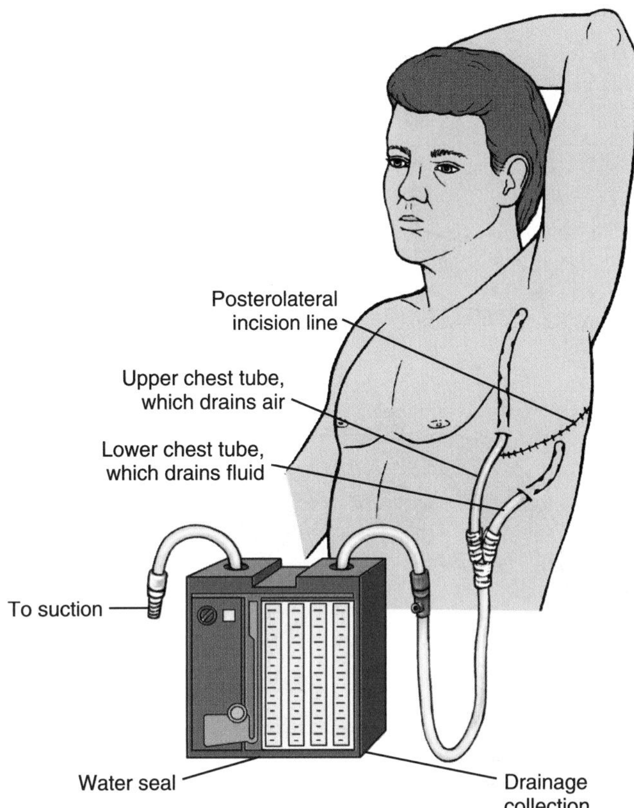

Figure 21-5 Closed chest drainage system.

lung abscesses, benign tumors, fungal infections, and TB. For a lobectomy to be successful, the disease must be confined to one lobe, and the remaining lung tissue must be capable of overexpanding to fill the space of the resected lobe. One or two chest tubes are connected to a closed drainage system for postoperative drainage.

In a segmental resection one or more segments of the lung are removed. This procedure is used in an attempt to preserve as much functioning lung tissue as possible. It is an extremely taxing procedure for the surgeon, because the dissection between segments must be performed carefully and slowly, and the identification of the segmental pulmonary artery and vein and bronchus is more difficult than when a lobe is involved. Because there are 10 segments in the right lung and 8 segments in the left lung, only a portion of a lobe or lobes may need to be removed. The most common indication for segmentectomy is bronchiectasis. Chest tube(s) and a closed drainage system are necessary after surgery. Because of air leaks from the segmental surface, the remaining lung tissue may take longer to reexpand.

In a wedge resection a well-circumscribed diseased portion is removed without regard to the segmental planes of the lung. The area to be removed is clamped, dissected, and sutured or stapled. Chest tube(s) and a closed drainage system are used after surgery. With decortication, a fibrinous peel is removed from the visceral pleura, allowing the encased lung to reexpand and obliterate the pleural space (see earlier discussion under Empyema). Chest tube(s) and chest suction are used to facilitate the reexpansion of the lung. If the lung has been encased for a long time, it may be incapable of reexpanding after decorticaton. In this situation, thoracoplasty may be necessary.

Diet. The diet for a patient with lung cancer varies with the stage of the cancer and the therapy prescribed. However, good nutrition is always important for healing, so the patient is encouraged to eat well as tolerated throughout the course of the disease (see Chapter 15).

Activity. Activity may vary with the patient's ability, strength, and therapy.

Referrals. Most patients with cancer are referred to local cancer support groups and assistive agencies for information,

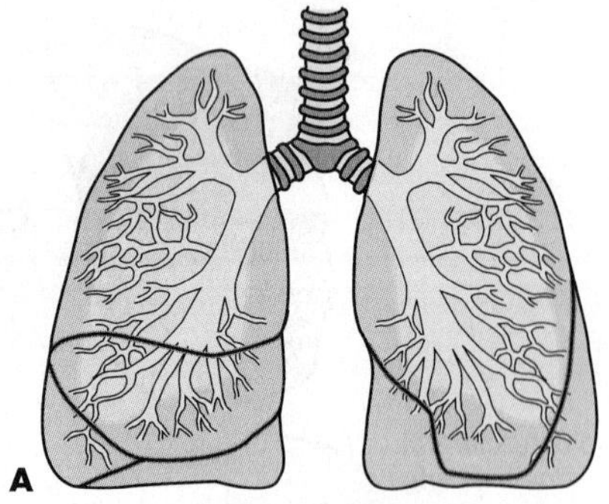

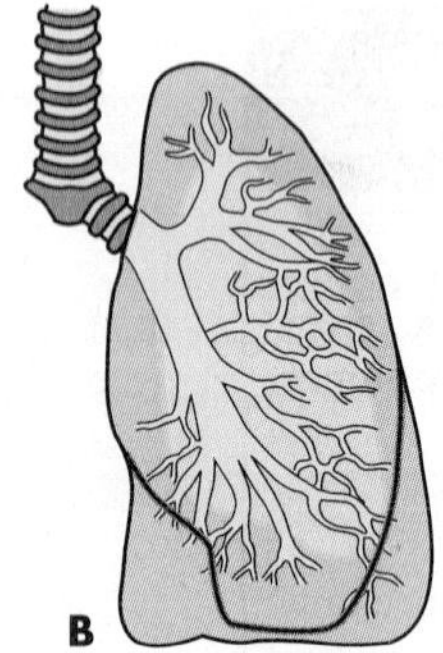

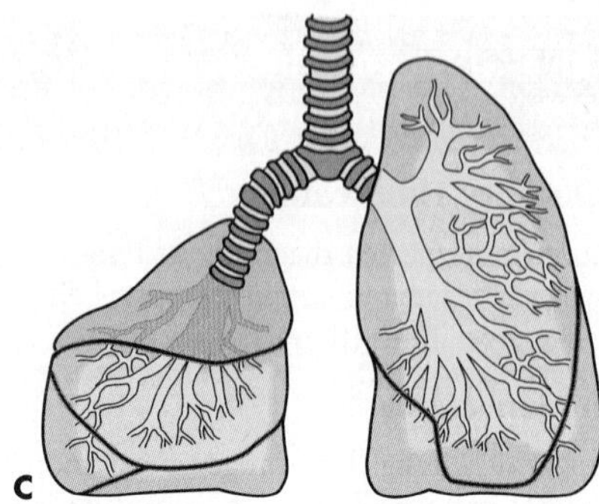

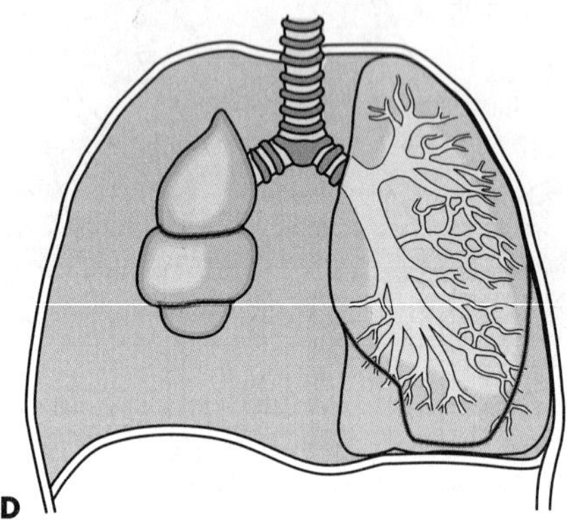

Figure 21-6 **A**, Normal lungs. **B**, Surgical absence of the right lung after a pneumonectomy. **C**, Surgical absence of the right upper lobe after a lobectomy. **D**, Complete collapse of the right lung as a result of air in the pleural cavity (pneumothorax.)

support, and other needs the patient and family are experiencing. If surgical intervention is necessary, referral is made to a thoracic surgeon. Referrals may also be made to an oncologist and radiation therapist.

NURSING MANAGEMENT OF PATIENT UNDERGOING THORACIC SURGERY

PREOPERATIVE CARE

The proposed surgery is discussed with both the patient and the family. The goal of teaching is to prepare the patient for what he or she is expected to do after surgery. Patients may be admitted to the hospital the day of surgery. To be effective, the responsibility for preoperative teaching is shared by primary care clinicians and home care and acute care nurses. In some hospitals nurses from the operating room, recovery room, or ICU participate in the preoperative teaching. The goal is that the patient understands about the impending surgery and has an opportunity to ask questions and express concerns. Topics to be addressed in the teaching plan are found in the Patient Teaching box.

> **Patient Teaching**
> **Thoracic Surgery**
>
> Begin by ascertaining the patient's understanding of the procedure to be performed and its purpose. Also assess the amount of information desired by the patient. Adjust teaching about the following topics accordingly:
>
> 1. Patient's knowledge of procedure
> 2. Explanation of procedure as necessary, including intubation for anesthesia, site of incision, and chest tube(s) and drainage system
> 3. Oxygen
> 4. Blood administration and intravenous infusions
> 5. Pain medication, including patient-controlled analgesia if used
> 6. What patient will be asked to do
>   a. Coughing and deep breathing
>   b. Arm exercises
>   c. Ambulation
> 7. Where patient will be taken after surgery
>   a. To recovery—for how long
>   b. To intensive care unit—for how long
> 8. Where family can wait during surgery

POSTOPERATIVE CARE

The care of the patient after thoracic surgery centers on promoting ventilation and reexpansion of the lung by maintaining a clear airway, maintaining the closed drainage system if one is used, promoting arm exercises to maintain full use of the patient's arm on the operative side, promoting nutrition, and monitoring the incision for bleeding and subcutaneous emphysema. In most hospitals the patient is taken from the recovery room to the ICU. The patient is usually attached to a cardiac monitor. A Swan-Ganz catheter and central venous pressure line are used for hemodynamic monitoring. Oxygen is attached to the endotracheal tube in the immediate postoperative period. After extubation, humidified oxygen is given by cannula, usually at 6 L/min. An oxygen mask is not used because of the need to have the patient cough and raise secre-

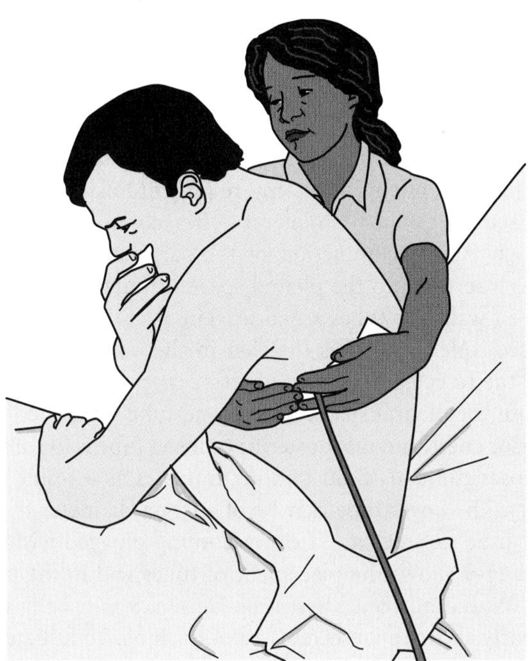

Figure 21-7 The nurse helps the patient cough by splinting the incision with firm support using her hands. This lessens muscle pull and pain as the patient coughs. Note that the nurse keeps her head behind the patient while he coughs, and the patient uses tissue to cover his mouth.

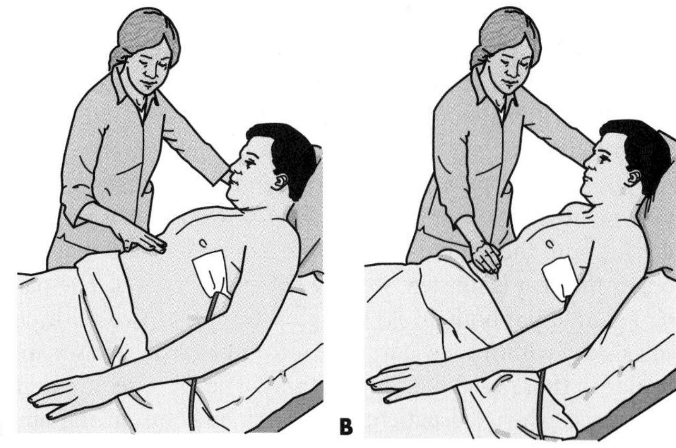

Figure 21-8 A, The physical therapist assists the patient in learning augmented abdominal breathing. The patient is instructed to inhale through the nose, using abdominal muscles, and to concentrate on moving the lower ribs under the therapist's hands. This exercise improves ventilation of the base of the lungs. **B,** The physical therapist places a hand on the upper abdomen while helping the patient to exhale fully.

tions frequently. Vital signs are checked every 15 minutes until the patient is well recovered from anesthesia, every hour until the patient's condition has stabilized, and then every 2 to 4 hours. It is not unusual for blood pressure to fluctuate during the first 24 to 36 hours, and close monitoring of the patient is essential. Acute changes or disturbing trends (hypotension, hypertension) are reported to the surgeon.

Positioning of the Patient in Bed

The patient is kept flat in bed or with the head elevated slightly (20 degrees) until blood pressure is stabilized to preoperative levels. Once blood pressure is stabilized, the patient can usually breathe best in semi-Fowler's position with a pillow under the head and neck but not under the shoulder and back because of the subscapular incision.

Initiating Coughing and Deep Breathing Exercises

The patient should be helped to cough as soon as he or she is conscious and extubated. If the blood pressure is stable, the patient is assisted to a sitting position, and the incision is supported anteriorly and posteriorly by the nurse's hands. Firm, even pressure over the incision with the open palm of the hands or a surgical pillow is effective. The nurse's head should be behind the patient when the patient is coughing (Figure 21-7). The patient is encouraged to use the huff coughing technique

Deep breathing and coughing keep the airway patent, prevent atelectasis, and facilitate reexpansion of the lung. The patient should be helped to cough every hour for the first 24 hours and then every 2 to 4 hours around the clock. The patient should cough until the chest sounds clear. Otherwise, secretions accumulate in the tracheobronchial tree. The patient is urged to use incentive spirometry 10 times every hour to help inflate the lungs and mobilize secretions. The patient can cough most effectively 20 to 30 minutes after receiving pain medication, and this should be a priority when planning the nursing care.

When a patient is unable to cough effectively, tracheobronchial suctioning is performed. If suctioning fails to clear the airway, fiberoptic bronchoscopy may be necessary, because it is crucial that the airway is kept clear. In these situations, bronchoscopy is performed at the bedside with a fiberoptic bronchoscope.

Promoting Abdominal Breathing

Abdominal breathing exercises are a valuable adjunct to the care of the patient with chest surgery, because abdominal breathing improves ventilation without increasing pain and assists in coughing more effectively (Figure 21-8). The exercises should be taught preoperatively so that the patient has time to practice them before surgery.

Promoting Comfort by Pain Relief

Medication for pain should be given as needed and may be required as often as every 1 to 4 hours during the first 48 to 72 hours. The patient is often extremely uncomfortable and is reluctant to cough or turn unless there is relief from pain. The tubes in the chest cause pain, and the patient may attempt rapid, shallow breathing to splint the lower chest and avoid motion of the catheters. This impairs ventilation, makes coughing ineffective, and causes secretions to be retained. It is a nursing responsibility to make the patient comfortable, because this facilitates deep breathing and coughing. Patient-controlled analgesia pumps and epidural catheters are widely used for pain medication management. Rarely an intercostal nerve block may be required.

Promoting Arm Exercises

Passive arm exercises are usually started the evening of surgery. The purpose of putting the patient's arm through range of motion (ROM) is to prevent restriction of function. Most patients are reluctant to move the arm on the operative side, but with proper pain control, preoperative instruction, and postoperative follow-through, they do so readily. It is important for both the patient and the nurse to understand that the longer the arm is unexercised, the stiffer it becomes. The patient should put both arms through active ROM two or three times a day within a few days. The recommended exercises are similar to those used after mastectomy. The exercises are best performed when the patient is upright or lying on the abdomen. Exercises such as elevating the scapula and clavicle, "hunching the shoulders," bringing the scapulae as close together as possible, and hyperextending the arm can be performed only in these positions. Because lying on the abdomen may not be possible at first, these exercises are performed with the patient sitting on the edge of the bed or standing.

Promoting Nutrition

The patient is encouraged to take fluids postoperatively and to progress to a general diet as soon as it is tolerated. Fluids help liquefy secretions and make them easier to expectorate. A diet adequate in protein and vitamins, especially vitamin C, facilitates wound healing.

Monitoring the Incision for Bleeding or Subcutaneous Emphysema

The dressing is checked periodically for bleeding. Blood on the dressing is unusual and should be reported to the surgeon at once. The time and amount of blood are recorded in the patient's record. The surgeon may reinforce the dressing. In the rare instance when bleeding persists, the patient may be taken back to surgery, the chest wall reopened, and the source of bleeding located and ligated.

Subcutaneous emphysema is not unusual after chest surgery. In subcutaneous emphysema, air leaks from the pleural space through the thoracotomy incision or around the chest tubes into the soft tissues. The presence of air under the skin is readily detected and has been described as feeling like "tissue paper" or "Rice Krispies" under the skin. Subcutaneous emphysema is most notable in the neck and chest, and if considerable air is leaking, the patient's face and neck become swollen. Small amounts of air will reabsorb over time and cause no problem. However, if subcutaneous emphysema is worsening, the chest tube may be changed by the surgeon and one with a larger diameter inserted, because air is leaking into the tissues faster than it is being removed by the tube. Additional suction may also be applied to the chest tube(s) in an attempt to remove air more rapidly. Rarely a patient needs to return to surgery for closure of air leaks.

The patient with a pneumonectomy should have only a small amount (if any) of subcutaneous emphysema. Progressive subcutaneous emphysema after pneumonectomy is very serious and should be reported to the surgeon immediately because it could indicate a major leak in the bronchial stump. This is a rare occurrence, requiring immediate return to surgery for reclosure of the stump.

Maintaining Chest Tube(s) and Drainage

All patients who have resectional surgery of the lung, except those having a pneumonectomy, require drainage of the pleural space by one or two chest tubes connected to closed drainage. At the completion of the surgical resection, each tube is inserted into the pleural space through an incision in the chest wall. The tubes are sutured in place. When two tubes are used, one catheter is inserted in the anterior chest wall above the resected area. This anterior or upper tube removes air from the pleural space. The second tube is inserted in the posterior chest, and this posterior or lower tube is for drainage of serosanguineous fluid that accumulates as a result of the surgery. The lower tube may be of a larger diameter than the upper tube to prevent it from becoming plugged with clots. Figure 21-9 shows the placement of tubes within the pleural space. When only one chest tube is used, it is usually placed anteriorly above the resected area of the lung. To initiate chest tube drainage, the chest tubes are connected to a closed-chest drainage system.

Water-Seal Drainage System

Each chest tube must be connected to a closed system that allows for removal of fluid and air from the intrapleural space to promote lung reexpansion. The most commonly used system is the Pleur-Evac. The water in a water-seal chest drainage system acts as a one-way valve, permitting the unidirectional flow of air or fluid out of the pleural space. As air and fluid drainage begins, the pressure in the pleural space becomes more negative. The more negative this pressure is, the more the lung expands. Lung expansion, in turn, forces more fluid and air out of the pleural space. This cycle continues until the lung is fully expanded and intrathoracic negative pressure returns to its normal (subatmospheric) level. A water-seal drainage system must be airtight between the pleural space and the water seal. Any air leak is an entry for atmospheric air into the pleural space, creating a positive

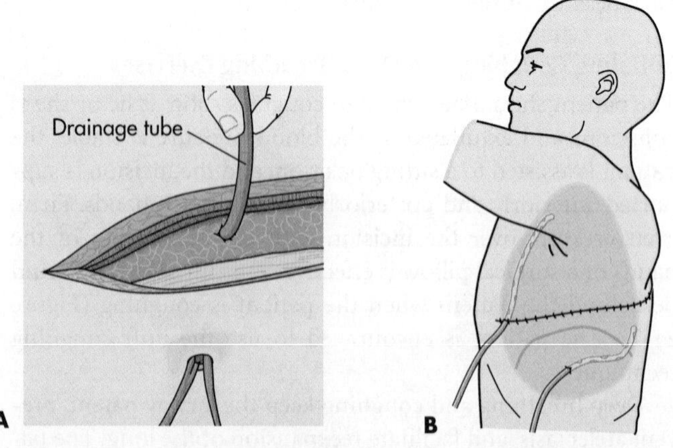

Figure 21-9 **A,** Drainage tube being inserted into the pleural space. **B,** Note that both tubes are placed well into the pleural space.

pressure that collapses the lung. Suction may be applied to water-seal systems to encourage drainage. Suction must be maintained at the prescribed level for the patient. The water in the suction chamber of the drainage system bubbles when suction is present. A gentle, continuous level of bubbling is desired. If the water fails to bubble, the desired level of suction is not being attained, and the tubing should be checked for air leaks. If there are no leaks, the surgeon should be notified at once, because the air leak in the pleural surface may be so great that the amount of negative pressure is not sufficient to overcome it. Chest tubes and closed drainage are shown in Figure 21-9.

Maintaining Patency of Chest Tubes

In the past, chest tubes were "milked" or "stripped" every hour to prevent the formation of clots that could plug the tubes. However, studies have shown that stripping the tube greatly increases the negative pressure exerted on the pleural space. Undesirable side effects of increased levels of pressure include (1) lung entrapment in the chest tube eyelets and focal tissue infarction and (2) persistent pneumothorax. The persistent pneumothorax occurs when the pleural surface of the lung, which normally has air leaks at the close of the procedure, does not seal off. Fibrin usually seals the air leaks; however, the presence of an increased amount of negative pressure may prevent the air leaks from sealing and may even increase the size of the air leaks. This is why some thoracic surgeons do not attach suction to the closed drainage system for the first 24 hours or more after surgery. They believe that this amount of time is sufficient in most instances to allow the pleural surface to seal off.

Because the anterior (upper) tube evacuates mainly air, there is less reason to believe that this tube will clot off. Posterior tubes, which are inserted lower in the chest, drain more fluid and blood and are more likely to clot off. However, gentle squeezing of the tube is usually sufficient to move the bloody drainage along in the tubing.

Removing Chest Tubes

Chest tubes are removed when there is no tidaling of fluid in the water-sealed chamber and when x-ray films confirm the full reexpansion of the lung. Most patients have their chest tube(s) removed within 48 to 72 hours after surgery. If there is a persistent air space in the apex of the lung, the upper tube may be left in longer. Surgeons are concerned about leaving tubes in for long periods of time because of the risk of an ascending tube track infection. The patient should receive medication for pain 15 to 30 minutes before removal of the tube. Physicians vary in the exact procedure used to remove the tube, but generally a sterile suture set, 4 × 4 inch gauze squares, and 2-inch tape are required. The suture holding the tube in place is cut, the patient is asked to take a deep breath and hold it, and the tube is removed. If a purse-string suture was used, it is retied, and a dry sterile dressing is placed over the site. Some physicians cover the site with petroleum gauze or a Telfa dressing instead of gauze squares to ensure an airtight dressing.

Care After Pneumonectomy

The postoperative care discussed previously applies to all patients with resectional surgery except those undergoing pneumonectomy. The special care required after a pneumonectomy is outlined in the Guidelines for Safe Practice box.

GERONTOLOGIC CONSIDERATIONS

Many older persons with lung cancer are not candidates for thoracic surgery, and some receive radiation as palliative therapy. For those who have surgery, adjunctive therapy with radiation or antineoplastic drugs, or both, may be necessary. The side effects of both radiation and chemotherapy may be more severe in older adults than in younger persons. Radiation therapy is usually given on an outpatient basis at the hospital, and chemotherapy may be administered in an outpatient clinic or at home. Special emphasis for the older adult is on fluid, dietary, exercise, and sleep requirements, all of which will be affected by the therapy the patient receives.

SPECIAL ENVIRONMENTS FOR CARE

Critical Care Management

Care in the initial postoperative period takes place in an ICU. The patient remains in the ICU until successfully extubated and hemodynamically stable.

Home Care Management

Patients with cancer of the lung treated with thoracic surgery are discharged from the hospital less than a week after surgery. Most require a family member or a home health aid to assist them until they regain strength and can care for themselves. Those who must leave their home to receive chemotherapy or radiation therapy need someone to drive them to treatments and to care for them after therapy. Both chemotherapy and radiation therapy can be extremely debilitating. Many patients become nauseated and require antiemetics to avoid becoming dehydrated.[76]

Because of the poor prognosis for most patients with lung cancer, available hospice services should be discussed with the patient and family. If the patient and family opt to use this service, a hospice nurse is responsible for managing the care of the patient, and the emphasis is on keeping the patient as comfortable as possible. Some patients are able to remain at home with hospice services; others need to go to the hospital or a long-term care facility for management of ongoing problems and progressive debilitation.

COMPLICATIONS

In the immediate postoperative period (24 to 48 hours), hypotension, cardiac dysrhythmias, pulmonary edema, and subcutaneous emphysema may occur. Long-term complications include a residual air space, which results from failure of the remaining portions of the lung to reexpand and fill the space. If this space is small, no treatment is indicated. Two major complications of chest surgery that tend to occur later in the postoperative period and require treatment are empyema and bronchopleural fistula. Empyema may occur alone or with a bronchopleural fistula. The signs and symptoms and treatment of these two complications are outlined in Table 21-9.

Guidelines for Safe Practice

The Patient After Pneumonectomy

1. Chest tubes are not necessary because there is no lung left to reexpand on the operative side.
2. The patient may lie on the back or operated side only. The patient is not allowed to lie with the operative side uppermost because of fear that the bronchial stump may leak, allowing fluid to drain into the unoperated side and drown the patient.
3. Pressure in the operative side will be checked in the operating room after the chest is closed. A pneumothorax apparatus (which can instill or remove air) will be used to check the pressure in the operative space, and air will be removed or instilled as necessary to bring the pressure to slightly negative (slightly less than 760 mm Hg).
4. The surgeon will palpate the patient's trachea at least daily to determine if it is in midline. Deviation of the trachea toward either the operated or unoperated side is a sign of mediastinal shift. If pressure builds up in the operated side, the trachea will deviate toward the unoperated side. The treatment is to remove air (positive pressure) with a pneumothorax apparatus. Mediastinal shift toward the "good" lung can seriously compromise ventilation and needs to be treated promptly. Deviation of the trachea toward the operated side indicates that more pressure (air) needs to be instilled into the empty space.
5. The patient with a mediastinal shift resembles the patient in congestive heart failure. Neck veins are distended, the trachea is displaced to one side, pulse and respirations are increased, and dyspnea is present.
6. Serous drainage will collect in the operated space and over time will congeal to the consistency of axle grease. This is often sufficient to keep the mediastinum from shifting toward the operative side. Persistent mediastinal shift toward the operative side may have to be treated with thoracoplasty (removal of ribs) to reduce the size of the remaining space and assist in maintaining the mediastinum in midline. Thoracoplasty is described below.
7. The remaining lung needs 2 to 4 days to adjust to the increase in blood flow. For this reason the amount of fluids and blood given intravenously is monitored closely to prevent fluid overload. Central venous pressure monitoring is common. Crackles are often heard over the base of the remaining lung, and vascular markings will be more prominent on x-ray films. Any increase in crackles, in pulse or blood pressure, and in dyspnea may indicate circulatory overload and should be reported immediately. Treatment may include diuretics or digitalization along with discontinuing intravenous fluids.
8. Deep breathing, coughing, and arm exercises are the same as described earlier in this chapter.
9. Patients who have had a lung removed may have a lowered vital capacity, and exercise and activity should be limited to that which can be performed without dyspnea. Because the body must be given time to adjust to having only one lung, the patient's return to work may be delayed.
10. If the diagnosis is cancer, radiation therapy is usually given, and it may be started before the patient leaves the hospital. (See Chapter 15 for further discussion of nursing care for patients receiving radiation therapy.)
11. The patient who has had a pneumonectomy for cancer is urged to call the physician promptly if hoarseness, dyspnea, pain on swallowing, or localized chest pain develops, because these symptoms may be signs of complications.

TABLE 21-9 Long-Term Complications of Resectional Surgery

Complications	Signs and Symptoms	Treatment
Empyema		
Pus in pleural space is a dreaded complication of thoracic surgery. Pus may drain from chest tube(s), or if chest tubes are already removed, pus can be obtained on thoracentesis (insertion of a needle attached to a syringe with a three-way stopcock used to remove fluid, blood, or pus from pleural space).	Unexplained elevation in temperature Evidence of pleural exudate on x-ray film	Dependent drainage by thoracentesis, intercostal chest tube, or open drainage with rib resection. Chest tube may be connected to a closed drainage system or cut off and allowed to drain into chest dressings. Water seal not necessary if empyema space has a thick wall and there is no danger of lung collapse. Over time as empyema drains out tube, the space becomes smaller and smaller and fills in with granulation tissue. If space persists, a thoracoplasty is necessary.
Bronchopleural Fistula (BPF)		
Opening in sutured bronchus that permits communication between bronchus and pleural space. Space usually becomes infected, and empyema develops. Use of an automatic stapling machine to close bronchus has reduced the incidence of BPF.	Cough (usually nonproductive), fever, leukocytosis, anorexia, expectoration of purulent sputum, and evidence of pleural exudate on x-ray film	Chest tube connected to a water-seal chamber because there is a direct communication between bronchus (positive pressure being inspired) and pleural space. A persistent bronchopleural fistula is treated by thoracoplasty and a muscle implant to seal off bronchus.

ACUTE LUNG INJURY AND ADULT RESPIRATORY DISTRESS SYNDROME

Etiology

Acute lung injury (ALI) is a syndrome of severe, acute respiratory failure characterized by respiratory distress, a severe impairment of oxygenation, and noncardiogenic pulmonary edema. ALI is defined as a syndrome of inflammation and increased permeability. Components include acute onset, bilateral infiltrates on chest x-ray films; a ratio of PaO_2 to fraction of inspired oxygen (FiO_2) of less than 300, regardless of positive end-expiratory pressure (PEEP); and pulmonary artery occlusion pressure of less than 18 mm Hg or no clinical evidence of left arterial hypertension.[71]

Adult respiratory distress syndrome (ARDS), also known as *acute respiratory distress syndrome,* has similar criteria but reflects more severe hypoxemia. In ARDS the PaO_2/FiO_2 ratio must be less than 200 mm Hg. There has been much debate about the definitions, criteria, and names of these entities.

Epidemiology

The exact incidence of ALI and ARDS is not clear. The variability in diagnosis has made determination of incidence difficult. A 1998 review of epidemiologic data indicates that the incidence of ALI is 71 cases per 100,000 persons and that the incidence of ARDS is less than 5 cases per 100,000 persons annually.[75]

Pathophysiology

There are a number of risk factors for the development of ALI/ARDS that include both direct and indirect causes of lung injury.[77] These are listed in the Risk Factors box.

There are four phases of ALI/ARDS that have been recognized. These are described in Table 21-10.

Risk Factors

Clinical Disorders Associated With Acute Lung Injury/Adult Respiratory Distress Syndrome

DIRECT LUNG INJURY	INDIRECT LUNG INJURY
Aspiration of gastric contents	Severe sepsis
Severe thoracic trauma	Shock
Pulmonary contusion	Acute pancreatitis
Diffuse pulmonary infection	Severe nonthoracic trauma
Bacterial	Multiple long bone fractures
Viral	Hypovolemic shock
Fungal: *Pneumocystis carinii*	Drug overdose
Toxic gas (smoke) inhalation	Hypertransfusion (multiple transfusions)
Near drowning	Reperfusion injury
	Following lung transplant
	Following cardiopulmonary bypass

Adapted from Weinacker AB, Vaszar LT: Acute respiratory distress syndrome: physiology and new management strategies, *Annu Rev Med* 52:221-237, 2001.

Collaborative Care Management

Diagnostic Tests. No laboratory findings are specific for ALI/ARDS. Tests that are used to evaluate the patient and document the criteria for diagnosing the syndrome include PFTs, ABG studies, chest x-ray studies, lactic acid levels, and BAL.

Results of PFTs indicative of ALI/ARDS are a V/Q-oxygen gradient increased to 300 to 500 mm Hg, which indicates an increased number of alveolocapillary units with a low (V/Q) ratio; a shunt factor greater than 15% to 20% (normal is 6%); below-normal compliance; and a low to normal pulmonary capillary wedge pressure. ABGs are markedly abnormal, with a PaO_2 of 55 mm Hg or lower and a $PaCO_2$ that is normal to low but may increase. The blood pH is elevated at first in response to hyperventilation, but as ARDS worsens, the pH decreases. Lactic acid levels may increase with tissue hypoxia, and chest x-ray films show diffuse bilateral infiltrates consistent with pulmonary edema. Findings on BAL demonstrate a high neutrophil count and procollagen peptide III. The latter is a marker of pulmonary fibrosis and correlates with mortality.

Medications. There is no specific drug therapy for ALI/ARDS, but there are trials looking at new therapies aimed to interfere with the toxic mediators thought to trigger the cascade of events. The medications being investigated include monoclonal/polyclonal antibodies to endotoxins, antiinflammatory agents, antioxidants, vasodilators, antiproteases, cytokine inhibitors, and surfactant.[8,75]

Treatments

Oxygen. Supplemental oxygen is a basic tool and the first choice of treatment in the management of impaired oxygen exchange. Although there may be some response in arterial oxygenation to supplemental oxygen administration in patients with ALI/ARDS, more oxygen is not always necessarily better. Increasing the FiO_2 improves arterial oxygen saturation only when an intrapulmonary shunt is not responsible for oxygen desaturation. In ALI/ARDS, deoxygenated venous blood is shunted from the right side of the circulation to the left side. There is no alveolar contact; thus oxygen is not taken up in the shunted areas. Supplemental oxygen should be prescribed at the lowest concentration that will allow for adequate tissue oxygenation. The goal is to increase the hemoglobin saturation to 90% without risking oxygen toxicity.

Mechanical Ventilation. Mechanical ventilation is the central supportive intervention in the management of ALI/ARDS.[35] Traditional approaches to ventilatory management of patients with ALI/ARDS include achievement and maintenance of normal gas exchange, using a combination of inspired oxygen concentration, PEEP, and tidal volume to reach that goal. This has usually meant using high tidal volumes to prevent atelectasis and normalize $PaCO_2$, and using increasing levels of PEEP to reduce FiO_2 to the lowest possible concentration to prevent complications from oxygen toxicity.

PEEP is a ventilator mode that has been shown to increase the effectiveness of mechanical ventilation in certain patients. It involves the maintenance of positive pressure at the end of expiration, rather than allowing airway pressure to return to normal (atmospheric pressure), as usually occurs. With the maintenance of positive pressure, alveoli that would otherwise collapse on expiration are held open, thus increasing the opportunity for gas exchange across the alveolocapillary membrane. This is accomplished by the increase in functional residual capacity (FRC). The result is a decrease in physiologic shunting and the ability to achieve a higher level of PaO_2 with lower concentrations of delivered oxygen (FiO_2). PEEP has had its greatest use in the treatment of ARDS but is also used in treating any patient who would otherwise require unacceptably high concentrations of oxygen.

PEEP can be hazardous because of the increase in intrathoracic pressure. Most serious of the dangers related to PEEP is the increased incidence of pneumothorax, particularly in those with friable lung tissue, as seen in persons with emphysema or lung cancer. The sudden disappearance of breath sounds on one side and mediastinal shift, in conjunction with signs of respiratory distress, in the patient being ventilated with PEEP must be taken as an indication of a pneumothorax. Another serious consequence of PEEP may be a reduction in venous return, caused by the increased intrathoracic pressure and a subsequent fall in cardiac output. This effect seems to be particularly common in patients who are relatively dehydrated and can sometimes be avoided with careful fluid administration.

This traditional treatment approach results in elevated airway pressures. It is now recognized that normal lung tissue coexists with more severely injured lung tissue in patients with ALI/ARDS and that traditional ventilation strategies may result in further pulmonary inflammation and lung injury from barotrauma and volutrauma, secondary to alveolar overstretching. In poorly compliant lungs, intense shearing forces develop in the alveolar walls as a result of the high pressures required to separate the collapsed walls of small airways and alveoli during each inspiration.[77]

Newer ventilation strategies have been devised to prevent further lung injury. These are called lung-protective strategies. They include PEEP and low tidal volumes, pressure control ventilation, airway pressure release ventilation (APRV), inverse-ratio ventilation, permissive hypercapnia, liquid ventilation, and the use of prone positioning. As these strategies are discussed, it is important to note that although they show promise, to date no method has been shown to be superior in minimizing lung injury and resulting in a survival benefit.

PEEP has been central to decreasing FiO_2 levels in ALI/ARDS patients. It reopens collapsed alveoli by shifting fluid out of them and increasing the FRC. This decreases shunting and allows the lowering of FiO_2. Some studies suggest that higher PEEP levels may protect alveoli from injury by keeping them open during expiration and preventing repetitive alveolar collapse. PEEP levels as high as 20 cm H_2O may be necessary. This is significant, since the use of low tidal volumes has become an important aspect of lung-protective ventilation. This strategy treats ALI/ARDS patients as if they had "small" lungs, recommending tidal volumes of 5 to 8 ml/kg of body weight. Traditional tidal volumes are 10 to 15 ml/kg of body weight.[48]

TABLE 21-10 Phases of Acute Lung Injury/Adult Respiratory Distress Syndrome

Phase	Characteristics
Phase I: acute injury	Occurs within first 24 hours of injury Mild hypoxemia, dyspnea, tachypnea with or without evidence of pneumonia or pulmonary edema; clinically may see only respiratory alkalosis
Phase II: latent period	May last from several hours to 2 days Gradual development of patchy lung infiltrates (tend to be peripheral) Hypoxemia is resistant to increases in supplemental oxygen administration Mechanical ventilation requires higher concentrations of oxygen and positive end-expiratory pressure (PEEP) At the tissue level, endothelial cell swelling, capillary congestion, microvascular destruction, and microatelectasis
Phase III: exudative phase	Occurs 2-10 days after injury Onset of acute respiratory failure Progressive dyspnea, tachypnea, hypoxemia, decreasing lung compliance Diffuse rales are heard on examination Chest x-ray film shows patchy infiltrates coalesce to become diffuse alveolar infiltrates Hemodynamic instability; may have signs of other organ involvement Shows signs of systemic inflammatory response syndrome At the tissue level, edematous alveoli; edema accumulates in interstitial spaces, and alveolar consolidation occurs secondary to accumulation of cellular debris and fibrin; hyaline membranes develop; surfactant dysfunction impairs gas exchange; lungs show microthrombus formation and occlusion
Phase IV: fibroproliferative phase	Occurs 10 days following lung injury Onset of severe physiologic abnormalities Intrapulmonary shunting leads to refractory hypoxemia and metabolic and respiratory acidosis Development of multiorgan involvement Fever, systemic inflammation, refractory hypoxia, loss of responsiveness to PEEP Results in remodeling of pulmonary microvascular system

Adapted from Van Soeren MH et al: Pathophysiology and implications for the treatment of ARDS, *AACN Clin Issues* 11(2):179-197, 2000.

Pressure control ventilation prevents alveolar overdistention by setting inspiratory pressure limits below 30 to 35 cm H_2O and allowing tidal volumes to fluctuate. This strategy allows earlier and more even alveolar filling to occur. Preset levels limit alveolar pressure but can result in high shear stresses. Close observation is required, since kinks in endotracheal tubing can lower tidal volume delivery.

APRV is a relatively new mode of ventilation that is time triggered, pressure limited, and time cycled. APRV produces tidal ventilation using a release of airway pressure from an elevated baseline to simulate expiration. The elevated baseline facilitates oxygenation, and the timed releases promote carbon dioxide removal. It has shown significant advantage over other ventilation strategies in lowering airway pressures, lowering minute ventilation, having minimal effect on the cardiovascular system, and allowing the patient to spontaneously breathe throughout the ventilatory cycle. Disadvantages are that volumes change with alterations in lung compliance and resistance and that it is a very new strategy, requiring staff training and ventilators, that permits this approach.[27]

Inverse-ratio ventilation increases the proportion of time spent in inspiration, which increases the mean airway pressure and the end-expiratory volume, creating auto-PEEP. Auto-PEEP increases applied PEEP and maintains alveolar inflation. The goal is to improve oxygenation, but it may take several hours to achieve maximal benefits.[75,77] Hyperinflation and decreased cardiac output are risks of this technique, and it is often poorly tolerated by awake patients, thus requiring increased sedation and paralysis (see Nursing Care Plan).

Nursing Care Plan — *Patient on Mechanical Ventilation With Positive End-Expiratory Pressure*

DATA Mr. R. is a 28-year-old married man admitted to the surgical intensive care unit (ICU) after a motor vehicle accident. Injuries sustained include a ruptured spleen and liver laceration resulting in hypovolemic shock. Mr. R. was taken to the operating room, where his injuries were repaired and blood losses replaced. His early postoperative course was unremarkable. On Mr. R.'s third postoperative day, he began experiencing some respiratory difficulties with deterioration in his arterial blood gases (ABGs). Because of severe hypoxemia, Mr. R. was intubated. His chest x-ray film revealed diffuse interstitial and alveolar infiltrates. He developed adult respiratory distress syndrome (ARDS) and eventually required positive end-expiratory pressure (PEEP).

Mr. R.'s wife has visited her husband daily and has often attempted to communicate with him. She reassures and calms him when he becomes anxious and resists the ventilator. Mrs. R. has asked the nurse many questions about her husband's status.

The nursing history reveals:

- Mr. and Mrs. R. have been married 5 years; they have no children.
- Mr. R. has full hospitalization and medical coverage through his employer.
- Mr. R. is a nonsmoker.

Collaborative nursing actions include those to assist in improving oxygenation through evaluating FiO_2 and levels of PEEP, as well as techniques used to wean Mr. R. from the ventilator. Nursing actions include:

- Supporting oxygenation and ventilation to maintain PaO_2 over 60 mm Hg and to maximize functional residual capacity
- Evaluating FiO_2 and PEEP levels to gradually wean patient from ventilator while monitoring ABGs
- Monitoring the patient for signs of hypoxia

NURSING DIAGNOSIS **Impaired gas exchange related to ARDS**
GOALS/OUTCOMES Will remain oxygenated within normal parameters

NOC Suggested Outcomes

- Respiratory Status: Airway Patency (0410)
- Respiratory Status: Gas Exchange (0402)
- Respiratory Status: Ventilation (0403)
- Comfort Level (2100)

NIC Suggested Interventions

- Artificial Airway Management (3180)
- Airway Suctioning (3160)
- Respiratory Monitoring (3350)

Nursing Interventions/Rationales

- Assess and monitor ABGs to determine PaO_2. *Altered ABGs result from inadequate oxygenation. Early recognition allows for early correction of problems.*
- Suction only when essential to prevent loss of PEEP secondary to disconnection from ventilator. *Suctioning may be needed to clear the airway. However, disconnecting the ventilator places the patient at risk for inadequate oxygenation.*
- Monitor required levels of PEEP and FiO_2. *To maintain oxygenation and make corrections when needed.*
- Assess peripheral circulation for pulses, color of extremities, and warmth. *To detect changes that indicate inadequate oxygenation and to determine effectiveness of ventilation.*
- Monitor mixed venous blood oxygen levels. *ARDS is an acute lung injury that affects capillary permeability, which permits proteins and fluids to leak out into alveoli and interstitial spaces, thus preventing normal gas exchange. Mixed venous blood oxygen levels reflect adequacy of oxygenation.*

Continued

Evaluation Parameters

1. Pao_2 on ABG analysis >75 mm Hg
2. Color pink; no cyanosis
3. Peripheral pulses intact; extremities pink and warm

NURSING DIAGNOSIS **Decreased cardiac output related to decreased venous return**
GOALS/OUTCOMES Hemodynamic parameters will remain within normal limits for adult male

NOC Suggested Outcomes

- Circulation Status (0401)
- Cardiac Pump Effectiveness (0400)
- Tissue Perfusion: Abdominal Organs (0404)
- Tissue Perfusion: Peripheral (0407)
- Tissue Perfusion: Cerebral (0406)

NIC Suggested Interventions

- Acid-Base Monitoring (1920)
- Acid-Base Management (1910)
- Cardiac Care (4040)
- Electrolyte Management (2000)
- Fluid Management (4120)
- Hemodynamic Regulation (4150)

Nursing Interventions/Rationales

- Monitor vital signs hourly as needed. *To determine abnormalities and initiate treatment for changes.*
- Monitor hemodynamic parameters (cardiac output, mean arterial pressure, central venous pressure [CVP]). *To identify alterations in cardiac status and to help evaluate effectiveness of treatments. PEEP may cause decreased cardiac output by increasing intraalveolar pressures, thereby decreasing venous return to the heart.*
- Monitor intake and output. *To identify adequacy of urinary function and fluid status. Normally, output approximates intake.*
- Assess peripheral circulation every 2 to 4 hours and as needed. *To identify adequacy of peripheral circulation.*
- Perform passive range-of-motion exercises every 4 to 6 hours. *Encourages venous blood return to the heart.*
- Administer prescribed adrenergic agents. *To improve cardiac output.*
- Notify physician of hemodynamic changes/complications. *To initiate any corrective treatments early.*

Evaluation Parameters

1. Vital signs within normal limits
2. CVP, mean arterial pressure within normal limits
3. Extremities warm and pink with pulses present

NURSING DIAGNOSIS **Ineffective breathing pattern related to altered lung–thoracic pressure relationship**
GOALS/OUTCOMES Will remain free of pulmonary complications secondary to PEEP

NOC Suggested Outcomes

- Respiratory Status: Ventilation (0403)
- Respiratory Status: Gas Exchange (0402)

NIC Suggested Interventions

- Airway Management (3140)
- Mechanical Ventilation (3300)
- Mechanical Ventilation Weaning (3310)
- Ventilation Assistance (3390)

Nursing Interventions/Rationales

- Monitor respirations and assess breath sounds for adventitious findings hourly and more often as needed. *Respiratory rate increases initially as lung compliance decreases. Respiratory workload increases as compliance decreases.*
- Administer pulmonary toilet (turning, chest physiotherapy) every 2 hours and as needed. *To maintain patent airway and prevent complications.*
- Monitor for signs of pulmonary complications and respiratory distress (asymmetric chest excursion, sudden sharp chest pain, cyanosis, anxiety, subcutaneous emphysema). *When alveolar walls cannot withstand the positive pressure from PEEP, perforation can occur. As a result, air leaks into the pleural space, the mediastinum, or its subcutaneous space. The result may be a pneumothorax, pneumomediastinum, or subcutaneous emphysema, respectively.*
- Keep a chest tube set up at the bedside. *Emergency chest tube placement may be necessary if a pneumothorax occurs.*
- Monitor ABGs as needed. *If the patient becomes fatigued and cannot initiate own respirations, carbon dioxide may be retained, adversely affecting ABGs.*
- Notify physician of respiratory complications. *To facilitate the implementation of corrective treatments.*

Evaluation Parameters

1. Normal breath sounds
2. Absence of complications
3. ABGs within baseline (or normal) range

NURSING DIAGNOSIS **Risk for imbalanced nutrition: less than body requirements related to intubation**
GOALS/OUTCOMES Will remain within 5 pounds of ideal weight

NOC Suggested Outcomes
- Nutritional Status (1004)
- Nutritional Status: Food and Fluid Intake (1008)
- Nutritional Status: Nutrient Intake (1009)

NIC Suggested Interventions
- Nutrition Management (1100)
- Nutritional Monitoring (1160)
- Nutrition Therapy (1120)

Nursing Interventions/Rationales
- Administer hyperalimentation or enteral feedings as prescribed. *Nutritional status must be maintained for healing to occur, strength to be maintained, and successful weaning of the patient from ventilation.*
- Monitor intake and output. *Decreased urine output is an indication of decreased cardiac output and inadequate renal perfusion.*
- Weigh daily. *To determine if nutritional needs are being met and to evaluate the effectiveness of nutritional interventions.*
- Administer albumin and plasma expanders as prescribed. *Protein and volume expanders increase colloidal osmotic pressure, thus maintaining fluid within the intravascular compartment.*
- Monitor serum albumin levels. *Serum albumin levels reflect the adequacy of protein intake. Decreased levels are associated with peripheral edema resulting from loss of osmotic pull from within the vascular space.*

Evaluation Parameters
1. Serum albumin levels within normal limits
2. Muscle strength maintained
3. Successful weaning from ventilator
4. Absence of weight loss

NURSING DIAGNOSIS **Anxiety related to ARDS, intubation, and discomfort with PEEP**
GOALS/OUTCOMES Will remain free of anxiety related to intubation and PEEP

NOC Suggested Outcomes
- Anxiety Control (1402)
- Coping (1302)
- Psychosocial Adjustment: Life Change (1305)

NIC Suggested Interventions
- Anxiety Reduction (5820)
- Calming Technique (5880)
- Coping Enhancement (5230)
- Presence (5340)
- Communication Enhancement: Speech Deficit (4976)

Nursing Interventions/Rationales
- Assess for signs of anxiety. *Intensive care, mechanical ventilation, the inability to communicate, and fear of the unknown all contribute to feelings of stress and anxiety for the patient in the ICU, as well as the patient's significant other.*
- Explain the disease process to family, including the benefits of mechanical ventilation and PEEP. *Knowledge often reduces fear and corresponding anxiety.*
- Allow patient and wife to express their concerns and fears. *When patients/family members can communicate their fears, anxiety is often reduced.*
- Explain procedures before performing them. *Patients have less fear and anxiety when they know what to expect.*
- Provide a means of communication between patient and wife. *The ability to communicate allows some degree of control for the patient and allows him to communicate his needs to health care providers and his wife.*
- Attempt to anticipate patient's needs. *If the patient's needs are met before he has to ask, his fear of the situation and of not having his needs met will be reduced.*
- Administer prescribed light sedation/antianxiety medications if necessary. *Sedative and antianxiety medications produce relaxation, which reduces fighting or "bucking" of the ventilator and promotes sleep. Positive pressure exhalation is often uncomfortable for the patient, who may respond by resisting ventilation.*
- Provide distraction from ICU environment (soft music, television). *Distraction may minimize the perception of discomfort and reduce anxiety.*

Evaluation Parameters
1. Relaxed appearance
2. Cooperative with ventilator, procedures, personnel

Permissive hypercapnia is not really a treatment but an effect and may result from any ventilation strategy that limits the maximum airway pressure applied and subsequently limits the tidal volume. The reduction in minute ventilation permits an increased $PaCO_2$ and decreased pH. As long as the rate of increased carbon dioxide is gradual, the "permitted" hypercapnia is usually well tolerated. This strategy is not recommended in those patients with head injury or elevated intracranial pressure, marked cardiovascular dysfunction, pulmonary hypertension, or metabolic acidosis.[48]

Liquid ventilation uses perfluorocarbon to maintain open lung units and improve oxygenation. It may improve pulmonary compliance and lessen shear stresses.[75]

Prone positioning during mechanical ventilation has been found to improve oxygenation by opening consolidated, dependent lung regions. Ventral lung regions do not seem to be affected with atelectasis, as one might expect in the prone position, and ventilation is distributed more homogeneously with better ventilation of the dorsal lung areas. The prone position shifts the weight of the heart from the dorsal lung regions to the sternum and anterior rib cage and facilitates better pulmonary drainage of dorsal segments. Most trials have shown best advantage early in the course of ALI/ARDS. Disadvantages include loss of the endotracheal tube, loss of vascular access, facial edema, and difficulties with cardiopulmonary resuscitation.[75]

Additional information on mechanical ventilation and the requisite nursing care is included later in the chapter under Acute Respiratory Failure.

Fluid Management. Fluid management has been controversial in the treatment of ALI/ARDS. It requires a balance between providing enough fluids to maintain adequate perfusion and creating more edema. Current recommendations recommend a fairly conservative approach to fluid replacement therapy while maintaining adequate hemodynamics. In the exudative phase, red blood cells are recommended as volume expanders, since they also improve oxygen-carrying capacity. Later in the disease process, liberal amounts of fluid are needed to overcome increased pulmonary vascular resistance and alveolar pressures, to perfuse pulmonary capillaries, and to minimize dead space.[75]

Other new modalities to improve ALI/ARDS outcomes include the use of nitric oxide. Nitric oxide plays numerous roles in the physiology and pathophysiology of the lung, including decreasing neutrophil adhesion, acting as a molecular reactant, and signaling vasoconstriction. Inhaled nitric oxide is a vasodilator that reduces pulmonary artery pressure and, in high doses, reverses hypoxic pulmonary vasoconstriction without causing systemic hypotension. Some studies have shown that inhaled nitric oxide improves oxygenation in patients with ARDS by reversing hypoxic pulmonary vasoconstriction in ventilated lung units.[77] Larger studies have yet to show improvement in mortality for ALI/ARDS.[52]

Diet. The patient with ALI or ARDS is generally in a well-nourished but extremely hypermetabolic state.[60] The hypermetabolic stress response results in increased energy needs. Nutritional assessment and intervention is aimed at minimizing excessive protein losses, preserving lean body mass by providing adequate energy, and maintaining positive nitrogen balance. Nonintubated patients are able to maintain better spontaneous oral intake. Mechanically ventilated patients often require nutritional support. Nutritional support can be administered systemically by total parenteral nutrition or by enteral nutrition. General nutrition prescriptions include 20% protein, 60% to 70% carbohydrate, and 20% to 30% fat.[60] Enteral nutrition should be the mode unless the GI tract is not functioning. The patient needs to be observed closely for nutrition-induced hypercapnia.

Activity. During the most acute phase of illness the patient is placed on bed rest to minimize energy expenditure. With the establishment of clinical and hemodynamic stability, gradual activity progression is initiated.

Referrals. Referrals to a respiratory therapist, physical therapist, nutritionist, and social worker are appropriate.

NURSING MANAGEMENT OF PATIENT WITH ALI/ARDS

ASSESSMENT

Nursing assessment of the patient with ALI/ARDS must be tailored to maximize information obtained without increasing respiratory distress.

Health History

Background information and the history of the present illness may need to be obtained from family members, because the patient is usually too ill to give details.

Physical Examination

Important aspects of the physical examination of the patient with ALI/ARDS are the same as described for respiratory failure.

NURSING DIAGNOSES

Nursing diagnoses are determined from an analysis of patient data. Nursing diagnoses for the person with ARDS may include but are not limited to:

Diagnostic Title	Possible Etiologic Factors
1. Impaired gas exchange	Changes in pulmonary capillary permeability with edema formation, alveolar hypoventilation and collapse, intrapulmonary shunting
2. Ineffective breathing pattern	Decreased lung compliance
3. Risk for deficient fluid volume	Fluid mobilization to and from third space (interstitium and alveolar space)
4. Imbalanced nutrition: less than body requirements	Hypermetabolic state creates increased energy needs; may be unable to eat
5. Risk for infection	Invasive procedures, bypass of defense mechanisms
6. Anxiety	Threat of death, change in health status

EXPECTED PATIENT OUTCOMES

Although the overall mortality due to ALI/ARDS has declined in the past 2 decades, mortality remains high. Some ALI/ARDS survivors recover completely; however, most experience some decrease in lung and other organ function.[77] Desired patient outcomes for the person with ALI/ARDS may include but are not limited to:

1. Will demonstrate improved ventilation and oxygenation
1a. PaO_2 will be maintained at 50 to 60 mm Hg during acute phase of illness
1b. On resolution of ALI/ARDS, PaO_2, $PaCO_2$, and pH will return to acceptable preillness levels
1c. Sensorium will return to preillness level
1d. During acute phase of illness, will tolerate mechanical ventilatory assistance
1e. Inspiratory-expiratory ratio will be 5 : 10 seconds
1f. Respiratory rate and tidal volume will be within normal limits
1g. Will not complain of dyspnea
2. Will breathe effectively
2a. Respirations will be regular and between 16 and 20/min
3. Will maintain fluid volume at functional level
3a. Pulmonary capillary wedge pressure (measure of pulmonary capillary pressure) will be below 18 mm Hg
3b. Vital signs will be stable
3c. Urine output will be at least 30 ml/hr
3d. Peripheral pulses will be present, and extremities will be warm to touch
3e. Will have good skin turgor, moist mucous membranes
4. Will maintain stable body weight within 5 pounds of preillness weight
5. Will be free of infection
5a. Vital signs will be within normal limits; temperature will not be elevated
5b. Cultures of pulmonary secretions and urine will be negative
6. Will display increased physiologic and psychologic comfort and decreased anxiety
6a. Will tolerate ventilator and artificial airway
6b. Will acknowledge and express fears
6c. Will communicate personal needs effectively with staff and family
6d. Will cooperate and assist with care

INTERVENTIONS

Patients with ALI/ARDS are critically ill and are best cared for in an ICU. Their care centers around the following measures.

1. Improving Gas Exchange

Oxygen

Oxygen therapy is provided as ordered, and the patient is monitored for signs of hypoxemia and oxygen toxicity.

A patent airway is maintained, and the patient is positioned for optimal oxygenation, usually with the head of the bed elevated 45 to 90 degrees. If an artificial airway is present, the necessary care is provided. An endotracheal tube must be secured to avoid movement either in or out of the established position. Because of the risk of an endotracheal tube slipping into the right main-stem bronchus, the lungs must be auscultated hourly to check the tube's placement. The tube is kept patent by suctioning if needed. Bronchoactive medications are administered as ordered, and ventilator settings are checked frequently. Proper ventilator function is checked to ensure delivery of adequate tidal volume and oxygen concentration. If the patient appears to be in respiratory distress although the ventilator is functioning properly, ABG levels need to be assessed.

2. Maintaining Effective Breathing Pattern

In addition to the interventions noted above, the nurse positions the patient for maximal lung expansion, checks respirations regularly, and assesses for adequate tissue perfusion.

3. Maintaining Fluid Balance

The pulmonary capillary wedge pressure is monitored, and the physician is notified if the pressure is above or below the established range. If the pressure is below the established range, volume expanders or antihypotensive medications are administered as ordered. If the pressure is high, diuretics or vasodilators are administered as ordered. Urine output, vital signs, and extremities are monitored hourly.

4. Maintaining Adequate Nutrition

Fluid and caloric intake are checked hourly to ensure adequate intake. Tube feedings or hyperalimentation are maintained in collaboration with the physician and nutritionist. Excessive carbohydrate intake is avoided because metabolism of carbohydrates may result in the production of carbon dioxide. The patient is observed for signs of malnutrition resulting from the increased caloric requirements of labored breathing.

5. Preventing Infection

Hands are washed before any contact with the patient, and sterile procedures and equipment are used. The airway is suctioned only when necessary to avoid trauma to tissue and introduction of bacteria.

6. Decreasing Patient and Family Anxiety

The nurse should identify a method by which the patient can communicate concerns and express feelings (see Evidence-Based Practice box). It is difficult for patients to feel secure when they cannot communicate vocally.[31]

Simple explanations about procedures are provided.. The patient is oriented to the surroundings, and explanations are repeated regularly. Explanations about care routines and the environment are also offered to the family. The family is encouraged to approach, talk to, and touch the patient as they desire.

Patient/Family Education

The patient and family are kept informed about each aspect of treatment, with special attention to intubation and mechanical ventilation when they are necessary.

Evidence-Based Practice

Reference: Happ MH: Communicating with mechanically ventilated patients: state of the science, *AACN Clin Issues* 12(2):247-258, 2001.

Effective communication is the foundation of the nurse-patient relationship. Communicating with the patient on mechanical ventilation is recognized as a priority of care, yet studies demonstrating best practices are limited. Critical care nurses often have minimal education in nonvocal communication and augmentive communication (AC) techniques. Evidence has shown that the inability to communicate because of intubation and/or cognitive, sensory, or language deficits can result in feelings of fear, panic, and insecurity in the patient. This review identified clinical issues and technologic advancements to facilitate communication with the mechanically ventilated patient. Continuity in caregiver is fundamental to the interpretation of nonvocal communication. Using AC devices requires patience and consistency. Effective AC methods are eye blinks, writing, pointing to pictures, words, letters, computerized touch screens, and auditory scanning devices for visually impaired patients. Conclusions reached are that improved methods for communication are available but not routinely used, and clinical research and application have not kept pace with technologic advancements in AC devices.

Health Promotion/Prevention. Prompt treatment of the underlying cause of ARDS is the major focus of preventive care. In addition, judicious use of the mechanical ventilator and oxygen therapy is required to avoid inducing ALI and ARDS as untoward complications of these treatment modalities.

EVALUATION

To evaluate the effectiveness of nursing interventions, compare patient behaviors with those stated in the expected patient outcomes. Achievement of patient outcomes is successful if the patient:

- **1.** Maintains own ventilation without mechanical assistance.
- **1a-g.** Has $Pa\text{O}_2$, $Pa\text{CO}_2$, and pH within normal limits or at baseline level; has no complaints of dyspnea; has normal sensorium; has inspiratory-expiratory ratio of 5 : 10 seconds and respiratory rate and tidal volume within normal limits or at baseline level.
- **2.** Breathes effectively at a rate of 16 to 20 breaths/min.
- **3a-e.** Maintains adequate fluid volume; has good skin turgor; has urine output of 150 to 200 ml at each voiding; has stable vital signs; has capillary wedge pressure below 18 mm Hg; has peripheral pulses present and extremities warm to touch.
- **4.** Demonstrates an improved appetite and daily weight gain, although body weight may be below preillness level.
- **5a,b.** Is free of nosocomial infection; has normal vital signs; has negative cultures.
- **6.** Appears calm and relaxed.
- **6a-d.** Sleeps at night; tolerates ventilator and artificial airway; expresses any concerns freely; communicates personal needs; appears calm in interactions with family; cooperates and assists with care.

GERONTOLOGIC CONSIDERATIONS

Mortality is significantly higher for patients with ALI/ARDS who are older than 55 years of age. The older adult may have a reduced ability to respond adaptively to environmental changes, and the processes of tissue repair are slowed or impaired. Older patients may also have chronic underlying health problems that contribute to the severity of the disease process and may influence the decision to withdraw life-sustaining therapy. Despite this, there is some evidence that ALI/ARDS is less severe in older patients, as evidenced by lower levels of PEEP and $F\text{IO}_2$ required to maintain $Pa\text{O}_2$. The issue of age bias in treatment decisions deserves continued investigation, since studies have shown that older patients with underlying chronic illnesses survive more often than younger patients with chronic illnesses and many elderly ALI/ARDS survivors are not necessarily severely impaired following recovery.[72]

SPECIAL ENVIRONMENTS FOR CARE

Critical Care Management

ALI and ARDS are the most common illnesses requiring care in the ICU.

COMPLICATIONS

Many complications are possible, including dysrhythmias, pneumonia, GI bleeding, disseminated intravascular coagulation, renal failure, and respiratory arrest.

OBSTRUCTIVE LUNG DISEASES

CHRONIC OBSTRUCTIVE PULMONARY DISEASE

Chronic obstructive pulmonary disease (COPD) is not a disease entity but a complex of conditions that contribute to airflow limitation. The airflow obstruction is generally progressive, may be accompanied by airway hyperreactivity, and may be partially reversible. In 1995 the American Thoracic Society defined COPD as a disease state characterized by airflow obstruction resulting from chronic bronchitis or emphysema[5] (Figure 21-10). In the past, asthma was included as a type of COPD. Asthma is now discussed separately because of its unique characteristics of inflammation and degree of reversibility.

Most persons with COPD have one predominant disease entity, but there are often manifestations of both. Why some individuals develop bronchitis and others develop emphysema is unknown. Differences in susceptibility and the predominant type of disease are believed to be influenced by hereditary or environmental factors or factors in the patient's history.

Etiology

Cigarette smoking is the causative factor of COPD in more than 90% of patients. However, only 15% to 20% of heavy

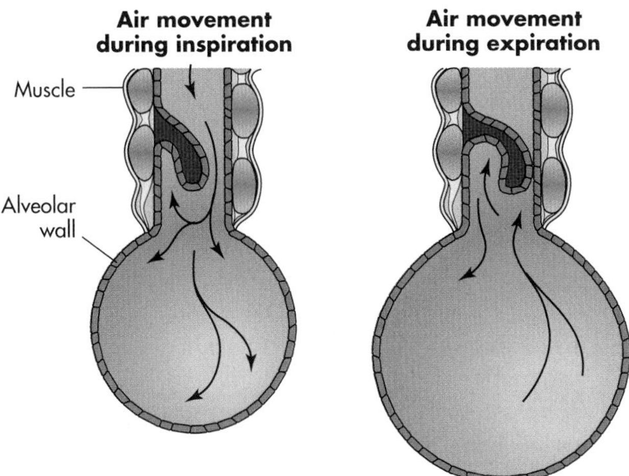

Figure 21-10 Mechanisms of air trapping in chronic obstructive pulmonary disease. Mucous plugs and narrowed airways cause air trapping and hyperinflation on expiration. During inspiration the airways enlarge, allowing gas to flow past the obstruction. During expiration the airways narrow and prevent gas flow. This mechanism of air trapping, known as ball valving, occurs in asthma and chronic bronchitis.

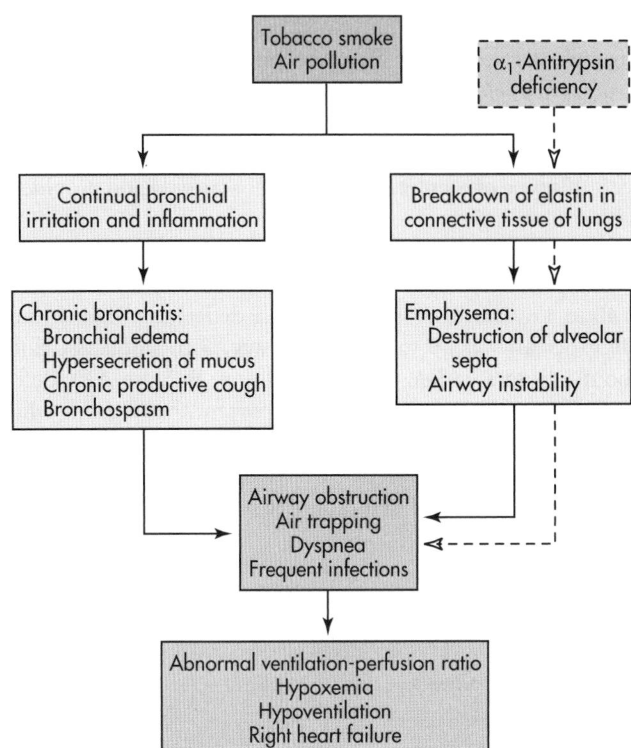

Figure 21-11 Pathogenesis of chronic bronchitis and emphysema. (*Dashed arrows* indicate role of alpha$_1$-antitrypsin deficiency, if present.)

smokers develop COPD.[73] This points to environmental and genetic factors as additional causal agents. Imbalances in the amounts of proteases and antiproteases are thought to play a major role in the development of COPD, especially emphysema. Deficiencies in antiproteases could lead to enhanced lung parenchymal destruction. Alpha$_1$-antitrypsin (AAT) deficiency is the only known genetic abnormality that leads to COPD, and it accounts for less than 1% of cases of COPD in the United States.[44] AAT is a serum protein produced by the liver and normally found in the lungs. Its main role is to protect the lungs from a breakdown product of WBCs called neutrophil elastase. Severe AAT deficiency leads to premature emphysema. The majority of persons with AAT deficiency are misdiagnosed or undiagnosed. A high index of suspicion is needed when emphysema occurs in patients under age 60, even when there is a significant smoking history.[7] Environmental tobacco smoke, also called secondhand smoke and passive smoking, is the exposure of nonsmokers to cigarette smoke and is a risk factor for COPD. High levels of urban air pollution and occupational exposure to toxins are also considered causative factors for a small percentage of patients with COPD.

Epidemiology

COPD is the fourth leading cause of death in the United States, and its incidence is increasing. It is estimated that 16 million adults have COPD, and it accounts for more than 110,000 deaths, 16 million physician office visits, and 500,000 hospitalizations.[70] The number of affected persons has doubled in the past 25 years, with more then 50% dying within 10 years of diagnosis.[9] Morbidity from COPD is rising also and accounts for more than $18 billion of direct health care costs in the United States and $23 billion if indirect costs such as lost productivity are included.[9]

Pathophysiology

The pathophysiologic hallmarks of COPD are destruction of the lung parenchyma (characteristic of emphysema) and inflammation of the central airways (characteristic of chronic bronchitis) (Figure 21-11).[73] The functional consequence of these abnormalities is expiratory airflow limitation.

Emphysema. Emphysema is defined in terms of anatomic pathology as abnormal permanent enlargement of the air spaces distal to the terminal bronchioles, accompanied by destruction of their walls and without obvious fibrosis. Recent data, however, have shown that the destructive process is accompanied by an increase in the mass of collagen, suggesting that there is alveolar wall fibrosis. The defining element of emphysema is, however, the destructive process. Depending on how the acinus is destroyed, emphysema is classified as centriacinar or panacinar. In centriacinar emphysema the destruction is restricted to respiratory bronchioles and central portions of the acinus surrounded by areas of grossly normal lung parenchyma. The whole acinus is uniformly involved in panacinar emphysema, and this type is less associated with smoking and more typically occurs in AAT-deficient persons.

As indicated above, evidence suggests that proteases released by polymorphonuclear leukocytes or alveolar macrophages are involved in the destruction of the connective tissue of the lungs. Connective tissue in the lungs is primarily composed of elastin, collagen, and proteoglycan, which can be damaged and destroyed by enzymes such as proteases and elastase. Protease-antiprotease imbalances and cigarette smoke destroy connective tissue. Cigarette smoke directly blocks the inhibitory capacity of AAT and promotes an excess of neutrophils through the attractant effects of alveolar macrophages. The neutrophils release elastases, which are capable of destroying the elastin structure of the lung. An established familial tendency to AAT deficiency indicates that relatives of persons with this type of emphysema should be screened and provided with counseling.

An estimated 1% of persons with COPD have AAT deficiency.[7] The mean age for onset of dyspnea related to COPD is 40 to 45 years in persons with AAT deficiency. Their mean life expectancy is 50 to 65 years of age, with smokers dying about 10 years earlier than nonsmokers. Because AAT deficiency cannot be prevented, it is important that persons who have it not smoke.

The clinical diagnosis of emphysema is inferred from the presence of signs and symptoms that are manifestations of known pathophysiologic changes associated with the disease. Physiologic abnormalities characteristic of emphysema include the following alterations:

- *Increased lung compliance.* Loss of elastic recoil resulting from destruction of elastin in lung parenchyma causes the lungs to become permanently overdistended (Figure 21-12). Thus compared with normal lungs, emphysematous lungs have a larger increase in volume relative to the pressure change that occurs during inhalation.
- *Increased airway resistance.* Destruction of elastic lung tissue causes the small airways to either collapse or narrow, particularly during expiration (Figure 21-13). Thus air becomes trapped in the distal air spaces, contributing to the lungs' overdistended state. The overdistended lungs press down against the diaphragm, diminishing its ventilatory effectiveness. Use of accessory muscles for

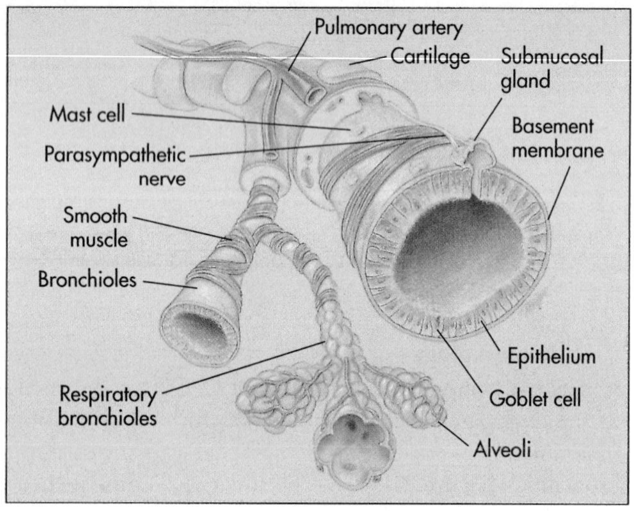

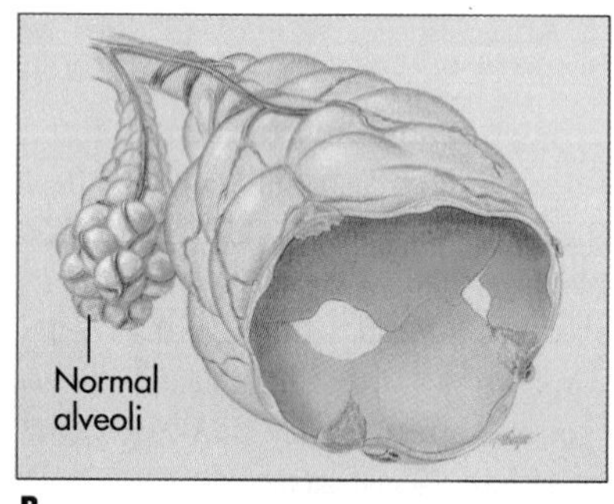

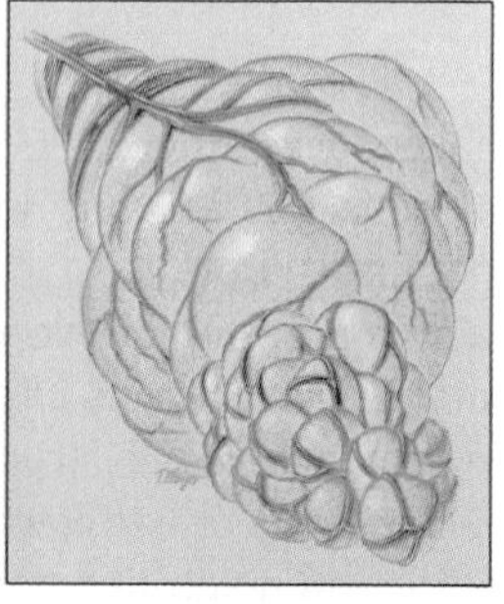

Figure 21-12 Airway obstruction caused by emphysema. **A,** Normal lung. **B,** Emphysema: enlargement and destruction of alveolar walls with loss of elasticity and trapping of air; *left,* panlobular emphysema showing abnormal weakening and enlargement of all air spaces distal to the terminal bronchioles (normal alveoli shown for comparison only); *right,* centrilobular emphysema showing abnormal weakening and enlargement of respiratory bronchioles in the proximal portion of the acinus.

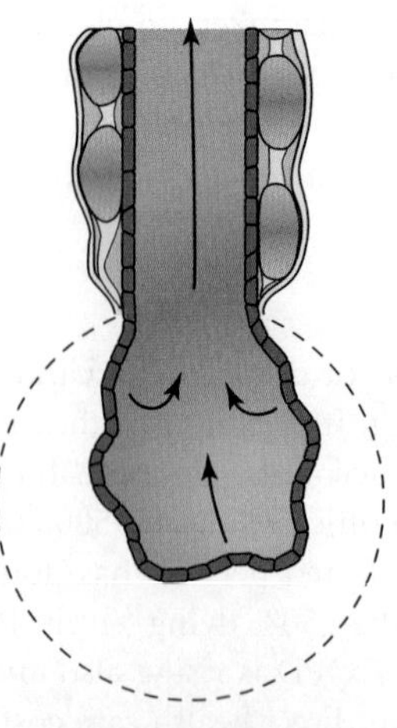

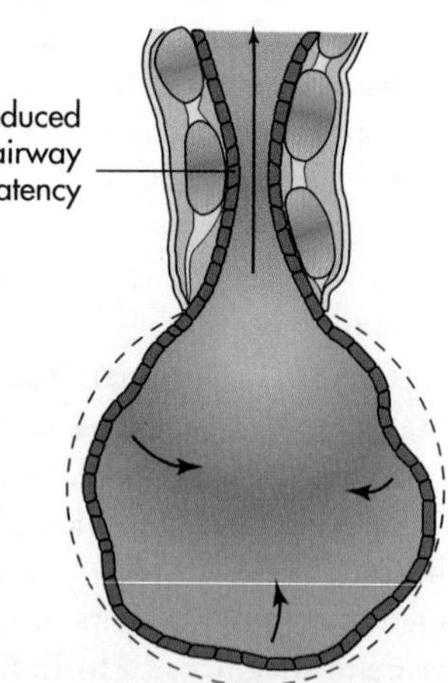

Figure 21-13 Mechanisms of air trapping in emphysema. Damaged or destroyed alveolar walls no longer support and hold airways open; alveoli lose their elastic recoil. Both of these factors contribute to collapse of alveoli during expiration.

breathing, which is a compensatory attempt to force the trapped air out of the lungs, causes an increase in intrapleural pressure, which further accentuates airway collapse.

- *Altered oxygen–carbon dioxide exchange.* Destruction of alveolar and respiratory bronchiole walls decreases alveolocapillary membrane surface area, which in turn may diminish diffusion of oxygen and carbon dioxide. Persons with emphysema are able to compensate for these destructive changes by increasing their respiratory rate. Thus ABGs remain relatively normal, although mild hypoxemia may be present. Late in the course of the disease, extensive surface area loss and V/Q inequalities usually cause respiratory acidosis and hypoxemia. The first sign of emphysema is an insidious onset of dyspnea, initially on exertion. Persons with predominant emphysema report first becoming aware of their breathing. With further disease progression, they become aware of difficulty exhaling and dyspnea becomes constant. There is minimal cough and sputum production. Persons with emphysema usually appear thin and manifest a "barrel chest" with an increased AP diameter from hyperinflation. The characteristic breathing pattern of the emphysematous individual includes accessory muscle breathing, an increased respiratory rate, and a prolonged expiratory phase resulting from airway narrowing or collapse on expiration. These individuals spontaneously exhibit pursed-lip breathing, which facilitates effective air exhalation (Figure 21-14).

Pulmonary function studies demonstrate an increased residual volume (RV), FRC, and total lung capacity (TLC). Diffusing capacity is significantly reduced because of lung tissue destruction. Diminished respiratory airflow is demonstrated by a decreased FEV_1 and maximum mid-expiratory flow rate. The vital capacity (VC) may be normal or only slightly reduced until late in the disease progression; thus the FEV_1/VC ratio is decreased.

ABGs are often near normal because of the individual's ability to compensate through an increased respiratory rate and tidal volume. Indeed, many people with emphysema overcompensate and develop a mild respiratory alkalosis from hyperventilation. Because resting hypoxemia is absent and ventilation is high, these individuals maintain a normal $PaCO_2$ despite abnormal gas exchange. Late in the course of the disease, the $PaCO_2$ is elevated, which promotes the development of cor pulmonale and respiratory failure.

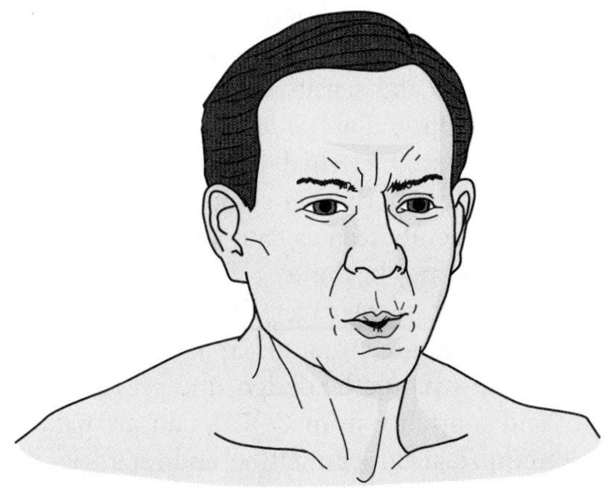

Figure 21-14 Pursed-lip breathing.

Chronic Bronchitis. Chronic bronchitis is defined in clinical terms as the presence of a chronic productive cough for 3 months in each of 2 successive years in a patient in whom other causes of chronic cough have been excluded.

The pathologic changes that typify chronic bronchitis are hypertrophy of mucus-secreting glands and chronic inflammatory changes in the small airways. Mucous gland hypertrophy and hyperplasia from chronic irritation cause excessive mucus production. The excessive mucus and impaired ciliary movement associated with chronic bronchitis increase susceptibility to infection. Bacteria, the most common of which are *Streptococcus pneumoniae* and *Haemophilus influenzae,* proliferate in the mucus secretions in the lumen of the bronchi. As bacteria multiply, they exert a neutrophilic chemotaxis, and pus cells migrate from between bronchial epithelial cells to produce a mucopurulent exudate in the lumen. The presence of granulation tissue and peribronchial fibrosis results in stenosis and airway obstruction. Small airways may be completely obliterated, and others may become dilated. This chain of events further traps secretions and promotes multiplication of bacteria. There is some evidence that the pathologic changes occur initially in small airways and move to larger bronchi. The disease may progress to ulceration and destruction of the bronchial wall (Figure 21-15).

Persons with chronic bronchitis develop increased airway resistance as a result of bronchial wall tissue changes, mucosal edema, and excessive mucus production. Excess mucus in the airways not only obstructs airflow but also often causes bronchospasm, which further increases airway resistance.

Oxygen–carbon dioxide exchange is altered. Airway obstruction results from all of the pathophysiologic changes that increase airway resistance and cause V/Q mismatching at the alveolocapillary membrane by decreasing the amount of

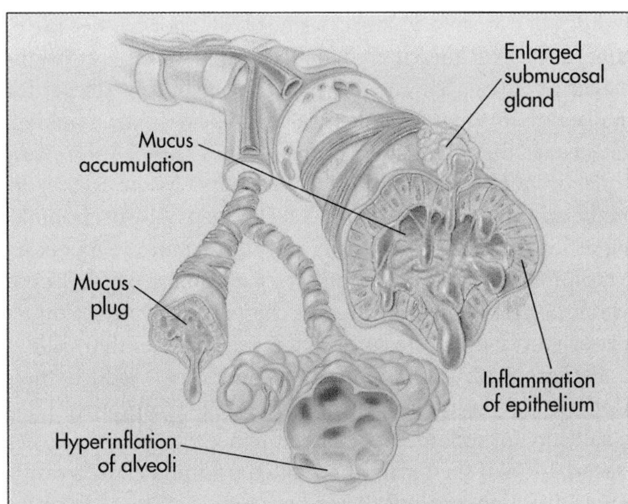

Figure 21-15 Airway obstruction caused by chronic bronchitis. Inflammation and thickening of mucous membrane with accumulation of mucus and pus, leading to obstruction; characterized by cough.

oxygenated air that reaches the alveoli. In addition, the obstructed airways may lead to atelectasis, which further diminishes the surface area available for respiration. The result of these pathophysiologic alterations is hypercapnia, hypoxemia, and respiratory acidosis.

Right ventricular decompensation (cor pulmonale) may develop. The hypercapnia and hypoxemia typically associated with chronic bronchitis cause pulmonary vascular vasoconstriction. The increased pulmonary vascular resistance results in pulmonary vessel hypertension that in turn increases vascular pressure in the right ventricle of the heart. The earliest symptom of chronic bronchitis is a productive cough, especially on awakening. This symptom is often ignored by cigarette smokers, who become so accustomed to an early-morning cough that they take it for granted; some of them even refer to it as their "cigarette cough."

Early in the course of chronic bronchitis, the symptoms tend to be episodic in nature. As the disease progresses in severity, the patient's symptoms are constantly present to some degree. The patient appears increasingly dyspneic, using accessory muscles to breathe. Chronic hypoxemia resulting in polycythemia causes the patient to appear cyanotic. Increased pulmonary vascular resistance caused by respiratory acidosis and hypoxemia increases pressure on the right side of the heart, ultimately resulting in right-sided heart failure (cor pulmonale). The person with late-stage chronic bronchitis and cor pulmonale appears stout or overweight from edema, and the skin appears dusky.

Patients with chronic bronchitis complicated by cor pulmonale often have chronic respiratory failure (gradual onset of Pa_{O_2} <50 mm Hg and a Pa_{CO_2} >50 mm Hg). They are also prone to develop acute respiratory failure as a complication of a respiratory infection superimposed on their already-diseased lung.

Clinical Manifestations

COPD progresses for about 30 years from inception to the development of clinical manifestations. Decline in lung function develops insidiously and is almost always caused by decades of exposure to tobacco smoke. The normal decline in lung function as measured by FEV_1 is 25 to 30 ml/year beginning at about age 35. The rate of decline of FEV_1 is steeper for smokers than for nonsmokers, and the heavier the smoking, the steeper the rate. Patients often do not complain of exertional dyspnea until their FEV_1 is between 40% and 50% of its predicted value.[5] Patients with COPD have usually been smoking at least 20 cigarettes per day for 20 or more years before symptoms develop. They commonly present in the fifth decade with productive cough or an acute chest illness. Dyspnea on effort usually does not occur until the sixth or seventh decade.

Persons with COPD often unconsciously reduce their ADLs to accommodate their respiratory symptoms. They usually do not seek medical help until they experience a severe exacerbation of their symptoms, often precipitated by a respiratory infection, or until their respiratory symptoms interfere significantly with ADLs, resulting in decreased quality of life.

Physical examination early in the disease may reveal only slowed expiration and wheezing on forced expiration. As obstruction progresses, hyperinflation becomes evident and the AP diameter of the chest increases. The diaphragm becomes limited in its motion. Breath sounds are decreased, expiration is prolonged, and heart sounds often become distant. Coarse crackles may be heard at the lung bases. Wheezes can often be elicited with forced expiration.

Collaborative Care Management

Diagnostic Tests

Pulmonary Function/Spirometry Tests. Pulmonary function/spirometry tests are used for diagnosis and to follow progression of disease. Spirometric testing can detect physiologic alterations that occur early in the disease. It measures airflow over time from fully inflated lungs. Although spirometry testing is sensitive in the identification of airflow obstruction, it does not identify the cause.

FVC is the entire exhaled breath; FEV_1 is the amount of air exhaled in the first second. Normally the FEV_1/FVC ratio is 70%. In COPD both of these measurements are reduced. Up to 30% of patients have an increase in FEV_1 following inhalation of a bronchodilator. Lung volumes (TLC, FRC, RV) are usually within normal limits until later in the course of the disease, when the lung volumes may be increased. There usually is no loss of diffusing capacity.

The Third National Health and Nutrition Examination Survey (NHANES III)[59] indicated a high prevalence of undiagnosed COPD. As a result, use of office spirometry to screen at-risk patients before symptoms appear and early intervention to preserve pulmonary function are recommended. This NHANES III recommendation for screening as a part of primary care has not, as yet, been fully embraced by clinicians because of concern about the cost of screening devices.

Chest X-Ray Films. Chest x-ray films of patients with COPD typically demonstrate a low, flat diaphragm, increased AP diameter of the thorax, and overdistention of the lungs. Bullae may be present, and patients with chronic bronchitis may have increased bronchovascular markings.

Arterial Blood Gas Studies. In the early stage of COPD, ABG studies show mild or moderate hypoxemia without hypercapnia. In the later stages there is more severe hypoxemia and hypercapnia, and values may worsen during exacerbations and during exercise and sleep.

Sputum and Hematology Studies. Sputum studies for Gram stain, culture, and sensitivity are done. The most frequent pathogens cultured are *S. pneumoniae* and *H. influenzae.* Neutrophils and bronchial epithelial cells usually are found in chronic bronchitis. On complete blood count, erythrocytosis is frequently seen as Pa_{O_2} levels fall below 55 mm Hg. AAT assay also may be done.

Effective health care management programs for persons who have COPD require a multidisciplinary approach. Management programs should be designed to prevent premature morbidity and mortality from COPD, educate patients and families, minimize airflow limitation and retard its progression, correct secondary physiologic problems, and optimize functional capabilities. A comprehensive management program benefits all patients, even those with severe disease.

Medications. The judicious use of appropriate medications in a stepwise approach is the recommended treatment strategy, with the goals of improving airflow and providing significant symptomatic relief.[23] Medications have yet to impact COPD mortality, so the focus is on improved morbidity outcomes.

Bronchoactive Medications. COPD is not completely reversible, but most patients experience some improvement in dyspnea with the inhalation of bronchodilating and antiinflammatory medications.

Anticholinergic Agents. Multiple cholinergic receptors are present in the lung. They stimulate muscle contraction and mucous gland secretion. Acute anticholinergic medication use in patients with COPD produces equal or greater bronchodilation than beta-agonists.[18] Long-term anticholinergic use provides sustainable effects. Anticholinergic agents are considered as first-line therapy for COPD.

Ipratropium (Atrovert) is currently the only anticholinergic available in the United States that is administered in an MDI. The usual dose is 2 puffs four times daily, but the dose may be increased to 3 to 4 puffs or more four times per day. Ipratropium is well tolerated. Some patients have a cough and dry mouth, which are side effects of anticholinergic agents.

Beta-Agonists. Inhaled $beta_2$-agonists are the second choice of therapy for COPD management. Beta-agonists have been shown to produce bronchodilation and improve hyperinflation, dyspnea, exercise capacity, and quality of life in patients with COPD. In addition to short-acting beta-agonists (albuterol, metaproterenol, pirbuterol), a long-acting agent, salmeterol, is now available in the United States. Beta-agonists may be delivered by inhaled, oral, subcutaneous, or IV routes. The preferred route is by inhalation to minimize side effects. Table 21-11 lists the commonly prescribed adrenergic agents that work at $beta_2$ sites located in smooth muscles of the airways.

Methylxanthines. Methylxanthines such as theophylline and caffeine have been used to treat patients with respiratory problems for decades. Theophyllines are known to increase respiratory muscle strength and prevent respiratory muscle fatigue. They are also mildly antiinflammatory and mitigate some lymphocyte responses. However, the role of theophylline in COPD management has been questioned, and use has fallen significantly. Theophylline has a narrow therapeutic range, interacts with numerous drugs, and is only a mild bronchodilator. Administering long-acting theophylline in the evening has been shown to reduce overnight decline in FEV_1 and morning respiratory symptoms. Current dosing recommendations include serum theophylline levels of 5 to 12 mg/L.[59] Close monitoring for side effects and toxicity is required. Seizures and arrhythmias remain high-risk complications. The more common side effects include tremor and GI distress.

Combination Therapy. Combinations of anticholinergics and beta-agonists have been shown to be of added benefit in patients with stable COPD. Combination therapy may be achieved with the use of separate MDIs, a single MDI with the two medications combined, or nebulizer delivery of medications. The addition of theophylline to this regimen appears to increase symptomatic relief.

Corticosteroids. More than 50% of patients with COPD are currently using inhaled steroids.[23] However, the use of corticosteroids in COPD is controversial. During acute exacerbations corticosteroids can improve patient symptoms and reduce the patient's hospital stay. Steroids may also reduce the incidence of relapses after acute exacerbations in patients with a history of frequent exacerbations, and regular use of inhaled steroids may improve quality of life and decrease exacerbations in patients with severe disease. Thus some COPD patients benefit from chronic steroid use, but it may require 6 months of use of inhaled steroids for these patients to be identified. Only 10% to 20% of COPD patients are steroid responders. Long-term treatment with oral corticosteroids should be prescribed only for patients who have documented improvement in airflow or exercise performance. When corticosteroids are used, every attempt should be made to keep the dose at the minimum level to achieve desired outcomes.

Mucolytics. Mucus hypersecretion is a risk factor for more rapid disease progression. It increases the likelihood for hospitalization and symptomatic limitations. Unfortunately, there is little evidence that currently available mucokinetic agents reduce mucus production or enhance the elimination of mucus in patients with COPD.

Antibiotics. Chronic or prophylactic antibiotics are not routinely recommended as part of the regular care of patients with COPD. In the presence of purulent sputum in conjunction with increasing sputum or dyspnea, antibiotics can shorten the course of acute exacerbations that involve purulent sputum in association with increased sputum production

TABLE 21-11 $Beta_2$-Agonists and Their Dosages for Metered-Dose Inhalers and Nebulized Solutions

Drug	Dose	mg/Puff	Nebulization
Albuterol (Proventil, Ventolin)	2-3 puffs q4-6h	0.09	0.3-0.5 ml 0.5% solution in 3 ml saline q4-6h
Bitolterol (Tornalate)	2-3 puffs q6-8h	0.37	
Metaproterenol (Alupent, Metaprel)	2-3 puffs q4-6h	0.65	0.3 ml 5% solution in 2.5 ml saline q4-6h
Pirbuterol (Maxair)	2-3 puffs q4-6h	0.20	
Salmeterol (Serevert)	2 puffs q12h	0.50	
Terbutaline (Brethaire)	2-3 puffs q4-6h	0.20	

or dyspnea. Lower-cost broad-spectrum antibiotics are preferred.

Alpha$_1$-Antitrypsin. Regular replacement of AAT in patients with deficiency may prevent the protease-antiprotease imbalance that damages the lungs of these patients. Although definitive proof of long-term benefits of AAT replacement therapy is still lacking, a growing body of evidence suggests that patients who are AAT deficient and receive replacement therapy have a slower rate of lung destruction as measured by spirometry and a chest CT scan. It may also reduce mortality.[5] IV infusion of AAT can be given on a weekly or biweekly basis but is most commonly administered on a monthly basis. Newer modes of delivery such as inhalation are under investigation.

Antidepressant and Antianxiety Medications. Depression is frequently unrecognized in patients with COPD and may manifest as insomnia or anxiety. Multiple medications can successfully treat depressed patients with COPD; however, serotonin selective reuptake inhibitors (SSRIs) are the most commonly prescribed.

Anxiety is also common in COPD patients, with panic attacks occurring in a significant number of these patients. SSRI medications, which provide effective therapy and relative patient safety, are the primary medications used to treat anxiety in patients with COPD. Buspirone is an example of an anxiolytic that does not have respiratory depressant effects. However, it has only mild antianxiety effects and may not be adequate.

Treatments

Smoking Cessation. Smoking cessation is essential to slow the rate of decline in pulmonary function in all patients with COPD, regardless of age.

Smoking cessation at any age is a challenge, but it is extremely difficult for older patients who have been smoking for years. Relapse rates are high among those who try to stop smoking. For each attempt, relapse rates approach 70% at 3 months and exceed 90% at 1 year.[45] The older adult may have tried many interventions, may have made multiple attempts to quit, and may have high expectations for failure. Older adults, however, are more likely to value advice from their physicians and health care providers and therefore more seriously contemplate smoking cessation. Some intervention studies have shown positive results from regular, brief calls and letters of encouragement from health care professionals. Counseling alone has been shown to result in a 3% to 5% sustained quit rate.[59] When using nicotine replacement strategies, older patients need to be monitored closely for signs of nicotine excess (nausea, tachycardia, dizziness). A lower dose may need to be prescribed.

Oxygen Therapy. Administration of supplemental oxygen is the only therapy proven to alter the course of advanced stages of COPD.

Hypoxemia in patients with COPD adversely affects patient mortality and function. Oxygen therapy is required for patients with COPD who are unable to maintain a Pao_2 greater than 55 mm Hg or an oxygen saturation greater than 85% or more at rest and for those who cannot carry out ADLs (breathing, eating, dressing, toileting) without becoming very short of breath. In these patients 1 to 2 L/min of oxygen is usually given via nasal prongs to relieve hypoxemia and decrease pulmonary hypertension, which in turn decreases the load on the right side of the heart. The goal of oxygen therapy is to provide oxygen to patients at rates sufficient to maintain oxygen saturations above 90% as close to 24 hours per day as possible. Studies have shown that patients receive the most benefit from oxygen therapy if the oxygen is used continuously. Detailed oxygen assessment at rest and with activity is recommended for all patients with moderate to severe COPD. Patients with COPD with adequate resting daytime oxygen levels may have significant hypoxemia during activity or at night. Oxygen supplementation during activity or at night can improve performance, quality of life, and sleep. It also may improve survival, especially if cor pulmonale or cardiac arrhythmias are present. Ambulatory oxygen is preferable to oxygen from stationary sources because it allows patients to exercise and improve cardiac output, thus improving tissue oxygenation.[59]

A common misunderstanding expressed by patients requiring ongoing oxygen therapy is that they should use their oxygen only when they are symptomatic (i.e., short of breath) to avoid becoming habituated to the oxygen and thus requiring higher levels of oxygen. The nurse needs to clarify that habituation to oxygen will not occur. The nurse also stresses the importance of continual oxygen use in order to receive maximal benefits of the therapy.

Because many patients with COPD have chronic carbon dioxide retention, their stimulus to breathe is their low Pao_2 level. Patients must understand that high flow rates of oxygen (greater than 6 L/min) and high concentrations (greater than 40%) may elevate their Pao_2 to a level that removes the stimulus by which they breathe, resulting in respiratory failure. Long-term oxygen therapy has been shown to be of substantial benefit in the management of patients with advanced COPD and chronic hypoxemia. Before discharge from the hospital, ABG and oxygen saturation levels at rest, with exercise, and during sleep need to be determined to evaluate the need for home use of oxygen. The Centers for Medicare and Medicaid Services (CMS), formerly called the Health Care Financing Administration (HCFA) funds Medicare and has established very specific criteria for reimbursement. Medicare coverage of home oxygen and oxygen equipment falls under the durable medical equipment (DME) benefit. Home oxygen therapy is considered reasonable and necessary only for patients with significant hypoxemia who meet the criteria related to medical documentation, laboratory evidence, and specified health conditions. Required medical documentation includes a diagnosis of the disease requiring home use of oxygen, the oxygen flow rate, and an estimate of the frequency, duration of use (e.g., 2 L/min, 10 minutes/hr, 12 hours/day), and duration of need (e.g., 6 months, lifetime). The required laboratory evidence includes the results of a blood gas study ordered and evaluated by a physician within 2 days of discharge. Covered blood gas values include:

- PaO_2 of 55 mm Hg or less or oxygen saturation of 88% or less taken on room air at rest
- PaO_2 of 55 mm Hg or less or oxygen saturation of 88% or less during exercise
- PaO_2 between 56 and 59 mm Hg or oxygen saturation of 88% or less in the presence of heart failure, pulmonary hypertension, cor pulmonale, or hematocrit more than 56%

Covered health conditions include severe lung disease (COPD, interstitial lung disease, cystic fibrosis, lung cancer), hypoxia-related symptoms or findings that might be expected to improve with oxygen therapy (pulmonary hypertension, heart failure due to cor pulmonale, erythrocytosis, impairment of cognitive processes, nocturnal restlessness, morning headaches).[33] Home oxygen accounts for about 45% of the total cost of DME.[58] Medical supply companies bring the oxygen to the home and show the patient and caregivers how to use it. They also check the equipment regularly. Oxygen for home use is available in three forms: liquid, tank, or oxygen concentrator. Either a mask or nasal cannula is used for home oxygen therapy. Oxygen concentrators are the most widely used stationary oxygen delivery system. Concentrators are fairly quiet, efficient, and low maintenance. The cost of electricity to operate these units is not reimbursable, and oxygen concentrators are inoperable during an electrical power failure. Liquid oxygen is stored in large, insulated canisters of 60 to 120 pounds as a stationary source of oxygen delivery in the home. The reservoir units must be refilled frequently, and even though liquid oxygen is relatively inexpensive, the cost of supplying liquid oxygen can be substantial, particularly in rural or remote areas.

Portable oxygen systems that weigh more than 10 pounds are mounted on wheels and allow for some mobility but are difficult to maneuver. Portable oxygen concentrators that can be operated from either a 12-volt battery or conventional AC electrical outlet are useful for travel. Ambulatory liquid oxygen systems that can be refilled in the home have vastly improved patient mobility and satisfaction. Technology advances continue to develop lighter-weight and longer-lasting units.

Oxygen-conserving devices reduce the cost of home oxygen therapy by reducing the frequency of renewing the supply of liquid or gaseous oxygen. Oxygen-conserving devices use a mechanical reservoir or an anatomic reservoir that fills with 100% oxygen during exhalation and empties the oxygen into the lungs early in inspiration. Mechanical reservoirs include a nasal reservoir cannula and a pendant reservoir cannula. Both empty on inspiration and fill during exhalation. In both systems the effective bolus of 100% oxygen is about 20 ml. The cannula is more visible, but the pendant is less comfortable.

Another system for oxygen conservation is the pulsation of a bolus of oxygen during the first one fourth to one half of inspiration, with which virtually all of the oxygen delivered goes to the oxygen-exchanging areas of the lung with minimal distribution to anatomic dead space. There are multiple manufacturers of these units, and each functions differently. Most are battery powered. The quantity of oxygen in each pulse may be variable or fixed, and the pulse may occur with each breath or have a variable frequency based on the flow setting. Patient acceptance has been excellent. All oxygen-conserving devices provide 50% or more oxygen savings at rest, but the degree of conservation may vary substantially during exercise.[58]

Another mode of oxygen delivery that may be used with COPD patients is transtracheal oxygen (TTO) delivery. TTO involves the insertion of a catheter percutaneously between the second and third tracheal interspaces; this is held in place by a necklace and transparent film dressing. Oxygen enters the trachea via this catheter, thus significantly reducing oxygen delivery to airway dead space. Patients have been reported to use 37% to 58% less oxygen during TTO delivery, compared with continuous-flow nasal oxygen. In all patients receiving TTO, it is standard practice to titrate the dose of oxygen to ensure adequate oxyhemoglobin saturation, both at rest and during exercise. Not all patients are candidates for TTO. The ideal candidate has a strong desire to remain active, is willing to follow the care protocol, is not experiencing frequent exacerbations, has a caregiver who is willing to assist with problem solving and details of care, and has access to good medical follow-up. Relative contraindications to TTO include high-dose steroids and conditions that predispose to delayed healing (diabetes, connective tissue disease, severe obesity). Absolute contraindications include subglottic stenosis or vocal cord paralysis, herniation of the pleura into the insertion site, severe coagulopathy, uncompensated respiratory acidosis, and inability to practice self-care. Complications of TTO include catheter displacement, bacterial cellulitis, subcutaneous emphysema, hemoptysis, a severed catheter, and mucous balls that can result in acute respiratory distress and, in some cases, acute respiratory failure (see Future Watch box).[63]

Aerosol Therapy. Aerosol therapy is one of the most effective ways to deliver bronchoactive medications with minimal

Future Watch
Options for Long-Term Oxygen Therapy

Long-term oxygen therapy (LTOT) has been a treatment option for patients with chronic hypoxemia for decades. Health care providers and medical suppliers have tried to match appropriately the prescription of the oxygen system to the physical and psychosocial needs of the person requiring LTOT. Because of the magnitude of use of home oxygen and its costs, the Centers for Medicare and Medicaid Services (CMS), formerly called the Health Care Financing Administration (HCFA), has concerns about the level of payment and possible abuse of this therapy. Changes in reimbursement policies have resulted in significantly decreased reimbursement to durable medical equipment (DME) vendors. One result of this has been that more expensive oxygen systems that enhance mobility are not made available to patients. Various organizations, including the Respiratory Nursing Society, have taken positions in support of persons needing LTOT to receive the services and oxygen system that best facilitate their mobility and activity within their developmental and functional capabilities, resulting in enhanced quality of life.

Reference: Respiratory Nursing Society: Position statement: long-term oxygen therapy, *Heart Lung* 28(2):143-144, 1999.

side effects. Directions for teaching patients to use an inhaler with a spacer are described in the Patient Teaching box.

Vaccination. Pneumococcal vaccination is recommended for all patients with COPD. All COPD patients are recommended to receive influenza vaccination on a yearly basis.

Surgical Management

Lung Transplantation. COPD is the most frequent indication for lung transplantation. The survival rate following transplantation for emphysema is the highest of any patient population with lung disease.[19] There is still debate as to when a transplant should be offered. Generally it is considered an option for those patients under age 65 with an FEV_1 below 30% of predicted, without evidence of pulmonary hypertension, and with consideration given to the patient's functional status and quality of life, assessed after pulmonary rehabilitation. Single-lung transplantation is done more often, since it is less rigorous for older and more tenuous patients. Infection is the most significant complication. Five-year survival is less than 50%, but quality-of-life scores have shown significant improvement following a lung transplant.[19]

Lung Volume Reduction Surgery. Lung volume reduction surgery (LVRS) is a surgical procedure for patients with severe emphysema. The hyperinflated portion of the lung or lungs is removed so that the patient's chest wall and diaphragm can return to normal positions, thereby easing breathing. Most often it is used as a bridge to transplantation that improves respiratory function for patients during the prolonged waiting time for donor organs.

Patient eligibility criteria for LVRS include:

- Severe limitation of pulmonary function, with FEV_1 less than 30% predicted, FVC less than 60%, and TLC greater than 8 L
- Impaired ADLs
- Maximally flattened diaphragm documented on chest x-ray examination
- No effective response to medical management
- Completion of 6 to 12 weeks of pulmonary rehabilitation
- Successful smoking cessation for at least 6 months

There are a number of surgical approaches used, with the most common being median sternotomy and bilateral stapling resection. Regardless of the approach, the goal is to reduce lung volume by approximately 25%.[53] The procedure involves deflating one lung by clamping one side of the bifurcated double-lumen endotracheal tube. Normal lung tissue turns gray, but the hyperinflated section of the lung remains pink from trapped air. The hyperinflated area is excised. The patient's chest cavity is then filled with saline to inspect for air leaks. If none are detected, the procedure is repeated on the opposite lung. After surgery one or two chest tubes are placed and connected to a water-seal drainage system. No suction is used unless an air leak develops. Postoperative emphasis is on monitoring of ABGs, early ambulation, and management of pain, usually with an epidural catheter.[66]

Researchers continue to examine outcomes of this new intervention. To date, most studies demonstrate improvement in pulmonary function, decreased dyspnea, and enhanced exercise capacity. There is some indication that these improvements may wane 36 months following surgery.[26] Other studies looking at LVRS and lung transplantation indicate that LVRS improves lung function beyond what is possible with pulmonary rehabilitation[13] and does not appear to jeopardize the chances for subsequent successful transplantation.[51] Of note, these studies also indicate that patients with emphysema are opting for surgical intervention, when possible, even with its increased risks, rather than continued medical management.

Diet. Improving nutrition is an important goal. (See discussion under Interventions.)

Activity. Patients should be up and about as much as possible. Some will have to use portable oxygen while walking or doing other tasks.

Referrals. Common referrals for the patient with COPD include respiratory therapy, physical therapy, dietary therapy, and social work. Hospice is considered also for its palliative care. COPD is a progressive and ultimately fatal disease. Palliative care should be the focus when physical or psychologic suffering becomes central. The provision of palliative care is not limited by the site of care (home, hospital, acute care, intensive care). The national hospice organization suggests the following criteria for patients with noncancerous conditions: disabling dyspnea at rest with progressive pulmonary disease, cor pulmonale, hypoxemia at rest ($Pa{O_2}$ less than 55 mm Hg or oxygen saturation less than 88) or hypercapnia ($Pa{CO_2}$ greater than 50 mm Hg), unintentional progressive loss of 10% of body weight in 6 months, or resting tachycardia (more than 100 beats/min).[24]

Patient Teaching
Using an Inhaler With a Spacer

1. Exhale fully.
2. Position nebulizer in mouth *without* sealing lips around it.
3. Take a deep breath while releasing a puff of medication into spacer.
4. Hold breath for 3 to 4 seconds at full inspiration.
5. Exhale slowly through pursed lips.
6. Take prescribed number of puffs–usually one or two.
7. Take number of breaths necessary to receive the entire prescribed dose from the spacer.
8. Rinse mouth after completing treatment.
9. Wash inhaler and spacer with warm soapy water, rinse, and dry thoroughly after each use.

NURSING MANAGEMENT OF PATIENT WITH CHRONIC OBSTRUCTIVE PULMONARY DISEASE

ASSESSMENT

Health History

Data to be collected to assess the patient with COPD include:

History, character, onset, and duration of symptoms

Dyspnea, including its effects on ADLs and whether it is associated with any specific illness or event

Cough
Sputum production (amount, color, consistency)
Pain in right upper quadrant (hepatomegaly)
Smoking history
Family history of COPD, respiratory illnesses
Disease history, especially influenza, pneumonia
History of respiratory tract infections, chronic sinusitis
Past or present exposure to environmental irritants at home or at work
Self-care modalities used to treat symptoms
Current pattern of activity and rest
Medications taken and their effectiveness in relieving symptoms

Physical Examination

Important aspects of the physical examination of the patient with COPD include:

Assessment of general appearance. Appearance and hygiene may be an indicator of symptom interference with ADLs. Patient may appear underweight, overweight, or bloated, and skin color may be dusky or pale.

Observation of the chest for an increased AP diameter ("barrel chest").

Checking for dependent edema and jugular vein distention.

Assessment of the abdomen for signs of hepatomegaly.

Measurement of vital signs to identify elevated temperature, tachycardia, tachypnea, or other abnormality.

Pulmonary examination, which includes inspection for use of accessory muscles of breathing, forward-leaning (tripod) posture, pursed-lip breathing, central cyanosis, clubbing of fingers, and signs of an altered sensorium (restlessness or lethargy), which may be the first indicator of hypoxia. Pulmonary examination also includes auscultation of breath sounds, which may be distant as a result of increased AP diameter and decreased airflow. Crackles (rales) are likely, especially in dependent lung fields, as are rhonchi (gurgles) and wheezes, especially on forced exhalation.

Relevant laboratory findings include an elevated hemoglobin, hematocrit, and WBC count and alterations in arterial bleed gases. PFTs typically report decreased FEV_1, decreased VC, normal diffusing capacity, and normal to increased lung volumes (TLC, FRC, RV).

NURSING DIAGNOSES

Nursing diagnoses are determined from assessment of patient data. Nursing diagnoses for the person with chronic bronchitis may include but are not limited to:

Diagnostic Title	Possible Etiologic Factors
1. Impaired gas exchange	Altered oxygen delivery and alveoli destruction
2. Ineffective airway clearance	Bronchospasm, hypersecretion, tracheobronchial infection, decreased energy/fatigue
3. Ineffective breathing pattern	Decreased energy/fatigue, airway changes
4. Activity intolerance	Imbalance between oxygen demand and requirement
5. Imbalanced nutrition: less than body requirements	Dyspnea, anorexia, sputum production, fatigue
6. Risk for infection	Decreased lung defenses, increased mucus production
7. Ineffective coping (individual)	Long-term illness and disability, change in role functioning

EXPECTED PATIENT OUTCOMES

Expected patient outcomes for the patient with COPD may include but are not limited to:

1. Will demonstrate improved ventilation and oxygenation
1a. Arterial blood PaO_2, $PaCO_2$, and pH will return to patient's baseline
1b. Will explain how and when to use oxygen therapy
2. Will demonstrate adequate airway clearance
2a. Will use effective methods of coughing
2b. Will appropriately use bronchoactive medications, including MDIs, DPIs, nebulizers, and humidifiers
3. Will demonstrate effective breathing pattern
3a. Inspiratory-expiratory ratio will be 5 : 10 seconds
3b. Will use controlled breathing techniques (pursed-lip breathing) (see Figure 21-14), forward-leaning postures (Figure 21-16), and diaphragmatic breathing (abdominal muscle breathing [Figure 21-17])
3c. Will exhale with exertion
3d. Respiratory rate will be within near-normal limits, with moderate tidal volume
4. Will maintain or work toward an optimal activity level
4a. Will pace activities
4b. Will plan for simplification of activities
4c. Will participate in planned muscle-conditioning program
4d. Will demonstrate how to carry out the exercise program to be followed at home, including specific exercises to be completed, frequency of each exercise, and criteria for monitoring physical response to exercises, such as heart rate increase, perceived fatigue
5. Will explain dietary changes required after discharge
5a. Will maintain optimal weight for height, age, and gender
5b. Will explain food and fluid requirements and daily plan for achieving them
5c. Will list specific foods to be avoided
5d. Will explain plan for frequent, small feedings that are easily chewable, allowing increased time for eating, and use of supplemental oxygen as indicated
6. Will remain infection free
6a. Temperature will remain normal
6b. Sputum will return to baseline in color, amount, and consistency
6c. Will inform health care provider if signs of infection occur

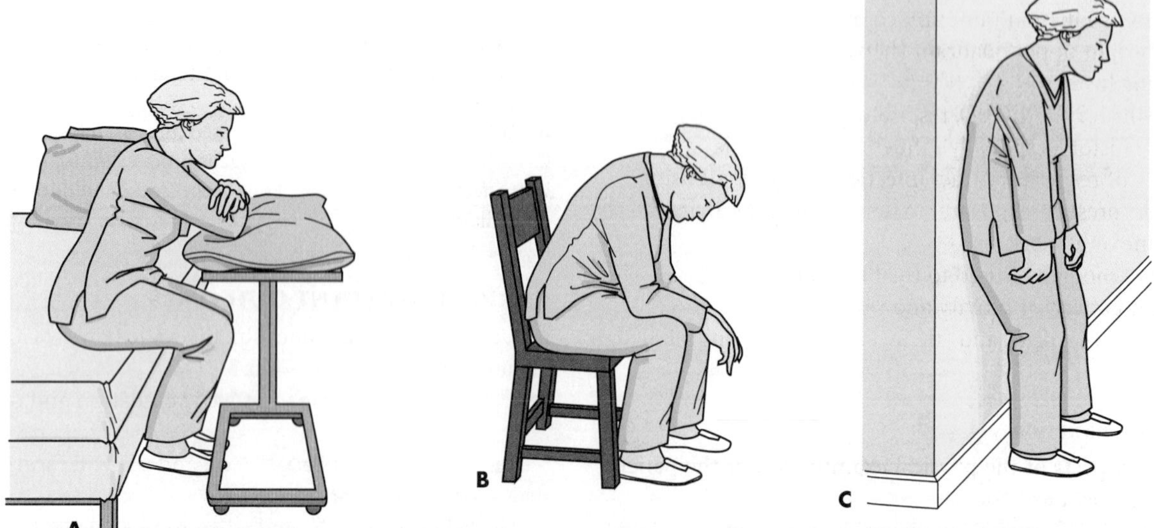

Figure 21-16 Forward-leaning position. **A**, The patient sits on the edge of the bed with arms folded on a pillow placed on the elevated bedside table. **B**, Patient in three-point position. The patient sits in a chair with the feet approximately 1 foot. apart and leans forward with elbows on knees. **C**, The patient leans against a wall with feet spread apart, allowing shoulders to sag forward with arms relaxed.

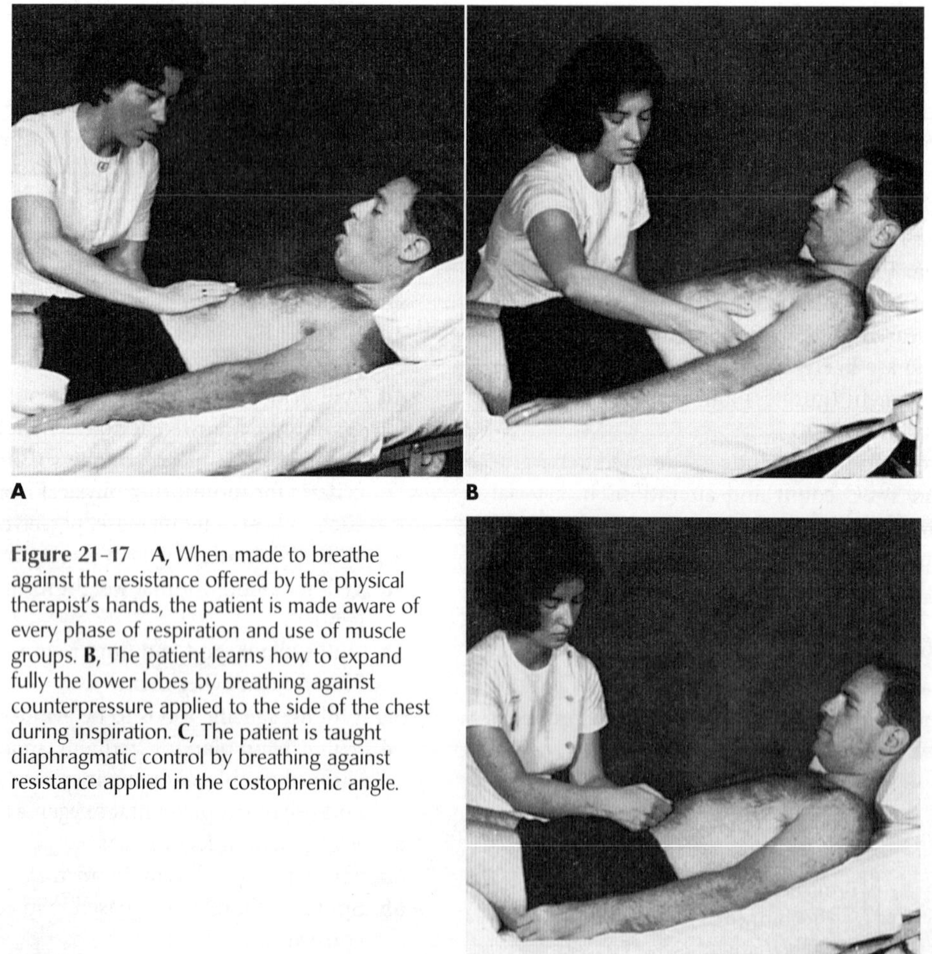

Figure 21-17 **A**, When made to breathe against the resistance offered by the physical therapist's hands, the patient is made aware of every phase of respiration and use of muscle groups. **B**, The patient learns how to expand fully the lower lobes by breathing against counterpressure applied to the side of the chest during inspiration. **C**, The patient is taught diaphragmatic control by breathing against resistance applied in the costophrenic angle.

7. Will identify own coping mechanisms, both effective and ineffective
7a. Will identify stressors, threats to role
7b. Will use effective coping mechanisms (discussion with family, health care providers)
7c. Will set realistic personal goals
7d. Will participate in ADLs and therapeutic regimens
7e. Will list names and telephone numbers of appropriate community support services, such as home health provider, Visiting Nurse Association, home medical equipment supplier

INTERVENTIONS

Pulmonary rehabilitation attempts to return patients to their highest possible functional capacity. The rehabilitative approach to the care of COPD patients has been shown to result in improved independence and quality of life, decreased hospital days, and improved exercise capacity. Lung function is usually not improved.[12] Pulmonary health care teams consist of physicians, nurses, respiratory therapists, occupational therapists, physical therapists, dietitians, social workers, and psychologists or psychiatrists. The complex multidisciplinary rehabilitation team is the ideal, but the nurse functioning in a small community hospital or community health agency can provide effective rehabilitation activities for the person with COPD.

1. Improving Gas Exchange

ABGs are monitored for indications of hypoxemia, respiratory acidosis, and respiratory alkalosis. Hypoxemia and hypercapnia often occur simultaneously, and the signs and symptoms of each are similar. These include headache, irritability, confusion, increasing somnolence, asterixis (flapping tremors of extremities), cardiac dysrhythmias, and tachycardia. Morning headache is a frequent sign of hypercapnia. If hypocapnia is developing, tachypnea, vertigo, tingling of the extremities, muscular weakness, and spasm are often present. The presence of signs and symptoms associated with altered levels of PaO_2 and $PaCO_2$ depend more on the rate of change than on the degree of change in the levels. Rapidly changing signs usually indicate a rapid worsening of the patient's condition. At the same time, patients with long-standing hypoxemia and hypercapnia may be relatively asymptomatic because they have physiologically accommodated to increased levels of $PaCO_2$ and decreased levels of PaO_2.

Oxygen Therapy

The nurse is in a key role to assess the need for supplemental oxygen, to assess the response to therapy and acceptance of therapy, and to ensure that criteria for home oxygen therapy are met. Patient and family education about oxygen therapy is essential. It is important that the patient and family know the following points:

- Oxygen is to be delivered at the prescribed flow rate. Adjustments need to be discussed with the health care provider.
- Oxygen is drying to the membranes of the nose. Applying a water-soluble lubricant (K-Y jelly) to the inside of the nose may reduce dryness and cracking. Petroleum jelly (Vaseline) should not be used because it may be inhaled.
- If humidification is used, the amount of water in the humidifier bottle must be checked every 6 to 8 hours and refilled as needed with sterile or distilled water.
- A new supply of oxygen must be ordered when the oxygen source reads one-quarter full.
- Safety precautions must always be observed. Oxygen is not flammable itself, but it supports combustion. No one should smoke in the room where oxygen is being used; patients using oxygen should stay away from gas stoves, gas space heaters, or kerosene heaters or lamps; the container should always be kept upright to prevent leakage; and an all-purpose fire extinguisher should be readily available in the home.
- The health care provider should be notified if breathing is more difficult or if restlessness, anxiety, tiredness, drowsiness, difficulty waking up, persistent headache, slurred speech, confusion, or cyanosis of the fingernails or lips occurs.

2. Improving Airway Clearance

Clearing of the airways is of utmost importance in meeting tissue demands for increased oxygen during periods of rest and periods of increased activity.

Effective coughing maneuvers must be taught. Patients should sit upright and use the huff coughing technique described earlier.

To thin secretions, a fluid intake of 3 to 4 L has traditionally been encouraged unless contraindicated. However, evidence suggests that this quantity of fluids may not be needed to keep secretions mobile. Although expectorants are sometimes prescribed, some experts believe they do more harm than good. Water is still considered the best expectorant, and adequate hydration without fluid overload should be encouraged.

Pulmonary physiotherapy techniques may be helpful to some patients with COPD, but many are not able to tolerate this intervention because of hypoxemia, age, debilitation, and other factors. (These techniques are discussed under Cystic Fibrosis.)

3. Improving Efficiency of Breathing

Controlled breathing techniques include pursed-lip breathing, the forward-leaning position, and abdominal breathing. The benefits of these methods include control of dyspnea and anxiety. The goal is a reduced respiratory rate and enhanced expiratory tidal volume, thus decreasing air trapping.

Pursed-lip breathing has been shown to decrease dyspnea when it is used with activities that produce tachypnea, which leads to progressive air trapping. Pursed lip breathing decreases the respiratory rate, increases tidal volume, decreases $PaCO_2$, and increases PaO_2 and SaO_2. Some patients use pursed-lip breathing intuitively, and others need to be taught. It is taught by asking the patient to (1) inhale through the nose for several seconds with the mouth closed and (2) exhale slowly (taking twice as long as inhalation) through pursed lips held in a narrow slit. One method of teaching this technique is by using a child's soap bubble wand and blowing one big soap bubble. Benefits of this approach are that it combines an enjoyable activity with a measurable means of visualizing a pursed-lip exhalation, provides immediate patient feedback, and promotes relaxation of the patient's upper body and decreased use of accessory breathing.[14]

Use of the forward-leaning (tripod) position for exhalation is also taught. A forward-leaning position of 30 to 40 degrees with the head tilted at a 16- to 18-degree angle effectively improves exhalation (see Figure 21-16). As mentioned earlier, patients with emphysema have increased TLC and RV with the diaphragm in a fixed, flattened position. Therefore the diaphragm cannot assist in exhalation as it does normally. Leaning forward allows more air to be removed from the lungs on exhalation. The forward-leaning position can be achieved with the patient in either a sitting or standing position. The patient can sit on the edge of the bed or a chair and lean forward on two or three pillows placed on a table or overbed stand, or sit in a chair with the legs spread apart shoulder width (or wider, if the patient is obese) with the elbows on the knees and the arms and hands relaxed, or stand with the back and hips against the wall with the feet spread apart and about 12 inches (30 cm) from the wall. The patient then relaxes and leans forward. In these positions the patient cannot use the accessory muscles of respiration, and the upward action of the diaphragm is improved.

Abdominal breathing improves the breathing efficiency of persons with COPD because it assists the patient in elevating the diaphragm. Abdominal breathing can be done in the sitting or lying position. In the sitting position, the patient sits on the side of the bed or in a chair and holds a small pillow or a book against the abdomen. The patient then exhales slowly while leaning forward and pressing the pillow or book against the abdomen. In the lying position, the patient's hand is placed on the abdomen and the patient is asked to "puff out" the abdomen and raise the hand as high as possible. The patient then exhales slowly through pursed lips while pulling in on the abdominal muscles. Manual pressure on the upper abdomen during expiration facilitates this maneuver (see Figure 21-17). In addition to abdominal breathing, exercises to strengthen the abdominal muscles help patients use their abdominal muscles more effectively in emptying their lungs. This controlled breathing pattern is to be used while performing various ADLs, from sitting, standing, walking, and climbing stairs to more complex activities. As this pattern becomes natural, the patient uses it automatically during periods of increased shortness of breath.

Environment plays a significant role in ease of breathing. Humidity of 30% to 50% is ideal and can be achieved by a humidifier as necessary. An air conditioner may reduce dyspnea by controlling the temperature and preventing entrance of pollutants from outside air. The cost of an air conditioner is a medically deductible expense for persons with COPD. The movement of cool air with a fan has also been shown to reduce dyspnea. This may result from the stimulation of receptors on the face or decreased temperature of facial skin. Wearing a scarf over the nose and mouth in cold weather helps warm the air and prevent bronchospasm. Masks for this purpose are also available. Smoking cessation is essential, as is minimal exposure to air pollution and the avoidance of environmental tobacco smoke.

4. Improving Activity Tolerance

Exercise conditioning is the single most important aspect of rehabilitation and has been repeatedly shown to improve exercise capacity and endurance in COPD patients.[67] Patients should undertake both general exercises and specific muscle training.

For general exercise conditioning, graded leg exercises performed by stationary cycling, stair climbing, and walking are safe and well tolerated. Oxygen during exercise is recommended for patients who both have significant exercise desaturation and show improved exercise tolerance while using oxygen.

Leg-raising exercises, with each leg being raised alternately as the patient exhales, is one way to strengthen abdominal muscles. Another way is to have the patient raise the head and shoulders from the bed while he or she exhales. With practice and encouragement, the patient can do the exercises 10 times each morning and evening after clearing the lungs of secretions as completely as possible.

The term *muscle reconditioning* refers to a variety of muscle-toning exercises. For patients who are able to be out of bed, walking, using a treadmill, or riding a stationary bicycle is helpful. The exercise period is started slowly, with 10 minutes twice daily three times a week, increasing to 20 minutes twice daily three times a week. The patient needs to be assessed for his or her ability to carry out such an exercise program, and a staff member should be present during the exercise period.

Patients need to be encouraged not to rush (i.e., to allow ample time for activities). Supplemental oxygen may be needed before and during activities. Activities such as walking should be gradually increased. Positive feedback on progress should be provided, and new endeavors encouraged when the patient is ready. Patients should be assisted in balancing work, rest, and recreation to regulate energy expenditure.

5. Improving Nutrition

Persons with COPD, particularly those with a predominance of emphysema, often demonstrate excessive weight loss. The weight loss is mainly caused by a 15% to 25% increase in resting energy expenditure secondary to increased work of breathing. Other contributing factors are the feeling of satiety that occurs with small amounts of food because the flattened diaphragm compresses abdominal contents; dyspnea, which interferes with eating; and the gastric irritation that is associated with the use of bronchodilators and steroids. Diminished total weight is correlated with a dramatic decrease in size and strength of respiratory muscle (especially the diaphragm).

To help the patient with COPD maintain adequate nutrition, the nurse explores the patient's and family's usual dietary habits and counsels the patient to select foods that provide a high-protein, high-calorie diet. It is important to counsel the patient to select foods that provide higher calorie levels through higher fat content rather than high carbohydrate levels. Persons with advanced chronic bronchitis or emphysema are unable to exhale the excess carbon dioxide that is a natural end product of carbohydrate metabolism. Therefore calories obtained from high-carbohydrate foods may elevate $PaCO_2$ levels in persons with COPD. The patient is also advised to take supplemental vitamins and to take prepackaged food supplements such as milk shakes or snack bars between meals because they are an excellent source of protein and calories. The patient is taught that smaller, more frequent meals are often tolerated better than three larger meals. Larger meals require more energy to digest and limit the downward movement of the diaphragm during inspiration. Patients are encouraged to select foods that are easy to chew and swallow to further conserve energy.

6. Preventing Infection

The most common complication of COPD, and the cause of most hospital readmissions, is respiratory infection. Pulmonary response to the infectious process includes increased respiratory rate, mucosal irritation, and increased mucus production. Because of these localized responses, patients may have bronchospasm and a change in their pattern of sputum production. If the infection remains untreated, the result is overall increased work of breathing with eventual respiratory failure. Thus the person with COPD should be instructed in measures to decrease the risk of respiratory infections. Instructions to be given are:

- Avoid large crowds, especially during known influenza seasons.
- Avoid contact with people who have an upper respiratory tract infection.
- Obtain influenza and pneumonia immunizations.
- Contact the health care provider if the following common signs and symptoms occur: change in sputum color, amount, and consistency; more frequent or productive cough; elevated temperature; change in behavior (e.g., more argumentative than usual) that indicates an increase in $PaCO_2$; increased fatigue; increased dyspnea; weight gain; or peripheral edema.

The nurse should also evaluate the person's knowledge of the care, cleansing, and use of inhalant and nebulizer equipment. Contaminated MDIs, DPIs, and nebulizer equipment are common sources of infection.

7. Promoting Effective Coping

Persons who are short of breath are usually anxious and frightened. The patient should be encouraged to talk about anxiety and fears with family members and health care professionals. A realistic assessment of abilities and limitations, with a focus on those activities that the patient is still able to do, should be fostered. Positive body responses should be stressed without negating the seriousness of the health issues involved. Vocational rehabilitation may be an option for some patients. Enrollment in pulmonary rehabilitation programs can also help lessen the sense of isolation and encourages ongoing involvement. The patient should be encouraged to try new coping behaviors and gradually master them. Referral to professional counseling should be initiated if indicated.

Patient/Family Education

Persons with COPD play a major role in monitoring their condition and in maintaining their physical and psychologic functioning at the maximum possible level. For these reasons, it is imperative that the nurse thoroughly assesses the patient's knowledge of COPD, including its cause and treatment. Individualized teaching plans based on the patient's knowledge level can then be developed.

Health Promotion/Prevention. The cornerstone of prevention of COPD is education. Public education must focus on the pulmonary health risks associated with inhaled irritants, regardless of their source. Increased public awareness of the vital role that clean air plays in pulmonary health is essential for the success of any legislative actions promoting air quality standards. Individuals must also be educated to understand the importance of personal responsibility to decrease their own health risk through smoking cessation.

Persons with a family history of emphysema should be screened for AAT deficiency. It is imperative that persons with this enzyme deficiency take active measures to prevent progressive lung damage from smoking, air pollution, and infection. Persons identified as being at high risk for emphysema may require vocational counseling if their current work environment is known to have inhaled irritants. These individuals should also be counseled to receive the influenza vaccine yearly and the pneumococcal vaccine every 3 to 5 years.

EVALUATION

To evaluate the effectiveness of nursing interventions, compare patient behaviors with those stated in the expected patient outcomes. Achievement of patient outcomes is successful if the patient:

1. Demonstrates improved ventilation and oxygenation.

1a,b. Has PaO_2, $PaCO_2$, and pH at baseline levels; verbalizes need to use oxygen therapy continuously, or at least while sleeping and exercising.

2a,b. Demonstrates improved airway clearance; has effective coughing; uses inhaler with bronchoactive medications as necessary to clear secretions; is well hydrated; uses humidifier as needed.

3a-d. Demonstrates effective breathing pattern; takes twice as long to exhale as to inhale (5:10 seconds); uses pursed-lip breathing when exhaling; leans forward on an overstuffed chair to increase ability to exhale; concentrates on abdominal breathing when lying in bed and when up and about; inhales before beginning an activity and exhales while doing activity; has respiratory rate of 24 to 28 breaths/min and moderate tidal volume.

4a-d. Maintains or works toward improving activity level; paces activities, using oxygen most of the time; participates in individualized exercise program.

5a-d. Verbalizes dietary changes after discharge; maintains optimal weight; eats several small meals daily because small, frequent meals cause less shortness of breath; explains food and fluid requirements; verbalizes that gas-producing foods such as cabbage, baked beans, and raw green pepper and radishes are to be avoided because they cause discomfort and bloating.

6a-e. Remains infection free; maintains normal temperature; has clear sputum; states need to call health care provider if sputum changes in color, consistency, amount, or odor.

7a-e. Demonstrates effective coping mechanisms; identifies stressors; sets realistic personal goals; participates in ADLs and therapeutic regimes; lists names and numbers of support services.

GERONTOLOGIC CONSIDERATIONS

Many patients with COPD are older and may require additional time and support in learning how to take their medications, perform breathing exercises, and use oxygen properly. A multidisciplinary team including social services, nutritional services, and physical therapy may be necessary to assess the patient and assist the nurse with teaching the patient. The patient's significant others need to be involved in each teaching activity so that they will be able to assist the patient as necessary.[47]

SPECIAL ENVIRONMENTS FOR CARE

Home Care Management

Before the patient goes home, an assessment is made of the home environment. A home health nurse should meet with the family at home to help determine whether they can care for the patient without assistance. If the patient is on Medicare, visits by the nurse and physical therapist are covered for a specified number of visits. If the family desires the assistance of a home health aide, the patient will have to pay for this service. Agencies such as the Visiting Nurse Association provide services on a sliding fee scale determined by the patient's financial resources. The main emphasis of home care is on determining the patient's understanding of his or her treatment plan and how well it is being carried out. It is important that the patient is taking medications as ordered and is able to manage any equipment needed to administer medications, oxygen, and so on. Another major emphasis is determining whether the patient and family know how to protect the patient from infection, because infection is the most common reason for admission to the hospital.

COMPLICATIONS

Infection and respiratory failure are the major complications.

ASTHMA

Asthma is a chronic inflammatory disorder of the airways that is characterized by an exaggerated bronchoconstrictor response to a wide variety of stimuli. Airway hyperresponsiveness leads to clinical symptoms of wheezing and dyspnea after exposure to allergens, environmental irritants, viral infections, cold air, or exercise.

Etiology

Asthma results from complex interactions among inflammatory cells, mediators, and other cells and tissues that reside in airways. An initial trigger in asthma may be the release of inflammatory mediators from bronchial mast cells, macrophages, T lymphocytes, and epithelial cells. These substances direct the migration and activation of other inflammatory cells to the airway, where they cause injury, abnormalities in autonomic neural control of airway tone, mucus hypersecretion, change in mucociliary function, and increased airway smooth muscle responsiveness. Common asthma triggers are listed in Box 21-6.

In sensitive individuals the inflammatory response causes recurrent episodes of wheezing, breathlessness, chest tightness, and cough, particularly at night and in the early morning. Early-phase reactions appear seconds after exposure and last about 1 hour. About half of all patients with asthma also experience a delayed, or late-phase, reaction. Symptoms of late-phase reactions are the same as those of early-phase reactions, but these reactions begin 4 to 8 hours after exposure and can last for hours or days. These episodes are usually associated with widespread but variable airflow obstruction that is often reversible either spontaneously or with treatment.[40]

Epidemiology

Increases in the prevalence of asthma and in its mortality and morbidity rates have been seen in the past two decades. Asthma affects 14 to 15 million people in the United States,[62] with costs in excess of $6 billion.[54] Asthma accounts for approximately 500,000 hospital admissions, with an average length of stay of 5 days and 2 million emergency visits. Both

BOX 21-6 Common Factors Triggering an Asthma Attack

Environmental factors
- Change in temperature, especially cold air
- Change in humidity: dry air

Atmospheric pollutants
- Cigarette and industrial smoke, ozone, sulfur dioxide, formaldehyde

Strong odors: perfume

Allergens
- Feathers, animal dander, dust mites, molds, allergens; foods treated with sulfites (beer, wine, fruit juices, snack foods, salads, potatoes, shellfish, fresh and dried fruits)

Exercise

Stress or emotional upset

Medications
- Aspirin and nonsteroidal antiinflammatory drugs (NSAIDs), beta-blockers (including eyedrops), cholinergic drugs (to promote bladder contraction and as eyedrops for glaucoma)

Enzymes, including those in laundry detergents

Chemicals: toluene and others used in solvents, paints, rubber, and plastics hospitalizations for the treatment of asthma and deaths from it have been increasing. Most of the morbidity and all of the mortality involve acute exacerbations of asthma, and treatment of these events accounts for the majority of expenditures in money and health care resources. Asthma begins most frequently in childhood and adolescence, but it can develop at any time in life. The reasons for the increase in morbidity and mortality are not well understood. They may be related to lack of access to primary care, overuse and incorrect use of medications, or the inability to recognize the severity of symptoms.

Pathophysiology

Airflow limitation in asthma is recurrent and caused by a variety of changes in the airway (Figure 21-18). These changes include bronchoconstriction, edema, chronic mucous plug formation, and airway remodeling,

Acute Bronchoconstriction. Allergen-induced acute bronchoconstriction results from an IgE-dependent release of mediators from mast cells. These mediators include histamine, tryptase, leukotrienes, and prostaglandins that directly contract airway smooth muscle. Aspirin and other nonsteroidal antiinflammatory drugs can also cause acute airflow obstruction in some patients, and this also involves mediator release from airway cells. Other stimuli, including exercise, cold air, and irritants, can cause acute airflow obstruction, but these mechanisms are less well defined.

Airway Edema. Airway wall edema, even without smooth muscle contraction or bronchoconstriction, limits airflow in asthma. Increased microvascular permeability and leakage caused by released mediators contribute to mucosal thickening and swelling of the airway. As a consequence, swelling of the airway wall causes the airway to become more rigid and interferes with airflow.

Chronic Mucous Plug Formation. In severe, intractable asthma, airflow limitation is often persistent. This change may arise as a consequence of mucus secretion and the formation of mucous plugs.

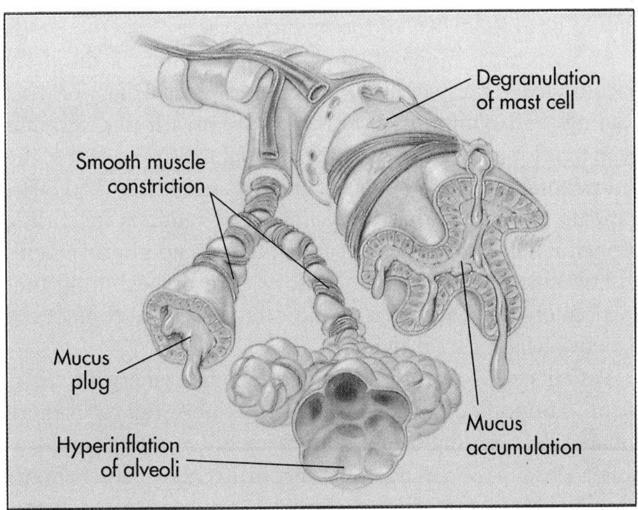

Figure 21-18 Bronchial asthma; thick mucus, mucosal edema, and smooth muscle spasm cause obstruction of the small airways; breathing is labored, and expiration is difficult.

Airway Remodeling. In some patients with asthma, airflow limitation may be only partially reversible because of structural changes in the airway that accompany long-standing and severe airway inflammation. There is evidence that a histologic feature of asthma in some patients is an alteration in the amount and composition of the extracellular matrix in the airway wall. The importance of airway remodeling and the development of persistent airflow limitation suggest a rationale for early intervention with antiinflammatory therapy.

To help standardize asthma management with the hope of improving outcomes, the National Asthma Education and Prevention Program (NAEPP) developed Guidelines for the Diagnosis and Management of Asthma. Under these guidelines asthma is classified into four categories:

1. Mild intermittent — Symptoms occur less than twice a week
2. Mild persistent — Symptoms occur more than twice a week but less than daily
3. Moderate persistent — Daily symptoms occur, including exacerbations more than twice a week
4. Severe persistent — Symptoms occur continually, along with frequent exacerbations, limiting the patient's physical activity

For each category a stepwise approach to symptom management has been outlined[18] (Table 21-12).

Persons who are severely affected by asthma and who have attacks that cannot be controlled with the usual medications have status asthmaticus. In status asthmaticus, the symptoms of an acute attack continue despite measures to relieve them. Air trapping in the distal air spaces ultimately leads to respiratory muscle exhaustion and severe V/Q abnormalities with resultant respiratory failure and hypoxemia. Repeated attacks of status asthmaticus may cause irreversible emphysema, resulting in a permanent decrease in total breathing capacity.

Patients with status asthmaticus often demonstrate such severe respiratory distress that they are unable to talk. They may be moving minimal amounts of air into and out of the lungs; thus audible wheezing and adventitious lung sounds may not be present. During this phase of the attack, the patient appears cyanotic and may demonstrate both pulsus paradoxus and sensorium changes. This is a medical emergency, and the patient requires immediate therapy. Most patients arrive in the emergency department, where treatment is begun. Patients remain in the emergency department until their condition is stabilized. Most patients are then admitted to the hospital for ongoing therapy and observation.

Collaborative Care Management

The major focus in asthma treatment is education for an active partnership with the patient. It begins at the time of asthma diagnosis and is integrated into all aspects of care. Patients learn to treat inflammation and day-to-day symptoms themselves through a program of provider-guided comanagement or partnership that stresses collaboration. This self-management program is developed according to the needs of each patient, with sensitivity to cultural beliefs and

TABLE 21-12 Stepped Approach to Asthma Management

Long-Term Control	Quick Relief (Rescue)
Step 1	
No daily medication needed	Short-acting bronchodilator: inhaled beta$_2$-agonist Use of above more than twice a week indicates need for long-term control therapy
Step 2	
Daily antiinflammatory: either inhaled low-dose corticosteroid, or cromolyn or nedocromil; sustained-released theophylline is an alternative but not preferred; zafirlukast or zileuton may be considered	Inhaled beta$_2$-agonist, short acting Use of above on a daily basis or increasing use indicates need for additional long-term therapy
Step 3	
Daily antiinflammatory: either inhaled medium-dose corticosteroid or inhaled low- to medium-dose corticosteroid plus long-acting bronchodilator—either long-acting inhaled beta$_2$-agonist or oral agent; if needed, inhaled medium- to high-dose corticosteroid and long-acting bronchodilator—either long-acting inhaled beta$_2$-agonist, sustained-release theophylline, or long-acting beta$_2$-agonist tablets	Inhaled beta$_2$-agonist, short acting Again, daily or increasing use of above indicates need for improved long-term control agent
Step 4	
Daily antiinflammatory: inhaled high-dose corticosteroid and long-acting bronchodilator—either long-acting inhaled beta$_2$-agonist, sustained-release theophylline, or long-acting beta$_2$-agonist tablets and corticosteroid tablets long term (2 mg/kg/day)	Inhaled beta$_2$-agonist, short acting

practices. Desired outcomes include effective symptom management, quality of life, and the ability to engage in usual activities.

Diagnostic Tests. Pulmonary function/spirometry tests, which include FEV_1 and peak expiratory flow (PEF), serve as diagnostic tools for assessing the degree of obstruction and its reversibility. They also establish baseline ventilatory function. ABGs are obtained and typically indicate mild to severe hypoxemia and mild to severe respiratory acidosis. Induced sputum specimen examinations show marked eosinophilia. Allergy testing may be done in an attempt to identify the allergen or other trigger responsible for the onset of asthma symptoms. Exhaled breath testing is being studied for use as a noninvasive measure of airway inflammation. This testing involves the measurement of a volatile mediator in exhaled breath, specifically, nitric oxide. Other potential markers include ethane, pentane, and carbon monoxide.[54]

Treatments. The objectives of medical management of asthma are to promote normal functioning of the individual, prevent recurrent symptoms, prevent severe attacks, and prevent side effects from medication. The chief aim of various medications is to afford the patient immediate, progressive, ongoing bronchial relaxation. Common asthma medications are listed in Table 21-13.

Patients, families, and health care professionals need an objective measure of airflow obstruction to guide them in managing asthma attacks promptly. Numerous clinical and experimental studies show that many patients with asthma cannot accurately evaluate the severity of airflow obstruction. Many patients are being encouraged to manage their asthma with the aid of peak flow meters. Peak expiratory flow rate (PEFR) is the greatest airflow velocity that can be produced during a forced expiration that starts from fully inflated lungs. Peak flow monitoring is used to audit daily response to treatment, detect a buildup in airflow obstruction, assess the severity of an attack, evaluate response to therapy, and aid decisions about the need for hospitalization. PEFR monitoring devices cost from $15 to $40 and are portable and easy to use. The normal range for peak flow is 500 to 700 L/min for men and 380 to 500 L/min for women. Peak flow rates vary with age, sex, race, height, smoking history, respiratory muscle strength, and effort. The NAEPP recommends that the peak flow value should be at least 70% of the predicted value.[39,40]

Patients with moderate and severe persistent asthma are encouraged to measure PEFR daily and to keep a diary of their readings and symptoms. A system based on a traffic light has been developed—the green zone is equal to 80% or better, the yellow zone is 50% to 79%, and the red zone is less than 50%. Patients are taught that the yellow zone requires increasing bronchodilator use as needed and, if there is no improvement, adding either the antiinflammatory dose or beginning oral corticosteroids. The red zone indicates a need to contact the patient's health care provider.

Patients with status asthmaticus require emergent treatment. Humidified oxygen is given to achieve full saturation. Inhaled short-acting beta$_2$-agonists are given in large and frequent doses. Subcutaneous epinephrine may help patients who do not respond after several hours of inhaled beta$_2$-agonists. Treatment with bronchodilators is given continuously until the desired clinical effect is achieved or until toxic side effects limit continued use. Noninvasive positive-pressure

TABLE 21-13 Common Medications for Asthma

	Administration	Action	Adverse Effects
Maintenance Medications			
Nonsteroidal Antiinflammatory Drugs	Metered-dose inhaler (MDI) or nebulizer	Decrease airway inflammation and irritation	Cough or throat irritation, headaches, bad taste in mouth
Cromolyn (Intal) Nedocromil (Tilade)			
Corticosteroids	MDI	Antiinflammatory	Sore throat, hoarseness, cough, oral thrush
Beclomethasone (Vanceril, Beclovent) Triamcinolone acetonide (Azmacort) Flunisolide (AeroBid) Fluticasone (Flovent)			
Leukotriene Inhibitors/Receptor Antagonists	Oral	Antiinflammatory	Headache, nausea, diarrhea, dizziness, myalgia, fever, dyspepsia, elevated alanine aminotransferase level
Zafirlukast (Accolate) Zilenton (Zyflo) Montelukast sodium (Singulair)			
Theophylline	Oral, parenteral	Long-acting bronchodilator	Nausea, vomiting, stomach cramps, diarrhea, headache, muscle cramps, tachycardia, irritability, restlessness; serum blood levels should be checked for therapeutic ranges
Theophylline (Theo-Dur, Slo-bid, Uniphyl, Theo-24, Uni-Dur, Slo-Phyllin) Theophylline ethylenediamine (Aminophylline)			
Anticholinergic	MDI, nebulizer, nasal spray	Short-acting bronchodilator	Nervousness, dizziness, headache, palpitations, cough, blurred vision, nausea, gastrointestinal distress, dry mouth
Ipratropium (Atrovent)			
Beta$_2$-Agonist	MDI	Long-acting bronchodilator	Headache, tremor, tachycardia, palpitations, nasopharyngitis, stomachache, cough, rash
Salmeterol (Serevent)			
Rescue Medications			
Corticosteroids	Parenteral, oral	Antiinflammatory	Increased appetite, fluid retention, weight gain, gastrointestinal irritation
Prednisone Methylprednisolone (Medrol) Prednisolone (Prelone) Prednisolone sodium phosphate (Pediapred)			
Beta-Agonists	MDI, nebulizer Albuterol is also available for parenteral administration	Short-acting bronchodilators	Nervousness, tremors, tachycardia, headache, dizziness, vomiting
Albuterol (Proventil, Ventolin) Metaproterenol (Alupent, Metaprel) Pirbuterol (Maxair) Bitolterol (Tornalate) Terbutaline (Brethaire) Epinephrine			

ventilation (NIV) is preferable to intubation and mechanical ventilation. If mechanical ventilation is required, MDIs and nebulizers may be used to deliver bronchodilators. MDIs require the use of a spacing device on the inspiratory limb of the ventilator to optimize drug delivery. A minimum of 4 puffs and up to 10 to 20 puffs may be given. Patient-ventilator synchrony is essential, and an inspiratory pause may be useful. Nebulizers may increase barotrauma because they require added gas flow (8 L/min) when used with mechanical ventilation. This can be minimized by decreasing the minute ventilation, placing the nebulizer close to the ventilator, raising the tidal volume above 500 ml, and decreasing the inspiratory flow to 40 L/min.[54] Corticosteroids are administered as early as possible. The minimum dose is 40 mg of methylprednisolone every 6 hours. Theophylline does not add to bronchodilation but may be helpful for its antiinflammatory and diaphragmatic effects.

Diet. The diet for the patient with asthma is as tolerated. Increased fluids may be beneficial.

Activity. Activities are not restricted unless the patient is having respiratory distress or if the particular activity is an asthma trigger.

Referrals. Referrals may be made to a respiratory therapist and to an allergy specialist for allergy testing.

NURSING MANAGEMENT OF PATIENT WITH ASTHMA

ASSESSMENT

Health History

Data to be collected to assess the patient with asthma include:

- History of asthma onset and duration
- Precipitating factors
- Any recent changes in medication regimen
- Medications used to relieve asthma symptoms
- Other medications
- Self-care methods used to relieve symptoms

Physical Examination

Important aspects of the physical examination of the patient with asthma include:

- General appearance
- Does patient appear apprehensive?
- Precipitating factors
- Any recent changes in medication regimen
- Medications used to relieve asthma symptoms
- Other medications
- Self-care methods used to relieve symptoms

Important aspects of the physical examination of the patient with asthma include:

- Assessment of general appearance and mental status. It is particularly important to observe for signs of altered sensorium or apprehension, which may be indicative of hyoxemia.
- Measurement of vital signs to identify tachycardia; pulsus paradoxus (diminished pulse with inspiration, confirmed by a 6 to 8 mm Hg drop in systolic blood pressure during inspiration); tachypnea; or other abnormality.
- Pulmonary examination, which includes inspection for dyspnea, use of accessory muscles for breathing, forward-leaning (tripod) posture, prolonged expiration, and cyanosis; palpation for decreased lateral expansion of the chest and decreased fremitus; and percussion for hyperresonance and decreased diaphragmatic excursion. Pulmonary examination also includes auscultation of breath sounds, which, as the patient approaches exhaustion from the increased work of breathing, may be absent or faint. Inspiratory and expiratory wheezing and rhonchi (gurgles) are common.

Relevant laboratory findings include ABGs, which, during a short-term or moderate asthma attack indicate respiratory alkalosis with mild hypoxemia and during a prolonged or severe attack demonstrate respiratory acidosis with severe hypoxemia. PFTs document a decreased FEV_1 and VC, and sputum examinations show eosinophilia.

NURSING DIAGNOSES

Nursing diagnoses are determined from analysis of patient data. Nursing diagnoses for the person with asthma may include but are not limited to:

Diagnostic Title	Possible Etiologic Factors
1. Deficient knowledge: predisposing factors	Lack of exposure to information; unfamiliarity with information prevention, treatment sources; lack of receptivity
2. Ineffective airway clearance	Ineffective technique, decreased energy, fatigue, impaired mucociliary clearance mechanism, inadequate fluid intake
3. Ineffective breathing pattern	Bronchoconstriction, underuse of medications
4. Impaired gas exchange	Mucous plugs, V/Q imbalance
5. Anxiety (mild, moderate, or severe)	Acute onset of dyspnea, threat of unknown or death

EXPECTED PATIENT OUTCOMES

Expected outcomes for the person with asthma may include but are not limited to:

1. Patient or significant other will describe the "stepped plan" and partnership approach to asthma management
1a. Will identify asthma triggers (e.g., allergens, infections, stress)
1b. Will describe strategies for avoiding asthma triggers
1c. Will state the importance of keeping a diary of symptoms and medications (time and dose)
1d. Will explain home medication program
1d(1) Will give name, dose, action, and side effects of each medication
1d(2) Will state conditions under which medications might be increased (e.g., infection: start or increase antibiotics; increased stress or worsening of symptoms: increase corticosteroids)
1e. Will demonstrate how to take inhaled medications, use of MDI, inhaler
1f. Will verbalize steps to take when an acute attack is beginning
1g. Will use peak flow meter to determine changes in medication regimen and when to call a health professional
1h. If receiving corticosteroid therapy, will show card to be carried at all times giving data about the drug,

dose of the drug, and name of the physician; an alternative is to wear a Medic-Alert bracelet

1i. Will state plans for ongoing follow-up care, including plans for desensitization if appropriate

2. Will demonstrate effective airway clearance

2a. Will cough effectively

2b. Will have breath sounds that are clear or at baseline

3. Will demonstrate effective breathing pattern

3a. Will have inspiratory-expiratory ratio of 5:10 seconds

3b. Will have respiratory rate within near-normal limits

4. Will demonstrate improved ventilation

4a. Arterial blood pH and $Paco_2$ will return to or be at acceptable limits

4b. Pao_2 will be at optimal level for the patient

5. Will demonstrate activities to control anxiety response to symptoms

5a. Progressive muscle relaxation (see Patient Teaching box)

5b. Meditation

5c. Appropriate use of medications

INTERVENTIONS

1. Patient/Family Education

The nurse assesses the patient's knowledge of asthma and teaches the information needed to enable the patient to become an effective partner in the management of the disease. Information that the patient needs to understand is:

Signs and symptoms of an attack: tightness in chest; restlessness or vague feeling of uneasiness; dyspnea; increased wheezing; productive cough

Importance of keeping a symptom diary in which is recorded timing of attacks, symptom patterns, possible precipitating factors, time and dose of self-administered medications and their effectiveness

Self-treatment of signs and symptoms:

Importance of taking bronchoactive medications as ordered

Conditions under which medication might be increased (e.g., change in peak flow readings, infection, increased stress or worsening of symptoms)

Need to call someone in the event of an attack so as not to be alone

Importance of remaining calm, breathing slowly, and using relaxation techniques at the first sign of an attack

Need to call a physician or go to the nearest emergency facility if symptoms do not dissipate

Use of equipment such as an MDI, inhaler with a spacer, and peak flow meter if one is prescribed (The patient should demonstrate use of the inhaler with each visit to the health care provider to reinforce correct technique.)

Importance of smoking cessation and avoidance of environmental tobacco smoke

Need to avoid large crowds during flu season

Importance of obtaining influenza and pneumococcal vaccines

Patient Teaching
Progressive Relaxation Exercises

1. Contract each muscle to a count of 10 and then relax it.
2. Do exercises in quiet room while sitting or lying in a comfortable position.
3. Do exercises to relaxing music, if desired.
4. Have another person serve as a "coach" by giving command to contract specific muscle, count to 10, and relax muscle.
5. The following are examples of exercises helpful to some persons with chronic obstructive pulmonary disease.
   a. Raise shoulders, shrug them, and relax for 5 seconds; then relax them completely.
   b. Make a fist of both hands, squeeze them tightly for 5 seconds, and then relax them completely.

Health Promotion/Prevention

Healthy people 2010 asthma-related goals focus on reducing hospitalizations for asthma, reducing deaths from asthma, and reducing hospital emergency department visits for asthma.[74] There is perhaps no disease in which an effective partnership between the patient and the health care professional is more important than in asthma. Knowing about the person's attitudes toward health and his or her lifestyle, such as his or her type of work, leisure-time activities, social supports, learning style, and interest in participating in self-care management, is an essential element in developing an effective management plan. The identification of asthma triggers requires involvement of both the patient and the health care professional. Avoidance of triggers can be an important component in preventing exacerbations. (See Chapter 3 for more information about the Healthy People 2010 document and the leading health indicators and goals for air quality [environmental health].)

2. Improving Airway Clearance

During an asthma attack, secretions tend to become viscous and can plug airways, causing increased airway obstruction. Mobilizing secretions often prevents the need for intubation and artificial ventilation. To promote mobilization, adequate systemic fluid intake should be ensured. Overhydration is not necessary, since research findings suggest that it may not increase secretion clearance above levels obtained by normal hydration. It is also important to provide extra humidity, teach effective cough maneuvers, provide adequate nutrition for energy, and medicate with short-acting rescue medications.

3. Improving Breathing Patterns

The nursing role in improving breathing patterns and gas exchange is to help the patient assume a position of comfort, administer medication as ordered, and monitor for both therapeutic and adverse effects of medications. The nurse must also assess for possible medication overuse. Table 21-13 lists medications, administration, action, and adverse effects of medications typically used to treat asthma. The nurse also encourages the patient to exercise and monitors the need for an inhaled $beta_2$-agonist 15 to 30 minutes before exercise.

4. Improving Gas Exchange

Blood gas results should be monitored carefully. If respiratory alkalosis is present, the patient should be encouraged to breathe more slowly. If respiratory acidosis and hypoxemia are present, oxygen is administered as prescribed. If oxygen and other therapeutic measures do not relieve the attack, intubation and ventilatory assistance may be required.

5. Providing Emotional Support and Preventing Anxiety

Never leave the patient alone during an asthma attack. Guide the patient in the use of relaxation techniques and respiratory maneuvers.

EVALUATION

To evaluate the effectiveness of nursing interventions, compare patient behaviors with those stated in the expected patient outcomes. Achievement of patient outcomes is successful if the patient:

1. Demonstrates knowledge of the stepped plan of asthma management and active partnership with the health care team.
1a. States factors most likely to precipitate an asthma attack; for example, attacks are frequently exercise induced and are more likely to occur during times of increased stress.
1b. Describes ways to avoid asthma triggers.
1c. Keeps a symptom diary to review and share with the health care team to manage symptoms.
1d. States name, dose, and adverse effects of prescribed medications.
1e. Demonstrates correct use of an MDI.
1f. Describes steps to take when an acute attack is beginning.
1g. Uses a peak flow meter to determine changes in the medication regimen and when to call a health care professional.
1h. Wears a Medic-Alert bracelet or carries a card indicating that he or she takes steroids.
1i. Describes plans for ongoing medical follow-up.
2. Demonstrates effective airway clearance.
2a. Uses huff coughing technique.
2b. Breath sounds are clear or at baseline level.
3. Breathing pattern is effective.
3a. Uses pursed-lip breathing to increase time of exhalation to twice that of inhalation by counting to 5 seconds for inhalation and 10 seconds for exhalation.
3b. Respirations are quieter and slower at 28/min.
4. Ventilation and perfusion are improving.
4a. $Pa{O_2}$, $Pa{CO_2}$, and pH are returning to patient's baseline levels.
4b. $Pa{O_2}$ is at optimal level for patient.
5. Is less anxious; demonstrates activities to control anxiety.
5a. Uses relaxation techniques.
5b. Uses meditation as needed.
5c. Uses medications appropriately.

GERONTOLOGIC CONSIDERATIONS

Although the goals of treatment of asthma are the same for persons of all ages, they may be more difficult to achieve in older adults. The Cardiovascular Health Study is one of the largest population-based examinations of heart and lung disease in older persons in the United States. This sample explored the associations of asthma in older adults with quality of life, morbidity, and use of asthma medications. Results of the study indicated that asthma in older persons is associated with a lower quality of life. Participants who had asthma were much more likely to rate their general health as fair or poor and report their activity as less than the previous year. Results also indicated that asthma is underdiagnosed in older adults and is often associated with allergic triggers. Inhaled corticosteroids are underused.[21] This study provides considerable impetus for health care providers to prioritize the diagnosis and treatment of asthma in the older population.

SPECIAL ENVIRONMENTS FOR CARE

Critical Care Management

The person with status asthmaticus usually requires intubation and ventilatory support and is cared for in an ICU.

Home Care Management

Most persons with asthma are able to manage their asthma well at home. Patients who adhere to their prescribed therapy and avoid allergens to which they are sensitive may not have an asthma attack for years unless they develop a severe respiratory infection.

COMPLICATIONS

Complications of asthma include status asthmaticus and respiratory failure.

CYSTIC FIBROSIS

Cystic fibrosis (CF) is a multisystem disorder characterized by chronic airway obstruction and infection and by exocrine pancreatic insufficiency, with its effects on GI function, nutrition, growth, and maturation.

Etiology

CF continues to be the most common fatal genetic disease among Caucasians. Numerous mutations of a single gene are responsible for CF. The gene encodes a membrane protein known as the CF transmembrane regulator (CFTR), and mutations of CFTR protein result in reduced secretion of chloride from epithelial cells. It is an autosomal-recessive disease. When both parents are carriers (heterozygotes), there is a one-in-four chance with each pregnancy that the child will have CF (Figure 21-19).

Epidemiology

In Caucasian populations 2% to 5% are carriers of a CF gene mutation. Approximately 25,000 individuals with CF live in the United States. The number of adults with CF continues to increase steadily because of increased life expectancy and

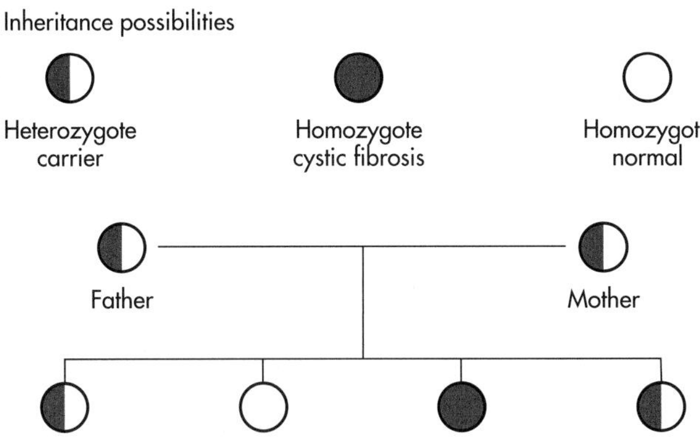

Figure 21-19 Inheritance of cystic fibrosis (CF) when both mother and father are carriers of the CF gene.

diagnostic advances. Two groups make up this adult CF population: (1) those diagnosed when infants or children and (2) those diagnosed as adolescents or adults. Statistics indicate that approximately 20% of the adult CF population is diagnosed after age 15.[20]

Reaching adulthood is now a realistic expectation for infants and children with CF. The average life expectancy in 1998 was 32.3 years.[20] The major contributing factors to this increased life expectancy include advancements in antibiotic therapies, new treatments, more aggressive management, and the availability of a network of about 115 comprehensive CF referral centers sponsored by the Cystic Fibrosis Foundation.

Pathophysiology

CF is an exocrine gland disease involving various systems (pulmonary, pancreatic/hepatic, GI, reproductive). Obstruction of the exocrine gland ducts or passageways occurs in nearly all adult patients with CF. Exocrine gland secretions are known to have a decreased water content, altered electrolyte concentration, and abnormal organic constituents (especially mucous glycoproteins); however, the specific biochemical or physiologic defect that leads to obstruction is not known.

Pulmonary Involvement. Disease of the conducting airways in CF is acquired after birth. Either hypersecretion or failure to clear secretions at an early age accounts for mucus accumulation in bronchial regions. Failure to clear secretions from the airway probably initiates infection because mucous plaques and plugs serve as media for growth of bacteria.[54] Chronic airway infection is rarely eradicated. As lung disease progresses, bronchiolitis and bronchitis are evident, submucosal glands hypertrophy, and goblet cells increase. Bronchiectasis is a consequence of persistent obstruction-infection cycles. Bronchiectatic cysts occupy as much as 50% of the late-stage CF lung. *Pseudomonas aeruginusa* and *Staphylococcus aureus* are the organisms most frequently causing infection.[65] The earliest manifestation of lung involvement is generally cough, at first intermittent and then daily. It is often worse at night and on arising in the morning. Cough becomes productive, then paroxysmal, and is associated with gagging and emesis. Sputum is usually tenacious, purulent, and often green. Recurrent pulmonary infections erode blood vessels such as the bronchial arteries, which branch from the aorta and the lung at high pressures and can lead to bleeding with hemoptysis.

Gastrointestinal and Pancreatic Involvement. Intestinal obstruction occurs in 20% of adult patients with CF. Generally, pancreatic insufficiency predisposes to intestinal obstruction. Cramps and abdominal pain in adults with CF should arouse suspicion of intestinal obstruction. Pancreatic insufficiency is reported in 80% to 90% of adults with CF. The pathologic lesions in the pancreas decrease pancreatic enzyme production and lead to malabsorption of fat.

Other Involvement. In older children and young adults CF may be manifested by heat exhaustion after exercise or exposure to hot weather, or by dehydration after fever. In some young adults the only clinical manifestation of CF may be infertility. The varied signs and symptoms of CF are summarized in the Clinical Manifestations box.

> ## *Clinical Manifestations*
> **Cystic Fibrosis**
>
> Specific clinical manifestations by system are listed below. Pulmonary signs and symptoms of cystic fibrosis include:
> - Chronic productive cough and/or recurrent bronchitis or pneumonia
> - Crackles and rhonchi, decreased pulmonary compliance, digital clubbing
> - Shortness of breath and dyspnea on exertion, wheezing, and weight loss—occur with respiratory complications and usually indicate need for vigorous therapy
>
> Gastrointestinal signs and symptoms include:
> - Frequent, bulky, greasy stools
> - Weight loss
> - Cramps and abdominal pain—should arouse suspicion of obstruction
>
> Glucose intolerance signs and symptoms include:
> - Polyuria, polydipsia, polyphagia
> - Absence of ketoacidosis even with above signs

Collaborative Care Management

Management of CF often involves extensive and complicated treatment regimens that require many hours daily.

Diagnostic Tests. The diagnosis of CF is confirmed by the presence of at least two of the following:

1. A positive sweat test with a chloride level greater than 60 mEq/L
2. Chronic sinopulmonary disease
3. Chronic chest x-ray abnormalities: hyperinflation of the lung; mucoid impaction of bronchi, which is seen as branching fingerlike shadows; or atelectasis of the right upper lobe
4. Pancreatic exocrine insufficiency
5. Obstructive azoospermia in males
6. Laboratory evidence of CFTR dysfunction
7. Positive family history of CF

Medications. Lung infection is the major source of morbidity and mortality. By age 18, 80% of CF patients are chronically infected with *P. aeruginosa,* 40% with *S. aureus,* and 50% with *Burkholderia cepacia.*[18] Antibiotic therapy is a mainstay designed not to eradicate the bacteria from the airways but to reduce the number of bacteria and to control progression of disease. Best results have been shown with early and vigorous use of antibiotics. Dosages need to be higher than in non–CF-related chest infections, and the choice is based on sputum culture and sensitivity. Combination therapy with two or three antibiotics is recommended to prevent bacterial resistance and is usually prescribed for 10 to 14 days. Shorter courses of antibiotic therapy are associated with reexacerbation of symptoms. Studies evaluating the benefit of inhaled antibiotics indicate that they are more effective in the suppression of chronic infections than in the treatment of acute exacerbations.[49] Organisms with multiple resistance profiles such as *B. cepacia* have emerged in the CF population. This reinforces the need for close monitoring of antibiotic susceptibility and strict adherence to isolation policies for infection control.

Dornase-alfa (Pulmozyme), a recombinant form of the naturally occurring human enzyme deoxyribonuclease I (DNase I), which is responsible for the breakdown of extracellular deoxyribonucleic acid (DNA), was released in 1994.[22] In patients with CF the viscosity of airway secretions is abnormally high because of an increased number of neutrophils and DNA in cellular breakdown products. Inhalation of dornase-alfa may provide a modest improvement in lung function and decreased pulmonary exacerbation in patients with mild to moderate lung disease. The dosage is 2.5 mg aerosolized daily. Best effects are achieved when the drug is used daily.

Bronchodilators are frequently used in CF as an adjunct to chest physiotherapy. Airway reactivity is a component of CF, but airway obstruction is complex and often not improved by an inhaled beta-agonist or anticholinergic agent. In some patients a paradoxical response may occur.

Treatments. Treatment goals include the control of infection, promotion of mucus clearance, and improved nutrition.

Pulmonary Physiotherapy (Chest Physiotherapy). Cough clears mucus from large airways, and chest vibration moves secretions from small airways to large ones. Daily pulmonary physiotherapy is one of the most important preventive and therapeutic aspects of care in patients with CF.

Pulmonary physiotherapy activities (segmental postural drainage, percussion, and vibration) may be performed by a physical therapist, nurse, or family member, or by the patient using new modalities. Pulmonary physiotherapy is physically demanding and time consuming but essential to care. The frequency and duration of treatment is individualized.

Segmental postural drainage with percussion and vibration combines the force of gravity with the natural ciliary activity of the small bronchial airways to move secretions upward toward the main bronchi and the trachea. From this point the patient can cough secretions up, or they can be suctioned. Drainage of all segments is usually accomplished by placing patients in various postural drainage positions. Treatment may also be directed at draining specific areas of the lung. For example, if the right middle lobe of the lung is affected, drainage is accomplished best by way of the right middle bronchus. The patient lies supine with the body turned at approximately a 45-degree angle. The angle can be maintained by pillow supports placed under the right side from the shoulders to the hips. The foot of the bed is raised about 30 cm (12 inches). This position can be maintained fairly comfortably by most patients for half an hour at a time. If the lower posterior area of the lung is affected, the foot of the bed can be raised 45 to 50 cm (18 to 20 inches) with the patient assuming a prone position for drainage. Table 21-14 summarizes the positions for segmental postural drainage.

While the patient is in each position, percussion with a cupped hand is performed over the area being drained. This

TABLE 21-14 Positions for Segmental Postural Drainage, Percussion, and Vibration

Area of Lung	Position of Patient	Area To Be Percussed or Vibrated
Upper lobe		
Apical bronchus	Semi-Fowler's position, leaning to right, then left, then forward	Over area of shoulder blades with fingers extending over clavicles
Posterior bronchus	Upright at 45-degree angle, rolled forward against a pillow at 45 degrees on left and then right side	Over shoulder blade on each side
Anterior bronchus	Supine with pillow under knees	Over anterior chest just below clavicles
Middle lobe (lateral and medial bronchus)	Trendelenburg's position at 30-degree angle or with foot of bed elevated 35-40 cm (14-16 inches), turned slightly to left	Anterior and lateral right chest from axillary fold to midanterior chest
Lingula (superior and inferior bronchus)	Trendelenburg's position at 30-degree angle or with foot of bed elevated 35-40 cm (14-16 inches), turned slightly to right	Left axillary fold to midanterior chest
Apical bronchus	Prone with pillow under hips	Lower third of posterior rib cage on both sides
Medial bronchus	Trendelenburg's position at 45-degree angle or with foot of bed raised 45-50 cm (18-20 inches) on right side	Lower third of left posterior rib cage
Lateral bronchus	Trendelenburg's position at 45-degree angle or with foot of bed raised 45-50 cm (18-20 inches) on left side	Lower third of right posterior rib cage
Posterior bronchus	Prone Trendelenburg's position at 45-degree angle with pillow under hips	Lower third of posterior rib cage on both sides

maneuver helps loosen secretions and stimulates coughing (Figure 21-20). After the area is percussed for approximately 1 minute, the patient is instructed to breathe deeply. Vibration (pressure applied with a vibrating movement of the hand on the chest) is performed during the expiratory phase of the deep breath. This helps the patient to exhale more fully. The procedure is repeated as necessary. When the patient cannot tolerate a head-down position, a modified position is used.

Positions that provide gravity drainage of the lungs can be achieved in several ways, and the procedure selected usually depends on the age and general condition of the person, as well as the lobe or lobes of the lungs where secretions have accumulated. Electric hospital beds can be tilted into a head-down position with little difficulty. If an electric bed is not available (e.g., in the home), blocks can be placed under the casters at the foot of the bed, or a hydraulic lift can be used under the foot of the bed.

Newer techniques such as positive expiratory pressure, a flutter valve, a ThAIRapy* vest and autogenic drainage, or active cycle breathing are alternatives to traditional chest physiotherapy. They are used with varying degrees of success to facilitate mucus mobilization.

*Website: www.cff.org/clinical04.

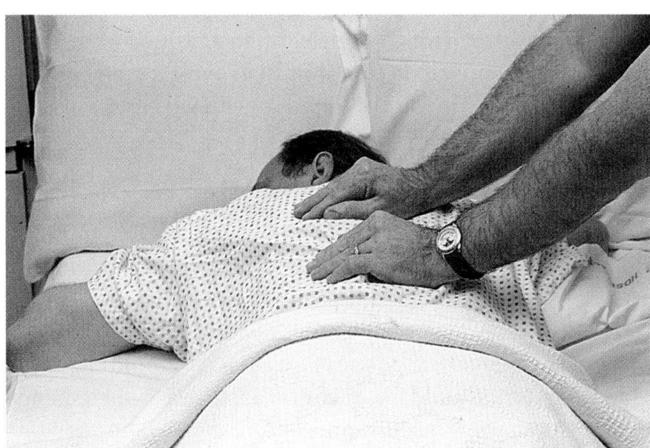

A

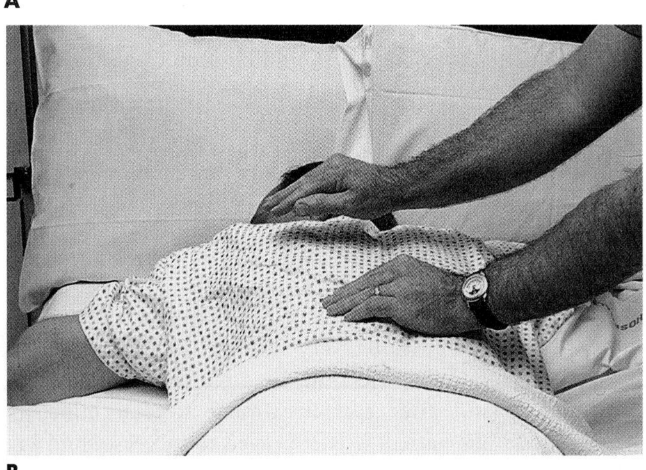

B

Figure 21-20 **A,** Hand position for chest wall percussion during physiotherapy. **B,** Chest wall percussion; alternating hand motion against the patient's chest wall.

Postural drainage and percussion should be planned so as to achieve maximal benefit. Some patients spend up to 8 hours per day involved with this treatment. The frequency of treatments depends on each person's needs, but care should be taken to avoid exhaustion, which results in shallow ventilation and negates the positive effects of the treatment. Because the patient may feel nauseated because of the odor and taste of sputum, the procedure should be timed so that it comes at least 1 hour before meals. A short rest period after the treatment often improves postural drainage. Chest percussion is contraindicated in patients with pulmonary emboli, hemorrhage, exacerbation of bronchospasms, or severe pain and also over areas of resectable carcinoma.

Lung Transplantation. Lung transplantation has become accepted therapy for respiratory failure secondary to CF. Patients should be referred when their prognosis is about equal to the waiting time for donor lungs, currently about 2 years. The best indicator thus determined is an FEV_1 of less than 30% of predicted, although women and younger children may need a transplant before reaching this level. The transplanted lungs remain free of CF but are subject to secondary infection and acute or chronic rejection. Survival rates are 73% at 1 year and 48% at 5 years.[82]

Diet. The diet may be as tolerated, but since GI problems can occur, the diet may be altered. (See discussion of complications later in this section.)

Activity. The patient is encouraged to be as active and independent as possible.

Referrals. Common referrals include pulmonary physiotherapy, respiratory therapy, social services, and genetic counseling. It is important to promote compliance with therapy. Approaches that promote a positive self-concept and foster the ability of the patient to take control of the medical management have been successful. Care that provides continuity and fosters trust is essential to achieving expected patient outcomes.

NURSING MANAGEMENT OF PATIENT WITH CYSTIC FIBROSIS

ASSESSMENT

Health History

Information essential to the assessment of the patient with CF relates to pulmonary, nutritional/GI, and psychosocial status. It includes:

- Description of symptoms such as shortness of breath, dyspnea on exertion, fatigue, and wheezing
- Patient's understanding of CF pathophysiology and treatment regimens, including postural drainage and percussion; antibiotics; aerosol therapy with dornase-alfa, bronchodilators, and antibiotics; and nutritional supplements such as pancreatic enzymes and vitamins
- Color, consistency, and frequency of stools
- Color, smell, and frequency of urination
- Description of appetite and ability to swallow food
- Daily eating pattern
- Medications taken at home and their effectiveness in decreasing stool frequency

Onset, duration, intensity, and type of any abdominal discomfort
Signs or symptoms of gastric reflux
History of weight loss, including amount and time of onset
Description of daily routine as it relates to work or school, pulmonary regimen, medications, and leisure activities
Description of current coping strategies and support network
Concerns about sexuality or fertility
Method of financial support (job, family, other forms of assistance)
Patient's and family's understanding of CF
Symptoms and stage of grieving: anxiety, sleeplessness, hallucinations
Patient and family strengths
Patient support structure
Normal adult developmental needs
Need for genetic counseling, career counseling, or social services

Physical Examination

Important aspects of the physical examination of a patient with CF are:

Auscultation for diminished breath sounds, wheezes, and adventitious breath sounds, which are most often heard in the upper lobes. The patient must be examined for chest pain on inspiration, cyanotic mucous membranes, digital clubbing, presence of a productive cough (observe color of sputum if possible), and presence of fever or tachypnea. ABGs are reviewed for indications of a falling PaO_2 or rising $PaCO_2$ and results of PFTs (decrease in tidal volume and FEV_1).

Assessment for adverse effects of medications, such as renal toxicity from antibiotics and tachycardia from bronchodilators.

Assessment of nutritional and GI status. The patient's weight must be obtained, and the abdomen auscultated for the presence of bowel sounds.

NURSING DIAGNOSES

Nursing diagnoses are determined from analysis of patient data. Nursing diagnoses for the adult with CF may include but are not limited to:

Diagnostic Title	Possible Etiologic Factors
1. Risk for infection	Increased mucus in airway, stasis of respiratory secretions
2. Ineffective airway clearance	Thick secretions, decreased ciliary action, tracheobronchial infection
3. Imbalanced nutrition: less than body requirements	Pancreatic insufficiency resulting in malabsorption, glucose intolerance/weight loss; shortness of breath makes eating difficult
4. Dysfunctional grieving	Loss of fertility/loss of independence/loss of job or role/loss of control of one's life; unhealthy grief work/withdrawal, preoccupation, sleeplessness

EXPECTED PATIENT OUTCOMES

Expected patient outcomes for the person with CF may include but are not limited to:

1. Will evidence a decreased risk for infection
1a. Will demonstrate decreased mucus in the airway
1b. Will maintain an environment free of pathogenic bacteria
1c. Will identify ways of reducing risk of infection
1d. Will verbalize knowledge of when to take influenza and pneumococcal vaccines
2. Will demonstrate improved airway clearance
2a. Will demonstrate decreased mucus production
2b. Will have clear breath sounds
2c. Will report decreased fatigue and shortness of breath
3. Will demonstrate improved nutrition
3a. Will maintain weight within 20% of ideal weight
3b. Will maintain normal blood glucose level
3c. Will eat small, frequent feedings
4. Will manifest enhanced grieving skills
4a. Will verbalize actual and potential losses
4b. Will identify own strengths and personal goals
4c. Will identify support person to assist with coping and achievement of goals

INTERVENTIONS

Because the adult with CF is most often admitted to the hospital when the airway is compromised, considerable nursing care is necessary. The care of the adult with CF centers around the following measures.

1. Decreasing Risk of Infection

Because the adult with CF is extremely vulnerable to infection, the environment should be kept as free of pathogens as possible. The patient should wash his or her own hands frequently, especially after coughing, and frequent mouth care, especially after postural drainage, should be provided. Visitors should be encouraged to wash their hands before touching the patient, and exposure to persons with upper respiratory tract infections should be minimized.

The patient's temperature should be monitored regularly, as should the color, volume, and consistency of sputum. Sputum specimens must be collected correctly and sent for culture and sensitivity as indicated. Care must be taken to administer antibiotics on time to ensure that an adequate blood level is maintained.

2. Improving Airway Clearance

The patient should be assisted with coughing, postural drainage, and percussion every 2 to 4 hours, depending on the severity of the infection. Breath sounds are auscultated before and after each treatment to determine its effectiveness. The patient is encouraged to increase fluid intake to 3 to 4 L every 24 hours unless contraindicated, and the room is kept cool, with the temperature below 21.1° C (70° F).

3. Promoting Adequate Nutrition

Because the patient with CF often has difficulty in maintaining nutrition, the nurse may need to be ingenious in promoting nutrition. Baseline and periodic assessments of nutrition, including food history, recording of daily intake and output, and recording of daily weight are performed. Blood glucose levels are monitored so that insulin can be given as prescribed according to blood glucose findings. The nurse needs to work with the dietitian and the patient to provide small, frequent feedings that are appealing to the patient. Pancreatic enzymes and vitamins are administered as ordered.

4. Helping the Patient Cope With Grief

The nurse can play a major role in helping the patient work through the grieving process by identifying the stage of grieving; allowing time for the patient to verbalize feelings, hopes, and fears; and supporting expressions of hope, but avoiding false reassurance. The nurse supports both the patient and the family through grief work and recommends CF support groups as indicated. The nurse may also refer the patient for genetic counseling, career counseling, or social services. The nurse intervenes for pathologic symptoms of grief, such as anxiety, sleeplessness, and hallucinations.

Patient/Family Education

Because the adult patient has had CF for several years, teaching is more in the form of review and reinforcement. Information to be reviewed includes:

- Daily nutrition requirements, vitamins, and the need to check weight daily
- Daily pulmonary exercises and treatments, including postural drainage and percussion, as well as use of bronchoactive medication before postural drainage
- Usual dose, expected effects, and side effects of medications
- Clinical symptoms that indicate that the health care provider should be notified, such as signs of an acute respiratory tract infection (fever, increased fatigue, shortness of breath, increased production of sputum, or change in color of sputum), hemoptysis, and sudden, sharp chest pain
- Patient's knowledge and understanding of fertility, genetic testing, and contraceptive methods
- Patient's and family's knowledge of community and social resources for assistance with health care reimbursement programs, disability insurance, and finding an appropriate support group.

Health Promotion/Prevention. Because CF is a genetically inherited disease, identification of carriers who may pass on the defect and disease to offspring remains the most important preventive strategy. Early identification of carriers combined with genetic counseling minimizes the chance of offspring inheriting this lethal genetic disease. Family histories of possible incidences of CF should be followed up by genetic testing.

EVALUATION

To evaluate the effectiveness of nursing interventions, compare patient behaviors with those listed in expected patient outcomes. Achievement of patient outcomes is successful if the patient:

1a,b,c,d. Is free of clinical signs of infection; has decreased mucus; states ways to reduce infection and verbalizes when vaccines are needed.

2a,b,c. Mobilizes secretions and clears own airway; has decreased mucus; has clear breath sounds; reports decreased fatigue and shortness of breath.

3a,b,c. Maintains adequate hydration and weight at baseline; maintains normal blood glucose level; eats small, frequent meals.

4a,b,c,e. Verbalizes feelings about disease, treatments, hospitalization, and impact on life plans; identifies strengths and goals; identifies support person(s).

GERONTOLOGIC CONSIDERATIONS

A few patients will live into the sixth or seventh decade of life. Only 50% of patients can expect to survive beyond age 30.[49]

SPECIAL ENVIRONMENTS FOR CARE

Critical Care Management

When patients with CF develop respiratory failure, they may be placed in an ICU. However, most of these patients have do-not-resuscitate (DNR) orders and are not moved to an ICU.

Home Care Management

The goal in the care of persons with CF is to care for them at home, with admission to the hospital being limited to life-threatening conditions that should respond to hospital treatment. The care discussed under Interventions would be given at home by either a family member or a nurse from a home health care agency. The Cystic Fibrosis Foundation is very helpful to patients and families in terms of supplying names of health care resources and providing support to family members who are caregivers.

COMPLICATIONS

Complications of CF include pneumothorax, hemoptysis, airway problems, GI problems, and respiratory failure. Patients with CF eventually succumb to progressive respiratory and cardiac failure. Because these patients have a fatal disease, they usually have DNR orders and are not intubated or placed on mechanical ventilation. The patient and family have to be involved in the DNR decision, and nurses play an important role in supporting the patient and family in their decision.

Pneumothorax. A pneumothorax occurs secondary to rupture of a subpleural bleb. The incidence is 1% per year but increases with age. It occurs more frequently in the right side of the chest. It should be suspected any time a patient with CF experiences the acute onset of shortness of breath, chest pain, and/or hemoptysis. When a pneumothorax occurs, a stab wound is made between the ribs, and a chest tube connected to a closed drainage system is inserted. After the lung is reexpanded, pleural sclerosis using doxycycline or talc may be induced. This procedure causes the visceral pleura to adhere to parietal pleura, obliterating the pleural space. If there is a persistent air leak or pleural sclerosis fails, a partial pleurectomy may be performed. In a partial pleurectomy the portion of the pleura overlying the cysts that ruptured is removed.

Hemoptysis. Hemoptysis occurs when a blood vessel is eroded as a result of pulmonary disease. It is more common in older CF patients and correlates with the presence of bronchiectasis. It is caused by chronic airway inflammation. Patients with large-volume hemoptysis may describe a bubbling or gurgling sensation in one area of the chest. The patient may expectorate as much as 300 to 500 ml of blood in 24 hours. The patient is very anxious and should not be left alone.

During episodes of hemoptysis the head of the bed is elevated 45 to 90 degrees, and the patient's head is turned to the left side to facilitate expectoration of blood. Tissues and an emesis basin are provided, and the basin is emptied frequently so that the patient is not made more anxious by the amount of blood. The amount of hemoptysis is measured, and the time and amount are recorded.

Hemoptysis usually subsides with conservative measures. Postural drainage and percussion are withheld during acute episodes of bleeding, usually for at least 24 hours. Vitamin K_1 (Mephyton) may be given orally or subcutaneously. Bronchoscopy with endobronchial tamponade is another option and is most successful for patients with minimal bleeding. If hemoptysis becomes life threatening, surgical intervention, such as removal of the bronchiectatic lobe, may be necessary. Unfortunately, in most patients the pulmonary disease is too extensive to permit surgery.

Airway Problems. Allergic bronchopulmonary aspergillosis is an allergic immune reaction to aspergillus organisms that is characterized by airway inflammation and edema. This complication occurs in 1% to 10% of patients with CF. It should be considered when new lung infiltrates appear on x-ray films or increased cough, respiratory distress, wheezing, and the expectoration of rusty brown plugs of sputum occur. Treatment is with corticosteroids and oral antifungal agents for several months.[24]

Gastrointestinal Problems. GI problems are common, and treatment includes vitamin and pancreatic enzyme supplements. Supplemental fat-soluble vitamins are used to aid digestion and improve weight. Most patients take multivitamins and vitamin E. Pancreatic enzyme supplement doses are individualized and titrated by patients to control fatty stools to less than three per day. Approximately 90% of patients with CF require mealtime pancreatic enzyme supplements. The number and dose is prescribed on the basis of weight gain, the presence or absence of abdominal cramping, and the number of stools. When a patient can take nothing by mouth (is NPO), minimal doses of pancreatic enzyme supplements are necessary. If adequate intake cannot be maintained orally, IV feedings or gastrostomy may be necessary.

Respiratory Failure. Respiratory failure leads to death in more than 90% of CF patients. Hypoxemia develops during exertion or sleep and progresses over years. Hypercapnia reflects severe airway obstruction. The principal mechanism underlying hypoxemia is a V/Q mismatch causing hypercapnia.

RESPIRATORY FAILURE

Etiology

Respiratory failure is impairment of the lung's ability to maintain adequate oxygen and carbon dioxide homeostasis. Analysis of ABGs and pulse oximetry are required for diagnosis. Respiratory failure is classified as acute (ARF), chronic (CRF), or acute-on-chronic (AOCF). ARF is any rapid change in respiration resulting in hypoxemia, hypercarbia, or both. It occurs over hours to days, and the term *acute respiratory failure* connotes a sense of urgency. CRF develops over months to years, allowing compensatory mechanisms to improve oxygen transport and buffer respiratory acidemia. AOCF is an ARF that is superimposed on CRF, as in a patient with COPD who experiences an acute exacerbation.

Respiratory failure may also be classified according to the underlying pathophysiology as hypoxemic respiratory failure or hypoxemic-hypercapnic respiratory failure. Patients often demonstrate characteristics of both during the course of the illness. Hypoxemic respiratory failure is characterized by a low Pa_{O_2} (less than 55 mm Hg) and a normal or low Pa_{CO_2}. It is the result of V/Q mismatch best demonstrated by ARDS. Hypoxemic-hypercapnic respiratory failure is characterized by a low Pa_{O_2} (less than 55 mm Hg) and an elevated Pa_{CO_2} (greater than 50 mm Hg). An elevated Pa_{CO_2} normally increases ventilatory drive, so this form of respiratory failure indicates that the patient is not able to sense the elevated Pa_{CO_2} (COPD) or the lungs and chest are not able to respond (parenchymal or muscular inefficiency).[10]

Epidemiology

Many disorders can lead to or are associated with respiratory failure. Some of these are listed in Table 21-15.

Pathophysiology

The respiratory system is made up of two basic parts: the gas exchange organ (the lungs) and the pump (the respiratory muscles and the respiratory control mechanisms). Any alteration in the function of the gas exchange unit or the pump can result in respiratory insufficiency or failure. Regardless of the underlying condition, the resultant events or processes that occur in respiratory failure are the same. With inadequate ventilation, the arterial oxygen falls and tissue cells become hypoxic. Carbon dioxide accumulates, leading to a fall in pH and respiratory acidosis.

ARF is defined by predetermined physiologic criteria. These criteria are sudden onset of:

- Pa_{O_2} of 50 mm Hg or less (measured on room air)
- Pa_{CO_2} of 50 mm Hg or more
- pH of 7.35 or less

Hypercapnia and hypoxemia are present in CRF. In CRF the pH usually stays within the range of 7.35 to 7.40 because of compensation. Patients with CRF develop acute-on-CRF as a result of a secondary insult to their already-compromised pulmonary system, usually in the form of a respiratory infection. The individual can no longer compensate for the altered lung function, and a dramatic decrease in pH (below 7.35), accompanied by severe hypoxemia, occurs. Because carbon

TABLE 21-15 Disorders Associated With Respiratory Failure

Pulmonary Disorders	Nonpulmonary Disorders
Severe infection Pulmonary edema Pulmonary embolism (PE) Chronic obstructive pulmonary disease (COPD) Cystic fibrosis (CF) Adult respiratory distress syndrome (ARDS) Cancer Chest trauma (flail chest) Severe atelectasis Airway compromise secondary to trauma, infection, or surgery	Central nervous system disturbance secondary to drug overdose, anesthesia, head injury Neuromuscular disorders (e.g., Guillain-Barré syndrome, myasthenia gravis, multiple sclerosis, poliomyelitis, muscular dystrophy, spinal cord injury) Postoperative reduction in ventilation following thoracic and abdominal surgery Prolonged mechanical ventilation

dioxide retention (hypercapnia) preexists in these individuals, the $PaCO_2$ is less relevant than pH and PaO_2 in determining respiratory status. In fact, these patients often display few clinical signs or symptoms, even though they may have major blood gas derangements.

Underlying blood gas alterations are the basis for the clinical signs and symptoms associated with respiratory failure. The Clinical Manifestations box identifies the common signs and symptoms associated with hypoxemia, hypercapnia, and respiratory acidosis. The signs and symptoms are presented together because the blood gas derangements causing them usually occur simultaneously.

It is important for the nurse to recognize that the signs and symptoms associated with hypoxemia and hypercapnia depend more on the rate of change in value than on absolute value. The patient with COPD may show few signs until severe ARF occurs.

Collaborative Care Management

Medical therapy is based on the severity of the failure, ventilation needs, and determination of the underlying cause.

Diagnostic Tests. Usual diagnostic tests are ABGs, chest x-ray studies, pulmonary spirometry, and sputum for culture and sensitivity. Additional tests are based on other needs the patient may develop.

Medications. The medications prescribed vary, depending on the patient's symptoms and the underlying cause.

Treatments. Oxygen therapy and support ventilation are usually prescribed. Other complications the patient experiences are treated as needed.

Diet. Diet is as tolerated. However, the patient may be NPO, depending on the acuity and severity of the respiratory failure.

Activity. Activity is usually restricted because of the respiratory difficulties.

Referrals. Referrals may be made to pulmonary specialists, social services, and respiratory therapy.

Clinical Manifestations
Respiratory Failure

SECONDARY TO HYPERCAPNIA, HYPOXEMIA, AND RESPIRATORY ACIDOSIS

Headache
Irritability
Confusion
Increasing somnolence, coma
Asterixis (flapping tremor)
Cardiac dysrhythmia
Tachycardia
Hypotension
Cyanosis

SECONDARY TO INCREASED WORK OF BREATHING

Dyspnea
Exhaustion

SECONDARY TO PRESSURE ON THE RIGHT SIDE OF THE HEART

Peripheral edema
Neck vein distention
Hepatomegaly

NURSING MANAGEMENT OF PATIENT WITH RESPIRATORY FAILURE

ASSESSMENT

Health History

Data to be collected to assess the patient with respiratory insufficiency or failure include:

History of past or present associated disorders, recent change in respiratory status, change in sputum (color, viscosity, odor), increased dyspnea, change in mental status, complaints of chest tightness or pain

Current medications and any recent changes in medication regimen

Self-care modalities used

If available, a family member or friend may be able to provide objective information about changes in the patient.

Physical Examination

Important aspects of the physical examination of the patient in respiratory failure include:

Assessment of general appearance

Assessment of mental status, which may vary from agitation to somnolence

Measurement of vital signs to identify tachycardia, tachypnea, bradypnea, or apnea (respiratory rates less than 8/min result in alveolar hypoventilation; rates over 35/min cannot be sustained), hypotension, or other abnormality

Pulmonary examination, the extent of which will depend on what the patient can tolerate (Findings will depend on the underlying cause of respiratory failure.)

Relevant laboratory studies include ABGs for blood gas derangements associated with ARF, as well as sputum culture and sensitivity, and bedside spirometry typically shows a VC less than 15 ml/kg ideal body weight.

NURSING DIAGNOSES

Nursing diagnoses are determined from analysis of patient data. Nursing diagnoses for the person with respiratory failure may include but are not limited to:

Diagnostic Title	Possible Etiologic Factors
1. Impaired gas exchange	V/Q imbalance
2. Ineffective airway clearance	Fatigue, tracheobronchial infection, airway obstruction
3. Decreased cardiac output	Increased pulmonary vascular resistance
4. Imbalanced nutrition: less than body requirements	Unable to maintain intake large enough to balance increased metabolic needs from increased work of breathing

EXPECTED PATIENT OUTCOMES

Expected patient outcomes for the person with respiratory failure may include but are not limited to:

1. Will demonstrate improved ventilation and oxygenation
   - 1a. PaO_2, $PaCO_2$, and pH will be within acceptable baseline limits
   - 1b. Sensorium will return to or be maintained at pre–respiratory failure level
   - 1c. Respiratory rate will be within or near normal levels, with moderate tidal volume
   - 1d. Dyspnea will be absent or will return to pre–acute illness level
2. Will demonstrate effective airway clearance
   - 2a. Will use effective coughing maneuvers
   - 2b. Breath sounds will be clear or at baseline level
   - 2c. Will use nebulizers, MDIs, and humidifiers appropriately
3. Will maintain adequate cardiac output
   - 3a. Blood pressure will remain within acceptable limits
   - 3b. Heart rate and rhythm will remain within acceptable limits
   - 3c. Pulses will be equal and present in all extremities
   - 3d. Urine output will be greater than 30 ml/hr
4. Will maintain nutritional intake adequate to balance metabolic needs
   - 4a. Weight will stabilize at preacute illness weight
   - 4b. If preillness weight is outside acceptable limits for size and age, weight will progress toward an established goal weight

INTERVENTIONS

The level of nursing interventions for ARF depends on the patient's immediate status. The patient's condition may vary from critically ill, requiring immediate life support measures (cardiopulmonary resuscitation), to less urgent, in which aggressive nursing interventions can prevent further deterioration of physical status.

1. Improving Gas Exchange

Severe hypoxemia is incompatible with life. Thus it is imperative to initiate oxygen therapy rapidly if severe hypoxemia is present. The effectiveness of oxygen therapy is evaluated with ABG measurements and pulse oximetry. Supplemental oxygen should be provided to maintain a PaO_2 of 60 to 90 mm Hg. Persons without underlying pulmonary disease can receive oxygen by either high-flow or low-flow systems. However, hazards are associated with prolonged exposure to high concentrations of oxygen.

Oxygen toxicity is the term used to describe the damage to lung tissue that results from prolonged exposure to high oxygen concentrations. Although the exact effects of oxygen in any one individual may depend on the person's underlying pathologic condition, exposure to greater than 60% oxygen for more than 36 hours or exposure to 90% oxygen for more than 6 hours may result in atelectasis and alveolar collapse. Breathing very high concentrations of oxygen (80% to 100%) for prolonged periods (24 hours or more) is often associated with the development of ARDS. Thus a firm general principle is to use the lowest amount of oxygen necessary to achieve an acceptable PaO_2.

Special precautions must be taken when administering oxygen to patients with COPD who are carbon dioxide retainers to avoid further elevation of their $PaCO_2$ levels, resulting in carbon dioxide narcosis or coma. Patients with COPD (who are carbon dioxide retainers) must receive supplemental oxygen via a controlled oxygen therapy system. The preferred mode is a nasal cannula or Venturi mask. A nasal cannula has the advantage of allowing the patient to talk, eat, and drink. However, the actual concentration of oxygen delivered to the lungs by cannula depends on the patient's ventilatory pattern. The Venturi mask provides oxygen at controlled ranges of 24% to 40% (Figure 21-21) but may be poorly tolerated. Regardless of the oxygen delivery system used, the patient's response to oxygen therapy can be accurately assessed only by ABG measurements or pulse oximetry. The goal is to achieve a PaO_2 of 60 mm Hg, which allows an arterial saturation of 90% or greater.

Adequate oxygenation is essential for life. Therefore if adequate oxygenation cannot be maintained without a concurrent rise in $PaCO_2$ (hypercapnia), oxygen therapy must be provided by alternative delivery modes. Although carbon dioxide narcosis might be precipitated if a chronically hypoxemic person receives high concentrations of oxygen, treatment of the hypoxemia is the first priority in the patient's care.

Mechanical Ventilation

When respiratory failure progresses despite medical therapy, mechanical ventilation often becomes necessary.

The goals of mechanical ventilation are to correct potentially life-threatening blood gas and acid-base abnormalities; provide support during bronchoactive pharmacologic therapy; and rest the muscles of respiration, allowing them to recover from fatigue. In respiratory failure, adjustments are made to the ventilator to promote respiratory muscle rest.

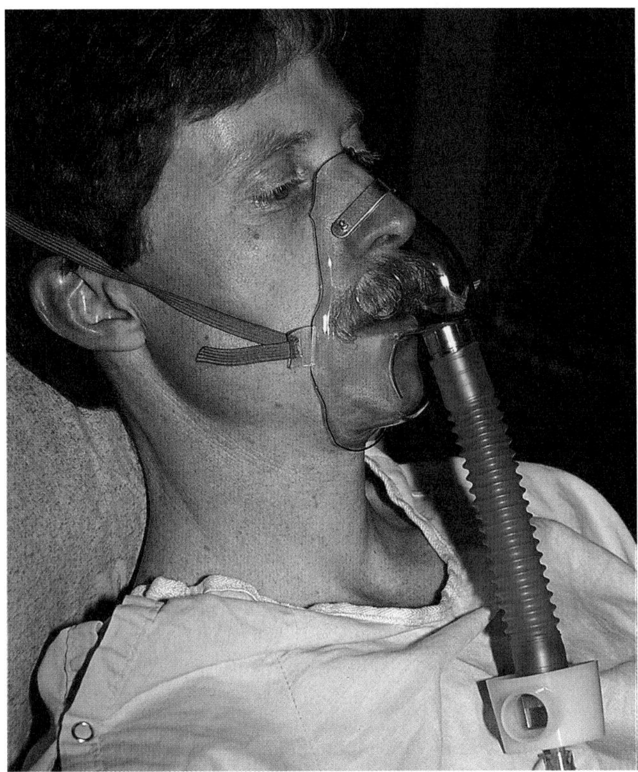

Figure 21-21 Venturi mask.

Respiratory muscles require 48 to 72 hours to achieve full recovery. Rest can be achieved in any mode of ventilation as long as settings are chosen to minimize patient effort. Mechanical ventilation can be provided noninvasively by face or nasal mask or by intubation.

Noninvasive Modes. Noninvasive mechanical ventilation (NIV) is the delivery of mechanical ventilation without the use of an invasive airway. It is becoming the treatment of choice for respiratory failure, although the specific indications are still somewhat controversial. The methods include negative-pressure ventilation and nasal and face mask intermittent positive-pressure ventilation (IPPV). Most centers use a face or nasal mask and pressure support ventilation (PSV), also called noninvasive positive-pressure ventilation (NPPV). Ventilation is delivered via a volume- or pressure-cycled ventilator or a continuous positive airway pressure (CPAP) or bilevel positive airway pressure (BiPAP) ventilation device. A tight-fitting mask allows ventilatory assistance and provides for brief periods off the ventilator, during which the patient can speak, inhale nebulized medications, expectorate, and swallow liquids. NIV methods may be used for up to 1 week. They have been effective in relieving symptoms, decreasing respiratory rate, increasing tidal volume, improving gas exchange, decreasing the length of the hospital stay, and decreasing in-house mortality.[35] Complications are few compared with other methods of ventilatory support and include local skin breakdown and aspiration; also, some patients cannot tolerate the mask.

With NIV the positive pressure is applied during the patient's inspiration via IPPV or PSV or throughout the respiratory cycle at a constant pressure (CPAP). The NPPV may also be set to different levels during patient inspiration and expiration through the use of BiPAP. These positive-pressure modes reduce the work of breathing, decrease respiratory muscle fatigue, and increase minute ventilation. NIV requires an alert, cooperative, hemodynamically stable patient. Relative contraindications include the presence of copious secretions, aspiration risk, and impaired mental status. This approach to ventilatory support requires careful attention to a properly fitting mask and time from the clinician(s) to stay with the patient to explain the device, titrate pressures, troubleshoot problems, and provide support and ongoing close assessment.[10]

Intubation. If the patient with respiratory failure is not a candidate for NIV or if NIV is not maintaining adequate ventilation, intubation is required for mechanical ventilation.

Ventilator Modes. Ventilator modes determine whether breaths are controlled by the machine and, if so, how many, or whether breaths are to some degree controlled by patient effort with assistance from the machine. The most common modes are assist/control (A/C), synchronized intermittent mandatory ventilation (SIMV), and CPAP.

In the A/C mode the ventilator senses each time the patient begins to inspire and delivers a breath. If the patient is unable to trigger the machine, the ventilator delivers the preset number of breaths at the set tidal volume. The A/C mode is also called continuous mechanical ventilation (CMV) and gives the patient complete ventilatory support. This mode is the most frequently used in respiratory failure to ensure respiratory muscle rest. Tidal volumes of 5 to 7 ml/kg are used with respiratory rates of 20 to 24.

SIMV allows the patient to take additional breaths over the set rate of the ventilator. The volume of extra breaths is determined by the patient's ability and effort to breathe spontaneously. In SIMV the number of ventilator breaths can be gradually reduced until the patient is breathing on his or her own.

In the CPAP mode the machine delivers a set airway pressure throughout inspiration and exhalation and the patient determines respiratory rate, tidal volume, inspiratory flow, and inspiratory time. Additional pressure can be added to assist the inspiratory muscles. A summary of ventilator modes is presented in Table 21-16.

Different kinds of ventilators are available to deliver these modes (Table 21-17; Figures 21-22 and 21-23). In adults there are two basic types: pressure-cycled and volume-limited ventilators. Volume-cycled ventilators are used most often. With a volume-cycled machine a constant volume of air is delivered with each breath. The volume is preset and delivered to the patient at whatever pressure is necessary to attain that volume. A volume-cycled machine should have a pressure cutoff valve. Such a mechanism allows a pressure limit to be set. If the pressure required to deliver the set volume exceeds the pressure limit, the machine will turn off before the entire volume is delivered. The pressure limit on a volume-cycled machine usually has an audible alarm. The nurse can set the limit slightly

TABLE 21-16 Ventilator Modes

Assist/control (A/C)	Each breath is ventilator assisted. If patient is unable to trigger machine, the ventilator continues to deliver preset number of breaths at the set tidal volume.
Bilevel CPAP (BiPAP)	Positive pressure applied to spontaneous breathing, allowing inspiratory positive pressure and expiratory positive pressure to be set independently.
Continuous positive airway pressure (CPAP)	Positive pressure applied during respiration and maintained throughout entire respiratory cycle. Decreases intrapulmonary shunting.
Controlled mandatory ventilation (CMV)	Ventilator delivers a preset volume at a fixed rate regardless of patient's effort to breathe.
Independent lung ventilation (ILV)	Each lung is ventilated separately. Used in unilateral lung disease. Requires intubation with double-lumen tube.
Intermittent mandatory ventilation (IMV)	Ventilator delivers preset number of breaths. Patient may take unassisted breaths.
Positive end-expiratory pressure (PEEP)	Applies positive pressure at end of expiration. Decreases intrapulmonic shunting.
Pressure support ventilation (PSV)	Selected amount of positive pressure applied to airway during patient's spontaneous respiratory efforts. Amount of pressure gradually reduced until patient is receiving no assistance.
Synchronized intermittent mandatory ventilation (SIMV)	Intermittent ventilator breaths synchronized with patient's spontaneous breaths. Reduces competition between patient and ventilator.
High-frequency ventilation	Special positive-pressure ventilator used in some patients.
High-Frequency Ventilators	
High-frequency positive-pressure ventilation (HFPPV)	Extremely short inspiratory times with a total volume equivalent to dead space. Rate 60-100 cycles/min.
High-frequency jet ventilation (HFJV)	Small volumes less than anatomic dead space are pulsed through jet injector catheter at 100-600 cycles/min.
High-frequency oscillation ventilation (HFO)	Small volume of gas is continuously vibrated in airways at rates up to 4000 cycles/min.

Adapted from Stillwell SB: *Mosby's critical care nursing reference,* ed 2, St Louis, 1996, Mosby.

TABLE 21-17 Types of Mechanical Ventilators

Types		Basic Function Mode
Positive-pressure ventilator	Require intubation	Types of positive-pressure ventilators are based on how inspiratory phase is ended.
Pressure-cycled ventilator	Require intubation	Inspiration ends at a preset pressure limit; time and volume are variable.
Time-cycled ventilator	Require intubation	Inspiration is preset for a given time interval; volume and pressure are variable.
Volume-cycled ventilator	Require intubation	Preset volume of air is delivered. Time and pressure are variable. However, volume-cycled ventilators often have pressure- and time-cycled capacities.
Negative-pressure ventilator (intubation not required)		Thorax, at least, is encapsulated. When ventilator expands, it creates negative pressure by pulling the thorax outward. Air rushes into the airways because of the pressure gradient created.
High-frequency ventilation (requires intubation)		There are several variants of this system. All high-frequency ventilators use high respiratory rates to deliver small tidal volumes at low pressures.

above the pressure required to ventilate the patient (approximately 5 cm of water). The alarm will then go off if the patient coughs, accumulates secretions, or starts to resist the machine. Box 21-7 describes the functionality of the volume-cycled ventilator.

Pressure-cycled ventilators deliver a volume of gas to the airway using positive pressure during inspiration. The positive pressure is delivered until the preselected pressure has been reached; the machine then cycles off. Exhalation occurs passively. The disadvantage of pressure-cycled ventilators is that a varying tidal volume may be delivered as a result of changes in airway resistance or compliance.

Suctioning the Patient. When the patient on a ventilator needs suctioning, a closed system is preferred. In closed-system endotracheal suctioning, an adaptor is inserted at the endotracheal tube–ventilatory circuitry interface. This allows

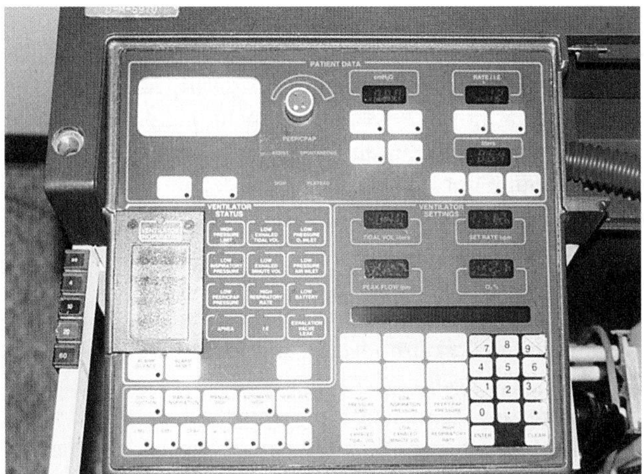

Figure 21-22 Front display panel of a ventilator for monitoring airway pressures and volumes.

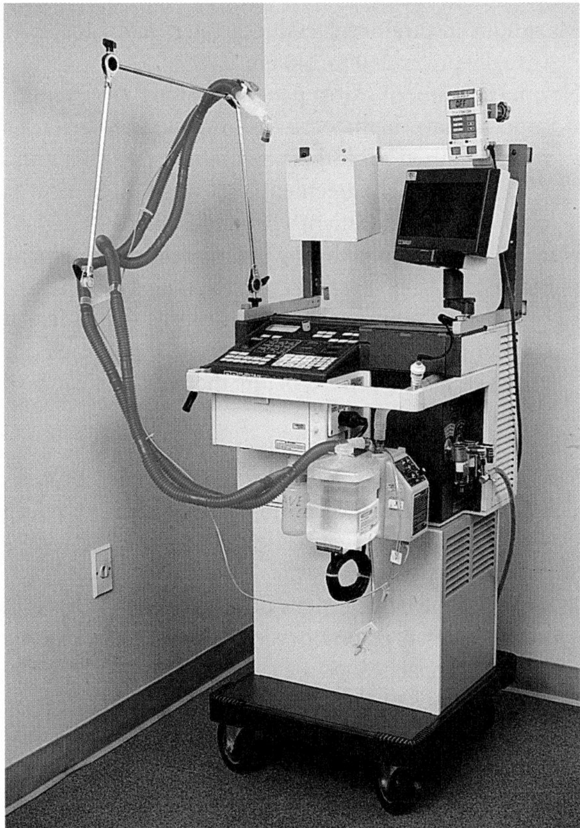

Figure 21-23 Mechanical ventilator.

patients to be suctioned without disconnecting them from the ventilator. The benefits of this form of suctioning are (1) continuation of the oxygen supply, (2) the stability of PEEP, and (3) a reduced incidence of ventilator-assisted pneumonia. See the Guidelines for Safe Practice box for the steps in closed-system suctioning. Also see Figure 21-24.

General Care of the Patient on a Ventilator. When care is planned for the patient on a mechanical ventilator, knowing the patient's ability to breathe spontaneously in the event of

BOX 21-7 Functions That Can Be Adjusted with Volume-Cycled Ventilators

Tidal volume: volume of air in a normal breath
FiO_2: oxygenation concentration delivered through the ventilator
Alarm systems: vary from machine to machine; basic alarms usually present
- High-pressure alarm: increased resistance somewhere in system from lungs to machine
- Low-pressure alarm: system not reaching minimal pressure required for ventilation
- Low-volume alarm: when volume of ventilation does not equal the amount set

Control modes: degree of ventilation that is controlled by the ventilator; can vary from complete ventilator control to almost total patient control

Guidelines for Safe Practice

Closed-System Suctioning

1. Wash hands for 10 seconds as recommended by the Centers for Disease Control and Prevention (CDC).
2. Glove.
3. Select a catheter that is one half the diameter of the artificial airway. The catheter has a suction valve at one end, a patient connector at the other end, and is enclosed in a plastic sheath.
4. Attach suction valve to suction source. Select suction pressure between −80 mm Hg and −120 mm Hg. Set maximum pressure by pinching suction tubing closed.
5. Attach patient connector to ventilator tubing and the endotracheal tube (ET).
6. Use the ventilator to hyperoxygenate and hyperinflate the patient's lungs before suctioning.
7. Open access valve and advance catheter through the connector into the ET and trachea.
8. Using the suction valve, apply suction for not more than 10 seconds as the catheter is withdrawn. Repeat as necessary.
9. Provide 100% oxygen and deep breaths while suctioning.
10. Withdraw catheter and close access valve.
11. Clean suction tip by attaching a normal saline unit-dose vial or syringe containing normal saline to irrigation port. Squirt the saline on the catheter tip and apply suction until the catheter is clean and saline is sucked out of the catheter.
12. Remove gloves and wash hands for 10 seconds.

accidental disconnection from the ventilator is imperative. In most facilities respiratory therapists regularly monitor ventilator function and settings, but the nurse is also responsible for ensuring that the ventilator settings are maintained. Usually a checklist is used to verify the ventilator settings on an hourly basis.

The patient should be assessed on a regular basis and any time a ventilator alarm sounds. The cause of an alarm sounding can be a dysfunction anywhere from the person's lungs to the machine. Troubleshooting should be carried out in a systematic manner, starting with the patient and moving toward the machine. Assessment should include:

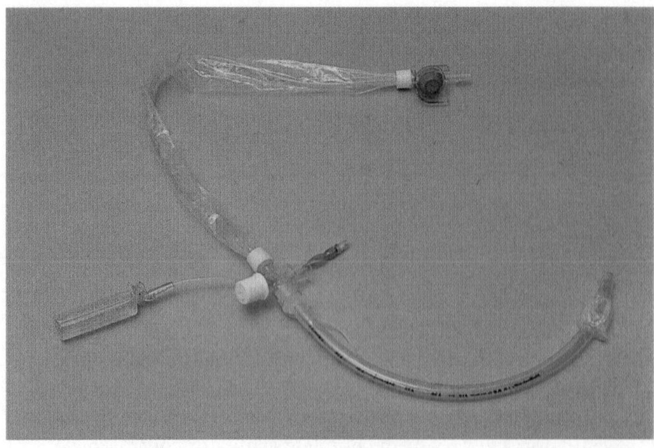

Figure 21-24 Closed-system suctioning tube.

Patient assessment

Inspection

Does the person appear to be in respiratory distress?

Is the person's chest moving with machine-cycled inspiration?

Is the chest moving bilaterally?

Auscultation

Are breath sounds present?

Are adventitious sounds present?

Are breath sounds coordinated with ventilator inspiration?

Assessment of tubing to machine: inspection

Is there an air leak around the endotracheal cuff?

Is there excess condensation in the tubing? (Always remove water from the tubing system. Do not empty back into the humidifier reservoir.) NOTE: Not all ventilators have humidifiers.

Check all ventilator settings and readouts.

If the alarm continues to sound and the cause cannot be determined or the patient is in respiratory distress, the patient is disconnected from the machine and manually ventilated with an Ambu bag (or anesthesia bag) with oxygenated air until the problem can be resolved.

Patients who have a prolonged course of mechanical ventilation need to be evaluated for tracheostomy. If a course of mechanical ventilation is projected to go beyond 2 weeks, a tracheostomy is usually placed for patient comfort and communication and to avoid the complications associated with prolonged endotracheal tube placement.

Weaning From the Ventilator. Prolonged mechanical ventilation is dangerous and expensive. The incidence of pneumonia increases with each day on mechanical ventilation. Most patients can be extubated once the precipitating cause of ARF resolves and the patient is medically stable. The decision to wean a person from the ventilator is based on clinical evidence of improved physical status. Weaning is most successful when it is planned by the health care team in partnership with the patient. Weaning protocols are used in a number of settings and are overseen by clinicians highly skilled in the art of weaning.

Some nurse experts divide the weaning process into three phases: preweaning, weaning, and extubation. During the preweaning stage, special attention is given to ensuring that the patient has normal electrolytes, including phosphate, calcium, and magnesium. Malnutrition is to be avoided, but the patient should not be overfed. Overfeeding with carbohydrates and extra calories may result in increased carbon dioxide production and increased ventilatory demand. The recommended 24-hour caloric intake is 1500 to 2500 calories, which should ensure adequate calories for energy expenditure. Protein intake is important, and 1 to 1.5 mg/kg has been suggested. Tube feedings containing these requirements are given to prepare the patient for weaning.

Weaning is initiated when the patient meets certain physiologic criteria. These are:

Acceptable ABGs

Tidal volume greater than 10 ml/kg

VC greater than 15 ml/kg

FiO_2 less than 0.5

Maximum inspiratory pressure greater than 220 cm H_2O (usually prefer 230 to 240 cm H_2O)

Normal hematocrit (Most patients on long-term ventilator support have hematocrits below 30. They are usually not transfused until their hematocrit falls to about 25. There is general agreement that weaning is most successful when the patient's hematocrit is 30 or higher.)

Nursing interventions during the weaning process include:

Before initiating weaning, prepare the patient. Teach effective breathing techniques. Inform the patient that weaning may require several attempts, each for a longer period of time, before the ventilator can be disconnected.

Obtain baseline vital signs, tidal volume, and VC.

Stay with the patient during the initial weaning process.

Coach the patient as needed to breathe slower and deeper, with emphasis on increasing the time of exhalation.

Suction as needed.

Monitor for the clinical signs of hypoxemia and hypercapnia (increased respiratory rate, tachycardia, dysrhythmias, increased blood pressure, agitation, diaphoresis, or increased somnolence).

If the patient cannot breathe on his or her own, reconnect to the ventilator.

The weaning process is individualized to meet the patient's needs. The three most common methods of weaning are T-piece weaning, SIMV weaning, and PSV weaning.

For T-piece weaning, the patient is placed in an upright position and disconnected from the ventilator, and a T-piece is connected to the endotracheal tube cuff to provide oxygenated humidified air. The patient is observed for signs of respiratory distress and is reconnected to the ventilator when he or she indicates fatigue. Some patients may be able to breathe for only a few minutes on their own; others may do well for 30 minutes. Time off the ventilator is gradually increased. With SIMV weaning, the patient remains connected to the ventilator. The number of synchronized mandatory breaths delivered by the machine is gradually reduced, allowing the patient to take an increasing number of breaths independently. The patient is disconnected from the ventilator when predetermined physiologic criteria are maintained. With PSV weaning, the patient also remains connected to the ventilator, and the level of preset positive pressure during inspiration is gradually reduced until the patient is receiving no assistance. This mode helps reduce airflow resistance of artificial airways, making breathing easier.

Noninvasive ventilation modes are being used more often in weaning protocols. Patients who are able to breathe comfortably after weaning and have satisfactory ABGs are extubated. Some patients may receive supplemental oxygen by face mask for 24 hours. The patient is observed closely for signs of respiratory distress and increased efforts to breathe (e.g., respirations less than 8/min or more than 30/min; increase in respiratory rate of 10 or more from starting rate; increase or decrease in heart rate by 20 beats/min; increase or decrease in blood pressure by 20 mm Hg; decrease in PaO_2 or increase in $PaCO_2$; or pH less than 7.35). If a patient develops respiratory distress, reintubation may be necessary.

Patients who have a projected course of mechanical ventilation beyond 2 weeks usually have a tracheostomy done to facilitate comfort and communication, and to avoid complications from the endotracheal tube. Patients with a prolonged course may be transferred to a transitional ventilator unit for specialized but less intensive care.

Failure to Wean Successfully. Some patients cannot be weaned from a ventilator. Reasons include underlying obstructive lung disease, severe chest wall deformities, neuromuscular disease, and patients with prolonged hospitalizations secondary to multisystem organ failure. Additional factors that have been shown to contribute to weaning failure include malnutrition, recurrent aspiration, electrolyte abnormalities, occult infection, and steroid myopathy.[56]

Because of the number of patients who require long-term ventilatory support and thus may be difficult to wean, the North American Nursing Diagnosis Association (NANDA) has approved two new nursing diagnoses: dysfunctional ventilatory weaning response and impaired spontaneous ventilation. Dysfunctional ventilatory weaning response is divided into three types: mild, moderate, and severe. Impaired spontaneous ventilation has two categories: major and minor. With either of the diagnoses, related factors are noted. For dysfunctional ventilatory weaning response, the related factors are pathophysiologic, such as muscle weakness; situational, such as fear of separation from the ventilator; and treatment errors, such as rushing the weaning process. Related factors for impaired spontaneous ventilation include physiologic, such as respiratory muscle fatigue, and psychosocial, such as depression.[11]

Care of the Patient Who Cannot Be Weaned. Patients who require prolonged mechanical ventilation may be cared for in a specialized respiratory unit of a hospital or long-term care facility or at home. Chronic ventilator units have a larger nurse-patient ratio than critical care units. Thus the patient's acute care needs must be resolved before transfer. These units usually continue weaning efforts, often using a slower, more individualized approach. Few patients find it possible to go home on a ventilator, because of the lack of suitable space and the lack of a significant other who can assume responsibility for the ventilator 24 hours a day for 7 days a week. If the patient and significant others decide that the patient will be discharged home, careful planning is required to ensure that the home can accommodate the patient and the necessary equipment. The assessment of the home is best made by a nurse from the health care agency that will be following the patient and monitoring care at home.

Patients and families also have the option of choosing to be taken off the ventilator. Once the patient indicates that this is his or her choice, the care team meets to discuss how the patient's wishes can best be accommodated. To ease the patient's anxiety, sedation, usually a morphine infusion, is started before the ventilator is disconnected. A comfort measures–only approach to care is then adopted. Hospice involvement is encouraged.

Additional Interventions for Improving Gas Exchange

Nursing interventions for patients in ARF must be implemented in a firm but empathetic manner. The patient may be agitated or nearly exhausted from hypoxemia, hypercapnia, and the increased work of breathing. It is imperative that the patient be gently guided in respiratory maneuvers to improve breathing. The nurse must be alert for signs and symptoms indicating that the patient's condition has changed from acutely ill but adequately ventilating to critically ill with insufficient ventilation to maintain body functions. Nursing interventions include:

- Frequent assessment of respiratory status, vital signs, level of consciousness, tolerance of ventilatory support, ventilator settings
- Facilitation of use of controlled breathing techniques
- Review of pertinent laboratory data, especially electrolytes, hematocrit
- Judicious administration of analgesia, especially opiates

2. Improving Airway Clearance

Airways clogged with excess mucus are one of the most reversible precipitating components of ARF. Causes of mucus clogging are many, and positive-pressure ventilation itself may contribute to increased mucus production. Monitoring is basic to effective intervention, and patients' breath sounds need to be auscultated at least every 1 to 2 hours in the acute phase of respiratory failure. Nursing interventions designed to promote airway clearance include helping patients to cough effectively using the huff technique; changing the patient's position every 2 hours; elevating the patient's head and chest; guiding the patient in frequent deep breathing exercises or using the sigh mechanism on the ventilator; encouraging the patient to be out of bed as tolerated; and promoting sufficient fluid intake to mobilize secretions (3 to 4 L, unless contraindicated, has traditionally been encouraged, but some evidence suggests that this quantity may not be needed). In addition, humidification of the airway is maintained to further help liquefy secretions, and nasotracheal suctioning is done if the patient is unable to cough effectively.

3. Improving Cardiac Output

Decreased cardiac output may be a complication of ARF or may be a precipitating factor related to underlying cor pulmonale. Diminished cardiac output causes tissue hypoxia, which creates a metabolic acidosis in addition to the respiratory acidosis caused by the respiratory failure. Thus vital signs and hemodynamic parameters (arterial, central venous, pulmonary, and left atrial pressures) must be assessed at least every hour during the acute phase of respiratory failure. In addition, the patient must be monitored for signs of inadequate tissue perfusion (urine output less than 30 ml/hr, cool extremities with decreased peripheral pulses) and for cardiac arrhythmias.

4. Maintaining Adequate Nutrition

Individuals with ARF are at increased risk for nutritional deficits because of the increased work of breathing. The overall focus of nutritional interventions is to prevent or correct malnutrition. Nutritional intake affects ventilatory drive, respiratory muscle function, and the amount of oxygen consumed and carbon dioxide produced from metabolic processes. Nutritional status can have a major impact on the individual's ability to be successfully weaned from the ventilator. Actions must focus on providing appropriate nutrition to meet the patient's specific metabolic needs while on the ventilator and during and after weaning from it. Nutritional support by either enteral supplementation or parenteral hyperalimentation may be necessary. Whenever feasible, the enteral route should be used because it poses fewer risks and is more economical. It is advisable to supply at least 50% of total calories in the form of lipids to minimize high levels of carbon dioxide production.

Patient/Family Education

The patient and family are kept apprised of the patient's status and all procedures and treatments that are instituted.

Health Promotion/Prevention. Prevention of respiratory failure is focused on early identification of persons at high risk for developing ARF. In the inpatient setting, a preventive plan of care should be developed for every person with an increased risk of developing respiratory failure. A preventive plan of care should include the following actions:

Keeping the airway clear by instituting regularly performed deep breathing and coughing maneuvers and using nasotracheal suctioning if necessary
Maintaining an optimal activity level
Using sedatives or analgesics judiciously
Assessing regularly for signs and symptoms indicating deterioration of respiratory status

EVALUATION

To evaluate the effectiveness of nursing interventions, compare patient behaviors with those listed in the expected patient outcomes. Achievement of patient outcomes is successful if the patient:

1. Demonstrates improved ventilation and oxygenation.
1a. PaO_2, $PaCO_2$, and pH have returned to baseline level.
1b. Level of consciousness is at baseline.
1c. Verbalizes how and when to use oxygen therapy (when exercising; when feeling very fatigued).
1d. Dyspnea is greatly improved.
2. Demonstrates effective airway clearance.
2a. Coughs effectively and does not tire self with ineffective coughing.
2b. Respiratory rate and depth has returned to baseline level.
2c. Uses inhaler correctly.
3. Maintains adequate cardiac output.
3a. Has stable blood pressure.
3b. Has heart rate and rhythm within acceptable limits.
3c. Has pulses that are equal and present in all extremities.
3d. Has urine output of at least 30 ml/hr or that has returned to baseline level.
4. Maintains nutritional intake adequate to balance metabolic needs
4a. Has weight that is returning to preacute illness level.
4b. Has weight that is progressing to an established goal weight.

GERONTOLOGIC CONSIDERATIONS

Care for older adults with respiratory failure is similar to that for older adults with COPD.

SPECIAL ENVIRONMENTS FOR CARE

Critical Care Management

The patient with respiratory failure requires care in an ICU or transitional ventilator unit.

Home Care Management

The patient who requires prolonged ventilator support may be discharged home on ventilator support if a family caregiver is willing to accept the responsibility for the patient's care. Before the patient can be discharged, the designated caregiver must be taught basic skills by the hospital nursing staff. These skills include clean technique for tracheostomy care and for suctioning; cuff management; tracheostomy tube changing; how to recognize breathing problems; medications; and ADLs.

The home ventilator company is contacted as soon as the decision is made to discharge the patient. The home ventilator company reviews the financial obligations of the patient and family for home ventilation care; investigates the patient's insurance coverage; and evaluates the patient's home to determine if a ventilator and other electrical equipment can be operated safely.

The home ventilator company is asked to deliver a portable ventilator and suction machine to the hospital and coordinate ventilator instruction time with the patient, family, and nurse. The ventilator company is responsible for instruction on the safe use, setup, maintenance, and troubleshooting of the ventilator, circuits, oxygen, and suction machine; home visits by respiratory therapists for equipment evaluation, cleaning, and maintenance; written reports to the patient's physician about results of home visits; backup equipment service 24 hours a day, 7 days per week; and notification of the fire department, electric company, police, and ambulance service about the patient's arrival home and potential need for their services.

The nurse from the home health agency evaluates the patient's home nursing requirements and insurance coverage for home nursing visits, home health aides, and physical and occupational therapy.

The diagnosis-related group (DRG) for ventilator-dependent patients is 30 days. This amount of time allows for the teaching and supervised practice of the designated caregiver and other family members with the ventilator and suction machine that go home with the patient. The caregiver must also become certified in cardiopulmonary resuscitation (CPR) before the patient can be discharged.

COMPLICATIONS

Complications of respiratory failure and mechanical ventilation include impaired gas exchange from a plugged tube, kinked tube, or cuff herniation; fluid volume excess; electrolyte imbalance; stress ulcer and GI bleeding; infection; increased intracranial pressure secondary to altered cerebral perfusion; tissue hypoxia; and cardiopulmonary arrest.

One-year survival following respiratory failure is 28% to 72%. The prognosis is best for those with hyphoscoliosis or neuromuscular disease and worst for those with pneumoconiosis and pulmonary fibrosis. Men with COPD who require mechanical ventilation have a survival rate of about 50% at 1 year.[41]

PULMONARY VASCULAR DISEASES

PULMONARY EMBOLISM AND PULMONARY INFARCTION

Etiology

Pulmonary embolism (PE) is not a disease per se; it is a complication of venous thrombosis. PE is caused by the lodging of a clot or clots in a pulmonary arterial vessel. Commonly the clot is from a deep vein thrombosis (DVT). Pulmonary emboli can cause massive occlusion of a major part of the pulmonary circulation and may be chronic or recurrent. Pulmonary infarction results when an embolus is large enough to interfere with the blood supply to a part of lung tissue, causing necrosis of lung parenchyma. Embolism without infarction occurs when the embolus does not cause permanent lung injury.

Epidemiology

Emboli rarely occur without the presence of certain risk factors, although in some cases it may be difficult to identify the cause (see Risk Factors box). Pulmonary emboli result from damage to blood vessel walls (surgery, trauma), blood stasis (varicosities), or hypercoaguability of blood (estrogen therapy). They are the most common cause of acute pulmonary disease in hospitalized patients, cause 100,000 deaths yearly, and are thought to contribute to another 100,000 deaths each year. Interestingly, the trend toward early discharge has been accompanied by an increased incidence of postdischarge venous thromboembolism. Thromboembolic risk does not end at discharge.[54] About 50% of the deaths from PE occur within 2 hours of the event, and the PE is often undetected.

Pathophysiology

Emboli travel from their site of origin through the right side of the heart and lodge in the pulmonary vasculature. The size of the pulmonary artery and the number of emboli determine the severity of symptoms. Blood flow is obstructed, causing localized tissue hypoxia and ultimately a decrease in the pulmonary vascular bed. Pulmonary vessels vasoconstrict in response to the hypoxia. The resultant V/Q inequality (ventilation greater than perfusion) causes arterial hypoxemia. The pathophysiology and clinical picture of a patient with PE are presented in Table 21-18.

If the embolus blocks a larger vessel, the person may complain of sudden dyspnea, sharp upper abdominal or thoracic pain, and cough, and may have hemoptysis; shock may develop rapidly. If the area of infarction is smaller, the symptoms are much milder. The patient may have dyspnea, unexplained tachypnea, cough, pleuritic chest pain, slight hemoptysis, tachycardia, elevation of temperature, and an increased leukocyte count. An area of dullness or crackles may be detected when checking breath sounds.

Collaborative Care Management

Diagnostic Tests. The diagnosis of PE is not easy to make. Clinical history, changes in blood chemistries, and plain chest x-ray films are often not definitive in establishing the diagnosis. Pulmonary angiography is the ultimate standard diagnostic test for PE because an abrupt cutoff of a vessel or a filling defect indicates the presence of an embolus. However, V/Q scanning is the recommended first test when PE is suspected because of the exclusionary value of a normal scan. High-probability scans have 87% specificity and sensitivity. Low-probability and intermediate probability scan results indicate that more testing is needed. V/Q scanning is not a helpful diagnostic tool for patients with COPD.

D-dimer is a relatively new test used in the diagnosis of PE, and its sensitivity is still being reviewed.[43] The advantage of this test is that it is safe, noninvasive, rapid, and inexpensive. It measures fibrin cross-links that are cleaved and released into

Risk Factors

Pulmonary Emboli

Thrombophlebitis (deep vein thrombosis)
Immobility
Recent surgery (especially orthopedic or gynecologic)
Obesity
Congestive heart failure/myocardial infarction
Recent fracture
Estrogen therapy (oral contraceptives)
Pregnancy

TABLE 21-18 Normal Function, Primary Pathophysiology, and Clinical Manifestations of Pulmonary Embolism

Normal Function	Pathophysiology	Clinical Manifestations
Pulmonary Vasculature		
Carry venous blood received from right side of heart to alveolocapillary membrane in lung for oxygen–carbon dioxide exchange	Occlusion of pulmonary vessels because of increased vascular resistance, decreased cardiac output (usually occurs only in massive emboli), decreased lung perfusion	Elevated pulmonary artery pressure Dyspnea Hypotension Tachycardia High ventilation-perfusion ($\dot{V}/\dot{Q}$) ratio as shown on lung scan Hypocapnia and elevated arterial blood pH
Airways		
Carry oxygenated air to alveolocapillary membrane for exchange and deoxygenated air out of lung	Airway constriction from lowered alveolar carbon dioxide levels	Underventilated lung areas as shown on lung scan Hypoxemia Tachypnea Cough
Alveoli		
Lung site where gas exchange takes place (alveolocapillary membrane)	Infarction of alveolar tissues caused by complete obstruction, resulting in extravasation of blood cells into alveoli (NOTE: Occurs only in more severe cases)	Hemoptysis Radiologic opacity
Pleura		
Maintain close approximation of lungs and chest wall Minimize friction during lung expansion and contraction	Transudate from damaged vascular structures (pleural effusion)	Pleural friction rub Chest pain during inhalation/exhalation

the circulation by the action of plasmin during fibrinolysis. This normally occurs within 1 hour after thrombus formation. D-dimers have a half life of 4 to 6 hours, but the continued fibrinolysis of a PE increases the level for about 1 week.

Dead-space determination is another type of testing in use. A pulmonary embolus causes a decrease in blood flow to the alveoli, thus increasing alveolar dead space, which, in turn, decreases the carbon dioxide content of expired breath. Efforts are being directed to improve the sensitivity of testing measures to increases in dead-space to aid in the diagnosis of PE.[43]

Echocardiography is 90% specific and sensitive with PE of the pulmonary trunk and right and left pulmonary arteries. It shows an unexplained increase in right ventricular volume or pressure. Spiral CT is a test under investigation for use in the diagnosis of PE. Because it can be completed in 20 to 30 seconds,[43] if its sensitivity is strong, it will offer great advantage over traditional CT. Spiral CT is most helpful in diagnosing a centrally located PE rather than one in the periphery of the lung field. It is not useful in patients with COPD.

Medications. A focus of medical treatment of PE is the prevention of venous thromboembolism. Anticoagulant therapy may either be prophylactic for persons at risk for DVT or curative for persons with an actual pathologic event. When the patient is not responsive to anticoagulant therapy or when it is contraindicated, surgical intervention may be necessary.

Anticoagulant Therapy. The goal of anticoagulant therapy is to limit the growth of the embolized thrombus and prevent reembolization by inhibiting coagulation and preventing deposition of new clots. Heparin is the mainstay of therapy for pulmonary emboli without hemodynamic compromise or bleeding. It substantially reduces morbidity and mortality by preventing further fibrin deposition on the thrombus.[64] When there is strong suspicion of PE, heparin therapy should be started immediately while awaiting diagnostic confirmation. Heparin is most effective when given as a bolus followed by continuous IV infusion to achieve therapeutic concentration within a few hours of treatment. Standard protocols are being developed using weight-based dosing or standardized parameters to hasten achieving therapeutic levels. The patient is monitored by activated partial thromboplastin time (aPTT) every 4 to 6 hours. The goal is to achieve an aPTT of 1.5 to 2.5 times the control. Heparin may be given subcutaneously to patients with poor venous access. It is more difficult to achieve and maintain therapeutic values, however. For the patient with a major PE, current recommendation is heparin therapy for at least 1 week.[64]

Low-molecular-weight heparins (LMWHs) are progressively replacing heparin in the treatment of DVT and being used with greater confidence to treat PE. LMWHs are being used to decrease the complexities involved in heparin administration and thromboplastin aPTT monitoring. They may be given subcutaneously once or twice per day. The specific agents used most often include aldeparin, dalteparin, and enoxaparin; enoxaparin is the only one currently indicated for treatment of PE.[17,37] Advantages of these medications include increased bioavailability, longer half-life, and simplified administration. Dosing adjustments are needed in patients with renal insufficiency because they are renally excreted. Disadvantages include lack of a specific means to reverse the effect, difficult monitoring of their anticoagulant effect, and high cost.

Warfarin, 5 to 10 mg daily, is begun once the patient's condition is stable. Warfarin is monitored by prothrombin time (PT). The goal is to achieve a PT of 2 to 3 international normalized ratio (INR). Heparin and warfarin are continued until the PT is at the desired level. The length of anticoagulation treatment is 3 to 6 months. A small population of patients need lifelong anticoagulation, including those with irreversible acquired or genetic predisposition to venous thrombosis, major V/Q scan defects, and a history of recurrent thromboembolic events.

Inferior vena cava filters (see Chapter 25) are recommended if anticoagulants are contraindicated or if the patient has had a recurrent PE while receiving anticoagulation therapy. They may also be placed if the PE is severe (right ventricular failure, hypotension). A filter may be placed percutaneously to protect the vascular bed from embolization. The filter does not lessen the occurrence or extension of venous thrombosis. There is no evidence that filters have any advantages over anticoagulation. Complications associated with vena cava filters include perforation of the vessel wall, thrombosis at the access site, and leg edema.[64]

Thrombolytic Therapy. This therapy promotes immediate dissolution of the embolus and prompt return of pulmonary function in a patient who is hemodynamically unstable or severely hypoxic. It is not recommended for routine treatment of PE, and current evidence does not indicate a change in mortality. One of the thrombolytic agents (urokinase, streptokinase, or recombinant tissue-type plasminogen activator [rt-PA]) is used. Therapy can be delivered either systemically or directly into the pulmonary artery via selective catheterization, although systemic therapy appears to be superior. This therapy is often not applicable to many postsurgical patients because of the increased risk of bleeding complications at the surgical site.

Treatments

Pulmonary Embolectomy. A small group of patients with PE may be considered for surgical removal of the thrombus from the pulmonary vasculature. This intervention is reserved for those patients with hemodynamically massive PE who have contraindications to anticoagulant or thrombolytic therapy, or cardiopulmonary arrest, and fail to respond to immediate aggressive medical support. This procedure is usually performed with the patient under general anesthesia, although it may be performed with a special IV suction catheter with the patient under local anesthesia.

Diet. Diet is as tolerated; the patient is usually started with fluids and progressed to soft foods.

Activity. The patient is confined to bed initially. Activity increases as the patient heals and is able to tolerate it.

Referrals. The patient may be referred to a vascular surgeon and also to social services.

NURSING MANAGEMENT OF PATIENT WITH PULMONARY EMBOLISM

ASSESSMENT

Health History

Information to be collected as part of the health history when assessing the patient with PE relates to the presence of risk factors and recent onset of any of the following symptoms: dyspnea, substernal chest pain, hemoptysis, chest palpitations, pleuritic pain, cough, apprehension (sense of foreboding), or diaphoresis.

Physical Examination

General appearance is assessed. Specifically, color, signs of dyspnea or chest pain, and an appearance of being apprehensive are noted, since these are common findings in patients with PE. Vital signs are checked for tachypnea, tachycardia, and elevated temperature. A pulmonary examination is done, although findings on inspection, palpation, and percussion are usually normal with PE unless there is an underlying pulmonary disease. The chest is auscultated for pleural friction rub and localized, decreased breath sounds and crackles.

NURSING DIAGNOSES

Nursing diagnoses are determined from analysis of patient data. Nursing diagnoses for the person with PE may include but are not limited to:

Diagnostic Title	Possible Etiologic Factors
1. Ineffective breathing pattern	Tracheobronchial obstruction
2. Impaired gas exchange	Ventilation-perfusion imbalance
3. Ineffective tissue perfusion (in pulmonary vascular lung)	Interruption of blood flow
4. Anxiety (moderate, severe)	Change in health status, threat of death

EXPECTED PATIENT OUTCOMES

Expected patient outcomes for the person with PE may include but are not limited to:

1. Will establish effective breathing pattern
1a. Will have respiratory rate of 16 to 20 breaths/min
1b. Breath sounds will be clear; no use of accessory muscles
2. Will demonstrate improved gas exchange; $Pa{O_2}$, $Pa{CO_2}$, and pH will be within normal limits or will have returned to baseline level with no cyanosis

3. Will demonstrate adequate tissue perfusion
3a. Extremities will be warm and dry to touch; pulses will be present
3b. Coagulation studies (PT, INR, PTT) will be within normal limits
3c. No bleeding will be present
4. Will report anxiety is at manageable level and will verbalize concerns, ask questions about prognosis, plan of care

INTERVENTIONS

1. Establishing Effective Breathing Pattern

Respiratory rate, depth, and pattern, as well as breath sounds, are monitored. The head of the bed is elevated to promote physiologic and psychologic ease of maximal inspiration. Use of controlled breathing techniques is encouraged.

2. Promoting Gas Exchange

The patient is helped to deep-breathe and cough every 4 hours and to use an incentive spirometer every hour. Oxygen therapy is administered as ordered and monitored with pulse oximetry. Prescribed activity is maintained, whereas overexertion is avoided.

3. Promoting Tissue Perfusion

Lower extremities are elevated and monitored for adequate pulses. Leg size is measured. Legs are not massaged, nor the bed gatched. Pneumatic compression devices are applied as ordered.

Anticoagulants are administered as ordered. PT, INR, and aPTT are monitored, and the physician is notified if PT or aPTT is below or above the desired therapeutic range. Opiates are used cautiously for pain if the patient is hypotensive.

4. Reducing Anxiety

The patient is encouraged to verbalize fears and concerns. All treatments and procedures are explained. Support is offered, and the patient is made comfortable. The patient may also be guided in the use of relaxation therapy strategies.

Patient/Family Education

Patient and family teaching focuses on the prescribed anticoagulant therapy and prevention of future embolic events. In regard to the anticoagulant therapy, the patient should be taught the dose, side effects, and time of administration and the need to wear a Medic-Alert bracelet or carry a card stating that he or she is taking an anticoagulant. Precautions to be observed to prevent bleeding while on anticoagulant therapy must be stressed. These include using a soft toothbrush, not going barefoot, applying pressure to cuts to stop bleeding, and not taking any medication containing aspirin without conferring with a health care professional. The patient is also instructed to seek immediate medical attention if dyspnea, substernal chest pain, hemoptysis, chest palpitations, cough, diaphoresis, or feelings of unexplained apprehension occur.

In regard to prevention, the patient is taught about risk factors associated with PE and how to avoid them. The patient is instructed to avoid wearing constrictive clothing such as rolled garters; avoid standing or sitting for prolonged periods; move about at least every 2 hours; and actively dorsiflex the feet while sitting. The importance of not smoking is also stressed, and referrals to smoking cessation resources are made if needed.

EVALUATION

To evaluate the effectiveness of nursing interventions, compare patient behaviors with those stated in the expected patient outcomes. Achievement of patient outcomes is successful if the patient:

1. Manifests a breathing pattern that is normal or at baseline level.
1a. Has respiratory rate of 16 to 20 per minute.
1b. Has breath sounds that are clear; does not use accessory muscles.
2. Demonstrates adequate gas exchange; has $Pa{O_2}$, $Pa{CO_2}$, and pH at normal or baseline level; has no evidence of cyanosis.
3. Demonstrates adequate tissue perfusion
3a. Extremities warm and dry, pulses present
3b. Coagulation studies: PT, INR, and PTT within therapeutic limits
3c. No indication of bleeding
4. Manifests calm demeanor, using effective coping mechanisms; verbalizes concerns and asks questions about pronosis and plan of care.

GERONTOLOGIC CONSIDERATIONS

Older persons are at higher risk for developing DVT and PE because they are more likely to have surgery, such as knee and hip replacements, and they may be less active than younger persons. Diagnosis of PE in older adults is difficult because clinical and laboratory findings can be nonspecific and atypical. D-dimer studies may have a more limited role in the management of PE because values increase with age and many older patients suffer from multiple medical problems that influence D-dimer values.[50]

SPECIAL ENVIRONMENTS FOR CARE

Critical Care Management

Patients with PE who are hemodynamically unstable are cared for in an ICU.

Home Care Management

Patients with PE are hospitalized for evaluation and initiation of therapy. Ongoing anticoagulation therapy is managed in the home. Home care nurses are responsible for monitoring response to therapy, following laboratory data, and doing follow-up preventive teaching.

COMPLICATIONS

Complications of PE include pulmonary infarction, pleural effusion, right ventricular failure, GI bleeding, and bleeding from other sites.

BOX 21-8 Penetrating and Nonpenetrating (Blunt) Chest Injuries

Penetrating

Open pneumothorax (sucking chest wound)	Pulmonary contusion
Hemothorax	Diaphragm rupture
Tracheobronchial injury	Mediastinal injury

Blunt (Nonpenetrating)

Fractured ribs	Tracheobronchial injury
Flail chest	Diaphragm rupture
Closed pneumothorax	Mediastinal injury
Tension pneumothorax	

CHEST TRAUMA

Chest trauma is a major problem most often seen first in the emergency department. A chest injury may affect the rib cage, pleurae and lungs, diaphragm, or mediastinal contents. Chest injuries are broadly classified into two groups: blunt and penetrating (Box 21-8). Blunt, or nonpenetrating, injuries damage the structures within the chest cavity without disrupting chest wall integrity. Penetrating injuries disrupt chest wall integrity and result in alteration in intrathoracic pressures.

Trauma is the leading cause of death in those younger than 45 years of age and the fifth leading cause of death for those older than 65 years of age. Blunt chest trauma is second only to head and spinal cord trauma as the leading cause of death among trauma victims, and for almost 25% of all trauma patients who die, blunt chest trauma is reported as a predominant or contributing factor.[42] Penetrating wounds usually result from gunshot or stabbing injuries.

BLUNT INJURIES

Etiology/Epidemiology

Blunt chest trauma is associated with three mechanisms of injury: rapid acceleration/deceleration, direct impact, and compression. An acceleration/deceleration injury is most commonly caused by a motor vehicle or motorcycle crash, a pedestrian injury, or a fall. These injuries create a shearing force during which tissue, organs, or blood vessels are stretched beyond their capacity, resulting in tear, leak, or rupture. Direct-impact injuries are caused by motor vehicle and motorcycle crashes and from a blunt object striking the chest. Direct-impact injuries can cause rib, sternal, or scapular fracture and injuries to the lung parenchyma, heart, or thoracic cage. Compression injuries are caused by blunt chest trauma resulting from the force of the rapid deceleration as the tissues strike a fixed object such as the sternum and ribs. Compression injuries can result in organ rupture, contusions, or bleeding.[42]

Rib Fractures

Pathophysiology

Bony fractures are the most common type of blunt chest trauma. Fractures of ribs 1 and 2 are called the "hallmark of severe trauma" because these ribs are short, thick, and well protected by the thoracic musculature. It requires tremendous force to cause a fracture of these bones. Ribs 4 through 9 are most often fractured, because they are less well protected by the chest muscles. The ribs usually fracture at the point of maximum impact, but they may fracture at a site distant from the impact.[42] Rib fractures are caused by blows, crushing injuries, or strain caused by severe coughing or sneezing spells. If the rib is splintered or the fracture displaced, sharp fragments may penetrate the pleura and lung, resulting in a hemothorax (blood in the pleural space) or pneumothorax (air in the pleural space), which are penetrating injuries.

Common signs and symptoms of rib fracture include pain at the site of injury that increases on inspiration, localized tenderness and crepitus on palpation, splinting of the chest, and shallow breathing.

Collaborative Care Management

Diagnosis of rib fractures can be difficult. Fractures are confirmed by chest x-ray findings but often are not visible. They may be diagnosed by clinical assessment alone with acute pain over a specific location along the rib. Uncomplicated rib fractures require no treatment except pain relief to ensure adequate ventilation.

Close assessment of breathing and airway status is a priority. The patient is observed for splinting of the chest and shallow breathing, which could lead to atelectasis. To improve breathing, the patient is placed in a position of comfort—usually Fowler's or semi-Fowler's position. Analgesia is given to relieve pain so that the patient can breathe more deeply. Epidural anesthesia may be used, or an intercostal nerve block may be required for those patients with severe discomfort.

Patient/Family Education. The patient is instructed to use an incentive spirometer every hour, to rest and avoid strenuous activities for several days, and to take prescribed oral analgesics as needed for pain. The patient is also directed to contact the health care provider if pain relief is inadequate and to return to the emergency department immediately if shortness of breath, sudden sharp chest pain, or coughing up of blood occurs. If the patient is discharged with an epidural catheter for pain management, specific care is taught and a home health follow-up is arranged.

Flail Chest

Flail chest is a thoracic injury resulting in paradoxical motion of the chest wall segments.

Etiology/Epidemiology

The etiology and epidemiology of flail chest are the same as those for other blunt injuries discussed previously.

Pathophysiology

Fracture to at least four consecutive ribs in two or more places is usually required to cause a flail chest, which is categorized by location as sternal, anterior, lateral, or posterior. With a flail, the chest wall no longer provides the rigid bony support that is necessary to maintain the bellows function required for normal ventilation. The result is paradoxical breathing, or paradoxical respiratory movement. During inspiration the dislocated segment is pulled inward by the subatmospheric intrapleural pressure (Figure 21-25, *C*). During expiration the dislocated segment bulges outward as intrapleural pressure becomes less negative (Figure 21-25, *D*). Flail chest is often the result of a direct-impact, high-speed mechanism of injury.

Flail chest usually causes localized atelectasis secondary to decreased ventilation, resulting in hypoxemia. Because of the increased work of breathing, the individual may also develop hypercapnia and respiratory acidosis. Pulmonary contusion is also a common occurrence. The signs and symptoms of flail chest are summarized in the Clinical Manifestations box.

Collaborative Care Management

Chest x-ray studies are done to determine the extent of trauma, and ABGs are obtained to determine PaO_2 and $PaCO_2$. Oxygenation saturation is maintained at 90% or above with the use of supplemental oxygen if needed. In addition, management focuses on pain control and other measures to promote good ventilation, such as incentive spirometry and aggressive pulmonary physiotherapy, humidification of air, and early mobilization.

Treatment of patients in severe distress includes intubation and mechanical ventilation. In these patients the focus of care is the maintenance of proper gas exchange and observation for signs of hypovolemic shock that would require aggressive fluid resuscitation. Stabilization of the flail chest with surgical fixation has demonstrated improved long-term pulmonary function, fewer cases of pneumonia, and less ventilator time.[42] Complications of flail chest include pneumonia, tension pneumothorax, ARDS, and shock secondary to hemothorax.

Health history data to be collected include the nature of the injury and when it occurred. Often the patient is too badly injured to answer questions, and data are obtained from those accompanying the patient. Pain is severe and increases with each respiratory movement. Thus the flail segment should be splinted with the hands during coughing and deep breathing (see Figure 21-7). On physical examination the mediastinum is found to oscillate or flutter with each respiration, and breath sounds are decreased. If there is severe interference with cardiac function, neck veins will be distended. Pulse and respiratory rates are increased, and blood pressure falls if paradoxical motion is not relieved.

Patient/Family Education. The patient needs to be encouraged to request pain medication as needed to promote deep breathing and early mobilization. The patient also should be encouraged to promptly report changes in respiratory status to the nurse or other health care professional. Additional patient education focuses on the importance of wearing seat belts, since motor vehicle accidents account for the majority of chest trauma, and on follow-up care at home.

Gerontologic Considerations

Older persons account for 12% of trauma admissions but consume 33% of each health care dollar spent on trauma patients.[3] Older adults are potentially more vulnerable to thoracic injury and increasing mortality. Aging frequently results in osteoporosis, exaggerated thoracic kyphosis, decreased muscle mass, thinning of intervertebral disks, shortening of vertebral bodies, and decreased chest wall compliance. Postmenopausal women are particularly susceptible to age-related loss of bone density. These factors can predispose the older adult to rib fractures in traumatic situations and increase the morbidity of such injuries. Age is a strong predictor of outcome with flail chest and is associated with increased mortality.[3]

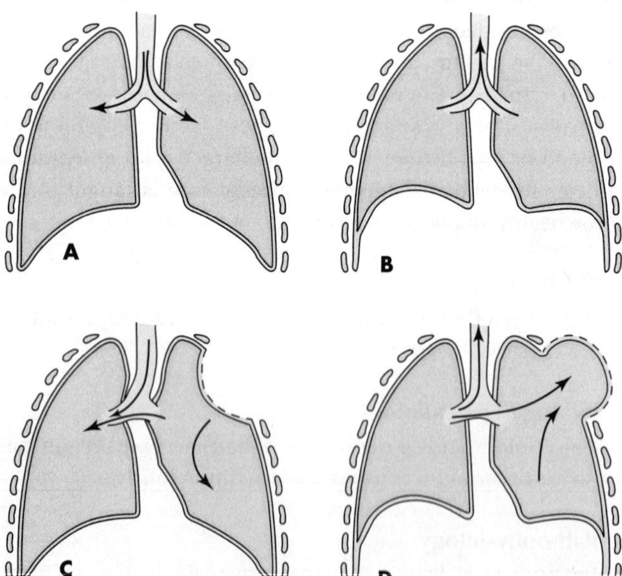

Figure 21-25 Normal respiration. **A**, Inspiration. **B**, Expiration. **C** and **D**, Paradoxical motion. **C**, Area of lung underlying unstable chest wall sucks in on inspiration. **D**, Same area balloons out on expiration. Note movement of mediastinum toward opposite lung on inspiration.

Clinical Manifestations

Flail Chest

- Severe chest pain
- Paradoxical breathing (asymmetric chest movement)
- Oscillation of mediastinum
- Increasing dyspnea
- Rapid shallow respirations
- Accessory muscle breathing
- Restlessness
- Decreased breath sounds on auscultation
- Cyanosis
- Anxiety related to difficult breathing

PULMONARY CONTUSION

Etiology/Epidemiology

A pulmonary contusion is a serious injury to the lung parenchyma. It leads to interstitial hemorrhage with resulting alveolar collapse, atelectasis, and consolidation of the uninjured areas of the lung.

Pathophysiology

As edema forms around the area of initial injury, a decrease in ventilation begins to occur. The resulting hypoxia is due to shunting of blood through the unventilated lung (see Clinical Manifestations box).

Collaborative Care Management

Chest x-ray films show patchy infiltrates or nonsegmental areas of opacification. This reflects the mechanical forces applied to the lung, resulting in the tearing of tissues.[42] These findings usually appear within 4 to 6 hours of injury and typically occur in areas that underlie rib, clavicular, or sternal fractures. Chest CT is the gold standard for diagnosis because it is more specific and sensitive. A pulmonary contusion appears on a CT scan as an ill-defined area of consolidation.

Treatment is supportive and includes supplemental oxygen to prevent hypoxemia (oxygen saturation is maintained at 90% or greater); incentive spirometry to promote adequate chest expansion; coughing and deep breathing to promote good ventilation; and repositioning in bed with aggressive activity progression to promote perfusion of all lung areas. Pain control is critical for adequate chest expansion, and epidural or patient-controlled analgesia may be needed. Chest wall splinting techniques are also used to facilitate coughing and deep breathing exercises.

Patient/Family Education. The nurse educates the patient about the cause and treatment for pulmonary contusion. The emphasis is on preventing injuries/accidents and thus further pulmonary contusions.

PNEUMOTHORAX

Etiology/Epidemiology

In pneumothorax there is air in the pleural space between the lung and the chest wall. A pneumothorax can occur spontaneously or as a result of penetrating or nonpenetrating chest injuries.

Pathophysiology

A closed pneumothorax is caused by fractured ribs that pierce the pleura. It can also occur when there is a sudden compression of the rib cage. Air enters the pleural space, increasing intrapleural pressure and collapsing the lung (Figure 21-26, *B*). A variant of closed pneumothorax is a spontaneous pneumothorax that results from the rupture of an emphysematous bleb on the lung surface. A spontaneous pneumothorax may also follow severe bouts of coughing in persons with a chronic pulmonary disease such as asthma. It commonly occurs as a single or recurrent episode in an otherwise healthy young man.[80] If large enough and left untreated, a closed pneumothorax can become a tension pneumothorax.

A tension pneumothorax occurs when air enters the pleural space on inspiration but cannot leave it on expiration. Although usually a result of a closed pneumothorax, a tension pneumothorax can be caused by a penetrating chest injury. The accumulating air builds up positive pressure in the chest cavity, resulting in lung collapse on the affected side; mediastinal shift toward the unaffected side; and decreased venous return due to compression of mediastinal contents (heart, great vessels).

An open pneumothorax occurs when a penetrating chest wound opens the intrapleural space to atmospheric pressure. Each time the person inspires, air is sucked into the intrapleural space, increasing intrapleural pressure. This is a life-threatening injury and can severely compromise breathing and lead to a tension pneumothorax. Blood also may leak into the pleural cavity, creating a hemothorax.

Collaborative Care Management

The clinical manifestations and medical management of the various types of pneumothorax are presented in Table 21-19. Nursing interventions associated with the specific types of pneumothorax are presented in Table 21-20.

Patient/Family Education. The nurse supports and informs the patient about the treatments and procedures for restoring lung function.

Clinical Manifestations

Pulmonary Contusion

Pulmonary contusion may vary from total absence of symptoms to the full spectrum of symptoms associated with noncardiogenic pulmonary edema. Signs and symptoms (some of which may be delayed) include:

- Increasing dyspnea
- Tachypnea
- Increasing restlessness
- Crackles noted on auscultation
- Hemoptysis

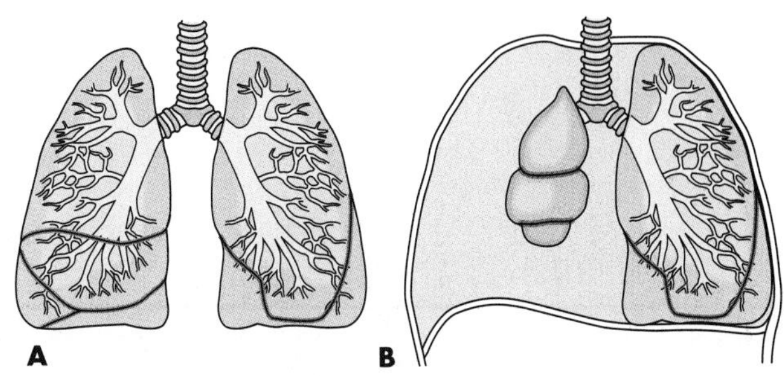

Figure 21-26 **A,** Normal expanded lungs. **B,** Complete collapse of right lung caused by air in pleural cavity (pneumothorax).

TABLE 21-19 Clinical Manifestations and Medical Management of Pneumothorax

Pneumothorax	Clinical Manifestations	Medical Management
Closed (spontaneous)	Small or slowly developing pneumothorax may produce no symptoms. Larger or rapidly developing pneumothorax results in: Sharp pain on inspiration Increasing dyspnea Increasing restlessness Diaphoresis Hypotension Tachycardia Absence of chest movement on affected side Absence of breath sounds on affected side Hyperresonance on affected side	Observation on outpatient basis Supplemental oxygen Needle aspiration of air from pleural space, if present; insertion of chest catheter connected to a flutter valve or closed drainage system If frequent recurrences, doxycycline or talc instilled into pleural space to cause adhesions between pleurae; if this procedure fails, lung portion with defect resected and parietal pleura abraded
Tension	Severe dyspnea Agitation Trachea deviated from midline toward unaffected lung—mediastinal shift Jugular venous distention Absence of chest movement on affected side Hypotension, tachycardia Breath sounds absent on affected side Hyperresonance on affected side Diminished heart sounds Shock Subcutaneous emphysema Ineffective ventilation	True emergency Defect in chest wall covered with a sterile dressing Insertion of chest tube connected to a flutter valve or closed drainage system
Open	Sucking sounds at wound site with respiration Tracheal deviation (trachea moves toward unaffected side during inspiration and returns toward midline with expiration)	Occlusion of open wound Same as for closed pneumothorax

TABLE 21-20 Nursing Interventions for Pneumothorax

Pneumothorax	Interventions
Closed (spontaneous)	Perform the following: Place in semi-Fowler's position. Administer oxygen. Obtain thoracentesis tray and closed drainage equipment. For outpatient or for patient after chest tube removal, instruct to: Report any increased dyspnea to physician. Avoid strenuous exercise or activity that increases rate and depth of breathing. Avoid holding breath. Follow physician's instructions about resuming normal activity.
Tension	Life-threatening event; imperative that interventions be carried out immediately to relieve increased intrapleural pressure; interventions same as those listed for closed pneumothorax Perform the following: Monitor vital signs frequently. Observe for cardiac dysrhythmias. Palpate for subcutaneous emphysema in upper chest and neck. Sample discharge instruction as for patient with closed pneumothorax
Open	Perform the following: Occlude wound with nonporous covering. Same interventions as for closed pneumothorax. Same discharge instructions as for closed pneumothorax.

Critical Thinking Questions

1. A patient has just been admitted to your unit with a history of chronic obstructive pulmonary disease. She is developing respiratory complications. What nursing interventions are appropriate for this patient? What laboratory tests do you want to review?
2. Consider the trend of increasing the life expectancy for patients with cystic fibrosis. What ethical issues arise from this trend? What is the nurse's responsibility when these issues are discussed?
3. A patient with asthma is on your unit. This patient has had many episodes of status asthmaticus in the past. What preparations should you make in case she has another episode while hospitalized? What nursing assessments are important?
4. You are caring for a 67-year-old patient with lung cancer. His wife is always at his bedside. What nursing interventions are important to institute with this patient? What are your responsibilities to his family? What referrals might be appropriate for this patient?
5. You have cared for several patients lately who are rather heavy smokers and also have respiratory disorders. What can you do to help convince them to join a smoking cessation program? What are the benefits of such program? What strategies are used to help people quit smoking? Does age or gender make a difference in the strategies used?

References

1. Adatsi G: Health going up in smoke: how can you prevent it? *Am J Nurs* 99(3):63-66, 68-69, 1999.
2. Adjei AA: Primary lung cancer. In Rakel RE, Bope ET, editors: *Conn's current therapy 2001,* Philadelphia, 2001, WB Saunders.
3. Albaugh G et al: Age-adjusted outcomes in traumatic flail chest injuries in the elderly, *Am Surg* 66(10):978-981, 2000.
4. Altorki N, Kent M, Pasmantier M: Detection of early-stage lung cancer: computed tomographic scan or chest radiograph, *J Thorac Cardiovasc Surg* 121(6):1053-1057, 2001.
5. American Thoracic Society: COPD: definitions, epidemiology, pathophysiology, diagnosis and staging, *Am J Respir Crit Care Med* 152(5, Pt. 1):1713-1735, 1995.
6. American Thoracic Society: Statement on sarcoidosis, *Am J Respir Crit Care Med* 160(2):736-755, 1999.
7. Banasik J: Diagnosing alpha 1-antitrypsin deficiency, *Nurse Pract* 26(1):58-62, 64, 67, 2001.
8. Bernard GR et al: The American-European Consensus Conference on ARDS, *Am J Respir Crit Care Med* 149(3 pt 1):818-824, 1994.
9. Boyle AH, Waters HF: COPD: focus on prevention, *Heart Lung* 29(6):446-449, 2000.
10. Bryan CL, Homma A: Acute respiratory failure. In Rakel RE, Bope ET, editors: *Conn's current therapy 2001,* Philadelphia, 2001, WB Saunders.
11. Carpenito LJ: *Nursing diagnosis: application to clinical practice,* ed 8, Baltimore, 2000, JB Lippincott.
12. Celli BR: Pulmonary rehabilitation for patients with advanced lung disease, *Clin Chest Med* 18(3):521-534, 1997.
13. Criner GJ et al: Prospective randomized trial comparing bilateral lung volume reduction surgery to pulmonary rehabilitation in severe chronic obstructive pulmonary disease, *Am J Respir Crit Care Med* 160(6):2018-2027, 1999.
14. Custodio LM: Blowing soap bubbles: teaching pursed lip breathing, *Chest* 114(4):1224, 1998.
15. Deslauriers J: Should screening for lung cancer be revisited? *J Thorac Cardiovasc Surg* 121(6):1031-1032, 2001.
16. De Souza A et al: Optimal management of complicated empyema, *Am J Surg* 180(6):507-511, 2000.
17. Didomenico RJ: New antithrombotics for the intensive care unit setting: GP IIb/IIIa inhibitors, low molecular weight heparins, direct thrombin inhibitors, *Crit Care Nurs Q* 22(4):61-74, 2000.
18. Dipiro JT et al: *Pharmacotherapy,* Norwalk, Conn 1999, Appleton & Lange.
19. Edelman JD, Kotloff RM: Lung transplantation, *Clin Chest Med* 18(3):627-644, 1997.
20. Elpern EH, Cheatham J: Inpatient care of the adult with an exacerbation of cystic fibrosis, *AACN Clin Issues* 12(2):293-304, 2001.
21. Enright PL et al: Underdiagnosis and undertreatment of asthma in the elderly, *Chest* 116(3):603-613, 1999.
22. Feldman C: Pneumonia in the elderly, *Clin Chest Med* 20(3):563-573, 1999.
23. Ferguson GT: Update on pharmacologic therapy for chronic obstructive pulmonary disease, *Clin Chest Med* 21(4):723-738, 2000.
24. Ferrin M et al: Palliative care and lung transplantation: conflict or continuum, *Am J Nurs* 101(2):61-66, 2001.
25. File TM, Tan JS, Plouffe JF: Bacterial pneumonia: community-acquired and nosocomial in immunocompetent hosts. In Rakel RE, Bope ET, editors: *Conn's current therapy 2001,* Philadelphia, 2001, WB Saunders.
26. Flaherty KR et al: Short-term and long-term outcomes after bilateral lung volume reduction surgery, *Chest* 119(5):1337-1346, 2001.
27. Frawley PM, Nader NM: Airway pressure release ventilation: theory and practice, *AACN Clin Issues* 12(2):234-246, 2001.
28. Grap MJ, Muro CL: Ventilator-associated pneumonia: clinical significance and implication for nursing, *Heart Lung* 26(6):419-429, 1997.
29. Han LL, Alexander JP, Anderson LJ: Respiratory synctial virus pneumonia among the elderly, *J Infect Dis* 179(1):25-30, 1999.
30. Hannon MM et al: Hospital infection control in an era of HIV infection and multidrug resistant tuberculosis, *J Hosp Infect* 44(1): 5-11, 2000.
31. Happ MB: Communicating with mechanically ventilated patients: state of the science, *AACN Clin Issues* 12(2):247-258, 2001.
32. Harrington J: The deadly return of tuberculosis, *Int Nurs Rev* 46(6):176-177, 180, 1999.
33. Health Care Financing Administration: *Coverage issues manual,* Washington, DC, 1999, US Government Printing Office.
34. Henschke CI et al: Early Lung Cancer Action Project: overall design and findings from baseline screening, *Lancet* 354(9173):99-105, 1999.
35. Hill N: Non-invasive mechanical ventilation for post-acute care, *Clin Chest Med* 22(1):35-54, 2001.
36. Hirshberg B et al: Factors predicting mortality of patients with lung abscess, *Chest* 115(3):746-750, 1999.
37. Hovanessian HC: New generation anticoagulants: the low molecular weight heparins, *Ann Emerg Med* 34(6):768-779, 1999.
38. Hyer JD, Silvestri G: Diagnosis and staging of lung cancer, *Clin Chest Med* 21(1):95-106, 2000.
39. Jain P, Kavuru MS: A practical guide for peak expiratory flow monitoring in asthma patients, *Cleve Clin J Med* 64(4):195-202, 1997.
40. JAMA Asthma Information Center: *Guidelines for the diagnosis and management of asthma,* 1998, website: jama.ama-assn.org.
41. Kanner RE: Chronic obstructive pulmonary disease. In Rakel RE, Bope ET, editors: *Conn's current therapy 2001,* Philadelphia, 2001, WB Saunders.
42. Keough V, Pudelek B: Blunt chest trauma: review of selected pulmonary injuries focusing on pulmonary contusion, *AACN Clin Issues* 12(2):270-281, 2001.
43. Kline JA et al: New diagnostic tests for pulmonary embolism, *Ann Emerg Med* 35(2):168-180, 2000.

44. Knebel A, Leidy NK, Sherman S: When is the dyspnea worth it? *Image J Nurs Sch* 30(4):339-343, 1998.
45. Lantz MS, Gianbuco V: Smoking cessation: the key to treating older smokers? Don't quit helping, *Geriatrics* 56(5):58-59, 2001.
46. Lynch JP, Kazerooni EA, Gay SE: Pulmonary sarcoidosis, *Clin Chest Med* 18(4):755-785, 1997.
47. Lynn J et al: Living and dying with chronic obstructive pulmonary disease, *J Am Geriatr Soc* 48(5 suppl):S91-S100, 2000.
48. Marion BS: A turn for the better: "prone positioning" of patients with ARDS, *Am J Nurs* 101(5):26-34, 2001.
49. Marshall BC, Samuelson WM: Basic therapies in cystic fibrosis: does standard therapy work? *Clin Chest Med* 19(3):487-504, 1998.
50. Masotti L et al: Plasma D-dimer levels in elderly patients with suspected pulmonary embolus, *Thromb Res* 98(6):577-579, 2000.
51. Meyers BF: Outcome of bilateral lung volume reduction in patients with emphysema potentially eligible for lung transplantation, *J Thorac Cardiovasc Surg* 122(1):10-17, 2001.
52. Morrissey BM, Albertson TE: To just say NO or I don't inhale? *Crit Care Med* 29(6):1284-1285, 2001.
53. Morse CJ: Volume lung reduction surgery: a review, *Crit Care Nurs Q* 21(1):1-7, 1998.
54. Murray JF, Nadal JA, editors: *Textbook of respiratory medicine,* ed 3, Philadelphia, 2000, WB Saunders.
55. Naughton BJ, Mylotte JM: Treatment guidelines for nursing home–acquired pneumonia based on community practice, *J Am Geriatr Soc* 48(1):82-88, 2000.
56. Nevins ML, Epstein SK: Weaning from prolonged mechanical ventilation, *Clin Chest Med* 22(1):13-33, 2001.
57. O'Brien RJ, Nunn PP: The need for new drugs against tuberculosis, *Am J Respir Crit Care Med* 163(5):1055-1058, 2001.
58. O'Donohue WJ: Home oxygen therapy, *Clin Chest Med* 18(3):535-545, 1997.
59. Petty TL: COPD: interventions for smoking cessation and improved ventilatory function, *Geriatrics* 55(12):30-32, 35-39, 2000.
60. Pingleton SK: Nutrition in chronic critical illness, *Clin Chest Med* 22(1):149-163, 2001.
61. Rau JL: Recent developments in respiratory care pharmacology, *J Perianesth Nurs* 13(6):359-369, 1998.
62. Reinke LF, Hoffman L: Asthma education: creating a partnership, *Heart Lung* 29(3):225-236, 2000.
63. Respiratory Nursing Society: Position statement: long term oxygen therapy, *Heart Lung* 28(2):143-144, 1999.
64. Riedel M: Acute pulmonary embolism. II. Treatment, *Heart* 85(3):351-360, 2001.
65. Rosenstein BJ: What is a cystic fibrosis diagnosis? *Clin Chest Med* 19(3):423-441, 1998.
66. Schedel EM, Connolly MA: Lung volume reduction surgery: new hope for emphysema patients, *Dimens Crit Care Nurs* 18(1):28-34, 1999.
67. Scherer YK, Schneider LE, Shimmel, S: The effects of education alone and in combination with pulmonary rehabilitation on self-efficacy in patients with COPD, *Rehabil Nurs* 23(2):71-77, 1998.
68. Sepkowitz KA: Tuberculosis control in the 21st century, *Emerg Infect Dis* 7(2):259-262, 2001.
69. Skerrett SJ: Diagnostic testing for community-acquired pneumonia, *Clin Chest Med* 20(3):531-548, 1999.
70. Snow V, Lascher S, Mottur-Pilson C: The evidence base for management of acute exacerbations of COPD: clinical practice guidelines, part 1, *Chest* 119(4):1185-1189, 2001.
71. Steinberg KP, Hudson LD: Acute lung injury and acute respiratory distress syndrome, *Clin Chest Med* 21(3):401-417, 2000.
72. Suchyta MR et al: Increased mortality of older patients with ARDS, *Chest* 111(5):1334-1339, 1997.
73. Turato G, Zuin R, Saetta M: Pathogenesis and pathology of COPD, *Respiration* 68(2):117-128, 2001.
74. US Department of Health and Human Services: *Healthy people 2010: understanding and improving health,* Washington, DC, 2000, USDHHS.
75. Van Soeren MH et al: Pathophysiology and implications for the treatment of ARDS, *AACN Clin Issues* 11(2):179-197, 2000.
76. Walker WC, Glassman SJ, Rashbaum IG: Cardiopulmonary rehabilitation and cancer rehabilitation, *Arch Phys Med Rehabil* 82(3 suppl 1):S56-S62, 2001.
77. Weinacker AB, Vaszar LT: Acute respiratory distress syndrome: physiology and new management strategies, *Annu Rev Med* 52:221-237, 2001.
78. Wheat J et al: Practice guidelines for the management of patients with histoplasmosis, *Clin Infect Dis* 30(4):688-695, 2000.
79. Williams PL: Coccidioidomycosis. In Rakel RE, Bope ET, editors: *Conn's current therapy 2001,* Philadelphia, 2001, WB Saunders.
80. Woodruff DW: Pneumothorax, *RN* 62(9):62-65, 1999.
81. World Health Organization: Revised international definitions in TB control, *Int J Tuberc Lung Dis* 5(3):213-215, 2001.
82. Zuckerman JB, Kotloff RM: Lung transplantation for cystic fibrosis, *Clin Chest Med* 19(3):535-554, 1998.

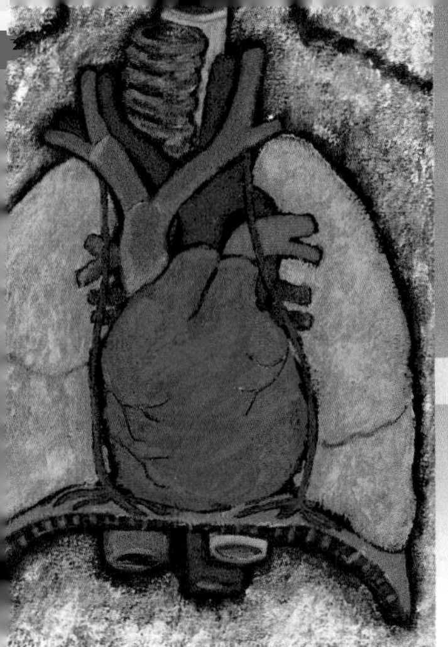

Assessment of the Cardiovascular System

22

Shelley Yerger Huffstutler

Objectives

After studying this chapter, the learner should be able to:

1. Describe the health history and physical examination data relevant to a cardiovascular examination.
2. Discuss the basic structure and function of the heart and peripheral vasculature.
3. Explain the conduction system of the heart in relation to the cardiac cycle.
4. Analyze factors that affect cardiac output.
5. Discuss physiologic changes that occur in the cardiovascular system with aging.
6. Differentiate common manifestations of altered cardiac functioning.
7. Explain the significance of various diagnostic tests used to assess cardiac functioning.
8. Compare nursing care of patients undergoing various cardiovascular diagnostic testing.

Cardiovascular disease (CVD) continues to rank first among all disease categories and is the leading cause of death in the United States. According to current estimates, one or more types of CVD afflict nearly 61 million Americans, and approximately 41% of all deaths in 1998 were attributable to CVD.[1] The American Heart Association reports that one in five males and females have some form of CVD. Even though CVD mortality rates from 1998 indicated that female deaths exceeded male deaths, 53.1% to 46.9%, respectively, misperceptions still exist that CVD is not a significant problem for women.

Given the aforementioned data, it is not surprising that the cost of CVD in the United States in 2001 was estimated at $252.8 billion. This figure is a reflection of both health care expenditures and lost productivity resulting from morbidity and mortality.[1] Therefore, even though the mortality rate from CVD has declined more than 20% in the last 25 years, statistics strongly support the need for ongoing public education. Continued emphasis must be placed on recognizing signs and symptoms of various types of CVD along with risk factor reduction including diet, exercise, and smoking cessation. Research to enhance medical management, improve surgical techniques, and advance technology and pharmacotherapy will contribute significantly to a reduction in mortality and morbidity from CVD.

This chapter is the first of four chapters that focus on the heart and vascular system. Initially, a review of anatomy and physiology of the cardiovascular system is presented. This content is followed by a discussion of the health history and physical examination; a description of various cardiovascular diagnostic tests along with nursing care is provided.

ANATOMY AND PHYSIOLOGY OF THE HEART

Basic Structure

The heart is a relatively small organ that weighs 300 g and is approximately the size of a fist. It is located in the middle of the mediastinum, where the lungs partially overlap it. This pulsatile four-chambered pump beats approximately 72 times per minute, pumping more than 5 L of blood each minute, or about 2000 gallons per day. It continually propels oxygenated blood into the arterial system and receives poorly oxygenated blood from the venous system. The heart muscle rests on the diaphragm and is tilted forward and to the left so that the apex of the heart is rotated anteriorly.

The heart is enclosed by the pericardium, which consists of two layers: the inner layer (visceral pericardium) and the outer layer (parietal pericardium). The two pericardial surfaces are separated by a pericardial space that normally contains approximately 10 to 20 ml of thin, clear pericardial fluid. This lubricating fluid moistens the contacting surfaces of the pericardial layers and reduces the friction produced by the pumping action of the heart. The visceral pericardium encases the heart and extends several centimeters onto each of the great vessels. The parietal pericardium is attached anteriorly to the manubrium and xiphoid process of the sternum, posteriorly to the vertebral column, and inferiorly to the diaphragm.

The three layers of cardiac tissue are (1) epicardium, the outer layer of the heart, which is the same structure as the visceral pericardium; (2) myocardium, the middle layer of the heart, which is composed of striated muscle fibers and is responsible for the heart's contractile force; and (3) endocardium, the innermost layer of the heart, which consists of endothelial tissue. The endocardium lines the inside of the heart's chambers and covers the heart valves.

Chambers

The heart is divided into two halves by a muscular wall (septum) (Figure 22-1). Each half has an upper collecting chamber (atrium) and a lower pumping chamber (ventricle). Oxygen-poor venous blood enters the right atrium, flows from the right atrium to the right ventricle (mainly by gravity) when the tricuspid valve is opened, and is pumped into the pulmonary artery to the lungs. Oxygen-rich blood returns from the lungs to the left atrium, enters the left ventricle when the mitral valve is opened, and is ejected into the aorta for distribution to the peripheral tissues.

The right atrium is a thin-walled structure that serves as a reservoir for venous blood returning to the heart. Venous blood returns to the heart via the superior and inferior vena cavae and the coronary sinus, which drains venous blood from the heart muscle. Blood is temporarily stored in the right atrium during right ventricular systole (contraction). During ventricular diastole (filling), approximately 80% of the venous return to the right atrium flows by gravity into the ventricle through the tricuspid valve. The remaining 20% of the venous return is delivered to the ventricles during atrial systole. This additional 15% to 20% of the venous return, which is actively propelled into the ventricles, is called the atrial kick.

The right ventricle is normally the most anterior structure of the heart and is situated immediately beneath the sternum. The right ventricle receives venous blood from the right atrium during ventricular diastole. During ventricular diastole this blood is propelled through the pulmonic valve into the pulmonary artery and then to the lungs. Because the pulmonary system is a low-pressure system, the overall workload of the right ventricle is much lighter than that of the left ventricle. The right ventricle has a crescent-shaped chamber and a thin outer wall that is 4 to 5 mm thick. This thin structure is suitable for right ventricular systole because the right ventricle contracts against low resistance.

The thin-walled left atrium receives oxygenated blood from the four pulmonary veins and serves as a reservoir during left ventricular systole. Blood flows by gravity from the left atrium into the left ventricle through the opened mitral valve during ventricular diastole. Left atrial contraction then propels the remaining 20% of the venous return and provides a significant increment of blood volume to the left ventricle. This atrial kick stretches the ventricle preparing for ventricular ejection.

The left ventricle receives blood from the left atrium through the opened mitral valve during ventricular diastole. Blood is then ejected through the aortic valve into the systemic arterial circulation during ventricular systole. The left ventricle must contract against a high-pressure systemic circulation to deliver blood flow to the peripheral tissues. Therefore the left ventricular chamber is surrounded by 8 to 15 mm of thick muscle, which is approximately two to three times the thickness of the right ventricle. The thick muscle and

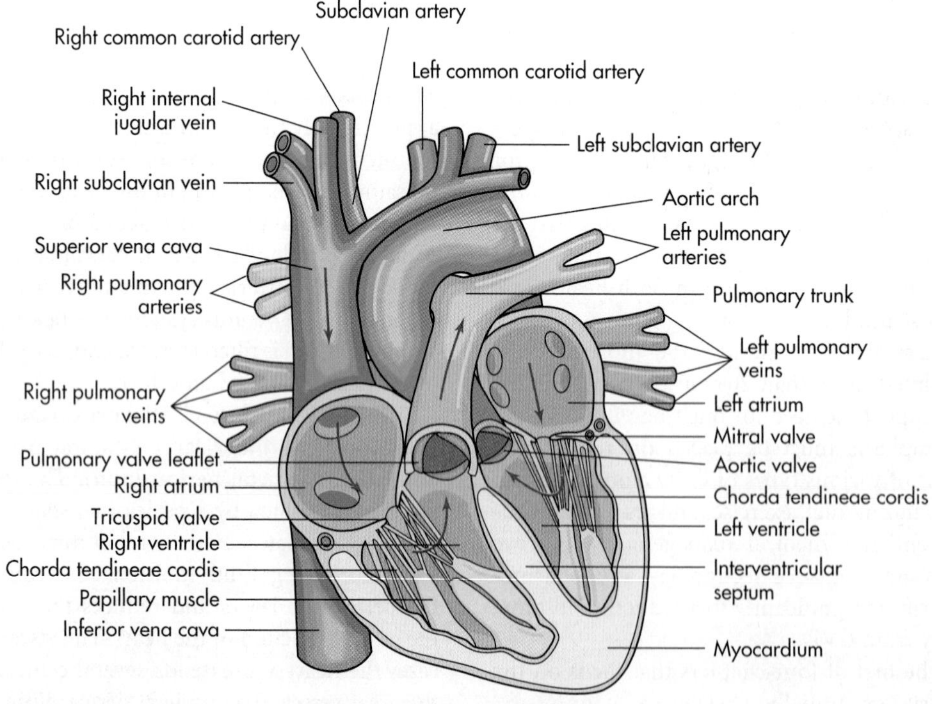

Figure 22-1 Heart in frontal section; course of blood through the chambers.

ellipsoidal-sphere shape contribute to the powerful expulsive ability of the left ventricular chamber during systole.

Valves

The four cardiac valves are flaplike structures that function to maintain unidirectional (forward) blood flow through the heart chambers. These valves open and close in response to pressure and volume changes within the cardiac chambers. The cardiac valves can be classified into two types: the atrioventricular (AV) valves, which separate the atria from the ventricles, and the semilunar valves, which separate the pulmonary artery and the aorta from their respective ventricles.

Atrioventricular Valves

The AV valves are the tricuspid valve, located between the right atrium and the right ventricle, and the bicuspid (or mitral) valve, located between the left atrium and left ventricle. The tricuspid valve contains three leaflets held in place by fibrous cords called the chorda tendineae cordis, which in turn are anchored to the ventricular wall by the papillary muscles. The mitral valve on the left side of the heart is a bicuspid valve with two valve cusps or leaflets. It also is attached to chorda tendineae cordis, which extend to the papillary muscles (Figure 22-2). The chorda tendineae cordis are extremely important because they support the AV valves during ventricular systole to prevent valvular prolapse into the atrium. Some leaflet overlapping occurs during closure of the AV valves, which helps prevent the backward flow of blood. Damage to the chorda tendineae cordis or to the papillary muscles allows valvular regurgitation of blood back into the atrium during ventricular systole, resulting in increased pressure and volume. During diastole the AV valves serve as a type of funnel inasmuch as they allow blood to flow from the atria to the ventricles. The diameter of the AV cusps is almost double that of the orifice occluded by the valve. In general, the AV valves are structurally much more complex than the semilunar valves.

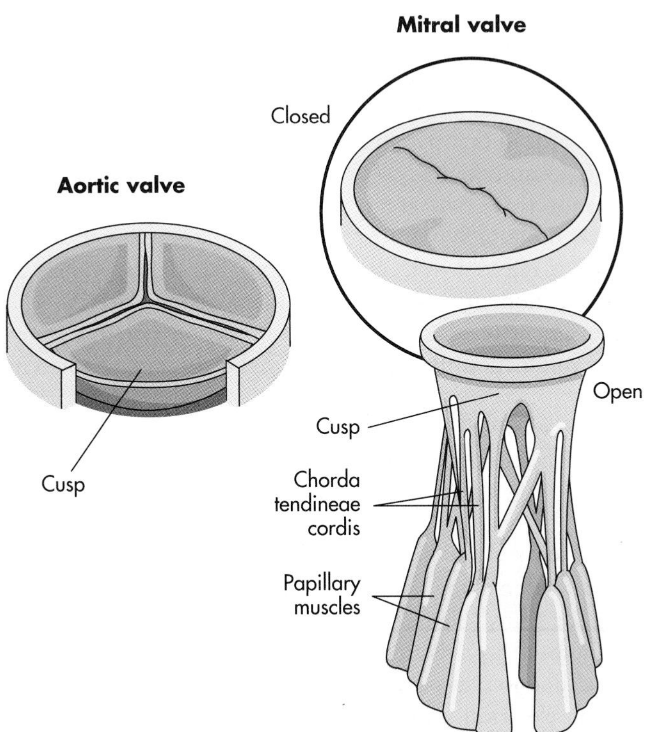

Figure 22-2 Aortic and mitral (bicuspid) valves.

Semilunar Valves

The semilunar valves are the pulmonic and aortic valves. The structural design of the semilunar valves is quite different from the AV valves; each consists of three cuplike cusps. (see Figure 22-2). The pulmonic valve lies between the right ventricle and the pulmonary artery. The aortic valve lies between the left ventricle and the aorta. These valves are open during ventricular systole (contraction) to permit blood flow into the aorta and the pulmonary artery. They are closed during diastole (relaxation) to prevent retrograde flow from the aorta and the pulmonary artery into the ventricles.

Coronary Arteries

The coronary arteries arise from the aorta (just behind the cusps of the aortic valve) in an area known as Valsalva's sinus. The function of the coronary artery system is to provide an adequate blood supply to the myocardium.

There are two main coronary arteries, the left and the right (Figure 22-3). The left coronary artery (LCA) divides into two branches: the left anterior descending (LAD) artery and the circumflex coronary artery (CCA). The LAD branch supplies the left ventricular myocardium, septum, anterior papillary muscle, and parts of the right ventricle. In addition, the LAD artery usually supplies the anterior apex and some part of the posterior apex. The CCA typically emerges at a sharp 90-degree angle from the LCA and is then directed toward the lateral left ventricle and apex. The CCA and its branches supply most of the left atrium, the lateral wall of the left ventricle, and part of the posterior wall of the left ventricle. Diagonal branches arise between the LAD artery and the CCA and are distributed along the free wall of the left ventricle.

Two important external landmarks are used in tracing coronary circulation. These anatomic landmarks are sulci, or grooves. The first is the atrioventricular groove, which encircles the heart between the atria and the ventricles. The second is the interventricular groove, which divides the right and left ventricles. The meeting of the two anatomic grooves on the posterior side of the heart is known as the crux of the heart. The location of the crux is significant because this is where the AV node is located. The terms *dominant left circulation* and *dominant right circulation* refer to whether the left or the right coronary artery turns at the crux of the heart and supplies the posterior interventricular groove. Therefore, if the CCA extends as far as the posterior interventricular groove, the circulation is considered to be dominant left. This condition occurs in only 10% to 15% of the population.

The right main coronary artery (RCA) arises from the right Valsalva's sinus off the aorta and courses around the right AV groove. Its branches supply the right ventricle, a portion of the septum, and in more than 50% of all persons, the sinoatrial

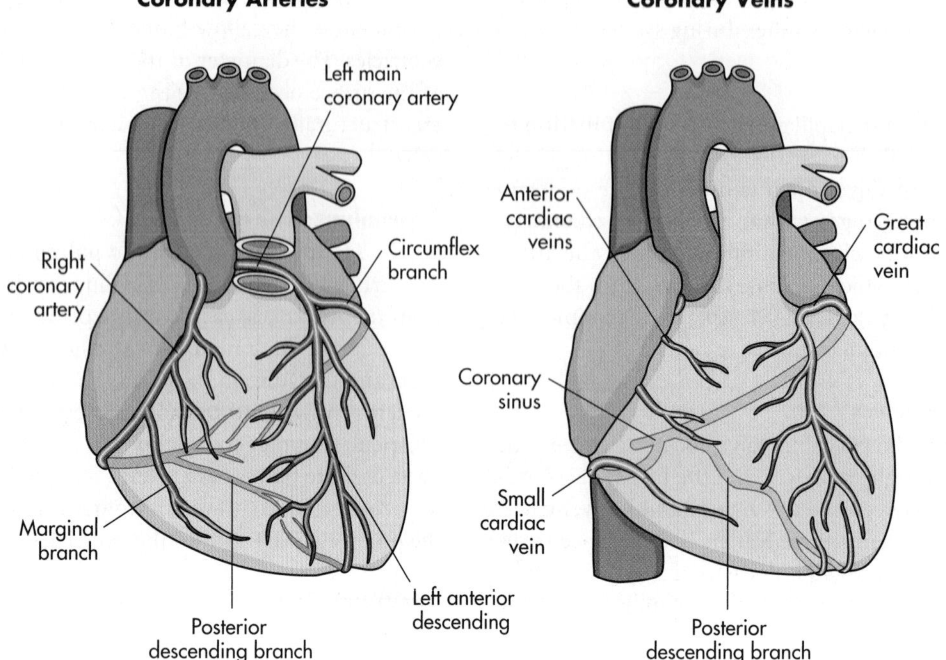

Figure 22-3 Coronary blood vessels.

(SA) node. In approximately 67% of all persons, the RCA turns at the crux of the heart and descends in the posterior interventricular groove. These hearts are classified as dominant right. The posterior descending branch of the RCA then supplies the posterior aspect of the septum and the posterior left papillary muscle before terminating in several branches to the left ventricular wall.

Great variation exists in the branching pattern of the coronary arteries. In approximately 18% of the population, the CCA reaches the crux of the heart with the RCA; this is the "balanced" coronary artery pattern. In the remaining persons, no true posterior interventricular branch exists; rather, many branches from either main coronary artery supply the posterior septum.

Blood flow to the myocardium occurs almost exclusively during diastole, when coronary vascular resistance is diminished. During systole, coronary vascular resistance is increased because of the increased ventricular wall tension produced by ventricular contraction. During diastole, blood enters the coronary arteries at the pressure that exists at that moment in the aortic arch. This is termed aortic diastolic pressure.

Coronary venous drainage is accomplished via three subdivisions of the heart's venous system: (1) the thebesian veins drain a portion of the right atrial and right ventricular myocardium; (2) the anterior cardiac veins drain a large portion of the right ventricle; and (3) the coronary sinus and its branches drain the left ventricle and most myocardial venous return.

Conduction System

Properties of Cardiac Muscle

The mechanical contraction of the heart is the product of a stimulus-response process. The four properties of automaticity, excitability, conductivity, and contractility are integral components of the electromechanical events in the heart.

Automaticity. The ability of the heart to initiate impulses regularly and spontaneously is known as automaticity, or rhythmicity. Although most cardiac cells have this ability; it is the prominent property of the SA node, making it the dominant pacemaker in the normal heart. Pacemaker cells are known to have lower resting membrane potentials than other myocardial cells and exhibit spontaneous depolarization.

Excitability. The ability of cardiac cells to respond to a stimulus by initiating a cardiac impulse is known as excitability. It should be noted that excitatory cells differ from pacemaker cells in that pacemaker cells do not require a stimulus to initiate an impulse.

Conductivity. The ability of cardiac cells to respond to a cardiac impulse by transmitting the impulse along cell membranes is referred to as conductivity. Cells that specialize in this function are found in the conduction system. The arrangement of cells outside the conduction system ensures rapid conduction through intercalated disks joining adjacent cells.

Contractility. The ability of cardiac cells to respond to an impulse by contracting is known as contractility. Contractile cells compose the largest mass of the myocardium.

Anatomy of Conduction System

The pacemaking center of the normal heart is the SA node, or sinus (Figure 22-4). It is composed of a group of highly specialized tissues located in the right atrium adjacent to the superior vena cava. Automatically and at regular intervals, an electrical impulse is emitted from the SA node at a rate of 60 to 100 beats/min. The atria are then depolarized, and the impulse travels to the AV node via three tracts desig-

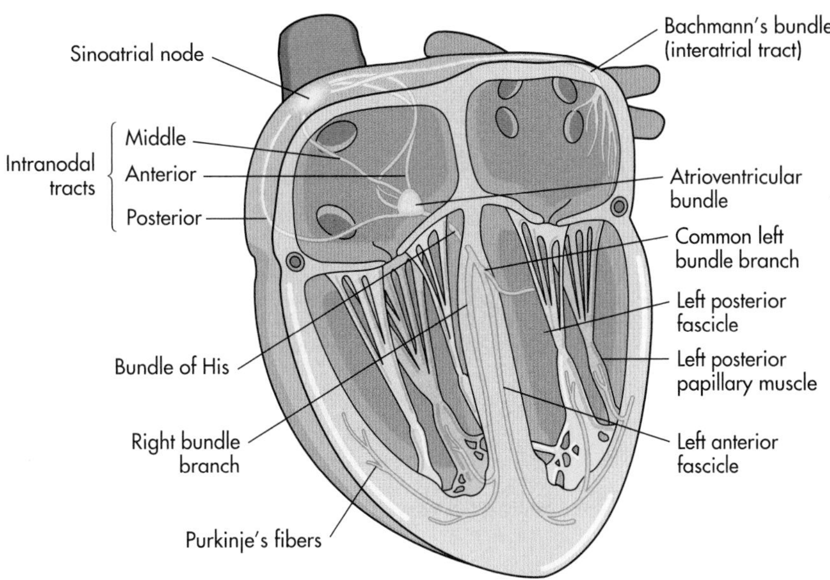

Figure 22-4 Schematic diagram of heart illustrating the conduction system.

nated as anterior, middle, and posterior internodal tracts. A fourth tract, called Bachmann's bundle, branches off the anterior nodal tract and transmits the impulse to the left atrium.

The three internodal tracts meet at the atrionodal junction. The junctional area refers to the region where atrial and ventricular tissues merge. This junction contains the AV node. The junctional cells above and below the AV node are capable of pacemaking activity under many circumstances (e.g., failure of the SA node to fire).

The AV node itself is located on the right side of the interatrial septum. These cells lack the ability to initiate electrical impulses (i.e., automaticity), but they are uniquely responsible for a brief physiologic delay in the conduction of the impulse to the ventricles.

The bundle of His begins anatomically at the "tail" of the AV node. It is a short, thick cable of fibers separated by collagen septa that bifurcates into the right bundle branch (RBB) and the left bundle branch (LBB).

The RBB extends down the right side of the interventricular septum and is covered by a connective tissue sheath. It extends to reach the anterior papillary muscle of the right ventricle, where it merges with the Purkinje system. It lies close to the septal surface for much of its length, and therefore its functional ability is vulnerable to right ventricular pressure changes.

The LBB bifurcates into anterior and posterior fascicles. The anterior fascicle extends anteriorly down the left side of the interventricular septum to reach the anterior papillary muscle. The posterior fascicle is shorter and thicker and extends to the posterior papillary muscle of the left ventricle. Both fascicles connect with the Purkinje system and share equally in the spread of the impulse to the left ventricle.

Purkinje's fibers lie as a network on the endocardial surface and penetrate the myocardium of both ventricles. They are responsible for the transmission of the impulse to both ventricular free walls. Purkinje's cells are elongated and contain intercalated disks, which contribute to the superiority of conductivity in myocardial tissue.

Cells outside the conduction system also play a role in the conduction of an impulse. A surface membrane, the sarcolemma, surrounds each cell and acts as a selectively permeable barrier to sodium and potassium ions. Adjacent myocardial cells are connected end to end by a thickened portion of the sarcolemma known as an intercalated disk. These disks act as low-resistance pathways to the transmission of an impulse between cells.

Sequence of Cardiac Activation

Depolarization (activation of the cardiac muscle) is initiated by an impulse from the SA node. The impulse first spreads through the right atrium and then activates the left atrium. Atrial activation normally is accomplished in 0.11 second or less.

Shortly after the impulse reaches the left atrium, it also activates the junctional region and subsequently the AV node. The AV node delays the impulse about 0.1 second before the impulse enters the bundle of His.

On reaching the bundle of His, the impulse is transmitted along the bundle branches. Within the ventricles, the first structure to be activated is the ventricular septum. The septum is activated by the impulse traveling from the left side to the right side (Figure 22-5).

The impulse then continues down the remaining length of the bundle branches and into the Purkinje network, thus activating the ventricular walls almost simultaneously. Activation of the ventricular muscle then proceeds from the apex back toward the base of the heart to complete the process.

Depolarization of cardiac musculature proceeds from endocardium to epicardium. Repolarization in the atria follows this same pathway. In contrast, repolarization of ventricular musculature proceeds from epicardium to endocardium.

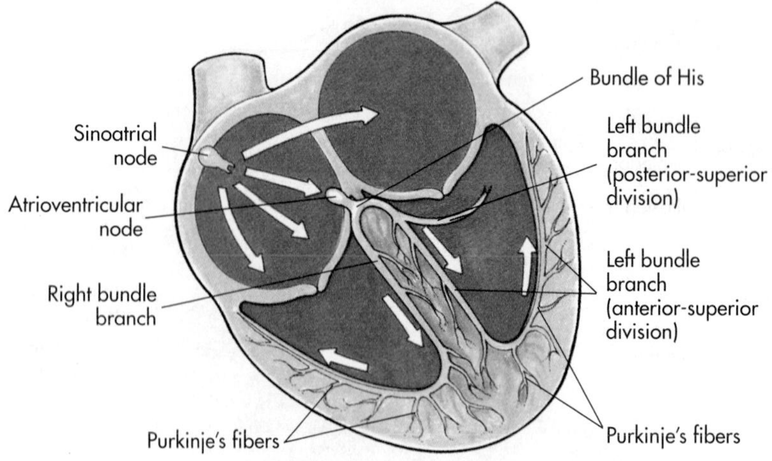

Figure 22-5 Sequence of electrical activation in the heart.

Knowledge of the sequence of activation is fundamental to analysis of the electrocardiogram (ECG).

Action Potential. The resting myocardial cell has a membrane potential (i.e., an electrical charge) as a result of the relative distribution of sodium and potassium ions extracellularly. Whenever the cell is stimulated, the membrane potential undergoes a change. A graphic record of this change forms the basis for an ECG. The change in electrical potential in response to a stimulus is known as the action potential. The two components of the action potential are depolarization and repolarization.

Resting Membrane Potential. In the resting state the inside of the cell is negative with respect to the outside (Figure 22-6). Initiation and conduction of cardiac impulses depend on the cell's ability to maintain an electrical potential gradient when the cell is at rest. The main factor that contributes to the 290 mV resting membrane potential is the cell's permeability to potassium and not to sodium. The sodium-potassium exchange pump is responsible for actively transporting sodium out of the cell and potassium into the cell. The hydrolysis of adenosine triphosphate (ATP) provides the energy for the functioning of this pump. Because more sodium is pumped out of the cell than potassium is moved in, a net outward current of positive ions further enhances the cell's negativity during the resting phase.

Depolarization. The initiation of a cardiac impulse begins with the process of depolarization. Depolarization indicates the rapid reversal of the resting membrane potential, which results from the following sequence of events: (1) the cell membrane permeability to sodium increases spontaneously (as in pacemaking cells) or in response to a stimulus; (2) a rapid influx of sodium occurs; and (3) potassium moves out of the cell. This movement of ions across the membrane creates an electrical current. When the amount of sodium entering the cell reaches a critical level, an electrical impulse is generated. The impulse may spread as a wave of depolarization to adjacent cells.

Repolarization. Repolarization is the process by which the cell is returned to the resting state. The cell membrane permeability to sodium decreases, and sodium leaves the cell. Potassium returns through an active ion transport system.

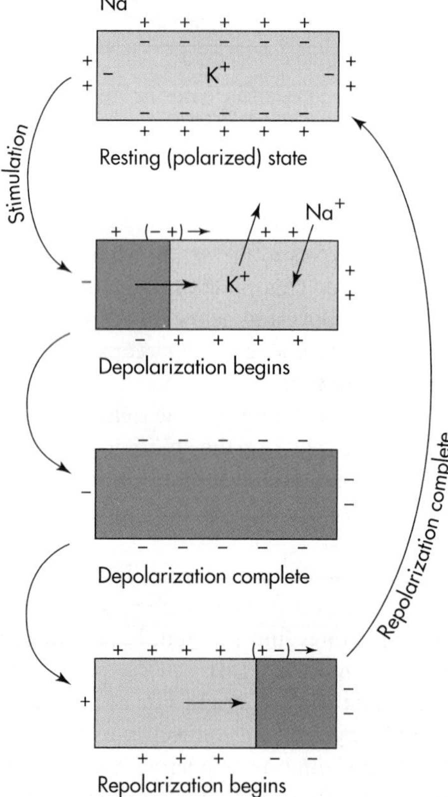

Figure 22-6 Schematic diagram illustrating process of depolarization and repolarization.

Phases of Action Potential

Phase 0. Phase 0 is the tall upstroke of the action potential that occurs when the cell is stimulated, causing the cell membrane to become permeable to sodium ions. Fast sodium channels open to allow sodium to rush into the cell, creating a positive intracellular membrane potential of 0 to 120 mV (Figure 22-7).

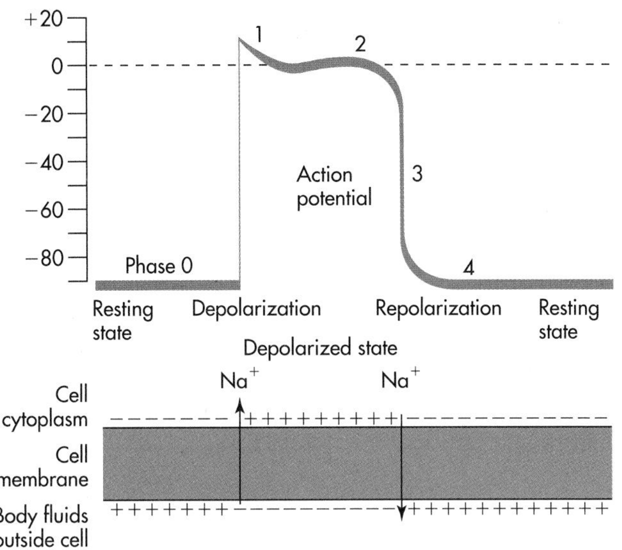

Figure 22-7 Phases of the action potential of cardiac muscle.

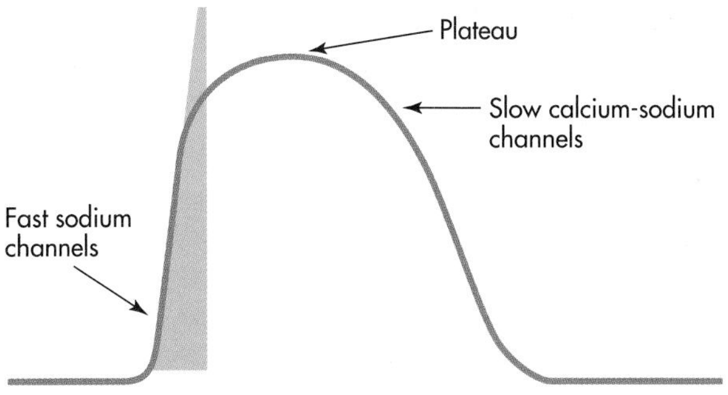

Figure 22-8 The differing effects of the fast sodium channels and the slow calcium-sodium channels on the action potential. The flow of sodium throughout the fast sodium channels initiates the action potential, and then these channels close *(shaded area)*. The flow of current through the slow calcium channels is responsible for the plateau and duration of the action potential.

Phase 1. Phase 1 represents a brief period of rapid repolarization secondary to an outward positive current carried mainly by potassium ions. Sodium influx is abruptly terminated as soon as the cell depolarizes. These two factors cause a slight decline in intracellular positivity.

Phase 2. Phase 2 of the action potential is often referred to as the plateau phase. It is sustained by an influx of positive ions, primarily calcium, through the slow calcium channels into the cell (Figure 22-8). This supplies the cell with the calcium needed for contraction. This inward current results in a prolonged refractory period by maintaining the cell in a depolarized state, allowing time for completion of muscular contraction.

Phase 3. During phase 3 the sodium pump, along with the increased loss of intracellular potassium, causes a rapid restoration of negativity to the cell.

Phase 4. Phase 4 is the return of the cell to the resting membrane potential.

Refractoriness. The inability of cardiac cells to respond to successive stimuli is known as refractoriness. During the absolute refractory period, no stimulus will produce a response. This period begins with depolarization and extends through a portion of the repolarization period until the sodium ion carrier sites are again free to transport the sodium ions necessary for depolarization (Figure 22-9).

Refractoriness progressively diminishes in the relative refractory period, which occurs in the final stage of repolarization. During this interval a stimulus of sufficient strength will produce a response. When the resting state is attained, the cell is no longer refractory and a mild stimulus will initiate a cardiac impulse. This is known as the supernormal period.

Cardiac Cycle

The action potential itself does not cause the myofibrils to contract. The electrical stimulation initiates muscular contraction by stimulating the release of calcium ions in the sarcoplasmic reticulum of the muscle. Calcium ions then catalyze

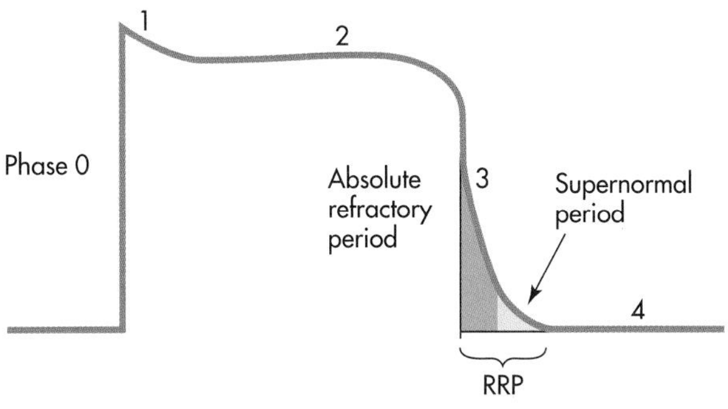

Figure 22-9 Schematic of the action potential showing the absolute and relative refractory period (RRP). A strong stimulus will produce a response in the first part of the RRP and a mild stimulus in the latter (supernormal period).

the chemical reaction that promotes the interdigitating and sliding of the actin and myosin filaments along each other, producing muscle contraction (see Chapter 45).

The cardiac cycle has two phases, diastole and systole. Relaxation and filling of both atria and then both ventricles take place during diastole. Contraction and emptying of both atria and then both ventricles occur during systole.

Diastole. The diastolic phase of the cardiac cycle is subdivided into the following phases: (1) isovolumetric ventricular relaxation, (2) rapid ventricular filling, (3) slow ventricular filling, and (4) atrial systole (Table 22-1 and Figure 22-10, *A*).

Isovolumetric ventricular relaxation begins as soon as the aortic and pulmonic valves close. During this time the myocardial muscle relaxes, and ventricular pressure falls. However, the falling ventricular pressure is still higher than atrial pressure; therefore the AV valves remain closed, and, as a result, a large amount of blood collects in the atria. As ventricular pressure begins to drop more rapidly to its low diastolic level, the higher pressure in the atria pushes the AV valves open and allows blood to flow rapidly into the ventricular cavity. This second phase of diastole, rapid ventricular filling, lasts for approximately the first third of diastole and causes intraventricular pressures to rise. As ventricular pressure increases, it

TABLE 22-1 Events During the Cardiac Cycle

Phase	Valves: Pulmonary and Aortic	Valves: Mitral and Tricuspid	Actions	Pressure (P) Changes
Diastole				
Isovolumetric relaxation	Closed	Closed	Blood collects in atria	Atrial P increases until greater than ventricular P
Rapid ventricular filling	Closed	Open	Blood flows rapidly into ventricles from pressure differential	Atrial P decreases; ventricular P increases
Slow ventricular filling	Closed	Open	Blood flows passively into ventricles	Same as for rapid filling
Atrial systole	Closed	Open, then closed	Atrial contraction pushes additional blood into ventricles	Ventricular P becomes greater than atrial P
Systole				
Isovolumetric contraction	Closed	Closed	Myocardial tension increases	Ventricular P increases; aortic P decreases until ventricular P greater than aortic P
Maximal ventricular ejection	Open	Closed	Blood is pumped from ventricles into pulmonary artery and aorta	Ventricular P decreases
Reduced ventricular ejection	Open, then closed	Closed	Some blood ejected	Ventricular pressure decreases rapidly when ventricles relax

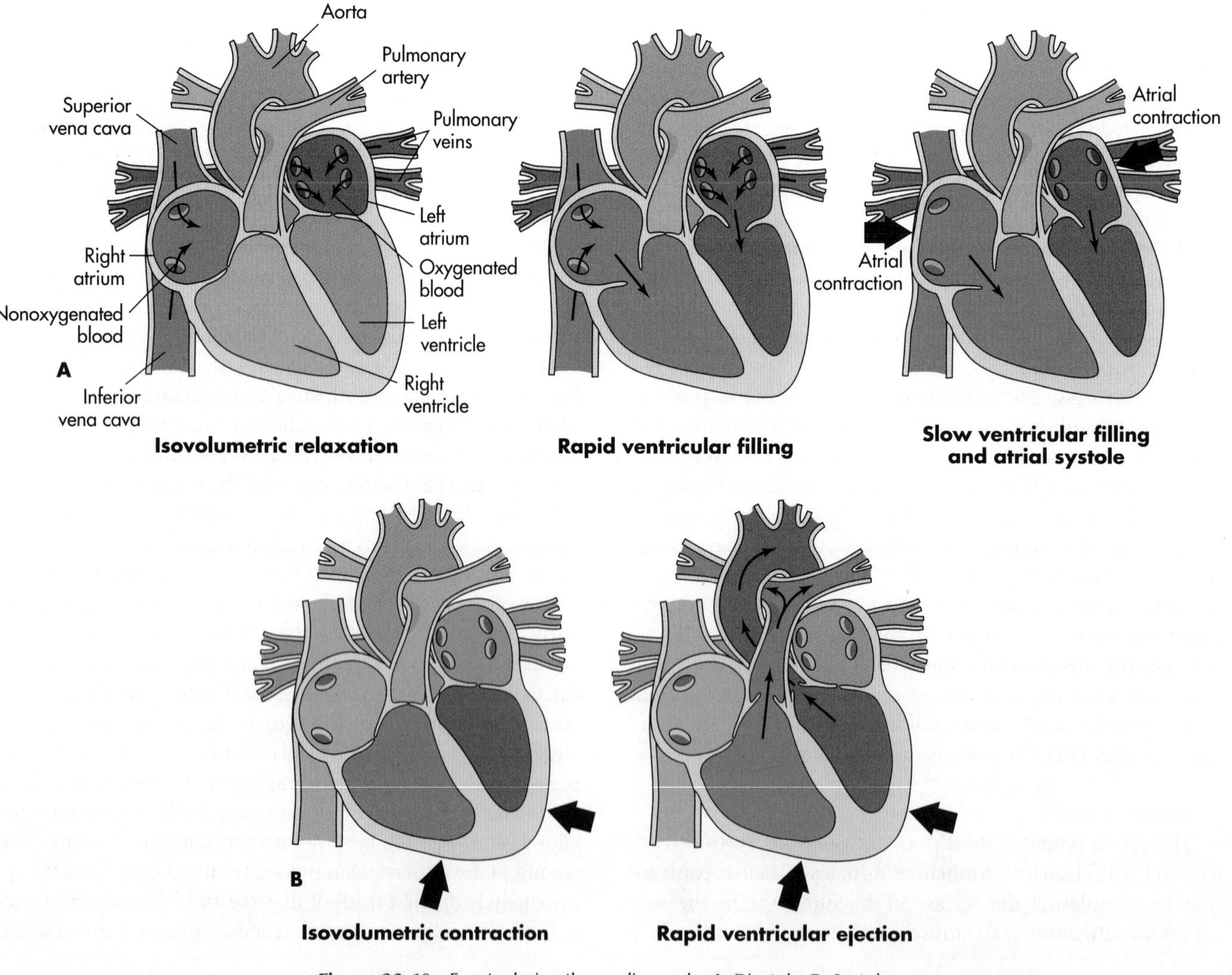

Figure 22-10 Events during the cardiac cycle. **A**, Diastole. **B**, Systole.

impedes further rapid filling, and the resultant slowing of ventricular filling marks the third phase of diastole. This phase of slow ventricular filling is referred to as diastasis. Both the atrial and the ventricular chambers are relaxed, and blood entering the atria flows passively into the ventricles. During the phase of atrial systole, electrical depolarization spreads through the atria and pauses at the AV node for 0.10 second. The atrial musculature then contracts, propelling an additional 20% to 30% of blood into the ventricle before ventricular contraction.

Systole. The ventricular systolic phase of the cardiac cycle is subdivided into phases of isovolumetric ventricular contraction, maximal ventricular ejection, and reduced ventricular ejection (see Table 22-1 and Figure 22-10, *B*).

During the isovolumetric ventricular contraction phase, myocardial tension and intraventricular pressure increase, whereas no change occurs in blood volume or muscle fiber length. At this time the aortic valve is closed because pressure in the aortic root exceeds left ventricular pressure. The higher pressure in the aortic root is the result of a previous systole that has just ejected blood into the aorta. As this aortic blood is distributed to the periphery, aortic pressure falls slowly. At the same time, intraventricular pressure and tension are increasing. When intraventricular pressure exceeds aortic root pressure, the aortic valve opens and maximal ventricular ejection begins. Blood from the ventricles is pumped into the pulmonic and systemic circulations. As the ejection rate starts to slow, the phase of reduced ventricular ejection, or protodiastole, begins. The ventricles remain contracted, but little blood is being ejected from the ventricle into the aorta. Ventricular pressure actually falls slightly below aortic root pressure, but some blood is still being ejected simply because of the momentum built up by the contraction. At the end of systole, ventricular relaxation begins suddenly, and a rapid decrease in intraventricular pressure occurs. The higher pressure in the large arteries and in the aortic root immediately pushes blood back toward the ventricles, thus snapping shut the semilunar valves.

Cardiac Output

The amount of blood ejected from the left ventricle into the aorta per minute is called the cardiac output (CO). Although the right ventricle ejects an equivalent amount of blood into the pulmonary artery, it is not included in the measurement of total CO. Rather, CO is equivalent to stroke volume (SV) (volume of blood ejected from the left ventricle with each contraction) times heart rate (HR) (number of heartbeats per minute):

$$\text{CO} = \text{SV} \times \text{HR}$$

The average CO ranges from 4 to 8 L/min in the adult male. However, during periods of strenuous exercise, the CO may reach 20 to 25 L/min. Because cardiac requirements vary according to individual body size, a more accurate means of assessing tissue perfusion is to compute the cardiac index. The cardiac index is obtained by dividing the CO by the patient's total body surface area:

$$\text{Cardiac index} = \text{CO (L/min)/Body surface area (m}^2\text{)}$$

Therefore the cardiac index represents the CO in terms of liters per minute per square meter of body surface. This corrects an individual's CO to match body size. The normal range for cardiac index is 2.4 to 4.0 L/min. For example, the average 70-kg man has an approximate cardiac index of 3 L/min.

Stroke Volume. Stroke volume is the amount of blood ejected by the left ventricle into the aorta per beat. At the completion of each filling phase, or diastole, the ventricle contains approximately 120 ml of blood (end-diastolic volume [EDV]) (Figure 22-11). Under normal circumstances, the heart ejects approximately two thirds of the EDV. The blood that is ejected is called the ejection fraction. The volume of residual blood in the ventricle at the end of systole is known as the end-systolic volume (ESV). Therefore stroke volume can be defined as the difference between the volumes of blood contained in the ventricle at the end of diastole and the volume of blood remaining at the end of systole:

$$\text{SV} = \text{EDV} - \text{ESV}$$

Control of Cardiac Output. Cardiac output depends on the relationship between two important variables: stroke volume and heart rate. Despite fluctuations in one of these two variables, CO can be maintained at relatively constant levels by compensatory adjustments in the other variable. For example, if the heart rate slows, the time for ventricular filling (diastole) is lengthened. This lengthened period allows for an increase in preload and a subsequent increase in stroke volume. Conversely, if the stroke volume falls, the heart rate can increase to compensate temporarily and maintain CO. Therefore the actual determinants of CO are the mechanisms regulating stroke volume and heart rate.

Control of Stroke Volume. Stroke volume, and ultimately CO, is determined by three factors: preload, contractility, and afterload.

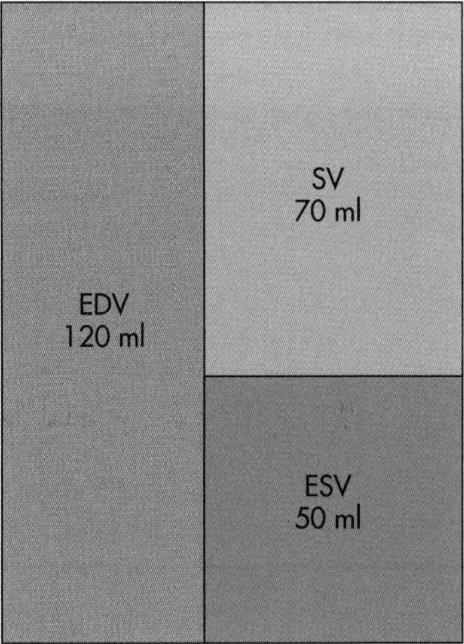

Figure 22-11 Representation of normal ventricular function, illustrating relationship between end diastolic volume *(EDV)*, stroke volume *(SV)*, and end-systolic volume *(ESV)*.

Preload. Starling's law of the heart states that myocardial fibers respond with a more forceful contraction when they are stretched. An example of this phenomenon is increasing the stretch of a rubber band to obtain a more forceful recoil when the rubber band is released. Myocardial fibers can be stretched by increasing the volume of blood delivered to the ventricles during diastole. The degree of myocardial stretch before contraction is expressed in terms of preload. Preload is defined as the volume of blood distending the ventricles at the end of diastole. Preload is based on the amount of venous return and the ejection fraction, which determines the amount of blood left in the ventricle at the end of systole.

According to Starling's law, increasing venous return and thereby increasing left ventricular EDV (preload) facilitates ventricular contraction and promotes increased ventricular function by stretching the myocardial fibers. Stretching of the sarcomeres increases the number of interaction sites for actin-myosin linkages and therefore increases ventricular contraction. Under normal conditions the sarcomere is stretched to 2 mm during ventricular diastole. Maximal ventricular force is developed at a sarcomere length of 2.2 mm. At this length, actin and myosin are able to use the most interaction sites. When myocardial stretching exceeds 2.4 mm, the myofilaments become partially disengaged, and fewer contractile sites are activated. Because Starling's length-tension relationship is functional only within physiologic limits, it is important to note that prolonged, excessive stretching of the myocardial fibers eventually will lead to a decrease in CO by reducing the stroke volume (as in ventricular hypertrophy).

Contractility. Contractility is another major determinant in stroke volume. By definition, contractility refers to a change in the inotropic state of the muscle without a change in myocardial fiber length or preload. Increased contractility (inotropism) is a function of the increased intensity of interaction at the actin-myosin linkages. Contractility can be increased by sympathetic stimulation or by administration of medications such as calcium or epinephrine. Increased contractility improves ventricular emptying during systole, thereby increasing the stroke volume.

Afterload. Another factor involved in the control of stroke volume is afterload. Afterload is defined as the amount of tension the ventricle develops during contraction to eject blood from the left ventricle into the aorta. The major impedance against which the left ventricle must pump is peripheral vascular resistance. Increase in pressure resulting from hypertension or vasoconstriction produces increased resistance to pumping and requires an increase in ventricular tension to eject blood. The afterload on the heart is affected not only by the amount of aortic pressure but also by the size of the heart. This relationship between ventricular tension, arterial pressure, and ventricular size is known as Laplace's law:

$$\text{Ventricular tension} = \text{Arterial pressure} \times \text{Ventricular radius}$$

Both hypertension and dilation of the ventricular chamber increase ventricular tension (increase afterload). Therefore, if arterial pressure increases, the ventricle must pump against higher resistance to empty adequately. Also, if ventricular radius increases, ventricular volume will increase. Thus at the same level of aortic pressure, the afterload against which an enlarged or dilated left ventricle must work is greater than that encountered by a normal-sized ventricle. This would result in an impaired ventricular emptying, thereby reducing stroke volume and CO.

Control of Heart Rate. The autonomic nervous system (ANS) regulates the heart rate through the sympathetic and the parasympathetic nervous systems.

The sympathetic fibers arise from the thoracic spinal cord and reach the entire atria and ventricles, as well as the SA and the AV nodes. Control of the heart by the ANS is mediated by neurotransmitters. The sympathetic neurotransmitter is norepinephrine. The sympathetic fibers have both positive chronotropic (increase rate) and inotropic (increase force) effects. Therefore with an increase in sympathetic stimulation, the neurotransmitter norepinephrine is released from the nerve endings and increases heart rate, atrial and ventricular contractility, and the speed of electrical conduction through the AV node.

The parasympathetic fibers originate in the medulla and have their innervation primarily in the atrial musculature and the SA and AV nodes; however, parasympathetic stimulation has been shown to reach the ventricles. The parasympathetic fibers have a negative chronotropic effect and may exert a slightly negative inotropic effect; however, in the healthy circulatory system, the increased filling that occurs as a result of a lengthened diastole compensates for this negative inotropic effect. Stimulation of the parasympathetic system causes the release of the neurotransmitter acetylcholine at the vagal nerve endings, which has basically the opposite effect of norepinephrine. Parasympathetic stimulation causes a decrease in the rate of discharge of the SA node, a decrease in the rate of conduction from the atria to the ventricles, and a decrease in the force of atrial contraction and probably also of ventricular contraction. The final effect of ANS control of the heart is a balance between these two opposing nervous systems. Normally, the heart is under the control of vagal inhibition and maintains a resting heart rate of 60 to 90 beats/min.

The effects of the ANS can be greatly influenced by several additional factors, such as the central nervous system (CNS) and pressoreceptor reflexes. Impulses from the cerebral cortex can have a significant effect on heart rate. Pain, fear, anger, and excitement can cause substantial increases in heart rate. Also, reflex changes caused by stimulation of the pressoreceptors can influence heart rate. The baroreceptor reflex, with afferent branches in the aortic arch, carotid sinus, and other pressoreceptor zones, functions as a negative feedback mechanism to regulate both pressure in the arteries and resistance of vessels in the vasculature. Consequently, an episode of hypotension would cause a sudden drop of blood pressure in the aorta or carotid sinus and would stimulate the pressoreceptors less intensely. Subsequently, stimulation of the cardiac inhibitory center would decrease in frequency resulting in a reflex increase in heart rate.

Other important factors involved in the control of heart rate include body temperature, medication, catecholamines, arterial blood gas tensions, hormones other than epinephrine, and plasma electrolyte concentrations. However, these are beyond the scope of discussion for this chapter.

ANATOMY AND PHYSIOLOGY OF THE PERIPHERAL VASCULAR SYSTEM

The vascular system is a closed circuit consisting of the systemic and pulmonary circulations. Blood circulates from the left side of the heart to the tissues and back to the right side of the heart. It then flows through the lungs and back to the left side of the heart. The main components of the vascular system are the arteries, capillaries, and veins.

Arteries

Arteries are thick-walled vessels that transport oxygen and blood via the aorta from the heart to the tissues. Figure 22-12 shows the principal arteries. As the arteries approach the tissues, they branch into smaller vessels called arterioles. Arteries are composed of three tissue layers:

1. Inner layer of endothelium (intima)
2. Middle layer of connective tissue, smooth muscle, or elastic fibers (media)
3. Outer layer of connective tissue (adventitia)

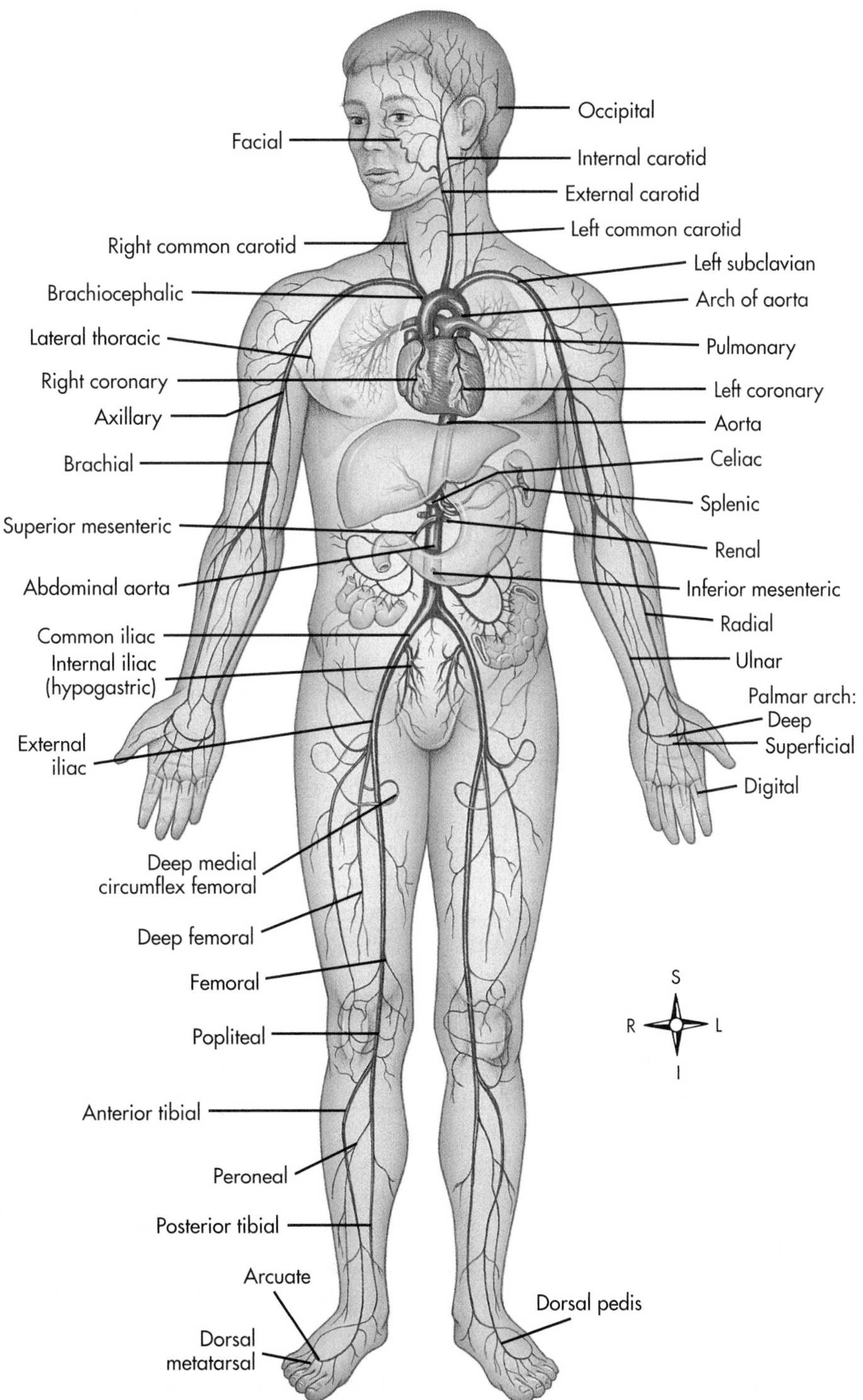

Figure 22-12 Principal arteries of the body.

The media forms the major portion of the vessel wall and in larger arteries is composed primarily of elastic and connective tissue. This enables the artery to respond to alterations in blood volume while maintaining a constant flow. In the smaller arteries and arterioles there is much less elastic fiber; the smooth muscle contracts and relaxes by nervous, chemical, and hormonal factors.

Capillaries

Capillaries, composed of a single layer of cells, are minute, thin-walled vessels located in the tissues. The capillaries connect the arterioles to the smallest veins and venules, allowing for the exchange of essential cellular products. Nutrients, oxygen, and regulatory substances move into the cells; waste products, carbon dioxide, and cellular secretions move from the cells into the blood.

Veins

Veins are thin-walled vessels that transport deoxygenated blood from the capillaries back to the right side of the heart. Veins are composed of the same three layers as arteries (intima, media, and adventitia), but in contrast to arterial walls, venous walls have little smooth muscle and connective tissue. This makes the veins distensible, enabling them to accumulate large volumes of blood. The sympathetic nervous system innervates the veins, causing venoconstriction, decreased venous volume, and increased circulating blood volume. Major veins, particularly those in the lower extremities, have one-way valves that promote blood flow against gravity and thereby prevent retrograde flow. Additionally, the squeezing action of skeletal muscle contraction creates an opposing force against gravity. Figure 22-13 shows the major veins in the body.

Principles of Blood Flow

Blood flow is brought about by a pressure difference between the various parts of the circulatory system. Multiple factors influence blood flow including vessel length, vessel radius, viscosity of the blood, pressure difference between the two ends of the vessel, cross-sectional area of the vessel, and wall tension. The rate of flow is directly related to pressure differences between the two ends of the vessel and inversely related to vessel length, vessel radius, and blood viscosity. The cross-sectional area of a vessel influences the velocity of flow; therefore, as the cross-sectional area decreases, the velocity increases and vice versa. The relationship between wall tension, pressure, and radius is described by the law of Laplace, which states wall tension becomes greater as the radius increases. Wall tension is also inversely related to wall thickness; therefore the thicker the wall of the vessel, the less tension that exists, and the thinner the wall of the vessel, the greater the tension that exists.

Physiologic Changes With Aging

The number one cause of death in people 65 years of age and older is cardiovascular disease. Age-related changes take place in the chemical composition, cells, and tissues of the heart and blood vessels that influence many aspects of cardiovascular functioning. Despite the physiologic changes of aging, however, the heart is able to meet day-to-day demands and function adequately. Only under unusual circumstances or increased stress is the changing function of the heart apparent. Coronary atherosclerosis is more prevalent in elders, but it commonly manifests as an occult (hidden) condition.

Heart

Progressive left ventricular hypertrophy occurs with aging and is accompanied by a rise in systolic blood pressure. Heart weight increases in women but not in men. Ventricular septal thickness and the circumference of all four cardiac valves increase. By age 40 years, the circumference of the aortic valve generally surpasses that of the pulmonic valve. In both genders the leaflet thickness and calcification of the mitral and aortic valves increase progressively and significantly with advancing age. These rigid valves can lead to audible systolic murmurs, usually of an ejection nature.

An increase in average myocyte (muscle cell) size explains the increase in heart mass; however, the simultaneous change in the amount and functional properties of myocardial collagen plays a key role in the development of aging-related cardiovascular abnormalities. The increased connective tissue contributes to myocardial stiffness and decreased cardiac compliance. The amount of subendocardial fat increases, and the endocardium undergoes fibrosis, thickening, and sclerosis.

A decreased peak-systolic left ventricular wall stress occurs with aging. Increasing left ventricular wall thickness and increasing body surface area with age are presumed to be contributing factors. The isovolumetric relaxation period also is prolonged, resulting in incomplete relaxation during early diastolic filling. However, enhanced ventricular filling occurs later in diastole as a result of a compensatory, augmented atrial contribution to ventricular filling.

Arteries

The degenerative changes that occur in the walls of the blood vessels as part of normal aging cause problems in the transport of blood and nutrients to the tissues. Increased thickness in the intimal wall results from fibrosis and is further affected by the accumulation of collagen and calcium.

The elastic fibers of the media become thin and calcified, greatly decreasing the elasticity and flexibility of the vessels and increasing peripheral vascular resistance. The result is a rise in blood pressure and less flow through the vessels. This results in a decreased supply of oxygen and nutrients to the tissues coupled with an accumulation of cellular secretions, waste products, and carbon dioxide.

Both the aorta and its branches and the large pulmonary arteries and their branches undergo progressive dilation and elongation with age. Because the enlargement is both transverse and longitudinal, the aorta tends to become tortuous. However, the large pulmonary arteries do not dilate longitudinally because the vessels are anatomically shorter and maintain a considerably lower pressure. The generalized loss of elasticity in the arterial system can also lead to a sluggish baroreceptor response. The baroreceptors are then less able to

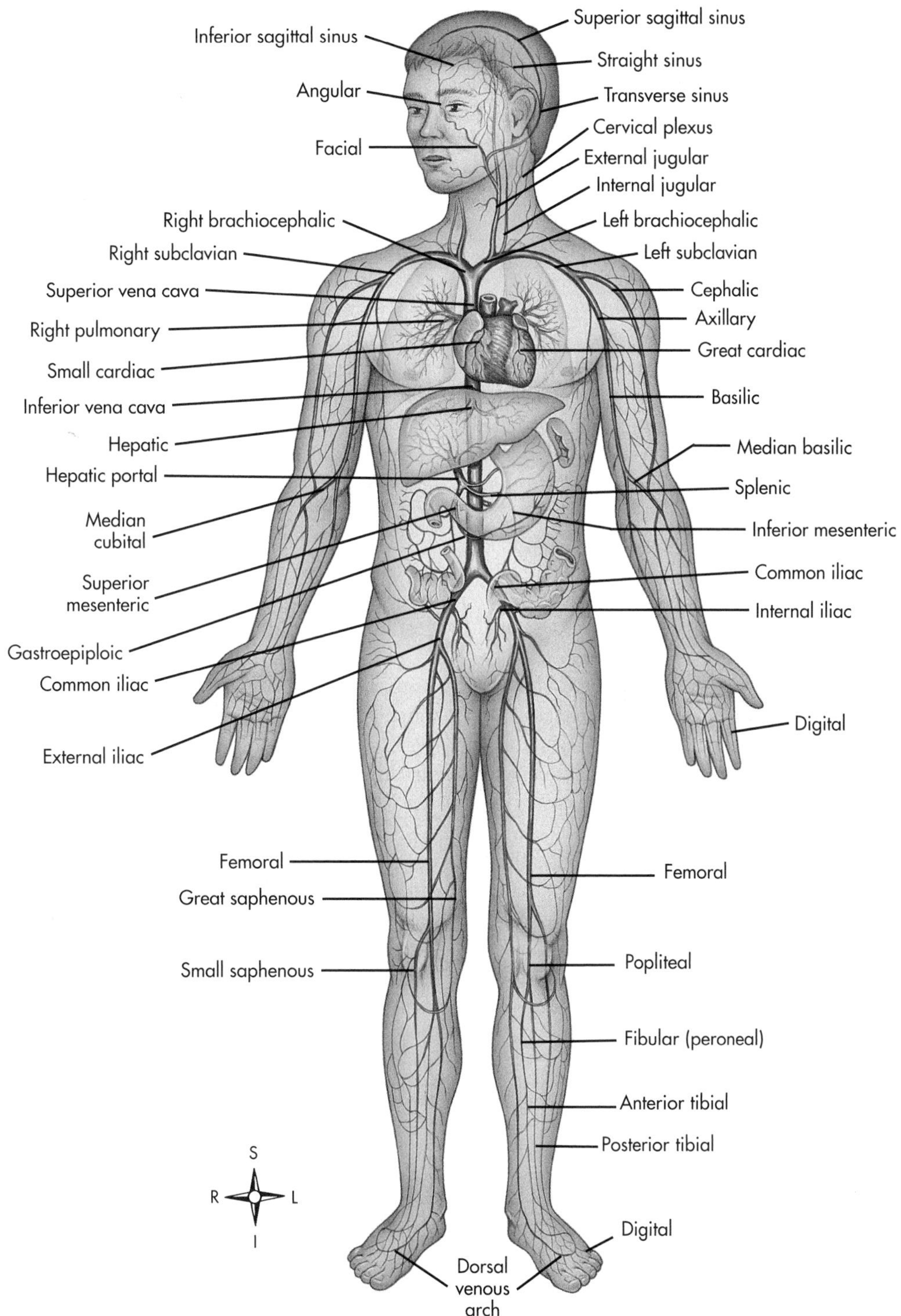

Figure 22-13 Principal veins of the body.

modulate blood pressure, particularly during rapid postural change.

Conduction System

Prolonged AV conduction with disturbances in cardiac rate and rhythm occurs in healthy aging persons as a result of fibrosis and fatty infiltration. Fibrotic changes occur predominantly in the ventricular system, whereas fatty deposits tend to occur in the SA and AV nodes, as well as in the atria.

Exercise and Cardiovascular Response

Age-related changes in the cardiovascular system are significantly more pronounced in response to exercise. The overall increase in heart rate during vigorous exercise is less in elderly persons. Older persons without significant coronary artery disease may demonstrate greater stroke volume increases compared with younger adults to compensate for the lesser increases in heart rate. Persons of all ages exhibit comparable increases in left ventricular EDV during upright exercise at low workloads. At higher workloads, in older persons whose heart rate increase is less, increases in left ventricular volume and stroke volume may continue throughout physical exercise.

Left ventricular ejection fraction has been shown to decrease, or fail to increase, with more exercise in persons with coronary artery disease. Similarly, reductions in left ventricular ejection fraction from rest to exercise also could be attributed to aging.

CARDIOVASCULAR ASSESSMENT

Systematic cardiovascular assessment provides the nurse with baseline data useful in identifying the physiologic and psychosocial needs of the patient and for planning appropriate nursing interventions to meet these needs. One must be aware that patients often present somewhat differently from one another; this is particularly true of women, who often have an "atypical" presentation associated with heart disease, with an absence of the "classic" subjective and objective presentation.

Health History

Data obtained by means of a detailed patient history can be as diagnostically significant as laboratory data and ECG recordings in the assessment of the patient with suspected cardiac disease. Accurate assessment attempts to identify both alterable and nonalterable cardiovascular risk factors pertinent to the individual and to determine the psychodynamic family relationships that must be addressed during treatment.

Classic symptoms of heart disease include dyspnea, chest pain or discomfort, edema, syncope, palpitations, and fatigue. Cardiovascular function, which may be adequate at rest, may be insufficient during exercise or exertion. Therefore careful attention is directed to the effects of activity on the patient's symptoms.

Personal Habits

The collection of data regarding nutrition, smoking, alcohol, exercise, and medications is essential. It is particularly important to assess the diet related to calorie and cholesterol content and sodium consumption. A smoking and alcohol consumption history, including the frequency and duration of consumption, is also critical. Exercise participation, both type and amount, as well as medication use, both prescription and over the counter (including herbals) are also important considerations.

Cardiovascular History: Self and Family

It is important to inquire if the patient has any significant cardiovascular history including hypertension, hyperlipidemia, congestive heart failure, coronary artery disease, murmurs, aneurysms, DVT, Raynaud's disease, and/or venous ulcers. A personal history of other diseases such as diabetes mellitus, renal disease, and/or blood dyscrasias should also be explored. If any family members have a significant cardiovascular history, it is important to obtain a detailed account of their experience and treatment if possible.

Dyspnea

Dyspnea, one of the most common and distressing symptoms of cardiopulmonary disease, is described as an abnormally uncomfortable awareness of breathing. The patient complains of shortness of breath. Dyspnea is a subjective experience and is associated with anxiety, as well as a variety of disease processes.

Assessment of dyspnea must include factors that precipitate and relieve dyspnea and data regarding the patient's body position when dyspnea occurs.

Dyspnea on exertion is a common symptom of cardiac dysfunction. In the early stages of heart failure, dyspnea usually is provoked only by effort and is relieved promptly by rest. It is important to identify the amount of exertion necessary to produce dyspnea, because the lower the cardiac reserve (heart's ability to adjust and adapt to increased demands), the less effort is required to precipitate dyspnea.

Orthopnea refers to dyspnea in the recumbent position. It is usually a symptom of more advanced heart failure than is exertional dyspnea. Patients relate that they require two or more pillows to sleep restfully. When the person assumes the recumbent position, gravitational forces redistribute blood from the lower extremities and splanchnic bed, increasing venous return. The augmentation of intrathoracic blood volume elevates pulmonary venous and capillary pressures, resulting in a transient pulmonary congestion. Orthopnea usually is relieved in less than 5 minutes after the patient sits upright.

Paroxysmal nocturnal dyspnea, also known as cardiac asthma, is characterized by severe attacks of shortness of breath that generally occur 2 to 5 hours after the onset of sleep. This condition is commonly associated with sweating and wheezing. Classically, the person awakens from sleep, arises, and quickly opens a window with the perception of needing fresh air. These frightening attacks are precipitated by the same physiologic mechanisms that cause orthopnea. The diseased heart is unable to compensate for this increase in blood volume by pumping extra fluid into the circulatory system, and pulmonary congestion results. Paroxysmal nocturnal dyspnea is relieved by the patient sitting on the side of the bed or getting out of bed. However, unlike simple orthopnea, 20 minutes or more may be required for the patient with paroxysmal nocturnal dyspnea to obtain relief.

Chest Pain

Although pain or discomfort in the chest is one of the cardinal symptoms of cardiac disorders, chest pain can also be precipitated by various noncardiac conditions such as anxiety, acute musculoskeletal injuries, pulmonary disorders (e.g., pleurisy and pulmonary embolism), esophageal spasm or reflux, and peptic ulcer disease (see Future Watch box). To evaluate chest pain accurately the following factors should be addressed during the assessment[3]:

1. Onset: When was the chest pain first noticed? (e.g., date, time)
2. Manner of onset: Did the pain or discomfort start suddenly or gradually? (e.g., quick, slow, vacillation)

Future Watch

Facial Expressions Used To Diagnose Myocardial Infarctions?

The purpose of this study was to determine whether facial expressions of patients complaining of chest pain could assist in the diagnosis of myocardial infarctions. On admission to the emergency department, patients were videotaped during physical examination. Videotapes were reviewed to code the facial action units exhibited by the patients. The presence or absence of creatine kinase enzymes were determined; however, these results were blinded to the coders until after all facial actions were coded.

An exploratory design was used for the study that occurred in a Southeastern university medical center emergency department. Twenty-eight patients who presented with chest pain were included in the study with ages ranging from 40 to 84 years. By using the Facial Action Coding System, four facial expressions were found to be associated with true myocardial infarction: lowering the brow, pressing the lips, parting lips, and turning the head left. The authors concluded that additional research with a larger sample size presenting with chest pain is needed to validate the findings of the study. However, if these findings are supported, instruction regarding assessment of specific facial expressions in clinical settings may be warranted.

Reference: Dalton JA et al: An evaluation of facial expression displayed by patients with chest pain, *Heart Lung* 28(3):168, 1999.

3. Duration: How long did the pain last? (e.g., seconds, minutes, hours)
4. Precipitating factors: What factors were associated with the onset of pain? (e.g., exertion, food, anxiety, emotions)
5. Location: Where did the pain originate? Did it radiate? To what area? (e.g., shoulder, jaw, neck, arms)
6. Quality: What did the pain feel like? Can the patient describe it? (e.g., sharp, dull, ache, pressure)
7. Intensity: How severe was the pain? (assess based on 1 to 10 scale)
8. Chronology and frequency: Has this pain occurred in the past? If so, how often? (e.g., establish timeline)
9. Associated symptoms: Did any other signs or symptoms occur at the same time? (e.g., nausea, sweating, dizziness, shortness of breath)
10. Aggravating factors: What made the pain worse? (e.g., activity, positioning, stress)
11. Relaxing factors: What made the symptoms less intense? (e.g., rest, nitroglycerin, oxygen use)

The same list of factors can also be used to evaluate leg pain. The nature of the responses can assist the examiner in establishing a diagnosis of peripheral vascular disease. Furthermore, the analysis can help to differentiate arterial from venous disease.

Syncope

Syncope is defined as a generalized muscle weakness with an inability to stand upright, accompanied by loss of consciousness. The most common cause of syncope is decreased perfusion to the brain. Any condition that results in a sudden reduction of CO and thus reduced cerebral blood flow could potentially cause a syncopal episode. In patients with cardiovascular disorders, conditions such as orthostatic hypotension, hypovolemia, or a variety of dysrhythmias (e.g., heart block and severe ventricular dysrhythmias) may precipitate syncope.

Palpitations

Palpitation is a common subjective phenomenon defined as an unpleasant awareness of the heartbeat. It may be precipitated by a change in cardiac rate or rhythm or by an increase in myocardial contractility. Patients may describe their heartbeat as "pounding," "racing," or "skipping." Palpitations that occur either during or after strenuous activity are considered physiologic. Palpitations that occur during mild exertion may suggest the presence of heart failure, anemia, or thyrotoxicosis. Other noncardiac factors that may precipitate palpitations include nervousness, heavy meals, lack of sleep, and a large intake of caffeine-containing beverages, alcohol, or tobacco.

Fatigue

Fatigue and lassitude have many causes, and therefore these symptoms are not diagnostic of cardiovascular disorders. However, fatigue may be a direct consequence of heart failure. The exact physiologic mechanism is not known, but it is probably a consequence of an inadequate CO. Such fatigue can occur during effort or at rest and generally worsens as the day progresses. Fatigue that occurs after mild exertion may indicate a low cardiac reserve if the heart is unable to meet even small increases in metabolic demands.

Physical Examination

Physical examination of the cardiovascular system includes the standard assessment techniques of inspection, palpation, percussion, and auscultation. Before beginning the cardiovascular examination, vital signs should be obtained. Respiration, pulse, temperature, and blood pressure provide initial information about the patient's baseline physiologic status.

Inspection

Skin Color. The color of the patient's skin and mucous membranes is noted. A person's "normal" color depends on race, ethnic background, and lifestyle and is an indication of adequate CO and circulation. Pallor may indicate anemia, hypoxia, or peripheral vasoconstriction. Cyanosis, a bluish discoloration of the skin, is most easily observed by examining the earlobes, oral mucosa at the base of the tongue, lips, and nailbeds. (Refer to Chapter 61 for more detail on assessment of skin color.)

There are two types of cyanosis: central and peripheral. In central cyanosis the tongue is characteristically cyanotic. This form of cyanosis is caused by low arterial oxygen saturation and generally is seen in patients who have congenital heart defects or in those with pulmonary diseases that interfere with ventilation or diffusion.

Peripheral cyanosis results from low CO and generally is accompanied by decreased skin temperature and mottling. In contrast to central cyanosis, no cyanosis of the tongue is present.

Skin color of the extremities is also assessed. It is important to note any erythema or pigmentation changes, as well as the presence of shiny or dry, scaly skin, which may indicate a vascular disorder. Hair distribution, venous pattern, and size of the extremities should be assessed.

Neck Vein Distention. A general estimate of venous pressure can be obtained by observation of the neck veins (Figure 22-14). Normally, when a person is supine, the neck veins are distended. However, when the head of the bed is elevated to a 45-degree angle, the neck veins are collapsed. If jugular distention is present, jugular venous pressure can be assessed by measuring from the highest point of visible distention to the sternal angle. Measurements above 3 cm are considered elevated.

The jugular veins reflect venous tone, blood volume, and right atrial pressure. Therefore distended neck veins suggest increased venous pressure, which may be caused by right-sided heart failure, circulatory volume overload, superior vena caval obstruction, or tricuspid valve regurgitation.

Respirations. The rate and character of the patient's respirations are important to assess. Normally an adult breathes comfortably at a rate of 12 to 20 times per minute. Particular attention is paid to the ease or difficulty in breathing and the patient's general demeanor.

Pulsations. Inspection of the anterior chest is best accomplished with the patient lying supine, either flat or with the head slightly elevated. The precordium is observed for the apical impulse, which is a pulsation of the chest wall caused by the forward thrusting of the left ventricle during systole. When visible, the apical impulse occupies the fourth or fifth intercostal space, at or inside the midclavicular line. The apical impulse was formerly known as the point of maximal impulse. The apical impulse is not always visible, but it is palpable in about half of adults.

Clubbing and Capillary Refill. The nails are assessed for clubbing and capillary refill. The exact cause of clubbing is not known; however, clubbing of the fingers is common in congenital heart defects and pulmonary arteriovenous (A-V) fistulas with right-to-left shunting. Capillary filling, or blanching, is an indicator of peripheral circulation to the fingers and toes and can be tested in all nailbeds. The examiner presses a thumbnail against the edge of a patient's fingernail or toenail and then quickly releases it. The normal response is whitening (blanching) of the area when pressure is applied and brisk return of color when pressure is released. Lack of the blanching response may indicate lack of circulation to the finger or toe because of arterial insufficiency secondary to atherosclerosis or spasm; however, severe vasoconstriction may be the causative factor.

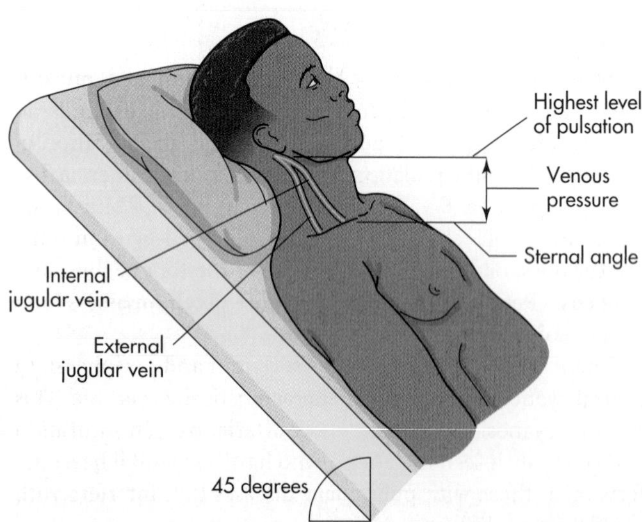

Figure 22-14 Position of internal and external jugular veins used in measuring venous pressure.

Palpation

Peripheral Pulses. One method for evaluating the arterial flow of the vascular system is palpation of the extremities simultaneously to determine skin temperature. A second method is palpation of the peripheral pulses, which are evaluated bilaterally on the basis of their absence or presence, rate, rhythm, amplitude, quality, and equality. Each pulse, except the carotids, is palpated on the left and right side simultaneously to evaluate contralateral symmetry (Figure 22-15).

Pulses are rated on a scale of 0 to +4 as follows:

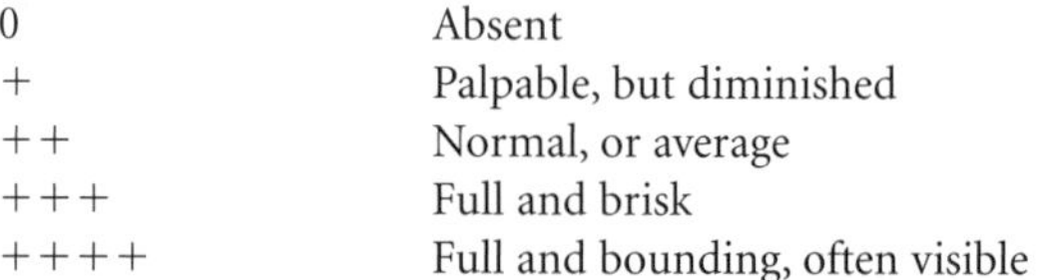

0	Absent
+	Palpable, but diminished
++	Normal, or average
+++	Full and brisk
++++	Full and bounding, often visible

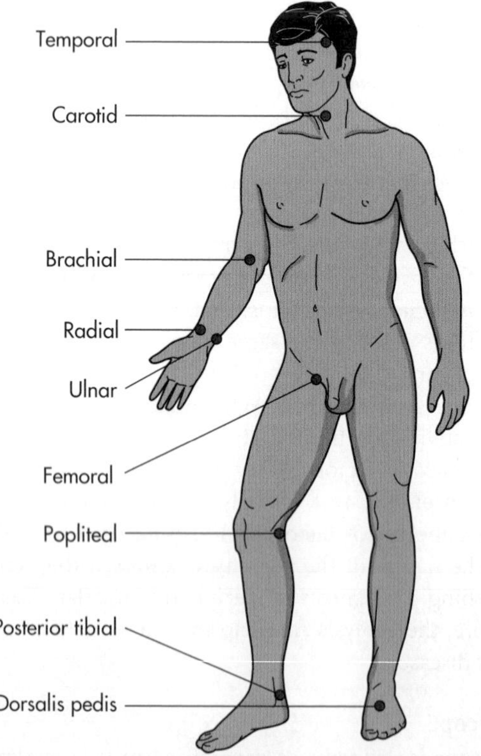

Figure 22-15 Body sites at which peripheral pulses are most easily palpated.

Several abnormalities may be detected during palpation of pulses. A hypokinetic (weak) pulse signifies a narrowed pulse pressure, a decreased difference between the systolic and diastolic pressures. It usually is produced by a low CO and is associated with increased peripheral vascular resistance. This type of pulse is often detected in such conditions as severe left ventricular failure, hypovolemia, or mitral and aortic valve stenosis.

A hyperkinetic (bounding) pulse represents a widened pulse pressure. It usually is associated with an increased left ventricular stroke volume and a decrease in peripheral vascular resistance. This type of pulse is often found in hyperkinetic circulatory states caused by exercise, fever, anemia, or hyperthyroidism.

Pulsus alternans is a condition in which the heart beats regularly, but the pulses vary in amplitude. It is caused by an alternating left ventricular contractile force and usually indicates severe depression of myocardial function. Pulsus alternans may be detected by palpation but is more accurately assessed by auscultation of the blood pressure.

Pulsus paradoxus signifies a reduction in the amplitude of the arterial pulse during inspiration. Variations in pulse strength can be palpated, but a paradoxic pulse is most readily detected by sphygmomanometry. Pulsus paradoxus is an accentuation of the normal decrease in systolic arterial pressure with inspiration. This is a result of decreased left ventricular stroke volume and the transmission of negative intrathoracic pressure to the aorta. Pulsus paradoxus may occur in conditions such as cardiac tamponade and constrictive pericarditis, but it also may occur in patients with chronic obstructive airway disease who have wide swings of intrapleural pressure during respiration.

Normally the apical impulse is felt as a single, light tap. The presence of anything other than a single, light tap may suggest a myocardial pathologic condition and should be reported to the physician. A thrill, or palpable murmur, indicates the presence of significant turbulent blood flow across an intracardiac shunt or a severely stenotic valve. A thrill is often described as a vibration similar to that of a cat's purr and is more readily palpated after the patient exhales forcefully. Having the patient in a left lateral position or leaning forward may accentuate the vibration.

Edema. Edema is defined as an accumulation of fluid in the interstitial spaces. It may be localized to one particular body part, organ, or tissue; or there may be a generalized distribution. Retention of considerable amounts of extracellular fluid may occur without associated edema. In fact, weight gains of up to 7 kg of water can occur before the abnormality is detected. Because early manifestations of edema may be subtle, careful comparison of daily weights is required to determine weight gains resulting from fluid retention. Normally, basal body weight varies little from day to day; therefore subtle weight gains resulting from fluid retention are readily detectable.

An important indicator of cardiovascular function is the presence or absence of peripheral edema, especially in the feet, ankles, legs, and sacrum. Non-pitting peripheral edema is caused by gravity flow or by interruption of the venous return to the heart as a result of constricting clothing or pressure on the veins of the lower extremities. This edema often disappears on elevation of the body part.

In contrast, pitting edema does not disappear with elevation of the extremity or body part, and it may indicate fluid overload or a pathologic condition (e.g., heart failure). Pitting edema is described as an indentation left in the skin after a thumb or finger has been used to apply gentle pressure. See Table 22-2 for a scale that is commonly used to assess pitting edema.[8]

Percussion

The use of percussion for detecting cardiac enlargement generally has been replaced by the chest x-ray study, which is much more accurate. Therefore the use of percussion in the

TABLE 22-2 Pitting Edema Scale

Scale	Description	Measurement
1+	A barely perceptible pit	2 mm (3/32 in)
2+	A deeper pit; rebounds in a few seconds	4 mm (5/32 in)
3+	A deep pit; rebounds in 10-20 seconds	6 mm (1/4 in)
4+	A deeper pit; rebounds in >30 seconds	8 mm (5/16 in)

From Wilson S, Giddens J: *Health assessment for nursing practice*, ed 2, St Louis, 2001, Mosby.

cardiovascular examination is somewhat limited. Usually only the left border of cardiac dullness can be determined, inasmuch as this is located near the apical impulse, or within the midclavicular line. Cardiac dullness is characteristic of cardiac hypertrophy. Unfortunately, mild to moderate degrees of cardiac hypertrophy are not usually detectable by percussion.

Auscultation

Heart Sounds. The first heart sound (S_1), called lub, generally is thought to be produced by the almost simultaneous closures of the mitral and tricuspid valves. S_1 lasts approximately 0.10 second and signals the onset of ventricular systole. S_1 is generally loudest at the apex but can be heard over the entire precordium. S_1 is longer and lower pitched than the second heart sound (S_2), called dub (the first and second heart sounds together are referred to as lub-dub), and S_1 corresponds to the beat of the carotid pulse. S_2 is caused mainly by the closure of the semilunar valves (aortic and pulmonic) and is loudest at the base of the heart and described as shorter, higher pitched, and "snappier" than S_1. The sounds of the cardiac cycle are depicted in Figure 22-16.

The diaphragm chest piece of the stethoscope is most useful for listening to high-pitched sounds and murmurs. These include S_1, S_2, ejection sounds, and clicks. The diaphragm is placed firmly on the chest wall so that an indentation is present on the patient's skin when the diaphragm is removed. The bell chest piece is most useful in detecting low-pitched sounds and murmurs. These include the third heart sound (S_3), the fourth heart sound (S_4), and mitral and tricuspid diastolic rumbles. The bell is placed lightly on the chest wall, barely creating an airtight seal. If the bell is placed firmly on the skin it acts as a diaphragm.

Splitting of S_1 and S_2. The two main components of S_1 (closure of the mitral and tricuspid valves) are asynchronous, because left ventricular systole usually occurs slightly ahead of right ventricular systole. The S_1 may be split in persons who have RBB block, left-sided mechanical defects (e.g., mitral stenosis) or tricuspid valve dysfunction associated with pulmonary hypertension.

Because left ventricular contraction slightly precedes right ventricular contraction, the aortic valve also normally closes slightly before the pulmonic valve. On inspiration, intrathoracic pressure decreases and facilitates an increase in venous blood return to the right side of the heart. This increased blood return delays the closure of the pulmonic valve and results in a normal physiologic split S_2. On expiration, closure of the aortic and pulmonic valves occurs almost simultaneously and therefore is heard only as a single sound. In conditions of increased blood flow or increased right ventricular pressure there may be a "fixed" splitting of S_2; that is, both components of S_2 are heard on both inspiration and expiration. A fixed split is considered abnormal and may occur in RBB block, pulmonary hypertension, and right ventricular failure related to atrial or ventricular septal defects.

Extra Heart Sounds. Extra heart sounds include ejection sounds (systolic clicks), opening snaps, S_3, and S_4. The two most common extra heart sounds are S_3 and S_4, or ventricular gallop and atrial gallop, respectively (Figure 22-17).

Ventricular diastolic gallop, or S_3, is a faint, low-pitched sound produced by rapid ventricular filling in early diastole. It occurs when the volume of early filling is increased or a decrease occurs in ventricular compliance. Ventricular "gallop" recalls the gallop of a horse, which is mimicked at heart rates greater than 100. When this sound is present in healthy children and young adults, it is almost always a normal condition and is referred to as a physiologic S_3. An S_3 heard in an older person usually is a pathologic sign and commonly is one of the first signs of serious heart disease or cardiac decompensation. S_3 is typically present in such conditions as left-to-right shunts, mitral regurgitation, heart failure, and constrictive pericarditis.

Atrial diastolic gallop, or S_4, is a low-frequency sound that occurs under circumstances of altered ventricular compliance, either left or right. S_4 occurs late in diastole when atrial systole ejects blood into a noncompliant ventricle. Because the presence of an audible S_4 is related to a decrease in left ventricular compliance and an increase in left ventricular end-diastolic pressure, it is often heard in hypertensive cardiovascular disease and idiopathic hypertrophic subaortic stenosis. An S_4 commonly is identified in patients with acute myocardial infarction and in patients with coronary artery disease, especially during an attack of angina pectoris. In addition, an S_4 may be present when CO and stroke volume are increased, such as in severe anemia, thyrotoxicosis, and large A-V fistulas. Although the S_4 sound occurs close to S_1, it can be easily differentiated because S_4 is lower pitched than S_1.

Murmurs. Murmurs are audible vibrations of the heart and great vessels that occur because of turbulent blood flow. They may be produced by hemodynamic events or by structural alterations occurring in the heart or in the walls of the great vessels. In general, murmurs are heard most distinctly over the area of the valve or altered cardiac structure respon-

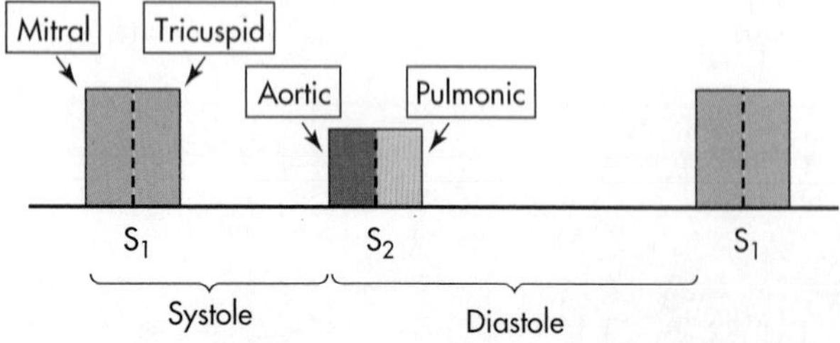

Figure 22-16 Heart sound S_1 is the closure of mitral and tricuspid valves: S_2 is the closure of the aortic and pulmonic valves. Systole is the interval between S_1 and the start of S_2; diastole is S_2 to the start of S_1. Diastole is longer than systole.

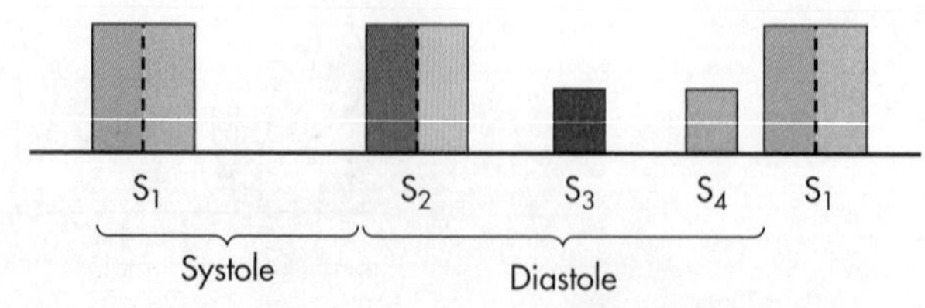

Figure 22-17 Location of extra heart sounds during cardiac cycle.

sible for the vibrations. The major factors involved in the production of cardiac murmurs include the following: (1) increased velocity of blood flow through normal or abnormal valves; (2) forward flow through a stenotic or irregular valve orifice; (3) backward (regurgitant) blood flow through an incompetent valve, septal defect, or patent ductus arteriosus; and (4) turbulent blood flow produced in a dilated chamber, such as in a ventricular or aortic aneurysm.[4]

Murmurs generally are characterized according to timing (position in the cardiac cycle), intensity, quality, pattern, posture, pitch, location, and direction of radiation. These characteristics provide data concerning the location and nature of the cardiac abnormality.

Pericardial Friction Rub. A pericardial friction rub is an extra heart sound originating from the pericardial sac as the heart moves. It is often a sign of inflammation, infection, or infiltration The sound is high pitched and scratchy, similar to sandpaper being rubbed together. The sound is best heard with the diaphragm of the stethoscope while the patient is in an upright position and leaning forward.

Assessment measures and variations in normal findings relevant to the care of older adults are presented in the Gerontologic Assessment box. Also identified are disorders common in older adults, which may be responsible for abnormal assessment findings.

Diagnostic Tests

Cardiovascular diseases usually are diagnosed by reviewing diagnostic test results combined with findings from the patient interview and the physical examination. The diagnostic tests ordered most commonly in patients with heart disease include blood tests, urinalysis, electrocardiography, invasive hemodynamic monitoring, sonic studies, dynamic studies, radiography, scintigraphic studies, and angiography.

The nurse may be directly or indirectly involved in these tests and procedures. It is essential that the nurse possess an understanding of the various tests or procedures and the importance of the data to an accurate diagnosis. This information enables the nurse to prepare the patient adequately before any diagnostic procedure and to document relevant signs and symptoms while caring for the patient.

Laboratory Tests

A complete blood cell count is ordered for all patients with documented or suspected heart disease. Data concerning red blood cells (RBCs) and white blood cells are helpful in diagnosing infectious heart disease and myocardial infarction (Table 22-3). The RBC count may be elevated as a physiologic response to inadequate tissue oxygenation. The erythrocyte sedimentation rate is a measurement of the rate at which RBCs "settle out" of anticoagulated blood in 1 hour. The rate of settling is increased if the proportion of globulin to albumin increases or if fibrinogen levels are excessively increased. Nonspecific increases in globulin and fibrinogen levels occur when the body responds to injury or inflammation, as seen with infectious heart disorders and myocardial infarction.

Blood coagulation tests, including prothrombin time, international normalized ratio, and activated partial thromboplastin time, indicate the rapidity of blood clotting.[5] These tests are useful during anticoagulation therapy (Table 22-3) A blood urea nitrogen (BUN) determination is a useful indicator of renal function. Decreased CO leading to a low renal blood supply and reduction in glomerular filtration rate will elevate the BUN.

Blood Lipids. The blood (plasma) lipids are composed mainly of cholesterol, triglyceride, phospholipid, and free fatty acids, all of which are insoluble in water and require a "carrier" to transport them. The carriers for plasma lipids are the proteins to which they are bound, thus the name lipoproteins. There are four major classes of lipoproteins: chylomicrons, very low–density lipoproteins, low-density lipoproteins, and high-density lipoproteins, all of which contain varying levels of cholesterol, triglycerides, and phospholipids.

Gerontologic Assessment

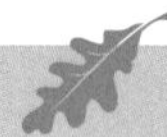

ASSESSMENT

Count the pulse for a full minute at rest and after exertion.
- The pulse is often slower and may be irregular because elders are more prone to decreased cardiac output and dysrhythmias.

Monitor changes in blood pressure.
- Systolic blood pressure in elders may normally be as high as 160 mm Hg (as compared with 140 mm Hg in younger adults). A widened pulse pressure also may be observed.
- Check blood pressure in a lying, sitting, and standing position to detect postural hypotension because vasomotor control is decreased in older adults.

Auscultate carefully.
- Murmurs are common from thickening and calcification of the valves. Also, extra heart sounds may be present on auscultation. S_4 often occurs in older people with no known cardiac disease. However, detection of an S_3 is associated with congestive heart failure and is always abnormal over age 35. When assessing the heart, note that the apical impulse may be harder to locate.

Monitor for signs of mental confusion, lethargy, indigestion, and weakness in the elderly person.
- These may be early signs of cardiac disease. Angina is common with ischemic heart disease.

Always use caution when palpating and auscultating the carotid artery because pressure in the carotid sinus area can cause a reflex slowing of the heart rate.
- Creating pressure on this area is a particular risk with older adults because circulation may already be compromised by atherosclerosis.

COMMON DISORDERS IN OLDER ADULTS

Atherosclerosis
Congestive heart failure
Angina pectoris
Myocardial infarction
Dysrhythmias
Valvular disorders
Left ventricular hypertrophy
Hypertension
Peripheral vascular disease

TABLE 22-3 Selected Laboratory Tests for Cardiovascular Disorders

Test	Normal Values	Significance in Heart Disorders
Serum red blood cell count	Men: 4.6-6.2 million/mm³ Women: 4.2-5.4 million/mm³	Decreased in subacute endocarditis Increased with inadequate tissue oxygenation Decreased in some congenital heart disease with right-to-left shunt
Serum white blood cell count	4,500-11,000/mm³	Increased in acute and chronic heart inflammations and in acute myocardial infarction
Erythrocyte sedimentation rate (ESR)	Men: up to 15 mm/h Women: up to 20 mm/h	Increased in acute myocardial infarction and infectious heart disease
Prothrombin time	12-14 sec 100% compared to control	Indicates rapidity of blood clotting; used to monitor anticoagulant therapy with warfarin (Coumadin)
International normalized ratio	2-3	Ratio of patient's prothrombin time to the normal standard prothrombin time of the testing laboratory; used to monitor anticoagulant therapy with warfarin (Coumadin)
Activated partial thromboplastin time	20-35 sec	More sensitive than PT; used to monitor heparin therapy
Blood urea nitrogen	11-23 mg/dl	Increased with decreased cardiac output
Serum proteins	6-8 g/dl	Levels below 5 g/100 ml seen with edema

Chylomicrons are composed mainly of triglycerides and originate in the intestine after the absorption of dietary fat. Chylomicrons should not be found in the plasma after 12 to 14 hours of fasting. Elevated chylomicron levels do not appear to be associated with heart disease.

Very-low-density lipoproteins (VLDLs) are composed primarily of triglycerides and are synthesized in the liver. Sustained elevations of VLDLs are associated with the development of both atherosclerosis and coronary artery disease.

Low-density lipoproteins (LDLs) are composed of approximately 50% cholesterol and are thought to have the greatest correlation with coronary artery disease. The LDLs are believed to enter the arterial intima and produce arterial endothelial injury. This process can result in progressive atherosclerotic plaque formation and eventually ischemic heart disease. Lipoprotein (a), or Lp(a), is a protein associated with LDL. High plasma levels of Lp(a) have been correlated with an increased risk for atherothrombotic cardiovascular disease. Structurally Lp(a) is similar to plasminogen, which explains its ability to interfere with the processes involved in plasmin generation and clot lysis.

High-density lipoproteins (HDLs) are composed of mostly protein with a modest amount of cholesterol and a considerable amount of phospholipids. This lipoprotein appears to have the lowest atherogenic potential. In fact, studies have demonstrated that HDLs are inversely associated with coronary heart disease. The HDLs are believed to carry cholesterol away from tissues, including atheromatous plaques and provide some protection against coronary heart disease.

The National Cholesterol Education Program Expert Panel on Detection, Evaluation, and Treatment of High Blood Cholesterol established and updates criteria for cholesterol and lipid assessment that includes total cholesterol, LDL, HDL, and triglyceride levels (Table 22-4). Adjustments in target levels are made for individuals with coronary artery disease risk factors such as hypertension, diabetes mellitus, or family history of premature coronary disease.[7]

Evaluation of individual components is important, but the most significant predictor of coronary artery disease is the ratio of total cholesterol to HDL. Before blood lipid tests are performed the patient must fast for 12 hours. No alcoholic beverages or lipid-influencing drugs (e.g., estrogens, oral contraceptives, steroids, salicylates) should be taken. Because lipid levels may fluctuate greatly from day to day, repeated blood samples are obtained before a definitive diagnosis of hyperlipidemia is made.

Blood Cultures. Blood cultures are crucial in the diagnosis of infectious diseases of the heart such as endocarditis. Culture results help identify the organism responsible for the infectious process and its sensitivity to various antibiotics.

Enzyme Studies. Enzymes, which are located in all tissues, catalyze the biochemical reactions of the body. When cell membranes are damaged, such as in myocardial infarction, enzymes leak out of the damaged myocardial cell and escape into the serum. The different enzymes are released into the blood at varying times after a myocardial infarction. It is crucial to evaluate the enzyme level in relation to the time of onset of the chest pain or other symptoms. Refer to Chapter 23 for a detailed description of the time course of cardiac enzymes after a myocardial infarction.

The serum enzyme measurements that are used to detect myocardial necrosis are serum aspartate aminotransferase (AST), creatine kinase (CK), troponin I, lactic dehydrogenase (LDH), and hydroxybutyrate dehydrogenase (HBD). Because these enzymes are located in various body tissues, numerous conditions other than myocardial damage may produce enzyme elevations; for example, the brain, pancreas, and liver are all rich sources of AST. If a person were to develop chest pain concurrently with pancreatic or liver disease, an elevated AST level may be mistaken for myocardial necrosis. Fortunately, three of the enzymes, CK, troponin I, and LDH, have isoenzymes that are thought to be present almost exclusively in myocardial muscle.

The CK molecule has two subunits, which have been identified as follows: M, associated with muscle; and B, associated

TABLE 22-4 Initial Classification of Total, Low-Density Lipoprotein, and High-Density Lipoprotein Cholesterol and Triglycerides

Classification	Total Cholesterol	Low-Density Lipoprotein Cholesterol	High-Density Lipoprotein Cholesterol	Triglycerides
Optimal	<200 mg/dl	<100 mg/dl	>60 mg/dl	—
Normal/Near Optimal	200 mg/dl	100-129 mg/dl	>40 mg/dl	<150 mg/dl
Borderline high	200-239 mg/dl	130-159 mg/dl	—	150-199 mg/dl
High	≥240 mg/dl	160-189 mg/dl	—	200-499 mg/dl
Very high		≥190 mg/dl	—	>500 mg/dl

with brain. The brain and gastrointestinal tract contain modest amounts of the BB dimer, and skeletal muscle contains large amounts of the MM form. Heart muscle contains huge quantities of MM, but it also contains the MB hybrid form of CK. Because CK-MB is not found in any other tissue, its presence in the serum is a sensitive indicator of myocardial damage.

Cardiac troponin I is the newest enzyme study. Troponin is normally present in minuscule amounts and is specific to heart muscle. It is immediately released from damaged myocardial cells and is present in the blood for about 1 week after release. Of the five LDH isoenzymes, LDH1 has been found to be the most sensitive indicator of myocardial damage; however, the use of LDH isoenzymes has largely been replaced by troponin and CK-MB.

Serologic Tests. Syphilis can play an important role in the development of aortic disorders. The patient may have aortic insufficiency, aortic aneurysms, or disease of the orifices of the coronary arteries. Because of the relationship between syphilis and heart disease, a routine Venereal Disease Research Laboratories (VDRL) test is performed on all cardiac patients.

Urinalysis. A routine urinalysis is performed to determine the effects of cardiovascular disease on renal function. Mild to moderate proteinuria (usually albuminuria) may be seen in patients with malignant hypertension and venous congestion of the kidneys secondary to heart failure or constrictive pericarditis. The presence of RBCs in the urine may indicate infective endocarditis or an embolic kidney disease.

Detection of myoglobin in the urine (myoglobinuria) has been useful in the diagnosis of myocardial infarction. Clinical experience with this test remains limited; however, it may prove to be a sensitive indicator of myocardial damage. Destruction of striated muscle by infarction liberates myoglobin, and because of its small size, the molecule can filter through the glomerulus and be excreted in the urine.

Radiologic Tests

Chest Radiography. A radiograph (x-ray film) of the chest may be taken to determine overall size and configuration of the heart, as well as individual cardiac chamber size. Most abnormalities of heart size and calcification in the heart muscle, valves, and great vessels can be detected with standard posteroanterior and lateral views of the chest.

Cardiac Fluoroscopy. Cardiac fluoroscopy facilitates observation of the heart from varying views while the heart is beating. Fluoroscopy can be used to detect ventricular aneurysms, monitor prosthetic valve movement, or assess the position of cardiac calcifications during the cardiac cycle. Because of the radiation risk associated with fluoroscopy, many institutions no longer use this diagnostic technique.

BOX 22-1 Diagnostic Uses for the Electrocardiogram

The ECG may be used to evaluate the following:
- Tachycardia, bradycardia, or dysrhythmias
- Sudden onset of dyspnea
- Pain occurring in the upper part of the trunk and in the extremities
- Syncopal episodes
- Shock state or coma
- Preoperative status
- Postoperative hypotension
- Hypertension, murmurs, or cardiomegaly
- Artificial pacemaker function

Special Tests

Electrocardiogram. The ECG is a graphic representation of the electrical forces produced within the heart. The ECG is an essential tool for cardiac evaluation, but it must be combined with other data sources for accurate diagnosis. A resting ECG may be normal, even in the presence of heart disease. Conversely, abnormal variances may be seen in the ECG of a normal heart.

An ECG may be used for a wide variety of diagnostic purposes (Box 22-1). The patient should be informed of the step-by-step procedure and assured of its safe, painless nature.

Standard 12-Lead ECG. The ECG tracing represents the net electrical activity or electrical potential variations of the atria and ventricles as each depolarizes and repolarizes. The electrical currents passing through the heart can be detected by electrodes and measured when they reach the surface.

The conventional 12-lead ECG machine uses several electrode sites to measure the electrical potential differences between a series of locations on the body surface. Each pair of electrodes, consisting of a positive and a negative terminal, constitutes an ECG lead. Representative tracings obtained from the 12 leads are shown in Figure 22-18. The standard lead sites are right arm, left arm, right leg, and left leg. The

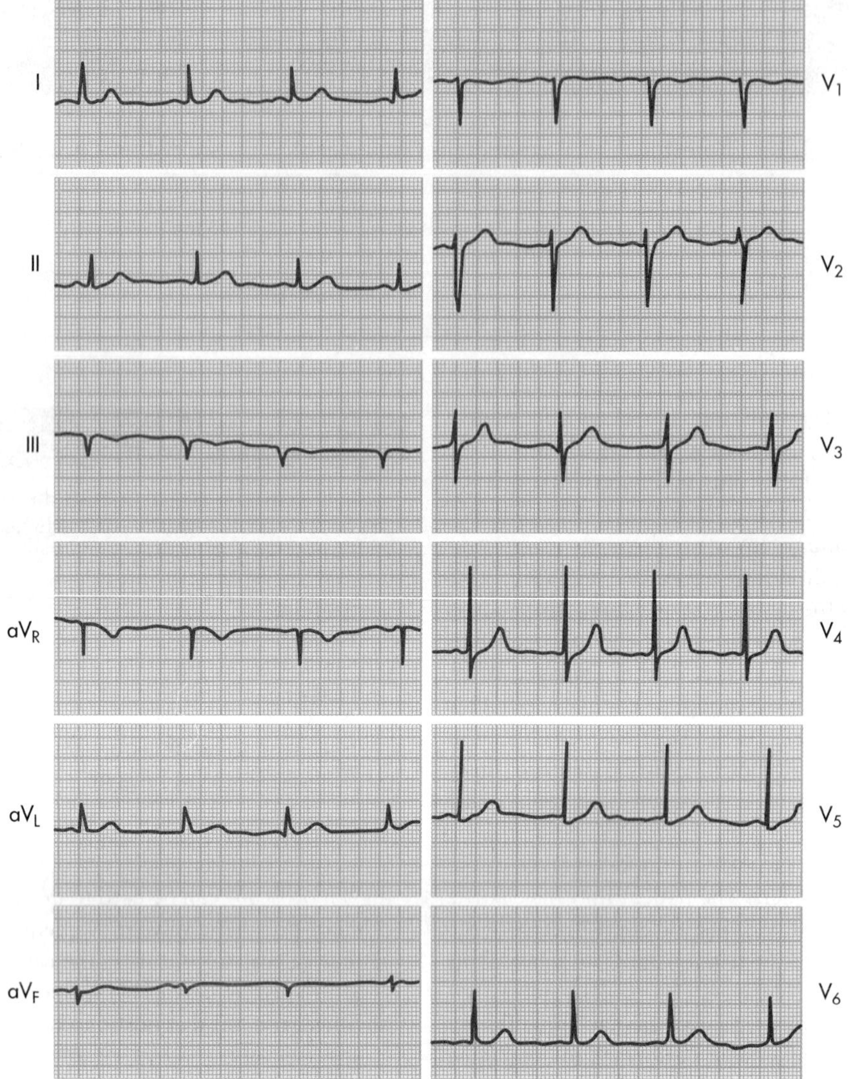

Figure 22-18 Twelve-lead ECG showing normal sinus rhythm.

chest (or precordial) electrodes are placed across the chest wall in six different locations. These 10 sites are combined in pairs through a switching network in the ECG machine. Effective contact between the skin and electrode is established by the use of electrode jelly, which contains electrolytes and an abrasive capable of penetrating the waterproof layer of the skin.

Limb Leads. The standard bipolar limb leads, designated by Roman numerals I, II, and III, are created by electrodes applied to the right arm (RA), left arm (LA), and left leg (LL) (Figure 22-19). The right leg (RL) electrode acts as a grounding electrode. Lead I records the difference between the RA and LA potentials. Lead II records the difference between the RA and LL potentials. Lead III records the difference between the LA and LL potentials.

The augmented unipolar limb leads are designated by the abbreviated forms aV_R, aV_L, and aV_F. For these leads the right arm (R), left arm (L), and left leg (F) become the respective positive electrodes (Figure 22-20).

For clinical purposes the amplitude of the recordings from these electrodes is augmented by approximately 50% to produce a tracing that is easier to interpret. Together, the augmented and standard limb leads provide the six frontal plane leads.

Precordial Leads. There are six precordial or chest leads designated by the symbols V_1 through V_6. These leads register the electrical variations of the heart in the horizontal plane (Figure 22-21). The positive electrode is placed on six different sites across the chest (Figure 22-22).

Monitoring. To perform continuous cardiac monitoring, the conventional ECG leads have been modified to eliminate cumbersome wiring. The most popular leads for continuous cardiac monitoring are lead II and lead V_1. The patient wears two, three, or five electrodes, which are attached by small lead wires to a cable connected to a wall-mounted monitor with an oscilloscope screen.

An alternative type of continuous monitoring is known as telemetry. The telemetry system requires no cables that would

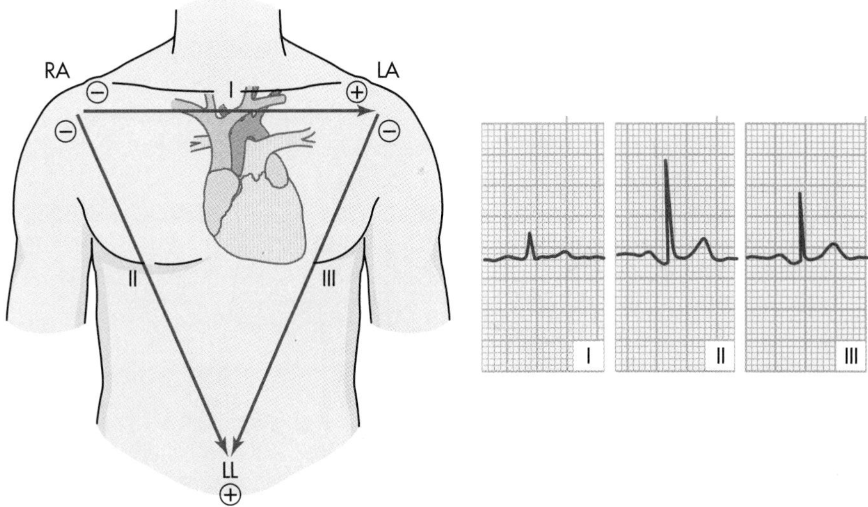

Figure 22-19 Schematic representation of standard limb lead system.

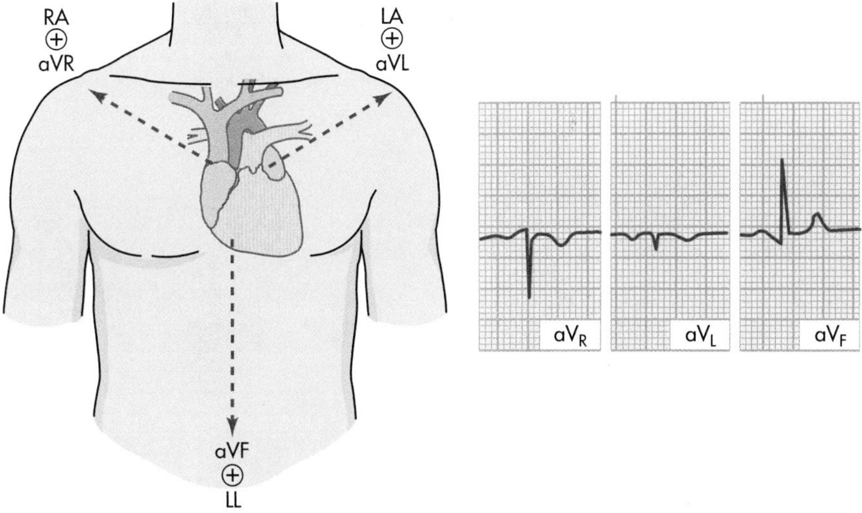

Figure 22-20 Schematic representation of augmented unipolar limb lead system.

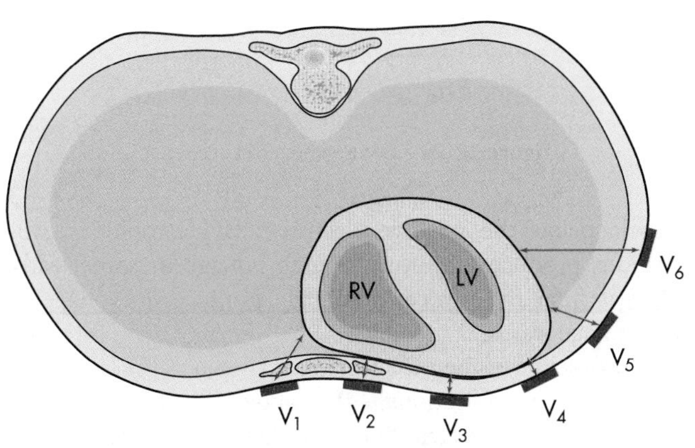

Figure 22-21 Cross-section of heart showing precordial leads V_1 through V_6 in a horizontal plane.

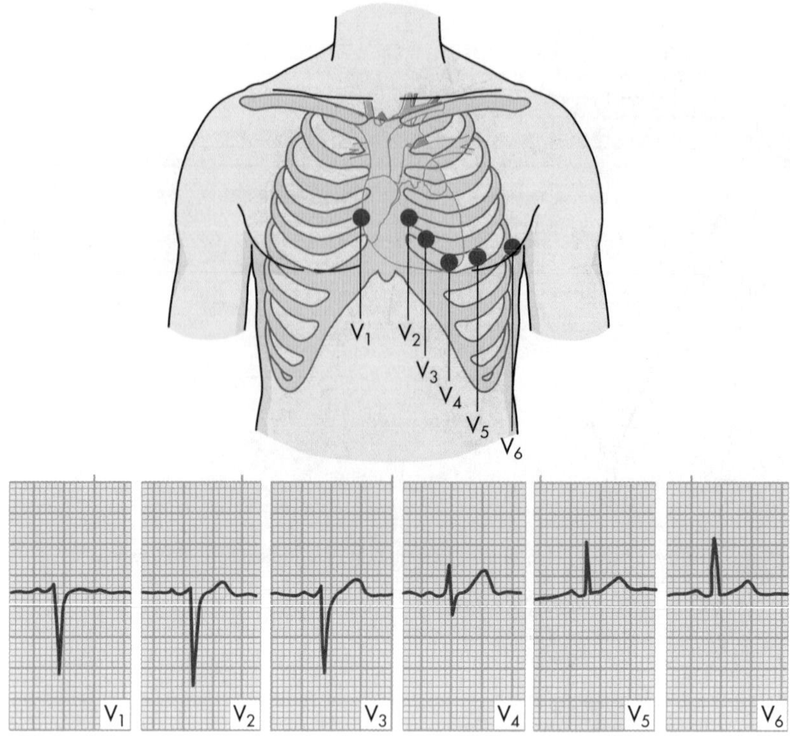

Figure 22-22 Anatomic placement of precordial leads.

restrict patient mobility. The electrical impulses are transmitted through an antenna to an oscilloscope at another location.

Lead II is produced by placing the negative electrode on the right arm (modified and placed near the right shoulder below the clavicle) and the positive electrode on the left leg (modified and placed on the lower left rib cage eighth intercostal space).

Lead V_1 is produced by placing the negative electrode on the left arm (modified and placed near the left shoulder below the clavicle) and the positive electrode at the fourth intercostal space to the right of the sternum. With these modifications, V_1 is known as MCL_1. The MCL_1 lead is the most helpful lead for determining the origin of premature beats and determining the presence of bundle branch blocks.

***Electrocardiographic Tracing*.** The ECG tracing is recorded on graph paper that is divided into millimeter squares. The millimeter squares are grouped and divided into larger squares by thick lines that occur every fifth square (Figure 22-23).

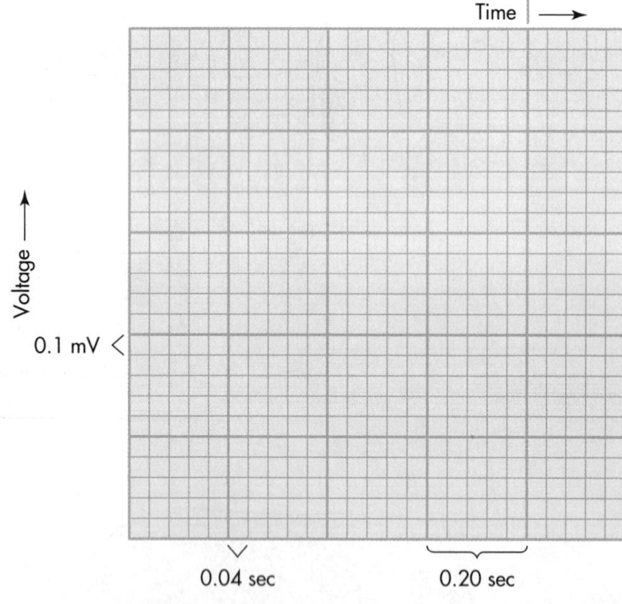

Figure 22-23 Components of ECG paper.

Horizontally each millimeter square represents 0.04 second of time elapsed. Each thick line denotes the passage of 0.20 second. Fifteen hundred (1500) small, or 300 large, squares represent 1 minute. With this information, the duration of any complex or interval on the ECG can be determined by counting the number of small squares and multiplying by 0.04 second. Heart rate may be measured or estimated by various methods (Box 22-2).

Vertically each small square is 1 mm in height and represents 0.1 mV of voltage. Thus each large square represents 5 mm or 0.5 mV. The voltage or amplitude of a wave or complex in a given lead indirectly indicates the electrical activity of the muscle below the positive electrode. Hypertrophied myocardium produces abnormally high voltage in some leads, whereas infarcted myocardium may produce no voltage or low-voltage waves.

The baseline of the ECG tracing is known as the isoelectric line. Waves are deflections, either above (positive) or below (negative) the isoelectric line. The direction of deflection is determined by (1) the direction in which the electrical im-

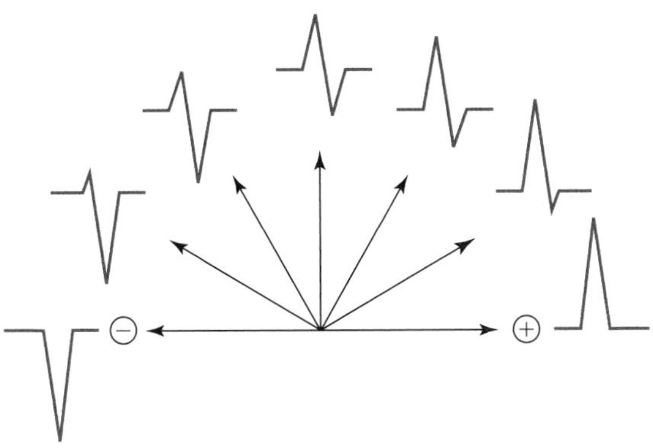

Figure 22-24 Several vectors and their resultant ECG complex. Note: (1) a current perpendicular to the axis produces an equiphasic deflection, and (2) a current parallel to the axis results in the tallest or deepest complex possible.

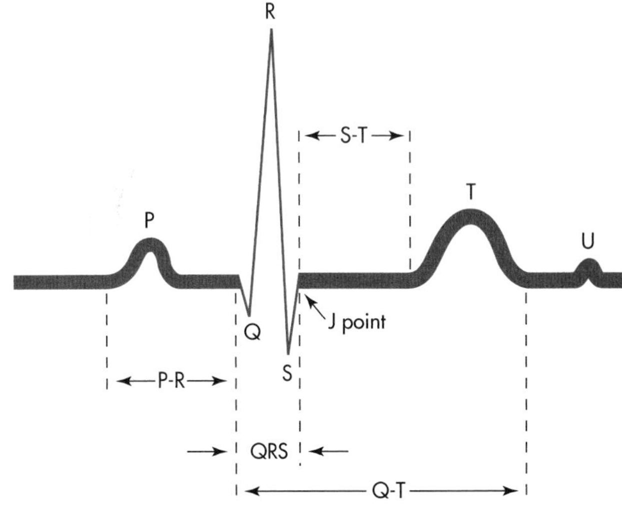

Figure 22-25 Schematic drawing of ECG waves produced by the cardiac cycle.

BOX 22-2 Three Methods for Estimating Heart Rate From the Electrocardiogram Tracing

1. Measure the interval between consecutive QRS complexes, determine the number of small squares, and divide 1500 by that number. This method is used only when the heart rhythm is regular.
2. Measure the interval between consecutive QRS complexes, determine the number of large squares, and divide 300 by that number. This method is used only when the heart rhythm is regular.
3. Determine the number of RR intervals within 6 seconds and multiply by 10. The ECG paper is conveniently marked at the top with slashes that represent 3-second intervals. This method can be used when the rhythm is irregular. If the rhythm is extremely irregular an interval of 30 to 60 seconds should be used.

TABLE 22-5 Electrical Activity of the Heart and Resultant Electrocardiogram Findings

Electrical Activity of Heart	Electrocardiogram Events
SA node fires	Not recorded
Wave of depolarization spreads through atria	P wave
Slight pause at AV node	Isoelectric baseline between P wave and QRS complex
Atrial repolarization	Not recorded; overpowered by electrical activity of ventricles
Ventricular depolarization	QRS complex
Ventricular repolarization	T wave

pulse flows, (2) the distance between the source of the impulse and the positive electrode, and (3) the site of the electrode. As a rule, when the flow of electrical current is directed toward the positive electrode, the deflection will be positive, and when the flow of current is directed away from the positive electrode, the deflection will be negative (Figure 22-24).

The waves recorded by the ECG have been arbitrarily designated by the letters P, Q, R, S, T, and U (Figure 22-25). The P wave represents the depolarization of the atria (Table 22-5). Normally the P wave is gently rounded, does not exceed 2 to 3 mm in amplitude, and is 0.11 second or less in duration. It is normally positive in leads I, II, aV_F, and V_4 to V_6. It is negative in lead aV_R and variable in all other leads. Repolarization of the atria also produces a wave, but it generally is hidden within the QRS complex.

The PR interval is a measurement of the amount of time it takes for the impulse to travel from the SA node to the ventricular musculature. It includes the normal physiologic delay of impulse conduction by the AV node. This interval is measured from the beginning of the P wave to the beginning of the QRS complex. Normally the PR interval measures from 0.12 to 0.20 seconds.

The QRS complex represents depolarization of the ventricles and is often the most significant portion of the ECG. The Q wave is a negative initial deflection from the isoelectric line and may not always be present. A small Q wave of less than 0.04-second duration is a normal finding in leads I, II, III, aV_L, aV_F, and V_4 to V_6. The first positive deflection from the isoelectric line is an R wave. The negative deflection following an R wave is an S wave. The full duration of the QRS complex is measured from the first deflection from the isoelectric line (whether it is a Q or an R wave) to the point where the QRS complex ends and the ST segment begins. The normal QRS complex is 0.05 to 0.10 seconds.

The ST segment represents the plateau (phase 2) of the action potential. It is normally isoelectric because all cells are at zero potential and no current flows. Slight elevation no greater than 1 mm or a subtle depression no greater than 0.5 mm is considered normal. Abnormal elevations or depressions of the ST segment can occur as a result of myocardial muscle injury, conduction disturbances, hypertrophy, and the effect of digitalis.

The T wave represents phase 3 of the action potential, when the ventricles are being rapidly repolarized. It is normally rounded, slightly asymmetric, and of the same polarity as the QRS complex. The height of the T wave should not exceed 5 mm in a limb lead or 10 mm in a precordial lead. It is normally a positive wave in leads I, II, and V_3 to V_6. The T wave is a negative deflection in lead aV_R and variable in all other leads.

The effective refractory period is present during the beginning of the T wave. At the peak of the T wave, more of the fast sodium channels have recovered and therefore a stronger-than-normal stimulus can produce a successful action potential. However, some fibers are still unresponsive, and electrical chaos and subsequent ventricular fibrillation may occur. The approximate location of this vulnerable period is illustrated in Figure 22-26.

The QT interval is measured from the beginning of the QRS complex to the end of the T wave. It represents the entire duration of ventricular depolarization and repolarization. The normal QT value varies with age, gender, and heart rate but generally should be less than half the preceding RR interval.

The termination of the T wave is sometimes difficult to determine, and measuring the QT interval accurately is not always easy.

The U wave is a small wave sometimes seen after the T wave. It usually deflects in the same direction as the T wave and is best seen in lead V_3. It has been suggested that the U wave represents late repolarization of papillary muscle.

Normal Sinus Rhythm. The term normal sinus rhythm implies that cardiac electrical activity is within normal limits. This means that the following criteria are met (Figure 22-27):

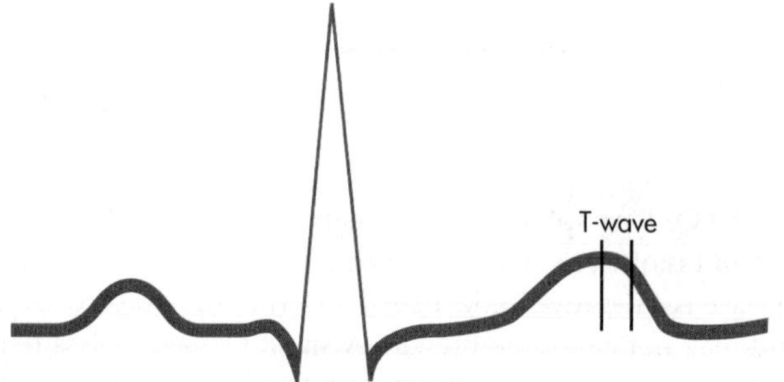

Figure 22-26 Approximate location of the vulnerable period of ventricular repolarization.

- P waves are present and regular.
- The atrial rate (P waves) is between 60 and 100 beats/min.
- Each P wave is followed by a QRS complex.
- The PR interval and QRS duration are within established norms.

Electrocardiographic Signal Averaging. Electrocardiographic signal averaging involves amplification of electrical signals from the heart that have a voltage too small to be recorded by a standard ECG. It is used to detect low-amplitude, high-frequency signals in the terminal portion of the QRS complex to identify patients at risk for ventricular tachycardia. Approximately 200 identical QRS complexes are grouped and averaged, resulting in a waveform that appears smooth and continuous. Signal averaging minimizes the noise that contaminates the ECG signal and thereby exposes signals of a microvolt level normally hidden within the noise.

The rate of postinfarction sudden death precipitated by ventricular tachycardia that degenerates into ventricular fibrillation is approximately 10% to 15%. Thus early identification of this life-threatening complication is essential.

Dynamic Studies

Holter Monitor. Resting ECGs supply valuable information about a person's cardiovascular status. However, for patients who experience chest pain or palpitations only during exertion, a more dynamic method for studying the ECG may be necessary.

The Holter monitor is used to obtain a continuous graphic tracing of a patient's ECG during daily activities. It is helpful in documenting episodic dysrhythmias. The Holter monitor is a small, portable ECG monitor about the size of a large transistor radio that can be carried with a shoulder strap. The patient is attached to the Holter monitor for approximately 24 hours. During this time the patient keeps a log or diary of daily activities. The log includes activities, medications taken, and unusual sensations the person experiences while attached to the monitor. At the end of the monitoring period, the physician compares the ECG with the patient's log to determine whether any correlations exist between the ECG and the patient's activities.

Stress Testing. The exercise stress test evaluates cardiovascular response to a progressively graded workload. The stress test may be invasive or noninvasive. Stress testing may be performed for a variety of reasons and is often combined with an

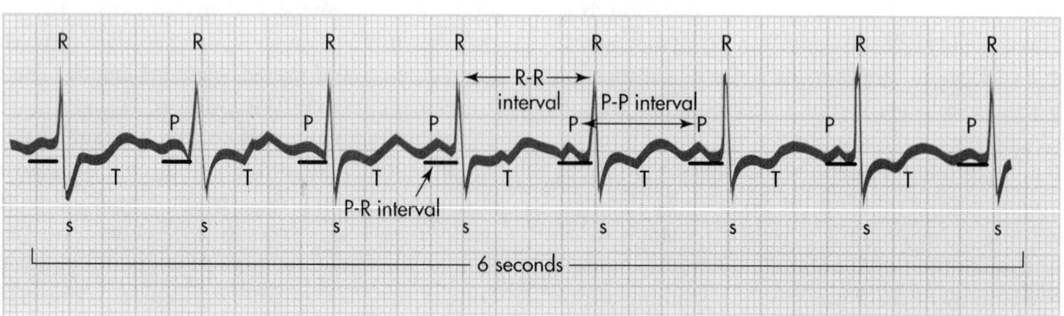

Figure 22-27 Normal sinus rhythm showing R-R, P-P, and PR intervals.

echocardiogram to obtain additional information about heart function (Box 22-3).

The exercise test can be performed using a treadmill or a stationary bicycle with adjustable resistance to pedaling. Various protocols are used during the procedure, but the patient's blood pressure and ECG are monitored closely during and after the test. Because the stress test is designed to progressively increase myocardial oxygen demand, some patients may experience untoward effects (e.g., ventricular tachycardia, a significant change in peak systolic blood pressure, premature ventricular contractions, or chest pain), and the test may need to be terminated.

Adequate preparation for stress testing is important. Although the procedure is not painful, it can be fatiguing; patients may be anxious because they will be exercising at a level that might produce symptoms such as dyspnea, palpitations, and chest pain. The nurse reviews the purpose and method of stress testing and encourages the patient to do the following:

1. Avoid coffee, tea, and alcohol the day of the test.
2. Avoid smoking and taking nitroglycerin 2 hours before the test.
3. Wear comfortable, loose-fitting clothes. (Women are advised to wear a brassiere for support.)
4. Wear sturdy, comfortable walking shoes.
5. Consult with the physician about taking any medications before the test.[6]

BOX 22-3 Indications for Performing a Stress Test

- Evaluation of the patient with symptoms suggestive of coronary artery disease
- Determination of the patient's physical work capacity and aerobic capacity
- Determination of the patient's functional capacity after a myocardial infarction and as an aid in planning an exercise rehabilitation program
- Evaluation of exercise-induced dysrhythmias
- Evaluation of the symptom-free person older than 40 years old who is at risk for coronary artery disease
- Evaluation of pharmacologic interventions for dysrhythmias, angina, or ischemia

Scintigraphic Studies

Various types of myocardial imaging can be used to identify myocardial infarctions, evaluate myocardial perfusion, and assess left ventricular function. Myocardial imaging studies are relatively safe and noninvasive techniques for evaluating myocardial function. Techniques of myocardial imaging are occasionally combined with stress testing to improve the depth and accuracy of information about myocardial function.

Stannous Pyrophosphate Scan. The pyrophosphate scan, referred to as "hot spot" imaging, typically uses technetium 99m stannous pyrophosphate. A minute dose of the radioisotope is injected into an antecubital vein, and the heart is visualized after about 2 hours. The healthy myocardium shows a homogeneous distribution of the radioisotope, whereas the damaged heart shows an increased uptake of the radioactive material. A gamma scintillator camera is used to identify the area of increased uptake (hot spot). The test is best performed 1 to 3 days after the infarction.

Thallium Imaging. Thallium imaging is referred to as "cold spot" imaging because the uptake of the isotope is greater in healthy myocardial tissue than in the infarction area; thus this area remains a cold spot. A gamma scintillator is used to detect the distribution of the radioisotope. Thallium imaging, which most often is combined with exercise testing, can provide valuable information about the extent and severity of myocardial infarction.

Thallium scanning can be helpful in quantifying the amount of myocardium at risk during acute infarction by use of two resting scans to localize the affected area. The resting scan is obtained very early in the infarction, and a redistribution scan is obtained 3 to 4 hours later. The total area of ischemia and infarction is visible on the initial scan. A smaller cold spot is visible during the redistribution scan if the ischemic tissue has successfully extracted the isotope. This technique is useful in evaluating the efficacy of therapeutic interventions such as thrombolytic therapy, as well as providing direction for further treatment based on the degree of myocardium still in jeopardy. Risk is minimal because the amount of thallium injected is small.

Pharmacologic Myocardial Perfusion Imaging. Dipyridamole is a potent coronary vasodilator. By blocking cellular reuptake of adenosine, dipyridamole acts to increase blood and tissue concentrations of adenosine, which in turn promotes optimal coronary vasodilation. In normal coronary arteries, dipyridamole increases blood flow three to four times that of baseline values. In stenosed arteries the increase in flow is less, and with severe stenosis a flow increase may not occur.

Adenosine perfusion imaging can be used as an alternative to dipyridamole perfusion imaging because of its significantly shorter half-life (2 to 10 seconds for adenosine vs. several minutes for dipyridamole). Furthermore, adenosine elicits more consistent maximal coronary vasodilation over a shorter period than does dipyridamole. Side effects are common and include headache, dyspnea, chest pain, and facial flushing. Side effects generally disappear within 1 to 2 minutes and rarely require the administration of aminophylline as an antagonist.

Technetium 99m Sestamibi Myocardial Perfusion SPECT Imaging. Technetium 99m sestamibi (Cardiolite) is a nonredistributing radionuclide agent used to evaluate outcomes of thrombolytic and other interventional therapy for acute myocardial infarction. Typically technetium 99m sestamibi is administered in the emergency department, followed by thrombolytic or interventional therapy. Once hemodynamic stability has been established, perfusion imaging is performed. Because minimal redistribution occurs with this agent, delayed images still delineate the initially nonperfused myocardial region. Improvements noted in repeat scintigraphy provide accurate assessment of salvaged myocardium.

Multiple Gated Acquisition Scanning. Multiple gated acquisition scanning has the ability to demonstrate cardiac wall motion to enable assessment of injury and residual cardiac function. The technique lends itself well to the portable imaging techniques required to scan acutely ill patients.

Gated blood pool imaging is a noninvasive radionuclide technique. ECG leads are applied, and the ECG is synchronized to a computer and a gamma scintillator camera. A small amount of technetium 99m is injected intravenously. After the radioactivity reaches a state of equilibrium (approximately 3 to 5 minutes), the patient is placed supine with the gamma scintillator camera positioned over the precordium. The computer then constructs an average cardiac cycle that represents the summation of several hundred heartbeats. Enough data are generated so that an outline of the left side of the heart in all phases of the cardiac cycle can be seen.

Gated blood pool imaging offers several advantages. Because all RBCs are tagged, their counts reflect blood volume. Thus, if the heart can be positioned to isolate the left ventricle on the scan, the left ventricular ejection fraction can be determined. The ejection fraction may provide an early indicator of deteriorating cardiovascular functioning. This information is extremely useful in patients with heart failure or low CO.

Right ventricular ejection fraction also can be determined but is less accurate. The effects of pharmacotherapeutics (e.g., nitroglycerin, vasodilators) on ventricular function can also be evaluated.

Stress-testing ventriculography can be performed to evaluate the ejection fraction during exercise. Some patients with coronary artery disease demonstrate a normal ejection value at rest but experience a decline under the stress of exercise.

Positron Emission Tomography. Positron emission tomography (PET) is a radionuclide-based imaging technique that uses short-lived radionuclides as tracers to report both perfusion and metabolic events. The tracers are administered by intravenous injection or inhalation. Myocardial uptake is proportional to the quantity of tracer delivered by the blood flow. The tracer elements readily pass through the tissues and are detected by counters placed on opposite sides of the body.

Under normal circumstances the well-perfused, aerobically metabolizing myocardium prefers free fatty acids for energy production. When ischemia is present, more glucose and less fatty acid tends to be used. PET is particularly useful in demonstrating this process because the radioisotopes are incorporated into biochemically relevant components. It also provides the basis for medical management of asymptomatic coronary atherosclerosis and is useful in evaluating the effectiveness of interventions such as thrombolysis and percutaneous transluminal coronary angioplasty.

Sonic Studies

Echocardiography. Echocardiography uses ultrasound to assess cardiac structure and mobility noninvasively. It is useful in the diagnosis of a variety of cardiac conditions (Box 22-4). A small transducer is placed on the patient's chest at the level of the third or fourth intercostal space near the left lower sternal border. The transducer transmits high-frequency sound waves and then receives these waves back from the patient as they are reflected from different structures. The ultrasonic beam that is reflected back from the patient's heart produces "echoes" that are viewed as lines and spaces on an oscilloscope. These lines and spaces represent bone, cardiac chambers and valves, the septum, and muscle. A copy of the echocardiogram is recorded on paper.

BOX 22-4 Conditions Detected or Evaluated by Echocardiography

- Abnormal pericardial fluid
- Valvular disorders, including prosthetic valves
- Ventricular aneurysms
- Cardiac tumors, such as atrial myxomas
- Some forms of congenital heart disease, such as atrial septal defects
- Cardiac chamber size
- Stroke volume and cardiac output
- Some myocardial abnormalities, such as idiopathic hypertrophic subaortic stenosis
- Wall motion abnormalities

BOX 22-5 Clinical Indications for Transesophageal Echocardiography

- Aortic dissection/aneurysm
- Mitral valve prosthetic dysfunction
- Mitral valve regurgitation
- Infective endocarditis
- Congenital heart disease
- Intracardiac thrombi (especially left atrium and left atrial appendage)
- Cardiac tumor
- Intraoperative assessment: left ventricle function, adequacy of valve repair/replacement

Because echocardiography is a noninvasive procedure, it is safer than cardiac catheterization and is usually performed first. There are virtually no contraindications to the echocardiogram, and it can be performed at the bedside of critically ill patients. No special preparation is necessary for the test; the patient can eat and medications can be administered without interruption. Patient teaching regarding the echocardiogram should include the purpose of the test and the facts that the test is painless and takes approximately 30 to 60 minutes. The patient lies quietly in a supine position during the test with the head elevated 15 to 20 degrees. The patient may resume normal activities as soon as the test is completed.

Transesophageal Echocardiography. Transesophageal echocardiography (TEE) allows high resolution ultrasonic imaging of the cardiac structures and great vessels via the esophagus. It permits echocardiography to be used effectively with patients who have chronic pulmonary disease or are mechanically ventilated and poor candidates for ultrasound testing. This technique uses a transducer affixed to the tip of a modified, flexible endoscope that is advanced into the esophagus and manipulated to produce clear posterior images of the heart. The left atrium, left atrial appendage, and the aortic and mitral valves are easily visualized with TEE. It is, however, unable to visualize the aortic arch and arch vessels. Indications for TEE are summarized in Box 22-5. This procedure can be performed at the bedside without contrast dye.

The procedure is performed with the patient under local anesthesia and sedation. The patient receives nothing by mouth for at least 4 to 6 hours before the test. Preprocedure assessment includes any history of esophageal dysfunction or surgery.

Initially the patient assumes a chin-to-chest position to facilitate passage of the endoscope through the oropharynx. The scope is advanced 30 to 35 cm to allow posterior visualization of the left atrium by the transducer. To view the left ventricle, the scope is advanced into the stomach and flexed upward for an inferior view. The procedure usually takes about 5 to 20 minutes.

Suction and resuscitation equipment are kept readily available. Cardiac rhythm, vital signs, and oxygen saturation (SaO_2) are monitored throughout the procedure. The patient is given a topical anesthetic by spray or gargle to reduce coughing or gagging during probe insertion. Additional sedation, usually diazepam (Valium) or midazolam (Versed), may be given.

The priority for posttest monitoring is the prevention of aspiration. The patient is given nothing by mouth until the gag reflex fully returns. The patient is kept in an upright or side-lying position to support ventilation. Throat lozenges and saline rinses can help alleviate throat discomfort. Other potential complications include esophageal perforation, pharyngeal bleeding, dysrhythmias, and transient hypoxemia.

Phonocardiography

Phonocardiography involves the use of electrically recorded amplified cardiac sounds. Special microphones attached to the patient's chest pick up cardiac sounds produced by pressure changes in the heart and great vessels. The sounds are graphically recorded on special phonograph paper. Phonocardiography can be helpful in determining the exact timing and characteristics of murmurs and extra heart sounds. Phonocardiograms may be used in conjunction with echocardiograms so that a comparison can be made between sound (phono) and motion (echo). Patient preparation is similar to that described for the echocardiogram.

Cardiac Catheterization

Cardiac catheterization is an extremely valuable diagnostic tool for obtaining detailed information about the structure and function of the cardiac chambers, valves, and coronary arteries. Cardiac catheterization may include studies of the right side of the heart, the left side of the heart, and the coronary arteries. Indications for cardiac catheterization are summarized in Box 22-6.

BOX 22-6 Indications for Cardiac Catheterization

- Confirmation of the presence of suspected heart disease, including congenital heart disease, valvular disease, and myocardial disease
- Determination of the location and severity of the disease process
- Preoperative assessment to determine if cardiac surgery is indicated
- Evaluation of ventricular function after surgical revascularization
- Evaluation of the effect of medical treatment modalities on cardiovascular function
- Performance of specialized cardiac interventions such as internal pacemaker placement

Right-Sided Heart Catheterization. Right-sided heart catheterization is performed to evaluate congenital heart disease and valvular disorders. Blood samples and pressure readings are taken, and cineradiographs of the right chambers of the heart and the pulmonary arterial circulation are made. A cardiac biopsy may be obtained in a heart transplant patient to assist in determining whether the body is rejecting the new heart.

To perform a catheterization of the right side of the heart, a catheter is inserted via cutdown or percutaneously into a large vein (e.g., the medial cubital, brachial, or internal jugular). The catheter is then threaded with the use of fluoroscopy into the superior vena cava, the right atrium, the right ventricle, the pulmonary artery, and pulmonary capillaries. As the catheter is passed through the various chambers and vessels, blood samples are taken to determine the oxygen content and saturation. Blood pressure measurements also are recorded (Figure 22-28). The pressure is highest in the right ventricle because of the stronger ventricular contractions. Normally the pulmonary artery pressure is approximately 25/10 mm Hg or approximately one-fifth the systemic blood pressure. Elevations in chamber pressures such as an elevated right atrial pressure can indicate valvular problems or possibly right ventricular failure.

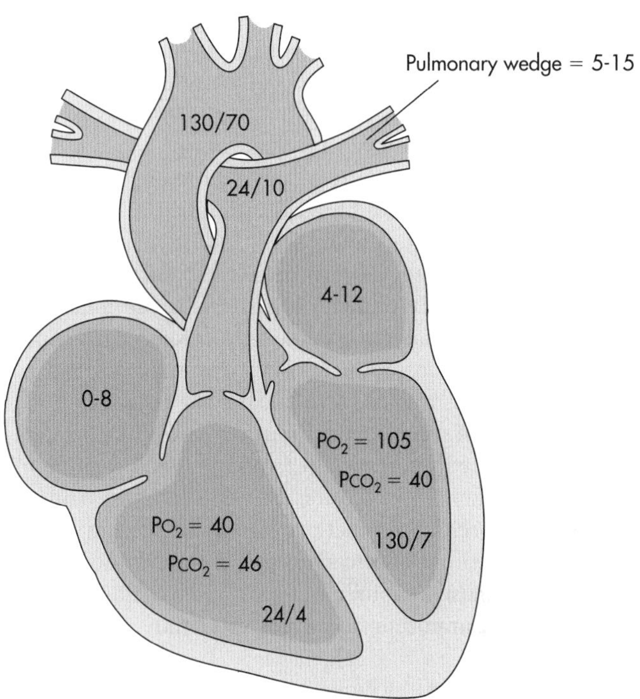

Figure 22-28 Pressure readings and blood gases in millimeters of mercury (mm Hg) in chambers of heart and major blood vessels.

Left-Sided Heart Catheterization. Left-sided heart catheterization is performed to evaluate pressures on the left side of the heart, valvular competency, and left ventricular function.

A catheter is passed into the aorta from either the brachial or the femoral artery with the use of fluoroscopy. After reaching the aorta, the catheter is manipulated around the aortic arch, down the ascending aorta, and through the aortic valve into the left ventricle. Pressure-gradient measurements are obtained to detect pressure changes across the valves.

Ventricular angiography may be performed during left-sided heart catheterization. This involves the injection of contrast material into the ventricle while radiographs are taken. Information about contractility, aneurysm formation, valvular disorders, and ejection fraction can be obtained.

Selective coronary arteriography also may be performed during left-sided heart catheterization. The catheter is threaded to the aortic root, and the tip of the catheter is then advanced into the right and left coronary arteries. Contrast medium is injected into each coronary artery, which outlines the entire coronary circulation, and cineangiographic films are taken to monitor the progression of the dye. This outlines the number and severity of stenotic segments and the presence of collateral vessels.

Introduction of the dye may temporarily displace blood flow in the coronary arteries and may produce transient ischemia and chest pain. Sublingual nitroglycerin may be administered to relieve the discomfort. In addition, medications such as isosorbide (Isordil) may be given to dilate the vessels so that greater visualization may be achieved. Occasionally, injection of contrast material into the right coronary artery may suppress the SA node, producing bradydysrhythmias, and administration of intravenous atropine may be required.

Patient Preparation. Preparation for cardiac catheterization is extremely important. Preparation should include information about the procedure, care after the test, and the more common sensations that may be experienced during the catheterization. Even after careful preparation most patients remain apprehensive about both the procedure and the possible results. It is important to include the family in all pretest teaching if possible.

Instruction should include a brief description of the room environment during the test. The patient is questioned concerning any history of allergy, especially to iodine, shellfish, and contrast media. The meal before the procedure is usually withheld. If the procedure is scheduled for later in the day, the patient may be permitted a clear liquid breakfast. A mild sedative may be given before the procedure, and an antibiotic may be ordered as a prophylactic measure. The presence and quality of peripheral pulses are assessed and marked before the test.

A local anesthetic is injected over the artery or vein to be used, and a small cutdown is performed. Relatively little discomfort is involved in a right-sided heart catheterization, although the patient may feel pressure in the femoral or antecubital area. During a left-sided heart catheterization, the patient may experience a warm, flushing sensation as the contrast medium is injected. This flushing sensation lasts for approximately 30 seconds. The patient also may experience nausea and "fluttering" sensations produced by catheter manipulation or from catheter advancement through the heart.

The body's physiologic responses to cardiac catheterization are numerous and vary with each person. Therefore, it is essential that the patient understand the importance of reporting any unusual sensations that might occur during and after the catheterization.

Nursing Care After Catheterization. The postprocedure nursing care following both types of heart catheterization is similar. These procedures generally last from 1 to 3 hours and can be tiring for the patient. Many patients prefer to rest or sleep after the examination.

The patient's pulse and blood pressure are monitored every 15 minutes for 1 hour and then every 30 minutes for 3 hours. It is essential to check the pulses distal to the catheter insertion site to determine the patency of the cannulated artery. The amplitude of the pulse may be slightly diminished for approximately 24 hours because of arterial spasm or edema at the site. At times thrombus formation may totally obliterate the distal pulse, and surgery may be necessary to restore circulation.

If a femoral approach was used, the patient is kept on bed rest for approximately 3 to 4 hours and monitored for signs of bleeding, inflammation, tenderness, or edema at the cutdown site. Various modalities are presently being used to prevent hemorrhage at the insertion site. Historically, sandbags or weights were used; however, these have been replaced by mechanical devices called Fem Stops, which are an external mode of compression. Invasive devices referred to as hemostatic plugs may also be used. Frequent puncture site observation is a priority in any post procedure monitoring protocol.[2] The patient should not have the head of the bed elevated more than 30 degrees and should keep the affected leg extended.

If the brachial site is used, the arm is kept straight for several hours, usually with an armboard, but the patient can be up in the room as soon as vital signs are stable. If any bleeding occurs from the cutdown site, firm pressure is applied directly over the site and the physician is notified.

Intake and output are monitored in all patients regardless of the approach used to ensure an adequate intake to flush the dye from the circulation and to monitor the patient's renal status. Hypotension may develop as a result of the diuretic effect of the contrast material used during angiography.

Complications of cardiac catheterization are not common; however, cardiac dysrhythmias such as ventricular fibrillation can occur. The development of tachycardia or any dysrhythmia is reported to the physician immediately.

Electrophysiologic Study

The electrophysiologic (EP) study systematically assesses the electrical stability of the heart. This procedure requires electrode placement within the heart to record intracardiac electrical activity. The degree of invasiveness depends on the area of the heart to be studied. More detailed information about the heart's electrical activity can be obtained with the EP study than with the surface ECG because of the proximity of the catheters to the cardiac conduction system. The test demonstrates the exact sequence of atrial and ventricular activation, localizes areas of conduction disturbances (such as accessory pathways, areas of ischemia and infarction, and dysrhythmia foci), and evaluates the effectiveness of antidysrhythmic management. Although EP studies are used more often than in the past, they are not routinely ordered. Use is currently reserved for persons not responding to standard treatment.

An EP study is performed under laboratory conditions with fluoroscopy to guide the pacing electrodes into position. The electrodes are typically inserted through the femoral, brachial, and basilic veins. Arterial cannulation is performed only when left ventricular stimulation is necessary.

Before the test antidysrhythmic drugs usually are discontinued for approximately five half-lives to prevent pharmacologic interference with the study. Three to six intracardiac pacing catheters are inserted and connected to a multichanneled electrogram. A surface ECG is recorded simultaneously for comparison and evaluation. When indicated, dysrhythmias may be initiated by applying a series of programmed extra stimuli to areas of the heart, and the effects of various antidysrhythmic drugs are evaluated. Pacing also may be used to terminate a tachycardia by inhibiting impulse transmission in conduction pathways.

The EP study usually lasts 2 to 4 hours. At the completion of the test, catheters are removed and pressure is applied at the insertion site, followed by application of a pressure dressing. Patients may be monitored in a telemetry or intensive care unit after the test, where they can be closely observed. Complications of EP studies are similar to those of cardiac catheterization. Patients should be closely monitored for hemorrhage, perforation, hematoma, pulmonary emboli, deep vein thrombus, infection, cerebrovascular accident, angina, and dysrhythmia.

Nurses play a key role in preparing patients for an EP study. Reinforcing physician information about the indications for the test, the procedure itself, and risks may allay anxiety for the patient and family. A description of the equipment used and the room's appearance also may be helpful. It is important to inform patients that they will be awake throughout the procedure.

Postprocedural monitoring includes vital signs; peripheral pulses; insertion site; and color, warmth, and sensation of extremities. Initially these observations are performed every 15 minutes and then gradually increased to every 4 hours. The affected extremity is immobilized, and the patient is placed on bed rest for 4 to 6 hours. Documentation of any changes in rhythm and frequency of ectopy is essential.

Invasive Hemodynamic Monitoring

Invasive hemodynamic monitoring is not a typical diagnostic test, but it is used to evaluate the hemodynamic status of the critically ill patient and has greatly increased the database on which health professionals can plan and evaluate therapeutic modalities. Numerous devices are used in hemodynamic monitoring.

Central Venous Pressure. Central venous pressure (CVP) measurements reflect the pressures in the right atrium and provide information regarding changes in right ventricular pressure. The CVP is used to monitor blood volume and the adequacy of venous return to the heart. The primary factors affecting CVP are the circulating blood volume, right-sided ventricular function, and the degree of peripheral vasoconstriction. Because the CVP reflects the pressure in the great veins as blood returns to the right side of the heart, a low (or falling) reading may indicate an inadequate blood volume (hypovolemia). A high (or rising) CVP usually is secondary to left-sided pump failure. Unfortunately, the patient's hemodynamic status may be severely altered before representative changes in the CVP are evident.

Normal values for CVP vary with different equipment; however, a range of 5 to 15 cm H_2O is acceptable. It is important to note that a change or a trend in the CVP is more important than the actual numerical value.

Intraarterial Blood Pressure Measurement. In the critically ill patient, the CO may be decreased to such an extent that standard blood pressure readings may be inaccurate. As the stroke volume falls, Korotkoff's sounds become increasingly more difficult to auscultate. Invasive arterial blood pressure monitoring may be implemented, which will more accurately reflect actual blood pressure.

Arterial catheters may be placed in various arteries; however, the radial, brachial, and axillary arteries are used most often. The arterial catheter is attached to a transducer that converts the mechanical pressure of the pulses to electrical impulses, which can be viewed as waveforms on an oscilloscope. In addition, the arterial catheter provides easy accessibility for obtaining blood samples for blood gas analysis.

The patient with an arterial line requires frequent observation. It is essential that the extremity with the arterial line be kept uncovered so that the insertion site can be monitored for bleeding. The pulse, color, sensation, and temperature of the extremity distal to the catheter are assessed every 2 hours.

Pulmonary Artery and Pulmonary Capillary Wedge Pressures. A balloon-tipped catheter (Swan-Ganz catheter) may be introduced into the pulmonary artery to obtain essential information regarding left ventricular function. The pulmonary artery catheter permits the measurement of the pulmonary artery end-diastolic pressure (PAEDP) and the pulmonary capillary wedge pressure (PCWP) (Table 22-6).

The best indicator of left ventricular function is the left ventricular end-diastolic pressure (LVEDP). Elevations in LVEDP result from impaired left ventricular contractility that does not permit adequate emptying of the ventricles.

The PAEDP and the PCWP are similar in a healthy person. However, in the presence of increased peripheral vascular resistance such as that found in pulmonary embolism, the PAEDP will rise while the PCWP remains normal. Therefore, to evaluate the true LVEDP accurately, the PCWP must be monitored.

Insertion of the pulmonary artery catheter is accomplished using several different approaches. These include a small incision (cutdown) made in an antecubital vein or percutaneously through the internal jugular or subclavian veins. The catheter is threaded through the superior vena cava, through the tricuspid valve, and into the pulmonary artery. This allows for

TABLE 22-6 Pulmonary Artery and Capillary Wedge Pressures

Type	Common Abbreviation	Normal Values
Left ventricular end-diastolic pressure	LVEDP	12-15 mm Hg (elevations result from inadequate emptying of the ventricles)
Pulmonary artery end-diastolic pressure	PAEDP	4-12 mm Hg (elevations result from increased peripheral vascular resistance)
Pulmonary capillary wedge pressure	PCWP	4-12 mm Hg (levels >25 mm Hg indicate imminent pulmonary edema)

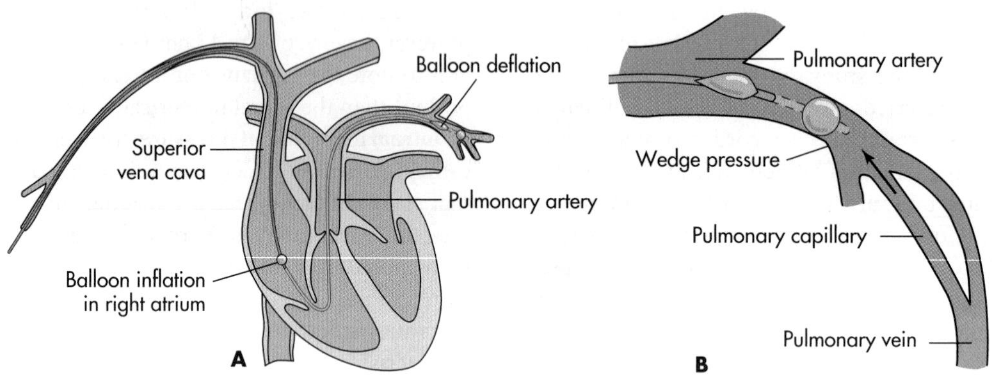

Figure 22-29 **A,** Flow-directed, balloon-tipped catheter showing inflation of balloon in right atrium and consequent "floating" of catheter through the right ventricle and out to distal pulmonary artery branch. Balloon is deflated, advanced slightly, and reinflated slightly to obtain pulmonary capillary wedge pressure (PCWP). **B,** During the initial positioning of the balloon-tipped catheter in pulmonary artery, balloon is deflated. Catheter is then advanced and balloon is reinflated just long enough to obtain PCWP.

continuous measurement of the PAEDP. One of the lumens of the catheter is attached to a monitor that records a numerical reading and a display of waveforms that indicate the location (capillary bed, pulmonary artery, or right ventricle) of the catheter. The balloon is then inflated, which causes the catheter to wedge in a distal branch of the pulmonary artery (Figure 22-29). The reading obtained when the balloon is inflated is the PCWP and reflects pressures in the pulmonary capillary bed and left-sided heart function. When the balloon is inflated, it occludes the flow from the right side of the heart; therefore it should never be left inflated for more than a few seconds in order to prevent damage to the pulmonary circulation. The nurse usually obtains measurements of the PCWP every 2 to 4 hours; however, readings should be obtained more frequently if the patient's condition is unstable.

Various types of pulmonary artery catheters may be used that allow measurement of additional hemodynamic parameters. Some catheters have a third lumen that contains a thermistor that is used to determine cardiac output by the thermodilution technique. A fourth lumen that ends at the level of the right atrium can be used to monitor CVP and to obtain blood samples. A four-lumen thermodilution catheter is illustrated in Figure 22-30.

Vascular Diagnostic Studies

Both noninvasive and invasive vascular diagnostic studies are conducted to evaluate vascular blood flow throughout the body. Most vascular studies require pretest or posttest interventions by the nurse. Other studies simply require an adequate explanation of the procedure.

Noninvasive Tests

Ankle-Brachial Index. Ankle-brachial index is the most commonly used parameter for overall evaluation of arterial vascular status in the lower extremity. Blood pressure measurements are obtained over both the dorsalis pedis and posterior tibial arteries using a regular blood pressure cuff. The Doppler probe is then placed over the pulse, and the cuff is inflated to above systolic pressure. The point at which the pulse returns as the cuff deflates is recorded as the systolic endpoint number. Typically the higher of the two pressures is used as the indication of vascular status. This number is divided into the higher of two brachial artery pressures (e.g., an ankle pressure of 70 mm Hg with a brachial pressure of 140 mm Hg gives an index of 0.5). Normal foot arteries have an index of 1.0 to 1.2. Indexes below 1.0 indicate arterial obstruction.

Impedance Plethysmography. Venous outflow in the lower extremities is measured by inflation and deflation of pneumatic cuffs around the thighs. The assumption is that because blood is a good conductor of electricity, the electrical resistance will change as blood volume is altered. Electrodes are attached to obtain measurements and determine quality of blood flow. Sharp rises in venous volume suggest venous occlusion, such as blood clots. If a deep vein thrombosis (DVT) is present in a major vessel, the increase in blood volume during the test is less than expected because the veins are already

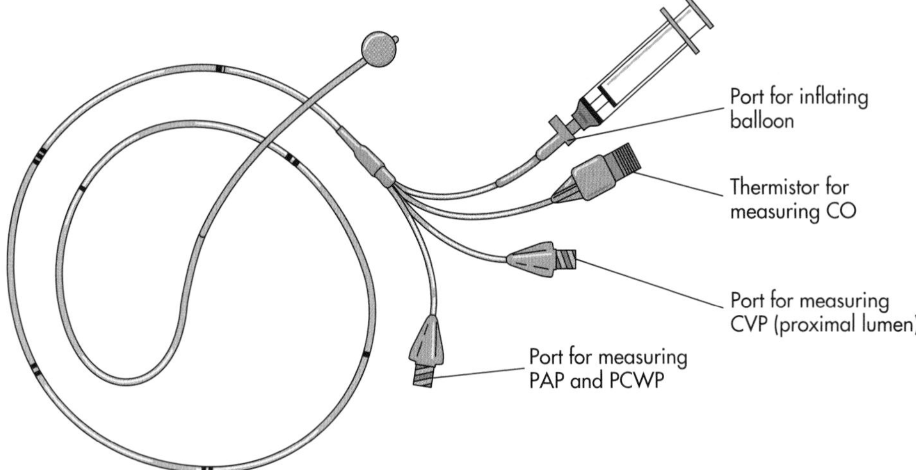

Figure 22-30 Four-lumen thermodilution pulmonary artery catheter for measuring cardiac output (*CO*), central venous pressure (*CVP*), pulmonary artery pressure (*PAP*), and pulmonary capillary wedge pressure (*PCWP*).

full.[5] During the procedure the patient is kept supine with the leg elevated and knee flexed.

Doppler Ultrasound. Doppler ultrasound, or ultrasound imaging, aids in the diagnosis of carotid artery disease, peripheral artery disease, venous occlusive disease, valvular insufficiency, and DVT. Ultrasonic waves directed at an artery or vein reflect off red blood cells, producing a waveform or audible sound. Arterial waveforms should be pronounced, with peaks and valleys reflective of the systolic and diastolic pressures; a flattened waveform indicates obstruction. Venous waveforms are in phase with respirations and are of continuous amplitude.

Exercise Testing. The treadmill test is used to obtain an objective measurement of the severity of intermittent claudication. This test is similar to the test used for coronary patients, except the walking speed is usually 1.5 to 2 miles per hour with a grade elevation of 10% to 20% and a time limit of 5 minutes. Walking tolerance of 5 minutes suggests mild disease, and 1 minute indicates severe disease. Patients should wear loose-fitting clothing and good walking shoes. The exercise is stopped at the maximal level of exertion or when symptoms become disabling.

Magnetic Resonance Imaging. Magnetic resonance imaging (MRI) capabilities include evaluation of the vascular network, measurement of blood flow velocities, and assessment of stages of vascular disease. Radiofrequency pulses excite the protons, which give a signal creating a three-dimensional image of the vessels. This test does not require ionizing radiation or any injections into the vascular system; therefore it may be preferred to arteriography. However, MRI is expensive and time consuming, which makes it a less likely choice for routine screening and follow-up monitoring. The patient should be informed that the noise level during the test may be high and require use of earplugs. Additionally, confinement to a relatively small space is sometimes problematic for patients who have a tendency toward claustrophobia.

Invasive Tests

Contrast Angiography and Venography. Contrast angiography, or arteriography, is a standard in vascular diagnostic imaging. It is the most invasive test used in evaluation of peripheral disease and has the greatest risk for the patient. Angiography assists in the diagnosis of arterial emboli, arterial trauma, aneurysm, Buerger's disease, and reevaluation of the patency of arteries after grafting. The procedure involves insertion of a radiopaque catheter into the vessel with the patient under local anesthesia followed by injection of a contrast medium. X-ray films are obtained that visualize the arterial system.

Venography is performed in a similar manner except that the venous system is examined. It is the definitive test in the diagnosis of DVT; another common use of this test is with patients suspected of having incompetent vein valves. The test takes about an hour and is uncomfortable for the patient.

The procedure and nursing interventions are similar to a cardiac catheterization, but the peripheral system is being examined instead of the coronary vessels (see discussion on p. 640). The patient must be assessed for allergies to contrast media before the procedure. Informed consent is obtained, and the patient is told that it is common to experience a flushing or burning sensation after injection of the contrast medium. There is disagreement regarding the need to abstain from food and fluids before the test; some physicians prefer patients to have nothing by mouth for 6 to 8 hours, but others recommend a clear liquid diet to prevent possible dehydration and concomitant hemoconcentration.

A pressure dressing may or may not be placed at the insertion site after the procedure. However, the extremity must be kept straight while the site is closely monitored for hemorrhage, hematoma, and inflammation. Postprocedure protocols vary; but vital signs, distal pulses, skin temperature, and the insertion site are usually monitored every 15 minutes for the first hour, every 30 minutes for the second hour, and hourly for the remaining time. Assessment of motor and sensory function is important. Mild analgesics may be administered for pain at the insertion site. The physician is notified if the patient experiences severe pain.

Potential complications include an allergic reaction to the contrast medium, thrombi, perforation of the vessel, emboli, renal failure, and pseudoaneurysms. Creatinine levels should be monitored to evaluate renal function.

Digital Subtraction Angiography. Digital subtraction angiography, or digital vascular imaging, is a computerized fluoroscopic procedure that visualizes the vascular system. It is less expensive and quicker than angiography. Again contrast medium is injected through a catheter, and x-ray films are taken with the patient under local anesthesia. A state-of-the-art video system displays the vessels on a television monitor while a computer subtracts images that are not necessary. Separate injections are required for different views of the limb. Patients must be assessed for allergies to contrast media before the procedure. Posttest nursing care is similar to that provided after arteriography.

References

1. American Heart Association Cardiovascular Statistics, 2001, website: http://amhrt.org/heartg/cvdstats.html.
2. Botti M, Williamson B, Steen K: Coronary angiography observations: evidence-based or ritualistic practice? *Heart Lung* 30(2):138, 2001.
3. Hill B, Geraci S: A diagnostic approach to chest pain based on history and ancillary evaluation, *Nurse Pract* 23(4):20, 1998.
4. Jarvis C: *Physical examination and health assessment,* ed 3, Philadelphia, 2000, WB Saunders.
5. McCabe S, Fowler S: Neurotrauma and deep vein thrombosis: the signs of DVT are elusive, *Am J Nurs* 101(Suppl):45, 2001.
6. Meyer N: Using physiologic and pharmacologic stress testing in the evaluation of coronary artery disease, *Nurse Pract* 24(4):70, 1999.
7. National Cholesterol Education Program: Summary of the third report of the National Cholesterol Education Program (NCEP) Expert Panel on Detection, Evaluation, and Treatment of High Blood Cholesterol in Adults (Adult Treatment Panel III), 2001, website: http://www.nhlbi.nih.gov/index.htm.
8. Wilson S, Giddens J: *Health assessment for nursing practice,* ed 2, St Louis, 2001, Mosby.

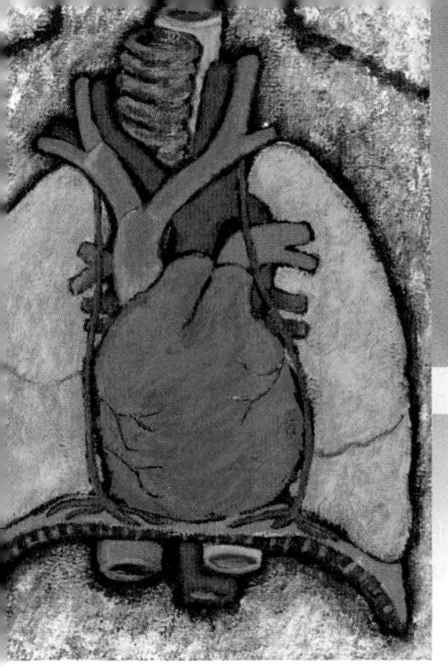

http://www.mosby.com/MERLIN/medsurg_phipps

Coronary Artery Disease and Dysrhythmias

23

Kathy Henley Haugh, Arlene Keeling

Objectives

After studying this chapter, the learner should be able to:

1. Discuss the role of risk factors in the pathogenesis of coronary artery disease.
2. Recognize the signs and symptoms of coronary artery disease.
3. Explain the collaborative management of angina pectoris, unstable angina, and myocardial infarction.
4. Discuss the nursing role in the care of the patient with coronary artery disease.
5. Recognize common dysrhythmias associated with the cardiac conduction system.
6. Discuss the collaborative care management of patients with cardiac dysrhythmias.
7. Describe the basic components of cardiopulmonary resuscitation.

Patients with coronary artery disease (CAD) often seek health care after experiencing angina or myocardial infarction (MI). CAD is directly implicated in other cardiovascular diagnoses such as dysrhythmias, heart failure, and cardiomyopathy. All nurses need to be familiar with the collaborative care management of CAD because of its high prevalence in the industrialized world. This chapter discusses the origins and management of CAD and its progression along the continuum of angina, unstable angina, and MI. It also discusses the recognition and management of common dysrhythmias.

CORONARY ARTERY DISEASE

Etiology

CAD is a generic designation for many different conditions that involve obstructed blood flow through the coronary arteries. The two most prevalent etiologies of CAD are atherosclerosis and coronary vasospasm. Atherosclerosis is by far the most common and is the focus of the presentation.

Epidemiology

Coronary atherosclerosis is the leading cause of death in the industrialized Western world, accounting for 40.6% of all deaths in 1998. It is estimated that 12,400,000 Americans have coronary heart disease, 7,300,000 have experienced MI and 6,400,000 have angina. Approximately 1,100,000 Americans experience a new or recurrent MI each year, and 40% of these individuals die during the attack. CAD remains the number one health problem in the United States, and coronary heart disease is the leading cause of premature, permanent disability.[1]

Both individual risk factors and the presence of concurrent disease states influence the incidence of CAD. Some populations have an increased occurrence of CAD because of definable characteristics or risks. Risk factors are classically categorized as nonmodifiable and modifiable. Nonmodifiable risk factors include age, gender, race, and family history/genetics. Modifiable risk factors include diabetes, hypertension, the use of tobacco, sedentary lifestyle, obesity, and stress (see Risk Factors box.) Table 23-1 links the major risk factors for CAD with their specific physiologic effects.

Age and Gender

Clinical evidence of CAD is rarely apparent before the second and third decades of life, but CAD is already a leading cause of mortality in men 35 to 45 years old. Overall, 50% of deaths in men and 49% of deaths in women can be attributed to CAD. It is the leading cause of death in both men and women, exceeding that of cancer. The incidence of CAD in women significantly increases after menopause, and one in three women over age 61 has some form of CAD. The mortality rate from CAD is actually 11% higher for women than men after age 65. With increasing longevity in the Western world, the incidence of CAD among both male and female octogenarians and nonagenarians also will increase.

Race

CAD is nondiscriminatory, affecting all races, but the independent role of race in the development of CAD is unclear. Other risk factors such as hypertension, obesity, lifestyle

Risk Factors

Coronary Artery Disease

Age and gender
Family history
Diabetes
Hypertension
Tobacco use
Sedentary lifestyle
Diet
Stress management

TABLE 23-1 Role of Risk Factors in Coronary Artery Disease

Risk Factor	Physiologic Effect
Age and gender	Decrease in elasticity of arteries with age Estrogen in females lowers serum cholesterol, decreases systemic vascular resistance, and improves endothelium-dependent vasodilation
Heredity: family history of coronary artery disease	Undetermined—genetic research pending
Diabetes	Damage to intima Insulin modifies lipid metabolism
Hypertension	Decreased elasticity of blood vessels Tearing effect on arteries Increased resistance to ejection of ventricular volume
Tobacco use (nicotine)	Decreased high-density lipoproteins Displacement of oxygen from hemoglobin Increased catecholamines in response to nicotine, increasing heart rate, and blood pressure Increases platelet adhesiveness Accelerates atheroma formation Coronary spasm
Sedentary lifestyle	Alters lipid metabolism Alters insulin sensitivity
Hypercholesterolemia, familial hyperlipidemia	Provide more substrate for lesion formation Increase levels of low-density lipoproteins, increasing atherogenesis

(including cultural practices), ethnic traditions, access to health care, and individual choices, may play a more significant role in the development of CAD than race alone.

Family History/Genetics

The likelihood that an offspring will have CAD increases if the biologic parent manifests CAD before the age of 55, but it is difficult to determine the independent role of genetics in the pathogenesis of CAD. Confounding variables include environmental factors and individual lifestyle choices that significantly influence the development of CAD. Genetics may directly affect the incidence of CAD through differential coding of genes responsible for lipid metabolism (apolipoprotein E), cardioprotective nitric oxide levels, angiotensin-converting enzyme (ACE) levels, and estrogen sensitivity in males.[2]

Diabetes

The incidence of CAD in individuals with diabetes mellitus is two to four times higher than in nondiabetic individuals,[8] and the incidence of type 2 diabetes is increasing epidemically in developing and developed countries. Hyperinsulinemia, a consequence of peripheral insulin resistance, can occur up to a decade before hyperglycemia is even diagnosed. Elevated levels of circulating insulin may begin the process of atheroma formation by initiating damage to the arterial intima. Impaired insulin regulation is associated with a variety of atheromatous processes, including elevated triglycerides, decreased high-density lipoprotein (HDL) levels, elevated very-low-density-lipoprotein (VLDL) levels, coagulation disorders, increased vascular resistance, obesity, and hypertension.[3]

Hypertension

Hypertension, defined as a measured elevation in blood pressure above 140/90 on at least three occasions, increases the incidence of CAD twofold to threefold. Hypertension affects the ability of the blood vessel to constrict and dilate. In addition, shearing forces on the intimal lining from hypertension predispose the artery to atherosclerosis. Adequate control of hypertension with medication and lifestyle modifications may decrease the incidence of CAD in the hypertensive population.

Tobacco

The risk of death from CAD is significantly higher in smokers than in nonsmokers, and the risk is proportional to the amount of tobacco used. About one in five deaths from cardiovascular disease can be attributed to smoking.[1] Cigarette smokers have the highest incidence of CAD; however, pipe and cigar smokers, as well as tobacco chewers, also have an increased risk of developing CAD compared with nonusers.

Sedentary Lifestyle

In 1996 the Surgeon General released a report on physical activity and health. This report noted that the incidence of CAD is higher in individuals who do not participate in regular physical activity compared with those who exercise. Exercise is associated with a decrease in total cholesterol, LDL cholesterol, and triglycerides. A total of 60% of U.S. adults report no pattern of regular exercise.[21]

Dyslipidemia

An estimated 100,870,000 American adults have total blood cholesterol levels of 200 mg/dl and higher, and research findings consistently report an association between elevated blood cholesterol levels and CAD.[1] LDLs are the most atherogenic of the lipid compounds, transporting 60% to 70% of the body's cholesterol. An increased triglyceride level, in combination with a high LDL level is also a strong predictor of heart disease and MI. Current research also indicates that elevated plasma lipoprotein (a) levels are predictive of premature CAD in men.[4] Hyperlipidemia may be either primary (familial) or secondary to some other process, such as concomitant disease states (diabetes) or lifestyle factors, such as diet, sedentary activity levels, and smoking. Excess cholesterol in the circulation results in endothelial injury and increases the available substrate for foam cell production, an early step in the development of atherosclerotic lesions (see Pathophysiology below).

Obesity

Obesity is associated with an almost threefold higher risk of cardiovascular disease.[22] Of particular concern are the 5 million children ages 6 to 17 who are considered to be overweight.[1] Although obesity is commonly cited as a significant coronary risk factor, the extent to which it has an independent effect in predisposing a person to CAD is controversial. Obese persons are more prone to glucose intolerance, hypertension, elevated triglycerides, and low levels of HDL. In addition, obese individuals often demonstrate other behaviors, such as sedentary lifestyles, that are known risk factors for CAD.

Stress

Much discussion has taken place over the years about the relationship between stress and CAD. Catecholamines, released during the stress response, increase platelet aggregation and may also precipitate vasospasm. A complete understanding of the effects of stress on circulation, lipid metabolism, and coagulability requires additional research.

Pathophysiology

CAD refers to the development and progression of plaque accumulation in the coronary arteries. Figure 23-1 illustrates the dynamic nature of CAD. The three stages along the continuum are stable angina, unstable angina, and MI. The newer term *acute coronary syndrome* (ACS) encompasses both unstable angina and MI. A patient with CAD may seek treatment at any point along this continuum and may move back and forth along the continuum over time. A designation is made based on the nature and severity of the patient's clinical presentation, but a firm diagnosis of unstable angina versus myocardial infarction cannot be made until after diagnostic testing is complete.

Stable Angina

The coronary arteries are small arteries that provide oxygen to the beating heart, a surface that is constantly moving (see Chapter 22). The arteries lie on the epicardial surface and branch often. The small size of the arteries, constant tension, and turbulence that is created at the bifurcations all contribute to the development of atherosclerotic lesions.

Normally the endothelium of the coronary artery allows for unrestricted blood flow to the myocardium. Any kind of

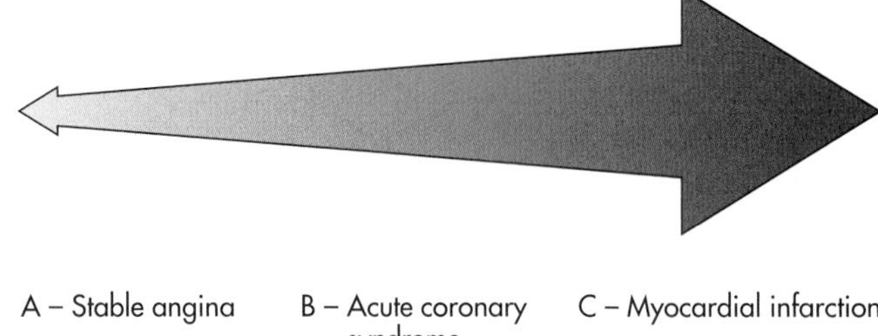

Figure 23-1 The continuum of CAD. Large arrow depicts the increased severity of the continuum to the right.

trauma or irritant, including high levels of cholesterol, hypertension, and smoking, can disrupt this protective endothelium. Infectious pathogens such as *Chlamydia pneumoniae*, hepatitis A virus, *Helicobacter pylori*, and cytomegalovirus have also been implicated in endothelial injury. The body's response to the injury involves a complex interplay of chemical mediators designed to protect the area. Platelets adhere to the collagen and release adenosine diphosphate (ADP). Circulating platelets with ADP-specific surface receptors become activated and bind to the released ADP. Endothelial injury also triggers the release of thromboxane A_2, which causes local vasoconstriction to minimize the extent of injury and further stimulates platelet aggregation (Figure 23-2). Endogenous nitric oxide acts to protect the artery through vascular relaxation.

The intima also releases prostacyclin in response to the effects of thromboxane A_2. Prostacyclin works to restore equilibrium through local vasodilation and by opposing platelet aggregation. With repeated injury, however, the deteriorating intima cannot produce sufficient prostacyclin to balance the process, and platelet aggregation forces predominate. Activation of the various platelet factors also causes the glycoprotein IIb/IIIa receptor sites to change shape and build fibrinogen bridges with adjacent platelets. Platelets and accumulating monocytes also release powerful growth factors into the arterial wall that stimulate the proliferation and migration of medial smooth muscle cells into the intima. This increases the permeability of the vessel wall to cholesterol. The accumulation of cholesterol produces a fatty streak that protrudes into the lumen of the artery. Smooth muscle cells and fibrous tissue then form a fibrous cap over the fatty streak.

The fatty streak continues to grow, invading both the intima and media. Involvement of the media affects the ability of the vessel wall to vasodilate and vasoconstrict. The artery continues to supply oxygen and nutrients to the myocardium as long as the blockage is less than 70% of the arterial lumen. Stable plaques may even occlude the coronary artery by more than 70% and still not cause symptoms.

The presence of risk factors appears to accelerate the atherogenesis, decreasing the oxygen supply. The presence of risk factors can also increase the myocardium's demand for oxygen (see Table 23-1). Concomitant conditions such as anemia, smoking (carbon monoxide displaces oxygen in the bloodstream), and hypovolemia further compromise delivery of oxygen to the myocardium. The demand for oxygen can be

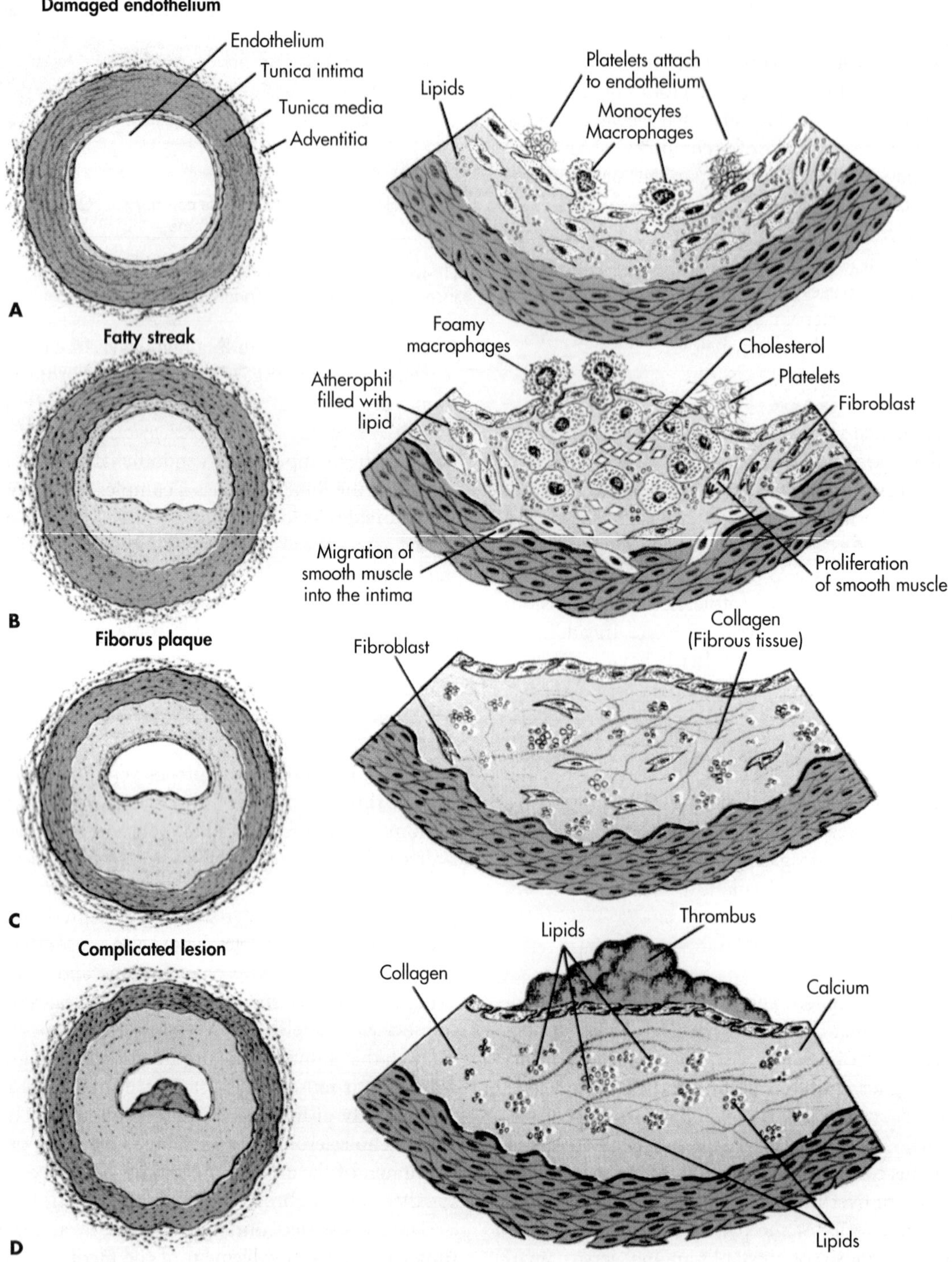

Figure 23-2 Progression of atherosclerosis. **A,** Thromboxane stimulates platelet aggregation. **B,** Medial smooth muscle migrates into the intima, increasing permeability of the wall to cholesterol. **C,** Fibrous cap seals plaque. **D,** Rupture of the plaque stimulates thrombus formation and acute coronary syndrome.

met only by an adequate blood supply. As long as supply is greater than or equal to demand, aerobic metabolism occurs. When demand is greater than supply, the myocardium must switch to anaerobic metabolism for nourishment. Anaerobic metabolism produces lactic acid, which is believed to be responsible for ischemic anginal pain. This pain is the most common initial symptom of CAD, but it does not have to be present for the diagnosis of CAD to be made (see Clinical Manifestations box on p. 651). With stable angina the patient usually experiences a known threshold beyond which myocardial oxygen demand exceeds supply. Myocardial oxygen demand increases with any condition causing an increase in heart rate, resistance to ejecting blood volume, or myocardial size.

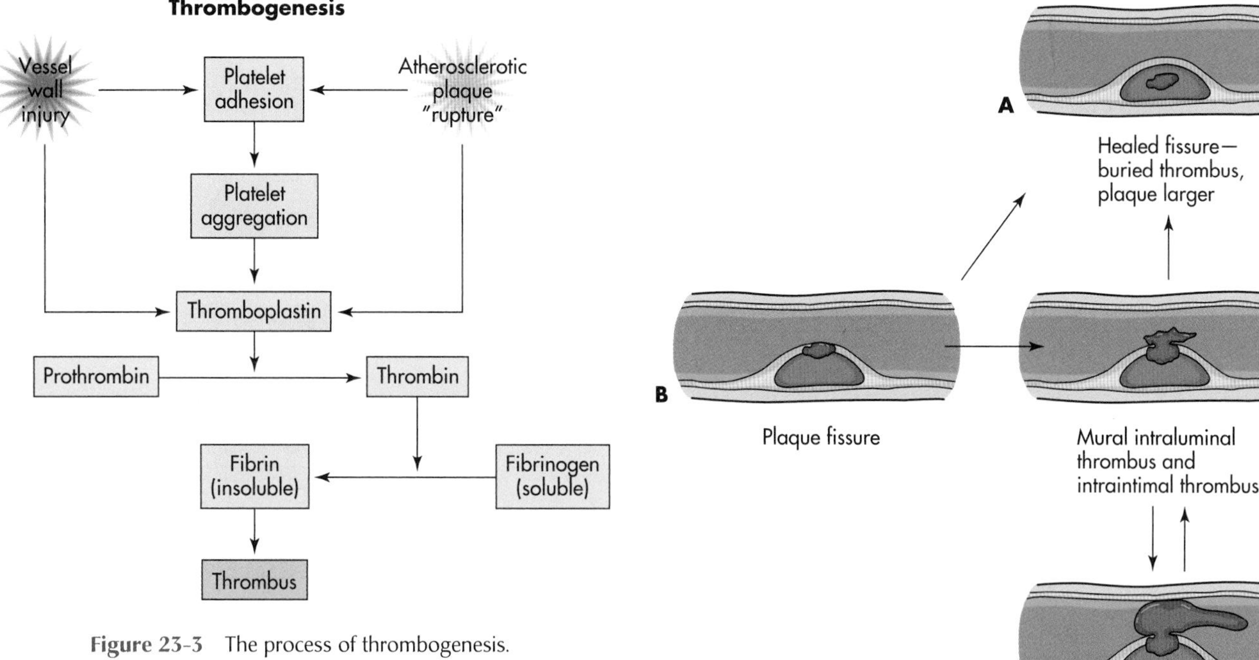

Figure 23-3 The process of thrombogenesis.

Figure 23-4 Possible pathophysiologic scenarios following plaque fissure. **A,** Clot is resorbed into plaque, healing over area of fissure, but with a smaller lumen resulting. **B,** Clot remains at site of fissure, decreasing lumen diameter. **C,** Clot extends into lumen, completely obstructing lumen (myocardial infarction).

Acute Coronary Syndrome

Atherosclerosis may remain stable if the blockage in the coronary artery does not progress beyond 70%; if collateral (alternate) vessels develop to supply the myocardium; and most importantly, if the fibrous cap remains intact. However, pressure within the lesion (plaque) can increase to the point of plaque rupture. Smaller, soft, lipid-rich, lesions appear to be the most likely to rupture. Rupture of the fibrous cap exposes the inner plaque to the circulating blood, activating clotting factors and causing both collagen accumulation and smooth muscle cell proliferation (Figure 23-3). The process of platelet activation is once again initiated to seal the rupture.

Risk factors contribute to this pathophysiology. Nicotine from tobacco use increases platelet adhesion and increases the potential for clotting at the site of disruption. Catecholamines released during the stress response also increase platelet aggregation.

Plaque rupture has several possible outcomes (Figure 23-4, *A* and *B*). The area can heal over with the platelet plug absorbed into the plaque under a new cap in which case the larger plaque further narrows the vessel lumen and may initiate symptoms. The second outcome leaves a residual fibrous clot extending into the lumen, partially obstructing the artery. A third possible outcome is complete obstruction of the coronary artery with the fibrous clot. This is termed coronary thrombosis or coronary occlusion and is the first stage of myocardial infarction (Figure 23-4, *C*). Acute coronary occlusion triggers a rapid series of physiologic events. Myocardial ischemia distal to the occlusion occurs immediately. Ischemia alters the integrity and the permeability of the myocardial cell membrane to vital electrolytes. This instability depresses myocardial contractility and predisposes the patient to sudden death from dysrhythmias. Figure 23-5 illustrates the spiraling series of events that occur in the cardiovascular system from myocardial ischemia.

The body activates the process of fibrinolysis to lyse the clot and restore blood flow. However, if clot lysis does not immediately restore blood flow, ischemia continues in the area of myocardium distal to the obstruction. Time is a critical factor in this scenario. Ongoing myocardial ischemia for 20 minutes or longer can result in death of tissue. This is termed *acute myocardial infarction* (AMI). A zone of ischemia, made up of potentially viable tissue, surrounds the infarcted area of myocardium. The final size of an infarct depends on whether this marginal area in the ischemic zone succumbs to the effects of prolonged ischemia (Figure 23-6).

The entire thickness of the myocardium may not become ischemic or infarcted if some blood is able to reach the area. If this is the case the MI that results is termed a subendothelial or non-Q wave infarction, as pathologic Q waves do not develop on the electrocardiogram (ECG). (See Chapter 22 for a discussion of the normal ECG.) A non-Q wave infarction involves less muscle damage and therefore fewer complications. However, the potential for further damage remains as long as the coronary artery lumen is atherosclerotic. Q wave infarctions extend through the full thickness of the ventricular wall and exhibit pathologic Q waves on the ECG.

In addition to distinctions between Q wave (full-thickness) and non-Q wave (subendothelial) infarctions, infarctions are also usually classified according to their anatomic location

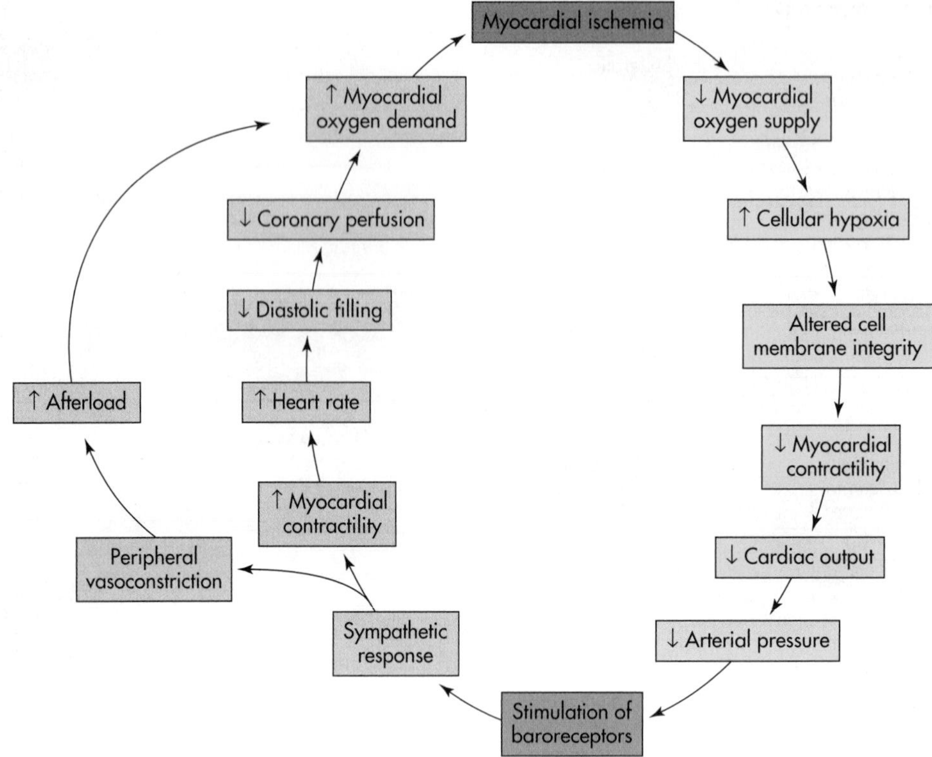

Figure 23-5 Effects of prolonged myocardial ischemia.

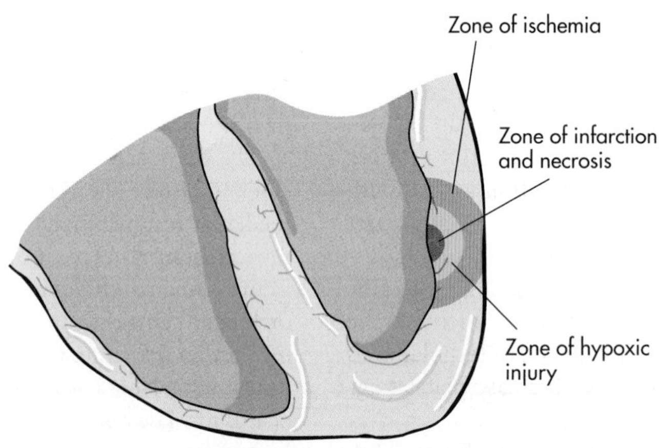

Figure 23-6 Zones of myocardial ischemia and infarction.

(Table 23-2). The left anterior descending (LAD) artery supplies the anterior surface of the left ventricle and the bundle branches of the conduction system. This area of the heart is responsible for most of the contractility necessary to eject blood into the aorta. This portion of the heart requires a substantial source of oxygen to generate the force needed to pump against the aorta's high-pressure system. Lesions in the LAD that lead to anterior infarctions are often associated with a decrease in contractility and cardiac output that results in heart failure. Sudden death secondary to ventricular dysrhythmias may also occur (see discussion on dysrhythmias later in this chapter).

The circumflex artery most often supplies the lateral surface of the left ventricle. Obstruction affecting only this area is often well tolerated. Most patients with a lateral MI experience few complications.

The right coronary artery supplies the inferior surface of the left ventricle, the entire right ventricle, and both the sinoatrial (SA) and atrioventricular (AV) nodes in most individuals. Inferior infarctions or right ventricular infarctions may be

TABLE 23-2 Correlation of Coronary Artery with Affected Myocardium

Coronary Artery	Structure Supplied	Potential Complications
Left anterior descending	Anterior surface of the left ventricle Ventricular septum Bundle branches of the conduction system Left atrium	Bundle branch blocks Left-sided heart failure Rupture of septum
Circumflex	Lateral and posterior surfaces of the left ventricle Sinoatrial (SA) node (45% of people) Atrioventricular (AV) node and bundle of His (10% of people)	When the circumflex artery supplies the SA node, bradydysrhythmias may result
Right coronary artery	Right atrium Right ventricle Posterior surface of the left ventricle SA node (55% of people) AV node (90% of people)	Bradydysrhythmias and heart blocks Right-sided heart failure

complicated by transient or permanent heart blocks or right-sided heart failure.

Clinical Manifestations

The patient with CAD usually seeks health care during an episode of ischemia or after an ischemic event. Many patients experience the classic midsternal chest pain; however, a considerable number of patients instead complain of indigestion, "heartburn," left arm pain, or pain radiating from the chest to the scapula, neck, jaw, or the left or right arm. Women often experience "atypical" symptoms such as chest heaviness, heartburn, fatigue, or shortness of breath. The differences in presentation that may occur with stable angina, acute coronary syndrome, and MI are summarized in the Clinical Manifestations box. The occurrence of angina is often perceived as sudden; however, some individuals may perceive it as gradual, especially if the initial intensity was mild.

Symptoms of stable angina are often of short duration, ending when the demand for oxygen is decreased. Symptoms of unstable angina are of longer duration and usually require intervention. Symptoms of MI continue until blood flow is restored or the myocardium dies.

Precipitating factors for stable angina include any circumstance that increases myocardial oxygen demand, such as exercise, stress, sexual intercourse, and smoking. Precipitating factors for acute coronary syndrome can include similar activities, or there may not be an identifiable precipitating event. The onset of acute coronary syndrome can occur at rest or on awakening if platelets are stimulated.

The classic location of ischemic pain is retrosternal. The pain may radiate down the left arm or both arms, upward to the neck or jaws, or backward to the scapular region. Some patients do not experience pain, termed *silent ischemia.* This is especially true for elderly patients or patients with diabetes owing to alterations in sensory perception. Therefore the quality and intensity of pain may be unreliable indicators of the severity of ischemia. For example, some patients with MI describe the pain as "mild indigestion" or "tightness," whereas others describe the pain as excruciating and viselike.

In addition to chest pain, patients may complain of dizziness, dyspnea, nausea, vomiting, or anxiety. Patients experiencing an acute MI often report a feeling of doom or feeling as though they are "going to die."

Changes in vital signs may include tachycardia or bradycardia, increased or decreased blood pressure, and shortness

> ***Clinical Manifestations***
> **Coronary Artery Disease**
>
> The following may occur with stable angina or acute coronary syndrome:
> - Chest pain or anginal equivalent (jaw pain, left arm pain)
> - Nonverbal indicators of pain: clutching, rubbing, or stroking the chest
> - Increase or decrease in heart rate
> - Increase in blood pressure
> - Dysrhythmias
>
> The following is unique to stable angina:
> - Angina that occurs with predictable level of exertion
>
> The following are unique to acute coronary syndrome:
> - Angina not necessarily associated with activity
> - ECG: ST depression
>
> The following are unique to myocardial infarction:
> - Angina not relieved by rest or nitroglycerin therapy
> - Associated symptoms: dizziness, dyspnea, nausea, vomiting, feeling of impending doom
> - Altered neurologic status, if decreased cardiac output
> - Rales, if decreased contractility creates left ventricular failure
> - Presence of S_3 or S_4 gallop
> - Diminished pulses
> - Pallor
> - ECG: ST elevation, Q waves, T wave abnormalities
> - Laboratory values: elevated CK-MB, elevated troponin 1, elevated glucose, leukocytosis, elevated erythrocyte sedimentation rate

of breath. Dysrhythmias may develop from myocardial ischemia, and decreased cardiac output can result in classic "shocky" symptoms such as pale, cool, diaphoretic skin.

Collaborative Care Management

Diagnostic Tests

When a patient has signs or symptoms of CAD, diagnostic tests help determine whether the patient has stable angina, unstable angina, or MI.

Electrocardiography. The ECG remains a critical tool in diagnosing CAD and is most useful while the patient is symptomatic. Because the ECG represents only one point in time, serial 12 lead ECGs and/or continuous monitoring are the standard of care for the evaluation of chest pain. Ischemia is most clearly reflected in the ST segment of the ECG.

ST segment elevation is the hallmark of acute myocardial ischemia that is progressing toward infarction (Figure 23-7). ST elevation resolves when blood flow is restored or the MI is complete. If the full thickness of the myocardium becomes necrotic, significant Q waves evolve over the next week. Future ECGs continue to show the Q wave, indicating that the patient suffered an MI in the past. When only the subendocardial surface infarcts (non-Q wave MI), Q waves do not develop. T wave abnormalities such as T wave inversion may also occur at the time of acute infarction. ST depression on the ECG represents ischemia and resolves with improved perfusion. Non-ST-segment elevation MI (NSTEMI) refers to an acute coronary syndrome that does not cause ST elevation, but produces elevated troponin levels.[5]

The 12-lead ECG represents 12 different anatomic views of the myocardium. (See Chapter 22.) ST changes occur in leads that are specific to the area of myocardium involved. Table 23-3 shows the relationship of leads to the affected area of myocardium. It is necessary to use 15-18 leads to reveal damage to the right ventricle or posterior wall of the left ventricle. The use of a 15-18 lead ECG is becoming more common in order not to overlook these less frequent infarctions.

Blood Tests. Biomarkers provide definitive information about the presence and severity of myocardial damage and are drawn immediately in patients experiencing unrelenting chest pain. Biomarkers are especially valuable in evaluating patients who present for possible fibrinolytic therapy. The most specific biomarker for MI is serum troponin, which is composed of three proteins: troponin C, troponin I, and troponin T. Cardiac troponin I rises within 3 hours of myocardial damage and the elevation persists up to 7 days. Cardiac troponin I that is already elevated on admission is associated with an increase in both complications and mortality. Because the serum troponin level in normal individuals is usually undetectable, any elevation of serum troponin indicates myocardial cell damage. The normal serum level of troponin T is 0.0 to 0.1 ng/ml; troponin I is 0.0 to 3.1 ng/ml.

Another biomarker, the enzyme creatine kinase (CK), confirms the presence of myocardial damage. Injured myocardial cells release CK during AMI. CK elevation begins within 3 to 9 hours after MI, peaks in 12 to 18 hours, and returns to normal in 2 to 3 days (Table 23-4). Brain tissue and skeletal muscle also release CK with injury, but the isoenzyme CK-MB is

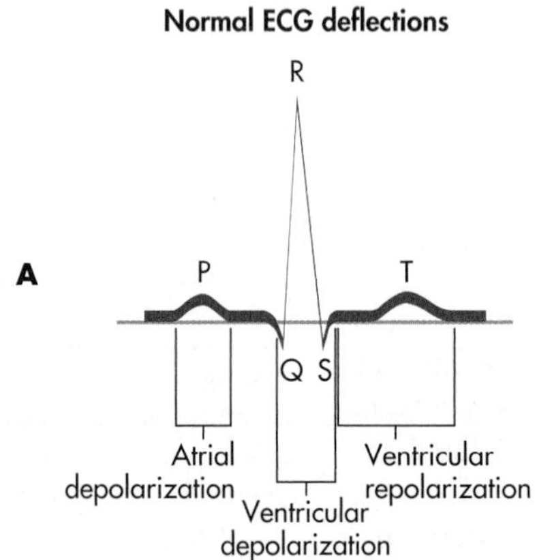

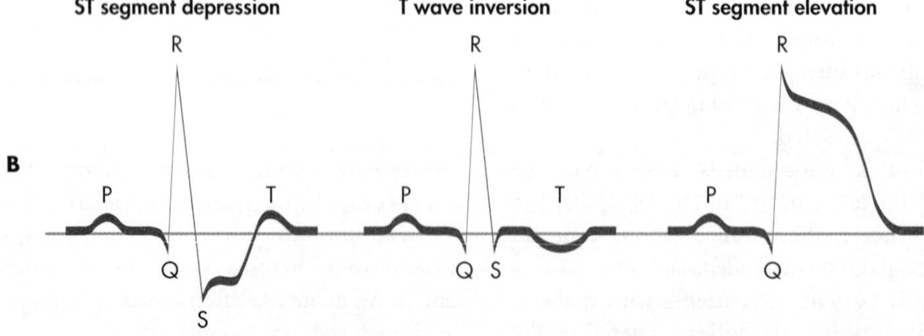

Figure 23-7 ECG and ischemia. **A,** Normal ECG. **B,** Electrocardiographic alterations associated with ischemia.

specific to the myocardium. Because levels of CK-MB decrease at 12 hours, CK-MB levels are useful in determining the endpoint of myocardial damage, and are clear indicators of the presence of reinfarction.

Myoglobin, an oxygen-binding protein found in cardiac and skeletal muscle, is another early biomarker for MI. Levels increase within 1 hour after MI, reach peak levels in 4 to 6 hours, and return to normal within 24 to 36 hours.

Blood chemistry tests and a complete blood count (CBC) are performed to determine concurrent disease states and help with differential diagnosis. Patients with AMI may have elevated blood glucose levels secondary to the stress response. The white blood cell (WBC) count may also increase (leukocytosis). Leukocytosis begins within a few hours after the onset of symptoms as an inflammatory response to the injured cardiac tissue. The WBC count can reach 12,000 to 15,000/mm^3 and the elevation lasts for approximately 3 to 7 days. The erythrocyte sedimentation rate also rises during the first week after infarction and remains elevated for several weeks. C-reactive protein, another measure of inflammation, may also be determined in patients presenting with ACS.

Stress Testing. With the introduction of managed care, risk stratification of CAD has taken on increasing importance. Risk stratification refers to the use of diagnostic tests and physical assessment to determine prognosis and guide patient management. Cardiologists must decide which diagnostic tests to use, and when, to maximize quality patient care and minimize health care costs.

TABLE 23-3 Correlation of ECG Findings with Cardiac Anatomy

Acute Changes in Leads	Anatomic Location of Infarct
2, 3, aV_F	Inferior
1, aV_L	Lateral
V_1-V_3	Anteroseptal
V_4-V_6	Anterolateral
Tall R waves in V_1, V_2	Posterior
V_4R, V_5R, V_6R (right precordial lead placement)	Right ventricular

TABLE 23-4 Cardiac Biomarker Levels in Acute Myocardial Infarction

Cardiac Enzyme	Elevation (hours)	Peak Elevation (hours)	Duration (days)
Creatinine kinase MB (CK-MB)	4-8	8-16	2-3
Troponin T	3.5	2-5	10-14
Troponin I	4-6	2-5	7
Myoglobin	1	4-6	1-2

Typically the patient with stable angina completes an exercise stress test with or without nuclear imaging. Stress testing, often of modified intensity, may also be safely performed with patients after infarction. Stress testing is safe and cost-effective for use in emergency department chest pain centers with patients who have been identified as having low risk/low likelihood of ACS. An exercise stress test reveals the significance of coronary artery blockages in regard to the patient's functional status. This noninvasive test indicates areas of the myocardium that do not receive adequate perfusion at peak exercise. Use of nuclear imaging allows comparison between images of underperfused areas at peak exercise with images taken at rest. Differences between the images indicate infarction (fixed defect) or ischemia (redistribution). The ECG tracings recorded during the exercise component of the test can also indicate which coronary arteries might be involved. When a patient cannot exercise because of arthritis, peripheral vascular disease, or general debility, pharmacologic agents (e.g., adenosine, dobutamine) can be administered intravenously to simulate the exercise response in the coronary arteries.

Echocardiography is another noninvasive test that may be used. Variations include echocardiography with exercise and dobutamine stress echocardiography. Echocardiography is also used to identify abnormal ventricular wall motion in select patients presenting with chest pain. However, its usefulness for this purpose is limited, as it cannot distinguish old from new damage.

Cardiac Catheterization. Cardiac catheterization is an invasive cardiac procedure used to assess coronary anatomy, ventricular function, and hemodynamic status. In the United States, an estimated 1,291,000 inpatient cardiac catheterizations were performed in 1998 at an average cost of $12,450. An additional 472,000 outpatient catheterizations were performed.[1] Cardiac catheterization is indicated for patients who have recurrent symptoms despite maximal medical management and for patients with one or more recurrent, severe, or prolonged (longer than 20 minutes) ischemic episode. Patients who may also benefit from catheterization include those with prior angioplasty, bypass surgery, or MI; those with high-risk clinical findings or noninvasive test findings; and those with significant heart failure or left ventricular dysfunction.

Right-sided heart catheterization provides information on the hemodynamic status of the heart. Left-sided heart catheterization includes coronary angiography and left ventriculography. Coronary angiography visualizes the coronary arteries using radiopaque dye and provides an indirect estimate of the severity of blockage in the coronary arteries and their branches (Figure 23-8).

Ventriculography, often done at the same time as arteriography, involves injection of dye into the left ventricle. Cardiac output can be calculated from the amount of dye ejected from the left ventricle during systole.

Fluoroscopic imaging allows direct visualization of the contractility of the left ventricle. Areas of poor contractility (hypokinesis), overcompensation (hyperkinesis), nonmovement (akinesis), and asynergy (dyskinesis) can be identified with ventriculography. An infarcted area is usually akinetic.

Medications

Risk factor modification is one of the most important components of the management of stable angina, but drug therapy also plays a major role in the management of CAD. Box 23-1 provides an easy acronym for the guidelines used to manage chronic stable angina. Figures 23-9 and 23-10 outline treatment algorithms for the management of stable angina and ACS that incorporate both drug therapy and risk factor modification. Clinical research continues at a rapid pace to determine the ideal combination of medications for the management of patients with acute coronary syndromes.[9] Table 23-5 presents an overview of drugs commonly used. Hormone replacement therapy, once advocated for post-MI management in postmenopausal women is no longer routinely prescribed (see Research box). The role of gene therapy in the treatment of CAD is just beginning to evolve (see Future Watch box).

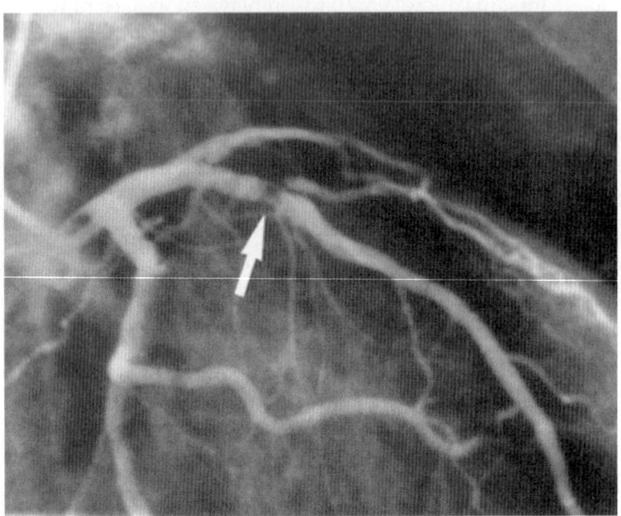

Figure 23-8 Coronary arteriogram showing a coronary artery thrombus *(arrow)* in a patient with unstable angina.

Antiplatelet Agents. Aspirin is the primary antiplatelet agent used in the prevention and treatment of CAD. Aspirin is given in the emergency department (or in the prehospital setting) to any patient suspected of having an MI. Aspirin blocks the formation of thromboxane A_2, inhibiting platelet aggregation, and research has demonstrated that a single daily dose of

BOX 23-1 Guidelines for Management of Stable Angina

Aspirin and antianginals
Beta-blocker and blood pressure
Cholesterol and cigarettes
Diet and diabetes
Education and exercise

From Gibbons RJ et al: ACC/AHA/ACP-ASIM pocket guidelines for management of patients with chronic stable angina: a report of the American College of Cardiology/American Heart Association Task Force on Practice Guidelines, Bethesda, Md, 2000, American College of Cardiologists.

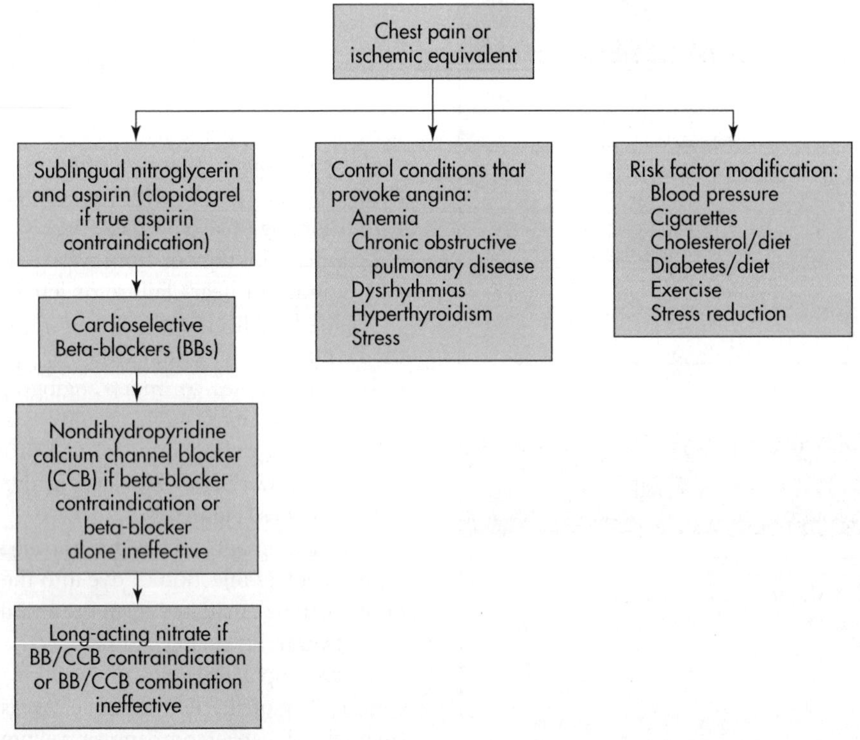

Figure 23-9 Management of chronic stable angina.

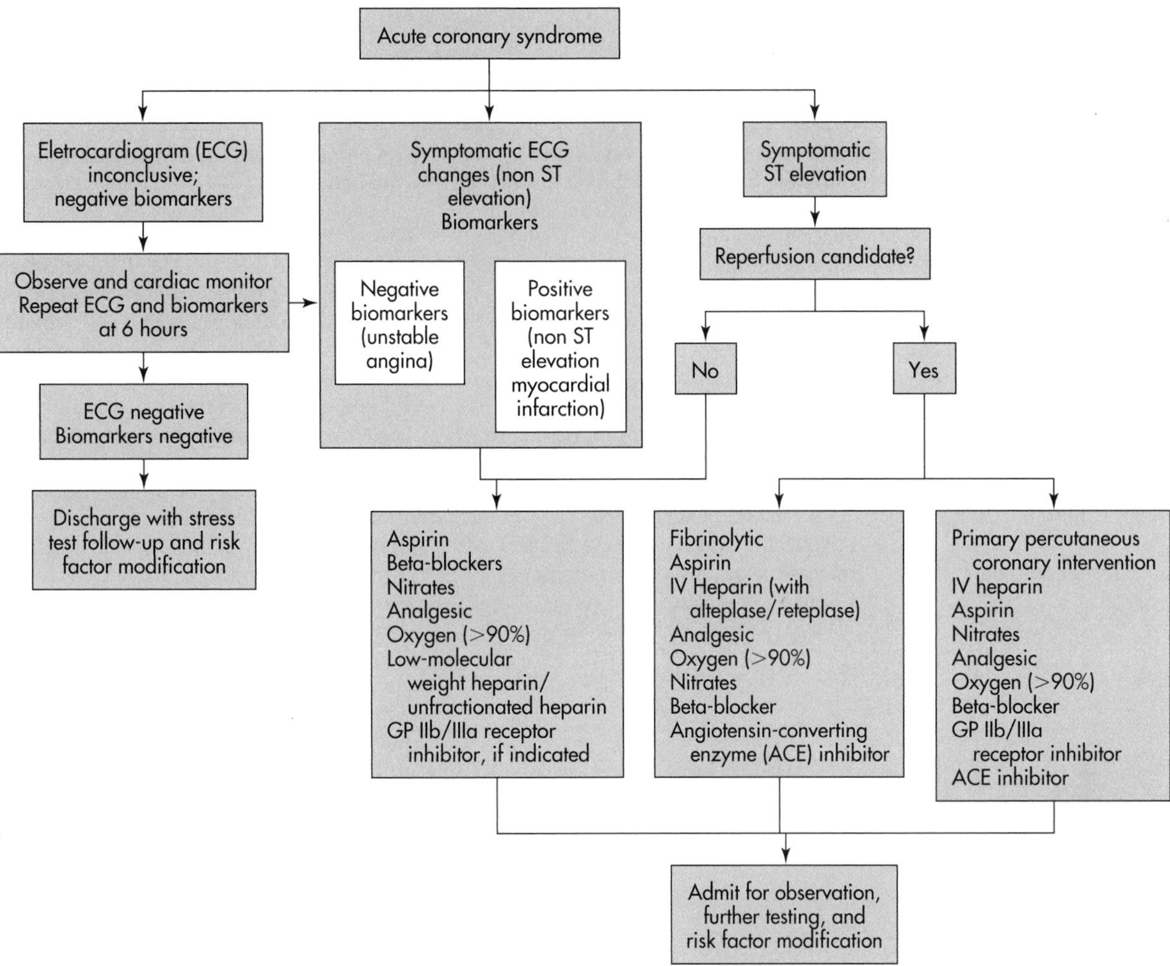

Figure 23-10 Management of acute coronary syndrome.

TABLE 23-5 Common Medications for Coronary Artery Disease

Drug	Action	Intervention
Antiplatelet agents (Aspirin, clopidogrel)	Aspirin inhibits thromboxane-induced platelet aggregation Clopidogrel prevents platelet activation by blocking ADP-induced platelet binding.	Aspirin should be prescribed unless a true hypersensitivity reaction is present or the patient has a severe risk of bleeding.
Fibrinolytics Alteplase (recombinant t-PA) Reteplase (r-PA) Tenecteplase (TNK-tPA) Streptokinase	Activate fibrinolytic processes to lyse the clot associated with plaque rupture and vessel occlusion of MI. Streptokinase activates the conversion of plasminogen to plasmin, which degrades fibrin and fibrinogen into fragments. Tissue plasminogen activators (t-PA) also activate plasmin, but preferentially at the site of occlusion.	Patients must be carefully screened before administration of fibrinolytic agents. The nurse monitors for reperfusion, reocclusion, and bleeding complications with fibrinolytic administration. Interventions are directed toward preventing bleeding complications.
Glycoprotein IIb/IIIa receptor inhibitors Tirofiban Eptifibatide Abciximab	Affect the final pathway in platelet-thrombus formation by binding to the GP IIb/IIIa receptor site.	Patients should be observed for bleeding complications. Care should be given to correct weight-based dose.

Continued

TABLE 23-5 Common Medications for Coronary Artery Disease—cont'd

Drug	Action	Intervention
Anticoagulants Unfractionated heparin Low-molecular-weight heparin	Prevent propagation of an established thrombus by rapidly inhibiting thrombin. Low-molecular-weight heparin (LMWH) affects predominantly factor Xa, with less effect on thrombin.	With unfractionated heparin, heparin partial thromboplastin times (PTTs) should be measured 6 hours after any change in dose. Dose is weight based. Therapeutic levels should be maintained between 50 and 70 sec. LMWH does not require heparin PTTs. Hemoglobin, hematocrit, and platelets should be followed for downward trends. Platelets should be followed for heparin-induced thrombocytopenia. Recurrent ischemia, active bleeding, and hypotension may signify subtherapeutic or supratherapeutic dosages and should be evaluated immediately.
Nitrates Isosorbide dinitrate Isosorbide mononitrate Nitroglycerin	Decrease myocardial oxygen demand: Venodilate (decrease preload) Peripherally vasodilate (decrease afterload) Increase myocardial oxygen supply Coronary vasodilate	Patients should be lying or sitting with administration of sublingual nitrates. Intravenous nitroglycerin is titrated to relief of symptoms or limiting side effects such as headache or systolic BP <90 mm Hg. Intravenous preparations are usually replaced with oral or topical preparation when the patient has been symptom free for 24 hours. Cautious use with known aortic stenosis. Anticipate headache, administer analgesics as appropriate. Tolerance to nitrates can develop within 24 hours. A nitrate-free interval of 6 to 8 hours may improve responsiveness to therapy. Topical nitrates must be cleaned from the skin surface before applying new dose. Appropriate areas of application include any hair-free area, preferably in noticeable areas when the initial dose is being determined. Application areas should be rotated. Gloves should be worn when applying topical preparations.
Beta-blockers Atenolol Metoprolol	Decrease myocardial oxygen demand: Decrease contractility Slow heart rate Slow impulse conduction Decrease BP (through renin interaction) Slow heart rate, thereby increasing diastolic filling time and coronary perfusion Decrease incidence of morbidity and mortality after acute MI	Intravenous metoprolol is given in 5-mg increments over 1 to 2 minutes. Atenolol may be prescribed intravenously instead of metoprolol. Intravenous preparations are followed by oral preparations after the patient is stabilized. Monitor for atrioventricular block (including measuring PR interval), symptomatic bradycardia, hypotension, left ventricular failure (rales, decreased cardiac output), and bronchospasm. Target heart rate for beta blockade is 50 to 60 beats/min.
Calcium channel blockers Diltiazem Verapamil	Decrease afterload and preload, thereby decreasing the workload of the heart. This decreases remodeling of the left ventricle. Long-term consequences of remodeling are increased oxygen demand and heart failure	Often prescribed when vasospasm is considered part of the pathology or if significant hypertension exists. Monitor for symptomatic bradycardia, prolonged PR intervals, advanced heart blocks, hypotension, heart failure.
Angiotensin-converting enzyme inhibitors Captopril Enalapril Benazepril Lisinopril Fosinopril	Decrease myocardial oxygen demand Venodilate (decrease preload)	Monitor for adverse effects: angioneurotic edema, cough, hypotension, hyperkalemia, pruritic rash, renal failure. First doses require BP before and 30 minutes after administration.

TABLE 23-5 Common Medications for Coronary Artery Disease—cont'd

Drug	Action	Intervention
Morphine sulfate	Blunts the deleterious consequences of sympathetic stimulation with pain Vasodilates, creating decreased preload	Establish baseline vital signs, level of consciousness, and orientation. Monitor for hypotension, respiratory depression, changes in level of consciousness. Doses are usually given in increments of 2 to 5 mg.
Oxygen	Increased arterial oxygen saturation	Monitor for adequate arterial oxygenation with finger pulse oximetry. Maintain saturation levels above 90%.
Cholesterol-lowering agents Atorvastatin Lovastatin Pravastatin Simvastatin Gemfibrozil Nicotinic acid	Reduce the substrate for lipid deposition in the coronary artery	Side effects vary with drug class. Intolerance to side effects may limit the usefulness of certain medications. Lipid levels should be obtained at regular intervals to monitor for success in effecting changes. Patients must be educated that cholesterol-lowering agents do not substitute for dietary modifications (see Table 23-6).

Research

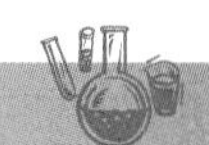

Reference: Hulley S et al: Randomized trial of estrogen plus progestin for secondary prevention of coronary heart disease in postmenopausal women, *JAMA* 280(7):605, 1998.

A total of 2763 postmenopausal women with heart disease (mean age 66.7 years) participated in a randomized, blinded, placebo-controlled secondary prevention trial. Treatment groups received 0.625 mg of conjugated equine estrogens plus 2.5 mg of medroxyprogesterone acetate in 1 tablet daily (hormone replacement therapy [HRT]) or a placebo of identical appearance (control). There was a significant decrease in low-density lipoprotein (LDL) and increase in high-density lipoprotein (HDL) level in the HRT group compared to the control group. Overall, there was not a significant difference between groups in the occurrence of myocardial infarction or coronary heart disease (CHD) death, or in the occurrence of secondary outcomes of coronary revascularization, unstable angina, heart failure, resuscitated cardiac arrest, stroke or transient ischemic attack, and peripheral arterial disease. There was a statistical time trend such that those treated with HRT had more CHD events in the first year of follow-up and fewer events than the control group in years 4 and 5 of follow-up. More women in the HRT group experienced thromboembolic events and gallbladder disease. The researchers concluded that HRT did not reduce the overall rate of CHD events in postmenopausal women with known coronary artery disease (CAD). With the pattern of increased events at 1 year, the recommendation followed not to start HRT for the purpose of secondary prevention in postmenopausal women with CAD; however, for women already on HRT, it could be favorable for them to continue treatment in light of the 4- to 5-year follow-up findings.

Future Watch

Gene Therapy in Treating Cardiovascular Disease

Genetic therapy is fast becoming a distinct nursing specialty. It used to be that "talking genetics" was reserved for those in obstetrics and gynecology, but not for nurses in the next millennium. Increasingly, links are being found between coronary artery disease, heart failure, and dysrhythmias and genetics. Therefore nurses must gain an appreciation of gene therapy and what the future may hold. Angiogenesis, or the growth of new blood vessels, has obvious indications for treating coronary artery disease. Collateralization is a benefit that naturally occurs with exercise, but can we produce new vessels from genes? Presently, gene therapy products are being studied for just that purpose. Gene therapy products to stimulate angiogenesis, and thereby decrease anginal events, are being introduced into the coronary circulation during routine catheterization. Catheterization personnel and patients must protect themselves with goggles, gown, gloves, and special masking. The product is directly injected into the coronary circulation using a viral vector for transport, in this case an adenovirus. All material used in the procedure is considered biohazard waste products. Patients are monitored for dysrhythmias overnight and discharged the next day. Side effects from the treatment relate most directly to the adenovirus and the growth factor component of the genetic product. These effects include myocarditis, hepatitis, upper respiratory infections, vascular changes, accelerated atherosclerosis, rising platelet levels, and proteinuria.

Reference: Coombs, VJ: Gene therapy for the treatment of cardiovascular disease, *Crit Care Nurs Clin North Am* 11(3):349, 1999.

81 mg (one baby aspirin) can effectively sustain the desired antiplatelet effect. Enteric-coated forms can be prescribed for individuals who cannot tolerate pure aspirin. Clopidogrel (Plavix), a thienopyridine, prevents platelet activation by blocking ADP-induced platelet binding. It is used for individuals who cannot tolerate aspirin and for patients undergoing percutaneous coronary interventions (PCIs). Ticlopidine (Ticlid), also a thienopyridine, is rarely used because of the associated risk of neutropenia.

Fibrinolytics. Fibrinolytic agents are the standard of care for patients treated within 6 to 12 hours of the onset of MI. These agents are used with symptomatic patients with ST elevation and/or new onset left bundle branch block (LBBB). Fibrinolytics activate fibrinolytic processes to lyse the clot that is occluding the lumen of the coronary artery. Fibrinolytics are administered intravenously when the ECG confirms the diagnosis of acute MI. Commonly used fibrinolytics include tissue plasminogen activators such as alteplase (recombinant t-PA), reteplase (r-PA), tenecteplase (TNK-tPA), and streptokinase (Streptase). Streptokinase activates the conversion of plasminogen to plasmin, which degrades fibrin and fibrinogen into fragments. Tissue plasminogen activators also activate plasmin, but preferentially at the site of occlusion. The risk of bleeding associated with the use of clot dissolution agents necessitates thorough screening of all patients for bleeding risks (see Guidelines for Safe Practice box on p. 671). When contraindications to fibrinolytic therapy exist, primary PCI are initiated without delay. The reperfusion of previously ischemic myocardium results in numerous biochemical and cellular events, which can include myocyte necrosis, dysrhythmias, and depressed myocardial contractility. Reperfusion injury of the ischemic myocardium is a phenomenon under continued investigation.[6] Researchers report the feasibility and benefit of prehospital administration of fibrinolytics in decreasing hospital mortality.[14]

Glycoprotein IIb/IIIa Receptor Inhibitors. GP IIb/IIIa antagonists have been used successfully to affect the final pathway in platelet-thrombus formation in both acute coronary syndromes and in conjunction with PCI. By binding to the GP IIb/IIIa receptor site, these drugs block the binding of fibrinogen to the platelet, thereby preventing platelet aggregation and clot formation. Approved agents currently include tirofiban (Aggrastat), eptifibatide (Integrelin), and abciximab (ReoPro).

Anticoagulants. Anticoagulants are often prescribed for the patient with acute coronary syndrome. Intravenous unfractionated heparin binds to antithrombin III, inactivating coagulation factors Xa, IXa, and thrombin, thereby blocking the conversion of fibrinogen to fibrin. Weight-adjusted doses are administered to achieve activated partial thromboplastin (aPTT) levels of 50 to 70 seconds. Low-molecular-weight heparins (LMWH) have a more predictable dose-response curve and an increased plasma half-life compared with unfractionated heparin. LMWHs include enoxaparin (Lovenox), dalteparin (Fragmin), and ardeparin (Normiflo). Current guidelines call for the use of enoxaparin for patients with ACS and ST elevation who are not candidates for fibrinolytic therapy or acute PCI.

Hirudin, a specific inhibitor of thrombin, affects the final step in the coagulation cascade. By binding to thrombin, Hirudin prevents further platelet aggregation and clot formation. Research continues to investigate the role of direct thrombin inhibitors in ACS.

Nitrates. Nitrates are effective in the treatment of both stable and unstable angina, and MI. Nitrates cause vasodilation, reducing the amount of blood returning to the heart from the venous system, thus decreasing preload. This decreases both the workload of the heart and the demand of the myocardium for oxygen. Nitrates also dilate the peripheral arteries, decreasing the resistance against which the left ventricle must pump. This decrease in systemic blood pressure contributes to a decreased afterload. Because the left ventricle can pump with less force, there is again a decrease in myocardial oxygen demand. In addition, nitrates act specifically to dilate coronary arteries that are not atherosclerotic. As a result, collateral flow increases to the ischemic parts of the myocardium.

Many nitrate preparations are available for use. Sublingual nitroglycerin is used most commonly for acute episodes of angina. The tablets, absorbed within minutes from beneath the tongue, are highly effective in relieving the acute symptoms of angina by increasing oxygen supply to the myocardium while simultaneously decreasing oxygen demand. Intravenous nitroglycerin is recommended for patients experiencing prolonged chest pain associated with acute MI and heart failure, large anterior infarctions, persistent ischemia, or hypertension.[15] Nitrates are also available as topical preparations. Both ointments and patches provide a sustained therapeutic effect. Shorter-acting ointment preparations are used during the hospitalization as medications are initiated and adjusted. An advantage of the ointment is the ability to quickly remove it from the skin surface if hypotension occurs. Patches and oral preparations, such as isosorbide dinitrate and Imdur, are usually prescribed for long-term management.

Beta-Blockers. Most beta-blockers used to treat stable angina and ACS are cardioselective, blocking predominantly the beta-1 receptor. Blockade of beta-1 receptors causes a decrease in the force of contraction, a slowing of heart rate, and a slowing of impulse conduction. These three mechanisms of action combine to decrease myocardial oxygen demand. In addition, by slowing the heart rate, beta-blockers indirectly increase the supply of blood to the myocardium by increasing diastole, thus increasing the time available for coronary artery perfusion. Beta-blockers also decrease blood pressure (thereby decreasing both afterload and myocardial oxygen demand) through their effect on the renin-angiotensin system.

The use of beta-blockers is associated with a decreased incidence of morbidity and mortality when they are administered within 48 hours of MI and continued for 2 to 3 years after AMI. For this reason, beta-blockers may be administered intravenously in the emergency department to individuals with probable MI. After the patient with AMI is stabilized, beta-blockers are administered orally. Metoprolol (Lopressor) and atenolol (Tenormin) are commonly used cardioselective beta-blockers.

Calcium Channel Blockers. The role of calcium channel blockers in the management of CAD is limited. Nondihydropyridine calcium channel blockers (diltiazem [Cardizem] or verapamil [Calan]) may be used when beta-blockers are contraindicated. These agents inhibit the influx of calcium through the slow calcium channels, which must open and allow calcium to enter the cell before an electrical impulse can occur. By slowing the heart rate, diltiazem and verapamil decrease myocardial oxygen demand and indirectly increase myocardial oxygen supply by increasing the time for coronary perfusion during diastole. These agents also block the calcium used for myocardial contractility, decreasing the force of contraction (and hence oxygen demand).

Angiotensin-Converting Enzyme Inhibitors. ACE inhibitors may be used in the management of CAD to decrease preload and afterload. ACE inhibitors are routinely administered, at least short term, to patients with MI to decrease the overall workload of the heart. Decreasing workload prevents "remodeling" of the left ventricle, which involves the compensatory development of hypertrophy in the unaffected left ventricle. The hypertrophy attempts to compensate for the loss of function in the infarcted area. The long-term consequence can be a steady increase in myocardial oxygen demand for the enlarged muscle and the onset of heart failure.

Analgesics. Even though fibrinolytics, ASA, and heparin may open the coronary arteries and decrease chest pain, severe chest pain often persists. Pain activates the sympathetic nervous system, increasing heart rate and producing vasoconstriction. These changes decrease myocardial oxygen supply and increase myocardial oxygen demand. The immediate administration of intravenous opioid analgesics interrupts the deleterious effects of pain. The drug of choice is morphine sulfate, which not only blunts the sensation of pain, but also promotes vasodilation, thereby decreasing preload.

Oxygen. Oxygen is administered to the patient experiencing ACS to maintain arterial oxygen saturation levels above 90%. This simple but effective intervention is key to increasing myocardial oxygen supply. Oxygen may be administered by nasal cannula or mask.

Cholesterol-Lowering Agents. Because considerable evidence links hypercholesterolemia to atherosclerosis, drugs that can reduce plasma lipids and lipoproteins are often prescribed in the treatment of patients with CAD. Drug classes include HMG CoA reductase inhibitors, bile acid sequestrants, nicotinic acid, and fibric acids. The "statin" group of drugs (HMG-CoA reductase inhibitors) predominantly block the production of LDLs and increase receptor activity that removes LDL. These lipid-lowering agents are especially useful as adjuncts to dietary management for patients with familial hypercholesterolemia. Atorvastatin (Lipitor) has been most successful in decreasing total cholesterol and LDL and has fewer side effects than the other drugs in this group (Table 23-6.)

Treatments

Intraaortic Balloon Pump. Patients experiencing MI with hemodynamic instability may benefit from placement of an intraaortic balloon pump (IABP). The IABP, inserted into the descending thoracic aorta, inflates during diastole, augmenting early diastolic pressure and coronary artery perfusion. The balloon deflates rapidly at the end of diastole, decreasing afterload, resulting in an increase in cardiac output. A more complete description of the IABP can be found in Chapter 24.

Percutaneous Coronary Interventions. More than half a million PCI procedures are performed each year in the United States.[1] These procedures can be performed in conjunction with diagnostic cardiac catheterization or as a separate procedure. The patient is sedated and a local anesthetic is injected at the femoral artery insertion site. The brachial or radial artery may also be used. A sheath is inserted into the artery, and a catheter is guided up the aorta, where radiopaque dye is injected directly into the coronary arteries. The coronary anatomy is viewed, and blockages can be identified under fluoroscopy. Adjunctive procedures such as cardiac electromechanical mapping[17] help to evaluate myocardial viability and determine the appropriateness of PCI vs. bypass surgery. The cardiologist determines the technical feasibility of various PCI procedures, including percutaneous transluminal coronary angioplasty (PTCA), stenting, atherectomy, and laser angioplasty. PTCA is used alone in less than 30% of cases; coronary stenting is used in more than 70% of cases.[16]

Percutaneous Transluminal Coronary Angioplasty. With balloon angioplasty a guide wire is first inserted across and beyond the lesion. A catheter with a cylindric balloon is then

TABLE 23-6 Drugs Used to Lower Blood Lipids

Drug Class	Lipid/Lipoprotein Effects	Side Effects
HMG CoA reductase inhibitors: Atorvastatin, cerivastatin, fluvastatin, lovastatin, pravastatin, simvastatin	↓ LDL 18%-55% ↑ HDL 5%-15% ↓ TG 7%-30%	Myopathy Increased liver enzymes
Bile acid sequestrants: Cholestyramine, colesevelam, colestipol	↓ LDL 15%-30% ↑ HDL 3%-5% TG: no change or ↑	Bloating Constipation Decreased absorption of other drugs
Nicotinic acid: Immediate release, extended release, sustained release	↓ LDL 5%-25% ↑ HDL 15%-35% ↓ TG 20%-50%	Flushing Hyperglycemia Hyperuricemia Upper GI distress Hepatotoxicity
Fibric acids: Clofibrate, fenofibrate, gemfibrozil	↓ LDL 5%-20% (may increase if high TG) ↑ HDL 10%-20% ↓ TG 20%-50%	Dyspepsia Gallstones Myopathy

From US Department of Health and Human Services: *National Cholesterol Education Program: Third Report of the Expert Panel on Detection, Evaluation, and Treatment of High Blood Cholesterol in Adults (Adult Treatment Panel III)*, NIH Pub No 01-3305, 2001, U.S. Department of Health and Human Services, Public Health Service, National Institutes of Health, National Heart, Lung, and Blood Institute.[20]

advanced over the guidewire, and the balloon is positioned centrally in the blockage. The balloon, filled with radiopaque dye and saline, is inflated at pressures great enough to reconfigure the blockage. This reconfiguration includes both controlled dissection (splitting) of the intima and to a lesser extent vessel dilation (Figure 23-11). The controlled dissection creates a wider passage for the arterial blood flow. At times, the dissection may create enough turbulence to stimulate clot formation or actually interfere with blood flow by obstructing the coronary lumen. In these situations, GP IIb/IIIa receptor inhibitors and/or additional interventional measures (such as intracoronary stenting) may be necessary.

The major limitation of PTCA is the strong chance of lesion recurrence or restenosis, usually within 6 months. Restenosis occurs in response to the controlled injury caused by balloon inflation. In approximately 30% of procedures, the arterial wall continues to heal with smooth muscle proliferation into the arterial lumen. Although this is not the same lipid accumulation that caused the original blockage, it nevertheless compromises myocardial blood flow and results in myocardial ischemia. Research continues to explore ways to prevent restenosis, including current trials with tranilast, a medication believed to decrease inflammation and hyperplasia.

PTCA can be used in most situations, including small distal branches of the coronary arteries, multiple lesions in one or more grafts, and long lesions. Primary angioplasty is now considered to be a first-line treatment for AMI when appropriate facilities and personnel are readily available.[9] The decision to use PTCA occurs after physician-patient consultation regarding coronary anatomy, symptoms, coexisting disease states, surgical risks associated with coronary artery bypass graft surgery, and the patient's feelings regarding open heart surgery. Care of the patient undergoing PCI is summarized in the accompanying Guidelines for Safe Practice box.

Stents. Placement of intracoronary stents helps to maintain the patency of the treated coronary arteries and decrease the incidence of restenosis (see Figure 23-11). Stents may be either balloon-expandable, requiring a balloon to deploy the stent, or self-expanding. The stent remains in the coronary artery as a scaffold and endothelializes over a period of 3 weeks, gradually decreasing the risk of thrombus formation on the foreign material. The incidence of stent thrombosis is also decreased with the administration of aspirin and loading doses of platelet ADP-receptor inhibitor therapy before the procedure; aggressive heparinization during the procedure; the use of intravenous GP IIb/IIIa receptor blockers during and postprocedure; and the administration of oral platelet ADP-receptor inhibitor therapy for 30 days after the procedure.

Despite aggressive preventive measures, the potential for restenosis still exists after stent placement. Brachytherapy, the localized delivery of ionized radiation to reduce intimal hyperplasia, is the most promising therapy available for treating restenosis at this time.[16] After repeat PCI, radioactive seeds are delivered by catheter to the restenotic area and left to "dwell"

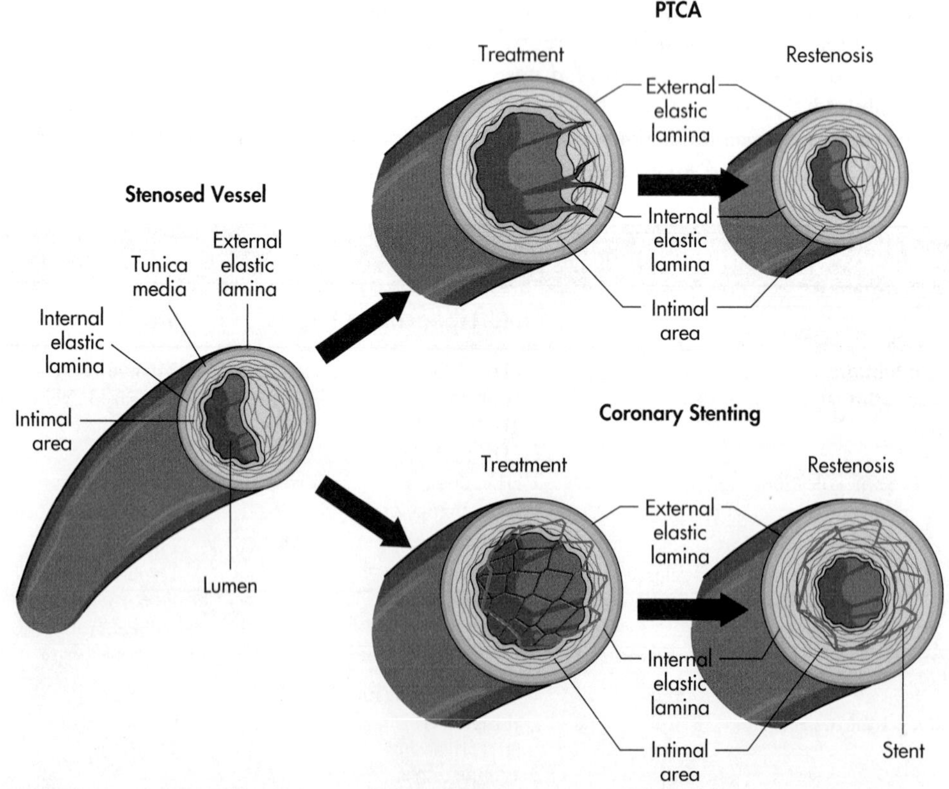

Figure 23-11 Possible mechanisms of restenosis after PTCA and coronary stenting. Left figure illustrates atherosclerosis. Upper figure illustrates PTCA to the left and restenosis following PTCA on right. Bottom figure illustrates coronary stenting to the left and restenosis of stent to the right.

for 20 to 25 minutes. Complications include late thrombosis from delayed endothelialization, perforation, and a "candy-wrapper" effect of ineffective vessel treatment at the ends of the restenotic area. Antiplatelet therapy is continued into the future. Long-term effects are still not known, but could include a small risk of radiation-induced malignancy or cardiomyopathy.

Other PCIs. Less commonly used PCI procedures include directional coronary atherectomy (DCA), laser therapy, transluminal extraction catheters, and rotablators. These procedures are especially beneficial for specific types of lesions. For example, rotablators are useful in the treatment of calcified lesions in the coronary arteries. These devices pulverize lesions, creating microemboli of insignificant size.

The patient undergoing interventional procedures requires close monitoring for complications such as vessel occlusion, bleeding and hematoma formation at the arterial access site, thromboembolism, pseudoaneurysms, and contrast dye reactions. A Clinical Pathway for PCI is presented on pp. 662 to 665. The pathway addresses both monitoring and nursing care during the preprocedure and postprocedure phases. Nurse researchers have positively impacted care for the patient undergoing PCI through research on standards of care and managing patient discomfort (see Research and Evidence-Based Practice boxes).

Enhanced External Counterpulsation. Enhanced external counterpulsation is a noninvasive computerized method of altering blood flow to improve coronary circulation. Three pairs of inflatable cuffs are secured around the patient's calves, lower thighs, and upper thighs. The computer interprets the ECG and initiates inflation of the cuffs sequentially during diastole,

Text continued on p. 666.

Guidelines for Safe Practice

The Patient Undergoing Percutaneous Coronary Intervention

GENERAL CONCEPTS TO REINFORCE

- Indication for the procedure
- Review of rationale for percutaneous coronary intervention (PCI) versus other interventions
- PCI is not a surgical intervention: no incisions, no general anesthesia
- Risk factors associated with procedure, including <1% chance of emergency surgery in noncomplicated PCIs

PREPROCEDURE PREPARATION

- Tests performed before procedure: laboratory work, electrocardiogram (ECG)
- Anxiolytics for anxiety
- Intravenous access started to give medications/fluids; if radial access, use contralateral arm
- NPO after midnight, except medications, clear liquid breakfast if late procedure
- If groin access, groin will be shaved and scrubbed
- Pedal pulses marked (femoral access)/Allen's test documented as normal/abnormal (radial access)
- Cardiac monitor placed

INTRAPROCEDURE EXPECTATIONS

- Catheter laboratory environment–cool, sterilely draped, staff with masks and gowns, camera close to body
- Anxiolytics for anxiety
- Cardiac monitor at all times
- Local anesthetic to access site; arm support if radial access
- Back or arm discomfort might occur from positioning–notify staff
- Chest pain or anginal equivalent may occur with intervention
- Fluoroscopy used to visualize all interventions
- Need to cough to clear dye and deep breathe to provide a better picture of anatomy
- Duration of procedure varies from 30 minutes to 2 hours

POSTPROCEDURE EXPECTATIONS

Access Site

- Groin: need to keep affected leg still until 4 hours after sheath removed; clear dressing over access site; while femoral sheath is in, head of bed (HOB) should be less than 30 degrees; flexible sheaths allow HOB up to 60 degrees; after sheath is removed, HOB needs to be flat with patient on bed rest for 4 additional hours; Vital signs and neurovascular assessments every 15 minutes ×4, every 30 minutes ×2, then every hour until stable.
- Radial: sheath removed immediately and dressing applied; may receive medication to decrease arterial spasm for sheath removal; wristband applied to obtain hemostasis and armboard positioned to minimize mobility. Vital signs and neurovascular assessments every 15 minutes while wristband on. Wristband removed after 1 to 2 hours and pressure dressing applied (×24 hours). Immobilize wrist for 2 to 4 hours after wristband removed. Keep arm at heart level ×24 hours. Can walk after sheath removal with care taken to evaluate for effects of sedation and fluid shifts before ambulation.
- Back pain (most often occurs with femoral approach); may logroll with assistance; back rubs, pain medication available
- ECG: routine ECG after procedure
- Notify staff if feels warm or wet at access site; any pain: anginal, back, leg; inability to void with abdominal fullness
- NPO until sheath pulled; fluids encouraged, unless contraindicated, to flush dye from system

DISCHARGE EXPECTATIONS

All teaching relevant to angina or myocardial infarction patient (see Nursing Management) plus the following:

Femoral site: groin restrictions–no heavy lifting, no tub baths for 2 days

Radial site: for 2 days–no driving, avoid wrist movement, do not lift >1 pound; for 5 days avoid strenuous arm movement; no tub baths for 3 days.

PCI not a cure–should carry nitroglycerin and use as instructed in coronary artery disease teaching

Restenosis can occur per no fault of patient; restenosis represents ineffective, inefficient healing at PCI site; most likely time of occurrence is within 6 months; need to contact cardiologist or primary care provider for symptoms similar to those experienced during PCI

Aspirin must be taken daily; if stent, clopidogrel also taken bid for 30 days

clinical pathway *Left Cardiac Cath/PTCI*

	WORK UP PHASE ⟶		PROCEDURE PHASE	RECOVERY PHASE ⟶		
DATE:	**PRE-PROCEDURE (CATH CLINIC/UPON ADMIT)**	**IMMEDIATELY PREPROCEDURE**	**INTRA-PROCEDURE**	**POST PROCEDURE SHEATH IN**	**POST PROCEDURE SHEATH OUT**	**DAY OF DISCHARGE**
Assessment	Adult Screening Tool • Emotional/spiritual Needs • Financial Needs • Nutritional Needs • Discharge Needs • Cardiac Rehab Height/Weight Bilateral BP History/Physical or Cath/PTCI Work Up Advanced Directives Addressed Cath films reviewed if applic.	Clinical Data Flow Sheet/Critical Care Systems Assessment Cath Lab Receiving Assessment Cardiac Monitoring	Cath Lab Procedure Assessment Cardiac Monitoring/O2 sats	F/U Consultations as indicated Post Procedure Assessment–pain control ◆❤ Cardiac Monitoring	Post Procedure Assessment–pain control DC Cardiac monitoring 6 hrs post sheath removal for short stay PTCI (◆❤) Orthostatic BP and HR prior to ambulation	CDFS/CCSA–Discharge Criteria met D/C Cardiac Monitoring
Tests	ECG w in 30 days CBC/plt. w in 30 days Basic Chem Panel w in 30 days PT/PTT per guidelines		(◆❤) ACT after heparin bolus to maintain level >300-350 seconds (◆❤) 2 B/3A pts. ACT to adjust to maintain level >200 seconds Lipid profile 1 (for pt w unknown lipid status or not on lipid-lowering therapy) (◆❤) ACT at end of the procedure	(◆❤) EKG and prn pain Consider CK for prolonged pain Hep PTT q 6 hr as ord. (◆❤) Consider Basic Chem Panel and CBC w plts. in am (◆❤) 2 B/3A pts: CBC w plts. 2 hrs after bolus and in the am	ACT as ordered may pull sheath when </= 180 seconds	Review all labs as ord.
Activity	As tolerated	As tolerated	Bed rest	Bed rest with affected limb straight, may roll w assist, no chin to chest/, may raise HOB </= 30 degrees	Bed rest with affected limb straight 4 hrs after sheath removal, may roll w assist, no chin to chest then OOB at completion of bedrest 2B/3A pts. ortho check 4 hrs after sheath removal w bed to chair and BRP only, may fully ambulate 2 hrs after drip is d/c'd	Up as tolerated with restriction for 2 days post procedure (refer to activity restriction form)

Medications/ Treatments	Continue all meds except: • Hold oral anticoagulant 48-72 hours prior to procedure	ASA 325 mg prior to the procedure as indicated (CP, known CAD) as ord. Hold all oral hypoglycemic on the day of procedure as ord.	Prep and drape Sheath placement Sedative as ordered Pain meds (Morphine, Fentanyl) as ordered	Resume scheduled meds as ord. Pain meds as ordered	Resume scheduled meds as ord. Pain meds as ordered	Continue scheduled meds as ord. D/C pain meds
	For Contrast Allergy: Prednisone 60 mg po p.m. before the procedure	Hold Regular insulin the am of the procedure as ord.	IV Anticoagulation as ord.	IV/sub q/po Anticoagulation as ord.	IV/sub q/po Anticoagulation as ord.	D/C IV/sub q Anticoagulation as ord.
	Clopidogrel 300 mg po as ordered (loading dose for elective PTCI's w stent)	Give $^{1}/_{2}$ dose of long acting insulin the am of the procedure as ord.	NTG as ord.–SI, IC, IV	NTG as ordered	NTG as ord.	D/C
		For pts at high risk for contrast induced renal insufficiency–(diabetics, creat. >1.5) follow renal protection protocol	Verify contrast type per policy/guidelines Beta-Blockers IV as ord. Arterial line flush as ord./dressing to site	Clopidogrel 300 mg (loading dose) as ord. Arterial Line flush/dressing to site	DC arterial line and remove dressing at completion of bedrest	Band-Aid to puncture site
		Increase IV rate to 150 cc's an hr once pt. arrives in the Cardiac Cath Lab receiving For Contrast Allergy: Prednisone 60 mg po/Benadryl 50 mg po am of the procedure on call Pre Med on call as ord: Vallum 5-10mg po Hold am dose of Enoxaparin as ord.	2B/3A as indicated	2B/3A as ordered Pre Med for sheath removal: • Lidocaine 2% 10 cc's for groin infiltration • MS 2-4 mg and Atropine 0.5 mg prn as ord.	2B/3A as ordered	D/C
		Insert saline lock and/or Start 1000 cc's 0.9 NS to KVO IV on call	NS IV	Maintain IV fluids	Maintain IV fluids or saline lock	D/C
Nutrition	Clear liquids after 00:01 until 0600 Encourage po fluids the night before the Cath/PTCI	Clear liquids until 0600 then NPO except for meds	NPO	For early sheath removal NPO (may have ice chips) then advance to Heart Healthy If Sheath overnight, NPO (may have ice chips) after midnight then advance to Heart Healthy	Heart Healthy–encourage po fluids	Heart Healthy

Courtesy University of Virginia Health System, Charlottesville, Va.
❤ PTCA/DCA
◆ Stent

Continued

clinical pathway *Left Cardiac Cath/PTCI—cont'd*

	WORK UP PHASE →		PROCEDURE PHASE	RECOVERY PHASE →		
DATE:	**PRE-PROCEDURE (CATH CLINIC/UPON ADMIT)**	**IMMEDIATELY PREPROCEDURE**	**INTRA-PROCEDURE**	**POST PROCEDURE SHEATH IN**	**POST PROCEDURE SHEATH OUT**	**DAY OF DISCHARGE**
Discharge Planning/ Instruction	Identify discharge needs by adult screening tool–initiate appropriate support service Designate person to drive pt. home after procedure Identify referring MD Preprocedure teaching using Cath/PTCI educational folder • Procedural booklet • Patient/family pathway • Discharge instructions • Offer procedural video • Answer any questions • Tell family where to wait during the procedure Informed consent for procedure and/Research protocols signed and witnessed Screen for Jehovah Witness	Identify discharge needs by adult screening tool–initiate appropriate support service Communicate any reason for delay to the lab Verify location of family Verify home transportation for short stay pts.	Orient to lab • Instruct pt. to communicate needs/ questions to CCL personnel • Instruct regarding deep breathing, cough on command and need for arms in overhead position prn Update family on decision to perform PTCI MD to MD/NP/family communication of preliminary results CCL RN to unit RN report	Identify discharge needs by adult screening tool–initiate appropriate support service Designate person to drive pt. home Reinforce immediate post cath/PTCI groin protection and activity progression Reinforce all teaching using Cath/PTCI Ed. package	Identify discharge needs by adult screening tool–initiate appropriate support service Designate person to drive pt. home Reinforce immediate post cath/PTCI groin protection and activity progression Reinforce all teaching using Cath/PTCI Ed. package	Verify phone number and approximate time for f/u phone call by high risk criteria MIS med instructions given ◆ Stent card given/Pictures if applicable ◆ Medic Alert Application given Follow-up physician identified MD Discharge summary to referring MD (◆❤) Reinforce signs and symptoms of Restenosis Pts with dx. of CAD: • Goals for lifestyle modifications, lipid control, BP control, BS control • Review interventions for chest pain using NTG and when to call 911 Ensure pt/family have Cath/PTCI educational folder for reference after discharge.

Outcomes	Recognizes and verbalizes any fears Describes briefly and is able to follow pre procedure care Understands purpose for the procedure Identify and treat for potential complications (ex. Coagulopathy)	Denies anxiety level that might interfere with ability to follow plan of care.	Hemodynamic/ Neurological Stability Pain/Anxiety Control Skin Integrity Intact Transfer to CCU/AC/23 Hr. unit	Hemodynamic/ Neurological Stability Pain/Anxiety Control Skin Integrity Intact	Hemodynamic/ Neurological Stability Pain/Anxiety Control Skin Integrity Intact Ability to progress activity w comfort Have no significant BP and HR change first time out of bed	Meets discharge criteria: 1. Vital signs, LOC, distal pulses and urinary output at baseline 2. No evidence of unresolved complications: • Allergic reaction • Bleeding or complete loss of circulation in cannulated extremity • No new bruit • Unrelieved chest discomfort • Unexplained abdominal pain • Free of s/s of infection at cannulation site • Free of s/s of UTI • No expanding pulsatile mass, pseudoaneurysm or hematoma • No significant BP and pulse change first time out of bed • Resolution of transient rhythm changes

Research

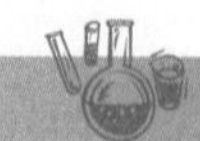

Reference: Botti M, Williamson B, Steen K: Coronary angiography observations: evidence-based or ritualistic practice? *Heart Lung* 30(2):138, 2001.

Nurse researchers at three university hospitals randomized 1075 patients undergoing coronary angiography into two groups; one group received pressure-bandaging (n = 519) after the procedure, and one group did not (n = 556). The pressure bandage consisted of 8 gauze squares wadded and placed over the femoral site and held firmly in place with a 2-m, elasticized, nonadhesive bandage, applied in a figure 8 around the leg, across the lower abdomen, and lower back. All patients received manual compression for 10 minutes to achieve hemostasis. Both groups were monitored at 30-minute intervals for 4 hours. Patients remained in bed for these 4 hours with the bed elevated at 30 degrees.

Fifty-five patients (5.1%) experienced femoral bleeding, defined as any incident of bleeding requiring manual compression: 6.7% (n = 37) without pressure dressing, 3.5% (n = 18) with pressure dressing. There was no statistical difference among demographics, risk factors, or catheter-insertion technique between the group that bled and the nonbleeding group.

There was a significant difference between the bandage and no-bandage group in the time that elapsed to bleeding occurrence. For all patients who bled, bleeding occurred at a median of 2.02 hours: 1.32 hours for the no-bandage group; 4.75 hours in the bandaged group. Within the no-bandage group 46% of patient bleeds occurred within 1 hour postprocedure, 24% occurring during the transfer from stretcher to bed. For those who were bandaged, 16.6% of bleeds occurred within 1 hour after angiogram, without reference to the number that occurred at transfer. Patient observations were recorded on average 23.7 minutes before the bleeding incident. In 59% of cases, bleeding was detected by the nurse; in 41% of cases, by the patient. Implications from this study include the timing of postprocedure observations to patient care practices (use of pressure bandages), the importance of patient education, and the minimization of patient transfers postprocedure.

thereby increasing coronary perfusion pressure and venous return. The cuffs rapidly deflate during systole, decreasing afterload. Patients undergo 1- to 2-hour treatments for 35 sessions. The patient wears seamless "tights" to protect the legs from abrasion. The procedure is believed to stimulate angiogenesis over time and improve angina. It is generally used for individuals who are not candidates for traditional PCI or surgery, or for patients who have not had success with traditional therapy.

Transmyocardial Laser Revascularization. Transmyocardial laser revascularization uses laser energy to create channels through the left ventricular free wall into ischemic myocardium. The procedure is used to treat refractory angina and is believed to increase blood flow to the myocardium through the channels and stimulate angiogenesis to increase the collateral blood flow.[12] It can be performed percutaneously, similar to other PCIs, or surgically, through a median sternotomy or left thoracotomy approach. Depending on the type of laser used, myocardial channels are created from thermal ablation or by breaking molecular bands within the myocardial cells. Complications may include cardiac tamponade and heart failure.

Evidence-Based Practice

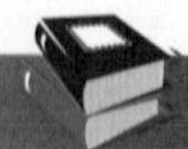

Reference: Fulton TR et al: Effects of 3 analgesic regimens on the perception of pain after removal of femoral artery sheaths, *Am J Crit Care* 9(2):125, 2000.

Nurse researchers compared the effects of three treatment regimens on patients' pain perceptions after removal of a femoral artery sheath. A total of 130 patients undergoing a percutaneous coronary intervention (PCI) procedure were randomized to one of four groups: control (intravenous 0.9% sodium chloride), intravenous morphine 0.05 mg/kg; subcutaneous lidocaine (2% without epinephrine) 5 ml, and intravenous fentanyl 0.5 μg/kg. IV medications were diluted and premixed by the pharmacy, creating double blind conditions. For breakthrough pain, nurses administered open-label intravenous fentanyl. Study medications were administered as a bolus 10 minutes before sheath removal. The cardiac fellow administered subcutaneous lidocaine to that treatment group within 10 minutes of sheath removal. Pain assessments were made at three points: at the time of medication administration, 1 minute after sheath removal and 20 minutes after sheath removal. Patients rated their pain using a 100-mm visual analog scale. The mean pain rating for combined groups was 23.5 mm, with the greatest pain occurring immediately after sheath removal. There were no significant differences between the four groups in pain perception and frequency of side effects. Only 12 requests for breakthrough pain management occurred. The researchers conclude that analgesics should be administered to PCI patients for pain on an as-needed basis.

Surgical Management

Coronary artery bypass graft (CABG) surgery bypasses the obstruction in a coronary artery by grafting an artery or vein to the coronary artery beyond the blockage, reestablishing blood flow (Figure 23-12). The decision to operate considers the location of the coronary lesion and the surgical risks and benefits. CABG is indicated for patients with significant left main CAD; for patients with three-vessel disease and a left ventricular ejection fraction (LVEF) <0.50; and for patients with two-vessel disease with significant proximal left anterior descending CAD and either an LVEF <0.50, or evidence of significant ischemia with stress testing. Although CABG surgery is not curative because the grafts can and do occlude, it improves the quality of life for many patients. Chapter 24 presents information related to CABO surgery in detail.

Diet

The patient being evaluated for acute chest pain is given nothing by mouth (NPO) until the diagnosis of MI is ruled out. Keeping the patient NPO prevents blood from being redirected to the gastrointestinal system at a time when the heart is ischemic and demanding an increased blood flow. Keeping the patient NPO also prevents vomiting, which commonly accompanies chest pain from vagal effects. Patients may also be NPO before cardiac procedures. When not NPO, the diet recommended for patients with cardiac disease is low fat and low cholesterol.

Because of the role of cholesterol and lipids in plaque formation, most patients with a diagnosis of CAD will be offered diet counseling. Counseling begins with careful assessment of the patient's usual daily diet and knowledge of the relation-

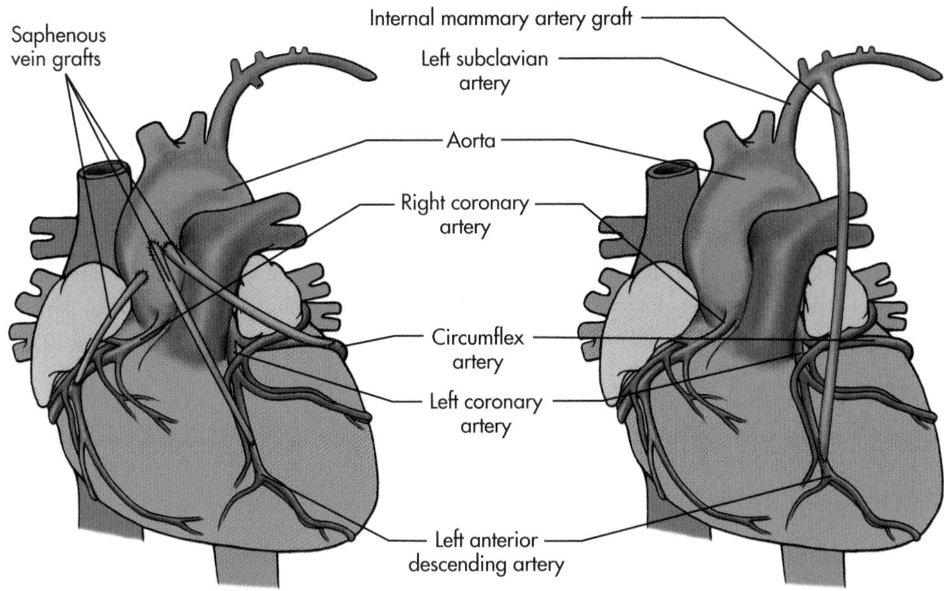

Figure 23-12 Coronary artery bypass surgery. Common grafts: saphenous vein and internal mammary artery.

TABLE 23-7 2001 Adult Treatment Panel Target Lipoprotein Values and Management Guidelines for Patients with CAD

Lipoprotein	ATP Classification	Treatment
LDL	100-129: Near optimal/above optimal 130-159: Borderline high 160-189: High ≥190: Very high	Diet: saturated fat <7% of calories: cholesterol <200 mg/day, soluble fiber 10-25 g/day, plant stanols/sterols 2 g/day Weight management Increased physical activity
Total cholesterol	<200: Desirable 200-239: Borderline high ≥240: High	Reach LDL goal
HDL Cholesterol	<40: Low ≥60: High	First reach LDL goal, then: intensify weight management and increase physical activity, If TG <200 mg/dl, consider nicotinic acid or fibrate
Triglycerides	<150: Normal 150-199: Borderline high 200-499: High ≥500: Very high	Primary aim is to reach LDL goal Intensify weight management Increase physical activity If TG 200-499 after LDL goal is reached: intensify LDL drug therapy or add nicotinic acid or fibrate If TG ≥500, initiate ≤15% calories from fat, fibrate or nicotinic acid; when TG <500, return to LDL therapy

From US Department of Health and Human Services: *National Cholesterol Education Program: Third Report of the Expert Panel on Detection, Evaluation, and Treatment of High Blood Cholesterol in Adults (Adult Treatment Panel III),* NIH Pub No 01-3305, 2001, US Department of Health and Human Services, Public Health Service, National Institutes of Health, National Heart, Lung, and Blood Institute.[26]
HDL, High-density lipoprotein; *LDL,* low-density lipoprotein; *TG,* triglyceride.

ship between diet and CAD. Diet teaching usually includes reducing the fat content of the diet, substituting polyunsaturated fat for saturated fat, and maintaining body weight at normal levels. When the LDL is elevated in the patient with CAD, dietary changes are initiated (Table 23-7). These include saturated fat <7% of calories, cholesterol <200 mg/day, soluble fiber 10 to 25 g/day, and plant stanols/sterols 2 g/day (soybean oil, tall oil, rapeseed oil).[20]

Studies indicate that dietary intake of large amounts of saturated fat raises the serum cholesterol level. When polyunsaturated fats replace saturated fats the blood cholesterol level tends to fall. Sources of polyunsaturated fats include corn, cottonseed, soy, and safflower oils; and margarines incorporating these oils in liquid form. Hydrogenated oils contain more saturated fat, as do tropical oils, butterfat, and animal fats. Transfatty acids are created when oil is hydrogenated, a process that makes an oil more solid at room temperature, extending the shelf life of the product. When an unsaturated fat converts to a transfatty acid, it then acts in the body in much the same way as a saturated fat. Transfatty acids increase LDLs and total cholesterol and may even decrease high-density lipoproteins (HDLs). Patients should avoid transfatty acid products such as stick margarines, shortenings, and foods prepared with these products. Fatty acids from fish oil decrease triglyceride levels and decrease platelet aggregation and blood pressure. The nurse and dietitian work collaboratively with the patient and family to plan realistic changes in the diet.

Activity

Initially the patient experiencing angina is restricted to bed rest. This activity restriction decreases myocardial oxygen demand until biomarkers peak and a definitive diagnosis of MI can be made. After the patient is hemodynamically stable and free of chest pain, activity can be increased gradually (see Guidelines for Safe Practice box). Assessment for activity tolerance includes monitoring for orthostatic changes in the blood pressure, dysrhythmias, appropriate changes in blood pressure and heart rate, and the presence of symptoms such as dyspnea or chest pain. The presence of symptoms or hemodynamic changes necessitates cessation of activity until the patient stabilizes and the potential for cardiac ischemia decreases.

Before discharge or soon thereafter, most postinfarction patients undergo stress testing to determine a safe individual exercise level. Patients ideally enroll in outpatient cardiac rehabilitation programs. These programs supervise the progression of activity and offer variety in modes of exercise (bicycle, steps, weights). Unfortunately, not all insurance companies recognize the benefit of structured rehabilitation programs, and financial constraints may prevent enrollment. In these situations standardized home exercise programs are recommended (see Patient Teaching box). Activity prescriptions consider the location and extent of myocardial damage, results of stress testing when available, and specific patient needs.

The importance of exercise in preventing disease progression is significant and cannot be overstated. A regular exercise regimen can decrease LDLs, increase collateral circulation, decrease resting heart rate, and decrease blood pressure. Despite these benefits, patients with known cardiac disease must take precautions to prevent overtaxing the already compromised balance of myocardial oxygen supply and demand. Activity guidelines promote conditioning and simultaneously prevent overexertion that could further increase myocardial oxygen demand.

Referrals

Managing the care of the patient with CAD requires collaboration among members of the cardiac health care team. For the patient newly diagnosed with stable angina, referrals

Guidelines for Safe Practice

Advancing Activity Levels

ACTIVITY PROGRESSION—ADMISSION

- 0 to 12 hours: bed rest with bedside commode
- 12 to 24 hours: orthostatic check; out of bed to chair with meals, ad lib in room

ACTIVITY PROGRESSION—DAY 2 TO DISCHARGE

- Duration: first session, ambulate 1 to 2 minutes; increase duration 1 to 2 minutes per session if patient tolerates (see Criteria)
- Frequency: initially 1 to 4 times per day, duration less than 10 minutes
- Intensity: maintain heart rate no greater than 20 beats/min over baseline; patient should be able to converse on ambulation without shortness of breath

CRITERIA FOR PROGRESSING ACTIVITY

- Heart rate* within 20 beats/min of standing baseline heart rate
- Systolic blood pressure* within 20 mm Hg of standing baseline blood pressure
- Absence of chest pain, pressure, or anginal equivalent; shortness of breath; dysrhythmia; fatigue; light-headedness; diaphoresis

*Blood pressures and heart rate checks are taken in a standing position preambulation and immediately postambulation. Postambulation heart rate should be measured by taking pulse for 10 seconds and multiplying by 6.

Patient Teaching

Home Walking Program

COUNT PULSE

- Take your pulse before, during, and immediately after your walk. Stop and rest if your heart rate is higher than 20 beats over resting heart rate, and then continue at a slower pace.

SAFETY

Carry your nitroglycerin with you and use as directed if symptoms occur.

WARM-UP

- Start with 1 minute of arm/chest exercises followed by 4 or 5 minutes of stationary walking. Purpose: to gradually increase blood flow to the muscles, preventing injury

WALK

- Walk at moderate intensity for 5 to 10 minutes. Increase your time by 1 to 2 minutes each time you walk with a goal of a 30- to 45-minute walk. Intensity: stay within a heart rate not higher than 20 beats above your resting heart rate and less than 120 beats/min initially. If you are taking beta-blockers, you must stay within 20 beats of your baseline.

COOL DOWN

- Cool down with 5 to 10 minutes of low-intensity walking followed by stretching. Purpose: to gradually decrease effort and prevent a drop in blood pressure causing dizziness.

GENERAL GUIDELINES

- Preferably walk on a level surface. If you must walk uphill, go more slowly.
- Walk at least three times per week.
- In the summer do not walk if the temperature is higher than 85° F or if the humidity is higher than 75%.
- Wear loose clothing. Drink plenty of water to prevent dehydration.
- In the winter do not walk outside if the temperature is lower than 40° F. Wear a hat and a face scarf.
- Avoid exercise for 1 to 2 hours after eating. Patients with diabetes should have a light snack before walking.
- Do not use tobacco for 1 hour before exercise.

may be made to cardiologists, nutritionists, stress management therapists, and exercise physiologists. For the patient admitted with an MI, referrals most often include members of inpatient and outpatient cardiac rehabilitation staffs: RNs, exercise physiologists, nutritionists, and social workers. Other professionals who may be consulted include vocational rehabilitation workers, chaplains, marriage counselors or sex therapists, and stress reduction therapists. Given the decreased length of hospital stay for patients with MI, much of the care provided occurs after discharge from the hospital.

NURSING MANAGEMENT

ASSESSMENT

Health History

Assessment data to be collected as part of the health history of a patient with CAD includes:

Chest pain: location, severity, intensity, quality, duration, time of onset; patient may be asymptomatic; classic pattern is retrosternal pain that may radiate down the left arm or both arms, upward to neck or jaw, or backward to scapular region; may be described as crushing, or worst pain ever experienced

Precipitating factors (e.g., exercise, stress, smoking)

Measures attempted to control pain (e.g., nitroglycerin, lying down, eating or drinking, using antacids); effectiveness

Other symptoms (e.g., indigestion, heartburn, nausea, abdominal pain, malaise, dizziness, dyspnea, anxiety and/or feeling of doom)

Risk factors for CAD (e.g., positive family history, lipid profile, tobacco use, history, stress levels, exercise pattern)

Other illnesses (e.g., diabetes, hypertension, bleeding disorders, recent trauma or surgery); current management regimens and allergies

Medications in use—prescription, over the counter, herbal products, nutritional supplements

Support systems, insurance coverage, financial resources for rehabilitation

Current employment, activity level

Physical Examination

Important aspects of the physical examination of a patient with CAD include:

Posture indicating presence of chest pain (e.g., clutching or rubbing chest, leaning forward)

Changes in vital signs: tachycardia or bradycardia, hypertension or hypotension

Dyspnea or shortness of breath, rales (crackles)

Presence of S_3 or S_4

Dysrhythmias

Altered level of consciousness, syncope

Vomiting

Declining urine output

Pale, cool, diaphoretic skin

NURSING DIAGNOSES

Nursing diagnoses are determined from the analysis of patient data. Nursing diagnoses for the patient with CAD may include but are not limited to:

Diagnostic Title	Possible Etiologic Factors
1. Acute pain (chest)	Myocardial ischemia, imbalance between myocardial oxygen supply and demand
2. Risk for ineffective tissue perfusion	Decrease in cardiac output, hypoxemia
3. Risk for injury (bleeding)	Altered clotting factors, use of fibrinolytics—decrease in platelet adhesiveness
4. Anxiety	Threat of death; threat to or change in health status, socioeconomic status, role functioning, interaction patterns; lack of information about cardiac procedures; general uncertainty
5. Activity intolerance	Deconditioning associated with bed rest, imbalance of myocardial oxygen supply and demand
6. Ineffective sexuality patterns	Illness, medical treatment, lack of information about safe guidelines for sexual activity, medication side effects, altered relationship with significant other

Additional diagnostic categories that may be applicable to specific patients with CAD include impaired adjustment, disturbed body image, ineffective coping, ineffective denial, ineffective role performance, ineffective therapeutic regimen management, and caregiver role strain.

EXPECTED PATIENT OUTCOMES

Expected patient outcomes for the patient with CAD may include but are not limited to:

1. Will be free of chest pain or pain will be reduced or controlled effectively by medication
2. Will have perfusion to all organs restored to baseline and maintained
3. Will not experience bleeding or bleeding will be effectively controlled and treated if it occurs
4. Will experience only manageable levels of anxiety, permitting patient to seek and process information
5. Will tolerate gradually increasing levels of activity
6. Will verbalize the guidelines for resuming sexual activity, will discuss concerns with partner, or will seek counseling as needed

INTERVENTIONS

In managing the care of patients with CAD, the nurse has numerous opportunities to collaborate with other health care professionals in determining appropriate interventions. Some interventions depend on physician's orders, such as the administration of oxygen, fibrinolytics, opioids, and intravenous fluids. The nurse may initiate others, such as the provision of psychologic support and specific information. Interventions should always address the patient's specific needs.

1. Controlling Chest Pain

Because ischemic cardiac pain results from an imbalance between myocardial oxygen supply and demand, treatment of pain attempts to increase myocardial oxygen supply while reducing myocardial oxygen demand (see Guidelines for Safe Practice box). Immediate interventions include the administration of oxygen, opioids, nitrates, and fibrinolytics. Before medication administration, the nurse validates the absence of allergies and bleeding risks and establishes baseline vital signs, level of consciousness, and orientation. The nurse observes the patient for deviations from baseline after the administration of nitrates, fibrinolytics, and opioids. It is helpful to have the patient rate the pain on a scale of 0 to 10, where 0 is no pain and 10 is the worst pain ever. The patient's pain ratings provide a baseline from which to evaluate the effectiveness of the immediate interventions of fibrinolytics, nitrates, and analgesics.

Sublingual Nitrates

Because of the vasodilatory effects of nitrates, the patient is instructed to lie down before administration. An ECG may also be obtained before the first dose of nitroglycerin. When the patient has documented CAD and the treatment strategy has already been determined, nitroglycerin administration can be initiated before a diagnostic ECG. This prevents additional delays in treatment. Because of the vasodilator effects of nitroglycerin on cerebral arteries, many patients receiving nitroglycerin complain of headache that may be severe enough to require analgesic administration. Detailed information about the safe and effective use of sublingual nitroglycerin is provided in the Patient Teaching box.

Topical Nitrates

Topical nitrates, supplied as ointments, creams, and pastes, may also be used. The nurse administering the medication must handle these preparations carefully and use clean gloves when applying the topical nitrate. The nurse places the topical nitrate on the chest or upper arm avoiding areas with excess hair. The site of application is rotated with each dose. Topical nitrates can be easily removed if untoward effects develop, and this advantage proves useful during dose adjustments in the early phases of treatment. Oral nitrates typically replace topical nitrates for long-term therapy. Nitrate tolerance develops with ongoing use and nurses should ensure nitrate-free intervals, usually at night, to minimize the development of nitrate tolerance.

Guidelines for Safe Practice

The Patient Experiencing Angina

- Stay with patient. Ask for assistance in obtaining needed equipment (e.g., 12-lead electrocardiogram [ECG] and oxygen setup).
- Assess the presence of chest pain (or anginal equivalent). Document baseline intensity.
- Obtain baseline vital signs. Continue to monitor vital signs every 5 minutes during interventions.
- Apply oxygen when available.
- Ensure intravenous access.
- Obtain an ECG as soon as possible. For diagnostic purposes an ECG should be performed before administration of nitroglycerin. If patient has known coronary artery disease, nitroglycerin may be administered before ECG. Set-up continuous ST-segment monitoring. Obtain serial ECGs as indicated.
- Ensure that patient has received aspirin.
- Administer nitroglycerin and morphine per orders until pain resolves. If pain is not responsive to sublingual nitroglycerin and morphine, anticipate additional interventions such as intravenous nitroglycerin.
- Treat alterations in vital signs with appropriate medications. If ECG indicates acute myocardial infarction, anticipate and prepare for fibrinolytic therapy or primary percutaneous coronary intervention.
- Obtain laboratory specimens as indicated. Specimens may include complete blood count, chemistry, coagulation studies, and cardiac biomarkers (troponin and CK-MB).
- Assess patient's level of anxiety and offer realistic reassurance. Explain all interventions. Approach patient and family in a calm, confident manner. Minimize environmental stimulation.

Patient Teaching

Use and Storage of Nitroglycerin

USE OF SUBLINGUAL NITROGLYCERIN

- Sit or lie down at onset of angina/chest pain.
- Place tablet under the tongue and allow tablet to dissolve; do not chew.
- If pain is not relieved within 5 minutes, take a second tablet. A third tablet can be used after an additional 5 minutes if pain persists. Continuing pain after 3 tablets and 15 minutes indicates a need to receive immediate medical evaluation.
- Tablet will cause a tingling sensation under the tongue.
- Rest for 15 to 20 minutes after taking nitroglycerin to avoid faintness.
- A tablet may, with the physician's permission, be taken 10 minutes before an activity known to trigger an anginal attack.
- Anticipate the occurrence of hypotension, tachycardia, and headache in response to the medication.
- Headache may persist for 15 to 20 minutes after administration.
- Keep a record of the number of anginal attacks experienced, the number of tablets needed to obtain pain relief, and the precipitating factors if known.
- NOTE: Sublingual spray is administered following the same guidelines as above.

STORAGE OF NITROGLYCERIN

- Carry tablets for immediate use if necessary. Do not pack in luggage when traveling.
- Keep tablets in tightly closed, original container. Tablets need to be protected from exposure to light and moisture.
- Tablets should be stored in a cool, dry place.
- Check expiration date on prescription. Tablets should be discarded after 6 months once the bottle has been opened. Plan for replacement of supply.

Intravenous Nitroglycerin

Intravenous nitroglycerin may be used to treat acute coronary syndrome. During the administration of intravenous nitroglycerin, the nurse frequently monitors the patient's blood pressure. Intravenous nitroglycerin is titrated to keep the patient pain free while maintaining a systolic blood pressure above 90 mm Hg.

Fibrinolytic Therapy

Fibrinolytics are used emergently to open the blocked coronary artery, increase the blood supply to the myocardium, and relieve pain. Before fibrinolytic administration, all members of the health care team participate in screening the patient for bleeding risks (see Guidelines for Safe Practice box). No question can be asked too often in this situation. Fibrinolytic therapy must be administered without delay, preferably within 4 to 6 hours of symptom onset, although benefits are still possible up to 12 hours. The nurse assisting in the administration of fibrinolytics must be knowledgeable of all current treatment protocols to minimize the preparation time. The nurse obtains baseline vital signs and completes a physical examination for signs and symptoms of overt or covert bleeding. During the administration of fibrinolytics, the nurse monitors the patient's pain status and assesses the ECG for resolution of ST segment elevation. Should increasing pain or further signs of myocardial injury develop, the nurse anticipates the possibility of emergency interventional cardiac procedures (PCI or bypass surgery) and helps mobilize the cardiac team.

Treatment efforts also address the need to decrease the patient's myocardial oxygen demand. The nurse modifies the environment to decrease myocardial oxygen demand. Examples include restricting visitors who increase the patient's anxiety or prevent the patient from getting adequate rest, and adjusting the room temperature. In addition, the nurse attempts to decrease the patient's anxiety level. The patient is approached in a calm and quiet manner (often quite the opposite occurs in the hectic setting of the emergency department or coronary care unit), and explanations are offered about care and procedures that affect the patient. MI patients may also be started on intravenous beta-blockers in the emergency room to decrease myocardial oxygen demand and the incidence of mortality.

2. Monitoring Tissue Perfusion

Patients with acute MI may experience alterations in tissue perfusion to the skin, brain, kidneys, and other organs in addition to alterations in myocardial perfusion. These alterations occur from a decrease in cardiac output that results from impaired myocardial contractility. Monitoring for altered perfusion is a critical nursing intervention for patients with MI. Frequent measurement of vital signs is essential. The nurse performs head-to-toe assessments that include level of consciousness and orientation, breath sounds, heart sounds, dysrhythmias, pulse amplitude, bowel sounds, urine output, and skin turgor and hydration. Abnormal findings require nurse-physician collaboration to prevent further complications.

3. Preventing/Monitoring for Bleeding

The patient who receives fibrinolytic therapy has an increased risk of bleeding, and the nurse frequently assesses the patient for any indications of bleeding. Relevant findings include the onset of unexplained hypotension or tachycardia, the presence of a rigid abdomen, frank blood in the urine, and guaiac-positive stools. Subtle changes such as headache and visual disturbances may be indicative of cerebral hemorrhage and should be carefully monitored. The CBC and blood coagulation studies are performed at prescribed intervals and monitored for trends indicative of bleeding.

Guidelines for Safe Practice

The Patient Receiving Fibrinolytic Therapy

PATIENT ELIGIBILITY

- Within 6-12 hours of symptom onset
- Symptom duration of at least 30 minutes
- Electrocardiogram (ECG) pattern strongly suggestive of acute myocardial infarction (ST elevation and/or new left bundle-branch block)

PATIENT SCREENING

- Screen for bleeding risks: history of cerebral hemorrhage at any time, other stroke or cerebrovascular event within 1 year, intracranial neoplasm, active bleeding, suspected aortic dissection, severe hypertension, known bleeding disorders, current anticoagulation therapy, recent surgery or trauma (including cardiopulmonary resuscitation), arteriovenous malformation
- Establish baseline vital signs and physical examination for overt/covert bleeding, such as unexplained hypotension or tachycardia, rigid abdomen, subtle neurologic changes

MONITOR FOR SUCCESSFUL REPERFUSION

- Resolution of chest pain
- Resolution of ECG ST changes
- Presence of reperfusion dysrhythmias, such as accelerated idioventricular rhythm
- Early peak of cardiac biomarkers

MINIMIZE RISK OF BLEEDING

- Continue assessment for bleeding, including intracranial, internal, retroperitoneal, and puncture sites.
- Monitor for frank and occult blood (heme/guaiac).
- Monitor laboratory values for therapeutic ranges.
- Use caution with patient transfers.
- Limit and coordinate venipunctures; avoid establishing noncompressible intravenous access sites
- Apply pressure to all venous and arterial access sites.
- Avoid arterial punctures after fibrinolysis.
- Maintain a safe, clean environment.

MONITOR FOR REOCCLUSION

- Recurrence of chest pain
- Return of ST abnormalities
- Evidence of hemodynamic compromise

SUPPORT PATIENT AND FAMILY DURING CRISIS

- Approach in a calm, quiet manner.
- Provide simple explanations of procedures and care.
- Offer realistic reassurance.
- Encourage family presence when interventions permit.

In addition to monitoring for bleeding complications, the nurse acts to prevent patient injury. The nurse assists in all transfers to ensure minimum abrasion to skin surfaces. The nurse limits the number of venipunctures and applies direct manual pressure to the puncture site until complete hemostasis is obtained. Arterial punctures are avoided once fibrinolytic therapy is begun, especially at sites that cannot easily be compressed to control bleeding.

Anticoagulation therapy is often used in the treatment of patients with acute coronary syndrome. Anticoagulation prevents future clot formation but does not lyse existing clots. Nursing interventions for the patient receiving anticoagulants (e.g., heparin) are the same as those for the patient receiving fibrinolytics. During the administration of intravenous unfractionated heparin, the nurse monitors the patient's partial thromboplastin time (PTT) to evaluate the effectiveness of therapy. The nurse follows established algorithms and adjusts the dosage of heparin to keep the PTT in the therapeutic range of 50 to 70 seconds. Patients receiving low-molecular-weight heparin do not need PTT monitoring. If patients are receiving warfarin (Coumadin), it is important to ensure that their INR (international normalized ratio) is less than 1.6 before they undergo any invasive procedure.

Antiplatelet therapy (beyond aspirin) is often used for acute coronary syndrome and with PCIs. The purpose of antiplatelet therapy is to minimize clot formation, especially in the area of unstable plaque or at the site of coronary intervention. Nursing interventions include physical assessment for bleeding, prevention of physical injury, and ensuring hemostasis of puncture sites.

4. Relieving Anxiety

Nursing interventions to relieve anxiety are best directed at the etiology. For the MI patient, the threat of death is real and a common source of severe anxiety (see Research box). Psychologic support, realistic reassurance, brief explanations about care (to the extent desired by the patient), and family visiting should be priorities for patients with MI.

After the patient's condition stabilizes, the nurse makes appropriate referrals for inpatient cardiac rehabilitation and initiates discharge planning. The experienced staff nurse recognizes when she or he is able to meet the needs of the patient and when it is more appropriate to refer the patient to someone with greater expertise, ability, or time for either immediate crisis intervention or long-term follow-up. Nursing research continues to explore different ways in which nurses can intervene to holistically help the patient experiencing acute MI (see Complementary & Alternative Therapies box).

Anxiolytics may be prescribed to decrease patient anxiety. The use of anxiolytic agents is especially important during the acute phase of MI. Severe anxiety is common and increases the patient's myocardial oxygen demand at a time of decreased oxygen supply. Persistent anxiety may be managed with stress reduction techniques alone or in combination with anxiolytics. Stress reduction techniques include relaxation therapy, guided imagery, music therapy, and exercise. Supportive listening is a simple but effective intervention, especially when combined with the use of realistic reassurance and appropriate sharing of information. All of these interventions are beneficial, but research indicates that an exercise program may offer the best overall outcomes for the patient with CAD.

Research

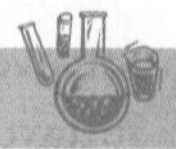

Reference: O'Brien JL et al: Comparison of anxiety assessments between clinicians and patients with acute myocardial infarction in cardiac critical care units, *Am J Crit Care* 10(2):97, 2001.

Nurse researchers compared the self-reported anxiety levels of 101 patients admitted with myocardial infarction (MI) to the anxiety levels recorded by health care professionals for the same patients. Patients rated their anxiety using the established Spielberger State Anxiety Index. The medical record was reviewed for documentation of patient anxiety in the 12 hours before and after the patient's completion of the SAI. Possible scores range from 20 to 80, with higher scores indicating greater levels of anxiety. In all, 30% of patient scores were between 20 and 29; 48% between 30 and 44; and 22% between 45 and 77 (mean: 37.2). Nurses documented anxiety in 39% of the enrolled patients; physicians noted the presence of anxiety for 6% of patients. For nine patients, anxiety was noted by a second health care provider; however, in two cases, the ratings conflicted. Clinicians did not use objective measures for documenting anxiety. When the patient's self-reported level of anxiety was compared against the health care documentation, no association was found between the two. The researchers concluded that clinicians do not routinely evaluate and document anxiety in MI patients, and when they do assess anxiety, the assessment is subjective and often does not match the patient's perception. The researchers urge nurses to adopt a standardized, objective approach to assessing and documenting anxiety in MI patients.

Complementary & Alternative Therapies

Patient Spirituality

The stress of hospitalization can be overwhelming for patients diagnosed with myocardial infarction. Spirituality has been theorized to play an extremely important role in recovery from illness. Nurses are not always comfortable in intervening with patients spiritually or even performing an assessment of what spirituality means to the patient. The researchers in this study posed two questions: (1) What does spirituality mean to patients recovering from acute myocardial infarction (AMI)? and (2) What are patients' perceptions of how spirituality influences their recovery from an AMI? Thirteen patients were interviewed within 7days of an AMI. The researchers concluded that spirituality was a life-giving force that was specific for each patient. This force was nurtured by a "receiving presence" from God, Nature, friends, family, and community. This life force was based on faith, discovering meaning and purpose, and giving the gift of self. Patients found spirituality within themselves as positively affecting their recovery through decreasing fear and anxiety, providing comfort and peace, enhancing coping, developing inner strength, courage, positivity, and hope; and by providing a sense of wellness and wholeness. Nurses need to increase their own comfort with addressing the spiritual needs of patients to enhance their spiritual well-being and effectively influence their recovery from AMI.

Reference: Walton J: Spirituality of patients recovering from an acute myocardial infarction: grounded theory study, *J Holistic Nurs* 17(1):34, 1999.

5. Improving Activity Tolerance

After MI the contractility of the infarcted area diminishes, and cardiac output often decreases. As a result, many MI patients experience activity intolerance. Overexertion leads to further damage because the myocardium must contract more forcefully than its weakened state can support. Guidelines for activity progression exist to increase patient conditioning without negatively affecting the balance of myocardial oxygen supply and demand. Bed rest also results in deconditioning. A structured rehabilitation program is ideal for patients with ACS and begins in the acute care setting. The nurse monitors the patient for activity tolerance and makes decisions about advancing the activity level (see Guidelines for Safe Practice box on advancing activity levels). Before ambulation, blood pressure and heart rate are checked while the patient stands. Readings are obtained before ambulation, immediately after ambulation, and 5 minutes after ambulation. Heart rate is measured for 10 seconds and then multiplied by 6. This method of heart rate calculation allows the nurse to determine an accurate postambulation heart rate before the heart rate returns to baseline. Additional monitoring parameters include symptoms of pain, dyspnea, fatigue, or light-headedness; oxygen saturation; and the presence of dysrhythmias. The nurse may collaborate with an exercise physiologist in advancing the patient's activity after MI.

After discharge from the acute care setting, patients benefit most from a structured monitored cardiac rehabilitation program. Exercise sessions include warm-up, aerobic exercise, and cool down; and both the equipment used and the intensity and duration prescribed are individualized for each patient. Once the patient safely exercises in a monitored program without experiencing adverse effects, the patient advances to an unmonitored program.

Some patients may not be able to enroll in a structured program because of inaccessibility, finances, time constraints, or other reasons. The nurse reviews with these patients the components of exercise and safe programs, the benefits and limitations of exercise, and the dangers of exercise. Stress test results, when available, can be used to individualize the patient's exercise program. In different settings, the nurse, exercise physiologist, or physician may be responsible for establishing such a program. Patients with stable angina are also encouraged to begin a home walking program or other individualized exercise program.

The nurse includes information about returning to work and sexual activity as part of the overall activity guidelines. Return to work is individualized to the patient's occupation. A patient with a desk job and low stress levels receives different guidelines than the patient with high occupational stress or heavy labor demands.

Medications often improve a patient's tolerance of activity. Nitroglycerin taken before an activity that is known to cause angina may allow the patient to complete the activity without experiencing chest pain. Beta-blockers decrease the sympathetic response to exercise, allowing patients to exercise at an increased intensity but with a safer heart rate. Both myocardial oxygen demand and efficiency improve with the use of beta-blockers.

Fatigue commonly limits the patient's exercise tolerance and can be related to medications. The most often cited medications are the beta-blockers. The nurse informs the patient about potential fatigue and what to do if it occurs. The patient taking beta-blockers is cautioned not to discontinue the medication abruptly, because this can result in rebound angina and hypertension. The nurse encourages the patient to discuss concerns with a primary care provider. Interventions for medication-induced fatigue include altering the dose, prescribing another type or class of medication, and offering counseling or referral, particularly if the fatigue is associated with depression.

6. Facilitating Return to Normal Sexual Patterns

Patients with CAD may have many concerns related to sexuality. They may be concerned about the occurrence of chest pain during sexual intercourse or their ability to perform sexually. In addition, patients may have concerns about aging or self-concept. If a therapeutic relationship has been established between the patient and the nurse, it is usually possible for the nurse to address these concerns with the patient. The nurse reassures the patient that concerns about sexuality after MI or with the diagnosis of CAD are normal and that it is important to discuss them with their partner.

The patient with acute coronary syndrome requires additional guidance about resuming sexual activity safely. For the patient with unstable angina, nitroglycerin may be taken before intercourse if intercourse causes angina. For the post-MI patient, guidelines for sexual activity are based on successful progression through a home walking or structured outpatient exercise program. As a general rule, patients with uncomplicated MIs may resume sexual intercourse after 7 to 10 days.[15] Traditional parameters for resuming intercourse include climbing two flights of stairs or walking at 3 to 4 miles per hour without dyspnea or chest pain. The patient's spouse or partner may also have fears about the effects of sexual activity on the patient's heart. Therefore he or she should be included in all counseling and educational sessions. See the Patient Teaching box for additional specific information about the safe resumption of sexual activity after MI.

Beta-blockers cause impotence in some men. This is a very real problem that must be addressed. The nurse is honest in communicating the side effects of these drugs. The patient who is aware of the possibility of impotence will perhaps be better able to cope with the problem should it occur. Herbal supplements, marijuana, and cocaine are additional drugs that may alter sexual function and place the myocardium at risk. Patients should consult with their primary care provider before using sildenafil (Viagra) because of its vasodilatory effects.

Patient/Family Education

Educational plans specific to interventional procedures have been previously discussed. For patients with CAD, the nurse develops an educational plan based on the individual's unique risk factors. An overview of educational guidelines for patients with CAD is presented in the Patient Teaching box.

Patient Teaching
Guidelines for Sexual Activity After Myocardial Infarction

STAGES OF SEXUAL RESPONSE

- Arousal: flushed; breathing and heart rate increase; blood pressure (BP) goes up slightly
- Plateau: increase in respirations, BP, and heart rate
- Orgasm (15 to 20 seconds): pulse and blood pressure increase further
- Resolution: return to resting state within seconds; angina or palpitations most likely to occur during resolution.

GENERAL GUIDELINES

- Sexual foreplay at a relaxed pace allows your heart rate and BP to increase more slowly.
- Hugging, stroking, and touching are safe ways to get back in touch with your partner.
- Talk with your partner. Express your feelings.
- Extramarital affairs or sex with new partners may produce more stress.
- Avoid positions for sex that you find uncomfortable.
- Have sex in a pleasant, comfortable environment.
- Do not take very hot or cold baths or showers before or after sex.
- Be rested before sex.
- Do not have sex after a heavy meal or drinking alcohol.
- If you have any questions about side effects of any drug, do not stop taking the drug, but talk to your health care provider.
- Masturbation and manual or oral stimulation are not harmful to your heart. Anal intercourse may lead to an irregular heartbeat. Avoid this choice unless you clear it with your health care professional.

Patient Teaching
The Patient With Coronary Artery Disease

RISK FACTOR MODIFICATION

- Provide specific verbal and written instructions on smoking cessation, stress management, and diet modification.
- Consider referral to a smoking cessation program or outpatient cardiac rehabilitation program.
- Encourage adherence to a diet low in calories, saturated fats, and cholesterol.
- Discuss the benefits of stress management techniques in decreasing negative effect on oxygen demand. Refer to individual or group counseling as needed.

RESUMPTION OF ACTIVITY

- Discuss guidelines for resuming sexual relations.
- Provide specific instructions on activities that are permissible and those that should be avoided.
- Discuss resumption of driving and return to work.
- Discuss the benefits of exercise and encourage a regular exercise program.

MEDICATIONS

- Ensure understanding of the role of aspirin.
- Instruct patient that recurrent symptoms lasting more than 1 to 2 minutes should prompt the patient to stop all activities, sit down, and take a sublingual nitroglycerin tablet. This may be repeated at 5-minute intervals for two additional tablets if needed. If symptoms persist, access emergency medical services (call 911).
- Teach correct use and storage of nitroglycerin (see Patient Teaching box on p. 670).
- Instruct patient in purpose, dose, and major side effects of each medication prescribed.

Before the patient's hospital discharge, all medications are reviewed with the patient and family. The nurse reviews the purpose of the medication, dose, and possible side effects and establishes a medication schedule suited to the patient's lifestyle. This collaborative effort promotes adherence to the medical regimen. The nurse reminds patients of the need to discuss drug side effects with their health care providers and not to discontinue any medications without consultation.

The family is included in discussions of activity progression after MI. Disagreements over acceptable activity are a major source of conflict between spouse and patient, adding to the stress of this crisis situation.

The nurse also facilitates discussion regarding the stress of this illness on children of all ages, who commonly exhibit behavior changes, sleep disturbances, and somatic complaints in response to the stress of MI involving a parent.[11]

Low-cholesterol, low-fat diets are also reviewed with patients and their families before discharge and the nurse explains the results of the patient's lipid profile. Patients who have sustained an MI should have lipid profiles drawn 6 weeks after the MI to ensure an accurate baseline. The nurse teaches the patient about cholesterol-lowering agents, including the potential for unpleasant side effects such as insomnia and myositis (muscle inflammation) commonly associated with these medicines. The nurse emphasizes that lipid-lowering medications do not eliminate the need for the patient to follow recommended dietary guidelines.

Health Promotion/Prevention. Many of the Healthy People 2010 goals are targeted at the prevention of CAD. Highlights of the national health objectives related to CAD are presented in the Healthy People 2010 box.[19]

EVALUATION

To evaluate the effectiveness of nursing interventions, compare patient behaviors with those stated in the expected patient outcomes. Achievement of outcomes is successful if the patient with CAD:

1. Is free of chest pain or anginal equivalent, or effectively able to control angina through the use of medications.
2. Has adequate cardiac output to maintain perfusion to all organs.
3. Is free of bleeding or initiates appropriate treatment when bleeding occurs despite precautionary measures.
4. Has ability to seek and process information.
5. Progressively increases activity back toward baseline.
6. Discusses concerns, including sexuality issues, and develops a plan to explore resolution of issues.

Healthy People 2010

Objectives Related to Heart Disease

1. Reduce coronary heart disease deaths to no more than 166 per 100,000 people.
2. Increase the proportion of adults ages 20 years and older who are aware of the early warning symptoms and signs of a heart attack and the importance of accessing rapid emergency care by calling 911.
3. Increase the proportion of eligible patients with heart attacks who receive artery-opening therapy within an hour of symptom onset.
4. Increase the proportion of adults ages 20 years and older who call 911 and administer cardiopulmonary resuscitation when they witness an out-of-hospital cardiac arrest.
5. Increase the proportion of eligible persons with witnessed out-of-hospital cardiac arrest who receive their first therapeutic electrical shock within 6 minutes after collapse recognition.
6. Reduce the mean total blood cholesterol levels among adults to 199 mg/dl.
7. Reduce the proportion of adults with high total blood cholesterol levels to no more than 17%.
8. Increase to at least 80% the proportion of adults who have had their blood cholesterol checked within the preceding 5 years.
9. Increase the proportion of persons with coronary heart disease who have their LDL-cholesterol level treated to a goal of less than or equal to 100 mg/dl.

From U.S. Department of Health and Human Services: *Healthy People 2010: understanding and improving health,* Washington, DC, 2000, USDHHS.

GERONTOLOGIC CONSIDERATIONS

The prevalence of CAD increases with advancing age. In assessing chest pain in the older adult, the nurse is aware that these patients may have atypical signs and symptoms and may delay seeking care. Older patients often experience "silent MIs," and come to the emergency department with shortness of breath, heart failure, or pulmonary edema, but without chest pain. Absence of chest pain as a classic symptom often impedes recognition of the fact that the older person is experiencing a heart attack. Elderly patients may therefore delay seeking medical care for the evaluation of their "heart condition," especially when they have a long history of angina. Older adults also may delay seeking care because they are reluctant to go to the hospital, do not want to "bother" anyone, or are experiencing loneliness and depression. Diminished cardiac reserve and altered response to inotropic medications place the older patient at risk for the development of heart failure or cardiogenic shock.

Older adults may also be especially sensitive to certain medications. The nurse carefully observes for side effects and drug interactions and anticipates that the elderly patient may require higher doses of vasoactive agents to achieve desired effects.

SPECIAL ENVIRONMENTS FOR CARE

Critical Care

The critically ill MI patient is kept in the coronary care unit (CCU) for 24 hours or until stabilized. The care provided in the CCU is as outlined in the collaborative care discussion. Patients who are not critically ill are admitted directly to monitored units designed specifically for cardiac patients. Today, with the routine use of fibrinolytic agents and PCI, the average hospital stay after MI has significantly decreased.

Research

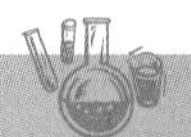

Reference: Stewart M et al: Myocardial infarction: survivors' and spouses' stress, coping, and support, *J Adv Nurs* 31(6):1351, 2000.

The researchers conducted a qualitative study to determine stressors, coping, and perceived support among myocardial infarction (MI) patients and their spouses. Fourteen MI survivors and their spouses participated in a 12-week support group intervention. Only one of the MI survivors was female; all were Caucasian. Data were collected regarding stressors, coping, and support systems from weekly field notes and participant diaries. Stressors identified by patients included (most to least) emotional impact, requisite lifestyle changes, dealing with health professionals, reactions of spouse, dependent role, return to work, financial concerns, and changes in social routines, intimacy, and other roles. Spouses identified four demands related to caring for the MI spouse: monitoring and managing lifestyle changes, dealing with emotional and behavioral reactions of the patient, interacting with the health care system, and vigilance associated with caregiving. Secondary demands included dealing with their own reactions and feelings and with the impact of the MI on family activities and relationships, finances, marital relationship, and other roles. Spouses and survivors reported inadequate informational support from health professionals. Support was perceived as lacking by both spouses and patients.

Community-Based Care

The trend of earlier hospital discharge has shifted much of the recovery from ACS into the community. Before discharge the patient and family must receive sufficient information about what to expect during this recovery period so that they can safely manage the patient's care at home (see Research box). Of particular importance is information about medications, activity progression, what to do for recurrent chest pain, and what to do if bleeding from an arterial catheter insertion site should occur. Many patients and families have questions about their care when they get home that they did not think to ask in the hospital. The nurse ensures that patients are knowledgeable about who to call in case of complications; have appointments for follow-up care; and are aware of the supports and resources available in their home community.

COMPLICATIONS

The most common complications of CAD are heart failure, dysrhythmias, and pericarditis. The likelihood of complications increases with severe multivessel CAD and with AMI. Additional complications include cardiogenic shock, ventricular septal defect, free wall rupture, ventricular aneurysms, and ischemic cardiomyopathy.

Heart Failure. Heart failure in CAD occurs in response to a decrease in contractility secondary to an ischemic myocardium. A hypokinetic or akinetic myocardium does not generate the inotropic action needed to sustain an adequate cardiac output. The amount of ischemic or infarcted myocardium determines the onset and severity of heart failure. Heart failure is most often seen in patients having large MIs, particularly MIs involving the anterior surface of the myocardium. Nursing management of the patient with heart failure is presented in Chapter 24.

Dysrhythmias. Dysrhythmias often occur secondary to the ischemic processes of CAD. Ischemia alters the stability of the myocardial cell membrane. Ischemia of the specialized conduction pathways (SA node, AV node, and bundle branches) can result in heart blocks. Individuals with right coronary artery blockages and inferior MIs may experience heart block and bradycardia because the right coronary artery most often supplies the SA and AV nodes. Patients with left anterior descending artery blockages may have complete or incomplete bundle branch blocks and ventricular dysrhythmias, because the left anterior descending artery supplies the bundle branch system and a disproportionately large surface of the anterior myocardium. Direct damage to the myocardial cell creates electrolyte imbalances that alter the action potential. Management of common dysrhythmias is presented in the next section.

Pericarditis. After AMI the pericardial lining of the heart can become inflamed and fluid may accumulate between the parietal and visceral layers. The patient complains of severe precordial chest pain that closely resembles that of AMI. The presence of a characteristic pericardial friction rub is helpful in the differential diagnosis. Pericarditis is usually treated with nonsteroidal antiinflammatory drugs or occasionally corticosteroids. Pericarditis is presented in greater detail in Chapter 24.

CARDIAC DYSRHYTHMIAS

Etiology/Epidemiology

Normal sinus rhythm begins with the spontaneous depolarization of the SA node. The impulse passes through the atria to the AV node and then through the bundle of His and bundle branches to the Purkinje fibers (see Figure 22-4). A rhythm is classified as "normal" when it meets the following criteria: presence of one upright and consistent-appearing P wave before each QRS complex, all PR intervals between 0.12 and 0.20 seconds, a consistent-appearing QRS complex of less than 0.12 seconds, a consistent RR interval, and a heart rate between 60 and 100 beats/min (Figure 23-13; all rhythm strips are Lead II).

Cardiac dysrhythmias are the result of alterations in impulse formation or propagation. The anatomic site of the dysfunction helps to classify the dysrhythmia, but the underlying etiology varies with each specific dysrhythmia. Common etiologies include underlying cardiac disease, sympathetic stimulation, vagal stimulation, electrolyte imbalances, and hypoxia.

Benign dysrhythmias such as sinus bradycardia and occasional premature beats are common in the general population, but dysrhythmias are more prevalent in patients with cardiac disease. In patients with CAD, a benign rhythm may have negative consequences because the myocardium is already compromised. Common dysrhythmias and their management are presented in the collaborative care management section.

Pathophysiology

An understanding of normal cardiac electrophysiology, presented in Chapter 22, is necessary to grasp the pathophysiology of dysrhythmias. Alterations in impulse formation and ropagation arise from one of three main pathophysiologic processes: altered automaticity, altered conduction resulting in delays or blocks, and reentry mechanisms.

Alterations in Automaticity

Automaticity, the ability to depolarize spontaneously without external stimulation, is a property that normally is confined to the cells of the SA node. Depolarization, however, is not unique to the SA node, and it occurs all along the electrical impulse pathway (Figure 23-14). These nonpacemaker cells may be responsible for dysrhythmias. The SA node usually depolarizes at a faster rate than other potential pacemaker cells because of the steep slope of phase 4, allowing sinus cells to reach threshold at a faster rate (Figure 23-15). A variety of conditions can alter the automaticity of the SA node and produce faster or slower than usual heart rates. Vagal stimulation decreases this slope, resulting in a slower heart rate (Figure 23-16). Sympathetic stimulation and hypoxia steepen phase 4, resulting in faster heart rates (Figure 23-17).

If the rate of phase 4 depolarization found in the AV node or ventricular conduction system increases, enhanced automaticity is said to exist. The result may be premature beats or tachycardias. Some causes of enhanced automaticity are hypoxia, catecholamines, atropine, hypokalemia, hypocalcemia, heat, trauma, and digitalis toxicity.

Even cells that do not normally have automaticity may develop abnormal automaticity if the resting membrane potential or threshold potential is altered. Increasing the threshold potential slows the heart rate (Figure 23-18). If the resting membrane potential is made less negative, automaticity

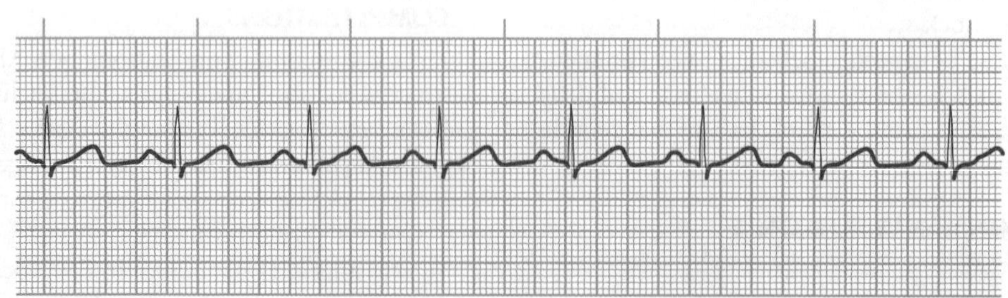

Figure 23-13 Normal sinus rhythm; heart rate, 80 beats/min.

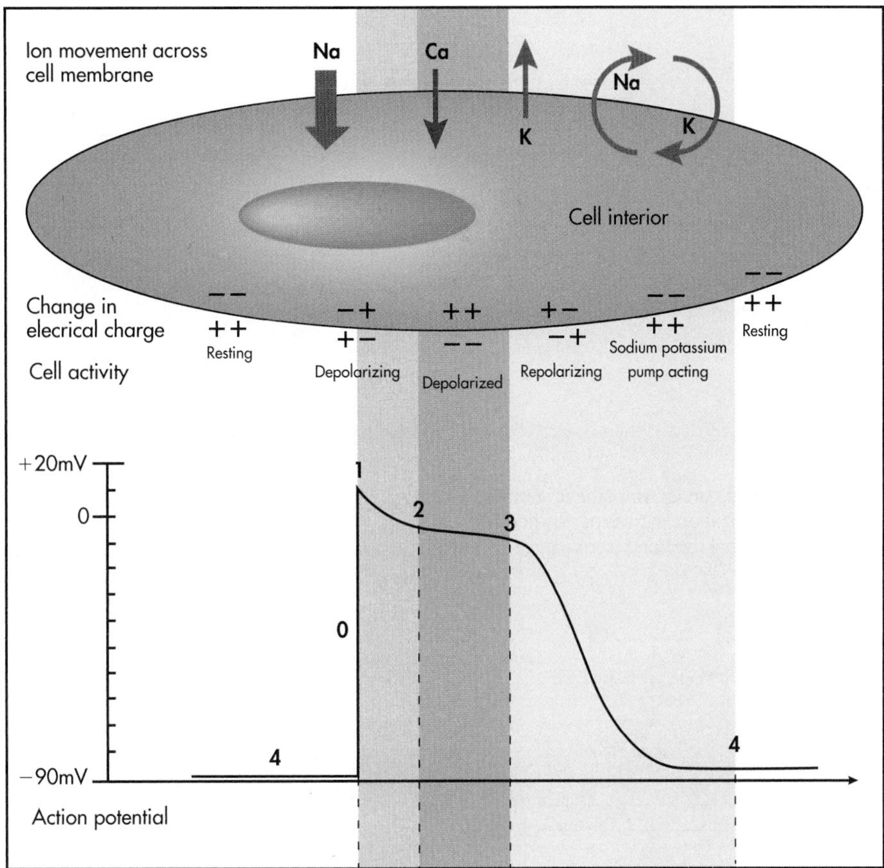

Figure 23-14 Phases of the action potential of a cardiac cell. In the resting phase (*4*), the cell membrane is polarized. The cell's interior has a net negative charge and the membrane is more permeable to potassium ions than to sodium. When the cell is stimulated and begins to depolarize (*0*), sodium ions enter the cell, potassium leaves the cell, calcium channels open, and sodium channels close. In its depolarized phase (*1*), the cell's interior has a net positive charge. In the plateau phase (*2*), calcium and other positive ions enter the cell and potassium permeability declines, lengthening the action potential. Then (*3*), calcium channels close and sodium is pulled from the cell by the sodium-potassium pump. The cell's interior then returns to its polarized, negatively charged state (*4*).

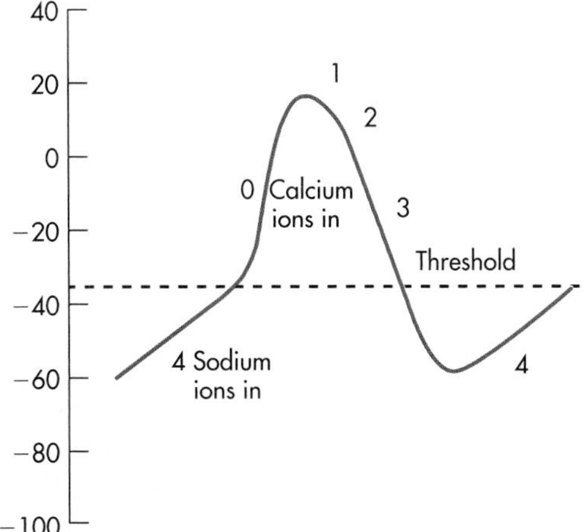

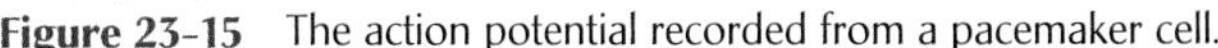

Figure 23-15 The action potential recorded from a pacemaker cell.

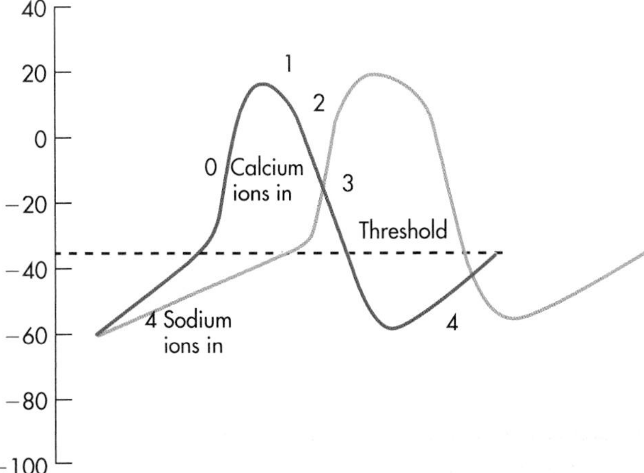

Figure 23-16 Decreased automaticity. Left curve: The normal action potential recorded from a pacemaker cell. Right curve: Vagal stimulation decreases the rate of phase 4 depolarization, decreasing the heart rate.

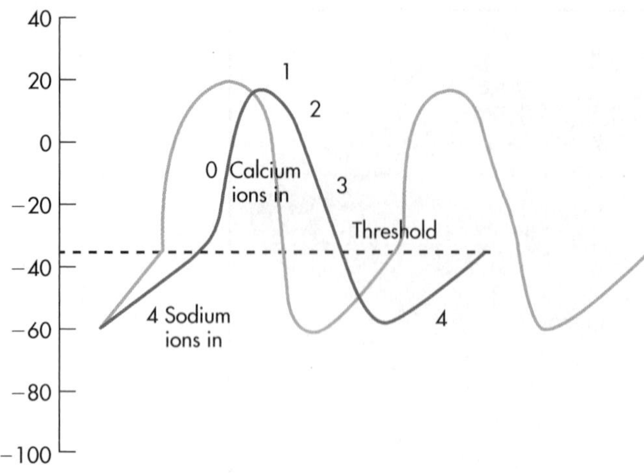

Figure 23-17 Increased automaticity. Left curve: Sympathetic stimulation and hypoxia steepen phase 4 depolarization, increasing the heart rate. Right curve: The normal action potential recorded from a pacemaker cell.

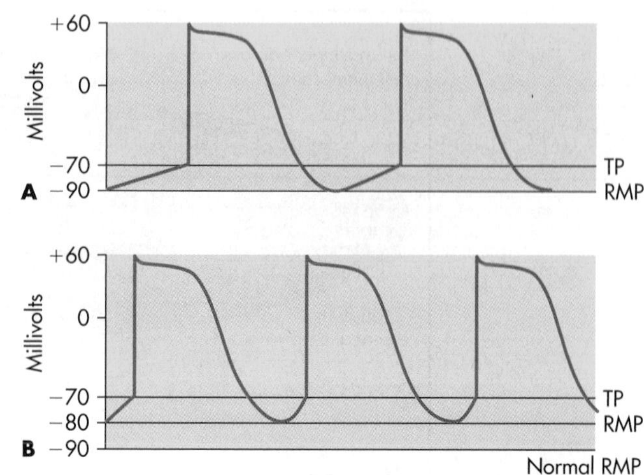

Figure 23-19 Increased automaticity. **A,** Normal action potential recorded from a nonpacemaker cell. **B,** Making the resting membrane potential less negative makes it easier to reach threshold, increasing heart rate.

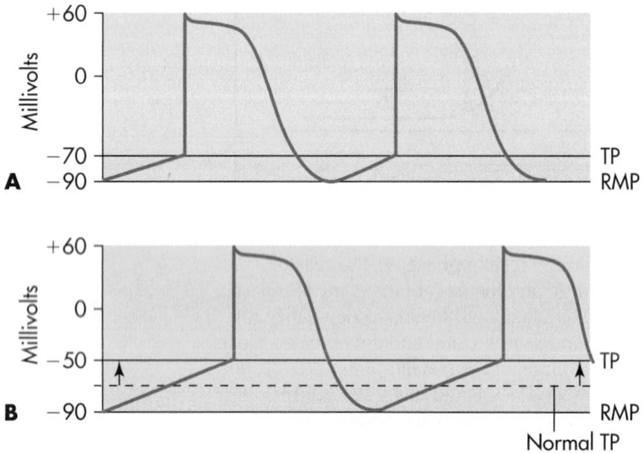

Figure 23-18 Decreased automaticity. **A,** Normal action potential recorded from a nonpacemaker cell. **B,** Making the threshold potential less negative increases the time needed to reach threshold, decreasing heart rate.

increases because it is easier to reach threshold (Figure 23-19). Abnormal automaticity is not easily suppressed by the activity of the usual pacemakers.

Alterations in Conduction

When the rate or amplitude of depolarization decreases, conduction also decreases. Any condition that decreases the amplitude of the action potential, such as ischemia, hypercalcemia, or calcification of the conducting fibers, can cause cardiac conduction disturbances. Abnormalities in conduction can occur anywhere in the conduction system, including the SA node, AV node, and the bundle branches. The severity of impaired conduction ranges from a slight delay to complete cessation or block of impulse transmission.

Reentry

Reentry involves impulse transmission around a unidirectional block. Reentry occurs when an impulse is delayed within a pathway of slow conduction long enough that the impulse is still viable when the remaining myocardium repolarizes. The impulse then reenters surrounding tissue and produces another impulse. This typically occurs when two different pathways share an initial and final segment. The first impulse travels down the faster pathway, leaving behind its refractory tail. Should a second, early impulse follow, it is blocked because that path is refractory. The second impulse then enters the slow pathway and can return retrograde through the fast path, initiating a circuitous pattern (Figure 23-20).

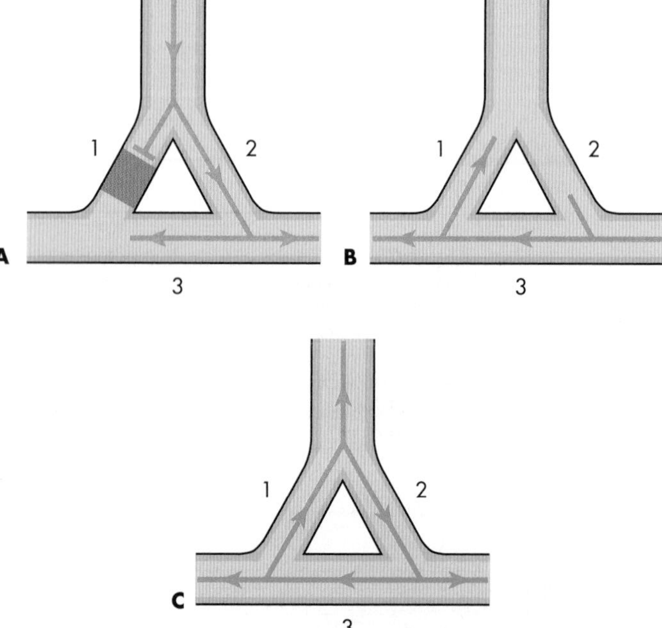

Figure 23-20 Reentry. **A,** Shaded area shows refractory area after the first impulse passes down path 1. Premature impulse is then blocked from entering path 1 but can travel down path 2. **B,** Path 1 is no longer refractory to stimulation; therefore, a premature impulse can travel backwards up path 1. **C,** Reentry down path 2 establishes circuitous pathway.

Clinical Manifestations

Cardiac Dysrhythmias

GENERAL

Palpitations (racing heart, skipped beats)
Anxiety
Fatigue

ALTERED CARDIAC OUTPUT

Pallor
Cool, clammy skin
Cyanosis
Shortness of breath
Rales
Decreased blood pressure
Confusion
Dizziness
Weakness
Presyncope
Syncope with loss of consciousness
Chest pain
Atrial thrombi (may dislodge to cause systemic emboli)

Clinical Manifestations

Many patients with dysrhythmias are asymptomatic as long as cardiac output meets the body's metabolic demands. The clinical manifestations associated with most dysrhythmias relate to decreases in cardiac output from slow or fast heart rates. Significant changes in heart rate may not allow adequate time for the ventricles to fill and empty. Clinical manifestations include those listed in the Clinical Manifestations box. In addition, patients may complain of palpitations (e.g., a "racing heart" or "skipping beats") related to changes in heart rate and stroke volume. These symptoms often create acute anxiety.

Collaborative Care Management

The diagnosis of dysrhythmias begins with the 12-lead ECG. Each dysrhythmia exhibits characteristic changes in the ECG tracing. A systematic approach to analyzing the ECG rhythm helps distinguish the different dysrhythmias (Box 23-2). Table 23-8 outlines the rhythm criteria that define each common dysrhythmia and their common associated etiologies. Some rhythms, especially fast rhythms, seem to defy interpretation using the ECG alone. Additional diagnostic tests are often needed to determine the dysrhythmia itself, and most important, its etiology. Electrophysiology studies (see Chapter 22) are used to determine the electrophysiologic properties of the various dysrhythmias. Management is then determined based on an understanding of the mechanism responsible for the dysrhythmia.

Medical and nursing management of dysrhythmias focuses on alleviating symptoms from altered cardiac output and eliminating or reversing the etiology. Common interventions specific to each dysrhythmia are included in the discussion that follows. The mechanism of the dysrhythmia, as determined by electrophysiology studies, determines the exact treatment.

BOX 23-2 Systematic Interpretation of ECG Tracing

Rate (atrial and ventricular)
Rhythm (atrial and ventricular)
Presence or absence of P waves
PR interval 0.12-0.20 sec
QRS complex 0.06-0.12 sec
Relationship of QRS to P wave
QT interval, 0.55 sec
Interpretation

NOTE: A normal sinus rhythm has an atrial (P) and ventricular (QRS) rate of 60 to 100 beats/min, a regular rhythm (constant PP and RR intervals), and a P wave before every QRS.

Sinus Bradycardia

Sinus bradycardia is characterized by atrial and ventricular rates of less than 60 beats/min (Figure 23-21), but in all other respects is a normal sinus rhythm. It may develop gradually or occur suddenly for a brief period.

Bradycardia generally results from increased vagal tone or decreased sympathetic tone. It is commonly seen in athletes and may also be associated with sleep, vomiting, and MI. Carotid sinus stimulation and drugs such as digoxin, morphine sulfate, and sedatives induce sinus bradycardia in many patients.

Generally sinus bradycardia is a benign rhythm. In association with MI it may even be a beneficial rhythm because it reduces myocardial oxygen demand. If the heart rate is too slow to maintain adequate cardiac output, however, the patient may be predisposed to syncope and congestive heart failure. Administration of atropine, isoproterenol, or dopamine is usually effective in increasing the heart rate.[13]

Sinus Tachycardia

Sinus tachycardia is characterized by an atrial and ventricular rate of 100 beats/min or more (Figure 23-22). Generally the upper limit of sinus tachycardia is 150 beats/min. The P waves are sinus in origin, but they may be buried in the T wave with very high heart rates. Intervals and complexes are within normal limits. The onset of sinus tachycardia usually is gradual as the sinus node rate increases in response to higher metabolic needs.

Sinus tachycardia is associated with the ingestion of alcohol, caffeine, and tobacco and is a normal physiologic response to exertion, fever, fear, excitement, acute pain, or any condition that requires a higher basal metabolism. Clinically sinus tachycardia can be a short-term compensatory response to heart failure, anemia, hypovolemia, and hypotension. Sinus tachycardia is also seen with hyperthyroidism and may be produced by drugs such as atropine and amphetamines.

Generally, sinus tachycardia is a benign rhythm that slows with resolution of the etiology. The patient may complain of palpitations or have no symptoms. In the patient with a compromised myocardium, the tachycardia increases myocardial oxygen demand and may cause a decrease in cardiac output with resultant light-headedness, chest pain, and heart failure. Sinus tachycardia can usually be slowed with digoxin, beta-blockers, or diltiazem if necessary.

TABLE 23-8 Comparison of Select Cardiac Dysrhythmias

Dysrhythmia	ECG Diagnostic Criteria	Etiologic Factors
Dysrhythmias of Sinus Node		
Sinus bradycardia	P waves present followed by QRS Rhythm regular Heart rate <60	Athletes Vagal stimulation Digitalis, beta-blockers, sedatives
Sinus tachycardia	P waves present followed by QRS Rhythm regular Heart rate 100 to 150 beats/min	Increased metabolic demands Compensatory mechanism for heart failure, shock, hemorrhage, anemia
Sinus dysrhythmia	Phasic shortening of PP and RR intervals with inspiration, lengthening with expiration	Respiratory variation in impulse initiation by SA node
Sick sinus syndrome	Sinus bradycardia alternating with sinus tachycardia	SA node ischemia, degeneration Hypertension Ischemia Digoxin
Sinus exit block/sinus arrest	Isoelectric line (pause) without P or QRS; P wave returns in synchrony (exit block) or asynchronous (sinus arrest)	Hypoxia Ischemia SA node ischemia, degeneration Digoxin
Atrial Dysrhythmias		
Premature atrial beats	Early P wave QRS may or may not be normal Pause follows QRS	Stress, ischemia, atrial enlargement, caffeine, nicotine
Wandering atrial pacemaker	P waves of different appearances or buried in QRS; varying PR intervals	Cardiac disease Drug toxicity
Atrial tachycardia	P wave present (may be hidden in previous T wave), QRS usually normal, heart rate usually >150 beats per minute	Sympathetic stimulation, caffeine, nicotine, drug toxicity Pulmonary disease Heart disease
Atrial flutter	Atrial rate 250 to 350; F waves usually in a ratio to QRS complexes such as 2:1, 3:1; QRS complexes normal	Pulmonary disease Valve disease Cardiac surgery
Atrial fibrillation	Rapid, indiscernible P waves (>350/min) Ventricular rhythm irregularly irregular Ventricular rate varies	Rheumatic heart disease Atrial ischemia Coronary atherosclerotic disease Hypertension Thyrotoxicosis Cardiac surgery Alcohol
Junctional Dysrhythmias		
Premature junctional beat	Early beat P before, during, or after QRS P inverted or retrograde PR interval <0.12 if P before QRS QRS normal	Increased metabolism Nicotine Caffeine Ischemia Electrolyte imbalance
Junctional rhythm	P before, during, or after QRS P inverted or retrograde PR interval <0.12 if P before QRS QRS normal Rate 40-60, junctional rhythm Rate 60-100, accelerated junctional rhythm Rate >100, junctional tachycardia	Accelerated: Heart disease Caffeine Pain Digoxin

TABLE 23-8 Comparison of Select Cardiac Dysrhythmias—cont'd

Dysrhythmia	ECG Diagnostic Criteria	Etiologic Factors
Ventricular Dysrhythmias		
Premature ventricular beats	Early, wide, bizarre QRS, not associated with a P wave Rhythm irregular	Stress, acidosis, ventricular enlargement Electrolyte imbalance Myocardial infarction Digitalis toxicity Hypoxemia, hypercapnia
Accelerated idioventricular rhythm (AIVR)/ventricular tachycardia (VT)	P not associated with QRS, QRS wide and bizarre VT: ventricular rate >100, usually 140-240 AIVR: rate 40-100	VT: hypoxemia, drug toxicity, electrolyte imbalance, bradycardia, CAD AIVR: reperfusion of ischemic myocardium
Torsades de Pointes	No associated P waves Wide, bizarre QRSs twist along isoelectric line Heart rate >100	Medications Electrolyte imbalance Congenital prolonged QT interval
Ventricular fibrillation	No recognizable complexes Wavy line of varying amplitude	Myocardial infarction Electrocution Drowning
Ventricular asystole	No complexes "Straight line"	Myocardial infarction Chronic diseases of conducting system
Impulse Conduction Deficits		
First-degree AV block	PR interval prolonged, >0.20 sec	Rheumatic fever Myocardial infarction Cardiac medications
Second-degree AV blocks		
Mobitz I	P waves usually occur regularly at rates consistent with SA node initiation. PR interval lengthened before nonconducted P wave; QRS may be widened	Acute myocardial infarction Increased vagal tone Electrolyte imbalance Infection
Mobitz II	Constant PR intervals Nonconducted P waves at random or patterned intervals	Coronary artery disease Myocardial infarction Rheumatic heart disease Digoxin
Complete third-degree AV block	Atria and ventricles beat independently P waves have no relation to QRS Ventricular rate may be as low as 20-40/min if ventricular; 40-60 if junctional	Digitalis toxicity Coronary artery disease Myocardial infarction
Bundle branch block	Same as normal sinus rhythm except QRS duration >0.12	Hypoxia, acute myocardial infarction, heart failure, coronary atherosclerosis, hypertension

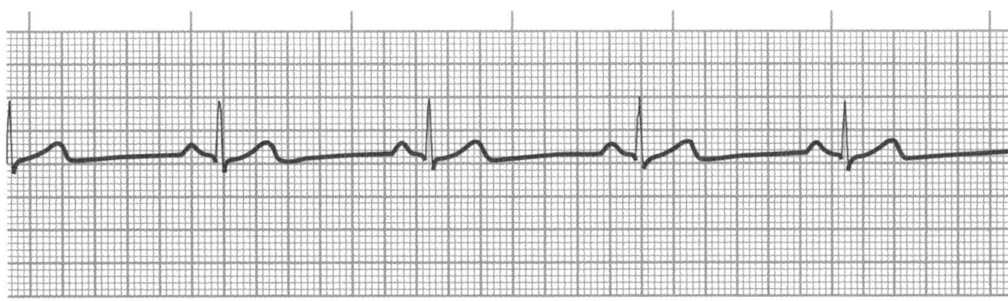

Figure 23-21 Sinus bradycardia; heart rate, 40 beats/min.

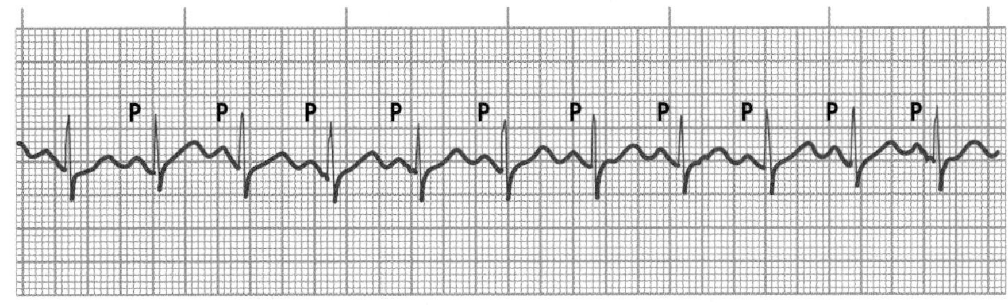

Figure 23-22 Sinus tachycardia; heart rate, 110 beats/min.

Sinus Dysrhythmia

Sinus dysrhythmia is typically found in young adults and elderly persons. Sinus dysrhythmia is an irregular rhythm in which PP intervals vary by more than 0.16 second. The P waves have a consistent shape, and the PR interval and QRS duration are within normal limits. Changes in PP intervals are accompanied by changes in RR intervals (Figure 23-23).

The cyclic pattern of changing PP or RR intervals often correlates with the patterns of inspiration and expiration. During inspiration the intervals shorten as the heart rate increases. Conversely, the intervals lengthen during expiration.

Sinus dysrhythmia is not treated unless the bradycardic phase is marked, causing symptoms. With slower heart rates, some patients may experience palpitations or dizziness if the PP intervals are unusually long. Atropine may be effective in treating symptomatic bradycardia.

Sick Sinus Syndrome

Tachycardia-bradycardia syndromes are characterized by the presence of bradycardia with intermittent episodes of tachydysrhythmias. The episode of tachydysrhythmia often is followed by a long pause before returning to bradycardia. Sick sinus syndrome (SSS) is one type of tachycardia-bradycardia syndrome. In SSS, the bradycardia and tachycardia are both sinus in origin. Complications of this inefficient rhythm include heart failure and cerebrovascular accident resulting from thromboembolism. In addition, cerebral blood flow may be decreased, producing confusion in the elderly. Sick sinus syndrome is associated with ischemia or degeneration of the SA node.

Some patients may remain free of symptoms or complain only of palpitations. For the patient with severe symptoms, the heart rhythm is stabilized with a permanent implantable pacemaker for the slow phase and the administration of digoxin or beta-blockers to control the ventricular rate of the tachycardic phase.

Sinus Exit Block and Sinus Arrest

Sinus exit block occurs when an impulse originates in the SA node but is immediately blocked (Figure 23-24). No P wave or QRS complex is generated, resulting in a long pause. The next impulse occurs in a time interval representing the normal PP interval. The term *sinus arrest* infers that the SA node never fired; therefore there is no P or QRS complex. The next impulse is asynchronous to the normal PP interval.

Sinus exit block and sinus arrest may occur as a result of medications such as digoxin, hypoxia, myocardial ischemia, and injury to the SA node. The patient becomes symptomatic from a decrease in cardiac output when the pauses are long or frequent. The patient may feel palpitations from the increased stroke volume that accompanies the next beat after the pause. When the patient is symptomatic, atropine may be administered to increase the heart rate and cardiac output. Definitive therapy includes the insertion of a permanent pacemaker.

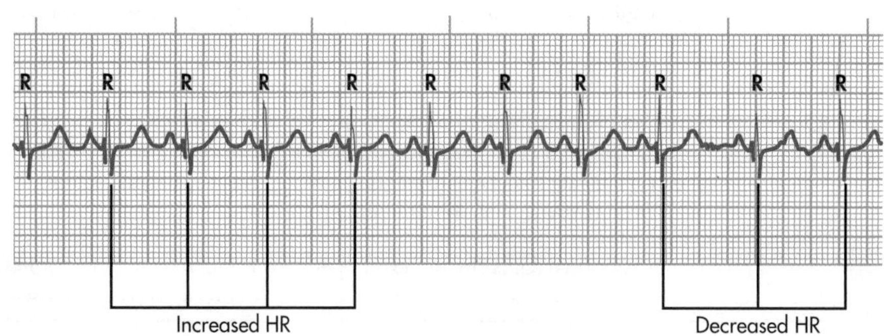

Figure 23-23 Sinus dysrhythmia. Heart rate increases with inspiration and decreases with expiration; overall heart rate, 100 beats/min.

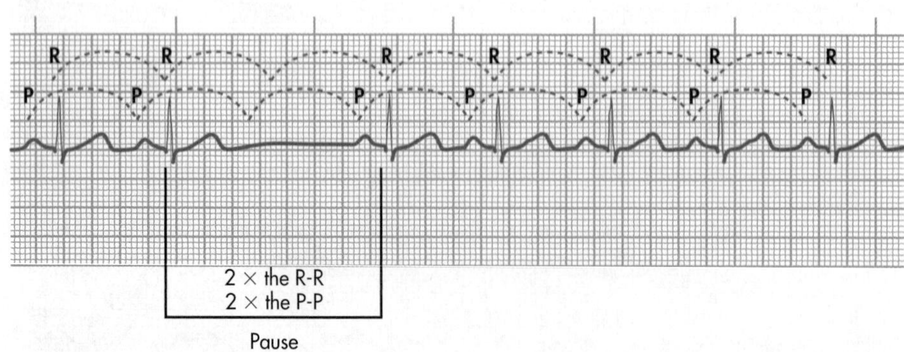

Figure 23-24 Sinus exit block. Pause equal to two complete cardiac cycles; overall heart rate, 70 beats/min.

Premature Atrial Beat

A premature atrial beat (PAB) is initiated by an ectopic focus in the atria (Figure 23-25) and is characterized by a premature P wave with a contour different from that of a sinus P wave. The location of the ectopic focus within the atria determines its shape. The QRS complex may or may not be normal. The PAB is often followed by a pause. The atrial impulse may be nonconducted (blocked) because of refractoriness of the AV node at the time the impulse arrives. The nonconducted atrial beat (blocked PAB) is a common cause of irregularity in the heart rhythm.

The PAB may be associated with stress or the use of caffeine or tobacco products. It also is seen in the clinical setting with hypoxia, atrial enlargement, infection, inflammation, and myocardial ischemia. Frequent PABs may warn of impending atrial fibrillation or tachycardia. In the absence of organic disease, no treatment is required. Often the elimination of caffeine and tobacco will suppress the atrial focus. Premature atrial beats may produce palpitations, but cardiac output is generally not affected unless PABs are frequent or there is a high occurrence of blocked beats.

Wandering Atrial Pacemaker

Wandering atrial pacemaker occurs when at least three ectopic sites create impulses for the cardiac rhythm (Figure 23-26). The ECG shows P waves of different shapes and PR intervals of different lengths. The impulse can originate from the area around the AV node, which creates inverted P waves from retrograde conduction. Impulses from this lower area may also cause stimulation of the atria at the same time as or after the ventricle. The P waves then appear to be buried in the QRS or even occur inverted after the QRS.

Wandering atrial pacemakers usually signify underlying heart disease or drug toxicity. The patient is usually asymptomatic unless the heart rate increases or decreases enough to affect cardiac output. The nurse monitors for changes in the rhythm and in the patient's symptoms.

Atrial Tachycardia

In atrial tachycardia, the atrial rate is approximately 150 to 250 beats/min. P waves are present but may be hidden in the T waves of the preceding beats when the ventricular rate is high. When the P waves vary in appearance, the rhythm is called multifocal atrial tachycardia (MAT). The QRS complex generally is normal, and the ventricular rhythm is regular (Figure 23-27). Transient episodes of AT occur in young adults in the absence of heart disease. The dysrhythmia is associated with rheumatic heart disease and pulmonary disorders.

The patient may complain of palpitations and experience anxiety during a tachycardic episode. Short, infrequent episodes require no treatment. Generally, hemodynamic changes are not severe unless the episode is prolonged, the rate is greater than 200 beats/min, or underlying disease exists. Lengthy episodes may respond to carotid sinus pressure or vagal stimulation. Some patients can be taught to perform Valsalva maneuvers to slow the rate. Depending on the electrophysiology associated with the atrial tachycardia, adenosine, intravenous calcium channel blockers, procainamide, and beta-blockers may be used to attempt to control the rhythm. For long-term management, symptomatic atrial

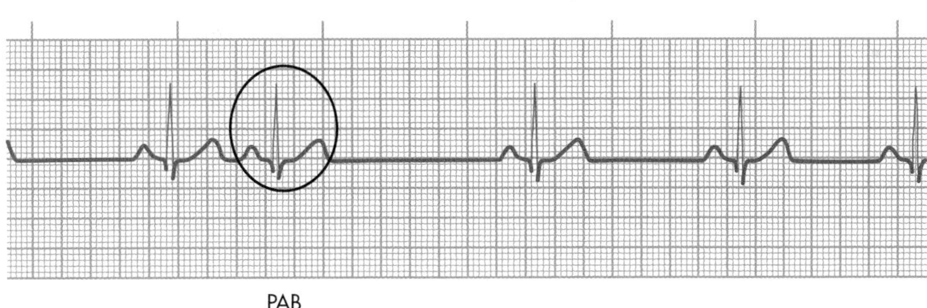

Figure 23-25 PAB in a sinus bradycardic rhythm; heart rate, 40 beats/min.

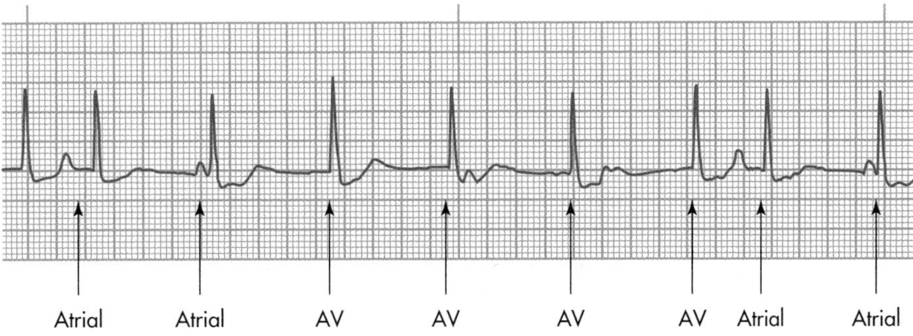

Figure 23-26 Wandering atrial pacemaker. Sites of origin; heart rate, 90 beats/min.

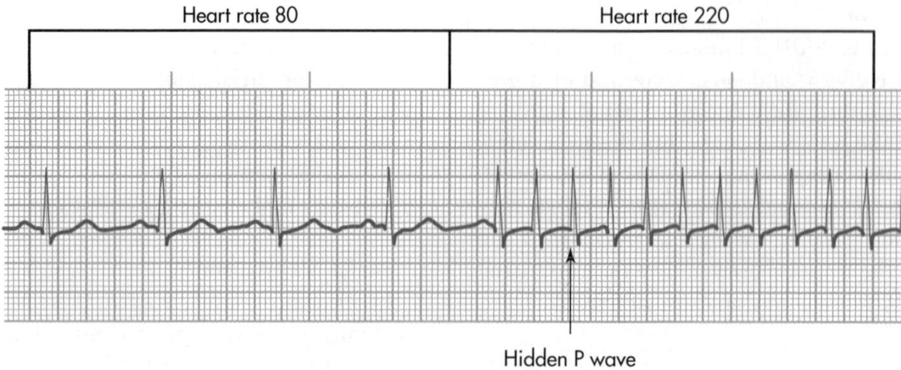

Figure 23-27 Normal sinus rhythm; heart rate, 80, progressing to AT; heart rate, 220 beats/min.

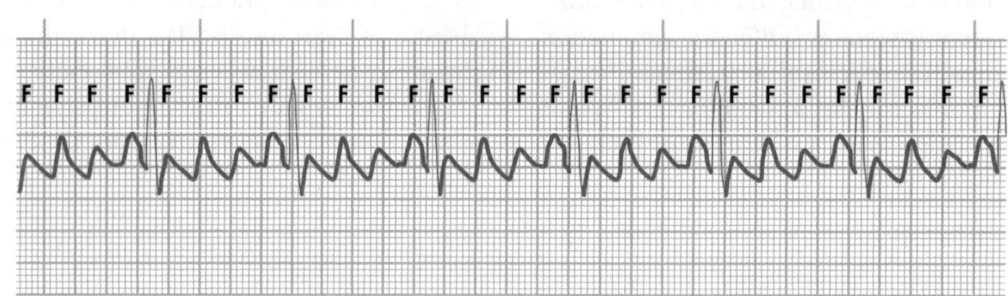

Figure 23-28 Atrial flutter, 4:1 block. Atrial heart rate, 260; ventricular heart rate, 60 beats/min.

tachycardia arising from reentry is treated with beta-blockers or calcium channel blockers. If these agents do not control the dysrhythmia, ablation of the ectopic focus with or without pacemaker insertion may be recommended instead of additional antidysrhythmic drugs.

Atrial tachycardia with block is characterized by the same rapid atrial rate, but some impulses are not conducted into the ventricles (i.e., they are blocked). The AV nodal conduction ratio is usually 2:1, producing a ventricular rate of 75 to 125 beats/min. This dysrhythmia is associated with organic heart disease and both digitalis toxicity and potassium deficit can cause it. Treatment depends on the clinical picture and often is aimed at correcting the underlying cause. Digitalis antibody may be indicated for hemodynamic compromise secondary to digitalis toxicity.

Atrial Flutter

In atrial flutter the atria depolarize at a rate of 250 to 350 beats/min. The atrial depolarizations produce flutter (F) waves that give the baseline a sawtooth appearance (Figure 23-28). The QRS configurations are normal. There is no measurable PR interval because it is difficult to determine electrocardiographically which atrial impulse actually is conducted to the ventricles. With rapid atrial rates, the AV node physiologically prevents conduction of each atrial impulse. The ventricles often respond to the impulses at a regular rate. The number of flutter waves to QRS complexes is expressed as a ratio (e.g., atrial flutter, 3:1 block).

Atrial flutter usually indicates underlying disease. It is associated most commonly with CAD, pulmonary embolism, mitral valve disease, thoracic surgical procedures, and chronic obstructive pulmonary disease.

The potentially rapid or slow ventricular rate of atrial flutter may result in a decrease in cardiac output. The major goal of treatment is control of the ventricular rate. Diltiazem, digoxin, or beta-blockers usually succeed in slowing the ventricular rate. Atropine may be used to augment the heart rate when the ventricular response is slow.

Cardioversion is highly successful in converting atrial flutter to sinus rhythm. Atrial pacing or catheter ablation may be used when pharmacologic intervention and external cardioversion have been unsuccessful.

Atrial Fibrillation

Atrial fibrillation (AF) is the most rapid atrial dysrhythmia (Figures 23-29 and 23-30). It is generated and perpetuated by one or more rapidly firing ectopic foci. The atria depolarize chaotically at rates of 350 to 600 beats/min. The baseline is composed of irregular undulations without definable P waves. The QRS complex usually is normal, but the ventricular rhythm is irregularly irregular.

Atrial fibrillation affects more than 2 million Americans, most of whom are 65 years of age or older.[1] Atrial fibrillation may be paroxysmal and transient, or chronic. The latter generally indicates underlying heart disease. It is typically associated with pericarditis, thyrotoxicosis, cardiomyopathy, CAD,

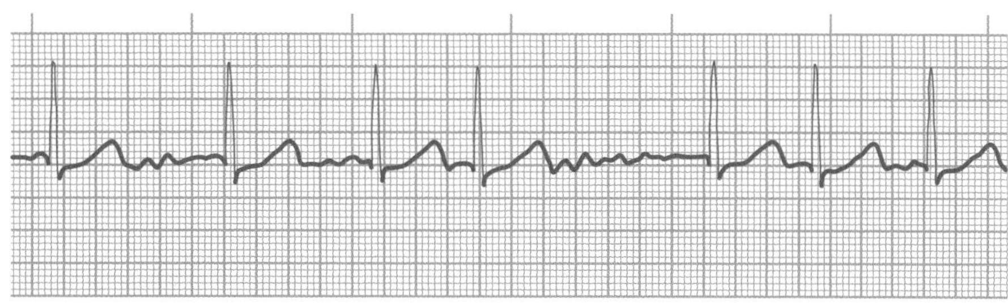

Figure 23-29 Rate controlled atrial fibrillation. Ventricular heart rate, 70 beats/min.

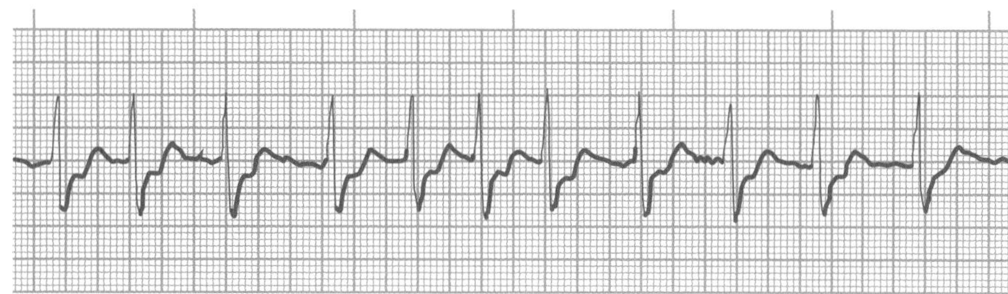

Figure 23-30 Atrial fibrillation with a rapid ventricular response. No distinguishable P waves. Ventricular heart rate, 110 beats/min.

hypertensive heart disease, rheumatic mitral valve disease, cardiac surgery, heart failure, and excessive alcohol intake ("holiday heart").

Atrial fibrillation causes irregularity in the ventricular rhythm and impairs the ventricular filling that normally occurs with synchronous atrial contractions (atrial kick), thus decreasing cardiac output. Symptoms include fatigue, dyspnea, and dizziness. Thrombi may form in the stagnant blood in the atria and cause emboli, which can lodge in the pulmonary or peripheral blood vessels. The goal of therapy is to prevent complications through control of the ventricular rate and the restoration of normal sinus rhythm (NSR).

Drugs used to control fast ventricular rates include diltiazem (Cardizem), verapamil (Calan), digoxin, and beta-blockers. Digoxin is not as effective in controlling the heart rate variations that occur with exercise. In atrial fibrillation with a slow ventricular response, atropine may be necessary to increase the heart rate and cardiac output. When medications are ineffective in controlling the rate and the patient is symptomatic from an ineffective cardiac output, cardioversion may be necessary to restore NSR and a more normal heart rate.

The severity of the patient's symptoms and hemodynamic instability guide treatment decisions. Several antidysrhythmics may be successful in converting AF to NSR, including ibutilide (Corvert), dofetilide (Tikosyn), amiodarone (Cordarone), sotalol (Betapace), procainamide (Pronestyl), and disopyramide (Norpace). These drugs can have a prodysrhythmic effect, and patients require careful monitoring.

External cardioversion is the most commonly used nonpharmacologic approach for restoring NSR. Internal atrial defibrillation is another treatment option. The maze procedure may also be used. In this procedure, sinus impulses travel down channels created by multiple atrial incisions to reach the AV node. Radiofrequency catheter ablation isolates and treats specific areas of atrial activity and has been successful in selected situations. Permanent pacemakers and implantable atrial defibrillators may also have a role. The risk of systemic emboli is high with persistent AF, and patients ideally are stabilized on warfarin therapy before any pharmacologic or electrical conversion attempts.

If the patient is hemodynamically unstable or has refractory symptoms, however, the need to electrically cardiovert may take priority. Transesophageal echocardiography (TEE) may be helpful in determining the presence of atrial thrombi. If no thrombi are found, the patient may be electrically cardioverted. Even after conversion to NSR, thrombi may still form until the atria contract effectively and in synchrony. Therefore anticoagulation therapy is continued for at least 4 weeks after conversion to NSR. If conversion to NSR is unsuccessful, the patient is maintained indefinitely on warfarin therapy. If the patient cannot tolerate warfarin, aspirin therapy may be used. A daily aspirin dose of 325 mg is recommended.

Premature Junctional Beats

Premature junctional beats (PJBs) arise from an ectopic focus either (1) at the junction of the atria and the AV node or (2) at the junction of the AV node and the bundle of His. If the PJBs arise from the first junction, the P wave will be inverted and premature and will precede the QRS complex. In the second case, the P wave is either hidden in the QRS or is inverted and follows the QRS (Figure 23-31). The abnormal timing and the inversion of the P wave are caused by depolarization of the atria in a retrograde fashion. The QRS is normal, but the PR interval is less than 0.12 second.

Premature junctional beats may occur in the normal heart. They also may result from digitalis toxicity, ischemia, hypoxia, pain, fever, anxiety, nicotine, caffeine, or electrolyte imbalance. Treatment, when needed, is directed toward correcting the underlying cause.

Junctional Rhythms

When the SA node fires at a rate less than 40 to 60 beats/min, the automatic cells in the AV junction may initiate impulses (escape beats) to stabilize the rhythm. A succession of beats from the junction is a junctional escape rhythm.

The P waves may occur before, during, or after the QRS. The QRS is normal, and the ventricular rhythm is regular. A junctional escape rhythm occasionally is found in the well-trained athlete or as a complication of an acute inferior wall MI. Junctional escape rhythm generally is not treated unless the loss of atrial kick produces symptoms of low cardiac output. These patients may require artificial pacing.

When the automaticity of a junctional pacemaker increases to a rate greater than 60 beats/min, it may usurp the SA node as the pacemaker of the heart. A rate of 60 to 100 beats/min is called an accelerated junctional rhythm (Figure 23-32). Accelerated junctional rhythm may be due to heart disease, pain, anemia, caffeine, or amphetamines.

A junctional tachycardia exists when the rate exceeds 100 beats/min. Junctional tachycardia is associated with digitalis toxicity, acute rheumatic fever, and heart disease; and treatment is aimed at alleviating the underlying cause. If the rate is interfering with cardiac output, vagal maneuvers may be attempted followed by digoxin, beta-blockers, or diltiazem administration.

Both junctional tachycardia and AT may be collectively referred to as supraventricular tachycardia (SVT), indicating that the rhythm originates above the ventricles. Symptomatic SVT from reentry may be treated with beta-blockers or calcium channel blockers. If these agents do not control the dysrhythmia, ablation of the irritable focus with or without pacemaker insertion may be recommended instead of antidysrhythmics.

Premature Ventricular Beats

A premature ventricular beat (PVB) is an early beat arising from an ectopic focus in the ventricles. The characteristic wide, bizarre QRS (usually greater than 0.12 second) makes the PVB readily identifiable on the ECG tracing. There is no associated P wave, and the T wave records in the opposite direction from the main QRS deflection. Most PVBs are followed by a pause until the next normal impulse originates in the SA node.

If PVBs are of different configurations on the ECG tracing, they are said to be multifocal. This indicates the presence of more than one ectopic focus in the ventricles, or one ectopic focus with multiple reentry pathways, each producing complexes of differing forms. Premature ventricular beats also may exhibit varying degrees of prematurity. The relationship of the PVB to the Q, R, S, and T waves of the preceding beat is important. An electrical impulse of any kind that stimulates the heart near the peak of the T wave (thereby preventing full repolarization of the ventricles) may precipitate a more dangerous or lethal dysrhythmia. The frequency and morphology of PVBs determine their importance. When every other beat is a PVB, the term

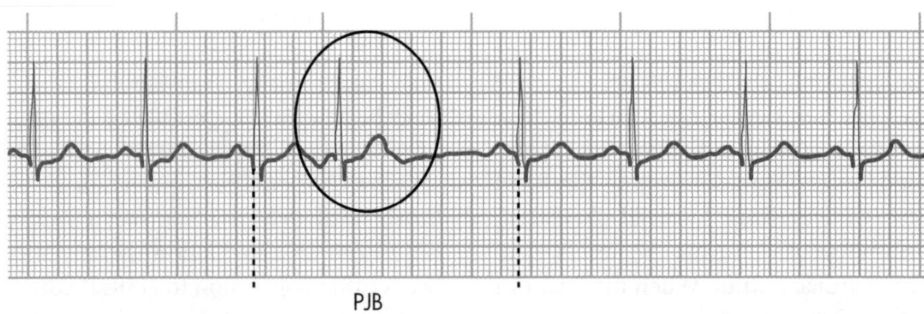

Figure 23-31 Sinus rhythm with a PJB; heart rate, 80 beats/min.

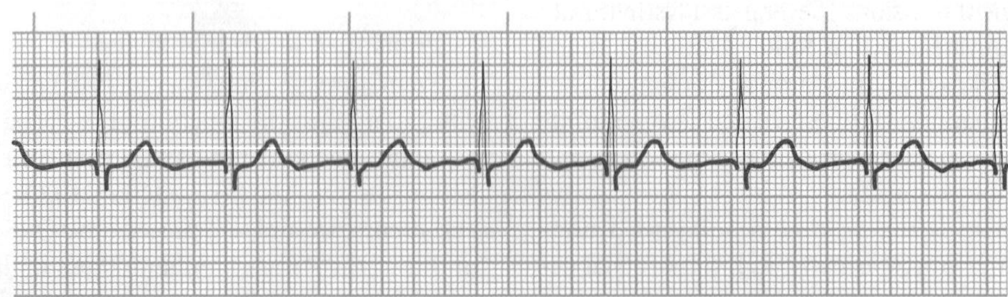

Figure 23-32 Accelerated junctional rhythm with hidden P waves; heart rate, 70 beats/min.

bigeminy is used; every third beat, *trigeminy,* and so forth (Figure 23-33). Two PVBs together are termed a *couplet.*

Premature ventricular beats occur in the absence of heart disease and increase in number with age. However, the incidence and frequency of occurrence are higher in the population with heart disease. Clinically, PVBs are associated with acute MI, heart failure, digitalis toxicity, hypoxia, stimulants, catecholamines, and electrolyte imbalances. In the latter cases treatment of the underlying cause may abolish the dysrhythmia.

Ventricular Rhythms and Tachycardia

If the SA node and AV junction fail to initiate impulses, a ventricular pacemaking cell automatically begins to initiate impulses at a rate of 20 to 40 beats/min. This is known as an idioventricular rhythm (Figure 23-34). P waves, when seen, are not associated with the ventricular rhythm and the QRS complex is greater than 0.12, wide, and bizarre.

If the rate of the ventricular-initiated rhythm increases to 40 to 100 beats/min, it is known as an accelerated idioventricular rhythm (AIVR). An AIVR may be seen in hypoxia, in digitalis toxicity, as a complication of an AMI, and as a reperfusion dysrhythmia after fibrinolytic therapy. Suppression of the heart's dominant and perhaps only rhythm could be hazardous. Therefore idioventricular rhythms are not treated except to correct underlying abnormalities.

If the cardiac output is low and symptoms of heart failure, syncope, or hypotension develop, the patient may require a temporary or permanent pacemaker. Atropine may be helpful in stimulating the return of SA node activity.

By definition, three or more successive PVBs constitute ventricular tachycardia (VT) (Figure 23-35). The ventricular rate is regular or slightly irregular, and is greater than 100 beats/min, usually 140 to 240 beats/min. P waves may be present but are not associated with the QRS complexes. Ventricular tachycardia may complicate any form of heart disease and may be a direct result of a PVB striking during the heart's action potential vulnerable period. Conditions that favor its occurrence include hypoxemia, drug toxicity, electrolyte imbalance, and bradycardia. Abnormal automaticity can occur in the postinfarction period from the loss of fast depolarizing sodium

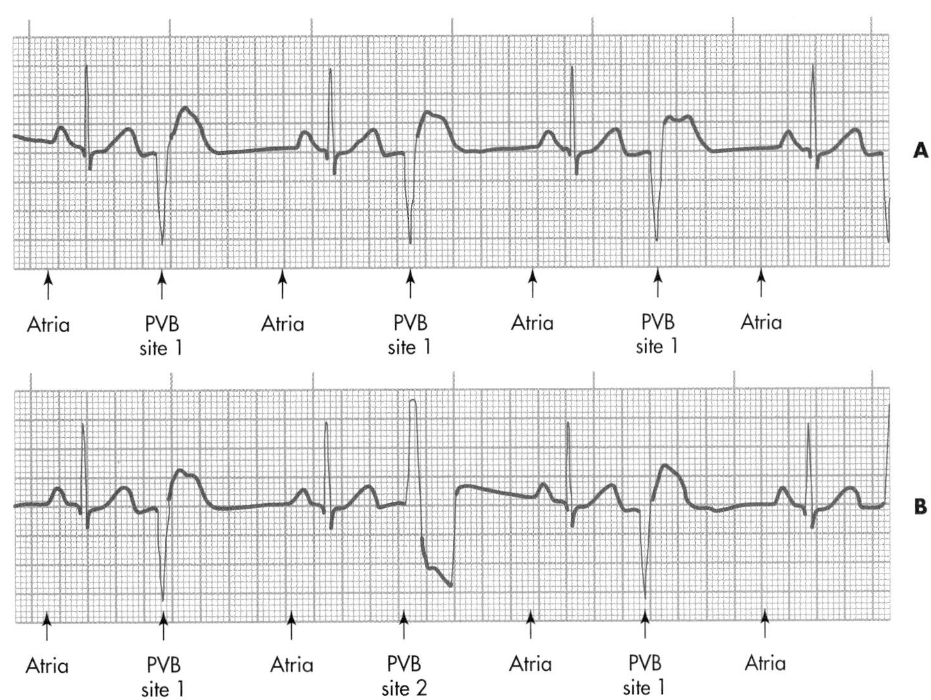

Figure 23-33 Bigeminy. **A,** Sinus rhythm with unifocal bigeminy PVBs; heart rate, 70 beats/min. **B,** Sinus rhythm with multifocal bigeminy PVBs; heart rate, 70 beats/min.

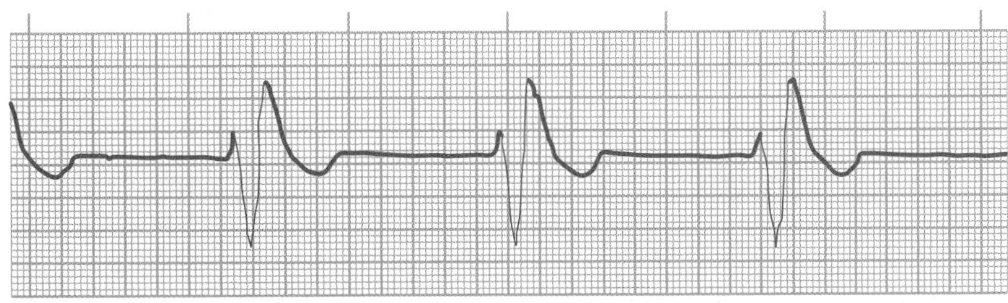

Figure 23-34 Idioventricular rhythm; ventricular heart rate, 30 beats/min.

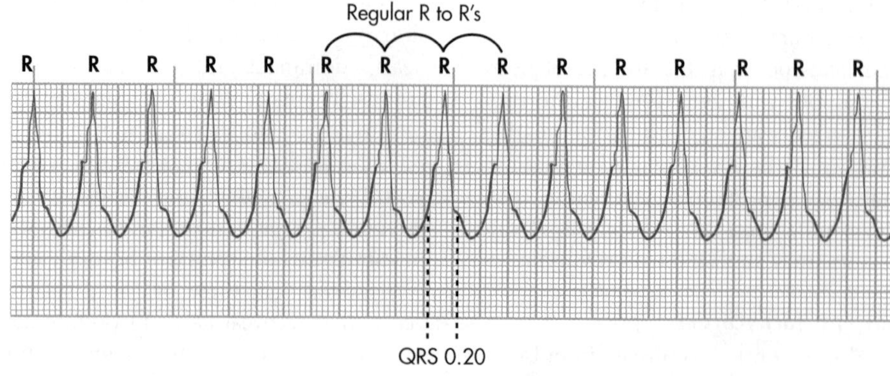

Figure 23-35 Ventricular tachycardia with regular R-to-R intervals and QRS greater than 0.12 second; heart rate, 150 beats/min.

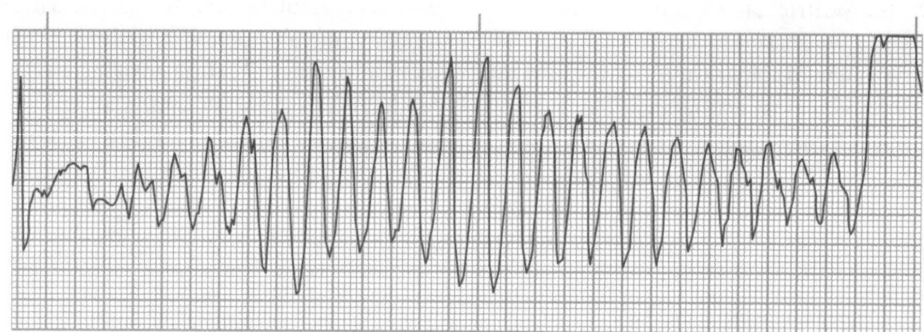

Figure 23-36 Torsades de pointes; heart rate, 240-250 beats/min.

channels, contributing to the development of VT. VT can also be attributable to ischemia, nonischemic heart disease, and drugs, and can even be found in the structurally normal heart (e.g., long QT syndrome). Treatment is based on the underlying electrophysiology of the dysrhythmia, which may be difficult to establish.

Ventricular tachycardia is classified as sustained (lasting more than 30 seconds) or nonsustained. Nonsustained VT may occur in patients with or without cardiac disease and is associated with palpitations or recurrent syncope. In the presence of severe ventricular dysfunction, nonsustained VT may be a precursor to sustained VT and sudden death. As the heart rate increases, cardiac output decreases as the ventricles do not have sufficient time to fill and empty. Symptoms vary depending on the length of the VT and the rate.

Intravenous lidocaine administration was standard therapy for VT for many years, but more efficacious antidysrhythmics are now available. If pharmacologic measures are unsuccessful, cardioversion is attempted. With pulseless VT, defibrillation is the standard of care. Intravenous amiodarone (Cordarone) and vasopressin have been added to advanced cardiac life support (ACLS) protocols to treat VT refractory to defibrillation. Long-term VT suppression is obtained with oral antidysrhythmic medications such as amiodarone or special procedures such as radiofrequency ablation.

Torsades de Pointes

Torsades de pointes, a variation of VT, can also progress to ventricular fibrillation (VF) if not managed appropriately. A long QT interval (over half of the corresponding RR interval) commonly precedes torsades de pointes. P waves, when seen, are dissociated from the QRS complexes. The QRS complexes are longer than 0.12 second and bizarre. The QRS complexes "twist" along the isoelectric baseline, varying in size and direction (Figure 23-36).

The rhythm may result from prolonged repolarization, represented on the ECG as a prolonged QT interval. Prolongation may occur secondary to various medications or electrolyte abnormalities, or it may be congenital in origin. Alterations in ion movement secondary to genetic mutations have been shown to be responsible for slightly more than 50% of researched cases of long QT syndromes.[2] Cardiac output decreases from inadequate ventricular filling and emptying that result from the increased heart rate.

Magnesium sulfate is administered to stabilize the electrical membrane. Lidocaine may be administered or other agents that do not prolong the QT interval may be tried. Cardioversion is commonly necessary. After resolution, the etiologic factors are eliminated or corrected, if possible.

Ventricular Fibrillation and Asystole

In VF the ventricular activity of the heart is chaotic, and the ECG tracing consists of unidentifiable waves. The fibrillatory waves may be coarse or fine (Figure 23-37). In the absence of depolarization there can be no effective ventricular contraction. The most common cause is coronary artery disease, and VF is frequently the terminal event in sudden cardiac death. It can also occur without warning after reperfusion.

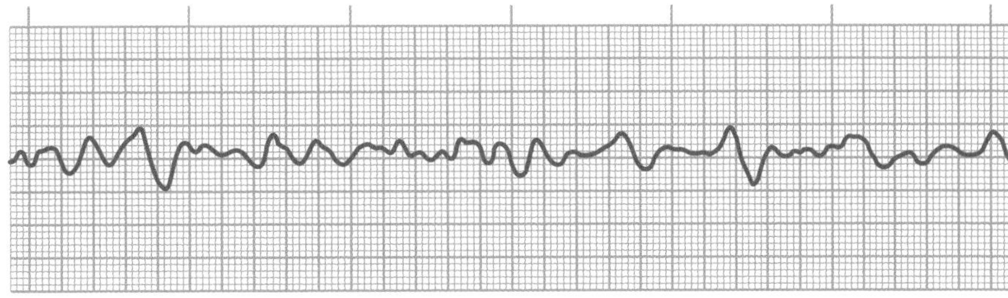

Figure 23-37 Coarse ventricular fibrillation; heart rate, not measurable.

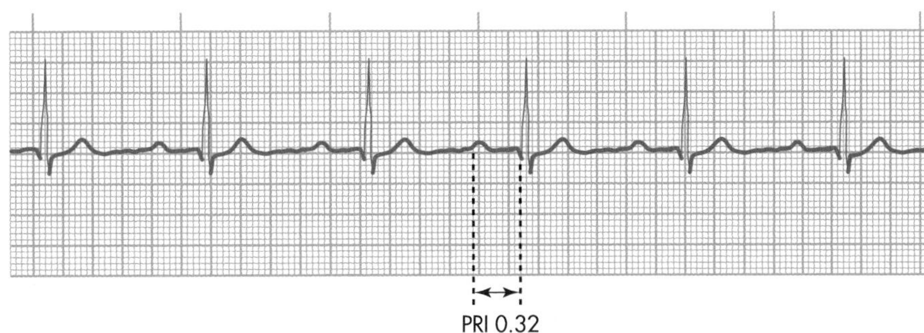

Figure 23-38 First-degree heart block. PR interval greater than 0.20 second.

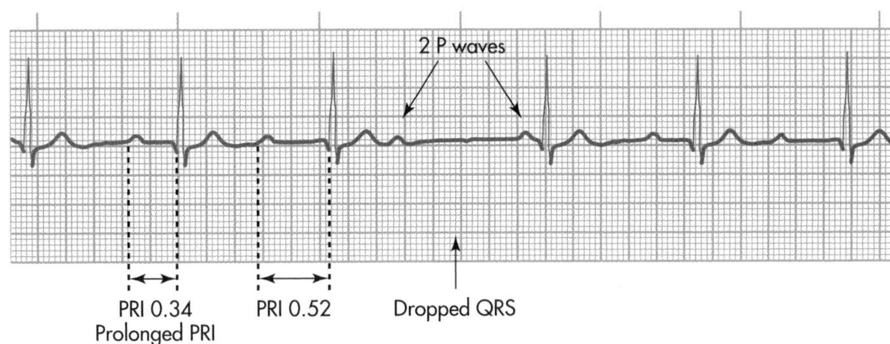

Figure 23-39 Mobitz I heart block. Atrial heart rate, 60 beats/min; ventricular heart rate, 50 beats/min.

Defibrillation is the only treatment for VF, and it must be performed as soon as possible. The administration of epinephrine may increase the effectiveness of defibrillation. Intravenous amiodarone (Cordarone) and vasopressin have also been added to the ACLS protocol for VF that is refractory to defibrillation.

In asystole the ECG tracing is a flat line and no electrical activity is noted; all pacemaking cells have failed. The patient has no blood pressure, pulse, or audible heartbeat; respirations quickly cease. Cardiopulmonary resuscitation (CPR) must be instituted immediately. Epinephrine, atropine, and external pacing are all used in the effort to restore cardiac excitability.

Pulseless electrical activity (PEA) is the term used to describe the presence of electrical activity in the absence of a heartbeat. CPR is instituted immediately along with measures to restore contraction. These may include pericardiocentesis, if tamponade is inhibiting contraction, or the administration of calcium to stimulate contractile force.

Atrioventricular Block

A block to impulse conduction can occur at any point along the conduction pathways. One common area is the AV junction. The severity of the block is identified by degrees, that is, first-, second-, or third-degree AV block. First-degree AV block is present when the PR interval is prolonged to greater than 0.20 second, indicating a conduction delay in the AV node (Figure 23-38). It usually is found in association with rheumatic fever, digoxin, beta-blockers, acute inferior MI, and increased vagal tone. When a first-degree AV block occurs in isolation, the patient is usually asymptomatic and no treatment is necessary.

Second-degree AV block may be subdivided into two categories. Type I (Wenckebach or Mobitz type I) is characterized by a PR interval that progressively lengthens until a P wave is not followed by a QRS complex (Figure 23-39). The nonconducted impulse arrives at the AV node during the refractory period. The ratio of P waves to QRS complexes may be 5:4, 4:3, 3:2, or 2:1 and creates a clustered appearance.

The pathology is usually within the AV node and produces QRS complexes of less than 0.12 second.

Any drug that slows AV conduction may cause a type I block, but such blocks are most often seen in the patient with an acute inferior wall MI, digitalis toxicity, increased vagal tone, electrolyte imbalance, acute myocarditis, or after cardiac surgery. Type I blocks often are transient and reversible and treatment is required unless the patient becomes symptomatic. Atropine may be effective in increasing cardiac output.

Type II (Mobitz type II) second-degree AV block is less common but more serious. A type II block is characterized by nonconducted sinus impulses despite constant PR intervals for the conducted P waves. The nonconducted P waves may occur at random or in patterned ratios (e.g., 2:1, 3:1) (Figure 23-40). The QRS complexes are widened unless the block is within the bundle of His.

Type II blocks may occur in CAD, MI, rheumatic heart disease, cardiomyopathy, and chronic fibrotic disease of the conduction system. If cardiac output is decreased, a temporary pacemaker usually is inserted prophylactically until the conduction stabilizes. If the block is persistent, the patient benefits from a permanent pacemaker.

In third-degree AV block (complete heart block) all the sinus or atrial impulses are blocked, and the atria and ventricles beat independently. Either a junctional or a ventricular pacemaker cell drives the ventricles. The lesion is usually in the bundle of His or the bundle branches but may also be at the AV junction. The rate and dependability of the ventricular rhythm are related to the level of the lesion. If a junctional pacemaker drives the ventricles, the ventricular rate will be at least 40 to 60 beats/min and the QRS complexes are narrow. This block may be a transient complication of inferior posterior MI or digitalis toxicity, or it may result from severe heart disease.

If a ventricular pacemaker drives the ventricles, the rate will be 20 to 40 beats/min, and the patient may experience syncope, heart failure, altered mentation, or angina. The QRS complex is abnormally wide, indicating that the block lies below the AV junction (Figure 23-41). The prognosis is more serious if complete heart block accompanies anterior MI. Generally the patient requires a permanent pacemaker. Epinephrine or isoproterenol administered intravenously may increase the ventricular rate temporarily until artificial pacing can be instituted.

Bundle Branch Block

In bundle branch block (BBB), one or both bundle branch paths of the conduction system are blocked. The impulse must travel a different path to stimulate the ventricle; therefore the QRS is prolonged to greater than 0.12 second. Instead of a synchronous QRS complex, each ventricle independently depolarizes, creating characteristic jagged QRS complexes (Figure 23-42). A BBB occurs as a permanent defect or as a transient block secondary to tachycardia, heart failure, AMI, pulmonary embolus, hypoxia, or metabolic derangements.

The right bundle branch is the more delicate of the two bundles and has a longer refractory period in some persons. In the younger patient right BBB often results from right ventricular hypertrophy, whereas CAD usually is the cause in the older patient. One classic ECG pattern is an M-shaped QRS in

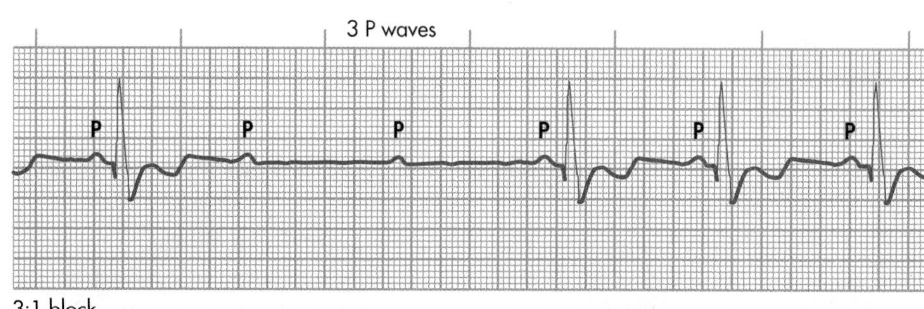

Figure 23-40 Mobitz II with a 3:1 heart block.

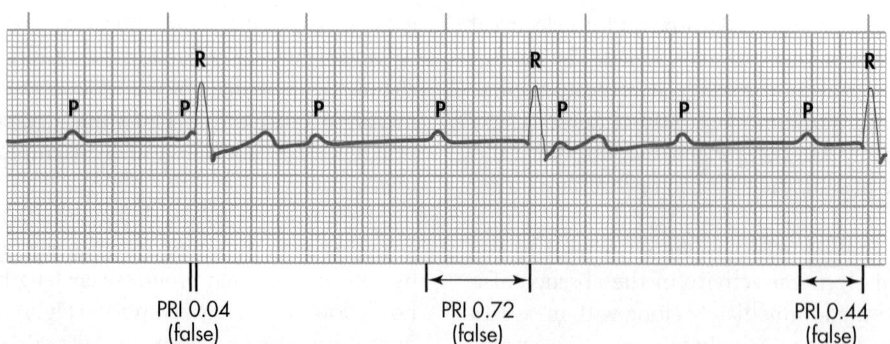

Figure 23-41 Separate P waves and QRS complexes of third-degree heart block. Atrial heart rate, 70 beats/min.; ventricular heart rate, 30 beats/min.

V_1 and V_2. In the absence of other conduction defects, no intervention is necessary.

The left bundle branch has a main trunk that bifurcates into the left anterior and left posterior divisions. A block may occur in the main trunk or in either of the divisions. (Blocks of the anterior or posterior division are known as left anterior hemiblock or left posterior hemiblock, respectively.) A block in the main trunk produces a complete left BBB resulting in a QRS greater than 0.12 second, large R waves in V_5 and V_6, and deep, wide S waves in V_1 through V_3. Left BBB is associated with severe CAD, valvular disease, hypertensive disease, cardiomegaly, and acute anterior wall MI. It also may occur as a result of degenerative changes in the conduction system. Whenever sufficient blockage is present to leave the heart dependent on just one fascicle for conduction to the ventricles, the patient is a candidate for a permanent pacemaker.

Treatment Options for Dysrhythmias

Collaborative care for the patient with a dysrhythmia includes diagnosing the specific dysrhythmia and its associated etiology and treating the disorder with medications or interventional procedures. Medications commonly used to manage dysrhythmias are presented in Table 23-9. The nurse must be knowledgeable about the mechanism of action of specific drugs and their associated nursing interventions. Careful attention is paid to potential drug interactions and synergistic effects when combination therapy is used. The metabolism and excretion of medications may be impaired in older adults and in patients with decreased perfusion to the kidneys and liver. The nurse must be aware of new agents approved for the management of cardiac dysrhythmias and how to monitor their safe use.

Nursing management of the patient experiencing dysrhythmias focuses on interventions to decrease oxygen demand. The nurse spaces activities and encourages frequent rest periods. While medication therapy is being adjusted, patients are on continuous monitoring (telemetry). Rhythms are documented every 4 to 8 hours and as needed. Skin care is provided to minimize the irritation of the monitoring electrodes.

The nurse must be alert to changes in the patient's rhythm. Assessments for changes in cardiac output are documented. Emergency drugs should be available, and intravenous access is ensured. Ancillary equipment such as defibrillators, oxygen, suction, and temporary pacemakers are kept readily available and in good working condition.

Interventions such as cardioversion, defibrillation, coronary ablation, pacemaker therapy, automatic implantable

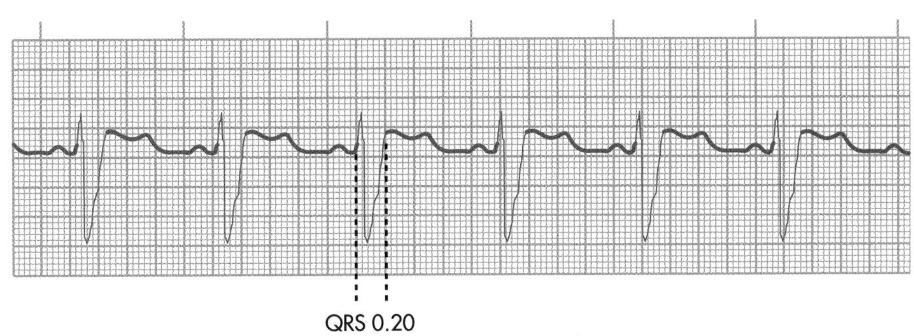

Figure 23-42 Sinus rhythm with a BBB; heart rate, 60 beats/min.

TABLE 23-9 Common Medications for Dysrhythmias

Drug	Action	Intervention
Quinidine Procainamide Disopyramide*	Inhibit sodium influx during phase 0 depolarization Prolong action potential and effective refractory period in atrium, bundle of His, and ventricle Indications: Atrial flutter, AF, SVT, VT	Quinidine: monitor QTc, PR, QRS; may cause tinnitus. Procainamide: administered PO or slow IV push followed by maintenance infusion; monitor for hypotension with IV initiation; monitor PR and QTc; may cause systemic lupus symptoms Disopyramide: monitor PR, QTc, QRS; may cause anticholinergic effects
Lidocaine Mexiletine Tocainide Moricizine†	Moderately inhibits sodium influx during phase 0 depolarization, decreasing automaticity; increases electrical stimulation threshold of ventricle, His-Purkinje system; shortens repolarization and action potential Indications: VT	Lidocaine: administered by IV push followed by maintenance infusion; toxic effects include confusion, psychosis, decreased hearing, seizures.

AF, Atrial flutter; *AP,* action potential; *AV,* atrioventricular; *BP,* blood pressure; *HF,* heart failure; *IV,* intravenous; *LV,* left ventricular; *PO,* by mouth; *PR,* pulse rate; *SA,* sinoatrial; *SVT,* supraventricular tachycardia; *VF,* ventricular flutter; *VT,* ventriciular tachycardia.
*The use of quinidine, procainamide, and disopyramide is decreasing due to newer, safer, and more efficacious drugs.

Continued

TABLE 23-9 Common Medications for Dysrhythmias

Drug	Action	Intervention
Flecainide Propafenone	Decreases sodium influx during phase 0 depolarization; reduces membrane responsiveness; inhibits automaticity; increases effective refractory period with little effect on action potential duration Indications: life-threatening dysrhythmias—not first-line drugs	Propafenone: significantly decreases inotropic activity; use with caution in LV dysfunction.‡
Propranolol Acebutalol Esmolol Metoprolol	Inhibit beta adrenoreceptors and slow ventricular rate through action on slow calcium channels of AV node that are coupled with beta-1 receptors Indications: dysrhythmias of abnormal automaticity, triggered activity, or reentry	Administer PO or slow IV push Monitor PR and BP Teach patient not to discontinue abruptly Monitor for HF in susceptible patients
Amiodarone Sotalol	Block outward potassium channels or facilitate the slow inward sodium current; lengthen refractory period Depress SA node automaticity and conduction in AV node Indications: VF and VT, Atrial flutter and AF (but not FDA approved for atrial dysrhythmias)	Amiodarone§: increases warfarin effect. May cause thyroid dysfunction, pulmonary toxicity, blue-gray skin discoloration Half-life: 15-100 days with PO onset 1-3 weeks Monitor PR and QTc Sotalol§: normalize potassium and magnesium before therapy. Monitor PR and QTc
Ibutilide Dofetilide	Block outward potassium channels or facilitate the slow inward sodium current; lengthen repolarization by prolonging action potential. Indications: atrial flutter and AF	Ibutilide: for intravenous cardioversion of AF in critical care unit. QTc should be less than 0.44 before infusion. Dofetilide: dose adjusted to creatinine clearance and QTc
Diltiazem Verapamil	Increase effective refractory period in AV node; inhibit calcium ion influx across cell membrane during cardiac depolarization; slow SA and AV node conduction times. Indications: atrial flutter, AF, SVT	Administer PO or slow IV push Avoid in patients with accessory pathways or wide-complex tachycardia May cause hypotension Direct depressant effect on contractility, use with caution in LV dysfunction
Adenosine	Depresses SA node and slows conduction through the AV node; can interrupt reentry pathways through AV node Indications: SVT	Administered rapid IV push followed by 20-ml flush Half-life 10 seconds Transient side effects include flushing, labored breathing, chest pain Effects blocked by methylxanthines and caffeine
Atropine	Increases heart rate by blocking vagal stimulation, increasing automaticity of SA node and conduction in AV node Indications: symptomatic bradydysrhythmias	May be given IV or endotracheally Increases oxygen demand with increased heart rate
Calcium chloride	Cation needed for cardiac contractility Indications: asystole	Give slow IV push: extravasation will result in necrosis
Digoxin	Direct suppression of the AV node Indications: AF, atrial flutter, SVT	Check apical pulse for 1 minute; if less than 50 notify primary care provider Hypokalemia increases risk of digoxin toxicity Monitor for therapeutic drug levels Administered PO or slow IV push Will increase contractility
Epinephrine	$Beta_1$ and $beta_2$ agonist increasing automaticity Indications: asystole, refractory VT/VF	Given intravenously or endotracheally Increases oxygen demand
Isoproterenol	Causes increased contractility and heart rate by acting on $beta_1$ and $beta_2$ receptors in heart Indications: symptomatic bradydysrhythmias	Given intravenously
Magnesium sulfate	Reduces SA node impulse formation, prolongs conduction time in myocardium Indications: documented hypomagnesemia with dysrhythmias, torsades de pointes	Monitor magnesium levels

†The use of these drugs, including lidocaine, (historically a first line choice for VT), is gradually decreasing in favor of safer, more efficacious antidysrhythmics.
‡These drugs are not recommended for use in patients with coronary artery disease due to an increased incidence of mortality and nonfatal cardiac arrest in patients after myocardial infarction.
§Among the most widely used antidysrhythmics.

cardioverter-defibrillators, and cardiopulmonary resuscitation are also part of the collaborative care strategies used for patients with dysrhythmias.

Patient/Family Education. The nurse directly addresses the patient's and family's fears and concerns, recognizing that living with a potentially life-threatening dysrhythmia is a challenge for the patient and family (see Research box). Patients are taught about the specific dysrhythmia, the treatment plan, and the importance of seeking medical attention promptly if symptoms recur. They should also know how to take the patient's pulse and the types of pulse changes that need to be reported. The nurse reviews the common side effects of the antidysrhythmic agents with the patient and encourages the patient to discuss the incidence and severity of side effects with a health care professional. Patients are cautioned not to adjust the dose or discontinue the use of any prescribed medication. Follow-up is essential in monitoring medication therapy and response.

Cardioversion and Defibrillation. Cardioversion and defibrillation use electrical energy to convert a cardiac dysrhythmia to a rhythm that is hemodynamically stable, preferably a sinus rhythm. Electrophysiologically the electrical countershock produces a simultaneous depolarization of a critical mass of cardiac fibers, thus halting the asynchronous chaos of a fibrillation or the rapid firing of a tachycardia. In some cases, especially in elective cardioversion, the shock will be delivered more than once until the required level of voltage is reached.

Research

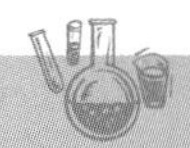

Reference: Cowan MJ et al: Psychosocial nursing therapy following sudden cardiac arrest: impact on two-year survival, *Nurs Res* 50(2):68, 2001.

Nurse researchers studied the effectiveness of psychosocial therapy as an intervention to decrease cardiovascular mortality for sudden cardiac arrest (SCA) survivors. These patients had electrocardiographic documentation of out-of-hospital ventricular fibrillation or asystole arrests. A total of 129 patients were randomized into two groups. The treatment group received 11 individual sessions composed of cardiovascular health education, physiologic relaxation with biofeedback, and cognitive behavioral therapy aimed at self-management and coping strategies for depression, anxiety, and anger. The second group received only conventional cardiovascular education. Two cardiovascular nurses conducted the therapy sessions. Researchers made follow-up phone calls to participants every 6 months for 2 years to determine mortality, implantable defibrillator firing incidence, recurrent SCA, and recurrent myocardial infarction (MI). Eight patients died, 7 in the control group and 1 in the treatment group. Six of the 7 deaths in the control group were associated with SCA with documented ventricular fibrillation or asystole. The remaining two deaths (one in each group) were due to strokes. Therapeutic benefits were consistent even after controlling for other predictors of mortality, including depression, hypertension, low ejection fractions, heart failure, medications, and heart rate variability. Researchers believe this is the first prospective randomized study to demonstrate efficacy of a psychosocial therapy on secondary prevention of sudden cardiac death. They encourage study replication to validate the findings.

Once the heart is fully depolarized, the SA node is better able to resume control.

Defibrillation applies an unsynchronized electrical countershock during a ventricular fibrillation emergency or pulseless ventricular tachycardia. The paddles from the defibrillator are placed at the third intercostal space to the right of the sternum and the fifth intercostal space on the left midaxillary line. Conducting gel or saline pads are applied between the paddles and the skin to ensure conductance and to minimize skin burning. The button on each paddle is depressed simultaneously to release 200 to 360 watt-seconds (joules) to the patient. Defibrillation must be performed quickly for ventricular fibrillation and most cases of ventricular tachycardia.

Cardioversion differs from defibrillation in that the electrical discharge is synchronized with the R wave to avoid triggering ventricular fibrillation from accidental discharge during the vulnerable period. Indications for cardioversion include hemodynamically unstable atrial flutter, atrial fibrillation, and atrial tachycardia. Patients are prepared psychologically for what to expect during cardioversion and are reassured that they will be sedated with intravenous diazepam (Valium), midazolam (Versed), or fentanyl.

The procedure is performed in a special laboratory and not the patient's room. The defibrillator is synchronized so that the impulse is not initiated until the next R wave occurs. This eliminates the danger of entering the vulnerable period. For most elective procedures, the amount of watt-seconds or joules required for conversion is lower than that required for defibrillation. The patient is monitored after cardioversion until vital signs are stable.

Internal atrial cardioversion may be an alternative when external cardioversion fails. Two small electrode catheters are placed in the right atrium and coronary sinus to accomplish the cardioversion. A bipolar catheter is placed in the right ventricle to precisely time the cardioversion. The patient is under conscious sedation during the procedure.[18]

Radiofrequency Catheter Ablation. An estimated 15,000 catheter ablation procedures are performed annually in the United States.[18] The procedure involves the insertion of a catheter, usually through the patient's femoral or jugular vein, that delivers programmed electrical stimulation to recreate the patient's dysrhythmia and localize the area for ablation. The site of origin for the dysrhythmia, or the pathway necessary for its propagation is then destroyed using radiofrequency energy, a form of high-frequency electromagnetic waves. The thermal energy causes coagulation necrosis in the area selected for ablation. The amount of damage caused by the catheter is relatively small because the energy used can be precisely regulated and focused. The patient remains in the electrophysiology laboratory for a short interval after the procedure for observation. Attempts are then made to reinitiate the dysrhythmia, using electrical or pharmacologic stimulation. If the dysrhythmia recurs, additional ablation bursts are administered until the site is destroyed. Indications for catheter ablation include AV node reentry tachycardias, accessory pathways (such as Wolff-Parkinson-White), focal atrial tachycardia, atrial flutter, and bundle-branch reentry.[7] Atrial fibrillation may also be treated by ablation of the AV node with pacemaker insertion. Ablation is also an alternative in select cases of ventricular tachycardia. Complications related to the procedure are rare but may include vascular access problems (hematomas, femoral pseudoaneurysms), the formation of catheter-induced thrombi, and myocardial perforation. The most common complication of AV node associated dysrhythmias is heart block.[18] Patient teaching is a major focus of nursing intervention because the procedure is not widely known and preprocedure anxiety is often high (see Patient Teaching box).

Pacemakers. Indications for pacemakers include the presence of symptomatic chronic or recurrent dysrhythmias unresponsive to pharmacologic therapy (Box 23-3). Pacemakers may be permanent, temporary, or external. Permanent pacemakers use a pulse generator as the "control center" for the pacemaker's functions (Figure 23-43). The generator attaches to one or two leads that are positioned in the right ventricle or right atrium (Figure 23-44). These leads are flexible, insulated wires with electrodes for sensing the heart's rhythm and delivering electrical impulses when necessary. The leads are introduced into the myocardium transvenously under fluoroscopic visualization through the subclavian or jugular vein. A guidewire facilitates correct placement of the leads against the atrial or ventricular endocardium. A surgically created subcutaneous pocket encloses the generator, most often infraclavicularly.

The procedure can be performed under local anesthesia. Before insertion of a permanent pacemaker, the patient receives information about the indication for the pacemaker, potential complications, the procedure itself, and pacemaker care (see Patient Teaching box on p. 695). Complications of pacemaker therapy include pacemaker malfunction, cardiac perforation and tamponade, pneumothorax and hemothorax, and infection. The nurse teaches the patient about permanent pacemakers and addresses any concerns over device failure. Nursing responsibilities before and after permanent pace-

Patient Teaching
The Patient Undergoing Radiofrequency Catheter Ablation

PREPROCEDURE

- Indication for procedure
- Potential complications
- Withholding of antidysrhythmics per physician orders
- Avoid caffeine and alcohol 24 hours before procedure
- NPO for 8 hours before the procedure
- Intravenous access for fluids, sedation, and cardiac medications
- Shaving and scrub of femoral site and right neck
- Potential for indwelling urinary catheter
- Preprocedure tests: clotting studies, chest x-ray study, baseline electrocardiogram

INTRAPROCEDURE

- Sedation throughout procedure
- Possible discomfort in groin and neck–local anesthetic used
- Cardiac monitor at all times
- Sterile drapes to prevent infection at access sites
- Medications readily available to test effectiveness of procedure or to treat dysrhythmias should they occur.

POSTPROCEDURE

- Access sheath pulled immediately after procedure
- Vital signs, access site, and neurovascular checks q15min ×4, then q30min until patient stabilized
- Baseline 12-lead electrocardiogram obtained
- Bed rest usually for 4 to 6 hours; analgesic and backrubs for back pain
- Need to report any pleuritic or chest pain

DISCHARGE

- May be discharged same day
- Daily aspirin
- Avoid prolonged sitting for first day
- Avoid strenuous activity for 72 hours
- Avoid driving for 24 hours
- Signs and symptoms of infection or complications at access site
- Signs and symptoms of dysrhythmia recurrence

BOX 23-3 Indications for Cardiac Pacing: American Heart Association Guidelines 2000

Hemodynamically unstable bradycardia (less than 50 beats/min)
Mobitz type II second-degree atrioventricular block (atropine may precipitate a third-degree block)
Third-degree heart block
Bilateral bundle-branch block (alternating BBB or RBBB with alternating LBBB)
Left anterior fascicular block
Newly acquired or age-indeterminate LBBB
RBBB or LBBB and first-degree atrioventricular block
Early-onset asytole

BBB, Bundle-branch block; *RBBB*, right bundle-branch block; *LBBB*, left bundle-branch block.

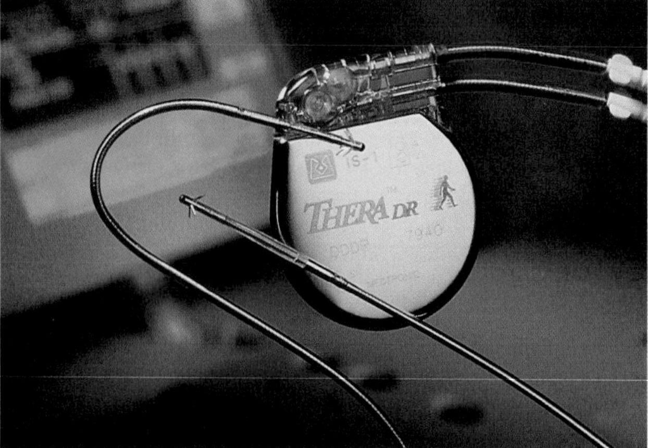

Figure 23-43 A permanent pacemaker (pulse generator) that can be implanted in subcutaneous tissue below the patient's clavicle or in the abdomen. The pacing wires are then threaded to the patient's heart.

maker implantation are summarized in the Guidelines for Safe Practice box.

The pacemakers in use today have multiple capabilities that can be identified through a 5-letter pacemaker code (Table 23-10). The last two letters of the code describe specific features such as antitachycardic pacing and rate-responsive pacing. When an antitachycardic pacemaker senses a heart rate above its programmed limit, it paces at a heart rate just above the patient's tachycardia to take control of the heart. The pacemaker then slows the rhythm to an acceptable rate. Rate-responsive pacemakers allow pacing at accelerated heart rates when the pacemaker senses programmed indicators of increased activity such as changes in oxygen saturation, cardiac output, or blood temperature.

Figure 23-45 shows the ECG appearance of pacemaker-stimulated heartbeats. Paced beats are readily identifiable by the sharp spike that precedes the ECG complex. The paced QRS complex is wide because initiation of the impulse occurs in the ventricle (as with a PVB).

If a pacemaker should malfunction, the patient usually experiences a recurrence of symptoms. However, the nurse must be able to diagnose the following ECG indicators of pacemaker malfunction: loss of sensing, loss of capture, and failure to pace. Table 23-11 describes common pacemaker problems and interventions to troubleshoot them. A Nursing Care Plan for a patient undergoing pacemaker insertion is on pp. 697 to 699.

Temporary pacemakers are indicated for the short-term management of dysrhythmias until the patient's rhythm stabilizes or a permanent pacemaker can be inserted. The pacer wire is advanced transvenously to the right ventricle and the leads are attached to an external pulse generator box (Figure 23-46, p. 699). The environment must be kept free from electrical hazards that could trigger dysrhythmias. Temporary epicardial pacing is used after cardiac surgery. The epicardial wires are attached to the right atrium and right ventricle during the surgical procedure, and are brought out through the chest wall and sutured to the skin. Care of the patient with a temporary pacemaker is summarized in the Guidelines for Safe Practice box on p. 700.

External cardiac pacing requires the application of two electrodes to the chest wall, one over the cardiac apex and the other on the back beneath the left scapula (Figure 23-47, p. 700). An electrical current flows between the electrodes and is controlled by the device operator. Most external pacing devices function in the demand mode. An oscilloscope allows monitoring of the pacemaker activity. External pacers are primarily used for patients with unstable rhythms in emergency

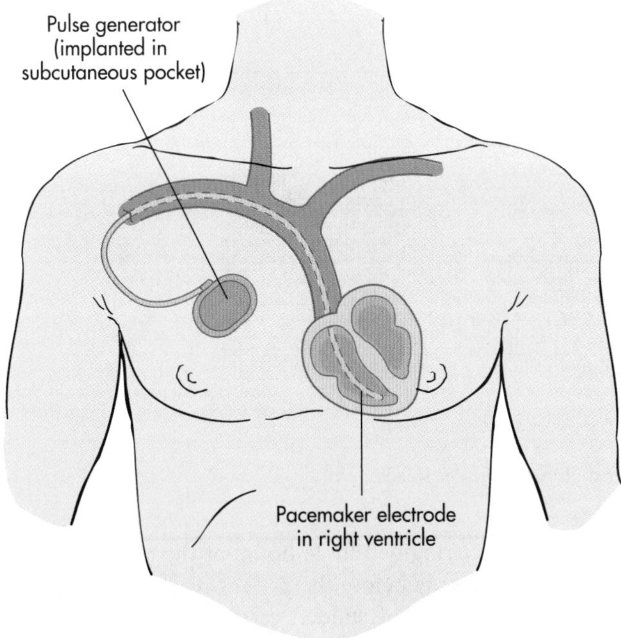

Figure 23-44 Permanent pacemaker placement.

Patient Teaching
The Patient With a Permanent Pacemaker

PERMANENT PACEMAKERS–PROCEDURAL

- Indication for pacemaker
- Potential complications
- NPO for 8 hours before the procedure
- Pretests, including baseline 12-lead ECG and bleeding function studies
- Cardiac monitor at all times during the procedure
- IV access for fluids, cardiac medications, and sedation
- Prep and shave area where generator will be implanted
- Anesthesia of access sites
- Sterile field during procedure
- Analgesics offered postprocedure
- Restricted movement of affected arm for 48 hours
- Routine chest x-ray to check placement

PERMANENT PACEMAKER–DISCHARGE

- Monitor site for infection and bleeding the first week.
- Avoid immersion of site in water for 3 days (tub bath OK).
- Steri-strips will come off in about 1 week.
- Limit range of motion of affected arm and wear loose covering over incision for 1 week.
- Avoid lifting more than 10 pounds until cleared by physician.
- Avoid contact sports.
- Contact health care professional with fatigue, palpitations, or recurrence of symptoms (may indicate battery depletion or pacemaker malfunction).
- Importance of follow-up via transtelephonic means or office visits.
- Carry pacemaker information at all times; can trigger alarms with some airport security.
- Pacemaker may need to be programmed to fixed mode.
- Special grounding precautions taken for certain medical procedures (electrocautery, radiation therapy, MRI, lithotripsy).
- Place cellular phones on the ear opposite the pacemaker. Carry cellular phones away from pacemaker site. (Newer cellular phones may not cause concern. Check individually.)
- Move away from electrical devices if dizziness experienced.
- Avoid working over large, running motors.
- How to take radial pulse–notify health care professional for rates outside those programmed (may indicate pacemaker malfunction or battery depletion).

Guidelines for Safe Practice

The Patient Undergoing Permanent Pacemaker Insertion

PREPROCEDURE

- Establish assessment baselines: vital signs, 12-lead electrocardiogram (ECG), peripheral pulses, heart and lung sounds, mental status.
- Teach patient per patient/family education guidelines.
- Maintain NPO status for 8 hours.
- Establish intravenous (IV) access for IV administration of fluids, sedation, and emergency drugs.
- Assess anxiety level and intervene appropriately with active listening, reassurance, education, and sedation as needed.

INTRAPROCEDURE

- Shave and scrub access site.
- Maintain sterile field.
- Cardiac monitor at all times.
- Assess patient's anxiety level and intervene appropriately with reassurance and sedation as needed.

POSTPROCEDURE

- Monitor for complications of insertion such as pneumothorax, hemothorax, perforation, tamponade.
- Be alert to lead dislodgement, manifested by ECG changes or hiccups if diaphragm is being paced.
- Control pain: provide analgesics and nonpharmacologic interventions (positioning, distraction) as needed.
- Obtain baseline ECG and monitor for loss of sensing, loss of capture, or failure to pace.
- Assess insertion site for bleeding and infection.
- Ensure bed rest for 12 hours.
- Limit range of motion of affected arm for 12 to 24 hours.
- Apply ice pack to minimize pain and swelling for first 6 hours.
- Do not administer aspirin or heparin for 48 hours.
- If defibrillation is necessary, anterior-posterior placement is preferable; avoid area surrounding generator site.
- If patient is symptomatic from pacer malfunction, enforce bed rest, follow safety precautions for syncope potential, monitor vital signs frequently, and obtain a 12-lead ECG to diagnose malfunction.
- Monitor continuous telemetry, obtain IV access (with atropine at bedside), provide oxygen if needed, perform chest x-ray study to check lead position, and use pacemaker magnet to convert pacemaker to fixed mode if indicated.
- Provide discharge teaching per patient/family teaching guidelines.

TABLE 23-10 Intersociety Commission for Heart Disease (ICHD) Codes for Pacemakers

Chamber(s) Paced	Chamber(s) Sensed	Mode of Responses (sensing function)	Programmable Functions	Special Tachydysrhythmia Functions
V: ventricle A: atrium D: double (dual)	V: ventricle A: atrium D: double (dual) O: none	T: triggered I: inhibited (demand) D=Double (dual function: T and I) O: none (continuous) R: reverse	P: programmable M: multiprogrammable O: none (permanent pacemakers only)	B: bursts N: normal rate competition (dual demand) S: scanning E: external

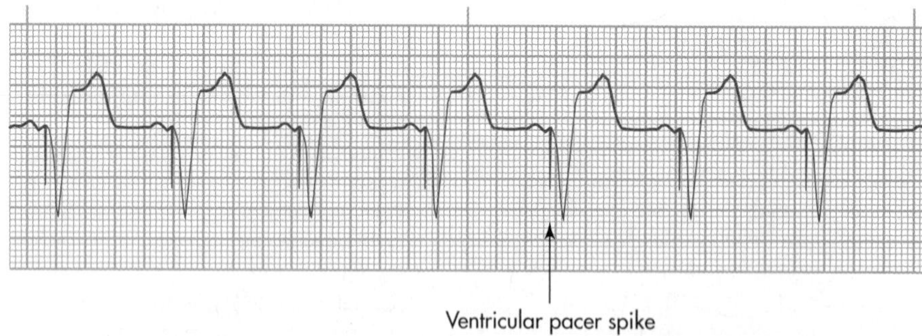

Figure 23-45 Ventricular pacemaker rhythm with pacer spikes.

situations. The nurse anticipates patient discomfort when the patient requires external pacing and offers supportive care and pain management.

Implantable Cardioverter Defibrillators. More than half the deaths from CAD in the United States each year are sudden deaths occurring within 24 hours of the onset of symptoms and commonly before the patient reaches the hospital. The pathophysiology of sudden cardiac death remains obscure, with only 20% of sudden deaths associated with MI. Researchers theorize that the cause of sudden cardiac death is

TABLE 23-11 Troubleshooting Pacemaker Malfunction

Problem	Definition	ECG Finding	Physiologic Effect	Nursing Action
Loss of sensing—oversensing	Pacemaker senses an extraneous signal as an impulse and therefore does not pace	Pause	Decreased cardiac output	Decrease sensitivity of pacemaker Check for electromagnetic interference and proper grounding of equipment (temporary pacemaker)
Loss of sensing—undersensing	Pacemaker does not sense heart's own impulse and therefore thinks it has to pace the heart	Inappropriate pacing (extra beats)	Danger of pacing in the vulnerable period causing ventricular tachycardia	Increase sensitivity to heart's rhythm
Loss of capture	Pacemaker fires but does not depolarize the ventricle	Spike present but without QRS complex	Decrease in cardiac output	Increase milliamperes (energy delivered); turn to left side (bring lead in better contact with endocardium) Check all connections (temporary pacemaker) Determine etiology of ventricle not responding and correct electrolyte abnormality, ischemia, lead dislodgement
Failure to pace	Electrical impulse never initiated	Pause without spikes	Decrease in cardiac output	External/temporary pacemaker at bedside Assess response and treat symptoms until etiology determined and corrected (dislodged lead, battery depletion, malfunctioning pulse generator)

Nursing Care Plan *Patient Receiving a Permanent Pacemaker*

DATA Ms. P. is a 75-year-old woman who was admitted with shortness of breath, chest pain, and heart failure. Past medical history includes a coronary artery bypass graft of the right coronary artery 10 years ago and a non–Q wave myocardial infarction 2 years ago. Noncardiac history includes type 2 diabetes mellitus of 20 years' duration. Ms. P's admitting medical diagnosis was unstable angina. Cardiac catheterization revealed native right coronary and left anterior descending coronary artery disease and 90% occlusion of the graft to the right coronary artery. After cardiac catheterization, Ms. P. experienced symptomatic junctional bradycardia requiring placement of a temporary pacemaker. Because of the potential for heart failure from her bradycardia and the alchemic blood supply to her conduction system, the decision was made to proceed with permanent pacemaker placement. Ms. P. underwent DDD pacemaker placement 6 days after admission to the hospital. Her postoperative course has been uncomplicated and plans are being made for her discharge to home. Ms. P's daughter will be assisting her at home. Ms. P. and her daughter voice concern that the pacemaker will fail and they will not know what to do.

NURSING DIAGNOSIS **Fear related to deficient knowledge of pacemaker function and care**
GOALS/OUTCOMES Patient/family will verbalize understanding of cardiac pacemaker function and decreased feelings of fear regarding pacemaker care

NOC Suggested Outcomes
- Fear Control (1404)
- Anxiety Control (1402)
- Coping (1302)
- Comfort Level (2100)

NIC Suggested Interventions
- Anxiety Reduction (5820)
- Coping Enhancement (5230)
- Emotional Support (5270)
- Teaching: Procedure/Treatment (5618)

Continued

Nursing Care Plan *Patient Receiving a Permanent Pacemaker—cont'd*

Nursing Interventions/Rationales

- Provide teaching/information. *To prevent distortions. Misinterpretation can increase fear and anxiety.*
- Teach patient how to problem solve. Have patient verbalize symptoms experienced during dysrhythmic event. *Knowing when to worry vs. appropriate expectations helps the patient identify areas requiring medical attention and/or follow up care.*
- Teach skills to enhance control. Instruct patient how to self-monitor for symptoms of pacemaker malfunction (daily pulse checks, trans-telephonic recordings). *Understanding home care (including monitoring for pacemaker malfunction) increases the patient's confidence in her ability to comply with treatment recommendations.*
- Provide written materials that reinforce teaching. *Written information provides a later resource for information that may have been forgotten or misunderstood.*
- Initiate referral for skilled home health nursing until first follow-up visit with cardiologist to monitor the surgical site, assess knowledge retention and application. *The availability of follow-up provides positive reinforcement of the patient's actions for self-care and decreases the patient's fears and anxiety.*
- Arrange for the patient to meet with another patient who successfully lives at home independently with a permanent pacemaker. *Learning from the successes of others helps the patient to identify misconceptions, areas where assistance may be needed and builds self-confidence.*

Evaluation Parameters

1. Reports feelings of comfort with functioning of pacemaker
2. Verbalizes understanding of symptoms that indicate pacemaker malfunction and need to be reported immediately
3. Accurately demonstrates pulse checks, trans-telephonic recording

NURSING DIAGNOSIS **Impaired physical mobility related to incisional site pain, activity restrictions, and fear of lead displacement**

GOALS/OUTCOMES
1. Will verbalize prescribed restrictions
2. Will perform activities of daily living (ADLs) with minimal complaints of discomfort
3. Will describes resources to assist with ADLs until physical mobility improves

NOC Suggested Outcomes

- Mobility Level (0208)
- Adherence Behavior (1600)
- Knowledge: Prescribed Activity (1811)

NIC Suggested Interventions

- Positioning (0840)
- Self-Care Assistance (1800)
- Teaching: Prescribed Activity/Exercise (5612)
- Pain Management (1400)

Nursing Interventions/Rationales

- Provide analgesics before activity while hospitalized. Encourage patient to self-administer analgesics at home before activities requiring arm movement. *Appropriate timing of pain medication allows the patient to perform ADLs with less pain and more independence. Controlling pain decreases the risk for complications caused by immobility.*
- Explore with patient activities requiring assistance and community resources to help during times of physical immobility (family, friends, church, neighbors, home health aides). *Encouraging the patient to list activities requiring assistance (meals, shopping, bathing) helps the patient identify the most appropriate community resources for her needs.*
- Reinforce the need to limit activities that stress the incision site for 4 weeks (lifting more than 25 pounds or activities that require placing the arms over the head). *Limiting activities that overuse the affected arm will help stabilize the pacemaker by fibrosis around the pacemaker and electrodes, which decreases the risk of electrode displacement.*

Evaluation Parameters

1. Verbalizes understanding of need to maintain prescribed activity restrictions
2. Remains active while maintaining prescribed restrictions
3. Remains free of complications of decreased mobility

Nursing Care Plan *Patient Receiving a Permanent Pacemaker—cont'd*

NURSING DIAGNOSIS **Risk for infection related to surgical implantation of foreign device**

GOALS/OUTCOMES Will exhibit no indications of systemic or localized infection (fever, elevated white blood cell count, redness, swelling or drainage at incisional site)

NOC Suggested Outcomes
- Risk Control (1902)
- Knowledge: Infection Control (1807)
- Immune Status (0702)

NIC Suggested Interventions
- Infection Control (6540)
- Infection Protection (6550)
- Surveillance (6650)
- Wound Care (3660)

Nursing Interventions/Rationales
- Assess insertion site for signs of infection (redness, swelling, tenderness, warmth). *To recognize the presence of wound infection so that treatment can be initiated.*
- Assess for signs of systemic infection (fever, fatigue, elevated white blood cell count). *To recognize the presence of systemic infection so that treatment can be initiated.*
- Teach patient how to maintain sterile technique when changing dressing or cleaning incisional site. *Microorganisms can readily penetrate through non-intact skin as occurs with a surgical incision. Sterile technique reduces the risk of contamination and subsequent wound infection.*
- Teach patient the signs and symptoms of localized and systemic infection. *So the patient will recognize impending infection and seek assistance quickly.*
- Encourage patient to avoid handling of or unnecessary contact with surgical site. *To decrease the risk of wound contamination and subsequent wound infection.*
- Encourage a high protein, high calorie diet. *Proteins and calories are necessary for wound healing.*

Evaluation Parameters
1. Remains free of signs of wound infection
2. Remains free of signs of systemic infection
3. Accurately demonstrates sterile technique in caring for surgical incision
4. Accurately lists symptoms associated with infection

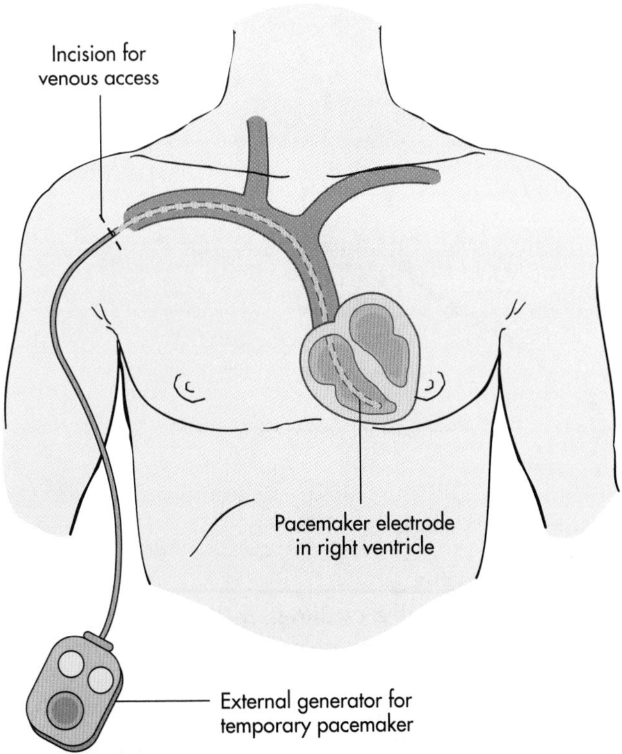

Figure 23-46 Transvenous temporary pacemaker placement.

Guidelines for Safe Practice

The Patient With a Temporary Pacemaker

ASSESS PATIENT'S TOLERANCE OF HEART RHYTHM

- Patient assessment: mental status, blood pressure and rhythm, urine output, skin color and warmth, pulses, heart sounds, and lung sounds
- Continuous ECG monitoring

CHECK SYSTEM FOR PROPER FUNCTIONING

- Check pacing threshold (the minimum amount of milliamperes needed to pace the heart every 8 hours); set milliampere level two to three times the threshold as a safety margin; adjust as needed and notify physician.
- Replace battery in generator or connecting cable for failure to pace as necessary.
- Adjust sensitivity for undersensing or oversensing; notify physician.
- Secure all connections; secure generator box to patient preferably or bed.

MAINTAIN ELECTRICAL SAFETY

- Maintain insulation cover over uninsulated ends.
- Wear rubber gloves when handling exposed terminals.
- Do not touch the patient and electrical equipment at the same time.
- Prevent liquids from coming in contact with the generator, cables, or insertion site.
- Keep ungrounded electrical equipment from contact with the patient.

MONITOR FOR COMPLICATIONS AT THE INSERTION SITE

- Inspect site daily for infection.
- Change dressing every 48 hours using central line dressing sterile technique.

ASSESS PATIENT SAFETY AND COMFORT

- Explain the purpose of the pacemaker to decrease anxiety.
- Position patient comfortably, avoiding accidental tension on external wires and generator.
- When mobility is limited, assist the patient to find diversional activities.

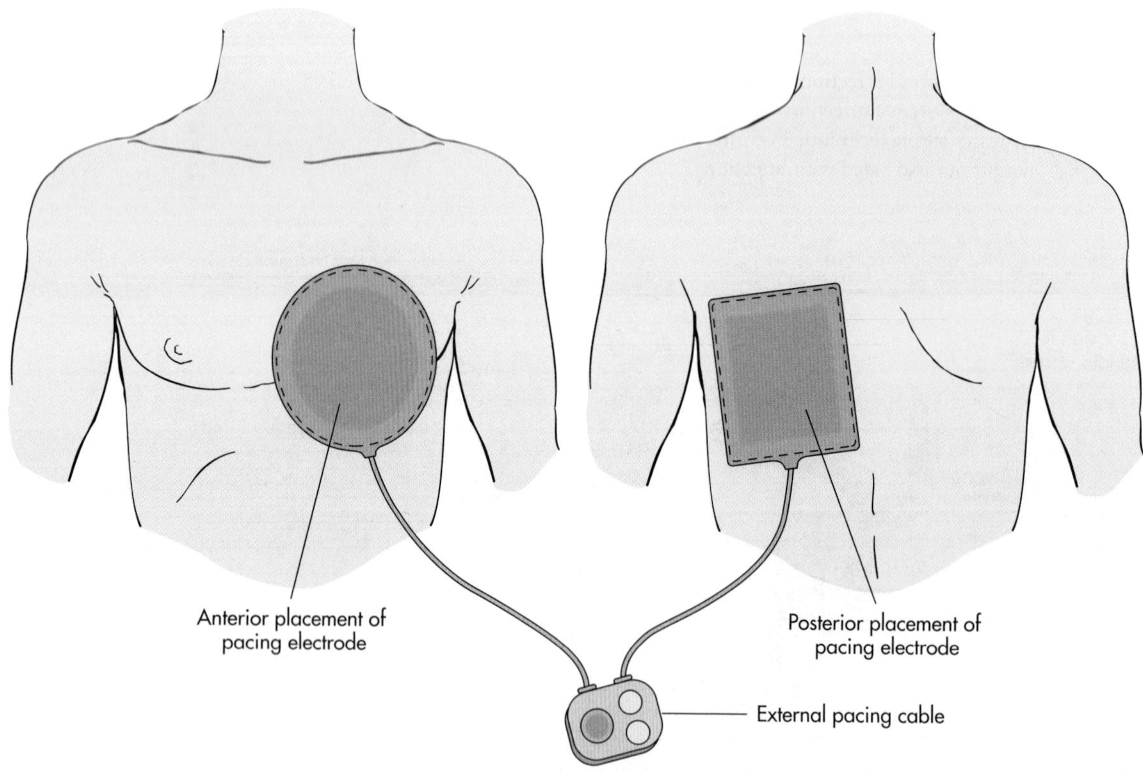

Figure 23-47 Transcutaneous external pacing.

not occlusive thrombosis or myocardial damage but a derangement in the heart's electrical stability, most often deteriorating into VF. The incidence of sudden death is greater in patients with cardiomyopathy, long QT intervals, myocarditis, prodysrhythmic medications, and electrolyte imbalance.

The implantable cardioverter-defibrillator (ICD) is indicated for the treatment of cardiac arrest due to VF or VT that is not caused by a transient or reversible cause; spontaneous sustained VT; syncope of undetermined origin with clinically relevant, hemodynamically significant sustained VT or VF in-

Patient Teaching

The Patient With an Implantable Cardioverter Defibrillator

IMPLANTABLE CARDIOVERTER-DEFIBRILLATOR–PROCEDURAL

- Indication for implantable cardioverter defibrillator (ICD)
- Potential complications
- NPO for 8 hours before the procedure
- Pretests, including baseline 12-lead ECG and bleeding function studies
- Cardiac monitor at all times during the procedure
- Intravenous access for fluids, cardiac medications, and sedation
- Prep and shave area where generator will be implanted
- Anesthesia of access sites
- Sterile field during procedure
- Analgesics available after procedure
- Restricted arm movement for 24 to 48 hours if implant site is infraclavicular
- Routine chest x-ray to check placement

ICD–DISCHARGE

Insertion Site

- Monitor site for infection and bleeding the first week
- Avoid immersion of site in water for 3 days
- Steri-strips will come off in about 1 week
- Wear loose covering over incision for 1 week

Activity

- Avoid contact sports
- Increase activity gradually after implantation of device (should be at full preimplant activity level once incision has healed)
- Driving restrictions individualized and must be discussed with cardiologist

Health Care Follow-up

- Importance of follow-up via office visits
- If experience signs or symptoms of decreasing cardiac output with dysrhythmia, sit or lie down
- Notify health care professional for:
  - Signs or symptoms of dysrhythmia similar to those before ICD
  - Rapid, irregular heart rate
  - Chest pain or shortness of breath

Safety

- Patient and others in physical contact with patient will experience a mild sensation with shock delivery.
- Carry ICD information at all times—will alarm some airport security.
- Consult with cardiologist before undergoing diagnostic or surgical interventions.
- Move away from devices if dizziness experienced.
- Avoid working over large, running motors.
- How to take radial pulse—notify health care professional for rates outside those programmed.

duced at electrophysiologic study; nonsustained VT with coronary disease, prior MI, LV dysfunction, and inducible VF or sustained VT at electrophysiologic study not suppressible with antidysrhythmics.[10]

The ICD consists of a pulse generator and two or three lead systems that continuously monitor heart activity and automatically deliver a countershock to correct a dysrhythmia. The pacemaker-cardioverter-defibrillator models can pace patients out of tachycardic rhythms as well as pace bradycardic rhythms. The devices can override the heart's pacemaker to gain control or cardiovert the heart at different energy outputs if overpacing is ineffective. Event records can be retrieved to evaluate the sequence of events and the appropriateness of ICD therapy.

The device is implanted via the subclavian transvenous lead system approach similar to permanent pacemaker insertion. A subcutaneous pocket is created for the generator infraclavicularly or intraabdominally. The nurse teaches the patient about situations that may cause malfunction of the ICD, such as magnetic resonance imaging or diathermy. Special precautions are also necessary during procedures such as lithotripsy and radiation therapy. Electrical interference may occur with stereo systems, high-powered motors, and arc welders. Emotional support is critical because patients and family members commonly respond to the ICD with anxiety, depression, fear, and anger. Teaching guidelines are included in the Patient Teaching box.

CARDIOPULMONARY RESUSCITATION

The American Heart Association estimates that one American suffers a coronary event every 29 seconds and that someone dies from a coronary event every minute. Approximately 220,000 people die of coronary heart disease each year without ever reaching a hospital. Most of these are sudden deaths caused by cardiac arrest, usually resulting from VF.[1] Sudden death from ischemic heart disease is one of the most serious and most important medical emergencies, and it seems reasonable to assume that many of these deaths might be prevented by prompt and appropriate intervention. Lay rescuers are increasingly being trained to use automatic external defibillators (AEDs), as the time from collapse to defibrillation is the single greatest determinant of survival. Access to AEDs is increasing at sites with concentrated populations (e.g., sporting events, airlines, and shopping malls).

Cardiopulmonary arrest is characterized by the cessation of breathing and circulation and signifies a state of clinical death. Unresponsiveness, cessation of respiration, development of pallor and cyanosis, absence of heart sounds and blood pressure, loss of palpable pulse, and dilation of the pupils are present. Immediate and definitive action must be instituted within 4 to 6 minutes after the arrest or biologic death occurs.

Basic life support is an emergency procedure that consists of recognizing an arrest and initiating proper CPR techniques to maintain life until the victim either recovers or is transported to a medical facility where advanced life-support measures are available. The "ABCD" mnemonic of CPR stands for airway, breathing, circulation, and defibrillation/definitive treatment (Table 23-12). Safe implementation of CPR involves five steps.

Step I: Assess Level of Consciousness

Persons who appear to be unconscious may be asleep, deaf, or possibly intoxicated. Unconsciousness is confirmed by shaking the victim's shoulders and shouting, "Are you OK?" If the person does not respond, the emergency response system (911) is activated immediately and the victim is cautiously placed in the supine position on a firm surface, remembering the potential for head injury.

Step II: Open the Airway

The tongue is the most common cause of airway obstruction in the unconscious person. The head tilt–chin lift method and the jaw thrust are the two recommended methods for opening and maintaining the airway (Figures 23-48 and 23-49). Jaw thrust (without head tilt) is the safest approach to use with a victim with a suspected neck injury. The head must be carefully supported to avoid turning or tilting it backward. While maintaining an open airway, the rescuer takes 3 to 5 seconds to look, listen, and feel for spontaneous breathing. The rescuer places an ear over the victim's nose and mouth while looking at the victim's chest to see if the chest moves with respiration, listens for air escaping during exhalation, and feels for air movement against the face.

Step III: Initiate Artificial Ventilation

Mouth-to-Mouth Ventilation

To initiate artificial ventilation give two breaths lasting 2 seconds each, and observe for adequate ventilation. If the patient does not resume breathing, continue mouth-to-mouth ventilation. One breath is delivered every 5 seconds.

1. Maintain victim in head tilt-chin lift position.
2. Pinch nostrils.
3. Take a deep breath and place mouth around outside of victim's mouth, forming a tight seal. Use a rescue airway if available.
4. Blow into victim's mouth.
5. Adequate ventilation is demonstrated by
   a. Rise and fall of chest
   b. Hearing and feeling air escape as victim passively exhales.
   c. Feeling the resistance of the victim's lungs expanding.

Mouth-to-Nose Ventilation

Mouth-to-nose ventilation is indicated when the mouth is seriously injured or if a tight seal cannot be established around the mouth. The rescuer places one hand on the forehead to tilt the head back and uses the other hand to lift the lower jaw and close the mouth. After taking a deep breath, the rescuer seals the mouth around the victim's nose and begins blowing until the lungs expand. Occasionally, when mouth-to-nose ventilation is used, it may become necessary to open the victim's mouth or lips to allow air to escape on exhalation because the soft palate may produce nasopharyngeal obstruction.

Mouth-to-Stoma Ventilation

Direct mouth-to-stoma artificial ventilation is performed for the laryngectomy patient. For the patient with a temporary tracheostomy tube, mouth-to-tube ventilation should be initiated after the cuff is inflated.

Mouth-to-Barrier Ventilation

An alternative to direct mouth-to-mouth ventilation is use of a barrier device such as a face shield and mask device. Most mask devices have a one-way valve so that exhaled air does not enter the rescuer's mouth; many face shields have no exhalation valves, which cause air leakage around the shield. The barrier device (face mask or face shield) is positioned over the victim's mouth and nose, ensuring an adequate air seal.

Step IV: Assess Circulation

The carotid pulse is palpated to determine whether cardiac compression is needed. The carotid pulse is located by finding the larynx and sliding the fingers laterally into the groove between the trachea and the sternocleidomastoid muscle (Figure 23-50). If the carotid pulse is not palpable in 5 to 10 seconds, cardiac compressions are initiated. The carotid pulse is palpated because it is accessible and the carotid arteries are cen-

TABLE 23-12 Sequence of Cardiopulmonary Resuscitation

Findings	Action	ABCs of Action	Timing
No response	Activate Emergency Medical Services	A—Open *airway*	3 to 5 sec to assess for respiration
Absence of respirations; cyanosis, dilated pupils	Open airway		
Respirations still absent	Initiate artificial ventilation	B—Restore *breathing*	Deliver 1 breath every 5 sec, 2 sec per breath, (12/min)
Carotid pulse not palpable (omitted with lay rescuers)	Initiate external cardiac compressions	C—Restore *circulation*	10 sec to establish pulselessness (lay rescuers omit)
ECG; ventricular fibrillation	Drug therapy; defibrillation	D—Provide *definitive* treatment	Compression rate of 80 to 100/min Compression depth 1.5 to 2 in

tral. Sometimes these pulses persist when more peripheral pulses are no longer palpable. If the pulse is absent, cardiac arrest is confirmed and external chest compression is initiated. Lay rescuers are no longer being taught to check for a pulse because their accuracy in pulse assessment was only about 65%. Other indicators of circulation are checked instead, including breathing, coughing, and movement.

Step V: Initiate External Cardiac Compression

External cardiac compression (sometimes called external cardiac massage) is the rhythmic compression of the heart between the lower half of the sternum and the thoracic vertebra. This intermittent pressure compresses the heart, raises intrathoracic pressure, and produces an artificial pulsatile circulation. Correctly performed cardiac compressions can produce a peak systolic blood pressure of more than 100 mm Hg. The diastolic pressure is close to zero, however, and the mean blood pressure in the carotid arteries is approximately 40 mm Hg, or about one-fourth normal. The technique for performing external cardiac compression consists of four steps:

1. The rescuer takes a position close to the victim's side. Using the middle finger of one hand the rescuer locates the xiphoid process (Figure 23-51, *A*). The index finger of the same hand is placed on the sternum directly next to the middle finger. Using the index finger as a landmark, the heel of the opposite hand is placed on the sternum next to the index finger (Figure 23-51, *B*). The first hand is then placed on top of the hand on the sternum (Figure 23-51, *C*). Fingers may be interlocked to avoid pressure on the patient's ribs (Figure 23-51, *D*).
2. To perform effective external cardiac compression, the rescuer needs to be positioned directly over the victim's shoulders keeping the elbows locked in a straight

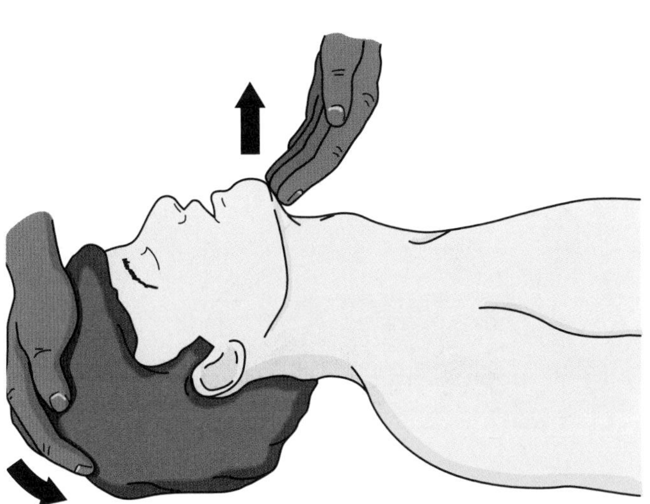

Figure 23-48 Head tilt-chin lift maneuver for opening airway. Place one hand on forehead and place tips of fingers of other hand under lower jaw near chin. Bring chin forward while pressing forehead down

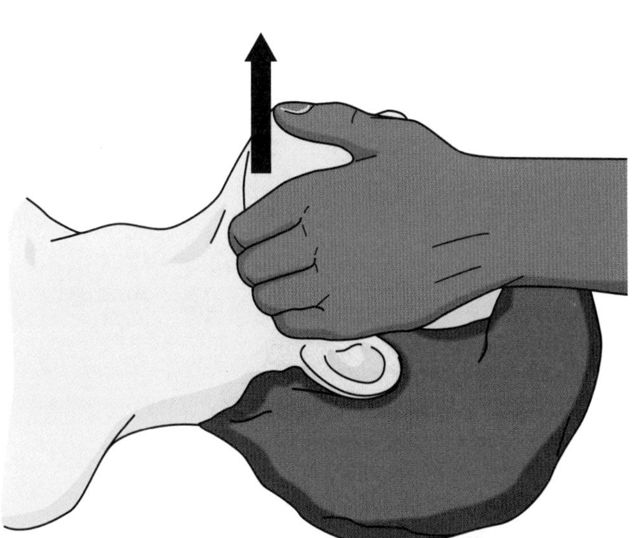

Figure 23-49 Jaw thrust maneuver for opening airway.

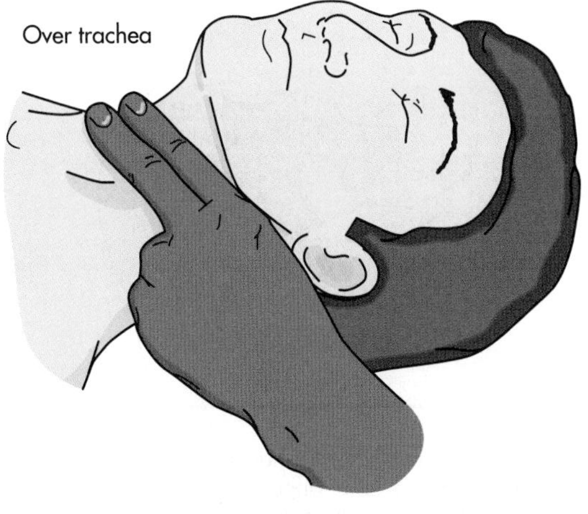

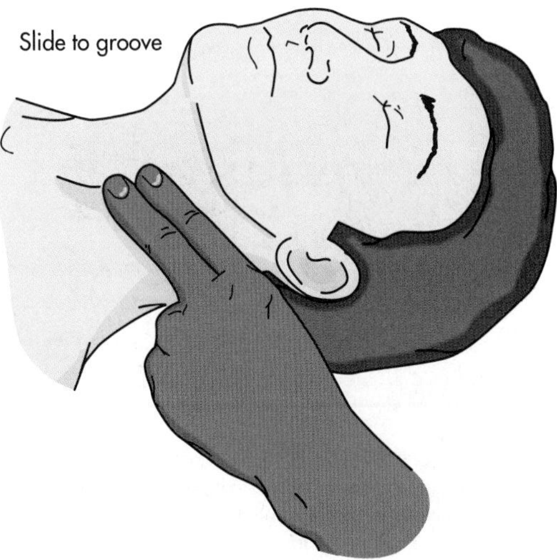

Figure 23-50 Locating carotid artery.

position, and depressing the lower sternum $1\frac{1}{2}$ to 2 inches. The compressions are regular, smooth, and uninterrupted. After each compression the rescuer releases the pressure completely to allow the heart to refill. A compression rate of 80 to 100 per minute is established with a ratio of compressions to breaths of 15:2. The rescuer delivers 2 full breaths after every 15 compressions (Figure 23-52).

3. When two rescuers are available to administer CPR, one rescuer is positioned at the victim's side and performs external cardiac compression while the second rescuer remains at the victim's head to perform artificial ventilation. If two rescuers are available, the cardiac compression rate remains the same but a 5:1 ratio of cardiac compressions to ventilation is established. The rescuer who is ventilating the victim quickly delivers one full breath (2 seconds) after every five compressions; compressions are paused to allow for a full breath to be delivered. Two-rescuer CPR is advocated only for skilled providers because of the coordination required to appropriately time the interventions.
4. After the first minute of CPR, the carotid pulse is again palpated to assess the effectiveness of CPR and to check for the return of spontaneous circulation. If two rescuers are performing CPR, the person ventilating the victim also assesses pulses and monitors for the return of spontaneous breathing. Rescuers continue to perform CPR until one of the following takes place:
   a. Spontaneous circulation and ventilation return.
   b. Another rescuer takes over basic life support.
   c. The victim is transported to an emergency facility.
   d. The victim is pronounced dead by a physician.
   e. The rescuer is exhausted and unable to continue.

For a summary of CPR steps, see the Guidelines for Safe Practice box.

Advanced Cardiac Life Support

Most hospitals have trained teams of personnel, including physicians, nurses, anesthesiologists, and technicians, who provide immediate care in the event of a cardiac arrest. Equipment needs include an ECG machine, suction device, oxygen, defibrillator, breathing bag, laryngoscope, a variety of endo-

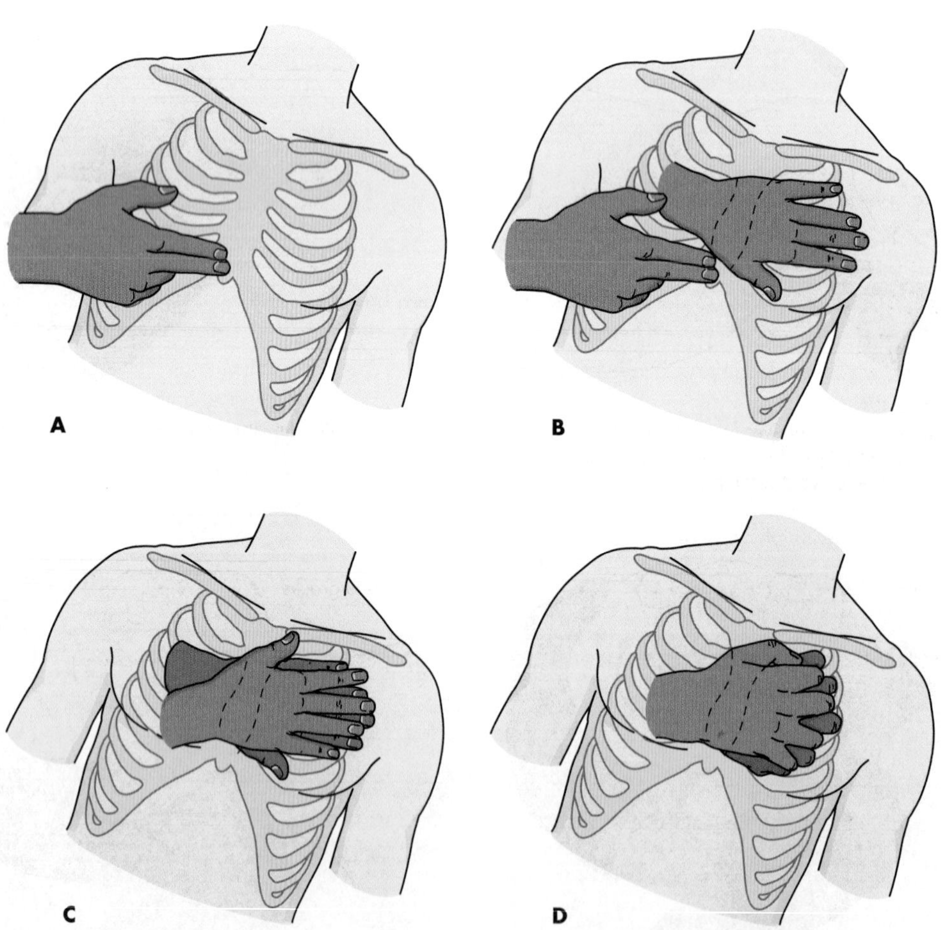

Figure 23-51 Positioning of hands on sternum in external cardiac compression. **A,** Middle finger locates xiphoid process; index finger is positioned next to middle finger. **B,** Heel of opposite hand is placed on sternum next to index finger. **C,** First hand is removed from landmark position and placed on top of other hand so that heels of both hands are parallel and the fingers point away. **D,** Fingers may be interlocked to avoid pressure on the ribs.

tracheal tubes, cutdown set, intravenous fluids, and a tracheostomy set. Medications administered during a cardiac arrest are usually stored on an emergency cart. Algorithms for advanced life support are reviewed and updated regularly by the American Heart Association (AHA). A local AHA office can provide the most current practice guidelines and information about available training sessions for advanced cardiac life support.

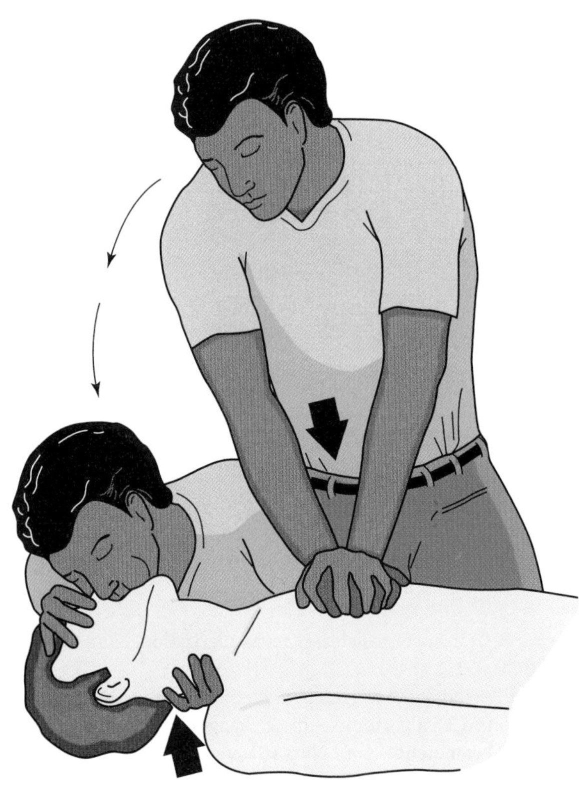

Figure 23-52 One-person rescuer CPR. The person delivers two effective ventilations after every 15 compressions.

Guidelines for Safe Practice

Cardiopulmonary Resuscitation for the Adult Victim

- Activate Emergency Medical Services after establishing unresponsiveness

AIRWAY

- Assess for respirations (3 to 5 seconds)
- Rescue breaths per minute: 1 every 5 seconds (12 per minute)
- Rate of breaths: 2 seconds

CIRCULATION

- Assess for carotid pulse (up to 10 seconds)—lay rescuers use other indicators of circulation
- Determine hand position
- Achieve compression rate of 80 to 100 per minute
- Compression depth: 1.5 to 2 inches
- Ratio of compressions to breaths, one-person CPR: 15:2
- Ratio of compressions to breaths, two-person CPR: 5:1

CPR, Cardiopulmonary resuscitation.

Complications of Cardiopulmonary Resuscitation

The most common complication of external cardiac compression is fracture of the ribs. This may occur even when external cardiac compression is performed correctly. Other possible complications include fractured sternum, costochondral separation, and lung contusions. Any indication of labored respiration, paradoxic pulse, muffled heart sounds, tachycardia, decreased breath sounds, or drop in blood pressure may indicate pericardial tamponade from the injection of intracardiac medications and is reported to the physician immediately. Laceration of the liver also may occur as a result of compressions performed over the xiphoid process.

Critical Thinking Questions

Mr. Lewis, age 49, is admitted through the emergency department to the CCU to rule out MI. His chest pain began at an intensity of 3 out of 10 at approximately 7:45 AM? this morning on his drive to work. He reported that he had to make a presentation for which he did not feel adequately prepared and had gotten little rest the night before. Once at work, he drank some coffee and took ibuprofen for the pain. He tried to give the ibuprofen time to work, but the unrelenting pain finally caused him to confide in a co-worker at approximately 9 AM. He asked his co-worker if he thought Maalox or "something else might get rid of the pain." It took an additional 30 minutes before the co-worker was able to convince him that he should go to the emergency department. He tried to "tough it out" with pain rated at an 8 out of 10. On arrival in the emergency department, his pain had reached 10/10, radiated to his left arm and up into his jaw. It was described as "gnawing and unrelenting."

1. What diagnostic tests will be done in the emergency department to rule out MI? What is being looked for on these diagnostic tests to confirm or rule out MI?
2. The patient is being considered for fibrinolytic therapy. What collaborative interventions are indicated for patients experiencing MI and being screened for fibrinolytic therapy?
3. Mr. Lewis undergoes a low-level stress test that validates redistribution in the inferior wall of his left ventricle (LV). Cardiac catheterization is planned with coronary stenting if appropriate. You are the evening shift nurse and must explain the procedure to him and his wife. What will you teach?
4. Mr. Lewis is to be discharged today after successful stenting. He lives with his wife of 22 years, his 17-year-old son, and a 13-year-old daughter. He works at a local company that has been downsizing. He is considered "middle management." His wife works as a physical therapist at a long-term nursing facility. Their home is two stories and has all modern conveniences. Mr. Lewis and his family attend church weekly and are involved in various activities (although "sometimes the kids have to be made to go"). A cholesterol screen was done on admission and showed a total cholesterol of 202. He does not routinely take any medications. He smokes ½ to 1 pack a day but only at the office since his wife cannot stand it and does not wish him to smoke in their home. He used to smoke 1½ packs a day until 5 years ago. He does not use alcohol. As the nurse responsible for his discharge *today,* develop a comprehensive teaching plan based on what you would *expect* the medical orders to be for this patient. Consider specifically diet, medications, activity, and risk factor modification.

5. The following rhythm strip shows sinus rhythm with conversion to
   a. Atrial fibrillation
   b. Paroxysmal atrial tachycardia
   c. Ventricular tachycardia
   Discuss possible causes and treatment.

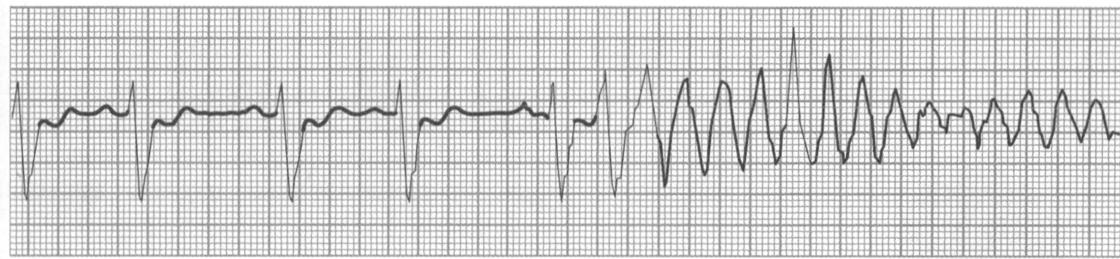

6. The following rhythm strip shows

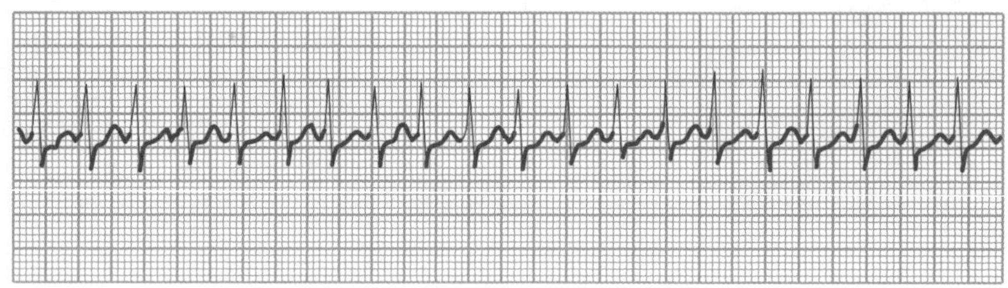

   a. Sinus tachycardia
   b. Atrial tachycardia
   c. Ventricular tachycardia
   Discuss possible causes and treatment indicated.

References

1. American Heart Association. *2001 Heart and Stroke Statistical Update,* Dallas, 2000, American Heart Association.
2. Beery TA: The evolving role of genetics in the diagnosis and management of heart disease, *Nurs Clin North Am* 35(4):963, 2000.
3. Beller GA: Coronary heart disease in the first 30 years of the 21st century: challenges and opportunities: The 33rd Annual James B. Herrick Lecture of the Council on Clinical Cardiology of the American Heart Association, *Circulation* 103(20):2428, 2001.
4. Botti M et al: Coronary angiography observations: evidence-based or ritualistic practice? *Heart and Lung* 30(2):138, 2001.
5. Braunwald et al: ACC/AHA guidelines for the management of patients with unstable angina and non-ST segment elevation myocardial infarction: executive summary and recommendations: a report of the American College of Cardiology/American Heart Association Task Force on Practice Guidelines (Committee on Management of Patient with Unstable Angina), *Circulation* 102(10):1193, 2000.
6. Brennan J: Reperfusion injury of cardiac myocytes: mechanisms, treatment, and implications for advanced practice nursing, *AACN Clinical Issues* 11(2):252, 2000.
7. Calkins H: Catheter ablation for cardiac arrhythmias, *Med Clin North Am* 85(2):473, 2001.
8. National Institute of Diabetes & Digestive & Kidney Diseases: *Diabetes Statistics,* NIH Publication 99-3926, Bethesda Md, 1999, National Diabetes Information Clearinghouse.
9. Fullwood J et al: New strategies in the management of acute coronary syndromes, *Nurs Clin North Am* 35(4):877, 2000.
10. Gregoratos G: ACC/AHA Pocket guidelines for implantation of cardiac pacemakers and antiarrhythmic devices (report of the American College of Cardiology/American Heart Association Task Force on Practice Guidelines) developed in collaboration with the North American Society of Pacing and Electrophysiology, Bethesda, Md, 1999, Amercan College of Cardiology.
11. Keeling A: *The family experience after acute myocardial infarction, doctoral dissertation,* Charlottesville, 1992, University of Virginia.
12. Leeper B: Transmyocardial laser revascularization, *Nurs Clin North Am* 35(4):933, 2000.
13. Madrid P, Sendelbach S: Heart-smarter drugs for resuscitation: an update on ACLS algorithms – drug changes introduced at the historic 2000 conference, *Am J Nurs* 101(suppl):42, 2001.
14. Morrison LJ et al: Mortality and prehospital thrombolysis for acute myocardial infarction, *JAMA* 283(20):2686, 2000.
15. Ryan TJ et al: ACC/AHA Practice Guidelines: 1999 update. ACC/AHA Guidelines for the management of patients with acute myocardial infarction: executive summary and recommendations, *Circulation* 100:1016, 1999.
16. Smith SC et al: ACC/AHA Guidelines for percutaneous coronary intervention (revision of the 1993 PTCA guidelines): executive summary, *J Am Coll Cardiol* 37(8):2215, 2001.
17. Taylor B: Putting some color in the heart, *Helix* Fall:3-4, Fall 2000.
18. Tracy CM et al: American College of Cardiology/American Heart Association clinical competence statement on invasive electrophysiology studies, catheter ablation, and cardioversion: a report of the American College of Cardiology/American Heart Association/American College of Physicians-American Society of Internal Medicine Task Force on Clinical Competence, *Circulation* 102(18):2309, 2000.
19. US Department of Health and Human Services: *Healthy People 2010: understanding and improving health,* Washington, DC, 2000, USDHHS.
20. US Department of Health and Human Services: National Cholesterol Education Program: *Third report of the expert panel on detection, evaluation, and treatment of high blood cholesterol in adults (Adult Treatment Panel III),* NIH Pub No 01-3305, Washington, DC, 2001, USDHHS.
21. USDHHS: *Physical activity and health: a report of the Surgeon General,* Washington, DC, 1996, USDHHS.
22. Wei M et al: Relationship between low cardiorespiratory fitness and mortality in normal weight, overweight, and obese men, *JAMA* 282:1547, 1999.

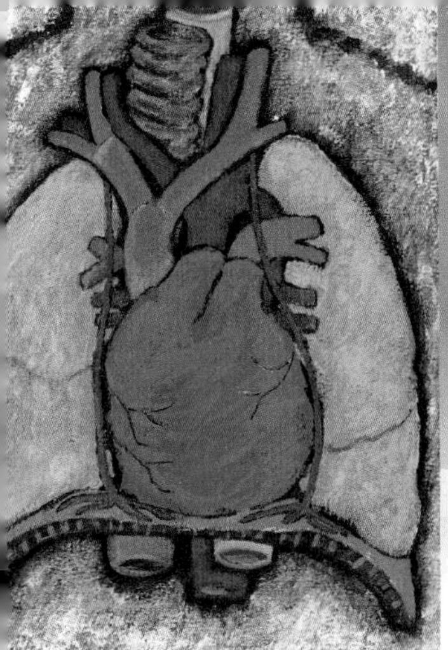

Heart Failure, Valvular Problems, and Inflammatory Problems of the Heart

24

Kathy Henley Haugh, Kathryn Ballenger Reid

Objectives

After studying this chapter, the learner should be able to:

1. Discuss the collaborative care management of patients with heart failure, pericarditis, endocarditis, and myocarditis.
2. Explain the pathophysiology that produces the clinical manifestations associated with heart failure.
3. Develop a plan of care for the patient with progressive heart failure.
4. Differentiate between the various forms of cardiac valve problems in terms of etiology, impact on the heart's function, clinical manifestations, and treatment.
5. Identify at least three important aspects of patient and family education for patients with cardiac valve disorders.
6. Describe six indications for cardiac surgery.
7. Discuss the nursing management of patients after heart surgery.

Heart disease can be divided into two general types: congenital and acquired. Congenital heart disease is caused by some error in the embryologic development of the heart's structures. Acquired heart disease results from inflammation, infection, chemical agents, or a diminished blood supply. Its onset may be sudden or gradual. Heart disease can also be classified according to its specific etiologic agent (e.g., rheumatic fever, infective endocarditis, valvular scarring). Any of these problems can eventually lead to cardiac failure.

INFLAMMATORY HEART DISEASE

Pericarditis

Etiology/Epidemiology

Pericarditis is an inflammatory process of the visceral or parietal pericardium. It can be acute or chronic and can spread from or to the myocardium. Pericarditis can develop as bacterial, viral, or fungal infection and can also occur as a complication of a systemic disease process such as rheumatoid arthritis, systemic lupus erhythematosus, malignancy, uremia, or myocardial infarction. Pericarditis also occurs secondary to trauma or interventions such as surgery, radiation, or chemotherapy.

Pathophysiology

In acute pericarditis the membranes surrounding the heart become inflamed and rub against each other producing the classic pericardial friction rub. The friction rub sounds scratchy and harsh on auscultation and persists throughout both systole and diastole. The patient complains of severe precordial chest pain, which may closely resemble that of acute myocardial infarction. The pain intensifies when the person is lying supine and decreases in a sitting position. The pain also may intensify when the patient breathes deeply. The pain of pericarditis often radiates to the trapezius muscle.

Fever typically occurs accompanied by leukocytosis and a rise in the erythrocyte sedimentation rate (ESR). Malaise, myalgias, and tachycardia are common. The onset of bacterial pericarditis is associated with high fevers, shaking chills, and night sweats. The electrocardiogram (ECG) shows PR depression and diffuse nonspecific ST segment abnormalities. These changes reflect pericardial inflammation over the entire surface of the heart. Computed tomography, magnetic resonance imaging, and echocardiography are useful tools in the diagnosis of pericardial disorders. Thickening and calcification of the pericardium, which can be seen on echocardiography, occur more commonly with bacterial or fungal pericarditis.

The acute inflammation causes an accumulation of fluid within the pericardial sac called a pericardial effusion. The fluid may be serous, purulent, or hemorrhagic in nature. Serous effusions usually accompany heart failure; purulent effusions indicate disorders such as tuberculosis or neoplasms. Hemorrhagic effusions usually occur from trauma, aneurysm rupture, or coagulation abnormalities. An echocardiogram provides the most definitive diagnosis of the effusion. The ECG may exhibit bradycardia with low-voltage QRS complexes. When fluid accumulation is gradual, the patient may not develop symptoms until as much as 1 L of clear or serosanguinous fluid is present.

Excessive fluid in the pericardial sac can cause compression of the heart (cardiac tamponade), which decreases venous return to the heart, resulting in a decrease in ventricular filling and ultimately a decrease in stroke volume. These events can rapidly lead to cardiac failure, shock, and death. The three classic symptoms of tamponade, referred to as Beck's triad, include hypotension, jugular venous distention, and muffled heart sounds. Additional signs include tachycardia, paradoxic pulse, and a narrowed pulse pressure.

Chronic pericarditis can also occur. Adhesive pericarditis occurs when the pericardial layers adhere to each other, restricting movement of the heart. Chronic constrictive pericarditis results from fibrosis of the pericardial sac that can develop secondary to surgery, uremia, or radiation. The thick fibrous pericardium tightens around the heart, decreasing cardiac filling and output. Patients exhibit symptoms of heart failure from the diminished ability of the heart to pump.

Collaborative Care Management

Treatment is specific to the underlying cause of the pericarditis. It is critical to differentiate the pain of pericarditis from that of myocardial infarction, because thrombolytic administration in the presence of pericardial effusion may result in hemorrhage. If the pericardial effusion is small, therapy is primarily supportive and includes administration of nonsteroidal antiinflammatory drugs (NSAIDs), including aspirin or indomethacin. Corticosteroids are prescribed if the inflammation is refractory to nonsteroidal agents. The pericarditis can recur after the antiinflammatory drug therapy is completed.

A pericardiocentesis (pericardial tap) may be performed to remove excess fluid from large effusions. A small anterolateral thoracotomy may be performed, or a pericardial fenestration (pericardial window) can be created to allow for continuous drainage of pericardial fluid when necessary. Complications include atelectasis and the introduction of infection. The nurse monitors the amount and quality of the drainage and reports increases or changes to the physician.

In chronic pericarditis removal of the pericardium (pericardiectomy) may be necessary to restore cardiac function. Postoperative care is similar to that for other open cardiac surgeries (see p. 749). Treatment may also include medications to restore the heart's pumping efficiency.

With both acute and chronic pericarditis, the nurse monitors vital signs and heart sounds for changes that suggest cardiac tamponade. Analgesics are used as needed to control pain and facilitate lung expansion. Antiinflammatory medications and comfort measures are used to treat fever and general malaise. Nursing interventions include encouraging adequate fluid intake, spacing activities to allow rest periods, and using distraction or other nonpharmacologic methods to manage discomfort.

Patient/Family Education. The nurse teaches the patient and family about the nature of the disease and the purpose and correct use of all medications including the management of side effects. The nurse teaches measures to decrease fatigue and provides information on how to minimize the risks of complications. The nurse emphasizes that a return of symptoms can indicate recurrent pericarditis and needs to be promptly reported to the primary care provider.

Infective Endocarditis

Etiology/Epidemiology

Infective endocarditis (IE) involves the endocardium, most often of the heart valves. Acute IE develops rapidly, often on otherwise normal heart valves, and if untreated may result in death within days to weeks. Subacute infective endocarditis develops gradually, usually on previously damaged heart valves, and responds well to treatment.

Infective endocarditis is classified by the causative organism. Hemolytic streptococci are the most common causative organisms, especially for the subacute form. Other infective agents include staphylococci, such as *Staphylococcus aureus, Staphylococcus epidermidis,* and enterococci.

Individuals at high risk for IE are those with underlying pathologic cardiac conditions, including rheumatic valve disease, congenital heart disease, and degenerative heart disease. Mitral valve prolapse is a leading risk factor.[27] Endocarditis develops in 1% to 4% of persons who have prosthetic heart valve implants. In some cases IE occurs after invasive procedures such as oral surgery, gynecologic procedures, implantation of internal cardiac devices, and insertion of indwelling urinary catheters or renal shunts. Intravenous (IV) drug users are also at high risk because of the possibility of bacteremia from contaminated needles and syringes. Human immunodeficiency virus (HIV) infection is also a risk factor for infective endocarditis. Box 24-1 identifies specific patient populations at risk for infective endocarditis.

Pathophysiology

A damaged cardiac valve or a ventricular septal defect produces turbulent blood flow that allows bacteria to settle on the low-pressure side of the valve or defect. Infective endocarditis from IV drug abuse most commonly affects the tricuspid valve.

BOX 24-1 Patient Populations at Risk for Infective Endocarditis

High Risk

Some clinical presentations of mitral valve prolapse*
Prosthetic heart valves
Previous history of endocarditis
Complex congenital cyanotic heart disease
Surgically constructed systemic pulmonary shunts or conduits

Moderate Risk

Patent ductus arteriosus
Ventricular septal defect
Primum atrial septal defect
Coarctation of aorta
Bicuspid aortic valve
Acquired valvular dysfunction
Hypertrophic cardiomyopathy

*See complete American Heart Association guidelines in Dajani et al.[8] for specific indications.

The hallmark of IE is a platelet-fibrin-bacteria mass on the valve called a vegetation (Figure 24-1). The organisms surround the heart valve, become embedded in the valve matrix, and cause vegetative growths that may scar and perforate the leaflets. Emboli occur if the vegetative growths break free of the valves and enter the bloodstream. If the emboli become trapped in organs such as the spleen or kidney, abscesses may form.

In acute IE the onset is swift, with septicemia and fevers above 38° C. The patient with subacute IE has a more insidious onset, with vague complaints of malaise and general achiness. Low-grade fever is usually present, although a high fever may occur with *S. aureus* infection. Other commonly reported symptoms include headache, arthralgias, arthritis, low back pain, myalgias, anorexia, weight loss, chest pain, night sweats, and occasional hemoptysis. Physical examination may reveal splenomegaly, clubbing of the fingers, the presence of Osler's nodes (small, raised, tender, bluish areas) on the fingers or toe pads, and small capillary hemorrhages (petechiae) in the conjunctiva, in the mouth, and on the extremities. Janeway lesions (nontender lesions on the palms or soles) and Roth spots (retinal lesions) are additional findings unique to IE. Auscultation reveals murmurs over the affected cardiac valves.

Diagnostic tests include blood cultures to guide antibiotic therapy, echocardiography (preferably transesophageal in the higher risk patient) to demonstrate valvular vegetations and function and occasionally cardiac catheterization to evaluate ventricular and valvular function. The Duke Criteria are used as an objective mode of diagnosis (Box 24-2). Using the Duke Criteria, definite IE requires either the presence of two major criteria, one major criterion with three minor criteria, or five minor criteria.[10] Laboratory tests usually reveal an increased white blood count and ESR. A normocytic normochromic anemia may also be present.

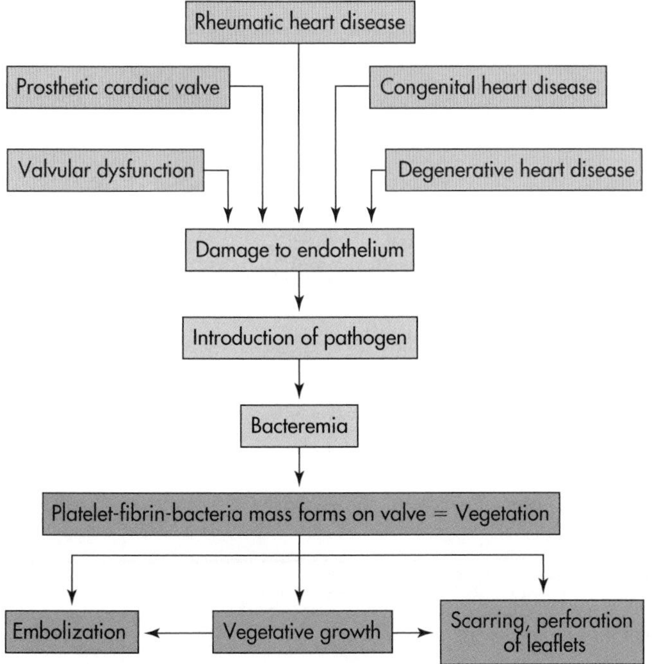

Figure 24-1 Infective endocarditis. Relationship of endothelial damage, bacteria introduction, and subsequent vegetative growth.

Collaborative Care Management

The major aim of therapy is to eliminate all microorganisms from the vegetative growths and prevent complications. Cellular and humoral host defenses are impaired over affected areas because the colonized bacteria are embedded in the valve matrix, preventing host defenses from reaching the bacteria. If IE goes untreated for weeks or months, the incidence of embolic complications and progressive involvement of the heart valves greatly increases. Therefore antibiotic therapy is initiated after three blood cultures are obtained to identify the infecting organism. Antibiotic therapy continues even after symptoms abate, usually for 4 to 6 weeks. Outpatient IV antibiotic administration may be considered when barriers to adherence are low, therapeutic regimens are uncomplicated, and support systems are in place. Outpatient management is contraindicated for IV drug abusers and those with prosthetic heart valves. Peak and trough drug levels are evaluated to ensure the desired therapeutic outcomes of antibiotic administration and avoid adverse patient outcomes. The nephrotoxic effects of many antibiotics necessitate ongoing assessment of renal function throughout treatment. Deteriorated heart valves are surgically repaired or replaced with prostheses when IE is refractory to medical therapy or in the presence of cardiac and hemodynamic compromise.

The nurse monitors the patient for new murmurs or changes in preexisting murmurs. With impaired valve function, the patient is at risk for developing heart failure. Changes in breath sounds and fluid status can alert the staff to early signs of heart failure. The patient is continuously assessed for signs and symptoms of embolic events and dysrhythmias. Decreased tissue perfusion also affects the peripheral vasculature and alters the person's activity tolerance. When bed rest is necessary, active or passive range-of-motion exercises are performed regularly. The nurse encourages rest periods of 30 to 60 minutes between all activities.

BOX 24-2 Duke Criteria for the Diagnosis of Infective Endocarditis

Major Criteria

Positive blood culture
Endocardial involvement
Echocardiographic confirmation of mass, abscess, or prosthetic valve damage
New murmur or change in previous murmur

Minor Criteria

Risk factor for IE
Fever
Vascular changes consistent with IE, such as emboli, Janeway lesions
Immunologic changes consistent with IE, such as Osler's nodes, Roth spots
Blood culture, supportive of, but not confirmatory for IE
Echocardiographic evidence supportive of, but not confirmatory for IE

IE, Infective endocarditis.

Patient/Family Education. The nurse teaches the patient to avoid excessive fatigue and to stop activity immediately if chest pain, dyspnea, light-headedness, or faintness occurs. Patients are taught to avoid infection. The nurse initiates referrals for outpatient IV management and begins the necessary patient education. The nurse instructs the patient to inform all primary care providers, including physicians and dentists, about their history of IE so that antibiotic therapy, if clinically indicated, can be administered before intrusive procedures. American Heart Association recommendations for the use of prophylactic antibiotics are presented in Box 24-3. The patient is instructed to use a soft-bristled toothbrush and floss regularly to protect the gums from infection and prevent dental caries. Good dental hygiene is of utmost importance in decreasing the risk of recurrent IE in susceptible patient populations. A sample Nursing Care Plan for the person with IE follows.

BOX 24-3 American Heart Association Recommendations for Antibiotic Prophylaxis of Infective Endocarditis

Dental, Oral, Respiratory Tract, or Esophageal Procedures

Pathogen: *Streptococcus viridans*
Antibiotic of choice: amoxicillin 2 g 1 hour before procedure; alternatives if unable to take oral preparation or if allergic to penicillin:
Ampicillin, intravenous (IV)
Clindamycin, oral or IV
First-generation cephalosporins—cefazolin IV
Azithromycin or clarithromycin

Genitourinary and Nonesophageal Gastrointestinal Procedures

Pathogen: *Enterococcus faecalis*
Antibiotic of choice: parenteral ampicillin or oral amoxicillin

Nursing Care Plan *Patient With Ineffective Endocarditis*

DATA Mr. B. is a married, 73-year-old retired man with a history of aortic regurgitation first noted 4 years ago. He also has a history of irritable bowel syndrome for which he underwent a colonoscopy and polyp removal 6 weeks before this admission. After the colonoscopy, Mrs. B. noticed a decrease in Mr. B's normal activity level. He complained of muscle aches and the need to rest after simple yard work. Two nights ago Mr. B. began experiencing night sweats. He visited his physician who noted that Mr. B. had a low-grade fever of 100° F, small, raised, tender, bluish areas on his fingers, multiple petechiae over his extremities, and an increase in intensity from the baseline aortic murmur. A transesophageal echocardiogram confirmed the presence of vegetations on the aortic valve. Blood cultures were quickly obtained and antibiotic therapy initiated. Mr. B. responded well to treatment and will be discharged in another week with plans for ongoing administration of IV ampicillin at home. The nursing history also revealed:

- Mr. B. recalls being instructed about antibiotic prophylaxis before invasive procedures but had been doing so well over the years that he failed to mention his valve while being evaluated for his gastrointestinal pain.
- Mrs. B. finds it hard to help Mr. B. in dependent situations because of his need for facts and to feel in control of his health.
- Mr. B. is used to being active and on the go. Being confined and resting for any time are difficult for him to accept.

NURSING DIAGNOSIS **Activity intolerance related to imbalances between oxygen supply and demand secondary to infective process**

GOALS/OUTCOMES Will report decreased fatigue; pulse, respiration, and blood pressure will return to normal for patient after increased activity

NOC Suggested Outcomes
- Activity Tolerance (0005)
- Endurance (0001)
- Energy Conservation (0002)
- Cardiac Pump Effectiveness (0400)

NIC Suggested Interventions
- Energy Management (0180)
- Teaching: Prescribed Activity/Exercise (5612)
- Cardiac Care: Rehabilitative (4046)
- Progressive Muscle Relaxation (1460)

Nursing Interventions/Rationales
- Assess and monitor patient's response to exercise (vital signs before and after exercise, dyspnea, signs of exertion). *Activity intolerance depends on the ability to physiologically adapt to changes in demand. Heart rate and blood pressure should increase with increasing demand but decrease to near baseline within 3 minutes after activity ceases.*
- Teach the patient to report dyspnea, chest pain, palpitations, and fatigue during activity. *Abnormal subjective responses indicate intolerance of activity.*
- Teach the patient to perform activities more slowly. *Energy conservation minimizes the risk of exceeding the heart's oxygen requirements.*

Nursing Care Plan — Patient With Ineffective Endocarditis—cont'd

- Assist the patient in sequencing activities to provide for rest periods. *Rest decreases myocardial oxygen consumption, allowing intervals of low energy demand.*
- Provide an environment conducive to rest. *Environmental stimulation inhibits the patient's ability to enter a state of relaxation and subsequent rest.*

Evaluation Parameters

1. Balances activity with rest
2. Performs only essential activities until endurance achieved
3. Explains physiologic basis for fatigue
4. Reports decreased fatigue
5. Vital signs return to normal within 3 minutes after activity

NURSING DIAGNOSIS **Risk for ineffective family management of therapeutic regimen related to complexity of therapeutic regimen, deficient knowledge**

GOALS/OUTCOMES Will practice preventive behaviors to minimize future episodes of endocarditis; Will verbalize understanding of the importance of maintaining therapeutic regimen

NOC Suggested Outcomes

- Adherence Behavior (1600)
- Compliance Behavior (1601)
- Knowledge: Treatment Regimen (1813)

NIC Suggested Interventions

- Behavior Modification (4360)
- Family Support (7140)
- Self-Modification Assistance (4470)
- Referral (8100)

Nursing Interventions/Rationales

- Provide verbal and written instructions for pathophysiology of endocarditis, treatment plan, medications, and signs and symptoms of endocarditis that need to be reported. *Teaching reinforces the need to comply with recommended management. Written material provides additional resource for home reference.*
- Teach the importance of appropriate antibiotic prophylaxis as recommended by the American Heart Association. *Adhering to recommendations helps decrease the risk of recurrence of disease.*
- Emphasize the importance of good oral care, avoidance of trauma to the gums, and the need for regular dental checkups. *Proper oral hygiene decreases the risk of pathogen entry via the oral mucosa. Trauma provides an opening in the oral mucosa for pathogenic entry.*
- Teach the importance of wearing an identification bracelet or necklace to inform health care providers of heart condition. *Proper identification can decrease the risk of inadvertent exposure to pathogens without appropriate prophylaxis.*
- Stress the importance of compliance with follow-up care recommendations. *Repetitive explanations may help improve adherence behaviors. Follow-up care is essential to prevent further cardiac compromise.*

Evaluation Parameters

1. Verbalizes understanding of therapeutic regimen
2. Reports adherence to therapeutic regimen
3. Reports for follow-up appointments as scheduled
4. Seeks assistance with therapeutic regimen as needed

NURSING DIAGNOSIS **Acute pain related to arthralgia and myalgia secondary to endocarditis**

GOALS/OUTCOMES Will report relief of pain from use of management strategies

NOC Suggested Outcomes

- Comfort Level (2100)
- Pain Control (1605)
- Pain Level (2120)

NIC Suggested Interventions

- Analgesic Administration (2210)
- Pain Management (1400)
- Coping Enhancement (5230)
- Medication Management (2380)

Nursing Interventions/Rationales

- Administer analgesics to relieve pain as prescribed. *Analgesics may lower pain level to tolerance, working synergistically with other nonpharmacologic strategies.*

Continued

Nursing Care Plan — Patient With Ineffective Endocarditis–cont'd

- Teach patient regarding self-administration of prescribed pain medications, including correct dosage, intervals between dosing, and potential side effects. *Allows patient to be in control and decreases the risk for over or under dosing.*
- Assess and document patient response to analgesic medications. *The effectiveness of medications needs to be evaluated to minimize risk of side effects and tolerance. Ineffective strategies need to be replaced with more effective alternatives.*
- Encourage adequate rest. *Sleep deprivation lowers pain threshold.*
- Monitor for signs of decreased tissue perfusion secondary to embolization. *Patients with endocarditis are at increased risk for embolism. Complete physical assessments are done every 8 hours to establish a baseline. Early detection of problems enables prompt intervention to minimize serious complications.*
- Teach patient the importance of maintaining antibiotic schedules. *Treating the underlying cause will reduce the pain associated with the disease.*

Evaluation Parameters

1. Reports progressive decrease in pain
2. Takes analgesic medications as prescribed
3. Maintains prescribed antibiotic schedule

Myocarditis

Etiology/Epidemiology

Myocarditis is an inflammatory disease of the myocardium that causes an infiltrate in the myocardial interstitium and injury to adjacent myocardial cells. Myocarditis may be a primary disease with an unknown etiology or occur secondary to an identifiable cause such as drug hypersensitivity or toxicity, connective tissue disease, sarcoidosis, or infection. The inflammatory process often develops secondary to endocarditis or pericarditis. Myocarditis may be classified as acute or chronic.

Viral infection is the most common cause of myocarditis. Picornaviruses as a group are the most common viral agents. The subset of coxsackie virus B accounts for nearly 50% of the cases, and coxsackie virus A, echovirus, and poliovirus account for most of the remainder. Other viruses include influenza A and B, rubella, mumps, rabies, Epstein-Barr, and hepatitis. Myocarditis can also be caused by several other infections, by noninfectious agents, or by an autoimmune reaction. Myocarditis has been associated with acquired immunodeficiency syndrome possibly related to opportunistic viral infection or HIV itself. The detection of the enterovirus genome in patients with suspected myocarditis supports the need for further study of a possible genetic basis for myocarditis.[11]

Pathophysiology

Both humoral and cell-mediated immune responses contribute to the damage of myocarditis. Direct damage to the myocardium through cytotoxic mechanisms probably occurs. An autoimmune response causes persistent myocardial disease. The clinical presentation varies with the extent of hypertrophy, fibrosis, and inflammation present within the myocytes and conduction system. During the acute phase symptoms are flulike and include fever, lymphadenopathy, pharyngitis, myalgias, and gastrointestinal complaints. Hepatitis, encephalitis, nephritis, and orchiitis also can occur. The most common cardiac symptom during the acute phase is pericardial pain, which may be associated with a friction rub. Other cardiac manifestations include signs of heart failure, syncope, pericardial effusion, and ischemia. Pulmonary rales (crackles) may be auscultated. Electrocardiogram changes include ST segment elevation, T wave flattening or inversion, appearance of Q waves, and QT interval prolongation. These abnormalities may disappear after recovery or persist for several years. Ventricular ectopy can include multiple forms of premature ventricular beats and ventricular tachycardia.

Preliminary laboratory findings are nonspecific and include elevation of the ESR, viral titers, and levels of various enzymes (such as lactic dehydrogenase, creatine kinase, and the transaminases). Mild to moderate leukocytosis with atypical lymphocytes may be seen. Chest radiographs may show the heart size to be normal or enlarged. Echocardiography shows dilated chambers, depressed systolic function, and mild or no pericardial effusion. Although the diagnosis of myocarditis may be suspected clinically, it must be confirmed histologically by endomyocardial biopsy while lymphocytic infiltration and myocyte damage are present (within 6 weeks of the acute illness). Autoimmune myocarditis is diagnosed through additional testing for autoimmune serum markers or the presence of intercellular adhesion molecules on cardiac myocytes.

Collaborative Care Management

Postbiopsy monitoring focuses on the potential for hematoma or bleeding at the cannulation site, cardiac tamponade, or pneumothorax. The site is inspected for bleeding, ecchymosis, or swelling. Shortness of breath, changes in breath sounds, dyspnea, and alterations in respiratory rate and pattern of breathing are reported. Vital signs are monitored closely to assess for continued hemodynamic stability.

Digitalis, once routinely used, is now prescribed with caution owing to a reported increase in mortality associated with its use.[11] Immunosuppressive therapy may be used to prevent irreversible myocardial damage in persons with autoimmune myocarditis. Medical therapy includes antibiotics, treatment of heart failure, and management of dysrhythmias. Monitoring for heart failure is an important nursing responsibility. Anticoagulation therapy is often prescribed to prevent intraventricular thrombi and embolic events. Ventricular assist devices may be indicated for patients progressing to dilated cardiomyopathy.

Supportive care is the cornerstone of management, including bed rest to decrease metabolic demand. Measures to decrease cardiac workload include frequent rest periods, a quiet environment, and the use of semi-Fowler's position. Patients are commonly anxious about the sudden onset of heart disease and its implications for the future. The nurse provides emotional support and encourages patients to verbalize their concerns.

Patient/Family Education. The nurse emphasizes the importance of an extended period of energy conservation. The risk of myocardial damage increases with exercise. The nurse teaches the need for slow progression in activity, with frequent rest periods. The use of NSAIDs in viral myocarditis appears to increase the myocardial damage, and the nurse emphasizes the need to avoid the use of NSAIDs. The patient is instructed about a heart-healthy diet and the early symptoms of heart failure that need to be reported promptly.

HEART FAILURE

Etiology

Heart failure occurs when the myocardium cannot maintain a sufficient cardiac output to meet the metabolic needs of the body. Failure can result from either systolic or diastolic dysfunction. The progression of heart failure depends in large part on the degree of ventricular remodeling that occurs after myocardial injury. Remodeling involves an increase in the intraventricular dimension, an increase in collagen formation leading to fibrosis, and myocyte changes that adversely affect contractility. Remodeling increases myocardial oxygen demands, decreases myocardial perfusion, and increases the potential for dysrhythmias.

Systolic dysfunction causes inadequate pumping of blood from the ventricle and decreases cardiac output. Any process that alters myocardial contractility can produce systolic dysfunction. Many disease processes are implicated, but ischemic heart disease and hypertension are the most prevalent causes (Box 24-4).

Diastolic dysfunction (stiff heart syndrome) occurs when the ventricle does not fill adequately during diastole. Inadequate filling decreases the amount of blood available in the ventricle for cardiac output. Systolic function is often normal. Hypertension and coronary artery disease (CAD) are again the primary causes of diastolic dysfunction, but it also occurs secondary to aging, infiltrative diseases (such as myocarditis), and constrictive pericarditis (Box 24-4).

BOX 24-4 Common Etiologies of Heart Failure

Systolic	Diastolic
Coronary artery disease	Coronary artery disease
Hypertension	Hypertrophy
Metabolic disorders	Fibrosis of advanced age
Myocarditis	Constrictive pericarditis
Alcohol	Myocarditis
Cocaine	Hypertension
Cardiac valve disease	Aortic stenosis
Dilated cardiomyopathy	Ventricular remodeling
	Collagen diseases
	Cardiomyopathy

The etiologies for both systolic and diastolic dysfunction are similar, but they affect the ventricles in different ways. Systolic dysfunction is the more common form of heart failure; however, the percentage of patients with chronic heart failure and preserved left ventricular systolic function is increasing. Nearly all patients with systolic dysfunction develop some degree of diastolic dysfunction over time.

Additional classifications of heart failure include right- or left-sided heart failure, biventricular failure, forward or backward failure, high- and low-output failure, and acute or chronic failure (Box 24-5). Such terms are useful for descriptive purposes, but they do not explain the underlying dysfunction.

Epidemiology

Approximately 4.7 million Americans have heart failure, and 550,000 new cases are diagnosed each year. Heart failure is the most common cause of cardiac disease related death in the United States. A total of 50% of all patients with heart failure die within 5 years of diagnosis.[1] Heart failure is the only major cardiovascular disorder that is increasing in incidence, prevalence, and mortality rate.

The most common cause of chronic heart failure is no longer hypertension or valvular heart disease, but CAD.[13] An increase in the number of survivors of myocardial infarction is in part responsible for this increase in patients with heart failure. Hypertension contributes to both systolic and diastolic dysfunction. Additional contributors to heart failure include diabetes, cigarette smoking, obesity, an elevated total cholesterol–to–high-density lipoprotein cholesterol ratio, an abnormally high or low hematocrit level, and proteinuria.

Morbidity from heart failure has made this diagnosis the number 1 reason for hospital admission. Management of heart failure is also extremely expensive. Inpatient costs for 1999 were estimated to be in excess of $23 billion, and outpatient costs added an additional $14.7 billion.[21] The prevalence of heart failure and its associated morbidity create multiple socioeconomic dilemmas for the health care system.

BOX 24-5 Categories of Heart Failure

Left-Sided vs. Right-Sided Heart Failure	
Left-sided heart failure	Left ventricular CO is less than volume received from the pulmonary circulation; blood accumulates in LV, LA, and pulmonary circulation
Right-sided heart failure	Right ventricular CO is less than volume received from the peripheral venous circulation; blood accumulates in the RV, RA, and peripheral venous system
Forward versus Backward Failure	
Forward failure	Decreased CO results in inadequate tissue perfusion
Backward failure	Blood remains in ventricle after systole, increasing atrial and then venous pressure; rise in venous pressure forces fluid out of capillary membranes into extracellular spaces
High-Output vs. Low-Output Failure	
High-output failure	Occurs in response to conditions that cause the heart to work harder to supply blood; the increased oxygen demand can be met only with an increase in CO; systemic vascular resistance decreases to promote CO
Low-output failure	Occurs in response to high blood pressure and hypovolemia; results in impaired peripheral circulation and peripheral vasoconstriction
Acute vs. Chronic Failure	
Acute failure	Occurs in response to a sudden decrease in CO; results in rapid decrease in tissue perfusion
Chronic failure	Body adjusts to decrease in CO through compensatory mechanisms; results in systemic congestion

LV, Left ventricle; *LA,* left atrium; *RV,* right ventricle; *RA,* right atrium; *CO,* cardiac output.

Pathophysiology

Systolic and diastolic heart failure both occur secondary to myocardial injury. The injury initiates ventricular remodeling, which is associated with myocyte hypertrophy, interstitial fibrosis, and changes in the genetic expression of cardiac cells and sarcomeric proteins. The ventricle changes shape and dimensions, decreasing its effectiveness as a pump. Increases in diastolic pressure may further change the shape of the left ventricle, resulting in papillary muscle rearrangement and mitral insufficiency. Accelerated programmed cell death (apoptosis or cell "suicide") decreases the number of myocytes available for pumping and occurs for as yet undetermined reasons. Geneticists continue to explore why the myocytes prematurely eliminate themselves without being damaged or diseased. Mutations in mitochondrial DNA have also been implicated in myocardial dysfunction.[3]

In most cases heart failure begins with left ventricular systolic dysfunction. Common causes of decreased left ventricular contractility include CAD, aortic stenosis, and systemic hypertension. CAD decreases contractility by diminishing the oxygen supply to the myofibrils. In aortic stenosis the left ventricle (LV) must increase its pumping force to deliver blood through the tight valve. Hypertension also causes the LV to contract more forcefully to eject blood into the aorta. Over time, the muscle fibers thicken (hypertrophy) and increase the myocardial oxygen consumption. Failure occurs when the heart's need for oxygen can no longer be met.

The diminished pumping power of the LV results in ejection fractions (EFs) of less than 40%. Blood remains in the LV at the end of systole. Left atrial pressure must increase to empty its volume into the LV. When the left atrium (LA) cannot completely empty its volume, blood backs up into the pulmonary circulation and increases the pressure within the fragile pulmonary capillaries. The increased pressure drives fluid out of the smaller pulmonary capillaries into the interstitium and alveoli. High pulmonary pressures then impede the flow of blood from the right ventricle (RV) to the lungs. The RV must generate more force to move blood into the pulmonary system. The remaining blood backs up into the (RA) and ultimately the peripheral venous circulation.

Right ventricular dysfunction most often results from LV dysfunction. Primary pulmonary hypertension and chronic obstructive pulmonary disease are other possible causes. The high pulmonary pressures impede the ability of the RV to pump blood to the pulmonary vessels, and the RV must generate higher pressures to overcome the resistance.

With left ventricular diastolic dysfunction, the LV is abnormally "stiff" (noncompliant) during diastole and does not fill at the normal lower pressures. Myocardial fibrosis and ventricular hypertrophy are possible causes of ventricular noncompliance. Fibrotic changes prevent the ventricle from expanding and occur with aging, myocardial infarction, and constrictive pericarditis. Hypertrophy results from hypertension, cardiac valve disease, and the compensatory changes that follow myocardial infarction. The increased muscle mass is often thick, stiff, and noncompliant. Elevated calcium concentrations also inhibit diastolic relaxation. Calcium concentrations rise when the sarcoplasmic reticulum is unable to remove calcium from the myofibril, as occurs with ischemia, hypertrophy, and advanced age.

A stiff LV is not able to expand effectively to receive additional blood volume. With higher preloads, congestion of blood within the heart may develop, as atrial pressures must increase to overcome the higher ventricular pressures. With low preload, the net result is a decrease in stroke volume (the actual volume pumped per beat), although the EF in diastolic heart failure may be normal.

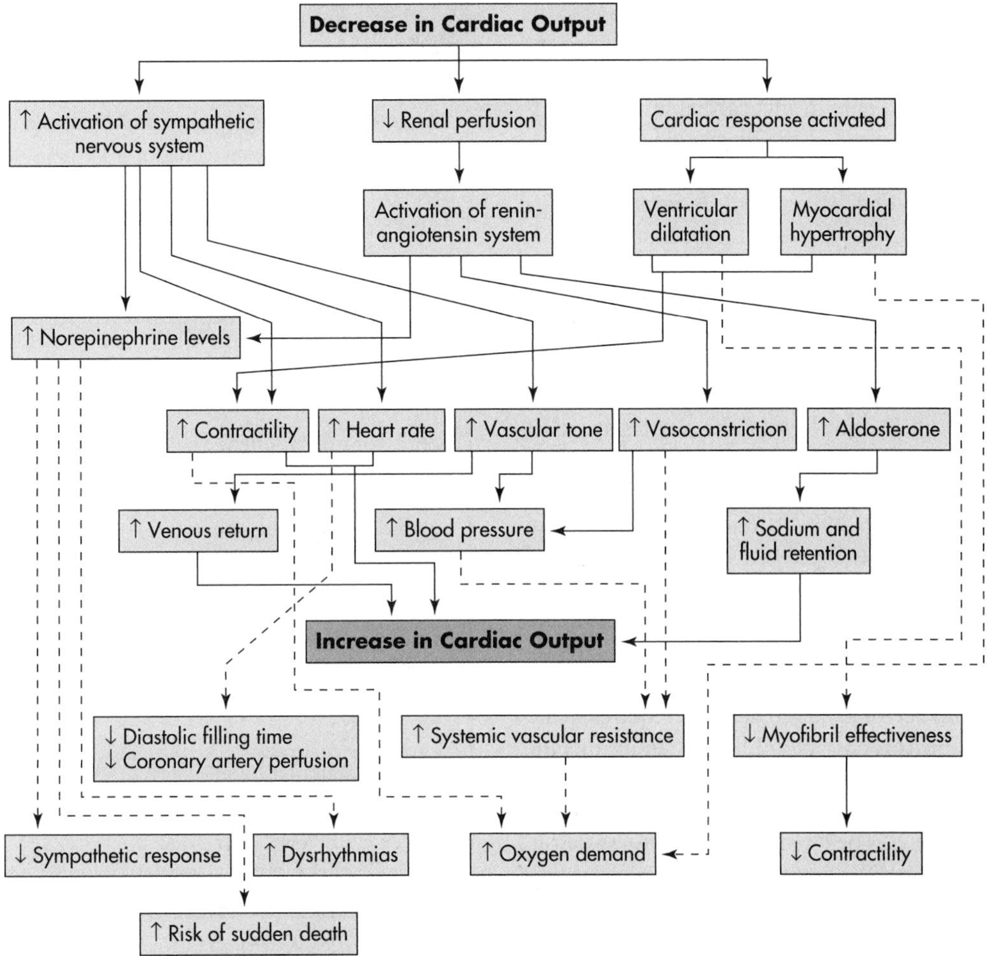

Figure 24-2 Compensatory mechanisms seen in response to the decreased cardiac output and blood pressure of heart failure. Dotted lines represent the negative effects of sustained compensatory mechanisms.

Compensatory Mechanisms. Altered myocardial contractility and filling result in hemodynamic instability. The body compensates for this instability through complex neurohormonal and endocrine responses. These "compensatory mechanisms" arise from the sympathetic nervous system, kidneys, and the heart itself (Figure 24-2).

Sympathetic Nervous System. The sympathetic nervous system responds to a drop in cardiac output by releasing more catecholamines, thereby increasing stimulation of both beta and alpha$_1$ receptors. Beta stimulation increases both heart rate and contractility and also causes the release of renin from the kidneys, increasing vascular tone. Alpha stimulation increases systemic arteriolar tone, causing a rise in blood pressure. The concomitant rise in venous tone increases the amount of blood returning to the right side of the heart. This increase in heart rate, contractility, and venous return initially all work to increase cardiac output.

Unfortunately these compensatory mechanisms lose their effectiveness over time. With increasing heart rates, the time for diastole shortens and less time is available for ventricular filling. Coronary blood flow (and oxygen delivery) decreases because the coronary arteries are perfused only during diastole. An increase in contractility requires more oxygen, and an increase in blood pressure raises the systemic vascular resistance (SVR). The SVR is the pressure the LV must overcome to eject its blood volume. The additional work required of the LV again increases myocardial oxygen demand. High levels of norepinephrine eventually decrease the heart's ability to respond to sympathetic stimulation and may cause cardiac dysrhythmias and sudden death. As heart failure progresses the ratio of alpha and beta receptor sites is altered. Excessive levels of norepinephrine can become directly cardiotoxic, increasing myocyte hypertrophy and fibrosis, and worsening the failure.

Renal System. Insufficient cardiac output decreases renal perfusion and activates the renin-angiotensin system to correct a perceived hypovolemia. Increased secretion of renin converts angiotensinogen to angiotensin I. Converting enzymes then change angiotensin I to angiotensin II, a potent vasoconstrictor. Angiotensin II also increases myocyte hypertrophy and fibrosis and promotes the release of norepinephrine from cardiac nerve endings. Aldosterone secretion is also increased, resulting in sodium and fluid retention. The increases in fluid volume and blood pressure increase cardiac output but quickly outlive their usefulness. In systolic dysfunction, any additional fluid volume increases the amount of fluid the failing ventricle must pump. Vasoconstriction increases SVR, which requires the ventricle to increase its pressure to eject its volume. Increased levels of angiotensin II may play a role in myocardial apoptosis. Aldosterone has been implicated in the fibrotic changes of advanced heart failure.[23]

Ventricular Dilation and Myocardial Hypertrophy. The heart tries to compensate for its failing performance in two additional ways: ventricular chamber dilation and myocardial hypertrophy. With increasing venous return from sympathetic stimulation and fluid retention, the ventricle dilates to accommodate the larger volumes. This dilation causes the myocardial fibers to stretch, resulting in an increased force of contraction. The Frank-Starling law of the heart states that continued overstretch of the myocardial fibers decreases their effectiveness. The fibers can no longer respond with an increase in force. Hence, in systolic dysfunction the additional increments in volume eventually result in more myocardial failure.

The heart also compensates by increasing the muscle mass. The hypertrophy results in a more forceful contraction. However, increasing numbers of myofibrils require more oxygen, and the increase in myocardial oxygen demand requires a corresponding increase in coronary blood flow; without this increase, subendocardial ischemia occurs.

Other. Additional neurohormonal influences occur in progressive heart failure. It is believed that excessive neurohormonal activation may increase myocyte apoptosis, hypertrophy, and endothelial dysfunction. Heart failure activates the release of endothelin, produced by vascular endothelial cells, and arginine vasopressin, released by the posterior pituitary gland. These neurohormones cause additional vasoconstriction and increases in preload. Research continues to explore the cardioprotective roles of atrial and brain natriuretic hormones, endothelium-derived relaxing factor, prostaglandins, and bradykinins. The levels of these protective substances may decrease as heart failure progresses. The deleterious role of cytokines, such as tumor necrosis factor-alpha and interleukin-6, have been implicated in the pathophysiology of progressive heart failure and future therapy directed toward these substances may positively affect the course of heart failure.

Decompensation. Compensatory mechanisms are beneficial in the short term. Stabilization of heart failure occurs through these compensatory mechanisms, as well as through therapeutic interventions. However, each compensatory mechanism also works against the heart to further increase myocardial oxygen demand (Figure 24-2). A patient with compensated heart failure may become decompensated when new insults or stresses to the heart occur (Box 24-6). Triggers include infections (e.g., pneumonia, active ischemia from CAD, tachydysrhythmias such as atrial fibrillation, surgery, and ineffective control of chronic conditions such as hypertension, pulmonary disease, or diabetes). These triggers increase the metabolic demand of the myocardium or interfere with its ability to contract or fill and can undo the fragile balance temporarily achieved through compensatory mechanisms and therapeutic modalities. Exacerbations of heart failure frequently require stabilization within the hospital setting and a reevaluation of management.

BOX 24-6 Precipitating Events in Decompensated Heart Failure

Factors Increasing Myocardial Demand

Additional Increases in Ventricular Volume to Be Pumped

Hypervolemia from high-output states (e.g., pregnancy, anemia, hyperthyroidism, infection)
Aortic regurgitation
Mitral regurgitation
Excessive sodium intake
Excessive administration of fluids
Renal failure

An Increase in the Ventricular Force Needed To Eject Blood

Poorly controlled systemic hypertension
Pulmonary hypertension
Significant aortic stenosis
Significant pulmonic stenosis

Factors Interfering With the Heart's Ability To Contract or Fill

Myocardial ischemia
Myocardial infarction
Cardiomyopathy
Myocarditis
Ventricular aneurysm
Excess alcohol intake
Mitral stenosis
Cardiac tamponade
Restrictive pericarditis
Dysrhythmias

Clinical Manifestations. Symptoms of heart failure occur secondary to elevated filling pressures and tissue hypoperfusion. Classic symptoms include dyspnea with exertion, orthopnea, nocturnal dyspnea, a dry hacking cough, and unexplained fatigue. When volume overload contributes to the pathology, the following additional signs and symptoms occur: rales (crackles), a third heart sound, peripheral edema, unexplained weight gain, jugular venous distention, hepatic engorgement, ascites, and worsening dyspnea. Compensatory mechanisms account for many of the clinical signs and symptoms of heart failure. Common symptoms as well as symptoms encountered with progressive heart failure are summarized in the Clinical Manifestations box.

Dyspnea, an abnormally uncomfortable awareness of breathing, occurs when high pulmonary pressures force fluid out of the pulmonary capillaries into the alveoli. The fluid in the alveoli interferes with effective gas exchange. Dyspnea may occur at rest or only with physical exertion when oxygen requirements increase.

Orthopnea, dyspnea in the recumbent position, is often present in heart failure. In the recumbent position, chest expansion diminishes, resulting in decreased ventilation. In addition, venous return to the right heart increases with elevation of the legs. Patients experiencing orthopnea must often

Clinical Manifestations

Heart Failure

RESPIRATORY

Dyspnea
Orthopnea
Paroxysmal nocturnal dyspnea
Persistent hacking cough
Alternating periods of apnea and hyperpnea
Rales (crackles)

CARDIOVASCULAR

Angina
Jugular venous distention
Tachycardia
Decrease in systolic blood pressure with increase in diastolic blood pressure
S3 or S4 heart sounds

GASTROINTESTINAL

Enlargement and tenderness in the right upper quadrant of the abdomen
Ascites
Nausea
Vomiting
Bloating
Anorexia
Epigastric pain

CEREBRAL

Altered mental status (confusion, restlessness)

GENERALIZED

Fatigue
Decrease in activity tolerance
Postural dizziness
Edema (peripheral, pitting)
Cool extremities
Weight gain

PSYCHOSOCIAL

Anxiety

BOX 24-7 New York Heart Association Classification of Heart Failure

Class I: No symptoms, tolerates ordinary physical activity
Class II: Comfortable at rest; ordinary physical activity results in symptoms
Class III: Comfortable at rest; less than ordinary physical activity results in symptoms
Class IV: Symptoms may be present at rest; symptoms with any physical activity

sleep using several pillows or sitting in a semi-Fowler's position.

Although orthopnea may occur immediately after the patient lies down, it typically does not occur for 2 to 5 hours. The patient awakes suddenly with severe shortness of breath, often in panic, a condition called paroxysmal nocturnal dyspnea. The severe dyspnea resolves after being upright for 10 to 30 minutes.

With severe heart failure the patient may experience alternating periods of apnea and hyperpnea (Cheyne-Stokes respiration). Poor gas exchange causes an inadequate delivery of oxygen to the brain, and makes the respiratory center in the brain insensitive to subtle changes in the amount of carbon dioxide in the arterial blood. Respirations cease until stimulation of the respiratory center occurs from either a dramatic increase in the carbon dioxide content or critically low levels of oxygen. The patient then experiences hyperpnea. The rapid respirations decrease the carbon dioxide content of the arterial blood, resulting in apnea.

A persistent hacking cough is a common symptom of heart failure. Coughing results from the congestion of trapped fluid, which is irritating to the mucosal lining of the lungs and bronchi. On auscultation, rales (crackles) are heard as a moist popping and crackling sound at the end of inspiration.

Patients with heart failure commonly become fatigued after activities that ordinarily are not tiring. The fatigue results from inadequate tissue perfusion as a result of the decreased cardiac output. The reduction in tissue oxygen decreases the aerobic production of adenosine triphosphate, the immediate energy source for muscle contraction. Inadequate perfusion also decreases removal of metabolic waste products, further decreasing muscle function. Activity intolerance is common in both systolic and diastolic dysfunction. It is often the initial symptom with diastolic dysfunction because (1) stroke volume cannot increase when the LV prevents an adequate end diastolic volume and (2) exercise-induced tachycardia decreases the diastolic filling time further. The severity of activity intolerance, while subjective, is often recorded in objective terms. One of the most widely used classification systems for activity intolerance is the New York Heart Association classification shown in Box 24-7.

Angina can occur from decreased blood flow to the myocardium. The balance of myocardial oxygen supply and demand is precarious in even the most stable, compensated patient with heart failure. When factors occur that can precipitate decompensation (see Box 24-6), the likelihood of angina increases. Angina is most likely to occur in patients with preexisting CAD.

Engorgement of the low-pressure peripheral venous system results from pressure increases in the right heart. Distention of the internal jugular vein (jugular vein distention) is often observed with the patient in a semi-Fowler's position. With sharply elevated venous pressure, pulsations of the earlobes may occur when the patient sits upright.

High venous pressures force fluid into the extravascular tissue. The patient often notices this as pitting, nontender edema in dependent areas, usually the lower extremities. As the edema becomes more pronounced, it progresses up the legs into the thighs, external genitalia, and lower portion of the trunk. If the tissue becomes extremely engorged, the skin may crack and fluid may "weep" from the tissues. Increasing fluid volume is most often responsible for the unexplained weight gain experienced by patients in heart failure. Fluid volume increases as urine output diminishes from poor renal perfusion.

The liver also becomes engorged with intravascular fluid, resulting in enlargement and tenderness in the right upper quadrant of the abdomen. Altered hepatic blood flow adversely affects liver function. Among its many functions, the liver metabolizes aldosterone and antidiuretic hormone and many of the medications used to treat heart failure. Pressure increases within the portal system can force fluid through the blood vessels into the abdominal cavity. The resulting ascites can create nausea, vomiting, bloating, and epigastric pain and put pressure on the diaphragm, resulting in respiratory distress.

Tachycardia is often present as the sympathetic nervous system attempts to compensate for the low cardiac output. The skin becomes cool and clammy as the sympathetic nervous system triggers vasoconstriction and stimulates the sweat glands. Additional physical assessment findings include a decrease in systolic blood pressure with an increase in diastolic blood pressure. S3 and S4 heart sounds are often heard over the mitral or right ventricular area. These sounds reflect the resistance to ventricular filling. Confusion and restlessness can occur if cerebral blood flow diminishes.

TABLE 24-1 Common Laboratory Value Abnormalities with Heart Failure

Laboratory Value	Alteration	Rationale
Sodium	Decreased	An increase in total body water dilutes body fluid
Chloride	Decreased	Associated with sodium loss
Potassium	Increased	Depressed effective renal blood flow and low glomerular filtration rate
Blood urea nitrogen	Increased	Decreased renal perfusion
Creatinine	Increased	Impaired renal function
Red blood cell count	Decreased	Decreased production of erythropoietin with renal involvement
Liver function tests	Increased	Hepatic congestion
Pao_2	Decreased	Fluid in alveoli limits exchange of oxygen
$Paco_2$	Decreased	Compensatory increase in respiratory rate decreases CO_2

Collaborative Care Management

Diagnostic Tests

Chest Radiograph. When blood backs up into the pulmonary vasculature, the congestion appears on the chest film as whitened dense areas. Dilated upper lobe vessels are a common finding. A normal size heart with pulmonary congestion suggests acute new-onset heart failure or diastolic dysfunction. An enlarged heart (cardiomegaly) signals chronic heart failure with hypertrophy or dilation. An additional feature is the appearance of Kerley's B lines on the x-ray film, which occur at the bases of the lungs and extend to the pleura. Kerley's B lines reflect lymphatic drainage of the overloaded pulmonary vasculature. The presence of liver congestion on x-ray study may signify right-sided heart failure.

Laboratory Blood Tests. Blood tests can be useful in determining the precipitating factors of heart failure. Common blood tests include studies for anemia or hyperthyroidism. Heart failure directly alters many laboratory findings as well. Table 24-1 lists common laboratory findings in heart failure with a brief rationale for the abnormal values.

Brain natriuretic peptide may be released as a consequence of vascular volume changes. It is a cardioprotective compensatory mechanism, and its levels are highest in early heart failure. Levels decrease with progressive, chronic heart failure. Currently, brain natriuretic peptide is being evaluated as a diagnostic marker for heart failure; it is not specific to heart failure, however, and is also elevated in myocardial infarction, ventricular hypertrophy, and chronic obstructive pulmonary disease.[7]

Electrocardiography. The electrocardiogram (ECG) may be normal in heart failure. However, the ECG of a patient with substantial left ventricular dysfunction is usually abnormal and reflects the etiology of the failure (e.g., ischemia, infarction, tachydysrhythmias, hypertrophy, tamponade).

Echocardiography. Echocardiography provides data about left and right ventricular function, valve function, and abnormal areas of contractility. A nondilated, normally contracting LV rules out systolic dysfunction. Left ventricular EF and cardiac size reflect the severity and progression of heart failure. An EF below 40% often confirms left ventricular dysfunction. However, patients with EFs above 40% may still have heart failure from valvular disease or diastolic dysfunction. Doppler echocardiography analyzes blood flow and may reveal a reduction in early filling of the LV.

Cardiac Catheterization. In patients with known CAD, cardiac catheterization provides additional information to guide the management of heart failure. With diastolic dysfunction, cardiac catheterization of the right side of the heart reveals an elevated end-diastolic pressure at normal or decreased left ventricular volumes. A summary of hemodynamic findings characteristic of heart failure is provided in Table 24-2.

Other. In patients without ECG evidence of CAD, exercise stress testing is sometimes helpful in ruling out CAD as a factor in heart failure. Radionuclide ventriculography (multiple gated acquisition [MUGA]; see Chapter 22) uses radioactive dye to determine the EF. MUGA is superior to echocardiography for obtaining quantitative data and assessing the right ventricle.

Medications. Pharmacologic agents play a central role in the management of heart failure. Prescribed agents include diuretics, angiotensin-converting enzyme (ACE) inhibitors, and inotropes. These medications decrease the pressure generated by the volume of blood that the heart must pump (preload), decrease the resistance the heart must overcome to eject its volume (afterload), or increase the force of myocardial contraction (positive inotropic action). Beta-blockers blunt the neurohormonal mechanisms responsible for the downward

TABLE 24-2 Altered Hemodynamic Findings in Heart Failure

Hemodynamic Variable	Finding in Heart Failure	Rationale
Cardiac output (CO)/index	Decreased	Systolic or diastolic dysfunction
Systemic vascular resistance	Increased	Compensate for decreased CO
Pulmonary artery wedge pressure	Increased when left side of heart affected	End-diastolic pressure or volume in left ventricle rises due to inadequate emptying or inability to relax during diastole
Central venous pressure	Increased when right side of heart affected	Reflects increased pressure and volume within right side of heart

spiraling nature of heart failure. Most protocols that outline the treatment of heart failure evolved from research about systolic heart failure. Diastolic heart failure is managed using many of the same medications, but the approach to managing pulmonary congestion is individualized to the patient's preload. Box 24-8 outlines the pharmacologic management of heart failure endorsed by the expert group on Heart Failure for Quality of Care and Outcomes Research.[14] Figure 24-3 is an algorithm for the pharmacologic management of systolic heart failure. Table 24-3 lists commonly used pharmacologic agents and the mechanism of action for each.

Angiotensin-Converting Enzyme Inhibitors. ACE inhibitors block the enzyme that converts angiotensin I to angiotensin II, thereby blocking both vasoconstriction and the production of aldosterone. The resulting decrease in SVR reduces afterload. The resulting mild hypotension is usually well tolerated because of the accompanying increase in cardiac output. The decrease in aldosterone production causes less sodium and water to be retained, resulting in a decrease in preload. Renal blood flow increases, promoting natriuresis. ACE inhibitors also block the catabolism of bradykinins, promoting further vasodilation, and they inhibit remodeling by decreasing hypertrophy and collagen formation. Because of their combined effects on afterload, preload, and remodeling, ACE inhibitors are considered to be the drugs of choice for all patients with heart failure. ACE inhibitor therapy is the only therapy that has been conclusively shown to reduce mortality and morbidity in heart failure.[13]

ACE inhibitors are prescribed for patients who are asymptomatic but are known to have low EFs, and for patients who require long-term therapy after experiencing an acute episode of heart failure. Research indicates that ACE inhibitors remain underprescribed and underdosed despite their proven effectiveness. Side effects such as hypotension, cough, and renal impairment may deter clinicians from maximizing their use of these important drugs.

BOX 24-8 Quality Indicators Endorsed by the American Heart Association/American College of Cardiology for the Management of Heart Failure

Medication Measures

Patients with heart failure, left ventricular systolic dysfunction, and no contraindications to angiotensin-converting enzyme (ACE) inhibitors should be prescribed ACE inhibitors. Angiotensen-receptor blockers or a hydralazine-nitrate combination should not be substituted for ACE inhibitors in patients who tolerate ACE inhibitors.

Patients hospitalized with heart failure and left ventricular systolic dysfunction should be treated with digoxin.

Patients with NYHA class II and III heart failure, left ventricular systolic dysfunction, and no contraindication to beta-blockers should be prescribed beta-blockers.

General Medical Interventions

Vaccinations against influenza and pneumonia

Anticoagulation to prevent emboli associated with atrial fibrillation

Evaluation of ischemia

Treatment of hyperlipidemia for coronary artery disease

Reference: Krumholz HM et al: American Heart Association/American College of Cardiology First Scientific Forum on Assessment of Healthcare Quality in Cardiovascular Disease and Stroke: Conference Proceedings, Measuring and Improving Quality of Care: a report of the Quality of Care and Outcomes Research Working Group on Heart Failure, *Circulation* 101(12):1483, 2000.

Diuretics. Diuretics are administered when clinical signs of volume overload exist. Commonly administered diuretics include loop diuretics, thiazides, and potassium-sparing diuretics. Diuretics increase urinary output, causing a decrease in blood volume, preload, and ultimately cardiac workload. Diuretics can be administered intravenously to treat acute heart failure and orally for long-term management of fluid overload. Patients with chronic heart failure are likely to benefit from combination diuretic therapy.

Loop diuretics act in the ascending limb of the loop of Henle to enhance the excretion of sodium, chloride, potassium, calcium, and magnesium. The loop diuretics, including furosemide (Lasix), bumetanide (Bumex), and torsemide (Demadex), are powerful diuretics that can be administered intravenously or orally. Electrolyte imbalance is a common adverse side effect in many patients and can predispose them to dysrhythmias.

Thiazide diuretics block the resorption of sodium, potassium, and water in the proximal portion of the distal tubule, but they lose their effectiveness when renal function is impaired. Thiazide diuretics are often combined with loop diuretics for increased diuresis. Metolazone (Diulo) is a commonly prescribed combination. Electrolyte abnormalities remain a significant concern.

Potassium-sparing diuretics include spironolactone (Aldactone), amiloride (Midamor), and triamterene (Dyrenium). Spironolactone inhibits aldosterone, causing sodium

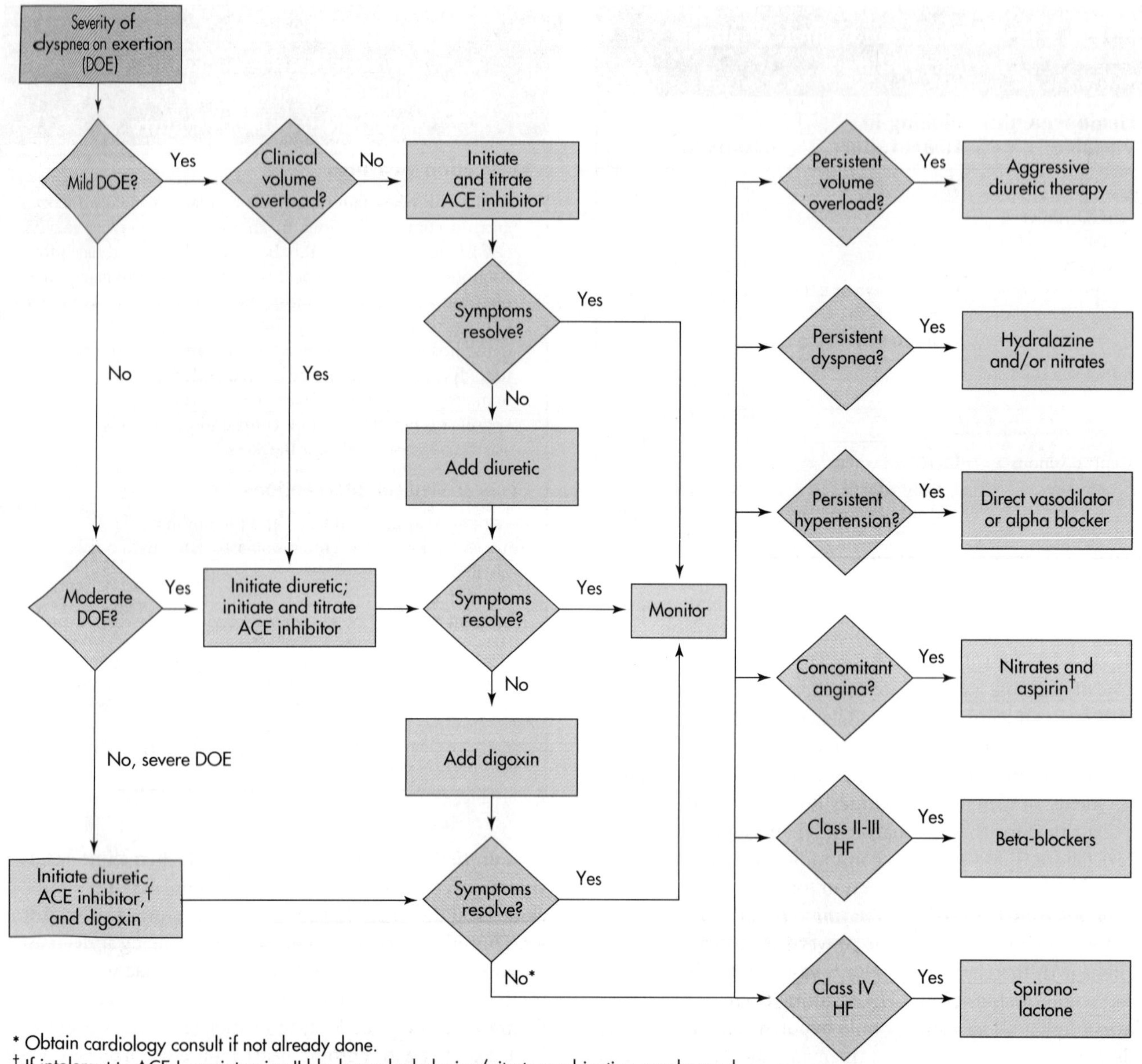

Figure 24-3 Pharmacologic management of patients with systolic heart failure.

to be excreted in the distal tubule, but sparing potassium. Spironolactone also blocks the remodeling and fibrotic effects of aldosterone on the myocardium, and the drug is considered to be cardioprotective for NYHA III and IV heart failure patients when used as an adjunct to conventional therapy.[23]

Inotropes. Digitalis preparations remain the most widely prescribed inotropic agents. Digoxin, the most common form of digitalis, inhibits the sodium-potassium pump, causing an increase in intracellular sodium levels. Concentration gradients force the excess sodium out of the cell in exchange for calcium. Higher intracellular calcium levels increase the force of contraction, increasing cardiac output and decreasing the end-diastolic pressure. Digoxin also blocks the slow calcium channels of the atrioventricular nodes, slowing the heart rate and increasing time for ventricular filling. In addition digoxin blunts the neurohormonal compensatory mechanisms of heart failure, and this action is now believed to be the key to its effectiveness rather than its ability to increase contractile force. Digoxin does not benefit all patients and can even be deleterious in diastolic dysfunction. The use of digoxin has not been shown to influence mortality rates.

Dobutamine (Dobutrex), a sympathomimetic agent, acts primarily on beta-1 receptors, stimulating cyclic adenosine monophosphate (cAMP), which increases intracellular calcium and results in a greater contractile force. The increase in cardiac output causes the body's own compensatory sympathetic stimulation to decrease, slightly decreasing afterload. In severe heart failure dobutamine therapy can be used continuously or intermittently until alternatives such as heart transplant become available. However, dobutamine may gradually

TABLE 24-3 Common Medications for Heart Failure

Drug	Action	Intervention
Angiotensin-Converting Enzyme Inhibitors		
Captopril, enalapril, fosinopril, lisinopril, quinipril, ramipril	Block vasoconstriction and aldosterone, decreasing systemic vascular resistance, afterload, and preload	Be alert to the presence of volume depletion from diuretics before initiating ACE inhibitor therapy (may need to correct hypovolemia before ACE inhibitor therapy) Closely monitor for hypotension at initiation of therapy; maintain patient on bed rest for 3 hours after initial dose Monitor lab values for development of hyperkalemia, renal insufficiency (increasing blood urea nitrogen and creatinine) and neutropenia (decreasing white blood cell count) Be alert to side effects limiting compliance: cough, rash, and angioedema
Diuretics	Decrease volume overload Increase urinary output Decrease preload	
Loop diuretics (furosemide, bumetanide, torsemide)	Enhance the excretion of sodium, chloride, potassium, calcium, and magnesium	Loop diuretics, thiazides: monitor labs for hypokalemia, hyperglycemia, hyperuricemia; observe for postural hypotension and rashes
Thiazides (hydrochlorothiazide); thiazide-related (metolazone)	Block resorption of sodium, chloride, water in distal tubule	
Potassium sparing (spironolactone)	Inhibit action of aldosterone, interferes with sodium reabsorption in distal tubule	Monitor for increasing potassium levels, especially when administered with ACE inhibitors
Inotropes	Increase contractility Increase cardiac output Decrease left ventricular end-diastolic pressure	
Digoxin	Inhibits sodium-potassium pump, increasing intracellular calcium; slows heart rate by slowing conduction through the atrioventricular node, blunts neurohormonal mechanisms	Be alert for cardiac dysrhythmias and clinical manifestations of toxicity (confusion, nausea, anorexia, visual disturbance); monitor for hypokalemia, which can increase potential for toxicity
Dobutamine	Stimulates beta-1 receptors, increases intracellular calcium and contractility; increases myocardial oxygen demand; decreases afterload; increases cardiac output	Record accurate weight for correct dose; communicate signs and symptoms of hypovolemia when therapy initiated; be alert to dysrhythmias that may require decrease in dose or discontinuation of therapy; be aware of safe intravenous administration including knowledge of onset of action within 1 to 2 minutes, titrating dose to blood pressure and heart rate, tapering drip when discontinuing therapy, monitoring site for infiltration
Phosphodiesterase Inhibitors		
Milrinone	Vasodilates by relaxing vascular smooth muscle, decreasing afterload and preload; increases cardiac output by increasing cyclic adenosine monophosphate levels	Observe for chest pain, hypotension, dysrhythmias, hypotension; administer loading dose over 10 minutes; note onset within 5 to 15 minutes
Beta Blockers		
Metoprolol	Blunts neurohormonal mechanisms Decrease oxygen demand	Should be initiated only after patients have been stabilized with conventional therapy (ACE inhibitors, diuretics, and digoxin). Monitor for bradycardia, heart block, and hypotension. Anticipate initial worsening of heart failure upon initiation of therapy. Patient education to include support through initiation period and warnings not to stop medication abruptly.
Carvedilol	Vasodilates by alpha-1 blockade	

ACE, Angiotensin-converting enzyme.

Continued

TABLE 24-3 Common Medications for Heart Failure—cont'd

Drug	Action	Intervention
Angiotensin II Receptor Blockers		
Losartan	Produces direct antagonism of angiotensin II receptors	Monitor for adverse effects: dizziness, upper respiratory infection, hyperkalemia
Vasodilators	Decrease cardiac workload Improve stroke volume and cardiac output	
Nitrates (isosorbide dinitrate)	Venodilate, reducing preload	Monitor for headache and hypotension
Hydralazine	Directly dilate arterioles, decreasing afterload	Monitor for headache, nausea, tachycardia, and lupuslike syndrome
Nitroprusside	Dilates arteries and veins; decreases left ventricular filling pressure	Monitor for severe hypotension
Prazosin	Dilates arteries and veins	Monitor for dizziness, headache, and hypotension
Dopamine	At low doses: stimulates dopaminergic receptors in renal vessels, increasing renal blood flow, increasing diuresis; increases myocardial contractility; vasodilates peripheral arterioles	Note onset of action within 10 minutes; monitor site for infiltration; if extravasation occurs, prepare Regitine to infiltrate site; titrate drip to blood pressure and urine output; taper dose when discontinuing
Morphine Sulfate	Decreases anxiety Promotes venous pooling, decreasing preload and workload	Monitor vital signs before and after administration, with special attention to respiration depression; evaluate effect on anxiety
Anticoagulants	Patients with a history of systemic or pulmonary embolism or recent atrial fibrillation should be anticoagulated to an INR of 2 to 3	Communicate bleeding precautions and safety measures to all caregivers; teach importance of follow-up coagulation studies, minimizing changes in intake of vitamin K, and need for safety to prevent bleeding occurrences

become ineffective as downregulation of the beta-receptor sites occurs. Downregulation reflects a decline in the number of responsive beta-receptor sites that occurs from overstimulation of the receptors. Beta blockers are now a recommended component of heart failure management; dobutamine's future role is therefore uncertain.

Milrinone (Primacor) blocks the activity of phosphodiesterase, which breaks down cAMP, resulting in an increase in contractility that improves stroke volume and cardiac output. Milrinone also increases vasodilator activity and relaxes smooth muscle, thereby decreasing both afterload and preload. Milrinone is usually prescribed short term for refractory heart failure.

Dobutamine and milrinone are most often used for treatment of acute episodes of heart failure. They can also be administered intermittently at outpatient clinics, although the benefits of intermittent or home therapy have not been substantiated. Current evidence suggests that intermittent dosing is associated with symptom improvement and increased functional status, but also with an increase in mortality.[16]

Beta-Blockers. Beta-blockers halt the negative effect of the sympathetic nervous system on the failing heart. They decrease heart rate and allow more complete emptying of the LA, thereby improving left ventricular volume. Myocardial oxygen demand decreases along with the decrease in heart rate and contractility. Beta-blockers were once believed to be detrimental in heart failure because of their negative inotropic properties, and numerous studies of their effects in heart failure have been conducted. These studies confirm that beta-blockers blunt neurohormonal mechanisms, decrease remodeling, improve overall myocardial function, and decrease dysrhythmias. Beta-blocker therapy is initiated once the patient is stabilized with ACE inhibitors and diuretic therapy. Treatment begins at very low doses and is increased only if tolerated. An initial worsening of heart failure is anticipated. Carvedilol (Coreg) has vasodilatory properties in addition to its beta-blocking effects and is the only beta-blocker currently approved for heart failure management.

Angiotensin II Blockers. Angiotensin II blockers are direct antagonists of the angiotensin II receptor. By blocking the binding of angiotensin II to its receptor site, the vasoconstrictor and aldosterone effects of angiotensin II are interrupted. Preload and afterload are decreased. Angiotensin II blockers do not block the catabolism of bradykinin and do not cause the angioedema or cough associated with the bradykinin-mediated effects of ACE inhibitors. However, the beneficial effects of bradykinin on vasodilation and remodeling are also absent. Research does not support the use of angiotensin II antagonists over ACE inhibitors for heart failure. ACE inhibitors remain the drugs of choice for all heart failure patients. Angiotensin II blockers are prescribed for patients who cannot tolerate ACE inhibitors.

Vasodilators. Arterial and/or venous dilation causes a reduction in cardiac workload. Nitrates dilate both arteries and veins when given intravenously; nonparenteral nitrates predominantly affect the systemic veins, reducing preload. Hydralazine (Apresoline) is a direct arteriolar vasodilator that reduces afterload and therefore cardiac workload. The decrease in afterload improves both stroke volume and cardiac output. Hydralazine may be given IV in conjunction with nitrates to stabilize acute heart failure. It can also be given orally with nonparenteral nitrates for long-term management, but its use in chronic failure is not well supported by research.

Nitroprusside (Nipride) also dilates both arteries and veins and can be administered intravenously for stabilization of acute heart failure. Prazosin (Minipress), an alpha-adrenergic blocker, also dilates both arteries and veins and can be administered orally.

Adjunctive Pharmacologic Agents. Dopamine hydrochloride (Intropin) in low doses (2 to 5 μg/kg/min) is often used in combination with inotropes, vasodilators, or diuretics to treat heart failure. Low-dose dopamine stimulates dopaminergic receptors in the renal vessels, resulting in an increased renal blood flow and a more effective diuresis. The net result is an increase in cardiac output. Doses between 5 and 10 μg may be used to increase myocardial contractility. Doses above 10 mg/kg/min stimulate alpha-receptors and cause profound vasoconstriction and are not used.

Morphine sulfate decreases anxiety and sympathetic stimulation and is used in acute episodes of heart failure. Morphine also promotes venodilation, reducing both preload and cardiac workload.

Supplemental oxygenation is appropriate when inadequate oxygenation and gas exchange occur, as often evidenced by oxygen saturation levels below 90%. Mechanical ventilation may occasionally be necessary to reduce the work of breathing.

Heart failure can increase the risk of blood clots occurring as a result of stagnant blood flow. Anticoagulation is currently recommended for heart failure patients with a history of systemic or pulmonary embolism, recent onset of atrial fibrillation, or existing left ventribular thrombi.[28] Low-dose aspirin therapy may be indicated for its antiplatelet activity. Higher doses of aspirin are associated with possible interference with the action of ACE inhibitors. The use of warfarin (Coumadin) and antiplatelet therapy in heart failure is currently being studied in a major clinical trial.[29]

Dysrhythmias are frequent, and at times fatal, complications of heart failure, but the routine use of antidysrhythmics is not supported through clinical research. Amiodarone (Cordarone) is the only antidysrhythmic agent that is not contraindicated for individuals with heart failure. Sotalol (Betapace) may have a role in the management of life-threatening dysrhythmias, but further investigation is required.

Research also does not support the use of calcium channel blockers in the management of heart failure. However, newer calcium channel blockers such as amiodipine (Norvasc) and felodipine (Plendil), which have predominantly vasodilatory action, may be used safely for afterload reduction in selected patients with heart failure. These agents decrease SVR and lower neurohormonal activity.

New agents are being investigated that can block the remodeling process. Etanercept (Enbrel) is an investigational agent currently being studied for its role in blocking tumor necrosis factor-alpha, which is implicated in the pathology of progressive heart disease. Additional studies will continue to investigate ways to interrupt the numerous compensatory pathways involved in heart failure pathophysiology.

Treatments. The goal of treatment for heart failure is to improve cardiac performance without increasing cardiac workload. Medications are the mainstays of treatment; however, adjunctive therapies are effective in specific patient populations. Treatment guidelines continue to evolve in response to ongoing clinical trials.[28]

Patients with both heart failure and renal failure may benefit from ultrafiltration (hemofiltration) or hemodialysis to reduce blood volume. Vascular access is established, and blood flows through a hemofilter within an extracorporeal circuit that removes fluid and metabolic wastes. The two primary methods of ultrafiltration are continuous arteriovenous hemofiltration (CAVH) and continuous arteriovenous hemofiltration and dialysis (CAVHD). Patients who are hypotensive and are receiving maximal inotrope support can seldom tolerate removal of large fluid volumes through hemodialysis. For these patients, CAVH or CAVHD may be appropriate alternatives.

In chronic heart failure beta-receptor responsiveness diminishes (downregulation), causing the heart's compensatory mechanisms to fail and medications to become ineffective. It then becomes necessary to decrease cardiac workload through nonpharmacologic devices such as the intraaortic balloon pump (IABP) and ventricular assist devices (VAD). These devices are described in more detail later in the chapter (see p. 747). The IABP decreases afterload, thus decreasing the workload of the heart. It also increases coronary perfusion during diastole when the balloon inflates. Patients in low-output states or with a structural abnormality may require stabilization with a VAD. The VAD withdraws blood from the ventricle or atrium and infuses it directly into either the pulmonary or systemic circulation; this rests the failing ventricle. Currently approved VADs are preload driven, meaning they pump to the body what they receive from venous return. VADs are being used increasingly to support patients who are awaiting heart transplantation. It is theorized that VAD therapy may even replace transplantation as the preferred mode of therapy.[6] Patients can already be successfully managed at home with a VAD in place.

Surgical Management. Surgical interventions can reverse the course of heart failure arising from some etiologies. Corrective surgeries include pericardiectomy, valve replacements or valvuloplasty, surgical repair of septal defects, and ventricular aneurysmectomies. Revascularization through coronary artery bypass graft surgery may be of benefit for patients who also have severe angina, although the surgery is accompanied by significant morbidity and mortality. Revascularization does not play a role for patients with heart failure who do not have angina.

In progressive heart failure transplantation may be the only option. Ischemic heart disease and dilated cardiomyopathies account for the majority of cardiac transplant procedures. Survival rates are good and remain steady at 69% at 5 years. Criteria for heart transplantation continue to change as surgical experience improves. The primary limiting factor is the availability of donor hearts; only 2184 heart transplants were performed in the United States in 1999.[1] Transplantation is discussed in detail in Chapter 51.

Because of the shortage of donor hearts, new treatment strategies are continuously being researched (see Future Watch box). For the patient with heart failure secondary to cardiomyopathy, the Batista procedure that removes excess ventricular muscle may be beneficial. Cardiomyoplasty is another surgical option for end-stage heart failure. The procedure involves surgically wrapping the latissimus dorsi muscle around the heart, limiting additional dilation of the ventricle. Stimulating electrodes are also placed in the muscle and connected to a cardiomyostimulator. When muscle stimulation is initiated, the wrapped muscle supports left ventricular contraction.

Diet. A "no added salt" diet is recommended for patients with mild heart failure. This diet eliminates salt in food preparation and avoids obviously salted foods. Sodium-restricted diets of 2 g of sodium daily decrease extracellular water and blood volume. Sodium restrictions of less than 2 g are rarely ordered because the diet is unpalatable, resulting in poor patient adherence. The use of salt substitutes requires careful attention to potassium content if patients are taking potassium-sparing diuretics.

Fluid restrictions may also be necessary for patients with acute or chronic heart failure. Such restrictions consider weight fluctuations, intake and output ratios, and the electrolyte status of the patient. Fluid restrictions are often unnecessary. For patients with diuretic-induced thirst, an upper limit of 64 oz (2 L) daily is a valid guideline.

Supervised weight loss programs are indicated for obese patients with heart failure. Other patients may need nutritional supplementation owing to cachexia-related weight loss. Albumin levels may decrease as a result of nutritional deficiencies and fluid overload. Serum albumin levels below 3 g/dl indicate malnutrition and require further assessment and intervention. Alcohol use is restricted to one drink per day, defined as one glass of beer or wine, or a mixed drink containing no more than 1 oz of alcohol. Minimizing caffeine intake is advisable for patients with tachycardic heart rhythms.

Activity. Patients experiencing acute heart failure need to be on bed rest to minimize oxygen demands; however, activity increases as soon as blood pressure, heart rate, and oxygen saturation stabilize. In general, monitored aerobic exercise programs are most effective in improving exercise tolerance and performance. Patients with EFs as low as 13% can safely exercise without experiencing exercise-related complications or adversely affecting cardiac output or wall motion. Heart failure patients without ischemia receive detailed exercise prescriptions that include activity frequency, intensity, type, and duration. Patients with heart failure need to recognize their individual tolerance levels for physical activity and limit activity until their symptoms resolve. Patients with heart failure and ongoing ischemia may need to undergo revascularization before beginning a conditioning program.

Referrals. The complexity of heart failure requires a team approach to care. Multidisciplinary health care professionals work collaboratively with the patient and family to improve quality of life. Nutritionists, exercise physiologists, nurses, stress management professionals, chaplains, respiratory therapists, social workers, physicians, and psychosocial counselors may all be involved. Coordination of care is essential to decrease the frequency of hospital admissions, limit length of stay, and increase both the quality of care and patient satisfaction.

Future Watch
Arm Muscle Keeps Heart Pumping?

In May 2001, researchers at the University of California, Los Angeles successfully implanted arm muscle cells into the failing heart of a 62-year-old man. Physicians removed a small amount of bicep tissue from the man's arm in April. The cells were sent to a biotech company and replicated into hundreds of millions of cells. Surgeons injected the cells into the posterior wall of the myocardium at the same time a quadruple bypass was performed. The patient was discharged after 5 days. At his first follow-up visit, the patient reported a decrease in dyspnea and was angina-free. Researchers are careful to point out that these effects are most likely attributable to the concomitant bypass surgery. It will be months before cardiologists can determine whether the new cells have indeed strengthened the heart. At present, only about 3000 donor hearts become available for transplant each year, limiting the opportunity for an improved quality and quantity of life for the 400,000 Americans who suffer from severe heart failure each year. For patients with refractory heart failure, this and similar trials offer hope where hopelessness now exists.

Reference: *Los Angeles Times/Daily Progress,* May 30, 2001.

NURSING MANAGEMENT OF PATIENTS WITH HEART FAILURE

ASSESSMENT

Health History

The nurse collects patient data during the initial baseline assessment and in all subsequent interactions. Data include:

- History of current episode—onset, duration
- Paroxysmal nocturnal dyspnea—frequency, severity, duration
- Orthopnea—frequency, severity, self-treatment
- New-onset dyspnea on exertion—related activities, severity
- Fatigue
- Lower extremity edema
- Persistent cough
- Recent weight gain—documented or perceived
- Presence of comorbid health conditions, treatment

Medications in use, prescription, over the counter, natural products

The nurse records a diet and activity history to serve as a baseline and facilitate teaching. Additional areas for assessment include concerns and anxieties of the patient and significant others and the effectiveness of support systems.

Physical Examination

Physical signs are not unique to heart failure, but must be evaluated along with data from the health history. Data from the physical assessment may include:

Presense of third heart sound
Respiratory distress, including increased effort and respiratory rate
Presence of pulmonary rales
Elevated jugular venous pressure
Peripheral edema—severity
Increase in daily weight without increased intake
Abdominal distention
Cool extremities and decreased pulses
Alterations in level of consciousness
Decreased urine output

NURSING DIAGNOSES

Nursing diagnoses are determined from analysis of patient data. Nursing diagnoses for the patient with heart failure may include but are not limited to:

Diagnostic Title	Possible Etiologic Factors
1. Decreased cardiac output	Alteration in preload, afterload, or inotropic changes in heart
2. Impaired gas exchange	Alveolar capillary membrane changes
3. Excess fluid volume	Compromised regulatory mechanism
4. Activity intolerance	Imbalance between oxygen supply and demand
5. Hopelessness	Declining or deteriorating physiologic condition

Additional diagnostic categories that may be applicable to specific patients with heart failure include disturbed sleep pattern, impaired adjustment, anxiety, disturbed body image, ineffective coping, fatigue, impaired home maintenance, ineffective role performance, ineffective therapeutic regimen management, caregiver role strain, noncompliance, powerlessness, imbalanced nutrition: less than body requirements, sexual dysfunction, and risk for infection.

EXPECTED PATIENT OUTCOMES

Expected patient outcomes for the patient with heart failure may include but are not limited to:

1. Hemodynamic parameters (cardiac output, central venous pressure, pulmonary artery wedge pressure, blood pressure, and heart rate) will improve or remain at patient's baseline
1a. Urine output will be greater than 30 ml/hr (exception: renal failure)
1b. Peripheral pulses, capillary refill time, and skin temperature will improve or remain at patient's baseline
1c. Signs of systemic circulatory insufficiency (hepatomegaly, nausea, dependent edema) will be absent or at the patient's baseline
2. Pulse oximetry will be above 90% with activity
2a. Patient will not experience respiratory distress
2b. Adventitious breath sounds will resolve or be at the patient's baseline
2c. Skin and mucous membranes will be pink
3. Intake and output will balance
3a. Weight will stabilize
3b. Patient will adhere to sodium and fluid restrictions
4. Patient will tolerate a progressive increase in activity and accomplish activities of daily living with decreased dyspnea
4a. Patient will demonstrate appropriate heart rate and blood pressure responses to exercise
5. Patient will demonstrate initiative and self-direction in decision making and express confidence in the future

INTERVENTIONS

The Guidelines for Safe Practice box summarizes the care of the patient with heart failure. A discussion of interventions appropriate to each diagnosis follows.

Guidelines for Safe Practice
The Patient With Heart Failure

1. Support oxygenation:
   a. Administer oxygen by nasal cannula at 2 to 6 L/min for oxygen saturation greater than 90%.
   b. Give oxygen as needed for dyspnea.
   c. Patient should be well supported in a semi-Fowler's position.
   d. Encourage use of incentive spirometry q4h.
2. Balance rest and activity:
   a. Reinforce importance of conservation of energy and planning for activities that avoid fatigue.
   b. Encourage activity within prescribed restrictions; monitor for intolerance to activity (dyspnea, fatigue, increased pulse rate that does not stabilize).
   c. Assist with activities of daily living as necessary; encourage independence within patient's limitations.
   d. Provide diversional activities that assist in conservation of energy.
   e. Provide a calm, quiet environment.
3. Perform head-to-toe assessment each shift, including assessment of lab values, daily weights, and intake and output.
4. Provide skin care, particularly over edematous areas; use prophylactic measures to prevent skin breakdown.
5. Assist in maintaining an adequate nutritional intake while observing prescribed dietary modifications (offer smaller meals with supplements).
6. Monitor for constipation; give prescribed stool softeners.
7. Give prescribed medications and monitor for adverse effects.
8. Provide patient and family opportunities to discuss their concerns and time to learn about the diagnosis and plan of care.

1. Improving Cardiac Output

The nurse actively works to improve existing alterations in cardiac output by reducing cardiac workload, promoting venous return, and minimizing myocardial oxygen requirements. Interventions include positioning the patient in a semi-Fowler's position or position of comfort; avoiding the Valsalva maneuver, which triggers abrupt changes in venous return to the heart; and promoting a calm, quiet, and comfortable environment. Maintaining safe and effective IV access is important in the management of patients with heart failure who require cardioactive IV medications and frequent blood work analysis (see Evidence-Based Practice box). Ongoing assessments focus on identifying changes in cardiac output and include vital signs, hemodynamic parameters, telemetry monitoring, heart sounds, level of consciousness, presence and severity of edema, peripheral temperature, capillary refill, urine output, and laboratory values. With acute failure assessments occur hourly or even more frequently while medications are being adjusted. When the patient stabilizes, the frequency of assessments becomes a nursing judgment.

Patients with pitting edema may be at risk for skin breakdown caused by poor nourishment of the skin and cracks in the skin surfaces. The nurse appropriately positions the patient to minimize pressure points and shearing. Positioning is especially important for the patient confined to bed rest and at risk for the development of sacral edema. Skin care includes gentle cleansing and the application of lotion as needed to decrease disruptions in skin integrity. The use of 4-inch foam and other pressure-relieving mattresses is a standard preventive intervention.

Anorexia may occur when venous engorgement affects the gastrointestinal system. The nurse helps the patient select a diet that meets baseline nutrient needs so that catabolism does not occur. Smaller, more frequent meals reduce stress on the gastrointestinal tract. The use of stool softeners minimizes the risk of Valsalva maneuvers. Increasing fiber in the diet as a measure to avoid constipation may not be well tolerated in some patients with heart failure because of intestinal edema and bloating.

Evidence-Based Practice

Reference: Major BM, Crow MM: Peripherally inserted central catheters in the patient with cardiomyopathy: the most cost-effective venous access, *J Intravenous Nurs* 23(6):366, 2000.

The waiting period for a heart transplant varies depending on donor availability and may range from a few days to more than a year. During this period, reliable venous access is essential for medication administration, including intravenous inotropes and diuretics. This study was a 2-year comparative retrospective analysis that compared four types of venous placement: peripherally inserted central catheters (PICCs) inserted by an infusion nurse, PICC lines inserted in the interventional radiology department by a physician, peripheral IV catheters inserted by an infusion nurse, and Hickman catheters placed by a surgeon in an operating room. The final sample included the records of 47 patients with cardiomyopathy with a total of 70 PICC placements. The study found that therapy with PICC placement was completed 71% of the time without complications. The remaining 29% experienced complications such as dislodgment (13%), phlebitis (10%), and infection (6%). A comparison of costs found that bedside PICCs saved 77% of the cost of using a Hickman catheter, 53% of the cost of using a PICC placed by a physician in interventional radiology, and 40% of the cost of using two peripheral IV catheter sites for a mean time period of 54.4 days. The costs were calculated based on line insertion, weekly maintenance, and duration of catheter placement. The researchers conclude that bedside PICC placement is the most cost-effective method of providing ongoing venous access to patients with cardiomyopathy.

2. Improving Gas Exchange

The less effective oxygenation of the blood as it passes through the congested lungs greatly reduces the oxygen content of the blood. The patient may be more comfortable and better able to rest while receiving oxygen because it helps reduce dyspnea and fatigue. Oxygen is usually administered by nasal cannula at 2 to 6 L/min. The nurse positions the patient in a semi-Fowler's position, encourages the use of the incentive spirometer, and teaches relaxed, controlled breathing to improve gas exchange. The nurse also monitors the patient's respiratory rate, depth, and ease; breath sounds; skin color; and pulse oximetry to evaluate improvement or deterioration in gas exchange. Mechanical ventilation is necessary when the work of breathing significantly increases cardiopulmonary demands. However, because of the complications associated with mechanical ventilation in patients with heart failure, alternatives such as noninvasive positive pressure ventilation are under investigation.[20]

3. Restoring Fluid Volume Balance

To decrease excessive fluid volumes, nurses work with the patient to determine how to best manage fluid and sodium restrictions. The physician orders the total amount of fluid permitted, and the nurse and patient develop a schedule to divide the fluid allowance throughout the day according to patient preferences. Appropriate and safe concentrations of IV medications minimize unnecessary fluid intake. The assessment of fluid balance is ongoing. Parameters include peripheral edema; intake and output; laboratory values for sodium, potassium, blood urea nitrogen (BUN), and creatinine; and monitoring the diuretic response to administered medications. The nurse records the patient's weight daily in similar clothing, using the same scale, with an empty bladder, and before eating. Weight gain indicates fluid retention: 1 kg of weight gain represents 1 L of retained fluid. Again, the frequency of assessment decreases as the patient's condition stabilizes. With pure diastolic failure, intravascular volume depletion can trigger worsening heart failure. Therefore the nurse individualizes the assessment of fluid balance based on the patient's underlying pathophysiology.

4. Improving Activity Tolerance

Patients with heart failure often experience severe fatigue and have little ability to perform even basic ADLs. Bed rest reduces myocardial oxygen demand during acute episodes of heart failure while medications are being adjusted and until the severity of symptoms resolves. The nurse organizes the environment to limit myocardial oxygen demand by providing a bedside commode, placing toiletry and other items within reach, and assisting with ADLs as needed. Nursing interventions that promote sleep include offering back rubs, providing comfortable bedding, closing doors, turning off televisions and phones, decreasing alarm volumes, minimizing bright lights, and promoting quiet conversations. Sedatives may be beneficial in the acute care setting.

As the acute stage resolves, the patient progresses gradually to sitting, ambulating in the room, and finally ambulating in the hall. The nurse helps the patient space activities and avoids the 1-hour after meals when gastrointestinal perfusion needs are greatest. The ability to tolerate activity is monitored through the pulse and blood pressure response to activity and the absence of symptoms. Fatigue and dizziness may occur in some patients receiving aggressive diuretic therapy.

The patient's ability to tolerate activity while hospitalized guides the discharge activity prescription. An explanation of the importance of exercise can encourage patients to gradually return to daily activities. The nurse works with the patient to explore exercise and activity options (see Complementary & Alternative Therapies box). Cardiac rehabilitation programs are especially beneficial for patients who are anxious about exercising on their own. Walking on level surfaces at least four times a week is a reasonable alternative to a structured outpatient exercise program. The nurse teaches the patient to discontinue walking if the heart rate increases by more than 20 beats/min or if the patient experiences chest discomfort, excessive fatigue, severe shortness of breath, or syncope. Pacing activities to decrease myocardial oxygen demand is the guiding principle for all activity.

5. Instilling Hope

Heart failure is a chronic illness with a poor prognosis. Patients need counseling regarding the effects of heart failure on self-concept and role performance. Quality of life remains a priority for patients with heart failure. Nurses encourage patients to be active, using energy conservation guidelines to promote optimal functioning.[26] The patient with heart failure must learn to accept uncertainty in life and needs support in confronting that uncertainty (see Research box). Health care professionals need to encourage patients with heart failure to complete advance directives concerning their health care preferences. All individuals involved in the patient's care need updates on these preferences. The Quality of Care Working Group on Heart Failure[1,14] endorsed as an indicator of the quality of patient care, provides specific programs to address the end-of-life needs of patients with heart failure.

Patient/Family Education

The nurse performs an accurate assessment of the patient's knowledge base before implementing an education plan (see Patient Teaching box). A large amount of information must be provided and the nurse uses a variety of educational strategies to help the patient and family learn. An explanation of heart failure and its probable cause is the foundation for teaching. The nurse teaches the patient signs and symptoms, what to do if symptoms

Complementary & Alternative Therapies

T'ai Chi Chih

T'ai Chi is a form of mind-body discipline derived from spiritual, martial, and health exercises developed in China 2000 years ago. T'ai Chi is believed to affect the endogenous neurohormonal pathways, thereby explaining its purported link to achieving health benefits in patients with heart failure. T'ai Chi Chih is a modification of T'ai Chi for individuals unable to engage in traditional T'ai Chi movements because of physical or mental impairment. Five patients with a stable heart failure status completed biweekly T'ai Chi Chih classes over a 12-week period. The safety of the 20 movements was extrapolated after determining metabolic equivalents for 8 of the 20 movements (1.5-2.6 mets). The dependent variables were energy perception, heart failure symptoms, exercise tolerance, physical functioning, and well-being. Both qualitative and quantitative data were obtained. Four patients had a complete data set. For these patients, all decreased their heart failure symptom scores; three decreased dyspnea scores; all improved in at least one vigor score, and three improved in distances walked in 6 minutes. Qualitative themes included a sense of peace associated with participation and a sense of energy source from within the body core. The researchers noted possible biases that may have influenced the outcomes within this particular sample as an interest in supplements and herbs and a strong spirituality component of coping.

Reference: Fontana JA et al: T'ai Chi Chih as an intervention for heart failure, *Nurs Clin North Am* 35(4):1031, 2000.

Research

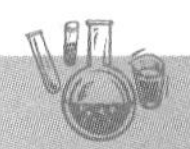

Reference: Winter CA: Heart failure: living with uncertainty, *Prog Cardiovasc Nurs* 14:85, 1999.

According to leading researchers in the field of uncertainty, uncertainty stems from illness ambiguity, complexity of therapeutic regimens, knowledge deficits, and unpredictability. For patients with chronic heart failure, all four of these criteria are present in their lives. This qualitative study sought to describe further the uncertainty experienced by men and women with heart failure. Qualitative data were gathered through interviews with 22 adult patients with class I-IV heart failure. Participants also completed the community form of the Mishel Uncertainty in Illness Scale. Three major themes emerged from the data and included the recognition and response to symptoms and treatments, the ability to stay well, and the quality of life and death. Uncertainty increased with changes in symptoms or treatments, incomplete information, a perceived loss of control over the illness, thinking of the future, and inability to discriminate symptoms from age-appropriate events. Uncertainty scores from the MUIS tool found the greatest uncertainty to be whether the physician would find anything else wrong with them. The researchers emphasize that from their findings nurses should continue ongoing educational emphasis on symptomatology and the unpredictable nature of heart failure. Open discussion and ongoing education by the nurse may help to decrease some of the uncertainty for patients with heart failure.

Patient Teaching
Heart Failure

1. Monitor for signs and symptoms of recurring heart failure, and report these signs and symptoms to the primary care provider:
   a. Weight gain of 1 to 1.5 kg (2 to 3 lb)
   b. Loss of appetite
   c. Shortness of breath
   d. Orthopnea
   e. Swelling of ankles, feet, or abdomen
   f. Persistent cough
   g. Frequent nighttime urination
2. Avoid fatigue and plan activity to allow for rest periods. Incorporate activities of daily living, occupational activity, and sexual activity into daily routine by pacing activities.
3. Plan and eat meals within prescribed sodium restrictions:
   a. Avoid salty foods.
   b. Avoid drugs with high sodium content (e.g., some laxatives and antacids, Alka-Seltzer); read all labels.
   c. Eat several small meals rather than three large meals per day.
4. Take prescribed medications:
   a. If several medications are prescribed, develop a method to facilitate accurate administration.
   b. Digoxin: check own pulse rate daily; report a rate of less than 50/min to primary care provider.
   c. Diuretics:
      (1) Weigh self daily at same time of day.
      (2) Eat foods high in potassium and low in sodium (such as oranges, bananas) if on potassium depleting diuretics.
   d. Vasodilators:
      (1) Report signs of hypotension (light-headedness, rapid pulse, syncope) to physician.
      (2) Avoid alcohol when taking vasodilators.
5. Adopt healthy lifestyle choices: establish a daily routine; develop support groups; smoking cessation; alcohol intake limited to no more than one drink per day; minimize risk of infections.
6. Comply with follow-up appointments.

worsen, and the importance of self-monitoring for symptoms (including daily weights). The nurse emphasizes the importance of preventive health measures, including healthy lifestyle modifications, avoiding individuals with infections, and receiving annual influenza vaccinations. Health care professionals involve the patient and family in the management plan and discussion of prognosis. Additional content areas for patient teaching include advance directives, stress management techniques, relaxation strategies, and the availability of support groups.

The nurse encourages the patient to be as active as possible and provides specific guidelines for aerobic exercise. Guidelines include the type of exercise, frequency, duration, and intensity. Alterations in sexual activity may occur as a result of the disease process (hypoperfusion, fatigue), medications, depression, fear, or altered body image. The nurse is proactive in supporting partner communication and provides honest information about drug side effects, counseling the patient concerning energy conservation measures, positioning, and the atmosphere for sexual intercourse.

The nurse or dietitian reviews recommended sodium and fluid restrictions if indicated. This review includes teaching the patient about the importance of abstinence from alcohol or limiting intake to one serving daily. Permitted foods on the sodium-restricted diet receive emphasis. A printed list of foods to avoid goes home with the patient and family. The nurse teaches the patient alternatives to satisfy thirst, such as sugarless hard candy, Popsicles, and ice chips. When teaching about fluid restrictions, the nurse educates the patient about what counts as fluid intake, including Jello, ice cream, pudding, and sauces.

The nurse carefully reviews the safe use of all medications, including purpose and side effects. The nurse works with the physician and patient to schedule medications in order to minimize their effect on daily routines. Administering diuretics in the morning minimizes sleep disturbances but may not be compatible with employment demands. Using individualized algorithms, many patients can be taught to adjust their diuretic (and electrolyte) dose to weight fluctuations. The patient on ACE-inhibitor or spironolactone therapy should avoid potassium-containing salt substitutes. The nurse also cautions the patient about the possible occurrence of gynecomastia with spironolactone therapy. The nurse teaches the patient taking digoxin about the signs and symptoms of toxicity. Because of the potential for heart failure to initially worsen with the initiation of beta-blocker therapy, the nurse provides the patient with established parameters for when to seek care. The nurse cautions all patients to avoid all over-the-counter, herbal, and prescription medications without first consulting their primary care provider, especially NSAIDs and alternative medications such as herbal products.

All health care professionals emphasize the importance of follow-up and regimen adherence. Patients must be able to recognize risks for decompensation and the early associated signs and symptoms Adherence directly affects mortality, and lack of adherence is a major cause of hospitalization. The nurse discusses the importance of adherence and assists the patient in removing barriers such as knowledge deficits, self-confidence, cost, side effects, and complexity of protocols (see Research box). Family and social support is critical in helping the patient sustain a commitment to heart failure management.

Health Promotion/Prevention. As part of the Healthy People 2010 initiative, 16 objectives were identified for heart disease and stroke. Decreasing the number of heart failure hospitalizations for older adults is one of the 16 objectives (see Healthy People 2010 box).

EVALUATION

1,2,3,4,5. On follow-up visits, the nurse asks about the presence of orthopnea, paroxysmal nocturnal dyspnea, edema, and dyspnea on exertion. Patients are likely to experience changes in symptoms before changes are evident on physical examination. Family members contribute important information about the patient's physical health and regimen adherence. A thorough evaluation includes an evaluation of physical functioning and quality of life. Achievement of outcomes is successful if the patient with heart failure:

Research

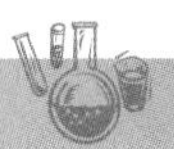

Reference: Bennett SJ et al: Heart messages: a tailored message intervention for improving heart failure outcomes, *J Cardiovasc Nurs* 14(4):94, 2000.

A pilot study using a pretest posttest design was conducted to evaluate the effect of tailored messages on beliefs about compliance with medication regimens and dietary sodium restrictions. A convenience sample of 16 patients with ejection fractions of <40% was recruited from a nurse-managed heart failure clinic. All participants completed the Beliefs about Medication Compliance Scale and The Beliefs about Dietary Compliance Scale. These scales consist of two subscale scores that measure the patient's degree of perceived benefits and barriers to compliance. Six patients received conventional care in the control group. Ten patients in the intervention group received individualized follow-up care based on their responses as to benefits and barriers to compliance. Experts in heart failure and patient education wrote a brief tailored educational message to increase the likelihood that a desired behavior would occur. These messages were attractively displayed on $5^1/_2$- × $8^1/_2$-inch stock paper. The individualized tailored messages were delivered to the participant (in most cases, the patient's home) by the investigator along with informal discussion lasting on average 20 to 30 minutes. The cards were then left with the patient. Change scores were computed for each patient's subscale scores to determine whether the patient's scores improved, remained the same, or decreased. The benefits subscales showed the least improvement. Most improvement was noted in intervention patients for the medication barriers subscale. In cases where the actual change had been negative, the researchers postulated that small group numbers, the strength of the intervention, or the degree of illness may have impacted the findings. This pilot study is one of many intervention studies designed to improve compliance in patients with heart failure. Much nursing research remains to be conducted to influence patient compliance and outcomes.

Healthy People 2010

Objective for Heart Failure

1. Reduce hospitalizations of older adults with congestive heart failure as the principal diagnosis

ADULTS AGES 65-74 YEARS

Reduce hospitalizations from the 1997 rate of 13.2 per 1000 population to a 2010 target of 6.5 per 1000 population

ADULTS AGES 75-84 YEARS

Reduce hospitalizations from the 1997 rate of 26.7 per 1000 population to a 2010 target of 13.5 per 1000 population

ADULTS AGES 85 YEARS AND OLDER

Reduce hospitalizations from the 1997 rate of 52.7 per 1000 population to a 2010 target of 26.5 per 1000 population

From US Department of Health and Human Services: *Healthy People 2010: understanding and improving health,* Washington, DC, 2000, USDHHS.

1. Has hemodynamic parameters (cardiac output, central venous pressure, pulmonary artery wedge pressure, blood pressure, heart rate) that are at baseline or improved from baseline.

1a. Maintains urine output of greater than 30 ml/hr (exception: renal failure).

1b. Has peripheral pulses, capillary refill time, and skin temperature that are at baseline or improved from baseline.

1c. Demonstrates adequate systemic circulation (edema at baseline or improved).

2. Manifests pulse oximetry above 90% with activity.

2a. Denies respiratory distress.

2b. Demonstrates resolution of adventitious breath sounds.

2c. Has skin and mucus that are free of cyanosis or pallor.

3. Has a balanced intake and output.

3a. Maintains desired weight.

3b. Eats diet within sodium and fluid restrictions.

4. Tolerates a progressive increase in activity and accomplishes ADLs with decreased dyspnea.

4a. Demonstrates acceptable responses in heart rate and blood pressure to exercise.

5. Demonstrates initiative and self-direction in decision making and expresses confidence in the future.

When necessary, the nurse alters the plan of care to include new diagnoses or new interventions negotiated with the patient and significant others.

GERONTOLOGIC CONSIDERATIONS

Heart failure is the most common cause of hospitalization in patients over 65 years of age. Older patients with heart failure may not exhibit the common clinical manifestations of dyspnea, rales (crackles), and edema. Confusion, fatigue, and failure to thrive may be the only clinical manifestations.

Primary health care providers make adjustments in medications that consider the physiologic changes seen in older patients. Nurses caution older patients to make position changes slowly while taking diuretics, because they may not be able to adapt quickly to venous pooling. Older patients are also especially sensitive to the first-dose hypotensive effect of ACE inhibitors. When even mild renal impairment is present, older adults may develop acute renal insufficiency. The nurse monitors BUN, creatinine, and potassium routinely for older patients taking ACE inhibitors and diuretics. The routine use of NSAIDs by the older population decreases the effectiveness of ACE inhibitors. All elderly patients taking digoxin must be carefully monitored for signs and symptoms of toxicity. Older adults are at an increased risk for toxicity because of a decrease in renal function and reduced lean body mass.

Older individuals may not be adherent to their medication regimen for a multitude of reasons, including cognition, sensory perception, lack of social support and financial resources, and lack of motivation. A multidisciplinary approach for follow-up care after discharge can reduce the rate of readmission for this population. This approach considers the impact of potential physiologic changes, including sensory and motor deficits and comorbid processes, on the willingness and capacity of the elderly patient to comply.

SPECIAL ENVIRONMENTS FOR CARE

Critical Care

Before admission to either a critical care or an inpatient unit, patients with acute heart failure may be managed in an observation unit, similar to chest pain centers for acute cardiac ischemia.[21] Patients admitted to critical care most often require one-on-one nursing for the titration of medications and ongoing assessment of fluid status and hemodynamic response. The use of adjunctive treatments for refractory heart failure, such as intraaortic balloon pumping, requires careful monitoring in the intensive care setting. Once stabilized, the cardiology step-down unit becomes the environment best suited for management of patients in heart failure. This transition allows for continued pharmacologic intervention along with appropriate monitoring, and it facilitates education and activity interventions.

Community-Based Care

Patients are discharged to the home environment only when their symptoms are controlled; comorbid problems (e.g., atrial fibrillation) have been treated; educational outcomes have been met; and arrangements are in place for needed care, support, and follow-up monitoring in the community. Plans for return to home begin on admission.

The nurse emphasizes the importance of consistent follow-up monitoring with primary care providers or nurse-managed heart failure clinics. Follow-up includes physical assessment, adherence evaluation, and ongoing education. Elderly patients with heart failure who follow up with nurse practitioner clinics and home health care nurses have significantly fewer exacerbations than patients not managed by these professionals.[24] Telephone follow-up can be a useful strategy to support medication and symptom management. Home-monitoring services through secure Internet web sites allow patients to enter data such as daily weights into a program that is monitored by health care professionals. Nurses or physicians then contact the patient if a change is indicated such as decreasing or increasing the diuretic dose (see Research box). At times, successful home management requires only the use of supportive systems such as individuals to deliver nutritional meals or supplemental education about the proper use of mobility aids (e.g., bedside commodes, shower seats) to decrease cardiac workload.

The increased prevalence of heart disease coupled with demands for cost-effective care has also introduced technology into the home setting that was once limited to critical care. Home care now routinely includes home inotrope or IV diuretic therapy administration, assessment of the environment to minimize cardiac workload, provision of support and education, and evaluation of outcomes. With the increasing use of left ventricular assist devices in the outpatient population, the home management of patients with end-stage heart failure has become increasingly challenging. There is significant need for nursing research regarding the role and nature of palliative care in the home setting for patients with end-stage heart failure.

Research

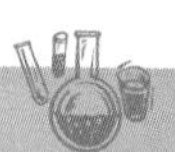

Reference: Bondmass M et al: The effect of physiologic home monitoring and telemanagement on chronic heart failure outcomes, *Internet J Adv Nurs Pract* 2000; 3(2):http://www.ispub.com/journals/IJANP/Vol3N2/chf.htm; Published March 27, 2000.

Transtelephonic monitoring is a means for patients to communicate physiologic variables over telephone lines to a network server for computer display to health professionals. The health professional then may communicate with the patient to intervene based on the objective data. This study measured the effects of physiologic home monitoring of daily weight, blood pressure, heart rate, and oxygen saturation and telemanagement of chronic heart failure outcomes, including hospital readmissions, length of stay, charges, and quality of life. Inclusion criteria included patients with systolic or diastolic heart failure, NYHA III or IV status who were responsive to diuresis; 60 patients met the inclusion/exclusion criteria. After discharge, patients transmitted their data one to two times daily for 2 to 3 months. The majority of medication interventions and patient education calls were made directly by an advance practice nurse following clinical guidelines. Outcomes were analyzed at 3, 6, and 12 months after enrollment. Readmissions, length of stay, and hospital charges all significantly decreased ($P \leq 0.001$) from baseline; and quality of life significantly improved ($P \geq 0.002$) from baseline. The researchers believe the major advantage to such a method is efficiency in both time and financial costs.

COMPLICATIONS

Acute Pulmonary Edema. Acute pulmonary edema is a medical emergency that may develop as a result of severe ventricular failure. Any of the events presented in Box 24-6 can cause decompensation in chronic heart failure, resulting in pulmonary edema.

Pulmonary edema arises from left ventricular overload. The volume overload increases left atrial pressure, resulting in increased pulmonary vein and pulmonary capillary pressures. Pulmonary capillary hydrostatic pressure quickly exceeds the intravascular oncotic pressure. The high pressure forces fluid and sodium into the interstitium. The high interstitial pressure then forces fluid into the alveoli. The surfactant that keeps the alveoli expanded loses its effectiveness. The fluid-filled alveoli collapse, preventing the exchange of oxygen and carbon dioxide, and unoxygenated blood returns to the left side of the heart. Red blood cells also enter the alveoli, producing the characteristic blood-tinged sputum. The fluid then rapidly moves into the bronchioles and bronchi, creating the acute life-threatening symptoms that characterize this medical emergency: profound dyspnea, pallor, audible wheezing, and cyanosis. Restlessness, anxiety, and tachycardia also develop from the acutely impaired gas exchange.

The acute anxiety that accompanies pulmonary edema must be quickly and effectively managed. Anxiety triggers catecholamine release that results in tachycardia and other events that increase oxygen demand and confound treatment. The nurse approaches the patient in a calm, reassuring manner. Morphine sulfate is the drug of choice because it blunts the sympathetic response and increases venous capacitance, thereby lowering left atrial pressure. It is not administered in heart failure for its analgesic effect. The "air hunger" of pulmonary edema triggers the anxiety. Nursing interventions such as raising the head of the bed and positioning the patient in the bed to maximize chest expansion decrease the air hunger.

Arterial blood gas or pulse oximetry results determine the need for supplemental oxygen. Oxygen may be administered at 40% to 70% by facemask to quickly achieve oxygen saturations above 90%. Humidification aids in the removal of secretions. Intubation is necessary for patients who do not respond to conventional measures. Mechanical ventilation ensures the delivery of adequate tidal volumes and oxygen concentrations to decrease the work of breathing. Intubation also facilitates the removal of secretions by suctioning. Aminophylline may be administered to dilate the bronchi, increase urinary output, and increase cardiac output.

Medications prescribed for pulmonary edema include inotropic agents, diuretics, afterload reducers, and supportive adjuncts such as dopamine hydrochloride to increase renal perfusion. The significant diuresis that typically occurs with treatment requires careful monitoring for electrolyte imbalance.

Dysrhythmias. Atrial fibrillation is a common complication of heart failure. The backup of blood into the atria causes atrial enlargement and ischemia. The ischemia alters the electrical stability necessary for impulse initiation and conduction and increases both the automaticity and irritability of the atrial tissue. Atrial fibrillation can provoke heart failure or trigger an exacerbation in a patient who is in compensated heart failure. The management of atrial fibrillation is presented in Chapter 23.

Ischemia and irritability in the ventricles can also result in premature ventricular beats. As the disease progresses, premature beats may lead to more lethal dysrhythmias that are difficult to manage owing to altered cardiac metabolism, but the prophylactic use of antidysrhythmics is not supported through clinical research. Amiodarone is used for symptomatic ventricular dysrhythmias. Implantable cardiac defibrillators may be beneficial for symptomatic ventricular dysrhythmias in select patients with heart failure.

Multisystem Failure. Heart failure affects every organ system and multiple organ system failure can occur. Clinical manifestations and treatment are specific to the organ that is underperfused. Renal failure is a common problem.

CARDIOMYOPATHY

Etiology/Epidemiology

Cardiomyopathy (CMP) causes specific progressive structural changes within the myocardium. There are three major categories of CMP: dilated CMP, hypertrophic CMP, and restrictive CMP (Figure 24-4). In dilated CMP the LV dilates but does not experience a proportional increase in contractility. Possible etiologies for dilated CMP include ischemia, damage from inflammatory processes, toxins such as ethanol and chemotherapy, or heredity. Long-standing hypertension and valve disorders also contribute to the development of dilated CMP. Hypertrophic CMP refers to a dilated, hypertrophied, and hypercontractile ventricle. Hypertrophic CMP may represent a defect of muscle development and therefore may have a hereditary component. Familial hypertrophic CMP seems to be an autosomal-dominant disorder, transmitted on the nonsex chromosomes, involving mutations of seven distinct genes.[3] Hypertrophic obstructive cardiomyopathy (HOCM) is the term used when the septum hypertrophies asymmetrically, obstructing left ventricular ejection. Restrictive CMP occurs when the LV is of normal or small size and the muscle mass is normal or increased (Table 24-4). Infiltrative and proliferative disorders such as amyloidosis and sarcoidosis are common etiologies for restrictive CMP. CMP is classified as idiopathic when a specific etiology cannot be identified.

Pathophysiology

In dilated CMP the ventricular chamber dilates in response to constant stress. Dilation of the LV increases its volume capacity (increased compliance). The stretching of the myocardial fibers, however, displaces the sarcomeres beyond the limits of the Starling curve. As a result, optimum cross-linkages for contractility do not occur, decreasing contractility. Fibrosis can also inhibit the ability to contract. Therefore in dilated CMP there is a larger capacity for ventricular volume but a decrease in contractility. These changes result in a decrease in cardiac output, stroke volume, and EF. Clinical manifestations reflect the decrease in cardiac output. Major signs and symptoms include fatigue, weakness, and overt manifestations of left-sided heart failure.

In hypertrophic CMP muscle mass increases but without an increase in LV chamber size. Fibrotic infiltrates of the myocardium increase the stiffness of the ventricle, creating additional hypertrophy. Compliance to LV filling decreases, and the LA dilates in an attempt to increase volume. When the

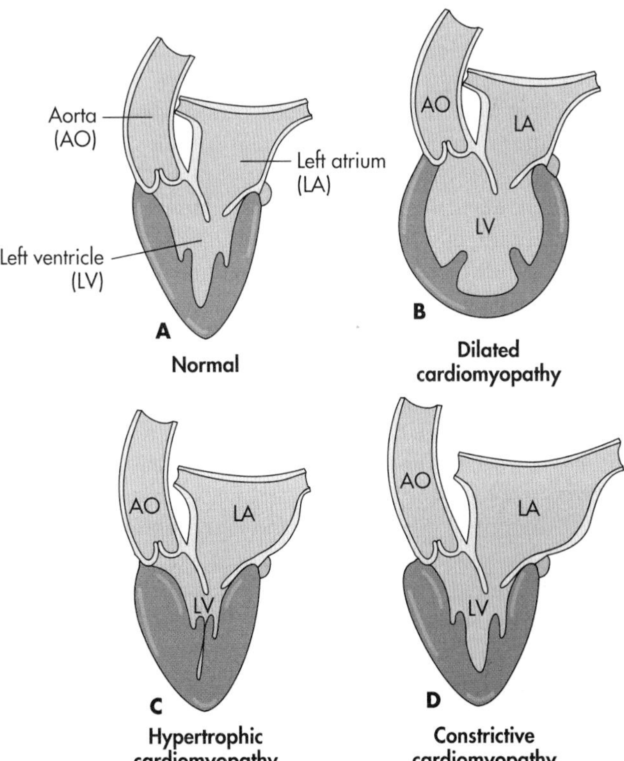

Figure 24-4 Diagram showing major distinguishing pathophysiologic features of the three types of cardiomyopathy. **A,** The normal heart. **B,** In the dilated type of cardiomyopathy, the heart has a globular shape and the largest circumference of the left ventricle is not at its base but midway between apex and base. **C,** In the hypertrophic type, the wall of the left ventricle is greatly thickened; the left ventricular cavity is small but the left atrium may be dilated because of poor diastolic relaxation of the ventricle. **D,** In the restrictive (constrictive) type, the left ventricular cavity is of normal size but, again, the left atrium is dilated because of the reduced diastolic compliance of the ventricle.

TABLE 24-4 Pathophysiologic Effects of the Cardiomyopathies

	Type of Cardiomyopathy		
Pathophysiology	**Dilated**	**Hypertrophic**	**Restrictive**
Major symptoms	Fatigue, weakness, palpitations	Dyspnea, angina pectoris, fatigue, dizziness (syncope), palpitations	Dyspnea, fatigue
Chamber size	Increased	Normal or decreased	Decreased or normal
Hypertrophy	Left ventricular myocardium	Left ventricular myocardium and interventricular septum	Left ventricular myocardium
Alterations of chamber volume	Volume increased	Volume decreased, particularly in left ventricle	Volume normal to decreased
Alterations of chamber compliance	Compliance increased	Compliance decreased, particularly in left ventricle	Compliance decreased, particularly in left ventricle
Ventricular filling pressure	Increased	Normal or increased	Increased
Alterations of systolic function (myocardial contractility)	Contractility decreased in left ventricle	Contractility increased or vigorous	None
Cardiac output	Decreased	Normal	Normal or decreased
Associated conditions	Alcoholism, pregnancy, infection, nutritional deficiency, exposed to toxins	Possible inherited defect of muscle growth and development	Infiltrative disease
Eventual cardiovascular event	Left-sided heart failure	Left-sided heart failure	Heart failure

Adapted from Huether SE, McCance KL: *Understanding pathophysiology,* St Louis, 1996, Mosby.

hypertrophied ventricle contracts, the ventricle easily ejects the small available volume of blood, but increases in demand, as would occur with exercise cannot be met by increasing cardiac output. This results in syncope, serious dysrhythmias, or sudden death. Heart failure is the eventual outcome as the disease progresses. Metabolic needs increase and create an imbalance between the high oxygen demand and the reduced cardiac output, and may precipitate angina. Clinical manifestations include those of dilated CMP plus an increased cardiac impulse, a high EF in the early stages, and a decreased EF when heart failure ensues.

In restrictive CMP the LV is fibrotic and thickened secondary to infiltrates. The ventricle loses its ability to stretch, thereby decreasing compliance; the heart cannot adequately fill, thereby decreasing cardiac output. Heart failure ensues. As in hypertrophic CMP, the LA often dilates. The patient may have symptoms of infection and amyloid infiltration.

Collaborative Care Management

Diagnostic tests for CMP include chest x-ray, echocardiogram, 12-lead ECG, and physical examination. The nurse monitors for subtle changes in systemic perfusion (e.g., mental status, heart rhythm, vital signs, peripheral perfusion, oxygenation, fluid status). The nursing assessment also seeks to determine how the illness has affected the patient's quality of life. The nurse considers the patient holistically, including the planned medical management and patient's special needs, such as those related to the disbelief and shock that follow the sudden onset of viral CMP.

Management focuses on decreasing the workload of the heart, improving contractile efficiency, and managing symptoms and complications. Medications include all those used in heart failure. Pacing of activities decreases workload, and restriction of activities with high metabolic equivalents may be beneficial. Even everyday conversation may create extreme dyspnea, and the nurse cautions the patient to pace even this activity to minimize cardiac workload. Proper positioning and supplemental oxygen facilitate breathing. Assessment for orthostatic blood pressure changes and the initiation of appropriate safety measures decrease the risk of injury. Complications include altered renal function and electrolyte imbalance from diuretic therapy, as well as thromboemboli from stagnant blood flow within the myocardium. Anticoagulation may be prescribed. Chapter 25 discusses nursing interventions for the patient receiving anticoagulant therapy. Dysrhythmias can occur if ischemia creates enhanced automaticity, reentry, or conduction defects. Ventricular dysrhythmias are the leading cause of mortality in hypertrophic CMP and implantable defibrillators are often recommended after one or more documented episodes of ventricular tachycardia or ventricular fibrillation.

The value of pacemaker therapy continues to be investigated with regard to improving cardiac output in dilated CMP and HOCM. In hypertrophic CMP removal of the septum (septal myotomy-myomectomy) or reduction of the left ventricular mass through a partial ventriculectomy (the Batista Procedure) have been used with success in select patients. Cardiac transplantation may be an appropriate intervention for the patient refractory to conventional management

Patient/Family Education. To facilitate adherence to the recommended regimen, the nurse provides appropriate explanations of all treatments and interventions. Many of the teaching guidelines appropriate to patients with heart failure are also appropriate for the patient with CMP. Patients with CMP are at an increased risk of sudden death owing to dysrhythmias, and the

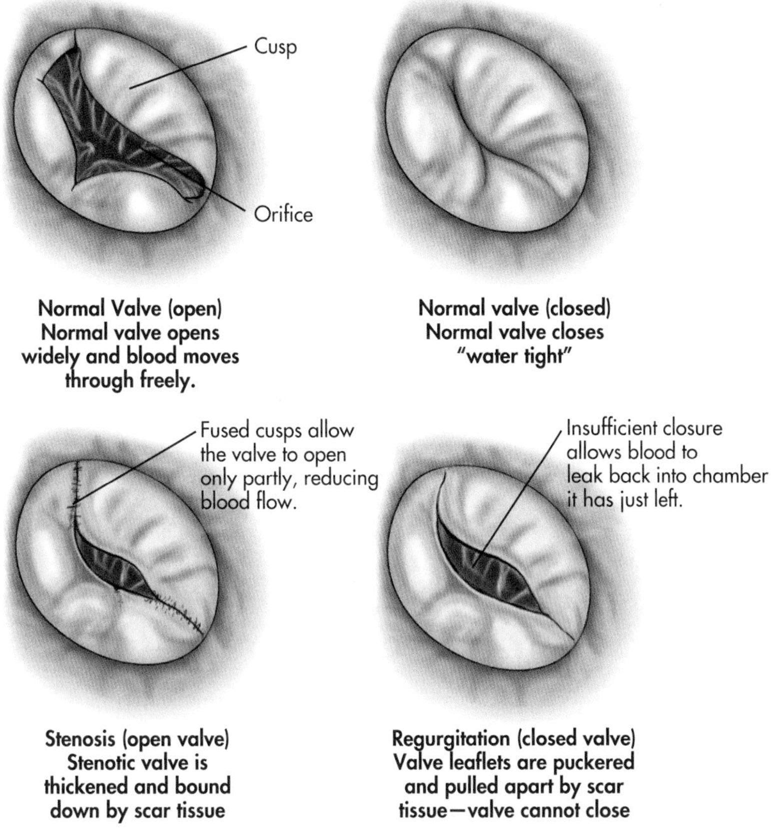

Figure 24-5 Valvular diseases.

nurse refers interested family members to an appropriate agency for instruction in cardiopulmonary resuscitation. Treatment options may seem limited to the patient and family but the nurse emphasizes the importance of follow-up care.

VALVULAR HEART DISEASE

The cardiac valves are responsible for ensuring unidirectional blood flow through the heart. Valvular stenosis produces narrowing of the valve lumen, which impedes blood flow through the valve. Valvular insufficiency causes incomplete valve closure, which leads to regurgitation or backward leaking of blood through the valve (Figure 24-5). See Chapter 22 for a review of valve structure and function.

When a cardiac valve is mildly stenotic or regurgitant, the heart is initially able to compensate and maintain function despite gradual chamber dilation and myocardial hypertrophy. However, over time the compensatory ability of the myocardium begins to fail. Excessive myocardial hypertrophy and chamber dilation result in decreased contractility, reduced EF, and ultimately ventricular failure. Medical therapy supports cardiac function with the use of inotropes, diuretics, dietary sodium restriction, and antibiotic prophylaxis (see the discussion of heart failure). If symptoms continue to worsen surgical valve repair or replacement may become necessary.

The next section reviews the major cardiac valve disorders. Symptoms and complications of valvular heart disease are primarily related to decreased cardiac input, and the general management follows the guidelines presented for patients with heart failure. Table 24-5 presents an overview of the specific valvular disorders, and the diagnostic findings associated with each. Table 24-6 compares the common clinical manifestations associated with each disorder.

Mitral Stenosis

Etiology/Epidemiology

Mitral stenosis impedes the blood flow from the LA to the LV during ventricular diastole (ventricular filling). It is usually caused by thickening or fibrotic changes in the mitral valve. Mitral stenosis is the most common disorder of the mitral valve. The primary etiology is rheumatic fever, which causes an inflammatory process on the mitral valve's chordae tendineae or commissures (leaflets). Less common causes of mitral stenosis include bacterial vegetation, thrombus formation, calcification of the mitral annulus, and atrial myxoma (tumor).

Forty percent of persons with rheumatic heart disease develop mitral stenosis, and two thirds of all persons with rheumatic mitral stenosis are women.[18] With the decreasing incidence of rheumatic fever in industrialized countries, the incidence of rheumatic mitral stenosis has substantially declined, although it remains a common disorder in developing countries.

Pathophysiology

In mitral stenosis the mitral valve leaflets become thickened and fibrotic from calcification and scar tissue formation.

TABLE 24-5 Findings in Valvular Heart Disorders

Disorder	Chest Radiograph	Electrocardiogram	Echocardiogram	Cardiac Catheterization
Mitral stenosis	Left atrial enlargement Mitral valve calcification Right ventricular enlargement Prominence of pulmonary artery	Left atrial hypertrophy Right ventricular hypertrophy Atrial fibrillation	Thickened mitral valve Left atrial enlargement	Increased pressure gradient across valve Increased left atrial pressure Increased PCWP Increased right heart pressure Decreased CO
Mitral regurgitation	Left atrial enlargement Left ventricular enlargement	Left atrial hypertrophy Left ventricular hypertrophy Atrial fibrillation Sinus tachycardia	Abnormal mitral valve movement Left atrial enlargement	Mitral regurgitation Increased atrial pressure Increased LVEDP Increased PCWP Decreased CO
Aortic stenosis	Left ventricular enlargement Aortic valve calcification May have enlargement of left atrium, pulmonary artery, right ventricle, right atrium	Left ventricular hypertrophy	Thickened aortic valve Thickened ventricular wall Abnormal movement of aortic leaflets	Increased pressure gradient across valve Increased LVEDP
Aortic regurgitation	Left ventricular enlargement	Left ventricular hypertrophy Tall R waves Sinus tachycardia	Left ventricular enlargement Abnormal mitral valve movement Increased movement of ventricular wall	Aortic regurgitation Increased LVEDP Decreased arterial diastolic pressure
Tricuspid stenosis	Right atrial enlargement Prominence of superior vena cava	Right atrial hypertrophy Tall peaked P waves Atrial fibrillation	Abnormal valvular leaflets Right atrial enlargement	Increased pressure gradient across valve Increased right atrial pressure Decreased CO
Tricuspid regurgitation	Right atrial enlargement Right ventricular enlargement	Right ventricular hypertrophy Atrial fibrillation	Prolapse of tricuspid valve Right atrial enlargement	Increased atrial pressure Tricuspid regurgitation Decreased CO

CO, Cardiac output; *LVEDP*, left ventricular end-diastolic pressure; *PCWP*, pulmonary capillary wedge pressure.

BOX 24-9 Relationship of Mitral Orifice Size to Emergence of Symptoms

$>2.6\ cm^2$	No symptoms with exertion
$2.1\text{-}2.5\ cm^2$	Symptoms with extreme exertion
$1.6\text{-}2.0\ cm^2$	Symptoms with moderate exertion
$<1.5\ cm^2$	Symptoms with minimal exertion

From Hurst JW, editor: *The heart*, ed 7, New York, 1990, McGraw-Hill.

As the valve leaflets become stiff and fused, the valve lumen progressively narrows and becomes immobile. The chordae tendineae may also shorten and thicken and the mitral valve orifice may decrease from its normal size of 4 to 6 cm to less than 1 cm (Box 24-9).

Progressive mitral stenosis causes the left atrial pressure to elevate as a result of incomplete emptying of the LA. This causes the myocardium to compensate with left atrial dilation and hypertrophy. In addition, high pressures in the LA lead to elevated pulmonary venous, capillary, and arterial pressures. Eventually, sustained elevation of the left atrial pressure can cause pulmonary hypertension and subsequent right ventricular hypertrophy. Increased pressure in the pulmonary vasculature causes fluid leakage across the pulmonary capillary membrane into the lung interstitium and can lead to pulmonary edema (Figure 24-6).

Persons with mitral stenosis experience a reduction in cardiac output that is directly related to the degree of mitral stenosis. Persons with mild to moderate stenosis can generally maintain a normal cardiac output at rest but may be unable to tolerate exercise.

Mitral stenosis also increases the risk for cardiac dysrhythmias. Atrial fibrillation develops in 50% of persons with mitral stenosis, causing a further decrease in cardiac output. In addition, atrial fibrillation may allow blood to pool in the LA, resulting in thrombus formation and possible embolization to vital organs.

Many persons with mitral stenosis remain symptom free for as many as 20 years after the initial attack of rheumatic carditis. Symptoms may develop gradually or abruptly depending on the severity of the stenosis (see Table 24-6). When acute symptoms develop, the disease progresses rapidly and death occurs within 5 to 10 years unless surgical correction takes place.

TABLE 24-6 Clinical Manifestations of Valvular Stenosis and Regurgitation

Manifestation	Aortic Stenosis	Mitral Stenosis	Aortic Regurgitation	Mitral Regurgitation	Tricuspid Regurgitation
Cardiovascular outcome*	Left ventricular failure	Right ventricular failure	Left-sided heart failure	Left-sided heart failure	Right-sided heart failure
General symptoms	Fatigue	Fatigue, weakness	Fatigue, weakness	Fatigue, weakness	Peripheral edema (with heart failure)
Respiratory effects	Dyspnea on exertion	Dyspnea on exertion, orthopnea, paroxysmal nocturnal dyspnea, predisposition to respiratory infections, hemoptysis, pulmonary hypertension, and edema	Dyspnea with effort	Dyspnea; occasional hemoptysis	Dyspnea
Central nervous system effects	Syncope, especially on exertion	Neural deficits only associated with emboli (e.g., hemiparesis)	Syncope	None	None
Gastrointestinal effects	None	Ascites; hepatic angina with hepatomegaly	None	None	Ascites, hepatomegaly (with heart failure)
Pain	Angina pectoris	Chest pain	Chest pain (anginal)	None	Palpitations
Heart rate, rhythm	Bradycardia, dysrhythmias (with heart failure)	Palpitations (atrial fibrillation)	Palpitations, water-hammer pulse	Palpitations	Atrial fibrillations
Heart sounds	Systolic murmur	Diastolic murmur, accentuated first heart sound, opening snap	Diastolic and systolic murmurs	Murmur throughout systole	Murmur throughout systole
Most common cause	Congenital, rheumatic fever	Rheumatic fever	Bacterial endocarditis; aortic root disease	Floppy valve; coronary artery disease	Congenital

Data from Braunwald E, editor: *Heart disease: a textbook of cardiovascular medicine,* ed 4, Philadelphia, 1992, WB Saunders; Hancock EW: Valvular heart disease, *Sci Am Med* 1(I-XI):1, 1992.
*If disease not treated.

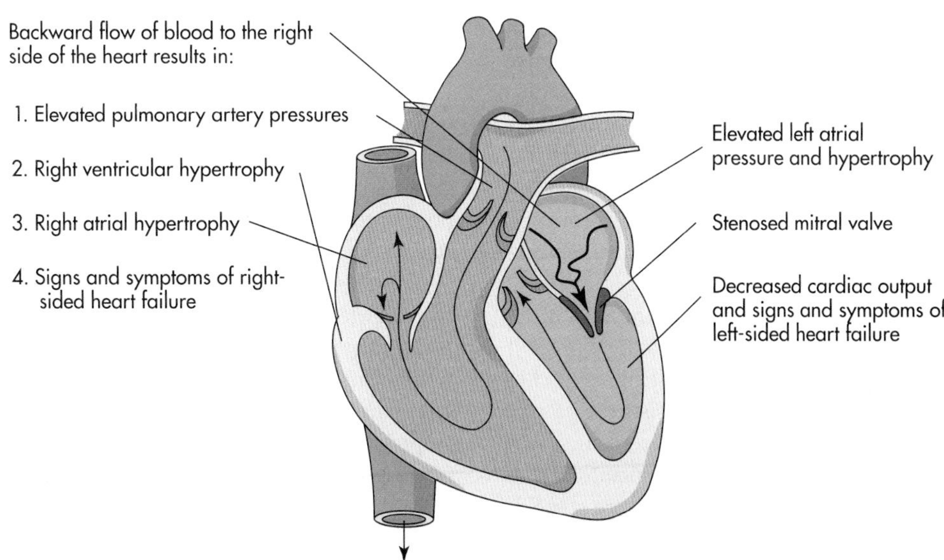

Figure 24-6 Effects of mitral stenosis.

The primary symptom of mitral stenosis is dyspnea, which is largely the result of reduced lung compliance. Dyspnea on exertion, paroxysmal nocturnal dyspnea, and orthopnea occur as a result of pulmonary hypertension. The symptoms may be precipitated by emotional stress, respiratory infection, sexual intercourse, or atrial fibrillation. Some persons experience a dry cough, dysphagia, or bronchitis because of bronchial irritation from the enlarged LA. Pressure exerted on the laryngeal nerve by an engorged pulmonary artery can cause hoarseness. Fatigue and weakness occur as a result of decreased cardiac output. Hemoptysis, usually a late sign, occurs from the rupture of a bronchial vein. Eventually right-sided heart failure leads to jugular vein distention, pitting edema, and hepatomegaly.

Collaborative Care Management

The diagnosis of mitral stenosis is established by the clinical symptoms, such as an opening snap, created by the forceful opening of mitral valve, followed by a diastolic rumbling or murmur that results from the increased velocity of blood flow. The diastolic murmur is absent when the valve is severely calcified. ECG changes indicate right ventricular hypertrophy, and chest x-ray films show left atrial enlargement. The most sensitive and noninvasive diagnostic test is the echocardiogram, which shows an impedance of flow, fusion of valve leaflets, and poor leaflet separation during diastole. Mitral stenosis also can be diagnosed with a cardiac catheterization (see Table 24-5).

Mildly symptomatic patients with mitral stenosis are treated with diuretics, and digitalis is used to control heart rate in the event of atrial fibrillation. Anticoagulation therapy with warfarin (Coumadin) is used to prevent thrombus formation in patients with moderate to severe mitral stenosis or those with a history of thromoembolism. Medical therapy also includes antbiotic prophylaxis before dental or surgical procedures to reduce the risk of bacterial endocarditis.

More definitive intervention is indicated when the disease causes either loss of exercise capacity or pulmonary hypertension. Percutaneous valvuloplasty using balloon dilation provides a nonsurgical alternative to reopen the valve. Surgical commissurotomy can also be performed while the valve leaflets remain mobile. Both commissurotomy and valvuloplasty allow patients to retain their natural valve and reduce the need for long-term anticoagulant therapy. Mitral valve replacement using open heart surgery and cardiopulmonary bypass is performed when the valve is severely fibrotic or calcified. In general, patients undergoing mitral valve replacement require permanent anticoagulation therapy.

Patient/Family Education. Patients with symptomatic mitral stenosis are prescribed a sodium-restricted diet to help prevent fluid retention and progressive heart failure. The nurse teaches the patient about the dietary restriction and assists the patient to adjust activity to his or her level of tolerance. Family involvement in both diet and activity teaching is encouraged to support adherence. Patients with moderate to severe stenosis are advised to avoid activities that require sudden increases in cardiac output. Patients receiving anticoagulant therapy receive instruction about the safe use of the drug and measures to follow to prevent bleeding. Patient teaching related to anticoagulant therapy is further discussed in Chapter 25.

Mitral Regurgitation

Etiology/Epidemiology

Mitral regurgitation (mitral insufficiency) occurs when the mitral valve fails to completely close during ventricular systole, allowing blood to flow backward into the LA. Mitral regurgitation can be either an acute or chronic condition.

Mitral regurgitation can be caused by rheumatic heart disease and is often present in conjunction with mitral stenosis. Mitral regurgitation occurs more commonly in men than in women and is the most prevalent lesion in patients who experience heart failure with active rheumatic carditis. With the exception of congenitally malformed mitral valves and connective tissue disorders, mitral regurgitation is primarily a disease of middle-aged and elderly persons. Other causes of mitral regurgitation include endocarditis, coronary heart disease, dilated cardiomyopathy, a leaky prosthetic mitral valve, mitral valve prolapse, congenital malformation of the mitral valve, and connective tissue disorders such as Marfan syndrome, amyloidosis, and ankylosing spondylitis.

Weakness, rupture, or fibrosis of a papillary muscle secondary to ischemic heart disease, ventricular aneurysm, or acute myocardial infarction can also cause acute mitral regurgitation. Papillary muscle dysfunction allows the valve leaflets to flop in the direction of the LA during systole, and the blood flows backward. In addition, rupture of the chordae tendineae or perforation of a mitral valve cusp can cause acute mitral regurgitation.

Pathophysiology

In chronic mitral insufficiency or regurgitation a variable amount of blood from the LV is shunted back through the mitral valve to the LA. This backflow of blood causes both the LA and LV to dilate and hypertrophy. Increasing preload and left atrial pressure also raise the pulmonary venous and arteriolar pressures and eventually cause right-sided heart failure (Figure 24-7). As the ventricle hypertrophies, it becomes dysfunctional and cardiac output decreases. Concurrently, the LA is often fibrillating, diminishing the cardiac output even further.

Fatigue and weakness are the primary symptoms of mitral regurgitation. Right-sided heart failure causes hepatic congestion, edema, ascites, and distended neck veins in severe cases. Some persons experience palpitations or paroxysmal nocturnal dyspnea.

Progressive dyspnea on exertion and pulmonary edema from an elevated left atrial pressure are the primary symptoms of acute regurgitation. The increased atrial pressure is transmitted immediately to the pulmonary veins, causing the congestive symptoms. Because the ventricle has not yet hypertrophied, the cardiac output remains sufficient and fatigue is not a problem. Although persons with mitral regurgitation commonly develop atrial fibrillation, thrombus formation in the atria is less common than with mitral stenosis because backflow and the resulting turbulence of the blood limit pooling.

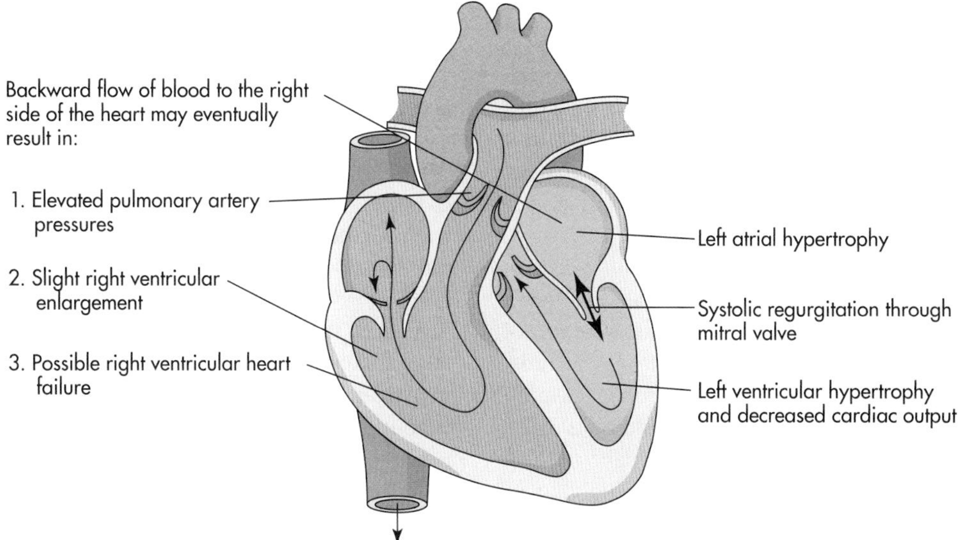

Figure 24-7 Effects of mitral regurgitation.

Collaborative Care Management

The diagnosis of mitral regurgitation is made from the clinical symptoms and auscultation of a blowing, high-pitched systolic murmur and third heart sound. The first heart sound (S1) may not be heard, depending on the severity of regurgitation. A chest x-ray reveals left atrial enlargement and occasional left ventricular dilation. The ECG tracings show left ventricular hypertrophy and, less commonly, right ventricular hypertrophy (Table 24-5). An echocardiogram may identify mitral valve cusp prolapse, ruptured chordae tendineae cordis, and enlargement of the LA and LV. Definitive diagnosis is made through cardiac catheterization (see Chapter 22), which assesses left ventricular function and the degree of regurgitation.

Patients with mild mitral regurgitation who develop new-onset atrial fibrillation may need to undergo controlled cardioversion to restore normal sinus rhythm and maximize cardiac output. Patients with long-standing atrial fibrillation or a history of thromboembolism receive long-term anticoagulation.

Mitral regurgitation that progresses despite medical therapy necessitates valve repair or prosthetic replacement. Individuals with intact left ventricular function and without other severe noncardiac disease may be candidates for open heart surgery and valve replacement.

Patient/Family Education. Patient/family teaching for patients with mitral regurgitation is directed primarily at symptom management, and is similar in most respects to the education provided to patients with mitral stenosis.

Mitral Valve Prolapse

Etiology/Epidemiology

Mitral valve prolapse occurs when abnormalities in the mitral valve leaflets, chordae tendinae, or papillary muscles allow prolapse of the mitral valve leaflets backward into the LA during ventricular systole. Mitral valve prolapse is also known as Barlow's syndrome, as well as a "floppy" or "billowing" mitral valve. Mitral valve prolapse is the most common valvular disorder in the United States. It occurs in approximately 4% to 7% of adults and is most common in young women.[18] In many patients, mitral valve prolapse is a benign, asymptomatic disorder and may remain undiagnosed.

Mitral valve prolapse may be caused by a variety of factors. Its incidence is possibly linked to an autosomal dominant inherited trait, and it is also associated with other inherited connective tissue disorders such as Marfan syndrome, Ehlers-Danlos syndrome, and osteogenesis imperfecta. Other causes of mitral valve prolapse include endocarditis, coronary artery disease, myocarditis, cardiomyopathy, cardiac trauma, and hyperthyroidism.

Pathophysiology

In mitral valve prolapse the leaflets of the mitral valve become enlarged or thickened, and the chordae tendineae may become elongated. These changes permit the valve leaflets to billow upward into the LA during ventricular systole. Depending on the degree of prolapse and the integrity of the valve leaflets, mitral regurgitation may occur. The subsequent pathophysiology parallels that of mitral regurgitation. In addition, research suggests that individuals with mitral valve prolapse may experience some autonomic nervous system dysfunction causing excessive catecholamine release, leading to a wide array of subjective complaints.

Many cases of mitral valve prolapse are asymptomatic. Individuals who are symptomatic report palpitations, which are secondary to dysrhythmias and tachycardia. Other symptoms include light-headedness, syncope, fatigue, lethargy, weakness, dyspnea, and chest tightness. In addition, hyperventilation, anxiety, depression, panic attacks, and atypical chest pain may occur. Many of the symptoms of mitral valve prolapse are vague and are not necessarily related to the degree of prolapse.

Although mitral valve prolapse is generally benign, as many as 15% of individuals develop mitral regurgitation and subsequent left ventricular failure. In addition, individuals with mitral valve prolapse are at increased risk for embolic stroke.

On physical examination most individuals with mitral valve prolapse have a mid-systolic click, and if mitral regurgitation is present, a late-systolic murmur is heard. In the absence of auscultatory findings, mitral valve prolapse may be detected on echocardiography.

Collaborative Care Management

Electrocardiograms of individuals with mitral valve prolapse are normal unless the person is symptomatic from dysrhythmias. The most common rhythm disturbances include premature ventricular contractions, supraventricular tachycardia, and atrial tachydysrythmias. Mitral valve prolapse is diagnosed principally by echocardiography, although cardiac angiography may be used to confirm the diagnosis. Individuals who experience palpitations require 24-hour ambulatory ECG monitoring to determine the severity of the dysrhythmia.

Asymptomatic individuals with mitral valve prolapse usually do not require treatment. Symptomatic individuals may require medications to control dysrhythmias (see Chapter 23). Beta-blockers are the treatment of choice for managing palpitations and chest pain.

All persons with mitral valve prolapse need regular follow-up care and should have an echocardiogram every few years to monitor disease progression. The severity of mitral regurgitation associated with the valve prolapse determines the necessity for surgical intervention.

Antibiotic prophylaxis against endocarditis is indicated before dental and surgical procedures for individuals who have a systolic murmur or echocardiographic evidence of mitral valve leaflet thickening. Asymptomatic individuals do not usually require antibiotic prophylaxis.

Patient/Family Education. Individuals with mitral valve prolapse are encouraged to avoid caffeine, which may exacerbate the incidence of tachycardia and atrial dysrhythmias. These episodes can be frightening for the patient and family, who need to thoroughly understand the nature of the problem and how to control or respond to it. No additional dietary restrictions are needed. Activity is also unrestricted, although symptomatic patients may need to adjust their activities in response to the nature and severity of their symptoms.

Aortic Stenosis

Etiology/Epidemiology

Aortic stenosis occurs when the aortic valve leaflets become stiff, fused, or calcified and impede blood flow from the left ventricle into the aorta during ventricular systole. Aortic stenosis is caused by congenital malformations of the aortic valve, inflammatory heart disease (endocarditis), or degenerative disease (calcification). Aortic stenosis generally impedes the outflow of blood from the left ventricle at the level of the aortic valve, although obstruction to flow can also occur above and below the valve itself. Conditions such as hypertrophic cardiomyopathy may lead to subvalvular aortic stenosis. Coarctation of the aorta is a supravalvular lesion that may mimic aortic stenosis.

The causes of aortic stenosis vary with the age of the patient. In patients less than 30 years old, aortic stenosis is typically caused by a congenitally stenotic aortic valve. Between the ages of 30 and 65 years, aortic stenosis is more commonly caused by progressive stenosis of a congenital bicuspid aortic valve, and less commonly by rheumatic heart disease. Although less than 2% of the general population have a congenital bicuspid aortic valve, 50% of these individuals develop aortic calcification and stenosis by the age of 50. In persons over 65 years old, aortic stenosis is caused by degeneration and sclerosis of the valve and the incidence is equally distributed between men and women.[18] Except in elderly persons, men are three to four times more likely to develop isolated aortic stenosis.

Pathophysiology

Aortic stenosis occurs when the aortic valve narrows and obstructs the flow of blood into the aorta during systole (Figure 24-8). Resistance to blood flow from the LV causes an in-

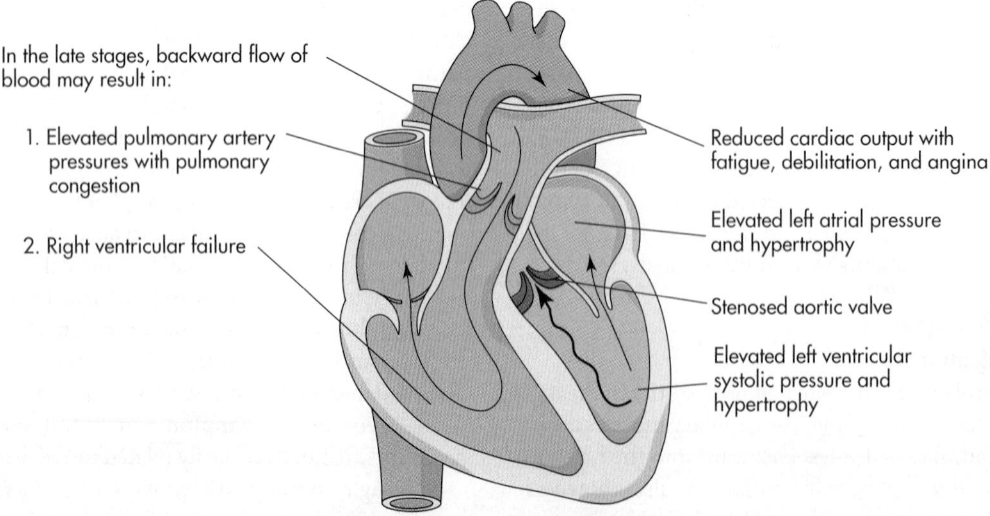

Figure 24-8 Effects of aortic stenosis.

crease in left ventricular systolic pressure. This pressure increase and the LV's compensatory efforts to increase cardiac output lead to left ventricular hypertrophy. Even though the LV pumps harder to meet the body's needs, the stenotic valve effectively blocks any increase in blood flow from the heart. Hence, in advanced aortic stenosis, cardiac output becomes fixed despite the LV's attempts to increase blood flow.

Worsening left ventricular hypertrophy leads to a constellation of problems late in the course of the disease, including pulmonary congestion, syncope, and myocardial ischemia. Pulmonary congestion occurs when the stenosis significantly interferes with the forward movement of the blood. Syncope and myocardial ischemia occur because of the fixed-flow condition and the inability of the LV to meet the changing needs of the body. The severity of aortic stenosis is determined by the pressure gradient between the LV and the aorta.

Aortic stenosis develops gradually, and symptoms do not appear until late in the course. Life expectancy without medical or surgical intervention is generally less than 4 years after the onset of symptoms. Early symptoms of aortic stenosis include fatigue and dyspnea. The combination of dyspnea, exertional angina, and syncope or near-syncopal episodes indicates severe aortic stenosis. Individuals who develop symptomatic heart failure survive less than 2 years, whereas patients with either syncope or angina survive longer (5 years and 3 years, respectively). In addition, 15% of those with symptomatic aortic stenosis and 5% of asymptomatic patients suffer sudden cardiac death.

In addition to the symptoms of dyspnea, fatigue, heart failure, angina, and syncope, an array of physical findings is present in individuals with aortic stenosis. The hallmark clinical findings include a grade III/VI or IV/VI systolic ejection murmur over the aortic area radiating upward into the carotid arteries and a pulse pattern that demonstrates a delayed systolic upstroke (Table 24-7). Other clinical findings depend on the degree of heart failure and pulmonary edema.

Collaborative Care Management

A diagnosis of aortic stenosis is made from the clinical symptoms and diagnostic tests (Table 24-5). Tests that aid in the diagnosis of aortic stenosis include the ECG, chest x-ray, echocardiogram, and cardiac catheterization.

The ECG is normal early in the course of aortic stenosis. Late changes include left ventricular hypertrophy, nonspecific ST depression, and T wave inversion, indicative of subendocardial ischemia. The chest x-ray may reveal aortic calcification. The echocardiogram reveals valve leaflet defects and increased ventricular wall thickness.

Cardiac catheterization definitively diagnoses aortic stenosis and quantifies the severity of the disease. A pressure difference of 50 mm Hg or greater between the LV and the aorta is evidence of hemodynamically significant disease. In addition, cardiac catheterization evaluates left ventricular function, coronary vessel patency, and the degree of associated aortic and mitral regurgitation before cardiac surgery.

Percutaneous balloon valvuloplasty may be used to alleviate aortic stensois. The technique involves cardiac catheterization and the introduction of a balloon catheter into the aortic valve orifice. The balloon is repeatedly inflated until the valve lumen is further opened, thus relieving some of the stenosis. Patients receive the same care provided to individuals undergoing cardiac catheterization but may also be monitored in an intensive care unit for 24 to 48 hours after the procedure. Although balloon valvuloplasty improves symptoms for some individuals, the procedure carries a high morbidity and mortality rate and is currently used primarily for individuals who are poor candidates for cardiac surgery and cardiopulmonary bypass.

The definitive therapy for patients with aortic stenosis is valve replacement with a prosthetic aortic valve. Although the surgery carries significant risks, most individuals experience substantial improvement in their general health and exercise tolerance.

Patient/Family Education. The diet for persons with aortic stenosis is unrestricted unless heart failure is present, in which case the nurse instructs patients to restrict their daily intake of sodium and fluid. Activity levels are carefully monitored because patients are at risk for sudden cardiac death. Patients are cautioned against undue physical exertion or stress, which may precipitate acute heart failure or dysrhythmia. Patients and families need ongoing teaching and support to effectively manage the disease in their daily lives. The nurse also reminds patients of the importance of seeking prophylactic antibiotic treatment against endocarditis before any invasive dental procedure or surgery.

Aortic Regurgitation

Etiology/Epidemiology

Aortic regurgitation occurs when an incompetent aortic valve allows blood to flow backward from the aorta into the left ventricle during diastole. An incompetent aortic valve may result from disease of the valve cusps or the aortic root.

TABLE 24-7 Auscultatory Differences in Valvular Heart Disease

Valvular Disorder	General Findings	Murmurs
Mitral stenosis	S_1 snapping, louder Palpable thrill at apex	Soft, low-pitched, rumbling Diastolic
Mitral regurgitation	S_1 soft or absent S_3 present Palpable thrill at apex	High-pitched, blowing Pansystolic
Aortic stenosis	S_2 soft Left-sided S_4 Systolic thrill at heart base	Low-pitched, harsh, rasping Midsystolic
Aortic regurgitation	S_3 present Systolic thrill over aortic area	High-pitched, blowing Diastolic
Tricuspid regurgitation	Systolic thrill at lower left sternal border	High-pitched, blowing Pansystolic

Common causes of aortic regurgitation include inflammatory diseases (rheumatic heart disease, bacterial endocarditis), the presence of a congenital bicuspid aortic valve, or idiopathic dilation of the aortic root (cardiomyopathy). Less common causes include traumatic rupture of an aortic valve cusp, rheumatoid arthritis, ankylosing spondylitis, Reiter's syndrome, connective tissue disorders (Marfan syndrome, Ehlers-Danlos syndrome, osteogenesis imperfecta), and syphilitic aortitis. The incidence of aortic regurgitation related to rheumatic heart disease has decreased significantly during the last 20 years. Except in cases of rheumatic heart disease, aortic regurgitation is more common in men than in women.

Acute aortic regurgitation occurs with sudden dilation of the aortic root and is most commonly associated with an ascending dissecting aortic aneurysm. The most common risk factor for acute aortic dissection is systemic hypertension. Selected connective tissue disorders, especially Marfan syndrome, also pose a risk for acute aortic dissection. Refer to Chapter 25 for further information relating to aortic aneurysms.

Pathophysiology

In chronic aortic regurgitation the backward flow of blood through the incompetent, leaky aortic valve increases the volume of blood in the LV (Figure 24-9). This increased blood volume and subsequent increase in left ventricular end-diastolic pressure increase stroke volume and sustain cardiac output. Over time, however, left ventricular dilation and hypertrophy occur. Ultimately, the LV loses its ability to compensate for the increased pressure and volume, leading to decreased stroke volume and cardiac output and finally left ventricular failure. Progressive aortic regurgitation can also lead to increased left atrial pressures, left atrial chamber dilation, pulmonary congestion, pulmonary hypertension, and possibly right-sided heart failure.

In acute aortic regurgitation the LV cannot compensate for the sudden dramatic increase in workload, and patients develop fulminant pulmonary edema. Left ventricular decompensation and failure occur rapidly, and these patients require emergent lifesaving care.

Individuals with chronic aortic regurgitation may remain asymptomatic for 20 years or report only mild dyspnea on exertion. With disease progression and gradual left ventricular decompensation, symptoms of heart failure and pulmonary edema develop, including progressively more severe dyspnea, orthopnea, paroxysmal nocturnal dyspnea, and angina. The development and progression of these symptoms reflect advanced disease. Other symptoms vary depending on the etiology.

The hallmark physical finding in individuals with aortic regurgitation is a diastolic murmur that is loudest over the aortic area (Table 24-7). The duration of the murmur reflects the severity of the regurgitation. Other classic physical findings of chronic aortic regurgitation include decreased diastolic pressure, widened pulse pressure, and subsequent water-hammer pulse. Pistol-shot pulse sounds can be auscultated over the femoral arteries, and some persons demonstrate a head bobbing with each heartbeat. Individuals with acute aortic regurgitation do not demonstrate the changes in pulse pressure because of the sudden onset of the disease.

Collaborative Care Management

The diagnosis of aortic regurgitation is made based on the presence of the diastolic murmur and the widened pulse pressure (Tables 24-4 and 24-6). Persons with chronic aortic regurgitation exhibit evidence of left ventricular hypertrophy on the ECG and cardiomegaly is usually apparent on the chest x-ray. Patients with acute aortic regurgitation may exhibit only nonspecific ST or T wave changes with a normal heart size. Echocardiography is useful in assessing left ventricular function, hypertrophy, and aortic root dilation.

Persons with asymptomatic aortic regurgitation do not require treatment beyond yearly follow-up with a chest x-ray, and ECG. Persons with symptomatic aortic regurgitation are managed medically until a decision can be made concerning

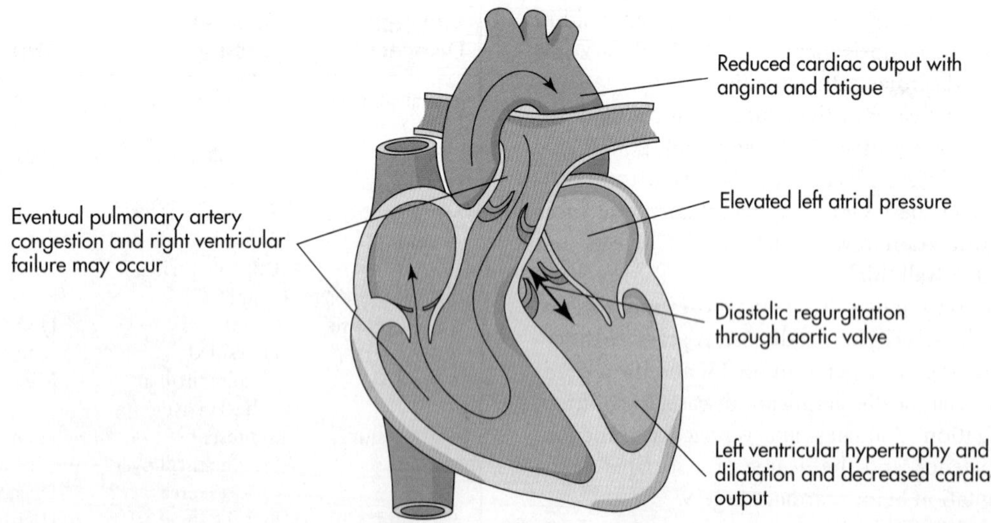

Figure 24-9 Effects of aortic regurgitation.

valve surgery. Digitalis and diuretic therapy are indicated for individuals who demonstrate heart failure. Afterload-reducing agents may also be used.

Because of the high mortality rate associated with symptomatic aortic regurgitation, all symptomatic individuals are evaluated for aortic valve replacement surgery. Operative mortality is significantly reduced when the surgery is performed before the development of left ventricular dysfunction. Early intervention is also associated with an improved quality of life.

Patient/Family Education. Patients with aortic regurgitation must understand the nature and potential seriousness of their disease and commit to regular medical follow-up care and evaluation. Asymptomatic patients do not need to restrict their diet or activity in any way. Symptomatic patients are instructed to reduce their intake of sodium to help control the symptoms of heart failure and to adapt their activity as needed to changes in their symptoms. Patients need to be knowledgeable about the safe use of any prescribed medications. The nurse reminds patients that it is very important to request prophylactic antibiotic therapy against endocarditis before undergoing any dental or surgical procedure.

Tricuspid and Pulmonary Valve Disorders

Etiology/Epidemiology

Tricuspid stenosis is a restriction of the tricuspid valve orifice that impedes blood flow from the RA to the RV during right ventricular diastole (filling). Conversely, tricuspid regurgitation involves an incompetent tricuspid valve that allows blood to flow backward from the RV to the RA during ventricular systole. Pulmonary stenosis is a restriction of the pulmonary valve orifice impeding blood flow out of the RV into the pulmonary vasculature during systole. Pulmonary regurgitation involves an incompetent pulmonary valve that allows blood to flow backward into the RV during diastole.

Disorders of the tricuspid and pulmonary valves are significantly less common than disorders of the valves on the left side of the heart. The right side of the heart is a low-pressure system, and the potential for inflammatory changes and calcification is much greater on the higher-pressure left side. Mitral and aortic valve diseases often also involve the tricuspid or pulmonary valves.

Disorders of the tricuspid valves are primarily caused by rheumatic fever. Less common causes include endocarditis or congenital malformations of the valve cusps. Tricuspid stenosis is generally seen in women with a history of rheumatic heart disease who suffer from mitral stenosis. Tricuspid regurgitation often accompanies triscuspid stenosis.

Pulmonary valve disorders are rare. Pulmonary regurgitation, like tricuspid valve disease, is caused by endocarditis or rheumatic fever. Congenital malformations and tumors may also cause pulmonary valve dysfunction.

Pathophysiology

All tricuspid and pulmonary valve disorders have similar effects on cardiac function. Tricuspid stenosis causes increased pressure in the RA and subsequent right atrial enlargement and hypertrophy (Figure 24-10). Over time, systemic venous congestion occurs and causes ascites, hepatomegaly, and edema. Because of reduced flow across the stenotic tricuspid valve, cardiac output is fixed and eventually diminished. Symptoms of tricuspid stenosis are generally overshadowed by those associated with mitral or aortic valve dysfunction. Fatigue is present and is related to decreased cardiac output. Tricuspid regurgitation involves the same pathologic consequences as tricuspid stenosis with the exception that the backward flow of blood into the RA during systole serves to increase the workload of the RV. Therefore right ventricular dilation, hypertrophy, and failure are present in tricuspid regurgitation but not in tricuspid stenosis. The pathophysiologic mechanisms affecting cardiac function in

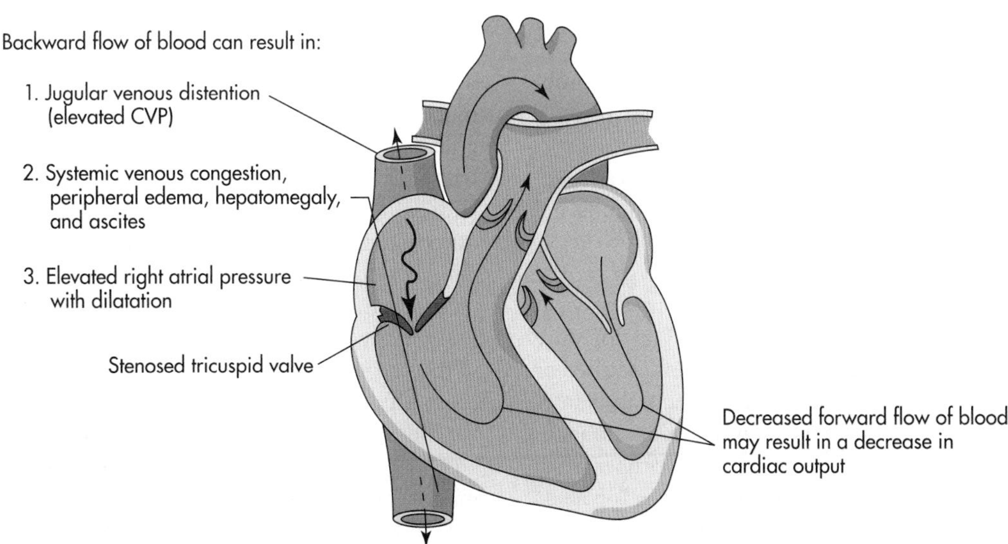

Figure 24-10 Effects of tricuspid stenosis.

pulmonary stenosis and pulmonary regurgitation are identical to those described for tricuspid disorders.

Disorders of the tricuspid and pulmonary valves ultimately lead to symptoms of right-sided heart failure and decreased cardiac output. The ECG shows tall, peaked P waves (atrial hypertrophy) in both tricuspid stenosis and tricuspid regurgitation. Right ventricular hypertrophy is evident on ECG with tricuspid regurgitation, pulmonary stenosis, and pulmonary regurgitation. Atrial fibrillation may also be present. In tricuspid stenosis, a high-pitched diastolic murmur can be auscultated along the left sternal border. In the other disorders of the tricuspid and pulmonary valves, the murmur is harsh and can be heard throughout systole. The chest x-ray shows right atrial enlargement, right ventricular enlargement (except in tricuspid stenosis), and a prominent shadow of the superior vena cava. Echocardiogram is used to determine the degree of valve dysfunction.

Collaborative Care Management

Care for patients with tricuspid and pulmonary valve disorders focuses on the management of right-sided heart failure and decreased cardiac output. The care is similar to that previously outlined for mitral and aortic valve disorders. One exception is that patients do not experience dyspnea and pulmonary consequences with tricuspid or pulmonary valve disease, unless these disorders occur concurrently with aortic and mitral valve disease.

Patient/Family Education. Teaching for patients with tricuspid and pulmonary valve disorders is targeted toward symptom management, which may vary substantially from patient to patient. Patients are encouraged to modify activities to match their tolerance level and to plan for the presence of chronic fatigue. Congestion within the gastrointestinal tract may lead to chronic anorexia, and the nurse emphasizes the importance of adequate nutrition. Patients are taught to monitor their edema at home and to protect the skin from breakdown. Patients are also instructed in the correct and safe use of all medications and the management of expected side effects.

CARDIAC SURGERY

Although the first attempts to surgically correct cardiac problems date back to the 1930s, favorable outcomes for patients did not occur until the 1950s with the development of cardiopulmonary (heart-lung) bypass and new surgical techniques. Today, numerous cardiac disorders in both adults and children can be effectively treated surgically.

The most common reason for an adult to undergo cardiac surgery is for myocardial revascularization (coronary artery bypass grafting). Patients also undergo cardiac surgery for valve repair or replacement, repair of structural defects (acquired or congenital), implantation of devices, and cardiac transplantation. Table 24-8 provides a list of the common indications for cardiac surgery. Cardiac surgery is classified as either open heart or closed heart, depending on whether the heart is "opened" during the course of the surgery. Cardiac surgery involving the repair of internal structural defects is open heart, whereas myocardial revascularization is a closed heart procedure.

TABLE 24-8 Indications for Cardiac Surgery and Associated Procedures

Problem	Procedure
Ischemic heart disease	Coronary artery bypass graft
Repair of structural abnormalities	Valve repair Valve replacement Atrial septal defect repair Ventricular septal defect repair Ventricular aneurysm resection Atrial tumor resection Aortic aneurysm (thoracic) repair
Implantation of devices	Automatic implantable cardioverter-defibrillator Ventricular assist device Artificial heart chamber
Transplantation	Replacement of diseased heart with healthy heart

Coronary Artery Bypass Graft

CAD is the most common indication for cardiac surgery. When a coronary artery becomes obstructed, a coronary artery bypass graft (CABG) may be performed. The graft allows blood to bypass the obstructed portion of the coronary artery and provides improved blood flow and increased oxygen to the myocardial tissue distal to the lesion. Although CABG does not cure the underlying heart disease, it does reduce the incidence of angina and prevents myocardial ischemia and infarction.

Patients can undergo a single bypass or simultaneously receive multiple bypass grafts, depending on the nature and severity of the coronary disease. Traditionally, the surgical procedure involved closed heart surgery via a median sternotomy, cold cardioplegia (heart activity is stopped), and extracorporeal circulation via a cardiopulmonary bypass machine. Recent advances in cardiac surgery have led to the development of the minimally invasive direct coronary artery bypass (MIDCAB) for individuals with only one diseased coronary artery. In this surgery, access to the heart is via a smaller incision at the left sternal border of the anterior thorax instead of the larger median sternotomy, and neither cardioplegia nor cardiopulmonary bypass is used. Also multiple coronary artery bypass grafts are now being performed via median sternotomy, but without the use cardioplegia and cardiopulmonary bypass ("off-pump") (see Future Watch box). These advances have reduced the incidence of complications after surgery and facilitate a speedier recovery. The average length of hospital stay for patients undergoing traditional CABG surgery is 4 to 5 days. Preliminary data for the less invasive MIDCAB and "off-pump" procedures show even shorter recovery times with an estimated length of hospital stay of 2 to 3 days (Box 24-10).[9,22]

The graft used to bypass the affected coronary artery must be either a vein or artery. Although vein grafts have been the mainstay of bypass procedures in the past, arterial grafts provide improved long term patency and perfusion of the myocardium. Therefore arterial grafts are being used with increasing frequency.

Future Watch

Cardiac Surgery Without Cardiopulmonary Bypass

Traditional open-heart surgical procedures have been dependent on cardiopulmonary bypass to provide a quiet heart to permit accurate surgery. Increasingly, however, surgeons have been attempting to develop ways to perform these technically difficult procedures without the need for cardiopulmonary bypass, which is accompanied by multiple risks for the patient. Minimally invasive procedures are achieving wide acceptance for certain types of cardiac problems. Another option is the off-pump coronary bypass (OPCAB) that uses a plastic and metal device with two stabilizer arms that can be positioned and manipulated. When it touches an area of the heart it causes it to "still" while the rest of the heart keeps beating. The surgeon is then able to precisely suture the bypass grafts to the coronary arteries in the desired location.

The procedure is not appropriate for all patients (e.g., it is inappropriate for use with the main circumflex artery because of its inaccessibility), but it can support the placing of multiple bypass grafts and is often useful for patients who are considered to be poor surgical risks. It is associated with a lower need for surgical transfusion, fewer postoperative pulmonary problems, and fewer fluid imbalance problems in the immediate postoperative period. It also costs less than traditional bypass procedures that involve cardiopulmonary bypass. Patient recovery appears to be facilitated, but more data are needed to verify this conclusion.

Reference: Taylor B: Heart surgery without the pump, *Helix* 18(3):5, 2001.

The most common donor vein is a long portion of the saphenous vein, although occasionally a cephalic vein from the forearm is used. After vein harvesting, the graft is anastamosed to the coronary artery distal to the obstructive lesion, and the proximal end is anastomosed to the acscending aorta. The donor graft is reversed before insertion because of the presence of directional valves (see Figure 23-12). Preoperative Doppler studies of venous flow help pinpoint optimal segments of veins for use as grafts. This enables the surgeon to use minimally invasive vein harvesting in which only the necessary segments, rather than the entire length of the vein, are removed.

The artery most commonly used for CABG is an internal mammary artery (right or left). Only the distal end of the artery is dissected away from the tissues and anastomosed to the coronary artery distal to the obstructive lesion. The proximal segment is left in place. A more recent trend involves using the radial artery from the forearm or occasionally the gastroepiploic artery.

Long-term patency rates for internal mammary artery grafts exceed those for saphenous vein grafts. Studies have shown that 40% to 50% of saphenous vein grafts close within 2 years, whereas 90% of internal mammary artery grafts remain patent 10 years after surgery.[25] However, internal mammary artery grafts are contraindicated for use in patients with diabetes mellitus (because of the impact of reduced arterial circulation to the chest wall), as well as in obese or large-breasted individuals.

Correction of Structural Defects

Cardiac valve dysfunction is the most common structural repair in adults. Options include either valve repair (annuloplasty, valvuloplasty, or commisurotomy) (Box 24-11) or replacement with a valve prosthesis. Less commonly, adults undergo cardiac surgery to repair structural defects such as a ventricular aneurysm or septal defect, to remove a cardiac tumor, or to repair the heart after trauma.

The repair of intracardiac structural defects requires open heart surgery, cardioplegia, and cardiopulmonary bypass. Surgery involving extracardiac structures such as repair of a

BOX 24-10 Minimally Invasive Coronary Artery Bypass Graft

A surgical technique allows for coronary artery bypass graft surgery to be performed without the use of a median sternotomy, cardiopulmonary (heart-lung) bypass, or cardioplegia. In this procedure, a small left chest incision allows the surgeon to directly visualize the heart and complete an internal mammary artery–to–left anterior descending coronary artery bypass. Preliminary data suggest that operative time and postoperative complications are reduced, and hospital stay averages 2 days as opposed to 5 days for traditional heart surgery.

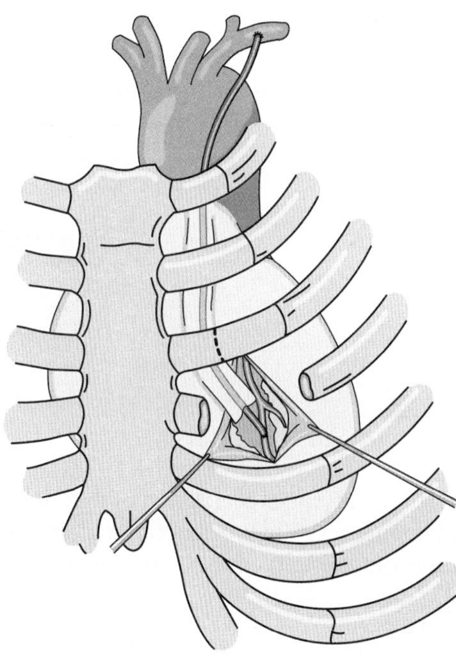

Through a pericardial window anastomosis of the left internal mammary artery to the left anterior descending coronary artery is performed under direct vision.

BOX 24-11 Types of Valve Repair

Annuloplasty

Repair of ring or annulus of incompetent or diseased valve

Valvuloplasty

Repair of valve, suturing of torn leaflets

Commissurotomy

Dilation of valve; repair of a leaflet or commissure, fibrous bond or ring

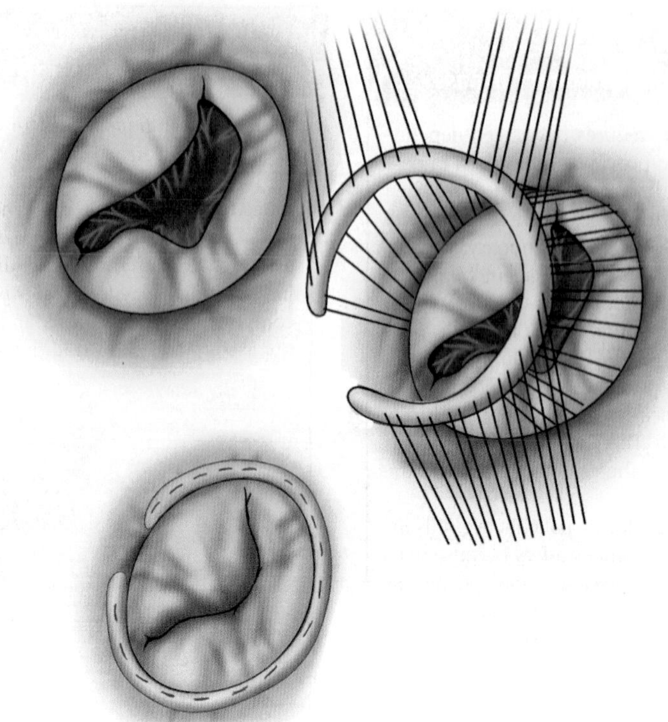

Figure 24-11 Annuloplasty.

thoracic aortic aneurysm or coarctation of the aorta may also include cardiopulmonary bypass and cardioplegia, depending on the location and severity of the lesion.

Valve Repair

Annuloplasty. Annuloplasty is a procedure to reduce an enlarged annulus (fibrous ring surrounding the valve). A prosthetic ring is sutured into the circumference of the mitral or tricuspid annulus, and the stitches are pulled together toward the prosthesis, reducing the size of the valve orifice (Figure 24-11).

Valvuloplasty. Valvuloplasty involves direct repair of torn leaflets or clefts by open heart surgery. The advantages of operative valve repair over valve replacement include (1) higher survival rates, (2) fewer cardiac complications (especially thromboembolism), (3) lower operative mortality and morbidity rates, (4) potential improvement in left ventricular function, (5) reduced need for anticoagulation, and (6) lower cost. Mitral valvuloplasty has gained increasing acceptance as the surgery of choice for mitral regurgitation, including cases of rheumatic etiology.

Commissurotomy. Mitral commissurotomy is the separation or incision of the stenosed valve leaflets at their borders or commissures. Either an open or a closed technique may be used, although open commissurotomy is currently the procedure of choice. An open commissurotomy usually is performed through a median sternotomy or a right anterolateral thoracotomy incision to allow for proper visualization of the mitral valve. Cardiopulmonary bypass is initiated, the LA is opened, and the commissures are incised with a scalpel. The newly mobilized leaflets are attached to the chordae tendineae cordis. Disadvantages of this approach include those associated with open heart surgery in general. Advantages include fewer thrombotic and embolic complications and fewer atrial tears with resultant hemorrhage. If the valve disease appears to be too advanced to repair, valve replacement can be performed immediately.

A closed commissurotomy (without bypass) is performed through a left posterolateral thoracotomy. The fifth rib is removed and the atrium is palpated to detect the presence of any thrombi. If a thrombus is present, the procedure is converted to an open procedure to allow for clot removal. Otherwise, the surgeon inserts a finger through a small incision, dividing the papillary muscle longitudinally from the apex toward the base as shown in Figure 24-12. The atrium is digitally examined for thrombi, and the valve is examined for calcium particles. Some surgeons digitally open the fused commissures and use a dilator to open the valve and relieve the stenosis. The advantages of the closed approach include a shorter operating time, a simpler procedure, and less blood replacement. Systemic emboli, atrial wall tears, inadequate alleviation of the stenosis, and mitral regurgitation are risks associated with this approach.

Valve Replacement

Valve replacement is considered when the valve is so stenosed and calcified that repair would not achieve long-term relief of the stenosis. The decision carefully considers the patient's general health status and level of myocardial functioning because valve replacement carries a significant operative mortality.

The heart usually is approached by a median sternotomy and cardiopulmonary bypass is initiated. The diseased valve leaflets are excised at the annulus, and the remaining annuli

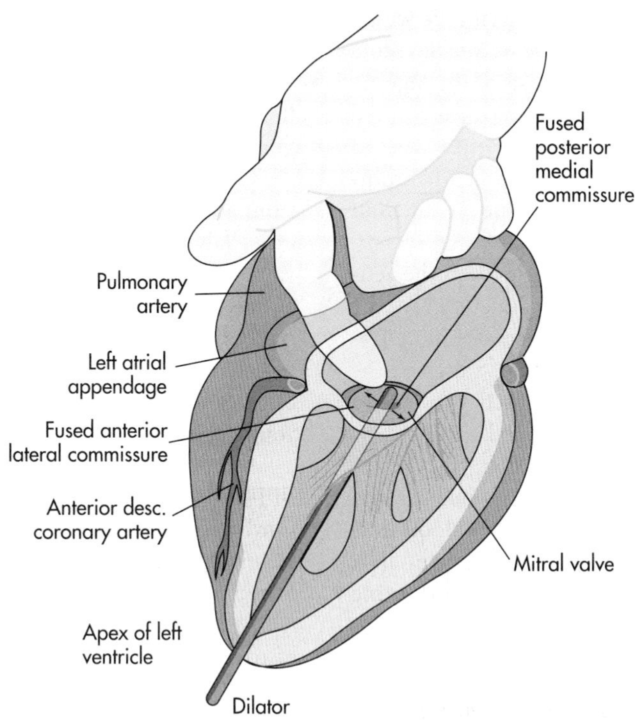

Figure 24-12 Technique of closed mitral commissurotomy using mitral dilating instrument.

TABLE 24-9 Types of Prosthetic Valves

Type	Examples	Advantages	Disadvantages
Caged ball	Starr-Edwards Smeloff Braunwald-Cutter McGovern-Cromie	Durable, low incidence of endocarditis	Large size that may create obstruction to blood flow
Caged disk	Beall Hufnagel Cross-Jones Kay-Shiley	Low incidence of thromboemboli	Disk may stick, causing severe obstruction of blood flow
Tilting disk	Bjork-Shiley Wada-Cutter St. Jude	Central blood flow, low incidence of hemolysis	Higher incidence of thrombus
Stenting allograft	Lillehei-Kaste	Central blood flow, low incidence of hemolysis, no thromboemboli	High incidence of regurgitation
Xenograft	Porcine	Silent valves, low incidence of thromboembolism or hemolysis	High incidence of calcification over time

are sized with an obturator. The loose chordae are excised to avoid their becoming tangled in the new valve, and the prosthetic valve is sutured into the new annulus. The operative mortality rate for aortic valve replacement is less than 5% but 10% for mitral valve replacement.[19] Risk factors include physiologic and chronologic age, chronicity, type of valvular lesion, and left ventricular function. Mortality rates for valvular replacement surgery increase in persons older than 70 years.

The Ross procedure is an alternative method of aortic valve replacement using the patient's own pulmonary valve, which has all the characteristics of the patient's aortic valve. This procedure is specifically indicated for young patients with a long life expectancy. Primary indications include isolated aortic valve disease, severe aortic stenosis, and severe aortic regurgitation with or without dilation of the aortic root. A routine midline sternotomy is performed and cardiopulmonary bypass is initiated. Extreme care is taken in removing the pulmonary valve to avoid damage to the left main coronary artery. A homograft valve cadaver graft is carefully inserted into the pulmonary position and the patient's pulmonary valve is inserted into the aortic root and sutured in place.

Types of Valves. The ideal replacement valve has the following characteristics: durable, hemodynamically accurate, nonhemolytic, nonthrombogenic, easily inserted, and anatomically suitable. A wide variety of prosthetic valves are available, and the advantages and disadvantages of each are listed in Table 24-9.

Caged-ball prosthetic valves consist of a metal cage with a synthetic, freely moving ball inside; the cage is attached to a sewing ring (Figure 24-13). The ring and struts of the cage are covered by a synthetic cloth. The cloth-covered ring is sutured carefully into the existing valve annulus. Within 2 to 3 months, tissue covers the cloth and the incidence of thromboembolism decreases. Caged-ball valves come in different sizes and various designs and materials.

Caged-disk prosthetic valves occupy less space in the ventricles than do other valves and require less force to move the occluding disk. However, this type of valve creates more obstruction to blood flow than do other types of valves. If the disk "sticks" in the cage, causing total obstruction of blood flow, hemodynamics are seriously compromised.

Tilting-disk prosthetic valves have occluders that tilt or pivot within a ring rather than balls or disks that pop back and forth. This type of valve produces nearly central blood flow through its orifice, which more closely approximates flow through a normal valve; however, the areas under the pivoting points are more susceptible to thrombus formation as a result of blood stasis.

Stenting allografts are human heart valves that are supported or "stented" by an underlying frame. Allografts provide relatively normal hemodynamic characteristics with central flow, no thromboemboli, and little hemolysis; however, allografts are not readily available.

Xenograft bioprosthetic valves are composed of valves from nonhuman species. They are more readily available than other valves and can be obtained in all sizes. Porcine xenograft valves are most commonly used. The hemodynamic performance is similar to that of human heart valves. Patients with this type of valve may not require anticoagulants. Porcine valves remain patent for about 10 years but then begin to experience calcification. Therefore they are not recommended for use in young people.

Implanted Devices

Cardiac surgery may involve the implantation of a variety of technologic devices designed to prevent sudden death from fatal dysrhythmias, prevent end-organ damage in individuals with severe heart failure, and offer temporary support to the heart to augment the circulatory system. Automatic im-

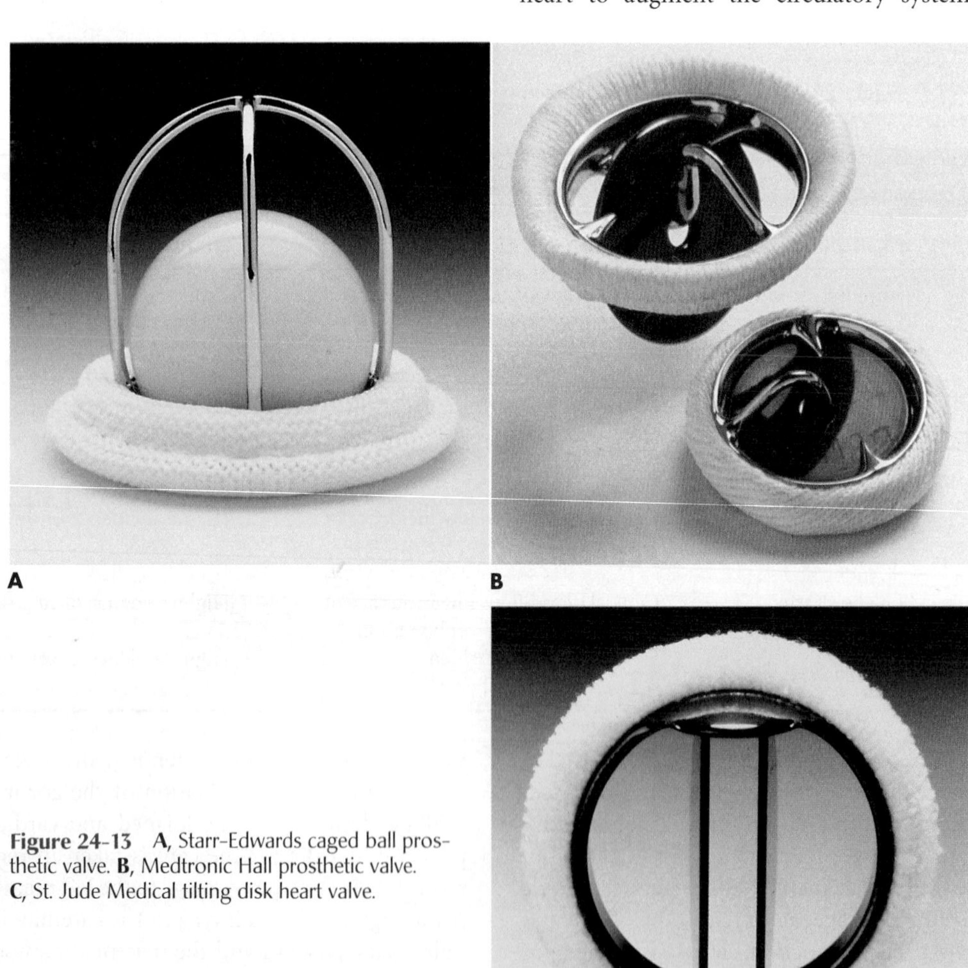

Figure 24-13 **A,** Starr-Edwards caged ball prosthetic valve. **B,** Medtronic Hall prosthetic valve. **C,** St. Jude Medical tilting disk heart valve.

plantable cardioverter-defibrillators (AICD), ventricular assist devices (VADs), and artificial heart chambers are all in use. Work also continues on the artificial heart. The AICD is discussed in Chapter 23, and cardiac transplantation is discussed in Chapter 51.

The IABP is a counterpulsation device that augments the circulation by pumping when the heart is in diastole. Indications for use of an IABP are summarized in Box 24-12. When the balloon inflates during diastole, it causes an intraaortic pressure rise known as diastolic augmentation. This heightened diastolic pressure forces blood in the aortic arch to flow in a retrograde fashion, increasing coronary artery perfusion. When the balloon deflates at the end of diastole, it reduces pressure in the aorta, and blood from the aortic arch moves into the space that was occupied by the balloon. This reduces the resistance the ventricle must overcome during systole (afterload). The left ventricle empties more effectively, leaving more space for ventricular filling, which also reduces preload.

The intraaortic balloon is inserted percutaneously or by cutdown into the right or left femoral artery and advanced into the thoracic aorta. It is sutured into place after the balloon tip has been correctly positioned just distal to the left subclavian artery. The balloon catheter is attached to a pump that inflates and deflates it with helium. The timing of the inflation-deflation sequence is extremely important in obtaining maximal counterpulsation effect. The ECG is used to trigger the balloon, which inflates just at the beginning of ventricular diastole, immediately after closure of the aortic valve. The balloon remains inflated during diastole and then deflates immediately before the next ventricular systole, just before the aortic valve reopens (Figure 24-14).

The IABP is used to provide temporary assistance to the patient's circulation until the underlying condition can be corrected. It is not indicated for persons whose underlying disease is so severe that eventual weaning from the IABP is considered impossible. Although patients have been maintained on the pump from several hours to several months, the usual time interval is 2 to 3 days.

The patient undergoing intraaortic balloon counterpulsation requires intensive nursing observation and care. Guidelines for care are summarized in the Guidelines for Safe Practice box.

BOX 24-12 Intraaortic Balloon Counterpulsation: Indications for Use

- Cardiogenic shock secondary to acute myocardial infarction
- Other low cardiac output states
- During emergency diagnostic procedures on unstable cardiac patients
- In unstable cardiac patients before and during open heart surgery
- Assistance in removing patients from cardiopulmonary bypass postoperatively
- Drug-resistant, life-threatening dysrhythmias
- Unstable angina pectoris
- Severe acute myocardial infarction

Guidelines for Safe Practice

The Patient With an Intraaortic Balloon Pump

1. Monitor vital signs and cardiac indices per protocol.
2. Titrate vasopressor and antidysrhythmic agents to keep patient values within established parameters.
3. Monitor peripheral pulses and circulation hourly until balloon is removed.
4. Position patient to keep affected leg extended, avoiding hip flexion.
   a. Keep HOB elevated to no more than 30 degrees to prevent balloon migration.
5. Tilt patient to alternate sides every 2 hours to prevent skin breakdown.
   a. Ensure that appropriate pressure-relieving devices are in place on the bed.
6. Monitor the insertion site regularly.
   a. Keep dressing clean and dry.
   b. Change dressing every 24-72 hours per protocol using sterile technique
7. Provide teaching to patient and family about the purpose and function of IABP.
   a. Provide reassurance and support as needed.
   b. Reinforce that the IABP is assisting the patient's heart, not replacing it.

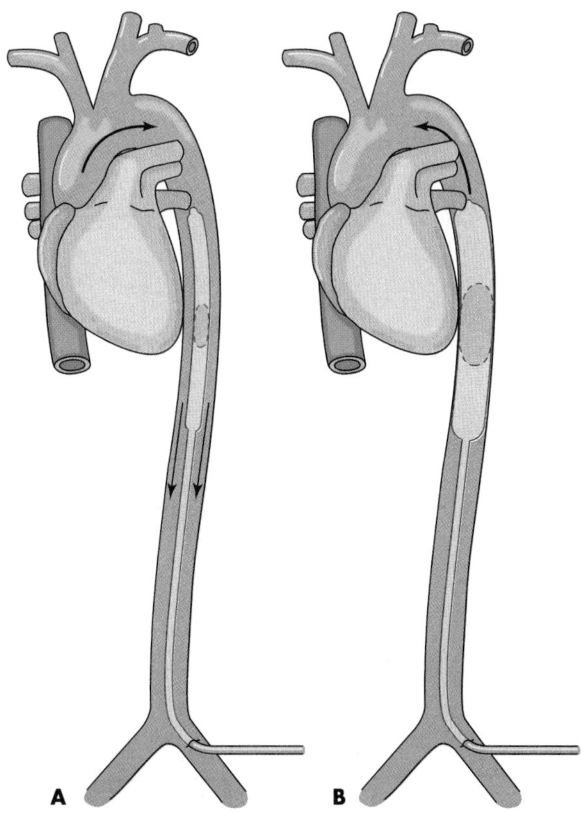

Figure 24-14 Representation of intraaortic balloon positioned just distal to left subclavian artery. **A,** Balloon is deflated, allowing forward blood flow during systole. **B,** Balloon is inflated to increase coronary perfusion during diastole.

Both left and right VADs are also available to support the failing heart. These devices provide rest for the ventricles while artificially replacing systemic pumping. They are used for patients with progressive late stage heart failure and patients who experience profound intraoperative myocardial depression with failure to wean from the cardiopulmonary bypass. Patients requiring this type of assistance are critically ill and require care in an intensive care unit.

Cardiopulmonary Bypass

Some heart surgery procedures can be performed without artificial circulation, but most require either partial or total cardiopulmonary bypass. In partial, or left heart, bypass, blood is drained from the LA and LV and passed through a pulsatile or roller pump, which returns the blood to the common femoral artery or the descending aorta. In this type of bypass, the pulmonary circulation is not interrupted.

In total cardiopulmonary bypass the heart-lung bypass machine provides artificial oxygenation and circulation of the blood during the surgical procedure. Venous blood is removed from the body through large cannulas placed in either the RA or the inferior or superior vena cavae (Figure 24-15). The blood passes through an oxygenating mechanism and is then pumped back into the arterial circulation through large cannulas placed either in the ascending aorta (most common) or the femoral artery. In addition to providing artificial oxygenation and circulation, the cardiopulmonary bypass machine also provides a way to administer medications and control body temperature during the procedure. The cardiopulmonary bypass machine is primed for use with approximately 2500 ml of crystalloid fluid, which dilutes the patient's blood and causes the hematocrit to fall. If necessary, blood can be transfused during the procedure to sustain an adequate hematocrit. Autotransfusion is commonly used. Bypass circuits used to be primed with cross-matched blood, but nonblood primer has been shown to provide several advantages, including decreased blood viscosity, limited hemolysis, and no risk of transfusion reaction or disease transmission from the primer solution.

Systemic anticoagulation with heparin is required during the surgery to prevent thrombus formation within the bypass machine. Anticoagulation also prevents the patient from developing a thrombus during periods of reduced blood flow and cardiac output. Anticoagulation is reversed with protamine sulfate at the end of cardiopulmonary bypass. The bypass machine also induces systemic hypothermia by cooling

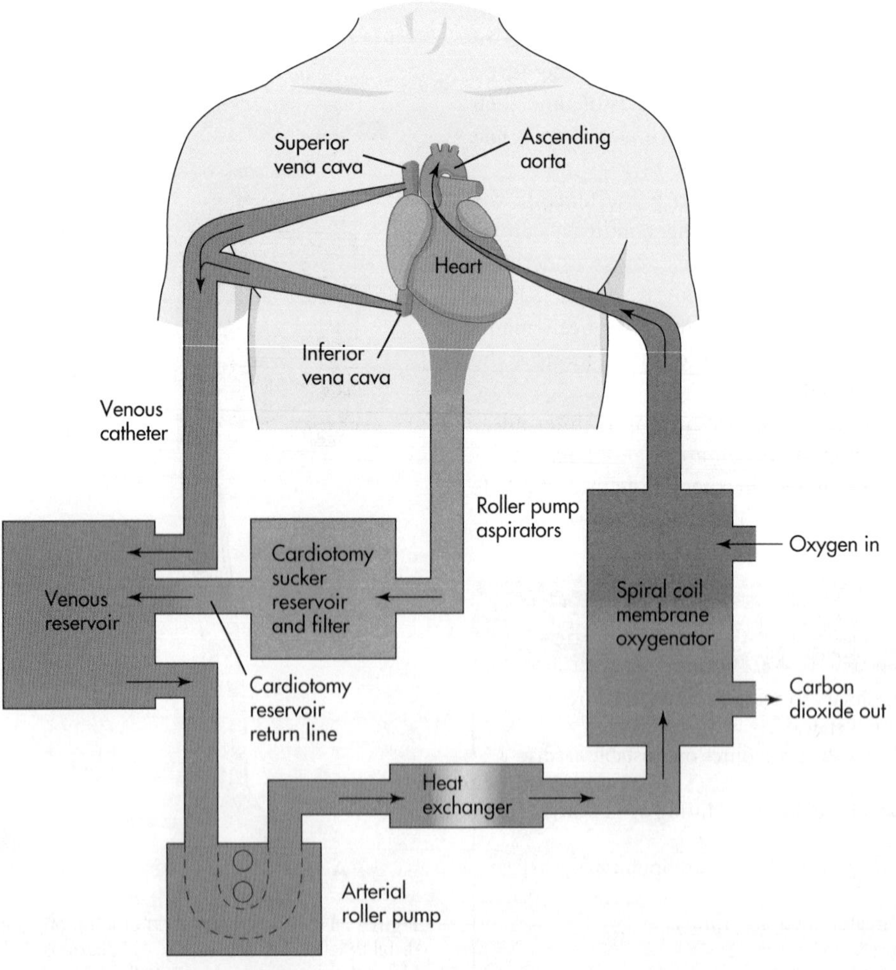

Figure 24-15 Set-up for cardiopulmonary bypass.

the perfusion solution mildly (30° to 35° C) or profoundly (15° C). Hypothermia lowers the metabolic needs and oxygen consumption of the body's vital organs and tissues, helping to preserve the tissues during the period of aortic cross-clamping and reduced cardiac output.

Cardioplegia is the intentional arrest of the heart during bypass surgery. The aorta is clamped and a cold cardioplegic solution is infused into the heart and coronary arteries, causing the heart to stop beating. This induced cardiac arrest provides the surgical team with a quiet heart on which to operate. The cardioplegic solution is chilled to reduce myocardial oxygen demand and contains an alkaline solution that helps to preserve the myocardial tissue. Advances in cold cardioplegic techniques have significantly improved the outcomes of open cardiac surgery.

Once the surgical repair is complete, the cardioplegia infusion is terminated and the blood in the bypass machine is rewarmed, slowly bringing the patient's core body temperature back to near normal. The heart is restarted, the lungs are reexpanded, and weaning from cardiopulmonary bypass begins. The autologous blood from the bypass machine is collected and returned to the patient and the systemic anticoagulation is reversed.

Cardiopulmonary bypass has allowed dramatic advancements in heart surgery, but its use is accompanied by a number of potentially devastating complications. Cardiopulmonary bypass creates a shocklike state with a low hematocrit and decreased systolic blood pressure and perfusion of the body's organs and tissues. This state can contribute to neurologic, myocardial, and renal ischemia and damage. Both platelet destruction and red blood cell hemolysis occur during bypass, predisposing the patient to postoperative coagulation complications. Thrombus formation and arterial embolism can lead to infarction of vital organs and tissues. Some patients experience difficulties in being weaned from bypass and may require circulatory assistance (e.g., IABP) to temporarily augment their circulatory system.

NURSING MANAGEMENT OF PATIENT UNDERGOING CARDIAC SURGERY

Care of the person undergoing cardiac surgery involves a multidisciplinary team approach. Clinical pathways are frequently used to guide and coordinate the patient's care. A sample Clinical Pathway for a person undergoing cardiac surgery is shown on pp. 750 to 752.

Cardiac surgery patients are generally admitted to the hospital either the day before or the morning of surgery. After surgery most patients spend 24 to 36 hours in the intensive care recovery area and are transferred to the floor on the first or second postoperative day. Rapid recovery allows for discharge on the fourth through sixth postoperative day.

PREOPERATIVE CARE

Much of the preoperative care provided to patients undergoing cardiac surgery occurs before their admission to the hospital. Important goals for the preoperative period include obtaining an accurate and complete patient history, ensuring that preoperative teaching has been provided to the patient and family, reinforcing that teaching as needed, and preparing the patient for surgery.

Before admission the patient undergoes extensive testing to establish the medical diagnosis and evaluate the severity of the disease process. Information is obtained from the chest x-ray, cardiac catheterization and coronary angiography, echocardiography, stress testing, and serum blood analyses. Particular attention is given to assessing the degree of cardiac impairment and its impact on the patient's ADLs and preferred lifestyle, as well as identifying factors that may impede the recovery process.

Significant risk factors include a history of myocardial infarction, bacterial endocarditis, pulmonary embolism, or coagulation abnormalities. Cigarette smoking, diabetes mellitus, and obesity also increase the risk of complications. Information about the patient's support systems, coping patterns, and level of understanding help the nurse anticipate the patient and family's needs related to preoperative teaching, postoperative recovery, and care after discharge.

Preoperative teaching for cardiac surgery patients has been well researched and standardized. The Patient Teaching box on p. 753 summarizes the elements covered in preoperative teaching. Ideally patients and their families receive printed, taped, or video information about the surgery well before admission. The nurse provides additional information as needed and reinforces the patient and family's understanding of the planned procedure. Patients are aware that they are facing a potentially life-threatening situation. The nurse plays a vital role in addressing specific questions, fears, and concerns that the patient and family may express.

A baseline database is completed before surgery. Baseline vital signs (including apical and radial heart rates and bilateral arm blood pressures), integrity of all pulses (both proximal and distal), neurologic status, height, weight, nutritional status, elimination patterns, and psychologic status are assessed and recorded. Patients continue with their normal medical and activity routines before surgery, with the exception of withholding aspirin for 1 to 3 days before the day of surgery. Patients receive nothing by mouth after midnight the night before surgery.

POSTOPERATIVE CARE

Postoperative care initially focuses on stabilizing the patient and preventing complications. Initial care takes place in an intensive care setting. The Guidelines for Safe Practice box on p. 754 summarizes the major aspects of postoperative care after cardiac surgery.

Promoting Cardiac Output and Perfusion

Patient care in the immediate postoperative period focuses on promoting cardiac function, tissue perfusion, and stabilization of vital signs. Heart rate and arterial pressures are monitored continuously and recorded every 15 minutes until stable, and then hourly thereafter. Central venous pressure, pulmonary artery pressure, pulmonary capillary wedge

clinical pathway *Coronary Artery Bypass Graft*

PREOP VISIT	DAY OF SURGERY	POSTOPERATIVE DAY #1	POSTOPERATIVE DAY #2	POSTOPERATIVE DAY #3	POSTOPERATIVE DAY #4 THROUGH DISCHARGE
Interdisciplinary communication (Consults)	Anesthesia		Respiratory care smoking cessation consult (prn)		
Cardiology	→	→	→	→	→
Chaplain prn	Respiratory care →	Respiratory care prn	→	→	→
		PT consult prn	→	→	→
		Nutrition consult prn	→	→	→
		Pharmacy consult prn	→	→	→
Assessments					
Adult screening tool (Multidisc.)	• Pt systems assessment q1° →	q 2°-4° in TCVPO			
Ht/Wt (Nsg)		Systems assessment q 4-8° →	→	→	→
H&P (MD)					
Emotional needs (Nsg)	• ICU VS Policy →	4 W VS Policy →	→	→	→
Financial needs (SW)	• Wt post-op then q AM	→	→	→	→
Discharge needs (Nsg, SW)	• Cardiac monitoring	→	→	D/C Cardiac monitoring Assess need for home O_2	
Diagnostics (LAB, RADIOL)					
Cardiac Cath EKG CXR Wt	• EKG • CXR • Cardiac indices q 1°-2° and change in status or med adjustment	EKG CXR after CT removal		CXR PA + LAT	EKG
Labs: CBC, u/a, Chem 10, pt/ptt T/X 4u PRBC (8 U if Redo) ABG if Pulmonary Hx	• ACT at bedside • CBC, plats, pt/ptt, chem 6, mg,$^{++}$ • Glucose q2°-4° • ABGs on admission and prn • CBC after PRBC, pt/ptt after FFP	Chem 10, CBC with plts q AM until disch.	→	→	→

Medications D/C as a 48° preop D/C Coumadin 3 days pre-op Pre-op cardiac antibiotic orders Continue preop meds	• Ancef o.c. to OR → administ. within 1° of incision, then q 8° • IV H_2 blockers → • ASA supp. within 6° postoperative → • Administer/titrate → vasoactive/inotropic infusion per order set • Fluid resuscitation per order • Replace K+/Ca^{++}/Mg^{++} per orders • Treat glucose per orders • IV opiates for pain →	D/C IV abx after 3 doses D/C H_2 blockers when extubated unless pre-op indication ASA q AM D/C vasoactive/inotropic infusions • Restart pre-op meds except antianginals PO pain meds	Initiate bowel regimen → → →	→ → →	→ → →
Dressings tubes/drains	• Pulmonary artery → • A-line → • NGT → • Epicardial wires → • Chest tubes → • Foley → • IV/CVP → • ETT → D/C when awake and stable	D/C D/C D/C 2° after extubation D/C ½ hr before MCT removed D/C (*see activity) → → Incision care: →	D/C Foley D/C IV when taking po Incision care BID →	• Remove CT dressing 48° after CTs D/C'd → →	→ →
Interventions/Treatments Antibacterial scrub PM before surgery and AM of surgery Incentive spirometer Cardiac skin prep/clip guidelines	• Mechanical ventilation and weaning • O_2 therapy • Continuous pulse oximetry • Heat lamps • Extubation	• Initiate O_2 via cannula • Incentive spirometry q2° • Deep breath/cough q2° • Knee-high teds • Support bra for women	• Wean O_2 per policy → → Deep breath/cough q4° →	D/C O_2 per policy → → → →	→ → → →

*This form is a documentation and decision support tool only.

H&P, History and physical examination; *TCVPO,* thoracic cardiovascular postoperative unit; *o.c.,* on call; *abx,* antibiotics; *MCT,* mediastinal chest tube.

Continued

clinical pathway *Coronary Artery Bypass Graft—cont'd*

PREOP VISIT	DAY OF SURGERY	POSTOPERATIVE DAY #1	POSTOPERATIVE DAY #2	POSTOPERATIVE DAY #3	POSTOPERATIVE DAY #4 THROUGH DISCHARGE
Activity Up ad lib	OR ——→ TCVPO Bedrest; HOB 30° IF VS within parameters and stable rhythm	TCVPO ——→ 4W acute Raise HOB for comfort • *Prior to MCT removal; turn patient side to side; or sit patient on side of bed • OOB to chair with assistance	• Ambulate in room and hall with assistance • Physical therapy exercises ——→	• Ambulate in room without assistance ——→	——→ ——→
Nutrition NPO after MN	NPO except ice	• Advance diet as tolerated to ice chips ——→ Clear liquids ——→ Traditional diet	• Advance from transitional diet ——→ ♥ Healthy or ♥ Healthy, limited sucrose, if diabetic • Patient should have BM by discharge	——→	——→
Discharge preparation Identify discharge need via adult screening tool (multi-D)		• Review D/C plans with patient/S.O. Initiate appropriate support services per D/C planning: • D/C Coordinator • Social work • Dietitian • Nursing • Respiratory care • Physical therapy • Pharmacy • M.D.	• Reinforce need for patient/S.O./family to learn self-care measures ——→ Evaluate patient for cardiac rehabilitation	——→ ——→	——→ ——→
Educational activities Initiate: • Pre-op teaching • Incentive spirometry • Effective coughing techniques • Introduce teaching folder • Patient pathway		Initiate discharge patient education plan	Patient/S.O. observe incision care Teach cardiac exercises ——→	Patient/S.O. perform incision care Patient/S.O. describe home management	

Patient Teaching

Preoperative Teaching for the Patient Undergoing Cardiac Surgery

1. General information
   a. Places of care during hospitalization
      (1) CCU or ICU after surgery
      (2) Return to general patient care unit in 2 to 3 days
   b. Visiting hours and location of waiting rooms
2. Description of surgery
   a. Simple explanation of anatomy of heart and effect of the patient's cardiovascular disorder (e.g., incompetent valve, obstructed coronary artery)
   b. Explanation of surgical procedure, including planned incision
   c. Definition of any unfamiliar terms: bypass, extracorporeal
   d. Length of time in surgery: 2 to 4 hours
   e. Length of time until able to see family (usually 1½ to 2 hours after surgery)
3. Preparation for surgery
   a. Shower or bath night before surgery with special antimicrobial soap
   b. Surgical shave: shaving of entire chest and abdomen, neck to groin and left midaxillary line to right
   c. Legs shaved if saphenous vein grafts will be used
   d. Preoperative medication
4. Explanation of monitors
   a. Round patches on chest connected to a cardiac monitor that records patient's heartbeats
   b. Monitor makes beeping sound all the time
5. Explanation of lines
   a. Intravenous routes for fluid and medications
   b. Central venous line in neck or chest to monitor fluid status
   c. Pulmonary artery catheter in chest or neck to measure pulmonary pressures and monitor fluid status
   d. Plastic connector line to obtain blood samples without a needle stick
6. Explanation of drainage tubes
   a. Indwelling urinary catheter
   b. Chest tube: bloody drainage is expected
7. Explanation of breathing tube
   a. Tube in windpipe connected to machine called ventilator
   b. Unable to speak with tube in place but can mouth words and communicate in writing
   c. Tube is removed when patient is fully awake and stable
   d. Secretions in lungs or tube removed by nurse using a suction catheter
   e. Food and oral fluids not permitted until breathing tube is removed
8. Explanation and demonstration of activities and exercises
   a. Purpose of activity is to promote circulation, keep lungs clear, and prevent infection
   b. Activity includes:
      (1) Turning from side to side in bed
      (2) Sitting on edge of bed
      (3) Sitting in chair the night of or the morning after surgery
   c. Range-of-motion exercises
   d. Deep breathing using sustained maximal inspiration
   e. Tubes and lines will restrict movement somewhat, but nurse will assist patient
9. Relief of pain
   a. Some pain will be experienced, but it will not be excruciating (different pain than original angina if this was present)
   b. Frequent pain medication will be given to help relieve the pain, but patient should always tell nurse when pain is present

pressure, and cardiac output measurements are obtained as indicated by the patient's condition. Peripheral pulses are monitored for bilateral strength and symmetry. Apical and radial pulses are compared for evidence of a pulse deficit. Skin color, temperature, and capillary refill are assessed for evidence of adequate tissue perfusion. Urine output, a reliable indicator of cardiac output, is assessed hourly. Chest tube drainage is assessed and recorded hourly to monitor for postsurgical bleeding.

Heart Rate and Rhythm

The patient's ECG is monitored continuously and compared with the preoperative baseline. Cardiac dysrhythmias are common and may be caused by operative trauma, anesthesia, extracorporeal circulation, alterations in potassium values, hypotension, hypovolemia, and hypoxia. See Chapter 23 for a discussion of the pharmacologic management of dysrhythmias.

Temporary epicardial pacing may be used to manage cardiac dysrhythmias and low cardiac output. Supraventricular tachycardia commonly occurs after cardiac surgery because of edema or inflammation of the atrial tissue. Atrial flutter, atrial fibrillation, or other supraventricular tachycardias produce decreased left ventricular diastolic filling and a subsequent deterioration in cardiac output. Atrial pacing can effectively restore a normal sinus rhythm. Bradydysrhythmias after cardiac surgery are transient and may be associated with low cardiac output. Temporary pacing may be required to increase the heart rate and augment cardiac output. Temporary pacing wires are a potential source of lethal ventricular dysrhythmias if they come in contact with a ground current. The electrodes must be insulated with either a rubber cap or glove when not in use.

Blood Pressure

Maintenance of a stable blood pressure is critical to the patient's recovery, and pharmacologic agents are used aggressively to keep the patient's blood pressure within the desired range. Postoperative hypertension can lead to excessive postsurgical bleeding, cardiac tamponade, and excessive oxygen demand in the weakened myocardium. IV nitroglycerin or sodium nitroprusside infusions may be administered to reduce hypertension, reduce SVR, and ease the myocardial workload and oxygen demand. Postoperative hypertension

Guidelines for Safe Practice

The Patient Who Has Undergone Cardiac Surgery

I. Monitoring
  A Cardiovascular
    1. Blood pressure and pulse (rate, pulse deficit)
    2. Pulmonary artery pressure (PAP), pulmonary capillary wedge pressure (PCWP), cardiac output (CO), central venous pressure (CVP), left atrial pressure (LAP)
    3. ECG of signs of dysrhythmias
    4. Body temperature
    5. Skin color, temperature, capillary filling
    6. Signs of hypovolemic shock (decreased CVP, decreased LAP, decreased PCWP, decreased cardiac output)
    7. Signs of cardiac tamponade (cessation of chest drainage, restlessness, decreased blood pressure, increased CVP, increased PAP, increased LAP)
  B. Respiratory
    1. Respirations: rate, depth, quality
    2. Breath sounds
    3. Chest tubes for patency and drainage
    4. Autotransfuse chest tube drainage
  C. Neurologic
    1. Level of consciousness
    2. Pupillary size and reaction
    3. Orientation
    4. Movement and sensation of extremities
  D. Gastrointestinal
    1. Nausea
    2. Anorexia
  E. Urinary
    1. Output (amount)
    2. Color
    3. pH and specific gravity
  F. Fluid and electrolyte balance
    1. Intake/output balance
    2. Daily weights
    3. Serum potassium and calcium levels
  G. Presence of discomfort: pain, fatigue
  H. Ability to sleep
  I. Behavior: depression, fear, disorientation, hallucinations

II. Promoting oxygen/carbon dioxide exchange
  A. Preoxygenation and suction during intubation; suction as necessary after extubation
  B. Position with head only slightly elevated; turn side to side
  C. Encourage breathing exercise; incentive spirometry
  D. Give analgesics before breathing and coughing exercises
  E. Encourage range-of-motion exercises and progressive activity

III. Promoting fluid and electrolyte balance
  A. Record accurate intake and output
  B. Maintain prescribed flow rates of parenteral fluids
  C. Give prescribed supplemental IV potassium chloride

IV. Promoting comfort
  A. Give opioid analgesics every 3 hours during the first 24 hours, then as needed
  B. Give frequent mouth care
  C. Control environment for comfort
  D. Change bed linens when diaphoresis is present (assure patient that this is common)
  E. Plan activities to permit periods of sleep
  F. Provide back rubs for backache
  G. Splint incision during coughing
  H. Encourage patient to share feelings and experiences
  I. Support family visiting

V. Promoting activity
  A. Provide for passive then active range-of-motion exercises
  B. Encourage ambulation when permitted

VI. Teaching
  A. Progressive return to physical activity as recommended by the physician
  B. Rehabilitation exercise program
  C. Sexual activity usually permitted in 3 to 4 weeks
  D. Signs of overexertion include fatigue, dyspnea, pain
  E. Eat a balanced diet with any prescribed modifications (such as no added salt or low cholesterol)
  F. Medications
    1. Name, dosage, schedule, action, and side effects of prescribed medications
    2. Use of prescribed medications as needed
  G. Signs that may persist: dyspnea, pain, night sweats
  H. Signs requiring medical attention (fever, increasing dyspnea, or chest pain with minimal exertion)
  I. Need for ongoing medical care

can also result from the patient awakening from anesthesia and experiencing anxiety and acute pain. Appropriate pain management and patient reassurance assist in the management of postoperative hypertension.

An unstable low blood pressure must also be aggressively treated. Causes include hypovolemia and shock. Hypovolemia may be caused by third space fluid shifts that occur during cardiopulmonary bypass, or excessive blood loss. Cardiogenic shock can result from myocardial depression secondary to anesthesia, trauma from surgery, preexisting heart disease, dysrhythmias associated with an inadequate stroke volume, or cardiac tamponade. Treatment of postoperative hypotension includes fluid resuscitation and gentle rewarming of the patient's core body temperature. IV infusion of inotropic agents such as dobutamine help stimulate myocardial performance. Dysrhythmias are aggressively managed with antidysrhythmic agents or temporary cardiac pacing. Refer to Chapter 14 for further discussion of hypovolemic and cardiogenic shock management.

Persistent cardiogenic shock that is unresponsive to these measures may be treated with the use of a temporary mechanical assist device. Intraaortic balloon counterpulsation can be used at any point during the preoperative, perioperative, or postoperative period. The use of a VAD may also provide circulatory assistance if the myocardial performance is insufficient to meet the body's needs.

Maintaining Blood Volume and Chest Drainage

During cardiac surgery mediastinal chest tubes and possibly pleural chest tubes are placed to drain the surgical area. Refer

Clinical Manifestations

Cardiac Tamponade

Diminished or absent point of maximal impulse
Diminished heart sounds
Tachycardia
Paradoxic pulse
Narrowed pulse pressure
Distended neck veins (increased central venous pressure)

to Chapter 21 for further information about care of the patient with a chest tube. Excessive postsurgical bleeding is evidenced by increased drainage of blood from the mediastinal or pleural chest tube. Chest tube drainage should not exceed 100 ml/hr during the first 2 postoperative hours and should be approximately 500 ml during the first 24 hours. A sudden increase or cessation in drainage from the chest tubes may signify a postoperative bleeding problem, and the surgeon is notified immediately. Excessive blood loss through the chest tubes can lead to hypovolemic shock unless the patient's blood volume is maintained. Fluid resuscitation with IV crystalloid fluids or blood products is essential to correct the patient's hypovolemic state. Ideally the chest drainage system allows for the collection of bloody chest drainage for later autotransfusion in the event of a bleeding complication. In this way, the risks of transfusion reaction and disease transmission are avoided. Postoperative bleeding may require correction of clotting abnormalities or surgical reexploration of the chest.

A sudden decrease or cessation of drainage from the chest tubes can indicate clotting of the chest tubes. Clotting predisposes the patient to cardiac tamponade, as the drainage builds up around the heart. The Clinical Manifestations box lists the symptoms of cardiac tamponade. Cardiac tamponade is corrected through emergent reexploration of the mediastinum by the surgeon.

Normalizing Body Temperature

Although patients are rewarmed before cardiopulmonary bypass is terminated, body temperature frequently remains unstable, leading to postoperative hypothermia. Persistent hypothermia causes shivering, increases myocardial workload, and increases carbon dioxide and lactic acid production. Measures to gently rewarm the patient include the use of heat lamps, thermal blankets, perfusion blankets, and vasodilation with IV sodium nitroprusside. Once the patient's body temperature has rewarmed, cool or diaphoretic skin can be an indication of shock.

Promoting a Patent Airway and Effective Gas Exchange

Intubation and mechanical ventilation are maintained until the patient is stable and fully recovered from anesthesia. The rate, depth, and quality of respirations are monitored and recorded; and the patient's breath sounds are assessed. The effectiveness of coughing efforts and sputum production are monitored. Arterial blood gas and oxygen saturation monitoring provide evidence of effective gas exchange. A postoperative chest x-ray verifies proper lung reexpansion and chest tube placement after the surgical procedure. In general, patients are awake and extubated within 4 to 18 hours after cardiac surgery.

The lack of alveolar expansion and ventilation during cardiopulmonary bypass leads to decreased surfactant production and alveolar collapse in the postoperative period. Therefore the nurse promotes aggressive pulmonary hygiene every 1 to 2 hours while the patient is awake. Administration of adequate pain medication helps the patient cough, deep breathe, and use an incentive spirometer more effectively. Splinting the surgical incision with a small pillow or blanket provides extra support during coughing. Patients unable to clear excessive pulmonary secretions may require nasotracheal suctioning. Frequent position changes while in bed and early ambulation are also critical interventions to prevent pulmonary complications after cardiac surgery.

Preventing Infection

Cardiac surgery patients receive prophylactic antibiotic therapy to prevent infection during the perioperative period. A broad-spectrum antibiotic is administered intravenously for 2 to 4 days. Although any initial postoperative fever is likely to be pulmonary in origin, the nurse assesses the patient's skin and all incisions for evidence of infection. Incision care is provided based on the hospital's protocol.

Monitoring Neurologic Status

Patients usually awaken within 1 to 2 hours after surgery. Failure to awaken may be the result of unusually deep anesthesia or embolization of air, calcium, fat, or thrombotic particles to the brain. A sluggish return of consciousness may be caused by poor cerebral perfusion or microembolization during cardiopulmonary bypass.

Pupil size, equality, and reaction to light are checked frequently in the immediate postoperative period. Pupil dilation may be caused by excessive carbon dioxide in the blood or by cardiac medications such as atropine. Constricted pupils may be caused by opioids or dopamine. Disorientation and restlessness may be signs of hypoxia or embolization in addition to being symptoms of pain, fatigue, fear, or sensory overload.

Monitoring Fluid Balance

Accurate recording of intake and output is essential for the first few postoperative days. Careful observation of hourly urinary output, as well as urine color, pH, and specific gravity, provides essential information about renal function. Urine output should be at least 30 ml/hr. Red blood cells may be present initially as a result of cardiopulmonary bypass. Fluids are limited at first to reduce the chance of fluid overload and increased cardiac workload. Daily weights are obtained, and diuretics are administered if fluid retention occurs.

Renal insufficiency after heart surgery is caused by complications of cardiopulmonary bypass. The destruction of red blood cells can cause obstruction in the kidneys. If low-perfusion states occurred during the surgical procedure, the kidneys themselves may have been damaged, resulting in acute tubular necrosis. If acute renal failure is severe and prolonged, temporary hemodialysis is initiated. Up to 25% of cardiac surgery patients may experience some form of renal failure after bypass.

Serum electrolyte levels are checked several times during the first 24 hours and at least daily thereafter. Supplemental potassium may be needed in the immediate postoperative period, particularly if diuretics are in use. The serum glucose may be initially elevated from the stress of surgery and cardiopulmonary bypass, but this is temporary and usually does not require intervention.

Hemoglobin and hematocrit values and prothrombin times are obtained daily to assess the extent of blood loss and the effect of replacement therapy. Plasma and plasma expanders are given to avoid hypovolemia and to maintain a normal osmotic gradient in the blood. Crystalloid solutions are administered to ensure adequate circulating volume.

Promoting Comfort, Rest, and Sleep

Pain management is critical in the postoperative period, and patients are kept as comfortable as possible. In addition to patient comfort, pain management reduces stress on the heart, decreases the need for oxygen, and promotes healing. Other comfort measures are routinely used, such as positioning, controlling environmental temperature, frequent oral hygiene, and visiting from concerned family or friends.

Supporting Nutrition

Gastrointestinal symptoms, such as anorexia and nausea, may occur after cardiac surgery. Contributing factors include preexisting gastrointestinal disease, drug therapy, perioperative hypoperfusion or hypotension, systemic hypothermia, stress, and anxiety. Although anorexia occurs more commonly than nausea, the latter is more distressing. Comfort measures to decrease nausea are instituted, and antiemetics are administered if needed. Small amounts of food may be more palatable than a large meal.

Promoting Activity

After cardiac surgery the patient is weak and tires easily. Activity periods are organized so that rest periods are frequent (even if brief) and uninterrupted.

Passive arm exercises are started shortly after surgery, followed by active exercises as the patient gains strength. The nature and extent of activity depend on the patient's individual situation, but most patients are assisted out of bed the first day after surgery.

Activity progresses steadily from dangling at the bedside to sitting in a chair. Ambulation begins in the room and if tolerated progresses to walking in the halls. Close supervision is necessary during ambulation; and activity that causes excessive fatigue, dyspnea, or an increased pulse or respiratory rate is discontinued. If any of these symptoms appear, the patient is returned to bed, and the physician is consulted before further activity is attempted. Many patients experience a prompt and satisfying improvement in their activity tolerance after corrective cardiac surgery.

Monitoring Anticoagulation

Patients with mechanical or bioprosthetic valves are at high risk for developing systemic emboli. Anticoagulation is necessary to prevent thrombus formation on the surface of the valves. Warfarin (Coumadin) is the most commonly used anticoagulant and its use is continued long term. The maintenance dose of warfarin is based on the prothrombin time (PT); a therapeutic PT is 1.2 to 1.5 times the control value. Use of the INR (international normalized ratio) allows for greater standardization in anticoagulant monitoring. Bleeding is a major risk of long-term anticoagulation with warfarin. See Chapter 25 for a discussion of the patient teaching associated with anticoagulant use.

Promoting Psychologic Adaptation

The psychologic ramifications of heart surgery, sleep deprivation, and sensory overload can be overwhelming. Some patients experience a period of depression or disorientation after surgery, and others may become unreasonably fearful or hallucinate. The disorientation can even progress to panic. The nurse is alert to subtle behavioral changes and reassures the patient and family that these reactions are common and do not mean that the patient is "losing his or her mind." Physiologic causes of the behavior must be ruled out.

It is helpful to the patient and family if the nursing staff members attempt to personalize the patient's experience as much as possible. It is easy to lose sight of the person behind the monitoring equipment in an intensive care unit. Calling the patient by his or her preferred name, using frequent physical contact, orienting the patient to time and place, and including the patient in any discussions that are held at the bedside help to decrease the sense of isolation.

Patient/Family Education

In preparation for discharge the patient is asked to describe normal daily activities. The activities are discussed with the physician to determine their safety and appropriateness. The person is allowed to do anything that does not cause fatigue or pain but must be advised against attempting too much too soon. Patients are advised to start activities slowly and progress gradually to more energy-consuming tasks. Sexual intercourse usually is permitted within 3 to 4 weeks after surgery. The physician will want the patient to return for frequent medical follow-up care, at which time advice will be given regarding additional activities. Definite instructions are provided about climbing stairs. Only two or three steps should be attempted the first time, and the patient is instructed to climb slowly. The patient should rest two or three times while climbing one flight of stairs.

The family is also instructed about the patient's activity guidelines. Because the patient may have been an invalid before surgery, the family may be fearful about any increase in activity.

The patient and family need to be cautioned that no major improvement may be noticed immediately after the operation. It can take at least 3 to 6 months before the full result of the surgery can be evaluated. Many patients are able to return to work, but the physician needs to provide them with specific directions regarding timing and intensity. Patients are informed that some dyspnea and pain may still be present after discharge. Discharge instructions for cardiac surgery patients and a list of symptoms to report are presented in the Patient Teaching box.

GERONTOLOGIC CONSIDERATIONS

As the population ages, the number of very old patients (between 80 and 100 years old) undergoing cardiac surgery continues to increase. Advanced age alone is not a contraindication to cardiac surgery, but consideration of the special needs of the older patient is essential to postoperative recovery after cardiac surgery.

Cardiovascular age-related changes include decreased cardiac output, decreased vasomotor responsiveness, decreased cardiac conduction tissue, and increased aortic calcification. These changes can predispose the very old patient to a decreased tolerance of sudden fluctuations in fluid volume status, orthostasis, dysrhythmias, and arterial embolism. Age-related changes in renal and hepatic function can alter the pharmacokinetics of drugs; endocrine and immune system dysfunction can contribute to impaired skin integrity and wound healing. Changes in mobility, functional status, and neuropsychologic status can impair postoperative progress and slow recovery. In addition, very old patients often have significant coexisting medical problems that can complicate recovery from surgery.

SPECIAL ENVIRONMENTS FOR CARE

Critical Care

All patients undergoing cardiac surgery are cared for at least temporarily in an intensive care unit to ensure in-depth physiologic monitoring. The care provided in this setting has been discussed in the nursing management section. The ICU stay may be brief and measured in hours until the patient is successfully stabilized and extubated. Patients requiring IABPs or VADs may be extremely unstable and require more long-term management. This is especially true of patients in severe heart failure who are waiting for a donor heart.

Community-Based Care

Hospital stays after cardiac surgery have been dramatically reduced, and it is expected that a significant part of the patient's recovery from surgery will take place in the home environment. Careful adherence to clinical pathway elements guides the nurse in evaluating the patient's resources, self-care abilities, and family supports and permits timely referral for home health supervision and monitoring. The nurse ensures that the patient and family are knowledgeable and capable of providing care (see Patient Teaching box). Discharge planning is particularly important for older patients, who can expect a longer convalescence and may have limited social supports available to them in the community.

Patient Teaching
Discharge Instructions After Cardiac Surgery

INCISION CARE
Clean twice a day
Care of sterile strips, staples, sutures
Incision massage with cocoa butter after 10 days

SHOWERING
Wash with soap that is unscented, gentle, bactericidal
No tub baths until incisions completely healed

ACTIVITY
No lifting greater than 10 pounds
No driving for 6 weeks
No prolonged sitting
Activity as tolerated, cardiac rehabilitation if ordered
May resume sexual activity when comfort level allows

NUTRITION
Low-sodium, low-fat, heart-healthy diet
Increase protein intake for 4 to 6 weeks

MEDICATIONS
Pain medications: do not drive or operate machinery if taking narcotics

SYMPTOMS TO REPORT
Incision is red (like a sunburn)
Area around incision feels warm
Incision is swollen
Incision has increased or different drainage (pus)
Fever above 100.5° F
Unusual pain
Return of presurgical symptoms (if angina occurs, rest and take nitroglycerin); seek medical attention for angina unrelieved by three nitroglycerin or for frequent occurrence of angina
Shortness of breath
Palpitations (skipping of heart beat)
Heart beating too fast or too slow
Severe bruising or bleeding
Worsening fatigue
Flu symptoms (aches, chills, fever, loss of appetite)

MISCELLANEOUS
Women should wear a bra to help support chest
TED stockings
Daily weights—notify physician for gain of 6 pounds in 2 days
Incentive spirometer three times a day
Prevent constipation with fiber, fluids, and stool softeners

COMPLICATIONS

Many factors can complicate the patient's recovery after cardiac surgery. Pulmonary complications are most common and include atelectasis, pleural effusion, and pneumonia. Cardiovascular complications include hemodynamic instability and dysrhythmias. Neurologic changes, fluid imbalance, fever, immobility, and sleep disturbances are all common complications that can impede recovery from cardiac surgery. Late complications from cardiac surgery include mediastinitis and the postpericardiotomy syndrome.

Mediastinitis. Mediastinitis can occur after cardiac surgery from separation of the sternal wound and infection. It involves the anterior mediastinal space. The incidence of mediastinitis is 0.5% to 5% of cardiac surgery patients and occurs from 4 to 30 days after the surgery. Signs and symptoms include pain, erythema, and tenderness of the incisional area; serous or purulent wound drainage; grating of the sternum with coughing; fever; elevated white blood cell count; and positive wound vultures. The most common infecting organisms are normal skin flora such as *S. epidermidis, S. aureus, Candida albicans, Pseudomonas, Klebsiella, Enterobacter,* and *Aspergillus.* Risk factors for the development of mediastinitis include nutritional deficiency, diabetes, obesity, smoking, and the use of the internal mammary artery for CABG. Stress to the sternal wound may also predispose the patient to mediastinitis. Such stressors include vomiting, coughing, external cardiac massage, and lifting heavy objects.

Treatment of mediastinitis depends on the depth of the infection and ranges from parenteral antibiotic therapy to surgical debridement of the sternum, mediastinal irrigation, and subsequent sternal dressing changes. Severe cases of mediastinitis may require muscle or omental flaps to revascularize and support the affected area. Mediastinitis is prevented through hand washing, meticulous aseptic technique, and antibiotic prophylaxis during the perioperative period. Prevention is clearly the most effective intervention.

Postpericardiotomy Syndrome. Postpericardiotomy syndrome is a form of a postcardiac injury syndrome that affects between 10% and 40% of patients undergoing cardiac surgery. Symptoms may appear 1 week to several months after surgery and include fever, malaise, and pleuropericardial pain. An important physical finding is the presence of a pericardial friction rub on auscultation. Diagnostic studies may reveal nonspecific ST-T wave changes on ECG, bilateral pleural effusions on chest x-ray, and pericardial effusion on echocardiogram. Laboratory values include an increased eosinophil count, increased white blood cell count, and possible anemia.

Although the cause of postpericardiotomy syndrome is not completely clear, the most accepted explanation is that it is an immune-mediated reaction. An autoimmune reaction to cardiac injury during surgery leads to the production of anticardiac antibodies. This autoimmune reaction leads to the inflammatory changes seen in the typical patient. Treatment is directed toward reducing the symptoms of fever and pain and consists of administering aspirin, NSAIDs, or corticosteroids. Postpericardiotomy syndrome generally resolves spontaneously within several days to several weeks.

Critical Thinking Questions

1. A 59-year-old woman was discharged 2 weeks ago with the diagnosis of heart failure after her second myocardial infarction in 18 months. She now comes to the emergency department with acute shortness of breath, chest pain, a positive S3, and significant bilateral rales. Her ECG shows new onset atrial fibrillation at 150 and evidence of her prior anterolateral myocardial infarction. Her serum electrolytes are normal, except for a potassium level of 3.2. Her hemoglobin (Hgb) and hematocrit (Hct) are 7.3 g/dl and 25%, respectively. Her discharge levels were Hgb 11.2 g/dl and Hct 30.3% Discuss the likely precipitating events for her heart failure exacerbation including the pathophysiology.
2. A 49-year-old man was diagnosed with an asymptomatic heart murmur at age 45. While shopping one day with his wife, he suffered an acute cardiac arrest. Bystanders immediately provided basic cardiopulmonary resuscitation. Emergency personnel arrived quickly and provided advanced cardiac life support. He was successfully resuscitated and transported to a nearby hospital. Diagnostic studies revealed aortic stenosis with associated left ventricular hypertrophy.
   - What precipitating physiologic event caused this patient's sudden cardiac arrest?
   - Discuss the relationship between aortic stenosis, left ventricular hypertrophy, and coronary blood flow.
   - Identify the symptoms, physical findings, and diagnostic findings you would most likely expect him to exhibit.
3. The patient's physician recommends that he undergo aortic valve surgery to correct his aortic stenosis. The patient is talking with you, his nurse, about his fears and whether he should proceed with the open heart surgery. What information will you base your response on?
4. A 27-year-old woman has been diagnosed with symptomatic mitral valve prolapse. She now needs education about her condition. Using lay terminology, provide her with:
   - A description of mitral valve prolapse and the associated changes in heart function.
   - The relationship between mitral valve prolapse and the symptoms she has experienced or may experience in the future.
   - Home monitoring actions she will need to take when symptoms occur.
   - Aspects of lifestyle management that can lessen the symptoms of her condition.
   - Symptoms that require immediate notification of her physician
5. A 72-year-old man has undergone a triple coronary artery bypass graft operation without complications and is preparing for discharge tomorrow. What factors do you need to assess about his home situation to appropriately plan for his discharge? What factors would either impair or facilitate his recovery after discharge?

References

1. American Heart Association: 2001 Heart and Stroke Statistical Update, http://www.americanheart.org/statistics/othercvd.html
2. "Arm muscle keeps heart pumping?" *Los Angeles Times/Daily Progress,* May 2001.
3. Beery TA: The evolving role of genetics in the diagnosis and management of heart disease, *Nurs Clin North Am* 35(4):963, 2000.
4. Bennett SJ et al: Heart messages: a tailored message intervention for improving heart failure outcomes, *J Cardiovasc Nurs* 14(4):94, 2000.
5. Bondmass M et al: The effect of physiologic home monitoring and telemanagement on chronic heart failure outcomes, *Internet J Adv Nurs Pract* 2000; 3(2): website: http://www.ispub.com/journals/IJANP/Vol3N2/chf.htm; Published March 27, 2000.
6. Christensen DM: The ventricular assist device: an overview, *Nurs Clin North Am* 35(4):945, 2000.

7. Collins AS: More than a pump: the endocrine functions of the heart, *Am J Crit Care* 10(2):94, 2001.
8. Dajani AS et al: Prevention of bacterial endocarditis. recommendations by the American Heart Association, *JAMA* 277(22):1794, 1997.
9. Doering LV et al: Determinants of intensive care unit length of stay after coronary artery bypass graft surgery, *Heart Lung: J Acute Crit Care* 30:9, 2001.
10. Durack DT et al: New criteria for diagnosis of infective endocarditis: utilization of specific echocardiographic findings, *Am J Med* 96:200, 1994.
11. Feldman AM, McNamara D: Medical progress: myocarditis, *N Engl J Med* 343(19):1388, 2000.
12. Fontana JA et al: T'ai Chi Chih as an intervention for heart failure, *Nurs Clin North Am* 35(4):1031, 2000.
13. Gheorghiade M et al: Current medical therapy of advanced heart failure, *Heart Lung* 29(1):16, 2000.
14. Krumholz HM et al: American Heart Association/American College of Cardiology First Scientific Forum on Assessment of Healthcare Quality in Cardiovascular Disease and Stroke: Conference Proceedings, Measuring and Improving Quality of Care: a report of the Quality of Care and Outcomes Research Working Group on Heart Failure, *Circulation* 101(12):1483, 2000.
15. Lasater M: Impedance cardiography: a method of noninvasive cardiac output monitoring, *AACN News* 17(5):12, 2000.
16. Levine BS: Intermittent positive inotrope infusion in the management of end-stage, low-output heart failure, *J Cardiovasc Nurs* 14(4):76, 2000.
17. Major BM, Crow MM: Peripherally inserted central catheters in the patient with cardiomyopathy: the most cost-effective venous access, *J Intravenous Nurs* 23(6):366, 2000.
18. Massie BM, Amidor TM: Valvular heart disease. In *Current medical diagnosis and treatment*, ed 40, Los Altos, Calif, 2001, Lange Medical Publications.
19. Michalopoulos A et al: Determinants of hospital mortality after coronary artery bypass grafting, *Chest* 115:1598, 2001.
20. Parsons CL et al: Noninvasive positive-pressure ventilation: averting intubation of the heart failure patient, *Dimens Crit Care Nurs* 19(6):18, 2000.
21. Peacock WF, Albert NM: Observation unit management of heart failure, *Emerg Med Clin North Am* 19(1):209, 2001.
22. Piatek Y, Atzori M: PTM, *Am J Nurs* 99:64, 1999.
23. Pitt B et al: The effect of spironolactone on morbidity and mortality in patients with severe heart failure, *N Engl J Med* 341(10):709, 1999.
24. Quaglietti SE et al: Management of the patient with congestive heart failure using outpatient, home, and palliative care, *Prog Cardiovasc Dis* 43(3):259, 2000.
25. Reger TB, Vargtas G: The return of the radial artery in CABG. *Am J Nurs 99*:26, 1999.
26. Scott LD: Caregiving and care receiving among a technologically dependent heart failure population, *Adv Nurs Sci* 23(2):82, 2000.
27. Thornton SE: Differential diagnosis of infective endocarditis, *J Am Acad Nurse Pract* 12(5):77, 2000.
28. Williams JF et al: Evaluation and management of heart failure: report of the American College of Cardiology/American Heart Association Task Force on Practice Guidelines, *JACC* 26:1376, 1995.
29. Winter CA: Heart failure: living with uncertainty, *Prog Cardiovasc Nurs* 14:85, 1999.

http://www.mosby.com/MERLIN/medsurg_phipps

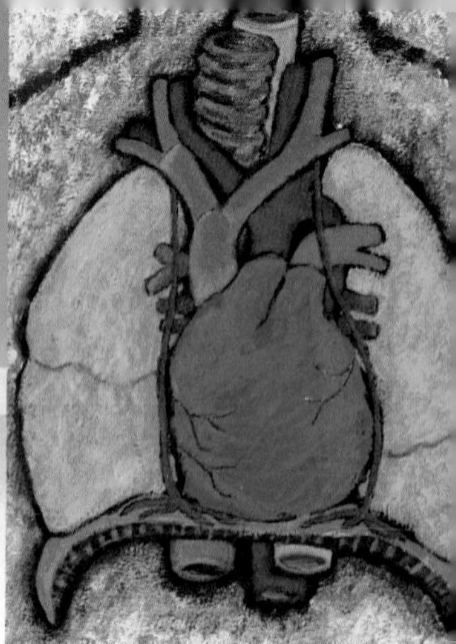

25 Vascular Problems

Carol Lynn Maxwell-Thompson, Kathryn B. Reid

Objectives

After studying this chapter, the learner should be able to:

1. Discuss the pathophysiology of arterial and venous disease.
2. Prepare a teaching plan for a person with primary hypertension.
3. Discuss the use of pharmacologic agents in the management of vascular diseases.
4. Identify the risk factors associated with the development of vascular disease.
5. Compare the collaborative management of arterial and venous disease.
6. Describe the preoperative and postoperative nursing care for patients undergoing vascular surgery.
7. Develop a plan of care for a patient undergoing amputation related to the complications of vascular disease.

HYPERTENSION

Etiology

Hypertension is defined as a consistent elevation of the systolic blood pressure above 140 mm Hg, a diastolic blood pressure above 90 mm Hg, or report of taking antihypertensive medication.[16] Early diagnosis and effective management of hypertension are essential because it is a major modifiable risk factor for cerebrovascular, cardiac, vascular, and renal diseases.

There are two major types of hypertension: essential (primary) and secondary. Primary hypertension accounts for more than 90% of all cases and has no known cause, although it is theorized that genetic factors, hormonal changes, and alterations in sympathetic tone all may play a role in its development. Secondary hypertension develops as a consequence of an underlying disease or condition. Common examples of conditions that can precipitate secondary hypertension are outlined in Table 25-1. Treatment for secondary hypertension focuses on correcting or controlling the underlying disease process, although only 1% to 2% of cases are curable.

Epidemiology

It is estimated that more than 60 million people in the United States have hypertension, but barely half of these individuals are actually diagnosed with the condition. Because hypertension is largely asymptomatic, it is often called "the silent killer," as the condition may proceed undetected and uncontrolled, leading to irreparable end-organ damage. Therefore the importance of hypertension as a health problem in the United States is reflected in several specific Healthy People 2010 goals, which are summarized in the Healthy People 2010 box.[22]

A wide variety of risk factors for hypertension have been identified and are summarized in the Risk Factors box. Both modifiable and nonmodifiable factors are important. In general, the risk of hypertension increases with age and is particularly important in African-Americans of both genders.[9] The exception is the rare condition of hypertensive crisis, which typically occurs in patients 40 to 50 years old.

Hypertension is more common among men than women until after menopause, when the incidence in women increases. The incidence of hypertension also varies significantly among different races and cultural groups. Hypertension is twice as prevalent among African-Americans as among Caucasians and is also usually more severe. For reasons that are not fully understood, the incidence and severity of hypertension are particularly high among African-Americans living in the southeastern United States as compared with other areas.

Pathophysiology

Blood pressure is controlled by a complex set of interrelated mechanisms that involve the control of cardiovascular tone and sodium and water balance. The sympathetic nervous system and the renal renin-angiotensin system provide overall control (Figure 25-1). Cardiac output and peripheral vascular resistance are the primary regulating factors. Baroreceptors within the carotid sinus and the aortic arch sense changes in blood pressure along with chemoreceptors in the medulla oblongata and cause the vasomotor center to respond through the sympathetic and parasympathetic nervous systems. The

TABLE 25-1 Causes of Secondary Hypertension

Cause or Contributing Factor	Mechanism
Renal Causes	
Renal parenchymal disease	Most often causes a renin- or sodium-dependent hypertension
Chronic glomerular nephritis or pyelonephritis	
Polycystic renal disease	
Collagen disease of the kidney	
Obstructive uropathy	
Renovascular disease	Decreased renal perfusion activates the renin-angiotensin-aldosterone system
Renal artery stenosis	
Adrenal and Endocrine Causes	
Cushing's syndrome	Increased aldosterone levels stimulate sodium and water retention and lead to an increase in the blood volume
Primary aldosteronism	
Pheochromocytoma	Benign adrenal tumor that secretes excessive amounts of catecholamines
Hyperthyroidism	Excessive adrenergic stimulation
Myxedema	Progressive atherosclerosis
Other Associated Factors	
Excessive alcohol intake	Effects not clearly known
Oral contraceptives	
Sympathomimetics	
Corticosteroids	
Cocaine	
Licorice	
Head trauma or cranial tumor	Increased intracranial pressure reduces cerebral blood flow; resultant ischemia stimulates medullary vasomotor center to raise blood pressure
Pregnancy-induced hypertension	Cause unknown; generalized vasospasm may be a contributing factor
Coarctation of the Aorta	Decreased perfusion to the kidney causes activation of the renin-angiotensin-aldosterone system

Healthy People 2010

Goals Related to Hypertension

1. Reduce the proportion of adults with high blood pressure to less than 28%.
2. Increase the proportion of adults with high blood pressure whose blood pressure is under control to greater than 18%.
3. Increase the proportion of adults with high blood pressure who are taking action (for example, losing weight, increasing physical activity, or reducing sodium intake) to help control their blood pressure to greater than 82%.
4. Increase proportion of adults who have had their blood pressure measured within the preceding 2 years and can state whether or not their blood pressure was normal or high to greater than 90%.

From US Department of Health and Human Services: *Healthy People 2010: understanding and improving health*, Washington, DC, 2000, USDHHS.

renin angiotensin system contributes to the control of blood pressure through release of angiotensin II (a potent vasoconstricting agent) and the production of aldosterone that leads to sodium and water retention. Despite a detailed understanding of the mechanics and regulation of blood pressure, the exact cause of hypertension remains unknown.

Risk Factors

Hypertension

NONMODIFIABLE RISK FACTORS

Age >60 years
Male gender
African-American race
Postmenopausal status
History of diabetes, high cholesterol
Positive family history

MODIFIABLE RISK FACTORS

Obesity
Smoking
Sedentary lifestyle
Excessive sodium intake, alcohol use
Chronic emotional stress
Atherosclerosis

ASSOCIATED CONDITIONS

Coronary artery disease–angina, myocardial infarction
Heart failure, left ventricular hypertrophy
Peripheral vascular disease
Cerebrovascular disease, stroke
Nephropathy
Retinopathy

Hypertension usually occurs without any symptoms, yet can be profoundly damaging to the blood vessels of major organ systems, including the brain, heart, and kidneys. In the early phases of hypertension, few pathologic changes can be found in the structure of the blood vessels. Over time, however, chronically elevated blood pressure causes the development of widespread pathologic changes that interfere with effective blood flow, especially to the body's vital organs. Most important, shearing forces from the elevated blood pressure damage the intimal layers of the blood vessels, leading to increased fibrin accumulation and vessel edema. Both the large and small arteries in the body may become atherosclerotic, tortuous, and weak. These changes result in narrowing of the vessel lumen, thereby decreasing blood flow to the organ or tissue supplied. As the damage progresses, the vessel can become occluded or can rupture, causing an abrupt cessation of blood flow to the area. Finally, these pathophysiologic changes decrease local autoregulatory controls of blood flow, as the vessels are less able to constrict and dilate in response to tissue needs. Over time, these changes greatly increase the person's risk for developing coronary artery disease, cerebrovascular disease, renal artery and parenchymal disease, and peripheral vascular disease.

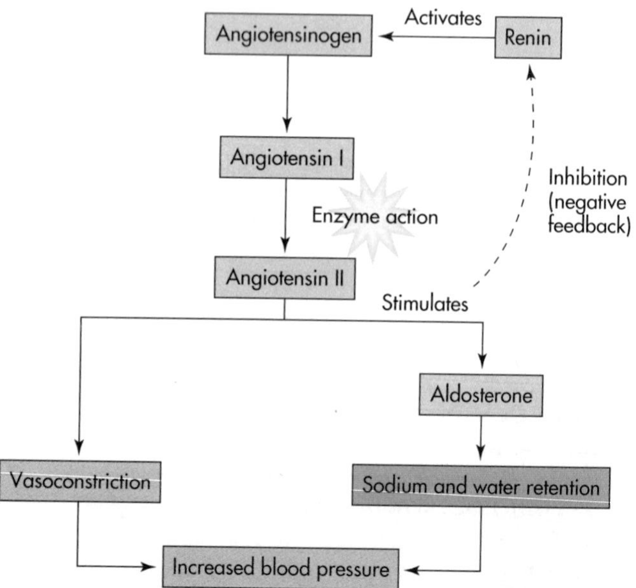

Figure 25-1 Diagram of the effect of the renin-angiotensin system on blood pressure.

Although hypertension in itself is largely asymptomatic, symptoms of end-organ damage become evident as the disease progresses. Symptoms of coronary artery disease and cerebrovascular disease may not be evident until the affected blood vessel is more than 80% occluded or an acute occlusion or vessel rupture occurs. The signs and symptoms of hypertension are summarized in the Clinical Manifestations box.

Collaborative Care Management

Diagnostic Tests

The initial diagnosis of hypertension is made on the basis of two or more elevated blood pressure readings, supine and sitting, obtained on at least two separate occasions. At the time of diagnosis, the hypertension is classified based on the degree of blood pressure elevation (Table 25-2).[16] If the systolic and diastolic blood pressures fall into different categories, the higher category is used to classify the person's disease.

Once hypertension is diagnosed, specific diagnostic tests will be ordered to: (1) rule out an underlying cause, (2) evaluate the presence and extent of organ damage and cardiovascular disease, and (3) identify other risk factors or disorders that will affect the person's treatment.[16] The Joint National Committee (JNC) on Prevention, Detection, Evaluation and Treatment of High Blood Pressure[16] has identified three risk factor categories, described in Table 25-3. Group A is the hypertensive patient with no risk factors. Group B is the patient with one risk factor. Group C includes all hypertensive pa-

Clinical Manifestations

Hypertension

Advanced disease:
- Headache, especially early-morning headache
- Blurred vision
- Spontaneous nosebleed
- Depression

NOTE: Hypertension is usually asymptomatic in its early stages.

TABLE 25-2 Classification of Blood Pressure for Adults Ages 18 and Older*

Category	Systolic (mm Hg)	Diastolic (mm Hg)
Optimal	<120	<80
Normal	<130	<85
High-normal	130-139	85-89
Hypertension		
Stage 1	140-159	90-99
Stage 2	160-179	100-109
Stage 3	≥180	≥110

Source: NIH: *Sixth report of the Joint National Committee on prevention, detection, evaluation and treatment of high blood pressure,* NIH publication No. 98-4080, Washington, D.C., 1997, National Institutes of Health, National Heart, Lung & Blood Institute.
*Not taking antihypertensive drugs and not acutely ill.

tients with clinical cardiovascular disease, end-organ damage, and/or diabetes, whether or not they have other risk factors.

Routine diagnostic tests ordered for a person diagnosed with hypertension include a complete blood count, urinalysis, serum analysis (sodium, potassium, glucose, blood urea nitrogen (BUN), creatinine, and a lipid profile, and an electrocardiogram. Other tests may be ordered to assess for secondary causes of hypertension.

Medications

Lifestyle modification is the first line intervention for all patients with hypertension, but pharmacologic therapy is the cornerstone of disease treatment. The initiation of drug therapy is guided by the patient's risk stratification as presented in Table 25-3. Treatment goals for hypertension are summarized in Box 25-1.

Drug selection is made on an individual basis with consideration of the patient's age, gender, cultural background, and lifestyle. In general, treatment is started with a low dose of a drug from one drug category that ideally can be administered once a day to support patient adherence. Either the frequency of administration or the dose may be increased later based on the patient's therapeutic response. Adjustments are based on a series of blood pressure readings obtained over several weeks. Other classes of drugs may be added or a new drug substituted if the previous medication is unsuccessful in controlling the patient's hypertension after approximately 2 to 3 months of treatment. Figure 25-2 illustrates the sites of blood pressure regulation and the action of major categories of antihypertensive drugs. The vast array of drug categories and combinations used in the treatment of hypertension are presented in Tables 25-4 and 25-5.

The JNC report recommends diuretics and beta-blockers as first-line therapy in uncomplicated stage 1 and 2 hypertension. Angiotensin-converting enzyme (ACE) inhibitors, calcium antagonists, alpha-blockers, and alpha-beta blockers are used as first-line therapy only when diuretics and beta-blockers are contraindicated.[9,13] Age and cultural differences in response to certain classes of blood pressure medications are important considerations in treatment decisions. ACE inhibitors are most effective in the Caucasian young adult population, who tend to have higher levels of renin than African-Americans and older patients. ACE inhibitors have also proven to be effective with diabetic patients experiencing proteinuria and patients with a history of heart failure.[18] On the other hand, diuretics are highly effective in the African-American and older populations because these groups tend to have higher levels of intracellular sodium. Diuretics are also the preferred agents for treating older adults with isolated systolic hypertension. Patients with a history of myocardial infarction (MI) are treated with beta-blockers to reduce the risk of another MI or sudden cardiac death. Calcium channel blockers may be used to reduce the risk of stroke.

Often two or more agents from different pharmacologic classes are needed for adequate blood pressure control. Single dose combination therapy is now an option with convenient once daily dosing to improve adherence. Combination antihypertensive agents include diuretics and potassium-sparing diuretics, beta- blockers and diuretics, ACE inhibitors and

BOX 25-1 Principles of Treatment for Hypertension

1. Treat hypertension based on total cardiovascular risk (not just BP).
2. Systolic hypertension in the elderly is an important determinant of cardiovascular disease.
3. More aggressive goals are warranted for persons with comorbid conditions such as diabetes mellitus and renal insufficiency.
4. Tailor the antihypertensive regimen to the individual's specific risks.
5. Simultaneously reduce other cardiovascular risk factors.
6. Home and ambulatory BP monitoring enhance adherence to treatment.

Adapted from Carretero OA, Oparil S: Essential hypertension. Part II: treatment, *Circulation* 101(4):446, 2000.

TABLE 25-3 Risk Stratification and Treatment of Hypertension*

Blood Pressure Stages (mm Hg)	Risk Group A (No Risk Factors–No TOD/CCD)	Risk Group B (At Least One Risk Factor, not Including Diabetes–No TOD/CCD)	Risk Group C (TOD/CCD and/or Diabetes, With or Without Other Risk Factors)
High-normal (130-139/85-89)	Lifestyle modification	Lifestyle modification	Drug therapy‡
Stage 1 (140-159/90-99)	Lifestyle modification (up to 12 months)	Lifestyle modification† (up to 6 months)	Drug therapy
Stages 2 and 3 (≥160/≥100)	Drug therapy	Drug therapy	Drug therapy

Source: NIH: Sixth report of the Joint National Committee on prevention, detection, evaluation and treatment of high blood pressure, NIH publication No. 98-4080, Washington, DC, 1997, National Institutes of Health, National Heart, Lunch & Blood Institute.

TOD/CCD, Target organ disease/clinical caradiovascular disease.

*Lifestyle modification should be adjunctive therapy for all patients recommended for pharmacologic therapy.

†For patients with multiple risk factors, clinicians should consider drugs as initial therapy plus lifestyle modifications.

‡For those with heart failure, renal insufficiency, or diabetes.

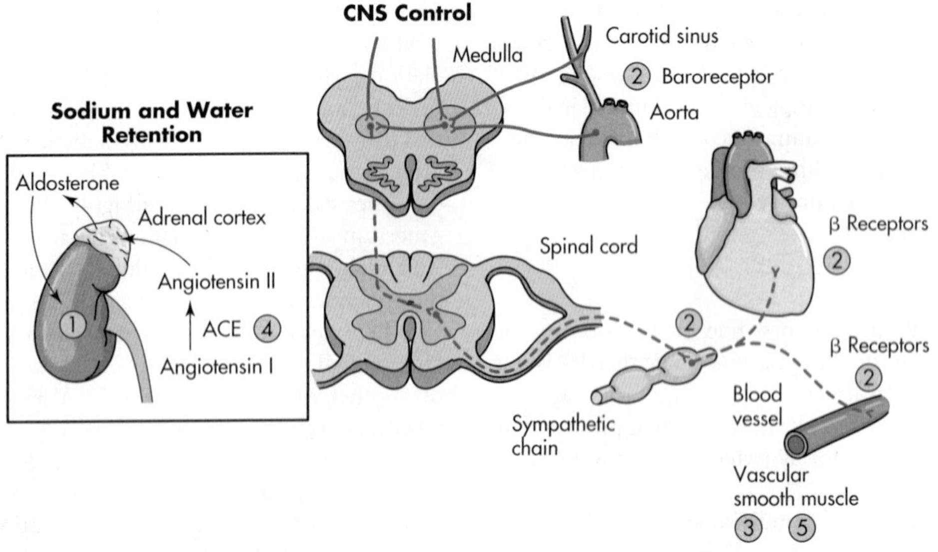

Figure 25-2 Sites of blood pressure regulation and action of antihypertensive drugs. *1,* Diuretics. *2,* Adrenergic inhibitors. *3,* Vasodilators. *4,* ACE inhibitors. *5,* Calcium antagonist. *ACE,* Angiotensin-converting enzyme.

TABLE 25-4 Common Medications for Hypertension

Drug	Action	Intervention
Diuretics		
Thiazide/Thiazide-Like Diuretics		
Bendroflumethiazide (Naturetin) Benzthiazide (Aquatag, Exna) Chlorothiazide (Diuril) Chlorthalidone (Hygroton) Cyclothiazide (Fluidil, Anhydron) Hydrochlorothiazide (Esidrix, HydroDIURIL) Hydroflumethiazide (Saluron) Indapamide (Lozol) Methyclothiazide (Enduron) Metolazone (Zaroxolyn) Polythiazide (Renese) Quinethazone (Hydromox) Trichlormethiazide (Diurese, Metahydrin)	Block sodium resorption in cortical part of ascending tubule; water excreted with sodium, producing decreased blood volume. NOTE: Thiazides ineffective in renal failure	Check vital signs before administering in early days of treatment. Monitor laboratory values of electrolytes, particularly potassium. Monitor patient's weight. Teach patient to: • Take drug early in the day. • Maintain a liberal fluid intake. • Take drug with food if GI upset occurs. • Eat a potassium-rich diet (e.g., fruits, legumes, whole grains, cereals, potatoes) • Expect an increased frequency and volume of urination • Report the incidence of muscle weakness, cramping, fatigue, nausea • Change positions slowly
Loop Diuretics		
Bumetanide (Bumex) Ethacrynic acid (Edecrin) Furosemide (Lasix)	Block sodium and water resorption in medullary portion of ascending tubule; cause rapid volume depletion	Same as above, but potassium loss can be severe. Monitor daily weight to assess response to treatment. Monitor laboratory values for increases in uric acid, glucose, BUN.
Potassium-Sparing Diuretics		
Amiloride (Midamor) Spironolactone (Aldactone) Triamterene (Dyrenium)	Inhibit aldosterone; sodium excreted in exchange for potassium	Monitor laboratory values for potassium excess. Weigh patient daily. Teach patient to: • Expect an increased volume of urine. • Avoid potassium-rich foods. • Report incidence of drowsiness or GI side effects.

ACE, Angiotensin-converting enzyme; *BP,* blood pressure; *BUN,* blood urea nitrogen; *CHF,* congestive heart failure; *COPD,* chronic obstructive pulmonary disease; *GI,* gastrointestinal.

TABLE 25-4 Common Medications for Hypertension—cont'd

Drug	Action	Intervention
Adrenergic Inhibitors		
Beta-Adrenergic Blockers		
Acebutolol (Sectral) Atenolol (Tenormin) Betaxolol (Kerlone) Carteolol (Cartrol) Metoprolol (Lopressor) Nadolol (Corgard) Penbutolol (Levatol) Pindolol (Visken) Propranolol (Inderal) Timolol (Blocadren)	Block beta-adrenergic receptors of sympathetic nervous system, decreasing heart rate and BP NOTE: Beta-blockers should not be used in patients with asthma, COPD, CHF, and heart block; use with caution in diabetes and peripheral vascular disease	Establish baseline vital signs and lab values before treatment. Check BP and pulse before administration. Teach patients to: • Change positions slowly. • Take drug as prescribed. • Avoid abruptly discontinuing use. • Report any decline in sexual responsiveness. • Report incidence of fatigue, drowsiness, difficulty breathing. • Be alert to signs of hypoglycemia if diabetic because drugs mask the symptoms.
Centrally Acting Alpha-Blockers		
Clonidine (Catapres) Guanabenz (Wytensin) Guanfacine (Tenex) Methyldopa (Aldomet)	Activate central receptors that suppress vasomotor and cardiac centers, causing a decrease in peripheral resistance NOTE: Rebound hypertension may occur with abrupt discontinuation of drug (except with Aldomet)	Check vital signs before administration. Teach patient to: • Change positions slowly. • Avoid hot baths, steam rooms, saunas. • Use gum or hard candies to counteract dry mouth. • Be cautious driving or operating machinery if drowsiness or sedation occur. • Report any decline in sexual responsiveness.
Peripheral-Acting Adrenergic Antagonists		
Guanadrel (Hylorel) Guanethidine (Ismelin) Rauwolfia serpentina (Raudixin) Reserpine (Serpasil, Serpazide)	Deplete catecholamines in peripheral sympathetic postganglionic fibers Block norepinephrine release from adrenergic nerve endings	Check vital signs before administration. Teach patient to: • Change positions slowly (dizziness is common). • Avoid hot baths, steam rooms, saunas. • Use stool softeners as needed to prevent constipation. • Report incidence of edema in hands or feet. • Use gum or hard candy to relieve dry mouth. • Report any decline in sexual responsiveness.
Alpha$_1$-Adrenergic Blockers		
Doxazosin mesylate (Cardura) Prazosin (Minipress) Terazosin (Vasocard, Hytrin)	Block synaptic receptors that regulate vasomotor tone; reduce peripheral resistance by dilating arterioles and venules	Monitor closely for first-dose syncope occurring 30–90 min after first administration. Give first dose at bedtime. Monitor BP and pulse. Syncope may be preceded by tachycardia. Other interventions as described for other adrenergic blockers.
Combined Alpha- and Beta-Adrenergic Blockers		
Labetalol (Normodyne, Trandate)	Same as for beta blockers	Interventions are same as for beta blockers.
Vasodilators		
Hydralazine (Apresoline) Minoxidil (Loniten)	Dilate peripheral blood vessels by directly relaxing vascular smooth muscle NOTE: Usually used in combination with other antihypertensives as they increase sodium and fluid retention and can cause reflex cardiac stimulation	Check BP and pulse before each dose. Palpitations and tachycardia are common during first week of therapy. Teach patient to: • Change positions slowly because dizziness is common. • Avoid hot baths, steam rooms, saunas. • Take drug with meals. • Be prepared for nasal congestion and excess lacrimation. • Report incidence of constipation or peripheral edema.

Continued

TABLE 25-4 Common Medications for Hypertension—cont'd

Drug	Action	Intervention
ACE Inhibitors		
Benazepril (Lotensin) Captopril (Capoten) Enalapril (Vasotec) Fosinopril (Monopril) Lisinopril (Prinivil, Zestril) Ramipril (Altace) Quinapril (Accupril)	Inhibit conversion of angiotensin to angiotensin II, thus blocking the release of aldosterone, thereby reducing sodium and water retention	Monitor for first-dose syncope in patients with congestive heart failure. Monitor renal function through laboratory work, potassium levels. Check BP before administering. Teach patient to: • Change positions slowly. • Report incidence of fatigue, skin rash, impaired taste, chronic cough.
Angiotensin II Receptor Antagonist		
Losartan (Cozaar)	Selectively blocks the binding of angiotensin II to the angiotensin II receptors found in many tissues and vascular smooth muscle, which blocks its vasoconstrictive and aldosterone-secreting effects	Monitor for first-dose syncope, especially in volume-depleted patients. Check BP before administering. Teach patient per ACE inhibitor teaching. Check vital signs before administering (bradycardia is common).
Calcium Antagonists		
Amlodipine besylate (Norvasc) Diltiazem (Cardiazem, Dilacor XR) Felodipine (Plendil) Isradipine (DynaCirc) Nifedipine (Procardia, Adalat) Nisoldipine (Sular) Verapamil (Calan, Calan SR, Isoptin, Isoptin SR)	Inhibit influx of calcium into muscle cells; act on vascular smooth muscles (primary arteries) to reduce spasms and promote vasodilation	Monitor renal and liver function tests Teach patient to: • Take drugs before meals. • Change positions slowly. • Report incidence of peripheral edema, fatigue, and headache,

diuretics, angiotensin II antagonists and diuretics, and calcium channel blockers and ACE inhibitors (see Table 25-5).[20]

Drug interactions are important considerations in the treatment of hypertension. Studies have shown that nonsteroidal antiinflammatory drugs (NSAIDs) can elevate the blood pressure in the normotensive population. Antihypertensive agents that act via the renal prostaglandin pathway are affected by NSAID use. These include the thiazides, loop diuretics, beta-blockers, alpha-blockers and ACE inhibitors. The combination of calcium channel blockers and NSAIDs appear to have little or no adverse effect on blood pressure.[12]

Adherence is the primary concern with hypertension management. Hypertension is usually completely asymptomatic, and the medications prescribed often represent a substantial financial outlay. It is therefore desirable to keep the regimen as simple as possible and to make adjustments in dosage gradually to minimize adverse side effects. It is occasionally possible to reduce drug dosages slightly after a year of successful hypertension control.

Treatments

The primary treatment for all stages of hypertension involves lifestyle modification to both lower blood pressure and decrease the risk of cardiovascular disease. Box 25-2 presents the goals of lifestyle modification proposed by the JNC.[16] Avoidance of tobacco in any form is essential. Cigarette smoking causes direct vasoconstriction of blood vessels and significant increases in blood pressure, thereby counteracting the benefit of antihypertensive therapy and increasing the risk of developing cardiovascular disease. The role of stress is less clear, but the use of relaxation and stress management strategies is often helpful in blood pressure control.

Surgical Management

Surgery does not play a role in the treatment of primary hypertension. It can be used to treat secondary causes such as the adrenal tumor, pheochromocytoma, which secretes excessive amounts of catecholamines, or to correct selected renal problems.

Diet

Diet plays an important role in hypertension management. Excess body weight is closely correlated with high blood pressure, and weight reduction of as little as 10 pounds can reduce blood pressure in many overweight persons.[7] Weight reduction also reduces other cardiovascular risk factors. Therefore

TABLE 25-5 Common Examples of Combination Agents for the Treatment of Hypertension

Drug Combination	Brand Name
Diuretic Combinations	
Amiloride and hydrochlorothiazide	Moduretic
Spironolactone and hydrochlorothiazide	Aldactazide
Triamterene and hydrochlorothiazide	Dyazide
Triamterene and hydrochlorothiazide	Maxzide
Beta Blockers and Diuretics	
Atenolol and chlorthalidone	Tenoretic
Bisoprolol and hydrochlorothiazide	Ziac
Metoprolol and hydrochlorothiazide	Lopressor HCT
Nadolol and bendroflumethazide	Corzide
Propranolol and hydrochlorothiazide	Inderide
Propranolol ER and hydrochlorothiazide	Inderide LA
Timolol and hydrochlorothiazide	Timolide
ACE Inhibitors and Diuretics	
Benazepril and hydrochlorothiazide	Lotensin HCT
Captopril and hydrochlorothiazide	Capozide
Enalapril and hydrochlorothiazide	Vaseretic
Lisinopril and hydrochlorothiazide	Prinzide, Zestoretic
Moexipril and hydrochlorothiazide	Uniretic
Angiotensin-II Receptor Antagonists and Diuretics	
Losartan and hydrochlorothiazide	Hyzaar
Valsartan and hydrochlorothiazide	Diovan HCT
Calcium Channel Blockers and ACE Inhibitors	
Amlodipine and benazepril	Lotrel
Diltiazem and enalapril	Teczem
Felodipine and enalapril	Lexxel
Verapamil and trandolapril	Tarka
Miscellaneous Combinations	
Clonidine and chlorthalidone	Combipres
Hydralazine and hydrochlorothiazide	Apresazide
Methyldopa and hydrochlorothiazide	Aldoril
Proazosin and polythiazide	Minizide

all patients with hypertension who are above their ideal body weight should be assisted to develop a daily regimen that includes caloric restriction and increased physical activity.

Because dyslipidemia is a major independent risk factor for the development of cardiovascular disease, dietary management of dyslipidemia is an important adjunct to antihypertensive therapy. In general, fat intake does not increase blood pressure, and large of amounts of omega-3 fatty acids may actually play a role in lowering blood pressure. A recent study indicated that the use of olive oil contributed to a significant reduction in total and saturated fatty acid levels and decreased both blood pressure and the amount of antihypertensive drug required for a study population of hypertensive patients.[4]

BOX 25-2 Lifestyle Modification Goals for Hypertension

Reduce body weight to within 10% of ideal body weight.
Limit alcohol intake to no more than 1 drink per day.
Limit sodium intake to no more than 2 to 4 g/day.
Reduce dietary fat intake to heart-healthy levels.
Increase intake of fruits and vegetables rich in potassium and magnesium.
Increase intake of low fat milk products rich in calcium.
Exercise for 30 to 40 minutes at least 4 days per week—moderate aerobic exercise is preferred.
Implement stress reduction strategies.

High levels of sodium intake lead to higher blood pressure, although there is a wide degree of variability in the blood pressure increase. Therefore, moderate sodium limitation of 2 to 4 g of sodium per day is recommended for all persons with high blood pressure. Because most dietary sodium is contained in processed foods, effective dietary counseling includes assisting patients and families to learn how to read food labels and select lower sodium choices.

Recent evidence indicates that there may be an inverse relationship between serum levels of potassium, calcium, and magnesium and blood pressure. Although there is insufficient evidence to support offering supplements, high dietary levels of these three important electrolytes may help lower blood pressure and protect against hypertension. Therefore dietary counseling also focuses on helping patients to identify foods rich in potassium, calcium, and magnesium. Potassium-rich food sources are also an essential component of patient teaching for patients taking potassium-wasting diuretics.

Alcohol consumption is a risk factor for both hypertension and stroke, and all persons with hypertension are advised to limit alcohol intake to no more than one beverage equivalent per day.

Activity

Patients with hypertension are encouraged to develop a pattern of regular aerobic exercise, which may help control their hypertension, but also contributes to weight loss and reduces cardiac risk factors. Patients are cautioned to avoid strenuous exercise, particularly activities that involve heavy lifting or the Valsalva maneuver. Weight lifting should be avoided, and sustained moderate exertion is preferable to bursts of effort. Current activity guidelines recommend that the person with hypertension should engage in moderately intense physical activity, such as 30 to 45 minutes of brisk walking, on at least 4 days of each week.

Referrals

Patients with hypertension do not require referral to other professional services as part of their primary treatment plan. The disease is self-managed in the community and home setting. Patients may profit from information concerning community resources that are available to support efforts in smoking cessation, stress management, diet modification, or aerobic exercise. The nurse encourages the patient and family to take advantage of these services as available.

NURSING MANAGEMENT OF PATIENT WITH HYPERTENSION

ASSESSMENT

Health History

Data to be collected to assess the patient with hypertension include:

- Presence of risk factors: family history of heart disease, hypertension, stroke, diabetes, hyperlipidemia
- History of hypertension: treatment prescribed; adherence and follow-up care
- History or symptoms of cardiovascular, cerebrovascular, or renal disease; diabetes; hyperlipidemia
- Smoking history, alcohol use
- Usual diet, history of weight gain or loss
- Activity and exercise pattern
- Occupation, stress level, and stress management
- Patient's knowledge of hypertension and its treatment
- Social and environmental factors that may influence understanding of and compliance with treatment

Physical Examination

Data to be collected during the physical examination include:

- Two or more blood pressure measurements taken in both arms at different times
- Height and weight
- Funduscopic eye examination; presence of arteriolar narrowing or hemorrhage
- Examination of the neck for carotid bruits, distended neck veins, or enlarged thyroid gland
- Auscultation of heart for murmurs, S3, S4, increased rate, or evidence of left ventricular hypertrophy
- Examination of the abdomen for bruits, aortic pulsations, masses, or organomegaly
- Examination of the extremities for warmth, color, edema; palpation of peripheral pulses; auscultation over femoral arteries for bruit
- Laboratory tests (CBC, chemistries, lipids, BUN, creatinine), ECG, urinalysis

NURSING DIAGNOSES

Nursing diagnoses are determined from analysis of patient data. Nursing diagnoses for the patient with hypertension may include but are not limited to:

Diagnostic Title	Possible Etiologic Factors
1. Deficient knowledge: hypertension risk factors, medications	Lack of exposure/recall, misinterpretation, unfamiliarity with information sources
2. Ineffective therapeutic regimen management	Patient value system, treatment side effects, prescription costs

EXPECTED PATIENT OUTCOMES

Expected patient outcomes for the patient with hypertension may include but are not limited to:

1. Will verbalize knowledge about the disease process and its effective management
1a. Will accurately describe hypertension and its effects on vital organs
1b. Will identify lifestyle modifications to reduce risk factors
1c. Will accurately describe action of prescribed medications and expected side effects
2. Will adhere to the therapeutic regimen, as evidenced by
2a. Weight reduction as specified in the individual care plan
2b. Dietary modifications that reflect decreased sodium, alcohol, and fat intake, as well as increased potassium, calcium, and magnesium intake
2c. Moderate level exercise at least 4 days per week
2d. Cessation of use of all tobacco products
2e. Use of antihypertensisve medication as prescribed

INTERVENTIONS

1. Patient/Family Education

The effective treatment of hypertension requires the patient to make a commitment to lifelong therapy and lifestyle modifications. Nursing interventions focus on teaching the patient and family about the disease, its associated risk factors, and the importance of adherence to the medical regimen. Although drug therapy plays a central role in hypertension management, effective treatment is also clearly based on lifestyle modification to reduce major risk factors. The nurse focuses patient teaching on the major areas of smoking cessation, diet modification, weight control, exercise, and stress management.

Cigarette smoking is a major risk factor for cardiovascular disease and is an important target of any health promotion effort. Nicotine causes constriction of the blood vessels, which increases peripheral vascular resistance and contributes to a chronic elevation in blood pressure. The nurse explores the issue of smoking cessation directly and openly with the patient and ensures that the patient and family have the information they need about options to support quitting and community resources available to assist them with this difficult challenge.

The primary diet modifications recommended for patients with hypertension mirror those recommended for heart-healthy living in general. The nurse encourages the patient to reduce the intake of dietary fats and use only moderate amounts of sodium. Dramatic changes are not necessary. Excess sodium elevates blood pressure because it contributes to fluid retention. Saturated fats have no direct effect on blood pressure and are targeted primarily because of their etiologic role in cardiac disease. A patient with both hypertension and hyperlipidemia has an increased risk of major adverse cardiovascular events such as heart attack and stroke. Reduction of saturated fat intake also makes it easier for the patient to achieve goals related to weight reduction and the maintenance of a stable body weight. Blood pressure typically but not always drops as the patient loses weight, and less medication may be required. Alcohol use is also discussed as part of the overall plan. Alcohol has little direct effect on hypertension and moderate alcohol intake can be continued, but alcohol potentiates the effects of certain antihypertensive medications and can increase the risk of adverse reaction. The negative effects of alcohol on major target organs such as the liver and heart are also well documented.

Regular aerobic exercise helps reduce resting blood pressure, improves the response of the heart to exercise and physical exertion, and assists the patient in effective weight control. The nurse encourages the patient to begin an exercise plan gradually and slowly work up to a regular program of 30 to 45 minutes of aerobic exercise at least three to four times a week. The nurse cautions the patient to avoid weight lifting and other forms of exercise that involve bursts of activity or the Valsalva maneuver.

The nurse also explores the role of stress in the patient's life and the patient's interest in or willingness to use stress reduction strategies. Patients may need help in identifying their sources of life stress and recognizing their own unique responses to stress. Simple measures such as relaxation techniques and improved coping mechanisms can be suggested to any patient. Patients who are interested in self-management strategies may be encouraged to explore the use of biofeedback as part of their hypertension treatment plan.

Medication teaching is the final major area of regimen education. Lifestyle modifications are a critical component of management, but the vast majority of patients also depend on drugs to control their hypertension, and they need to know how to use these medications safely. Once initiated, drug therapy is usually required for life.[17] Patients need to know the name, dosage, action, and side effects of each blood pressure medication prescribed; and the nurse provides the patient and family with this information in written form for home reference. The nurse encourages the patient to keep an updated list of all medications with his or her health insurance information for easy reference in case of emergency. Family members, especially the spouse or partner, are included in the medication education process if possible. Significant others play an essential role in adherence, particularly for elderly persons. Many antihypertensive medications cause a variety of side effects and the nurse discusses these side effects and their management with the patient and family. The nurse also encourages the patient to discuss any severe adverse effects with the health care provider. Numerous options are available in the antihypertensive drug arsenal (Table 25-4), and patients can be switched to a different drug if their prescribed agent is unacceptable.

Common side effects of antihypertensive medications include potassium depletion and orthostatic hypotension. Potassium depletion occurs primarily with the use of diuretics and can usually be managed by eating foods high in potassium or taking a potassium supplement. Orthostatic hypotension occurs with the use of many drugs. It is often worse in the morning when blood pressure is normally lower, after alcohol use, and after active exercise. The nurse instructs the patient to change positions slowly and sit down immediately if feeling faint. The nurse advises the patient to avoid standing in one position for long periods because this promotes venous pooling. Hot showers and baths, hot tubs, saunas, and steam baths all promote vasodilation and should be used with caution.

2. Supporting Treatment Adherence

Adherence is a major multidimensional concern that is neither easily understood nor accomplished. The absence of symptoms associated with hypertension makes adherence a greater challenge, especially when financial constraints and troublesome drug side effects are present. The nurse encourages the patient to be involved in the plan of care and to actively participate in all decisions about disease management. The nurse also encourages patients to take advantage of opportunities to have their blood pressure regularly checked at community sites such as health fairs, grocery stores, walk-in clinics, and so on. A log of blood pressure readings can be kept and brought to the health care provider's office on each visit. These records give the provider more information about the status of the patient's blood pressure control than can be obtained in a single office measurement. The nurse also stresses the importance of keeping regular follow-up visits for ongoing disease management.

EVALUATION

To evaluate the effectiveness of nursing interventions, compare patient behaviors with those stated in the expected patient outcomes. Achievement of outcomes is successful if the person with hypertension:

1. Is knowledgeable about the disease process and its effective management.
1a. Correctly describes the disease process of hypertension and its effects on vital body organs.
1b. Identifies the expected side effects of prescribed drugs and measures to minimize adverse effects.
1c. Makes lifestyle adaptations to reduce risk factors.
2. Demonstrates commitment to antihypertensive regimen by:
2a. Maintaining weight within recommended range.
2b. Consuming a heart-healthy diet.
2c. Exercising regularly.
2d. Successfully eliminating the use of tobacco.
2e. Taking antihypertensive medication as prescribed.

GERONTOLOGIC CONSIDERATIONS

Hypertension can occur at any point in the adult life span, but it clearly becomes increasingly prevalent with aging. Therefore the entire overview of hypertension and its management is relevant to older adults. Lifestyle changes can be particularly difficult for this age-group and the nurse needs to be sensitive to these challenges in teaching. Economic issues frequently become extremely important for older adults as medication costs chip away at fixed incomes. Polypharmacy issues are also common and the nurse reviews all medications in use and explores the use of generic alternatives or combinations where possible.

Older adults are also more vulnerable to the side effects of hypertension medication, and the development of orthostatic hypertension can pose a significant risk for falls. Failing memory may also interfere with medication compliance, and patients may profit from the use of medication boxes that can be filled for the week by family, friends, or visiting nurses. Hypertension is a community-managed problem, and the nurse who manages care for the elderly must plan holistically to meet the patient's needs for safe medication, side effect management, and follow-up care.

SPECIAL ENVIRONMENTS FOR CARE

Critical Care

Most patients with essential hypertension have a chronic stable disease that can be successfully managed on an outpatient basis. In rare cases, however, systolic blood pressure rises to a critical level above 210 mm Hg and requires immediate emergency treatment. When severe hypertension presents a serious risk of irreversible organ damage or stroke, the patient may be admitted to a critical care unit, where drug therapy can be administered intravenously with continuous monitoring. Sodium nitroprusside and nitroglycerine are two of the most commonly used drugs for hypertensive emergencies. The goal of therapy is to lower the blood pressure gradually, because rapid drops in pressure can lead to organ ischemia and stroke. As the blood pressure begins to respond to these powerful vasodilator medications, the oral drug regimen is gradually resumed and adjusted. Once the patient's blood pressure is under control, therapy with oral medication is continued as an outpatient. The patient gradually resumes their precrisis lifestyle.

Community-Based Care

Hypertension is typically managed in the community with the support and supervision of the primary care provider. The entire discussion of hypertension presented previously therefore addresses management of the disease in the community. Multiple outreach and education programs are available in most communities to assist patients to successfully manage hypertension. The nurse encourages the patient to explore programs offered by the American Heart Association, senior centers, and health providers on topics as varied as smoking cessation, heart-healthy cooking, and exercise. This again underlines the importance of careful and thorough patient education, particularly related to issues of adherence with the drug regimen.

COMPLICATIONS

Progressive damage to major body organs is the most common complication of essential hypertension. It primarily occurs when control is ineffective or erratic due to regimen adherence problems. End-organ damage can eventually lead to encephalopathy, renal failure, left ventricular failure, and retinal hemorrhage. Hypertensive crisis produces significant and immediate risks of acute complications such as MI and cerebrovascular accident. Untreated hypertensive crisis results in significant morbidity and mortality, as high as 90% within 2 years. When hypertensive crisis is treated successfully, however, the survival rate approaches 94% at 1 year. Appropriate ongoing follow-up monitoring appears to be the key variable and is clearly linked to the effectiveness of the patient education provided.

ARTERIAL DISORDERS

Arterial disease can affect any artery of the body and can manifest as either an acute or chronic condition. Disruption of the arterial blood flow can result from narrowing or complete obstruction of the wall of the vessel from a variety of causes (Box 25-3). The symptoms of arterial disease are directly related to the severity of interruption in blood flow, which impedes the delivery of oxygen and nutrients to the tissues and causes accumulation of waste products and carbon dioxide. If the tissue needs for oxygen and nutrients exceed the supply, ischemia and necrosis can result.

Chronic Arterial Occlusive Disease

Etiology

Chronic arterial occlusive disease (also commonly referred to as peripheral vascular disease or PVD) involves the progressive narrowing, degeneration, and eventual obstruction of the arteries of the extremities. The lower extremities are most frequently involved and arteriosclerosis obliterans is the most common form. The process of atherosclerosis combines with the process of diffuse arteriosclerosis or calcification to produce widespread, slowly progressive narrowing of the arteries. The superficial femoral, iliac, and popliteal arteries are the most common sites of involvement. Plaque typically develops at points of arterial branching or bifurcation (Figure 25-3).

Epidemiology

Risk factors known to predispose individuals to chronic arterial occlusive disease are the same as those identified for

BOX 25-3 Causes of Decreased Arterial Blood Flow

- Atherosclerotic plaque
- Arterial spasm
- Embolus or thrombus
- Changes in blood pressure
- Increased blood viscosity or hypercoagulability
- Arterial venous fistula
- Trauma
- Heart failure
- Compartment syndrome

other forms of cardiovascular disease. Nonmodifiable risk factors include increasing age, male gender, and a positive family history. Chronic occlusive disease is strongly associated with aging, and symptoms usually develop between the ages of 50 and 70 years. Approximately 10% of adults over the age of 70 are believed to experience symptoms of arterial occlusive disease.[10] The disease is more prevalent in men than in women. Modifiable risk factors include smoking, obesity, stress, and a sedentary lifestyle. The presence of other related diseases, including hypertension, atherosclerosis, diabetes, and hyperlipidemia, also increases the risk for arterial occlusive disease.[8] Risk factors for chronic arterial occlusive disease are listed in the Risk Factors box.

Pathophysiology

The atherosclerotic plaque formation that occurs with arteriosclerosis obliterans causes thickening of the intima and media of the artery, resulting in partial or complete obstruction of the vessel lumen. The calcification of arteriosclerosis further weakens the arterial wall and increases the chance for both thrombus and aneurysm formation. The disease usually occurs segmentally, with lengths of normal vessel interspersed with diseased portions. As blood flow to the affected tissues decreases, the body attempts to compensate by vasodilating the arteries to improve blood flow to the area, as well as by developing and enhancing other sources of blood supply, known as collateral circulation.[23]

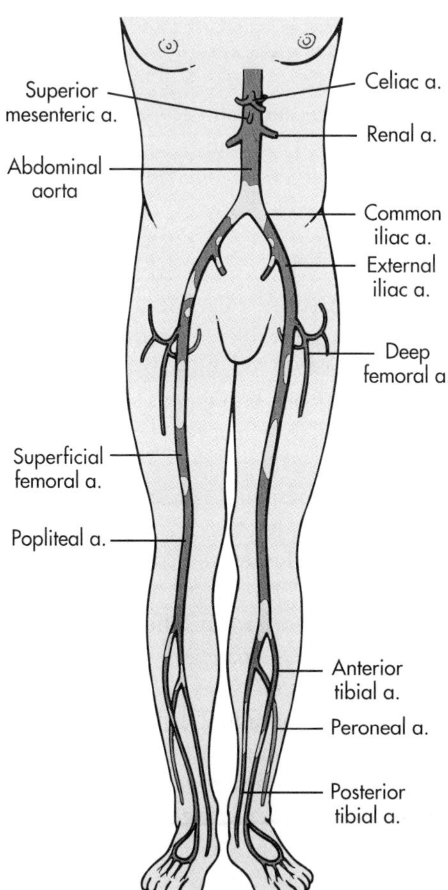

Figure 25-3 Common sites of atherosclerosis.

Symptoms develop as the disease progresses and the compensatory mechanisms become inadequate. Intermittent claudication, an aching pain or cramping sensation that occurs in the muscle with activity or exercise, is the classic symptom. The pain is usually distal to the site of obstruction and disappears within 1 to 2 minutes after cessation of exercise.[23] Muscles of the calf are commonly involved when disease affects the femoral artery. Muscles of the lower back, buttocks, thigh, and foot are also commonly affected. Symptoms initially occur when the individual has walked one half to two blocks and appear even more rapidly when the person walks uphill. Exercise tolerance decreases as the disease worsens. The affected vessel is frequently more than 70% occluded before the onset of symptoms.[5] The body attempts to bypass the obstruction by developing additional blood vessels in the affected areas. In slowly progressive disease this collateral circulation may successfully reduce the overt symptoms.

Sedentary patients may not develop claudication if they do not ambulate enough to cause ischemia. Pain that occurs at rest, termed rest ischemia, indicates severe disease. Rest pain typically occurs at night and is accompanied by coldness, numbness, and tingling of the extremity.[10] Any factor that decreases cardiac output and peripheral arterial blood flow such as elevating the extremities can trigger the pain. The patient may be awakened at night and need to sit up or walk around. Gravity improves perfusion of the tissues and relieves or lessens the pain. In advanced arteriosclerosis obliterans, rest ischemia may lead to necrosis, ulceration, and gangrene, particularly in the toes and distal foot. Ischemic ulcers are pale, round, painful, and crusty in appearance. Either eschar or black necrotic tissue may be present.

Other symptoms of chronic occlusive disease include hair loss on the affected extremity; thick, brittle, and slow-growing nails; and impaired motor function. The skin typically appears shiny and taut and is fragile, dry, and scaly. It also feels cooler than normal to the touch. The extremity becomes extremely pale when elevated above the level of the heart for 5 minutes and then exhibits reactive hyperemia or redness when lowered, which persists for more than 15 seconds.[10] Reddish

Risk Factors

Peripheral Vascular Disease

- Increasing age
- Smoking
- Hypertension
- Atherosclerosis
- Obesity
- Diabetes mellitus
- Stress
- Family history of PVD or atherosclerosis
- Sedentary lifestyle
- Hyperlipidemia

discoloration or rubor may be present whenever the extremity is in a dependent position. Bruit, a blowing sound, may be auscultated over the obstructed vessel where the blood flow is turbulent. A Doppler ultrasound may be necessary to hear either pulses or bruit in obstructed vessels. The signs and symptoms of chronic arterial occlusive disease are summarized in the Clinical Manifestations box.

Collaborative Care Management

Diagnostic Tests. Chronic arterial occlusive disease is initially diagnosed through the history and physical examination. The ankle-brachial index (ABI) may be used to confirm the diagnosis. The ABI measures the difference in blood pressure and blood flow in the upper and lower extremities and is an objective measurement of the degree of stenosis present in the vessel. The test is described in more detail in Chapter 22. In a healthy person the pressure in the leg should be the same or slightly higher than the pressure in the arm, yielding an ABI of about 1. Patients with arterial insufficiency have an ABI of 0.5 to 0.95. Patients experiencing ischemic rest pain typically exhibit an ABI of 0.5 or less, and in the presence of severe tissue damage and ischemia the ABI can be 0.25 or lower. Other noninvasive tests include ultrasonography, segmental limb pressure, pulse volume recordings, and exercise testing. Arteriography, an invasive procedure, is used to localize the site and severity of the disease process and is an essential part of any plan for surgical intervention.

Medications. Therapy for chronic arterial occlusive disease follows the general outline of cardiovascular disease management and includes lifestyle modification (diet, exercise, and smoking cessation) and pharmacologic therapy. Pharmacologic therapy is used in PVD to improve blood flow and prevent thrombus formation in affected extremities. Vasodilators have no proven effectiveness in treating chronic arterial occlusive disease, although they are commonly prescribed. Their effectiveness is limited because the dilating capabilities of the affected vessels are already maximized by the time symptoms appear.

Clinical Manifestations

Chronic Arterial Occlusive Disease

- Intermittent claudication
- Rest pain in advanced disease
- Diminished hair growth on affected extremities
- Thick, brittle, slow-growing nails
- Shiny, thin, fragile, taut skin
- Dry and scaly
- Cool temperature
- Diminished or absent pulses
- Pale, blanched appearance with extremity elevation
- Reddish discoloration, rubor with extremity in dependent position
- Reactive hyperemia
- Decreased motor function
- Ulcer formation with advanced disease
- Ankle-brachial index of 0.5 to 0.95

Pharmacologic agents helpful in treating patients with chronic arterial occlusive disease include pentoxifylline (Trental) and thromboxane A_2 inhibitors such as aspirin. Pentoxifylline increases erythrocyte flexibility and reduces blood viscosity, directly improving the supply of oxygenated blood to the ischemic tissue. Antiplatelet agents inhibit the formation of arterial thrombi that are composed primarily of platelets. Aspirin is the classic antiplatelet drug, but dipyridamole (Persantine) and ticlopidine (Ticlid) are also commonly prescribed. The effectiveness of antiplatelet agents in improving circulation through diseased arteries has not been proven and continues to be studied. Antiplatelet and anticoagulant medications are also used after surgical bypass interventions to prevent reocclusion. Drugs commonly used to treat chronic arterial occlusive disease are presented in Table 25-6.

Treatments. A variety of interventional radiologic procedures may be used in the management of PVD, including percutaneous transluminal angioplasty (PTA), laser surgery, atherectomy, and intravascular stent placement. These procedures are used when the disease has become incapacitating.

Percutaneous Transluminal Angioplasty. This interventional procedure is an adaptation of the well known coronary balloon angioplasty procedure (see Chapter 23). It can be used for both diagnostic and treatment purposes. PTA can be used to dilate any artery of the body except for the carotids. Angioplasty has been used to successfully treat stenosis in the coronary, aortic, iliac, femoral, popliteal, tibial, mesenteric, and renal arteries; but calcified and fibrous lesions cannot be treated in this manner. A catheter is inserted into a major artery and advanced under fluoroscopic guidance to the site of obstruction. If a red thrombus (deep vein thrombus or embolus) is found, it can be treated with either thrombolytic therapy or thrombectomy. If a white or yellow-white atherosclerotic plaque is seen, the vessel is either dilated with the balloon to increase blood flow, or treated with a surgical bypass or recanalization procedure.[14] Patients are typically anticoagulated after the procedure to reduce the risk of immediate restenosis and then placed on long-term antiplatelet therapy.

Laser-Assisted Balloon Angioplasty. Laser energy is used to vaporize the obstructive plaque and open the occluded artery so that balloon angioplasty can be effectively performed. The use of the laser is designed to reshape the artery and reduce the incidence of restenosis.

Intravascular Stents. Restenosis is a persistent problem after any revascularization procedure. Stents have been developed that can be inserted into the affected artery to provide structure and support vessel patency.

Intravascular Ultrasound. This procedure is used as a diagnostic adjunct with other more definitive treatment strategies. Ultrasound accurately measures the stenotic area to allow for the safe removal of the atheroma without vessel injury. It may also be used to assist in placing stents or to evaluate their placement.

Peripheral Atherectomy. This is a percutaneous procedure that directly removes the obstructing atheroma or plaque from the diseased artery.

None of the described interventions is without risk. Rethrombosis, embolism, vasospasm, and both local and systemic bleeding are all possible complications, especially when patients are also anticoagulated.

Surgical Management. Surgical procedures are typically used in the management of arterial disease that is disabling, does not respond to other more conservative treatment, or threatens the patient with loss of the limb. Surgery may be the treatment option of choice for severe occlusion, or it may be used when more conservative interventions fail to reverse the severe ischemia. Bypass grafting is the most commonly used and successful surgical option (Box 25-4). An autologous graft of the patient's own saphenous vein is the preferred graft option because there is less risk of restenosis and graft failure.

BOX 25-4 Options for Surgical Repair of Acute Arterial Occlusion

Endarterectomy: a direct opening is made into the artery to remove the obstruction.
Embolectomy: removal of an embolus from an artery.
Femoral-femoral bypass: a graft from one femoral artery to the other.
Axillofemoral bypass: a graft from the axillary artery to the femoral artery. It is created subcutaneously on the side of the chest.
Femoral-popliteal bypass: a graft from the femoral artery to the popliteal artery.
Aortoiliac bypass: a graft from the aorta to the iliac arteries; the incision is made from the xiphoid process to the pubis.

Synthetic grafts such as polytetrafluoroethylene (PTFE), commonly known as Gore-Tex grafts, have also been successfully used for many years. Grafts from human umbilical cord veins have also been used.

The aorta, renal, iliac, femoral, popliteal, and anterior and posterior tibial arteries are common sites of severe obstruction. The surgeon determines the optimal graft placement to reestablish patent arterial flow. Grafting from the femoral to the popliteal artery is common (Figure 25-4). Patients with occlusion of the distal aorta may undergo aortoiliac bypass. A femoral-femoral bypass shifts blood from one femoral artery to the other and may be a procedure of last resort for patients who have had prior aortic surgery and are no longer candidates for further surgery on the aorta. Grafts can also be placed subcutaneously from the axillary artery to the femoral artery. Procedures involving the aorta tend to be more extensive and carry a higher risk of complications. Inability to restore necessary blood flow to the affected area can ultimately result in amputation when gangrene is extensive or infection invades the bone.

Diet. A heart-healthy, low-fat, low-cholesterol diet is recommended to slow further progression of the disease process. Additional dietary needs are based on the presence of other comorbid conditions, such as obesity, diabetes, dyslipidemia, and hypertension.

Activity. A sedentary lifestyle is an identified risk factor for atherosclerosis. Increasing daily activity in a carefully planned way can decrease blood lipids, help control hypertension, and improve arterial blood flow by stimulating development of collateral circulation in the occluded regions. A

TABLE 25-6 Common Medications for Arterial Occlusive Disease

Drug	Action	Intervention
Antiplatelet Medications		
Aspirin Ticlopidine (Ticlid) Dipyridamole (Persantine)	Inhibit platelet aggregation, prolong bleeding time	Administer with food to reduce GI distress. Monitor coagulation times. Assess for signs of bleeding.
Xanthine Derivatives		
Pentoxifylline (Trental)	Increases flexibility of the RBCs, thereby facilitating passage through microcirculation; decreases RBC aggregation; increases fibrinolytic activity	Monitor for side effects—GI upset, tremor. Monitor for effect on claudication and exercise tolerance. Therapeutic effect may take 2-4 weeks.
Dihydropyridines		
Nifedipine (Adalat, Procardia) Isradipine (DynaCirc) Felodipine (Plendil) Nimodipine (Nimotop) Amlodipine besylate (Norvasc)	Selectively block influx of calcium ions across cell membrane of vascular smooth muscle; decreased peripheral resistance increases blood flow; primarily indicated for Raynaud's phenomenon	Monitor blood pressure. Teach patient to change position slowly and report the incidence of edema, fatigue, or headache.
Vasodilators		
Hydralazine (Apresoline) Minoxidil (Loniten, Minodyl)	Cause vasodilation and decrease peripheral vascular resistance; useful in peripheral vascular disease only if small vessels can dilate in response to stimulation	Monitor blood pressure and pulse. Teach patient to change positions slowly, take drug with meals, and report the incidence of constipation or peripheral edema.

RBC, Red blood cell; *GI,* gastrointestinal.

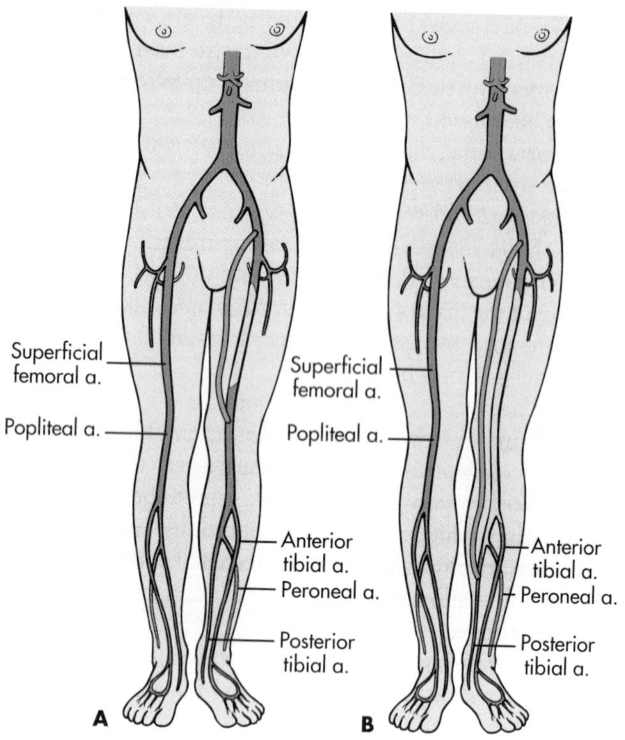

Figure 25-4 **A,** Femoral-popliteal bypass graft around an occluded superficial femoral artery. **B,** Femoral-posterior tibial bypass graft around occluded superficial femoral, popliteal, and proximal tibial arteries.

daily walking program is suggested for patients with arterial occlusive disease and discussed further under nursing interventions. Participation in a structured rehabilitation program is recommended if possible because the patient can receive the professional support and monitoring that can ensure safety.

Referrals. A variety of professionals may be included in the plan of care for the patient with arterial occlusive disease. Diet counseling is often needed. A nutritionist can provide assistance and guidance in making the needed diet changes to both reduce body weight and overall disease risk factors. Diet teaching is especially important with diabetic patients. Referral for physical therapy can assist the patient to develop an appropriate exercise plan and regain the strength and endurance to manage activities of daily living independently. Referral to community support groups may also be essential, particularly for patients who are attempting smoking cessation.

NURSING MANAGEMENT OF PATIENT WITH ARTERIAL OCCULSIVE DISEASE

ASSESSMENT

Health History

Data to be collected from the health history include:

- Presence, severity, and location of intermittent claudication; presence of rest pain, if any
- Exercise/walking tolerance
- History of hypertension, diabetes, coronary artery disease; treatment used, adherence to regimen
- Smoking history, attempts to quit, if any
- Dietary patterns
- Impact of disease on activities of daily living (ADLs)
- Effect of disease on family, work, social activities
- Effects of disease on sexuality—impotence
- Home living situation and effect on mobility
- Daily activities and usual exercise routine, if any

Physical Examination

Data to be collected as part of the physical examination include:

- Peripheral pulse assessment by palpation (1 to 4) or Doppler
- Appearance of skin, nails, hair on extremities
- Signs of skin breakdown
- Postural color changes, presence and severity of reactive hyperemia
- Presence and severity of muscle wasting
- Skin temperature
- Presence, location, and severity of numbness/tingling in extremity
- Body weight
- Ankle-brachial index
- Cholesterol and triglyceride levels

NURSING DIAGNOSES

Nursing diagnoses are determined from analysis of patient data. Nursing diagnoses for the patient with arterial occlusive disease may include but are not limited to:

Diagnostic Title	Possible Etiologic Factors
1. Ineffective tissue perfusion	Decreased arterial blood flow (lower extremity)
2. Risk for impaired skin integrity	Ischemia, immobility
3. Chronic pain	Imbalance between oxygen supply and demand

EXPECTED PATIENT OUTCOMES

Expected patient outcomes for the patient with chronic arterial occlusive disease may include but are not limited to:

1. Will promote tissue perfusion through daily exercise, temperature control, clothing modifications, positioning, and smoking cessation
2. Will maintain skin integrity and avoid injury and infection
3. Will minimize pain by balancing activity and rest

INTERVENTIONS

Most of the nursing interventions that are appropriate for patients with chronic arterial occlusive disease fall into the category of patient/family education. The disease is chronic and progressive and is best managed by lifestyle modifications that support peripheral perfusion and prevent injury. The patient needs to incorporate these measures into her or his daily lifestyle in a way that is comfortable and acceptable.

1. Promoting Tissue Perfusion

The nurse encourages patients to incorporate lifestyle modifications into their daily activities to improve oxygen delivery to the tissues. Maintaining an environmental temperature of about 21° C (70° F) is recommended. Avoiding exposure to the cold is critical because cold triggers vasoconstriction and is likely to induce ischemia and pain. Socks, layered clothing, and blankets should be used for warmth, but the nurse cautions patients about the dangers associated with heating pads and hot water bottles. The nurse encourages the patient to avoid constrictive or restrictive clothing such as girdles, rolled garters, tight shoes or shoelaces, tight waistbands, and socks with tight banding that could impede circulation.

Positioning is also an important intervention to support perfusion. The patient maintains the legs in a position of slight dependency, which uses gravity to enhance tissue perfusion. If the patient experiences rest pain at night the head of the bed is elevated 4 to 6 inches. The legs are not elevated above the level of the heart because this would impede arterial flow. The patient is encouraged to avoid crossing the legs at the knees, which places pressure on the arteries of the leg, and to avoid sitting in a slumped or slouched posture that could cause acute constriction of the arteries in the pelvis.[19] Both pressure on and massage of the extremities should be avoided. The skin is fragile and breaks down easily. Vigorous massage can also promote embolus formation.

Eliminating smoking can also improve perfusion. Nicotine causes vasoconstriction and promotes vasospasm, and inhaled carbon dioxide reduces the oxygen carrying capacity of the blood. The importance of smoking cessation in PVD cannot be overestimated. The nurse explores the patient's knowledge about the effects of smoking, prior efforts to quit, interest in quitting, and knowledge of options available to support quitting. Referral for community support is an important strategy.

Alternative and complementary therapies have also demonstrated some possible effectiveness in managing the pain associated with intermittent claudication. Agents with proven effectiveness are described in the Complementary & Alternative Therapies box.

2. Maintaining Skin Integrity and Preventing Injury and Infection

The skin of the extremities is at high risk for breakdown because of decreased tissue oxygenation. The nurse teaches the patient to carefully inspect the skin daily for dryness, redness, and injury. A mirror can be used to inspect areas that are difficult to see such as the heels and the plantar surfaces of the toes. If the patient is hospitalized, the nurse performs a complete skin assessment at least once each day and equips the bed with antipressure devices to prevent skin breakdown. The feet are cleaned daily using a mild soap. The skin is gently dried and a moisturizing lotion such as lanolin is applied as necessary to counteract dryness. Cotton nonconstricting socks are recommended and should be changed daily to prevent moisture buildup and irritation. Properly fitted shoes are extremely important, and the nurse recommends the use of soft leather shoes that allow the feet to breathe.

Complementary & Alternative Therapies
Vascular Disease

Complementary and alternative therapies have a long history in the management of vascular disease. Vitamin E has long been known to be useful in improving the pain of intermittent claudication. Studies have confirmed its effectiveness and clarified that positive outcomes are associated with the use of daily doses of 400 to 800 mg/day. About 3 months of treatment are required before positive outcomes are seen. Other approaches have less clear outcomes. Gingko biloba appears to have a minimally positive effect on the discomfort of intermittent claudication. Garlic has also shown promise, but the doses required are too high to be palatable for most individuals.

Horse chestnut seed extract appears to have a positive effect on chronic venous insufficiency, and in early studies may have equal effectiveness with the use of compression stockings. The extract is being widely used in Europe with acceptable side effects.

Patient Teaching
Teaching Points for the Patient With Peripheral Vascular Disease

- Avoid trauma to the feet.
  - Wear properly fitted shoes; avoid going barefoot; wear socks, preferably cotton, with your shoes.
  - Avoid the use of heating pads and hot water bottles; use layered clothing for warmth.
  - Do not self-treat any calluses, corns or ingrown toenails; see a podiatrist or nurse specialist for care.
- Avoid use of all medications on the feet unless prescribed by the health care provider.
- Care for the feet daily.
  - Wash feet with mild soap.
  - Dry feet well.
  - Inspect the feet daily for injury or abrasion using a mirror to visualize hard to access places.
- Exercise regularly; 20 minutes of daily walking is recommended.
- Prevent vasoconstriction.
  - Avoid the use of any tobacco products.
  - Avoid wearing tight or constrictive clothing.
  - Avoid crossing the legs.
- Maintain control of other related chronic conditions.
  - Control blood pressure.
  - Keep diabetes under control.
  - Follow a low fat diet.
  - Monitor blood lipids with health care provider.

Sensation may be decreased in the feet, particularly in diabetic patients, and this increases the chance for injury. It is important for the patient to learn how to protect the feet from abrasion and irritation as much as possible. The use of direct heat is contraindicated. Toenails are trimmed straight across using nail clippers. Corns, calluses, and other minor foot problems should be evaluated by a podiatrist and not self-treated. The patient is encouraged to contact the health care provider immediately if ulceration, infection, or skin breakdown is detected. A summary of relevant patient teaching is included in the Patient Teaching box.

3. Reducing Pain and Increasing Exercise Tolerance

Activity improves circulation through rhythmic muscle contraction and stimulates the formation of collateral circulation that can increase blood flow to the ischemic area. The patient is encouraged to exercise or walk frequently to the point of pain to decrease the incidence and severity of claudication. The exercise should be slow and progressive. Walking is the preferred exercise, but swimming and use of a stationary bicycle can also be incorporated into the plan. The patient is instructed to avoid bed rest as much as possible. The goal is an exercise tolerance of 30 to 45 minutes of steady walking twice a day. Exercise is halted immediately when pain occurs. The patient rests and resumes walking when the pain has completely subsided. If initial walking tolerance is poor, the nurse encourages the patient to walk and rest repeatedly as needed until the cumulative 30 to 45 minutes of activity is achieved.

Buerger-Allen exercises can also be recommended to patients with advanced disease. These exercises can be used by those with minimal exercise tolerance. The patient lies flat with the legs elevated above the heart for 2 to 3 minutes and then relaxes with the legs in a slightly dependent position for an additional 2 to 3 minutes. The patient then proceeds to exercise the feet (flexion, extension, inversion, eversion), ankles (rotations and pumps), and knees (flexion, extension) for 30 seconds in each position. The exercises are repeated several times a day.

EVALUATION

To evaluate the effectiveness of nursing interventions, compare patient behaviors with those stated in the expected patient outcomes. Achievement of outcomes is successful if the patient with arterial occlusive disease:

1. Successfully incorporates measures to promote tissue perfusion into daily lifestyle.
2. Keeps the lower extremities and feet free of infection and skin breakdown.
3. Increases walking tolerance and is free of claudication pain.

GERONTOLOGIC CONSIDERATIONS

Chronic arterial occlusive disease is primarily a disease of later life and almost exclusively affects older adults. All of the interventions discussed apply to this population. Several factors make interventions with this population more challenging. Lifestyle patterns and habits are usually deeply entrenched and change is difficult to achieve. The presence of arthritis and other chronic diseases can make it difficult for older adults to increase their activity, and diabetes frequently complicates disease management. None of the measures are curative in nature and a great deal of damage has already occurred before diagnosis. The presence of adequate social support can often determine the success or failure of the interventions presented. Patients are carefully assessed for the presence of vision or hearing losses that may make it more difficult for them to learn the self-care regimen. Potential obstacles in the home environment also need to be considered and modified if possible.

SPECIAL ENVIRONMENTS FOR CARE

Critical Care

Critical care management would not be routinely needed in the management of chronic arterial occlusive disease. This is a slowly progressive problem that only rarely causes acute complications. Acute obstruction can occur, however, and cause an acute limb-threatening emergency. Acute arterial obstruction is presented on p. 784.

Community-Based Care

Virtually all of the care described for the patient with chronic arterial occlusive disease takes place in the community setting. The patient requires hospitalization only for complications of the disease. All of the teaching that is discussed in the section on nursing interventions is addressed toward successful self-management by the patient at home. Care planning, especially for older adults, is based on thorough assessment of the home setting and the support network available to assist the patient in managing the disease.

COMPLICATIONS

The major complications of chronic arterial occlusive disease include injury, infection, gangrene, and acute occlusion. Many of these problems, if not identified and treated promptly, can result in the loss of the limb through amputation.

Arterial ulcers may also develop as a result of the decreased blood supply. Arterial ulcers are typically located on or between the toes or on the upper surface of the foot over the metatarsal heads, and are extremely painful (Figure 25-5). The diabetic patient is particularly vulnerable to the development of ulcers, which may become chronic. Necrotic tissue must be removed before healing can occur. This is accomplished by mechanical debridement, chemical debridement with an enzymatic agent such as Varidase, or autolytic debridement with hydrocolloid and film dressings. Nonrestrictive bandages are used to support circulation and healing. Treatment is difficult, and outcomes are unpredictable. Prevention through the previously discussed strategies is the focus of intervention.

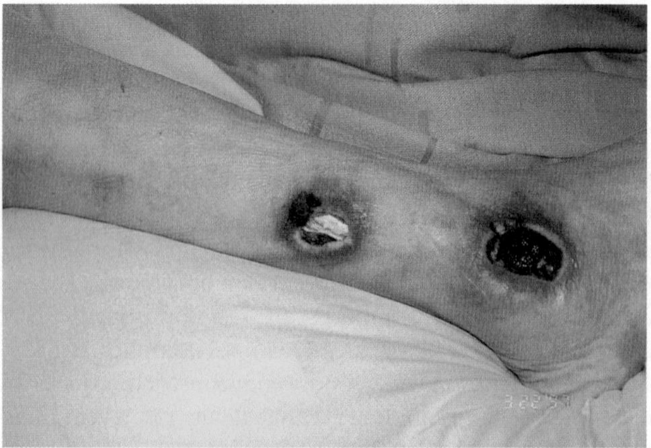

Figure 25-5 Arterial ulcers of the lateral malleolus and distal lateral portion of the leg. Note round, smooth shape.

Buerger's Disease (Thromboangiitis Obliterans)

Etiology/Epidemiology

Buerger's disease is an obstructive vascular disorder caused by segmental inflammation in the arteries and veins that was first described by Leo Buerger, an American surgeon, in 1908. It typically occurs in men between 20 and 40 years old and is rare in women. An increased incidence of the disease in women that has occurred since the 1980s is attributed to the increased prevalence of smoking. Although Buerger's disease occurs worldwide, its incidence is much higher in the Middle East and Asia and in persons of Jewish heritage. The incidence of Buerger's disease is directly related to cigarette smoking—the disease does not occur in nonsmokers.[21] The underlying cause remains unknown. It primarily affects the vessels of the lower extremities, and the tibial arteries and vessels of the foot are the most common sites. Usually more than one limb is involved. Only 30% of patients with Buerger's disease have upper extremity involvement, primarily in the vessels of the forearm and hand. In rare cases the disease can affect the aorta, cerebral, coronary, pulmonary, iliac, or renal arteries.

Pathophysiology

Buerger's disease is characterized by an inflammatory response in the arteries, veins, and nerves. It is theorized that the inflammation is an autoimmune response that is triggered by nicotine in genetically susceptible persons. The affected area is infiltrated by white cells and becomes fibrotic as healing occurs. The presence of inflammatory thrombi causes occlusion of the veins and arteries. The pathology differs from atherosclerotic disease because small and medium-sized arteries and veins are involved. Arteriogram findings reveal a classic tapering or abrupt occlusion of peripheral vessels with collateral vessels exhibiting a corkscrew appearance.

Symptoms of Buerger's disease include slowly developing claudication, cyanosis, and coldness in the affected extremity. Rest pain is common. Recurrent superficial thrombophlebitis occurs in both the upper and lower extremities and necrotic lesions form at the tips of the finger and toes. The risk of gangrene increases in the presence of collagen disease or atherosclerosis and in response to stress or cold weather.

Collaborative Care Management

The goals of treatment are to halt disease progression and avoid amputation. Buerger's disease is difficult to treat, and management is focused on assisting the patient to quit smoking. Smokeless tobacco such as snuff or chewing tobacco, nicotine replacement gums and patches, and exposure to large amounts of secondary passive smoke can all aggravate the disease process. Anticoagulants, vasodilators, and antiplatelet agents have no proven effectiveness. Calcium channel blockers can be beneficial in reducing the severity of vasospastic episodes. Daily intravenous infusions of Iloprost, a prostacyclin analog, has achieved some success in Europe, and intraarterial thrombolytic therapy with low-dose streptokinase has also achieved modest success. Surgical revascularization is seldom effective because of the diffuse nature of the disease and the involvement of distal vessels. Gene therapy has been successful in stimulating the development of collateral circulation in controlled research studies.

Spinal cord stimulators have been used in select cases to control chronic ischemic pain. Sympathectomy may be needed to eliminate vasospasm and improve healing of superficial ischemic ulcerations, but to be effective it must be performed early in the disease process. Amputation of the involved extremity may be the end result of treatment.

Patient/Family Education. It is crucial to help the patient and family to understand the direct relationship between cigarette smoking and the disease process. Complete abstinence from smoking is essential if the disease is to be successfully controlled. Most patients improve when they stop smoking. In addition to supporting the patient's smoking cessation efforts, the nurse teaches the patient to avoid exposure to the cold and to protect the extremities from injury and trauma.

Raynaud's Disease

Etiology/Epidemiology

Raynaud's disease is an episodic vasospastic disorder of the small cutaneous arteries, usually involving the fingers and toes. It affects an estimated 5% to 10% of the population and 93% of those affected are women. When Raynaud's disease occurs in isolation it is called Raynaud's syndrome. When it occurs in conjunction with another disease process, such as systemic sclerosis, systemic lupus erythematosus, rheumatoid arthritis, hematologic disorders, trauma, and arterial obstruction, it is termed Raynaud's phenomenon. The disease is characterized by bilateral, intermittent vasospasm of the small arteries in the digits. The symptoms are commonly precipitated by exposure to the cold, emotional upset, caffeine ingestion, and tobacco use and occur more frequently in winter and in damp, cool climates. Other contributing factors include occupation-related trauma and pressure to the fingertips such as that experienced by typists, pianists, and workers who use handheld vibrating equipment.

Pathophysiology

Vasoconstriction occurs as the result of activation of the alpha-2 receptors in the blood vessels by norepinephrine. Persons with Raynaud's disease may have an increased number of alpha-2 receptors or a decreased number of beta-receptors and calcitonin, which are responsible for vasodilation. The pathologic sequence of Raynaud's disease/phenomenon is not completely understood.

Symptoms of Raynaud's disease are symmetric and occur bilaterally in two distinct phases. In the ischemic phase the fingers are cold, pale, and numb. This is followed by a hyperemic phase in which redness, swelling, and throbbing pain in the fingers develop from rebound vessel dilation. The vasospasm is confined to the digits and does not usually include the thumb. Only the tip of the finger distal to the metacarpophalangeal joint is typically affected. Toes may also be affected in the same pattern.

The classic triphasic color changes of pallor, cyanosis, and rubor of one or more digits of both hands is considered to be diagnostic for Raynaud's disease (Figure 25-6), although the

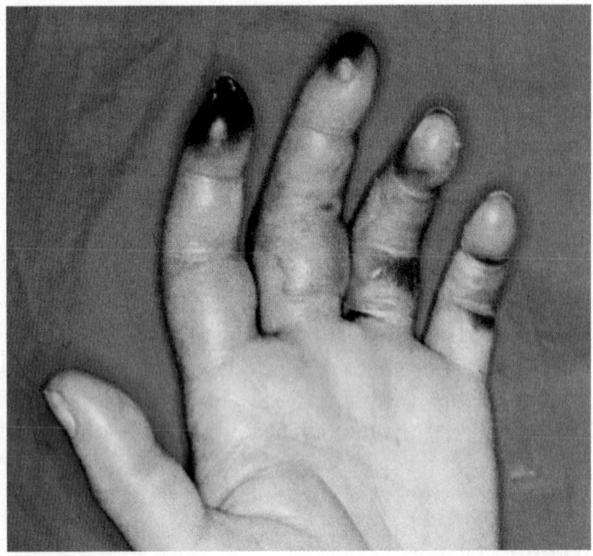

Figure 25-6 Raynaud's phenomenon.

cyanotic phase is not always present. Normal radial and ulnar pulses are usually preserved. Episodes typically last just minutes, but in severe cases they can persist for hours. Lesions and gangrenous ulcers on the fingertips can develop from persistent ischemia. A positive antinuclear antibody (ANA) is present in 25% of patients.

Collaborative Care Management

Raynaud's disease has no known cure and in mild cases does not require treatment because the episodes are self-limiting, but it is important to rule out the presence of an underlying treatable condition. Treatment for primary Raynaud's disease focuses on preventing vasospasm and includes keeping the extremity warm and advising the patient to avoid tobacco, as both cold and nicotine are frequent vasospasm triggers. Drug therapy includes the use of calcium channel blockers, vascular smooth muscle relaxants, and vasodilators, although their effectiveness is highly variable. A prostacyclin analog, iloprost, has been successfully used to improve circulation and decrease pain in research subjects. Biofeedback techniques to increase skin temperature and prevent spasm have been used successfully with selected patients. Sympathectomy may be necessary in severe cases. Persistent uncontrolled spasms can cause gangrene and necessitate amputation.

Patient/Family Education. Patient education focuses on reassuring the patient that episodes of vasospasm can be effectively managed in most cases. The nurse explores ways to help the patient minimize exposure to the cold through the use of layered clothing. The use of mittens is encouraged because they do not constrict the fingers and allow the fingers to touch and warm each other. The use of socks can also be important. The nurse cautions the patient to avoid direct contact with ice and frozen food and to use gloves when handling cold products. Stress management and relaxation techniques can often be effective in decreasing the frequency of vasospastic episodes and preventing the need for surgical intervention.

BOX 25-5 Types of Amputations

- Below-the-knee amputation (BKA)
- Above-the-knee amputation (AKA)
- Amputation of the foot and ankle (Syme's)
- Amputation of the foot between metatarsus and tarsus (Hey's or Lisfranc's)
- Hip disarticulation—removal of the limb from the hip joint
- Hemicorporectomy—removal of half of the body from the pelvis and lumbar areas

NURSING MANAGEMENT OF PATIENT UNDERGOING AMPUTATION

Amputation is a surgical intervention commonly used in the treatment of advanced peripheral vascular disease. Amputation is usually considered to be a last resort treatment used when other medical and surgical interventions have failed to preserve the limb. Amputation, although radical and traumatic for the patient, can provide relief from chronic pain, the potential to walk again with the use of a prosthesis, and an improved quality of life.

More than 110,000 amputations are performed each year in the United States, and 91.7% of them are lower extremity amputations. Diabetes is the underlying pathology that results in severe peripheral vascular disease in more than 50% of all cases. Amputation occurs in patients with diabetes 15 times more frequently than in other patients with chronic arterial occlusive disease. Birth defects, trauma, and malignancy are other possible causes of amputation.

Chronic tissue ischemia that results in necrosis and then gangrene is the most common pathologic sequence that results in amputation. Peripheral pulses become decreased or absent as the ischemia worsens and the patient experiences progressive pain. Gangrene in diabetics is typically the dry type. The tissues dry, become cold and black, and actually begin to separate from the body. The toes are usually affected first, and then the gangrene moves steadily upward toward the knee. Moist gangrene is more common after limb trauma when the area is filled with blood and infectious material.

The goal of amputation is to preserve as much of the functional length of the extremity as possible while removing all infected or ischemic tissue. Lower extremity amputations are roughly classified as below the knee (BKA), or above the knee (AKA) as described in Box 25-5. Before the 1960s most leg amputations were performed above the knee to increase the chance for successful wound healing. As diagnostic testing has improved, clinicians are able to more accurately assess the adequacy of perfusion to the extremity. This enables BKAs to be performed more frequently and with greater success. Below-knee amputations preserve the knee joint, which allows the patient an increased range of motion and improves the likelihood of successful prosthesis fitting after surgery. A BKA is usually made at the lower third of the leg, leaving a 12 to 18 cm stump. An AKA can be made at any level, although a longer stump makes it easier to fit a prosthesis.

The two major techniques for amputation are closed and open. With the closed method the bone is cut approximately 2 inches shorter than the skin flap. This creates a stump that is suitable for weight bearing with a prosthesis. The incision is closed with the sutures placed in a posterior position to avoid the weight-bearing area. This reduces the chances of irritation from the prosthesis. Drains are inserted to prevent excessive swelling and to allow for the removal of old blood, fluid, and infectious matter. The open amputation is used most commonly when infection is present in the limb. The bone and muscle are cut at the same level, and the wound is left open to allow for drainage. Wound closure is usually achieved at a future point through a second surgical procedure.

PREOPERATIVE CARE

The preoperative period focuses on the careful evaluation and preparation of the patient for surgery. The medical goal is to ensure that the patient is in the best possible physical state to undergo extensive surgery. Diagnostic testing is completed using Doppler ultrasound, thermography, radioisotope clearance, and arteriogram to accurately assess the circulation in the limb and determine the likelihood of successful healing after surgery. Stabilization of diabetes is critical but may be difficult if infection is present in the affected limb. A physical therapy consultation is initiated to plan an effective exercise program that can begin to strengthen the muscles needed for crutch walking and postoperative rehabilitation. Teaching about transfer techniques and the safe use of crutches and walkers is initiated before surgery when pain is not as distracting for the patient. An over-bed trapeze increases the patient's independence in self-care activities.

The nurse focuses on teaching and patient support in the preoperative period. Amputation can have tremendous psychologic implications for the patient. This radical change in body image can evoke feelings of loss, anger, fear, shock, and denial. A period of anger and depression is expected, and the nurse validates the appropriateness of these emotions and encourages the patient to express the feelings. The nurse assesses the patient's coping resources and the support systems available. The patient's family should be involved in this process to the degree that it is comfortable for the patient. A thorough home assessment is an important step in beginning the process of discharge planning.

Preoperative teaching focuses on the care that will be delivered in the postoperative period, pain management strategies, plans for prosthesis fitting, and a basic introduction to stump care routines. The patient is told to anticipate the occurrence of phantom limb sensation, a sensation of aching, tingling, itching, or simple "awareness" of the amputated part. Phantom limb sensation is an expected but still extremely disconcerting aspect of amputation. Sensations typically decrease over time but initially can be quite strong. If chronic pain has been present in the extremity, the patient is also taught about the possibility of phantom limb pain. Phantom limb pain is similar to the ischemic pain experienced before surgery and represents a complex management problem. Phantom sensation occurs in most patients, but fortunately phantom pain is much less common.

POSTOPERATIVE CARE

Maintaining Physiologic Stability

Monitoring for complications is an important aspect of initial postoperative nursing care. Vital signs and pulse oximetry values are closely monitored until the patient stabilizes. The wound dressing and drainage systems are assessed at least every 2 hours to monitor for excessive bleeding because hemorrhage is the primary immediate complication of amputation. A surgical tourniquet is kept available at the bedside in case of acute bleeding. Some serosanguineous drainage is expected, but the appearance of bright red blood should be reported immediately. Tachycardia and hypotension are classic indicators of bleeding and early shock. The stump dressing is not usually disturbed for the first 2 to 3 days, but the nurse assesses the operative site as thoroughly as possible. Careful intake and output records are maintained, as well as flow rates for all intravenous lines. Respiratory care and assessment are also critical. The patient is encouraged to begin deep breathing, position changes, and coughing as needed to clear the airway, as soon as he or she is alert. Effective pain management is a critical intervention because severe pain can adversely affect the patient's vital signs, decrease the ability to deep breathe and clear the airway, and compromise the patient's ability to participate in self-care.

Maintaining Appropriate Stump Positioning

The stump is elevated on pillows to reduce postoperative pain and swelling for the first 24 hours. Stump positioning and exercise become critical interventions after this initial period. The stump is supported but not elevated because of the risk of flexion contractures. The flexor muscles in the extremities are stronger than the opposing extensors, and the patient needs to counteract the flexion pull effectively if hip and knee contractures are to be prevented. Position changes are made at least every 2 hours, and the patient is encouraged to lie prone for at least 20 to 30 minutes twice a day to stretch the hip flexor muscles. Positioning is also used to prevent both the abducted and adducted position. Any change in normal hip alignment makes it difficult for the patient to achieve an acceptable prosthesis fit and normal gait. The patient continues to work with the physical therapist to build strength in the muscles needed for ambulation and is encouraged to be out of bed for increasing intervals each day.

Conditioning the Stump

Stump care is a critical nursing intervention in the early postoperative period, and it remains a major management concern throughout the healing and rehabilitation period. Some surgeons apply an immediate temporary prosthesis after amputation. These devices are composed of a rigid plastic bandage that is applied around the closed stump and attached to a prosthetic pylon with an ankle and foot assembly. The device is applied in the operating room while the patient is still anesthetized. Its main advantages are the potential for early weight bearing and reduction of edema. The major disadvantage is the inability to directly assess wound healing in the stump. If delayed prosthesis fitting is planned, the stump is initially wrapped snugly in dressings and Ace wraps to provide compression and minimize edema. Examples of standard prostheses are illustrated in Figure 25-7.

Proper stump bandaging supports shaping of the stump for eventual prosthesis fitting and weight bearing. A compression bandage is worn at all times, except for needed skin care, and needs to be correctly reapplied whenever it becomes loose or wrinkled. The shrinker bandage typically is reapplied at least daily, and the nurse teaches the patient how to correctly apply the bandage as soon as possible. The bandages need to be washed and changed regularly, and the nurse instructs the patient in the importance of keeping these wrappings clean. Figure 25-8 illustrates the correct method of applying compression or shrinker bandages to above-knee and below-knee amputations.

Daily stump care is also part of the conditioning process. The healing of the incision is closely monitored, and the patient is instructed to carefully assess the stump each day for signs of redness or irritation. The stump is washed daily after healing is complete and thoroughly air dried before rewrapping. No lotion, oil, or powder should be applied to the stump surface without specific orders from the surgeon or rehabilitation specialist. The goal is to achieve a well-healed and appropriately shaped stump whose surface skin is tough enough to absorb the pressures of weight bearing with a prosthesis. Guidelines for care of a patient following an amputation are summarized in the Guidelines for Safe Practice box.

Supporting Independence in Self-Care

The physical therapist continues to work with the patient on range of motion, ambulation with an assistive device, and general conditioning. Building upper body strength, particularly triceps strength, is emphasized because these muscles are critical to crutch walking. The therapist teaches the patient the principles of safe transferring, and this skill is practiced on the unit under the nurse's supervision. The loss of the weight and mass of the amputated limb can significantly alter the patient's center of gravity, and the nurse is alert to the patient's need for support while relearning upright balance. A fall can have serious adverse consequences on wound healing.

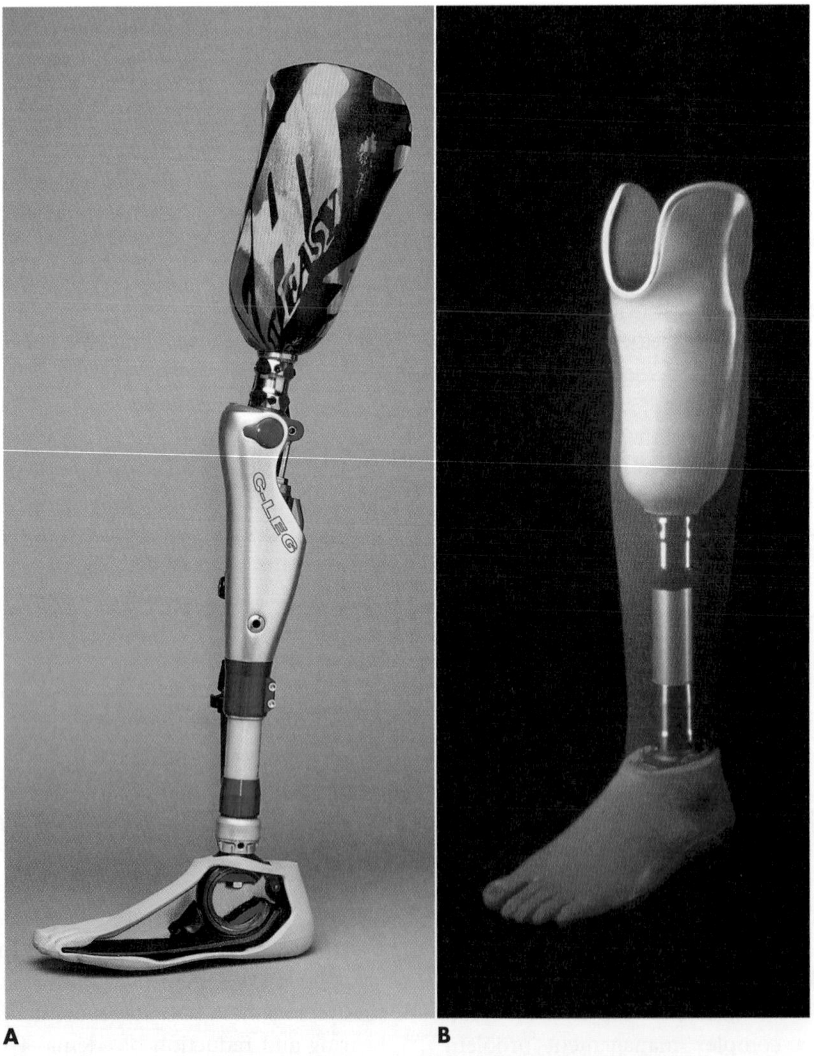

Figure 25-7 Permanent lower-extremity prostheses. **A**, Above-knee prosthesis. **B**, Below-knee prosthesis.

Patient/Family Education

Hospitalizations for all conditions are being steadily shortened, and planning for discharge must begin before surgery. The nurse creates a teaching plan that includes time for the patient to learn stump care, transfer techniques, safe ambulation, prevention of complications and contractures, and the importance of follow-up care from the multidisciplinary care team. Referral to a prosthetist may not occur until after discharge, and achieving a good prosthetic fit can take as long as 2 years because the healing stump continues to shrink and alter in shape. The process is slow and often frustrating, and the nurse needs to help the patient and family anticipate the long-term nature of the rehabilitation period. A Nursing Care Plan for a patient with a lower extremity amputation is found on pp. 782 to 784.

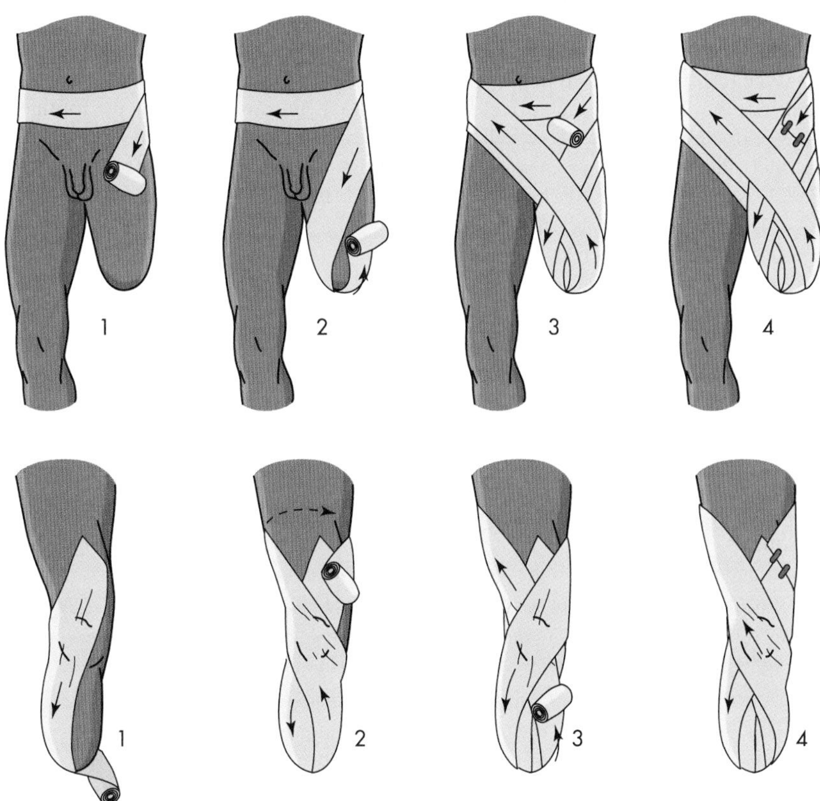

Figure 25-8 *Top,* Correct method for bandaging midthigh amputation stump. Note that bandage must be anchored around patient's waist. *Bottom,* Correct method for bandaging midcalf amputation stump. Note that bandage need not be anchored around the waist.

Guidelines for Safe Practice

Care of the Patient After an Amputation

- Assess stump and monitor drainage for color and amount; report signs of increased drainage.
- Position patient with no flexion at hip or knee to avoid contractures; encourage prone position.
- Maintain patient in low-Fowler's or flat position after AKA.
- Support stump with pillow for first 24 hours (according to physician preference and avoiding flexion); place rolled bath blanket along outer aspect to prevent external rotation.
- Encourage exercises to prevent thromboembolism:
  - Active ROM of unaffected leg, ankle rotations and pumps
  - Use of overhead trapeze when moving in bed
  - Push-ups from sitting position in bed
  - Quadriceps sets (see Chapter 18)
  - Lifting stump and buttocks off bed while lying flat on back to strengthen abdominal muscles
- Teach care of stump:
  - Inspect for redness, blister, and abrasions.
  - Wash stump with mild soap, rinse with water, and pat dry.
  - Avoid use of alcohol, oils, and creams.
  - Remove stump bandage or stump sock and reapply as needed; use firm smooth figure-of-8 Ace wrapping (Figure 25-8) to reduce swelling and shape stump (if rigid dressing not used).
- Encourage patient to ambulate using correct crutch-walking technique.:
  - Keep elbows extended; limit elbow flexion to 30 degrees or less.
  - Avoid pressure on axilla.
  - Bear weight on palms of hands, not on axilla.
  - Maintain upright posture (head up, chest up, abdomen in, pelvis in, foot straight).
  - Monitor patient's ability to use a prosthesis.

AKA, Above-knee amputation; *ROM,* range of motion.

Nursing Care Plan — *Patient Undergoing Amputation*

DATA Mr. L. is a 68-year-old man who has a long history of type 2 diabetes mellitus, hypertension, and peripheral vascular disease. He has been experiencing progressively increased levels of claudication in his right leg over the past 6 months. He is unable to walk across a room without pain and has begun experiencing pain at rest during the night, which forces him to get out of bed and put his legs in a dependent position. One month ago he developed an ulcer on his great toe that has progressed to gangrene despite aggressive treatment. Yesterday, he underwent a right below-the-knee amputation. Mr. L. tolerated the surgery well, although both he and his wife indicate that the idea of the amputation is terrifying and he is concerned about becoming disabled and a burden to his family. Mrs. L. is employed and concerned about being available to help Mr. L. when he returns home.

His routine care orders are:
- Out of bed to chair with assistance
- Patient-controlled analgesia with morphine for pain, basal administration plus bolus
- Elevating stump when out of bed; avoiding use of pillows beneath the stump when in bed
- Stump monitoring for edema, bleeding; evaluation of Hemovac drainage every shift
- Blood glucose monitoring per routine with sliding-scale insulin coverage as needed
- Physical therapy referral for evaluation of crutch walking
- Prosthetic referral for prosthetic limb

NURSING DIAGNOSIS **Anticipatory grieving related to loss of limb**
GOALS/OUTCOMES Will verbalize grief over loss of limb

NOC Suggested Outcomes
- Coping (1302)
- Family Coping (2600)
- Grief Resolution (1304)

NIC Suggested Interventions
- Emotional Support (5270)
- Grief Work Facilitation (5290)
- Support System Enhancement (5440)

Nursing Interventions/Rationales
- Assess significance of loss to patient and family. *The significance of loss varies among individuals and families. Plans to facilitate grief are dependent on the patient's reaction to the loss.*
- Encourage patient/family to verbalize feelings. *Allows the opportunity for patient/family to ventilate feelings of anger and grief in a safe environment. Recognizing and verbalizing feelings is an essential step in working through grief.*
- Allow privacy for the expression of grief. *Grief is a personal experience that many individuals choose to deal with privately, at least initially. The patient may be reluctant to cry or demonstrate other expressions of grief unless privacy is provided.*
- Refer to mental health Clinical Nurse Specialist (CNS), support group, or rehabilitated amputee for counseling as needed. *Effective support and resolution of grief are necessary for the patient to successfully cope with needed lifestyle adjustments and changes.*

Evaluation Parameters
1. Expresses grief verbally
2. Verbalizes plan for resocialization

NURSING DIAGNOSIS **Acute pain related to tissue trauma and phantom limb sensation**
GOALS/OUTCOMES Will report satisfaction with pain control measures; will achieve pain-free status by discharge

NOC Suggested Outcomes
- Pain Control (1605)
- Comfort Level (2100)
- Pain Level (2102)

NIC Suggested Interventions
- Analgesic Administration (2210)
- Pain Management (1400)
- Coping Enhancement (5230)

Nursing Interventions/Rationales
- Assess and monitor character, intensity, and location of pain. *To establish baseline for later comparisons.*
- Administer prescribed analgesics. *Analgesics decrease the transmission and perception of pain stimulus. Adequate pain control is essential for optimal physical therapy and rehabilitation.*
- Explain the causes, sensations, and methods of treatment for phantom pain. *Phantom pain is similar to pain experienced before the amputation. Warning the patient about the possibility of phantom pain helps the patient cope with the sensations.*
- Encourage use of nonpharmacologic measures to control/reduce pain (relaxation exercises or distraction). *Many nonpharmacologic measures minimize pain perception.*

Nursing Care Plan *Patient Undergoing Amputation—cont'd*

Evaluation Parameters

1. Verbalizes relief of stump pain
2. Verbalizes understanding of phantom pain
3. Uses nonpharmacologic pain relief strategies

NURSING DIAGNOSIS **Risk for impaired physical mobility related to lack of experience with crutch walking, skill, and lack of physical endurance**

GOALS/OUTCOMES Will perform ADLs independently and without injury

NOC Suggested Outcomes

- Mobility Level (0208)
- Adherence Behavior (1600)

NIC Suggested Interventions

- Self-Care Assistance (1800)
- Activity Therapy (4310)
- Exercise Therapy: Balance (0222)
- Amputation Care (3420)

Nursing Interventions/Rationales

- Assess upper extremity strength, cardiopulmonary status and endurance. *Upper body strength and optimal conditioning are essential to achieve mobility and perform bed-to-chair transfers.*
- Teach ROM and strengthening exercises. *To build endurance, strength, and flexibility.*
- Teach positioning and exercises to prevent flexion and abduction contractures. *Contractures will prevent proper fitting of prosthesis and thus limit rehabilitation progress.*
- Dangle or assist up to chair 12-24 hours after surgery. *To prevent loss of muscle strength from disuse or bed rest.*
- Teach the purpose and benefits of exercise and interventions. *Understanding why exercise is necessary and beneficial helps with exercise compliance.*

Evaluation Parameters

1. Maintains baseline range of motion
2. Uses assistive devices for ambulation
3. Remains free of contractures

NURSING DIAGNOSIS **Risk for impaired skin integrity related to incision and effects of diabetes on wound healing**

GOALS/OUTCOMES Patient will remain free of skin breakdown

NOC Suggested Outcomes

- Tissue Integrity: Skin & Mucous Membranes (1101)
- Wound Healing: Primary Intention (1102)

NIC Suggested Interventions

- Incision Site Care (3440)
- Infection Protection (6550)
- Skin Surveillance (3590)
- Amputation Care (3420)

Nursing Interventions/Rationales

- Assess stump for drainage or bleeding, edema, proximal pulses, and tissue perfusion. *Drainage or bleeding may indicate lack of healing or presence of complications such as infection. Edema, absent proximal pulses, and decreased tissue perfusion indicate compromised circulation, which predisposes the patient to skin breakdown.*
- Maintain dressing without wrinkles or constriction. *To prevent compromised circulation and resultant skin breakdown.*
- Teach patient on stump care, hygiene, and prosthesis care as indicated. *Meticulous skin care helps prevent infection and loss of skin integrity.*
- Teach signs and symptoms of decreased stump perfusion that need to be reported. *If tissue compromise occurs, it must be quickly recognized and reported so that immediate correction treatments can be implemented.*
- Monitor blood glucose levels before each meal and at bedtime. *Stress of surgery and infection can result in increased hyperglycemia and decreased healing, which predispose to skin breakdown.*

Evaluation Parameters

1. Wound shows evidence of healing
2. Demonstrates wound care, stump care, and prosthesis care accurately
3. Maintains blood glucose within normal limits

Continued

Nursing Care Plan — Patient Undergoing Amputation—cont'd

NURSING DIAGNOSIS **Risk for situational low self-esteem related to loss of limb and change in functional abilities**

GOALS/OUTCOMES Self-esteem will remain intact as evidenced by acceptance of body changes and participation in socialization.

NOC Suggested Outcomes
- Psychological Adjustment: Life Change (1305)
- Acceptance: Health Status (1300)
- Body Image (1200)
- Self-Esteem (1205)

NIC Suggested Interventions
- Coping Enhancement (5230)
- Emotional Support (5270)
- Body Image Enhancement (5220)
- Self-Esteem Enhancement (5400)

Nursing Interventions/Rationales
- Assess patient's view of self and role relationships. *Data regarding the patient's view of self is essential to plan appropriate interventions for supporting self-esteem.*
- Encourage expression of feelings about self. *Allows the opportunity for patient to verbalize feelings in a safe environment.*
- Assess significant other's view of loss. *To determine if intervention is necessary and to determine the degree of support the significant other will be able to provide the patient.*
- Clarify misconceptions. *Patient may be needlessly stressed due to misunderstandings about treatments or prognosis, which can impact self-esteem and coping abilities.*
- Facilitate use of prosthesis as early as possible. *Increased mobility and ability to perform self-care fosters independence and positive self-esteem.*
- Assist patient to identify personal strengths. *Identifying strengths helps the patient focus on present and future possibilities rather than losses.*
- Refer for counseling as needed. *Counseling may be necessary to help the patient cope with his loss.*

Evaluation Parameters
1. Verbalizes feelings about impact of loss
2. Regains confidence in his ability to accomplish goals (physical, social, emotional)
3. Identifies positive characteristics about self

GERONTOLOGIC CONSIDERATIONS

Lower limb amputations are commonly performed on older patients. The patient's previous ability to ambulate and perform self-care profoundly affect the ability to make a successful transition to independence after amputation. Use of a prosthesis for ambulation requires strength and energy. If the older adult is already weakened from the presence of other debilitating health problems, it may not be possible to fit a prosthesis, even if the stump heals adequately. Wheelchair mobility may be a more realistic option. Most older adults also require at least short-term admission to a rehabilitation facility after discharge to continue with needed therapy.

SPECIAL ENVIRONMENTS FOR CARE

Critical Care

Patients who undergo lower extremity amputation usually do not require postoperative management in a critical care unit unless serious complications develop. After the initial stabilization and recovery from anesthesia in the postanesthesia care unit, the patient returns to a general surgical floor.

Community-Based Care

Patients are not able to complete their recovery and rehabilitation in the acute care setting and planning for ongoing management and rehabilitation after discharge is an important consideration that needs to be addressed early in the hospitalization. The degree and duration of support needed by the patient are determined by age, baseline health status, financial and social resources, and living situation. The nurse is responsible for initiating the careful assessment of these variables and then making referrals as indicated through social services, home health agencies, and community physical therapy to ensure that the patient receives all needed support. The family is involved in all planning if possible because significant modifications may need to be considered or implemented in the home environment to accommodate the patient's mobility limitations and establish a safe environment. An occupational therapist can often assist with this needed planning.

Acute Arterial Occlusive Disease

Etiology

Acute arterial occlusion can occur in both healthy and diseased arteries. The occlusion can result from an arterial thrombus that forms in an atherosclerotic artery, an embolism in a healthy artery, or trauma. The occlusion typically occurs suddenly and without warning. An embolus that forms in the heart or an atherosclerotic aneurysm is the most common etiology. The embolus dislodges and travels to the lungs if it originates in the right side of the heart or to anywhere in the systemic circulation if it originates in the left side of the heart. The occlusion typically occurs at sites of vessel bifurcation or narrowing.

Epidemiology

Acute arterial occlusion can occur in any patient in the presence of appropriate risk factors. Patients with rheumatic heart disease, artificial heart valves, myocardial infarction, and atrial fibrillation are at particular risk because the incidence of thrombus formation with these conditions is high. Postoperative vascular surgery patients, patients who have undergone invasive arterial procedures, and trauma patients with lacerated or compressed arteries are also at risk.

Pathophysiology

When an acute arterial occlusion occurs, the blood supply distal to the obstruction is abruptly interrupted. The extent and severity of the resulting symptoms depend on the location and size of the obstruction and the patency of the surrounding vessels. When peripheral vascular disease is already present in the extremity, symptoms are likely to be much more severe. Acute embolic occlusion usually occurs suddenly, and the pain is severe and unrelenting. Neither rest nor activity relieves it. The primary symptoms of acute occlusion can be clearly described through the "six Ps" of neurovascular assessment. The limb exhibits pain, pallor, pulselessness, paresthesia, paralysis, and poikilothermia (coolness to the touch). Development of paralysis in the affected limb is considered to be a late and ominous sign that usually reflects the ischemic death of nerve cells supplying the extremity. Patients are often unable either to rest or sleep due to the severity of the pain. Severe ischemia rapidly progresses to necrosis and gangrene and will require limb amputation if prompt intervention does not successfully restore perfusion. The window of opportunity for successful treatment can be mere hours in severe cases. The classic signs and symptoms of acute occlusion are summarized in the Clinical Manifestations box.

Clinical Manifestations

Acute Arterial Occlusion

Pain: when the obstruction is complete, the pain is severe and constant and is not relieved by rest.
Pallor: the limb typically appears pale or mottled.
Pulselessness: the peripheral pulses are either diminished or completely absent over the path of the affected vessel.
Paresthesia: numbness, tingling, and burning in the extremity are common when ischemia is severe.
Poikilothermia: the limb is typically cool, if not frankly cold, to the touch.
Paralysis: mobility of the part is limited. Development of frank paralysis is an ominous sign because it may indicate the ischemic death of nerves in the extremity.
If perfusion is not rapidly restored, the limb will develop signs of necrosis and gangrene, often in a matter of hours.

NOTE: Symptoms typically occur suddenly and are severe.

Collaborative Care Management

Diagnostic Tests. The diagnosis of acute occlusion is primarily established through physical assessment of the affected limb. Noninvasive tests such as Doppler ultrasonography and ankle-brachial index measurements are commonly used. Magnetic resonance imaging (MRI) or angiography may be used to map the location and severity of the obstruction before surgical intervention.

Medications. Drug therapy may be used as a primary treatment modality or as a follow-up to interventions such as embolectomy. The goal of drug therapy is to dissolve the clot and prevent further clot formation. Anticoagulant therapy with continuous intravenous heparin is usually initiated immediately to prevent further enlargement of the thrombus. However, heparin does not dissolve existing clots. Emboli may be treated with thrombolytic agents when the risks associated with ischemia outweigh the risk of bleeding. Thrombolytics can also prevent the occurrence of complications associated with the more invasive procedures. Urokinase is the most commonly used drug. Its effectiveness depends on the severity and location of the obstruction.

A percutaneous arterial catheter is inserted into the femoral artery and advanced to the site of obstruction. This allows the drug to be directly administered to the thrombus. The thrombus is dissolved over 24 to 48 hours. The risk of bleeding complications is high; therefore patients need to be carefully selected and screened.

Arterial thrombi and emboli can also trigger severe vessel spasm. Spasmolytic agents such as papaverine, tolazoline, and calcium channel blockers may be administered to relieve or prevent arterial spasm. Blood pressure control is also important for any patient with an acute arterial condition, especially if surgical intervention is planned. Drug therapy is used as needed to manage the patient's blood pressure.

Anticoagulant therapy may also be initiated after successful treatment of the thrombus. Any patient considered to be at risk for future embolization is usually prescribed long-term anticoagulant therapy with an oral agent such as warfarin (Coumadin) to prevent future episodes.

Treatment. Treatment of an acute arterial occlusion may involve the use of an endovascular procedure that allows for treatment within the artery itself to remove blockages. Possible procedures include balloon angioplasty or PTA, intraluminal ultrasound, laser angioplasty, mechanical atherectomy, and stent placement (see the descriptions on p. 772).

Surgical Management. Surgery is indicated in the event of life or limb-threatening arterial occlusion when other measures have failed to restore blood flow. An open embolectomy or thrombectomy may be performed to remove the obstructive clot from the vessel lumen. Bypass graft procedures previously discussed may also be performed.

Diet. Diet does not play a major or direct role in the treatment of acute arterial occlusion. Patients usually receive nothing by mouth (NPO) while the workup is completed and treatment decisions are made. An empty stomach minimizes aspiration risks associated with both interventional and surgical procedures. The NPO status is extremely important when general anesthesia is used, particularly with abdominal procedures. Patients are gradually advanced to a normal diet after surgery. Ileus is common after surgery on the aorta, and meticulous abdominal assessment is important. Once a normal oral diet is resumed, attention is again directed toward encouraging the patient to adhere to a heart-healthy diet of low-fat, low-cholesterol foods. Diet is particularly important when diabetes complicates the management of vascular problems.

Activity. After interventional procedures patients are kept on bed rest until the invasive arterial lines and thrombolytic agents can be discontinued. Protocols vary based on the nature and extent of the intervention, but bed rest is commonly maintained for 6 to 24 hours. Early ambulation is important after vascular surgery and helps prevent the complications of immobility. Patients are assisted out of bed the first day after surgery as long as they are hemodynamically stable. Activity is then steadily progressed. A daily walking program is usually recommended at discharge. If possible, the patient is referred to a structured vascular rehabilitation program. Exercise helps support blood flow, improves overall functioning, and increases the patient's general sense of well-being. Heavy lifting is restricted for at least 6 weeks after surgery. Sexual activity may be resumed as soon as the patient's comfort level permits.

Referrals. A pain service may be consulted in the preoperative period to help manage the patient's severe ischemic pain. Both patient-controlled analgesia and epidural administration are commonly used. A nutrition referral may be appropriate for diet teaching before discharge. Both physical and occupational therapists are essential collaborative partners in the patient's management. They assist the patient to develop a manageable exercise plan and adapt daily activities to maintain independence in self-care. Home health referrals may be appropriate for patients who experience complications, or for older adults who live alone.

NURSING MANAGEMENT OF PATIENT UNDERGOING VASCULAR BYPASS SURGERY

PREOPERATIVE CARE

Preoperative care focuses on the physical, emotional, and psychosocial preparation of a severely stressed patient. The patient may be undergoing a variety of emergency tests and procedures and is likely to have extensive needs for teaching and support. This is a very high stress situation for the patient and family. Pain, medication effects, anxiety, and uncertainty all influence the ability of the patient and family to absorb the information being presented. The nurse performs frequent vital sign and neurovascular assessments to monitor for changes in patient status. The nurse is an important liaison between the patient and the rest of the treatment team and attempts to keep the channels of communication open.

POSTOPERATIVE CARE

The patient receives meticulous general surgical care because the complications of vascular surgery can affect virtually any organ system. The more invasive the procedure, the greater the risk of complications. Surgery involving the aorta creates the greatest risk. Potential complications include bleeding, infection at the graft site, heart failure, myocardial infarction (MI), dysrhythmias, stroke, renal failure, and injury to adjacent organs and tissues (e.g., ureters, bowel, nerves). The nurse is responsible for meticulous postoperative monitoring of all major body systems. A sample Clinical Pathway that outlines care provided to a patient undergoing bypass graft surgery follows on pp. 787 and 788. Care of the patient undergoing surgery for an acute vascular occlusion is summarized in the Guidelines for Safe Practice box.

Supporting Circulation and Perfusion

Patients with vascular disease also frequently have problems with coronary artery disease or hypertension. Cardiac monitoring, vital signs, and peripheral vascular assessments are all critical nursing interventions. The nurse monitors for the development of dysrhythmias or heart failure. The nurse integrates data from vital sign measurements, pulse oximetry, arterial blood gases, cardiac enzymes, electrolytes, and Swan-Ganz catheter measurements.

Graft patency is a priority concern in the postoperative period because the risk of reocclusion from thrombosis, restenosis, or debris is significant. The nurse monitors the patient's

Guidelines for Safe Practice
The Patient With an Acute Arterial Occlusion

- Monitor the patient for any change in circulatory status to the affected limb. Monitor temperature, color, sensation, and pain. A change in these parameters may indicate worsening occlusion.
- Monitor peripheral pulses bilaterally for presence, strength, quality, and symmetry.
- Keep the extremity warm, but do not apply direct heat or heat lamps.
- Avoid chilling.
- Maintain bed rest unless activity is specifically ordered.
- Keep the extremity flat or in a slightly dependent position to promote perfusion.
- Use an overbed cradle to protect a painful extremity from the pressure of linens.
- Use a sheepskin and 4-inch foam mattress beneath the extremity.
- Do not use the knee gatch on the bed; instruct the patient not to cross the legs at the knee or ankle.
- Do not apply any restraint to the affected limb.
- Keep the head of the bed low to support circulation to the lower extremities.
- Monitor the effects of anticoagulant and thrombolytic therapy. Monitor INR, partial thromboplastin time, platelets, and other coagulation studies.
- Assess for local and systemic bleeding.

INR, International normalized ratio.

clinical pathway *Agram + Peripheral Bypass Surgery*

DATE:	PREOPERATIVE/DAY OF AGRAM	DAY OF SURGERY	POD #1	POD #2	POD #3	POD #4	POD #5
Assessment	Adult Screening Tool H&P and Surgical Consent Emotional/Financial Needs Discharge Needs Ht./Wt.	Cardiac Monitoring if history of CAD VS per 4W guideline Vascular Checks q1° × then Systems assessment per 4W guideline	Cardiac Monitoring if history of CAD VS per 4W guideline Vascular checks Systems Assessment per 4W guideline Assess need for consults: PT/OT/ Rehab/Nutrition/ Speech/SW ________ if needed Daily weight	VS and vascular checks per 4W guideline Systems Assessment per 4W guideline Consults as appropriate Daily weight	VS and vascular checks per 4W guideline Systems Assessment per 4W guideline Daily weight	VS and vascular checks per 4W guideline Systems Assessment per 4W guideline Daily weight	VS and vascular checks per 4W guideline Systems Assessment per 4W guideline Daily weight
Tests	Peripheral Agram EKG, CXR Labs: CBC, Plt & diff, Pt & Ptt, Comp. Metab., Mg & Phos, UA, T&C 2 Units	Labs: per PVD order set	Labs: per PVD order set	Labs: per PVD order set PVRs	Labs: per PVD order set	Labs: per PVD order set	Labs: per PVD order set
Activities	Flat bedrest 6 hours after agram then bedrest	OR→4 West Bedrest	OOB to chair→ slouch sit Ambulate with PT as tolerated Leg elevation to decrease swelling	OOB to chair 2-3 × Daily Ambulate with assistance in room or hallway Leg elevation	OOB to chair 2-× 3 daily Walk in hallway with assistance 2-3 × daily Leg elevation	OOB to chair 2-3 × daily Walk in hallway with minimal help 2-3 × daily Leg elevation	OOB to chair 2-3 × daily Walk in hallway with minimal help 2-3 × daily Leg elevation
Medications/ Treatments	Hibiclens shower PM before and AM of surgery Sheepskin and foot cradle to foot of bed Continue all meds DOS except: • Coumadin D/C 4 days prior • Glucophage, NSAIDS 48 hr prior • Insulin dose per TCV MD Foley catheter IVF	IVF ASA Ancef on call to OR Meds per TCV order set PCA for pain Foley catheter O_2 Incentive Spirometer q1° Electrolyte Replace per TCV order set	D/C IVF ASA Resume home meds PCA for pain D/C Foley Wean O_2 Incentive Spirometer q2° Electrolyte Replace per TCV order set	ASA Continue Home meds D/C PCA and transition to pain pills D/C O2 Incentive Spirometer q2° while awake Incision Care with NSS BID Ace wrap operative leg per MD order Electrolyte Replace per TCV order set	ASA Continue Home Meds Pain Pills Incentive Spirometer q2° while awake Incision Care with NSS BID Ace wrap per MD order Electrolyte Replace per TCV order set	ASA Continue Home Meds Pain Pills Incentive Spirometer q2° while awake Incision Care with NSS BID Ace wrap per MD order Electrolyte Replace per TCV order set	ASA Continue Home Meds Pain Pills Incentive Spirometer q2° while awake Incision Care with NSS BID Ace wrap per MD order

References: Tucker, SM et al: *Patient care standards: collaborative practice planning guides,* ed 6, St Louis, 1996, Mosby; Perry AG, Potter PA: *Clinical nursing skills & techniques,* ed 4, St Louis, 1998, Mosby; Wooldridge-King, M: *AACN procedure manual for critical care,* ed 3, Philadelphia, 1993, WB Saunders; Finkelmeier BA: *Cardiothoracic surgical nursing,* 1997, St Louis, Mosby; Fahey V: *Vascular nursing,* ed 3, St Louis, 1998, Mosby.

Continued

clinical pathway *Agram + Peripheral Bypass Surgery–cont'd*

DATE:	PREOPERATIVE/DAY OF AGRAM	DAY OF SURGERY	POD #1	POD #2	POD #3	POD #4	POD #5
Nutrition	Regular diet NPO after midnight w/ sips of H_2O for meds	NPO Clear liquids when awake and alert then advance as tolerated	Heart Healthy diet as tolerated	Heart Healthy Diet	Heart Healthy Diet	Heart Healthy Diet	Heart Healthy Diet
Discharge Planning/ Instruction	Pre-op Teaching: • Care Map • Ed. Folder • Incentive Spirometer	Orient family to 4W visitors lounge Reinforce Preop Teaching	Begin Disch Teaching: • Activity Restrictions • New Meds • Heart Healthy Diet Review Disch Needs	Continue Disch. Teaching • Incision Care • Ace wrap to affected extremity Plan for Disch. Needs	Review Disch. Teaching Home Health Referral prn Pt/family return demonstrates incision care	Reinforce Disch. Teaching Vascular Rehab Referral or information given Home Health Referral prn	
Outcomes	Ready for Surgery Stable s/p Agram	Recovery from Anesthesia and Vascular Surgery Hemodynamic Stability including intact pulse exam Pain Control	Hemodynamic Stability Vascular Stability Pain Control Skin Integrity Increase ADL Increase Mobility Discharge Teaching	Hemodynamic Stability Vascular Stability Pain Control Skin Integrity Increase ADL Increase Mobility Discharge Teaching	Hemodynamic Stability Vascular Stability Pain Control Skin Integrity Increase ADL Increase Mobility Discharge Teaching	Hemodynamic Stability Vascular Stability Pain Control Skin Integrity Increase ADL Increase Mobility Discharge Teaching May meet disch. criteria: disch. home w/ home care instruc. & orders	ADL Independence Independent or Minimal Assist Mobility Meets discharge criteria: disch. Home w/ home care instructions & orders Return clinic appt made

ALTERNATIVE PATHWAY OR PLAN OF CARE INITATED FOR THIS PATIENT ON DATE ____ INITIALS ____

peripheral pulses and limb temperature, as well as the degree of pain, pallor, sensation, and movement.

The initiation of anticoagulant therapy increases the risk of bleeding from the suture line and graft anastamoses. The nurse closely monitors appropriate laboratory values such as hemoglobin, hematocrit, and coagulation studies. These values can alert the clinician to potential bleeding. Body excretions, particularly nasogastric secretions, are tested for blood. The nurse also monitors all incision and arteriogram sites for signs of bleeding. Measuring the patient's abdominal girth and limb circumferences provides an objective means to assess for distention from either internal bleeding or edema.

Preventing Respiratory Complications

Atelectasis is the most common cause of fever in the first 24 hours after surgery. Atelectasis can progress rapidly to pulmonary infection if aggressive pulmonary toilet measures are not instituted. The nurse encourages the patient to deep breathe and cough to clear the airway as needed and to use an incentive spirometer frequently. Early ambulation is a critical intervention. Patients with abdominal and chest incisions need lots of encouragement plus effective pain management to assist them in complying with essential respiratory and ambulation protocols. Chest percussion and postural drainage are initiated if needed.

Supporting Fluid Balance

The kidneys are at particular risk after bypass surgery because many of the procedures involve the aorta or femoral arteries. Hypotension, hypovolemia, and trauma to the kidneys or ureters during surgery can all lead to acute postoperative renal failure. The nurse carefully measures and records the patient's intake and output and daily weight, and monitors laboratory values of BUN, creatinine, and serum electrolytes. The urine is assessed for signs of myoglobinuria, indicative of tissue damage.

Promoting Wound Healing

Wound healing problems and infection are common after vascular surgery, particularly in diabetic and malnourished patients. The incision is cleaned with saline solution at least twice daily, and this technique is taught to the patient or a family member. With the surgeon's approval the patient may shower a few days after surgery. An antibacterial soap without lotions or perfume is suggested. Tub baths are not recommended because of the risk of contamination from standing water. The patient and family are taught the signs and symptoms of wound infection, complications to monitor for after discharge, and the importance of promptly reporting any complications to the surgeon. Infection in the graft is an extremely serious complication with a high mortality rate. Graft infection is usually accompanied by high fever, prolonged ileus, and a rapidly rising white blood cell count.

Patient/Family Education

Hospitalization is brief, and the patient and family need to receive adequate education for self-care at home. If the ability of the patient and family to provide adequate care is questioned by either the nurse or the family, a home health referral is promptly initiated. Patients receive standard discharge teaching concerning diet, activity, wound care, and resumption of normal activities. The nurse also provides the patient with information about risk factor reduction to decrease the risk of vascular problems and future complications. A summary of discharge instructions for the patient after vascular surgery is presented in the Patient Teaching box.

GERONTOLOGIC CONSIDERATIONS

Most individuals with vascular disease are older and have multiple health care needs. The presence of diabetes, coronary heart disease, poor nutrition, and other chronic illnesses and conditions may complicate surgical recovery. An acute arterial occlusion is an abrupt emergency situation that disrupts the patient and family's normal patterns of support and interaction. The older person's sudden need for significant support and physical assistance can have a tremendous impact on all concerned. The nurse uses the multidisciplinary care team to coordinate the patient's care and effectively plan for needed care and support after discharge. Discharge planning needs to be proactive, especially when the need for home care can be anticipated.

SPECIAL ENVIRONMENTS FOR CARE

Critical Care

Patients with multiple health problems may need close monitoring in an intensive care unit after vascular surgery. This is particularly true after abdominal and aortic procedures. A 1- to 2-day stay is standard to ensure hemodynamic stability, and successful extubation from ventilator support.

Patient Teaching

Discharge Teaching After Bypass Graft Surgery

- Shower daily, cleaning the incision gently with a mild or antibacterial soap without lotion or perfume added. Pat dry. Use a shower chair or stool to prevent falling if any instability is present. Avoid tub baths until healing is complete.
- Monitor the incision daily for signs of infection– redness, swelling, increased pain, discharge, or suture or staple separation. Report any of these symptoms to the surgeon promptly.
- Advance activity gradually as tolerated. Initiate a daily walking regimen. Expect to feel fatigued, and plan for rest periods throughout the day. Avoid lifting anything heavier than 10 pounds until approved by surgeon.
- Resume a low-fat, low-cholesterol diet as tolerated. Use supplements as needed to ensure adequate calories, protein, and vitamin C during the healing period. Four to six small meals a day are often better tolerated than three large ones.
- Avoid constipation and straining at stool. Eat a high-fiber diet with plenty of fluids to avoid constipation. Remain active. Take a stool softener daily plus a bulk-forming laxative if constipation cannot be managed through diet and fluids alone.
- Use prescribed pain medications as needed to ensure adequate rest and activity. Take oral medication with food to prevent gastric irritation.

Community-Based Care

The home is the primary site of postoperative care and recovery for all patients as hospital stays continue to shorten. The needs for discharge teaching have been outlined in the Patient Teaching box. The unique needs of the older patient have also been addressed. The nurse needs to be alert to the need for temporary or long-term care and support in the home. Referrals to social services are initiated early in the patient's hospital stay so the patient can be discharged with all needed supports in place.

COMPLICATIONS

Acute arterial occlusions are serious medical emergencies that can be accompanied by a wide variety of complications. Most of the complications have been discussed during the general care presentation. Infection, reocclusion, and a wide variety of respiratory, circulatory, and renal complications may occur. Whenever acute or chronic arterial occlusion occurs, the possibility exists that treatment will be ineffective. In these situations the ischemia leads to necrosis and gangrene. Therefore amputation must be considered as one of the potential complications of vascular occlusion.

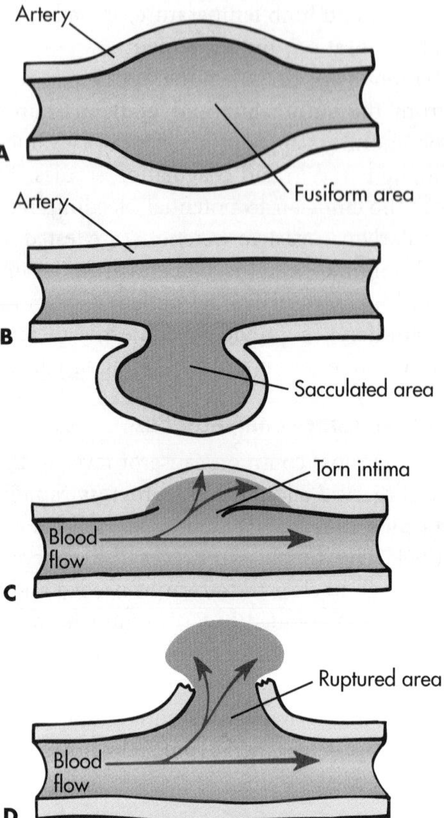

Figure 25-9 Types of aneurysms. **A**, Fusiform. **B**, Saccular. **C**, Dissecting. **D**, Ruptured.

Aneurysms

Etiology/Epidemiology

Aneurysms are points of weakness, dilation, or outpouching of arteries to at least 1.5 times their normal size. The word aneurysm comes from the Greek word *aneurysma* meaning widening. Aneurysms occur most commonly in the aorta, but they can occur in any artery of the body. Other common sites include the femoral and popliteal arteries. Aneurysm disease is the thirteenth leading cause of death in the United States.[11] It is more common in men than women and typically occurs between the ages of 50 and 70 years. Aneurysms are caused by atherosclerotic disease, trauma, syphilis, congenital abnormalities of the vessel, infection, and connective tissue disorders that cause weakness in the wall of the vessel. Cigarette smoking, hypertension, and a genetic predisposition to aneurysm formation are all linked to the development of aneurysms. The steady aging of the population and improved diagnostic tools have increased the frequency with which aneurysms are diagnosed.

Pathophysiology

The abdominal aorta is the most common site for aneurysm formation. Risk factors that weaken the vessel wall act in combination with the forceful turbulent blood flow in this region to gradually dilate the vessel. The four primary types of aneurysms are illustrated in Figure 25-9. A fusiform aneurysm involves a circumferential dilation of the vessel wall and is relatively uniform in shape. A saccular aneurysm is a localized outpouching that occurs on just one side of the artery. A narrow neck connects the aneurysm sac to the vessel wall. Saccular aneurysms have a higher incidence of rupture. A dissecting aneurysm develops from a tear in the intima of the artery that causes an accumulation of blood in the newly formed cavity between the intima and the media. Dissecting aneurysms are further classified by the type of tear and the degree of hematoma or bleeding. Dissecting aneurysms are strongly associated with arterial hypertension and hemodynamic instability and are most common in the thoracic aorta. Aneurysms can even affect the aortic valve. The growth rate of aneurysms is unpredictable, but in general the larger the aneurysm, the greater the risk of rupture. An estimated 50% of all aneurysms larger than 6 cm in diameter rupture within 1 year.

Patients with aneurysms are commonly asymptomatic. Abdominal aneurysms may be felt as a palpable mass, and a systolic bruit may be heard. The patient may complain of abdominal or back pain. If the aneurysm leaks or ruptures, the patient develops severe pain, signs of shock, decreased red blood cell count, and increased white blood cell count. Symptoms of thoracic aneurysms vary and depend on the size and placement of the aneurysm and its effect on surrounding tissues. Most patients are again asymptomatic. Patients may experience anterior chest wall, back, flank, or abdominal pain or may develop signs of shock if the aneurysm leaks. Symptoms such as dyspnea, cough, and wheezing may develop if the aneurysm puts pressure on the trachea or bronchus.[24]

Collaborative Care Management

Most aneurysms are discovered on routine physical or x-ray examination. Once the diagnosis is established, the primary therapeutic goal is to prevent aneurysm rupture

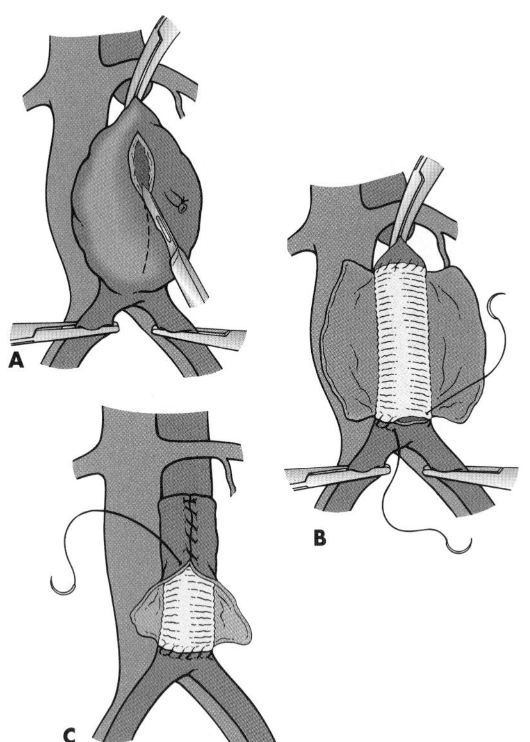

Figure 25-10 Surgical repair of an abdominal aortic aneurysm. **A**, Incising the aneurysmal sac. **B**, Insertion of synthetic graft. **C**, Suturing native aortic wall over synthetic graft.

through control of blood pressure and smoking cessation. The only definitive treatment for an aneurysm is surgical repair, but surgery on the abdominal or thoracic aorta is complex and dangerous, and potentially affects all body systems.[26] The decision to operate is made collaboratively with the patient after a careful workup is completed and all risks and benefits have been discussed. Patients who are symptom free and have small aneurysms may be treated conservatively with careful monitoring. The risk of rupture with aneurysms greater than 6 cm outweighs the risks of surgical intervention.[1,25] Regardless of whether surgery is attempted, maintenance of blood pressure in an optimal range is a high priority of care. Surgical repair involves the use of a synthetic graft to support the weakened area (Figure 25-10). Care of the patient undergoing aneurysm repair surgery is similar to that for patients who undergo vascular bypass surgery.

Patient/Family Education. The decision regarding whether to undergo surgical repair of the aneurysm is one of the most difficult aspects of patient care. The nurse can play an essential role in helping the patient and family to sort through the available data and make an informed choice. The nurse helps ensure that the patient's decision is respected and supported. The nurse reinforces the importance of blood pressure control and careful medical follow-up, especially if surgery is not planned. Discharge education for patients undergoing aneurysm repair is similar to that provided to patients after vascular bypass surgery. Teaching highlights are summarized in the Patient Teaching box on p. 789.

VENOUS DISORDERS

The most common venous disorders result from incompetent valves in the veins and obstructions of venous return to the heart, usually as a result of a thrombus.

Deep Vein Thrombosis

Etiology

A variety of different terms are used to describe the disorder that results from the formation of a thrombus within a vein (Figure 25-11). The term *phlebothrombosis* refers to the actual process of clot formation. Thrombus formation is commonly accompanied by some degree of vein wall inflammation, and the terms *phlebitis* and *thrombophlebitis* are used to reflect this inflammation. Thrombus formation occurs in either the superficial or deep veins of the body. Superficial thrombophlebitis occurs in the majority of patients receiving intravenous (IV) therapy. Deep vein thrombosis (DVT) is more serious, often necessitates hospitalization, and carries the risk of potentially fatal embolization.

Venous thrombosis typically results from at least one element of Virchow's triad: venous stasis, damage to the endothelial lining of the vein, and hypercoagulopathy. Venous return to the heart is supported by the action of the vein valves in conjunction with the rhythmic contractions of the muscles in the extremities, which compress the veins and help move the blood toward the heart. Any period of relative or partial inactivity or immobility, such as prolonged sitting, surgery, or bed rest, impairs venous return. A decrease in muscle tone and activity in the legs causes pooling and venous distention. The distention causes minor damage to the endothelial lining of the veins and valves, and platelets are attracted to the site.[15] This can result in the development of a thrombus. The presence of IV catheters, central lines, and pacemaker wires; and the irritation of drugs and IV solutions contribute to endothelial damage. Any increase in viscosity or hypercoagulability of the blood increases the likelihood of thrombus formation. Dehydration, pregnancy, clotting disorders, sickle cell anemia, malignancy, polycythemia, systemic lupus erythematosus, and oral contraceptive use are all examples of conditions that can contribute to the subtle alteration in coagulability that results in thrombus formation. The presence of atherosclerosis and varicosities also increases the risk. Travel, especially air travel and journeys longer than 4 hours, has been theorized to contribute to the development of DVT and/or pulmonary emboli (see Research Box).[4] Risk factors for DVT are summarized in the Risk Factors box.

Most thrombi form in the veins of the pelvis and lower extremities, but they can also form in the vessels of the upper extremities and those leading directly to the heart. A venous thrombus that becomes dislodged is called an embolus. An embolus can travel from the site where it formed through the larger veins and into the right side of the heart, where it may be ejected into the pulmonary arteries. The development of a pulmonary embolus is an extremely dangerous condition that carries a significant mortality risk. The pulmonary arteries become partially or totally obstructed depending on the size of the embolus, and the circulation to a lung segment or the

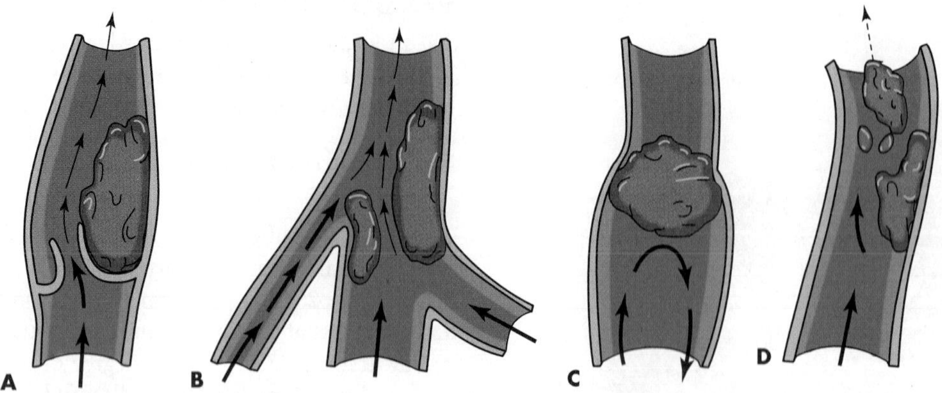

Figure 25-11 Development of deep vein thrombosis with arrows indicating direction of blood flow. **A,** Thrombus in a valve pocket of a deep vein with blood flowing beside thrombus. **B,** Thrombi tend to form at bifurcations of deep veins with some slowing of blood flow. **C,** Complete occlusion of the vein by a thrombus forcing backflow of blood. **D,** An embolus that has broken off from a thrombus and is floating in the bloodstream could migrate to the lungs and cause pulmonary embolus.

Research

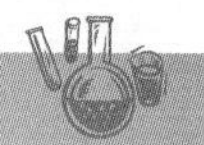

Reference: Ferrari, E: Travel as a risk factor for venous thromboembolic disease: a case control study, *Chest* 115(2):440, 1999.

This study explored the link between travel and the development of deep vein thrombosis (DVT) or pulmonary embolus (PE). All patients admitted with the diagnosis of DVT/PE at the institution were included in the study and questioned about the incidence of travel lasting greater than 4 hours in the previous 4 weeks.

Data analysis confirmed that travel lasting more than 4 hours constituted a risk for DVT/PE, and the risk was increased with prolonged air travel as a result of a variety of circulatory changes that occur with immobility at high altitudes.

The study confirmed the risk of DVT/PE associated with prolonged travel, especially air travel. It is hypothesized that the number of confirmed DVTs may represent only a small portion of the total number that occur after travel.

entire lung may be affected. If the area of obstruction is large, the lung may undergo severe infarction with massive tissue loss. Pulmonary embolism is clearly the most serious outcome of deep vein thrombosis and is the major reason that treatment is immediate and aggressive.

Epidemiology

Approximately 2 million Americans are diagnosed with DVT each year, and as many as 50% of these patients develop pulmonary emboli. It is estimated that 90% of pulmonary emboli begin as thrombi in the lower extremities, usually in the popliteal, femoral, and pelvic veins.[3] Calf thromboses rarely embolize, although the reason is unknown. DVT is a relatively common occurrence in both hospital and community settings, and it is the third most common form of cardiovascular disease. DVT occurs more commonly in women and persons over 40 years old. No racial prevalence has been identified. The multiple risk factors for DVT are presented in the Risk Factors box.

Risk Factors

Deep Vein Thrombosis

Age—the elderly typically have a number of risk factors, which increases the incidence of DVT in this population
Gender—deep vein thrombosis occurs more often in women
Positive history of thromboses
Immobility/stasis
Surgery, bed rest, paralysis
Prolonged sitting (automobile or air travel), especially >4 hrs
Obesity and pregnancy
Increased viscosity
Dehydration, fever
Polycythemia
Intimal damage
Central and peripheral intravenous catheters, pacemaker wires
Intravenous drug abuse
Associated conditions/disorders
Malignancy
Varicose veins
Inherited coagulation disorders
Hemolytic anemias (sickle cell anemia)
Trauma
Fractures, especially involving the pelvis and long bones
Burns
Use of oral contraceptives (risk is primarily related to estrogen content)
Chronic lung and heart disease

Pathophysiology

Thrombi develop from platelets, fibrin, and both red and white blood cells. They form in areas where the blood flow is slow or turbulent. Three primary factors, called Virchow's triad, trigger the formation of DVT: vessel wall damage, venous stasis, and hypercoagulability. Muscle spasm and changes in intravascular pressure can cause the developing thrombus to dislodge and move toward the heart and lungs.

The lungs are rich in heparin and plasmin activators and can effectively dissolve some thrombi. If the thrombus is not successfully dissolved, however, it can lodge in an artery and obstruct perfusion to the lung segment. A major pulmonary embolism can be rapidly fatal.

Clinical manifestations of DVT vary substantially according to the size and location of the thrombus and the adequacy of the collateral circulation. Approximately 80% of all patients with DVT are completely asymptomatic.[3] Possible symptoms include pain or tenderness in the affected area, unilateral edema or swelling of the affected extremity, and redness or warmth if the phlebitis is extensive (Figure 25-12). Superficial thrombophlebitis produces a palpable, firm, cordlike vein; and the area surrounding the affected vessel is usually tender, reddened, and warm. Fewer than 20% of all patients exhibit the classic Homans' sign (calf tenderness with dorsiflexion of the foot). Possible signs and symptoms of deep vein thrombosis are summarized in the Clinical Manifestations box.

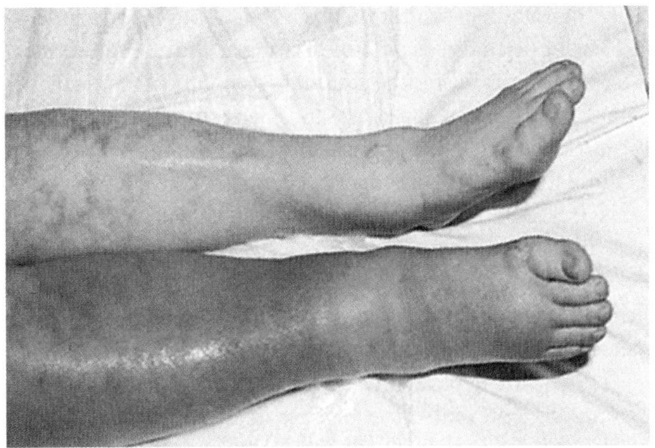

Figure 25-12 Deep vein thrombosis with phlebitis.

Clinical Manifestations

Deep Vein Thrombosis

Local pain or tenderness
Unilateral edema or swelling
May be bilateral if DVT is located in the vena cava
Local warmth, redness
Mild fever
Tender, palpable venous cord in the popliteal fossa
Fewer than 20% of all patients with DVT have a positive Homans' sign.
NOTE: Approximately 50% of all patients are asymptomatic.

DVT, Deep vein thrombosis.

Collaborative Care Management

Diagnostic Tests. The venogram is the gold standard for the diagnosis of DVT, but even this test is not infallible. It may mistakenly identify filling defects in the vein as the presence of a DVT. Venogram is more accurate in diagnosing peripheral thrombi and is less effective in diagnosing pelvic, renal, or vena caval thrombi. The test itself is irritating to the veins and can trigger phlebitis and thrombus formation. Radiolabeled fibrinogen scans may also be used in diagnosis. The fibrinogen becomes visible at the site of thrombosis, but there is a lag time of 24 to 36 hours before sufficient fibrinogen reaches the site.

Noninvasive testing with impedance plethysmography and ultrasonography is being increasingly used. Plethysmography measures changes in electrical resistance to blood flow, and ultrasonography evaluates the sound of blood flowing through the veins. Duplex scanning combines traditional Doppler scanning with B-mode ultrasonography, which determines the compressibility of the vein. The presence of a deep vein thrombosis renders the vein noncompressible. D-dimer testing is also being combined with plethysmography. This newer agglutination assay blood test uses venous blood to assess the degree of agglutination occurring. Additional information about these diagnostic tests can be found in Chapter 22.

Medications. Drug therapy plays a major role in both the prevention and treatment of DVT. Heparin has long been the drug of choice for preventing DVT in high-risk patients. Heparin works by binding with antithrombin III and inactivating thrombin and other clotting factors. Unfractionated heparin is administered by subcutaneous injection, usually twice a day. Low-molecular-weight heparins (LMWHs) were first introduced for the treatment of DVT and have recently been approved by the Food and Drug Administration for prevention as well.[3] LMWH is also administered subcutaneously once or twice a day. Three drugs are currently approved for this purpose:

Enoxaparin (Lovenox): following hip, knee and abdominal surgery
Dalteparin (Fragmin): following hip or abdominal surgery
Ardeparin (Normiflo): following knee surgery

Research

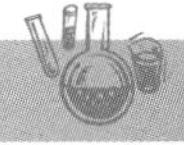

Reference: Harrison, L: Assessment of outpatient treatment of deep-vein thrombosis with low-molecular-weight heparin, *Arch Intern Med* 158(18):2001, 1998.

This study examined the efficacy, safety, and feasibility of home treatment with low-molecular-weight heparin (LMWH). A total of 113 patients with confirmed deep vein thrombosis were included in the study. Eligible patients were treated with either LMWH or warfarin and monitored for the occurrence of complications and patient satisfaction with treatment. Adverse reactions occurred in both groups with no significant differences found. Patients treated with LMWH were discharged earlier and expressed greater satisfaction with a regimen that allowed for home treatment.

LMWH has quickly become the option of choice for treating existing DVT.[2] The dose is administered subcutaneously, but does not require ongoing blood coagulation monitoring and is safe for use in the home setting (see Research Box). Examples of LMWHs approved for DVT treatment include enoxaparin, dalteparin, and tinzaparin (Innohep). These drugs are administered in weight-based doses (1 mg/kg subcutaneously every 12 hours), which allows for much greater accuracy in establishing adequate levels of anticoagulation with minimal fluctuations. Blood levels are quickly established and easily maintained without constant laboratory monitoring, and earlier discharge is possible as long as the patient is able to successfully administer the drug at home.[6] Studies indicate that LMWH can be used safely as a long-term preventive measure, but most patients are still gradually converted to oral warfarin (Coumadin) for long-term treatment. In contrast, most patients treated with conventional unfractionated heparin require hospitalization for intravenous administration, frequent blood drawing, and ongoing dosage adjustments to maintain the activated partial thromboplastin time (APTT) at the therapeutic level of 1.5 to 2 times the control.

The goal of heparin therapy is to prevent new clots from forming and prevent the extension or growth of the existing thrombus. Heparin does not dissolve existing thrombi, but it does block the conversion of fibrinogen to fibrin. Bleeding is the major adverse consequence of heparin administration, although thrombocytopenia also occurs. The platelet count is therefore monitored throughout therapy. Heparin-induced thrombocytopenia (HITT), or white clot syndrome, is diagnosed when the platelet count falls below 100,000 or more than 50% from the onset of therapy. This serious complication of heparin therapy occurs in 5% to 10% of patients receiving heparin and can result in life-threatening thrombosis in either the arteries or veins. Heparin therapy is discontinued and the effects of the drug are reversed through the administration of protamine sulfate. Plasmapheresis is also used to remove the thrombi. The LMWH alternatives appear to have a lower associated incidence of HITT.

Oral anticoagulation with warfarin (Coumadin) is initiated along with the LMWH or intravenous heparin therapy to prevent the recurrence of thrombi. There is little consensus about when warfarin therapy should be started. Because warfarin takes several days to reach a therapeutic concentration, some authorities recommend starting it immediately. Others advocate beginning warfarin administration after 3 to 5 days of heparin therapy. A standard beginning dose of 5 to 10 mg is administered and is then gradually adjusted until a therapeutic international normalized ratio (INR) of 2.0 to 3.0 is achieved. Warfarin therapy is usually continued for at least 6 months after an initial episode of thrombosis.

Thrombolytic therapy with streptokinase, urokinase, or tissue plasminogen activator is also used to treat deep vein thrombosis and pulmonary embolus. These agents activate the conversion of plasminogen to plasmin and actively dissolve existing thrombi. Thrombi in the veins of the lower extremities are usually older and larger than those that cause acute arterial occlusions and often do not respond as well to the administration of thrombolytics.

Treatments. DVTs are common complications of routine hospital admissions and are usually attributed to the effects of immobility. Therefore several preventive interventions are in common use. Preventive interventions include the use of antiembolic stockings, graduated compression stockings (GCS), and external pneumatic compression (EPC) sleeves. Frequent leg and ankle exercises also help to prevent DVT. Each of these devices is designed to increase the venous return from the lower extremities and prevent venous stasis.

Antiembolic stockings provide moderate consistent compression to the legs from the toes to either the knees or thighs. Graduated compression stockings apply different degrees of compression to different parts of the legs. The highest degree of compression is applied at the ankle. The pressure is recorded as 100% at the ankle and then decreases to 70% compression at midcalf and 40% at midthigh. Pneumatic compression devices consist of soft plastic sleeves that are applied to the legs. The sleeves are attached to an air pump that regulates the flow of air into the sleeves. This provides gentle intermittent compression by inflating and deflating the sleeves at regular intervals to stimulate venous return (Figure 25-13). Both GCS and EPC devices are contraindicated in patients with arterial disease, severe edema, phlebitis, leg fractures, or skin breakdown. Early ambulation remains one of the most effective preventive measures.

Surgical Management. Surgery does not play a major role in the management of a DVT, although the thrombus may be removed via thrombectomy if the circulation of the extremity is compromised. Surgical intervention may be used, however, for patients who do not respond well to anticoagulant therapy or who experience recurrent DVT and pulmonary emboli. The primary surgical option is a transvenous filtration device placed in the vena cava to trap emboli before they reach the heart and pulmonary vessels. The two types of devices in current use are the Greenfield filter and the bird's nest filter. The Greenfield filter (Figure 25-14) is inserted either surgically or by interventional radiology through an incision in the jugular or femoral vein and is then advanced to the superior vena cava. The bird's nest filter is a web of stainless steel wires that is inserted percutaneously through the femoral vein or occasionally through the subclavian or jugular veins. Both filters intercept and trap emboli and are permanently implanted. They rarely become dislodged or occluded. Safety guidelines for a patient with a vena cava filter are summarized in the Guidelines for Safe Practice box.

Diet. There are no dietary restrictions for a person with a DVT. Patients receiving warfarin need to restrict their intake of foods high in vitamin K because the vitamin acts as an antidote to the action of warfarin and can disrupt its therapeutic blood level. Obese patients may also be advised to attempt to achieve a more optimal body weight.

Activity. Patients with DVTs have traditionally been restricted to bed rest for 5 to 7 days while therapeutic blood levels of unfractionated heparin were being established. Activity restriction is generally not ordered for patients receiving LMWH. These patients are usually permitted to ambulate as tolerated and may be allowed to continue employment while on LMWH therapy. Some physicians, however, still prefer to order bed rest for the initial treatment of DVT. If severe edema or pain is present in the extremity, the patient is kept on bed rest, with the leg elevated. Warm wet compresses may be applied to the affected area.

Referrals. Patients who will receive long-term oral anticoagulation with warfarin may be referred to a home health agency for follow-up blood drawing and assessment for complications such as recurrent thrombi, pulmonary emboli, or medication side effects. Home health referral is particularly appropriate for older adults, who may have restricted mobility, live alone, suffer visual or other sensory impairments, or are on multiple drug protocols for other chronic health problems. Advanced practice nurses are commonly responsible for

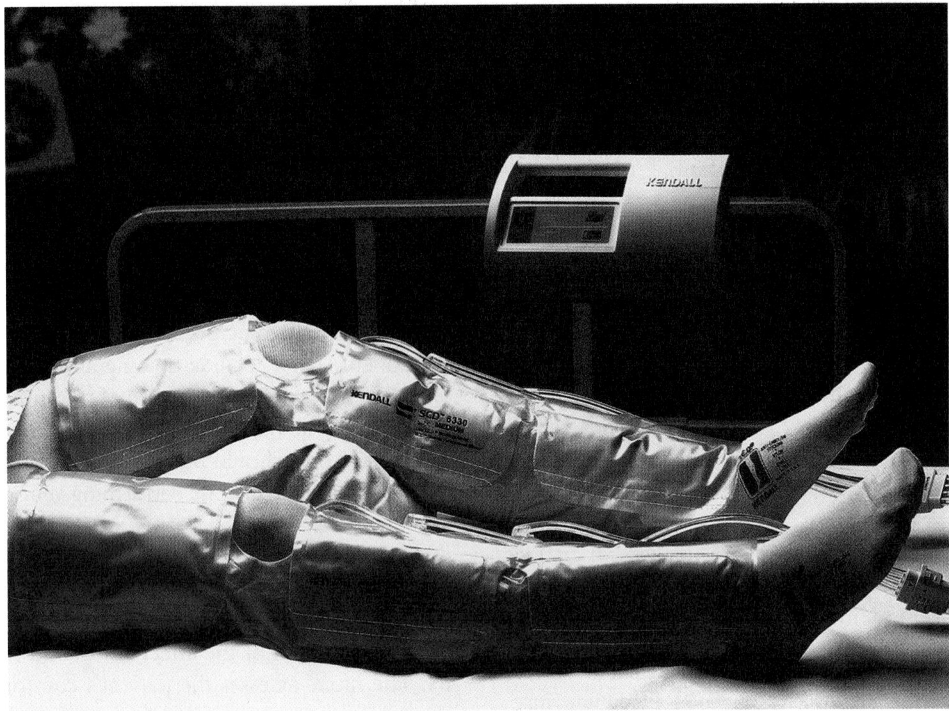

Figure 25-13 Pneumatic compression devices, such as the Kendall sequential compression device, are commonly used to prevent deep vein thrombosis in high risk patients.

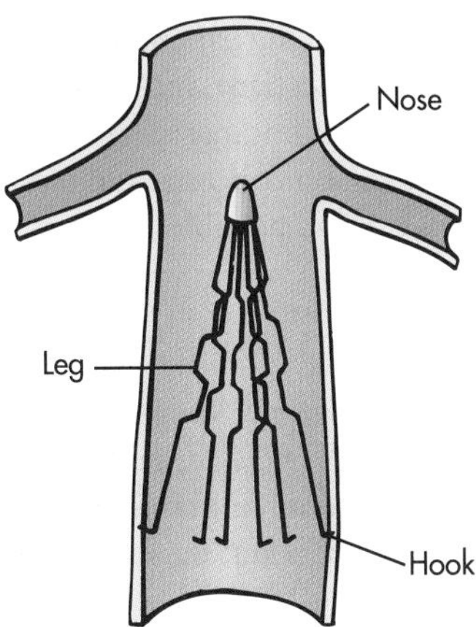

Figure 25-14 Greenfield filter placed in the vena cava.

managing anticoagulation clinics, and their services and expertise are consulted as indicated.

NURSING MANAGEMENT OF PATIENT WITH DEEP VEIN THROMBOSIS

ASSESSMENT

Health History

Data to be collected during the health history include:
- Previous history of deep vein thrombosis, treatment
- Presence of significant risk factors (e.g., female, advancing age, prolonged sitting or immobility, recent extensive air travel)
- History of oral contraceptive use, duration

Guidelines for Safe Practice

The Patient With a Vena Caval Filter

- Assess venipuncture site for signs of bleeding or infection. Maintain an adhesive covering over the insertion site.
- Immobilize the extremity after the procedure per institution protocol or physician's order.
- Assess peripheral pulses, temperature, color, and sensation in affected extremity per protocol. Assess for pain and presence of positive Homans' sign.
- Assess respiratory status and monitor pulse oximetry or blood gases as indicated. Position in partial or high Fowler's position.
- Implement bleeding precautions and associated safety measures if systemic anticoagulation is to be continued. Monitor appropriate laboratory test results (e.g., PTT, platelets, Hgb, Hct, INR).
- Teach the patient to monitor for:
  - Signs of infection at insertion site; signs of systemic bleeding (e.g., blood in urine, stool, gums; nosebleeds; easy bruising);
  - Bleeding precautions for home use if anticoagulation is to be continued (e.g., use of soft toothbrush, electric razor, stool softeners);
  - Symptoms to report to health care provider (bleeding and infection;
  - DVT; swelling and warmth in extremity;
  - Sudden chest pain, dyspnea, tachypnea, restlessness;
  - Filter occlusion—localized pain, venous stasis or swelling, unusual symptoms).

DVT, Deep vein thrombosis; *Hct*, hematocrit; *Hgb*, hemoglobin; *INR*, international normalized ratio; *PTT*, partial thromboplstin time.

Physical Examination

Data to be collected during the physical examination include:

- Pain or tenderness in calf or thigh muscle at rest or with exercise
- Tenderness over affected area with palpation
- Abrupt pain on attempted dorsiflexion of the foot (Homans' sign)
- Warmth or redness over affected area
- Engorgement of collateral veins in affected area
- Unilateral or bilateral extremity edema, increase in leg circumference over the affected area
- Positive results from Doppler ultrasonography, venography, or plethysmography
- Sudden onset of chest pain, dyspnea, or tachypnea, which may indicate pulmonary embolus

NURSING DIAGNOSES

Nursing diagnoses are determined from analysis of patient data. Nursing diagnoses for the patient with deep vein thrombosis may include but are not limited to:

Diagnostic Title	Possible Etiologic Factors
1. Ineffective tissue perfusion	Decreased venous blood flow, immobility
2. Acute leg pain	Inflammation, edema
3. Deficient knowledge: pharmacotherapy, support stockings, surgery	Lack of exposure/recall, unfamiliarity with information

EXPECTED PATIENT OUTCOMES

Expected patient outcomes for the patient with a DVT may include but are not limited to:

1. Will have adequate circulation to lower extremity: palpable distal pulses and warm, pink extremity
2. Will report decreased pain; increased comfort and decreased edema
3. Will correctly explain rationale for medical therapy: will be able to state the major action and side effects of anticoagulants and thrombolytics; will adhere to activity guidelines in treatment regimen

INTERVENTIONS

1. Supporting Tissue Perfusion

The nurse monitors the adequacy of perfusion to the affected extremity through regular neurovascular assessment, including all pulses distal to the site of the obstruction, the degree of pain and paresthesia if any, temperature changes, and degree of swelling. Calf and thigh circumferences are recorded each shift. When leg circumference is being monitored, the nurse marks the exact site to be used directly on the skin to ensure that the tape measure is consistently placed on the same site for each measurement.

The presence and severity of the pain, edema, and redness of the involved extremity determine the patient's activity level. If the extremity is red, edematous, and painful, bed rest with the leg elevated is usually prescribed. Patients receiving LMWH often have no activity restrictions, although some physicians are hesitant to allow patients to ambulate because of the perceived risk of pulmonary embolus. Patients receiving traditional heparin therapy may be kept in bed for 5 to 7 days. Once out of bed the patient is encouraged to ambulate frequently, avoid prolonged standing and sitting, and avoid crossing the legs at the knee or ankle. Compression stockings are applied to both legs unless contraindicated.

The nurse also carefully monitors the patient for signs of complications related to anticoagulant therapy or pulmonary embolus. The nurse monitors all laboratory results, assesses the patient for signs of bleeding, and tests urine, stool, and any emesis for blood. Bleeding precautions are implemented to protect the patient. These include holding all venipuncture sites for at least 5 minutes, avoiding the use of intramuscular medications, and checking all body excretions for the presence of blood. The patient's records should be clearly marked to indicate the anticoagulated state to anyone performing venipuncture.

2. Promoting Comfort

Patients with DVT experience both physical and psychologic discomfort. Leg pain is managed with mild analgesics as needed, elevation of the affected leg, and restriction of activity. The nurse assesses the patient's comfort level frequently. Warm soaks may be applied to the affected leg for comfort if active phlebitis is present. NSAIDs are frequently used for both their pain relieving and antiinflammatory effects. The patient is likely to be extremely anxious during the early days of treatment because the risk of pulmonary embolus is very real. The nurse encourages the patient to participate in all care decisions and keeps the patient and family informed about laboratory results and test findings. The nurse encourages the patient to express fears and concerns and offers realistic comfort and reassurance where possible.

3. Patient/Family Education

Patients who experience DVT need extensive education because they are likely to require long-term anticoagulation at home. Patients need to be knowledgeable about how to monitor their anticoagulant therapy and prevent complications. The nurse instructs the patient about the major action and side effects of the anticoagulants, the rationale for long-term management, and the planned schedule for laboratory monitoring of coagulation levels. The nurse instructs the patient to assess for and report the incidence of any excessive bruising or bleeding. Major elements of patient teaching related to the safe use of anticoagulants are summarized in the Patient Teaching box.

The patient may also be instructed to wear compression stockings after discharge, and the nurse provides instruction about their safe and appropriate use. The patient needs more than one pair of the stockings so that they can be washed regularly. The correct fit of any pair of compression stockings is ensured by careful ankle, calf, and thigh circumference measurement before purchase. The stockings should be smoothly applied before getting out of bed in the morning and worn throughout the day. The skin is carefully inspected for bruising and signs of irritation or breakdown whenever the stockings are removed. Routine cleansing of the legs and feet should be maintained.

Patient Teaching
Patients Receiving Oral Anticoagulant Therapy

- Teach patient the action, dosage, and side effects of medication.
- Consult with pharmacist about the concurrent use of any other medications because many drugs display strong interactions with anticoagulants.
- Instruct patient not to take aspirin or any aspirin-containing over-the-counter (OTC) preparation. Aspirin will increase the anticoagulant effect. Teach patient to read all OTC medication labels carefully for aspirin content.
- Instruct patient to take the drug at the same time each day and to never discontinue the drug without specific instruction from the health care provider.
- Teach the patient to monitor for signs of bleeding and report them to the health care provider (bleeding gums, nosebleeds, blood in the urine or stool, bruising, cuts that do not stop bleeding despite prolonged direct pressure).
- Teach patient the importance of follow-up blood tests to monitor anticoagulant levels.
- Teach patient to do the following:
  - Eat dark green and yellow leafy vegetables moderately because these are rich sources of vitamin K, which can counteract the effect of warfarin (Coumadin).
  - Use alcohol only in moderation because it increases the anticoagulant effect.
  - Wear a Medic-Alert tag or bracelet that identifies the use of anticoagulants.

Health Promotion/Prevention

Preventing the incidence of DVT is a major nursing concern for all hospitalized patients. Early ambulation remains the single best preventive measure available, and the nurse needs to explain the rationale for frequent ambulation to both the patient and family to increase adherence with this measure. High-risk patients are identified and more aggressive preventive measures are implemented, such as low-dose heparin and the use of compression stockings or sequential compression devices. All patients need instruction about the risks associated with prolonged sitting and the importance of taking breaks for walking every 1 to 2 hours during long car trips. Exercising on airplanes is more difficult but equally important. Patients are also instructed to maintain a high fluid intake to avoid dehydration when traveling, to avoid sitting with the ankles or knees crossed, to consider the use of compression stockings when traveling, and to perform ankle and leg exercises every hour if possible. Young women are informed about the risks of DVT associated with the use of estrogen-containing oral contraceptives, particularly if they also smoke cigarettes. Not all episodes of DVT can be prevented, but the risks can be decreased with the use of some of these basic measures (see Guidelines for Safe Practice box).

EVALUATION

To evaluate the effectiveness of nursing interventions, compare patient behaviors with those stated in the expected patient outcomes. Achievement of outcomes is successful if the patient with DVT:

1. Maintains adequate circulation to lower extremity as indicated by palpable distal pulses and warm pink extremity.
2. States that pain is absent and leg edema has decreased.
3. Correctly explains safe use of all medications, incorporates activity guidelines into daily lifestyle.

Guidelines for Safe Practice
The Patient With Deep Vein Thrombosis

BED REST

The patient on traditional heparin therapy will be on bed rest for 5 to 7 days. Patients on low-molecular-weight heparin (LMWH) can be out of bed after 24 hours if pain level permits.

TREATMENTS

Use local heat to extremity when inflammation is acute. Fit the patient carefully for graduated compression stockings and teach correct use.

DRUG THERAPY

Administer bolus of heparin and begin heparin dosing: (1) IV drip with weight-based dosing and traditional heparin; (2) subcutaneous injection of low-molecular-weight heparin with weight-based dosing.

- Monitor APTT to establish desired heparin dosage.
- Monitor antifactor Xa to establish desired LMWH dosage; LMWH does not affect APTT or PT times.
- Begin warfarin (Coumadin) treatment on day 2. Monitor INR results to establish desired warfarin dosage. Administer stool softener as needed.

PATIENT TEACHING

- Risks and complications of DVT, signs and symptoms of complications
- Risks and complications of heparin administration, signs and symptoms of complications
- Bleeding precautions
- Need for ongoing laboratory follow-up of anticoagulation levels after discharge

APTT, Activated partial thromboplastin time; *PT*, prothrombin; *INR*, international normalized ratio; *DVT*, deep vein thrombosis.

GERONTOLOGIC CONSIDERATIONS

DVT is common in older adults, and preventive measures are particularly important for this age group. Early ambulation and avoidance of prolonged bed rest are important measures during any hospitalization, particularly after surgery. Compression stockings and the administration of subcutaneous heparin are essential preventive measures. Older adults are more likely to need home care assistance after discharge for teaching, follow-up, and support.

SPECIAL ENVIRONMENTS FOR CARE

Critical Care

Critical care placement is not required for the routine treatment of DVT, but it could become necessary if the patient were to develop a pulmonary embolus. Pulmonary embolus is a potentially life-threatening emergency that necessitates critical care placement for aggressive pulmonary therapy and monitoring.

Community-Based Care

Initial care for a patient with a DVT is provided in an acute care setting, but long-term management of the disorder takes place in the home. Patients are typically discharged on anticoagulant therapy and require all of the teaching and follow-up care previously outlined. The incidence of DVT predisposes an individual to a future occurrence of the problem, and patients are counseled about the importance of adherence to the general preventive measures outlined. These guidelines need to be incorporated into the patient's lifestyle far into the future.

■ COMPLICATIONS

Recurrence of DVT and the development of pulmonary embolus are the two most significant complications of the disorder. It is not always possible to prevent these complications, but the measures outlined under nursing interventions are the best available strategies for prevention.

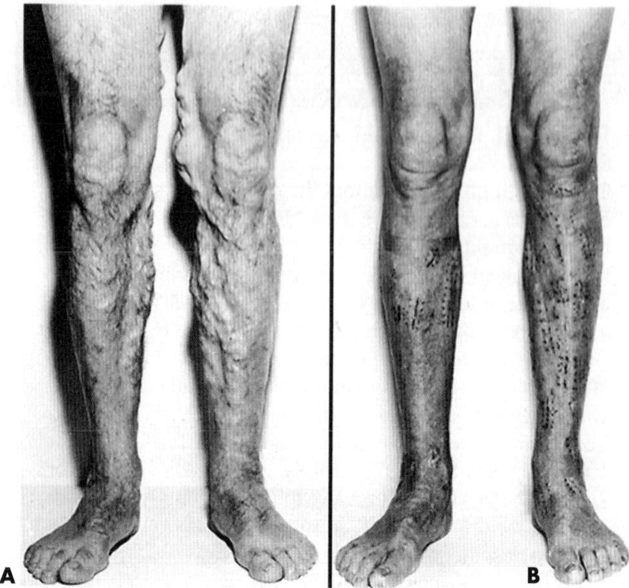

Figure 25-15 Extensive varicosities (incompetency of the greater saphenous systems). **A,** Appearance before surgery. **B,** Appearance 2 weeks after surgery.

Varicose Veins

Etiology/Epidemiology

Varicose veins are prominent, abnormally dilated veins that develop most often in the lower extremities because of the effects of gravity on venous pressure. In 1891 Trendelenburg first concluded that varicose veins were caused from vein valve incompetence combined with abnormally high hydrostatic pressure in the lower extremities. Few individuals younger than 25 develop varicose veins with the exception of young women who have had multiple pregnancies. By 40 years of age, 25% of men and more than 50% of women have some varicosities. The incidence rate increases to 50% of men and more than 64% of women by age 50. A hereditary component is theorized to play a role in the development of varicose veins, but obesity, prolonged standing, and the effects of chronic diseases such as cirrhosis and heart failure are also well documented.

Pathophysiology

Venous blood flow in the legs begins in the capillaries and moves through the superficial veins that lie next to the skin. The blood then moves into the penetrating or communicating veins to the deep veins, which return the blood to the heart. Venous blood flow from the lower extremities is constantly working against gravity and is assisted by the unidirectional intraluminal valves in the veins that help move the blood toward the heart. Activity causes intermittent compression of the veins by the leg muscles and also supports venous blood flow. Over time, the accumulated pressure on the vein valves can cause them to become incompetent. Risk factors such as obesity, prolonged standing, pregnancy, and chronically elevated intraabdominal pressure can significantly contribute to the elevated pressure within the veins. As the valves fail, the veins appear progressively swollen and enlarged and may become hard and tortuous (Figure 25-15). The patient may be asymptomatic or may develop swelling and a feeling of heaviness, pressure, or chronic fatigue in the legs, particularly after standing for any length of time.

Collaborative Care Management

The Trendelenburg test is commonly used to evaluate valve competence. The patient lies supine and elevates the leg. A tourniquet is then applied to the upper thigh and the patient is assisted to a standing position. If the veins fill immediately, varicosities are present.

Treatment depends on the severity of the disease. Primary interventions include teaching the patient about the importance of regular exercise, leg elevation, and avoidance of prolonged standing. Elastic stockings or another form of external support is usually recommended. Custom-fitted stockings are prescribed to be worn whenever the legs cannot be elevated. The appearance and weight of these stockings have improved over time, but they still may be unacceptable to many women. They are also somewhat difficult to put on, which makes them challenging for older patients and those with arthritis.

Sclerotherapy is an option for patients with small, localized varicosities. A sclerosing agent, usually 1% to 3% sodium tetradecyl, is injected into the vein. Ligation, stripping, and excision of veins are surgical options for more severe disease and can usually be performed as outpatient surgery if no untoward complications develop.

Patient/Family Education. Teaching is an important component of the conservative management of varicose veins. The patient needs to understand the relationship between gravity and varicose filling. The nurse assists the patient to find ways to minimize prolonged sitting or standing during daily activities, and ways to elevate the legs above the level of the heart at intervals throughout the day. The nurse also encourages the patient to maintain an optimal body weight and explore whether symptom improvement can be obtained through weight loss. The nurse also encourages the patient to wear compression stockings. The patient may need to experiment with different types and brands until a style and weight can be found that provide the needed support and are acceptable to the patient for daily use. The nurse reinforces the importance of applying compression stockings before getting out of bed in the morning. Discharge teaching after vein surgery includes monitoring wound healing, assessing for signs of infection, and resting with the legs elevated at intervals throughout the day. Walking is encouraged; prolonged sitting and standing should be avoided.

Venous Ulcers

Etiology/Epidemiology

Leg ulcers can be caused by many conditions, including venous hypertension, infection, diabetes mellitus, malignancy, connective tissue disorders, rheumatoid arthritis, and damage from DVT or venous stasis. External insults such as trauma, pressure, and insect bites are other possible causes. Although ulcers may be either arterial or venous in nature, more than 85% of all ulcers are venous. One in four Americans over the age of 65 (more than 1.5 million people annually) develop extremity ulcers. Treatment is prolonged and is estimated to cost from $750 million to $1 billion each year. Most ulcers result from a coexisting disease process or trauma, but risk factors for ulcers include a positive family history, pregnancy, obesity, and an occupation that requires prolonged standing.

Pathophysiology

Venous ulcers typically develop from a pattern of increased venous tension and valve incompetence that leads to venous stasis, poor venous return, edema, and ultimately ulceration. The pattern is similar in most ways to the pathology of other venous disorders. It is theorized that fibrin cuffs may develop around the dermal capillaries in response to prolonged venous hypertension. These cuffs prevent sufficient oxygen and nutrients from reaching the tissue. The decreased circulation results in ulceration. An alternative theory suggests that capillaries are damaged from prolonged venous stasis and cellular permeability increases owing to the release of inflammatory substances from the white cells.

Chronic venous hypertension causes varicosities, stasis eczema, and lipodermatosclerosis. The varicosities are the direct result of the incompetent valves, but only 3% of patients with varicosities develop ulcers. Stasis eczema or dermatitis occurs from edema and blistering. Eczema is often the first sign of ulcers. Lipodermatosclerosis occurs when fibrotic tissue develops in response to long-standing extremity edema. The fibrotic tissue replaces the normal tissue and fat in the legs. The leg becomes larger at the calf and smaller at the ankle, and the skin is tough and thick. Venous ulcers are often located over the medial or lateral malleolus but can develop on other parts of the leg.

The ulcers typically exhibit irregular margins and the ulcerated area ranges in appearance from red granulation tissue to fibrinous tissue to necrotic tissue (Figure 25-16). Venous ulcers usually produce copious serous exudate. The surrounding skin is brown or brawny in appearance because of the accumulation of waste products from hemolyzed red blood cells. Edema and distention of the veins on the medial aspect of the foot are also typical.

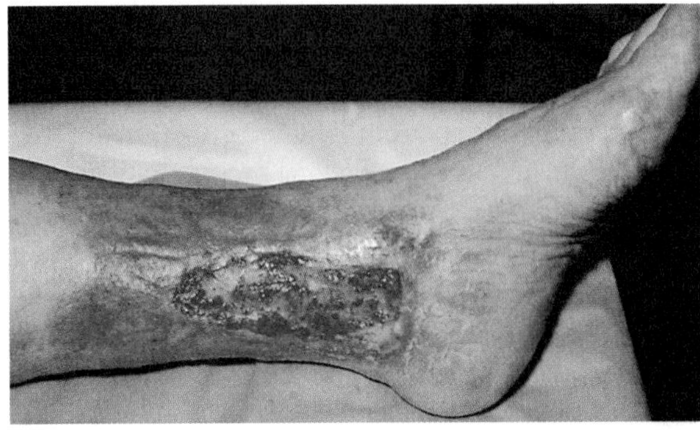

Figure 25-16 Classic venous ulceration in the malleolar region.

Collaborative Care Management

Venous ulcers are treated with a combination of compression, elevation, and topical wound care. Compression is directed at improving the blood flow and venous return to the heart. Compression also decreases the edema and therefore assists in the healing process. Two approaches to compression are typically used: the Setopress and Unna's boot. Elastic stockings may also be used as both a treatment and prevention tool. As with other conditions, compression hose are applied before getting out of bed and removed before going to bed. Intermittent compression devices can also be beneficial to patients with venous ulcers.

Unna's boot was developed by Dr. Paul Unna in the late 1800s. It is a continuous compression bandage that contains glycerol and zinc oxide with the option to include diphenhydramine lotion. The extremity is covered by an elastic compression dressing that is wet when applied and requires up to 12 hours to dry. Unna's boot disintegrates in water, so bathing is prohibited during treatment. Skin and circulatory assessments are essential components of care. Excessive boot pressure can cause arterial compression, and both peripheral pulses and capillary perfusion are carefully monitored after the boot is applied.

Patients with stasis dermatitis may be treated with a topical steroid cream. A hydrocolloid dressing such as Duoderm may be applied over the cream. An open wound needs to be kept clean. Normal saline is an appropriate choice for cleansing noninfected wounds. Infected ulcers may require topical or systemic antibiotics and daily wound care. Alginates, hydrocolloids, hydrogels, foams, and transparent films may all be used on the infected ulcer. Ideally, a wound care specialist develops the overall plan for wound care to be implemented by the patient and family at home. A compression wrap is usually applied over the base dressing.

Surgical intervention may be necessary to prevent the recurrence of venous ulcers and promote healing. Thrombosed veins may be surgically removed. Split-thickness skin grafting may be necessary to cover the wound after excision of the ulcer.

Patient/Family Education. Venous ulcers are difficult and time consuming to heal. From 70% to 80% of them recur, so their management becomes a lifelong process. Patients may be admitted to an acute care institution for portions of their care, but most of the wound management takes place in the home. The wound cleansing and dressing routines can be complex and time consuming. Home health assistance may be indicated initially, but most patients are expected to manage their ongoing wound care with the help of the family. The nurse plays an essential role in teaching the patient and family about needed wound care techniques and the rationale for all interventions. The patient and family also need to know where to find wound care supplies in their community and how to effectively compare the wide range of wound care products that are available on the market. Compression, elevation, and optimal skin care are the essential components for healing. The nurse also discusses supportive measures such as weight loss or control, rest, optimal nutrition, and avoiding prolonged standing.

Critical Thinking Questions

1. A 62-year-old woman is recovering from a recent myocardial infarction. She is in atrial fibrillation. She suddenly complains of a severe pain in her left leg. The nurse notes that pulses are absent, and the leg is cool to the touch. On further questioning she states that her leg feels somewhat numb. What is the likely cause of her symptoms? What are the appropriate next steps in her care?
2. What criteria would you use to help distinguish between a chronic venous and a chronic arterial disorder?
3. You have been told that a 70-year-old widower who lives alone in a rural community has been noncompliant with his drug regimen for control of his hypertension. What additional assessment would you complete to gain sufficient understanding of his situation to begin to formulate a teaching plan for him related to his hypertension?
4. You are addressing a community group of young pregnant women. One of them raises the issue of varicose veins and asks you if it is true that they are inevitable. What information would you provide these women about varicose veins and their prevention?

References

1. Aragon D et al: Variables influencing patients' outcomes after elective aortic reconstruction surgery, *Am J Crit Care* 9(4):279, 2000.
2. Boccalon H et al: Clinical outcome and cost of hospital vs. home treatment of proximal deep vein thrombosis with low-molecular-weight heparin, *Arch Intern Med* 160(12):1769, 2000.
3. Breen P: DVT: What every nurse should know, *RN* 63(4):58, 2000.
4. Ferrari E, Chevallier T, Baudouy M: Travel as a risk factor for thromboembolic disease: a case-control study, *Chest* 155(2):44, 1999.
5. Gorton ME: Current trends in peripheral vascular disease, *Postgrad Med* 106(3):87, 92, 1999.
6. Harrison L et al: Assessment of outpatient treatment of deep vein thrombosis with low-molecular weight heparin, *Arch Intern Med* 158(18):2001, 1998.
7. He J et al: Long term effects of weight loss and dietary sodium reduction on the incidence of hypertension, *Hypertension* 35(2):544, 2000.
8. Hooi JD et al: Incidence of and risk factors for asymptomatic peripheral arterial occlusive disease: a longitudinal study, *Am J Epidemiol* 153(7):666, 2001.
9. Hurley M: New hypertension guidelines, *RN* 61(3):25, 1998.
10. Karch A, Karch F: When a blood pressure isn't routine, *Am J Nurs* 100(3):23, 2000.
11. Keats TE: The emergency x-ray: aneurysm, *Emerg Med* 30(8):147, 1998.
12. Kozuh J: NSAIDs and antihypertensives: an unhappy union, *Am J Nurs* 100(6):40, 2000.
13. Kuncl N, Nelson KM: Antihypertensive drugs, *Nursing* 27(8):46, 1997.
14. Lips DL, Vacek JL: Catheter based methods for managing peripheral vascular disease, *Postgrad Med* 106(3):76, 1999.
15. Merli GJ: Low molecular weight heparins versus unfractionated heparin in the treatment of deep vein thrombosis and pulmonary embolism, *Am J Phys Med Rehabil* 79(5 suppl):S9, 2000.
16. NIH: *Sixth report of the Joint National Committee on prevention, detection, evaluation, and treatment of high blood pressure,* NIH publication No. 98-4080, Washington, DC, 1997, National Institutes of Health, National Heart, Lung, and Blood Institute.
17. Ogden L et al: Long-term absolute benefit of lowering blood pressure in hypertensive patients according to the JNC VI risk stratification, *Hypertension* 35(2):544, 2000.
18. Pahor M et al: Therapeutic benefits of ACE inhibitors and other antihypertensive drugs in patients with type 2 diabetes, *Diabetes Care* 23(7):888, 2000.
19. Powers KB, Vacek JL, Lee S: Noninvasive approaches to peripheral vascular disease, *Postgrad Med* 106(3):70, 1999.
20. Skolnik N, Beck J, Clark M: Combination antihypertensive drugs: recommendations for use, *Am Fam Physician* 61(10):3049, 2000.
21. Sparks RD: The answer is Buerger's disease, and the question is, *West J Med* 168(4):286, 1998.
22. US Department of Health and Human Services: *Healthy People 2010: understanding and improving health,* Washington, DC, 2000, USDHHS.
23. Vacek JL: Peripheral vascular disease, *Postgrad Med* 106(3):51, 1999.
24. Varadarajulu S, Stephenson TF: Thoracic aortic aneursym: indications for surgery, *Consultant* 40(2):241, 245, 2000.
25. Varon J, Marik P: The diagnosis and management of hypertensive crisis, *Chest* 118(1):214, 2000.
26. Willmitch B: FDA approves stent-grafts for aortic aneurysms, *Nurs Spectrum* 12A:NJ12, 2000.

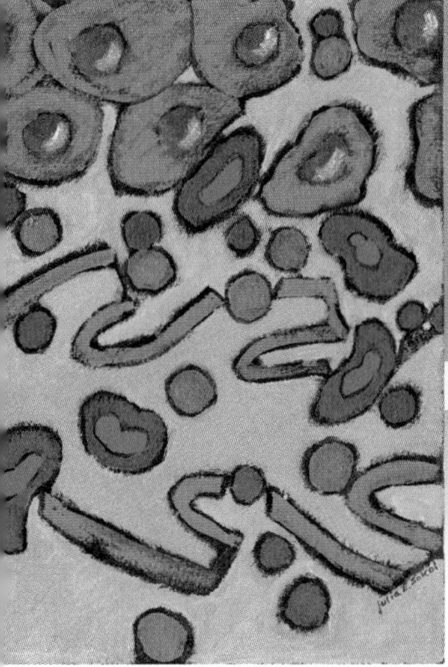

Assessment of the Hematologic System 26

Peggy Ellis

Objectives

After studying this chapter, the learner should be able to:

1. Recall the structure and function of the organs, tissues and cells of the hematologic system.
2. Discuss changes that occur within the hematologic system as a result of normal aging.
3. Identify essential data to be collected as part of the assessment of the hematologic system.
4. Describe common diagnostic tests used in the assessment of the hematologic system.
5. Explain the nursing implications of hematologic-related diagnostic tests.

ANATOMY AND PHYSIOLOGY

Diseases associated with the hematologic system are diverse in their underlying pathologic manifestations, disease course, and response to treatment. Most often the accompanying symptoms result from altered hematopoiesis (blood cell production) or interference with the normal development and function of the blood components: erythrocytes (red blood cells [RBCs]), thrombocytes (platelets), and leukocytes (white blood cells [WBCs]). Normally a balance is maintained between the rate of production of normal blood cells and the rate of destruction. Disorders of the blood occur when this balance is lost. Disturbances in the coagulation mechanism also result in blood disorders.

Components of the Hematologic System

The hematologic system includes blood and its components and bone marrow, as well as the mononuclear phagocyte system (MPS), previously known as the reticuloendothelial system (RES), which is located throughout the body. The MPS function is phagocytizing foreign materials and lysing (breaking down) RBCs.

Blood

Blood is an aqueous solution (plasma) that contains water, proteins, electrolytes, and inorganic and organic constituents. Cells make up 7% to 9% of the blood.

The cell components of blood include erythrocytes, leukocytes, thrombocytes, and plasma cells. All normal cells are derived from a single stem cell that can divide into lymphoid and myeloid stem cells. These stem cells can, in turn, become progenitor cells that divide along a specific single pathway (Figure 26-1). This process is known as hematopoiesis and takes place in the bone marrow of the flat bones in adults. This activity is highest in the iliac crests, the sternum, the ribs, and the proximal epiphysis of long bones. Production may occur in all the long bones during periods of increased demand, such as with hemorrhage or during cell destruction (hemolysis).

Erythrocytes. An erythrocyte (RBC) is a nonnucleated biconcave disk that is soft and pliable. These characteristics enable the RBC to change its shape during passage through the microcirculation and to function efficiently as a gas carrier (O_2 and CO_2). The major component of the RBC is hemoglobin (Hgb), a protein that transports oxygen and carbon dioxide and maintains normal pH through a series of intracellular buffers. The Hgb molecule contains globin (two pairs of polypeptide chains) and four heme groups, each containing an atom of ferrous iron. Thus each Hgb molecule can unite with four oxygen molecules to form oxyhemoglobin (a reversible reaction). Carbon dioxide is carried by the globin portion of the Hgb molecule. In a normal person 99% of the hemoglobin molecules are saturated with oxygen.

Immature RBCs are called reticulocytes. They are released in the bloodstream where they circulate until they mature. Reticulocytes make up approximately 1% of the normal number of RBCs. Production of RBCs in the bone marrow requires adequate amounts and use of vitamin B_{12}, folic acid, proteins, enzymes, and minerals (iron, copper). Erythropoiesis (RBC formation) can be greatly stimulated by the secretion of the hormone erythropoietin from the kidneys; this occurs when the numbers of RBCs falls below normal (such as with severe blood loss) or when demand for oxygen increases (tissue hypoxia). The RBCs circulate for 120 days and are then destroyed by the macrophages of the MPS. Most of the iron is removed from the heme and can be used to form new heme groups. Small amounts of iron lost daily in urine and feces and through menstrual flow must be replaced by iron ingestion.

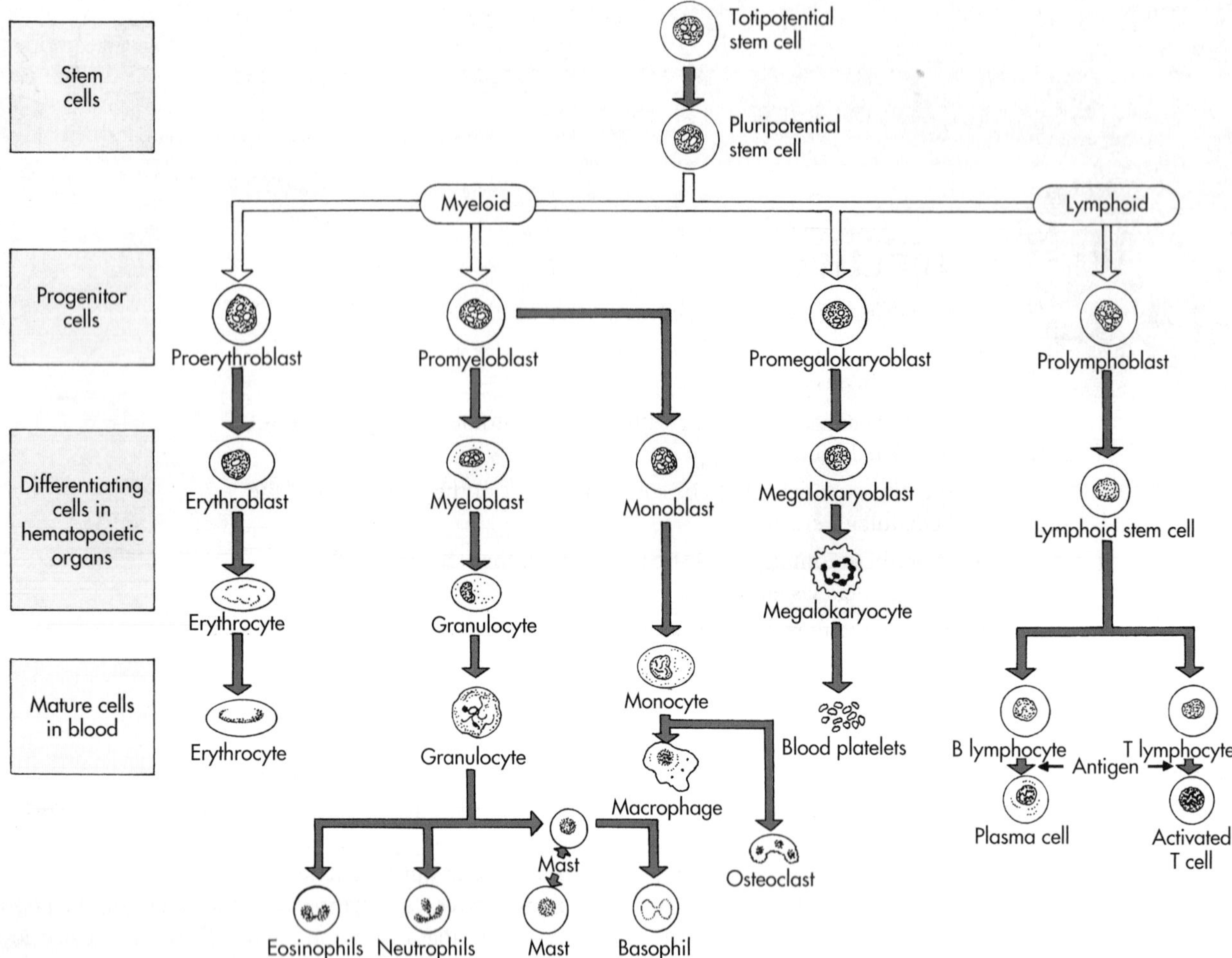

Figure 26-1 Scheme of stem cell differentiation.

The remainder of the heme is broken down to form bilirubin and is secreted into the bile. Energy in the form of adenosine triphosphate is required to maintain cell membrane integrity and the relatively low sodium and high potassium content of the RBC.

Leukocytes. The leukocytes make up the body's mobile defense system against foreign invaders. These cells are formed both in the bone marrow (granulocytes, monocytes, and some lymphocytes) and in the lymphatic tissue (lymphocytes). These cells are classified into two groups: polymorphonuclear granulocytes (neutrophils, basophils, and eosinophils) and nongranular leukocytes (monocytes and lymphocytes). The average life span of a leukocyte is 4 to 5 days, but once activated it lives only 6 to 8 hours in circulation. Monocytes that lodge in tissue become macrophages and can live months to years until they are destroyed in the process of phagocytosis.

Neutrophils, also referred to as segmented neutrophils or SEGS, make up 50% to 70% of circulating leukocytes. Immature forms are called bands or stabs. In response to inflammation or infection transient increases in neutrophils occur (neutrophilia). Neutrophils provide defense in two ways. First, they release the contents of their granules, which contain enzymes to kill and digest bacteria. Second, they are capable of direct phagocytosis of foreign organisms (see Chapter 11).

Eosinophils constitute about 4% of circulating leukocytes. Although not significant in bacterial infections, eosinophils are active in parasitic infections by attaching to the organism and releasing chemicals to aid in destruction of the invader. Eosinophils also participate in the allergic response by preventing local inflammation from spreading throughout the body.

Basophils are less than 1% of circulating leukocytes. The granules of the basophil contain heparin and histamine, as well as small quantities of bradykinin and serotonin. These substances are released during the process of inflammation. In the allergic response, the immunoglobulin E (IgE) antibody attaches to the basophil, causing the release of chemicals and resulting in the localized tissue reaction commonly seen with the allergic response.

Circulating monocytes make up 2% to 8% of the total number of leukocytes. These cells are larger than granulocytes and have a kidney-shaped nucleus. The majority of monocytes are tissue-based and become macrophages as they leave the circulation. The tissue macrophage is the first line of defense against infection. These tissue macrophages participate in phagocytosis of dead and injured cells, cell fragments, and microorganisms.

Lymphocytes make up the remaining 20% to 40% of leukocytes. These cells have a round to oval nucleus. The majority of lymphocytes originate in lymphoid tissue but some are made in the bone marrow. The two types of lymphocytes are circulating T lymphocytes originating from the thymus and noncirculating B lymphocytes. The function of lymphocytes is discussed in Chapter 11.

Thrombocytes. Thrombocytes (platelets) are not cells but granular, disk-shaped, nonnucleated cell fragments. Their production is regulated by thrombopoietin which is produced in the liver and kidneys. They are important in the blood clotting process. Approximately two thirds of all platelets are within the circulatory system, and the remaining one third are present in the spleen as a reserve pool. The life span of a platelet is approximately 6 to 10 days. Platelets also originate from the stem cells and are essential to hemostasis and coagulation (see Figure 26-1).

The coagulation process occurs in stages and usually takes about 5 to10 minutes. An individual with a shorter clotting time than this may be prone to develop intravascular thrombi, and an individual with a longer clotting time may have a tendency to bleed more than normal. In the first stage, platelets along with plasma proteins agglutinate at the injury site. Platelet factors are released and thromboplastin is formed. In the second stage, the thromboplastin activates the conversion of prothrombin to thrombin in the presence of calcium. In the third stage, thrombin and fibrinogen form fibrin. With the presence of calcium, a fibrin clot forms. In the fourth stage, the clot breaks into fibrin and split products and is removed, a process called fibrinolysis (Figure 26-2).

Mononuclear Phagocyte System

The MPS, previously known as the RES, includes circulating monocytes and their precursor cells in the bone marrow. Also included are more or less fixed mononuclear phagocytic cells (also called macrophages) found in blood channels in the spleen and liver (Kupffer's cells), in the lymphatic system, in serosal cavities of the body, in the lungs, in general connective tissue, and in the bone marrow.[4]

The MPS is primarily responsible for phagocytosis, the process of engulfing and removing "wasted" white blood cells. In addition to phagocytosis, the MPS processes the Hgb of RBCs that has reached the end of its life span, splitting Hgb into an iron-containing substance and bilirubin.

Lymphatic System

The lymphatic system is an alternative pathway in which fluid can flow between the interstitial spaces and the blood. Its chief function is to remove proteins from the tissue spaces. All tissues of the body contain lymph channels with the exception of the central nervous system, bone, and the superficial skin layers. Lymph fluid circulates throughout the body at a rate of 120 ml/hr. The lymphatic system also plays an important role in the regulation of tissue volume and interstitial fluid pressure.

The normal lymph node consists of connective tissue encapsulating a fine mesh of reticular cells. The reticuloendothelial cells function chiefly in the phagocytosis of cellular debris. The chief function of lymphocytes, which are the main cells constituting the lymph nodes, is to provide an immune response to antigens presented to the node from the structure being drained by the node.

Lymph node enlargement, or lymphadenopathy, results from an increase in the number and size of lymphoid follicles with proliferation of lymphocytes and reticuloendothelial cells. Lymphadenopathy also may occur when the node is invaded by cells normally not present (leukemic cells, cancer cells) or when lymph channels and nodes are surgically removed. In the lymphomas the actual nodal structure is destroyed by the malignant cells.

Normally lymph nodes are not palpable. With disease and the consequent increase in size, the nodes become palpable.

Physiologic Changes With Aging

The effect of aging on hematopoiesis is under study, but to date there have been no clear, clinically significant findings. There is some indication that the cellularity of human marrow decreases with age perhaps as a result of an increase in fat from osteoporosis. In addition some research demonstrates a decrease in bone marrow production of cells.[1-3]

In human beings the total number of leukocytes and differential counts show no variation through middle age and no gross changes in old age. In general, however, the leukocyte count does not rise as high in response to infection for the elderly, and studies suggest that elderly persons have a diminished marrow granulocyte reserve.

The Hgb level decreases after middle age, although the decrease in women seems to be relatively less than that in men. Unexplained anemia in older adults has been noted, but iron absorption is not impaired. This anemia does not appear to be solely a function of age[2] and may be related to reduced use of orally administered iron because of the side effect of constipation. Serum iron and iron-binding capacity decrease in elders, and low serum vitamin B_{12} and folic acid levels occur in a significant number of elderly persons—but without anemia. Obvious signs and symptoms of hematologic disorders in a younger individual may be mistaken for normal aging in an elderly person. Fatigue, activity intolerance, and pallor may be attributed to advanced age. It is important when assessing an elderly patient to be aware of the normal physiologic changes and to discern those from pathologic changes related to hematologic dysfunction (see Gerontologic Assessment box). The elderly are also more likely to have a chronic illness, as well as a higher risk for malignancy. Both of these situations may cause an anemia of otherwise unexplained origin.

No age-related changes in platelets have been reported. Some of the plasma coagulation factors have been reported to increase with age (factors I, V, VII, and IX). Partial thromboplastin time (PTT) may be shortened. The RBC sedimentation rate increases significantly, but this rate is of limited value in detecting disease in older adults.

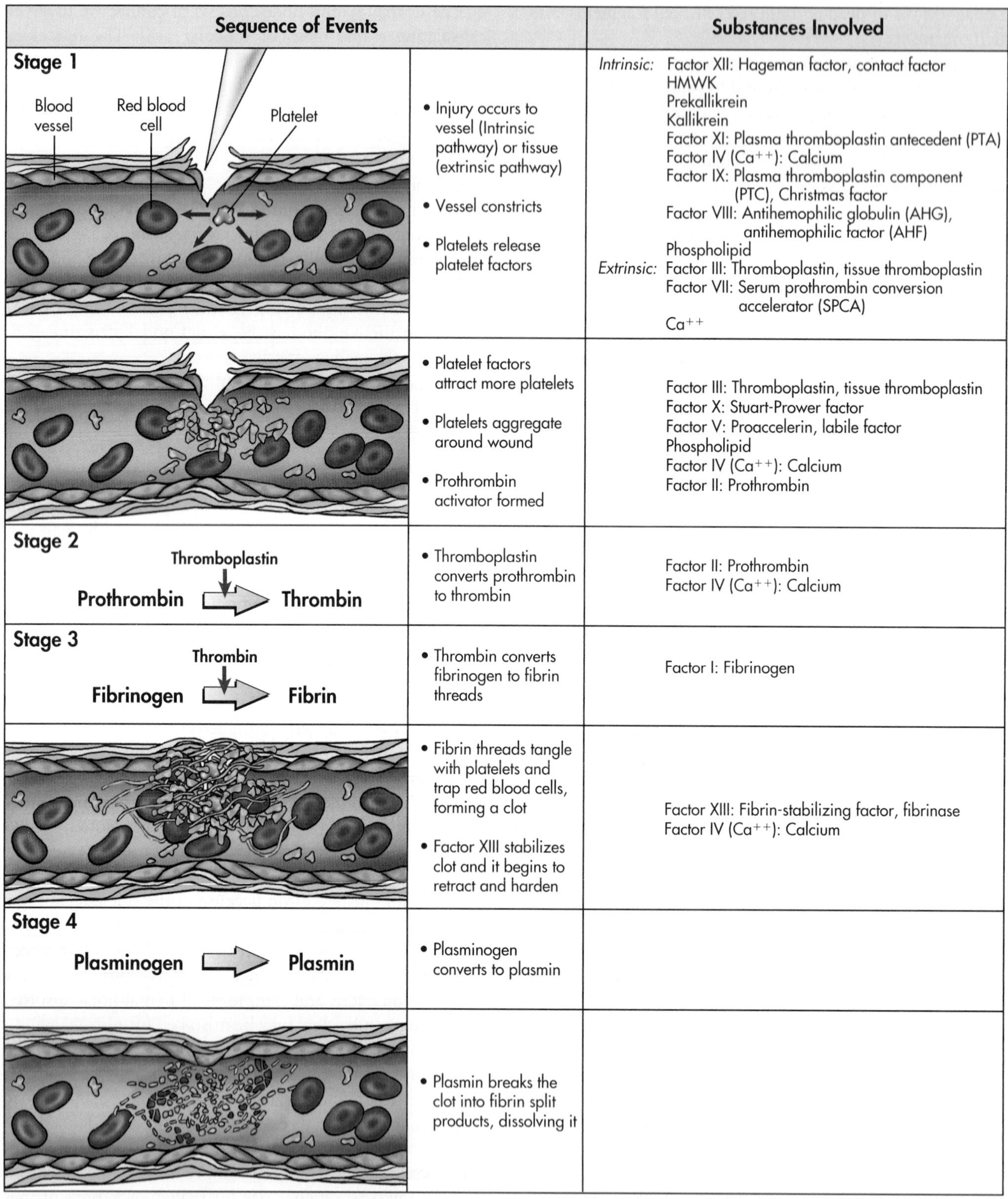

Sequence of Events		Substances Involved
Stage 1 Blood vessel Red blood cell Platelet	• Injury occurs to vessel (Intrinsic pathway) or tissue (extrinsic pathway) • Vessel constricts • Platelets release platelet factors	*Intrinsic:* Factor XII: Hageman factor, contact factor HMWK Prekallikrein Kallikrein Factor XI: Plasma thromboplastin antecedent (PTA) Factor IV (Ca^{++}): Calcium Factor IX: Plasma thromboplastin component (PTC), Christmas factor Factor VIII: Antihemophilic globulin (AHG), antihemophilic factor (AHF) Phospholipid *Extrinsic:* Factor III: Thromboplastin, tissue thromboplastin Factor VII: Serum prothrombin conversion accelerator (SPCA) Ca^{++}
	• Platelet factors attract more platelets • Platelets aggregate around wound • Prothrombin activator formed	Factor III: Thromboplastin, tissue thromboplastin Factor X: Stuart-Prower factor Factor V: Proaccelerin, labile factor Phospholipid Factor IV (Ca^{++}): Calcium Factor II: Prothrombin
Stage 2 Thromboplastin **Prothrombin** → **Thrombin**	• Thromboplastin converts prothrombin to thrombin	Factor II: Prothrombin Factor IV (Ca^{++}): Calcium
Stage 3 Thrombin **Fibrinogen** → **Fibrin**	• Thrombin converts fibrinogen to fibrin threads	Factor I: Fibrinogen
	• Fibrin threads tangle with platelets and trap red blood cells, forming a clot • Factor XIII stabilizes clot and it begins to retract and harden	Factor XIII: Fibrin-stabilizing factor, fibrinase Factor IV (Ca^{++}): Calcium
Stage 4 **Plasminogen** → **Plasmin**	• Plasminogen converts to plasmin	
	• Plasmin breaks the clot into fibrin split products, dissolving it	

Figure 26-2 Formation of a blood clot.

HEALTH HISTORY

A thorough health history is essential to assessment of hematologic status because there is a variety of primary hematologic disorders and many of their symptoms are nonspecific and common to many diseases. This diverse array of symptoms includes shortness of breath, fatigue, bruising, tarry stool, constipation, lymphadenopathy, flulike illness, pallor, and musculoskeletal pain. Further complicating the assessment is the fact that secondary effects from disease of another body system may manifest in abnormal hematologic findings. For example, the anemia associated with renal insufficiency is the consequence of disease outside the hematopoietic system.

Gerontologic Assessment

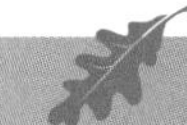

Obtain a thorough history of chronic illness such as diabetes, heart disease, renal failure. These diseases can cause hematologic abnormalities.
Gather detailed information about diet and nutritional status. Older adults are at risk for malnutrition and vitamin deficiency which can cause hematologic problems.
Question about changes in usual activity tolerance and ability to perform activities of daily living; muscular and skeletal pain, which often is attributed to arthritis; and changes in taste, smell, and vision. These diverse, nonspecific symptoms can all reflect hematologic disorders.
Obtain orthostatic vital signs. Changes in vital signs are systemic manifestations of hematologic disorders.
Inspect the skin for lesions and note color. Platelet dysfunction can cause petechiae, ecchymoses, and purpura. Jaundice can be indicative of hemolytic disease or pernicious anemia. Despite the popular belief, pallor is not a reliable indicator of anemia.

COMMON DISORDERS IN OLDER ADULTS

Mental status (dehydration and hypoxia may be attributed to dementia)
Iron deficiency anemia
Anemia of chronic disease
Folic acid and pernicious anemia
Chronic leukemia
Lymphoma

Patient Teaching
Hematologic Health

To maintain the hematologic system health, adults should:

- Eat a well-balanced diet, including 4 to 6 small meals per day, following the guidelines of the food pyramid.
- Seek early treatment when symptoms of infection are present.
- Report continued weakness, dyspnea or extreme fatigue unrelated to excessive work, straining or sleeplessness.
- Report excessive bruising or bleeding.
- Report excessive joint and bone pain.
- Maintain good hygiene, especially oral hygiene.
- Wash hands frequently.
- Avoid contact with individuals who have diagnosed infections.

A thorough history includes detailed information about the person's symptoms and a thorough review of systems. Other key areas are family history, drug history, exposure to chemicals, and general nonspecific complaints offered by the patient. Since the history not only assists in assessing the patient's health status but also in identifying needs for health information and instruction, assessing for good health practices relating to hematologic system function is essential (see Patient Teaching box).

Family History

The existence of inherited hematologic disorders such as sickle cell disease and malignant tumors requires a detailed family history. Questions regarding disease or presence of symptoms among relatives should include reference to parents and siblings (a genogram is an excellent tool to visualize the family's history). More specific disorders such as hemophilia may involve questions to grandfathers, uncles, and nephews. Female relatives need to be considered for other disorders. Questions should explore instances of severe or prolonged bleeding after minor trauma, dental extractions, or surgery. The occurrence of jaundice or anemia in relatives also should be ascertained.

BOX 26-1 Selected Drugs Implicated in Hematopoietic Suppression*

Acetophenetidin (1, 3)
Acetylsalicylic acid (aspirin) (1, 2, 3)
Acetyl sulfisoxazole (3)
Aminosalicylic acid (3, 4)
Ammonium thioglycolate (3)
Amodiaquin HCl (3)
Arsenicals (1, 2, 3, 4)
Arsphenamine (1, 2)
Atabrine (1, 2)
g-Benzene hexachloride (1, 3)
Benzene (1, 2, 3, 4)
Bishydroxycoumarin (3, 4)
Carbamide (2)
Carbon tetrachloride (1)
Carbutamide (Orabetic) (2)
Chloramphenicol (1, 2, 3, 4)
Chlordane (1)
Chlorophenothane (DDT) (1, 2)
Chlorothiazide (3)
Chlorpheniramine maleate (3)
Chlorpromazine (Thorazine) (3)
Chlorpropamide (2)
Chlortetracycline (1, 3)
Cinophen (3)
Coldricine (2, 3)
Cycloheximide (3)
Dextromethorphan HBr (2)
Diethylstilbestrol (2)
Diphenylhydantoin (Dilantin) (4)
Dipyrone (3)
Ethinamate (2)
Fumagillin (3)
Hair lacquer (3)
Imipramine HCl (3)
Iproniazid (1)
Isoniazid (1, 3, 4)
Lead (1)
Lithium carbonate (1)
Mephenytoin (Mesantoin) (1, 2)
Meprobamate (1, 2, 3)
Methaminodiazepoxide (Librium) (3)
Methapyrilene HCl (4)
Methylpromazine (3)
Mezapine (2)
β-Naphthoxyacetic acid (2)
Nitrofurantoin (4)
Novobiocin (4)
Nystatin (2)
Oxyphenbutazone (2)
Para-aminosalicylic acid (3, 4)
Penicillin (1, 2, 3, 4)
Phenobarbital (1, 2, 3, 4)
Phenylbutazone (Butazolidin) (1, 2, 3)
Pipamazine (1)
Primidone (1)
Prochlorperazine (Compazine) (2, 3)
Pyrimethamine (Daraprim) (1, 2, 3)
Quinidine (2)
Quinine (2, 3)
Reserpine (2)
Stibophen (2)
Streptomycin (1, 2, 3)
Sulfamethoxypyridazine (Kynex) (2, 3, 4)
Tetracycline (3)
Thenalidine tartrate (3)
Thioridazine HCl (3)
Tolazoline HCl (1, 2)
Tolbutamide (1, 2, 3)
Tolbutamide (Orinase) (2)
Trifluoperazine (1, 3)
Trifluoperazine (Stelazine) (3)
Trimethadione (Tridione) (1, 2)

*More than 500 are listed in a report of the American Medical Association subcommittee on blood dyscrasias. The drugs listed in this table are those that have produced dyscrasias when given alone. *1,* Pancytopenia; *2,* thrombocytopenia; *3,* leukopenia; *4,* anemia.

Drugs and Chemicals

Drugs may induce or potentiate hematologic disease (Box 26-1). Most notable are the hematologic effects of the cytotoxic drugs used in cancer chemotherapy and the neutropenia associated with chloramphenicol. A thorough history of drugs ingested by a person is a crucial part of assessment. Many persons regularly ingest "something to help me sleep," "something to calm me down," or "just aspirin." Analgesics, tranquilizers, laxatives, and sedatives often are overlooked by persons when asked about drugs. Specific, often rephrased questioning is necessary to obtain a complete drug history. The importance of obtaining information about over-the-counter medication is underscored because drugs such as aspirin and ibuprofen, as well as alcohol, delay coagulation. Long-term use of these drugs can cause additional bruising and bleeding.

Certain chemicals may also exert a potentially harmful effect on the hematopoietic system. To obtain a history of exposure to chemicals, an occupational history is useful.

Fever

Fever is a common manifestation of many hematologic disorders and is an important symptom to be explored during the history. Fever typically occurs in lymphoma, primarily Hodgkin's disease and leukemia. Severe chills may accompany hemolytic disorders. Night sweats commonly are associated with both lymphoma and leukemia.

Fatigue and Malaise

Fatigue and malaise are difficult symptoms to evaluate because they accompany many physical and emotional disorders. Information regarding the occurrence of these symptoms should be included in the history. When combined with physical and laboratory findings, they are of some diagnostic value. In addition, the person's subjective description of such symptoms lends some insight into perception of the illness, the extent to which the illness is affecting daily living, and the ability of an individual to adapt to changes in homeostasis.

PHYSICAL EXAMINATION

A thorough physical examination is performed in the assessment of a person with a hematologic disorder. Particular attention is given to target organs and alterations known to reflect hematologic disease.

Skin

Skin manifestations of hematologic disease are often readily visible. Petechiae, ecchymoses, and purpura are associated with decreased platelets (thrombocytopenia) and other bleeding disorders. Jaundice may be associated with pernicious anemia, hemolytic disease, or primary liver dysfunction. Pallor is typically associated by the layperson with disorders of the blood. Pallor as a criterion for assessment may be deceptive because many healthy persons have pale complexions, whereas some severely anemic patients may have ruddy complexions. It is important to look at the palms of the hands, conjunctivae, and oral mucosa for pallor. Other skin changes that appear pathologic may be normal for a particular patient. Therefore it is essential to establish norms for individual patients.

Changes in skin texture also may be observed. Except in severe cases, the patient most likely will not observe such changes. With iron deficiency anemia dry skin, dry hair, and brittle nails occur. Severe itching, especially on the palms, often is associated with Hodgkin's disease and also may occur with polycythemia vera, especially after bathing. In persons with leukemia and lymphoma, infiltrative lesions of the skin may be observed on any part of the body.

Head and Neck

The sclerae of the eyes are examined for jaundice and the conjunctivae for pallor. Retinal hemorrhages may occur in persons with severe anemia and thrombocytopenia. Questions also may elicit a history of visual disturbances.

The oral mucosa is observed for pallor, bleeding tendency, and ulceration. The tongue may be very smooth in association with both pernicious anemia and nutritional deficiencies.

The neck is observed primarily for evaluation of lymph nodes. Nodes may be so large as to be visible, but palpation is always used in their assessment. A "lump" on the neck often is the reason for seeking medical attention. Enlarged tumors may obstruct breathing or cause coughing or difficulty in swallowing.

Chest

Firm pressure with the fingertips is exerted along the sternum and ribs to elicit any tenderness that may be present. Such tenderness may reflect a leukemic process or multiple myeloma. Lung sounds are assessed for signs of pneumonia, another common occurrence with leukemia or multiple myeloma.

Abdomen

The abdomen is percussed and palpated with special attention to the liver and spleen. Both organs are prone to enlargement in association with hematologic disease. Ascites may be a late manifestation of liver failure that can be associated with a hematologic disease process.

Back and Extremities

The skeletal system is evaluated primarily for pain, joint deformity, and arthritis. Bone pain may be associated with malignant conditions of hematologic origin. In persons with hemolytic processes and in some hematologic malignancies, there is increased uric acid production and a corresponding increase in the incidence of gout. Joint deformities are associated with bleeding disorders, and pathologic fractures may be a late sign of a disorder.

Lymph Nodes

Lymph nodes are widely distributed in the body and are routinely examined by palpation. In the healthy adult the only palpable nodes are in the inguinal region and occasionally in the axilla. In a disease, cervical, supraclavicular, or other nodes may become palpable. Any enlarged lymph node may reflect a disease process and must be evaluated thoroughly. Enlarged lymph nodes may be painful if they impinge on other organs. Further evaluation of lymph nodes requires x-ray examination, lymphangiography, and/or biopsy.

Nervous System

Many neurologic abnormalities may develop in persons with hematologic disorders. These catastrophic complications are caused by bleeding or infection within the central nervous system. Infiltration of malignant leukemic or lymphomatous cells may produce signs and symptoms of a cerebral tumor or stroke. In addition, some of the lymphomas, especially Hodgkin's disease, may produce a dementia as a remote effect. Therefore initial physical examination should include assessment of mental status, cranial nerve function, sensory function (pain, touch, position, vibratory sensation), and motor function (strength, reflexes, plantar response). It is important to know an individual's baseline assessment. Deviations from the baseline should be noted.

Assessment measures and variations in normal findings relevant to the care of older adults are presented in the Gerontologic Assessment box. Also identified are disorders common in older adults, which may be responsible for abnormal assessment findings.

DIAGNOSTIC TESTS

Laboratory Tests

Extensive blood examinations are performed as part of the diagnostic workup of a person suspected of having a hematologic disorder. A list of these tests according to the blood cell under study along with reference intervals for adults is found in Table 26-1. The most common laboratory tests are Hgb and hematocrit (Hct) levels, RBC indices, reticulocyte count, and peripheral smear, which includes a WBC count and differential diagnosis. The information obtained from such studies provides important clues as to the pathology of the disorder. In addition to their diagnostic value, blood studies are used to monitor a patient's progress and response to treatment. The confirmation of a hematologic disease often depends on an examination of a peripheral blood smear and results of the bone marrow examination. Culture and sensitivity results are important to rule out other sources of fever, malaise, or abnormal CBC results.

Hemoglobin and Hematocrit

The Hgb test measures the amount of Hgb in the peripheral blood. The packed RBC volume, or Hct, is the ratio of RBC volume to the whole blood volume.

Red Blood Cell Indices

The RBC indices consist of the mean corpuscular volume (MCV), mean corpuscular hemoglobin (MCH), and the mean corpuscular hemoglobin concentration (MCHC). The MCV estimates the average size of the RBC. Both the MCH and the MCHC measure the content of the Hgb in RBCs. The MCHC is considered more accurate than the MCH because it measures the entire blood volume of Hgb rather than just that

TABLE 26-1 Laboratory Tests of Blood Cell Structure and Function

Laboratory Tests	Reference Intervals
Erythrocyte Tests	
Red blood cell count	Male: 4.6-6.1 million/mm^3 Female: 4-5.4 million/mm^3
Hemoglobin	Male: 13-18 g/100 ml Female: 12-16 g/100 ml
Hematocrit	Male: 45%-52% Female: 37%-48%
Reticulocyte count	1%-2% of the total RBC count
Mean corpuscular hemoglobin concentration	32%-36%
Mean corpuscular volume	80-95 mm^3
Red cell fragility	
Morphologic description in stained smear	
Thrombocyte (Platelet) Tests	
Platelet aggregation	60%-100%
Platelet count	150,000-400,000/mm^3
Bleeding time, Ivy	1-9 minutes
Leukocyte Tests	
White blood cell count with differential	5000-10,000/mm^3 Granulocytes Neutrophils (PMN, SEG) 55%-70% Eosinophils 1%-4% Basophils 0%-1% Monocytes 2%-6% Lymphocytes 25%-40%

PMN, Polymorphonuclear; *SEGs,* segmented neutrophils.

from a single cell. The RBC indices provide a differential diagnosis of the type of anemia.

Reticulocyte Count

The number of reticulocytes circulating in the blood provides useful information about the erythropoietic activity of the bone marrow. If bone marrow activity is increased as might occur in the early stages of anemia, the reticulocyte count may be increased before the actual total RBC count is decreased.

Peripheral Blood Smear

Each blood cell possesses microscopic features that identify and set the cell apart from other cell types. Examination of the peripheral blood smear provides information concerning the etiology of an anemia. The size and shape of the RBC is observed (Box 26-2). Alteration in the size of the RBC is classified as anisocytosis; alteration in shape of the RBC is noted as poikilocytosis. The WBC may be examined to provide information about adequate bone marrow production. A differential WBC count can provide useful information about what might be causing alterations in the WBC. A decreased platelet count may indicate a tendency for bleeding. Often results of a peripheral blood smear, when combined with data from the history, physical examination, and other laboratory tests, determine the medical diagnosis.

Coagulation Studies

Activated Partial Thromboplastin Time. Activated partial thromboplastin time (APTT) (normally 25 to 35 seconds) measures the number of seconds in which a clot forms. It is used to evaluate and identify congenital and acquired deficiencies in the coagulation system and to monitor the effectiveness of heparin therapy.

Prothrombin Time and International Normalized Ratio. The prothrombin time (PT), normally 10 to 13 seconds or 60% to 140% of normal clotting activity, also measures the time needed to form a clot, but specifically measures factors I, II, V, VII, and X in the coagulation cascade. The PT is used to monitor warfarin (Coumadin) therapy and to screen for vitamin K deficiency and disseminated intravascular coagulation (DIC).

The PT may be reported as time in seconds, as a percentage of normal clotting activity, or as an International Normalized Ratio (INR). The INR reports the relationship of the patient's PT to a normal control. This measurement is more accurate for anticoagulation control in the patient. The normal INR range for warfarin therapy is ≤2.5 for low-dose therapy and 2.5 to 3.5 for high-dose therapy. This may vary from patient to patient, depending on the reason for the anticoagulant therapy and specific treatment goals. The INR increases or decreases from the same conditions that increase the PT (see Research box).

Fibrin Split Products. During the process of fibrinolysis, fibrinogen is broken down into fragments called fibrin split products or fibrin degradation products. The normal split fibrin products test (protamine sulfate test) is negative. Increased levels of these products occur in DIC, deep vein thrombosis, pulmonary embolism, and infarcts. They are also a measure of rejection in patients with organ transplants.

Coagulation Factor Assay. To diagnose specific disorders of the coagulation pathway, it is necessary to isolate specific factor level abnormalities. The coagulation factor analysis facilitates identification of specific deficiencies (Box 26-3).

Hemoglobin Electrophoresis. Normal Hgbs found in the adult erythrocyte are types A, A_2, and F, with 96% to 98% of Hgb being type A. With electrophoresis, abnormal levels of Hgb (hemoglobinopathy) and abnormal types of Hgb (Hgbs S and C, hemoglobinopathy) can be detected. This test can be used to diagnose sickle cell disease and the thalassemias (Box 26-4).

Iron Studies. Serum iron measures the concentration of iron that is bound to transferrin, which is normally 50 to 150

Research

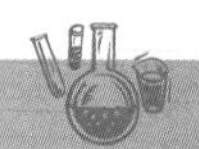

Reference: Murray D, Pennell B, Olson J: Variability of prothrombin time and activated partial thromboplastin time in the diagnosis of increased surgical bleeding, *Transfusion* 39:56, 1999.

One problem experienced by patients undergoing elective surgery is that of dilutional coagulopathy which is a coagulation disorder causing increased surgical bleeding. The prothrombin time and activated partial thromboplastin time are the main coagulation tests used to diagnose the cause of this disorder and guide the treatment. Variability in the results from these tests might effect the outcomes for these patients. The purpose of this study was to examine the use of prothrombin time (PT) and activated partial thromboplastin time (APTT) for diagnosis of causes for increased surgical bleeding. Various commercial PT and APTT tests were compared for sensitivity. Patients who had clinical signs of increased surgical bleeding during an elective surgery were identified and blood was obtained from those patients. Various commercial APTT, APTT ratio, PT, PT ratio, and International Normalized Ratio (INR) were compared. Sixteen patients were included in the study. The results demonstrated that PT and APTT test results varied significantly. When using the tests that were least sensitive, only two patients would have been identified as needing coagulation factor replacement. However, the most sensitive PT and APTT tests indicated a need for coagulation factor replacement in all of the patients. This suggests that the PT and APTT tests may not provide the specificity needed to identify the need for coagulation factor replacement. The use of PT ratio, APTT ratio, and INR did not decrease the variability among tests. This variability may influence the diagnosis and treatment of surgical patients with dilutional coagulopathy.

BOX 26-2 Descriptive Cell Characteristics in Anemia

Size

Macrocytic (large)
Normocytic
Microcytic (small)

Hemoglobin

Normochromic
Hypochromic (decreased)

mg/dl. The total iron binding capacity (TIBC) measures the amount of iron that could still bind to the receptor sites on the transferrin. The serum iron and TIBC should vary conversely and are both used to evaluate microcytic anemia. Serum vitamin B_{12} and serum folate, as well as bilirubin, are also useful in identifying causes and types of anemia (Table 26-2).

Radiologic Tests

Lymphangiography

Lymphangiography is a radiologic technique used for visualization of the lymphatic system nodes to detect the presence of disease. This procedure is especially valuable in the assessment of para-aortic nodes that are anatomically too deep in the abdomen to allow for evaluation by palpation. For this procedure a small incision is made between the toes or fingers, and dye is instilled. After approximately 30 minutes the lymphatic system is outlined. An iodine-based dye is then injected; radiographs are taken then and again 24 and 48 hours after the procedure. In addition, because the dye remains in the lymph nodes for as long as 6 months after the initial study, disease status and response to therapy can be periodically evaluated with routine abdominal roentgenograms.

Patient preparation includes information regarding the type and length of procedure, associated sensations, and aftercare. The patient may or may not have food and fluids restricted before the procedure. A consent form is necessary. The patient may experience discomfort associated with needle puncture and lying still for the procedure, which may last up to 3 hours. An assessment of the patient's allergy status, particularly to iodine, is necessary because of the contrast media used.

The patient may experience a sensation of warmth and flushing as the iodine-based dye is injected. Local anesthesia is used before the needle insertion.

After the procedure the affected limb is elevated for 24 hours. The nurse assesses the patient for signs of bleeding or adverse reactions to the dye. The dissection site may require a few sutures, and mild analgesia (acetaminophen or nonsteroidal antiinflammatory) may be indicated.

The affected extremity should be carefully assessed for any changes in sensory-motor function, which suggest possible nerve damage. The nurse should inform the patient that a blue skin discoloration may result from the first dye injected. The stool and urine may also be discolored. Complications include infection, and rarely pneumonia if the dye migrates to the lung via the thoracic duct. The patient and family should be instructed to report any respiratory problems to the physician.

Computed Tomography

Computed tomography (CT) also is used to assess abdominal lymph nodes. The CT scan is used as a monitoring tool to evaluate the patient's disease process, remission during chemotherapy, and response after treatment. Assessment by periodic CT scans (every 6 to 12 months) helps evaluate the remission or detect a relapse. Lymph nodes may also be evaluated by biopsy or endoscopy (mediastinoscopy, laparoscopy).

Special Tests

Bone Marrow Examination

An adjunct to the peripheral blood smear is the bone marrow examination. Generally the bone marrow is examined when the diagnosis is not clearly established from the peripheral blood smear or when further information is needed. A bone marrow specimen is obtained by bone marrow aspiration or bone marrow biopsy.

Bone Marrow Aspiration

Aspiration is the most common procedure for obtaining a bone marrow sample. The procedure is possible because

BOX 26-3 Coagulation Factor Deficiencies

Vitamin K deficiency: decreased VII, IX, X
Liver disease: decreased II, V, VII, IX, X
Hemophilia A: decreased VIII
Hemophilia B: decreased IX
Disseminated intravascular coagulation: decreased V, VI

BOX 26-4 Abnormal Hemoglobins

Hemoglobin A_2: 0.7% beta thalassemia
Hemoglobin S: sickle cell disease
Hemoglobin C: hemolytic anemia
Hemoglobin F: 0.1% microcytic hypochromic red blood cells

TABLE 26-2 Laboratory Values in Anemia

	Anemia of Chronic Disease	Iron Deficiency	Vitamin B_{12} Deficiency	Folate Deficiency	Thalassemia
Mean corpuscular hemoglobin	Normal	Decrease	Increased	Normal	Decreased
Iron	Normal	Slight decrease	Elevated	Elevated	Elevated
TIBC	Slight decrease	Elevated	Normal	Normal	Normal
Bilirubin	Normal	Normal	Elevated	Elevated	Elevated
Vitamin B_{12}	Normal	Normal	Decreased	Normal	Normal
Folate	Slight decrease	Normal	Normal	Decreased	Slight decrease

TIBC, Total iron-binding capacity.

normal bone marrow is soft and semi-fluid and can therefore be removed by needle aspiration. Bone marrow aspiration is most likely to be performed in persons with severe anemia, neutropenia (decreased number of WBCs), acute leukemia, and thrombocytopenia (decreased number of platelets).

Education, preparation, and emotional support of the patient before bone marrow aspiration can reduce anxiety. Emotional support of the patient and family is necessary because of the potential life-threatening diagnoses that may result from the examination.

Procedure. The most common site for bone marrow aspiration is the posterior iliac crest (Figure 26-3). Other sites include the sternum and the anterior and posterior iliac spines. The skin surrounding the puncture site is shaved (if necessary) and cleansed with an antiseptic such as povidone-iodine complex (Betadine). Sterile towels are placed around the site. The skin and periosteum are anesthetized to decrease pain. First the most superficial layer of the skin is infiltrated with procaine. After a few seconds the needle is advanced until it meets bone. Procaine is then injected to anesthetize the periosteum.

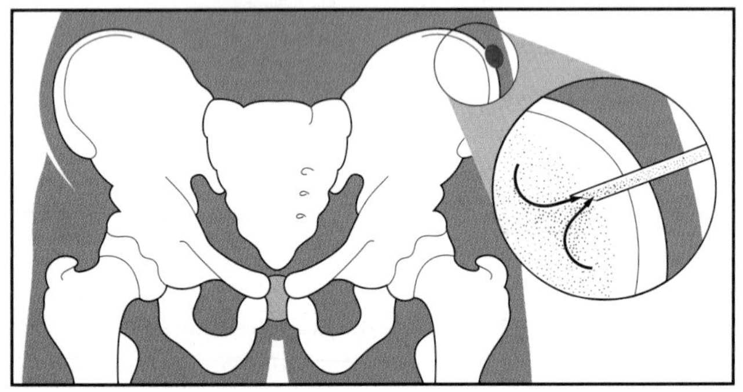

Figure 26-3 Most common site for bone marrow aspiration.

The marrow aspiration needle is inserted; when the marrow cavity is entered, the marrow stylet is removed from the needle, and a sterile syringe is attached. The syringe plunger is drawn back until marrow appears in the syringe. As the plunger is drawn back, the person will experience a brief, sharp pain, sometimes described as a burning sensation. The pain is caused by the suction exerted as the plunger is pulled back. At this point the nurse's hands placed gently on the patient's shoulder and a calm reminder to lie still might prevent a sudden jerk or movement.

After the needle is removed, a pressure dressing is applied over the aspiration site to stop the minimal bleeding that occurs. If the patient has thrombocytopenia, pressure is applied for 15 minutes. The site should be monitored every 15 minutes for 1 hour after the procedure.

Some persons may complain of tenderness at the aspiration site for a few days. Most often, no pain or discomfort is experienced after the procedure.

Bone Marrow Biopsy. A bone marrow biopsy is indicated when a large sample of bone marrow is needed. Persons most likely to undergo a bone marrow biopsy are those with pancytopenia (a decrease in more than one cell type), myelofibrosis, metastatic tumor, lymphoma, and multiple myeloma. The most common site for bone marrow biopsy is the posterior superior iliac spine. The sternum and proximal tibia may also be used. The initial steps in the biopsy procedure are similar to those outlined for bone marrow aspiration. The use of a Jamshidi needle allows for a core of marrow to be collected (Figure 26-4).

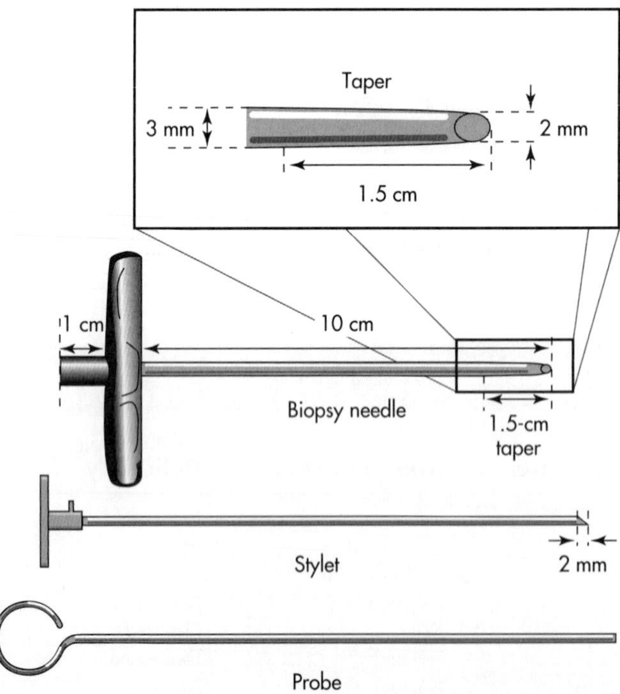

Figure 26-4 Bone marrow biopsy needle showing shape and size.

From microscopic examination of the bone marrow, iron stores can be determined, as can the morphology of the progenitor cell. Large immature cell changes may be observed; infiltration with leukemic cells and absence of cells, as in aplastic anemia, can be determined.

As mentioned with bone marrow aspiration, emotional support before, during, and after the procedure is indicated. Both the patient and family may be stressed and anxious while awaiting results.

• • •

Other diagnostic tests are discussed throughout the text along with the specific disorders to which they pertain.

References

1. Bagnara GP et al: Hemopoiesis in healthy old people and centurians: well-maintained responsiveness of CD34+ cells to hemopoietic growth factors and remodeling of cytokine network, *J Gerontol: Series A, Biolog Sci Med Sci* 55:361, 2000.
2. Beguin Y: Erythropoietin and platelet production, *Haematologica* 84:541, 1999.
3. Fernandez-Ferrero S, Ramos F: Dyshaemopoietic bone marrow features in healthy subjects are related to age, *Leukemia Res* 25:187, 2001.
4. McCance KL: Structure and function of the hematologic system. In McCance KL, Huether SE: *Pathophysiology: the biologic basis for disease in adults and children,* ed 3, St Louis, 1998, Mosby.

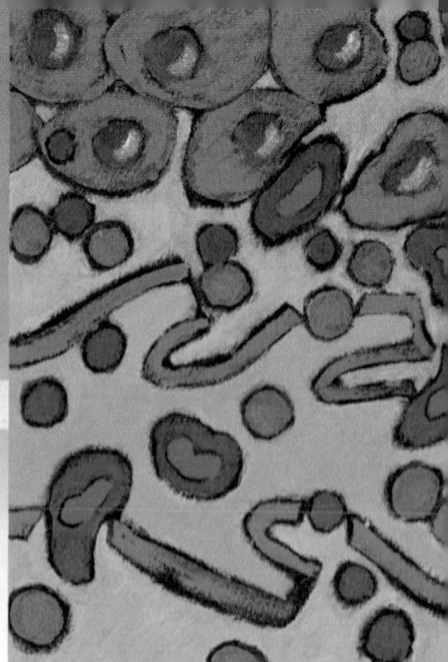

27 Hematologic Problems

Joyce A. McConaughy

Objectives

After studying this chapter, the learner should be able to:

1. Differentiate among types of anemias in terms of pathophysiology, assessment, and interventions.
2. Explain the genetics of sickle cell disease.
3. Describe the nursing care for patients with sickle cell disease.
4. Differentiate among disorders of hemostasis, platelets, and coagulation (thrombocytopenia, thrombocytosis, hemophilia, vitamin K deficiency, and disseminated intravascular coagulation) in terms of pathophysiology, treatment, and nursing interventions.
5. Describe the nursing interventions and therapeutic modalities for the four major types of leukemia.
6. Identify gerontologic considerations important to the assessment and treatment of hematologic disorders in older adults.
7. Explain the differences between Hodgkin's disease and non-Hodgkin's lymphoma and the management of each.

Management of persons with problems of the hematologic system presents challenges to the nurse because of the diversity and vagueness of the presenting symptomatology. Disease processes are as diverse as the components that make up the hematologic system. For this reason, a thorough assessment of the patient is necessary to determine the etiology of the patient's health concerns. Interventions are focused on supporting the patient's return to optimal function and resolution of the hematologic alteration. Treatment options vary, depending on the patient's age, health status, and previous history of illness.

DISORDERS ASSOCIATED WITH ERYTHROCYTES

Common disorders of erythrocytes include underproduction (anemias), overproduction (erythrocytosis), and impaired hemoglobin synthesis (hemoglobinopathies). The term *anemia* refers to a deficiency in the number of circulating red blood cells (RBCs) available for oxygen transport. This condition is determined by an overall decrease in the number of RBCs, the concentration of RBCs (hematocrit [Hct]), and the hemoglobin (Hgb) concentration of the RBCs. Anemias can be further subdivided by RBC size (macrocytic or microcytic) or by the concentration of Hgb (hyperchromic or hypochromic). Refer to Table 26-2 for normal values.

Anemias can also be classified by their causative factors. Some causative factors include blood loss, bone marrow dysfunction, nutritional deficits, hemolysis, hemoglobin defects, and chronic disease. The anemias are summarized in Table 27-1.

ANEMIA CAUSED BY BLOOD LOSS

Etiology/Epidemiology and Pathophysiology

Acute Blood Loss. The anemia associated with acute blood loss is the direct result of the decrease in circulating RBCs. The adult of average build has a total blood volume of approximately 6000 ml. Usually an adult can lose 500 ml of blood without serious or lasting effects because of the spleen's ability to release stored red cells. If the loss reaches 1000 ml or more, serious acute consequences may result.

Signs and symptoms of acute blood loss include those associated with hypovolemia and hypoxemia (see Table 27-1). Weakness, stupor, irritability, and cool, moist skin may be observed. Vital signs indicate hypotension and tachycardia. Decreased Hgb and Hct levels may not be evident until several hours after the blood loss has occurred. The severity of the patient's symptoms correlates with the severity of the blood loss. Acute blood loss is associated with trauma, surgery, platelet dysfunction, and coagulation disorders.

Chronic Blood Loss. The body has remarkable adaptive powers and can adjust fairly well to a severe reduction in RBCs and Hgb, provided the condition develops gradually. A person may remain asymptomatic even though the total RBC count drops to almost half its normal amount. For example, patients with chronic renal failure tolerate hemoglobin levels of less than 8.0 without difficulty. With chronic anemia, determinations of RBC counts, Hgb and Hct levels, mean corpuscular volume (MCV), mean corpuscular hemoglobin concentration (MCHC), and reticulocyte counts are important diagnostic tests. All indices usually are below normal (see Table 26-2 for normal values).

Chronic blood loss is the most common cause of iron deficiency anemia. When blood loss is continuous and moderate, the bone marrow compensates by increasing the production of RBCs. However, if the cause of chronic blood loss is not corrected, the patient becomes iron deficient and symptoms of anemia appear (see Table 27-1).

Collaborative Care Management

Successful treatment of anemia caused by blood loss requires immediate identification of the source of the loss and institution of appropriate treatment. In addition, transfusion therapy or iron supplements may be needed.

Blood transfusions are not indicated for the asymptomatic patient with chronic anemia because of the increased risks associated with them. Transfusions are used only in cases of severe symptoms. General guidelines for the use of transfusions in symptomatic patients are found in Table 27-2.

Transfusion of whole blood is rarely indicated even in situations of surgical hemorrhage. Instead, packed red blood cells (PRBCs) are used because they reduce the incidence of pulmonary edema and circulatory overload. If colloids and clotting factors are needed, plasma, platelets, and cryoprecipitate may be transfused as separate products.

Patients need to be educated about the risks and benefits of transfusion therapy. Concerns regarding acquired immunodeficiency syndrome (AIDS) and hepatitis may need to be addressed by the nurse. The nurse also needs to explore the patient's belief system regarding the use of blood products. Certain cultural and religious belief systems (e.g., Jehovah's Witness) prohibit the receiving of blood products. These beliefs need to be respected by the health care team, although this may create some ethical dilemmas for the nurse.

If transfusion therapy is indicated, the nurse must ensure that the patient is carefully monitored during the process. Transfusion reactions can occur even though laboratory testing was done to verify compatibility of the product. Because transfusion reactions generally occur within the first 15 to 20 minutes after the infusion is started, it is important for the nurse to observe hospital protocols for administering blood

TABLE 27-1 Types of Anemia and Clinical Manifestations

Type	Causes	Clinical Manifestations
Secondary to Blood Loss		
Acute	Hemorrhage	Early: weakness, cool moist skin, tachycardia, hypotension; late: decreased Hgb and Hct
Chronic	Gastrointestinal or other malignancy, bleeding ulcers, bleeding hemorrhoids, menorrhagia	Decreased RBCs, Hgb, Hct, MCV, and MCHC; fatigue
Secondary to Impaired Production of RBCs		
Aplastic anemia	Drugs, chemicals, radiation, chemotherapy, virus, congenital, autoimmune mechanism	Pallor of skin and mucous membranes, fatigue, palpitations, exertional dyspnea, pancytopenia, bleeding tendency, infection
Anemia of chronic disease	Chronic illness, renal disease, diabetes	Decreased serum iron concentration; fatigue
Hemolytic Anemias		
Hereditary spherocytosis	Genetic: inherited as autosomal dominant trait	Spherocytes and increased reticulocytes on peripheral blood smear; fatigue, exertional dyspnea
Thalassemia	Genetic: decreased synthesis of one of globin chains of Hgb	Microcytosis, hypochromic RBCs, decreased growth at pubescence, eventual cardiac failure
Sickle cell disease	Genetic hemoglobinopathy	Painful episodes; vasoocclusive crises; chronic leg ulcers, chronic renal and ocular problems; sickled cells on peripheral blood smears
Enzyme deficiency anemia	Genetic: deficiency of glucose-6-phosphate dehydrogenase (G6PD)	Episodic hemolytic episodes, decreased levels of G6PD
Hemolytic anemia	Drug-induced or autoimmune response	Splenomegaly, jaundice (may or may not be present depending on cause), pallor
Nutritional Anemias		
Iron deficiency anemia	Chronic blood loss, inadequate intake	Fatigue, exertional dyspnea, microcytosis, low serum iron concentration
Megaloblastic anemia	Deficiency in vitamin B_{12} or folic acid	Macrocytosis, glossitis, and neurologic abnormalities with vitamin B_{12} deficiency

Hct, Hematocrit; *Hgb,* hemoglobin; *MCHC,* mean corpuscular hemoglobin concentration; *MCV,* mean corpuscular volume; *RBCs,* red blood cells.

TABLE 27-2 Transfusion Guidelines for the Symptomatic Patient With Anemia

Component	Indications	Patient Symptoms
Red blood cells	Hgb <8	Shortness of breath, fatigue
Platelets	<20,000	Bleeding, petechiae, bruising
Granulocytes	<500	Sepsis; failure of antibiotic therapy
Fresh frozen plasma	Deficiency of coagulation factors	Hemorrhage
Cryoprecipitate	Deficiency of factors VII and XIII	Diagnosis of hemophilia; uncontrolled hemorrhage

Hgb, Hemoglobin.

products and to monitor the patient carefully for adverse reactions. The nurse should also teach the patient reportable signs and symptoms.

In addition to transfusion therapy, iron supplementation is used to replace depleted iron stores from increased blood cell production (see Iron Deficiency Anemia). Patients experiencing chronic blood loss are encouraged to eat a well-rounded diet that includes foods rich in iron and vitamins.

Patients with low hemoglobin levels may exhibit chronic fatigue and activity intolerance as a result of tissue hypoxia. Activities should be spaced at intervals, allowing the patient frequent rest periods. This optimizes the patient's limited energy reserves.

Routine screening for anemias may be done for high-risk populations by occupational health nurses. Fecal occult blood screening is recommended for persons over the age of 50. Most screening takes place during routine physical examinations and includes blood tests.

Patient/Family Education. Nurses in all settings teach about dietary needs for iron and vitamins. Persons with low incomes can be taught to identify inexpensive food sources of the vitamins and minerals necessary for hematologic health. Nurses can also become politically active to ensure adequate government funding for low-cost nutritional programs for persons with marginal incomes.

Women who have long-term blood loss because of heavy menstrual bleeding are at risk for anemias, as are other persons with long-term, slow blood loss. These women need to be informed of the risks and of the need for continued monitoring of RBC indices. Energy conservation techniques to decrease fatigue should also be taught.

APLASTIC ANEMIA

Etiology/Epidemiology

Aplastic anemia (anemia as a result of impaired erythrocyte production) affects all age-groups and both genders In approximately one half of patients with aplastic anemia in the United States, no etiologic agent is identifiable. Identified causes of aplastic anemia include antineoplastic drugs and exposure to certain drugs, including chloramphenicol, sulfonamides, phenylbutazone (Butazolidin), and anticonvulsant agents such as mephenytoin (Mesantoin). Insecticides such as DDT and chemicals, particularly benzene, also are thought to cause aplastic anemia. Infections associated with the pathogenesis of aplastic anemia include hepatitis (types B and C), Epstein-Barr virus infection, cytomegalovirus infection, and miliary tuberculosis. The defect leading to aplastic anemia is most likely injury or destruction of a common stem cell that affects all subsequent cell populations. Aplastic anemia may also be congenital (Fanconi's anemia).

Pathophysiology

Aplastic anemia usually is characterized by depression or cessation of activity of all blood-producing elements. There is a decrease in the number of white blood cells (WBCs) (leukopenia), a decrease in the number of platelets (thrombocytopenia), and a decrease in the formation of RBCs, which leads to an anemia (Table 27-3). The process may be chronic or acute, depending on the causative factor.

Symptoms of aplastic anemia usually develop gradually over weeks or months but in some cases can have an abrupt onset. Pallor of the skin and mucous membranes is characteristic, in addition to fatigue, palpitations, and exertional dyspnea. Infections of the skin and mucous membranes occur with severe granulocytopenia; hemorrhagic symptoms (bleeding into the skin and mucous membranes and spontaneous bleeding from the nose, gums, vagina, and rectum) occur with severe thrombocytopenia. Findings on physical examination are often unremarkable. The complete blood count (CBC) characteristically reveals a pancytopenia (a marked decrease in the numbers of all cell types) with a low reticulocyte count. Definitive diagnosis of aplastic anemia is made by bone marrow examination. Attempts at bone marrow aspiration may yield a "dry tap" because of hypocellularity and a decrease in active marrow, so a bone marrow biopsy is often necessary.

Fanconi's anemia is an autosomal recessive inherited disorder that is characterized by pancytopenia, or deficiency of all bone marrow elements. Heart, kidney, and skeletal abnormalities may also be present. It is usually lethal by age 20, but new treatment modalities using bone marrow transplantation (BMT) and stem cells to repopulate the patient's body with RBCs, lymphocytes, and platelets are being researched in such places as St. Jude's Hospital in Memphis, Tennessee.[9]

Collaborative Care Management

The immediate treatment for aplastic anemia is the removal of the causative agent, if known. In the past, treatment for aplastic anemia was aimed primarily at stimulating hematopoiesis through the administration of steroids and an-

TABLE 27-3 Normal Blood Cell Function Correlated With the Pathophysiology and Clinical Manifestations of Aplastic Anemia

Normal Function	Pathophysiology	Clinical Manifestations
Red Blood Cells		
Major component is Hgb, which transports oxygen to cells and carbon dioxide from cells to lungs	Reduction or depletion of hematopoietic stem cells, with decreased production of erythrocytes, platelets, and leukocytes Decreased tissue oxygenation	Pallor of skin and mucous membranes; fatigue and exertional dyspnea Low Hgb and Hct levels
Platelets		
Adhesion and aggregation capabilities to plug small breaks in small blood vessels Release of thromboplastin, which, in presence of calcium ions, converts prothrombin into thrombin in initial step of coagulation process	Fewer platelets available for blood coagulation	Bleeding tendency, as evidenced by ecchymosis, purpura, and petechiae Bleeding from nose, mouth, vagina, and rectum Low platelet count
White Blood Cells		
Neutrophils serve as primary defense against bacterial infection through phagocytosis Monocytes remove dead and injured cells, cell fragments, and microorganisms Lymphocytes participate in cellular immune response (T cell) and humoral immune response (B cell)	Fewer WBCs increase susceptibility to infection as a result of decreased phagocytosis and decreased immune response	Repeated infections; frequent sick days Low WBC count

Hct, Hematocrit; *Hgb,* hemoglobin; *WBCs,* white blood cells.

drogen therapy. Because these agents have proved to be of limited value and can produce toxic side effects, BMT from a donor with identical human leukocyte antigen (HLA) has emerged as the treatment of choice for persons with severe aplastic anemia who are younger than age 40 years. Other individuals are treated with immunosuppressive therapy. BMT centers are reporting strong survival rates, often up to 80%.[11] (See Chapter 51 for details on BMT.)

The prognosis for persons with aplastic anemia depends primarily on the severity of the anemia, the method of treatment, and general supportive care. In addition, a higher treatment success rate occurs in patients who receive BMT early and have not received blood products, especially from the potential bone marrow donor. Patients who have undergone transfusion have a higher mortality rate from development of graft-versus-host disease. If transfusions are essential, leukocyte-poor RBCs and platelets should be given. Patients who are not successfully treated often die of complications associated with repeated hemorrhage and infection.

Nursing care is based on careful assessment and management of the complications of pancytopenia and is primarily focused on preventing infection and monitoring for signs of bleeding. To prevent infection in the hospitalized patient who is immunosuppressed, the following interventions should be included in the plan of care:

- Provision of a private room
- Use of protective isolation
- Provision of and instruction of the patient on meticulous hygiene
- Assessment and maintenance of protective oral care regimens
- Monitoring of invasive lines for signs of infection
- Avoidance of bladder catheterization
- Instruction for family and visitors on careful hand washing

Nursing interventions aimed at the prevention of bleeding episodes include:

- Monitoring invasive line sites
- Testing urine and stool for blood
- Minimizing venipuncture and injections
- Avoiding rectal temperatures, medications, and enemas
- Instructing the patient on the use of soft sponges for oral care

Decreased oxygen-carrying capacity of the blood decreases oxygen supply to the tissues, leading to fatigue with activity. Measures to prevent fatigue include providing frequent rest periods, avoiding fatigue-producing activities, and monitoring the patient for signs of excessive fatigue or shortness of breath with activities.

Patient/Family Education. Education of the patient and family members is the cornerstone in the prevention of infection and the avoidance of bleeding episodes in the bone marrow–suppressed patient (see Guidelines for Safe Practice box). Patients are often hospitalized for several weeks, depending on the type of treatment received. The nurse needs to assist the patient in developing coping strategies to deal with the anxiety and isolation of prolonged hospitalization. Music and art therapies are helpful strategies to assist the patient in coping positively with the disease and treatment.

Guidelines for Safe Practice

Teaching the Patient With Aplastic Anemia

1. Prevent infection.
   a. Use good hand-washing technique.
   b. Avoid contact with those who have infections.
   c. Avoid sharing eating utensils and bath linens.
   d. Take a bath every day (or every other day if skin is dry); keep perineal area clean.
   e. Use good oral hygiene.
   f. Eliminate intake of raw meats, fruits, or vegetables.
   g. Report signs of infection immediately to health care provider.
2. Prevent hemorrhage.
   a. Observe for signs such as bloody urine, stool, and petechiae, and report these to physician.
   b. Use a soft toothbrush or swab for mouth care; avoid use of dental floss.
   c. Keep mouth clean and free of debris.
   d. Avoid enemas or other rectal insertions.
   e. Avoid picking or blowing the nose forcefully.
   f. Avoid trauma, falls, bumps, and cuts; avoid contact sports.
   g. Avoid use of aspirin or aspirin preparations (anticoagulant effect).
   h. Use an electric razor.
   i. Use adequate lubrication and be gentle during sexual intercourse.
3. Prevent fatigue.
   a. Take frequent rest periods between ADLs and activity.
   b. Avoid excessive workload or heavy lifting, and ask for assistance with strenuous activity.
   c. Increase time necessary for routine care.
   d. Decrease activity if shortness of breath, dizziness, or sensation of heaviness in extremities occurs.
   e. Report signs of increased fatigue with activity to health care provider.

HEMOLYTIC ANEMIAS

Hemolytic anemia is defined as the premature destruction of erythrocytes occurring at such a rate that the bone marrow is unable to compensate for the loss of cells. Hemolysis can occur either extravascularly or intravascularly. In the case of extravascular hemolysis, the spleen removes erythrocytes from the circulation at an accelerated rate, usually because of some perceived problem with the erythrocyte. Examples of this type of hemolytic anemia are the autoimmune anemias and hereditary spherocytosis.

Intravascular hemolysis, in which erythrocytes lyse and spill cell contents into the plasma, occurs as a result of an enzyme deficiency in the erythrocyte membrane or mechanical factors such as dialysis or prosthetic heart valves, which can prematurely weaken the erythrocyte.

Hemolytic anemias can also develop as a result of abnormal hemoglobin synthesis, as in thalassemia and sickle cell disease. In each case the spleen identifies the RBC as being "abnormal" and destroys it.

Autoimmune Hemolytic Anemia

Etiology/Epidemiology

Autoimmune hemolytic anemias are classified as warm-reacting, cold-reacting, and drug-induced forms.[6] Warm-reacting forms are usually idiopathic and are more commonly seen in women. Associated disease entities are systemic lupus erythematosus, rheumatoid arthritis, chronic lymphocytic leukemia, and myeloma. Immunoglobulin A has also been identified as an etiologic factor in warm-reacting hemolytic disease.

Cold-reacting disease is less common and affects mostly older adults, with an increased incidence in older women. An example of cold-reacting disease is Raynaud's phenomenon. Cold-reacting disease is associated with mononucleosis, *Mycoplasma pneumoniae,* Epstein-Barr virus, mumps, and Legionnaires' disease.

A reaction to drugs causes approximately one fifth of the autoimmune hemolytic anemias. Drugs causing this type of autoimmune reaction are methyldopa, penicillin, quinine, and quinidine.

Pathophysiology

In warm-reacting anemias, antibodies (IgGs) develop against an individual's own erythrocytes. These antibodies combine more readily at body temperature. Antibody-coated RBCs are destroyed by the reticuloendothelial system, particularly the spleen. In episodes of severe hemolysis, dyspnea, palpitations, and congestive heart failure can occur. Jaundice, pallor, and splenomegaly are common.

In cold-reacting disease, IgM antibodies react with antigens on the erythrocyte, optimally in cold temperatures (below 31° C). Ischemia occurs when red cells clump in the capillary beds, causing cyanosis, pain, and paresthesias. Hemoglobinuria also occurs.

Methyldopa (Aldomet, Dopamet) is associated with production of an autoantibody and a positive Coombs' test result in approximately 20% of patients and with a hemolytic anemia that is indistinguishable from an idiopathic autoimmune hemolytic anemia in 1% of patients. Infrequently, high-dose penicillin produces hemolysis through production of an antibody that requires the presence of penicillin on the RBC membrane for its effects to occur.

Collaborative Care Management

Diagnosis is confirmed by demonstrating the presence of the antibody or complement on the RBCs (direct Coombs' test) or in the serum (indirect Coombs' test). Additional laboratory findings show a decreased Hct, an increased reticulocyte count, and an increased bilirubin level. The treatment depends on the cause of the hemolysis.

Mild cases require no treatment. When treatment is indicated, 70% of persons respond to the administration of corticosteroids or danazol (Cyclomen, Danocrine), a gonadotropin inhibitor. Splenectomy is performed for those patients not sufficiently responsive to steroids or danazol and often is successful in controlling or ameliorating the disease. Transfusions may be given cautiously for life-threatening anemia, but this therapy may be difficult and dangerous because of the autoantibody reacting not only with the patient's RBCs but also with all donor cells. Plasmapheresis may be indicated for critically ill patients.

Patient/Family Education. Nursing management consists of teaching the patient about the drug therapy, preparing the patient for surgery if indicated, and helping the patient and family to cope with the illness. The patient and family need to be instructed regarding precipitating factors associated with autoimmune hemolytic anemia. Teaching includes preventive measures such as avoiding exposure to cold for persons with cold-reacting anemias.

Hereditary Spherocytosis

Etiology/Epidemiology

Hereditary spherocytosis (HS) is the most common problem of alteration in erythrocyte shape. This anomaly occurs in approximately 1 of every 5000 persons. It affects all races and both genders fairly equally.[5] HS, inherited as an autosomal dominant trait, is characterized by a membrane abnormality that leads to osmotic swelling of the RBC and susceptibility to destruction by the spleen. It usually is detected in childhood but may appear initially in adulthood.

Pathophysiology

In HS there is a defect in the proteins that form the structure of the erythrocyte. This malformation of proteins gives the cells a thick, spherical appearance. The abnormal cell becomes increasingly permeable to sodium, leading to increased energy demands by the cell. The circulating spherocytes become trapped in the spleen because of the cell's inability to traverse the spleen's microcirculation.[6] Hemolysis occurs in the spleen.

Collaborative Care Management

Diagnosis depends on observation of spherocytes on the peripheral blood smear and by laboratory demonstration of increased osmotic fragility of the RBCs. The reticulocyte count usually is elevated, as is the serum bilirubin level. Bilirubin is derived from the breakdown of the hemoglobin released by the destroyed RBCs. Occasionally, red cell survival time needs to be determined. This is accomplished by labeling the cells with radioactive chromium and measuring the rate of decrease of radioactivity for 1 to 2 weeks (chromium survival). Symptoms of spherocytosis include those typically associated with anemia (pallor, fatigue, exertional dyspnea), jaundice from the increased serum bilirubin level, and an enlarged spleen from the increased RBC destruction.

The treatment for HS is splenectomy. This corrects the hemolysis, but the underlying spherocytosis persists. The gallbladder is often also removed because of the increased incidence of gallstones (50%) in patients with HS. Patients should be given pneumococcal and *Haemophilus influenzae* vaccines before splenectomy.[6] In a recent study of the long-term beneficial effects of subtotal splenectomy for the management of HS, investigators found subtotal splenectomy to be beneficial as a treatment option for individuals with HS (see Research box). The study also showed the phagocytic function of the spleen to remain intact as opposed to the loss associated with total splenectomy.

Research

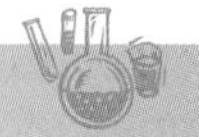

Reference: Bader-Muenier et al: Long-term evaluation of the beneficial effect of subtotal splenectomy for management of hereditary spherocytosis, *Blood* 97(2):399, 2001.

The clinical and biologic features of 40 patients who had undergone subtotal splenectomies were evaluated over a period of 1 to 14 years. Subtotal splenectomy was found to decrease the hemolytic rate while maintaining the phagocytic functions. Gallstone formation and aplastic crisis occurred in a small number of patients. Regrowth of the spleen did not have a major impact. Results indicated that subtotal splenectomy is a reasonable treatment option, especially in children.

Routine postoperative care is indicated for persons who have undergone splenectomy or cholecystectomy. Nursing management includes careful monitoring for infection and continuing monitoring for signs of anemia.

Patient/Family Education. Patient education should include wound management if splenectomy was performed. Genetic counseling is indicated for couples considering childbirth. Energy conservation techniques should be included in the teaching plan.

Enzyme Deficiency Anemia

Etiology/Epidemiology

Deficiency of enzymes in the pathways that metabolize glucose and generate adenosine triphosphate (ATP) (Embden-Meyerhof and pentose phosphate shunt pathways) commonly leads to premature RBC destruction, known as enzyme deficiency anemia. The most common clinically significant enzyme abnormality is that of glucose-6-phosphate dehydrogenase (G6PD). This defect is autosomal recessive and occurs in a mild form among African-Americans. A more severe form can occur in certain population groups in the Mediterranean area and may cause chronic hemolytic anemia.

Pathophysiology

The enzyme G6PD is responsible for the antioxidant reactions in the RBC. The lack of this enzyme causes the cell to be susceptible to oxidizing agents. Exposure to these agents results in damage to the hemoglobin on the RBC membrane and the subsequent release of hemoglobin into the circulation.

Hemolytic episodes in G6PD deficiency can be caused by viral and bacterial infection or oxidant drugs (antimalarials, antipyretics, sulfonamides, quinidine, vitamin K derivatives, and phenacetin). Diagnosis is established by laboratory confirmation of the lack of the G6PD enzyme.[6] Hemolytic episodes persist for 7 to 10 days after exposure to oxidating agents. Symptoms include back pain, jaundice, and hemoglobinuria.

Collaborative Care Management

Treatment is in the recognition of the disorder and cessation of the offending drugs. During a hemolytic episode, hydration and blood transfusions may be necessary. Prompt treatment of infections is also important in managing these patients.

Patient/Family Education. Nursing care centers on the education of patients and their families on the precipitating factors of the disorder and ways to prevent hemolytic episodes. Teaching should include the rationale for increasing oral fluids during bacterial and viral illnesses and avoiding precipitating drugs.

Thalassemia

Etiology/Epidemiology

Thalassemia is one of the most common inherited single-gene disorders in the world. This inherited disorder of hemoglobin synthesis primarily affects persons of Mediterranean descent, but it also occurs in Southeast Asians, Chinese persons, and persons of African descent.

Pathophysiology

Thalassemia is characterized by a decreased synthesis of one of the globin chains of Hgb. The beta (β) chain is most often affected (β-thalassemia). As a result, there is decreased synthesis of hemoglobin and an accumulation of the alpha (α) globin chain in the erythrocyte. These alterations result in decreased RBC production and a chronic hemolytic anemia.

There are two presentations of thalassemia.[5] The heterozygous state, thalassemia minor, is associated with a mild anemia (usually asymptomatic). No therapy is required. The homozygous condition, thalassemia major (also called Cooley's anemia), is characterized by a severe anemia. The RBCs are characteristically hypochromic (low MCHC) and microcytic (low MCV). Diagnosis is by hemoglobin electrophoresis. Growth failure usually begins between ages 10 and 12 years. Death usually occurs during the young adult years between ages 17 and 30[12] (Table 27-4).

Collaborative Care Management

The common treatment for thalassemia is transfusion therapy. BMT is usually considered in children with thalassemia major who are under 5 years of age. Transfusions may be administered either to alleviate severe symptoms or to maintain the Hgb at a near-normal level to allow for a more normal lifestyle. The latter approach incurs the risk of producing iron overload from frequent transfusions, a problem that can be ameliorated by the use of an iron-chelating agent such as deferoxamine. Splenectomy may help decrease transfusion requirements in some patients. Allogenic BMT has been successful in a small number of patients.[17]

The nurse must be familiar with transfusion therapy and sensitive to the emotional needs of patients receiving frequent transfusions. Because the average age at which death occurs is 17 to 30 years, the nurse should be aware of the hopelessness and depression that may occur in this population.

Patient/Family Education. Patients and their families need education about the disease process and rationales for treatment. Couples should be referred for genetic counseling.

Sickle Cell Disease

Etiology

Sickle cell disease (also called sickle cell anemia) is a hemoglobinopathy. Normal Hgb is composed of heme (related to iron) and globin (protein component). The globin part comprises two pairs of polypeptide chains: α and β. Each of the polypeptide chains has a specific amino acid sequence and number. Any deviation in the normal number or sequence of essential amino acids results in abnormal Hgb synthesis.[22]

Disorders of Hgb synthesis are categorized as hemoglobinopathies. They result from abnormalities in one or both of the polypeptide chains (α or β) or in any one of the more than 500 amino acids. One of the most common hemoglobinopathies is sickle cell anemia (hemoglobin SS disease [HbSS]).

Epidemiology

Sickle cell anemia is the most common genetic disorder in the United States. Sickle cell disease (Hb SS) is homozygous recessive (Table 27-5 and Figure 27-1) and is characterized by a chronic hemolytic anemia. Sickle cell anemia occurs predominantly in the black population. An estimated 70,000 African-Americans develop sickle cell disease, and 10% of African-Americans have sickle cell trait. To a lesser extent,

TABLE 27-4 Types of Thalassemia

Type	State	Symptoms	Therapy
Thalassemia minor	Heterozygous	Mild anemia; usually asymptomatic	None required
Thalassemia major	Homozygous	Severe anemia Low MCH Low MCV	Transfusion

MCH, Mean corpuscular hemoglobin concentration; *MCV,* mean corpuscular volume.

TABLE 27-5 Phenotypes for Sickle Cell

Genetic Relationship	Hemoglobin Alleles	Sickle Cell Disease
Homozygous dominant	Hb A, Hb A	No disease
Heterozygous	Hb A, Hb S	Sickle cell trait
Homozygous recessive	Hb S, Hb S	Sickle cell anemia

sickle cell disease also occurs in persons from Asia Minor, India, the Mediterranean area, and the Caribbean area.

Pathophysiology

The basic abnormality lies within the globin fraction of the Hgb, where a single amino acid (valine) is substituted for another (glutamic acid) in the sixth position of the β-chain. This single amino acid substitution profoundly alters the properties of the Hgb molecule (Table 27-6). Because of the intermolecular rearrangement, Hb S is formed instead of normal Hb A. Hb S has normal oxygen-carrying capacity. However, when the oxygen tension of RBCs decreases, Hb S polymerizes, causing the Hgb to distort and realign the RBC into a sickle shape (Figure 27-2). The sickle cell in circulation leads to increased blood viscosity, which prolongs circulation time. This decrease in circulation time causes an increase in the hypoxic time of the cell, promoting further sickling. The development of sickle cells leads to plugging of the small circulation, further decreasing cellular pH and oxygen tension (Figure 27-3).[7] Anaerobic metabolism occurs, with resulting

TABLE 27-6 Normal Hemoglobin, Primary Pathophysiology, and Clinical Manifestations in Sickle Cell Disease

Normal Hemoglobin	Pathophysiology	Clinical Manifestations
Hgb A is major Hgb fraction in adults and consists of two α- and two β-chains, which form a smooth, round shape	Inheritance of homozygous Hgb S interferes with function and structural integrity of Hgb molecule	Chronic hemolytic anemia classified as normochromic and normocytic; peripheral blood smears demonstrate sickled RBCs
Carries oxygen to tissues and carbon dioxide from tissues to lungs	When cellular oxygen tension decreases, RBC distorts itself into sickle shape Sickled cells increase viscosity of blood, slowing circulation and causing increased cellular hypoxia and plugging of circulation to organs; infarcts can occur in central nervous system, eyes, lungs, liver, spleen, kidney, joints, and bone	Vasoocclusive or "painful" crisis, cerebrovascular accident (CVA), retinal hemorrhage, pulmonary infarct, hepatomegaly, autosplenectomy, renal failure, enlarged heart, bone and joint abnormalities, leg ulcers

Hgb, Hemoglobin; *RBC*, red blood cell.

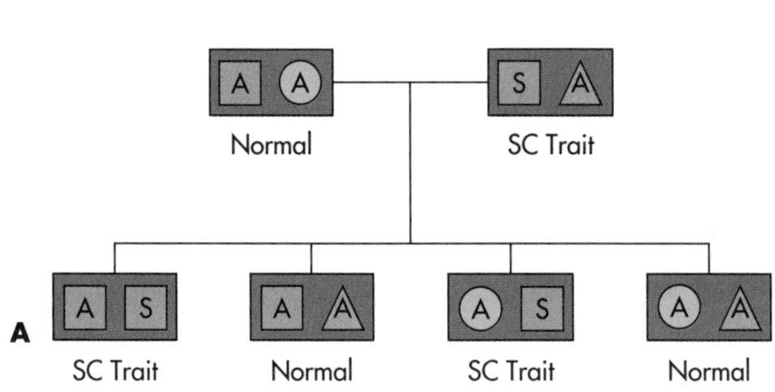

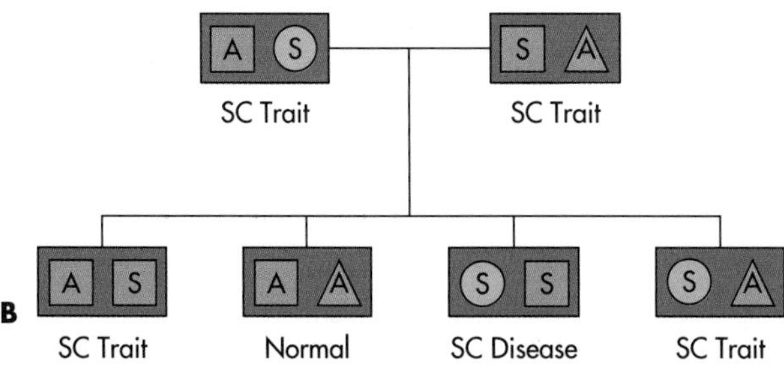

Figure 27-1 **A,** When one parent has sickle cell trait (Hb SA), a 50% probability (2/4) exists that a child will have sickle cell trait. **B,** When both parents have sickle cell trait, there is a 25% probability (1/4) that a child will have sickle cell disease and a 50% probability of sickle cell trait.

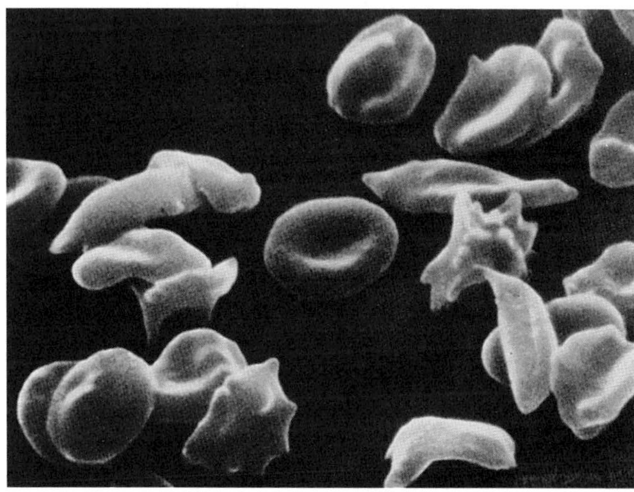

Figure 27-2 Sickled red blood cells.

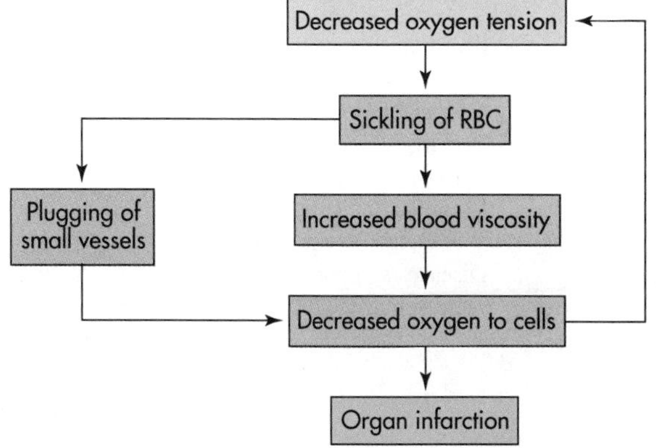

Figure 27-3 Physiologic effects of red blood cell sickling.

tissue ischemia in any organ. This cycle leads to further hypoxia, infarction of organs, and a painful crisis. The affected cells have a shortened life span. They survive in the circulation only 7 to 20 days, as compared with the normal 105 to 120 days, because they are identified as abnormal and destroyed by the spleen.

Different terminologies are used in discussions of sickle cell disease (Table 27-7). Only the homozygous condition of Hb SS describes the classic form of the disease, called *sickle cell anemia.* The heterozygous state, Hb SA, refers to the often asymptomatic condition called *sickle cell trait.* In addition, a category of sickling disorders, called *sickling syndromes,* is associated with the presence of Hb S.

Sickle cell disease is often diagnosed in early childhood and may be fatal by middle age. The gradations of sickling and symptoms vary both in occurrence and intensity. The complexity of this disorder and the problems that can arise from sickle cell disease make it a major health problem. It is usually severe, chronic, and hemolytic. When hospitalization is necessary, it is usually due to one of many complications inherent in sickle cell disease (see Clinical Manifestations box).

The painful vasoocclusive episode is the most common event in sickle cell disease. The pain is a manifestation of localized bone marrow necrosis affecting the juxtaarticular areas of the long bones, spine, pelvis, ribs, and sternum. The frequency of these episodes varies greatly. Some patients experience one or two episodes per month, whereas others have only one or two per year. The duration of the episode also varies and may last from 1 to 10 days. Physical and probably emotional factors (stress) precipitate painful episodes. Physical factors include events that cause dehydration or change the oxygen tension in the body, such as infection, fever, anesthesia, overexertion, exposure to cold or high altitudes, high Hgb levels, ingestion of alcohol, and smoking.

Periodic exacerbations of the anemia are also characteristic of sickle cell disease. Most often these are due to aplastic crises, which are transient periods of time during which erythropoiesis ceases and anemia worsens rapidly as a result of the shortened life span of the RBCs. Aplastic crises can be due to infection or bone marrow necrosis. Diagnosis of aplastic crisis can be made by bone marrow examination. Megaloblastic crisis can also occur with some cases as a result of the depletion of bone marrow stores of folic acid. In such cases the crisis may be treated or prevented by administration of folic acid. Another cause of exacerbation of anemia is acute splenic sequestration. This occurs when the spleen suddenly increases in size, blood pools in it, and hypovolemia with signs of shock develops.

Bacterial infection is a major cause of morbidity and mortality in patients with sickle cell disease. Persons with other hemoglobinopathies, such as Hb SC and Hb S, seem to be at lower risk for infection. Persons with sickle cell disease are particularly susceptible, primarily because most experience functional asplenia (no spleen function). Meningitis, sepsis, pneumonia, and urinary tract infections are potential risks for the person with sickle cell disease.

Collaborative Care Management

Diagnostic Testing. The diagnosis of sickle cell anemia should be considered when any African-American patient presents with hemolytic anemia. The common screening test for sickle cell is the metabisulfate test, or sickle cell solubility test ("sickle prep"). This test will be positive for both sickle cell trait and sickle cell disease. Examination of a peripheral blood smear shows target cells or sickle cell forms. Also seen are Howell-Jolly bodies and siderocytes. The confirmative test for sickle cell disease is hemoglobin electrophoresis. For the homozygous patient the usual pattern is 2% to 20% hemoglobin F, 2% to 4% hemoglobin A_2, and the remainder hemoglobin S. Routine screening should be performed on all newborns in high-risk populations.

Medications. Hydroxyurea is a part of current therapy because it has been shown to decrease the number and severity

TABLE 27-7 Types of Sickle Cell Disorders

Term	Characteristic	Hemoglobin Molecule
Sickle cell trait	Carrier of Hb S Persons are symptom free	Hb SA
Sickle cell disease	Presence of sickling with associated symptoms	Hb SS
Sickle cell syndromes	Diseases associated with presence of Hb S	Hb SC (sickle cell Hb C) Hb SD (sickle cell Hb D) Hb Sβ (sickle cell thalassemia)

Clinical Manifestations

Sickle Cell Disease

ACUTE EPISODES

Pain: usually in the back, chest, or extremities; may be localized, migratory, or generalized
Fever: low grade, 1 to 2 days after onset of pain
Vasoocclusive crises: occlusion of blood vessels by the sickled cells; may occur in areas such as the brain (CVA), chest, liver, or penis (priapism)
Jaundice: caused by increased RBC destruction and the release of bilirubin (Adams and colleagues[2] found that chronic blood transfusions in children with abnormal results on Doppler ultrasonography resulted in a significant decrease in risk for a first or subsequent stroke.)

CHRONIC PROBLEMS

Leg ulcers: usually of the medial malleolus
Renal problems: renal insufficiency from repeated infarctions
Ocular problems: microinfarctions of the peripheral retina leading to retinal detachment and blindness
Musculoskeletal: necrosis of the femoral head

CVA, Cerebrovascular accident; *RBC,* red blood cell.

of pain episodes, the need for transfusions, and episodes of acute chest syndrome and hospitalizations.[8] Erythropoietin, supplemental iron, folic acid, and vitamin B_{12} are given to promote RBC production. Antibiotics are given early in the course of infection to avoid precipitating a crisis.[16] Medications to manage both acute and chronic pain are individualized to the patient's current needs, so frequent reassessment is just as important as initial assessment. Opioids are titrated to give the best pain control for the individual; they are not given by a routine protocol. Drugs used in addition to the opioids include antihistamines, nonsteroidal antiinflammatory drugs, and ketorolac.

Treatments. The cornerstones of treatment continue to be hydration and pain management. Oxygen therapy should be administered during an acute crisis to prevent hypoxemia. Frequent blood transfusions (every 3 to 4 weeks) in children younger than 18 years of age have been shown to prevent both initial strokes and second or third strokes.[2,24] Exchange transfusions have been done with varying degrees of success during vasoocclusive crises.

Patients with sickle cell anemia can be considered for BMT. A problem is the lack of HLA-identical donors because of the genetic component of the disease. Research is continuing for the use of unrelated cord blood stem cell transplantation.

Genetic counseling is important in the prevention of sickle cell disease and is recommended for persons considering childbirth. Parents who both have the sickle cell trait should be informed that the risk of giving birth to an infant with sickle cell disease is one out of four births. Diagnosis of sickle cell disease can be done early in the first trimester of pregnancy.

Diet. A diet rich in protein, calcium, vitamins, and adequate fluids should be encouraged. Iced liquids should be avoided because they may precipitate a crisis.

Activity. Physical stress or overexertion may precipitate a sickle cell crisis. The patient should be taught to avoid activities such as contact sports that may cause joint injury or swelling. Nonstressful exercise such as walking or swimming is recommended to maintain muscle tone and stimulate circulation. Range-of-motion exercises and regular physical activity are important measures to maintain muscle tone and joint mobility.

Referrals. Referrals are indicated for genetic counseling, for chronic pain management, and to specialty clinics on the basis of manifestations of complications. For example, a referral to an orthopedic surgeon may be indicated in the case of severe joint trauma, hemarthrosis, or avascular necrosis.

NURSING MANAGEMENT OF PATIENT WITH SICKLE CELL DISEASE

ASSESSMENT

Health History

Assessment data to be collected as part of the health history include information about the person's present and prior symptoms, knowledge and feelings about the disease, and factors that appear to precipitate or exacerbate symptoms.

Physical Examination

Important aspects of the physical examination of the patient with sickle cell disease include vital signs, a check for blood in the urine, and observation for overt signs of pain and restlessness.

NURSING DIAGNOSES

Nursing diagnoses are determined from analysis of patient data. Prioritizing of nursing diagnoses depends on patient status and main concerns. Nursing diagnoses for the patient with sickle cell disease may include but are not limited to:

Diagnostic Title	Possible Etiologic Factors
1. Acute pain	Imbalance between oxygen supply and demand
2. Deficient fluid volume	Infection, overexertion, weather changes, high Hgb levels, alcohol, smoking
3. Risk for infection	Decreased immune response
4. Ineffective tissue perfusion	Decreased blood flow
5. Impaired gas exchange	Ventilation/perfusion imbalance
6. Activity intolerance	Imbalance between oxygen supply and demand
7. Ineffective individual coping; compromised family coping	Crisis, prolonged disability, genetic component of disease
8. Deficient knowledge	Unfamiliarity with disease and information given

EXPECTED PATIENT OUTCOMES

Expected patient outcomes for the person with sickle cell disease may include but are not limited to:

1. Will feel more comfortable and experiences a reduction in pain
2. Will have moist skin and mucous membranes
3. Will not develop infection
4. Will have warm skin; reports no tissue pain
5. Will breathe easily and regularly
6. Will not complain of fatigue or shortness of breath with activity
7. Will demonstrate coping strategies to deal with chronic illness and will make informed decisions with partner about family planning
8. Will describe the basis of the anemia, availability of genetic and regular counseling, measures to prevent infection, and events that may cause crisis

INTERVENTIONS

1. Promoting Comfort and Pain Reduction

The person who experiences weakness and fatigue from the anemia is assisted in planning daily activities to include rest periods. Pain medication is given before activities that may enhance discomfort. Nursing care for painful episodes involves all the principles of pain management.[8] The goal is to relieve the pain but not overmedicate. This usually involves the use of both narcotic and nonnarcotic analgesics. Astute evaluation of the effectiveness of pain medication is most important. Managing pain in a sickle cell crisis may include the use of patient-controlled analgesia.

2. Promoting Hydration

The vasoocclusive nature of painful episodes requires adequate hydration to decrease blood viscosity. Patients who are supposedly in a steady state of their disease are advised to drink 4 to 6 quarts of water daily; this requirement increases to 6 to 8 quarts of water daily during a painful episode. If intravenous hydration is necessary, careful attention must be given to venous access, with avoidance of multiple punctures and infiltration.

3. Preventing Infection

Because patients with sickle cell disease have a high risk for infection, monitoring for early signs is important. Persons with invasive lines and indwelling urinary catheters are at an increased risk for developing infection. Early signs of respiratory infection (cough, abnormal breath sounds) are reported to the health care provider.

4. Promoting Tissue Perfusion

The patient is monitored for signs of pain that indicate blood vessel occlusion. Changes in pain or mental status are reported to the physician. To avoid vasoconstriction, the patient should be encouraged not to smoke. Constrictive clothing should be avoided.

5. Promoting Oxygenation

Oxygen is given for dyspnea or excessive fatigue with exertion. Reducing activity strain lessens the demand for oxygen. Promoting frequent rest periods while assisting the patient with difficult activities also reduces the demand.

6. Promoting Activity Tolerance

Persons who are trying to maintain independence with activities of daily living (ADLs) are encouraged to take regular rest periods. Increased time may be needed for daily care because of the patient's fatigue or dyspnea.

7. Facilitating Coping, Family Planning, and Genetic Counseling

Patients with sickle cell disease are sometimes labeled as difficult or malingerers because of their behavior patterns, which are influenced by anxiety about their chronic illness. Counseling, use of support groups, and verbalization of fears and anxieties should be encouraged. The patient and family should be supported while implementing behavior and lifestyle changes necessary to cope with a chronic illness.

Many patients with genetic disorders such as sickle cell disease are now deciding when or if they want to have children. Some forms of birth control, such as the intrauterine device (IUD), are not as highly recommended as other forms, such as the diaphragm or spermicides, for persons with sickle cell disorders. An IUD has a higher incidence of infection than the diaphragm or spermicides. Tubal ligation, vasectomy, and oral contraceptives are other possible choices for birth control, but they are associated with significant risk. To make a wise decision about contraception, a couple must be provided with accurate information about side effects, risks, and options. Such family counseling must be performed by persons who are well versed and knowledgeable about the options.

Family planning for persons with sickle cell disease can be a most difficult issue. The fact that a person carries a gene for the disorder makes it possible that this gene will be carried into the next generation. Although moral and ethical arguments can be made, it is ultimately the personal decision of the involved couple.

8. Promoting Knowledge About the Disease

The nurse presents information about the disease, prognosis, and treatment plans in an understandable manner for the patient and family. Strategies for infection control and handling fatigue and pain are offered. Information and/or a referral for genetic counseling should be presented.

Patient/Family Education

See Patient Teaching box.

EVALUATION

To evaluate effectiveness of nursing interventions, compare patient behaviors with those stated in the expected patient outcomes. Achievement of outcomes is successful if a patient with sickle cell anemia:

1. States pain is at a manageable level.
2. Has moist skin and mucous membranes.
3. Has no infection.
4. Has warm skin and no tissue pain.
5. Breathes easily and regularly.
6. Has no complaints of fatigue or shortness of breath with activity.
7. Implements positive coping strategies to deal with chronic illness, including making informed decisions with partner about family planning.
8. Correctly describes the basis of the anemia, availability of genetic and regular counseling, measures to prevent infection, and events that may cause crisis.

Patient Teaching
The Patient With Sickle Cell Disease

The nurse should include the following information when teaching an individual with sickle cell disease:

1. Knowledge of the disease
2. Avoidance of situations that cause crises (infection, high altitudes, overexertion, emotional stress, alcohol, cigarette smoking); avoidance of trauma
3. Importance of adequate fluid intake
4. Availability of psychologic support services and social resources
5. Need for medical follow-up

SPECIAL ENVIRONMENTS FOR CARE

Critical Care Management

The individual experiencing a vasoocclusive episode or exacerbation of the anemia may be hospitalized in the critical care unit during the immediate phase of the crisis if symptoms are severe and respiratory status is compromised. Care is focused on restoring adequate ventilatory capacity, reducing pain and anxiety if present, and preventing complications.

COMPLICATIONS

Occlusion of the microvasculature causes hypoxia, which results in further sickling. This sickling process has major effects on many body systems. Infarction and thromboses resulting from anoxia may occur in the brain, kidneys, bone marrow, and spleen. Increased intracranial pressure may result. In younger patients death may occur from cerebral hemorrhage or shock. The incidence of first and subsequent strokes in children younger than 18 years of age has been significantly reduced through regular monthly transfusion therapy (chronic transfusion therapy).[2] A Nursing Care Plan for the patient with sickle cell crisis follows.

Infection is another complication, which usually occurs in tissues damaged from sickling, especially the lungs, urinary tract, and bones. Urinary tract infections may be a chronic problem. Alterations in skin integrity, such as leg ulcers, are common skin manifestations. Leg ulcers commonly occur on the malleoli and tend to heal poorly.

Bony complications involve the growth plates, resulting in uneven bone growth. Avascular necrosis, especially in the shoulders and hips, can lead to arthritis and eventually total

Nursing Care Plan — Patient With Sickle Cell Crisis

DATA Mr. S. is a 24-year-old married African-American who is the father of one child. He was diagnosed with sickle cell disease at age 10 but was largely symptom free until 2 years ago. He has been admitted with symptoms of sickle cell crisis, including severe joint pain in his upper and lower extremities, moderate fever (38.1° C), and shortness of breath. Sickle cell crisis with congestive heart failure has been diagnosed.

Physical examination reveals crackles in both lower lung lobes, cyanosis of the lips and nail beds, dry scaly skin on both legs, and 2+ pitting edema with a small (2-cm) reddened area over each medial malleolus. His hemoglobin (Hgb) level is 9 g/dl.

Physician orders include 4 L/min of oxygen by nasal cannula, bed rest with bathroom privileges, and morphine sulfate intravenously via patient-controlled analgesia (PCA). He received two units of packed red blood cells followed by intravenous (IV) fluids.

Nursing history identified:

- Mr. S. expresses concern about the outcome of the hospitalization, his ability to "catch his breath," his ability to support his family and care for his son, and his ability to take part in athletic events. His wife has assumed responsibility for some of the yard work, which was formerly his responsibility. He is also concerned about his sexual relationship with his wife because of his general fatigue.
- Mr. S. exercises and jogs several times a week. He admits that he has never been a good water drinker, although he does enjoy soft drinks and an occasional beer. He is unaware of the events that brought on his crisis.
- Mr. S. states that he had his son before understanding the genetic nature of his disease. He fears having more children because he does not want to pass on the sickle cell trait.
- Collaborative nursing actions include maintaining fluid and electrolyte balance, as well as peripheral and pulmonary oxygen/carbon dioxide balance, and preventing further vascular occlusion.

NURSING DIAGNOSIS **Anxiety related to threat to self-esteem, health status, and role functioning**
GOALS/OUTCOMES Will report reduction in anxiety following use of coping strategies

NOC Suggested Outcomes
- Anxiety Control (1402)
- Coping (1302)
- Acceptance: Health Status (1300)

NIC Suggested Interventions
- Anxiety Reduction (5820)
- Coping Enhancement (5230)
- Calming Technique (5880)

Nursing Interventions/Rationales
- Provide opportunities for patient to explore concerns about the effects of his disease. *Making known the unknown and correcting any misconceptions that may exist reduce anxiety.*
- Assess patient's knowledge of sickle cell anemia and sickle cell crisis and correct any misunderstandings. *Misinformation or misunderstandings often lead to fear and resultant anxiety that can be relieved by providing accurate information.*
- Teach relaxation measures and encourage patient to use them when feeling anxious. *Relaxation decreases the psychomotor responses to anxiety.*

Evaluation Parameters
1. Accurately verbalizes signs of anxiety
2. Demonstrates use of relaxation techniques
3. Demonstrates use of positive coping mechanisms

Continued

Nursing Care Plan — *Patient With Sickle Cell Crisis—cont'd*

NURSING DIAGNOSIS **Risk for infection related to spleen dysfunction, inadequate primary and secondary defense mechanisms**

GOALS/OUTCOMES Will remain free of infection

NOC Suggested Outcomes
- Risk Control (1902)
- Nutritional Status (1004)
- Immune Status (0702)

NIC Suggested Interventions
- Infection Protection (6550)
- Skin Surveillance (3590)
- Infection Control (6540)

Nursing Interventions/Rationales
- Monitor for signs of localized infection (redness, warmth, tenderness, swelling) and systemic infection (elevated white blood cell [WBC] count, fever, lethargy). *Treatment for infection can be instituted more quickly when signs of infection are recognized early.*
- Use good hand-washing techniques and maintain medical asepsis. *Aseptic technique decreases the patient's contact with pathogenic organisms. Infection is predicated on the type and number of organisms to which a person is exposed, as well as the patient's resistance to infection.*
- Restrict persons (staff members/visitors) with active infections. *Restricting persons with infections decreases the patient's exposure to infectious agents.*

Evaluation Parameters
1. WBC within normal limits
2. Temperature within normal limits
3. No signs of localized infection

NURSING DIAGNOSIS **Acute pain in joints and chest related to lack of understanding about pain management and sickle cell crisis**

GOALS/OUTCOMES Will achieve pain-free status

NOC Suggested Outcomes
- Comfort Level (2100)
- Pain Level (2102)
- Pain Control (1605)

NIC Suggested Interventions
- Pain Management (1400)
- Analgesic Management (2210)
- Coping Enhancement (5230)

Nursing Interventions/Rationales
- Assess effectiveness of analgesics at least every 4 hours. Consult physician if analgesia is not effective in reducing/controlling pain. *The pain from a sickle cell crisis can be excruciating, and large doses of medication may be necessary. Other medications need to be considered when ordered medication does not control pain.*
- Identify pain relief measures the patient has found useful for relieving pain in the past. *Often pain control methods that are effective for one kind of pain will be effective for other types of pain.*
- Support joints gently when assisting patient with range-of-motion (ROM) exercises. *Improper or lack of support increases stress on joints and exacerbates pain.*
- Use moist heat or massage, if helpful. *Heat dilates blood vessels and increases circulation to the area.*
- Use nonpharmacologic pain relief measures (relaxation, distraction, biofeedback, music, self-hypnosis). *Nonpharmacologic measures may decrease physiologic responses to pain and potentiate the effect of analgesics.*

Evaluation Parameters
1. Reports satisfaction with pain control measures
2. No evidence of pain (restlessness, facial grimace, complaints of pain)
3. Infrequent or nonuse of PCA

NURSING DIAGNOSIS **Risk for situational low self-esteem related to change in disease status, pain, and fear of future disability**

GOALS/OUTCOMES Will verbalize satisfaction with life and self

NOC Suggested Outcomes
- Psychologic Adjustment: Life Change (1305)
- Acceptance: Health Status (1300)
- Body Image (1200)
- Self-Esteem (1205)

NIC Suggested Interventions
- Coping Enhancement (5230)
- Emotional Support (5270)
- Body Image Enhancement (5220)
- Self-Esteem Enhancement (5400)

Nursing Care Plan — Patient With Sickle Cell Crisis—cont'd

Nursing Interventions/Rationales

- Provide opportunities for patient to discuss his feelings about the inability to fulfill his expected role at this time. *Verbalization of concerns decreases their impact and assists in problem solving.*
- Help patient to identify personal strengths. *Focusing on strengths and positive aspects of life provides a basis for personal growth.*
- Assist patient with exploring alternative ways to meet role expectations. *Concern over losses may immobilize the patient. Providing assistance in exploring alternatives helps the patient refocus and seek new methods of reaching desired goals.*
- Refer to a support group or for counseling. *To minimize dependent behaviors. Research shows that increased social support from family and groups increases recovery from disease and disability and facilitates rehabilitation.*

Evaluation Parameters

1. Initiates discussion about changes in health status
2. Identifies alternative means of reaching desired goals
3. Participates in support group discussions

NURSING DIAGNOSIS **Deficient knowledge related to lack of previous experience with sickle cell crisis and unfamiliarity with information sources**

GOALS/OUTCOMES Will accurately describe sickle cell crisis and methods to prevent its exacerbation

NOC Suggested Outcomes

- Knowledge: Health Resources (1806)
- Knowledge: Disease Process (1803)
- Knowledge: Energy Conservation (1804)
- Knowledge: Health Promotion (1823)

NIC Suggested Interventions

- Health System Guidance (7400)
- Teaching: Disease Process (5602)
- Teaching: Prescribed Activity/Exercise (5612)
- Teaching: Prescribed Medications (5616)

Nursing Interventions/Rationales

- Assess patient's knowledge regarding his disease. *The extent of the patient's knowledge about his disease should be acknowledged. It is necessary to determine what the patient does and does not know before teaching can be planned.*
- Teach patient the basis of sickle cell disease, sickle cell crisis, and genetic impact. *Knowledge of the disease helps ensure patient compliance with the medical regimen and adherence to preventive measures.*
- Teach patient to avoid situations that cause crises (see text). *Crises can often be avoided if the patient understands factors that promote crises and can learn to avoid them.*
- Provide resources for family planning and genetic counseling. *Persons and groups with in-depth knowledge of family-planning methods help the patient identify family-planning methods that conform to the patient's cultural and religious values.*
- Teach patient the importance of drinking 4 to 6 L of fluid daily. *Dehydration is a primary cause of red blood cell (RBC) sickling. If the patient understands this, compliance is more likely.*

Evaluation Parameters

1. Accurately describes the nature of the disease and factors that trigger a crisis
2. Asks questions and reads supplied materials
3. Increases oral intake of fluids to prescribed level

NURSING DIAGNOSIS **Sexual dysfunction related to fatigue, pain, and fear of pregnancy**

GOALS/OUTCOMES Will verbalize satisfaction with sexual functioning and relationship

NOC Suggested Outcomes

- Sexual Functioning (0119)
- Endurance (0001)

NIC Suggested Interventions

- Sexual Counseling (5248)
- Energy Management (0180)

Nursing Interventions/Rationales

- Discuss coital positions that require less energy for the patient. *Coitus requires energy and involves neuromuscular activity; side-lying or male-inferior position is less demanding for male patients.*
- Suggest coitus at times of day when the patient is less fatigued (morning, afternoon). *Fatigue increases with continued daily activities and demand on the cardiovascular system.*
- Discuss the need for genetic counseling and contraception. *Knowledge and use of reliable contraception methods to prevent pregnancy reduce fear that contributes to sexual dysfunction.*

Evaluation Parameters

1. Seeks sexual counseling
2. Verbalizes satisfaction with sexual functioning

joint replacement. The vertebrae are also susceptible to bony collapse.

Pulmonary complications include pneumonia, infiltrates, and pulmonary infarction. Fat embolism (arising from the bone marrow) may also occur. Long-term pulmonary complications include pulmonary hypertension and cor pulmonale. Multiorgan failure, including pulmonary, renal, neurologic, and hepatic involvement, may occur in the person with sickle cell disease.

Cardiovascular complications may result from an increased cardiac workload. The patient should be assessed for dysrhythmias and murmurs.

Priapism (prolonged, painful erection) can result from a sickle cell crisis. There is no effective therapy. The best treatment is avoidance of prolonged sexual activity, alcohol, and dehydration.

Although many patients may die during childhood from cerebral hemorrhage or shock, the mortality rate is decreasing and life expectancy is slowly increasing. In the older patient, death usually results from progressive renal damage and uremia.

IRON DEFICIENCY ANEMIA

Etiology/Epidemiology and Pathophysiology

Iron is a fundamental part of the Hgb molecule, and its deficiency leads to production of RBCs with a decreased amount of Hgb and ultimately to fewer RBCs. The average adult body contains approximately 4 g of iron, 3 g of which are in Hgb, 500 mg to 1 g in iron stores in the liver and bone marrow, and the rest in certain tissues and enzyme systems. The body loses approximately 1.5 mg of iron daily; this loss is usually compensated for with daily dietary intake. This tenuous balance may be compromised by chronic blood loss, either physiologic (such as menstruation) or pathologic (from gastrointestinal [GI] or other bleeding), as well as by poor nutrition, especially in older adults (Box 27-1). This compromise results in an iron deficiency anemia.

Gradual development of iron deficiency anemia may permit adaptation with few clinical signs of anemia. Some persons may develop fatigue and exertional dyspnea. Severe iron deficiency anemia causes the nails to become brittle and spoon shaped (concave) and to develop longitudinal ridges (see Clinical Manifestations box). The papillae of the tongue atrophy, and the tongue has a smooth, shiny, bright red appearance. The corners of the mouth may be cracked, reddened, and painful (cheilosis). The RBCs are characteristically hypochromic and microcytic, and the anemia is evident in a peripheral blood smear and blood cell indices. Diagnosis is confirmed by a low serum iron level and elevated serum iron-binding capacity or by a low serum ferritin level or absent iron stores in the bone marrow.

BOX 27-1 Identifying and Preventing Iron Deficiency Anemia in Older Adults

Since older adults may be prone to develop iron deficiency anemia, the nurse should include the following steps in the care plan:

- Observe for dyspnea, bleeding, paleness, clubbing.
- Check the patient's nutritional patterns.
- Listen carefully to the patient's comments about nutritional habits and general health status.
- Assess the dietary iron intake.
- Check if the patient is taking an iron supplement or vitamin with iron.
- Observe the patient's laboratory studies for Hgb and iron levels.
- Offer strategies on how to increase iron intake in the diet.
- Talk to the patient about the importance of preventing iron deficiency anemia.

Hgb, Hemoglobin.

Collaborative Care Management

The first step in medical therapy is to determine and correct the cause of the iron deficiency. Iron is then administered to replace iron stores in the body. Oral iron supplement usually is given in the form of ferrous sulfate.

Patient/Family Education. Patient teaching is the major nursing intervention, especially with a patient newly diagnosed with iron deficiency anemia. Because ferrous sulfate may be irritating to the GI tract, the patient is instructed to take it after meals and with orange juice or vitamin C to increase absorption. The person is told that the stools will be black or tarry and that symptoms of diarrhea or nausea should be reported to the health care provider. Constipation is a major side effect of iron supplementation, and a stool softener may be needed. When the patient cannot tolerate oral iron preparations or is unable to absorb iron properly, parenteral iron is administered intravenously and, rarely, with Z-track intramuscular injection.

Poor diet is rarely the sole cause of iron deficiency anemia but is usually a contributing factor. An assessment is made of the person's dietary habits and knowledge of principles of nutrition. Persons with insufficient financial means for food, medication, or medical attention may be referred to community resources, including a dietitian, social worker, or Meals-on-Wheels.

MEGALOBLASTIC OR MACROCYTIC ANEMIA

Megaloblastic anemia refers to anemias with characteristic morphologic changes caused by defective deoxyribonucleic acid (DNA) synthesis and abnormal RBC maturation. On the peripheral blood smear, macrocytic RBCs and hypersegmented neutrophils (increased number of nuclei) are present.

Clinical Manifestations

Iron Deficiency Anemia

MILD

Fatigue and exertional dyspnea

SEVERE

Brittle, spoon-shaped nails with longitudinal ridges
Smooth, shiny tongue
Cheilosis

In the bone marrow, erythroid precursors can be found that are two to three times larger than normal, with nuclei that are immature relative to their cytoplasmic development.

Etiology/Epidemiology

Most megaloblastic anemias are caused by deficiency of either vitamin B_{12} (cobalamin) or folic acid (Table 27-8). Deficiency of vitamin B_{12} can result from dietary deficiency, surgery, malabsorption, or pernicious anemia. Pernicious anemia is the most common cause of vitamin B_{12} deficiency. Vegetarians can develop vitamin B_{12} deficiency as a result of dietary habits. Both vitamin B_{12} and folic acid are essential in the synthesis of DNA, and their deficiency leads to impaired nuclear development in cells throughout the body. Deficiency of either leads to anemia and often leukopenia and thrombocytopenia. Administration of medication that interferes with DNA metabolism, such as chemotherapeutic agents and anticonvulsants, can also cause megaloblastic anemia. It is essential that the cause of the anemia be identified before medications are started. Failure to recognize a combined vitamin B_{12} and folate deficiency, plus treatment of the folate deficiency only, can result in worsening of neurologic problems for the patient as a result of failure to correct the vitamin B_{12} deficiency. A subacute neurologic syndrome can occur and may progress.[14]

Vitamin B_{12} Deficiency

Vitamin B_{12}, obtained from dietary sources, combines with intrinsic factor in the stomach and is carried to the ileum, where it is absorbed and transported by a carrier protein to the tissues of the body. Patients who have had a total gastrectomy or ileal resection will need parenteral vitamin B_{12} injections for life. Anemia is caused by a lack of intrinsic factor, which allows absorption of vitamin B_{12}.

Pathophysiology

Diagnosis of vitamin B_{12} deficiency is made by demonstration of a low serum vitamin B_{12} level in a patient with macrocytic anemia and megaloblastic bone marrow. In addition to the general symptoms associated with anemia, patients with vitamin B_{12} deficiency may manifest neurologic abnormalities; in particular, they may develop a peripheral neuropathy and a loss of balance resulting from an abnormality of the posterior and lateral columns of the spinal cord (subacute combined degeneration).

Loss of proprioception and diminished vibratory sense have been reported in up to 40% of persons with vitamin B_{12} deficiency. Other neurologic manifestations, including mental status changes, impaired memory, dementia, and depression, are often overlooked or mistaken for Alzheimer's disease in older adults. Diagnosis of pernicious anemia is confirmed by an abnormal Schilling test result, which demonstrates the inability to absorb vitamin B_{12} unless intrinsic factor also is administered.

Collaborative Care Management

Treatment of vitamin B_{12} deficiency consists of parenteral administration of vitamin B_{12}, usually once a month by a nurse in an outpatient setting for patients with any condition that interferes with absorption from the small bowel or who are not producing intrinsic factor. Oral administration is used only in cases of nutritional deficiency. Vitamin B_{12} is available in oral, intramuscular, subcutaneous, and intranasal forms. The most common cause of relapse in persons with pernicious anemia is their reluctance to continue therapy for life.

Patient/Family Education. Patient teaching is a focus of nursing care and discharge planning. The patient must be helped to understand the nature of the illness and the absolute necessity for continued treatment.

Folic Acid Deficiency

Folic acid deficiency anemia may be caused by dietary deficiency, often in association with chronic alcoholism, overcooking of vegetables, malabsorption syndromes, and medications that inhibit the enzyme involved in normal folate

TABLE 27-8 Etiology and Pathophysiology of Megaloblastic or Macrocytic Anemias

Anemia	Etiology	Pathophysiology
Vitamin B_{12} or cobalamin deficiency	Poor dietary intake Malabsorption syndrome Pernicious anemia	Deficiency results in impaired synthesis of DNA, resulting in morphologic changes in blood and marrow
Folic acid deficiency	Poor dietary intake Chronic alcoholism Malnutrition Pregnancy	Folic acid is an essential element required for DNA synthesis and RBC maturation; deficiencies result in morphologic changes in blood and marrow
Pernicious anemia	Autoimmune reaction Loss of parietal cells Overgrowth of intestinal organisms Gastrectomy Ileal resection Tapeworms Inflammatory bowel disease Celiac disease	Intrinsic factor produced by stomach is absent or deficient, resulting in malabsorption of vitamin B_{12}

DNA, Deoxyribonucleic acid; *RBC,* red blood cell.

absorption through the intestinal wall. Pregnancy causes an increase in the need for and use of folic acid. Deficiencies during pregnancy may result in neural tube defects.

Signs and symptoms are associated with the underlying disease and anemia in general. Laboratory findings include macrocytic anemia, megaloblastic changes in the bone marrow, and a low serum folate level.

Collaborative Care Management

Most persons respond promptly to oral folic acid and a well-balanced diet. Daily requirements for folic acid are 100 to 200 mg. The body is able to store approximately a 4-month supply of folic acid. Persons with anemia caused by dietary deficiency can be treated with 1 mg of folic acid for a 3-month period. Return visits to nurse clinics and community health nurse home visits help the person incorporate dietary modifications into daily life. Patients who drink alcohol excessively may be referred to Alcoholics Anonymous. Patients with financial limitations are referred to appropriate community resources.

Patient/Family Education. Patients should be given information about food sources of folic acid and instructed about proper preparation. Foods rich in folic acid include organ meats, eggs, cabbage, broccoli, citrus fruits, and brussels sprouts. Boiling, steaming, and canning of folic acid–rich foods reduces the amount of available vitamin. Persons who consume large amounts of fast foods are susceptible to folic acid deficiency.

ANEMIA OF CHRONIC DISEASE

Etiology/Epidemiology

Anemia of chronic disease (ACD) is one of the most common types of anemia, second only to iron deficiency anemia.[5] It is a normochromic, normocytic, hypoproliferative type of anemia. This anemia commonly accompanies such diseases as chronic inflammatory disorders, some infections, malignancy, AIDS, Crohn's disease, and other systemic disorders.

Pathophysiology

The pathophysiology of ACD is not fully understood but is thought to be related to the failure of erythropoietin (EPO) to stimulate RBC production. Immune activation contributes to the inability of EPO to stimulate the bone marrow. Also contributing to ACD are certain treatments such as chemotherapy, which suppress the marrow's ability to produce RBCs. Symptoms include fatigue, weakness, dyspnea, and anorexia, as well as symptoms of the underlying disease.

Collaborative Care Management

Diagnosis is based on findings of low serum iron, decreased total iron binding capacity, and increased serum ferritin. Treatment is supportive and related to appropriate management of the underlying disease process. The anemia is usually mild, but transfusions may be given in more severe cases. EPO therapy has also been shown to improve the anemia associated with chronic disease.

Patient/Family Education. Education of the patient and family should center on the relationship of the anemia to the underlying disease process. Patients also need to be taught to maximize periods of high energy and to allow frequent rest periods to avoid fatigue. Risks and benefits of transfusion therapy should also be presented to the patient. Instruction about the self-administration of EPO may also be required.

ERYTHROCYTOSIS

Erythrocytosis refers to an abnormal increase in erythrocytes. The increase may be a primary disorder (polycythemia vera) or occur secondary to hypoxia (from high altitudes or from pulmonary and cardiac disease) or certain EPO-producing tumors. With hypoxia, RBCs increase as a compensatory mechanism to carry additional oxygen. Principal laboratory tests to determine the nature of erythrocytosis include determination of the arterial oxygen concentration, RBC volume, and plasma volume.

Polycythemia Vera

Etiology/Epidemiology

Polycythemia vera is a myeloproliferative disorder of the pleuripotent stem cell. The etiology is unknown. The incidence is approximately 2 per 100,000.[23] Polycythemia vera affects both men and women of all ages, with a median age of 60 years. Without treatment, 50% of symptomatic patients die within 18 months.[18] The median survival time (MST) with treatment is 7 to 15 years. The disease is found mainly among Jewish men of European descent. Complications of polycythemia vera include thrombosis, hemorrhage, hyperuricemia, aquagenic pruritus, acid-peptic disease, splenomegaly, hepatomegaly, myelofibrosis, and acute leukemia. Only about 2% of patients develop leukemia unless the treatment includes leukemogenic therapies, in which case, the incidence increases. Death is usually a result of thrombosis, leukemia, or hemorrhage.

Pathophysiology

Polycythemia vera (primary polycythemia) is a bone marrow disorder characterized by erythrocytosis, usually with a simultaneous leukocytosis and thrombocytosis. Hypervolemia (increased blood viscosity from the increased RBC mass) and platelet dysfunction occur.

Symptoms usually are absent in the early stages. As hypervolemia develops, headaches, vertigo, tinnitus, and blurred vision occur. Thromboses with embolization may result from the increased blood viscosity, and the skin may develop a more reddened appearance. Platelet dysfunction may lead to nosebleeds, ecchymoses, and GI bleeding (see Clinical Manifestations box). Thromboembolic events occur in over one third of persons with polycythemia vera and include deep vein thrombosis, cerebral infarction, myocardial infarction, pulmonary embolism, arterial embolism, and splenic infarction. Causes of death are thrombosis (40%), hemorrhage (9%), and leukemia-myelofibrosis (10%).

On physical examination splenomegaly typically is found in persons with polycythemia vera, but it is not common in other types of erythrocytosis. Laboratory tests demonstrate an increased total RBC volume and a plasma volume that is ei-

Clinical Manifestations
Polycythemia Vera

EARLY STAGE
No symptoms

MODERATE STAGE
Headaches, vertigo, tinnitus, blurred vision

LATE STAGE
Thromboses, embolization
Nosebleeds, ecchymoses, gastrointestinal (GI) bleeding

ther increased or normal. The Hct at sea level is greater than 53%. Arterial oxygen concentration is usually normal.

Collaborative Care Management

The goal of therapy is to decrease the red cell mass. Treatment options are phlebotomy (use of alkylating agents), radioactive phosphorus, or interferon. Leukemia transformation may be a significant risk in younger persons treated with myelosuppressive therapy. Usual treatment is periodic phlebotomy aimed at maintaining the Hct and Hgb at a normal level. For patients with secondary erythrocythemia, treatment of the underlying cause is undertaken.

Patient/Family Education. Teaching for the person with polycythemia vera includes the following information:

1. Nature of the disorder
2. Importance of continued medical care, blood tests, and phlebotomy
3. Name, dosage, frequency, desired action, and side effects of prescribed medications
4. Signs of thromboembolic events that require immediate medical attention
5. Maintenance of hydration to decrease blood viscosity
6. Importance of quitting or avoiding smoking

DISORDERS OF PLATELETS AND COAGULATION

Normal hemostatic function requires vascular integrity, normal numbers and function of platelets, and normal clotting factors. Although each of the essential components arises separately and is independently regulated, the balanced interplay among these components is necessary to protect the body from excessive bleeding or excessive thrombi formation.

Primary hemostasis involves the formation of a platelet plug over a damaged area of endothelial cells lining a blood vessel. Primary hemostasis is completed with the formation of the platelet plug. Secondary hemostasis is the formation of a fibrin clot overlying the platelet plug. This process requires sequential activation in the cascade of clotting factors (see Chapter 26). The major steps are the formation of thrombin from prothrombin, leading to the formation of fibrin from fibrinogen.

A fibrinolytic mechanism exists to balance clot formation and leads to clot lysis. Two enzymes are involved in clot lysis: plasminogen and plasmin. Plasminogen is the inactive form that circulates in the blood. It is converted to plasmin by the action of active Hageman factor in addition to other factors. Plasmin then degrades and dissolves the clot. Streptokinase is a fibrinolytic enzyme.

Anticoagulants also help to balance clot formation. A naturally occurring anticoagulant is heparin, which acts by interfering with activation of several coagulation factors, including activation of thrombin. Coumarin derivatives interfere with synthesis of coagulation factors II, VII, IX, and X in the liver by interfering with vitamin K. Heparin interferes with the intrinsic mechanism, whereas warfarin interferes with the extrinsic mechanism.

DISORDERS OF PLATELETS

Disorders of platelet function (Box 27-2) include both increased and decreased numbers of platelets. The term *thrombocytosis* (Box 27-3) is defined as the presence of an abnormally high number of circulating platelets. Mild bleeding syndromes may be caused by quantitatively normal but functionally defective platelets. The most common cause of such platelet abnormalities is drugs, particularly aspirin. Aspirin inhibits the release of intrinsic platelet adenosine diphosphate (ADP) and produces a defect in platelet aggregation. The defect remains for the life span of the platelet. A variety of familial and nonfamilial platelet disorders also has been described, and defective platelet function typically occurs in persons with uremia. The abnormality may be detected by a test of bleeding time or, more sensitively, by platelet aggregation tests. Patients with disorders of platelet function have clinical manifestations and patient care needs similar to those of persons with thrombocytopenia, although the bleeding abnormality usually is mild.

Thrombocytopenia

Etiology/Epidemiology

Thrombocytopenia is defined as a lower than normal number of circulating platelets. Laboratory values for a normal adult platelet count range from 150,000 to 400,000/mm^3. The many types of thrombocytopenia may result from (1) decreased platelet production, (2) decreased platelet survival, (3) increased platelet destruction (most common form), (4) sequestration of blood in the spleen, (5) consumption of platelets, or (6) loss from hemorrhage.

The most common cause of increased destruction of platelets is idiopathic thrombocytopenic purpura (ITP). ITP can be divided into acute and chronic forms. Acute ITP is self-limiting, lasts less than 6 months, and generally follows a viral illness (usually in children). Chronic ITP occurs most often in the second and third decades of life, affects women two to three times more often than men, and is caused by production of an autoantibody (IgG) directed against a platelet antigen.[25] This disorder is named autoimmune thrombocytopenic purpura (ATP).

Platelet destruction may also be drug induced. Approximately 70 drugs (some of which are listed in Box 27-4) have

BOX 27-2 Disorders Associated With Platelets and Coagulation

Platelets

Thrombocytopenia	Decreased number of platelets
Thrombocytosis	Increased number of platelets
Bleeding syndromes	Disorders of platelet function

Coagulation

Congenital

Hemophilia A	Decrease of factor VIII
Hemophilia B	Decrease of factor IX
von Willebrand's disease	Decrease of factor VIII and defective platelet aggregation

Acquired

Vitamin K deficiency	Decrease of factors II, VII, IX, and X
Disseminated intravascular coagulation	Stimulates first the clotting process, then the fibrinolytic process

BOX 27-3 Thrombocytosis

Thrombocytosis can be categorized as reactive (hyperactive bone marrow) or essential (myeloproliferative syndrome).

Associated Conditions

Polycythemia vera
Myelofibrosis
Splenectomy
Iron deficiency anemia
Chronic inflammatory diseases
Hemorrhagic thrombocythemia (thrombocytosis)
Advanced carcinomas

Clinical Manifestations

Thrombosis
Increased bleeding tendencies
Platelet counts >1,000,000/ml

Collaborative Care

Control of underlying cause
Myelosuppressive drug therapy
Plasmapheresis to reduce circulating number of platelets
Antiplatelet agents (e.g., aspirin, dipyridamole)

BOX 27-4 Selected Drugs Typically Causing Thrombocytopenia

Alcohol	Oral hypoglycemic agents
Aspirin	Penicillin
Chemotherapeutic agents	Phenobarbital
Chloroquine	Quinidine
Digitoxin	Quinine
Gold salts	Rifampin
Heparin	Sulfonamides
Methyldopa	Thiazides
Nonsteroidal antiinflammatory agents	

been shown to induce thrombocytopenia. Platelet counts generally return to normal within 1 to 2 weeks after the drug is withdrawn; some drugs such as gold salts may require several months.

Secondary thrombocytopenia may result from aplastic anemia, acute leukemia, and conditions causing splenomegaly (such as cirrhosis or lymphomas, which lead to sequestration of blood in the spleen). Sequestration of blood in the spleen results in splenomegaly. Consumption of platelets is seen in conditions such as disseminated intravascular coagulation, where the platelet supply is simply used up. Hemorrhage from any cause also results in loss of large numbers of platelets.

Pathophysiology

The major signs of thrombocytopenia observable by physical examination are petechiae, ecchymoses, and purpura. Petechiae occur only in platelet disorders. The person may give a history of menorrhagia, epistaxis, and gingival bleeding. The patient is questioned about recent viral infections, which may produce a transient thrombocytopenia; drugs in current use; and the extent of alcohol ingestion.

Collaborative Care Management

Diagnostic tests include complete laboratory studies to ascertain the status of all blood components. The most commonly used tests for assessment of platelets are platelet count, peripheral blood smear, and bleeding time (Table 27-9). In addition, a bone marrow examination is performed to determine the presence of megakaryocytes (precursors of platelets in the bone marrow). Their presence suggests that the thrombocytopenia is caused by peripheral platelet destruction, and their absence or decrease suggests a failure of thrombopoiesis. Examination of the bone marrow also reveals the presence or absence of primary bone marrow abnormalities, such as neoplastic invasion, aplastic anemia, or fibrosis.

The most common treatments for ITP are corticosteroid and immunoglobulin therapy and splenectomy.[26] Steroids appear to decrease both antibody production and phagocytosis of the antibody-coated platelets. Splenectomy removes the principal organ involved in destruction of the antibody-coated platelets. Other therapeutic modalities include danazol or immunosuppressive drugs, but these are usually reserved for severe cases that have not responded to other therapies. Both danazol and immunosuppressive therapies have the potential for severe side effects. Plasma exchange may have some efficacy in acute ITP.

Platelet Transfusion. Transfusion with platelet concentrates may be used in persons with thrombocytopenic bleeding. It is not usually helpful for ITP because the transfused platelets have a short survival time and are rapidly destroyed by the same mechanism as the person's own platelets. When there is impaired platelet production, the platelet concentrates increase the platelet count for approximately 1 to 3 days.[26]

Platelets may be obtained from random or HLA-compatible donors. Random donors are logistically easier to obtain and often provide effective platelets for considerable periods, but use of these platelets may eventually lead to decreased ef-

TABLE 27-9 Common Bleeding/Coagulation Blood Tests

Test	Description	Normal Value
Bleeding time	Evaluation of vascular and platelet factors—the time it takes for a small stab wound to stop bleeding	2-9 min
Clotting time	Time required for solid clot to form (less sensitive test than PTT)	5-10 min
Prothrombin time (PT)	Indicates rapidity of blood clotting (indicative of adequacy of extrinsic coagulation pathway; factors I, II, V, VII, X)	11-15 sec; 100%, compared with control levels
Partial thromboplastin time (PTT)	More sensitive test than PT to evaluate adequacy of intrinsic coagulation pathway (fibrin clot formation)	60-70 sec
Activated partial thromboplastin time (APTT)	Modified PTT; more sensitive; quicker to perform; commonly used to monitor heparin therapy and hemophilia	25-35 sec
International normalized ratio (INR)	A mathematic calculation that corrects for variability in the PT; standardizes PT by correcting for the variability in sensitivities of thromboplastin reagents used in testing	Therapeutic range is 2.0-3.0 in most instances

ficacy because of antibody production. Because platelets are not always matched for ABO antigens and the infused platelets usually are contaminated with some erythrocytes, antibodies to these antigens may develop. When production of antibody impairs platelet transfusion effectiveness, an attempt should be made to obtain platelets from an HLA-compatible donor. The effectiveness of platelet transfusions may be monitored by performing a platelet count before and 1 hour after transfusion. No increase in the platelet count indicates that the transfusion was ineffective. Platelets must be transfused within several days of collection, or they lose their viability. Their survival in a recipient ranges from 48 to 72 hours, compared with a normal platelet life span of 10 days. Transfusions often must be administered twice weekly.

A primary concern in the nursing care of persons with decreased numbers of platelets is the concomitant bleeding tendency. Bleeding associated with trauma is likely with a platelet count less than 60,000/mm^3. Spontaneous hemorrhage may be a life-threatening possibility when the platelet count is below 20,000/mm^3.

Ongoing nursing assessment of the patient is essential and includes alertness for an increase in ecchymoses or petechiae, bleeding from other sites, and any change in mental status. The need for avoiding trauma is obvious. Persons with platelet counts below 20,000/mm^3 should have bleeding precautions instituted. These include:

1. Test all urine and stools for blood (guaiac).
2. Do not take temperatures rectally.
3. Do not administer intramuscular injections.
4. Apply pressure to all venipuncture sites for 5 minutes and to all arterial puncture sites for 10 minutes.

Patient/Family Education. Patient teaching is an important component of patient care. Points to be included in the teaching are listed in the Patient Teaching box.

Patient Teaching
The Patient With Thrombocytopenia

Patient teaching should include information about:

1. The nature of thrombocytopenia
2. Signs of decreased platelet count (petechiae, ecchymoses, gingival bleeding, hematuria, menorrhagia)
3. The name, dosage, frequency, and side effects of prescribed medications (corticosteroids) and the importance of not stopping corticosteroid medications abruptly
4. Guidelines for preventing injury, such as:
   a. Use a soft toothbrush or swab for mouth care.
   b. Do not use dental floss.
   c. Keep mouth clean and free of debris.
   d. Avoid intrusions into rectum (e.g., rectal medications, enemas).
   e. Use an electric shaver.
   f. Apply direct pressure for 5 to 10 minutes if any bleeding occurs.
   g. Avoid contact sports, elective surgery, and tooth extraction.
   h. Avoid blood-thinning drugs, such as aspirin, that decrease sticking ability of platelets.
   i. Increase knowledge of contents of over-the-counter (OTC) medications and effects on platelet functioning. Read labels on OTC medications.
5. The need for follow-up medical care.

Thrombotic Thrombocytopenic Purpura

Etiology/Epidemiology

Thrombotic thrombocytopenic purpura (TTP) is a rare disorder of young adults, occurring more commonly in women than in men. In the majority of cases, the etiology is unknown. The increased incidence within families suggests a genetic component. There is also an increased incidence in persons with an immune system disorder (rheumatoid arthritis, systemic lupus erythematosus, or sarcoidosis). Certain drugs have also been associated with TTP. These include iodine, sulfonamides, penicillin, oral contraceptives, and cyclosporine. Lymphoma, pregnancy, and bacterial endocarditis have also been associated with TTP.

Pathophysiology

The underlying problem in TTP relates to the depletion of circulating platelets as a result of abnormal clotting processes.

The cause of the abnormality in the clotting process is unknown but is thought to be related to vascular injury and hypercoagulability of circulating platelets. The resulting platelet aggregation results in thrombus formation; the thrombus then lodges in the microvasculature of susceptible organs, such as the heart, brain, kidneys, pancreas, and adrenal glands. Symptoms of the disease include fever (with no infection noted), anemia, nausea, anorexia, weakness, petechiae, and hematuria. Additional symptoms are related to the organ involved and include renal failure and neurologic changes.

Collaborative Care Management

Diagnosis of TTP is made by peripheral blood smear. Findings include low platelet counts and red cell fragmentation. Other laboratory features include anemia, reticulocytosis, increased serum lactic dehydrogenase (LDH), normal or increased blood urea nitrogen (BUN), and increased fibrin degradation products (FDPs).

Plasma exchange using fresh frozen plasma is the treatment of choice for TTP. Survival rates are over 80%.[23] Treatment is most effective if it is initiated as soon as TTP is suspected. Exchanges should be continued until platelet counts and serum LDH levels are near normal. Other therapies include vincristine, cyclosporine, azathioprine, immunoglobulin, and splenectomy. Monitoring the patient's mental status is important because coma associated with TTP is not uncommon. Monitoring renal and cardiac function is necessary for early treatment of complications. Renal dysfunction occurs in 50% to 75% of patients with TTP.

Patient/Family Education. Patients may require prolonged treatment with plasma exchanges and may require placement of central venous access devices. Patients and families need to be taught correct management of these devices. Patients should also follow the guidelines presented in the Patient Teaching box on p. 831.

DISORDERS OF COAGULATION

Hemophilia

Etiology/Epidemiology

Hemophilia is a hereditary coagulation disorder. Hemophilia A (factor VIII deficiency), hemophilia B (factor IX deficiency), and hemophilia C (factor XI deficiency) are inherited as sex-linked recessive disorders and are therefore almost exclusively limited to males. An example of the inheritance pattern of hemophilia is shown in Figure 27-4. The incidence of hemophilia A is 1 : 10,000 of the male population, and for hemophilia B, 1 : 100,000. Hemophilia C is rare, with an incidence of 2% to 3% of all hemophilias. The most common "other" form of hemophilia is von Willebrand's disease (vWD), which affects 1% to 3% of the U.S. population but is often overlooked or undertreated in women.[25] In vWD there is a lack of von Willebrand's factor or the factor does not function as it should in platelet adhesion or as a carrier of factor VIII.

Defective gene is found on X chromosome.
When faulty X chromosome is present in a male, he will be a hemophiliac.
(X) Y
When faulty X chromosome is present in a female, she will be a carrier of hemophilia.
(X) X
In conception between a normal male and a carrier female, four possibilities arise:
(X) X — XY
(X) Y Hemophiliac son (mother's carrier X)
XY Normal son (mother's normal X chromosome)
(X) X Carrier daughter (mother's carrier X and father's X)
XX Normal daughter (mother's normal X and father's X)
XX — (X) Y
XY
(X) X
In conception between a hemophiliac male and a normal female, son will be normal but daughter will be carrier.

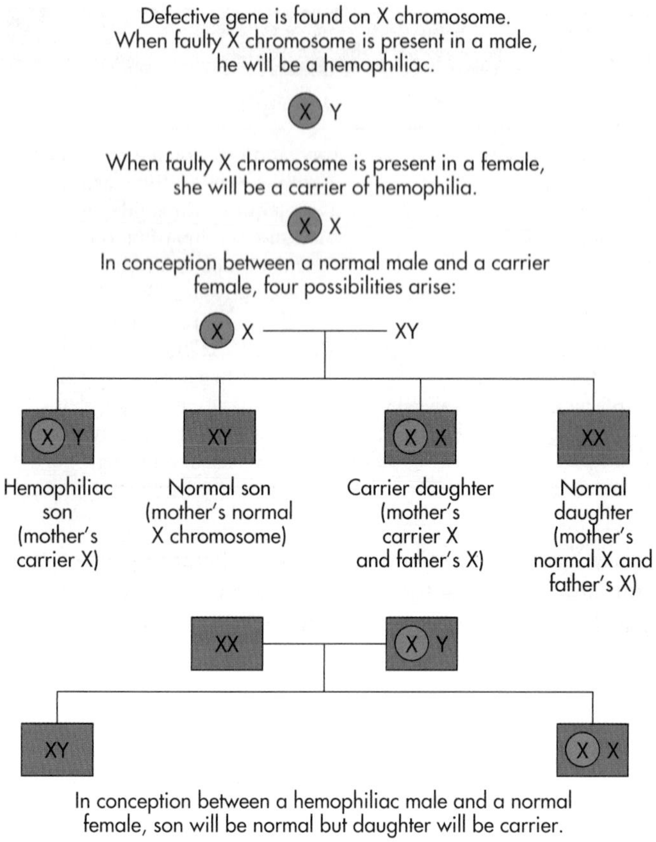

Figure 27-4 Pattern of inheritance of hemophilia.

Pathophysiology

The diagnosis of hemophilia usually is made in infancy or early childhood. The clinical history is one of lifelong bleeding tendency. A history of excessive bleeding after circumcision or dental extractions commonly is obtained. Persons with hemophilia may give a history of bleeding into any part of the body—spontaneously or after trauma (see Clinical Manifestations box). Women with vWD often have a history of easy bruisability, heavy menstrual flow, or postpartal hemorrhage.[25]

A diagnosis of hemophilia is made by specific assays for factors VIII, IX, and XI. The partial thromboplastin time (PTT), which reflects the intrinsic pathway of coagulation, is prolonged in hemophilia A, hemophilia B, and hemophilia C. The platelet count and prothrombin time (PT) are normal.

Complications associated with hemophilia are the direct result of the bleeding tendency. Commonly the person experiences repeated episodes of spontaneous bleeding into the joints, resulting in joint deformities. Life-threatening bleeding involves retroperitoneal, intracranial, and paratracheal soft tissue hemorrhages.

Collaborative Care Management

Treatment is replacement of the deficient coagulation factor when bleeding episodes do not respond to local treatment (ice bags, manual pressure or dressings, immobilization, elevation, or topical coagulants such as fibrin foam and thrombin). Because the deficient factors are contained in plasma, the treatment used for many years was fresh plasma and blood or fresh frozen plasma. In major hemorrhages adequate blood levels were difficult to maintain without overloading the per-

Clinical Manifestations

Hemophilia

History of lifelong bleeding tendency
Repeated episodes of spontaneous bleeding into joints
Excessive bleeding after dental extractions
Life-threatening hemorrhages: retroperitoneal, intracranial, paratracheal

son's circulation with large volumes of blood and plasma. The discovery of cryoprecipitate in 1964 led the way to the development of commercially prepared concentrated preparations such as fibrinogen, factor VIII, and a concentrate containing the four vitamin K–dependent factors (prothrombin and factors VII, IX, and X). Concentrates avoid the problem of circulatory overload and produce fewer adverse effects (e.g., urticarial or febrile reactions) in some patients. High cost and possible contamination with the virus of serum hepatitis or human immunodeficiency virus (HIV) have been drawbacks to the use of some of the concentrates from pooled blood. It has been estimated that at one time, up to 95% of patients with hemophilia developed hepatitis C and that 90% were infected with HIV by 1985.[25]

A number of persons with hemophilia A have developed AIDS from transfusions of factor VIII concentrate. This problem has been corrected with the testing of blood donors for evidence of HIV and with heat treatment of the factor VIII concentrates, which kills HIV. The ability to test for the hepatitis C virus has decreased the per-unit risk for developing the disease to 0.001%.[25]

In classic hemophilia the treatment of choice for an acute bleeding episode is infusion of concentrates of the antihemophilic factor (AHF) (factor VIII). One such concentrate is cryoprecipitate, with a concentration of AHF 15 to 40 times that of normal plasma. Two new recombinant products made from clones of factor VIII are now on the market (Recombinate and Kogenate).[25] In 1997 a recombinate factor IX was approved for use. The use of these recombinant factors has eliminated most, if not all, danger of transmission of HIV or hepatitis (viral) C (HVC) to patients.

DDAVP (D-amino-8-D-arginine vasopressin) has been demonstrated to increase the factor VIII level in persons with vWD and mild hemophilia A. It is given nasally for mild cases and intravenously for moderate or severe cases. DDAVP does not carry the risk of transmitting hepatitis, AIDS, or other disorders.

The outlook for the person with hemophilia has been greatly improved by the availability of transfusion therapy and recombinant therapy. In the past, many persons with factor VIII deficiency died in infancy or in the first 5 years of life. Surgical procedures can now be performed and joint deformity prevented, thus increasing quality of life. Today many persons with moderate or mild hemophilia live normal, productive lives.

Patient/Family Education. Adults with hemophilia generally are knowledgeable about their disease. They should be aware of the possibility of hemorrhage after dental extraction, injury, or surgery. Persons who have hemophilia should carry a card or wear a Medic-Alert tag that includes their name, blood type, physician's name, and disorder to avoid delay in medical treatment if they should accidentally sustain injury and lose consciousness.

Pain control and the threat of spontaneous bleeding episodes are ongoing stressors the person must confront. Those persons who are able to meet the demands of their illness and adapt their lifestyles accordingly are able to live productive lives. Genetic counseling, aimed at explaining the pattern of inheritance of hemophilia, may be of great value to adults contemplating having children. Such counseling can help potential parents realistically evaluate their ability to raise a child afflicted with hemophilia and to anticipate ways to meet the demands placed on both them and the child.

The National Hemophilia Foundation (http://www.hemophilia.org/splash.htm) is an organization established for persons with hemophilia and their families. The basic function of the national organization is hemophilia research. Other functions include the establishment of standards for chapters, publication of literature, production of films, and promotion of federal health care legislation. Local chapter services include special camps for children with hemophilia; parent, child, and adult counseling; group therapy sessions for parents; and a newsletter that reports advances in hemophilic care. A chapter may function as a liaison between hospitals and families with insurmountable bills for blood.

Vitamin K Deficiency

Etiology/Epidemiology

Vitamin K, a fat-soluble vitamin, is a cofactor in the synthesis of clotting factors II, VII, IX, and X. Approximately 50% of required vitamin K is obtained from a normal diet, and 50% is produced by intestinal bacteria. Vitamin K deficiencies can be anticipated in persons who have a decreased intake and who are given broad-spectrum antibiotics (such as neomycin sulfate) that decrease the growth of intestinal bacteria. Interference with vitamin K absorption occurs with primary intestinal disease (e.g., ulcerative colitis, Crohn's disease), biliary disease, and malabsorption syndromes. Drugs such as coumarin derivatives and large doses of salicylates, quinine, and barbiturates interfere with vitamin K function.

Pathophysiology

Symptoms of vitamin K deficiency are those of hypoprothrombinemia superimposed on the underlying disease. Bleeding is similar to other coagulation disorders (i.e., bleeding of the mucous membranes and into the tissues). Postoperative hemorrhage may be observed. In severe cases GI bleeding may be massive.

Collaborative Care Management

Diagnostic features of vitamin K deficiency are a prolonged PT and PTT. There is also a decrease in the levels of vitamin K–dependent clotting factors. Treatment consists of therapy for the underlying disorder and cessation of causative drugs. For mild disorders a water-soluble vitamin K preparation (menadione) is given orally or parenterally. In severe disorders a fat-soluble vitamin K preparation (phytonadione) may be given. Fresh frozen plasma will partially correct the disorder immediately, whereas vitamin K therapy, which does not have the complications of fresh frozen plasma, takes 6 to 24 hours to be effective.

Patient/Family Education. Nursing management includes monitoring of vital signs and patient teaching regarding safety precautions to prevent bruising or bleeding episodes. The patient should be instructed to avoid trauma, use a soft-bristled toothbrush, avoid intramuscular injections, and apply direct pressure immediately on any bleeding sites.

Disseminated Intravascular Coagulation

Disseminated intravascular coagulation (DIC) is a response of the body's hemostatic mechanisms to a variety of diseases or injury. DIC is a complicated and potentially fatal process characterized first by clotting and secondarily by hemorrhage.[15] It almost always occurs in response to a primary disease.

Etiology/Epidemiology

DIC is essentially an imbalance between the processes of coagulation and anticoagulation. Many disease states may alter the normal balance of clotting and fibrinolytic factors, which under normal conditions prevents bleeding while maintaining the fluidity of the blood. DIC may be directly or indirectly initiated by conditions that trigger at least one of three mechanisms: factor XII formation, activation of factors II and X, or tissue thromboplastin release.[23] A stimulus such as sepsis, anoxia, or a burn most likely causes activation of the intrinsic clotting system by the release of factor XII after endothelial cell wall damage and platelet aggregation. DIC may be caused by factor VII activation from massive trauma or the release of tissue thromboplastin from an amniotic fluid embolus entering the maternal circulation. Proteolytic enzymes in snake venom can cause direct activation of factors II and X (Box 27-5). Mortality rates vary because of the multiple precipitating factors associated with DIC. Death usually results from uncontrolled bleeding or multiple organ failure.

Pathophysiology

The primary disease initiates the clotting process. This response is generalized and occurs throughout the vascular system, creating a state of hypercoagulability. The fibrinolytic processes, which normally operate to limit clot extension and dissolve clots, are then stimulated (Figure 27-5). As clotting factors are depleted and fibrinolysis continues, a state of hypocoagulability develops.

The most common sequela of DIC is hemorrhage. This paradox is caused by (1) decreased platelets; (2) depletion of clotting factors II, V, VIII, and fibrinogen in the clotting process; and (3) the production of FDPs through fibrinolysis. The FDPs act as anticoagulants and increase the hemorrhagic tendency.

As the disorder progresses, clinical manifestations may include bleeding of the mucous membranes and tissues, manifested as petechiae and ecchymoses; oral, GI, genitourinary, and rectal bleeding; and bleeding after injections and venipunctures. Hypoxia, tachypnea, hemoptysis, hypotension, acidosis, and fever may also be present (see Clinical Manifestations box).

Collaborative Care Management

Clinical suspicion of DIC is confirmed by laboratory findings (Table 27-10). Abnormal RBCs may be found on a peripheral smear; fibrinolysis may be reflected in increased fibrin split products, increased D-dimers, and a prolonged thrombin time. The management of DIC always begins with treatment of the primary disease. Once this has been initiated, the goal is to control the bleeding and restore normal levels of clotting factors. Blood products such as fresh frozen plasma, platelet packs, cryoprecipitate, and fresh whole blood may be administered to replace the depleted factors. Heparin has been used to inhibit the underlying thrombotic process; however, it too often promotes rather than decreases bleeding, and its use is controversial.

Nursing management of the patient with DIC is extremely challenging. The person who develops DIC is critically ill and commonly has numerous sites of bleeding. The amount and nature of drainage from chest and nasogastric tubes, oozing from surgical incisions, and progressive discoloration of the skin should be noted and recorded.

Continual observation for new bleeding sites and for an increase or decrease in bleeding is an integral part of the nursing plan, especially if heparin therapy is being used. The susceptibility of these persons to bleeding presents special problems; medications should be given orally or intravenously

BOX 27-5 Common Precipitating Factors Associated With Disseminated Intravascular Coagulation

Infections
Hepatitis
Sepsis
Gram-negative infections
Glomerulonephritis

Neoplastic
Adenocarcinoma
Acute leukemias
Pheochromocytoma

Other
Snakebites
Blood transfusion reaction
Surgery
Anaphylaxis
Polycythemia vera
Shock

Obstetric
Retained dead fetus
Abruptio placentae
Amniotic fluid embolus
Toxemia
Septic abortion

Vascular
Aortic aneurysm
Fat embolus
Vasculitis

Trauma
Crush injury
Brain injury
Burns
Ischemia

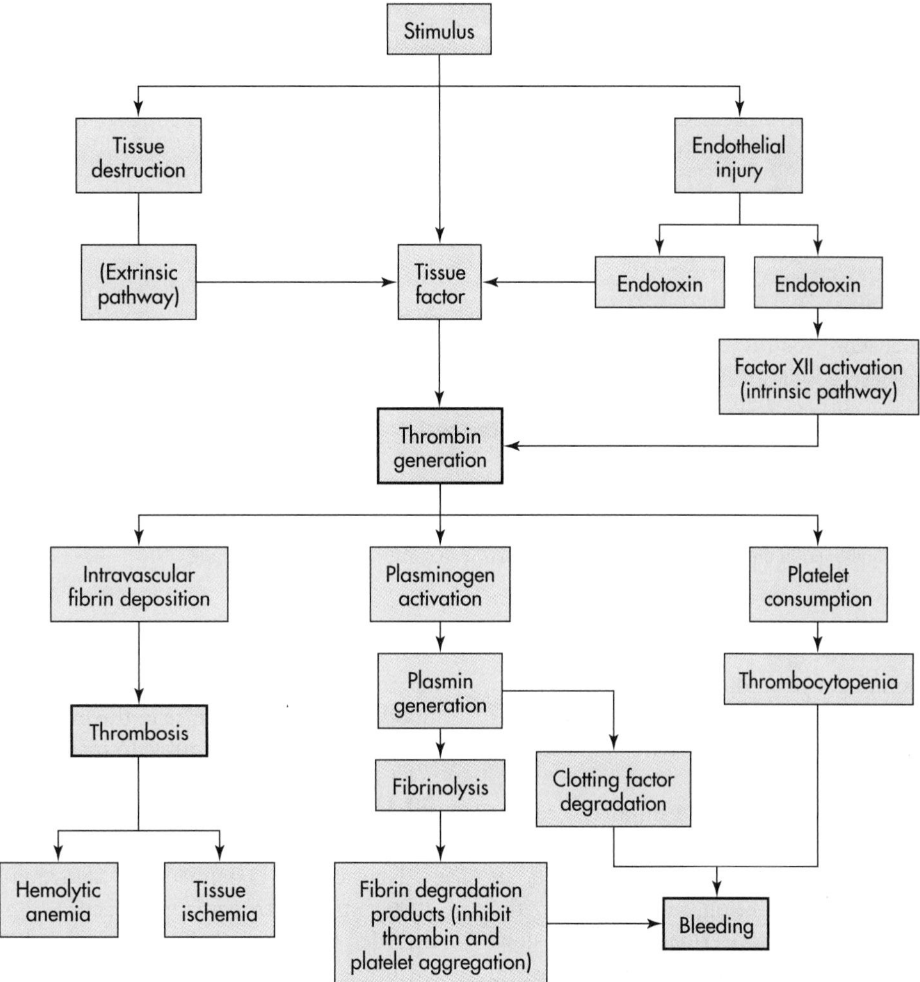

Figure 27-5 Pathophysiology of disseminated intravascular coagulation.

Clinical Manifestations

Disseminated Intravascular Coagulation

NEUROLOGIC
- Confusion
- Irritability
- Headache
- Dizziness
- Seizures
- Fevers
- Increased intracranial pressure
- Vertigo
- Decreased level of consciousness

SENSORY
- Blurred vision/intraocular hemorrhage
- Inner ear bleeding
- Conjunctival hemorrhage
- Epistaxis

CARDIOVASCULAR
- Tachycardia
- Chest pain
- Hypotension
- Absence of peripheral pulses
- Abnormal or increased bleeding from venipuncture or intravenous (IV) insertion sites

RESPIRATORY
- Hemoptysis
- Diffuse infiltrates on x-ray study
- Hypoxia
- Dyspnea
- Tachypnea
- Pulmonary embolus
- Pulmonary edema

GENITOURINARY
- Progressive oliguria
- Hematuria
- Renal failure
- Bleeding around indwelling Foley catheters
- Severe bleeding during menstruation
- Vaginal bleeding
- Proteinuria

Gastrointestinal
- Melena
- High-pitched bowel sounds
- Nausea
- Vomiting
- Abdominal distention
- Hematemesis

INTEGUMENTARY
- Cool, moist skin
- Cyanosis
- Petechiae
- Mottling
- Ecchymoses
- Purpura

GENERAL
- Acidosis
- Acral cyanosis

TABLE 27-10 Laboratory Profile of Disseminated Intravascular Coagulation

Diagnostic Test	Normal Value	Expected Value in DIC
Bleeding time	1-9 min (Ivy method)	Prolonged
Platelet count	150,000-400,000/mm³	Decreased
Prothrombin time (PT)	11-12.5 sec	Prolonged
Partial thromboplastin time (PTT)	PTT: 60-70 sec APTT: 30-40 sec	Prolonged
Factor assay (I, II, V, VII, VIII, IX, X, XI, XII, XIII)		Decreased levels of factors I, II, V, VIII, X, and XIII
Fibrinogen level	200-400 mg/100 ml	Decreased
Fibrinogin/fibrin degradation products (FDPs)	<10	Increased
Red blood cell (RBC) smear		Damaged RBC
Euglobulin lysis time	90 min-6 hr	Normal or prolonged
D-dimer	Qual-Negative Quan- <250 ng/ml	Increased
Thrombin time	10-12 sec	Usually prolonged

Source: Pagana KD, Pagana TJ: *Mosby's manual of diagnostic and laboratory tests,* St Louis, 1998, Mosby.
APTT, Activated partial thromboplastin time; *DIC,* disseminated intravascular coagulation; *RBC,* red blood cell.

if at all possible, and small-gauge needles should be used when other injections are necessary. The precautions previously described for patients with thrombocytopenia are applicable to the patient with DIC.

Maintaining fluid balance assumes great importance. Persons with DIC usually lose large quantities of blood and receive frequent transfusions and other fluid replacement. In addition to monitoring blood infusion rates carefully, the nurse must be alert to signs of fluid overload, such as a slow, bounding pulse and increasing central venous pressure. Hourly urine output is recorded not only as another indication of cardiac function but also because of the possibility of renal thrombi formation and subsequent renal failure.

Patient/Family Education. Commonly the patient is comatose, and the presence of purpura, numerous intravenous lines, and drainage tubes makes the patient's appearance especially upsetting to the family. Most of the primary conditions associated with DIC are of a sudden nature, and the family requires preparation and help in understanding this catastrophic occurrence, as well as support during treatment. Emotional support of the family is paramount because of the sudden and unexpected onset of DIC. Depending on the etiology and severity of DIC, the family may need support and referrals during the grieving process.

DISORDERS ASSOCIATED WITH WHITE BLOOD CELLS

The WBC (leukocyte) system is composed of neutrophils, lymphocytes, monocytes, basophils, and eosinophils. All but the lymphocytes are derived from a common stem cell. The primary function of WBCs is to provide for humoral and cellular response to infection. Neutrophils are primarily responsible for phagocytosis and the destruction of bacteria and other infectious organisms. Lymphocytes are the principal cells involved in immunity, which is responsible for the development of delayed hypersensitivity and the production of antibodies. Any compromise in the integrity of the WBC system renders a person susceptible to infection.

NEUTROPENIA

Etiology/Epidemiology and Pathophysiology

Neutropenia is defined as a neutrophil count of less than 2000/mm³. Neutropenia may occur as a primary hematologic disorder, but more often it is associated with other disorders, including malignant diseases of the bone marrow, aplastic anemia, megaloblastic anemia, use of chemotherapeutic agents, and hypersplenism. The degree of susceptibility to infection is in direct proportion to the degree of neutropenia. Persons with severe neutropenia are at risk of contracting a life-threatening infection.

Collaborative Care Management

Severe neutropenia, sometimes referred to as agranulocytosis, occurs as a reaction to a variety of drugs and chemicals, including sulfonamides, propylthiouracil, and chloramphenicol. Specific treatment consists of removing the offending agent. Granulocyte transfusion may be used for the patient with severe neutropenia whose condition is life threatening. Neutropenic precautions are instituted to protect the patient from infection.

Patient/Family Education. A person with a compromised WBC system is highly susceptible to life-threatening infections. Teaching focuses on avoidance of potential sources of infection and recognition of the earliest signs of infection. If infection is suspected, the patient should report to the primary health care provider.

Meticulous hand washing by hospital personnel and visitors is mandatory. The environment should be kept scrupulously clean and dustless, and persons with any type of infection should not be allowed contact with the patient. Family members and hospital personnel need frequent reminders of this. Mild colds and respiratory tract infections, taken for granted in daily life, are serious threats to patients with decreased numbers of WBCs.

Patients should be in private rooms with posted neutropenic precautions. When this is not possible, cautious screening of roommates for a potential source of infection is mandatory. The patient should be instructed to wear a mask whenever leaving his or her room. To decrease the risk of exposure to bacteria, fresh fruits, vegetables, and flowers are not permitted.

NEUTROPHILIA

Neutrophilia is defined as a neutrophil count greater than 10,000/mm^3. Such an increase is a normal response to infections, primarily bacterial infections. Prolonged elevation of the neutrophil count, especially in the absence of an apparent cause, demands a diligent search for the underlying cause. Persistent elevated neutrophil counts are associated with leukemia, polycythemia vera, myeloid metaplasia, and various systemic and inflammatory disorders.

LEUKEMIAS

Etiology/Epidemiology

Approximately 28,900 new cases of leukemia occur each year in the United States, and the numbers have been increasing over the past three decades.[17] Leukemia is most common in Caucasian males. Five-year survival rates are approximately 40% for acute myelogenous leukemia (AML) and 80% for acute lymphocytic leukemia (ALL).[4] For comparison, the survival rate 50 years ago was 0%. Leukemia is a malignant disorder of the hematopoietic system involving the bone marrow and lymph nodes; it is characterized by uncontrolled proliferation of leukocytes and myelocytes and their precursors. With rare exceptions the bone marrow is involved at the onset, with infrequent manifestations in other hematopoietic organs that lead to organ enlargement (splenomegaly, hepatomegaly). The proliferation of one type of cell often interferes with the normal production of other hematopoietic cells, resulting in the development of immature cells, thrombocytopenia, and anemia.[3] The immaturity of the WBCs leads to decreased immunocompetence and increased susceptibility to infections.

The etiology of leukemia is unknown, but some predisposing relationships have been discovered. Persons with specific chromosomal aberrations, such as occur with Down syndrome, von Recklinghausen's neurofibromatosis, and Fanconi's anemia, have an increased incidence of acute leukemia. Chronic exposure to chemicals such as benzene, drugs that cause aplastic anemia, and radiation exposure has been associated with an increased incidence of the disease. An increased risk for development of acute leukemia also has been noted after cytotoxic therapy for Hodgkin's disease, non-Hodgkin's lymphoma, multiple myeloma, polycythemia vera, and breast, lung, and testicular cancers.

The leukemias are classified as acute or chronic and are further subdivided according to cell type or maturity using the FAB (French, American, British) system devised in 1976. The FAB system sorts ALL into three subsets and AML into seven subsets. All of the types can be traced back to the pleuripotenial stem cell. Acute leukemias involve immature cells and are categorized according to the predominant cell in the bone marrow. They are subclassified as acute ALL or acute nonlymphocytic leukemia (ANLL) according to the specific morphology of the leukemic cell. Acute nonlymphocytic leukemia is further classified as acute AML, promyelocytic leukemia, monocytic leukemia, and other varieties according to cell type. Distinguishing among the various subclassifications of ANLL is difficult, but it is important to do so because newer chemotherapeutic agents appear to have more success against some types and almost none against others. Chronic leukemias may be lymphocytic, as in chronic lymphocytic leukemia (CLL), or granulocytic, as in chronic granulocytic or myelogenous leukemia (CML).

Acute leukemias have a rapid onset and a short course ending in death if untreated.[1] The paucity of normal WBCs leads to numerous infections such as pneumonia and septicemia. Early symptoms include fever and bruising from low WBC and platelet counts; lymphadenopathy; and pallor, malaise, and fatigue from anemia. The WBC count may be normal, decreased, or increased. Other symptoms include bone pain, increased abdominal girth from hepatosplenomegaly, oliguria, obstipation, dehydration, DIC, central nervous system symptoms of nausea and vomiting, headache, and blurred vision.

Chronic leukemias have a more insidious onset. The MST is 3 to 4 years for patients with CML and 2 to 10 years for those with CLL, depending on the stage at diagnosis.[11] Nonspecific flulike symptoms are the usual presentation of leukemia. Early signs include fatigue, weakness, anorexia, and weight loss characteristic of a hypermetabolic state. An enlarged spleen and liver usually can be palpated. The WBC count usually is considerably elevated. See Table 27-11 for a synopsis of the four types of leukemia, symptoms, cell type, and commonly used chemotherapeutics.

Acute Lymphocytic Leukemia

Etiology/Epidemiology

As mentioned earlier, the etiology of ALL is unknown. Eighty percent of persons affected by ALL are between 2 and 4 years of age. There is a decreased incidence of the disease past the age of 10 years.

Pathophysiology

ALL is a malignant disorder arising from a single lymphoid stem cell with impaired maturation and accumulation of the malignant cells in the bone marrow. Diagnosis is confirmed by bone marrow aspiration or biopsy, which typically shows different stages of lymphoid development, from very immature to almost normal cells. The degree of immaturity is a guide to the prognosis: the greater the number of immature cells (increased percentage of lymphocytes and presence of blast cells on a peripheral smear and bone marrow aspiration), the poorer the prognosis.

Signs and symptoms of ALL include anemia, bleeding, lymphadenopathy, and a predisposition to infection. A blood smear may show immature lymphoblasts. The platelet count and Hct level are reduced in most patients.

TABLE 27-11 Clinical Manifestations and Common Chemotherapeutic Agents Used in Different Leukemias

Leukemia	Peak Age (yr)	Characteristic Symptoms	WBC Level	Bone Marrow Cell Predominance	Common Chemo-therapeutic Agents
Acute lymphocytic leukemia (ALL)	2-4	Fever, infections of respiratory tract, anemia, bleeding of mucous membranes, ecchymoses, lymphadenopathy	Decreased, normal, or increased	Lymphoblasts	Regimens with vincristine and prednisone, 6-mercaptopurine, methotrexate
Acute myelogenous leukemia (AML)	12-20, after 55	Same as ALL except less lymphadenopathy	Normal, decreased, or increased	Myeloblasts	Cytarabine, 6-thioguanine, doxorubicin (Adriamycin), daunomycin
Chronic lymphocytic leukemia (CLL)	50-70	Weakness, fatigue, lymphadenopathy, pruritic vesicular skin lesions, thrombocytopenia, anemia, splenomegaly	Increased (20,000-100,000)	Lymphocytes	Alkylating agents (e.g., chlorambucil), glucocorticoids
Chronic myelogenous leukemia (CML)	30-50	Weakness, fatigue, anorexia, weight loss, splenomegaly	Increased (15,000-500,000)	Granulocytes	Hydroxyurea (Droxia) and imatinib (Gleevec) (Busulfan [Busulflex] rarely used now)

WBC, White blood cell.

Collaborative Care Management

Perhaps more dramatically than in any other malignant disorder, chemotherapy has improved the prognosis of children with ALL. Untreated patients have an MST of 4 to 6 months. With current chemotherapy regimens, the MST is close to 5 years, and approximately 50% of children with ALL can be cured.

Complete remissions are obtained in more than 90% of patients treated with chemotherapeutic regimens.[13] Chemotherapeutic protocols for ALL involve three phases: (1) induction, often using vincristine and prednisone; (2) consolidation, using a modified course of intensive therapy to eradicate any remaining disease; and (3) maintenance, usually a combination of drugs, usually including the antimetabolites 6-mercaptopurine and methotrexate. In most chemotherapeutic regimens, vincristine and prednisone are administered intermittently during the maintenance program. Appropriate duration of therapy in patients who remain disease free remains unsettled, but in most centers it is approximately 3 years. The use of "prophylactic" treatment of the central nervous system (e.g., intrathecal administration of methotrexate with or without craniospinal radiation) has greatly diminished recurrences. Because the blood-brain barrier does not allow parenterally infused chemotherapy to reach the leukemic cells, the central nervous system acts as a sanctuary for the leukemia. Intrathecal administration of chemotherapy and/or craniospinal radiation, or both, eradicates the leukemic cells (see Clinical Pathway).

Patient/Family Education. Patient and family teaching should include information about the principles of nutrition. The diet should be high in protein, fiber, and fluids. The patient and family should be taught methods to avoid infection (e.g., hand washing, avoiding crowds) and injury. It is stressed that any signs of bleeding or infection should be reported to the health care provider. Teaching also focuses on measures to decrease nausea and to promote appetite, oral hygiene and interventions to prevent stomatitis, and the need to avoid smoking and spicy, hot foods, which may alter taste or irritate buccal mucosa.

Teaching should also include the prescribed medication regimen. The patient and family should understand the desired and adverse effects of medications, especially chemotherapeutics and the importance of taking antibiotics as prescribed. Pain management is another important intervention. Both pharmacologic and nonpharmacologic methods should be taught. Finally, the patient and family should be aware of the support services available.

Acute Myelogenous Leukemia

Etiology/Epidemiology

AML is a disease of the pluripotent myeloid stem cell. The cause of the malignant transformation is unknown. AML can occur at any age but occurs most often at adolescence and after age 55. Other terms for AML include acute nonlymphocytic, acute granulocytic, and acute myelocytic leukemia.[4,18]

Pathophysiology

AML arises from a single myeloid stem cell and is characterized by the development of immature myeloblasts in the bone marrow. Clinical manifestations are the same as for ALL (see Table 27-11). The WBC count may be low, normal, or high. Bone marrow aspiration reveals a marked increase in myeloblasts.

Collaborative Care Management

Therapy includes the use of cytarabine, and doxorubicin or daunomycin. Elderly patients who cannot tolerate the severity

Text continued on p. 844.

clinical pathway *Acute Leukemia*

DATE	PROBLEM LIST	DISCHARGE CRITERIA
	1. Nausea	1. Vital signs stable (afebrile × 24 hrs)
	2. Pancytopenia	2. Labs stable (ANC >500)
	3. Infection/sepsis	3. Nausea controlled with antiemetics
	4. Pain	4. Able to tolerate 2L fluid/day
	5. Fluid & electrolyte imbalance	5. Pt has not required platelet transfusions for 48 hrs
	6. Bleeding	6. Pain absent/controlled
	7. Knowledge deficit	7. Absence of bleeding
		8. Patient/caregiver has knowledge, resources, and ability to safely provide care outside the hospital environment

4/02 (g:\cct\hem-oncology\leukemia.wpd) ACUTE LEUKEMIA © The Cleveland Clinic Foundation, 2002.* This is a guideline to *assist* in the management of patients. This guideline is not designated to replace clinical judgment or individual or individual patient needs.

Directions:
1. Review CCT approximately every shift.
2. Appropriate and completed interventions need no additional documentation.
3. Cross through any interventions which are not applicable.
4. Circle any items/outcomes which should have been but were not achieved.
5. The plan of care may be revised as necessary.

DRG 473 Expected LOS 17.3
Physician(s) ________________
____
Admit Date ________________
Discharge Date ________________
Surgery/Procedure ________________
____
____
Date of CVAD Placement ______
Surgeon ________________

Comorbid Conditions:
☐ HF ☐ COPD
☐ T1DM
☐ T2DM
☐ CAD

Leukemia type: _____
Date of Dx: ________
Induction:
1st ___ 2nd___
Consolidation:______
Salvage: ________
Risk Factors:
☐ Obesity ☐ ETOH/Substance Abuse ☐ Smoking ☐

Imprint/Label

Complications during this admission:
☐ ICU required ☐
☐ Failure to achieve remission ☐

Last course of chemo: ________

*Specific to Cleveland Clinic requirements.

Continued

clinical pathway *Acute Leukemia—cont'd*

ACUTE LEUKEMIA: DIAGNOSTIC PHASE (PRECHEMO)
PROCEED TO CHEMO PHASE WHEN CHEMO ORDERS ON CHART.

TIME FRAME LOCATION	HOSPITAL DAY DATE UNIT	HOSPITAL DAY DATE UNIT	HOSPITAL DAY DATE UNIT
Discharge Planning Patient Education	Pain education per routine care protocol Teaching re: Bone Marrow Bx Disease process Triple lumen central venous access device (CVAD) Catheter Give written material on Leukemia	Teaching re: Thrombocytopenia Review disease process Review CVAD catheter Review written material	Thrombocytopenia Precautions @ home
Tests/ Procedures/ Consults	Admission labs Bone Marrow Bx MUGA Scan/Echocardiogram WBC ____ K ____ PT/PTT ____ Hgb ____ Cr ____ Fibrinogen ____ Plt ____ Mg ____ Phos ____ DDimer ____ ANC ____ Weight _______	CVAD catheter (following defined diagnosis & treatment decided) WBC ____ K ____ PT/PTT ____ Hgb ____ Cr ____ Fibrinogen ____ Plt ____ Mg ____ ANC ____ Weight _______	WBC ____ K ____ PT/PTT ____ Hgb ____ Cr ____ Fibrinogen ____ Plt ____ Mg ____ ANC ____ Weight _______
Allied Health Interventions	☐ Social Work ☐ Pastoral Care ☐ Nutrition	☐ Case Manager for discharge needs	
Nursing/Medical Interventions	Pain assessment with VS Monitor fluid/electrolyte balance/replace as ordered Monitor blood cts/tx as ordered Monitor coagulation labs/correct as ordered	Pain assessment with VS Monitor fluid/electrolyte balance/replace as ordered Monitor blood cts/tx as ordered Monitor coagulation labs/correct as ordered	Pain assessment with VS Monitor fluid/electrolyte balance/replace as ordered Monitor blood cts/tx as ordered Monitor coagulation labs/correct as ordered
Outcome Criteria	Central venous access devicer site dry & intact Vital signs stable Patient verbalizes an understanding of the disease process and asking appropriate questions	Vital signs stable Patient verbalizes an understanding of the disease process and asking appropriate questions	Vital signs stable Patient verbalizes an understanding of the disease process and asking appropriate questions

Patient Education	Assess for understanding of treatment Pain education per routine care protocol				
Tests/ Procedures/ Consults	WBC ____ K ____ Hgb ____ Cr ____ Plt ____ Mg ____ ANC ____ Weight ________	WBC ____ K ____ Hgb ____ Cr ____ Plt ____ Mg ____ ANC ____ Weight ________	WBC ____ K ____ Hgb ____ Cr ____ Plt ____ Mg ____ ANC ____ Weight ________	WBC ____ K ____ Hgb ____ Cr ____ Plt ____ Mg ____ ANC ____ Weight ________	WBC ____ K ____ Hgb ____ Cr ____ Plt ____ Mg ____ ANC ____ Weight ________
Allied Health Interventions					
Nursing/Medical Interventions	Pain assessment with VS Antiemetics as ordered Monitor fluid/electrolytes/ replace as ordered Monitor blood cts/transfuse as ordered Continue mouthcare protocol CVAD dressing change Chemo Day 6 ________	Pain assessment with VS Antiemetics as ordered Monitor fluid/electrolytes/ replace as ordered Monitor blood cts/transfuse as ordered Continue mouthcare protocol CVAD dressing change Chemo Day 7 ________	Pain assessment with VS Antiemetics as ordered Monitor fluid/electrolytes/ replace as ordered Monitor blood cts/transfuse as ordered Continue mouthcare protocol CVAD dressing Change Chemo Day 8 ________	Pain assessment with VS Antiemetics as ordered Monitor fluid/electrolytes/ replace as ordered Monitor blood cts/transfuse as ordered Continue mouthcare protocol CVAD dressing change Chemo Day 9 ________	Pain assessment with VS Antiemetics as ordered Monitor fluid/electrolytes/ replace as ordered Monitor blood cts/transfuse as ordered Continue mouthcare protocol CVAD dressing change Chemo Day 10 ________
Outcome Criteria	Pain absent/controlled Tolerating chemo Electrolytes stable No evidence of bleeding	Pain absent/controlled Tolerating chemo Electrolytes stable No evidence of bleeding	Pain absent/controlled Tolerating chemo Electrolytes stable No evidence of bleeding	Pain absent/controlled Tolerating chemo Electrolytes stable No evidence of bleeding	Pain absent/controlled Tolerating chemo Electrolytes stable No evidence of bleeding

Continued

clinical pathway *Acute Leukemia—cont'd*

ACUTE LEUKEMIA: NEUTROPENIC PHASE
PROCEED TO DISCHARGE PHASE WHEN ANC >100

TIME FRAME LOCATION	HOSPITAL DAY DATE UNIT	HOSPITAL DAY DATE UNIT	HOSPITAL DAY DATE UNIT	HOSPITAL DAY DATE UNIT	HOSPITAL DAY DATE UNIT
Discharge Planning	Assess for Homecare needs				
Patient Education	Pain education per routine care protocol Teaching re: ATBs Blood products CVAD care				
Tests/ Procedures/ Consults	WBC ____ K ____ Hgb ____ Cr ____ Plt ____ Mg ____ ANC ____	WBC ____ K ____ Hgb ____ Cr ____ Plt ____ Mg ____ ANC ____	WBC ____ K ____ Hgb ____ Cr ____ Plt ____ Mg ____ ANC ____	WBC ____ K ____ Hgb ____ Cr ____ Plt ____ Mg ____ ANC ____	WBC ____ K ____ Hgb ____ Cr ____ Plt ____ Mg ____ ANC ____
Allied Health Interventions	Assess for PT/OT				
Nursing/Medical Interventions	Pain assessment with VS ATBs as ordered Monitor fluid/electrolytes/ replace as ordered Monitor blood cts/transfuse as ordered Continue mouthcare protocol CVAD dressing change	Pain assessment with VS ATBs are ordered Monitor fluid/electrolytes/ replace as ordered Monitor blood cts/transfuse as ordered Continue mouthcare protocol CVAD dressing change	Pain assessment with VS ATBs as ordered Monitor fluid/electrolytes/ replace as ordered Monitor blood cts/transfuse as ordered Continue mouthcare protocol CVAD dressing change	Pain assessment with VS ATBs as ordered Monitor fluid/electrolytes/ replace as ordered Monitor blood cts/transfuse as ordered Continue mouthcare protocol CVAD dressing change	Pain assessment with VS ATBs as ordered Monitor fluid/electrolytes/ replace as ordered Monitor blood cts/transfuse as ordered Continue mouthcare protocol CVAD dressing change
Outcome Criteria	Pain absent/controlled Afebrile Nausea & vomiting under control Electrolytes stable	Pain absent/controlled Afebrile Nausea & vomiting under control Electrolytes stable	Pain absent/controlled Afebrile Nausea & vomiting under control Electrolytes stable	Pain absent/controlled Afebrile Nausea & vomiting under control Electrolytes stable	Pain absent/controlled Afebrile Nausea & vomiting under control Electrolytes stable

Discharge Planning/ Patient Education	Pain education per routine care protocol Consult TPN Nurse for CVAD teaching Assess for Homecare needs Consult ASC as needed	CVAD Teaching begun or scheduled	Discharge Teaching re: Meds, Precautions, Dietary needs and CVAD care Written instructions given	Review Discharge Teaching and written Instructions	Review Discharge Teaching
Tests/ Procedures/ Consults	WBC ____ K ____ Hgb ____ Cr ____ Plt ____ Mg ____ ANC ____ Weight ________	WBC ____ K ____ Hgb ____ Cr ____ Plt ____ Mg ____ ANC ____ Weight ________	WBC ____ K ____ Hgb ____ Cr ____ Plt ____ Mg ____ ANC ____ Weight ________	WBC ____ K ____ Hgb ____ Cr ____ Plt ____ Mg ____ ANC ____ Weight ________	WBC ____ K ____ Hgb ____ Cr ____ Plt ____ Mg ____ ANC ____ Weight ________
Allied Health Interventions	Case Manager to see & evaluate home needs				
Nursing/Medical Interventions	Pain assessment with VS Monitor fluid/electrolytes/ replace as ordered Monitor blood cts/transfuse as ordered Continue mouthcare protocol CVAD dressing change	Pain assessment with VS Monitor fluid/electrolytes/ replace as ordered Monitor blood cts/transfuse as ordered Continue mouthcare protocol CVAD dressing change	Pain assessment with VS Monitor fluid/electrolytes/ replace as ordered Monitor blood cts/transfuse as ordered Continue mouthcare protocol CVAD dressing change	Pain assessment with VS Monitor fluid/electrolytes/ replace as ordered Monitor blood cts/transfuse as ordered Continue mouthcare protocol CVAD dressing change	Pain assessment with VS Monitor fluid/electrolytes/ replace as ordered Monitor blood cts/transfuse as ordered Continue mouthcare protocol CVAD dressing change
Outcome Criteria	Pain absent/controlled Afebrile Nausea & vomiting under control Electrolytes stable	Pain absent/controlled Afebrile Nausea & vomiting under control Electrolytes stable	Pain absent/controlled Afebrile Nausea & vomiting under control Electrolytes stable ANC >500 ATBs D/C'd	Pain absent/controlled Bleeding not present ANC >500 Afebrile IV hydations stopped Able to demonstrate CVAD care	Pain absent/controlled Afebrile × 48 hrs Pt has not required Plt Tx for 48 hours D/C criteria met

of the therapy may elect to take hydroxyurea (less cure, but less early death and better quality of life).[1] Complete remission occurs in 50% to 75% of treated patients, and the MST is approximately 2 to 3 years. Approximately 20% of patients are in complete remission at 5 years and are capable of prolonged disease-free periods (remission). Although patients in remission clearly have an improved quality of life, induction of therapy is arduous, often requiring weeks in the hospital with the need for intensive supportive care (blood component replacement and antibiotic therapy). BMT with the use of HLA-identical allogeneic bone marrow is being used with increasing frequency. Transplanting the patient's own (autologous) bone marrow obtained after a remission with chemotherapy or radiation therapy is another option. Several studies have shown the advantages of BMT with the benefits of colony-stimulating factor, as compared with salvage chemotherapy.[1] A newer method for obtaining stem cells is to retrieve them from the patient's blood (autologous peripheral stem cell transplantation), centrifuge them to remove cancerous clones, and store them for reinfusion after the patient's bone marrow has been destroyed.[6] In the untreated patient or the patient who is unresponsive to therapy, the MST is approximately 2 to 3 months.

Patient/Family Education. The patient and family should be instructed to avoid sources of potential infection. Signs of potential infection should be recognized and reported to the primary health care provider. Precautions to minimize bleeding are emphasized (e.g., soft-bristled toothbrush, electric razors). The patient should be instructed to avoid possible injury or tissue trauma (e.g., blow nose gently, avoid constipation). Dietary instructions should include the basics of a nutritionally adequate diet, particularly high-protein and high-fiber foods. Adequate amounts of fluids (2000 to 3000 ml/day) should be encouraged. The patient also needs instruction about medication protocols, side effects, and management of complications (e.g., nausea, vomiting, mouth care). The nurse should inform the patient and family about available support groups and services.

Chronic Lymphocytic Leukemia

Etiology/Epidemiology

As with other types of leukemia, the etiology of CLL is unknown. An estimated 9000 new cases occur annually. The incidence of CLL increases with age and is rare under age 35. Approximately 90% of CLL patients are younger than 50 years of age.[11] CLL is more common in men than in women.

Pathophysiology

CLL is characterized by a proliferation of small, abnormal, mature B lymphocytes, often leading to decreased synthesis of immunoglobulins and depressed antibody response. The accumulation of abnormal lymphocytes begins in the lymph nodes, then spreads to other lymphatic tissues and the spleen. The number of mature lymphocytes in the peripheral blood smear and bone marrow is greatly increased.

The onset is insidious, with weakness, fatigue, and lymphadenopathy. Symptoms include pruritic vesicular skin lesions, anemia, thrombocytopenia, and an enlarged spleen (see Table 27-11). The WBC count is elevated to a level between 20,000 and 100,000; this increases blood viscosity, and a clotting episode may be the first manifestation of disease. Bone marrow biopsy shows infiltration of lymphocytes.

Collaborative Care Management

The MST of persons with CLL is 4.5 to 5.5 years. As a general rule, persons are treated only when symptoms appear, particularly anemia, thrombocytopenia, or enlarged lymph nodes and spleen. Chemotherapeutic agents used in the treatment of CLL are most often one of the alkylating agents, such as chlorambucil, or one of the glucocorticoids. Although no treatment is curative, remissions may be induced by chemotherapeutics or radiation of the thymus, spleen, or entire body.

Patient/Family Education. Patient and family teaching is similar to that described for AML. Education is necessary regarding the course of the disease and benefits and possible side effects of treatment. This is especially important because of the age of the affected population and the advantages of conservative therapy. Some persons do well without treatment, especially if they are asymptomatic.

Chronic Myelogenous Leukemia

Etiology

Although the etiology of CML is unknown, benzene exposure and high doses of radiation have been associated with CML. In 80% to 95% of persons diagnosed with CML, the Philadelphia chromosome (translocation of chromosomes 22 and 9) has been identified.[11] This has led to research regarding a genetic component to this disease. Further study continues in this area.

Epidemiology

CML accounts for 15% to 20% of all cases of leukemia.[4] The incidence is about 5000 cases per year. The onset of this disease occurs in the third and fourth decades of life and is equally distributed between the sexes.[10]

Pathophysiology

The primary defect in CML is an abnormal stem cell leading to uncontrolled proliferation of the granulocytic cells. As a result of this proliferation, the number of circulating granulocytes increases sharply.

The classic symptoms of chronic types of leukemia also exist in CML. These include fatigue, weakness, anorexia, weight loss, and splenomegaly (Table 27-12). The WBC ranges from 15,000 to 500,000, depending on the stage of the disease. The peripheral blood smear demonstrates granulocytes in varying degrees of maturity, from blast cells to mature neutrophils, and granulocytic hyperplasia in the bone marrow.

CML commonly changes from a chronic indolent phase into an accelerated phase that progresses rapidly into a fulminant neoplastic process sometimes indistinguishable from an acute leukemia. The accelerated phase of the disease (blastic phase) is characterized by increasing numbers of granulocytes

TABLE 27-12 Symptomology of the Phases of Chronic Myelogenous Leukemia

	Stable	Accelerated	Blast Crisis
Presence of symptoms	None to minimal	Moderate	Pronounced
Splenomegaly	Mild	Increased	Marked
WBC count	Slight elevation	Erratic	Very high
Differential	<1% blasts	Increase immature cells	>25% blasts

WBC, White blood cell.

in the peripheral blood. Often there is a corresponding anemia and thrombocytopenia. Fever and adenopathy also may develop. Of patients with CML, 50% to 60% progress to the blastic phase. Once the CML enters the blastic phase, the chemotherapeutic regimen is similar to that of AML.

The overall survival rate for CML is poor. Only 30% of patients survive 5 years after diagnosis. After the onset of a blast crisis, the life expectancy decreases to 2 to 4 months, and the prognosis is grave. A new drug, imatinib (Gleevec), was approved by the Food and Drug Administration under its "accelerated approval" regulations in May 2001.[27] Imatinib is approved for the treatment of three stages of CML: CML myeloid blast crisis, CML accelerated phase, and CML in the chronic phase after failure of treatment with interferon.[19] Imatinib inhibits the translocation-created enzyme and works by blocking the rapid growth of WBCs. The long-term efficacy of the drug has not yet been tested, but individuals in the three stages of CML for which the drug is intended are often rapidly approaching terminal disease if standard treatments are not inducing remission. Clinical trials have indicated that improvement for many patients is possible.

Collaborative Care Management

Diagnostic Tests. The most distinguishing characteristic of CML is the WBC count, which may be greater than 100,000 at the time of diagnosis. The WBC differential count shows a shift to the left. The eosinophil and basophil counts are also elevated. A leukocyte alkaline phosphatase stain, which is low in CML, differentiates this from other types of leukocytosis.

The bone marrow aspirate is hypercellular with increased myeloid cells. CML is confirmed by verifying the presence of the Philadelphia chromosome by genetic karyotyping. In juvenile-onset CML (younger than 4 years of age), the Philadelphia chromosome is missing.

Medications. The goal of treatment for CML is to control the proliferation of WBCs. Two commonly used medications are hydroxyurea and busulfan. Of these two, hydroxyurea is most commonly used because of the high incidence of toxic side effects associated with busulfan. Patients taking hydroxyurea must be instructed about compliance with daily medications and have their blood counts monitored at frequent intervals.

Once CML has converted to the blast phase of the disease, aggressive therapy becomes necessary. Anthracyclines and cytosine arabinoside have been used, but with less than a 20% remission rate. Some success has been seen with the use of the biologic response modifier interferon-α, and current studies are being done to further evaluate the long-term effects of this medication. The newly approved drug imatinib (Gleevec) is given orally once daily and continued for as long as the patient benefits from it.[20] Like the other drugs used to treat CML, imatinib has side effects and adverse reactions that require careful monitoring of the patient. These include fluid retention and edema, GI irritation, hematologic toxicity, hepatotoxicity, and toxicities from long-term use (liver, kidney, immunosuppression seen in animal studies for the drug).

Treatments. The only potential curative therapy for CML is BMT. Transplants with HLA-matched sibling donors are the most successful if they are done early in the course of the disease in patients who are younger than 50 years of age and who are in good underlying health. Transplant-related complications include graft-versus-host disease, sepsis, and uncontrolled bleeding. These present significant risk to the patient.

Diet. Diet is generally unrestricted. Patients who are considered neutropenic (absolute neutrophil count less than 500) should be placed on a low-pathogen diet, which excludes fresh uncooked fruits and vegetables.

Activity. Activity, like the diet, is usually unrestricted. However, patients with platelet counts less than 20,000 should be instructed to avoid activities that may result in injury.

Referrals. The patient and family may benefit from referrals to social services and available community resources (see Patient Teaching box.).

Patient Teaching
The Patient With Leukemia

Patient teaching should include information about:

1. The nature of the disease process and its effects
2. How to prevent infection
3. The drug regimen: name, side effects
4. Arrangements for chemotherapy administration and periodic blood counts
5. Symptoms requiring immediate medical attention (fever, bleeding)
6. Available community resources (American Cancer Society, Leukemia Society)
7. The need for continual medical follow-up
8. How to do meticulous oral care to prevent stomatitis

NURSING MANAGEMENT OF PATIENT WITH CHRONIC MYELOGENOUS LEUKEMIA

ASSESSMENT

Health History

Assessment data to be collected as part of the health history of a patient with CML include:

Symptoms (onset; duration; severity; precipitating, aggravating, and alleviating factors; other characteristics):
- Presence of fatigue
- History of arthralgia, malaise
- Tenderness in the left upper quadrant
- Abnormal bruising or bleeding
- Weight loss
- Decreased exercise tolerance

Physical Examination

Important aspects of the physical examination of the patient with CML include checking for:

- Altered vital signs, including elevated temperature
- Splenomegaly
- Petechiae
- Presence of bruising
- Lymphadenopathy
- Abdominal tenderness
- Shortness of breath
- Pallor
- Hematuria

NURSING DIAGNOSES

Nursing diagnoses are determined from analysis of patient data. Nursing diagnoses for the patient with CML include:

Diagnostic Title	Possible Etiologic Factors
1. Risk for infection	Immunosuppressive therapy, nonfunctioning WBCs
2. Risk for injury	Decreased platelets, bone marrow suppression
3. Impaired oral mucous membrane	Breakdown of oral mucosa secondary to chemotherapy, neutropenia
4. Fatigue	Anemia, chronicity of disease
5. Deficient knowledge	Treatment options
6. Ineffective coping	Poor prognosis of disease

EXPECTED PATIENT OUTCOMES

Expected outcomes for the patient with CML may include but are not limited to:

1. Will maintain normal body temperature and is free of signs of infection
2. Will demonstrate measures to minimize the complications of thrombocytopenia
3. Will demonstrate measures to restore or maintain the integrity of oral mucosa
4. Will maintain level of independence without complaint of fatigue or shortness of breath
5. Will verbalize understanding of the signs of CML and treatment options available
6. Will participate in support groups and identifies effective coping strategies to deal with chronic illness

INTERVENTIONS

1. Preventing Infection

Patients who are neutropenic from either chemotherapy or leukemia are at an increased risk for infection and sepsis. Interventions aimed at reducing patient risk begin with careful hand washing before patient contact. Instructions must also be given to visitors and patients about the necessity of good hand washing. Proper perineal care after urination and bowel movements also decreases the risk of infection.

Patients should have private rooms and be placed in protective isolation. A low-pathogen diet eliminating raw fruits and vegetables is appropriate. Foods from outside sources (carryout, fast foods) and fresh plants and flowers should be discouraged.

The skin, oral cavity, phlebotomy sites, and invasive line sites should be carefully monitored for signs of infection. All invasive lines should be maintained aseptically. Patients should be instructed on the signs and symptoms of impending septic shock and to report any related symptoms immediately. The patient's temperature should be monitored.

2. Promoting Safety

Bleeding is a constant risk for the patient with CML. Platelet counts are monitored daily during hospitalizations. Platelet transfusions may be indicated for patients whose platelet counts are below 20,000 and who are exhibiting signs of bleeding.

The skin should be assessed daily for the presence of petechiae and ecchymosis. Intravenous lines and all invasive sites should be assessed for bleeding. The nurse should also monitor stool and urine for the presence of blood. Any changes in mental status, severe headache, changes in visual and pupillary response, restlessness, or widening pulse pressure should be reported immediately. All invasive procedures should be avoided. Electric razors should be used to avoid potential trauma, and soft-bristled toothbrushes should be provided to the patient for oral care. Stool softeners should be given to avoid constipation, and the patient should be instructed to avoid straining with bowel movements or blowing the nose forcefully.

3. Providing Oral Hygiene

Stomatitis, mucositis, and esophagitis are serious and painful complications related to depression of the immune system, particularly in patients receiving chemotherapy. Persistent comprehensive oral care should be maintained by the patient. Pain associated with breakdown and infection of the oral cavity can be severe. Narcotics may be administered to relieve the pain.

4. Preventing Fatigue

To minimize fatigue in patients with a chronic disease such as CML, it is important to minimize energy expenditure. The patient should be encouraged to prioritize activities and maximize energy potential to complete activities that are most valued. The nurse should assist the patient in delegating nonessential activities to others and provide assistance with ADLs as needed. The patient's activity level can be increased as tolerated. The day should be structured to allow for frequent rest periods.

Sleep deprivation also contributes to a patient's feelings of fatigue. Noise should be limited, and needless interruptions to the patient's sleep avoided. Vital signs and assessments should be performed before the patient is medicated for sleep, allowing for maximal periods of uninterrupted sleep.

5. Promoting an Understanding of the Treatment Options

Patients should be informed about the disease progression, complications, and the treatment options available. Information is given so that the patient can understand the terminology and make informed decisions about the care and treatment delivered.

6. Promoting Effective Coping

CML is a chronic disease with a poor prognosis. Patients and family members must cope with actual and potential losses, as well as with the fear of future treatments and possible side effects. Actively listening as patients and families verbalize their concerns while creating a nonjudgmental atmosphere facilitates coping. Helping the patient to establish personal goals helps promote feelings of self-worth despite chronic illness.

Additional strategies to facilitate coping include relaxation, guided imagery, and music therapy. Patients should also be encouraged to seek out support groups. Many organizations provide assistance to persons with cancer, and patients may need assistance locating available help. Sources of assistance include:

American Cancer Society
Leukemia Society of America
American Red Cross
National Coalition for Cancer Survivorship

Patient/Family Education

Patient and family education should initially focus on the disease process and typical course. Knowledge of specific drug therapy and anticipated side effects is also a component of the teaching plan. Of utmost importance is that the patient learn to identify signals that blood abnormalities exist. Petechiae, ecchymoses, and gingival bleeding (indicating infection) are warning signs indicating the need to seek prompt medical attention. Bone pain, often severe, may signal a blast crisis (acute proliferation of immature cells).

Persons whose illness runs the course of several months to years often become highly knowledgeable about their disease, blood components, related symptoms, and specific chemotherapeutic drugs. These persons sometimes discuss their progress in terms of changes in their blood counts. Many patients are quite knowledgeable about the significance of laboratory results and the effects on the body. For example, they often can predict their count by how they feel. Many such persons respond well to being included in their plan of care during hospitalization and in preparation for discharge.

Establishing a therapeutic relationship with the patient and family allows the patient to vent feelings and fears regarding living with the diagnosis of CML. Teaching sessions should include sufficient time for questions. The family should be included whenever possible (see Patient Teaching box on p. 845).

EVALUATION

To evaluate effectiveness of nursing interventions, compare patient behaviors with those stated in the expected outcomes. Achievement of outcomes is successful if a patient with CML:

1. Remains free of infection.
2. Demonstrates appropriate measures to prevent bleeding episodes.
3. Displays intact oral mucosa and demonstrates correct oral hygiene regimen.
4. Maintains typical level of function without fatigue or shortness of breath.
5. Verbalizes understanding of the disease process and makes informed choices regarding treatment.
6. Identifies coping strategies and develops a support group to assist in managing the stress of chronic disease.

GERONTOLOGIC CONSIDERATIONS

CML is a disease that primarily affects older adults. The typical symptoms of CML may be confused with characteristic changes of aging (Box 27-6). Some persons may be asymptomatic; others may report vague symptoms such as malaise, fatigue, headache, and weight loss.

SPECIAL ENVIRONMENTS FOR CARE

Home Care Management

Since most individuals with CML are managed on an outpatient basis and stay home or with family, helping the patient to become independent is important. During critical periods,

BOX 27-6 Chronic Myelogenous Leukemia in Older Adults

Assessment Findings in CML	Changes Associated With Aging
Skin changes: petechiae, ecchymoses	Increased fragility and decreased skin turgor
Oral cavity: swollen, irritated gums	Ill-fitting dentures
Neurologic: headache, confusion, decreased nerve response	Alzheimer's disease/dementia
Musculoskeletal: joint pain, inflammation, bone pain	Degenerative joint disease
Genitourinary: hematuria, urinary tract infection	Benign prostatic hypertrophy

CML, Chronic myelogenous leukemia.

when the patient is suffering from extreme fatigue, or when the patient is receiving a medication treatment regimen, home health care may be indicated. The home health nurse provides assistance with self-care needs, medication administration, and continued education for the patient.

COMPLICATIONS

Complications of CML include those associated with treatment options. Hemorrhage, infection, and mucositis can occur as a result of chemotherapy or the disease process. During the blast phase, lytic bone lesions, soft tissue infiltrates, and epidural tumors causing cord compression may complicate the course of the disease. As stated earlier, prognosis in this phase is grave. Widespread organ damage may occur, caused by large numbers of leukemic cells occluding the vasculature.

The major side effect of hydroxyurea is reversible myelosuppression. Busulfan toxicity includes potentially fatal myelosuppression, organ fibrosis (lung, heart, and bone marrow), and a wasting syndrome similar to Addison's disease. (Because of the toxicities associated with busulfan, it is rarely used.) Imatinib can cause sudden, severe fluid retention with ascites, effusions in the lungs and pericardium, and pulmonary edema.[20]

Toxicity associated with the use of interferon-α manifests as fever, chills, malaise, arthralgia, fatigue, and headache. These symptoms usually resolve after 2 weeks of therapy with interferon-α. Late signs of toxicity include hepatitis, proteinuria, hypothyroidism, depression, and psychosis.

DISORDERS ASSOCIATED WITH THE LYMPH SYSTEM

LYMPHEDEMA

Etiology

Lymphedema is an abnormal accumulation of lymph within the tissues that is caused by an obstruction in flow. Lymphedema can be classified as primary or secondary. Primary lymphedema results from hypoplastic, aplastic, or hyperplastic development of the lymphatic vessels. Symptoms may manifest at birth, during puberty, or in middle age. Secondary or acquired lymphedema most often develops from trauma to the lymph nodes. Common causes include surgical removal of lymph nodes, radiation-induced fibrosis, inflammation, lymphomas, and parasitic infections.

Epidemiology

Primary lymphedema affects women more commonly than men. Filarial infections, prevalent in tropical climates, are the most common worldwide cause of secondary lymphedema.

Pathophysiology

The lymphatic vessels carry lymph from the tissues back into the venous circulation. This system is made up of small, thin vessels that are found throughout the body in close proximity to the veins. The lymphatics begin as capillaries that drain the tissues of lymph (a fluid similar to plasma) and tissue fluid that contains cells, cellular debris, and proteins. The lymph flows through the lymph nodes, which remove noxious agents such as bacteria and toxins. The flow then drains into the thoracic duct and the right lymphatic duct, which empty into the bloodstream at the junction of the internal jugular vein and subclavian vein (Figure 27-6).

Pathophysiologic changes may include (1) roughening of the surface of the lymphatic vessel, (2) dilation of some lymph channels with thickening and edema of the lymphatic tissue, and (3) fibrosis and separation of elastic fibers that may be present in inflammatory states. Recurrent episodes of lymphedema may cause fibrosis and hyperplasia of lymph vessels, leading to a severe enlargement of the extremity, called *elephantiasis.*

Lymphedema of the lower extremities begins with mild swelling at the ankle, which gradually extends to the entire limb. Initially the edema is soft and pitting, but it then progresses to firm, rubbery, nonpitting edema. Left leg swelling is more common than right leg swelling. This condition is ag-

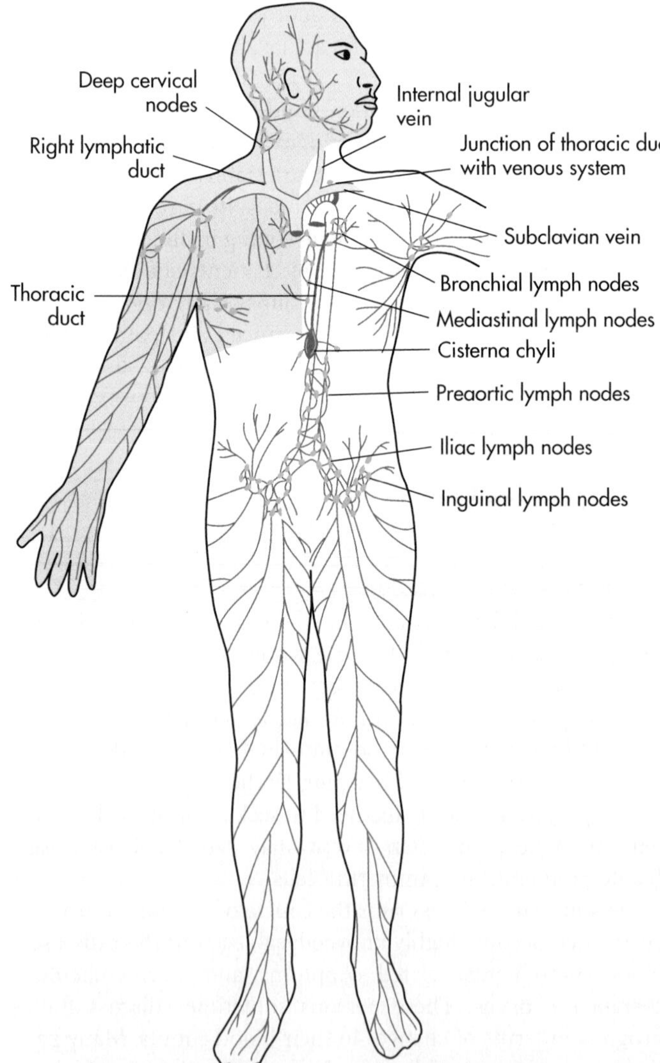

Figure 27-6 Lymph pathways of the lower limb drain into the subclavian vein.

gravated by prolonged standing, pregnancy, obesity, warm weather, and menstruation.

Collaborative Care Management

Diagnostic Tests. Diagnostic tests include the use of lymphangiography. Radioisotope lymphography involves injection of the isotope into the foot, with subsequent scanning. A computed tomography (CT) scan may show a honeycomb pattern in the subcutaneous compartment.

Medications. Diuretics can be prescribed to temporarily decrease the size of the limb. Long-term antibiotic therapy may be indicated to control recurrent cellulitis and infection.

Treatments. Treatment consists of elevating the foot of the bed on blocks at a height of 8 inches, wearing compression support stockings, and using an intermittent pneumatic compression device. Monitoring the circumference of the extremities can help in determining the effectiveness of treatments.

Surgical Management. Surgery is restricted to severe cases of lymphedema that are unsuccessfully treated by medical management. In general, surgery is directed at restoring lymphatic function or improving the patient's symptoms. The most common reason is to reduce the size and bulk of the limb. Surgery also may be used to decrease the incidence of recurrent infections and to improve the cosmetic appearance of the involved limb. The surgical approaches are varied. Microsurgery involving vein grafting to small lymph vessels has been successful.

Diet. There is no special diet to treat lymphedema; however, the patient receiving diuretic therapy requires adequate potassium. Salty and spicy foods that predispose to fluid retention and edema should be avoided.

Activity. Standing still for long periods of time is contraindicated. If infection is present, activity is restricted to bed rest with leg elevation. Otherwise, regular moderate exercise may improve lymph flow.

Referrals. A physical therapy consultation may be appropriate if the patient needs additional assistance with mobility. A wound care specialist may be of help if infection is present.

NURSING MANAGEMENT OF PATIENT WITH LYMPHEDEMA

ASSESSMENT

Health History

Assessment data to be collected as part of the health history of the patient with lymphedema include:

Onset of swelling in affected limb
Any history of surgical removal of lymph nodes, radiation therapy, recurrent inflammation, parasitic infection
Functional limitation of swelling
Association with prolonged standing, pregnancy, obesity, warm weather, and menstruation
Effectiveness of current therapy in decreasing swelling

Physical Examination

Important aspects of the physical examination of the patient with lymphedema include checking for:

Presence of edema: pitting or nonpitting
Location of edema: more common in left leg
Comparison in size of extremities
Texture of skin: firm, rubbery

NURSING DIAGNOSES

Nursing diagnoses are determined from analysis of patient data. Nursing diagnoses for the patient with lymphedema may include but are not limited to:

Diagnostic Title	Possible Etiologic Factors
1. Risk for infection	Lack of knowledge
2. Disturbed body image	Change in body appearance
3. Deficient knowledge	Lack of exposure/recall

EXPECTED PATIENT OUTCOMES

Expected patient outcomes for the person with lymphedema may include but are not limited to:

1. Will describe measures to prevent infection
2. Will express acceptance of body image changes
3. Will state measures to improve lymph circulation

INTERVENTIONS

1. Preventing Infection

The nurse monitors the skin daily for intactness, swelling, redness, and lesions. It is important to provide meticulous care to the skin, especially the feet. The patient should be reminded to complete the entire course of prescribed antibiotics and to avoid application of nonprescribed topical ointments and creams.

2. Promoting a Positive Body Image

The patient is encouraged to express concerns regarding swelling of the affected limb. The nurse presents strategies for altering clothing and shoes to accommodate the swelling. The nurse also should teach about the importance of adherence to measures that decrease edema.

3. Patient/Family Education

The nurse instructs the patient to:

Perform passive and active exercise of involved limb.
Elevate affected extremity.
Avoid standing still for long periods.
Wear compression support stockings.
Avoid constrictive clothing.
Elevate foot of bed on 8-inch blocks.
Use pneumatic external compression pump as ordered.
Take medications as prescribed.

The patient is also taught to exercise on a regular basis and how to adhere to any dietary restrictions that are indicated.

EVALUATION

To evaluate effectiveness of nursing interventions, compare patient behaviors with those stated in the expected patient outcomes. Achievement of outcomes is successful if the patient with lymphedema:

1. Correctly describes measures to prevent infection.
2. Expresses acceptance of body image change.

3. Correctly describes measures to improve lymph circulation (see Chapter 54 for further discussion of lymphedema associated with breast cancer).

GERONTOLOGIC CONSIDERATIONS

Older adult patients with lymphedema may be at increased risk for nonadherence to the prescribed regimen. If the patient has other chronic diseases, restricted mobility, lack of support systems, or difficulty with self-care activities the nurse should refer the patient to a home care agency for additional assistance after discharge. Meeting with family members or other patient caregivers is important for continuity of care. Teaching sessions may need to be extended to the home environment after discharge.

SPECIAL ENVIRONMENTS FOR CARE

Home Care Management

As noted above, the patient with lymphedema may be referred to a home care agency for continued assistance and teaching after discharge from the acute care hospital. The home health nurse works with both the patient and the family to educate them about the care necessary to manage the disease and prevent problems.

COMPLICATIONS

Complications of lymphedema include infection and deformity. These complications are infrequent and can usually be avoided with adherence to the treatment regimen.

HODGKIN'S DISEASE

Etiology/Epidemiology

Hodgkin's disease is a malignant disorder of lymph nodes first described by Thomas Hodgkin in 1832. The etiology is unknown, but there may be a genetic component to the disease.[21] An increased incidence among siblings has been reported. An infectious etiology is under debate. The Epstein-Barr virus has been associated with the development of Hodgkin's disease and is noted in the history of up to 40% of patients who develop Hodgkin's disease. The peak incidence of disease occurs in the third decade of life, with a second peak at ages 55 to 75 years. Men are more frequently affected. An estimated 7400 persons are diagnosed with Hodgkin's disease in the United States annually, causing 1500 deaths.[21]

Pathophysiology

The presence of the Reed-Sternberg cell is the pathologic hallmark of the disorder, but four histologic subtypes of Hodgkin's disease have been recognized: lymphocyte predominant, nodular sclerosis, mixed cellularity, and lymphocyte depletion. The lymphocyte predominant and nodular sclerosis types have the best prognosis, and lymphocyte depletion has the worst. Nodular sclerosis is the most common type and accounts for 40% to 70% of cases. Nodular sclerosis typically manifests in the supraclavicular and cervical nodes. The origin of the Reed-Sternberg cell is unclear, but it may originate from the B lymphocyte or macrophage. The most important prognostic indicator is the stage of the disease at the time of diagnosis. Accurate staging is crucial to the subsequent treatment regimen. The diagnostic workup is often arduous and difficult, and explanation of the many facets of the complex diagnostic procedures helps provide the emotional support so often needed during this time.

Systemic symptoms that may be associated with Hodgkin's disease include fatigue, weakness, anorexia, unexplained fever, night sweats, and generalized pruritus. Physical examination may show painless enlargement of the lymph nodes, liver, and spleen. Lymphadenopathy is most common in the cervical, axillary, and inguinal nodes. A chest roentgenogram may identify the presence of a mediastinal mass. A bone marrow biopsy is performed to determine if there is marrow involvement. The disease may spread via the lymph system to the liver, spleen, vertebrae, uterus, and bronchi. The liver and spleen are evaluated by radionuclide scanning or by a CT scan. Lymphangiography, which requires an experienced operator for accurate results, is performed to evaluate the intraabdominal nodes. A staging laparotomy is performed in some circumstances to obtain a biopsy specimen of retroperitoneal lymph nodes and both lobes of the liver and to remove the spleen. The classification of disease into stages allows for comparison of persons with similar disease involvement and their response to a given treatment regimen. Over time such comparisons have identified the treatment course most appropriate for a described disease. The revised Ann Arbor staging classification for Hodgkin's disease is shown in Box 27-7.

BOX 27-7 Ann Arbor Clinical Staging Classification of Hodgkin's Disease

Stage I

Involvement of a single lymph node region (I) or of a single extralymphatic organ or site (IE)

Stage II

Involvement of two or more lymph node regions on the same side of the diaphragm (II) or localized involvement of an extralymphatic organ or site and of one or more lymph node regions on the same side of the diaphragm (IIE)

Stage III

Involvement of lymph node regions on both sides of the diaphragm (III), which may also be accompanied by involvement of the spleen (IIIS) or by localized involvement of an extralymphatic organ or site (IIIE) or both (IIISE)

Stage IV

Diffuse or disseminated involvement of one or more extralymphatic organs or tissues, with or without associated lymph node involvement

The presence or absence of fever, night sweats, or unexplained loss of 10% or more of body weight in the 6 months preceding admission are denoted by the suffix letters *B* and *A*, respectively. Biopsy-documented involvement of stage IV sites also is denoted by letter suffixes: *M*, marrow; *L*, lung; *H*, liver; *P*, pleura; *O*, bone; *D*, skin and subcutaneous tissue.

Collaborative Care Management

Radiation therapy (Figure 27-7) is used for stages IA, IB, IIA, and IIB. This treatment yields a cure rate of approximately 90% for stage I and 80% for stage II. Combination chemotherapy is the treatment of choice for stages IIIB and IV. Therapy of stage IIIA is controversial and involves chemotherapy, radiation, or a combination of these therapies. The most commonly used chemotherapy combination is the MOPP regimen, which consists of mechlorethamine (nitrogen mustard), vincristine (Oncovin), procarbazine, and prednisone (Table 27-13). This regimen is administered in a 2-week course each month with prednisone added during the first and fourth courses. The drugs are administered for at least 6 months or for two or three courses after the attainment of complete remission. Complete remissions are achieved in approximately 80% of these patients; long-term, disease-free remissions and probable cures occur in half of this group.[21] Continuing chemotherapy beyond the attainment of complete remission has not been shown to improve survival.

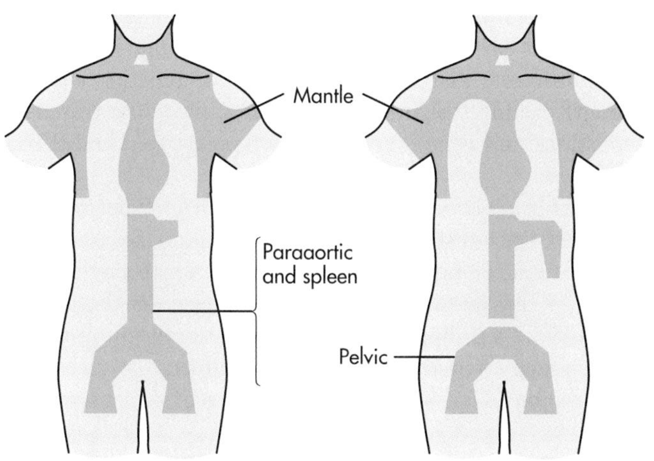

Figure 27-7 Diagram of mantle and inverted Y-fields used in total lymphoid radiotherapy of Hodgkin's disease.

Combinations such as ABVD (doxorubicin [Adriamycin], bleomycin, vinblastine [Velban], and dacarbazine; see Table 27-13) are likely to be added to the treatment regimen if relapse occurs, and complete remission can again be attained. Use of alternating courses of MOPP and ABVD has not significantly increased the complete remission rates, but at 8 years, freedom from progression increased from 36% with MOPP alone to 65% for the alternating therapy.[21] Unfortunately, the toxicity from the treatment was greater than from either therapy used alone. Omitting dacarbazine from the therapy greatly reduces the toxicity, and the death rate from stage IV Hodgkin's disease has been significantly reduced with this protocol.

Patient/Family Education. Teaching regarding methods to decrease the risk for infection and skin damage is important for the patient with Hodgkin's disease. The patient and family should be knowledgeable regarding the treatment regimen and potential side effects. As with other hematologic disorders, the patient should avoid all types of potential injury.

Refer to Chapter 15 for more information on the nursing care needs of patients with cancer.

NON-HODGKIN'S LYMPHOMA

Etiology/Epidemiology

The non-Hodgkin's lymphomas include a broad spectrum of lymphoid malignant diseases with different histopathologies, disease courses, and responses to therapy. The cause is unknown, although viruses have been implicated. An association between the development of non-Hodgkin's lymphoma and immunosuppressed status, particularly in persons with AIDS and organ transplant recipients, has been reported. An increased incidence has also been reported in persons with certain autoimmune disorders such as Sjögren's syndrome.

The incidence of non-Hodgkin's lymphoma has increased over the past 20 years.[21] Men are more commonly affected, with the greatest incidence occurring in persons over 60 years of age. Burkitt's lymphoma, a high-grade tumor, is most common in children and persons with AIDS.

TABLE 27-13 Chemotherapeutic Regimens for Treatment of Hodgkin's Disease

Drugs	Dosage	Method	Schedule	Cycle
MOPP				
Mechlorethamine (nitrogen mustard)	6 mg/m^2	IV	Days 1 and 8	2 wk with 2-wk rest period
Vincristine (Oncovin)	1.4 mg/m^2	IV	Days 1 and 8	
Prednisone	40 mg/m^2	PO	Days 1-14	
Procarbazine	100 mg/m^2	PO	Days 1-14	
ABVD				
Doxorubicin (Adriamycin)	25 mg/m^2	IV	Days 1 and 15	2 wk with 2-wk rest period
Bleomycin	10 mg/m^2	IV	Days 1 and 15	
Vinblastine (Velban)	6 mg/m^2	IV	Days 1 and 15	
Dacarbazine (DTIC-Dome)	375 mg/m^2	IV	Days 1 and 15*	

IV, Intravenous, *PO,* oral.
*NOTE: Dacarbazine may be omitted (MOPP/ABV).[20]

Pathophysiology

Accurate identification of the histopathology is crucial to the determination of the treatment plan. The classifications are briefly reviewed here so that familiarity with terminology will allow the reader to review charts and treatment plans.

One classification separates the non-Hodgkin's lymphomas into lymphocytic, histiocytic, and mixed-cell types, each of which may appear as nodular or diffuse on microscopic examination. These have been subdivided into "favorable" and "unfavorable" histology (Box 27-8). In general, a nodular pattern of cell structures conveys a more favorable prognosis than a diffuse pattern. A lymphocytic cytology is more favorable than a histiocytic one, and a mixed cellularity–histiocytic type is intermediate in its prognosis.

Patients most often have nontender peripheral lymphadenopathy that may appear bulky. The liver and spleen may be moderately enlarged. Other symptoms that may occur include unexplained fever, night sweats, and weight loss.

Collaborative Care Management

The diagnosis of non-Hodgkin's lymphoma is made by examination of pathologic lymph node tissue. Accurate histologic classification is of importance, and often slides are sent to major cancer centers for consultation regarding the classification. Once the diagnosis is made, the extent of the disease (staging) must be determined. As with Hodgkin's disease, accurate staging is a crucial factor in determining the treatment regimen. The staging workup is similar to that for Hodgkin's disease, except that staging laparotomies are less often needed. Explanations of the extensive workup and its importance in determining the treatment plan are an important focus of patient teaching during the diagnostic period.

The complexity of the disease and the array of treatment regimens used require nurse-physician discussion of the treatment plan. It is especially important that the goals of therapy be shared, whether the goals are for cure or only local or systemic palliation.

In general, radiotherapy is the initial treatment when the disease is localized. Local field radiation is used. Total nodal radiation is reserved for patients whose disease is more widespread. Chemotherapy is the mainstay of treatment of non-Hodgkin's lymphomas that are not localized (Table 27-14).

Nodular poorly differentiated lymphocytic lymphoma is the most commonly occurring non-Hodgkin's lymphoma.[21] In some patients, observation is reasonable until the disease shows signs of progression. Treatment with a single alkylating agent, most often chlorambucil, is effective in that it produces a response rate that extends survival. Combination chemotherapy produces higher response rates, including complete remissions, but is not yet shown to be curative. The MST is 7 to 10 years.

In diffuse histiocytic lymphoma, which includes most of the cases previously designated as reticulum cell sarcoma, combination chemotherapy has been superior to single-agent therapy. Survival is significantly prolonged in those who demonstrate a complete response, and a significant minority of this group is cured. Chemotherapy regimens produce complete responses in 40% to 60% or more of patients whose MST is well over 3 years.

In nodular histiocytic and nodular mixed histiolymphocytic types, complete responses have been achieved with single agents, and 50% to 70% of those treated with COP, COPP, MOPP, and other combinations have shown an MST of 55 months for those who attained a complete response and 13

BOX 27-8 Non-Hodgkin's Lymphomas

"Favorable" Histology

Nodular poorly differentiated lymphocytic lymphoma (NLPD)
Nodular mixed lymphocytic and histiocytic lymphoma (NML)
Well-differentiated lymphocytic lymphomas of the nodular (NLWD) or diffuse (DLWD) type

"Unfavorable" Histology

Nodular histiocytic lymphoma (NHL)
Diffuse poorly differentiated lymphocytic (DPDL)
Diffuse histiocytic lymphoma (DHL)
Diffuse mixed lymphoma (DML)
Diffuse undifferentiated lymphoma (DUL)

TABLE 27-14 Chemotherapeutic Regimens for Treatment of Non-Hodgkin's Lymphomas

Drugs	Dosage	Method	Schedule	Cycle
COP				
Cyclophosphamide (Cytoxan)	800-1000 mg/m²	IV	Day 1	3 wk
Vincristine (Oncovin)	2 mg	IV	Day 1	
Prednisone	60 mg/m²	PO	Days 1-5	
CHOP				
Cyclophosphamide (Cytoxan)	750 mg/m²	IV	Day 1	3 wk
Hydroxydaunomycin (doxorubicin, Adriamycin)	50 mg/m²	IV	Day 1	
Vincristine (Oncovin)	1.4 mg/m²	IV	Day 1	
Prednisone	100 mg/m²	PO	Days 1-5	

TABLE 27-14 Chemotherapeutic Regimens for Treatment of Non-Hodgkin's Lymphomas—cont'd

Drugs	Dosage	Method	Schedule	Cycle
CHOP-BLEO				
Cyclophosphamide (Cytoxan)	750 mg/m^2	IV	Day 1	3 wk or 4 wk
Hydroxydaunomycin (doxorubicin, Adriamycin)	50 mg/m^2	IV	Day 1	
Vincristine (Oncovin)	2 mg	IV	Days 1 and 5	4 wk
Prednisone	100 mg	PO	Days 1-5	
Bleomycin	15 U	IV	Days 1 and 5	
COPP				
Cyclophosphamide (Cytoxan)	400-650 mg/m^2	IV	Days 1 and 8	4 wk
Vincristine (Oncovin)	1.4 mg/m^2 (max, 2 mg)	IV	Days 1 and 8	
Procarbazine	100 mg/m^2	PO	Days 1-10	
Prednisone	40 mg/m^2	PO	Days 1-14	
BACOP				
Bleomycin	5 U/m^2	IV	Days 15 and 22	4 wk
Doxorubicin (Adriamycin) Cyclo-phosphamide (Cytoxan)	25 mg/m^2	IV	Days 1 and 8	
Vincristine (Oncovin)	650 mg/m^2	IV	Days 1 and 8	
Procarbazine	1.4 mg/m^2 (max, 2 mg)	IV	Days 1 and 8	
Prednisone	60 mg/m^2	PO	Days 15-28	
PRO-MACE				
Prednisone	60 mg/m^2	PO	Days 1 to 14	Follow with MOPP regimen (see Table 27-13); then restart Pro-MACE
Methotrexate	1.5 g/m^2	IV	One time	
Doxorubicin (Adriamycin)	25 mg/m^2	IV	Days 1 and 8	
Cyclophosphamide	650 mg/m^2	IV	Days 1 and 8	
Etoposide (VP 16)	120 mg/m^2	IV	Days 1 and 8	
Leucovorin	50 mg/m^2	IV	q6h for 5 days	
M-BACOD				
Methotrexate	200 mg/m^2	IV	Days 8 and 15	Repeat cycles every 3 wk
Bleomycin	4 U/m^2	IV	Days 1 and 21	
Doxorubicin (Adriamycin)	45 mg/m^2	IV	Days 1 and 21	
Cyclophosphamide	600 mg/m^2	IV	Days 1 and 21	
Vincristine (Oncovin)	1 mg/m^2	IV	Days 1 and 21	
Dexamethasone	6 mg/m^2	PO	Days 1-5 and 21-25	
Leucovorin rescue	10 mg/m^2	PO	q6h for 8 doses, beginning 24 hr after each methotrexate dose	
MACOP-B				
Methotrexate	100 mg/m^2, then 300 mg/m^2	IV IV/4 hr	Wk 2, 6, 10 Wk 2, 6, 10	Cycles may be repeated
Leucovorin rescue	15 mg	PO	q6h for 6 doses beginning 24 hr after methotrexate	
Doxorubicin (Adriamycin)	50 mg/m^2	IV	Wk 1, 3, 5, 7, 9, 11	
Cyclophosphamide	350 mg/m^2	IV	Wk 1, 3, 5, 7, 9, 11	
Vincristine (Oncovin)	1.4 mg/m^2	IV	Wk 2, 4, 8, 10, 12	
Prednisone	75 mg	PO	Daily doses tapered over last 15 days	
Bleomycin	10 U/m^2	IV	Wk 4, 8, 12	
NOTE: CNS prophylaxis is also given to patients with bone marrow involvement after bone marrow remission.				
Methotrexate	12 mg	IT	Wk 6-8	Cycles may be repeated
Cytarabine	30 mg/m^2	IT	Wk 6-8	

CNS, Central nervous system, *IV*, intravenous; *IT*, intrathecal; *PO*, oral.

months for those in whom only a partial response was attained (see Tables 27-13 and 27-14).

Patient/Family Education. Hodgkin's and non-Hodgkin's diseases most often affect young adults; therefore special attention needs to be given to minimizing the impact of the illness and its treatment on their lives, not only during the treatment period, but later as well. Before the initiation of treatment, therapy-induced sterility should be discussed. For young women receiving radiation therapy alone, surgical relocation of the ovaries outside the field of radiation may be performed. Sterility commonly occurs in association with chemotherapy. For women, this is often temporary, and the ability to conceive and bear normal children often returns after therapy is completed. For men, sterility is more commonly permanent. For this reason the option of sperm banking should be discussed before beginning either radiation therapy or chemotherapy.

To allow for work and career development, every effort should be made to schedule treatment at those times and days of the week that least interfere with work and other important events in the person's life. The nurse has a crucial role in helping patients to develop a realistic approach to the illness and to meet successfully the demands and limitations imposed by the illness and its treatment.

Persons with lymphomas have periods of remission and recurrence. Such peaks and valleys are stressful and disruptive. Many patients describe subsequent courses of treatment after a recurrence as more stressful than the initial treatment. Comments include, "Is it worth it? I don't have the same faith." Other patients, realistically encouraged by the initial response to treatment, are able to express an optimistic outlook: "It worked the first time. It will work again." Recognition of the stress involved in therapy requires that support systems be available to the patient. The health care team can provide some of the needed support and guidance as the person learns to incorporate the illness into daily life.

Patient teaching includes information about:

1. Knowledge of the disorder, its treatment, and prognosis
2. Name, dosage, frequency, and side effects of medications
3. Arrangements for chemotherapy or radiation treatments and for periodic blood cell counts
4. Symptoms requiring immediate medical attention (fever, bleeding)
5. Need for continued medical follow-up
6. Resources available in the community: financial assistance and local support groups (American Cancer Society)

INFECTIOUS MONONUCLEOSIS

Etiology/Epidemiology

Infectious mononucleosis is an acute disease caused by a herpeslike virus, the Epstein-Barr virus. It occurs more often in young persons, with the highest incidence occurring between 15 and 30 years of age.

Pathophysiology

Signs and symptoms of infectious mononucleosis are varied (see Clinical Manifestations box). It is a benign disease with a favorable prognosis. The onset may be subtle, appearing almost as flulike symptoms. Malaise is a common early complaint, and it is often accompanied by fever, lymphadenopathy, sore throat, headache, generalized aches and pains resembling those of influenza, and moderate enlargement of the liver and spleen. Pruritus, palatal petechiae, jaundice, and rash may be present. The mode of transmission is via intimate contact, with the spread of the virus through the saliva. Rupture of the spleen and encephalitis are rare complications.

> ***Clinical Manifestations***
> **Infectious Mononucleosis**
>
> MILD
> Fever, malaise
>
> MODERATE
> Enlarged lymph nodes, sore throat, headache, generalized aches, moderate enlargement of liver and spleen
>
> SEVERE (RARE)
> Rupture of spleen, encephalitis

Collaborative Care Management

Diagnosis is established by the heterophil agglutination or monospot blood test. This test is based on the presence of a substance in the blood of a person with infectious mononucleosis that causes clumping, or agglutination, of the washed erythrocytes (antigen) of another animal. The test result is almost always positive after 10 to 14 days of the illness. Other laboratory findings are a great increase in the number of mononuclear leukocytes, which is the basis of the name of the disease, and an increase in atypical lymphocytes. At the height of the disease, the WBC count may range between 10,000 and 20,000 cells/mm^3.

Infectious mononucleosis is self-limiting, and with rest, affected persons usually recover spontaneously within 2 to 3 weeks. Effectiveness of antiviral therapy has not been established. The use of corticosteroids may be indicated in severe cases with tonsillar enlargement and potential airway obstruction. Acetaminophen is effective in relieving fever, sore throat, and myalgias. Most persons can return to activities that do not require heavy exertion in 1 to 2 weeks and to normal activities in 4 to 6 weeks. Some persons have persistent fatigue for several months. Nursing management is supportive and focuses on the relief of symptoms and promotion of rest.

Patient/Family Education. The patient is instructed to avoid heavy lifting or contact sports for at least 1 month or until the splenomegaly is resolved. An enlarged spleen is susceptible to rupture. Additional teaching includes the need to increase fluids and to use appropriate hand washing to prevent the spread of disease.

Young adults should be educated regarding the mode of transmission and incubation period of mononucleosis. Persons with mononucleosis should be cautioned against donating blood for at least 6 months after the onset of illness. Reassurance should be given that isolation is not necessary, but that the oral secretions of a person with acute mononucleosis should be considered infectious

Critical Thinking Questions

1. You are administering a vitamin B_{12} injection to an older man in the outpatient clinic. He has recently had a gastrectomy. He asks you why he needs to have these injections and how long he will need them. How do you respond?
2. A young male patient is hospitalized with multiple injuries from a motorcycle accident. His history states that he has polycythemia vera. How will this affect his present care? Are there nursing responsibilities related specifically to this diagnosis?
3. A young woman hospitalized with sickle cell crisis asks you why she needs oxygen via a nasal cannula. How do you respond? What other interventions will promote comfort for this patient?
4. A 63-year-old man recently diagnosed with chronic myelogenous leukemia (CML) is extremely anxious about his diagnosis. He has heard many horror stories about chemotherapy. To relieve his anxiety, what would you explain to him regarding the initial therapy for CML? How does this treatment differ from treatment for acute types of leukemia?

References

1. Acute leukemia cancer. In *The CancerGroup,* North Miami Beach, Fla, 2001, The Cancer Group Institute, website: http://www.cancergroup.com.
2. Adams RJ et al: Prevention of first stroke by transfusions in children with sickle cell anemia and abnormal results on transdoppler ultrasonography, *N Engl J Med* 339(1):5-11, 1998.
3. *Adult acute lymphoblastic leukemia treatment—health professionals (PDQ®),* 2001, website: http://www.cancer.gov/cancer_information/doc_pdq.
4. *Adult acute myeloid leukemia (PDQ®),* 2001, website: http://cancernet.nci.nih.gov/cancer.
5. Anemias. In *The Merck manual,* Section 11, Chapter 127, website: http://www.merck.com.
6. Bacigalupo A: *Recent advances in the treatment of leukemias and aplastic anemia,* 1997, website: http://www.labfocus.com.
7. Bader-Muenier B et al: Long-term evaluation of the beneficial effect of subtotal splenectomy for management of hereditary spherocytosis, *Blood* 97(2):399-403, 2001.
8. Benjamin LJ, Swinson GI, Nagel RL: Sickle cell day hospital: an approach for the management of uncomplicated painful crisis, *Blood* 9(4):1130-1137, 2000.
9. *Bone marrow transplant:* website: http://www.stjude.org/medical/bone.hym, 2001.
10. Bosch X: Setbacks and hopes for patients with Fanconi's anemia, *Lancet* 355(9200), 2000, website: http://www.thelancet.com/search/search.isa.
11. Chronic leukemia cancer. In *The CancerGroup,* North Miami Beach, Fla, 2001, The Cancer Group Institute, website: http://www.cancergroup.com.
12. d'Onofrio G et al: *New parameters for diagnosis and management of anemia,* 2001, website: http://www.labfocus.com.
13. Drs acute leukemia cancer. In *The CancerGroup,* North Miami Beach, Fla, 2001, The Cancer Group Institute, website: http://www.cancergroup.com.
14. Green R: *The recognition and diagnosis of early, masked, subtle and atypical cobalamin and folate deficiency,* 1997, website: http://www.labfocus.com.
15. Harmening DM: *Clinical hematology and fundamentals of hemostasis,* ed 3, Philadelphia, 1997, FA Davis.
16. Koshy M et al: 2-Deoxy 5-azacytidine and fetal hemoglobin induction in sickle cell anemia, *Blood* 96(7):2379-2384, 2000.
17. Leukemias. In *The Merck manual,* Section 11, Chapter 127, website: http://www.merck.com.
18. Myeloproliferative disorders. In *The Merck manual,* Section 11, Chapter 130, website: http://www.merck.com.
19. National Organization for Rare Disorders: *Anemia, Fanconi's,* 2001, website: http://www.rarediseases.org.
20. Novartis Pharmaceuticals Corporation: *Gleevec™ (imatinib mesylate) capsules,* NDA 21-335, Package insert, East Hanover, NJ, 2001, The Corporation.
21. Physician's Hodgkin's and non-Hodgkin's review. In *The CancerGroup,* North Miami Beach, Fla, 2001, The Cancer Group Institute, website: http://www.cancergroup.com.
22. Platt A, Eckman J: *Sickle cell research.* Web update. The Sickle Cell Information Center, 1999, website: http://www.emory.edu./peds/sickle.
23. Rakel RE, Boke ET: *Conn's current therapy,* ed 3, Philadelphia, 1997, WB Saunders.
24. Rucknagel DL: Progress and prospects for the acute chest syndrome of sickle cell anemia, *J Pediatr* 138(2):160-162, 2001.
25. *Treatment of hemophilia and other bleeding disorders,* 2001, website: http://www.nhlb.nih.gov/health/prof.
26. US Department of Health and Human Services: *Facts about immune thrombocytopenic purpura,* NIH Pub No 90-2114, 2001, website: http://www.nhlbi.nih.gov/health/public.
27. US Department of Health and Human Services, Food and Drug Administration: FDA approves Gleevec for leukemia treatment, *FDA News,* 2001, website: http://www.cancer.gov/pressreleases.

28 Assessment of the Endocrine System

Margaret M. Ulchaker

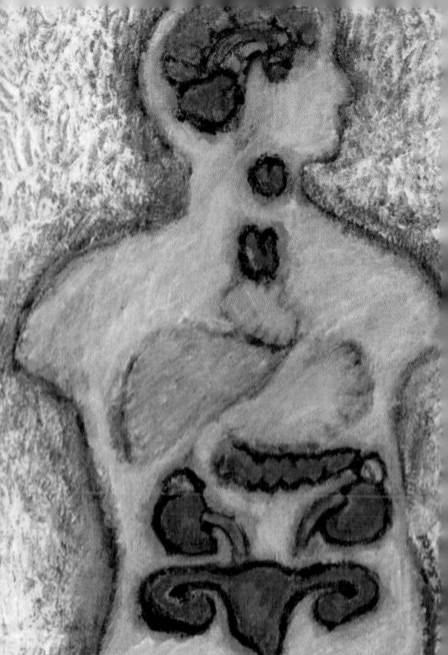

Objectives

After studying this chapter, the learner should be able to:

1. Describe the locations of endocrine glands and the mechanisms that control hormone synthesis and release from these glands.
2. Analyze the functions of the hormones secreted by the pituitary, thyroid, parathyroid, adrenal cortex, adrenal medulla, and the pancreas.
3. Compare the biologic effects of deficit and excess of each major hormone.
4. Relate the physiologic changes that occur within the endocrine system with aging.
5. Describe data essential to the assessment of patients with actual or potential health problems of the endocrine system.
6. Discuss the common diagnostic tests used to identify endocrine dysfunction and explain the meaning of the results.

The endocrine system is a cellular communication system involving hormones. A hormone is a molecule secreted from one organ that travels in the systemic circulation and has its effect(s) on a distant organ(s).

The endocrine system consists of the anterior and posterior pituitary, thyroid, parathyroid, adrenal cortex, adrenal medulla, pancreas, gonads, pineal body, and thymus glands. Specialized endocrine cells are also located along the gastrointestinal (GI) tract. The hormones from these endocrine glands are vital to the important life transactions of the organism, including differentiation, reproduction, growth and development, metabolism, adaptation, and aging. The neuroendocrine response to stressors, which involves the nervous system, the adrenal medulla, and other endocrine glands, is briefly discussed in Chapter 17; the GI hormones are discussed in Chapter 31; and the gonads are discussed in Chapter 52. The thymus, which is critical to development of immunocompetent T lymphocytes, is discussed in Chapters 11 and 48.

ANATOMY AND PHYSIOLOGY

General Endocrine Processes

A hormone may:

- Stimulate another endocrine gland to produce another hormone with specific tissue effects (e.g., thyroid-stimulating hormone [TSH] stimulates the thyroid gland to secrete thyroxine [T_4] and triiodothyronine [T_3])
- Inhibit another endocrine gland's production of a hormone (e.g., somatostatin inhibits growth hormone)
- Have a direct effect on specific tissues (e.g., insulin promotes glucose transport into insulin-sensitive cells)

The end-organ tissue effects of a hormone are mediated via several mechanisms, depending on the structure of the hormone (Table 28-1). Peptide hormones (e.g., insulin) bind to cell surface receptors and trigger a secondary cascade of intracellular signals resulting in the final event—the transportation of glucose into the cell. Steroid hormones bind to the nucleus of the target cell and result in altered protein synthesis.

Mechanisms of Hormone Action

The secretion and release of hormones do not occur at a uniform rate. Many hormones are secreted in a pulsatile fashion and may have diurnal variations. Physiological levels of hormones are determined by the amount of hormone produced, an intact transport system, adequate receptors, feedback systems, and metabolic degradation of the hormone.

Hormone Release

Hormone release is influenced by negative feedback systems, intrinsic rhythmicity, and the nervous system.

Understanding the Endocrine Axis/Feedback Loops. Understanding hormonal feedback loops is important not only for diagnosis, but also for therapeutic monitoring. In a negative feedback system, a gland responds to a low hormone level by releasing an additional hormone. As the level of this second hormone returns to normal, its further release is inhibited.

TABLE 28-1 Structural Categories of Hormones

Structural Category	Examples
Peptide Hormones	Growth Hormone
Prolactin	Parathyroid hormone
	Follicle-stimulating hormone
	Lutenizing hormone
	Thyroid-stimulating hormone
	Thyrotropin-releasing hormone
	Oxytocin
	Calcitonin
	Glucagon
	Adrenocorticotropic hormone
	Endorphins
	Melanocyte-stimulating hormone
	Hypothalamic hormones/factors (e.g., corticotropin-releasing hormone)
	Somatostatin
Amino acid derivatives	Epinephrine
	Norepinephrine
Steroid hormones	Estrogens
	Progestins
	Thyroxine
	Triiodothyronine

From McCance KL, Huether SE: *Pathophysiology: the biologic basis for disease in adults and children,* ed 4, St Louis, 2002, Mosby.

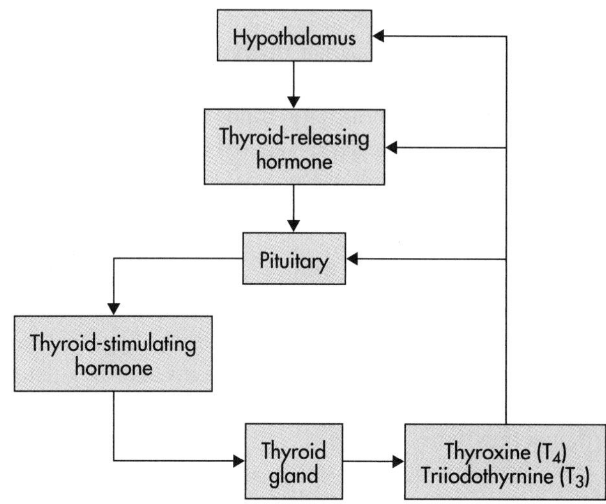

Figure 28-1 Endocrine axis feedback loop.

Thyroid hormone regulation is an example of a negative feedback system (Figure 28-1). In the example of the thyroid, it is important to recognize that (1) the earliest marker of excess thyroid hormone in the circulation is a suppressed TSH and (2) the earliest marker of deficiency of thyroid hormone is an elevated TSH. Changes in TSH normally occur before circulating thyroid hormone levels are out of the normal range and really reflect the pituitary's assessment of ambient thyroid levels. TSH levels return to normal very slowly (6 to 8 weeks) after correction of ambient thyroid hormone levels. Therefore, measuring TSH at time intervals shorter than this will not yield meaningful information.

Although negative feedback control is a distinguishing feature of the endocrine system, it does not control all hormones. Examples include estrogen in males, testosterone in females, placental hormones, and hormones produced by ectopic tumors.

Intrinsic Rhythmicity. A second factor regulating hormone levels is intrinsic rhythmicity. The intrinsic rhythms can vary over minutes, days, or weeks. For example, prolactin, cortisol, and growth hormone demonstrate daily circadian rhythms (Figure 28-2). These intrinsic rhythms are controlled by various factors.

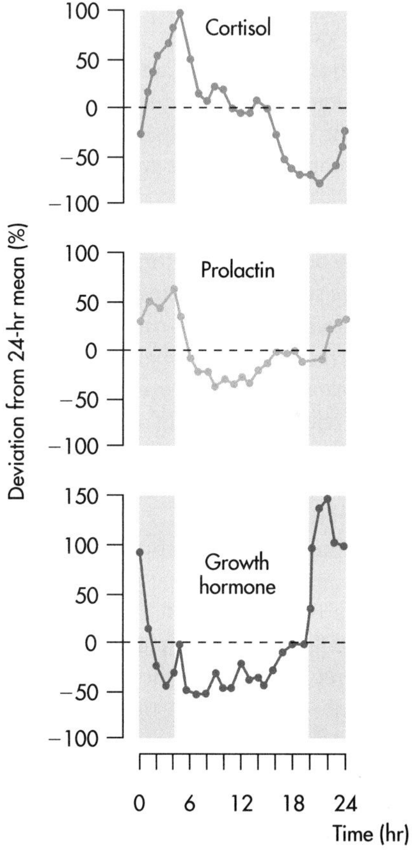

Figure 28-2 Intrinsic rhythms of cortisol, prolactin, and growth hormone.

The environmental factor of sleep-wake patterns influences the circadian rhythms of growth hormone, adrenocorticotropic hormone (ACTH), and cortisol. Age, growth, and development influence the intrinsic rhythmicity of gonadotropins and gonadal steroids. Neurogenic factors influence the intrinsic rhythm of other hormones such as prolactin (PRL). In addition to circadian rhythms, hormone secretion may demonstrate pulsatile or cyclic patterns.

Extrinsic factors such as pain, trauma, infection, or other stressors also influence levels of selected hormones. These extrinsic factors can override the normal feedback mechanisms or intrinsic rhythmicity and increase secretion of hormones above normal levels.

Nervous System. The central nervous system influences hormone release. The hypothalamus contains neurons and neurosecretory cells. Nerve tracts connect the hypothalamus with the posterior lobe of the pituitary. This neuroregulatory system is discussed in the section on endocrine structures and hormonal function.

The autonomic nervous system (ANS) is also involved in hormone release. As the ANS responds to a stressor, the adrenal medulla is stimulated to release epinephrine.

Excretion/Metabolism. Finally, the level of hormones is affected by excretion or metabolic inactivation. The liver and kidneys are primarily responsible for hormonal inactivation and excretion, and diseases of these organs can result in increased hormone levels.

In summary, hormone levels are controlled by multiple mechanisms. Understanding these mechanisms helps clarify the rationale for the various types of diagnostic testing used to assess pathologic conditions of the endocrine system.

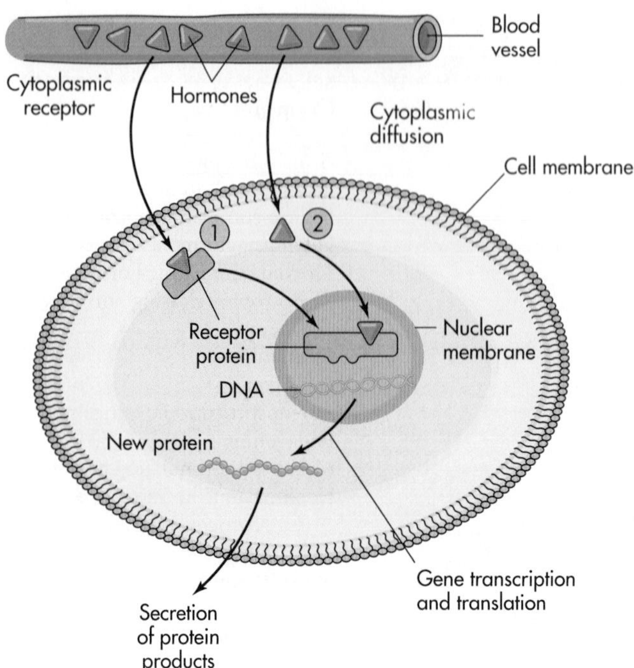

Figure 28-3 Lipid-soluble hormones receptor activity.

Hormone Transport

Hormones may be transported through the circulatory system either in a free state or bound to plasma proteins. Biologically active hormones are transported in the free state. The concentration of free hormones is balanced by the concentration of bound hormones. As the level of free hormones falls, plasma proteins release enough of the bound hormone to reach equilibrium.

Hormone Action

Hormones stimulate responses by binding either with cell surface receptors or intracellular receptors. Steroid hormones such as adrenal steroids, gonadal steroids, active derivatives of vitamin D, T_4, and T_3, which are lipid soluble, are believed to use intracellular receptors. These hormones freely cross the cell membrane and combine with their specific intracellular receptor. The steroid-receptor complex is changed in size and conformation and is translocated to the nucleus, where it combines with acceptor sites located in the nucleus near the deoxyribonucleic acid (DNA) sequences. The binding of the hormone-receptor complex initiates transcription of DNA, translation of ribonucleic acid, and synthesis of protein. A summary of this model of hormone activation is shown in Figure 28-3.

Water-soluble hormones (hypothalamic-releasing hormones, anterior and posterior pituitary hormones, parathyroid hormone [PTH], calcitonin, insulin, glucagon, and biogenic amines) are believed to use cell surface receptors. The hormone, acting as a first messenger, combines with its specific receptor on the cell membrane, and this hormone-receptor combination activates a second messenger located inside the cell. The second messenger then initiates a sequence of events in the cytoplasm that results in altered cell function. Cyclic adenosine monophosphate (cAMP) has been identified as the second messenger for several hormones. It is hypothesized that the combination of the hormone with the receptor activates adenyl cyclase, which causes the formation of 39,59-cAMP from adenosine triphosphate. The cAMP activates protein kinases. These activated kinases phosphorylate specific proteins in the stimulated cell and result in altered cell function.

Although cAMP has been identified as a second messenger for several hormones, other compounds serve as second messengers. Growth hormone (GH) is mediated by somatomedin-C (insulin-like growth factor-1), its second messenger. Calcium ions, calmodulin, adenosine, and prostaglandins are some of the other potential second messengers. A summary of this model of hormone activation is presented in Figures 28-4 and 28-5.

Endocrine Structures and Hormonal Function

The endocrine structures are located throughout the body. In addition to the glands depicted in Figure 28-6, there are endocrine cells throughout various parts of the GI tract.

Hypothalamus and Pituitary Gland

The hypothalamus, a part of the diencephalon, consists of numerous poorly defined nuclei. On its inferior surface the hypothalamus is continuous with the pituitary stalk. Although a very small area of the brain, the hypothalamus receives input directly or indirectly from almost every other part

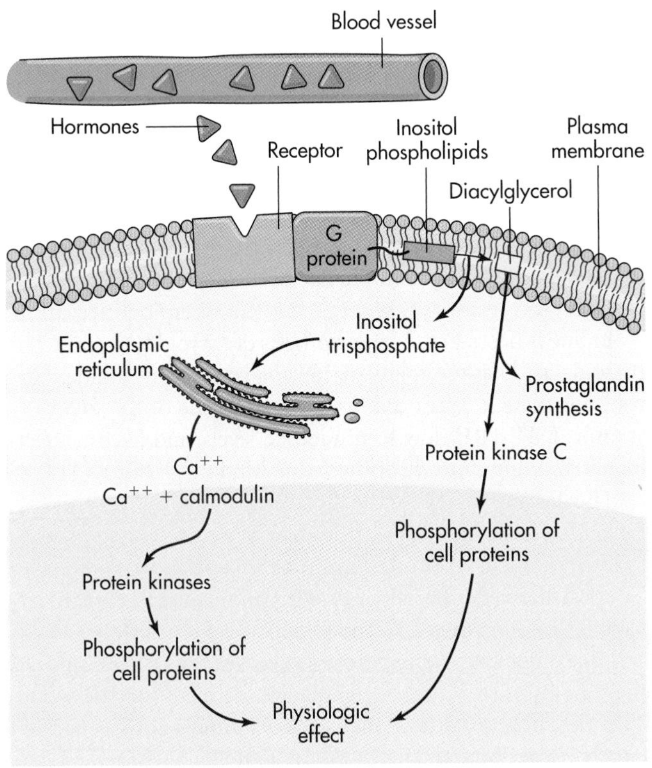

Figure 28-4 Calcium as a second messenger.

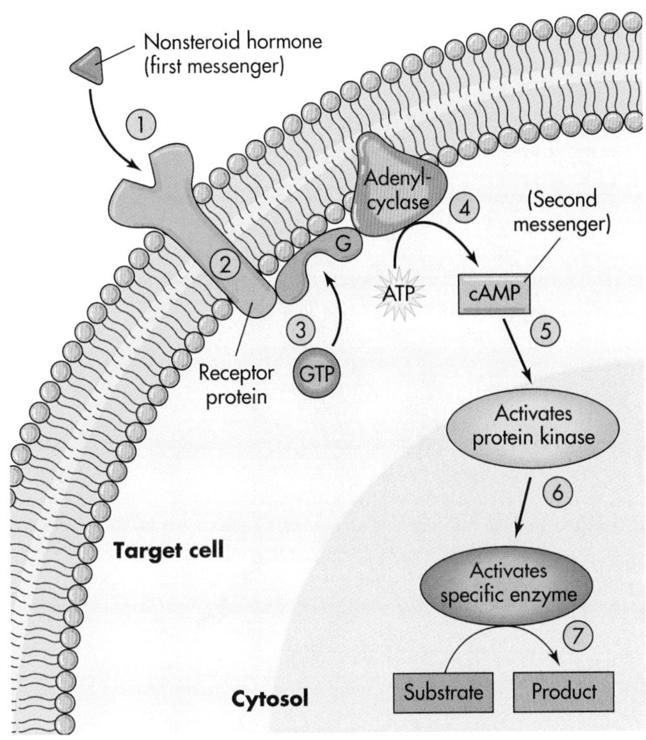

Figure 28-5 Cyclic AMP as a second messenger.

of the brain and is a major controller of the anterior and posterior pituitary gland.

The pituitary gland, which is approximately 1 cm in size, lies in the sella turcica of the sphenoid bone. This gland is composed of two functionally distinguishable components: the adenohypophysis (anterior pituitary) and the neurohypophysis (posterior pituitary). The posterior pituitary is a continuation of the pituitary stalk. The anterior pituitary, which makes up 75% of the total gland, arises embryonically from an outpouching of ectoderm and fuses with the posterior pituitary.

Hypothalamic-Pituitary Relationship. The hypothalamus serves as a critical link between the rest of the nervous system and the endocrine system, controlling both the posterior and anterior pituitary glands. By its control of the anterior pituitary gland, the hypothalamus exerts global control over the entire endocrine system. Figure 28-7 depicts the connections between the hypothalamus and pituitary gland.

The hypothalamus is connected to the posterior pituitary gland by nerve tracts that originate in the paraventricular and supraoptic nucleus of the hypothalamus. Posterior pituitary hormones are actually synthesized in the hypothalamus and transported along nerve axons to the posterior pituitary gland, where they are stored.

The hypothalamus and anterior pituitary glands are connected by the hypothalamic-hypophyseal portal blood supply. Blood entering the anterior pituitary gland has first passed through the hypothalamus. The hypothalamus regulates anterior pituitary function by the synthesis and secretion of

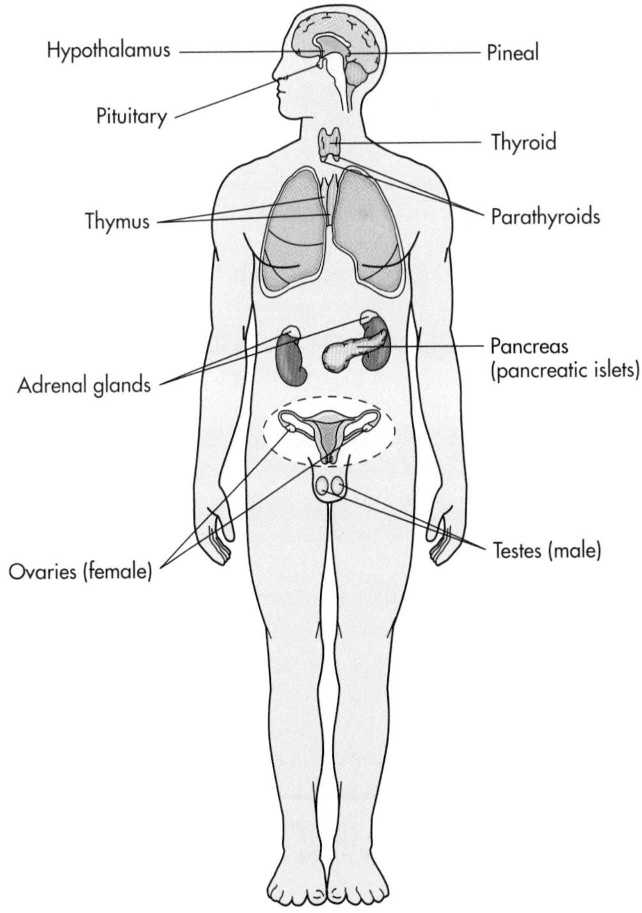

Figure 28-6 The endocrine system.

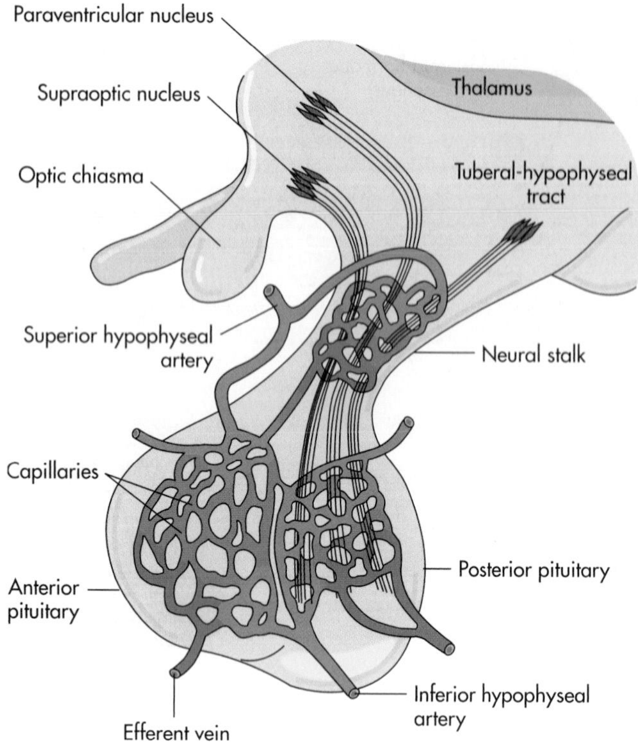

Figure 28-7 Hypothalamic pituitary connections. Hypothalamus connects to posterior pituitary gland by nerve tracts. Connection between hypothalamus and anterior pituitary gland is vascular.

releasing or inhibiting hormones into the hypothalamic-hypophyseal portal blood supply. These hormones are released in the anterior pituitary gland and stimulate or inhibit release of appropriate hormones.

Pituitary Hormones. Most trophic hormones from the pituitary are stimulated by hypothalamic factors. PRL is an exception and is under tonic inhibition via an inhibiting factor, dopamine. Therefore, interference with inhibition via pituitary stalk resections or compression or certain medications can raise PRL levels. Very high levels of thyrotropin-releasing hormone (TRH), such as are seen in severe hypothyroidism, can also stimulate prolactin.

The known releasing and inhibiting hormones/factors include growth hormone-releasing hormone and growth hormone-inhibiting hormone (or somatostatin) for GH, TRH for TSH, corticotropin-releasing factor for ACTH, gonadotropin-releasing hormone (GnRH) for follicle-stimulating hormone (FSH) and luteinizing hormone (LH), and prolactin-inhibiting hormone and prolactin-releasing hormone for PRL.

The posterior pituitary gland stores and releases two hormones: antidiuretic hormone (ADH) (vasopressin) and oxytocin. Both of these hormones are synthesized in the paraventricular and supraoptic nucleus of the hypothalamus. The blood levels of these two hormones are controlled by multiple factors that act either as stimulators or inhibitors. Table 28-2 defines the regulation and function of ADH and oxytocin.

The anterior pituitary gland produces six hormones. These hormones are produced in specific cells located throughout the anterior pituitary gland. Table 28-3 lists the hormones and their regulation and functions.

Thyroid Gland

The thyroid gland, consisting of two lobes connected by an isthmus, is located below the thyroid cartilage on the superior portion of the trachea (Figure 28-8). The gland weighs approximately 20 g and is composed of two distinct cell types: follicular cells and parafollicular cells. The thyroid is highly vascular and receives adrenergic and cholinergic innervation.

Iodine is necessary for the synthesis of thyroid hormone. The thyroid gland has the ability to trap and concentrate iodide. Thyroid hormone is produced in response to one of the following stimuli: TSH, TRH, low serum iodide levels, and factors affecting the binding capacity of thyroxine-binding globulin (TBG).

The follicular cell is the functional unit of the thyroid. Follicular cells are responsible for thyroxine (T_4) and triiodothyronine (T_3) production. The follicle consists of a ring of epithelial cells that surround a colloid-filled center. Thyroglobulin is produced by the follicular cells and stored in the colloid. When thyroid hormone is needed, the follicle converts thyroglobulin to T_4 and T_3, which are secreted into the blood. T_3 is the more potent of the two hormones and is generated largely by peripheral conversion of T_4 to T_3.

Thyroid hormone is transported via binding proteins; TBG is the protein with the greatest affinity for T_4 and T_3. Less than 1% of thyroid hormone is free and therefore active. The bound hormone acts as a reservoir to protect the cells against sudden large increases or shortages of thyroid hormone.

The parafollicular cells synthesize and secrete the hormone calcitonin, which is involved in calcium metabolism. Serum calcium levels influence the release of calcitonin. As the serum calcium level rises, calcitonin acts to maintain a normal level by opposing the action of PTH. Its physiologic significance in adults is unknown, as evidenced by the fact that no apparent adverse effects have been noted from the lack of calcitonin in patients who have had thyroidectomies. Table 28-4 lists the thyroid hormones, their regulation, and their function.

Parathyroid Gland

The parathyroid glands consist of four minute glands, located on the posterior aspect of the upper and lower poles of each lobe of the thyroid (Figures 28-6 and 28-8). Occasionally a fifth parathyroid gland is found on the thyroid, in the mediastinum, or behind the esophagus. The parathyroid gland produces PTH, which regulates calcium levels in the blood. As the serum calcium decreases, PTH secretion increases. This release of PTH is also influenced by serum phosphate and magnesium levels (Figure 28-9). Hypomagnesemia may result in failure of PTH secretion. Parathyroid hormone acts on bone and kidneys to maintain serum calcium levels. Calcitonin and vitamin D are also involved in calcium regulation.

Adrenal Gland

The adrenal glands cap the upper pole of each kidney. Each adrenal consists of two glands: the outer gland is the adrenal cortex, and the inner core is the adrenal medulla.

TABLE 28-2 Posterior Pituitary Hormones: Their Regulation and Function

Hormone/Regulation	Function
Antidiuretic Hormone (ADH, Vasopressin)	
Stimulators	
PRIMARY	Target organ: kidneys
Increased serum osmolality (as little as 1% increase) via hypothalamic osmoreceptors	Major regulator of osmolality and body water volume Increases permeability of collecting ducts in kidney to water, resulting in increased water resorption May stimulate water intake by stimulating perception of thirst
OTHERS	
Modest volume depletion via atrial volume receptors Modest hypotension via baroreceptors Stressors Psychological Pain Nausea and vomiting Chemicals Cholinergic agonist Beta-adrenergic agonist Barbiturates Morphine Nicotine	
Inhibitors	
PRIMARY	
Decreased serum osmolality (as little as 1%) via osmoreceptors Modest increased volume and blood pressure via atrial volume receptors and baroreceptors Chemicals Alcohol Alpha-adrenergic agonist	
Oxytocin	
Stimulators	
PRIMARY	Target organ: breast tissue and uterus
Suckling via neurogenic reflex conducted from afferent fibers in nipple to hypothalamus	Results in milk "let-down" in lactating breast Causes increased uterine contraction after labor has begun; role in initiating labor unclear
OTHERS	
Uterine contraction via neurogenic reflex from afferent fibers in uterus	
Inhibitors	
Stressors Psychologic Physical Alpha-adrenergic stimulation	

Adrenal Cortex. The adrenal cortex consists of three layers: the outer layer, the zona glomerulosa, produces the mineralocorticoid aldosterone; the mid-layer, the zona fasiculata, produces the glucocorticoid cortisol; and the inner layer, the zona reticularis, produces androgens. The glucocorticoids and mineralocorticoids are not only secreted and used daily, but are secreted as part of the physiologic response to stress. The mineralocorticoids and glucocorticoids are critical to maintain life. Lack of an adrenal cortex is synonymous with death if the missing hormones are not replaced. Figure 28-10 illustrates the feedback control of glucocorticoids, and Table 28-5 outlines the regulation and functions of the adrenal cortex hormones.

Adrenal Medulla. The adrenal medulla makes up approximately 10% of the total gland and produces two secretions: the catecholamines, epinephrine (Epi) and norepinephrine (NE). The adrenal medulla arises embryonically from the neural crest and is really a modified sympathetic ganglion innervated by preganglionic splanchnic nerves. As the sympathetic nervous system stimulates the adrenal medulla, Epi and NE are released. They travel via the blood to various organs and bind to receptors on target cells. Norepinephrine is also

TABLE 28-3 Anterior Pituitary Hormones: Their Regulation and Function

Hormone/Regulation	Function
Growth Hormone (GH)	
Controlled by GHRH/GHIH GH shows episodic secretion with increases after eating (particularly a high-protein diet) and after onset of deep sleep (usually within 1-2 hours after sleep) Other stimuli that increase GH Exercise (strenuous) Hypoglycemia Stressors Chemicals Arginine infusion L-dopa Clonidine TRH in acromegaly Adrenergic agonists Beta-adrenergic antagonists Hyperglycemia decreases GH	Target organ: whole body Possibly works on most tissue through action of somatomedin(s) Concerned with growth of cells, bones, and soft tissues Increases mitosis Affects carbohydrate, protein, and fat metabolism Increases blood glucose by decreasing glucose use; insulin antagonist Increases protein synthesis Increases lipolysis, free fatty acid levels, and ketone formation Increases electrolyte retention and extracellular fluid volume
Prolactin (PRL)	
Controlled by PRH and PIH; PRL chronically inhibited by hypothalamus PRL shows episodic secretions occurring during later hours of sleep Other stimulants Stressors Suckling Chemicals Estrogen TRH Dopamine antagonist Chlorpromazine Metaclopramide Selective serotonin re-uptake inhibitors Chemicals that are dopamine agonists (L-dopa, bromocriptine) inhibit PRL	Target organ: breast, gonads Necessary for breast development and lactation Regulator of reproductive function in males and females
Thyroid-Stimulating Hormone (TSH)	
Controlled by TRH and negative feedback from plasma T_4 and T_3 levels Increase $T_4 \rightarrow$ decrease TSH Decrease $T_4 \rightarrow$ increase TSH	Target organ: thyroid gland Necessary for growth and function of thyroid; controls all functions of thyroid
Adrenocorticotropin (ACTH)	
Controlled by CRH and negative feedback by cortisol levels ACTH shows episodic secretion with rhythm that peaks between 6 and 8 AM Circadian pattern (24-hour pattern) related to sleep-wake pattern and caused by increased CRH Physiologic and psychologic stressors (e.g., hypoglycemia, infections, pain, anxiety) increase ACTH caused by increased CRH (override negative feedback); changes in cortisol influence ACTH Increase cortisol $\rightarrow$ decrease ACTH Decrease cortisol $\rightarrow$ increase ACTH	Target organ: adrenal cortex gland Necessary for growth and maintenance of size of adrenal cortex Controls release of glucocorticoids (cortisol) and adrenal androgens Minor role in release of mineralocorticoids (aldosterone)
Gonadotropins **Follicle-Stimulating Hormone (FSH)** **Luteinizing Hormone (LH) (Also Previously Called Interstitial Cell-Stimulating Hormone [ICSH] in Males)**	
Secretion controlled by GnRH Amount of FSH secreted is decreased by inhibin in males Amount of LH secreted is decreased by testosterone in males Sex steroids in females exert positive feedback on FSH and LH at certain times in normal menstrual cycle and negative feedback at other times	Target organs: gonads Stimulates gametogenesis and sex steroid production in males and females

CRH, Corticotropin-releasing hormone; *FSH*, follicle-stimulating hormone; *GHIH*, growth hormone-inhibiting hormone; *GHRH*, growth hormone-releasing hormone; *GnRH*, gonadotropin-releasing hormone; *LH*, luteinizing hormone; *PIH*, prolactin-inhibiting hormone; *PRH*, prolactin-releasing hormone.

released from the terminal of postganglionic sympathetic fibers. Approximately 85% of the secretions of the adrenal medulla is Epi; the remaining 15% is norepinephrine. Epinephrine and NE stimulate alpha-adrenergic and beta-adrenergic receptors; NE is a potent stimulant of alpha adrenergic receptors, whereas Epi stimulates both alpha- and beta-adrenergic receptors (Table 28-6).

In the presence of major stressors (i.e., physiologic, psychologic, or pathologic) increased amounts of Epi and NE are released as an adaptive mechanism. In contrast to the life-threatening consequences of an absent or nonfunctioning adrenal cortex, the absence of an adrenal medulla is compatible with life.

Pancreas

The pancreas is both an exocrine and an endocrine gland. It lies retroperitoneally behind the stomach, with its head and neck in the curve of the duodenum, its body extending horizontally across the posterior abdominal wall and its tail touching the spleen. Endocrine function resides in the cells in the islets of Langerhans. There are more than 1 million islet cells spread throughout the pancreas; these cells make up 1% to 2% of the pancreatic mass. The islets of Langerhans consist of four cell types: (1) *alpha* cells, which secrete glucagon; (2) *beta* cells, which make up 70% of the cells and secrete insulin; (3) *delta* cells, which secrete somatostatin; and (4) cells that

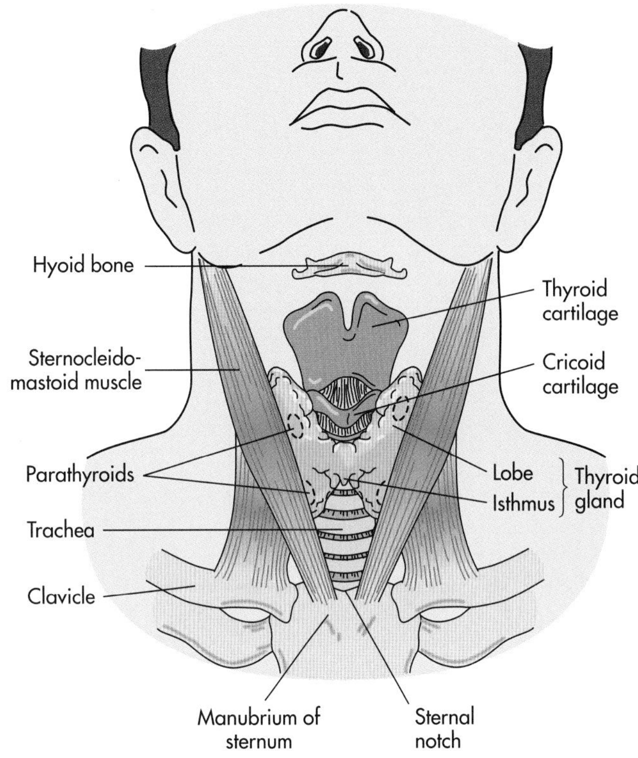

Figure 28-8 Midline neck structures; note thyroid gland in anterior aspect of neck.

TABLE 28-4 Thyroid Gland Hormones: Their Regulation and Function

Regulation	Function
Thyroxine (T_4) and Triiodothyronine (T_3)	
T_4 and T_3 levels controlled by TSH	Regulates protein, fat, and carbohydrates catabolism in all cells
Hormones show diurnal variation with peak during late evening	Regulates metabolic rate of all cells
Influences on amount secreted	Regulates body heat production
Gender	Acts as insulin antagonist
Pregnancy	Maintains growth hormone secretion, skeletal maturation
Gonadal steroid and adrenal corticosteroids; increased steroids = ↑ levels of T_4 and T_3	Affects central nervous system development
Exposure to extreme cold = ↑ levels	Necessary for muscle tone and vigor
Nutritional state	Maintains cardiac rate, force, and output
Chemicals	Maintains secretions of GI tract
Somatostatin (GHIH) = ↓ levels	Affects respiratory rate and oxygen utilization
Dopamine = ↓ levels	Maintains calcium mobilization
Catecholamines = ↑ levels	Affects red blood cell production
	Stimulates lipid turnover, free fatty acid release, and cholesterol synthesis
	Regulates sympathetic nervous system activity
Calcitonin	
Elevated serum calcium—major stimulant for calcitonin	Lowers serum calcium by opposing bone-resorbing effects of PTH, prostaglandins, and calciferols by inhibiting osteoclastic activity
Other stimulants	Also lowers serum phosphate levels
Gastrin	May also decrease calcium and phosphorus absorption in GI tract
Calcium-rich foods (regardless of serum Ca^{++} levels)	
Pregnancy	
Lowered serum calcium—suppresses calcitonin release	

GHIH, Growth hormone-inhibiting hormone; *GI,* gastrointestinal, *PTH,* parathyroid hormone.

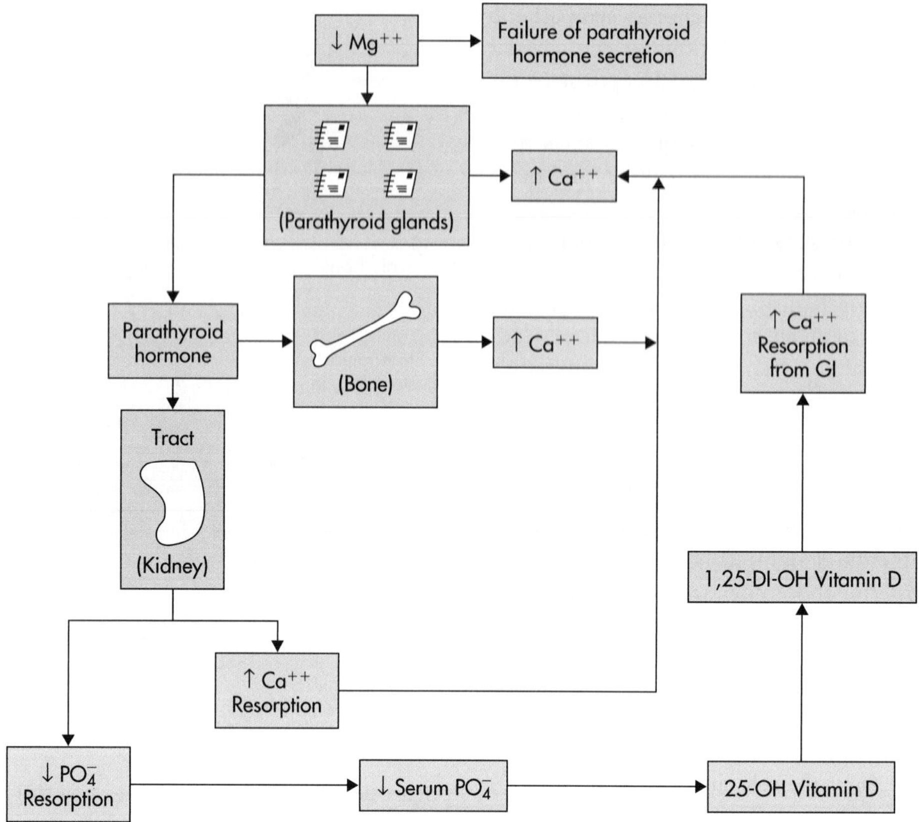

Figure 28-9 Regulation and function of parathyroid hormone. *Ca++*, Calcium; *Mg++*, magnesium.

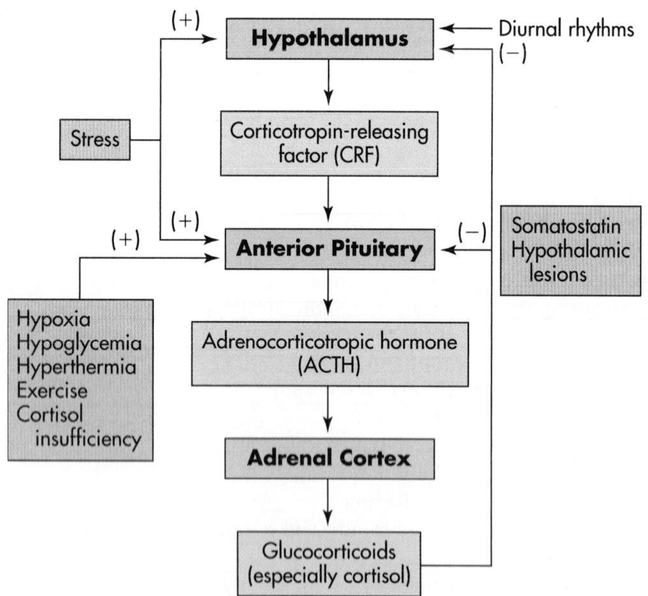

Figure 28-10 Feedback control of glucocorticoid synthesis and secretion.

secrete pancreatic polypeptide. Somatostatin inhibits gastric motility and emptying; gallbladder contraction; intestinal absorption of fats, amino acids, glucose, and other nutrients; and insulin and glucagon secretion. Pancreatic polypeptide inhibits pancreatic exocrine secretion and contraction of the gallbladder.

Insulin. Insulin, a peptide hormone, is secreted as a prohormone and an enzymatic reaction occurs to produce the active hormone, insulin. Insulin is an anabolic hormone and the only hormone that lowers blood glucose levels to maintain glucose homeostasis. (See Chapter 30 for detailed information on diabetes mellitus.)

Glucagon. The primary target of glucagon is the liver, where it stimulates glycogenolysis (breakdown of glycogen to glucose). When glycogenolysis fails to provide enough glucose, glucagon promotes amino acid transport from the muscle and stimulates gluconeogenesis (formation of glycogen from fatty acids and proteins, rather than carbohydrates). As a result of the autoimmune pancreatic destruction, individuals with type 1 diabetes mellitus lose glucagon secretion early in the course of the disease. In response to hypoglycemia, the individual with type 1 diabetes must rely on the effects of the adrenergic response and the secretion of catecholamines.

Somatostatin. Somatostatin is a natural inhibitor of glucagon and helps to maintain glucose homeostasis in the nondiabetic. Synthetic somatostatin analogs are used to successfully treat acromegaly, to reduce pancreatic polypeptide levels and prevent recurrent pancreatitis in patients with pseudocysts, and to treat gastrin-producing tumors and vasoactive intestinal peptide-producing tumors (VIPomas). When administered to an individual with type 1 diabetes, a somatostatin analog can increase the risk of hypoglycemia.

TABLE 28-5 Adrenal Cortex Hormones: Their Regulation and Function

Regulation	Function
Glucocorticoids (Cortisol)	
Level of cortisol is controlled by CRH/ACTH. Cortisol shows episodic secretion with a circadian rhythm that peaks between 6 and 8 AM; this circadian pattern follows the circadian pattern of CRH/ACTH. Physiologic and psychologic stressors (e.g., hypoglycemia, hypoxia, pain, infection, trauma, anxiety) result in increased cortisol via increased CRH and ACTH. This stress response overrides negative feedback cortisol normally exerts on ACTH.	Overall effect: maintain blood glucose level by increasing gluconeogenesis and decreasing rate of glucose use by cells Increases protein catabolism Promotes lipolysis Antiinflammatory Degrades collagen Decreases T-lymphocyte participation in cellular-mediated immunity by decreasing circulating level of T lymphocytes Increases neutrophils by increasing release and decreasing destruction Decreases new antibody release Decreases eosinophils, basophils, and monocytes Decreases scar tissue formation Increases red blood cell formation and possibly increases platelet formation Increases gastric acid and pepsin production Promotes sodium and water retention Maintains emotional stability
Mineralocorticoids (Aldosterone)	
Major regulator is renin-angiotensin system. When vascular volume or sodium is decreased, the renin-angiotensin system is activated (see Chapters 13 and 38, and angiotensin II stimulates release of mineralocorticoids. Other regulators Increased serum potassium (K^+) directly stimulates adrenal cortex to release mineralocorticoids. CRH/ACTH system is a weak regulator.	Maintains sodium and volume status Increases sodium resorption in distal tubules Increases potassium and hydrogen excretion in distal tubules
Adrenal Androgens	
Major regulator is CRH/ACTH system.	Responsible for some secondary sex characteristics in females; in males, acts as gonadal steroids

ACTH, Adrenocorticotropin hormone; *CRH,* corticotropin-releasing hormone.

TABLE 28-6 Effects of Adrenal-Medullary-Sympathetic Stimulation on Body Organs

Organ	Effect*	Organ	Effect*
Heart	Increased conduction velocity, automaticity, contractility, rate, and stroke volume caused by β_1-stimulation	Kidney	Increased renin secretion caused by β_2-stimulation
Blood vessels		Urinary bladder	Relaxation of detrusor muscle and contraction of sphincter
Coronary vessels, brain, lungs	Dilation caused by β_2-stimulation and autoregulatory phenomena	Skin	Pilomotor muscle contraction and localized sweating
Skin, mucosa, abdominal viscera, renal and salivary gland vessels	Constriction caused by α_1-receptor stimulation; renal vessels also have dopaminergic receptors	Liver	Glycogenolysis and gluconeogenesis caused by β_2-stimulation
Veins	Constriction caused by α_1-stimulation	Pancreas	Decreased secretion of exocrine cells; β_2-stimulation causes increased secretion of islet β-cells, but α-stimulation causes decreased secretion of islet cells; α-effect predominates
Bronchial muscles	Relaxation caused by β_2-stimulation	Fat cells	Lipolysis
		Brain	Increased alertness, restlessness
Gastrointestinal tract	Inhibition of production of gastrointestinal secretions; decreased motility and contraction of sphincters	Eyes	Dilation of pupils and relaxation of ciliary bodies
Gallbladder	Relaxation		

*These total effects would be seen in the physiologic responses to stressors.

Physiologic Changes With Aging

Changes in the endocrine system occur with normal aging. Signs and symptoms of endocrine dysfunction may be subtle, progress slowly, and often mimic normal changes associated with aging. In general, a pathologic process must always be searched for and ruled out before attributing hormonal alterations to aging.[25]

Types of hormonal changes associated with the aging process include the following:

- Reduction in hormone production
- Changes in hormone clearance
- Reduction in cellular responsiveness to a particular hormone
- A response to changes in nutritional status, physical activity, and body composition

Specific common endocrine changes associated with aging are the following:

- Menopause with loss of ovarian function is a naturally occurring event. The earliest hormonal signs of menopause are rising levels of gonadotropins (FSH and LH), which are trying to stimulate the failing ovaries. Ongoing controversy exists on the benefits versus risks of hormone replacement therapy.
- Androgen production in males declines with age but only within the normal reference range. Libido and sexual performance do not correlate well with absolute testosterone levels within the normal range. Sperm production may decrease somewhat with aging; however, fertility is well preserved in many octogenarians.
- Changes in PTH levels are not uncommon in older adults. In response to decreased intake of calcium (dietary and supplements) and vitamin D intake or production via decreased exposure to sunlight, many older patients have mild elevations in PTH levels and are in negative calcium balance. This has a negative impact on bone density and increases fracture risk.
- Reduced insulin sensitivity rather than reduced insulin secretion is responsible for the high prevalence of impaired glucose tolerance and type 2 diabetes mellitus in older adults. This is related to factors that worsen insulin resistance, including (1) physical inactivity, (2) altered body composition with increased fat mass and decreased lean muscle mass, (3) obesity, and (4) the use of certain medications such as thiazide diuretics, and beta-blockers.

HEALTH HISTORY

The health history must be comprehensive, with special attention given to growth patterns in children and altered reproductive function in adults (menstrual disturbances/infertility/impotence). Specific questions should be targeted to the suspected endocrine dysfunction. The health history should include the reason for seeking care, history of present illness, a review of systems, social history, and family history. Areas requiring particular focus are discussed in the following paragraphs.

Intake: Food/Fluid/Electrolytes

Endocrine dysfunction can result in an alteration of the patient's fluid/electrolyte status and nutritional status. A thorough assessment of food and fluid intake via an accurate 24-hour dietary recall is helpful. Changes in appetite can accompany endocrine dysfunction (hyperthyroidism can cause a voracious appetite). Part of the treatment plan for endocrine dysfunction may include very specific dietary recommendations for intake of food and fluids (carbohydrate consistency in diabetes mellitus, fluid restriction in syndrome of inappropriate antidiuretic hormone [SIADH]), in addition to vitamin and mineral supplementation (1,25-DIOH vitamin D supplementation in secondary hyperparathyroidism).

Elimination Pattern

The endocrine system regulates water and electrolyte homeostasis. The nurse should assess urine frequency, volume, and characteristics (color, turbidity, odor, specific gravity). Urine volume is excessive in diabetes insipidus (DI) and may be excessive in diabetes mellitus; it is subnormal in SIADH. Also the presence or absence of nocturia or dysuria should be noted. In conjunction with assessment of urine output, the volume and type of oral fluid intake should be assessed (patients with DI crave cold liquids).

Bowel habits may be affected by endocrine dysfunction. The color, characteristics, and frequency of bowel movements are all important to assess. Constipation can be a manifestation of hypothyroidism or dehydration secondary to DI.

Energy Level

Any factors, including endocrine function and dysfunction, affect energy levels. A confounding variable is the presence of depression or dysphoria, a common comorbid condition in individuals with chronic medical conditions. Multiple hormones such as T_4, T_3, testosterone, and GH can affect energy levels. Assessment of sleep patterns is also critical. Sleep patterns can be worsened by hyperthyroidism. However, poor sleep patterns unrelated to endocrine dysfunction also reduce energy levels.

Perceptions of Body Characteristics

Body image is a critical component of the ego. Endocrine dysfunction can be marked by numerous physical signs and symptoms such as hirsutism (polycystic ovarian syndrome [PCOS], Cushing's syndrome), hair loss (thyroid disease), hoarse voice (hypothyroidism), proptosis and ophthalmopathy (Graves' disease), darkening skin pigmentation (Addison's disease—primary adrenal insufficiency), excessive sweating (hyperthyroidism, acromegaly), and soft tissue/bony structure changes (acromegaly). Reviewing family photographs can reveal gradual changes in appearance, which can help define a rough date-of-onset of an endocrine disorder such as Cushing's syndrome or acromegaly.

Reproductive and Sexual Function

Endocrine dysfunction can both directly and indirectly affect reproductive and sexual function. Both are intimately integrated with body image and self-image. The reproductive history should include assessment data on menarche, menses patterns, and pregnancies in women; in men, onset of puberty, erectile function, and testicular size and volume are important to assess. The sexual history should assess partner issues, frequency and type of sexual contact, arousal capabilities, ability to achieve orgasm, and sexually transmitted diseases. Fertility potential is negatively affected by many endocrine disorders (mild hypothyroidism, PCOS). On the other hand, individuals may not desire conception and have specific concerns about contraception.

PHYSICAL EXAMINATION

A comprehensive physical examination, focusing on pigmentation, skin texture, growth patterns, and visual fields, should be performed. Special attention should be directed to endocrine glands suspected of being diseased.

Objective assessment begins during the professional nurse's initial encounter with the patient.

Observation of the patient's facies. Does the patient have:

- Facial plethora as seen in Cushing's syndrome?
- Facial hirsutism as seen in PCOS, Cushing's syndrome, and adrenal disorders?
- Ophthalmopathy of Graves' disease?

The handshake. Are the patient's hands:

- Large and "doughy" as in acromegaly?
- Sweaty and clammy as in hypoglycemia, hyperthyroidism, or pheochromocytoma?

Observation of the patient's demeanor. Is the patient:

- Anxious as seen in hyperthyroidism or pheochromocytoma?
- Lethargic as seen in hypothyroidism or hypopituitarism?

A thorough multisystem physical examination by a skilled clinician assists in narrowing the differential diagnosis (see Table 28-7).

TABLE 28-7 Physical Assessment Cues in Endocrine Dysfunction

System	Physical Assessment	Potential Endocrine Dysfunction
Dermatologic	Erythema, facial plethora, purplish striae, thin skin, moon facies, supraclavicular fat pads, thin hair or hair loss	Cushing's syndrome
	Hyperpigmentation, poor skin turgor, dry mucous membranes	Adrenal insufficiency
	Pallor, decreased perspiration, cool and dry skin, coarse skin texture, periorbital edema, nonpitting edema, thin hair or hair loss	Hypothyroidism Hypopituitarism
	Smooth warm skin, increased perspiration, flushing, onycholysis	Hyperthyroidism
Neurologic	Confusion	Hypoglycemia Cushing's syndrome Myxedema (severe hypothyroidism) Hyperglycemia with incipient diabetic ketoacidosis
	Decreased mentation	Hypoglycemia Myxedema Cushing's syndrome Hyperglycemia with incipient diabetic ketoacidosis
	Decreased neurologic tone, decreased deep tendon reflexes	Hypothyroidism
	Spasms, positive Trousseau's sign, positive Chvostek's sign	Hypoparathyroidism
	Seizures	Hypoglycemia Hypoparathyroidism Adrenal insufficiency
	Hoarseness, speech changes	Hypothyroidism
	Blurred vision	Hypoglycemia Hyperglycemia
	Exophthalmos, proptosis	Graves' disease
Cardiovascular	Bradycardia	Hypothyroidism
	Tachycardia, palpitations, increased blood pressure, angina	Hyperthyroidism
Respiratory	Dyspnea	Hyperthyroidism
	Kussmaul's respirations, acetone breath	Diabetic ketoacidosis
Gastrointestinal	Constipation, weight gain	Hypothyroidism
Genitourinary	Diarrhea, weight loss	Hyperthyroidism
	Polyphagia	Hyperglycemia Hyperthyroidism
	Polyuria, polydipsia	Diabetes mellitus Diabetes insipidus

SIADH, Syndrome of inappropriate antidiuretic hormone.

Continued

TABLE 28-7 Physical Assessment Cues in Endocrine Dysfunction—cont'd

System	Physical Assessment	Potential Endocrine Dysfunction
Genitourinary—cont'd	Salt craving, weight loss	Adrenal insufficiency
	Decreased urine output	Adrenal insufficiency SIADH
	Increased urine output	Uncontrolled diabetes mellitus Diabetes insipidus
Musculoskeletal	Weakness, fatigue	Hypoglycemia Hyperglycemia Hypothyroidism Hyperthyroidism Hypopituitarism Acromegaly
	Muscle cramps	Hypoparathyroidism Adrenal insufficiency
	Muscle wasting	Cushing's syndrome
	Fractures, osteoporosis	Cushing's syndrome Hyperparathyroidism Hyperthyroidism
Psychosocial	Depression	Hypothyroidism Diabetes mellitus Adrenal insufficiency
	Emotional lability	Cushing's syndrome Hyperthyroidism
	Anxiety	Hyperthyroidism
Nonspecific	Cold intolerance, decreased body temperature	Hypothyroidism
	Heat intolerance, increased body temperature	Hyperthyroidism

Assessment measures and variations in normal findings relevant to the care of older adults are presented in the Gerontologic Assessment box. Also identified are disorders common in older adults that may be responsible for abnormal assessment findings.

DIAGNOSTIC TESTS

Laboratory evaluation to assess endocrine function of the suspect gland is based on the history and physical examination. Laboratory tests should be ordered to confirm or refute a clinical suspicion. Routine screening for endocrine conditions is limited to a few situations such as congenital hypothyroidism and phenylketonuria. For any diagnostic testing, appropriate patient preparation for endocrine testing is critical to obtain accurate results (see Guidelines for Safe Practice box).

Principles of Laboratory Evaluation

1. Basal hormone output may be assessed by measuring serum values. Serum values of protein-bound hormones (e.g., T_4) may be elevated by high levels of binding proteins. In such situations, measurement of the active free or unbound hormone better reflects basal hormone production.
2. Timing of the hormone measurement may be very important in hormones with circadian rhythms such as cortisol.
3. The relationship to food ingestion is important where feeding may stimulate hormone production or suppress it (eating carbohydrate stimulates insulin production but suppresses GH production).
4. Many hormones, such as gonadotropins, are secreted in a pulsatile fashion, such that measuring the peak (highest) vs. the trough (lowest) levels may yield widely divergent values.
5. In some instances measuring a trophic hormone (one that stimulates organ growth) may be a more reliable marker of mild hyperfunctioning or hypofunctioning of an endocrine gland. An example is the measurement of TSH in the evaluation of the thyroid gland.

Dynamic Testing

In many instances of endocrine dysfunction, there is an overlap with the extreme ends of both the normal range and the pathologic range. When this scenario is encountered in clinical practice, dynamic testing is conducted. In suspected cases of hyperfunction of a gland one attempts to suppress the gland. For example, the dexamethasone suppression test is an attempt to suppress production of cortisol; a glucose-loading test is an attempt to suppress secretion of GH. Failure to normally suppress the elevated hormone indicates a pathologic state. On the other hand, in suspected cases of hypofunction, one attempts to stimulate the gland. For example, a Cortrosyn (a synthetic subunit of ACTH) stimulation test attempts to stimulate the adrenal glands to produce cortisol. Failure to normally stimulate the gland indicates a pathologic state.

Urine Assessment of Hormonal Status

A 24-hour urine collection of either the hormone itself or its metabolites can yield an integrated marker of hormone produc-

Gerontologic Assessment

NEUROLOGIC

Hoarseness, progressive deafness, unsteady gait, and muscle weakness may be caused by hypothyroidism.
Confusion, lethargy, and memory problems. May result from hypothyroidism, hyperthyroidism, hyponatremia, hypernatremia, or hypoglycemia.
Neurologic symptoms such as paresthesias, blurred vision, headache, and inability to sense temperature may be attributed to complications from diabetes.

CARDIOVASCULAR

Count the pulse for 1 full minute. Check for signs and symptoms of angina and congestive heart failure. Both may occur with hyperthyroidism.
Check for orthostatic hypotension, which may occur in hypernatremia.

EYES

Ophthalmopathy is rarely found in elderly who are newly diagnosed with hyperthyroidism.
Visual problems may be a result of complications of diabetes.

SKIN AND HAIR

Assess for dry skin, poor skin turgor, and thin or fine hair. Some of these may occur with thyroid dysfunction. Persons with frequent yeast or fungal infections may have diabetes mellitus.

MUSCULOSKELETAL

Assess ability to perform ADLs and other activities.
Lack of energy, muscle weakness, and apathy occur with hypernatremia and thyroid and pancreatic dysfunction.
Arthralgias may occur with adrenal insufficiency. Fractures and loss of height may occur from osteoporosis secondary to decreased estrogen.

GASTROINTESTINAL

Assess for changes in bowel habits.
Constipation may occur with hypothyroidism.
Diarrhea may occur with hyperthyroidism. Weight loss, nausea, and abdominal pain may occur with adrenal insufficiency. Anorexia and weight loss may occur with hypothyroidism and hyperthyroidism.

PSYCHOSOCIAL, INCLUDING APATHY AND NERVOUSNESS

Apathy is often the most apparent symptom of hyperthyroidism in an older adult. Depression and withdrawal are often found in persons with hypothyroidism. The cause of these psychologic symptoms is unclear.

COMMON DISORDERS IN ELDERS

Hypothyroidism
Type 2 diabetes mellitus

ADLs, Activities of daily living.

Guidelines for Safe Practice

Preparing the Patient for Diagnostic Tests

Explain the purpose of the test.
Explain what to expect before, during, and after the test.
Patient preparation as ordered, such as
- Fasting hormone assays are generally performed after an overnight fast with blood drawn at 8 AM due to circadian hormonal rhythms

Dietary preparation for certain tests is critical. Iodide-containing foods such as cabbage, as well as iodine supplements must be eliminated from the diet of a patient scheduled to undergo a radioiodine uptake scan.

tion. This is frequently used in suspected adrenal cortisol disorders (Cushing's syndrome) and adrenal medullary disorders (pheochromocytoma). In addition to measurement of the desired hormone/metabolite, it is common to measure the 24-hour urine creatinine as a marker of the completeness of the collection.

Imaging Studies in Endocrinology

There are a variety of imaging techniques for assessment of endocrine glands:

- Ultrasound (thyroid)
- Nuclear medicine scans (thyroid, parathyroid)
- Computed tomography (CT) and magnetic resonance imaging (MRI)

Plain-film x-ray studies have generally been replaced by the technologies in the preceding list.

Imaging studies should be ordered after a thorough history, physical examination, and chemical examination/hormonal evaluation of the patient. Incidental lesions (incidentalomas) are frequently encountered in otherwise normal people when scans are carried out for unrelated reasons such as trauma, or vague pain in the region. Autopsy studies show that 20% of individuals may have incidentalomas, benign nonfunctioning lesions in the pituitary gland or adrenal glands. An obvious diagnostic pitfall then arises in attributing clinical significance to incidentalomas and subjecting patients to unnecessary and perhaps major surgery. The opinion of the skilled experienced endocrinologist is of paramount importance in these diagnostic dilemmas.[2,10,28,29]

ASSESSING FUNCTION OF INDIVIDUAL ENDOCRINE GLANDS

Endocrine dysfunction is broadly categorized into hyposecretory and hypersecretory disorders. These may be further categorized. Diagnostic tests confirm suspicions: if underactivity is suspected, a stimulation test is indicated; if overactivity is suspected, a suppression test is indicated.

Using the thyroid gland as an example, categories of dysfunction are:

1. Primary dysfunction of the gland (hypothyroidism resulting from intrinsic disease of the gland)
2. Secondary dysfunction (secondary hypothyroidism due to pituitary disease and deficiency of biologically active TSH)

3. Tertiary dysfunction (tertiary hypothyroidism caused by hypothalamic dysfunction, resulting in deficiency of biologically active TRH with resultant deficiency of TSH and ultimately reduced T_4 and T_3 levels.

The disease process at each of these levels (the individual endocrine gland, the pituitary gland, or the hypothalamus) may be due to either an intrinsic destruction of that organ (autoimmune thyroid disease damaging the thyroid gland and causing primary hypothyroidism, autoimmune adrenal gland disease damaging the adrenal glands and causing primary adrenal insufficiency, hypophysitis damaging the pituitary gland and causing secondary hypothyroidism) or a secondary process such as metastatic disease (breast cancer metastasizing to the hypothalamic area and causing tertiary hypothyroidism, lung cancer metastasizing to the adrenal glands and causing primary adrenal insufficiency, chronic kidney failure causing failure of activation of vitamin D and causing secondary hyperparathyroidism). Uncommonly, hyperfunctioning of an endocrine gland can result from ectopic hormone production (ACTH production from carcinoma of the lung, growth hormone production from a pancreatic tumor).

Finally, one must always be cognizant of iatrogenic and factitious disease. Iatrogenic disease can consist of overdosing or underdosing of hormone replacement (e.g., levothyroxine). Occasionally iatrogenic disease may be related to a side effect of a concurrently administered medication (lithium-induced hypothyroidism; amiodarone-induced hypothyroidism or hyperthyroidism). Factitious disease can consist of a patient intentionally overdosing such as with levothyroxine in an attempt to lose weight.

Pituitary Gland

Pituitary Function Testing

Prolactin. The assessment of basal PRL levels generally suffices for evaluating PRL excess. Before further evaluation, it is critical to rule out hypothyroidism, renal disease, pregnancy, and adverse effects of medications (cimetadine, metoclopramide). Absolute PRL levels may be of value in distinguishing a tumor from other causes of hyperprolactinemia. A value in excess of 150 μg/L nearly always is diagnostic for a tumor. However, PRL levels lower than 150 μg/L may be associated with either a tumor or other causes. Prolactin deficiency is generally seen as a part of panhypopituitarism.[18]

Growth Hormone. Basal levels of GH do not suffice on their own for diagnosing either deficiency or excess (acromegaly). Patients with high GH levels usually have characteristic clinical features. Basal GH levels in the fasting state in the morning with concurrent somatomedin-C levels are usually the initial evaluation of a patient. In an individual with elevated basal GH levels, the next step in the evaluation process is a glucose suppression test, whereby a baseline GH level is measured, a glucose load is administered, and then a postglucose load GH level is measured. Failure to suppress GH levels with a glucose load confirms autonomous secretion of GH and is consistent with the presence of a tumor.[13]

Isolated GH deficiency in a prepubertal patient is associated with growth retardation. In the adult, GH deficiency is generally associated with panhypopituitarism, such that other hormonal deficiencies are also present. Stimulation of GH secretion may be performed via (1) insulin-induced hypoglycemia, (2) arginine stimulation, and (3) levadopa stimulation. Because no single stimulation test is 100% reliable, two tests are generally performed.

Adrenocorticotropic Hormone. ACTH measurements are typically performed in the fasting and basal state in conjunction with cortisol determinations (Table 28-5).

Gonadotropins: Follicle-Stimulating Hormone and Luteinizing Hormone. FSH and LH can be measured in the basal and stimulated state, the stimulation being measured via administration of GnRH (see Chapter 52 for discussion of ovarian function). In situations of progressive pituitary dysfunction, the first hormones lost are generally FSH and LH. Hence, measurement of FSH and LH is commonly part of the anterior pituitary workup in situations of suspected hypopituitarism.[22,26]

Antidiuretic Hormone. This hormone may be inappropriately produced to excess, as in SIADH, or may be deficient, related to posterior pituitary dysfunction. ADH deficiency results in DI, in which the patient is unable to concentrate the urine with resultant polyuria and increased thirst. Patients generally crave liquids, especially ice cold liquids, and report sleep disturbances owing to nocturia and thirst. An overnight water deprivation test is the test of choice to diagnose DI. When a diagnosis of DI is highly probable and a patient is undergoing an overnight water deprivation test, it is critical that the nurse closely monitor the patient for dehydration, hypotension, and vascular collapse. Assuming the patient is able to tolerate the test, fasting serum and urine osmolality, plasma ADH, and electrolytes are measured. A positive water deprivation test will reveal a serum osmolality in excess of 300 mOsm/L in the context of inappropriately dilute urine as reflected by a low urine osmolality. The serum sodium may be elevated. To determine whether the DI is central (posterior pituitary dysfunction) versus unresponsiveness of the kidneys to ADH (nephrogenic diabetes insipidus), a baseline urine osmolality and serum osmolality is taken. Then aqueous vasopressin at a subcutaneous dose of 5 U is administered. In central DI, in response to administration of vasopressin, the urine osmolality rises and serum osmolality falls. In nephrogenic DI there is no change in either urine or serum osmolality.[3,21]

Pituitary Imaging

Modern imaging of the anterior and posterior pituitary consists of contrast-enhanced CT or MRI, with MRI being generally the preferred approach. Plain film x-ray studies are generally not useful, but may be done in some cases to identify pituitary microadenomas.

Thyroid Gland

Thyroid Function Testing

The mainstay of screening for thyroid disease is the modern third-generation TSH assay, which can distinguish low-normal TSH levels from truly suppressed TSH levels as are seen in hyperthyroidism.[14] Measurement of a free thyroxine (free T_4)

level in turn complements the TSH. The American Thyroid Association recommends measurement of a third-generation TSH level and a free T_4 level as the initial tests to be performed in an individual with suspected thyroid disease.[19] Triiodothyronine (T_3) levels may be ordered in suspected cases of T_3 toxicosis; either a total T_3 or free T_3 level may be drawn. As a result of the great improvement in reliable free T_4 assays, there has been a switch away from ordering total T_4 levels. Measurement of free T_4 levels eliminates the confusion created by situations resulting in increased TBG proteins with resultant elevation in the total T_4 levels. Increased binding proteins in response, for example, to estrogen therapy or pregnancy yield an elevated total T_4 value but a normal free T_4 value. Thyrotropin-releasing hormone stimulation tests used to be carried out in the setting of equivocal hyperthyroidism. These tests are no longer needed in the context of the third-generation TSH assays and the modern free T_4 and free T_3 assays.[1,7,16,27]

Thyroid Imaging

Ultrasound. Ultrasound of the thyroid can accurately define the thyroid anatomy, including volume, echogenicity, and the presence and size of nodules and cysts. Thyroid ultrasound may also be used for guidance with fine needle aspirations of suspicious thyroid nodules. An endocrinologist experienced in ultrasonography should ideally perform thyroid ultrasound.

Radioactive Iodine Uptake Test. The thyroid has tremendous affinity for iodine; the normal 24-hour uptake of a tracer dose of ^{123}I is in the range of 5% to 35%. The radioactive iodine uptake test (RAIU) is generally ordered in hyperthyroid patients to enable calculation of a therapeutic ^{131}I dose. A low RAIU may be seen in thyroiditis, hypothyroidism, previous thyroid ablation, recent excess iodine uptake (diet, medication, iodinated contrast media), factitious hyperthyroidism, or malabsorption of the ^{123}I tracer dose secondary to illness.[7]

Nuclear Thyroid Scan. After a dose of labeled pertechnitate or radioactive iodine is given, a scintillation scan is carried out. The distribution of the radioactivity yields an image of the thyroid anatomy; however, the anatomic detail is not nearly as good as the ultrasound image. The nuclear medicine scan can yield information about the functioning of thyroid nodules. A "cold" nodule refers to a nodule that fails to pick up the radioactive material and thus raises the issue of the nodule being malignant. A "hot" nodule, on the other hand, concentrates the radioactivity within the nodule with little or no uptake throughout the rest of the gland. This is indicative of a hyperfunctioning benign nodule.[7]

Patient isolation is not necessary for RAIU or nuclear thyroid scans. Such isolation is necessary only for large ablative doses of ^{131}I such as those used in the treatment of thyroid cancer.

Parathyroid Glands

Parathyroid Function Testing

PTH may be produced in excess (hyperparathyroidism) or be deficient (hypoparathyroidism). The clinical history and physical examination as well as the baseline serum calcium and phosphorus yield important clinical information. The availability of sensitive intact PTH molecule assays versus the old C-terminal and N-terminal assays has greatly increased the ease of diagnosis. In individuals with normal renal function, PTH excess results in increased mobilization of calcium from bone, decreased renal calcium excretion, and increased phosphorus excretion. Primary hyperparathyroidism is generally the result of a solitary parathyroid adenoma, although occasionally it is related to hyperplasia of all four parathyroid glands. Either of these situations results in an elevated serum calcium level, normal to subnormal serum phosphorus level, and an elevated, intact PTH level (see Figure 28-9). The serum alkaline phosphatase levels may be elevated to varying degrees.[5, 23]

Secondary hyperparathyroidism occurs in response to a disorder that tends to cause hypocalcemia, such as (1) intestinal malabsorption, (2) failure of vitamin D hydroxylation associated with liver disease or kidney failure, or (3) with excessive catabolism of vitamin D as a side effect of certain medications. In secondary hyperparathyroidism, the intact PTH level is elevated in the context of a low normal or mildly subnormal serum calcium. The phosphorus level varies pending the primary cause of the disordered calcium balance; the alkaline phosphatase level is generally elevated to varying degrees.[23]

Tertiary hyperparathyroidism occurs in the setting of chronic sustained secondary hyperparathyroidism (most commonly chronic kidney failure) where adenoma formation occurs in one of the parathyroid glands. Intact PTH levels are generally very high in the setting of hypercalcemia in a patient with known prior secondary hyperparathyroidism.[23]

Hypoparathyroidism generally occurs in the setting of either previous surgery to the parathyroid/thyroid area or postradiation therapy to the region. Intact PTH levels are inappropriately low normal to subnormal in the context of a low serum calcium level.

Parathyroid Imaging

Attempts to identify hyperfunctioning adenomas are still problematic. The most common imaging techniques used are ultrasound or a sestamibi scan; however, even with these, the ability to obtain a diagnostic image meets with variable success. Reduced bone mineral density (osteopenia and osteoporosis), particularly involving cortical bone (assessed best in the forearm), may be an important parameter to consider when surgery is being contemplated for an otherwise asymptomatic patient.

Adrenal Cortex

Adrenocortical Function Tests

The principal parameters of cortisol metabolism that are used are ACTH level, serum cortisol level, and the 24-hour urinary free cortisol level (Table 28-8). The principal parameters of mineralocorticoid metabolism that are used are plasma aldosterone and plasma renin. Concurrent measurement of electrolytes and glucose are also generally carried out.

Cortisol

Suspected Pathologic Cortisol Excess. Initially a 24-hour urine free cortisol level is measured as a marker of integrated

TABLE 28-8 Diurnal Pattern of Serum Cortisol and Adrenocorticotropic Hormone (ACTH) Levels

Analyte	Time/Serum Level	
Cortisol	8 AM 4.3-2.4 μg/dl	4 PM 3.1-16.7 μg/dl
ACTH	7-10 AM 9-52 pg/ml	

TABLE 28-9 Urinary Adrenomedullary Secretions in Adults: 24-Hour Urine

Analyte	Normal Values
Epinephrine	2-24 μg//24 hr
Norepinephrine	15-10 μg/24 hr
Total metanephrines	Males: 110-480 μg/g creatinine Females: 150-510 μg/g creatinine
Dopamine	52-480 μg/24 hr
Vanillylmandelic acid	< 6.0 mg/24 hr

cortisol production. When results are elevated, an overnight dexamethasone suppression test is conducted. The patient takes an oral dose of 1 mg dexamethasone at 11 PM before sleep. The next morning at 8 AM a fasting serum cortisol is measured. Normally cortisol suppresses to <5 ng/dl.

If these tests are abnormal, additional testing is needed to clarify the primary mechanism involved in the cortisol excess. Is the issue ACTH-dependent pituitary Cushing's disease? An ectopic ACTH-dependent tumor? An adrenal adenoma? An adrenal carcinoma?

ACTH and cortisol values (serum and 24-hour urine) are measured after a patient takes dexamethasone, 0.5 mg four times a day for 48 hours. Patients with pituitary Cushing's disease will show some suppression of the 24-hour urine free cortisol level to less than 50% reduction from baseline, as well as some suppression of the ACTH level, indicating some responsiveness of the feedback loop.[12] Patients with either ectopic ACTH-dependent Cushing's or primary adrenal Cushing's syndrome will show no change in their 24-hour urine free cortisol levels after these doses of dexamethasone. In primary adrenal Cushing's syndrome the ACTH levels are low throughout the testing period, whereas in ectopic ACTH-dependent Cushing's syndrome, the ACTH levels are high. Occasionally 24-hour urine collections are ordered for 17-hydroxyketosteroids and 17-ketosteroids as markers of cortisol metabolism.[4,6]

Suspected Hypocortisolism. Declining cortisol reserve is readily assessed by the Cortrosyn stimulation test, generally done in the fasting state. A baseline serum cortisol level is drawn and then 250 μg of Cortrosyn is injected either intravenously (IV) or intramuscularly (IM). A follow-up serum cortisol is drawn 30 minutes after IV administration or 60 minutes after IM administration of Cortrosyn. The normal response is a peak stimulated cortisol level in excess of 20 μg/dl.[17]

Aldosterone Excess. Clinically the principal issue is the presence of hyperaldosteronism in a patient with (1) hypertension and (2) hypokalemia or borderline low potassium levels, unrelated to diuretic use.[24] Aldosterone can be measured in the basal state as a plasma aldosterone level; it can also be assessed via a 24-hour urine. If salt loading with resultant volume expansion fails to suppress aldosterone levels, there is high likelihood of autonomous secretion of aldosterone from an adenoma or tumor. Plasma renin levels are low in patients with autonomous aldosterone secretion; in patients with secondary hyperaldosteronism, renin levels are elevated.[11,15]

Adrenocortical Imaging

A CT scan with contrast is the most common imaging technique. Occasionally, right and left adrenal vein catheterization is needed to define the source of the hormonal excess when a neoplasm is not clearly imaged.

Adrenomedullary Assessment

Adrenomedullary Function Tests

These tests are performed to diagnose a pheochromocytoma, a tumor (benign or malignant) producing excess catecholamines in a patient with hypertension (intermittent or persistent). Caffeine, alcohol, and smoking should be discontinued during all assessments for catecholamine excess. The initial screening test is a 24-hour urine determination for catecholamine metabolites: vanillylmandelic acid and metanephrines. In individuals with a true pheochromocytoma, the 24-hour urine results are generally elevated considerably outside of the reference range and not just "borderline-high" (Table 28-9).

In equivocal situations plasma catecholamines may be assessed. Fasting before the test is required. The patient is positioned comfortably in the supine position for at least 30 minutes in a dark quiet room. Blood is drawn from an indwelling heparinized catheter to assess plasma catecholamines. The combination of the 24-hour urine catecholamines and plasma catecholamines usually confirms or refutes the diagnosis of pheochromocytoma in most patients. Rarely a clonidine suppression test may need be required.[9,20,28]

Adrenomedullary Imaging

To detect a pheochromocytoma, most endocrinologists prefer MRI over CT scanning. In addition, specialized imaging may be necessary when the aforementioned adrenomedullary function testing is nondiagnostic and/or the neoplasm is thought to be extraadrenal.[8,9]

Endocrine Pancreas

Assessment of insulin secretory capacity is accomplished via a connective-peptide (C-peptide) test. When insulin is secreted by the *beta* cells in the islets of Langerhans, it is actually secreted as proinsulin. An enzymatic reaction occurs and cleaves each proinsulin molecule resulting in the production of one molecule of insulin and one molecule of C-peptide. Measurement of C-peptide provides an indirect marker of insulin secretory capacity because both the insulin user and nonuser metabolize it. If one were to measure insulin levels in an insulin user, both endogenous and exogenous insulin would be measured. In contrast, C-peptide measures only endogenous insulin production, as C-peptide is purified out of exogenous insulin. Glucagon levels are measured in cases of suspected glucagonomas.

Clinical measurement of somatostatin levels is rare. Diagnostic criteria for diabetes mellitus are discussed in detail in Chapter 30.

References

1. Bagachi N, Brown TR, Parish RF: Thyroid dysfunction in adults over age 55 years, *Arch Intern Med* 150:785, 1990.
2. Barzon L, Boscaro M: Diagnosis and management of adrenal incidentalomas, *J Urol* 163:398, 2000.
3. Bichet DG: Nephrogenic diabetes insipidus, *Am J Med* 105:431,1998.
4. Biller BMK et al: Cushing's syndrome. In Molitch ME, editor: *Atlas of clinical endocrinology,* vol 4: *Neuroendocrinology and pituitary disease,* Philadelphia, 1999, Current Medicine.
5. Bilezikian JKP et al: Clinical presentation of primary hyperparathyroidism. In Bilezikian JP, editor: *The parathyroids,* ed 3, New York, 2001, Raven.
6. Bornstein SR et al: Adrenocortical tumors: recent advances in basic concepts and clinical management, *Ann Intern Med* 130:759, 1999.
7. Braverman LE, Utiger RD, editors: *Werner and Ingbar's the thyroid,* ed 7, Philadelphia, 1996, JB Lippincott.
8. Bravo EL, Gifford RW: Pheochromocytoma: diagnosis, localization and management, *N Engl J Med* 311:1298, 1984.
9. Canizares Hernandez F et al: A five-year report on experience in the detection of pheochromoctyoma, *Clin Biochem* 33:649, 2000.
10. Chidiac RM, Aron DC: Incidentalomas: a disease of modern technology, *Endocrinol Metab Clin North Am* 26:233, 1997.
11. Conn JW: Presidential address: Part I. Painting background. Part II. Primary aldosteronism, a new clinical syndrome, *J Clin Lab Med* 45:3, 1955.
12. Cushing H: The basophil adenomas of the pituitary body and their clinical manifestation, *Bull Johns Hopkins Hospital* 50:137, 1932.
13. Etxabe J et al: Acromegaly: an epidemiologic study, *J Endocrinol Invest* 16:181, 1993.
14. Franklyn JA et al: Comparison of second and third generation methods for measurement of serum thyrotropin in patients with overt hyperthyroidism, patients receiving thyroid hormone, and those with non-thyroidal illness. *J Clin Endocrinol Metab* 78:1368, 1994.
15. Ganguly A: Primary aldosteronism. *N Engl J Med* 339:1828, 1998.
16. Gittoes NJ, Franklyn JA: Hyperthyroidism. Current treatment guidelines, *Drugs* 55:543, 1998.
17. Grinspoon S, Biller B: Laboratory assessment of adrenal insufficiency. *J Clin Endocrinol Metab* 79:923, 1994.
18. Katznelson L, Klibanski A: Prolactin and its disorders. In Becker KL, editor: *Principles and practice of endocrinology and metabolism,* ed 2, Philadelphia, 1995, JB Lippincott.
19. Ladenson PW et al: American Thyroid Association guidelines for detection of thyroid dysfunction, *Arch Intern Med* 160:1573, 2000.
20. Noshiro T et al: Changes in clinical features and long-term prognosis in patients with pheochromocytoma, *Am J Hypertens* 13:35, 2000.
21. Robertson GL: Diabetes insipidus, *Endocrinol Metab Clin North Am* 24:549-572, 1995.
22. Rolih C, Ober K: Pituitary apoplexy, *Endocrinol Metab Clin North Am* 22:29, 1993.
23. Silverberg SJ, Fitzpatrick LA, Bilezikian JP: Hyperparathyroidism. In Becker KL, editor: *Principles and practice of endocrinology and metabolism,* ed 3, Philadelphia, 2001, JB Lippincott.
24. Stewart PM: Mineralocorticoid hypertension, *Lancet* 353:1341, 1999.
25. Trivalle C et al: Differences in the signs and symptoms of hyperthyroidism in older and younger patients, *J Am Geriatr Soc* 44:50, 1996.
26. Vance M: Hypopituitarism, *N Engl J Med* 330:1651, 1994.
27. Weetman AP: Medical progress: Graves' disease, *N Engl J Med* 343:1236, 2000.
28. Young WF Jr: Pheochromocytoma: 1926-1993, *Trends Endocrinol Metab* 4:122, 1993.
29. Young WF Jr: Management approaches to adrenal incidentalomas: a view from Rochester, Minnesota, *Endocrinol Metab Clin North Am* 29:159, 2000.

http://www.mosby.com/MERLIN/medsurg_phipps

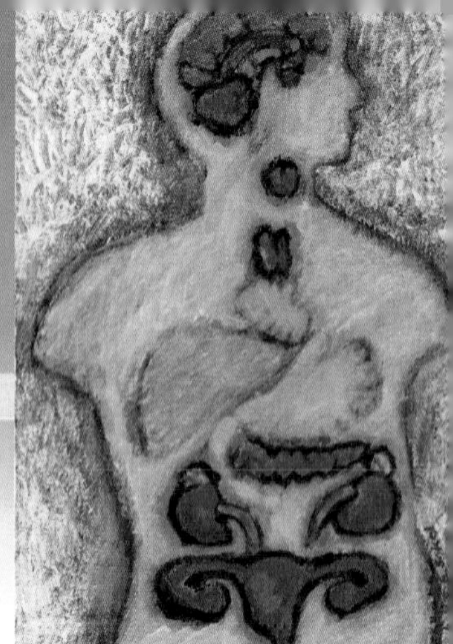

29 Pituitary, Thyroid, Parathyroid, and Adrenal Gland Problems

Margaret M. Ulchaker, Jane F. Marek

Objectives

After studying this chapter, the learner should be able to:

1. Differentiate between the pathophysiology of hypersecretion and hyposecretion of the anterior and posterior pituitary, thyroid, parathyroid, and adrenal glands.
2. Correlate the clinical manifestations, including history, physical examination, and diagnostic test findings, with hypersecretion and hyposecretion of the anterior and posterior pituitary, thyroid, parathyroid, and adrenal glands.
3. Synthesize a nursing plan of care, including identification of appropriate nursing diagnoses, patient outcomes, and interventions, for a patient with hypersecretion or hyposecretion of the anterior or posterior pituitary, thyroid, parathyroid, or adrenal gland.
4. Explain reasons for surgery of the pituitary, thyroid, parathyroid, or adrenal gland.
5. Formulate a nursing plan of care for an individual having surgery on the pituitary, thyroid, parathyroid, or adrenal gland.
6. Describe self-care skills needed by a patient receiving long-term hormonal replacement therapy for pituitary, thyroid, parathyroid, or adrenocortical insufficiency.
7. Develop a teaching plan for a patient receiving long-term hormonal replacement therapy for pituitary, thyroid, parathyroid, or adrenocortical insufficiency.

Endocrine dysfunction of the pituitary, parathyroid, thyroid, and adrenal glands generally results in hyposecretion or hypersecretion of the particular gland. Although the primary dysfunction may be localized in a particular gland, the effects are usually systemic. Clinical manifestations vary in severity from mild, which are usually treated on an outpatient basis, to medical emergencies, requiring surgical intervention. Types of pathologic processes involved in decreased hormone production include:

- Congenital (e.g., a biosynthetic defect such as in congenital adrenal hyperplasia)
- Inflammatory (e.g., autoimmune thyroid disease, infection)
- Ischemic (e.g., hemorrhagic infarction of the adrenals or pituitary, ischemic injury to the parathyroid glands during surgery)
- Destructive (surgical removal, radiation, or trauma of glands)
- Neoplastic (benign or malignant)
- Iatrogenic (e.g., medication-related side effects)

The pathologic processes involved in excess hormone production include:

- Hyperplasia or hypertrophy of endocrine glands
- Inflammation (e.g., acute or subacute thyroiditis resulting in acute discharge of preformed thyroid hormone from the gland causing transient thyrotoxicosis)
- Stimulation of receptors on the gland with resultant hormone release (e.g., stimulation of thyroid-stimulating immunoglobulin [TSI] in Graves' disease; stimulation of thyroid-stimulating hormone [TSH] receptors by a TSH-producing pituitary neoplasm, stimulation of adrenocorticotropic hormone [ACTH] receptors from ACTH produced from a carcinoma of the lung)
- Neoplasia (benign or malignant)
- Stimulation of hormone production secondary to administration of medications for cardiovascular, psychiatric, neurologic, and gastrointestinal disorders
- Exogenous administration of hormones

Disorders of the endocrine glands controlled by the hypothalamus and pituitary gland (thyroid and adrenocortical glands and gonads) that result in hyposecretion or hypersecretion are classified as *primary, secondary,* or *tertiary.* Disease of the thyroid and adrenocortical glands and gonads are classified as primary dysfunction. Secondary dysfunction occurs when the problem results from anterior pituitary dysfunction, and tertiary problems arise from hypothalamic dysfunction.

PITUITARY DISORDERS

Pituitary dysfunction may manifest as hypersecretion, hyposecretion, or nonfunctioning tumors. Function, as defined in endocrinology, refers to whether or not the gland or tumor is producing hormone.

ANTERIOR PITUITARY GLAND

Hyperfunction

Etiology/Epidemiology

Hyperfunction of the anterior pituitary gland may involve one or more hormones. Tumors and hyperplasia are common causes of anterior pituitary hyperfunction.

Pituitary hypersecretion can result from a discrete functioning tumor producing one hormone to excess with relative hyposecretion of the remaining gland secondary to compression from the tumor. Hypersecretion is occasionally related to idiopathic hyperplasia of cells producing one trophic hormone. The cause of pituitary tumors is generally unknown.

Pathophysiology

Pituitary Tumors. Pituitary tumors are classified by:

- Size
- Macroadenomas >10 mm in diameter
- Microadenomas ≤10 mm in diameter
- Hormone production
- Prolactin-secreting most common ~60%
- Growth hormone-secreting ~20%
- ACTH-secreting ~10%
- Other ~10%

Functioning pituitary tumors resulting in pituitary hypersecretion are usually benign. The clinical picture varies, depending on which hormone is secreted (see Clinical Manifestations box). Clinical manifestations may include neurologic symptoms as the tumor enlarges, compressing adjacent structures and blood vessels.

In addition to the manifestations of hormone excess or deficiency, patients may complain of headaches and/or visual

Clinical Manifestations

Pituitary Hormone-Secreting Tumors

NEUROLOGIC

1. Visual defects often first seen as losses in superior temporal quadrants with progression to hemianopia or scotomas and finally to total blindness
2. Headache
3. Somnolence
4. Rarely, signs of increased intracranial pressure (hydrocephalus, papilledema)
5. With very large tumors, disturbance in appetite, sleep, temperature regulation, and emotional balance because of hypothalamic involvement
6. Behavioral changes and seizures with expansion causing compression of the temporal or frontal lobe (very rare)

ENDOCRINE

Prolactin Hypersecretion

1. Females
   a. Menstrual disturbances, such as irregular menses, anovulatory periods, oligomenorrhea, or amenorrhea
   b. Infertility
   c. Galactorrhea
   d. Manifestations of ovarian steroid deficit, such as dyspareunia, vaginal mucosal atrophy, decreased vaginal lubrication, decreased libido
2. Males
   a. Loss of libido and erectile function
   b. Reduced sperm count and infertility
   c. Gynecomastia
   d. Galactorrhea (rare)
3. Decreased testosterone (men), decreased estradiol (women)

Growth Hormone (GH) Hypersecretion (Acromegaly)

1. Macroadenomas with resultant headache and visual changes
2. Changes in facial features (coarsening of features; increased size of nose, lips, and skinfolds; prominence of supraorbital ridges; growth of mandible resulting in prognathism and widely spaced teeth; soft tissue growth resulting in facial puffiness)
3. Increased size of hands and feet, weight gain
4. Deepening of voice from thickening of vocal cords
5. Increases in vertebral bodies resulting in thoracic kyphosis
6. Enlarged tongue, salivary glands, spleen, liver, heart, kidney, and other organs; cardiomegaly may result in increased blood pressure and signs and symptoms of congestive heart failure.
7. Elevated blood pressure
8. Snoring, sleep apnea, and respiratory failure
9. Dermatologic changes: acne, malodorous diaphoresis, oiliness, development of skin tags
10. Hypertrophy progressing to atrophy of skeletal muscles
11. Backache, arthralgia, or arthritis from joint damage and bony overgrowth
12. Nerve entrapment syndromes such as carpal tunnel syndrome from bony overgrowth and changes in nerve size
13. Impaired glucose tolerance progressing to diabetes mellitus
14. Changes in fat metabolism resulting in hyperlipidemia
15. General changes in mobility: presence of lethargy and fatigue
16. Radiographic findings indicative of bony proliferation in hands, feet, skull, ribs, and vertebrae
17. Electrolyte changes: increased urinary excretion of calcium; elevated serum phosphorus level

disturbances when the neoplasm extends out of the sella turcica and impinges on the optic chiasm. Sudden expansion of the tumor can occur as a result of hemorrhage into the tumor (*pituitary apoplexy*), and this can result in a severe headache and other neurologic symptoms. The abrupt loss of pituitary function is a medical emergency with resultant hypotension and vascular collapse resulting from loss of ACTH secretion. Pituitary apoplexy may occur years after surgery and/or radiation therapy for the original tumor.

Prolactin Hypersecretion. Prolactin (PRL) inhibits gonadotropin-releasing hormone and is necessary for lactation. Prolactin secretion by the pituitary is controlled primarily by the inhibitory factors of the hypothalamus, chiefly dopamine. Normal levels are usually less than 20 ng/ml. As mentioned previously, prolactin-secreting adenomas are a major cause of prolactin excess. Other pathophysiologic mechanisms responsible for prolactin excess include dopamine disorders, chronic kidney failure (decreased clearance), neurogenic secretion triggered by chest irritation (rib fracture, thoracotomy, herpes zoster), hypothyroidism, and medications (Box 29-1).

The clinical manifestations of PRL excess are the same, regardless of the cause. Classic manifestations are galactorrhea and amenorrhea in women and decreased libido or erectile dysfunction in men.

Growth Hormone Hypersecretion (Acromegaly). In most instances somatotropin or growth hormone (GH) hypersecretion is related to a pituitary tumor, generally a macroadenoma. In rare instances there may be an ectopic GH-producing tumor (e.g., in the pancreas) and also GH-releasing hormone (GHRH) producing tumors. The clinical features of acromegaly usually evolve slowly over time, and a review of old family photographs can often show changes evolving over periods in excess of 10 years before diagnosis (Figure 29-1). Men and women are equally affected.

Excess of GH affects all growing cells; if it occurs before the epiphyses close, *gigantism* results with excess growth of the skeleton and soft tissues. *Acromegaly,* which occurs after the epiphyses close, is distinguished by an increase in connective, soft tissue, and cartilage, giving the characteristic growth and thickening of the hands, face, and feet (see Clinical Manifestations box). The soft tissue features may regress slowly after the cessation of the high GH levels; however, the bony changes are permanent.

In addition to the local effects of the tumor (mass effect), which impinges on other brain/skull structures, and other effects of GH excess, especially diabetes mellitus, untreated acromegaly results in hypertension, cardiomegaly, and premature cardiovascular death. In addition, GH excess is associated with an increased risk of colon cancer.

Most of the adverse effects of chronic GH hypersecretion are caused by stimulation of excessive amounts of insulin-like growth factor 1 (IGF-1, secreted by the liver). The growth-promoting effects of IGF-1 lead to the characteristic proliferation of bone, cartilage, and soft tissue and increase in the size of other organs. The insulin resistance and carbohydrate intolerance seen in acromegaly appear to be direct effects of GH, not IGF-1 excess.

Pituitary ACTH Hypersecretion. A pituitary adenoma producing ACTH is the most common noniatrogenic cause of Cushing's syndrome (see discussion of Cushing's syndrome later in this chapter). In general, these tumors are microadenomas and the remaining pituitary function is normal. In the case of larger tumors, there may be compression of the normal

BOX 29-1 Stimulants of Prolactin Secretion

Physiologic

Sleep
Stress (physical and psychologic)
Pregnancy, lactation

Pathologic

Prolactinoma
Primary hypothyroidism
Chronic kidney failure
Polycystic ovarian syndrome
Cushing's disease
Hypothyroidism
Acromegaly
Chest wall trauma
Spinal cord injury
Idiopathic

Pharmacologic

Psychotropic agents
- Neuroleptics: phenothiazine, chlorpromazine, haloperidol

Antidepressants
- Tricyclics
- Imipramine
- Monoamine oxidase inhibitors

Anxiolytics
- Benzodiazepines

Antiemetics
- Metoclopramide

Opiates
- Methadone
- Morphine

H_2 blockers
- Ranitidine
- Cimetadine
- Famotidine

Antihypertensive agents
- Reserpine
- Methyldopa

Calcium-channel blockers
- Verapamil

Hormones
- Estrogens
- Thyrotropin-releasing hormone (TRH)

Selective serotonin reuptake inhibitors

pituitary gland with hypofunction and loss of several trophic hormones and varying degrees of hypopituitarism and/or other mass effect such as optic chiasm impingement with homonymous bitemporal hemianopsia. Occasionally, the microadenoma is not visualized with the usual imaging modalities such that inferior petrosal sinus sampling is needed to assess for the ACTH excess. This in turn is of immense value for the neurosurgeon undertaking the transsphenoidal surgery.[7]

Collaborative Care Management

Diagnostic Tests

Pituitary Adenoma. Diagnosis of pituitary tumor is made based on the history and physical examination, radiologic studies, and laboratory determination of hormone levels. Imaging studies, including magnetic resonance imaging (MRI) with contrast of the sella turcica, can detect pituitary tumors. Presence of a functioning tumor is indicated by elevated pituitary hormone levels.

Prolactin Hypersecretion. Evaluation of patients with galactorrhea or unexplained gonadal dysfunction with normal or low plasma gonadotropin levels should include a thorough history relating to menstrual status, pregnancy, fertility, sexual function, and symptoms of hypothyroidism or hypopituitarism. An accurate medication history is critical to accurate diagnosis. Prolactin levels in excess of 150 ng/ml are more likely caused by medication than by tumor. Although PRL levels greater than 150 ng/ml are considered diagnostic for adenoma, levels may exceed 3000 ng/ml. Basal PRL levels; gonadotropins; and thyroid, liver, and kidney function tests should be evaluated. Serum testosterone levels in men and pregnancy tests in women presenting with amenorrhea should also be performed.

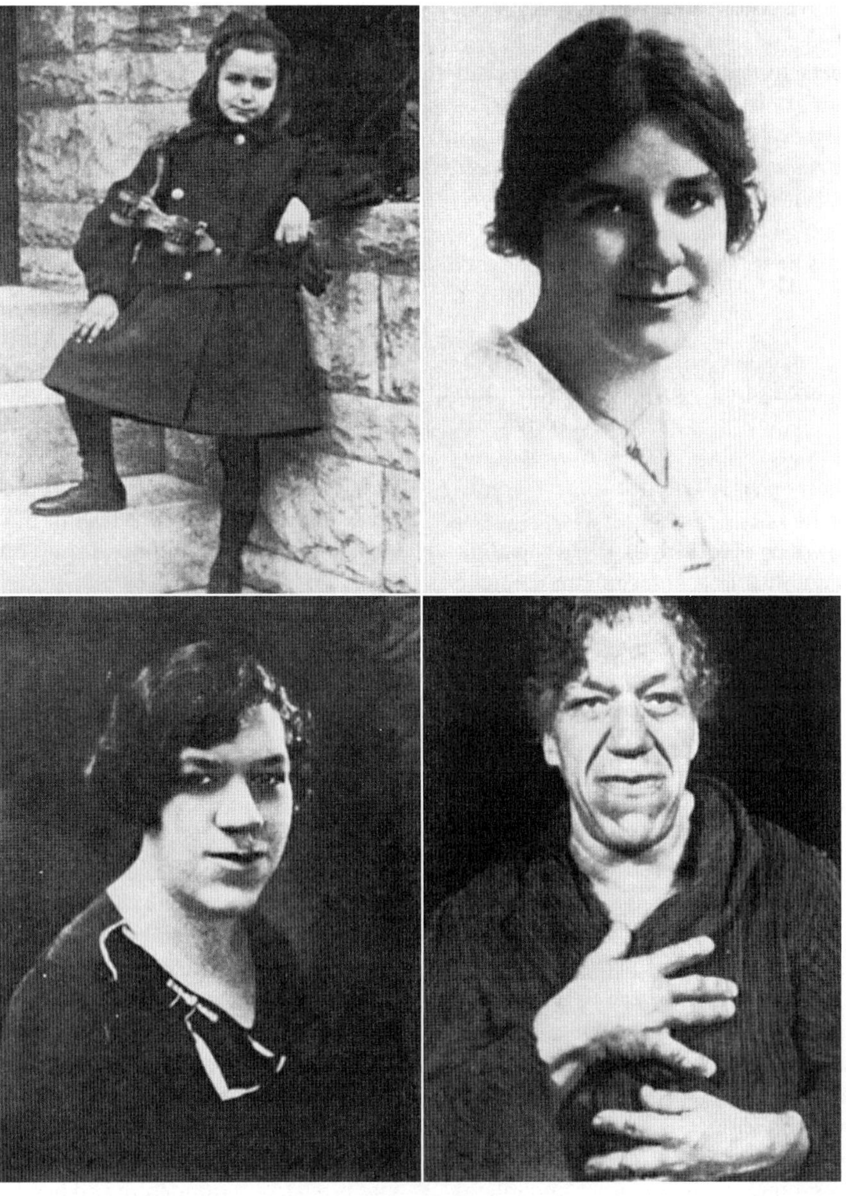

Figure 29-1 The progression of acromegaly in a woman from age 9 to 52 years.

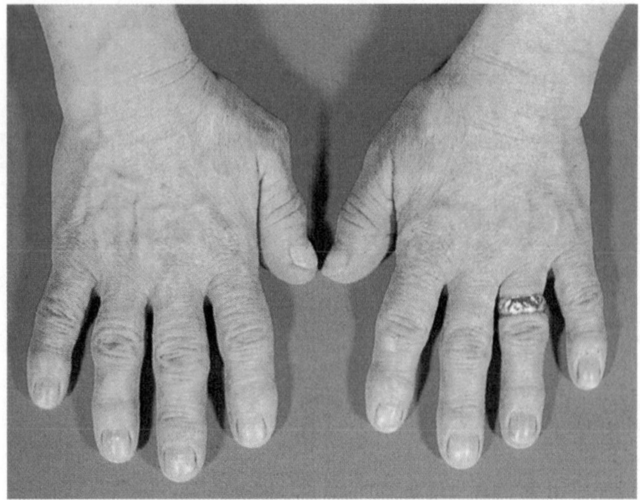

Figure 29-2 The hands of the patient with agromegaly may appear broad and spadelike.

Growth Hormone Hypersecretion. Diagnosis of acromegaly is usually clinically obvious and can be confirmed by assessment of GH secretion. Other tests that may be performed to confirm the diagnosis include suppression with oral glucose and IGF-1 measurement. Due to the effects of GH or IGF-1, elevated postprandial plasma glucose, elevated serum phosphorus, and hypercalciuria may be seen in persons with GH excess. Radiographs show evidence of enlargement of the frontal and maxillary sinuses and thickening of the soft tissues.

Medications. Prolactinomas are usually managed medically with dopaminergic medications such as bromocriptine (Parlodel), cabergoline (Dostinex), or pergolide (Pergonal). Cabergoline typically has fewer side effects than bromocriptine, which frequently causes nausea, and occasionally vomiting, dizziness, and hypotension.

In addition to acute lowering of PRL levels, these dopaminergic agents can have long-term effects on neoplasm size, with some neoplasm shrinkage and fibrosis. The natural history of microadenomas appears to be benign and most remain stable in size. Macroadenomas on the other hand are more problematic in terms of potential for progressive growth when patients are not treated with dopaminergic agents. Treatment with pergolide and transsphenoidal surgery is recommended for patients with larger neoplasms and extrasellar extension. Surgery is not commonly used as the primary treatment of microadenomas and macroadenomas simply because of the high recurrence rates; many patients are placed on medical therapy.[8,23]

Octreotide acetate, a somatostatin analog, is useful for the treatment of acromegaly and thyroid-stimulating adenomas. Originally octreotide acetate (Sandostatin) had to be dosed as subcutaneous injections three times a day; it can now be given as a monthly depot injection (Sandostatin LAR). This is the most effective adjunctive medical therapy for acromegaly, and response can be measured with serial IGF-1 and GH measurements.[25] Dopamine agonists paradoxically lower GH levels in some acromegalic patients; however, their efficacy and tolerability are inferior to those of octreotide acetate.[26] Recent development of an investigative GH receptor antagonist, pegvisomant, has been associated with normalization of IGF-1 levels in 97% of patients treated for more than 12 months in a recent clinical trial of 160 patients.[39]

Treatments. Treatment goals for patients with pituitary adenomas are to correct hypersecretion of the anterior pituitary hormones, preserve normal secretion of other anterior pituitary hormones, and remove or suppress the adenoma. Treatments include surgery, radiation, or medications. Patients with macroadenomas usually require a combination of therapies to achieve these goals.

Pituitary radiation is usually reserved for patients who have had incomplete resection of large pituitary adenomas. Conventional radiation using high-energy sources is most commonly used. Response to radiation therapy is usually slow. Hypopituitarism is a common complication following radiation therapy. Heavy particle radiation with alpha particles or protons is also used. Advantages of this type are the ability to precisely focus the beam of radiation, limiting the exposure of surrounding tissues and a more rapid response to therapy than to conventional radiation. Use of this type of radiation is usually limited to smaller tumors and those without extrasellar extension. Hypopituitarism also may occur after this treatment.

Goals of treatment for patients with PRL hypersecretion are control of PRL levels, cessation of galactorrhea, and return to normal gonadal function. All patients with PRL-secreting adenomas should be treated either medically or surgically to avoid the risk of further tumor expansion, hypopituitarism, and visual impairment. Treatment of patients with microadenomas is also recommended to prevent osteoporosis secondary to persisting hypogonadism and to restore fertility.

Treatment goals for patients with acromegaly are to halt progression of the disorder and to prevent complications and excess mortality. The objectives of therapy are removal or destruction of the tumor, reversal of GH secretion, and maintenance of normal anterior and posterior pituitary function. Many patients present with advanced manifestations of acromegaly (Figure 29-2). The soft tissue features may regress slowly after cessation of the high GH levels; however, the bony changes are permanent. Surgical intervention is less successful with larger tumors; adjuvant medical treatment may be required. Conventional radiation therapy is seldom used now because it is slow to take effect and ultimately results in panhypopituitarism. Other radiologic therapies include particle beam radiation and the gamma knife.

Surgical Management. Transsphenoidal removal of a pituitary adenoma is considered by some to be the primary form of treatment. Surgical success is related to tumor size and the amount of invasion into the sella turcica. Although the microsurgical approach is preferred, subfrontal approach via craniotomy (see Chapter 42) is sometimes required for patients with suprasellar tumor extension. If residual tumor is present, radiation or bromocriptine therapy may be indicated. The surgical outcome for patients with PRL-secreting adenomas is related to tumor size and basal PRL level. Surgery is indicated if severe visual field defects are present.

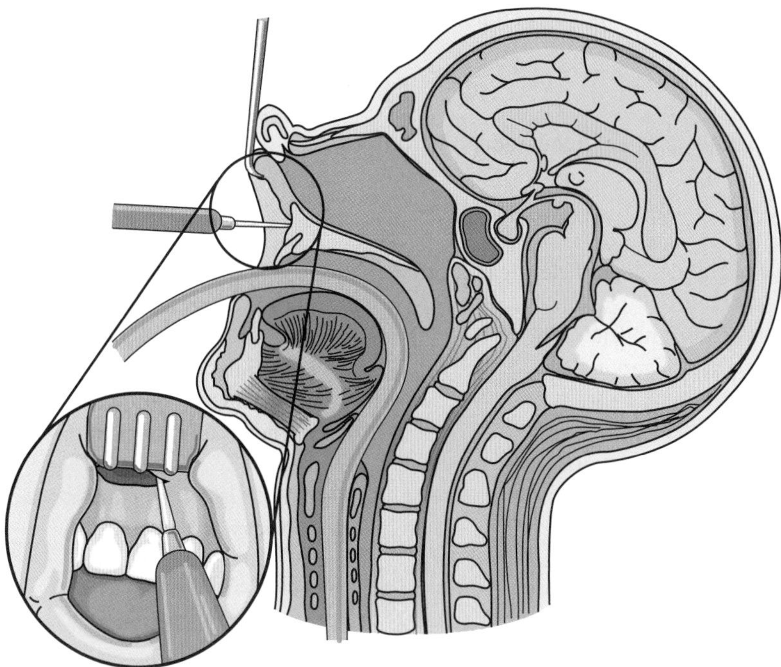

Figure 29-3 Transsphenoidal approach in anterior pituitary surgery with incision in the gingival mucosa.

In the transsphenoidal procedure the surgical approach to the pituitary is from the nasal cavity through the sphenoid sinus or from the mouth through a gingival incision (Figure 29-3). The microscope is used to incise the inferior sellar floor and dura and to remove the adenoma. Normal pituitary tissue is preserved when possible. Complications, more common in persons with large or invasive tumors, include postoperative hemorrhage, cerebrospinal fluid (CSF) leak, and visual impairment. The most common complication is transient diabetes insipidus (DI) lasting from days to weeks; permanent DI is rare. Other complications include syndrome of inappropriate antidiuretic hormone secretion with symptomatic hyponatremia, surgical hypopituitarism, infection, and meningitis.

Diet. Dietary changes may be necessary for patients with acromegaly or Cushing's syndrome. Carbohydrate intolerance or frank diabetes mellitus may be associated with both of these disorders (see Chapter 30 for dietary management of patients with diabetes). Congestive heart failure may occur in patients with acromegaly, and sodium, lipid, and fluid restrictions may be indicated. The subsequent decrease in calcium levels may place the patient at risk for osteoporosis; supplemental calcium may be required.

Activity. No specific activity is prescribed for persons with pituitary tumors. Persons with acromegaly should be encouraged to maintain joint mobility and range of motion. Kyphosis and arthritis may impose problems with balance and mobility.

Referrals. The patient with acromegaly may benefit from physical or occupational therapy. The patient with visual loss may benefit from occupational therapy and visual rehabilitative services. Social work services can be helpful when an acute crisis or the burdens of chronic illness stress financial, personal, and family resources. A referral to a mental health professional may be indicated if the patient is having difficulty coping with the physical changes in his or her appearance.

NURSING MANAGEMENT OF PATIENT WITH PITUITARY TUMOR

ASSESSMENT

Patient assessment focuses on the manifestations of hormone hypersecretion and the effects on the patient's total health. Assessment should also include the psychologic response of the patient to these major body changes.

Health History

Data to be collected to assess the patient with hypersecretion of the pituitary gland associated with pituitary tumor include:

- History of sensory alterations, particularly vision and visual fields, as well as other peripheral sensory changes
- Discomforts: temporal or frontal headache of moderate intensity, arthralgias, backache
- History of changes in body appearance: coarsening of facial features; increase in ring, glove, or shoe size; increase in sweating or oiliness of skin
- History of change in energy level (lethargy or fatigue) or decrease in mobility
- Psychosocial concerns: behavioral changes such as anxiety, irritability, concerns about self-image
- History of menstrual changes in females, erectile dysfunction in males, changes in libido; fertility concerns
- Drug history: use of oral contraceptives and/or psychotropic drugs

Knowledge level related to disorder, treatment, and potential outcome of treatment

Physical Examination

Physical examination of the patient with a pituitary adenoma should focus on assessment of/for:

Functioning of cranial nerves II, III, IV, and VI (see Chapter 41)
Retinal changes indicative of papilledema or elevated blood pressure
Mental status: alertness and emotional status
Peripheral nerve functioning (see Chapter 41)
Body appearance and description
Mobility and joint functioning (see Chapter 45)
Vital signs: blood pressure, pulse, respirations, and temperature
Body weight and height
Presence of organomegaly, particularly cardiac and hepatic, and signs associated with these changes

NURSING DIAGNOSES

Nursing diagnoses are determined from analysis of patient data. Nursing diagnoses for the patient with hypersecretion of the anterior pituitary gland associated with pituitary tumor may include but are not limited to:

Diagnostic Title	Possible Etiologic Factors
1. Situational low self-esteem	Uncertainty about cause of problem and outcomes of treatment; changes in body characteristics and functions associated with hormonal excess, visual disturbance, sexual dysfunction, impaired mobility
2. Risk for deficient fluid volume	Disruption in normal antidiuretic hormone (ADH) secretion or adrenocortical functioning associated with surgical trauma
3. Risk for infection	Surgical intervention; possible CSF leak
4. Deficient knowledge	Lack of exposure regarding diagnosis, treatment plan, surgery and perioperative routines (if indicated), expected outcomes of treatment, follow-up care

EXPECTED PATIENT OUTCOMES

Expected patient outcomes for the person with hypersecretion of the anterior pituitary gland associated with pituitary tumor may include but are not limited to:

1. Will talk positively about self when discussing body characteristics, changes, and functions
2. Will exhibit physical signs of fluid balance
2a. Will return to baseline weight
2b. Will have elastic skin turgor and moist mucous membranes
2c. Will have blood pressure and pulse within normal range
2d. Will have serum electrolytes and hematocrit within normal limits
2e. Will have urine specific gravity of 1.010 to 1.025
2f. Will have a fluid intake of 2.5-3 L/day, orally or parenterally (unless restrictions are prescribed)
2g. Will explain measures to prevent fluid deficit
3. Will remain free of infection, as evidenced by absence of persistent headache, CSF leak, and nuchal rigidity
4a. Will have adequate knowledge, as evidenced by patient's and family's ability to describe disease process, effects on bodily function, and goals of treatment
4b. Will explain nature of the disorder, medications, treatment regimen, surgical intervention, and expected outcomes of treatment, plan for follow-up care
4c. Will understand and participate in perioperative routines and care

INTERVENTIONS

1. Promoting Self-Esteem

The patient must be assessed for factors posing a threat to self-esteem and for statements of negative self-appraisal. The patient who has just been diagnosed with a pituitary tumor is faced with important decisions and may feel overwhelmed and/or helpless. Support must be provided for the patient to ask questions, seek information, obtain needed resources, and make decisions about care.

Threats to self-esteem can be increased by visual disturbances, infertility, immobility, or changes in body appearance. The patient's knowledge about the disease, its treatment, and anticipated effects on body appearance and functions must be clarified; and the patient and significant others need to know that although changes in body characteristics and vision are not always reversible, progressive changes can be stopped. Sexual dysfunction associated with prolactin excess is usually reversible. The nurse can assist the patient and family to cope with irreversible changes. Participation of the patient/family/significant others in a support group can provide an opportunity to learn how others have coped. It is also important to reassure the patient and family about the normalcy of individual responses to stressors. Enabling the patient to maintain an optimal level of independence in activities of daily living (ADLs) and personal control of his or her situation to the extent possible significantly support self-esteem.

2. Preventing Deficient Fluid Volume

Risk factors for deficient fluid must be regularly assessed. Weight is measured daily before breakfast with the patient wearing the same clothing, with an empty bladder, and on the same scale. The patient is assessed every 8 hours for signs of deficient fluid: decreased skin turgor, dryness of mucous membranes, postural hypotension, tachycardia, and extremes of specific gravity of urine. Laboratory reports of serum osmolality and sodium levels, and hematocrit should be monitored as available. Fluid intake of 2.5 to 3 L/day is encouraged unless contraindicated; this intake is facilitated by providing fluids of the patient's preference. Parenteral therapy is maintained as ordered. The patient and family are taught about diet and fluid needs and measures to prevent deficient fluid, as appropriate.

Deficient fluid volume is a potential problem in any patient during the postoperative period. However, the patient who has had a transsphenoidal surgery is at higher risk because inadequate release of ADH may cause DI. Diabetes insipidus usually develops within 24 hours and is usually temporary because ADH is produced in the hypothalamus, and adequate amounts can be released even if damage occurs to the posterior pituitary gland. Remissions may occur for up to 2 weeks, followed by a recurrence.

The signs and symptoms are similar to those exhibited by the patient with DI (see Diabetes Insipidus). Intake and output measurements every 4 to 8 hours, specific gravity checks, daily weights, and assessment for reports of thirst help identify the presence of DI. If a deficit in ADH does occur, treatment depends on the severity. Increasing intake of oral fluids sufficiently to satisfy thirst may treat mild deficits. In patients with severe ADH deficits or in those unable to tolerate oral fluids, desmopressin (synthetic vasopressin) is administered.

Before surgery intravenous cortisol administration is initiated. Postoperative ACTH deficiency is a potential problem and can result in severe deficient fluid volume (see Adrenal Cortex Hyposecretion). Cortisol replacement is necessary after surgery to prevent life-threatening adrenal crisis. All patients should be monitored for potential glucocorticoid deficiency and early signs and symptoms of adrenal insufficiency. Monitoring should include assessment of the adequacy of ADH, as well as vital signs every 4 hours and observation of energy level, alertness, appetite, and patient's stated feelings of well-being. If abnormalities in these data are found, serum sodium, potassium, and glucose levels may be obtained. Increased urine output; hypotension while lying down; or orthostatic hypotension, persistent nausea, vomiting, fatigue and tiredness, hyponatremia, hyperkalemia, hypoglycemia, and acidosis indicate inadequate ACTH and glucocorticoid secretion. Hydrocortisone or the equivalent and fluid replacement are provided. If the deficit in ACTH is permanent, the patient will require treatment as discussed later for persons with chronic adrenal insufficiency.

3. Preventing Infection

After transsphenoidal surgery preventing infection and maintaining the integrity of the surgical incision between the upper gum and lip are nursing priorities.

The patient must be assessed for signs of infection during every shift. These include elevated temperature, rhinorrhea, nuchal rigidity, and persistent headache. It is also important to teach the patient the importance and methods of mouth care. Oral incisional care consists of rinsing the mouth with saline or mouthwash and cleansing the teeth with a Toothette or cotton swab. Brushing the teeth and the use of dental floss are forbidden until the suture line heals.

Clear liquids are given as soon as the patient is alert and no longer nauseated from the anesthetic. The diet is advanced as tolerated. Foods that could irritate the mucous membranes and disrupt the suture line must be avoided because of the mouth incision.

Increased intracranial pressure (ICP) can disrupt the incision in the sella turcica and dura. After the tumor is resected, the sella turcica is packed with muscle or fat from the abdomen or thigh. (NOTE: It is important that the patient be prepared for this additional incision.) The floor of the sella turcica is reconstructed with bone or cartilage. This patching, although strong, can be disrupted by increased ICP, which causes pressure on the incisional site. Activities such as bending over, straining, coughing, sneezing, and nose blowing are forbidden. To reduce cerebral edema, the head of the bed should be elevated at least 30 degrees. In most cases, these interventions prevent disruption of the patch and incision.

After surgery the patient's nose is packed for 24 to 48 hours, and a gauze sling is worn under the nose to absorb drainage. CSF leakage occurs if the patching and incision in the sella turcica are disrupted. The professional nurse must monitor for signs and symptoms of such leakage. A CSF leak is indicated by:

- Complaints of postnasal drip, even with the packing in place
- Increased swallowing (observation or patient's report)
- Appearance of a halo ring on the gauze sling (CSF is clear and, when mixed with serous fluid on gauze, forms a halo surrounding the serous drainage.)

Nasal drainage can be differentiated from CSF based on glucose content. Although the nurse can assess the glucose content of nasal drainage with Test-Tape or a dipstick for glucose, fluid should be sent to a laboratory for confirmation. If a CSF leak occurs or is suspected, bed rest with the patient's head elevated is indicated until the leakage is ruled out or stops. Occasionally, patients must return to surgery for repair of the leakage site in the sella turcica.

If a documented CSF leak occurs, the patient is at high risk for infection, including meningitis. Besides restricting the patient's activities to prevent or control a CSF leak, the nurse should monitor the patient for signs of an infection. Monitoring includes temperature checks at least every 4 hours and evaluation for presence of nuchal rigidity. Antibiotics should be administered as prescribed.

4. Facilitating Learning

The first objective of patient education relates to basic preoperative and postoperative teaching and is similar to that for any surgical patient (see Chapter 16). The second objective of perioperative education is to prepare the patient for discharge, to resume self-care, and to assume responsibility for follow-up care. The patient should know when to return to see the endocrinologist (initially in 1 to 4 weeks, depending on postoperative hormone deficits and then every 3 to 6 months pending hormonal stability) and neurosurgeon (initially in 1 to 2 weeks and then in 6 weeks). At the first follow-up visit the patient's hormonal status and general recovery from surgery are assessed. At the other visits, recurrence of the tumor and any newly developing hormonal deficits are assessed.

The third objective of patient education is to prepare the patient to manage any hormonal deficiencies that have occurred. If ADH, ACTH, or glucocorticoid deficiency occurred after surgery, diagnostic tests are done before the patient leaves the hospital to identify whether the deficiencies are permanent. If they are permanent, the patient needs the same education required by any patient with diabetes insipidus (for ADH deficiency) or adrenocortical insufficiency (for ACTH deficiency) (see discussions later in this chapter).

If a deficiency of ACTH and glucocorticoid occurs, secretion of other hormones such as TSH or gonadotropins from the anterior pituitary gland may also be deficient. Adequacy of anterior pituitary secretion of these hormones is assessed before discharge and at return visits. Diagnostic tests to evaluate hormonal status are performed 4 to 6 weeks after surgery if no hormonal deficiencies develop.

The final objective of patient education is to reinforce care needs related to irreversible changes in body appearance, joint and back pain, and visual problems. Information shared may include ways to minimize body changes with makeup and clothes, frequent showers to help control increased sweating and oily skin, pain management techniques, modification of activities to decrease stress and strain on the joints and back, and referral to a society to aid the visually impaired.

Postoperative routines include management of incisional discomfort and headache and prevention of postoperative complications. After surgery, because of the caution against coughing and the nasal packing necessitating mouth breathing, patients are at some risk for ineffective gas exchange. Patients should be instructed about mouth breathing and deep breathing exercises before surgery, have an opportunity for practice and a return demonstration, and then be monitored for compliance with deep breathing exercises at least every 2 hours for the first 1 to 3 postoperative days. Assessment of vital signs and breath sounds every 4 to 8 hours helps identify any impairment of air exchange. Maintenance of adequate fluid intake helps prevent drying of mucus secretions and the formation of mucous plugs.

Persistent headaches may indicate meningitis and should be reported to the physician immediately. A firm mattress, range of motion exercises, back massage, frequent ambulation, and heat may be used to help decrease back and joint discomfort in persons with GH-secreting tumors. Early ambulation helps to prevent deterioration in mobility and joint movement. The patient's postoperative vision and visual fields should be monitored for changes. Rearranging the room so that necessary articles are placed in line with intact vision may be necessary. Although additional visual compromise after transsphenoidal resection is rare, the visual pathway can be damaged during surgery or as a result of hemorrhage.

Patient/Family Education

Patients with pituitary hypersecretion may exhibit high anxiety levels in response to the body changes induced by neurologic or endocrine alterations and uncertainty about diagnosis, treatment method, and effects of treatment. Particular stressors may include visual loss, infertility, sexual dysfunction, or immobility. Although some patients in whom neurologic symptoms are diagnosed require immediate surgical treatment, most patients have a diagnostic workup in the outpatient setting and time to learn about their illness and its implications. The professional nurse can help the patient reduce stress by attending to the emotional impact of the illness. The major need of the patient at this stage of the illness is education. The patient and significant others need to know:

- The relationship of the patient's symptoms to a pituitary tumor and hormone excess.
- Definition of a *tumor.* Many individuals assume that tumor means cancer. These tumors are usually not malignant.
- Planned diagnostic tests, which include skull x-ray, computed tomography (CT) or MRI, visual assessment.
- Available treatment for the tumor. On the basis of signs and symptoms, the physician has a high index of suspicion for the type of tumor and potential treatment. This information is initially provided by the physician and later reinforced by the professional nurse.
- Dietary instruction about prescribed changes as needed, and methods to meet dietary requirements.
- Medication therapy: hormonal agents used as replacement therapy.
- Step-by-step instruction on performing a subcutaneous injection if prescribed; the nurse should provide teaching and multiple opportunities for practice and return demonstration.
- Expected outcomes from the treatment, including reversibility or irreversibility of signs and symptoms.
- The importance of follow-up care. The nurse should clarify the plans for follow-up care.

Knowledge helps the patient cope with physiologic changes and should help to relieve uncertainty and decrease anxiety. Usually this education is done in an outpatient setting. The use of a model of a brain during the educational process will help the patient better understand the pathology and treatment of his or her illness. Written material should be provided as reinforcement. A telephone contact number for the physician and professional nurse should be provided in case the patient has additional questions.

EVALUATION

To evaluate the effectiveness of nursing interventions, compare patient behaviors with those stated in the expected patient outcomes. Achievement of outcomes is successful if the patient with hypersecretion of the anterior pituitary gland associated with pituitary tumor:

1. Comments positively about self-attributes, body characteristics and changes, abilities, and participation in activities to regain optimal functioning.
2. Demonstrates fluid balance as evidenced by:
2a. Maintains baseline weight.
2b. Demonstrates elastic skin turgor and moist mucous membranes.
2c. Has blood pressure and pulse within normal range.
2d. Has serum electrolytes and hematocrit within normal limits.

2e. Has urine specific gravity between 1.010 and 1.025.
2f. Achieves fluid intake of 2.5 to 3 L/day, unless restrictions are necessary.
2g. Verbalizes measures to prevent fluid deficit.
3. Is free from infection.
4. Patient and family/significant other verbalize knowledge of disease process, effects on bodily functioning, treatment and expected outcomes, surgical intervention (if indicated) and perioperative routines, and plan for follow-up care.

SPECIAL ENVIRONMENTS FOR CARE

Critical Care

The patient with a hypersecretory state of the pituitary gland requires critical care nursing only in the case of complications. If transsphenoidal resection of the tumor resulted in development of meningitis or increased ICP, monitoring of the patient's ICP and overall status in an intensive care unit would be necessary. If the tumor required resection by craniotomy, the patient would be routinely admitted to a critical care unit after surgery and then transferred to a regular nursing floor when his or her condition stabilizes (see Chapter 42).

Community-Based Care

If significant neurologic deficits develop as a result of tumor growth or surgical intervention, the patient may be transferred to a subacute unit or rehabilitation facility after discharge. Arthritic changes occur in the patient with long-standing acromegaly, and adaptations may need to be made to the home environment. A home health aide may be helpful on a temporary basis to assist with ADLs. Assistance may be needed in administration of medications, particularly if the patient has any visual deficits. Ensuring safety is a priority, especially if the patient has limitations in musculoskeletal functioning or neurologic deficits. The home environment should be assessed for potential safety hazards. In addition, the patient must have access to the physician or other health care provider for routing monitoring of hormonal levels.

COMPLICATIONS

Common complications of pituitary tumors and their management have been discussed previously and are summarized in Box 29-2. In addition, pituitary apoplexy or other types of pituitary hemorrhage can occur (see Hypopituitarism).

BOX 29-2 Complications of Pituitary Tumors

Neurologic

Compression of optic chiasm and/or other brain tissue; visual loss
After surgery: CSF leak, meningitis, increased ICP, neurologic deficit, visual impairment
Pituitary apoplexy
Increased ICP

Endocrine

Syndromes of excess hormone: acromegaly, Cushing's syndrome; suppression of gonadotropic hormones; infertility and/or sexual dysfunction
Iatrogenic syndromes of hormonal deficit: diabetes insipidus, adrenal insufficiency, hypopituitarism (deficit in one or more anterior pituitary hormones: ACTH, TSH, GH, or gonadotropin)
Recurrence of pituitary tumor

ACTH, Adrenocorticotropic hormone; *CSF,* cerebrospinal fluid; *GH,* growth hormone; *ICP,* intracranial pressure; *TSH,* thyroid-stimulating hormone.

Hyposecretion: Hypopituitarism

Hypopituitarism, or hyposecretion of the pituitary gland, may be congenital or related to tumor, infarction, autoimmune dysfunction, infection (bacterial or viral), or trauma (surgery or radiation).

Etiology/Epidemiology

The causes of hypopituitarism are summarized in Box 29-3. The spectrum can extend from missing all of the trophic hormones—*panhypopituitarism*—to isolated hormone deficiency. In some instances, the hypopituitarism may be reversible, such as occurs when a macroadenoma that had been compressing the normal pituitary is removed. Acute loss of anterior pituitary function is generally vascular with acute infarction of a pituitary tumor and ischemic damage to the surrounding normal pituitary gland (pituitary apoplexy) or simply an ischemic infarction of the pituitary as seen in Sheehan's syndrome (postpartum pituitary necrosis).

BOX 29-3 Causes of Hypopituitarism

Tumors: craniopharyngioma, primary central nervous system tumors, nonsecreting pituitary tumors
Ischemic changes: Sheehan's syndrome (ischemic changes following postpartum hemorrhage or infection resulting in shock)
Developmental abnormalities
Infections: viral encephalitis, bacteremia, tuberculosis
Autoimmune disorders
Radiation damage, particularly after treatment of secreting adenomas of pituitary gland
Trauma, including surgery

Sequelae of hypopituitarism related to individual hormonal deficiencies are outlined in Figure 29-4. The incidence of hypopituitarism is unknown.

Pathophysiology

Symptoms of hypopituitarism vary widely, depending on the cause and the endocrine dysfunction present (see Clinical Manifestations box). If a tumor is present, the patient may exhibit some of the symptoms previously described. If the tumor arises from regions surrounding the pituitary, such as the third ventricle or hypothalamus, the neurologic signs and symptoms are more severe and include manifestations of increased ICP (see Chapter 42).

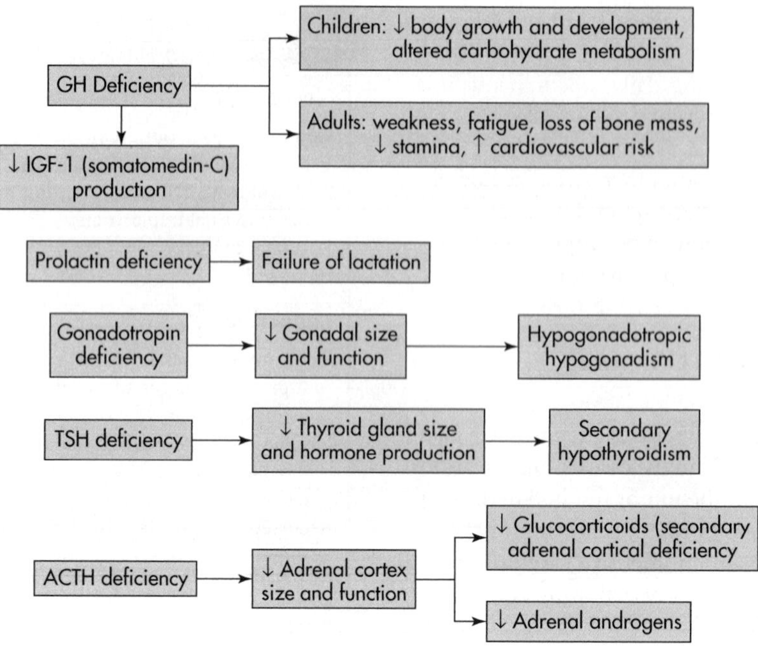

Figure 29-4 Sequelae of individual anterior pituitary hormone deficiency. *ACTH,* Adrenocorticotropic hormone; *GH,* growth hormone; *IGF,* insulin-like growth factor; *TSH,* thyroid-stimulating hormone.

Clinical Manifestations

Hypopituitarism

1. Manifestations based on cause, such as bacteremia, viral hepatitis, autoimmune disorders, and trauma
2. Manifestations such as vision changes, papilledema, or hydrocephalus if cause is tumor
3. Manifestations of gonadotropin deficiency
   a. Decreased serum levels of FSH, LH, and gonadal steroids
   b. Children-delayed puberty
   c. Adults
      (1) Women—oligomenorrhea or amenorrhea, uterine and vaginal atrophy, potential atrophy of breast tissue, loss of libido, decrease in body hair
      (2) Men—loss of libido, decreased sperm count, possible erectile dysfunction, decreased testicular size, decreased total body hair
4. Manifestations of GH deficiency
   a. Children
      (1) Stunted growth (below third percentile) with normal body proportions, excessive subcutaneous fat, poor muscle development
      (2) Immature facial features, immature voice
      (3) Slow growth of nails and thin hair
      (4) Delayed puberty but eventual normal sexual development
      (5) Decreased levels of GH
   b. Adults
      (1) Severe, short stature
      (2) Immature facies
      (3) Moderate obesity
      (4) Decreased muscle mass and weakness
      (5) Lassitude
      (6) Emotional lability
      (7) Decreased basal levels of GH or decreased response to provocative testing
      (8) Some persons may have normal GH levels with low level of somatomedins (IGF-I)
5. Manifestations of prolactin deficiency
   a. Failure to lactate in the postpartum woman
   b. Decreased serum levels of prolactin
6. Manifestations of TSH deficiency
   a. Signs and symptoms of secondary hypothyroidism
   b. Decreased serum level of TSH and thyroid hormone
7. Manifestations of ACTH deficiency
   a. Signs and symptoms of secondary ACTH insufficiency; *no hyperpigmentation*
   b. Decreased serum levels of ACTH, glucocorticoids, and adrenal androgens (aldosterone levels may be normal)

ACTH, Adrenocorticotropic hormone; *FSH,* follicle-stimulating hormone; *GH,* growth hormone; *LH,* luteinizing hormone; *TSH,* thyroid-stimulating hormone.

Endocrine dysfunction may be a result of hypothalamic damage or primary pituitary disease. The most frequent pathophysiologic change results from lack of synthesis and secretion of gonadotropins.

Collaborative Care Management

Medical management is focused on identifying patients with deficiency syndromes, treating the underlying problem, and supplying the appropriate hormonal replacement. Failure to provide appropriate hormonal replacement therapy results in increased mortality.[35] The target gland hormone (thyroid, cortisol, or gonadal steroids) is replaced as necessary. If a woman of childbearing age desires fertility, gonadotropins must be replaced. However, prolactin does not need to be replaced.

Growth Hormone Deficiency. Isolated GH deficiency is generally seen only in childhood and responds to GH therapy; GH deficiency in adults is usually part of panhypopituitarism.

Replacing GH in adults requires daily subcutaneous injections starting at a dose of 0.006 mg/kg of actual body weight/day and titrating upward to yield an IGF-1 level in the upper half of the normal range. Anticipated patient outcomes include increased general well-being, physical endurance, and improvement in body composition and bone mineral density. The use of GH outside of these scenarios is experimental. The high cost of GH therapy may be prohibitive for some, although most of the manufacturers do have compassionate need programs.

Thyroid-Stimulating Hormone Deficiency. Isolated TSH deficiency is uncommon and is generally part of panhypopituitarism; therefore, concurrent cortisol deficiency is to be anticipated and its replacement mandatory. TSH itself is not available for replacement therapy; therefore a thyroid hormone preparation is used. Replacement of thyroxine is similar to that for the primary hypothyroid patient. Thyroid hormone replacement accelerates the metabolism of glucocorticoids such that failure to replace glucocorticoids concurrently can precipitate an acute adrenal crisis. Monitoring of thyroxine levels, generally with the free T_4 blood test, is done on a regular basis as an evaluation of therapy. Because thyroxine is converted to triiodothyronine (T_3) in the periphery, circulating T_3 levels may also be monitored.

Adrenocorticotropic Hormone Deficiency. Glucocorticoid deficiency is replaced with hydrocortisone or one of the more potent synthetic analogs. Cortisone, prednisolone, and prednisone are also used for therapy. Replacement dose of hydrocortisone varies considerably, but averages 25 mg/day in divided doses. Because the normal diurnal secretion of cortisol peaks in the early morning, two thirds of the dose is generally given in the morning and one third at night. Side effects of therapy are similar to those of Cushing's syndrome.

Because cortisol is a primary stress hormone, it is imperative to augment these physiologic doses when the patient is ill, injured, or undergoing anesthesia and surgery. For mild stress, such as a viral illness, the dose should be doubled or tripled. With more severe stress, such as surgery, threefold to fivefold increments should be administered. The patient should be instructed to wear a Medic-Alert bracelet that states a need for hydrocortisone for emergency use (50 to 100 mg intravenously or intramuscularly). Intravenous hydrocortisone should be continued at doses of 50 to 100 mg every 6 hours until the acute condition resolves.

Gonadotropin Deficiency. Gonadotropin deficiency results in secondary hypogonadism, with estrogen deficiency and amenorrhea in women and erectile dysfunction and infertility in men. Testosterone and estrogen replacement is similar to that used in primary gonadal failure. Testosterone deficiency in men can lead to osteoporosis and therefore should be considered in elderly men even if sexual function is not a priority with the patient.

In the absence of pituitary destruction, the majority of patients with gonadotropin deficiency have hypothalamic gonadotropin-releasing hormone (GnRH) deficiency. Replacement of GnRH in a pulsatile fashion with a subcutaneous infusion pump can restore fertility as well as estrogen/androgen production.

Prolactin Deficiency. Failure of lactation in the postpartum woman is a useful clinical clue to PRL deficiency. There is no PRL replacement preparation available for clinical use, and there does not appear to be any long-term adverse sequelae from chronic PRL deficiency apart from the lactation issue.

Patient/Family Education. Nursing care focuses on assisting the patient to effectively cope with changes in body image and teaching about treatment protocols. Helping patients identify their strengths and coping strategies may help them deal with the disturbances in body image and self-esteem that may result from their illness.

Some symptoms are reversible once treatment is initiated. Treatment with sex steroids helps to initiate development of sexual characteristics in the adolescent entering puberty and restores secondary sexual characteristics in adults. Treatment with gonadotropins restores fertility in the woman with normal menstrual cycles.

Patient education is an important focus of care. The patient must be prepared for various diagnostic tests, including blood tests, and radiologic procedures such as CT scans or MRI. Hormone replacement therapy must be individualized and patients instructed about prescribed medications. Growth hormone therapy is administered via subcutaneous injections. The patient must learn proper self-injection technique. Patients should be taught that gonadal steroids are effective in preventing premature decrease in bone mass. Patients who decline sex hormone therapy, particularly women, need to be monitored periodically for the development of osteopenia or osteoporosis, must take adequate calcium, and should be offered other pharmacotherapy if osteopenia or osteoporosis develops.

POSTERIOR PITUITARY DYSFUNCTION

Diseases of the posterior pituitary may result in excess secretion as in syndrome of inappropriate antidiuretic hormone (SIADH) or undersecretion with resultant central diabetes insipidus.

Hypersecretion of Antidiuretic Hormone: Syndrome of Inappropriate Antidiuretic Hormone

Etiology/Epidemiology

Causes of SIADH are summarized in Box 29-4. The most common causes are small cell carcinoma of the lung (80% of cases) and medications, especially the sulfonylurea chlorpropamide.

Pathophysiology

Inappropriate free water retention for the volume status of an individual results in a hypoosmolar state with a dilutional hyponatremia. Despite the expansion in intracellular volume, edema is not present; this volume expansion causes enhanced glomerular filtration and decreased proximal tubular sodium reabsorption resulting in *natriuresis* (urinary sodium excretion). These features contrast with the volume overload of congestive heart failure and cirrhosis and the hyponatremia seen in Addison's disease. The hypoosmolality of the plasma

BOX 29-4 Etiologic Factors Associated With SIADH

Pulmonary disorders: malignant neoplasms (e.g., oat cell adenocarcinoma of lung), tuberculosis, ventilator patients receiving positive pressure, lung abscesses
Other malignancies: duodenum, pancreas, prostate lymphoma, sarcoma, leukemia, Hodgkin's lymphoma, non-Hodgkin's lymphoma
CNS disorders: tumors, infection, trauma, cerebrovascular accident, surgery
Drugs such as clofibrate, chlorpropamide, thiazides, vincristine, cyclophosphamide, general anesthetic agents, opioids, tricyclic antidepressants, carbamazepine
Stressors: fear, acute infections, pain, anxiety, trauma, surgery

CNS, Central nervous system; *SIADH,* syndrome of inappropriate antidiuretic hormone.

Clinical Manifestations

Syndrome of Antidiuretic Hormone

EARLY SIGNS/SYMPTOMS

Anorexia	Mild disorientation
Nausea	Malaise
Vomiting	Anger
Weight gain	Anxiety
Muscle weakness	Uncooperativeness
Irritability	

LATE SIGNS/SYMPTOMS

Lethargy	Coma
Headache	Seizures
Decreased deep tendon reflexes	

FLUID AND ELECTROLYTE CHANGES

Decreased plasma sodium and plasma osmolality
Increased urinary sodium and urinary osmolality
Decreased urinary volume
Absence of edema
Low normal/subnormal uric acid levels

creates an osmotic gradient across the cell membranes (including the blood-brain barrier) with resultant flow of water into all cells.

Severity of the clinical symptoms depends on the absolute serum sodium level and the rapidity of its fall (see Clinical Manifestations box). A rapid fall in serum sodium levels can result in rapid-onset cerebral edema and death, whereas a gradual fall over several weeks may result only in lethargy.

In general, the following serum sodium levels may be correlated with patient symptoms:

- Serum sodium level ≤125 mEq/L: nausea and malaise
- Serum sodium level 115 to 120 mEq/L: headache, lethargy, obtundation
- Serum sodium level 110 to 114 mEq/L: seizures and coma

Collaborative Care Management

Medical management of acute SIADH focuses on treating the etiologic factor (e.g., carcinoma or infection) and correcting, or at least restoring toward normal, the plasma sodium level and plasma osmolality. Water restriction is the first priority of management. Water may be restricted to as little as 500 ml/day. Oral salt intake is increased if the patient is able to take oral nutrients.

Chronic SIADH and hyponatremia are first treated with water restriction. If water restriction alone cannot prevent hypoosmolality, pharmacologic treatment is added. Demeclocycline, a tetracycline derivative, blocks the action of ADH on the renal tubule and collecting duct cells and decreases urine osmolality. Lithium carbonate and phenytoin have also been used to treat SIADH.

If the patient's plasma sodium level is less than 120 mEq/L and the patient is exhibiting central nervous system manifestations such as nausea, vomiting, lethargy, and headaches, more rapid correction of the low plasma sodium level is necessary. This severe hyponatremia is treated with hypertonic saline (3% sodium chloride) and a loop diuretic such as furosemide (Lasix) or ethacrynic acid. The goal of this therapy is not to return the plasma sodium level to normal but to increase it to 125 to 130 mEq/L or to administer enough sodium chloride to relieve symptoms or increase the plasma sodium by 25 mEq/L. This correction needs to be made cautiously because of potential complications from either too rapid or too slow correction.

Too rapid an increase in the plasma sodium level can produce a hypertonic plasma solution and a fluid shift from the intracellular to the extracellular compartment. A rapid fluid shift can result in central pontine myelinolysis, which is demyelination of the pons. This demyelination results in dysfunction of the nerve tracts that travel through or originate in the pons, causing bulbar palsies, quadriplegia, coma, and death. During treatment with hypertonic saline or loop diuretics, plasma osmolality and serum sodium are monitored every 2 to 4 hours. Note that 3% sodium chloride is used for sodium replacement, not for volume replacement.

Nursing care associated with SIADH includes identifying persons at risk and monitoring neurologic and fluid volume status. For high-risk patients, daily weights, intake and output, daily serum and urinary sodium levels and osmolality, vital signs, and neurologic status are monitored. Any decrease below normal in serum sodium, any signs of fluid retention (increased weight or decreased output), and any neurologic changes (complaints of headaches or nausea or decreased level of consciousness) must be reported. If the serum sodium level is below 125 mEq/L, laboratory results need to be reported immediately.

For patients with diagnosed SIADH being treated aggressively with hypertonic sodium or loop diuretics, the frequency of monitoring is increased to every 1 to 2 hours. Any deterioration in neurologic status is reported immediately.

For patients with chronic SIADH, weights are monitored daily to weekly and any increases not attributed to dietary changes or any reports of nausea, headache, or lethargy reported. Monitoring by the nurse in the outpatient department is the same as that described for high-risk patients.

The nurse should explain the rationale for fluid restrictions and methods to relieve discomfort from thirst. Fluid intake should be spaced throughout the 24-hour period. Ice chips should be encouraged to allow more frequent relief of thirst with less fluid intake. Mouth care should be provided frequently.

Patient/Family Education. Patient and family teaching should focus on the purpose and management of fluid restriction. The need for self-monitoring on a long-term basis must be stressed. Accurate measurement of intake and output and of weight change should be taught. In addition, information about drug therapy should be provided as needed.

Diuretics may be used long term, and a high-sodium diet may be continued. In some patients salt tablets are used with diuretics to replace urinary sodium losses and prevent volume depletion.

Clinical Manifestations

Diabetes Insipidus

1. Polyuria: as much as 20 L of urine/day may be excreted; urine is dilute, with a specific gravity of 1.005 or less or an osmolality of 200 or less
2. Polydipsia secondary to increased thirst
3. Only slightly elevated serum osmolality because water intake is usually maintained
4. Abnormal results of tests for urine concentration
   a. Water deprivation test (see Chapter 28): no increase in urine concentration with either pituitary or nephrogenic DI
   b. Antidiuretic hormone replacement: increase in urine osmolality with pituitary DI but no response with nephrogenic DI
5. Sleep disturbance from polyuria
6. Inadequate water replacement results in:
   a. Hyperosmolality: irritability, mental dullness, coma, hyperthermia
   b. Hypovolemia: hypotension, tachycardia, dry mucous membranes, poor skin turgor

Hyposecretion of Antidiuretic Hormone: Diabetes Insipidus

Etiology/Epidemiology

The etiology of DI may be either central (loss of production of ADH) or nephrogenic (lack of a renal response to ADH). The following discussion focuses on central DI, the endocrine cause of DI. Central DI may be transient (such as occurs after transsphenoidal surgery for anterior pituitary adenomas) or may be permanent. The permanent causes of central DI include sarcoidosis, posterior hypophysectomy, pituitary tumors, head trauma, encephalitis, and meningitis. In many instances no underlying causes is found such that many cases are labeled idiopathic.[29]

Pathophysiology

The lack of adequate ADH results in inadequate water resorption in the kidneys. The resulting loss of excessive water from the body (polyuria) produces dehydration and an increase in serum osmolality that stimulates thirst and polydipsia (see Clinical Manifestations box). Patients characteristically crave cold liquids and must drink copious amounts of liquids during the day and night to maintain some semblance of fluid balance. The amount needed varies depending on the severity of the deficiency of ADH. Long-standing DI can result in increased bladder capacity and hydronephrosis. When inadequate water replacement occurs, central nervous system and vascular changes from hyperosmolality and volume depletion can result.

Collaborative Care Management

The person with pituitary DI is treated with vasopressin replacement (Table 29-1). Vasopressin synthetic analog (Desmopressin or DDAVP) is the agent used to treat DI rather than vasopressin itself. Both DDAVP and vasopressin bind to the V2 receptors in the renal tubule. However, vasopressin also binds to the V1 receptors found in smooth muscle of arterioles and other tissues and causes pressor side effects of exogenous ADH (abdominal cramping, hypertension, and angina). In addition, DDAVP is much more potent in its antidiuretic effect and has a longer duration of action. For persons who have some residual pituitary function, chlorpropamide and clofibrate, which stimulate release of endogenous ADH, may be prescribed.[30]

Temporary DI associated with head trauma or surgery is treated with parenteral DDAVP. After transsphenoidal surgery, nasal packing and edematous nasal mucosa preclude using the nasal route for medications. The most common treatment for persons with nephrogenic DI is a low-sodium, low-protein diet and thiazide diuretics. The low-sodium diet and thiazide diuretics induce mild volume depletion. This volume depletion enhances sodium chloride and water reabsorption in the proximal part of the kidney tubule, resulting in less water being delivered to the collecting tubules where ADH should be; therefore, less water is excreted. The diuretic also increases the osmolality of the medullary interstitial space and thus promotes more water resorption in collecting tubules that are less permeable because of inadequate ADH. Protein restriction helps control water loss by decreasing solute excretion. Nephrogenic DI can also be treated by administration of nonsteroidal antiinflammatory agents, which impair prostaglandin production in the kidney and increase urinary concentrating ability.

For patients with clinical evidence of hypernatremia such as mental status changes and hyperthermia, replacement of water must be instituted. Fluid replacement is calculated by estimating the patient's water deficit and adding the insensible water loss and urinary loss. Fluid replacement must be done carefully over 48 hours to avoid cerebral edema, seizures, or even death. Too rapid correction of hypernatremia by fluid administration may result in the establishment of an osmotic

TABLE 29-1 Common Preparations of Desmopressin (DDAVP) Used for Treatment of Diabetes Insipidus

Medication	Dosage	Route of Administration
DDAVP nasal spray	10-40 μg/day administered in 1-3 doses/day	Intranasal
DDAVP tablets	Initial dose: 0.05 mg bid Optimal dose: 0.05-0.6 mg bid	Orally
DDAVP parenteral solution	1-2 μg bid	Subcutaneously

gradient, with plasma osmolality being less than intracellular osmolality and the entry of water into the brain. The exact fluid administered varies depending on the patient's needs.

Nursing interventions for the person with DI focus on maintaining fluid and electrolyte balance. Intake and output, daily weights, urine specific gravity, vital signs (orthostatic), skin turgor, and neurologic status are monitored every 1 to 2 hours during the acute phase, then every 4 to 8 hours until discharge, and again on return to physician or outpatient clinic.

Adequate fluid intake is provided. Because nocturia may disrupt sleep cycles, adequate rest periods during the day are also provided.

Patient/Family Education. Patient and family teaching should include information about diagnostic tests including their purposes, procedures, and required monitoring (see Chapter 28). Also important is teaching about the dosage, route, and frequency of prescribed medications. The patient must be taught that if nasal congestion occurs, drug effectiveness may decrease, and polyuria and thirst will occur. The need to observe for signs of volume excess (weight gain, edema) must also be stressed.

Research

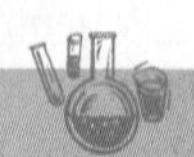

Reference: Auer J et al: Subclinical hyperthyroidism as a risk factor for atrial fibrillation. *Am Heart J* 142:838, 2001.

Atrial fibrillation is a well-known clinical manifestation of hyperthyroidism. The objective of this study was to determine whether subclinical hyperthyroidism increases the risk of atrial fibrillation. The authors studied 23,638 individuals and classified them according to their thyroid-stimulating hormone concentration. Group 1 consisted of individuals with normal thyroid function; group 2 consisted of individuals with hyperthyroidism; and group 3 consisted of individuals with subclinical hyperthyroidism. Rates of atrial fibrillation were: group 1 (euthyroidism), 2.3%; group 2 (hyperthyroidism), 13,8%; and group 3 (subclinical hyperthyroidism), 12.7%. The relative risk of atrial fibrillation in group 3 (subclinical hyperthyroidism) versus group 1 (euthyroidism) was 5.2: having subclinical hyperthyroidism increased the relative risk of atrial fibrillation by more than fivefold. There was no significant difference between the rates of atrial fibrillation in the hyperthyroid versus subclinical hyperthyroid groups. Implications include the importance of treating patients with subclinical hyperthyroidism to decrease the risk of atrial fibrillation with its inherent risks of cerebrovascular and pulmonary embolic events.

THYROID DISORDERS

Thyroid disease is relatively common, with a gender predisposition to females. Diseases of the thyroid may result in hypersecretion, hyposecretion, or simply thyroid enlargement (goiter). A goiter refers to any enlargement of the thyroid and does not indicate any particular pathologic process.

HYPERSECRETION: HYPERTHYROIDISM

Hyperthyroidism refers to elevated serum thyroid hormone levels and may be due to several causes. *Thyrotoxicosis* refers to the toxic effects/manifestations of excess thyroid hormone. The mildest form of hyperthyroidism is subclinical hyperthyroidism, which is generally devoid of symptoms and is characterized by normal free T_4 and free T_3 levels with a suppressed TSH. In addition to being a precursor of overt hyperthyroidism, thyrotoxicosis has been associated with a fivefold increased risk of atrial fibrillation in elderly individuals[2] (see Research box).

Etiology

The causes of hyperthyroidism are summarized in Table 29-2. Drug-induced hyperthyroidism is now more common, especially with the more widespread use of the antiarrhythmic agent amiodarone.[9,20,22]

Graves' disease is the most common cause of hyperthyroidism, accounting for more than 60% of all cases. In addition to the symptoms and signs of hyperthyroidism, Graves' disease is characterized by a smooth diffuse goiter, variable degrees of ophthalmopathy, and occasionally an infiltrative dermopathy. Graves' disease has an autoimmune basis and is seen more commonly in patients with other autoimmune diseases such as type I diabetes mellitus, systemic lupus erythematosus, rheumatoid arthritis, pernicious anemia, and/or Addisons' disease.

Toxic multinodular goiter, or Plummers's disease, does not have an autoimmune basis and is generally seen in patients over 50 years old. These patients generally have had longstanding progressively enlarging goiters. Solitary toxic nodules or hot nodules can also cause hyperthyroidism and selective overproduction of T_3. Solitary toxic nodules are essentially always benign.

Epidemiology

The incidence of hyperthyroidism in adults is estimated at 0.02% to 0.06%. Graves' disease, like other autoimmune disease, is more common in women. There is some familial predisposition to autoimmune thyroid disease.

TABLE 29-2 Etiology of Hyperthyroidism

Classification	Etiology
Graves' disease	Autoimmune; genetic component
Toxic multinodular goiter	Autonomous function of thyroid; multiple nodules
Toxic solitary adenoma	Single adenoma of follicular cells that secretes and functions independent of thyroid-secreting hormone (TSH) May selectively hypersecrete T_3 resulting in T_3 toxicosis
Hyperthyroidism caused by metastatic thyroid cancer	Rare; thyroid cancer cells do not usually concentrate iodine efficiently; may occur with large follicular carcinomas
TSH-secreting pituitary adenoma	A rare form of pituitary adenoma; treatment involves surgical removal
Chorionic hyperthyroidism	Chorionic gonadotropin has weak thyrotropin activity. Tumors such as choriocarcioma, embryonal cell carcinoma, and hydatidiform mole have high concentrations of chorionic gonadotropins that can stimulate T_4 and T_3 secretion; hyperthyroidism resolves with treatment of the tumor
Struma ovarii	Ovarian dermoid tumor made up partly of thyroid tissue that secretes thyroid hormone

BOX 29-5 Hyperthyroidism: Pathophysiologic Alterations and Clinical Manifestations

Increased metabolic rate, heat production and oxygen consumption due to the overall increase in metabolism

Common signs and symptoms include:

- Heat intolerance
- Increased body temperature
- Warm, moist skin
- Increased appetite
- Weight loss
- Muscle fatigue

Alteration in Protein, Fat, and Carbohydrate Metabolism

The entire cycle of synthesis, degradation, and clearance is accelerated. Because of the increased lipolysis and increased lipid metabolism, especially lipid degradation, serum cholesterol and triglyceride levels may decline. The patient with preexisting diabetes mellitus may experience rising blood glucose levels due to increased glycogenolysis, increased intestinal glucose absorption, and increased insulin degradation.

Alteration in Cardiovascular Function

The hypermetabolic state coupled with increased sensitivity to catecholamines increases myocardial oxygen consumption, shortens the systolic interval, and increases cardiac output. Signs and symptoms include tachycardia, palpitations, elevated blood pressure, atrial fibrillation, angina, dyspnea, and/or high output congestive heart failure.

Alteration in Central Nervous System Function

Thyroid hormone synergizes with other centrally acting hormones and neurotransmitters and this is accelerated in hyperthyroidism. Signs and symptoms may include nervousness, anxiety, restlessness, decreased attention span, insomnia, emotional lability, and fine rhythmic tremors of the hands, tongue, and eyelids.

Alteration in Reproductive Function

Secretion and metabolism of gonadotropins and gonadal steroids are altered. Signs and symptoms include delayed sexual development in the prepubertal patient and increased libido, decreased fertility, and altered menses in the postpubertal patient.

Alteration in Calcium and Phosphorus Balance

Thyroid hormone excess increases the mobilization of calcium from bone and the urinary excretion of calcium and phosphorus. Bone mass may decline and proximal muscle weakness may occur.

Alteration in Gastrointestinal Function

Increased motility of the gastrointestinal tract may lead to increased frequency of bowel movements.

Pathophysiology

Hypermetabolism. Hyperthyroidism results from autonomous production of thyroid hormone, independent of TSH from the pituitary gland. The first hormonal sign of emerging hyperthyroidism is therefore a suppressed TSH. The hyperthyroidism of Graves' disease results from an immunoglobulin that stimulates the TSH receptor on the thyroid gland, resulting in hypertrophy of the gland and overproduction of thyroid hormone. This immunoglobulin, thyroid-stimulating immunoglobulin (TSI) can be measured in the patient's serum as a marker of Graves' disease activity.[41]

Toxic solitary nodules and multinodular goiters are benign tumors autonomously overproducing thyroid hormone. The exact underlying cause of these entities is unknown.

Excess thyroid hormone in the circulation increases metabolic rate, increases activity of the sympathetic nervous system, and affects fat and carbohydrate metabolism (Box 29-5). The degree of thyroid hormone excess correlates fairly well with the clinical picture.

Severely toxic patients can have high output congestive heart failure, cardiac arrhythmias, and even thyroid storm, which is life threatening. Patients generally exhibit multiple manifestations of hyperthyroidism rather than a solitary sign or symptom. An exception would be atrial fibrillation in older adults as the sole manifestation of hyperthyroidism

Graves' Ophthalmopathy. Ophthalmopathy may have an infiltrative or noninfiltrative cause. Both types of ophthalmopathy may be present in a given patient (Box 29-6). In

BOX 29-6 Ophthalmopathy in Graves' Disease

Signs

Bright-eyed stare: results from retraction of upper eyelid
Lid lag: on downward gaze, upper lid lags behind globe movement, and sclera seen between lid and limbus
Globe lag: globe lags behind lid with upward gaze
Lid movement: jerky and spasmodic
Lid closure can be problematic when significant proptosis exists
Periorbital edema

Symptoms

Sense of irritation and excessive tearing
Feeling of pressure behind eyes
Complaints of blurred vision or diplopia, easy tiring of eyes

Complications

Corneal ulceration
Optic nerve involvement (optic neuropathy)
Myopathy of extraocular muscles

infiltrative ophthalmopathy, the retrobulbar connective tissue and extraocular muscle volume are expanded. This volume expansion occurs because of fluid retention resulting from the accumulation of glycosaminoglycans. The increase in tissue mass forces the eye forward *(proptosis)* up to the limits of the restraining action of the extraocular muscles *(exophthalmos)* (Figure 29-5). The pressure in the retrobulbar space increases because of the increased tissue and limited forward movement, causing periorbital and lid edema and pressure on the optic nerve. The stretched enlarged extraocular muscles do not function well and commonly result in diplopia.

Noninfiltrative changes occur as a result of the thyrotoxicosis and usually resolve when the hyperthyroidism is treated. These changes, including lid retraction and lid lag, are due to sympathetic nervous system overstimulation resulting in contraction of the eyelid levator muscle.

Glycosaminoglycans and fluid accumulation also occur in the connective tissue in other parts of the body. This accumulation is particularly seen in the pretibial area a condition called pretibial myxedema.

The risk of ophthalmopathy may be increased in cigarette smokers.[5,16] Patients with Graves' disease who have significant preexisting ophthalmopathy may be at risk for exacerbation of their ophthalmopathy by radioiodine (RAI) therapy. For this reason some endocrinologists prefer to treat such a patient with antithyroid drug therapy rather than RAI.[4]

Collaborative Care Management

The choice of therapy is individualized based on the age, sex, reproductive status, and cause and severity of hyperthyroidism. The most toxic patients are treated with antithyroid drugs initially and thereafter a decision is made to pursue RAI therapy or ongoing antithyroid drug therapy. The potential for permanent remission with antithyroid drugs exists only for patients with Graves' disease.

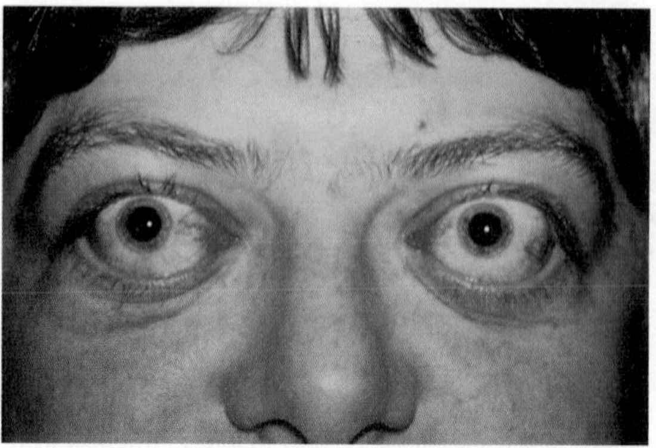

Figure 29-5 Classic Graves' ophthalmopathy.

Diagnostic Tests. After completion of a comprehensive history and physical examination, a TSH level should be the initial test ordered; TSH will be suppressed in all cases of hyperthyroidism. A free T_4 level confirms the magnitude of the hyperthyroidism. Triiodothyronine (T_3) levels may be ordered if T_3 toxicosis is suspected (solitary nodules). The free T_4 in T_3 toxicosis may be normal or mildly elevated.

Ultrasound is also used to define the size of the gland, pathology, and/or the presence of nodules. A 24-hour radioactive iodine uptake (RAIU) test is elevated in almost all cases of hyperthyroidism. A near-zero RAIU is found in subacute thyroiditis/painless thyroiditis and factitious disease. RAIU findings are inaccurate if the patient has received iodine in the weeks preceding the test. Other tests, such as the thyroid-binding globulin, can be used to calculate the free T_4 index if the patient has recently received iodine.

Medications. The two commonly used antithyroid drugs (thioamides) are propylthiouracil (PTU) and methimazole (Tapazole). These drugs block the synthesis of thyroid hormone within the gland and may have some immunomodulatory properties. PTU also may block the peripheral conversion of T_4 to T_3, which is of some additional value in severely toxic patients. Until the preformed thyroid hormone still stored in the thyroid gland is released and the excessive amounts of thyroid hormone in the circulation are metabolized, no significant clinical effects of the antithyroid drugs are seen. Given that the half-life of T_4 is 7 days, several weeks must elapse before seeing significant improvement. Propylthiouracil is generally dosed three times a day with a total daily dose of 300 to 450 mg. Methimazole is generally dosed twice a day or in daily doses of 10 to 60 mg/day. The dosage of antithyroid is gradually tapered as the patient becomes euthyroid, and treatment is generally maintained for 12 to18 months.

Twelve to 18 months after cessation of antithyroid drug therapy, approximately 50% of patients with Graves' disease are in remission. In an effort to increase the remission rate, it has been found that maintaining total thyroid suppression with antithyroid drug therapy and treating the then drug-induced hypothyroidism with concurrent thyroid hormone will increase the remission rate to in excess of 90%. This study was carried out in a Japanese population but was unable to be reproduced in other populations, suggesting that genetics may be important in the response to this approach.[19] However, many practitioners have adopted this protocol into routine clinical practice. In the event of patient relapse, options include a further course of antithyroid drug therapy, RAI therapy, or surgery.

Side effects of antithyroid drugs include agranulocytosis; hence, baseline and subsequent periodic monitoring of the white blood count (WBC) is recommended. It is important to note baseline values, as many patients with Graves' disease have borderline-low WBCs. Patients must be instructed to look for signs and symptoms of leukopenia (e.g., sore throat, fever, sepsis) and other side effects (e.g., jaundice) and notify the health care provider if these occur. In general, the best remission rates with antithyroid drug therapy in Graves' disease are seen in females with smaller goiters.

Beta-adrenergic blockers such as propranolol are used to treat the tachycardia, arrhythmias, tremors, and agitation associated with the sympathetic nervous system stimulation. The doses required are generally toward the high end of the dosing spectrum and give prompt symptomatic relief. The dose is titrated down as the hyperthyroidism is controlled. These drugs should be prescribed cautiously to patients with asthma or congestive heart failure, as worsening of symptoms can occur in response to the negative inotropic side effects of the beta-adrenergic blockers. If beta-adrenergic blockers are contraindicated or not tolerated, calcium channel blockers may be used.[14]

Treatments

Radioactive Iodine Therapy. Therapeutic RAI therapy with ^{131}I is a more definitive therapy for hyperthyroidism resulting from Graves' disease and is the only long-term therapy, other than surgery, for toxic multinodular goiter or solitary toxic nodules. Radioiodine therapy is contraindicated in pregnancy. The dose is individualized based on the thyroid size and 24-hour ^{123}I uptake. Hypothyroidism is to be anticipated, as it is impossible to titrate the dose of ^{131}I to achieve a euthyroid state without a high failure rate and the need for retreatment. The radiation dose for ^{131}I therapy for hyperthyroidism is usually 6000 to 7000 rads and is equivalent to the radiation exposure for an intravenous pyelogram radiologic study. Depending on the severity of the hyperthyroidism and the dose administered, a euthyroid state generally results sometime between 6 weeks and 6 months after therapy. Repeat treatment may be needed in 10% to 20% of patients. The RAI is gradually eliminated from the body over a few days, primarily via the urine. Therefore appropriate hygienic measures should be used. Small amounts of radioiodine appear in the saliva; patients should be instructed to not share food, drink, or utensils with others and should avoid kissing for several days after receiving radioiodine therapy. Close contact with children should be minimized. A woman who has received ^{131}I therapy should defer pregnancy for 6 months. Women who have received ^{131}I therapy postpartum should not breastfeed for 6 months.

Surgery. Hyperthyroidism is rarely managed surgically. Surgery is indicated for (1) failure of antithyroid drug therapy, (2) failure of or contraindication to RAI therapy, (3) large goiters with compressive symptoms, or (4) concurrent thyroid cancer.

Subtotal thyroidectomy, removal of approximately 80% of the thyroid gland, is generally the procedure of choice; total thyroidectomy is reserved for thyroid cancer. The rate of hypothyroidism is less with subtotal thyroidectomy versus RAI therapy; however, the relapse rate may be higher over time. Before surgery, patients are given antithyroid medication to achieve a euthyroid state. The risks of thyroidectomy include damage to the recurrent laryngeal nerve, hypoparathyroidism, tracheal and esophageal injury, as well as the usual postoperative issues.

Diet. Increased food intake and weight loss are characteristic of untreated hyperthyroidism. Increased nutrient and calorie intake are necessary to meet the increased metabolic requirements. Cessation of weight loss with treatment can signal the return of the euthyroid state in elderly patients. While hyperthyroidism is present, caloric intake needs to be increased, with attention to appropriate distribution of calories from macronutrients. Supplemental vitamins and trace minerals may be prescribed.

Activity. Activity may be self-limited because of the fatigue the patient experiences. Symptoms of fatigue and insomnia may help patients accept and plan for rest periods during the day; however, the sympathetic nervous system activation may make trying to rest at any one time very frustrating. Work requiring concentration for long periods may be difficult to perform. The patient may need assistance coping with activity restrictions that interfere with occupational and financial demands. Usually activity restrictions are not imposed unless the patient has symptoms of tachycardia, atrial fibrillation, or other cardiovascular problems. Thyroid storm mandates complete bed rest and admission to an intensive care unit.

NURSING MANAGEMENT OF PATIENT WITH HYPERTHYROIDISM

ASSESSMENT

As described, hyperthyroidism can affect almost every system of the body and cause major physiologic and psychosocial problems.

Health History

Information to be collected as part of the health history when assessing the patient with hyperthyroidism includes:

- History of emotional and mental status changes
- Reports of palpitations or chest pain
- Reports of dyspnea, with or without exercise
- History of changes in hair, skin, nails, or amount of sweating
- Reports of visual disturbances and irritations; reports of eye fatigue
- Appetite and history of nutritional intake and weight changes
- Sleep patterns (e.g., insomnia)
- Presence of muscle tremors
- History of increased stool frequency and stool bulk
- History of heat intolerance

Reports of weakness, fatigue, and decreased ability to complete ADLs
History of changes in menses or change in libido
Knowledge: disease, treatment, care needs

PHYSICAL EXAMINATION

Physical examination of the patient with hyperthyroidism focuses on:

Mental status changes: shortened attention span, emotional lability, hyperkinesia, tremors

Cardiovascular status changes: increased systolic blood pressure, decreased diastolic pressure, widened pulse pressure, tachycardia at rest, dysrhythmias, murmurs

Skin and hair changes: warm, flushed, sweaty skin; dermopathy; fine, thinning hair

Eye changes: lid lag, proptosis, exophthalmos, diplopia, injected conjunctiva, decreased acuity

Nutritional/metabolic changes: decreased weight, increased appetite and intake, decreased serum triglycerides and cholesterol levels

Musculoskeletal changes: proximal muscle weakness, decreased muscle tone, difficulty rising from sitting position

Diagnostic test findings include: decreased serum levels of TSH measured by a third-generation assay and elevated free T_4 and/or free T_3 levels.

NURSING DIAGNOSES

Nursing diagnoses are determined from analysis of patient data. Nursing diagnoses for the person with hyperthyroidism may include but are not limited to:

Diagnostic Title	Possible Etiologic Factors
1. Risk for activity intolerance	Proximal muscle weakness and wasting associated with altered metabolism, fatigue, sympathetic stimulation
2. Anxiety	Changes in appearance, restlessness, tremors, heat intolerance, increased metabolism
3. Deficient knowledge	Unfamiliarity with information

EXPECTED PATIENT OUTCOMES

Expected patient outcomes for the person with hyperthyroidism may include but are not limited to:

1a. Will demonstrate no further decrease in activity tolerance and will show a gradual increase in activity over 2 to 3 months

1b. Will show evidence of adequate tissue perfusion and cardiac output: no change in mental status, breath sounds clear, no edema formation, heart rate within 20 beats of baseline, and gradual decrease in resting heart rate

2. Will show signs of decreased anxiety and effective coping

2a. Will rate self as less anxious or less stressed on a scale of 0 to 10, with 0 meaning no stress and 10 meaning the worst stress

2b. Will list three ways to cope with feelings regarding body changes

2c. Will identify home maintenance difficulties and methods to deal with difficulties until health stabilizes

3. Will describe how hyperthyroidism causes the signs and symptoms present, will list treatment options available, expected outcomes of treatment with realistic time frames, signs and symptoms requiring self-monitoring (signs/symptoms of hypothyroidism, hyperthyroidism, agranulocytosis), and precautions to be observed if RAI therapy is used

INTERVENTIONS

A Nursing Care Plan for the patient with hyperthyroidism follows.

Nursing Care Plan — *Patient With Hyperthyroidism*

DATA Mrs. T. is a 28-year-old housewife admitted for diagnostic evaluation before thyroidectomy, which will be performed in 2 weeks. Graves' disease was diagnosed 2 days ago, at which time methimazole (Tapazole) and Lugol's solution were prescribed.

The nursing history reveals that Mrs. T.:

- Feels overwhelmed, cries frequently, and fears losing control
- Has lost 15 pounds in 2 months and is persistently hungry, even though she eats large quantities of food
- Is heat intolerant, noise intolerant, and feels clumsy
- Expects the medication to make her feel better and is dreading surgery

Physical examination reveals:

- Blood pressure, 140/60; pulse rate, 132; respirations, 24/min; sinus tachycardia at 32 beats/min confirmed by electrocardiogram
- Staring gaze of eyes with proptosis (equal bilaterally); lid lag and globe lag present; right eye slightly reddened
- Warm skin with perspiration present
- Increased muscle tone with weakness of lower extremities, quick muscle response to sudden noise; fine tremor of both hands
- Diffuse visible enlargement of the thyroid gland
- Bruit present over thyroid

Collaborative nursing actions include those to prevent further environmental stressors that could make Mrs. T. more uncomfortable or increase her symptoms.

Nursing Care Plan Patient With Hyperthyroidism—cont'd

NURSING DIAGNOSIS **Decreased cardiac output related to increased sympathetic stimulation**
GOALS/OUTCOMES Cardiac output will be within normal limits; will remain free of cardiac dysrhythmias

NOC Suggested Outcomes
- Cardiac Pump Effectiveness (0400)
- Circulation Status (0401)
- Vital Signs Status (0802)

NIC Suggested Interventions
- Acute Cardiac Care (4044)
- Cardiac Care (4040)
- Vital Signs Monitoring (6680)

Nursing Interventions/Rationales
- Assess vital signs, especially heart rate and rhythm, at least every 4 hours or more often as indicated. *To detect changes from baseline that indicate the development of cardiac compromise.*
- Teach patient to report palpitations, chest pain, or dizziness. *These symptoms are indicative of cardiac compromise and need to be evaluated.*
- Assess daily weight, intake and output, and for signs of edema, jugular vein distention, and lung crackles. *To detect fluid volume changes that may be related to cardiac compromise secondary to tachycardia.*
- Decrease known stressors; explain all interventions, and listen to patient. *Decreasing external stress decreases anxiety and the workload on the heart.*
- Balance periods of activity with periods of rest. *Activity can be better tolerated when the patient is well rested. Frequent rest periods decrease the workload of the heart.*
- Administer prescribed medications and monitor for drug effectiveness. *To control symptoms, prevent excessive cardiac workload, and determine if the selected medications are serving their intended purpose.*
- Report any changes in cardiac status to physician. *Early detection of atrial fibrillation or thyroid storm allows for prompt treatment and prevents cardiac crisis.*

Evaluation Parameters
1. Pulse rate less than 20 beats above baseline during first 72 hours
2. Pulse rate gradually decreases after first 72 hours
3. Absence of cardiac dysrhythmias

NURSING DIAGNOSIS **Ineffective coping related to personal vulnerability and environmental stimuli**
GOALS/OUTCOMES Will identify and use coping mechanisms effectively

NOC Suggested Outcomes
- Coping (1302)
- Decision Making (0906)

NIC Suggested Interventions
- Coping Enhancement (5230)
- Decision-Making Support (5250)
- Calming Technique (5880)

Nursing Interventions/Rationales
- Discuss reasons for emotional lability. *If the patient understands that her emotional lability is part of her disease process, she may be better able to cope with her current situation.*
- Maintain a calm, relaxed environment. *Excessive external stimuli produce anxiety, which interferes with the patient's ability to cope with the current situation.*
- Provide privacy (e.g., a private room). *To reduce external stimuli and stress.*
- Explain all procedures and interventions. *Knowledge reduces fear, which reduces anxiety, allowing the patient to better cope with the stressful situation.*
- Encourage avoidance of all stimulants (coffee, tea, caffeine-containing colas, alcohol). *To reduce physiologic stressors that can further accelerate the metabolic rate and prevent sleep or rest.*
- Encourage patient to identify previous coping mechanisms or explore new ones. *Mechanisms that have been beneficial in the past may be present in her current situation.*
- Encourage patient to use relaxation techniques. *Relaxation promotes rest. A well-rested person is better able to use coping strategies than one who is fatigued.*

Evaluation Parameters
1. Accurately explains reason for changes in behavior
2. Identifies at least one coping strategy that is helpful when nervous or stressed
3. Uses relaxation techniques accurately

Continued

Nursing Care Plan — Patient With Hyperthyroidism—cont'd

NURSING DIAGNOSIS **Imbalanced nutrition: less than body requirements related to increased metabolic needs**
GOALS/OUTCOMES Weight will remain within 5 pounds of ideal weight

NOC Suggested Outcomes
- Nutritional Status (1004)
- Nutritional Status: Food and Fluid Intake (1008)
- Nutritional Status: Nutrient Intake (1009)

NIC Suggested Interventions
- Nutritional Monitoring (1160)
- Nutritional Management (1100)
- Nutrition Therapy (1120)

Nursing Interventions/Rationales
- Monitor weight at least weekly and more often if needed. *To determine if nutritional needs are being met.*
- Monitor serum albumin, hemoglobin, and lymphocyte levels. *To determine if nutrition is adequate to meet metabolic and bodily needs or if further intervention is needed.*
- Encourage high-calorie, high-protein, high-carbohydrate diet with selections from all food groups. *Increased nutrient intake is needed in order to meet increased metabolic demands.*
- Encourage intake of six small meals per day and between-meal supplements when tolerated. *To provide adequate nutrients consistently throughout the day to meet metabolic demands.*

Evaluation Parameters
1. Intake provided per prescribed diet
2. No further weight loss

NURSING DIAGNOSIS **Risk for disturbed sensory perception (visual) secondary to Graves' disease**
GOALS/OUTCOMES Will remain free of visual loss

NOC Suggested Outcomes
- Vision Compensation Behavior (1611)
- Risk Control: Visual Impairment (1916)

NIC Suggested Interventions
- Eye Care (1650)
- Environmental Management (6480)
- Emotional Support (5270)

Nursing Interventions/Rationales
- Assess visual acuity, ability to close eyes, and for photophobia. *To determine the extent of injury (if any) that has occurred and to prevent any further damage.*
- Protect eyes from irritants: use patches or glasses, artificial tears; elevate head of bed at night. *Protective measures can prevent corneal injury and minimize the risk of loss of vision.*
- Teach patient to avoid lying prone at night and to wear an eye shield if eyes do not close completely. *To protect the eyes from injury while sleeping.*

Evaluation Parameters
1. Vision remains stable when compared with baseline
2. Accurately explains measures to protect eyes

NURSING DIAGNOSIS **Activity intolerance related to generalized muscular weakness and increased metabolic rate secondary to Graves' disease**
GOALS/OUTCOMES Will report ability to perform activities without experiencing fatigue

NOC Suggested Outcomes
- Activity Tolerance (0005)
- Energy Conservation (0002)
- Nutritional Status: Energy (1007)

NIC Suggested Interventions
- Energy Management (0180)
- Nutrition Management (1100)
- Sleep Enhancement (1850)

Nursing Interventions/Rationales
- Assess severity of fatigue and patient's understanding of the physiologic cause. *A baseline assessment of the patient's fatigue is essential for later comparisons.*
- Encourage patient to prioritize daily activities and let go of unessential tasks. *Fatigue compromises one's ability to participate in daily activities. It is important that the patient's available energy be used to complete priority activities.*
- Explore strategies to modify existing activities, conserving energy when possible; seek assistance or delegate activities; and pace activities throughout the day to allow a balance between activity and rest. *Many daily activities can be modified to consume less energy, but this requires the patient's willingness to think*

Nursing Care Plan Patient With Hyperthyroidism—cont'd

about routine activities in a different way. Accepting the reality of fatigue may allow the patient to consider ways of seeking assistance or delegating activities that would not usually be considered acceptable.

- Encourage patient to obtain at least 8 hours of uninterrupted sleep at night. *Effective nighttime sleep patterns may decrease daytime fatigue.*

Evaluation Parameters

1. Balances activity with rest
2. Explains physiologic reason for fatigue
3. Performs only essential activities
4. Reports obtaining adequate nighttime sleep

NURSING DIAGNOSIS **Deficient knowledge related to lack of prior experience and/or access to information about disease**

GOALS/OUTCOMES Will accurately describe disease process and treatments

NOC Suggested Outcomes

- Knowledge: Diet (1802)
- Knowledge: Disease Process (1803)
- Knowledge: Energy Conservation (1804)
- Knowledge: Health Resources (1806)

NIC Suggested Interventions

- Teaching: Disease Process (5602)
- Teaching: Prescribed Diet (5614)
- Teaching: Prescribed Activity/Exercise (5612)
- Teaching: Prescribed Medication (5616)

Nursing Interventions/Rationales

- Teach patient how and when to take prescribed medications. *To increase the likelihood of compliance with medication routine to achieve a euthyroid state.*
- Teach patient regarding side effects of medications that need to be reported. *To prevent injury from drug side effects that may further complicate the existing condition.*
- Teach patient regarding signs and symptoms that need to be reported immediately (e.g., increased tachycardia, lightheadedness). *To detect complications quickly so that corrective action can be taken.*
- Teach patient about required care needs (diet, activities, rest). *To maintain maximal health and to prevent complications while becoming regulated on medications and awaiting surgery.*
- Repeat teaching frequently. *Stress interferes with learning. There is too much information to learn at one time. Therefore repetitive teaching enhances learning.*
- Provide written materials to enforce verbal teaching. *A patient who is ill or stressed does not always remember information taught. Written materials allow the patient to review important information and to proceed at her own pace.*
- Provide information about community resources that may be useful to patient and family. *The patient may not be aware of available community resources.*

Evaluation Parameters

1. Expresses interest in learning
2. Accurately describes at-home care, including medications and possible complications

1. Promoting Activity Tolerance

A balance of activity and rest should be promoted. The first step is assessing the patient's baseline energy level and tolerance to activity. Baseline vital signs and vital signs in response to activity should be documented and the patient's response to and ability to tolerate activity monitored. Periods of rest should be planned before activity. A relaxing environment should be provided to allow the patient rest periods during the day, especially if the patient is unable to sleep at night.

2. Decreasing Anxiety

Information should be provided regarding the physiologic reasons for changes in appearance, fatigue, activity intolerance, heat intolerance, and sleep disturbances. Providing symptomatic relief can decrease anxiety and feelings of frustration and powerlessness. The patient needs to be assisted to identify coping strategies to deal with feelings. Use of previously effective coping methods may be successful again. The environment should be supportive and allow the patient to participate in his/her care to the fullest extent possible. The patient should be helped to explore relaxation techniques as a means to decrease anxiety.

3. Patient/Family Education

The nurse can help the patient learn to incorporate the therapeutic regimen into ADLs. In addition, the patient needs to plan how to achieve rest, adequate nutrition, and energy conservation at home and at work. The patient may explore with the physician the appropriate and recommended options for definitive treatment. The nurse can support information seeking about risks, benefits, consequences of the treatment, and the requirements for follow-up care. The patient's beliefs and desires need to be valued, and the patient should be supported in expressing any concerns to the physician. A common concern is the effect of environmental radiation if RAI therapy is an option.

The teaching plan should include information to allow the patient to:

Describe the disease and how it causes signs and symptoms.
Clarify treatment options.
List the expected outcomes, such as relief of symptoms in 4 weeks if the patient is receiving drug therapy, the need for drug therapy for extended periods, and the potential complications of therapy.
State purpose, dose and schedule, and side effects to report for each prescribed medication.
List precautions to be observed if treated with RAI.
List signs and which must be self-monitored.

EVALUATION

To evaluate the effectiveness of nursing interventions, compare patient behaviors with those stated in the expected patient outcomes. Achievement of outcomes is successful if the patient with hyperthyroidism:

1a. Reports increased energy level, activity endurance, and activity completion.
1b. Tolerates physical activity without signs of cardiac decompensation.
1c. Reports adequate rest and sleep.
2. Rates anxiety as reduced and tolerable.
3a. Verbalizes knowledge of disease process, rationales for treatment, expected outcomes of treatment, and plan for follow-up care.
3b. Describes dosage schedule, rationale, and importance of drug therapy.

GERONTOLOGIC CONSIDERATIONS

Older adult patients have less clear-cut clinical findings of hyperthyroidism.[36] There may be weight loss, fatigue, and irritability; but goiter, tachycardia, eye changes, or tremor may be absent. In fact, subclinical hyperthyroidism, or "apathetic" or "masked" hyperthyroidism, is typical in elderly persons and needs to be treated. Radioiodine therapy is the treatment of choice in elderly patients.

When caring for an older adult with hyperthyroidism, it is important to remember that hyperthyroidism can cause new onset atrial fibrillation and also increases metabolism of drugs such as digoxin, theophylline, and warfarin, which are frequently taken by older persons. Research has also shown that elderly Caucasian women with low serum TSH concentrations have increased risk of vertebral and hip fractures (see Research box).

Nonthyroid disease may or may not raise the serum T_3 and/or T_4 in older persons and may suppress serum TSH. This is an important consideration because older persons typically have more than one chronic illness.

Research

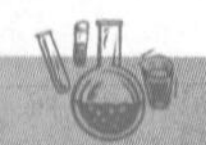

Reference: Bauer DC et al for the Study of Osteoporotic Fractures Research Group: Risk for fracture in women with low levels of thyroid-stimulating hormone, *Ann Intern Med* 134:561, 2001.

From 1986 to 1988, 9704 Caucasian women over the age of 65 were enrolled in a prospective study of risk factors for fracture. Baseline serum samples, spine radiographs, and bone mass of the calcaneus by single-photon absorptiometry were done. Approximately 80% of these women had bone mineral density measurements of the proximal femur performed 2 years later and spine x-ray studies performed 3.7 years later. These women were then grouped by subsequent fracture into four groups: those with hip fractures, those with vertebral fractures, those with nonspine fractures, and those without fracture. After the observation period baseline values for thyroid-stimulating hormone (TSH) levels were performed, the mean TSH was similar in all groups. The women in each of the fracture groups had lower baseline calcaneal and femoral neck bone mineral density values. Results indicated that women with a TSH $\leq$ 0.1mIU/ml had a 3.6-fold increased risk of hip fracture and a 4.5-fold increased risk of vertebral fracture. The authors concluded that elderly Caucasian women with low serum TSH levels have an increased risk of hip and vertebral fractures. Limitations of the study include that not all women had TSH levels assayed and serum thyroxine levels were not measured.

SPECIAL ENVIRONMENTS OF CARE

Critical Care

The patient with hyperthyroidism with atrial fibrillation is treated in the critical care unit (see Clinical Pathway and Nursing Care Plan) as is the patient with thyroid crisis or storm. Thyroid storm is managed in the critical care unit because it is a medical emergency in which patients develop severe manifestations of the signs and symptoms of hyperthyroidism. These include an elevated temperature, increased tachycardia or onset of dysrhythmias, worsening tremors and restlessness, worsening mental status including a delirious or psychotic state or coma, and sometimes reports of abdominal pain. Blood pressure and respiratory rate increase above baseline.

Thyroid storm is a rare, severe manifestation of hyperthyroidism, usually seen in an individual with Graves' disease. Symptoms result from a severe increase in metabolism and are usually precipitated by a major stressor such as infection, trauma, or surgery. The use of medications to suppress thyroid activity before surgery decreases the risk of thyroid storm, because less hormone is available to be released into the circulation with manipulation of the gland. Thyroid crisis also may occur in a person who has been inadequately treated or who stops taking prescribed therapy.

Patients with thyroid storm are critically ill. The immediate focus of care is to lower the metabolic rate as fast as possible, treat the precipitating cause, and support physiologic function-

clinical pathway *The Patient With Hyperthyroidism and Atrial Fibrillation*

EXPECTED LENGTH OF STAY: 3 DAYS WITH ADDITIONAL DEPENDING ON PROGRESS

	DAY OF ADMISSION DAY 1	DAY 2	DAY 3
Diagnostic Tests	CBC; UA; CMP*; serum TSH free T_4 concentration; total T_4 or T_3 concentrations as necessary; ECG; C&S blood/UA/sputum if necessary; O_2 saturation on room air, ABGs if necessary	CBC; O_2 saturation on room air, ABGs if necessary	CMP* ECG
Medications	IV (rate pending hydration/cardiac status); propylthiouracil; antiatrial fibrillation medication (possibly including coumadin, propranolol, or calcium channel blockers); medication for CHF as necessary; eye drops OU q2h prn for dryness; multivitamins; medication for rest/sleep if necessary; stool softener	IV (same); propylthiouracil; antiatrial fibrillation medication; medication for CHF as necessary; eye drops OU q2h prn for dryness; multivitamins; medication for rest/sleep if necessary; stool softener	IV (same); propylthiouracil; antiatrial fibrillation medication; medication for CHF as necessary; eye drops OU q2h prn for dryness; multivitamins; medication for rest/sleep if necessary; stool softener
Treatments	I&O q4hr; continuous VS; O_2 prn; cardiac monitor; weight; record food intake; assess moisture to eyes q2hr; assess neuro-cardio-pul-circ systems q2h 4 times then q4hr	I&O q8hr; continuous VS; cardiac monitor; weight; record food intake; assess moisture to eyes q2h; assess neuro-cardio-pul-circ systems q4hr	I&O q8hr; continuous VS; cardiac monitor; weight; record food intake; assess moisture to eyes q2h; assess neuro-cardio-pul-circ systems q4h
Diet	Soft diet with high calories, protein, and CHO; serve 6 meals; NO STIMULANTS	Soft diet with high calories, protein, and CHO; serve 6 meals; NO STIMULANTS	Soft diet with high calories, protein, and CHO; serve 6 meals; NO STIMULANTS
Activity	Bed rest with BRP; minimize environmental stressors (keep room cool, calm, quiet; provide rest periods)	Bed rest with BRP; minimize environmental stressors	Up to chair qid; minimize environmental stressors
Referral/ Consultations	Social services	Dietary, home health if necessary	

*Serum, creatinine, blood urea nitrogen (BUN), total bilirubin, alkaline phosphate, aspartate aminotransferase (AST) (formerly serum glutamic oxaloacetic transaminase [SGOT]), total protein, albumin, sodium, potassium, chloride, total CO_2, glucose, globulin.
ABGs, Arterial blood gases; *BRP,* bathroom privileges; *C&S,* culture and sensitivity; *CBC,* complete blood count; *CHF,* congestive heart failure; *CHO,* carbohydrates; *OU,* each eye.

ing. The typical therapeutic regimen is outlined in the Guidelines for Safe Practice box. The doses of medications used to treat thyroid storm are higher than those used in less critically ill patients because of accelerated metabolism of the drugs. Doses of drugs are adjusted according to patient response. Patients may require continual monitoring during rapid treatment.

Priority interventions are focused on the management of the cardiovascular status of the patient as well as any present hyperthermia. Atrial fibrillation is often the first cardiac alteration noted; other dysrhythmias are possible. Angina and high output congestive heart failure may occur in hyperthyroid patients, often in patients with underlying heart disease. Interventions for these patients are designed to normalize cardiac output. Cardiovascular status is monitored every hour and any changes, such as increased tachycardia, dysrhythmias, or signs of congestive heart failure, are reported to the physician (see Chapter 24). Cardiac workload is decreased by decreasing physical and emotional stressors. Temperature is also monitored every hour and any elevations are reported. Room temperature is maintained in the cool range and external cooling devices are used as ordered.

As the acute crisis subsides, continued attention should be paid to normalizing cardiac output and normal temperature.

Community-Based Care

Home care management is generally reserved for the patient with hyperthyroidism who had a hospital admission for atrial fibrillation and/or thyroid storm. The nurse focuses on assessment of the patient's and family's ability to manage the therapeutic regimen and to adapt resources to meet patient needs. The patient and family need to understand the therapy and expected results and to decide how to incorporate therapeutic requirements into daily life. The nurse can help the patient and family to:

- Increase resources for home maintenance while fatigue is present.
- Ensure adequate nutrition; monitor weight weekly.
- Plan for increased rest periods during the day.
- Plan strategies to manage insomnia, hyperkinesis, increased stool frequency, visual changes, and heat intolerance.

Understand the importance of adherence to therapy and follow-up monitoring.

HYPOSECRETION: HYPOTHYROIDISM

Etiology

Hypothyroidism refers to low levels of thyroid hormone and may result from:

- Congenital hypothyroidism (cretinism), which is detected through routine screening at birth
- Primary thyroid failure (i.e., Hashimoto's disease, other types of thyroiditis)
- Secondary thyroid failure (pituitary disease causing TSH deficiency)
- Tertiary thyroid failure resulting from thyrotropin-releasing hormone [TRH] deficiency with resultant TSH deficiency
- External thyroid gland destruction (i.e., postsurgery, post-^{131}I therapy, antithyroid drugs, medication side effects such as those from amiodarone or lithium)
- Miscellaneous (i.e., environmental iodine deficiency and peripheral resistance to thyroid hormone, both of which are rare)

In primary autoimmune thyroid failure, declining T_4 production results in increased TSH production with resultant hypertrophy of the remaining functioning thyroid tissue. Progressive thyroid enlargement over time can ensue with resulting clinical goiter. A goiter is any enlargement of the thyroid gland (Figure 29-6). If this enlargement is not associated with hyperthyroidism or hypothyroidism, cancer, or inflammation, it is referred to as a *simple goiter. Endemic goiters* refer to those that occur in a particular geographic region and from a common cause, such as iodine deficiency. *Sporadic goiter* describes those that occur sporadically in regions that are not the locus of endemic goiters. (See Box 29-7 for goitrogenic factors.) In many instances mild iodine deficiency is responsible for thyroid enlargement in pregnancy.

The most common cause of primary hypothyroidism in the United States is Hashimoto's disease. Patients are generally euthyroid or hypothyroid at presentation. Some may be asymptomatic with mild elevations in TSH, a condition called mild thyroid failure. Goiter formation in Hashimoto's disease is common in younger patients, and the goiter tends to enlarge over time if the patient is not on suppression therapy with exogenous thyroid hormone. Elderly individuals frequently have an atrophic form of the disorder with thyroid atrophy (atrophic thyroiditis).

Guidelines for Safe Practice
The Patient With Thyroid Storm

Monitor the patient's temperature, intake and output, neurologic status, and cardiovascular status every hour.
Initiate an IV line for medications and fluids.
Administer increasing doses of oral propylthiouracil (PTU) as ordered (200 to 300 mg every 6 hours may be given) after a loading dose of 800 to 1200 mg orally. PTU is the preferred antithyroid drug in this situation because it also inhibits the conversion of T_4 to T_3.
Administer iodide preparations as ordered. Sodium iodide given IV twice daily or an oral preparation may be ordered.
Administer dexamethasone, 2 mg IV every 6 hours. Glucocorticoids help to inhibit the release of thyroid hormone.
Administer β-adrenergic blockers IV, as ordered. Noncardioselective β-adrenergic blockers can worsen asthma or congestive heart failure because they constrict bronchial smooth muscles and cause a decrease in cardiac output.
Initiate measures to lower body temperature, including external cooling devices, cold baths, and acetaminophen. Salicylates are contraindicated because they inhibit thyroid hormone binding to protein carriers and thus increase free thyroid hormone levels.
Initiate other supportive therapy as ordered, including oxygen, cardiac glycosides, and treatment measures for the precipitating event.
Maintain a quiet, calm, cool, private environment until the crisis is over.
Maintain continuity of care.
Decrease stressors by use of patient education, comfort measures, or family support.

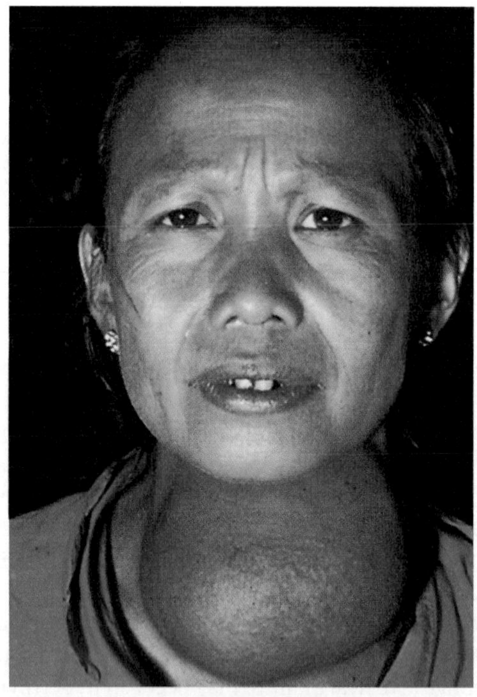

Figure 29-6 Simple goiter.

BOX 29-7 Goitrogenic Factors

- Iodine deficiency
- Foods with goitrogenic factors (cabbage, turnips, soybeans)
- Lithium
- Intrinsic abnormality in thyroid hormone synthesis

Epidemiology

Hypothyroidism affects an estimated 1% of the general population. In elderly persons, the prevalence rates may be in excess of 10%; routine screening for hypothyroidism has been advocated. Hypothyroidism has a gender predisposition to females. Congenital hypothyroidism is detected in 1 of every 4000 to 5000 newborns (see Risk Factors box).

Pathophysiology

Thyroiditis. Thyroiditis may be classified as acute, subacute, or chronic (Table 29-3). Hashimoto's disease is the most common form of chronic thyroiditis; most patients have thyroid enlargement owing in part to the trophic effects of the compensatory increase in TSH. Secondary and tertiary hypothyroidism are associated with low levels of TSH such that thyroid growth is not stimulated. The characteristic histologic picture includes infiltration with lymphocytes and varying degrees of fibrosis. Progressive glandular destruction results in an initial decline in T_4 levels and subsequent elevation in TSH.

Triiodothyronine levels fall into the subnormal range after T_4 levels. Thyroid autoantibodies (antimicrosomal [thyroid peroxidase] and antithyroglobulin) are present in more than 90% of patients with Hashimoto's disease.

Hypometabolism. Regardless of the cause, a lack of thyroid hormone results in a general depression of the basal metabolic rate and slows the development or functioning of almost every system of the body. Alterations in the integumentary, cardiovascular, nervous, musculoskeletal, alimentary, and reproductive systems are often seen. Manifestations of hypothyroidism in infants are not usually seen until several months after birth, when signs such as retardation of mental and physical development occur and are usually irreversible.

In adults early signs and symptoms are vague and may go unrecognized. Symptoms cover a wide range of body systems and present a challenge for diagnosis. Symptoms include menorrhagia, infertility, hoarseness, carpal tunnel syndrome, constipation, hair loss, xeroderma, bradycardia, depression, and macrocytic anemia.

Early reports of symptoms may consist of tiredness, lethargy, and weakness resulting in the inability to carry out a normal day's activities. Intolerance to cold and constipation develop. Menstrual cycle irregularity, menorrhagia, and inability to conceive may occur. Both men and women may note loss of libido. The majority of patients have multiple symptoms and signs, depending on the severity of the hypothyroidism (Box 29-8).

As the disease progresses, mental dysfunction occurs, appetite decreases, and changes in physical characteristics are noted. One major physical change is an accumulation of hyaluronic acids and alteration of ground substances producing mucinous edema *(myxedema)* and third-space fluid effusions. Figure 29-7 illustrates the puffiness characteristic of myxedema facies. In the periphery the edematous tissues feel thickened or "doughy." The patient may report muscle and joint discomforts, and chest pain may occur. Severe hypothyroidism with markedly elevated TSH levels, secondary in part to the elevated TRH, results in concurrent elevation in prolactin and potentially galactorrhea and amenorrhea.

Occasionally patients with undiagnosed severe hypothyroidism present for coronary artery bypass graft (CABG) with advanced coronary artery disease. The dilemma then arises as to what to treat first—the hypothyroidism or the coronary artery disease. Clinical studies have documented the safety and efficacy of CABG in known hypothyroid patients, with thyroid hormone replacement therapy being deferred until after

Risk Factors

Hypothyroidism

- History of thyroid disease
- History of radiation to neck
- Presence of other autoimmune disorders
  - Type I diabetes mellitus
  - Pernicious anemia (vitamin B_{12} deficiency)
  - Vitiligo
  - Addison's disease
- Family history of thyroid disease
- Family history of other autoimmune disorders
- Amiodarone treatment[9,20]

TABLE 29-3 Thyroiditis: Types and Characteristics

Type	Characteristics
Chronic thyroiditis Hashimoto's thyroiditis	Autoimmune process characterized by inflammation and fibrosis
Subacute thyroiditis Silent, painless thyroiditis/ lymphocytic thyroiditis	A form of thyroiditis of increasing frequency. Etiology unknown, but possible autoimmune factor. Symptoms include self-limiting form of hyperthyroidism and nontender, enlarged thyroid gland, which may be followed by hypothyroidism. Symptomatic treatment during the hyperthyroid phase consists of use of beta-adrenergic blockers, but not antithyroid medications. Patient should be monitored annually for development of hypothyroidism.
Postpartum thyroiditis	Occurs within a few months after delivery in 1% to 5% of pregnancies. Clinical course is similar to silent painless thyroiditis with transient toxic and hypothyroid phases that may be so mild as to go unnoticed in some patients. Permanent hypothyroidism may occur more frequently after postpartum thyroiditis than after painless, silent thyroiditis.

BOX 29-8 Hypothyroidism: Pathophysiologic Alterations and Clinical Manifestations

Decreased metabolic rate, heat production, and oxygen consumption

Because of the overall decrease in metabolism, common signs and symptoms include:

- Cold intolerance and perhaps decreased body temperature
- Cool, dry skin
- Decreased appetite
- Weight gain
- Myxedema facies with facial and periorbital edema, enlarged tongue, deepened or hoarse voice
- Fatigue
- Anemia

Alteration in Protein, Fat, and Carbohydrate Metabolism

The entire cycle of synthesis, degradation, and clearance is slowed. Because of decreased lipolysis and decreased lipid metabolism, especially lipid degradation, serum cholesterol and triglyceride levels may increase. The patient with preexisting diabetes mellitus may experience a decrease in blood glucose levels due to decreased glycogenolysis, decreased intestinal glucose absorption, and decreased insulin degradation.

Alteration in Cardiovascular Function

The hypometabolic state, coupled with decreased sensitivity to catecholamines, decreases the inotropic and chronotropic effects on the heart resulting in decreased cardiac output. Additionally, polysaccharide infiltration can occur in the myocardium. Signs and symptoms may include bradycardia, cardiomegaly, pericardial and pleural effusions, hyponatremia, decreased free water excretion, hypotension, and/or low output congestive heart failure.

Alteration in Central Nervous System Function

Thyroid hormone is synergized with other centrally acting hormones and neurotransmitters; this is decreased in hypothyroidism. Signs and symptoms may include apathy, lethargy, depression, slowed slurred speech, somnolence, paresthesias, hypoactive deep tendon reflexes, and coma.

Alteration in Reproductive Function

Secretion/metabolism of gonadotropins and gonadal steroids is altered. Signs and symptoms include decreased libido, decreased fertility, altered menstrual patterns with or without anovulation, erectile dysfunction, and oligospermia

Alteration in Gastrointestinal Function

Decreased motility of the gastrointestinal tract may lead to constipation.

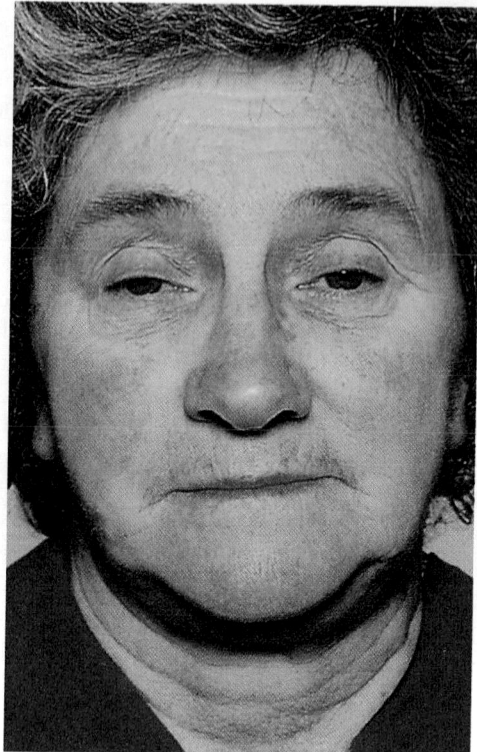

Figure 29-7 Adult with hypothyroidism.

surgery. If hypothyroidism is not treated, myxedema coma develops.

Myxedema Coma. *Myxedema coma* represents the most severe form of hypothyroidism and ultimately can occur in any patient with untreated prolonged hypothyroidism. Precipitating factors include sedatives, opioids, exposure to cold, surgery, infections, and trauma. The patient has all the classic symptoms of hypothyroidism and also is comatose and has severe hypothermia. Therapy focuses on treating the underlying cause or precipitating event. See section on Critical Care Management for further discussion.

Collaborative Care Management

Diagnostic Tests. Studies of thyroid function to diagnose hypothyroidism include the free T_4 index and serum TSH assay. Decreased levels of T_4 and T_3 and an elevated TSH level confirm the diagnosis of a patient who has primary hyposecretion and no other disease.

Acute illness and presence of nonthyroid disease may alter levels of T_3, T_4, and TSH. Free T_4 levels and TSH levels may fall significantly in severe illness, a condition called *euthyroid sick.* As the illness resolves, the TSH may rise slightly as normal homeostasis is established. The professional nurse must be aware of these adaptive changes to illness and not be confused by the fluctuations in TSH, T_4, and T_3.

Thyroid antibody tests and fine-needle biopsy may be done to confirm the presence of chronic thyroiditis, Hashimoto's disease, or to identify other pathology. If a goiter in a hypothyroid patient shows progressive growth on optimum replacement therapy, then concurrent thyroid cancer needs to be ruled out. The best way to assess change in thyroid size over time is with serial ultrasound determinations.

Medications

Goiter Suppression. Apart from the unusual situations of iodine deficiency and goitrogenic drugs, most goiters are of unknown etiology, manifesting as euthyroid Hashimoto's disease, colloid nodules, or euthyroid multinodular goiters. The principle of suppression therapy is to exogenously supply thyroid hormone, thus rendering the thyroid redundant with a

Research

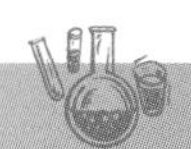

Reference: Bunevicius R, et al: Effects of thyroxine as compared with thyroxine plus triiodothyronine in patients with hypothyroidism, *N Engl J Med* 340(6):424, 1999.

Patients diagnosed with hypothyroidism are generally treated with thyroxine monotherapy. However, in an individual with a normally functioning thyroid gland, thyroxine and triiodothyronine are cosecreted. This study compared the effects of monotherapy with thyroxine to combination therapy with thyroxine and triiodothyronine.

The sample consisted of 33 subjects (31 women) with a mean age of 46 ± 13; efficacy was evaluated using a series of physical, psychologic, and cognitive function tests/scales. Subjects were treated for two 5-week periods. During period A, each subject received thyroxine monotherapy at his or her usual dose. In period B, each subject received combination therapy in which 50 μg of thyroxine was replaced with 12.5 μg of triiodothyronine. The order of the periods was randomly assigned. During period B with combination therapy, subjects had lower serum-free and total thyroxine levels and higher triiodothyronine levels.

Subjects underwent assessment of cognitive function, mood, and subjective physical symptoms. Statistically significant results revealed that when treated with thyroxine-triiodothyronine combination therapy, subjects demonstrated improved mood and neuropsychologic functioning, thereby suggesting the benefits of combination therapy.

decrease in TSH to the lower end of normal. This facilitates shrinkage of the goiter or at least cessation of growth. Goiter shrinkage tends to occur most readily in Hashimoto's disease. In some instances, because of the autonomous nature of the thyroid disorder, exogenous thyroid supplementation results in elevated free T_4 levels and a suppressed TSH rendering suppression therapy ineffective.

Replacement Therapy. Standard replacement therapy for hypothyroidism is daily oral sodium levothyroxine (L-thyroxine); the replacement dose is generally 1.6 to 1.8 (μg/kg) of body weight. The dosage should be titrated slowly, particularly in elderly individuals and those with coronary artery disease, until a normal metabolic rate is attained. The optimal dose is determined based on clinical parameters and a normal TSH and free T_4. It is important to note that the free T_4 is normalized long before the TSH, which may take in excess of 8 weeks. Patient teaching should emphasize taking L-thyroxine on an empty stomach to ensure consistent bioavailability. Failure to follow this guideline may be the reason for a patient suddenly requiring progressively larger doses of L-thyroxine. The interfering compounds include fiber, calcium, and iron.[33] The use of triiodothyronine in conjunction with L-thyroxine is under investigation (see Research box).[10]

Symptoms of hypothyroidism generally start to improve within a few days of replacement therapy. Complete resolution of all symptoms may take a couple of months in some patients, depending on the severity of the baseline hypothyroidism and the rapidity of replacement to euthyroid hormone levels.

The major side effects of therapy relate to either underreplacement or overreplacement, with resultant symptoms of either hypothyroidism or hyperthyroidism. Inappropriately rapid dose titration can precipitate angina, myocardial infarction, and tachyarrhythmias (e.g., atrial fibrillation) in predisposed individuals. These sequelae can also occur with chronic overdosing of L-thyroxine as well as accelerated bone loss with reduced bone mineral density and fracture predisposition.

Surgical Management. Pharmacologic therapy is the treatment of choice for patients with hypothyroidism. Surgery is indicated for large goiters producing persistent compression symptoms despite being euthyroid on replacement therapy. The degree of shrinkage of very large goiters is generally limited with optimum thyroid hormone replacement. Patients should be informed that surgical intervention might be needed to relieve symptoms.

Subtotal thyroidectomy is indicated for (1) compression symptoms and (2) concerns about the possibility of concurrent thyroid cancer due to progressive growth of the goiter on thyroid hormone replacement therapy or to fine-needle aspiration of a suspicious lesion. Compression symptoms many manifest as choking sensations, dysphagia, or inspiratory stridor related to compression and/or deviation of the esophagus and trachea. These compression symptoms may be accentuated by asking the patient to raise his or her arms above the head. This is known as Pemberton's sign.

Diet. Adequate nutrition in the form of well-balanced meals is advocated for patients with hypothyroidism. Patients may be advised to follow a weight-reduction diet. If iodine deficiency or excessive intake of goitrogenic foods (such as cabbage) has been identified, pertinent dietary instructions are given. In severe hypothyroidism, apathy, anorexia, and self-care deficit may combine to limit food intake, and attention must be given to achieve adequate intake. Fluid restriction and occasionally sodium modifications are necessary in severe hyponatremia.

Activity. Fatigue limits endurance in persons with hypothyroidism. Symptoms such as angina and dyspnea on exertion may occur with severe fatigue. Patients should be encouraged to increase activity gradually, building endurance and tolerance.

Referrals. Hospitalization, most likely for the treatment of myxedema coma, is generally the only indication for referrals. Appropriate referrals might include home care nursing, physical therapy, and social services if family or personal resources are limited.

NURSING MANAGEMENT OF PATIENT WITH HYPOTHYROIDISM

Assessment

Health History

Hypothyroidism affects every body system. Early manifestations will most likely be identified by a thorough history that addresses:

- Changes in physical energy level and activity or mental/neurological status
- Changes in skin, hair (head or body), nails
- Presence of chest pain; occurrence of syncope

Changes in appetite and weight with typical nutritional intake
Changes in bowel elimination
Presence of discomfort: headache, muscle, or joint pain; intolerance to cold
Changes in sexual function:
Women: changes in menses or libido, infertility
Men: changes in libido

Physical Examination

Data are collected using a head-to-toe approach, with particular emphasis on the followiing assessments:

Mental status: intellectual functioning; memory; speech pattern; presence of somnolence, lethargy, or confusion
Body weight and temperature
Skin: pigmentation, temperature, presence of nonpitting edema
Neck/hair: quality and quantity of head and body hair, thyroid examination
Cardiovascular: pulse rate and blood pressure
Respiratory: rate, breath sounds
Abdomen: bowel sounds
Motor: muscle strength, tone, and mass; range of motion; deep tendon reflexes; joint movement

NURSING DIAGNOSES

Nursing diagnoses are determined from analysis of patient data. Nursing diagnoses for the person with hypothyroidism may include but are not limited to:

Diagnostic Title	Possible Etiologic Factors
1. Activity intolerance	Reduced work capacity associated with decreased cardiac function, decreased breathing capacity, and muscle stiffness
2. Disturbed body image	Change in appearance (weight gain, hair and skin changes), changes in sexual functioning, decreased mental and physical function
3. Constipation	Decreased peristaltic action, decreased physical activity
4. Risk for impaired skin integrity	Mucinous deposits in skin, xeroderma, decreased elasticity
5. Deficient knowledge	Pharmacologic therapy, signs and symptoms, treatment plan

EXPECTED PATIENT OUTCOMES

Expected patient outcomes for the patient with hypothyroidism may include but are not limited to:

1. Will show a gradual increase in activity tolerance over 2 to 3 months
2a. Will relate body image changes to hypothyroidism and will verbalize that most changes are reversible
2b. Will understand that sexual function will increase as thyroid status returns to normal
3. Will attain and maintain a bowel pattern that was typical before onset of illness
4. Will have intact skin
5. Patient and significant others will be able to:
5a. Explain the disease
5b. Explain that treatment is lifelong oral medication therapy
5c. Explain that treatment should reverse most signs and symptoms
5d. Describe self-monitoring needs and planned follow-up care

INTERVENTIONS

Nursing interventions required by the patient with hypothyroidism vary greatly, depending on the severity of disease. Because the hypothyroid state is reversed slowly, the patient will not return to his or her baseline health state for 2 to 3 months.

1. Promoting Activity Tolerance

Increasing activities gradually promotes activity to the level of patient tolerance. Cardiovascular response to new activities must be monitored. If the patient complains of chest pain or develops an unacceptable heart rate, the activity must be stopped and then resumed at a slower rate. Blood pressure, pulse, and respirations should be monitored before, during, and after each new activity.

2. Promoting a Positive Body Image

Information that helps the patient and significant others understand the relationship of body changes to hypothyroidism should be provided. Information about reversible body changes should be provided, and the patient should be helped to understand the relationship between the sexual problems and the hypothyroidism.

3. Promoting Normal Bowel Elimination

The patient's normal pattern of bowel function should be determined and current bowel elimination monitored. Adequate fluid intake and a diet high in fiber should be encouraged along with ambulation and adequate exercise to promote peristalsis and bowel motility. Stool softeners may be prescribed as needed.

4. Maintaining Skin Integrity

Skin should be assessed at least daily to monitor for areas of redness and pressure. A tool such as the Braden Scale is helpful in assessing patients at risk for alterations in skin integrity. Emollients should be applied daily and after bathing. The number of baths should be limited to avoid overdrying the skin. Tepid water should be used because hot water depletes skin of moisture, especially in elderly patients. Superfatted soaps should be used and the skin patted dry to avoid friction.

Preventive care measures such as use of sheepskin pads, soft sheets, and padding of bony prominences should be instituted as indicated. If the patient is unable or does not turn, he or she is assisted in turning every 2 hours. Ambulation is encouraged when possible. Fluid intake is increased unless contraindicated by cardiac or renal disease to increase moisture in the skin. Use of a humidifier in the home increases moisture in the air and thus in the skin. A diet with adequate protein, carbohydrates, and vitamins is essential to promote optimal nutritional status.

5. Patient/Family Education

The nurse must assist the patient and family/significant others to learn how to continue the plan of care after discharge. The importance of compliance with medications and follow-up care should be stressed. The teaching plan should include:

- Nature of the disorder, diagnostic tests, and treatment; need for lifelong thyroid hormone replacement therapy
- Medications: dosage, method of administration, and side effects of hypothyroidism and hyperthyroidism
- Self-monitoring of vital signs, weight, skin integrity, and bowel function
- Measures to prevent skin breakdown and constipation
- Need for periods of rest alternating with activity
- Need for continued follow-up care

The patient with a large goiter may need help with altered body image related to disfigurement. The goiter may be concealed by the use of scarves and high collared shirts. An open and trusting relationship is necessary so that the patient can share feelings and concerns.

Health Promotion/Prevention

Primary prevention of hypothyroidism focuses on the identification and treatment of dietary iodine deficiency. Dietary iodine deficiency results from living in an area with low iodine levels in the water and soil. In the United States, the Great Lakes region has been an area of dietary iodine deficiency; however, the use of iodized salt has been successfully used to essentially eliminate the problem. Elsewhere in the world, however, dietary iodine deficiency is still problematic, and the World Health Organization has estimated that 200 million people have goiters related to iodine deficiency.

Secondary prevention of hypothyroidism has focused mainly on routine newborn screening and prompt treatment to prevent the irreversible brain damage, growth retardation, and other sequelae of hypothyroidism. The case for routinely screening the elderly for hypothyroidism has significant merit. Screening of patients, especially women, with risk factors for hypothyroidism is reasonable[15] (see Research box).

Research

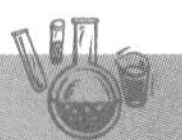

Reference: Danese MD et al: Screening for mild thyroid failure at the periodic health examination: a decision and cost-effectiveness analysis, *JAMA* 276:285, 1996.

This study used computer decision analysis to estimate the cost-effectiveness of routine periodic screening for mild thyroid failure via measurement of thyroid-stimulating hormone (TSH). The computer model simulated TSH screening every 5 years beginning at age 35 over a 40-year follow-up period. Positive cases, diagnostic costs, medical consequence, and costs were computed. Cost-effectiveness of TSH screening in women was $9223 per quality adjusted life year; in men it was $22,595. The costs compare favorably to the costs of other generally accepted medical practices. Hence, TSH screening every 5 years is a cost-effective intervention.

Tertiary prevention of hypothyroidism focuses on ongoing iodine replacement of the iodine-deficient patient, as well as encouraging compliance with thyroid hormone replacement therapy.

EVALUATION

To evaluate the effectiveness of nursing interventions, patient behaviors should be compared with those stated in the expected patient outcomes. Achievement of outcomes is successful if the patient:

1. Demonstrates increasing ability to ambulate and participate in ADLs.
2a. Attributes body changes to disease and its treatment.
2b. Explains how therapy should improve sexual function.
3. Reports resumption of usual elimination patterns.
4. Demonstrates intact skin and measures to prevent breakdown.
5a. With significant others accurately explains disease and need for lifelong intake of a thyroid drug, even though symptoms will be alleviated.
5b. With family is knowledgeable regarding symptoms of hypothyroidism and hyperthyroidism and need for follow-up care and monitoring of thyroid function.

GERONTOLOGIC CONSIDERATIONS

Older adult patients must be assessed for decreased alertness, decreased mobility, or increased susceptibility to cold, which are signs and symptoms more typically found with hypothyroidism in elderly persons. They also must be assessed for signs of myxedema, as seen with untreated hypothyroidism, and for signs of drug toxicity because of decreased metabolic activity.

Elderly patients need to be helped to plan a way for remembering to take replacement therapy appropriately—first thing in the morning and on an empty stomach. They need to be taught to monitor for drug side effects and to report signs of angina or congestive heart failure, which may result from initial doses of thyroid hormone replacement. The need to take measures to prevent constipation, which often occurs with hypothyroidism and especially in older persons, also needs to be stressed.

SPECIAL ENVIRONMENTS FOR CARE

Critical Care

The patient with myxedema coma is frequently in both respiratory and cardiac failure and requires close monitoring in an intensive care unit. Manifestations are those of severe hypothyroidism with marked emphasis on:

- Hypothermia
- Respiratory dysfunction related to respiratory muscle weakness (myopathy), sleep apnea, and decreased ventilatory drive in response to hypoxia and hypercapnia
- Reduced cardiac output due to bradycardia and decreased stroke volume. Overt congestive cardiac failure can occur in patients with underlying cardiac disease
- Slowed drug metabolism and clearance resulting in potential drug toxicity (e.g., digoxin toxicity)

Concurrent adrenal insufficiency, which may require stress doses of glucocorticoids

Therapy for the patient with myxedema coma includes supportive care (cardiovascular, respiratory, and fluid balance support) and administration of thyroid hormone. Intubation and mechanical ventilation may be necessary for patients in respiratory failure. The hypothermic patient needs to be gradually rewarmed and additional heat loss prevented; however, rapid rewarming can cause vascular collapse. Treatment protocols vary; options for thyroid hormone therapy include levothyroxine, liothyronine, or T_3 and T_4. Some patients with myxedema coma may also have adrenal insufficiency, intravenous hydrocortisone in stress doses should be maintained until the cortisol value is greater than 20 μg/dl or the cosyntropin test is within normal limits.

Nursing interventions include care of the comatose patient; surveillance of respiratory, cardiovascular, and fluid status; care of the patient with respiratory insufficiency; preventive care for problems of immobility; and assistance with the institution of the medical regimen.

Community-Based Care

Hypothyroidism is a lifelong condition requiring ongoing hormone replacement with L-thyroxine and ongoing medical management. Most patients with hypothyroidism are managed as outpatients. When beginning pharmacologic therapy, the patient should be monitored every 4 to 6 weeks for response to treatment. After the dosage of medication is stabilized, the patient should be monitored every 6 to 12 months, including serum TSH levels. The patient should be taught to recognize and report the signs and symptoms of hypothyroidism and hyperthyroidism. Persons with subclinical hypothyroidism should be periodically evaluated to detect progression to overt hypothyroidism. In elderly women, subclinical hypothyroidism has been shown to be an independent risk factor for atherosclerosis and myocardial infarction.[18]

Family involvement is usually necessary to ensure appropriate care and compliance with the therapeutic regimen in the elderly patient with myxedema. Fatigue may necessitate rearrangement of the home environment to avoid stair climbing until the patient regains endurance. A bedside commode can be obtained if the bathroom is a significant distance from the patient's room.

COMPLICATIONS

Myxedema coma, previously discussed, is a rare, but life-threatening complication of untreated hypothyroidism. The patient with hypothyroidism who remains hypothyroid either from lack of treatment or under-treatment with L-thyroxine is at increased risk for dyslipidemia and cardiovascular disease. As with all patients, any angina, chest pain, or dyspnea should be reported to the health care provider immediately.

THYROID CANCER

Etiology/Epidemiology

Thyroid cancer is less prevalent than other forms of cancer and generally has a much better prognosis. Papillary thyroid cancer is the most common type and is linked to prior radiation exposure to the head and neck. Some cancers may be familial (e.g., medullary thyroid cancer) and are associated with other endocrine neoplasms (multiple endocrine neoplasia [MEN]). Most thyroid cancers arise in a solitary nodule and the risk of a solitary nodule being malignant is greater in younger patients and in men.[11,12]

Pathophysiology

Five types of primary thyroid cancer can occur, with the majority arising from thyroid follicular epithelium. Papillary thyroid cancer is generally diagnosed on the basis of a fine-needle aspiration biopsy where characteristic papillary structures can be seen. A follicular neoplasm, on the other hand, may be hard to classify as benign or malignant on the basis of fine-needle aspiration alone; further histologic analysis is needed for definitive diagnosis. Follicular cancers may spread via the bloodstream to the bone, lung, or liver. Malignant follicular and papillary lesions may produce some thyroid hormone, but generally not enough to cause hyperthyroidism. Medullary cancer of the thyroid (MCT) arises in the parafollicular or C-cells. MCT may spread early to cervical nodes and metastasize to the liver, lungs, or bone. Anaplastic thyroid cancer and thyroid lymphomas are uncommon (Table 29-4).[11,12]

Collaborative Care Management

Diagnostic Tests. Thyroid nodules may be discovered by the patient or on routine examination. Additionally, nodules may be discovered during diagnostic imaging for other diseases (e.g., MRI of the cervical spine for cervical disk disease

TABLE 29-4 Characteristics of the Five Types of Thyroid Cancer

	Cancers of Follicular Epithelium				Cancer of Parafollicular Tissue
Characteristics	**Papillary**	**Follicular**	**Anaplastic**	**Thyroid Lymphoma**	**Medullary**
Incidence of all thyroid cancers	65%	20%	5%	5%	5%
Age	Young persons	After 40	After 60	After 40	After 50
Female/male ratio	2-3 : 1	2-3 : 1	F > M	F > M	F = M

TABLE 29-4 Characteristics of the Five Types of Thyroid Cancer—cont'd

Characteristics	Cancers of Follicular Epithelium: Papillary	Follicular	Anaplastic	Thyroid Lymphoma	Cancer of Parafollicular Tissue: Medullary
Metastasis	By intraglandular lymphatics; slow-growing tumor	By blood vessels to distant sites (bone, lung, liver); occurs early	By direct invasion to adjacent structures; highly malignant	By lymphatic system; gland fixed to other structures	By intraglandular lymphatics and blood vessels
Prognosis	Good; rarely causes death in young persons if occult or intrathyroidal	Good if minimally invasive lesion	Prognosis varies with cell type; for giant cell, very poor (<6 months from diagnosis); for small cell, better (5-year survival rate of 20%–50%)	Good	Moderate; 10-year survival is estimated at 60%; multiple endocrine neoplasia (MEN) type IIb has the worst prognosis
Symptoms	Asymptomatic	Nodule may have been present for years	Hoarseness, inspiratory stridor, pain, dysphagia (signs of invasion of adjacent areas)	May have long history of previous goiter; rapid enlargement of goiter, hoarseness, dysphagia, pressure sensation, dyspnea, some pain	Tumors can produce adrenocorticotropic hormone resulting in Cushing's syndrome. Serotonin, prostaglandins and other hormones may be produced, resulting in flushing and diarrhea.
Tumor	Occult (<1.5 cm in diameter), intrathyroidal (>1.5 cm in diameter but does not extend through thyroid surface), and extra-thyroidal (extends through thyroid surface); well differentiated; psammoma body found in 40% of tumors and virtually diagnostic of malignant nature; tumors appear as "cold" spots on thyroid scan	Well differentiated to poorly differentiated; cyst formation and calcification possible	Two cell forms: giant cell and small cell	Usually of nodular histiocytic form	Tumors may vary in size from 1-2 mm in diameter to masses several centimeters in diameter
Other	Growth partially dependent on thyroid-stimulating hormone; thyroid hormone can cause regression of metastatic lesions; ^{131}I may be used for nonresectable lesions; may have history of radiation therapy to head and neck	Suppressive thyroid therapy can cause regression of metastatic lesions; radiation therapy with ^{131}I may be used when vascular invasion or metastasis present	—	Strong association with Hashimoto's thyroiditis; may have lymphoma at other sites	80% of cases are sporadic Occurs as a familial form as part of MEN type IIa or MEN IIb; in MEN IIa, there is medullary carcinoma, pheochromocytomas and hyperparathyroidism; in MEN IIb, there is medullary carcinoma, pheochromocytomas, intestinal ganglioneuromas, mucosal neuromas, marfanoid habitus; skeletal abnormalities; also occurs as a non-MEN familial form

or trauma). A thorough history should be carried out, focusing on any history of radiation exposure to the head/neck, history of compression symptoms (e.g., dysphagia), or symptoms of hypothyroidism/hyperthyroidism. Physical examination should document the size of the nodule, whether or not any additional nodules are palpable, and any lymphadenopathy.

Thyroid function is assessed via a TSH to confirm a euthyroid state. A suppressed TSH suggests a benign hyperfunctioning nodule. A thyroid ultrasound is done to identify anatomy and any lesions. This procedure can be performed in the office.[27] If a solitary nodule is hyperfunctioning there is suppression and atrophy of the contralateral lobe. Ultrasonography cannot definitively classify nodules as being benign or malignant; fine-needle aspiration is required. Ultrasound may be helpful for needle guidance to ensure accurate needle placement in fine-needle aspiration of smaller thyroid nodules. Ultrasonography may readily differentiate a solid from a cystic lesion; after aspiration of a cystic lesion ultrasonography can assist with needle guidance for fine-needle aspiration of the cyst wall. Cystic lesions containing clear fluid on aspiration are generally benign; those with a bloody aspirate may be malignant.

Radionuclear imaging of malignant thyroid nodules shows absence of uptake of the radioiodine isotope—the so-called cold nodule; however, only approximately 20% of cold nodules are malignant. A hyperfunctioning or hot nodule on radionucleide scanning demonstrates uptake of the radioiodine in the nodule with suppression of the uptake in the rest of the gland. Hot nodules are always benign. Fine-needle aspiration of the thyroid consists of insertion of a 22-gauge needle, with or without ultrasound guidance, into the nodule. The patient is generally placed in the supine position with the neck extended. Usually several needle insertions into the nodule are made to ensure that a representative and adequate sample is obtained and submitted to the pathologist for cytologic evaluation. Most patients describe the discomfort as comparable to a routine phlebotomy and the professional nurse should reassure the patient. Lesions are classified as one of the following: (1) diagnostic or highly suspicious for malignancy, (2) indeterminate, or (3) benign. Lesions that are diagnostic or highly suspicious for malignancy must be removed. Indeterminate lesions are generally removed. Occasionally physicians elect to monitor indeterminate lesions while treating them with exogenous thyroid hormone suppression therapy. A thyroid nodule that shrinks on serial ultrasound examinations is usually benign. A thyroid nodule that expands while on suppression therapy is highly suspicious of malignancy. Sudden expansion of a benign thyroid nodule can occur as a result of hemorrhage into the nodule. Most benign nodules are simple colloid nodules and do not need to be removed unless causing compressive symptoms.[13]

Medications. After thyroidectomy or ablation therapy with radioiodine, patients require lifelong thyroid hormone replacement therapy. Dosages should be high enough to suppress serum TSH levels. Monitoring of T_4 and TSH levels should be done 6 to 12 weeks after surgery.

Treatments

The lowest risk of recurrence of thyroid cancer (papillary and follicular) results from total thyroidectomy with ^{131}I ablation of any thyroid remnants. The dosage of ^{131}I is much higher than that used to treat hyperthyroidism. After such ablation therapy, the patient must be placed in isolation in the hospital, usually in a corner room. All urine and feces must be collected and disposed of into a radiation sewage disposal system. The patient must use disposable plates, cups, and utensils. The patient is not allowed visitors and contact with health care professionals is strictly minimized. The isolation must continue until the total-body ^{131}I burden falls to less than 30 mCi as measured by a Geiger counter. In the patient with normal renal function, this ordinarily is achieved within 3 days. For the next several days, the patient needs to follow the radiation safety instructions for the patient with hyperthyroidism undergoing ^{131}I for hyperthyroidism.

Thyroid hormone replacement with L-thyroxine is started the day after the ^{131}I treatment with the goal being a TSH suppressed slightly below the lower limits of the reference range. Serum thyroglobulin can then be measured and monitored as a marker of residual autonomously functioning thyroid tissue. A measurable serum thyroglobulin may indicate neoplastic tissue either in the thyroid bed or elsewhere. A radioiodine body scan is done for further evaluation. There are two methods of performing the scan. The conventional way calls for withdrawal of thyroid hormone replacement and a low iodine diet for several weeks until the TSH becomes frankly elevated. An elevated TSH is needed to obtain radioiodine uptake into any remnant of neoplastic thyroid tissue. Patients naturally complain of fairly severe symptoms of hypothyroidism throughout this whole process. The alternative approach is to use recombinant TSH injections (Thyrogen) to facilitate stimulation of thyroglobulin levels and/or uptake of radioiodine. This approach is much more comfortable for the patient; however, the radioiodine scan yield may be somewhat less than with the conventional approach. If the radioiodine scans prove positive, repeat ablative doses of ^{131}I may be administered, or if the recurrence is localized to the neck, repeat surgical removal may be carried out. Generally, after the patient has had two consecutive negative scans, most physicians are comfortable to monitor either basal or thyrogen-stimulated thyroglobulin levels.[1]

For smaller papillary neoplasms, some physicians advocate a more conservative surgical approach consisting of a lobectomy to include the neoplasm and thyroid isthmus. Long-term suppression therapy with L-thyroxine follows. Patients with lymphoma of the thyroid are rarely treated with surgery. Radiotherapy is the treatment of choice; compressive symptoms usually respond rapidly to treatment.

Surgical Management

Total thyroidectomy is the treatment of choice for patients with bilateral disease, large unilateral tumors, papillary tumors, or a history of neck radiation. Advantages of total thyroidectomy include the ability to treat recurrences or metastases outside the thyroid with RAI. Minimally the procedure for a malignant or suspicious nodule is total ipsilateral thyroid lobectomy and isthmusectomy; this procedure eliminates the need for ipsilateral reoperation. Serum thyroglobulin is used to monitor therapy after surgery. Neck dissection is indicated for patients with palpable metastases in cervical nodes. Radioablation of the remaining thyroid tissue is performed with ^{131}I 1 month after surgery while the patient is hypothyroid.

Treatment for the patient with MCT is total thyroidectomy with removal of the lymph nodes in the center of the neck. The prognosis for anaplastic thyroid cancer is extremely poor. Invasion of local structures may make curative surgical resection impossible; radiation or chemotherapy may be offered as palliation.

NURSING MANAGEMENT OF PATIENT UNDERGOING THYROID SURGERY

Care of the patient with a thyroid nodule first focuses on helping the patient through the diagnostic process. Thyroid nodules occur frequently and most are not malignant. No single diagnostic test is completely reliable. Depending on patient characteristics and physician philosophy, various tests may be performed. The nurse prepares the patient for each test, focusing particularly on education.

PREOPERATIVE CARE

The patient having thyroid surgery needs care focused on producing and maintaining a euthyroid state. The patient with a diagnosis of cancer may be experiencing a major disruption in coping as a result. Patient teaching regarding general preoperative and postoperative care (see Chapters 16 and 18) is provided on an outpatient basis. The patient also needs to learn how to cough and to move the head and neck postoperatively without placing strain on the suture line. Thus the patient is taught preoperatively to support the neck by placing both hands behind the neck when moving the head or when coughing.

POSTOPERATIVE CARE

Immediate postoperative interventions are listed in the Guidelines for Safe Practice box. In addition to routine monitoring, the patient is checked for major complications that can occur after thyroid surgery: recurrent laryngeal nerve injury, hemorrhage, transient hypocalcemia, and respiratory obstruction. Signs of these complications are reported immediately to the health care team.

Sore throat or hoarseness after surgery may be related to intubation during surgery; such hoarseness should clear gradually. If hoarseness persists or worsens, it is reported immediately to the surgeon. Hoarseness may be a first sign of laryngeal nerve damage, which can result in vocal cord spasm and respiratory distress. Unilateral nerve injury usually causes hoarseness; bilateral injury may result in airway obstruction. An emergency tracheostomy may be necessary, and equipment for this should be available at the patient's bedside.

Guidelines for Safe Practice

Care of the Patient After Thyroid Surgery

1. Monitor for and report signs of complications.
   a. Laryngeal nerve damage; hoarseness, weak voice
   b. Hemorrhage or tissue swelling
      (1) Bleeding on dressing: check back of dressing by slipping hand gently under neck and shoulders
      (2) Choking sensation
      (3) Difficulty in coughing or swallowing
      (4) Sensation of dressing being too tight even after it is loosened
   c. Calcium deficiency (tetany)
      (1) Early signs: tingling around mouth or of toes and fingers, decreasing serum calcium levels
      (2 Later signs: positive Chvostek's and Trousseau's signs (see Chapter 13), grand mal seizures
   d. Respiratory distress associated with any of signs just listed
2. Provide emergency care.
   a. Keep emergency supplies readily available:
      (1) Tracheostomy set (for laryngeal nerve damage), oxygen and suction equipment, suture removal set (for respiratory obstruction from hemorrhage)
      (2) IV calcium gluconate or calcium chloride (for tetany)
   b. For acute respiratory distress:
      (1) Call for immediate medical help.
      (2) Raise head of bed.
      (3) Loosen dressing over incision.
      (4) Give calcium as ordered, if signs and symptoms of tetany are present.
      (5) If loosening the dressing does not relieve symptoms of respiratory distress and if medical help is not readily available, remove clips or sutures as instructed.
3. Provide comfort.
   a. Avoid tension on suture lines; encourage patient to support head when turning by placing both hands behind neck.
   b. Give prescribed analgesics as necessary.
4. Maintain nutritional status.
   a. Start soft foods as soon as tolerated (only fluids may be tolerated initially).
   b. Encourage a high-carbohydrate, high-protein diet.
5. Teach patient:
   a. Range-of-motion exercises to neck when suture line is healed to prevent permanent limitations
   b. Need for lifelong thyroid hormone replacement therapy after a total thyroidectomy
   c. Any special care measures related to the underlying disease
   d. Need for follow-up care

The patient is monitored for hemorrhage for the first 12 to 24 hours after surgery. Hemorrhage can result in incisional bleeding or in compression of the trachea or surrounding tissue. If hemorrhage causes compression, the patient exhibits signs of respiratory distress. If these signs occur, the dressing is loosened. If this does not relieve the respiratory distress, the surgeon may need to remove surgical clips or sutures. The patient may have to be taken back to surgery for ligation of the blood vessels and wound closure.

Although the occurrence of hypocalcemia or tetany is minimal, the parathyroid glands can be injured during surgery, or inflammation may block the normal release of parathyroid hormone (PTH). If the level of PTH drops, symptoms of calcium deficiency can occur. If not treated promptly, calcium deficiency can result in tetany with contraction of the glottis and respiratory obstruction leading to death. Tetany typically appears 24 to 48 hours after surgery. Treatment for calcium deficiency is calcium carbonate or calcium gluconate given intravenously. Oral calcium is then necessary until normal parathyroid function returns. Permanent hypoparathyroidism is uncommon after total thyroidectomy.

The nurse must know that respiratory obstruction can occur from (1) recurrent laryngeal nerve damage causing vocal cord spasms that close off the larynx, (2) tracheal compression from hemorrhage, (3) tissue swelling, or (4) tetany. The nurse should be prepared to assist in the management of all these problems.

The patient who has undergone a total thyroidectomy must immediately initiate L-thyroxine replacement therapy. Dosage should be calculated as per the guidelines for the patient with hypothyroidism based on actual body weight (see Hypothyroidism).

GERONTOLOGIC CONSIDERATIONS

Thyroid nodules have been identified in 5% of persons older than age 60 years, and 90% of these nodules are found to be benign. The elderly person needs special consideration when undergoing surgical intervention (see Chapters 16 through 18).

SPECIAL ENVIRONMENTS FOR CARE

Critical Care

The person recovering from thyroidectomy or thyroid resection only needs critical care nursing if complications such as hemorrhage or respiratory distress develop. The patient may require invasive monitoring to adequately assess fluid volume and cardiac status or may require ventilator support.

COMPLICATIONS

As previously discussed complications after thyroid surgery include hemorrhage, recurrent laryngeal nerve damage, hypocalcemia, and respiratory distress. Other complications associated with the procedure or anesthesia may also occur (see Chapters 17 and 18).

PARATHYROID GLAND DISORDERS

HYPERSECRETION: HYPERPARATHYROIDISM[4]

Primary Hyperparathyroidism

Etiology

Hyperparathyroidism refers to elevated serum calcium levels caused by inappropriate release of PTH from the parathyroid glands. Primary hyperparathyroidism and hypercalcemia of malignancy are the most common causes of elevated serum calcium, accounting for approximately 90% of cases. Secondary hyperparathyroidism results from malabsorption syndrome or a defect in mineral homeostasis, such as kidney failure, with a resultant increase in parathyroid function.

The most frequent cause of primary hyperparathyroidism is a solitary adenoma (85%) involving one of the four parathyroid glands. The remaining 15% of patients usually have hyperparathyroidism of all four glands, and in rare instances, primary parathyroid cancer.

It is postulated that the "set point" for negative feedback on PTH secretion by ambient ionized calcium levels is elevated. In essence, this means that PTH secretion is not "switched off" in the adenoma/hyperplastic cells when serum calcium levels are at the upper limit of normal. Parathyroid adenomas are thought to represent clonal expression of mutant cells, in turn related to loss of function of tumor suppressor genes.

Primary hyperparathyroidism may also be part of a MEN syndrome. The type I syndrome or MEN I consists of pituitary adenoma, pancreatic islet cell tumor, and primary hyperparathyroidism. The type II syndrome or MEN II consists of pheochromocytoma, medullary thyroid cancer, and primary hyperparathyroidism. An appropriate workup for these entities is prompted by family history and relevant symptomatology/physical findings.

Epidemiology

The incidence of primary hyperparathyroidism is approximately 1 in 500 to 1000 individuals, with women being affected more often than men by 3:1. The majority of the patients are postmenopausal and in the sixth decade of life. Some patients may be diagnosed after a workup for osteoporosis or osteopenia.

Pathophysiology

Elevation in PTH levels raises serum calcium via several mechanisms:

- Increased bone resorption
- Enhanced activation of vitamin D to 1,25-hydroxy vitamin D, with resultant enhanced calcium absorption from the gastrointestinal tract
- Enhanced renal resorption of calcium from the glomerular filtrate

In addition, PTH enhances the renal excretion of phosphate with resultant decrease in the serum phosphate level. Thus the constellation of hypercalcemia with low/subnormal serum phosphate is characteristic of primary hyperparathyroidism. Excess bone resorption results in declining bone mass, especially in cortical bone. This is best assessed with bone density measurements in the forearm. Although rare, in severe cases of hyperparathyroidism cysts may form in the bone, giving rise to osteitis fibrosa cystica.[31]

Most patients with mild hyperparathyroidism are asymptomatic. In contrast, patients with more advanced disease present with renal calculi, bone pain, and vague generalized arthralgias (Box 29-9).

Collaborative Care Management

Diagnostic Tests. The initial diagnostic tests for primary hyperparathyroidism are serum calcium, phosphorus, and

BOX 29-9 Hypersecretion of Parathyroid Hormone: Pathophysiologic Alterations and Clinical Manifestations

Increase in calcium resorption from bone resulting in hypercalcemia, decreased bone mass, bone cysts, and fractures that can be characterized by bone pain and arthralgias
Alteration in urinary calcium excretion during course of the disease
Early: disease: hypocalciuria
Later: hypercalciuria with polyuria, polydipsia, nephrolithiasis, and kidney failure
Decreased renal bicarbonate and phosphate reabsorption
Symptoms include hyperchloremic acidosis, anorexia, nausea, and vomiting.
Increased gastrin secretion may cause peptic ulcer disease.
Increased renal activation of vitamin D produces calcitriol, increasing gastrointestinal calcium absorption, thereby adding to the hypercalcemia.
Depression of nerve and muscle activity from hypercalcemia
Cardiac muscle signs and symptoms include hypertension and electrocardiographic changes such as shortened QT intervals and dysrhythmias.
Neuromuscular signs and symptoms may include impaired mentation, apathy, lethargy, somnolence, hypoactive deep tendon reflexes, fasciculation of the tongue, muscle weakness, and myalgias (lower limbs more than upper limbs).
Gastrointestinal signs and symptoms include anorexia, nausea, vomiting, and constipation.
Hypercalcemia may cause pancreatitis.

PTH levels. Various PTH assays have evolved over the last several years, including C-terminal, N-terminal, midmolecule, and intact PTH. The most reliable and clinically useful assay is the intact PTH assay.[32] The combination of an elevated serum calcium, low normal/subnormal serum phosphate, and elevated intact PTH level generally confirms the diagnosis (see Chapter 28).

Results of tests indicative of primary hyperparathyroidism include:

- Blood: elevated serum calcium, decreased serum phosphate, elevated PTH levels
- Urinary: elevated 24-hour urinary calcium excretion
- Radiographic: reduced bone mineral density, presence of renal calculi

When the results do not meet the preceding criteria, an alternative explanation for hypercalcemia must be sought (Box 29-10). Malignancy is the most common alternative explanation for hypercalcemia when primary hyperparathyroidism is not present. In general, patients with hypercalcemia of malignancy usually have obvious features of malignancy such as cachexia and weight loss, with many indeed having a previously diagnosed malignancy. Malignant cells can produce a PTH-like compound, parathyroid hormone-related protein, which can bind to and stimulate PTH receptors with resultant hypercalcemia. This so-called humoral hypercalcemia of malignancy is usually seen in patients with a large tumor burden,

BOX 29-10 Causes of Hypercalcemia (Other Than Hyperparathyroidism)

Malignancy
Leukemia, lymphoma, multiple myeloma
Vitamin D intoxication
Granulomatous diseases (sarcoidosis)
Other endocrine disorders: thyrotoxicosis, adrenal insufficiency
Milk-alkali syndrome
Immobilization
Medication-induced (thiazides, lithium, aminophylline, gonadal steroids, vitamin D)

and patients generally have a poor prognosis related to the underlying malignancy.[6]

Medications/Treatments. Acute medical intervention to lower serum calcium is reserved for patients who are symptomatic from the hypercalcemia (anorexia/nausea/vomiting) and generally occurs in persons with serum calcium levels greater than 13 mg/dl. Long-term medical management is rarely undertaken except when patients are poor surgical candidates.[6, 31]

The immediate treatment is to correct any dehydration and promote fluid intake of 2 to 3 L/day unless contraindicated. Activity should be encouraged to promote resorption of calcium by the bone. Thiazide diuretics promote renal calcium retention and are contraindicated in this setting. Loop diuretics such as furosemide reduce renal calcium resorption, but should be used cautiously because of the long-term risk of worsening bone disease. If given to a patient with dehydration, furosemide may worsen prerenal kidney failure.

Diuresis results in significant lowering of serum calcium and symptomatic patient improvement. Effects are temporary and cease when treatment is discontinued. Bisphosphonates have been used to control the hypercalcemia of primary hyperparathyroidism with intravenous pamidronate or oral alendronate. Effects are also transient.

Estrogen therapy in postmenopausal women has been used as adjunctive therapy with modest effects on the serum calcium. The rationale behind estrogen therapy is that it somewhat antagonizes the bone resorbing action of PTH. Oral and intravenous phosphate is seldom used because of concerns about ectopic calcifications in soft tissues. Phosphate can interfere with the absorption of calcium, renal hydroxylation of vitamin D, and bone resorption.

Patients who are not surgical candidates should be monitored regularly to monitor disease progress. The patient's serum calcium and electrolytes, albumin, creatinine, and alkaline phosphatase levels should be evaluated at regular intervals. Bone densitometry and renal ultrasound should be done every 1 to 2 years.

Surgical Management. Surgery is the definitive therapy for primary hyperparathyroidism and is usually curative. Surgical intervention is used to[24]:

Prevent progression of preexisting complications of the disease (renal calculi, overt bone disease, fracture, life-threatening hypercalcemia)

Prevent development of complications in high risk patients, with high risk defined as:

Serum calcium >1 mg/dl above the upper limit of normal

Age <50 years

Marked hypercalciuria (>400 mg/24 hr)

Bone mineral density at the distal radius more than 2 standard deviations below age and sex-matched subjects Z-score ≤ −2.0)

In most cases the procedure is removal of a solitary adenoma. In the case of four-gland hyperplasia, the approach is to remove 3½ glands, leaving the half-gland remnant in the neck or autotransplanting it in the nondominant forearm. The half-gland is left because if all the parathyroid glands were removed, permanent hypoparathyroidism would result. Operative success can be readily confirmed by intraoperative PTH assay; results are available within 15 minutes. This intraoperative assay has clearly assisted in reducing the need for repeat surgery for hyperparathyroidism.

In some centers parathyroidectomy is routinely being carried out with the patient under local anesthesia, and results are comparable to those completed with the patient under general anesthesia. Minimally invasive surgery using perioperative radioisotope localization of abnormal parathyroid tissue with a gamma probe holds additional promise of success.[6]

Preoperative Localization Testing. In the patient with no prior neck surgery, an experienced parathyroid surgeon finds the abnormal parathyroid gland(s) in more than 90% of instances without any prior localization procedure. In the patient who has had prior neck surgery with resultant distortion of anatomic landmarks, however, most physicians support the use of preoperative localization to reduce the length of surgery and increase operative success. Several preoperative localization tests have been used including ultrasonography, CT, MRI, and radioisotope (technetium-sestimibi) scintigraphy. This latter dual isotopic method is currently the most preferred method in clinical practice. It is not uncommon for studies to be falsely positive, and two different studies are frequently ordered to increase the confidence in the localization.[31]

Diet. Dietary calcium intake for the patient with hyperparathyroidism should be moderate, with high intake being clearly undesirable. Low calcium intake may also be undesirable, as this will potentially cause further stimulation of PTH secretion and worsening bone disease.

The patient with significant hypercalcemia managed medically needs careful monitoring to ensure adequate hydration, normal electrolytes, normal blood urea nitrogen and serum creatinine, and normal serum phosphorus with optimum control of the serum calcium. Patients need a fluid intake of at least 2 L/day assuming the absence of underlying/limiting cardiac/renal processes and must further increase their fluid intake when outside temperatures are high because of increased insensible fluid losses via sweat.

Activity. Because of the myopathy, myalgia, and arthralgia patients often experience, range of motion exercises and ambulation are encouraged to prevent muscle atrophy and further deterioration of mobility. Walking and weight-bearing exercise should be encouraged to promote bone calcification. Safety measures should be instituted to prevent falls and injury that may result in fracture.

Referrals. Referrals to physical therapy may be indicated for muscle strengthening and progressive ambulation, particularly if bony deformities are present. Assessment of the patient's and/or family's ability to manage the therapeutic regimen at home is necessary.

NURSING MANAGEMENT OF PATIENT UNDERGOING PARATHYROID SURGERY

PREOPERATIVE CARE

Routine preoperative assessment and teaching are discussed in Chapter 16. The patient having parathyroid surgery requires explanations regarding the pathophysiology of hyperparathyroidism and hypercalcemia. If renal damage has occurred, some changes may not be reversible. The family should be involved if possible, particularly if mental status changes are present. The nurse should assess the home environment and availability of caregivers after surgery.

Patients with primary hyperparathyroidism have an increased risk of fall injuries as a result of musculoskeletal weakness and/or altered mental status. The patient with altered mental status should be placed in an environment where he or she can be observed closely, measures to increase orientation are used, and side rails of the bed are kept raised. Patients with weakness need assistance for changing positions and ambulating and should wear nonskid slippers for ambulation. The room should be free of unnecessary equipment. A gradual increase in activity and the incorporation of isometric exercise may increase endurance.

Hypercalcemia associated with primary hyperparathyroidism presents a risk for decreased cardiac functioning. The patient's vital signs should be monitored every 2 to 4 hours, and the patient should be instructed to report any palpitations or vertigo. If cardiac dysfunction occurs, the patient may need continuous cardiac monitoring. The patient treated with digitalis therapy must be monitored closely for digitalis toxicity because the myocardium is unusually sensitive to digitalis in the presence of hypercalcemia; the dosage of digitalis may need to be decreased.

If the patient is hospitalized before surgery, increasing fluid intake before imposing "nothing by mouth" restrictions is important. Increasing the fluid intake to decrease the urinary mineral concentration helps prevent formation of renal calculi formation. A fluid intake of at least 2 L/day should be the goal unless other physiologic alterations such as cardiac or renal problems are present. The urine should be strained through a gauze mesh to collect any small renal calculi that pass. The patient is monitored continually for renal calculi (see Chapter 39). Intake and output are measured and the patient is observed for flank pain, hematuria, and nausea and

BOX 29-11 Foods High in Calcium

Almonds	332 mg/1 cup
Blackstrap molasses	137 mg/1 tbsp
Brazil nuts	260 mg/1 cup
Broccoli spears	132 mg/1 cup
Cabbage (cooked)	220 mg/1 cup
Canned mackerel	221 mg/3 oz
Cheese (blue cheese, cheddar, American)	About 100 to 150 mg/1 oz
Collard greens (cooked)	289 mg/1 cup
Custard	280 mg/1 cup
Dandelion greens (cooked)	252 mg/1 cup
Egg	27 mg/1 egg
Green beans	80 mg/1 cup
Ice cream	175 mg/1 cup
Ice milk	292 mg/1 cup
Kale (cooked)	147 mg/1 cup
Lima beans	75 mg/1 cup
Macaroni (enriched) and cheese, baked	398 mg/1 cup
Milk (whole, 2%, skim, buttermilk)	290 mg/1 cup
Mustard greens (cooked)	193 mg/1 cup
Oranges	50 mg/1 orange
Oysters	226 mg/1 cup
Peanut halves	107 mg/1 cup
Pizza (cheese)	107 mg/1 slice
Raisins	124 mg/1 cup
Rhubarb (cooked)	212 mg/1 cup
Salmon, pink, canned	167 mg/3 oz
Sardines	372 mg/3 oz
Spinach (drained solids)	212 mg/1 cup
Turnip greens (cooked)	250 mg/1 cup
White sauce, medium	305 mg/1 cup
Yogurt	295 mg/1 cup

vomiting. The patient is advised to avoid foods high in calcium (Box 29-11) to limit hypercalcemia.

POSTOPERATIVE CARE

Postoperative care requirements specific to parathyroid surgery are detailed in the Guidelines for Safe Practice box. Potential physiologic complications include hemorrhage, hypocalcemia, and airway obstruction. The patient's respiratory, cardiovascular, neurologic, and fluid volume states are monitored routinely. A tracheostomy set should be at the patient's bedside for emergency use. The serum calcium level decreases within 24 hours, and the patient should be monitored for tetany. Parathyroid function usually returns to normal within 5 to 7 days after a partial parathyroidectomy because the remaining tissue resumes normal functioning.

If mild hypocalcemia occurs, oral calcium is given. Severe hypocalcemia can occur if there has been extensive decrease in bone mass. As the PTH level declines, the calcium-deficient bones extract larger-than-normal quantities of calcium from the extracellular fluids—the "hungry bone syndrome." For patients with severe hypocalcemia, calcium chloride or calcium gluconate is given intravenously. These calcium preparations

Guidelines for Safe Practice

Care of the Patient After Parathyroidectomy

Care for the patient after parathyroidectomy is similar to that after thyroid surgery. Priorities of care are lowering serum calcium levels and preventing renal complications. In most patients serum calcium levels will return to normal within 24 hours. However, mild hypocalcemia may occur after a rapid decrease in serum calcium levels. This transient decrease in serum calcium is usually treated with intravenous calcium infusion.

In patients with significant parathyroid bone disease, the risk of postoperative hypocalcemia is increased. Treatment is usually intravenous calcium infusion and frequent monitoring of serum calcium levels. These patients may require supplemental calcium and an active vitamin D metabolite for weeks or months after surgery.

Monitor respiratory status and vital signs every 2 to 4 hours to detect changes in neurologic status and neuromuscular and cardiac function; provide explanations for frequent vital signs and neurologic assessments.

Have tracheostomy tray and intravenous calcium preparations readily available.

Report any signs of respiratory obstruction, laryngeal stridor, recurrent laryngeal nerve damage, or hemorrhage.

Assess patient for quality of voice, dyspnea, choking sensation; tracheal obstruction may occur with vocal cord spasm or hemorrhage.

Assess mental status and motor strength; implement safety interventions if signs of decreased mental status or weakness are present.

Keep head of bed elevated 30 degrees to facilitate respirations. Encourage deep breathing, coughing, and turning.

Monitor serum calcium, magnesium, and electrolytes; assess for presence of tetany and paresthesias.

Encourage fluids, at least 3 L/day unless contraindicated to maintain fluid balance and promote calcium excretion; avoid dehydration.

Monitor and record input and output; weigh patient daily; assess for signs of fluid volume imbalance.

Strain urine for renal calculi; teach patient signs of renal colic (see Chapter 39).

Encourage early ambulation to promote bone resorption, decrease muscle atrophy, and decrease complications associated with immobility; inactivity will decrease the rate of calcium deposition in the bone

Teach the patient and family to recognize signs of hypercalcemia (anorexia, nausea, vomiting, constipation, weakness, apathy, somnolence, coma), hypocalcemia (paresthesias, muscle cramps, irritability, convulsions), and infection and to notify physician if these signs occur.

Avoid medications that may cause increase serum calcium levels, including thiazides, vitamin D preparations.

Provide information regarding calcium in the diet: recommendations for dietary intake of calcium will depend on serum levels; hypercalcemia is to be prevented, but intake must be allow for sufficient serum levels to promote bone recalcification.

Provide information for follow-up care; stress importance of periodic assessment of serum calcium levels.

should be readily available for immediate administration if necessary. If permanent hypoparathyroidism results because the remaining tissue does not resume normal secretion or because a total parathyroidectomy is done, the patient will need continued treatment.

Patient/Family Education

Patient and family teaching begins with assessment of their current knowledge of the disease, diagnostic tests, and therapeutic measures; identification of barriers to learning; and determination of the type and amount of information wanted. Dietary instruction about calcium is provided as needed, and the patient and family are helped to plan ways of meeting dietary requirements. For every prescribed medication, the name, purpose, dosage, special administration requirements, side effects, and signs and symptoms to report immediately need to be taught. This information should be explained, and written instructions provided for reference. The need for follow-up care must be stressed, and plans for it clarified with the patient and family.

Teaching can help the patient cope more effectively with changes. Frequent reexplanations may be required for the person with altered mental functioning. Anxiety may also interfere with the person's ability to learn and process information.

The family is included in the teaching. Patients receiving medical therapy need written and verbal instructions about comfort measures, safety, diet, activities, increased fluid intake, prevention of constipation, medications, and planned follow-up care.

SPECIAL ENVIRONMENTS FOR CARE

Critical Care

Indications for critical care management for the patient with hyperparathyroidism are similar to those for the patient recovering from thyroid surgery. Intensive care monitoring and nursing are needed if complications develop, such as hemorrhage, respiratory distress, or significant electrolyte imbalance.

COMPLICATIONS

Complications of parathyroid resection are rare in the hands of a skilled surgical team. Rare but significant acute complications include vocal cord spasm, hemorrhage, tracheal obstruction, and laryngeal stridor. Chronic complications include hoarseness from recurrent laryngeal nerve damage and permanent hypoparathyroidism.

After surgery there is usually adequate parathyroid tissue to maintain calcium and phosphorus metabolism. The patient should be monitored for development of hypocalcemia. If the remaining parathyroid gland(s) is/are too small or nonfunctioning, some of the tissue removed can be implanted into the forearm. The excised gland must have been cryopreserved at the time of surgery to allow reimplantation.

Secondary/Tertiary Hyperparathyroidism

Etiology and Pathophysiology

Failure to absorb adequate amounts of calcium and vitamin D from the gastrointestinal tract, failure to activate vitamin D in the liver or the kidney, and excessive catabolism of vitamin D result in downward drift in serum calcium. To maintain normal serum calcium, a compensatory increase in PTH secretion *(secondary hyperparathyroidism)* occurs to maintain serum calcium levels. Secondary hyperparathyroidism is therefore a situation of hyperplasia in response to compromised calcium balance most commonly caused by gastrointestinal or renal disease. Chronic secondary hyperparathyroidism can occasionally result in *tertiary hyperparathyroidism* where a PTH-producing adenoma is formed and is unresponsive to the normal feedback loop. Exceptionally high PTH levels ensue with resultant hypercalcemia. In both secondary and tertiary hyperparathyroidism, a marked decrease in bone mass is to be expected.

Collaborative Care Management

Treatment of secondary hyperparathyroidism revolves around treating the underlying disease responsible for the derangement of calcium balance. If the disease is progressive and irreversible (e.g., chronic kidney failure), augmentation of calcium intake and supplementation with 1,25-hydroxy vitamin D in addition to normalizing the serum phosphate elevation will minimize the secondary hyperparathyroidism.[6]

In the case of tertiary hyperparathyroidism, surgical therapy is needed to remove the autonomously functioning adenoma. This will ultimately revert the patient to a state of secondary hyperparathyroidism, previously discussed. Postoperative nursing measures are the same as for the patient with primary hyperparathyroidism who has undergone surgical excision.

Patient/Family Education. Care of patients with secondary hyperparathyroidism primarily involves teaching about the pathophysiology of the disease and the prescribed medication regimen. Teaching needs of patients with tertiary hyperparathyroidism who have undergone surgical excision of an adenoma are the same as those of the patient with primary hyperparathyroidism. After surgery, the patient will exhibit secondary hyperparathyroidism and will need medication instruction.

HYPOSECRETION OF PARATHYROID HORMONE: HYPOPARATHYROIDISM

Etiology/Epidemiology

Hypoparathyroidism is an uncommon endocrine disorder in which hypocalcemia occurs as a result of inadequate PTH secretion or impaired PTH action in target tissues. Transient hypoparathyroidism is often a complication of neck surgery. The risk of transient hypothyroidism after parathyroid or thyroid surgery is approximately 1% to 10%. Recovery often occurs within days to weeks after surgery. Permanent hypoparathyroidism can be the result of congenital absence of the parathyroids as in DiGeorge syndrome, or of destruction of the glands. Gland destruction can occur secondary to surgery, particularly radical head or neck surgery; infarction; infiltrative disorders such as hemochromatosis and Wilson's disease; or autoimmune disease. Hypoparathyroidism can also result from impaired secretion as in hypomagnesemia, or from impaired action as with pseudohypoparathyroidism.

Pathophysiology

Most cases of hypoparathyroidism are diagnosed when hypocalcemia occurs after neck surgery. Symptoms vary, depending on the onset, duration, and extent of hypocalcemia (see Clinical Manifestations box). Mild cases may be relatively asymptomatic. Patients with pseudohypoparathyroidism have additional skeletal and developmental abnormalities most characteristically being unilateral or bilateral shortening of the fourth and fifth metacarpals. In addition, mental retardation, short stature, stocky body, and short neck are commonly present. In contrast to other hypoparathyroid entities, these patients have elevated PTH levels in addition to hypercalcemia and hyperphosphatemia.[21]

Collaborative Care Management

Parathyroid hormone replacement therapy for PTH-deficient patients is not a clinically viable option. Dietary measures to increase calcium intake and decrease phosphate intake have a negligible therapeutic effect and are not recommended. Thus the generally used treatment is calcium supplementation (either as calcium carbonate or calcium citrate) coupled with vitamin D supplementation, generally in the form of calcitriol (1,25-hydroxy vitamin D) for ease of adjustment/titratability. Because the loss of PTH action at the level of the kidney results in renal calcium wasting or hypercalciuria, augmenting calcium and vitamin D to achieve a midnormal serum calcium causes significant hypercalciuria and risk of renal calculi. Hence the goal of therapy is to maintain low-normal levels of serum calcium to control symptoms and minimize the risk of hypercalciuria and renal stone formation. Fluid intake should be increased to decrease the urinary mineral concentration and decrease formation of renal calculi. A fluid intake of at least 2 L/day is recommended unless contraindicated. Fluid intake must be increased in hot weather due to an increase in insensible fluid losses.

Patients need an eye examination every 1 to 2 years to screen for cataracts, as well as careful clinical follow-up monitoring to ensure adherence to and success of their therapeutic regimen. Nonadherence can have serious sequelae including tetany, seizures, and mental status changes. Presence of a positive Chvostek's sign or Trousseau's sign during a patient follow-up examination is indicative of a subtherapeutic regimen.

Patient/Family Education. Patient teaching is a critical component of therapy. The patient needs to understand:

- Basic pathophysiology of the disease
- Medication administration
  - Calcium is administered in divided doses
    - Carbonate formulation taken with food as hydrochloric acid is needed for absorption
    - Citrate formulation can be taken irrespective of food intake
  - Vitamin D and phosphate binders
- The need for on-going medical follow-up care every 3 to 6 months
- Self-monitoring for signs of
  - Hypocalcemia (muscle spasms, tetany, declining mental status)
  - Hypercalcemia (thirst, polyuria, decreased muscle tone, constipation)
  - Complications (renal calculi manifesting as renal colic [i.e., flank pain with or without radiation to the groin])
- Importance of diet: foods high in calcium but low in phosphorus (processed cheese, yogurt, milk)
- Importance of wearing a Medic-Alert bracelet

Clinical Manifestations

True Hypoparathyroidism

1. Neuromuscular manifestations: changes in nerve activity affect peripheral motor and sensory nerves
   a. Paresthesias around mouth, tips of fingers, and sometimes in the feet
   b. Tetany with positive Chvostek's and Trousseau's signs (see Chapter 13), spasms of wrists, fingers, forearms, feet, and back
   c. Seizures that may consist of syncopal spells, tonic spasms of the total body, or the more typical tonic-clonic activity
   d. Hyperventilation/laryngospasm/bronchospasm/respiratory alkalosis
   e. Other neurologic signs: headache, papilledema, elevated cerebrospinal fluid pressure, local signs that mimic a cerebral tumor; extrapyramidal neurologic signs and symptoms, including gait changes, tremors, rigidity and spasms. These symptoms are seen almost exclusively in patients with calcification of the basal ganglia.
2. Emotional-mental manifestations: irritability, depression, anxiety, emotional lability, impairment of memory and cognitive function, confusion, frank psychosis
3. Cardiovascular manifestations (effect of hypocalcemia)
   a. Prolonged QT and ST intervals and occasional dysrhythmias
   b. Resistance to effects of digitalis preparations
   c. Decreased cardiac output from congestive heart failure
4. Eye manifestations: cataract formation
5. Dental manifestations (depending on age of onset)
   a. Enamel defects seen on the tooth crown
   b. Delayed or absent tooth eruption
   c. Defective dental root formation
6. Integumentary manifestations: fragile nails, thin patchy hair, dry scaly skin, mucocutaneous candidiasis, impetigo herpetiformis
7. Gastrointestinal manifestations: malabsorption

ADRENAL GLAND

Disorders of the adrenal gland may be classified as disorders of the cortex, medulla, or glomulerosa. Hyperfunction gives rise to distinct clinical syndromes: Cushing's syndrome, hyperaldosteronism, and pheochromocytoma with symptoms occurring as a result of excess hormone production. Hypofunction of the adrenal cortex in terms of cortisol production is fatal if untreated. In contrast, lack of the adrenal medulla, which occurs after bilateral adrenalectomy, is compatible with normal bodily function.

ADRENAL CORTEX

Hypersecretion of Cortisol: Cushing's Syndrome

Etiology

Excess circulating glucocorticoids can occur as a result of disorders at different levels of the hypothalamic-pituitary-adrenal axis (Figure 29-8). Clinical manifestations of glucocorticoid excess are illustrated in Figure 29-9 and are readily identified on a careful clinical examination. Milder degrees of glucocorticoid excess pose a diagnostic challenge as well as the pseudo-Cushings' syndrome seen in some depressed patients and patients with obesity. Additionally, diagnostic dilemmas occur in the patient with an incidentally discovered adrenal nodule on abdominal CT scanning for other reasons (adrenal incidentaloma).[3]

Epidemiology

The most common cause of noniatrogenic Cushing's is a pituitary adenoma (approximately 60% of cases) in which excess ACTH production results in excess glucocorticoid production. Second to pituitary adenoma is primary adrenal neoplasm/hyperplasia (approximately 25% of cases), with ectopic ACTH or corticotropin-releasing hormone (CRH) accounting for the remaining 15%. The most common ectopic source is an ACTH-producing pulmonary neoplasm such as a bronchial carcinoid or lung cancer. Cushing's syndrome, whether of pituitary or primary adrenal origin, is more common in women than in men. The estimated incidence of pituitary Cushing's (Cushing's disease, in which there is a tumor producing excess ACTH) is estimated at 5 to 25 cases per 1 million persons per year. The incidence of iatrogenic Cushing's syndrome is unknown, but because more than 10 million patients in the United States are on chronic glucocorticoid therapy, the incidence has to be relatively high.

Pathophysiology

Regardless of the etiology of noniatrogenic Cushing's syndrome, the first discernible abnormality is the loss of diurnal variation in cortisol secretion. The morning serum cortisol levels may be at the high end of the normal range, but the evening level may not show the normal decline. Therefore a single fasting serum cortisol is not a reliable marker of cortisol excess.

The pathophysiologic sequelae of cortisol excess involve multiple systems and are outlined in Box 29-12. In many instances patients may be treated for the secondary metabolic dysfunction such as diabetes mellitus or hypertension before a diagnosis of Cushing's syndrome is considered. Emotional lability and psychiatric changes may dominate the clinical picture in some patients. Anterior pituitary dysfunction is also common where secretion of gonadotropins and other hormones may be altered with resultant secondary organ hypofunction (e.g., amenorrhea). Adrenal androgen overproduction concurrent with cortisol excess is common, with resultant hirsutism and acne.

Collaborative Care Management

Diagnostic Tests. The most important initial diagnostic test in the patient with suspected Cushing's syndrome is confirmation of excess glucocorticoid production. The 24-hour urine free cortisol is probably the single best test for making a diagnosis of Cushing's syndrome. The false-positive rate is less than 4% and the false-negative rate less than 6%. The 1-mg overnight dexamethasone suppression test is also a useful screening test; it has a false-negative rate less than 2%, but a high false-positive rate (see Chapter 28).

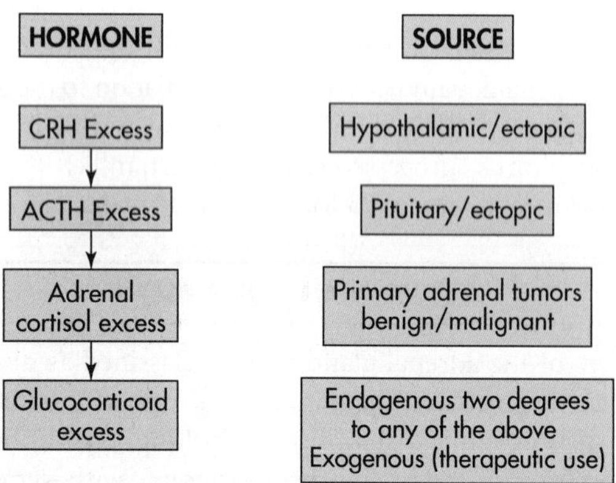

Figure 29-8 Hypothalamic-pituitary-adrenal axis and Cushing's syndrome: possible pathways to cortisol excess. *ACTH,* Adrenocorticotropic hormone; *CRH,* corticotropin-releasing hormone.

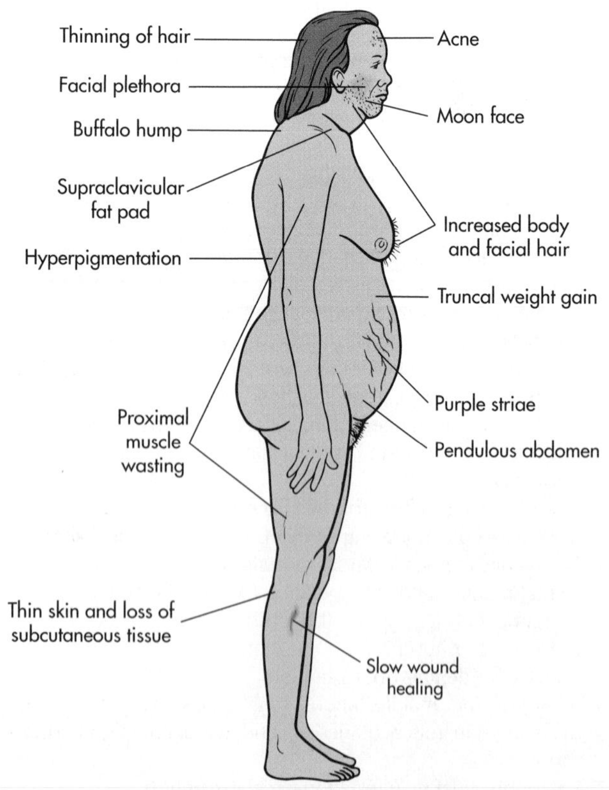

Figure 29-9 Common characteristics of Cushing's syndrome.

Once glucocorticoid excess has been documented, it must be determined whether or not it is ACTH-dependent (pituitary/ectopic) or ACTH-independent (adrenal neoplasm). In ACTH-independent Cushing's syndrome, the ACTH is appropriately low/subnormal secondary to pituitary suppression, whereas in the ACTH-dependent Cushing's syndrome, the ACTH is high normal/frankly elevated.

Pituitary Cushing's syndrome can be evaluated by an 8-mg overnight dexamethasone suppression test (see Chapter 28), in which 8 mg of dexamethasone are taken at 11 PM and the fasting serum cortisol is measured at 8 AM the next day. The patient with pituitary Cushing's syndrome exhibits a more than 50% reduction in the morning serum cortisol measurement. This test carries a sensitivity of 89% and a specificity of 100% and has clear advantages over some of the other diagnostic tests.[7]

If results of ACTH levels are borderline, a CRH stimulation test is of value. Corticotropin-releasing hormone is administered as an intravenous bolus, and serum values for cortisol and ACTH are drawn at 15-, 30-, 60-, 90-, and 120-minute

BOX 29-12 Hypercortisolism: Pathophysiologic Alterations and Clinical Manifestations

Alteration in Protein, Fat, and Carbohydrate Metabolism

Altered Protein Metabolism

Excessive catabolism of proteins results in loss of muscle mass, causing the following symptoms:

1. Proximal muscle wasting and weakness, which may be characterized by difficulty getting up from low chairs, difficulty climbing stairs, or generalized weakness and fatigue
2. Depletion of protein matrix of bone, resulting in osteoporosis, compression fractures of spine, backache, bone pain, and pathologic fractures
3. Loss of collagen support of skin, resulting in thin, fragile skin that bruises easily, ecchymosis at trauma sites, and purple striae
4. Poor wound healing

Altered Fat Metabolism

Changes in fat metabolism with abnormal deposition of fat in the face producing moon face (see Figure 29-9), in the interscapular area producing a "buffalo hump" and in the mesenteric bed producing truncal obesity. Redistribution of fat with these characteristic features may be seen in patients without overt obesity. Body weight usually is increased.

Altered Carbohydrate Metabolism

Increased hepatic gluconeogenesis and impaired insulin utilization result in postprandial hyperglycemia and occasionally frank diabetes mellitus with all its signs and symptoms (see Chapter 30). Patients with concurrent diabetes mellitus may experience worsening hyperglycemia.

Alteration in Inflammatory and Immune Response

Cortisol excess results in decreased lymphocytes, particularly T lymphocytes, decreased cell-mediated immunity, increased neutrophils, and altered antibody activity. These changes make persons particularly vulnerable to viral and fungal infections. Depression in inflammatory and immune responsiveness results in opportunistic infections such as *Pneumocystis carinii* or other fungal infections. Early signs of infection, such as fever, may not be seen. Poor wound healing may also be related to infections.[17]

Alterations in Water and Mineral Metabolism

Cortisol itself possesses mineralocorticoid activity; therefore, cortisol excess results in characteristic signs and symptoms of increased mineralocorticoid activity even though the level of aldosterone is normal. These include:

1. Sodium and water retention, which may accentuate body weight increase, may cause edema, and may expand blood volume; serum sodium usually normal
2. Hypertension, which is found in almost every patient with excessive cortisol and may be caused by increased volume or increased sensitivity of arterioles to circulating catecholamines
3. Hypochloremia and metabolic alkalosis (with severe cortisol excess) due to increased excretion of potassium and chloride (most often seen with ectopic Cushing's syndrome). Hypokalemia is unusual except with ectopic adrenocorticotropic hormone (ACTH).
4. Increased calcium resorption from the bones and renal calculi from hypercalciuria, resulting in renal colic

Alteration in Emotional Stability

Various emotional changes may occur: from irritability and anxiety, mild depression and poor concentration and memory, to severe depression and psychosis. Euphoria and sleep disorders are frequently noted. These may be the presenting signs and symptoms.

Hematologic Alterations

1. Various changes in blood components, which occur as the result of excessive cortisol
2. Normal to high red blood cell count, hemoglobin, and hematocrit (may account in part for facial plethora)
3. Leukocytosis, lymphopenia, eosinopenia
4. Increases in various clotting factors and platelets, resulting in thromboembolic phenomena

Excessive Androgen Activity

If excessive androgens are present, female patients exhibit virilization, which includes the following signs:

1. Hirsutism, manifested initially as fine, downy coat of hair on face and body
2. Male pattern hair loss
3. Acne
4. Changes in menstrual cycle, varying from irregularities to oligomenorrhea to amenorrhea
5. Changes in libido

Other Findings

Hyperpigmentation on the skin and mucous membranes may be present and indicates elevation of ACTH, which may be from an ectopic site or the pituitary. ACTH (which has melanotrophic activity) levels are higher and therefore hyperpigmentation is more common and significant from ectopic sources than from the pituitary.

intervals. Pituitary-dependent Cushing's syndrome will result in a rise in ACTH levels; in ectopic and adrenal Cushing's syndrome, there is no significant change in the ACTH level. False-positive tests for cortisol excess can occur (Box 29-13). Imaging studies are indicated if there is clear documentation of cortisol excess and dynamic tests to indicate the source (i.e., pituitary versus adrenal versus ectopic) (Table 29-5). If the lesion is not visible by imaging techniques, bilateral inferior petrosal sinus sampling for ACTH levels is of value in lateralizing the tumor for the transsphenoidal surgeon.

Medications. Medical therapy for Cushing's syndrome is reserved for patients failing surgical therapy, cases in which surgical therapy is not feasible, or when the effects of radiation therapy are still pending. All these therapies revolve around inhibition of cortisol production in the adrenal glands. Medications used include ketoconazole, metyrapone, aminoglutethemide, and mitotane.[7]

Treatments

Pituitary irradiation for failed transsphenoidal surgery for pituitary Cushing's syndrome has the serious disadvantages of delayed effectiveness, perhaps for several years; the risk of panhypopituitarism; and potential neurologic damage. Conventional irradiation induces remission in 20% to 50% of adults, although other forms of radiation such as alpha particle or proton beam may potentially have higher success rates. The role of stereotactic irradiation such as the gamma knife is under investigation.

Surgical Management. Definitive management of noniatrogenic Cushing's syndrome revolves around identifying the cause; surgical cure is possible. In the case of pituitary Cushing's, transsphenoidal surgery should result in cure for 80% to 90% of patients. Morbidity is low and mortality is less than 1%. Complications include permanent diabetes insipidus and panhypopituitarism.

In the case of adrenal tumors, adrenalectomy is the treatment of choice; adrenalectomy can now be carried out laparoscopically in select patients. Bilateral adrenalectomy is the second line of management for patients who have failed transsphenoidal surgery for pituitary Cushing's syndrome. The mortality rate from adrenalectomy is 4% to 10% with a 1% risk of recurrent Cushing's syndrome as a result of growth of an adrenal remnant. In the case of bilateral adrenalectomy for failed transsphenoidal surgery, there is a 10% to 20% risk of Nelson's syndrome. Nelson's syndrome involves progressive enlargement of an ACTH-secreting pituitary tumor and associated hyperpigmentation and mass effects, including visual field compromise and headache. Definitive therapy for ectopic tumors producing ACTH involves resection of the primary neoplasm, (generally the lung) if feasible.

After surgery, patients with unilateral solitary adrenal tumors, ACTH-producing pituitary tumors, or ectopic ACTH-producing tumors have suppression of the normal ACTH-adrenal axis and require temporary physiologic cortisol replacement. Recovery of the normal ACTH-adrenal axis may take 6 to 24 months with gradual tapering of the cortisol replacement dose. Bilateral adrenalectomy patients require lifelong glucocorticoid and mineralcorticoid replacement (see section on Addison's disease for discussion of glucocorticoids and mineralcorticoids).[7]

BOX 29-13 Causes of a False-Positive Elevation of Cortisol

Persons with acute or chronic illnesses: Acute stressors may result in high cortisol levels and abnormal dexamethasone tests; these tests must be repeated after patient's condition is stable.

Obesity: This results in high levels of urinary 17-OHCS and 17-KGS and abnormal screening suppression tests, but urine free cortisol, serum cortisol, and response to standard suppression test are normal.

Pregnancy, estrogen therapy, and oral contraceptives: Elevated estrogen associated with these states can increase serum cortisol and give abnormal results on a screening cortisol suppression test, but urine free cortisol and response to standard suppression test are normal.

Alcoholism: Alcoholics may have both clinical and diagnostic characteristics of Cushing's syndrome, but abstinence from alcohol reverses signs, symptoms, and abnormal test results.

Depression: Endogenous depression results in increased cortisol levels, loss of diurnal rhythm, increased urine free cortisol, increased urine 17-OHCS and 17-KGS, and abnormal suppression tests; however, patients with depression have increased cortisol in response to insulin-induced hypoglycemia, whereas patients with true Cushing's syndrome do not.

TABLE 29-5 Diagnostic Imaging for Cortisol Excess

Suspected Source	Diagnostic Imaging	Disadvantage
Pituitary	Magnetic resonance imaging	The pituitary lesion that is the source of the adrenocorticotropic hormone (ACTH) excess is not seen in 50% of patients, owing to the small size of the lesion. The pituitary lesion that is noted may be an incidentaloma and not the source of the ACTH excess.
Adrenal	Adrenal computed tomography (CT)	The adrenal lesion noted may be an incidentaloma and not the cause of the cortisol excess.
Ectopic ACTH	Chest CT Abdominal CT	The CT scan may miss a lesion that is actually present.

Diet. Diet modifications are prescribed according to individual patient needs. Calories, sodium, lipids, and cholesterol are commonly restricted. If the patient becomes hyperglycemic or indeed develops diabetes mellitus, dietary management of blood glucose levels is indicated.

Activity. The patient with untreated Cushing's syndrome is usually obese with chronic fatigue. Patients may have muscle weakness and/or pathologic bone conditions. Maintenance of optimal activity is encouraged; activity restrictions are related to particular complications.

Referrals. Referrals to physical therapy may be helpful in assisting the patient with muscle strengthening and conditioning. The patient may need support in dealing with his or her feelings regarding changes in appearance associated with Cushing's syndrome. A referral to social service or a psychologist may be indicated.

NURSING MANAGEMENT OF PATIENT WITH CUSHING'S SYNDROME

ASSESSMENT

Health History

Information to be collected as part of the health history when assessing the patient with cortisol excess includes:

- Changes noted in body proportions, weight, hair distribution, pigmentation, bruising, delayed wound healing
- History of discomfort, particularly back pain
- History of frequent infections: skin, respiratory, yeast infections
- Neurologic data: changes noted in behavior, concentration, memory
- Nutritional data
  - Usual 24-hour food/fluid intake
  - History of increase in thirst
- Musculoskeletal data: complaints of weakness, fatigue, or difficulty doing normal activities
- Elimination data: changes in urine output
- Sexuality data: changes in menstrual history, secondary sexual characteristics, libido, or feelings about self
- Knowledge level: condition, treatment, diagnostic tests

Physical Examination

Physical examination of the patient with cortisol excess focuses on:

- General body appearance (presence of moon facies, buffalo hump, truncal obesity, proximal muscle wasting, hyperpigmentation, purple striae, ecchymoses, thin skin, facial plethora, unhealed wounds)
- Neurologic status: affect and its appropriateness to situation, short-term memory, concentration
- Cardiovascular status: blood pressure, pulse, presence of edema, jugular vein distention
- Nutritional status: intake and output, weight
- Musculoskeletal status: muscle mass and tone, strength, ability to stand up from a sitting position
- Elimination status: urine output, presence of glycosuria
- Sexuality in the female: secondary sexual characteristics, body and scalp hair distribution, presence of acne

NURSING DIAGNOSES

Nursing diagnoses are determined from analysis of patient data. Nursing diagnoses for the person with cortisol excess may include but are not limited to:

Diagnostic Title	Possible Etiologic Factors
1. Disturbed body image	Changes in body characteristics and functioning
2. Risk for infection	Decreased immune resistance caused by relative immunosuppression of hypercortisolism
3. Risk for injury (trauma)	Falls associated with muscle weakness and decreased bone mass, risk of pathologic fractures
4. Deficient knowledge	Lack of information regarding treatment plan

EXPECTED PATIENT OUTCOMES

Expected patient outcomes for the patient with cortisol excess may include but are not limited to:

1. Will have improved body image, as evidenced by speaking about self in positive terms; will participate in ADLs, leisure activities as tolerated

2a. Will detect early signs and symptoms of infections

2b. Will verbalize measures to prevent infection

3a. Will not fall or injure self

3b. Will verbalize measures to decrease risk of injury

4. Will verbalize knowledge of treatment plan, complications, need for long-term follow-up care

INTERVENTIONS

The patient with hypercortisolism can be critically ill. During the acute period, the primary focus of care is on the high-priority needs of supporting coping, restoring fluid balance, and preventing infections and injuries. In the more stable patient, these needs are still a focus of care.

1. Promoting Positive Body Image

A major focus of care is helping the patient deal with changes in body image, sexuality, and self-concept. Patients should know that some body changes are reversible with treatment. To help increase self-concept, patients are assisted in setting realistic goals. Clear explanations about changes in sexual characteristics and changes that will occur with treatment help patients to cope better. Including the patient's significant other can help alleviate anxiety regarding roles and relationships.

Helping the patient resume his or her usual activities can be beneficial to restoring a positive body image. This may require assisting with some activities that expend energy such as bathing. In addition, the nurse should space the patient's activities and provide rest periods between them. When electrolyte and fluid balance and glucose metabolism have been stabilized, the patient's energy level will increase, and therefore the activity level will increase. The patient can then assume a more active role in self-care activities. The patient should be reassured that symptoms should subside with treatment.

2. Preventing Infection

Temperature is taken every 4 hours, and the white blood cell is monitored. The mouth, lungs, and skin are checked every shift for early signs of infection; and, if present, they are reported immediately. Also the patient should be taught to self-assess the skin daily for signs of pressure or injury. Protective pads and an alternating air pressure mattress can be used to prevent skin breakdown, a source of potential infection. It is important to remember that the usual signs of inflammation may be masked by excess cortisol production.

The patient's exposure to possible pathogens must be minimized. The patient and family are taught proper handwashing techniques. Staff and visitors with signs and symptoms of upper respiratory infections are limited as is visitation by young children. Invasive procedures are avoided when possible, and aseptic technique is used when they must be done.

Routine turning, coughing, and deep breathing are instituted every 2 hours; oral hygiene is given before breakfast, after meals, and at bedtime.

3. Preventing Injury

The patient with excess cortisol production is at risk for injury due to decreased bone mass. The patient should be assisted in identifying potential sources of trauma and ways to minimize the risk of injury. Walking is recommended to promote bone calcification and shoes with nonskid soles should be encouraged. Exercises to increase muscle tone and strength should be encouraged. Avoidance of injury is important because of the risk of increased bleeding. The skin should be inspected for areas of ecchymosis. Isometric leg exercises and ambulation are important interventions to decrease the risk of thromboembolic events.

4. Patient/Family Education

Education of patients and significant others is ongoing. The patient needs basic information regarding the care being given and restrictions such as diet and preventing infection. Many diagnostic tests may be necessary, and careful explanations are given. Over time the patient needs information about the disease process and planned treatment, long-term care needs related to the disease process, and specific care for complications such as adrenal insufficiency, which can occur with some treatments. The patient should be taught to recognize the signs and symptoms of both adrenal insufficiency and excess.

Teaching should include information regarding diet: low sodium, encouraging foods rich in vitamin K, and limiting carbohydrates; a weight-reduction diet may be indicated. The patient should be taught to monitor body weight and to look for signs of fluid retention.

Instructions regarding prescribed medication should include the name, dosage, side effects, desired effects, interactions, and any necessary precautions. Persons with bilateral adrenalectomy require lifelong hormone replacement. The patient should be encouraged to obtain a Medic-Alert bracelet outlining diagnosis and treatment.

An explanation regarding the relationship between stress and hormone levels is vitally important. Consulting with the health care provider during times of great emotional or physical stress is beneficial; adjustment in medication dosages may be necessary. Assisting the patient to develop effective coping and relaxation methods to manage stress is an important intervention.

Health Promotion

Most causes of excessive cortisol production are not preventable. One exception is the ectopic secretion of ACTH from bronchogenic carcinoma, which could be prevented by decreasing the occurrence of bronchogenic carcinoma through elimination of smoking. No screening tests are available for secondary prevention. Evaluation of adrenal function depends on the clinical suspicion of the primary health care provider. Tertiary preventive activities should be a major focus of nursing care. Nurses should help patients deal with their chronic health problems, carry out self-monitoring practices to identify exacerbations early, and maintain their therapeutic regimens. These practices help prevent progression of problems. Patients receiving long-term glucocorticoid therapy are an important group for nurses to target for teaching. Through the role of patient educator, nurses can help patients carry out their therapy in the safest manner possible.

EVALUATION

To evaluate the effectiveness of nursing interventions, compare patient behaviors with those stated in the expected patient outcomes. Achievement of outcomes is successful if the patient with cortisol excess:

1. Demonstrates acceptance of changes in body image, role; speaks of self in positive terms; participates in ADLs and leisure activities to fullest extent possible.
2. Is free from infection; uses measures to prevent or minimize risk of infection.
3. Is free from injury; explains methods to reduce risk of injury.
4. Verbalizes knowledge of disease process, treatment plan, and plan for follow-up care.

SPECIAL ENVIRONMENTS FOR CARE

Critical Care

The patient who has undergone adrenal surgery is usually managed in the intensive care unit after surgery (see Guidelines for Safe Practice box). The high risk for adrenal crisis and need for invasive monitoring to maintain fluid and electrolyte balance after adrenalectomy necessitates intensive care nursing.

Hemodynamic monitoring (central venous pressure, blood pressure, pulse, and at times pulmonary wedge pressure) is done continuously. In addition, daily serum electrolyte concentrations, blood glucose levels every 4 hours, daily weights, and hourly intake and output are monitored.

Guidelines for Safe Practice

The Patient Undergoing Adrenal Surgery

Preoperative
1. Provide supportive care.
2. Assist patient with usual preoperative care.
3. Maintain nutritional status with a high-protein, prescribed-calorie diet with adequate minerals and vitamins.
4. Assist with correction of fluid and electrolyte imbalance.
5. Assist with hormonal therapy as prescribed.
6. Assist with measures used to prevent or treat crisis of adrenal hormonal excess or deficit.
7. Administer prescribed IV fluids and glucocorticoids before surgery.

Postoperative
1. Establish monitoring schedule to detect complications of surgery and:
   a. Adrenal crisis
   b. Blood pressure alterations
   c. Blood glucose alterations
   d. Fluid and electrolyte imbalances
2. Because the patient may have unusual activity intolerance, pace postoperative activities with alternate periods of rest and a gradual increase in self-care.
3. Provide measures to minimize effects of postural hypotension:
   a. Supply Ace bandages or elastic stockings.
   b. Assess effects of posture on blood pressure.
   c. Assist or accompany the patient during ambulation while blood pressure remains labile.
4. Provide measures to decrease risk of infection in the immunosuppressed patient (e.g., strict surgical asepsis, deep breathing, and avoiding contact with persons with infections).
5. Administer cortisol replacement as typically prescribed:
   a. IV route for the first 24 to 48 hours
   b. Oral route when patient is able to tolerate food by mouth
6. Administer mineralocorticosteroid (fludrocortisone) replacement, if prescribed; this is typically prescribed when cortisol replacement is less than 40 to 50 mg/24 hours in the patient with bilateral adrenalectomy.
7. Assist patient and family in learning about required hormonal replacement:
   a. Bilateral adrenalectomy–maintenance dose of cortisol and mineralocorticoids
   b. Unilateral adrenalectomy–doses of cortisol dependent on degree of suppression of hypothalamic-pituitary-adrenal

Intravenous cortisol replacement is continued for 24 to 48 hours after surgery. Fluids are given based on the clinical data and usually include saline/dextrose solutions. On the second postoperative day, mineralocorticoids may be started. By the third postoperative day, the patient is usually able to tolerate oral glucocorticoids and a normal diet. If unusual weakness or anorexia, nausea, or vomiting occurs, glucocorticoids are increased. If unusual hypotension occurs, mineralocorticoids and fluids are adjusted appropriately.

A major complication of surgery is poor wound healing and infection caused by the effects of excess cortisol. Strict aseptic technique is used with wound care. Other postoperative needs are similar to those described for the patient with adrenal insufficiency. Replacement therapy is necessary throughout life.

For the patient who has had a unilateral adrenalectomy, monitoring, hormonal support, fluid therapy, and other care needs are the same during the immediate postoperative period as for the patient with a bilateral adrenalectomy. After the patient's condition has stabilized and physiologic and psychologic crises have been successfully avoided, the glucocorticoid support is slowly withdrawn because eventually a single gland can maintain enough hormonal secretion for both daily living and additional stressors. When glucocorticoids are withdrawn, monitoring for signs and symptoms of adrenal insufficiency and crisis must be continued because the remaining gland may have atrophied. If signs and symptoms occur, glucocorticoids are restarted and then again slowly withdrawn.

COMPLICATIONS

Persons with Cushing's syndrome caused by pituitary adenoma and treated by transsphenoidal resection may experience complications described for hyperpituitarism. Persons treated with bilateral adrenalectomy require lifelong glucocorticoid and mineralocorticoid replacement therapy. Adrenal crisis is a potential complication. Occasionally severe side effects are associated with treatment of ectopic ACTH-secreting tumors with radiation or chemotherapy. If pituitary irradiation is used, panhypopituitarism or pituitary dysfunction may result. Effects of excess cortisol on the musculoskeletal system may result in (1) corticosteroid-induced osteoporosis with resultant pathologic fractures and (2) avascular necrosis, necessitating total joint replacement in some patients.

In addition, a patient who has chronic adrenal insufficiency and who needs surgery for an unrelated adrenal problem will require perioperative stress doses of steroids. This information should be included in discharge instructions.

Hypersecretion of Aldosterone

Etiology

Primary aldosterone excess is characterized by high levels of aldosterone with suppressed renin levels, hypertension, and hypokalemia. This must be distinguished from secondary aldosterone excess, which results from a variety of conditions (Box 29-14) causing hypoperfusion of the juxtoglomerular apparatus cells and therefore elevated renin levels. The most common cause of secondary hyperaldosteronism is congestive heart failure.

Epidemiology

Primary aldosteronism (PA) affects up to 12% of the hypertensive population and is twice as common in women as men for unknown reasons. It is now the most common cause of secondary hypertension. Findings suggestive of PA include:

BOX 29-14 Exogenous Causes of Secondary Aldosteronism

Cardiac failure
Liver disease
Hypovolemic states
Pregnancy
Idiopathic cyclic edema
Renal artery stenosis
Bartter's syndrome (hypertrophy and hyperplasia of the juxtaglomerular cells)

- Hypertension with hypokalemia
- Hypertension that is difficult to control
- Hypertension with an adrenal incidentaloma

Pathophysiology

Primary aldosteronism is due to bilateral angiotensin-responsive adrenal hyperplasia (also known as idiopathic hyperaldosteronism) in 70% of patients and unilateral aldosterone-producing adrenal cortical adenoma in 25% of patients. The remaining patients have rare causes: unilateral zona glomerulosa hyperplasia, glucocorticoid-suppressible aldosteronism, and aldosterone-producing adrenal cortical carcinoma.

The excess aldosterone produced stimulates the resorption of sodium in the renal tubules in exchange for potassium. The resultant volume expansion raises blood pressure without creating edema. Serum sodium levels tend to be at the upper end of the normal range or slightly elevated. Most persons have hypokalemia, except those with rare familial forms of PA. Most patients are asymptomatic; however, occasional neuromuscular complaints related to hypokalemia are reported. Excessive urinary loss of hydrogen ions results in mild alkalosis.[34,38]

Collaborative Care Management

In the patient suspected of having primary aldosteronism (hypertension and hypokalemia), diagnostic testing should be done with the patient not taking hypertensive medication for 2 to 4 weeks. Many antihypertensive agents affect the renin-angiotensin system, especially spironolactone and angiotensin-converting enzyme (ACE) inhibitors. Peripheral alpha-1 adrenergic blockers have the least potential to interfere with diagnostic testing for primary aldosteronism. A fasting early morning plasma aldosterone concentration (PAC) and plasma renin activity (PRA) are generally the fist approach to document excess PAC with suppressed PRA.[34]

After primary aldosteronism has been confirmed, adrenal CT or MRI scanning is performed. The scan may show unilateral adrenal adenoma or bilateral hyperplasia, or be near normal. When unilateral hyperplasia is suspected, bilateral adrenal vein sampling for aldosterone levels may be carried out. The result of adrenal vein sampling will show which adrenal gland is overproducing aldosterone.

Definitive therapy for primary aldosteronism is surgical removal of a unilateral adenoma, unilateral hyperplastic adrenal gland, or adrenal cancer. Aldosterone-producing adenomas can be removed laparoscopically. Patients may have residual hypertension on the basis of underlying essential hypertension even after successful removal of an adrenal tumor.

Pharmacologic therapy is used for all other etiologies. Spironolactone is the mainstay of drug therapy and, when not tolerated, ameloride may be used.[38] Alternatives for patients intolerant to spironolactone also include a diuretic with the addition of a calcium-channel blocker, beta-blocker, or ACE inhibitor.

Dietary sodium restriction (less than 100 mEq sodium/day), alcohol avoidance, regular aerobic exercise, and weight control are important in successful patient management. Evaluation and consultation with a registered dietitian are helpful. Spironolactone and/or ameloride correct the hypokalemia, and long-term potassium supplementation is frequently not needed.

Patient/Family Education. Nursing care, including teaching needs, for the care of the patient following adrenal surgery was discussed earlier. For patients who have had unilateral adrenalectomy, lifelong steroid replacement is not necessary. Patients treated nonsurgically need instructions regarding medications, including dosage, side effects, therapeutic effects, drug interactions, and any special precautions necessary. A consult with a dietitian may be helpful to provide instructions for a low-sodium, high-potassium diet. The patient should be taught to recognize the signs and symptoms of hypokalemia. Symptoms that warrant medical attention include weight gain, edema, weakness, palpitations, headache, or dyspnea.

Hyposecretion of the Adrenal Cortex: Hypocortisolism

Etiology

Cortisol deficiency results from alteration in any step in the hypothalamic-pituitary-adrenal axis (CRH deficiency, ACTH deficiency, or primary adrenal disease). Dysfunction may be temporary (transient ACTH deficiency after removal of an ACTH-producing pituitary adenoma) or permanent (adrenal suppression resulting from chronic glucocorticoid therapy).

Epidemiology

Permanent primary adrenal insufficiency is most commonly (70% of cases) due to acute autoimmune destruction *(Addison's disease)* of the adrenal glands. Patients with autoimmune adrenal failure may also have other autoimmune disease with endocrine gland failure. Tuberculosis of the adrenal gland accounts for 20% of cases of primary adrenal failure. The remaining 10% of cases are due to metastatic cancer, adrenal hemorrhage, surgical removal, acquired immunodeficiency syndrome, fungal infections, congenital adrenal hypoplasia, and other rare disorders.

Pathophysiology

The major distinguishing feature between primary and secondary adrenal insufficiency lies with the degree of skin pigmentation and mineralocorticoid deficiency. In terms of skin pigmentation, patients with primary adrenal failure have a compensatory large increase in ACTH and concurrent increase in melanocyte-stimulating hormone with resultant increase in skin pigmentation. In contrast, pallor is present in secondary adrenal failure where ACTH secretion is low. In terms of mineralocorticoid deficiency, patients with primary adrenal insufficiency are mineralocorticoid deficient; in contrast, patients with secondary adrenal insufficiency are not mineralocorticoid deficient and therefore do not exhibit electrolyte disturbances.

Slight hemodilution may be seen in secondary adrenal deficiency due to water retention as a result of increased ADH secretion; the patient may have a mild decrease in serum sodium. In the patient with primary adrenal failure, loss of mineralocorticoid action results in enhanced sodium excretion with characteristic hyponatremia, hyperkalemia, and dehydration. Progressive dehydration can lead to adrenal crisis *(Addisonian crisis)* with shock, kidney failure, and death.

The pathophysiologic changes and clinical manifestations of adrenal insufficiency are outlined in Box 29-15. The clinical presentation depends on the severity of the adrenal insufficiency and the rate of decline of adrenal function. In the majority of patients with primary autoimmune adrenal insufficiency, the rate of decline in adrenal function is gradual and the early symptoms, such as fatigue, may be vague and nonspecific. The clinical manifestations outlined in Box 29-15 represent advanced adrenal insufficiency.

BOX 29-15 Hypocortisolism: Pathophysiologic Alterations and Clinical Manifestations

Alteration in Metabolism of Protein, Carbohydrate, and Fats

As a result of decreased glucocorticoids, carbohydrate metabolism is particularly affected due to decreased gluconeogenesis and glycogenesis. Signs and symptoms include hypoglycemia, inability to tolerate prolonged fasts, weakness, lightheadedness, and fatigue.

Alteration in Hypothalamic-Pituitary-Adrenal Axis

Adrenocorticotropic hormone (ACTH) levels increase as a result of a diminished negative feedback on secretion of ACTH. ACTH stimulates melanocyte-stimulating hormone. As a result, a generalized hyperpigmentation occurs. An increase in pigmentation in skinfold creases and the buccal mucosa may be early clues.

Alteration in Catecholamine Activity

As glucocorticoids potentiate the catecholamine response, diminished catecholamine activity yields a poor response to endogenous and exogenous stressors. Hypovolemic shock as characterized by hypovolemia, hypotension, and tachycardia may occur.

Alteration in Emotional Stability

Glucocorticoids in normal amounts assist in maintaining emotional stability. Glucocorticoid deficiency may lead to dysphoria, apathy, or depression.

Alteration in Water and Mineral Metabolism

Aldosterone is the primary adrenal mineralocorticoid and deficiency results in loss of both water and sodium. Potassium is abnormally conserved. Signs and symptoms may include dehydration and hypovolemia (decreased weight, increased blood urea nitrogen, increased hematocrit, decreased skin turgor), hyponatremia, hyperkalemia, decreased bicarbonate with acidosis, muscle weakness, fatigue, postural hypotension, and hypovolemic shock. Glucocorticoid deficiency has similar, but milder, effects on water and mineral metabolism.

Collaborative Care Management

Diagnostic Tests. A random serum cortisol level does not definitively diagnose adrenal insufficiency, as it may be in the low normal range and does not reflect physiologic reserves to combat stress. Serum cortisol levels may be inappropriately normal during the stress of acute illness; normally levels should be elevated above 20 μg/dl.

In suspected acute adrenal insufficiency with advancing shock, serum cortisol levels should be drawn, then stress doses of intravenous hydrocortisone given until the crisis is over or the diagnosis is excluded. In persons with chronic adrenal insufficiency, the rapid Cortrosyn (synthetic CRH) stimulation test is most useful (see Chapter 28). However, this test does not distinguish between primary and secondary adrenal insufficiency, as it may take weeks or months after loss of ACTH secretion for the adrenal glands to atrophy. A 24-hour urinary free cortisol determination is not useful in the diagnosis of adrenal insufficiency, as approximately 20% of patients have normal results and the test gives no indication of the physiologic reserve in response to stress.

Medications

Acute Adrenal Crisis Management. Management includes prompt rehydration, administration of stress doses of intravenous hydrocortisone, and correction of electrolyte disturbances. Additional intravenous glucose may be needed if the patient is hypoglycemic. Aggressive treatment of any underlying precipitating illness is, of course, mandatory.

Chronic Adrenal Insufficiency. Traditional glucocorticoid therapy is cortisone acetate, 25 mg every morning and 12.5 mg every evening, or hydrocortisone, 20 mg every morning and 15 mg every evening. As an alternative, prednisone, 5 mg every morning and 2.5 mg every evening, may be given as glucocorticoid replacement. Because of the negligible mineralocorticoid activity of these glucocorticoids, concurrent use of the mineralocorticoid fludrocortisone is needed in primary adrenal insufficiency. Doses are adjusted to maintain the patient symptom-free with normal electrolytes. There are no reliable laboratory tests to assess optimum replacement therapy. It has been suggested that the usual empiric replacement glucocorticoid dose may be too high for optimum skeletal health.[28]

Stress Steroid Dosing. The body's increased demand for glucocorticoids during periods of stress must be met with increased glucocorticoid administration. It is difficult to precisely define stress; however, most would agree on a fever above 100° F (38° C), vomiting and diarrhea secondary to gastroenteritis, major trauma, and surgical procedures. Doubling of the glucocorticoid dose is generally advocated during minor stress such as low-grade fever and vomiting/diarrhea. If oral replacement is not feasible, parenteral administration is necessary. Patients may be taught intramuscular glucocorticoid administration when living in remote areas or where access to an emergency room is not available. For major stress such as major trauma and major surgical procedures, parenteral hydrocortisone at a dose of 200 mg/day is generally given in divided doses. This, in turn, is rapidly tapered to the maintenance dose as the patient recovers.

Diet. Fluids are encouraged, and the patient's hydration status is continually monitored. Nursing interventions should include measures to decrease nausea, vomiting, and diarrhea in an effort to maintain fluid/electrolyte and nutritional balance. The patient should be weighed daily. A high-sodium, low-potassium diet is indicated.

Activity. The patient's activity level depends on the severity of the adrenal failure. Patients experiencing severe and/or abrupt decline in adrenal function will have muscular weakness until hormonal balance is restored. Adequate rest should be encouraged and activities increased gradually. Range of motion and isometric exercises should be encouraged until the patient is fully ambulatory. Assistance may be needed with ADLs.

NURSING MANAGEMENT OF PATIENT WITH ADRENAL INSUFFICIENCY

ASSESSMENT

Health History

Information to be collected as part of the health history when assessing the patient with adrenal insufficiency includes:

History of weakness, fatigue, muscle pain, dizziness, changes in behavior, lethargy, depression; attention or ability to do work and activities; symptoms of hypoglycemia
Skin: history of changes in skin pigmentation
Nutrition: history of anorexia, nausea, vomiting, salt craving, weight loss, and abdominal pain; usual 24-hour food/fluid intake
Elimination: history of changes in bowel habits; urine output
Sexual: Females: menstrual history, history of changes in body/ axillary hair
Knowledge: disease, treatment, expectations

Physical Examination

Physical examination of the patient with adrenal insufficiency focuses on:

Emotional-mental status: affect, attention, activity level
Integumentary status: hyperpigmentation, axillary/body hair distribution, skin turgor
Cardiovascular status: blood pressure and pulse, especially with postural changes; heart rhythm
Gastrointestinal status: weight, 24-hour intake and output, abdominal tenderness
Musculoskeletal status: muscle strength; presence of muscle wasting; ability to do ADLs, muscle strength

NURSING DIAGNOSES

Nursing diagnoses are determined from analysis of patient data. Possible nursing diagnoses for the patient with adrenal insufficiency include but are not limited to:

Diagnostic Title	Possible Etiologic Factors
1. Deficient fluid volume	Sodium and water loss associated with deficiency of glucocorticoids and mineralocorticoids
2. Deficient knowledge regimen	Disease process, therapeutic

EXPECTED PATIENT OUTCOMES

Expected patient outcomes for the person with adrenal insufficiency may include but are not limited to:

1. Will maintain fluid balance
2. Will verbalize knowledge of disease process and treatment plan, expected outcomes of treatment, and plan for follow-up care

INTERVENTIONS

1. Promoting Fluid Balance

A Nursing Care Plan for the patient with adrenal insufficiency follows.

Nursing interventions include monitoring the patient for signs of hypovolemia, including weakness, muscle cramps, and changes in vital signs. Daily weights and hourly and daily intake and output should be closely monitored. Minimum hourly urine output should be greater than 30 ml. If the patient has had vomiting and/or diarrhea, monitoring for electrolyte imbalance is important. Vital signs indicating fluid volume deficit are hypotension, tachycardia, decreased pulse volume, and temperature increase or decrease. The patient should also be monitored for postural hypotension. Other assessments suggestive of fluid volume deficit include dry mucous membranes, thirst, decreased urine output, decreased skin turgor, sunken eyeballs, weakness, and confusion. Laboratory data should be evaluated for hemoconcentration and fluid replacement administered as ordered. Fluid intake should be encouraged, up to 3 L/day, unless contraindicated. A diet with normal sodium content (approximately 3 g/day) should be encouraged. Discharge instructions should include measures to prevent excessive fluid losses during periods of strenuous exercise, hot temperatures, and vomiting or diarrhea. Sodium intake should be increased when excessive diaphoresis is expected; potassium intake (depending on baseline values) may need to be increased to compensate for gastrointestinal losses.

2. Patient/Family Education

The initial teaching during the acute phase relates to proposed diagnostic tests and immediate interventions. After the patient's condition is stable, information is given about the disease and long-term needs. Instructions about replacement therapy are similar to those given to patients taking therapeutic doses of glucocorticoids, but some important differences

Nursing Care Plan Patient With Adrenal Insufficiency

DATA Mr. L. has been admitted from the emergency department with complaints of feeling so tired that he is unable to get out of bed. For the past 2 months he has experienced loss of appetite, nausea, vomiting, and diarrhea with increasing fatigue. Mr. L. thought he was having relapses of the flu, which had been prevalent during the winter months. He is an accountant and believes that his job has been interfering with his ability to recover fully.

Physical examination reveals:

- Tan-appearing Caucasian man who looks ill
- Cool, sweaty skin
- Respirations, 20 breaths/min with lungs clear bilaterally
- Temperature, 36.5° C orally; heart rate, 110 beats/min; blood pressure lying, 98/60; blood pressure sitting, 72/50
- Poor skin turgor; dry mucous membranes
- Weight, 70 kg (states 3-kg weight loss during past month)
- Complains of lightheadedness when head of bed is elevated

Laboratory findings include:

- White blood cell count, 16,000
- Blood glucose, 60 mg/dl
- Sodium, 130 mEq/L
- Chloride, 86 mEq/L
- Hemoglobin, 15 g/dl; hematocrit, 46%
- Blood urea nitrogen (BUN), 39 mg/dl
- Creatinine, 0.8 mg/dl
- Potassium, 5.4 mEq/L

NURSING DIAGNOSIS **Activity intolerance related to postural hypotension secondary to adrenal insufficiency**
GOALS/OUTCOMES Will remain free of fatigue during performance of usual activities

NOC Suggested Outcomes
- Activity Tolerance (0005)
- Energy Conservation (0002)
- Nutritional Status: Energy (1007)

NIC Suggested Interventions
- Energy Management (0180)
- Sleep Enhancement (1850)
- Nutrition Management (1100)

Nursing Interventions/Rationales
- Provide bed rest for first 24 hours. *To conserve energy and reduce metabolic demands until corticosteroid levels are normalized.*
- Avoid any unnecessary activities, such as bathing, for first 12 hours. *To conserve energy and reduce metabolic demands until corticosteroid levels are normalized.*
- Offer patient support by explaining that energy will return when hormone levels return to normal. *To reduce anxiety and fear, which increase metabolic demands and contribute to fatigue.*
- Gradually increase activities after hormone levels are returned to normal. *The patient has been ill for several months and may be much weaker than normal. Activities should be gradually increased until endurance improves.*

Evaluation Parameters
1. Progressively requires less assistance with activities of daily living
2. Reports feeling less fatigued
3. Blood pressure returns to normal range for age
4. No significant change in blood pressure between lying and standing

NURSING DIAGNOSIS **Ineffective coping related to inability to respond to stressors normally secondary to adrenal insufficiency**
GOALS/OUTCOMES Will demonstrate adequate coping as evidenced by absence of signs of stress (tachycardia, restlessness, lack of attention, increased blood pressure)

Nursing Interventions/Rationales
- Decrease environmental stressors (noise, lights, temperature changes). *The patient has reduced ability to respond to any stressors. External stressors can be controlled or eliminated.*
- Explain all procedures and interventions. *Understanding reduces fear and anxiety, both of which contribute to stress.*
- Maintain consistency of care providers for first 24 hours. *Consistency of personnel increases the patient's trust and reduces stress.*
- Provide care in a calm, unhurried manner. *Stress can be readily transferred from the nurse to the patient. If the nurse is calm, the patient is more likely to be calm.*
- Encourage family members to remain with patient if they are comforting to him. *The presence of family members can increase comfort and security and reduce stress. If the patient does not find family members comforting, their presence will increase stress.*

Continued

Nursing Care Plan Patient With Adrenal Insufficiency–cont'd

Evaluation Parameters
1. Reports feeling relaxed
2. Vital signs within normal parameters
3. Participates in decision making

NURSING DIAGNOSIS **Deficient fluid volume related to inability to conserve fluid secondary to glucocorticoid deficiency**
GOALS/OUTCOMES Will have normal fluid status as evidenced by blood pressure within normal parameters and absence of hemoconcentration

Nursing Interventions/Rationales
- Monitor intake and output hourly. *Loss of fluid volume predisposes the patient to renal compromise and, possibly, acute kidney failure. Intake should approximate output.*
- Monitor blood pressure and heart rate hourly until normal. *To compare with the patient's baseline to detect increasing problems or determine the effectiveness of interventions.*
- Weigh daily. *To determine fluid and nutritional needs. Fluid deficit results in weight loss. Fluid restoration results in weight gain.*
- Administer intravenous fluids as prescribed (usually 5% dextrose in normal saline) and monitor fluid status. *Surveillance allows for early identification of problems with replacement therapy so that solutions or infusion rates can be adjusted or changed. Deficient fluid volume results from excessive loss of sodium and water from glucocorticoid deficiency.*
- Monitor hematocrit, hemoglobin, BUN, and serum creatinine daily. *To determine the presence of hemodilution/concentration and to monitor renal function.*
- Administer cortisol as prescribed. *Replacement cortisol is the primary treatment for cortisol deficiency.*

Evaluation Parameters
1. Gradually increases fluid intake to 3000 ml/day
2. Signs of fluid deficit resolve (decreased blood pressure, hemoconcentration)

NURSING DIAGNOSIS **Risk for injury (trauma) related to weakness and hypoglycemia**
GOALS/OUTCOMES Will remain free of injury

NOC Suggested Outcomes
- Risk Control (1902)
- Safety Behavior: Fall Prevention (1909)
- Symptom Control (1608)

NIC Suggested Interventions
- Environmental Management: Safety 6486)
- Fall Prevention (6490)
- Surveillance: Safety (6654)

Nursing Interventions/Rationales
- Keep bed in lowest position. *To increase the ease with which the patient can get into bed and decrease the possibility of falling.*
- Keep side rails up at all times unless patient refuses. *Side rails provide protection from falling out of bed when sleeping. If the patient refuses side rails, they must be left down because they are considered restraints.*
- Monitor blood glucose levels every 4 hours. *Hypoglycemia and weakness can lead to injury.*
- Instruct patient to call for assistance when getting into or out of bed. *The patient is weak and fatigued. The assistance of another person is needed in order to decrease the risk for falls and injury.*

Evaluation Parameters
1. Calls for assistance when getting into and out of bed
2. Experiences no injuries

NURSING DIAGNOSIS **Deficient knowledge related to lack of previous experience with new problem**
GOALS/OUTCOMES Will verbalize understanding of disease and its treatment

- Explain all care to patient and family so that no unexpected events occur. *To decrease stress so that the patient is capable of hearing and understanding information provided.*
- Focus on immediate care rather than home care at this time. *The patient is capable only of handling information about what is happening now. He will not likely retain information regarding home care until he is stable and less fatigued.*

Nursing Care Plan *Patient With Adrenal Insufficiency—cont'd*

- Repeat teaching frequently. *Stress interferes with learning. There is too much information to learn at one time, and the patient is very fatigued. Therefore repetitive teaching enhances learning.*
- Provide written materials to enforce verbal teaching. *A patient who is ill or stressed does not always remember information taught. Written materials allow the patient to review important information and proceed at his own pace.*
- Provide information about community resources that may be useful to patient and family. *The patient may not be aware of available community resources.*

Evaluation Parameters

1. Is able to explain expectations for the next 24 hours
2. Asks questions about his disease and its treatment
3. Reads written resources provided

exist (see Patient Teaching box). Additional teaching should include the effect of stressors on the disease and methods to reduce or eliminate stress. The patient and significant others should be able to describe:

Discharge medication regimen, the need for continued treatment, and situations that require an increase in medication dosage
Medical follow-up plan
Symptoms indicating adrenal crisis and the need for medical attention
Need for continual medical follow-up care
Need to wear a Medic-Alert bracelet
Need to carry identification card with information concerning physician and current medication

EVALUATION

To determine the effectiveness of nursing interventions, patient behaviors should be compared with those stated in the expected patient outcomes. Achievement of outcomes is successful if the patient with adrenal insufficiency:

1a. Describes need for intake of 3 L/day, strategies to monitor fluid intake and output, and measures to prevent excess fluid loss.
1b. Demonstrates fluid balance by balanced intake and output, moist mucous membranes, elastic skin turgor, laboratory values within expected normal range, and stable vital signs.
2. Verbalizes knowledge of disease process, medications, the need for lifelong therapy, signs of addisonian crisis, and follow-up care.

GERONTOLOGIC CONSIDERATIONS

Feedback mechanisms involved in maintaining glucocorticoid levels are not affected by age. However, the decrease in the metabolic rate of the glucocorticoids is age related. The amount of fibrous tissue in the gland increases, and the gland loses some weight after the age of 50. As liver and kidney function decline with age, metabolic clearance of cortisol decreases.

Patient Teaching

The Patient Taking Replacement Doses of Glucocorticoids and Mineralocorticoids

1. Follow medication regimen.
   a. Take drugs with meals or snacks.
   b. Glucocorticoids: take as directed.
   c. Mineralocorticoids: take medication in the morning.
   d. Do not omit a drug dose.
   e. Keep sufficient medication on hand on person and at home.
   f. If unable to retain oral form of drug, take parenteral form as instructed.
   g. Carry drugs on person or in carry-on luggage when traveling; do not ship drugs with luggage; make sure traveling companion knows how to give the injectable form of glucocorticoid.
   h. Carry extra doses in case of delays or illness.
2. Wear a Medic Alert bracelet or necklace that lists condition, drugs and dosage, and name and phone number of physician.
3. Monitor self for presence of increased stressors (fever, infections, dental work, accidents, or family or personal crises) and increase dose of glucocorticoids as instructed.
4. Monitor self daily for signs and symptoms of insufficient drug therapy (anorexia, nausea, vomiting, weakness, depression, dizziness, polyuria, and weight loss) and report immediately (larger drug dose may be necessary).
5. Monitor self daily for signs and symptoms of excessive drug therapy (rapid weight gain, round face, edema, or hypertension) and report immediately (smaller drug dose may be necessary).
6. Eat a well-balanced diet, choosing foods from all food groups.
7. Maintain a regular schedule with adequate sleep, regular meals, and regular exercise (irregular health habits increase glucocorticoid needs).
8. See physician as instructed; consult as necessary if questions arise concerning therapy.

SPECIAL ENVIRONMENTS FOR CARE

Critical Care

Acute adrenal crisis (Addisonian crisis) is a potential life-threatening critical care issue for both the undiagnosed and the previously diagnosed patient (see Collaborative Care section on acute adrenal crisis). Frequent monitoring of the patient is necessary to detect changes, to evaluate effectiveness of therapy, to detect side effects of therapy (e.g., fluid overload), and to prevent or detect complications. Of particular concern are changes in mental status and respiratory depression. Monitoring for fluid status may include vital signs taken as often as every 15 minutes, hourly intake and output, and daily weights. Hemodynamic monitoring may be used to help determine the exact amount of fluids needed. The fluid deficit is usually corrected in 4 to 6 hours.

Until the patient's condition is stabilized, serum values are monitored daily or more frequently as necessary. During the early phase of illness, a neurologic assessment is made at least every 4 hours for signs of hyponatremia (dizziness, confusion, or neuromuscular irritability); this assessment can be done while the nurse is taking vital signs.

If serum potassium levels are elevated, cardiac monitoring should be instituted to assess for changes in T wave or QRS complexes or for changes in rhythm. The hyperkalemia usually disappears with glucocorticoid and mineralocorticoid therapy, and the patient may actually need potassium after the acute period. Until the serum potassium level returns to normal, the nurse should make sure the patient does not inadvertently receive potassium in intravenous fluids or medications. Measures to prevent infections and trauma, which can increase cell death and the release of potassium into the extracellular space, are incorporated into the nursing care plan.

Monitoring for signs and symptoms of hypoglycemia and monitoring of blood glucose levels are done on a routine basis, such as every 4 hours. Glucose is given in intravenous fluids as prescribed and, when food is allowed, snacks may be incorporated between meals to avoid long periods of fasting. If symptoms of hypoglycemia occur, the blood glucose is checked, if possible, and treatment is initiated for hypoglycemia (see Chapter 30).

A focus of care is avoiding additional stressors. These patients should do nothing for themselves and should be protected from all stimuli and from exposure to infection. To decrease stressors, the same nurse should provide care for the first several hours, during which time the patient's condition stabilizes. One-on-one care may be necessary. To prevent aspiration, the patient is given nothing by mouth until nausea and vomiting subside and until mental status has returned to baseline. After several hours, oral liquids may be given, and oral glucocorticoids may be started within 48 hours. The patient may experience a severe headache; comfort measures should be provided.

After the patient's condition is stabilized, attention is focused on achieving an improved state of well-being and preparing for discharge; the plan of care is modified as the patient recovers from crisis to a state of chronic adrenal insufficiency.

Community-Based Care

The patient requires lifelong therapy with both mineralocorticoids and glucocorticoids. If the medication is unable to be taken orally, then the patient or caregiver must learn to administer the medication intramuscularly. Wearing a Medic-Alert bracelet is advised. As described earlier, medication doses must be increased in times of physiologic or psychologic stress.

COMPLICATIONS

The major complication of adrenal insufficiency, acute adrenal crisis, was discussed previously. Patients who present with unexplained weakness or confusion and a history of chronic disease that may be managed with corticosteroids should be assessed for the possibility of adrenal crisis. The patient may be unable to give an accurate medical history that would alert the health care team into the possibility of adrenal insufficiency.

ADRENAL MEDULLA HYPERSECRETION: PHEOCHROMOCYTOMA

Etiology/Epidemiology

Pheochromocytoma is a catecholamine-producing tumor arising from cells of the adrenal medulla and sympathetic ganglia: 90% of tumors occur within the adrenal gland and 10% are extraadrenal; 10% of the adrenal tumors are bilateral; 10% of all tumors are malignant. Pheochromocytomas may be part of the type IIa MEN syndrome (hyperparathyroidism, medullary thyroid cancer) or type IIb MEN syndrome (medullary thyroid cancer, multiple mucosal neuromas). The prevalence of pheochromocytomas may be up to 0.3% of the hypertensive population.[40] Familial tumors account for approximately 10% of pheochromocytomas.[40]

Both men and women are affected equally; the usual age at diagnosis is 40 to 60 years. Pheochromocytomas are usually benign and curable but, if unrecognized or untreated, can be fatal.

Pathophysiology

Pheochromocytomas release excessive amounts of catecholamines, mainly norepinephrine, with associated symptoms to include the five Ps:

1. Pressure: paroxysmal increases in blood pressure
2. Palpitations
3. Pallor
4. Perspiration: profuse and generalized
5. Pain: paroxysmal pulsatile headaches, chest and abdominal pain

Most patients present with hypertensive crises; the hypertension may be resistant to standard treatment for essential hypertension. In tumors secreting mainly epinephrine, paroxysmal hypotension, shock, tremors, anxiety, epigastric pain, diaphoresis, and chest pain are common manifestations. Labile hypertension is characteristic. Episodes may be spontaneous or precipitated by maneuvers that increase intraabdominal pressure such as lifting, straining, or bending. Episodes may also be precipitated by anesthesia and diagnostic tests. Tumor manipulation and induction of anesthesia can cause hypertensive crisis, arrhythmias, or stroke as a result of extensive catecholamine release. The clinical signs of pheochromocytoma include:

- Hypertension: paroxysmal (50%) or treatment-resistant
- Orthostatic hypotension
- Weight loss: obesity very uncommon
- Constipation
- Tremors
- Pallor
- Hypertensive retinopathy
- Hyperglycemia
- Hypercalcemia

Collaborative Care Management

The most useful screening test is a 24-hour urine total metanephrines. Twenty-four hour vanillylmandelic acid (VMA) has a false-positive rate greater than 15% and is the least specific test. The 24-hour urine collection should be started at the onset of a hypertensive episode. Plasma catecholamine determinations are not as sensitive or specific as the 24-hour measurements. Radiologic imaging is best achieved with MRI or CT of the adrenals and abdomen. If MRI and CT are negative, ^{123}I metaiodobenzylguanidine (MBG) scintigraphy may be carried out.[40]

Laparoscopic removal of both adrenal and extraadrenal pheochromocytomas is the treatment of choice. Laparoscopic partial adrenalectomy has been successful in preserving adrenal cortical function in persons with hereditary forms of pheochromocytoma.

Surgery without catecholamine blockade is associated with a 24% to 50% mortality rate.[40] Catecholamine blockade is best accomplished with the administration of the alpha-adrenergic blocker phenoxybenzamine, followed by beta-adrenergic blockers. Phenoxybenzamine is started 2 weeks before surgery. The most common side effect is nasal congestion. Metyrosine (Demser), recently added to preoperative protocols, decreases catecholamine tumor content by 50% to 80%.[40]

The addition of metyrosine has resulted in the use of less vasoactive medication to control blood pressure and less intraoperative blood loss. Calcium channel blockers have been used as an alternative in some centers.[37] Correction of volume depletion with a liberal salt diet and, if necessary, intravenous normal saline is critical to prevent postoperative hypotension.

Before surgery nursing care is focused on instituting measures to help stabilize the patient's hemodynamic status, monitor the clinical state, prepare the patient for tests and surgery, and prevent episodes of hypertension. Patients experiencing hypertensive crises should be in an intensive care unit because frequent cardiac, blood pressure, and neurologic monitoring is required. If phentolamine infusion is necessary, the blood pressure is checked every 15 minutes, and the drug is given by controlled infusion at a rate to keep the blood pressure at a prescribed level. During this time the patient must be informed about planned diagnostic tests and treatments and be prepared for surgery. Activities that precipitate paroxysms, such as bending, Valsalva maneuver, palpating the abdomen, and lifting, should be limited. Hypertension can also occur with inadequately treated postoperative pain.

After surgery the patient needs close monitoring of blood pressure, pulse, cardiac rhythm, neurologic status, and the effectiveness of treatment. Blood glucose levels should be monitored until homeostasis returns, as elevated catecholamine levels lead to increased insulin production. After the hypertensive period, hypotension may occur; thus nursing care is focused on continual monitoring and administration of fluids or plasma expanders as prescribed.

Patient/Family Education. For patients treated medically or surgical patients without remission of symptoms, nursing care is focused on helping the patient attain the skills necessary for self-care. Patient teaching includes:

- Information about the disease and its relationship to the signs and symptoms
- Medication regimen: purpose, dosage, expected effects, and side effects
- Blood pressure self-measurement
- Measures to prevent paroxysms: preventing constipation, avoiding Valsalva maneuver, and avoiding bending or flexing the body
- Importance of follow-up care
- Need to wear Medic-Alert bracelet and carry wallet card

Catecholamine levels should return to normal baseline approximately 6 weeks after surgery. Surgery results in complete remission of symptoms in most patients; therefore discharge teaching for most patients is focused on helping the patient plan for resumption of normal activities, maintain an adequate diet, and follow-up with the physician.

Critical Thinking Questions

1. A 52-year-old Caucasian male presents with hypertension with a BP of 190/102 mm Hg, tachycardia, and diaphoresis. What endocrine abnormalities could be responsible for his hypertension? What questions would you ask him? What diagnostic tests might his physician order?
2. Endocrine disorders may cause a number of physical changes that can adversely affect body image and self-esteem. As you consider several endocrine disorders and their physical sequelae, formulate a plan to help a patient cope with changes in body image and self-esteem.
3. A 72-year-old woman has just been diagnosed with hypothyroidism. She has a history of rheumatoid arthritis and has been taking prednisone for several years. Devise a plan of care for this patient. What teaching is needed?

References

1. American Association of Clinical Endocrinologists/American Association of Endocrine Surgeons Thyroid Carcinoma Task Force: AACE/AAES medical/surgical guidelines for clinical practice: management of thyroid cancer, *Endocr Pract* 7(3):202, 2001.
2. Auer J et al: Subclinical hyperthyroidism as a risk factor for atrial fibrillation, *Am Heart J* 142(5):838, 2001.
3. Bailey RH, Aron D: The diagnostic dilemma of incidentalomas: working through uncertainty, *Endocrionl Metab Clin North Am* 29(1):91, 2000.

4. Bartelana L et al: Relation between therapy for hyperthyroidism and the course of Graves' ophthalmopathy, *N Engl J Med* 338(2):73, 1998.
5. Bartelena L et al: Cigarette smoking and treatment outcomes in Graves' ophthalmopathy, *Ann Intern Med* 129(8):632, 1998.
6. Bilezikian JP, Marcus R, Levine MA, editors: *The parathyroids,* ed 2, San Diego, 2001, Academic Press.
7. Biller BMK et al: Cushing's syndrome. In Molitch ME, editor, *Atlas of clinical endocrinology,* vol 4, Philadelphia, 1999, Current Medicine.
8. Blackwell RE: Hyperprolactinermia: evaluation and management, *Endocrinol Metab Clin North Am* 21(1):105-124, 1992.
9. Bogazzi F et al: The various effects of amiodarone on thyroid function, *Thyroid* 11(5):511, 2001.
10. Bunevicius R et al: Effects of thyroxine as compared with thyroxine plus triiodothyronine in patients with hypothyroidism, *N Engl J Med* 340:424, 1999.
11. Burman KD: Thyroid cancer I. *Endocrinol Metab Clin North Am* 24(4):663-883, 1995.
12. Burman KD: Thyroid cancer II. *Endocrinol Metab Clin North Am* 25(1):1-211, 1995.
13. Carmeci C et al: Ultrasound-guided fine needle aspiration biopsy of thyroid nodules, *Thyroid* 8:283, 1998.
14. Cooper DS: Antithyroid drugs for the treatment of hyperthyroidism caused by Graves' disease, *Endocrinol Metab Clin North Am* 27(1):225, 1998.
15. Danese MD et al: Screening for mild thyroid failure at the periodic health examination: a decision and cost-effectiveness analysis, *JAMA* 276:285, 1996.
16. Glinoer D, de Nayer P, Bex M for the Belgian Collaborative Study Group on Graves' Disease: Effects of l-thyroxine administration, TSH-receptor antibodies and smoking on the risk of recurrence in Graves' hyperthyroidism treated with antithyroid drugs: a double-blind prospective randomized study, *Eur J Endocrinol* 144(5):475, 2000.
17. Gordon CB et al: Impaired wound healing in Cushing's syndrome: the role of heat shock proteins, *Surgery* 116(6):1082, 1994.
18. Hak AE et al: Subclinical hypothyroidism is an independent risk factor for atherosclerosis and myocardial infarction in elderly women: the Rotterdam Study, *Ann Intern Med* 132:270, 2000.
19. Hashizume K et al: Administration of thyroxine in treated Graves' disease: effects on the levels of antibodies to thyroid stimulating hormone receptors and on the risk of recurrence of hyperthyroidism, *N Engl J Med* 324:947, 1991.
20. Martino E et al: The effects of amiodarone on the thyroid, *Endocr Rev* 22(2):240, 2001.
21. Marx SJ: Hyperparathyroid and hypoparathyroid disorders, *N Engl J Med* 343:863, 2000.
22. Mechlis S et al: Amiodarone-induced thyroid gland dysfunction, *Am J Cardiol* 59:833, 1997.
23. Molitch ME, Thorner MO, Wilson C: Therapeutic controversy: management of prolactinomas, *J Clin Endocrinol Metab* 82:996, 1997.
24. National Institutes of Health Consensus Development Conference Panel: Diagnosis and management of asymptomatic primary hyperparathyroidism: consensus development conference statement, *Ann Intern Med* 114(7):593, 1991.
25. Newman CB et al: Octreotide as primary therapy for acromegaly [see comments], *J Clin Endocrinol Metab* 83:3034, 1998.
26. Newman CB: Medical therapy for acromegaly, *Endocrinol Metab Clin North Am* 28(1):170-190, 1999.
27. Ortiz R et al: Effect of early referral to an endocrinologist on efficiency and cost of evaluation and development of treatment plan in patients with thyroid nodules, *Ann Intern Med* 87:265, 1977.
28. Peacey S et al: Glucocorticoid replacement therapy: are patients over treated and does it matter? *Clin Endocrinol (Oxf)* 46:255, 1997.
29. Robertson GL: Diabetes insipidus, *Endocrinol Metab Clin North Am* 24(3):549-572, 1995.
30. Robinson AG, Verbalis JG: Diabetes insipidus. In Bardin W, editor: *Current therapy in endocrinology and metabolism,* ed 6, St Louis, 1997, Mosby.
31. Silverberg SJ, Bilezikian JP: Primary hyperparathyroidism. In DeGroot L, Jameson JL, editors: *Endocrinology,* ed 4, Philadelphia, 2001, WB Saunders.
32. Silverberg SJ et al: A new highly sensitive assay for parathyroid hormone in primary hyperparathyroidism, *J Bone Min Res:* 15(suppl I):S167, 2000.
33. Singh N et al: Effect of calcium carbonate on the absorption of levothyroxine, *JAMA* 283:2822, 2000.
34. Stewart PM: Mineralcorticoid hypertension, *Lancet* 353:1341, 1999.
35. Tomlinson J et al: Association between premature mortality and hypopituitarism, *Lancet* 357:425, 2001.
36. Trivalle C et al: Differences in the signs and symptoms of hyperthyroidism in older and younger patients, *J Am Geriatr Soc* 44:50, 1996.
37. Ulchaker JC et al: Successful outcomes in pheochromocytoma surgery in the modern era, *J Urol* 161(3):764, 1999.
38. Vallotton MB: Primary hyperaldosteronism: Parts I- II, *Clin Endocrinol* 45:47, 53, 1996.
39. van der Lely AJ et al: Long-term treatment of acromegaly with pegvisomant, a growth hormone receptor antagonist, *Lancet* 358(9295);1754, 2001.
40. Walther MM: Pheochromocytoma. In Rakel RE, Bope ET, editors: *Conn's current therapy,* Philadelphia, 2002, WB Saunders.
41. Weetman AP: Medical progress: Graves' disease, *N Engl J Med* 343(17):1236, 2000.

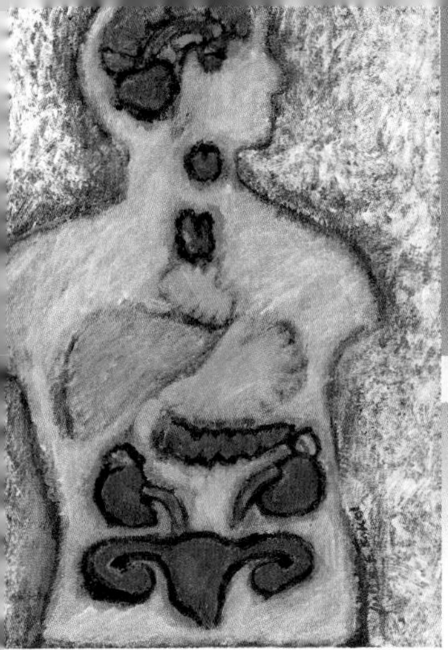

Diabetes Mellitus and Hypoglycemia

30

Margaret M. Ulchaker

Objectives

After studying this chapter, the learner should be able to:

1. Differentiate among type 1, type 2, and gestational diabetes mellitus (DM).
2. Contrast the epidemiologic and etiologic factors of type 1 and type 2 DM.
3. Differentiate the pathophysiologic basis for type 1 DM from that for type 2 DM.
4. Describe the common manifestations of uncontrolled type 1 and type 2 DM.
5. Compare the comprehensive care of the individual with type 1 DM with the care of the individual with type 2 DM.
6. Describe the pivotal role of dietary management and education in type 1 and type 2 DM.
7. Discuss the role of exercise in the treatment of type 1 and type 2 DM.
8. Describe physiologic insulin regimens in type 1 DM.
9. Analyze the oral agents used in the treatment of type 2 DM in terms of mechanism of action, dosage ranges, metabolic effects, side effects, and contraindications.
10. Develop a nursing care plan, including nursing diagnoses, patient outcomes, and interventions, for an individual with stable DM.
11. Discuss sick-day management guidelines for the individual with DM.
12. Describe the surgical considerations for the individual with DM.
13. Discuss hypoglycemia as a consequence of diabetes management, including causes, signs and symptoms, treatment, and prevention.
14. Differentiate the pathophysiology, clinical manifestations, and management of persons with diabetic ketoacidosis from those of persons with hyperglycemic hyperosmolar nonketotic coma.
15. Describe the chronic complications of DM, the relationship between metabolic control and the chronic complications, and the management of the complications.
16. Differentiate fasting and reactive hypoglycemia on the basis of causes, clinical manifestations, and management.

DIABETES MELLITUS

"Diabetes mellitus is a group of metabolic diseases characterized by hyperglycemia resulting from defects in insulin secretion, insulin action, or both."[7] The basis of the abnormalities in carbohydrate, protein, and fat metabolism in diabetes is the deficient action of insulin on the target tissues of skeletal muscle, adipose tissue, and the liver. Uncontrolled diabetes mellitus (DM) may result in long-term damage, dysfunction, and failure of various organs. Diabetes cannot be cured, but it can be controlled. Elliott Joslin, MD,[47] who is regarded as the father of diabetes care, stated, "Diabetes is a serious disease and deserves the best effort of doctor and patient from beginning to end."

By its very nature, DM can be significantly influenced by daily self-care. No other disease demands so much of the patient's own self-knowledge and skills. Thus the professional nurse has the challenge and responsibility of helping patients gain the knowledge, skills, and attitudes necessary for self-care.

National (American Diabetes Association[6]) and international (World Health Organization/St. Vincent Declaration) standards of care for DM have been in existence for several years. These standards of care encompass diabetes evaluation, management, and education. Despite their publication and dissemination to both the health care community and patients alike, these protocols have yet to become standard practice. Fewer than 10% of patients with diabetes in the United States go to endocrinologists for diabetes care. Thus primary care physicians provide the bulk of diabetes care, although the standards recommend that care be delivered by an endocrinologist. Numerous studies demonstrate a large gap between current recommendations for diabetes care and actual practice patterns of primary care physicians.* Diabetes care by a dedicated specialty team has been demonstrated to confer a survival advantage of up to 15 years.[56,109]

CLASSIFICATION

The current diagnostic and classification system for diabetes was first published by the Expert Committee on the Diagnosis and Classification of Diabetes Mellitus of the American Diabetes Association (Table 30-1) in July 1997. This system reflects the etiology and pathophysiology of diabetes, with the two major categories being type 1 DM (previously termed *insulin-dependent diabetes mellitus* or *juvenile-onset diabetes mellitus*) and type 2 DM (previously termed *non–insulin-dependent diabetes mellitus* or *maturity-onset diabetes mellitus*).[7]

This chapter focuses on type 1 and type 2 DM, which are the two most common types of the disease. Table 30-2 compares the characteristics of type 1 and type 2 DM. Both the classifications and their characteristics are important for the professional nurse in understanding this chapter.

ETIOLOGY

Table 30-3 summarizes the known etiologic factors of type 1 and type 2 DM; however, the etiology of each type of DM is still unfolding. In relation to type 1 DM, genetics seem to have a permissive role that allows environmental factors, perhaps viruses, to trigger the onset of diabetes by stimulating an autoimmune response. In regard to type 2 DM, individuals with a family history of diabetes are at high risk. Other risk factors for type 2 DM are a prior history of impaired glucose tolerance (IGT) or gestational diabetes mellitus (GDM), particularly in obese individuals. The conversion rate from IGT to type 2 DM is 7% per year. Seventy percent of individuals with prior GDM develop type 2 DM later in life. *Glucotoxicity,* the toxic effects of hyperglycemia on the pancreatic islets, may be another causal factor in precipitating type 2 DM. *Insulin resistance,* or the inability of the insulin-sensitive tissues (skeletal muscle, liver, and adipose tissue) to respond normally to insulin-stimulated glucose uptake, also has a role in the pathogenesis of type 2 DM.

*References 38, 42, 57, 58, 70, 111.

EPIDEMIOLOGY

In the United States approximately 16 million individuals (5.9% of the population) have diabetes, with one third of them being undiagnosed. DM is the seventh leading cause of death by disease in the United States. The prevalence of diabetes varies with race and ethnicity, is slightly greater in women, and increases significantly with age (Table 30-4). Each year approximately 798,000 new cases are diagnosed; approximately 95% of new cases are type 2 DM. Each day approximately 2200 individuals are diagnosed with diabetes.[64]

Figure 30-1 depicts the risks of major complications of diabetes when persons with diabetes are compared with nondiabetic persons. In addition, as many as 50% of men with diabetes and 35% of women with diabetes have sexual problems from neuropathy.

Diabetes is a disease that kills women more readily than men. A woman with diabetes has four times the risk of cardiovascular disease as compared with her nondiabetic counterpart. A man with diabetes has only twice the risk of cardiovascular disease as compared with his nondiabetic counterpart.[27]

Diabetes is a costly disease in terms of morbidity and mortality, and also in dollars and cents. The average annual cost per patient ranges from 2.3 times to 7.8 times higher for an individual with diabetes as compared with a nondiabetic individual.

PATHOPHYSIOLOGY

The hallmark of diabetes is insulin deficiency, either absolute or relative. In *absolute* insulin deficiency, the pancreas produces either no insulin or very little insulin, as is seen in type 1 DM. In *relative* insulin deficiency, the pancreas produces either normal or excessive amounts of insulin, but the body is unable to use it effectively, and glucose levels remain elevated. This latter defect is known as insulin resistance and is seen in type 2 DM (Figure 30-2). Fundamentally, it is failure of the pancreas to produce enough insulin to overcome this insulin resistance that precipitates clinical type 2 DM in predisposed individuals.

This absolute or relative insulin deficiency results in significant abnormalities in the metabolism of the body fuels. The body needs fuel for all its functions, including growth and repair of tissues. The fuel comes from the food that is ingested, which is composed of carbohydrates, proteins, and fats. It is important to understand and emphasize to patients that diabetes is not a disease of glucose alone, although the diagnostic criteria that have been devised use the serum glucose level as the marker for the diagnosis and control of the disease. Because the most common word used in the diabetes vocabulary is *sugar,* it is understandable how patients with long-standing or new diabetes can believe that if sugar is eliminated from the diet, the battle is won. It is important that nurses help patients understand that diabetes is a disease that affects how the body utilizes all foods (carbohydrates, fats, and proteins).

Hormones

The hormones involved in glucose metabolism include those from the pancreas (insulin and glucagon) (Table 30-5),

TABLE 30-1 Classification of Diabetes Mellitus and Other Disorders of Glucose Tolerance

Type	Defining Characteristics
Type 1 diabetes mellitus (DM)	
Immune mediated	Insulinopenic (insulin deficient) and dependent on exogenous insulin to sustain life Onset generally before age 30, but may occur at any age, including the geriatric years Generally lean, rarely obese Variable rate of beta-cell destruction Clinical presentation usually rapid In 85%-90%, one or more of the following autoantibodies are present at the time when fasting hyperglycemia is initially detected: Islet cell autoantibodies Insulin autoantibodies Glutamic acid decarboxylase autoantibodies Tyrosine phosphatase IA-2 or IA-2β autoantibodies Strong human leukocyte antigen (HLA) associations Linkage to DQA and B genes Influenced by DRB genes
Idiopathic diabetes	No immunologic evidence for beta-cell destruction No HLA association Strongly inherited Most individuals affected are of African or Asian origin Episodic ketoacidosis with varying degrees of insulin deficiency between episodes The absolute requirement for exogenous insulin is episodic
Type 2 DM	No requirement for exogenous insulin to sustain life at least initially Ranges from a picture of predominantly insulin resistance with mild relative insulin deficiency to a picture of more severe insulin secretory defects with insulin resistance Usually obese; those who are not obese by traditional criteria usually have abdominal adiposity Onset usually after age 40, but may occur at any age No autoimmune or HLA association
Other	
Genetic defects of beta-cell function	Previously termed *maturity-onset diabetes of youth*—impaired insulin secretion without defects in insulin action Autosomal-dominant inheritance Abnormalities in three genetic loci have been determined to date
Genetic defects in insulin action	N/A
Diseases of the exocrine pancreas	Pancreatitis, trauma, infection, pancreatectomy, pancreatic carcinoma, cystic fibrosis, hemochromatosis
Endocrinopathies	Acromegaly, Cushing's syndrome, glucagonoma, pheochromocytoma
Drug-induced	Permanent destruction of beta cells (Vacor [rat poison], IV pentamidine) Impairment of insulin action (nicotinic acid, glucocorticoids, thiazide diuretics) Impairment of insulin secretion, thereby precipitating DM in an individual with insulin resistance (e.g., drug-induced hypokalemia)
Infections	Congenital rubella, cytomegalovirus
Uncommon forms: immune mediated	Stiff-man syndrome, anti-insulin receptor antibodies
Genetic syndromes associated with DM	Turner's syndrome, Down syndrome, Klinefelter's syndrome
Gestational DM	Pregnancy related
Impaired glucose tolerance (IGT)	Glucose levels are higher than normal but do not meet diagnostic criteria for DM 21 million individuals in United States Generally obese 7% per year progression to overt type 2 DM Insulin resistant and are at increased cardiovascular risk
Impaired fasting glucose	Fasting glucose levels higher than normal but lower than those in IGT or DM

Adapted from American Diabetes Association, Expert Committee on the Diagnosis and Classification of Diabetes Mellitus: Report of the Expert Committee on the Diagnosis and Classification of Diabetes Mellitus, *Diabetes Care* 24(suppl 1):S55, 2001.
N/A, Not applicable.

TABLE 30-2 Characteristics of Type 1 and Type 2 Diabetes Mellitus

Characteristics	Type 1 Diabetes Mellitus	Type 2 Diabetes Mellitus
Insulin status	Insulin secretion ↓	Insulin secretion ↑, ↓, or normal
Age	Usually under 30 but may occur at any age	Usually over 40 but may occur at any age
Clinical presentation	Rapid	Slow
Body build	Lean or normal usually	80%-90% overweight
Family history	Weak	Strong
Islet cell antibodies	Present at onset in 85%-90%	Absent
Human leukocyte antigen (HLA) association	Positive (DQA, B)	Negative
Incidence	10% of total	90% of total
Symptoms	Polyuria, polydipsia, polyphagia, weight loss	No symptoms or may have same symptoms as type 1 May have symptomatic complications when diagnosed
Ketones	Prone	Resistant except during infection or with stressors
Complications	Related to degree and duration of hyperglycemia	Related to degree and duration of hyperglycemia
	Not present at time of diagnosis	May be present at diagnosis in 20% or more because of delay in diagnosis
Treatment	Insulin, diet, exercise	Diet, exercise, oral agents, insulin
Racial distribution	More common in Caucasians	More common in African-Americans and Hispanics Highest in Native Americans

TABLE 30-3 Etiologic Factors in Type 1 and Type 2 Diabetes Mellitus

Factors	Type 1 Diabetes Mellitus	Type 2 Diabetes Mellitus
Genetic	Human leukocyte antigen (HLA) association (particularly DQA and B genes)	Not associated with HLA antigens
Heredity	Unknown Familial aggregates rare Less than 50% concordance in monozygotic twins Greater risk for child to develop type 1 if father has type 1 (6%) than if mother has type 1 (3%)	Unknown except for class of genetic defects of beta-cell destruction, which is inherited dominantly
Autoimmune basis	Strong autoimmune basis as seen by: Insulitis (inflammation of islets of Langerhans with lymphocytic infiltration) Presence of autoantibodies to islet cells, insulin, glutamic acid decarboxylase, or tyrosine phosphatase	None
Environmental basis	Viral infections may be an environmental trigger; as counterregulatory hormones increase in response to stress of illness, islets are unable to respond with needed increased insulin secretion to maintain euglycemia	Modern lifestyle of poor eating and nutritional habits resulting in obesity and inactivity provides stimuli for those who are predisposed

TABLE 30-4 Prevalence of Diabetes by Race/Ethnicity

Race/Ethnicity	Diagnosed and Undiagnosed (%)
Non-Hispanic Caucasian Americans	7.8
Non-Hispanic African-Americans	10.8
Mexican-Americans	24.0
Other Hispanic/Latino Americans	Ranges from 16% to 26%
North American Indians/Alaska Native Americans	Ranges from 3% among Native Americans in Alaska to 50% among Pima Indians in Arizona
Asian-Americans/Pacific Islanders	Ranges from 16% to 20%
Pacific Islanders	Limited data but reported to be high among Hawaiians and Samoans

Adapted from National Diabetes Data Group: *Diabetes in America,* ed 2, NIH Pub No 95-1468, Baltimore, 2000, National Institutes of Health, US Department of Health and Human Services.

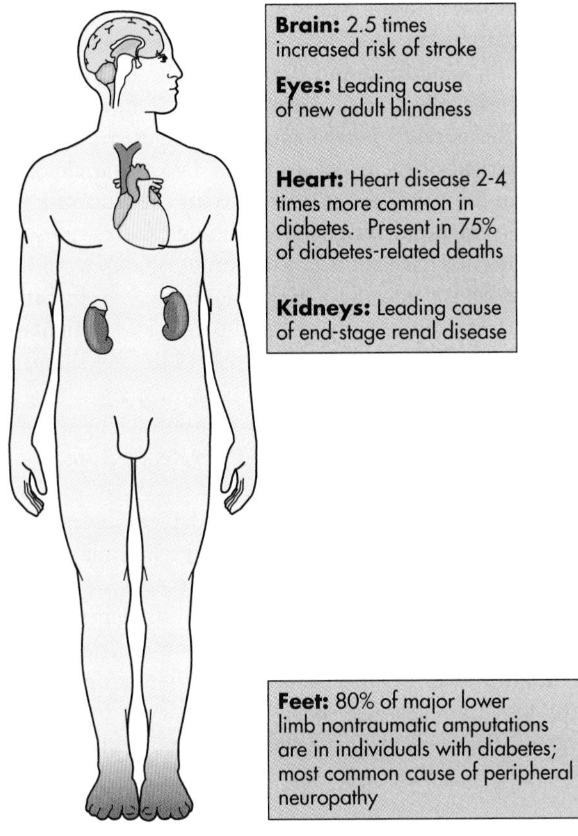

Figure 30-1 Diabetes complications.

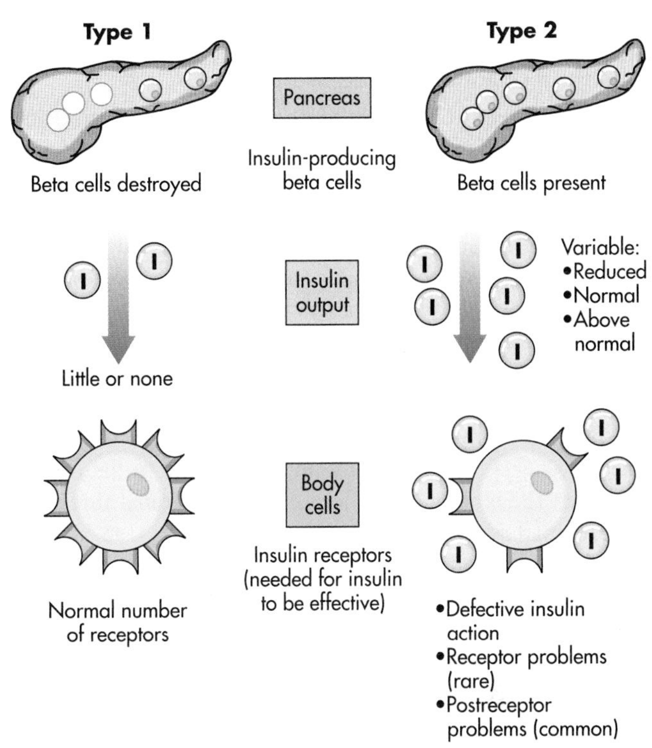

Figure 30-2 Insulin defects in type 1 and type 2 diabetes mellitus.

TABLE 30-5 Pancreatic Hormones

Insulin Promotes, Glucagon Inhibits	Insulin Inhibits, Glucagon Promotes
Glucose uptake into skeletal muscle and liver	Hyperglycemia
Glycogenesis (glycogen synthesis)	Gluconeogenesis (conversion of amino acids into glucose)
	Glycogenolysis (glycogen breakdown)
Protein anabolism (protein synthesis)	Protein catabolism (protein breakdown)
Lipogenesis (fat synthesis and deposition)	Lipolysis (fat breakdown)

NOTE: Insulin is the only hormone that lowers blood glucose levels.

TABLE 30-6 Extrapancreatic Glucose-Elevating Hormones

Cortisol	Catecholamines	Growth Hormone
Gluconeogenesis	Glycogenolysis	Gluconeogenesis
Lipolysis	Lipolysis	Lipolysis
Secretion is controlled by pituitary adrenocorticotropic hormone; deficiency or excess affects glucose control	Inhibition of insulin release	Decreases glucose uptake into skeletal muscle

pituitary gland (growth hormone and adrenocorticotropic hormone), adrenal cortex (cortisol), autonomic nervous system (norepinephrine), and adrenal medulla (epinephrine) (Table 30-6). Insulin is the only hormone that lowers blood glucose levels. The other hormones, called counterregulatory hormones, elevate blood glucose levels. Insulin is synthesized by the beta cells in the islets of Langerhans within the pancreas. Insulin ensures that the body is able to use glucose for energy. Insulin binds to insulin receptors on the surface of the insulin-sensitive tissues (skeletal muscle, liver, and adipose tissue). In response, a cascade of events (postreceptor events) occurs that allows glucose to move from the bloodstream into the cell.

Consequences of Insulin Deficiency: Absolute or Relative

The insulin-requiring organs are the liver, skeletal muscle, and adipose tissue. The consequences of either absolute or relative insulin deficiency at the level of these organs are as follows: (1) liver—hyperglycemia, hypertriglyceridemia, and ketone production; (2) skeletal muscle—failure of glucose uptake and amino acid uptake; and (3) adipose tissue—lipolysis resulting in elevated free fatty acid levels in the circulation (Figure 30-3). This situation is worsened by the consumption of dietary carbohydrate, which is metabolized into glucose and fails to be utilized by the liver and skeletal muscle, with resultant progressive hyperglycemia (elevated blood glucose levels) and glycosuria (abnormal amounts of glucose in the urine).

When the blood glucose level reaches the renal threshold (approximately 180 mg/dl) in normal kidneys, the kidneys cannot keep up with resorbing the glucose from the glomerular filtrate, and glycosuria results. Glucose attracts water, and an osmotic diuresis occurs, resulting in *polyuria* (increased urination). This polyuria results in the loss of water and electrolytes, particularly sodium, chloride, potassium, and phosphate. The loss of water and sodium results in thirst and increases fluid intake *(polydipsia)*. Losses of electrolytes such as potassium, magnesium, and phosphorus occur with the osmotic diuretic effect of glycosuria. Extreme hunger and increased food intake *(polyphagia)* are triggered as the cells become starved of their fuel. In type 1 DM this cycle of glucose loss in the urine and the inability to use glucose for energy results in rapid weight loss. Patients with type 2 DM generally do not have sufficient insulin deficiency to result in pathologic ketosis and the major weight loss seen in patients with type 1 DM. In both type 1 and type 2 DM patients, dehydration and electrolyte disturbance lead to fatigue and listlessness.

Serum lipids (triglycerides, very-low-density lipoproteins, and sometimes cholesterol) may be elevated. Serum ketones may also be elevated. Total body levels of electrolytes (sodium, potassium, chloride, phosphate) can be depleted, even though the serum levels may be elevated (e.g., hyperkalemia). This results from transcellular shifts secondary to acidosis (from ketones). The severity of this altered metabolism depends on the severity of the absolute or relative insulin deficiency. Early recognition of symptoms and diagnosis (before dehydration, weight loss, and ketogenesis) is best achieved by increased awareness of diabetes by both the public and health care professionals.

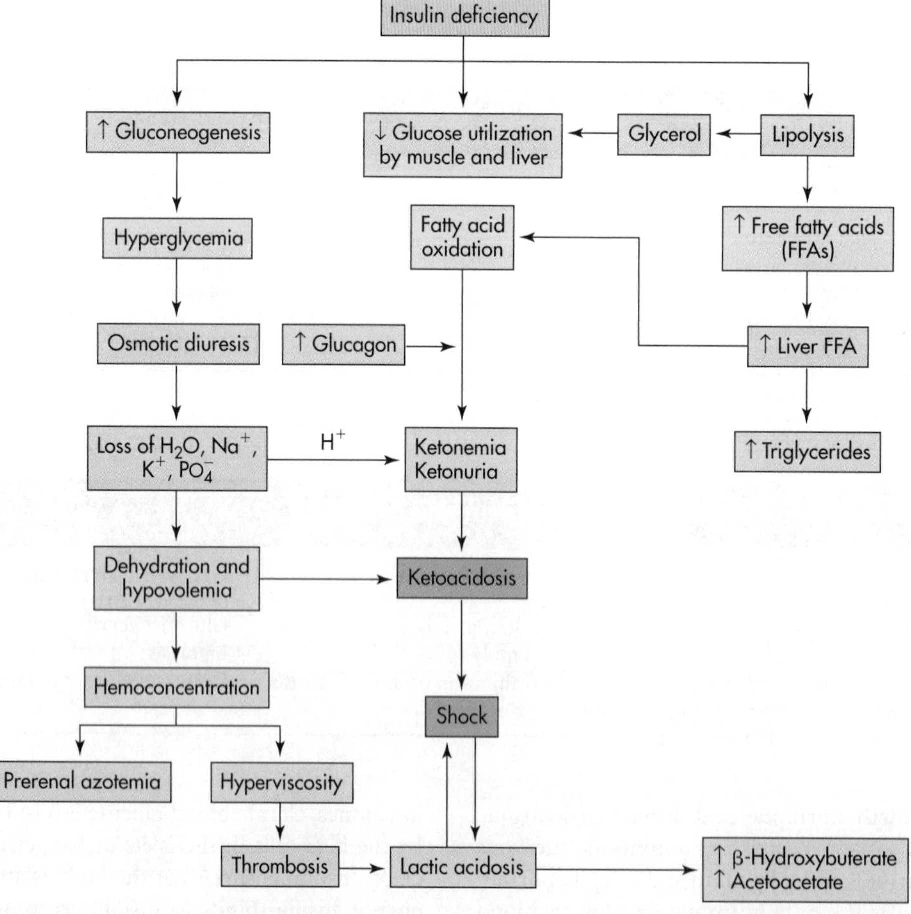

Figure 30-3 Pathophysiology of insulin deficiency.

In mildly insulin-deficient conditions, altered glucose metabolism with hyperglycemia and glycosuria may occur only after meals. Glucose levels and protein metabolism may be normal in the fasting state. As the deficiency increases in severity, hyperglycemia, glycosuria, and protein catabolism are present all of the time. Altered lipid metabolism resulting in elevated levels of triglycerides occurs even in mildly insulin-deficient states. Abnormally high production of ketones may be seen only in markedly insulin-deficient states and is usually present only in persons with type 1 DM.

If the alterations just described are not corrected or adequately controlled, acute and chronic complications can occur. Acutely, the patient can develop nausea and vomiting and other alterations, fluid and electrolyte problems worsen, and the patient's condition can advance to hyperglycemic hyperosmolar nonketotic coma (HHNC) or diabetic ketoacidosis (DKA). The mortality rate in DKA approaches 10%, and the mortality rate in HHNC reaches 70%. Chronically, the patient can develop microvascular (small blood vessel) and macrovascular (large blood vessel) complications or neuropathy. These conditions are described later in this chapter.

The classic symptoms of diabetes are polyuria, polydipsia, and polyphagia. These "polys" are nearly always present in individuals with newly diagnosed type 1 DM and can be present in individuals with newly diagnosed type 2 DM (see Clinical Manifestations box). However, many persons with type 2 DM have very subtle symptoms of acute metabolic changes or chronic complications.

When differentiations are being made between type 1 and type 2 DM, most individuals are readily classified on the basis of age, body weight, and family history. Some elements of a patient's history may make diagnosis difficult (e.g., age 30 to 40 years, unavailable family history [adopted], and weight loss to less than 120% of ideal body weight). However an understanding of the basic pathophysiology readily clarifies the situation. Pancreatic islet cell antibodies are positive in 85% to 90% of type 1 DM patients, and insulin levels are low or subnormal. In a patient already being treated with insulin (before a definitive diagnostic classification has been made), a C-peptide level can provide clarification of endogenous insulin production. A molecule of C-peptide is generated when the insulin precursor molecule proinsulin, produced in the islet cells, is converted to insulin. Hence for every molecule of insulin secreted by the pancreatic islets, a molecule of C-peptide is produced.

An important clue to the correct classification of type 2 DM patients is the presence of other components of the cardiodysmetabolic syndrome—a syndrome encompassing varying degrees of glucose intolerance, hypertension, hypertriglyceridemia, low high-density lipoprotein (HDL) cholesterol, abdominal obesity, hyperuricemia, and elevated levels of plasminogen activator inhibitor type 1. All are mediated and modulated by the control of insulin resistance.[77-79] Insulin resistance essentially blocks the normal uptake of glucose into these insulin-sensitive tissues. The earliest abnormality in glucose metabolism occurs in skeletal muscle as insulin-mediated glucose uptake decreases. A compensatory hyperinsulinemia develops as the pancreatic islets try to increase production and secretion of insulin in an effort to maintain euglycemia (normal blood glucose levels). Eventually, pancreatic exhaustion occurs, and the necessary insulin production falls off. Once the pancreas is no longer able to secrete enough insulin to overcome the insulin resistance, type 2 DM occurs.

Clinical Manifestations
Diabetes

EARLY SYMPTOMS

Polyuria
Polydipsia
Polyphagia
Visual blurring
Fatigue
Weight loss

LATE SIGNS AND SYMPTOMS

Coma
Chronic complications

COLLABORATIVE CARE MANAGEMENT

In the past, patients with diabetes were often hospitalized to initiate management. Hospitalization now occurs only if the patient is experiencing acute metabolic decompensation. Patients need to establish goals with their health care team members for management of their diabetes. The foci of collaborative care include:

- Using diagnostic tests to determine the presence of DM or complications
- Establishing goals related to the level of daily control
- Using medications, treatments, diet, and activities to manage diabetes on a day-to-day basis
- Using medications, treatments, and diet to manage acute and chronic complications of diabetes
- Working as a multidisciplinary team

Achievement and maintenance of metabolic control requires the judicious use of medications, diet, activity, monitoring, and education. By its very nature, diabetes can be significantly influenced by each of these management components (Figure 30-4).

Diagnostic Tests

Diagnostic criteria for diabetes are found in Box 30-1. Frequent monitoring of diagnostic tests (blood glucose, lipids) is a method of assessing glycemic control.

The definition of *control* has changed dramatically over the years. Before the discovery of insulin in 1921, control was defined as the avoidance of early death or coma. The current definition is normalcy—normalization not only of glucose levels but also of other metabolic parameters, such as lipids and blood pressure (Table 30-7).

The relationship of glycemic control to the development of microvascular complications of diabetes was debated for years, despite evidence gathered in a large retrospective study

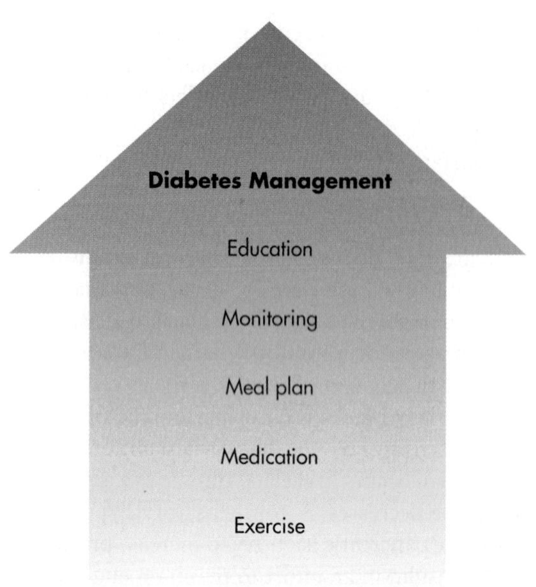

Figure 30-4 Diabetes management.

TABLE 30-7 Goals for Control: Normalization of Metabolic Parameters

Time	mg/dl
Target Blood Glucose Levels in the Nonpregnant State: Euglycemia	
Fasting	70-110
1 hour postprandially	<120
2 AM-4 AM	70-110
Target Lipid Levels (Adults)*	
Total Cholesterol	<200
HDL cholesterol	>45
Triglycerides	<150
LDL cholesterol	<100
Target Blood Pressure (Adults)†	<130/80 mm Hg

HDL, High-density lipoprotein; *LDL,* low-density lipoprotein.
*NCEP III Guidelines.[29]
NOTE: These guidelines are the result of an expert panel and do not reflect the data from randomized clinical trials and evidence-based medicine.
†National High Blood Pressure Working Group.[65]

BOX 30-1 Diagnostic Criteria for Diabetes Mellitus, Impaired Glucose Tolerance, and Gestational Diabetes

Nonpregnant Adults

Diabetes mellitus: Diagnosis of diabetes mellitus in nonpregnant adults should be restricted to those who have one of the following:

1. Fasting plasma glucose level of 126 mg/dl. *Fasting* is defined as no caloric intake for at least 8 hours.
2. Symptoms of diabetes mellitus (such as polyuria, polydipsia, unexplained weight loss) coupled with a casual plasma glucose level of 200 mg/dl. *Casual* is defined as any time of day, without regard to the time interval since the last meal.
3. Two-hour postprandial plasma glucose level of 200 mg/dl during an oral glucose tolerance test. The test should be performed according to World Health Organization criteria, using a glucose load containing the equivalent of 75 g of anhydrous glucose dissolved in water.

In the absence of unequivocal hyperglycemia with acute metabolic decompensation, these criteria should be confirmed by repeat testing on a second occasion. The oral glucose tolerance test is not recommended for routine clinical use. A normal glycosylated hemoglobin does not rule out the presence of diabetes, because the earliest defect is in postprandial control. Hence the glycosylated hemoglobin is not part of the diagnostic package.

Impaired glucose tolerance: Two-hour postprandial plasma glucose level of 140 mg/dl and less than or equal to 200 mg/dl during an oral glucose tolerance test. The test should be performed according to World Health Organization criteria, using a glucose load containing the equivalent of 75 g of anhydrous glucose dissolved in water.

Gestational diabetes: After an oral glucose load of 100 g, gestational diabetes is diagnosed if two plasma glucose values equal or exceed the following:

- Fasting: 105 mg/dl
- 1 hour: 190 mg/dl
- 2 hour: 165 mg/dl
- 3 hour: 145 mg/dl

Impaired fasting glucose: Fasting plasma glucose level greater than 110 mg/dl and less than 126 mg/dl.

Adapted from American Diabetes Association, Expert Committee on the Diagnosis and Classification of Diabetes Mellitus: Report of the Expert Committee on the Diagnosis and Classification of Diabetes Mellitus, *Diabetes Care* 24(suppl 1):S55, 2001.

by Pirart[72] and in smaller controlled studies (the KROC[50] and Steno II[51] studies) that demonstrated a definite relationship. The control and complications issue, however, was proved beyond doubt when results of the landmark Diabetes Control and Complications Trial (DCCT) were published in 1993.[23] The purpose of the DCCT was to examine the effect of two treatment regimens on the development and progression of complications. The DCCT was a 10-year, nationwide, multicenter, randomized prospective clinical trial of over 1400 individuals with type 1 DM. Subjects were randomized to either conventional therapy or intensive therapy. Conventional therapy consisted of one or two insulin injections daily, random home blood glucose monitoring (HBGM), and clinic follow-up every 3 months. In contrast, intensive therapy consisted of three or more insulin injections daily or insulin pump therapy, HBGM before meals and at bedtime, and a more precise carbohydrate-consistent meal plan. Follow-up with the study diabetes team was every 1 to 2 months.

The DCCT was terminated 1 year early because the intensive therapy group had a statistically significant reduction in both (1) the development of and (2) the progression of microvascular complications (Table 30-8). The DCCT found that the lower the hemoglobin A_{1c} (HbA_{1c}) (a marker of diabetes control), the lower the risk of complications. At no point did better blood glucose control not result in fewer complications. As a result of this landmark study, the American Diabetes Association (ADA) recommends intensive therapy for all

TABLE 30-8 Diabetes Control and Complications Trial Research Group: Reduction in Complication Risk With Intensive Therapy

Complication	% Risk Reduction
Clinically significant retinopathy	76
Severe retinopathy/laser surgery	45
Microalbuminuria	35
Albuminuria	56
Clinically significant neuropathy	60

Source: Diabetes Control and Complications Trial Research Group: The effect of intensive treatment of diabetes on the long-term complications in insulin-dependent diabetes mellitus, *N Engl J Med* 329:977, 1993.

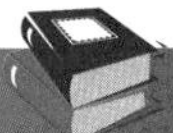

Evidence-Based Practice

Reference: UK Prospective Diabetes Study Group (Stratton IM et al): Association of glycaemia with macrovascular and microvascular complications of type 2 diabetes (UKPDS 35): prospective observational study, *BMJ* 321:405, 2000.

The United Kingdom Prospective Diabetes Study (UKPDS), conducted at 23 centers in England, Scotland, and Northern Ireland, was a prospective clinical trial of the intensive control of blood glucose and blood pressure in patients with newly diagnosed type 2 diabetes. A total of 4585 Caucasian, Asian Indian, and African-Caribbean subjects participated in the trial. In the glucose control part of the study, subjects were randomized to conventional therapy (diet and exercise) versus intensive therapy (sulfonylureas, metformin, or insulin treatment). The UKPDS concluded that intensive glucose therapy resulted in a reduced risk of development of diabetic complications. In addition, complete data were obtained on 3642 subjects to enable analysis in the epidemiologic portion of the trial that analyzed the effect of hemoglobin A_{1c} lowering on the risk of developing complications.

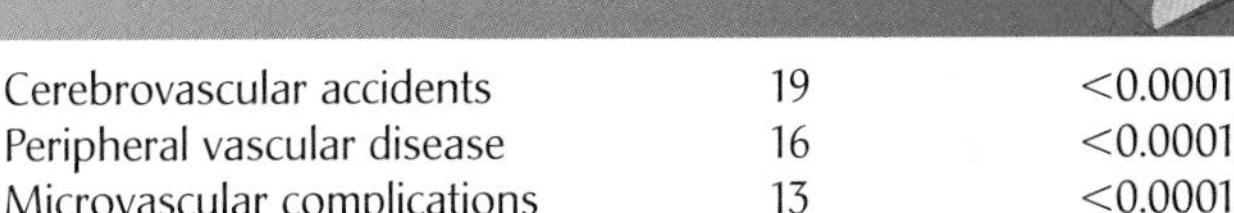

Evidence-Based Practice

Reference: UK Prospective Diabetes Study Group (Adler et al): Association of systolic blood pressure with macrovascular and microvascular complications of type 2 diabetes (UKPDS 36): prospective observational study, *BMJ* 321:412, 2000.

Of the 4585 subjects in the glucose control study, 4801 Caucasian, Asian Indian, and African-Caribbean subjects were eligible for the blood pressure control study. Of these, complete data were obtained on 3642 subjects to enable analysis in the epidemiologic part of the study. A total of 1148 patients with hypertension were randomized to tight blood pressure control (<150/85) versus less tight blood pressure control (<180/105) using a beta-blocker or an angiotensin-converting enzyme (ACE) inhibitor. Additional agents were prescribed as necessary to meet the blood pressure goals.

The intensively treated group had a significant decrease in risk of events as compared with the conventionally treated group. However, regardless of whether a subject was randomized to the intensive treatment or the conventional treatment group, for every 10 mm Hg decrease in systolic blood pressure, the following risk reductions were noted:

COMPLICATION	RISK REDUCTION (%)	P-VALUE
Any diabetes endpoint	12	<0.0001
Diabetes-related death	17	<0.0001
All-cause mortality	12	<0.0001
Myocardial infarction	12	<0.0001
Cerebrovascular accidents	19	<0.0001
Peripheral vascular disease	16	<0.0001
Microvascular complications	13	<0.0001
Congestive heart failure	15	<0.0001

There was no threshold at which a lower blood pressure did not reduce complications; the lower the systolic blood pressure, the lower the risk of complications. The trial also noted that beta-blockers and ACE inhibitors may have additional benefits in reducing complications over and above that related to blood pressure lowering.

For every 1% reduction in the mean hemoglobin A_{1c} (HbA_{1c}), the following risk reductions were noted:

COMPLICATION	RISK REDUCTION (%)	P-VALUE
Any diabetes endpoint	21	<0.0001
Deaths related to diabetes	21	<0.0001
Myocardial infarction	14	<0.0001
Microvascular complications	37	<0.0001

There was no threshold of diabetes control for risk reduction: there was no level below which a lower HbA_{1c} did not result in a lower risk of complications, nor was there a level above which a higher HbA_{1c} did not result in a higher risk of complications. In other words, the lower the HbA_{1c}, the lower the risk of complications.

individuals with type 1 DM, with few exceptions, such as advanced age and end-stage complications.[4,5]

The control and complications issue in type 2 DM was answered by two clinical trials. Intensive therapy for type 2 DM, however, involves different regimens, aimed both at reducing insulin resistance and augmenting insulin secretion. The Kumamoto study of intensive insulin therapy in type 2 DM patients demonstrated a statistically significant relationship between control and complications comparable to the DCCT findings in type 1 DM patients.[67] The United Kingdom Prospective Diabetes Study (UKPDS), a 20-year prospective study in type 2 DM demonstrated that both intensive glycemic control and intensive blood pressure control reduced the risk of microvascular and macrovascular complications of DM (see Evidence-Based Practice boxes).[98-103]

Blood Parameters

Short-Term Control. HBGM is a critical component of the treatment regimen for individuals with either type 1 or type 2

DM. Glucose levels are "vital signs" to individuals with diabetes. HBGM is the only accurate method of monitoring glucose control on a daily basis and allows the person with diabetes to make any necessary changes in the diabetes regimen. Results should be recorded in a logbook. Minimally, nonpregnant individuals with type 1 DM should perform HBGM before meals and at bedtime. Patients using an insulin pump perform HBGM up to 12 or more times per day. The frequency of HBGM in type 2 DM patients is determined by the treatment regimen and varies from once per day to several times per day. Postprandial HBGM is critical even in the diabetic patient with a normal HbA_{1c}. Approximately 50% of individuals with diabetes who have a normal HbA_1c have a 2-hour postprandial glucose level in excess of 200 mg/dl. The higher the HbA_{1c}, the more likely it is that a patient will have an elevated postprandial glucose level. Unfortunately, according to Healthy People 2010, only 42% of individuals with diabetes 18 years of age or older perform HBGM at least once daily.[107,110]

HBGM uses capillary whole blood obtained by a fingerstick and correlates well with laboratory values when accurate techniques are used. Serum glucose values are approximately 10% lower than whole blood values (see Guidelines for Safe Practice box). The majority of available glucose meters use a "no blot" technique—the user does not blot or wipe the blood off the test strip. A test strip is inserted into the meter, and a drop of capillary blood is applied to the strip, which is impregnated with either glucose oxidase or another chemical. A chemical reaction occurs, and the result is displayed on the meter. Test time varies among manufacturers, ranging from 5 to 45 seconds. Some blood glucose meters are approved for alternate site testing—obtaining capillary blood at a site other than the finger, such as the forearm. All marketed glucose meters must be approved by the U.S. Food and Drug Administration (FDA) and yield accurate results when proper technique is used. Meters must be calibrated to each test strip lot according to manufacturers' specifications. The most common source of errors in HBGM results is user technique, followed by problems with the test strips. Because a chemical is embedded in the test strip, any factors that can affect the chemical—light, heat, cold, humidity—will alter the result. Use of control solution is the only manner in which to test the accuracy of the strips. Control solution, produced by the meter's manufacturer, is glucose solution in a known concentration that yields a standard result. Unfortunately, control solution is often not readily available in pharmacies and is an additional cost to the individual, the insurance company, or both. New technologies for home glucose monitoring are increasing (see Future Watch box).

Long-Term Control. Long-term glycemic control is monitored by the HbA_{1c}. The HbA_{1c} reflects the average blood glucose level over a period of time. Glucose in the blood readily attaches to hemoglobin. Once attached, it remains so throughout the life span of the erythrocyte (90 to 120 days). The HbA_{1c} provides an objective measure of control and is not influenced by age, sex, duration of diabetes, or very recent blood glucose levels. The HbA_{1c} reflects glycemic control over the past 3 months but can be affected by hemoglobin variants, such as hemoglobin S found in sickle cell anemia. High-performance liquid chromatography reveals patients with variants. The HbA_{1c} should be used in conjunction with HBGM results to assess glycemic control. Unfortunately, in the United States the majority of individuals with diabetes fall far short of having the ADA-recommended quarterly HbA_{1c} measurements; only 24% of individuals with diabetes have an HbA_{1c} measurement done at least once per year.[107]

Guidelines for Safe Practice

Procedure for Capillary Blood Glucose Monitoring

1. Verify meter calibration. If the meter is not calibrated to the current lot of strips, calibrate before using.
2. Use control solution when opening a new box or bottle of test strips or any time the glucose result does not make sense in the context of the clinical setting.
3. Cleanse finger with either soap and water or alcohol. If alcohol is used, wait for the finger to dry.
4. Place lancet in a fingerstick device.
5. Prick finger.
6. Gently squeeze finger to obtain an adequate sample of blood. NOTE: If alcohol was used to cleanse the finger, the first drop of blood must be discarded.
7. Follow manufacturer's instructions to perform the test.
8. Discard lancet, cap of lancing device, and any other part of the equipment that may have been contaminated by blood in a hazardous waste receptacle.
9. Record glucose result, noting date, time, result, and action taken.

Future Watch

Monitoring Blood Glucose Levels

Until recently the only way for individuals with diabetes to monitor their glucose levels was to do a capillary fingerstick. However, new methods have arrived, and more are on the horizon. Several glucose meters now have approval for alternate site testing–obtaining the "stick" from the forearm. The U.S. Food and Drug Administration has recently approved the GlucoWatch Biographer by Cygnus, which is a watchlike device that creates a low-voltage electric current with an AAA battery, causing wicking of glucose from the interstitial fluid that is read by a sensor worn on the forearm. The GlucoWatch does not replace the need to perform blood glucose monitoring with a meter. Its role is to provide additional blood glucose trend data to the wearer. Disadvantages of this device include a 3-hour warm-up period for each sensor (which can be used for only 12 hours of data collection) and the potential for skin irritation. Technologies of the future include near-infrared light or other light sources to measure blood glucose via the skin and measurement of interstitial glucose by shining a light in the eye of an individual wearing a special contact lens. One of the most promising technologies is measurement of interstitial glucose via a sensor inserted every 48 to 72 hours, with the glucose level being "read" by a small device via radiofrequency or other methods.

Urine Parameters

Glucose Monitoring. Urine glucose monitoring should not be used to assess glycemic control. Glucose spills into the urine when serum glucose reaches the renal threshold (approximately 180 mg/dl). A urine glucose result always gives retrospective data, never current blood glucose levels. It only reflects blood glucose levels hours before, when the renal threshold is exceeded.

Ketone Monitoring. Individuals with type 1 DM should perform urine ketone monitoring when ill and when HBGM results exceed 300 mg/dl. Ketone monitoring is performed by using test strips impregnated with acetoacetate, which are dipped into the urine. Test time varies, depending on the manufacturer. Negative results are indicated by a beige color on the test strip. Urine ketones are positive at the trace level; as ketone levels rise, the color turns to deeper shades of purple. The Precision Xtra is a combination blood glucose/blood ketone meter. Blood ketone monitoring is useful in children and in individuals with insulin pumps, both of whom can become rapidly ketotic at lower than typical glucose levels. In addition, individuals who have color blindness cannot successfully read urine ketone strips accurately. In individuals with type 1 DM, the presence of ketones in the blood or urine is a dangerous sign and requires prompt attention to insulin, diet, and fluid intake to avoid DKA. Individuals with type 2 DM should monitor urine ketones during periods of illness. Ketones can be present in a type 2 DM patient if there is significant hyperglycemia, hypertriglyceridemia, dehydration, and/or electrolyte depletion. As in a type 1 DM patient, positive urine ketones require prompt attention.

Ankle-Brachial Indices

Ankle-brachial indices (ABIs) are part of clinical recommendations for assessment of vascular disease and risk.[68] A sphygmomanometer cuff of appropriate size is placed on the upper arm, and using a handheld Doppler, the systolic pressure is auscultated at the radial artery. This procedure is repeated for the opposite arm. Then a cuff of appropriate size is placed on the lower leg proximal to the ankle. Using the Doppler, the systolic pressure is auscultated at both the dorsalis pedis and the posterior tibial. The procedure is repeated on the opposite leg, and an index is calculated for each pedal site (ankle pressure divided by brachial artery pressure).

An index greater than 1.2 is indicative of calcific disease. Calcification of blood vessels is common as a consequence of long-standing diabetes, which may be complicated by hypertension and dyslipidemia. An index below 0.9 signifies diminished blood flow and implies arterial disease. Abnormal results require a complete noninvasive lower extremity evaluation consisting of segmental pressures, pneumoplethysmography, and photoplethysmography for further assessment. The clinical importance of an ABI extends beyond the peripheral arterial tree; a reduced ABI is a marker of systemic cardiovascular risk. An isolated posterior tibial index carries a threefold higher risk of all-cause mortality and a fourfold higher risk of coronary heart disease mortality.[21]

Medications and Treatments

Type 1 DM and type 2 DM are two separate and distinct pathophysiologic entities. As a result, the pharmacologic treatment regimen of type 1 DM differs significantly from that of type 2 DM.

Type 1 Diabetes Mellitus: Insulin

Treatment of type 1 DM involves a triad: insulin, diet, and exercise. Because type 1 DM is characterized by insulinopenia, physiologic insulin replacement is the first management component.

The discovery of insulin by Banting and Best in 1921 occupies a major place in medical history. Their "extract of pancreatic origin" became the *eau de vivre* of individuals with diabetes. Insulin products over the years have become increasingly pure and plentiful since January 11, 1921, when Leonard Thompson became the first individual treated with insulin.[11,89]

Properties of Insulin. Three properties of insulin preparation may be identified in the prescription: source, strength, and type or kinetics. Animal-source insulins, extracts from pancreases of pigs or cows, have been discontinued from the U.S. market. Human insulin is derived by recombinant DNA technology (Humulin from *Escherichia coli;* Novolin from *Saccharomyces cerevisiae* [bakers' yeast]). The strength of insulin in the United States is U-100: 100 units of insulin per milliliter of volume. A rare patient requiring very large doses of insulin may need U-500 insulin, which must be specially ordered. Insulins used to treat diabetes are detailed in Table 30-9.[71]

Insulins differ in their speed of onset, peak, and duration of action and are classified as quick, intermediate, or long acting. Dietary carbohydrate and activity must be coordinated with insulin action so that (1) insulin is available for optimal metabolism when the food that was eaten is absorbed, and (2) food is available while insulin is acting to prevent hypoglycemic reactions.

Two principles are useful in coordinating food and insulin:

1. Carbohydrate intake must be coordinated with insulin kinetics (action).
2. Regular insulin and intermediate-acting insulins (NPH and Lente) require that a supplemental snack of 15 g of carbohydrate be given to match the peak action of the insulin; for example, a 10AM snack would be given after a 7 AM injection of regular insulin.

When the insulin prescription is changed, careful patient monitoring is necessary to identify the clinical effect.

Physiologic Replacement of Insulin

Normal Glucose Metabolism. In an individual without diabetes, insulin is secreted by the pancreas in two fashions: basal and prandial (Figure 30-5). Insulin is secreted in a basal fashion in the fasting state and between meals to control hepatic glucose output and disposal. In individuals without diabetes who live a "day life" (awake during the day and asleep at night), counterregulatory hormones are at their nadir between midnight and 2 AM; therefore blood glucose levels are at their lowest point. After 3 to 4 AM the counterregulatory

TABLE 30-9 Common Insulins for Diabetes Mellitus

Type	Onset (hr)	Peak (hr)	Duration (hr)	Retarding Agent	Appearance
Quick-Acting Insulin					
Lispro	0-0.2	1	3	None	Clear
Aspart	0-0.2	0.75-1.5	3	None	Clear
Regular	0.5	2.5-3.5	6-8	None	Clear
Intermediate-Acting Insulin					
NPH	1.5	4-12	22	Protamine sulfate	Cloudy suspension
Lente	2.5	7-15	22	Zinc	Turbid solution
Long-Acting Insulin					
Ultralente	4	None	28	Zinc	Turbid solution
Glargine	1-2 hours	None	24+	None	Clear
Combination Insulin					
Humulin 50/50 50% NPH 50% regular	0.5	2-5	22	Protamine sulfate	Cloudy suspension
Humulin or Novolin 70/30 70% NPH 30% regular	0.5	1.5-16	22	Protamine sulfate	Cloudy suspension
Humalog Mix 75/25 75% NPH 25% Lispro	0-0.2	1-6.5	22	Protamine sulfate	Cloudy suspension
Humalog Mix 50/50 50% NPH 50% Humalog	0-0.2	1-4.5	22	Protamine sulfate	Cloudy suspension

hormones rise, causing an increase in hepatic glucose output, which can continue until 10 or 11 AM. In a nondiabetic person, to maintain euglycemia, the pancreas responds by increasing secretion of insulin by approximately 50%. This is the concept of "the happy liver"—the liver needs to "see" insulin continuously to control glucose output and production in the fasting state. Prandial insulin is secreted by the nondiabetic pancreas in response to the ingestion of dietary carbohydrate. Native prandial insulin is secreted biphasically, with the first phase or peak occurring in 1 minute and the second phase or peak occurring in 60 minutes. First-phase insulin secretion serves to shut off hepatic glucose output in the context of an anticipated glucose load from a meal. The pancreas tailors the amount of insulin to the amount of carbohydrate ingested.

Intensive Insulin Therapy Regimens. The challenge in the treatment of type 1 DM is physiologic insulin replacement: one must "think like a pancreas." Joslin[47] aptly described the challenge: "Insulin . . . is primarily a remedy for the wise and not the foolish, be they patients or doctors. Everyone knows it requires brains to live long with diabetes, but to use insulin successfully requires more brains."

Intensive therapy using multiple daily insulin injections has become the gold standard since the publication of the DCCT. Conventional therapies, which use once- and twice-daily insulin injection programs, were shown to be less effective in the management and control of diabetes. The "split-mix" insulin regimen is one such intensive therapy regimen. It uses premixed insulin, which is a mix of two types of insulin in a preset proportion. For example, 1 U of Humulin or Novolin 70/30 provides 0.7 U of NPH insulin and 0.3 U of Regular insulin. A disadvantage of premixed insulins is that they do not allow fine tuning of the insulin regimen. Thus if one strives for fasting blood glucose levels consistently within the euglycemic range of 70 to 100 mg/dl with the split-mix regimen, an unacceptable incidence of nocturnal hypoglycemia occurs because the predinner intermediate-acting insulin has its peak effect during the counterregulatory nadir (approximately 12 midnight to 2 AM) (Figure 30-6).

Three Injections per Day: Regular or Lispro and Intermediate-Acting Insulin. An example of this regimen with a prescribed daily insulin dose of 60 U follows. Approximately two thirds of the total daily insulin dose (40 U) is given in the morning before breakfast, with one third of that dose (13 U) being given as Regular or Lispro insulin; the remaining two thirds of the prebreakfast dose (27 U) is given as NPH or Lente. In the evening the remaining one third of the total daily dose (20 U) is delivered: 50% (10 U) as Regular or Lispro insulin before dinner and 50% (10 U) as NPH or Lente at bedtime. This moving of the predinner NPH/Lente to bedtime (10 PM to 1 AM) moves the insulin peak to dawn and can reduce nocturnal

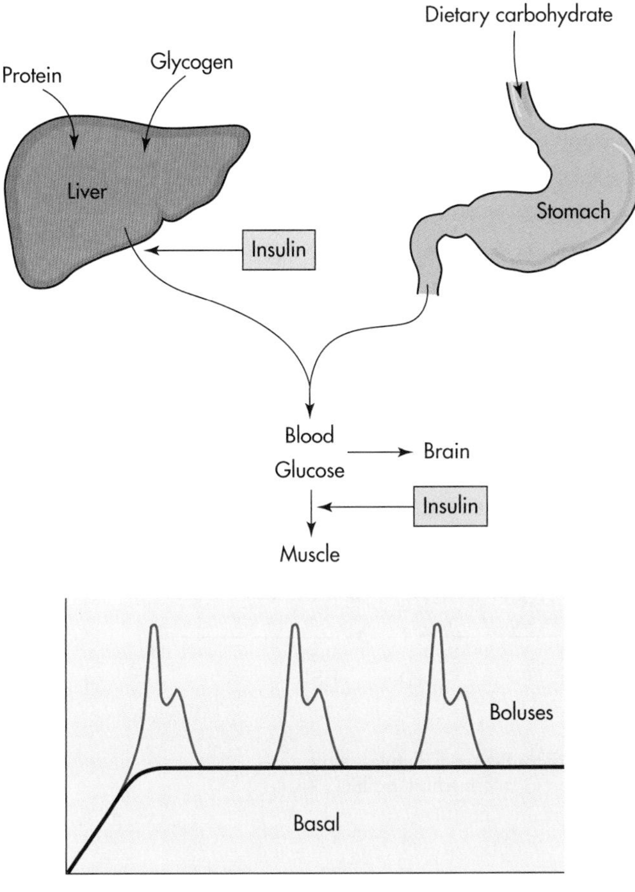

Figure 30-5 Glucose metabolism.

hypoglycemia as much as fivefold. Therefore the dose is 13 U of Lispro and 27 U of NPH/Lente before breakfast, 10 U of Lispro before dinner, and 10 U of NPH/Lente at bedtime. The drawback of this insulin regimen is the lack of flexibility with regard to the timing of lunch because of the emerging peak effect from the prebreakfast dose of NPH/Lente insulin (see Figure 30-6).

Three Injections per Day: Ultralente Basal With Premeal Regular or Lispro Insulin. In this regimen approximately 50% of the total daily insulin dose is given as Ultralente, divided into two injections given before breakfast and before dinner, respectively. The Ultralente insulin acts as basal insulin to control hepatic glucose output and disposal in the fasting state, and it is given regardless of whether or not dietary carbohydrate is consumed. Then Regular or Lispro insulin is given before each meal (before snacks also if using Lispro insulin), with the dosage titrated to the amount of carbohydrate planned. This regimen provides a significant amount of flexibility in meal timing, and patients may compensate for addition or deletion of carbohydrate at each meal with the adjustment of the premeal insulin dose. Because of these advantages, this regimen is commonly known as "the poor man's pump." It is not useful for treating individuals with a pronounced dawn hormonal surge (adolescents and pregnant women) or individuals with long-standing diabetes, in whom insulin kinetics may be erratic (see Figure 30-6).

Four Injections per Day: Premeal Lispro and Bedtime Glargine Insulin. Glargine is a new basal insulin analog with no peak effect and over 24 hours' duration of action. Glargine insulin injected once daily at bedtime controls hepatic glucose output and production in the fasting state. Premeal Lispro insulin is taken before consuming carbohydrates, with the dosage titrated to the amount of carbohydrate planned. Approximately 40% to 60% of the total daily dose is Glargine, with the remaining being Lispro. This regimen is another example of "the poor man's pump." Because Glargine insulin has a low pH, it can never be mixed in an insulin syringe with any other insulin or precipitation will occur.

Four Injections per Day: Premeal Regular and Overnight NPH/Lente Insulin. Typically, about 20% of the total daily dose is given as NPH/Lente at bedtime (10 PM to 1 AM), with the remaining 80% of the total daily dose given as Regular insulin and distributed proportionately between the carbohydrate load at each of the three meals. This regimen is especially suited to patients with extremely labile diabetes in whom other regimens fail. It must be remembered that the overnight NPH/Lente insulin dose does not cover the full 24-hour basal requirements. Therefore a portion of the premeal regular insulin dose is covering the basal requirements. If individuals have longer than a 6-hour time span between injections of regular insulin, they generally experience "insulin runout hyperglycemia," because if the liver does not "see" insulin, it uncontrollably releases more glucose (see Figure 30-6).

Four Injections per Day: Prebreakfast Ultralente and Lispro, Prelunch and Predinner Lispro, and Overnight NPH/Lente Insulin. This regimen is ideal for individuals who use Lispro insulin, require flexibility, and have a significant dawn hormonal surge. The substitution of Lispro for Regular insulin in the previously described regimen would result in significant insulin runout hyperglycemia because of the very short duration of action of Lispro. The insulin runout issue with Lispro can be managed by the addition of a small dose of Ultralente insulin before breakfast to control hepatic glucose output and disposal during the day, with the bedtime NPH/Lente insulin providing coverage of hepatic glucose output and disposal during the night (see Figure 30-6). This regimen allows flexibility in dosages and the interval between injections and mealtimes to best control postprandial glucose levels.

Continuous Subcutaneous Insulin Infusion/Insulin Pump Therapy. Insulin pump therapy using a portable external insulin infusion pump offers the most physiologic insulin delivery. The pump holds only quick-acting insulin, with the majority of patients using Lispro insulin. The pump is preprogrammed to deliver varying hourly basal rates. For example, the pump can be programmed to deliver less insulin during the 12 midnight to 2AM counterregulatory nadir and then to increase insulin delivery in the dawn hours, thus matching the individual's needs. Before consuming carbohydrates, the patient delivers a bolus of insulin matched to the carbohydrate content of the meal. In addition to being the most physiologic insulin delivery system, an insulin pump is also the most flexible (see Figure 30-6).

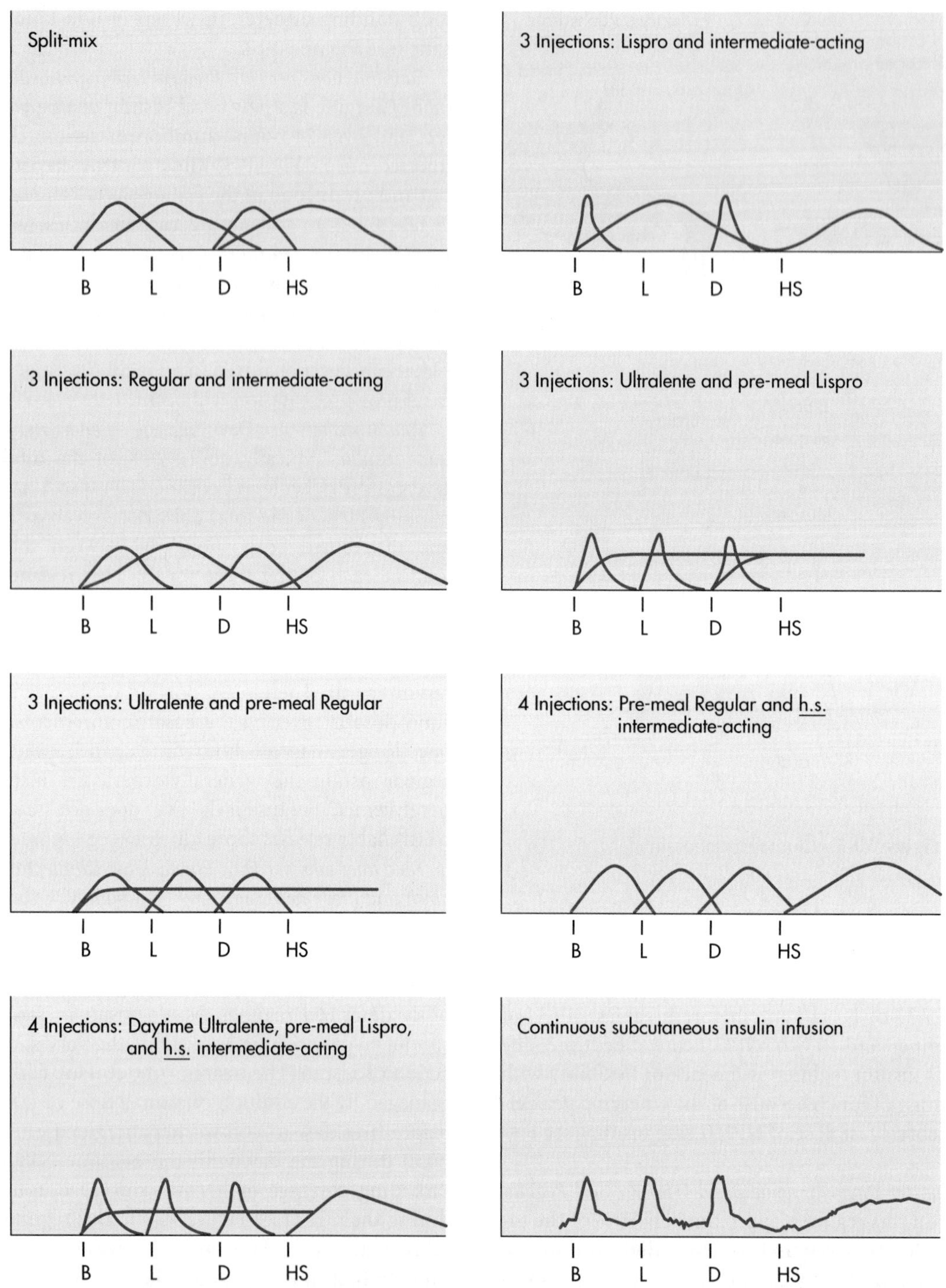

Figure 30-6 Insulin delivery programs.

Current insulin pumps are no larger than a pager (see Figure 30-7). The ideal candidate for the pump is an individual who has failed to control diabetes on one of the aforementioned insulin regimens, someone who is pregnant or contemplating pregnancy, or someone who desires increased daily flexibility. Disadvantages include the initial capital outlay ($5300) and cost of maintenance supplies (although most insurance companies cover 70% to 100%), the continual presence of a needle or Teflon-like cannula placed subcutaneously in the abdomen, and the potential risk of sepsis. Attention to sterile technique and changing the infusion site every 24 to 48 hours minimize the risk of sepsis. The greatest risk is the potential for rapid-onset DKA if there is any interruption of insulin delivery via partial occlusion of the tubing, needle, or cannula or accidental removal of the needle or cannula. Because the pump uses only quick-acting insulin, the patient is at risk for rapid-onset DKA if insulin delivery is interrupted for any reason. A good safety net is to have patients with pumps change the infusion site if the capillary blood glucose level is greater than 300 mg/dl and they are unable to account

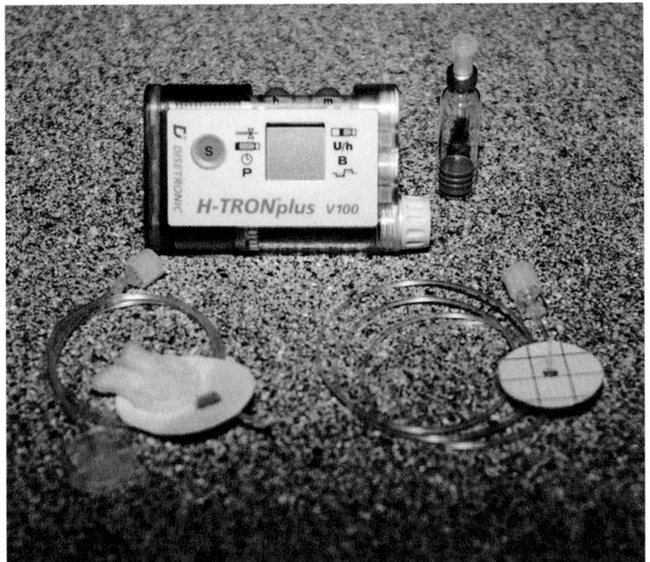

Figure 30-7 Insulin infusion pump and supplies.

for the elevation because of excess carbohydrate intake. Insulin pump therapy should be initiated only in an educated, motivated patient under the care of a diabetes team educated and skilled in pump therapy and offering 24-hour support for the patient.[2] Exercise with a pump is facilitated by the ability to program a temporary basal reduction for planned physical activity, thus removing the need for individuals to consume additional carbohydrates before exercise.

Insulin Algorithms as a Component of Intensive Therapy. An insulin algorithm is a plan for additional insulin to be administered for episodes of hyperglycemia; each patient should have an individualized plan. Via an algorithm, additional insulin is given over and above the baseline or usual insulin dose on the basis of fingerstick blood glucose levels. For example, in a patient taking 0.5 to 0.8 U/kg of body weight, an additional unit of Lispro or Regular insulin would be expected to lower blood glucose levels by approximately 50 mg/dl (Box 30-2).[86]

Insulin algorithms must be differentiated from "sliding scales." In a sliding scale no baseline insulin is administered to control either hepatic glucose output and disposal or prandial needs; insulin is administered on a contingency basis every 4 to 6 hours on the basis of the prevailing fingerstick blood glucose level (Box 30-3). In other words, with a sliding scale, quick-acting insulin is given only after hyperglycemia has already occurred. Sliding-scale insulin dosing makes no physiologic sense and results in an "unhappy liver" manifested by hyperglycemia and perhaps ketosis. A health care team can readily precipitate nosocomial DKA by using sliding-scale insulin dosages.[75,84,104]

Inhaled quick-acting insulin is under clinical investigation, and early results have been promising in terms of glycemic control. In the trials, inhaled quick-acting insulin is administered to cover prandial requirements; intermediate-acting or long-acting insulin is injected to cover basal requirements.[15] However, there are concerns with inhaled insulin. These concerns center on the vasodilatory properties of insulin and the theoretic potential for pulmonary hypotension and pulmonary edema, especially in patients with cardiac dysfunction.

BOX 30-2 Sample Algorithm for Hyperglycemia

Premeal, for every 50 mg/dl elevation in blood glucose above 120 mg/dl, add 1 U of Lispro/Regular insulin to the baseline dose:

Blood Glucose	Add Lispro/Regular Insulin SQ
≥170 mg/dl	1 U
≥220 mg/dl	2 U
≥270 mg/dl	3 U

At bedtime, for every 50 mg/dl elevation in blood glucose above 150 mg/dl, add 1 U of Lispro/regular insulin to the baseline dose:

Blood Glucose	Add Lispro/Regular Insulin SQ
≥200 mg/dl	1 U
≥250 mg/dl	2 U
≥300 mg/dl	3 U

SQ, Subcutaneously.

BOX 30-3 Sample Sliding Scale

Give no baseline insulin. Give regular insulin every 4 hours based on fingerstick blood glucose values as follows:

Blood Glucose	Give Regular Insulin SQ
≥200 mg/dl	2 U
≥250 mg/dl	6 U
≥300 mg/dl	10 U

SQ, Subcutaneously.

Medications: Type 2 Diabetes Mellitus

Pharmacotherapy for type 2 DM can be directed at (1) decreasing insulin resistance and increasing insulin sensitization (metformin hydrochloride and the thiazolidinediones), (2) interfering with the digestion and absorption of dietary carbohydrate (alpha-glucosidase inhibitors), (3) augmenting insulin secretion and action (sulfonylureas, repaglinide, and nateglinide), or (4) providing exogenous insulin (Table 30-10).

Decreasing Insulin Resistance/Increasing Insulin Sensitivity. Metformin (Glucophage) and the thiazolidinediones work via different mechanisms. Metformin primarily inhibits uncontrolled hepatic glucose production, whereas the thiazolidinediones enhance skeletal muscle glucose uptake—the earliest defect in evolving type 2 DM.

Metformin, a true insulin sensitizer, decreases hepatic glucose production and enhances peripheral glucose use. Because it is an antihyperglycemic agent and does not stimulate insulin secretion, it cannot induce hypoglycemia when used as monotherapy. Ideal candidates for treatment with metformin are overweight or obese patients with type 2 DM. The potentially fatal side effect of lactic acidosis generally occurs only when metformin is used in contraindicated patients—those

TABLE 30-10 Common Oral Medications for Type 2 Diabetes Mellitus

Parameter	Metformin	Pioglitazone	Rosiglitazone	Sulfonylureas
Mode of action	↓Hepatic glucose ↑ Skeletal muscle glucose utilization	↑ Skeletal muscle glucose utilization ↓Hepatic glucose	↑ Skeletal muscle glucose utilization ↓ Hepatic glucose	↑Insulin secretion ↓Hepatic glucose production
Glucose effects	Fasting and postprandial	Fasting and postprandial	Fasting and postprandial	Fasting and postprandial
Hypoglycemia as monotherapy	No	No	No	Yes
Weight gain	No	Possible	Possible	Possible
Insulin levels	↓	↓	↓	↑
Side effects	GI (self-limiting symptoms of nausea, diarrhea, anorexia)	? elevation in hepatic transaminases	? elevation in hepatic transaminases	Potential allergic reaction if sulfa allergy Potential drug interactions (first-generation agents) SIADH
Lipid effects	↓	↑ HDL, ↓ triglycerides LDL concentration unaltered	Increase in total cholesterol, LDL, and HDL concentration ? change in particle composition	↑ or ↓
Usual starting dose for a 70-kg man	500 mg bid with meals or XR 500 mg with the evening meal	15 mg qd	4 mg daily either single or divided dose Better results with divided dose	Varies with each agent Glyburide 2.5 mg qd Glucotrol XL 5 mg qd Glynase 3 mg qd Amaryl 2 mg qd
Maximum dose	850 mg tid with meals or XR 2000 mg with the evening meal	45 mg qd	8 mg daily as either single or divided dose Better results with divided dose	Varies with each agent Glyburide 10 mg bid Glucotrol XL 20 mg qd Glynase 6 mg bid Amaryl 8 mg qd
Contraindications	Type 1 diabetes Renal or hepatic dysfunction History of ETOH abuse Chronic conditions associated with hypoxia (asthma, COPD, CHF) Acute conditions associated with potential for hypoxia (CHF, acute MI, surgery) Situations associated with potential renal dysfunction (e.g., IV contrast)	Type 1 diabetes	Type 1 diabetes	Type 1 diabetes

CHF, Congestive heart failure; *COPD,* chronic obstructive pulmonary disease; *ETOH,* ethanol; *GI,* gastrointestinal; *HDL,* high-density lipoprotein; *IV,* intravenous; *LDL,* low-density lipoprotein; *MI,* myocardial infarction; *SIADH,* syndrome of inappropriate antidiuretic hormone; *XR,* extended release.

with renal insufficiency, liver disease, alcohol excess, or underlying hypoxic states (congestive heart failure, chronic obstructive pulmonary disease, significant asthma, acute myocardial infarction). Metformin should be discontinued on the morning of an elective surgical procedure that may require general anesthesia because risks of general anesthesia include hypoxia, which can cause lactic acidosis. Metformin should also be discontinued on the morning of any elective procedures using contrast materials (e.g., intravenous [IV] pyelogram, cardiac catheterization), because contrast materials can directly cause renal shutdown and drug accumulation. In both of the above situations, metformin should not be restarted for 48 to 72 hours after the surgery/procedure, pending documentation of a normal serum creatinine level. Adjustments in the individual's diabetes regimen will have to be made for this time period to maintain glycemic control. In the UKPDS, despite similar levels of glycemic control, the subset of obese type 2 DM patients treated with metformin had a statistically significantly lower cardiovascular event and death rate than the other groups.[100] Thus metformin must be modulating other aspects of the cardiodysmetabolic syndrome.

Thiazolidinediones, better known as the glitazones (pioglitazone [Actos] and rosiglitazone [Avandia]), are antihyperglycemic insulin-sensitizing agents that bind to the PPAR nuclear receptor and amplify the insulin signal. Glitazones stimulate skeletal muscle glucose uptake directly; in addition,

TABLE 30-10 Common Oral Medications for Type 2 Diabetes Mellitus—cont'd

Parameter	Repaglinide	Nateglinide	Acarbose	Miglitol
Mode of action	↑ Insulin secretion	↑ Insulin secretion	Alpha-glucosidase inhibition ↓ Carbohydrate digestion and absorption from GI tract	Alpha-glucosidase inhibition ↓ Carbohydrate digestion and absorption from GI tract
Glucose effects	Postprandial and fasting	Postprandial	Postprandial	Postprandial
Hypoglycemia as monotherapy	Yes; less than that seen with sulfonylureas	No	No	No
Weight gain	No	No	No	No
Insulin levels	↑	↑	↓ or no change	↓ or no change
Side effects	Rare hypoglycemia	Very rare hypoglycemia, since effects are glucose dependent	GI (flatulence, abdominal distention, diarrhea)	GI (flatulence, abdominal distention, diarrhea)
Lipid effects	No change	No change	↓ or no change	↓ or no change
Usual starting dose for a 70-kg man	0.5 mg before meals	120 mg tid	25 mg TID with first bite of each meal	25 mg TID with first bite of each meal
Maximum dose	16 mg daily in divided doses at meals/snacks	120 mg tid	100 mg tid with first bite of each meal	100 mg tid with first bite of each meal
Contraindications	Type 1 diabetes	Type 1 diabetes	Type 1 diabetes Inflammatory bowel disease Bowel obstruction Cirrhosis Chronic conditions with maldigestion or malabsorption	Type 1 diabetes Inflammatory bowel disease Bowel obstruction Cirrhosis Chronic conditions with maldigestion or malabsorption

and perhaps more important, they may do so indirectly via effects on adipose tissue with reduction in circulating free fatty acids. Free fatty acids induce insulin resistance. In addition to glucose-lowering properties, glitazones have purported beneficial effects on the other components of the cardiodysmetabolic syndrome. These agents may also assist in preservation of beta-cell function via reduction in lipid deposition within the islets of Langerhans—a concept known as lipotoxicity and a finding documented in animals. These agents can be safely used in patients with renal insufficiency without the need for dosage adjustment. A contraindication to their use is liver disease or elevations in hepatic transaminases. Although the risk of transaminase elevation is rare, monitoring should be done every 2 months for the first year and periodically thereafter. These agents are contraindicated in patients with New York grade III or grade IV congestive heart failure. The most common adverse effect is edema. Clinically, glucose lowering is very gradual with these agents.

Interference With Carbohydrate Digestion and Absorption. Alpha-glucosidase inhibition by acarbose (Precose) and miglitol (Glyset) have a primary mode of action of decreasing postprandial blood glucose levels via direct interference with the digestion and absorption of dietary carbohydrate. These agents are most commonly used as adjunctive therapy rather than as monotherapy. Both of these agents need to be dosed with the first bite of the meal. Increased intestinal gas formation, the most common side effect, is minimized with slow dose titration and does improve with continued administration.

Augmentation of Insulin Secretion. Sulfonylureas enhance insulin secretion and action. First-generation sulfonylureas (chlorpropamide, tolazamide, tolbutamide), although efficacious, have a higher risk of side effects, such as sustained hypoglycemia, the chlorpropamide flush (an Antabuse-like reaction), protein-binding interference with certain medications, and the syndrome of inappropriate diuretic hormone secretion. The second- and third-generation sulfonylureas are preferred because of their increased milligram potency, shorter duration of action, and better side effect profile.

Prior concerns about possible cardiotoxicity of sulfonylureas related to the University Group Diabetes Program Study have generally disappeared, given the emergence of data to support the safety of these agents from the cardiovascular prospective in the UKPDS. Glimepiride, a third-generation sulfonylurea, has benefits in terms of a reduced risk of hypoglycemia, potentially lower risk of adverse cardiovascular effects, and perhaps reduced potential for secondary failure.

One of the meglitinides, repaglinide (Prandin), is dosed before meals to lower blood glucose levels by stimulating the release of insulin from the islet cells. Because there is a risk of hyperglycemia, the patient must be monitored carefully.

Nateglinide (Starlix), a phenylalanine derivative, is given before meals to produce an abrupt spurt of insulin. Hypoglycemia is very rare. Switching from a sulfonylurea to nateglinide can result in a slight rise in fasting glucose levels; however, since postprandial glucose levels are significantly improved, the HbA_{1c} may be maintained or lowered. This is due to the fact that postprandial glucose contributes more to the HbA_{1c} than fasting or premeal glucose levels do.

To achieve the ADA goal HbA_{1c}, the vast majority of type 2 DM patients require combination therapy. Beginning pharmacotherapy with an insulin-sensitizing agent appears physiologically logical and hopefully will help delay or prevent sulfonylurea failure, which is frequently seen after 5 to 6 years of sulfonylurea monotherapy. In addition, it is hoped that insulin sensitization will decrease many of the other components of the cardiodysmetabolic syndrome and reduce macrovascular disease. This hypothesis is currently being tested in several clinical trials.

Insulin Therapy in Type 2 Diabetes Mellitus. Insulin therapy in patients with type 2 DM remains controversial. Insulin therapy is indicated when patients are in a state of acute metabolic decompensation and are more insulin resistant because of the stress of illness. In these individuals short-term insulin therapy can reestablish glycemic control and metabolic stability. Reevaluation of insulin secretory capacity via a C-peptide test is important so that patients do not remain on a regimen of insulin unnecessarily.[91-93]

In the individual with type 2 DM and a low-normal C-peptide level or the lean individual with a normal C-peptide level, insulin therapy will probably be needed, along with maintenance of diet, exercise, and oral agents. The use of bedtime insulin therapy with a single daily dose of intermediate-acting insulin or Glargine insulin may be sufficient. The theory is that this bedtime dosage will maximally affect and control both the dawn hepatic glucose output and disposal and the peak insulin resistance. The bedtime insulin dose assists in achieving the best possible fasting blood glucose level and minimizes glucotoxicity. Minimizing glucotoxicity maximizes the daytime pancreatic insulin secretory capability and minimizes the daytime insulin dose. In addition, the appetite-stimulating effect of insulin is minimized, which assists weight control. Occasionally individuals may require multiple injections similar to a patient with true type 1 DM. The exact needs of each patient can be determined on the basis of the premeal and bedtime blood glucose levels.[91-93]

In contrast, insulin therapy in the C-peptide–positive overweight patient with type 2 DM should be avoided if possible. Insulin is lipogenic, and the weight gain may further exacerbate the insulin-resistant state. Diet, exercise, and appropriate oral agents should be aggressively used before insulin therapy is contemplated. In such a patient requiring insulin, a bedtime dose of intermediate-acting insulin or Glargine insulin is the ideal starting point, along with the continuation of oral agent therapy. Combination therapy with oral agents usually helps maintain glycemic control with a lower insulin dosage.[91-93] Insulin therapy must not be viewed as a substitute for diet and exercise, but as an adjunct. Commonly, insulin therapy in the obese C-peptide–positive patient not only fails to improve glycemic control on a sustained basis but also increases appetite, resulting in weight gain, increased hyperglycemia, and increased hyperinsulinemia, thus perpetuating the insulin-resistant state and the components of the cardiodysmetabolic syndrome.[77-79]

Insulin therapy is necessary for the type 2 DM patient who becomes C-peptide negative. Such individuals are usually lean and look phenotypically more like an individual with type 1 DM. In these individuals, just as in type 1 DM patients, intensive insulin therapy with carbohydrate gram counting is needed. It is also important to note that in the geriatric years, 10% of newly diagnosed individuals will have bona fide type 1 DM, again requiring intensive therapy and carbohydrate gram counting.[91-93]

Complications of Medications

Insulin Hypersensitivity. Hypersensitivity to insulin itself is uncommon. Rarely a sulfa allergy cross-reacts with NPH insulin, which contains protamine sulfate. A rare patient who is allergic to zinc may react to the Lente insulins. Patients may react to preservatives within insulin. A switch in insulin manufacturer may eliminate the latter problem. Insulin hypersensitivity reactions are generally local reactions, consisting of wheals at injection sites. However, systemic symptoms and anaphylaxis can occur. When systemic reactions occur, local reactions may also be present. Formal desensitization is an option for patients with true insulin allergy.

Hypoglycemia. Hypoglycemia, or a blood glucose level ≤60 mg/dl, is a potential complication of therapy with insulin or oral hypoglycemic agents. Hypoglycemia is caused by a disturbance in the balance between insulin or secretagogues, carbohydrates, and activity (Box 30-4).

BOX 30-4 Causes of Hypoglycemia During Treatment With Exogenous Insulin or Sulfonylureas

Unphysiologic insulin regimen
Overdosage of insulin or sulfonylureas
Inconsistent carbohydrate intake
Omission of meal
Omission of planned snack
Uncompensated exercise
End-stage renal disease
End-stage liver disease
Alcohol consumption

BOX 30-5 Signs and Symptoms of Hypoglycemia

Adrenergic Symptoms

Pallor
Diaphoresis
Tachycardia
Piloerection
Palpitations
Nervousness
Irritability
Sensation of coldness
Weakness
Trembling
Hunger

Neuroglycopenic Symptoms

Headache
Mental confusion
Circumoral paresthesia
Fatigue
Incoherent speech
Coma
Diplopia
Emotional lability
Convulsions

Signs and Symptoms. The common signs and symptoms of hypoglycemia may be adrenergic (caused by activation of the sympathetic nervous system) or neuroglycopenic (caused by depression of central nervous system activity as the brain receives an insufficient supply of glucose) (Box 30-5).

Adrenergic symptoms generally precede neuroglycopenic symptoms. The particular signs and symptoms in a given individual may vary with the absolute blood glucose level, the rapidity of the decrease in blood glucose level, and the duration of hypoglycemia. In addition, signs and symptoms commonly vary throughout a given individual's life.

A rapid drop in plasma glucose results primarily in manifestations from increased sympathetic nervous system activity. In slow-developing hypoglycemia, as might be seen with long-acting insulin or with oral hypoglycemic agents, the central nervous system signs and symptoms predominate. If a rapid drop occurs and is allowed to persist, all signs and symptoms usually occur.

Hypoglycemia may occur during sleep. The only symptoms may be nightmares, sweating, restless sleep, headache on awakening, elevated fasting blood glucose value, or feeling totally exhausted on awakening. Nighttime hypoglycemia may be part of the Somogyi effect (see p. 966).

Individuals with long-standing diabetes may become less sensitive to hypoglycemia and may have very low blood glucose levels before some, if any, symptoms occur. Sustained recurrent hypoglycemia results in an increase in glucose transporter numbers at the blood-brain barrier to maintain the cerebrospinal fluid glucose level as close to normal as possible. This is why patients with recurrent hypoglycemia can maintain consciousness at lower blood glucose levels without experiencing significant adrenergic symptoms as compared with individuals without diabetes. Euglycemia with elimination of hypoglycemia results in a reduction of the glucose transporter number at the blood-brain barrier to a normal level. Consequently, when glucose levels fall slightly into the hypoglycemic range, the patient experiences adrenergic symptoms.[20]

Patients with DM who are treated with beta-adrenergic antagonists (beta-blockers) may be at special risk for hypoglycemia. These beta-adrenergic antagonist agents block or inhibit the appearance of early signs and symptoms of hypoglycemia by blocking the sympathetic nervous system. In addition, these drugs prevent or block gluconeogenesis and glycogenolysis, thus inhibiting the normal endogenous response to hypoglycemia, making it more difficult to reverse the problem.

Signs and symptoms similar to those of hypoglycemia may occur when the blood glucose level is elevated and drops rapidly to a level that is still in an elevated range. The sudden rapid drop in blood glucose is a stimulus for the physiologic neuroendocrine response to stressors to come into play. Thus a patient whose glucose level drops rapidly from 500 to 300 mg/dl may demonstrate the same signs and symptoms as a patient whose glucose drops to 30 mg/dl. Patients with uncontrolled diabetes may complain of feeling hypoglycemic, even though their plasma glucose levels are high.

This phenomenon should be discussed with patients with uncontrolled diabetes. They should be reassured that this "relative hypoglycemia" associated with improved glycemic control generally lasts only a few weeks.

Most hypoglycemia is mild and easily self-treated. The majority of cases of severe hypoglycemia result from patient error: inadequate carbohydrate intake at meals, missed snacks, or uncompensated activity.

Diagnosis and Treatment. A fingerstick blood glucose value should be obtained to verify hypoglycemia (blood glucose level of 60 mg/dl or lower). In a conscious patient, treatment consists of 15 g of quick-acting carbohydrate (e.g., three glucose tablets, 4 ounces of juice [no added sugar], or three hard candies). The fingerstick blood glucose value should be rechecked in 15 minutes. If the blood glucose level remains at 60 mg/dl or lower, the patient should self-treat again. If a glucose meter is not readily available, treatment should be taken

BOX 30-6 Target Nutritional Goals for Patients With Diabetes

Calories

Sufficient to achieve and maintain as close to desirable body weight as possible

Carbohydrate

Varies in relation to assessment and protein and fat intake; usually 45% to 60% of total calories

Liberalized individualized emphasis on total carbohydrate intake versus eliminating simple sugars only

Carbohydrate consistency at meals

Modest amounts of sucrose and other refined sugars may be acceptable contingent on metabolic control and body weight

Protein

Usual dietary intake of protein is double the amount needed

Exact ideal percentage of total calories is unknown; however, usual intake is 12% to 20% of total calories

Recommended Dietary Allowance (RDA) is 0.8 g/kg body weight for adults; RDA is modified for children, pregnant and lactating women, older adults, and those with special medical conditions

Avoidance of excess dietary protein intake is important in renal disease

Fat

Usually ≤30% of total calories, but may be as high as 40%
Polyunsaturated fats, 6% to 8%
Saturated fats, 10%
Monounsaturated fats, remaining percentage
Cholesterol <300 mg/day
May need to be further modified, depending on lipid profile

Fiber

Up to 40 g/day
25 g/1000 kcal for low-calorie intakes

Alternative Sweeteners

Use of various nutritive and nonnutritive sweeteners is acceptable

Sodium

≤3000 mg/day
Modified for special medical conditions (e.g., hypertension, edema)

Alcohol

≤2 equivalents per day

1 equivalent = 1.5 ounces distilled liquor, 4-ounce glass of wine, or 12-ounce glass of beer{

Vitamins/Minerals

Although there is no scientific evidence that individuals with diabetes mellitus (DM) who eat a well-balanced diet require vitamin/mineral supplementation, the RDAs were developed and based on a healthy population. Also, given that many vitamins/minerals are excreted in excess in the urine of individuals with DM, supplementation with a general multivitamin is prudent and rarely harmful.

regardless. In an unconscious patient, oral administration of glucose should never be attempted. In the hospital setting one ampule of 50% dextrose should be given by IV push. Recovery is usually within 1 minute. In the outpatient setting a significant other should inject 1 mg of glucagon subcutaneously; this causes the liver to release its glycogen store. The unconscious patient given subcutaneous glucagon generally regains consciousness in 10 to 20 minutes. After recovery, the patient should be given a snack of 45 g of carbohydrate to aid in replacing glycogen stores. Patients commonly are nauseated after receiving glucagon and may vomit. Seizures can occur when hypoglycemia is severe.

Side Effects of Oral Agents. Oral agents may cause hypoglycemia. Potential adverse effects of the oral agents are noted in Table 30-10.

Surgical Management

Pancreas transplantation has been shown to be effective in improving the quality of life in persons with diabetes by eliminating the need for exogenous insulin, frequent blood glucose monitoring, and dietary restrictions. However, there is no evidence that a pancreas transplant prevents or slows progression of long-term complications of diabetes or that it prolongs life. A pancreas transplant is indicated for persons with end-stage renal disease who are planning to or have had a kidney transplant. A pancreas transplant may be done at the time of the kidney transplant or after the kidney transplant. See Chapter 51 for further discussion of pancreas transplantation.

A group of investigators in Edmonton, Alberta, Canada, have treated seven patients with type 1 DM with islet cell transplantation. Further research is needed to explore the relationship between immunosupressants and glucose metabolism.[88]

Diet

Overview

Nutritional management is the cornerstone of therapy in all types of DM. Patients need to be referred early to a registered dietitian, preferably one who is also a certified diabetes educator (CDE), for nutritional education and the development of meal plans that are flexible and fit their lifestyles. Food issues are never simple for patients, and an initial understanding can often determine the success of their management. If no dietitian is available, the professional nurse should be able to give basic nutritional information that will suffice until the patient can talk with a dietitian.

The current nutritional management for diabetes is to maintain a reasonable weight and control blood glucose and lipid levels without compromising health. Current nutritional recommendations for people with diabetes are similar to those for healthy individuals without diabetes, as developed by the National Research Council, the American Heart Association, and the American Cancer Society (Box 30-6).[32,33,43,106]

Most persons need 25 kcal/kg of desired body weight to maintain their weight and meet basic metabolic needs. With this as the basis, calories are added or subtracted, based on the

TABLE 30-11 Guidelines for Estimating Calorie Requirements

Level	Activities	Calorie Requirements
Light, >55 years, obese, or inactive	Less than for "light" below	10 calories/lb (22 kcal/kg) Desired body weight (DBW)
Light	Ambulating in hospital, washing clothes, walking 2.5 to 3 miles per hour, carpentry, electrical work, golfing, sailing	10-12 calories/lb (22-26 kcal/kg) DBW
Moderate	Weeding and hoeing, bicycling, dancing, tennis, walking 3.5 to 4 miles per hour, scrubbing floors, work involving loading and stocking	12-14 calories/lb (26-32 kcal/kg) DBW
Heavy	Climbing, walking uphill with a full load, basketball, football, swimming	14-16 calories/lb (31-35 kcal/kg) DBW
Weight reduction		Subtract 500 calories from total calories for the day for a 1 lb weight loss per week

patient's activity level, age, and need to lose or gain weight (Table 30-11).

Another dietary component that is manipulated is fiber. A high-fiber, high-carbohydrate diet has been shown to decrease insulin requirements and cholesterol, both fasting and postprandial glucose serum levels. Fiber can increase satiety, which might help with weight reduction. Fiber delays gastric emptying and decreases peak blood glucose, so when fiber is introduced into the diet, blood glucose should be monitored, and insulin or any oral agents may need to be adjusted. Adding fiber gradually helps minimize abdominal discomfort and flatulence. Increasing water intake also helps.

Principles of Dietary Management

Recommendations need to be made with the awareness that eating habits are difficult if not impossible to change overnight. Changes should be instituted gradually as the nurse helps the patient adopt a diet that is as close to ideal as possible.

To increase success, dietary planning should consider:

- Religious, cultural, and personal preferences of the patient
- Lifestyle components: family eating patterns, finances, and work schedule
- Activity/rest patterns: amount, timing, and level of exercise, work, and sleep
- Actions of prescribed medications: onset, duration, and peak
- Self-perception of desired body weight

Carbohydrates must be distributed on a consistent basis so that the blood level of nutrients matches the blood level of insulin or any oral hypoglycemic agent. Relative consistency in timing of meals is also important for the person who needs to lose weight. Distribution of carbohydrates helps prevent large increases in postprandial blood glucose and allows the blood glucose to return to the preprandial level before the next meal regardless of whether the patient is receiving insulin or oral agents.

Systems for Learning and Maintaining Dietary Plans

Once the goals of nutritional therapy are established, patients are taught one of several methods for manipulating calories and food.

Exchange System. Historically the exchange system has been the most widely used method. The American Dietetic Association and the American Diabetes Association (ADA) have divided foods into six groups with exchange lists (or choices).[32,33,43] Each list is based on the amount of carbohydrate, protein, and fat contained in foods. There are six exchange lists: starch/bread, meat and meat substitutes, vegetables, fruit, milk, and fat. Each exchange list contains foods in specific serving sizes that contain approximately equal amounts of carbohydrates, proteins, fats, and calories. Because of this, these foods can be substituted or exchanged for one another. For example, in the fruit list, one 4-ounce apple equals 12 cherries equals 4 ounces of orange juice. Using the suggested serving size is an important point. Foods should be weighed and measured. The exchange system offers a wide variety of foods and combinations of foods that can be eaten. Implementation of the system requires knowing the caloric, carbohydrate, protein, and fat content of different foods. Labels on food products, convenience foods, and special foods and recipe books list carbohydrate, protein, and fat content. The total number of exchanges for each day is determined from the total calorie, carbohydrate, fat, and protein prescription.

Once the dietary prescription has been made and the caloric amount decided, a meal plan such as the one shown in Figure 30-8 can be made. There are resources other than the one depicted in the figure. Some are simple and have pictures of foods and a place to write in the number of exchanges from each group to be used. Examples of other plans can be obtained from the ADA.

It is important to maintain consistency with the distribution of exchanges and not "borrow from lunch and add to dinner." The nutritional information in Box 30-7 is an example of what can be found on cereal boxes. In terms of carbohydrate,

My Meal Plan

Meal plan for: *John Doe* Date: *8/16/98*
Dietitian: *Jane Smith* Phone: ______

	Grams	Percent
Carbohydrate	*199*	*55*
Protein	*79*	*20*
Fat	*44*	*25*
Calories *1580*		

Time	Meal plan	Menu ideas	Menu ideas
Breakfast	*2* Starch	*1/2 Cup oatmeal, 1 slice whole grain toast*	
	___ Meat		
	___ Vegetable		
	1 Fruit	*1/2 Banana*	
	1 Milk	*1 Cup skim milk*	
	1 Fat	*1 Tsp margarine*	
	___ ___		
	___ ___		
	___ ___		
Lunch	*2* Starch	*2 Slices whole grain bread*	
	2 Meat	*2 Slices turkey breast (2oz)*	*Lettuce leaf, tomato slice (free)*
	1 Vegetable	*1/2 Cup broccoli/cauliflower*	*marinated in 1 tbsp low-calorie Italian dressing (free food)*
	1 Fruit	*Apple*	
	___ Milk		
	1 Fat	*1 Tsp mayonnaise*	
Afternoon snack	*1* *Starch*	*3 Graham crackers*	
	1 *Meat*	*1 Tbsp peanut butter*	
	___ ___		
Dinner	*2* Starch	*1 Large potato*	
	2 Meat	*Meatloaf (2oz)*	*Tossed salad with 1 tbsp low-calorie Italian dressing (free food)*
	1 Vegetable	*1/2 Cup green beans*	
	1 Fruit	*1 1/4 Cups fresh strawberries*	
	___ Milk		
	1 Fat	*1 Tsp margarine*	
Bedtime snack	*1* *Starch*	*1/2 Bagel*	
	1 *Fat*	*1 Tbsp lite cream cheese*	
	1 *Milk*	*1 Cup skim milk*	

Figure 30-8 Sample meal plan.

BOX 30-7 Nutrition Information per Serving

Serving size: 1 ounce ($1\frac{1}{4}$ cup)
Serving per package: 20 (1-ounce servings)
Calories: 110
Protein: 4 g
Carbohydrate: 20 g
Sodium: 320 mg
Percentage of vitamins and minerals listed next
Ingredients: whole-oat flour, wheat starch, salt, sugar, calcium carbonate, etc.

protein, and fat content, one serving of cereal is equal to about $1\frac{1}{3}$ bread exchanges.

Total Gram Counting of Carbohydrate. Total gram counting of carbohydrate is now the most popular meal-planning system for both individuals with type 1 DM and those with type 2 DM. This system counts the total amount of carbohydrate available in the meal/snack. Only carbohydrates are initially tracked. Insulin is then matched to the carbohydrate planned. Carbohydrate gram counting helps individuals understand the relationship between food ingested and blood glucose levels.[32,43] One disadvantage of this method is that patients may minimize carbohydrate intake and increase their intake of fat and protein, which is clearly undesirable. Successful focus on carbohydrate gram counting occurs in the context of an overall healthy meal plan.

Food Guide Pyramid. Another system that can be used to help patients with meal plans is the Food Guide Pyramid (Figure 30-9).[105] This guide recommends less meat and poultry than does the exchange list.

Point System. Another system is point counting. With this system, foods are assigned points for the number of calories and carbohydrate, protein, and fat content. The total daily food allowance is written as the number of calorie and carbohydrate points, and the person is instructed to select foods according to a point distribution. This system is similar to the exchange list but is less well known.

Dietetic Foods, Sweeteners, and Alcohol

The diabetic diet does not require the use of special or dietetic foods. If used, these foods must be counted into the

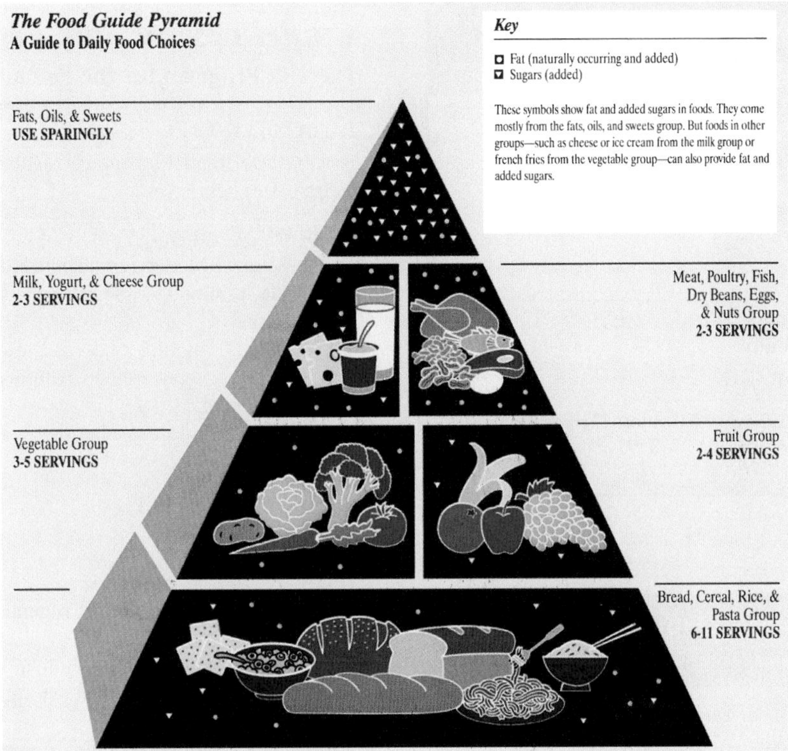

Figure 30-9 Food Guide Pyramid.

meal plan, because they are products that have had a substitution made and the substitution does not necessarily mean that the product is low in calories or useful for people with diabetes. Foods that are labeled "sugar free" are only "sucrose free"—not carbohydrate free. These foods frequently are sweetened with alternative sweeteners such as fructose or maltose, or one of the sugar alcohols such as sorbitol, mannitol, or xylitol. Sugar alcohols are not absorbed or digested as well as other carbohydrates and therefore contribute only 2 kcal/g as compared with the 4 kcal/g of other carbohydrates. Intake of large amounts of foods containing sugar alcohols can produce a significant osmotic diarrhea.

Various sweeteners other than sugar are available in the United States, including saccharin, aspartame (Equal), acesulfame-K (Sunette), and sucralose (the first sugar substitute made from sugar). All of these products are called low- or no-calorie sweeteners. Patients commonly ask how much of the sweeteners can be consumed safely. The accepted daily intake (ADI) is generous and is usually reported as an amount per kilogram of body weight (2.2 pound = 1 kg). For example, 50 mg/kg is the ADI for aspartame. For a 110-pound person this represents twelve 12-ounce cans of 100% aspartame-sweetened soda pop or 71 packets of Equal per day for a lifetime.

Alcohol does not furnish carbohydrate, protein, or fat, but it yields 7 kcal/g when metabolized and must be included in caloric calculations if weight loss is necessary. Some alcohol may be permitted, but the patient must be instructed about the caloric value of pure alcohol; the high carbohydrate content of beer, cordials, wine, and mixed drinks; the inhibiting effect of alcohol on gluconeogenesis with the possible precipitation of hypoglycemia; and the alcohol-induced increase in triglyceride levels.

The general rule is to allow a maximum of two drinks per day (1 drink = $1\frac{1}{2}$ ounces of liquor, 5 ounces of wine, or 12 ounces of beer) and to consume alcohol with food. Lower-carbohydrate alcohol (light beer, rum with diet cola) is preferable. Alcohol should never be calculated as part of the carbohydrate load of a meal. Hypoglycemia is especially common if alcohol is consumed without food, because the liver's priority is to metabolize alcohol and liver glucose output is then reduced.[10]

Activity

In all persons with diabetes, activity is an important part of the medical management and deserves careful and thorough explanation before implementation. Physical activity has important physiologic and psychologic implications.

Exercise is a wonderful insulin sensitizer, enhancing glucose uptake into skeletal muscle. The exact mechanism is unknown, but it occurs in both type 1 and type 2 DM. An excellent example of insulin sensitization as a result of exercise is seen in children going away to summer camp. As a consequence of the insulin sensitization resulting from exercise, insulin doses can be decreased by 25%.

Insulin resistance and excess weight are present in many persons with type 2 DM. Any type of therapy that decreases resistance and promotes weight loss has potential benefit. Exercise helps in both cases. Both clinical experience and various studies have shown exercise to be of value in both insulin resistance and weight loss. For maximal benefit, the exercise

BOX 30-8 Benefits of Exercise for the Patient With Diabetes

Improves insulin sensitivity
Lowers blood glucose during and after exercise
Improves lipid profile
May improve some hypertension
Increases energy expenditure
Assists with weight loss
Preserves lean body mass
Promotes cardiovascular fitness
Increases strength and flexibility
Improves sense of well-being

From Horton ES: Exercise. In Lebovitz HE, editor: *Therapy for diabetes mellitus and related disorders,* Alexandria, Va, 1991, American Diabetes Association.

BOX 30-9 Risks of Exercise for the Patient With Diabetes

Precipitation or exacerbation of cardiovascular disease, angina, dysrhythmias, sudden death
Hypoglycemia, if taking insulin or oral agents
Exercise-related hypoglycemia
Late-onset postexercise hypoglycemia
Hyperglycemia after very strenuous exercise
Worsening of long-term complications
Proliferative retinopathy
Peripheral neuropathy
Autonomic neuropathy

From Horton ES: Exercise. In Lebovitz HE, editor: *Therapy for diabetes mellitus and related disorders,* Alexandria, Va, 1991, American Diabetes Association.

program should be done on a regular basis. Even then, the effect on glucose may be short lived.

Exercise plans for persons with diabetes cannot be discussed without exploring the risks and benefits of such programs.[9] Box 30-8 lists some of the benefits of exercise for persons with diabetes. Entering into an exercise plan can also pose certain risks for patients with diabetes (Box 30-9).

Exercise is contraindicated during periods of hyperglycemia (fingerstick blood glucose value of 250 mg/dl or higher) and ketosis. The combination of hyperglycemia, ketosis, and exercise exerts a physiologic stress on the body, resulting in progressive hyperglycemia.

Both benefits and risks must be carefully investigated before an exercise prescription is launched. The exercise prescription may look something like Figure 30-10 and consists of the following parts: type of exercise, intensity, duration, and frequency. Before entering into any type of exercise program, all patients should have a complete history and physical examination, with particular attention to the cardiovascular system and any existing long-term complications. An exercise stress electrocardiogram (ECG) is recommended for all patients over 35 years of age. By doing this test, silent ischemic heart disease and exaggerated hypertensive responses to exercise can be identified. Once the patient has been cleared for an exercise program, special precautions may be indicated. General guidelines for exercise are listed in the Guidelines for Safe Practice box.

Guidelines for Safe Practice

Exercise Program for the Patient With Diabetes

EXERCISE TYPE

Aerobic (low impact for type 2 diabetes mellitus)
Start with light level.

EXERCISE SESSION

Each session should eventually include:

1. 5 to 10 minutes of warm-up stretching and limbering exercises
2. 20 to 30 minutes of aerobic exercise with heart rate in target zone (as defined by physician) or perceived exertion rating
3. 15 to 20 minutes of light exercise and stretching to cool down

EXERCISE FREQUENCY

3 to 5 times per week

Special Precautions

1. Consider insulin/oral agent regimen (may need to decrease insulin).
2. Consider the plan for food intake. Discuss with health care provider. May need to take extra carbohydrate before exercise.
3. Check blood glucose before, during, and afterward (for baseline).
4. If glucose level is higher than 250 mg/dl, check urine ketones. If negative, okay to exercise. If positive, take insulin; do not exercise until ketones are negative.
5. Exercise should not cause shortness of breath and should be stopped with any onset of chest pain or dyspnea.
6. Carry diabetes identification card and bracelet.
7. Carry a source of easily absorbed carbohydrate (three glucose tablets or hard candies).
8. Do not exercise in extreme heat or cold.
9. Inspect feet daily and after exercise.

PRECAUTIONS FOR SELECTED PERSONS

1. Persons with insensitive feet should choose good shoes for walking and avoid running and jogging. Swimming and cycling may be included in the exercise program.
2. Persons with proliferative retinopathy should avoid exercises associated with Valsalva's maneuver or that cause jarring and jolting of the head and exercises with the head in a low position.
3. Persons with hypertension should avoid exercises associated with Valsalva's maneuver and intense exercises involving the torso and arms. (Exercises involving the lower extremities are preferred.)

Referrals

In some settings the nurse assumes responsibility for making referrals and consultations to other services. Referrals may be

Name: ______________________ Date: ____________

Mode: (type of exercise)*

( ) Cycling ( ) Jumping rope
( ) Walking
( ) Swimming ( ) Other ____________
* Can change/rotate

Intensity: (how hard)

Perceived exertion scale

6	
7	Very, very light
8	
9	Very light
10	
11	Fairly light
12	
13	Somewhat hard
14	
15	Hard
16	
17	Very hard
18	
19	Very, very hard
20	

Duration: (how long)*

Slow	(stretch-warm up)	____________
Faster	(training)	____________
Slow	(cooling down)	____________

* Start slow and build up

Frequency: (how often)

	Type of exercise	How often
Aerobic:	____________	____________
Other:	____________	____________

Physician: ____________

Figure 30-10 Sample exercise prescription.

indicated to ophthalmologists, CDEs, registered dietitians who are CDEs, psychologists, and podiatrists. In addition, the ADA and the Juvenile Diabetes Foundation and local diabetes organizations may provide support and information.

Depression commonly occurs with any chronic illness. Prevalence rates in individuals with diabetes may be as high as 32%.[64] The contributions of a behavioral psychologist or psychiatric clinical nurse specialist are important to assist in the many psychosocial aspects of DM.

Economic issues are a key concern to persons with diabetes. Many persons with diabetes do not have adequate insurance coverage. Reasons are that the cost of private insurance may be prohibitive; some companies will not insure people with diabetes; and group plan benefits may be limited. A referral to a social worker may be indicated to help the patient obtain information regarding available insurance plans.

NURSING MANAGEMENT OF PATIENT WITH DIABETES MELLITUS

A Nursing Care Plan for a patient with type 2 DM is found on pp. 954 to 957.

ASSESSMENT

Establishing a therapeutic relationship with the patient with diabetes is challenging as the professional nurse interacts with the patient at some time and place in the "diabetes life span." Having diabetes for 30 years does not imply 30 years of optimal management. People can be "experienced" at doing the wrong thing. Many patients and health care professionals alike believe myths about diabetes (Box 30-10). These myths must be dispelled through education. The professional nurse is in an ideal position to educate patients and peers and dispel the myths of diabetes; it is imperative that the professional nurse

Nursing Care Plan Patient With Diabetes Mellitus

DATA Mrs. F. is an obese, 62-year-old married woman diagnosed with type 2 diabetes mellitus 8 years ago. She has been referred to a short-term ambulatory diabetes education program for instruction on insulin administration because blood glucose control has not been adequately achieved with diet and oral hypoglycemic agents.

The nursing history reveals that Mrs. F.:

- Maintains an inconsistent sleep/activity schedule
- Has accurate knowledge of dietary modifications and has successfully lost between 20 and 40 pounds on more than one occasion
- Performs regular foot checks and wears well-fitted shoes
- Does not exercise consistently
- Has performed glucose monitoring on herself once or twice but has no monitoring equipment at home
- Regards church activities as important, since they meet her socialization needs

Objective data include:

- Fasting blood glucose of 220 mg/dl
- Weight, 200 pounds; height, 5 feet 4 inches
- Blood pressure, 134/84; heart rate, 92 beats/min; respirations, 24/min
- Urine negative for microalbuminuria
- Peripheral pulses, 1+
- Legs warm and dry, color even with rest of body
- Patellar and Achilles tendon reflexes, 3+ (on scale of 0 to 4)
- Decreased perception to touch in lower extremities
- Decrease in vibration and pinprick sensation to great toes bilaterally
- 20/20 vision on Snellen chart

Collaborative nursing actions include teaching Mrs. F. measures that will help her achieve control of blood glucose (diet, insulin, exercise) and teaching her to detect, prevent, and treat hypoglycemic reactions.

NURSING DIAGNOSIS **Risk for deficient fluid volume related to hyperglycemia**
GOALS/OUTCOMES Will remain free of fluid imbalance

NOC Suggested Outcomes

- Fluid Balance (0601)
- Hydration (0602)
- Electrolyte and Acid-Base Balance (0600)

NIC Suggested Interventions

- Fluid Monitoring (4130)
- Fluid Management (4120)
- Hypovolemia Management (4170)
- Intravenous (IV) Therapy (4200)

Nursing Interventions/Rationales

- Assess and monitor for fluid volume deficiency. *Diabetic patients are at increased risk for hypovolemia because of osmotic diuresis secondary to hyperglycemia. The earlier fluid volume deficiencies are identified, the more quickly fluid balance can be restored.*
- Encourage intake of 2000 to 3000 ml of fluid per day. *To replace fluid losses and prevent hypervolemia and cellular dehydration.*
- Teach patient the relationship between high blood glucose levels and fluid loss. *To help the patient understand the need for blood glucose control and to increase the likelihood of compliance with the therapeutic regimen.*
- Teach patient the signs and symptoms of fluid volume depletion and the need to report such manifestations quickly. *To facilitate early recognition and treatment.*

Evaluation Parameters

1. Skin turgor elastic and mucous membranes moist
2. Blood pressure and pulse within normal range
3. Blood glucose within normal range
4. Verbalizes means of preventing fluid volume deficiencies

NURSING DIAGNOSIS **Imbalanced nutrition: more than body requirements**
GOALS/OUTCOMES Will maintain weight within 5 pounds of ideal weight

NOC Suggested Outcomes

- Nutritional Status (1004)
- Nutritional Status: Food and Fluid Intake (1008)
- Nutritional Status: Nutrient Intake (1009)

NIC Suggested Interventions

- Eating Disorders Management (1030)
- Nutrition Management (1100)
- Weight Reduction Assistance (1280)
- Weight Management (1260)

Nursing Interventions/Rationales

- Obtain a thorough diet history. *To assess the patient's current dietary intake so that dietary alterations to maintain blood glucose control can be planned.*
- Encourage patient to become involved in setting goals for dietary changes, documenting food intake, and planning meals. *There is a greater probability that changes will be made when the patient is involved*

Nursing Care Plan Patient With Diabetes Mellitus—cont'd

in planning those changes. Patients know their own likes and dislikes, financial resources, and ability to make dietary changes. Participation allows the patient greater control over her situation.

- Help patient identify an acceptable weight loss schedule. *Permanent weight loss is generally gradual weight loss based on sound dietary principles. Fad diets should be avoided. The patient's agreement with the weight loss plan ensures a greater probability of compliance.*
- Teach or reinforce earlier teaching about the selected system of dietary management. *Knowledge increases the likelihood of compliance.*
- Teach patient the signs and symptoms of hypoglycemia and how to treat it. *Patients receiving insulin must be concerned about hypoglycemia; they need to know how to identify and handle it.*
- Teach patient how to handle sick days and unplanned social events. *To prepare the patient to deal appropriately with unusual dietary events or inability to take in food.*
- Teach patient the need for maintaining food intake distribution throughout the day. *To maintain consistency of blood glucose levels following the administration of insulin.*

Evaluation Parameters

1. Loses weight gradually after making dietary modifications
2. Blood glucose, glycosylated hemoglobin, and lipid measurements move toward normal
3. Food intake is distributed throughout the day

NURSING DIAGNOSIS **Activity intolerance related to fatigue**
GOALS/OUTCOMES Will perform activities without experiencing fatigue

NOC Suggested Outcomes

- Activity Tolerance (0005)
- Energy Conservation (1804)
- Endurance (0001)

NIC Suggested Interventions

- Energy Management (0180)
- Sleep Enhancement (1850)
- Teaching: Prescribed Activity/Exercise (5612)

Nursing Interventions/Rationales

- Teach patient that improvement in metabolic control will decrease fatigue. *Understanding the relationship between metabolic abnormalities and fatigue increases the likelihood of compliance with the prescribed treatment regimen.*
- Assess severity of patient's fatigue. *A baseline assessment is necessary for later comparisons and to determine treatment effectiveness.*
- Encourage patient to prioritize daily activities when feeling fatigued and to let go of unessential tasks. *Fatigue compromises one's ability to participate in daily activities. It is important that the patient's available energy be used to complete priority activities until blood glucose levels are regulated.*
- Explore strategies to modify existing activities, conserving energy when possible; seek assistance or delegate activities; and pace activities throughout the day to allow a balance between activity and rest. *Many daily activities can be modified to consume less energy, but this requires the patient's willingness to think about routine activities in a different way. It may not be possible for the patient to perform all desired activities until she is metabolically stable.*
- Encourage patient to obtain at least 8 hours of uninterrupted sleep at night. *Effective nighttime sleep patterns help decrease daytime fatigue.*

Evaluation Parameters

1. States fatigue is reduced and energy is returning to normal
2. Performs daily activities without becoming fatigued
3. Maintains blood glucose levels within normal limits

NURSING DIAGNOSIS **Risk for infection related to altered tissue perfusion secondary to chronic hyperglycemia**
GOALS/OUTCOMES Will remain free of infection

NOC Suggested Outcomes

- Immune Status (0702)
- Knowledge: Infection Control (1807)
- Tissue Integrity: Skin and Mucous Membranes (1101)

NIC Suggested Interventions

- Surveillance (6650)
- Teaching: Disease Process (5602)
- Skin Surveillance (3590)

Continued

Nursing Care Plan Patient With Diabetes Mellitus–cont'd

Nursing Interventions/Rationales

- Teach patient the relationship between infection and metabolic control. *If the patient understands that good metabolic control decreases the risk for infection, she is more likely to comply with prescribed treatments.*
- Monitor for signs of localized (heat, redness, warmth, pain) and systemic infections (elevated white blood cell count, fever, lethargy). *Early detection of infection results in treatment being implemented more quickly.*
- Teach patient the signs of localized and systemic infections. *The patient is usually the first to identify early infections. The earlier the infection is detected, the more quickly treatment can be instituted.*
- Teach patient to inspect feet daily for signs of infection. *Diabetic neuropathy (sensory loss) increases the patient's risk for foot infections. The need for foot care cannot be overemphasized.*

Evaluation Parameters

1. Verbalizes need to do regular blood glucose monitoring
2. Accurately verbalizes relationship between poor blood glucose control and risk for infection
3. Accurately lists signs and symptoms of infection

NURSING DIAGNOSIS **Deficient knowledge of self-administration of insulin, care of equipment, home monitoring of blood glucose related to lack of previous exposure to information**

GOALS/OUTCOMES Will accurately verbalize disease process, need for blood glucose control, signs of infection, and signs of hyperglycemia and hypoglycemia; will demonstrate correct self-insulin administration

NOC Suggested Outcomes

- Knowledge: Diabetes Management (1820)
- Knowledge: Medication (1808)
- Knowledge: Treatment Regimen (1813)

NIC Suggested Interventions

- Teaching: Individual (5606)
- Teaching: Prescribed Medication (5616)
- Teaching: Psychomotor Skill (5620)

Nursing Interventions/Rationales

- Support and encourage patient as necessary to self-inject insulin. *Adults who perform self-injections have minimal discomfort and come to realize they are capable of performing this skill.*
- Demonstrate and have patient return demonstrate home blood glucose monitoring (HBGM), correcting technique as needed. *The patient needs to be taught the skill before performing the skill. Evaluation of the patient's skill is necessary to ensure accuracy.*
- Teach patient about the effects of activity, dietary intake, and insulin on blood glucose; instruct patient on timing of blood glucose monitoring. *To help the patient understand that all aspects of care are interrelated. HBGM provides immediate feedback about previous behaviors and reinforces the value of therapeutic measures.*
- Teach patient the signs and symptoms and treatment measures for hyperglycemia and hypoglycemia. *This knowledge ensures that the patient can safely administer own insulin, decreases fear of reactions, and allows for quick intervention if hyperglycemia or hypoglycemia do occur.*
- Teach patient regarding care of insulin and supplies. *To ensure that insulin remains stable and equipment is sterile.*
- Refer to dietitian for further teaching regarding any dietary modifications that need to be made now that the patient is receiving insulin. *The dietitian enforces previous teaching, assesses for new dietary needs, and teaches new information.*

Evaluation Parameters

1. Correctly demonstrates insulin injections, including correct insulin and correct dose
2. Lists signs and symptoms of infection, hyperglycemia, and hypoglycemia
3. Consistently monitors blood glucose levels

NURSING DIAGNOSIS **Ineffective health maintenance related to ineffective coping skills**

GOALS/OUTCOMES Will independently maintain blood glucose control via diet, monitoring, and self-administration of insulin

NOC Suggested Outcomes

- Health-Promoting Behavior (1602)
- Knowledge: Health Resources (1806)
- Knowledge: Treatment Regimen (1813)
- Participation: Health Care Decisions (1606)

NIC Suggested Interventions

- Health System Guidance (7400)
- Teaching: Disease Process (5602)
- Self-Modification Assistance (4470)
- Coping Enhancement (5230)

Nursing Care Plan — Patient With Diabetes Mellitus—cont'd

Nursing Interventions/Rationales

- Counsel patient regarding effects of stress, lack of exercise, and activity pattern on blood glucose levels. *Change in behavior is more likely to occur if the patient understands the relationships between stress, activity, and diet and glucose control.*
- Explore patient's willingness and ability to change behaviors: sleep/activity, ways of coping, and exercise. *Goals are more likely to be achieved if the patient agrees that the changes will be beneficial.*
- Engage patient in mutual problem solving as opposed to prescribing. *Increasing a patient's sense of control can help with self-esteem and enhance attitudes toward change.*
- Explore sources for long-term support in learning more effective ways of coping (e.g., weight loss, exercise, diabetes management). *Changing lifestyle, eating behaviors, and ways of coping is very difficult; support over long periods is usually required.*

Evaluation Parameters

1. States at least one change that will help her improve her blood glucose control
2. Maintains prescribed diet and insulin administration
3. Reports ability to take control of her illness

BOX 30-10 Myths of Diabetes

1. Diabetes is just a touch of sugar.
2. My diabetes will always control me.
3. *Symptom free* means complication free.
4. Complications are inevitable.
5. If you have diabetes, you are doomed to illness and early death.

Research

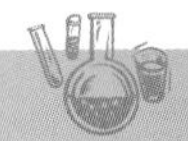

Reference: Baxley SG et al: Perceived competence and actual level of knowledge of diabetes mellitus among nurses, *J Nurs Staff Dev* 13(2):93, 1997.

Staff nurses in a rural 62-bed acute care hospital in the southeastern United States were surveyed regarding their perceived and actual level of knowledge of diabetes mellitus. Perception of diabetes knowledge was assessed by the Diabetes Self-Report Tool, a Likert-type scale; the mean knowledge score was 88%. The Diabetes Basic Knowledge Test measured actual knowledge; the mean score was 75%. Such a discrepancy between perceived and actual knowledge raises questions regarding competency validation in diabetes management.

be knowledgeable regarding current diabetes management (see Research box).

Health History

Health history information to be collected when assessing the patient with diabetes includes:

Psychosocial/emotional status: perception of the meaning of the diagnosis and how it affects the patient's life, future plans, day-to-day activities (e.g., work, social activities, family role, meals); identification of life stressors; current coping strategies; support systems; level of education, literacy

Knowledge level: concept of diabetes, effect of uncontrolled metabolic state, potential treatment

Family history: food buying, cooking, history of diabetes

Cardiovascular status: drugs, history of blood pressure problems, chest pain or leg pain with exercise

Respiratory status: smoking history, environmental hazards

Neuromuscular status: history of changes in vision or speech, dizziness, confusion, headache, symptoms of neuropathy (tingling, numbness, pain at rest that disappears with activity)

Gastrointestinal status: weight changes, history of gastrointestinal problems (indigestion, diarrhea, constipation)

Urinary status: history of changes in urinary frequency or incontinence

Sexual function: women—menstrual history, history of changes noted with intercourse (if sexually active); men—problems with erectile dysfunction or amount of ejaculate (if sexually active)

Vision: history of blurring, decreased acuity, most recent eye examination

Financial security, insurance

Physical Examination

Important data to be collected as part of the physical examination of the patient with diabetes include:

General: weight and height

Emotional/mental: emotional state, responsiveness, attention, alertness, comprehension, appropriateness of response

Neuromuscular: eyes—visual acuity (with and without glasses); motor—range of motion, muscle strength (both upper and lower extremities); sensory—touch, temperature, pain, vibratory sense (especially lower extremities), position sense, deep tendon reflexes

Cardiovascular: blood pressure (both lying and standing), peripheral pulses, ankle and brachial indices

Gastrointestinal: bowel sounds, masses

Urinary: output and fluid intake

Vagina: discharge, irritation

Skin: intactness, temperature, presence of lesions, moisture, hair distribution, texture (especially in lower extremities), turgor

Diagnostic test findings:

Blood/plasma glucose levels in the fasting state or postprandial state may be normal (euglycemia), high (hyperglycemia), or low (hypoglycemia).

HbA_{1c} may be normal or elevated.

Serum lipids may be normal or abnormal.

Urine ketones may be negative or positive.

Urine microalbumin-creatinine ratio and serum creatinine, as markers of renal function, may be normal or abnormal. Many individuals with type 2 DM have diabetes of 10 or more years' duration at the time of "diagnosis" as a result of the insidious onset of the disease.

NURSING DIAGNOSES

Nursing diagnoses are determined from analysis of patient data. Possible nursing diagnoses for the person with DM may include but are not limited to:

Diagnostic Title	Possible Etiologic Factors
1. Risk for deficient fluid volume	Excess urination, limited access to fluids, inadequate knowledge
2. Fatigue	Inadequate nutrition (from glycemic state), muscle weakness
3. Risk for infection	Elevated blood glucose levels
4. Imbalanced nutrition: less or more than body requirements	Alteration in metabolism, decreased nutrition, lack of knowledge
5. Fear	Long-term illness, taking insulin, lifestyle change (loss of job)
6. Deficient knowledge: disease, drugs, self-care skills (insulin injection, HBGM), diet needs, activity needs	New information and skills; lack of exposure

EXPECTED PATIENT OUTCOMES

Expected patient outcomes for the patient with diabetes may include but are not limited to:

1. Will exhibit physical signs of fluid balance
1a. Will return to baseline weight
1b. Will have elastic skin turgor and moist mucous membranes
1c. Will have blood pressure and pulse within normal range
1d. Will have serum electrolytes and hematocrit within normal limits
1e. Will have urine specific gravity of 1.010 to 1.025
1f. Will have a fluid intake of 2.5 to 3 L/day, orally or parenterally (unless restrictions are prescribed)
1g. Will explain measures to prevent fluid deficit
2. Will experience less fatigue
2a. Will state that fatigue level is decreased by a lower rating on a scale of 1 to 10 (1 = no fatigue; 10 = most fatigue)
3. Will demonstrate knowledge of information needed to decrease the risk for infection
3a. Will verbalize the need to do HBGM, the frequency of which is prescribed by the health care team
3b. Will identify factors that increase blood glucose
3c. Will list signs and symptoms of infection
4. Will exhibit signs of nutritional adequacy
4a. Will maintain weight, or lose or gain weight as appropriate
4b. Will have blood glucose, HbA_{1c}, and lipid measurements that are moving toward normal
4c. Will have food intake distributed throughout the day
4d. Will verbalize dietary plan and ways to achieve dietary modifications
5. Will manifest decreased fear
5a. Will express feelings about having diabetes
5b. Will state coping strategies
6. Will evidence a level of knowledge adequate for self-care
6a. Will verbalize that diabetes is a disease in which the body is unable to use all foods properly because of lack of insulin or inability to use insulin
6b. Will demonstrate correctly how to give insulin (if necessary)
6c. Will verbalize how to take medications and effects to report
6d. Will demonstrate correctly how to monitor for blood glucose and urine ketones (will know when and whom to call for help)
6e. Will verbalize the definitions of hypoglycemia and hyperglycemia
6f. Will verbalize symptoms and treatment of hypoglycemia
6g. Will verbalize exercise plan, safety precautions, and what to report

INTERVENTIONS

1. Improving Fluid Status

To improve fluid status, the patient's metabolic status needs to be improved, and the patient needs to ingest an adequate amount of fluid. Possible causes of loss of fluid (dehydration) must be explored with the patient, and the relationship of fluid loss to high blood glucose levels reinforced. This can be done by using terminology such as "glucose attracts water, and when blood glucose is high, glucose goes out in the urine, pulling water with it, thus increasing urination." It should be stressed that increased thirst is nature's way of telling the person to drink more fluids and that if the person is not drinking, fluid losses will not be controlled. This illustration can help the patient visualize how to manage the diabetes using tools such as HBGM and testing for urine ketones. The patient and family also need teaching about diet, medications, HBGM, and urine testing for ketones. Also, telephone numbers of the physician and diabetes team must be provided for emergencies.

2. Decreasing Fatigue

Measures that improve metabolic control also improve fatigue. However, if the patient is deconditioned and has lost muscle mass, metabolic control usually improves before the fatigue. Therefore the patient will need help in developing a schedule to promote gradual increase in activity and adequate rest and sleep. The nurse should explain that with regular exercise and metabolic control, feelings of fatigue can dissipate.

3. Preventing Infection

Improvement in metabolic control is the primary way to prevent infections. The patient and significant others must understand the relationship of poor blood glucose control to infection. They must also understand that infection can worsen glycemic control. Awareness of the signs and symptoms of infections and management of sick days is critical (Box 30-11).

4. Promoting Adequate Nutrition

Both the nurse and the dietitian are involved in nutritional education for the patient and family. A dietary history should be part of the professional nurse's initial assessment. Information about cultural or social food habits that are identified in the dietary history needs to be incorporated into the dietary plan. For example, it may be necessary to make accommodations for a vegetarian diet or for incorporation of fast foods into the diet.

Because of the difficulty in changing food habits, the patient should be involved in setting goals for dietary changes. Compromises that may be necessary include:

Identifying an acceptable weight loss schedule for the obese person

Incorporating an alcoholic beverage into the daily plan, if desired

Distributing food in a different pattern (e.g., a large noon meal and a small evening meal)

Adding desserts to some meals

The system for maintaining the dietary plan should be identified by the patient and the registered dietitian. The selected system is documented in the nursing care plan so that everyone involved uses the same terminology and food groupings. The mutually established goals, including compromises and sociocultural practices, are also documented so that the patient is not given conflicting information. Significant others should be included in the teaching.

After dietary goals are established, the nurse should help the patient apply dietary knowledge. This can be done through simulations in which the person chooses foods from the hospital menu, food models, or other learning tools and through patient participation in documenting food intake, blood and urine results, activity, and medications, and in discussing how these interrelate.

Patient and family satisfaction with the plan must be evaluated. Skills that the patient should possess after the initial management period are (1) ability to manage the diet for 1 week, (2) knowledge of whom to contact if unusual events requiring adjustments occur, and (3) knowledge of how to handle sick days.

Ultimately patients should be able to:

Manage dietary needs on a daily basis, making adjustments for normal life changes.

BOX 30-11 Sick-Day Guidelines

When to call your physician/nurse about being sick or "out of sorts" (just go through the checklist and check what you have):

_____ Unable to keep down fluids/food
_____ Unable to eat regular foods for more than 1 day
_____ Signs of infection: redness, warmth, swelling, pus, tenderness any place
_____ Symptoms of dehydration: dry mouth, fever, thirst, dry flushed skin, vomiting, abdominal pain, severe nausea, diarrhea, rapid breathing
_____ Vomiting more than three times or diarrhea lasting longer than 3 hours
_____ Increased urination and increased thirst
_____ Have cough and bring up yellow or green material
_____ Any symptoms getting worse
_____ Home blood glucose monitoring consistently shows elevated blood glucose beyond specified levels
_____ Fever present
_____ Ketones present
_____ Have any questions about how to take care of yourself and control your diabetes
_____ Have questions about adjusting insulin/oral agents

Information to have ready for physician/nurse when you call:

_____ Length of time you have been sick
_____ Your temperature
_____ What's bothering you (a list of symptoms)
_____ Test results: urine ketones and blood glucose
_____ Diabetes medication: type, time you take, and amount, as well as what you have taken
_____ Other medications you take; medication allergies; type, amount, time of medications recently taken
_____ Pharmacy phone number

Remember:

1. Always take your insulin or oral agent.
2. Drink plenty of fluids, including broth.
3. Test urine ketones and blood glucose every 4 hours; record results.
4. Eat carbohydrates according to your meal plan; replace with liquids if necessary.
5. Know all your caregivers' phone numbers and names.

(When you get better, return to your normal eating plan and medication dosage. This information applies to short-term illness [1 to 2 days]. If you are unable to eat, or have vomiting or diarrhea, call immediately.)

Select appropriate foods from restaurant menus or at social occasions.

Manage dietary needs while traveling or for shift work.

Manage dietary needs at unplanned social events (e.g., "happy hour" after work, unexpected business dinner, unexpected company).

Evaluate success in dietary management through evaluating weight changes and HbA_{1c} or through HBGM.

Eliminate excess salt, decrease saturated fat intake, decrease caffeine intake, and make a conscious effort to include adequate vitamins and minerals.

Keep up-to-date on new findings about dietary management and consult health team members about the new recommendations.

Avoid "quack" recommendations.

Manipulate diet, exercise, and medications together to cover a variety of daily situations.

Work with others in the household to help them incorporate principles of healthy eating into the diet.

5. Decreasing Fear

Before the patient is ready to accept self-care, the patient must learn to control his or her fears. The nurse should anticipate the presence of fears by asking straightforward questions about the patient's fears concerning the impact of the diagnosis on his or her job, giving self-injections, or relationships with others. Possible conflicting factors such as lifestyle changes should be identified. The nurse needs to eliminate misconceptions that can increase fear. Patients must have permission to grieve for losses being experienced, must know that many individuals feel like they are "falling apart," and must know that with time they will get better and feel better. Referrals to clinical nurse specialists, psychologists, counselors, or clergy for emotional support may be necessary.

6. Facilitating Learning

Adjustment to a chronic illness such as diabetes is ongoing. The degree to which individuals with DM adjust, as evidenced by taking control of the disease management, often depends on how well they adapt emotionally to their diagnosis. Helping the person begin to cope with chronic illness may be one of the first nursing care priorities. Patients must have a chance to work through their feelings of loss, shock, disbelief, identity change, or anger in response to the crisis. They need to feel accepted, regardless of their behavior.

A major responsibility of the professional nurse is helping individuals gain self-management skills for any chronic health problem through teaching and counseling. Self-management skills are probably the major determinant of how well the health problem is controlled and the quality of life maintained. This is particularly true for individuals with diabetes. Research supports the idea that patient education has a positive effect on patient outcomes. Teaching and management are instituted in a manner to avoid overwhelming the patient.

The major problem confronting the professional nurse when dealing with the problem of knowledge deficit in the person with DM is, "What do I teach, and how much do I teach?" A pretest is an ideal format by which to assess what the patient knows, or does not know, about diabetes. The bottom line is that patients have to survive in the real world. Hence the patient's ability to perform day-to-day survival skills should always be validated.

The ADA has suggested that diabetes education take place in three stages and be continuous:

- Survival/initial stage
- In-depth stage
- Continuous stage

Stages 2 and 3 place emphasis on knowledge and skills needed to be completely self-sufficient in daily management and on knowledge and skills needed to gain flexibility in management, insight, and self-determination. A tool such as the Professional Prompter Worksheet for Diabetes Education (Box 30-12) can help facilitate learning.[25] This tool provides the survival/initial knowledge that must be mastered by the person with type 1 or type 2 DM; it also contains teaching strategies. Other areas, such as dealing with complications and in-depth knowledge about hyperglycemia and ketoacidosis, are left for stages 2 and 3 teaching.

Other teaching tools are available from pharmaceutical companies, the ADA, and health care institutions with a diabetes center. It is important to assess the patient's education and reading level before giving out educational materials. Streiff[94] evaluated various written materials for diabetes education and found that a high school reading level was required, but an evaluation of 106 adults revealed an average reading level of less than seventh grade (6.8). The CDEs and the diabetes clinical nurse specialist are also sources of information and assistance.

6a. Managing Medications: Insulin Knowledge

Patients taking insulin should be able to name their prescribed type of insulin, their doses and the peak effects, and how the exercise regimen and diet are coordinated with the insulin. They should know insulin measurement (units) and the need for similarly calibrated syringes. In addition, they must know how to handle insulin needs on sick days.

6b. Insulin Self-Administration

For safe insulin administration, patients must know how to draw insulin into the syringe, mix two insulins (if pertinent), select and prepare the injection site, use consistent injection sites, rotate within those sites, and inject insulin. The essential teaching points are summarized on the Professional Prompter Worksheet for Diabetes Education (see Box 30-12). Most persons have some fears related to self-injection. Repeated practice is necessary, so patients should start practicing self-injection as soon as insulin treatment is deemed necessary.

Preparing the Insulin Dose

The patient is taught to rotate or roll the vial of cloudy insulin to return any precipitated particles to solution and to draw the required dose of insulin into the syringe using correct technique. Current insulin syringes have little or no dead

BOX 30-12 Professional Prompter Worksheet for Diabetes Education

SI = Survival information/skills for type 1
SII = Survival information/skills for type 2

Survival/Initial Teaching

Survival/Initial Skills

1. Concentrate on survival. These are the skills every patient must know before discharge. It is necessary, and patient cannot go further without this foundation.
2. Assess patient's knowledge via a pretest.

Type 1 Survival/Initial Skills

1. Psychologic and family.
2. Can patient give insulin correctly (i.e., see the increments, inject correctly, use proper sites, reuse syringe, know time, action of insulin)?
3. Monitor blood glucose and urine ketones.
4. Recognize and treat hypoglycemia.

Type 2 Survival/Initial Skills

1. Psychologic and family.
2. Explanation of what diabetes is—insulin resistance versus insulin deficiency.
3. Treatment with diet, oral agent, and insulin if necessary, or combination therapy.
4. Monitor blood glucose and urine ketones.
5. Recognize and treat hypoglycemia if taking sulfonylureas or insulin.

Tools to Use for Survival/Initial Teaching

- Barrier check
- Initial assessment
- Take-home instruction sheet
- American Diabetes Association Curriculum Guidelines
- Refer to group class in local hospital
- Refer to specialty practice/center

Assessment (SI and SII)

Complete assessment, including diabetes knowledge

Barriers (SI and SII)

Define Barrier

1. Fatigue/pain
2. High anxiety
3. Blindness

Teaching Tools

1. Give instructions another time.
2. Identify why and work on anxiety before proceeding.
3. Audio material and devices.
4. Referral to specialty center.

Overview of Diabetes (SII)

Patient Can Verbalize/Demonstrate

1. Diabetes is a disease in which the body is unable to utilize carbohydrate foods properly because of lack of insulin or inability to use insulin.
2. Defines high blood sugar in terms of blood glucose: normal versus diabetes. Lists symptoms.
3. Defines which type of diabetes the patient has.
4. Describes essential parts of diabetes management: knowledge, self-care, meal planning, exercise, and medication. Knows the effect each of these has on the blood glucose level.
5. Knows effect of activity on blood glucose.
6. Knows effect of illness/stress on blood glucose.

Stress and Psychologic Adjustment (SI and SII)

Patient Can Verbalize/Demonstrate

1. Has adapted to having diabetes.
2. Expresses feelings about having diabetes.
3. Acknowledges losses—grief process (fear, anxiety, denial, anger, bargaining, depression, acceptance). Discussion with nurse or social worker.

Family Involvement and Social Support (SI and SII)

Patient Can Verbalize/Demonstrate

1. Family can identify one feeling a person with diabetes may experience.
2. Ways diabetes has affected the family.
3. A support person.

Nutrition (SI and SII)

Patient Can Verbalize/Demonstrate

1. Individualized meal plan.
2. Reason for maintaining consistency (if appropriate) of meal spacing, proper mealtimes, and snacks to avoid hypoglycemia/hyperglycemia.
3. Relationship of insulin or oral agent, activity, and caloric intake.
4. Diet changes for sick-day management, exercise, use of alcohol, change in meal schedule, and restaurant dining.
5. The importance of attaining and maintaining ideal body weight.
6. Effects of dietary fiber.

Data from Eaks GA: *Professional prompter worksheet,* Kansas City, 1993, University of Kansas Medical Center, Cray Diabetes Education Center.

Continued

BOX 30-12 Professional Prompter Worksheet for Diabetes Education—cont'd

Exercise and Activity

Patient Can Verbalize/Demonstrate

1. How exercise affects diabetes control.
2. Cautions and risks of exercise.
3. When one should not exercise.
4. Patient's personal exercise program.

Medications (SI and SII)

Patient Can Verbalize/Demonstrate

Insulin

1. What is function of insulin (quick, intermediate, or long acting)?
2. Differentiation of insulin types.
3. Medication schedule—amounts and times taken.
4. Correct technique for insulin preparation:
   a. Insulin to be injected is at room temperature.
   b. Rotates bottle to mix (cloudy insulin).
   c. Injects air.
   d. Withdraws proper amount of insulin.
   e. Rids syringe of air bubbles.
5. Correct technique for drawing up insulin, two types:
   a. Rotates bottle to mix (cloudy) insulin.
   b. Injects air into both bottles.
   c. Withdraws clear (regular) insulin first.
   d. Adds proper amount of second insulin.
6. Correct technique for insulin administration:
   a. Cleans site with alcohol.
   b. Gathers skin and inserts needle all the way.
   c. Injects insulin, holding needle steady (needle should go in at 90-degree angle unless person is very thin).
   d. Use of consistent sites, rotates within those sites (abdomen, arm, leg, buttocks).
7. Storage of insulin:
   a. Best to store in refrigerator.
   b. For travel, insulin can be stored at room temperature up to 1 month (57° to 85° F).
8. Discards syringes in sealable can or special disposal unit.
9. Knows that insulin can cause hypoglycemia.

Oral Agents

1. Action of oral agent.
2. Medication schedule—amount and time to be taken.
3. Need to eat three carbohydrate-consistent meals a day.
4. Can cause hypoglycemia.

Relationships Among Nutrition, Exercise, Medication, and Blood Glucose Levels (SI and SII)

Patient Can Verbalize/Demonstrate

1. Effect of food on blood glucose.
2. Effect of insulin oral agents on blood glucose.
3. Effect of oral agents on insulin resistance.
4. Effect of physical activity on blood glucose.
5. Effect of illness on blood sugar.

Monitoring and Use of Results (SI and SII)

Patient Can Verbalize/Demonstrate

1. Explains need for monitoring glucose.
2. Normal range of blood glucose and acceptable targets.
3. Capillary blood glucose monitoring:
   a. Loads and operates lancing device.
   b. Holds arm down to the side to get better drop of blood.
   c. Obtains large hanging drop of blood.
   d. Places blood on strip properly.
   e. Waits appropriate amount of time according to directions.
   f. Reads visual and records results.
   g. Uses meter (knows name of meter, strips to use; how to calibrate and use control solutions; how to clean, insert battery; and understands readout).
4. Checking urine ketones:
   a. Knows how to do.
   b. Knows when to do.
5. Knows when and whom to call for help.

Acute Complications: Hyperglycemia

Patient Can Verbalize/Demonstrate

1. Definition and cause of hyperglycemia.
2. Symptoms of hyperglycemia.
3. Illness and sick-day rules:
   a. What to do about insulin/oral agents when ill.
   b. How often to check sugar and ketones.
   c. When to call physician.
   d. Sick-day eating.

Acute Complications: Hypoglycemia (SI and SII)

Patient Can Verbalize/Demonstrate

1. Definition and cause of hypoglycemia.
2. Symptoms of hypoglycemia.
3. Treatment of hypoglycemia (wears diabetes identification).
4. When to call physician, nurse practitioner.

Chronic Complications

Patient Can Verbalize/Demonstrate

1. Possible long-term complications.
2. Importance of prevention; primary role of glycemic control.
3. The organs/body systems at risk in diabetes:
   a. Eyes
   b. Blood vessels
   c. Blood pressure
   d. Feet
   e. Kidneys
   f. Neurologic
   g. Reproductive
4. Reasons for good foot care, including daily cleansing and inspection/appropriate footwear
5. Reason for yearly dilated fundoscopic examination (and last date).
6. Need for blood pressure control. Knows blood pressure goal.

BOX 30-12 Professional Prompter Worksheet for Diabetes Education—cont'd

Foot, Skin, and Dental Care

Patient Can Verbalize/Demonstrate

1. Importance of good health habits:
   a. Dental
   b. Skin
   c. Feet
   d. Signs of infection
   e. Effect of smoking, alcohol, and drug abuse

Behavior Change Strategies, Goal Setting, and Problem Solving

Patient Can Verbalize/Demonstrate

1. The need for a planned system of medical care, including follow-up and education.
2. The benefits and responsibilities of goal setting for self-help care.
3. The importance of being well informed, equal partner to make choices.

Use of Health Care System and Community Resources

Patient Can Verbalize/Demonstrate

1. Resources that can help:
   a. American Diabetes Association
   b. Self-management classes
   c. Services for the blind
   d. Juvenile Diabetes Foundation
   e. Local diabetes associations

Necessary Take-Home (SI and SII)

Patient Can Verbalize/Demonstrate

1. Feels comfortable doing all skills under survival.
2. Knows the skills and is able to simulate them in a normal day (i.e., take you through a day and list all diabetes-related activities as patient would do them).
3. Knows whom to call, the telephone number, and when to call.
4. Has a return appointment card with health care provider's name and phone number listed.
5. Has instructions written on:
   a. *Take Home Instruction* form
   b. *Choice to Better Daily Living* form
6. Has a schedule of the diabetes classes if patient chooses to attend them.
7. Has a meal plan—have patient seen by dietitian. If dietitian is unavailable and you must instruct on meal plan, refer to section on nutrition.

space, thus eliminating a potential source of error. The procedure can be practiced using saline solution and a syringe.

Patient fear is greatly reduced if the nurse self-injects sterile saline (rather than the traditional orange or sponge), thus demonstrating no discomfort with injection. Given the superior insulin absorption from the abdomen, patients can be taught to give their first injection in the upper abdomen. This overcomes the patient's fears that abdominal injections are very painful.

For the first injection, the nurse may elect to delay teaching about the preparation and focus first on self-injection. Adults may be better able to focus on preparing the syringe after experiencing self-injection.

Mixing Two Insulins

If the patient is using two insulins, they may be mixed in one syringe so that only one injection is necessary (see Guidelines for Safe Practice box). As mentioned earlier, Glargine can never be mixed in a syringe with any other insulin, since its lower pH will result in precipitation. A relative contraindication is mixing a crystalline zinc insulin (Lente or Ultralente) with other types of insulins. Most practitioners permit patients to mix other insulins with Lente and/or Ultralente and inject immediately. The mix–and–inject immediately routine is the recommendation, regardless of which insulins are being mixed together.

Mixing two insulins in the same syringe is one of the more complex psychomotor skills the patient has to learn; therefore it needs to be started early. A major risk of mixing two insulins in one syringe is contamination of the two vials of insulin. Cross-contamination can be avoided by always withdrawing from the Lispro or Regular insulin vial first, because injecting minute amounts of Lispro or Regular insulin into a vial of longer-acting insulin is less problematic than the Lispro or Regular insulin being contaminated with the longer-acting insulin.

Guidelines for Safe Practice

Mixing Two Insulins in One Syringe

1. Gather equipment.
2. Wash hands.
3. Roll vial of longer-acting insulin. NEVER MIX GLARGINE INSULIN IN A SYRINGE WITH ANY OTHER INSULIN!
4. Cleanse tops of vials with alcohol.
5. Draw up air equivalent to the dose of the longer-acting insulin and inject the air into that vial. (Do not draw up this insulin.) Remove needle from vial.
6. Draw up air equivalent to the dose of the Lispro/Aspart/regular insulin, inject the air into the bottle, and withdraw the Lispro/Aspart/Regular insulin to the correct dose. Remove all air, and readjust to the correct dose. Remove needle.
7. Insert needle into the vial of the longer-acting insulin, and draw up the correct dose.
8. If an error is made, discard the insulin in the syringe and start over.

If there is difficulty mastering the skill of mixing two insulins, the patient may take two separate injections each time or have a family member, significant other, or friend prefill the syringes. A week's supply of insulin (including mixed insulin) can be predrawn for up to 1 week.

Injection Sites

Two principles govern injection sites: consistency and rotation. Consistent use of sites is critical because insulin absorption varies dramatically depending on the anatomic site. The upper abdomen provides the quickest absorption, followed by the arms, legs, and lower buttocks. The abdominal site is also not affected by exercise. Consistency with use of a specified injection site for a specified injection time helps eliminate some variability in glucose levels. For example, the patient could use the abdomen for the prebreakfast injection, the arm for the predinner injection, and the buttocks for the bedtime injection. Then, rotation of injections among the designated anatomic sites helps prevent the development of lipodystrophy. Ideally, injections should be given 1 inch apart while trying not to reuse an injection site within a 2- to 4-week period of time. The injection site should be cleansed with 70% isopropyl alcohol before use.

Lipodystrophy can occur with repeated injections, causing poor absorption of medication. Two forms of lipodystrophy can occur: hypertrophy and atrophy. Hypertrophy is thickening of an injection site from the development of fibrous scar tissue as a result of repeated injections. A hypertrophic area is usually devoid of nerve endings, and the patient likes to reuse it because injections are painless, but absorption is erratic. Atrophy is loss of subcutaneous fat from unknown causes; however, an immunologic process has been implicated. Lipodystrophies may be partially caused by impurities in insulin; the development of purified insulins has decreased this problem, but rotation of sites is still important (Figure 30-11). Recommended sites for subcutaneous injection are illustrated in Figure 30-12.

Injection of Insulin

Insulin should be administered subcutaneously. Historically the subcutaneous tissue was pinched up before injection. With the current insulin syringes, with needles from 0.25 to 0.5 inch long, there is no need to pinch up the subcutaneous tissue unless the patient is very thin or cachectic. Rather, the subcutaneous tissue should be gently gathered or, if the patient is obese, stretched tautly. With these shorter-needle syringes, the needle should be inserted at a 90-degree angle. There is no need for routine aspiration. Injections should produce little, if any, discomfort. Use of the techniques described in the Patient Teaching box can minimize painful injections.

Although disposable syringes are designed for single use, many individuals with diabetes reuse their own insulin syringes until the needle dulls. Insulin has bacteriostatic additives that inhibit bacterial growth. With reuse of the syringe, however, the light coating of lubrication on the needle is lost and injections may be more uncomfortable. Some studies also demonstrate physical damage to the bevel of the needle after even single use, thereby creating the potential for inaccurate drawing up of insulin and perhaps incomplete insulin delivery when syringes are reused. In patients who practice good hygiene and good injection technique, however, the reuse of syringes is safe and practical.

Safe disposal of syringes and lancets used at home is critical. Sharps disposal containers are available for purchase at

Patient Teaching

Steps to Eliminate Painful Insulin Injections

1. Inject insulin that has been at room temperature for 15 minutes. Do not inject cold insulin.
2. Wait until the topical alcohol has dried before injecting insulin.
3. Keep muscles in the area of injection relaxed, not tensed.
4. Penetrate the skin quickly. Use the hingelike action of the wrist to "dart" the needle in.
5. Do not change the direction of the needle on insertion or withdrawal.
6. Do not use dull needles.

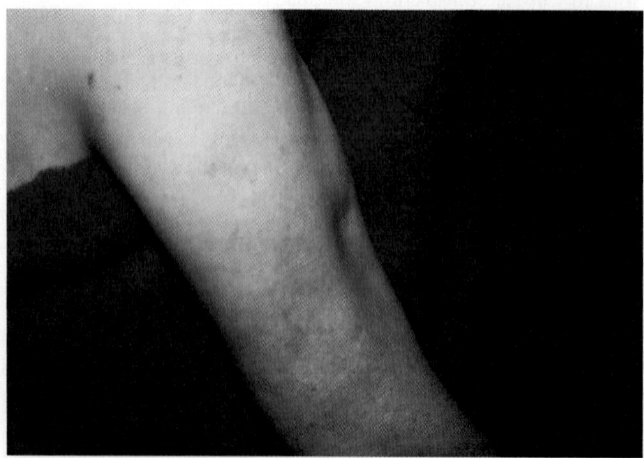

Figure 30-11 Lipodystrophy of the arm.

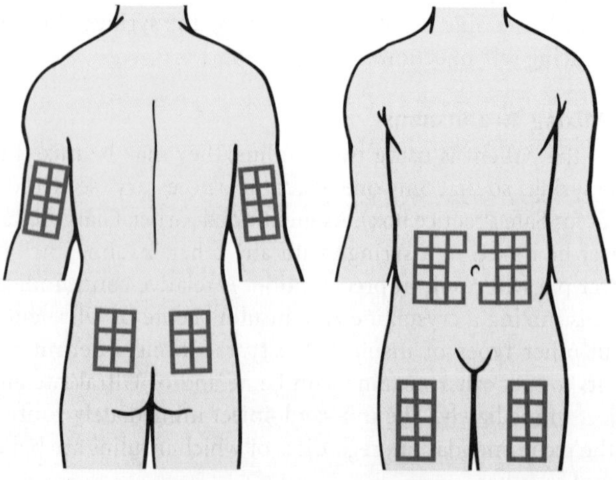

Figure 30-12 Insulin injection sites.

drugstores, or needles and syringes can be placed in a hard-sided receptacle, such as a detergent or bleach bottle. Patients should call their local government office for information on disposal.

Storage of Insulin and Other Supplies and Care of Syringes

Patients need to develop a home storage system for insulin and equipment. Insulin is stable for 30 days at room temperature; however, it is a good idea to have patients refrigerate extra insulin. Prefilled syringes should be stored in the refrigerator with the needles facing upward. All equipment should be stored out of the reach of children.

Patients should always have an extra bottle of each type of insulin they use. Insulin has an expiration date, which should be checked at purchase; patients should purchase only the amount that can be used before the expiration date. When traveling, insulin and supplies should be hand-carried to prevent loss. It is also recommended to bring twice as many supplies as one anticipates using.

For persons unwilling or unable to use syringes, a variety of injection aids are available (Figure 30-13). Pen devices for insulin delivery facilitate taking injections away from home. The Autojector by Ulster, an insulin injection aid, not only injects the needle but also injects the insulin; it gives a virtually pain-free injection and retails for approximately $60. Jet-spray injectors are also available but are expensive, retailing for approximately $400. Although jet-spray injectors are designed to reduce discomfort and enhance insulin absorption, some patients actually find them more uncomfortable and report inconsistencies with insulin delivery as a result of the variable pressure settings needed in different anatomic sites.

Measures to Assist the Sensory-Impaired Person

Adaptation of equipment may be necessary for the sensory-impaired person. A number of aids available for the visually handicapped are advertised in diabetes publications or are available from the American Federation of the Blind or local agencies for the visually impaired. Special syringes with plunger locks, attachable devices for locking the plunger, and attachable needle and insulin bottle guides to facilitate entry of the needle into the bottle can be purchased. Persons who have failing vision may also use a small magnifying adapter that can be clipped to a syringe.

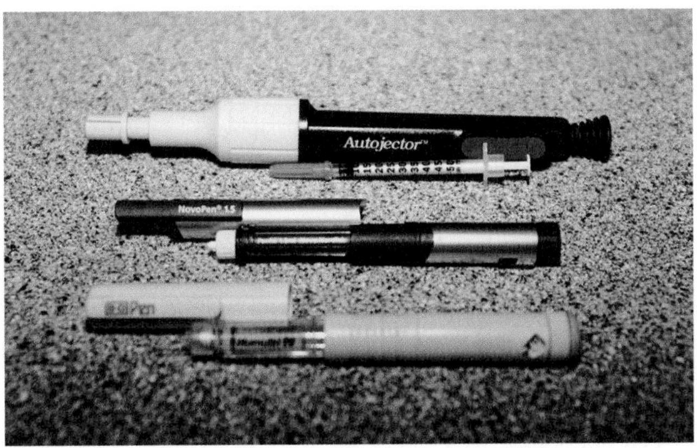

Figure 30-13 Insulin injection aids.

Persons with poor vision may draw air instead of insulin into the syringe and should be cautioned to invert the vial completely and insert the needle only a short distance. Visually impaired persons are often advised to use only about two thirds of a vial of insulin. Some persons have a family member or a friend draw the last doses from a bottle of insulin. Another option is to know how long to use a vial before the level gets so low that the needle is not covered (e.g., if there is 1000 U in a vial, and if the person is taking 40 U/day, he or she should stop using the vial on the twenty-second day unless assisted by a sighted person).

6c. Managing Oral Agents

Patients taking oral agents must be equally prepared to handle their medication. Each patient must know the name of the medication, dose, peak effects, and how the diet and exercise regimens are coordinated with medication therapy. If taking sulfonylureas, patients must be educated about hypoglycemia symptoms and treatment. Patients must know how to handle illness. Oral agents should be kept out of the reach of children, at room temperature, and not exposed to direct sunlight. The medication should be hand-carried when traveling to decrease the risk of loss.

6d. Self-Monitoring of Metabolic Status

All individuals with diabetes should perform HBGM if possible. Meters are very affordable (less than $80), and most manufacturers provide discount coupons or no-cost meters with the purchase of test strips. Home blood glucose meters correlate well with venous samples when correct technique is used (see Guidelines for Safe Practice box on p. 938).

Although health care professionals emphasize the use of physiologic parameters to monitor glucose status, patients continue to use symptoms as guides for self-regulation. Health care providers must emphasize to patients the importance of performing a home blood glucose test to correlate a subjective symptom with an objective measure.

All patients should use a diary or log to record the date, time, and monitoring results. Other diary notations may include medications, food intake, activity level, and illnesses so that the person can begin to see the relationship between blood glucose or urine ketone levels and the treatment regimen.

As patients gain flexibility and self-determination, they may manipulate insulin, diet, and exercise independently on the basis of monitoring results. Patients gain increasing independence on the basis of ability, interest, and encouragement by caregivers.

6e,f. Managing Hypoglycemia

Patients receiving insulin or sulfonylureas must be educated about hypoglycemia (plasma blood glucose level of 60 mg/dl or lower). Patients must know:

Causes of hypoglycemia (see Box 30-4)
Signs and symptoms of hypoglycemia (see Box 30-5)

Knowledge of appropriate treatment of hypoglycemia (Most hypoglycemia is mild and easily treated.)
How to obtain an identification card/Medic-Alert bracelet/necklace and the importance of carrying or wearing it at all times
Importance of carrying a quickly absorbed glucose source
Methods to prevent further episodes of hypoglycemia

Because hypoglycemia can occur suddenly, family members and friends also should learn the symptoms and how to handle a reaction. If a patient is awake but groggy, another person can be taught to assist with oral treatment. This consists of putting corn syrup, honey, or cake icing in the patient's mouth between the gum and cheek. This will be absorbed through the oral mucosa, and the patient will usually be aroused sufficiently to take a glass of juice, milk, or sugar-sweetened coffee or tea (Box 30-13).

Glucagon should be prescribed for all individuals with type 1 DM. Significant others should be educated in its proper use. All patients should strive for prevention of hypoglycemia. Information about hypoglycemia should be included as part of the survival skills during the initial management phase. A good time to teach about hypoglycemia is after teaching about insulin injection and self-monitoring has been completed. It is helpful to illustrate survival teaching using simulation and going through a typical day with patients, letting them take the lead in going through all the diabetes-related activities in sequence. At this time, information about insulin reaction can be taught in relationship to time and action of insulin.

Somogyi Effect

The Somogyi effect is characterized by hyperglycemia after hypoglycemia. As is true with healthy persons without diabetes, the hypoglycemia in persons with diabetes stimulates the production of counterregulatory hormones (glucocorticoids, growth hormone, epinephrine). These hormones promote glycogenolysis and gluconeogenesis. In individuals without diabetes, the blood glucose level remains in the normal range because with minimal elevations, insulin secretion is stimulated. In individuals with diabetes, the blood glucose rises to abnormally high levels because insulin secretion is absent or altered. In some instances the signs and symptoms of hypoglycemia are subtle and may not be recognized. Or, hyperglycemia following the hypoglycemia is recognized in the early morning and may be mistaken for the dawn phenomenon. The assumption is made that the patient needs higher doses of insulin, but this treatment worsens the problem. Figure 30-14 illustrates this cycle.

The signs and symptoms of the Somogyi effect can be any of those normally associated with hypoglycemia but commonly consist only of nighttime sweats, nightmares, restless sleep, and a headache on arising. With both the Somogyi effect and the dawn phenomenon, there may be glycosuria, relatively normal blood glucose levels with positive ketones (remember that counterregulatory hormones stimulate lipolysis and beta-oxidation of fats), and wide fluctuations in blood glucose unrelated to meals.

To differentiate the Somogyi effect from the dawn phenomenon, the patient should perform overnight HBGM at 2AM and 4 AM. In the Somogyi effect hypoglycemia will be identified and then followed by hyperglycemia. In the dawn phenomenon there is no overnight hypoglycemia; rather, there is a consistent rise in blood glucose levels overnight. Decreasing the dose of insulin precipitating the hypoglycemia treats the Somogyi effect. Treatment of the dawn phenomenon consists of increasing the dose of the insulin, which is affecting nocturnal glucose levels.

A primary nursing role is to document reports of hypoglycemia, glucose intake, and laboratory results and to assess for the presence of night sweats, nightmares, and early-morning headaches. The nurse should also correlate these complaints and laboratory results with mealtimes. Such data help identify the phenomenon.

6g. Providing Exercise Knowledge

Exercise is another major area of patient education for persons with DM. Nursing activities include obtaining an exercise history, helping the person understand and obtain a preexercise examination, and planning an enjoyable and safe exercise program. The nurse should:

1. Help select an exercise that will not cause problems if conditions such as neuropathy or proliferative retinopathy are present.

BOX 30-13 Carbohydrates for Relief of Hypoglycemia*

½ cup pure fruit juice
6 ounces carbonated soda drink (regular, not diet)
½ cup regular gelatin dessert, not diet
4 cubes or 2 packets of sugar
3 pieces of hard candy
3 glucose tablets

*Items listed will provide 10 to 15 g of carbohydrate.

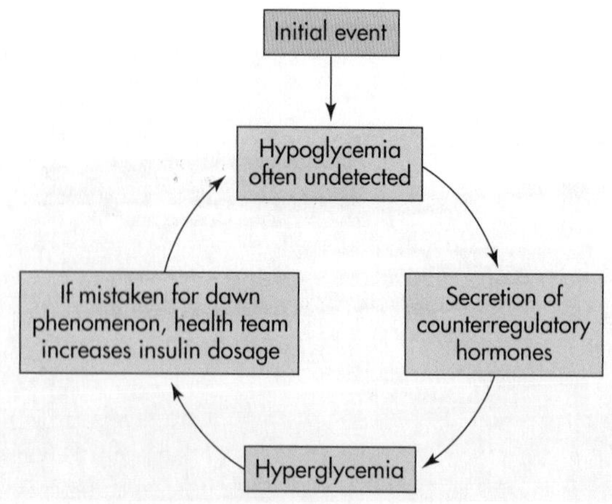

Figure 30-14 Somogyi effect.

2. Refer the patient to a podiatrist for correct footwear for the chosen exercise if applicable.
3. Help establish a regular exercise routine to reduce the risk of hypoglycemia.
4. Explain the components of a safe exercise program and the special needs of the person with diabetes.
5. Teach how to monitor cardiovascular tolerance (e.g., by pulse rate or level of exertion).
6. Identify the parameters to monitor before daily exercise (blood glucose level, ketone level, environmental temperature).
   a. The patient should not exercise if the blood glucose level is greater than 300 mg/dl or if there are ketones in the urine.
   b. If the weather is hot, to avoid dehydration suggest exercising in an air-conditioned area, such as a shopping mall or gymnasium, or using an exercise bicycle.

Hygiene and Foot Care

Hygiene. Persons with uncontrolled diabetes are at increased risk of infection. The effectiveness of the skin as a first line of defense can be diminished. Uncontrolled diabetes leads to loss of fat deposits under the skin, loss of glycogen, and catabolism of body proteins. Hyperglycemia can hamper the inflammatory response and wound healing and impair leukocyte function, migration of leukocytes to the site of infection, phagocytosis, and bacterial killing, all of which are involved in combating infection. Circulatory impairments can also delay healing. The skin must be kept supple and as free of pathogenic organisms as possible. This is especially true in warm, moist areas that encourage growth of organisms (between the toes, under the breasts, and in the axillae and groin). It is extremely important that persons with diabetes carry out hygienic measures for prevention of infection daily, with special emphasis on foot care. They should seek medical attention immediately if an infection occurs.

Foot Care. Three major factors interact in foot problems in diabetes: neuropathy, ischemia, and sepsis. The need for foot care cannot be overemphasized. The patient's feet should be visually assessed at every follow-up visit (Box 30-14). Thorough assessment is required to identify patients at risk. Peripheral neuropathy must be assessed objectively by measuring sensation to pinprick, vibration, and temperature and by assessing deep tendon reflexes (see Box 30-14). Subjective sensations of paresthesias, pain, and numbness appear only after years of damage. The decreased ability to perceive a standard nylon filament pressure on the foot is a sign of advanced neuropathy with predisposition to foot ulceration.

Once protective sensory loss is determined, the risk of the patient's foot being injured can be categorized. The National Hansen Disease Program in Baton Rouge, Louisiana, developed a system for risk stratification.[18] The risk categories used by the team are listed in Table 30-12.

Each individual with diabetes is responsible for practicing preventive care on a daily basis through a thorough foot examination (see Patient Teaching box). Podiatric consultation may be necessary for orthotics to relieve pressure areas and to treat calluses and corns. Extra-depth and custom-made shoes may be necessary and can be purchased in specialty stores. Medicare reimburses patients who meet certain foot problem criteria for a percentage of the cost of the shoes.

Managing Concurrent Illnesses

All illnesses influence the status of diabetes control. In most instances the person with diabetes needs increased insulin during a concurrent illness. A patient taking oral agents may need an increased dosage or even temporary insulin therapy during a concurrent illness.

Unfortunately, many people mistakenly believe that if they cannot eat, they do not need to take the prescribed insulin or oral hypoglycemic agent. Patients with type 1 DM who fail to

BOX 30-14 Assessment of the Feet of the Patient With Diabetes

Color: Compare one foot with the other.
Temperature: Compare both feet with upper legs; assess for lines of demarcation.
Sensory function: Test for pinprick and vibratory sense.
Reflexes: Test Achilles and quadriceps tendon reflexes.
Pulses: Check dorsalis pedis and posterior tibial pulses (ankle-brachial indices should be performed by diabetes team).
Lesions: Examine for calluses, cuts, bruises, cracks, or infection.
Self-care: Discuss self-care regimen being used.

TABLE 30-12 Risk Categories and Associated Footwear Guidelines

	Clinical Findings	Footwear Changes
Category 0	Has protective sensation	Education on proper footwear
Category 1	Has lost protective sensation	Add soft insole to shoe of proper contour and fit
Category 2	Has lost protective sensation and has foot deformity	Depth footwear or custom shoe for severe deformity, molded insoles
Category 3	Has lost protective sensation and has history of foot ulcer	Inspect type and condition of footwear and insoles at every visit

From Coleman W: Foot care and diabetes mellitus. In Haire-Joshu D, editor: *Management of diabetes mellitus—perspectives of care across the life span,* St Louis, 1992, Mosby.

Patient Teaching
Foot Care for the Patient With Diabetes

1. Never soak feet.
2. Wash feet daily and dry them well, paying attention to the area between the toes.
3. Inspect feet daily. Look for:
   a. Color changes
   b. Swelling
   c. Cuts
   d. Cracks in the skin
   e. Redness
   f. Blisters
   g. Temperature changes
4. Never walk barefoot. Always wear shoes or slippers.
5. Wear well-fitting shoes and clean socks.
6. After bathing, when toenails are soft, cut nails straight across. Do not cut into the corners. File edges smooth with an emery board. If you have visual problems, have someone else cut your toenails for you.
7. If feet are dry, apply lotion or cream; do not put lotion between the toes.
8. Do not perform "bathroom surgery."
9. Do not self-treat corns, calluses, warts, or ingrown toenails. Consult a podiatrist.
10. Bathwater should be no warmer than 90° F. Test water temperature on your inner forearm, just as you would a baby's bottle, before immersing hands or feet.
11. Do not use heating pads or hot water bottles.
12. Enhance your circulation by:
    a. Not smoking
    b. Avoiding crossing legs when sitting
    c. Protecting your hands and feet when exposed to cold
    d. Avoiding tight elastic on socks
    e. Exercising
    f. Using sunscreen
13. ANY FOOT PROBLEM IS A MEDICAL EMERGENCY. Consult your primary care provider, podiatrist, or diabetes team immediately if any foot problem arises. Delay in seeking care can cost you your feet.

Research

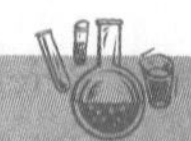

Reference: Coonrod BA, Betschart J, Harris MI: Frequency and determinants of diabetes patient education among adults in the U.S. population, *Diabetes Care* 17(8):852, 1994.

The authors surveyed 2405 individuals at least 18 years of age with diabetes regarding attendance at a diabetes education class or program since diagnosis. Only 35.1% had ever attended such a class or program. Of individuals with insulin-dependent diabetes, 58.6% had done so; the percentages were 48.9% of insulin-treated individuals with type 2 diabetes and 23.7% of non–insulin-treated individuals with type 2 diabetes. Positive associations with diabetes education in individuals with type 2 diabetes, regardless of insulin administration, were younger age, African-American race, residence in the Midwestern United States, higher educational level, and presence of diabetes complications. Positive associations with diabetes education in non–insulin-treated individuals with type 2 diabetes were increasing income, living alone, and not having a diabetes physician or not visiting one in the last year. Despite the fact that patient education has been recognized for its contribution to the reduction in morbidity and mortality of diabetes, many individuals, especially those with type 2 diabetes, still do not receive such education.

take insulin when they are sick commonly develop ketoacidosis. These persons must take carbohydrates in some form. See Box 30-11 for data that patients must be taught in relation to managing concurrent illnesses.

Patient/Family Education. Joslin[47] summarized the critical importance of patient education: "There is no disease in which an understanding by the patient of the methods of treatment avails as much." Joslin[47] told his patients, "Therefore face the facts, accept the situation, study the disease, and become master of your fate" (see Research box).

Ideally patient education is integrated with traditional medical care of patients with diabetes. The ADA and the American Association of Diabetes Educators (AADE) have worked closely over the past decade to improve the quality of diabetes education and management. The AADE and its certifying body, the National Certification Board for Diabetes Educators, are responsible for the certification of health care professionals as CDEs. Local chapters of the AADE are present in many major U.S. cities. To locate the nearest chapter, call 1-800-TEAM-UP-4 or, on the Internet, go to the following website: www.aadenet.org. The ADA has two accreditation programs. The ADA Provider Recognition Program recognizes physicians who have documented the delivery of exemplary diabetes care to patients on both a clinical and an educational basis. The ADA also has a Diabetes Education Recognition Program that recognizes programs that deliver comprehensive diabetes education. Some states also have state-specific accreditation programs.[4] The content areas of patient education programs accredited by the ADA Recognized Providers and ADA are outlined in Box 30-15.

Health Promotion/Prevention

Primary Prevention of Type 1 Diabetes Mellitus. Primary prevention of type 1 DM is under active research in both basic science and clinical care. All type 1 DM prevention programs are experimental and focus on arresting the autoimmune process.

Primary Prevention of Type 2 Diabetes Mellitus. Primary prevention of type 2 DM takes on a very different focus. Abdominal obesity and a high waist-hip ratio (>1.0) are significant risk factors for type 2 DM. Individuals with abdominal obesity are hyperinsulinemic and are at increased risk not only for type 2 DM, but for all components of the cardiodysmetabolic syndrome, as previously described.[77-79,108]

Primary prevention of type 2 DM involves identification and modification of risk factors (see Risk Factors box). Primary prevention should be directed toward lifestyle changes that include exercise, weight loss or weight control, and knowledge of risk factors. It is important that persons with diabetes

BOX 30-15 Fifteen Content Areas of Diabetes Education

1. *Overview of diabetes mellitus*
    - Definition of diabetes mellitus
    - Effects of alterations in metabolism of carbohydrates, proteins, and fats
    - Classification of diabetes (e.g., type 1, type 2, gestational)
2. *Stress and psychologic adjustment*
    - Grieving and adaptation to living with a chronic disease
    - Expressing feelings openly
    - Unrealistic expectations
    - Effect of stress on metabolic control
    - Recognizing the need for professional help
    - Stress management
3. *Family involvement and social support*
    - Diabetes as a family challenge
    - Learning to recognize and work with adverse family dynamics
    - Need for support
4. *Nutrition*
    - Individualized meal plan to control weight, glucose, and lipids
    - Composition of the diet
    - Achieving and maintaining desired body weight and glucose control
    - Advice on alcohol use
    - Eating on special occasions
    - Reading and interpreting nutrition labels
5. *Exercise and activity*
    - Benefits/risks
    - Effects of exercise on therapeutic plan
    - Preparing for exercise (food and medication; companion)
    - Heart rate monitoring
    - Monitoring necessary before starting exercise
    - Monitoring necessary when establishing an exercise program
6. *Medications*
    - Goals of treatment
    - Oral agents
        - Action on blood glucose
        - Side effects
        - Drug interactions
    - Insulin
        - Action on blood glucose
        - Cautions (especially Somogyi effect)
        - Strengths/purities
        - Injection techniques
        - Complications of treatment: hypoglycemia, antibodies, lipodystrophy
        - Glucagon
        - How to buy, store, and use
7. *Monitoring and use of results*
    - Goals
    - Types of blood glucose monitoring available
    - Quality control of monitors
    - How to use blood glucose monitoring to achieve and maintain good glucose control: performing tests accurately, interpreting test results, frequency of testing, taking action appropriate to test results
    - Urine ketone testing
    - Glycosylated hemoglobin test: how to relate to average blood glucose level
8. *Relationships among nutrition, exercise, medication, and blood glucose levels*
    - Balancing nutrition, exercise, and medications
    - Adjusting each factor in relation to the others
    - Adjusting times of monitoring
    - Identifying times for snacks
    - Effects of exercise on blood glucose
9. *Acute complications: hyperglycemia and hypoglycemia*
    - Definitions of hyperglycemia and hypoglycemia
    - Prevention of each
    - Early recognition/treatment/record keeping
    - Hypoglycemia unawareness
    - Dawn phenomenon and Somogyi effect
    - What to do for diabetic ketoacidosis/hyperosmolar coma
    - Effects of illness on diabetes
    - Monitoring glucose/ketones
    - Sick-day guidelines (including diet)
10. *Chronic complications: prevention, detection, and treatment*
    - Kinds of complications—microvascular and macrovascular, neuropathy
    - Examples of each kind of complication (especially those likely to occur in your population)
    - Possible causes of complication
    - Self-care for prevention or delay of complications
    - Coping strategies (support groups, counseling, stress management)
11. *Foot, skin, and dental care*
    - Daily self-care measures
    - Relationship of problems to diabetes care
    - The need for regular evaluation of feet and teeth
12. *Behavioral change strategies, goal setting, risk factor reduction, and problem solving*
    - Changing behaviors through goal setting
    - Rights of patient
    - Responsibility of patient
    - Patient-professional partnership in planning care
    - Taking care of self when sick
13. *Benefits, risks, and management options for improving glucose control*
    - Diabetes Control and Complications Trial (DCCT) results
    - Therapeutic care plans—maps to good health and quality of life
14. *Preconception care, pregnancy, and gestational diabetes*
15. *Use of health care systems and community resources*
    - Planned follow-up
    - Patient's responsibility
    - Names and telephone numbers of health care team members
    - Emergency care
    - Community resources
    - Planning for travel
    - Educational resources and need for continuing educa
    - Insurance and employment regulations and reimbursement

From American Diabetes Association: *Goals for diabetes education, clinical education program: national standards for diabetes self-manageme grams,* ed 2, Alexandria, Va; Updated in American Diabetes Association: Clinical practice recommendations 2001, *Diabetes Care* 24(suppl

Risk Factors
Type 2 Diabetes Mellitus

Family history of diabetes
Obesity
Race (Native American, Hispanic, or African-American)
Age
Previously identified impaired glucose tolerance
Hypertension or hyperlipidemia
History of gestational diabetes mellitus or delivery of babies >9 pounds
Reactive hypoglycemia

TABLE 30-13 Estimated Risk of Developing Diabetes Mellitus

Relationship to Person With Diabetes	Approximate Rate of Developing Diabetes
No diabetes in family	Type 1: 0.3%
Identical twin with type 1	Type 1: 36%
One parent with type 1	Type 1: 3%
Sibling with type 1	Type 1: 3%
No diabetes in family	Type 2: 14%
Identical twin with type 2	Type 2: almost 100%
One parent with type 2	Type 2: 20%-30%
Both parents with type 2	Type 2: 35%-55%

Adapted from American Diabetes Association, Expert Committee on the Diagnosis and Classification of Diabetes Mellitus: Report of the Expert Committee on the Diagnosis and Classification of Diabetes Mellitus, *Diabetes Care* 24(suppl 1):S5, 2001.

be made aware of the familial tendencies and risks for siblings of the individual with either type of diabetes (Table 30-13).[107]

Prevention of type 2 DM is being studied. Results of the Diabetes Prevention Program, a study of primary prevention of type 2 DM in individuals with IGT, were released in August 2001. The 3200 subjects were randomized to one of three groups: (1) intensive lifestyle changes (including diet and exercise), (2) treatment with metformin, or (3) a control group receiving a placebo. The intensive lifestyle group had a 58% risk reduction in the development of type 2 DM; in individuals ages 60 and older, the risk reduction was a dramatic 71%. The metformin-treated group experienced a 31% risk reduction. In the Heart Outcomes Prevention Evaluation (HOPE) trial for nondiabetic patients at high risk for developing cardiovascular disease, individuals who were treated with ramipril 10 mg daily had a 34% risk reduction in the development of type 2 DM.[39,40] In the West of Scotland trial the use of pravastatin reduced the risk of developing type 2 DM by 30%.[34] A recent Finnish lifestyle modification study demonstrated a 58% risk reduction in the development of type 2 DM patients with IGT who were randomized to a program of nsive diet and exercise.[97]

Healthy People 2010
Diabetes Mellitus

Prevent diabetes: reduce new cases to 2.5 per 1000 people per year (age-adjusted baseline: 3.5 new cases per 1000 people in 1994 to 1996) and reduce the overall rate of diabetes that is clinically diagnosed to 25 overall cases per 1000 people (age-adjusted baseline: 40 overall cases, including new and existing cases, of diabetes per 100,000 people).[107]

Reduce complications among people with diabetes: end-stage renal disease, blindness, and lower extremity amputation.[107] Reduce deaths from cardiovascular disease in persons with diabetes to 309 deaths per 100,000 persons with diabetes (age-adjusted baseline: 343 per 100,000 persons with diabetes).[107]

Reduce the diabetes death rate to more than 45 deaths per 100,000 people (age-adjusted baseline: 75 per 100,000 in 1997) and the diabetes-related death rate to 7.8 per 1000 persons with diabetes (age-adjusted baseline: 8.8 per 1000 persons with diabetes listed anywhere on the death certificate in 1997).

From US Department of Health and Human Services: *Healthy people 2010: understanding and improving health,* Washington, DC, 2000, USDHHS.

Healthy People 2010. The surgeon general's report Healthy People 2010[107] has established several goals that give the previously discussed primary prevention recommendations more momentum. One goal is to reduce overweight prevalence to not more than 15% among people ages 20 or older (baseline: 23% for people ages 20 through 74 in 1988 to 1994). Another goal from Healthy People 2010 that has relevance for prevention of type 2 DM pertains to exercise. The goal is to increase to at least 30% the proportion of adults ages 18 years and older who engage regularly, preferably daily, in moderate physical activity for at least 30 minutes per day (baseline: 15% of people ages 18 and older were active for at least 30 minutes five or more times per week in 1992). Other objectives specifically related to diabetes are outlined in the Healthy People 2010 box.

The importance of patient education is clear, and the need for its availability is outlined in Healthy People 2010.[107] The goal is to increase to at least 60% the proportion of people with chronic and disabling conditions who receive formal patient education, including information about community and self-help resources, as an integral part of the management of their condition (age-adjusted baseline: 45% of persons with diabetes in 1998).[107]

Secondary Prevention of Type 1 Diabetes Mellitus. Screening for type 1 DM is not recommended. From 85% to 90% of individuals with type 1 DM have autoantibodies at the time of initial fasting hyperglycemia. The ADA does not recommend screening for type 1 DM in either the general population or in higher-risk individuals (siblings of type 1 DM individuals) until clinical trials demonstrate the efficacy and safety of treatments to prevent or delay type 1 DM.[7]

Secondary Prevention of Type 2 Diabetes Mellitus. On the other hand, the prevalence of undiagnosed type 2 DM is high, with as many as 8 million individuals in the United States un-

BOX 30-16 Screening for Diabetes in Asymptomatic Individuals

Screening for diabetes mellitus (DM) may be done via an oral glucose tolerance test or with a fasting plasma glucose (FPG). In clinical settings the FPG is preferred because of ease of testing, patient acceptance, convenience, and lower cost.

Screening for DM should be considered in any individual ≥45 years of age. If normal, screening should be repeated every 3 years.

Screening for DM should be considered at a younger age or be carried out more frequently in individuals who:

- Have a first-degree relative with DM
- Are obese
  - Weight ≥120% of desirable body weight or
  - Body mass index (BMI) >25—Weight (kg) ÷ Height (meters squared)
  - Belong to a high-risk DM ethnic population (Hispanic, Native American, African-American)
- Are women with previously diagnosed gestational diabetes mellitus or those who have delivered a baby ≥9 pounds
- Have hypertension
- Have a triglyceride level ≥200 mg/dl or a high-density lipoprotein (HDL) cholesterol ≤35 mg/dl
- On previous testing have had impaired glucose tolerance or impaired fasting glucose

Adapted from American Diabetes Association, Expert Committee on the Diagnosis and Classification of Diabetes Mellitus: Report of the Expert Committee on the Diagnosis and Classification of Diabetes Mellitus, *Diabetes Care* 24(suppl 1):S55, 2001.

TABLE 30-14 Prevention of Long-Term Complications of Diabetes Mellitus

Complications	Early Detection	Early Intervention
Retinopathy	Dilated funduscopic examination	Care by an ophthalmologist or retinal specialist Control of hyperglycemia Control of hypertension
Nephropathy	Examination of urine for albumin or protein excretion Measurement of serum creatinine and creatinine clearance	Control of hyperglycemia Control of hypertension and other cardiovascular risk factors Limiting protein intake Avoiding nephrotoxic agents
Atherosclerosis	History of risk factors and symptoms Examination: electrocardiogram and serum lipid measurements, peripheral pulses	Control of hyperglycemia Control of hypertension Weight control Exercise Control of lipids
Neuropathy	History of symptoms of pain, numbness, etc. Examination: orthostatic blood pressures, muscle strength, reflexes, and sensory function	Control of hyperglycemia Avoidance of neurotoxic agents Education about importance of routine evaluation, foot care, and specific treatment of neuropathy
Foot problems	History of symptoms of numbness, infection, and peripheral vascular insufficiency Complete foot examination Ankle-brachial indices	Control of hyperglycemia Control of atherogenic risk Education about importance and methods of foot care Referral to a podiatrist Referral for orthotics/custom shoes

Source: Herman W: *The prevention and treatment of complications of diabetes mellitus—a guide for primary care practitioners,* Washington, DC, 1992, US Department of Health and Human Services.

diagnosed. Individuals with components of the cardiodysmetabolic syndrome are in the high-risk group. Box 30-16 outlines the ADA recommendations for screening for the presence of undiagnosed type 2 DM.[7]

Tertiary Prevention of Diabetes. Tertiary prevention is the major focus of diabetes management. Both chronic and acute complications occur often, and nurses who work with persons who have diabetes must be involved in tertiary prevention to reduce severe complications of diabetes (Table 30-14). Cardiovascular disease is the leading cause of death among people with diabetes, accounting for more than half of all deaths. Health behaviors aimed at modifying the risk of cardiovascular disease by reducing cardiovascular disease risk factors could have a major effect on morbidity and mortality from DM. The major emphasis of tertiary preventive education will be on the ability of nurses to counsel the patient about the early detection and interventions listed in Table 30-15.

Complementary and Alternative Therapy

Chromium and vanadium are two trace elements that positively affect glucose tolerance. Chromium picolinate has been studied in humans. Trials with vanadium have been limited to animals at this time (see Complementary & Alternative Therapies box).

TABLE 30-15 Classification of Diabetic Neuropathy

Type	Signs and Symptoms
Peripheral sensory polyneuropathy	Classic symmetric glove-and-stocking distribution Paresthesia Hyperesthesia Pain (characteristics vary; may be sharp, stabbing, lancinating, aching, etc.) Loss of sensation to pinprick, vibration, temperature Loss of deep tendon reflexes Muscle wasting and weakness
Autonomic	Orthostatic hypotension Cardiac denervation Anhidrosis Gustatory sweating Gastroparesis, with delayed gastric emptying, nausea, emesis Diarrhea Bladder atony Erectile dysfunction
Mononeuropathy	Cranial nerve palsy (III, IV, VI, and VII) Ulnar nerve palsy Carpal tunnel syndrome
Amyotrophy	Acute anterior thigh pain or numbness Weakness to hip flexion on examination Quadriceps wasting
Radiculopathy	Follows a dermatomal distribution on trunk Paresthesia Hyperesthesia Pain Numbness

Complementary & Alternative Therapies
Chromium Picolinate

Chromium increases (1) insulin binding to the insulin receptor, (2) insulin receptor numbers, and (3) phosphorylation of the insulin receptor. Studies have demonstrated that supplementation with chromium picolinate improves blood glucose and hemoglobin A_{1c} levels in individuals with type 2 diabetes mellitus. The safe effective dosage appears to be in the 200 to 800 μg/day range.

EVALUATION

To evaluate the effectiveness of nursing interventions, compare patient behaviors with those stated in the expected patient outcomes. Achievement of patient outcomes is successful if the patient:

- **1.** Demonstrates improved fluid balance.
- **1a.** Has weight that has increased or decreased by about 2 pounds/week back to baseline.
- **1b.** Has elastic skin turgor with no tenting and moist mucous membranes.
- **1c.** Has blood pressure and pulse within normal range and without orthostatic changes.
- **1d.** Has sodium, chloride, and hematocrit levels within normal limits.
- **1e.** Has urine specific gravity between 1.010 and 1.025.
- **1f.** Has fluid intake of 2.5 to 3 L/day.
- **1g.** Describes measures to prevent dehydration.
- **2.** Experiences less fatigue.
- **2a.** States that no fatigue is present.
- **3.** Exhibits knowledge of information needed to decrease the risk for infection.
- **3a.** States importance of checking glucose on a regular basis.
- **3b.** Correctly describes how infections affect blood glucose.
- **3c.** Correctly lists signs and symptoms of infection.
- **4.** Exhibits signs of nutritional adequacy.
- **4a.** Maintains weight changes as listed previously.
- **4b.** Has an HbA_{1c} measurement that has decreased and serum lipid levels that have decreased.
- **4c,d.** Appropriately describes food type, amount, and distribution.
- **5.** Manifests decreased fear.
- **5a.** States that fears about having diabetes are lessened.
- **5b.** Uses effective coping strategies.
- **6.** Evidences a level of knowledge adequate for self-care.
- **6a.** Correctly describes the disease process of diabetes.
- **6b.** Correctly demonstrates how to inject insulin and rotate sites.
- **6c.** Correctly describes dosage, time, and effects of oral hypoglycemic agents.
- **6d.** Correctly demonstrates BGM and urine ketone monitoring; describes plan to report abnormal results.
- **6e.** Correctly defines hypoglycemia and hyperglycemia.
- **6f.** Correctly describes signs, symptoms, and treatment of hypoglycemia.
- **6g.** Correctly describes exercise plan, foot care and hygiene, sick-day guidelines, and safety precautions.

GERONTOLOGIC CONSIDERATIONS

The prevalence of DM increases with age because insulin resistance increases with advancing age. In the age-group 65 years and older, 18.4% of individuals have DM; 10% have type 2 DM.[64] DM prevalence estimates in individuals over 80 years of age are as high as 40%. An estimated 42% of individuals with type 2 DM are 65 years of age or older, rendering diabetes a major clinical problem. In addition, when persons with IGT are included, the prevalence of abnormal glucose tolerance (IGT and DM) rises to 40% of the geriatric population.[46]

Accurate diagnosis of diabetes is a problem. Because of the insidious onset of type 2 DM, the initial diabetes presentation in an older adult is often painful diabetic neuropathy or other diabetic complications without prior documentation of hyperglycemia.

The etiology of geriatric insulin resistance is complex and may include genetic factors, obesity (increase in the ratio of fat body mass to lean body mass),[31,81] physical inactivity,[62] renal insufficiency, infections or illness, medications (corticosteroids, thiazide diuretics), and perhaps nutritional factors (increase in carbohydrate intake).[22] Insulin resistance at the cellular level may be due to decreased receptor numbers, receptor binding, and postreceptor defects.[31,81]

Worsening insulin resistance is not an inevitable consequence of aging and may be prevented by physical fitness,[96] control of obesity, good nutritional habits, and avoidance of medications that exacerbate insulin resistance (thiazide diuretics, beta-blockers, corticosteroids).[16] Clearly, lifestyle changes need to be made before the geriatric years as the primary preventive strategy. However, improvements are clearly attainable in later life, even in individuals who have developed overt diabetes. The evidence to date supports glycemic control in older adults to reduce the risk of chronic complications of diabetes.

Special considerations must be used when approaching the elderly patient (Box 30-17). Therapeutic principles need to be tailored to the elderly patient (Box 30-18).

BOX 30-17 Special Considerations for the Elderly Patient With Diabetes

1. Accuracy of diagnosis
2. Accuracy of classification of diabetes; C-peptide level needed
3. Mental status; presence of depression or dementia
4. Visual acuity
5. Fine motor skills
6. Social support systems
7. Diabetes knowledge and education potential
8. Blood glucose monitoring: patient, family, friend
9. Diet and meal planning: may have poor or variable intake or compulsive overeating
10. Activity level: inactivity leads to weight gain and decreased insulin sensitivity
11. Increasing ratio of fat to lean body mass
12. Diabetic complications
13. Concurrent illnesses
14. Concurrent pharmacotherapy
15. Increased risk of adverse drug reaction

BOX 30-18 Therapeutic Principles in the Elderly Patient With Diabetes

1. Set realistic goals for glycemic control in the context of age, general condition, and diabetic complications.
2. Patients with true type 1 diabetes mellitus should be treated with intensive therapy (i.e., multiple daily insulin injections and carbohydrate-consistent meal plan).
3. Avoid unnecessary insulin therapy.
4. Review potential for diet therapy with patient and family. A 5% to 10% weight reduction may be highly significant.
5. Increase physical activity safely whenever possible.
6. Use antihyperglycemic agents such as metformin, troglitazone, or acarbose if not contraindicated.
7. Consider nateglinide, with its negligible risk of hypoglycemia. If using a sulfonylurea, consider glimepiride, since its reduced risk of hypoglycemia may result in more safety. Use sulfonylureas at low doses.
8. Combination therapy with oral agents and insulin may be of value with selected patients.

NURSING MANAGEMENT OF PATIENT WITH DIABETES WHO IS UNDERGOING SURGERY

Most nurses working in acute care settings will provide care to the individual with diabetes who is undergoing surgery. Understanding patient concerns and the metabolic consequences of surgery will facilitate patient recovery. In many instances the greatest concern of the individual with diabetes who is admitted to the hospital is not the admitting medical problem; rather, it is concern regarding diabetes management.

The perioperative management of the individual with diabetes may be complicated by poor control of blood glucose levels and the presence of complications such as hypertension, diabetic nephropathy, autonomic neuropathy, coronary artery disease, and systemic atherosclerosis. Counterregulatory hormones increase during anesthesia, surgery, and recovery and result in hyperglycemia.

Poor control of blood glucose levels can negatively affect the patient's recovery. Hyperglycemia may precipitate DKA and retards wound healing. Hyperglycemia also promotes thrombosis as a result of hypercoagulability.

EFFECTS OF SURGERY ON METABOLIC CONTROL OF DIABETES

The person with DM faces the risk of developing hypoglycemia or hyperglycemia during the perioperative period. During the perioperative period, persons are not usually given anything by mouth and are given IV fluids. This decreases total carbohydrate intake and also decreases insulin needs; however, the effects of surgery on counterregulatory hormones usually increase the need for insulin. The stressors of surgery cause the release of glucocorticoids and catecholamines, which elevates blood glucose levels.

MANAGEMENT OF GLUCOSE CONTROL IN PERSONS TREATED WITH INSULIN

Various protocols may be used to maintain glucose control in the person receiving insulin. Neither hyperglycemia nor hypoglycemia should be allowed to occur. One of the most commonly used perioperative protocols involves starting an IV infusion of dextrose the morning of surgery and giving one-half the usual insulin dose subcutaneously as intermediate-acting insulin. This insulin covers hepatic glucose production during the intraoperative period and prevents hyperglycemia. If the surgery is long, blood glucose levels are checked during surgery, and insulin or extra glucose is given as needed.

During the postoperative period the person is maintained by IV glucose infusion until food can be taken. Insulin is given either by dividing the normal daily dose equally over a 24-hour period and giving it subcutaneously or by having a separate IV infusion of insulin fluids. If a standard dose of insulin is being given, extra insulin may be given via an algorithm based on fingerstick blood glucose checks every 4 to 6 hours.

MANAGEMENT OF GLUCOSE CONTROL IN PERSONS NOT RECEIVING INSULIN

Persons with diabetes who are not normally managed with insulin receive an IV infusion of dextrose on the morning of surgery, after fasting during the night. Such patients may be able to meet their usual insulin needs with their endogenous insulin supply, but in times of stress they may require exogenous insulin. As mentioned earlier, patients with type 2 DM who are treated with metformin should have the drug discontinued 48 to 72 hours before elective surgery that may require general anesthesia. After surgery, blood glucose and urine ketone levels are checked every 4 to 6 hours; if hyperglycemia is present, exogenous insulin may need to be given.

RESUMPTION OF DIET

All persons with diabetes, whether or not they are treated with insulin, should receive 125 to 250 g of carbohydrate per day until their normal diet is resumed. Fewer grams of carbohydrate than this may result in starvation ketosis. The patient's normal diabetes regimen should be resumed as soon as possible. Blood glucose and urine ketone levels should be monitored frequently, even after the patient's usual diet and medication are resumed. The increase in catabolism because of the surgery remains for some time, and additional insulin may continue to be needed. By the time patients are discharged, they should be back on their normal regimens.

SPECIAL ENVIRONMENT FOR CARE

Critical Care Management

Patients experiencing HHNC or severe DKA may need to be managed in a critical care environment. Both of these conditions are discussed in the following sections.

Community-Based Care

Given the current short hospital lengths of stay, some patients, such as those with severe visual impairment, may need short-term home care to learn diabetes care survival skills. The individual with diabetes should be immediately referred to the diabetes team for outpatient follow-up. The individual with diabetes also may require home care services for issues not pertaining to diabetes control, such as a nonhealing foot ulcer. The ultimate goal is to help the individual with diabetes maintain as much independence as possible while optimizing metabolic control and quality of life.

COMPLICATIONS

The complications of diabetes are classified as acute or chronic. Acute complications include hypoglycemia, DKA, and HCNC. Information on hypoglycemia in individuals with diabetes is presented earlier in the chapter.

Acute Complications

Diabetic Ketoacidosis

Diabetic ketoacidosis (DKA) is the extreme consequence of severe insulin deficiency at the insulin-sensitive tissues: adipose tissue, skeletal muscle, and liver (see Figure 30-3). DKA can be precipitated by illness or omission of insulin. Lack of insulin in adipocytes results in failure to suppress lipolysis, with resultant release of free fatty acids into the circulation and weight loss. The free fatty acids in turn serve as a substrate for the liver to synthesize triglyceride and ketone bodies. Lack of insulin in skeletal muscle results in failure to take up glucose from the plasma and protein catabolism with amino acid release into the circulation. These amino acids may then be used by the liver to make glucose (gluconeogenesis). Lack of insulin in the liver results in glycogen breakdown to glucose (glycogenolysis) and accelerated gluconeogenesis. This results in an outpouring of glucose into the circulation that cannot be used by skeletal muscle. Early in the course of insulin deficiency, this hyperglycemic state may be compounded by ingestion of dietary carbohydrate, which gets digested into glucose and is unable to be eliminated.

Progressive hyperglycemia rapidly exceeds the renal threshold for glucose, resulting in glycosuria. The blood glucose level in hyperglycemia may be as high as 1500 mg/dl. Glycosuria acts as an osmotic diuretic, resulting in dehydration, with water and electrolyte losses. An increase in thirst and oral fluid intake tends to minimize the severity of the dehydration early on; however, nausea and vomiting associated with progressive ketosis lead to rapidly worsening dehydration.

With insulin deficiency, high levels of free fatty acids, and high levels of counterregulatory hormones (especially glucagon), the liver produces excessive amounts of ketone bodies. Ketone bodies are acidic and must be cleared from the circulation or buffered with alkali (bicarbonate) to prevent progressive lowering of the arterial pH and systemic acidosis. Early on, the ketones are cleared in the urine; however, with progressive dehydration and decreasing urine output, the production of ketone bodies rapidly exceeds renal clearance. Progressive ketosis is therefore associated with ketones in the urine, with rising plasma ketones, with lowering of plasma bicarbonate, and with declining arterial pH. Systemic acidosis is also associated with transcellular shifts of ions, especially potassium, as potassium leaves the cells and the serum potassium value rises, despite total body potassium depletion. Potassium depletion caused by renal losses may be compounded by gastrointestinal losses (vomiting and diarrhea).

Failure to recognize emerging and worsening DKA results in progressive dehydration, ketosis, acidosis, circulatory collapse, tissue hypoxia, and shock. The advent of tissue hypoxia results in lactate accumulation and lactic acidosis, which dramatically decrease the rate of survival.

Treatment of DKA involves rehydration, insulin administration, and electrolyte repletion. Each medical institution has its own protocol for DKA management. Basic principles are found in the Guidelines for Safe Practice box.

Hyperglycemic Hyperosmolar Nonketotic Coma

Hyperglycemic hyperosmolar nonketotic coma (HHNC) is the acute complication of type 2 DM. The pathophysiology and clinical issues are similar to those of DKA, with the following exceptions. In HHNC:

Guidelines for Safe Practice

Diabetic Ketoacidosis: Management Principles and Priorities

I. Monitoring
   A. Fingerstick blood glucose determinations every hour.
   B. Serum potassium initially and then every hour.
   C. Bicarbonate initially and then every 2 hours.
   D. Arterial blood gas studies initially and then every 2 to 4 hours.
   E. Electrocardiogram initially and then as needed.
   F. Additional monitoring may be needed pending patient status: continuous cardiac tracing, central venous pressure, Swan-Ganz catheter, nasogastric intubation, and indwelling urinary catheter.
   G. Intake and output.

II. Intravenous rehydration
   A. Fluid deficit may be in excess of 6 L.
   B. Normal saline at 500 ml/hr for the first hour; then 250 ml/hr.
   C. Avoid hypotonic solutions (0.45% normal saline) because they may increase the risk of cerebral edema.

III. Intravenous (IV) insulin to control gluconeogenesis, lipolysis, and ketogenesis and to promote skeletal muscle glucose uptake
   A. Should be given as constant infusion. Start at rate of 0.1 U/kg of body weight. If no concern about IV volume (i.e., congestive heart failure), a more dilute solution is easier to titrate. Dilute as 50 ml regular insulin in 500 ml normal saline; then 1 U = 10 ml. Titrate drip hourly by 0.1-U (1-ml) increments until glucose reaches goal of 70 to 150 mg/dl.
   B. IV bolus of regular insulin has a half-life of 5 minutes and is of no value.
   C. When the patient begins to take oral fluids with carbohydrates, additional insulin must be given subcutaneously to match the carbohydrate load.
   D. When the patient is recovering and ready to eat, resume routine insulin program. Do not discontinue IV insulin infusion until 2 hours after subcutaneous insulin dosage to prevent loss of control of hepatic glucose output and disposal.

IV. Electrolyte repletion
   A. Give IV potassium once renal output is established.
      1. If serum potassium is ≤3 mEq/L, give 40 to 60 mEq/hr.
      2. If serum potassium is 3 to 4 mEq/L, give 30 mEq/hr.
      3. If serum potassium is 4 to 5 mEq/L, give 20 mEq/hr.
      4. If serum potassium is ≥6 mEq/L, withhold potassium replacement until serum potassium is ≤6 mEq/L.
   B. May give half as potassium chloride and half as potassium phosphate to also replace phosphate losses.
   C. May need magnesium replacement pending serum values.
   D. IV bicarbonate indicated only if arterial pH is ≤7.0 and patient has complicating medical problems such as hypotension, shock, or dysrhythmia. If given, should be by slow IV infusion. Goal is an arterial pH ≥7.0. Concern with bicarbonate is association with the potentially fatal complication of cerebral edema.

V. White blood count with differential
   A. A leukocytosis may be present.
      1. Differentiate whether leukocytosis is indicative of underlying sepsis or is the leukocytosis with left shift that is commonly seen in diabetic ketoacidosis.

VI. Treatment of underlying cause (sepsis, myocardial infarction)
   A. In an individual with diabetes who acutely loses glycemic control, silent myocardial infarction must be ruled out.

VII. Patient education
   A. Educate patient about prevention and early intervention.

- Dehydration is profound, with fluid deficit as high as 8 to 9 L.
- The degree of hyperglycemia is greater, with serum glucose levels in the range of 600 to 2000 mg/dl.
- The serum osmolarity is 350 mOsm/L or higher.
- Ketosis is absent because individuals with type 2 DM have adequate insulin secretion.
- An underlying central nervous system problem (e.g., underlying cerebrovascular disease) is usually present, which impairs the patient's thirst perception.
- A concurrent illness is usually present.

Because of the aforementioned impairment in thirst perception, the patient does not have adequate oral fluid intake, resulting in the primary defect of profound dehydration. As a consequence of the profound dehydration, hemoconcentration and severe hyperglycemia occur. Polyuria disappears early because of the severe dehydration. Lethargy and somnolence may result.

HHNC is a medical emergency. The primary management of HHNC involves IV rehydration with hypotonic solutions (0.45 normal saline). Hypotonic solutions are indicated because the patient is hyperosmolar. As the patient is rehydrated, the hyperglycemia resolves. IV insulin is generally not needed. In addition, treatment of the precipitating illness is critical to patient survival, because the mortality rate approaches 70%.

Chronic Complications

Chronic complications of diabetes are classified as microvascular or macrovascular. These changes are a consequence of the duration and degree of hyperglycemia and result in diabetic retinopathy, diabetic nephropathy, peripheral and autonomic neuropathy, peripheral vascular disease, cerebrovascular disease, and coronary artery disease. The DCCT demonstrated that intensive therapy resulted in a decreased risk of the development and progression of complications.[23] Therefore glycemic control should be a priority in both prevention and treatment.

Microvascular complications of diabetes rarely occur within the first 5 to 10 years after diagnosis of type 1 DM. They may, however, be present at the time of diagnosis of type 2 DM because of the slow, insidious onset of type 2 DM and the resultant delay in diagnosis. Cigarette smoking increases the risk of the development and progression of every known complication of DM. Aggressive attempts at smoking cessation are critical.

Microvascular Complications

Diabetic Retinopathy. Diabetic retinopathy is the leading cause of new blindness among adults 20 to 74 years of age in the United States. Between 12,000 and 24,000 new cases of blindness from diabetic retinopathy occur each year.[64] A diagnosis of diabetic retinopathy results in an elevenfold increased risk of blindness as compared with the risk in the general population.[45] The DCCT demonstrated that intensive therapy resulted in a statistically significant decreased risk in the development and progression of retinopathy. Good visual acuity does not exclude significant retinopathy.

The earliest lesion is the microaneurysm in the retinal vessels. Having one dot-blot hemorrhage results in a twentyfold increased risk of blindness as compared with the risk in the general population.[45] Soft exudates ("cotton-wool spots,") are areas of ischemia in the retina resulting from reduced retinal blood flow. Hard exudates are deposits of lipid on the retina, resulting from leaking retinal blood vessels. Early retinal changes (background retinopathy) may progress to a more serious state—proliferative retinopathy.[48]

Proliferative retinopathy, or neovascular disease, results when the ischemic retina responds with the formation of new, fragile blood vessels on the retina. These fragile vessels bleed, causing vitreous hemorrhage (hemorrhage into the vitreous fluid of the eye) and can sometimes result in retinal detachment. This hemorrhage can be repetitive and lead to permanent visual loss. Early laser photocoagulation to seal off the leaking retinal vessels to preserve vision is now the standard treatment and is based on the results of the Diabetic Retinopathy Study (DRS).[24] The DRS demonstrated a 60% reduction in severe visual loss with the use of argon laser treatment. However, laser photocoagulation does destroy some normal retina in the process; peripheral and night vision are most affected. Without laser photocoagulation, progressive hemorrhage and subsequent blindness are inevitable. Laser photocoagulation is an outpatient surgical procedure performed in the ophthalmologist's office.

In severe cases the extent of vitreous hemorrhage necessitates a vitrectomy. In a vitrectomy, surgical instruments are placed into the eyeball and the hemorrhagic fluid is removed by suction and replaced with fluid. This inpatient surgical procedure is also vision preserving[48] (see Chapter 58 for further discussion of vitrectomy).

Macular edema is a form of nonproliferative disease. The macula is the part of the retina responsible for central vision. Macular edema results from the leaking of fluid and lipid into the macula of the eye, resulting in edema and loss of vision. The Early Treatment Diabetic Retinopathy Study established the benefit of laser photocoagulation in macular edema with a 50% reduction in severe visual loss.[26]

The ADA recommends an annual ophthalmologic examination for early detection, diagnosis, and treatment of retinopathy.[4,6] One goal of Healthy People 2010 is to increase the proportion of adults with diabetes who have an annual dilated eye examination to 75% (age-adjusted baseline: 47% of adults ages 18 or older in 1998).[107,110] The DCCT demonstrated that intensive therapy resulted in a significant decrease in the risk of development and progression of diabetic retinopathy. In addition, blood pressure control is critical, because hypertension accelerates the development and progression of retinopathy.

Diabetic Nephropathy. Diabetic nephropathy is the leading cause of end-stage renal disease in the United States, accounting for approximately 40% of new cases. In 1995 alone, 27,851 new cases were diagnosed.[3] Unless aggressively treated, nephropathy rapidly progresses. End-stage renal disease may develop, requiring dialysis, transplantation, or both. In 1995, 98,872 individuals with diabetes were undergoing dialysis or transplantation treatment.[64]

The characteristic renal lesion is nodular glomerulosclerosis, or Kimmelstiel-Wilson syndrome. This syndrome involves nodular masses of laminated hyaline material that occur randomly throughout the kidney and is associated with proteinuria, edema, and hypertension. Kimmelstiel-Wilson lesions are seen only in DM and occur in 10% to 35% of individuals with DM.

Laboratory abnormalities of renal disease generally do not occur until 10 years or more after the onset of type 1 DM, but they may be present at diagnosis in persons with type 2 DM. The natural history of diabetic nephropathy begins with early glomerular hypertrophy and hyperfiltration with an elevated glomerular filtration rate. Microscopic amounts of albumin in the urine, or microalbuminuria, is the earliest laboratory abnormality and is asymptomatic. Microalbuminuria can be assessed via a radioimmunoassay on either a spot or a timed urine collection. Microalbuminuria is present if the urinary albumin level is greater than or equal to 30 μg/mg creatinine on a random urine specimen or if the excretion rate is 20 μg/min (30 mg/24 hours) on a timed specimen.[1] Dipstick results are also available but are much less accurate. The development and progression of microalbuminuria can be reduced through meticulous glucose control[23] and blood pressure control, especially with angiotensin-converting enzyme (ACE) inhibitors.

Microalbuminuria has additional significance. Individuals with microalbuminuria are at increased risk for retinopathy and autonomic neuropathy.[60] Microalbuminuria has poor prognostic implications in regard to both cardiovascular disease and mortality in both type 1[69] and type 2 DM patients.[59]

Microalbuminuria may progress to albuminuria or clinical proteinuria (300 mg albumin/24 hours, which is equivalent to 500 mg total protein/24 hours) and end-stage renal disease. Proteinuria also has poor prognostic implications in terms of cardiovascular disease and the mortality rate in both type 1[13,14] and type 2 DM patients.[55,66] Renal disease, even at this point, can remain asymptomatic, detectable only by objective measures. Glycemic control still plays a role in reducing risks of progression. The ADA recommends an annual laboratory examination for urine microalbumin/protein.[41]

A unifying hypothesis in microalbuminuria, albuminuria, proteinuria, and cardiovascular disease and mortality is the Steno hypothesis. The Steno hypothesis is based on the common cause, which appears to be endothelial dysfunction in a multitude of vascular beds in the body, with the resultant end-stage disease depending on the vascular bed involved.[22]

Hypertension is the factor that most often accelerates diabetic nephropathy. Aggressive blood pressure control decreases the rate of deterioration and improves survival.[17,35,83] Studies demonstrate that in an individual with diabetes, the lower the blood pressure within the normal range, the lesser the albuminuria.

ACE inhibitors also have an important role in clinical proteinuria. The ACE inhibitor captopril is approved by the FDA for use in patients with clinical proteinuria to slow progression to end-stage renal disease, even in the absence of hypertension.[54] The use of ACE inhibitors in microalbuminuria is well studied with promising results, and FDA approval is pending.

Reduction in dietary protein intake may be of additional benefit, although clinical trials have not been conclusive. In patients with renal disease, a restriction of protein to 0.8 mg/kg of actual body weight is recommended.[61]

Neuropathy. Diabetic neuropathy affects 60% to 70% of individuals with diabetes.[64] The most common forms of neuropathy are peripheral and autonomic (see Table 30-15).

Symmetric Sensory Peripheral Polyneuropathy. In symmetric sensory peripheral polyneuropathy, sensory changes and subsequent sensory loss occur symmetrically in a glove-and-stocking distribution. The lower extremities are generally affected first because they contain the longest nerves in the body; upper extremity involvement may follow. Comprehensive assessment of neuropathy is critical because most patients with mild to moderate neuropathy are asymptomatic; even the patient with severe damage can remain asymptomatic. A thorough neurologic examination assessing sensation, vibration, and deep tendon reflexes should be performed. Routine assessment with a monofilament is widely performed during follow-up examinations. Monofilament testing assesses only a patient's risk of foot ulceration. Once a patient has an abnormal monofilament examination, extensive nerve damage has already occurred. When patients do get symptoms, they can experience abnormal sensations such as paresthesias, numbness, and pain. Pain can range from minimal in the toes to sharp, stabbing, lancinating pain in a glove-and-stocking distribution. Abnormal sensations tend to worsen in the evening and may make it difficult for the patent to fall asleep. Even the light pressure of the bedsheet may be uncomfortable for the patient. Commonly patients are unaware of sensory loss, so proper foot care is critical. In addition to sensory involvement, motor neurons may also be affected. The impairments occur slowly and are progressive.

Painful Peripheral Neuropathy. The glove-and-stocking distribution of pain is common in persons with painful peripheral neuropathy (PPN). Patients may exhibit loss of vibratory sense, increased or decreased temperature sensation, loss of fine motor skills, and gait changes due to dorsiflexion weakness. Pain management of PPN involves the use of antidepressants, anticonvulsants, topical agents, opioids, and other therapies. Other medications used include clonidine and mexiletine. Nonpharmacologic therapies include the use of heat and cold, massage, relaxation, biofeedback, physical therapy, and psychotherapy. See Chapter 12 for further discussion of PPN.

Autonomic Neuropathy. Damage to the autonomic nervous system may also occur, resulting in alterations in many body systems (see Table 35-14). An easy and quick assessment of autonomic function is the R-R trend analysis. Using a special electrocardiograph machine, R-R trend analysis measures the variation in heart rate with deep breathing. In an individual with intact autonomic function, there is great variability in the heart rate with deep breathing. Individuals with autonomic neuropathy lose that heart rate variability. A patient may experience none, some, or all of the dysfunctions. Commonly the only symptom a patient may have is fatigue with exercise resulting from an inability to increase the heart rate to increase cardiac output. Another common symptom is dizziness on postural change. Autonomic neuropathy carries a poor prognosis, with up to a 50% 5-year mortality rate, generally because of silent ischemia resulting in silent myocardial infarctions or cardiac dysrhythmias.[28,76] Improvement in glycemic control can improve autonomic function.

Other Neuropathies. Cranial nerve palsies (of the third, fourth, sixth, and seventh cranial nerves) occur more commonly in individuals with diabetes than in nondiabetic individuals. The onset is acute, and the course is self-limiting. Ulnar nerve palsies may be a result of a mononeuritis of acute onset or from nerve entrapment. Carpal tunnel syndrome is twice as common in individuals with diabetes as in nondiabetic individuals (see Chapter 46 for further discussion). Diabetic amyotrophy is an acute event involving anterior thigh numbness or pain, which can be excruciating. Quadriceps muscle wasting and resultant weakness on hip flexion may occur within a few days. No specific diagnostic tests are indicated. Supportive therapy with analgesics and maintenance of walking are critical. Amyotrophy generally resolves spontaneously in 6 to 8 weeks, although severe cases may require 6 to 12 months.

Macrovascular Complications

Statistics of macrovascular disease comparing diabetic individuals with nondiabetic individuals are stunning. Cardiovascular disease is two to four times more prevalent in individuals with diabetes and is present in approximately 75% of diabetes-related deaths. Middle-aged individuals with diabetes have coronary disease death rates two to four times higher than those of their nondiabetic peers. The stroke risk in individuals with diabetes is two to four times higher.[64]

Individuals with diabetes develop the same macrovascular changes as individuals without diabetes. However, these changes occur at an earlier age, are more severe, and are more extensive in the vascular tree. Patients with type 2 DM have a higher rate than those with type 1 DM. Risk factors involved in the pathogenesis of macrovascular disease that must be aggressively addressed include dyslipidemia and hypertension.[63,112]

Dyslipidemia. Dyslipidemia affects an estimated 50% of individuals with diabetes. Elevated low-density lipoprotein cholesterol, elevated triglycerides, and low HDL cholesterol are risk factors for atherosclerosis. Because of insulin resistance, the lipid profile in the patient with type 2 DM is commonly characterized by hypertriglyceridemia and a low HDL cholesterol level with varying degrees of hypercholesterolemia.[36,95] In type 1 DM, lipid disorders are generally seen only if there is a familial dyslipidemia or in the presence of renal disease. Evidence-based medical data are available from clinical trials to support aggressive diagnosis and treatment of dyslipidemia in the individual with DM.[74,82,85,90] Aggressive screening, diagnosis, and treatment are critical to reduce morbidity and mortality.

Hypertension. Hypertension affects 60% to 65% of individuals with diabetes.[64] Hypertension in the patient with type 1 DM implies renal disease, microalbuminuria, or proteinuria, until proven otherwise. In contrast, hypertension in the patient with type 2 DM can result from either coexistent renal disease or essential hypertension. Regardless of the etiology, blood pressure must be aggressively monitored and hypertension diagnosed early because it exacerbates retinopathy, nephropathy, and macrovascular disease. In the individual with DM, hypertension is diagnosed at a blood pressure of 130/85. The goal blood pressure in the individual with diabetes is less than 130/80 mm Hg.[71]

Lifestyle modification (weight loss, sodium restriction, exercise) should be the primary modality of treatment. When lifestyle modification fails, the pharmacologic agent chosen should be metabolically neutral (i.e., not worsen insulin resistance or dyslipidemia or cause electrolyte disturbance). ACE inhibitors are the antihypertensives of choice, unless contraindicated, given the data not only in nephropathy but also in retinopathy. The recent HOPE study demonstrated a reduced risk of microvascular and macrovascular events in individuals with DM treated with the ACE inhibitor ramipril[39,40] In patients intolerant of ACE inhibitors because of cough, angiotensin receptor blockers and calcium channel blockers are good alternatives in light of data that show decreasing proteinuria with the use of these agents. Beta-blockers have an important role in the post–myocardial infarction/angina patient and in the patient with heart failure. The benefits of beta-blockade in these patients outweigh the theoretic problems of the masking of hypoglycemia, delay in recovery from hypoglycemia, and worsening of insulin resistance.[91-93] Monotherapy of hypertension is frequently unsuccessful, especially in persons with nephropathy.[1,91-93]

The Diabetic Foot. Three major factors play a role in the diabetic foot: neuropathy, ischemia, and sepsis. More than half of lower limb amputations in the United States occur in individuals with diabetes.[64] Diabetes is responsible for almost 80% of major lower limb nontraumatic amputations in the United States.[49]

Sensory impairment leads to painless trauma and the potential for ulceration. Motor impairment contributes to wasting of intrinsic muscles in the feet, resulting in foot deformity. Foot deformities alter the normal gait and pressure distribution. Friction and resultant callosities may develop and result in pressure necrosis and ulceration. Painless trauma can result in fractures in the ankle or forefoot and ultimately in significant deformity known as Charcot's arthropathy. Anhidrosis (decreased or absent sweat secretion) as a manifestation of autonomic neuropathy can result in excessive dryness and cracking of the skin, which also contributes to infection. Macrovascular and microvascular alterations produce tissue ischemia and may lead to sepsis. This triad of neuropathy, ischemia, and sepsis can result in gangrene and ultimately amputation.[52] Aggressive glycemic control and hospitalization for IV antibiotics to limit the spread of infection are necessary. Amputation of affected toes is often necessary. The area must be kept dry to prevent wet gangrene. Wet gangrene is gangrene coupled with inflammation; septicemia and shock may occur.

Podiatric care is critical to attaining and maintaining foot health. Proper toenail trimming and the use of orthotic, extra-depth, extra-width, or custom-molded shoes can prevent ongoing trauma and ultimately amputation associated with the diabetic foot.[52]

HYPOGLYCEMIA IN THE INDIVIDUAL WITHOUT DIABETES MELLITUS

Hypoglycemia in the nondiabetic person is characterized by subnormal plasma glucose levels, generally less than 50 mg/dl. It may be asymptomatic, may cause adrenergic symptoms (anxiety, irritability, palpitations, diaphoresis, pallor), or may cause neuroglycopenic symptoms with more severe hypoglycemia. Neuroglycopenic symptoms include mental confusion, seizures, and coma and may be associated with severe trauma (e.g., motor vehicle accidents). A firm diagnosis rests with the documentation of Whipple's triad: (1) appropriate signs and symptoms, (2) a documented subnormal blood glucose level, and (3) response to normalization of blood glucose with carbohydrate ingestion.[30]

Classification

Hypoglycemia may be broadly classified as either fasting or nonfasting (reactive) hypoglycemia. Fasting hypoglycemia generally results in neuroglycopenic symptoms, whereas reactive hypoglycemia is usually associated with more adrenergic symptoms.

Etiology

The etiology of fasting hypoglycemia is presented in Box 30-19.

Reactive hypoglycemia generally occurs 3 to 5 hours after meals, in relation to either a primary delay in insulin secretion (idiopathic) or a rapidly rising postprandial glucose value as a result of rapid gastric emptying (postgastric surgery). Failure of the pancreas to keep pace with this rapidly rising postprandial glucose level results in later insulin hypersecretion and hypoglycemia. Individuals with true idiopathic reactive hypoglycemia, reflecting an insulin secretory defect, are at increased risk for developing type 2 DM.

Collaborative Care Management

Diagnosis of fasting hypoglycemia is performed in the hospital via a 72-hour fast to document a subnormal glucose level with a simultaneous increased insulin level and increased C-peptide level. Insulinomas (insulin-secreting tumors of the pancreas) are the most common organic cause of fasting hypoglycemia. Management of fasting hypoglycemia is accom-

BOX 30-19 Etiology of Fasting Hypoglycemia

Insulin Excess

Exogenous insulin surreptitiously
Sulfonylurea ingestion (accidental in individual without diabetes mellitus, surreptitious use, pharmacy dispensation error)
Insulin-producing islet cell tumor (insulinoma)—benign or malignant
Islet hyperplasia

Decreased Hepatic Glucose Production

Advanced renal disease
Advanced liver disease
Ethanol use, especially in the setting of poor nutrition
Severe sepsis
Severe malnutrition

Counterregulatory Hormone Deficiencies

Hypopituitarism
Adrenocorticotropic hormone deficiency
Growth hormone deficiency
Primary adrenal failure (Addison's disease)

Hypothyroidism

Rare

Non–islet Cell Tumors

Mesenchymal tumors, generally clinically obvious, with limited life expectancy

Autoimmune Disease

Antibodies that stimulate the insulin receptor (rare)

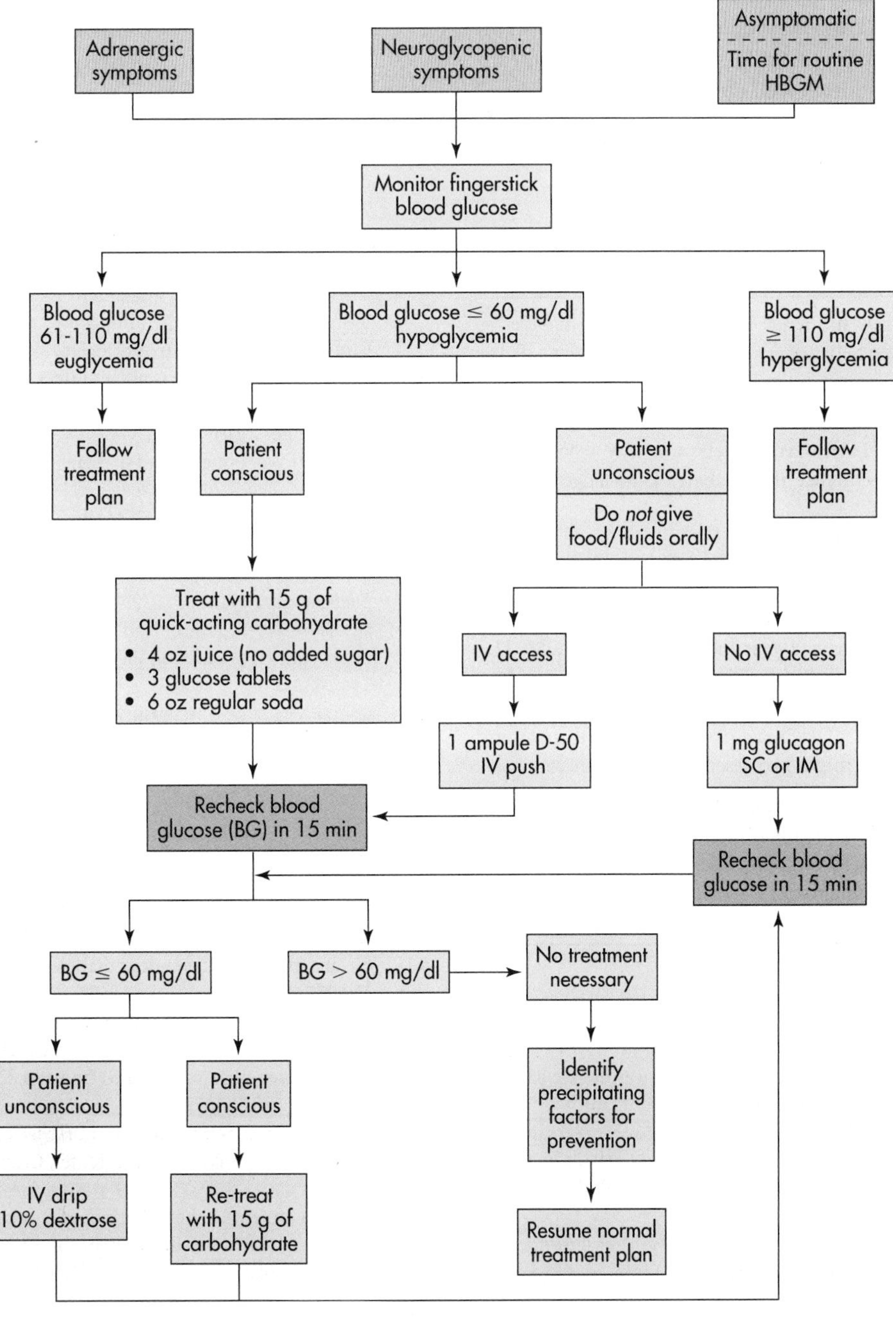

Figure 30-15 Algorithm for treating hypoglycemia.

plished by surgical removal of the neoplasm, management of the underlying disease, or both.

Reactive hypoglycemia is overdiagnosed as a result of Whipple's triad not being documented. The diagnosis is best made by randomly documenting a blood glucose level of less than 50 mg/dl in association with signs and symptoms and prompt response to carbohydrate ingestion.[30,87] Many individuals with underlying anxiety states are misdiagnosed with "hypoglycemia" with no documentation of a truly low blood glucose level and are placed on unnecessarily strict diets, usually low in carbohydrates and high in proteins and fats, with resultant weight gain and an adverse lipid profile. In persons with true idiopathic hypoglycemia, this dietary approach is even more deleterious given these individuals' propensity to develop type 2 DM and the cardiodysmetabolic syndrome (Figure 30-15).

Patient/Family Education. Patient teaching needs focus on prevention of hypoglycemic episodes. The most logical management approach revolves around (1) delaying the postprandial glucose rise through increased dietary fiber and the use of complex carbohydrates and (2) enhancing insulin sensitivity through exercise and weight reduction toward a desirable body weight.

Critical Thinking Questions

1. How can you positively influence your patients with diabetes to take a more active participatory role in the management of the disease?
2. You are a professional nurse working on a busy medical-surgical or intensive care unit. During your hectic workday, what specific things can you do to enhance the "diabetes knowledge" of your patients with diabetes?
3. Develop a teaching plan to help at-risk patients reduce their risk of developing type 2 diabetes mellitus (DM).
4. You are caring for an obese woman (height, 5 feet 3 inches; weight, 210 pounds) with a 2-year history of type 2 DM. Her home blood glucose monitoring results show fasting glucose levels of 130 to 160 mg/dl and a hemoglobin A_{1c} of 8.2% on her regimen of diet and exercise. Develop a plan of care for this patient. What pharmacotherapy might be prescribed for her treatment?
5. You are performing the assessment and preoperative teaching for a 55-year-old female patient with a long history of type 1 DM. She is scheduled for surgery for an open cholecystectomy. What data are essential to best plan her care? Develop a teaching plan for this patient. What are some perioperative concerns for this patient?

References

1. ALLHAT Collaborative Research Group: Major cardiovascular events in hypertensive patients randomized to doxazosin vs. chlorthalidone: the antihypertensive and lipid-lowering treatment to prevent heart attack trial (ALLHAT), *JAMA* 283:1967, 2000.
2. Alzaid AA: Microalbuminuria in patients with NIDDM: an overview, *Diabetes Care* 19(1):79, 1996.
3. American Diabetes Association: *Diabetes—1996 vital statistics,* Alexandria, Va, 1996, ADA.
4. American Diabetes Association: Clinical practice recommendations 2001, *Diabetes Care* 24(suppl 1):S1, 2001.
5. American Diabetes Association: Implications of the Diabetes Control and Complications Trial, *Diabetes Care* 24(suppl 1):S25, 2001.
6. American Diabetes Association: Standards of medical care for patients with diabetes mellitus, *Diabetes Care* 24(suppl 1):S33, 2001.
7. American Diabetes Association, Expert Committee on the Diagnosis and Classification of Diabetes Mellitus: Report of the Expert Committee on the Diagnosis and Classification of Diabetes Mellitus, *Diabetes Care* 24(suppl 1):S55, 2001.
8. Baxley SG et al: Perceived competence and actual level of knowledge of diabetes mellitus among nurses, *J Nurs Staff Dev* 13(2):93, 1997.
9. Bell DS: Exercise for patients with diabetes: benefits, risks, precautions, *Postgrad Med* 92:183, 1992.
10. Bell DS: Alcohol and the NIDDM patient, *Diabetes Care* 19:509, 1996.
11. Bliss M: *The discovery of insulin,* Chicago, 1982, University of Chicago Press.
12. Reference deleted in proofs.
13. Borch-Johnsen K, Kragh AP, Deckert T: The effect of proteinuria on relative mortality in type 1 diabetes mellitus, *Diabetalogia* 28:540, 1985.
14. Borch-Johnsen K, Kreiner S: Proteinuria: value as predictor of cardiovascular mortality in insulin-dependent diabetes mellitus, *BMJ* 294:1651, 1987.
15. Chan NH et al: Inhaled insulin in type 1 diabetes, *Lancet* 357:2001.
16. Chen M, Bergman RN, Porte D Jr: Insulin resistance and beta cell dysfunction in aging: the importance of dietary carbohydrate, *J Clin Endocrinol Metab* 67:951, 1988.
17. Christensen CK, Mogensen CE: Effect of antihypertensive treatment of progression of incipient diabetic nephropathy, *Hypertension* 7(suppl 2):109, 1985.
18. Coleman W: Foot care and diabetes mellitus. In Haire-Joshu D, editor: *Management of diabetes mellitus—perspectives of care across the life span,* St Louis, 1992, Mosby.
19. Coonrod BA, Betschart J, Harris MI: Frequency and determinants of diabetes patient education among adults in the U.S. population, *Diabetes Care* 17(8):852, 1994.
20. Cranston I et al: Restoration of hypoglycemia awareness in patients with long-duration insulin-dependent diabetes, *Lancet* 344:283, 1974.
21. Criqui MH et al: The sensitivity, specificity, and predictive value of traditional clinical evaluation of peripheral arterial disease: results from noninvasive testing in a defined population, *Pathophysiology and Natural History—Periph Vascular Dis* 71:516, 1985.
22. Deckert T et al: Albuminuria reflects widespread vascular damage: the Steno hypothesis, *Diabetalogia* 32:219, 1989.
23. Diabetes Control and Complications Trial Research Group: The effect of intensive treatment of diabetes on the long-term complications in insulin-dependent diabetes mellitus, *N Engl J Med* 329:977, 1993.
24. Diabetic Retinopathy Study Group: Photocoagulation treatment of proliferative diabetic retinopathy: clinical application of Diabetic Retinopathy Study (DRS) findings, DRS Report No 8, *Ophthalmology* 88:583, 1981.
25. Eaks GA: *Professional prompter worksheet,* Kansas City, 1993, University of Kansas Medical Center, Cray Diabetes Education Center.
26. Early Treatment Diabetic Retinopathy Study Research Group: Photocoagulation for diabetic macular edema, *Arch Ophthalmol* 103:1796, 1985.

27. Eastman RC, Keen H: The impact of cardiovascular disease on people with diabetes: the potential for prevention, *Lancet* 350(suppl 1):29, 1997.
28. Ewing DJ, Campbell IW, Clarke BF: The natural history of diabetic autonomic neuropathy, *Q J Med* 49:95, 1980.
29. Expert Panel on Detection, Evaluation, and Treatment of High Blood Cholesterol in Adults: Executive summary of the third report of the National Cholesterol Education Program (NCEP) Expert Panel on Detection, Evaluation, and Treatment of High Blood Cholesterol in Adults, *JAMA* 285:2486, 2001.
30. Field JB: Hypoglycemia: definition, clinical presentation, classification, and laboratory tests, *Endocrinol Metab Clin North Am* 18:27, 1989.
31. Fink RI et al: Mechanisms of insulin resistance in aging, *J Clin Invest* 71:1523, 1983.
32. Franz MJ, Bantle JP: *The American Diabetes Association guide to medical nutrition therapy,* 1999, Alexandria, Va, American Diabetes Association.
33. Franz MJ et al: Nutrition principles for the management of diabetes and related complications (technical review), *Diabetes Care* 17:490, 1994.
34. Freeman DJ et al: Pravastatin and the development of diabetes mellitus: evidence for a protective treatment effect in the West of Scotland Coronary Prevention Study, *Circulation* 103:346, 2001.
35. Gall MA et al: Albuminuria and poor glycemic control predict mortality in NIDDM, *Diabetes* 44:1303, 1995.
36. Garber AJ: Dyslipidemia as a risk factor for coronary artery disease in patients with diabetes, *Endocr Pract* 3:244, 1997.
37. Reference deleted in proofs.
38. Hayes TM, Harries J: Randomised controlled trial of routine hospital care versus routine general practice care for type 2 diabetics, *BMJ* 289:728, 1984.
39. Heart Outcomes Prevention Evaluation (HOPE) Study Investigators: Effects of an angiotensin-converting enzyme inhibitor, ramipril, on cardiovascular events in high risk patients, *Lancet* 342:145, 2000.
40. Heart Outcomes Prevention Evaluation (HOPE) Study Investigators: Effects of ramipril on cardiovascular and microvascular outcomes in people with diabetes mellitus: results of the HOPE study and MICRO-HOPE sub-study, *Lancet* 345:253, 2000.
41. Herman W: *The prevention and treatment of complications of diabetes mellitus—a guide for primary care practitioners,* Washington, DC, 1992, US Department of Health and Human Services, Public Health Service, Centers for Disease Control and Prevention, National Center for Chronic Disease Prevention and Health Promotion, Division of Diabetes Translation, US Government Printing Office.
42. Ho M et al: Is the quality of diabetes care better in a diabetes clinic or in a general medicine clinic? *Diabetes Care* 20:472, 1997.
43. Holler HJ, Pastors JG: *Diabetes medical nutrition therapy: a professional guide to management and nutrition education resources,* Alexandria, Va, 1997, American Dietetic Association/American Diabetes Association.
44. Horton ES: Exercise. In Lebovitz HE, editor: *Therapy for diabetes mellitus and related disorders,* Alexandria, Va, 1991, American Diabetes Association.
45. Huang S: *Diabetic retinopathy: prevention, diagnosis and vision preservation.* Presented at the Symposium on Multidisciplinary Management of Diabetes Mellitus in the Post-DCCT Era for Primary Care Physicians and Healthcare Providers; sponsored by the Departments of Family Medicine and Medicine, Case Western Reserve University School of Medicine and University Hospitals of Cleveland, June 7, 1995, Cleveland, Ohio.
46. Johnson KC et al: Prevalence of undiagnosed non–insulin-dependent diabetes mellitus and impaired glucose tolerance in a cohort of older persons with hypertension, *J Am Geriatr Soc* 45:695, 1997.
47. Joslin EP: *Diabetic manual,* ed 10, Philadelphia, 1959, Lea & Febiger.
48. Klein R, Klein BEK: Diabetic eye disease, *Lancet* 350:197, 1997.
49. Kozak GP, Rowbotham JL: Diabetic foot disease: a major problem. In Kozak GP et al, editors: *Management of diabetic foot problems,* Philadelphia, 1984, WB Saunders.
50. KROC Collaborative Study Group: Blood glucose control and the evolution of diabetic retinopathy and albuminuria, *N Engl J Med* 311:364, 1984.
51. Lauritzen T et al: Continuous subcutaneous insulin (2-year Steno study data), *Lancet* 1:1445, 1983.
52. Lehto S et al: Risk factors predicting lower extremity amputation in patients with NIDDM, *Diabetes Care* 19:607, 1996.
53. Reference deleted in proofs.
54. Lewis EJ et al for the Collaborative Study Group: The effect of angiotensin-converting enzyme inhibition on diabetic nephropathy, *N Engl J Med* 329:1456, 1993.
55. MacLeod JM, Lutale J, Marshall SM: Albumin excretion and vascular deaths in NIDDM, *Diabetalogia* 38:610, 1995.
56. Mandrup-Poulson T: Personal communication, Gentofte, Denmark, 1992, The Steno Diabetes Center.
57. Marrero DG: Current effectiveness of diabetes health care in the U.S: how far from ideal? *Diabetes Rev* 2:292, 1994.
58. Marrero DG: Evaluating the quality of care provided by primary care physicians to people with non–insulin-dependent diabetes mellitus, *Diabetes Spect* 9:30, 1996.
59. Mogensen CE: Microalbuminuria predicts clinical proteinuria and early mortality in maturity-onset diabetes, *N Engl J Med* 310:356, 1984.
60. Molgard H et al: Early recognition of autonomic dysfunction in microalbuminuria: significance for cardiovascular mortality in diabetes mellitus, *Diabetalogia* 37:788, 1994.
61. Mudaliar SR, Henry RR: Role of glycemic control and protein restriction in clinical management of diabetic kidney disease, *Endocr Pract* 2:220, 1996.
62. Myllynen P, Koivisto VA, Nikkila EA: Glucose intolerance and insulin resistance accompany immobilization, *Acta Med Scand* 222:75, 1987.
63. Nathan DM, Meigs J, Singer DE: The epidemiology of cardiovascular disease in type 2 diabetes mellitus: how sweet it is . . . or is it? *Lancet* 350(suppl 1):4, 1997.
64. National Diabetes Data Group: *Diabetes in America,* ed 2, NIH Pub No 95-1468, Baltimore, 2000, National Institutes of Health, US Department of Health and Human Services.
65. National High Blood Pressure Education Program Working Group: National High Blood Pressure Education Program Working Group report on hypertension in diabetes, *Hypertension* 23:145, discussion 159, 1994.
66. Niskanen LK et al: Evolution, risk factors, and prognostic implication of albuminuria in NIDDM, *Diabetes Care* 19:486, 1996.
67. Ohkubo Y et al: Intensive insulin therapy prevents the progression of diabetic microvascular complications in Japanese patients with non–insulin-dependent diabetes mellitus: a randomized prospective 6-year study, *Diabetes Res Clin Pract* 28:103, 1995.
68. Orchard TJ, Strandness DE Jr: *Assessment of peripheral vascular disease in diabetes.* Report and recommendations of an international workshop sponsored by the American Heart Association and the American Diabetes Association, New Orleans, Sept 18-20, 1992, *Diabetes Care* 16(8):1199, 1995.
69. Parving HH et al: Prevalence of microalbuminuria, arterial hypertension, retinopathy, and neuropathy in patients with insulin-dependent diabetes, *BMJ* 296:156, 1988.
70. Peters AL et al: Quality of outpatient care provided to diabetic patients: a health maintenance organization experience, *Diabetes Care* 19:601, 1996.

71. *Physicians' desk reference,* ed 55, Montvale, NJ, 2001, Medical Economics.
72. Pirart J: Diabetes mellitus and its degenerative complications: a prospective study of 4400 patients observed between 1947 and 1973, *Diabet Med* 3(2):97; 3(3):173; 3(4):245, 1977; *Diabetes Care* 1:168, 1978.
73. Reference deleted in proofs.
74. Pyorala K et al and the Scandinavian Simvastatin Survival Study (4S): Cholesterol lowering with simvastatin improves prognosis of diabetic patients with coronary heart disease: a subgroup analysis of the Scandinavian Simvastatin Survival Study (4S), *Diabetes Care* 20:614, 1997.
75. Queale WS, Seidler AJ, Brancati FL: Glycemic control and sliding scale insulin use in medical inpatients with diabetes mellitus, *Arch Intern Med* 157:545, 1997.
76. Rathmann W et al: Mortality in diabetic patients with cardiovascular autonomic neuropathy, *Diabet Med* 10:820, 1993.
77. Reaven GM: Role of insulin resistance in human disease, Banting lecture 1988, *Diabetes* 37:1595, 1988.
78. Reaven GM: Role of insulin resistance in human disease (syndrome X): an expanded definition, *Annu Rev Med* 440:121, 1993.
79. Reaven GM: Syndrome X, *Clin Diabetes* 12:32, 1994.
80. Reference deleted in proofs.
81. Rowe JW et al: Characterization of the insulin resistance of aging, *J Clin Invest* 71:1581, 1983.
82. Sacks FM et al for the Cholesterol and Recurrent Events Trial Investigators: The effect of pravastatin on coronary events after myocardial infarction in patients with average cholesterol levels, *N Engl J Med* 335:1001, 1995.
83. Sawicki PT et al: Intensified antihypertensive therapy is associated with improved survival in type 1 diabetic patients with nephropathy, *J Hypertension* 13:933, 1995.
84. Sawin CT: Action without benefit: the sliding scale of insulin use, *Arch Intern Med* 157:489, 1997.
85. Scandinavian Simvastatin Survival Study Group: Randomised trial of cholesterol lowering in 4444 patients with coronary heart disease: the Scandinavian Simvastatin Survival Study (4S), *Lancet* 344:1383, 1994.
86. Schade D et al: Intensive insulin therapy, *Excerpta Medica,* 1983.
87. Service FJ: Hypoglycemia, including hypoglycemia in neonates and children. In DeGroot LJ, editor: *Endocrinology,* Philadelphia, 1995, WB Saunders.
88. Shapiro AMJ et al. Islet transplantation in seven patients with type 1 diabetes mellitus using a glucocorticoid-free immunosuppressive regimen, *N Engl J Med* 343:230, 2000.
89. Sheehan JP: The gift of insulin, *J Lab Clin Med* 115:267, 1990.
90. Shepherd J et al for the West of Scotland Coronary Prevention Study Group: Prevention of coronary heart disease with pravastatin in men with hypercholesterolemia, *N Engl J Med* 333:1301, 1995.
91. Smith KC, Sheehan JP, Ulchaker MM: Diabetes mellitus. In Taylor RB, editor: *Fundamentals of family medicine,* New York, 1996, Springer.
92. Smith KC, Sheehan JP, Ulchaker MM: Diabetes mellitus. In Taylor RB, editor: *Family medicine: principles and practice,* ed 5, New York, 1997, Springer.
93. Smith KC, Sheehan JP, Ulchaker MM: Diabetes mellitus. In Taylor RB, editor: *Manual of family practice,* Boston, 1997, Little, Brown.
94. Streiff LD: Can clients understand our instructions? *Image J Nurs Sch* 18:48, 1986.
95. Syvanne M, Taskinen M: Lipids and lipoproteins as coronary risk factors in non–insulin-dependent diabetes mellitus, *Lancet* 350(suppl 1):20, 1997.
96. Tonino RP: Effect of physical training on the insulin resistance of aging, *Am J Physiol* 256(3 pt 1):E352, 1989.
97. Tuomilehto J et al. Prevention of type 2 diabetes mellitus by changes in lifestyle among subjects with impaired glucose tolerance, *N Engl J Med* 344:1343, 2001.
98. UK Prospective Diabetes Study Group: UK prospective diabetes study XI: biochemical risk factors in type 2 diabetic patients at diagnosis compared with age-matched normal subjects, *Diabet Med* 11:533, 1994.
99. UK Prospective Diabetes Study Group: UK prospective diabetes study XVI: overview of 6 years' therapy of type 2 diabetes: a progressive disease, *Diabetes* 44:1249, 1995.
100. UK Prospective Diabetes Study Group: Effect of intensive blood-glucose control with metformin on complications in overweight patients with type 2 diabetes (UKPDS 34), *Lancet* 352(9131):854, 1998.
101. UK Prospective Diabetes Study Group: Intensive blood-glucose control with sulphonylureas or insulin compared with conventional treatment and risk of complications in patients with type 2 diabetes (UKPDS 33), *Lancet* 352:837, 1998.
102. UK Prospective Diabetes Study Group (Stratton et al): Association of glycaemia with macrovascular and microvascular complications of type 2 diabetes (UKPDS 35): prospective observational study, *BMJ* 321:405, 2000.
103. UK Prospective Diabetes Study Group (Adler et al): Association of systolic blood pressure with macrovascular and microvascular complications of type 2 diabetes (UKPDS 36): prospective observational study, *BMJ* 321:412, 2000.
104. Ulchaker MM, Sheehan JP: Iatrogenic brittle diabetes: the hold-the-insulin decision, *Diabetes Educ* 17:111, 1991.
105. US Department of Agriculture/Human Nutrition Information Service: *Food guide pyramid—a guide to daily food choices,* Washington, DC, 1992, US Department of Agriculture/Human Nutrition Information Service.
106. US Department of Agriculture/Human Nutrition Information Service: *Nutrition and your health: dietary guidelines for Americans,* ed 4, Hyattsville, Md, 1995, US Department of Agriculture/Human Nutrition Information Service.
107. US Department of Health and Human Services: *Healthy people 2010: understanding and improving health,* Washington, DC, 2000, USDHHS.
108. Vague J: The degree of masculine differentiation of obesities: a factor determining predisposition to diabetes, atherosclerosis, gout and uric calculous disease, *Am J Clin Nutr* 4:20, 1956.
109. Verlato G et al: Attending the diabetes center is associated with increased 5-year survival probability of diabetic patients: the Verona Diabetes Study, *Diabetes Care* 19:211, 1996.
110. Vinicor F et al: Healthy people 2010: diabetes, *Diabetes Care* 23:853, 2000.
111. Weiner JP et al: Variation in office-based quality: a claims-based profile of care provided to Medicare patients with diabetes, *JAMA* 273:1503, 1995.
112. Zimmet PZ, Alberti KGMM: The changing face of macrovascular disease in non–insulin-dependent diabetes mellitus: an epidemic in progress, *Lancet* 350(suppl I):1, 1997.

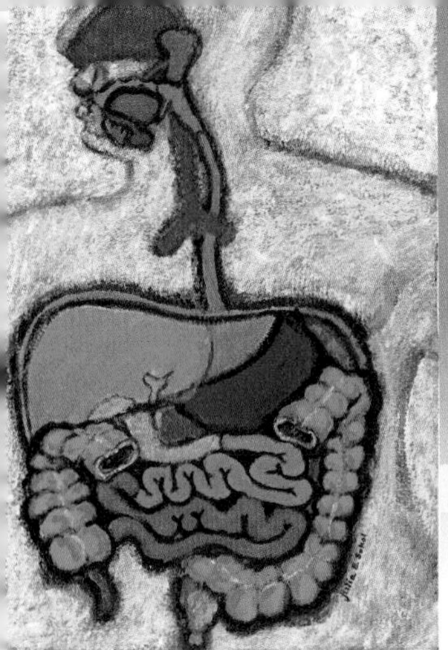

Assessment of the Gastrointestinal, Biliary, and Exocrine Pancreatic Systems

31

Shelley Yerger Huffstutler

Objectives

After studying this chapter, the learner should be able to:

1. Explain the anatomy and physiology of the gastrointestinal system and its accessory organs.
2. Discuss age-related physiologic changes that occur in the gastrointestinal system.
3. Identify health history and physical examination data essential to the nursing assessment of the gastrointestinal system.
4. Describe data obtained from diagnostic tests for various problems of the gastrointestinal tract.
5. Explain the rationale for nursing interventions associated with various diagnostic tests of the gastrointestinal biliary and exocrine pancreatic systems.

The gastrointestinal (GI) system, also termed the digestive system and alimentary canal, consists of the GI tract and its accessory organs. Its primary function is to convert ingested nutrients and fluids into a form that can be used by the cells of the body. This goal is accomplished through the processes of ingestion, digestion, and absorption. The second major function of the GI system is the storage and final excretion of the solid waste products of digestion. Proper functioning of the GI system is essential to the maintenance of proper nutrition and health.

ANATOMY AND PHYSIOLOGY

The upper portion of the GI tract consists of those structures that aid in the ingestion and digestion of food. These structures include the mouth, esophagus, stomach, and duodenum, plus the related organs of the biliary system and exocrine pancreas. The lower GI tract consists of the small and large intestines, the rectum, and the anus. The structures of the GI system are illustrated in Figure 31-1. The GI system is primarily composed of a hollow, muscular tube approximately 9 m (30 feet) long that stretches from the mouth to the anus.

Although this muscular tube is located within the body, it is actually an extension of the external environment. The walls of the GI tract successfully prevent most harmful agents from entering the body and essential body fluids and materials from leaving the body. The composition of the walls is predominantly smooth muscle; however, the mouth and upper esophagus, along with a portion of the rectum and anus, consist of voluntary muscle.

Mouth

The mouth is made up of the lips, cheeks, tongue, hard and soft palates, teeth, and salivary glands (Figure 31-2). These structures begin the digestive process by mechanically breaking down and lubricating the food. Because digestive enzymes can function only on the exposed surfaces of food particles, the teeth must begin the breakdown of food. No other portion of the GI system can perform the function of the teeth in their absence.

The lubrication of food is accomplished by the action of the watery and mucous secretions of the salivary, parotid, sublingual, and submandibular glands of the mouth. Saliva also contains ptyalin (amylase), which hydrolyzes starch to maltose. Small amounts of saliva, which contain immunoglobulin A (IgA) antibodies to many normal environmental microorganisms, are produced continually to keep the tissues of the mouth moist and clean. After chewing and moistening are completed, the muscular tongue pushes the food bolus back to the pharynx to initiate swallowing (deglutition).

Esophagus

The esophagus begins at the lower end of the pharynx. It is a hollow, muscular tube 10 inches (25 cm) in length that lies behind the trachea, passes through the thorax, and connects the mouth and stomach. The upper third is composed of skeletal muscle, and the lower two thirds are smooth muscle. Both ends of the esophagus are protected by sphincters that help prevent the reflux of gastric contents. Both sphincters are normally closed, except during the act of swallowing.

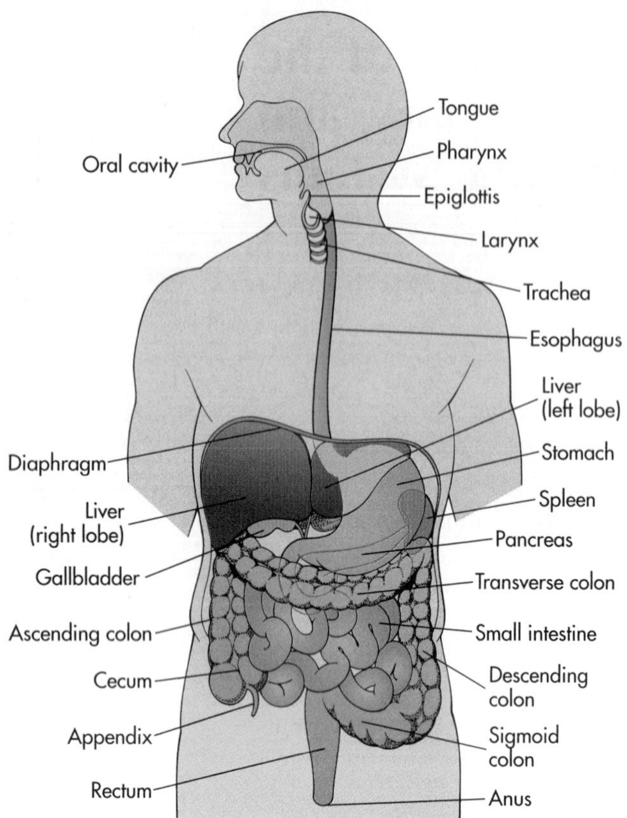

Figure 31-1 The organs of the gastrointestinal system and related structures.

The primary function of the esophagus is to move the food bolus by peristalsis from the pharynx to the stomach. No enzymes are secreted by the esophagus, and only mechanical digestion takes place. The secretion of mucus assists in the movement of the food bolus and protects the walls of the esophagus from abrasion by partially digested food.

Swallowing is a complex physiologic mechanism that must be accomplished without compromising respiration. It consists of three phases: (1) the voluntary phase, in which the tongue forces the bolus of food into the pharynx; (2) the involuntary pharyngeal phase, in which the food moves into the upper esophagus; and (3) the esophageal phase, during which food moves down into the stomach. The esophageal muscles are activated by the glossopharyngeal and vagal nerves, which create rhythmic peristaltic waves that propel the food toward the stomach. Food is prevented from passing into the trachea by the closing of the epiglottis and the opening of the esophagus.

Stomach

The stomach is roughly J shaped and lies in the upper abdomen to the left of midline. It is positioned to the left of the liver, to the right of the spleen, and posterior to both organs. It is a muscular pouch whose shape changes with its contents. Its three major regions are the fundus, body, and antrum. The cardiac sphincter protects the opening from the esophagus, and the pyloric sphincter protects the exit to the duodenum. The rugae, or longitudinal folds, of the stomach enable it to quadruple in size and increase from a resting volume of 50 ml

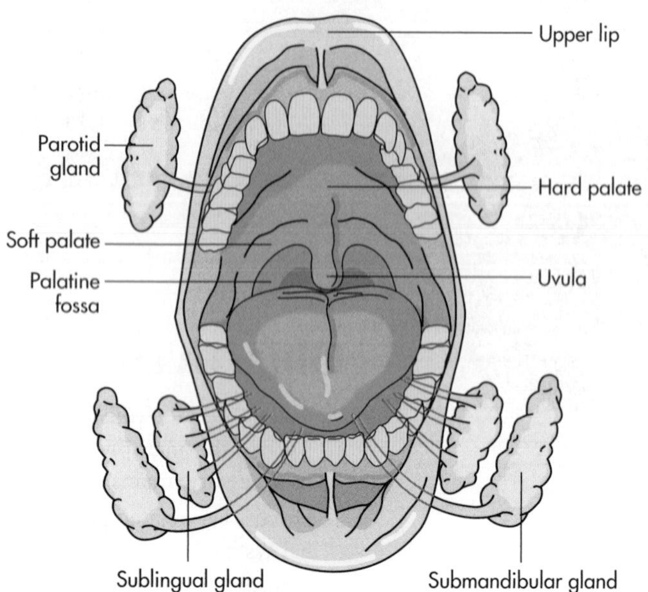

Figure 31-2 The structures of the mouth.

to a capacity of approximately 1500 ml for food digestion without major changes in pressure. The stomach has an outer serous layer and three layers of smooth muscle. The outermost layer of smooth muscle is longitudinal, the middle layer is circular, and the inner layer is oblique (Figure 31-3). The rugae are found on the inner mucosal layer.

The stomach primarily serves as a reservoir but also has digestive and secretory functions. Food is stored in the stomach until partially digested. The fundus contains chief cells, which secrete digestive enzymes, and parietal cells, which secrete water, hydrochloric acid (HCl), and the intrinsic factor that is essential for the absorption of vitamin B_{12}. The HCl is responsible for the highly acidic medium of the stomach (pH of 0.9 to 1.5), which is needed to activate the enzymes that initiate protein digestion. This highly acidic pH also serves as a protective barrier, destroying most ingested microorganisms. Gastric acid secretion is under the control of parasympathetic stimulation via the vagus, as is the secretion of gastrin and histamine. Gastrin is a hormone secreted from endocrine cells in the gastric glands of the stomach in response to vagal stimulation and mechanical distention of the stomach. The secretion of histamine 2 (H_2) also increases gastric acid secretion. Approximately 2 to 2.5 L of gastric secretions are produced each day.

The gastric mucosa is covered by a thick mucous gel layer produced by the densely packed epithelial cells of the mucosa. The mucous layer is almost completely impermeable to hydrogen ions. The mucosal epithelial cells also secrete bicarbonate, which acts as a buffer and helps neutralize the acidic secretions. The combined actions of these two mechanisms are so effective that, although the gastric secretions have a pH of less than 2.0, the intraluminal pH of the mucosa is maintained at about 7.0.

Gastric emptying is controlled by both hormonal and autonomic nervous system activity. Parasympathetic stimulation by the vagus nerve increases both peristalsis and secretion.

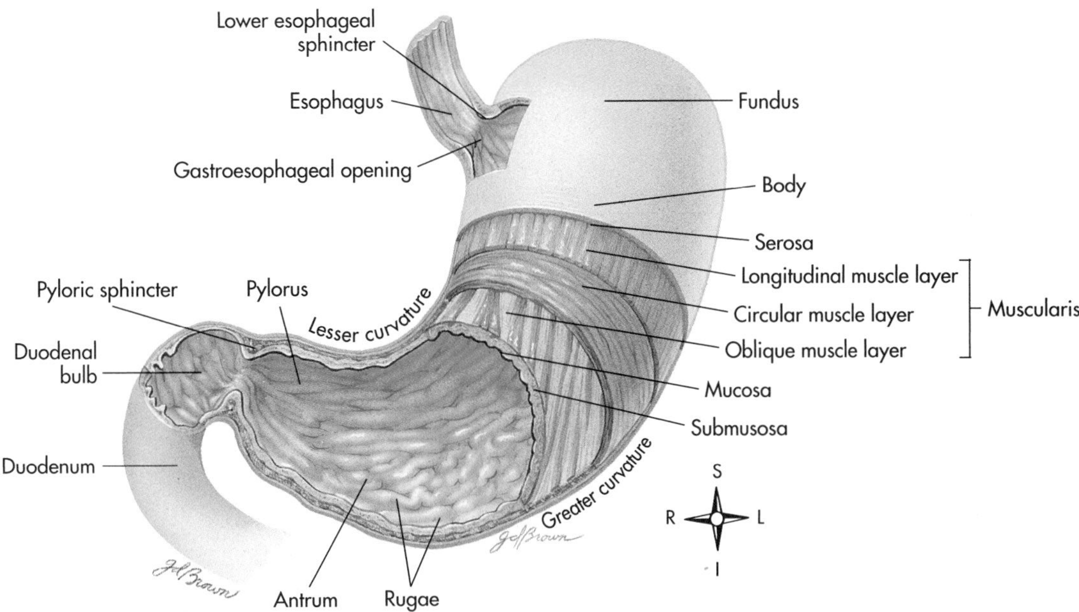

Figure 31-3 The stomach.

Sympathetic stimulation inhibits them. The peristaltic contractions of the stomach propel the chyme toward the antrum and occur at a frequency of about three to five contractions per minute. The pylorus closes during antral contraction, and larger food particles are propelled back toward the body of the stomach for further mixing. Gastric contents are emptied into the duodenum between peristaltic contractions. Although the pylorus is not a true anatomic sphincter, it does help prevent the backflow of duodenal contents and bile salts into the stomach.

Gallbladder and Biliary Ductal System

The gallbladder is a pear-shaped organ that lies on the inferior surface of the liver. It is composed of serous, muscular, and mucus layers and has a usual capacity of 50 ml, although it can increase in size under normal conditions. Innervation of the gallbladder is from the parasympathetic and sympathetic nervous system. The cystic duct connects the gallbladder with the remaining structures of the ductal system—the hepatic ducts and common bile duct.

The major function of the gallbladder is to store and concentrate bile. Bile, which is formed in the liver, is excreted into the hepatic ducts, which unite to form the common bile duct. It passes behind the pancreas, is joined by the pancreatic duct, and empties into the duodenum. The sphincter of Oddi regulates the flow of bile into the duodenum. A second sphincter is located above the junction with the pancreatic duct and controls the flow of bile in the common bile duct. When this sphincter is closed, bile moves back into the gallbladder, where it is concentrated fivefold to tenfold. Because bile can be released directly into the duodenum from the liver, the gallbladder is not essential to life. Bile salts facilitate fat digestion by emulsifying fats for action by intestinal lipases and facilitate the absorption of fats, fat-soluble vitamins, and cholesterol.

The release of bile from the gallbladder or liver is controlled by cholecystokinin (CCK). Approximately 600 to 800 ml of bile is produced daily. CCK is released from the walls of the duodenal intestinal mucosa when lipids, amino acids, and hydrogen ions enter the duodenum from the stomach. It travels via the blood to the gallbladder and causes contraction of the gallbladder's smooth musculature and relaxation of the sphincter at the end of the common bile duct (the sphincter of Oddi), so that bile can be emptied into the duodenum.

Most of the bile salts are reabsorbed from the intestine into the enterohepatic circulation and returned to the liver, where they can be recirculated. The system is so efficient that only 15% to 25% of the bile salt pool needs to be replaced by the liver each day.

Pancreas

The pancreas is an elongated, flattened organ located in the posterior abdomen, with its head lying within the curve of the duodenum and its tail resting against the spleen. The pancreas has both exocrine and endocrine functions. The exocrine functions are carried out by the acini cells and duct system, and the endocrine functions are carried out by islets of Langerhans cells (Figure 31-4). Exocrine functions will be discussed in this chapter. The endocrine functions have been previously discussed in Chapter 28.

The pancreas is divided into three parts, which are composed of lobules. The lobules are formed from groups of secretory cells termed acini, which drain into a ductal system that ultimately reaches the main pancreatic duct of Wirsung. This major duct extends the entire length of the gland. At the head of the pancreas the ductal secretions enter the duodenum through the ampulla of Vater. The sphincter of Oddi controls its opening.

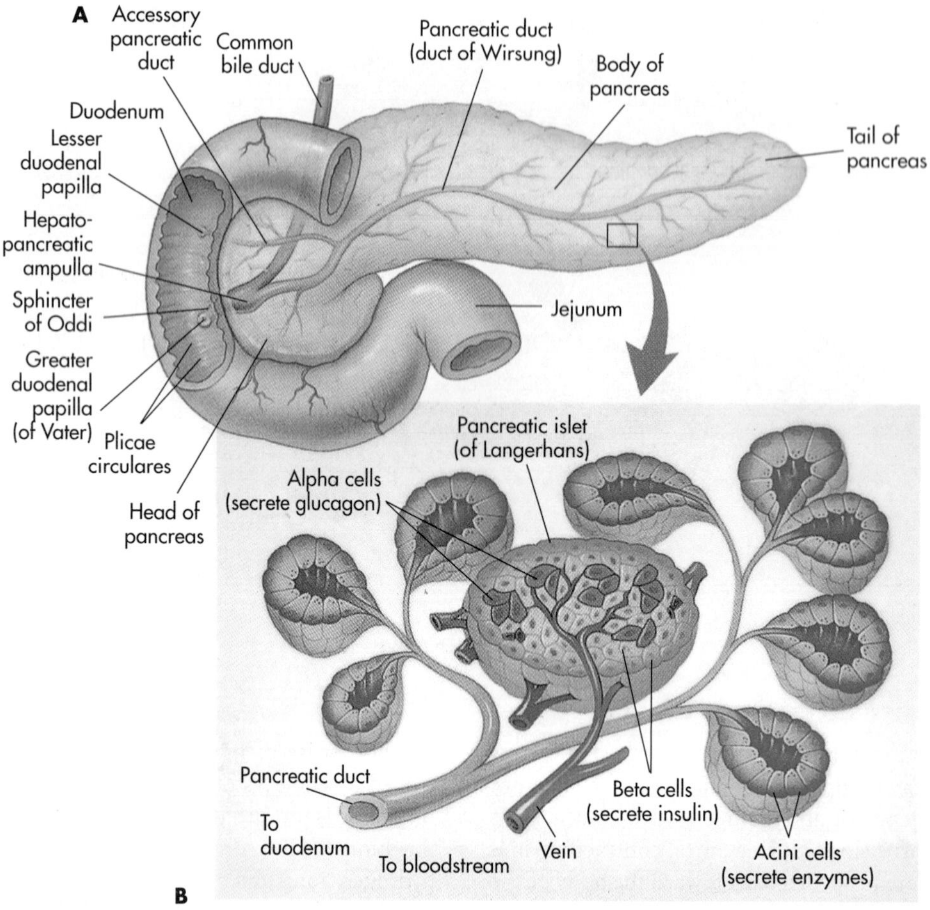

Figure 31-4 **A,** The pancreatic ductal system. **B,** Note both the endocrine and exocrine glandular cells of the pancreas.

Approximately 2 L of pancreatic secretions are produced daily. The ductal epithelium produces a balanced electrolyte secretion, and the acini secrete digestive enzymes in an inactive precursor state. The pancreatic secretions contain trypsin, a proteolytic enzyme, which breaks down protein; pancreatic amylase, which breaks down starch; and lipase, which hydrolyzes fat into glycerol and fatty acids. The pancreatic acini also produce an enzyme inhibitor that prevents the activation of the secretions before they reach the duodenum. The production of the pancreatic secretions is controlled by the action of the parasympathetic nervous system, gastrin, and hormones released from the duodenum during digestion.

Intestines

The small intestine is about 2.5 cm (1 inch) wide and 6 m (20 feet) long and fills most of the abdomen. It consists of three parts: (1) the duodenum that connects to the stomach, (2) the jejunum, or middle portion, and (3) the ileum that connects to the large intestine (see Figure 31-1).

The large intestine is about 6 cm (2.5 inches) wide and 1.5 m (5 feet) long. It also consists of three parts: (1) the cecum that connects to the small intestine, (2) the colon, and (3) the rectum. The ileocecal valve prevents backward flow of fecal contents from the large intestine to the small intestine. The vermiform appendix, which has no known function, is an appendage close to the ileocecal valve. The colon is subdivided into four sections: the ascending, transverse, descending, and sigmoid colons. The points at which the colon changes direction are named for adjacent organs: the liver (hepatic flexure) and the spleen (splenic flexure). The rectum is 17 to 20 cm (7 to 8 inches) long, ending in the 2- to 3-cm anal canal. The opening of the anus is controlled by a smooth muscle internal sphincter and a striated muscle external sphincter.

Table 31-1 summarizes the major digestive enzymes. The actions and stimuli for secretion of the major gastrointestinal hormones are presented in Table 31-2.

Small Intestine

The primary functions of the small intestine are the digestion of food and the absorption of nutrients. This process occurs primarily in the jejunum and ileum. The duodenum contains the opening for the bile and pancreatic ducts, which allow bile and pancreatic secretions to enter the intestine. Mucus-producing glands are concentrated where gastric contents are emptied and digestive secretions enter the duodenum. The mucus helps protect the duodenum from the acids in the gastric chyme and the actions of the digestive enzymes.

Digestion begins in the mouth and stomach, but it takes place primarily in the small intestine. The intestinal mucosa is impermeable to most large molecules, so proteins, fats, and

TABLE 31-1 Digestive Enzymes

Source	Action
Mouth	
Pytalin (salivary amylase)	Breaks starch into maltose (polysaccharides to disaccharides)
Stomach	
Gastric pepsin	Breaks protein into polypeptides
Gastric lipase	Digests butterfat
Pancreas	
Pancreatic amylase	Breaks starch into maltose (polysaccharides to disaccharides)
Trypsin	Splits polypeptide chains
Pancreatic lipase	Splits emulsified fat into monoglycerides
Small Intestine	
Maltase	Breaks maltose into glucose
Dextrinase	Breaks alpha-limit dextrin to glucose
Lactase	Breaks lactose into galactose and glucose
Sucrase	Breaks sucrose into glucose and fructose
Enterokinase	Activates trypsin
Peptidases	Splits polypeptides into amino acids
Intestinal lipase	Splits neutral fats into glycerol and fatty acids

TABLE 31-2 Major Gastrointestinal Hormones

Hormone	Action	Stimulus for Secretion
Gastrin	Stimulates secretion of gastric acid and pepsinogen; increases gastric blood flow; stimulates gastric smooth muscle contraction and motility	Secreted from antrum of stomach and duodenum in response to vagal stimulation, epinephrine, solutions of calcium salts, and alcohol; inhibited by an antral stomach pH of less than 2.5
Secretin	Stimulates secretion of bicarbonate-containing solution by the pancreas and liver; inhibits gastric acid secretion and motility	Secreted by duodenum in response to low pH chyme (less than 3.0) entering the duodenum
Cholecystokinin	Stimulates the contraction of the gallbladder and the secretion of pancreatic enzymes; slows gastric emptying	Secreted in duodenum and jejunum in response to the presence of fatty and amino acids
Enterogastrone	Inhibits gastric secretion and motility; relaxes sphincter of Oddi	Secreted in duodenum in response to the presence of partially digested proteins and fats

complex carbohydrates must be broken down into small particles before they can be absorbed. The intestinal mucosa also secretes surface enzymes that aid in digestion and about 2 L/day of serous fluid that acts as a diluting agent to facilitate absorption.

Carbohydrate digestion, which begins in the mouth, is completed in the small intestine as disaccharides are broken down into monosaccharides (glucose, fructose, and galactose) by the action of intestinal enzymes and pancreatic amylase. Protein digestion, which begins in the stomach, is completed as polypeptides are broken down into peptides and amino acids by the action of pancreatic trypsin. Fat digestion is accomplished by emulsification into small droplets by the action of bile and pancreatic lipase. The droplets are then further broken down into glycerol and fatty acids. The release of digestive secretions is stimulated by the hormones secretin and CCK (also called pancreozymin), as well as by the action of the parasympathetic nervous system.

The inner mucosal surface of the small intestine is covered with millions of villi, which are the functional units for absorption. Each villus is equipped with a blind-end lymph vessel (lacteal) in its center, which is surrounded by capillaries, venules, and arterioles (Figure 31-5). These structures bring blood to the surface of the intestine and provide a network for absorption into the portal blood or lymphatic system. Ninety percent of absorption occurs within the small intestine by either active transport or diffusion. Active transport requires a metabolic energy expenditure and is used to absorb amino acids, monosaccharides, sodium, and calcium. Fatty acids and water diffuse passively, primarily into the lymphatics.

The contents of the small intestine (chyme) are propelled toward the anus by regular peristaltic movements. Both segmental

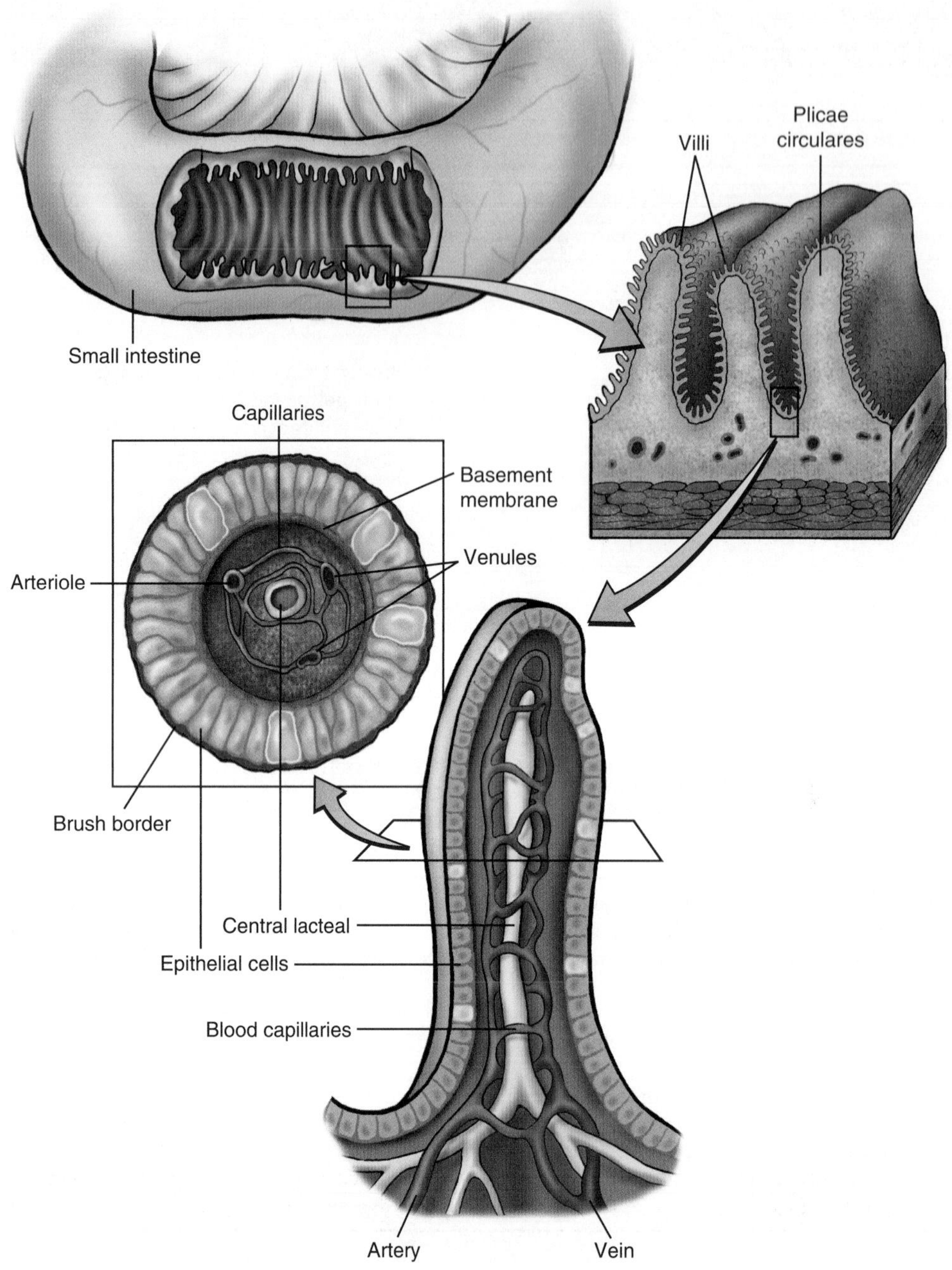

Figure 31-5 Adaptations in the wall of the small intestine assist digestion and absorption of foods. Note the plicae circulares covered with villi, the capillary bed and central lacteal in each villus, and the brush border of microvilli.

and propulsive movements occur. The segmental movements involve primarily the circular muscles of the intestine. Slow contractions move the chyme back and forth in small segments of the intestine (1 to 4 cm). This movement mixes the chyme and facilitates digestion and absorption. Segmental peristaltic movements increase after meals. The propulsive peristaltic movements involve intestinal segments 10 to 20 cm long. Contraction occurs in the proximal segment, with relaxation in the distal segment. Chyme advances slowly and normally takes 3 to 10 hours to move from the stomach to the colon. Parasympathetic stimulation, primarily through branches of the vagus nerve, increases peristaltic activity. Sympathetic stimulation is primarily inhibitory.

Large Intestine

Minimal chemical digestion takes place in the large intestine. It functions primarily to absorb water and electrolytes from the chyme and store the food waste (feces) until defecation. Reabsorption occurs predominantly in the right or ascending colon. The colon can absorb six to eight times more fluid than is delivered to it daily, and only approximately 100 ml of fluid is left in the colon to be mixed with the fecal residue.

The large number of microorganisms found in the large intestine further break down the residual proteins that were not digested or absorbed in the small intestine. The breakdown of amino acids produces ammonia, which is converted to urea by the liver. These intestinal bacteria also play a vital role in the synthesis of vitamin K and some of the B vitamins. The only significant secretion of the colon is mucus, which protects the walls and helps the fecal matter adhere into a mass.

Approximately 450 ml of chyme reaches the cecum each day. The transit time in the large bowel is slow, taking about 12 hours to reach the rectum. The fecal contents in the colon are pushed forward by mass movements that occur only a few times each day. These mass movements are stimulated by gastrocolic reflexes initiated when food enters the duodenum from the stomach, especially after the first meal of the day.

The rectum is well innervated with sensory fibers. Parasympathetic fibers are responsible for the contraction of the rectum and relaxation of the internal sphincter of the anus. The defecation reflex occurs when feces enter the rectum. Afferent impulses are transmitted to the sacral segments of the spinal cord; subsequently, reflex impulses are transmitted back to the sigmoid and rectum, initiating relaxation of the internal anal sphincter.

Physiologic Changes With Aging

Gastrointestinal complaints are extremely common in elderly persons. Distinct changes occur in the GI system with aging, although these changes are incompletely understood. Although most of the aging-related changes do not interfere with normal functioning, it is important for nurses to be cognizant of the changes and incorporate appropriate modifications when planning care for elders. In addition, the GI effects of other chronic illnesses such as diabetes require careful consideration because they are usually more important than the effects of aging itself.

In the mouth, teeth darken and may loosen or fracture, and the gums recede. Salivary gland output decreases, which causes mouth dryness and increased susceptibility to infection and tissue breakdown. Aging causes decreased motility and strength of peristalsis in the esophagus, but these changes appear to have minimal significance in healthy persons. Some deterioration in the lower esophageal sphincter may increase the frequency of esophageal reflux.

Gastric motility and emptying diminish slightly but progressively with age, and gastric acid secretion also decreases steadily after age 50. Achlorhydria (absence of free HCl) is relatively common. These changes can produce minor problems in digestion but are usually asymptomatic. Chronic gastritis is common in elderly persons, but the condition is usually the result of bacterial colonization by *Helicobacter pylori* and not aging.

No significant changes in biliary system morphology are associated with aging. However, the composition of the bile becomes increasingly lithogenic (likely to produce calculi), possibly related to an increase in biliary cholesterol; therefore the incidence of gallstones increases with each decade.

The pancreas exhibits ductal hyperplasia and fibrosis with aging, but these changes are not necessarily associated with altered functioning. The output of pancreatic secretions steadily declines after age 40, but related problems with absorption have not been documented.

Age-related changes in small intestinal function are important and can lead to poor nutrition even with adequate intake. Nutrient absorption is impaired, particularly the absorption of carbohydrates. Absorption of water-soluble vitamins remains intact, but the absorption of vitamin D is defective in many elderly persons, and the active transport of calcium is also impaired. Decreased production of secretory IgA can lead to an increase in the frequency and severity of infections.

Chronic constipation is one of the most common complaints in elderly persons. Yet the segmental mass movements and contractions of the large intestine have been found to be unchanged as long as the individual remains physically active. The incidence of both diverticula and polyps in the colon increases with age. There is a decrease in elasticity in the rectum and a steady decrease in the rectal volume, which can result in sphincter failure. However, the sensation of rectal fullness remains intact, and most problems with bowel incontinence in elderly persons are not attributable to the effects of aging.

HEALTH HISTORY

A thorough health history is necessary to adequately assess the health status of persons with potential dysfunction of the GI system.

Patient/Family History

The nurse asks the patient about previous GI problems, hospitalizations, and surgeries. This includes past and current medication use, both over-the-counter and prescribed. The use of antacids and laxatives is particularly important. The nurse inquires about the presence of GI problems in the nuclear or extended family, including cancer and disorders such as inflammatory bowel disease, which have a documented hereditary link.

Diet and Nutrition

The adequacy of the diet, in terms of both quality and quantity, can be quickly estimated through comparison of the diet with recommended food intake patterns. Nutritional assessment has particular significance in GI disorders, because it may reveal changes in eating patterns characteristic of specific illnesses or disorders. The nutritional assessment includes an exploration of usual eating patterns and any changes that may be the result of illness or specific symptoms. The assessment explores changes in appetite, food preferences and intolerances, food allergies, planned and unplanned changes in weight, adherence to special or therapeutic diets, and the use of dietary or vitamin supplements. A 24-hour dietary recall may be a useful tool to approximate caloric and specific nutrient intake and analyze the overall adequacy of the diet. Symptoms related to food intake should also be carefully assessed. Changes in appetite and the presence of such symptoms as dysphagia, nausea, and discomfort are carefully explored.

Lifestyle, economic, and cultural factors affecting nutrition are also assessed. Food has multiple social and emotional values for individuals that are distinct from its role in nutrition. Financial resources, access to food preparation and storage facilities, and religious or social beliefs may all influence both the quality and quantity of the diet. Lifestyle factors can have a direct or indirect effect on GI function. Gastrointestinal symptoms commonly develop or worsen in response to life stressors. Open-ended questions are most effective for exploring beliefs and feelings about food.

A complete nutritional assessment includes an evaluation of the patient's use of sugar and salt substitutes, coffee, alcohol, and tobacco (both chewing and smoking). The presence of dentures is an essential consideration because dentures may significantly influence food selection and chewing.

Abdominal Pain

Although pain is not an early or common manifestation of GI disease, it is frequently the reason individuals seek medical attention. The nurse assesses its onset, duration, character, location, and relationship to meals, stressful events, activity, or medications.[8] The patient is asked to point to the site of pain in the abdomen. Pain may be experienced anywhere along the length of the GI tract in a specific localized pattern, a general nonspecific pattern, or referred to another somatic or skeletal region that shares the same nerve innervation (Figure 31-6). Abdominal pain may be continuous, episodic, or associated with eating. The pain sensation is thought to arise from the distention or sudden contraction of a hollow viscus; therefore, local stretching or traction on pain-sensitive structures will elicit the pain stimulus. The painful area may exhibit local muscle guarding, which serves as a protective mechanism. The pain associated with pancreatic or biliary dysfunction is usually severe.

Food Intolerance

Abdominal pain or discomfort may also be reported as heartburn, indigestion, belching, or bloating and requires further clarification. The discomfort may interfere with chewing or swallowing food. Specific foods, such as those that are spicy, very hot, or very cold, may precipitate the discomfort; smoking and/or alcohol consumption may also trigger abdominal discomfort. The patient may have already self-treated the abdominal pain with a variety of over-the-counter preparations such as antacids and H_2 receptor antagonists. Difficulties in swallowing (dysphagia) can also result in abdominal discomfort.

Nausea and Vomiting

Nausea and vomiting are commonly associated with GI problems, and the nurse assesses for onset, frequency, duration, patterns of occurrence, relationship to meals, and the quantity and character of the emesis. Nausea and vomiting are commonly associated with medication administration. Emesis may contain red blood indicative of recent bleeding. "Coffee-ground" emesis may indicate old bleeding in the stomach. The presence of bile produces a green color and has a bitter taste; brown vomitus may contain fecal matter.

Fatigue and Weakness

Persons with GI system problems often complain of fatigue or weakness. Inadequate nutrient intake, abnormal fluid and electrolyte status, and increased metabolic demands may all contribute to the problem. It is important for the nurse to carefully consider other problems that may be contributing to the symptoms, including cardiac, respiratory, renal, and other metabolic disorders.[2] These complaints may be present in a wide variety of situations, but their careful assessment is essen-

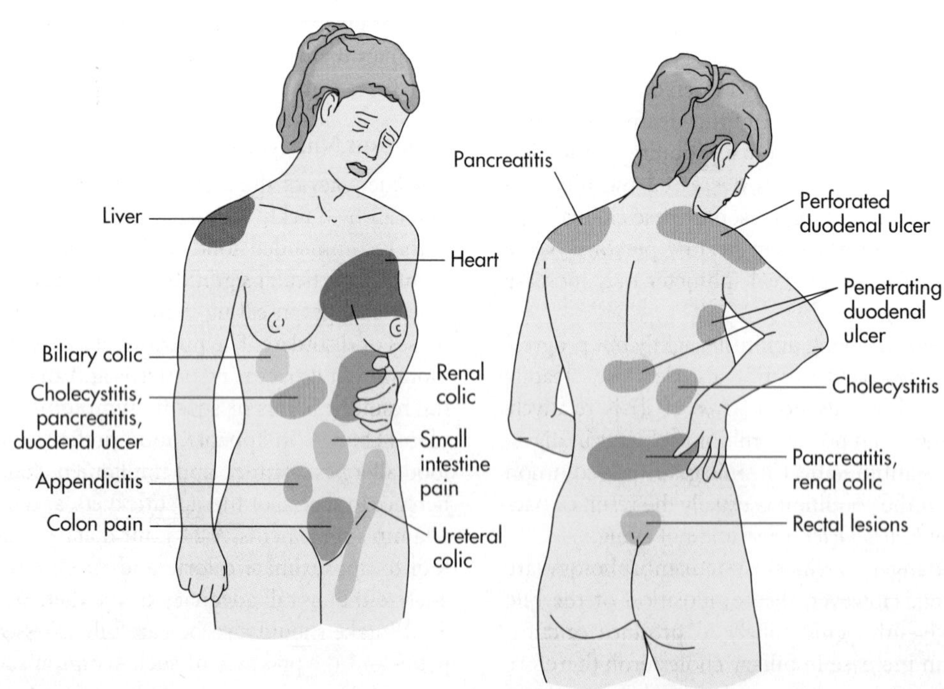

Figure 31-6 Common sites of referred pain. Note that the location of the pain may not be directly over or even near the site of the organ.

tial for planning an overall approach to care. Resolution of these problems usually takes time. Fatigue and weakness may also contribute to weight loss, particularly when associated with persistent anorexia, nausea, vomiting, or abdominal pain.

Elimination Patterns

Patterns of bowel elimination vary significantly among healthy individuals, and these patterns are commonly altered by GI system disorders. The nurse assesses the individual's usual elimination pattern and explores any changes that have occurred. The use of laxatives, suppositories, or other products to support bowel elimination is carefully assessed.

Changes in the normal pattern of bowel elimination may represent a physiologic alteration, a pathologic condition, or simply a change in normal diet and activity patterns. Constipation, defined as the presence of small, hard stools that are passed with difficulty at infrequent intervals, is a classic example. Constipation may be a temporary response to a change in diet or activity, or it may be a sign of bowel obstruction. Constipation may also result from the administration of opioids that slow peristalsis, whereas diarrhea can be the result of surgical interventions that remove significant bowel segments. Diarrhea and stools containing mucus, pus, and possibly undigested food may indicate enteritis or invasion by a parasite. Obstruction in the descending colon may produce small, ribbon-shaped stools, or no stool if the obstruction is complete.

When fat absorption is abnormal, steatorrhea (bulky, foul-smelling, fatty stools) may occur. If biliary obstruction is present, the patient may give a history of clay-colored (grayish) stools. Bright red blood in the stool indicates lower GI bleeding. Blood from the upper GI tract is broken down by digestive secretions, and the stool appears black and sticky (tarry). Sometimes the presence of blood in the GI tract acts as a powerful cathartic and may produce abrupt, severe diarrhea. Blood in the stool (melena) may be a recent or a chronic symptom and may result from erosion of the mucosa, leading to perforation of the muscle wall or rupture of a blood vessel (see Table 31-6 on p. 996). All cases of melena and/or rectal bleeding should be immediately explored since both are symptoms associated with colorectal cancer.

PHYSICAL EXAMINATION

Information gained from the physical examination helps the nurse determine the patient's baseline status and develop an appropriate plan of care.

Mouth

Assessment of the mouth provides data about the patient's ability to salivate, masticate, and swallow. The lips are observed for symmetry, color, moisture, swelling, cracks, or lesions. If asymmetry is noted, the ability to masticate and swallow is assessed. A tongue blade and penlight are needed to improve visualization, and gloves should be worn for all examinations of the mouth. In certain situations, a mask and eye shield may also be appropriate.

The lips are normally reddish in color and are good indicators of pallor or cyanosis. Dryness may indicate dehydration, and cracks or fissures can occur with excessive dryness, exposure to cold, poorly fitting dentures, or a riboflavin deficiency. When cracks occur in the corners of the mouth they are referred to as angular stomatitis. Swelling of the lips is usually the result of an inflammatory response. Lesions on the lips may be benign or malignant. A commonly encountered benign lesion is herpes simplex (cold sore, fever blister), which is caused by a virus and can create enough discomfort to limit mastication.

The enamel surface of the teeth should be white but will darken with surface stains (tea, coffee, tobacco). Commonly found abnormalities of the teeth include caries, loose or broken teeth, and absence of some or all teeth. The gums or gingivae are normally pink, attach to the teeth, and fill the interdental surfaces. Recession of the gum line is not uncommon in older individuals. If the person is partially or completely edentulous (without teeth), the gingivae are examined for areas of redness caused by improperly fitting dentures, partial plates, or implants. The person is then asked to insert the dentures so their correct fit and comfort for chewing can be assessed.

The buccal mucosa is light pink, although patchy pigmentation is seen in dark-skinned individuals. The mucosa is examined for moisture, white spots or patches, debris, areas of bleeding, or ulcers resulting from ill-fitting dentures or braces. Dryness and debris may indicate dehydration. White, curdy patches, which are removable with some effort, may be caused by candidiasis (thrush). White, nonremovable patches (leukoplakia); white plaques within red patches; or red, granular patches (erythroplakia) may be premalignant lesions and should be reported to the physician. A round or oval white ulcer surrounded by an area of redness is indicative of an aphthous ulcer (canker sore) (see Chapter 32).

While the tongue is depressed with a tongue blade and the person says "Ah," the soft palate is observed for symmetry and the effective functioning of cranial nerve X, the vagus, which is necessary for effective swallowing. The uvula, soft palate, tonsils, and posterior pharynx are observed for signs of inflammation. Tongue mobility and function are essential to mastication, taste, and swallowing. Normally there is no limitation to movement in any direction, but the tongue deviates toward the paralyzed side with paralysis of the twelfth cranial nerve (hypoglossal). A thin, white coating and presence of large papillae on the dorsum of the tongue are normal findings. A thick coating indicates poor oral hygiene; and a smooth, red surface suggests a nutritional deficiency. The ventral surface is examined for leukoplakia, ulceration, or nodules, any of which may indicate malignancy.

Any distinctive odor of the breath is noted. A foul odor may occur after the ingestion of certain foods, with poor hygiene or oral infections, and with some metabolic dysfunctions such as diabetic ketoacidosis, liver disease, and bowel obstruction. Normally the mandible slides forward and down without difficulty, and a "cracking" sound is audible when the mouth is opened widely. The interior of the mouth is also carefully examined with a gloved finger to check for areas of tenderness, ulcers, and lumps.

Abdomen

Examination of the abdomen determines the presence or absence of (1) tenderness, (2) organ enlargement, (3) masses, (4) spasm or rigidity of the abdominal muscles, and (5) fluid or air in the abdominal cavity. Physical examination of the abdomen is performed in the following order: inspection, auscultation, percussion, and palpation. Auscultation is performed before percussion and palpation, because the latter two may alter the frequency and intensity of bowel sounds.

The surface of the abdomen can be divided anatomically into either four quadrants or nine regions (Figure 31-7). The patient is placed in a supine position and kept as relaxed as possible. Bending the patient's knees slightly, placing a small pillow under the head, and positioning the patient's arms flat on the bed can help the patient to relax the abdominal muscles and make palpation easier. Good lighting should be available.

Inspection

The skin of the abdomen is inspected for color, texture, scars, rashes, lesions, symmetry, contour, and the presence of visible peristalsis. The abdomen is normally flat but will be rounded in an obese person and may appear scaphoid in the thin or emaciated person. The integrity and turgor of the skin are reliable indicators of total body hydration.

Abdominal distention may be caused by air or fluid in the GI tract or fluid in the peritoneal space (ascites). Air may collect from swallowing or from gas produced by bacterial action in the bowel. Decreased peristalsis prevents the accumulated air from moving through the GI tract. Fluid may also accumulate from decreased peristalsis and be a symptom of partial or complete bowel obstruction. Ascites usually results from increased portal hypertension secondary to liver or heart disease.

Measurement of abdominal girth provides a baseline for the evaluation of any increase or decrease in size related to distention. A measuring tape is placed around the abdomen at the level of the umbilicus or 2.5 cm below, and the reading is taken. It is important to lightly mark the site for measurement on the patient's skin with a waterproof pen so that all subsequent measurements are taken at the same level for accurate evaluation.

Inspection incorporates assessment for the presence of jaundice, which is a common symptom in biliary tract or liver disease. A slight aortic pulsation may be present in the epigastric area, but peristalsis is not normally visible. A summary of common findings from abdominal inspection is included in Table 31-3.

Auscultation

Auscultation is used primarily to determine the presence or absence of peristalsis. In the normal abdomen, bowel sounds caused by fluid and air movement can always be heard. Their intensity and frequency depend mainly on the phase of digestion. Most intestinal sounds occur at a rate of 5 to 34 per minute (although some may not be audible for up to 5 minutes) and are high pitched and gurgling in quality. A normal peristaltic wave produces audible sounds of air and fluid movement through the intestine. The sounds are the loudest to the right and below the umbilicus.[6]

Abnormalities may include either extreme. A virtual absence of normal sounds occurs when bowel motility is inhibited by inflammation or paralytic ileus. Exaggerated peristalsis produces waves of loud, gurgling sounds called borborygmi, which may result from infection or obstruction. Bowel sounds are auscultated by placing the diaphragm of the stethoscope lightly

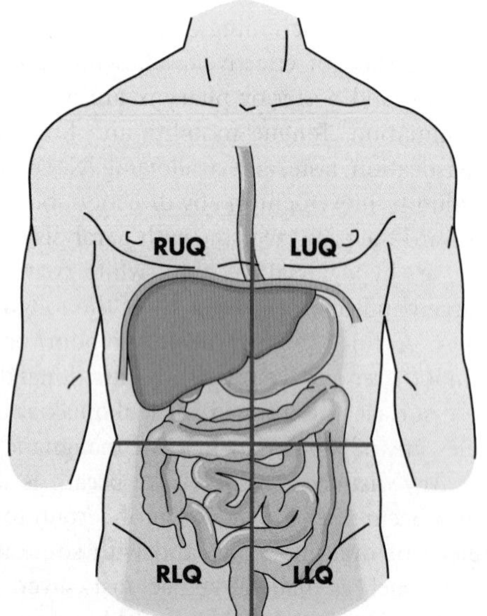

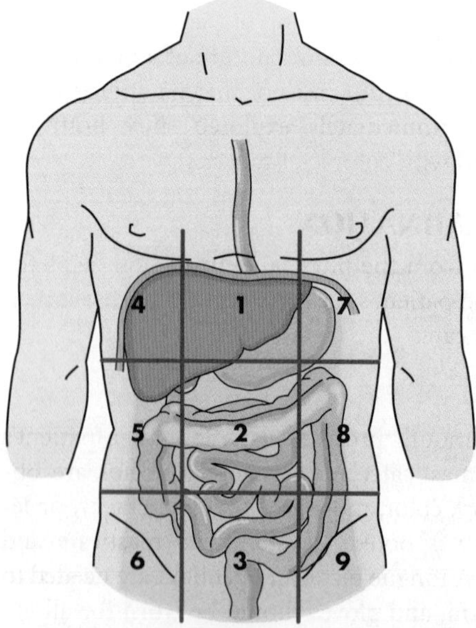

Figure 31-7 Anatomic divisions of the abdomen. **Left,** The abdomen divided into four quadrants. **Right,** The abdomen divided into nine topographic regions: *1,* Epigastrium; *2,* umbilical; *3,* suprapubic; *4,* right hypochondrium; *5,* right lumbar or flank; *6,* right inguinal or iliac; *7,* left hypochondrium; *8,* left lumbar or flank; *9,* left inguinal or iliac.

against the abdomen and listening to all quadrants systematically. It may take 5 full minutes to determine that bowel sounds are completely absent, but the absence of any bowel sounds in 2 minutes clearly indicates a problem. Sounds that occur at a rate of about 1 per minute are hypoactive. The bell of the stethoscope may be used to auscultate for vascular sounds, such as bruits over the aorta and renal and iliac arteries. These sounds are not considered to be normal assessment findings. Box 31-1 outlines the location of the organs within the quadrants of the abdomen. A summary of common findings from auscultation is found in Table 31-4. Optimal areas for auscultation of vascular sounds are illustrated in Figure 31-8.

Percussion

Percussion of the abdomen is used primarily to confirm the size of various organs and to determine the presence of excessive amounts of fluid or air. Normally, percussion over the abdomen is tympanic because of the presence of a small amount of swallowed air within the GI tract. A dull or flat percussion note is found over a solid structure. Dull sounds normally occur over the liver and spleen or a bladder filled with urine. Abnormal percussion findings occur because of the presence of ascites or abnormal masses. Ascites classically produces a shifting dullness, which is caused by fluid movement to dependent areas. Interpreting the sounds of abdominal percussion may be difficult in obese individuals.

The four quadrants are percussed beginning with the thorax and moving downward systematically. The degree of tympany, from soft to pronounced, is recorded. Tympanic sounds should be heard beginning at the ninth interspace in the left upper quadrant of the abdomen.

Palpation

Palpation is of value in determining the outlines of abdominal organs, the presence and characteristics of any abdominal masses, and the presence of direct tenderness, guarding, rebound tenderness, and muscular rigidity. In the presence of gallbladder disease, normal palpation of the liver elicits sharp pain and a positive inspiratory arrest (Murphy's sign). The acute onset of pain causes the patient to stop inspiration abruptly, midway through the breath.

Abnormal findings from palpation may include (1) direct tenderness over an organ capsule, (2) rebound tenderness, (3) muscular rigidity, or (4) masses that may be felt if they are large enough or close enough to the surface. Distinction

TABLE 31-3 Common Findings From Abdominal Inspection

Finding	Interpretation
Scars or striae	May be result of pregnancy, obesity, ascites, tumors, edema, surgical procedures, or healed burned areas
Engorged veins	May be caused by obstruction of vena cava or portal vein and circulation from abdomen
Skin color variation	May be caused by jaundice (yellow), inflammation (red), or intraabdominal hemorrhage (blue)
Visible peristalsis	May be caused by pyloric or intestinal obstruction; normally peristalsis not visible except for slow waves in thin persons
Visible pulsations	Normally slight pulsation of aorta, visible in epigastric region
Visible masses and altered contour	Observe for hernias, distention of ascites, and obesity; instructing patient to cough may bring out hernia "bulge" or elicit pain or discomfort in the abdomen; marked concavity may be caused by malnutrition
Spider angioma	Appear on upper part of body and blanch with pressure; commonly result from liver disease

BOX 31-1 Anatomic Locations of Organs Within Each Abdominal Quadrant

Right Upper Quadrant (RUQ)
- Liver
- Gallbladder
- Duodenum
- Right kidney
- Hepatic flexure of colon

Left Upper Quadrant (LUQ)
- Stomach
- Spleen
- Left kidney
- Pancreas
- Splenic flexure of colon

Right Lower Quadrant (RLQ)
- Cecum
- Appendix
- Right ovary and tube

Left Lower Quadrant (LLQ)
- Sigmoid colon
- Left ovary and tube

TABLE 31-4 Common Findings From Abdominal Auscultation

Finding	Interpretation
Absence of bowel sounds in 5 minutes	Peritonitis, paralytic ileus, and hypokalemia
Repeated, high-pitched bowel sounds occurring at frequent intervals	Increased peristalsis caused by gastroenteritis, early pyloric obstruction, early intestinal obstruction, or diarrhea
Bruit	Presence of abnormal sound caused by turbulence of blood flow through partially occluded or diseased aorta or renal artery
Hum and friction rub	Heard over liver and splenic areas, indicating an increased venous blood flow, possibly related to peritoneal inflammation

should be made between a distended abdomen that is firm to the touch and one that is soft to the touch.

Light palpation is used to elicit tenderness and cutaneous hypersensitivity. The nurse uses the pads of the fingertips, with the fingers together, and presses gently, depressing the abdominal wall about 1 cm. All quadrants are palpated using smooth movements.[7]

Deep palpation is used to delineate organs and masses and should be performed only by properly trained persons because improper technique can result in injury. The nurse again uses the palmar surface of the fingers but presses more deeply using a single- or two-handed technique. Known tender or painful areas should be assessed last. Rebound tenderness is tested by pressing slowly but firmly over the painful site. The fingers are then quickly withdrawn. Acute pain on withdrawal reflects peritoneal inflammation (positive Blumberg's sign). This maneuver (Figure 31-9) can be extremely painful and should never be performed unnecessarily.

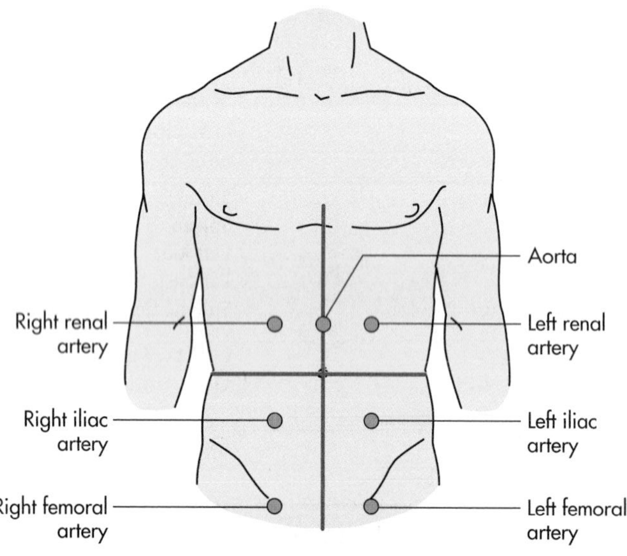

Figure 31-8 Sites for auscultation of vascular sounds in the abdomen.

Rectum

The normal perineal and perianal skin resembles the skin on the rest of the body with no breaks in integrity. Abnormal findings may include pruritus ani, coccygeal or pilonidal sinus tract openings, fistulas, fissures, external hemorrhoids, or rectal prolapse. Internal hemorrhoids may appear when the patient bears down.

Assessment measures and variations in normal findings relevant to the care of older adults are presented in the Gerontologic Assessment box. Also identified are disorders common in older adults, which may be responsible for abnormal assessment findings.

DIAGNOSTIC TESTS

Many of the examinations and tests performed for diagnosis of problems of the GI system are both time consuming and

Gerontologic Assessment

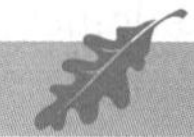

Inspect Abdomen

Peristalsis may be more easily observed because the abdominal musculature is thinner and has less tone.

There are usually increased deposits of subcutaneous fat on the abdomen because the ratio of fat to water increases with aging.

Palpate Abdomen Gently

Abdominal palpation is often easier because the abdominal wall is softer and thinner. The liver and kidneys are usually palpable if the patient is not obese.

Assess Thoroughly for Pain

Older adults often verbalize less pain than younger adults when experiencing an acute abdomen.

Obtain a Week-Long Diary of Dietary Intake

Food patterns may vary during the course of the month based on monthly income.

COMMON DISORDERS IN OLDER ADULTS

Gastroesophageal reflux disease
Gastritis
Gallstones

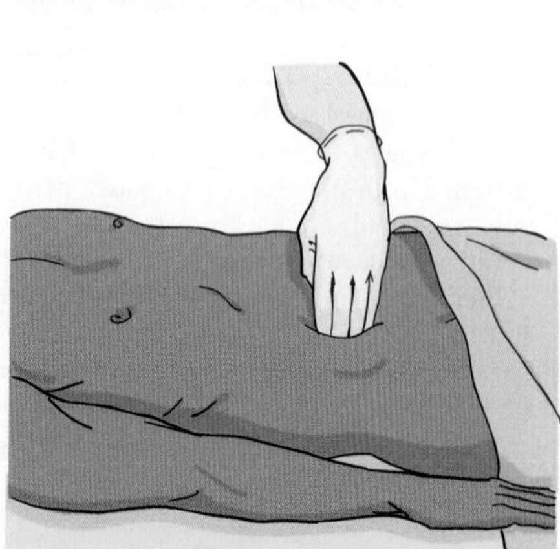

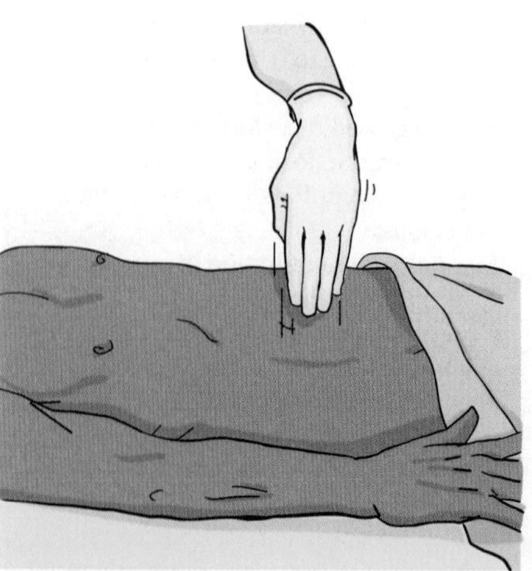

Figure 31-9 Palpating for rebound tenderness.

unpleasant. Several of the tests are intrusive procedures that are uncomfortable and embarrassing, which results in added stress for the patient. Representatives from the radiology department or laboratory may assume responsibility for instructing patients about diagnostic tests, because the tests are usually performed on an outpatient basis. Most institutions also have printed educational material for the patient and family. It remains the nurse's responsibility to meet the educational and psychologic needs of the patient by answering questions concerning the test procedure, rationale for its use, and specific test preparation in a caring manner. Diagnostic tests are sequenced to make the most effective use of time and equipment. The nurse ensures that the patient is prepared physically and mentally to avoid the preventable repetition of time-consuming and expensive tests.

Laboratory tests

Numerous tests may be used as part of the evaluation of GI, biliary, and exocrine pancreas function.[1] Major blood and urine tests that may be ordered are summarized in Table 31-5.

TABLE 31-5 Major Gastrointestinal, Biliary, and Exocrine Pancreas Blood and Urine Tests

Blood Test	Reference Interval	Description and Purpose
Stomach		
Stomach gastrin (fasting serum)	0-100 pg/ml (0-1 mg/L)	Gastrin is a gastric hormone that is a powerful stimulus for gastric acid secretion. Elevated levels are found in those with pernicious anemia and Zollinger-Ellison syndrome.
Helicobacter pylori	None	*Helicobacter pylori* detected in serum is a highly sensitive but less specific indicator of an active infection; *H. pylori* infection predisposes to peptic ulcer disease.
Biliary System		
Total bilirubin	0.3 to 1 mg/dl	Bilirubin is excreted in the bile. Obstruction in the biliary tract contributes primarily to a rise in conjugated (direct) values.
Conjugated (direct)	0.1-0.4 mg/dl	
Alkaline phosphatase	35-150 U/L	Alkaline phosphatase is found in many tissues with high concentrations in bone, liver, and biliary tract epithelium. Obstructive biliary tract disease and carcinoma may cause significant elevations.
Pancreas		
Amylase	25-125 U/L	Amylase is secreted normally by the acinar cells of the pancreas. Damage to these cells or obstruction of the pancreatic duct causes the enzyme to be absorbed into the blood in significant quantities. It is a sensitive yet nonspecific test for pancreatic disease.
Lipase	10-140 U/L	Lipase is a pancreatic enzyme normally secreted into the duodenum. It appears in the blood when damage occurs to the acinar cells. It is a specific test for pancreatic disease.
Calcium	8.4-10.6 mg/dl	Calcium levels may be low in cases of severe pancreatitis or steatorrhea, because calcium soaps are formed from the sequestration of calcium by fat necrosis.
Intestine		
Total protein (albumin/globulin)	Total protein: 6-8 g/dl Albumin: 3.5-5.5 g/dl Globulin: Alpha$_1$ 0.2-0.4 g/dl Alpha$_2$ 0.5-0.9 g/dl Beta 0.6-1.1 g/dl Gamma 0.7-1.7 g/dl	Although primarily a reflection of liver function, serum protein level is also a measure of nutrition. Malnourished patients have greatly decreased levels of serum protein.
D-xylose absorption test	Blood levels of 25-40 mg/dl 2 hr after ingestion	D-xylose is a monosaccharide that is easily absorbed by the normal intestine but not metabolized by the body. It does not require biliary or pancreatic function. D-xylose is administered orally and assists in the diagnosis of malabsorption.
Lactose tolerance test	Rise in blood glucose level of >20 mg/dl	An oral dose of lactose is administered. In the absence of intestinal lactase, the lactose is neither broken down nor absorbed and plasma glucose levels do not rise. The test assists in the diagnosis of lactose intolerance.
Carcinoembryonic antigen (CEA)		CEA is a protein normally present in fetal gut tissue. It is typically elevated in persons with colorectal tumors. Although not useful as a screening tool, it is useful in determining prognosis and response to therapy.

Continued

TABLE 31-5 Major Gastrointestinal, Biliary, and Exocrine Pancreas Blood and Urine Tests—cont'd

Blood Test	Reference Interval	Description and Purpose
Urine		
5-hydroxyindoleacetic acid (5-HIAA)		Carcinoid tumors are serotonin secreting and are derived from neuroectoderm tissue. This neurohormone is metabolized to 5-HIAA by the liver and excreted in the urine.
Quantitative	<5 ng/ml 2-6 mg/24 h	
Qualitative	Negative	
Urine bilirubin	Negative	Bilirubin is not normally excreted in the urine. Biliary stricture, inflammation, or stones may cause its presence.
Urobilinogen	0.5-4 mg/24h	A sensitive test for hepatic or biliary disease. Decreased levels are seen in those with biliary obstruction and pancreatic cancer.
Urine amylase	<17 U/h	A rise in level usually mimics the rise in serum amylase. However, the level remains elevated for 7-10 days, which allows for retrospective diagnosis.

TABLE 31-6 Interpretation of Feces Color

Color	Interpretation
White	Barium
Gray, tan (clay)	Lack of bile, biliary obstruction
Red	Lower GI bleeding
Black	
Tarry	Rapid peristalsis with bile present
Dry	Upper GI bleeding
Green	Rapid peristalsis with bile present

NOTE: Stool color may also vary in response to food intake and artificial colors in foods. For example beets may cause red stool, and licorice green-black stool.
GI, Gastrointestinal.

Stool Examination

Stool specimens are collected for culture, determination of fat content, and examination for the presence of ova, parasites, and fresh or occult blood.[9] Special collection procedures may be necessary to enhance the identification of bacteria (*Salmonella, Shigella,* and *Staphylococcus aureus*), ova, and parasites. A fresh, warm stool specimen is optimal for laboratory analysis.

Fecal urobilinogen is responsible for the brown color of the stool. Biliary obstruction may cause decreased amounts to be present and turns the stool light or clay colored. These specimens should also be sent promptly to the laboratory because urobilinogen breaks down rapidly. Table 31-6 identifies other fecal color changes that may occur.

Detection of occult blood in the stool is useful in identifying bleeding in the GI tract. Occult blood may be identified by one of three tests: guaiac (Hemoccult), benzidine, or orthotoluidine (Occultest). The guaiac test is the least sensitive test and is often used to determine whether additional study is indicated. It does not require any special preparation. Meat, poultry, or fish eaten within 3 days before testing can cause a false-positive test as well as aspirin or antiinflammatory drugs taken within 7 days; vitamin C in quantities of greater than 500 mg/day may cause a false-negative test if consumed 3 days before testing with benzidine or orthotoluidine. Determination of fecal fat may be done as part of a workup for malabsorption. Elevations in fecal fat will be present with biliary or pancreatic obstructions and many intestinal malabsorption disorders.

Radiologic Tests

Visualization of the GI tract may be performed by barium swallow, upper GI series, or barium enema. Barium is a radiopaque substance that, when ingested or given by enema, outlines the passageways of the GI tract for viewing by fluoroscopy or x-ray films.

Nursing responsibilities commonly involve cleansing of the GI tract with enemas and laxatives. It is important for the nurse to monitor the patient's fluid and electrolyte status because extensive bowel cleansing may cause significant fluid losses, particularly in elderly persons. The nurse should provide psychologic support to the patient because the procedures can be intrusive and uncomfortable. The nurse must also address the educational needs of the patient, explaining the procedure, the rationale for use, and procedural steps, which will assist in reducing anxiety.

Upper Gastrointestinal Series

An upper GI series involves visualization of the esophagus, stomach, duodenum, and upper jejunum through the use of a contrast medium. It is a fluoroscopic x-ray test that permits the examination of the structure, position, peristaltic activity, and motility of the organs. It can assist in the detection of tumors, ulceration, inflammation, abnormal anatomy, or malposition. The upper GI series used to be the foundation of a diagnostic workup for many GI disorders, but the ready availability of endoscopy has now relegated the test to a seldom used status.

An upper GI series involves swallowing the contrast medium (usually barium), which is prepared in a flavored milk shake form. The barium is unpleasant tasting and may cause vomiting. It is administered cold. The barium outlines the structures as it flows by gravity through the esophagus and stomach into the intestinal loops. Films are taken at intervals during the test, and the entire test takes about 45 minutes. The procedure is termed a barium swallow if only the function of the esophagus is to be evaluated and takes about 15 minutes. If the small bowel is the primary focus of the test, it may be termed a small bowel series. No special preparation is necessary before a GI series; however, the patient maintains nothing-by-mouth (NPO) status for at least 6 hours before the test. After an upper GI series, the patient is prescribed a laxative to hasten elimination of the barium; barium that remains in the colon may become hard and difficult to expel, leading to fecal impaction. The stool should return to its normal color (barium is white) after the barium is expelled.

Barium Enema

A barium enema clearly outlines most of the large intestine through the use of a contrast medium. It is used to detect colon polyps, tumors, and chronic inflammatory bowel disease. If both an upper GI series and a barium enema are to be performed, the barium enema is done first, before barium from the upper GI series reaches the colon.

The procedure involves the instillation of barium through a rectal tube with an inflatable balloon to hold the barium in the colon. The patient is then placed in various positions while the radiologist observes on a monitor as the barium flows through the colon. The procedure takes about 30 minutes, and the instillation and retention of the barium can cause the patient considerable embarrassment and discomfort.

Preparation for a barium enema involves thorough cleansing of the bowel by laxatives, enemas, or both. Thorough preparation is essential because retained fecal material obscures the normal bowel anatomy. The patient may be asked to restrict dairy products, follow a liquid diet for 24 hours before the test, and remain NPO for at least 8 hours before the test. Laxatives are frequently administered after the test to facilitate the removal of the barium. The stools may be white tinged for several days. Inpatients are closely monitored for complications after the test, such as perforation of the bowel. Outpatients are instructed to report the development of abdominal pain and to monitor carefully for constipation.

Ultrasonography

Ultrasonography involves the use of high-frequency sound waves that are transmitted into the abdomen and create echoes that vary with tissue density. The echoes bounce back to a transducer and are electronically converted into pictorial images of the organs. This reveals organ size, shape, and position and is extremely useful in diagnosing cysts, tumors, and stones. Ultrasonography has gradually become the procedure of choice for diagnosing gallbladder disease because it does not expose the patient to radiation. The procedure is both painless and safe.

Patient preparation is straightforward. The patient remains NPO for 8 to 12 hours before the test, because gas in the bowel may interfere with the results. If the gallbladder is the focus of the test, the patient is instructed to eat a low-fat meal the evening before the test so that bile will accumulate in the gallbladder, thereby enhancing visualization. The patient resumes a normal diet and activity after the test.

Computed Tomography

Computed tomography (CT) can also be used to assess patients with gallbladder, biliary ductal system, or pancreatic problems. It is helpful in identifying problems similar to those described for ultrasonography. Multiple x-rays are passed through the abdomen. A computer reconstructs the data into two-dimensional images on a television screen. Still photographs can also be taken of the images. Contrast medium can be used with the CT scan to better visualize the biliary tract or to accentuate differences in tissue density of the pancreas. The test is comparable to ultrasonography in effectiveness. It is used less often because of its significantly higher cost and moderate radiation exposure for the patient. It is extremely useful with obese individuals, however, because increased tissue density limits the effectiveness of ultrasound transmission.

The patient should remain NPO for 8 to 12 hours before the test. If contrast medium is to be used, the patient should be assessed for allergies to iodine, seafood, or contrast medium. Barium studies, if necessary, should be done at least 4 days before CT scan or after the scan, because the barium can interfere with test results. There are no special after-care considerations. The patient may resume pretest diet and activity.

Radionuclide Imaging

GI scintigraphy may be used to localize the site of GI bleeding. Endoscopy provides excellent visualization of gastric or esophageal bleeding, but other areas of the GI tract are much more difficult to visualize and pinpoint. An intravenous injection of ^{99m}Tc sulfur colloid is administered. Pooling of the radionuclide will occur at the bleeding site. No pretest preparation is required, and no discomfort is experienced. Patients in unstable condition may not be candidates for this test if they are unable to travel safely to the nuclear medicine department for the 30 minutes required for the test.

Cholecystography

Oral cholecystography involves the radiographic examination of the gallbladder after the administration of a contrast medium. A normal liver will remove radiopaque drugs, such as iodoalphionic acid (Priodax), iopanoic acid (Telepaque), and iodipamide methylglucamine (Cholografin Meglumine), from the bloodstream and store and concentrate them in the gallbladder. The dye-filled gallbladder shows on x-ray examination as a dense shadow. If no shadow is seen, this indicates a nonfunctioning gallbladder. Stones, which are not radiopaque, show as dark patches on the film. Ultrasonography has largely replaced this once commonly used test in the diagnosis of gallbladder disease. Cholecystography is primarily used today when the ultrasound picture is inconclusive.

Patient preparation involves instruction to eat a fat-free meal the evening before the test. The radiopaque substance (usually iopanoic acid) is administered orally 2 to 3 hours after the evening meal. The dose is based on body weight, and the tablets are administered one at a time at 5- to 10-minute intervals with several swallows of water after each pill. The patient then maintains NPO status until the test. The patient is carefully assessed for allergies to contrast dyes, seafood, or iodine.

Cholangiography

Cholangiography involves x-ray examination of the bile ducts to confirm the presence of stones, strictures, or tumors. The radiopaque substance may be administered intravenously or injected directly into the common bile duct with a needle or catheter during surgery or endoscopy. After surgery on the common bile duct, a radiopaque drug such as iodipamide methylglucamine is instilled through a drainage tube such as the T tube to determine the patency of the duct before the tube is removed (T tube cholangiography). The dye also may be injected through the skin and abdominal wall directly into a bile duct within the main substance of the liver (percutaneous transhepatic cholangiography). The technique is useful in visualizing the location and extent of a pathologic process, such as obstructive jaundice, and permits decompression of the liver. Complications from the test are rare, but include bile leakage leading to bile peritonitis or bleeding caused by accidental rupture of a blood vessel.

The patient remains NPO for about 8 hours before the test. The injection of the contrast medium may cause temporary pain or a feeling of pressure or epigastric fullness. The patient is carefully monitored for bleeding or adverse reactions to the dye. Vital signs are monitored, and the patient typically rests in bed for about 6 hours after the test, lying on the right side as much as possible. The needle insertion site is carefully monitored for signs of bleeding or infection.

Special Tests

Esophageal Function Tests

Several diagnostic tests may be used to evaluate the functioning of the esophagus and aid in the diagnosis of esophageal reflux or motility problems. These tests can be performed by having the patient swallow two or three tiny tubes that are attached to an external transducer. Once the tubes are located in the stomach, they are slowly pulled back into the distal esophagus at varying levels. Lower esophageal sphincter pressure, swallowing activity, pH, and effectiveness of clearance can all be measured in about 30 to 45 minutes. However, 24-hour pH monitoring may be performed because it is considered the “gold standard” for the accurate diagnosis of esophageal reflux.

In preparation for these tests, it is important to provide the following instructions to the patient: (1) remain NPO for 8 hours before the procedure(s), (2) avoid alcohol and smoking the day before, and (3) do not take medications such as antacids, H_2-receptor antagonists, proton pump inhibitors and anticholinergics before the test(s). Sedation is not required but may be used if the patient experiences persistent choking or gagging during the procedure. After removal of the tubes, a mild sore throat is common.

Manometry. This test is used to measure the pressure in the lower esophageal sphincter and record the duration and sequence of peristaltic movements within the esophagus. Readings are taken at various levels in the esophagus with the patient at rest and during swallowing. Baseline sphincter pressure is normally about 20 mm Hg. The test is used primarily to diagnose esophageal reflux, but the graphic record of muscular activity during swallowing may also help document the presence of achalasia or esophageal spasm.

pH Monitoring. This test evaluates the competency of the lower esophageal sphincter (LES) by obtaining a single measurement of the esophageal pH. An electrode is placed above the LES and attached to a manometry catheter. Normally, the esophagus maintains a pH of more than 6.0. Serial measurements may be obtained by maintaining the electrode in place for 24 hours. The probe must be inserted transnasally and connected to a recording box similar to a Holter monitor that is worn about the waist. The patient can then be monitored at home while eating a normal diet; 24-hour pH monitoring is the most sensitive and specific diagnostic test for the presence of abnormal acid reflux.

Esophageal Clearance Test. In conjunction with the previous two tests, esophageal clearance tests evaluate the function of both the upper and lower esophageal sphincters along with the body of the esophagus in response to swallowing. Normally, esophageal function allows for the complete clearance of acid material from the esophagus in less than 10 swallows. Readings are recorded from the catheter tip to determine the rate and efficiency of acid clearance.

Acid Perfusion Test (Bernstein Test). Confusion surrounding the origin of heartburn symptoms is often resolved with the Bernstein test, which attempts to reproduce the pain. Small quantities of HCl are instilled into the distal esophagus by nasogastric tube. The test is positive if the acid produces pain. Saline is instilled to rinse out the acid, and an antacid may be administered to relieve the discomfort.

Tests of Gastric Function

Gastric Analysis (Basal Gastric Secretion and Gastric Acid Stimulation Tests). Examination of the fasting contents of the stomach may be helpful in establishing a diagnosis of gastric disease. The purpose is to quantify gastric acidity in the fasting and stimulated states. Abnormal secretion may be related to ulcers, malignancy, pernicious anemia, or Zollinger-Ellison syndrome. A nasogastric tube is inserted, and gastric contents are aspirated. Gastric contents may then be aspirated every 15 minutes for 90 minutes.

The patient is instructed to restrict food, fluid, and smoking for 8 to 12 hours before the test. The flow of gastric acid is then stimulated by betazole hydrochloride, histamine phosphate, or pentagastrin given subcutaneously. The person may experience side effects from the medication, including flushing, a feeling of warmth, slight headache, or itching. Epinephrine is given to counteract the effects of histamine if sensitivity occurs.

Tubeless Gastric Analysis (Diagnex Blue Test). Tubeless gastric analysis may be used for detection of gastric achlorhydria.

The test will indicate the presence or absence of free hydrochloric acid but cannot be used to determine the amount of free hydrochloric acid that is present. A gastric stimulant such as caffeine is given and then a cation exchange resin containing azure A is given orally an hour later. If free hydrochloric acid is present in the stomach, introduction of the resin will cause a substance to be released in the stomach that will be absorbed from the small intestine and excreted by the kidneys as blue dye within 2 hours. Absence of detectable amounts of blue dye in the urine indicates that free hydrochloric acid probably was not secreted.

Schilling Test. The Schilling test evaluates vitamin B_{12} absorption. In the normal GI tract, vitamin B_{12} combines with the intrinsic factor that is produced by the parietal cells in the gastric mucosa and is absorbed in the distal portion of the ileum. Pernicious anemia develops if intrinsic factor is lacking or malabsorption exists. This is a concern in patients who have had the terminal ileum removed for diseases such as Crohn's disease.

The patient is kept NPO for 8 to 12 hours before the test and then administered an oral preparation of radioactive vitamin B_{12}, followed by an intramuscular injection of nonradioactive vitamin B_{12} to saturate the tissue-binding sites. Urinary B_{12} levels are measured after urine is collected for 24 to 48 hours. With normal absorption of vitamin B_{12}, the ileum absorbs more vitamin B_{12} than the body needs and excretes the excess into the urine. With impaired absorption of vitamin B_{12}, little or no vitamin B_{12} is excreted into the urine. Intrinsic factor preparations may also be administered to differentiate intestinal problems from pernicious anemia.

Urea Breath Test. Testing for *H. pylori* has been both technically difficult and expensive. The urea breath test (UBT) is based on the principle that the *H. pylori* organism is able to produce large amounts of urease, a surface enzyme that catalyzes the urea in gastric secretions into bicarbonate and ammonia. Patients are administered an oral solution of carbon isotope-labeled urea in water. If *H. pylori* is present in the stomach the urea is metabolized. The labeled bicarbonate is excreted in the form of labeled carbon dioxide, which can be collected and measured. The patient exhales into a balloon or other receptacle, and the carbon dioxide is measured with a scintillation counter. The sample can be collected 20 minutes after the solution is ingested. The test has minimal risks associated with radioactivity and is estimated to be 97% sensitive for *H. pylori* and 100% specific.

Biopsy

Upper Gastrointestinal Biopsy. A biopsy of the oral cavity or tongue may be done on any lesion or ulcerated area that requires a differential diagnosis. This procedure is usually performed with a local anesthetic. After the biopsy, the biopsy site is assessed for bleeding. Biopsy of the stomach is typically performed during fiberoptic endoscopy.

Intestinal Biopsy. Biopsy of the small or large bowel may also be performed during the course of endoscopic examination to allow tissue analysis of lesions, polyps, or masses. A knife blade or snare is typically used to obtain the tissue sample. The procedure is not usually painful, although a feeling of pressure may be experienced. Bleeding from the site of the biopsy is uncommon. If bleeding does occur, the patient is instructed to report this to the physician and to curtail physical activity until examined by a physician.

Endoscopy

Endoscopy allows for direct visualization of portions of the GI tract by means of a long, flexible, fiberoptic scope (Figure 31-10). Images are seen through an eyepiece or projected onto a video screen. The remote control tip moves in multiple directions. Endoscopy may be used for direct inspection, biopsy and removal of polyps and stones. In addition, GI bleeding may be controlled endoscopically through laser, photocoagulation, or the injection of sclerosing agents. The upper GI tract may be visualized as far as the duodenum by insertion of a fiberscope through the mouth. A fiberscope inserted through the rectum is used for visualization of the rectum (proctoscopy), sigmoid colon (sigmoidoscopy), or the entire colon (colonoscopy).

Today most endoscopic procedures are performed on an ambulatory basis, even with the elderly. Oral fiberscope insertion is uncomfortable and may precipitate gagging or choking despite the use of topical anesthetic sprays or gargles. Premedication with an IV sedative such as midazolam (Versed) or diazepam (Valium) or an analgesic such as meperidine (Demerol) is used. Thus the patient is conscious but sedated; amnesia is often experienced when high doses of these drugs are used.

Esophagogastroduodenoscopy. Upper GI endoscopy may be limited to the esophagus (esophagoscopy), stomach (gastroscopy), or duodenum (duodenoscopy); or it may involve examination of the entire region (esophagogastroduodenoscopy [EGD]) (Figure 31-11). It is particularly useful for identifying the source of upper GI bleeding and for differentiating gastric malignancies from benign ulcers, and gastric ulcers from duodenal ulcers. Other uses include visualization of

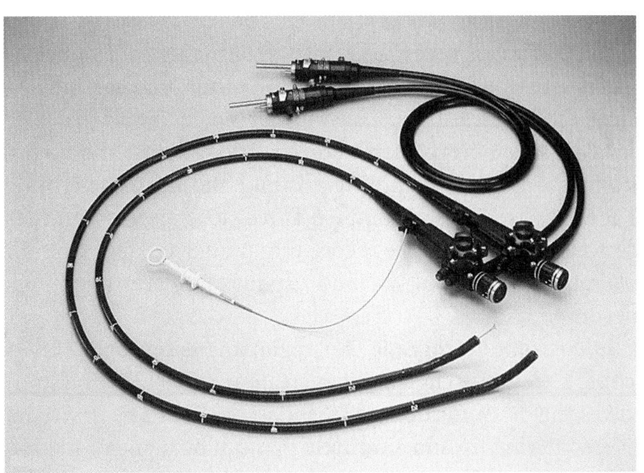

Figure 31-10 Flexible colon fiberscopes.

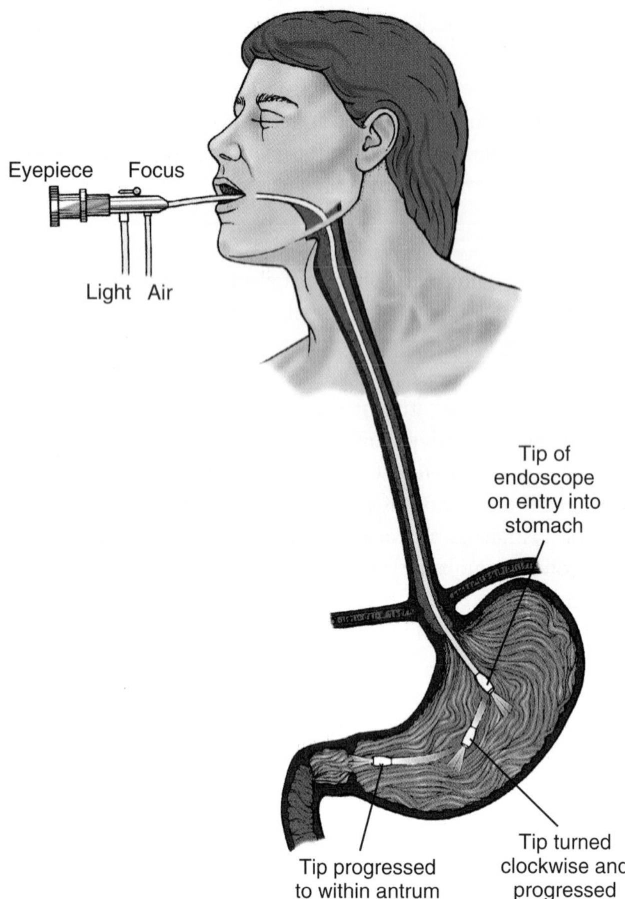

Figure 31-11 Flexible endoscope shown passing through the mouth and the esophagus to the stomach. Dotted lines show how the endoscope is moved to allow visualization of all areas of the stomach.

esophageal strictures, varices, tumors, achalasia, and hiatal hernias; and surgical removal of gastric polyps.[3]

Preparation for an EGD involves instructing the patient to remain NPO for 8 hours before the test. Because air is typically introduced as the endoscope is advanced to improve visibility, the patient should be told that a feeling of pressure or fullness will likely be experienced. The entire test lasts about 15 to 30 minutes unless additional treatments are planned.

After the procedure the patient is monitored carefully for signs of dyspnea, pain, bleeding, or acute dysphagia. Vital signs are taken every 30 minutes for 3 to 4 hours, and no oral food or fluids are administered until the nurse determines that the gag reflex is fully intact. Throat lozenges or saline gargles may be used to relieve sore throat after the test. Complications are rare but include aspiration, perforation, and bleeding.

Endoscopic Retrograde Cholangiopancreatography. Endoscopic retrograde cholangiopancreatography (ERCP) also involves the oral insertion of an endoscope, but this device has a side-viewing tip and a cannula that can be maneuvered into the ampulla of Vater (Figure 31-12). Dye may be injected to outline the pancreatic and biliary ducts. The procedure may be combined with papillotomy to enlarge the sphincter and

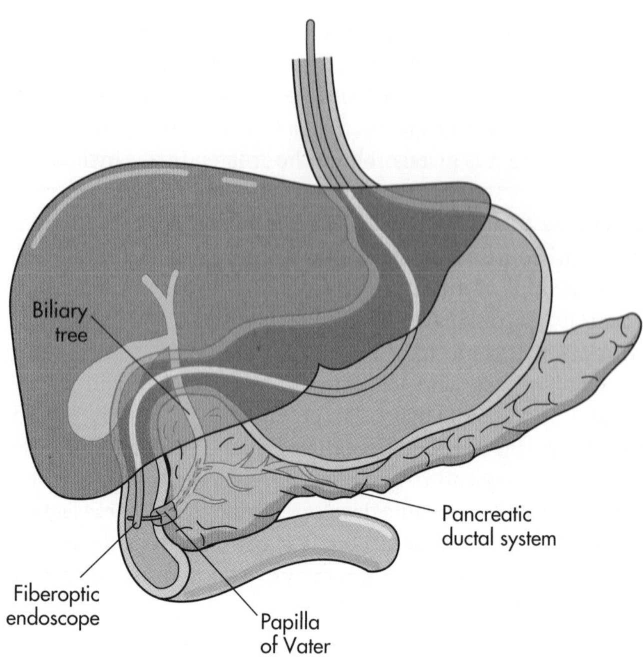

Figure 31-12 Endoscopic retrograde cholangiopancreatography (ERCP).

release gallstones. Glucagon may be administered to minimize spasm in the duodenum and sphincter.

Care after the procedure is similar to that previously described for an EGD. The patient is monitored carefully for signs of abdominal pain, nausea, and vomiting, which might indicate the development of pancreatitis.

Colonoscopy. Fiberoptic colonoscopy allows the examination of the entire colon in most patients. It is used to evaluate benign and malignant growths, remove polyps, take biopsy specimens, and localize sites of bleeding. A colonoscopy is the current "gold standard" for diagnosing colorectal cancers.[4] Screening colonoscopies for colorectal cancer are recommended after age 50.

Thorough bowel preparation is essential before the test, which is especially difficult for elderly persons. A 1-day preparation with an oral osmotic solution is now standard because it reduces overall fluid and electrolyte loss. A gallon of polyethylene glycol (Colyte) solution is administered rapidly (8 ounces every 15 minutes) and induces a profuse watery diarrhea within 30 to 60 minutes, which lasts about 4 hours. In some cases, the patient may receive a 2- to 3-day preparation consisting of a clear liquid diet, strong laxatives, and an enema the day of the test. All patients are NPO for about 8 hours before the test.

Patients are sedated before the colonoscopy. The fiberoptic colonoscope, which is 105 to 185 cm (42 to 72 inches) long, is advanced through the colon and the colon is visualized simultaneously. Air is introduced as the colonoscope is inserted to increase visualization of the mucosa. The air commonly causes abdominal cramping. The procedure lasts from 20 to 60 minutes.

Afterward the nurse assumes responsibility for carefully monitoring the patient and ensuring full recovery from sedation. Any changes in vital signs or development of severe abdominal pain, rectal bleeding, or fever should be immediately reported to the physician. In addition, arrangements for transportation home are important because the patient should not drive.

Sigmoidoscopy may be performed rather than colonoscopy. The cost of a sigmoidoscopy is considerably less than a colonoscopy but only allows for visualization of the anus, rectum, and distal sigmoid colon.[5] Approximately 75% of all polyps and tumors of the large intestine can be visualized with a flexible sigmoidoscope. Pretest preparation instructions vary widely. The patient may be instructed to prepare with a 2-day clear liquid diet and pretest fasting. Fleet enemas may be ordered, or a cleansing enema may be preferred. The knee-chest position and a strong urge to defecate that is produced by the larger-diameter sigmoidoscope make this an uncomfortable and unpopular procedure for patients. Sedation is not usually used. Aftercare involves monitoring for distention, increased tenderness, and bleeding. The patient may initially pass large amounts of flatus from the instillation of air during the procedure. Slight rectal bleeding may occur if biopsies have been taken.

References

1. Bates J, Saver B: Finger-stick vs laboratory serological testing for *H. pylori* antibody, *J Fam Pract* 49(3):205, 2000.
2. Chene BL, Decker AP: Battling hepatitis C, *RN* 64(4):54, 2001.
3. Flynn CA: The evaluation and treatment of adults with gastroesophageal reflux disease, *J Fam Pract* 50(1):57, 2001.
4. Griffith S, Kane K: What is the most cost-effective screening regimen for colon cancer? *J Fam Pract* 50(1):13, 2001.
5. http://www.acs.org
6. Jarvis C: *Physical examination and health assessment,* ed 3, Philadelphia, 2000, WB Saunders.
7. Mattice C: When assessing the abdomen: look, listen, feel, *RN* 64(2):79, 2001.
8. Metules TJ: ACE inhibitors may cause abdominal pain, *RN* 64(3):77, 2001.
9. Weber TS: When are stool cultures indicated for hospitalized patients with diarrhea not caused by *Clostridium difficile* (*C-diff*)? *J Fam Pract* 50(4):300, 2001.

http://www.mosby.com/MERLIN/medsurg_phipps

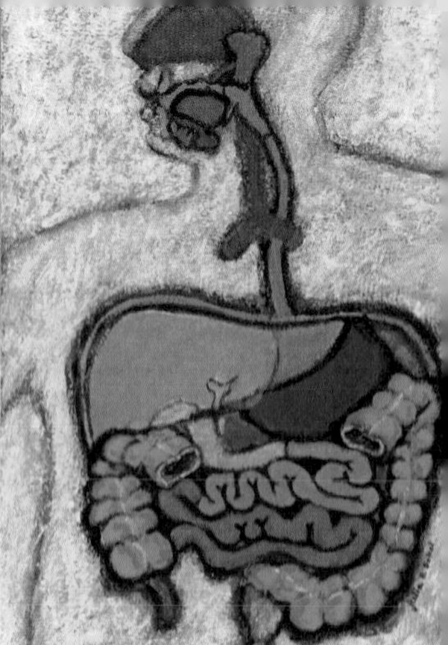

32 Mouth and Esophagus Problems

Judith K. Sands

Objectives

After studying this chapter, the learner should be able to:

1. Describe lifestyle modifications for the prevention of common oral and esophageal disorders.
2. Discuss the pathophysiology underlying common problems of the mouth and esophagus.
3. List the major clinical manifestations of common oral and esophageal disorders.
4. Discuss the collaborative care management of common problems of the mouth and esophagus.
5. Use the nursing process to describe nursing care of patients with major esophageal disorders.

Problems involving the mouth and esophagus include a number of common disorders that affect millions of adults. The majority of the disorders are managed by the individual in the home and rarely involve admission to the acute care setting. The nurse's role includes patient and family education directed toward prevention and health promotion, as well as self-care management.

PROBLEMS OF THE MOUTH

TOOTH AND GUM DISEASE

Progressive tooth loss used to be considered a virtually inevitable consequence of aging. Advances in our understanding of dental health and new approaches to tooth maintenance have changed these perspectives substantially, and the preservation of natural teeth is now a primary goal. This heavy emphasis on prevention is clearly reflected in the Healthy People 2010 goals for oral health (see Healthy People 2010 box).

Etiology/Epidemiology

Tooth decay is by far the most common problem affecting the teeth. Plaque formation is the most important factor in tooth decay, but familial tendency, poor oral hygiene, poor health, and perhaps a diet high in simple or refined sugars also play a role.

The periodontium is the tissue that surrounds and supports the teeth. Disease of the peridontium is the most common cause of tooth loss in adults after age 50. At any time, an estimated 25% to 75% of the adult population with natural teeth have some evidence of the disease. Bacterial plaque is again the most important contributor to the problem, but dental malocclusion, caries, dietary deficiencies, and systemic diseases such as diabetes may also play a role.

Pathophysiology

Dental plaque is a soft colorless mass composed of proliferating bacteria that adheres to the teeth. Acids produced by these bacteria slowly destroy the enamel and dentin of the teeth creating cavities, which are the visible evidence of decay. Food, particularly carbohydrates, stimulates bacterial acid production. Simple sugars have the greatest effect. Plaque begins to collect on the teeth within 2 hours of eating, and the more frequently carbohydrates are ingested, the longer it takes for the pH of the mouth to return to normal.

Gingivitis, the earliest form of periodontal disease, is characterized by reddened gums, swelling, and easy bleeding. Inflammation causes the gingivae to separate from the tooth surface and pockets form that can collect bacteria, food particles, and pus. Progressive gingivitis can result in receding gums, resorption of alveolar bone, and loosening of the teeth (Figure 32-1). Bleeding of the gums with normal tooth brushing is a common early sign. There is usually no pain.

Collaborative Care Management

Prevention is the most appropriate management strategy for both dental decay and periodontal disease. It should start in childhood and continue throughout life. Widespread fluoridation of water supplies has significantly decreased the incidence of tooth decay. Fluoride makes tooth enamel more resistant to acids and is widely available in toothpastes, dental rinses, and mouthwashes. Fluoride may also be applied in concentrated forms by a dentist. Sealants and bonding preparations are routinely applied in childhood to increase tooth resistance to decay.

Healthy People 2010

Objectives Related to Oral Health

GOAL

Prevent and control oral and craniofacial diseases, conditions and injuries and improve access to related services.

1. Reduce the proportion of children, adolescents, and adults with untreated dental decay.
2. Increase the proportion of adults who have never had a permanent tooth extracted because of dental caries or periodontal disease.
3. Reduce the proportion of older adults who have had all their natural teeth extracted.
4. Reduce periodontal disease.
5. Increase the proportion of the U.S. population served by community water systems with optimally fluoridated water.
6. Increase the proportion of adults and long-term care residents who use the oral health system each year.
7. Increase the proportion of local health departments and community-based centers, including community migrant, and homeless health centers, that have an oral health component.
8. Increase the number of states and the District of Columbia that have an oral and craniofacial health surveillance system.
9. Increase the number of tribal, state (including the District of Columbia), and local health agencies that serve jurisdictions of 250,000 or more persons that have in place an effective public dental health program directed by a dental professional with public health training.

From US Department of Health and Human Services: *Healthy people 2010: understanding and improving health,* Washington, DC, 2000, USDHHS.

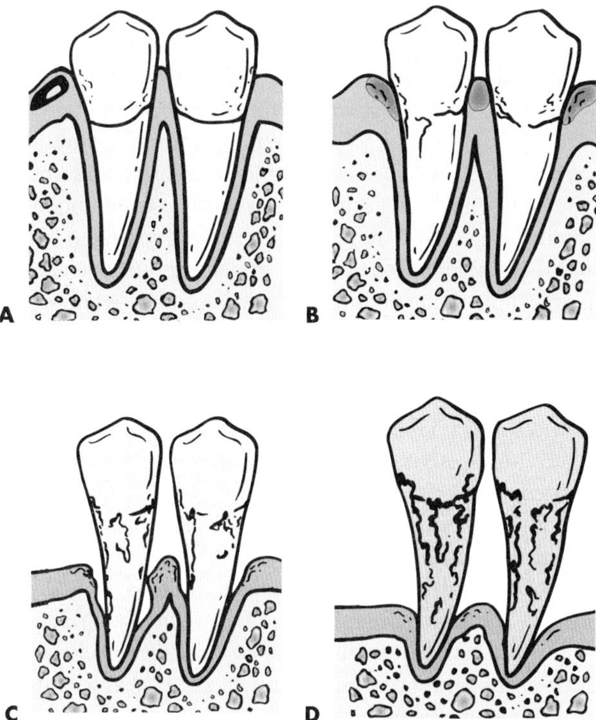

Figure 32-1 The progression of periodontal disease. **A**, Calculus (calcification of dental plaque) deposited on teeth at gum line. **B**, Gingivae become swollen and tender. **C**, Inflammation spreads, pockets develop between gums and gingivae, and gums recede. **D**, Alveolar bone is destroyed and teeth loosen.

Treatment of periodontal disease routinely includes the removal of decayed tooth structures and their replacement with restorative barriers. The presence of progressive gingivitis may require aggressive measures such as scaling or root planing to control or correct the problem. If control is not possible the individual may face the need for tooth extraction and the fitting of dentures.

Patient/Family Education. Good oral hygiene with frequent brushing and regular flossing is the mainstay of prevention for tooth and gum disease, and health care providers should take every opportunity to reinforce this principle and instruct individuals in correct techniques. Regular checkups and professional cleaning facilitate early identification and intervention. Restricting the amount of simple sugar in the diet is a standard recommendation, and adequate or supplemental vitamin C is believed to reduce plaque. It is increasingly recognized that access to affordable dental care is a significant obstacle to the achievement of public health goals related to oral health.

MOUTH INFECTIONS

Any of the structures of the mouth may develop infection, and the presence of infection can seriously affect the individual's ability to eat and drink.

Etiology/Epidemiology

A wide variety of primary oral infections can develop triggered by various bacteria and viruses. Oral infections may also occur secondary to vitamin deficiencies, other systemic diseases or treatments, or in response to local trauma or stress. Common examples include the following infections.

Aphthous stomatitis (canker sore) produces well-circumscribed ulcers on the soft tissues of the mouth, including the lips, tongue, insides of the cheeks, pharynx, and soft palate. The lesions are acutely painful but noncontagious and are of uncertain, although perhaps autoimmune, origin. Aphthous ulcers are a chronic problem. They affect 17% of the population and usually first appear in the teenage years. Healing usually occurs in 1 to 3 weeks.

Herpes simplex is a viral infection that produces characteristic blisters referred to as cold sores or fever blisters. The virus is usually acquired in early childhood, and it is estimated that as much as 80% of the adult population may be infected. The virus is harbored in a dormant state by cells in the sensory nerve ganglia. Reactivation of the virus can occur with emotional stress, fever, or exposure to cold or ultraviolet light. The lesions typically appear on the mucocutaneous border junction of the lips in the form of small vesicles, which then erupt and form painful, shallow ulcers.

Acute necrotizing ulcerative gingivitis, also called trench mouth, is an acute inflammatory gum disease caused by a tremendous proliferation of normal mouth flora, such as spirochetes and fusiform bacilli. It is commonly triggered by poor oral hygiene, nutritional deficiencies, alcoholism, infection, or immunocompromise. The disease is not infectious.

Candidiasis (thrush) is caused by an increase in the number of *Candida albicans,* a yeastlike fungus normally found in the gastrointestinal (GI) tract, vagina, oral cavity, and on the skin. Overgrowth of the organism may result from antibiotic depletion of normal flora or immunosuppression from steroid therapy, chemotherapy, or human immunodeficiency virus infection. The condition is painful and, if widespread, can interfere with oral nutrition.

Parotitis is an inflammation of the salivary or parotid glands. The viral infection known as mumps occurs primarily in the pediatric population, although it can occur in unimmunized adults. Acute bacterial parotitis typically occurs in debilitated or elderly patients in whom poor oral hygiene, dehydration, minimal oral intake, or medications have resulted in chronic dry mouth.

As the natural secretions diminish, bacteria invade the gland. The causative organism is often *Staphylococcus,* and the infection may be serious. Sudden-onset pain and acute swelling occur, and the infection can become chronic and recurrent. An acute form of the inflammation can also occur in postoperative patients as surgical mumps.

Pathophysiology

Most of the infectious diseases of the mouth have similar signs and symptoms. The mucosa throughout the mouth is thin, and evolving vesicles and bullae break open rapidly forming ulcers. These ulcers may be further traumatized by the teeth and can readily become infected by the abundant oral flora. Many of the causative organisms are the same as those that cause common skin infections. Clinical manifestations of common disorders are summarized in Table 32-1.

Collaborative Care Management

Most oral infections are self-limiting and will heal spontaneously without the need for direct intervention. Supportive or palliative care includes brushing and flossing, rinsing with mouthwashes, and diet modification to reduce irritation.

Patient/Family Education. Teaching is directed at self-care management because virtually all mouth infections are treated at home. The proper use of antibiotics, rinses, and anesthetic ointments is discussed, as well as the importance of maintaining regular oral hygiene despite discomfort. Herpes virus lesions can be spread by direct contact to other areas of the body, as well as to others, and the importance of good hand washing is stressed. The patient is also provided with specific information about symptoms that indicate complications requiring medical intervention.

CANCER OF THE MOUTH

Etiology/Epidemiology

Cancer may develop on the lips, tongue, palate, floor of the mouth, or other portions of the oral cavity. With the exception of cancer of the tongue, the development of oral cancer is clearly linked to a history of smoking and alcohol consumption, and the risk increases with heavy use.[13] It has proven to be difficult to separate the unique effects of smoking and alcohol use, but their combined effects are theorized to cause a breakdown in the body's defense mechanisms as evidenced by a decrease in immunoglobulin A levels. The role of viruses, particularly the herpes viruses, is also being thoroughly researched. The precise etiology of oral cancer remains unknown, and the etiologic factors discussed are theorized to act as co-carcinogens with as yet unidentified primary factors.

Oral cancers account for approximately 4% of cancers in men, 2% of cancers in women, and 3.5% of cancers overall.[16] More than 90% of these cancers occur in persons over 45 years

TABLE 32-1 Mouth Infections

Infection	Clinical Manifestations	Collaborative Management
Aphthous stomatitis (canker sore)	Painful, small mucosal ulcerations occurring anywhere in the oral cavity; heal in 1-3 weeks	Palliative: mouthwashes, hydrocortisone-antibiotic ointment; fluocinonide (Lidex) ointment in Orabase
Herpes simplex stomatitis (cold sore, fever blister)	Painful vesicles and ulcerations of mouth, lips, or edge of nose; may have prodromal itching or burning; fever, malaise, lymphadenopathy may occur	Palliative: mouthwashes, fluids, soft diet, topical or systemic acyclovir (Zovirax) in severe cases
Acute necrotizing ulcerative gingivitis (trench mouth)	Painful hemorrhagic gums with ulceration, foul mouth odor, fever, lymphadenopathy	Oral antibiotics, analgesics, topical hydrogen peroxide, good oral hygiene, referral to dentist for removal of plaque or tartar
Candidiasis (thrush)	Creamy white, curdlike patches closely adherent to mucosa; mucosa bleeds and ulcerates when patches scraped off; condition is painful	Oral nystatin, ketoconazole, clotrimazole; amphotericin B for the immunocompromised person
Parotitis	Fever, swelling, and pain in the glands with an abrupt onset	Local heat and cold, frequent oral hygiene, adequate hydration; broad-spectrum antibiotics occasionally needed Salivary secretion is stimulated with lozenges, hard candies, and lemon slices

old, and the incidence increases with age. Many oral cancers are believed to be preventable through lifestyle changes (e.g., long-term use of smokeless tobacco is associated with a 50-fold increase in cancers of the cheek and gums).[13] The importance of prevention is reflected in The Healthy People 2010 objectives[22] (see Healthy People 2010 box).

Pathophysiology

The vast majority of oral cancers arise from squamous cells that line the surface oral epithelium; epidermoid, basal cell, and other carcinomas also may occur. The majority of tumors appear on the lateral or ventral surfaces of the tongue. They are often asymptomatic and frequently go unnoticed by the patient. A single lesion is typical.

The tongue has an abundant supply of blood vessels and lymphatic drainage channels, so spread of the cancer to adjacent structures may be rapid. Although frequently curable in the early stages, metastasis has already occurred in 60% of patients at the time of diagnosis and the mortality rate is high.[1] The cure rate for cancer involving the lips, on the other hand, is high, because the lesion is so readily apparent. Early metastasis is rare, although rapid extension to the mandible or floor of the mouth is possible. Tumors of the parotid gland are usually benign, whereas those arising in the submaxillary glands have a high rate of malignancy and tend to grow rapidly. Clinical manifestations of parotid and submaxillary gland tumors may include palpable masses, enlarged lymph nodes, dysphagia, chronic ear pain, or visible lesions.

Red and white mouth lesions are frequently found in smokers who are at risk for oral cancer. The vast majority of these lesions are asymptomatic, and the primary concern is their degree of cancer-causing potential. The term *leukoplakia* refers to white lesions that occur on the mucosa of the cheeks, lips, gingivae, and palate (Figure 32-2). They may take varied forms but are commonly associated with smoking and *Candida* infection. They are more common in men and those more than 60 years old. One classic variety, stomatitis nicotina (also called smokers' patch), is clearly linked to heavy smoking, especially pipe smoking. These grayish-white lesions appear on the palate and are theorized to be related to high heat exposure from the smoke. The lesions disappear if the person stops smoking, and they do not appear to be related to an increased cancer risk unless found on the floor of the mouth. Snuff dippers' lesion is another classic form of leukoplakia. Similar lesions may develop from chronic cheek or lip biting and from friction trauma associated with ill fitting dentures. Erythroplasia or erythroplakia are similar lesions in many respects but are bright red and velvety in appearance. They are associated with a significantly higher risk of cancer and need to be clearly differentiated from inflammatory lesions.[13]

Healthy People 2010

Objectives Related to Oral Cancer

1. Reduce the oropharyngeal cancer death rate from a baseline of 3 per 100,000 to 2.7 per 100,000.
2. Increase the proportion of oral and pharyngeal cancers detected at the earliest stage.
3. Increase the proportion of adults who, in the last 12 months, report having had an examination to detect oral and pharyngeal cancers.

From US Department of Health and Human Services: *Healthy people 2010: understanding and improving health,* Washington, DC, 2000, USDHHS.

Collaborative Care Management

Biopsy is the primary diagnostic test used in cases of suspected oral cancer. It may be used to evaluate lymph nodes, leukoplakia or erythroplakia lesions, ulcers, or neck masses that do not resolve spontaneously within 1 to 2 weeks. Ultrasonography is an excellent adjunct for evaluating masses that are close to the surface. Computed tomography scans may be used to evaluate deeper, less defined masses; magnetic resonance imaging is most useful for evaluating deep masses.

Treatment of oral cancer depends on the location and stage of the tumor. Early-stage cancer is usually treated by either radiation or surgery, depending on the size and accessibility of the tumor. More invasive cancers may require both modalities, and advanced oral cancers are treated palliatively. Early lesions are highly curable with radiation if they are confined to the mucosa, and the use of radiation prevents widespread tissue destruction. Radiation may be delivered by external beam or through the insertion of needles or seeds. If both radiation and surgery are planned, the radiation therapy is usually administered after the surgery, because irradiated tissue is more susceptible to infection and breakdown. Care of the patient being treated with radioactive needle implants is summarized in the Guidelines for Safe Practice box.

Several surgical options exist. Confined local excision is possible in some situations, but many of the procedures are radical in nature and involve extensive resection. Examples include partial mandibulectomy, partial (hemiglossectomy) or total (glossectomy) removal of the tongue, and resections of the floor of the mouth or buccal mucosa. Because many oral cancers metastasize early to the cervical lymph nodes, the surgery usually also includes functional or radical neck dissection, with removal of the regional and deep cervical lymph

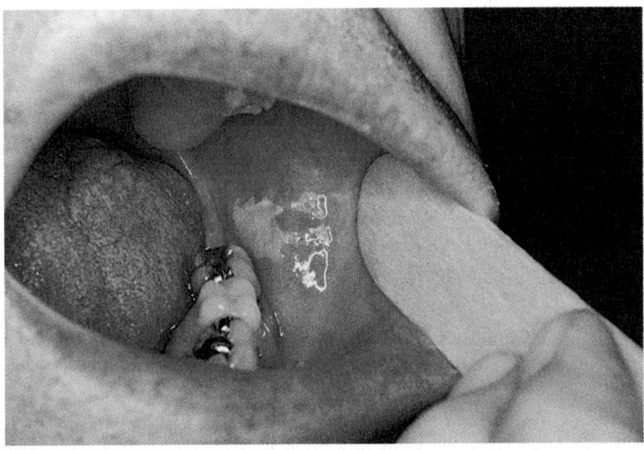

Figure 32-2 Leukoplakia.

nodes and their channels.[5] In advanced cases the surgical procedure may also include removal of the sternocleidomastoid muscle or other neck muscles, internal jugular vein, thyroid gland, submaxillary gland, and spinal accessory nerve. A more complete discussion of radical neck dissection can be found in Chapter 20 in the discussion of laryngeal cancer.

The extent of excision can create significant aesthetic and functional problems for the patient, including problems with speech, chewing and swallowing, and airway management. High-dose radiation therapy commonly causes stomatitis, xerostomia, and dental decay as well as changes in taste, which may be long term. The xerostomia (severe dry mouth) begins 1 to 2 weeks after treatment is started and may persist throughout life. Dental decay, especially at the gingival margins, results from decreased salivary secretion and altered pH of the saliva.

Patient/Family Education. Depending on the aggressiveness of the treatment, the patient may need to acquire significant new self-care skills. Good mouth care is essential to minimize tooth decay and infection, and promote healing. The mouth care regimen may include mouth irrigations or a soft toothbrush and fluoride treatment. Sterile water, dilute peroxide and saline, and bicarbonate solutions are initially prescribed and commercial mouthwashes are avoided.

Adaptations in food consistency and feeding method may be necessary, and the nurse encourages the patient to be independent in feeding as quickly as possible. Privacy is essential during the initial learning period. The patient should not be hurried and is observed carefully to determine how much assistance is needed. Forks are not used, because they may traumatize healing tissues. Both very hot and very cold foods are avoided because they may irritate healing tissue or produce facial pain. Patients are instructed to carefully rinse the mouth with clear water or with a prescribed solution after finishing each meal.

Patients may need to adapt to significant changes in body image and function after treatment for oral cancer. Patients need honest information about the changes to expect and their degree of permanence. Family members are included in all teaching and the nurse encourages them to assist the patient to avoid social isolation. Referrals are made as necessary for speech therapy and ongoing dental care.

Guidelines for Safe Practice

The Patient With Radioactive Needle Implants in Oral Tissue

IMPLANT CARE

1. Do not pull on the strings. Any movement could alter the placement or direction of the radiation or cause the needles to loosen.
2. Check needle patency several times each day.
3. Monitor linens, bed areas, and emesis basin for needles that may dislodge.
4. Ensure that a protective container is present in the room to contain any needles that might dislodge.

PATIENT CARE

1. Assist with gentle oral hygiene q2h while awake.
2. Encourage the patient to avoid hot and cold foods and beverages, as well as smoking.
3. If the patient has dentures, encourage their removal at night for comfort. Assess gums for irritation and bleeding whenever dentures are removed.
4. Provide viscous lidocaine (Xylocaine) solutions or lozenges as needed when oral discomfort interferes with nutrition.
5. Provide the patient with an alternate means of communication; talking around implanted needles is usually difficult or impossible.
6. Assist the patient to implement the mouth care regimen prescribed by the physician.

PROBLEMS OF THE ESOPHAGUS

GASTROESOPHAGEAL REFLUX DISEASE

Etiology

Gastroesophageal reflux disease (GERD) is a heterogeneous syndrome resulting from esophageal reflux. Most cases are attributed to the inappropriate relaxation of the lower esophageal sphincter (LES) in response to an unknown stimulus. Reflux allows gastric and duodenal contents to move back into the distal esophagus. The presence of a hiatal hernia, which displaces the LES into the thorax, was formerly believed to be the primary cause of GERD. However, hiatal hernia has now been found to be a common condition in the adult population and, although most persons with hiatal hernias do experience reflux, the reverse has not been found to be true.[3] A number of environmental and physical factors appear to influence the tone and contractility of the LES, and these may play an etiologic role in some cases of GERD. The pressure of the LES is lowered by fatty foods, chocolate, cola, coffee, and tea; nicotine; drugs such as calcium channel blockers, theophylline, and possibly nonsteroidal antiinflammatory drugs; elevated levels of estrogen and progesterone; and conditions that elevate intraabdominal pressure, such as obesity, pregnancy, or heavy lifting.[15] Population studies of the link between lifestyle factors and reflux, however, continue to provide conflicting results.[3] Genetic factors may also be important. Reflux is much more common after a meal, and more than 60% of reflux sufferers have delayed gastric emptying.

Epidemiology

GERD is a common disorder in all age groups and occasional heartburn is estimated to affect more than 60 million Americans, with 15% to 20% of the population experiencing heartburn at least weekly.[3] Daily symptoms occur in about 10% of the population and treatment costs exceed $1 billion annually.[15,18] It is theorized that the actual incidence of mild disease may be even higher, because many individuals simply accept reflux as an occasional mild problem that can be effectively self-treated. Fewer than 25% of all reflux sufferers ever consult a health care provider about it.[15] There are no documented gender or cultural patterns associated with reflux, but older adults experience decreased esophageal peristalsis and a higher incidence of hiatal hernia, which together increase the likelihood of reflux in this population.

Pathophysiology

Two zones of high pressure, one at each end of the esophagus, normally prevent the reflux of gastric contents. The zones maintain a constant pressure and relax only during swallowing. Although they are termed the upper and lower esophageal sphincters, they are not really distinct anatomic structures. Esophageal reflux occurs when either gastric volume or intraabdominal pressure is elevated or when LES sphincter tone is decreased. Periodic reflux occurs in most persons and is usually asymptomatic.

The normal physiologic response to occasional reflux is immediate swallowing. One or more rapid swallows induce peristaltic contractions to clear the reflux and neutralize the acid with the bicarbonate-rich saliva. However, the esophagus has only a limited ability to withstand the damaging effects of acid reflux, and GERD develops when frequent episodes of reflux break down the mucosal barrier and initiate an inflammatory response.

The degree of esophageal inflammation is related to the number, duration, and acidity or alkalinity of the reflux episodes. The effectiveness and efficiency of esophageal clearance also are important. Esophageal clearance is particularly important at night when the swallowing rate and salivation decrease by two thirds and a recumbent position interferes with clearance. An inflamed esophagus gradually loses its ability to clear refluxed material quickly and efficiently, and the duration of each episode gradually lengthens.

Chronic reflux causes hyperemia and inflammation. Minor capillary bleeding is common, although frank bleeding is rare. Repeated episodes of inflammation and healing can gradually produce a change in the epithelial tissue that makes it more resistant to acid. However, the presence of this new tissue, termed Barrett's epithelium, is also associated with a higher risk of adenocarcinoma.[20] Over time, fibrotic tissue changes can also occur and produce esophageal stricture.

The clinical manifestations of GERD are consistent in their nature, but they vary substantially in severity. The irritation of chronic acid reflux produces the primary symptom of heartburn (pyrosis). The pain is described as a substernal or retrosternal burning sensation that tends to radiate upward and may involve the neck, jaw, or back. The pain typically occurs 20 minutes to 2 hours after eating. An atypical pain pattern that closely mimics angina may also occur and needs to be carefully differentiated from true cardiac disease. The second major symptom of GERD is regurgitation, which is not associated with either belching or nausea. The individual experiences a feeling of warm fluid moving up the throat. If the fluid reaches the pharynx, a sour or bitter taste is perceived. Water brash, a reflex salivary hypersecretion that does not have a bitter taste, occurs less commonly.

In severe cases GERD can produce dysphagia or odynophagia (painful swallowing). Belching and a feeling of flatulence are other common complaints. Nocturnal cough, wheezing, or hoarseness all may occur with reflux, and it is estimated that greater than 80% of adult asthmatics may experience reflux.[10] The frequency and severity of reflux episodes usually determine the severity of the symptoms. The clinical manifestations of GERD are summarized in the Clinical Manifestations box.

Collaborative Care Management

Diagnostic Tests. Mild cases of GERD are diagnosed from the classic symptoms, and treatment is initiated without further diagnostic workup. Millions of people self-diagnose and treat occasional heartburn without consulting a primary care provider. More severe and persistent cases may require other screening tools. The "gold standard" for diagnosis is 24-hour pH monitoring, which accurately records the number, duration, and severity of reflux episodes and is considered to be 85% sensitive. The esophageal motility and Bernstein tests can be performed in conjunction with pH monitoring to evaluate LES competence, quantify reflux episodes, and evaluate the response of the esophagus to acid infusion. These tests are described in more detail in Chapter 31. The barium swallow with fluoroscopy is widely used to document the presence of hiatal hernia, but it can demonstrate only gross reflux disease. Endoscopy is rarely necessary to establish the diagnosis, but it is routinely performed to evaluate the presence and severity of esophagitis and to rule out malignancy.

Medications. Drug therapy is the cornerstone of GERD management, and it usually begins with the occasional use of over-the-counter agents to treat heartburn. Antacids were the mainstay of GERD treatment until the 1980s and are still effective for symptom management in mild disease. Antacids are effective in dealing with occasional heartburn and usually produce prompt relief of symptoms. The choice of antacid is usually based on palatability and patient preference. Alginates may be used as an alternative. Alginates (Gaviscon) combine alginic acid with an antacid, which forms a viscous foam that floats on top of the gastric contents. This theoretically creates a mechanical barrier to reflux and limits acid contact with the mucosa when reflux occurs.

Since their release for over-the-counter purchase, histamine (H_2) receptor antagonists have been heavily marketed as

Clinical Manifestations

Gastroesophageal Reflux Disease

Heartburn: substernal or retrosternal burning sensation that may radiate to the back or jaw
NOTE: In some cases the pain may mimic angina
Regurgitation (not associated with nausea or belching): a sour or bitter taste is perceived in the pharynx
Water brash: reflex hypersecretion of the salivary glands that does not have a bitter taste
Frequent belching, flatulence
Dysphagia or **odynophagia** (difficult or painful swallowing): usually occurs only in severe cases
Nocturnal cough, wheezing, hoarseness

first-line agents for occasional heartburn. Ease of use and absence of side effects have ensured their popularity. Although these drugs do not influence reflux directly, they reduce gastric acid secretion and provide symptomatic improvement. They also support tissue healing, although resolution of esophageal inflammation is exceedingly difficult to achieve and sustain (see Evidence-Based Practice box).

Severe GERD is routinely treated with proton pump inhibitors. A single daily dose decreases acid secretion by 90% to 95% and supports healing within 4 to 6 weeks.[7,19] Mild concern still exists regarding the long-term effects of such complete acid suppression, but these agents have been in use for decades in Europe without evidence of adverse effects.[19] Ongoing use of proton pump inhibitors appears to be necessary to sustain healing in severe cases.

Prokinetic drugs that increase the rate of gastric emptying have always been a logical part of GERD therapy, but both bethanechol (Urecholine) and metoclopramide (Reglan) are associated with multiple side effects that make them inappropriate for long-term use. Cisapride (Propulsid) appeared to be an effective and well-tolerated drug but caused unexpected cardiac problems in follow-up studies and has been withdrawn from the market. New prokinetic agents are currently in development. Drug therapy for GERD is summarized in Table 32-2.

Treatments. There are no specific treatments included in the standard medical plan of care.

Surgical Management. Antireflux surgery is usually performed in patients with severe GERD who do not respond to aggressive medical management. As more is learned about the difficulties in healing esophagitis and the discouragingly high relapse rates, however, the use of surgery is again being explored as an earlier primary intervention for GERD.[11] The question of long-term cost effectiveness is also being raised because it appears that drug therapy must be maintained at high dosage levels almost indefinitely to prevent relapse. The proliferation of laparoscopic techniques for fundoplication is making surgical intervention for GERD an increasingly viable option in the hands of a skilled surgeon[21] (see Research box). The surgical procedures involve fundoplication, the wrapping and suturing of the gastric fundus around the esophagus to reinforce the LES and anchor it below the diaphragm. These

Evidence-Based Practice

Reference: Richter JE et al: Lansoprazole compared with ranitidine for the treatment of nonerosive gastroesophageal reflux disease, *Arch Intern Med* 160(12):1803, 2000.

This study compared the safety and symptom relief efficacy of lansoprazole and ranitidine in the treatment of more than 900 patients with symptomatic reflux disease. Proton pump inhibitors have proven effectiveness in patients with severe erosive disease, but this form is the exception in clinical practice. This study attempted to determine if a benefit is also present in more typical patients who experience frequent heartburn symptoms but do not have endoscopic evidence of esophageal erosion.

Patients who reported moderate to severe heartburn for more than 50% of days in the last 6 months were randomly assigned to one of the two treatment groups. None of the patients had endoscopic evidence of esophageal erosion, and all of them were treated for 8 weeks with recommended doses of each drug.

Patients treated with lansoprazole experienced significantly fewer days and nights with heartburn compared with the group treated with ranitidine. Patients also reported less severe daytime and nighttime heartburn, and required fewer antacids to treat pain during the first weeks of treatment. Treatment-related side effects were rare in both groups.

TABLE 32-2 Common Medications for Gastroesophageal Reflux Disease

Drug	Action	Intervention
Antacids		
Aluminum or magnesium-based product	Neutralize gastric acids	Evaluate effectiveness Monitor frequency of use Monitor for constipation or diarrhea, and assist patient to adjust product use as needed
Antacid Plus Alginic Acid		
Gaviscon	Neutralizes gastric acid; forms viscous foam that prevents reflux or buffers its effects	Same as for antacids
Histamine (H_2) Receptor Antagonists		
Cimetidine (Tagamet) Ranitidine (Zantac) Famotidine (Pepcid) Nizatadine (Axid)	Reduce gastric acid secretion and support tissue healing	Instruct patient to take drugs with meals if ordered at intervals Monitor for common side effects: fatigue, headache, diarrhea
Proton Pump Inhibitors		
Omeprazole (Prilosec) Lansoprazole (Prevacid)	Inhibit enzyme system of gastric parietal cells and suppress gastric acid secretion by more than 90%	Instruct patient to take the drug before meals; monitor for side effects: abdominal cramping, headache, diarrhea

procedures are also used to correct hiatal hernia and are discussed on p. 1012.

Diet. The modification of diet and eating patterns may relieve symptoms in mild GERD. Certain foods have been shown to affect LES pressure, although no studies have proven their role in reflux disease. Fatty foods, cola, coffee, tea, chocolate, onions, tomato-based products, and alcohol all decrease LES pressure and patients are usually encouraged to avoid them. Adequate dietary protein stimulates the release of gastrin and cholecystokinin, which increase LES pressure. Spicy and acidic foods are usually restricted until healing occurs and then may be eaten if they do not produce heartburn. Weight loss and avoidance of overeating may also reduce the frequency of reflux episodes.

Activity. Activities that increase intraabdominal pressure and the likelihood of reflux are restricted. Lifting heavy objects, straining, wearing constrictive clothing, and working in a stooped or bent-over position are all contraindicated.

Referrals. Referrals are rarely necessary for persons with uncomplicated GERD, but the nurse may encourage the patient to seek assistance for weight loss or smoking cessation as indicated.

NURSING MANAGEMENT OF PATIENT WITH GASTROESOPHAGEAL REFLUX DISEASE

ASSESSMENT

Health History

Assessment data to be collected as part of the health history of a patient with GERD include:

Symptoms (onset, duration, severity, precipitating, aggravating, and alleviating factors, other characteristics):
- Heartburn
- Regurgitation or water brash
- Dysphagia and odynophagia
- Belching or flatulence
- Nocturnal cough
- Hoarseness or wheezing—day or night

Diet and meal pattern
- Relationship of symptoms to food intake, meal pattern, and activity
- Use of over-the-counter medications, particularly antacids and H_2-receptor antagonists

Physical Examination

Important aspects of the physical examination of the patient with GERD include:

- Measurement of body weight
- Auscultation of lungs for signs of reflux aspiration

NURSING DIAGNOSES

Nursing diagnoses are determined from analysis of patient data. Nursing diagnoses for the person with GERD may include but are not limited to:

Diagnostic Title	Possible Etiologic Factors
1. Acute pain	Irritation of the esophagus from acid reflux
2. Deficient knowledge	Lifestyle and diet modifications needed to control reflux

EXPECTED PATIENT OUTCOMES

Expected patient outcomes for the patient with GERD may include but are not limited to:

1. Will report few or no episodes of heartburn

2a. Will incorporate lifestyle changes to reduce reflux in daily activities

2b. Will list diet changes that can control reflux

INTERVENTIONS

1. Promoting Comfort

The nurse discusses the medication regimen with the patient and ensures that written information about the safe use and expected side effects of all medications is provided. Proton pump inhibitors are taken once a day before breakfast and rarely induce mild GI side effects. Patients need to be aware of the cost of these drugs, which may be prohibitive without prescription coverage. Adherence to the daily drug regimen is essential to achieve and sustain healing. Antacids may be used on an as-needed basis until the heartburn is controlled.

The nurse also explores the patient's use of other medications. Anticholinergics, calcium channel blockers, xanthine derivatives, and diazepam all appear to lower the LES pressure and may need to be avoided. Their use should be discussed with the primary care provider.

2a. Patient/Family Education

Lifestyle changes have always been the foundation of treatment for GERD. However, few of these recommendations

Research

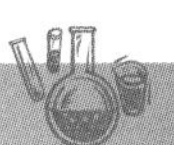

Reference: Rantenen T et al: Functional outcome after laparoscopic or open Nissen fundoplication: a follow-up study, *Arch Surg* 134(3):240, 1999.

This study compared the functional outcomes of a group of about 60 patients with severe symptomatic GERD who underwent laparoscopic or open Nissen fundoplication. Outcomes were evaluated 3 years after surgery.

Interviews were conducted with the patients to determine the incidence, frequency, and severity of heartburn symptoms; the ability to belch and vomit; the degree of gas and bloating; the presence and severity of dysphagia; and the degree of patient satisfaction. The state of the fundic wrap was confirmed by endoscopy.

The study concluded that success in controlling heartburn symptoms was comparable in both groups, with 97% to 100% of patients experiencing mild or no reflux symptoms. The incidence of persistent dysphagia (20%) and excess gas and bloating (>60%) were also comparable in both groups. Temporary dysphagia after the surgery was more common after the laparoscopic surgery. Patient satisfaction scores for both groups were comparable at 3 years after the surgical procedure.

have proven efficacy through research, and it is easy to minimize their value with the development of newer and more potent pharmacologic agents. Because GERD is a chronic disease with a great tendency to relapse, lifestyle modifications continue to offer the potential for improved disease control.

Teaching the patient to elevate the head of the bed 6 to 12 inches for sleep is the highest priority lifestyle change. Nighttime reflux is the most difficult to manage. Wooden blocks used to be recommended, but research has shown that the use of thick foam wedges can also achieve satisfactory results. The nurse must introduce this crucial intervention with tact, because a change affects both the patient and his or her sleeping partner.

Other recommended lifestyle changes include avoiding increases in intraabdominal pressure caused by constrictive clothing, straining, weight lifting, or working in a bent-over or stooped position. Smoking cessation is another critical lifestyle change because smoking causes a rapid and significant drop in LES pressure. Evening smoking, particularly while resting in bed, is of greatest concern, especially when combined with snacking.

2b. Modifying the Diet

The patient is encouraged to reduce consumption of foods that have been shown to lower LES sphincter pressure. A low-fat diet with limited use of caffeine-containing beverages, alcohol, and chocolate is ideal. Adequate protein intake is encouraged for its LES sphincter–enhancing ability. The nurse explores barriers to adherence in the patient's usual diet pattern and involves the family if possible to support needed changes.

Patients are also encouraged to modify their basic meal pattern. Eating four to six small meals a day is recommended. Large meals increase gastric pressure and volume and delay gastric emptying. These factors increase the frequency and severity of reflux episodes. Avoiding evening snacking is particularly important. The patient should not eat for at least 3 hours before bedtime. Nighttime reflux, when both recumbency and inactivity dramatically decrease the effectiveness of esophageal clearance, is a serious problem in GERD that is significantly worsened by evening snacking.

Weight reduction can lower intraabdominal pressure and may reduce the severity of reflux in obese patients. Simple strategies such as eating slowly and chewing thoroughly facilitate digestion and reduce belching. The nurse works with the patient to identify strategies that most effectively reduce the incidence and severity of symptoms.

Recommended diet and lifestyle changes for patients with GERD are summarized in the Patient Teaching box.

Health Promotion/Prevention

Primary prevention does not play a major role in GERD because the condition does not have readily identifiable preventable etiologic factors. Standard preventive measures might include maintaining an optimal body weight and avoiding episodes of overeating, particularly at night. The most significant issue in secondary prevention is the need for health care professionals to directly inquire about a patient's experience with heartburn. Studies have shown that patients rarely report heartburn to their health care provider unless directly asked or until the symptoms have become severe.[3] If identified and recognized early, the disease may be more responsive to treatment.

Patient Teaching

Diet and Lifestyle Modifications to Manage Gastroesophageal Reflux Disease

DIET

Eat 4-6 small meals daily.
Follow a low-fat, adequate-protein diet.
Reduce intake of chocolate, tea, and all foods and beverages that contain caffeine.
Limit or eliminate alcohol intake.
Eat slowly, chew food thoroughly.
Do not eat for 2-3 hr before bedtime.
Remain upright for 1-2 hr after meals when possible; never eat in bed.
Avoid any food that directly produces heartburn.
Reduce body weight if indicated.

LIFESTYLE

Eliminate or reduce smoking.
Avoid evening smoking; never smoke in bed.
Avoid constrictive clothing over the abdomen.
Avoid activities that involve straining, heavy lifting, or working in a bent-over position.
Elevate the head of the bed at least 6-8 inches for sleep.
Never sleep flat in bed.

EVALUATION

To evaluate the effectiveness of nursing interventions, compare patient behaviors with those stated in the expected patient outcomes. Achievement of outcomes is successful if a patient with GERD:

1. Experiences no heartburn episodes.
2a. Adopts specific lifestyle factors that reduce the incidence of reflux.
2b. Knows dietary factors that increase reflux.

GERONTOLOGIC CONSIDERATIONS

Esophageal function continues effectively into advanced age, but some decline in esophageal peristalsis is expected, and a decrease in saliva production impairs the efficiency of esophageal clearance. Even routine reflux becomes protracted and increases the risk of irritation. Elderly individuals need to be assessed for heartburn, because they typically underreport their symptoms. They also appear to be particularly vulnerable to alkaline reflux from the duodenum. Acid combined with bile and pancreatic juice is believed to be more damaging to the mucosa than acid alone. Alkaline reflux typically occurs at night and causes respiratory symptoms such as choking, paroxysmal coughing, and wheezing. Patients with frequent nighttime awakenings from coughing should be evaluated for

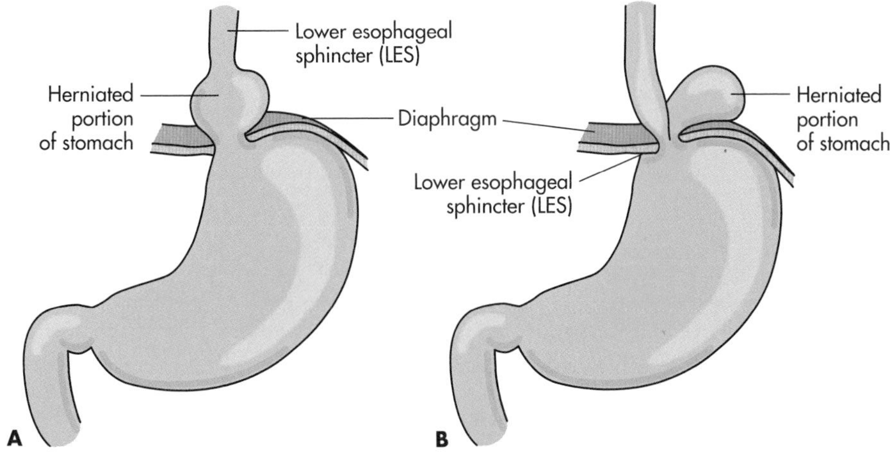

Figure 32-3 Hiatal hernia. **A**, Sliding hernia. **B**, Paraesophageal hernia.

GERD. The risk of aspiration is high. Treatment approaches are the same as those outlined for other forms of GERD.

SPECIAL ENVIRONMENTS FOR CARE

Critical Care

Gastroesophageal reflux disease does not ordinarily require critical care management. Critical care management would be needed only in the case of severe complications such as aspiration pneumonia or hemorrhage.

Community-Based Care

GERD is self-managed almost exclusively in the home. Written instructions are provided about all aspects of the treatment plan to reinforce verbal teaching. The nurse involves the spouse or partner and family where possible, because changes in diet and meal patterns affect the entire family. Major lifestyle changes are not necessary, but even relatively minor changes require planning and support if they are to be successful.

COMPLICATIONS

If GERD is not successfully controlled, it can progress to serious and even life-threatening problems.

Esophageal ulceration and hemorrhage may result from severe erosion, and chronic nighttime reflux is accompanied by a significant risk of aspiration. Adenocarcinoma can develop from the premalignant tissue called Barrett's epithelium. Gradual or repeated scarring can permanently damage esophageal tissue and produce stricture.

HIATAL HERNIA

Etiology

The opening in the diaphragm that allows the esophagus to pass from the thorax to the abdomen is called the esophageal hiatus. Hiatal hernias (also called diaphragmatic hernias) develop when the distal esophagus, and possibly a portion of the stomach, move into the thorax through the hiatus. There are two major types. The first is the sliding hernia, which accounts for 90% of the total.[12] In these hernias the distal esophagus, gastric junction, and often a part of the stomach are simply displaced upward into the thorax (Figure 32-3, *A*). The hernia is freely movable and slides back and forth in response to changes in position or abdominal pressure. Sliding hernias are believed to develop from muscle weakness in the esophageal hiatus. Aging may contribute to the weakness, although a congenital defect, trauma, surgery, or prolonged increases in intraabdominal pressure may also play a role.

The second and relatively unusual form of hiatal hernia is the paraesophageal, or rolling, hernia. The gastric junction remains anchored below the diaphragm, but the fundus of the stomach, and possibly portions or even all of the greater curvature, rolls into the thorax next to the esophagus (Figure 32-3, *B*). An anatomic defect may be the cause, but muscle weakening does not appear to play a major role.

Epidemiology

Hiatal hernias are common in the adult population. Their incidence is roughly estimated at 25% to 30% in the general population and as high as 60% in the over-60 age group.[2] Hiatal hernias affect women much more commonly than men, although their incidence increases in both sexes with aging.

Pathophysiology

Most individuals with hiatal hernias are completely asymptomatic. Development of symptoms is rare before middle age. Hiatal hernias are usually small, but their relative size is not necessarily related to the presence or severity of symptoms.

Sliding hernias cause no functional problems. The symptoms produced are directly related to chronic reflux. Reflux occurs from the exposure of the LES to the low-pressure environment of the thorax where sphincter function is significantly impaired. The clinical manifestations mimic GERD (see Clinical Manifestations box on p. 1007).

Reflux is rarely a concern with paraesophageal hernias, because the LES remains anchored below the diaphragm. However, the anatomic risks of volvulus, strangulation, and obstruction are high. In addition, venous obstruction in the herniated part of the stomach may cause the mucosa to become engorged and ooze. Slow bleeding leads to the development of iron deficiency anemia, but significant bleeding or hemorrhage is rare.

Collaborative Care Management

Diagnostic Tests. Unless acute complications develop, most hiatal hernias are diagnosed as part of a workup for GERD, and the diagnostic tests are similar (see p. 1007). The barium swallow with fluoroscopy is the most useful test. Paraesophageal hernias are usually clearly visible, and sliding hernias can be easily demonstrated when the individual is moved into positions that increase intraabdominal pressure. Additional findings in individuals with paraesophageal hernias may include low hemoglobin and hematocrit levels from chronic low-grade bleeding, which will be evident on routine blood tests.

Medications. Antacids, histamine receptor antagonists, and proton pump inhibitors are used as needed to manage the reflux that may accompany hiatal hernia. See the discussion on p. 1007 under GERD.

Treatments. There are no specific treatments used in the management of hiatal hernia.

Surgical Management. Surgical correction of paraesophageal hernias is mandatory because the risk of serious complications is significant. The surgery consists of straightforward anatomic repair because there is no need to correct or modify LES function.

The repair of sliding hernias is more complex, because simple repair of the defect in the diaphragm rarely corrects the reflux problem. Restoring LES competence becomes a major consideration. Several different surgical procedures exist, but each involves LES reinforcement through fundoplication, or wrapping of the stomach fundus around the LES.

The Nissen fundoplication (Figure 32-4) is the most commonly used procedure. The fundus of the stomach is wrapped a full 360 degrees around the lower esophagus to reinforce the LES. Surgeons traditionally have used both abdominal and thoracic approaches; there are advantages and disadvantages associated with each. The first laparoscopic fundoplication was performed in 1991, and it has rapidly become the surgical treatment of choice for both patients and physicians.[21] A variety of other surgical approaches are in use that involve various degrees of fundoplication, posterior vs. anterior wrapping, and fixation to the diaphragm vs. the abdominal wall for stability. Physician preference plays a major role in the decision.

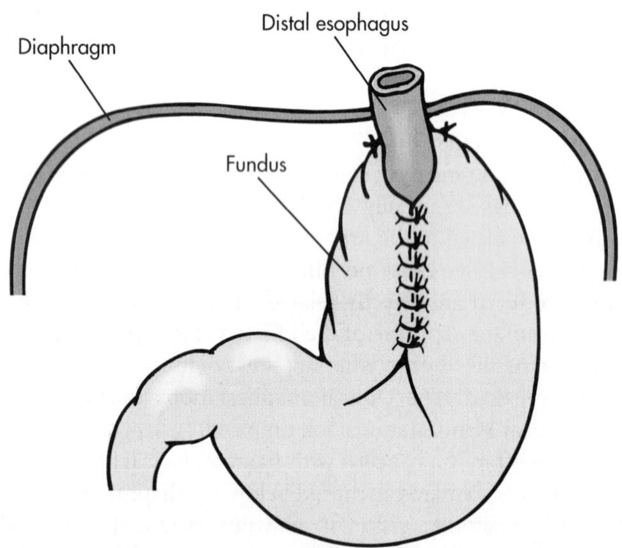

Figure 32-4 Nissen fundoplication for repair of hiatal hernia.

Diet. The recommended diet modifications for hiatal hernia follow the general guidelines outlined in the section on antireflux therapy. The diet also focuses on reducing obesity if possible. Obesity can significantly increase intraabdominal pressure and worsen the severity of both the hernia and the symptoms of reflux.

Activity. Activities that increase intraabdominal pressure and reflux are restricted as discussed under GERD (see p. 1009).

Referrals. Referrals are rarely necessary for the management of hiatal hernia, except possibly to assist the individual with weight loss and smoking cessation, which are critical components in managing reflux.

NURSING MANAGEMENT OF PATIENT WITH HIATAL HERNIA SURGERY

PREOPERATIVE CARE

Preoperative teaching focuses on instructing the patient in deep breathing, the correct use of an incentive spirometer, and splinting the incision effectively for coughing. All surgical approaches involve the diaphragm, and pulmonary hygiene is essential in preventing respiratory complications. The high, long incisions of open procedures make pulmonary hygiene painful, and it is essential to discuss the pain management plan with the patient. If a thoracic approach is used, teaching also includes management of chest tubes. The small incisions, decreased pain, and brief hospital stay associated with laparoscopic fundoplication readily support its popularity with patients.

Individuals who are overweight are encouraged to lose weight if possible before surgery, and smokers are encouraged to significantly reduce or eliminate their use of tobacco. The nurse also teaches about the nasogastric (NG) tube that is inserted during surgery and the planned time frame for resuming oral feedings.

POSTOPERATIVE CARE

Facilitating Airway Clearance

Prevention of respiratory complications is the primary postoperative consideration. The head of the bed is elevated 30 degrees to facilitate lung expansion. The nurse assists the patient out of bed as soon as possible and supports the incision for coughing. Regular lung auscultation, incentive spirometry, and chest physiotherapy are routinely used. Adequate analgesia is essential to the success of the respiratory protocol. It should be provided via patient-controlled analgesia or through aggressive nursing management, particularly before ambulation or chest physiotherapy. Patients with a smoking or pulmonary disease history need to be managed even more aggressively.

Patients treated laparoscopically may remain in the hospital only overnight. Although their pain is usually significantly less than that experienced by patients with major incisions, it is still essential that they be instructed in the importance of frequent deep breathing and effective coughing.

Facilitating Swallowing

A large-diameter NG tube is usually inserted during surgery to prevent the fundoplication from being too tight. The nurse monitors the tube postoperatively for secure anchoring and patency and regularly assesses the drainage, which should consist of normal yellowish-green gastric secretions within the first 8 hours after surgery. It should not contain fresh blood. It is essential that the stomach remain decompressed to prevent vomiting, which could disrupt the fundoplication sutures.

The NG tube is carefully placed by the surgeon and is usually neither moved nor repositioned. Orders concerning irrigation are carefully followed. Sterile solutions are generally preferred for irrigation in the early postoperative period. Frequent oral and nasal hygiene are important for comfort because the large tube is irritating. An NG tube may not be used with the laparoscopic procedures.

The patient is offered oral fluids after peristalsis has been reestablished. Some surgeons prefer to use gastrostomy feedings to facilitate healing, but most patients progress to a near-normal diet within 6 weeks. Temporary dysphagia is almost universal because of the tight wrap around the LES. The food storage area of the stomach is also decreased. The nurse encourages the patient to eat multiple small meals throughout the day, gradually exploring tolerance to different foods and consistencies. Few foods need to be completely restricted. An upright position is also helpful. Support and encouragement during early feeding attempts are essential.

Many patients also experience temporary or persistent gas bloat from a decreased ability to belch as needed.[17] The nurse teaches the patient to avoid carbonated beverages and gas-producing foods. Patients who swallow a lot of air during meals need to eat and drink slowly and chew food thoroughly. Excess air in the stomach that cannot be relieved by belching produces significant abdominal discomfort. Frequent position changes and ambulation are often effective strategies for clearing air from the GI tract.

A Nursing Care Plan for a patient undergoing hiatal hernia repair follows.

Nursing Care Plan — *Patient Undergoing Hiatal Hernia Repair*

DATA Mr. K. is a 56-year-old man with a 5-year history of progressively worsening heartburn. His pain is most severe at night. Recently he began experiencing regurgitation, sometimes consisting of water and sometimes consisting of a sour, acidic fluid. He has self-treated the problem with liquid antacids, which are no longer beneficial. Other than his current problem, Mr. K.'s medical history is unremarkable and he considers himself in good health.

Nursing history revealed that Mr. K.:

- Has abdominal obesity and is 40 pounds overweight.
- Takes aspirin and ibuprofen for headaches, which he feels are due to his stressful job.
- Smokes about one pack of cigarettes per day.
- Is a moderate social drinker.
- Snacks at night while watching television.
- Is anxious about the surgery because this is his first major illness.

After esophageal studies and barium swallow under fluoroscopy, Mr. K. was diagnosed with severe reflux and a large sliding hiatal hernia that shifts into the thorax with minimal position change. His esophagus is inflamed and minimally ulcerated with no signs of cancer. His surgeon recommended surgical repair owing to the size of the hernia and the rapid progression of his symptoms.

Mr. K. was scheduled for hiatal hernia repair via Nissen fundoplication. Collaborative nursing actions before surgery included preparing him for imminent surgery and:

- Clarifying knowledge and expectations concerning surgery.
- Preparing him for expected postoperative care.
- Implementing preoperative orders and providing Mr. K. with support and reassurance.

Mr. K. was returned to his room directly after surgery, which was uneventful and successful. He has an NG tube in place connected to low suction. He is receiving intravenous fluids, cimetidine, and antibiotics. His incision is intact, with a Jackson-Pratt drain. The planned abdominal approach was successful and no chest tubes are in place. He is groggy but alert when addressed by name. He is complaining of incisional pain.

NURSING DIAGNOSIS **Acute pain related to surgical incision**
GOALS/OUTCOMES Will achieve pain free status

NOC Suggested Outcomes
- Pain Level (2102)
- Pain Control (1605)
- Comfort Level (2100)

NIC Suggested Interventions
- Pain Management (1400)
- Analgesic Management (2210)
- Coping Enhancement (5230)

Nursing Interventions/Rationales
- Administer prescribed analgesics to prevent pain from becoming severe. *Analgesics decrease the transmission and perception of pain stimuli.*

Continued

Nursing Care Plan Patient Undergoing Hiatal Hernia Repair—cont'd

- Encourage patient to report pain before it is severe. *Administering pain control medications during the early stages of pain prevents the pain from becoming severe. It is more difficult to control severe pain than moderate pain.*
- Encourage patient to use PCA if prescribed. *Allows patient control over the pain process and the administration of pain medications.*
- Encourage nonpharmacologic measures to reduce pain. *Relaxation, music, and other nonpharmacologic measures minimize pain perception.*

Evaluation Parameters

1. Reports satisfaction with pain control methods
2. Reports pain of 2 or less on a 1 to 5 scale with 5 being severe pain
3. No evidence of pain (facial grimace, withdrawn behavior, complaints of pain)

NURSING DIAGNOSIS **Risk for ineffective airway clearance related to incisional pain, temporarily limited mobility, and history of cigarette smoking**

GOALS/OUTCOMES Patient will remain free of airway compromise

NOC Suggested Outcomes

- Respiratory Status: Airway Patency (0410)
- Aspiration Control (1918)
- Respiratory Status: Gas Exchange (0402)

NIC Suggested Interventions

- Respiratory Monitoring (3350)
- Aspiration Precautions (3200)
- Cough Enhancement (3250)
- Positioning (0840)

Nursing Interventions/Rationales

- Maintain bed in semi-Fowler's position (at least 30 degrees). *Positions diaphragm and lungs in most effective position to facilitate breathing.*
- Perform pulmonary assessment q2-4h and more often as needed. *To detect retained secretions or atelectasis so that treatment can be implemented early.*
- Provide adequate opioid analgesia for incisional pain (or monitor PCA use if prescribed). *Adequate pain control facilitates pulmonary hygiene and mobility.*
- Supervise pulmonary hygiene (incentive spirometry, chest percussion and vibration) at least every 4 hours. *Prevents atelectasis and facilitates expulsion of secretions.*
- Reposition and encourage deep breathing exercises at least every 2 hours. *Movement and position changes facilitate expulsion of secretions and prevent atelectasis.*
- Splint incision for deep breathing exercises, coughing, and position changes. *Splinting of incision controls pain. Pain control facilitates the ability to breathe deeply, cough, and move.*
- Medicate patient ½ hour before ambulating. *Patient will be able to ambulate better if pain is controlled by analgesia before ambulation.*

Evaluation Parameters

1. Maintains clear breath sounds
2. Coughs up secretions (if present)

NURSING DIAGNOSIS **Impaired swallowing related to functional changes of fundoplication surgery**

GOALS/OUTCOMES Patient will remain free of aspiration or choking

NOC Suggested Outcomes

- Swallowing Status (1010)
- Swallowing Status: Esophageal Phase (1011)
- Aspiration Control (1918)

NIC Suggested Interventions

- Surveillance (6650)
- Positioning (0840)
- Aspiration Precautions (3200)

Nursing Interventions/Rationales

- Maintain initial nothing-by-mouth status and monitor for patency of nasogastric tube. *NG tube must remain patent to prevent fluid accumulation in the stomach and vomiting.*
- Do not irrigate or reposition the NG tube. *Stomach must remain decompressed to prevent vomiting.*
- Report fresh blood occurring in drainage after the first 8-hour postoperative period. *Tube movement or vomiting can disrupt sutures and cause fresh bleeding.*
- Offer frequent oral and nasal hygiene. *To increase comfort while the NG tube is in place.*

Nursing Care Plan Patient Undergoing Hiatal Hernia Repair—cont'd

- Initiate feedings with 30 ml of clear liquids after peristalsis is reestablished. *The capacity of the stomach is significantly reduced. Therefore, initial feedings must be smaller volumes until it is tolerated.*
- Evaluate presence and severity of dysphagia. *Fundoplication and reduced stomach capacity make swallowing difficult initially.*
- Advance feedings to multiple small feedings and from liquids to solids as tolerated. *The ability to swallow will improve slowly but steadily.*
- Encourage techniques to prevent gas bloating (chew thoroughly; eat slowly; sit up to eat; avoid air swallowing, use of straws, carbonated beverages, gas-producing foods, and excessive talking while eating). *Fundoplicaton may make belching difficult if not impossible. Retained air and gas can produce significant abdominal discomfort.*
- Ambulate after meals. *To stimulate peristalsis and movement of food and fluids into the intestines.*

Evaluation Parameters

1. Intakes food/fluid without choking or aspiration
2. Progresses from clear liquid to normal diet
3. Does not complain of abdominal discomfort from gas

NURSING DIAGNOSIS **Deficient knowledge of reflux management related to lack of previous exposure or access to resources**

GOALS/OUTCOMES Will accurately describe dietary and lifestyle measures to prevent reflux; participates in self-care measures to prevent reflux

NOC Suggested Outcomes

- Knowledge: Health Resources (1806)
- Knowledge: Diet (1802)
- Knowledge: Disease Process (1803)
- Knowledge: Health Behaviors (1805)

NIC Suggested Interventions

- Teaching: Disease Process (5602)
- Teaching: Prescribed Diet (5614)
- Teaching: Individual (5606)

Nursing Interventions/Rationales

- Teach patient about necessary dietary modifications (low-fat; avoid excess tea, coffee, chocolate, caffeine-containing foods; strictly limit or eliminate alcohol intake; eat 4-6 small meals daily; eat slowly and chew thoroughly; remain in upright position 1-2 hours after eating; avoid eating in bed, nighttime snacking, foods that induce heartburn; reduce overall body weight). *Fundoplication reduces the severity of reflux but does not eliminate it. Foods that lower the LES pressure need to be avoided. Overloading the stomach increases the occurrence of reflux. Reflux is worse at night, so the stomach needs to be empty before retiring for the night.*
- Discuss lifestyle habits that promote reflux (smoking, straining, lifting, stooping, constrictive clothing) and modifications that can help reduce those habits. *Smoking decreases LES pressure significantly and can induce reflux. Heavy lifting and straining increase intraabdominal pressure and reflux. Reflux is more common and severe at night when the patient is in a recumbent position and has a full stomach.*
- Encourage use of antacids for occasional heartburn. *Antacids reduce acid formation and may decrease pain associated with reflux.*
- Encourage patient to report frequent or severe reflux episodes. *Surgical repair rarely eliminates acid reflux completely. Alternative treatments may be necessary.*
- Repeat teaching frequently and provide written information about home care. *Stress interferes with learning. Repetitive teaching enhances learning. Written materials provide a resource for later review as needed.*

Evaluation Parameters

1. Expresses interest in assuming self-care
2. Accurately verbalizes measures to reduce acid reflux
3. Participates in decision making and self-care

GERONTOLOGIC CONSIDERATIONS

Muscle weakness develops in the esophageal hiatus with aging. It is estimated that 60% of the over-60 age group is affected by hiatal hernia.[14] The development of reflux symptoms in older individuals should be investigated and the possibility of hiatal hernia determined. The management, as outlined in the preceding discussion, is applicable to the elderly as well as the younger adult population and the refinement of laparoscopic fundoplication techniques reduces the risk of surgery in this population. Open procedures are associated with an increased risk of surgical complications, particularly respiratory complications and meticulous nursing management is essential.

SPECIAL ENVIRONMENTS FOR CARE

Critical Care

Critical care placement is rarely needed for patients undergoing hiatal hernia repair. However, high-risk patients, particularly older adults, can easily experience complications whenever major surgery is undertaken, particularly if a thoracic approach is used. In addition, although rare, esophageal hemorrhage accounts for up to 7% of all massive upper GI bleeding and can be life threatening.

Community-Based Care

Minimal ongoing care is required after hiatal hernia surgery, but lifting and stair climbing are restricted until healing is complete. Relatively few dietary restrictions are in place at discharge, but the patient should continue to incorporate measures designed to facilitate swallowing, prevent gastric distention, and minimize air retention. Even with successful surgery, reflux may continue to be a problem, and the antireflux diet, medications, and lifestyle modifications may need to be continued. This can be discouraging to the individual who anticipated a complete cure from the procedure.

COMPLICATIONS

Routine complications of hiatal hernia surgery include persistent dysphagia and gas bloat.[17] In some cases esophageal dilation may be necessary to support effective swallowing.

MOTILITY DISORDERS

Motility disorders of the esophagus are conditions in which the normal motor function of the esophagus is disturbed. The disorder may be a primary esophageal problem or secondary to another systemic disease. Selected regions or the entire length of the esophagus may be affected. The classic motility disorder, achalasia, is a failure of the esophageal muscle to relax in synchrony, which can result in mechanical or functional obstruction to food passage. Failure to close adequately after swallowing can also occur, resulting in chronic reflux or regurgitation. Esophageal spasm is a common component of motility disorders, and the spasm is often intense enough to mimic angina. Common neuromuscular disorders that can affect esophageal motility are summarized in Box 32-1.

BOX 32-1 Motility Disorders Resulting in Dysphagia

Primary Esophageal Disorders

Achalasia
Esophageal spasm
Tumor or stricture

Neuromuscular Disorders

Cerebrovascular accident
Multiple sclerosis
Myasthenia gravis
Parkinson's disease
Amyotrophic lateral sclerosis
Muscular dystrophy
Myopathies
Cranial nerve disease or trauma (V, IX, X)

Achalasia

Etiology/Epidemiology

Achalasia is a primary motility disorder of the esophagus in which the lower esophageal muscles and sphincter fail to relax appropriately in response to swallowing. It is characterized clinically by slowly progressive dysphagia and regurgitation of swallowed food. The cause of the disorder is unknown, although a familial link is possible. Achalasia usually develops between 20 and 40 years of age, although it also occurs in both children and older adults.[4] Both sexes are affected about equally, and there appear to be no cultural differences in incidence.

Pathophysiology

Achalasia is theorized to result from a neuromuscular defect in the inner circular muscle layer of the esophagus. Resting pressure in the LES is elevated and the sphincter fails to relax with swallowing. Degeneration and loss of ganglion cells cause a defect in the innervation of the esophagus with resultant aperistalsis.[4] Considerable functional obstruction results and, as the disease progresses, the portion of the esophagus surrounding the constriction becomes dilated and the muscle walls hypertrophy. Although the severity of achalasia varies widely, the obstruction may be so severe that little or no food can enter the stomach. In extreme cases the esophagus may hold 1 L or more of food and fluid above the constricted area. Slowly progressive dysphagia and regurgitation are the classic symptoms. Spasm may be provoked by cold or hot liquids or foods and is often worsened by stress or overeating. Dysphagia is present with both liquids and solid foods. A foul mouth odor from retention of food in the esophagus may become a chronic problem. The classic "rat tail" narrowing is readily observable with barium studies (Figure 32-5). Esophageal manometry reveals an elevated resting LES pressure, combined with diminished or absent peristaltic waves.

Collaborative Care Management

Conservative treatment is usually successful for patients with mild disease. Various categories of medications have been used

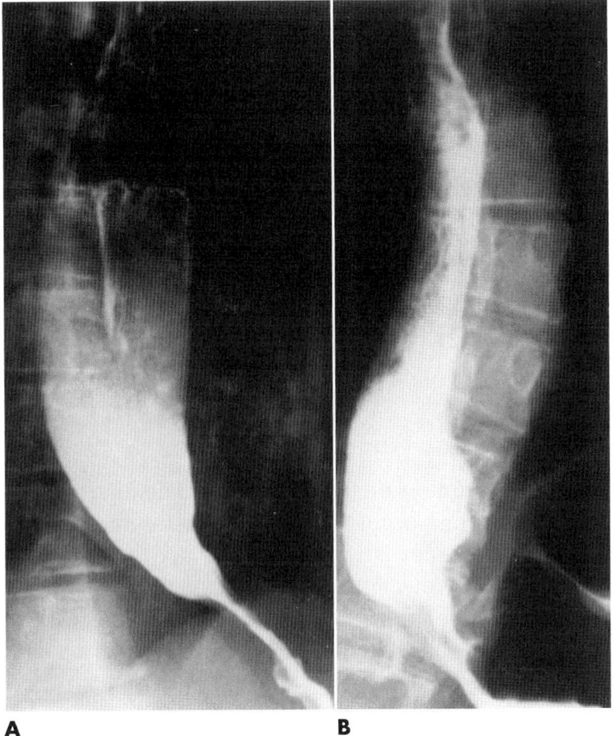

Figure 32-5 A, Achalesia with a narrowed, elongated esophagogastric junction (rat tail sign). B, Widening of the esophagogastric junction in a patient with achalasia after balloon dilation.

to try to lower esophageal pressure and relax the LES. Anticholinergics, sublingual nitrates, and calcium channel blockers have all been used, but none have proven to be consistently valuable or effective.[9] Analgesics may be needed for severe pain.

Esophageal dilation has been a mainstay of treatment for achalasia for centuries. Various techniques have been used, but pneumatic balloon dilation is currently believed to be the most effective.[12] The procedure involves passing polyurethane balloons on a catheter across the lower esophagus and then inflating the balloon to a predetermined volume. The procedure is repeated as needed. Esophageal tearing is the primary concern, and the risk of perforation is small but serious. The success rate is 60% to 85%, and long-term relief is obtained for many patients.[12] Dilation is an outpatient procedure that can be repeated in 2 to 3 months if needed.

Severe unrelieved achalasia may require surgical intervention with esophagomyotomy, which releases the stricture through longitudinal incisions. A success rate of 90% is reported with the surgery, which may involve either a thoracic or abdominal approach. Antireflux fundoplication may be included, based on surgeon preference. Surgery is usually recommended after two or three dilations have failed to provide lasting relief.

Patient/Family Education. Dysphagia is the primary challenge of motility disorders, and the nurse works with the patient and family to explore diet and lifestyle modifications that will best control it. Education begins with careful assessment of the scope and severity of the dysphagia, including:

- Swallowing ability with liquids vs. solids
- Response to foods of differing textures and temperatures
- Variability of the dysphagia (intermittent or constant)
- Response to stress, fatigue, and other activities
- Approaches used by the patient to manage the dysphagia and the degree of success

The nurse encourages the individual to experiment with various types and consistencies of foods and meal sizes to evaluate their influence on swallowing. Small, frequent, semisoft meals that are eaten slowly are usually best tolerated. Warm liquids are recommended, and extremes of temperature should be avoided because they usually worsen the spasm. The nurse also advises the patient to experiment with changing positions during eating. Some individuals can swallow more effectively if they arch their back. Use of the Valsalva's maneuver (bearing down with a closed glottis) while swallowing may help propel food beyond the LES.[8] Nocturnal reflux of retained food and fluid presents a significant risk for aspiration. The nurse instructs the patient to sleep on a foam wedge or with the head of the bed elevated.

ESOPHAGEAL CARCINOMA

Etiology

Both benign and malignant tumors occur in the esophagus. Benign tumors, usually leiomyomas, are extremely rare and usually asymptomatic; they require no intervention unless symptoms necessitate local excision. Malignant tumors of the esophagus are relatively rare but very virulent, with a 5-year survival rate of just 12%.[6]

In the United States alcohol intake and tobacco use have been identified as the primary risk factors for esophageal cancer, and there is a clear dose-response and duration-of-use relationship.[6] Heavy alcohol use increases the risk threefold even without the synergistic effect of smoking, which can drive the incidence to six times that of the rest of the population. The carcinogenic effects are clearly cumulative because the cancer typically appears in persons between 60 and 70 years old. In areas of the world where esophageal cancer is common, the development of the tumor is linked to high levels of nitrosamines and other contaminants in the soil and foods. Diets that are chronically inadequate in fresh fruits, vegetables, and vitamins are also implicated.

Esophageal cancer is extremely common in regions of Asia where none of the major risk factors are applicable (see Risk Factors box). The effects of opium smoking and the practice of consuming extremely hot beverages are also under investigation.

Epidemiology

Despite statistically significant annual increases in the incidence of cancer of the esophagus over the last several decades, particularly among the African-American population, the tumor still accounts for less than 2% of all newly diagnosed cancers and 7% of GI tract cancers in the United States. However, low incidence statistics for esophageal cancer are unique to the United States and the Western world. Localized areas of

Risk Factors
Esophageal Cancer

SQUAMOUS CELL CARCINOMA
Tobacco use
Alcohol use
Dietary nitrates
Poor nutrition
Vitamin deficiency
Mucosal irritants
Ethnicity
  Risk is higher in African-Americans
Sex
  Risk is higher in men

ADENOCARCINOMA
Chronic gastroesophageal reflux disease
Barrett's esophagus
Lack of dietary intake of fresh fruits and vegetables
Ethnicity
  Risk is higher in Caucasians
Sex
  Risk is higher in men

Clinical Manifestations
Esophageal Cancer

Early disease: largely asymptomatic
Gradually progressive dysphagia
  Usually not present until >90% of diameter is obstructed
  Progresses from solids to liquids
  Continuous, not intermittent
Weight loss: up to 40 lb in 2-3 months is common
Odynophagia: typically a steady, dull substernal pain
Regurgitation: foul breath from retained food in esophagus
Heartburn
Anorexia

China, the former Soviet Union, Iran, and southern Africa have such high incidence that 25% of all cancer deaths can be attributed to cancer of the esophagus in some regions.[6]

The disease typically affects men between the ages of 50 and 80 years. It occurs in men four times as often as in women and in African-Americans four times as often as in Caucasians. The most disturbing recent epidemiologic finding has been the steady rise in the incidence of adenocarcinoma, which has previously been rare. This cancer now accounts for between 20% and 40% of all cases and does not appear to be linked to the classic risk factors. It is theorized to arise from Barrett's epithelium, which forms in response to the irritation of chronic reflux.[20]

Cancer of the esophagus is almost always fatal, and this is particularly true in the African-American population. The tumor is theoretically curable in its earliest stage but is rarely diagnosed early enough to allow for effective treatment. Disease is confined to the mucosa or submucosa in less than 10% of cases.

Pathophysiology

Tumors may develop at any point along the length of the esophagus, but the majority occur in the middle and lower two thirds of the esophagus. Squamous cell tumors tend to develop in the middle third and are clearly related to the risk factors of smoking and alcohol use. Adenocarcinomas, believed to evolve from Barrett's epithelium, tend to develop in the lower third of the esophagus.

Barrett's epithelium is an acquired condition. Tissue changes occur in response to acid irritation over a period of months to 1 to 2 years. Barrett's epithelium is typically present for 20 to 30 years before malignant change occurs, but its presence increases the risk of cancer from 30 to 400 times.[20]

Esophageal tumors of all types appear to develop as part of a slow process that begins with benign tissue changes. Local growth of the tumor is rapid, however, and early spread is common because of the rich lymphatic supply found in the esophagus and the absence of a serosal membrane. Tumors are characteristically intraluminal and ulcerating, with a tendency to encircle the esophageal wall, as well as extend up or down the length.

Spread of the carcinoma is by local invasion or through the bloodstream or lymphatics. Neoplasms of the upper and middle esophagus may extend into the pulmonary system and those of the lower esophagus into the diaphragm, vertebrae, or heart. Metastasis is present in about 80% of esophageal cancers at the time of diagnosis.

Ninety percent of the circumference of the esophagus is commonly involved before symptoms develop, and early diagnosis is rare. Tumors of less than 10 cm are considered to be small. Progressive dysphagia and abrupt weight loss are the most common presenting symptoms. Dysphagia begins with solid foods but progresses to include liquids. Pulmonary complications such as fistula formation or aspiration are common, and complete obstruction is inevitable without successful therapy. Common clinical manifestations of esophageal cancer are summarized in the Clinical Manifestations box.

Collaborative Care Management

Diagnostic Tests. Barium swallow with fluoroscopy and endoscopy are the two primary diagnostic tools. The barium swallow clearly outlines large masses and endoscopy allows for direct visual inspection and biopsy for cytologic analysis. Computed tomography may be used to assess for regional and distant metastasis. Endoscopic ultrasound may be used to accurately assess the depth of tumor invasion before treatment decisions are made.

Medications. Primary treatment of esophageal cancer increasingly combines chemotherapy, radiation, and surgery. The use of preoperative chemotherapy alone does not improve survival. Combination therapy is also used for palliation in advanced disease, but quality of life issues are important to consider in treatment decisions.

Treatments. Treatment decisions are based on the location and size of the tumor, degree of metastasis, and the individ-

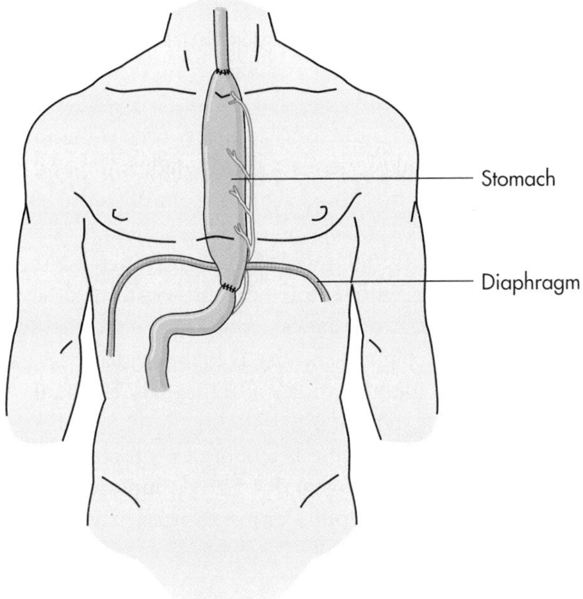

Figure 32-6 Esophagogastrostomy for esophageal cancer.

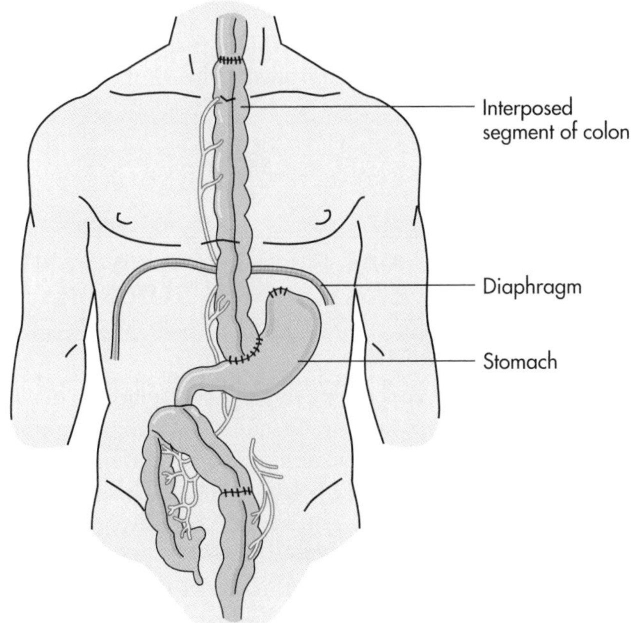

Figure 32-7 Esophagectomy with colon interposition.

ual's health status. Nonsurgical options are usually selected when the individual is unable or unwilling to undergo radical surgery. They focus on palliation of symptoms. Options include radiation therapy, dilation of strictures, and prosthesis insertion, as well as chemotherapy.

Radiation Therapy. External beam radiation is extremely effective in rapidly relieving symptoms of obstruction. It reduces tumor size and gives consistent long-term symptom relief, but it can lead to debilitating stricture or stenosis, because esophageal tissue is extremely sensitive to radiation. The treatment is spread over 6 to 8 weeks to minimize the edema and epithelial desquamation, which often lead to acute esophagitis and odynophagia. Anorexia, nausea, and vomiting may also occur. Combining radiation and chemotherapy is thought to improve the results.

Laser Therapy. Palliative treatment of the tumor may also be accomplished by use of the neodymium:yttrium-aluminum-garnet (nd:YAG) laser, which vaporizes a portion of the tumor to open the esophageal lumen. The treatment is performed endoscopically and offers substantial relief of obstruction in more than 90% of cases.

Dilation. Esophageal dilation is performed as needed throughout therapy to relieve dysphagia resulting from either tumor obstruction or radiation stricture (see the discussion under Achalasia on p. 1017). The beneficial effects are brief, however, and repeated dilations may be necessary. Metal stents are being used successfully to maintain the patency of the esophageal lumen.[6]

Prosthesis Insertion. A semirigid prosthesis can be inserted into the esophagus to bypass an obstruction or fistula. The procedure preserves swallowing and a patent esophagus, but it creates a significant risk of aspiration, dislodgement, or esophageal perforation, which occur in about 20% of those treated. The prosthesis disrupts the function of the LES and permits free reflux of gastric contents.

Surgical Management. Radical surgery is the only definitive treatment for esophageal cancer, and it is the treatment of choice for otherwise healthy individuals with early stage disease. The surgeries are extensive and have a high mortality rate, especially for patients with concurrent health problems. Subtotal or total esophagectomy is usually required. Although several options exist, the preferred surgery is the esophagectomy with either gastric pull through (Figure 32-6) or colonic interposition (Figure 32-7). Colonic interposition is usually necessitated by spread of the tumor into the stomach. The surgeries are complex and may involve either a thoracotomy or laparotomy or both.

In addition to the usual surgical risks of shock, hemorrhage, and infection, these procedures also create a serious risk of leakage at the site of anastomosis, particularly with colon interposition. Anastomosis leakage occurs in up to 20% of cases and operative mortality is about 7%.[6] Even when surgical healing is successful, the patient remains at serious risk for reflux and aspiration from the elimination of the sphincter protection of the LES.

Diet. Maintaining adequate nutrition as the disease progresses is the primary consideration. The diet is modified as needed as dysphagia worsens. Tube or gastrostomy feedings and short-course hyperalimentation may all be needed at some point in the disease process. Malnutrition significantly increases the risk of treatment complications.

Activity. The individual is encouraged to remain as active as the symptoms and treatment allow. Positioning and activity restrictions are important for individuals experiencing frequent reflux or regurgitation. The nurse teaches the patient to remain upright for several hours after meals; to avoid all bending, stooping, and lifting; and to never lie down in a flat position. The head should always be elevated at least 30 to 45 degrees.

Referrals. In some settings the nurse assumes responsibility for making referrals to other services. Nutritional support services are frequently needed. Patients also commonly need significant assistance at home, particularly after radical surgery, and the nurse coordinates these referrals as part of the discharge planning process.

NURSING MANAGEMENT OF PATIENT WITH ESOPHAGECTOMY SURGERY

PREOPERATIVE CARE

The duration of preoperative preparation is largely determined by the patient's nutritional status. Nutritional support is provided as needed via tube feedings or hyperalimentation. Most of this preparation takes place in the home setting. Intake and output, total daily calories, and body weight are all carefully monitored. The nurse encourages the patient to perform frequent mouth care to reduce the risk of postoperative infection, because the patient may be regurgitating retained food particles, blood, or pus from the tumor. Mouthwashes can help control foul mouth odors and make oral intake more palatable. Dental problems are usually corrected before surgery, particularly if adjunctive radiation is planned.

The nurse ensures that the patient and family are knowledgeable about the planned surgery and its expected outcomes. Specific teaching includes the purpose, number, and location of all incisions, lines, and tubes. Wound drainage, chest and NG tubes, and intravenous lines may all be in place. Pulmonary hygiene is a major focus of postoperative care, and the nurse instructs the patient about the importance of turning and deep breathing regimens and other aspects of chest physiotherapy. Practice time is provided. The possibility of temporary ventilator support is also introduced. If a colon interposition procedure is planned, a complete bowel preparation is also completed in the preoperative period.

The nurse encourages the patient to verbalize feelings and concerns related to this extensive surgery. It is natural for the patient to be both extremely anxious and ambivalent about the surgery. Family members are encouraged to be involved in all teaching sessions, and all caregivers should be familiar with the patient's wishes as expressed through advance directives. Quality of life issues are extremely relevant when the prognosis is poor and deserve careful discussion.

POSTOPERATIVE CARE

Protecting the Airway

The patient receives routine but meticulous postoperative care, because the extensive nature of the surgery increases the risk of serious complications. Respiratory care is the highest priority. The patient may remain intubated for the first 24 hours. Respiratory assessment is documented every 1 to 2 hours, and vigorous turning, deep breathing, coughing, and chest physiotherapy routines are initiated. Tracheal suctioning is avoided if possible. Adequate analgesia is essential to the achievement of respiratory goals. The nurse assists the patient to adequately splint major incisions for turning and coughing and ensures that appropriate opioid analgesia is provided, usually through patient-controlled (PCA) or epidural analgesia.

The patient is placed in a semi-Fowler's or high Fowler's position to support ventilation and prevent regurgitation and reflux. Supplemental oxygen is administered, and blood gases or O_2 saturation is monitored. The nurse ensures the patency of the chest tubes and water seal drainage system.

Multiple incisions and drains significantly increase the potential for problems with wound healing. Anastomosis leakage is a serious complication that can compromise the airway and pulmonary gas exchange. The risk is highest 5 to 9 days after surgery. Prompt identification of leakage is essential. The nurse monitors for signs of inflammation, fever, or fluid accumulation. Pulmonary edema is a common problem, and the patient may be kept somewhat dry. Early symptoms of shock, such as tachycardia, tachypnea, or restlessness, may be the first warning signs.

Promoting Adequate Nutrition

The patient is usually allowed nothing by mouth for 4 to 5 days until GI motility is fully reestablished, and frequent oral hygiene is provided to improve patient comfort. The NG tube is carefully secured and monitored to prevent movement or dislodgement, which might disrupt the sutures at the anastomosis sites. The tube is not routinely irrigated or repositioned. The initial NG drainage is bloody, but it should gradually resume a normal greenish-yellow color by the end of the first postoperative day. The continued presence of blood usually indicates oozing at the anastomosis.

After this initial period of stabilization, the patient is given 3 to 5 ml of water every 15 to 30 minutes throughout the day. The quantity is gradually increased as tolerated. The nurse supervises the patient during all initial swallowing efforts and ensures that an upright position is maintained. The NG tube remains in place while oral fluids are introduced because esophageal tissue is friable and bleeds easily. The surgical area needs to remain decompressed to protect the anastomoses.

Nutritional support is essential in the postoperative period, particularly if the patient was severely dysphagic before surgery and losing weight. Adequate nutrition is also critical for effective wound healing, particularly if radiation or chemotherapy has been used or is planned. Nutrition has also been found to be an important element in supporting effective ventilator weaning and preventing nosocomial infection. Nutrition support includes attention to an adequate calorie and protein intake. Serum albumin levels should remain above 3.5.

The patient is slowly progressed to a pureed or semisolid diet if problems do not develop. The nurse assists the patient to carefully determine the amount and type of foods and fluids that can be safely and comfortably swallowed. Small meals are essential because the food storage area of the stomach is drastically reduced. Initially patients may experience a feeling of fullness in the chest or shortness of breath with meals. Adjusting meal size and eating slowly usually alleviates these problems. The process of gradually resuming oral nutrition continues into the postdischarge period and requires patience. Calorie counts and daily weights assist in the ongoing evaluation of the patient's nutritional status. The nurse also stresses the importance of eating only in an upright sitting position because the loss of the LES leaves the patient continually vulnerable to reflux aspiration.

Promoting Coping

Despite the radical surgery, the patient with esophageal cancer still has a potentially terminal illness and dramatically shortened life expectancy. Considerable psychologic support is needed by the patient and family in their efforts to cope with the prognosis and physical limitations of the disease. Realistic planning is important, because the patient's condition will inevitably worsen. The nurse encourages the patient and family to talk about the situation together, make realistic plans, and seek out supports available in the community.

Guidelines for care of the patient undergoing esophagectomy are summarized in the Guidelines for Safe Practice box.

GERONTOLOGIC CONSIDERATIONS

Cancer of the esophagus is usually identified in late middle age or in the older population. These patients have a high incidence of chronic health problems, which increase the risk of radical surgery. Postoperative complications are more common and more severe. Older adults are also less likely to have family and support networks to help them manage their care after discharge. The nurse must be vigilant in assessing the need for postdischarge assistance and initiating needed referrals.

SPECIAL ENVIRONMENTS FOR CARE

Critical Care

The radical surgery performed to treat cancer of the esophagus carries an extremely high risk of complications, particularly if the patient is frail and has chronic diseases affecting the cardiovascular or pulmonary systems. Critical care placement may be necessary while the patient is intubated and ventilated or for close monitoring of hemodynamic stability. It may also be needed if the patient experiences anastomosis leakage in the postoperative period.

Community-Based Care

Most patients with cancer of the esophagus require a significant amount of assistance after discharge. Even without major postoperative complications, the patient will need to deal with ongoing respiratory care, wound healing concerns, and nutritional support. The care initiated in the hospital continues after discharge, and both the patient and family need to be well informed about its components. Essential concerns include pulmonary hygiene, which may include chest physiotherapy. Any surgery that removes or disrupts the LES necessitates precautions with positioning to protect the airway and prevent reflux or regurgitation. No anatomic protection remains, and the risk of aspiration is high and constant. Wound healing also remains a concern, and the incisions need to be inspected regularly for signs of infection. Nutritional recovery is ongoing. The patient and family will slowly explore the patient's range of food tolerance to meet nutrient needs. Home preparations of milk shakes or other supplements may be used to support nutrient intake. The family may also need to learn to manage

Guidelines for Safe Practice

The Patient Undergoing Esophagectomy

PREOPERATIVE CARE

1. Encourage improved nutritional status
   a. High-protein, high-calorie diet if oral intake is possible
   b. Tube feedings or total parenteral nutrition may be necessary for severe dysphagia or obstruction
2. Assist with frequent oral hygiene to minimize breath odor
3. Teach appropriate techniques for effective deep breathing and coughing and the importance of frequent pulmonary hygiene; have patient demonstrate respiratory exercises and how to splint the incision for coughing
4. Teach patient about all tubes and drains that will be used postop and how surgical pain will be managed

POSTOPERATIVE CARE

1. Promote good pulmonary ventilation
   a. Hourly deep breathing and coughing if needed
   b. Incentive spirometry and chest physical therapy as ordered
   c. Auscultate lung fields q2h (avoid tracheal suctioning if possible)
2. Maintain chest drainage system as prescribed
3. Provide for adequate analgesia by PCA or epidural catheter; monitor respiratory and neurological response
4. Maintain gastric drainage system
   a. Small amounts of blood may drain from nasogastric tube for 6 to 12 hr after surgery
   b. Do not disturb nasogastric tube (to prevent traction on suture line)
5. Maintain nutrition
   a. Start clear fluids at frequent intervals when oral intake is permitted
   b. Introduce soft foods gradually, and slowly progress to several small meals of bland foods
6. Prevent aspiration if LES is removed or disrupted
   a. Always raise the head of the bed for swallowing food or liquid
   b. Head of the bed must be elevated for sleeping
   c. Bending or stooping should be avoided
   d. Keep suction apparatus available at the bedside

PCA, Patient-controlled analgesia; *LES*, lower esophageal sphincter.

tube feedings or hyperalimentation. The nurse encourages the family to seek out and use supports such as those available from the American Cancer Society and makes referral to community home care agencies as needed. Hospice referrals may be appropriate for patients needing palliative care.

COMPLICATIONS

Esophageal cancer is commonly a terminal illness, and complications are expected. Tumor regrowth may cause recurrent dysphagia and obstruction, and dilation may be required. Weight loss may persist. The high risk of aspiration from regurgitation makes pulmonary complications common. Tumor regrowth, invasion, and metastasis can create problems with chronic pain, bleeding, and fistula development.

Critical Thinking Questions

1. A 79-year-old woman has come to the medical clinic with a 6-month history of heartburn, which has been steadily increasing in both frequency and severity. She also reports frequent regurgitation of acidic fluid into the mouth. She has self-medicated with antacids and H_2 blockers, but they are no longer controlling the discomfort. She is 5 feet 4 inches tall and weighs 180 pounds. She is an avid gardener and spends long hours weeding and pruning. She laughs as you ask her to put on a gown for a physical examination, saying that it will take a few moments to get out of her corset.
   a. *What specific factors in her presentation will you target to teach her how to better control esophageal reflux?*
   b. *What other data do you need to improve your understanding of her situation?*
2. A 33-year-old mother of five has come to the clinic for a prenatal examination for her sixth pregnancy. She is a single mother on Medicaid and does not have family in the area. As part of the oral examination you note that her teeth are in poor repair, her gums are reddened and receding, and there is a smoker's patch leukoplakia on the dorsal surface of her tongue plus an ulcer on her inner cheek near a broken tooth.
   a. *What specific assessment data do you need to complete your understanding of this situation?*
   b. *Review the Healthy People 2010 guidelines for oral health. What services are available in your community, and which services might be lacking to enable a patient such as this one to meet those goals?*
3. Design a nursing research study to evaluate the effectiveness of the lifestyle modifications recommended for patients with GERD.
4. Lobbying efforts are underway to allow proton pump inhibitors to be sold over the counter because of their excellent safety record. What would be the major advantages and disadvantages of such a policy decision?

References

1. Armstrong WB, Giglio MF: Is this lump in the neck anything to worry about? *Postgrad Med* 104(3):63, 1998.
2. Boyce GA, Boyce HW: Esophagus: anatomy and structural anomalies. In Yamada T, editor: *Textbook of gastroenterology,* ed 3, Philadelphia, 1999, JB Lippincott.
3. Castell DO: A practical approach to heartburn, *Hosp Pract* 34(12):89, 1999.
4. Castell DO, Katz PO: Approach to the patient with dysphagia and odynophagia. In Yamada T, editor: *Textbook of gastroenterology,* ed 3, Philadelphia, 1999, JB Lippincott.
5. Correa AJ, Burkey BB: Current options in management of head and neck cancer patients, *Med Clin North Am* 83(1):235, 1999.
6. Fox JR, Kuwada SK: Today's approach to esophageal cancer: what is the role of the primary care physician? *Postgrad Med* 107(5):109, 2000.
7. Galmiche JP, Letessier E, Scarpignato C: Treatment of gastro-oesophageal reflux disease in adults, *BMJ* 36(7146):1720, 1998.
8. Galvan TJ: Dysphagia: going down and staying down, *Am J Nurs* 101(1):37, 2001.
9. Goroll AH: Evaluation of dysphagia and suspected esophageal chest pain. In Goroll AH, Mulley AG, editors: *Primary care medicine,* ed 4, Philadelphia, 2000, JB Lippincott.
10. Harding SM, Guzzo MR, Richter JE: The prevalence of gastro-esophageal reflux in asthma patients without reflux symptoms, *Am J Respir Crit Care Med* 162:34, 2000.
11. Isolauri JK et al: Long-term comparison of antireflux surgery versus conservative therapy for reflux esophagitis, *Ann Surg* 225(3):295, 1997.
12. Kahrilas PJ: Motility disorders of the esophagus. In Yamada T, editor: *Textbook of gastroenterology,* ed 3, Philadelphia, 1999, JB Lippincott.
13. Kelly JP: Screening for oral cancer. In Goroll AH, Mulley AG, editors: *Primary care medicine,* ed 4, Philadelphia, 2000, JB Lippincott.
14. Landreneau RJ et al: Success of laparoscopic fundoplication for gastroesophageal reflux disease, *Ann Thorac Surg* 66:1886, 1998.
15. Locke GR et al: Risk factors associated with symptoms of gastro-esophageal reflux, *Am J Med* 106(6):642, 1999.
16. Prisco MK: Evaluating neck masses, *Nurse Pract* 25(4):30, 2000.
17. Rantenen TK, Salo JA, Salminen JT, Kellokumpo I: Functional outcome after laparoscopic or open Nissen fundoplication: a follow up study, *Arch Surg* 134(3):240, 1999.
18. Resto MA: Gastroesophageal reflux disease, *Am J Nurs* 100(9):24-D, 2000.
19. Richter JE et al: Lansoprazole compared with ranitidine for the treatment of non-erosive gastroesophageal reflux disease, *Arch Intern Med* 160(12):1803, 2000.
20. Sampliner RE: Practice guidelines on the diagnosis, surveillance and therapy of Barrett's esophagus, *Am J Gastroenterol* 93(7):1028, 1998.
21. US Department of Health and Human Services: *Healthy people 2010: understanding and improving health,* Washington, DC, 2000, USDHHS.
22. Velanovich V: Comparison of symptomatic and quality of life outcomes of laparoscopic versus open antireflux surgery, *Surgery* 126(4):782, 1999.

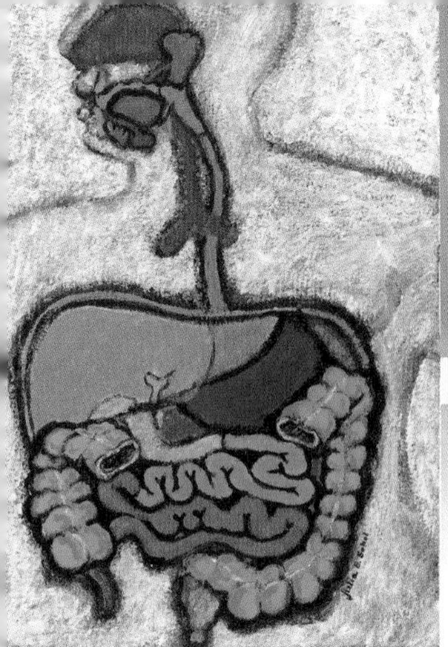

Stomach and Duodenum Problems 33

Judith K. Sands

Objectives

After studying this chapter, the learner should be able to:

1. Discuss the etiology and epidemiology of common problems affecting the stomach and duodenum.
2. Describe the mechanisms of mucosal defense and breakdown and the roles of *Helicobacter pylori,* nonsteroidal antiinflammatory drug administration, and other risk factors in the development of peptic ulcer disease.
3. Compare the advantages and disadvantages of the medical and surgical management of peptic ulcer disease and its complications.
4. Describe appropriate nursing interventions for the management of peptic ulcer disease and its complications.
5. Outline the medical and nursing management of gastric cancer.
6. Identify the essential nursing care associated with gastric surgery.

Problems related to the stomach are extremely common in American society. Many of these problems are episodic in nature and can easily be managed through temporary diet modification or self-medication in the home setting. Other stomach problems require aggressive medical or surgical intervention. Peptic ulcer disease (PUD) and its complications is the primary focus of this chapter, but it also discusses the management of gastric cancer.

GASTRITIS AND DYSPEPSIA

The terms *gastritis* and *dyspepsia* are used in an imprecise manner by both laypersons and health care professionals. The term *gastritis* refers to a diffuse or localized response of the gastric mucosa to injury or infection and primarily is a histologic diagnosis.[33] The term *dyspepsia,* on the other hand, refers to a group of symptoms that include belching, heartburn, bloating, and possibly nausea that is typically experienced after eating and is frequently not accompanied by any histologic changes in the stomach.[3,12] Dyspepsia is reported to affect up to 25% of the adult population on a regular or occasional basis.[3] It can occur in conjunction with specific clinical problems such as gastroesophageal reflux disease (GERD) (see Chapter 32) gastritis, PUD, or gastric cancer; but in many patients a definite cause is never established. Classic symptoms associated with dyspepsia are summarized in Box 33-1.

Acute Gastritis

Etiology/Epidemiology

Acute gastritis is a short-term inflammatory process that can be initiated by numerous factors such as excess alcohol ingestion, drug effects, severe physical stress or trauma, ingestion of caustic or noxious substances, radiation exposure, and bacterial contamination of food or water. Acute gastritis is predominantly an erosive process and is believed to be responsible for up to 10% to 30% of all episodes of gastrointestinal (GI) bleeding.

Pathophysiology

Acute gastritis develops when the protective mechanisms of the stomach mucosa are overwhelmed by the presence of bacterial toxins or irritating substances. Mucus provides little protection against chemical injury. Regeneration of the gastric mucosa after injury is both prompt and efficient, however, and the disorder usually is self-limiting after the irritating agent is removed. Common symptoms, which may be severe, include anorexia, nausea and vomiting, abdominal cramping or diarrhea, epigastric pain, and fever. Painless GI bleeding may occur and is more likely if the person regularly uses aspirin or nonsteroidal antiinflammatory drugs (NSAIDs).

Collaborative Care Management

Most cases of acute gastritis are managed by removing the causative agent and supporting the patient while the mucosa heals itself. The person is usually put on nothing-by-mouth (NPO) status to support healing of the mucosa and then slowly advanced to liquids and a normal diet. Antacids, histamine 2 (H_2) receptor antagonists, or proton pump inhibitors may be administered to reduce acid secretion and increase comfort. Temporary intravenous fluid and electrolyte replacement may be indicated in severe cases, and the patient is monitored carefully for signs of bleeding.

BOX 33-1 Dyspepsia Syndrome

A syndrome of chronic dyspepsia is one of the most common GI complaints encountered in primary practice. It is characterized by persistent or recurrent discomfort centered in the upper abdomen. There is no evidence of structural or biochemical abnormality, and the cause is unknown. Research findings to date indicate that individuals with dyspepsia syndrome have:

- Normal rates of acid secretion
- Postprandial hypomotility and delayed gastric emptying in 25% to 50% of cases; cause unknown
- Increased sensitivity to gastric distention; cause unknown
- No identified link with life stress or personality profiles

Symptoms

- Epigastric discomfort or pain
- Feeling of fullness or flatulence
- Early satiety
- Bloating or nausea

Treatment

There is no approved drug treatment.

- Histamine receptor antagonists may be used for ulcer-like pain.
- Antacids may be used for occasional heartburn or bloating symptoms.
- Prokinetic agents are frequently helpful.
- Diet and lifestyle changes are suggested:
  - Reducing dietary fat (fat prolongs digestion and may worsen bloating)
  - Eating smaller, more frequent meals
  - Avoiding foods that precipitate symptoms

Patient/Family Education. Teaching is targeted to the etiology of the acute gastritis and may include counseling about alcohol abuse or a review of food safety guidelines. The nurse suggests that the patient resume a normal diet slowly, eating only foods that minimize symptoms. A pattern of four to six small meals a day may initially be best tolerated. The nurse also encourages the patient to avoid irritating foods, alcohol, and smoking until recovery is complete. Follow-up care with a health care provider is strongly recommended if the symptoms persist.

Chronic Gastritis

Etiology/Epidemiology

Chronic gastritis is a separate clinical entity that can be further subdivided into type A and type B. Its presence is usually a sign of some underlying disease process.

Type A is believed to be autoimmune in nature and involves all of the acid-secreting parietal cells of the fundus. Circulating antibodies are produced that attack the gastric parietal cells and eventually may cause pernicious anemia from loss of the intrinsic factor.

The vast majority of cases are type B. Type B chronic gastritis is caused primarily by infection with *Helicobacter pylori* bacteria. The infection is usually acquired from contaminated food and water, and fecal-oral/oral-oral transmission is theorized. An estimated 30% to 50% of the U.S. population is infected with the organism and the incidence increases with age.[27,28] The prevalence of *H. pylori* infection is inversely proportional to socioeconomic status, and the infection rate is more than 90% in developing countries.[23] People typically contract *H. pylori* infection during childhood and remain infected for life unless treated. *H. pylori* is now the most common chronic bacterial infection in adults.[30] It plays a pivotal role in the development of PUD.

Pathophysiology

Type A chronic gastritis results in a decrease in gastric secretions from an autoimmune attack on the parietal cells. The gastric glands gradually atrophy, and the mucosa thins and deteriorates. The disease is usually nonerosive and is diagnosed by the histologic appearance of the gastric mucosa. The progressive decline in parietal cell function leads steadily to pernicious anemia. There are usually no symptoms until the destructive process is well advanced.

Type B chronic gastritis involves primarily the fundus and antrum of the stomach. There is minimal reduction in acid secretion, gastrin levels remain normal, and vitamin B_{12} absorption is rarely impaired. As the condition progresses the mucosa atrophies, and acid secretion is reduced.

The diagnosis of type B chronic gastritis can be confirmed only by histologic evaluation of a biopsy specimen. The diagnosis is challenging because the endoscopic appearance of the mucosa does not necessarily correlate with the histology. The diagnosis cannot be made on the basis of symptoms because most persons are asymptomatic after the initial acute infection, but even asymptomatic persons have some evidence of gastric tissue reaction to H. pylori.[30] Persons who experience symptoms report simply general dyspepsia (Box 33-1). There is no apparent causal relationship between the presence of dyspepsia and the severity of the disease.[2]

Collaborative Care Management

Treatment of type A chronic gastritis focuses on management of the underlying systemic disease. Vitamin B_{12} is administered if pernicious anemia occurs. The treatment of type B is less clear. Although the infection is caused almost exclusively by *H. pylori* infection, routine treatment remains controversial unless the person is symptomatic or develops an ulcer.[23,28,30] Treatment of *H. pylori* infection has undergone continuous change, but currently involves the use of triple or quadruple combinations of antibiotics, bismuth, and proton pump inhibitors.[23,28] Drug treatment of *H. pylori* is further discussed under Peptic Ulcer Disease later in this chapter.

Patient/Family Education. The nurse instructs the patient in the safe use of any prescribed medications and how to manage expected side effects. The nurse stresses the importance of not using any over-the-counter medications, such as antacids and histamine receptor antagonists, in addition to, or instead of, those prescribed by the health care professional. If antibiotic treatment is prescribed the nurse stresses the importance of completing the entire course of medications. Relapse is common with inadequate treatment, and drug-resistant strains of *H. pylori* are already a concern.[2]

The nurse encourages the person to experiment with minor diet and lifestyle modifications that may reduce the incidence and severity of symptoms. These include reducing the intake of dietary fat to reduce postprandial bloating, eating smaller and more frequent meals, and avoiding known precipitators. Stress management techniques also may be helpful for some individuals. The nurse emphasizes the importance of seeking prompt care if symptoms recur after treatment or if any symptoms of PUD develop.

PEPTIC ULCER DISEASE

PUD is an extremely common health problem that has undergone dramatic shifts in incidence and prevalence over the last century. The last two decades have revolutionized understanding of the etiology of PUD, and the development of effective new pharmacologic agents has enabled cure to become a reasonable goal for a traditionally chronic disease. Enormous progress has been made, but PUD still consumes billions of dollars annually in direct care costs, and the cost of medications has skyrocketed.[23] The importance of the disease is reflected in the Healthy People 2010 objective to "reduce hospitalizations caused by PUD in the United States from the baseline of 71 per 100,000 to a target of 46 per 100,000 population."[34]

Etiology

At the turn of the nineteenth century peptic ulcers were believed to be caused by diet and stress. As industrialization progressed, thinking shifted toward acid oversecretion as the primary cause, probably in response to stress and dietary factors. This was reflected in the traditional treatment approaches, which emphasized acid reduction and neutralization. Beginning with the discovery of *H. pylori* infection in the early 1980s and its critical role in histologic gastritis, research has increasingly focused on the role of *H. pylori* in ulcer etiology. Today the Centers for Disease Control and Prevention estimates that *H. pylori* may be the causative agent in as many as 90% of all peptic ulcers.[30] The remainder are primarily attributed to the effects of chronic NSAID use. Both factors target the mucosal defenses of the stomach and duodenum and lead to ulceration in vulnerable persons. The relationship between *H. pylori* infection and the development of ulcers is clearly causal, but current knowledge cannot explain why only 1 or 2 of every 20 persons who are infected with *H. pylori* actually develop ulcers; clearly other factors are operational that influence host resistance.

There is also an unequivocal causal association between NSAID use, mucosal injury, and the development of gastric ulcers (and, to a lesser degree, duodenal ulcers).[11] The GI complications of NSAID use are increasingly being recognized as one of the most common and severe drug side effects in the United States.[17] NSAIDs cause both local and systemic damage. Within 1 hour of taking a single dose of aspirin, multiple subendothelial hemorrhages can be found in the stomach, and gastric erosion will develop within 24 hours if use is continued. No relationship, however, has been established between the presence and severity of these superficial lesions and the development of ulcers. Although dramatic, these lesions appear to have little clinical significance in most patients.

The risk of ulcers associated with NSAID use is not predictable, and most NSAID users can derive benefit from their use without experiencing complications. The risk appears to be dose related, but problems can occur with even the smallest doses, especially with aspirin use. Ulcer risk is low in the under-50 age-group but rises rapidly over age 60. The prevalence of PUD among long-term NSAID users is 10% to 30%, a percentage that is 10 to 30 times higher than in the general population.[11] The concurrent presence of *H. pylori* infection in NSAID users does not appear to add to the risk of ulceration caused by the NSAIDs.[17]

Other Factors. Although *H. pylori* infection and chronic NSAID use are clearly the critical etiologic factors in PUD, other factors may play a role. Twin studies point to a genetic role in ulcer development, but its specific nature is unknown. Ulcers appear to demonstrate a familial clustering, but this effect may be related to *H. pylori* exposure and infection. An observed link between duodenal ulcers and blood group O is theorized to be associated with the improved ability of *H. pylori* to attach to the gastric epithelium when blood group antigens A and B are not present.

It would appear that a strong positive association exists between smoking and ulcer incidence, complications, recurrence, and mortality.[30] Current smokers are twice as likely as nonsmokers to develop ulcers, and the effects appear to be related to the amount smoked and duration. The pathology is not well identified, but smoking may increase the risk of infection with *H. pylori,* thereby acting as a cofactor. Smoking also plays a significant role in ulcer relapse. Although heavy smokers appear to have a higher incidence of peptic ulcer, quitting smoking has not been proven to affect the long-term course of the disease.

Alcohol is known to cause direct surface irritation of the gastric mucosa and can cause acute gastritis, but its role in ulcer development, if any, is unclear. Wine and beer are known to be potent secretagogues for acid secretion, but no etiologic role in ulcers has been identified.

Diet has received a great deal of attention over the years, but no data currently support any etiologic role of diet in PUD despite the frequent occurrence of dyspepsia symptoms in response to food. Tea, coffee, cola, and milk have all been identified as potent secretagogues, but no causal link to ulcers has been found. The same appears to be true for spices. The role of dietary fiber in ulcer development is being explored in some regions of the world where the use of rice-based vs. wheat-based diets appear to be associated with a lower incidence of peptic ulcers.

The role of stress in ulcer etiology, once believed to be pivotal, is also unknown. The relationship between intense physiologic stress and acute hemorrhagic gastritis is well documented, but there is definitely no "ulcer personality" that plays an identifiable etiologic role in ulcer development. The role of stress continues to be discussed as an etiologic factor in PUD, but current research has been unable to prove a link. Risk factors for PUD are summarized in the Risk Factors box.

Risk Factors

Peptic Ulcer Disease

Major
- *Helicobacter pylori* infection
- Chronic use of nonsteroidal antiinflammatory drugs

Minor
- Age
  - Ulcer incidence clusters in middle age
  - Gastric ulcers are more common in older adults
- Smoking is implicated in both ulcer incidence and recurrence
- Race
  - Gastric ulcers are more common in African-Americans and extremely common in Hispanics
- Sex
  - Ulcers are more common in men, but the ratio is approaching 1:1

Zollinger-Ellison Syndrome. Zollinger-Ellison syndrome is an ulceration syndrome of the duodenum or jejunum caused by a gastrinoma (gastrin-producing tumor). The tumor is commonly found in the noninsulin-producing islet cells of the pancreas. Most patients have a single tumor that eventually becomes malignant. This rare syndrome occurs more commonly in men, usually in early or middle adulthood.

The tumor produces an enormous quantity of gastrin, which massively overstimulates gastric acid secretion. The resulting ulcers usually do not respond to conventional therapy, and complications are common. Diarrhea is a common symptom, caused by a relative lack of the pancreatic lipase needed for fat digestion. The diagnosis of Zollinger-Ellison syndrome is differentiated from standard duodenal ulcers by radioimmunoassay measurements of high serum gastrin levels. A computed tomography (CT) scan may be used to localize the pancreatic tumor, and the tumor is removed if possible. The ulcers are treated as outlined for PUD.

Epidemiology

The incidence of PUD increased rapidly in the early 1900s and became one of the most common human ailments. Ulcer prevalence peaked in the 1950s, declined until 1980 and now appears to have stabilized at about 2% of the population. Up to 10% of the population will be affected at some point in their lives.[23] Most of the decline has occurred in the incidence of duodenal ulcers, whereas the incidence of gastric ulcers has remained fairly stable.[13] In fact, the progressive aging of the population is pushing the statistics for gastric ulcer steadily higher. Physician visits, hospitalizations, and the incidence of complications all declined by more than 50% during this period, and ulcer-related mortality has declined by more than 30%.[13,26] No satisfactory explanation exists for these dramatic swings in incidence and prevalence in such a short period.

The changes in sex ratios have also been dramatic and baffling, and wide variation can still be found worldwide. The incidence of duodenal ulcers in men was about four times that of women during the peak period of the 1950s.[25] This incidence supported the theory that ulcer etiology was related to social and occupational stress. The current sex ratio is approaching 1:1. The ratio of duodenal to gastric ulcers has also steadily declined since the 1950s, from nearly 4:1 to almost 1:1. The prevalence for both types of ulcers increases steadily with age, peaking in the sixth decade. The overall mortality rate for ulcer is low, but it increases dramatically in persons over 75 years old, particularly in older adults who have gastric ulcers. Racial and cultural variations have also been noted, with gastric and duodenal ulcers occurring about equally in Caucasians, but gastric ulcers being more common in African-Americans and extremely common in Hispanics. An increased incidence is also found in persons with chronic systemic diseases such as chronic obstructive pulmonary disease, end-stage renal disease, and cirrhosis.

Pathophysiology

The integrity of the gastric mucosa is maintained when a balance exists between the acid-secreting functions and mucosal protective functions of the stomach and duodenum. Peptic ulcers are present when a distinct crater is visible radiologically or endoscopically. The actual ulcer represents the end point of mucosal disruption.

Acid Secretion. Acid secretion is controlled by endocrine, neural, and paracrine factors. Gastric acid is secreted by the parietal cells of the fundus of the stomach in response to (1) gastrin, which is secreted by cells in the pyloric region of the stomach; (2) acetylcholine, which is secreted by cholinergic activation of the vagus; and (3) histamine, which is found in cells throughout the gastric mucosa.

There are two types of cellular receptors to histamine in the body. Histamine 1 (H_1) receptors are found in the cells of smooth muscle and capillaries, and they mediate smooth muscle contraction and capillary dilation. H_2 receptors are found in cells of the stomach and mediate secretion of hydrochloric acid (HCl). The process of stimulation and inhibition of gastric acid is illustrated in Figure 33-1.

Acid oversecretion was long assumed to be the major pathophysiologic factor in ulcer development. Although some patients with duodenal ulcers demonstrate increases in both basal and peak acid secretion, the vast majority of duodenal ulcer patients have gastric acid secretory responses both at rest and after meals that are identical to those in so-called normal individuals. Patients with gastric ulcers typically have lower levels of acid secretion, and *H. pylori* infection often decreases overall acid secretion.[23] The most commonly encountered abnormality in acid secretion in PUD patients is a slight increase in the duration of acid secretion that is particularly apparent after meals, and at night.[13] A slight increase in parietal cell mass may also be found that can increase both gastric acid and peptic activity. Neither *H. pylori* infection nor NSAIDs increase the aggressive forces of acid secretion. Some patients also exhibit an increased rate of gastric emptying. The ability of protein to buffer gastric acid is therefore impaired, and more unbuffered acid moves into the duodenum. These changes typically become significant only when the mucosal defenses are impaired. Acid oversecretion alone rarely if ever plays a role in gastric ulcers. Figure 33-2 illustrates the classic lesions formed by PUD.

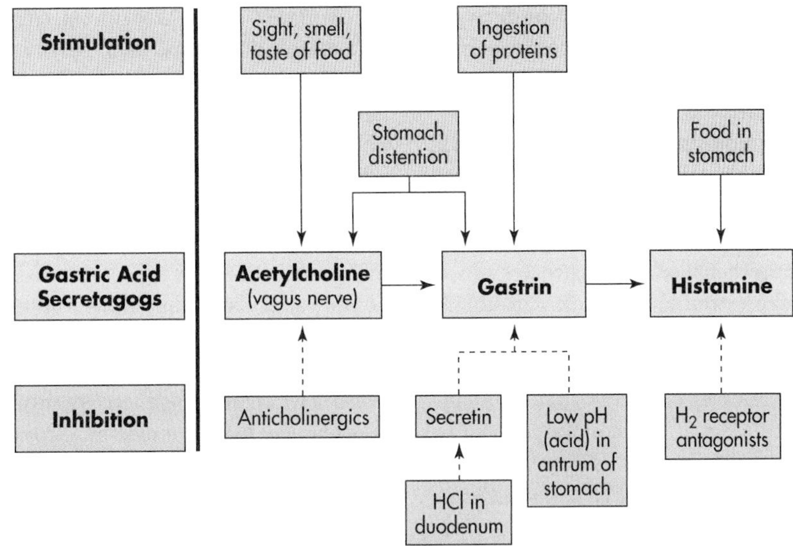

Figure 33-1 Stimulation and inhibition of gastric acid.

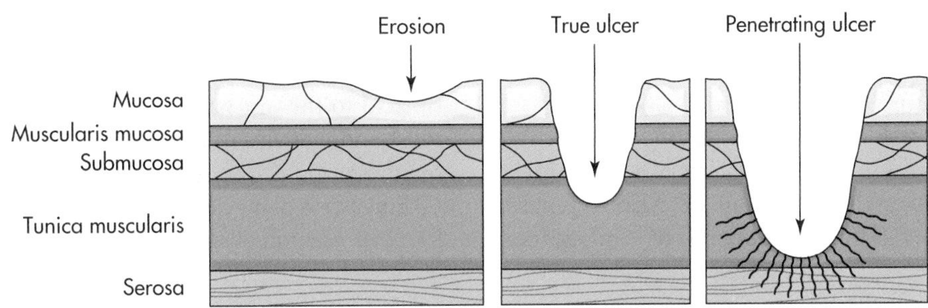

Figure 33-2 Lesions caused by peptic ulcer disease.

TABLE 33-1 Mechanisms of Gastroduodenal Mucosal Defense

Level of Defense	Mechanism or Effect
Preepithelial	
Mucus/bicarbonate barrier	Provides a modest barrier to H^+ diffusion and other molecules
Mucoid cap	Develops in response to mucosal injury and provides a juxtamucosal alkaline or neutral microenvironment
Epithelial	
Restitution	Prompt reconstitution of surface epithelium by movement of existing cells over damaged area; impeded by ischemia, reduced Ca^{++}, and acidosis
Acid-base transporters	Transport HCO_3^- into the pH/mucous barrier and subepithelial tissues and extrude acid to prevent cellular acidification
Release of growth factors, prostaglandins, nitric oxide	Growth factors promote cell division; prostaglandins stimulate mucus and HCO_3^- secretion and increase mucosal blood flow; nitric oxide increases mucosal blood flow
Subepithelial	
Mucosal blood flow	Delivers nutrients and buffers, especially HCO_3^-, to the surface epithelial cells

Modified from McCance KL, Huether SE: *Pathophysiology: the biologic basis for disease in adults and children,* ed 3, St Louis, 1998, Mosby.

Mucosal Defenses. The entire stomach and duodenum are covered by a 100-μm thick layer of gel-like mucus that is 95% water and 5% glycoproteins. This layer is continuously both degraded and replaced. The gel protects the mucosa against shearing and mechanical injury, assists in the transport of food particles, retains water near the mucosa, and blocks the back diffusion of hydrogen ions. The epithelial cells of the stomach are densely packed and secrete bicarbonate into the mucous layer, which helps maintain a neutral pH immediately adjacent to the mucosa. The mucosa is therefore remarkably resistant to physical injury. The epithelial cells are less dense in the duodenum making it slightly more susceptible to injury. When minor injury occurs the epithelium is capable of quick repair by creating a "cap" of mucus and fibrin that raises the mucosal pH and repairs the damage. An adequate mucosal blood flow at a normal pH is critical to the support of normal epithelial cell function. These defenses are so powerful that mucosal pH is maintained at a level greater than 6, even when the gastric luminal pH is as low as 1.5. Table 33-1 summarizes the major components of mucosal defense.

Effects of *Helicobacter pylori* Infection and Nonsteroidal Antiinflammatory Drugs. *H. pylori* is a gram-negative bacterium with a curved or spiral shape. Once in the stomach it uses flagella to imbed itself into the mucous layer. The bacterium produces significant amounts of urease at the epithelial cell surface. The urease catalyzes the hydrolysis of urea into ammonia and carbon dioxide. The ammonia forms a cloud around the bacterium and both neutralizes the gastric acid and has a toxic effect on the epithelial cells. This process allows the bacterium to thrive in the extremely hostile environment of the stomach.[23] Figure 33-3 illustrates the penetration of the mucosal layer by *H. pylori.*

The *H. pylori* bacterium releases cytokines that cause inflammatory changes in the mucosa. It also contains proteases that degrade mucus. Bicarbonate secretion is eventually impaired. It is theorized that various strains of *H. pylori* differ in the virulence of their cytotoxins, which could explain the relatively small number of people infected with *H. pylori* who actually develop ulcers.[13] The presence of chronic *H. pylori*–related gastritis causes slow metaplastic changes to take place in the adjacent cells of the duodenum. These cellular changes facilitate the movement of *H. pylori* into the duodenum with subsequent colonization.

Most NSAIDs are weak acids that can cause local mucosal irritation and inflammation, but their primary adverse effect on the stomach involves the inhibition of cyclooxygenase, an enzyme essential for the production of endogenous prostaglandins in the plasma and mucosa. Prostaglandins are critical in maintaining normal mucosal defenses. A deficit in prostaglandins results in decreased mucus and bicarbonate secretion, decreased mucosal blood flow, and a failure to inhibit gastric acid secretion. It also prevents the formation of the mucous "cap" that supports epithelial regeneration in the event of injury. The adverse consequences are profound. Approximately 2% to 4% of long-term NSAID users develop serious complications each year, and approximately 25% of NSAID users will develop ulcers. The NSAID-induced ulcers are believed to be directly responsible for 30% of upper GI bleeding episodes and approximately 30% of all ulcer-related deaths.

The major elements involved in the pathophysiology of peptic ulcers are presented in Figure 33-4. Peptic ulcers usually occur at or near mucosal transition zones that are believed to be particularly vulnerable to the effects of acid, pepsin, and enzymes. Most gastric ulcers are localized in an area about 2 cm long on the antral side of the stomach along the lesser curvature where muscle fibers are prominent and blood supply is decreased. Duodenal ulcers are concentrated at the junction of the antrum and duodenum.

Symptoms reported by patients with gastric and duodenal ulcers often overlap and may be nonspecific. Pain is the classic symptom associated with PUD, but its sensitivity and specificity as a disease marker are very low. The pain traditionally has been attributed to the irritation of gastric acid over the eroded mucosa. During endoscopy, however, rubbing, cutting, burning, and even directly applying hydrochloric acid to the mucosa produce little or no perceived pain in most individuals. A complication may be the first clinical manifestation in about 25% of persons with PUD.

Epigastric pain, described as "burning" or vague discomfort, is present in 60% to 80% of patients. The pain is episodic in nature, lasting 30 minutes to 2 hours, and occurs 1 to 3 hours after meals. Pain that occurs between 12 and 3 AM and awakens the person from sleep is a common symptom with duodenal ulcers. The pain may radiate and commonly is relieved by ingestion of food or antacid.[13] Anorexia and weight loss are more commonly associated with ulcers than are hunger and weight gain.

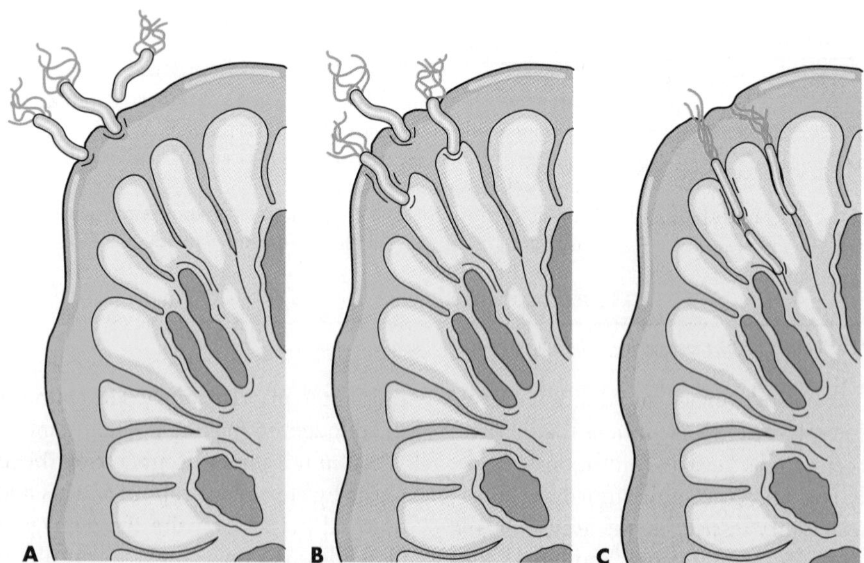

Figure 33-3 Penetration of the mucosal layer by *H. pylori.* **A,** After penetration, *H. pylori* forms clusters near membranes of surface epithelial cells. **B,** Some attach to the cell membrane. **C,** Others lodge between the epithelial cells.

Dyspepsia is also commonly reported, but because this is such a common complaint in the general population, it is not very helpful in distinguishing the presence of an ulcer. Fewer than 30% of persons who experience chronic and severe dyspepsia are found to have ulcers on endoscopy, but many ulcer sufferers experience dyspepsia.[12]

No special features clearly distinguish gastric ulcers from duodenal ulcers, although patients with gastric ulcers are more likely to be asymptomatic, particularly older adults and NSAID users. Pain may or may not be present and tends to be localized to the epigastrum but may radiate to the back. The pain is described as "dull," and relief from food or antacid is less common. Anorexia, early satiety, nausea, and weight loss may all occur. Symptoms may cluster for a few days or weeks and then disappear and recur. Symptoms may also persist after the ulcer crater has healed. Clinical manifestations associated with PUD are summarized in the Clinical Manifestations box.

Collaborative Care Management

Diagnostic Tests. The diagnosis of PUD cannot be made from the symptoms alone because they are nonspecific. Although an ulcer crater is usually readily identifiable with an upper GI series, a definitive diagnosis involves endoscopy with biopsy to accurately differentiate between benign and malignant ulcers. Gastric cancer frequently presents with ulcer symptoms.

H. pylori screening is increasingly being included in the diagnostic workup for ulcers. Both invasive and noninvasive screening options are available. Invasive tests include gastric biopsy with culture, histology, DNA analysis, and the rapid urease test, which assesses a biopsy sample for urease activity.[24] Nonendoscopic options include serologic testing, which identifies specific *H. pylori* immunoglobulin G (IgG) antibodies. The test is both sensitive and specific, but cannot differentiate between active and inactive infection.[28] The urea breath

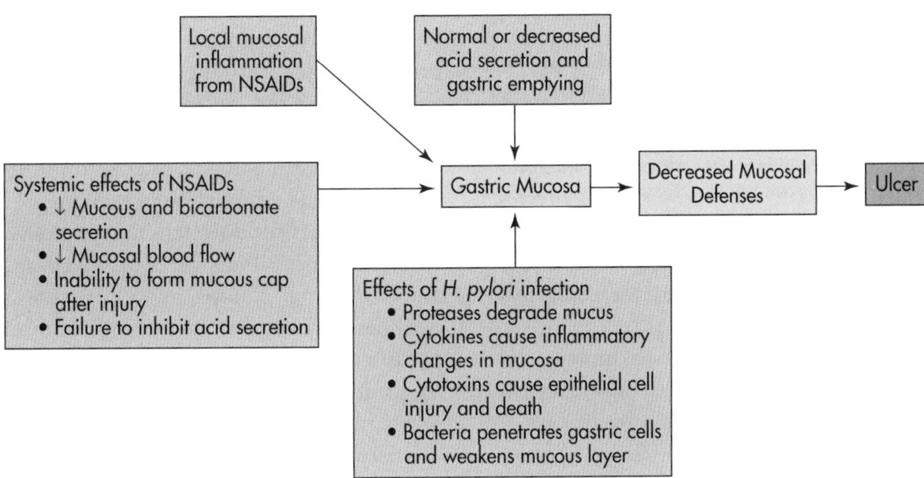

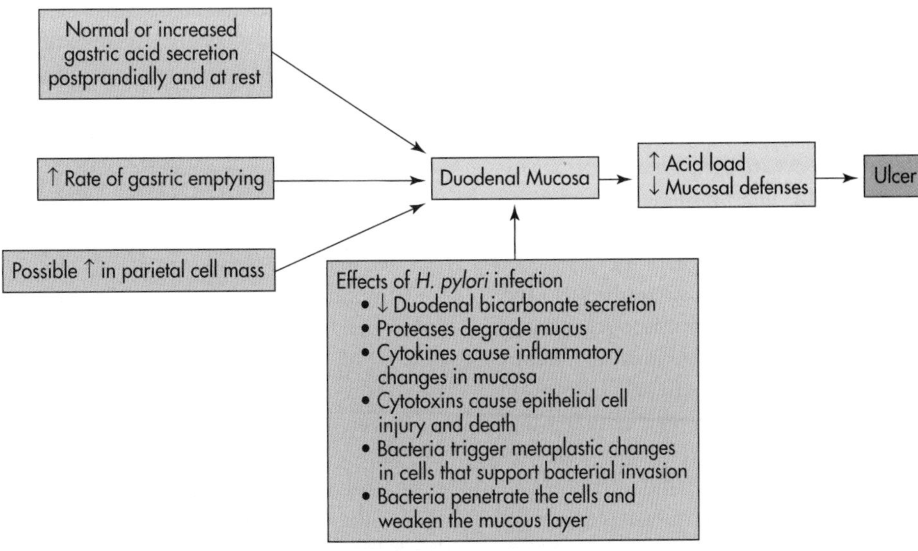

Figure 33-4 Pathophysiologic components of peptic ulcer.

Clinical Manifestations

Duodenal and Gastric Ulcers

Ulcers may be completely asymptomatic.

DUODENAL ULCER

Pain

- Episodic in nature lasting 30 min-2 hr
- Epigastric location near midline; may radiate around costal border to back
- Described as gnawing, burning, aching
- Occurs 1-3 hr after meals and at night (12-3 AM)
- Often relieved by food or antacid

GASTRIC ULCER

Pain

- Dull epigastric location near midline
- Early satiety
- No usually relieved by food or antacid

BOTH

Dyspepsia syndrome: fullness, epigastric discomfort, vague nausea, distention, and bloating

Anorexia

Weight loss

test is a measure of current *H. pylori* infection. The bacteria hydrolyze urea that is labeled with radioactive carbon and release labeled carbon dioxide in the breath.[32]

The newest approach involves stool antigen testing and also identifies active infection. See Chapter 31 for additional information about diagnostic testing.

Medications. Advances in drug therapy have dramatically changed the management of PUD. Drug therapy controls peptic ulcer symptoms effectively, often in a matter of days. It heals most ulcers completely within 8 weeks. However, ulcer relapse remains a significant problem, and long-term control is difficult. It has become increasingly apparent that any successful ulcer treatment must also consider eradication of the underlying *H. pylori* infection. The major objectives of drug therapy are to facilitate healing, eliminate symptoms, and prevent complications and recurrences, all at reasonable cost with minimal side effects.[13]

Antacids, H_2-receptor antagonists, proton pump inhibitors, and cytoprotective agents are the primary options for pharmacologic management of ulcers. All are effective to some degree, but they vary substantially in cost, ease of administration, side effects, and patient acceptability.

Antacids. Antacids are weak bases that neutralize free hydrochloric acid to prevent irritation and permit mucosal healing. Antacids usually play a supporting role in ulcer therapy today and are used primarily for symptomatic relief; however, they can also heal ulcers, although at a slower rate than other products. The main disadvantage to antacid therapy is the frequency with which the antacids must be administered. Their effect is transitory, and they need to be administered 1 and 3 hours after meals and at bedtime. This is not a practical schedule for most patients, who are usually encouraged to use antacids during treatment on an as-needed basis. These drugs are available over the counter.

Aluminum hydroxide antacids are the preferred preparations. In addition to neutralizing acid, they appear to decrease pepsin activity and possibly stimulate prostaglandin synthesis. Administration in tablet rather than liquid form prolongs the buffering effect slightly and is recommended. Antacids should never be given concurrently with other ulcer drugs such as H_2 blockers because they decrease drug absorption by 10% to 20%. Because aluminum hydroxide products used alone commonly cause constipation, they typically are combined with magnesium hydroxide for its laxative effect. Table 33-2 summarizes the commonly used antacids.

Histamine Receptor Antagonists. H_2-receptor antagonists inhibit HCl secretion by binding to the H_2 receptors on stomach cells and blocking the release of histamine, which is a secretagogue for HCl. Basal and postprandial acid production is reduced 50% to 80% and gastric emptying is unaffected by their use.[13]

Several different generations of H_2-receptor antagonists have been developed, but there is no clear evidence that one is best. They vary in potency and cost but are equally effective in healing peptic ulcers after an average of 4 weeks of therapy.

Recommended dosage schedules have varied over the years. Most are now administered twice a day in divided doses or in one bedtime dose. Suppression of nocturnal acid secretion appears to support rapid healing.

H_2 blockers produce few side effects and have an excellent record of safety. Potential side effects may include diarrhea and abdominal cramps, as well as confusion, dizziness, and weakness, which are more common in elderly patients. The predominant difference in the drugs is their relative cost. The drugs in current use include the following:

- Cimetidine (Tagamet) is the oldest and least expensive drug. It also has the potential for multiple drug interactions and is not recommended in situations that necessitate multiple drug administration. Cimetidine has also been shown to have antiandrogenic effects that may cause gynecomastia, decreased libido, and impotence in some men. It may also cause confusion in older adults.
- Ranitidine (Zantac) is more potent and usually has no side effects.
- Famotidine (Pepcid) is the drug of choice when the possibility of adverse reactions with other prescribed medications is a concern.
- Nizatidine (Axid) is the newest and most costly of the H_2-receptor antagonists.

Cimetidine, ranitidine, and famotidine are all available in intravenous forms to address acute and emergency situations. Several of the H_2-receptor antagonists are also now available in nonprescription strength for over-the-counter purchase.

Proton Pump Inhibitors. Proton pump inhibitors reduce 24-hour acid production by more than 90% with a single daily dose, and they are significantly more effective in healing ulcers than other medications (see Evidence-Based Practice box). With higher doses, acid secretion is virtually eliminated and clinically significant side effects are rare. These drugs also ap-

TABLE 33-2 Common Medications for Ulcer Discomfort (Antacids)

Drug	Action	Intervention
Aluminum Products		
Amphojel AlternaGEL Alu-Cap Basaljel	All antacids act by buffering excess acidity in the stomach to neutralize the pH.	All aluminum hydroxide antacids are constipating. Patients need to be taught to maintain regular bowel elimination. Teach patient to use as needed for ulcer discomfort, but not at the same time as an H_2-receptor antagonist.
Combinations of Aluminum and Magnesium		
Maalox Gaviscon Riopan		As above, but nonconstipating.
Calcium Products		
Alka-Mints Tums Rolaids		As above, but only for short-term use. Often severely constipating. May cause acid rebound.
Antacids With Simethicone		
Mylanta Maalox Plus Gelusil		Simethicone is non–gas forming and can be recommended to patients with gas problems. Nonconstipating.

NOTE: Antacid tablets have a longer duration of effect than liquids and are recommended.

pear to have some antibacterial effect on *H. pylori* infection and are increasingly being included in treatment protocols. Available drugs include omeprazole (Prilosec), lansoprazole (Prevacid), pantoprazole (Protonix), rabeprazole (Aciphex), and esomeprazole (Nexium). Prohibitive cost is the major drawback to these drugs.

Mucosal Protective Agents. Improved understanding of the etiology of peptic ulcers has shifted attention to the development and use of drugs designed to support the mucosal barrier. These include sucralfate (Carafate) and misoprostol (Cytotec).

- Sucralfate is a complex of aluminum hydroxide and sulfated sucrose that is believed to coat an ulcer crater and provide a sealant barrier against acid irritation. Additional research has indicated that it also acts as a cytoprotective agent and increases prostaglandin synthesis. It neither inhibits acid secretion nor neutralizes gastric acid, but it is comparable to H_2 blockers in its ability to heal ulcers. Its only common side effect is constipation. The drug comes in a large tablet and must be taken orally several times a day, which limits its acceptability to patients. A liquid form has been developed for use in critical care. Combining sucralfate with an acid-suppressing agent does not significantly improve healing and is not recommended.
- Misoprostol and the newer enprostil are synthetic prostaglandin analogs that offer a new dimension to ulcer management. They enhance mucosal defenses by replacing gastric prostaglandins and also appear to have some antisecretory properties. Therefore they can be used for both treatment and prophylaxis of NSAID-induced ulcers.[13] In low doses they have a protective effect on the stomach but not the duodenum. They are used primarily for the prevention of gastric ulcers in high-risk elderly patients who need to continue to take NSAIDs. The pain-relieving effectiveness of NSAIDs does not appear to be lessened by their use. Misoprostol frequently causes diarrhea and crampy abdominal pain, which are usually dose dependent. Administration after meals decreases side effects in many patients. The drug can induce abortion, and it is rarely used in women of childbearing age. The increased use of selective COX-2 NSAIDs for managing arthritis pain is expected to decrease the incidence of NSAID-related ulceration.

Evidence-Based Practice

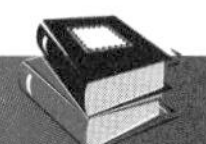

Reference: Yeomans ND et al: A comparison of omeprazole with ranitidine for ulcers associated with NSAIDs, *N Engl J Med* 338(11):719, 1998.

This study was an international multicenter evaluation of omeprazole and ranitidine for the healing and prevention of recurrence of gastric ulcers in more than 500 patients receiving long-term NSAID therapy. Only patients with endoscopic evidence of ulcers or erosions in the stomach were included in the study. Patients were randomly assigned to treatment with standard doses of each drug for 4 to 8 weeks or until evidence of healing was endoscopically confirmed. Patients who were successfully treated entered a maintenance phase and were monitored for recurrence for an additional 6 months.

Both ulcers and erosions healed faster in patients treated with omeprazole. Most patients obtained relief of symptoms within 4 weeks, but the omeprazole group achieved significantly faster relief of symptoms. During maintenance, patients receiving omeprazole were significantly more likely to have sustained remission at 6 months. All patients continued to receive NSAIDs during the study period.

BOX 33-2 *H. Pylori* Treatment Options

FDA-approved treatment options include:

- Omeprazole QD plus clarithromycin TID for 2 weeks followed by omeprazole QD for another 2 weeks
- Ranitidine bismuth citrate BID plus clarithromycin TID for 2 weeks followed by ranitidine bismuth citrate BID for another 2 weeks
- Bismuth subsalicylate QID plus metronidazole QID and tetracyline QID for 2 weeks followed by a histamine-receptor antagonist BID for another 4 weeks
- Lansoprazole TID plus amoxicillin TID for 3 weeks
- Ranitidine bismuth citrate BID plus clarithromycin BID for 2 weeks followed by ranitidine BID for another 2 weeks
- Omeprazole BID plus clarithromycin BID plus amoxicillin BID for 10 days
- Lansoprazole BID plus clarithromycin BID plus amoxicillin BID for 10 days

Helicobacter pylori *Drug Treatment*. *H. pylori* infection is now recognized as the main determinant of ulcer relapse. Controversy continues, however, over exactly which patients need to be treated for the infection. Treatment advocates contend that immediate treatment of documented *H. pylori* infection in ulcer patients is cost-effective because the vast majority of ulcers will otherwise eventually relapse. Others recommend that *H. pylori* treatment be reserved for refractory lesions or patients who experience frequent relapses.[13,28]

Drug protocols for the treatment of *H. pylori* infection continue to evolve with research and testing. Drug regimens in use involve three or four drugs and are associated with multiple side effects that make patient adherence a serious concern. Treatment with any single agent has proven to be ineffective, and the development of antibiotic-resistant strains of the organism are an increasing concern.[23]

Box 33-2 summarizes current recommended treatment protocols. Successful treatment of the *H. pylori* infection reduces the incidence of ulcer relapse to well below 10%, and maintenance therapy with H_2-receptor antagonists or other drugs is usually unnecessary.

Treatments. There are no routinely ordered treatments because most peptic ulcers are responsive to an aggressive pharmacologic approach. If an ulcer bleeds, obstructs, or perforates, however, the management shifts dramatically. Treatments for these problems are discussed under Complications (see p. 1037).

Surgical Management. The emergence of effective drug therapy for PUD has also changed the role of surgery in disease management. As effective treatment of *H. pylori* reduces the incidence of ulcer reoccurrence, it is anticipated that the need for elective surgery for ulcer management will be rare. Surgery is used primarily for the management of complications such as perforation and the treatment of the occasional intractable ulcer that is resistant to all standard therapy. Patients who require surgery to manage acute complications are usually older and frailer and commonly have significant comorbid conditions.

Vagotomy, with or without drainage procedures, is the most commonly performed ulcer surgery today. Vagotomy procedures reduce gastric acid production by decreasing cholinergic stimulation of the parietal cells and limiting the response to gastrin. The vagotomy procedure of choice is the highly selective vagotomy, which preserves the pylorus and almost abolishes the negative outcomes of dumping syndrome, diarrhea, and bilious vomiting. More aggressive procedures that include various forms of partial gastrectomy are rarely recommended today. Vagotomy procedures are being successfully adapted for laparoscopic approaches, which appear to significantly minimize morbidity and recovery time, although data concerning long-term outcomes are not yet available. All vagotomy procedures are highly technical, and the results are strongly related to the skill and experience of the surgeon. The various approaches to vagotomy are described in Box 33-3 and illustrated in Figures 33-5 and 33-6.[31]

Diet. The role of diet in PUD management has changed dramatically over the last 40 years. The Sippy and Hurst milk-based therapy was used for years in the belief that constantly diluting and neutralizing acid would facilitate ulcer healing.

BOX 33-3 Vagotomy Procedures for Management of Intractable Ulcers

Truncal Vagotomy

Severs the vagus nerve on the distal esophagus:

- Removes the cholinergic drive
- Reduces parietal cell sensitivity to gastrin
- Creates gastric stasis and poor gastric emptying and requires a drainage procedure (pyloroplasty)
- Affects motility of duodenum, biliary tract, and pancreas and is associated with multiple digestive complications

Selective Vagotomy

Divides and severs the vagal nerve branches to confine the effects to the stomach and preserve the function of the biliary tract, pancreas, and small intestine:

- Removes the cholinergic drive to the parietal cells
- Creates gastric stasis and poor gastric emptying and requires a drainage procedure (pyloroplasty)
- Technically difficult and outcomes are not significantly better than the truncal approach

Highly Selective Vagotomy

Divides and severs the specific vagal nerve branches that supply the stomach while preserving those that supply the antrum and pylorus, biliary tract, pancreas, and intestine:

- Removes the cholinergic drive to the parietal cells
- Preserves innervation of the antrum and pylorus and does not require a drainage procedure
- Preserves extragastric function
- Minimizes digestive side effects
- Technically extremely difficult

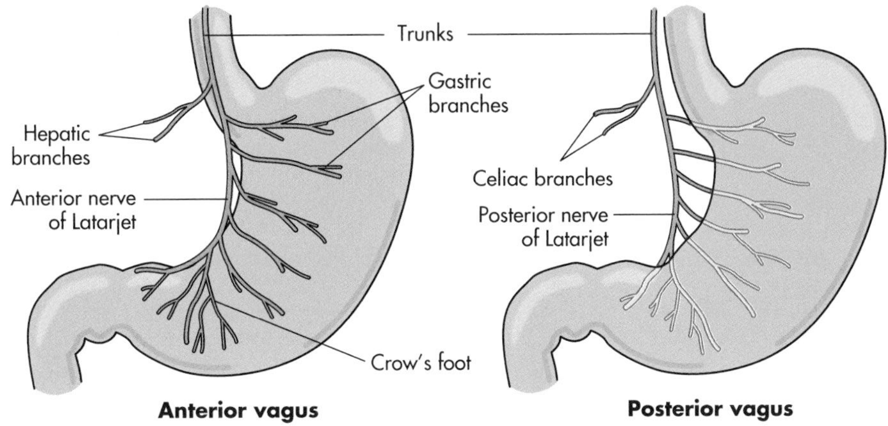

Figure 33-5 Normal vagal anatomy.

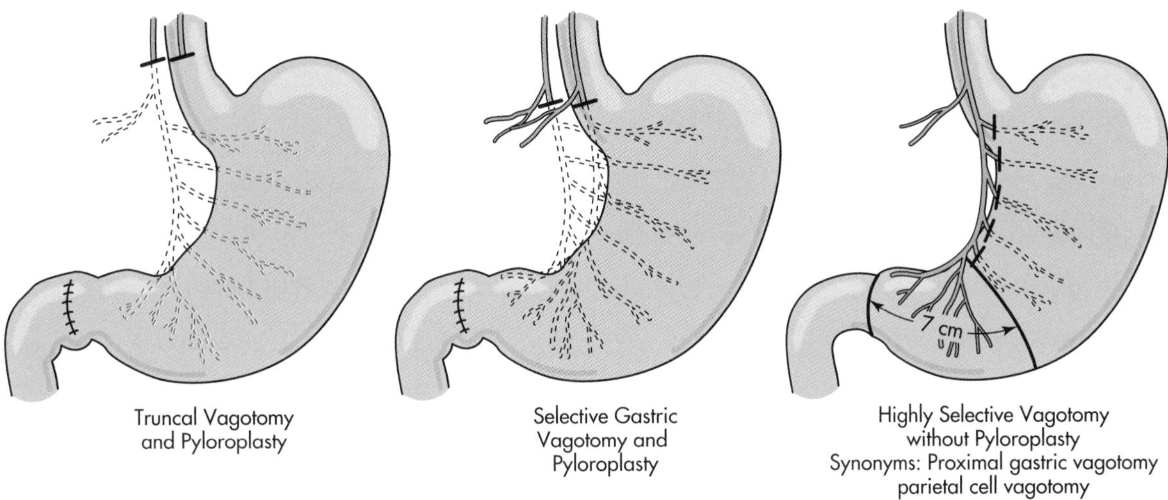

Figure 33-6 Types of vagotomy with and without pyloroplasty.

Although milk-based diets provide symptomatic relief, they do not influence healing. In fact, research has shown that the amino acids and calcium in milk actually act as secretagogues and increase acid secretion. Current management reflects the understanding that diet plays no defined role in ulcer etiology. Bland diets do not facilitate healing, and patients are simply encouraged to eliminate or restrict specific foods that cause discomfort until healing occurs.

Activity. Patients with ulcers do not need to restrict their activity in any particular way to support the healing of the ulcer. Most care is managed at home, and patients are able to continue with their usual activities while undergoing treatment. Adequate rest, however, is encouraged because it appears to promote healing.

Referrals. Consultation usually is not needed for management of uncomplicated ulcers. The nurse may encourage patients to seek community support for smoking cessation and stress management. Surgical consultation may be indicated if ulcer complications develop.

NURSING MANAGEMENT OF PATIENT WITH PEPTIC ULCER DISEASE

ASSESSMENT

Health History

Assessment data to be collected as part of the health history of a patient with PUD include:

- Pain: presence, location, severity, nature, and relationship to eating and sleeping
- Medications (prescription , OTC, and herbal preparations) used, particularly aspirin, NSAIDs, and other ulcerogenic drugs; frequency/pattern of use; effectiveness for symptom control
- Dietary habits, meal patterns, and alcohol history
- Smoking history
- General lifestyle: work, leisure, exercise, stressors, usual coping measures
- Knowledge of PUD: causes, treatment, complications

Physical Examination

Important aspects of the physical examination of the patient with PUD include:

Evidence of GI bleeding including occult blood in stool
Changes in hemoglobin, hematocrit, and red blood cell (RBC) counts
Weight loss or gain from baseline

NURSING DIAGNOSES

Nursing diagnoses are determined from analysis of patient data. Nursing diagnoses for the person with PUD may include but are not limited to:

Diagnostic Title	Possible Etiologic Factors
1. Acute pain	Mucosal irritation and ulceration
2. Risk for ineffective health maintenance	Lack of knowledge of disease process, treatment regimen, and signs and symptoms of complications

EXPECTED PATIENT OUTCOMES

Expected patient outcomes for the patient with PUD may include but are not limited to:

1. Will describe pain as decreased, minimal, or absent
2. Will accurately describe components of disease management

2a. Medication schedule and control of side effects
2b. Plans for follow-up care
2c. Lifestyle factors that may facilitate ulcer healing and prevent recurrence:
Smoking cessation
Stress reduction
Diet modification
2d. Symptoms that indicate presence or development of complications

INTERVENTIONS

1. Relieving Pain

Taking prescribed medications as ordered is the major strategy for relieving ulcer pain. Drug therapy will control or eliminate the pain within a few days to a week, but peptic ulcer control is a long-term process. Successful self-care depends on a clear understanding of the purpose of each drug and the importance of adherence to the complete ulcer regimen, including follow-up care. Most cases of ulcer relapse can be traced to nonadherence unless the initial treatment is inadequate or does not include treatment of *H. pylori.*

2. Patient/Family Education

The nurse teaches the patient how to take prescribed medications and discusses the management of common side effects. Elderly patients and their families are encouraged to monitor and report the incidence of any mental confusion or dizziness that may occur with cimetidine use. Patients are taught to never abruptly discontinue their use of antiulcer medications because of the danger of severe acid rebound. Antacids should never be taken with H_2-receptor antagonists because they significantly block drug absorption.

The patient is strongly encouraged to substitute the use of acetaminophen for other NSAIDs in routine pain and fever management. Patients with chronic arthritis who need to continue daily NSAID use should be encouraged to explore with their physician the use of misoprostol (Cytotec) or a switch to a COX-2 inhibitor NSAID that might decrease the risk of gastric ulceration. This is particularly important for older patients.

The nurse teaches the patient and family that no special diet is needed to promote ulcer healing. The nurse encourages the patient to avoid any food that causes discomfort and to avoid overdistention of the stomach and binge eating. There is no research evidence that a pattern of small, frequent feedings is any more effective in ulcer healing than a standard three meal-a-day pattern, but overeating should be avoided.[7] Eating slowly and chewing thoroughly prevent overdistention and reflux. Bedtime snacking may promote nighttime acid secretion and should be avoided.

The nurse may encourage the patient to limit the use of foods that have been shown to have a strong acid-stimulating effect, at least during the initial treatment period. These include coffee, tea, cola, beer, and chocolate. Direct irritants such as spices and red and black pepper also should be limited.

Promoting Successful Disease Management

The role of lifestyle or psychologic stress in PUD is unclear, although mental and physical rest do appear to facilitate ulcer healing. The nurse encourages the patient to establish a pattern of regular exercise and to explore appropriate approaches to stress reduction at home and work. The Patient Teaching box summarizes the major points involved in teaching self-care management to the patient with PUD.

Although the initial peptic ulcer cannot usually be prevented, it is often possible to minimize the risk of relapse by effective *H. pylori* treatment. Many patients are unaware of the role of *H. pylori* in ulcer development, and the nurse teaches the patient about the causal role of *H. pylori* and the importance of completing recommended treatment to prevent relapse.[7]

The nurse cautions the patient about the use of over-the-counter H_2-receptor antagonists once therapy is completed. The return of pain may indicate that the ulcer treatment has been inadequate or that further *H. pylori* treatment is indicated. Use of over-the-counter ulcer medications to manage symptoms could delay treatment or mask the development of complications.

The role of cigarette smoking in ulcer relapse is also clearly documented, and the nurse strongly encourages the patient to quit smoking. Referral to community smoking cessation programs should be made in consultation with the health care provider about the appropriateness of the various nicotine replacement systems. The role of alcohol in ulcer relapse is less clear, but moderation is encouraged, and alcohol should never be ingested on an empty stomach because of its irritating ef-

Patient Teaching
Managing a Peptic Ulcer

MEDICATIONS
- Know the dosage, administration, action, and side effects of all drugs in use.
- Take all of prescribed drug, even when pain is relieved. It is essential to complete the full treatment to eradicate *H. pylori* and prevent recurrence.
- Keep antacids available for use as needed, but do not take them at the same time as an H_2-receptor antagonist or proton pump inhibitor. Antacids should be taken 1 to 3 hours after meals, at bedtime, and as needed for pain.
- Avoid the use of over-the-counter H_2-receptor antagonists.
- Use acetaminophen for routine pain relief during treatment if needed. Avoid the use of all NSAIDs, including aspirin and ibuprofen.
- If the treatment of arthritis or other chronic illness requires the ongoing use of NSAIDs, explore the use of misoprostol or a COX-2 inhibitor with health care provider.
- Know the symptoms of ulcer recurrence and report them promptly to the health care provider.

DIET
- Eat three balanced meals a day.
- Eat between-meal snacks if this helps control pain.
- Avoid bedtime snacking because it increases nighttime acid secretion.
- Eat slowly and chew foods thoroughly. Do not overeat.
- Avoid any foods that increase discomfort.
- Avoid the use of alcohol during treatment if possible.
- Never drink alcohol on an empty stomach.

SMOKING
- Stop smoking if possible.
- Explore community support for smoking cessation or use of nicotine withdrawal patches.

STRESS REDUCTION
- Participate in recreation and hobbies that promote relaxation.
- Participate in a moderate aerobic exercise program for promotion of well-being.
- Provide for increased rest during healing.

NSAID, Nonsteroidal antiinflammatory drug.

fects on the mucosa. A Nursing Care Plan for a patient with a peptic ulcer is found on pp. 1036 and 1037.

EVALUATION

To evaluate the effectiveness of nursing interventions, compare patient behaviors with those stated in the expected patient outcomes. Achievement of outcomes is successful if a patient with PUD:

1. States that ulcer pain is no longer present.
2. Correctly describes components of disease management:
2a. Medication schedule and control of side effects.
2b. Plans for follow-up care.
2c. Lifestyle modifications to prevent relapse.
2d. Symptoms indicating complications.

GERONTOLOGIC CONSIDERATIONS

Although the incidence of PUD in the general population has been steadily declining, the incidence in elderly persons has shown a slight increase as the population ages. Older adults are also much more likely to be colonized by *H. pylori,* which contributes to an increased incidence of peptic ulcers.

Hospitalization rates for older adults with PUD also have risen steadily in the face of a continuing overall decline in hospitalization for the disease. Most of the complications and mortality associated with ulcers occur in elderly patients, with more than 80% of ulcer-related deaths occurring in the over-65 age-group.

Older adults experience frequent dyspepsia, which makes the diagnosis of ulcers more difficult. They are also less likely to seek medical attention for their symptoms. The frequent use of NSAIDs in this population for the management of chronic arthritis is another significant contributor to ulcer incidence. An estimated 1% to 2% of the total U.S. population uses NSAIDs daily, and the elderly are the most frequent users. From 2% to 4% of long-term NSAID users develop serious complications each year, and 30% of ulcer-related deaths can be directly attributed to NSAID use. If GI hemorrhage occurs, its seriousness is potentiated by the platelet inhibition associated with NSAID use.

PUD often manifests in an atypical manner in older adults. Symptoms tend to be more poorly defined, and the classic pain is frequently not present. If discomfort is present at all, it often is poorly localized and vague, radiating in ways that cause confusion and overlap with the presentations of angina, gallbladder disease, and dysphagia. Because early accurate diagnosis is rare, ulcers in older adults tend to be larger at diagnosis, or are already causing complications. PUD is clearly a more serious problem in older adults, and the elderly are more prone to complications. The risk of serious complications is four times higher in the elderly, and most patients are completely asymptomatic until complications develop. Older women appear to be at particular risk.

The diagnosis and treatment of PUD in older adults follow the same general guidelines outlined in the prior discussion. Older adults are more likely to require aggressive *H. pylori* treatment to heal the ulcer and minimize relapse, and they are more likely to need maintenance ulcer therapy. Older adults should be thoroughly assessed concerning their use of both prescription and over-the-counter NSAIDs and cautioned to eliminate use of these drugs if possible. Acetaminophen is considered to be a much safer alternative for occasional use than aspirin and most NSAIDs. Consideration should be given to the use of a COX-2 inhibitor NSAID

Nursing Care Plan Patient With a Peptic Ulcer

DATA Mr. J. is a 42-year-old computer programmer with a 4-year history of duodenal ulcers. For the past month he has experienced gastric distress with partial relief from Maalox and over-the-counter cimetidine. He was admitted 2 days ago with hematemesis, tarry stools, faintness, and blood pressure of 96/54 (usual BP 124/84).

Intravenous fluids were initiated, and an NG tube inserted for lavage. When the bleeding persisted, an endoscopic examination was performed for local treatment of the recurrent duodenal ulcer. Antacids were administered hourly through the NG tube after endoscopy. Cimetidine was administered intravenously.

Mr. J.'s blood pressure is now stable, and the NG tube has been removed. He is taking oral fluids and has been started on a soft diet. He is taking 30 mg of cimetidine with meals and at bedtime. Maalox, 30 ml, is ordered 1 hour and 3 hours after meals as needed. The nursing history identified that Mr. J.:

Lacks knowledge about the nature of peptic ulcer disease, its treatment, and potential complications.
Takes aspirin fairly regularly for headaches caused by eye strain.
Smokes 1½ packs per day; he has tried to quit several times.
Drinks three or four beers on an average of three times weekly.

Collaborative nursing actions include monitoring for:

Signs of further hemorrhage; hematemesis; decreased blood pressure; restlessness; cool, clammy skin; guaiac positive stools.
Signs of perforation: severe, sudden, sharp abdominal pain.

NURSING DIAGNOSIS **Acute pain related to duodenal mucosal irritation and ulceration**
GOALS/OUTCOMES Will report decreased or absence of pain

NOC Suggested Outcomes
- Comfort Level (2100)
- Pain Level (2102)
- Pain Control (1605)

NIC Suggested Interventions
- Analgesic Administration (2210)
- Pain Management (1400)
- Coping Enhancement (5230)

Nursing Interventions/Rationales
- Administer cimetidine with meals and at bedtime as prescribed. *Cimetidine facilitates ulcer healing by decreasing gastric acid secretion; it is given with meals to inhibit food-stimulated HCl secretion.*
- Administer antacids as prescribed. *Antacids neutralize HCl and quickly reduce pain; they interfere with absorption of cimetidine if given concurrently. They must be administered frequently because they are cleared rapidly from the stomach.*
- Monitor pain quality and duration. *To differentiate ulcer pain from perforation and to determine the effectiveness of medications*

Evaluation Parameters
1. Reports control of pain
2. Free of indications of pain (facial grimace, withdrawn behavior, complaints of pain)

NURSING DIAGNOSIS **Ineffective health maintenance related to lack of resources and knowledge of disease process, treatment regimen, and complications**
GOALS/OUTCOMES Will make lifestyle modifications necessary to facilitate ulcer healing

NOC Suggested Outcomes
- Health Promoting Behavior (1602)
- Knowledge: Health Resources (1806)
- Knowledge: Treatment Regimen (1813)
- Participation: Health Care Decisions (1606)

NIC Suggested Interventions
- Health System Guidance (7400)
- Teaching: Disease Process (5602)
- Smoking Cessation Assistance (4490)
- Self-Modification Assistance (4470)

Nursing Interventions/Rationales
- Encourage patient to avoid any food that causes pain, acid-stimulating foods (tea, coffee, chocolate, cola, milk). *Dietary elements do not cause and cannot heal ulcers, but they can cause increased discomfort.*
- Teach patient the relationship between aspirin use and smoking on peptic ulcer disease. *Aspirin and ibuprofen contribute to mucosal breakdown. Smoking appears to exacerbate ulcer relapse.*
- Refer to community smoking cessation program. *Greater success with smoking cessation may be achieved when support systems are available and used.*
- Encourage the use of acetaminophen instead of aspirin or ibuprofen for headache relief. *Acetaminophen does not contribute to mucosal breakdown.*
- Avoid use of over-the-counter cimetidine unless prescribed. *May mask ulcer relapse symptoms.*
- Suggest eye examination and/or environmental modification to reduce eyestrain. *Correcting cause of eye strain may result in fewer headaches, which require drug intervention and potential exacerbation of ulcer disease.*

Nursing Care Plan — *Patient With a Peptic Ulcer–cont'd*

- Encourage the use of stress-reduction techniques. *Ulcer recurrence is more common in patients with chronic anxiety and poor coping skills.*
- Explain side effects of prescribed medications and potential effect on bowel elimination. *Antacids may have either a cathartic or constipating effect depending on their constituents. Bowel elimination may need to be supported through dietary changes.*
- Reinforce the importance of *H. pylori* treatment to prevent relapse. *H. pylori drug treatment creates multiple GI side effects that adversely affect treatment adherence. Failure to adhere contributes to drug resistance.*
- Teach patient to monitor for and report persistent epigastric pain, sudden severe abdominal pain, tarry stools, persistent vomiting, and bloody or brown vomitus. *These symptoms may indicate ulcer complications such as GI bleeding, perforation, or obstruction.*

Evaluation Parameters

1. Accurately describes components of disease process, treatment, and complications
2. Participates in self-care activities to reduce ulcer formation
3. Begins making lifestyle modifications to promote ulcer healing
4. Adheres to prescribed medication regimens

or a synthetic prostaglandin such as misoprostol in this population.

SPECIAL ENVIRONMENTS FOR CARE

Critical Care

Critical care is rarely indicated in PUD management. The vast majority of patients are successfully managed in a community or home setting. When complications occur, however, they tend to be emergent and potentially life threatening, and sophisticated critical care management may be essential. This is particularly true for older adults. Common complications include upper GI bleeding or hemorrhage and perforation (discussed later). These complications commonly require critical care management.

Community-Based Care

The standard treatment of PUD is managed by the individual patient and family in a home-based self-care regimen. Adherence issues are important as they relate to medication administration and smoking cessation. The severity of symptoms provides an initial impetus for regimen compliance, but this effect is difficult to sustain once symptom control has been achieved. The nurse's teaching concerning the regimen and its rationale is essential to long-term success.

COMPLICATIONS

The major complications of PUD are hemorrhage, perforation, and obstruction of the pyloric outlet.

Hemorrhage. Acute upper GI bleeding results in more than 300,000 hospital admissions each year, and PUD is responsible for about 50% of all cases.[9] The 5% to 10% associated mortality rate has generally remained stable throughout the years despite vast improvements in endoscopic techniques for treatment.[18] The mortality rate reflects the vulnerability of the elderly population and the fact that most upper GI bleeding–related deaths are the result of comorbid conditions and not the bleeding itself. Increasingly effective pharmacologic treatment of PUD has had little if any effect on hospitalization rates for GI bleeding, as most patients report no prior ulcer history or symptoms. Gastric ulcers bleed more often and more severely than duodenal ulcers. NSAID use plus alcohol ingestion greatly increase the risk and men experience bleeding twice as often as women. Aging is the most critical risk factor as the risk of bleeding is three to five times greater for older adults.[9,18,29] Although close to 80% of all bleeding episodes are self-limiting and resolve spontaneously with only supportive care, bleeding is a serious complication that must be handled in an appropriate and timely manner. Massive bleeding is always treated in an intensive care unit (ICU) setting if possible.

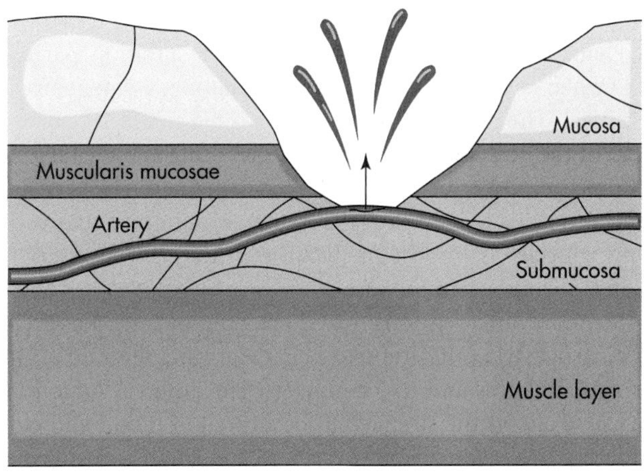

Figure 33-7 Bleeding vessel at ulcer base occurs when ulcer erodes into artery.

The severity of ulcer bleeding ranges from slight oozing to frank profuse hemorrhage (Figure 33-7). Emesis that is dark or of coffee-ground appearance indicates that the blood has been in the stomach long enough for HCl to alter it. Bright-red bleeding indicates a recent onset. Significant bleeding is almost always arterial in nature and usually originates from a single eroded vessel in the base of the ulcer. Small arteries typically are involved, but deep erosion (>1 mm) may affect the larger arterial trunks.

Rapid assessment and resuscitation are the keys to successful treatment of an upper GI bleed. Careful vital sign assessment can yield early cues. Postural blood pressure changes of 10 mm Hg or an increase in pulse rate of more than 20 beats/min indicate at least a 20% blood loss.[18] Clinical manifestations vary with the extent of the bleeding. The most common sign is hematemesis, although patients with duodenal ulcers may not exhibit any overt bleeding signs even with gastric aspiration if the pylorus successfully prevents duodenal reflux. They may experience melena. Anxiety and altered alertness may also be present. Shock will not occur until blood loss approximates 40% of the total volume. (See Chapter 14 for a more detailed discussion of shock assessment.) A large-bore IV catheter is inserted, and normal saline or Ringer's solution is infused rapidly to sustain the systolic pressure above 100 mm Hg. Supplemental oxygen is provided.

Hematemesis presents a serious risk for aspiration, particularly when large clots are present. Maintaining a patent airway is critical. The nurse turns the patient to the side and keeps the head of the bed elevated about 45 degrees unless the vital signs become unstable. Suction should be present at the bedside and used as needed to help clear the mouth. Mouth care after vomiting episodes is important. Intubation may be necessary to protect the airway in the case of massive bleeding.[18]

Standard interventions for GI bleeding include placement of a nasogastric (NG) tube to help determine the rate of ongoing blood loss and to facilitate gastric lavage. A large-bore NG tube allows the stomach to be cleared of blood and clots and prepares it for diagnostic endoscopy. Fluid is instilled in 500 to 1000 ml volumes and removed by gentle suction. This process is repeated until the returns are clear. Room temperature tap water is commonly used for lavage, although some centers still advocate the use of saline to minimize the risk of electrolyte washout.[9]

Iced saline or water is not advised because it is extremely uncomfortable, can significantly lower the patient's core body temperature, particularly in elderly persons, and does not result in vasoconstriction or a reduction in bleeding.[9] Also the chilling may trigger cardiac dysrhythmias. The addition of epinephrine or other medications to lavage solutions has not been shown to reduce bleeding.

Transfusion with packed RBCs may be ordered to help stabilize the patient hemodynamically and to provide a buffer in case of rebleeding. Efforts are usually made to keep the hematocrit above 30 in older adults, especially if cardiac or respiratory comorbid conditions are present. Younger healthy people can tolerate much lower hematocrit values and may not require transfusion.[29]

Acute bleeding can be terrifying for the patient. The nurse maintains a calm and confident approach and remains at the bedside to provide reassurance to the patient. All interventions should be carefully explained. Ensuring warmth also is important. Gastric lavage, IV solutions, and chilled blood products can induce chilling and shivering, which can significantly increase the body's need for oxygen.

Drug therapy during an active bleeding episode usually involves the IV administration of an H_2-receptor antagonist or a proton pump inhibitor, although there is little research evidence that they affect either mortality or the incidence of rebleeding. It is assumed that reducing the acid load will promote healing. Antacids and sucralfate are not used initially because they interfere with endoscopic evaluation.[9]

Most bleeding episodes resolve spontaneously, and situations that will require more definitive interventions cannot be accurately predicted. Concern exists for both the control of the initial bleeding episode and the risk of rebleeding. Endoscopic evaluation has dramatically reduced morbidity associated with GI bleeding and is essential to isolate and evaluate the bleeding site. It is generally agreed that actively bleeding ulcers, either oozing or spurting, or the presence of visible vessels in the ulcer crater warrant further intervention. A clean white ulcer bed presents a very low risk of rebleeding, and most patients can be discharged and monitored on an outpatient basis.[18]

Therapeutic endoscopy may incorporate thermal coagulation of the bleeding vessel or injection therapy. Both approaches are consistently effective, and the choice is a clinical one. Thermal coagulation may be achieved through bipolar electrodes, heater probes, or laser therapy (Figure 33-8). Lasers produce excellent results, but they are extremely expensive pieces of equipment that can rarely be brought directly to the bedside, and require a highly skilled operator. Thermal coagulation is more efficient and cost-effective.[18]

Injection therapy—with epinephrine, absolute alcohol, or other sclerosing agent—is an alternative primary or adjunct therapy. It is also the easiest and least expensive approach. Angiographic techniques that embolize the bleeding vessel with

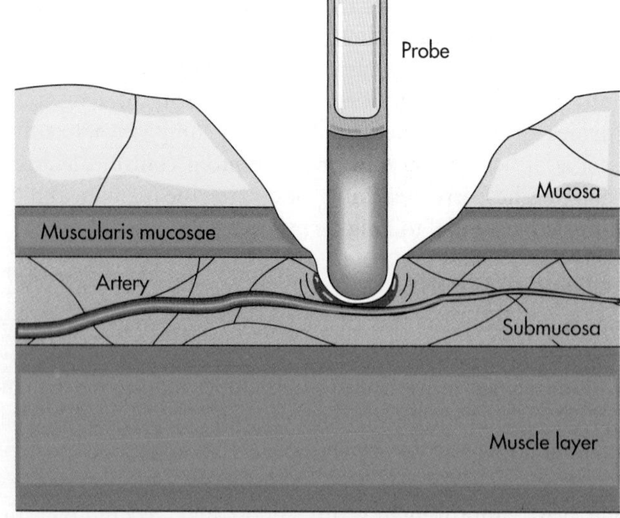

Figure 33-8 Heater probe or bipolar electrode is used first for tamponade of bleeding vessel, then to bring about coagulation.

foreign materials can produce dramatic results, but they require extremely experienced and skilled angiographers.

Surgery is used only when all nonsurgical methods have been tried. However, results are directly linked to the promptness of the decision to operate, with outcomes deteriorating rapidly when surgery is delayed. Operative mortality ranges between 30% and 40%. The dilemma is compounded by reported success with repeat endoscopic treatment (see Research box). Agreement does not exist concerning the procedure to use. Simple oversewing of the ulcer is quick and effective, but many surgeons advocate performing an acid reduction procedure (vagotomy) at the same time to reduce the risk of future bleeding. Laparoscopic approaches show early promise in decreasing operative mortality rates.[31]

The nursing role in the management of GI hemorrhage is largely collaborative and involves careful ongoing patient assessment, prevention of complications, and support of the patient and family. The nurse establishes IV access and implements the fluid resuscitation and ongoing vital sign monitoring. The nurse may be responsible for the gastric lavage. Management of the patient with GI bleeding is summarized in the accompanying Guidelines for Safe Practice box, and a Clinical Pathway for the patient with a GI bleed is found on pp. 1040 to 1043.

Perforation. Perforation involves the erosion of a peptic ulcer through the muscular wall of the stomach or duodenum, with spillage of gastric secretions into the abdominal cavity. It may occur spontaneously or as a complication of therapeutic endoscopy. It occurs six to eight times more often with duodenal ulcers than with gastric ulcers. A chemical peritonitis quickly develops from contact with the GI contents, and a bacterial peritonitis develops within 12 hours. The clinical presentation of perforation usually is dramatic in younger adults, but it may be subdued in elderly persons. This fact typically causes delays in seeking treatment and contributes to the high mortality rate associated with perforation in older patients, which runs as high as 35%. Perforations commonly seal spontaneously in younger adults but are less likely to do so in elderly persons.[18]

The classic clinical picture of ulcer perforation includes (1) severe, sharp abdominal pain; (2) an abdomen that becomes rigid, with rebound tenderness; (3) tachycardia, tachypnea, and diaphoresis; and (4) decreased bowel sounds. A perforation usually is diagnosed by the symptom pattern and supported by the finding of subdiaphragmatic free air on abdominal x-ray film.

Immediate care consists of establishing IV access to replace fluids and inserting an NG tube for drainage of the GI tract. High-dose antibiotics are usually administered in anticipation of sepsis. Effective management of pain is crucial.

The patient is kept in a low Fowler's position to attempt to contain the escaped secretions in a limited area of the abdomen. The nurse provides the patient with emotional support and reassurance, offers comfort measures, and prepares the patient for surgery.

Emergency surgery is the definitive treatment for perforation. Controversy exists over whether the surgery should simply repair the defect with oversewing and use of an omental patch or include definitive ulcer correction. Truncal vagotomy and pyloroplasty may be performed in stable elderly patients in whom the risk of recurrence is believed to be high.

Research

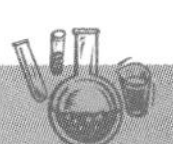

Reference: Lau JYW et al: Endoscopic retreatment compared with surgery in patients with recurrent bleeding after initial endoscopic control of bleeding ulcers, *N Engl J Med* 340(10):751, 1999.

Endoscopic treatment is the first choice for treating bleeding ulcers, but controversy exists over the appropriate treatment for patients who experience rebleeding, which occurs in 15% to 20% of all patients. The question has been difficult to answer because delay in initiating surgical intervention is associated with a significantly higher surgical mortality rate.

This study compared endoscopic retreatment with surgery for more than 100 patients who experienced rebleeding after initial control of their ulcer bleeding with endoscopic therapy. Patients were randomly assigned to one of the two treatment groups. Long-term hemostasis was achieved in about 75% of patients in the endoscopic retreatment group, significantly reducing the need for surgery with its attendant morbidity and mortality. Surgical outcomes for patients needing surgical intervention after endoscopic treatment failure did not differ from those of the primary surgical treatment group. There is early evidence that the success of endoscopic retreatment is dependent to some degree on the size of the bleeding vessel, with larger vessels being more difficult to seal.

Guidelines for Safe Practice

The Patient With Gastrointestinal Bleeding

- Establish at least one large-bore IV access:
  - Infuse normal saline or Ringer's lactate as ordered
- Monitor vital signs frequently for signs of shock.
- Start oxygen by nasal cannula as ordered:
  - Extremely important in elderly persons
- Draw blood for CBC, type, and crossmatch.
- Insert NG tube and institute gastric lavage:
  - Instill 250 ml room-temperature tap water
  - Allow a 2 min dwell time
  - Aspirate and evaluate the returns using a piston type of syringe
  - Repeat as needed until returns are light colored and free of clots
- Measure and record all output.
- Raise head of bed 45 degrees if vital signs remain stable.
- Turn vomiting patient on side to protect the airway.
- Maintain the patient NPO.
- Provide oral suction at bedside to help clear blood.
- Provide mouth care after vomiting episodes.
- Reassure patient and maintain a calm manner.
- Administer IV H_2-receptor antagonist as ordered.
- Administer blood products as ordered.
- Prepare patient for therapeutic endoscopy.

CBC, Complete blood count; *IV,* intravenous; *NG,* nasogastric; *NPO,* nothing by mouth.

clinical pathway *Gastrointestinal Hemorrhage*

	DAY 1	DAY 2	DAY 3	DAY 4	DAY 5	DAY 6
Assessment						
Neurological/ psychological	Mental status • LOC • restlessness • subjective statement of fatigue & weakness • explore anxiety/coping skills • begin assessment of knowledge of health care problem & potential modifiable risk factors (smoking, diet, alcohol, stress, & exercise) • identify available & needed family/human/economic resources to resume independent self-care activities	Mental status • LOC • restlessness • subjective statement of fatigue & weakness • anxiety/coping skills • continue assessment of knowledge of health care problem & potential modifiable risk factors (alcohol, smoking, diet, stress, exercise) • collaborate w/social services re: available & needed family/human/economic resources to resume independent self-care activities	Mental status • restlessness • subjective statement of fatigue & weakness	Mental status • restlessness • subjective statement of fatigue & weakness	Mental status	Mental status
Pulmonary:	RR & pattern	RR & pattern	RR & pattern	RR & pattern	RR	RR
Cardiovascular:	HR & BP for hypovolemia & tachycardia • rhythm for dysrhythmias • narrow pulse pressure • pulses & capillary refill	HR & BP for hypovolemia & tachycardia • rhythm for dysrhythmias • narrow pulse pressure • pulses & capillary refill	HR & BP for hypovolemia & tachycardia • narrow pulse pressure • pulses & capillary refill	HR & BP for hypovolemia & tachycardia • BP for orthostatic changes • pulses & capillary refill	BP for orthostatic changes • pulses	BP for orthostatic changes • pulses
Gastrointestinal:	Mucous membranes for dryness • bowel sounds • abdominal pain (location, stage, level, & duration), cramps, distention • nausea • vomiting • stool for frequency, color, & form • daily wgt	Mucous membranes for dryness • bowel sounds • abdominal pain (location, stage, level, & duration), cramps, distention • nausea • vomiting • stool for frequency, color, & form • daily wgt	Mucous membranes for dryness • bowel sounds • abdominal pain (location, stage, level, & duration), cramps, distention • nausea • vomiting • stool for frequency, color, & form • daily wgt	Appetite & food tolerance • stool for frequency, color, & form • daily wgt	Appetite & food tolerance • stool for frequency, color, & form • daily wgt	Appetite and food tolerance • stool for frequency, color, & form • daily wgt

Genitourinary:	I & O • UO > 30 ml/hr	I & O • UO > 30 ml/hr	I & O • UO > 30 ml/hr	I & O • UO > 30 ml/hr	UO qs	UO qs
Integumentary:	Skin turgor, temp, color, & integrity • presence of diaphoresis, petechiae, or spider angiomata	Skin turgor, temperature, color, & integrity • presence of diaphoresis, petechiae, or spider angiomata	Skin turgor, temp, color, & integrity • presence of diaphoresis, petechiae, or spider angiomata	Skin turgor, temp, color, & integrity • presence of diaphoresis, petechiae, or spider angiomata	Skin turgor & integrity	Skin turgor & integrity
Focus	Fluid resuscitation/ volume replacement • identify source of bleeding	Fluid resuscitation/ volume replacement • initiate PO fluid intake	Increase in PO fluid • progressive increase in activity • teaching	Teaching • increased independence in ADL • increased activity & diet tolerance	Discharge plan & teaching	Self-care & discharge
Diagnostic Plan	Chemistries • monitor Hct & hemoglobin q2-4h until stable • hemolytic profile w/platelets • coagulation studies • liver function tests • blood grouping & crossmatch • stool for occult blood • specific gravity qs *Consider:* urgent anoscopy, sigmoidoscopy, colonoscopy, or endoscopy (esophageal, stomach, duodenal) w/cautery/injection or biopsy • gastric secretion pH & occult blood q4h • Sa_{O_2} pulse oximeter • cardiac monitor	CBC w/differential • continue monitoring Hct, hemoglobin, & electrolytes q6-8h until stable • repeat abnormal lab tests *Consider:* visceral (mesenteric) angiography • nuclear bleeding scan w/labeled red blood cells • gastric secretion analysis	Repeat any abnormal lab test(s) *Consider:* contrast x-ray to rule out underlying pathology • further coagulation studies	CBC w/differential • repeat abnormal lab tests	Repeat Hct & any lab study w/abnormal value	None
Therapeutic Interventions	Large-bore IV access • give 2 L IV NS/RL in 1-2 hr then 150-200 ml/hr (as tolerated) to keep UO > 30 ml/hr until stable • irrigate NGT q2h w/30 ml NS • NPO w/frequent oral care	Clamp NGT for 12 hrs • give sips of H_2O PO • discontinue NGT if clamping tolerated • continue IV fluid hydration • start on clear fluids once	Discontinue NGT • decrease IV fluids as PO fluid intake increased to maintain UO > 30 ml/hr • progress diet from fluids to soft • change to PO meds	Discontinue IV • increased walking in hall • soft diet	Encourage activity & independence in ADL	Discharge • encourage lifestyle modifications

From Birdsall C, Sperry SP: *Clinical paths in medical surgical practice,* St Louis, 1997, Mosby.
LOC, Level of consciousness; *NGT,* nasogastric tube; *ASA,* aspirin; *NS,* normal saline; *RL,* Ringer's lactate.

Continued

clinical pathway *Gastrointestinal Hemorrhage—cont'd*

	DAY 1	DAY 2	DAY 3	DAY 4	DAY 5	DAY 6
Therapeutic Interventions—cont'd	• bed rest • cardiac monitor • O_2 prn *Consider:* antacids • histamine H_2 receptor blocker • sucralfate • antibiotics (if ulcers suspected) • IV vasopressin • packed red blood cells (if Hct <25%)	NGT removed & no nausea • BRP w/assistance • assist w/hygiene	• get OOB to chair tid • walk in hall w/help bid • discontinue cardiac monitor & specific gravity *Consider:* oral iron, stool softener, & fiber supplement			
Patient/Family Teaching/ Discharge Planning	Explain initial treatment/ meds/fluids • instruct to call nurse for chest pain, SOB, dizziness, fast HR, diaphoresis, vomiting, diarrhea • explore potential precipitating factors (ASA, NSAID, smoking, alcohol, corticosteroids, family history, anticoagulants, prolonged retching) & document same • identify available & needed family/ human/economic resources to resume independent self-care activities • identify Pt/family coping mechanisms • initiate discharge plan • discuss plan for daily review of plan of care w/Pt/family	Explain need for adequate hydration • explain disease process • identify learning needs related to disease syndrome & document same • discuss potential lifestyle changes prn (alcohol, smoking cessation, diet, stress management, wgt reduction, exercise program) • reassure that responses (anxiety, subjective feelings of emotional lability or inability to concentrate, etc.) are a normal reaction • encourage verbalization of anxiety/fear • review, clarify, & confirm information given to date	Collaborate w/dietitian & initiate diet teaching • teach to get up slowly from lying position • teach signs of intestinal bleeding (hematemesis, melena, hematochezia) • review meds & food/drug interactions	Teach S & S of bleeding (thirst, frequent lip licking, lightheadedness, dizziness, weakness/ fatigue, impaired mental status, irritability, pallor, tremors, decrease in uo, dry skin & mucous membranes) • review meds, food/ drug interactions, appropriate health-seeking behaviors, & when to seek medical care	Review discharge plan, disease process, exercise plan, meds & drug/food interactions • value of relaxation techniques & health-seeking behaviors by modifying lifestyle prn (smoking, stress, alcohol, diet, aspirin, other meds, etc.)	Review appointment dates for physician visit & discharge plan

Expected Outcomes	W/volume replacement, hemodynamic stability is restored • active bleeding stopped • UO > 30 ml/hr • verbalizes treatment plan	Tolerating PO fluids • plan for encouraging PO fluids documented • fluid & potassium in balance as evidenced by UO > 30 ml/hr, stable VS, & stable Hct & hemoglobin • decrease in anxiety	No parenteral therapy • increased tolerance of PO fluids & diet • nutritional assessment documented & calorie/protein needs identified • well hydrated • no bleeding • no abdominal distress • formed stools • independent ADL • verbalizes disease process & potential lifestyle changes	Ambulates without assistance & independent in ADL • verbalizes meds information • demonstrates improved appetite • states signs of intestinal bleeding (hematemesis, melena, hematochezia) & to report same (red or brown-tinged vomitus & maroon, red, bloody, or tarry stools)	Verbalizes diet restrictions (avoid foods that previously caused discomfort, high-acid foods, hot pepper, caffeine, highly spiced food, & alcohol) & need to prevent constipation while on oral iron • denies subjective feelings of anxiety • verbalizes appropriate concerns & fears • states S & S of bleeding (thirst, frequent lip licking, light-headedness, dizziness, weakness/fatigue, impaired mental status, irritability, pallor, tremors, decrease in urine output, dry skin & mucous membranes) & when to seek medical care	Verbalizes risk factors & health-seeking behaviors • states appointment date w/physican
Trigger(s)	S & S of new bleeding w/ hypotension, tachycardia, & UO <30 ml/hr	Persistent hypotension, tachycardia, or UO <30 ml/hr • nausea/vomiting/abdominal pain	Persistent hypotension, tachycardia, or UO <30 ml/hr • nausea/vomiting/abdominal pain	Pain, new bleeding, anorexia, decreased output • inability to maintain fluid & food intake needed for hydration & to meet caloric needs	Inadequate fluid or dietary intake	Inadequate fluid or dietary intake • unable to be independent in ADL

Obstruction. Improved treatment of peptic ulcers has caused the incidence of gastric outlet obstruction to decline to the point of being rare. Obstruction can result from scar tissue formation but also from muscle obstruction and narrowing caused by spasm and inflammatory edema. It is usually associated with long-standing PUD.

The obstruction usually develops slowly, and the patient may initially experience dyspepsia symptoms, including anorexia and nausea, as the stomach fails to empty completely. Weight loss and malnutrition develop if the diagnosis is delayed, and this is a common occurrence in elderly persons. Vomiting occurs when the chyme is completely unable to pass into the duodenum, which usually represents a narrowing of the normally 10- to 20-mm pyloric channel to less than 6 mm.

Diagnosis of obstruction can be established by aspiration of stomach contents or abdominal x-ray films that show gastric distention and large fluid levels. Endoscopy is performed to rule out the presence of an obstructing tumor and may be used to treat uncomplicated obstructions.

Initial management of obstruction involves fluid and electrolyte replacement and gastric decompression with an NG tube. Aggressive therapy for the ulcer may be initiated first because obstruction is rarely an emergent condition. The obstruction may resolve sufficiently with ulcer healing to eliminate the need for surgical intervention. When surgery is needed a vagotomy-plus-drainage procedure is the procedure of choice to minimize postoperative digestive problems. Even high-risk older adults can generally tolerate this surgery if attention has been paid to careful preoperative stabilization.

STRESS ULCERS

Etiology/Epidemiology

The terms stress-related mucosal damage and stress ulcer refer to a syndrome characterized by the development of multiple diffuse gastric lesions and ulceration shortly after the onset of acute illness, trauma, or sepsis. The problem used to be almost universal among patients in critical care settings. The incidence of stress ulcers reported in the 1970s was in excess of 80% of the critical care population, and the incidence of clinically significant bleeding was nearly 20%. Because GI hemorrhage in the critically ill is accompanied by a high mortality rate, these statistics served as the basis for the development of aggressive prevention protocols that were implemented with virtually every critically ill patient. The incidence of significant bleeding has declined dramatically over the last 15 to 20 years, probably primarily in response to significant overall improvements in the care of the critically ill.[10] Clinically important bleeding is now considered to be a rare event.

It is now accepted that not all ICU patients are at equal risk for stress ulcer bleeding. Efforts are ongoing to identify the factors that place patients at risk and conditions where the association with bleeding is high. Respiratory failure requiring mechanical ventilation and the presence of coagulopathies are the two most frequently identified risks, and advanced age complicates the situation. Research is now focusing on accurate identification of patients in need of aggressive stress ulcer prophylaxis and the cost effectiveness of various prevention protocols.[10] Significant risk factors are summarized in the Risk Factors box.

Pathophysiology

The major factor that causes stress ulceration is a loss of the ability to maintain the integrity of the mucosa. The maintenance of mucosal homeostasis is a complex process involving mucus production, mucosal blood flow, prostaglandin secretion, bicarbonate production, and maintenance of the needed pH gradient. The severe stress state decreases gastric mucosal blood flow and triggers a series of changes that can ultimately result in mucosal breakdown. The epithelial cells of the mucosa are extremely sensitive to hypoxia, and the process of cellular necrosis can begin within minutes. Stress ulceration cannot occur without the presence of acid and pepsin, but overproduction of acid is rarely the cause of stress ulcers. In fact, acid secretion commonly is temporarily diminished in the acute stress state. Mucosal resistance therefore is believed to be the key. The notable exceptions are Cushing's and Curling's ulcers, which are associated with massive increases in acid output, often exceeding 3 to 4 L/day.

Stress ulcer lesions tend to be more shallow than standard peptic ulcers and develop in multiple sites rather than as a single well-defined lesion. The proximal acid-secreting areas of the stomach are the prime targets. The classic presentation of stress ulcers is the development of painless GI bleeding within 3 to 7 days of admission to a critical care unit.

Collaborative Care Management

The focus of the clinical management of stress ulcers is prevention because the mortality rate associated with significant bleeding is high. The challenge lies in identifying which patients to treat prophylactically and in what way.[10] The traditional approach has been to treat all critical care patients aggressively with antacids, histamine-receptor antagonists, or sucralfate. Frequent monitoring of gastric pH is usually performed either by intermittent aspiration of gastric secretions or through the use of special NG tubes with the capability for

Risk Factors

Stress Ulcer Bleeding

MAJOR

Respiratory failure/intubation with mechanical ventilation for longer than 48 hours
Coagulopathy
Hypotension/Shock

RELATED

Sepsis
Multiple trauma
Neurologic injury/surgery
Severe burns over 30% of the body surface
Hepatic/renal failure

NOTE: The presence of more than one risk factor significantly increases the likelihood of bleeding.

continuous pH monitoring. The pH is usually kept above 3.5, although some sources recommend a pH of at least 4.0.[5]

Increased individualization of care is now recommended. Patients with multiple risk factors, and particularly patients who will need mechanical ventilation for longer than 48 hours and those with demonstrable coagulopathies are recommended for preventive treatment. Treatment options include H_2-receptor antagonists, proton pump inhibitors, and sucralfate. Repeated clinical studies (see Research box) continue to present contradictory findings.[8,10,15] The issue has significant cost implications, especially with the increased popularity of proton pump inhibitors, and continues to be studied.

Concern arose that the prophylactic neutralization of gastric secretions might be leaving ICU patients vulnerable to nosocomial infection, particularly in the form of gram-negative pneumonias. In the absence of gastric acid these organisms can colonize the stomach within 2 to 5 days.[15] Research has again produced conflicting results concerning the development of pneumonia and remains ongoing. Sucralfate is recommended for prophylaxis by some authorities because of its low cost and ability to prevent stress ulcer without altering the gastric pH. Much remains to be learned about the origins, prevention, and treatment of stress ulcers, but it is clear that meticulous bedside monitoring of patient status by skilled ICU nurses will continue to play an essential role.

Patient/Family Education. Critically ill patients and families need to be kept informed about all aspects of the plan of care. This includes all measures aimed at the identification, prevention, or treatment of stress ulcers. The nurse is the primary liaison with the family and informs them about the rationale for all planned interventions.

Stress ulcer is not a problem that is familiar to most laypersons, and the nurse will need to lay the foundation for understanding all relevant care. The stresses of the situation may make it difficult for the patient and family to hear and process information, and time for reteaching should be planned as needed.

Research

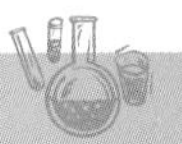

Reference: Cook D et al: A comparison of sucralfate and ranitidine for the prevention of upper GI bleeding in patients requiring mechanical ventilation, *N Engl J Med* 338(12):791, 1998.

This study compared the use of sucralfate and ranitidine to prevent upper GI bleeding in 1200 patients requiring mechanical ventilation. Successful prevention of stress ulcer bleeding is a critical goal, but insufficient evidence is available about which regimens are most effective and cost efficient. Patients needing prolonged mechanical ventilation are considered to be at particular risk. Studies have reported greater success for sucralfate at lower cost and a belief that the risk of nosocomial infection is less with sucralfate than with agents that change the pH environment of the stomach.

In this study patients receiving ranitidine had a significantly lower risk of GI bleeding than those receiving sucralfate. There was no difference in the incidence of pneumonia between the two groups, but a nonsignificant trend in favor of the group treated with sucralfate was found.

CANCER OF THE STOMACH

Etiology

The cause of cancer of the stomach remains unknown and it appears to have a complex, multifactorial etiology. Its highly erratic worldwide incidence pattern strongly suggests the involvement of powerful environmental and cultural factors, but their exact nature remains unclear. Diet has received a great deal of attention, but no single dietary element explains the great variations in incidence. High nitrate content in soil and water and diets high in smoked and preserved foods are believed to be important factors. Nitrates and nitrites in foods are reduced to nitrosamines in the body, and a cascade of DNA changes can then occur that lead to cancer. Improved refrigeration and the availability of fresh foods appears to have decreased the risk in industrialized societies despite vegetables being a major source of nitrates in some diets.[20] Vitamins C and E appear to interfere with nitrate metabolism in the body and may play a protective role.[4] The sharp decline in incidence rates for gastric cancer in the United States since the 1950s is largely believed to be attributable to these factors. No strong links have been found with alcohol or caffeine consumption, and although a link with heavy smoking is present, it is not significant. An inverse relationship appears to exist between incidence and socioeconomic status. Familial clusters are occasionally seen but no genetic link has been isolated at this time.

The development of gastric cancer is related to the presence of achlorhydria and pernicious anemia. Approximately 10% of persons with chronic gastritis develop gastric cancer within 15 years and the link with *H. pylori* infection is apparent. *H. pylori* infection is now considered to be a major carcinogen for gastric cancer despite the confounding data that demonstrate that the vast majority of persons infected with *H. pylori* never develop either ulcers or cancer.[19] Multiple factors clearly play a role.

Epidemiology

Cancer of the stomach was the most common malignant disease in the United States as recently as the 1940s, and it remains the second leading cause of cancer death worldwide.[4,6] Since that time it has undergone a steady decline in incidence in the United States that is not readily explainable. The mortality rate from gastric cancer has declined from 22.5 to 6 per 100,000 population in the United States, and the incidence declined almost 70% between 1950 and 1980.[6] The disease exhibits tremendous variation among different regions of the world and is 10 times more common in Japan where the incidence is in excess of 70 per 100,000 population, the highest in the world.[4] Environmental factors are clearly pivotal, as the incidence in immigrants to the United States drops sharply by the second generation. Gastric cancer is rare before age 40, and the incidence increases sharply with age. The male/female ratio is about 2:1. Risk factors for gastric cancer are summarized in the Risk Factors box.

Pathophysiology

Gastric cancers are virtually all primary adenocarcinomas that are derived from the epithelium. They may occur anywhere

Risk Factors
Gastric Cancer

Chronic infection with *H. pylori*
Diets high in smoked and preserved foods, which contain nitrites and nitrates
Diets low in fresh fruits and vegetables
High nitrate content in the soil and water
History of heavy smoking
Presence of chronic gastritis and achlorhydria (10% of patients develop cancer within 15 years)
Age and sex (incidence increases steadily after age 40, male-to-female ratio is 2:1)

Clinical Manifestations
Gastric Cancer

Dyspepsia: early satiety, bloating, anorexia
Epigastric pain or burning (usually mild and relieved by antacids or over-the-counter H_2-receptor antagonists)
Mild nausea
Weight loss (may be rapid and severe)
Fatigue and weakness

NOTE: Gastric cancer typically is asymptomatic in early stages.

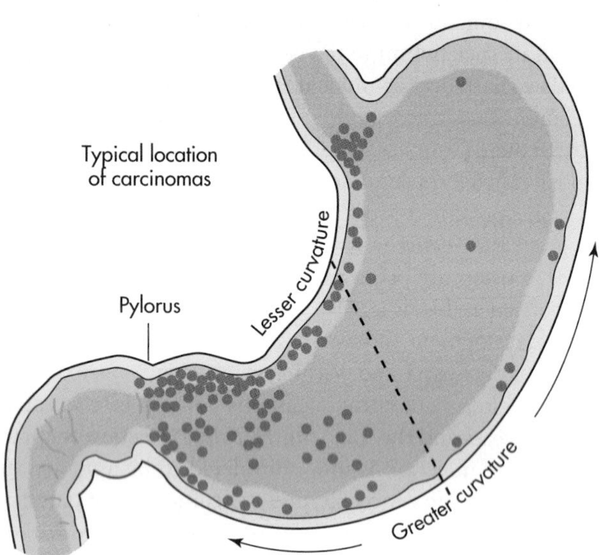

Figure 33-9 Typical sites of gastric cancer.

in the stomach, but about 50% occur in the antrum. Typical sites are illustrated in Figure 33-9. A significant proximal shift has been occurring over the last 30 years, with more than 40% of gastric cancers now originating in the fundus, cardia, and gastroesophageal junction.[4] Histologically, the cancers are classified as diffuse or intestinal. The intestinal form is associated with the presence of intestinal metaplasia in the stomach. This type of gastric cancer has been declining in incidence. The diffuse forms have shown little change in incidence. Early gastric cancer is confined to the mucosa or submucosa and exhibits a long latency period.

Gastric cancer may spread directly through the stomach wall into adjacent tissues; to the lymphatics; to the regional lymph nodes of the stomach; to the esophagus, spleen, pancreas, and liver; or through the bloodstream to the lungs or bones. Involvement of regional lymph nodes occurs early. Prognosis depends on the depth of invasion, extent of metastasis, and location. Cancer that occurs in the upper third of the stomach is associated with a poor prognosis.[4] Three fourths of patients with gastric carcinoma have metastases at the time of diagnosis.

Gastric cancer has an insidious onset. It is accompanied by vague nondescript dyspeptic symptoms that overlap with multiple benign disorders, including nonulcer dyspepsia and PUD.[20] Early diagnosis is therefore extremely rare. Pain does not usually develop until late in the disease. Concern exists that the ready availability of H_2-receptor antagonists over the counter may further delay treatment because early ulcerative lesions frequently respond to acid reduction, at least temporarily. Marked cachexia and a palpable mass in the abdomen may be present at diagnosis. Common clinical manifestations are presented in the Clinical Manifestations box.

Collaborative Care Management

Diagnostic Tests. Upper endoscopy with biopsy has proven to be extremely accurate in diagnosing gastric cancer. Multiple biopsy specimens are obtained. Many gastric cancers can be located by barium contrast upper-GI x-ray films, but only biopsy can confirm the diagnosis. Computed tomography scanning and endoscopic ultrasonography also may be used to define the tumor and to search for distant metastasis. Mass screening programs have been implemented in Japan that have significantly increased the identification of gastric cancer in early treatable stages.

Medications. Medications do not play a role in the management of gastric cancer. The role of chemotherapy remains controversial and continues to be studied. Chemotherapy is the mainstay of treatment for nonresectable tumors, but only partial responses have been achieved and chemotherapy has had no significant effect on survival. Adjuvant chemotherapy after surgery offers no proven benefit at this time.

Treatments. Radiotherapy is being researched as a treatment option for gastric cancer, but at present it shows little proved effectiveness. When used, it is in combination with chemotherapy for nonresectable or recurrent cancer cases, or for palliation of bone metastases. Intraoperative radiation is being used in Japan and shows initial promise in increasing 5-year survival rates.[4] There is insufficient experience with this approach in the United States at this time to begin to evaluate its potential.

Endoscopic treatment may be used for palliation of symptomatic unresectable or recurrent tumors. Endoscopic laser treatment and bipolar probe coagulation can both be used to control bleeding and relieve obstructive symptoms.

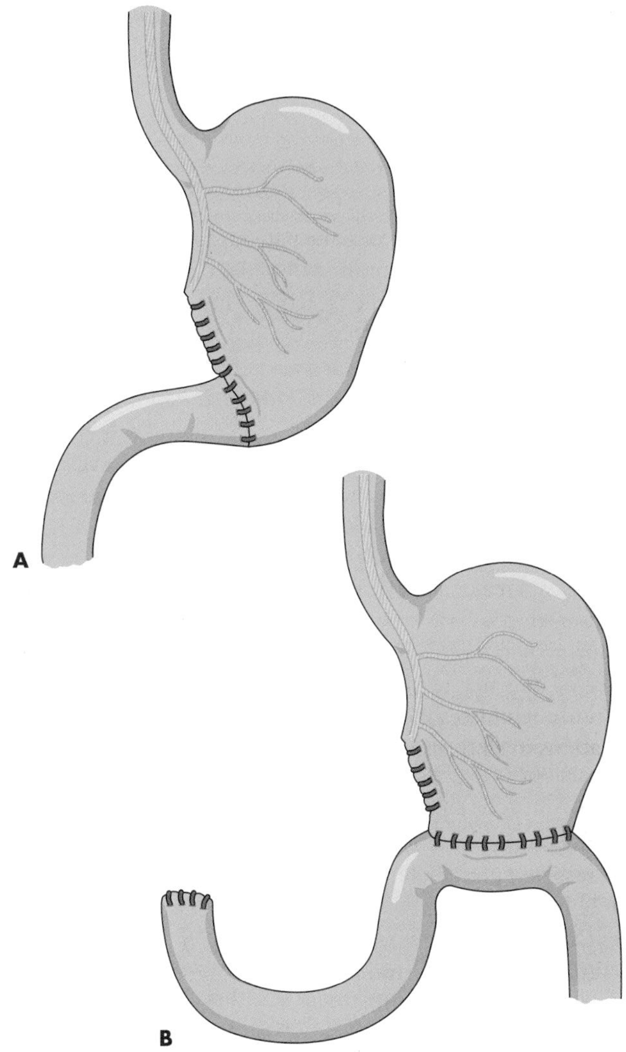

Figure 33-10 Types of gastric resections with anastomoses. **A,** Billroth I anastomosis of gastric segment to duodenum. **B,** Billroth II, anastomosis of gastric segment to the proximal jejunum.

Surgical Management. The only potentially curative treatment for gastric cancer is surgical resection. The procedure of choice depends on the location and extent of the tumor. There is debate concerning the value of routine total gastrectomy. Total gastrectomy is no longer commonly used in the United States because of the serious digestive difficulties and quality of life issues that may result. Five-year survival statistics are only 5% to 15% and operative mortality is high.[14] Most surgeons perform subtotal gastrectomies (Figure 33-10) and attempt to remove all of the tumor. Surgical margins of 5 to 10 cm beyond the cancer are recommended, but difficult to achieve. The extensive experience of Japanese surgeons with gastric cancer indicates the importance of performing more extensive lymph node dissections than have been standard in the United States. Physicians have been reluctant to adopt this aggressive approach and question its applicability for the U.S. population. Tumors that are high in the cardia present more technical challenges to resection and anastomosis. Removal of other abdominal organs appears to have no positive impact on survival.

Diet. There are no specific dietary considerations for the treatment of gastric cancer. Patients may experience severe weight loss and cachexia and eventually require nutritional support. If a patient experiences ulcer-related pain, the standard recommendations for avoiding spicy and irritating foods are made. The patient is encouraged to work within the scope of individual preferences to maintain adequate nutrition. Patients who undergo gastric resection may develop significant problems with dumping syndrome and malabsorption. Management of these disorders is discussed on pp. 1049 to 1050.

Activity. The patient with gastric cancer does not need to restrict activity in any way. Patients are encouraged to remain as active in their usual lifestyles as possible. Treatment for gastric cancer is rigorous and may take a significant toll on the patient's energy level and stamina. The nurse encourages patients to make any necessary modifications in their daily activities to accommodate the demands of the treatment protocol. Quality of life issues play a significant role in treatment decisions.

Referrals. The treatment of resectable gastric cancer is primarily surgical. Referral to consultants usually is not necessary in the early period. The primary ongoing concerns are maintenance of desired weight and nutritional status. If digestion and absorption problems become severe, the patient may be referred to a nutritional support team for guidance and management.

NURSING MANAGEMENT OF PATIENT UNDERGOING GASTRIC SURGERY

PREOPERATIVE CARE

Preoperative care focuses on both ensuring that the patient is in the best nutritional state to support healing and on patient teaching. Correction of nutritional deficits may involve short-term parenteral nutrition if the patient is severely cachectic.

A high abdominal incision is standard with gastric surgery. This incision limits respiration and creates a high risk of postoperative respiratory complications. The nurse focuses preoperative teaching on pulmonary hygiene and the importance of deep breathing, effective coughing, splinting the incision, frequent position changes, incentive spirometry, and chest physiotherapy if indicated. These teaching interventions are even more critical if the patient has a history of smoking. Planned methods for postoperative pain control are also discussed.

Most patients undergoing gastric surgery have an NG tube in place for several days after surgery. The NG tube prevents trauma, reduces pressure on the suture lines, and minimizes gas and fluid accumulation from decreased postoperative peristalsis. The nurse teaches the patient about the NG tube and its purpose, the necessity for an initial NPO status, and the planned use of any other wound-drainage device.

Anxiety is another important area to be addressed by the nurse in the preoperative period. Gastric cancer carries an extremely poor prognosis, and the threat of death affects the patient's ability to attend to teaching and participate in self-care. Accurate staging of the cancer is commonly not possible until surgical exploration is completed, and this adds an additional element of uncertainty to an already stressful situation. The nurse provides support and encourages the patient to verbalize any concerns.

POSTOPERATIVE CARE

Maintaining a Patent Airway and Ventilation

A patient who undergoes gastric surgery tends to lie still and breathe shallowly to limit incisional pain. Pain management is critical and is ideally accomplished through patient-controlled or epidural analgesia. Adequate pain management is essential to achieving respiratory goals. Turning, deep breathing, incentive spirometry, and ambulation are essential postoperative activities, and the nurse must ensure that the patient is comfortable enough to participate actively in them. A semi-Fowler's position assists with natural chest expansion. The nurse routinely auscultates the lungs to monitor pulmonary status and consistently encourages the patient in all pulmonary hygiene routines.

Supporting Adequate Nutrition

The patient is given nothing by mouth until peristalsis resumes and initial surgical healing occurs. Drainage from the NG tube usually contains some blood for the first 6 to 12 hours, but the presence of bright-red blood, large amounts of blood, or excessive bloody drainage is reported to the surgeon at once. If the NG tube stops draining, the surgeon also is notified immediately because a buildup of gas or fluid can put pressure on the suture line, resulting in rupture or dislodgement.

To protect the healing suture line, the nurse does not routinely irrigate or reposition the NG tube. Fluids are given parenterally until the tube is removed and the patient is able to drink sufficient fluids. The nurse offers or provides the patient with frequent mouth care. It is important for gastric drainage and urinary output to be accurately measured and recorded.

Fluids by mouth may be restricted for 12 to 24 hours after the NG tube is removed. Small amounts of fluid are then given frequently, and the patient is observed for signs of leakage, such as difficulty in breathing, pain, or a rise in temperature. Foods are added as tolerated by the patient. The dietary regimen must be adapted to the individual, because some persons tolerate increasing amounts of food and fluids better than others.

When the cardia of the stomach has been removed, the patient may complain of nausea and experience vomiting. This problem is usually caused by irritation of the esophageal mucosa by the gastric juices or duodenal fluids that reflux into the esophagus when the patient lies down. The patient should never lie flat in bed and should avoid bending and stooping.

Early satiety is a common problem after gastric surgery. Regurgitation after meals also occurs and may be caused by eating too fast, eating too much, or postoperative edema around the suture line that prevents the food from passing into the intestines. If regurgitation occurs, the patient is encouraged to eat more slowly and to temporarily decrease the size of each meal. The dumping syndrome and malabsorption may cause serious problems after significant resection, and weight loss may occur. The ongoing involvement of a dietitian or nutritionist may be necessary.

Patient/Family Education

Subtotal gastrectomy is associated with a variety of digestive complications that may cause the patient significant problems with eating, nutritional status, and maintaining a stable body weight. The nurse assists the patient to understand the physiologic basis for these complications and the appropriate diet and lifestyle modifications aimed at minimizing their severity. These problems are discussed later under complications.

Patients with gastric cancer are facing the likelihood of a dramatically shortened life expectancy and a steady decline in self-care abilities. The nurse ensures that the patient and family are aware of resources available for support in their community, particularly the services of the American Cancer Society and Hospice, and makes appropriate referrals as needed. Patients are encouraged to clearly articulate their wishes for future care in the form of advance directives, living wills, and health care power of attorney to support their family's decision making. The nurse reinforces the appropriateness of quality of life considerations in all treatment decisions.

Monitoring for Complications

Bleeding at the anastomosis site is a common problem that may resolve spontaneously. Major risk periods include the first 24 hours after surgery and again between the fourth and seventh days when clot breakdown occurs. The nurse carefully monitors the NG tube drainage for blood and avoids irrigating or repositioning the tube unless specifically ordered.

Any of the anastomosis sites are at risk for leakage in the early postoperative period. The blind-end duodenal stump that is created with a Billroth II (Figure 33-11) procedure appears to be particularly vulnerable. The nurse monitors for classic peritonitis symptoms such as severe abdominal pain, rigidity, and fever. Surgical drainage and closure are often necessary.

The Guidelines for Safe Practice box summarizes the nursing care provided to a patient undergoing gastric surgery.

GERONTOLOGIC CONSIDERATIONS

Gastric cancer is rare before the age of 40 years and typically occurs in persons between 50 and 70 years old. Therefore the entire discussion related to the collaborative management of gastric cancer is targeted primarily toward older persons who are most likely to be affected by this deadly disease process. The presence of comorbid conditions increases the challenge of managing gastric cancer in older adults and increases the risk of postoperative complications.

SPECIAL ENVIRONMENTS FOR CARE

Critical Care

Critical care is rarely needed in the management of gastric cancer. The disease prognosis is extremely poor, especially for advanced invasive disease, and only palliative treatment may be undertaken. Treatment may be restricted to relieving obstruction or treating bleeding. Anastomosis leakage is a se-

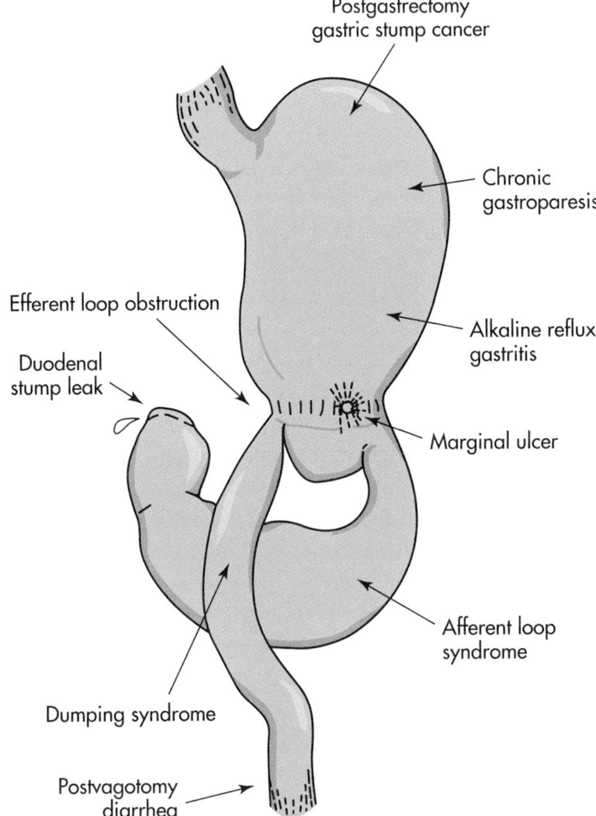

Figure 33-11 Complications of gastric surgery.

rious complication of gastrectomy surgeries, and its occurrence might require critical care monitoring, particularly if patients have other chronic illnesses that increase their risks.

Community-Based Care

Returning home after treatment presents a series of ongoing challenges for the patient and family. The dumping syndrome is the most common complication of the surgical treatment of gastric cancer, and the patient will need to make multiple dietary adjustments to control its symptoms. Nutritional support may become necessary in certain situations and is essential if further active treatment is planned.

Pain control is a common community care issue for patients with advanced disease. The appropriate use of long-acting oral opioids, transdermal patches, epidural catheters, and infusion pumps can make it possible for patients to remain comfortably in their home environments with home health or hospice support.

The greatest ongoing challenge for both the patient and family is the knowledge of the terminal prognosis. They need support and encouragement to deal effectively with a progressive and deteriorating situation. In many cases the disease is fatal within 1 year of diagnosis, and the patient's physical decline can be both rapid and frightening.

COMPLICATIONS

Gastrectomy is associated with several major digestive complications that require ongoing management. These include

Guidelines for Safe Practice
The Patient Undergoing Gastric Surgery

PREOPERATIVE CARE

Teach deep breathing exercises.
Explain special postoperative measures: nasogastric tube and parenteral fluids until peristalsis returns.

POSTOPERATIVE CARE

Promote pulmonary ventilation.
- Position patient in mid or high Fowler's position.
- Encourage patient to turn and breathe deep at least q2h (or more frequently until ambulating well); splint or support incision with hands or folded towel during coughing if needed to clear secretions.
- Provide adequate analgesics during first few days; patient-controlled analgesia is effective.
- Encourage ambulation.
- Provide good mouth care until oral fluids can be resumed.

Promote nutrition.
- Measure nasogastric drainage accurately; monitor for blood in drainage. Do not irrigate or reposition tube unless ordered.
- Monitor for signs of leakage of anastomosis (dyspnea, pain, fever) when oral fluids are resumed.
- Add food in small amounts at frequent intervals until well tolerated.
- Monitor for early satiety and regurgitation.
- If regurgitation occurs, tell patient to eat less food at a slower pace.
- Report signs of dumping syndrome to physician (weakness, faintness, palpitations, diaphoresis, nausea, diarrhea).
- Monitor weight.

Provide patient/family education.
- Gradually increase amount of food each meal until able to eat 3 to 6 meals per day, if possible.
- If discomfort occurs after eating, decrease size of meals and amount of fluids with meals; eat more slowly.
- Avoid eating simple carbohydrates and concentrated sweets.
- Avoid stress during and immediately after meals; plan a rest period after eating. Lie on left side.
- Elevate head when lying down (if cardia of stomach removed).
- Monitor weight regularly.
- Report signs of complications: vomiting after meals, increasing feelings of abdominal fullness or weakness, hematemesis, tarry stools, persistent diarrhea.

dumping syndrome and malabsorption (see Figure 33-11). Vitamin B_{12} deficiency may also develop.

Dumping Syndrome. *Dumping syndrome* is the term used for a group of unpleasant vasomotor and GI symptoms that occur after gastric resection and vagotomy surgery in as many as 50% of patients.[31] It is a complex process with several contributing causative factors. One major element is believed to be the rapid entry of hyperosmolar food directly into the upper small intestine without first undergoing the usual breakdown and dilution in the stomach. This causes distention, stimulates motility, and produces both an intense feeling of fullness and discomfort plus diarrhea.[14] The undiluted chyme is highly hyperosmolar and causes an osmotic shift of fluid from the intravascular compartment into the intestine. This worsens the distention and triggers a systemic response of weakness, sweating, tachycardia, and flushing. This reaction is called the early dumping syndrome and typically occurs within 15 to 30 minutes of eating. Common features of the dumping syndrome are included in the Patient Teaching box.

A second "late" dumping syndrome follows. Rapid absorption of glucose from the chyme results in hyperglycemia and provokes insulin secretion. The insulin secretion outlasts the hyperglycemia, which then swings to hypoglycemia and its associated anxiety, weakness, diaphoresis, palpitations, and faintness. These symptoms develop about 2 hours after eating.

Prevention is the most effective means of controlling dumping syndrome. The nurse instructs the patient to follow a moderate-fat, high-protein diet with limited carbohydrates. Simple sugars should be avoided completely. Fluids with meals are discouraged because they increase total volume. Lying down on the left side for 20 to 30 minutes after eating to delay gastric emptying is helpful for some patients. Anticholinergic or antispasmodic drugs may be effective in certain cases. Management of the dumping syndrome is summarized in the Patient Teaching box.

Diarrhea/Malabsorption. Malabsorption of fat may occur after gastric resection from decreased acid secretion, decreased availability of pancreatic enzymes, and increased upper GI motility, which prevents adequate mixing of the chyme with biliary and pancreatic secretions. It is particularly troublesome after Billroth II procedures. The patient experiences steatorrhea, diarrhea, and weight loss. Deficiencies in fat-soluble vitamins may occur. Diet adjustments are made to evaluate the patient's response to varying amounts of dietary fat. Pancreatic enzymes or antispasmodic agents may be helpful.

The combined effects of dumping syndrome and steatorrhea can result in significant weight loss over a relatively short time. The patient is encouraged to monitor body weight at least weekly and to experiment with food supplements as tolerated to meet nutritional needs.

Vitamin B_{12} Deficiency. Gastrectomy procedures result in a partial or total loss of the intrinsic factor that is secreted by the parietal cells of the stomach. Intrinsic factor is essential to the absorption of vitamin B_{12} in the intestine. Without its presence, the patient gradually develops the symptoms of pernicious anemia, which can be fatal if not treated. The nurse teaches the patient about the vitamin deficiency and explains why oral vitamin replacement is not possible. Lifelong replacement therapy with a 100 to 200 mg monthly injection of vitamin B_{12} prevents the deficiency. The digestive changes associated with gastrectomy also impair absorption of both calcium and iron. Iron deficiency anemia commonly develops, and ferrous sulfate may be prescribed if tolerated. Over time the calcium deficiency can result in bone demineralization, especially in older postmenopausal women. Calcium supplementation has minimal effect.

Alkaline Reflux Gastritis/Esophagitis. Excessive reflux of duodenal or jejunal secretions may occur after gastric resection and cause severe irritation of the stomach or distal esophagus, depending on the extent of resection. Bile acids are believed to be the primary cause. Chronic abdominal pain and vomiting may result. The syndrome is difficult to treat; it does not respond well to pharmacologic intervention. In severe cases a surgical bypass procedure may be indicated.

Patient Teaching
Dumping Syndrome

CLINICAL MANIFESTATIONS

- Weakness
- Dizziness
- Diaphoresis
- Tachycardia
- Palpitations
- Feeling of fullness or discomfort
- Nausea
- Diarrhea
- Onset of symptoms occurs first within 1 hour of eating and may recur after 2 hours

MANAGEMENT

Prevention is the key:
- Small frequent meals
- Moderate-fat, high-protein diet
- Limited carbohydrates, no simple sugars
- Minimal liquids with meals
- Avoid very hot and very cold foods and beverages
- Rest on left side for 20-30 min after eating
- Anticholinergic or antispasmodic medications

NAUSEA AND VOMITING

Etiology/Epidemiology

Nausea and vomiting, which often occur together but may occur independently, are extremely common GI symptoms. They are part of the body's protective mechanisms and are usually a response to chemical, bacterial, or viral insults to the body's integrity. They are present in a wide array of disorders and, if persistent, can lead to serious consequences. Chronic problems with nausea and vomiting may develop during pregnancy, in severe metabolic imbalances associated with uremia or alcoholism, and during cancer chemotherapy. Some of the many causes of nausea and vomiting are presented in Box 33-4.

Pathophysiology

Nausea is a subjective sensation of an impending urge to vomit. It may be accompanied by weakness, hypersalivation, and diaphoresis. Gastric tone and peristalsis are typically slowed or absent. The neural pathways that control nausea are not well identified but probably are the same general pathways that control vomiting.[16]

Vomiting is a complex phenomenon that begins with rhythmic contractions of the respiratory and abdominal muscles and culminates in the forceful expulsion of gastric contents from the mouth. It may be accompanied by retching or dry heaves and should be distinguished from the classic regurgitation that may accompany gastroesophageal reflux.

The vomiting center, located in the medulla adjacent to the respiratory and salivary control centers, can be stimulated directly by both the vagus nerve and sympathetic nervous system. Receptors can be found throughout the GI tract and internal organs that, when triggered by spasm or inflammation, can directly produce vomiting. Indirect stimulation can come from the chemoreceptor trigger zone (CTZ), which is located on the floor of the fourth ventricle and appears to respond to chemical stimuli in the blood. A wide variety of medications and other substances can act on the CTZ. The CTZ may also mediate the response to nonchemical stimuli such as radiation and motion sickness.

There is strong evidence that dopamine receptors in the CTZ play a role in mediating vomiting. Serotonergic pathways also play pivotal roles in mediating the effects of peripheral stimuli. Gastrointestinal serotonin is synthesized by enterochromaffin cells found throughout the abdomen, and is believed to activate 5-hydroxytryptamine$_3$ (5-HT$_3$) receptor sites on afferent vagal fibers. This pathway plays a crucial role in the severe protracted vomiting commonly associated with chemotherapy. Activation of the CTZ causes a reflex loss in gastric tone and peristalsis resulting in delayed gastric emptying. The CTZ may also play a role in psychogenic vomiting, which occurs in response to specific sensations and situations.

Short-term episodic nausea and vomiting is distressing, but prolonged vomiting can have serious physiologic effects. Prolonged and severe vomiting interferes with nutrition and causes fluid and electrolyte imbalances—specifically dehydration and metabolic alkalosis, with loss of potassium, chloride, and hydrogen ions. The act of vomiting strains the abdominal muscles and in postoperative patients may cause wound dehiscence. It can also result in Mallory-Weiss lacerations in the esophagus or stomach and trigger severe bleeding.

Vomiting is especially dangerous for anesthetized patients and persons with decreased alertness because they are at risk for aspiration of the vomitus. Aspiration may cause atelectasis, pneumonitis, or asphyxia, especially in elderly persons whose protective reflexes work less efficiently.

BOX 33-4 Common Causes of Nausea and Vomiting

- Infectious
  - Gastroenteritis
    - Viral (e.g., rotaviruses, adenoviruses, Norwalk agent)
    - Bacterial (e.g., *Staphylococcus, Salmonella, Clostridium, Bacillus cereus*)
- Medications
  - Chemotherapy (e.g., cisplatinum, methotrexate, nitrogen mustard)
  - Analgesics (e.g., opioids, nonsteroidal antiinflammatory drugs)
  - Antibiotics (e.g., tetracycline, erythromycin)
- Early pregnancy
- Postoperative state
- Gastrointestinal disturbances
  - Obstruction
  - Dyspepsia
  - Gastroparesis
  - Alcohol abuse
  - Inflammations (e.g., cholecystitis, pancreatitis, appendicitis)
- Labyrinthine disorders
  - Motion sickness
  - Meniere's disease
- Central nervous system disorders
  - Increased intracranial pressure
  - Tumors
  - Meningitis
  - Migraine headache

Collaborative Care Management

Treatment of nausea and vomiting depends on the cause and severity. Short-term problems resolve without intervention, but protracted vomiting requires intervention. Medications or other substances known to cause nausea and vomiting are discontinued if possible, and fluid and electrolyte imbalances are corrected. Fluids may be given intravenously if vomiting persists.

Antiemetic medications may be necessary. Drugs that are classified as antiemetics are theorized to act as a pharmacologic blockade to stimuli that may trigger nausea and vomiting. Most of the drugs also are believed to have some direct sedative action on the CTZ. Antiemetics are prescribed orally if the patient is able to retain the tablets, but they often need to be given by rectal, intramuscular, or IV routes. The choice of drug is governed by the specific clinical situation. Table 33-3 summarizes some of the great variety of available medications. Drug categories include the following.

Antihistamines. These drugs are believed to act on neurons in the vomiting center and in the vestibular pathways. They are effective in controlling motion sickness but have little effect on GI disorders. These drugs cause drowsiness and sedation.

Anticholinergics. These drugs are useful in the management of motion sickness, but the common side effects of dry mouth, urinary retention, and drowsiness limit their use.

Dopamine-Receptor Antagonists. These drugs are believed to act by antagonizing dopamine receptors in the CTZ. They also have antihistamine and anticholinergic effects. They are effective in managing mild symptoms and are often first-line therapies. They have significant side effects, including drowsiness and sedation.

Prokinetic Agents. These drugs are useful with gastroparesis and motor dysfunction of the upper GI tract. Metoclopramide also blocks dopamine receptors in the stomach.

Serotonin Antagonists. This highly effective group of drugs avoids the central nervous system effects of many antiemetics and is extremely effective in controlling severe chemotherapy-induced and postoperative vomiting. They bind 5-HT$_3$ receptor sites throughout the GI tract.

Miscellaneous Agents. Cannabis derivatives are a controversial option. Their antiemetic site of action is uncertain, but the active ingredient in marijuana is often useful in controlling chemotherapy-related nausea and vomiting. Drowsiness and dry mouth are common side effects. Dexamethasone, a synthetic glucocorticoid, appears to increase the effect of other antiemetics when administered in combination. Its mechanism of action is unknown.

TABLE 33-3 Common Medications for Nausea and Vomiting

Drug	Action	Intervention
Antihistamines		
Meclizine (Antivert) Diphenhydramine hydrochloride (Benadryl) Dimenhydrinate (Dramamine, Dimetabs) Hydroxyzine hydrochloride/hydroxyzine pamoate (Atarax, Vistaril)	Act on neurons in the vomiting center and the vestibular pathways Used in morning sickness and motion sickness	Monitor for drowsiness. Teach patient to use caution with all activities that require alertness. Driving may be hazardous.
Promethazine (Phenergan)	Phenothiazine with strong antihistaminic activity	Same as above.
Antidopaminergics		
Prochlorperazine (Compazine) Thiethylperazine (Torecan) Droperidol (Inapsine) Chlorpromazine	Antagonize dopamine receptors in the CTZ; also have antihistamine and anticholinergic effects	Monitor severity of drowsiness and sedation. Teach patient to avoid all hazardous activities and driving during use. Avoid alcohol use and sun exposure.
Prokinetic Agents		
Metoclopramide (Reglan) Domperidone (Motilium)	Complex actions in both CNS and GI tract; stimulate gastric emptying; domperidone does not cross blood-brain barrier	Monitor for side effects: diarrhea, mild sedation.
Anticholinergics		
Scopalamine (Transderm-Scōp)	Reduce neuron transmission; useful in motion sickness and postoperative nausea	Teach patient to apply to dry surface behind the ear. Use in advance of anticipated need.
Serotonin Receptor Antagonists		
Ondansetron (Zofran) Granisetron (Kytril)	Bind serotonin receptor sites along GI tract and afferent nerves	Monitor for side effects: diarrhea, headache.
Cannabis Derivatives		
Dronabinol (Marinol)	Site of antiemetic action unknown	Teach patient to be alert to mood and behavior change. Drowsiness is common so driving should be avoided. Avoid concurrent alcohol use.
Miscellaneous		
Trimethobenzamide (Tigan)	Believed to act on CTZ; has weak antihistaminic action, similar to phenothiazines	Monitor for side effects: hypotension, diarrhea, irritation at injection site. Drowsiness is common.
Benzquinamide (Emete-Con)	Inhibits stimulation of the CTZ; similar activity to antihistamines and phenothiazines	Monitor for side effects: drowsiness, fluctuations in blood pressure.
Corticosteroids (Dexamethasone)	Mechanism of action is unknown; useful in combination with chemotherapy-induced vomiting	Monitor for side effects: mood changes.

CNS, Central nervous system; *CTZ,* chemoreceptor trigger zone; *GI,* gastrointestinal.

Patient/Family Education. Nausea and vomiting can be extremely distressing and debilitating problems that severely interfere with quality of life. Effective management includes drug therapy but may also include exploration of daily lifestyle strategies, including environmental modification and stress management. There are rarely quick answers or easy fixes. Acupuncture and acupressure techniques can produce dramatic results for some people. Control and prevention of dehydration are important because dehydration appears to worsen the cycle of nausea and vomiting. Liquids are usually better tolerated because they exit the stomach rapidly. Overdistention of the stomach should usually be avoided. Creamy and milk-based liquids are rarely well tolerated, and starches are generally better tolerated than fatty foods. Lean poultry is usually the recommended source of protein. Guidelines for the management of nausea and vomiting are summarized in the accompanying Patient Teaching box.

Patient Teaching
Nausea and Vomiting

SAFETY AND COMFORT

Keep head of bed elevated and emesis basin handy.
Protect airway with suction and positioning if patient is not alert.
Provide frequent mouth care.
Control sights and odors in room.
Reduce anxiety if possible.
Provide quiet or distraction on the basis of patient response.
Modify environmental stimuli (cool cloth, dim light), and evaluate response.
Provide ongoing patient support. Explore new strategies.

DIET MODIFICATIONS

Maintain NPO if vomiting is severe.
Explore use of clear liquids:
- Serve liquids cool or room temperature.
- Try effervescent drinks and evaluate effect.
- Encourage adequate fluids to prevent dehydration.

Avoid fatty foods.
Avoid highly sweetened foods and milk products.
Keep meals small, avoid overdistention.

DRUGS

Administer medications before vomiting occurs, if possible.
Evaluate patient response to medications.
Maintain patient safety and assess for sedation or confusion.

NPO, Nothing by mouth.

PROBLEMS OF NUTRITION AND ABSORPTION

The importance of adequate sustained nutrition to the maintenance and restoration of health is increasingly recognized in health care. Adequate nutrition is acknowledged to be critical to wound healing, resistance to infection, ventilator weaning, and organ function. Acutely and chronically ill patients may experience social and environmental problems related to food access and preparation as well as complex problems related to the structure and function of various organs of the GI tract and related structures.

Malabsorption

Etiology/Epidemiology

The GI tract must be able to both break down ingested food and transport nutrients across the mucosa to the bloodstream. Approximately 7 to 10 L of liquid chyme move through the GI tract daily, but resorption is so efficient that all but 600 to 800 ml are resorbed before reaching the ileocecal valve. The term *malabsorption* refers to a heterogeneous category of disorders that share the common feature of failure to assimilate one or more essential ingested nutrients. It can result from impaired function of any of the primary or accessory organs of digestion and may be structural in nature, involve a digestive alteration, or result from impairment of nutrient transport across the mucosa. The problem with absorption may be caused by a primary disorder such as celiac disease or lactase deficiency; or it may develop secondary to gastric or bowel surgery, inflammatory diseases, infections, or the administration of specific medications. Examples of common causes of malabsorption are presented in Box 33-5.

BOX 33-5 Primary and Secondary Causes of Malabsorption

Primary Causes

Lactase deficiency
Celiac disease, tropical sprue

Secondary Causes

Subtotal gastrectomy, gastric bypass
Ileal resection or bypass greater than 3 feet
Pancreatic disease: chronic pancreatitis, cancer, cystic fibrosis
Liver or biliary disease or obstruction
Inflammatory bowel disease
Bacterial, viral, or parasitic infection of the bowel
Radiation enteritis
Drug side effects: antibiotics, colchicine

Pathophysiology

Malabsorption syndrome is a group of signs and symptoms resulting from inadequate absorption of fat, protein, and/or carbohydrates. Fat malabsorption is the most common problem, but malabsorption can occur with any nutrient. The symptoms vary somewhat based on the specific problem. Because fat-soluble vitamins (A, D, E, and K) require fat for absorption, decreased absorption of fat also typically results in a deficiency of these vitamins.

The classic sign of malabsorption is steatorrhea, excess loss of fat in the stool. The range of severity can be from minimal to overwhelming. The fat gives the stool a greasy, bulky, mushy appearance and a foul odor. The stools float because of their low specific gravity and high gas content. Stools may be limited to one bulky stool a day or may occur frequently. Steatorrhea also causes flatulence with borborygmus (loud bowel sounds) and abdominal distention. Decreased fat absorption leads to weight loss, weakness, fatigue, and anorexia.

Signs and symptoms of concurrent fat-soluble vitamin deficiencies can include bleeding (ecchymosis and hematuria), bone pain, fractures, hypocalcemia, anemia, glossitis, cheilosis, muscle tenderness, peripheral neuritis, and dermatitis. Protein deficiency results in edema, hypoalbuminemia, and loss of muscle mass. The person with malabsorption syndrome usually appears pale and emaciated and has dry, scaly, hyperpigmented skin.

Major primary malabsorption disorders in adults follow.

Gluten-Sensitive Enteropathy (Celiac Disease). This familial disorder involves a permanent intolerance to fractions of gluten (wheat protein). It primarily affects Caucasians, and about 30% to 40% of those affected develop diarrhea, which is the primary symptom. Effective treatment involves the rigid and lifelong exclusion of gluten.

Tropical Sprue. This syndrome primarily affects residents of and visitors to tropical areas. The cause is unknown, although an infectious origin is theorized. Affected persons develop severe malnutrition and vitamin deficiencies from protracted diarrhea, that can be life threatening. Effective treatment involves both antibiotic therapy and folic acid replacement.

Disaccharide Malabsorption. Congenital lactase deficiency is the most common form of genetic deficiency syndrome in humans. It affects more than 50% of the world's population and is particularly prevalent among non-Europeans. The milk intolerance may be mild or severe and is treated by diet restriction and/or enzyme supplement.

Short Bowel Syndrome. The small intestine has a tremendous functional reserve, but loss of more than 50% of its length significantly reduces the amount of mucosal surface area available for absorbing nutrients and produces a condition called "short bowel syndrome." Symptom severity depends on the site and extent of bowel loss. Treatment is complex and may involve long-term parenteral nutrition, enteral feedings, and drugs to decrease peristalsis.

Secondary malabsorption problems can accompany a wide variety of GI disorders and treatments. Protein-losing gastroenteropathy involves the excess loss of serum proteins and is a common component of disorders such as inflammatory bowel disease, pancreatic disease, and cystic fibrosis. Treatment is directed at effectively controlling the primary disorder.

Collaborative Care Management

Medical treatment for malabsorption is based on the underlying cause. Nutrition is the major concern, and dietary intervention is the primary approach to management. Diet modifications and supplements are often successful in compensating for the malabsorption on a routine basis, but more aggressive management with enteral or parenteral (total parenteral nutrition [TPN]) feedings may be necessary during disease exacerbations.

Patient/Family Education. The nurse assists the patient to incorporate needed dietary changes into the daily lifestyle and works with the family on strategies to promote adherence. The nurse ensures that the patient understands the rationale for all prescribed dietary and drug interventions. The severely malnourished person may require frequent gentle mouth care to increase comfort and prevent oral inflammations as well as skin care to prevent skin breakdown.

Protein-Calorie Malnutrition

Etiology/Epidemiology

Acute and chronic illness, trauma, infection, and wound healing put enormous strain on the body's nutritional reserve. A poor nutritional state is a common problem in both acute and long-term care settings, and the problem of protein-calorie malnutrition has received increasing attention as the importance of nutrition to factors such as wound healing, immunocompetence, and ventilator weaning is acknowledged. The actual incidence of protein-calorie malnutrition is unknown, but it is a particularly severe problem in older adults. Some authors estimate that it occurs in up to 60% of hospitalized older adults, 80% of older adults in nursing homes, and 20% of older adults living in the community. Box 33-6 identifies some of the typical causes of malnutrition in hospitalized patients.

BOX 33-6 Causes of Malnutrition in Hospitalized Patients

Decreased Intake

Anorexia and nausea	Self-care deficits
NPO status	Dysphagia
Pain	Depression
Medication effects	

Increased Losses

Vomiting	Open wounds
Diarrhea	GI suctioning

NOTE: Patients can lose 50 g of protein daily through an open pressure ulcer.

Increased Needs

Fever	Trauma
Infection	Surgery

Pathophysiology

If a diet provides adequate carbohydrates and fats, the body uses these nutrients to meet its energy needs. When intake of these nutrients is inadequate, however, the body uses its own stores to meet its energy needs. Most severely ill hospitalized adults experience a deficiency of all dietary elements, but the deficiency of protein is most significant. The process of protein synthesis occurs continuously, and although the body can synthesize certain amino acids from its stored pools, it depends on ingested protein sources for others. Dietary amino acids that are not used are excreted. Negative nitrogen balance occurs when more nitrogen (which is an end product of amino acid breakdown) is excreted than is ingested via dietary proteins and indicates that body tissue is being broken down faster than it is being replaced.

Ongoing severe protein deficit leads to decreases in both muscle and visceral mass. Cardiac output decreases, respiratory muscles weaken, and malabsorption occurs in the GI tract. Immunocompetence is impaired, and the risk of infection increases. The greatest impairment is noted in cell-mediated immunity as the number of T cells declines. Weight loss, decreased muscle mass, and weakness are common, but the affected person may exhibit few overt signs and appear physically robust.

Collaborative Care Management

The primary approach to malnutrition management is identifying persons at risk, monitoring physical and laboratory parameters, and intervening with oral supplements, tube feedings, or TPN as indicated. Weight loss typically exceeds 15% of usual body weight. Serial measurements of serum albumin and transferrin levels are important. Albumin is a major protein synthesized by the liver, and levels less than 3.5 g/dl indicate early malnutrition. Prealbumin levels are monitored during treatment because they provide an indication of protein changes occurring during the previous 48 hours. Serum transferrin is a beta-globulin synthesized by the liver that transports iron in the plasma. Levels lower than 100 mg/dl indicate severe depletion. The total lymphocyte count reflects a basic measure of immunity and should remain greater than 16% of the total. A nutrition-support team, if available, guides decision making concerning dietary supplements or replacements (see discussion of tube feedings and TPN later).

Patient/Family Education. The nurse teaches the patient and family about the disorder and its planned management. Anemia-induced fatigue is common, and the nurse provides the patient with frequent rest periods and spaces needed treatments and activities throughout the day. A high-calorie, high-protein diet is encouraged if the patient can tolerate an oral diet. The nurse ensures that the environment is conducive to eating and arranges for small frequent feedings rather than large meals. It is essential that all nutritional planning incorporate the patient's food preferences and cultural habits as much as possible. The goal is to modify the diet enough to meet the body's needs for tissue growth and repair. The nurse keeps an accurate record of the patient's weight and records calorie counts if ordered. Care for the patient receiving tube feedings or TPN is discussed in the next section.

ENTERAL AND PARENTERAL NUTRITION

Enteral Nutrition

Enteral nutrition involves the delivery of nutrients directly into the GI tract via tube feeding. It can be used to either supplement or replace oral nutrition in patients who cannot take in adequate amounts of nutrients by mouth. Enteral nutrition is used primarily for patients who have both structural and functional integrity of the GI tract, although enteral feedings are increasingly being used successfully with critically ill patients who would not previously have been considered good candidates. Enteral nutrition is a safer and more cost-effective alternative to TPN, and is also significantly less likely to cause sepsis and other complications. Other advantages of enteral feedings include:

- Preservation of the normal sequence of intestinal and hepatic metabolism
- Maintenance of normal insulin/glucagon ratios
- Maintenance of lipoprotein synthesis by the intestinal mucosa and liver

Tube feedings may be delivered to the stomach (nasogastric) or to the distal duodenum or proximal jejunum (nasointestinal). Nasointestinal feedings have become increasingly popular since it was learned that the adynamic ileus that frequently occurs with acute illness or trauma primarily affects the stomach and the colon. The small intestine frequently retains both motility and the ability to absorb nutrients. Early feeding after major surgery and trauma has now become routine. Long-term enteral nutrition is usually delivered with a permanent access, either into the stomach or jejunum.

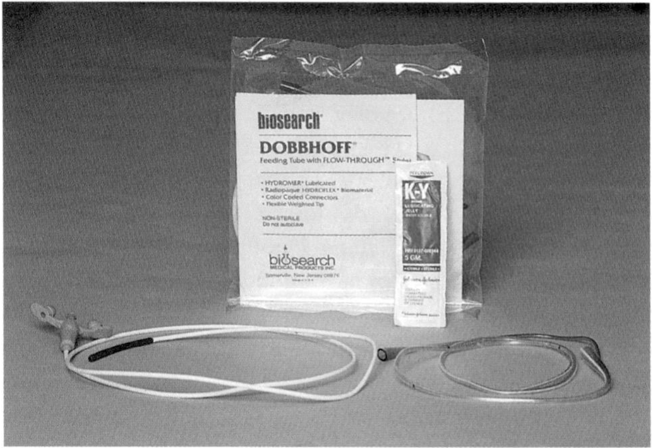

Figure 33-12 Typical small-bore feeding tube.

Enteral Feeding Tubes

A wide variety of containers, tubes, catheters, and delivery systems are available for use in enteral feedings. Enteral tubes are classified according to their composition, external diameter, length, and the presence or absence of a weighted tip. Most tubes are constructed of either polyurethane or silicone. The polyurethane tubes have a larger internal diameter, which facilitates fluid flow. Enteral feeding tubes vary in diameter from 8 to 10 F (small bore), to 12 to 14 F (medium bore), to16 to 18 F (large bore).

Nasogastric feeding tubes can be used with patients who have intact gag and swallow reflexes and a competent lower esophageal sphincter to minimize reflux. Nasointestinal tubes are used for patients who are at risk for aspiration or who are experiencing acute stress-related gastric ileus. They are typically small bore and have a weighted tip to help the tube move through the pylorus into the duodenum or jejunum. A monofilament or stainless steel stylet may be used with small bore tubes to guide insertion. A typical small bore feeding tube is shown in Figure 33-12.

Gastrostomy

Insertion of a gastrostomy tube is an alternative approach to enteral nutrition for patients who are unable to take oral nutrients for long periods. The gastrostomy tube is inserted surgically through an incision in the abdominal wall or endoscopically.

The percutaneous endoscopic gastrostomy (PEG) does not require incision into the abdominal cavity and is a safe and rapid method of creating a gastrostomy. It is performed via endoscopy and local anesthesia. A small incision is made on the skin of the abdomen, and a cannula is pushed through the abdominal and gastric walls into the stomach while the site is observed through a gastroscope. A long suture is threaded through the cannula, grasped, and pulled up through the endoscope, which is then removed. A specially prepared catheter is attached to the suture thread, and the catheter is then pulled back through the esophagus and stomach and out the abdominal wall. Internal and external dams hold the catheter in place. A jejunostomy tube may be inserted by a similar method (Figure 33-13). A "low-profile" version of the PEG is available, which lies close to the surface of the abdomen.

The catheter used to create a gastrostomy usually is large in diameter (18 to 24 F). A Foley catheter can be used, which allows the balloon to serve as an anchor against the stomach wall. PEG tubes are smaller (12 to 16 F) and usually are anchored by a 1- to 2-inch cross-linked latex tube placed inside the stomach. A dressing is not generally used. Keeping the site open helps to prevent skin laceration, breakdown, and infection. The skin around the gastrostomy may be cleaned with hydrogen peroxide solution to remove crusts and rinsed with normal saline or water.

The "button" gastrostomy does not require a tube and lessens the chance of complications from tube irritation or obstruction. The "button" is constructed by making a small tube from the wall of the stomach and then pushing it in to form an intussusception valve. The "valve" is brought out flush with the skin surface to create a flat stoma and prevents leakage of stomach contents; therefore no skin care or dressings are needed. A tube is inserted through the valve for feedings.

Enteral Feeding Solutions

A variety of feeding solutions are available to meet multiple and diverse patient needs. All enteral formulas contain the essential nutrients, but they differ in the balance of those nutrients as well as in the amount of digestion and absorption required to use them.

Protein is considered to be the most critical component of any formula. Patients who have normal levels of pancreatic enzymes available to breakdown the protein for absorption may receive a solution of intact nutrients that resembles a pureed diet. Formulas also may contain hydrolyzed proteins derived from meat, soy, and lactalbumin. These proteins have

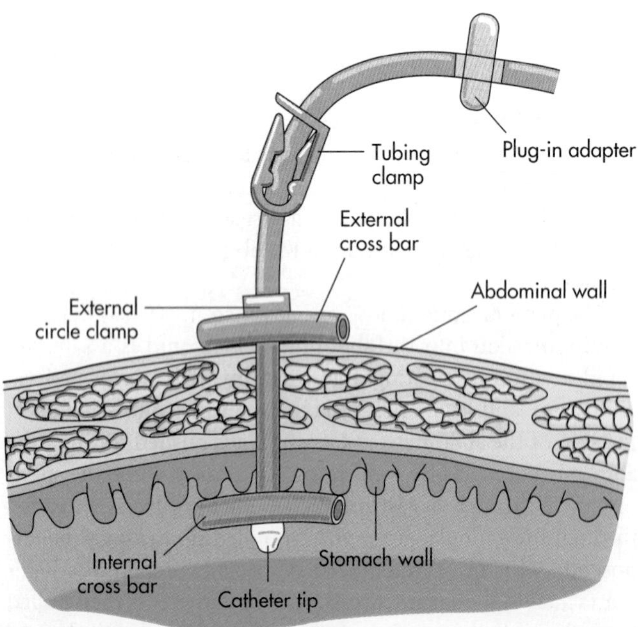

Figure 33-13 A percutaneous endoscopic gastrostomy (PEG) tube in place in the stomach.

been predigested to dipeptides and free amino acids and do not require further digestion by the patient; however, GI absorption must be intact. Crystalline amino acid formulas are composed of amino acids that require no digestion and readily move across the intestinal mucosa for absorption.

The major concerns in the carbohydrate content of feeding solutions relate to lactose content and total calorie needs. Increasing awareness of the pervasiveness of partial lactose intolerance has stimulated the development of formulas without a milk base. Carbohydrates in standard formulas are easily utilized as long as intestinal absorption remains intact. Formula components include starch and polysaccharides, disaccharides, and monosaccharides. Effective carbohydrate utilization also depends on the person having adequate amounts of insulin, glucagon, norepinephrine, and vitamins. Any imbalance or deficiency in these elements can impair absorption and produce watery diarrhea.

Fats in the formula provide a source for concentrated calories and essential fatty acids and serve as a carrier for fat-soluble vitamins. Fat digestion depends on pancreatic enzymes, bile salts, and normal intestinal flora. Short-, medium-, and long-chain fatty acids may be included in both saturated and polyunsaturated forms.

Caloric density (the number of calories per unit volume) is an extremely important consideration. High-density formulas tend to be more hypertonic and may contribute to diarrhea. Lower-density formulas require a larger volume of solution to provide needed nutrients, which may be an issue if fluids must be restricted.

Osmolality is another essential consideration for enteral solutions. Isotonic formulas approximate the osmolality of plasma (280 to 300 mOsm/kg) and can be administered at full strength with the rate adjusted to patient tolerance. Adequate amounts of hypotonic fluids such as water are also essential to maintain the desired osmolality. The osmolality of enteral solutions is primarily a reflection of the concentration of proteins and carbohydrates. Hypertonic formulas typically have osmolalities ranging from 400 to 1100 mOsm/kg and need to be diluted or administered at an extremely slow rate until patient tolerance increases. Formulas with simple (predigested) proteins often have a higher osmolality, and patients receiving them need careful monitoring. Table 33-4 compares the various components of a few sample formulas. All formulas are supplemented with substantial amounts of essential vitamins and minerals.

Enteral Feeding Techniques

Feeding schedules may be planned on a continuous, intermittent, or bolus basis. Continuous feedings are used for most short-term nutrition support because the volume of fluid delivered can be kept very low, which increases patient tolerance. This is ideal for nasointestinal delivery because the small intestine normally receives nutrients from the stomach in small volumes over several hours after each meal. Intermittent or bolus scheduling significantly increases the risk of dumping syndrome and diarrhea. When long-term support is planned, an intermittent schedule with delivery of the feeding to the stomach best replicates a normal eating pattern. It also permits the patient to be free of the tube feeding for intervals throughout the day. Clinical decisions are based on the unique patient circumstances.

Residual volumes are checked before each intermittent feeding and at specified intervals, usually at least once a day, for patients receiving continuous feedings. Most institutional protocols direct that an intermittent feeding be held if the residual is greater than 100 to 150 ml. Lower parameters are set for gastrostomies. With continuous feedings a residual of two times the amount of feeding delivered over the last hour would usually require notification of the physician. Consensus does not exist over whether the aspirated fluid should be refed to the patient, although this is frequently recommended. The bag and tubing are thoroughly washed after each intermittent feeding and are discarded every 24 to 48 hours per institutional policy. Care of the patient receiving an enteral feeding is summarized in the Guidelines for Safe Practice box.

Managing Complications

Tube Obstruction. Feeding tube obstructions are relatively common problems. Pill fragments, formula residue adhering to the tube lumen, and formula/medication incompatibilities are common causes. Thoroughly flushing tubes with 20 to 30 ml of tepid water before and after feedings and medication administration, or every 4 to 6 hours during continuous administration, is the best prevention. The Guidelines for Safe Practice box on p. 1058 summarizes strategies to prevent or relieve tube obstruction.

Regurgitation/Aspiration. Pulmonary complications are the most dangerous problems associated with enteral feedings. A tube of any size may enter the tracheobronchial tree on insertion or migrate there with vigorous coughing or suctioning. Patients who are obtunded and have impaired cough or gag reflexes are at particular risk.

No method except chest x-ray is foolproof in verifying correct tube placement. Most institutions use several tests of tube placement. Proper taping of the tube to secure it in position and verifying the external length of the tube should be routinely performed. Instilling a small amount of air while simultaneously auscultating the abdomen is a recommended test of tube placement even though sounds are readily transmitted throughout the abdomen, and this does not guarantee that the tube is located where the sounds are heard. Aspirating tube contents is more accurate, and pH testing of the aspirate can help to verify accurate placement; however, small bore tubes often collapse easily, making aspiration difficult or impossible. The head of the bed is kept elevated 30 to 40 degrees at all times if possible to decrease the risk of aspiration. The use of nasointestinal tubes with weighted tips for patients at risk for aspiration appears to decrease the incidence of reflux.

Diarrhea. Diarrhea is the most commonly encountered complication of enteral feedings, and it may be caused by a variety of factors. Diarrhea may be directly related to the formula used. Formulas containing lactose, a high-fat content, or a low-fiber content have all been implicated in the development of diarrhea. High osmolality also appears to be important, particularly with severely malnourished patients. Diarrhea may also be caused by prescribed medications, such as antibiotics, H_2-receptor antagonists, and elixirs containing sorbitol. Methods of combating this diarrhea include the use of bulking agents, slow delivery rates, and formula dilution during the initial administration period. It is also essential that dehydration be prevented through the administration of adequate amounts of

TABLE 33-4 Sample Tube Feeding Composition

Formula	Carbo-hydrate	Proteins	Osmolality (mOsm)
Liquid Whole Food			
Ensure, Isocal, Sustacal, Osmolite	Complex carbohydrates	Intact proteins	300-600
Supplemental			
Precision, Vital	Complex carbohydrates	Peptides	450-600
Predigested/Elemental			
Vivonex, Flexical, Pregestimil	Simple carbohydrates	Amino acids	500-800

Guidelines for Safe Practice

The Patient Receiving Enteral Tube Feedings

Keep the head of the bed elevated at least 30 degrees during all feedings and for at least 1 hour after discontinuation.
- Use high Fowler's position for intermittent feedings if permitted.

Verify tube placement.
- Check the length of tube that protrudes from the nose.
- Inject 10 to 30 ml of air into the tube and auscultate over the left upper quadrant of the abdomen.
- Aspirate secretions if possible and check the pH of the aspirate.
- Check the volume of the residual against ordered parameters.
- Refeed aspirated fluid per institution protocol.

Flush tube with 30 to 50 ml of water before initiating and at the end of the feeding or every 4 hours for continuous feedings.

Always flush the tube before and after medication administration.

Verify rate settings on the delivery pump.

Ensure that the tube is properly and securely taped and check for the presence of nasal irritation.

Record all administered volumes and residuals, including irrigation fluids, on intake and output records.

Cleanse delivery equipment after each use and discard per institution protocol (usually 24 to 48 hours).

INTERMITTENT (BOLUS) FEEDINGS

Attach syringe to feeding tube.
- Elevate syringe 18 inches above the patient's head.
- Fill syringe with formula.
- Allow feeding to empty by gravity.
- Keep syringe filled to avoid infusion of air.

Guidelines for Safe Practice

Preventing Feeding Tube Obstruction

Use a polyurethane feeding tube if possible.

Flush the tube with at least 30 ml of water every 4 hours; do this before and after administering medications and before and after checking gastric residual volumes.

Use a controller pump to maintain a steady flow.

Administer all medications with care.

- Do not administer medications with the tube feeding running. Always flush first.
- Do not administer any enteric-coated, chewable, or sublingual drugs through the tube. Obtain liquid forms of medications if possible.
- Do not crush slow-release tablets. The beads from slow-release capsules may be flushed through the tube if size permits.
- Crush all tablets thoroughly into a fine powder. Do not open the package before crushing. Mix with 15 to 100 ml of water before administering.
- Time the administration of antacids around the other medications.
- Administer each drug separately; do not combine.
- Stop feedings for 15 to 30 minutes before administration if a drug needs to be given on an empty stomach.

Irrigate clogged tubes with water. If this is ineffective, Viokase or a declogging stylus may be used per institution policy. There is no evidence that cranberry juice is effective, and water is as effective as cola products.

Guidelines for Safe Practice

Preventing Bacterial Contamination of Tube Feeding Formulas

Use prefilled, ready-to-use sets if available.

Follow strict aseptic technique in handling all components; good hand washing is essential.

Use full-strength ready-to-use formula; dilution and reconstitution increase the chances of contamination.

Rinse the delivery set with water before adding new formula.

Hang commercially prepared formulas for no more than 8 to 12 hours (hospital-prepared formulas for no more than 6 hours).

free water. The greater the osmolality of the formula, the more water is needed.

Malnutrition, particularly hypoalbuminemia, is associated with a decrease in intestinal absorption and can contribute to diarrhea. This problem resolves as the patient's nutritional status improves, but it may require formula readjustment or direct replenishment of the serum albumin.

Bacterial contamination is another significant cause of diarrhea. Formula can become contaminated at any point in the preparation and delivery process. Formulas with higher osmolalities appear to be less likely to support bacterial growth. The length of time the formula hangs at room temperature also is a factor. Hospital-prepared formulas that contain milk are the most vulnerable. The Guidelines for Safe Practice box at right summarizes measures to help reduce the risk of bacterial contamination of formula.

Hyperglycemia. Hyperglycemia may become a problem for patients who are receiving high-caloric density formulas, especially those who are also taking corticosteroids. Elderly persons are also at increased risk. Blood glucose monitoring may be ordered, and administration of sliding-scale insulin may be necessary.

Parenteral Nutrition

Parenteral nutrition is a method of giving concentrated solutions intravenously to maintain or supplement a patient's nutritional balance when oral or enteral nutrition is inadequate or not possible. Parenteral nutrition is indicated for patients whose GI tract is not functioning as a result of obstruction, acute inflammation, or malabsorption. It is also used for patients who are extremely hypermetabolic from trauma or sepsis, need to be given nothing by mouth for more than 5 to 7 days, are unable to take adequate amounts of nutrients orally, or experience severe GI side effects from radiation therapy or chemotherapy. The increased recognition of the importance of adequate nutrition for healing has resulted in physicians initiating parenteral nutrition as a therapeutic tool much earlier in the management process.

Parenteral nutrition is commonly administered through the central venous route, but it can be administered by peripheral vein as well. Peripheral solutions differ primarily in their glucose content, which generally does not exceed 10%. Strongly hypertonic solutions can be extremely irritating to the peripheral veins. Peripheral solutions rely more heavily on isotonic lipid emulsions as the main nonprotein calorie source.

Central Venous Catheters

A variety of options exist for the delivery of parenteral nutrition solutions. Central venous catheters allow for rapid mixing and dilution of strongly hypertonic solutions. Subclavian, tunneled, and implantable port catheters are available in single-lumen and multilumen forms. Central venous catheters and venous access devices are discussed and illustrated in Chapter 15. Infection is the primary concern related to the administration of parenteral nutrition. It is believed that catheter contamination at the point of entry into the skin and migration of bacteria along the catheter are the major sources of sepsis. Rigorous dressing care is essential, but there are wide variations in institutional protocols. Research is ongoing to determine the optimal interval for dressing changes and the effectiveness of the various dressing materials.

Solutions

Parenteral nutrition solutions are complex formulas that provide all known essential nutrients in quantities that will support wound healing, anabolism, weight gain or maintenance, and growth in children. All such solutions contain water, protein, carbohydrates, fat, vitamins, and trace elements.

The various proportions of each element are individualized to the patient's unique clinical situation and needs.

Solutions used to deliver parenteral nutrition usually consist of 25% to 35% dextrose, 3% to 5% amino acids, electrolytes, minerals, and vitamins. Intravenous fat emulsions in 10% to 20% concentrations also may be added. Dextrose and fat are given for their caloric value. The body uses them to meet its energy needs. This permits the administered amino acids to be used for tissue building. Fat provides twice the caloric value of dextrose, exerts minimal osmotic pressure, and prevents fatty acid deficiency. Regular insulin may be added to the solution or administered subcutaneously to support glucose utilization.

Parenteral nutrition solutions provide good culture media for bacteria. They are therefore prepared under strict aseptic conditions in the pharmacy under a laminar airflow hood. The solutions are kept refrigerated until ready for use and are left at room temperature for 30 minutes before administration. Prepared formulas ideally should be used within 24 hours to minimize the risk of contamination, but institutional protocols may vary slightly.

Parenteral nutrition solutions are administered slowly and increased as patient tolerance permits. Blood glucose levels are checked frequently at the beginning of treatment while endogenous insulin production adjusts to the increased glucose load. An infusion pump is used to ensure a steady infusion rate. If administration needs to be interrupted for any reason, infusions of 10% dextrose are substituted to prevent rebound hypoglycemia. Parenteral nutrition administration is gradually tapered before it is discontinued to allow the body time to make the necessary metabolic adjustments. Lipid emulsions may be mixed with the solution, given through a separate peripheral IV line, or given through a Y-connector in the main IV line.

The use of a 0.2-μm filter is recommended for administering all parenteral nutrition solutions, but if lipids are also administered their large molecules require the use of a filter of at least 1.2 μm or larger. The effectiveness of filters in reducing the risk of bacterial contamination remains unproven, but they do trap crystals and air from the solution and tubing.

COMPLICATIONS

Complications of parenteral nutrition include problems with the catheter, infection, and metabolic imbalances. Correct insertion and placement of the catheter are extremely important. Proper insertion prevents most problems related to pneumothorax or hemothorax, air embolism, brachial plexus injury, and thromboembolism.

Catheter-related sepsis is a serious complication of parenteral nutrition that cannot always be prevented. Strict aseptic technique during catheter insertion and subsequent care is essential. Vital signs are monitored regularly, and the insertion site is assessed for tenderness, redness, and drainage. The catheter site is the most common source of infection. The onset of sepsis may be preceded by the development of unexplained hyperglycemia.

The major metabolic alteration associated with the use of parenteral nutrition is glucose intolerance. Blood glucose levels are carefully monitored through finger sticks. Insulin may be added to the solution or administered on a sliding scale if needed. Severe osmotic diuresis can result from uncontrolled hyperglycemia and can lead rapidly to dehydration. Hypoglycemia is also a potential problem when the patient is being weaned from parenteral nutrition or whenever the continuous infusion of solution is interrupted for any reason.

Other possible complications associated with parenteral nutrition include fluid and electrolyte imbalances, and acid-base imbalances (primarily acidosis). Vitamin D deficiency and vitamin A excess also may occur. Serum electrolyte levels are monitored several times a week. Carbohydrate metabolism yields water and carbon dioxide. The increased production of carbon dioxide caused by concentrated glucose solutions can induce respiratory distress in patients with compromised pulmonary status. Abnormalities in liver function may also occur when patients receive high volumes of carbohydrate calories. The body converts the calories into intrahepatic fat, which can cause liver dysfunction.

Care of the patient receiving parenteral nutrition is summarized in the Guidelines for Safe Practice box.

Home-Based Parenteral Nutrition

Administration of IV therapy in the home has become routine as home care agencies have worked to adapt high-technology interventions to the home setting. The cost savings can be dramatic. Antibiotics, hydration, and parenteral nutrition are the most common interventions. They may be a continuation of care initiated in a hospital or be initiated in the outpatient setting. To qualify for insurance or Medicare coverage, these interventions must usually be needed long term. See Box 33-7 for sample Medicare requirements.

Home administration of parenteral nutrition has enabled thousands of patients to remain in their homes and out of the acute care setting. Advanced inflammatory bowel disease is the most common medical indication, but acquired immunodeficiency syndrome and cancer are other common diagnoses. Cost constraints put significant pressure on patients and families to learn to safely administer the parenteral nutrition without the ongoing supervision of a home health nurse. With a well-structured teaching plan and initial supervision, most families are able to successfully provide the needed care.

A nutrition-support team, if available, usually initiates the educational process before the patient's discharge. The nurse typically coordinates the home care team, which may include the physician, dietitian, social worker, pharmacist, and counselor or psychiatrist. Successful management demands a team approach. Patient teaching includes basic information about parenteral nutrition; discussion about symptoms, problems, and complications; and practical planning concerning the acquisition of equipment, location and storage of supplies, and

Guidelines for Safe Practice

The Patient Receiving Parenteral Nutrition

If possible, do not use the catheter for other purposes.

PREVENTING INFECTION

Maintain strict aseptic technique.
Keep solutions cold until ready for use, but allow solution to warm to room temperature before administration; use solutions within 24 to 36 hours.
- All additions to parenteral solutions should be performed in laminar flow areas.

Change dressing according to institutional protocol.
- Follow strict aseptic technique in handling catheter, dressing, tubing, and solution.

Change administration sets every 24 hours or by institution protocol.
Monitor for signs of redness, swelling, or drainage at insertion site.
- Suspect sepsis if afebrile patient develops a fever.

PREVENTING AIR EMBOLISM

Tape all connections securely.
Clamp catheter before opening system.
Cover subclavian catheter insertion site with an air-occlusive dressing (covered with adhesive tape) or transparent polyurethane (Op-site) dressing.
Position patient as flat as possible for dressing and tubing changes.
Instruct patient to perform Valsalva's maneuver whenever catheter hub is open to the air.

MAINTAINING FLUID AND ELECTROLYTE BALANCE

Maintain a uniform infusion rate. Never abruptly discontinue solution administration.
- Use a pump for controlled delivery rates.
- Never exceed prescribed rate of administration; do not attempt to "catch up" if infusion falls behind schedule.
- Monitor for signs of *overhydration* (neck vein distention, cough, weight gain):
  - Weigh patient daily.
  - Record accurate intake and output.

PREVENTING METABOLIC IMBALANCE

Monitor and report to physician signs of *hypoglycemia* (pallor, diaphoresis, tachycardia, hunger, trembling, behavioral changes):
- Administer 10% glucose solution if solution must be interrupted for any reason

Monitor for signs of *hyperglycemia* (nausea, weakness, thirst, headache, rapid respirations):
- Check fingerstick blood glucose as ordered (every 6 hours initially and every day once stable).
- Administer sliding scale insulin as ordered.

PROMOTING COMFORT

Provide for good oral hygiene.
Encourage ambulation and activities of daily living.
Monitor for "refeeding syndrome" when parenteral nutrition is initiated (first 24 to 48 hours).
- Symptoms include respiratory depression, lethargy, confusion, and weakness.
- Syndrome results from the abrupt shift of electrolytes from the plasma to the intracellular compartment.

BOX 33-7 Sample Medicare Criteria for Home IV Therapy

The patient must be homebound (i.e., unable to leave the home for work, shopping, or other self-care activities).
The planned parenteral nutrition therapy must be at least 90 days long.
Parenteral nutrition must be the patient's sole source of nutrition.
Documentation must exist that the patient is unable to absorb nutrition from the enteral route.

NOTE: Coverage is provided by Medicare Part B—Durable Medical Equipment Benefit.

Patient Teaching

Sample Teaching Plan for Home Parenteral Nutrition

Review purpose and procedures for the home nutrition regimen.
Validate presence of detailed written instructions for each procedure and piece of equipment.
Validate understanding of all home equipment:
- Provide additional instruction as needed inasmuch as equipment and supplies used in the hospital frequently differ from those available through home health care.

Validate aseptic technique and skills.
Evaluate adequacy of home refrigeration and supply storage.
Teach patient/family about ordering replacement supplies.
Establish record-keeping system for body weights, temperatures, finger sticks, and sliding-scale insulin if ordered.
Reinforce importance of aseptic technique and safe disposal of equipment.
Discuss troubleshooting of common equipment problems.
Review symptoms related to infection, air embolism, and other complications; provide written instructions of actions to be taken in the event of a complication.
Provide list of emergency telephone numbers.

special telephone service to cover emergencies. A sample teaching plan for home parenteral nutrition is outlined in the Patient Teaching box.

Recognizing and managing complications are important aspects of the care plan. Common complications and their management are outlined in Table 33-5. The nurse needs to offer support and encouragement to the patient and family, as home parenteral nutrition is a demanding therapy that requires a major time commitment. It is easy for caregivers to feel isolated and alone with the demands of the task.

Caregivers are provided with appropriate written materials to guide their interventions and problem solving. It is critical that they be able to recognize symptoms that indicate a potential complication and have 24-hour phone numbers to access in the event of problems.

TABLE 33-5 Potential Problems of Home Parenteral Nutrition

General guidelines to prevent home parenteral nutrition problems:
- Wash hands thoroughly before any procedures.
- Wear gloves for all procedures, particularly if cuts, scrapes, or rashes are present on the hands.
- Keep all supplies dry and sterile during storage.
- Use aseptic technique for any procedures.

Problem	Symptoms	Patient Instructions
Possible leak in internal catheter	Swelling of skin over catheter insertion site; sensations of pain, heat, burning near site	Call home health nurse or physician. Do not use catheter to give fluids. Tape the catheter securely to the skin so that it does not dangle. Avoid rough contact or sports that could dislodge catheter.
Possible loose cap or leak in external catheter	Leak of blood from injection cap or catheter	Clamp catheter. Change cap and heparin lock. Call physician or go to emergency room for catheter repair.
Water intoxication	Puffy eyes, neck vein distention, increased urination, confusion	Contact physician and go to emergency room for laboratory tests.
Possible air embolism—air may be drawn into the vein if catheter is not clamped during cap change	Cough, shortness of breath, chest pain	If giving fluids, stop and place heparin lock on catheter. Lie on left side. Call physician or go to emergency room.
Skin infection or irritation	Redness, swelling, drainage, tenderness at exit site	Call home health nurse or physician. Change bandage and clean daily.
Possible infection within the bloodstream	Chills, fever, fatigue, aches, weakness, hyperglycemia	Change the bandage and clean around the catheter if bandage gets wet or soiled. Go to emergency room for tests.

Critical Thinking Questions

1. Your neighbor confides in you that he is afraid to go to the doctor because he fears he has stomach cancer. On further questioning you learn that he has had frequent episodes of indigestion and increased flatulence. He also comments that he has been under a lot of pressure at work, which has caused him to become nauseated on a few occasions. He does not have a family history of stomach cancer. What approach would you take to respond to his concerns?
2. You are having lunch with a co-worker and observe him taking an over-the-counter H_2-receptor antagonist. He tells you that he's been experiencing frequent abdominal pain that often wakes him up at night. You ask him if he has seen his primary care provider and he replies that he doesn't think that's necessary. He's been watching his diet, eating bland foods, and drinking lots of milk; and he is sure the symptoms will go away as soon as he successfully meets his deadline for a major project.
   a. *What other information might you want to obtain from him?*
   b. *What teaching will you try to provide?*
3. You are visiting your elderly grandmother over the holidays and notice that her osteoarthritis appears to have worsened. You ask her what she is doing to treat it and she admits that she has started using a long-acting NSAID twice a day. You have serious concerns about her risk for gastric ulcers and hemorrhage. What actions will you take to address your concerns?
4. You are a nurse in a busy medical ICU where routine stress ulcer prophylaxis is the standard of care. Design a research project to test the effectiveness of routine prophylaxis. What patient criteria would you use for selection? How will you measure your outcomes?

References

1. Agrawal NM et al: Superiority of lansoprazole vs ranitidine in healing nonsteroidal, anti-inflammatory drug-associated gastric ulcers: results of a double-blind, randomized, multicenter study, *Arch Intern Med* 160(10):1455, 2000.
2. Malcolm MC: *Helicobacter pylori, Postgrad Med J* 76:141, 2000.
3. Bazaldua OV, Schneider FD: Evaluation and management of dyspepsia, *Am Fam Physician* 60(6):1773, 1999.
4. Boland CR, Savides TJ: Tumors of the stomach. In Yamada T, editor: *Textbook of gastroenterology,* ed 3, Philadelphia, 1999, JB Lippincott.
5. Bradley JS et al: Clinical utility of pH paper versus pH meter in the measurement of critical gastric pH in stress ulcer prophylaxis, *Crit Care Med* 26(11):1905, 1998.
6. Centers for Disease Control and Prevention (CDC): *Helicobacter pylori and peptic ulcer disease, 2001,* website: http://www.cdc.gov/ulcer/md.htm.
7. Centers for Disease Control and Prevention (CDC): Knowledge about causes of peptic ulcer disease—United States, *JAMA* 278(21):1731, 1997.
8. Cook D et al: A comparison of sucralfate and ranitidine for the prevention of upper gastrointestinal bleeding in patients requiring mechanical ventilation, *N Engl J Med* 338(12):791, 1998.

9. Elta GH: Approach to the patient with gross gastrointestinal bleeding. In Yamada T, editor: *Textbook of gastroenterology,* ed 3, Philadelphia, 1999, JB Lippincott.
10. Erstad B et al: Impacting cost and appropriateness of stress ulcer prophylaxis at a university medical center, *Crit Care Med* 25(10):1678, 1997.
11. Gerritz S, Newton WP: Prevention of NSAID-induced GI muscosal injury, *J Fam Pract* 44(2):130, 1997.
12. Glaser V: Empiric therapy for nonulcer dyspepsia, *Patient Care* 34(1):35, 2000.
13. Goroll AH: Management of peptic ulcer disease. In Goroll AH, Mulley AG, editors: *Primary care medicine,* ed 4, Philadelphia, 2000, JB Lippincott.
14. Hartgrink HH, Bonenkamp HJ, van de Velde CJ: Influence of surgery on outcomes in gastric cancer, *Surg Oncol Clin North Am* 9(1):97, 2000.
15. Hanisch EW et al: A randomized, double-blind trial for stress ulcer prophylaxis shows no evidence of increased pneumonia, *Am J Surg* 176(5):453, 1998.
16. Hasler WL: Approach to the patient with nausea and vomiting. In Yamada T, editor: *Textbook of gastroenterology,* ed 3, Philadelphia,1999, JB Lippincott.
17. Hawkey CJ et al: Omeprazole compared with misoprostol for ulcers associated with nonsteroidal antiinflammatory drugs, *N Engl J Med* 338(11):727, 1998.
18. Hines SE: Current management of upper GI tract bleeding, *Patient Care* 34(2):20, 2000.
19. Hundahl S et al: The national cancer data base report on gastric carcinoma, *Cancer* 80:2333, 1997.
20. Kodama M, Kodama T: In search of the cause of gastric cancer, *In Vivo* 14(1):125, 2000.
21. Khuroo MS et al: A comparison of omeprazole and placebo for bleeding peptic ulcer, *N Engl J Med* 336(15):1054, 1997.
22. Lau JYW et al: Endoscopic retreatment compared with surgery in patients with recurrent bleeding after initial endoscopic control of bleeding ulcers, *N Engl J Med* 340(10):751, 1999.
23. McManus TJ: *Helicobacter pylori:* an emerging infectious disease, *Nurse Practitioner* 25(8):40, 2000.
24. Misra SP et al: Evaluation of the one-minute ultra-rapid urease test for diagnosing *Helicobacter pylori, Postgrad Med J* 75:154, 1999.
25. Mulley AG: Evaluation of nausea and vomiting. In Goroll AH, Mulley AG, editors: *Primary care medicine,* ed 4, Philadelphia, 2000, JB Lippincott.
26. Munnangi S, Sonnenberg A: Time trends of physician visits and treatment patterns of peptic ulcer disease in the United States, *Arch Intern Med* 157(13):1489, 1997.
27. National Digestive Diseases Information Clearinghouse: Digestive diseases statistics, 2000, website: http://www.niddk.nih.gov/health/digest/pubs/ddstats.htm.
28. Peterson WL et al: *Helicobacter pylori*–related disease: guidelines for testing and treatment, *Arch Intern Med* 160(9):1285, 2000.
29. Richter JM: Evaluation of gastrointestinal bleeding. In Goroll AH, Mulley AG, editors: *Primary care medicine,* ed 4, Philadelphia, 2000, JB Lippincott.
30. Saunders CS: *H. pylori* infection: simplifying management, *Patient Care* 33(23):118, 1999.
31. Seymour NE, Anderson DK: Surgery for peptic ulcer disease and postgastrectomy syndromes. In Yamada T, editor: *Textbook of gastroenterology,* ed 3, Philadelphia, 1999, JB Lippincott.
32. Stone MA: Transmission of *Helicobacter pylori, Postgrad Med J* 75:198, 1999.
33. Talley NJ, Holtman, G: Approach to the patient with dyspepsia and related functional gastrointestinal complaints. In Yamada T, editor: *Textbook of gastroenterology,* ed 3, Philadelphia,1999, JB Lippincott.
34. US Department of Health and Human Services: *Healthy People 2010: understanding and improving health,* Washington, DC, 2001, USDHHS.
35. Yeomans ND: A comparison of omeprazole with ranitidine for ulcers associated with nonsteroidal antiinflammatory drugs, *N Engl J Med* 338(11):719, 1998.

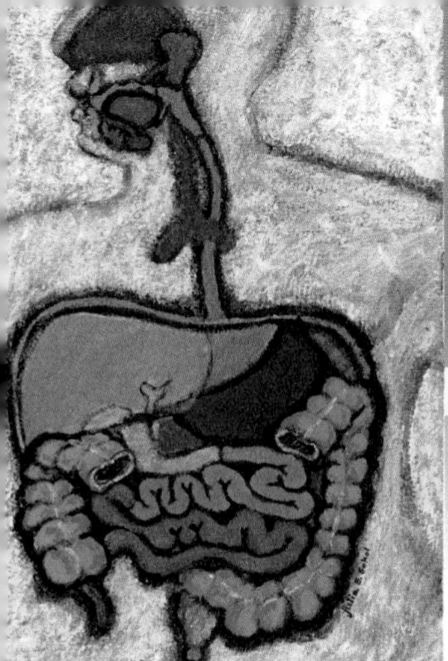

Intestinal Problems 34

Judith K. Sands

Objectives

After studying this chapter, the learner should be able to:

1. Discuss lifestyle modifications for the management of constipation and diarrhea, and the prevention of foodborne illness.
2. Compare the common forms of intestinal inflammation and their management.
3. Describe current pharmacologic and nursing management of inflammatory bowel disease.
4. Compare the pathophysiology of hernias, cancer, and volvulus as causes of bowel obstruction.
5. Discuss the nursing management of the patient with an ostomy.
6. Differentiate among the various surgical approaches to the management of common anorectal disorders.
7. Discuss preoperative and postoperative care of the patient undergoing bowel surgery.

Disorders that affect the intestines are major health problems in the United States. The scope of problems ranges from mild to life threatening, and digestion, absorption, and elimination may be affected. The categories of intestinal disorders discussed in this chapter include problems of elimination, inflammatory bowel diseases, bowel obstructions, and anorectal disorders.

FUNCTIONAL BOWEL DISORDERS

Constipation

Etiology/Epidemiology

The act of defecation, which is initiated when feces enter the rectum, is voluntarily controlled by contraction of the external anal sphincter. Most people have a regular pattern of defecation, but the pattern varies widely, from three times a day to once every 3 or more days. The term *constipation* refers to an abnormal infrequency of defecation or the passage of abnormally hard stools, or both. The term lacks precise definition because it has different meanings for different people. Almost everyone experiences occasional constipation, and it is considered an almost universal problem in Western countries. It is particularly common among older adults. Constipation accounts for millions of physician visits each year, and more than $500 million is expended annually on products to cause or support defecation.[41] Many of these products are unnecessary; some are even harmful.

Constipation can be a functional consequence of numerous disorders. Endocrine and neurologic diseases such as diabetes, hypothyroidism, multiple sclerosis, and Parkinson's disease are commonly associated with chronic constipation. Constipation is also a frequent side effect of the use of opioids, anticholinergics, and a wide variety of specific drugs such as anticonvulsants and calcium channel blockers. In many adults, however, occasional constipation can be attributed to physical inactivity, stress, dietary changes, lack of fluids, and failure to respond to the urge to defecate.[41]

Overuse of laxatives is a common problem in older adults, who can become laxative dependent, which worsens their chronic constipation. If the urge to defecate is not promptly heeded, it is quickly suppressed, and the feces remain in the rectum and harden. The urge to defecate occurs most often after meals, particularly breakfast, as a result of stimulation of the gastrocolic reflex from food entering the stomach. Common risk factors for constipation are summarized in the Risk Factors box.

Pathophysiology

Constipation may result from decreased motility of the colon or from retention of feces in the lower colon or rectum. The longer the feces remain in the colon, the greater the amount of water reabsorbed and the drier the stool becomes. The stool is then more difficult to expel. Occasional constipation is not detrimental to health, but habitual constipation leads to decreased intestinal muscle tone, increased use of Valsalva's maneuver as the person bears down in an attempt to pass the hardened stool, and an increased incidence of hemorrhoids. Dietary fiber increases the water content of the stool and promotes colonic motility through bacterial degradation.

Risk Factors
Constipation

FUNCTIONAL DISORDERS
Diabetes mellitus
Hypothyroidism
Multiple sclerosis
Parkinson's disease
A wide variety of other neurogenic and collagen disorders

MEDICATIONS
Aluminum-based and calcium-based antacids
Opioids
Anticholinergics
Antidepressants/antipsychotics
Iron, calcium, and bismuth salts
Anticonvulsants
Calcium channel blockers

DIETARY FACTORS
Dehydration
Lack of dietary fiber

PHYSICAL AND PSYCHOLOGIC FACTORS
Immobility
Confusion, disorientation
Interruption of normal bowel routines, stress

BOX 34-1 Fiber Content in Common Foods

Fruits
Raspberries: 6 g per cup
Apples: 3 g each
Tangerines: 3 g each
Peaches: 1 g each

Vegetables
Carrots: 2 g each
Peeled potatoes: 2 g each
Broccoli: 1 g per ½ cup
Cauliflower: 1 g per ½ cup
Lettuce: 1 g per cup
Spinach: 1 g per ½ cup

Starchy Vegetables
Lima beans: 4 g per ½ cup
Kidney beans: 3 g per ½ cup
Black-eyed peas: 4 g per ½ cup

Grains
Whole-wheat bread: 2 g per slice
White rice: 1 g per cup
Brown rice: 3 g per cup
Oatmeal: 3 g per ⅔ cup

Fecal impaction is a significant negative outcome of chronic constipation in institutionalized older adults in whom mental confusion and immobility may complicate the effective management of elimination. The rectum overdistends and is unable to respond to normal sensory stimulation from the anus, leading to damaging cycles of impaction, rebound diarrhea, and eventually, fecal incontinence.

Collaborative Care Management

The treatment of constipation begins with a careful assessment of the nature, severity, and duration of the problem. Treatment is individualized to the unique needs of the patient and generally includes dietary and fluid modifications, increased activity, establishment of regular toileting patterns, and the use of fiber supplements as needed. Adherence to this regimen successfully manages the problem for most individuals. Nonabsorbable saccharides (e.g., sorbitol or lactulose) may be added if needed. Numerous laxative agents are available over the counter, but the chronic use of stimulant laxatives is avoided if possible. Stool softeners are a popular option, but there is little concrete research documenting their effectiveness.[51] Drugs commonly used in the management of constipation are presented in Table 34-1.

Hospitalization inevitably interferes with a person's normal patterns of exercise and eating. The nurse monitors all hospitalized patients for constipation and records all bowel elimination. For greatest success, preventive bowel programs need to be initiated before problems with constipation arise. Initiation of a plan to prevent constipation should be a priority for any patient on bed rest or receiving frequent doses of opioids.

Patient/Family Education. Teaching begins with ensuring patient understanding of the relationship between diet, fluids, activity, stress, and the development of constipation. The nurse encourages patients to eat a high-fiber diet and to limit highly refined foods. (See Box 34-1 for the fiber content of selected foods.) Bran may be used as a supplement in a limited way. Patients should attempt to drink at least 2000 ml of fluid daily unless their medical condition contraindicates a liberal fluid intake. Regular exercise and a planned daily time for defecation are important measures. The patient is instructed to manage occasional episodes of constipation with bulk-forming laxatives if needed and to avoid the regular use of harsh laxatives or any type of enema.

Diarrhea/Foodborne Illness

Etiology/Epidemiology

Diarrhea is a major cause of morbidity in this country and remains a leading cause of death in developing nations, especially among infants and small children. Diarrhea is also one of the classic symptoms of gastrointestinal (GI) disease and can be caused by a wide variety of agents and disorders. Diarrhea involves an increase in stool number and/or a change to a more fluid consistency, but the diagnosis is based primarily on the consistency of the stool rather than the number of stools per day. Diarrhea has a wide range of etiologies, which include infectious and inflammatory processes, autoimmune disease, malabsorption, and secretory diarrhea. Acute diarrhea, continuing for less than 2 to 3 weeks, is usually self-limiting, although supportive intervention may be necessary. Chronic diarrhea is usually related to changes in the GI tract that alter the transport of fluids, electrolytes, and solids. See Box 34-2 for some of the common causes of diarrhea.

TABLE 34-1 Common Medications for Treatment of Constipation

Drug	Action	Intervention
Bulk Formers		
Psyllium (Metamucil) Methylcellulose (Citrucel)	Polysaccharides and cellulose derivatives mix with intestinal fluids, swell, and stimulate peristalsis	Ensure adequate fluid intake to prevent impaction or obstruction. Instruct patient to take separately from prescribed drugs to avoid problems with absorption.
Stool Softeners (Emollients)		
Docusate sodium (Colace) Docusate calcium (Surfak)	Act as detergents in intestine, reducing surface tension, which facilitates incorporation of liquid and fat, softening stool	Preparations lose effectiveness with long-term use; patient should not rely on this measure alone. Patient should discontinue use if abdominal cramping occurs.
Lubricants		
Mineral oil	Soften fecal matter by lubricating intestinal mucosa, facilitating easy stool passage Excessive use interferes with absorption of fat-soluble vitamins A, D, E, and K, leading to deficiency	Patient should not take with meals or drugs because oil can impair absorption; instruct patient to swallow carefully to prevent lipid aspiration.
Hyperosmolar Laxatives		
Lactulose (Cephulac) Polyethylene glycol (GoLYTELY) Sorbitol	Nonabsorbable sugars are degraded by colonic bacteria and increase stool osmolarity; fluid is drawn into the intestine, stimulating peristalsis	Adjust dose and frequency of administration to control side effects and regulate defecation. Monitor for fluid and electrolyte imbalance if response is severe.
Saline Laxatives		
Magnesium citrate Magnesium sulfate (epsom salts) Magnesium hydroxide (Milk of Magnesia)	Cause osmotic retention of fluid, which distends colon and increases peristalsis	Liquid preparations are more effective than tablets. Instruct patient to take with full glass of water. Monitor for fluid and electrolyte imbalance if response is severe.
Stimulant/Irritant Laxatives		
Cascara sagrada Senna (Senokot) Bisacodyl (Dulcolax) Castor oil	Directly stimulate and irritate intestine, promoting peristalsis	Cramps and diarrhea can occur; monitor for fluid and electrolyte imbalance if reaction is severe.

Acute diarrhea is by far the most frequent type and is usually caused by infectious agents. Despite improvements in sanitation, hygiene, and food-handling practices that have decreased the incidence of acute diarrhea in developed countries, it is still a common occurrence. The Centers for Disease Control and Prevention (CDC) estimates that at least 33 million people develop food poisoning each year, about 1 in every 10 Americans; millions of cases are probably wrongly attributed to an episode of "stomach flu."[29] The annual cost of care exceeds $28 billion.[36] Raw and undercooked eggs and undercooked chicken are two of the prime sources of infection.[11] It is estimated that up to 20% of commercially sold eggs are contaminated with *Salmonella.*[11] *Campylobacter jejuni* is considered the leading cause of bacteria-induced diarrhea in the United States, and most hens are believed to be contaminated with the organism.[11] The contamination of food preparation surfaces has also been identified as a prime source of infection. Organisms proliferate rapidly when food is either inadequately cooked or inadequately refrigerated. Risk factors for

Box 34-2 Common Causes of Diarrhea

Infections

Bacteria (*Escherichia coli, Salmonella, Shigella, Staphylococcus, Campylobacter jejuni*)
Viruses (rotavirus, human immunodeficiency virus [HIV])
Parasites (*Giardia, Cryptosporidium, Trichinella, Etamoeba histolytica,* hookworm)

Hypersensitivity

Food allergy

Autoimmune Disease

Ulcerative colitis, Crohn's disease
Graft-versus-host disease

Effects of Cytotoxic Agents

Chemotherapy-induced mucositis
Radiation enteritis

infectious diarrhea are identified in the Risk Factors box, and Table 34-2 provides an overview of some of the major causes of foodborne illness.

Pathophysiology

Large-volume diarrhea is caused by a hypersecretion of water and electrolytes by the intestinal mucosa. This secretion occurs in response to the osmotic pressure exerted by non-absorbed food particles in the chyme or from direct irritation of the mucosa. Peristalsis is increased, and the transit time through the intestine is significantly decreased. Increased peristalsis may also result from inflammation as mucosal cells hypersecrete water in the presence of infectious organisms. Diarrhea may be accompanied by severe abdominal cramping, tenesmus (persistent spasm) of the anal area, abdominal distention, and borborygmus (loud bowel sounds).

Risk Factors

Acute Diarrhea

Recent travel to developing nations
Outdoor camping
Ingestion of raw meat, seafood, or shellfish
Eating at banquets, restaurants, picnics, or fast-food establishments
Day care placement or employment
Residence in institutions, nursing homes, prisons, or mental institutions
Homosexual lifestyle
Prostitution
Intravenous drug abuse

Fluid and electrolyte imbalances can quickly result from diarrhea, depending on its severity. Mild diarrhea in adults can lead to losses of sodium and potassium, causing metabolic alkalosis. Severe diarrhea causes dehydration, hyponatremia, hypokalemia, and metabolic acidosis from the loss of large amounts of bicarbonate. Malnourished, immunosuppressed, and older persons tolerate severe diarrhea less well than do younger or well-nourished persons. Persistent diarrhea also readily leads to skin breakdown in the perianal region.

Collaborative Care Management

The management of diarrhea focuses on preventing fluid and electrolyte imbalance, controlling symptoms, and treating the underlying cause if possible. The risk of a serious outcome or death is usually directly attributable to dehydration, and short-term hospitalization may be necessary to ensure adequate fluid replacement. Aggressive rehydration with oral replacement solutions is used if the person is alert and able to take oral fluids. Solutions such as the World Health Organization solution, Pedialyte, Resol, and Rehydralyte are preferred over fruit juices, soda, or even Gatorade because they contain a balanced electrolyte composition plus glucose.

Bowel rest is no longer routinely recommended in most cases of acute diarrhea, since malnutrition can develop rapidly, but bed rest can support recovery and ease the discomfort of cramps. Clear liquids are provided along with a diet low in fiber but rich in sodium and glucose. The use of antidiarrheal agents is variable. Motility-altering drugs are rarely given in infectious diarrhea because these drugs interfere with clearance of the bacteria from the GI tract. Antidiarrheal agents may be appropriate to manage other kinds of diarrhea. Bismuth subsalicylate is usually safe and effective, but kaolin-pectin preparations are rarely helpful. Drugs that act systemically are

Table 34-2 Foodborne Illness

Causative Agent	Clinical Manifestations	Treatment
Staphylococcus aureus	Nausea, vomiting, diarrhea, and cramps within 1-6 hr of eating	Supportive care; IV fluids if needed
Bacillus cereus enterotoxin	Watery diarrhea and cramps within 8-16 hr of eating or nausea and vomiting within 1-6 hr of eating	Supportive care
Clostridium perfringens	Diarrhea and intense cramps within 8-16 hr of eating	Supportive care; IV fluids if needed
Escherichia coli (toxigenic)	Profuse watery diarrhea, cramps, low fever, and nausea within 16-24 hr of eating	Supportive care; bismuth subsalicylate (Pepto-Bismol) may be helpful; IV fluids if needed
E. coli (invasive)	Cramps, fever, vomiting, and bloody diarrhea within 6-48 hr of eating	Supportive care, antibiotics
E. coli (0157:H7)	Cramping and bloody diarrhea within 3-5 days of eating; hemolytic uremic syndrome if fever develops	Supportive care; plasma exchange if uremic syndrome develops
Shigella	Cramps, vomiting, fever, and diarrhea within 6-48 hr of eating	Supportive care, fluids, antibiotics
Salmonella enteritidis	Diarrhea, nausea, vomiting, cramps, and fever within 6-48 hr of eating	Supportive care, bland diet
Campylobacter jejuni	Diarrhea, cramps, fever, and nausea within 6-48 hr of eating	Supportive care, antibiotics
Vibrio cholerae	Cramps and watery diarrhea within 16-72 hr of eating	Fluid replacement, tetracycline
Vibrio parahaemolyticus	Diarrhea, cramps, nausea, vomiting, fever, and headache within 4 hr-4 days of eating	Supportive care
Clostridium botulinum	Nausea, vomiting, diarrhea, and paralysis, including respiratory failure and death, within 18-36 hr of eating	Antitoxin, mechanical ventilation

IV, Intravenous.

usually required to significantly affect motility. Antibiotic therapy is also controversial and is reserved for patients with infections caused by specific agents (e.g., *Escherichia coli* or *Campylobacter*).[11] The decision is based on the nature of the causative organism. Commonly used antidiarrheal medications are summarized in Table 34-3.

When patients are hospitalized with acute diarrhea, the nurse maintains an accurate record of incidence and severity, estimates fluid losses, assesses for fluid and electrolyte disturbances, and promotes patient comfort. The prevention of perianal skin breakdown is an important nursing intervention. The nurse may need to assist a weakened patient in keeping the area clean and dry. Skin ointments and barriers (e.g., zinc oxide) are reapplied as needed after each episode of diarrhea. Sitz baths can be extremely comforting when perianal skin becomes irritated.

Patient/Family Education. Patient teaching primarily focuses on measures related to the preventable causes of acute diarrhea. Strategies for ensuring food safety are summarized in Box 34-3. Strict cleanliness in regard to all food preparation surfaces and utensils is critical. Care should be taken in defrosting and handling uncooked meat and ensuring prompt and adequate refrigeration of all foods. Avoiding raw meats and seafood and thoroughly cooking ground beef are essential. Travelers are cautioned to exercise caution in consuming local water, uncooked fruits, and raw vegetables. Thorough hand washing and meticulous personal hygiene practices are helpful preventive strategies for all forms of infectious diarrhea. Reducing the incidence of foodborne illness is an important goal of Healthy People 2010.[54] The objectives related to food safety are summarized in the Healthy People 2010 box.

Fecal Incontinence

Etiology/Epidemiology

Fecal incontinence is the involuntary release of stool. It is a complex problem that has a variety of causes. The mechanisms

Box 34-3 Prevention of Foodborne Illness

Food Buying

Do not buy cans or jars that are damaged or have bulging lids.
Refrigerate all perishable and frozen foods promptly.
Never buy raw, unpasteurized milk.
Buy eggs that are clean and without cracks.
Do not buy fish that has a strong odor, cloudy eyes, or discolored skin.

Food Handling

Wash hands before handling food and after contact with raw meat or poultry.
Do not thaw foods on the kitchen counter; keep meat, fish, poultry, mayonnaise, and cream-filled foods refrigerated.
Store eggs in the refrigerator, and use within 3 to 5 weeks; use hard-boiled eggs within a week.
Cook hamburger thoroughly and all the way through.
Do not place cooked meat or poultry on boards or platters used for uncooked foods.
Make sure your refrigerator is 40° F or colder and that the freezer is 0° F or colder.
Wash vegetables and fruits thoroughly or peel off skin.
Clean the wheel of the can opener after every use.
Change dishcloths and towels frequently.
Use a meat thermometer for cooking large pieces of meat.
Avoid slow cooking.
Stuff poultry immediately before cooking, and remove stuffing after the meal.

Eating

Do not eat raw eggs in any form. Do not consume uncooked pancake, cake, or cookie batter.
Cook eggs well.
Do not eat raw fish, oysters, or clams.
Do not eat ground beef raw.
Order hamburger or meatloaf well done without a pink middle.
Verify that Caesar salad and hollandaise sauce have not been made with raw eggs.

TABLE 34-3 Common Medications for Treatment of Acute Diarrhea

Drug	Action	Intervention
Local Acting		
Bismuth subsalicylate (Pepto-Bismol)	Mechanism not known, may bind bacterial toxins	Shake liquids well before using. Bismuth products may turn stool black.
Kaolin and pectin (Kaopectate)	Soothes intestinal mucosa and increases absorption of water, nutrients, and electrolytes	Shake liquids well before using. No significant side effects exist.
Systemic Acting		
Loperamide (Imodium) Tincture of opium (paregoric) Diphenoxylate hydrochloride with atropine (Lomotil)	Acts systemically to reduce peristalsis and gastrointestinal motility	Be aware that these drugs are part of the opioid family; potential for dependence exists with paregoric. Loperamide has few side effects and no associated physical dependency. Lomotil has a low potential for dependency. Monitor patient response. Can enhance bacterial invasion and prolong excretion of the pathogen. Monitor for opioid side effects: central nervous system depression or respiratory depression.

Healthy People 2010

Goals and Objectives Related to Food Safety

GOAL: REDUCE FOODBORNE ILLNESSES

1. Reduce infections caused by key foodborne pathogens (e.g., *Campylobacter* species, *Escherichia coli* 0157:H7, *Listeria monocytogenes, Salmonella* species, *Cyclospora cayetanensis, Toxplasma gondii*).
2. Reduce outbreaks of infections caused by key foodborne bacteria (e.g., *E. coli* 0157:H7, *Salmonella, Staphylococcus*).
3. Prevent an increase in the proportion of isolates of *Salmonella* species from humans and from animals at slaughter that are resistant to antimicrobial drugs.
4. Reduce deaths from anaphylaxis caused by food allergies.
5. Increase the proportion of consumers who follow key food safety practices.
6. Improve food employee behaviors and food preparation practices that directly relate to foodborne illnesses in retail food establishments.
7. Reduce human exposure to organophosphate pesticides from food.

GOAL: PROMOTE HEALTH FOR ALL THROUGH A HEALTHY ENVIRONMENT

1. Reduce waterborne disease outbreaks arising from water intended for drinking among persons served by community water systems.

From US Department of Health and Human Services: *Healthy People 2010: understanding and improving health*, Washington, DC, 2000, USDHHS.

of anal competence are complex, and incontinence can result from a breakdown of any of the individual components.[3] The external or internal anal sphincters may be relaxed; voluntary control of defecation may be interrupted in the spinal cord or brain; anal sensation may be impaired; or structural damage may be present. The disorders that cause a loss of conscious control of defecation include neurologic disorders, diarrheal illnesses, trauma to the anal sphincter (e.g., from a fistula, an abscess, or surgery), loss of mobility, and psychiatric disorders.[3] Perineal relaxation and damage to the anal sphincter often result from vaginal delivery. Relaxation of the sphincter occurs as part of the general loss of muscle tone in aging, but the normal changes that occur with aging are not of sufficient significance to cause incontinence unless concurrent health problems are present. Statistics about incidence and prevalence of fecal incontinence are difficult to obtain because of the social stigma associated with the problem, but it is estimated that as much as 18% of the population has experienced some occurrence of fecal incontinence, and the problem is pervasive among nursing home residents.

Pathophysiology

Normally the contents of the bowel are propelled by mass movements toward the rectum. The rectum stores the feces until defecation. Distention of the rectum by feces triggers stretch receptors in the walls that initiate the urge to defecate. The external sphincter then tightens to maintain continence until voluntary defecation can take place. The rectum quickly accommodates to the increased volume, and the urge to defecate subsides. With voluntary defecation, relaxation of the internal anal sphincter is followed by relaxation of the external anal sphincter, and Valsalva's maneuver helps to expel the stool. Voluntary control of defecation is learned in early childhood, and control typically lasts throughout life.

Reflex defecation continues to occur even in the presence of most upper and lower motor neuron lesions, because the musculature of the bowel contains its own nerve centers that respond to distention through peristalsis. Reflex defecation therefore often persists or can be stimulated even when motor paralysis is present. Reflex defecation occurs primarily in response to mass peristaltic movements that follow meals. Any physical, mental, or social problem that disrupts any aspect of this complex learned behavior can result in incontinence.

Collaborative Care Management

Treatment of incontinence is multifaceted and depends on the cause. Correction of the underlying problem is crucial. This may involve control of diarrheal illnesses, treatment of impaction, prevention of constipation (which can weaken the sphincter and damage the nerve plexus as a result of chronic pressure in the rectum), or correction of structural problems.

Bowel training is the major approach used with patients who have cognitive and neurologic problems resulting from stroke or other chronic diseases. If a person can sit on a toilet, it may be possible to achieve automatic defecation when a pattern of consistent timing, familiar surroundings, and controlled dietary and fluid intake can be achieved. This approach allows many patients to defecate predictably and remain continent throughout the day.

Biofeedback training is the cornerstone of therapy for patients who have motility disorders or sphincter damage that causes fecal incontinence. The patient learns to tighten the external sphincter in response to manometric measurement of responses to rectal distention. This technique has demonstrated effectiveness with alert, motivated patients.

Patient/Family Education. Bowel training requires significant amounts of time and effort on the part of the nursing staff, family, and patient. The nurse teaches the family about the training program and how they can assist and support the effort. Incontinence is a major issue in home care and often is cited as the most common reason for older persons to be admitted to nursing homes.

To plan the most effective approach, the nurse gathers specific information concerning the person's general physical and cognitive condition, ability to contract the abdominal and perineal muscles on command, and awareness of the need or urge to defecate. Data are also collected about the nature and frequency of the incontinence problem, particularly its relationship to meals or other regular activities.

The nurse teaches the family about the importance of a high-fiber diet and ensuring that the patient consumes at least 2500 ml of fluid daily. The need for a regular stool softener or bulk former is evaluated. When an optimal time for defecation has been established, usually after breakfast, a glycerin suppository may be inserted to stimulate defecation.

Despite honest efforts by family members, staff, and the patient, the fecal incontinence may remain uncontrolled. Efforts then shift toward odor control, preventing skin breakdown, and supporting the patient's psychologic integrity. Commercially available protective pants are expensive, but they can substantially reduce the burden of care for the family and provide the patient with a sense of security and dignity. Construction of a colostomy may be a more manageable option for a small group of patients with unremitting fecal incontinence problems.

Irritable Bowel Syndrome

Etiology/Epidemiology

Irritable bowel syndrome (IBS) is one of the most common chronic disorders, affecting about 25% of the population at some time.[19] The disorder shows widespread variation among cultural groups but can be found worldwide. It is most common in Western countries and in the United States, and primarily affects women.[19]

IBS is classified as a functional disorder because no demonstrable sign of disease can be found during a routine diagnostic workup. It was considered a stress-related psychosomatic disease for many years, and only recently has the presence of an underlying physiologic abnormality been acknowledged. IBS is defined by the American Gastrointestinal Association as a combination of chronic and recurrent GI symptoms, usually including abdominal pain, distention, and disturbed defecation that cannot be explained by structural or biochemical abnormalities. It is usually mild and annoying, but in severe cases it can be incapacitating.

Pathophysiology

IBS is theorized to result from disturbances in nervous system control of the intestines that cause visceral hypersensitivity and abnormal bowel motility. The bowel wall is extremely sensitive to distention and normal motor events such as peristalsis. Patients with IBS consistently experience increased discomfort related to distention at lower volumes than do control subjects.[19] The role of serotonin is under active investigation. Serotonin causes a variety of mechanical and neurohormonal responses that are closely related to IBS symptoms.

Classic symptoms include abdominal pain; diarrhea or constipation or an alternating pattern of the two; mucus in the stool; a sensation of incomplete evacuation; and relief of discomfort with defecation. Some persons also experience a wide range of general dyspepsia symptoms, including excessive gas and bloating.

Collaborative Care Management

The diagnosis of IBS is made by eliminating other potential causes of the symptoms. At present there are no definitive tests or biologic markers. Nonpharmacologic treatment approaches focus on thorough dietary analysis and elimination of any irritating substances. Limiting gas-producing foods may be helpful, and adding fiber to the diet improves symptoms in many patients. Cognitive behavioral strategies to more effectively manage stress are also frequently helpful. A number of pharmacologic options exist, depending on the person's symptoms. Antidiarrheal agents, bulk-forming laxatives, and antispasmodics are routine options (see Tables 34-1 and 34-3). Newer drug therapies are under development to improve motility or target the specific classes of serotonin primarily responsible for intestinal hypersensitivity.

Patient/Family Education. Patient teaching and reassurance are critical aspects of the care of a person with IBS. The absence of a demonstrable structural cause of the symptoms can quickly lead to suspicions of malingering. The physiologic basis of IBS is difficult to understand, but patients need reassurance that it is not "all in their head" or a hidden symptom of some other deadly disease process. The nurse assists the person in analyzing his or her diet and lifestyle to identify factors that minimize or worsen symptoms, and also assists in designing a regimen that effectively blends pharmacologic and nonpharmacologic strategies for improved symptom control.

ACUTE INFLAMMATION OF THE INTESTINES

Appendicitis

Etiology/Epidemiology

The vermiform appendix is a small, fingerlike projection attached to the cecum just below the ileocecal valve (Figure 34-1). The appendix is approximately 10 cm (4 inches) long and has no clearly identified function. It is an integral part of the cecum and fills with chyme and empties by peristalsis along with the rest of the bowel.

Appendicitis is an acute inflammation of the appendix and is one of the most common surgical emergencies. The cause rarely is clear-cut, but the lumen of the appendix is quite small, making it vulnerable to incomplete emptying, distention by accumulated mucus, or obstruction, which can lead to infection. Obstruction by fecaliths (hardened feces) or foreign bodies is believed to be the most common etiology of acute appendicitis.

Appendicitis occurs most commonly in teenagers and young adults between the ages of 10 and 30 years. Although only 10% of cases occur after age 50, appendicitis can occur at any age and is an extremely serious condition in older adults. Males are affected more commonly than females during the teenage and young adult years. Approximately 7% of the population is affected by the disorder at some point. Appendicitis increased steadily in incidence from the late nineteenth century to a peak in the 1950s. The incidence since 1950 has been steadily declining for poorly understood reasons. Appendicitis appears to occur more commonly in Western societies, in which the diet is low in fiber and high in refined carbohydrates. The higher incidence of constipation associated with this dietary pattern is theorized to increase the chance of developing obstructive fecaliths.

Pathophysiology

The inflammatory process of appendicitis can involve all or part of the appendix. Intraluminal pressure increases, leading to occlusion of the capillaries and venules and vascular engorgement. Bacterial invasion follows, and microabscesses may

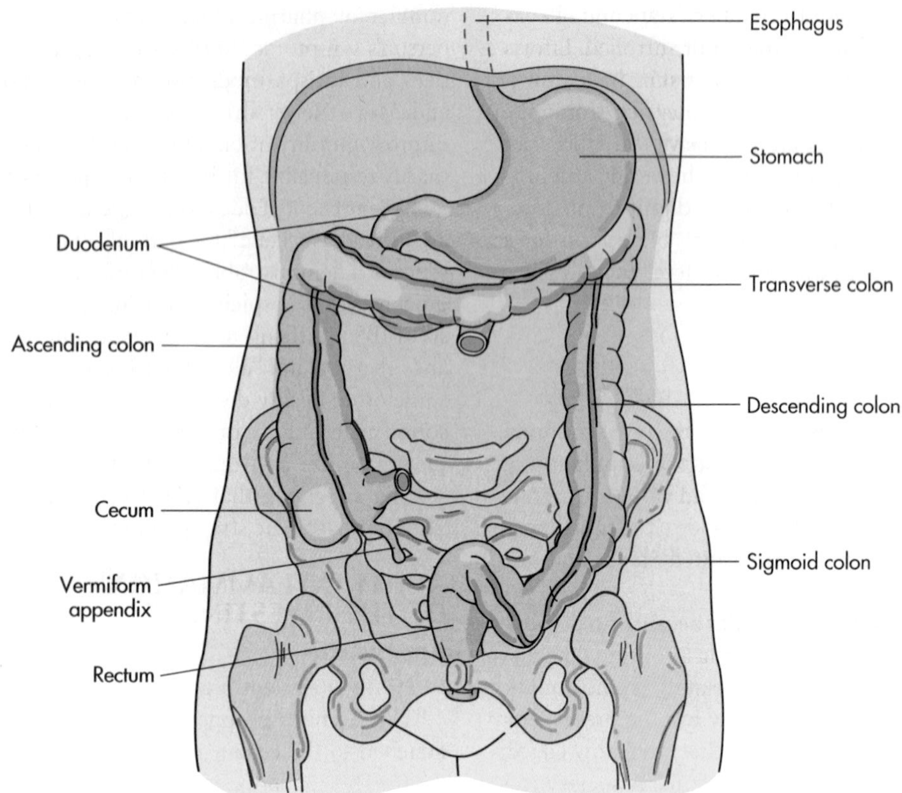

Figure 34-1 The appendix at the beginning of the ascending colon.

develop in the appendiceal wall or surrounding tissue, which, unless treated, can progress to gangrene and perforation within 24 to 36 hours. If the inflammatory process develops fairly slowly, the infection may be successfully walled off in a local abscess. In more rapidly developing cases, the risk of rupture and acute peritonitis is quite high.

The classic clinical manifestation of appendicitis is abdominal pain that comes in waves. The pain starts in the epigastric or umbilical region but gradually becomes localized in the right lower quadrant of the abdomen. Localization at McBurney's point, halfway between the umbilicus and the anterior spine of the ileum (Figure 34-2), is considered classic. The pain is intermittent at first but becomes steady and severe over a short period of time. Pain is often accompanied by anorexia, nausea, and vomiting. Light palpation of the abdomen elicits acute pain in the right lower quadrant. Rebound tenderness is a common finding (see Chapter 31). The abdominal muscles overlying the area of inflammation may feel tense as a result of voluntary rigidity. The person with appendicitis often lies on the side or back with knees flexed in an attempt to decrease muscle strain on the abdominal wall. Other symptoms may include temperature elevations in the range of 38° to 38.5° C (100.5° to 101.5° F), accompanied by an elevation in the white blood cell (WBC) count to more than 10,000/mm^3 and a neutrophil count of more than 75%.

Patients with appendicitis may experience less well defined local symptoms that can make prompt and accurate diagnosis a challenge. Elderly patients are less likely to experience classic

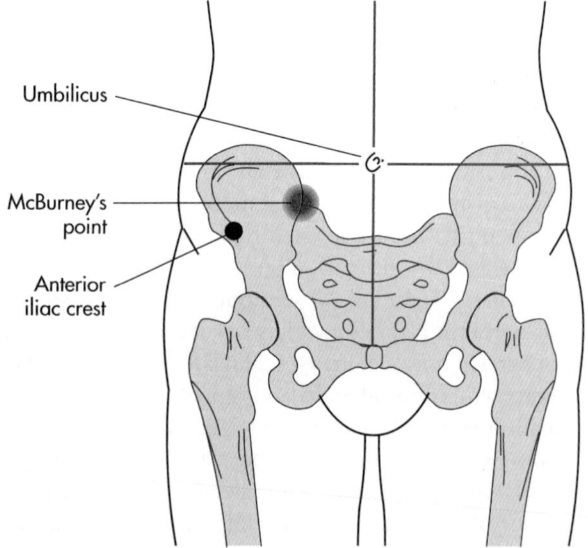

Figure 34-2 McBurney's point, located halfway between the umbilicus and the anterior iliac crest in the right lower quadrant of the abdomen.

acute symptoms at all. Their response to pain is decreased, and their symptoms may be mild or vague. Because appendicitis is relatively rare in this age-group, the diagnosis may be delayed or missed. Perforation also occurs more often in older adults, and mortality is greater.

Delay or confusion about the diagnosis of appendicitis can lead to perforation, which is associated with substantial morbidity and mortality, particularly in children and older adults. In adults a perforation generally results in a localized abscess. Local containment of the perforation is less effective in children, who often experience generalized peritonitis. Perforation is believed to occur early in the disease process in older adults, increasing the incidence of complications.

Collaborative Care Management

The diagnosis of appendicitis is made from the classic physical and laboratory indicators when they are present. Many other diseases can produce symptoms similar to those of appendicitis, and these problems may need to be ruled out before a positive diagnosis can be made. Related disorders include ureteral stones, acute salpingitis, regional ileitis, ovarian cysts, and biliary colic. Ultrasonography may be used to identify the inflamed appendix and the presence of perforation or abscess.

During the diagnostic period the nurse focuses on keeping the patient as comfortable as possible, relieving anxiety, and preparing the patient for surgery. The patient is placed on bed rest and given nothing by mouth. Intravenous (IV) fluids are administered to maintain fluid and electrolyte balance, and antibiotic therapy may be initiated. To avoid masking critical changes in symptoms, pain medication is usually withheld until a definite diagnosis of appendicitis has been made. The nurse explains the need for withholding analgesics and uses nonpharmacologic methods such as positioning and environmental management to increase the patient's comfort. Unnecessary movement, which typically increases the patient's pain, is avoided. Heat is not applied to the abdomen because the increased circulation to the appendix can lead to rupture.

The appendix is removed surgically (appendectomy) as soon as possible to prevent rupture with subsequent peritonitis. When surgery is performed promptly, mortality is less than 0.5%. If the diagnosis is not made promptly, however, the incidence of complications rises dramatically. Traditional surgery removes the appendix through a small incision over McBurney's point or through a right paramedial incision. The incision usually heals with no need for external drainage. Drains are inserted when an abscess is discovered, when the appendix has ruptured, or when the appendix is severely edematous and surrounded by a pocket of clear fluid. Bowel function usually returns to normal soon after surgery, and convalescence is short. Appendectomies can also be successfully performed laparoscopically, but the cost is greater and the length of stay is not significantly reduced, although patients do report less pain. Laparoscopic appendectomy does not appear to offer any significant improvement over traditional surgery at this time.

Patient/Family Education. The nurse provides the patient with an overview of the planned surgery and postoperative care. Postoperative nursing care after an appendectomy is similar to that provided to any surgical patient. Oral fluids and foods are restarted as tolerated, and discharge is rapid. The patient usually can resume all normal activities within 2 to 4 weeks. The nurse provides the patient with instructions concerning monitoring for wound healing, avoidance of strenuous activities and heavy lifting, and the importance of promptly reporting the development of any symptoms indicative of complications.

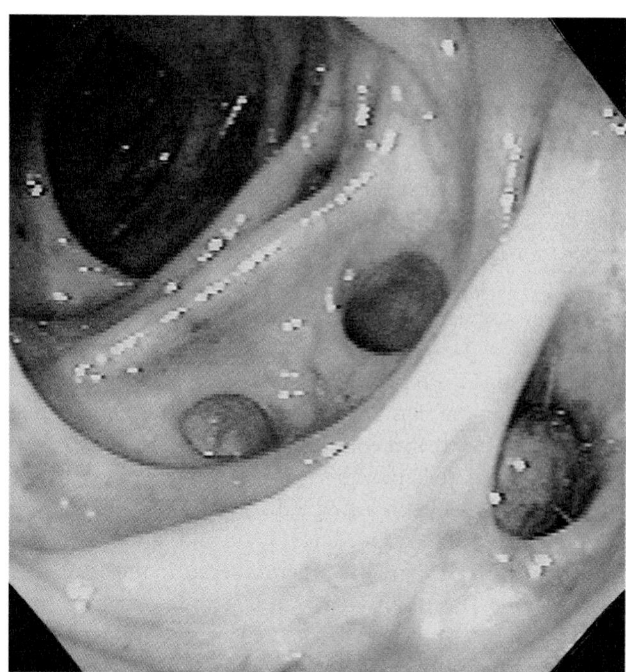

Figure 34-3 Diverticular disease.

Diverticular Disease/Diverticulitis

Etiology/Epidemiology

Diverticula are small outpouchings or herniations of the mucosal lining of the colon (Figure 34-3). They are regarded by many as part of the normal aging process. Thirty percent of individuals older than 50 years of age are estimated to have diverticula, and the incidence increases to about 70% in persons over 70 years of age.[14] Diverticula develop primarily in the left colon and rarely occur alone. The number of diverticula is also believed to increase with age. The vast majority of diverticula are never formally diagnosed, and the person remains completely asymptomatic. Patients typically seek medical care only if diverticulitis occurs. Diverticulitis is an episode of acute inflammation that can occur from local obstruction of a diverticulum by mucus or fecal matter. About 15% of persons with diverticula experience an episode of diverticulitis at some point.[14]

Diverticulosis (the condition of having uninflamed diverticula) has been described as a disease of Western civilization because of its high incidence in developed countries. The disease shows wide geographic variations in incidence that are at least partly attributable to the quantity of nonabsorbable fiber in the daily diet. The increased incidence of diverticular disease parallels the changes in Western diet that have occurred since the 1850s when the refinement of grains became standard. The steady aging of the population is also reflected in these figures. Low-fiber diets have been shown to increase intraluminal pressure in the bowel, but aging also appears to change the composition of the bowel and decreases its tensile strength.

Pathophysiology

The development of intestinal diverticula is believed to be related to increased intraluminal pressure in the colon and decreased muscle strength in the colon wall. Diverticula tend to form at points in the wall where blood vessels penetrate the mucosal and muscular layers, creating points of relative weakness.

Diverticula are commonly found in the sigmoid colon where the lumen is narrowest and pressure is highest. Muscle contractions in the sigmoid increase the thickness of the muscle and cause the weaker connective tissue to herniate between the circular muscle bands and form the diverticula.[12] Diverticulitis often develops in a single diverticulum in response to irritation initiated by trapped fecal material. The blood supply to the area decreases, and bacteria proliferate in the obstructed diverticulum. The diverticular sac is a thin structure composed entirely of mucosal tissue, which is easily perforated. Microperforations usually quickly and effectively wall off because they are directly adjacent to the mesocolon. Larger perforations may progress to abscess formation or general peritonitis. Generalized inflammation can result in thickening and scarring of the bowel wall.

Diverticular disease is usually asymptomatic, but mild inflammation can trigger a nonspecific bowel dysfunction that resolves in a matter of hours or days. The clinical manifestations of diverticulitis reflect the inflammation of the diverticula or the development of complications. Crampy lower left quadrant abdominal pain accompanied by low-grade fever is a classic sign. The pain is triggered by muscle spasms of the sigmoid colon and is acute and persistent in nature. Nausea, vomiting, and a feeling of bloating are also common. The inflammatory process also often involves the bladder and may cause urinary symptoms. The development of an abscess initiates the symptoms of localized peritonitis (see the following section). The traditional symptoms tend to be less pronounced or underreported by older adults.

Diverticular Bleeding. Diverticular disease is also one of the most common causes of lower GI bleeding.[20] The diverticula develop around a rich network of blood vessels, and as the vasa recta passes over the dome of the diverticulum, it may be separated from the lumen of the colon only by a thin layer of mucosa. Episodes of acute bleeding occur in about 15% of persons with diverticular disease. The bleeding is abrupt and copious and not related to any identifiable precipitating event in most cases. The bleeding is self-limited and stops spontaneously in more than 80% of patients.

Meckel's Diverticulum. Meckel's diverticulum is a congenital abnormality in which a blind tube, similar in structure to the appendix, is present and opens into the distal ileum near the ileocecal valve. The tube may be attached to the umbilicus by a fibrous band. It occurs in about 2% of the population and is more common in men. The anomaly usually remains asymptomatic but can become grossly inflamed later in life and require surgical excision.

Collaborative Care Management

The preliminary diagnosis of diverticulitis may be made from the history and presenting symptoms. A computed tomography (CT) scan reveals the presence of both diverticula and an abscess. A barium enema clearly reveals the classic diverticular pouches and thickened muscle layers but is usually not performed until after the inflammation subsides. A proctosigmoidoscopy may be performed to rule out other serious colon pathologies such as inflammatory bowel disease and cancer.

An episode of diverticulitis is managed by resting the bowel. Hospitalization may be required in acute episodes.[14] The patient is kept NPO or restricted to clear liquids, and a regimen of IV fluids, antibiotics, and analgesics is begun. Anticholinergics (e.g., propantheline bromide [Pro-Banthine]) may be administered to reduce bowel spasm. Symptoms should subside within 48 to 72 hours. Mild cases can be effectively managed in the home.

Acute diverticulitis usually resolves with conservative medical management. In about 25% of patients, however, surgical intervention may be needed to deal with complications. Surgical resection of the involved part of the bowel may be necessary, particularly if abscesses need to be drained. An end-to-end anastomosis is performed if possible. A temporary colostomy is occasionally necessary.

Nursing care during an acute episode is largely supportive and focuses on patient comfort. The nurse teaches the patient the rationale for bed rest and bowel rest and the role that these interventions play in bowel healing. The nurse monitors fluid and electrolyte balance and the status of the patient's pain. The patient is regularly assessed for signs of complications.

Patient/Family Education. Asymptomatic diverticulosis is managed by the prevention of constipation through the use of a high-fiber diet. Bulk-forming laxatives may be used to increase the mass and water content of the stool. The nurse encourages the patient to maintain a liberal fluid intake of 2500 to 3000 ml/day and to ingest a diet that contains soft foods high in fiber, such as fruits, vegetables, and whole grains. The American Dietetic Association recommends 20 to 35 g of fiber daily. Patients used to be advised to avoid eating foods such as nuts or seeds, which could become trapped in the diverticula and trigger inflammation. No evidence exists that these foods represent actual risks for obstruction, and avoidance is no longer suggested. Small amounts of bran may be added to regular foods, or bulk-forming agents may be used daily to increase stool mass and softness, increase the diameter of the colon, and prevent straining at hard stool. High-fiber foods should not be consumed when symptoms of inflammation are present because they can be highly irritating to the mucosa. The fiber content of selected foods is presented in Box 34-1. The patient is also encouraged to avoid activities that increase intraabdominal pressure. Weight loss may be recommended in an attempt to lower the resting intraabdominal pressure.

Peritonitis

Etiology/Epidemiology

Peritonitis involves either a local or generalized inflammation of the peritoneum, the membranous lining of the abdomen that covers the viscera. Peritonitis may be primary or secondary, aseptic or septic, and acute or chronic. Primary peritonitis usually is caused by bacterial infection, whereas secondary peritonitis often results from trauma, surgical injury, or chemical irritation.[24]

A ruptured appendix, perforated peptic ulcer, diverticulitis, pelvic inflammatory disease, urinary tract infection or trauma, bowel obstruction, and surgical complications are possible causes of primary peritonitis. Secondary bacterial invasion occurs within hours of the initiating event and is an important component of all forms of peritonitis. Common organisms for bacterial invasion include *Escherichia coli,* streptococci, staphylococci, pneumococci, gonococci, *Klebsiella,* and *Pseudomonas.*

Pathophysiology

The body creates natural barriers to attempt to control the inflammation associated with peritonitis. Adhesions form rapidly and may be successful in limiting involvement to only a portion of the abdominal cavity. The end result may be abscess development. Adhesions are more likely to develop in the lower part of the abdomen. As healing progresses, the adhesions may shrink and virtually disappear, or they may persist as constrictions that bind the involved structures together, possibly creating intestinal obstruction.

The peritoneum is a semipermeable membrane that allows the flow of water and electrolytes between the bloodstream and peritoneal cavity. When peritonitis occurs, fluid can shift into the abdominal cavity at a rate of 300 to 500 ml/hr in response to the acute inflammation.[7] The inflammatory process also shunts extra blood to the inflamed areas of bowel to combat the secondary bacterial infection, and peristalsis slows or ceases. The bowel increasingly becomes distended with gas and fluid. The circulatory, fluid, and electrolyte changes can rapidly become critical. Local reactions of the peritoneum include redness, inflammation, and the production of large amounts of fluid containing electrolytes and proteins. Hypovolemia, electrolyte imbalance, dehydration, and finally shock can develop. The loss of circulatory volume is proportional to the severity of peritoneal involvement. The fluid usually becomes purulent as the condition progresses and as the bacteria become more numerous. The bacteria may also enter the blood and cause septicemia.

The clinical manifestations of peritonitis are both local and systemic. They depend to some degree on the site and extent of the inflammation. Abdominal findings include local or diffuse pain and rebound tenderness. Guarding and rigidity are classic signs. Distention and paralytic ileus develop as the inflammation progresses. Systemic signs may include fever; an elevated WBC count; nausea and vomiting; and symptoms of early shock such as tachycardia, tachypnea, oliguria, restlessness, weakness, pallor, and diaphoresis. The symptoms initially are much less severe in older persons, and the diagnosis may be overlooked until the condition is extremely serious. Patients receiving high doses of corticosteroids also may exhibit mild or ambiguous symptoms, making early diagnosis difficult.

Collaborative Care Management

The diagnosis of peritonitis is made primarily on the basis of the symptom pattern, laboratory findings, and x-ray studies, which may show abnormalities in gas and air patterns in the abdomen. Free air or fluid in the abdominal cavity is indicative of perforation. Specimens of blood and peritoneal fluid are obtained for culture before the initiation of antibiotic therapy. WBC counts often are elevated to 20,000/mm^3 or higher. Electrolyte values are carefully monitored.

The primary curative intervention for peritonitis is surgery to correct the underlying cause and remove infected material. Surgical healing is impaired if sepsis or ischemia occurs, and complications associated with wound healing are common. Peritoneal lavage with warm saline may be performed during surgery, followed by the insertion of drainage tubes to facilitate healing. Surgery may have to be delayed until the patient's condition can be medically stabilized.

The patient with peritonitis is critically ill and requires careful monitoring of all vital parameters. Placement in a critical care environment may be indicated. The nurse monitors vital signs and intake and output frequently and adjusts IV lines and medications as ordered. Fluid, electrolyte, and colloid replacement is the major focus of medical care. The fluid shifts that cause massive hypovolemia and shock need aggressive management. Broad-spectrum antibiotics against suspected organisms are administered and then adjusted as needed in response to culture and sensitivity reports.

A nasogastric (NG) tube is inserted to help relieve abdominal distention. Bed rest in a semi-Fowler's position is maintained to support ventilation and increase patient comfort. The nurse encourages the patient to deep breathe frequently because pain and distention can significantly impair ventilation. The nurse also provides comfort measures, including frequent mouth care, basic hygiene, and measures to reduce anxiety. Nutritional management with parenteral nutrition may be necessary when sepsis is severe and recovery is expected to be prolonged. The overall mortality of patients with severe peritonitis is about 40%.[24]

Patient/Family Education. Peritonitis typically develops rapidly and creates a serious and frightening situation for the patient and family. The nurse reinforces teaching about the nature of the problem and its treatment and provides ongoing support and encouragement. The nurse teaches the patient the importance of routine respiratory care and encourages ambulation when tolerated. If the abdominal involvement is extensive, the patient may have multiple drains in place, and wound healing is complex. Careful teaching about wound management is important, since recovery is often prolonged, and the patient is likely to be discharged with ongoing needs for wound care support from home health care services. Careful discharge preparation and referrals are critical.

Inflammatory Bowel Disease

The term *inflammatory bowel disease (IBD)* is an umbrella term used to describe conditions that are characterized by bowel inflammation. Crohn's disease and ulcerative colitis are the two major forms. They have distinctly different pathologies but share many overlapping features. Their management is therefore presented together.

Etiology

The etiology of IBD remains unknown despite extensive research. It is believed that both Crohn's disease and ulcerative colitis occur in response to some complex interplay of genetic, immune system, and environmental factors.[39] Simply stated, it is theorized that IBD develops when genetically susceptible individuals mount a sustained immune reaction causing bowel inflammation in response to exposure to a viral or bacterial antigen.[17] Persons with IBD have a high prevalence of antibodies to intestinal epithelial antigens, and persons with Crohn's disease exhibit high levels of selected T-cell populations. First-degree relatives have a significantly increased risk of developing IBD, and familial aggregations of cases have been found.

The dramatic shifts that have occurred in disease incidence over time also point to a strong environmental influence in IBD etiology, but few clear directions have emerged from the extensive research.[52] Diet has been an obvious focus of research, especially with the concentration of IBD in industrialized countries, but none of the extensive studies performed thus far supports a role for diet in the etiology of IBD.[27] Other environmental factors have also not been proven to play an etiologic role. Smoking is a striking exception. Smokers have a two to four times greater risk of developing Crohn's disease than nonsmokers, and the risk does not appear to be dose dependent. Smoking is believed to play a causal role in susceptible persons.[49] Nonsmokers, however, appear to be at greater risk of developing ulcerative colitis, and the apparent protective effect of cigarette smoking against ulcerative colitis does appear to be dose dependent. Similar contradictory evidence confounds research into infectious etiologies of IBD as well. An apparent increased risk in women using oral contraceptives is seen in the statistics but remains an unproven link.

Stress and emotional factors once were believed to play an important etiologic role in IBD, but research has not supported a psychogenic cause.[17] IBD is clearly multifactorial in origin, and at this point it can simply be said that IBD occurs in susceptible people; genetic factors and immune system dysfunction probably play a role, with environmental agents acting as triggers to produce inflammation in the bowel wall. Other environmental factors may influence the disease presentation and severity, as well as the tendency for relapse.

Epidemiology

IBD occurs worldwide, with an annual incidence of approximately 3 to 20 new cases per 100,000 population. The incidence is significantly higher in the United States, northern Europe, and the United Kingdom, and approximately 1 million Americans deal with the problem on a daily basis.[27]

IBD used to be extremely rare or nonexistent in many parts of the world, but its incidence accelerated during the twentieth century. Ulcerative colitis used to occur much more commonly than Crohn's disease, but the incidence of Crohn's disease now equals, and in some areas such as the United States and northern Europe even exceeds, that of ulcerative colitis.[17] Incidence rates for both major forms of IBD are still increasing around the world but appear to have stabilized in the areas of highest risk.[27] It is difficult to know to what degree the steady increases in incidence can be attributed, at least in part, to improved disease recognition and diagnosis.

IBD is common among Caucasians but less common in African-Americans and Native Americans. One of the most unusual aspects of the incidence statistics is the higher incidence among American and European Jews. This higher incidence does not occur among native-born Israelis and appears to point to some as yet unidentified genetic and environmental interaction.

No gender pattern is evident in racially mixed groups, but Caucasian women appear to be at particular risk. Although IBD can occur at any age, its peak period of onset is in young adulthood between the ages of 15 and 25 years. A second smaller peak occurs between the ages of 55 and 60 years, and ulcerative colitis appears to preferentially affect a small subset of older men.[27] Risk factors for IBD are summarized in the Risk Factors box.

Pathophysiology

Although inflammation is the hallmark of both Crohn's disease and ulcerative colitis, the two disorders have markedly different effects on the bowel. The diseases are distinguished largely by the nature of the inflammation, the location of lesions in the GI tract, the pattern of distribution, and the degree of mucosal penetration. See Table 34-4 for a comparison of the major pathophysiologic features of each disease process.

Both forms of IBD are characterized by exacerbations and remissions. Although there is a great deal of overlap in the presenting symptoms, ulcerative colitis and Crohn's disease have different characteristic features. There is also a great deal of overlap in the clinical picture of IBD and that of IBS.

Ulcerative Colitis. Ulcerative colitis targets the bowel mucosa and creates a diffuse continuous process of inflammation characterized by edema and shallow ulceration (Figure 34-4). It primarily affects the distal colorectal area, and about 30% of patients experience disease that is confined to this region.[22] More extensive disease is described as left sided and affects

Risk Factors
Inflammatory Bowel Disease

- Age 15 to 25 years
- Caucasian race
  - Women at slightly higher risk
- Jewish ancestry, but does not apply to native-born Israelis
- First-degree relative of person with inflammatory bowel disease
- Residence in the United States, Great Britain, northern Europe, or Scandinavia
- History of smoking (Crohn's disease)
- Nonsmoking status (ulcerative colitis)
- Use of oral contraceptives (among Caucasian women)

about 40% of patients. It involves the colon up to the splenic flexure. In severe disease the inflammatory process extends all the way to the hepatic flexure or ileocecal junction. A fortunate subset of patients with ulcerative colitis develop a less virulent disease variant that is confined to the rectum and referred to as ulcerative proctitis. Although relapses are common with ulcerative proctitis, the disease rarely progresses and is associated with a low risk for the development of cancer and other long-term complications.

In ulcerative colitis the mucosa is very fragile and bleeds spontaneously or in response to minimal trauma. Over time it becomes increasingly thickened and edematous. The ulceration and healing process gradually result in scar tissue formation that can cause the colon to lose its normal elasticity and absorptive capability. As normal mucosa is gradually replaced by scar tissue, the colon becomes thickened, rigid, and pipelike. The mucosa may also undergo structural changes over time, forming pseudopolyps that can become malignant.

Bloody diarrhea and abdominal pain are the classic symptoms of ulcerative colitis. The diarrhea ranges in severity from three to four times daily to hourly; it is small in volume, mushy in consistency, and liberally mixed with blood, mucus, and pus.[22] The inflammatory exudate and mucus secretion increase both the fecal solutes and water. The diarrhea is associated with significant urgency and left-sided abdominal pain that is colicky in nature and relieved by emptying the bowel. Severe diarrhea may result in significant losses of fluids, sodium, potassium, bicarbonate, and calcium. As scarring within the bowel occurs, the sensation of the urge to defecate can be lost, leading to involuntary leakage of stool.

Crohn's Disease. Crohn's disease can affect any portion of the digestive tract with any degree of severity but is found most often in the proximal colon and ileocecal junction, making it a right-sided disease. Fifty percent of patients experience disease confined to the colon and ileum.[17] More than one site may be affected. The presentation of Crohn's disease is so variable that speculation exists that the disease will eventually be found to be a cluster of disorders rather than a single disease entity.[17]

The inflammation of Crohn's disease is transmural, affecting all layers of the intestinal wall. It follows a "skip" or "cobblestone" pattern in which affected areas are separated by normal tissue. Mucosal granulomas, luminal narrowing, thickening of the intestinal wall, mucosal nodularity, and ulceration are characteristic features.[38] The lesions may perforate and form fistulas that connect with the bladder, vagina, or other segments of the bowel or mesentery. Scar tissue may form as the lesions heal, preventing the normal absorption of nutrients, and stricture bands may form, causing intestinal obstruction. Figure 34-5 illustrates several of the common complications of Crohn's disease.

Diarrhea and abdominal pain are also classic features of Crohn's disease, but the symptoms vary according to the location and severity of the inflammation. The diarrhea is likely to consist of three to five daily large, semisolid stools that contain mucus and pus but no blood. Steatorrhea may be present if the inflammation extends high into the small intestine. Fat-soluble vitamins—A, D, E, and K—may be poorly absorbed.

TABLE 34-4 Comparison of Ulcerative Colitis and Crohn's Disease

Ulcerative Colitis	Crohn's Disease
Usual Area Affected	
Left colon, rectum	Distal ileum, right colon Can occur anywhere in gastrointestinal tract
Extent of Involvement	
Diffuse areas, contiguous	Segmental areas, noncontiguous
Inflammation	
Mostly mucosal	Transmural
Mucosal Appearance	
Shallow mucosal ulcerations, edematous, superficial bleeding	Cobblestone effect, granulomas Thickened walls, narrowed lumen
Complications	
Loss of absorption and elasticity Replacement of mucosa by scar tissue Development of pseudopolyps that may become malignant Toxic megacolon Hemorrhoids Bleeding	Fistulas Perianal disease Strictures Abscesses Perforation Anemia Malabsorption of fat and fat-soluble vitamins

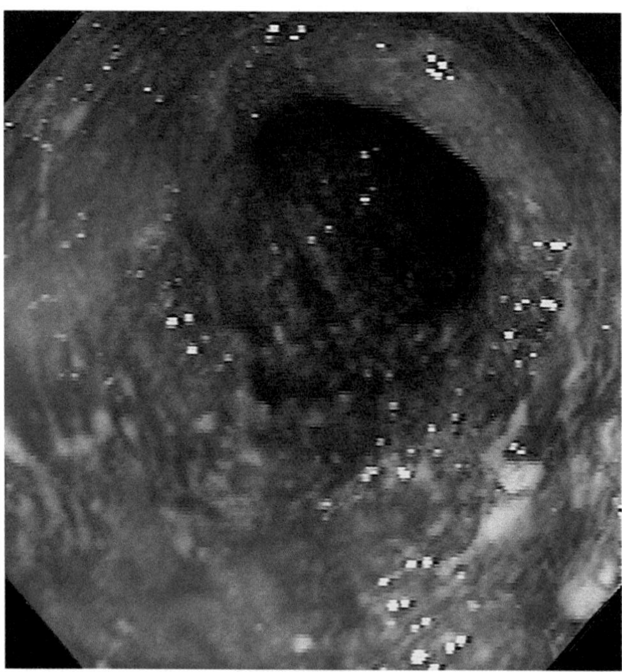

Figure 34-4 Severe ulcerative colitis.

Severe abdominal pain that is colicky in nature and tenderness that is diffuse or localized in the right lower quadrant are also characteristic of Crohn's disease. A tender mass of thickened intestine may be palpable in the area. During an acute episode the symptoms may closely resemble those of appendicitis.

Extraintestinal and Systemic Symptoms of Inflammatory Bowel Disease. Extraintestinal and systemic symptoms of IBD occur commonly and often complicate the patient's disease management. IBD can involve virtually every organ system. Although it is generally accepted that extraintestinal symptoms are separate systemic disorders, their etiology is not understood. They appear to reflect some type of generalized tissue vulnerability and are considered immunologic phenomena. They may precede or accompany the underlying bowel disorder. A patient with one extraintestinal manifestation has an increased risk of developing others.

Peripheral arthritis is the most common extraintestinal manifestation and occurs in 4% to 23% of patients with IBD.[17] It is migratory in nature, affects single joints in an asymmetric pattern, and primarily targets the hips, ankles, wrists, and elbows. A wide range of ocular problems may occur (e.g., uveitis, corneal ulceration, and retinopathy). The incidence is about 4% to 10%.[41] Skin lesions are also common. A grouping of small bowel–related problems appears to be associated with Crohn's disease. Cholelithiasis, for example, has an incidence of 13% to 34% in patients with Crohn's disease versus 10% to 15% in the general population.[38]

In addition to the classic symptoms, IBD often causes anorexia, nausea, weakness, and malaise from the chronic inflammation. Weight loss is common and may result in nutritional deficiencies if the absorption capability of the bowel is significantly impaired. Intermittent fever and leukocytosis often accompany an exacerbation, and iron deficiency anemia may develop from both chronic mucosal bleeding and poor iron absorption. Patients are often pale and thin and look chronically ill. The course of IBD is highly unpredictable and cannot be determined from the initial presentation. In most patients the course is chronic and recurrent, but occasionally patients are able to achieve and sustain long-term remissions. Classic clinical and extraintestinal manifestations of IBD are summarized in the Clinical Manifestations box.

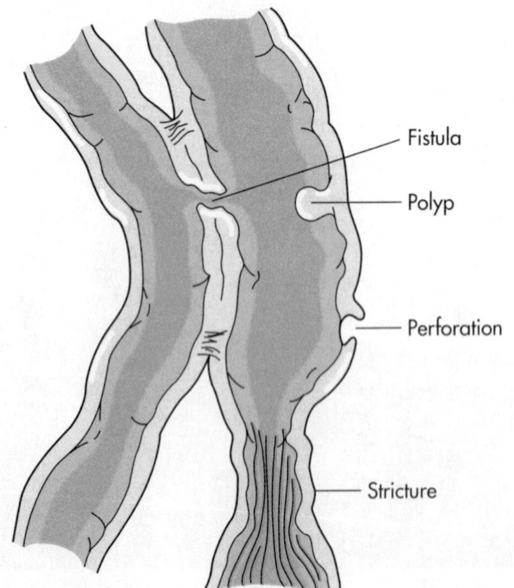

Figure 34-5 Common complications of Crohn's disease.

Collaborative Care Management

Diagnostic Tests. The diagnosis of IBD begins with a careful health history that includes the symptom pattern and its severity and duration. A stool examination for leukocytes, parasites, blood, and culture is performed to rule out an in-

Clinical Manifestations

Inflammatory Bowel Disease

GENERAL

Anorexia, nausea, and weight loss
Weakness and malaise
Fever and leukocytosis (a high fever and white blood cell count >15,000/mm^3 suggest an abscess)
Iron deficiency anemia

SPECIFIC TO ULCERATIVE COLITIS

Profuse diarrhea (15 to 20 stools per day)
Stools containing blood, mucus, and possibly pus
Abdominal cramping can be present before the bowel movement
Losses of fluid, sodium, potassium, bicarbonate, and calcium

SPECIFIC TO CROHN'S DISEASE

Three to five large, semisolid stools per day
Stools containing mucus and possibly pus but rarely blood
Steatorrhea if small bowel affected
Right lower quadrant cramping: may be severe and mimic appendicitis; diffuse rather than localized pain

EXTRAINTESTINAL MANIFESTATIONS

***Arthritis** (4% to 23%)*

Involvement of large joints: hips, ankles, wrists, and elbows
Migratory and asymmetric incidence, nondeforming

***Ocular** (4% to 10%)*

Uveitis, episcleritis
Serous retinopathy

***Skin** (3% to 6%)*

Erythema nodosum: raised, red, tender nodules on anterior tibial surfaces
Pyoderma gangrenosum: painful, necrotizing ulcerations; most common on legs

***Hepatobiliary** (4% to 5%)*

Cholelithiasis
Fatty liver, cirrhosis
Cholangitis (70% of patients with cholangitis have ulcerative colitis)

***Renal** (4% to 23%)*

Kidney stones
Ureteral obstruction

fectious origin for the symptoms. Laboratory tests may include a complete blood count, erythrocyte sedimentation rate, and serum albumin measurement, although no laboratory study is diagnostic by itself. New antibody assay tests are showing promise in differentiating between Crohn's disease and ulcerative colitis,[16] but at present there is no definitive diagnostic tool for either form of IBD.

A barium enema usually is performed to evaluate the physical changes in the bowel; it provides accurate data about the structure of the colon, can be performed rapidly, and provides a permanent record for future disease comparison. The classic "string lesions" representing the typical strictures of Crohn's disease are readily visible on barium enema. They are caused by extensive bowel narrowing and are often found in the terminal ileum. These asymmetric segmental lesions help to distinguish Crohn's disease from ulcerative colitis. An upper GI series may be performed to evaluate small bowel involvement.

Transabdominal ultrasound is being successfully used to identify the presence of abscesses and fistulas. CT scanning provides even greater accuracy but is much more expensive. New imaging techniques using labeled leukocytes and erythrocytes are providing a noninvasive way of identifying sites of disease activity or bleeding.[39] Endoscopy procedures such as sigmoidoscopy or colonoscopy may be used to directly examine the nature and pattern of the inflammation and obtain biopsies if necessary. The presence of major perianal complications such as abscesses and fistulas is characteristic of Crohn's disease. The classic cobblestone, skip pattern of Crohn's disease is also readily apparent on endoscopy, with focal patches of ulcerative lesions. In ulcerative colitis there is often a small zone where the mucosa makes a distinct transition back to normal, and no evidence of disease is found above this point.

Medications. Medications are a cornerstone of the treatment of IBD and are used to relieve symptoms, induce remission, postpone the need for surgery, and improve the quality of life. Since the cause of IBD remains basically unknown, the components of drug therapy are empirically based on a combination of clinical trials and practical experience. Medications commonly used to treat IBD are summarized in Table 34-5.

TABLE 34-5 Common Medications for Treatment of Inflammatory Bowel Disease

Drug	Action	Intervention
Aminosalicylates (Oral)		
Sulfasalazine (Azulfidine)	Converted in colon to sulfapyridine and 5-aminosalicylic acid, which may exert an antiinflammatory effect, possibly through prostaglandin inhibition	Assess for allergy to sulfonamides or aspirin. Monitor for common side effects: anorexia, nausea and vomiting, headache. Teach patient to: Take in divided doses. Take with full glass of fluid or with food. Maintain a liberal fluid intake (2500-3000 ml daily). Report incidence of skin rash or other adverse effects.
Olsalazine (Dipentum)	As above without antibacterial action of sulfapyridine	Monitor for common side effects as above. Drug may also cause mild to moderate diarrhea. Teach patient to: Take in divided doses. Take with full glass of fluid or with food. Maintain a liberal fluid intake (2500-3000 ml daily).
Mesalamine (Asacol, Pentasa)	Same as olsalazine	Teach patient to: Take in divided doses. Maintain a liberal fluid intake (2500-3000 ml daily). Swallow tablets whole; do not chew or break outer coating.
Aminosalicylates (Rectal)		
Mesalamine in suspension for retention enema	As above	Administer enema while patient is positioned on left side, and teach patient to retain as long as possible.
Mesalamine suppository	As above	
Corticosteroids (Oral/IV)		
Prednisolone/ prednisone	Potent systemic antiinflammatory action	Teach patient to: Take with food or fluid. Monitor weight gain; assess for edema. Have blood pressure checked regularly. Be alert to signs of infection and report promptly. Be aware that mood swings occur commonly. Do not change dose or schedule or abruptly discontinue drug. Maintain good personal hygiene; keep perianal area clean and dry.

IV, Intravenous.

Continued

TABLE 34-5 Common Medications for Treatment of Inflammatory Bowel Disease—cont'd

Drug	Action	Intervention
Corticosteroids (Rectal)		
Hydrocortisone	As above	As for oral/IV corticosteroids
Intrarectal foam (Cortifoam)		
Retention enema (Cortenema)		
Budesonide enema	As above; rapid presystemic metabolism minimizes absorption	Administer enema while patient is positioned on left side, and teach patient to retain as long as possible. Other interventions as above; side effects should be less.
Immunosuppressive Agents		
6-Mercaptopurine (Purinethol)	Potent systemic suppression of immune response; may take 4-6 mo for full effect	Teach patient to: Report any signs of infection. Be alert to easy bruising. Return for laboratory work as scheduled. Maintain liberal daily fluid intake (2500-3000 ml daily). Take with food or after meals.
Azathioprine (Imuran)	As above	As above
Cyclosporine (Sandimmune)	As above; effects seen after several days "	Oral solution may be mixed in glass and given with milk or orange juice at room temperature; avoid refrigeration. Teach patient to: Monitor blood pressure. Report hematuria or any change in urinary function.
Monoclonal Antibodies		
Infliximab (Remicade)	Binds to TNF-α, blocking its activity and decreasing inflammation	Monitor for infusion-related problems: pruritus, hypotension, dyspnea, headache, fatigue. Teach patient to promptly report any signs of infection.
Antibiotics		
Metronidazole (Flagyl)	No apparent effect on ulcerative colitis but useful in colon-based Crohn's disease; action not clear	Teach patient to: Report side effects: diarrhea, peripheral neuropathies, strong metallic taste. Avoid alcohol use; alcohol use with drug can cause disulfiram (Antabuse) reaction.

TNF-α, tumor necrosis factor-alpha.

Aminosalicylates. Sulfasalazine (Azulfidine) was developed in the 1930s and first used for treating arthritis. Arthritis was believed to have an infectious origin, and sulfasalazine combined the proven effectiveness of aspirin with a sulfonamide antibiotic. Its use was quickly broadened to include IBD, and it has been a mainstay of treatment ever since. The exact mechanism of action of sulfasalazine is unknown, but its effectiveness is primarily attributed to its antiinflammatory effects. It successfully induces and sustains remission in most patients with mild to moderate ulcerative colitis and mild Crohn's disease affecting the colon. Sulfasalazine is split by bacteria in the colon into its two components. The first component, 5-acetylsalicylic acid (5-ASA) is poorly absorbed and thus maintains prolonged contact with the inflamed mucosa. Sulfapyridine, the second component, has no proven effectiveness against IBD and accounts for most of the troubling side effects.

Therefore efforts have focused on developing 5-ASA products that can be delivered intact to the colon without an additional carrier drug. Options include olsalazine (Dipentum), which is poorly absorbed in the small intestine and broken down in the colon by the action of the intestinal bacteria; and mesalamine (Pentasa, Asacol), which is coated with a pH-sensitive resin that dissolves only in a pH greater than 7 in the terminal ileum and proximal colon.[27] Sustained-release granules of this product are also available. The pH-sensitive coating allows these drugs to be delivered to the small intestine and increases their effectiveness with Crohn's disease.

These drugs are generally well tolerated if prescribed in increasing doses and taken buffered with food. Toxicity appears to be minimal. The most common side effects include nausea, vomiting, and diarrhea. No particular agent has been shown to be superior. Sulfasalazine retains the advantage of being significantly less costly than the other preparations for patients who respond to and can tolerate the drug.

Aminosalicylates can also be used topically for the 25% or more of patients with ulcerative colitis whose disease is confined to the rectal and sigmoid area. The drugs can be administered by enema, which provides for homogeneous delivery to the inflamed lower colon. Enemas provide high local concentrations of the drug, with minimal systemic absorption, and have been shown to be as effective as steroids in many situations. Suppository forms of the drugs also have been developed in an attempt to increase patient acceptability. Patients often find daily enemas to be unacceptable for long-term therapy.

Corticosteroids. Corticosteroids also have played an important role in IBD management for many years. The potent anti-inflammatory effects of steroids have proved to be effective in inducing remission in patients with moderate to severe Crohn's disease and severe ulcerative colitis. Oral steroids remain the quickest and most effective way to treat active disease.[27] Both local and systemic steroids are used, but their widespread and severe side effects limit their long-term use; and, although they are extremely effective in achieving remission, they cannot sustain it. Steroids can be administered rectally, but most forms absorb readily from the rectal mucosa and produce systemic effects. Prednisone remains the most commonly prescribed steroid, but budesonide (Entocort) offers the advantages of high topical potency, poor absorption, and rapid first-pass metabolism. It can now also be administered in a pH-sensitive coating for delivery to the distal ileum and cecum.[27]

Immunosuppresive Agents. Potent immunosuppressive agents such as azathioprine (Imuran) and mercaptopurine (Purinethol) may be used in selected patients with extensive disease who cannot be successfully weaned from steroids. These potent immunosuppressive drugs have a slow onset of action and may take up to 4 months to demonstrate effectiveness. They are not useful in acute situations but are effective in prolonging remission and are usually well tolerated.

Methotrexate has been shown to improve symptoms in patients with steroid-dependent Crohn's disease, but its side effect of bone marrow depression requires careful ongoing patient monitoring. Cyclosporine (Sandimmune) has not proved to be effective in the management of IBD, but trials with other immunosuppressants developed for use in managing transplants are underway.

Antibiotics. Antibiotics have also been extensively explored. They do not appear to be effective in the treatment of ulcerative colitis, but metronidazole (Flagyl) has been shown to be effective for mild Crohn's disease that is confined to the colon. Frequent adverse effects such as a strong metallic taste and peripheral neuropathy limit its effectiveness. Antibiotics are appropriate for severely ill patients at risk for infection and in situations in which bowel stricture causes stasis and bacterial overgrowth in the bowel.

Monoclonal Antibodies. Infliximab, a monoclonal antibody against tumor necrosis factor–alpha (TNF-α), represents the beginning of a new era in the drug treatment of IBD (see Future Watch box). TNF-α is an inflammatory agent found in high amounts in patients with Crohn's disease. By binding to TNF-α, the drug blocks its activity, leading to decreased inflammation and healing of complications such as fistulas.[16]

Other. Drug therapy for IBD may include the use of antidiarrheal medications when a high degree of disease activity is present. Codeine and loperamide are frequent choices. These drugs are administered for symptomatic relief, and an accurate record of their administration and effectiveness in controlling symptoms needs to be maintained. Fat-soluble vitamin supplements are often necessary.

Treatments. No specific treatments are indicated for IBD management. Patients with primarily rectal involvement may follow a regimen of daily enema administration. Other prescribed treatments may be related to the management of skin breakdown or excoriation that may accompany severe diarrhea.

Surgical Management. Surgery plays important but very different roles in the management of Crohn's disease and ulcerative colitis. Surgery is indicated for patients whose disease is refractory to medical therapy and for the management of complications. It plays a curative role in ulcerative colitis.

Crohn's Disease. Surgical intervention is avoided in Crohn's disease because recurrence of the disease process in the same region is virtually inevitable.[27] Nevertheless, more than 50% of patients will need surgery at least once during the course of their disease.[17] Improved surgical techniques, however, are making surgical intervention to improve patients' quality of life (rather than simply treating complications) a reasonable therapeutic option.[34] The major management challenge with Crohn's disease is the fact that it is stubbornly incurable even with aggressive medical or surgical intervention. Therefore surgical approaches to Crohn's disease focus on sparing and conserving as much of the bowel as possible, particularly when the small bowel is involved. The loss of more than 100 cm of bowel almost inevitably results in short bowel syndrome and persistent problems with malabsorption and diarrhea (see Chapter 33). Segmental resection with reanastomosis has been the primary surgical approach. Surgeons typically resect the bowel 5 to 10 cm above and below the macroscopically visible disease. Symptoms recur at a rate of approximately 10% per year,[38] but they do not always necessitate repeat surgery. The primary indications for surgery include bowel obstruction, fistula, abscess, perforation, and hemorrhage. Laparoscopic approaches show promise in significantly reducing the morbidity associated with these procedures.

Future Watch

Monoclonal Antibody Treatment for Crohn's Disease

Inflammatory bowel disease involves complex inflammatory mechanisms that are just beginning to be understood. With this new understanding, new drug approaches are being developed that can selectively target specific points in the inflammatory pathway. A variety of agents are being researched. Infliximab is a potent inhibitor of tumor necrosis factor–alpha and has already demonstrated effectiveness in inducing remission in patients who have become refractory to other therapies. The major drawback of this new therapy is cost, which averages $3000 to $4000 per infusion. With the success of infliximab, a variety of other approaches are being tried, including anti-CD4 and cellular adhesion molecule antibodies, interleukin 10 and 11, antisense oligonucletides, and nuclear transcription factors. Multiple drugs may be used in the not-distant future to induce and sustain remission.

Bowel strictures are a common complication of Crohn's disease that can cause acute bowel obstruction. The development of strictureplasty (Figure 34-6), which is analogous to pyloroplasty, enables surgeons to release the strictures without the need for major surgery, especially when a laparoscopic approach is used. The procedure can correct the obstruction without the loss of the involved bowel segments. Strictured segments tend to be fibrous in nature rather than acutely inflamed and rarely obstruct again. It is theorized that the obstruction, rather than the stricture, triggers the acute inflammation and that the bowel is able to resolve the inflammation once the obstruction is relieved.[55] The procedure has now been adapted to allow for the release of "long" strictures (as much as 25 cm), making bowel conservation a reasonable goal for difficult cases.[48] The nursing management of patients undergoing bowel resection is presented on p. 1108.

Ulcerative Colitis. Surgical intervention may be selected for patients with ulcerative colitis whose disease cannot be satisfactorily controlled with standard medical management. The procedures are curative in nature and involve the removal of the entire colon. Surgery is also undertaken when acute complications such as hemorrhage or toxic megacolon develop or when the presence of cellular dysplasia indicates an unacceptably high risk of bowel cancer.[30] Most patients are able to achieve a high quality of life after surgery, and the successful development of continent procedures has made the lifestyle challenges much less daunting (see Research box).

Ileostomy. The Brook ileostomy procedure is the oldest colectomy procedure and remains the standard against which other procedures are measured.[17] The Brook procedure involves the removal of the colon, rectum, and anus, with permanent closure of the anus. The ileostomy is created by bringing the end of the terminal ileum out through the abdominal wall to form a stoma (Figure 34-7). Any colectomy

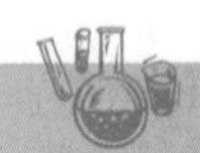

Research

Reference: Farouk R et al: Functional outcomes after ileal pouch–anal anastomosis for chronic ulcerative colitis, *Ann Surg* 231(6):1-11, 2000.

This study assessed long-term functional outcomes in 1450 patients who underwent ileal pouch construction for chronic ulcerative colitis between 1981 and 1994, with particular attention to the impact of aging, childbirth, and pouch failure. Functional outcomes were comparable between men and women. Stool frequency and continence were similar in both men and women. Aging was found to be related to more frequent pouch evacuation and a slightly increased risk of incontinence. Patients who were younger than 45 years of age at the time of surgery experienced increased fecal spotting as they aged, but incontinence remained uncommon.

Earlier studies had found a significantly increased risk of pouch problems following pregnancy and vaginal delivery, including anal sphincter injury, pelvic floor denervation, and incontinence. This study did not uncover any patterns of functional compromise with childbirth. Pelvic pain and soiling during intercourse were significant concerns for a small number of participants. Pelvic sepsis was the major cause of pouch failure in this population, but the incidence was extremely low.

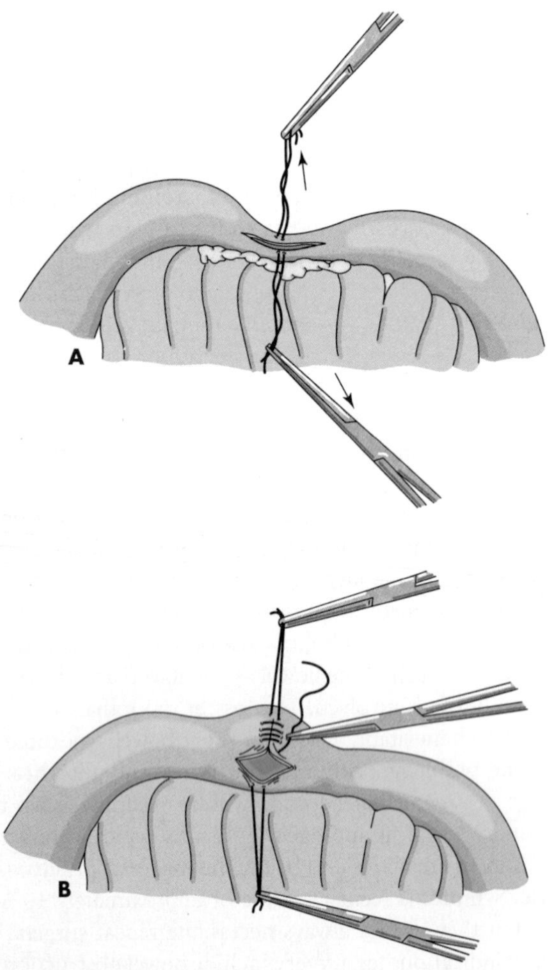

Figure 34-6 Strictureplasty. **A,** A linear incision is made at and beyond the stricture site. The site is spread open. **B,** The widened site is sutured closed.

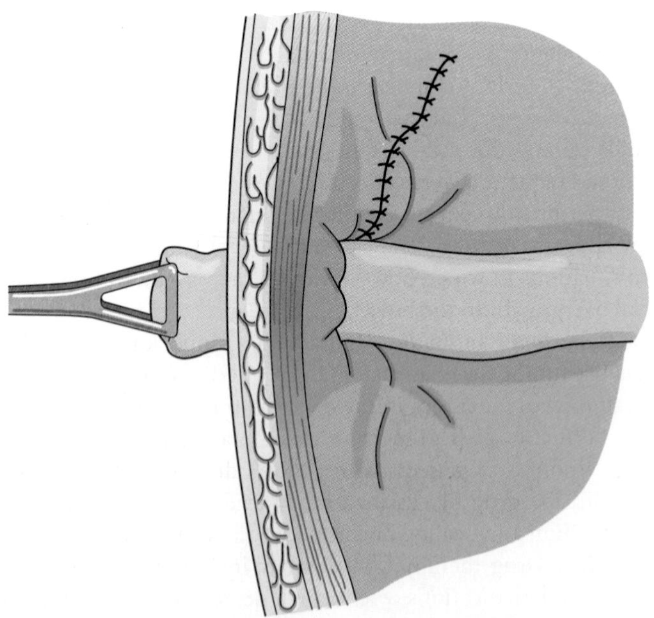

Figure 34-7 Construction of an ileostomy.

procedure decreases the bowel's ability to reabsorb fluid and electrolytes, and the ileostomy drainage is profuse and watery; but the terminal ileum dilates over time and assumes some of the functions of the cecum. The volume of stool decreases, but about 300 to 800 ml of fluid is still lost in the stool each day along with substantial amounts of electrolytes, particularly sodium. The person experiences chronic fluid deficit as the small intestine is unable to fine-tune fluid balance, and any increase in fluid intake simply increases the volume of the ileostomy drainage.

The surgery cures the ulcerative colitis and eliminates the risk of colon cancer. However, the permanent ileostomy creates both physical and emotional challenges for the patient. Malfunctioning of the ostomy is relatively common, since poorly digested foods can easily obstruct the narrow lumen. Fears of leakage, embarrassment from noise and odor, and negative effects on self-concept, body image, and sexuality are common problems. Impotence can also occur after the surgery unless the surgeon is able to successfully dissect around the autonomic nerves in the pelvis.

Continent Ileostomy. In the late 1960s Dr. Nils Kock developed a surgical procedure to spare patients some of the challenges of traditional ileostomy. The procedure (the Kock pouch) involves the creation of an abdominal reservoir from a piece of terminal ileum to store the feces. The end of the ileum is intussuscepted to form a nipple valve that lies flush with the abdomen (Figure 34-8). A catheter is used to drain the pouch, and a small dressing or adhesive bandage is worn over the stoma between emptyings. The pouch eventually can expand to hold about 500 ml of drainage. Problems with the nipple valve are common and often require surgical repair. Valve failure plus the incidence of chronic inflammation in the pouch limits the usefulness of the procedure, and it is rarely recommended any longer as a primary intervention.

Ileoanal Anastomosis (Ileorectostomy). The ileoanal anastomosis was the first colectomy procedure developed that does not require any type of ileostomy. A 12- to 15-cm rectal stump is left after the colon is removed. The small intestine is inserted inside this rectal sleeve and anastomosed (Figure 34-9). The procedure is technically easier than the anal reservoir surgeries (see following section) but requires a large, compliant rectum, which makes it inappropriate for some older adults. Complications related to the rectal stump are the primary drawback to the procedure. Ulcerative colitis can recur in the rectal stump, which is also at significant risk for rectal cancer. Five percent to 50% of patients with ulcerative colitis who undergo ileoanal anastomosis will need surgery at some point in the future to remove the rectal segment. If the rectum remains disease free, however, its ability to reabsorb water and electrolytes results in a decreased volume of stool and an increased quality of life. The procedure can also be used successfully for patients with Crohn's disease who have pancolitis.

A new approach is attempting to decrease the complications of the anastomosis procedure while maintaining its benefits. The ileoneorectal anastamosis focuses on meticulous stripping

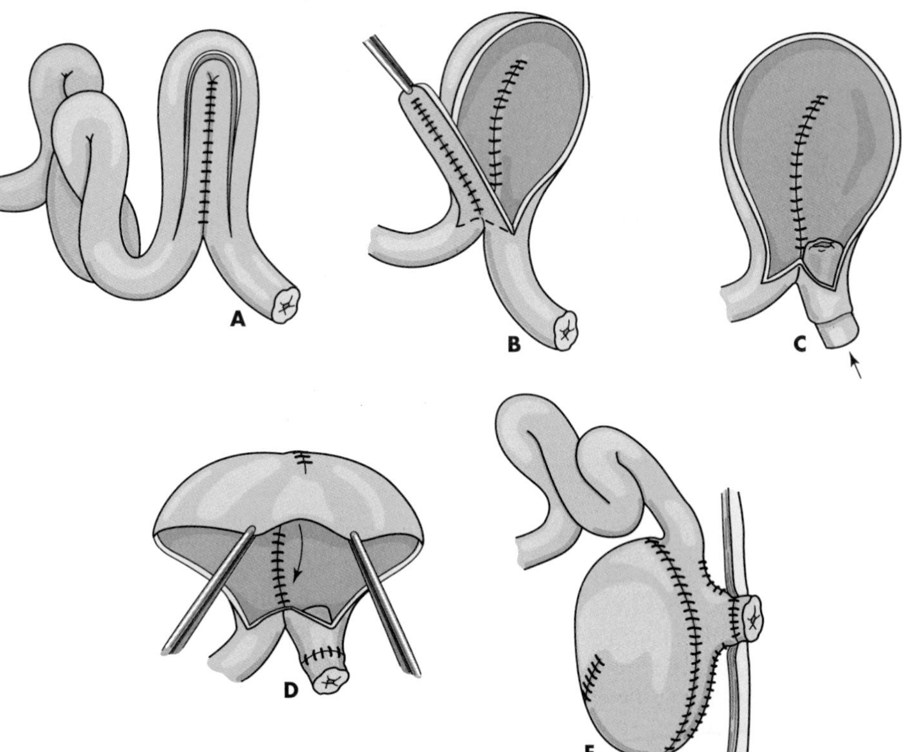

Figure 34-8 Continent ileostomy (Kock pouch). **A,** Loop of bowel sewn together. **B,** Removal of anterior portion. **C,** Nipple valve made by pushing bowel back on itself. **D,** Pouch formation. **E,** End brought through stoma.

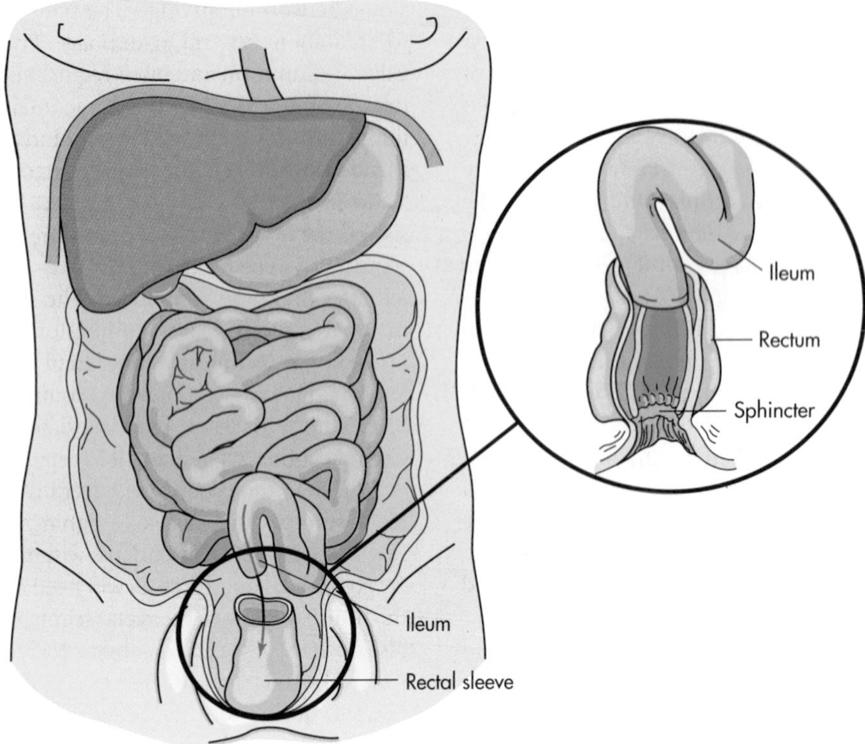

Figure 34-9 Ileoanal anastomosis.

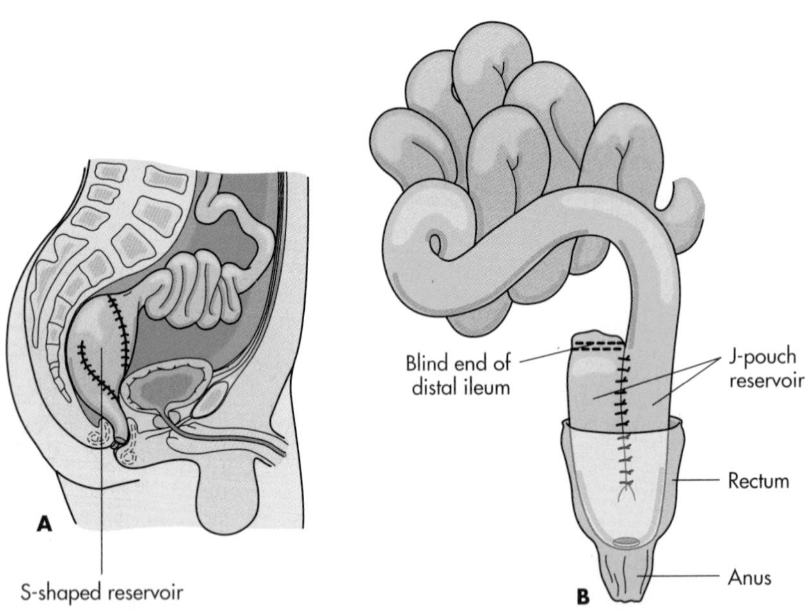

Figure 34-10 Ileoanal reservoir. **A**, S-shaped reservoir. **B**, J-shaped reservoir.

of the mucosa, the target of ulcerative colitis, from the rectum. Mucosal transplantation is then performed from the disease-free ileum, and direct anastamosis can take place without the need for the sleeve. Original rectal function is preserved.[10]

Ileoanal Reservoir. The current procedure of choice for colectomy involves the creation of a pouch from the terminal ileum that is sutured directly to the anus.[30] The anal sphincter is left intact, which preserves continence, plus approximately 1 inch of rectum that is stripped of its mucosa to remove the last vestige of ulcerative colitis. A temporary loop ileostomy is usually created until healing of all anastamoses is complete, making this a two-stage procedure. The loop ileostomy can be closed within 3 to 4 months. Single-stage procedures without a diverting ileostomy are being researched with promising early results.[33] Several different approaches to reservoir construction have been developed. A J-shaped anastomosis is commonly chosen because of its ease of construction. It is shown in Figure 34-10. W- and S-shaped pouches also are

Research

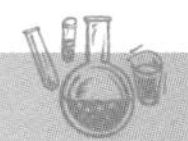

Reference: Meagher AP et al: J ileal pouch–anal anastomosis for chronic ulcerative colitis: complications and long-term outcomes in 1310 patients, *Br J Surg* 85:800-803, 1998.

This study explored the long-term outcomes of J–ileal pouch construction for more than 1000 patients who underwent surgery for ulcerative colitis between 1981 and 1994. The procedure has been performed for 25 years and is well accepted, but it is technically difficult and can be associated with serious complications. The study focused on the effect of increasing surgical experience and expertise with the procedure and its relationship to long-term outcomes.

Ninety-one percent of patients who were followed for 10 years had a functioning pouch. The mean stool frequency was 6 per 24 hours, and about 90% reported either no incontinence or rare fecal spotting. Bowel function was relatively stable in most patients. The number of patients who developed pouchitis increased with time, and it was especially prevalent in patients who developed their first episode within the first 2 years of pouch construction. Small bowel obstruction was a problem in 12% to 24% of patients. These complications did not demonstrate a statistically different incidence with increasing surgical experience, but the number of cases of pelvic sepsis did decrease significantly with increasing surgical experience.

used, but the S-shaped pouch is large, and the distal limb may not empty effectively.

Functional results continue to improve for up to 12 months after surgery, and most patients have three to eight bowel movements per day. Slight fecal incontinence is a problem—sometimes a persistent one and especially at night—but the normal manner of defecation makes this a popular procedure.[2] It usually is not used in persons older than 55 years of age, who may experience anal sphincter deterioration related to aging.

The procedure is not without complications, and "pouchitis," acute inflammation within the reservoir, is a common chronic problem.[30] Pouchitis creates discomfort, bleeding, and increased output that is similar in many ways to the original disease process. It is attributed by some researchers to faulty diagnosis of the colitis and the possibility that Crohn's disease is the primary pathologic process. Others attribute this inflammatory reaction to a general propensity of these patients for inflammatory disease. The Research box presents findings concerning long-term outcomes for a large group of patients undergoing J–ileal pouch construction.[37]

Nursing management of the patient undergoing ostomy surgery is presented on p. 1087.

Diet. Diet does not cause IBD and cannot influence the course of the disease, but diet is an important consideration in patient comfort. Nutritional concerns become extremely important during exacerbations of the disease when diarrhea may be severe, and the presence of anorexia and nausea makes it difficult for the patient to meet nutritional needs through an oral diet.

Dietary recommendations are tailored to the needs of the individual patient, but as a general rule patients with diarrhea or abdominal pain are encouraged to restrict their intake of raw fruits and vegetables, as well as fatty and spicy foods. Constipation may be a problem in distal colon or rectal disease and usually can be controlled with the use of bulk hydrophilic laxatives such as psyllium (Metamucil). The general guideline for IBD is that when patients feel well, they can eat almost anything, but when they feel sick, they should limit what they eat.[21] Bowel rest plays a role in Crohn's disease management, and elemental diets or supplements may be used. These preparations are completely digested and absorbed in the duodenum and ileum and place no demands on the large bowel. Recent attention has been focused on the possible suppressive effect of fish oil on the inflammatory process. Lactose intolerance is often a problem in persons with IBD, and patients are encouraged to evaluate whether restricting dairy products has a positive effect on their symptoms.

Acute exacerbations of IBD make it difficult to maintain adequate nutrition. Short-term parenteral nutrition may occasionally be necessary to ensure minimal amounts of essential nutrients. Nutritional support is particularly important when the patient requires surgery.

Activity. Activity levels may be restricted during acute exacerbations of IBD in response to fever, fatigue, and malaise. Reduced activity also may be useful in slowing peristalsis and decreasing the frequency of diarrhea episodes. When remission is established, patients are encouraged to resume all aspects of their normal lifestyles, and no activity restrictions apply.

Referrals. In some settings the nurse assumes responsibility for making referrals to other services. Common referrals for persons with IBD include nutritional support and counseling.

Nutritional Support. The assessment of nutritional status and determination of the most appropriate approach to improving or maintaining nutrition may involve a skilled nutritionist. Dietary modifications, supplement selection, and management of enteral or parenteral nutrition may be coordinated through this service.

Counseling. Although it has been clearly established that neither stress nor personality plays a role in the etiology of IBD, coping with the effects of IBD can put a tremendous strain on a person's adaptive abilities. Disease exacerbations may leave the patient particularly vulnerable to depression and even despair. The disease typically affects young adults who are just beginning their education, careers, or families. The stress of this unpredictable and potentially incapacitating disease cannot be ignored. Support services in this area can be extremely important. Patients and families should be routinely referred to the services of the National Foundation for Ileitis and Colitis.*

*National Foundation for Ileitis and Colitis, 386 Park Avenue South, New York, NY 10016-7374; (800) 932-2423.

NURSING MANAGEMENT OF PATIENT WITH INFLAMMATORY BOWEL DISEASE

ASSESSMENT

Health History

Data to be collected to assess the patient with IBD include:

- Patient's knowledge base and understanding of the disorder
- Pain: location, nature, severity, frequency; relationship to eating; measures used to self-treat
- Bowel elimination pattern: constipation or diarrhea; frequency and character of stools
- Nutritional status: usual meal pattern and intake; recent weight changes, food intolerances and allergies, appetite, fatigue or weakness, nausea
- Social relationships: support network; impact of illness on family, employment, lifestyle, and sexuality
- Perceived life stress and usual coping patterns
- Medications in current use: prescribed and over the counter; dosage and side effects; perceived effectiveness in managing disease and symptoms

Physical Examination

Data to be collected during the physical examination include:

- Body weight
- Skin turgor and condition of mucous membranes
- Presence of fever
- Bowel sounds: presence and character
- Condition of perianal skin
- Composition of stools: presence of blood, fat, mucus, and/or pus

NURSING DIAGNOSES

Nursing diagnoses are determined from analysis of patient data. Nursing diagnoses for the patient with IBD may include but are not limited to:

Diagnostic Title	Possible Etiologic Factors
1. Chronic pain	Inflammatory process in intestine
2. Diarrhea	Chronic inflammation in intestine
3. Imbalanced nutrition: less than body requirements	Anorexia and nausea, abdominal cramping with meals, malabsorption of food
4. Ineffective coping	Persistent symptoms and lack of curative treatment
5. Ineffective health maintenance	Lack of knowledge of condition, treatment, or recognition of complications

EXPECTED PATIENT OUTCOMES

Expected patient outcomes for the patient with IBD may include but are not limited to:

1a. Will relate an improvement in frequency and severity of abdominal discomfort
1b. Will use dietary and nonpharmacologic pain relief measures to manage pain
2a. Will have fewer episodes of diarrhea
2b. Will identify dietary and activity factors that improve or worsen diarrhea
2c. Will list the major signs and symptoms of dehydration and electrolyte imbalance
3a. Will follow a balanced, high-nutrient diet, avoiding foods that increase symptoms
3b. Will maintain desired weight or regain weight to desired goal at a rate of ½ to 1 pound/week
3c. Will achieve a positive nitrogen balance as evidenced by a serum albumin level greater than 4 g/dl
4a. Will identify factors that increase disease-related anxiety and stress
4b. Will verbalize coping strategies and support mechanisms to handle problems
5a. Will describe the nature of the illness, prescribed therapy schedule, and side effects of all medications
5b. Will list symptoms requiring medical attention
5c. Will identify plans for ongoing medical follow-up

INTERVENTIONS

1. Promoting Comfort

The nurse encourages the patient to document the character and severity of the pain and to record its relationship to eating, drinking, and passing stool or flatus. Anticholinergic or antispasmodic medications such as propantheline bromide (Pro-Banthine) may be prescribed to reduce the cramping, but opioids are rarely used because of their negative effect on peristalsis. A warm heating pad applied to the abdomen often is comforting but should not be used during acute exacerbations. The nurse assists the patient with position changes and encourages the use of diversional activities and relaxation strategies. The nurse documents the patient's pain pattern and response to all interventions.

2. Controlling Diarrhea

Chronic diarrhea often becomes a focus of care during exacerbations of the disease process. Patients may feel trapped by the frequency and urgency of their need to defecate. The nurse encourages the person to keep accurate records of the frequency, severity, and character of each diarrheal episode, particularly if blood or pus is present.

The medication regimen is designed to control the inflammation and eventually the diarrhea, but this process may take days or weeks. Antidiarrheal agents such as loperamide may be used to slow peristalsis, and mucilloids such as Metamucil may add bulk to the stool and help reduce the frequency of defecation. The patient is encouraged to limit activity when diarrhea is severe and to lie down for 20 minutes after meals to limit peristalsis. Patients are encouraged to use the toilet or commode whenever possible, but a weak, acutely ill person may need to have a bedpan readily accessible. Room deodorizers may be necessary for odor control.

The anal region often becomes excoriated from the frequent stools. Painful anal fissures and fistulas may develop, and the anal area needs to be kept clean and dry. Medicated wipes (such as Tucks) and sitz baths three times a day can provide both comfort and cleanliness. Ointments such as Desitin or zinc oxide can create a barrier to protect the perianal skin.

Profuse diarrhea can lead to severe losses of fluids and electrolytes. If the patient is consuming an oral diet, the nurse encourages a liberal fluid intake (at least 2500 to 3000 ml daily) and explores the patient's tolerance to solutions such as Gatorade, which can help replace lost electrolytes. It is important for the patient to understand that any increase in fluid intake will also increase output, since the bowel is limited in its ability to reabsorb fluids. The nurse records accurate intake and output, assesses the skin and mucous membranes for signs of dehydration, and monitors the patient's weight daily.

3. Promoting Nutrition

During acute exacerbations of IBD, the patient may be malnourished from anorexia, inflammation of the bowel, and malabsorption. The method of feeding depends on the type and extent of the disorder. With severe or extensive disease, especially when complications are present, the patient may be kept NPO, and parenteral nutrition may be instituted. Bowel rest can be very helpful in Crohn's disease but has no proven therapeutic benefit in ulcerative colitis.

Elemental feedings, similar to those given in tube feedings, are started as soon as possible. These feedings are absorbed rapidly in the upper GI tract, causing minimal demand on the colon. Palatability is a problem with elemental diets, and serving the fluids chilled and offering a variety of flavors may increase patient acceptance. A low-residue, high-protein, high-calorie diet is then gradually reintroduced.

During periods of remission, patients are advised to eat a well-balanced, high-calorie diet with a liberal fluid and salt intake to compensate for daily losses. Only those foods that are known to cause problems are restricted. The person with ulcerative colitis may need to avoid intestinal stimulants such as alcohol, caffeinated beverages, high-fat foods, and very high fiber foods such as raw fruits and vegetables (cooked fruits and vegetables are usually better tolerated). Milk products are often poorly tolerated, since lactose intolerance is common in persons with IBD, and the nurse encourages the patient to evaluate the effect of milk product restriction on the severity of symptoms. Multivitamin and mineral supplements are used regularly.

4. Promoting Effective Coping

IBD is characterized by periods of exacerbation and remission throughout the patient's adult life. It can significantly disrupt the patient's preferred lifestyle. Although emotions and stress do not play a role in disease etiology, they are believed to influence the severity and frequency of disease exacerbations. Frustration, depression, and a sense of powerlessness are common responses to the disease and may precipitate hostile or dependent behaviors. Patients often become preoccupied with their physical symptoms.

The nurse encourages the patient to become an active participant in all decisions related to disease management and to verbalize concerns and feelings related to the disease and treatment. The nurse provides the patient with information about local support groups and encourages involvement with the National Foundation for Ileitis and Colitis.

Fatigue is a common problem with IBD and can worsen the patient's psychologic response to the disease. Fatigue results from the combination of increased energy demands secondary to the inflammatory process and the decreased energy supply from inadequate nutrition, anemia, and depression. Planned rest periods should be included in daily activities. When the acute episode begins to subside, progressive activity is encouraged. During periods of remission, the person is encouraged to participate in social activities but should not overexert to the point of fatigue. Sexual response also may be affected by IBD. Malnutrition and frequent diarrhea often lead to decreased libido, and the presence of an ileostomy may be associated with a sense of diminished sexual attractiveness. The nurse encourages the patient to express sex-related concerns and explore them openly with the spouse or partner. IBD support groups can be excellent resources for strategies to manage concerns over odor and leakage during sexual activity, particularly after a colectomy.

5. Promoting Effective Self-Care

Accurate knowledge about the disease process and therapeutic modalities can be extremely influential in helping the patient achieve a sense of control. The nurse explores the patient's existing knowledge base about the cause, course, and prognosis of the disease; treatment options; and the identification and management of complications. Patient education materials are available from the National Foundation for Ileitis and Colitis and the National Institutes of Health (NIH). The nurse ensures that the patient understands the importance of careful adherence to the medication regimen and has a plan for scheduled medical follow-up. Guidelines for teaching the patient with IBD are summarized in the Patient Teaching box.

EVALUATION

To evaluate the effectiveness of nursing interventions, compare patient behaviors with those stated in the expected patient outcomes. Achievement of patient outcomes is successful if the patient:

- **1a.** States that abdominal pain is absent or less frequent and severe.
- **1b.** Successfully uses nonpharmacologic pain relief strategies to manage abdominal pain.
- **2a.** Reports fewer or no episodes of diarrhea.
- **2b.** Successfully modifies the diet to reduce diarrhea.
- **2c.** Correctly identifies major warning signs of fluid and electrolyte imbalance (see Chapter 13).
- **3a.** Adheres to a high-calorie, well-balanced diet.
- **3b.** Maintains optimal body weight.
- **3c.** Achieves serum albumin levels within the normal range.
- **4a.** Identifies personal lifestyle factors that increase stress.
- **4b.** Uses community support mechanisms to enhance coping strategies.

5a. Accurately describes the nature of the illness and prescribed therapy, schedule, and side effects of medications.
5b. Correctly lists symptoms needing medical attention.
5c. Schedules appointments for follow-up care.

GERONTOLOGIC CONSIDERATIONS

Although both forms of IBD typically begin in young adulthood, the onset can occur after age 60 years. The presentation, clinical course, and response to treatment generally are similar in both age-groups. The disease often takes the form of proctitis in older adults, and local treatment is usually effective. Complications are more likely to be related to comorbidity problems than to the primary IBD, but toxic megacolon occurs often. Once the disease process is controlled, an older adult with ulcerative colitis is less likely to have a relapse, and the risk of disease-related cancer is minimal. Crohn's disease in older adults tends to be localized in the distal colon and rectum, and generalized involvement is unusual. Because both forms of IBD tend to concentrate in the distal colon and rectum, the differential diagnosis may be unclear in older patients. This is particularly true if the disease does not have an acute onset.

Surgical intervention is avoided, if possible, because older patients tend to experience an increased incidence of complications, although recurrence of Crohn's disease after surgery is not common in older adults. Sphincter-sparing colectomy procedures are used less commonly in this population because it is more difficult to achieve successful wound healing and adequate continence, particularly at night.

Patient Teaching
The Patient With Inflammatory Bowel Disease

DIET AND FLUIDS

Eat a high-calorie, well-balanced diet.
Avoid any foods that increase symptoms (e.g., fresh fruits and raw or uncooked vegetables, fatty foods, spicy foods, and alcohol).
Assess the effect of dairy products on disease symptoms, and limit use if appropriate.
Take a multivitamin/mineral supplement daily.
Ensure a liberal fluid intake–2500 to 3000 ml daily:
- Drink Gatorade or other commercial products, if tolerated, during flare-ups to replace lost electrolytes.

Use salt liberally during disease flare-ups.

ELIMINATION

Take medication as prescribed.
Keep the rectal area clean and dry; use analgesic rectal ointment or sitz baths for rectal discomfort.
Consult with physician about the appropriateness of antidiarrheal agents or bulk-forming laxatives when diarrhea is present.
Monitor weight daily during disease flare-ups.

REST AND COPING

Maintain a regular sleep schedule.
Schedule daily activities to avoid fatigue; take rest periods as necessary.
Use relaxation strategies when stress levels rise.
Discuss concerns with family or support person.
Attend a local support group for inflammatory bowel disease if available.

HEALTH MAINTENANCE

Report signs requiring medical attention:
- Change in pattern or severity of abdominal pain or diarrhea
- Development of constipation
- Change in stool character
- Unusual discharge from rectum
- Fever

Plan for regular follow-up care.

SPECIAL ENVIRONMENTS FOR CARE

Critical Care

Critical care is not an expected part of the treatment of IBD. Most disease flare-ups can be successfully managed in the community setting. The development of complications may require hospitalization for replacement of fluids and electrolytes, provision of nutritional support through parenteral nutrition, initiation of high-dose steroid or immunosuppressive therapy, and surgery. It is conceivable that critical care intervention would be needed in the management of such crises as perforation or toxic megacolon, especially in older patients, but this intervention would not be a standard part of disease management.

Community-Based Care

The patient with IBD has a chronic, lifelong condition that is primarily managed in the home with family support. Two particular situations may necessitate the involvement of home care support. Patients may need short- or long-term home administration of parenteral nutrition. IBD is one of the most common reasons for long-term parenteral nutrition administration. This therapy necessitates supervision by home health nurses. In addition, patients who undergo ileostomy procedures are referred to community enterostomal therapy services for ongoing teaching and follow-up. The patient needs to know where ostomy supplies can be purchased in the local community and is encouraged to contact a local ostomy support group for peer assistance.

COMPLICATIONS

The primary complications of IBD are hemorrhage, obstruction, perforation, toxic megacolon, and cellular dysplasia that can lead to cancer. The management of the first three is similar to that discussed under Collaborative Care Management. Toxic megacolon involves an extreme dilation of a segment of the diseased colon (often the transverse colon) that results in complete obstruction. The patient is at risk for toxic megacolon during acute exacerbations. The problem may develop after bowel preparation for a barium enema or other diagnostic test, or from the negative effects of opioids and anticholinergic drugs on peristalsis. Bacteria rapidly invade the inflamed tissue, creating the acute state. The condition may respond to conservative management or require surgical correction.

The development of cellular dysplasia and eventually carcinoma from the chronic irritation of ulcerative colitis has been a concern for many years. Patients who have had the disease for 7 to 10 or more years need routine surveillance inasmuch as dysplasia develops often. The risk of cancer increases exponentially after 10 years and is estimated to be 30 times that of the average 40- to 60-year-old person.[22] The risk of cancer is also greater with widespread disease than with localized disease. Colectomy eliminates the risk and may be recommended even when medical management is satisfactorily controlling the disease. Generally, patients who developed ulcerative colitis at a young age and who experience ongoing inflammation are at greatest risk. Dysplasia is estimated to be present in 50% to 80% of patients before the development of the cancer. Sigmoidoscopy and colonoscopy are the primary tools for detecting dysplasia. Colonoscopy allows for improved visualization and greater accuracy of diagnosis. In general, it is recommended that colectomy be performed if mass lesions or high-grade dysplasia is found; conservative management consists of repeat colonoscopy at least every 3 months.

It was formerly believed that patients with Crohn's disease did not have an increased risk of cancer. This premise is no longer accepted, and research indicates a cancer incidence six times that of normal populations. The risk increases with the duration of the IBD disease process, and dysplasia usually appears at sites of severe disease involvement or at sites of stricture formation. Standards for the early detection of cancer in patients with Crohn's disease are still under study, and recommendations for routine cancer surveillance in this population do not currently exist.

NURSING MANAGEMENT OF PATIENT UNDERGOING FECAL OSTOMY SURGERY

The word *ostomy* refers to a surgical procedure in which an opening is created to drain either urine or feces. A fecal ostomy may be created as a temporary or permanent approach to the management of a wide variety of bowel problems. Ostomies can be created from the ileum or at various sites within the large bowel (Figure 34-11; see also Figure 34-7). Loop colostomies are generally temporary and allow for easy closure at a future point. Although each type of ostomy presents its own unique management problems, all ostomies challenge patients to maintain skin integrity and achieve effective self-care.

PREOPERATIVE CARE

Preoperative care focuses on patient teaching. The nurse assesses the patient's knowledge and understanding of the proposed surgery and its outcomes. This includes a brief overview of GI tract structure and function and the nature and functioning of an ostomy. Written materials also are provided that reinforce the teaching and outline the postoperative plan of care. Comprehensive ostomy care involves a team approach

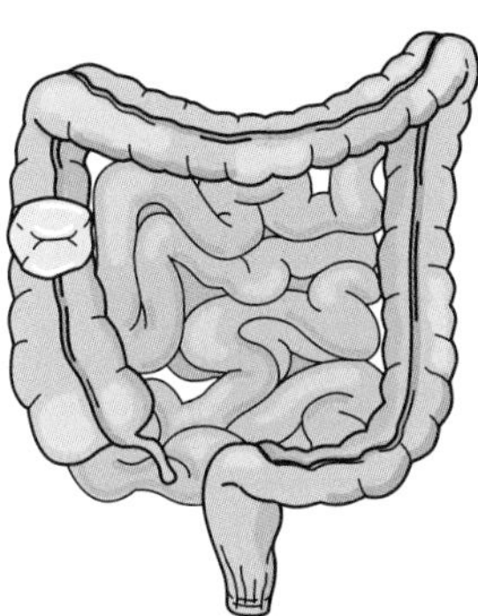

The **ascending colostomy** is done for right-sided tumors.

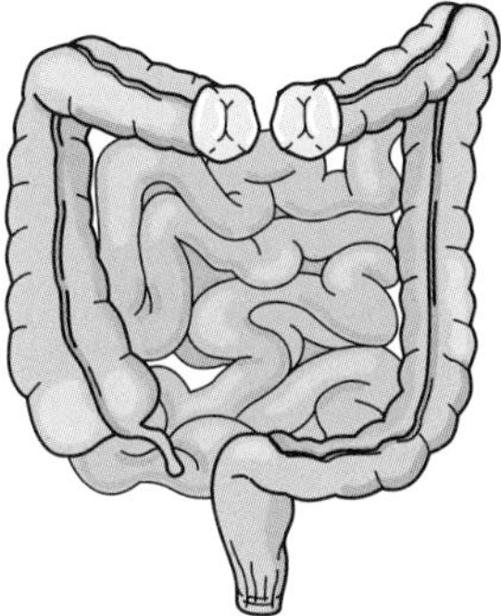

The **transverse (double-barreled) colostomy** is often used in such emergencies as intestinal obstruction or perforation because it can be created quickly. There are two stomas. The proximal one, closest to the small intestine, drains feces. The distal stoma drains mucus. Usually temporary.

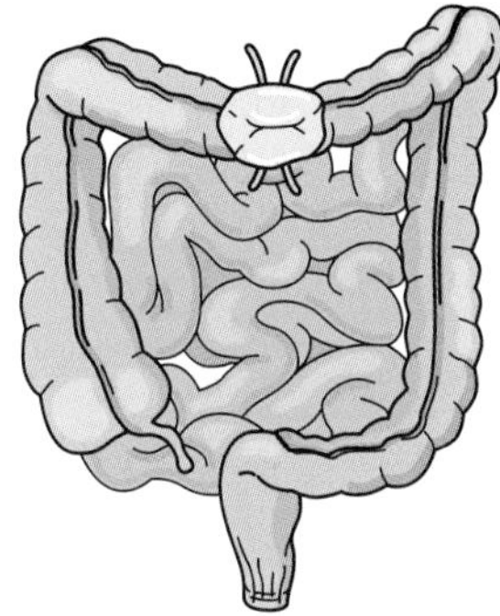

The **transverse loop colostomy** has two openings in the transverse colon, but one stoma. Usually temporary.

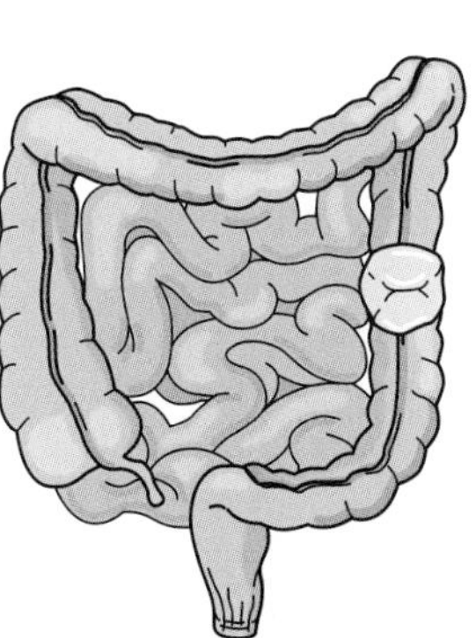

Descending colostomy

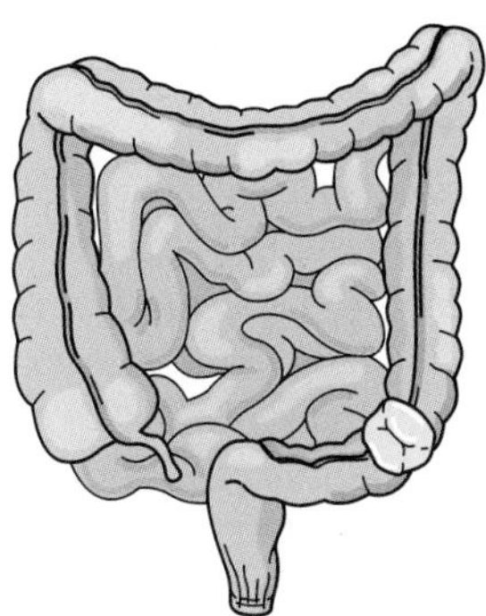

Sigmoid colostomy

Figure 34-11 Types of colostomies.

and ideally includes an enterostomal therapy nurse, dietitian, and discharge planner in addition to the surgeon and staff nurses. Early involvement of the enterostomal therapy nurse provides structure for the teaching plan and ensures that an ostomy specialist is involved in selecting the site for the stoma. Many common stoma complications can be avoided by appropriate site selection with consideration for the shape and contour of the skinfolds of the patient's abdomen in both a sitting and an upright position.[50] The site should be visible and accessible to the patient when sitting or standing, lie within the rectus muscle, and avoid scars, bony prominences, skinfolds, and the patient's belt line. The site selected for the stoma plays a significant role in the patient's ability to maintain a good pouch seal and manage the ostomy independently after surgery.

Emotional preparation for ostomy surgery is extremely important. The nurse encourages the patient to verbalize feelings related to this radical change in body image and function. Validating the appropriateness of these concerns lays the foundation for an effective working relationship with the patient. The patient will need to work through the grieving process, and specific factual teaching may be ineffective if the patient is in the shock and disbelief stage. The nurse offers acceptance of all feelings and reinforces the importance of open communication.

The preoperative preparation phase may include nutritional support, possibly with parenteral nutrition, if the patient's nutritional state is inadequate for surgery. The patient should know what to expect in the postoperative period. The nurse discusses the management of postoperative pain, the nature and appearance of all incisions and drains, and the purpose of the NG tube and IV lines. Thorough bowel cleansing is performed and may include the use of enemas, laxatives, and antibiotics to reduce intestinal bacterial flora.

POSTOPERATIVE CARE

The nurse provides general postoperative care. Nasogastric suction is usually maintained for a few days after surgery, and the patient is kept NPO to prevent distention and pressure on the suture lines. Careful attention paid to pain management ensures patient comfort and supports the patient's ability to follow the deep breathing and early ambulation protocols.

Maintaining Fluid and Electrolyte Balance

Attention to fluid and electrolyte balance is crucial for all ostomy patients but particularly for the person with an ileostomy. After surgery the fecal drainage from the ileostomy is liquid and may be constant. Fecal outputs range from 1000 to 1500 ml every 24 hours. This amount begins to decrease slightly within 10 to 15 days as the terminal ileum absorbs more water and the stool thickens. The losses are still significant, however, and careful intake and output records are essential. The ileostomy patient becomes dehydrated easily. The stool may not thicken if the patient has had previous small bowel resections for Crohn's disease. The more intestine that has been resected, the greater the chance for a high-volume output of liquid stool. Loperamide (Imodium) or diphenoxylate hydrochloride–atropine (Lomotil) may be used to control the output and the fluid loss in severe cases.[2]

The pouch may initially need to be emptied every 1 to 2 hours. Volumes in excess of 1500 ml in 24 hours are considered excessive. Fluid and electrolyte problems are usually not a major concern after colostomy surgery, although it may take time to reestablish a normal pattern of elimination.

Stoma Monitoring

The patient who has undergone ostomy surgery typically returns from surgery with an ostomy pouch system in place. The nurse observes the stoma regularly for color and edema. Color reflects perfusion, and the stoma should be bright red and moist. A dark, dusky, or brown-black stoma indicates ischemia and necrosis and should be reported immediately to the surgeon. A small amount of bleeding from the stoma is expected because it has a rich blood supply, but any significant bleeding should be reported to the surgeon immediately. Initial stoma edema is an expected response to surgical manipulation. Edema typically resolves in 5 to 7 days, but the stoma continues to decrease in size slowly over 6 to 8 weeks.[9] The shape of the stoma also changes slightly throughout the day in response to peristalsis, and the pouch opening must be able to accommodate the changing stoma size.

The abdominal incision and the sutures anchoring the stoma are inspected for intactness. Some of the stoma mucosa may pull away from the abdominal skin before healing is complete. Superficial separations heal by granulation, but deeper separations may require packing or resuturing. The stoma drainage consists initially of mucus and serosanguineous secretion. As peristalsis returns, flatus and fecal drainage begin, usually in 2 to 4 days.

A loop colostomy may be opened during surgery or in the patient's room 48 to 72 hours later. A cautery is used to create two openings, one proximal and one distal, in the one stoma (see Figure 34-11). The nurse reassures the patient that the procedure causes no pain because the bowel has no sensory nerve endings for pain sensation. The procedure creates a distinct burning smell, however, and can be quite frightening. The nurse offers support and reassurance during the loop opening. The supporting rod for the loop is removed after 7 to 10 days, when adhesions prevent the stoma from retracting into the surrounding skin.

Managing a Perineal Wound

The abdominal perineal resection (formation of a permanent colostomy with removal of the rectum and anus using both an abdominal and a perineal incision) has been the gold standard for the treatment of rectal cancer for many years and is still the treatment of choice for managing highly invasive disease. Postoperative care is more complex because of the presence of a major perineal wound that may require up to 6 months to heal completely. The patient's convalescence is prolonged.

The perineal wound is created by the removal of the entire rectum and anus plus muscle and fatty tissue. The wound may be left open and loosely filled with packing. The large gap that is created gradually fills with granulation tissue. Wound irrigations and absorbent dressings are used until the wound closes. Alternatively, the perineal wound may be sutured with stab wounds formed for drainage and irrigation. The remaining pelvic organs shift slightly to fill the remaining space.

The perineal wound makes it difficult for the patient to sit or find a comfortable position. Foam pads or soft pillows may increase comfort while the patient is sitting. The nurse instructs the patient to avoid the use of air or rubber rings that separate the buttocks and put stress on the healing wound. The side-lying position is usually preferred. Phantom rectal sensations and itching may occur after healing. The origin of these sensations is unknown. Serosanguineous wound drainage initially is copious and must be effectively removed to prevent infection and abscess formation. The drainage tubes may work passively by gravity or be attached to suction. Wound irrigations, usually with normal saline, are initially done with a catheter, but the patient gradually may progress to a handheld shower massage or Water Pik. The dressings are changed as needed. A T-binder may be useful in holding the dressings in place over the perineum. Sitz baths may be substituted for irrigations once the patient is ambulatory, but a free flow of water on the perineal wound is preferred.

Teaching for Self-Care

It is essential that the patient acquire basic ostomy self-care skills during the postoperative period. Successful self-care provides the foundation for both independence and a reintegration of body image that includes the ostomy. The nurse teaches the patient the principles of ostomy care and encourages the patient to handle, assemble, and use all equipment. Allowing time for practice is imperative. The process can rarely be completed during the hospitalization, particularly with older persons, and the nurse initiates referrals to appropriate home health care and community ostomy services. Involvement of a family member or supportive friend can be helpful if it is acceptable to the patient.

Stoma Care

An ostomy pouch is placed over the new stoma at the conclusion of the surgery. Teaching begins with the first pouch change. The patient may or may not be ready to view the stoma, but the nurse gently encourages the patient to look at and touch it. The nurse briefly and factually explains each step of the procedure. The nurse reminds the patient that the stoma has no touch sensation but that the rest of the abdomen will be painful from the surgery. Surgical pain should be adequately controlled before any teaching session takes place.

A systematic plan should be in place to guide teaching of the colostomy regimen. Teaching sessions should be spaced throughout the hospitalization to allow for repetition and assimilation. Pouches are changed more frequently than needed to allow for practice time. Written instructions and resource materials are invaluable supplements to instruction by the nurse.

Pouch Selection. An effective pouch system protects the skin, contains stool and odor, molds to the body's contours, allows for movement, and is inconspicuous under clothing. It is the most important aspect of ostomy management. Choices are based on the ostomy type, the size and contour of the abdomen, the peristomal skin condition, financial considerations, and individual preferences.

Products for ostomy care are available in a variety of styles, shapes, and sizes. Disposable pouches are available in one- and two-piece systems, with skin barriers attached, and in a variety of materials (Figure 34-12). Reusable pouches are worn, cleaned, and worn again. Drainable pouches are easier to keep clean and are more economical than closed, nondrainable pouches. They are available in one- and two-piece systems in a variety of materials. Drainable colostomy pouches are changed every 3 to 7 days if there are no problems with leakage. The usual wearing time for an ileostomy pouch is 5 to 7 days, with the pouch emptied and rinsed every 4 to 6 hours.

A properly applied pouch system is odor free except during changes. Persistent odor is usually the result of inadequate cleansing of the drainage spout or a poor pouch seal. Pinholes in a pouch destroy its odor-proof quality and should not be used to release gas. Fecal odor is caused by the action of bacteria in the colon. Therefore the drainage from an ileostomy should not be foul smelling. A foul odor may indicate a problem such as infection or obstruction.

It is essential that the patient learn to properly measure the stoma to ensure a proper pouch fit. The pouch should closely surround the stoma but not press or rub against it. The stoma may shrink dramatically during the first week after surgery, and it will continue to change in size slightly throughout the first several months. It is important for the patient to measure the stoma accurately during each pouch change in the first weeks after surgery. Cutouts of various diameters are included in the box of pouches. The skin barriers are cut approximately $\frac{1}{16}$- to $\frac{1}{8}$-inch larger than the stoma to accommodate stoma swelling. Once the stoma has stabilized in size, only occasional checks are needed to maintain proper fit. The pouch change procedure is outlined in more detail in the Guidelines for Safe Practice box on p. 1091, top right.

The nurse teaches the patient to change the pouch immediately if leakage occurs and to establish a routine in which pouches are changed before stool leakage occurs. The pouch should be emptied when it is one-third to one-half full. The pouch is changed during inactive times and before meals to minimize the chance of the intestine emptying during the change. The nurse instructs the patient to use each pouch change as an opportunity to carefully assess the stoma and peristomal skin.

The nurse ensures that the patient has adequate temporary supplies before discharge, a complete list of supplies needed for home management, and information about where supplies can be obtained in the local community. A prescription for supplies may be needed for Medicare or insurance reimbursement.

Skin Care. The drainage from an ileostomy is both continuous and erosive, and it is essential that the pouch be secure and properly fitted. Ileostomy drainage contains residual digestive enzymes that will break down the peristomal skin if they are allowed to make contact with it. Skin care is also

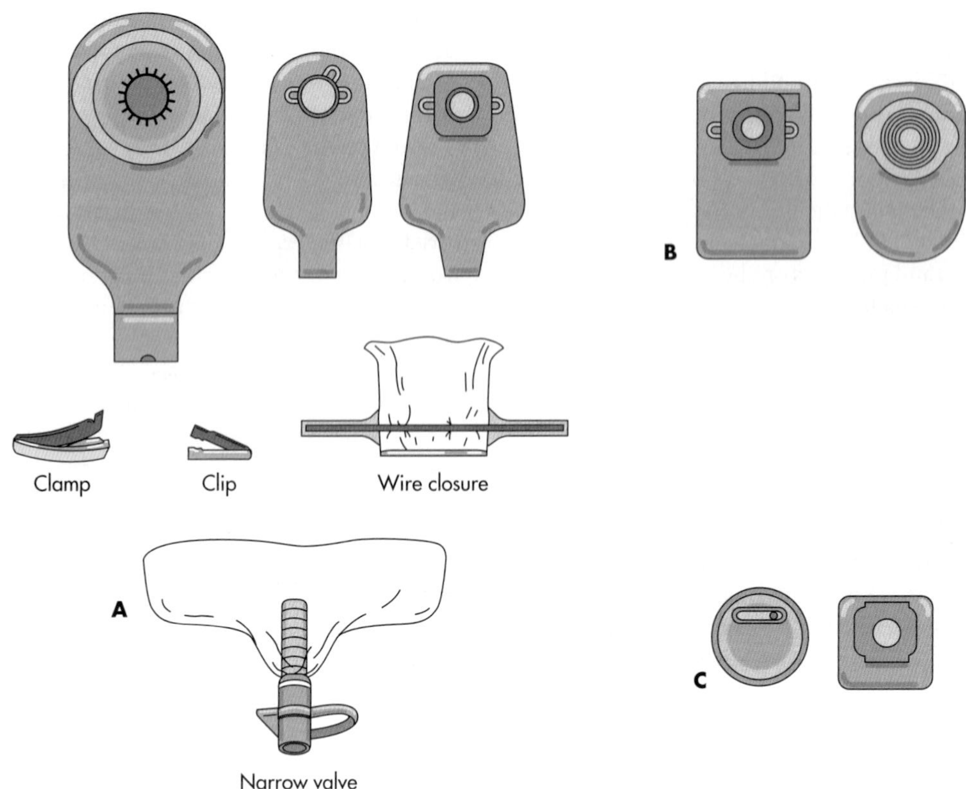

Figure 34-12 Common ostomy pouch products, closures, and patches. **A**, Drainable pouches and pouch closures. **B**, Nondrainable pouches. **C**, Patches for regulated colostomies.

important with colostomies. In addition to irritation from stool, the skin can also be damaged by an allergic reaction to the tape or skin barrier product, rough or frequent removal of pouch adhesives, or infection. The skin around the stoma should appear as healthy and normal as the remainder of the skin on the abdomen. Prevention of skin problems is always easier and less expensive than treatment. The most common peristomal skin infection is a bright red rash with papular lesions caused by *Candida albicans.* Dryness and scaling develop if the condition persists. It can be treated by applying an antifungal powder with each pouch change.[50]

The use of a skin barrier is an important means of protecting the peristomal skin. Skin barriers come in several basic forms: powder, paste, washer, or wafer (Figure 34-13). Skin barriers include products such as karaya, Stomahesive (ConvaTec), Hollihesive (Hollister), ReliaSeal (Bard), Coloplast Skin Barrier, and Mason Colly-Seal Disc. They come already attached to the pouch for both one- and two-piece systems or as single-use items that can be used with any pouch.

Powder. A pouch will not adhere to powder, cream, or ointment. If powder is applied to the skin, it must be sealed before applying the pouch. Karaya powder releases an acid that may sting irritated skin, but Stomadhesive powder is well tolerated.

Paste. Paste barriers are available for use around the stoma, to fill in creases or folds, and to extend the life of the seal. The use of paste has made it easier to keep a pouch seal intact in poor locations.

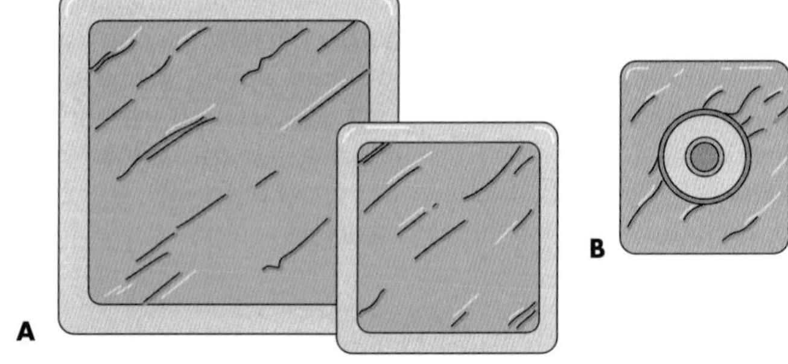

Figure 34-13 Skin barrier products. **A**, Skin barriers. **B**, Wafer.

Skin Barrier Wafers. Skin barrier wafers may be used with a variety of pouches and protect the skin from stool. The opening in the wafer is carefully measured so that it fits around the base of the stoma without rubbing into or onto the stoma.

Skin Sealants. Skin sealants come in sprays, liquids, gels, and wipes and are used to seal in powders and coat the skin with a clear film; they are useful under pouch adhesives. When adhesive is removed from the skin, the stratum corneum layer of the skin is also pulled off. If a skin sealant is used under the adhesive, the underlying skin remains intact.

• • •

Guidelines for skin care are summarized in the Guidelines for Safe Practice box on p. 1091, top left. If the peristomal skin becomes irritated, barrier powder may be applied to help dry

Guidelines for Safe Practice

Changing an Ostomy Pouch

Gather all needed supplies.

STOMA MEASUREMENT

Use the measuring guide and sample diameters, and cut the ostomy appliance to fit—pattern should be $^1/_8$ to $^1/_4$ inch larger than the stoma.

Use the same procedure to prepare the skin barrier. NOTE: The pouch opening is cut slightly larger than the skin barrier to prevent the paper from cutting the stoma.

Apply a ring of stoma adhesive paste if needed.

REMOVAL OF OLD POUCH

Put on clean gloves.

Empty the drainable pouch to prevent spills.

Disconnect the pouch from the skin wafer if a two-piece system is used.

Beginning at the top, gently peel the wafer away from the skin by pushing the skin and peeling downward.

SKIN CARE

Cleanse the skin with warm water; use soap only if stool adheres to the skin. Rinse with water, and dry thoroughly.

Assess the peristomal skin and stoma carefully for signs of irritation or infection.

Pat the peristomal skin dry thoroughly.

Apply a layer of skin sealant and paste if needed to fill spaces.

APPLICATION OF NEW POUCH

Label the template top, bottom, right, and left.

Place the opening of the template over the stoma to ensure fit.

Center the pouch opening over the stoma. Ask patient to tense abdominal muscles to make application easier.

Gently press into place, and hold for at least 30 seconds to seal.

If a two-part system, apply the pouch to the flange until it snaps in place.

moist irritation. The addition of barrier powder or a wafer to the usual pouching system allows for rapid healing. An enterostomal therapist should be consulted for the management of severe skin problems. The use of antacids or products that contain alcohol should be avoided because they dry the skin and alter the pH, leaving it vulnerable to infection.

Managing Odor. Ostomy pouches are made of odor-proof plastic, but a leaking seal or improperly cleaned pouch can emit an unpleasant odor. The inside of the pouch is rinsed with tepid water after emptying, and the pouch outlet is wiped with toilet paper. Oral deodorizing agents exist, and deodorizing solutions and tablets may be placed in the pouch if the patient so desires. Attention to diet can also be helpful.

The nurse encourages the patient to eat a balanced diet and to chew foods slowly and thoroughly. No special diet is required once healing has occurred; however, patients need to be informed about foods that increase gas and odor. Dairy products, highly seasoned foods, fish, and a variety of vegetables are known to increase the odor of the stool. Individual responses to gas-producing foods tend to be variable, with known exceptions such as beans, cabbage, and brussels sprouts. The patient

Guidelines for Safe Practice

Ostomy Skin Care

Change pouch when two-thirds full to avoid leakage. Stool held against the skin can quickly cause severe skin irritation.

Apply clean gloves.

Remove pouch gently, with one hand holding the skin in place to decrease pulling.

Gently but thoroughly clean the skin, rinse it, and pat it dry.

Trim peristomal hair, but do not shave it to prevent folliculitis.

Use a skin barrier to protect the peristomal skin from contact with stool.

Use a skin sealant under all tape.

Encourage patient to consult an enterostomal therapist for specific care guidelines if skin problems occur.

will need to experiment with dietary modifications that reflect individual food preferences and tolerances. Closed pouches usually have a charcoal filter at the top that releases and deodorizes gas. Pouches can be opened to release accumulated gas but should never be pricked. A puncture in the pouch would create a constant odor problem.

Ostomy Irrigation

An ostomy irrigation is an enema given through the stoma to stimulate bowel emptying at a regular and convenient time. The procedure is no longer routinely recommended and is used only with sigmoid colostomies that expel formed stool. Irrigation is never a part of the routine management of an ileostomy because the drainage is continuous and semiliquid in nature. A patient who uses irrigations successfully may be able to dispense with a standard pouch and wear a stoma cap—a small adhesive pouch with an absorbent dressing. Because the ostomy continues to secrete mucus and release flatus, a gas filter is desirable.

If irrigations are planned, they are initiated about 5 to 7 days after surgery. The procedure is described in the Patient Teaching box. A variety of equipment is commercially available, and most sets include irrigating sleeves, a cone tip for insertion into the stoma, a bag to hold the solution, and clips to close the sleeve.

Preventing Ileostomy Complications

Excessive loss of fluid can be a serious concern after ileostomy surgery, and the nurse explains to the patient that diarrhea accompanied by nausea and vomiting can rapidly progress to dehydration. The nurse provides the patient with a list of signs of dehydration and electrolyte imbalance. Losses of sodium and potassium are of particular concern. The patient needs to know how to safely replace lost fluids and when to seek medical attention. Patients with an ileostomy also may become dehydrated if they are given laxatives in preparation for diagnostic procedures.

Enteric-coated, time-released medications or hard tablets may not be absorbed by a patient with an ileostomy and should

Patient Teaching
Colostomy Irrigation

Assemble all equipment:
- Water container, irrigating sleeve, and belt
- Skin care items
- New pouch system, ready for use

Apply clean gloves.
Remove the old pouch, and dispose of it.
Clean the stoma and peristomal skin with water and assess.
Apply the irrigating sleeve and belt. Place the open end of the sleeve in the toilet.
Fill the irrigating container with 500 to 1000 ml of lukewarm tap water, and suspend the container at shoulder height.
Run water through the tubing to remove air.
Gently insert the irrigating cone into the stoma, and slowly start the flow of water. Catheters are inserted no more than 2 to 4 inches. Do not force. If cramping occurs, stop the irrigation and wait.
Allow approximately 15 to 20 minutes for stool to empty.
Rinse the sleeve, dry the bottom, roll it up, and close off the end. Patient should go about regular activities for 30 to 45 minutes.
Remove the sleeve, clean the stoma, and apply a new pouch.
Clean and store the irrigating equipment.

not be used. Liquid or chewable forms of medications are preferred. Because the remaining ileum develops a bacterial flora, antibiotic therapy can cause diarrhea. Supplementation of vitamins A, D, E, and K is a standard measure inasmuch as colon absorption and synthesis are eliminated.

Ileostomy patients should be aware of the potential for obstruction. Obstruction usually is caused by a large mass of undigested food that becomes lodged at a narrow point in the bowel and blocks the intestinal lumen. Dietary changes are essential. Patients are encouraged to eat a soft diet divided into six small meals a day. New foods are added gradually. Raw fruits and foods with nuts, skins, or seeds are all potential problems. Chewing all food thoroughly (20 to 25 times) is a helpful strategy. Obstructions typically present with crampy abdominal pain, bloating, constipation, and an inability to pass flatus (see p. 1094). Rest and a liquid diet are sufficient to resolve minor obstructions, but if the symptoms persist beyond 24 hours or become severe, the individual should contact the physician.[2] Adhesions are also a common cause of obstruction. Gentle irrigation of the stoma may be successful in relieving mild obstructions related to food boluses.

Supporting a Positive Self-Concept

The formation of a stoma often is viewed as mutilating, and most patients need time and the support of others to work through their feelings. Removal of any part of the body involves a sense of loss and grief. The nurse encourages the patient to express these feelings of loss and makes no attempt to suppress them or minimize their validity. The nurse acknowledges the work involved in grief resolution and explores the patient's usual coping strategies. The resolution of grief is not a quick or easy process, and it will not be accomplished during the hospitalization. Both the patient and the family need to be aware that grief resolution can take as much as a year or more and that grief can make a return to independence in self-care more difficult.

The nurse encourages the patient to view the stoma and care for it in a matter-of-fact manner. Emotional support is incorporated into all self-care sessions, and the nurse encourages the patient to verbalize concerns and feelings about the stoma and its anticipated effects on daily life. The nurse provides positive support and reinforcement for all self-care efforts. The nurse encourages the patient to use the services of the United Ostomy Association* and to involve family members in the teaching-learning process.

Patients are encouraged to gradually resume all of their usual activities. No clothing restrictions are necessitated by the stoma except the avoidance of tight belts or garments directly over it. Pouches hold well in baths and showers, and normal hygiene patterns may be resumed as soon as the incision is healed. There are no specific restrictions on exercise or recreational activities.

The nurse reminds the patient to always carry ostomy supplies when traveling and to not place them in checked luggage. Traveler's diarrhea can create serious problems, and the patient is encouraged to carefully consider the quality of local water when traveling.

Preventing Sexual Dysfunction

Many patients do not directly verbalize their concerns about sexuality after ostomy surgery; thus it is usually necessary for the nurse to address the topic directly. The nurse provides the patient with specific suggestions for dealing with sexual concerns such as:

- Explore positions for sexual activity that minimize stress and pressure on the pouch.
- Empty and clean the pouch before sexual activity.
- Use a smaller-sized pouch or a pouch cover during sexual activity.
- Use a binder or special underwear to hold the pouch secure.

The nurse encourages the patient to discuss sexual concerns with his or her partner. Silence and emotional distancing are common reactions, but they can be very destructive to the patient's sexual relationship. Role playing or visualizing worst-case scenarios helps some patients to acknowledge their fears. The use of a community support group can be particularly helpful for getting practical advice about sexual matters. About 15% of male ostomates report a decrease in sexual activity after surgery. Female patients should be reassured that ostomy surgery does not interfere with contraception, pregnancy, or delivery; and pregnancy seldom produces stoma complications. A pamphlet entitled *Sex and the Ostomate* is available from the United Ostomy Association.*

*36 Executive Park, Suite 120, Irvine, CA 92714; (800) 826-0826.

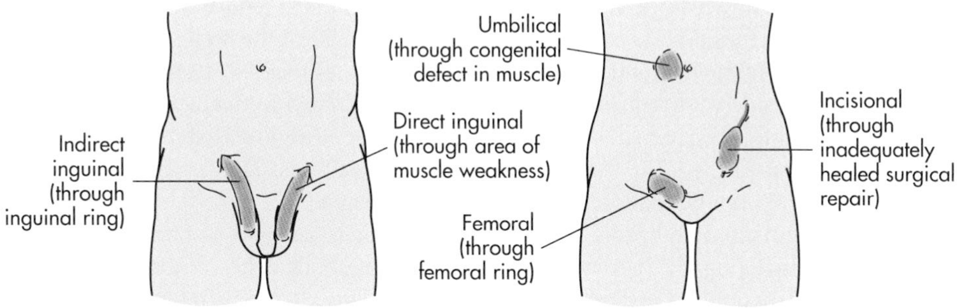

Figure 34-14 Common sites of abdominal herniation.

GERONTOLOGIC CONSIDERATIONS

Ostomy surgery may be required at any age, but a majority of ostomy procedures are performed on elderly patients as part of treatment for colorectal cancer. An ostomy is difficult to adjust to at any age but can be particularly difficult for older adults, who may need to simultaneously cope with the need for this radical surgery and the shock of a diagnosis of cancer. Older adults can clearly learn to manage an ostomy successfully but may take longer to reach a point of readiness than can be supported by shortened hospital stays. Teaching and learning principles for older adults need to be incorporated into the plan of care, allowing for additional time, repeat presentations of information, and consistent caregivers if possible. Arthritis and sensory problems may make manipulation of equipment and regimen mastery more difficult. Discharge planning is particularly important for older adults, who often live alone and may not have adequate assistance in the home or community.

SPECIAL ENVIRONMENTS FOR CARE

Critical Care

Critical care is rarely needed following ostomy surgery except to deal with serious complications. Ostomy surgery is complex and requires a significant recovery period for adequate wound healing, but it is rarely associated with the need for ventilatory assistance or the development of shock. Profound wound infection and peritonitis are the obvious exceptions.

Community-Based Care

Acquiring sufficient confidence and expertise to manage an ostomy effectively requires time and practice. Adequate amounts of either of these elements can only rarely be provided in the acute care setting. Discharge planning for continuity of care and teaching is therefore essential. Most patients will appropriately be referred to community home health and ostomy support services for ongoing teaching and supervision. Support groups are available in most larger cities and are a good source of information about day-to-day management problems related to acquiring supplies and coping with ostomy challenges.

COMPLICATIONS

Most of the more common complications of ostomy surgery have been discussed in a preventive framework under the discussion of postoperative care. Common problems include skin breakdown or infection, obstruction, and day-to-day problems with leakage, diet, and gas. Prevention is the key to management. All of these complications are easier to prevent than to treat. Nursing interventions are discussed on p. 1089.

OBSTRUCTIVE DISORDERS

Abdominal Hernias

Etiology/Epidemiology

A hernia is a protrusion of an organ or structure from its normal cavity through a congenital or acquired defect, usually in the muscle of the abdominal wall. Depending on its location, the hernia may contain peritoneum, omentum, a loop of bowel, or a section of bladder. Inguinal and umbilical hernias usually result from congenital weakness of the muscle, whereas incisional hernias are usually a complication of surgery. Hernias can occur at any age and are more common in men and older adults.

Hernias of the groin account for more than 80% of all hernias and are the result of primary muscular defects.[32] Indirect hernias represent more than 50% of all hernias and are much more common in men than in women. The higher incidence is probably explained by the need for the testes to pass through the inguinal ring during fetal development. Indirect inguinal hernias develop from weakness of the abdominal wall at the point where the spermatic cord emerges and are bilateral in about 12% of men.[32] A parallel weakness is found in women from the emergence of the round ligament. Figure 34-14 illustrates the indirect inguinal hernia. The protruded bowel may rest in the inguinal canal or move down into the scrotum in men and, on rare occasions, into the labia in women.

Direct inguinal hernias pass through the posterior inguinal wall at a point of muscle weakness. They typically are caused by increased intraabdominal pressure. These hernias occur most often in older men and are technically difficult to repair. They often recur after surgery. Femoral hernias occur almost exclusively in women. They develop when a loop of intestine passes through the femoral ring and down the femoral canal. The hernia creates a round bulge below the inguinal ligament and is thought to be caused by pressure and changes in the ligaments that are related to pregnancy.

Several other terms are used to describe the severity of the hernia obstruction. A sliding hernia moves freely in and out of the hernia sac. If the protruding structure requires manipulation to return it to its proper position, the hernia is considered reducible. If the protruding structure cannot be returned to its proper position, the hernia is considered irreducible. The term *incarcerated* is usually reserved for an irreducible hernia in which bowel obstruction occurs. The size of the defect largely determines whether the hernia can be reduced. When the blood flow to the trapped segment is compromised by pressure from the surrounding muscle ring, the hernia is said to be strangulated. Intestinal obstruction occurs, and gangrene of the viscera can develop rapidly.

Pathophysiology

Hernias typically form as a result of increased abdominal pressure, decreased resistance of the tissues of the abdominal wall, and the presence of spaces in the abdominal cavity. Aging usually results in a loss of muscle strength and tone, and obesity increases intraabdominal pressure. Both elements are significant contributors to the herniation process.[32] The major pathologic concern associated with hernias is the risk of strangulation and bowel obstruction. Once present, hernias tend to extend, and the risk of complications increases.

The person with a hernia typically has a mass in the groin, around the umbilicus, or protruding from an old surgical incision. The mass may always have been present, or it may have appeared suddenly after coughing, straining, lifting, or other vigorous exertion. There may be no other symptoms. The protrusion usually disappears when the person lies down and reappears with standing, coughing, or lifting.

The person may perceive a vague feeling of discomfort as the hernial contents slide in and out of the abdominal defect, but little actual pain is experienced as long as the hernia is freely reducible. A "dragging" sensation or feeling of heaviness is common, especially with groin hernias. An irreducible hernia may become strangulated, causing severe pain and symptoms of intestinal obstruction such as nausea, vomiting, and distention. These complications require emergency surgery, and a portion of bowel may have to be resected.

Collaborative Care Management

A diagnosis of hernia is readily established by reviewing the patient's history and the results of the physical examination. The contents of the hernia sac may feel soft and nodular to palpation (omentum) or smooth and fluctuant (bowel). Fingertip palpation is used to feel the edges of the hernia ring and its contents by inserting the examining fingertip into the ring and feeling for the surge of the intestine into the hernia sac as the person coughs.

Hernias are repaired by elective surgery if at all possible. Strangulation is an ever-present risk, and if it should occur, the surgical repair would have to be performed on an emergency basis. The herniated tissues are returned to the abdominal cavity, the hernia sac is excised, and the defect in the fascia or muscle is closed with sutures (herniorrhaphy). To prevent recurrence of the hernia and to facilitate closure of the defect, a hernioplasty may be performed. This procedure uses fascia or a variety of synthetic materials to strengthen the muscle wall. Attempts to reduce strangulated hernias are generally not made because of the high risk of rupture. The emergency surgery is accompanied by a high incidence of postoperative complications. Elective hernia surgery is often performed in ambulatory surgical centers with the patient under local or spinal anesthesia. The patient is discharged directly home after the repair.

Hernia repair may be performed by either open or laparoscopic methods. The results appear to be quite similar, although laparoscopic surgery causes less pain and allows a more rapid return to normal activities. However, laparoscopic surgery is also significantly more expensive and necessitates the use of general anesthesia. The benefits of a laparoscopic approach are less clear with hernia repair than with many other laparoscopic surgeries, and the use of this approach is not routine at this time.[26]

Recovery from hernia repair usually is rapid and without incident. Standard postoperative interventions are used, but the nurse encourages the patient to deep breathe rather than cough. Fluid and food are resumed as tolerated. Ice bags are applied after inguinal hernia repair to minimize edema, particularly in the scrotum. A scrotal support or "jockey" style underwear may make initial ambulation less painful. Fluids are encouraged, and IV infusions are continued until the patient is able to successfully empty the bladder.

Patient/Family Education. Discharge teaching includes the avoidance of any heavy lifting, pushing, or pulling for about 6 weeks. Driving and stair climbing are initially restricted. The nurse instructs the patient to monitor the incision for signs of infection. Postoperative ecchymosis should disappear in a few days. Stool softeners or bulk-forming laxatives are prescribed to prevent straining at defecation. The nurse also reassures the patient that sexual functioning is not affected by the surgery and that sexual activity may be resumed once healing is complete.

Bowel Obstruction

Etiology/Epidemiology

Normal functioning of the small and large intestines depends on an open lumen for the movement of intestinal contents, as well as adequate circulation and nervous innervation to sustain rhythmic peristalsis. Any factor or condition that either narrows the intestinal lumen or interferes with peristalsis can result in bowel obstruction. Bowel obstruction occurs in both genders, in all races, and at any point in the life span. It is the cause of about 20% of all cases of acute abdominal pain. Because bowel obstruction usually is a secondary effect of a variety of primary problems, accurate incidence statistics are unavailable. Obstruction is more common in older adults, particularly in relation to bowel cancer, but it can occur at any age. Bowel obstructions are commonly classified as either mechanical (affecting the intestinal lumen) or nonmechanical (related to peristalsis) and can be either partial or complete.

Mechanical Obstruction. A wide variety of conditions and disorders can result in mechanical bowel obstruction. The problem may arise outside the bowel or within the lumen.

Adhesions. Adhesions are the most common cause of small bowel obstruction, accounting for more than 70% of all cases.[47] Adhesions typically develop after gynecologic procedures or surgeries involving the small or large bowel. They may occur from just a few days to 10 to 20 years after the procedure. Their cause is unknown but may be related to the inflammatory response. In some persons the adhesions may become massive. The fibrous bands of scar tissue can loop over bowel segments, contract with time, and compress a segment of bowel. The resultant obstruction often creates a closed loop, which is associated with strangulation (Figure 34-15).

Hernias. A hernia can result in bowel obstruction if the abdominal wall defect through which the hernia protrudes becomes so tight that the bowel segment becomes strangulated.

Volvulus. A volvulus is a twisting of the bowel on itself, usually at least a full 180 degrees, that obstructs the intestinal lumen both proximally and distally (Figure 34-16). It involves the sigmoid colon in 70% to 80% of cases and the cecum in 10% to 20% of cases.[47] The acute obstruction can quickly result in bowel infarction and can be life threatening in the presence of bowel necrosis, perforation, and peritonitis.

Tumors. A tumor mass gradually restricts the internal lumen of the bowel from within as it enlarges. Eventually a fecal mass may be unable to pass through the constricted area, leading to partial or complete obstruction. Bowel cancer accounts for approximately 60% of obstructions of the large intestine, with most obstructions occurring in the sigmoid colon.

Intussusception. Intussusception occurs when a leading segment of bowel invaginates into an adjacent segment (Figure 34-16). The invagination occurs with peristalsis and in the adult is often triggered by the presence of a tumor mass. The bowel segment containing the mass is propelled by peristalsis into the adjacent bowel segment. The inner walls of the trapped segment rapidly become edematous, and venous obstruction, infarction, and necrosis can occur rapidly.

Other possible causes of mechanical obstruction include fecal impaction, gallstones, and the strictures produced by chronic inflammatory bowel disease.

Nonmechanical Obstruction

Ileus. Ileus is a state of impaired or absent peristaltic motility. Adynamic or paralytic ileus is a common temporary problem after abdominal surgery, particularly if the bowel has been extensively handled. The diagnosis is made when the absence of peristalsis persists for longer than 72 hours. Conditions associated with ileus are well recognized, but the origins of the disorder remain unclear. Neurogenic impairment, drug effects, reflex inhibition, and metabolic abnormalities are all believed to play a role.[3]

Other. A variety of other chronic disorders can cause a form of nonmechanical obstruction from failure to propel the intestinal contents. Most cases result from a failure of nervous innervation (e.g., multiple sclerosis, Parkinson's disease, or Hirschsprung's disease). Primary collagen or muscle disorders can affect bowel propulsion and cause obstruction. Endocrine disorders such as diabetes mellitus are commonly associated with problems of GI motility. Although constipation is the more common manifestation of all of these disorders, chronic problems with bowel obstruction also may occur. Thrombosis of the mesenteric arteries is a possible complication of heart disease in older adults. It can cause an abrupt ischemic episode that may necessitate surgical intervention to remove the affected area of the bowel.

Pathophysiology

Approximately 7 to 10 L of electrolyte-rich fluid is secreted into the small intestine each day. In the normal bowel all but approximately 600 to 800 ml is reabsorbed before the chyme enters the cecum. About 200 ml is lost daily in the stool. Even when the forward movement of chyme is obstructed, GI secretion continues, at least initially. Intestinal obstruction

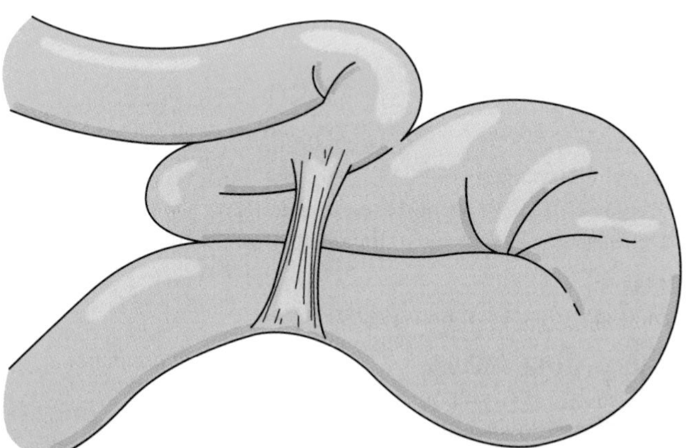

Figure 34-15 A band of adhesions causing intestinal obstruction in the small bowel.

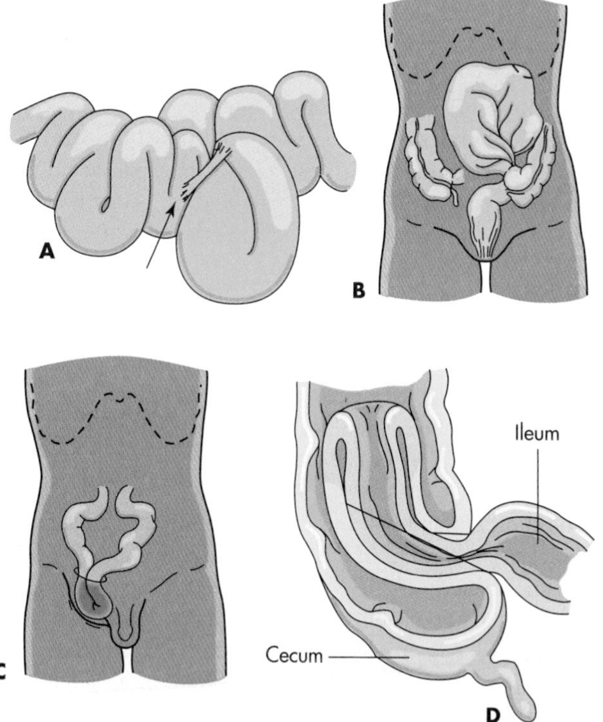

Figure 34-16 Common causes of intestinal obstruction. **A,** Constriction by adhesions. **B,** Volvulus of the sigmoid colon. **C,** Strangulated inguinal hernia. **D,** Ileocecal intussusception.

triggers a series of GI tract events whose clinical manifestations depend largely on the location of the obstruction and the degree of circulatory compromise.

In the presence of obstruction, a steadily worsening imbalance between secretion and absorption develops, and fluid and air accumulate proximal to the site of the obstruction. The outcomes are the result of changes in blood flow, motility, bowel contents, and bowel flora. The mediators that control secretion in the presence of obstruction have not been clearly identified. Progressive distention occurs with an increase in intraluminal pressure. The bowel wall becomes increasingly edematous, and venous drainage is impeded. Increased capillary permeability allows massive amounts of isotonic fluid to move from the plasma into the distended bowel, which begins to weep fluids from its surface into the peritoneum.[3] Gas accumulates in the bowel from both air swallowing and the action of intestinal bacteria on stagnant bowel contents. This worsens the abdominal distention.

Vascular compromise is the most serious aspect of obstruction. Closed-loop obstruction impairs blood flow and causes local mucosal ischemia. Visible changes occur in the villi within 30 to 60 minutes, and basic transport functions are impaired. Bowel ischemia breaks down the normal protective barriers, and the stagnant and distended bowel becomes increasingly permeable to bacteria. Organisms can enter the peritoneal cavity and cause peritonitis. Bacteria are normally sparse in the small bowel but accumulate rapidly during obstruction. Normal motility effectively clears both nutrients and organisms from the bowel, and tremendous bacterial overgrowth can occur in the presence of stasis.[3] Within hours of a complete bowel obstruction, the proximal bowel contents become fetid and foul smelling from the rapid proliferation of anaerobic organisms. *Escherichia coli, Klebsiella,* and *Pseudomonas* organisms are particularly prevalent, and the release of toxins can result in septic shock. The ischemic process can progress to gangrene and perforation. Submucosal hemorrhage and sloughing can be a source of substantial blood loss. Unlike mechanical obstruction, the intraluminal pressure generated by paralytic ileus is rarely significant enough to impair mucosal blood flow.

The loss of extracellular fluid can range from 2 to 6 L within 2 to 3 days of a mechanical bowel obstruction. The resulting hypovolemia may be mild or severe enough to compromise renal perfusion and induce dehydration, electrolyte imbalance, and shock. The resultant concentration of the blood can even cause vascular thrombosis. Mortality rates rise to greater than 30% in the presence of strangulation, peritonitis, and acute sepsis.[3]

The clinical manifestations of bowel obstruction depend on the exact site and extent of the obstruction, but crampy abdominal pain, distention, and vomiting are common symptoms. Simple obstruction produces crampy and poorly localized pain. Its onset parallels an initial increase in peristalsis proximal to the obstruction that raises intraluminal pressure in an attempt to clear the blockage. Frequent, loud, high-pitched bowel sounds are often heard on auscultation. The pain intensifies as the obstruction becomes complete. Smooth muscle atony decreases peristalsis, and bowel sounds gradually diminish. The pain associated with bowel strangulation is constant and severe. Pain is much less intense with ileus than with mechanical obstruction and may be described as pressure or fullness.

Nausea and vomiting are also common features, especially with obstructions that occur in the small intestine. Depending on the level of the obstruction, vomiting can be profuse. Vomiting temporarily relieves the pain in proximal but not distal obstructions. Abdominal distention usually develops slowly, although severe constipation is common. Rising fever usually indicates the presence of necrotic bowel. Laboratory values typically reflect the progressive nature of the dehydration and fluid losses through vomiting. The range of clinical manifestations that can occur with bowel obstruction is summarized in the Clinical Manifestations box.

Collaborative Care Management

Intestinal obstruction is diagnosed primarily from its clinical manifestations. In addition, abdominal x-ray films generally show clear patterns of air and fluid entrapment in the obstructed area. Obstruction cannot be ruled out, however, by the presence of apparently normal x-ray findings.

There are no laboratory tests that can confirm or rule out a diagnosis of bowel obstruction. WBC counts and a variety of enzymes may be elevated in the presence of strangulation but otherwise are normal. Once hypovolemia becomes severe, he-

Clinical Manifestations
Bowel Obstruction

PAIN

Crampy in nature
Poorly localized
Severe, continuous pain with strangulation of the bowel

NAUSEA AND VOMITING

Presence and severity depend on the level of the obstruction
Can be profuse with proximal small bowel obstructions
May have fecal odor if the obstruction is in the distal small bowel
Occurs late if at all in most large bowel obstructions

OBSTIPATION

ABDOMINAL DISTENTION

Usually nontender
Slow to develop especially with large bowel obstructions

BOWEL SOUNDS

Frequent and high pitched early in the obstructive process
Decreased or absent late in the obstructive process

FEVER

Indicates necrosis of bowel tissue

LABORATORY VALUES

Reflective of dehydration and fluid shifts
- Decreased urine output
- Hemoconcentration
- Hypokalemia and hyponatremia

moconcentration elevates the hemoglobin and hematocrit values and the serum potassium level typically falls.

Once the diagnosis has been established, the treatment of bowel obstruction is directed toward correcting the fluid and electrolyte imbalances, decompressing the GI tract, and preventing infection. Correction of fluid, electrolyte, and acid-base imbalances is the highest priority and is guided by clinical estimates of prior and ongoing losses plus daily maintenance needs. Acute complete bowel obstruction is considered a surgical emergency, and a decision about the need for surgical intervention is made as quickly as possible. Bowel resection with end-to-end anastamosis is the usual procedure.

Decompression of the bowel reduces gaseous distention, relieves pressure on organs, and reduces pain. Decompression also typically relieves associated vomiting and reduces the risk of aspiration. In patients with partial obstruction, decompression alone may be sufficient to relieve the problem. Decompression is generally accomplished with NG intubation and suction.

The use of long nasointestinal tubes such as the Cantor tube or Miller-Abbott tube used to be a standard intervention for bowel decompression, but their use is no longer recommended. These weighted tubes are difficult to insert, are very uncomfortable for patients, and appear to increase the risk of a variety of complications. They have also not been proven to be any more effective than an NG tube for achieving decompression.[3]

Analgesics are used sparingly, even in the presence of moderate to severe abdominal pain. The negative effects of opioids on peristalsis mitigate against their use, and the pattern and severity of the pain may be important in establishing an accurate diagnosis. Antibiotics may be administered to counter the effects of the significant bacterial overgrowth in the bowel.

A variety of newer nonoperative treatments also may be used to treat obstruction. Endoscopy allows treatment with balloon catheters to dilate obstructed bowel segments, and lasers, cautery devices, or heater probes may be used to reduce or remove obstructing tumor. The gentle instillation of barium has been routinely successful in reversing sigmoid colon volvulus.

The treatment of nonmechanical obstruction and paralytic ileus is generally conservative and supportive. Temporary ileus is initially expected in the postoperative period but needs to be addressed if it persists for more than a few days. An NG tube may be inserted to decompress the stomach and relieve nausea and bloating, and careful attention is paid to restoring and maintaining the balance of fluids and electrolytes. Careful monitoring for complications is ongoing. Promotility drugs are most likely to be useful in treating nonmechanical obstructions.

Nursing management focuses on careful monitoring of all physical parameters. The nurse monitors the patient's vital signs, urine output, and NG output frequently. Changes are compared with the symptoms of early shock (see Chapter 14). The nurse administers IV fluids as ordered and monitors for symptoms of electrolyte imbalance. Fluid replacement is provided for all patients with intestinal obstruction because fluid losses usually are significant. Supplemental potassium is added to the IV infusions as needed to compensate for losses through vomiting and fluid shifts.

Third spacing of fluids is typical with intestinal obstruction. The nurse assesses for edema and measures abdominal girth every 2 to 4 hours. Fluid losses trigger nagging thirst, and small amounts of ice chips may be comforting.

General comfort measures include positioning the patient with the head of the bed elevated to relieve abdominal pressure and providing frequent position changes. A side-lying position often is the most comfortable. The patient may be encouraged to be out of bed and ambulate frequently to promote peristalsis. Oral and nasal care is offered every 2 to 4 hours to counter the drying and irritating effects of the NG tube and NPO status.

The nurse regularly assesses the patient's pain. Opioids are rarely given to patients with bowel obstruction until the diagnosis is established, and it is critical for the nurse to explore nonpharmacologic measures to increase the patient's comfort. If the pain increases significantly or shifts from cramping to a constant character, it should be reported promptly, since this may indicate strangulation or perforation of the bowel. A Nursing Care Plan for a patient with a bowel obstruction is found on pp. 1098 and 1099.

Surgical correction of mechanical bowel obstruction is often necessary after bowel decompression. Specific surgical procedures depend on the nature and location of the obstruction. Release of adhesions, bowel resection with reanastomosis, and temporary colostomy may all be used. The existence or development of bowel strangulation or vascular compromise necessitates that corrective surgery be performed on an emergency basis. Postoperative care is the same as that provided to any patient who undergoes major abdominal surgery. See the discussion on p. 1108.

Patient/Family Education. The patient may be extremely anxious during the initial treatment period. It is important for the nurse to explain all tests, procedures, and planned care thoroughly. Support and reassurance are important, especially if corrective bowel surgery is planned.

The majority of large bowel obstructions affect older patients and are often related to the presence of cancer. The nurse needs to assist the patient in dealing with the discomfort and anxiety of the obstruction, as well as the diagnosis of cancer and the possible need for ostomy surgery. Both the patient and the family are likely to feel overwhelmed and need teaching and reteaching as they attempt to understand the diagnosis and treatment options.

Discharge planning is tailored to the unique needs of the patient. Recovery from intestinal obstruction may be swift or prolonged, depending on the location and severity of the obstruction and whether or not surgery was performed. Home care issues include wound healing, reestablishing a normal diet, and restoring regular bowel habits. Teaching is provided concerning the prevention of constipation through a fiber-rich diet, adequate fluids, and exercise.

Patients who undergo colostomy surgery because of cancer or complications of obstruction need ongoing support and supervision as they adjust to new self-care patterns. Referral to a home health care agency is initiated.

Nursing Care Plan Patient With a Bowel Obstruction

DATA Mrs. L. is a 62-year-old woman who was admitted last night with probable small bowel obstruction. Yesterday she developed cramping upper abdominal pain, which steadily worsened. She felt bloated and increasingly nauseated and thought that she was probably getting the flu. Her condition did not improve with rest. She vomited, which did improve her symptoms, but the cycle repeated itself several times. Her family became frightened and insisted that she go to the emergency department.

Mrs. L. has been in good health. She has a stable, caring family and a job she enjoys. Her health history is unremarkable and includes an appendectomy in her teens, the uncomplicated births of three children, and a vaginal hysterectomy for dysfunctional uterine bleeding 5 years ago.

On admission Mrs. L. had a temperature of 100° F (37.8° C), blood pressure of 110/60, and pulse rate of 88 beats/min. She reported continued abdominal pain and a tight, bloated feeling in her abdomen. Auscultation of her abdomen revealed diminished bowel sounds in the lower quadrants but high-pitched sounds in the upper quadrants. She is not passing gas per rectum and has not had a bowel movement for 2 days. She voided 90 ml of concentrated urine on admission. Abdominal x-ray films revealed significant accumulation of gas and fluid in the intestine. Her blood work is normal except for her hematocrit, which is 40%, and low-normal sodium and potassium levels. Adhesions are suspected as the cause of her bowel obstruction.

An intravenous (IV) line is present for hydration, and Mrs. L. is given nothing by mouth (is kept NPO) except for small amounts of ice chips. She has bathroom privileges, but intake and output are being strictly recorded. A nasogastric (NG) tube is in place for decompression. A decision about the need for surgery will be made within 48 hours.

NURSING DIAGNOSIS **Acute pain related to distention of the bowel with fluid and gas**
GOALS/OUTCOMES Will achieve pain-free status

NOC Suggested Outcomes
- Pain Level (2102)
- Pain Control (1605)
- Comfort Level (2100)

NIC Suggested Interventions
- Pain Management (1400)
- Analgesic Management (2210)
- Coping Enhancement (5230)

Nursing Interventions/Rationales
- Assess patient's pain level at least every 4 hours. *Pain presence and severity are important cues for identifying subtle changes in patient status. Worsening pain can indicate bowel ischemia or peritonitis.*
- Assist patient with developing a pain-related scale for evaluating changes. Record patient's pain ratings on the bedside flow record. *Pain scales assist the patient with evaluating and communicating pain status. Pain records demonstrate pattern changes over time.*
- Administer prescribed analgesics and antiemetics as ordered. *Analgesics are often withheld until the diagnosis is established. Aggressive comfort measures are needed to help the patient gain control of the pain. Nausea and vomiting contribute significantly to general discomfort.*
- Use nonpharmacologic comfort measures that are acceptable to the patient (hygiene and linen changes, oral care, back care and repositioning, relaxation techniques, distraction). *Analgesic administration is limited because of the adverse effect on peristalsis. Adjunct pain relief measures are therefore critical.*
- Maintain patency and proper functioning of NG suction (attach to low, intermittent suction as prescribed; irrigate or reposition the NG tube as needed to maintain drainage). *Effective decompression of the gastrointestinal (GI) tract will reduce both fluid and gas distention and reduce pain.*
- Position in semi- to high Fowler's position. *An upright position relieves pressure in the abdomen and facilitates ventilation.*
- Encourage frequent position changes and ambulation once the condition is stabilized. *Activity is important to help reestablish peristalsis.*
- Provide frequent oral care and lip lubrication. *NG intubation causes significant dryness and irritation of the oral mucous membranes. Oral care decreases thirst and helps relieve irritation and bad tastes.*

Evaluation Parameters
1. States that pain is steadily decreasing
2. Reports satisfaction with pain control measures
3. Absence of pain indicators (complaints of pain, facial grimace, crying)

NURSING DIAGNOSIS **Risk for deficient fluid volume related to vomiting, NG suction, NPO status, and fluid shifts in the GI tract**
GOALS/OUTCOMES Will return to normal fluid volume balance

NOC Suggested Outcomes
- Fluid Balance (0601)
- Hydration (0602)
- Electrolyte and Acid/Base Balance (0600)

NIC Suggested Interventions
- Fluid Monitoring (4130)
- Fluid Management (4120)
- Intravenous (IV) Therapy (4200)

Nursing Care Plan — Patient With a Bowel Obstruction—cont'd

Nursing Interventions/Rationales
- Maintain accurate intake and output. *To provide initial data about the patient's fluid needs and degree of third spacing*
- Maintain IV fluids at prescribed rate and flow. *Obstruction causes significant fluid and electrolyte losses. Steady replacement helps prevent stressful fluid swings and decreases nausea.*
- Monitor weight daily. *Body weight is the most accurate method of assessing fluid gains and losses.*
- Measure abdominal girth each shift until stabilized. *Fluid and gas accumulation in the GI tract can result in significant abdominal distention.*

Evaluation Parameters
1. Maintains stable body weight
2. Maintains good skin turgor
3. Urine output >30 ml/hr
4. Stable vital signs

NURSING DIAGNOSIS **Anxiety related to lack of knowledge concerning cause of bowel obstruction and uncertainty over need for surgery**

GOALS/OUTCOMES Will report reduced anxiety following use of coping mechanisms

NOC Suggested Outcomes
- Anxiety Control (1402)
- Coping (1302)

NIC Suggested Interventions
- Anxiety Reduction (5820)
- Presence (5340)
- Calming Technique (5880)

Nursing Interventions/Rationales
- Provide reassurance and comfort by spending time with the patient and family. *Communicates a feeling of empathy and willingness to support the patient through a crisis situation.*
- Listen attentively. *Demonstrates concern and empathy.*
- Provide simple explanations of all tests and procedures. Correct misconceptions as needed. *Accurate, understandable information reduces unnecessary fears and restores a sense of control.*
- Encourage supportive involvement of the family. *When relationships are supportive, family involvement decreases fear and increases active coping.*
- Set aside time to address family concerns. *The family can transfer their anxiety to the patient. Addressing and reducing their anxiety will help reduce the patient's anxiety.*

Evaluation Parameters
1. Communicates concern about the illness and treatments
2. Verbalizes understanding of planned interventions
3. Uses coping strategies

Colorectal Cancer

Etiology

The knowledge base about bowel cancer has expanded tremendously over the past decade, but the precise origins of bowel cancer remain elusive. The importance of genetics has become increasingly apparent, and the development and gradual cancerous transformation of bowel polyps and adenomas can often be traced to specific gene mutations. The incidence of bowel cancer varies substantially in different parts of the world, and these variations have pointed to the importance of environmental factors in its etiology.

The role of genetics in bowel cancer was first recognized in a rare disorder, familial adenomatous polyposis. This autosomal dominant disorder causes the early development of hundreds of polyps in the colon and rectum. The incidence of bowel cancer in individuals with this disorder is nearly 100% by midlife.[23] Gardner's syndrome is one small subtype of this disorder that causes osseous, as well as soft tissue, tumors. A second disorder, familial nonpolyposis syndrome, is also an autosomal dominant disorder. It causes the development of only a small number of bowel polyps, but they demonstrate an extremely strong tendency to undergo malignant change in affected persons at a very young age. The malignant change is attributed to the presence of a mutant gene that promotes mutations in other genes. The polyposis syndromes account for only 10% of all bowel cancers, but genetics is also believed to play an important role in the remaining 90% of so-called sporadic cases of colorectal cancer, perhaps contributing to at least 25% to 50% of them.[23] Persons who have one first-degree relative with colorectal cancer have nearly twice the normal risk of developing the disease.[1] The risk is even greater if the cancer was diagnosed before age 45.

Colorectal cancer usually develops as part of a slow and orderly change process in the bowel mucosa from polyp development to gradual malignant transformation in response to genetic signals. Most of the genetic changes involve the deletion of chromosome fragments, but the total number of mutations appears to be more significant than their specific placement or sequence. A number of the mutations have been identified, but none of them can currently be used for general screening. Although virtually all colon cancers appear to develop from polyps that gradually transform into adenomas, only about 5% of all colon adenomas ever become malignant.

Environmental factors are believed to function as stimulants or enablers that initiate the gene mutations that result in bowel cancer. The high risk of colorectal cancer associated with chronic irritation of the mucosa such as that associated with ulcerative colitis has been recognized for years.[35] Diet has received significant attention in recent years. Because bowel cancer is more common in industrialized societies, research has focused on the potentially detrimental role of a diet that is low in fiber and high in fat, protein, and refined carbohydrates. It has been theorized that processed foods are converted into metabolic and bacterial end products that act as carcinogens in the bowel. Low-fiber diets have been implicated because they increase colon transit time and increase the overall time in which the bowel mucosa is in contact with carcinogenic agents. Dietary research is difficult to control and conduct, but recent studies have not supported any positive outcomes from the implementation of high-fiber diets with reduced red meat content.[13,43] The roles of smoking and alcohol have also been extensively studied, but it is currently believed that neither plays a major role in colorectal cancer development.[8]

Several elements have shown evidence of a protective effect, reducing the risk of colorectal cancer. The long-term use of aspirin and nonsteroidal antiinflammatory drugs (NSAIDs) has been the most significant.[45,46] Extensive follow-up studies have noted a strong protective effect. The benefits appear to be related to cumulative use over a period of about 5 years and not to the magnitude of the daily dose. The specific nature of the protective effect is unknown but is theorized to be related to prostaglandin inhibition. Prostaglandins influence cell growth and proliferation in poorly understood ways and may be associated with tumor promotion. The effects appear to operate before the development of adenomas. A similar but more modest effect has also been noted among women taking postmenopausal hormone replacement.[15] Isolated studies have also indicated small benefits associated with calcium and lutein supplementation.[4,44] Risk factors for colorectal cancers are summarized in the Risk Factors box.

Epidemiology

Cancer of the colon and rectum is the second most common cause of death from cancer in adults of both sexes. Approximately 130,000 new cases are diagnosed each year, and 56,000 deaths are attributed to the disease annually.[40] In the United States approximately 1 in 17 persons will develop colorectal cancer at some point. When bowel cancer is diagnosed in its early stage, 5-year survival rates of 90% or greater can be expected, but unfortunately many cases are diagnosed in advanced invasive stages, for which 5-year survival rates hover around 40%. Bowel cancer therefore is theoretically amenable to significant decreases in mortality through early diagnosis. This possibility and the importance of early diagnosis are reflected in the objectives presented in the Healthy People 2010 box.

The incidence of bowel cancer is clearly age related. Incidence rates rise slightly after age 40, more sharply after age 50, and the mean age at onset is 63 to 67 years. All adults older than age 50 are believed to be at average risk for the disease.[40] The incidence of colorectal cancer rose steadily throughout the second half of the twentieth century with the steady aging of the population. It also occurred slightly more often in men. The incidence in Caucasians peaked in the 1980s and has since declined slightly, which is possibly related to increasingly widespread screening and removal of polyps. A similar decline in African-Americans has not occurred, and the rate in African-American men has increased from 50.8 to 60.1 per 100,000 population from 1975 to 1994, compared with a decline in Caucasian men from 56.6 to 53.9 per 100,000 in the same time period.[53] The incidence rates continue to be significantly higher in the industrialized Western world than in Asia and Africa. However, the rates in immigrant families rapidly increase to match those of the larger society, again indicating an as yet unidentified environmental link.

Risk Factors
Colorectal Cancer

Age over 50 years
Family history
- Colon cancer in two or more first-degree relatives
- Familial adenomatous polyposis syndrome

History of ulcerative colitis
- Risk increases 8 to 12 years after diagnosis

Colon polyps or adenomas
Cigarette smoking
- High pack-year history important

Diet low in fiber, high in fat
Obesity (nature of the risk is currently unknown)

Healthy People 2010
Goals and Objectives Related to Colorectal Cancer

1. Reduce the colorectal cancer death rate from a baseline of 21.2 per 100,000 to a target of 13.9 per 100,000.
2. Increase the proportion of adults who receive a colorectal cancer screening examination:
   a. The proportion of adults 50 and over who have had a fecal blood test in the last 2 years
   b. The proportion of adults 50 and over who have ever had a sigmoidoscopy

From US Department of Health and Human Services: *Healthy People 2010: understanding and improving health,* Washington, DC, 2000, USDHHS.

Figure 34-17 illustrates the pattern of incidence of colon cancer by site. A steady shift toward cancer development in the proximal colon has been occurring in recent years. The decline in incidence for Caucasians has primarily been for distal colon and rectal sites. Presently almost 40% of cancers develop in the proximal colon, with about 55% developing in the distal colon and the rectum.[53] This "shift to the right" appears to be more pronounced with advancing age.[42] The development of cancer in the small intestine is extremely rare and accounts for less than 1% of all GI tract malignant tumors.

Pathophysiology

There is strong evidence that almost all bowel cancers arise from preexisting benign adenomatous colon polyps.[23] Polyps occur in about 15% to 20% of the adult population and are increasingly common after age 50. All adenomas are dysplastic by definition and are considered premalignant lesions even though only about 5% actually become malignant. At present there are few indicators to predict which small polyps are likely to mutate, but the severity of the dysplasia is clearly related to the size of the polyp. Malignancy is found in less than 1% of polyps that are less than 1 cm in diameter but is found in 10% of those greater than 2 cm in diameter. The process of transformation is slow. It is theorized that it can take 10 to 12 years for a polyp to undergo malignant transformation[1] (Figure 34-18).

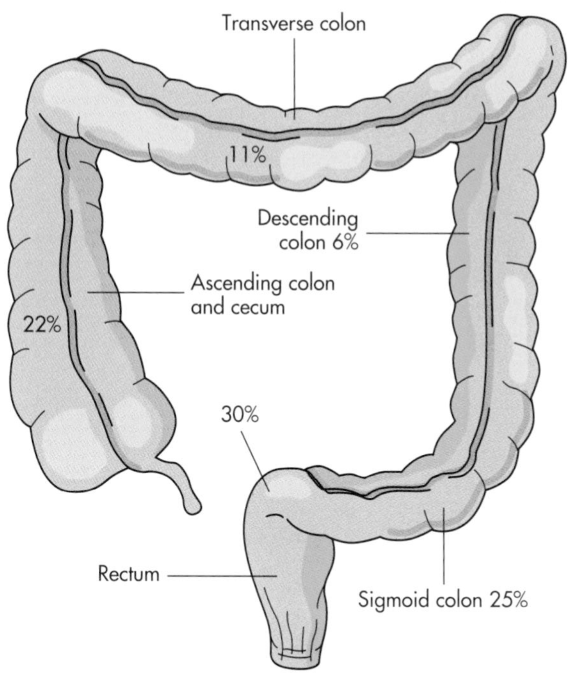

Figure 34-17 Incidence of cancer in various segments of the colon and rectum.

Adenomas may present in various shapes and configurations (Figure 34-19). They are typically round and polypoid (sessile) but may be more elongated and have stalks (pedunculated). Infrequently they appear flat or even depressed. Over time the lesions penetrate the colon wall and extend into the surrounding tissue.

Cancer of the colon may spread by direct extension or through the lymphatic or circulatory system. It may seed at distant points in the peritoneum or the colon. The liver and lungs are the major organs of metastasis. Box 34-4 summarizes Dukes' classification system for staging colorectal cancer. Note that the stage is determined by the degree of invasion of the tumor and not by its size. Staging is used to determine the appropriate treatment. Persons with stage A disease have a 90% 5-year survival rate; those with stage D disease have less than a 5% 5-year survival rate.[35]

The clinical manifestations of colon cancer vary with the location of the tumor. There are usually no early symptoms, and the disease is often diagnosed incidentally.[35] Cancer in the distal colon and rectum typically produces symptoms related to partial obstruction because the left colon is narrower than the right. The lesions are more likely to be annular and grow circumferentially, encircling the colon wall. The lumen becomes narrow and constricted. Obstruction occurs when formed stool is unable to pass through the narrowed lumen.

The patient may experience a change in bowel habits, a feeling of incomplete bowel emptying, or blood in the stool. Obstruction in the right colon is less common because of the larger lumen in this area and the semiliquid nature of the stool. Abdominal pain usually accompanies larger lesions.

BOX 34-4 Dukes' Classification of Colorectal Cancer

Stage A: a small tumor confined to the bowel mucosa; no evidence of lymph node involvement or metastasis
Stage B: progressively larger lesions invading the muscle wall; no evidence of lymph node involvement or metastasis
Stage C: a lesion of any size with lymph node involvement; no evidence of metastasis
Stage D: a lesion of any size with evidence of both lymph node involvement and metastasis; the lesion may be locally unresectable

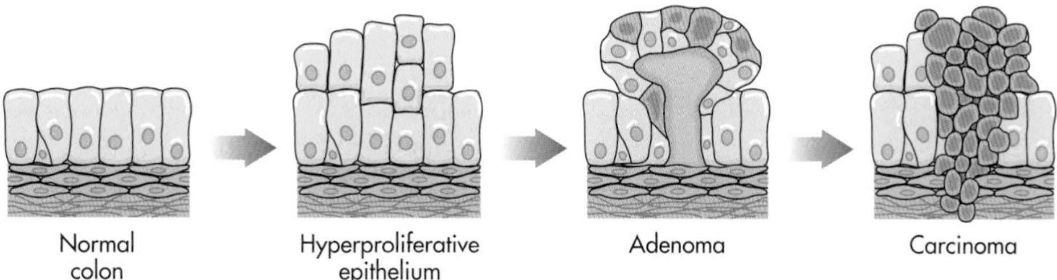

Figure 34-18 Progression to malignancy in bowel cancer.

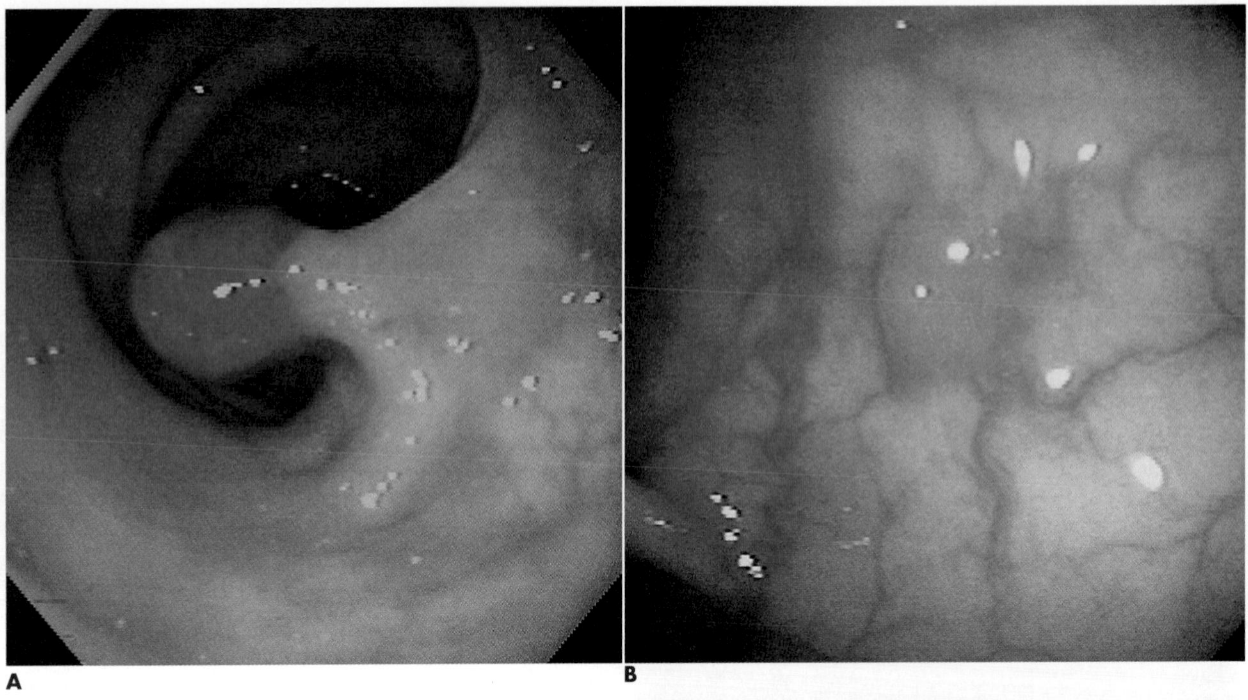

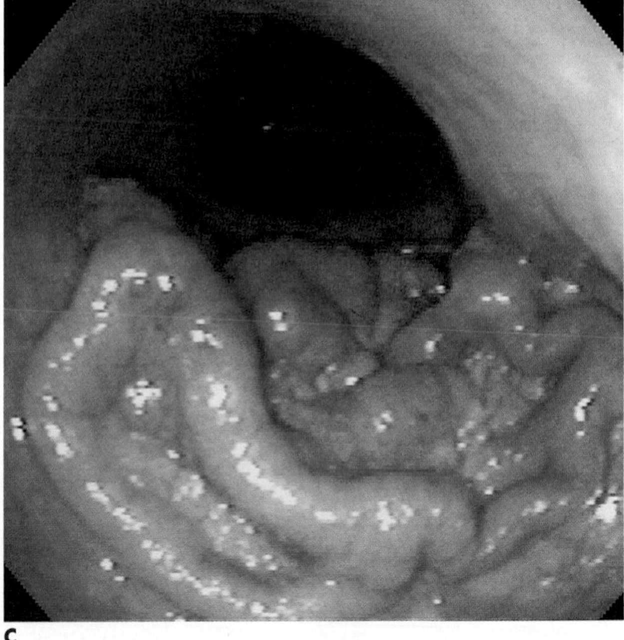

Figure 34-19 **A**, Typical polyp. **B**, Hyperplastic polyp. **C**, Villous adenoma.

Clinical Manifestations

Bowel Cancer

Often asymptomatic and diagnosed incidentally
Symptoms of partial bowel obstruction
- Change in bowel habits (e.g., constipation or diarrhea)
- Pencil- or ribbon-shaped stool
- Sensation of incomplete bowel emptying

Gas or bloating
Occult blood in the stool or rectal bleeding
Weakness, fatigue, malaise, and anorexia
Weight loss
Abdominal pain

Iron deficiency anemia may be present from slow chronic blood loss.

Weakness, malaise, anorexia, and weight loss are nonspecific symptoms that occur often in patients with colorectal cancer. The occurrence of weight loss often accompanies metastases. The tumor occasionally may perforate into the peritoneal cavity, and acute peritonitis occurs before the person notices any other signs of illness. The clinical manifestations of bowel cancer are summarized in the Clinical Manifestations box.

Collaborative Care Management

Diagnostic Tests. Diagnostic technology is currently available that has the theoretic capability to eliminate bowel cancer

BOX 34-5 U.S. Agency for Health Care Policy and Research Guidelines for Colorectal Cancer Screening

It is recommended that the following guidelines be followed in screening adults at average risk for colorectal cancer, beginning at age 50 years:

1. Fecal occult blood testing annually
2. Flexible sigmoidoscopy every 5 years
3. A combination of fecal occult blood testing annually and flexible sigmoidoscopy every 5 years
4. Double-contrast barium enema every 5 to 10 years
5. Colonoscopy every 10 years

From US Agency for Health Care Policy and Research: *Guide to clinical preventive services*, ed 2, Baltimore, 1996, Williams & Wilkins.

as a major cause of death. However, the scope, nature, and effectiveness of colorectal cancer screening remains a topic of significant controversy. Early and accurate diagnosis to enable prompt treatment is the primary goal, since most bowel cancers are slow growing and easily removed in their early stages. The challenge of early diagnosis is obviously enormous, however, since virtually all adults over age 50 are believed to be at average risk and would need to be included in any mass screening program. Research is ongoing to attempt to determine the optimal tests and time intervals for bowel cancer screening, and the literature presents conflicting viewpoints.[40] The issue is of tremendous importance from a cost perspective, since some of the diagnostic options are extremely expensive and their costs are not reimbursed by most private insurance companies. Medicare currently pays for fecal occult blood tests, sigmoidoscopy, and barium enema studies, but not colonoscopy.[40] Screening guidelines developed by the U.S. Agency for Health Care Policy and Research (AHCPR) and endorsed by the American Cancer Society are presented in Box 34-5.

Digital Rectal Examination. Digital rectal examination (DRE) is an integral part of colorectal cancer screening because of its simplicity, low cost, and general acceptability to patients. It is usually performed as part of a routine gynecologic or prostate examination. Figure 34-17 reinforces the fact that up to 30% of all colorectal cancers are found in the rectal region and may be within the reach of the examiner's finger.

Fecal Occult Blood Test. The use of fecal occult blood testing is based on the premise that evolving adenocarcinomas routinely bleed in amounts that are too small to be visible but can be readily detected in laboratory tests. The sensitivity and predictability of these tests are believed to be no more than 50% for cancerous lesions and less than 25% for adenomatous polyps. Both false-positive and false-negative results are often found.[25] Occult blood tests yield false-negative results by missing cancers that were not bleeding at the time of testing and yield false-positive results for which no bleeding source is ever found. Diet and medication can both cause false-positive results. Accurate sampling requires patients to eliminate red meat, aspirin, NSAIDs, turnips, horseradish, and vitamin C from their daily diet for 2 days before and throughout the 3 days of stool sample collection. This is important from a cost perspective, since patients with positive test results are referred for screening via colonoscopy. Fecal occult blood tests are included on most screening guidelines at least partly because of their relatively low cost and general acceptability to patients. The widespread acceptance of fecal occult blood testing despite its limitations is reflected in its inclusion in the Healthy People 2010 objectives, along with sigmoidoscopy (see Healthy People 2010 box on p. 1100). Research is ongoing and shows early promise for a new diagnostic test that identifies the presence of specific antibodies in the stool (see Future Watch box).

Sigmoidoscopy. Flexible fiberoptic sigmoidoscopy allows for good endoscopic visualization of the rectum and descending colon, but it cannot visualize the proximal colon. More than half of all bowel cancers occur within the range of sigmoidoscopy, however, and the bowel preparation is milder and better tolerated than that required for colonoscopy. The cost of sigmoidoscopy is also much lower, since sedation is not required. Sigmoidoscopy remains unacceptable to many patients, however, because of the associated discomfort and the fact that they are awake and aware during the procedure, and its unacceptability decreases its usefulness as a mass screening tool. Research is ongoing to identify the appropriate time interval between screenings for low- and average-risk patients. Five-year intervals are currently recommended.

Barium Enema. High-quality double-contrast barium enemas permit screening of the entire colon and can produce results that are comparable to those of colonoscopy at a significant cost savings. Barium enemas are extremely unpopular with patients, however, because of their significant discomfort. Barium enemas are excellent for outlining large polyps but are relatively ineffective for polyps less than 1 cm in size.

Future Watch

New Screening Test to Detect Bowel Cancer?

Little agreement exists over the appropriate screening to be performed for adults over age 50 in relation to the early diagnosis of colorectal cancer. The current screening programs, which include fecal occult blood testing, sigmoidoscopy, barium enema, and colonoscopy, are prohibitively expensive to consider implementing for the entire adult population, who are all believed to be at least at average risk for developing bowel cancer. A new testing approach may provide an alternative to existing screening modalities. A variety of known DNA mutations associated with colon cancer have been isolated from stool specimens. This new test can detect many of the known DNA mutations and has shown a 90% accuracy in initial testing, which is far above the accuracy rate for fecal occult blood testing.

Colonoscopy is still considered the gold standard for early detection, but this new test could become a mass screening tool that offers greater accuracy and patient acceptability at a reasonable cost. It is anticipated that the test may be commercially available in a few years.

Colonoscopy. Colonoscopy is considered to be the gold standard for colorectal cancer diagnosis, but it is extremely expensive, must be performed by highly trained professionals, requires patients to be sedated, and is associated with an uncomfortable bowel preparation. A major advantage of colonoscopy is the fact that if small lesions are found, they can be immediately removed by a snare that is built directly into the endoscope (Figure 34-20). Screening with fecal occult blood tests and barium enemas requires a second stage to treat any lesions that are discovered. However, at present it would be virtually impossible from a resource perspective to offer colonoscopy screening to the entire adult population. The optimal interval and frequency of screening by colonoscopy has not been proven, but the current recommendation is once every 10 years. Some authorities believe that enormous diagnostic gains could be achieved by screening the entire bowel just once or perhaps twice in a lifetime. A new diagnostic tool that incorporates a miniature camera in a pill is under development as an alternative to colonoscopy (see Future Watch box).

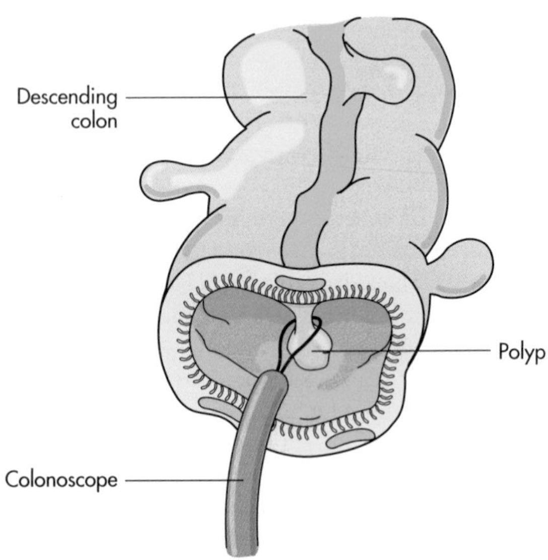

Figure 34-20 Colonoscopy allows for both diagnosis and treatment during the same procedure. A built-in snare attachment can remove any polyps found during the examination.

Future Watch
Endoscopy in a Pill?

Israeli scientists have invented a new approach for endoscopy screening that can visualize the small intestine. The patient is administered a capsule that contains a tiny video camera that transmits images to a receiver that the patient wears on his or her wrist. The physician can then download the images and view them as still images or film. At present the battery pack transmits for up to 6 hours, enough time to film the small intestine. The capsule is expelled from the body within 24 to 48 hours. Current costs are equivalent to routine endoscopy but much less invasive. The future holds the promise of extending the technology to the large bowel as well.

• • •

Any of the diagnostic tests discussed would eventually have to be implemented with the entire over-50 population at what could be a staggering cost. Acceptability of the screening tool to the population is also critical if compliance with guidelines is to be achieved (see Research box). Recommendations concerning colorectal cancer screening clearly have both health care and social policy implications.

Medications. Chemotherapy is primarily palliative in nature and is not used as a primary treatment modality for bowel cancer. It has been shown to improve survival in patients with stage III disease (see Box 34-4).[28,31] 5-Fluorouracil (5-FU) is the drug with the most established record of effectiveness. Current research protocols combine 5-FU with levamisole to stimulate immune system function and minimize the damage to healthy cells. 5-FU is also used routinely as an adjunct to the newer sphincter-sparing surgeries, and the incidence of recurrences is significantly reduced. Because the liver is the most common site of metastasis, portal venous infusion therapy is being researched with small positive outcomes.[31] Chemotherapy may also be administered in combination with radiotherapy, although outcomes have so far been mixed.

Treatments. Radiation is rarely used in the treatment of colon cancer, but it plays an important role in the management of rectal cancer. Anatomic constraints make the rectum less accessible surgically than the colon, and wide excision is rarely possible. Radiation can be used after surgery to reduce the chance of recurrence but appears to be much more effective before surgery. External beam radiation or endocavitary irradiation, in which the radiation source is placed directly on the tumor, may be used. Radiation enteritis is a common complication during treatment, but the incidence of serious complications is only 5% to 6% at major centers.

Research

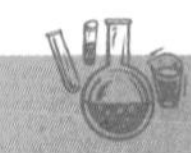

Reference: Centers for Disease Control and Prevention: Screening for colorectal cancer—United States, 1997, *JAMA* 281(17):1581-1582, 1999.

This study attempted to estimate the proportion of the U.S. population that received colorectal screening tests–a home-administered fecal occult blood test, sigmoidoscopy, or proctoscopy. The data were collected as part of the 1997 Behavioral Risk Factor Surveillance System questionnaire. A total of 52,754 persons over 50 years of age were asked whether they had ever had a colorectal screening test and when the test was performed.

Overall, only 39% of respondents reported ever having had a fecal occult blood test and only 41% reported ever having had a sigmoidoscopy or proctoscopy. Women were more likely to have had a fecal blood test, and men were more likely to have had a sigmoidoscopy. African-Americans, Native Americans, and Hispanics were less likely to have had a screening test than were Caucasians. The proportion of respondents who reported having had a test increased with increasing age and was significantly related to health care coverage. The rates for individuals without insurance coverage were 8% for fecal occult blood tests and 16% for sigmoidoscopy.

Surgical Management. Surgery is the definitive treatment for colorectal cancer.[8] It typically involves removal of the tumor, surrounding colon, and lymph nodes (Figure 34-21). When the tumor is located in the ascending, transverse, or descending colon, it usually is possible for the surgeon to perform a resection with end-to-end anastomosis that preserves the natural process of defecation. The specific type of surgery performed depends on the exact location and size of the tumor and the overall condition of the patient. The use of laparoscopic techniques for bowel resection has been shown to be technically difficult but feasible, with the ability to perform all needed local and lymph node dissection.[5] Outcomes of open and laparoscopic surgery appear to be quite similar after 2 to 3 years, but the benefits of decreased length of hospital stay and decreased postoperative morbidity have not been as clear as with other laparoscopic procedures.[6] Right colon disease has been most amenable to treatment laparoscopically.

There are no clear guidelines at this time concerning the use of local versus wide excision and whether or not extensive lymph node dissection should be performed. Local excision is used for Dukes' stage A and some stage B tumors. Wide excision plus adjuvant therapy is used for more aggressive disease.

Patients with tumors in the rectum were previously managed exclusively by removing the entire rectum and anus through a dual-incision procedure called an abdominoperineal resection. The procedure necessitates a permanent colostomy and leaves a significant perineal wound that heals slowly by granulation. The anus is sutured closed. Patients with early localized rectal cancers are now routinely offered the option of a sphincter-sparing procedure. Regional rectal resection is performed, and the rectum is reconstructed with the creation of a pouch from the descending colon.[56] The use of an anastomotic stapler has made these technically difficult procedures feasible. The surgery is performed in two stages with the creation of a temporary ileostomy while adjuvant treatments and healing are completed. The risk of rectal recurrence of the cancer is greater with this type of surgery. Therefore adjuvant therapy with chemotherapy and external beam radiation is also provided. Complications and challenges are similar to those described for patients undergoing a colectomy for ulcerative colitis.

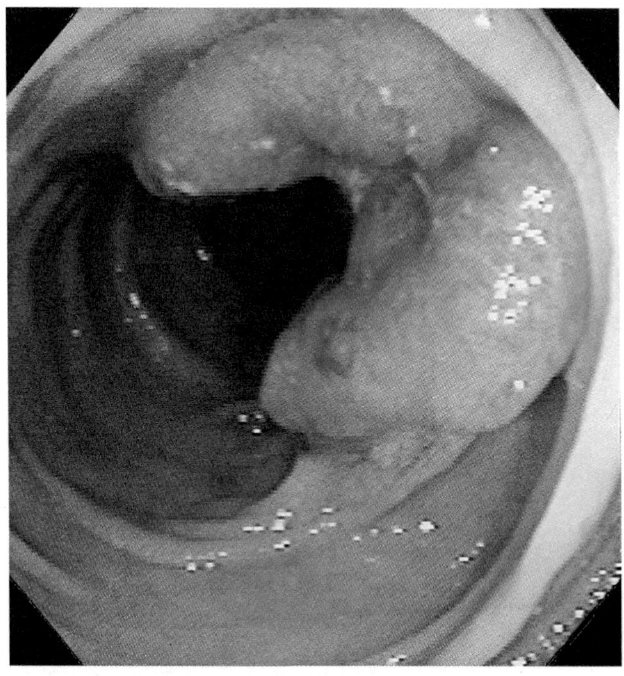

Figure 34-21 Adenocarcinoma of the sigmoid colon.

The newer procedures have significantly reduced the need for permanent colostomies, but temporary colostomies are often created to allow for bowel rest and healing, particularly if bowel obstruction with inflammation occurred preoperatively. Examples of various colostomy procedures are illustrated in Figure 34-11. General nursing care associated with abdominal surgery and ostomy management are discussed on p. 1088.

Diet. No special dietary restrictions are needed for patients with colorectal cancer. Anorexia and weight loss are common early symptoms, and concern may develop over the adequacy of the patient's nutritional status, especially with older adults. The standard treatment approaches also may compromise the patient's nutritional status. Bowel surgery necessitates a period of limited oral intake; aggressive chemotherapy may be accompanied by nausea and/or vomiting; and both external beam and endocavitary irradiation can trigger radiation enteritis.

Low levels of serum albumin are associated with a higher incidence of postoperative complications, especially in older adults. It is essential to consider the patient's nutritional status during all planned treatments.

Activity. The diagnosis of bowel cancer may affect the patient's activity level in several ways. Anemia and fatigue are common early signs of colon cancer. Severe anemia and fatigue often accompany aggressive chemotherapy and radiotherapy. Traditional bowel surgery is very painful and significantly restricts the patient's activity. The patient is encouraged to modify and space activities throughout the day to remain involved in the usual activities of daily living and is encouraged to remain as active as possible throughout all phases of treatment.

Referrals. In some settings the nurse assumes responsibility for making referrals to other services, which commonly include enterostomal therapy and nutritional support.

Enterostomal Therapy. Some patients are treated with surgical procedures that result in permanent ostomies, and it is essential that an enterostomal therapy specialist be involved in the patient's care from the point of admission.

Nutritional Support. The involvement of a nutrition support team may be appropriate at any point in the treatment plan. The team may perform a detailed nutritional assessment and plan for the appropriate use of scheduled meals and supplements to meet the varying needs of the patient. Ensuring adequate protein and calories for healing is essential.

• • •

A sample Clinical Pathway for a patient undergoing colon resection is presented on pp. 1106 and 1107. It summarizes the general care discussed under collaborative and nursing

clinical pathway *Colectomy*

HOSPITAL DAY	CONSULTS	TESTS	ACTIVITY/REST	MEDICAL INTERVENTIONS	MEDICATIONS	NUTRITION	NURSES' SIGNATURES
PTA or Day of Admittance Date: ______	Anesthesia	CBC Urinalysis	Up ad lib		Own, if any	NPO	______
Surgery Date: ______		Lytes if NG H&H or CBC	Up in PM to bathroom with help If A-line: bedrest, turn, cough, deep breathe q2hr Bedside commode with help	IV JP tube(s) NG suction Foley Possible A-line	Analgesics IM, IV, epidural Antibiotics	NPO, I&O	______ ______ ______
Day 1 Date: ______		Lytes if NG H&H or CBC	Walk in hall 4 times with assistance If A-line: turn, cough, deep breathe q2hr when in bed Up in chair	IV JP tube(s) NG to suction Foley A-line	Analgesics IM, IV, epidural Antibiotics	NPO, I&O	______ ______ ______
Day 2 Date: ______	If ordered, internist for resumption of usual meds	Lytes if NG H&H or CBC	Walk in hall at least 4 times with help	JP tube(s) NG to suction Possible to go to clamping schedule, if ordered	Analgesics PO, IM, IV, epidural Antibiotics	NPO, I&O Possible clear liquid (if ordered) If total clamping scheduled (if ordered)	______ ______ ______
Day 3 Date: ______			Walk in hall at least 4 times with help	Possible discontinue NG if ordered Clamping schedule for NG if ordered JP IV	Analgesics IV, PO, IM, epidural Antibiotics	I&O Clear liquid → full liquid late in day if tolerated clear liquids.	______ ______ ______
Day 4 Date: ______			Walk in hall at least 4 times (self-ambulation)	Possible heparin well JP tubes Colostomy or ileostomy	Analgesics PO or IM Antibiotics	Full liquid to diet as tolerated	______ ______ ______
Day 5 Date: ______			Walk in hall at least 4 times (self-ambulation)	Possible heparin line JP tube(s) Colostomy or ileostomy	Analgesics PO Antibiotics	Diet as tolerated	______ ______ ______
Day 6 Date: ______				Heparin line Colostomy/ileostomy			______

PTA or Day of Admittance Date: ______	Lung status Location and nature of pain		Reinforce preop teaching Reassure and encourage patient that numerous people have ostomies and still enjoy active, happy and productive lives	Assess anxiety level	ADL	______ ______ ______
Surgery Date: ______	Lung status Bowel sounds		Reinforce postop teaching	Continue to assess anxiety level Inform of colostomy/ileostomy immediately postop if one was constructed	Assisted ADL	______ ______ ______
Day 1 Date: ______	Lung status Bowel sounds	Assess at home needs	Continue to reinforce postop teaching	Continue to assess anxiety level Patient to look at ostomy area during AM care and ostomy care; if no ostomy, look at incision area/dressing	Assisted ADL	______ ______ ______
Day 2 Date: ______	Lung status Bowel sounds	Assess at home needs Ostomy to see patient if has ostomy.	Continue to reinforce postop teaching Begin ostomy self-care teaching if has ostomy	Continue to assess anxiety level Begin handling ostomy equipment, possibly refer patient to ostomy client if available to decrease sense of isolation	Assisted ADL	______ ______ ______
Day 3 Date: ______	Lung status Bowel sounds	Assess at home needs	Continue to reinforce postop and ostomy teaching If path report indicates malignancy give 1-800-4-CANCER number to patient for access to more information	Continue to assess anxiety level Patient may choose to look at incision when dressing is changed Empty own ostomy pouch	Self ADL	______ ______ ______
Day 4 Date: ______	Lung status Bowel sounds	Assess at home needs	Continue to reinforce postop teaching Continue ostomy teaching and assess patient response	Continue to assess anxiety level Patient may choose to look at incision when dressing is changed Empty own ostomy pouch	Self ADL	______ ______ ______
Day 5 Date: ______	Lung status Bowel sounds	Assess at home needs Continue ostomy teaching, assess pt. response	Continue to reinforce postop teaching	Continue to assess anxiety level Begin/continue self-care of stoma incl. changing bag, skin care per ostomy if appl.	Self ADL	______ ______ ______
Day 6 Date: ______	Lung status Bowel sounds	Assess at home needs Continue ostomy teaching, assess pt. response	Ascertain that patient and family are competent to handle ostomy care (if applicable)	Continue to assess anxiety level Continue assisted/self-care of stoma if appl.	Self ADL	______ ______ ______

From: Cohen EL, Cesta TG: *Nursing case management,* ed 2, St Louis, 1997, Mosby.
ADL, Activities of daily living; *CBC,* complete blood count; *H&H,* hemoglobin and hematocrit; *I&O,* intake and output; *JP,* Jackson Pratt; *Lytes,* electrolytes; *NG,* nasogastric tube; *PTA,* prior to admission.

management. Patients with uncomplicated cases are successfully restarted on oral feedings as soon as peristalsis is reestablished and may be discharged as early as postoperative day 4. When a colostomy is necessary, the patient's care will follow the principles discussed on p. 1088.

NURSING MANAGEMENT OF PATIENT UNDERGOING SURGERY FOR COLORECTAL CANCER

PREOPERATIVE CARE

Most preoperative care is completed in the community before the patient's admission. The diagnosis of cancer adds additional anxiety to the preoperative period and may make it difficult for the patient to understand and retain information about the planned surgery and the care that will be provided in the postoperative period. The nurse ensures that the patient has been adequately prepared for abdominal surgery and general anesthesia.

Bowel cleansing is required. This is accomplished by dietary modifications, mechanical cleansing, and pharmacologic suppression of colon bacteria that might lead to infection in the postoperative period. The patient is placed on a low-residue diet and then a clear liquid diet as surgery approaches. Boluses of vitamins K and C may be given to support clotting and wound healing in the postoperative period because the synthesis and absorption of these vitamins are impaired by the vigorous bowel preparation.

Immediate preparation of the bowel for surgery involves the use of laxatives, enemas, or both. Bowel preparation is performed to cleanse the colon and suppress bacterial growth that might lead to infection in the postoperative period. A solution such as sodium sulfate plus polyethylene glycol (GoLYTELY) provides for an osmotic cleansing of the entire bowel. Up to 4 L is administered orally in divided doses 10 to 15 minutes apart. The cleansing usually is complete in about 4 hours. Systemic or oral antibiotics may be administered to reduce colonic bacteria. Oral neomycin is a standard preparation. If the patient is in good physical condition, bowel preparation is performed at home before admission.

Teaching is another focus of preoperative nursing care. The nurse teaches the patient about the planned surgery and its expected outcomes, including incisions, NG and wound drainage, and the need for an ostomy if applicable. Most patients are extremely concerned about the severity of postoperative pain, and the nurse discusses the plan for postoperative pain management, including the use of patient-controlled analgesia if indicated (see Chapter 12). Pulmonary hygiene is extremely important in the early postoperative period, and the nurse reviews the correct technique for deep breathing, splinting for effective coughing, and the use of an incentive spirometer. The nurse also stresses the importance of early ambulation in preventing respiratory and circulatory complications.

POSTOPERATIVE CARE

Maintaining Fluid and Electrolyte Balance

The patient is kept NPO for brief or extended periods after surgery, and NG suctioning may be in use. NG suctioning was formerly a standard intervention after any bowel surgery, but it is increasingly being either omitted entirely or terminated very quickly, since studies have failed to demonstrate any difference in outcomes for patients who do not develop prolonged ileus.[18] If an NG tube is used, the output from the tube is carefully assessed and recorded, and the tube is irrigated as needed to maintain patency. The nurse evaluates intake and output balance, maintains IV fluids as ordered, records daily weight, and monitors for electrolyte imbalance. Monitoring continues as the patient is gradually advanced to a normal diet.

Early feeding has also become fairly standard, and patients may be kept NPO for the first 24 hours only (see Evidence-Based Practice box). The success of early feeding after laparoscopic surgery has supported this change. The importance of adequate nutrition for wound healing lends support to a policy of limiting the time the patient is kept NPO. The nurse carefully assesses the adequacy of the patient's oral intake as oral feeding is resumed.

Promoting Ventilation

Incisional pain typically is severe with abdominal surgery, and pain can interfere with lung expansion. The nurse monitors the effectiveness of the patient-controlled analgesia system or ensures that adequate opioid analgesia is provided to allow for early ambulation and regular deep breathing. The nurse auscultates regularly for signs of atelectasis and encourages the use of incentive spirometry to keep the alveoli open. Deep

Evidence-Based Practice

Reference: Hartsell PA et al: Early postoperative feeding after elective colorectal surgery, *Arch Surg* 132:518-521, 1997.

The routine use of a nasogastric (NG) tube for decompression after abdominal surgery is being increasingly challenged in clinical practice. Postoperative motility is typically delayed after surgery, and it has been assumed that NG decompression is necessary to manage the problem. This study involved 58 patients undergoing elective colorectal surgery who were randomly assigned to either an early-feeding or traditional-feeding group. The early-feeding group was started on a liquid diet on the first postoperative day. Patients in the traditional-feeding group were not offered liquids until postoperative ileus had resolved. Both groups were advanced to a regular diet when they were able to consume 1000 ml in a 24-hour period.

No significant differences were seen in the rates of nausea or vomiting that occurred in 55% of the early-feeding group and in 50% of the traditional-feeding group. All patients were treated with antiemetics. No significant differences or patterns were noted in the pattern of complications, which were rare in both groups. In this study there was no difference in the hospital length of stay, but patient comfort and satisfaction were increased with the early feeding.

breathing must be performed hourly in the early postoperative days to prevent pulmonary complications.

Supporting Peristalsis

Temporary ileus is an expected complication of bowel surgery resulting from manipulation of the intestines. Prolonged ileus may indicate an abdominal abscess or obstruction. The passage of gas rectally indicates the beginning return of peristalsis. The nurse auscultates the patient's abdomen for bowel sounds every 4 hours and assesses for the movement of gas or presence of distention. Ambulation facilitates the return of peristalsis, and the nurse encourages the patient to be as active as possible. The diet and activity changes plus loss of bowel tissue that accompany resection may make it difficult for the patient to resume a normal elimination pattern. Diarrhea may occur initially, but it usually is temporary and self-limiting. The nurse teaches the patient to avoid constipation through regular exercise, adequate fluids, and adjustment of the fiber content of the diet. Laxatives should be avoided if possible. Patients who undergo coloanal pouch construction, especially older patients, may experience significant problems reestablishing continence.[56]

GERONTOLOGIC CONSIDERATIONS

The incidence of cancer of the bowel is strongly skewed toward the older adult population, and the entire discussion of the disease is targeted at that population. The issues of comorbidity and general health therefore become extremely important. Healthy older adults can withstand the rigors of treatment well, but the concurrent existence of other chronic health problems increases the risk for postoperative complications.

Early diagnosis is often difficult in the older population. Symptoms tend to be underreported and attributed to the effects of aging. This is particularly true concerning symptoms related to digestion and elimination. Chronic constipation is a frequent complaint in this population, and changes in bowel habits may not be reported until the disease is well established.

The challenges of learning an ostomy self-care regimen also may be more significant for older persons, who may have difficulty processing new information and learning new tasks. The presence of arthritis or failing vision may make it difficult for older adults to acquire the psychomotor skills necessary for self-care. The teaching plan needs to be structured to address these concerns and needs to move at a slower pace. Referral for home health follow-up or community based services is appropriate.

SPECIAL ENVIRONMENTS FOR CARE

Critical Care

The standard diagnosis and treatment of bowel cancer do not necessitate the involvement of the critical care team unless serious complications develop. Advancing age has not been shown to be a factor in surgical management unless significant comorbid conditions complicate the patient's care. The rapid proliferation of laparoscopic approaches to bowel surgery can lessen the pain and immobility associated with surgery and further decrease the incidence of complications. The use of sphincter-sparing surgeries lessens the complexity of postoperative wound management even though these surgeries are extremely difficult from a technical point of view.

Community-Based Care

As the acute care hospitalization phase of treatment continues to get shorter, home care considerations for patients with colorectal cancer become increasingly important. It is extremely unlikely that sufficient time will be available for the hospital-based nurse to ensure that the patient can be safely independent in self-care before discharge, especially if the patient is older and has a new ostomy.

Discharge planning must begin at admission. The nurse assesses the patient's home environment and the supports that are available to meet the patient's physical and emotional needs. For older adults, particularly those who live alone, this assessment includes extended family and friendship networks. The involvement of a social worker is helpful to determine insurance and financial qualifications for home care assistance.

Referral for postdischarge assistance may be necessary. Plans for adjuvant treatment with radiation or chemotherapy further deplete the patient's physical and emotional resources. The American Cancer Society can provide much-needed services and support, and direct referral should be made.

COMPLICATIONS

Immediate complications related to bowel cancer are primarily surgical. The surgeries are extensive, and wound complications are a real risk, particularly for elderly patients and those with diabetes. Complications include infection, bleeding, anastomosis leakage, and fistula development. Close monitoring is required in the initial days and weeks.

Patients who undergo extensive lymph node dissection in the pelvic region often experience difficulties with urinary control and may develop sexual dysfunction from disruption of the nerve pathways. These problems may resolve with time or cause permanent disruption in the patient's lifestyle. The use of radiotherapy as an adjuvant therapy is often accompanied by mucosal inflammation that may result in severe and protracted diarrhea. When the patient has a coloanal pouch, this inflammation can result in fecal incontinence. These problems are not easily or quickly resolved, and the patient and family need ongoing support as they attempt to address these challenges in their daily lives.

Long-term concerns are primarily related to the risk of disease recurrence and metastasis. Ongoing disease surveillance is extremely important. Carcinoembryonic antigen is a tumor marker produced in the body in response to the presence of cancer and secreted into the circulation. Its levels can be used to monitor for recurrence, especially when the original cancer is more advanced at the time of diagnosis. Surveillance colonoscopy is typically performed at 3-year intervals unless the patient's clinical status warrants a shorter time interval. The prognosis is primarily related to the degree of invasiveness of the cancer at the time of diagnosis and initial treatment.

This fact reinforces the importance of early diagnosis at the polyp/adenoma stage. Recurrent colorectal cancer is often accompanied by chronic and severe pain, which makes patient comfort an ongoing and challenging goal.

ANORECTAL DISORDERS

A variety of common disorders can affect the perianal area. Persons who experience anorectal disorders typically seek medical care for symptoms such as pain, tenderness, itching, or the development of rectal bleeding. Many of the disorders can be treated on an outpatient basis.

Hemorrhoids

Etiology/Epidemiology

Hemorrhoids are masses of dilated blood vessels that lie beneath the lining of the skin in the anal canal. They result from dilation of the superior and inferior hemorrhoidal veins, which form a plexus, or cushion, in the submucosal layer of the lower rectum.[3] Because this cushion is a normal anatomic feature, virtually all adults are at risk for hemorrhoids, and they are estimated to be present in up to 50% of the population by age 50. Hemorrhoids affect persons of all ages, but they cause increasing problems with age. The exact cause of hemorrhoids remains unclear, but pregnancy is a common initiating condition. Other conditions associated with the development of hemorrhoids include obesity, congestive heart failure, and chronic liver disease with portal hypertension. These conditions are all associated with persistent elevations in intraabdominal pressure. Sedentary occupations that involve long periods of sitting or standing also are implicated, although the exact mechanism is not known. Chronic constipation has long been considered a risk factor, but the presence of diarrheal diseases such as IBD has actually been shown to be a greater risk factor.[3]

Hemorrhoids usually are classified into two types. Those that occur above the anal sphincter are classified as internal hemorrhoids, and those that occur below the anal sphincter are classified as external hemorrhoids (Figure 34-22). Internal hemorrhoids are further classified by size, since size determines both the nature and severity of symptoms and the appropriate management. Individuals often have both forms of hemorrhoids at the same time. Box 34-6 presents the grading scale for hemorrhoids. Although hemorrhoids usually are a chronic health problem, they may cause acute episodes.

Pathophysiology

Hemorrhoids traditionally have been viewed as varicose veins of the rectum. The superior hemorrhoidal veins contain no valves and are vulnerable to overdistention when the person is in an upright position. Age and other predisposing factors are theorized to promote deterioration of the anchoring and connective tissue, allowing the vessels to bulge and descend.[3] Additional studies have documented that hemorrhoids actually are composed of spongy vascular tissue and share similarities with arteriovenous malformations. The oxygen content of the blood is much higher than would be expected in a simple dilated vein.[3]

External hemorrhoids are seen most often in young and middle-aged adults and can be detected by the affected person. The classic "skin tag" consists of small lumps of fibrous tissue and folds of anal skin that have been stretched by bulging of the hemorrhoids (Figure 34-23). They rarely bleed and become truly symptomatic only when they become thrombosed or rupture subcutaneously with hematoma formation. A thrombosed external hemorrhoid may occur suddenly after vigorous exercise or after a severe episode of diarrhea or constipation. The intense pain accompanying thrombosis is caused by the presence of multiple sensory nerve endings in the epithelial tissue that composes the hemorrhoid. Bluish skin-covered lumps are readily visible in the anal region, and the thrombosed hemorrhoids are quite large and may encompass the entire anus.

Box 34-6 Hemorrhoidal Grading Scale

First degree: the hemorrhoid bulges into the lumen of the anorectal canal but does not protrude through the anus.

Second degree: the hemorrhoid prolapses out of the anus with defecation or straining but spontaneously returns to its normal anatomic position.

Third degree: the hemorrhoid prolapses out of the anus with defecation or straining and requires manual reduction to return it to its normal anatomic position.

Fourth degree: the hemorrhoid prolapses out of the anus, is irreducible, and is at risk for strangulation.

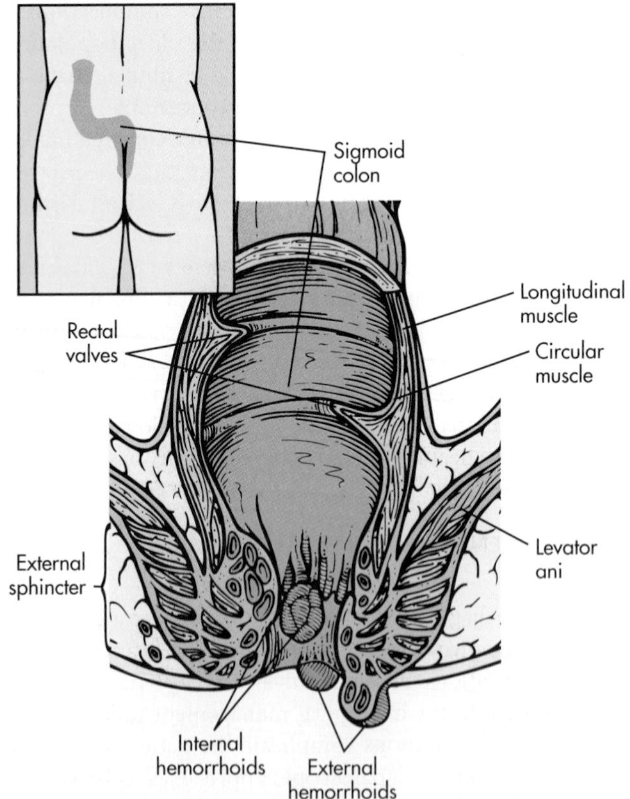

Figure 34-22 Internal and external hemorrhoids.

Internal hemorrhoids are usually asymptomatic. Excessive engorgement and prolapse occur, but painless rectal bleeding is their most common feature. The person may notice spotting on the toilet tissue or occasional episodes of spurts of blood that accompany defecation. Hemorrhoids are the most common cause of rectal bleeding, and the development of bleeding usually causes the person to seek treatment. Although the blood loss typically is small, it can deplete iron reserves if it persists over a long period. Internal hemorrhoids can be uncomfortable but rarely cause significant pain unless strangulation and prolapse occur. These conditions interfere with the blood supply to the area and require immediate surgical correction.[3]

Hemorrhoids of both types are basically asymptomatic unless complications occur. Routinely painful defecation accompanied by rectal bleeding is more commonly associated with anal fissure than with uncomplicated hemorrhoids. Perianal itching may occur with higher-grade internal hemorrhoids, but other causes should also be explored. If the hemorrhoids cause pain or bleeding, the patient may develop constipation in an effort to limit defecation.

Collaborative Care Management

The diagnosis of hemorrhoids is fairly straightforward. The person's presenting symptoms establish the initial diagnosis, which usually can be confirmed by inspection and digital palpation. Proctoscopy or sigmoidoscopy may be used to confirm the diagnosis, and middle-aged or older patients who are experiencing rectal bleeding may undergo colonoscopy to rule out cancer. Occult blood in the stool is not associated with hemorrhoids.

Both forms of hemorrhoids can be managed conservatively if the symptoms are not severe. Conservative management includes a high-fiber diet, bulk-forming laxatives, warm sitz baths, and gentle cleansing. If severe pain, bleeding, or thrombosis is present, however, more definitive management may be indicated. A variety of treatment options are available, including sclerotherapy, cryotherapy, bipolar diathermy, rubber band ligation, and surgical hemorrhoidectomy. Currently grades 2 and 3 internal hemorrhoids are treated with rubber band ligation, and complicated grades 3 and 4 hemorrhoids are treated with surgery. Patients with thrombosed external hemorrhoids that are diagnosed promptly can be treated with surgical evacuation or excision with the patient under local anesthesia. The wound is left open to heal by secondary intention. Most thrombosed external hemorrhoids resolve spontaneously after 48 to 72 hours.[3] Complicated prolapses may require surgery.

Rubber Band Ligation. Internal hemorrhoids may be treated with ligation with latex bands. No anesthesia is required, the treatment can take place in a physician's office, and the procedure is both cost-effective and extremely successful.[3] The hemorrhoid is grasped with forceps and pulled down into a special instrument that slips a latex band over the hemorrhoid and onto the rectal mucosa above it (Figure 34-24). The band constricts the circulation and causes necrosis, and the tissue usually sloughs off within a week. Submucosal scarring and fibrosis prevent the development of new hemorrhoidal tissue. An enema is given before the treatment to prevent a bowel movement for the first 24 hours, thus preventing straining that could cause the band to break or slip off. Local discomfort is usually minimal and can be successfully relieved by NSAIDs or acetaminophen and the use of sitz baths.

Sclerotherapy. The injection method can be effective for treating first- and second-degree small, bleeding internal hemorrhoids. A sclerosing solution such as 5% phenol in oil is injected into the hemorrhoidal tissue, producing an intense inflammatory reaction. Fibrous induration occurs at the site of the injection, adhering the mucosa to the underlying muscle. The procedure is palliative and not curative, and repeat injection may be required in the future. However, it is extremely

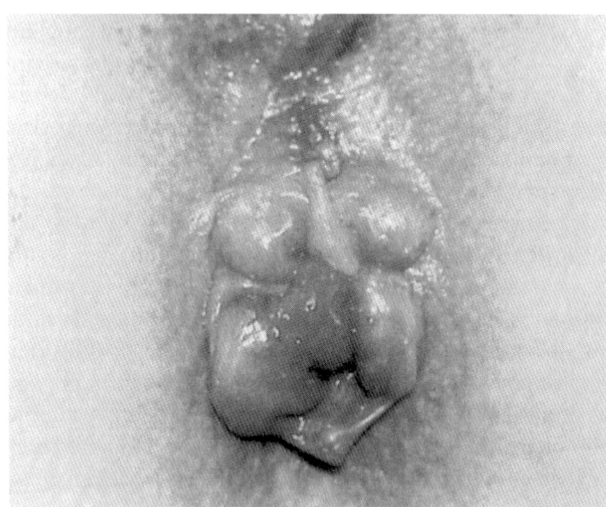

Figure 34-23 External hemorrhoids.

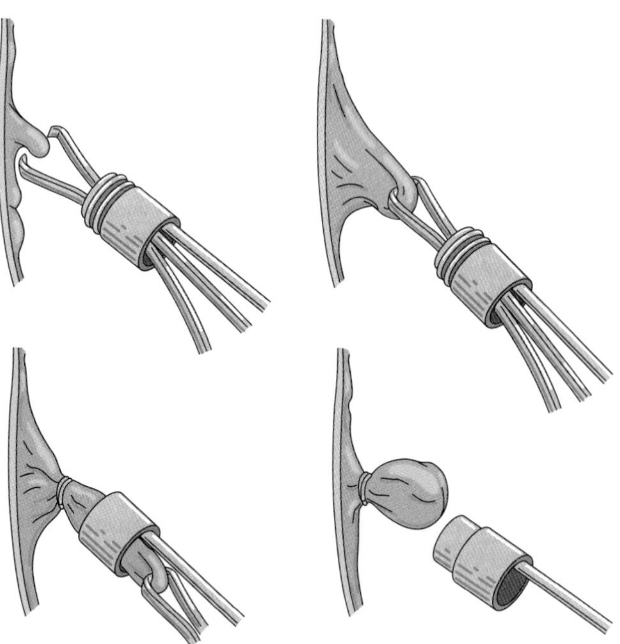

Figure 34-24 Rubber band ligation of an internal hemorrhoid.

Guidelines for Safe Practice

The Patient Undergoing Anorectal Surgery

PREOPERATIVE CARE

Bowel preparation is standard, but an enema may not be prescribed if rectal pain is acute.
Stool softeners may be given to promote a soft stool before surgery.

POSTOPERATIVE CARE

Promotion of Comfort

Administer analgesics as prescribed, especially before initial defecation (considerable rectal discomfort may be present).
Provide emotional support before and after first defecation.
Suggest a side-lying position.
Provide sitz baths as ordered (monitor for hypotension secondary to dilation of pelvic blood vessels in early postoperative period).

Promotion of Elimination

Administer prescribed stool softeners.
Encourage patient to defecate as soon as inclination occurs (prevents strictures and preserves the normal anal lumen). Considerable anxiety is usually present.
Monitor for hypotension, dizziness, and faintness during first defecation.
If an enema must be given, use a small-bore rectal tube.

Patient Teaching

Clean the rectal area after each defecation until healing is complete (a sitz bath is recommended).
Avoid constipation with a high-fiber diet, high-fluid intake, regular exercise, and regular time for defecation.
Use stool softeners until healing is complete.
Seek medical consultation for rectal bleeding, suppurative drainage, continued pain on defecation, or continued constipation despite preventive measures.

economical and is rarely associated with complications, making it an appropriate choice for selected patients.

Cryosurgery and Photocoagulation. Cryosurgery and photocoagulation use a probe to expose the hemorrhoidal tissue to liquid nitrogen, radiation, or another agent. Local tissue destruction occurs, and the tissue then gradually necroses and sloughs off, causing a foul-smelling discharge for several days or more. The drainage limits the acceptability of the treatment, which is also very expensive because of the complexity of the equipment.

Hemorrhoidectomy. Surgical excision (hemorrhoidectomy) is the treatment used for most third-degree hemorrhoids, all fourth-degree and strangulated hemorrhoids, and other hemorrhoids that have not responded to more conservative therapy. It is usually necessary in less than 10% of persons with symptomatic hemorrhoids.[3] The procedure involves the excision of all involved tissue with careful preservation of the anal sphincter. Care of the patient after anorectal surgery is summarized in the Guidelines for Safe Practice box.

Patient/Family Education. Minor problems with hemorrhoids often can be successfully managed through a combination of strict personal hygiene and prevention of constipation and straining. The nurse encourages the patient to follow a high-residue diet rich in fruit and vegetable fiber. Bran may be added to the diet to ease stool passage. A liberal intake of fluids and regular exercise also are encouraged to promote normal bowel function. If necessary, a bulk-forming hydrophilic laxative may be added to the person's daily routine.

Local treatment promotes comfort during symptom flare-ups. The patient is instructed to apply ice, warm compresses, or analgesic ointments such as dibucaine (Nupercaine) to provide temporary relief from pain and reduce the edema around external or prolapsed internal hemorrhoids. Sitz baths also are extremely helpful in relieving pain and supporting cleanliness. The nurse stresses the importance of good personal hygiene after defecation and thorough cleansing of the bathtubs or containers used for sitz baths.

Anal Fissures, Abscesses, and Fistulas

Etiology/Epidemiology

Anal fissures, fistulas, and abscesses are relatively common problems that develop from trauma or infection in the anorectal area. An anal fissure is a painful elongated tear between the anal canal and the perianal skin. Fissures may be primary or secondary. Most primary fissures are idiopathic and occur in young and middle-age adults. Ninety percent are found along the posterior midline.[3] Secondary fissures are associated with chronic constipation and the passage of hard stool, trauma, or the presence of chronic ulceration from IBD. Anal abscesses result most often from the obstruction of gland ducts in the anorectal region by feces, but they also may complicate the presence of a fissure. They occur twice as often in men, usually during the third and fourth decades. Stasis of duct contents results in acute infection that can spread to adjacent tissue. An anal fistula involves the development of an abnormal communication between the anal canal and skin outside the anus. The rupture and drainage of infected material from an abscess often causes the fistula.

Pathophysiology

Most acute anal fissures are superficial and heal spontaneously or in response to conservative therapy. If healing does not occur, however, the fissure may cause significant bleeding or become infected. The infection of an abscess may be relatively minor and confined to a single rectal crypt or become widespread. Widespread infection or sepsis may develop in patients with immunodeficiencies. The development of a fistula may necessitate extensive surgical repair.

Pain is the primary problem associated with anal fissures and abscesses. It can be severe and prolonged from pressure on the somatic nerves in the perianal area. Any position can be painful, since the pain often is widespread. Constipation is inevitable because the patient attempts to avoid pain by preventing defecation. Local swelling, erythema, and acute tenderness accompany abscess development. Pruritus in the anal region often accompanies both fissures and fistulas. When a fistula is present, the patient notices periodic purulent drainage, which stains undergarments.

TABLE 34-6 Treatment Options for Anal Fissure, Abscess, and Fistula

Lesion	Clinical Manifestations	Medical Management
Fissure		
Slitlike ulceration in epithelium of anal canal	Pain with defecation; bleeding; pruritus; constipation	Stool softeners; analgesic ointments; sitz bath; sphincterotomy or fissurectomy if medical therapy ineffective
Abscess		
Abscess in tissue around anus	Persistent throbbing; anal pain with walking, sitting, defecation; systemic signs of infection	Incision and drainage of abscess
Fistula		
Hollow track leading through anal tissue from anorectal canal through skin near anus	Purulent discharge near anus; pain; pruritus	Fistulotomy or fistulectomy

BOX 34-7 Selected Websites

Crohn's and Colitis Foundation of America
http://www.ccfa.org
National Digestive Diseases Information Clearinghouse
http://www.niddk.nih.gov
United Ostomy Association
http://www.uoa.org

Collaborative Care Management

The degree of medical intervention necessary for anal fissures, abscesses, and fistulas depends on the exact nature and severity of the problem. Medical treatment options are outlined in Table 34-6. Prompt surgical treatment is extremely important because the risk of overwhelming sepsis from an abscess is extremely high. Initial nursing interventions for anal disorders focus on improving the patient's comfort level. These may include analgesics, sitz baths, and the local application of heat, cold, or astringent preparations such as witch hazel. Analgesics are often required. These interventions are also important if the patient is undergoing surgical excision or repair. The repair of fistulas is technically more involved, and nursing interventions focus on restoring and maintaining skin integrity and ensuring adequate nutrition for healing.

Patient/Family Education. Patient education focuses on the prevention of recurrences. The nurse teaches the patient the importance of careful perianal hygiene and of avoiding constipation. All standard measures are presented, including a diet rich in fiber, the selective addition of bran to the diet, adequate intake of fluids, exercise, and the use of stool softeners or bulk-forming laxatives to prevent straining. See Box 34-7 for additional information.

Critical Thinking Questions

1. A woman has been admitted to the hospital with a diagnosis of acute diverticulitis. She has experienced mild episodes in the past, but this one is severe and has quickly led to perforation. She has developed acute peritonitis and is now extremely ill. While you are administering an antibiotic, she asks you how she became so sick. It is obvious that she is worried that she may not get better. How could you best explain the complication of peritonitis and its treatment to her?
2. An 18-year-old first-year nursing student was recently diagnosed with ulcerative colitis. She has lost 20 pounds in the past 8 weeks from persistent, severe diarrhea, which occurs every 1 to 2 hours and causes occasional fecal incontinence at night. She is fatigued and anorexic, but she desperately wants to continue with her education. What specific concerns would you anticipate that she would have about her disease and treatment regimen? What modifications would you recommend that she make in her lifestyle to attempt to meet her goal? What resources would you refer her to?
3. A 34-year-old woman has been successfully managing her ulcerative colitis since its diagnosis 12 years ago. She has experienced only occasional exacerbations, which have thus far responded promptly to short courses of high-dose steroids. Her physician told her recently that it is about time for her to think seriously about having a complete colectomy. She is very upset at the prospect of surgery and wants things to continue "as they are." What is the rationale for the physician's recommendation? How important is it to her future health and well-being? What alternatives, if any, exist?
4. Early diagnosis is clearly critically important in the management of colorectal cancer. Consider our current state of knowledge, and take and defend a position concerning the appropriate mass screening for adults over age 50. Consider economics, effectiveness, high-risk groups, and resources in your answer.

References

1. Ahsan H et al: Family history of colorectal adenomatous polyps and increased risk for colorectal cancer, *Ann Intern Med* 128(11):900-905, 1998.
2. Ball EM: A teaching guide for continent ileostomy, *RN* 63(12):35-40, 2000.
3. Barnett JL: Anorectal diseases. In Yamada T, editor: *Textbook of gastroenterology,* ed 3, Philadelphia, 1999, JB Lippincott.
4. Baron JA et al: Calcium supplements for the prevention of colorectal adenomas, *N Engl J Med* 340(2):101-107, 1999.
5. Bokey EL et al: Laparoscopic resection of the colon and rectum for cancer, *Br J Surg* 84:822-825, 1997.

6. Bouvet M et al: Clinical, pathologic, and economic parameters of laparoscopic colon resection for cancer, *Am J Surg* 176(6):554-558, 1998.
7. Breitfeller JM: Peritonitis, *Am J Nurs* 99(4):33, 1999.
8. Breuer-Katschinski B et al: Alcohol and cigarette smoking and the risk of colorectal adenomas, *Dig Dis Sci* 45(3):487-493, 2000.
9. Bryant D, Fleischer I : Changing an ostomy appliance, *Nursing* 30(11):51-53, 2000.
10. Cees JHM et al: Ileoneorectal anastomosis, *Ann Surg* 230(6): 757-758, 1999.
11. Cerrato PL: When food is the culprit, *RN* 62(6):52-54, 1999.
12. Ferzoco CB, Raptopoulos V, Silen W: Acute diverticulitis, *N Engl J Med* 338(21):1521-1526, 1998.
13. Fuchs CS et al: Dietary fiber and the risk of colorectal cancer and adenoma in women, *N Engl J Med* 340(3):169-176, 1999.
14. Goroll AH: Management of diverticular disease. In Goroll AH, Mulley AG, editors: *Primary care medicine,* ed 4, Philadelphia, 2000, JB Lippincott.
15. Grodstein F et al: Postmenopausal hormone use and risk for colorectal cancer and adenoma, *Ann Intern Med* 128(9):705-712, 1998.
16. Hanauer SB et al: Advances in the management of Crohn's disease: economic and clinical potential of infliximab, *Clin Ther* 20:1009, 1998.
17. Hanauer SB et al: Updating the approach to Crohn's disease, *Hosp Pract* 34(8):81-83, 87-93, 1999.
18. Hartsell PA et al: Early postoperative feeding after elective colorectal surgery, *Arch Surg* 132:518-521, 1997.
19. Heitkemper M, Jarrett M: Irritable bowel syndrome, *Am J Nurs* 101(1):26-32, 2001.
20. Kamen BJ: Battling lower GI bleeding, *Nursing* 29(8):32 hn1-hn6, 1999.
21. Klonowski E, Masoodi J: The patient with Crohn's disease, *RN* 62(3):32-37, 1999.
22. Kornbluth A, Sachar DB: Ulcerative colitis practice guidelines in adults: American College of Gastroenterology practice parameters committee, *Am J Gastroenterol* 92:204-210, 1997.
23. Kuwada SK: Colorectal cancer 2000, *Postgrad Med* 107(5):96-107, 2000.
24. Levin B, Hess K, Johnson C: Screening for colorectal cancer, *Arch Intern Med* 157:970-976, 1997.
25. Lewis AM: Gastrointestinal emergency, *Nursing* 29(4):52-54, 1999.
26. Liem MS et al: Comparison of conventional anterior surgery and laparoscopic surgery for inguinal hernia repair, *N Engl J Med* 336(21):1541-1544, 1997.
27. Logan RFA: Inflammatory bowel disease incidence: up, down or unchanged? *Gut* 42:309-311, 1998.
28. Mahoney T et al: Stage III colon cancers: why adjuvant chemotherapy is not offered to elderly patients, *Arch Surg* 135(2):182-185, 2000.
29. Mead PS et al: Food-related illness and death in the United States, *Emerg Infect Dis* 5(5):1-39, 2000.
30. Meaghr AP et al: Jileal pouch–anal anastomosis for chronic ulcerative colitis: complications and long term outcomes in 1310 patients, *Br J Surg* 85:800-803, 1998.
31. Midgley RS, Kerr DJ: Adjuvant therapy of colorectal cancer, *Hosp Pract* 35(5):55-62, 2000.
32. Moody FG, Calabuig R: Abdominal cavity: anatomy, structural anomalies, and hernias. In Yamada T, editor: *Textbook of gastroenterology,* ed 3, Philadelphia, 1999, JB Lippincott.
33. Mowschenson PM, Critchlow JF, Peppercorn MA: Ileoanal pouch operation: long-term outcome with or without diverting ileostomy, *Arch Surg* 135(4):463-466, 2000.
34. Nissan A et al: A more liberal approach to the surgical treatment of Crohn's disease, *Am J Surg* 174(3):339-341, 1997.
35. Pontieri-Lewis V: Colorectal cancer: prevention and screening, *MedSurg Nurs* 9(1):9-13, 2000.
36. Prier R, Solnick JV: Foodborne and waterborne infectious diseases, *Postgrad Med* 107(4):245-255, 2000.
37. Provenzale D et al: Health related quality of life after ileoanal pull through, *Gastroenterology* 113(1):7-14, 1997.
38. Rampton DS: Management of Crohn's disease, *BMJ* 319:1480-1485, 1999.
39. Rayhorn N: Understanding inflammatory bowel disease, *Nursing* 29(12):57-61, 1999.
40. Read TE, Kodner IJ: Colorectal cancer: risk factors and recommendations for early detection, *Am Fam Physician* 59(11):3083-3092, 2001.
41. Richter JM: Approach to the patient with chronic constipation. In Goroll AH, Mulley AG, editors: *Primary care medicine,* ed 4, Philadelphia, 2000, JB Lippincott.
42. Saltzstein SL, Behling CA, Savides TJ: The relation of age, race, and gender to the subsite location of colorectal carcinoma, *Cancer* 82(7):1408-1410, 1998.
43. Schatzkin A et al: Lack of effect of a low-fat, high-fiber diet on the recurrence of colorectal adenomas, *N Engl J Med* 342(16):1149-1155, 2000.
44. Slattery ML et al: Carotenoids and colon cancer, *Am J Clin Nutr* 71(2):575-582, 2000.
45. Smalley W et al: Use of nonsteroidal anti-inflammatory drugs and incidence of colorectal cancer: a population-based study, *Arch Intern Med* 159(2):161-166, 1999.
46. Standler RS et al: Aspirin and nonsteroidal anti-inflammatory agents and risk for colorectal adenomas, *Gastroenterology* 114:441-447, 1998.
47. Summers RW: Approach to the patient with ileus and obstruction. In Yamada T, editor: *Textbook of gastroenterology,* ed 3, Philadelphia, 1999, JB Lippincott.
48. Taschieri AM et al: Description of new "bowel-sparing" techniques for long strictures of Crohn's disease, *Am J Surg* 173(6):509-512, 1997.
49. Thomas GAO et al: Role of smoking in inflammatory bowel disease: implications for therapy, *Postgrad Med J* 76:273-279, 2000.
50. Thompson J: A practical ostomy guide, *RN* 63(11):61-66, 2000.
51. Tramonte SM et al: The treatment of chronic constipation in adults: a systematic review, *J Gen Intern Med* 12:15-20, 1997.
52. Tremaine WJ, Sandborn WJ: Practice guidelines for inflammatory bowel disease: an instrument for assessment, *Mayo Clin Proceed* 74:495-499, 1999.
53. Troisi RJ, Freedman AM, Devesa SS: Incidence of colorectal carcinoma in the U.S., *Cancer* 85(8):1670-1676, 1999.
54. US Department of Health and Human Services: *Healthy People 2010: understanding and improving health,* Washington, DC, 2000, USDHHS.
55. Yamamoto T et al: Outcome of strictureplasty for duodenal Crohn's disease, *Br J Surg* 86:259-262, 1999.
56. Young M: Caring for patients with coloanal reservoirs for rectal cancer, *Med Surg Nurs* 9(4):193-197, 2000.

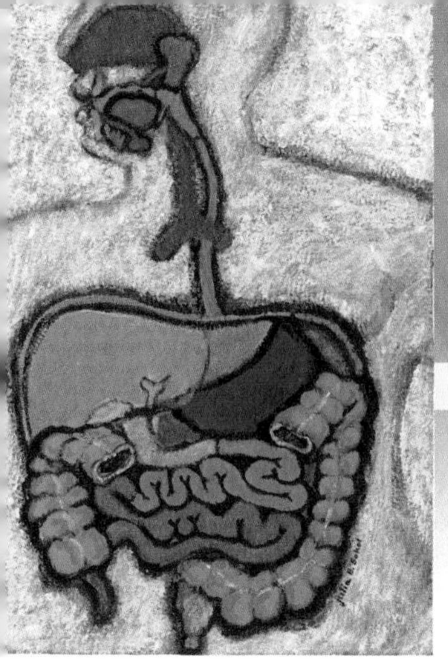

Gallbladder and Exocrine Pancreatic Problems

35

Judith K. Sands

Objectives

After studying this chapter, the learner should be able to:

1. Describe the etiology, epidemiology, and pathophysiology of cholelithiasis, cholecystitis, and cancer of the biliary tract.
2. Compare treatment alternatives for biliary tract disease.
3. Describe the nursing care needs of patients with disorders of the biliary system.
4. List the causes of acute and chronic pancreatitis.
5. Explain the pathophysiologic basis for signs and symptoms of acute and chronic pancreatitis.
6. Discuss management approaches for acute and chronic pancreatitis, and pancreatic tumors.
7. Develop nursing diagnoses, patient outcomes, and nursing interventions for patients who have acute or chronic pancreatitis or cancer of the pancreas.

PROBLEMS OF THE GALLBLADDER

Problems of the biliary system include obstruction, inflammation, infection, and cancer. Gallbladder disorders are extremely common and affect millions of adults every year.

Cholelithiasis/Cholecystitis/Choledocholithiasis

Etiology

Gallstones can occur anywhere in the biliary tree. The term *cholelithiasis* refers to stone formation in the gallbladder and represents the most common biliary disorder. Either acute or chronic inflammation, termed *cholecystitis,* can result and is usually precipitated by the presence of stones. When stones form in or migrate to the common bile duct, the condition is termed *choledocholithiasis.* Figure 35-1 illustrates common sites for gallstones.

More than 80% of gallstones are composed of cholesterol.[20] The remaining are pigmented stones, which are further classified as black or brown. Although the precise etiology of gallstones remains unknown, it is theorized that an imbalance in bile components that leads to supersaturation and crystallization plays a major role.[20] Because most healthy individuals experience supersaturation of the bile at various times without developing gallstones, it is clear that other factors such as gastrointestinal (GI) motility are also involved. Risk factors for gallstones are well known and are listed in the Risk Factors box. They include various clinical states associated with changes in cholesterol formation and excretion. The development of pigmented stones is linked to disease states such as cirrhosis, hemolytic disease, and chronic small bowel disease. Prevention of gallstone disease is not yet a realistic goal, but the Future Watch box presents some options that are currently being explored.[8,17]

Epidemiology

Cholelithiasis is an extremely common health problem in the United States. An estimated 20 to 25 million adults have gallstones, but since only about 20% of them ever develop symptomatic disease, these figures are simply estimates.[7,20] About 1 million new cases are diagnosed each year, and the overall incidence appears to have increased in the past 30 years.[1]

The prevalence of gallstones varies widely around the world and among various ethnic groups. In the United States the disease is more common in Caucasians and Hispanics and rare in African-Americans.[20] Gallstones are two to three times more common in women than in men, and the incidence increases steadily with age.[7] Obesity appears to be a significant factor.

Symptomatic gallbladder disease is one of the most common GI disorders requiring hospitalization, and 700,000 gallbladder surgeries are performed each year.[7] Treatment costs exceed $5 billion annually.[20] Once the disease becomes symptomatic, the risk of complications is 1% to 3% annually.

Pathophysiology

Bile is primarily composed of water plus conjugated bilirubin, organic and inorganic ions, small amounts of proteins,

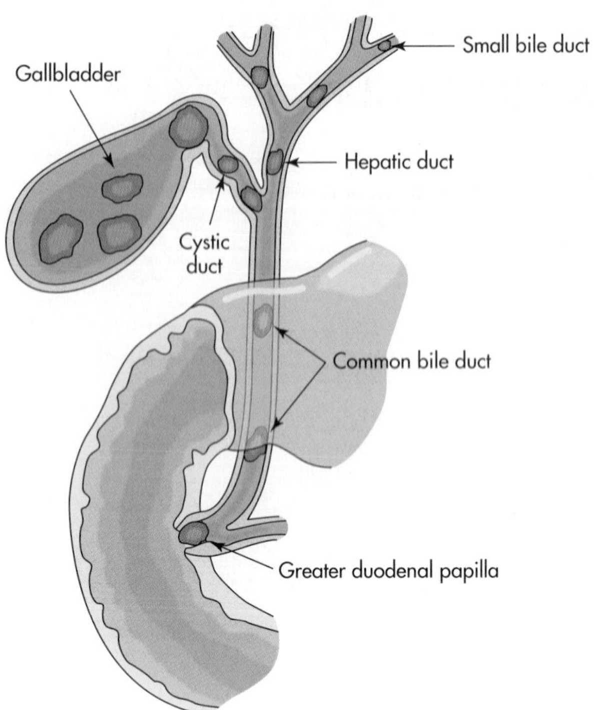

Figure 35-1 Common sites of gallstones.

Risk Factors

Cholesterol Gallstones

Gender: two to three times as common in women
Obesity: particularly in women; risk increased by 45% in morbidly obese patients
Middle age: risk increases with age
Rapid weight loss (~5 pounds/week)
Caucasian, Native American, Hispanic race
Pregnancy, multiparity, use of oral contraceptives
Hypercholesterolemia, use of anticholesterol medications
Diseases of the ileum

Future Watch

Preventing Gallstone Disease?

Gallbladder disease is a pervasive problem among adults in the United States, and until recently there was no indication that the development of gallstones might be preventable through lifestyle changes. Recent studies, however, show early evidence that exercise may play an important role in delaying the development of symptomatic gallstone disease. Thirty minutes of endurance-type physical exercise significantly reduced the risk of symptomatic gallstones in a trial group of men, and there was indication that moderate-intensity exercise might also have a beneficial effect.

Coffee consumption is also theorized to prevent symptomatic gallstone disease, possibly because it triggers the release of cholecytokinin, which promotes gallbladder emptying. It is unclear whether this effect is attributable to caffeine or to another component of coffee.

and three lipids—bile salts, lecithin, and cholesterol. When the balance of these three lipids remains intact, cholesterol is held in solution. If the balance is upset, cholesterol can begin to precipitate. Cholesterol gallstone formation is enhanced by the production of a mucin glycoprotein, which traps cholesterol particles. Twenty percent of biliary cholesterol comes from new synthesis, but the association with serum cholesterol levels remains unclear. Excess secretion is associated with aging, obesity, and the effects of certain drugs and hormones.[20] Supersaturation of the bile with cholesterol also impairs gallbladder motility and contributes to stasis. The gallbladder has the ability to absorb excess water and concentrate bile, which further complicates the picture of supersaturation and stasis.[20]

Cholesterol stones are soft, yellowish green, and radiolucent. They range in size from 1 mm to 2.5 cm.[4] The stones most commonly occur in multiples but can be solitary. The process of stone formation is slow. Stones are theorized to grow steadily for 2 to 3 years and then stabilize in size. Eighty-five percent are less than 2 cm in diameter. Most are found in the gallbladder, but 15% to 60% of persons older than age 60 who undergo surgery for gallstones are also found to have stones in the common bile duct.[7]

Black-pigmented stones result from an increase in unconjugated bilirubin and calcium with a corresponding decrease in bile salts. Impaired gallbladder motility may also be a factor. Black stones are very small, hard, and usually numerous. Brown stones develop in the intrahepatic and extrahepatic ducts and are usually preceded by bacterial infection.

Although most persons with gallstones are asymptomatic, cholecystitis can develop at any time, usually from obstruction of the cystic duct by the stone or from edema and spasm initiated by the presence or passage of the stone.[7] In acute cholecystitis the gallbladder is enlarged and tense. A secondary bacterial infection can occur within several days and is the cause of most of the serious consequences of the disease.

Biliary colic is the classic clinical manifestation of symptomatic gallstones in 70% to 80% of persons.[20] It is caused by spasm of the gallbladder or transient obstruction but is not associated with inflammation of the mucosa.[7] Biliary colic causes sudden-onset sharp pain that may occur anywhere in the upper abdomen or epigastrium. The pain may be steady or intermittent, may last for minutes to hours, and may localize to the right upper quadrant (RUQ) or radiate to the back or right shoulder. It may awaken the patient at night or occur after a heavy, fatty meal.[20] Vomiting, diaphoresis, and fever may also occur.

Acute cholecystitis begins with stone-related obstruction in over 90% of cases[7] but then progresses to mucosal inflammation and damage. The patient usually has a history of biliary pain. The pain localizes in the RUQ, and chills and fever are common.[3] Symptoms are typically milder in older adults. Palpation of the abdomen causes a severe increase in pain and temporary inspiratory arrest (Murphy's sign). The episode of cholecystitis usually subsides in 1 to 4 days. Clinical manifes-

Clinical Manifestations

Cholecystitis/Cholelithiasis

- Sudden-onset pain in the right upper quadrant (RUQ) of the abdomen
  - Severe and steady in quality
  - Frequently radiates to the right scapula or shoulder
  - Persists for about 1 to 3 hours
  - May awaken the patient at night
  - May be associated with consumption of a large or fatty meal
- Anorexia, nausea, and possibly vomiting
- Mild to moderate fever
- Decreased or absent bowel sounds
- Acute abdominal tenderness and a positive Murphy's sign
- Elevated white blood cell count, slightly elevated serum bilirubin and alkaline phosphatase levels

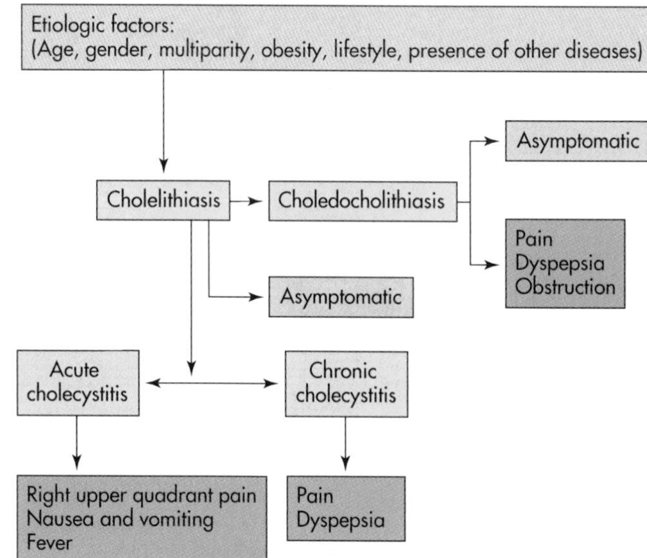

Figure 35-2 Development of uncomplicated cholecystitis.

tation of both symptomatic gallstones and cholecystitis are summarized in the Clinical Manifestations box.

When gallstones pass into the common bile duct, they may obstruct the flow of bile and cause jaundice and pruritus. Cholangitis is a serious potential complication, as is the development of acute pancreatitis if the stone obstructs the sphincter of Oddi.

Diagnosis of gallstones is fairly straightforward when the classic symptoms are present but is more difficult when the symptoms are milder and mimic other common GI conditions. It is estimated that up to 25% of patients with irritable bowel syndrome or peptic ulcer disease also have gallstones, and the exact etiology of the patient's symptoms needs to be determined if possible.[3] Researchers have theorized that many patients who experience "poor outcomes" after gallbladder surgery may not have been experiencing symptomatic gallbladder disease at all.[20]

Cholecystitis may become chronic after several acute attacks. Chronic cholecystitis is usually the result of stone injury to the gallbladder wall that causes scarring, thickening, and possibly ulceration. Bacterial infection may also be present. Patients with chronic disease often do not seek help until jaundice or other complications develop. Figure 35-2 shows the relationship between stone formation and associated outcomes in uncomplicated gallbladder disease.

Collaborative Care Management

Diagnostic Tests. Ultrasonography is the primary diagnostic tool for identifying cholelithiasis. This inexpensive test provides for precise visualization of the gallbladder and bile ducts and has greater than 95% accuracy in identifying all types of stones.[20] A gallbladder radionuclide scan may be useful in diagnosing cholecystitis.[3] Liver function tests and serum amylase may be ordered to evaluate the functional effects of obstruction, and endoscopic retrograde cholangiopancreatography (ERCP) may be performed to identify or treat stone obstruction in the ducts. Oral cystography is rarely used these days.

Medications. Surgery is the treatment of choice for symptomatic gallstones, but oral dissolution therapy with ursodeoxycholic acid (ursodiol [Actigall]) may be prescribed for patients who are poor surgical risks or who refuse surgical treatment. Drug therapy has significant limitations and side effects and is used only when absolutely necessary. The drug gradually dissolves cholesterol stones by expanding the pool of bile acids and altering cholesterol metabolism. The treatment is effective only when stones are less than 1.5 cm in diameter. A full course of treatment takes from 1 to 3 years and is extremely expensive. Up to 50% of treated patients experience stone recurrences within 5 years.[6]

Direct dissolution therapy with methyl-tert-butyl ether is occasionally used in high-risk surgical patients. The drug is instilled through a percutaneous catheter, which is monitored fluoroscopically. Multiple drug instillations are required over 12 to 24 hours, which makes the treatment both labor intensive and extremely expensive.

Treatments. Extracorporeal shock wave lithotripsy was pioneered in Germany and has been adapted to the treatment of gallstones. Lithotripsy uses shock waves to disintegrate the stones. Less than 10% of patients are candidates for this type of treatment, after which oral dissolution therapy is given to dissolve residual stone fragments. Recurrence is a common problem, and the treatment, including follow-up drug therapy, is much more expensive than surgery.[20]

Endoscopic bile duct stone removal may be used in selected high-risk patients when choledocholithiasis is suspected. Sphincterotomy may be performed to allow obstructing stones to spontaneously pass into the duodenum, or basket or balloon retrieval may be undertaken (Figure 35-3). Stones can be trapped and then pulled down through the bile duct.[20]

Surgical Management. Cholecystectomy provides definitive treatment for gallstones and has proved to be safe and effective. Laparoscopic cholecystectomy was first performed in

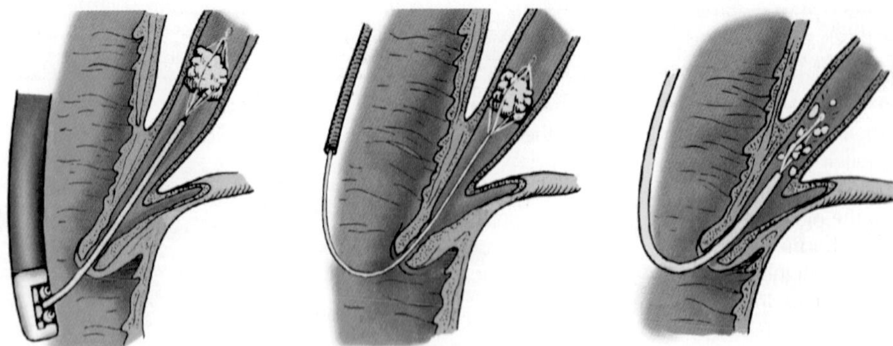

Figure 35-3 A basket contained in a flexible cord spring sheath is used to trap a stone and crush it.

Research

Reference: Chandler CF et al: Prospective evaluation of early versus delayed laparoscopic cholecystectomy for treatment of acute cholecystitis, *Am Surg* 66(9):896-900, 2000.

Timing of surgical intervention for patients experiencing acute cholecystitis has been a controversial topic. It has been assumed that the surgical risk is increased if surgery is scheduled before a period of medical stabilization has been completed. This study compared the safety and cost-effectiveness of early versus delayed intervention with laparoscopic surgery in patients with acute cholecystitis. Patients were randomly assigned to an early or delayed treatment group on admission. All patients were treated with bowel rest and antibiotics until surgery was completed. The early intervention group underwent surgery as soon as an operating room could be scheduled, usually within 24 hours. The delayed group underwent surgery after a period of stabilization or within 5 days of admission.

No advantage could be found for patients whose surgery was delayed. Operating time, conversion rates to an open procedure, and complications were all equivalent in both groups. However, the early surgical intervention group had a decreased length of stay with corresponding lower costs for total care.

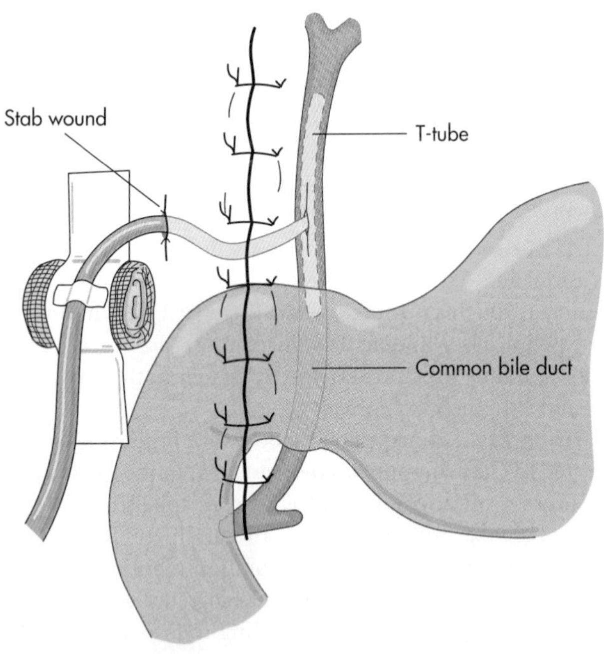

Figure 35-4 A section of T-tube emerging from a stab wound may be placed over a roll of gauze anchored to the skin with adhesive tape to prevent its lumen from being occluded by pressure.

France in 1987 and in the United States in 1988 and by the early 1990s had revolutionized the care of patients with gallbladder disease.[7] Laparoscopic cholecystectomy has become the standard of care for the treatment of gallstones and offers several real advantages over traditional laparotomy surgery. It is less invasive, which allows a shorter healing and recuperation time; there is less scarring; and most important, the pain associated with the procedure is significantly reduced. The hospital stay is less than 24 hours, and patients can return to normal activities in 2 to 3 days. An estimated 95% of patients can now be considered good candidates for laparoscopic surgery.[20] The need to revert to an open operation occurs in less than 5% of cases. When the laparoscopic approach was first introduced, the ability to explore the common bile duct was limited. This limitation necessitated the use of open cholecystectomy procedures with placement of a T-tube for drainage whenever stones were present or suspected to be present in the common bile duct (Figure 35-4). Surgical techniques have continued to improve, however, and laparoscopic approaches are now being successfully combined with endoscopic exploration and sphincterotomy to effectively treat patients with common bile duct stones. Open surgery is generally reserved for patients with multiple previous surgeries, extremely inflamed gallbladders, or gallbladder cancer (see Research box).

Laparoscopic cholecystectomy is performed with the patient under general anesthesia. Four ½-inch incisions are made—at the umbilicus, midline in the epigastric region, in the RUQ at the midclavicular line, and at the anterior axillary line. Carbon dioxide (CO_2) gas (3 to 4 L) is introduced to insufflate the abdomen and permit adequate visualization and the introduction of instruments. The operative field is magnified and projected onto a videoscreen, and a laser or cautery is used to dissect the gallbladder. The gallbladder is deflated and removed through the umbilical incision. The CO_2 gas is removed at the end of the procedure. If problems should develop during the procedure, it can be rapidly converted to an open cholecystectomy.

The skill of the surgeon is the primary determinant of outcomes. The slightly higher rate of bile duct injury that is associated with the procedure is usually attributable to inexperience with the technique.[7] Laparoscopic cholecystectomy takes about 90 minutes and is more expensive than traditional open surgery. The short hospital stay and tremendous patient satisfaction with the procedure, however, clearly outweigh the higher surgical costs. The mild shoulder pain that patients may experience for up to 1 week is attributed to nerve irritation from distention with the CO_2 gas, but the discomfort is easily managed with mild analgesics.

Diet. No diet is known to prevent the formation of gallstones. Patients who are experiencing symptoms are encouraged to follow a low-fat diet and eat small meals until definitive therapy is completed. After treatment they may resume a normal diet.

Activity. There are no activity restrictions for persons with cholelithiasis, cholecystitis, or choledocholithiasis.

Referrals. Referrals would not generally be required for the management of uncomplicated gallstones unless a serious comorbid condition necessitated the involvement of additional professionals.

NURSING MANAGEMENT OF PATIENT UNDERGOING LAPAROSCOPIC CHOLECYSTECTOMY

PREOPERATIVE CARE

Patients complete their preoperative preparation at home before their arrival on the day of surgery. The nurse verifies that the patient has had nothing by mouth and has completed any required bowel preparation. Preoperative teaching includes reviewing the scope and nature of the surgical procedure and the care that will be provided in the immediate postoperative period. The nurse also ensures that the patient understands that postoperative pain is expected to be mild and can be successfully managed with standard analgesics.

POSTOPERATIVE CARE

The patient is closely monitored in the immediate postoperative period, and pain management receives priority attention. A left side–lying Sims position can help move the retained pocket of CO_2 gas away from the diaphragm and decrease irritation. Deep breathing is encouraged. As soon as the patient is sufficiently alert, he or she is encouraged to sip clear fluids and get out of bed. Dressings over the small incisions are monitored for bleeding. Healthy patients with adequate home support may be discharged when they are fully alert and have successfully voided. A clinical pathway for a patient undergoing laparoscopic cholecystectomy is shown below.

Patient/Family Education

Discharge instructions are straightforward. The patient is instructed to slowly resume normal activity over the next 2 to 3 days and consume a light diet. The patient is advised to limit the intake of fatty and fried foods for the first few weeks after surgery until tolerance is established. The incisions require minimal care, and the dressings can usually be removed the next day. The patient is instructed to report the development of redness, swelling, or discharge from any incision, as well as the onset of fever, pain, or tenderness in the abdomen. Heavy lifting should be avoided.

The Guidelines for Safe Practice box on p. 1120, top left, summarizes the care provided to a patient who undergoes traditional open cholecystectomy.

clinical pathway Laparoscopic Cholecystectomy Without Complications

	DAY OF SURGERY DAY OF ADMISSION DAY 1	DAY OF DISCHARGE DAY 2
Diagnostic Tests	Preoperative: CBC, UA Postoperative: Hgb and Hct	
Medications	PAR: IVs decreased to saline lock after nausea subsides; IV analgesic, then PO	Disc saline lock; PO analgesic
Treatments	PAR: I&O q shift; VS q4h x 4, then q8h; assess bowel sounds q4h; check drainage on bandages q2h	Disc I&O; VS q8h; assess bowel sounds q8h; remove bandages and reapply after shower if necessary
Diet	NPO until nausea subsides, then clear liquids; advance to full liquids, low fat	Regular diet, low fat
Activity	Up in room with assistance about 6 to 10 hr after surgery; T & DB q2h	Up ad lib, OK to shower
Consultations		

CBC, Complete blood count; *DB,* deep breathing; *Hct,* hematocrit; *Hgb,* hemoglobin; *I&O,* intake and output; *IV,* intravenous; *NPO,* nothing by mouth; *PAR,* postanesthesia recovery; *PO,* oral; *T,* turn; *UA,* urinalysis; *VS,* vital signs.

Guidelines for Safe Practice

The Patient Undergoing Open Cholecystectomy

PREOPERATIVE

Teach patient the importance of frequent deep breathing and use of incentive spirometer because the high incision and right upper quadrant (RUQ) pain predispose the patient to atelectasis and right lower lobe pneumonia.

Explain the types of biliary drainage tubes that are anticipated, if any.

Teach patient about the pain control plan to be used in the postoperative period.

POSTOPERATIVE

Place patient in low Fowler's position; assist to change position frequently.

Urge patient to deep breathe at regular intervals (every 1 to 2 hours) and to cough if secretions are present until ambulating well. Assist patient to effectively splint the incision. Encourage use of incentive spirometer.

Give analgesics fairly liberally the first 2 to 3 days.

Use patient-controlled analgesia if possible. Meperidine (Demerol) has been the drug of choice because it is believed to minimize spasms in the bile ducts, but morphine is being used with increasing frequency.

Maintain a dry, intact dressing; usually a drain is inserted near the stump of the cystic duct; some serous fluid drainage is normal initially.

Encourage progressive ambulation when permitted.

Increase diet gradually to regular with fat content as tolerated (appetite and fat tolerance may be diminished if there is external biliary drainage).

BILIARY DRAINAGE

Connect any biliary drainage tubes to closed gravity drainage.

See Figure 35-4 and Guidelines for Safe Practice box at right for care of a T-tube.

Attach sufficient tubing so the patient can move without restriction.

Explain to patient the importance of avoiding kinks, clamping, or pulling of the tube.

Monitor the amount and color of drainage frequently; measure and record drainage at least every shift.

Report any signs of peritonitis (abdominal pain, rigidity, or fever) to the physician immediately.

Monitor color of urine and stools; stools will be grayish white if bile is flowing out a drainage tube, but the normal color should gradually reappear as external drainage diminishes and disappears.

GERONTOLOGIC CONSIDERATIONS

Gallbladder disease occurs more commonly with advancing age but is treated in the same manner. Older adults may experience more subtle symptoms in the presence of cholecystitis. Thus they can develop bacteremia before they seek help. Because of the normal decrease in immune function with aging, they are also at greater risk for septic shock. Older patients are at higher surgical risk, and laparoscopic cholecystectomy has been particularly effective in this age-group because it decreases the period of immobility and recovery substantially. Wound healing needs to be carefully monitored.

Guidelines for Safe Practice

Managing a T-Tube

PURPOSE

A T-tube may be placed after surgical exploration of the common bile duct to preserve patency of the common duct and ensure drainage of bile until edema resolves and bile is effectively draining into the duodenum. The tube is usually connected to gravity drainage and can be converted to a leg bag to limit its restrictiveness and visibility. The patient may be discharged with the T-tube in place (see Figure 35-4).

GENERAL CARE

Attach the tube to gravity drainage. Ensure that sufficient tubing is in place to prevent pulling and restriction of movement.

- Check drainage every 2 hours on the first day and at least once per shift on subsequent days.
- Record output carefully. Initial drainage may be as much as 500 to 1000 ml/day, but this amount should steadily decrease as healing occurs.

Follow the physician's order for initiating clamping of the tube.

Monitor the patient's response to clamping, and record any indication of distress.

- Unclamp the tube promptly if distress occurs.

Monitor the color of the stool. Stool is initially clay colored but regains pigmentation as bile again flows into the duodenum.

Keep the skin clean and protected from bile drainage, since bile is extremely irritating to the skin.

Teach the patient to empty the bag and convert it to a leg bag if discharge with the T-tube is planned.

Provide self-care teaching:

- A daily shower is usually permitted.
- A sterile dressing should be reapplied to the T-tube entry site each day.
- Zinc oxide may be used to protect the skin from irritation.
- Redness, swelling, or drainage from the site and the development of fever should be promptly reported to the physician.

SPECIAL ENVIRONMENTS FOR CARE

Critical Care

Critical care would not be anticipated for any phase of routine gallstone management. The surgical procedures have an excellent safety record and are associated with a less than 7% incidence of morbidity from any cause.

Community-Based Care

Cholecystectomy is the foundation of care for gallstones, and the procedure has become same-day/overnight surgery. Self-care management at home is therefore expected. Most patients have no specific home care needs beyond routine monitoring of wound healing and the progressive return to usual activities. Patients undergoing open cholecystectomy may be discharged from the hospital with a T-tube in place. The Guidelines for Safe Practice box above summarizes the appropriate care of a T-tube. These instructions are modified for home care and provided to the patient and family along with needed supplies such as a leg drainage bag. Older adults may require temporary home health support, and the nurse finalizes these arrangements before discharge.

COMPLICATIONS

Transient mild diarrhea is the only adverse outcome that has been consistently linked to cholecystectomy. The most common complication of nonsurgical management of gallstone disease is recurrence, and it is clear that undiagnosed or inadequately treated gallbladder disease can result in serious and even life-threatening complications, including overwhelming sepsis and peritonitis. Chronic dyspepsia and subclinical malabsorption are often included as possible complications of cholecystectomy, but there is no concrete evidence that reduction in the pool of bile salts and loss of the reservoir function of the gallbladder increase the incidence of duodenal reflux or an alkaline shift in the gastric pH. Some researchers suggest that these so-called complications may actually reflect situations in which the patient's original digestive symptoms were never related to the presence of gallstones and therefore were not improved by their removal.

Primary Sclerosing Cholangitis

Etiology/Epidemiology

The term *sclerosing cholangitis* refers to a variety of pathologic processes that cause bile duct injury from inflammation, fibrosis, thickening, or strictures.[10] Gallstones and infection are common causes. When no cause for the injury can be found, the process is called *idiopathic* or *primary sclerosing cholangitis (PSC).*

The etiology of PSC is unknown, but genetic, immune, and infectious mechanisms are suspected in its development. The disease occurs alone but is often associated with other disorders, most of which have a strong immunologic component. The most important link is with chronic ulcerative colitis. Of patients with PSC, 50% to 75% have ulcerative colitis, although PSC occurs in only 3% to 7% of all patients with ulcerative colitis.[10] The PSC may precede the diagnosis of inflammatory bowel disease (IBD) or follow it from 1 to 20 years later. Patients with PSC are usually men, and the disease is diagnosed in early or middle adulthood, typically by the age of 45. PSC is the third most common reason for liver transplant in adults.[10]

Pathophysiology

With PSC, inflammatory and fibrotic changes occur in and around the large bile ducts, gradually resulting in obstruction. Bile duct strictures can usually be found in multiple locations. The strictures alternate with normal or dilated segments of the ducts to create a beadlike appearance on x-ray examination. The disease does not usually involve the gallbladder or cystic duct. Liver biopsy documents the classic inflammation, fibrosis, proliferation, and ductal obliteration that confirm the presence of the disease. PSC is rarely diagnosed early, and in later stages biliary cirrhosis is also usually present (see Chapter 37), making the diagnosis complex.

Many patients are asymptomatic in early stages. Common complaints include fatigue, fever, jaundice, abdominal pain, and weight loss. Persistent severe pruritus can be a particularly difficult aspect of the disease. Patients may experience recurrent attacks of cholangitis.

Patient Teaching
Strategies To Control Pruritus

- Avoid irritating clothing (wool or restrictive clothing).
- Use tepid water for bathing rather than hot water.
  - Experiment with nonirritating soaps and detergents.
  - Pat skin dry after bathing or showering; do not rub.
- Apply emollient creams and lotions to dry skin regularly.
- Maintain a cool environment and ensure adequate amounts of humidity in the air.
- Avoid activities that increase body temperature or cause sweating.
- Experiment with treatments such as oatmeal baths.
- Keep the fingernails short, and consider use of cotton gloves at night to minimize skin damage from scratching.
- Use antipruritic medications as ordered.

Collaborative Care Management

PSC is slowly progressive and difficult to diagnose. The classic symptoms overlap with other, more common GI disorders. PSC causes elevated liver enzymes and serum bilirubin levels, but elevation in alkaline phosphatase is considered the hallmark feature of the disease. ERCP (see Chapter 31) is used to visualize the biliary tree and reveals the characteristic structural problems. Liver biopsy helps rule out other causes of the symptoms and assists in estimating the severity of the liver damage.

The prognosis of PSC largely depends on its clinical course, which is variable. The aggressiveness of the disease is influenced by the presence of infection and the development of complications related to cirrhosis and cholangiocarcinoma.[10] Survival is typically about 10 years after diagnosis unless a liver transplant is performed.

Drug therapy is aimed at reducing biliary tree inflammation and preventing the scarring that leads to obstruction. Steroids and other immunosuppressive agents have not proved to be effective, but the use of ursodeoxycholic acid has been shown to clearly improve the biochemical abnormalities of PSC. The mechanism of action of ursodeoxycholic acid is unknown. Endoscopic treatment to remove stones, relieve obstruction, dilate ducts, and place stent tubes is used but primarily in the form of clinical trials. Liver transplantation is the only curative option.

Patient/Family Education. The uncertain course of PSC is one of its most difficult aspects. Patients are instructed about the disease and its possible outcomes and are prepared for the possibility of the eventual need for liver transplant. Persistent jaundice may negatively affect body image, and chronic severe pruritus can be a daily nightmare. Some patients respond to cholestyramine resin, which theoretically binds the itch-triggering elements in the bile. The nurse also suggests that the patient experiment with common interventions that may lessen itching. Possible strategies are summarized in the Patient Teaching box. A low-fat diet is recommended to patients who develop problems with diarrhea or steatorrhea, and the fat restriction usually promptly corrects the problem. Fat-soluble vitamin replacement is often needed.

Carcinoma of the Biliary System

Etiology/Epidemiology

Primary tumors of the gallbladder are extremely rare in clinical practice, and their incidence may be declining because of prompt surgical intervention for gallbladder disease. Their etiology is unknown. Gallbladder cancer occurs almost exclusively in persons older than 60 years of age and is twice as common in women. High-risk groups for gallbladder disease such as Native Americans have a slightly increased risk of gallbladder cancer.[16]

Cancer can also develop in the bile ducts. Cholangiocarcinoma also typically affects patients between 50 and 70 years of age. It is strongly associated with PSC and certain parasitic infections that affect small populations in various places in the world.

Pathophysiology

Carcinoma can occur anywhere in the biliary system. It has an insidious onset and metastasizes by direct extension and through the lymphatics and blood. Most patients have no symptoms that are directly referable to the gallbladder. The symptoms are similar to those seen with cholelithiasis and cholecystitis.

Intermittent pain in the upper abdomen is the most common symptom. Anorexia, nausea, vomiting, weight loss, and jaundice may also be present. The patient may have a palpable abdominal mass. Signs and symptoms indicative of metastasis to the liver or pancreas may also be present. The development of jaundice indicates spread beyond the gallbladder. By the time gallbladder cancer produces symptoms, it is usually incurable.

Collaborative Care Management

Surgery is the primary treatment for cancer of the gallbladder. When the disease is found incidentally, it may be confined to the gallbladder and be curable with surgery. Cholecystectomy with wedge resection into the liver plus lymph node dissection is usually performed. Survival for those with invasive disease is usually less than 2 years. Neither radiotherapy nor chemotherapy has thus far improved patient outcomes.

Treatment of cholangiocarcinoma focuses on maintaining the patency of bile flow. Surgery may be used to divert bile flow to the jejunum, or stent tubes may be placed to attempt to maintain duct patency. When bile flow can be maintained, patients may live for several years after diagnosis.

Patient/Family Education. Nursing intervention is focused on helping the patient to self-manage the symptoms and possibly care for bile drainage systems (see Guidelines for Safe Practice box on p. 1120, top left). The remainder of care and teaching is generally supportive in nature as the patient and family face an uncertain future and poor prognosis. General care of the cancer patient is discussed in Chapter 15.

PROBLEMS OF THE PANCREAS

Acute Pancreatitis

Etiology

Acute pancreatitis is a clinical syndrome of pancreatic inflammation with varying amounts of injury to the gland and adjacent organs.[19] The defining characteristics of the syndrome are abdominal pain and elevated pancreatic enzyme levels. The two major causes of acute pancreatitis in the United States are biliary stones and alcohol abuse. Together they account for more than 80% of all cases.[19] Acute pancreatitis may be similar in presentation to chronic pancreatitis, but it represents a very different pathologic process. Other, less common causes of pancreatitis include trauma, cancer, drug toxicities, infectious diseases, and other chronic diseases of the GI tract. In more than 10% of cases no underlying cause can be identified.[14]

Alcohol-Related Pancreatitis. The role of alcohol in the development of acute pancreatitis is well recognized clinically but remains poorly explained. Alcohol is presumed to have a direct toxic effect on the pancreas in selected persons, probably through some increased susceptibility to injury. Alcohol is theorized to interfere with pancreatic function in several ways. Alcohol both stimulates pancreatic secretions and triggers spasm in the sphincter of Oddi, a combination that can result in obstruction. Alcohol may also change the composition of proteins secreted by the pancreas, possibly causing protein plugs to form in the small ducts. Alcohol weakens cell membranes and makes the acinar cells more vulnerable to injury and is also known to decrease the amount of trypsin inhibitor available, which increases the risk of injury. Alcohol alters both systemic and pancreatic lipid metabolism and can exacerbate hyperlipidemia.[19] All of these factors are believed to contribute to the development of alcohol-related pancreatitis, but none of them adequately explains the disease.

Biliary Pancreatitis. Although gallstone disease is clearly linked to acute pancreatitis, only a small number of patients with gallstones ever develop the disease. It is likely that most cases of biliary pancreatitis are caused by transient obstruction of the ampulla of Vater. Stones have been recovered from the stool of more than 90% of patients with gallstone pancreatitis in some studies.[19] The obstruction does not have to be prolonged to initiate acute inflammation. How the obstruction activates the pancreatic enzymes is not known. The presence of tiny gallstones (microlithiasis or biliary sludge) too small to be identified by imaging studies is believed to play a role. There is also considerable evidence that structural abnormalities that lead to narrowing at the sphincter of Oddi can be considered a cause of biliary pancreatitis. It is theorized that obstruction can temporarily reverse the normal pancreatic pressure gradient and permit reflux of bile or duodenal contents into the pancreatic ducts.

Risk factors for acute pancreatitis are summarized in the Risk Factors box.

Epidemiology

The incidence of acute pancreatitis has increased in recent years, but this increase may represent improved diagnostic

Risk Factors

Acute Pancreatitis

MAJOR

Biliary stones
Alcohol use/abuse

MINOR

Age

55 to 65 years for biliary pancreatitis
45 to 55 years for alcohol-related pancreatitis

Sex

Female for biliary tract pancreatitis
Male for alcohol-related pancreatitis

Other Gastrointestinal Tract Problems

Trauma
Infectious disease
Cancer
Chronic diseases (e.g., inflammatory bowel disease)
Drug toxicities

NOTE: 10% of cases cannot be attributed to any identifiable risk factors.

capabilities rather than a true increase in the number of cases. The current annual incidence is estimated to be one to five cases per 10,000 population.[19] Patients with biliary pancreatitis are likely to be 55 to 65 years of age and predominantly female, whereas patients with alcohol-related pancreatitis are usually slightly younger and predominantly male.

Acute pancreatitis may take a mild, severe, or fulminant course. Pancreatitis has a fulminant course in approximately 5% to 15% of all patients, and 20% to 60% of these patients will either die or face potentially lethal complications. The overall mortality rate for pancreatitis remains at about 10% despite improved diagnosis and more aggressive treatment. The disease may be recurrent, and repeated episodes can lead to chronic pancreatitis.[15]

Pathophysiology

The two major pathologic varieties of acute pancreatitis are (1) the acute interstitial form and (2) the acute hemorrhagic form. Although either form can be fatal, the interstitial form is often a milder disease.

In acute interstitial pancreatitis the gland is diffusely swollen and inflamed but retains its normal anatomic features. Neither hemorrhage nor necrosis is present. The interstitial spaces become grossly swollen by extracellular edema, and the ducts may contain purulent material. The acute hemorrhagic disease has a very different presentation. The gland is acutely inflamed, and both hemorrhage and marked tissue necrosis are present. Extensive fat necrosis is evident in patients with fulminant disease, not just in the pancreas but throughout the abdominal and thoracic cavities and subcutaneous tissues.[19] Necrosis of blood vessels can cause significant loss of blood, and abscesses and infection form in areas of walled-off necrotic tissue. Systemic complications such as fat emboli, hypotension, shock, and fluid overload are common.

Pancreatic juice normally contains only inactive forms of the proteolytic enzymes. The pancreas secretes a trypsin inhibitor specifically to prevent activation within the gland, because once trypsinogen is activated to trypsin, it can then activate the other enzymes as well. Activation of the pancreatic enzymes before they reach the duodenum has long been recognized as a major component of the disease process. The mystery of acute pancreatitis is how that pathologic sequence is initiated. The etiologic roles of alcohol and biliary disease have been discussed, but they fail to fully explain the disease process. Enzyme activation overwhelms all of the normal protective mechanisms of the pancreas and initiates a massive attack on the pancreatic tissues. Pancreatic autodigestion is initiated. Other systemic effects of the activated enzymes include:

- Activation of complement and kinin, producing increased vascular permeability and vasodilation
- Increased stickiness of the inflammatory leukocytes with the formation of emboli, which plug the microvasculature
- Initiation of consumptive coagulopathy, leading to disseminated intravascular coagulation
- Increased vascular permeability, causing massive movement of fluids, which leads to circulatory insufficiency
- Release of myocardial depressant factor, which further compromises cardiac function
- Activation of the renin-angiotension network, which impairs renal function in conjunction with circulatory insufficiency

Figure 35-5 outlines the major pathologic events that can occur in acute pancreatitis. The clinical manifestations of acute pancreatitis vary somewhat according to the severity of the attack. Acute pain in the epigastric region is the hallmark feature of the disease and occurs in 95% of all patients.[19] The pain is usually steady in nature and may radiate to the low thorax and back. It is typically worsened by lying supine, and patients may curve their backs and draw their knees up toward the body in an attempt to diminish its intensity. The classic pain is deep and visceral and may persist for hours or days. In severe cases the pain is agonizing. The pain is variously attributed to stretching of the pancreatic capsule, obstruction of the biliary tree, and/or chemical burning of the peritoneum by activated enzymes.

Nausea and vomiting occur in 85% of patients.[19] The severity of the vomiting varies and is typically worsened by the ingestion of food or fluid. Vomiting does not relieve the pain and may become protracted. Physical findings for patients with severe pancreatitis include abdominal tenderness and rigidity, progressive abdominal distention, and decreased bowel activity. Fever is common, but it rarely exceeds 39° C. Fulminant disease may progress to hypovolemic shock, ascites, acute tubular necrosis, and respiratory failure with adult respiratory distress syndrome (ARDS). The clinical manifestations of mild and severe pancreatitis are summarized in the Clinical Manifestations box.

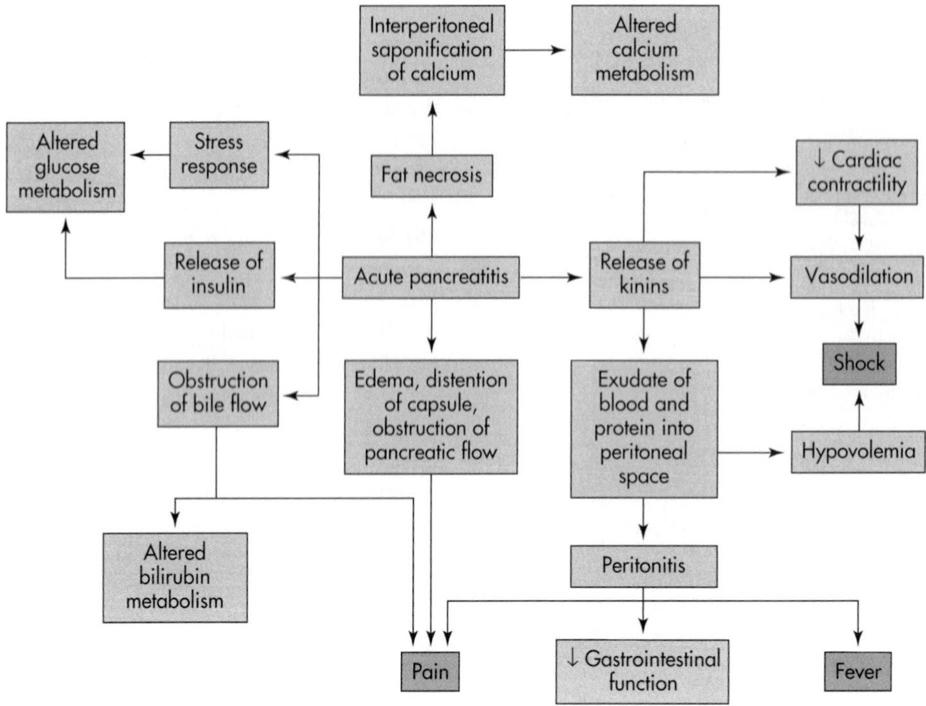

Figure 35-5 Summary of major pathologic events that occur in acute pancreatitis.

Clinical Manifestations

Acute Pancreatitis

PAIN

Steady and severe in nature; excruciating in fulminant cases
Located in the epigastric or umbilical region; may radiate to the back
Worsened by lying supine; may be lessened by flexed knee, curved-back positioning

VOMITING

Varies in severity but is usually protracted
Worsened by ingestion of food or fluid
Does not relieve the pain
Usually accompanied by nausea

FEVER

Rarely exceeds 39° C

ABDOMINAL FINDINGS

Rigidity, tenderness, guarding
Distention
Decreased or absent peristalsis

ADDITIONAL FEATURES OF FULMINANT DISEASE

Symptoms of hypovolemic shock
Oliguria: acute tubular necrosis
Ascites
Jaundice
Respiratory failure
Grey Turner's sign (bluish discoloration along the flanks)*
Cullen's sign (bluish discoloration around the umbilicus)*

*NOTE: These signs indicate the accumulation of blood in these areas and represent the presence of hemorrhagic pancreatitis.

Collaborative Care Management

Diagnostic Tests. The diagnosis of acute pancreatitis is based on the presence of acute abdominal pain and an elevated serum amylase level, which rises within a few hours of the onset of the disease. In mild disease amylase may remain elevated for only a few days. There is no apparent relationship between the severity of the disease and the height of the enzyme levels. The levels of urinary amylase may also be measured if the patient has adequate kidney function. Serum lipase elevations are also diagnostic and persist for up to 7 days. Lipase levels are more reliable indicators than amylase if the patient is not seen for several days after the onset of illness. Neither amylase nor lipase elevations are exclusive to pancreatic disease, which complicates diagnosis in questionable cases.

Other laboratory findings commonly seen with acute pancreatitis include leukocytosis and other inflammatory markers; hyperglycemia, which may reach levels as high as 500 to 900 mg/dl; and elevated liver function tests. Hypocalcemia may develop from the sequestering of calcium by fat necrosis in the abdomen, and this is usually a poor prognostic sign. It may occur in conjunction with low levels of both albumin and magnesium, especially in patients with chronic alcoholism.

Abdominal x-ray studies are performed on all patients with acute abdominal pain to rule out causes such as perforation. Ultrasonography is quite sensitive and can reveal pancreatic edema if the gland can be visualized. However, it is often obscured by gas and ileus. Ultrasonography remains the best noninvasive method of determining the presence of gallstones. Computed tomography (CT) scanning is a useful tool for diagnosing acute pancreatitis, although it is usually not needed except for patients with severe disease and suspected complications. CT scans can estimate the size of the pancreas; can identify cysts, abscesses, and masses; and with a contrast medium can clearly diagnose hemorrhagic disease.

Medications. There is no effective drug treatment for acute pancreatitis. Drug therapy to reduce pancreatic secretion has not been shown to have any therapeutic effect. Pain management is the primary consideration, and patients may require substantial amounts of opioids. Synthetic opioids such as meperidine (Demerol) have traditionally been used because they do not cause spasm in the sphincter of Oddi. Morphine, however, is now believed to have minimal effects on the sphincter and is a more effective analgesic.

Treatments. There are no known treatments for pancreatitis. Most patients with mild to moderate disease receive general supportive care. Nasogastric (NG) suctioning has often been used, but it is probably not necessary unless the patient develops ileus or experiences persistent vomiting.

Fluid and electrolyte replacement is critical. Pancreatitis often leads to "third spacing," and the loss of intravascular fluid through membrane leakage averages 4 to 6 L and can easily exceed these levels in severe cases. Prevention of hypovolemic shock necessitates aggressive fluid management. Urine output should remain at or above 30 to 50 ml/hr. Potassium losses can also be significant in both vomitus and pancreatic fluids, and serum levels need to be supported. Hypocalcemia often develops and is carefully monitored. Replacement of calcium is initiated if the patient becomes symptomatic. Exogenous insulin may be needed in severe disease, but it is used cautiously because these patients are very vulnerable to severe hypoglycemia from decreased glycogen and glucagon reserves.[19]

More aggressive and invasive interventions are used with patients who are at high risk for complications. The course of acute pancreatitis is not always apparent, and bedside assessment alone is often inadequate. Several clinical prognostic rating scales have been developed to help clinicians identify patients at greatest risk. The Ranson scale tracks 11 separate criteria that are applied at admission and again within the first 48 hours. The simplified Glasgow scale tracks just eight criteria and appears to be equally accurate. These prognostic scoring systems are presented in Table 35-1.

Peritoneal lavage has been used in patients with severe pancreatitis in the attempt to remove toxic substances. Clinical trials have involved small numbers of patients, and results have been somewhat inconsistent, so a clear benefit of this intervention cannot yet be proved. The removal of retained gallstones by ERCP reduces overall morbidity in the select group of patients in whom an obstructing stone can be identified.

Surgical Management. Surgery is not a routine part of the management of acute pancreatitis, but some procedures may be necessary to control related gallbladder problems such as pseudocyst, or abscess. Necrotic tissue may also be resected. Patients requiring surgery typically have fulminant disease and are acutely ill. The discussion of surgical intervention is included under Complications on p. 1128.

Diet. The patient is kept NPO until the abdominal pain has subsided and amylase levels have returned to normal. This practice, in theory, rests the pancreas and limits the secretion of enzymes. Most patients recover without complications or sequelae. Oral fluids and feedings can usually be resumed within 3 to 7 days and gradually advanced to a normal diet once peristalsis is reestablished. Hunger is a good indicator of readiness for eating.[19] There is no clinical proof of the need for a low-fat diet or any other dietary restrictions during recovery except for abstinence from alcohol.

Total enteral or parenteral nutrition may be implemented for patients who are unable to eat for extended periods of time (see Research box). The early use of parenteral nutrition does not appear to affect the outcome of patients with mild pancreatitis.[9] Parenteral nutrition is appropriate when patients have been NPO for 7 to 10 days, but the risk of sepsis is very real. Increased attention is being focused on the safer

TABLE 35-1 Two Representative Prognostic Scoring Systems Used in Acute Pancreatitis

Ranson	Glasgow
Admission	**Within 48 Hours of Admission**
Age >55 years	Age >55 years
WBC count >16,000 cells/mm³	WBC count >15,000
LDH >350 IU/L	Glucose >180 mg/dl
AST >250 IU/L	BUN >45 mg/dl
Glucose >200 mg/dl	Po_2 <60 mm Hg
	Albumin <3.2 g/dl
Initial 48 Hours	Calcium <8 mg/dl
Hematocrit decrease >10%	LDH >600 IU/L
BUN increase >5 mg/dl	
Calcium <8 mg/dl	
Po_2 <60 mm Hg	
Base deficit >4	
Estimated fluid sequestration >6 L	

Modified from Agarwal N, Pitchumoni CS: Assessment of severity in acute pancreatitis, *Am J Gastroenterol* 85:356, 1990; and Marshall JB: Acute pancreatitis: a review with an emphasis on new developments, *Arch Intern Med* 153:1185, 1993.
AST, Aspartate transaminase; *BUN,* blood urea nitrogen; *IU,* international units; *LDH,* low-density lipoprotein; Po_2, partial pressure of oxygen; *WBC,* white blood cell.

Research

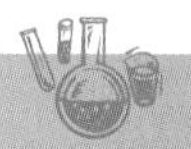

Reference: Lobo DN et al: Evolution of nutritional support in acute pancreatitis, *Br J Surg* 87(6):695-707, 2000.

Nutritional support, either enteral or parenteral, has been a standard part of the care of patients with acute pancreatitis for many years. This study reviewed 25 years of research related to nutritional support and concluded that there is no evidence that nutritional support affects the underlying disease process of acute pancreatitis in any way. However, it is effective in preventing undernutrition or starvation in protracted cases. The preponderance of evidence indicates that if a patient can tolerate enteral feeding, this route is preferable to parenteral nutrition in terms of efficacy and safety.

alternative of tube feeding, delivered into the intestine.[11] Efforts are made to keep plasma albumin levels above 3.5 g/dl and total protein values above 6.5g/dl, thereby maintaining a positive nitrogen balance.

Activity. Bed rest is maintained during the acute phase of disease management to decrease the body's overall metabolic demands. Once the patient's condition has stabilized, activity can be gradually increased according to the patient's tolerance. There are no long-term restrictions.

Referrals. Patients with acute pancreatitis are severely ill and may require the expertise of a variety of specialists during the treatment and recovery periods. Fulminant illness may necessitate critical care monitoring and consultation. This is particularly true for patients who develop respiratory complications such as ARDS or respiratory failure and require intubation and mechanical ventilation. The nutrition support team will be involved if parenteral nutrition is initiated.

Any number of medical specialists may be consulted to manage emergency complications. The surgeon is often needed to drain abscesses, relieve obstruction, or debride necrotic tissue. An enterostomal therapist may be consulted if draining wounds are left open to heal by secondary intention.

In many patients alcohol abuse is the etiologic stimulus of acute pancreatitis, and continuation of alcohol use will increase the risk of recurrent acute pancreatitis and chronic pancreatitis in the future. The nurse needs to be knowledgeable about resources available in the local community for supporting individuals who want to become and remain abstinent from alcohol. The severe nature of acute pancreatitis may serve as a stimulus for lifestyle change in some individuals. It is important to use this opportunity to refer the person for alcohol treatment if possible.

NURSING MANAGEMENT OF PATIENT WITH ACUTE PANCREATITIS

ASSESSMENT

Health History

Assessment data to be collected as part of the health history of a patient with acute pancreatitis include:

History of gallbladder disease, treatment

History of other GI diseases (e.g., peptic ulcer disease, inflammatory bowel disease)

History of alcohol use: amount and duration

Medications in use: prescription, over-the-counter, and herbal preparations

Onset and progression of symptoms such as:

Pain, which is often steady and severe in nature and quality; located in the epigastric or umbilical region or may radiate to back; worsens when patient is supine

Nausea and vomiting, which is usually severe and protracted and worsens with ingestion of food or fluid; vomiting does not relieve pain

Physical Examination

Important aspects of the physical examination of the patient with acute pancreatitis include:

Vital signs indications of hypovolemia: tachycardia, tachypnea, normal to low blood pressure, restlessness, and anxiety

Palpation for abdominal rigidity, distention, guarding, and tenderness

Auscultation for diminished or absent bowel sounds

Temperature measurement to check for fever, which is generally no higher than 39° C

Assessment for signs of third spacing: falling urine output, decreased skin turgor, dry or sticky mucous membranes, increased abdominal girth

Observation of general affect: patient appears distressed; lies with knees pulled toward abdomen

Inspection for presence of Turner's or Cullen's sign: bluish discoloration on flanks and/or around umbilicus

NURSING DIAGNOSES

Nursing diagnoses are determined from analysis of patient data. Nursing diagnoses for the person with acute pancreatitis may include but are not limited to:

Diagnostic Title	Possible Etiologic Factors
1. Acute pain	Inflammation of pancreas or peritoneum
2. Deficient fluid volume	Vomiting, fluid shifts in abdomen
3. Imbalanced nutrition: less than body requirements	Nausea and vomiting; pain
4. Risk for impaired home maintenance	Lack of knowledge about disease process and therapeutic regimen
5. Risk for ineffective health maintenance	Unhealthy lifestyle patterns, including alcoholism

EXPECTED PATIENT OUTCOMES

Expected patient outcomes for the person with acute pancreatitis may include but are not limited to:

1a. Will state that pain is controlled and will not display a distressed appearance

1b. Will not guard or limit activity or movement

2. Will maintain adequate fluid volume as demonstrated by normal blood pressure, absence of orthostatic blood pressure changes, normal skin turgor, moist mucous membranes, and adequate urine output

3. Will gradually resume a normal oral diet and regain lost weight

4a. Will be able to describe the disease process and the purpose of various interventions

4b. Will be able to explain the relationship between the etiologic factor (e.g., alcoholism or biliary disease) and pancreatitis

4c. Will be able to explain plans for follow-up care

5. Will adopt optimal health practices and control alcohol intake as appropriate

INTERVENTIONS

1. Controlling Pain

Control of pain is a major priority, and either morphine or meperidine (Demerol) may be used. Critically ill patients may receive a continuous infusion of intravenous (IV) opioids supplemented by boluses as needed for breakthrough pain.

Patient-controlled analgesia should be used if feasible to allow for successful pain management. The nurse regularly and frequently assesses the patient's level of pain using a scale of 1 to 10 and evaluates the patient's response to interventions. The physician is consulted for needed changes in the regimen. Staff occasionally exhibit the attitude that patients with alcohol-induced pancreatitis are "getting what they deserve," especially on repeat admissions for recurrent disease. The nurse must serve as the patient's advocate in the system, documenting the severity of the patient's pain and ensuring that an effective plan is in place to manage it.

Some patients find that the pain decreases if they assume a sitting position with the trunk flexed or a side-lying, knee-chest position with their knees drawn up to the abdomen. Epidural analgesia may be considered if the pain persists and is not relieved by routine opioid administration. Although the research is currently inconclusive, most patients are kept NPO to "rest" the pancreas and decrease the autodigestive process. An NG tube is inserted to keep the stomach decompressed if vomiting is severe.

The nurse also explores the use of a variety of nonpharmacologic pain relief strategies with the patient, such as distraction, imagery, massage, and back rubs. The environment should also be kept quiet, comfortable, and conducive to rest. These measures are used in addition to, and not in place of, opioid administration for pain control.

2. Maintaining Fluid and Electrolyte Balance

As soon as the patient is admitted, the nurse institutes monitoring related to fluid and electrolyte status, cardiac output, and renal status. Monitoring includes intake and output, vital signs, daily weights, abdominal girth, and all routine laboratory values with particular emphasis on hematocrit, potassium, and calcium levels. Physical assessment includes checking for signs of hypokalemia and hypocalcemia (see Chapter 13).

An indwelling Foley catheter may be inserted to monitor renal function that can be impaired by hypotension and shock. Monitoring parameters and frequency of monitoring depend on the stability of the patient's condition. Fluids, electrolytes, colloids, or blood is administered as necessary.

Aggressive fluid replacement necessitates establishing and maintaining adequate IV access. The nurse is responsible for administering the fluids and monitoring the patient's response. The development of hypovolemic shock is of particular concern in the early days of the disease, and the nurse watches carefully for early signs that could indicate the development of shock (see Chapter 14). The patient is also monitored for hyperglycemia, and blood glucose levels are checked four times a day. If severe hyperglycemia occurs, it may be treated with insulin.

3. Promoting Adequate Nutrition

The patient is kept NPO and may have an NG tube in place. Good oral hygiene is necessary to decrease discomfort from dry mouth and irritation from the NG tube. Enteral or parenteral feedings may be used during the critical phase of the illness. When the acute symptoms subside, oral fluids and food are restarted. The patient is given clear liquids and then slowly advanced toward a regular diet. Tolerance for oral feedings is carefully monitored, and the patient is regularly assessed for the return of pain. Frequent small meals are usually better tolerated in the early refeeding period. The only dietary restriction that needs to be followed after discharge is the avoidance of alcohol.

Restriction of fat in the diet has no proven effect on healing.

4. Patient/Family Education

Education for the patient and family is ongoing. At the beginning of hospitalization, the patient and significant others need basic information about acute pancreatitis, planned diagnostic tests, and the rationale for the proposed treatment. Because of the pain and distress that acute pancreatitis causes and the seriousness of the disease process, the patient and family may be experiencing tremendous anxiety. Therefore explanations and instructions need to be brief and as simple as possible and may need to be repeated frequently. Support and continuity of care also need to be provided to help decrease anxiety. Education is directed toward preventing future attacks and maintaining a nutritious diet. The patient must know that any recurrence of signs and symptoms should be reported immediately. Follow-up care is explained in detail.

5. Health Promotion/Prevention

If unhealthy lifestyle patterns such as alcoholism are a cause of acute pancreatitis, the nurse must help the patient to realistically address the problem. This care is not begun until the patient's condition is stabilized, but it must be introduced before the patient leaves the hospital. See Chapter 3 for further information about promoting a healthy lifestyle.

If the patient's pancreatitis is related to biliary disease, it is important to discuss treatment for gallstones. The episode of pancreatitis is frightening and could make the patient reluctant to undergo any further medical or surgical treatment. The nurse reinforces the etiologic role of biliary disease in acute pancreatitis and encourages the patient to follow through on recommended treatment.

EVALUATION

To evaluate the effectiveness of nursing interventions, compare patient behaviors with those stated in the expected patient outcomes. Achievement of patient outcomes is successful if the patient:

- **1a.** States that pain is absent; does not appear distressed.
- **1b.** Moves freely without guarding or grimacing.
- **2.** Has hemodynamic measures within normal limits; has balanced intake and output.
- **3.** Consumes a well-balanced diet without nausea, vomiting, or pain by discharge; and returns to normal weight.
- **4a.** Accurately describes the disease, tests, and planned interventions.
- **4b.** Accurately describes the relationship between etiologic factors and disease development.
- **4c.** Makes plans for follow-up.
- **5.** Makes a commitment to treatment for alcoholism as appropriate.

GERONTOLOGIC CONSIDERATIONS

Biliary disease becomes increasingly common as people age, and biliary disease–related pancreatitis is most likely to occur in the elderly patient. The severity of the disease is difficult to predict, but older adults with acute pancreatitis may become critically ill faster because of comorbid conditions.

Older adults are also more likely to develop complications from both the pancreatitis and the disease-enforced immobility. Respiratory complications are of particular concern, and the elderly patient needs frequent respiratory assessment and aggressive pulmonary hygiene during the acute stage of the disease.

Infection is a common complication of pancreatitis (see discussion under Complications), and elderly patients are less able to withstand the stress imposed on the body by sepsis. The same is true for the development of hypovolemia and fluid shifts. These factors strain the cardiovascular system and may overwhelm the elderly patient's ability to adapt and respond.

SPECIAL ENVIRONMENTS FOR CARE

Critical Care

Although most patients with pancreatitis recover without any residual dysfunction, a minority experience life-threatening disease. These patients are managed in a critical care unit. The nurse's major role is collaborative with the physician and involves ongoing monitoring of all systems and the prevention or identification of complications.

Routine interventions include hemodynamic monitoring and aggressive fluid support. Critically ill patients may also need cardiac support with drugs such as dopamine. A pulmonary artery catheter may be inserted to assess perfusion adequacy. Left ventricular dysfunction is a common problem.

The airway can be compromised in several ways. Severe pain limits diaphragmatic excursion, and both shock and sepsis place extraordinary metabolic demands on the respiratory system that can progress into ARDS in some patients. Prompt intubation and mechanical ventilation are crucial. Hypercoagulability increases the risk of pulmonary embolism. Management includes supplemental oxygen, suctioning as needed, and aggressive chest physiotherapy. Assessment is performed hourly. Respiratory failure accounts for a disproportionate number of pancreatitis-related deaths.

In addition to the concerns addressed in the preceding paragraphs, the critically ill patient with pancreatitis often receives parenteral nutrition to support a positive nitrogen balance and may undergo peritoneal lavage. Other interventions are directed at specific complications as they arise.

Community-Based Care

Most patients with acute pancreatitis recover spontaneously and can be discharged from the hospital within 1 to 2 weeks. Patient needs for home care are minimal if complications do not develop. Normal activities can be gradually resumed as strength and activity tolerance increase.

Patients with alcoholism present a unique challenge because even the pain and anxiety of acute pancreatitis may not be sufficient motivation for them to abstain from alcohol. The nurse discusses the importance of abstinence with the patient and makes referrals to community programs for alcohol treatment if the patient agrees. It is important to recognize, however, that the decision to continue drinking is a matter of personal choice. The nurse's role is to be certain that the patient has all of the information that he or she needs to make an informed decision about the future. A positive outcome cannot be guaranteed.

COMPLICATIONS

About 25% of patients who experience acute pancreatitis develop complications, and most deaths associated with the disease occur in that group of patients. Complications may be local or systemic. The systemic complications tend to occur within the first week and have largely been discussed within the context of the fulminant disease process. These include complications such as hypovolemic shock, sepsis, renal failure, and ARDS. The major complications of acute pancreatitis are summarized in Box 35-1.

Pseudocysts. Pancreatic fluid or exudate forms in up to 50% of patients with acute pancreatitis. Pseudocysts are localized collections of fluid enclosed in a fibrous capsule, and they occur in only 5% to 10% of all patients.[19] Pseudocysts may resolve over time, and intervention is not always warranted. However, pseudocysts can also become life threatening if they obstruct neighboring structures, rupture or hemorrhage, or become infected. A "wait and see" policy is generally followed, and the cysts are monitored regularly. Progressive enlargement of the pseudocyst or signs of early infection are indications for drainage. Inflammatory exudate from the pancreas

BOX 35-1 Major Complications of Acute Pancreatitis

Cardiovascular

Hypotension/shock from hypovolemia or hypoalbuminemia

Hematologic

Leukocytosis from generalized inflammation or secondary infections, anemia from blood loss, disseminated intravascular coagulation (DIC) from unknown causes

Respiratory

Atelectasis, pneumonia, pleural effusion, adult respiratory distress syndrome (ARDS)

Gastrointestinal

Gastrointestinal bleeding

Pancreatic

Pancreatic pseudocysts, pancreatic necrosis or phlegmon, pancreatic abscesses, pancreatic ascites

Renal

Oliguria and acute tubular necrosis

Metabolic

Hyperglycemia, hypocalcemia, hyperlipidemia

may form into an inflamed mass, which is called a phlegmon. Again, intervention is not indicated unless bleeding or infection develops. Pseudocysts and phlegmons can be drained endoscopically, percutaneously, or surgically depending on their size and location.[19]

Pancreatic Infection. Pancreatic infection is the most frequent cause of serious morbidity and mortality associated with acute pancreatitis. Infection typically appears 8 to 20 days after the onset of pancreatitis and has a 100% mortality rate if untreated. Infection usually develops in the areas of necrosis created by fulminant disease and then spreads into adjacent tissue. The initial diagnosis of infection can be complicated by the fact that acute pancreatitis itself manifests with the common symptoms of inflammation and infection. Infection-related fever, however, typically exceeds 39° C, and the patient's clinical condition deteriorates.

CT scanning allows for the accurate identification of areas of necrosis, which can then be aspirated by CT-guided needle aspiration. Gram stain and culture of the aspirate can identify the specific organisms responsible for the infection. Broad-spectrum antibiotics are initiated immediately, but definitive therapy requires percutaneous drainage or surgical debridement. Attempts to prevent the development of infection with the prophylactic use of antibiotics have not proved to be consistently effective, but IV prophylactic antibiotics do appear to reduce the incidence of complications in patients with severe disease and extensive necrosis.[19]

Percutaneous drainage is used most effectively with infected pseudocysts because there is minimal particulate matter present that can clog the tubes. The traditional surgical approach had been to excise as much necrotic material as possible and then place multiple large-bore sump drains in the operative areas to remove infected material. Continuous saline infusion and suction are needed to maintain tube patency. Many surgeons now use an open method in which the resected areas are packed, and the dressings are changed with the patient under anesthesia every 2 to 3 days until granulation is well underway. The abdomen is left open and eventually closes over an absorbable mesh barrier. A feeding tube can be placed once granulation is underway. The development of fistulas can complicate the healing process.

Chronic Pancreatitis. Patients with alcohol-induced acute pancreatitis are believed to already have asymptomatic chronic disease when they experience their first acute episode. If the patient continues to drink, the likelihood of recurrence is extremely high.

Chronic Pancreatitis

Etiology/Epidemiology

Chronic pancreatitis is a separate disorder from recurrent acute pancreatitis. In acute pancreatitis the gland gradually returns to normal as the inflammation resolves. Chronic pancreatitis is characterized by persistent and progressive functional and morphologic damage to the tissue. Fibrosis and scar tissue gradually replace the normal pancreatic tissue.[12]

Alcohol consumption accounts for more than 70% of cases of chronic pancreatitis in the United States, and the disease is more common in men.[12,13] Both the amount and duration of alcohol consumption appear to be contributory, and it generally takes at least 10 years of heavy drinking to produce symptomatic disease. Research is indicating, however, that alcohol can be toxic to the pancreas in any quantity, and there appears to be no threshold for toxicity.[12] Since alcohol use is pervasive and chronic pancreatitis is rare, there are obviously other factors at work as well. The actual prevalence of the disease is unknown, and subclinical pancreatic drainage may be more common than currently recognized. Other potential causes of chronic pancreatitis include obstruction, trauma, and metabolic disturbances. Twenty percent of cases are considered idiopathic. Malnutrition is the most common cause of chronic pancreatitis in underdeveloped countries.

Pathophysiology

The basic pathologic change of chronic pancreatitis is destruction of the exocrine parenchyma and replacement with fibrous tissue. This process is associated with varying degrees of duct dilation. Scarring and fibrotic changes may occur throughout the pancreas or be limited to selected areas. Calcium salts may be deposited in both the ducts and the parenchyma, and the factors that influence the solubility of calcium in the calcium-rich pancreatic secretions are not well identified. As the process becomes increasingly severe, the islets of Langerhans are also involved and destroyed. The disease therefore can lead to insufficiency or failure of both the exocrine and endocrine functions of the gland.

The patient with chronic pancreatitis may exhibit symptoms that are similar to those of acute pancreatitis. Abdominal pain is again the major symptom, and it is described as severe in intensity, dull in quality, and constant. The pain is epigastric, may radiate to the back or both upper quadrants, and is immediately worsened by eating. Over time the pain of chronic pancreatitis may persist, diminish, or even disappear as the disease progresses.[2,12] The mechanisms underlying the pain are unclear but may include inflammation, increased pressure, and nerve inflammation.

Nausea, vomiting, anorexia, and weight loss are also common symptoms of chronic pancreatitis. Weight loss occurs primarily from decreased caloric intake related to pain, but malabsorption may also play a role.

Pancreatic insufficiency begins once 80% of the pancreatic tissue has been destroyed. Diarrhea and steatorrhea develop when the secretion of pancreatic enzymes is too low to support normal digestion. Diabetes is common and may precede other clinical symptoms. Unique impairments in glucose metabolism make these patients extremely vulnerable to hypoglycemia, and their need for insulin is smaller than expected. Oral hypoglycemic agents are not effective. Malabsorption also leads to clinical deficiencies in vitamins E and B_{12} and other fat-soluble vitamins, but patients rarely develop overt symptoms of deficiency.

Collaborative Care Management

The diagnosis of chronic pancreatitis is suggested by the history and presenting symptoms and then confirmed by diagnostic tests. Serum enzyme levels may be elevated, normal, or low. Diffuse calcification can be seen on abdominal x-ray and ultrasound studies, and CT scanning reveals dilation of the pancreatic ducts and the presence of cystic lesions. Stool analysis can quantify the severity of the steatorrhea and estimate the degree of pancreatic insufficiency.

Treatment of chronic pancreatitis is directed at pain control and the correction of malabsorption. Effective management of abdominal pain is the greatest challenge. Patients who continue to consume alcohol usually continue to experience pain, and eventually even abstinence is no guarantee of relief. Patients can usually adapt to the malabsorption and steatorrhea, but the persistent pain can be incapacitating and lead to drug dependence.

Flare-ups of chronic pancreatitis are managed similarly to the acute disease. Bowel rest is maintained, and attention is paid to managing the acute pain. Nonopioid analgesics are used if possible, but the pain is often severe enough to necessitate opioid administration. Octreotide is a synthetic analog of somatostatin that inhibits pancreatic secretion and may be useful for patients who do not respond to conventional treatment. Ongoing care involves the use of a low-fat diet and supplemental pancreatic enzymes. These enzymes increase the patient's body weight and improve absorption, increasing the patient's general sense of well-being. The recommended diet is high in protein and carbohydrates and may provide as much as 3000 to 6000 calories/day. The use of medium-chain triglycerides to improve the patient's nutritional state is being evaluated. Fat-soluble vitamin replacement may also be indicated, and the management of diabetes often requires the use of insulin.

Chronic pancreatitis affects the small ducts of the pancreas and is usually not amenable to surgical correction. However, surgical intervention may be used to relieve ductal obstruction, bypass obstructed parts of the gland, or resect small or large parts of the diseased pancreas. Outcomes of these procedures are not predictable. A celiac plexus block is occasionally used to interrupt pain transmission.

The nurse serves as the patient's advocate in the search for comfort. Concerns about drug dependence must not be allowed to prevent the patient from receiving adequate and necessary analgesia. Health care providers can easily become exasperated with patients who are unable or unwilling to stop drinking and may begin to consider the pain of chronic pancreatitis as appropriate retribution for the patient's addiction. This attitude can seriously compromise the patient's care.

In some instances the patient has had negative experiences with pain management during previous hospitalizations for exacerbations and thus believes that analgesics are not being given because the health care team does not care about him or her. The involvement of a pain management team is appropriate if such services are available. See Chapter 12 for further discussion of pain management.

Patient/Family Education. The role of alcohol in the etiology and progression of chronic pancreatitis is unequivocal, and yet many of these patients find themselves unable or unwilling to abstain from alcohol use. The nurse consults with a substance abuse specialist to develop a consistent and appropriate approach for the patient's care and ensures that the patient has all of the information necessary to make informed decisions about his or her present and future. Information concerning community resources for alcohol treatment should be current and accurate and offered to the patient. The involvement of the family is encouraged if the family dynamics are supportive. Family members and health care workers need to be helped to understand and accept that ultimately it is the patient's right to make fundamental decisions about his or her own care, even when those decisions do not appear to be in the patient's own best interests.

The patient also needs to learn how to modify the diet and use pancreatic enzyme replacement effectively to control diarrhea and maintain a stable weight. Timing of the medications is critical. The nurse teaches the patient to take the capsules 1 to 2 hours before, during, or after meals. Powders can be mixed directly with food. Patients are informed that these products often have a bad taste and may alter the taste of foods. The patient is instructed to monitor the body's response to the supplements and consistently track weight changes. The anorexia and poor eating habits commonly associated with long-term alcohol use make adherence to a high-protein, high-calorie diet difficult. The use of vitamin supplements is encouraged if recommended by the physician.

Patients who continue to drink alcohol will always be just one step away from their next flare-up or complication. The nurse provides the patient with written material that outlines the symptoms of complications and encourages the patient to adhere to the plan for continued follow-up. A Nursing Care Plan for the patient with chronic pancreatitis is found on pp. 1131 to 1133.

Cancer of the Pancreas

Etiology/Epidemiology

Cancer of the pancreas is a malignant disease of the exocrine pancreas, and more than 85% of cases are ductal adenocarcinomas.[15] About two thirds of these adenocarcinomas develop in the head of the pancreas; the remainder occur in the body or tail of the gland. Both benign and malignant tumors can also arise from the islet cells, but these are extremely rare.

Pancreatic cancer is rare before middle age but increases sharply with age.[5] It occurs more commonly in men. About 28,000 new cases are diagnosed each year in the United States.[18] The etiology is unknown, but cigarette smoking is believed to be an important causative agent. Incidences of familial clustering of the disease point to a hereditary component. A diet high in fresh fruits and vegetables shows early evidence of playing a protective role. Despite the proven link between alcohol abuse and pancreatitis, no link has been found between alcohol ingestion and pancreatic cancer.

Pathophysiology

Pancreatic cancers can vary dramatically in size at the time of diagnosis. The tumor is usually deeply encased in normal tissue and is poorly demarcated. The common duct is often obstructed and distended by the presence of the tumor.

Nursing Care Plan Patient With Chronic Pancreatitis

Mr. T. is a 52-year-old man with a 12-year history of acknowledged alcoholism. He experienced his first attack of acute pancreatitis 4 years ago, and chronic pancreatitis has since been diagnosed. He has been admitted for an acute episode of the disease.

Mr. T. has tried to stop drinking and has even undergone inpatient alcohol treatment. His longest period of sobriety has been about 6 months. Some life stressor has always precipitated his return into alcohol dependency. His wife accompanied him to the hospital but made it clear that she is frustrated and cannot stand watching him "kill himself."

Mr. T.'s assessment reveals a thin, poorly nourished man who appears older than his stated age. He reports the presence of:

- Acute abdominal pain that is generally localized in the mid-epigastric region and radiates to his back. He rates the pain as 8 in severity on a 10-point scale.
- Steady and protracted vomiting that began late yesterday afternoon. He has had nothing to eat or drink for more than 12 hours.
- Large, soft, and foul-smelling stools that have been increasing in frequency and severity over the past few weeks. He has lost 12 pounds.
- A history of decreased alcohol use over the past 3 months.

Other admission data include:

- Blood pressure 94/60, pulse 92, respirations 22 and shallow, temperature 99.8° F orally
- Hemoglobin 10.2 g, red blood cell count 2.9 million, serum potassium 3.0 mg/dl, serum calcium 8.2 mg/dl, glucose 162 mg/dl

Initial care orders are:

- Administer intravenous (IV) infusion of 1000 ml 5% dextrose in one-half normal saline with 20 mEq potassium chloride at 125 ml/hr.
- Keep patient NPO.
- Monitor intake and output routinely, weight and abdominal girth once daily.
- Give meperidine (Demerol) 100 mg intramuscularly q3h prn for pain.
- Insert NG tube with to low intermittent suction if vomiting persists.
- Check blood glucose level four times daily per protocol; call if blood glucose level >160.
- Monitor closely for hypovolemic shock, electrolyte imbalance, and delirium tremors (DTs).
- Institute DT protocols if needed.

NURSING DIAGNOSIS **Acute pain related to distention of pancreatic capsule and activation of pancreatic enzymes**
GOALS/OUTCOMES Will voice control of pain at acceptable (or tolerable) level

NOC Suggested Outcomes

- Pain Level (2102)
- Pain Control (1605)
- Comfort Level (2100)

NIC Suggested Interventions

- Pain Management (1400)
- Analgesic Management (2210)
- Coping Enhancement (5230)

Nursing Interventions/Rationales

- Assess pain levels frequently, especially before and after administration of analgesics. *Frequent assessment is essential to validate the nature and severity of the patient's pain experience.*
- Document pain levels on a flow record. *Recording on a flow record allows for a pattern of pain to be established and the effectiveness of pain control methods to be evaluated.*
- Administer meperidine q3h as needed. *Synthetic opioids are effective analgesics and do not cause sphincter of Oddi spasms.*
- Encourage patient to use analgesics on a regular rather than as-needed basis. *A regular time schedule of drug use allows for a steady blood level to be established and for better pain control.*
- Validate your acceptance of the reality of the patient's pain and its severity. *Patients with chronic pancreatitis are often labeled "drug seekers" by staff.*
- Evaluate the effectiveness of the opioid analgesic. Collaborate with physician to make adjustments in dose or drug as needed. *Acute pain can be immobilizing. Morphine may be substituted for meperidine (some patients will experience sphincter of Oddi spasms from morphine).*
- Collaborate with wife to determine which nonpharmacologic methods have helped reduce pain in the past. *Nonpharmacologic methods allow the patient a degree of control of the pain experience and may augment pharmacologic pain control methods.*
- Explore his experience with strategies such as distraction, massage, relaxation, and guided imagery. *These methods can be effective in reducing pain, but the patient must be open minded and willing to experiment with new strategies.*
- Position patient in a mid to high Fowler's position with his knees flexed. *This position is theorized to reduce tension on the abdomen.*

Evaluation Parameters

1. States pain is effectively controlled
2. Requests pain medication before severe pain
3. Uses nonpharmacologic measures to control pain

Continued

Nursing Care Plan Patient With Chronic Pancreatitis—cont'd

NURSING DIAGNOSIS **Risk for deficient fluid volume related to vomiting, NPO status, hyperglycemia, and increased capillary permeability secondary to acute pancreatitis**

GOALS/OUTCOMES Will maintain fluid and electrolyte balance within normal limits

NOC Suggested Outcomes
- Fluid Balance (0601)
- Hydration (0602)
- Electrolyte and Acid/Base Balance (0600)

NIC Suggested Interventions
- Fluid Monitoring (4130)
- Fluid Management (4120)
- Intravenous (IV) Therapy (4200)

Nursing Interventions/Rationales
- Assess fluid and electrolyte status each shift. *The patient is at risk for hypovolemic shock and dehydration. May lose 4 to 14 L of fluid into the abdomen (ascites).*
- Maintain accurate intake and output. *Urine output of 30 to 50 ml/hr is essential to prevent acute tubular necrosis. Fluid replacement is based on fluid losses.*
- Monitor weight daily. *Body weight is the most accurate method of assessing fluid gains and losses.*
- Assess skin turgor and status of mucous membranes each shift. *Skin turgor and mucous membranes are good indicators of hydration or lack of hydration.*
- Maintain IV fluids at prescribed rate and flow. *To replace fluid losses and prevent hypovolemia and dehydration. Steady replacement helps prevent fluid swings and decreases nausea.*
- Measure abdominal girth each shift until stabilized. *Fluid and gas accumulation in the gastrointestinal tract can result in significant abdominal distention.*
- Monitor blood glucose level four times daily, and administer sliding-scale insulin as prescribed. *Destruction of beta cells and islets of Langerhans produces severe hyperglycemia. Because of the risk of labile hypoglycemia, insulin is not given unless the blood glucose level continues to rise.*
- Monitor for hypokalemia (muscle weakness, cramping) and hypocalcemia (numbness and tingling in fingertips or around mouth; positive Chvostek's and Trousseau's sign). *Large amounts of potassium are lost through vomiting and in the pancreatic secretions. Calcium is believed to bind with free fats and can drop to levels that increase neural excitability.*
- Monitor cardiovascular response to fluid replacement. *Fluid replacement can overload the intravascular space and put stress on the heart.*

Evaluation Parameters
1. Intake and output are balanced
2. Weight remains stable

NURSING DIAGNOSIS **Imbalanced nutrition: less than body requirements related to vomiting, NPO status, and malabsorption secondary to chronic pancreatitis**

GOALS/OUTCOMES Will maintain body weight within 5 pounds of baseline

NOC Suggested Outcomes
- Nutritional Status (1004)
- Nutritional Status: Nutrient Intake (1009)
- Electrolyte and Acid/Base Balance (0600)
- Fluid Balance (0601)

NIC Suggested Interventions
- Nutrition Management (1100)
- Fluid Monitoring (4130)
- Fluid/Electrolyte Management (2080)
- Nausea Management (1450)

Nursing Interventions/Rationales
- Maintain NPO status and bed rest until patient's condition stabilizes. *NPO status reduces the secretion of pancreatic enzymes. Bed rest decreases the body's metabolic rate.*
- Assess current nutritional and elimination status. *Patients with chronic pancreatitis are often malnourished before the attack from alcoholism and subsequent malabsorption.*
- Monitor daily weight, serum albumin, and serum protein levels. *These parameters provide the best ongoing data about nutritional status.*
- Initiate enteral/parenteral nutrition as prescribed if NPO status is prolonged. *The rapid catabolism of the disease must be counteracted by enteral/parenteral nutrition to prevent life-threatening complications.*
- Reinitiate oral feedings once abdominal pain is controlled and amylase/lipase levels stabilize. *Once pain and enzyme levels are stable, there is no contraindication to oral feeding, and the malnourishment needs to be corrected.*
- Offer small, frequent feedings to patient's tolerance and assess patient's response. *This feeding pattern minimizes distention and malabsorption symptoms.*
- Restrict fat in the diet if steatorrhea persists. *Malabsorption primarily affects the digestion of fats.*
- Evaluate composition and volume of stools. Adjust dose of pancreatic enzymes to achieve normal elimination. *Malabsorption manifests itself as large-volume, greasy, foul-smelling stools. Adequate enzyme replacement will restore the stool to near normal.*

Nursing Care Plan — *Patient With Chronic Pancreatitis—cont'd*

Evaluation Parameters

1. Receives sufficient nutrients to maintain body weight
2. Albumin levels remain above 3.8 g/dl
3. Vomiting slows and ceases
4. Produces normal stools

NURSING DIAGNOSIS **Risk for ineffective therapeutic regimen management related to inability to abstain from alcohol and inadequate knowledge of management of malabsorption and hyperglycemia**

GOALS/OUTCOMES Will participate in self-care and control intake of alcohol

NOC Suggested Outcomes

- Health-Promoting Behavior (1602)
- Participation: Health Care Decisions (1606)
- Knowledge: Treatment Regimen (1813)

NIC Suggested Interventions

- Teaching: Disease Process (5602)
- Self-Modification Assistance (4470)
- Coping Enhancement (5230)

Nursing Interventions/Rationales

- Assess patient's current understanding of the disease process and the role of alcohol in its recurrence. *To establish a baseline for planning and intervention.*
- Assess patient's interest and commitment to abstain from alcohol. *The patient must be committed to change before change can successfully occur.*
- Assess knowledge of community resources for treatment and support. Refer as appropriate. *The patient has previously tried to abstain from alcohol without success. Assistance and support are necessary for success to occur.*
- Assess for symptoms of DTs during first 48 to 72 hours. Follow DT protocols as needed. *The patient may not be truthful about current level of alcohol use. Withdrawal carries a high mortality in acutely ill patients and necessitates specialized care.*
- Teach patient correct use of pancreatic enzymes (take with each meal and snack; monitor weight and stool consistency to judge need for dosage adjustment). *Malabsorption is permanent, and the patient will develop serious nutrient deficiencies if enzymes are not adequately replaced. A well-informed patient can safely make dosage adjustments.*
- Teach patient about the nature and planned management of hyperglycemia, including symptoms to report (frequent urination, thirst, lethargy, abdominal cramping). *Insulin may be needed to control hyperglycemia associated with pancreatitis. The patient needs to know how to recognize ketoacidosis.*
- Teach patient about hypoglycemia and symptoms to report (anxiety, tachycardia, diaphoresis). *The patient will likely remain hyperglycemic but must know how to prevent and recognize hypoglycemia.*

Encourage patient to make commitment to changing his lifestyle and gaining control of his disease and his life. *Patients with chronic pancreatitis often have given up hope in themselves and their ability to influence the future.*

Evaluation Parameters

1. Verbalizes understanding of disease process, role of alcohol, and pharmacologic management of symptoms
2. Refrains from the intake of alcohol

Metastasis has almost always occurred before the tumor produces its first symptoms, because there is no capsule surrounding the pancreas to contain its growth and extension. Direct extension of the lesion may cause its spread to the posterior wall of the stomach, the duodenal wall, the colon, the common bile duct, and lymph nodes. Vital blood vessels in the area are also commonly involved.

Pain and jaundice are the most common symptoms of pancreatic cancer.[18] The pain is usually described as epigastric in location and steady and severe in character. It occurs or is worsened by lying down and bears no relationship to meals. The pain is relentlessly progressive in nature. Jaundice is a presenting symptom in 80% to 90% of patients with cancer in the head of the pancreas. The cancer produces jaundice by compressing and obstructing the bile duct. Light-colored stools and dark urine may also occur. Weight loss is also common, usually from pain-related anorexia. Diarrhea and steatorrhea may also occur if pancreatic duct obstruction is severe.

Collaborative Care Management

The diagnosis of pancreatic cancer is often initially made on the basis of the pattern of symptoms and then is confirmed through CT scanning. Guided needle biopsy may be performed to obtain histologic data.

Cancer of the pancreas is almost universally fatal, and the median survival time is only 18 to 20 months.[18] Surgical resection provides the only hope of cure, but it does not always improve survival.

Surgeons who are attempting curative resection typically use the aggressive Whipple procedure or total pancreatectomy (Figure 35-6). This is a complex surgical procedure that entails a prolonged recovery period. It includes a partial gastrectomy;

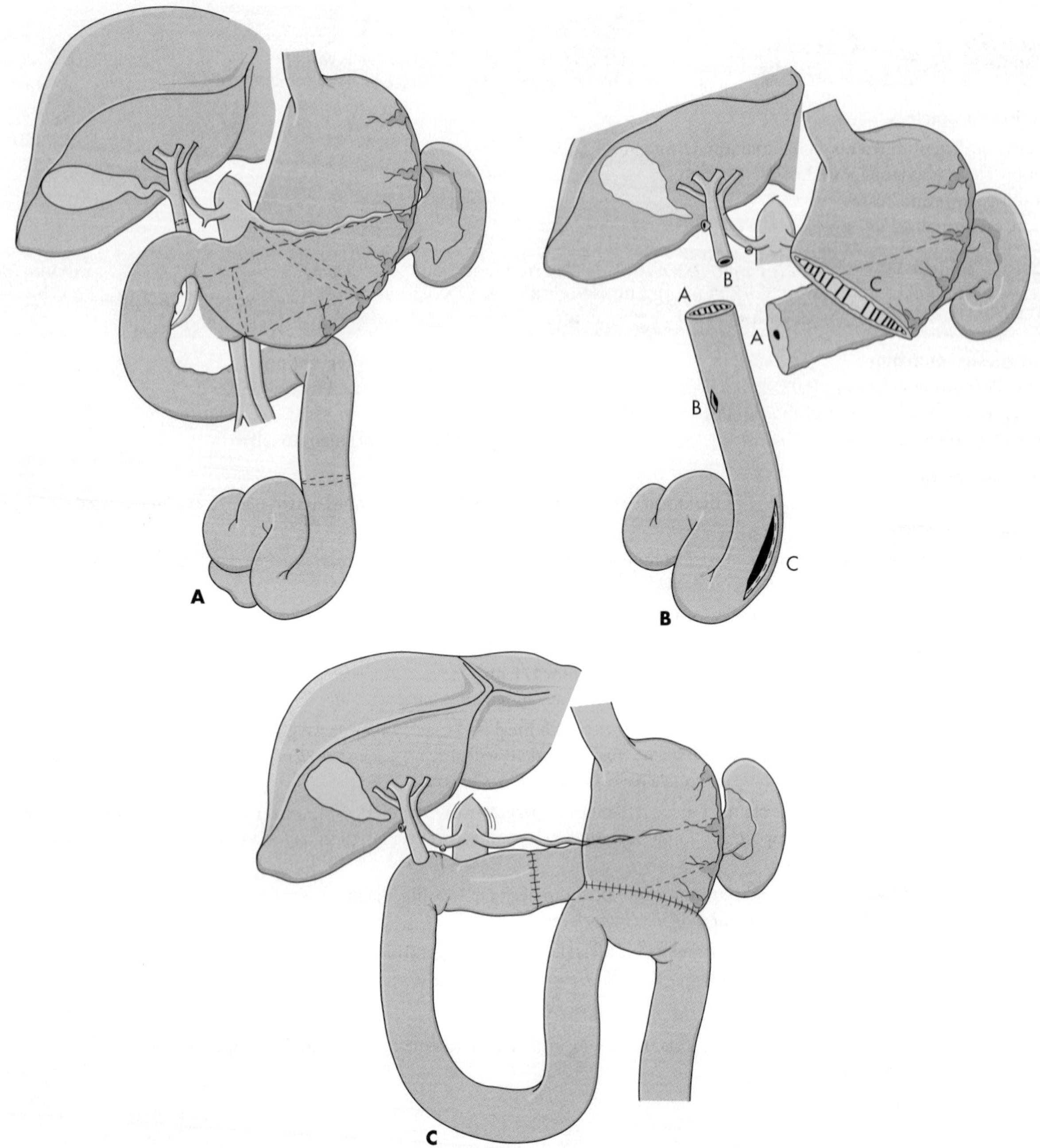

Figure 35-6 Standard Whipple pancreatic duodenectomy. **A,** Dotted lines indicate margins for resection. **B,** Tissue has been resected. Sites for anastomoses are labeled *A, B,* and *C.* **C,** Anastamoses are complete.

cholecystectomy; and removal of the distal common bile duct, head of the pancreas, duodenum, proximal jejunum, and regional lymph nodes. Some surgeons prefer to modify the procedure by preserving the stomach, pylorus, and first portion of the duodenum. This adaptation maintains gastric emptying at a near-normal level. Although the operative mortality is now less than 2% with a highly skilled surgeon, the procedure is used ideally only when cure is at least a possibility.

Obstruction is a common problem with large tumors involving the pancreatic head, and surgical bypass is often necessary even when curative resection is not feasible. Procedures include gastrojejunostomy to bypass the duodenum and choledochojejunostomy to relieve biliary obstruction. Endoscopic placement of stent tubes to support biliary drainage is increasingly being considered as an alternative to surgery. Stents may be placed internally or inserted for external drainage. Neither radiotherapy nor chemotherapy alone has had any positive effects on the course of the disease, but combination protocols show early promise of extending life expectancy by nearly a year.

Patient/Family Education. Pain management is an ongoing challenge with pancreatic cancer and is often the primary determinant of quality of life. The nurse serves as the patient's advocate in the health care system to establish an effective pain management protocol and continuously adapt it to changes in the patient's condition. The nurse provides careful teaching about the use of opioid analgesics and the inevitable development of tolerance and physical dependence (see Chapter 12).

Guidelines for Safe Practice

The Patient Undergoing Pancreatic Surgery

PREOPERATIVE CARE

Provide thorough teaching about planned surgical procedure and expected postoperative care.

Monitor prothrombin time and other clotting studies; vitamin K and other clotting factors may be administered.

Assess nutritional status. Administer nutritional support if ordered.

POSTOPERATIVE CARE

Monitor vital parameters every hour. Critical care placement is usually necessary.
- Check vital signs, intake and output, and hemodynamic parameters.
- Perform blood gas, oxygen saturation, and routine blood studies.
- Be alert to signs of bleeding or shock.
- Maintain urine output at 30 to 50 ml/hr.

Initiate pulmonary hygiene every hour with deep breathing, coughing as needed, and use of incentive spirometry.

Establish effective pain management regimen. Monitor every hour.

Monitor dressings and drainage tubes. Keep skin clear of drainage.

Maintain nutritional support with enteral or parenteral nutrition.
- Initiate oral feedings with clear liquids. Advance as tolerated.
- Monitor blood glucose and administer insulin as ordered.
- Monitor patient's weight and the development of steatorrhea.
  - Administer pancreatic enzyme replacement as ordered.
  - Assess for signs of dumping syndrome (see Chapter 33).

Provide support for patient and family, and initiate discharge planning.

Instruction is also provided about expected side effects and their management. Other general measures are those provided to any patient with invasive cancer (see Chapter 15). Nursing care of the patient undergoing pancreatic surgery is summarized in the Guidelines for Safe Practice box.

Critical Thinking Questions

1. A 57-year-old Caucasian woman has been experiencing frequent episodes of right upper quadrant abdominal pain and nausea after large meals. Her physician has identified the presence of gallstones on ultrasound examination and is recommending laparoscopic cholecystectomy. You know the woman slightly from your church, and she approaches you for advice. She confesses that she is terrified of surgery—her mother died during a surgical procedure—and asks, "Isn't there a way to treat this without surgery?"
   a. *How would you respond to her concerns?*
   b. *What are the pros and cons of the various treatment options for this situation?*
2. A 70-year-old married man was just diagnosed with acute pancreatitis and is extremely ill. His wife takes you aside and says, "I simply don't understand. I thought pancreatitis was something alcoholics got! How did my husband get this disease?" How will you answer her?
3. You work on an acute medical unit in a large urban hospital and care for a steady stream of patients with acute and chronic pancreatitis. You are interested in studying the question of enteral versus parenteral feeding for this population. Design a clinical study to compare the efficacy and cost-effectiveness of the two approaches. How will you select your sample, and what variables will you study?
4. A woman has been diagnosed with unresectable cancer of the pancreas and has a grim prognosis. Her family is clear that they want everything possible to be done for her. She is extremely ambivalent and expresses the desire to not pursue aggressive treatment. How will you address this "quality of life" issue? Who should be involved in the planning?

References

1. Bateson MC: Gallstones and cholecystectomy in modern Britain, *Postgrad Med J* 76:700-703, 2000.
2. Brodsky A et al: Laparoscopic cholecystectomy for acute cholecystitis: can the need for conversion and the probability of complications be predicted? *Surg Endosc* 14(8):755-760, 2000.
3. Farrar JA: Acute cholecystitis: recognizing the signs and symptoms and preventing complications, *Am J Nurs* 101(1):35-36, 2001.
4. Goroll, AH: Gallstone disease. In Goroll AH, Mulley AG, editors: *Primary care medicine,* ed 4, Philadelphia, 2000, JB Lippincott.
5. Hart AR: Pancreatic cancer: any prospects for prevention? *Postgrad Med J* 75:521-526, 1999.
6. Howard DE, Fromm H: Nonsurgical management of gallstone disease, *Gastroenterol Clin North Am* 28:133-144, 1999.
7. Lee SP, Ko CW: Gallstones. In Yamada T, editor: *Textbook of gastroenterology,* ed 3, Philadelphia, 1999, JB Lippincott.
8. Leitzman MF et al: The relation of physical activity to risk for symptomatic gallstone disease in men, *Ann Intern Med* 128:417-425, 1998.
9. Lobo DN et al: Evolution of nutritional support in acute pancreatitis, *Br J Surg* 87(6):695-707, 2000.
10. Lu SC: Diseases of the biliary tree. In Yamada T, editor: *Textbook of gastroenterology,* ed 3, Philadelphia, 1999, JB Lippincott.
11. McClave SA, Ritchie CS: Artificial nutrition in pancreatic disease: what lessons have we learned from the literature? *Clin Nutr* 19(1):1-6, 2000.
12. Owyang C: Chronic pancreatitis. In Yamada T, editor: *Textbook of gastroenterology,* ed 3, Philadelphia, 1999, JB Lippincott.
13. Richter J: Acute and chronic disease of the pancreas. In Goroll AH, Mulley AG, editors: *Primary care medicine,* ed 4, Philadelphia, 2000, JB Lippincott.
14. Sakorafas GH, Tsiotou AG: Etiology and pathogenesis of acute pancreatitis, *J Clin Gastroenterol* 30(4):343-356, 2000.
15. Somogyi L et al: Recurrent acute pancreatitis: an algorithmic approach to identification and elimination of inciting factors, *Gastroenterology* 120(3):708-717, 2001.
16. Strasberg SM, Drebin JA: Tumors of the biliary tree. In Yamada T, editor: *Textbook of gastroenterology,* ed 3, Philadelphia, 1999, JB Lippincott.
17. Sterling RK, Shiffman ML: Nonsteroidal anti-inflammatory drugs and gallstone disease: will an aspirin a day keep the gallstones away? *Am J Gastroenterol* 93:1405-1407, 1998.
18. Todd KE, Gloor B, Reber HA: Pancreatic adenocarcinoma. In Yamada T, editor: *Textbook of gastroenterology,* ed 3, Philadelphia, 1999, JB Lippincott.
19. Topazian M, Gorelick FS: Acute pancreatitis. In Yamada T, editor: *Textbook of gastroenterology,* ed 3, Philadelphia, 1999, JB Lippincott.
20. Trotto NE: Contemporary management of gallstone disease, *Patient Care* 33(20):90-106, 1999.

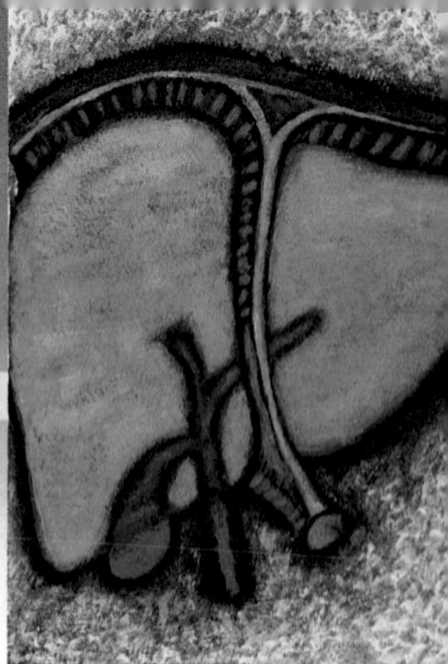

36 Assessment of the Hepatic System

Sally A. Brozenec

Objectives

After studying this chapter, the learner should be able to:

1. Describe the normal anatomy and physiology of the liver.
2. Describe the role of the liver in metabolism and maintenance of energy balance.
3. Explain the basis for data that must be collected to identify problems of the hepatic system.
4. Relate the various laboratory and diagnostic tests used in identifying the pathophysiologic states of the liver.
5. Synthesize a plan of care for patients undergoing the radiologic and special tests used in diagnosing hepatic dysfunction.

The liver is the largest gland in the body and has 500 identified functions. Because the liver has so many functions, pathologic conditions in this organ can cause a variety of problems that have an impact on the entire body. Of primary importance is its role in metabolism and the maintenance of normal energy stores.

ANATOMY AND PHYSIOLOGY

Anatomy

The liver is one of the most complex organs in the body and weighs approximately 1.3 to 1.8 kg. The falciform ligament divides the liver into right and left lobes and provides attachment to the anterior abdominal wall (Figure 36-1).

The round ligament is a remnant of the umbilical vein and extends from the umbilicus to the inferior surface of the liver. The Glisson capsule, a fibroelastic capsule containing blood vessels, lymphatics, and nerves, covers the liver.

Anatomically the liver extends up under the ribs and is 4 to 8 cm in height at the midsternal line and 6 to 12 cm in height at the midclavicular line. The liver normally extends from the fifth intercostal space.

The liver is served by two separate blood supplies, and at any one time contains about 13% of the total blood. Approximately 75% of the blood flow to the liver is through the portal vein, which carries nutrient-rich blood from the stomach and intestines (Figure 36-2). The remaining 25% of the blood flow is through the hepatic artery, which carries oxygenated blood from the lungs to the hepatic cells.

The portal system is a venous pathway through the liver. Blood from the portal vein flows to the large capillaries called sinusoids, which separate the layers of hepatic cells. From the sinusoids the portal blood, along with the oxygenated blood from the hepatic artery, progresses to the hepatic vein from which it is emptied into the inferior vena cava for return to the right atrium. The portal vein brings 75% of the blood supply to the liver, whereas the hepatic artery delivers about 25% (Figure 36-3).

Pressure in the portal system is normally 3 mm Hg. Portal hypertension is a rise in portal pressure to at least 10 mm Hg and can be caused by any disorder that obstructs or impedes blood flow through any portion of the portal system or vena cava. Elevated pressures in the portal system cause collateral vessels to open between the portal veins and the systemic veins, avoiding the obstructed portal vessels. These collateral vessels may develop in the esophagus, anterior abdominal wall, or rectum. The liver is innervated by the sympathetic and parasympathetic nervous systems. Sympathetic fibers innervate the hepatic artery branches and the bile ducts, while parasympathetic nerve fibers supply the intrahepatic and extrahepatic biliary tract system. Stimulation of the sympathetic and parasympathetic nervous systems affects both blood flow and the flow of bile within the biliary tract, but the function of the hepatic cells or parenchymal cells is not influenced.

The functional unit of the liver is the liver lobule (Figure 36-4). Each lobule is composed of multiple plates of hepatic cells. Between the individual cells of the cellular plate are biliary canaliculi, which empty into the bile ducts. The terminal bile ducts join to form the hepatic duct, which merges with the cystic duct of the gallbladder to form the common bile duct. Each side of the cellular plate contains a venous sinusoid, which receives blood from branches of the portal vein and hepatic artery. As blood flows through the sinusoids, substances can be exchanged between the hepatic cells and the blood.

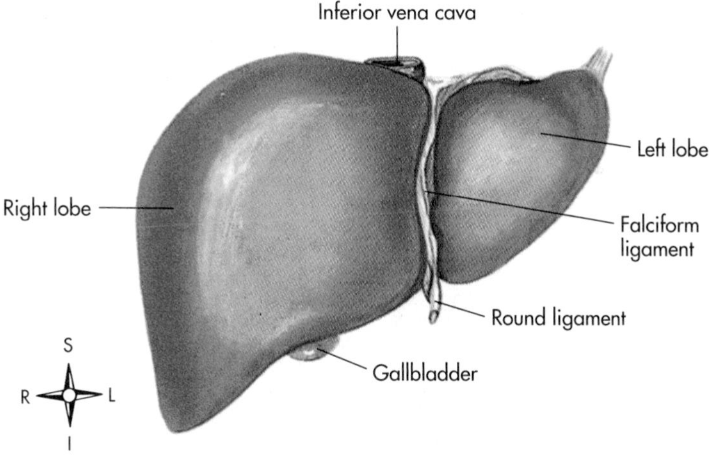

Figure 36-1 Gross structure of the liver, anterior view.

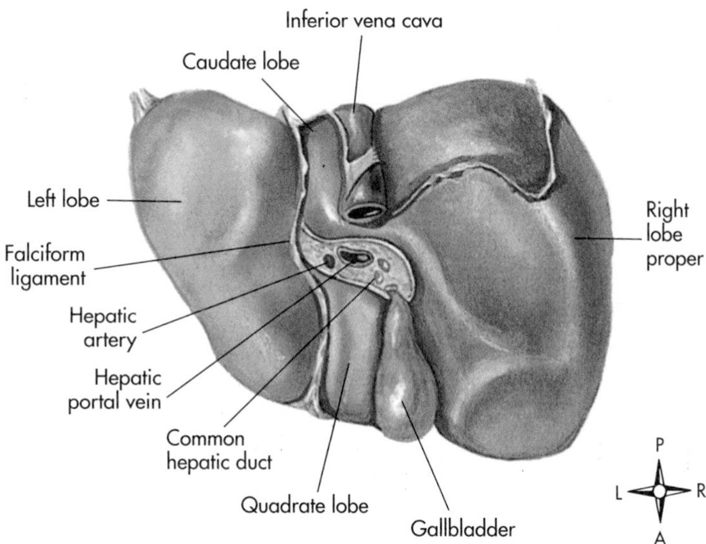

Figure 36-2 Gross structure of the liver, inferior view.

The sinusoids are lined with phagocytic cells of the reticuloendothelial system (Kupffer cells). These cells remove bacteria and other foreign substances from the blood. Because the portal blood originates in the gastrointestinal (GI) tract, some bacteria or other foreign substances need to be removed. The blood from the venous sinusoids empties into the central vein and then into the hepatic vein. The hepatic vein empties into the inferior vena cava.

Physiology

The liver can be thought of as a metabolic factory and a waste disposal plant. As should be evident from the anatomic description of the blood and bile flow, the liver is ideally structured to carry out its multiple metabolic and waste disposal functions. The major functions of the liver are summarized in Box 36-1 and presented in more detail in the following sections.

Carbohydrate, Protein, and Fat Metabolism

The liver has a significant role in the metabolism of each of the three major nutrients. It either oxidizes the nutrients for energy, uses them to synthesize storage forms of substances for future use, or uses them to synthesize other essential compounds.

Carbohydrates. Immediately after meals, the liver extracts glucose, fructose, and galactose from the blood. These simple sugars are metabolized into glycogen (glycogenesis) to replenish liver stores. If the diet ingested is low in carbohydrates, the liver converts protein to glucose to replenish glycogen stores. If more carbohydrate is ingested than is needed to replenish glycogen stores or to supply energy, the excess carbohydrate is converted to fat (lipogenesis). Between meals and during other fasting states, the liver assists in maintaining the blood glucose concentration by breaking down glycogen (glycogenolysis) or forming new glucose (gluconeogenesis). The new glucose is made from amino acids, glycerol, and lactic acids. Through

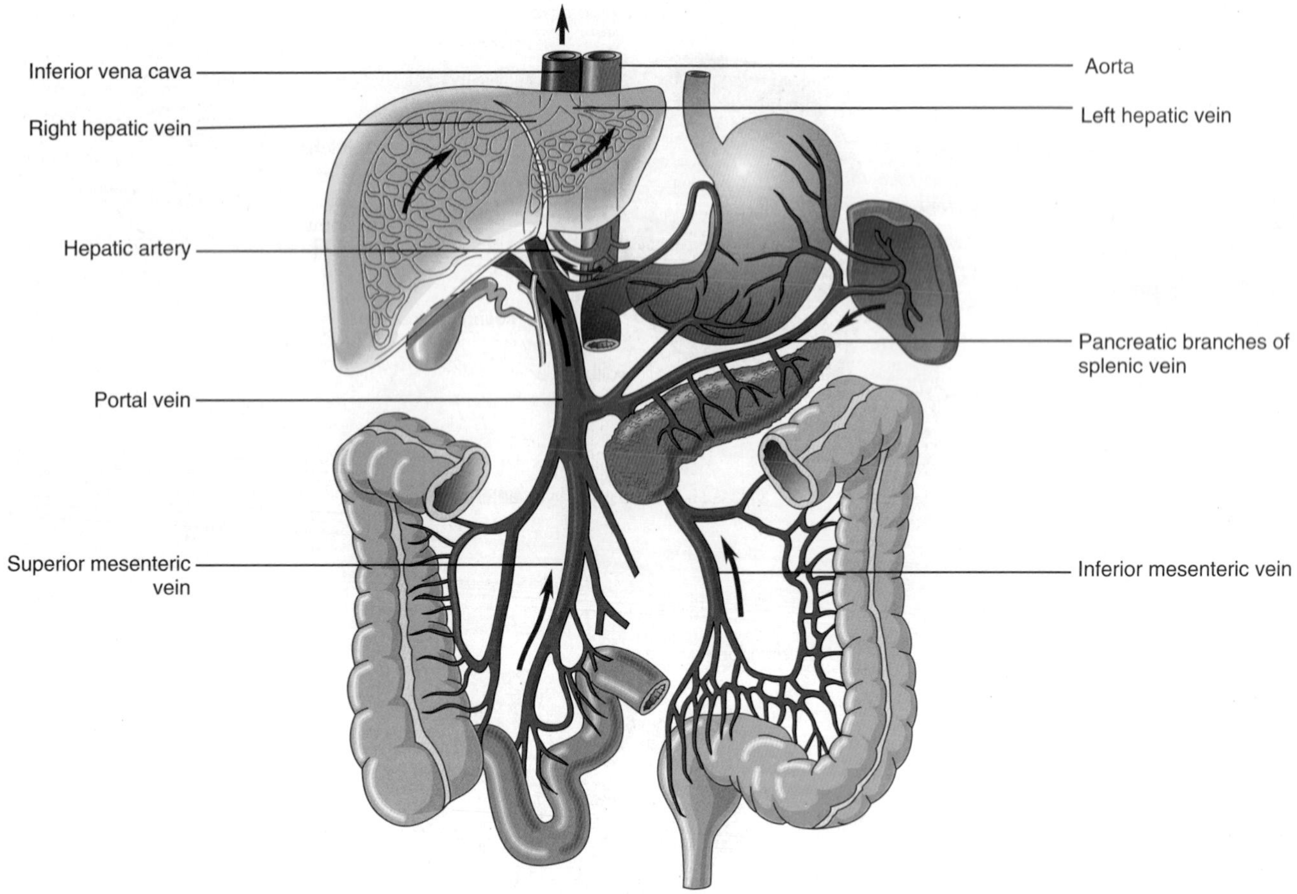

Inferior vena cava
Aorta
Right hepatic vein
Left hepatic vein
Hepatic artery
Pancreatic branches of splenic vein
Portal vein
Superior mesenteric vein
Inferior mesenteric vein

Figure 36-3 Diagram of normal portal circulation.

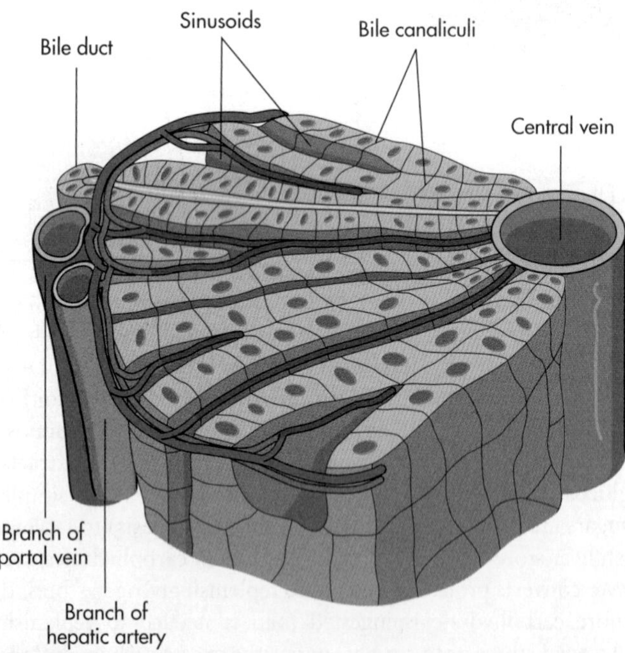

Figure 36-4 Diagrammatic representation of a liver lobule. A central vein is located in the center of the lobule with plates of hepatic cells disposed radially. Branches of the portal vein and hepatic artery are located on the periphery of the lobule, and blood from both perfuses the sinusoids. Peripherally located bile ducts drain the bile canaliculi that run between the hepatocytes.

glycogenesis, lipogenesis, glycogenolysis, and gluconeogenesis, which are under hormonal control, the liver helps to maintain a normal blood glucose level, preventing high levels immediately after eating (postprandial) and hypoglycemia between meals or during other periods of fasting.

Proteins. The liver is vital to normal protein metabolism. It provides needed amino acids through transamination. Transamination is the process of nitrogen metabolism in which the liver transfers an amino group (NH_2) to form nonessential amino acids. The liver also is the only source of some of the major plasma proteins. One of these major proteins is albumin, which is necessary for the maintenance of a normal internal environment and for fluid and electrolyte balance. Albumin is responsible for maintaining colloid osmotic pressure and thus the proper distribution of fluids between the vascular and interstitial compartments.

The liver is the source of several clotting factors. It produces fibrinogen (factor I), prothrombin (factor II), factor V (proaccelerin), factor VII (serum prothrombin conversion accelerator or Proconvertin), factor IX (Christmas factor), and factor X (Stuart or Stuart-Prower factor). The production of factors II, VII, IX, and X requires vitamin K. Vitamin K is a fat-soluble vitamin and therefore requires adequate production and excretion of bile for its absorption. In addition to protein synthesis, the liver catabolizes proteins as necessary for energy or glucose production.

BOX 36-1 Summary of Liver Functions

1. Carbohydrate, protein, and fat metabolism
   a. Carbohydrate metabolism
      (1) Glycogen formation and storage
      (2) Glucose formation from glycogen (glycogenolysis) and from amino acids, lactic acids, and glycerol (gluconeogenesis)
   b. Protein metabolism
      (1) Protein catabolism
      (2) Protein synthesis
         (a) Albumin
         (b) α- and β-Globulins
         (c) Clotting factors
         (d) C-reactive protein
         (e) Transferrin
         (f) Enzymes
         (g) Ceruloplasmin
      (3) Formation of needed amino acids
   c. Fat metabolism
      (1) Oxidation of fatty acids for energy
      (2) Ketone formation
      (3) Synthesis of cholesterol and phospholipids
      (4) Formation of triglycerides from dietary lipids and excessive dietary carbohydrates and proteins
      (5) Formation of lipoproteins
2. Production of bile salts
3. Bilirubin metabolism
4. Detoxification of endogenous and exogenous substances
   a. Ammonia
   b. Steroids
   c. Drugs
5. Storage of minerals and vitamins
6. Blood reservoir

Fats. The liver is involved in multiple aspects of fat metabolism. Triglycerides in the diet are absorbed in chylomicrons. The chylomicrons are taken up by the liver and metabolized to fatty acids. These fatty acids may be (1) oxidized and used for energy by the liver and other body tissues; (2) metabolized to ketones; (3) converted to phospholipids; (4) combined with cholesterol, which is synthesized in the liver, to form cholesterol esters; or (5) reesterified to triglycerides and combined with protein, cholesterol, and phospholipids to form lipoproteins. The liver also uses fatty acids released from adipose tissue storage sites for these same processes.

Production of Bile Salts

Bile production is one of the major functions of the liver. Bile is a complex compound composed of cholesterol, phospholipids, bile salts, bile pigments (bilirubin), and very small amounts of proteins and electrolytes; 97% of bile is water. Metabolites of drugs and other substances that need to be excreted may also be found in bile. Bile salts are necessary for the absorption of fats, cholesterol, and fat-soluble vitamins, particularly vitamin K. Bile is released from the liver and concentrated and stored in the gallbladder. The liver secretes approximately 700 ml of bile daily. The bile salts released during each meal are reabsorbed into the enterohepatic circulation and recycled two or three times during a meal. Bile itself is resorbed along the total intestinal tract, but the terminal ileum has a major role in its active resorption. If the terminal ileum is diseased or resected, resorption of bile does not occur and abnormal fat absorption results.

Bilirubin Metabolism

Bilirubin is a byproduct of the heme portion of red blood cells and is released when these cells are destroyed. The released bilirubin is not water soluble (unconjugated). Unconjugated bilirubin is carried in the blood bound to albumin and other proteins. The liver extracts the unconjugated bilirubin from the blood and combines it with glucoronide into a water-soluble form (conjugated). The conjugated bilirubin is secreted into the bile and then enters the duodenum. In the GI tract bilirubin is metabolized to urobilinogen. Urobilinogen is excreted in feces as stercobilin, which gives feces its brown color, or it is resorbed. Most of the resorbed urobilinogen is extracted from the blood by the liver and recycled; some is excreted in the urine.

Metabolic Detoxification

The liver has a prime role in metabolic detoxification or biotransformation of endogenous and exogenous substances. Ammonia (NH_3) is a major toxic product processed by the liver. Ammonia is produced in the gut and the liver from the deamination of amino acids (the removal of NH_2 from amino acids). Bacteria in the GI tract are responsible for the ammonia formation in the gut. Peripheral blood ammonia levels are kept very low because the ammonia from the gut is extracted from the enterohepatic circulation by the liver and it, along with the ammonia produced in the liver, is detoxified by conversion into urea, which is then excreted by the kidneys.

Steroids and hormones (estrogen, progesterone, testosterone, corticosterone, antidiuretic hormone, and aldosterone) are inactivated by the liver. Liver diseases may depress this inactivation, resulting in pathologic levels of these hormones.

The liver detoxifies many drugs; barbiturates (except phenobarbital and barbital), amphetamines, and many sedatives are metabolized by the liver. Detoxification decreases intestinal or renal tubular resorption of potentially harmful substances and facilitates intestinal or renal excretion. Pathologic states of the liver may impair the effectiveness of detoxification.

Storage of Minerals and Vitamins

The liver stores reserves of various minerals and vitamins. This storage prevents abnormal internal levels from occurring, although the oral intake may be very irregular. Vitamins A, D, and B_{12} are stored in sufficient quantities to prevent deficiencies for months. Vitamins E and K are also stored. Iron in the form of ferritin is stored and can be used to resupply iron for hemoglobin formation as needed; copper is stored as well.

Blood Reservoir

The liver, because of its tremendous vascular supply and sinusoidal system, can act as a reservoir for blood. When the venous vascular volume becomes greater than can be handled by the right side of the heart, the excess blood can be stored in the liver. In the event of hemorrhage, the liver can release blood to maintain systemic circulatory volume.[2]

Physiologic Changes With Aging

As the body ages, the number and size of hepatic cells decrease, which results in an overall decrease in the size and weight of the liver by about 37%. There is also a 35% decrease in hepatic blood flow with increasing age. Despite this, common liver function tests usually show normal results in elderly persons unless a pathologic condition exists. One of the most serious concerns about the aging liver is the decreased synthesis of enzymes that assist in the metabolism of drugs, particularly anticonvulsants, psychotropic drugs, and oral anticoagulants. Research indicates that the metabolic reactions associated with drug clearance decrease 5% to 30% with age. Thus, the nurse should be alert to the signs and symptoms of drug toxicity even when the drugs are administered in normal doses because the decreased metabolism in the liver can cause an accumulation of the drug. There is also some evidence that normal aging may adversely affect liver tissue regeneration, resulting in prolonged recovery time.

ASSESSMENT

Health History

A thorough history is necessary to assess the health status of people with dysfunction of the hepatic system. Assessment focuses on comfort status; nutritional status; fluid and electrolyte status; elimination patterns; energy level; perception, motion, and cognition; and potential exposure to toxins, as well as general living conditions and lifestyle. Information related to previous history of hepatic disease or family history of disease is collected.

Comfort Status

Two major sources of discomfort associated with hepatic disease are abdominal pain and pruritus (itching). The person may complain of continuous upper abdominal discomfort or a dull ache in the upper right quadrant. This discomfort does not usually alter normal functioning, although it can cause shallow breathing. The discomfort is most significant in that it verifies the presence of a pathologic process. General body aching may be present in cases of acute viral infections of the liver. Pruritus, which may cause significant discomfort, is usually associated with jaundice. The pruritus results from a combination of two factors. One is the capillary dilation caused by the elevated serum bilirubin that occurs with jaundice. The second is the irritating effect of the bilirubin on the chemosensitive area of the skin. The history should include a description of any discomfort stated in the patient's own words as well as information about factors that worsen itching and measures that help relieve it.

Nutritional Status

People with hepatic dysfunction often experience alterations in nutritional status. Some hepatic problems result in anorexia, nausea, and vomiting. The patient should be questioned about the occurrence of such episodes, and information about onset, precipitating factors, association with food or alcohol intake, and measures that provide relief should be obtained.

Poor nutritional habits and malnutrition resulting from lifestyle patterns or food intolerances may be present. A useful method to assess the patient's nutritional status is to ask the patient what he or she has eaten in the past 24 hours and ascertain whether this is the typical eating pattern.

Alcohol use should also be explored. Alcohol exerts a toxic effect on liver cells and provides calories but no nutrition. Malnutrition, often associated with alcoholism, may aggravate the tissue injury. In the case of chronic alcohol use, muscle mass may have decreased while the overall weight remained stable. In addition, weight loss may be masked by water retention.

People with chronic problems of the hepatic system often require treatment with special diets, such as low sodium, altered protein intake, and water restriction. The history should include information about food intolerances and food preferences.

Fluid and Electrolyte Status

Hepatic dysfunction can be associated with either fluid volume deficit or excess. Fluid volume deficit can result from nausea and vomiting or from acute bleeding with cirrhosis. Fluid volume excess (edema) typically occurs in people with hepatic dysfunction as a result of renal retention of sodium and water that is initiated by peripheral vasodilation. This expansion of the vascular space effectively decreases the circulating blood volume, which results in the release of renin, angiotensin, and aldosterone. These hormones increase sodium and water retention. Also contributing to fluid volume excess is the hypoalbuminemia that is associated with liver disease. Albumin is the primary source of osmotic pressure in the vasculature; decreased albumin causes fluid to leave the vascular space and enter the interstitial space, resulting in edema and/or ascites. Levels of electrolytes, particularly sodium, potassium, hydrogen, and bicarbonate, can be elevated or decreased.

To assess fluid and electrolyte status, the history collected should include information about:

- Normal fluid and food intake and output.
- Abnormal fluid and electrolyte losses, such as vomiting, diarrhea, or bleeding.
- Changes in weight, both losses and gains.
- Occurrence of signs and symptoms of fluid or electrolyte deficit, such as weakness, dizziness, syncope, and weight loss.
- Occurrence of signs and symptoms of fluid or electrolyte excess, such as edema in hands, feet, and legs; an increase in abdominal girth; and weight gain.

Elimination Patterns

Intestinal and urinary elimination may be altered in people with liver problems. If there is an obstruction of bile flow, the person may give a history of grayish-white or clay-colored stools and have dark amber, brown, or mahogany-colored urine. Urine bilirubin levels will be elevated. Blood in the urine or stools may be present. The nurse can test for occult blood in the urine by using a reagent strip and test the stool by performing a Hematest or guaiac test. A reported decrease in urine output or the occurrence of nocturia may result from sodium and water retention.

Energy Level

Because of altered nutrient intake, abnormal fluid and electrolyte status, and increased metabolic needs, people with hepatic problems often report an activity intolerance to normal daily activities or simply fatigue. Weakness also may be reported. If the patient has developed ascites, the increased fluid in the abdomen pushes up on the diaphragm and can result in respiratory distress. As the underlying liver condition resolves, the fatigue and weakness may resolve; however, the patient and family must understand that the energy level may take a long time to return to normal.

Perception, Motion, and Cognition

Chronic health problems of the hepatic system can cause changes in neurologic functioning, particularly in relation to the peripheral nervous system and higher cognitive functions. The patient should be asked about alterations in sensation in extremities, any noticeable changes in memory, episodes of forgetfulness or blackouts, and alterations in coordination or in the ability to do fine motor tasks. The onset of any alterations, pattern of changes (continuous or intermittent), and duration of any changes should be determined.

Exposure to Toxins

Hepatic dysfunction can be caused by various agents, such as alcohol, drugs, industrial chemicals, and viruses. A history of exposure to any toxins must be elicited. A drug and alcohol history is necessary to determine whether the patient has been exposed to these two hepatotoxins.

The drug history should focus on prescription, over-the-counter, and street drugs. For example, acetaminophen is a drug often used by adolescents to commit suicide and can cause severe liver damage in doses 10 times greater than the recommended dose. The liver damage is intensified by the combination of acetaminophen and alcohol. The alcohol history should focus on normal amount of intake and time since last intake. An occupational history helps to identify potential toxins in the work environment such as methylene chloride solvents. An environmental/social history might identify potential sources of viruses (Box 36-2). The environmental/social history also can help identify particular persons, factors, or places associated with substance abuse, if a problem exists. Data about persons, factors, or places associated with drug or alcohol abuse are needed for its long-term management.

BOX 36-2 Health History Information Needed to Identify Exposure to Hepatitis Viruses

- Contact with persons with jaundice
- Travel or visits to environments with poor sanitation (e.g., camping trips, travel to developing countries)
- Ingestion of shellfish or raw fish
- History of recent ear or body piercing or tattooing
- History of recent blood transfusions
- Intravenous drug abuse (sharing of contaminated needles)
- Occupational exposure (e.g., health service personnel with frequent blood contact, personnel in day care centers, personnel in centers of custodial care)
- History of hemodialysis
- History of multiple sex partners; male bisexual or male homosexual lifestyle

Physical Examination

To assess the functioning of the hepatic system completely, a thorough assessment of the total body is required. First, a general survey of the patient is necessary. Does the patient appear chronically or acutely ill? Is the individual attentive, restless, or lethargic? Does the person appear nourished or malnourished? Is there obvious jaundice of the skin or sclera or in a dark-skinned person, of the palms of the hands? One should also observe for other signs of hepatic dysfunction such as enlarged abdomen, palmar erythema, change in secondary sexual characteristics, bruises, muscle wasting, or edema. Petechiae and spider angiomas, usually on the nose, cheeks, or upper thorax, may be present.

After the general inspection, assessment should focus on fluid status. Vital signs, including orthostatic changes, weight, temperature, skin turgor, mucous membrane moisture, presence of edema, and behavior changes, should be assessed. To assess energy level and nutritional status, the patient's total muscle mass and muscle strength should be examined. The patient's current weight, as well as his or her usual weight, should be determined.

While performing the assessment, note the patient's mental status, affect, and alertness. Note changes in facial expression, responsiveness, and level of consciousness. Are there periods of confusion or disorientation? Is the affect appropriate for this situation? Because handwriting or the ability to draw a box, triangle, or square deteriorates with decreasing liver function, a sample of handwriting or a drawing of a geometric figure may be obtained from the patient.

Next the assessment should focus on the abdomen. The abdomen is inspected for enlargement, presence of distended or dilated periumbilical veins (caput medusae), and ascites. Ascites is characterized by distention of the abdomen with tight, glistening skin, protruding umbilicus, and bulging flanks. Palpation and percussion are used to ascertain the presence of a fluid wave and shifting dullness, which are indicative of ascites, as well as to assess for hepatic tenderness, size, and consistency and the presence of hepatic masses. The spleen often is enlarged in the patient with chronic hepatic dysfunction and should be percussed to determine the size and location; palpation should be deferred because of the fragility of the enlarged spleen. Last, abdominal girth should be measured. Hemorrhoids caused by prolonged elevations in portal system pressure may be present.[4]

Assessment measures and variations in normal findings relevant to the care of older adults are presented in the Gerontologic Assessment box. Also identified are disorders common

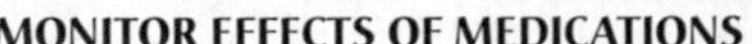

Gerontologic Assessment

MONITOR EFFECTS OF MEDICATIONS

- Older patients seem to have more problems with both the therapeutic effects of medications and drug toxicity. This may be due in part to the decrease in hepatic circulation that accompanies aging, as well as to the decrease in the enzyme activity of the liver.
- Standard doses of medication published in a formulary may be too high for elderly patients. Most drug dosages are calculated for healthy white adult men.
- Polypharmacy occurs when the elderly patient receives multiple medications from multiple prescribers.

ASSESS NUTRITIONAL STATUS

Because the liver has many functions that aim to maintain energy stores and metabolism, the elderly patient may show signs of fatigue if liver function has diminished enough to limit the available energy needed to support activities of daily living.

COMMON DISORDERS IN OLDER ADULTS

Increased risk for drug toxicity
Polypharmacy
Malnutrition

in older adults that may be responsible for abnormal assessment findings.

Diagnostic Tests

Laboratory Tests

Multiple tests may be necessary to determine the extent and seriousness of hepatic disease. To be of benefit many tests require serial readings. The procedure, preparation, and interpretation of blood, stool, and urine studies used to evaluate liver function are summarized in Table 36-1.[1,3] The nursing care responsibilities are listed under the column "Procedure and Preparation." In addition, the nurse explains the test to the patient and answers questions the patient my have regarding the preparation and/or specific test.

Radiologic Tests

Radiographic tests are used to assist in identifying the cause of hepatic dysfunction. Besides specific liver tests, abdominal films, barium swallow, barium enema, and gastroscopy may be ordered. These tests help identify the presence of pathologic GI conditions that may cause signs and symptoms similar to those found in hepatic dysfunction.

TABLE 36-1 Laboratory Tests of Liver Function

Function and Test	Procedure and Preparation	Interpretation
Fat metabolism Serum total cholesterol and cholesterol esters	Venipuncture; fasting may be required	Desirable range is <200 mg/dl of blood; approximately 70% is cholesterol ester; in hepatocellular disease, amount of total serum cholesterol and cholesterol ester may be decreased; in obstructive biliary tract disease, total serum cholesterol is increased, but amount of esterified cholesterol is decreased; normal cholesterol levels rise with age
Serum phospholipids	Venipuncture; no special preparation	Normal level is 150-250 mg/dl; serum phospholipids tend to be low in severe hepatocellular disease and high in obstructive biliary tract disease
Protein metabolism Total serum protein	Venipuncture; no special preparation	Normal level is 6-8 g/dl; measures all serum protein; may be normal in hepatocellular disease because increased serum globulin will replace decreased serum albumin; increased serum globulin is seen in chronic inflammatory disease, neoplastic diseases, and biliary obstruction
Albumin	Venipuncture; no special preparation	Normal level is 3.5-5.5 g/dl; albumin made only in liver; in hepatocellular disease may be decrease in serum albumin level
Protein electrophoresis	Venipuncture; no special preparation; protein fraction of blood will migrate in characteristic directions in electrical field; after separation of fractions, specimen stained, and densitometer used to measure amounts of various serum protein	Normal fractions in relation to total serum protein (100%): albumin, 52%–68%; α-globulins, 12%–17%; β-globulins, 7%–15%; and immune serum globulins (γ-globulins), 9%–19%; in severe hepatocellular damage, amount of albumin may be decreased; inflammatory processes of liver may produce increased amounts of α_1-globulins, neoplastic disease is associated with increased levels of α_2-globulins; some patients with obstructive biliary tract disease may have high levels of β-globulins
Immunoglobulins	Venipuncture; no special preparation	Five classes of antibodies: IgA, IgG, IgM, IgF, and IgD; IgA and IgG often increased in presence of cirrhosis; IgG elevated in presence of chronic active hepatitis; biliary cirrhosis and hepatitis A cause increase in IgM component
Blood urea nitrogen (BUN)	Venipuncture; no special preparation	Normal is 11-23 mg/dl; in severe hepatocellular disease if portal venous flow is obstructed, level may decrease; varies with dietary protein intake and fluid volume

Sources: Gopal DV, Rosen HR: Abnormal findings on liver function tests, *Postgrad Med* 107:100, 2000; Moseley RH: Approach to the patient with abnormal liver chemistries. In Kelley WN, editor: *Textbook of internal medicine,* ed 3, Philadelphia, 1997, Lippincott-Raven.

TABLE 36-1 Laboratory Tests of Liver Function—cont'd

Function and Test	Procedure and Preparation	Interpretation
Serum prothrombin time (PT)	Venipuncture; no special preparation; reflects activity of extrinsic and common coagulation pathways, including prothrombin, fibrinogen, and factors V, VII, IX, and X	Normal PT is 12-14 sec; it is compared with a control level; the normal PT is calculated based on the institution's control and therefore may differ among institutions; may be expressed as International Normalized Ratio (INR); PT reflects activity of extrinsic and common coagulation pathways, including prothrombin, fibrinogen, and factors V, VII, IX, and X; PT may be increased in hepatocellular disease because of the inability of liver to produce clotting factors or in obstructive hepatic or biliary tract disease because of the malabsorption of vitamin K; persistence of abnormal PT after parenteral administration of vitamin K indicates hepatocellular damage
Serum partial thromboplastin time (PTT) and activated partial thromboplastin time (APTT)	Venipuncture; no special preparation; reflects activity of intrinsic and common coagulation pathways	Normal PTT is 68-82 sec with standard technique, APTT is 20-35 sec; as with the PT, the normal value may differ among institutions, depending on control used; PTT reflects activity of intrinsic and common coagulation pathways; PTT and APTT will be increased in hepatocellular disease because of inability of liver to produce clotting factors
Blood ammonia levels	Venipuncture; may require fasting	Normal level is <75 mg/dl; may be elevated in severe hepatocellular disease because of obstruction of portal blood flow and rarely because of decreased urea synthesis
Bilirubin metabolism Total bilirubin Conjugated (direct) Unconjugated (indirect)	Venipuncture, no special preparation	Total serum bilirubin measures both conjugated and unconjugated bilirubin; normal total serum bilirubin values range from 0.3-1.1 mg/dl; conjugated bilirubin acts directly with diazo reagents; unconjugated bilirubin requires addition of methyl alcohol; thus the terms direct and indirect; conjugated bilirubin increases in presence of hepatocellular or obstructive biliary tract disease; unconjugated bilirubin is elevated in presence of increased hemolysis of red blood cells or hepatocellular disease
Urine bilirubin	Spot urine specimen; no special preparation	Normally no bilirubin is excreted in urine; urine with abnormal bilirubin is mahogany colored and has a yellow foam when shaken (foam test); unconjugated bilirubin even in excess is not excreted in urine because it is not water soluble; conjugated serum bilirubin levels >0.4 mg/dl will lead to conjugated bilirubin being excreted in urine because it is water soluble and indicates hepatocellular or obstructive biliary tract disease; bilirubinuria may be present before jaundice.
Urine urobilinogen	24-hr urine collection or 2-hr afternoon collection	Normally 0.2-1.2 U found in specimen; fresh urine urobilinogen is colorless; decreased amounts of urine urobilinogen found in obstructive biliary tract disease; increased amounts found in hepatocellular disease; alterations in intestinal flora by broad-spectrum antibiotics may change test.
Fecal urobilinogen	Stool specimen; no special preparation	Normally 90-280 mg/day; presence of fecal urobilinogen (stercobilin) gives stool brown color; absence of stercobilin causes stools to become clay (grayish white) to white colored; increased amounts of stercobilin found with increased hemolysis of red blood cells; absence of fecal stercobilin indicates obstructive biliary tract disease.
Serum enzymes Asparate aminotransferase (AST), formerly called serum glutamic-oxaloacetic transaminase (SGOT) Alanine aminotransferase (ALT), formerly called serum glutamic pyruvic transaminase (SGPT) Lactic dehydrogenase (LDH) γ-Glutamyl transpeptidase (GGT) (γ-glutamyltransferase)	Venipuncture; no special preparation	Normal values vary, depending on measurement used; these enzymes are present in hepatic cells; with necrosis of hepatic cells, enzymes are released and elevated serum levels will be found; GGT is found in high levels in liver cells as well as kidneys; ALT is primarily present in liver cells; AST is also present in high levels in skeletal and heart muscle; LDH is also present in heart cells, kidney cells, skeletal muscle cells, and erythrocytes, but in each tissue the LDH enzyme has characteristic composition: thus tissue source of elevated serum LDH levels can be determined by isoenzyme tests; with other three enzyme tests, necrosis of other organs must be ruled out; GGT is elevated early in liver disease, and elevation persists as long as cellular damage continues; GGT is routinely elevated in alcohol-induced liver disease, and increased levels are often seen before other abnormal test results occur.

Continued

TABLE 36-1 Laboratory Tests of Liver Function—cont'd

Function and Test	Procedure and Preparation	Interpretation
Alkaline phosphatase	Venipuncture; no special preparation	Normal values vary, depending on measurement used; originates in liver, bone, intestine, and placenta; alkaline phosphatase is slightly to moderately elevated in hepatocellular disease but extremely elevated in obstructive biliary tract and bone disease.
Antigens and antibodies of viral hepatitis	Venipuncture; no special preparation	Normally no hepatitis antigens are found in serum or other body fluids; hepatitis A virus (HAV) can be found in stool during last part of incubation period and early prodromal phase; IgM-class anti-HAV appears in the acute and early convalescent period and is used to diagnose hepatitis A; IgG-class anti-HAV becomes detectable during convalescent period and confers immunity; hepatitis B has many associated serum particles; complete hepatitis B virus (HBV) is also called Dane particle; core antigen (HBcAg) can be found in liver, an antibody (anti-HBc) can be found in blood, and presence of anti-HBc indicates past infection with HBV at some undefined time; a surface antigen (HBsAg) and several subtypes and antibody (anti-HBs) are also measurable; HBsAg is one of the antigens measured to diagnose hepatitis B, and its presence indicates infectivity; presence of anti-HBs indicates past infection and immunity to HBV, presence of passive antibodies from HBIG, or immune response from HBV vaccine; hepatitis Be antigen (HBeAg) indicates high infectivity and its antibody (anti-HBe) chronic infectivity; enzyme-linked immunosorbent assay (ELISA) has detected antibodies to hepatitis C (anti-HCV) in people who have been exposed to hepatitis C; however, antibodies do not appear in most people until at least 5 months after exposure to virus; an enterically transmitted virus that was previously related to hepatitis non-A non-B has been identified and labeled hepatitis E (HEV); anti-HEV has been detected using ELISA but is not available in United States at this time.

Ultrasonography. Ultrasonography of the liver is used to assess jaundice of unknown etiology, hepatomegaly, or suspected tumors. Information obtained from ultrasound includes liver size, shape, and location; cysts; abscesses; and filling or dilation defects.

Preparation of the patient for ultrasonography is relatively simple. Usually the patient is not allowed to eat for 8 to 12 hours before the procedure, because gas in the GI tract can interfere with the test. Also any residual barium from other tests needs to be eliminated from the GI tract. Finally the patient must be well hydrated, because dehydration can decrease the ability of ultrasonography to distinguish between the liver and surrounding tissues.

Computed Tomography. Computed tomography (CT) scanning can also be used to assess the liver. It can identify problems similar to those described for ultrasonography and in addition, can be used with the use of a contrast medium to intensify the appearance of vascular structures and hepatic parenchyma. The patient takes no food or drink by mouth for 8 to 12 hours before the test and, if contrast medium is to be used, is assessed for allergies to iodine or contrast media. Adequate hydration is also necessary when a contrast medium is used. Barium studies should be done at least 4 days before the CT scan or after the scan because the barium can interfere with test results.

Magnetic Resonance Imaging. Magnetic resonance imaging (MRI) is used to detect liver tumors. Because magnetic fields are used instead of radioactive isotopes to produce the image, no special preparation of the patient is necessary. It is important to inform the patient that this test is painless. The patient should be instructed to remove any jewelry, dentures, and partial dentures if they contain metal, or any other item that contains metal, such as hairpins or limb prostheses. Patients should be assessed for claustrophobia before the procedure, because the test may elicit this type of response. Contraindications to MRI include a pacemaker and titanium or stainless steel prosthetic implants or prosthetic heart valves.

Radionuclide Imaging. The liver may be outlined by radionuclide imaging techniques. Selected radioisotopes are given intravenously. After injection of the radioisotope, the patient is placed in the supine position, and a scintillation detector is passed over the abdomen in the area of the liver. The radiation coming from the isotopes immediately beneath the probe of the scanner is detected, amplified, and recorded. Scanning helps differentiate nonfunctioning areas from normal tissue and to identify hepatic tumors, cysts, and abscesses. Usually a nonfunctioning area appears as an area of decreased activity. However, gallium-67 (^{67}Ga) is preferentially taken up by hepatocellular carcinomas and abscesses, and hence these areas will appear as areas of very heavy radioactivity. Adverse reactions to the radioisotopes used for radionuclide imaging are unusual, and the procedure is relatively safe. Discomfort is minimal. Only small amounts of radioactive material are given, and radiation precautions are not necessary. Only ^{67}Ga scanning requires special preparation. ^{67}Ga is excreted by the GI tract. To avoid absorption of the radioisotope by the GI contents, laxatives and enemas are prescribed. The toilet should be flushed twice for bowel movements after the ^{67}Ga scanning to ensure the safety of the patient and others. Ultrasonography, CT scanning, and MRI have replaced radionuclide imaging in most instances of hepatic dysfunction.

Angiography and Portal Pressure Measurements. Catheterization of the hepatic artery, portal venous system (by various routes), and hepatic vein allows injection of a contrast medium and the visualization of the vascular supply of the hepatic system. Angiography determines the patency of the system and the presence of tumors, abscesses, collateral circulation, varices, and bleeding.

Portal and hepatic vein pressure (wedged hepatic vein pressure) can be measured. These readings may be done in conjunction with angiography or as a separate study. These measurements help in determining the degree of portal hypertension.

The presence of allergy to contrast media must be ascertained before angiography is done. After both angiography and pressure readings, the insertion site is observed for bleeding, and the patient's vital signs are checked every 15 minutes for 1 hour, every 30 minutes for 1 hour, every hour for 4 hours, and then if the patient is stable, every 4 hours. Bed rest is maintained for 24 to 48 hours after the test.

Special Tests

Liver Biopsy. A liver biopsy may be used to aid in establishing the cause of liver disease. In this procedure a specially designed needle is inserted through the chest or abdominal wall into the liver, and a small piece of tissue is removed for study. Liver biopsy is contraindicated for patients with infection of the right lower lobe of the lung, ascites, a blood dyscrasia, or a problem with blood clotting, as well as those unable to cooperate by holding the breath. To avoid hemorrhage, vitamin K may be given parenterally for several days before and after the biopsy is performed. A biopsy usually is not done if the prothrombin time is below 40% of normal. The importance of holding one's breath and remaining absolutely still when the needle is introduced should be explained to the patient, as movement of the chest may cause the needle to slip and to tear the liver covering. Most hospitals require that the patient sign a written permission form for the procedure to be done. In preparation for the biopsy, food and fluids may be withheld for several hours and a sedative given about 30 minutes before the procedure. For the procedure itself, the patient lies supine and the skin over the area selected (usually the eighth or ninth intercostal space) is cleansed and anesthetized with procaine hydrochloride. A nick is made in the skin with a sharp scalpel blade. Next the patient is instructed to take several deep breaths and then to hold his or her breath while the needle is introduced through the intercostal or subcostal tissues into the liver. The special needle assembly is rotated to separate a fragment of tissue and then is withdrawn. The specimen is placed into an appropriate container, which is labeled and sent to the pathology laboratory. A simple dressing is placed over the wound.

The dangers of liver biopsy are accidental penetration of blood vessels, causing hemorrhage, or accidental penetration of a biliary canniculi, causing a chemical peritonitis from leakage of bile into the abdominal cavity. After the procedure the nurse should assess the patient for signs of hypovolemia and shock. The nurse monitors the patient's pulse and blood pressure every 30 minutes for the first few hours after the procedure and then hourly for 24 hours. The patient's temperature should be taken at least every 4 hours to determine a baseline and detect the development of fever, which could indicate peritonitis. The physician may order pressure applied to the biopsy site to help stop any bleeding. An effective way to apply pressure is to have the patient lie on the right side with a small pillow or folded bath blanket placed under the costal margin for several hours after the biopsy. Bed rest is maintained for 24 hours after the test.

Paracentesis. A paracentesis, or peritoneal tap, is done to obtain peritoneal fluid (ascitic fluid) for cytologic or other laboratory studies or to drain large volumes of ascitic fluid. When conditions such as respiratory distress, severe abdominal discomfort, or cardiac dysfunction are present because of the ascites, a paracentesis may be necessary. Repeated paracenteses are not the treatment of choice for controlling chronic, recurring ascites because of complications.

Paracentesis is a sterile procedure. When paracentesis is performed, the skin is cleansed, and the abdominal wall is anesthetized. A long aspiration needle is inserted, and fluid is aspirated for diagnostic tests or drained. In preparation for the procedure, the patient is given a complete explanation and signs a consent form. Also, to diminish the risk of puncturing the bladder, the patient should void immediately before the procedure.

Complications of paracentesis include peritonitis and peritoneal bleeding resulting from trauma to blood vessels. When large amounts of fluid are removed from the peritoneal space, hypovolemia and shock can occur because additional fluid can shift from the intravascular compartment into the peritoneal cavity. (This risk is minimal in the patient with cirrhosis and edema.) Hence the patient's vital signs, including temperature, urine output, and skin temperature and moisture, are monitored after the procedure and the patient's abdomen is assessed for rigidity and his or her sensorium for confusion. Serum levels of protein and potassium are also monitored, as these substances are commonly lost during paracentesis.

Peritoneal Lavage. Peritoneal lavage may be used to assess damage to the liver from abdominal trauma in persons with altered states of consciousness who cannot give a satisfactory history. It may also be used in patients with abdominal trauma when unexplained hypotension is present, when unreliable physical examination results are present, or when the patient requires general anesthesia for other injuries.

Peritoneal lavage can be done by either the closed or open method. In the closed method a peritoneal dialysis catheter is inserted, and the peritoneal space is aspirated for gross blood. If no gross blood is found, lavage is carried out with normal saline. In the open method the peritoneum is exposed completely and then opened enough to allow entry of a dialysis catheter. Again, gross blood is aspirated first, and if no blood is found, lavage is carried out.

Peritoneal lavage requires a complete explanation to the patient and significant others and informed consent. The nurse inserts a nasogastric tube and Foley catheter before the procedure to prevent penetration of the intestines or bladder. In the closed method a local anesthetic is used, whereas in the open method general anesthesia is necessary. Postprocedural nursing care of patients who have closed peritoneal lavage involves monitoring for peritonitis and bleeding in. Patients who have open peritoneal lavage require general postanesthetic care.

Endoscopy

The hepatic system and gallbladder can be examined by several types of endoscopic procedures. The endoscope can be inserted directly through the peritoneum (peritoneoscopy), thus allowing direct visualization of the abdominal organs and the taking of biopsy specimens. Esophagoscopy and gastroscopy can be used to diagnose esophageal varices or to perform injection sclerotherapy. An endoscopic retrograde cholangiopancreatography (ERCP) can be done to visualize and provide radiographic examination of the liver, gallbladder, and pancreas. All these procedures require that the patient fast for at least 12 hours before the test. Before initiating ERCP the patient should be asked about allergies or sensitivities to x-ray dye.

After the procedure the nurse should assess the patient's ability to swallow. The patient's gag reflex may not return for 1 to 2 hours. After ERCP the patient should be monitored for signs of complications, which include perforation, sepsis, and pancreatitis. Vital signs are usually taken every 30 minutes and then hourly for 4 hours. Intravenous sedation is frequently used during endoscopic procedures.

References

1. Gopal DV Rosen HR: Abnormal findings on liver function tests, *Postgrad Med* 107:100, 2000.
2. Johnson, LJ: *Gastrointestinal physiology,* St Louis, 1997, Mosby.
3. Moseley RH: Approach to the patient with abnormal liver chemistries. In Kelley WN, editor: *Textbook of internal medicine,* ed 3, Philadelphia, 1997, Lippincott-Raven.
4. Seidel HM et al: *Mosby's guide to physical examination,* ed 4, St Louis, 1999, Mosby.

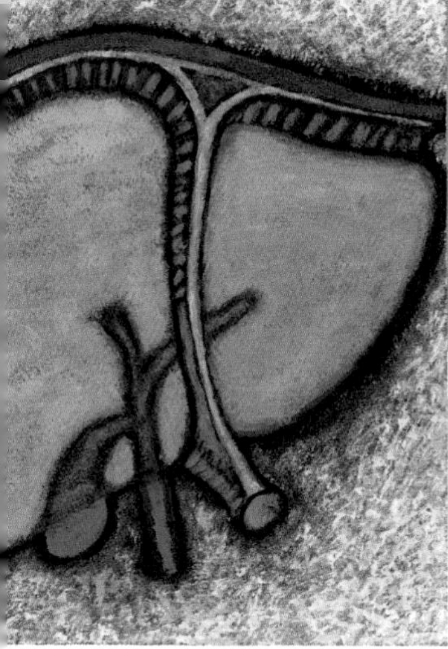

Hepatic Problems 37

Sally A. Brozenec

Objectives

After studying this chapter, the learner should be able to:

1. Explain signs and symptoms of a variety of hepatic disorders based on the pathophysiology.
2. Anticipate the nursing care needs of patients with focal hepatocellular disorders.
3. Differentiate among hepatitis A, B, C, D, and E.
4. Differentiate among toxic, autoimmune, and viral hepatitis.
5. Describe the pathophysiologic basis for the clinical manifestations of cirrhosis and its complications.
6. Develop plans of care for patients with diffuse hepatocellular disorders.

Because the liver is so complex and has so many functions, it is affected in many disorders and produces a variety of physiologic and psychosocial problems for patients. The degree of illness in people with liver disease ranges from critical, requiring intensive nursing care, to chronic, requiring home care.

CLINICAL MANIFESTATIONS OF LIVER DISEASE

Severe liver problems can be caused by a variety of factors including infection, neoplastic growths, toxic agents, and trauma. Regardless of cause, clinical manifestations of liver problems are similar and reflect alterations in normal liver function (Table 37-1). An overview of these clinical manifestations is presented here in preparation for the study of specific liver diseases. Nursing care related to each of these major clinical manifestations is presented under cirrhosis, a disorder in which all of them can occur.

JAUNDICE

Jaundice is a major problem for patients with hepatic disorders. It is caused by a disturbance in bilirubin metabolism. (See Chapter 36 for an explanation of bilirubin metabolism.) When the liver is diseased, problems with the uptake, conjugation, and/or excretion of bilirubin may occur, resulting in increased serum bilirubin levels (both conjugated and unconjugated). This excess bilirubin in the blood is distributed to the skin, mucous membranes, sclerae, and other body fluids and tissues, causing a yellow pigmentation. Because conjugated bilirubin is water soluble and is excreted in urine, darkening of the urine may also be seen. The presence of bilirubin in the skin causes pruritus (itching) in about 20% to 25% of the patients who have jaundice. The changes in concentration of bilirubin and bilirubin metabolites in the serum, urine, or stool help in determining the type of jaundice. Serum bilirubin levels must be combined with other laboratory and diagnostic tests and interpreted in view of the history and clinical findings.

Jaundice may also result from hemolysis (increased destruction of red blood cells) and/or obstruction of extrahepatic and intrahepatic biliary ducts. Table 37-2 compares the different causes of jaundice. Clay-colored (grayish-white) stools indicate that bile is not reaching the intestines and suggest extrahepatic obstruction. Frequent causes of extrahepatic obstruction are gallstones lodged in the common bile duct, pancreatitis, and carcinoma of the head of the pancreas, all of which are discussed in Chapter 35. The level of jaundice does not correlate with disease severity in hepatitis, but in persons with cirrhosis, jaundice suggests a poorer prognosis.

ASCITES

Ascites is the accumulation of fluid in the peritoneal cavity. It is the result of changes in the hemodynamics of the abdominal circulation. Increased pressure in the portal circulation from liver congestion increases capillary plasma hydrostatic pressure, and impaired production of albumin by the liver decreases capillary plasma oncotic pressure. Both of these events combine to facilitate movement of serous fluid out of the vessels into the peritoneum.

PORTAL HYPERTENSION

As hepatic damage occurs, the portal vascular system may become obstructed. Obstruction to portal blood flow increases portal venous pressure and results in portal hypertension. It

TABLE 37-1 Relationship Between Normal Liver Functions and Altered Functions Associated with Liver Disease

Normal Liver Functions	Altered Physiologic Functions
Maintenance of normal size and drainage of blood from GI tract	Liver inflammation ↓ Venous congestion of GI tract → Altered GI function ↓ GI symptoms
Metabolism of carbohydrates	Increased glycogenesis and decreased glycogenolysis and gluconeogenesis ↓ Altered glucose metabolism ↓ Decreased energy
Metabolism of fats	Increased fatty acid and triglyceride synthesis and decreased fatty acid oxidation and triglyceride release ↓ Fatty liver ↓ Hepatomegaly; ↓ Decreased energy production; weight loss
Protein metabolism	Decreased production of albumin → Decreased colloidal osmotic pressure → Edema and ascites Decreased production of clotting factors ↓ Altered clotting studies ↓ Bleeding tendencies ↓ Blood loss → Anemia Decreased protein synthesis in general ↓ Alteration in immune function and alteration in healing
Detoxification of endogenous substances	Decreased metabolism of sex steroids (estrogen, progesterone, and testosterone) ↓ Male ↓ Loss of masculine characteristics and development of some feminine characteristics from excessive estrogen; ↓ Female ↓ Loss of feminine characteristics and development of some masculine characteristics from excessive testosterone Decreased metabolism of aldosterone ↓ Sodium and water retention ↓ Edema, ascites; ↓ Increased potassium and hydrogen excretion ↓ Hypokalemia and alkalosis Decreased metabolism of ammonia (usually resulting from blood bypassing liver rather than loss of parenchymal cell function) → increased ammonia levels → Hepatic encephalopathy ↓ Changes in coordination, memory, orientation; coma
Detoxification of exogenous substances	Decreased metabolism of drugs ↓ Altered drug effects and potential increase in toxicities and side effects
Metabolism and storage of vitamins and minerals	Decreased stores of vitamins and minerals ↓ Decreased red blood cell production ↓ Anemia; ↓ Decreased energy production
Bile production and excretion	Obstruction to bile flow ↓ Decreased fat absorption ↓ Decreased vitamin K absorption ↓ Decreased clotting factors ↓ Bleeding/blood loss

TABLE 37-1 Relationship Between Normal Liver Functions and Altered Functions Associated with Liver Disease—cont'd

Normal Liver Functions	Altered Physiologic Functions
Bilirubin metabolism	Decreased uptake of bilirubin from circulation → Increased unconjugated bilirubin → Jaundice, pruritus, scratching, and skin lesions Decreased conjugation and release of bilirubin → Increased conjugated bilirubin and increased urine bilirubin → Jaundice, pruritus, scratching, and skin lesions Decreased excretion of bilirubin to bowel → Light-colored stools (clay or grayish white) Decreased reuptake of urobilinogen →↑ Urine urobilinogen → Dark urine

TABLE 37-2 Types of Jaundice

Category	Pathology	Possible Findings
Obstructive Intrahepatic	Suppression of bile flow in canaliculi or small biliary ductiles (cholestasis)	Direct* bilirubin elevated; alkaline phosphatase elevated; no enlargement of bile ducts seen on scan or ultrasound
Extrahepatic (bile duct obstruction)	Obstruction of bile flow in large bile ducts, as in gallbladder disease	Direct* bilirubin elevated; alkaline phosphatase elevated; enlargement of bile ducts documented by scan, ultrasound; absence of urobilinogen in urine
Hepatocellular	Hepatocyte injury from toxins (toxic hepatitis), from viruses (viral hepatitis), cancer, or as part of syndrome of cirrhosis (all types)	Transaminases (ALT, AST) elevated 10- to 15-fold; both direct* and indirect† bilirubin may be elevated (direct more than indirect); prolonged prothrombin time
Hemolytic	Excessive amounts of bilirubin are released from red blood cells as would be seen in sickle cell anemia or other hemolytic anemias; liver is unable to excrete bilirubin as rapidly as it forms	Usually mild elevation of total bilirubin (indirect more than direct)

*"Direct" measures conjugated bilirubin.
†"Indirect" measures unconjugated bilirubin.

also causes splenomegaly because of increased vascular pressure and venous congestion in the spleen, contributes to ascites by increasing hydrostatic pressure, and results in the development of collateral circulation to bypass the obstruction. These collateral vessels are most likely to form in the paraumbilical and the hemorrhoidal veins (causing hemorrhoids), and at the cardia of the stomach extending into the esophagus. The collateral vessels in the upper stomach and esophagus are called varices, and they are very thin-walled and fragile, and have limited ability to withstand increases in pressure. The presence of this collateral circulation places the individual at high risk for a massive upper gastrointestinal bleeding episode (Figure 37-1).

PORTAL-SYSTEMIC ENCEPHALOPATHY

Portal-systemic encephalopathy (PSE), also called hepatic encephalopathy or hepatic coma, is one of the major complications of severe liver disease. The onset of the condition may be acute or chronic.

PSE results from several metabolic derangements. A major cause is the liver's inability to metabolize and cleanse the

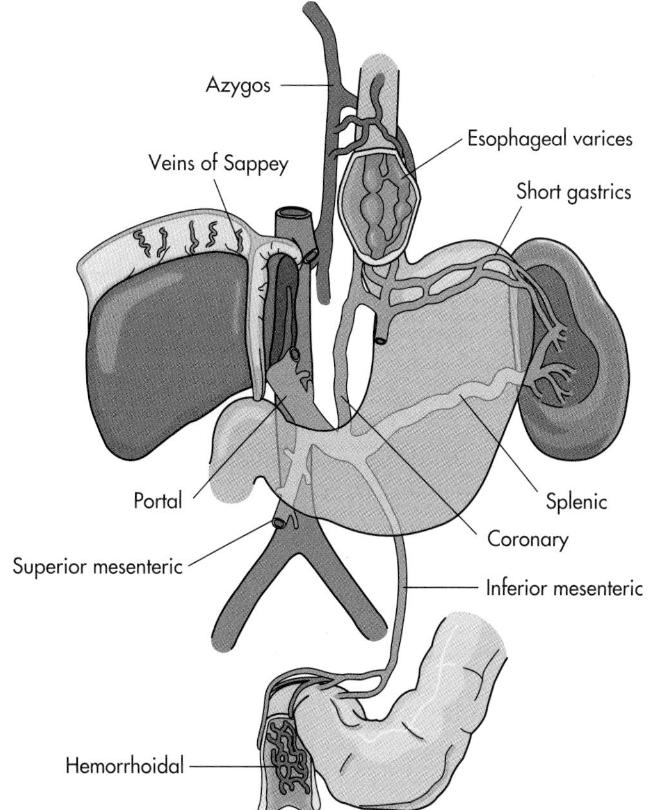

Figure 37-1 Varices related to portal hypertension. Portal vein, its major tributaries, and the most important collateral veins between the portal and caval systems.

blood of ammonia and mercaptions. Ammonia is an end product of protein metabolism, whereas mercaptans are toxins produced from the metabolism of sulfur-containing compounds. These metabolic activities occur in the intestines, and the end-products are normally carried to the liver where they are metabolized and excreted. The manifestations of PSE vary and may occur quickly or gradually over the course of a few days. There are alterations in the level of consciousness, intellectual function, behavior and personality, and neuromuscular function.

HEPATORENAL SYNDROME

Hepatorenal syndrome is a poorly understood complication of end-stage liver disease. It is characterized by sudden kidney failure for no known cause in a patient with progressively worsening liver failure. The patient with hepatokidney failure has oliguria and azotemia. The onset of hepatorenal syndrome is a grave sign in a patient with liver failure.[13]

ACUTE AND CHRONIC LIVER DISEASE

The most dreaded outcome of any liver disorder is the development of liver failure. This general term implies a degree of tissue necrosis such that all liver function is lost. It is believed that there is a minimum mass of well-functioning hepatocytes required to meet the basic metabolic needs of the body, and once this critical threshold is lost, organ failure occurs. Liver failure may occur as an acute presentation, or develop over time.

ACUTE LIVER FAILURE

Acute liver failure (ALF), also called fulminant hepatic failure (FHF), is an uncommon condition in which previously healthy persons develop severe liver dysfunction evidenced by the rapid onset of encephalopathy and/or bleeding. It is a highly complex clinical syndrome that arises within a few days or weeks. A total of 75% of patients with acute liver failure die within days of symptom onset.

Etiology/Epidemiology

There are numerous etiologies of ALF, including hepatitis B infection, especially with concurrent infection with the delta virus. The major cause of ALF in persons without another liver disease is acetaminophen overdose. This may be deliberate overdose as in suicide attempts or it may be inadvertent. Individuals are at high risk for ALF if they combine acetaminophen with chronic alcohol intake, some anticonvulsants, or antituberculosis (TB) drugs. In a large number of cases of acute liver failure, the etiology is unknown. Less common causes are poisoning with aminita muscaria (mushrooms) and liver failure associated with eclampsia or preeclampsia of pregnancy.

Pathophysiology

A sudden, massive necrosis of hepatocytes results in dramatic clinical manifestations of liver failure and multiple organ dysfunction syndrome involving the kidneys, lungs, and circulatory system. Hallmarks of this disorder are clinical encephalopathy, rapid decrease in coagulation ability, cerebral edema, and multiorgan failure. The pathogenesis of multiple organ dysfunction is complex and poorly understood. In addition to the loss of hepatocyte function, key mediators such as interleukin 1, tumor necrosis factor, and others have been identified. Microvascular obstruction with cellular debris from the damaged liver may impair tissue oxygen extraction and lead to lactic acidosis and circulatory failure. Although ammonia levels are high in ALF, the encephalopathy appears to be more related to hypoxia. Cerebral edema may result from fluid overload. Failure of the liver to manufacture the coagulation factors I, II, V, VII, IX, and X causes severe bleeding disorders, and there is also great risk of disseminated intravascular coagulapathy (see Chapter 27). Patients with ALF are susceptible to severe infections, and cerebral edema and septicemia are the most frequent causes of death.

Typically most of the damage to the liver has been done by the time symptoms present. A prolonged prothrombin time is characteristic, and the decline of the prothrombin time is closely related to the severity of organ damage. Values of more than 4 seconds secure the diagnosis of ALF, especially if mental status changes are also present. Jaundice is common, especially when hepatitis is the cause.

Collaborative Care Management

The primary treatment for ALF is organ transplantation (see Chapter 51). The patient is maintained on life-support systems until a donor is found. Recent research on the use of extracorporeal liver assist devices as a support for liver function during the waiting period for transplantation has been promising. These devices, similar to hemodialysis, use hepatocytes from pigs or humans to provide liver function. They have been successful in improving neurologic parameters, liver function tests, cardiovascular status, renal function tests, and coagulation factors.[7,18,19]

Nursing care of the patient in ALF involves the intensive care monitoring of a patient in need of life support. The areas of concern are the monitoring of neurologic changes, especially increasing intracranial pressure; hemodynamic status; and cardiovascular, renal, and coagulation function. Other major concerns include the development of sepsis and shock.

Patient/Family Education. The family is kept apprised of the patient's status during this critical period. Discussions about liver transplantation occur when appropriate.

CHRONIC LIVER FAILURE

Chronic liver failure represents the progressive, irreversible destruction of liver function over time. It is often referred to as end-stage liver disease. Cirrhosis of the liver is the prototypical presentation of chronic liver disease, and will be discussed later.

FOCAL HEPATOCELLULAR DISORDERS

Focal hepatic disorders are those that are localized to one portion of the liver. This classification is opposed to diffuse disorders, which are spread through a major portion of the liver (Box 37-1).

BOX 37-1 Common Liver Disorders

Focal Hepatocellular Disorders

Abscess
Trauma
Tumors

Diffuse Hepatocellular Disorders

Hepatitis
Cirrhosis
Sequelae of chronic diffuse hepatocellular disorders
Portal hypertension
Ascites
Esophageal varices
Portal-systemic encephalopathy
Hepatorenal syndrome

LIVER ABSCESS

Etiology

Liver abscesses may result from a variety of organisms; however, *Escherichia coli* and *Klebsiella pneumoniae* are the most common. *Staphylococcus, Streptococcus, Pseudomonas,* and *Proteus* spp. may also be found. In patients with depressed immune functioning, such as those with neutropenia or leukemia, systemic candidiasis with multiple hepatic abscesses has developed. Many people with abscesses have multiple bacteria involved.

Epidemiology

Hepatic abscesses are uncommon in the United States but are associated with a high mortality rate. Amebic liver abscesses are common worldwide, particularly in countries with tropical and subtropical climates. In the United States, amebic liver abscesses occur occasionally in the temperate regions and in people who have traveled to tropical climates.

Pathophysiology

Pyogenic abscesses can occur as either a singular large abscess or multiple small and/or microscopic abscesses. Amebic liver abscesses are typically large and singular and are usually a secondary site of infection. Pyogenic organisms originating in various areas of the body reach the liver through the biliary, vascular, or lymphatic systems. In addition, pyogenic organisms may be introduced by penetrating injuries to the liver or by direct continuous extension. The organisms cause necrosis of the liver tissue and abscess formation. In amebic abscesses, the vegetative form of the organism moves from the gut to the small portal vessels and into the hepatic tissue, where it becomes activated.

If liver abscesses are not identified, they continue to grow in size and can perforate into the pleural cavity, the peritoneal cavity, or the pericardial cavity. Fistulas from the abscess to other abdominal organs or through the abdominal wall may also develop. The major manifestations of liver abscess are caused by the infection rather than by changes in hepatic functioning (see Clinical Manifestations box). The patient with pyogenic abscesses, particularly multiple small or microscopic abscesses, may have clinical manifestations of sepsis and septic shock. Fever and constitutional symptoms such as malaise, anorexia, and weight loss are common. The patient with amebic abscesses may have signs and symptoms of intestinal amebiasis or give a history of previous intestinal signs and symptoms such as bloody, mucoid diarrhea, generalized abdominal pain, rectal tenesmus, dehydration, and hypotension. However, many patients with amebic abscess report no previous history of intestinal signs and symptoms.[15]

Clinical Manifestations

Liver Abscess

SIGNS AND SYMPTOMS RESULTING FROM INFECTIOUS PROCESS

Fever and chills (temperature between 102° F [38.8° C] and 106° F [41.1° C])
Cough
Diaphoresis
Difficulty breathing
Abnormal breath sounds from pleural involvement
Right upper quadrant abdominal pain and tenderness
Anorexia
Nausea and vomiting
Clinical manifestations of peritonitis (see Box 37-3, p. 1183)

SIGNS AND SYMPTOMS RESULTING FROM HEPATIC DYSFUNCTION

Hepatomegaly
Jaundice and pruritus
Splenomegaly
Abdominal distention and ascites

Collaborative Care Management

Diagnostic tests usually reveal leukocytosis and an elevated erythrocyte sedimentation rate caused by the infection, and moderate elevation of serum alkaline phosphatase and minimal elevation of serum transaminases (AST and ALT) from liver cell damage. Hyperbilirubinemia and hypoalbuminemia result from impaired liver function (see Chapter 36). In patients with amebic liver abscesses, serologic laboratory tests such as immunoglobulins against antigens, indirect hemagglutination titers, complement fixation tests, and latex agglutination tests are highly diagnostic for amebic infection. Hepatic radioisotope scans, ultrasonic scanning, and computed tomography (CT) scans also are used in diagnosis and follow-up evaluation and reveal the presence of abscesses. Scanning is also useful for guided drainage procedures.

Empiric antimicrobial therapy is used initially for pyogenic abscesses with the specific type of antibiotic determined from the culture and sensitivity of the aspirate of the abscess. Metronidazole (Flagyl), chloroquine, and dehydroemetine or emetine are the drugs of choice for amebic abscesses. Acetaminophen is used to control fever, and fluid and electrolyte replacement is initiated as supportive therapy when needed.

For pyogenic abscesses, surgical drainage or needle aspiration may be necessary because the necrotic tissue walls off the abscess from the healthy liver tissue and makes it more difficult for antimicrobial therapy to reach the infection. Drainage of a pyogenic abscess is usually attempted only when there is a single abscess. After an abscess has been located by ultrasound, arteriography, or CT scan, percutaneous aspiration can be attempted, usually under ultrasound guidance. After the application of a local anesthetic agent, the physician inserts a large-bore needle into the abscess, and the contents are aspirated. Complications of this procedure are similar to those of a liver biopsy, with hemorrhage being the most common. In the case of amebic abscesses, aspiration is not usually indicated because medications alone are effective.

Patients with liver abscesses commonly complain of abdominal pain in the right upper quadrant. However, the pain may be experienced in the shoulders. The patient may report nausea, vomiting, and anorexia. There may be few objective signs of a liver abscess. Fever is common. A palpable mass in the right upper quadrant may be felt in some patients. Weight loss may result from the nausea, vomiting, and anorexia and the increased metabolic needs. Some patients may exhibit dyspnea and pleural pain if there is involvement of the diaphragm.[14]

Nursing management focuses on (1) assisting with fluid and nutritional deficits, (2) controlling discomfort including dealing with pruritus if jaundice is present, (3) assisting with the medical regimen (diagnostic tests and therapeutic measures), and (4) helping the patient attain appropriate knowledge for self-management. In the acute situation nursing management may incorporate the care needs described for a patient with sepsis and septic shock (see Chapter 14) or severe intestinal colitis, appendicitis, and megacolon (see Chapter 34).

The first priority of care is to help with treatment of fluid volume deficit or shock, if present. The next priority is to provide comfort measures. The high temperature, episodes of chills and diaphoresis, pruritus, anorexia, and abdominal pain all cause discomfort. During periods of chills, adequate blankets to provide comfort without increasing temperature are necessary. Cool sponge baths may help lower the temperature. The gown and bed linens should be changed if the patient is diaphoretic. Pruritus can be controlled with cool sponge baths, use of soft linens, prevention of dry skin, and cool environmental temperatures.

Another aspect of care is to provide adequate fluids and nutrition. At first the patient may only tolerate intravenous (IV) fluids or at least require IV fluids to replace deficits. The effectiveness of these measures is evaluated by monitoring the patient's daily weight and skin turgor and assessing laboratory values for hemoconcentration or dilution. Food should be given in small amounts, with the patient's preferences considered to help overcome anorexia. Frequent oral hygiene (at least once every 2 hours) is necessary because fever and fluid loss cause drying of the mucous membranes and may worsen anorexia. The environment should be clean, free of odors, and relaxed.

In assisting with the medical regimen, the nurse is primarily involved with preparing patients physically for tests (instituting nothing by mouth status or other preparations as necessary, as described in Chapter 36 for the specific test). The patient and family also need appropriate education about the various tests. The nurse is involved in preparing those patients having surgical drainage of abscesses for surgery and providing appropriate postoperative care similar to that needed by any patient (see Chapters 16 and 18). The nurse also is involved in administering the prescribed antimicrobial and amebicidal agents. This involves not only appropriate administration but also monitoring for side effects.

Patient/Family Education. Patient education for long-term care is a major nursing responsibility. For some patients with liver abscesses, the medication may have to be taken for several weeks to several months. The patient must be instructed about the importance of continual adherence to the medication regimen. In addition, the patient should be instructed to immediately report any signs and symptoms of recurrence of infection (chills, fever, or diaphoresis), spread of infection (worsening abdominal pain or increased difficulty breathing), or deterioration of liver function (e.g., jaundice or ascites), as well as any side effects of the medication. Instructions about the need for continual follow-up care should be emphasized.

Health Promotion/Prevention. For the person with amebic abscesses, prevention of recurrence is important. The nurse should help the patient identify potentially contaminated sources of food and water, as well as ways to decontaminate or avoid these sources, such as using iodine-releasing tablets in water and scalding of vegetables or eating only peeled fresh fruit.

LIVER TRAUMA

Etiology/Epidemiology

Because of its location and size, the liver is frequently subjected to trauma, which may be either penetrating (gunshot wounds or stab wounds) or blunt (collision with steering wheel during automobile accidents or falls). If the injury is severe, the liver may rupture, with severe internal hemorrhage.

Pathophysiology

The pathophysiology depends on the type of liver injury. Injuries vary from a laceration and capsular tear with minimal parenchymal damage to liver rupture with extreme parenchymal damage and damage to the retrohepatic vasculature. Stab wounds often make a relatively superficial incision and may do no more damage than does a needle biopsy of the liver. Gunshot wounds and blunt trauma can result in severe hemorrhage leading to hypotension, shock, and peritonitis. Bile may also leak from the biliary canaliculi and contaminate the peritoneal cavity causing peritonitis. Less severe blunt trauma may result only in the development of a subcapsular hematoma.

The clinical manifestations of liver trauma also vary with type of injury (see Clinical Manifestations box). If peritoneal contamination from hemorrhage or bile has occurred, signs and symptoms of peritonitis (see Clinical Manifestations box) may be present.

Clinical Manifestations
Liver Trauma

SIGNS OF SHOCK
- Pale, cool, clammy skin
- Diaphoresis
- Hypotension
- Tachycardia
- Mental confusion

PENETRATING TRAUMA
- Entry and sometimes exit wounds

BLUNT TRAUMA
- Abdominal pain exaggerated by breathing
- Shoulder pain indicating diaphragmatic irritation

Clinical Manifestations
Peritonitis

- Abdominal tenderness
- Rebound tenderness
- Muscle rigidity or spasms
- Decreased or absent bowel signs
- Sometimes a fluid wave

Late complications of liver trauma may include:
- Severe hemorrhage resulting from disseminated intravascular coagulation that often accompanies shock during the total course of treatment
- Degeneration and sloughing of segments of the liver that have had disrupted circulation with resultant hemorrhage and microvascular damage
- Intrahepatic cyst or abscess formation
- Infections of other areas of body after the trauma
- Subphrenic abscess formation
- Biliary fistulas

The mortality for liver trauma has decreased over the years. The mortality depends on the type of injury (highest for blunt trauma because of the larger portion of liver damaged and because of other associated injuries), the severity of the injury (highest for those requiring resection of a large amount of liver), and the presence of associated injuries (increasing mortality with each additional injury to another organ).

Collaborative Care Management

In some instances the only sign of hepatic trauma is the presence of blood in peritoneal lavage. Useful diagnostic tools include CT and ultrasonography of the abdomen. Laboratory studies may reveal a decreasing hematocrit and hemoglobin from blood loss and leukocytosis from peritoneal infection and inflammation.

The immediate medical management for patients with suspected liver trauma is the same as that for any patient with intraabdominal trauma. Most penetrating abdominal injuries require surgical exploration to detect the presence of abdominal hemorrhage, trauma to the liver or other organs, presence of necrotic tissue, or presence of bile drainage. Management of the blunt hepatic injury, in which there is no abdominal penetration, has changed over the last 10 years. Studies have indicated that approximately 85% of all patients with blunt hepatic trauma are hemodynamically stable, and nonoperative management significantly improves the outcome over surgical management. These outcomes include decreased incidence of abdominal infection, decreased need for transfusions, and decreased length of hospital stay. Surgery remains the treatment of choice for individuals with blunt injury that are hemodynamically unstable. Other medical interventions relate to the stabilization of airway, fluid and electrolyte status, blood replacement, laboratory assessments, and the prevention and/or treatment of shock and peritonitis.[21,25]

Guidelines for Safe Practice
Assessing the Patient With Suspected Liver Trauma

- Respiratory status (rate, breath sounds, pulse oximetry, and blood gases)
- Vital signs every 15 minutes (blood pressure, pulse)
- Mean arterial pressure every hour
- Other hemodynamic monitoring such as intraarterial pressure monitoring and cardiac output measurements as ordered
- Urine output and other fluid losses documented hourly
- Intake documented hourly
- Serum and urinary electrolytes and osmolality at least daily
- Hematocrit and hemoglobin daily
- Neurologic checks for responsiveness and motion every hour
- Consciousness monitored every hour using Glasgow Coma Scale
- Skin temperature, color, and moisture checked every hour
- Bowel sounds, pain, and abdominal tenderness

The major focus of nursing care for the patient with suspected liver trauma is to establish and implement a systematic assessment of cardiovascular, fluid volume, and, neurologic status, along with observations for signs and symptoms of peritonitis (see Guidelines for Safe Practice box). This assessment is required from the moment the patient is first seen through the postoperative period. The nurse should anticipate the possibility of surgery and prepare the patient and family for this procedure.

Patient/Family Education. The major nursing focus is to help the patient and family control their fear and anxiety by using simple explanations of all activities and maintaining a calm environment. Continuity of care is essential to minimizing fear and anxiety.

Providing information and support for the patient's family or significant others are other important aspects of care. A specific time should be set aside for the family and significant others to ask questions and verbalize their fears. Spiritual support is extremely important to many patients and their families and should be considered when planning care.

After the acute/critical period, which includes the postoperative period for some patients, continual monitoring as already described plus provision of emotional support for the patient and family are still needed. The patient will also need help with self-care, a gradual increase in activity, and comfort measures. The patient will need to be educated about the signs and symptoms of recurrent liver dysfunction. The importance of complying with follow-up care should be stressed.

LIVER TUMORS

Liver neoplasms or tumors may be either benign or malignant. Benign lesions include hemangioma, cysts, and rarely adenoma. Most benign tumors are asymptomatic, but occasionally they enlarge enough to become symptomatic. If they become symptomatic, surgical intervention may be required. The focus of this section is malignant neoplasms.

Etiology

The incidence of primary liver cancer is increased in people with chronic liver disease, particularly those with chronic hepatitis B and C. Any chronic inflammatory liver disease has the potential to induce hepatocellular cancer, but the pathology most commonly associated with the disease is cirrhosis. The risk of developing hepatocellular cancer is approximately 40 times greater in persons with alcohol-induced cirrhosis. Certain environmental and hereditary causes of cirrhosis also have a strong correlation with hepatocellular cancer. Interestingly enough, a direct carcinogenic effect of alcohol of the liver has not been proved.

Epidemiology

Hepatocellular cancer is one of the most common cancers in the world and is also the most deadly, with a 5-year survival rate of less than 5% without treatment.[6] There is a marked geographic difference in incidence, with rates in Africa and Asia 20 times higher than in the United States. This disparity is probably related to endemic rates of viral hepatitis and nutritional deficits in these areas. Recently, however, the incidence of hepatocellular cancer in the United States has begun to increase.

Metastatic liver tumors occur 20 times more frequently than primary tumors. They rank second only to cirrhosis as a cause of fatal liver disease in the United States.

Pathophysiology

The liver is highly vascular and is a common site for metastasis from the cancers of gastrointestinal (GI) tract, lungs, breasts, kidneys, and malignant melanomas. Primary liver tumors arise in the liver cell (hepatocellular) or the bile duct cell (cholangiocellular), or they can be of mixed origin. The lesions are multiple or singular, diffuse or nodular, and may involve a lobe or the entire liver. The cancerous cells compress the surrounding normal liver cells and invade the portal vein branches. Some cells infiltrate the gallbladder, mesentery, peritoneum, and diaphragm by direct extension. Primary cancers also tend to cause hemorrhage by extension into the vascular tissue of the liver and necrosis by depriving normal hepatic tissue of adequate circulation. The most common site for metastasis of the primary liver lesion is the lung, but metastasis can occur to the adrenal glands, spleen, vertebrae, kidney, ovary, or pancreas. Primary lesions grow rapidly, sometimes without signs or symptoms, and often the patient lives only a short time after the diagnosis.

Metastatic carcinoma of the liver varies from a few small nodules to large growths. Adjacent nodules may eventually fuse and compress the surrounding liver tissue. Usually different parts of the liver are uniformly involved; thus liver biopsy may be a useful diagnostic aid.

The signs and symptoms of liver cancer depend on the size and extent of the tumor, the amount of hepatocellular damage, and the presence of liver failure (see Clinical Manifestations box). Unfortunately the disease is often clinically silent until it is well advanced.[28]

Collaborative Care Management

Diagnostic Tests. Diagnostic tests include blood studies, radioisotope scans, magnetic resonance imaging, liver biopsy, ultrasonography, and CT scans. The blood studies may show an increased erythrocyte sedimentation rate associated with generalized inflammation of the liver; anemia resulting from increased metabolism and decreased food intake; hyperbilirubinemia; elevated alkaline phosphatase, AST, and ALT; decreased blood glucose; and hypoalbuminemia. The number of abnormalities depends on the severity of hepatocellular damage. A special test that is useful in the diagnosis of primary

Clinical Manifestations
Liver Cancer

EARLY SIGNS
Right upper quadrant mass
Epigastric fullness
Pain
Fatigue
Weight loss
Changes in liver function tests

LATER SIGNS
Fatigue
Ascites
Liver failure
Fever
Hepatic bruits
Jaundice
Variceal bleeding

METASTATIC LIVER TUMORS
Fatigue
Anorexia
Weakness
Weight loss followed by weight gain resulting from ascites
Hepatomegaly
Hepatic bruits
Jaundice
Portal-systemic encephalopathy

liver carcinoma is serum concentrations of alpha-fetoprotein (AFP). AFP in concentrations of 500 ng/ml to 5 mg/ml is considered positive. High levels that occur in any adult without obvious GI tract tumors strongly suggest primary liver cancer. Note that the sensitivity of an elevated AFP is only 60%. More sensitive tests are presently in development.

Radioisotope and CT scans and ultrasonography may reveal lesions in the liver. Magnetic resonance imaging is less sensitive than CT scanning. A liver biopsy is necessary for definitive diagnosis of cancer.

Medications. High-dose chemotherapy has been used to induce regression of primary and metastatic liver tumors. These chemotherapeutic agents, usually 5-fluorouracil and fluorodeoxyuridine, are given directly into the hepatic artery via a surgically implanted infusion pump (Figures 37-2 and 37-3). Arterial infusion allows more drug to be delivered directly to the tumor and decreases systemic effects.

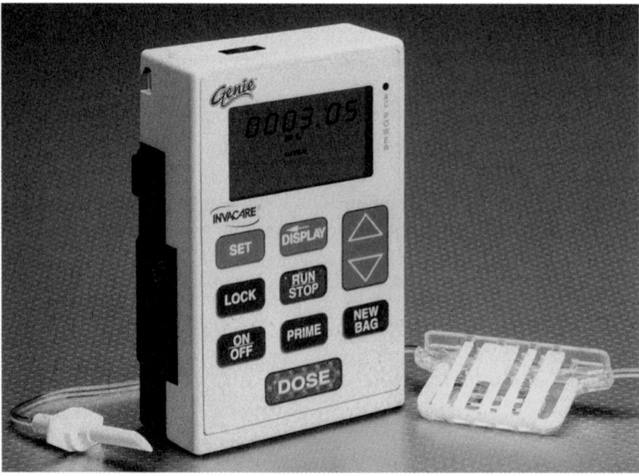

Figure 37-2 External infusion pump. Lightweight, battery-operated infusion pump for ambulatory patient. Flow rate is adjustable; power pack operates for 7 days before needing recharging.

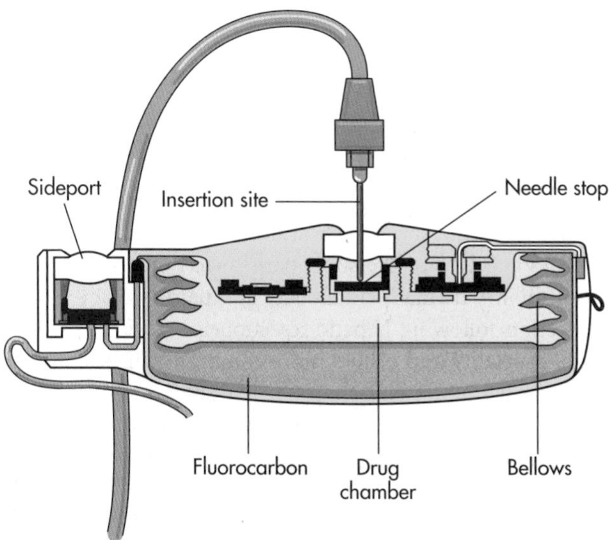

Figure 37-3 Implantable infusion pump (Infusaid pump).

Treatments. Radiation therapy may be used to control pain, but it does not improve survival rates. Ligation of the hepatic artery decreases the oxygen delivered to the tumor and may help control the pain and diminish the mass of the tumor.

Surgical Management. For solitary primary tumors and some solitary metastatic tumors, surgery may be performed. The liver has remarkable regenerative capacity, which allows as much as 90% resection. Orthotopic transplantation (removal of recipient's liver and replacement with a graft liver) has been performed for patients with primary liver tumors with varying success. In the United States, liver transplantation for hepatocellular carcinoma is indicated only in patients who have unresectable tumors, focal tumor recurrence after resection, or hepatic failure. Organ transplantation is discussed in Chapter 51.

Diet. A special diet is necessary only if signs and symptoms of cirrhosis occur.

Activity. Activity as tolerated is encouraged. The patient is encouraged to be as independent as possible.

Referrals. Common referrals for patients with hepatic tumors include social services, cancer support groups, and cancer specialists.

NURSING MANAGEMENT OF PATIENT UNDERGOING HEPATIC RESECTION

Patients with liver tumors often experience epigastric fullness, fatigue, weight loss, and abdominal pain early in the course of their illness. Later the fatigue becomes more pronounced, and patients may report weakness and anorexia.

Objective signs of liver tumors are minimal until the disease is well advanced. As the disease progresses, the patient may become jaundiced, have ascites, and show signs of liver failure, including variceal bleeding and portal-systemic encephalopathy (see Clinical Manifestations box on p. 1154).

PREOPERATIVE CARE

For the patient having a surgical resection of a hepatic tumor (hepatic resection), skilled perioperative care is necessary. Teaching about the preoperative preparation, the procedure itself, and postoperative care is needed (see Chapters 16 to18). The patient may need vitamin K for defects in clotting factors, as well as other vitamins if deficits are present. Preparation of the bowel is the same as for intestinal surgery (see Chapter 34). If a blood volume deficit is present, blood will be given. The goal is to make the patient's physical condition as stable as possible before surgery. Sometimes, preoperative total parenteral nutrition is initiated to improve the patient's status.

POSTOPERATIVE CARE

After surgery the patient requires close monitoring for complications, especially sepsis and hypovolemia from blood loss. Vital signs should be monitored every 15 minutes until stable and then every hour. Dressings should be checked for oozing or bleeding. Intake and output should be monitored every 4 to 8 hours, and weights should be recorded daily. Assessment of the cardiorespiratory system (cardiac rhythm, breath sounds, and pulse oximetry) is also necessary. Temperature should also be monitored at least every 4 hours. Laboratory values for serum electrolytes, liver function, and complete blood count with hematocrit and hemoglobin levels are carefully monitored.

Assessment also includes monitoring for decreased liver function. Thus blood glucose, coagulation status, serum albumin levels, and neurologic status are checked at regular intervals. The nurse should anticipate the possibility of administering glucose, albumin, and blood.

To promote turning and deep breathing, the nurse must ensure adequate pain control by giving the patient medications as ordered, splinting the incision, and positioning the patient properly (upright). Patient-controlled analgesia may be used to manage postoperative pain. Because most analgesics, narcotic and nonnarcotic, are metabolized in the liver, no "safe" analgesic exists for the patient with liver dysfunction, and the nurse should monitor closely for signs of toxicity.

The patient has nothing by mouth for several days and has a nasogastric tube attached to suction. Mouth care every 2 hours and monitoring of the suction device are indicated. Oral intake is started on approximately the fifth postoperative day. Initially ice chips and clear liquids are given, and then the diet is advanced as tolerated based on appetite and bowel function. The patient needs adequate calories, protein, vitamins, and minerals. Adequacy of intake may be monitored by daily calorie counts. The patient's tolerance to protein nitrogenous waste products must be monitored. If the patient cannot metabolize protein adequately because of loss of liver tissue, a low-protein diet is necessary. If the patient can adequately detoxify ammonium, a high-protein diet is given.

After surgery the patient initially dangles on the side of the bed and is out of bed by the first postoperative day. Close monitoring of vital signs, tolerance for activity, and respiratory status are required. Care of the patient undergoing hepatic resection is summarized in the Guidelines for Safe Practice box.

The patient should receive instructions concerning any dietary restrictions. The patient's liver function may be impaired for up to 6 months after surgery, and dietary protein and sodium are restricted accordingly. Corticosteroids may be given to enhance regeneration and prevent fibrosis. If steroids are to be continued after discharge, the patient should have written and verbal instructions regarding how to report dosage, purpose, administration, and side effects. The patient's activity tolerance will gradually increase. Activities such as heavy lifting should be avoided; generally, the patient should be instructed to lift no more than 5 to 10 pounds. Usually the patient uses his or her feeling of fatigue and tiredness as indicators of what can or cannot be done. The patient will not be able to assume all activities of daily living (ADL) immediately because of fatigue, and the nurse must assess whether self-care and home care needs can be met by the family or if outside help is necessary. Referrals for home health care should be made if necessary.

Jaundice is common after surgery, usually as a result of the inability of the remaining liver to use bile. Other causes of jaundice include multiple transfusions, vascular occlusion, and anoxia of hepatocytes during surgery. Jaundice usually resolves in approximately 10 days. If the jaundice persists, obstruction should be suspected.

Major postoperative complications after hepatic resection include hemorrhage; biliary fistula; infection; subphrenic abscess; respiratory complications such as pneumonia, atelectasis, and respiratory failure; portal hypertension; and clotting defects.

Hemorrhage is common because of the vascularity of the liver. This potentially fatal complication usually occurs within 24 hours of surgery and must be recognized early to prevent mortality. After hepatic resection, a T-tube (in the common bile duct) and subhepatic drain are usually in place. The T-tube normally drains approximately 400 ml of bile daily. If the drain becomes dislodged, the drainage decreases. Excessive drainage from the subhepatic drain can indicate a biliary fistula leaking bile into the subhepatic space. Other manifestations of biliary fistula include fever and pain.

Infection following hepatic resection is associated with increased mortality and occurs more commonly in persons who have cirrhosis. Subphrenic abscess may result because of insufficient drainage of the surgical defect and usually occurs later in the postoperative course. The placement and output of drainage tubes should be closely monitored in the postoperative period. An acute onset of sharp, piercing right upper quadrant pain with low-grade fever and the presence of adventitious sounds in the lung bases suggests a subphrenic abscess.

Guidelines for Safe Practice

The Patient Undergoing Liver Resection

PREOPERATIVE CARE

Explain special postoperative procedures (nasogastric intubation and parenteral fluids for several days).
Teach deep breathing exercises and leg exercises.
Teach use of side rails to facilitate turning in bed without exerting pull on the abdominal muscles.
Prevent hemorrhage.
Give prescribed vitamin K.
Complete bowel preparation.

POSTOPERATIVE CARE

Promote oxygenation.
Encourage turning and deep breathing exercises.
Encourage activity/ambulation as ordered.
Maintain fluid and electrolyte balance.
Check dressings for oozing or bleeding.
Maintain patency of GI tube.
Maintain prescribed rate of parenteral fluids.
Monitor for signs of fluid imbalance (daily weight changes, hematocrit, lung congestion, and dry skin and mucous membranes).
Promote comfort.
Give analgesics on a regular basis during the first 48 hours to minimize severe pain.
Give frequent oral hygiene until oral fluids are resumed.
Explain menu choices for a low-protein diet.
Reinforce information about a low-sodium diet.

Respiratory complications can arise because of the anatomic location of the surgical site. Persons are often reluctant to participate in pulmonary hygiene exercises due to incisional pain. Nursing care should be focused on preventing any respiratory complications.

Portal hypertension is another postoperative complication that results from the surgical alteration of venous blood flow in the remaining liver. This complication is usually transitory because the remaining liver has the potential to compensate and increase blood flow over time.

Coagulopathies usually develop during surgery, but may also occur after surgery. The patient should be closely monitored for bleeding and nursing care should focus on preventing episodes of bleeding. Monitoring of central venous pressure is a good indicator of the fluid volume status. The prothrombin time is generally prolonged in the first postoperative week, then gradually returns to normal.

GERONTOLOGIC CONSIDERATIONS

Surgical resection of a hepatic tumor poses a risk for all persons, but especially older adults. Changes in liver function associated with aging include decreased blood flow, decreased synthesis of cholesterol, and reduced ability to regenerate. These normal changes may be more evident with destruction of liver tissue associated with tumors. The older adult is also susceptible to drug toxicity. Patients with impaired liver function should be monitored for toxic and adverse effects, which may indicate a need for a reduced dosage of certain drugs. This is especially true if chemotherapeutic agents are used as treatment. Fatigue and weakness, which are common symptoms associated with hepatic cancer, may be increased in older patients, both as a result of aging and coexisting chronic disease.

SPECIAL ENVIRONMENTS FOR CARE

Home Care Management

Chemotherapy is increasingly being used to treat primary and metastatic tumors of the liver. Chemotherapy may be the treatment of choice if hepatic resection is not an option and may be given systemically or by infusion into the hepatic artery. Intraperitoneal chemotherapy has been used successfully in a limited number of patients. All chemotherapeutic agents have major side effects, and one of the major focuses of nursing is to help the patient and family deal with them. Patients receiving hepatic chemotherapy need to learn to care for an external infusion pump, as shown in Figure 37-2, or an internal pump as shown in Figure 37-3.

Patients receiving chemotherapy through the hepatic artery have additional needs. Hepatic arterial infusion can be accomplished by one of two methods. In the first method, a percutaneous catheter is inserted into the hepatic artery using fluoroscopy. The catheter is attached to an external infusion pump that is filled with the appropriate chemotherapeutic agent and programmed to deliver the agent over a desired period. The catheter is removed after each drug treatment cycle. In the second method, a catheter is surgically inserted into the hepatic artery and connected to an implanted infusion pump.

The implanted pump can be filled with the correct amount of drug and programmed to deliver the chemotherapeutic agent over a desired time and at a desired dosage. Generally pumps can deliver medication up to 14 days at a time. In chemotherapy-free intervals, the pump is filled with a heparin solution to maintain patency of the hepatic artery catheter. The chamber should be adequately filled to avoid complete emptying.

The implanted infusion pump allows the patient to be treated at home. The patient comes into an outpatient site at prescribed times for addition of drugs or heparin solution and a recheck of pump flow rate. The patient needs physical care before and after surgery similar to that for any patient having surgery and instructions regarding self-care needs related to the chemotherapeutic agent being used. The nurse also is involved in refilling the pump at the prescribed intervals.

COMPLICATIONS

The poor prognosis associated with liver cancer is partially due to the late onset of definitive signs of disease and hence advanced disease at the time of diagnosis. If the cancer is untreated, death usually occurs within 6 to 8 weeks of diagnosis. Nearly 50% of persons with hepatic cancer have distant metastases to the lungs, bone, adrenal glands, and brain. Tumors spread rapidly within the liver and occlusion of the portal vein is common. Occlusion of the portal vein can lead to necrosis, rupture, and hemorrhage. As the cancer progresses, multiple body systems are affected and complications arise. The cause of death in approximately 50% of patients with liver cancer is liver failure and hemorrhage. Other causes of death include pneumonia, malnutrition, and thromboemboli.

Care for persons with advanced liver cancer is primarily supportive. Persons with advanced disease will often experience liver failure, ascites, infection, bleeding, pain, weight loss, anorexia, vomiting, weakness, and pneumonia. Both the patient and family should be informed about treatment plans and be assured that care will focus on promoting comfort.

DIFFUSE HEPATOCELLULAR DISORDERS

HEPATITIS

Hepatitis is any acute inflammatory disease of the liver. Although the term hepatitis is most often used in conjunction with viral hepatitis, the disease can also be caused by bacteria, toxic injury, and autoimmune liver cell destruction.

Although some differences exist in the pathologic and clinical phenomena of these various causes of hepatitis, the clinical management is quite similar. Almost any form of hepatitis can result in postnecrotic cirrhosis, unless the hepatitis responds to treatment.

Toxic Hepatitis

Etiology

Because the liver has a primary role in the metabolism of foreign substances, many agents, including drugs, alcohol, industrial toxins, and plant poisons, can cause toxic hepatitis

(Table 37-3). Many health care workers are concerned about hepatic injury caused by adverse drug reactions from the drugs they handle (especially those needing to be mixed from powder).

Epidemiology

As many as 25% of all cases of acute hepatic failure are the result of adverse drug reactions, and drugs are responsible for 2% to 5% of all hospital admission for jaundice in the United States. Some plant sources used as alternative therapy also have been found to be hepatotoxic.[2]

The agents that produce hepatic injury are categorized into two major groups: predictable (intrinsic) and nonpredictable (idiosyncratic) hepatotoxins. The predictable hepatotoxins are further divided into two subgroups: direct and indirect (Box 37-2). Most drugs are nonpredictable (idiosyncratic) hepatotoxins; however, acetaminophen does produce a predictable hepatotoxic reaction. Examples of drug groups that cause unpredictable reactions include some antibiotics, monoamine oxidase inhibitors, anticonvulsants, and antitubercular medications.[20]

Pathophysiology

The morphologic changes produced in the liver by the toxins vary, depending on the specific hepatotoxin. For example, carbon tetrachloride, tetracycline, and ethanol cause fatty infiltration and/or necrosis. Oral contraceptives, cholecystographic dyes, and chlorpromazine produce cholestasis and portal inflammation. A major cause of toxic hepatitis is the use of acetaminophen, especially when used in conjunction with alcohol and other medications such as anticonvulsants and anti-TB drugs.[1] Regardless of the cause, some alteration in liver function occurs. The alteration may result in only minimal manifestations of altered liver function such as slightly elevated serum enzymes or major manifestations associated with acute liver failure (see Clinical Manifestations box).

Collaborative Care Management

Attention is focused on identifying the toxic agent and removing or eliminating it. Gastric lavage and cleansing of the bowel may be indicated to remove the hepatotoxin(s) from the intestinal tract. In some instances, there is a specific treatment for a particular hepatotoxin. For example, acetylcysteine, a mucolytic agent, can be given within 16 hours (immediately is preferred) of ingestion of an acetaminophen

TABLE 37-3 Selected Hepatotoxins

Agents	Source
Carbon tetrachloride and other chlorinated hydrocarbons	Dry-cleaning fluid
Chlorophenothane	Insecticide
Toluene	Glue
Yellow phosphorus	Rat poison, firecrackers
Plant Poisons	
Mushrooms	Aminita phalloides
Pyrrolizine alkaloids	Bush teas, Confrey
Guaiaretic acid	Chaparral
Drugs	Toxic effect
Acetaminophen	Causes liver cell necrosis
Acetylsalicylic acid	Elevates liver serum enzyme levels
Allopurinol	Cholestatic jaundice
Chlorpromazine	Impairs secretion of bile
Clorpropamide	Hepatotoxic
Diazepan	Long-term use alters liver function by unknown mechanisms
Erytromycin	Hepatotoxic
Isoniazid	Symptoms mimic viral hepatitis
6-Mercaptopurine	Hepatotoxic
Nitrofurantoin	Cholestatic jaundice
Oral contraceptives	May interfere with bile secretion
Phenobarbital	Lowers serum bilirubin levels
Phenytoin	May cause hepatitis

BOX 37-2 Classification of Hepatotoxins

Predictable Hepatotoxins

Agents cause toxic hepatitis with predictable regularity and produce injury in a high percentage of persons exposed to them; occurrence of toxic hepatitis is dose dependent.

Nonpredictable Hepatotoxins

Agents produce hepatic injury only in unusually susceptible persons and in only a small percentage of persons exposed to them; occurrence is not dose dependent.

Direct Predictable Hepatotoxins

Agents have direct effect on hepatic cells and organelles, producing structural changes that lead to metabolic defects.

Indirect Predictable Hepatotoxins

Agents first interfere with normal metabolic function, and this alteration in metabolic function produces structural changes.

Clinical Manifestations

Toxic Hepatitis

EARLY MANIFESTATIONS

- Anorexia
- Nausea and vomiting
- Lethargy
- Elevated alanine aminotransferase (ALT) and aspartate aminotransferase (AST) levels

LATER MANIFESTATIONS

- Jaundice
- Hepatomegaly
- Hepatic tenderness
- Dark urine
- Elevated serum bilirubin level
- Elevated urine bilirubin level

overdose. The drug may be given orally or intravenously, although only the oral form has been approved for use in the United States. However, in most instances of toxic hepatitis, medical treatment is supportive and focused on particular manifestations, such as treatment of cirrhosis, portal-systemic encephalopathy, or accompanying kidney failure.

Nursing care for the person with toxic hepatitis is supportive. The nursing management in the acute care setting is focused on promoting comfort, maintaining normal fluid and electrolyte balance, promoting a well-balanced diet when food and fluid are allowed, and promoting rest as discussed in the section on viral hepatitis. The nurse also assists with the implementation of any medical regimen.

Patient/Family Education. The major focus for nursing management is in the community or other outpatient setting and is centered on the nursing diagnosis, potential for injury related to improper use of chemicals at home, exposure to chemicals in the work environment, or injudicious use of drugs or other materials.

Health Promotion/Prevention

Primary Prevention. The nurse can assist in the prevention of toxic hepatitis by teaching the danger of injudicious use of materials that are known to be injurious to the liver. Emphasizing the need for a well-balanced diet with the recommended daily requirements of nutrients and with minimal or no consumption of alcohol should be encouraged.

Because cleaning agents, solvents, and related substances sometimes contain products that are harmful to the liver, the public should read instructions on labels and should follow them explicitly. Dry cleaning fluids may contain carbon tetrachloride, which can cause liver injury if warnings to avoid inhalation of the fumes and to keep windows open are not heeded. If people must use these agents inside the home, a good practice is to open the windows wide; use the cleaning materials as quickly as possible; and then vacate the room, apartment, or house for several hours, leaving the windows open.

Many solvents used to remove paint and plastic material and to stain and finish woodwork contain injurious substances and should be used outdoors and not in the basement, as dangerous fumes may spread throughout the house. Cleaning agents and finishes for cars should be applied outdoors or in the garage with the door open. Nurses in industry have a responsibility to teach the importance of observing regulations to avoid industrial hazards. Nitrobenzene, tetrachloroethane, carbon disulfide, and dinitrotoluane are examples of injurious compounds used in industry.

Secondary Prevention. Some drugs that are known to cause mild damage to the liver must be used therapeutically. However, the nurse should warn the public about the use of preparations available without prescription that can cause liver injury. Many drugs, prescription and nonprescription, reach the market before dangers resulting from their extensive use have been conclusively ruled out. An example is the prescription drug chlorpromazine, which was widely used as a tranquilizer, and then found to cause stasis of bile in the canaliculi of the liver, which can lead to serious hepatic damage. A safe rule to follow is to avoid taking any medication except that specifically prescribed by a physician.

Autoimmune Hepatitis

Autoimmune hepatitis is a chronic necroinflammatory liver disorder associated with circulating autoantibodies and high serum globulin levels.

Etiology/Epidemiology

The etiology of autoimmune hepatitis is unknown, although it is associated with a genetic predisposition to autoimmunity. It develops after exposure to some environmental agent. Familial studies have not proven whether there is a genetic basis for this response, or if the autoantibodies are an alternative way to show disease susceptibility. Autoimmune hepatitis is less common than chronic viral hepatitis, but its diagnosis is often missed because of vague early symptoms. It may occur at any age, but is most prevalent in girls and women between 15 and 40 years old.

Pathophysiology

The autoimmune response is directed at liver antigens, and causes progressive necrosis and inflammation of hepatocytes. Fibrosis and cirrhosis result. Clinical manifestations range from mild to those of clinically advanced cirrhosis. Some patients are asymptomatic. Early diagnosis is important, because this form of hepatitis responds very well to corticosteroid therapy.

Collaborative Care Management

There is no single diagnostic test for autoimmune hepatitis. Diagnosis is made by obtaining a detailed history and physical examination to rule out other causes of liver disease, and analyzing laboratory and biopsy results. The presence of circulating autoantibodies such as antinuclear antibodies, antimitochondrial antibodies, and others is useful, although it is not clear what role these antibodies play in the pathology. Corticosteroids are the mainstay of treatment for autoimmune hepatitis, and azathioprine (Imuran) has also proven useful. Medications such as cyclosporine, 6-mecaptopurine, and methotrexate are under investigation.[17]

Nursing care of the patient with autoimmune hepatitis centers around symptom management and varies, depending on the presentation of the disease. Of primary importance in this disorder is patient, family, and community education. Any individual who experiences chronic malaise, abdominal discomfort, and/or arthralgias should seek health care and not wait until the more obvious manifestations of liver disease (jaundice, ascites) appear. Clinicians also need to improve their understanding of autoimmune hepatitis. Often nurses are the first to be "consulted" about health care problems.

Patient/Family Education. Patients diagnosed with autoimmune hepatitis require follow-up care every 3 to 4 weeks to evaluate response to treatment. Once clinical and serologic responses are normalized, reevaluation should occur every 3 months.[14] The nurse should inform the patient and family about the need for this continuous care and evaluation.

Viral Hepatitis

Viral hepatitis is by far the most important liver infection and is a major health problem in the United States and in many other countries. The term *viral hepatitis* is used to refer to several clinically similar but etiologically and epidemiologically distinct infections.

Etiology

Five major categories of viruses have been identified as causing viral hepatitis: hepatitis A (HAV), hepatitis B (HBV), hepatitis C (HCV), hepatitis D (HDV or delta virus), and hepatitis E (HEV). Two other forms of hepatitis, F and G, have been identified but occur rarely. Table 37-4 provides a summary of the modes of transmission for each viral type.[22,24,29]

TABLE 37-4 Etiologic/Epidemiologic/Transmission Characteristics of Viral Hepatitis

Hepatitis A	Hepatitis B	Hepatitis C	Hepatitis D	Hepatitis E
Transmission				
Fecal-oral	Parenteral/sexual/perinatal	Parenteral/sexual/perinatal	Superinfection or coinfection with chronic HBV	Fecal/oral
Incubation Period				
2-6 wk	4-24 wk	2-20 wk	4-24 wk	2-8 wk
Virus Type				
RNA picornavirus	DNA hepadenavirus	RNA flavirs	Defective RNA virus	Unclassified RNA virus
Diagnostic Serologic Tests				
Acute phase: IgM anti-HAV	Acute phase: HBsAg, anti-HBc IgM, HBeAg	Acute phase: anti-HDV	Acute phase: anti-HCV	None
Lifetime: IgG anti-HAV	Lifetime: anti-HBs; anti-HBc	Life time: anti-HCV		
Secretions That Have Been Found to Contain Infective Agent				
Feces, blood	Blood/serous fluids, saliva, semen, urine, nasopharyngeal washings, feces, pleural fluid	Blood, semen	Blood	Feces
Indication of Protective Immunity				
IgG anti-HAV	anti-HBs, total anti-HBc	None	None	None
Chronicity				
None	90% infants, 6%-10% adults	50%-80%	2%-70%	None
Mortality				
<1%	1%-2%	1%-2%	2%-20%	1%-2% (as high as 20% in pregnant women)
High-Risk Groups				
Travelers to developing countries; staff and patients in custodial care institutions (prison, day care, nursing homes)	Household and sexual partners of HBV carriers; immigrants from HBV-endemic areas; IV drug users; patients and staff in custodial care institutions; sexually active gay men; patients on hemodialysis; health care workers with frequent contact with blood	Travelers to endemic areas; people receiving frequent blood transfusions; IV drug users; tattoos; organ transplant recipients; 40% report no risk factors	Same as for HBV	Immigrants and travelers to HEV-epidemic areas
Vaccine Available				
Yes	Yes	No	No	No

DNA, Deoxyribonucleic acid; *HAV*, hepatitis A virus; *HBc*, hepatitis B core antigen; *HBeAg*, hepatitis B early antigen; *HBsAg*, hepatitis B surface antigen; *HBV*, hepatitis B virus; *HCV*, hepatitis C virus; *HDV*, hepatitis virus, type D; *HEV*, hepatitis E virus; *RNA*, ribonucleic acid.

Epidemiology

Viral hepatitis is a reportable disease in all states in the United States. Statistics from the Centers for Disease Control and Prevention (CDC) indicate that viral hepatitis is one of the most frequently reported infectious diseases in the country. Native Americans and Native Alaskans have a high rate of endemic disease. The most common type of hepatitis worldwide is HAV, with 40% of the reported cases of hepatitis being caused by this virus.

The incidence of HBV infection is reported to be about 5% of the world's population. Approximately 59% of the reported cases of HBV infection in the United States occur in heterosexuals with multiple sex partners, homosexual men, and IV drug users. The incidence of HBV infection in health care workers is about 3% of all reported cases.

Of all cases of viral hepatitis reported to the CDC, 20% are caused by HCV infection, and 50% to 80% of these persons will develop chronic hepatitis. HDV is endemic among persons with HBV in areas around the Mediterranean and Middle East. HEV is extremely rare in the United States but occurs in epidemic proportions in areas of India. Cases of HEV have also been reported in Mexico, Asia, and Africa. The mortality rate is low, except for pregnant women, in whom it reaches 20%.

Hepatitis in the vast majority of patients seen clinically is caused by HAV or HBV. Most cases of all types of hepatitis occur in young adults. Factors such as the viral agent, transmission, and high-risk groups vary for the five types of hepatitis.[12,22,29]

Pathophysiology

Viral hepatitis causes diffuse inflammatory infiltration of hepatic tissue with mononuclear cells and local, spotty, or single cell necrosis. The liver cells may be very swollen. With typical acute viral hepatitis, there is no collapse of lobules, no loss of lobular architecture, and minimal or no fibrosis. Inflammation, degeneration, and regeneration occur simultaneously, distorting the normal lobular pattern and creating pressure within and around the portal vein areas and obstructing the bile channels. The pathologic changes in the hepatocytes is not always related to the effects of the virus itself, but rather the injurious response of the body's own immune system attempting to clear the virus. These changes are associated with elevated serum transaminase levels, prolonged prothrombin time, slightly elevated serum alkaline phosphatase level, and elevated bilirubin level.

Most patients recover from acute viral hepatitis, with normal liver function and no residual hepatic necrosis. Although chronic hepatitis can occur with all types of hepatitis, it is virtually unseen with HAV and HEV. Chronic hepatitis is defined as the presence of serum viral antigens 6 months after the acute episode. Persons with chronic hepatitis are carriers of the virus and remain contagious. Chronic hepatitis has been classified into active and persistent categories based on symptoms and histologic tissue changes on liver biopsy. However, the latest recommendation is to use terms that include the etiology and degree of hepatic injury, regardless of symptoms. Mild, moderate, or marked chronic presentations indicate the degree of hepatic damage and the risk of progression to cirrhosis or liver cancer. The patient with chronic hepatitis may be asymptomatic, except for minimal abnormalities in serum transaminase levels, or have mild to severe symptoms of liver disease. There is strong evidence of an association between chronic hepatitis B and the development of hepatocellular cancer. Chronic hepatitis C is the most common chronic liver disease in the United States and the leading indication for liver transplant.

The clinical manifestations of the various forms of acute viral hepatitis are generally not distinct from each other. The shorter incubation period of HAV infection results in a more abrupt onset and duration of symptoms is shorter. Clinical manifestations of viral hepatitis including abnormal values in diagnostic tests fall into three phases: preicteric, icteric, and posticteric (see Clinical Manifestations box).

Collaborative Care Management

Diagnostic Tests. Blood tests are checked for viral antibodies and antigens and for actual viral particles (see Table 37-4). Elevations in the serum liver enzymes ALT and AST are present in hepatitis A and B. Liver function tests are monitored until normal.

Medications. Because most medications are metabolized in the liver, only essential drugs should be given. Vitamin K may be necessary if the prothrombin time is prolonged. Analgesics are given only sparingly in people with liver dysfunction. Patients with chronic hepatitis C are treated with interferon, with some success. Combinations of interferon with antiviral drugs such as ribiviron are being studied. These medications have not worked well with chronic hepatitis B.[8]

Treatments. Most persons infected with hepatitis are not hospitalized. Rest is advised, but complete bed rest is not necessary. Persons requiring hospitalization include those with

Clinical Manifestations

Viral Hepatitis

PREICTERIC PHASE

- Nonspecific complaints of fatigue, anorexia, nausea, cough, joint pain, loss of appetite
- Laboratory values indicate elevated serum alanine aminotransferase (ALT) and aspartate aminotransferase (AST) and elevated urine bilirubin levels
- Presence of viral antibodies, antigens, or virus particles

ICTERIC PHASE

- Appearance of jaundice and darkening of urine; stools may be clay-colored due to decreased urobilinogen
- Preicteric symptoms subside, although appetite remains poor
- Right upper quadrant pain and increasing pruritis
- Laboratory studies show elevated direct bilirubin levels

POSTICTERIC PHASE

- Decreasing jaundice, return of normal color to urine and stool, improvement of appetite

LABORATORY

- Values return to normal
- Fatigue may continue

Reference: Shovein JT, Damazo RJ, Hyams I: Hepatitis A: how benign is it? *AJN* 100:43, 2000.

Complementary & Alternative Therapies
Alternative Therapy for Hepatitis

Natural therapies can be of great benefit in treating hepatitis. Several nutrients and herbs have been shown to inhibit viral reproduction, improve immune system function, and greatly stimulate regeneration of the damaged liver cells. During the acute phase of hepatitis, the focus should be on replacing fluids through consumption of vegetable broths, diluted vegetable juices, and herbal teas. Solid foods should be restricted to brown rice, steamed vegetables, and moderate intake of lean protein sources. Vitamin C in high doses (40 to 100 g orally) has been known to diminish acute viral hepatitis in 2 to 4 days, including the clearing of jaundice.

In chronic cases a diet that focuses on plant foods has been shown to increase elimination of bile acids, drugs, and toxic substances from the system. Liver extracts are said to promote hepatic regeneration and are especially useful in treatment of chronic hepatitis. Orally administered bovine thymus extracts have been used in both acute and chronic presentations, with decreases in liver enzyme studies, elimination of the virus, and a higher rate of formation of anti HBe antibodies. Plant medicines in the treatment of hepatitis include milk thistle (silymarin) and glycyrrhiza glabra (licorice).

MILK THISTLE

The seeds from the plant silybum marianum, a member of the daisy and thistle family, exerts hepatoprotective and antihepatoxic action over liver toxins, including the deadly mushroom *Amanita phalloides*. Silymarin alters the outer liver membrane cell structure so that toxins cannot enter the cell. It also stimulates RNA polymerase A, which results in activation of the regenerative capacity of the liver. It has been reported to be useful as an antidote for ingestion of poisonous mushrooms, viral hepatitis (both acute and chronic), and cirrhosis.

GLYCYRRHIZA

Glabra is derived from the roots of the licorice plant. Its main effect is to potentiate endogenous steroids. It has been useful in the treatment of hepatitis by enhancing the immune system, potentiating interferon, and promoting the flow of bile and fat to and from the liver.

Reference: Murray MT, Pizzorno JE: *Hepatitis: encyclopedia of natural medicine*, ed 2, Rocklin, Calif, 1997, Prima Publishing.

serum bilirubin concentrations 10 mg/dl or greater than 10 times the normal, and those with acute liver failure. There is evidence that some herbal preparations and vitamins may be beneficial in the treatment of hepatitis[23] (see Complementary & Alternative Therapies box).

Diet. If liver function is not impaired, a well-balanced diet is adequate. A low-fat, high-carbohydrate diet may be better tolerated. Protein and sodium are restricted if liver function is compromised. These decisions are based on laboratory values. Abstinence from alcohol is essential.

Activity. Rest is the foundation of treatment for viral hepatitis. Activity can be increased as tolerated by the patient.[21,29]

Referrals. Patients and their families may be referred to the local health department for information about viral hepatitis. It is important that they receive information about contagion and vaccination. Referral to a home health care agency may be indicated for persons not requiring hospitalization.

NURSING MANAGEMENT OF PATIENT WITH VIRAL HEPATITIS

ASSESSMENT

Nursing assessment focuses on identifying changes related to viral hepatitis and sources of transmission that are controllable.

Health History

Assessment data to be collected as part of the health history of a patient with viral hepatitis includes:

- Presence of discomfort: headache, right upper abdominal quadrant tenderness, arthralgia, and pruritus
- Presence of GI alterations: history of anorexia, nausea, vomiting, or dyspepsia
- Changes in nutritional intake of food and fluids
- History of changes in weight
- History of episodes of fever, chills, or adenopathy
- Reports of weakness/malaise not relieved by rest
- History of potential exposure to hepatitis virus: work environment, child-care facilities, recent international travel, injections of illegal drugs, recent blood transfusions, contaminated food and water, tattoos, recent sexual contact with infected person, homosexual or bisexual lifestyle
- Knowledge about the disease
- Length of time since onset of symptoms

Physical Examination

Important aspects of the physical examination of the patient with viral hepatitis include:

- Skin/sclerae: adequacy of skin turgor, presence of jaundice or lesions from scratching; if jaundice is present, the nurse should assess the patient for the presence of petechiae or bruises
- Lymph nodes: enlargement
- Abdomen: liver enlargement, tenderness or guarding in right upper quadrant
- Documented nutritional and fluid intake and output
- Temperature
- Weight/height
- Musculoskeletal: strength and ability to do activities

NURSING DIAGNOSES

Nursing diagnoses are determined from analysis of patient data. Nursing diagnoses for the patient with viral hepatitis may include but are not limited to:

Diagnostic Title	Possible Etiologic Factors
1. Fatigue	Imbalance between energy level and demand, decreased rest, feeling of malaise
2. Activity intolerance	Fatigue, weakness

3. Imbalanced nutrition: less than body requirements	Anorexia, inadequate intake, increased metabolic needs
4. Pain	Arthralgia, pruritis, headaches, abdominal tenderness
5. Deficient knowledge	Lack of knowledge relating to the spread of the disease and prevention
6. Risk for impaired skin integrity	Jaundice, pruritus, scratching
7. Social isolation	Physical isolation, fear of others catching disease

EXPECTED PATIENT OUTCOMES

Expected patient outcomes for the person with viral hepatitis may include but are not limited to:

1. Will indicate a decrease in fatigue, as evidenced by a lower rating on a scale of 1 to 5, with 1 indicating no fatigue
2. Will slowly increase activity until former activity level is achieved
3. Will increase food intake until adequate in amount and content for body size
4. Will verbalize that pain is controlled and/or will rate pain on a scale from 1 (no pain) to 10 (severe pain)
5. Will explain safe sex practices, the need for immunization, and the risk of needle sharing
6. Skin will be intact and free of lesions
7. Will express the feeling that isolation is not distressing and will share information that reveals he or she is being kept up to date about family affairs

INTERVENTIONS

1. Monitoring Fatigue

The patient with hepatitis needs considerable rest during the acute phase of the illness. The level of physical activity allowed is individually determined based on the amount of fatigue and severity of the disease. Rest periods should be interspersed throughout the day, and patient care should be scheduled to allow for uninterrupted periods for napping and relaxation.

2. Increasing Activity Tolerance

The patient should be instructed to increase activity slowly as tolerated. An adequate diet will provide needed energy for increasing activity. If hepatic enzyme levels increase with resumption of near-normal activities, limitations on activity will be imposed.

3. Maintaining Fluid Intake and Nutritional Status

During the acute phase of the illness, the patient needs 3000 ml/day of fluids because of the increased fluid needs associated with febrile illness and vomiting. Fluid can usually be given orally if nausea and vomiting are not severe. When nausea and vomiting are severe, IV infusions are given. Intake, output, and weight should be monitored to assess the patient for adequacy of intake. Fluids such as fruit juices and carbonated beverages that provide both volume and nutrients are encouraged.

No special dietary restrictions are required in most patients. The diet should be well balanced and provide adequate nutrients and calories based on the patient's size and age. Most of the calories should be from carbohydrate sources. The diet should be planned with the patient so that it is appealing. Frequent, small meals are usually better tolerated than larger meals. Fats are usually restricted, as they are poorly tolerated. Alcoholic beverages should be avoided because they are metabolized in the liver.

4,6. Providing Comfort Measures and Promoting Skin Integrity

During the early phase of the illness, the patient may have headaches and arthralgia, resulting in discomfort. General comfort measures—relaxing baths, backrubs, fresh linen on the bed, and a quiet, dark environment—may ease the patient's discomfort. During the icteric phase of the illness, the presence of bile pigments in the skin may cause severe pruritus. Pruritus can be exhausting and demoralizing to the patient.

Measures to control pruritus include:

- Use of cool, light, nonrestrictive clothing
- Avoidance of clothes or blankets made of wool
- Use of soft, dry, clean bedding
- Use of warm, not hot, tub baths
- Application of emollient creams and lotions to skin
- Use of superfat soaps
- Avoidance of activities that promote sweating and increase body temperature
- Maintenance of a cool environment
- Administration of antihistamines as ordered
- Use of diversional activities such as reading, television, and radio to reduce the patient's perception of pruritus

The major aim of care is to prevent scratching with resultant injury to the skin. It is impossible for people with pruritus not to scratch. Sometimes the person may be given a soft cloth with which to rub the skin. The patient's fingernails should be kept short, and the patient's hands should be kept clean to decrease the likelihood of excoriation or infection, if scratching occurs.

5. Correcting Deficient Knowledge

The nurse must provide an open and honest environment where frank discussions about dangerous sexual practices and drug use can be undertaken. The risk of contracting viral hepatitis through multiple sex partners should be addressed. Sharing of IV drug equipment should be discouraged, and alternatives, such as drug treatment, should be suggested. Explanations about immunization of close contacts should be given, along with information as to obtaining this service. Patients and their families should be educated about appropriate preexposure and postexposure prophylaxis. Teaching should include methods to avoid transmission of infection.

7. Promoting Social Interaction

The nurse must work with the patient and significant others so that they understand that the needed isolation does not prohibit social interaction and visiting. Fear of spread of the infection can lead others to avoid the patient. Proper teaching can ensure that both isolation and the patient's need for support from significant others are maintained.

Patient/Family Education

A major focus of care is patient education. Most patients are treated at home for the duration of their illness. The nurse must prepare these persons for adequate home care by teaching them about the measures previously described for the provision of adequate rest, provision of adequate fluid and nutritional intake, relief of discomfort, identification of signs and symptoms of bleeding, and maintenance of adequate isolation. The patient must be able to detect changes indicating a worsening of his or her condition (e.g., increasing fatigue, uncontrolled nausea and vomiting, onset of bleeding, worsening of upper quadrant discomfort, and water retention) and be instructed to report these changes immediately.

All patients, whether treated in the hospital or at home, should understand that it may take several months or longer for complete recovery, and that they must be evaluated frequently for repeated assessment of blood studies to monitor their progress. Blood studies may be performed weekly for several weeks and then monthly until results return to normal. If blood studies do not show the expected improvement from the care being given, more invasive procedures, such as a liver biopsy, may be necessary. The patient will be followed for at least 1 year after liver function tests have returned to normal to ensure that relapse does not occur.

Health Promotion/Prevention

Hepatitis A. Preexposure prophylaxis with the vaccine for hepatitis A virus is recommended for persons traveling to HAV-endemic countries, persons with occupational risk of infection (those who work with HAV-infected primates or with the virus in a laboratory), persons with chronic liver disease, chronic IV drug users, and individuals that engage in anal sex. Other high-risk groups are Native Americans and IV drug users. Postexposure prophylaxis with serum immunoglobulin (gamma globulin) is recommended for selected people who have had contact with a person known to be positive for HAV. Prophylaxis must be given within 2 weeks of exposure. Postexposure prophylaxis for the following people is recommended: close household and sexual contacts of people with HAV, staff and attendees of daycare centers, custodial care centers and hospital staff who have close contacts with patients with HAV, people exposed to a common source of infection (infected food or water), if identified within 2 weeks of exposure, and food handlers working with a handler in whom hepatitis A has been diagnosed.[27]

Hepatitis B. Hepatitis B is a vaccine-preventable disease. HBV vaccine is given as a series of three intramuscular injections (deltoid in adults and children; anterolateral thigh muscles in infants and neonates), with the second and third doses given 1 and 6 months after the first dose. The vaccine has shown an efficacy of 85% to 95%. The effect of the vaccine on the developing fetus is not known; however, pregnancy should not be considered a contraindication for its use in providing protection to the mother. Because HBV vaccine has no benefits for HBV carriers and because of the cost of the vaccination, prevaccination serologic screening for anti-HBc and anti-HBs may be done to identify both carriers and previously infected noncarriers who have adequate immunity. The cost of screening is weighed against the cost of unnecessary but harmless vaccination to identify whether screening before vaccinating should be performed.

Preexposure vaccination against hepatitis B is recommended for everyone, with highest priority to occupationally exposed workers, IV drug users, heterosexually active persons, and those that engage in anal sex. It is important to consider that health care workers include medical technologists, phlebotomists, nurses, physicians (especially surgeons), pathologists, dialysis unit staff, dentists, oral surgeons, dental hygienists, laboratory and blood bank technicians, emergency medical technicians, and morticians. Those who are frequently exposed to blood products, such as hemophiliacs and patients on hemodialysis, are also at high risk.

Postexposure prophylaxis involves the injection of hepatitis B immunoglobulin (HBIG), which contains high amounts of anti-HBs. HBIG should be given within 24 hours after exposure, and the individual should follow this injection with the routine 3-dose vaccination for HBV. Babies born to mothers with hepatitis B should receive HBIG and the first dose of the vaccination series at birth. If the exposed person has been vaccinated, he or she is checked for anti-HBs and given HBIG immediately plus a booster dose of HBV vaccination.

Postexposure prophylaxis should be considered for persons who have been exposed to HBsAg-positive blood, those who have sexual contact with HBsAg-positive persons, and infants younger than 12 months old exposed to a primary caregiver who has acute HBV.

Hepatitis C and E. Prophylaxis for HCV and HEV infections is not as effective as that for HBV. For travelers to countries where HEV occurs in endemic proportions, preventive health teaching is the best prophylactic measure. The value of immunoglobulin in this situation is unknown. For postexposure prophylaxis in persons exposed through breaks in the skin to blood from a patient with HCV, immunoglobulin may be given, but its value is questionable.

Hepatitis D. HDV requires the presence of HBV to be active; thus the preexposure and postexposure prophylaxes that are recommended for HBV should suffice to prevent delta hepatitis. Currently, no prophylaxis exists for preventing HDV infection in HBV carriers except health teaching.

Healthy People 2010 Goals (see Healthy People 2010 box). Vaccination against hepatitis A and B is the mainstay of these recommendations, especially the Vaccines for Children program. Until the goal of universal vaccination of newborns can be achieved, it continues to be important to find targeted high risk populations and provide vaccination services. A goal of Healthy People 2010 is to increase the proportion of international travelers who receive recommended preventive services for hepatitis A. There have been missed opportunities for the vaccination for individuals at high risk for hepatitis B. Studies indicate that as many as 70% of individuals at high risk for hepatitis B have been previously seen in settings such as drug

Healthy People 2010

Midcourse Review and Revisions

Reduce viral hepatitis as follows:

(Per 100,000 adults)	1997 Baseline	2010 Target
Hepatitis B	59.0	11.3
Hepatitis A (new cases)	11.3	4.4
Hepatitis C (new cases)	2.4 (1996)	1
SPECIAL POPULATION TARGETS		
Hepatitis B (number of cases)	1997 Baseline	2010 Target
Injecting drug users	7232	1808
Heterosexually active people	15,225	1240
Men who have sex with men	7232	1808
Occupationally exposed workers	249	62
Infants and young children	1682 (1995)	400

From US Department of Health and Human Services *Healthy People 2010: understanding and improving health,* Washington, DC, 2000, USDHHS.

Research

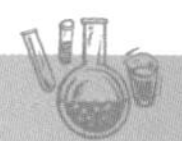

Reference: Chien et al: Seroprevalence of viral hepatitis in an older nursing home population, *J Am Geriatr Soc* 47(9):1110, 1999.

The purpose of the study was to investigate the prevalence of current or previous infection with viral hepatitis agents in nursing home residents. The 199 consenting subjects were from nursing homes in the St Louis area. Residents were asked for a history of hepatitis or liver disease and were also examined for symptoms of liver disease. Serum samples were tested for hepatitis B surface antigen, antibody to hepatitis B core, surface antigens, antibody to hepatitis A virus, antibody to hepatitis C virus, and hepatitis G virus RNA. Results showed that the frequency of HAV infection increased significantly with age, but HBV infection correlated with ethnic status and previous occupation as a manual laborer. A history of blood transfusion was correlated with a higher rate of anti-HAV. The study concluded that there is a high prevalence of anti-HCV in skilled nursing facilities and that new patients admitted to these institutions should be screened for anti-HCV.

treatment clinics, correctional facilities, or clinics for the treatment of sexually transmitted diseases. These facilities can be used for hepatitis B vaccination programs. Although there is no vaccine for hepatitis C, an important preventive strategy is to identify infected individuals. This provides an opportunity for counseling to prevent further transmission of the HCV, vaccination against HA and HBV to prevent additional liver damage, possible antiviral therapy, and counseling to avoid potential hepatotoxins. Community teaching about the spread of all types of hepatitis and the lifestyle changes that can reduce this spread are essential in the prevention and reduction of hepatitis.[29]

EVALUATION

To evaluate the effectiveness of nursing interventions, compare patient behaviors with those stated in the expected patient outcomes. Achievement of outcomes is successful if the patient with viral hepatitis:

1. States cause of fatigue, and that fatigue remains at a rating of 2 or less if rest periods are interspersed throughout the day.
2. Reports an increased activity level without an increase in fatigue.
3. Verbalizes knowledge of nutritionally adequate diet, demonstrates adequate intake, and uses measures to enhance appetite.
4. States that itching and arthralgia are controlled; that no scratching, restlessness, or grimacing is present.

5a. Describes isolation precautions for home, including using a separate bathroom from family if possible; flushing stool twice after using the toilet; handling own body secretions, not sharing razors, toothbrushes, and food or drinks; abstaining from sexual relationships until infection has subsided; and washing hands as appropriate.

5b. Verbalizes understanding of blood tests; explains why isolation is necessary; identifies persons in household who may have been exposed to same source of infection from contaminated foods and fluids, hygiene practices, sharing of needles, or sexual relationships; explains need for high-protein, high-calorie, well-balanced diet, adequate rest, and avoidance of alcohol; explains hygiene practices, safe sex practices, and avoidance of sharing of needles to avoid future infections; and states plans for obtaining vaccinations for self and others as appropriate.

6. States that skin remains intact.
7. Participates in social/family activities at level of ability.

GERONTOLOGIC CONSIDERATIONS

There has been a higher incidence of some types of hepatitis in the older adult population in some areas of the United States. Because of the depressed immunity of some of these individuals, mortality rates may increase. There is some ongoing research in this area, and recommendations for hepatitis antigen testing is available in the literature (see Research box). Nurses in long-term care facilities need to be astute in their initial and ongoing assessments of the residents, observing for early signs of viral hepatitis infections.[5]

COMPLICATIONS

Potential complications of viral hepatitis include chronic hepatitis and the possible development of cirrhosis, liver failure, or hepatocellular cancer.

CIRRHOSIS OF THE LIVER

Cirrhosis of the liver is the term applied to chronic disease of the liver characterized by diffuse inflammation and fibrosis resulting in drastic structural changes and significant loss of liver function. The basic changes with cirrhosis are liver cell death and replacement of normal tissue by scar tissue that results in nodules of normal liver parenchyma surrounded by fibrous tissue and fat. These changes result in distortion of the structure of the liver and loss of function.

Cirrhosis of the liver can be classified in various ways. Table 37-5 lists the major types of cirrhosis based on a pathologic classification.

Etiology

As can be seen from Table 37-5, cirrhosis can result from liver disease secondary to intrahepatic and extrahepatic cholestasis, viral hepatitis, and other hepatotoxins (drugs and chemicals). Alcoholism and malnutrition are two major predisposing factors for development of Laënnec's cirrhosis. Less common causes of cirrhosis are right-sided congestive heart failure, hemochromatosis, Wilson's disease, glycogen storage disease, cystic fibrosis, and small bowel bypass. In some patients the cause is idiopathic.

Epidemiology

Postnecrotic cirrhosis from hepatotoxins is the most common type of cirrhosis worldwide. Laënnec's cirrhosis is the most common type in North America and accounts for 75% of all cases of cirrhosis.

The role of alcohol in the development of cirrhosis is still under study. It is known, however, that approximately 15% of all alcoholics will develop cirrhosis and that the volume of alcohol rather than the type of alcohol is the important factor. Most persons with Laënnec's cirrhosis have a history of consumption of the equivalent of a pint of whiskey a day for 15 years. Healthy People 2010 indicates that sustained heavy alcohol consumption is the leading cause of cirrhosis and that changes in alcohol consumption patterns over time are associated with reduction in the death rate from cirrhosis. In 1998 there were 9.5 cirrhosis deaths per 100,000 population, and Healthy People 2010 has set a goal of 3 deaths per 100,000 by 2010. There is ongoing research to find drugs that may assist alcoholics to reduce or cease drinking alcohol. This should help prevent some cases of Laennec's cirrhosis in the future[3] (see Research box).

Cirrhosis as a cause of death in the United States now ranks fourth in middle-aged men and women, accounting for 350,000 deaths each year. Cirrhosis can occur in any age-group, but in the United States it is more common in 45- to 64-year-old Caucasian men and in non-Caucasians of both sexes.

Pathophysiology

In Laënnec's cirrhosis, fatty infiltration of the liver is the first alteration seen. This fatty infiltration is usually reversible if the causative factor (alcohol, malnutrition, or biliary ob-

Research

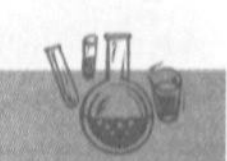

Reference: Bankole A et al: Ondansetron for reduction of drinking among biologically predisposed alcoholic patients, *JAMA*, 284(8):963-971, 2000.

Early-onset alcoholism differs from late-onset alcoholism in its association with greater serotoninergic abnormality and antisocial behaviors. The purpose of this study was to test the hypothesis that drinking outcomes associated with early versus late-onset alcoholism are differentially improved by the serotonin antagonist ondansetron (Zofran).

This was a double-blind, randomized, placebo-controlled clinical trial in which 271 patients with diagnosed alcoholism participated. Patients were randomly assigned to receive 11 weeks of treatment with ondansetron twice a day, or placebo. All patients also participated in weekly standardized group cognitive behavioral therapy.

Patients with early-onset alcoholism who received ondansetron had fewer drinks per day. Ondansetron was superior to placebo in increasing the percentage of days abstinent and total days abstinent per study week. Among patients with early-onset alcoholism, there was a significant difference in the mean log CDT ratio.

CDT, Carbohydrate-deficient transferrin.

TABLE 37-5 Types of Cirrhosis

Type	Etiology	Description
Laënnec's cirrhosis (nutritional, portal, or alcoholic cirrhosis)	Alcoholism, malnutrition	Massive collagen formation occurs; liver is fatty and in early hepatitis stages is large and firm; in late state, it is small and nodular.
Postnecrotic cirrhosis	Massive necrosis from hepatotoxins, usually viral hepatitis	Liver is decreased in size with nodules and fibrous tissue.
Primary biliary cirrhosis	Inflammation of intrahepatic bile ductules resulting in biliary obstruction in liver and common bile duct; cholangitis (destruction of the intrahepatic bile ducts) may occur; thought to be an autoimmune disorder; 95% are women between 30 and 60 years old.	Chronic impairment of bile drainage occurs; liver is first large, then becomes firm and nodular; there is increased skin pigmentation resembling a deep tan, jaundice, and pruritus.
Cardiac cirrhosis	Right-sided congestive heart failure (CHF)	Liver is swollen, and changes are reversible if CHF is treated effectively; some fibrosis occurs with long-standing CHF.
Nonspecific, metabolic cirrhosis	Metabolic problems, infectious diseases, infiltrative diseases, GI diseases	Portal and liver fibrosis may develop; liver is enlarged and firm.

struction) is halted or reversed. If the degenerative process continues, acute inflammation (alcoholic hepatitis) and cirrhosis result. Alterations in physiology are usually seen late in the progression of the disease because of the large reserve capacity of the liver. As much as three fourths of the liver can be destroyed before physiologic function is altered. The relationships between normal functions of the liver and alterations seen in liver disease such as in cirrhosis are presented in Table 37-1.

Fibrotic changes in the liver that result from continual destruction distort the hepatic structures and result in obstruction of the splanchnic veins and portal blood flow. This obstruction can result in additional problems with fluid retention, including increasing edema, ascites, and hydrothorax. Increased portal pressure and splanchnic venous congestion result in splenomegaly and altered spleen function, which can cause leukopenia, thrombocytopenia, and anemia. Portal hypertension causes increased venous pressure, vascular hemostasis, varicose veins, hemorrhoids, and esophageal varices. Figure 37-4, *A*, depicts the venous drainage of splanchnic organs, and Figure 37-4, *B*, depicts the massive ascites and gynecomastia (the enlarged breasts of this male patient, due to failure of the liver to metabolize estrogen) that can be seen in cirrhosis.

A variety of signs and symptoms can be seen in persons with cirrhosis; they reflect the diminishing capacity of the liver to function normally. The patient may exhibit any or all of the signs and symptoms. Most manifestations can be directly related to the pathophysiologic changes (see Table 37-1; Figure 37-5 and Clinical Manifestations box).

Collaborative Care Management

The goal for discharge of patients with cirrhosis as determined by diagnosis-related groups (DRGs) is 7 days. The nurse works collaboratively with the physician for implementation of prescribed medical therapy. Because the nurse has a major role in discharge planning and patient teaching, these are discussed under nursing management.

Diagnostic Tests. The patient with cirrhosis has various abnormalities in blood and urine laboratory data as depicted in Figure 37-5. Other studies, such as liver biopsy, CT scan, endoscopy, barium contrast, and angiography, may be done if the clinical manifestations are vague or inconsistent. The results of these later diagnostic tests depend on the complications the patient has developed.

Medications. Drug therapy varies, depending on the signs and symptoms. These include antihistamines to alleviate pruritus; potassium supplements to correct hypokalemia; diuretics (particularly aldosterone antagonists for edema because the patient with cirrhosis does not catabolize aldosterone appropriately and has hyperaldosteronism); and folic acid, thiamine, and other vitamins and minerals for deficiencies and anemia. Persons with alcoholism are particularly deficient in thiamine and folic acid because these water-soluble vitamins have been depleted, and thus deficits occur rapidly with lack of intake of nutrients. Sodium and fluids are also usually restricted. Occasionally albumin may be given for hypoalbuminemia; however, its effects last only a short time.

Treatments. No specific treatment exists for cirrhosis. Management is directed toward removal or treatment of causative factors such as alcoholism, biliary obstruction, infections, and cardiac problems and toward preventing additional liver damage. Symptom management is also important; for example, paracentesis may be done if ascites is causing respiratory distress.

Diet. Because alcoholism and malnutrition are major factors in the development of cirrhosis, supplying an adequate diet

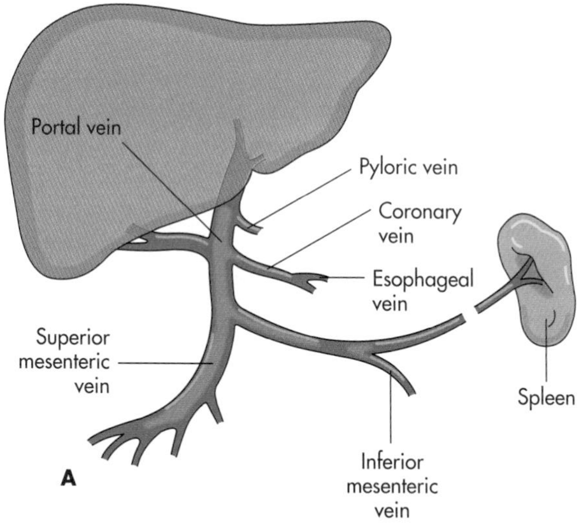

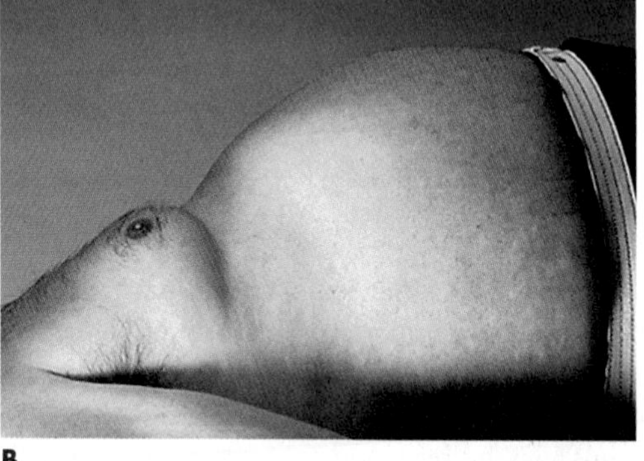

Figure 37-4 Splanchnic veins. **A**, Venous drainage of splanchnic organs. When portal hypertension develops, other vessels can become engorged, leading to stasis and hypoxia of the respective organs. **B**, Ascites and gynecomastia associated with cirrhosis of the liver. Photograph taken after a paracentesis was performed.

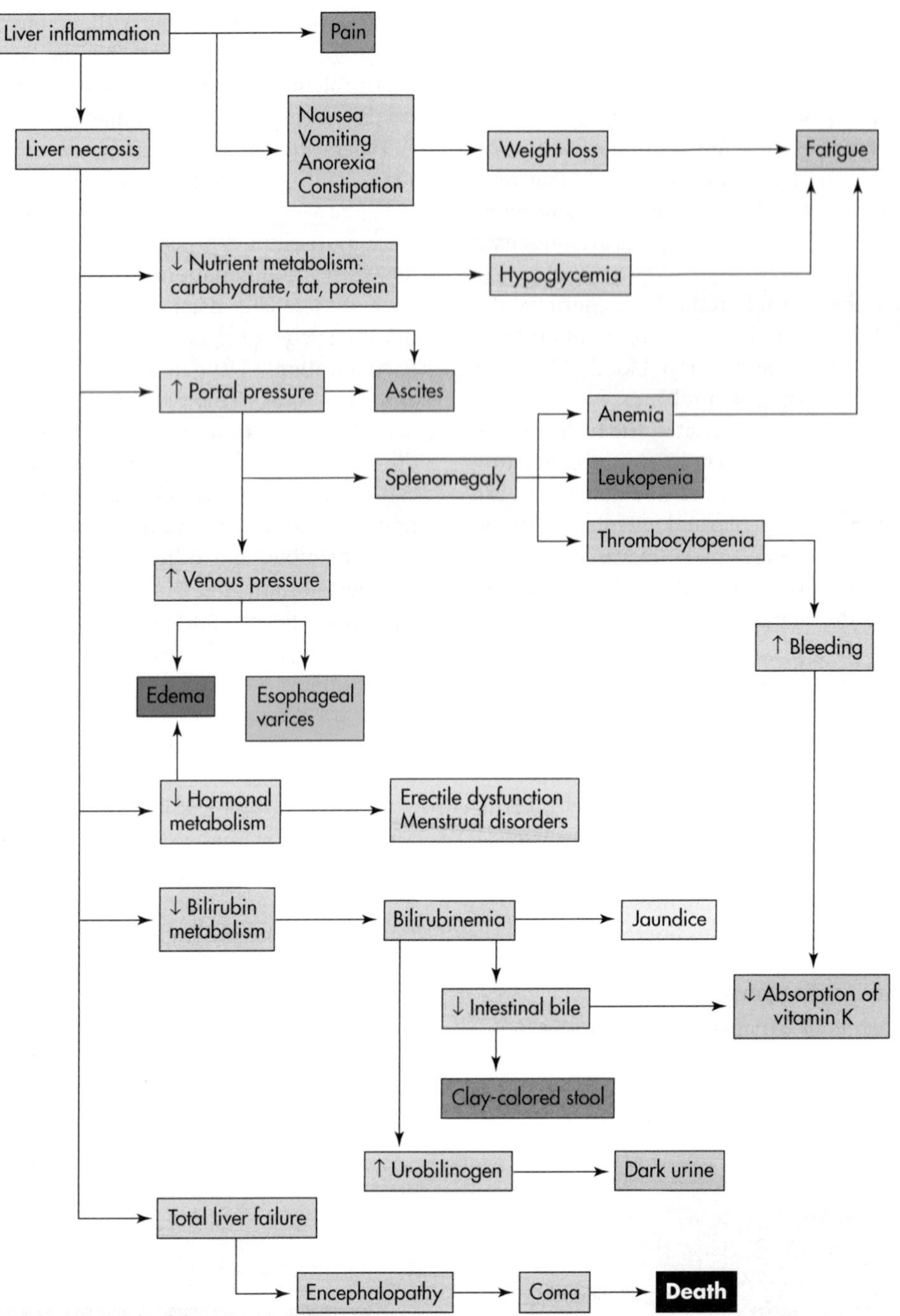

Figure 37-5 Progression of liver cell failure. Pathophysiology of signs and symptoms that occur in cirrhosis. NOTE: process can be arrested if adequate liver regeneration occurs. Regeneration is rarely complete, and there is always some liver cell deficiency.

(well-balanced with normal nutrients) and helping the patient control alcohol intake are important. Vitamin supplements are usually prescribed. In the presence of ascites, a low-sodium diet is recommended. Daily intake of sodium is limited to 500 to 1000 mg. Fluids may be restricted to prevent worsening fluid volume excess.

Activity. The patient is usually fatigued and does not tolerate activity well. The patient is encouraged to limit activity to what is comfortable.

Referrals. Common referrals for persons with cirrhosis include social services, dietary expertise, and home health agencies. Alcohol treatment groups such as Alcoholics Anonymous and Al-Anon may be consulted. The American Liver Foundation* provides information about primary biliary cirrhosis, alcohol-related liver problems, and liver transplantation.

*75 Maiden Lane, Suite 603, New York, NY 10038; website: www.liverfoundation.org.

Clinical Manifestations
Cirrhosis

History of failing health
Nausea
Vomiting
Anorexia
Indigestion
Flatulence
Constipation
Weight loss masked by water retention
Malnutrition
Abdominal pain (usually right upper quadrant)
Dull
Mild
Steady or wavelike
Late signs occurring gradually
Ascites
Jaundice
Edema
Anemia
Bleeding

NURSING MANAGEMENT OF PATIENT WITH CIRRHOSIS

ASSESSMENT

Health History

Assessment data to be collected as part of the health history of a patient with viral hepatitis includes:

Recent history of temperature elevations; frequent infections, recent weakness, or fatigue

General body characteristics: history of changes in color of skin or sclera; history of skin marks such as bruising and hematomas; history of changes in secondary sex characteristics (external genitalia, body hair distribution, or breast tissue); history of increase in abdominal girth (belt size); history of edema; any complaints of itching; muscle wasting

Social habits: drug and alcohol use, amount, factors that precipitate use, any attempts to quit, limitations on success, reasons for failure; last time patient had a drink; work environment

Nutritional history: daily 24-hour intake for past 1 to 3 days; history of recent change in appetite, anorexia, or weight loss

GI system: complaints of nausea, vomiting, anorexia, indigestion, flatulence, or abdominal tenderness

Elimination: history of any changes in amount or color of urine, changes in bowel movements, or changes in color of feces

Neuromuscular: any complaints of weakness or fatigue; history of decreased ability to do work; history of any changes in memory or coordination; any history of tremors

Sexuality: history of erectile dysfunction, decreased libido (men and women), or change in menstrual patterns

Physical Examination

Important aspects of the physical examination of the patient with viral hepatitis include:

Vital signs, including orthostatic blood pressure and pulse, temperature, and weight

Skin and sclerae: presence of jaundice, bruises, hematomas, petechiae, spider angiomas, palmar erythema, dilated vessels on upper body or lower extremities, loss of chest hair (men), gynecomastia, edema of lower extremities, and lesions from scratching

Respiratory: breath sounds and presence of dullness in right lower lobe

Abdomen: bowel sounds, presence of abdominal distention or guarding, presence of ascites (fluid wave or shifting dullness), abdominal girth, increased liver size, presence of hepatic bruits, enlarged spleen, and presence of dilated veins on abdomen (caput medusae)

Neuromuscular: muscle wasting, decreased muscle strength, presence of deficits in memory or coordination, presence of tremors, asterixis, exaggerated deep tendon reflexes, changes in orientation, behavior or emotional changes, presence of apraxia

Gastrointestinal/Genitourinary: volume of urine output, color of urine and stools, and presence of testicular atrophy

NURSING DIAGNOSES

Nursing diagnoses are determined from analysis of patient data. Nursing diagnoses for the person with cirrhosis may include but are not limited to:

Diagnostic Title	Possible Etiologic Factors
1. Ineffective breathing pattern	Restriction of chest movement from ascites or hydrothorax; decreased depth of breathing from limited mobility
2. Fatigue	Decreased energy production associated with anemia, altered metabolism, poor food intake, and electrolyte imbalance
3. Excess fluid volume	Abnormal fluid retention associated with increased circulating aldosterone, decreased colloidal osmotic pressure, or hepatorenal syndrome
4. Risk for infection	Decreased immune competence associated with altered protein metabolism and alcoholism; loss of normal phagocytic function of liver or decreased leukocytes secondary to splenomegaly; and alterations in external immune barriers (skin and GI mucosal integrity)
5. Risk for injury	Alteration in clotting mechanism, enhancing bleeding; alteration in neurologic function and strength that could lead to falls
6. Imbalanced nutrition: less than body requirements	Impaired metabolism, nausea, or decreased intake from appetite loss

7. Acute pain: itching	Liver inflammation and pruritus associated with jaundice
8. Risk for impaired skin integrity	Scratching, edema, or impaired mobility
9. Situational low self-esteem	Inability to accept physical changes of abdominal girth, jaundice, and change in secondary sexual characteristics; changes in roles and relationship

Many other nursing diagnoses result from the complications associated with cirrhosis. These vary from patient to patient.

EXPECTED PATIENT OUTCOMES

Expected patient outcomes for the patient with cirrhosis may include but are not limited to:

1. Will show no increase in dullness on percussion of thorax and will have normal breath sounds and normal chest x-ray films
2. Will demonstrate a gradual increase in activities, will meet self-care needs, and will ambulate an increased amount each day
3. Will have a urinary output that is greater than fluid intake until excess fluids are excreted, a daily decrease in weight, resolution of edema, a decrease of abdominal girth, and a return of electrolytes to normal
4. Will develop no new infection(s) and will have a return to normal temperature
5. Will not develop any bleeding, will maintain normal vital signs, and will have no falls or injuries
6. Will eat food from all food groups (unless restricted) in adequate amounts to meet caloric needs and will experience a decrease in signs of muscle wasting
7. Will report that itching is controlled and will not be observed scratching
8. Will maintain intact skin and will show healing of any lesions
9. Will describe self in positive terms, will discuss accomplishments, and will set realistic goals

INTERVENTIONS

The patient with cirrhosis may be acutely ill and may require critical nursing care or may be relatively free of acute problems and require teaching, counseling, and support. The nurse must set priorities for care on the basis of the patient's needs.

1. Supporting Respiration

The patient with cirrhosis has decreased resistance to infection and may be particularly prone to respiratory infection because of the presence of a hydrothorax and/or shallow breathing. The patient may experience dyspnea because of pressure on the diaphragm from ascites.

A high Fowler's position may assist respiratory exchange. The patient for whom bed rest is prescribed should be encouraged to turn frequently and to take deep breaths to prevent stasis of secretions. Hydrothorax is sometimes treated with thoracentesis (see Chapter 21). The nurse should prepare the patient for this procedure, assist with the procedure, and monitor the patient's response during and after the procedure.

2. Controlling Fatigue

Patients with cirrhosis have various levels of fatigue. The amount and type of activity encouraged depend on the individual's energy level, level of consciousness and coordination, and the presence of any complications of cirrhosis. If the patient has severe fluid excess and ascites or signs and symptoms of other complications, bed rest is usually required. In this case special attention to skin care is necessary, particularly if the patient also has severe peripheral edema. Alternating pressure mattresses or flotation pads may be helpful. If bed rest is not required, the patient should be ambulated within the room or hall as tolerated. Level of tolerance is based on the patient's statement about the level of fatigue and/or pulse changes. The pulse rate should not increase by more than 10 beats above baseline with activity.

3. Maintaining Fluid and Electrolyte Balance

Most patients with cirrhosis have sodium retention and hypokalemia. A great majority of patients have ascites, and some also have peripheral edema. The exact management of these depends on the patient's needs.

Potassium replacement is given for hypokalemia. It is usually given orally, and the nurse should monitor the patient's serum K^+ values to verify that the patient is not developing hyperkalemia. This is important because some patients with cirrhosis develop hepatorenal syndrome and have decreased renal function, which impairs the excretion of potassium, possibly resulting in hyperkalemia.

Sodium imbalance and ascites are treated in several ways. Restriction of sodium aids greatly in limiting the formation of ascitic fluid. The basis for determining the amount of dietary restriction necessary to reduce sodium and water retention may initially be a collection of urine for 24 hours to determine sodium loss. Sodium is generally restricted to 1 g daily. The sodium restriction along with bed rest may relieve the ascites and edema.[4]

If bed rest and sodium restriction do not improve ascites, diuretics may be used. Spironolactone A (Aldactone A), which inhibits the reabsorption of sodium in the distal tubules and promotes potassium retention by inhibiting the synthesis and renal effects of aldosterone, is frequently used. The therapy is adjusted on an individual basis. Sometimes furosemide (Lasix) or another diuretic is used with spironolactone. Because furosemide causes potassium excretion, serum potassium level is monitored frequently, and the patient is observed for signs and symptoms of hypokalemia such as abdominal distention, nausea, vomiting, anorexia, decreased bowel sounds, weakness, or irregular pulse.

Removal of ascitic fluid through the kidneys has the advantage of not also losing essential body proteins, which can occur when fluid is removed from the abdominal cavity by paracentesis. However, diuretic therapy may cause serious side effects for the patient with cirrhosis. An extremely rapid diuresis can precipitate oliguria and uremia caused by the rapidly diminished blood volume. Ascites should not be mobilized at rates greater than 500 ml/day or approximately 1 lb/day. Fluid losses in excess of 500 ml/day can result in the loss of nonascitic extracellular fluid. Infusions of albumin in 25-g units to promote retention of an adequate vascular volume may be given to prevent azotemia and encephalopathy by maintaining adequate perfusion of the kidneys and the brain and to promote diuresis. Administration of salt-poor albumin may expand the blood volume rapidly, and the patient should be monitored carefully for signs of congestive heart failure and pulmonary edema during and after administration.

Fluids are restricted if hyponatremia is caused by fluid retention. Fluid restriction is monitored closely because it may lead to decreased output and the hepatorenal syndrome. When fluids are restricted, the nurse must work with the patient to provide fluids that are tolerated best and to spread the allotted fluids throughout the total 24 hours. Fluids must be distributed so that some are available at each meal and for required medications. Some fluids should be given on all three shifts while the patient is hospitalized. At home the patient should distribute fluids over the waking hours.[4,9]

To evaluate further the effectiveness of therapy, daily weighing is required. Measurements of abdominal girth assist in determining the gross amount of abdominal swelling. Patients need to be taught the importance of monitoring and reporting weight gain or a rapid increase in abdominal girth after discharge. When ascites is intractable to the therapies mentioned, other procedures such as a peritoneal venous shunt may be used. Peritoneal venous shunts are described in the section on complications.

4. Preventing Infection

Loss of the normal phagocytic function of the liver and the leukopenia and malnutrition associated with cirrhosis require that precautions be taken to avoid infection. These precautions involve proper hand washing, observance of sterile technique with all invasive procedures, preventive respiratory care, and avoidance of contact with people with infections. The patient must be monitored carefully for the presence of infection, and any increase in temperature should be reported immediately so that appropriate measures can be taken.

5. Preventing Bleeding and Falls

The patient with cirrhosis is at great risk for bleeding because of poor vitamin K absorption, impaired production of clotting factors, and thrombocytopenia. Esophageal varices and hemorrhoids can easily rupture, causing excessive bleeding. Nursing care should focus on monitoring for the presence of bleeding and instituting measures that decrease the risk of bleeding from trauma or injury to varices (see Guidelines for Safe Practice boxes).

6. Promoting Nutrition

Most patients with cirrhosis require a well-balanced, high-calorie, high-carbohydrate diet with adequate vitamins to provide nutrients for repair of the liver. Protein intake may need to be limited and is determined by liver function tests.

Guidelines for Safe Practice

Monitoring for Bleeding in the Patient With Cirrhosis

Monitor urine and stool for blood.
Check the patient's body daily for purpura, hematomas, and petechiae.
Check mouth, especially gums, carefully for signs of bleeding.
Check vital signs at least every 4 hours.
Monitor prothrombin time, partial thromboplastin time, and thrombocyte count frequently.

Guidelines for Safe Practice

Decreasing the Risk of Bleeding

Avoid all intramuscular and subcutaneous injections, if possible.
Use the smallest-gauge needle possible when giving an injection.
Apply pressure to injection sites and venous puncture sites for at least 5 minutes and to arterial puncture sites for at least 10 minutes.
Give vitamin K as ordered.
Use or instruct patient to use a soft-bristled toothbrush or cotton swabs for oral hygiene.
Instruct patient not to strain on defecation and to avoid vigorous blowing of nose or coughing.
Instruct patient to avoid foods (e.g., spicy, hot, or raw) that can traumatize esophageal varices.
Provide assistance to avoid falls.
Make sure that room is free of clutter, that floors are dry, and that shoes or slippers are worn to avoid injuries.

When nausea is a problem, antiemetics should be given 30 minutes before meals to help increase food tolerance.

Sodium restriction is frequently necessary, and this restriction can make finding a palatable diet difficult. Salt substitutes and information on alternative seasonings may help.

Frequent oral hygiene and a pleasant environment should be provided to help increase food intake. The patient's food preferences should be incorporated into the diet. Food should be served in small, frequent amounts. Because persons with cirrhosis need increased calories but often have poor appetites, measures to increase calories without increasing the volume of food should be used. These measures include use of butter as a seasoning, adding dry milk to appropriate foods, and using gravies and sauces. The patient with cirrhosis has the same nutritional needs after discharge, and the person who shops and cooks for the patient must be included in the teaching. The patient's economic situation should be assessed to determine his or her ability to purchase the food required for the prescribed diet. A social service referral may be necessary to help the patient obtain financial assistance. For the person who eats out frequently, instruction about selecting appropriate meals from a restaurant menu is necessary. If the patient's meals are obtained through a service such as Meals on Wheels, arrangements can be made for some special dietary requirements.

7. Controlling Pruritus

Management of pruritus is similar to that discussed earlier in the chapter under care of patients with hepatitis.

8. Providing Skin Care

Because of pruritus, malnutrition, and the edema often associated with cirrhosis, the patient is prone to skin lesions and pressure ulcer formation. Preventive nursing care to avoid skin breakdown, such as use of air mattresses, frequent turning, backrubs, and massage of bony prominences, should be instituted. Measures to prevent pruritus assist in preventing damage to the skin resulting from the patient's scratching.

9. Promoting Positive Self-Esteem

The patient with cirrhosis may experience changes in body appearance and in roles and relationships. If the patient is not helped to establish or maintain positive self-esteem, this can add to the problem of alcoholism. The nurse is in a prime position to help promote positive self-esteem by giving the patient as much control as possible. Positive self-esteem can be facilitated by:

Involving the patient in goal setting
Allowing the patient to make as many decisions as possible
Giving positive feedback for accomplishments
Supporting the patient in times of failure, whatever the failure might be, including conflicts with family or friends or participation in drinking
Helping the patient recall past accomplishments
Helping significant others provide positive feedback
Helping the patient learn ways to disguise jaundice or ascites

Patient/Family Teaching

All patients need to be prepared for diagnostic tests, to understand their treatment, and to learn to meet long-term care needs. Information should be given verbally and supplemented with written information, depending on the patient's physical status; the information may need to be repeated several times and given in small increments. Family members or significant others should be included so that they can help reinforce the information or participate in the patient's care. Long-term care usually requires major changes in lifestyle (diet, fluid intake, and alcohol cessation), and thus continual support is necessary. Specific information that the nurse may want to include in the teaching plan is highlighted in the Patient Teaching box.

Health Promotion/Prevention. The goal of Healthy People 2010 is to reduce the number of deaths from cirrhosis to no more than 3 per 100,000 people, with African-American men, Native Americans, and Alaskan Inuits being targeted populations. Even though cirrhosis among African-American and Native-American men has decreased in the last decade, the death rate for non-Caucasian men is 70% higher than for Caucasian men.[29]

In the United States programs aimed at the prevention of cirrhosis are designed primarily to control the ingestion of alcohol. The loss of time from work related to alcoholism is estimated to cost billions of dollars annually. Many large corporations have or are organizing programs to help employees control their alcohol intake.

Since research has shown that the combination of acetaminophen and alcohol can impair liver function and increase the risk of cirrhosis, all over-the-counter acetaminophen must carry a warning label that reads "Alcohol Warning: If you consume three or more alcoholic drinks every day, ask your doctor whether you should take acetaminophen or other pain reliever/fever reducers. Acetaminophen may cause liver damage" (see Future Watch box).

Early detection of cirrhosis is difficult because three fourths of the liver can be destroyed before signs of cirrhosis become evident. For this reason, cessation of alcohol intake is the focus of secondary prevention. A sample Clinical Pathway and Nursing Care Plan follow on pp. 1174 to 1179.

Patient Teaching
The Patient With Cirrhosis

- Avoid further hepatic damage: abstain from alcohol; abstain from any drugs not prescribed by physician, including over-the-counter drugs, such as analgesics or cold remedies; avoid exposure to hepatotoxins in the work and home environments.
- Dietary regimen (may include sodium and/or protein restrictions) should be well balanced and include sources high in protein such as milk, eggs, fish, and poultry.
- Fluid restriction if required; how to incorporate restrictions throughout the day
- Signs and symptoms requiring immediate follow-up: weight gain; increased abdominal girth; recurrence of edema, fever, or bleeding (blood in urine, stool, or vomitus; epistaxis; cuts that continue to bleed); change in mental function or behavior
- Measures that lessen chance of bleeding
- Drug therapy (diuretics, potassium, and antihistamines)
- Activity plan that promotes adequate rest
- Care measures that help to control pruritus

■ EVALUATION

To evaluate the effectiveness of nursing interventions, compare patient behaviors with those stated in the expected patient outcomes. Achievement of outcomes is successful if the patient with cirrhosis:

1. Has clear breath sounds throughout lung fields and normal percussion results from thoracic cavity.
2. Increases involvement in daily self-care activities and ambulation in hospital hallways.
3. Loses 1 to 2 lb/day until dry weight is reached; has decreasing edema, decreasing abdominal girth, and urine output of 500 to 1000 ml greater than intake until dry weight is reached.

Future Watch

Food and Drug Administration Investigates Need for Stricter Acetaminophen Warnings

In 1998 the U.S. Food and Drug Administration announced that all over-the-counter acetaminophen must carry a warning label that reads "Alcohol Warning: If you consume three or more alcoholic drinks every day, ask your doctor whether you should take acetaminophen or other pain reliever/fever reducers. Acetaminophen may cause liver damage." Research conducted by Dr. William Lee at the University of Texas Southwestern Medical Center suggests that a more stringent warning may be needed to protect people from liver damage caused by acetaminophen overdoses.

In a study conducted at 22 hospitals, Dr. Lee linked 38% of more than 300 acute liver failure cases to acetaminophen. In another study conducted at six hospitals, he found 35% of 307 adult cases of severe liver injury to have been caused by acetaminophen. The studies suggest that acetaminophen overdoses may be a bigger cause of liver failure than some prescription medications. Other studies suggest that even small doses of acetaminophen could overwhelm people with hepatitis.

Recommended dosage of acetaminophen for adults is no more than 8 extra-strength pills in 24 hours. However, labels do not explicitly warn of liver damage resulting from overdoses. Some of the patients in Dr. Lee's study took maximum doses for days instead of just once or twice. Dr. Lee advises taking no more than four extra-strength pills per day.

Reference: http://liverfoundation.org/html/neweven.dir/newevenup.dir/.

4. Has normal body temperature and no indications of infections.
5. Shows normal prothrombin time and hematocrit; hemoglobin levels that are increasing; no orthostatic vital sign changes; and no falls, cuts, or other injuries.
6. Maintains adequate food intake to regain or keep weight as appropriate with incorporation of foods from all food groups and restriction of sodium and protein as necessary.
7. Shows no evidence of scratching and states that itching is decreased and controlled.
8. Makes positive statements about self and realistic statements about future goals.
9. Maintains intact skin and appropriate healing of any lesions.

GERONTOLOGIC CONSIDERATIONS

The incidence of primary biliary cirrhosis (PBC) increases with age and peaks at age 50; the disease progresses until most patients are 60 to 70 years old and thus is a serious problem in older adults. Liver transplantation is considered for persons with PBC when liver failure occurs. Advanced age is no longer an absolute contraindication for transplantation, but it is certainly controversial. Death usually results from complications of bleeding, ascites, or encephalopathy.

Diagnosis may be made in the last stage of the disease when the prognosis is poor because of the complications associated with cirrhosis. Early symptoms are vague or absent. Late symptoms include jaundice, diarrhea, bone pain, bruising, night blindness, and gradual weight loss. Many symptoms are attributed to malabsorption of vitamins and nutrients. Skin manifestations, including thickening and darkening of the skin and pruritus, are common manifestations of PBC.[16] Control of pruritus is especially important in the elderly patient because of skin changes associated with aging. The elderly person's skin is more fragile, and lesions may develop as a result from scratching. As the disease progresses, complications such as esophageal varices, ascites, and encephalopathy may develop. The elderly patient with anemia is at even greater risk from bleeding.

Blood flow to the liver decreases with aging. This physiologic change may worsen the effects of hypotension on the liver. An episode of severe hypotension in the elderly patient may result in shock liver. Patients with preexisting right-sided heart failure may experience severe liver complications with a hypotensive episode. Shock liver results from ischemia of hepatic tissues and elevated liver enzymes, progressing to liver failure. Lactic acid levels increase and clotting factors decrease, creating increased risk of metabolic imbalance and hemorrhage. Patients should be monitored closely to avoid episodes of hypotension.

Encouraging a nutritionally adequate diet is an important intervention for the elderly patient. A low-fat diet and vitamin supplements are recommended.

Emotional support is necessary to assist the patient in living with a chronic disease. An assessment of the patient's support system and coping methods can assist the nurse in formulating a plan to reduce the patient's anxiety.

SPECIAL ENVIRONMENTS FOR CARE

Critical Care Management

Persons with cirrhosis may need critical care management if complications such as hemorrhage, esophageal varices, and portal-systemic encephalopathy develop.

Home Care Management

The home environment should be assessed for any alterations needed to accommodate the patient's long-term needs. The patient's bedroom and bathroom should ideally be on the same floor. If this is not possible, a portable commode, bedpan, or urinal may be substituted. Incontinence pads or adult-sized briefs may be needed in the case of incontinence. If the patient has ascites, raising the head of the bed to a high Fowler's position may be necessary to facilitate respiration. The head of the bed may be elevated with pillows, or on bricks. The patient may be able to sleep in a reclining chair with a footrest. Alternatively, if resources permit, a hospital bed may be obtained.

Environmental hazards should be eliminated, especially if the patient has any mental status changes. Because of clotting defects, the patient should be protected from injury. Maintenance of normal bowel function should be encouraged, particularly to avoid constipation, which could lead to rupture of hemorrhoids. The patient may also need assistance in the preparation of nutritionally adequate meals.

clinical pathway *Cirrhosis of Liver With Gastrointestinal Bleeding*

DRG #: 202; expected LOS: 7

	ADMIT TO ICU DAY OF ADMISSION DAY 1	**DAY 2**	**DAY 3**
Diagnostic Tests	CBC, UA, SMA/18,* type and cross-match, PT/PTT, ABG	H&H, ABG, gastroscopy, hema-test stools	H&H, SMA/18,* hema-test stools
Medications	IVs, blood transfusions as indicated, IV cimetidine, antacids via NG tube after gavage	IVs, blood transfusions as indicated, IV cimetidine, acetaminophen PRN for fever and discomfort after sclerotherapy, antacids via NG tube	IVs, IV/PO cimetidine, Tylenol PRN for fever and discomfort, antacids, (?diuretics, K^+ replacement), multivitamins, folic acid, ferrous sulfate
Treatments	I&O q hr (including Foley and NG); VS q hr until stable, then q2hr; weight; measure abdominal girth; assess cardio-pul-neuro-circ systems q2hr; assess skin and mouth, give special care q2hr; NG gavage with NaCl for acute bleeding	I&O q hr (including Foley and NG); VS q2hr; weight; measure abdominal girth; assess cardio-pul-neuro-circ systems q2hr; assess skin and mouth, give special care q2hr; injection sclerotherapy as necessary	I&O q4hr (discontinue Foley and NG); VS q2hr; weight; measure abdominal girth; assess cardio-pul-neuro-circ systems q4hr; assess skin and mouth, give special care q2hr
Diet	NPO	NPO	Clear liquids and, as necessary, low sodium/protein and fluid restriction
Activity	Bedrest, T&DB q2hr	Bedrest, T&DB q2hr	Bedrest, up to bathroom with help, T&DB q2hr
Referral/Consultation	Gastroenterologist, other specialist as needed for other medical problems		Social services, home health, dietary

ABG, Arterial blood gases; *CBC,* complete blood count; *CHO,* carbohydrate; *H&H,* hemoglobin and hematocrit; *I&O,* intake and output; *NG,* nasogastric; *PT,* prothrombin time; *PTT,* partial thromboplastin time; *T&DB,* turning and deep breathing; *UA,* urinalysis.
*Serum, calcium, phosphorus, triglycerides, uric acid, creatinine, blood urea nitrogen (BUN), total bilirubin, alkaline phosphate, aspartate aminotransferase (AST) (formerly serum glutamic oxaloacetic transaminase [SGOT]), alanine aminotransferase (ALT) (formerly serum glutamic oxaloacetic transaminase [SGPT]), lactic dehydrogenase (LDH), total protein, albumin, sodium, potassium, chloride, total CO_2, glucose.

Before discharge the patient and family should be taught to recognize the signs and symptoms of worsening liver function including increased abdominal girth, rapid weight gain, edema, signs of bleeding, and deteriorating mental status, which should be reported to the physician or home health nurse. Loss of libido, erectile dysfunction, sterility, and amenorrhea may occur, and the patient and his or her sexual partner should be counseled about these possibilities. The patient and family should be assessed for the capability to deal with a chronic illness. If the patient requires much assistance in ADL, the primary caregiver may need periodic relief from care responsibilities. Home health care assistance may be possible. All persons involved in the care of the patient are encouraged to share feelings and fears concerning the patient's illness.

COMPLICATIONS

Persons with cirrhosis frequently develop portal hypertension that can result in ascites, esophageal varices, and/or portal-systemic encephalopathy.

Portal Hypertension

Pressures within the portal venous system become elevated as liver damage obstructs the free flow of blood through the organ. These elevated pressures can become high enough to cause a variety of problems.

Nursing and medical management of portal hypertension is directed first to treating its consequences: ascites and esophageal varices. The only way to achieve permanent lowering of portal pressure is surgical creation of a shunt to reduce blood flow through the obstructed part of the portal system. Because of the

TRANSFER OUT OF ICU DAY 4	DAY 5	DAY 6	DAY OF DISCHARGE DAY 7
Hema-test stools	H&H, hema-test stools	SMA/18*	CBC
IV to saline lock, PO cimetidine, Tylenol PRN for fever and discomfort, antacids, (?diuretics, K^+ replacement), multivitamins, folic acid, ferrous sulfate	IV saline lock, PO cimetidine, Tylenol PRN for fever and discomfort, antacids, (?diuretics, K^+ replacement), multivitamins, folic acid, ferrous sulfate	IV saline lock, PO cimetidine, discontinue acetaminophen, antacids, (?diuretics, K^+ replacement), multivitamins, folic acid, ferrous sulfate; adjust medications for home use.	Discontinue saline lock, continue cimetidine, antacids, vitamins, and other medications for home use
I&O q8hr; VS q6hr; weight; measure abdominal girth; assess cardio-pul-neuro-circ systems q8hr; assess skin and mouth, give special care q4hr.	I&O q8hr; VS q6hr; weight; measure abdominal girth; assess cardio-pul-neuro-circ systems q8hr; assess skin and mouth, give special care q4hr.	Discontinue I&O; VS q8hr; weight; measure abdominal girth; asses cardio-pul-neuro-circ systems q8hr; assess skin and mouth, give special care q6hr.	VS q8hr; weight; measure abdominal girth; assess cardio-pul-neuro-circ systems q8hr; assess skin and mouth, give special care q8hr.
Soft diet, high CHO and, as necessary, low sodium/protein and fluid restriction	Soft diet, high CHO and, as necessary, low sodium/protein and fluid restriction	Regular diet, high CHO and, as necessary, low sodium/protein and fluid restriction	Regular diet, high CHO and, as necessary, low sodium/protein and fluid restriction
Bedrest, up in chair twice with help	Up in chair 4 times with help, up walking in hall with help twice	Up ad lib, up walking in hallway with help 4 times	Up ad lib
	Chemical dependency counseling if appropriate		

risks of the surgery and the frequent fatalities from hepatic failure after surgical treatment, these shunting procedures are used only in persons who have developed esophageal varices, have had bleeding from the varices, and do not respond to other therapy. Surgical care is discussed later in this chapter.

Ascites

Ascites is one of the most frequent complications of cirrhosis of the liver and results in part from the portal hypertension. Other contributing factors are decreased hepatic synthesis of albumin, increased levels of aldosterone, and obstruction of hepatic lymph flow. Ascites may occur with or without peripheral edema. Because ascites is so frequently seen, the required therapy and nursing care were discussed on p. 1170. This section describes care related to treatments used when the previously discussed first-line therapies fail.

Large-Volume Paracentesis. Large volume paracentesis (LVP) is the removal of 5 liters or more of ascitic fluid during a single treatment. Because this fluid loss disrupts the individual hemodynamics, plasma expanders such as intravenous albumin are given simultaneously. Although this treatment resolves ascites in most patients, it is limited by a high frequency of recurrent ascites and the need for further paracentesis. LVP does not correct the underlying pathology or improve patient survival rates.

Peritoneal Venous Shunt. In chronic and resistant ascites, a LeVeen or Denver peritoneal venous (PV) shunt may be used (Figure 37-6). The shunt provides continuous reinfusion of ascitic fluid into the venous system through a silicone catheter with a one-way pressure-sensitive valve. One end of the catheter is implanted in the peritoneal cavity, and the tube is channeled through subcutaneous tissue to the superior vena

Nursing Care Plan Patient With Cirrhosis

DATA Mr. S. is a 55-year-old salesman with portal hypertension who was admitted to the hospital with upper GI bleeding. Endoscopy revealed enlarged esophageal and upper gastric veins and a bleeding ulcer. One unit of packed red blood cells was administered. Treatment orders include protein (20 g/day) and sodium (1000 mg/day) restrictions, fluid restriction (1000 ml/day), neomycin 1 g q4h, thiamine 1 ml IM, vitamin K subcutaneously daily, and spironolactone 25 mg twice a day. Physical examination reveals:

- Slight jaundice of the skin and sclera
- Ascites and peripheral edema
- Thin legs and arms and poor musculature
- Signs of increased estrogen
- Orientation to person, place, and time
- Blood pressure 116/60 mm Hg, pulse 60 bpm, respirations 32

Nursing history reveals that Mr. S:

- Participated in AA for 1 year; he has been sober since joining.
- Had influenza-like symptoms the past 2 weeks but continued with his busy schedule. He complains of fatigue, anorexia, and itching.

Collaborative nursing actions include interventions to prevent further impairment of physical status from hemorrhage and ammonia toxicity and assistance with treatment of his gastric ulcer and fluid excess. Nursing actions include monitoring for:

- Signs of hemorrhage: hematemesis, decreased blood pressure, tachycardia, restlessness, guaiac positive stools, and cool, moist skin
- Signs of hepatic encephalopathy; change in mental status, asterixis, tremors, and change in handwriting

NURSING DIAGNOSIS **Fatigue related to muscle wasting, blood loss, and anemia secondary to cirrhosis**
GOALS/OUTCOMES Will report decreased fatigue on a scale of 1 (no fatigue) to 10 (severe fatigue)

NOC Suggested Outcomes
- Activity Tolerance (0005)
- Endurance (0001)
- Energy Conservation (1804)

NIC Suggested Interventions
- Energy Management (0180)
- Teaching: Prescribed Activity/Exercise (5612)
- Sleep Enhancement (1850)

Nursing Interventions/Rationales
- Ensure or maintain bed rest as prescribed during the acute phase of illness or relapse. *Bed rest decreases metabolic rate and energy demands.*
- After acute phase, encourage increasing activity interspersed with rest periods as tolerated. *Resting between activities allows for greater energy availability for tasks that need to be performed. Activities can be increased as nutritional status is restored.*
- Intervene if patient shows fatigue after or during visits by family/friends. *Patients often feel that they must entertain visitors and expend more energy than is available to do so.*
- Encourage intake of well-balanced diet within prescribed restrictions. *A well-balanced diet will help restore nutritional balance and increase energy.*

Evaluation Parameters
1. Progressive decrease in complaints of fatigue
2. Demonstrates a gradual increase in ability to perform activities without experiencing fatigue

NURSING DIAGNOSIS **Imbalanced nutrition: less than body requirements related to anorexia and flulike symptoms secondary to cirrhosis**
GOALS/OUTCOMES Will maintain (or regain) weight within 5 pounds of baseline weight

NOC Suggested Outcomes
- Nutritional Status (1004)
- Nutritional Status: Food & Fluid Intake (1008)
- Nutritional Status: Nutrient Intake (1009)

NIC Suggested Interventions
- Nutrition Monitoring (1160)
- Nutrition Management (1100)
- Nutrition Therapy (1120)

Nursing Interventions/Rationales
- Assess nutrient needs. *Baseline data are needed to plan effectively for nutritional needs.*
- Encourage intake of well-balanced, high-carbohydrate, low-protein diet with adequate vitamins. *Food intake within prescribed limitations can influence liver regeneration.*
- Decrease dietary roughage. *Low-roughage diet is necessary to prevent irritation and possible bleeding of esophageal varices.*
- Encourage use of salt substitute or alternative seasonings. *To decrease sodium intake without discouraging food intake.*
- Administer antiemetics as prescribed and mouth care if nausea is present. *To decrease comfort and reduce nausea so that dietary intake is possible.*

Nursing Care Plan Patient With Cirrhosis–cont'd

- Encourage six small meals daily. *Large meals are overwhelming. Small meals encourage intake without producing distention or fatigue.*
- Use measures to encourage eating (clean environment, serve after patient has rested). *To increase the likelihood that the patient will intake sufficient food to meet dietary needs.*
- Support continuation in AA activities while patient is hospitalized. *To avoid breaking continuity of support system. AA representative should be allowed to see patient as condition permits.*

Evaluation Parameters

1. Ingests required nutrients and adequate calories on a daily basis
2. Decreased signs of muscle wasting

NURSING DIAGNOSIS **Excess fluid volume related to impaired metabolism of aldosterone**
GOALS/OUTCOMES Fluid volume status will return to baseline

NOC Suggested Outcomes
- Fluid Balance (0601)
- Electrolyte and Acid/Base Balance (0600)
- Nutritional Status: Food & Fluid Intake (1008)

NIC Suggested Interventions
- Fluid Monitoring (4130)
- Fluid Management (4120)
- Hypervolemia Management (4170)

Nursing Interventions/Rationales
- Monitor weight daily, blood pressure q4h, assess edema every shift, and measure abdominal girth daily. *To provide a baseline. To provide information about treatment effectiveness.*
- Monitor intake and output on every shift until excess fluid is excreted. *Diuresis in cirrhosis is undertaken slowly using very conservative measures due to the contracted intravascular fluid volume. Excessive diuresis can compromise renal perfusion and precipitate portal-systemic encephalopathy.*
- Teach patient the rationale for sodium restriction when able to comprehend teaching. *Understanding often increases the likelihood of compliance.*
- Provide bed rest until ascites is relieved. *To decrease metabolism and energy consumption.*
- Restrict fluids as prescribed and distribute those fluids throughout the 24 hours. *To prevent further fluid excess. Distributing fluids increases the patient's comfort by allowing small amounts of fluid throughout the day.*

Evaluation Parameters

1. Weight and abdominal girth decrease daily
2. Edema resolves

NURSING DIAGNOSIS **Ineffective breathing pattern related to ascites, immobility, and stasis of secretions**
GOALS/OUTCOMES Breath sounds will remain clear

NOC Suggested Outcomes
- Respiratory Status: Airway Patency (0410)
- Respiratory Status: Gas Exchange (0402)
- Immobility Consequences: Physiological (0204)

NIC Suggested Interventions
- Respiratory Monitoring (3350)
- Fluid Management (4120)

Nursing Interventions/Rationales
- Monitor respirations and breath sounds q4hr and more frequently if indicated. *To detect changes that require intervention.*
- Position patient in high Fowler's position. *This position may relieve pressure on diaphragm, which can decrease stasis of secretions.*
- Encourage frequent position changes and deep breathing exercises. *To prevent complications such as atelectasis.*
- Encourage ambulation when appropriate. *To prevent muscle weakness and complications such as atelectasis.*

Evaluation Parameters

1. Progressively decreasing dyspnea
2. Breath sounds progressively clear

Continued

Nursing Care Plan — Patient With Cirrhosis–cont'd

NURSING DIAGNOSIS **Risk for impaired skin integrity related to immobility, edema, poor nutrition, and pruritus**
GOALS/OUTCOMES Skin will remain free of breakdown or excoriation

NOC Suggested Outcomes
- Tissue Integrity: Skin & Mucous Membranes (1101)
- Fluid Balance (0601)
- Immobility Consequences: Physiological (0204)
- Tissue Perfusion: Peripheral (0407)

NIC Suggested Interventions
- Skin Surveillance (3590)
- Pressure Ulcer Prevention (3540)
- Exercise Promotion: Joint Mobility (0224)
- Pruritus Management (3550)

Nursing Interventions/Rationales
- Assess patient's skin daily for signs of breakdown or excoriation from scratching. *Patient has several risk factors for skin breakdown, including itching from jaundice. Early identification of potential skin breakdown leads to early intervention.*
- Use measures such as flotation mattress and routine turning schedule. *To prevent skin breakdown.*
- Keep skin clean and well moisturized. *Dry skin predisposes to cracking and excoriation. Unclean skin promotes bacterial growth, which predisposes to skin breakdown.*
- Keep finger and toenails short and clean. *To prevent accidental scratches or cuts. Jaundice can be irritating and lead to scratching.*
- Elevate extremities when feasible to reduce peripheral edema. *Aids in venous return of fluids from the periphery.*
- Avoid heat and heavy clothing; provide cool environment. *To reduce itching and promote comfort.*
- Apply antipruritic lotion as prescribed as needed. *To reduce itching and promote comfort.*
- Administer prescribed antihistamines. *Block the release of histamine to reduce itching.*
- Offer diversional activities such as music or television if acceptable to patient. *Distraction is often useful in blocking the perception of discomfort.*
- If patient must scratch, provide a soft cloth. *Itching may be intense. Use of a soft cloth will protect the skin from excoriation.*
- Use tepid water for bathing. *Tepid water does not generally exacerbate itching to the extent that hot water does.*
- Monitor for signs of localized skin infection. *Scratching can result in infections, which is characterized by redness, swelling, warmth, and tenderness.*

Evaluation Parameters
1. Verbalizes relief from itching
2. Patient not observed scratching
3. Skin free of redness and excoriation
4. Decreasing peripheral edema when compared with baseline

NURSING DIAGNOSIS **Risk for infection related to immunocompromise secondary to chronic illness.**
GOALS/OUTCOMES Will remain free of infection

NOC Suggested Outcomes
- Immune Status (0702)
- Risk Control (1902)

NIC Suggested Interventions
- Infection Protection (6550)
- Infection Control (6540)
- Surveillance (6650)

Nursing Interventions/Rationales
- Monitor for indications of infection every shift (fever, chills, lethargy, increased WBC). *To detect early signs of infection so that treatment can be implemented. Infections in a patient with cirrhosis can be life threatening since they can result in sepsis and liver failure.*
- Use sterile technique for all invasive procedures. *To decrease the risk for introduction of microorganisms and resultant infection.*
- Encourage pulmonary hygiene, such as turning and deep breathing every 2 hours. *To prevent stasis of secretions and increased risk for atelectasis and pneumonia.*
- Restrict exposure to persons with infection. *To decrease risk of transmitting infections to the immune compromised patient.*

Nursing Care Plan — Patient With Cirrhosis—cont'd

Evaluation Parameters

1. No evidence of systemic infection (fever, chills, lethargy)
2. No evidence of localized infection (redness, warmth, swelling, pain)
3. White blood cell count remains within normal limits

NURSING DIAGNOSIS **Ineffective coping related to health crisis**
GOALS/OUTCOMES Will use coping strategies to deal with health crisis

NOC Suggested Outcomes

- Coping (1302)
- Decision Making (0906)
- Information Processing (0907)

NIC Suggested Interventions

- Coping Enhancement (5230)
- Decision Making Support (5250)
- Distraction (5900)
- Support System Enhancement (5440)

Nursing Interventions/Rationales

- Assess patient's perception of health and present illness. *The nurse's perception of the illness may vary considerably from the patient's or family's perception. Misunderstandings can be corrected when the patient's perceptions are known.*
- Identify and support the patient's successful coping strategies (prayer, music, conversation). *Coping strategies that have been effective in the past are likely to be effective in new situations.*
- Listen actively if patient expresses feelings of powerlessness, fears, or spiritual distress. Plan times for active listening. *To demonstrate caring and empathy.*
- Assess and facilitate family support. Meet with the family/significant others on a scheduled basis. *The family must feel secure to provide support to the patient.*

Evaluation Parameters

1. Takes interest in diversional activities
2. Begins to participate in decision making about health
3. Uses coping strategies such as prayer or relaxation techniques

NURSING DIAGNOSIS **Risk for injury related to decreased metabolic function of the liver**
GOALS/OUTCOMES Patient will remain free of injury

NOC Suggested Outcomes

- Risk Control (1902)
- Risk Detection (1908)
- Safety Behavior: Fall Prevention (1909)

NIC Suggested Interventions

- Environmental Management: Safety (6486)
- Fall Prevention (6490)
- Surveillance: Safety (6654)

Nursing Interventions/Rationales

- Monitor for bleeding (stool, urine, skin, mucous membranes). *Patient's cirrhosis places him at increased risk for bleeding and falls.*
- Monitor vital signs q4h and prothrombin and partial thromboplastin levels daily. *To detect changes that place patient at increased risk for bleeding such as increased PT and PTT levels.*
- Avoid injections if possible; apply pressure at all injection sites for 5 minutes. *Patient has decreased clotting ability and may suffer significant bleeding from small puncture sites.*
- Administer prescribed vitamin K if bleeding occurs or as prophylaxis for bleeding. *Vitamin K promotes coagulation and inhibits bleeding.*
- Teach patient to use soft toothbrush, avoid use of dental floss and avoid coughing or straining at stool. *These activities can promote active bleeding.*
- Provide physical support when patient is ambulating. *To prevent falls.*
- Maintain safe environment. *A cluttered environment places the patient at increased risk for tripping and falling.*

Evaluation Parameters

1. No undetected bleeding occurs
2. Vital signs remain within normal limits
3. No falls or other injuries occur

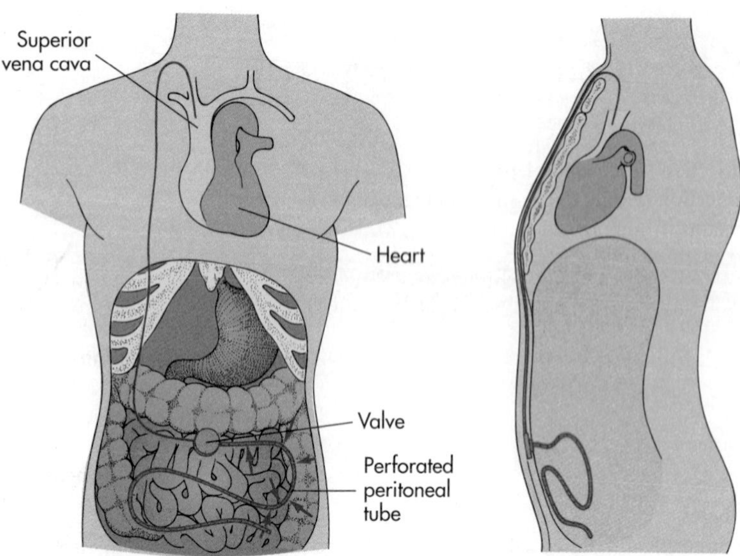

Figure 37-6 LaVeen shunt, showing placement of catheter.

cava, where the other end is implanted. The valve opens when there is a pressure differential greater than 3 mm of water between the peritoneal cavity and the vein in the thoracic cavity, allowing fluid to move from the peritoneal cavity into the superior vena cava. The Denver shunt is a variation of the LeVeen catheter and has a subcutaneous pump that can be compressed manually to irrigate the tubing to keep it patent. Although the efficacy of these shunts is comparable to that of LVP, there is high incidence of thrombus formation at the venous tip of the shunt, catheter occlusion, and infections. PV shunts also do not improve survival rates.[3,8,26]

Esophageal Varices

Bleeding esophageal varices are the most dangerous complication of portal hypertension. The mortality associated with variceal hemorrhage is 50%. In portal hypertension, the azygos vein and the vena cava become distended where they join the smaller vessels of the esophagus. Distention occurs because of the greater volume of blood flowing through these vessels as a result of higher pressure within the portal system. Normal portal pressure is about 9 mm Hg. The increased portal venous pressure causes the blood, which normally flows through the liver, to be forced into these other vessels (see Figure 37-4, *A*, for a diagram of the relationship between these various blood vessels). These small vessels cannot accommodate the increased blood volume, and they become tortuous and fragile. Changes in the structure of these vessels predispose them to injury whenever intraabdominal pressure is increased as a result of coughing, vomiting, sneezing, or straining during defecation (Valsalva maneuver). Bleeding may also be initiated by mechanical trauma from ingestion of coarse foods and acidic pepsin erosion.

Primary prophylaxis should be initiated for any patient diagnosed with cirrhosis. A screening endoscopy is done and repeated every 2 to 3 years. If large varices or other signs of increased risk of bleeding are found, treatment with nonselective beta-blockers should be initiated. Propranolol (Inderal) and nadolol (Corgard) have been used to reduce portal pressure and successfully prevent the first episode of bleeding. Nitrates are also used if the patient does not respond to beta-blockers alone.

The first priority in the medical management of an active bleeding episode is to establish the source of bleeding. Esophagoscopy is the major diagnostic tool, and, if this is not possible, angiography is used. If severe hemorrhage is not present, barium studies or scans may be used. It must be remembered that in patients with cirrhosis, bleeding may be from other causes such as peptic ulcers and gastritis.

Treatment goals are to control bleeding, restore and maintain hemodynamics, and replace blood volume as rapidly as possible. Bleeding may be controlled with:

- Gastric lavage
- Pharmacologic therapy
- Injection sclerotherapy
- Balloon tamponade of varices
- Surgery—ligation and shunts

The first priority of nursing care in the management of patients with bleeding esophageal varices is to establish monitoring for a patent airway; parameters of cardiac output; adequacy of vascular volume; effectiveness of tissue perfusion; adequacy of hemostasis treatment; and adequacy of fluid and electrolyte, respiratory, renal, and neurologic status.

Gastric Lavage. If not already present, a nasogastric tube is placed, and irrigation is initiated. The patient must be monitored frequently, every 15 to 30 minutes, because he or she can lose several units of blood within 1 hour if hemorrhage is severe.

Pharmacologic Therapy. Pharmacologic therapy is started, including administration of vasopressin, propranolol (Inderal), and octreotide (Sandostatin). Vasopressin is given intravenously mixed in 120 to 200 ml of dextrose either intermittently or as a continuous infusion. Vasopressin lowers portal pressure by causing splanchnic vasoconstriction and can thus

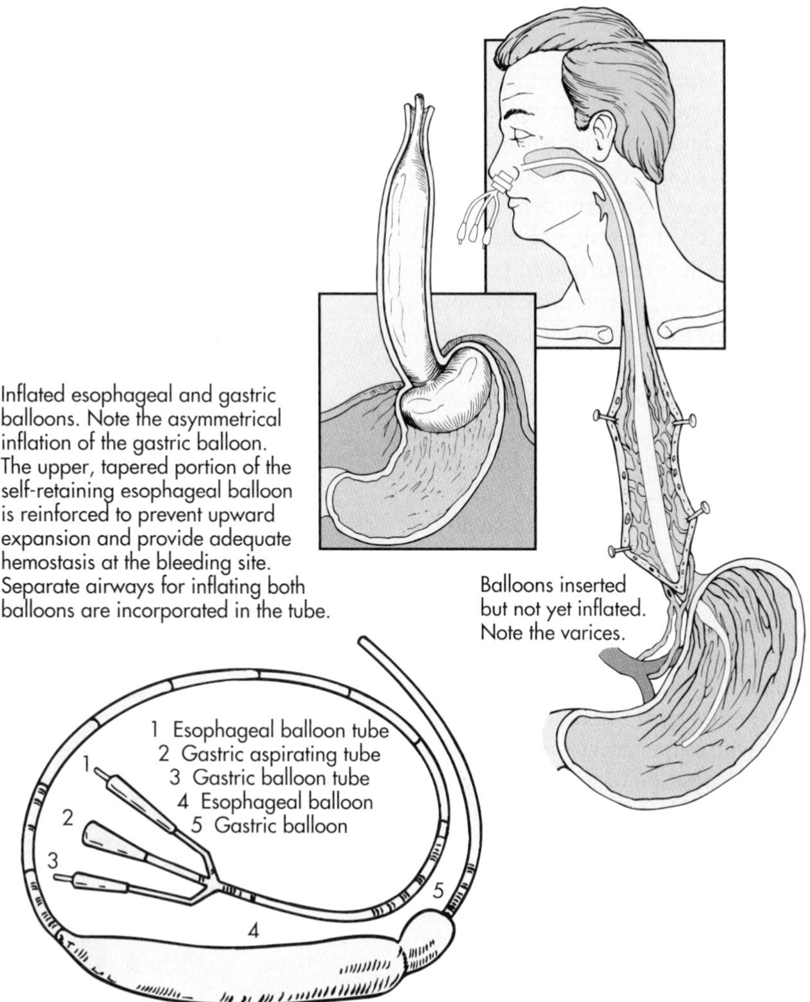

Figure 37-7 Esophageal tamponade accomplished with a Sengstaken-Blakemore tube.

stop or control esophageal bleeding. Side effects include abdominal cramping and pallor. Coronary artery vasoconstriction can occur, as well as mesenteric artery vasoconstriction; thus vasopressin must be used cautiously in persons with coronary artery disease and in elderly persons, and the length of this therapy is limited.

Propranolol (Inderal), a beta-adrenergic blocking agent, has been shown to reduce portal pressure and thus decrease esophageal bleeding in some people. Octreotide (Sandostatin) is frequently used to decrease total splanchnic flow and portal pressure. It is a long-acting octapeptide that mimics the action of the hormone somatostatin and is administered subcutaneously.

Endoscopic Sclerotherapy. Endoscopic sclerotherapy is the first-line treatment for active variceal bleeding. A fiberoptic endoscope is passed into the esophagus, the bleeding site is identified, and a sclerosing agent (sodium morrhuate, 5 ml) is injected into the varices. This agent causes thrombosis and sclerosis of the vessel and should result in hemostasis in 3 to 5 minutes. If hemostasis does not occur, a second injection may be given. The procedure may be repeated as necessary and can be performed while the varices are bleeding or as an elective procedure. Endoscopic therapy is ineffective in controlling bleeding from gastric varices. Endoscopic variceal ligation is an alternative to sclerotherapy, and there are fewer complications and similar efficacy in controlling bleeding.[9,30]

As after any endoscopic procedure, the nurse monitors the patient for complications of perforated esophagus, aspiration pneumonia, pleural effusion, and worsening of ascites. Respiratory support to ensure adequate air exchange is provided. Retrosternal pain is often present and is treated with analgesics; fever is common for several days.

Balloon Tamponade. If bleeding is not controlled by the preceding methods, balloon tamponade of varices may be instituted. Esophagogastric tubes (Sengstaken-Blakemore or Minnesota) are three- or four-lumen tubes with two balloon attachments. One lumen serves as an nasogastric (NG) suction tube, the second is used to inflate the gastric balloon, and the third is used to inflate the esophageal balloon (Figure 37-7). The Minnesota esophagogastric tamponade tube has a fourth lumen used for esophageal aspiration. The tube is passed by the physician through the nose into the stomach with the balloons deflated. When the tube is in the stomach, the gastric balloon is inflated and the lumen is clamped; the tube is then pulled out slowly so that the balloon is held tightly against the cardioesophageal junction. Studies have indicated that balloon tamponade controls bleeding as well as drugs and sclerotherapy, with no survival advantage. It should be reserved as a lifesaving temporary measure until the patient can undergo transjugular intrahepatic portosystemic shunt (TIPS) or surgical shunting.

The NG lumen is usually connected to intermittent gastric suction, which permits easy appraisal of cessation of bleeding and also keeps the stomach empty. It is important to remove all blood from the stomach, because its presence may precipitate portal-systemic encephalopathy from ammonia produced from the digestion of protein in the blood.

The esophageal balloon can be left inflated for up to 48 hours without causing tissue damage. The fully inflated gastric balloon with traction compresses the stomach wall between the balloon and the diaphragm, and can cause ulceration of the gastric mucosa and severe discomfort. To offset the possibility of necrosis, the physician may release traction on the gastric balloon and deflate the gastric balloon pressure periodically. If the gastric balloon ruptures (and the patient is not intubated), the entire tube may move and obstruct the airway. If this occurs, the tube is immediately removed. The major complication in the use of these tubes is esophageal ulceration.[29]

Nursing care of the patient with esophageal tamponade includes maintenance of the proper position of the tube, care to the mouth and nares, frequent oral suctioning as the patient is unable to swallow even saliva, and providing comfort measures, both physical and psychologic, to patient and family.

Shunts

Transjugular Intrahepatic Portosystemic Shunt. TIPS is a procedure in which, using radiography guidance, a shunt is created between the hepatic and portal veins and kept open by the placement of a metal stent. This decompresses the portal system and reduces portal hypertension enough to control active bleeding in most patients. Because there are long-term complications connected to TIPS, it is primarily used as rescue therapy when pharmacologic and endoscopic treatment of an acute bleed has failed. These complications include stent dysfunctions, such as thrombosis or stenosis, and right-sided heart failure. The advantage of TIPS is that it is relatively noninvasive and does not require anesthesia for a patient with a failing liver. TIPS may also be used as a prophylactic treatment for portal hypertension; however, the benefits of this procedure over other methods is debatable.[29]

Surgical Shunts. Surgery to shunt blood away from the portal circulation is one of the last measures used to treat esophageal varices. Portal decompression can be obtained by several procedures, most of them requiring open surgery. The mortality rate for shunt surgery is 5% to 15%, and if emergency shunt surgery is necessary, the mortality rate increases to 50%.

Various surgical procedures may be used (Figure 37-8) It must be remembered that, because the portal blood is being shunted away from the liver, toxins in the blood, especially ammonia, are not being metabolized and excreted. Therefore all patients who have had a portal-systemic shunt are at risk for portal-systemic encephalopathy. The incidence of PSE has been reported to be as high as 25% to 100% in patients undergoing these shunting procedures. Some patients require lifelong restriction of protein to limit ammonia toxicity.[11]

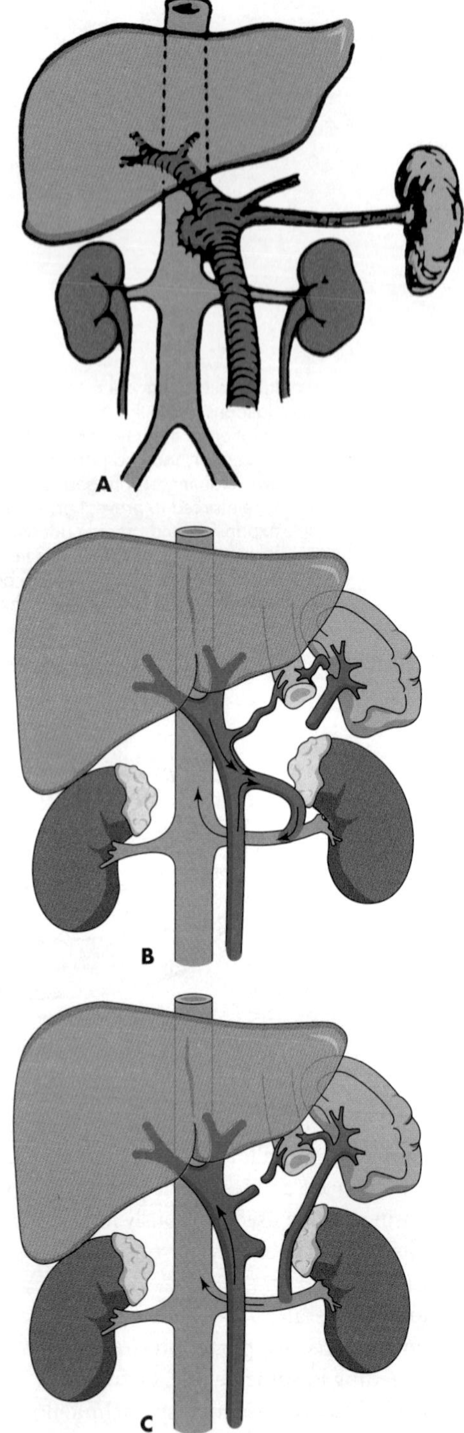

Figure 37-8 Decompression procedures for portal hypertension. **A**, Side-to-side portacaval shunt. **B**, Splenorenal shunt. **C**, Distal splenorenal shunt.

Before surgery the patient's vascular volume is stabilized with fluids and blood as necessary. Vitamin K may be given to correct coagulation problems, antibiotics may be given prophylactically, and nutritional status is improved as much as possible.

General needs of postoperative patients are discussed in Chapter 18. In addition, the patient recovering from shunt placement needs the following nursing interventions:

- Administration of narcotics for pain (the amount given is usually decreased because most narcotics are metabolized in the liver); avoidance of sedatives because of toxic effects on the diseased liver
- Careful observation for impending portal-systemic encephalopathy (beginning signs include mental confusion, slowness in response, and generally inappropriate behavior)
- Monitoring for hemorrhage and signs of shock
- Monitoring for signs of thrombosis at site of anastomosis (pain, distention, fever, and nausea)
- Encouragement of activity within the prescribed limits; starting leg and arm exercises on the first postoperative day
- Monitoring of the lower extremities for signs of edema; elevation of the lower extremities if ordered to prevent edema formation from the sudden increase of blood flow into the inferior vena cava

Liver transplantation remains a possible therapy for cirrhosis, although the indication for transplant is end-stage liver disease, and not variceal bleeding. TIPS procedures are often performed while the patient awaits liver transplantation.

In addition to the nursing care already mentioned, other nursing care responsibilities for the patient with bleeding esophageal varices include:

- Administration of fresh whole blood and IV infusions. Use of fresh blood avoids the increased ammonia and citrate of stored blood; fresh blood also has relatively more coagulation factors.
- Administration of saline cathartics through the NG lumen of the esophagogastric tube or through an NG tube to hasten expulsion of blood from the GI tract and to prevent an increase in the production of ammonia. Enemas may also be ordered to decrease gut content and bacterial action on the blood.
- Administration of lactulose or neomycin to prevent or decrease portal-systemic encephalopathy. Lactulose is a synthetic disaccharide degraded by bacteria in the lower intestines and is given either orally or by retention enema and promotes the excretion of ammonia in the stool by decreasing the pH of the bowel. Ammonia remains in its ionized state, which facilitates its movement from the blood to the stool. Bacterial growth is discouraged by the acidic environment.

Neomycin is a broad-spectrum antibiotic that destroys the normal flora of the bowel. Bacteria in the bowel normally break down protein, including blood protein in the GI tract, producing ammonia. Therefore neomycin is given to decrease the protein breakdown by bacteria in the bowel.[10]

Portal-Systemic Encephalopathy. Portal-systemic encephalopathy (PSE) is a major complication of cirrhosis, and is the result of rising levels of toxic substances normally metabolized and excreted by the liver. Common factors that precipitate PSE are summarized in Box 37-3. The manifestations of PSE vary and may occur quickly or gradually over the course of a few days. PSE results in alterations in the state of consciousness, intellectual function, behavior and personality, and neuromuscular function. These changes have been graded in four stages (Table 37-6).

BOX 37-3 Common Factors Associated With Portal-Systemic Encephalopathy

Factors Depressing Central Nervous System or Liver Function

Hypoxia
Secondary to hemorrhage and hypovolemic shock
Secondary to morphine and other sedatives
Infections
Exercise
In patients with chronic liver disease in whom coma is impending
Sedatives
Abdominal paracentesis
Resulting in reduction of plasma volume

Factors Increasing Level of Ammonia

Gastrointestinal (GI) ammonia (old blood in bowel from GI hemorrhage)
High-protein intake
Transfusions, especially with stored blood because it contains more ammonia
Hypokalemia
Secondary to thiazide diuretics
Secondary to potassium loss from the bowel
Alkalosis secondary to hyperventilation or hypokalemia
Shunting of blood into systemic circulation without passing through hepatic sinusoids
Natural collateral bypass of liver
Surgical bypass of liver
Constipation

Medical management of PSE involves identifying and treating precipitating factors such as hypokalemia, hemorrhage, and hypoxia; reducing serum ammonia levels; and providing supportive care. An elevated serum ammonia level provides the definitive diagnosis of PSE, but not all patients show an increase in ammonia. Therefore treatment is determined by the signs and symptoms and not the serum ammonia levels.

Lactulose and neomycin are given to decrease the serum ammonia levels. Lactulose also causes diarrhea, which helps eliminate blood from the GI tract in those patients with bleeding esophageal varices.

A low-protein diet may be prescribed, but this practice is controversial. Some researchers have found that increasing the calories and protein in patients with alcoholic liver disease does not worsen the encephalopathy.

Nursing management focuses on the following four goals:

1. Providing continual, regular monitoring of patients at high risk of PSE
2. Assisting with the therapeutic regimen
3. Providing supportive care
4. Providing long-term care

TABLE 37-6 Stages of Portal-Systemic Encephalopathy

Stage 1 (Prodromal)	Stage 2 (Impending)	Stage 3 (Stuporous)	Stage 4 (Coma)
Change in sleep pattern Slow response Shortened attention span Depressed or euphoric Irritable Tremors Slight asterixis Writing impaired	Lethargy Disorientation to time Impaired computation Decreased inhibition Anxiety or apathy Inappropriate behavior Speech slurred Decreased reflexes Ataxia Asterixis	Confused, somnolent Stupor, but arousable Disorientation to place Anger, rage, paranoia Increased reflexes Incoherent speech Asterixis (if patient can cooperate)	Unconscious No intellectual functioning Loss of deep tendon reflexes Unresponsive or responds only to deep pain Hyperventilation Fetor hepaticus (musty, sweet breath odor) Increased temperature and pulse rate

As can be seen from a review of Table 37-6, the early indications of PSE are subtle and can easily be missed if regular, objective assessments are not made. The nurse must (1) be as consistent and descriptive as possible; (2) assess skills such as handwriting or the ability to draw a circle, box, or square; and (3) maintain continuity of care so that the staff becomes familiar with the patient's behavior. Early detection of symptoms allows for more rapid treatment and consequently improves the patient's chance of recovery.

Monitoring should also focus on the patient's vital signs and overall status to detect deterioration of baseline functioning. The onset of fever or worsening results of laboratory studies (e.g., serum enzyme [ALT and AST] levels, prothrombin time, and bilirubin and albumin levels), and subtle mental status changes can indicate the onset of PSE.

If encephalopathy is present, a major focus of nursing is to implement the prescribed regimen. Treatment is focused on eliminating the causes of PSE, such as GI bleeding or hypokalemia, if known. The patient should be protected from sources of injury, as altered mental status increases the patient's potential for injury.

Other interventions focus on reducing ammonia levels and include:

- Eliminating or restricting protein intake
- Increasing carbohydrate intake to decrease metabolism of endogenous proteins
- Administering oral cathartics or enemas to empty the bowel and decrease ammonia formation
- Administering intestinal antibiotics such as neomycin to kill bacteria in the GI tract
- Administering lactulose
- Hemodialysis

The patient with PSE is very ill and requires care for the prevention of respiratory problems. Ventilatory support may be required. Coughing is prohibited if the patient has esophageal varices. The patient also needs care to prevent skin breakdown that may be worsened by malnutrition, pruritus, ascites, and frequent stools or incontinence. Infection must be prevented. If PSE progresses to hepatic coma, nursing care is similar to that of any unconscious patient.

Many patients with PSE die of kidney failure secondary to inadequate circulating blood volume (hypovolemia). In some patients, renal function progressively deteriorates without any apparent cause (hepatorenal syndrome). Treatment of PSE requires a careful balancing of fluid administration to maintain adequate perfusion of the kidney without creating an excessive load on the cardiovascular system. To monitor renal function adequately, an indwelling catheter is inserted, especially if the patient is being maintained on intravenous fluids. Central venous pressure monitoring is also frequently used to determine fluid volume status.

Because most narcotics and sedatives must be detoxified by the liver, their use is contraindicated in patients with impaired liver function. If a sedative must be used, drugs such as chlordiazepoxide (Librium), barbital, or phenobarbital, which are excreted by the kidney, are prescribed. If any sedatives, analgesics, or hypnotics are used, they should be given in less than normal doses, and the patient's response should be evaluated carefully.

Maintenance of adequate nutrition is a major nursing focus. A low-protein diet is often less palatable than a regular diet. Providing good oral hygiene, maintaining a pleasant clean environment, and serving small attractive meals may help increase appetite. A low-protein (20 to 40 g/day) diet may be prescribed indefinitely. Dietary or IV supplements that provide selected branch chain amino acids, which are metabolized in the muscle instead of the liver, may be used. Both oral and IV preparations are available commercially; these also contain carbohydrates. Vitamins and minerals are added as necessary.

The patient and family will need instructions regarding dietary restrictions and how to take medications. They also must be taught to be alert for subtle changes in the patient's behavior that indicate worsening or onset of PSE and to seek medical attention immediately if the patient shows any of these behaviors.

Hepatorenal Syndrome. The sudden onset of oliguria and azotemia in a patient with end-stage liver disease is a grave sign. The blood pressure may be elevated or decreased. The patient complains of anorexia, fatigue, and weakness. Fluid retention leads to hyponatremia and a decrease in urine osmolality. The continual accumulation of waste products and alterations in fluid and electrolytes cause neurologic changes that can resemble those of PSE. Blood pressure continues to drop. Hepatorenal syndrome has a poor prognosis, and its onset suggests impending death.

The focus of management is to determine whether the oliguria is caused by decreased cardiac output, hepatorenal syndrome, or acute tubular necrosis. Any of these processes can occur in the person with cirrhosis. Once the diagnosis of hepatorenal syndrome is made, management is designed to improve hepatic function and support renal function. Fluid and electrolytes are given to maintain hemodynamic status. Potentially nephrotoxic drugs such as neomycin are stopped. Some patients have shown improvement after a portacaval shunt has been performed. Liver transplantation is the major intervention for most patients with hepatorenal syndrome; however, it must be remembered that these patients are poor surgical risks. Liver transplantation and the related nursing care are discussed in Chapter 51. Hemodialysis has been successful in treating hyperkalemia and fluid overload. Note that these last treatments improve only symptoms and not the hepatorenal syndrome itself, because the basic problem is in the liver, not in the kidney.

Critical Thinking Questions

1. Examine the scientific principles underlying the nursing management of individuals with cirrhosis of the liver and determine those that could be applied or broadened to nursing care related to all types of liver disorders.
2. Distinguish between the characteristics of hepatitis A and hepatitis B. Identify principles of preventing transmission that are universal to all types of hepatitis.
3. A patient with cirrhosis is admitted for bleeding esophageal varices and ascites. A TIPS procedure is planned. What information should be included in preparing the patient and family for this procedure?
4. If a patient has lost considerable blood in an episode of bleeding esophageal varices, what changes in the hemoglobin and hematocrit values would you expect to see immediately?
5. What is the significance of a decrease in blood pressure and tachycardia in a patient immediately after blunt trauma to the liver?

References

1. Artnak KE, Wilkinson SS: Fulminant hepatic failure in acute acetaminophen overdose, *Adv Pract Nurs* 17:135, 1998.
2. Arguedas MR, Fallon MB: Prevention in liver disease, *Am J Med Sci* 321:145, 2001.
3. Bankole A et al: Ondansetron for reduction of drinking among biologically predisposed alcoholic patients, *JAMA* 284:963, 2000.
4. Bass M: Fluid and electrolyte management of ascites in patients with cirrhosis, *Crit Care Nurs Clin North Am* 10:459, 1998.
5. Bennett RG et al: Hepatitis B virus vaccination for older adults, *J Am Geriatr Assoc* 44:699-703, 1996.
6. Cance WG, Stewart AK, Menck HR: The National Cancer Data Base Report on treatment patterns for hepatocellular carcinomas, *Cancer* 88:912, 2000.
7. Demetriou A: Support of the acutely failing liver: state of the art, *Ann Surg* 228:14, 1998.
8. Dougherty AS, Heyward MD: Hepatitis C: current treatment strategies for an emerging epidemic, *Med Surg Nursing* 10:9, 2001.
9. Garcia N, Sanyal AJ: Minimizing ascites, *Postgrad Med* 109:91, 2001.
10. Hegab AM, Luketic VA: Bleeding esophageal varices: how to treat this dreaded complication of portal hypertension, *Postgrad Med* 109:75, 2001.
11. Henderson JM: Surgical management of portal hypertension. In Schiff ER, Sorrell MF, Maddrey WC, editors: *Schiff's diseases of the liver,* ed 8, vol 1, Philadelphia, 1998, Lippincott-Raven.
12. The Hepatitis Information Network, website: http://www.hepnet.com, 2001.
13. American Liver Foundation, website: http://www.liverfoundation.org, 2001.
14. Janotha B: Autoimmune hepatitis, *Adv Nurse Pract* 9:79, 2001.
15. Johannsen EC, Sifri DC, Madoff LC: Pyogenic liver abscesses, *Infect Dis Clin North Am* 14:547, 2000.
16. Klainberg M: Primary biliary cirrhosis, *AJN* 99:38, 1999.
17. Krawett EL: Can you recognize autoimmune hepatitis? *Postgrad Med* 104:145, 1998.
18. Lee WM, Schiodt FV: Fulminant hepatic failure. In Lee WM, Williams R, editors: *Acute liver failure,* Cambridge, 1997, Cambridge University Press.
19. Lee WM: Medical management of acute liver failure. In Lee WM, Williams R, editors: *Acute liver failure,* Cambridge, 1997, Cambridge University Press.
20. Letizia M, Noonan MA: Drug-induced hepatic injury, *Med Surg Nursing* 6:148, 1997.
21. Malhotra AK et al: Blunt hepatic injury: a paradigm shift from operative to nonoperative management in the '90s, *Ann Surg* 231:804, 2000.
22. Marx J: Understanding the varieties of viral hepatitis, *Nursing 98* 28:43, 1998.
23. Murray M, Pizzorno, J: Hepatitis. *Encyclopedia of natural medicine,* ed 2, Rocklin, Calif, 1997, Prima Publishing.
24. Perrillo T, Regenstein F: Viral and immune hepatitis. In Kelley W, editor: *Textbook of internal medicine,* ed 3, Philadelphia, 1997, Lippincott-Raven.
25. Richardson DJ et al: Evolution in the management of hepatic trauma: a 25-year perspective, *Ann Surg* 232:324, 2000.
26. Schiff ER, Sorrell MF, Maddrey WC: *Schiff's diseases of the liver,* Philadelphia, 1998, Lippincott-Raven.
27. Shovein JT, Damazo RJ, Hyams I: Hepatitis A: how benign is it? *AJN* 100:43, 2000.
28. Ulmer SC: Hepatocellular carcinoma, *Postgrad Med* 107:117, 2000.
29. US Department of Health and Human Services: *Healthy people 2010: understanding and improving health,* Washington, DC, 2000, USDHHS.
30. Vargus HE, Gerber D, Abu-Elmagd K: Management of portal hypertension-related bleeding, *Surg Clin North Am* 79:1, 1999.

http://www.mosby.com/MERLIN/medsurg_phipps

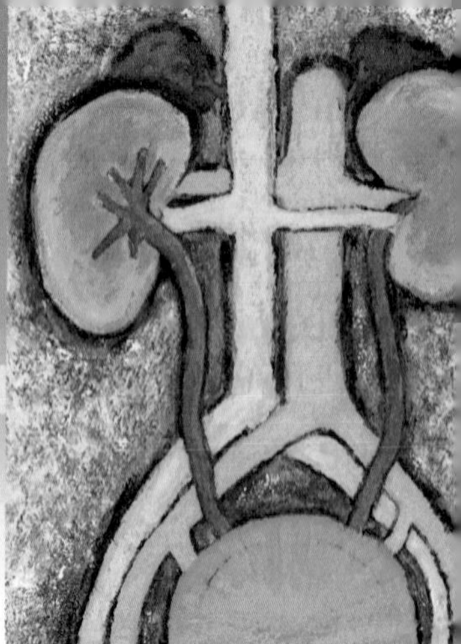

38 Assessment of the Renal System

Cynthia Hollamon, Carol Kelley, Kelly Weigel

Objectives

After studying this chapter, the learner should be able to:

1. List the major functions of the kidney.
2. Describe the anatomy of the kidney.
3. Identify subjective and objective data essential to the assessment of renal function.
4. Correlate significant urinary tract symptoms with common etiologies.
5. Describe common diagnostic tests used to identify renal alterations.
6. Explain guidelines for caring for patients after urologic diagnostic procedures.

The major organs of the renal system are the kidneys, retroperitoneal organs that are integral to the maintenance of the body's homeostasis. The kidneys produce and secrete hormones and enzymes that help regulate red blood cell production, blood pressure, and calcium and phosphate metabolism. By excreting metabolic end products and varying the excretion of water and solutes, the kidneys regulate body fluid volume, acidity, and electrolytes, thus maintaining normal body blood composition (Box 38-1).

ANATOMY AND PHYSIOLOGY

Anatomy

Upper Urinary Tract

The kidneys are two lima bean-shaped organs that lie outside the peritoneal cavity against the posterior abdominal wall (Figure 38-1). Each kidney is about 11 cm long, 5 cm wide, and 3 cm thick.[3] The kidneys lie on either side of the abdominal aorta, inferior vena cava, and lumbar spine between the twelfth thoracic and third lumbar vertebrae. The right kidney is displaced slightly inferiorly by the liver.

The kidneys are encased in a fibrous coat known as the renal capsule. Each kidney and capsule are embedded in a fatty layer that provides protection against injury. An adrenal gland lies above each kidney within the fatty layer. Renal fascia, a layer of connective tissue, and surrounding organs help hold the kidneys in place and protect them from trauma. On the medial aspect of each kidney is a concave notch known as the hilum. The renal arteries and nerves enter, and the renal veins, lymphatics, and ureters exit the kidney at the hilum.

When the kidney is cut longitudinally and opened, three distinct areas can be seen: the cortex, medulla, and renal sinus (Figure 38-2). The renal cortex, the outermost 1 cm, is pale and has a granular appearance. Most parts of the nephron, the functional unit of the kidney, lie in this area.

The inner 5-cm portion of the kidney is the renal medulla, which contains 8 to 10 triangular wedges or pyramids. The bases of the pyramids face the cortex, and their apices or renal papillae face the center of the kidney. The pyramids have a striated appearance because of the segments of the nephrons and collecting ducts located here.[3]

The third section of the kidney is the renal sinus. This is a cavity almost completely filled with blood vessels and structures formed by the expanded upper end of the ureter. Before entering the kidney, the ureter dilates to form the renal pelvis. The renal pelvis branches into two or three calyces. Each major calyx branches into several minor calyces. The minor calyces collect the urine that drains from the collecting ducts.

The nephron is the functional unit of the kidney. Each kidney contains approximately 1 million nephrons.[2,3] The two types of nephrons, cortical and juxtamedullary, are named according to their location within the renal parenchyma. The cortical nephrons account for 85% of the total nephrons and perform excretory and regulatory functions. The juxtamedullary nephrons make up the remaining 15% and play an important role in the concentration and dilution of urine by generating a steep osmotic gradient. The structures of the nephron involved in the process of urine formation include the renal corpuscle, the renal tubules, and the collecting duct (Figure 38-3). The renal corpuscle consists of the glomerulus and Bowman's capsule and is responsible for the formation of ultrafiltrate from the blood. The renal tubules consist of the proximal convoluted tubule, the loop of Henle, and the distal convoluted tubule and are responsible for the resorption and secretion that alter the volume and composition of the ultrafiltrate to form the final urine product. The collecting duct receives tubular fluid from many nephrons and transports the fluid from the cortex to the minor calyx.

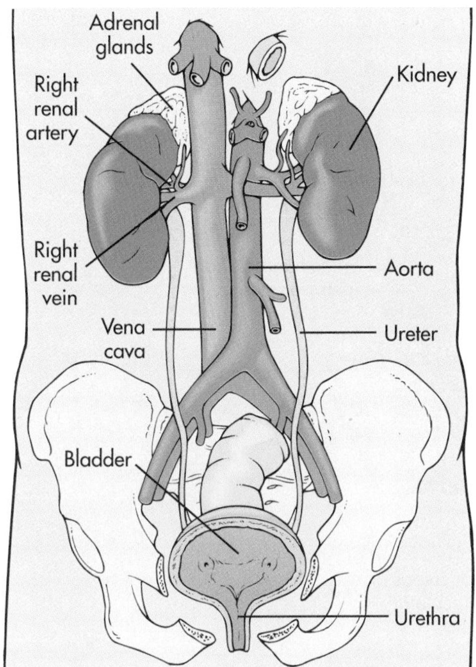

Figure 38-1 Organs and structure of the urinary system.

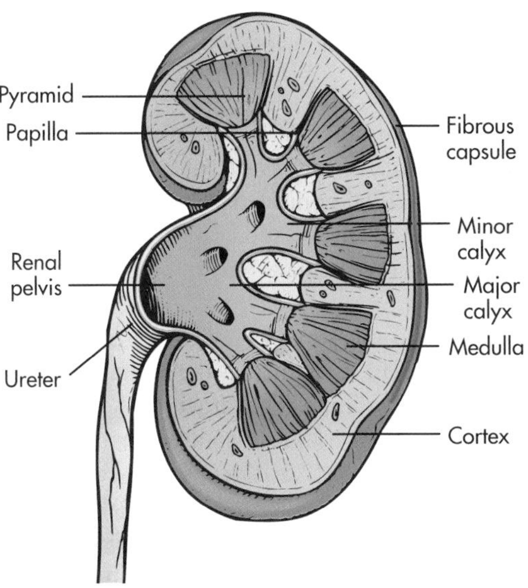

Figure 38-2 Frontal section of the kidney.

The kidneys are highly vascular organs, receiving about 20% of the cardiac output in the resting state, or about 1200 ml/min. Arterial blood is supplied by the renal arteries, which branch directly off the abdominal aorta (see Figure 38-1). Although 70% of human beings have one renal artery supplying each kidney, about 30% have one or more accessory renal arteries that also branch off the aorta and supply a part of the kidney.

The renal artery branches into approximately five segmental arteries, dividing the kidney into vascular segments. The segmental arteries branch to form the lobar arteries that supply each pyramid. The lobar arteries then branch several more times so blood can move efficiently through each nephron. Each nephron has its own blood supply; blood enters the glomerulus through the afferent arteriole and exits through the efferent arteriole. Blood then flows through the peritubular capillaries that surround the nephron's tubules. Ultimately the peritubular capillaries empty into venules that return the filtered blood to the general circulation via the renal venous system.[2]

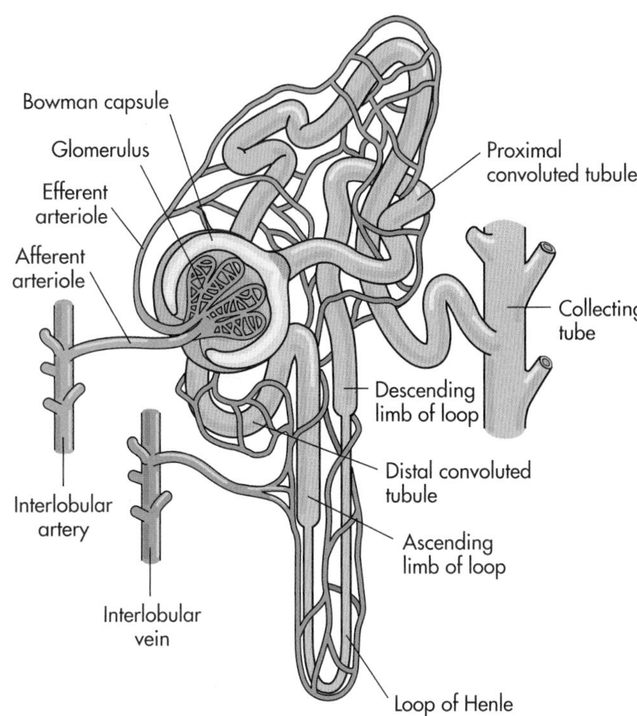

Figure 38-3 Nephron.

BOX 38-1 Functions of the Kidney

- Regulation of body fluid volume and osmolality
- Regulation of electrolyte balance
- Regulation of acid-base balance
- Excretion of metabolic waste products, toxins, and foreign substances
- Production and secretion of hormones

NOTE: Additional related functions such as blood pressure regulation and red cell production occur as the result of the above.

The ureters (see Figure 38-2), approximately 30 cm long, arise as extensions of the renal pelvis and empty into the bladder in an area known as the trigone (Figure 38-4). The trigone is a fold of mucous membrane that serves as a valve preventing the backflow or reflux of urine into the ureters when the bladder contracts. The ureters are composed of smooth muscle and are innervated by the sympathetic and parasympathetic nerves.[2] The function of the ureters is to propel urine from the renal pelvis to the bladder.

Lower Urinary Tract

The bladder, located behind the symphysis pubis (see Figure 38-1), serves as a collecting bag for the urine. The mucous membrane lining of the bladder is arranged in folds called rugae. These rugae, together with the elasticity of the muscular

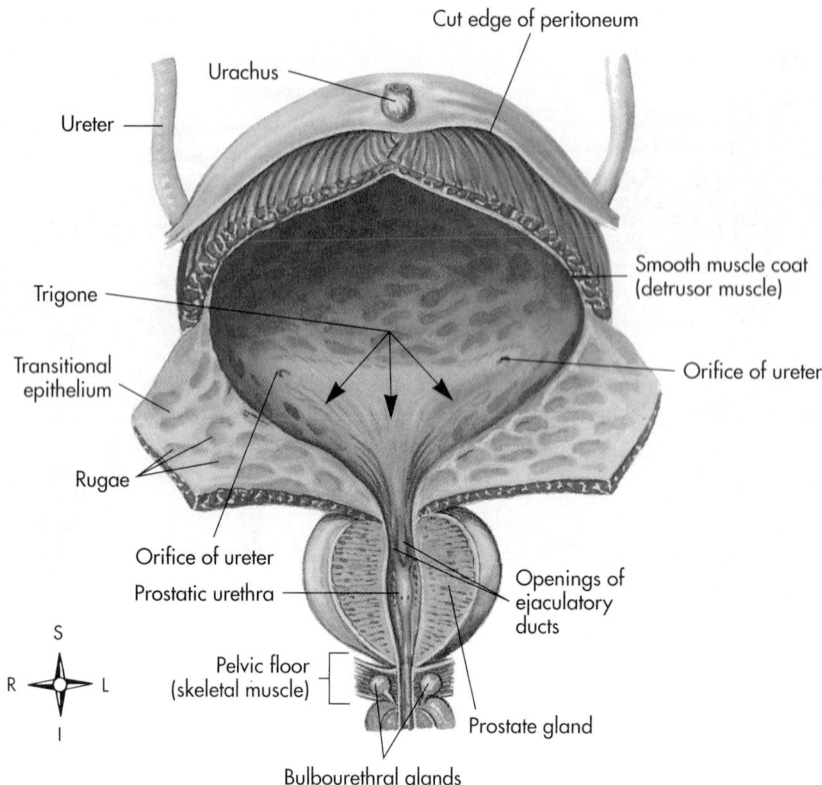

Figure 38-4 Interior of urinary bladder and associated structures in the male.

walls, enable the bladder to distend to hold large amounts of urine. A layer of skeletal muscle encircles the base of the bladder, forming the external urinary sphincter. Both the sympathetic and parasympathetic nervous systems innervate the bladder. The urethral sphincter, operating under voluntary control, allows the urine to pass into the urethra.

The urethra serves as the outlet for urine from the bladder. The male urethra is about 20 cm long, whereas the female urethra is about 4 cm long. The urinary meatus is the opening through which urine exits the body.

The walnut size prostate gland is a male reproductive gland that encircles the upper part of the male urethra (Figure 38-4). The gland is doughnut-shaped, with the urethra passing through the "hole." When the prostate is enlarged, the urethra is squeezed, obstructing the flow of urine. Numerous prostatic ducts empty into the urethra. Bacteria from urinary tract infections may travel up these ducts, causing inflammation and infection of the prostate.

Physiology

A clear understanding of the physiology of the kidneys is essential to mastering the constellation of physiochemical changes that occur with kidney failure. A short review of renal physiology follows.

Ultrafiltration

Ultrafiltration is the process by which the fluid part of urine is formed. As blood passes through the capillary bed of the glomerulus, the pressure of plasma forces fluid across the semipermeable membrane of the glomerulus into Bowman's capsule. The volume of this glomerular filtrate approximates 180 L/day. Of the total volume, 99% is resorbed by the kidneys. Because of the tremendous capacity of the kidneys for resorption, the average urinary output of an adult is only 1 to 2 L/day.

Ultrafiltration is measured as the glomerular filtration rate (GFR). Clinically GFR is defined as the amount of glomerular filtrate formed in 1 minute. The larger the body surface area, the greater the GFR. The GFR in an average-sized adult is approximately 125 ml/min (7.5 L/hr). At this rate, a volume of approximately 60 times the plasma volume is filtered each day. The average GFR of a woman is about 10% less than that of a man. Glomerular filtrate is formed by the same forces that affect fluid transport between vascular and interstitial spaces in other tissues of the body. These factors include hydrostatic pressure and oncotic pressure.

The rate of renal perfusion exceeds the metabolic and oxygen needs of the kidneys but facilitates efficient clearance of metabolic wastes. A severe or prolonged interruption in renal blood flow or cardiac output affects urine formation and cell viability.

Urine formation begins when blood enters the afferent arteriole of the nephron. It is in Bowman's capsule and the tubules that the ultrafiltrate begins to be transformed into urine. Table 38-1 presents the normal composition of urine.

The ability of the kidney to conserve water and electrolytes is essential for survival. If conservation were not possible, a person would be volume and electrolyte depleted in 3 to 4

TABLE 38-1 Normal Urine Values

Laboratory Test	Normal Adult Values
Calcium (24 hr)	100-250 mg/day (diet dependent; based on average calcium intake of 600-800 mg/24 hr)
Chloride	110-250 mEq/day
Creatinine	Men: 1-2 g/24 hr; women: 0.8-1.8 g/24 hr
Glucose	Up to 100 mg/24 hr
Osmolality	250-900 mOsm/kg
Protein	30-150 mg/24 hr (method dependent)
pH	4.5-8
Phosphorus	0.9-1.3 g/day (diet dependent)
Potassium	26-123 mEq/24 hr (markedly intake dependent)
Sodium	27-287 mEq/24 hr (diet dependent; output is lower at night)
Specific gravity	1.003-1.029 (range in SI units)
Urea nitrogen	6-17 g/day
Uric acid	250-750 mg/day
Volume	Men: 800-2000 ml/day; women: 800-1600 ml/day
Color	Pale to darker yellow
Clarity	Clear
Ketones	None
Red blood count	0-5/high-power field
White blood count	0-5/high-power field
Bacteria	None/occasional in voided specimen
Casts	0-4 hyaline casts/low-power field
Crystals	Interpreted by physician
Culture	Negative

Data from Thompson JM et al: *Mosby's clinical nursing,* ed 5, St Louis, 2002, Mosby.

TABLE 38-2 Average Filtration and Resorption Values for Several Common Substances

Substance	Amount Filtered (per day)	Amount Excreted (per day)	Percent Resorbed
Water (L)	180	1.8	99.0
Sodium (g)	630	3.2	99.5
Glucose (g)	180	0.0	100.0
Urea (g)	54	30.0	44.0
Potassium (g)	35	2.0	94.0
Calcium (g)	5	0.2	96.0
Amino acids (g)	10	0.3	97.0

minutes. Refer to Table 38-2 for a summary of the filtration and resorption values of common substances.

The proximal convoluted tubule resorbs 85% to 90% of the water in the ultrafiltrate; up to 80% of filtered sodium; and most of the filtered potassium, bicarbonate, chloride, phosphate, glucose, and amino acids. The distal convoluted tubule and collecting tubule produce the final urine.

Another mechanism that prevents water and electrolyte depletion is endocrine or hormonal response. Antidiuretic hormone (ADH or vasopressin) is an example of hormonal regulation of salt and water balance. ADH is produced by the hypothalamus and stored and released by the pituitary gland in response to changes in plasma osmolarity. Plasma osmolarity refers to the concentration of ions in the blood. If water intake is low or if water loss is high, ADH is released, causing the kidneys to retain water. ADH acts on the collecting ducts increasing their permeability to water. As a result more water is resorbed into the bloodstream.[1,4]

The kidneys maintain a stable internal environment by balancing the fluid and solute composition of the blood within narrow homeostatic ranges. Three intricate processes are used: filtration, resorption, and secretion. Each part of the nephron is anatomically constructed to perform one or more of these processes. Filtration occurs in Bowman's capsule and resorption and secretion in the tubules and collecting duct. See Box 38-2 for a summary of water and electrolyte regulation of the nephron.

Effective ultafiltration occurs as blood enters the glomerular capillaries, and water and small molecules begin to be filtered out into Bowman's capsule through tiny pores in the capillary wall. The pore size restricts the size of molecule that can leave the blood. For example, blood cells and proteins are

BOX 38-2 Water and Electrolyte Regulation of Nephron

Bowman's Capsule

Ultrafiltrate from plasma enters Bowman's capsule and flows into the proximal convoluted tubule

Proximal Convoluted Tubule

Passive resorption of 65% of glomerular filtrate with sodium, potassium, chloride, bicarbonate, magnesium, phosphate, glucose, amino acids, and urea

Secretion of hydrogen ions and some drugs and toxins

Loop of Henle

Resorption: 25% of the glomerular filtrate with sodium, calcium, potassium, magnesium, chloride and urea

Distal Convoluted Tubule

Resorption: 9% of the glomerular filtrate with sodium, chloride, bicarbonate, water, and urea

Secretion of hydrogen, potassium, and ammonia

Collecting Duct

Resorption of water dependent on presence of ADH Sodium resorbed and potassium secreted if aldosterone present.

Calcium is resorbed if PTH present.

Acid-base balance regulation continues.

ADH, Antidiuretic hormone; *PTH*, parathyroid hormone.

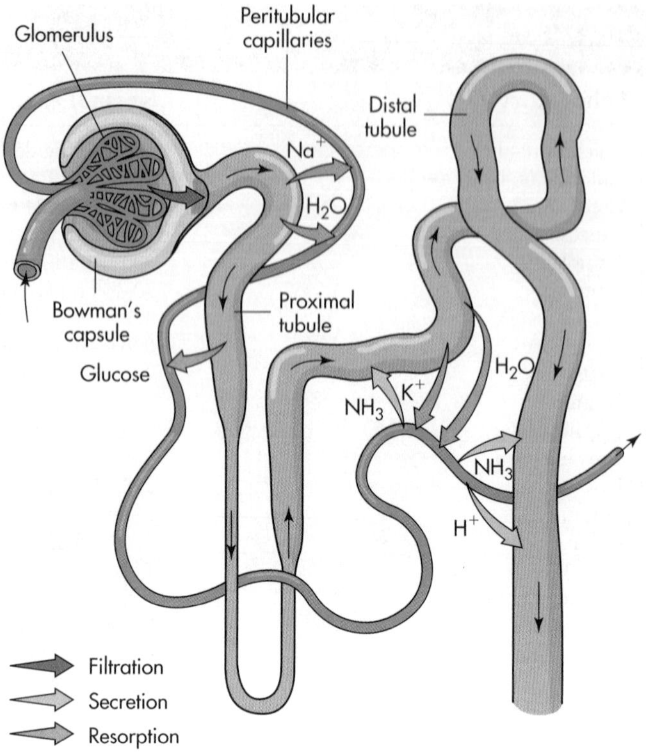

Figure 38-5 Mechanism of urine formation. Diagram shows the mechanisms of urine formation and where they occur in the nephron: filtration, resorption, and secretion.

too large, but urea is the correct size to be filtered out of the blood. From Bowman's capsule the ultrafiltrate moves into the proximal tubule where most of the water, sodium, potassium, calcium, chloride, and bicarbonate filtered out in the capsule originally are resorbed and returned to the blood. Body waste products such as hydrogen ions, phosphate, and drugs and their metabolites are secreted from the blood in the proximal tubules.[2,3,7]

In both the descending and ascending loops of Henle, the ultrafiltrate is further refined as more sodium and water is resorbed, and magnesium is reclaimed from the tubules. Final adjustment in urine composition is made in the distal nephron, which includes the distal convoluted tubule and the collecting ducts. The primary solutes affected in this area are potassium, bicarbonate, hydrogen ions, and again, sodium and chloride. This final refinement of the urine is accomplished primarily by feedback mechanisms regulated by the hormones aldosterone and ADH. The filtrate or eventual urine becomes increasingly concentrated and acidic as it moves from the proximal to the distal tubules and finally into the collecting ducts. The final pH of the urine is usually between 5 and 6, and the total amount of urine leaving the body is reduced to between 1 and 2 L. Considering the total blood volume filtered, an incredible amount of filtrate concentration occurs between the glomerulus and the ureter.[2] The nephron's intricate work successfully maintains the extracellular pH within a narrow range and finely tunes the fluid and electrolyte composition to sustain the complex delicate processes of the body. Figure 38-5 illustrates the mechanism of urine formation.

Electrolyte Balance

There is a constant ebb and flow of electrolytes (electrically charged particles) along the anatomic path of the ultrafiltrate. Electrolytes are filtered out in the capsule only to be mostly resorbed in the proximal tubules. Ultimately their concentration is adjusted in the distal nephron under the influence of hormones (primarily aldosterone and ADH). The specific mechanisms for moving electrolytes across the tubular membranes are both passive and active. Passive movement of electrolytes occurs when there is a concentration difference of molecules across the semipermeable membrane; molecules move from an area of greater concentration to one of lesser concentration. Active movement of electrolytes or active transport requires the expenditure of energy and enables the movement of molecules regardless of concentration gradients. Active and passive movement allows the kidney to maintain optimal electrolyte balance.

Maintenance of Acid-Base Balance

For normal cell function plasma pH must be maintained in a narrow range, between 7.35 and 7.45 for arterial blood. This balance is achieved by maintaining a blood bicarbonate to carbon dioxide ratio of 20:1. The respiratory system and the kidneys work together to maintain this ratio. The lungs contribute by varying the carbon dioxide content of the blood.

The kidneys principally secrete or retain bicarbonate and hydrogen ions in response to the pH of the blood. These two substances must move in or out of the blood at precisely the right time for the pH to remain stable. The exchange is accomplished in both the proximal tubules and in the collecting ducts of the nephron. See Chapter 13 for further discussion of acid base balance.

Erythropoiesis

The kidneys play a crucial role in red blood cell production. Decreased tissue oxygenation stimulates special cells in the kidneys (thought to be the epithelial cells of the peritubular capillaries) to produce about 90% of the body's erythropoietin or EPO.[3] EPO stimulates the bone marrow to produce proerythroblasts, which develop into erythrocytes. Hypoxia and anemia generally trigger an increase in production of erythropoietin. Treatment with genetically engineered erythropoietin (Epogen or Procrit) can improve the hematocrit and reduce the need for blood transfusions in patients with anemia secondary to chronic kidney failure, anemias associated with malignancies, and other disorders. With a synthetic form of erythropoietin, patients achieve a near-normal production of erythrocytes.

Calcium and Phosphorus Regulation

Serum calcium and phosphorus regulation is one of the kidney's most important functions. Calcium is crucial for bone formation, cell division and growth, blood coagulation, hormone response, and cellular electrical activity. Phosphate is a component of all intermediates of glucose metabolism, a part of the structure of all high-energy transfer compounds such as adenosine triphosphate (ATP), and an integral part of the crystalline structure of bones.

The kidneys influence the reciprocal calcium and phosphorous balance by converting the inactive form of vitamin D absorbed from the gut, to its active form, 1,25-dihydroxycholecalciferol. Parathyroid gland secretion of parathyroid hormone (PTH) is regulated by this form of vitamin D and calcium concentration. Under the influence of PTH, calcium reabsorption is increased and phosphate resorption is decreased.[1]

Blood Pressure Regulation

The kidneys play an active role in the regulation of blood pressure, primarily by regulating plasma volume and vascular tone. Blood pressure is manipulated through the kidneys' response to several mechanisms that alter the total volume of blood in the circulatory system. These mechanisms include ADH response, the renin-angiotensin system, and aldosterone response. As previously discussed, ADH release by the pituitary causes the kidneys to resorb water, increasing blood pressure.

The renin-angiotensin system and aldosterone response also influence the regulation of blood pressure. Renin is a hormone released by the juxtaglomerular apparatus of the nephron in response to sodium and potassium depletion, a drop in renal artery blood pressure, or sympathetic stimulation. Renin stimulates the conversion of angiotensinogen (a substance produced by the liver) to angiotensin I. Conversion of angiotensin I to angiotensin II by angiotensin-converting enzymes (ACE) from the lung produces a powerful vasoconstriction and release of aldosterone, resulting in increased blood pressure. Aldosterone is released from the adrenal glands and acts on the kidneys to resorb sodium and water, increasing circulating blood volume and pressure.

Prostaglandin and bradykinin, hormones produced by the kidney and other tissues, help elevate blood pressure and increase renal blood flow as well. They are released in response to renal ischemia, the presence of ADH and angiotensin II, and sympathetic stimulation.[4] Acting locally and rapidly inactivated, they provide an immediate mechanism for improving renal blood flow.[4]

Excretion of Metabolic Wastes and Toxins

Metabolic wastes are excreted in the glomerular filtrate. Creatinine contained in the glomerular filtrate is excreted unchanged in the urine. Other wastes, such as urea, are excreted unchanged in the glomerular filtrate but undergo resorption during passage through the nephron. The amount of waste material excreted in urine is only a portion of that which was originally contained in the glomerular filtrate. As electrolytes are reabsorbed by the nephron, so are most waste materials. It is important to remember that most drugs are either excreted directly by the kidneys or first metabolized by the liver to inactive forms and then excreted by the kidneys. Because of the role of the kidneys in drug excretion, some drugs are contraindicated and the dose of others must be adjusted when renal function is impaired. Examples include many antibiotics, salicylates, and long-acting barbiturates.

Micturition

Micturition (urination) is a complex sensory-motor process. Urine flows from the kidney pelvis and is propelled through the ureters by peristaltic action. About 200 to 300 ml of urine can collect in the bladder before the urge to void is felt. As the bladder wall is stretched, baroreceptors cause reflex stimulation of parasympathetic nerves to the bladder, resulting in bladder contractions. When the motor nerves to the external urinary sphincter are inhibited, the muscle relaxes, opening the sphincter and permitting urine to be expelled.

When the motor nerves to the external urinary sphincter are activated, the sphincter remains contracted. This allows for voluntary control of urination even if the bladder muscles are also contracting. The end products of ultrafiltration are finally eliminated in this last step and homeostasis is maintained.

Physiologic Changes With Aging

A variety of changes occur in the kidney and urinary tract in response to aging. A direct relationship exists between blood supply to the kidneys and renal function. The rate of blood flow to the kidneys is 5 to 10 times greater than that to the heart, liver, and brain. Glomerular capillary pressure, which is the force that promotes ultrafiltration, is controlled by blood flow to the kidneys. Therefore physiologic alterations in the vascular bed can lead to changes in renal function.

Arteriosclerotic changes in renal arteries are the most common form of renovascular pathologic condition. Arteriosclerotic changes occur to some extent in the normal aging process. The degree of morphologic change depends on the specific arteries affected and the extent of involvement within those arteries.

Aging is also known to cause predictable increases in both systolic and diastolic blood pressure. This slow increase in blood pressure begins early in life and continues through adulthood. This relationship between aging and increasing blood pressure is so well accepted that normal systolic blood pressure is commonly described as 100 mm Hg plus the person's age. Although not entirely accurate, this description does emphasize the effect of aging on blood pressure. Untreated hypertension further accelerates the development of atherosclerosis, which can lead to kidney failure.

Prostatic hypertrophy is a common physiologic change associated with aging discussed in detail in Chapter 55. Untreated prostatic hypertrophy results in urinary obstruction that can lead to kidney failure. Aging women frequently develop problems with stress incontinence as muscle tone weakens and the pelvic organs put increasing pressure on the bladder and urethra.

HEALTH HISTORY

Baseline subjective renal assessment begins with an assessment of the patient's overall state of health and perception of what constitutes good health, rather than a listing of documented health problems and comorbidities. The interview then explores any patient concerns or health problems, especially any urinary tract symptoms. See Table 38-3 for terms used to describe common urologic symptoms and their clinical significance. When a kidney problem is suspected, the nurse asks the patient directly about each of these symptoms.

Urination

Obtaining baseline data concerning the person's usual voiding patterns, such as the frequency and amount of urine with each void, is helpful when changes are anticipated. Persons who are admitted to a hospital or other nursing facility are questioned about their ability to carry out toileting independently. All persons should be questioned about any changes noted in voiding patterns. If changes have occurred, more detailed information must be obtained pertaining to onset, duration, and measures that the person has taken to deal with these problems.

When asking questions about urination, it is important to be aware that some persons may be somewhat reluctant to answer, either because of embarrassment or misunderstanding. A calm, matter-of-fact approach by the nurse helps put the person at ease. Many persons are not familiar with terms such as "voiding" or "urination," and more colloquial words may need to be used. The nurse should confirm that the person understands the questions.

The nurse asks specific questions to elicit information regarding the presence of abnormal conditions. Patients are asked directly in nonmedical terms if they have any of the signs or symptoms outlined in Table 38-3. The more descriptive the question, the more likely the clinician is to obtain accurate relevant information. For example, asking, "Do you

TABLE 38-3 Clinical Significance of Common Urinary Tract Symptoms

Symptom	Definition	Clinical Significance
Dysuria	Pain/burning with voiding	Urinary tract infection
Frequency	Voids multiple times during the day either in large or small amounts	Urinary tract infection, retention, hyperglycemia with increased fluid intake, prostatic hypertrophy
Urgency	The need to void immediately	Urinary tract infection, bladder irritation, trauma, tumor
Nocturia	Awakens to void; abnormal when it occurs multiple times during the sleep cycle	Diuretics, prostatic hypertrophy, kidney failure/insufficiency, increased fluid intake, congestive heart failure
Hesitancy	Difficulty initiating voiding	Partial urethral obstruction, neurogenic bladder
Incontinence	Loss of voluntary control of urination	Urinary tract infection, urethral obstruction, posturinary catheter removal, central nervous system or spinal cord disease, post-prostatectomy, laxity of perineal muscles in older women
Frothing	Excessive foaming of urine	Presence of protein in the urine
Foul odor	Foul smell associated with urine	Urinary tract infection
Polyuria	Urine output > 3000 ml/24 hr	Diabetes mellitis, hormonal abnormality, diabetes insipidus, high output kidney failure
Oliguria	Urine output < 400 ml/24 hr	Kidney failure, urinary retention/ obstruction
Anuria	Urine output < 100 ml/24 hr	Kidney failure, total obstruction (trauma, mass)
Myoglobinuria	Red-brown, at times black, pigment in the urine	Muscle tissue breakdown following extreme physical exertion or massive trauma (myoglobin is muscle hemoglobin); can result in kidney failure
Hematuria	Red blood cells in the urine; may be gross (visible to eye) or microscopic (detectable with urine screen and microscope)	Renal calculi, urinary tract infection, inflammation of the kidney or bladder, trauma to the kidney or urinary tract, posturinary catheter removal, menses

have any problems with urination?" is less likely to elicit useful diagnostic information than asking questions such as: "Do you experience burning when you pass urine?" or "Do you have to get up at night to urinate; if so, how many times?" Questions such as "How many times do you pass your water in 24 hours?" "Do you pass less than 2 cups of urine a day?" "Does your urine look cloudy or bloody?" are also helpful. See Box 38-3 for a review of health history guidelines related to upper urinary tract disorders.

BOX 38-3 Health History Related to Upper Urinary Tract Disorders

Change in Usual Voiding Pattern

Dysuria: pain or burning on urination
Frequency of urination: frequent voiding
Nocturia: need to void at night
Polyuria: excretion of unusually large amounts of urine
Oliguria: decreased capacity to form and pass urine
Anuria: inability to urinate, cessation of urine production
Questions: onset and duration, pattern, severity, associated symptoms, efforts to treat and their outcome
Pain
Location: kidney—flank, costovertebral angle; ureter—along course of ureter to groin
Questions: character, intensity, onset and duration, precipitating factors, relieving factors, accompanying symptoms

Change in Appearance of Urine

Hematuria: bright red bleeding, rusty brown, cola-colored; at beginning, end, or throughout voiding
Proteinuria: deep yellow color, foamy
Color changes may be caused by food or drugs
Passage of stone
May be a single stone or gravel-like material; may be associated with hematuria, fever, and pain

Patient's Perception of Problem

Degree of concern about the symptom and the patient's opinion as to its cause .

Patient History Relating To Upper Urinary Tract Disorders

Concurrent disorders
Medical history
Infancy—childhood
Previous disorders (urinary tract infection, kidney stones, other kidney disease)
Serious injuries
Hospitalizations, surgery
Gynecologic history
Medication history: current and recent prescription and nonprescription drugs taken
Family history: polycystic kidney disease, renal calculi, renal tubular acidosis, hypertension, diabetes mellitus, renal or bladder cancer
Diet and nutritional state
Sociocultural history
Psychosocial history

From Brundage D: *Renal disorders,* St Louis, 1992, Mosby.

Pain

Urinary tract pain deserves special emphasis, as the etiology can be medically serious and may require immediate attention to prevent complications. Pain associated with urinary tract disorders is referred to different anatomic locations depending on the etiology and the innervation of the area affected. (See Chapter 39 for a discussion of specific disease processes that cause urinary tract pain.) For example, pain from inflammation or infection of the kidney is commonly referred to the costovertebral angle (CVA) of the back and is often called "flank pain." Patients complaining of low back pain of renal etiology experience tenderness over the CVA area of the involved kidney when that area is percussed. The pain is often described as severe. If there is an infectious cause, these patients may also complain of lower urinary tract pain or dysuria.

Pain involving the ureter or upper urinary tract is also generally referred to the back and presents as vague chronic back pain. In contrast, bladder pain is often experienced as lower crampy, spasmodic midabdominal pain. This type of pain is typical of someone who has a bladder infection. It is important to remember that pain intensity varies from person to person. For example, patients with peripheral neuropathy commonly seen in advanced diabetes or patients with paresthesias from spinal cord lesions may experience remote, decreased, or even no pain from renal or urinary tract disease. The nursing implication of this deviation is that pain cannot be relied on as a warning sign of disease in these populations.

PHYSICAL EXAMINATION

Moderate or severe renal disease can cause significant observable pathologic changes. For example, the quantity of urine excreted in 24 hours offers critical diagnostic data. Polyuria, oliguria, and anuria as described in Table 38-3 are all clinically significant and require further evaluation.

Obtaining an accurate assessment of urinary output is often difficult in a hospital setting. Urine may be inadvertently discarded, or the patient may void into the toilet. The nurse explains the importance of accurate urine collection. All staff members need to be aware of patients whose output is being measured. In some cases, such as patients in shock or acute kidney failure, it is essential to accurately assess urinary output and an indwelling urinary catheter may be inserted. The risks and benefits of inserting an indwelling urinary catheter should always be assessed before placement.

The actual appearance of the urine is clinically important as well. The urine is inspected for gross variations from normal. Normal urine varies in color from pale to deep yellow, depending on specific gravity. A very dark color suggests that urine may be concentrated (high specific gravity) or that there may be an increased excretion of bilirubin. Certain medications and foods also can change the color of urine.

Hematuria (blood in the urine) may be detected overtly or may be present microscopically. In gross hematuria the urine may be pink-tinged to cherry red. If blood is observed in the urine of a woman having her menstrual period, the vaginal orifice can be blocked with cotton balls and another specimen

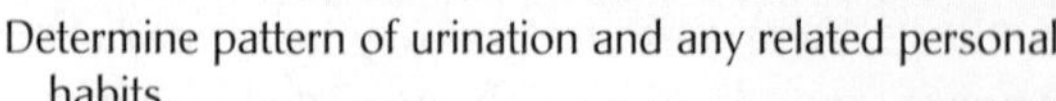

Gerontologic Assessment

Determine pattern of urination and any related personal habits.
Problems with urinary control are not unusual in older adults and individuals establish personal methods of coping such as use of incontinence products and timing of fluid intake.
Assess for contributing factors if functional (environmental) incontinence is a problem.
Mobility problems, diuretic use, or mental changes may be contributing factors.
Assess for signs of urinary tract infection that are commonly manifested in elderly persons.
Usual signs of fever and pain or burning with urination may be minimal or absent; confusion and anorexia may be the only symptoms.
Monitor kidney function during diagnostic testing.
When older adults undergo extensive testing that may lead to dehydration, marginal kidney function can be compromised.

COMMON DISORDERS IN OLDER ADULTS

Urinary incontinence
Urinary tract infections
Benign prostatic hyperplasia
Cancer of kidney, bladder, or prostate
Kidney failure
Dysuria

obtained to ascertain the source of the blood. Hematuria with pain may be the result of calculi, a clot from renal bleeding, or bladder infection.

Cloudy urine may result from precipitation of phosphate salts in alkaline urine or from bacterial growth. A urinary or vaginal discharge also may give the urine a cloudy appearance.

The physical appearance of the patient with kidney failure can change noticeably. For example, kidney failure commonly causes edema of the eyelids, hands, feet, and ankles (or even the sacrum in immobile bed-bound patients). The skin may be pale or even have a frosted appearance *(uremic frost)* when the kidneys stop functioning completely. The breath may have an ammonia-like odor as waste products accumulate in the body. Kidney failure is presented in detail in Chapter 40.

Assessment measures and variations in normal findings relevant to the care of older adults are presented in the Gerontologic Assessment box. Also identified are disorders common in older adults, which may be responsible for abnormal assessment findings.

DIAGNOSTIC TESTS

Special examinations of the urinary system are performed to identify the location and nature of existing disease. The accuracy of the test findings often depends on the cooperation of the patient in restricting or augmenting fluids and collecting specimens at designated times. The patient should be given clear, precise directions; written instructions are a valuable supplement to verbal directions for patients who can see and read.

Many of the diagnostic tests used to assess renal function can be performed on an ambulatory basis. Therefore it is important to make sure that the patient understands all instructions in preparation for the test. Some examinations must be performed with the patient under sedation; if so, the patient is instructed to make arrangements for someone to take him or her home after the procedure.

Laboratory Tests

Blood Tests

Several serum tests can be performed to evaluate kidney function. The two most common are tests for blood urea nitrogen (BUN) and creatinine levels. The kidney maintains serum levels of BUN and creatinine, by-products of protein breakdown and muscle metabolism, respectively, within a narrow range. Although they can fluctuate, the levels are still maintained within a predictable range as long as the kidneys function normally. Of the two, BUN varies the most because it can be influenced by a high-protein diet or events such as gastrointestinal bleeding.

Creatinine remains relatively constant. With severe renal disease (acute or chronic kidney failure or end-stage renal disease), the complete blood count, iron studies, and the complete blood chemistry analysis become altered as the kidney loses nephrons and the capacity to maintain homeostasis.

Blood tests used in the evaluation of renal function are summarized in Table 38-4.

Urine Tests

Urinalysis. A urinalysis is performed in two parts. The first part (the urine screen) consists of dipping a reagent strip into a clean-catch urine specimen and noting the color changes in each section of the strip. This may be followed by a microscopic examination, which is performed whenever the results from the urine screen are abnormal or abnormalities are suspected. The examination focuses on analysis of urine sediment, the solid matter found in the urine after centrifuging. Normal urine contains almost no sediment. Interpretation of abnormal sediment is difficult, and the findings are carefully correlated with data from the patient's history and physical examination. Table 38-5 summarizes normal and abnormal urinalysis findings.

Clean-Catch Urine Specimens. Ideally, all urinalysis specimens should be clean-catch specimens, but this is particularly important if a urinary tract infection is suspected. Guidelines for clean-catch urine collection are found in the Guidelines for Safe Practice box, p. 1196, left. Specimens should be transported to the laboratory within 30 minutes or promptly refrigerated. Clean-catch specimens are also obtained for toxicologic analysis (drugs or chemicals), cytology (abnormal cells), and pregnancy testing. A catheterized specimen may be indicated if midstream urine cannot be collected. However, catheterization should only be used if absolutely necessary. The risk of bacterial contamination is significant any time a catheter is introduced into the bladder.

Timed Urine Collection. A timed urine collection involves pooling all the urine a patient excretes over a specific period of time. This test is often required for urologic diagnosis. The duration of urine collections may vary from 2 to 24 hours, with

TABLE 38-4 Selected Renal Function Tests

Test	Normal Results	Purpose or Significance	Pretest Preparation/Posttest Care
Blood tests			
Serum creatinine	Men: 0.85-1.5 mg/100 ml Women: 0.7-1.25 mg/100 ml	Test indicates ability of kidneys to excrete creatinine. Serum creatinine gives rough estimate of glomerular filtration rate.	No specific preparation is needed for test. Diet and metabolic rate have little effect on serum creatinine value.
Blood urea nitrogen	5-20 mg/100 ml	Test indicates ability of kidneys to excrete nitrogenous wastes.	Blood urea nitrogen can be affected by high-protein diet, blood in gastrointestinal tract, hepatic disease, medications, hydration status, and catabolic state (injury, infection, fever, poor nutrition).
Urine tests			
Urine specific gravity	1.010-1.026	Test measures ability of kidneys to concentrate urine.	First morning void usually is in the high normal range in healthy person. False high is caused by presence of radiographic dyes.
Urine osmolality	500-800 mOsm/L	Test is excellent indication of renal function. Osmolality is total concentration of particles in solution.	No special preparation needed.
Fishberg concentration test	Urine volume: 300/ml/12 hr Specific gravity: 1.024 or greater Urine osmolality: 850 mOsm or greater	Test used to determine ability of kidney to conserve fluid and to establish differential diagnosis for diabetes insipidus and psychogenic polydipsia.	No fluid can be taken during test period. Test period is 8-12 hr, usually during night. First morning void ensures maximal concentration. Three hourly urine specimens are collected for volume, specific gravity, and osmolality after test period. Patient should be observed for signs of vascular collapse.
Urine chemistry	Sodium: 100-260 mEq/24 hr Potassium: 39-90 mg/24 hr Calcium: 100-300 mg/24 hr	Urine electrolytes reflect ability of kidney to excrete and resorb electrolytes	Abnormal results may be caused by disease processes other than renal disorders, for example, elevated urine calcium in hyperparathyroidism or prolonged immobilization.
Creatinine clearance	Men: 90-140 ml/min Women: 85-125 ml/min	Results provide rate at which kidneys remove creatinine from plasma. Because diet and metabolic state have little influence on it, creatinine clearance provides a rough estimate of glomerular filtration rate.	See Guidelines for Safe Practice box on p. 1196 for collecting a timed urine specimen.

24-hour collections being the most common. The pooled urine specimen is examined for sugar, protein, sediment (blood cells and casts), 17-ketosteroids, electrolytes, catecholamines, and breakdown products of protein metabolism. These tests provide information on (1) the ability of the kidneys to excrete and conserve various solutes, (2) the production of various hormones that are excreted in the urine, (3) changes in the body's regulation of glucose metabolism, (4) identification of organisms difficult to recognize through routine urine cultures, and (5) the presence of abnormal cells and debris in the urine.

The accuracy of findings in a timed urine collection depends on proper collection of the specimen. Whether the specimen is to be obtained in the hospital or in the home, the person needs to be told exactly how to collect it. Instructions for collecting a timed urine specimen are found in the Guidelines for Safe Practice box, p. 1196, right.

Timed urine tests also may involve collecting urine from more than one source. The person may pass urine from the urethra and also drain urine from a nephrostomy tube. In addition, urine may drain from ureteral catheters, with urine being collected separately from each kidney. Depending on the

TABLE 38-5 Urinalysis Findings

Test	Normal	Abnormal
Color	Amber-yellow	Red indicates hematuria (possibly urinary obstruction, renal calculi, tumor, kidney failure, cystitis).
Clarity	Clear	Cloudy: debris, bacterial sediment (UTI)
pH	4.6-8.0 (average 6.0)	Alkaline on standing or with UTI Increased acidity with renal tubular acidosis
Specific gravity	1.010-1.026	Usually reflects fluid intake; the less the fluid intake, the higher the specific gravity If specific gravity remains low (1.010-1.014), renal disease or pituitary disease (deficit of ADH) is suspected.
Protein	0-8 mg/dl	Proteinuria may occur with high-protein diet and exercise (particularly prolonged). Seen in renal disease
Sugar	0	Glycosuria occurs after high intake of sugar or with diabetes mellitus.
Ketones	0	Ketonuria occurs with starvation and diabetic ketoacidosis.
Red blood cells	0-4	Injury to kidney tissue (see Color above)
White blood cells	0-5	UTI
Casts	0	UTI, renal disease

UTI, Urinary tract infection.

Guidelines for Safe Practice

Collecting a Midstream Urine Specimen

EQUIPMENT NEEDED

Sterile container for the urine

Three sponges (cotton or gauze) saturated with cleansing solution

GENERAL DIRECTIONS

Touch only the outside of collecting container

Collect urine in container well after urinary stream is started

SPECIAL DIRECTIONS

Female

Keep labia separated throughout procedure

Cleanse meatus with one front-to-back motion with each of three cleansing sponges

Male

Retract foreskin if man is uncircumcised

Cleanse glans with each of three cleansing sponges

Guidelines for Safe Practice

Collecting a Timed Urine Specimen

1. Instruct the patient to empty the bladder and discard the urine at the appointed time to start the test.
2. Save the urine from all subsequent voidings.
3. Provide specific directions for storing the urine. Some specimens need to be kept cold during the collection period, some need preservatives, and some need no special care.
4. Instruct the patient to void into a separate receptacle before defecating to avoid contaminating the specimen.
5. Instruct the patient to empty the bladder and add the urine to the collection at the appointed time to end the test.
6. Send the designated amount (properly labeled) to the laboratory.
7. If an aliquot (5-10 ml sample of the total specimen) is the designated amount, measure the total amount collected and record, and mix the specimen well before the aliquot is removed.

purpose of the test, the urine collected from each source may be collected in separate containers or combined.

Clearance Tests. When renal disease is suspected, the physician will want to determine the amount of damage, if any, that has already occurred. Clearance tests are the most practical and efficient way to identify losses in renal function. These tests measure the amount of blood that a person's kidneys can "clear" of a substance in a given amount of time. When the results are compared with normal values, changes in renal function become apparent. Clearance tests also are used to monitor the direction of change and the rate of change in renal function over time.

The creatinine clearance test is the most practical and widely used of all clearance tests. Creatinine is a substance that results from the breakdown of muscle tissue. Produced at a relatively fixed and uniform rate throughout the day, creatinine can be measured readily in the blood, and it is not influenced by dietary intake. Creatinine is excreted through the kidneys; it is filtered in the glomerulus and passes practically unchanged through the renal tubules. Creatinine is an ideal naturally occurring substance that, when blood and urine values are compared, allows an estimation of changes in glomerular filtration rates and overall kidney function. A person's creatinine clearance value is expressed in terms of milliliters per minute and is determined according to the following formula:

$$\text{Creatinine clearance (ml/min)} = \text{Urine volume (ml/min)} \times \frac{\text{Urine creatinine concentration mg/ml}}{\text{Plasma creatinine concentration mg/ml}}$$

The Coclcroft and Gault equation (CGE) may also be used to assess kidney function. No urine collection is necessary for the CGE. The equation is

$$\text{Creatinine clearance (ml/min)} = \frac{(140\text{-age}) \times (\text{IBW}) \times 0.85 \text{ if female}}{72 \times \text{SCR}}$$

where IBW is ideal body weight (kg) (men = 50 kg + 2.3 kg/in over 5 ft; women = 45.5 kg + 2.3 kg/in over 5 ft) and SCR is serum creatinine.

A morning-to-morning 24-hour urine collection is obtained. Immediately after the final urine specimen is collected, a blood specimen is drawn to determine the serum creatinine level. Both blood and urine specimens are sent together for analysis. Analysis of the total urine volume for the test period is essential to accurately determine renal function. If one void is accidentally discarded, the test must be repeated. Accurate collection of all urine in the prescribed time is essential for the validity of the test. A shorter time period may be used in instances in which it is not possible to obtain an accurate 24-hour urine collection.

The sodium excretion test measures tubular function. Specifically this test provides information about the kidneys' ability to appropriately excrete or conserve sodium; in chronic kidney failure either inappropriate retention or excretion of sodium can occur. Knowledge of urinary excretion of this electrolyte is helpful in calculating the patient's sodium intake requirements. Current and past sodium excretion studies are compared to determine changes in tubular function. The test is performed by analyzing the sodium content of a 24-hour urine collection.

Radiologic Tests

A number of radiologic examinations are used to visualize the urinary tract (Table 38-6). Because the kidneys lie retroperitoneally, any accumulation of flatus or feces in the intestine can obstruct the view on the x-ray film. To ensure adequate visualization, bowel cleansing is necessary before the x-ray films are taken.

X-ray films of the urinary tract may be ordered in conjunction with other abdominal studies. Visualizing the urinary tract may be difficult if the patient has recently undergone barium studies. This problem can be prevented by performing urinary tract examinations before barium contrast studies of the gastrointestinal tract.

Special Tests

Evaluation of Bladder Function

Measurement of Residual Urine. Normally the bladder contains little or no urine after voiding; however, certain disease states prevent the bladder from emptying completely. Some common conditions associated with incomplete emptying of the bladder are benign prostatic hypertrophy, urethral strictures, and interruptions in bladder innervation (neurogenic bladder). Urine remaining in the bladder after voiding is called *residual* urine.

One way to determine the amount of residual urine is to catheterize the person immediately after voiding. This may be performed on a one-time basis or repeated with each void. If the residual volume is large, a Foley catheter may be left in place. Residual urine volumes of 50 ml or less indicate near-normal or returning bladder function.

To avoid inserting a catheter, an x-ray film examination of retained urine may be performed. A radiopaque substance is injected intravenously. As the dye is excreted in the urine, it passes into the bladder. A sufficient amount of urine containing the radiopaque material is allowed to accumulate in the bladder, and the person is then instructed to void. An x-ray film is taken and any urine retained in the bladder will be visualized on the x-ray film. This means of determining residual urine is used in conjunction with other studies requiring visualization of the urinary tract.

Cystometrography

Cystometric examination is performed to evaluate bladder tone. The examination is indicated in the presence of incontinence or evidence of neurologic dysfunction of the bladder. A Foley catheter is inserted before the examination. With the person in a supine position, a liter bag of normal saline or sterile distilled water and a cystometer are connected to the catheter. Fluid is instilled at a constant and specified rate; measurements of the pressure that the bladder musculature exerts on the fluid are recorded after the instillation of every 50 ml of fluid. The person is asked to report feelings of fullness, the need to void, and any urgency or discomfort. Fluid is instilled until urgency occurs or sensation is determined to be absent. During cystometric examination a cholinergic drug (bethanechol chloride or urecholine) may be administered to determine its effect on enhancing the tone of a flaccid bladder, or anticholinergic medication may be given to assess relaxation in a hyperactive bladder. No specific care is required after cystometric examination.

Other urodynamic tests may be used to evaluate the neuromuscular function of the urinary sphincter. Electromyography (EMG) aids in the assessment of functional or psychologic voiding disturbances. Electromyography may also be used to evaluate sphincter tone and determine whether nerve pathways are intact.

Kidney Biopsy

Kidney or renal biopsy is the most accurate diagnostic tool for determining the type and stage of a pathologic condition involving the kidneys. This test aids in differentiating diagnoses, following the progression of disease processes, assisting in selection of therapy, and determining prognosis of the illness. The biopsy can be performed either through a skin puncture (percutaneous) or through an incision (open renal biopsy) over the kidney.

Because the kidney is such a vascular organ, hemorrhage after a biopsy is a potential threat. Throughout the procedure, care is taken to prevent and detect early blood loss. Before biopsy is performed, a thorough medical evaluation with particular attention to any abnormality in bleeding or coagulation time is completed. Medications that alter clotting function are held. These include aspirin, nonsteroidal antiinflammatory

TABLE 38-6 Common Radiologic and Special Tests of the Urinary Tract

Purpose	Procedure	Pretest Preparation/Posttest Care
Retrograde Pyelography		
Visualization of urinary tract	1. Ureteral catheterization required 2. Radiopaque material (Hypaque, Renografin) gently injected 3. X-ray films taken of renal collecting structures	Patient may experience discomfort in region of kidneys as dye is injected. Pain may be experienced if too large a volume of dye is injected and renal pelvis becomes distended.
Intravenous Pyelography (IVP)		
Determination of size and location of kidneys, degree of obstruction Demonstration of presence of cysts, renal stones or tumors Outline of filling of renal pelvis Outline of ureters and bladder	1. X-ray film of abdomen (KUB) taken to identify size and position of kidneys 2. Radiopaque dye given intravenously 3. X-ray films of kidneys taken at 3-, 5-, 10-, and 20-min intervals	Bowel cleansing is required. Inform patient that a feeling of warmth, flushing of the face, and a salty taste in the mouth may occur as the dye is injected. Inform patient that numerous x-ray films are taken during the procedure; this does not indicate a problem. Patient is assessed before the test for any history of allergy to iodine, shellfish, or dyes and is carefully monitored for signs and symptoms of a reaction to the dye, including respiratory distress, diaphoresis, urticaria, instability of vital signs, or unusual sensations. Emergency equipment should be available. Fluids are forced after the test to help excrete the contrast material and prevent kidney failure.
Kidney, Ureter, and Bladder (KUB) X-Ray Films		
Gross visualization of KUB Location of calcifications and stones possible	X-ray plain film of abdominal region obtained	Bowel cleansing sometimes is ordered.
Computed Tomography (CT) Scan		
Visualization of kidneys and renal circulation using an x-ray beam rotated around body Gold standard for diagnosis of renal stones Stages and evaluates renal cell carcinoma and renal vein thrombosis	Whole body CT scanner segments kidneys Can be performed with IV contrast dye	If dye is used, the same implications apply as listed for IVP.
Magnetic Resonance Imaging (MRI)		
Gold standard for diagnosis of renal vein thrombosis	Uses electromagnetic energy to provide visualization of structures No dye needed No radiation	Contraindicated with cardiac pacemakers, implanted metallic clips, some heart valves, and life support devices. May need sedation. Patient must lie still in confined space for 30-90 minutes. Prepare patient for sounds from pulsing of magnetic field during scanning.
Renal Angiography		
Visualization of renal circulation Particularly useful in evaluating renal artery stenosis and polyarteritis nodosa	Similar to IVP; however, contrast dye is often injected directly into femoral artery by passing catheter through artery to level of renal arteries.	Nursing implications are the same as for IVP. Patient must be observed for dye-induced acute kidney failure and bleeding at arterial puncture site, especially within first 4 hr. The pressure dressing should be checked for fresh bleeding. The puncture site should be checked for tenderness or swelling. Vital signs and distal pulses must be assessed frequently (q15min for 3-4 hr). Bed rest should be maintained for 8 hr after the procedure.

TABLE 38-6 Common Radiologic and Special Tests of the Urinary Tract—cont'd

Purpose	Procedure	Pretest Preparation/Posttest Care
Isotope Glomerlular Filtration Rate		
Uses an isotope that is eliminated by kidney to accurately measure glomerular filtration rate	Radioisotope is injected and blood samples collected for 4-6 hr to track clearance of isotope.	Reassure the patient that only trace doses of the isotope are used, and there is no risk related to radioactivity.
Ultrasound		
Uses sound waves to determine size and texture of kidneys Test of choice to exclude urinary tract obstruction Can grossly differentiate cystic and solid masses	Sound waves reflect off kidneys and computer interprets different tissue densities.	Procedure is painless and noninvasive. A full bladder is required to delineate the abdominal structures.

drugs, platelet inhibitors, and warfarin. The patient's blood usually is typed and cross-matched for 2 units of blood. The risk of bleeding is greatest in the first 12 hours after biopsy.[5,6]

Preparation before either type of biopsy includes discussing the procedure with the patient and answering any questions the patient may have. Informed consent is required before any invasive procedure. The biopsy may be performed in the patient's room, the operating room, or in the radiology department.

The procedure for percutaneous (closed) renal biopsy is as follows. Before the biopsy, the patient is taken to the radiology department for localization of the kidney. This is accomplished with a plain film, a dye contrast film, or fluoroscopic location. The lower pole of the kidney is located and marked on the skin in ink. The lower pole is the site for obtaining the biopsy specimen because it contains the fewest blood vessels. The patient is then transported to the area where the biopsy will be performed. The biopsy may be performed blindly or with computed tomography to guide the placement of the biopsy needle.

Sedation usually is not required except for patients who are restless and unable to relax sufficiently to follow instructions during the procedure. The patient is placed in a prone position over a sandbag or firm pillow. The physician identifies the location for biopsy, and a local anesthetic agent is injected. As the biopsy needle is inserted, the patient is instructed to take a breath and hold it because the kidneys move up and down with respiration. Feelings of pressure or pain may be felt in the kidney region as the needle punctures the tough renal capsule. The needle is withdrawn immediately, and direct pressure is applied to the site for 20 minutes. A pressure dressing is then applied, and the patient is turned supine and kept flat for at least 4 hours. A small sandbag may be placed over the biopsy site to help prevent bleeding. The nursing care associated with renal biopsy is summarized in the Guidelines for Safe Practice box.

An open biopsy carries less risk of hemorrhage and provides better visualization of the kidney. However, it is a more invasive procedure with associated risks of anesthesia, wound infection, and longer recovery time.

The procedure for an open biopsy is similar to that used in kidney surgery. The nursing care for this type of surgery is discussed in Chapter 39. Most biopsies are performed by the percutaneous method.

Guidelines for Safe Practice

Care of the Patient After Percutaneous Renal Biopsy

1. Bed rest must be maintained with the patient flat, in a supine position, and motionless for 4 hours after the biopsy.
2. Coughing should be avoided for first 4 hours after the biopsy because it increases abdominal venous pressure.
3. Blood pressure and pulse should be taken on the following schedule:
   a. Every 15 minutes for 1 hour
   b. Every 30 minutes for 1 hour
   c. Every hour for additional 2 hours or until stable
   The responsible physician should be notified of increases in pulse of more than 10 to 20 beats/min above the baseline or decreases in blood pressure of more than 10 mm Hg, unless the physician instructs otherwise.
4. Bed rest should be maintained for 24 hours.
5. Urine is observed for hematuria for first 24 hours after the biopsy.
6. Patient should be instructed to:
   a. Avoid heavy lifting and strenuous activities for 10 to 14 days after the biopsy.
   b. Increase fluid intake unless contraindicated; and report any signs of renal bleeding or infection.

Endoscopy

Technologic advances make it possible to visualize the urinary tract directly and indirectly. Endoscopy allows for assessment of both structure and function of the organs and tissues of the urinary tract. Visualization of the urinary tract is used not only for diagnosis, but also for evaluation of the patient's response to therapy over time.

Cystoscopy

Cystoscopy is the direct examination of the bladder with an instrument called a cystoscope (Figure 38-6). The cystoscope relies on a flexible optic fiber to provide illumination in the urinary tract. The instrument is attached to the light source and then slowly passed through the urinary tract, enabling direct visualization of the urethra, ureteral orifices, and bladder. Informed consent is required before the procedure. The patient is asked to drink 2 to 3 L of fluid 2 hours before the procedure to ensure a continuous flow of urine in the event specimens need to be collected. If the patient is to receive general anesthesia, the fluids may be administered intravenously. If x-ray films are to be taken during the procedure, bowel preparation is ordered.

The cystoscopic examination may be performed with or without anesthesia. General anesthesia is rarely required for cystoscopy, but it may be used if the person is unable to cooperate and the procedure is absolutely necessary. The need for painful manipulation during the procedure may also necessitate general anesthesia. In these instances anesthesia reduces the possibility of urethral trauma or bladder perforation caused by the patient's sudden vigorous movement during the examination.

Much of the discomfort felt during this procedure is the result of contraction or spasm of the bladder sphincters; this can be decreased through deep-breathing exercises and general relaxation. A sedative such as diazepam (Valium) or midazolam (Versed) and an opioid such as morphine or meperidine hydrochloride (Demerol) usually are given an hour before the examination. This type of analgesia is the most common option.

If the patient is relatively comfortable, the cystoscope should be passed with little pain, provided there is no obstruction in the urethra. A local anesthetic such as procaine (usually 4%) may be instilled into the urethra before insertion of the cystoscope.

When the patient is awake, passing the instrument is followed immediately by a strong desire to void. This occurs as a result of the pressure the instrument exerts against the internal sphincter. During the examination the bladder is distended with normal saline for visualization. As the bladder becomes increasingly distended, the urge to void increases.

During cystoscopic examination a number of additional tests may be performed. *Cystography* involves the injection of a radiopaque dye such as methiodal (Skiodan) or air as a contrast medium to visualize the bladder and determine its size, shape, and irregularities. Bladder capacity can be measured through instillation of distilled water. A voiding *cystourethrogram* can reveal reflux of urine into the ureters on voiding, a bladder malfunction that can lead to pyelonephritis.

Ureteral catheterization (with a nylon, radiopaque, size 4 to 6 F catheter) can be performed through the cystoscope. The catheter is inserted into the ureteral opening in the bladder, carefully advanced up the ureter, and into the renal pelvis (Figure 38-7). This procedure may involve one or both ureters. Ureteral catheterization is performed (1) when culture and analysis of urine from individual kidneys is required, (2) when tests of renal function are to be performed on the kidneys separately, and (3) when visualization of the urinary tract is desired, and intravenous pyelogram visualization has been inadequate, obstruction is present, or sensitivity to intravenous radiopaque material is noted.

The nurse validates the person's understanding of the procedure as part of the pretest teaching. If local anesthesia is to be used, the nurse must be certain to describe what the patient can expect to feel during the procedure. The patient should not stand or walk alone immediately after cystoscopic examination. Prolonged lithotomy positioning can cause orthostatic hypotension.

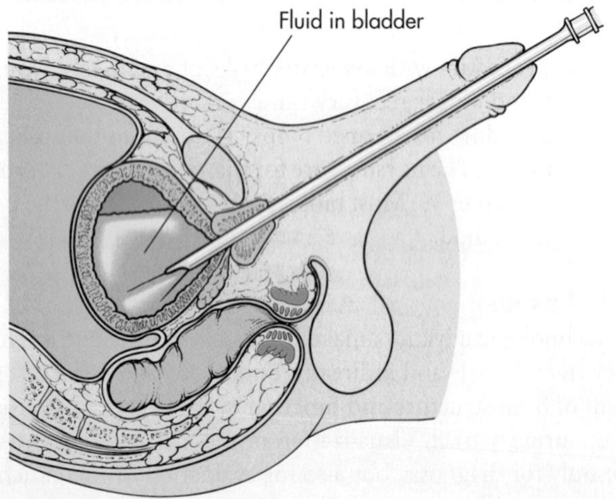

Figure 38-6 Cystoscope inserted for examination of the bladder.

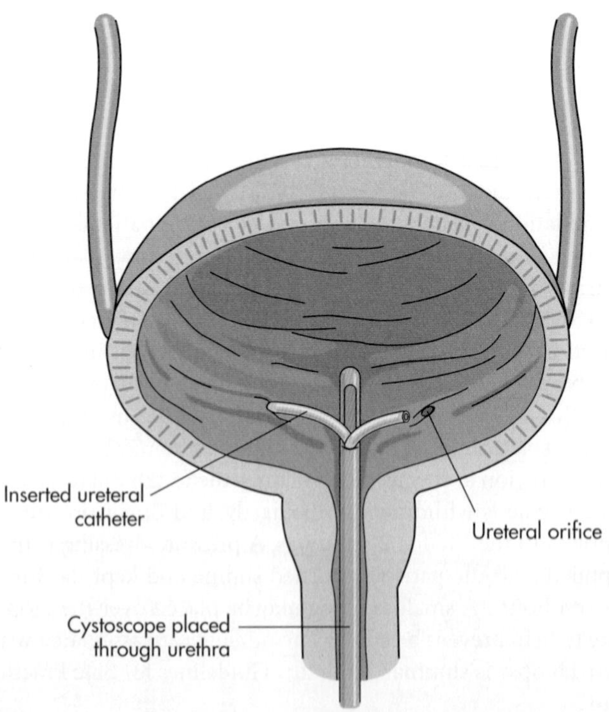

Figure 38-7 Ureteral catheterization through cystoscope. Note ureteral catheter inserted into left orifice. Right ureteral catheter is ready to be inserted.

Guidelines for Safe Practice

Care of the Patient After Cystoscopy

1. If the procedure was done under general anesthesia or if a medication such as midazolam (Versed) has been used for relaxation and sedation, the first priority is to ensure that vital signs are stable and that the patient has a patent airway immediately postprocedure.
2. Ensure a comfortable transition to the recovery area. If patient does not have an indwelling catheter ask if he or she needs to void. If the patient does not void, check the bladder for distention and discomfort. If a catheter is in place and no urine is flowing, check the bladder for distention and the catheter and tubing for clots or kinking.
3. If the patient has a full bladder follow physician's order for catheterization. If the catheter is obstructed follow standard guidelines and orders for irrigation or catheter change.
4. Once urine is flowing check for signs of frank bleeding from the bladder. If the urine is grossly bloody, recheck pulse and blood pressure (and hematocrit if possible) and have the urologist evaluate whether this is expected bleeding or excessive bleeding. NOTE: Some bleeding is normal but excessive continuous bleeding indicates serious trauma to the bladder wall, perhaps even bladder perforation, and should be recognized and treated promptly. This complication is rare but possible.
5. Medicate for pain as ordered if vital signs permit. Pain should not be severe but might be mild to moderate once sedation wears off.
6. Explain to the patient and family that anytime an instrument is passed into the bladder it is possible that an infection might develop. Tell them to report any signs of infection or bleeding. Describe these to the patient.
7. Monitor urine output and make sure that it is consistent with intake.
8. The patient is discharged when bleeding is minimal, and he or she is awake, voiding normally, and has stable vital signs. There may be mild pain with urination for a short time postprocedure.
9. Make sure that the patient has either a follow-up appointment or a number to call to reach the clinic or doctor.

The patient needs to be observed for three complications of cystoscopic examination: bleeding, bladder perforation, and infection. Observation for frank bleeding (pink-tinged urine is normal) is necessary. Urinary output and voiding pattern are monitored to detect obstruction, and fluid intake is increased to prevent urine stasis. Mild analgesics are given for discomfort, and warmth is provided if the patient complains of being chilled. Vital signs are monitored as necessary. The patient should be informed that the first void after cystoscopic examination may be uncomfortable. Warm sitz baths may provide comfort. See the Guidelines for Safe Practice box for a summary of associated nursing care.

References

1. Brenner BM, Rector FC: *Brenner's and Rector's the kidney,* ed 6, Philadelphia, 2000, WB Saunders.
2. Guyton AC, Hall JE: *Textbook of medical physiology,* ed 10, Philadelphia, 2000, WB Saunders.
3. Lancaster LE: *Core curriculum for nephrology nursing,* ed 4, Pittman, NJ, 2001, Anthony J. Jannetti.
4. McCance KL, Huether SE: *Pathophysiology: the biologic basis for disease in adults and children,* ed 4, St Louis, 2002, Mosby.
5. Post TW, Rose BD: Approach to the patient with renal disease including acute renal failure, 2001, website: http://www.uptodate.com.
6. Rose BD: Indications for and complications of renal biopsy, 2001, website: http://www.uptodate.com.
7. Schrier RW: *Renal and electrolyte disorders,* ed 5, Philadelphia, 1997, Lippincott-Raven.

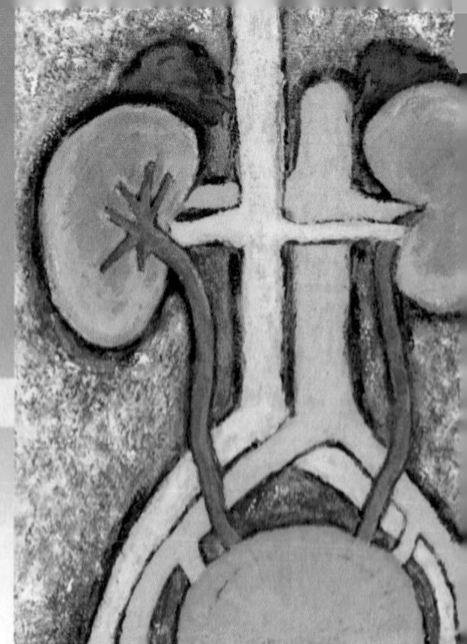

39 Kidney and Urinary Tract Problems

Carol Genet Kelley, Kelly A. Weigel, Cynthia Hollamon

Objectives

After studying this chapter, the learner should be able to:

1. Discuss the major health problems of the urinary system.
2. Discuss the pathophysiology and management of polycystic kidney disease.
3. Describe the etiology, pathophysiology, and management of lower urinary tract infections and pyelonephritis, including the importance of public awareness and patient teaching.
4. Compare glomerulonephritis and the nephrotic syndrome in relation to pathophysiology, clinical manifestations, and management.
5. Discuss the common vascular and obstructive problems of the kidney.
6. Discuss the common cancers of the urinary tract.
7. Implement management strategies for persons requiring urinary catheterization.
8. Explain the causes and treatments of renal calculi.
9. Differentiate types of urinary incontinence and their management.
10. Develop a plan of care for patients undergoing urinary diversion surgery.
11. Contrast the common types of urinary diversion procedures and management of urinary stomas.

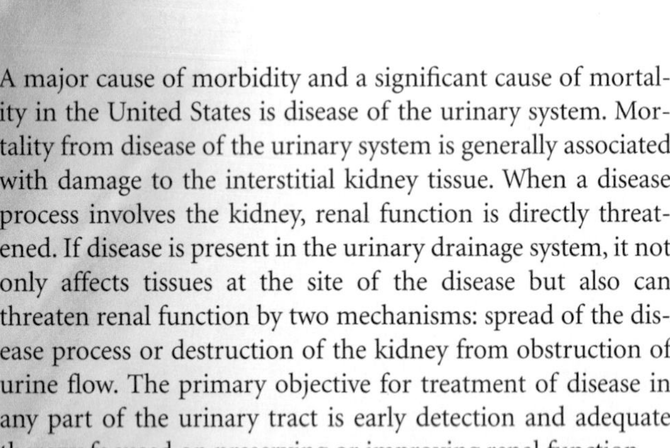

A major cause of morbidity and a significant cause of mortality in the United States is disease of the urinary system. Mortality from disease of the urinary system is generally associated with damage to the interstitial kidney tissue. When a disease process involves the kidney, renal function is directly threatened. If disease is present in the urinary drainage system, it not only affects tissues at the site of the disease but also can threaten renal function by two mechanisms: spread of the disease process or destruction of the kidney from obstruction of urine flow. The primary objective for treatment of disease in any part of the urinary tract is early detection and adequate therapy focused on preserving or improving renal function.

Nurses can provide valuable assistance in significantly reducing morbidity related to the urinary system. This can be achieved by (1) increasing public awareness of preventive measures, (2) assisting in early detection of signs and symptoms of renal disease, (3) providing ongoing health teaching for persons with renal disease, and (4) providing long-term care to the growing population of chronically ill individuals with diseases of the urinary system. This chapter describes common disorders of the urinary system and their management. Diseases of the prostate are covered in Chapter 55.

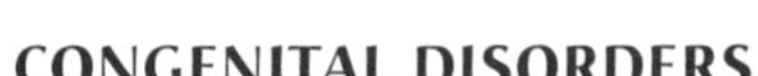

CONGENITAL DISORDERS

Approximately one third of all congenital abnormalities affect the genitourinary tract.[18] These deviations range in severity from minor anomalies that do not require correction to those that are incompatible with life. Box 39-1 lists some of the congenital malformations of the lower urinary tract. Details about the management of congenital disorders can be found in most pediatric nursing texts. However, renal cystic disorders, congenital conditions of the upper urinary tract, contribute to significant adult morbidity and are discussed in this chapter.

Polycystic Kidney Disease

Etiology

Renal cystic disorders encompass a relatively large group of diseases typified by the formation of one or more fluid-filled cavities within the kidneys. Cysts can arise in all parts of the kidney. Renal cysts may develop in utero, may be acquired after birth, or may be hereditary. Cysts may be slightly larger than a single nephron in their formative stage, or they may be so large as to compress the abdominal viscera.

Renal cysts may be benign or may compromise function, causing kidney failure. Cysts may be the primary renal disorder

BOX 39-1 Congenital Malformation of the Lower Urinary Tract

Duplication of ureters	Partial or complete
Hydroureters	Dilation of ureters
Exstrophy of urinary bladder	Eversion of bladder on outer abdominal wall
Hypospadias	Opening of urethra on underside of penis (Figure 39-1, *A*)
Epispadias	Opening of urethra on dorsum of penis (Figure 39-1, *B*)

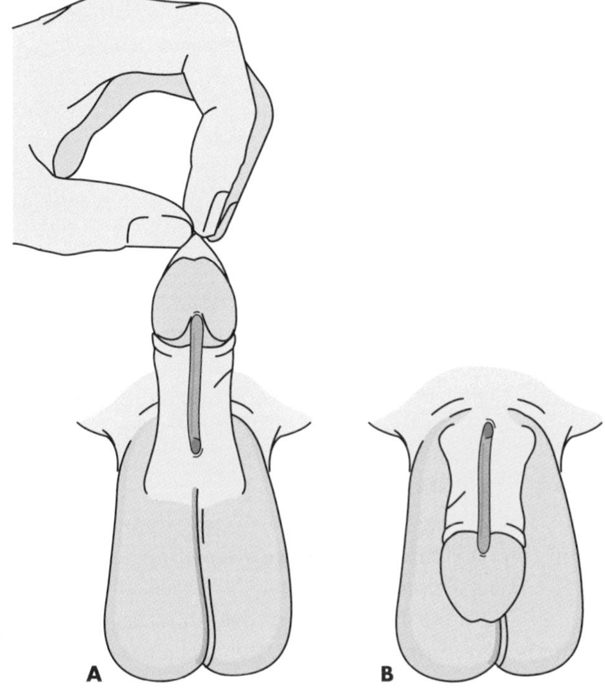

Figure 39-1 **A**, Hypospadias. **B**, Epispadias.

or may appear with nonrenal disorders. Cysts cause three major categories of diseases: polycystic, cystic, and medullary. Cystic kidney disease includes simple cysts, which are commonly seen in patients over 50 years and acquired cystic kidney disease seen in patients with either kidney disease (e.g., glomerulonephritis) or other disease that affects the kidney (e.g., diabetes). Medullary cystic kidney disease is a rare inherited disorder. Only polycystic kidney disease is discussed in detail here.

Epidemiology

There are two inherited forms of polycystic kidney disease (autosomal-dominant and autosomal-recessive) and one noninherited form (acquired cystic kidney disease). Autosomal-dominant polycystic kidney disease (ADPKD) is the most common form and is the focus of this discussion. The majority of cases of ADPKD are associated with a PKD1 gene located on chromosome 16. ADPKD is one of the five leading causes of kidney failure. It affects between 1:500 and 1:1000 live births in all racial groups, regardless of gender worldwide.

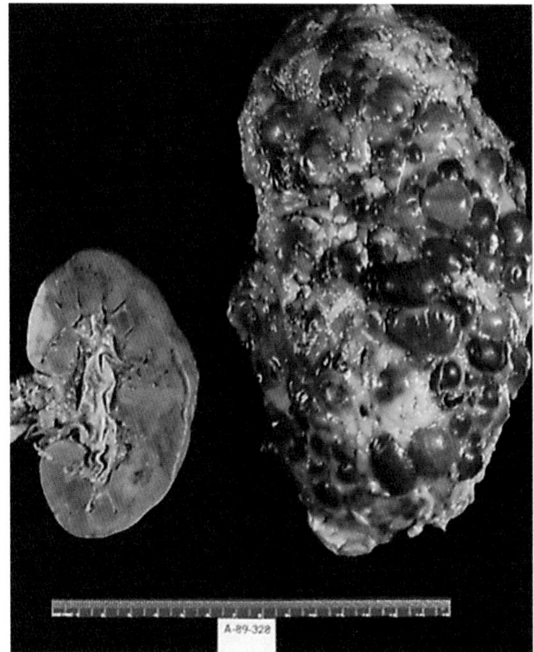

Figure 39-2 Polycystic kidneys.

In the United States about 500,000 people have ADPKD.[19] There is some variability in gene expression that accounts for some individuals developing symptomatic disease by age 20 and others who die of unrelated problems later in life.

Pathophysiology

ADPKD affects both kidneys in the majority of patients. Cysts are diffusely scattered through the renal parenchyma, with islands of normal tissue between them (Figure 39-2). The cysts arise from all segments of the nephron and collecting system. Cysts can range in size from a few millimeters to several centimeters. The kidneys can be five times normal size and are studded with cysts of various sizes. One of the most devastating features is that ADPKD undergoes relentless progression to end-stage kidney failure in a high percentage of patients, usually in the fourth or fifth decade of life. Loss of renal function occurs as the cysts enlarge and compress adjacent parenchyma, causing ischemia of surrounding tissue. The process of cyst formation begins with increased division of epithelial cells within a few renal tubule cells. This causes enlargement of the tubule and formation of "cysts." Cystic enlargement also causes occlusion of the normal tubules.

In addition to renal cysts, persons with ADPKD may develop cysts in the liver, pancreas, and spleen. As many as 10% to 20% of patients have cerebral and abdominal aneurysms.[20] Abdominal and inguinal hernias are relatively common in patients with ADPKD.

Abdominal or flank pain and hematuria are the most common early symptoms in patients with ADPKD. The pain is often caused by bleeding into the cyst. It may be a dull aching, a vague sense of heaviness, or knifelike and stabbing. Hematuria is seen when a cyst ruptures in the renal pelvis. Patients are prone to cyst infections and serious infections of the kidney parenchyma manifested by pain, fever, leukocytosis, pyuria, and positive blood and urine cultures. Hypertension develops in approximately 50% of patients at some time in the course of the disease. Hypertension often antedates measurable functional renal impairment by several years. If hypertension is uncontrolled, renal destruction is accelerated. Later in the disease, some patients notice increased abdominal girth and in many cases the kidneys can be palpated.

Collaborative Care Management

An ultrasound that shows five or more total cysts distributed through both kidneys can confirm the diagnosis in patients with a consistent family history. Computed tomography (CT) or magnetic resonance imaging (MRI) can be used for those patients when the results of the ultrasound are unclear.

Because there is no therapy directed at the disease process, the goals of management are to alleviate symptoms and slow the onset of renal dysfunction. Hypertension should be controlled since it has been shown to be associated with a more rapid decline in renal function compared with patients without hypertension. Diets limited in protein and salt, as well as the avoidance of nephrotoxic drugs, also appear to help in lengthening the functional duration of the kidneys.[19] Infections are treated vigorously with antibiotics because scarring may lead to further progression of the disease. Antibiotics are usually taken until renal pain resolves and the urine clears of pus, which may take several months. When infection is difficult to eradicate with oral antibiotics, parenteral antibiotics are started. When patients are admitted to the hospital, intake and output should be closely monitored.

Analgesics may be used to help control flank pain. Surgical aspiration or laparoscopic decompression of cysts has been found to improve discomfort, but not slow the progression of the disease. When urinary bleeding from ruptured cysts becomes severe, bed rest is often instituted. Bed rest and increased hydration are usually instituted for patients who have visible blood in their urine (gross hematuria).

Because polycystic disease leads to chronic kidney failure, ongoing support and health teaching are essential nursing interventions. The patient is instructed to be alert to signs and symptoms of infection and bleeding. The emotional overtones of this illness can be severe for both the individual and the family. Challenges exist in helping the person deal with an illness on an individual basis when relatives have died of the same disease, and children have not yet developed symptoms. Counseling may be required about family health care and the individual's role in passing on a potentially fatal disease to children. Patients are instructed to monitor urine output and report changes to their physician.

Most patients require no modification in physical activity or lifestyle until they approach the end stage of their illness. Because recurrent hematuria may be related to direct trauma and associated with a faster decline in renal function, patients should probably refrain from strenuous activity that could involve trauma to the abdomen.

Patient/Family Education. Patients and their families should be instructed on the long-term complications and typical disease progression of ADPKD. Although ADPKD cannot be prevented, persons should be informed that measures such as control of hypertension might slow the progression of disease. It is important that the patient be able to identify early signs of infection so that treatment can begin as soon as possible.

Prevention is the key to decreasing the incidence of ADPKD. Prevention occurs only by prospectively identifying those with the disorder so that they may have an opportunity to determine whether to bear children. Because it is an autosomal-dominant disorder, patients with the gene may expect that each child will have a 50/50 chance of having the disease.

The family history is a crucial part of the counseling process. Family members may be unwilling to reveal or may not know if other family members have had this disease. Often persons do not learn they have the ADPKD gene until beyond the childbearing period. Finally, the early discovery of a potentially disabling or life-threatening disease in a young person may affect future employability and insurability. These factors must be carefully discussed with the individual before screening for ADPKD.

INFLAMMATORY DISORDERS

The kidneys are susceptible to inflammation caused by bacterial infection, altered immune response, drugs and other chemicals, toxins, and radiation. Inflammation may be acute or chronic.

Urinary Tract Infections

Urinary tract infections (UTIs), the most common infections affecting humans throughout their lifespan, are an inflammation of some portion of the urinary tract usually caused by bacteria. UTIs are commonly described in terms of location, symptoms, and complications. A lower UTI affects the urinary bladder (cystitis), prostate (prostatitis), or urethra (urethritis). An upper UTI affects the renal parenchyma and renal pelvis (pyelonephritis). UTIs are considered uncomplicated in persons without structural or functional abnormalities of their voiding mechanisms and in those who respond readily to antibiotics. Complicated UTIs are seen in persons with anatomic or functional abnormalities of their voiding mechanisms and are difficult to treat because the organisms are less susceptible to antibiotics. Those with complicated UTIs also have a greater risk for spread of the infection to the blood (bacteremia) and damage to the kidneys.

Etiology

UTIs result from pathogenic bacteria invading one or more urinary tract structures. Although about 90% of UTIs are caused by a gram-negative rod, *Escherichia coli.*[34] Gram-positive cocci, such as *Staphylococcus* and *Streptococcus* also cause UTIs. There are many factors that place an individual at risk for a UTI (see Risk Factors box). Contrary to the beliefs of many, dietary practices, personal hygiene practices including wiping, and the use of tampons or tight clothing are not associated with a greater risk of development of a UTI.[41]

A major factor contributing to the development of a UTI in women is a short urethra, which facilitates the entry of or-

Risk Factors

Development of a Urinary Tract Infection

Obstruction to urinary flow
- Congenital anomalies
- Renal calculi
- Ureteral occlusion

Vesicoureteral reflux

Residual urine in the bladder
- Neurogenic bladder
- Urethral stricture
- Prostatic hypertrophy

Instrumentation of the urinary tract
- Indwelling urinary catheter
- Catheterization
- Urethral dilation
- Cystoscopy

Other
- Postmenopausal women
- Use of diaphragm and spermicide
- Pregnancy
- Sexual intercourse
- Delayed postcoital voiding

Guidelines for Safe Practice

Care of Indwelling Urinary Catheters

- Insert using proper sterile technique.
- Cleanse meatal catheter junction one to two times per day with an antimicrobial soap.
- Use a sterile closed drainage system and empty every 8 hours.
- Use sterile technique if the collecting system is opened for irrigations; however, do not irrigate regularly.
- Keep urine collection bags below the level of the bladder.
- Follow the institution policy for routine catheter change.

ganisms from the vagina and rectal area into the bladder. In men, the presence of zinc in the prostatic fluid acts as an antibacterial agent, which helps prevent UTIs. Men who are not circumcised have a greater incidence of developing a UTI than men who are circumcised

Bladder catheterization is responsible for a large number of hospital-acquired UTIs. Almost all persons with indwelling catheters develop a UTI within 3 to 4 days of catheterization.[41] New technologies such as antiinfective lubricants are currently being tested to decrease catheter-associated UTIs.[28]

Catheterization, even when performed without a break in aseptic technique, results in a significant rate of bladder infection (see Guidelines for Safe Practice box). Drug-resistant strains of *Staphylococcus* and *Pseudomonas* along with various other organisms typically found in hospitals are also frequently those involved in nosocomial UTIs. Prevention and control of all UTIs can be most significantly influenced through a lowering of the rate of nosocomial infection.

Epidemiology

UTIs account for more than 5 million office visits in the United States annually.[21] Because untreated UTIs can lead to more serious problems, they must be taken seriously. UTIs occur more frequently in women than men until after 50 years of age when the incidence for women and men is similar perhaps because of the age-related decrease in prostatic fluid that provides protection from a UTI for men.[26] Infection rates are approximately 1% in school-aged girls. This rate increases by approximately 1% per decade, up to almost 10% in elderly women.[21] The incidence increases to 30% for persons older than 80 years, either living at home or in a chronic care facility. Infection in the lower urinary tract increases the incidence of acute kidney infection (pyelonephritis) as the result of ascending microorganisms.

Pathophysiology

The mode of entry of bacteria into the genitourinary tract cannot always be traced with certainty; however, four major pathways exist:

1. *Ascending infection from the urethra.* This is the most common cause of genitourinary tract infection in men and women. Because the female urethra is short and rectal bacteria tend to colonize the perineum and vaginal vestibule, women are especially susceptible to ascending UTIs.
2. *Hematogenous spread.* This occurs infrequently, except in the case of tuberculosis, renal abscesses, and perinephric abscesses. Bacteremia is more likely to complicate a UTI when structural and functional abnormalities exist than when the urinary tract is normal.
3. *Lymphatogenous spread.* Rarely bacterial pathogens are thought to travel through lymphatics to the bladder, prostate, and female genitourinary tract.
4. *Direct extension from another organ.* This occurs with intraperitoneal abscesses, especially those associated with inflammatory bowel disease, fulminant pelvic inflammatory disease in women, paravesical abscesses, and genitourinary tract fistulae.

Structural and functional abnormalities of the urinary tract, obstruction to urine flow, and impaired bladder innervation increase risk of development of a UTI. Efficient emptying of the bladder decreases the number of bacteria and a protective layer within the bladder interferes with bacterial adherence. Whenever urinary stasis occurs, such as with incomplete emptying of the bladder, renal calculi, or genitourinary obstructions, the bacteria have a greater opportunity to grow. Urinary stasis also contributes to a more alkaline urine, which facilitates bacterial growth. During micturition, urine may flow back up the ureters (vesicoureteral reflux) and carry bacteria from the bladder up through the ureters to the kidney pelvis leading to pyelonephritis.

For bacteria to be able to colonize the urinary tract, organisms attach or adhere to the urothelium via rodlike structures called pili. In addition, bacteria may secrete a toxin that promotes their survival. Women who have a recurrent UTI may have receptors on the mucosa surface of their genitourinary tract; these receptors act as binding sites for bacteria and other pathogens.[33]

Symptoms that bring the person with a UTI to seek medical attention typically include frequency, urgency, dysuria (burning on urination), cloudy or foul-smelling urine, suprapubic discomfort, and hematuria. In asymptomatic persons, a UTI is identified only on routine examination of the urine.

Collaborative Care Management

Diagnostic Tests. Although a urine culture confirms the presence of infection, a urinalysis is useful for screening for a possible UTI in persons with symptoms (dysuria, urgency, and frequency). The presence of nitrites and leukocyte esterase indicates the presence of bacteria and white blood cells, respectively. A positive urine culture with colony counts in excess of 10^5 organisms/ml of urine in a properly obtained and stored midstream specimen (see Chapter 38) was considered the diagnostic standard for women with an uncomplicated UTI; however, 30% to 50% of women with an uncomplicated UTI have lower counts despite the presence of white blood cells (pyuria) on urinalysis.[37]

A urine culture is not routinely indicated in women with isolated episodes of frequency and dysuria. However a urine culture should be obtained for a first infection or for recurrent infection before drug therapy is initiated to confirm the organism's sensitivity to antimicrobials and to decrease the development of drug-resistant organisms. Because 24 to 48 hours are required to obtain results of urine cultures, an antibiotic that will cover the likely organisms may be prescribed until results are available. In most situations, it is not necessary to reculture the urine when the symptoms of a UTI have resolved after antibiotic therapy. A more extensive urologic workup is usually recommended for men with a first UTI episode, all patients with complicated infection or bacteremia, and those with suspected obstruction or renal stones. The rationale for the recommended workup in men is to assess for possible underlying anatomic problems because UTIs are not as common in men as they are in women. Ultrasound studies of the kidneys and pelvis are used during the initial workup if obstruction or other structural abnormalities are suspected. The intravenous pyelogram (IVP) had also been part of the urologic workup; however, CT with contrast has become the procedure of choice.

Medications. Antibiotics are not indicated for most asymptomatic bacteriuria (a condition in which large numbers of bacteria are present, but symptoms are not present) or those with indwelling catheters unless there are symptoms.[25] If a patient with a chronic indwelling catheter must be treated, the catheter should be replaced before antibiotics are started.[40] For uncomplicated UTIs antibiotics are usually given as a single dose or for 3 days. Persons who are pregnant, elderly, have diabetes, or have a recurrent UTI are usually treated for 7 days. Trimethoprim-sulfamethoxazole (Bactrim) and nitrofurantoin (Macrodantin) are considered first-line agents, as they are usually effective against the organisms that cause UTIs. These drugs have been the most widely used antibiotics for the treatment of an uncomplicated UTI in the outpatient setting.

Other agents may also be used to treat a UTI. The cephalosporins are usually reserved for culture-documented infections. Ampicillin and amoxicillin have fallen out of favor and are now ineffective against approximately 30% of common urinary pathogens. The fluoroquinolones (e.g., ciprofloxacin) are expensive and powerful antibiotics and should be reserved for the treatment of complicated UTIs and resistant organisms.[20]

Treatments. Additional treatment includes increasing fluid intake to 3 to 4 L/day unless contraindicated. Increased fluid intake helps to dilute the urine, lessen irritation and burning, and provide a continual flow of urine to minimize stasis and multiplication of bacteria in the urinary tract.

Diet/Activity. No special activity requirements are necessary. Cranberry juice (300 ml/day) is effective in decreasing asymptomatic bacteriuria in postmenopausal women.[42]

Referrals. Referrals are not indicated for uncomplicated UTIs. However, if UTIs are recurrent or complications develop, a urologist should be consulted for evaluation.

NURSING MANAGEMENT OF PATIENT WITH URINARY TRACT INFECTION

ASSESSMENT

Health History

The health history should focus on assessment of symptoms, specifically, frequency, urgency, dysuria, chills, and fever. Predisposing factors such as the use of diaphragms/spermicidals and a history of previous infections should also be explored.

Physical Examination

A urine culture is obtained because bacteriuria serves as the basis for diagnosis of a lower UTI. The urine should also be tested for occult blood. Palpation of the abdomen and costovertebral angle for tenderness is also indicated. The patient should be assessed for the presence of fever.

NURSING DIAGNOSES

Nursing diagnoses are determined from analysis of patient data. Nursing diagnoses for the person with a UTI may include but are not limited to:

Diagnostic Title	Possible Etiologic Factors
1. Impaired urinary elimination	Urinary infection
2. Deficient knowledge	Lack of exposure/recall

EXPECTED PATIENT OUTCOMES

Expected patient outcomes for the patient with a UTI may include but are not limited to:

1. Symptoms of frequency, urgency, and dysuria will resolve
2. Patient will describe:

2a. Signs and symptoms of a UTI

2b. Rationale for and means of increasing fluid intake to 3 to 4 L/day
2c. Risk factors for a UTI
2d. When and how to take prescribed medications
2e. Plan for follow-up care, including urine cultures

INTERVENTIONS

1. Patients should be encouraged to increase fluid intake.
2. Patients should be reminded to complete the course of antibiotic therapy even after symptoms resolve. Patient education concerning the specific problem and the requirements for drug therapy and follow-up care should increase compliance with drug regimens. Success depends directly on patient understanding and compliance and allows the patient to assist in overcoming this health problem.

The importance of follow-up care for patients with a complicated or recurrent UTI must be emphasized. Patients must be taught the sign and symptoms of a UTI and risk factors for developing a UTI.

Patient/Family Education: Health Promotion/Prevention

The most important defenses against a UTI are large urine volume, free urine flow, and complete emptying of the bladder to prevent urinary stasis. Patients should be advised to avoid a full bladder and increase fluid intake. Alcohol and caffeinated beverages should be avoided. Women should be instructed to void after intercourse. Estrogen replacement therapy (especially) vaginally may decrease the incidence of a UTI in postmenopausal women.[47] Urinary catheterization should be performed only when absolutely necessary, and when inserted, the catheter should be removed as soon as possible. Education of the public (Box 39-2) and efforts of the health care community can assist in decreasing the incidence of a UTI and its complications. See Figure 39-3 for an example of a patient education sheet and the Complementary & Alternative Therapies box for other preventive measures.

BOX 39-2 Information To Be Included in Public Education Programs About Urinary Tract Infections

- Symptoms of urinary tract infection
- Need to contact health care provider
- Need to continue antibiotics as prescribed, even if symptoms abate
- Need for follow-up care if urinary tract infections are recurrent
- Maintenance of fluid intake of 3 to 4 L/day if the person's health permits
- Need to void immediately before and after intercourse
- Void with the urge to void

EVALUATION

To evaluate the effectiveness of nursing interventions, compare patient behaviors with those stated in the expected patient outcomes. Achievement of outcomes is successful if the patient with a UTI:

1. Reports absence of pain, frequency, and urgency.
2. Correctly describes:

2a. Signs and symptoms of a UTI and need for prompt medical attention when they occur.
2b. Rationale for increasing fluids to 3 to 4 L/day.
2c. Risk factors for a UTI.
2d. Routine for taking prescribed medication with regard to dose, frequency, and length of therapy.
2e. Follow-up care, including return visit to health care professional and repeat urine culture.

GERONTOLOGIC CONSIDERATIONS

An estimated 10% to 20% of persons 65 years and older have bacteriuria. UTIs are the most common cause of bacterial sepsis in the older adult. Structural changes of the urinary system associated with aging add to susceptibility. Bladder muscles in the elderly woman may atrophy and weaken, and men may have prostatic hypertrophy, both of which lead to incomplete bladder emptying and retention. Decreased prostatic secretions in men and decreased estrogen that allows for vaginal colonization in women both predispose elderly individuals to development of UTIs.[5]

SPECIAL ENVIRONMENTS FOR CARE

Community-Based Care

UTIs are prevalent among persons who live in long-term care facilities perhaps owing in part to the presence of many comorbid illnesses that predispose them to UTIs. Most infections are asymptomatic. Several studies that compared therapy with no therapy found that antibiotic treatment had no benefits for asymptomatic persons.[36]

Many interventions for home care are aimed at preventing initial infections and/or recurrences. Patient education regarding risk factors is important. The patient with a UTI needs the resources to fill prescriptions and return for follow-up visits. The patient may also require instructions to obtain a sterile urine specimen (see Chapter 38).

COMPLICATIONS

Complications caused by an untreated UTI include sepsis and kidney failure. Recurrent UTIs can cause scar tissue, leading to

Complementary & Alternative Therapies
Urinary Tract Infection

- Cranberries and blueberries
- Vitamin C 1000 mg tid
- Beta carotene 25,000 to 50,000 IU/day
- Zinc 30-50 mg/day

Reference: http://home.md.consult.com.

JAMA PATIENT PAGE

Urinary Tract Infections

URINARY TRACT INFECTIONS

Water is the most vital substance your body requires. Water is very important for the basic chemical reactions that keep the body functioning. Many of the unusable by-products of these chemical reactions are then processed through the kidneys and eliminated from the body through the urinary tract as **urine**.

The normal function of the urinary system can be disrupted by structural abnormalities or disease. For example, infection can cause inflammation that can interrupt the normal operation of the urinary system. If you suspect you have a urinary tract infection or a problem with your urinary system, consult with your doctor, so that you can be tested and given proper treatment. Left untreated, an infection has the potential to cause more serious, even life-threatening, difficulties and permanent damage to your urinary tract.

An article in the March 22/29, 2000, issue of *JAMA* looks at the effectiveness of 2 different medications to treat a specific type of urinary tract infection, **pyelonephritis**, which is inflammation of the upper urinary tract and kidney. The article stresses the importance of testing and of receiving the correct medication.

TYPES OF URINARY TRACT INFECTIONS:

The most common types of urinary tract infections are:

- **Urethritis** – Inflammation of the **urethra** (the tube-like structure that allows urine to pass from the bladder to be eliminated outside the body)
- **Cystitis** – Inflammation of the **bladder** (the balloon-like structure that stores urine before elimination through the urethra)
- **Pyelonephritis** – A more serious condition that is characterized by inflammation of the upper urinary tract, which includes the kidneys and the **ureters** (the 2 tube-like structures that connect each kidney to the bladder)

If you are prescribed an antibiotic for an infection, it is important that you finish all of the pills even if the symptoms have gone away and you are feeling better.

COMMON SYMPTOMS:

- More frequent urge to urinate, even though only a small amount is eliminated
- Pain or burning sensation during urination
- Greenish-yellow or white discharge from, or itching in, your penis or vagina

If you have any of these symptoms see your doctor; you may have a urinary tract infection or a sexually transmitted disease. If you are diagnosed with a sexually transmitted disease you need to let your sex partner(s) know so that they can also be treated.

- Pain in the back that is just above the waist
- Pain in your side or groin area
- Fever, chills, nausea, and vomiting
- Pus or blood in the urine

If you have any of the above symptoms see your doctor immediately; you may have pyelonephritis or another serious problem

PREVENTING URINARY TRACT INFECTIONS:

- Drink plenty of fluids—at least 8 to 10 cups (64 to 80 ounces) of water a day. You need to increase your fluid intake beyond this if you are physically active or when you are in a warm environment.
- Urinate frequently
- Wash your genitals daily, especially before and after sexual relations
- Urinate after sexual relations
- Practice safer sex (e.g., wearing a condom during sexual relations)
- Women should always wipe from front to back after having a bowel movement
- Women should not use feminine hygiene products that contain deodorants

URINARY TRACT INFECTIONS IN CHILDREN:

Urinary tract infections can cause life-threatening and permanent damage to a child's urinary system. Therefore, it is important to receive treatment as soon as possible. Though the signs are similar for children and adults, they may not be as easy to observe in children. The child may have a fever and chills, experience nausea and vomiting, complain of pain in the abdomen, back, or pelvis, and complain about pain during urination. The child may also be irritable or not want to eat. For children with repeated urinary tract infections the child's doctor may suggest tests to determine if there are any abnormalities in the child's urinary system.

FOR MORE INFORMATION:

- National Kidney and Urologic Diseases Information Clearinghouse
  3 Information Way
  Bethesda, MD 20892-3580
  301/654-4415
  or www.niddk.nih.gov
- American Foundation for Urologic Disease
  Answers to Your Questions About Urinary Tract Infections
  (800) 242-2383
  or www.afud.org

INFORM YOURSELF:

To find this and previous *JAMA* Patient Pages, check out the AMA's Web site at www.ama-assn.org/consumer.htm.

From JAMA, March 22/29, 2000—Vol 283, No. 12

Figure 39-3 Sample patient education page for urinary tract infections.

strictures and distention. UTIs alone do not lead to deterioration of renal function.

PYELONEPHRITIS

Etiology/Epidemiology

Acute pyelonephritis is an infection of the upper urinary tract that involves both the parenchyma and kidney pelvis. It is one of the leading causes of infections in the blood (bacteremia) and accounts for more than 100,000 hospital admissions per year.[15] As discussed previously, this infection usually begins in the lower urinary tract and ascends into the kidneys. Lower UTIs may be asymptomatic, and kidney involvement may be the first indication of lower urinary tract disease. The diagnostic workup of a person with pyelonephritis often reveals previously unknown urinary tract obstruction or the presence of another chronic kidney disease. As in lower urinary tract infection, *E. coli* is the most common organism identified in pyelonephritis. Other causes are gram-negative bacilli and enterococci. Pregnant women with bacteriuria are at significant risk for developing pyelonephritis. Other risk factors that increase susceptibility to pyelonephritis include instrumentation of the urinary tract, diabetes, and female gender. Acute pyelonephritis may temporarily affect renal function, but rarely progresses to kidney failure. Chronic pyelonephritis permanently destroys renal tissue through repeated inflammation and scarring. The process of developing chronic kidney failure from repeated kidney infections occurs over a number of years or after several extensive and fulminant infections. Pyelonephritis is the original diagnosis in an estimated 13% of all persons with end-stage renal disease.[24]

Pathophysiology

The same bacterial adherence properties and toxins discussed for lower UTIs apply to pyelonephritis. Signs and symptoms of acute pyelonephritis may include those of lower UTIs in addition to the following typical signs of inflammation: chills and fever, malaise, flank pain, costovertebral angle tenderness, and leukocytosis. Urinalysis demonstrates presence of white blood cells, casts, and bacteria. In chronic pyelonephritis the only symptoms may be persistent bacteriuria until extensive scarring and atrophy result in renal insufficiency, as manifested by hypertension, increased blood urea nitrogen (BUN), and decreased creatinine clearance.

Collaborative Care Management

Optimal treatment of pyelonephritis includes early detection of the bacterial infection through urine culture, antibacterial therapy based on identified sensitivities, and detection and treatment of any underlying systemic disease or urinary tract abnormality. The course of antibiotic therapy usually lasts 10 to 14 days. Opioids or antiinflammatory drugs may be given for flank pain. Pain eases as the inflammation resolves. In chronic pyelonephritis, an evaluation is indicated to determine the cause of recurrent infections, such as obstruction caused by kidney stones. If structural abnormalities are found, surgery may be indicated. Antibiotic therapy is usually continuous with the goal of reducing and controlling the bacterial population of the urinary tract to prevent renal damage. The nursing interventions are the same as those for urinary tract infection.

Patient/Family Education. Persons with pyelonephritis may be treated at home; therefore patient teaching is important. Instruct the patient to:

- Continue the course of antibiotic therapy even after symptoms resolve.
- Drink 3 L/day of fluids unless otherwise indicated.
- Monitor urinary output; report to physician an output considerably less than fluid intake.
- Weigh self daily; report a sudden weight gain to physician.
- Take measures to prevent infection; if signs of urinary infection (increased flank pain, fever, chills, frequency, urgency) occur, report to the physician.
- Continue with medical follow-up care and follow-up urine cultures as instructed.

The most significant efforts to prevent pyelonephritis are through early detection and adequate treatment of lower UTIs.

Chemical-Induced Nephritis

Etiology/Epidemiology

Chemical-induced nephritis, also known as acute or chronic interstitial nephritis, is an idiosyncratic reaction that results in renal damage associated with interstitial edema and infiltration with inflammatory cells, T lymphocytes, and monocytes. Chronic lesions cause interstitial fibrosis. This disease process was first noted in patients sensitive to the sulfonamides. Many other substances are now associated with chemical-induced nephritis, including those listed in Table 39-1.

Pathophysiology

Chemical-induced nephritis usually begins within days or weeks of exposure to the chemical. The inflammatory process disrupts the ability of the glomeruli to filter. Furthermore, the capillary membrane becomes permeable to plasma proteins and red blood cells (RBCs), which results in mild to moderate proteinuria and hematuria. Eosinophils in the urine signify an allergic interstitial nephritis.

Signs and symptoms of nephritis include fever, eosinophilia, hematuria, mild proteinuria, and rash. A precipitous decrease in renal function results in an acute rise in serum creatinine. Oliguria or urine output of 400 ml or less in a 24-hour period may occur from interstitial inflammation severe enough to obstruct and impede urine flow. Kidney size is normal or slightly enlarged. Urinalysis is used to demonstrate protein, RBC, or white

TABLE 39-1 Substances Associated with Interstitial Nephritis

Antibiotics	Sulfonamides
	Methicillin, penicillin
	Cephalosporins
	Bactrim
	Rifampin
	Gentamicin
	Amphotericin B
Other Medications	Cimetidine
	Phenytoin
	Allopurinol
	Nonsteroidal antiinflammatory drugs (fenoprofen)
	Diuretics
Infections	Streptococcal
	Legionella
Solvents	Carbon tetrachloride
	Methanol
	Ethylene glycol
Heavy metals	Lead
	Arsenic
	Mercury
Pesticides	
Poisonous mushrooms	

cell casts in the urine. Lumbar pain is possible owing to distention of the renal capsule from diffuse kidney swelling. Serum toxicology screening may identify the source of the nephritis.

Collaborative Care Management

Medical management usually includes immediate withdrawal of the suspected chemical. Hemodialysis or charcoal kidney dialysis may be required to remove the nephrotoxins from the blood. Plasmapheresis may be indicated for treatment of some cases of idiopathic nephritis. Steroids are often administered because of their antiinflammatory effect. If renal function is severely compromised, dietary sodium and protein restrictions may be instituted.

The patient is assessed for signs of fluid and electrolyte imbalance, including the presence of edema, blood pressure changes, and adventitious breath sounds. The person needs to know the rationale for maintenance of fluid balance and any sodium restrictions. Care is similar to that for the patient with acute kidney failure (see Chapter 40).

Patient/Family Education. Education of the patient focuses on prevention. Patients should be instructed to keep solvents in well-ventilated areas. All household chemicals should be clearly labeled.

Identifying causative agents and removing them from the environment is the best method of preventing chemical-induced interstitial nephritis. Many people are exposed to these agents as a result of their medical regimen. The health care professional must be aware of these agents and the signs and symptoms associated with chemical-induced interstitial nephritis. The prognosis is improved with early detection and removal of the causative agent.

A major risk is industrial exposure to chemicals. Occupational health professionals should be aware of potential risks and should educate employees regarding appropriate preventive measures.

Acute Glomerulonephritis

Etiology

Glomerulonephritis is a disease that affects the glomerular capillaries. Etiologic factors are many and varied; they include immunologic reactions (systemic lupus erythematosus, streptococcal infection), vascular injury (hypertension), metabolic disease (diabetes mellitus), and disseminated intravascular coagulation. Glomerulonephritis exists in acute, latent, and chronic forms.

The most common form of acute glomerulonephritis occurs 1 to 3 weeks after a group A beta-streptococcal infection. Common sites of the primary infection include the pharynx or tonsils and the skin (impetigo).

Epidemiology

Preschool-age and grade school-age children (2 to 6 years old) are most likely to develop acute glomerulonephritis. Spontaneous recovery usually occurs after this acute illness. The severity of the acute illness does not relate to the prognosis. Less than 1% of children develop irreversible kidney failure.[7] Persons with mild illness may develop chronic disease, and those with severe illness may completely recover over a period of months and have no recurrence of the illness.[42]

Pathophysiology

Acute poststreptococcal glomerulonephritis is a result of an antigen-antibody reaction where insoluble immune complexes develop and become entrapped in glomerular tissue producing swelling and death of capillary cells. Renal function is depressed by scarring and obstruction of the circulation through the glomerulus.

Signs and symptoms reflect damage to the glomeruli, with leaking of protein and RBCs into the urine, and varying degrees of decreased glomerular filtration, with retention of metabolic waste products, sodium, and water (see Clinical Manifestations box). The patient typically reports shortness of breath, mild headache, weakness, anorexia, and flank pain. The usual signs associated with acute glomerulonephritis are proteinuria, hematuria, and azotemia.

Collaborative Care Management

Diagnostic Tests. Urinalysis provides important data, such as the presence of proteinuria, hematuria, and cell debris (red cells and casts). Hematuria and proteinuria can take several months to resolve. Serum BUN and urine creatinine clearance tests indicate renal function status. Tests to determine infection include white blood cell count, erythrocyte sedimentation rate, and antistreptolysin O titer.

Medications. Patients with poststreptococcal glomerulonephritis may be given a course of prophylactic antibiotics, with penicillin being the drug of choice. Prophylactic therapy may be continued for months after the acute phase of illness. Immunosuppressants and steroids may be indicated. Symptomatic salt and water retention is treated by diuretics and angiotensin-converting enzymes.[16] Hyperkalemia may need to be treated with potassium-binding resins, such as Kayexalate. Spontaneous diuresis usually occurs in 7 to 10 days. Diuretic therapy is implemented when severe fluid overload develops. Elevated blood pressure is controlled by antihyper-

Clinical Manifestations

Acute Glomerulonephritis

EARLY

- Hematuria
- Proteinuria
- Azotemia
- Increased urine specific gravity
- Elevated erythrocyte sedimentation rate
- Oliguria
- Elevated antistreptolysin O titer

LATE

- Circulatory congestion
- Hypertension
- Edema
- End-stage kidney failure

tensive drugs only after fluid control has proved to be unsuccessful.

Treatments. No specific treatment exists for acute glomerulonephritis. General management is focused on prevention.

Diet. Fluid retention is often a problem and is managed by dietary sodium restriction. Dietary protein is also restricted, usually to 1 to 1.2 g/kg/day when BUN and creatinine levels are elevated. It is important that the diet contain sufficient carbohydrates to prevent protein being used for energy, which will result in muscle wasting and nitrogen imbalance. Caloric requirements are 2500 to 3500 Cal/day. The patient should be monitored for weight loss, as loss of protein stores may occur. Potassium intake should be restricted if the glomerular filtration rate is less than 10 ml/min.

Activity. Bed rest is usually instituted until clinical signs of nephritis have resolved. Activity should be resumed gradually, as fatigue is common. To maintain muscle tone and to improve circulation, range of motion and isometric exercises should be performed while the patient is on bed rest.

Referrals. Prolonged bed rest during acute glomerulonephritis may cause fatigue and impair performance of activities of daily living (ADLs). Thus a referral for physical therapy for strengthening exercises may be beneficial after the acute phase of illness.

NURSING MANAGEMENT OF PATIENT WITH ACUTE GLOMERULONEPHRITIS

ASSESSMENT

Health History

The health history should focus on assessment of symptoms and predisposing factors. General questions to ask the patient include: Have you experienced shortness of breath, headaches, low back pain, weakness, nausea, vomiting, or loss of appetite? Have you noticed a change in your pattern of urination, either in frequency, color, or volume? Do you recall a recent infection or symptoms of a virus? Any recent weight gain or swelling?

Physical Examination

Key aspects of the physical examination of the patient with acute glomerulonephritis are assessment of vital signs for fever, hypertension, and edema. Measurement of intake and output and daily weights is also essential.

NURSING DIAGNOSES

Nursing diagnoses are determined from analysis of patient data. Nursing diagnoses for the person with acute glomerulonephritis may include but are not limited to:

Diagnostic Title	Possible Etiologic Factors
1. Excess fluid volume	Compromised regulatory mechanism, renal impairment
2. Risk for infection	Decreased immune response
3. Ineffective coping (individual)	Activity restrictions
4. Deficient knowledge	Lack of information

EXPECTED PATIENT OUTCOMES

Expected patient outcomes for the person with acute glomerulonephritis may include but are not limited to:

1. Will achieve fluid balance as indicated by fluid intake equaling output, decreased edema, stable weight, renal function tests within normal limits
2. Will exhibit no signs or symptoms of infection
3. Will express concerns and feelings about restricted activity; will not express boredom with prolonged bed rest
4. Will describe the rationale for therapy, dietary restrictions, medication program, measures to prevent infection, and signs and symptoms requiring medical attention

INTERVENTIONS

1. Promoting Fluid Balance

Edema and fluid overload are anticipated and treated initially with dietary sodium and fluid restrictions. Sodium intake is usually restricted to 2 to 4 g/day, but the amount varies with the severity of fluid retention. Sodium restriction is maintained until dependent edema and circulatory overload are no longer present. Strict recording of fluid intake and output is necessary to determine the extent of fluid retention. The nurse must be constantly alert for signs and symptoms of fluid overload. The patient is weighed daily using correct procedure (see Chapter 13). Vital signs are monitored every shift and the apical pulse checked for dysrhythmias. The patient is monitored for jugular vein distention, which is indicative of fluid overload and congestive heart failure, and for periorbital, pretibial, pedal, and sacral edema. The lungs are auscultated for adventitious sounds. Because antihypertensive and diuretic therapy is usually prescribed, serum potassium levels should be monitored closely. This is especially important for patients receiving diuretics that eliminate potassium because hyperkalemia may occur with uremic symptoms.

2. Preventing Infection

Mild infections may reactivate nephritis; therefore the patient must be protected from exposure to infection, particularly from persons with upper respiratory infections (URIs). If a URI is suspected, cultures are obtained, and when indicated, antibiotics are prescribed. When possible, any procedures such as catheterization that may lead to nosocomial infection must be avoided.

3. Facilitating Coping

Bed rest is prescribed during the acute phase of the illness. Ambulation is allowed when blood sedimentation rates and blood pressure are normal and edema abates. If ambulation causes an increase in proteinuria or hematuria, bed rest is reinstituted. Because the period of bed rest may be extensive, the nurse may need to continue to reinforce the importance of bed rest as the patient starts to feel better. The importance of diversional activities should not be ignored. When bed rest is resumed after a period of ambulation, the person may become depressed as a result of the perceived setback in recovery.

Helping the patient express concerns can serve as the impetus for making realistic plans about the illness and its sequelae.

4. Patient/Family Education

The recovery period for acute glomerulonephritis may be as long as 2 years; therefore patient teaching is important. Proteinuria, hematuria, and cellular debris may exist microscopically, even when other symptoms subside. Although fatigue may be present, these persons usually feel well; thus they often need to be convinced of the importance of follow-up care. Teaching includes:

- Nature of the illness and effect of diet and fluids on fluid balance and sodium retention.
- Diet teaching regarding prescribed sodium and fluid restrictions (provide written information regarding sodium content of foods).
- Medication regimen: dose, frequency, side effects, need to continue regimen as instructed by physician.
- Need to balance activities with rest if fatigue is present.
- Avoidance of infection, which may exacerbate the illness.
- Signs and symptoms indicating need for medical attention (hematuria, headache, edema, or hypertension).
- Importance of follow-up care.

Health Promotion/Prevention

Prevention of acute poststreptococcal glomerulonephritis involves prompt medical treatment of sore throats and URIs. Cultures should be obtained, and antibiotics prescribed when indicated.

EVALUATION

To evaluate the effectiveness of nursing interventions, compare patient behaviors with those stated in the expected patient outcomes. Achievement of outcomes is successful if the patient with acute glomerulonephritis:

1. Has intake equal to output, decreased edema, and stable weight.
2. Is free of signs or symptoms of infection.
3. Follows activity restrictions, participates in diversional activities, and does not express boredom.
4. Describes correctly the nature of the illness, dietary and fluid restrictions, the importance of preventing URI, signs and symptoms to be reported to physician, and the importance of follow-up care.

GERONTOLOGIC CONSIDERATIONS

Because of preexisting structural and age-related changes in the kidney, the elderly patient is at an increased risk for complications. Older adults are more likely to develop chronic glomerulonephritis. Treatment remains the same, regardless of age.

COMPLICATIONS

Besides the obvious complications such as sepsis from infection and kidney failure as a result of extensive kidney damage, other complications may arise as a result of fluid overload. These fluid-related complications include congestive heart failure, pulmonary edema, and, rarely, increased intracranial pressure. Each must be treated aggressively, and the patient may require critical care management. Cardiac glycosides may be prescribed to prevent congestive heart failure.

Chronic Glomerulonephritis

Etiology/Epidemiology

Although chronic glomerulonephritis (CGN) may follow the acute form of the disease, most persons have no history or source of predisposing infection, and evidence suggests the disease results from immunologic mechanisms.[10] The course of CGN is extremely variable. Some persons with minimal impairment in renal function continue to feel well and show little progression of disease. Progression of renal deterioration may be insidious or rapid, resulting in end-stage renal disease.

Pathophysiology

CGN, an autoimmune disease caused by loss of tolerance to self-antigens, is characterized by progressive destruction of glomeruli and gradual loss of renal function. The glomeruli have varying degrees of hypercellularity and become sclerosed (hardened). The kidney decreases in size. Eventually there is tubular atrophy, chronic interstitial inflammation, and arteriosclerosis (Figure 39-4).

Various symptoms of renal dysfunction may lead the person to seek health care, including headache, especially in the morning; dyspnea on exertion; blurred vision; lassitude; and weakness or fatigue. Other signs of CGN include edema, nocturia, and weight loss.

Early in the disease process urinalysis may reveal albumin, casts, and blood, despite normal renal function tests. The ability of the kidneys to regulate the internal environment will be-

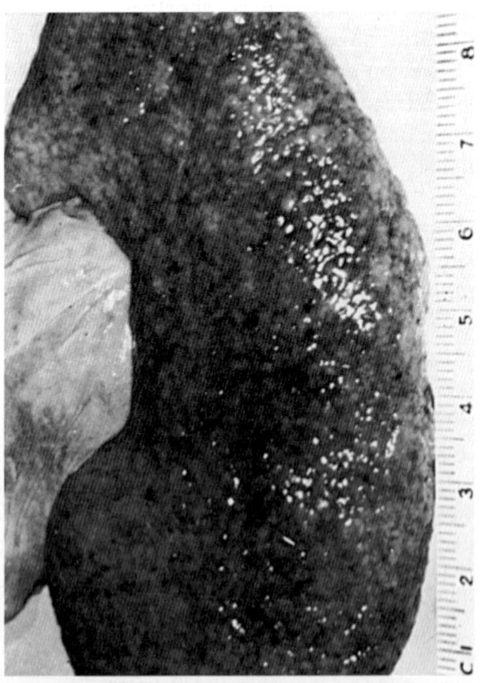

Figure 39-4 End-stage chronic glomerulonephritis. Note pebbly surface corresponding to surviving hypertrophied nephrons and atrophy.

gin to decrease as more glomeruli become scarred, resulting in fewer functional nephrons. When few nephrons remain intact, hematuria and proteinuria decrease, the specific gravity of the urine becomes fixed at 1.010 (equal to plasma), and the nonprotein nitrogen level in the blood increases.

Collaborative Care Management

No specific therapy exists to arrest or reverse this disease process. Treatment of kidney failure begins when the illness progresses to end-stage renal disease (see Chapter 40).

With any exacerbation of hematuria, hypertension, and edema, the patient is returned to bed rest, and treatment similar to that for acute glomerulonephritis is instituted. Signs of pulmonary edema and congestive heart failure are closely monitored.

Women with CGN who become pregnant appear to be susceptible to toxemia and to spontaneous abortion. The woman who has had nephritis of any nature should be urged to see a physician if she plans to become pregnant. When pregnancy does occur, she should be monitored closely by an obstetrician who specializes in high-risk pregnancies.

Care involves teaching the patient to maintain a healthy lifestyle, to avoid infections, to eat a balanced diet within prescribed limits, to take prescribed medications appropriately, to maintain follow-up health care, and to report any exacerbation in signs or symptoms to the physician or health care provider. If complications occur, specific treatment is symptomatic and supportive.

Patient/Family Education. Because predisposing factors have not been identified for CGN, no preventive measures can be instituted. To reduce the possibility of the acute disease progressing to CGN, infections should be treated promptly as discussed under acute glomerulonephritis. The patient should be encouraged to receive ongoing care for treatment of symptoms and to retard progression of disease.

Nephrotic Syndrome

Nephrotic syndrome (*nephrosis*) is not a single disease entity but a constellation of symptoms including albuminuria, hypoalbuminemia, edema, hyperlipidemia, and lipuria. Nephrotic syndrome causes damage to the glomeruli with resultant severe proteinuria, with losses of up to 3.5 g of protein daily.

Etiology

Nephrotic syndrome has been associated with allergic reactions (insect bites, pollen, and acute glomerulonephritis), infections (herpes zoster), systemic disease (diabetes mellitus, lupus, amyloidosis, Goodpasture's syndrome, and sickle cell disease), circulatory problems (severe congestive heart failure and chronic constrictive pericarditis), cancers (Hodgkin's, lung, colon, and breast), renal transplantation, and pregnancy. Many persons with chronic kidney failure develop nephrotic syndrome. Known glomerular disease is the most common precipitating event in adults. Some individuals have periods of remission and exacerbation. The etiology of nephrotic syndrome in children is usually idiopathic.

Epidemiology

Nephrotic syndrome is seen most often in children with minimal change nephropathy, which results in loss of negative charges in the basement membrane, thus allowing negatively charged proteins to pass through wasted into the urine. The prevalence is about 15 cases per 100,000 in the pediatric population, with 2 to 7 new cases per year.[44] In adults the most common cause of idiopathic nephrotic syndrome is membranous glomerulopathy.[44]

Pathophysiology

The initial physiologic change in nephrotic syndrome is damage to cells in the glomerular basement membrane from immune complex deposition, nephrotoxic antibodies, or other nonimmune mechanisms. These changes result in increased membrane porosity and permeability with significant proteinuria. As protein continues to be excreted, serum albumin is decreased (hypoalbuminemia), thus decreasing the serum osmotic pressure (Table 39-2). The capillary hydrostatic fluid pressure in all body tissues becomes greater than the capillary osmotic pressure, and generalized edema results (Figure 39-5). As fluid is lost into the tissues, the plasma volume decreases, stimulating secretion of aldosterone to retain more sodium and water, which decreases the glomerular filtration rate to retain water. This additional fluid also passes out of the capillaries into the tissue, leading to even greater edema.

Clinical manifestations of nephrotic syndrome include severe generalized edema *(anasarca)* pronounced proteinuria, hypoalbuminemia, and hyperlipidemia. Hyperlipidemia develops from increased hepatic production of lipids or perhaps from interference of lipid utilization. Urine volume and renal function may be either normal or greatly altered. Altered renal function and development of symptoms of kidney failure occur as a result of progressing glomerulonephritis. Loss of appetite and fatigue are common.

TABLE 39-2 Normal Function, Pathophysiology, and Clinical Manifestations in Nephrotic Syndrome

Normal Function	Pathophysiology	Clinical Manifestations
Glomerular capillaries are impermeable to serum proteins. Plasma proteins create colloid osmotic pressure to retain intravascular fluid.	Glomerular capillaries become permeable to serum proteins, resulting in proteinuria and decreased serum osmotic pressure. Glomerular filtration rate decreases.	Severe generalized edema; pronounced proteinuria; hypoalbuminemia; hyperlipidemia

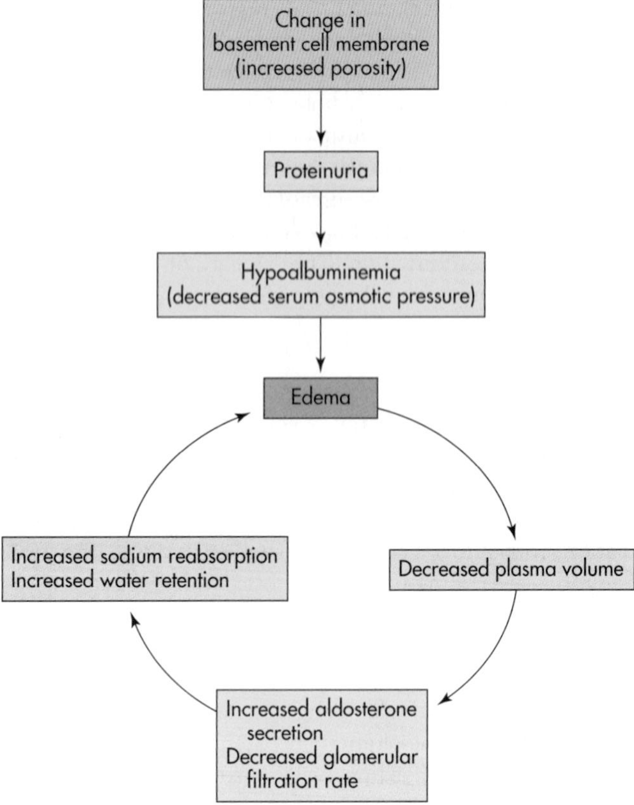

Figure 39-5 Pathophysiologic changes in nephrotic syndrome.

Collaborative Care Management

Treatment of nephrotic syndrome is focused on reducing albuminuria, controlling edema, and promoting general health.

Diagnostic Tests. Laboratory tests include urinalysis for protein, casts, and erythrocytes and serum tests for protein and lipid analysis. Dipstick urine protein may be as high as +3 or +4. Hyperlipidemia and elevated serum cholesterol, elevated triglycerides, and elevated low-density and very low–density lipid levels are common findings. Serum albumin can fall below 2 g/dl. Periodic determinations of proteinuria and measures of renal function are performed to monitor response to treatment and level of kidney function. Renal biopsy is sometimes used to obtain a definitive diagnosis or determine the extent of kidney damage. Biopsy may reveal minimal to extensive changes including hypercellularity, changes in the epithelium, fatty deposits in the tubules, sclerosing of the glomeruli, and deposition of immunoglobins along the capillary walls. Persons with extensive damage generally do not respond to treatment and develop end-stage renal disease.

Medications. Corticosteroids may be useful in controlling the illness, but responses vary. Even patients responsive to steroids may experience relapses for up to several years.[35] Prednisone is the drug of choice; cyclophosphamide or azathioprine is used for patients unresponsive to steroids.

Immunosuppressants are effective in stopping the proteinuria. Slow resolution of edema with diuretics and albumin may be indicated.

Treatments. No specific treatment exists for nephrotic syndrome. Prevention of infection is important because body defenses are impaired by protein losses and edematous tissues are susceptible to breakdown. Thoracentesis or paracentesis is indicated in patients with fluid accumulation in the pleural or abdominal cavities. Dialysis may be indicated for severe cases. Nephrotic patients with hypoalbuminemia are at risk for thromboembolism. Prolonged steroid therapy can lead to osteopenia or osteoporosis.

Diet. Dietary protein is usually prescribed at 1 g/kg body weight/day, depending on the glomerular filtration rate. Protein dietary supplements can be given with meals. Calories should be adequate to prevent catabolism. The caloric requirement varies with the individual; adults require 35 to 45 kcal/kg of ideal body weight/day. Sodium intake is restricted to 0.5 to 1 g/day to control edema. Patients receiving diuretics over prolonged periods should eat foods high in potassium. Supplements are prescribed only after attempts to increase serum potassium through dietary intake have failed.

Activity. Bed rest is indicated for patients with severe edema or those with infections. However, prolonged immobility is contraindicated to avoid complications.

Referrals. Consultation with a dietitian may be necessary to assist in meal planning. The patient may benefit from written lists of nutritional content of common foods.

NURSING MANAGEMENT OF PATIENT WITH NEPHROTIC SYNDROME

ASSESSMENT

Health History

The health history should focus on assessment of symptoms and predisposing factors as for glomerulonephritis. Intake and output should be determined and compared.

Physical Examination

Important aspects of the physical examination of the patient with nephrotic syndrome are assessment for edema with amount, location, and degree of pitting noted; daily weights; measurement of abdominal girth; and assessment of skin condition, because severe edema may lead to skin breakdown. Careful examination for signs and symptoms of infection and pulmonary edema is also essential.

NURSING DIAGNOSES

Nursing diagnoses are determined from analysis of patient data. Nursing diagnoses for the person with nephrosis may include but are not limited to:

Diagnostic Title	Possible Etiologic Factors
1. Imbalanced nutrition: less than body requirements	Anorexia, edema
2. Risk for infection	Decreased nutrition, immobility, edema
3. Deficient knowledge	Lack of exposure/recall

EXPECTED PATIENT OUTCOMES

Expected patient outcomes for the patient with nephrotic syndrome may include but are not limited to:

1a. Will eat a diet high in protein and calories and low in sodium
1b. Will maintain stable weight
2a. Will not exhibit signs or symptoms of infection
2b. Will maintain intact skin
3. Will describe dietary and drug therapy, measures to prevent infection, and symptoms requiring medical attention.

INTERVENTIONS

1. Promoting Nutrition

A sodium-restricted diet is usually prescribed. The protein prescription varies according to the amount of protein lost in the urine over 24 hours. Appetite is diminished as a result of fluid retention and decreased food palatability. Small frequent feedings may be better tolerated. Vitamin supplements with iron may be prescribed. After the patient's food preferences are assessed, a diet plan should be developed with the dietitian. Whenever possible, the protein should be of high biologic value (lean meat, fish, poultry, and dairy products).

Oral hygiene should be offered at regular intervals. Mouth care can help reduce the unpleasant metallic taste and breath odor that are partially responsible for the anorexia of renal failure.

Laboratory data, including serum protein, lipids, and calcium should be monitored to assess protein stores. The patient should be weighed daily.

2. Preventing Infection

Persons with nephrosis need to focus on preventing infection because urinary protein losses impair body defenses. It is important to remember that corticosteroid use may mask the signs of infection. When infection is suspected, it is important to address the problem immediately. Specimens for culture and sensitivity should be obtained. Antibiotics should be administered at prescribed times to maintain therapeutic blood levels. The importance of completing the prescribed course of medication should be stressed. The patient should be protected against sources of infection. Invasive procedures should be avoided; when necessary, they should be performed under strict aseptic technique.

Edematous tissue is particularly susceptible to skin breakdown and infection. Careful positioning and frequent position changes may increase comfort while also protecting the skin. Air or water mattresses may increase comfort and relieve skin pressure. Men may develop scrotal edema and, if so, a scrotal support provides comfort and aids in reducing swelling.

3. Patient/Family Education

Nephrosis is often progressive and an important aspect of health teaching relates to maintaining comfort. Teaching includes:

The effects of nephrotic syndrome on the kidneys and the possibility of the need for dialysis or renal transplant in the future.

Medication regimen: name, dose, actions, side effects, and the need to finish antibiotic prescription (as appropriate).

Nutritional need for increased calories, adequate protein, and decreased sodium and methods to meet nutritional needs.

Self-assessment of fluid status, including signs and symptoms of hypovolemia and hypervolemia.

Signs and symptoms requiring medical attention: increased edema, dyspnea, fatigue, headache, or infection.

Promotion of good health habits to prevent infection, including nutritionally adequate diet, exercise, adequate rest and sleep, and avoidance of sources of infection.

Need for follow-up care to monitor renal function.

EVALUATION

To evaluate the effectiveness of nursing interventions, compare patient behaviors with those stated in the expected outcomes. Achievement of outcomes is successful if the patient with nephrotic syndrome:

1a. Eats meals high in calories and low in sodium and follows the protein prescription.
1b. Maintains stable weight.
2a. Is free of signs of infection.
2b. Maintains skin integrity.
3. Describes medication regimen, nutrition prescription, measures to assess fluid status, signs and symptoms requiring medical attention, the need for follow-up care, and complications of nephrotic syndrome.

GERONTOLOGIC CONSIDERATIONS

With age, interest in eating may decline because of changes in the sensory organs, which alter the taste of food. A major component of the treatment for nephrotic syndrome is maintaining a high-protein, low-sodium diet. Elderly persons may lack the resources to comply with the prescribed diet. In addition, older adults are more likely to have complications related to steroid therapy because of excess levels of circulating free glucocorticoids.

COMPLICATIONS

Similar to glomerulonephritis, nephrotic syndrome can lead to kidney failure and complications involving fluid overload in the periphery owing to protein shifts. At the vascular level, the patient may become hypovolemic because of changes in osmotic pressure.

VASCULAR DISORDERS

Vascular renal disease results from one of two processes: (1) disease of the main renal arteries or renal artery stenosis and (2) sclerosis of renal arterioles or nephrosclerosis.

Renal Artery Stenosis

Etiology/Epidemiology

Renal artery stenosis is a narrowing of one or both renal arteries and their branches. It is the cause of approximately 2% to 5% of all cases of hypertension. Stenosis of the renal artery is usually caused by atherosclerosis in 90% of cases or fibromuscular dysplasia in about 10% of cases.[43] In either case, the end result is a narrowing of the lumen of the arteries supplying the kidneys. Patients at risk include those with severe hypertension, bruits, other vascular disease, and a history of smoking.

Pathophysiology

Renal artery stenosis results in a major reduction in blood flow to the kidneys. This change in renal perfusion causes increased secretion of renin and activation of the renin-angiotensin-aldosterone system.[43] The end result is acceleration of hypertension, which, if untreated, leads to further pathologic changes in the kidneys. See the Clinical Manifestations box for common clinical findings in persons with renal artery stenosis.

Collaborative Care Management

Diagnostic testing depends on the patient's clinical picture. Renal artery stenosis is usually diagnosed with renal arteriography, duplex Doppler ultrasound, and/or MRI.[50]

Medical treatment for patients with renal artery stenosis secondary to atherosclerotic disease includes antihypertensive therapy to control blood pressure, aspirin, cholesterol-lowering drugs, and smoking cessation. When significant stenosis exists in the renal artery, percutaneous angioplasty with or without stenting or surgical bypass of the stenotic area may be performed to improve circulation.[48] Complications after an angioplasty include hematoma at the puncture site, azotemia from the dye, and emboli. Nephrectomy may be indicated for persons unresponsive to medication and those with restenosis after percutaneous angioplasty.

Patients should be informed of the importance of follow-up care for regular blood pressure checks and measurement of renal function. In addition, patients need to undergo periodic noninvasive studies such as ultrasound to screen for restenosis. Because many patients have coexisting cardiac disease, they should be educated on behaviors that lower cholesterol, including maintaining a diet low in animal fat and increasing aerobic exercise. Patients should be instructed to monitor their blood pressure at home and to keep their health care provider apprised of their values. Patients should be taught to recognize the signs of decreasing renal function and report these symptoms promptly to their health care provider.

Nephrosclerosis

Etiology/Epidemiology

Whereas renal artery stenosis results in hypertension, hypertension can cause nephrosclerosis or damage to the renal arteries, arterioles, and glomeruli. Hypertension is the second major cause of end-stage renal disease.[14] An estimated 10% of individuals with essential hypertension develop severe renal damage, and approximately 1% develop end-stage renal disease and die unless supportive care is provided. It is thought that one's susceptibility to nephrosclerosis may be genetically based. Nephrosclerosis is more common in African-Americans.

Pathophysiology

The renal vasculature is affected in nephrosclerosis. The renal arterial vessels show thickening and narrowing of their lumina, and some glomerular capillaries are sclerosed and collapsed. Renal blood flow can be reduced as a result of these vascular changes causing ischemia. The renal tubules can also be affected, resulting in tubular atrophy. Proteinuria results from glomerular damage. Nocturia may occur from moderate loss of tubular concentrating ability. Urinary casts may be present from tubular injury.

Patients with nephrosclerosis resulting from hypertension often have target organ damage elsewhere such as left ventricular hypertrophy or retinopathy. Signs and symptoms of nephrosclerosis are the same as those for chronic kidney failure (see Chapter 40). By the time the signs and symptoms develop, the disease has progressed to an extreme point. Deterioration in renal function progresses gradually.

Collaborative Care Management

Renal biopsy confirms the diagnosis of hypertensive nephrosclerosis. Treatment of nephrosclerosis is focused on early detection and treatment of hypertension. Causative factors are sought, and treatment to lower blood pressure is initiated (see Chapter 25). When significant renal damage exists, stabilizing the person's current level of function or slowing deterioration of the kidney tissue is the goal while control of hypertension is continued.

Nursing management of patients with nephrosclerosis is the same as outlined for chronic kidney failure (see Chapter 40). The goals for nursing care center around providing comfort and maintaining self-care in daily living. During drug therapy, the patient must be monitored closely for tachycardia, hypotension, and marked sodium and water retention.

Patient/Family Education. Prevention is best accomplished by routine screening to detect hypertension and to provide adequate treatment and follow-up care. Identification of persons at risk for developing nephrosclerosis includes a history of hypertension and those with factors that increase the risk of hypertension (obesity, diabetes mellitus, positive family history, smoking history, and lack of exercise). Implementation of teaching programs to institute lifestyle modifications that prevent hypertension are important preventive strategies.

Persons with nephrosclerosis need to be taught about treatment strategies such as diet and medications and the need for continuous follow-up care. Skills to monitor the effectiveness of treatment should be taught, including taking vital signs, measuring fluid intake and output, and recording weights. The patient and family should also understand the possibility of the need for dialysis or transplant in the future if end-stage renal disease develops.

Clinical Manifestations

Renal Artery Stenosis

- Hypertension (usually abrupt onset)
- Abdominal bruits
- Disparity in kidney size
- Unexplained azotemia

OBSTRUCTIVE DISORDERS

Structural or functional changes in the urinary tract can impede the normal flow of urine. Obstruction can occur in any portion of the urinary tract from the meatus to the renal tubules. Patients with obstructions usually have characteristic signs and symptoms, depending on the location and extent of the obstruction. Less than 5% of the causes of acute kidney failure are due to urinary tract obstruction. This section describes the major concepts related to obstruction of the urinary system and the care of patients with obstructive disorders. Subsequent sections discuss specific obstructive disorders (renal calculi, urinary strictures, and tumors). Benign prostatic hypertrophy is discussed in Chapter 55.

Hydronephrosis

Etiology/Epidemiology

Hydronephrosis is the dilation of the renal calyces and pelvis proximal to the obstruction. Hydronephrosis may occur either unilaterally or bilaterally, depending on the site of the obstruction. Obstructive uropathy is the disruption in urine flow anywhere from the renal pelvis to the tip of the meatus. Hydronephrosis is more common in men after age 60 years because of prostate enlargement. It is more common in women between the ages of 20 and 60 years as a result of pregnancy and uterine cancer. Table 39-3 summarizes causes of obstruction of the urinary tract.

Pathophysiology

Obstruction of any part of the urinary system from the urethra to the kidney generates backflow of urine and pressure on the renal tubules causing tubular dysfunction. Partial obstruction may produce slow dilation of structures above the obstruction without functional impairment. As the obstruction increases, pressure builds up in the tubular system behind the obstruction, causing a backflow of urine and dilation of the ureter *(hydroureter)* (Figure 39-6). The urine backup eventually reaches the kidney, causing dilation of the kidney pelvis *(hydronephrosis)*. Pressure build-up in the renal pelvis leads to destruction of kidney tissue and eventually kidney failure.

With obstruction, urine flow is decreased, even to the point of stagnation. This stagnant urine provides a culture medium for bacterial growth; rarely is obstruction seen without some infection. The specific effects that occur with obstruction depend on the location, extent (partial or complete), and duration of the obstruction.

Obstruction in the lower urinary tract causes bladder distention. Obstruction of the upper urinary tract can progress rapidly to hydronephrosis because of the small size of the ureters and kidney pelvis. The increased pressure in the ureters extends into the kidney pelvis and results in increased pressure in the tubules; this along with progressive vasoconstriction in the kidney leads to decreased glomerular filtration rate. Urinary stasis in the dilated pelvis leads to infection and calculi, which add to the renal damage. The unaffected kidney then takes on increased elimination of waste products. With prolonged obstruction, the unaffected kidney hypertrophies and may function almost (80%) as effectively alone as both kidneys did before the obstruction; however, bilateral obstruction leads to kidney failure.

Symptoms of hydronephrosis depend on the onset and duration of the obstruction. Persons with a slowly developing obstruction may be asymptomatic. Pain radiating to the groin is common in persons with rapidly progressing obstruction (see Clinical Manifestations box). The pain is caused by stretching of the tissues and by hyperperistalsis. An acute upper urinary tract obstruction causes pain, nausea, vomiting, local tenderness, spasm of the abdominal muscles, and a mass in the kidney region. Because the amount of pain is proportional to the rate of stretching, a slowly developing hydronephrosis may cause only a dull flank pain, whereas a

TABLE 39-3 Causes of Urinary Obstruction

Location	Major Causes
Lower urinary tract	Benign prostatic hypertrophy Calculi Urethral strictures Tumors
Upper urinary tract	Calculi Trauma Tumor Aneurysms Congenital anomaly

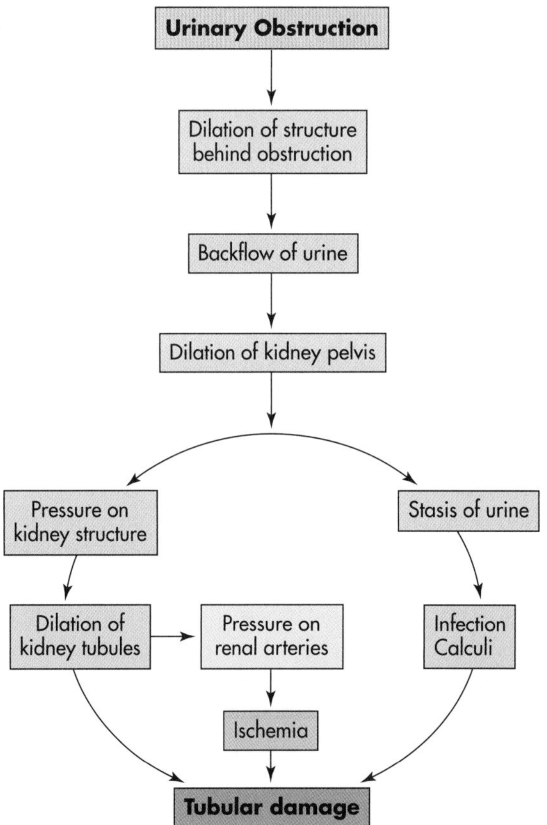

Figure 39-6 Pathophysiology of uncorrected urinary obstruction.

Clinical Manifestations

Urinary Obstruction

CHRONIC HYDRONEPHROSIS

- No symptoms
- Intermittent pain
- Elevated blood urea nitrogen and creatinine

ACUTE HYDRONEPHROSIS

- Renal colic
- Changes in urinary output
- Hematuria
- Palpable bladder
- Hypertension
- Hesitancy, urgency, incontinence, postvoid dribbling, decreased force of stream

sudden blockage of the ureter (e.g., from a stone) causes a severe stabbing (colicky) pain in the flank or abdomen. The pain may radiate to the genitalia and thigh and is caused by the increased peristaltic action of the smooth muscles of the ureter in an effort to dislodge the obstruction and force urine past the blockage.

The nausea and vomiting frequently associated with acute obstruction are caused by a reflex reaction to the pain and usually abate as soon as the pain is relieved. An extremely dilated kidney, however, may press on the stomach, causing continued gastrointestinal symptoms. If renal function has been seriously impaired, nausea and vomiting may indicate uremia. (See Chapter 40 for discussion of uremia and kidney failure.) The pain is caused by stretching of the tissues and by hyperperistalsis.

When the bladder is distended from lower urinary tract obstruction, the person experiences lower abdominal discomfort and feels the need to void, although voiding may not be possible. The bladder may be palpated above the symphysis pubis. With partial obstruction, as seen in benign prostatic hypertrophy, the patient first complains of increasing urinary frequency because the bladder fails to empty completely with each void and therefore refills more quickly to the amount that causes the urge to void (usually 250 to 500 ml). Nocturia, hematuria, and pyuria may also be present.

Collaborative Care Management

Early recognition and management are essential, as renal function is related to the duration and extent of the obstruction. Bladder outlet obstruction can be determined by placing a Foley catheter or by using an ultrasonic bladder scanner. If the cause is not determined by either of these two methods, an ultrasound or CT scan is used. Further diagnostic studies vary depending on whether an upper or lower tract obstruction is suspected. Urinalysis may lend important clues to the etiology and serum renal function studies help determine impairment in renal function.

Medical management is specific to the cause of the urinary obstruction. Treatment centers on preserving or restoring renal function. When an obstruction is relieved early, defects in function usually disappear completely. Complete obstruction warrants immediate action. If the obstruction is below the level of the bladder, an attempt should be made to insert a Foley catheter. Often relief of an obstruction is achieved by balloon dilation of the stenoses, placement of nephrostomy tubes, or stenting. Surgical relief of the obstruction is most often reserved for patients with fibrosis involving both ureters. Dialysis may be necessary before surgical interventions in patients with acute kidney failure.

Symptoms depend on the location (upper or lower), degree of obstruction (partial or complete), and duration and cause of the obstruction. For example, patients with an obstruction resulting from a kidney stone may present with severe pain (see next section). In contrast, patients with chronic or partial obstructions may be asymptomatic or have intermittent pain. Patients with acute, sudden obstruction are frequently acutely ill and may have severe colic. Opioids, such as morphine and meperidine, in combination with antispasmodic drugs, such as propantheline bromide (Pro-Banthine), and belladonna preparations are usually necessary to relieve severe colicky pain. When patients are relieved of a bilateral obstruction, initial urine output may be 200 ml/hr or greater, depending on their hydration status before the obstruction. This phenomenon is called *postobstructive diuresis.* During this diuresis, intake and output, body weight, and basic serum electrolytes should be monitored and fluid replacement given as indicated. Fluid is usually replaced with 0.45% normal saline with or without dextrose. Fluid replacement may be delayed in patients who are edematous or hypertensive at the beginning of diuresis.[46]

Nursing interventions for the person with urinary obstruction are specific for the underlying cause and are described in the following sections on calculi, tumors, and urinary strictures. Important foci of care for the person with a urinary obstruction include pain management, fluid balance assessment, prevention of urinary complications, and patient teaching. In addition, the patient should be monitored for signs and symptoms of infection and electrolyte imbalances.

Patient/Family Education. Patients and their families should be taught postoperative care of incisions and care and management of indwelling catheters if applicable. Information about the medication regimen, side effects of prescribed medications, and signs and symptoms of infection and recurrent obstruction should be included in the teaching plan.

Renal Calculi

Urinary stones *(urolithiasis)* may develop at any level in the urinary system but are most frequently found within the kidney *(nephrolithiasis)*. Nephrolithiases are commonly referred to as to renal calculi or kidney stones. These terms are often used interchangeably. Figure 39-7 illustrates the most common locations of calculi formation.

Etiology

A kidney stone forms when urine is supersaturated with a stone-forming salt. The mineral composition of renal calculi varies. The largest majority of kidney stones are composed of calcium oxalate or calcium phosphate. Approximately 75% of

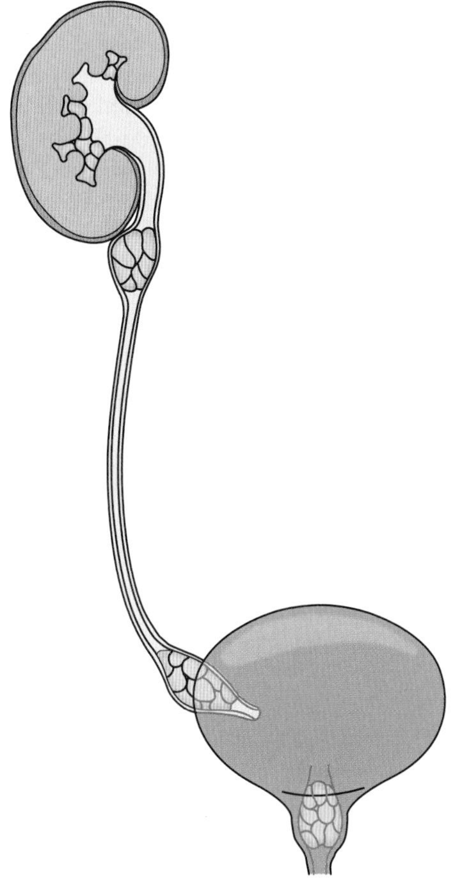

Figure 39-7 Most common locations of renal calculi formation.

renal stones consist of calcium salts (oxalates or phosphates) and the remaining stones are composed of struvite, uric acid, or cystine.

Risk factors can be identified in 90% of persons with kidney stones. In addition to inadequate hydration, risk factors for the development of calcium stones include hypercalciuria and high protein and sodium intake. UTIs increase the risk of developing struvite stones. Excess intake of dietary purine found in red meat, fish, and poultry and a disorder in purine metabolism (i.e., gout) are primary risk factors for formation of uric acid stones. Although rare, an autosomal-recessive inheritance of homocystinuria can cause development of cystine stones.

Epidemiology

Kidney stones affect 240,000 to 720,000 people in the United States each year[23] and account for 7 to 10 of every 1000 hospital admissions.[39] Renal calculi are 2.5 times more common in men than women and in persons between the ages of 20 and 50 years old. Approximately 50% of persons who develop renal calculi have a recurrence within 5 years.[23] Fortunately most stones pass without medical intervention.

Pathophysiology

Kidney stones are primarily made of a crystalline component. There are three major steps involved in this crystal formation: nucleation, growth, and aggregation. Nucleation starts or seeds the stone process and may be initiated by a variety of materials such as protein, foreign bodies, or crystals. The initial crystal serves as the core for further growth and aggregation. See Table 39-4 for the common contributing factors for each type of stone. It is now believed that persons who form stones may lack inhibitor substances in the urine that naturally slow or inhibit stone formation. Although it was once thought that a calcium-restricted diet would reduce the risk of recurrent calcium stone formation, past studies have shown that a low-calcium diet may even place some at increased risk for recurrent stone formation.[12,13]

TABLE 39-4 Renal Calculus Composition and Contributing Factors

Composition of Stone	Factors Contributing To Stone Formation
Calcium (oxalate and phosphate)	Low urine volume, hypercalciuria (resulting from primary hyperparathyroidism, renal tubular acidosis, immobilization, hyperthyroidism), hypocitruria (resulting from chronic diarrhea, renal tubular acidosis, and increased dietary protein loads), hyperuricosuria (resulting from inflammatory bowel disease, small bowel resection and dietary excess) (e.g., spinach, Swiss chard, rhubarb), medullary sponge disease
Uric acid	Low urine volume, high purine diet, gout
Struvite	Urinary tract infection
Cystine	Hereditary disorder of amino acid metabolism

Pain associated with the passage of a kidney stone (renal calculi) is referred to as *renal colic.* Pain is the primary symptom in an acute episode of renal calculi. The classic presentation is the sudden onset of severe flank pain usually combined with tenderness over the costovertebral angle. Radiation of the pain may indicate the location of the stone in the urinary tract. For example, if the stone is in the kidney pelvis, the pain is caused by hydronephrosis and is more dull and constant in character, occurring primarily in the costovertebral angle. As the stone moves down the ureter, excruciating and intermittent pain is caused by spasm of the ureter and anoxia of the ureter wall from the pressure of the stone. The pain follows the anterior course of the ureter down to the suprapubic area and radiates to the external genitalia. As the stone moves down the ureter closer to the bladder, there is often the urge to urinate or a burning sensation during urination. Pain can vary widely depending on the location of the stone, degree and acuity of obstruction, and variations in individual anatomy. Often a stone is "silent," causing no symptoms for years. This is especially true of very large stones that develop over a long period before resulting in symptoms. Extremely small, smooth stones may be passed asymptomatically. Hematuria is present in about 95% of persons. Many patients experience nausea and vomiting, but only a few have abdominal pain.

Collaborative Care Management

Diagnostic Tests. An x-ray called a flat plate of the abdomen or KUB (kidneys, ureters, and bladder) is often one of the first diagnostic studies obtained. It can reveal radiopaque stones larger than 2 mm. During the past decade, the spiral computed tomography has become the standard radiographic diagnostic test when available. An IVP is a radiographic study used to evaluate potential structural and anatomic abnormalities of the urinary tract. An ultrasound may be considered in patients allergic to contrast dye. Serum electrolytes (BUN and creatinine), a complete blood count, urinalysis, and urine culture should be obtained from patients who present with acute renal colic.

Because recurrence of renal calculi is common, stone composition should be analyzed to help direct preventive therapy for future stones. Additional studies are carried out after the acute episode has subsided. Successive determinations of serum calcium, phosphorus, protein, electrolytes, and uric acid levels may be performed to identify the underlying disease that may have influenced stone formation. The urine pH may be measured with a dipstick each time the patient voids to determine the urine acidity or alkalinity. The pH less is than 6 with calcium and uric acid stones; a pH greater than 7.2 is seen with struvite stones. A nitroprusside urine test may be performed to check for the presence of cystine. An accurate 24-hour urine specimen is collected to measure calcium, oxalate, phosphorus, and uric acid levels. A 24-hour urine specimen may be collected with the patient eating a normal diet or after a 3-day low-calcium, low-phosphorus diet.

Medications. Treatments are aimed at relieving pain, preserving renal function, preventing infection, and restoring fluid and electrolyte balance. The majority of stones less than 5 mm pass spontaneously. Patients who are unable to tolerate oral fluids or who have pain despite oral analgesics should be given IV fluid and IV medications for pain. IV opioids or nonsteroidals (ketorolac or Toradol) are good choices for analgesia. IV fluids may be necessary to restore fluid volume in patients who are dehydrated. Lastly, antiemetics may be indicated for patients with nausea and vomiting.[23]

Although management of kidney stones varies depending on the type of stone, there are certain recommendations for all patients with stones (Table 39-5). In general, fluid intake should be increased to 3 L/day and dietary oxalate and sodium should be limited. For calcium stones, a chelating agent such as cellulose phosphate is administered with meals if the problem is thought to be due to increased absorption of calcium in the bowel. The chelating agent binds to calcium and impedes absorption in the small bowel. Thiazide diuretics, particularly hydrochlorothiazide, decrease the calcium content in the urine by increasing reabsorption of calcium in the renal tubules. Because hyperparathyroidism is the second most common cause of calcium stones, a serum parathyroid level should be obtained. Those with hyperparathyroidism require surgical resection of the parathyroid adenoma (see Chapter 29).

Prophylaxis for uric acid stones consists of alkalinizing the urine by the administration of sodium bicarbonate or citrate solution. Allopurinol (Zyloprim) is usually prescribed to inhibit synthesis of uric acid. The gold standard treatment for struvite stones is complete surgical removal and treatment of the infection with antibiotics. Cystine stones can be treated with penicillamine, which acts by combining with cystine to form a soluble compound.

Treatments. Although 75% to 80% of urinary calculi are passed spontaneously,[38] if stones fail to pass and cause obstruction, ureteral stent(s) may be passed through a cystoscope up the ureter. This procedure relieves the obstruction in more than 85% of patients.

Over the past 15 years the interventional management of kidney stones has changed dramatically.[45] Treatments are now not only less invasive and safer for patients, but have hastened recovery and return to normal activities. In general there are four modalities available for interventional treatment: extracorporeal shock wave lithotripsy (ESWL), percutaneous nephrostolithotomy, rigid and flexible ureteroscopy, and open surgery.[29] ESWL has become the most commonly used treatment modality. Open surgical procedures have largely been replaced by less invasive techniques to fragment and remove stones and is used in less than 1% of patients; thus it is not included in this text.

Extracorporeal Shock Wave Lithotripsy. Although there are several categories of lithotripsy, the most common is ESWL. The overall success rate for ESWL is 90%. ESWL is performed by generating external shock waves that are transmitted through the skin and soft tissues and directed on the stone. In the past, the patient was submerged in water to transmit the shock; however, newer machines require only a cushion of water to transmit the shock. The energy delivered with the shock causes the stone to fragment into small pieces that are often passed spontaneously or can be removed with the use of an endoscope. An electrocardiogram (ECG) should be obtained on all patients before the procedure to determine abnormal rhythms because shock wave delivery is controlled by the patient's ECG. Patients with pacemakers may need reprogramming. Patients should be instructed to discontinue anticoagulants (warfarin, aspirin, and nonsteroidal antiinflammatory drugs) before the procedure to decrease the risk of bleeding.[29]

TABLE 39-5 Stone Clinic Recommendations for Conservative Therapy for Renal Calculi

High fluid intake	10 × 10-oz glasses of fluid (3 L) per day
Low-oxalate diet	Limit dark greens, nuts, chocolate, vitamin C
Low-sodium diet	Limit 2 g/day
Low purine	Limit 2 moderate meat servings per day
Citrus fruit juice intake	At least 10 oz/day; lemonade encouraged (2 L/day)
Moderate calcium intake	Limit 2 servings of dairy products per day (only if hypercalciuric)

From Rakel RE, Bope ET: *Conn's current therapy 2001,* Philadelphia, 2001, WB Saunders.

Pain and hematuria are the most commonly reported symptoms after the procedure. Immediately after the procedure, the patient may experience redness or bruising on the skin at the lithotripsy site. The patient can be discharged after the procedure if there are no complications. The patient should be informed that he/she might pass small particles in the urine for several days after lithotripsy. After lithotripsy, pain may occur from passing fragments of the pulverized stone through the lower urinary tract and persist for up to 3 days. Opioids may be prescribed for pain management. If large fragments of the stone are formed, a percutaneous nephrostomy may be performed to allow passage of the fragments.

Patient teaching focuses on monitoring urinary output, pain management techniques, and symptoms that need to be reported to the health care provider. These include flank pain, bleeding, decreased output, symptoms of obstruction, and fever.

Surgical Management

Percutaneous Nephrolithotomy. The procedure is carried out with the patient under general anesthesia. A fine needle with a guidewire is inserted into the renal pelvis under ultrasound guidance. A series of dilators are passed over the guidewire. When the stone is visualized it is broken up with ultrasound, electrohydraulic, laser, or pneumatic lithotripsy and the fragments are evacuated. A nephrostomy tube is then inserted and sutured to the skin. There are few complications and the risk of hemorrhage is low.

Ureteroscopy. This procedure is used most frequently to remove stones less than 2 cm in the distal and middle ureter. A ureteroscope is inserted directly to the level of the stone. Stones are removed with a basket or graspers and a stent is placed.

Diet. Specific dietary instructions depend on the composition of the stone. However, conservative measures that are recommended for all persons with kidney stones are discussed in Table 39-5. Because of potential adverse effects on the bones and the overall incidence of stones, calcium and protein restrictions are not recommended.[30]

Activity. A person who is up and moving is more likely to pass a stone than one who is in bed. The urine is strained and observed closely for stones. The person is permitted to carry out usual activities.

NURSING MANAGEMENT OF PATIENT WITH RENAL CALCULI

ASSESSMENT

Health History

A patient history is an important key to diagnosis as well as to stone location. The location of the stone may often coincide with pain. If the stone is in the kidney, the pain may be constant and in the area near the costovertebral angle. As the stone moves through the urinary tract, the pain may accompany it, presenting as renal colic. Dietary, medication, and family history may also be pertinent. Urinary patterns should be investigated to highlight the possibility of obstruction: dysuria or voiding in small amounts followed by urgency. The patient may also report episodes of nausea or vomiting.

Physical Examination

Important components of the physical assessment of the person with renal calculi are examination for flank and costovertebral angle tenderness and measurement of vital signs especially temperature. Volume of urinary output should be ascertained as well as the presence of stones in urine.

NURSING DIAGNOSES

Nursing diagnoses are determined from analysis of patient data. Nursing diagnoses for the patient with renal calculi include but are not limited to (see also Nursing Care Plan):

Diagnostic Title	Possible Etiologic Factors
1. Acute pain	Presence and/or movement of stones
2. Risk for infection	Urinary stasis, presence of stones
3. Impaired urinary elimination	Obstruction from calculi
4. Anxiety	Home care and pain management

Nursing Care Plan — *Patient With Renal Calculi Undergoing Nephrostomy Tube Placement for Obstruction*

DATA Mr. N. is a 55-year-old health care administrator who reported to the emergency department with sudden-onset severe right flank pain. Diagnostic evaluation led to the diagnosis of bilateral renal calculi with obstruction on the right side. A right nephrostomy tube has been placed and connected to gravity drainage. Mr. N. is married with two grown children living in distant states. His wife works full time. He is anxious about caring for his nephrostomy and voices concern about pain management. His wife is concerned that the remaining stones will block his other kidney.

Nursing assessment reveals that Mr. N.:

- Has a nephrostomy tube on the right midback connected to gravity drainage; urine in the bag is blood tinged with some clots
- Has a small amount of crusted drainage on the insertion site without erythema
- Has a blood pressure of 160/94, heart rate of 100 beats/min, and temperature of 98.2° F orally
- Guards his right flank during examination
- Has small pinpoint granules seen in strained voided urine

Continued

Nursing Care Plan *Patient With Renal Calculi Undergoing Nephrostomy Tube Placement for Obstruction—cont'd*

NURSING DIAGNOSIS **Acute pain related to renal calculi and placement of nephrostomy tube**
GOALS/OUTCOMES Will return to pain-free status

NOC Suggested Outcomes
- Pain Level (2102)
- Pain Control (1605)

NIC Suggested Interventions
- Pain Management (1400)
- Analgesic Administration (2210)

Nursing Interventions/Rationales
- Assess location, severity, frequency, duration, and quality of pain. Use a pain scale to rate patient's perception of pain. *Provides baseline data to assess effectiveness of pain control interventions.*
- Apply warm compresses to flank area. *Warmth decreases inflammation and promotes relaxation.*
- Administer prescribed analgesics. *Provides pain relief by altering the perception of pain and blocking pain pathways to the brain.*
- Encourage use of relaxation techniques such as focused breathing, music, and guided imagery if acceptable to patient. *Promotes comfort and decreases the need for narcotic analgesics by altering the perception of pain.*

Evaluation Parameters
1. Reports pain relief following pain control measures
2. Reports progressive decrease in pain

NURSING DIAGNOSIS **Risk for infection related to urinary stasis and break in skin integrity (insertion and presence of nephrostomy tube)**
GOALS/OUTCOMES Will remain free of infection

NOC Suggested Outcomes
- Immune Status (0702)
- Risk Control (1902)

NIC Suggested Interventions
- Infection Protection (6550)
- Wound Care (3660)
- Surveillance (6650)

Nursing Interventions/Rationales
- Assess temperature, nephrostomy site, urinary frequency and urgency, and abdomen for tenderness. *Changes from baseline data may indicate the presence of infection.*
- Maintain strict asepsis when changing nephrostomy dressing. *To decrease the potential for bacterial contamination of the surgical site.*
- Assess nephrostomy site for erythema, drainage, tenderness, induration, or swelling. *Indicates the presence of actual or developing infection.*
- Monitor for signs of systemic infection (chills, fever, diaphoresis). *Indicates the presence of actual or developing infection.*
- Obtain tissue/fluid sample for culture and sensitivity if indicated. *To identify the causative organism of infection and to monitor effectiveness of therapy.*
- Maintain hydration and voiding schedule. *To prevent bladder distention and urinary stasis.*
- Administer prophylactic antibiotics as prescribed. *To maintain steady blood levels to decrease the risk of infection.*

Evaluation Parameters
1. No evidence of localized (redness, swelling, tenderness, warmth) or systemic (fever, chills, increased white blood cell count) infection

NURSING DIAGNOSIS **Impaired urinary elimination related to presence of renal calculi and nephrostomy tube**
GOALS/OUTCOMES Will achieve normal urinary elimination pattern

NOC Suggested Outcomes
- Urinary Elimination (0503)

NIC Suggested Interventions
- Urinary Elimination Management (0590)
- Tube Care: Urinary (1870)

Nursing Care Plan Patient With Renal Calculi Undergoing Nephrostomy Tube Placement for Obstruction—cont'd

Nursing Interventions/Rationales

- Assess intake and output and presence of clots in nephrostomy collection bag. Strain all urine for calculi and send for analysis. *Deviations from normal indicate potential mechanical blockage. Data help determine treatment strategies.*
- Encourage high fluid intake (3500 to 4000 ml/24 hours). *Promotes passage of stones and dilutes urine.*
- Assess for dysuria, urgency, frequency, or incontinence. *These findings are indications of infection or altered renal function.*
- Maintain patency and position of nephrostomy tube, avoiding kinks in tubing and keeping urinary drainage bag in dependent position. *Prevents reflux of urine into the kidney and dislodging of the tube; allows for gravity drainage of urine.*

Evaluation Parameters

1. Urine output >30 ml/hr via voiding and nephrostomy tube
2. Urine flows freely from nephrostomy tube

NURSING DIAGNOSIS **Anxiety related to home management of nephrostomy tube**
GOALS/OUTCOMES Will perform self-care for nephrostomy tube without anxiety

NOC Suggested Outcomes

- Anxiety Control (1402)
- Coping (1302)
- Knowledge: Treatment Procedures (1814)

NIC Suggested Interventions

- Anxiety Reduction (5820)
- Coping Enhancement (5230)
- Teaching: Psychomotor Skill (5620)

Nursing Interventions/Rationales

- Assess level of anxiety. *Provides a baseline for planning interventions.*
- Encourage patient/family to express fears and concerns. *Provides opportunity to validate patient's/family's feelings. Identifies concerns/fears so that appropriate interventions can be planned and implemented.*
- Assist patient with identifying primary support systems. *Adequate support mechanisms reduce anxiety.*
- Teach (demonstrate and provide written instructions) patient and wife regarding care of nephrostomy tube. *Knowledge decreases anxiety. Written instructions provide a resource for later referral if needed.*
- Observe patient and wife performing nephrostomy care. *To ensure correct technique and to provide reinforcement of learning. Reinforcement builds self-confidence and decreases anxiety.*
- Provide emergency numbers for home support. *Knowledge of ready resources or support helps reduce anxiety.*

Evaluation Parameters

1. Uses resources and support systems effectively
2. Reports reduced anxiety
3. Independently cares for nephrostomy tube

EXPECTED PATIENT OUTCOMES

Expected patient outcomes for the patient with renal calculi may include but are not limited to:

1. Will report pain of 2 or less on a scale of 1 to 10
2. Will be free of the signs and symptoms of infection
3. Will maintain urine output equal to intake
4. Will use resources and support systems effectively

INTERVENTIONS

1. Controlling Pain

Renal colic is an excruciating type of pain. Morphine or other opiates are given in doses to control the pain. Relaxation techniques such as music therapy and guided imagery are also useful.

2. Preventing Infection

The presence of renal calculi can lead to an increased incidence of infection in susceptible patients. The nurse should monitor the patient for any signs of a UTI. Persons with renal calculi should be encouraged to increase fluid intake to at least 3500 to 4000 ml/day. Liquids should be caffeine-free as caffeine acts as a diuretic. Prophylactic antibiotics are frequently indicated and should be administered as directed.

3. Promoting Urinary Elimination

Input and output should be monitored. Urine output is normal in the presence of unilateral obstruction. Urinary diversion devices (nephrostomy or ureterostomy) should be assessed frequently for correct placement and patency. The tubing should be kept free of kinks to prevent reflux of urine.

The urine of all persons with relatively small stones should be strained. Urine can be strained easily by placing two opened gauze sponges over a funnel. Stones vary in size and may be no larger than the head of a pin. The stones are saved for inspection by the physician and sent to the laboratory for analysis.

4. Decreasing Anxiety

Because of the abrupt nature and severity of pain from renal calculi, fear and anxiety are commonplace. Careful assessment of the patient's anxiety level is necessary to guide future interventions and teaching. The patient should be encouraged to verbalize fears and concerns. The nurse should assist the patient in developing a support system and educate the patient on symptom management.

Patient/Family Education

Teaching for the person who has had urinary calculi should include:

- Drink at least 3000 ml of fluids/day and empty the bladder at regular intervals.
- Follow any dietary prescriptions.
- Know name, dosage, and side effects of medications prescribed to acidify or alkalinize the urine.
- Report to physician signs of recurrence of calculi (costovertebral pain or pain radiating to external genitalia).
- Report to physician signs of a UTI (burning on urination, frequency, urgency, or fever).

Health Promotion/Prevention. Measures can be taken to decrease the potential for renal stones in persons at high risk. Adequate hydration (intake of 3000 ml/day or more unless contraindicated) helps to prevent urinary stasis that can lead not only to stone formation but also to a UTI. Persons with indwelling catheters need scrupulous aseptic technique in catheter care to prevent infection and require adequate hydration and patent catheter drainage to flush away deposits at the catheter tip.

EVALUATION

To evaluate effectiveness of nursing interventions, compare patient behaviors with those stated in the expected patient outcomes. Successful achievement of patient outcomes for the patient with renal calculi is indicated by:

1. Reports pain as a 2 or less on a scale of 1 to 10.
2. Remains afebrile with no burning, urgency, or frequency of urination, and temperature within normal limits.
3. Has input equal to output.
4. Reports decrease in anxiety, has identified support systems, and is able to manage care independently.

COMPLICATIONS

Complications occur as a result of untreated obstruction. If urine flow is not reestablished, severe pain and hydronephrosis with resultant kidney failure may occur. In addition stasis of urine increases the risk of infection.

Urethral Strictures

Etiology/Epidemiology

A urethral stricture is a narrowing or constriction of the lumen of the urethra. Urethral strictures can be congenital or acquired. Congenital urethral strictures can occur in isolation or in combination with other urinary tract anomalies. The majority of acquired urethral strictures result from trauma secondary to accident or instrumentation (traumatic catheter placement/removal or a chronic indwelling Foley catheter), inflammation or pressure from the outside by adjacent structures, or by growing tumors. Urethral strictures occur more often in men than in women, primarily because of the length of the urethra.

Pathophysiology

Strictures are scars in the urethral epithelium. When the urethra is completely severed and anastomosed, strictures frequently occur at the surgical site. As the scar tissue contracts, the length of the urethra may shorten and the lumen of the urethra narrows. Inflammation causes a hyperplasia of the lining of the urethra, and the stricture develops. *Balanitis xerotica obliterans,* a chronic skin disease of the penis, is the major cause of inflammatory strictures.[3] Other causes include gonorrhea, chlamydia, and tumors that exert pressure against the exterior of the urethra.

The first symptoms of urethral stricture are usually a decrease in the urinary stream and difficulty initiating the stream. Other symptoms are those of a UTI and urinary retention. Severe urethral strictures result in complete urinary obstruction, leading to the signs and symptoms of hydronephrosis.

Collaborative Care Management

Special imaging studies (retrograde urethrography and voiding cystourethrography) are used to diagnose the length, location, and diameter of the stricture. Urethral strictures can be repaired with urethroplasty, dilation, or stent placement.[51] Dilation is accomplished by inserting splinting catheters of increasing size into the urethra past the area of the stricture.

Patient/Family Education. Education for the patient and family centers on recognition of early signs and symptoms of a decrease in urine stream and urine retention. Education should be focused on high-risk groups (persons with frequent bladder infections or a history of trauma to the pelvic region). If dilation is used as treatment, patients can be taught to perform this procedure.

Tumors of the Kidney

Etiology

Although the exact causes of renal cell carcinoma have not been identified, certain risk factors have been linked to the disease. The strongest risk factor is tobacco use (cigarette, pipe, or cigar). Obesity, exposure to analgesics, ADPKD, and occupational exposure to cadmium, asbestos, leather tanning, and certain petroleum products have been implicated in the development of renal cell carcinoma.[27] The majority of renal cell carcinomas start in the proximal convoluted tubule.

Epidemiology

In 2001 there were approximately 30,800 new cases of renal cell cancer and about 12,100 deaths from the disease.[1] Renal cell carcinomas account for approximately 3% of adult cancers and occur twice as often in men as in women. The onset is rarely before the age of 30 years, and this type of cancer is most commonly seen in persons 40 to 70 years old. At the time of diagnosis, about one third of persons have metastatic disease.[27] The most common sites of metastasis are the lung, lymph nodes, liver, and bone.

Pathophysiology

Renal carcinomas usually develop unilaterally but may occur bilaterally. There are five distinct cell types: clear cell, papillary, chromophobe, collecting duct, and "unclassified." Clear cell type is the most common type. Renal cell carcinoma is staged using the TMN system or the Robson system. The TMN system provides information about the tumor (T), regional lymph node involvement (N), and distant metastases (M). The Robson system, which is more widely used in the United States, categorizes tumors in stages. In stage I disease, the tumor margins are well defined (encapsulated) and compress the kidney parenchyma during growth, rather than infiltrating the tissue. The upper pole of the kidney is usually involved, and the tumor is usually large at the time of diagnosis. In stage II, the tumor invades the fat surrounding the kidney. Stage III consists of local metastasis either through direct extension or through the renal vein or lymphatics (lymph node involvement). Distant metastases during stage IV are primarily in the lungs or bone, but other areas, such as the liver, spleen, opposite kidney, or brain, may also be involved. Prognosis is based on the stage and advancement of the disease at diagnosis. Factors influencing the prognosis include the overall health and nutritional status of the patient.

Painless hematuria is the most frequent sign of renal cell carcinoma. Unfortunately, the hematuria is often intermittent, lessening the person's concern, which may cause a delay in seeking treatment. Any person with hematuria should have a complete urologic examination, as immediate investigation of the first signs of hematuria positively affects the prognosis. Other signs and symptoms include dull flank pain, palpable mass, unexplained weight loss, fever, and polycythemia. Some persons may be totally asymptomatic and are diagnosed by a radiologic abnormality detected on ultrasound or by abdominal CT scan. Hypertension may also be present as a result of stimulation of the renin-angiotensin system.

Collaborative Care Management

Diagnostic Tests. Most renal tumors are detected incidentally when an ultrasound or abdominal CT has been obtained for some other abdominal complaint. An IVP is usually done in the diagnostic workup of hematuria. If a mass is identified, further diagnostic imaging is usually indicated (ultrasound, CT scan, or MRI). Biopsy confirms the diagnosis.

Treatment. Unless the person is a poor surgical risk or has extensive metastases, the diseased kidney is removed (radical nephrectomy) through a transabdominal, flank, or extraperitoneal approach. Radical nephrectomy, performed to prevent metastases, includes the removal of the kidney, adrenal gland, proximal ureter, renal artery and vein, and surrounding fat and Gerota's fascia. Laparoscopic nephrectomy is a safe and minimally invasive alternative to a radical nephrectomy.[6] The laparoscopic technique offers a smaller incision, shorter length of stay, and a shorter recovery period.[31] See Figure 39-8 for incision sites using laparoscopic technique. Nephron-sparing surgery is indicated in those who have only one kidney or a small tumor and allows persons with only one kidney to maintain life without dialysis.

Neither standard chemotherapy nor radiation used before or after nephrectomy has been shown to be effective. Other therapies include the use of hormones, immunotherapy, alpha- interferon, and interleukin-2 therapy. The use of chemotherapeutic agents in combination with immunomodulation agents has shown some benefit. Interleukin-2 has shown some promise for the treatment of renal cell carcinoma with partial to complete regression of tumor in clinical trials. Five-year survival rates after treatment of stage I, II, and IIIA tumors are 70%.[1]

Patient/Family Education. If surgery is the treatment chosen, patient and family teaching focus on perioperative instructions (see Chapter 16). Management of the patient after nephrectomy is similar to that for persons undergoing major abdominal surgery (see Chapter 34) and urinary diversion (see p. 1229).

Education for persons with nonsurgical treatment should focus on the disease process, treatment options, and expected outcomes. Many therapies for renal cell carcinoma are experimental. It is imperative that patients fully understand the risks and benefits of each option. The diagnosis of cancer is frightening for patients and their families. Information on support groups such as "I Can Cope" through the American Cancer Society may be helpful to persons facing cancer.

Tumors of the Bladder

Etiology/Epidemiology

The bladder is the most common site of cancer in the urinary tract. An estimated 54,300 persons were diagnosed with cancer of the bladder in 2001.[1] Cancer of the bladder occurs three times more often in males than in females and is the fourth most common tumor in men. Most cases occur in men between 60 and 80 years old. Although environmental exposure to aromatic amines found in many industries (rubber, electric, paint, and textiles) had been a major risk factor in the development of bladder cancer, tobacco exposure is now the greatest risk factor. Other risk factors include previous exposure to certain chemotherapeutic agents, pelvic irradiation, and chronic infections.

There are three types of bladder tumors: transitional cell, squamous cell, and adenocarcinoma. Transitional cell carcinoma accounts for 90% of cases, followed by squamous cell (8%), and adenocarcinoma (1% to 2%). One of the earliest developments in transitional cell carcinoma is the loss of genetic material on the long arm of chromosome 9.

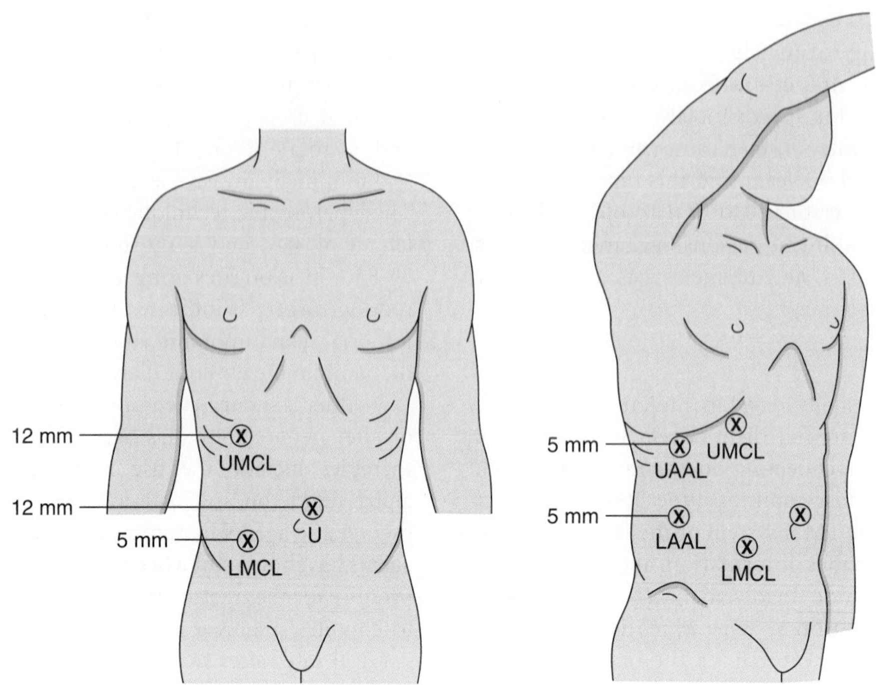

Figure 39-8 Port placement for laparoscopic nephrectomy. *LAAL*, Lower anterior-axillary line; *LMCL*, lower midclavicular line; *U*, umbilicus; *UAAL*, upper anterior-axillary line; *UMCL*, upper midclavicular line.

BOX 39-3 Grading and Staging of Advancement of Carcinomas of the Bladder

Grades	Differentiation
Grade I	Well differentiated
Grade II	Medially differentiated
Grade III	Poorly differentiated
Grade IV	Anaplastic

Stages	Tissue involvement
Stage 0	Mucosa
Stage A	Submucosa
Stage B	Muscle
Stage C	Perivesical fat
Stage D	Lymph nodes

Pathophysiology

Most neoplasms are of the transitional cell type because the urinary tract is covered with transitional epithelium. Most persons diagnosed with bladder cancer initially have superficial disease. Superficial bladder tumors develop via the papillary or invasive pathways. The majority of bladder tumors begin as papillomas. Although most papillomas are noninvasive, some infiltrate to deeper tissues; therefore all papillomas of the bladder are considered premalignant and are usually removed when identified. As the name implies, tumors that develop via the invasive pathway usually infiltrate deeper tissues and have a high risk of metastasis.

Carcinomas of the bladder are graded and staged according to the definitions in Box 39-3. Grading is done by the TMN classification system. Grade I and II bladder tumors are usually superficial, whereas grade III and IV tumors are usually invasive.

Painless hematuria is the first sign of a bladder tumor in most patients. As with renal cell carcinoma, the intermittent nature of the hematuria may cause delay in seeking treatment. Hematuria may be accompanied by urgency and dysuria. Some patients are asymptomatic until obstruction of the bladder outlet or ureters occurs. Painless hematuria may also be seen in nonmalignant urinary tract disease and in cancer of the kidney; therefore any hematuria should be investigated. Cystitis may also be an early sign of disease, because the tumor acts as a foreign body in the bladder, causing inflammation. Pain in the pelvic region may indicate regional or distant involvement.

Collaborative Care Management

Diagnostic Tests. Urinalysis that reveals blood for no apparent cause warrants further investigation. An IVP reveals filling defects in the bladder and upper tracts. A cystoscopy permits visual inspection and facilitates biopsy of suspicious lesions. Cytologic analysis on a total voided urine sample may reveal malignant cells before the lesion can be visualized by cystoscopy. Urine can also be tested for tumor markers. A chest x-ray study and bone scan maybe ordered to rule out metastases. A CT scan and MRI may be indicated to evaluate surrounding tissues and organs.

When a tumor is detected by cystoscopy, initial staging and treatment are done by transurethral resection of the bladder tumor. Clinical determination of the invasiveness of the tumor is important in establishing a therapeutic regimen and in predicting the prognosis.

Treatment. Treatment options include intravesical chemotherapy, surgery, and radiotherapy. In intravesical chemotherapy/immunotherapy, the agent is instilled directly into the bladder via a catheter. This technique is used in patients with superficial disease or to reduce recurrence in patients whose tumors have been surgically resected. Because of limited absorption of the drugs from the bladder, the main side effect is irritation with voiding. Mitomycin C, thiotepa, doxorubicin, and bacillus Calmette-Guérin are the most common agents used.[8]

Surgical Management. The most common surgical options include transurethral resection or laser photocoagulation and partial or radical cystectomy. Transurethral resection is used to grade and stage tumors and to remove superficial tumors. Laser photocoagulation is reserved for superficial bladder cancer. Cystectomy provides the best control of local disease. If the entire bladder is removed (radical cystectomy), diversion of the urinary tract is necessary. A long, vertical abdominal incision is present, along with one or more pelvic drains. A nasogastric tube is inserted in the operating room, and the patient is given nothing by mouth until gastrointestinal function returns. Radiotherapy or radiation directed at the bladder and standard chemotherapy are treatment options that are often used with the surgical treatments.

Partial removal of the bladder (segmental resection) is usually performed for tumors of the bladder dome. In the immediate postoperative period, bladder capacity is usually less than 60 ml. However, the elastic tissue of the bladder regenerates, increasing bladder capacity to 200 ml to 400 ml within several months.

Urinary diversion procedures are required for persons undergoing radical cystectomy. Other indications for diversion procedures include birth defects, neurogenic bladder, chronic progressive pyelonephritis, and irreparable trauma to the urinary tract. A urinary diversion establishes an uninterrupted flow of urine, most often via a stoma where the urine is collected in an appliance attached to the skin's surface. The flow of urine may be diverted at any level of the urinary system; however, the most common urinary diversion procedure in the United States is the ileal conduit, followed by the colon conduit.[9] With the *ileal conduit,* the ureters are excised from the bladder and transplanted into one end of a 15 to 20 cm segment of ileum resected from the intestinal tract. The remaining intestinal segments are anastomosed, and gastrointestinal function is expected to return to its normal preoperative state after healing. The end of the resected ileum into which the ureters are connected is sutured closed, and the other end is brought through the abdominal wall to the skin surface to create a stoma (Figure 39-9). The urinary bladder may be resected or left intact, depending on the reason for the diversion. The ileal segment functions as a passageway for urine, rather than as a reservoir.

The *colon conduit* (colonic loop) is performed similarly to an ileal conduit except that a segment of colon (ascending, descending, transverse, or sigmoid) instead of ileum acts as the conduit for the urine. The colon conduit has reduced the incidence of urinary reflux for some persons. Preoperative and postoperative nursing care and ongoing management are the same as those for ileal conduit surgery.

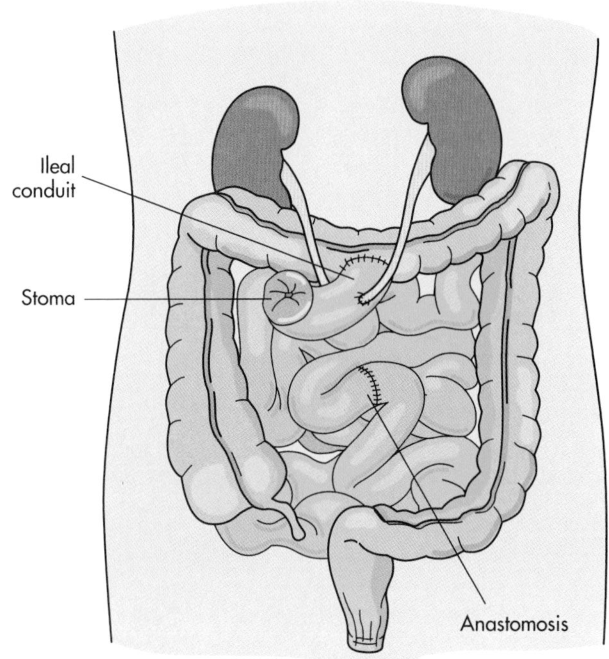

Figure 39-9 Ileal conduit or ileal loop.

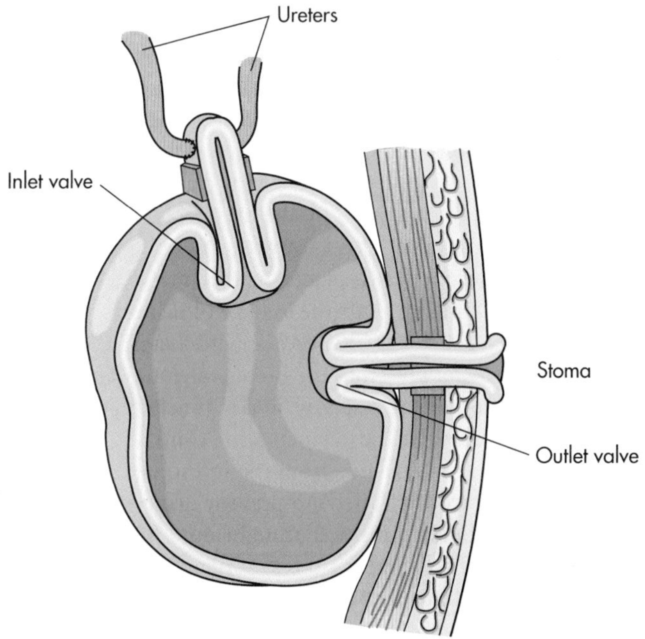

Figure 39-10 Kock continent ileal urinary reservoir.

The *continent urostomy* has an internal reservoir made from intestine that holds urine. The stoma must be catheterized at regular intervals to drain the reservoir. The *Kock continent ileal reservoir* (Figure 39-10) is formed from loops of the small intestine. The *ileocecal (or Indiana) pouch* consists of portions of large intestine and ileum (Figure 39-11).

Cutaneous ureterostomy is performed when the patient's physical condition prohibits more extensive surgical procedures and is rarely used as a permanent form of diversion.

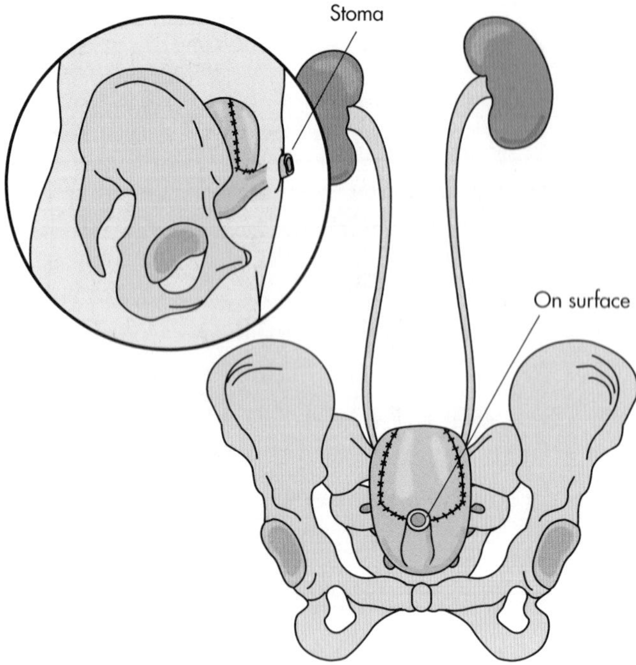

Figure 39-11 Ileocecal continent urinary reservoir (Indiana pouch).

One or both ureters are excised from the bladder and brought out through the skin, either on the flank or the anterior abdominal wall to create a small stoma. When both ureters are involved, each may be brought out to the skin surface separately, resulting in two stomas, or the ureters may be joined and brought out through the abdominal wall to form only one stoma.

In the Kock pouch procedure the ureters are connected to the pouch above a valve. This valve prevents reflux of urine to the kidney. A second valve placed in the intestinal segment leading to the stoma prevents the leakage of urine, thus maintaining continence. For the ileocecal or Indiana pouch, which incorporates the large bowel, the ureters are anastomosed to the colon portion of the reservoir in a manner to prevent reflux. The ileocecal valve is used to provide continence, and the section of ileum that extends from the intestinal reservoir to the skin is narrowed (plicated) to prevent urine leakage. The end of the intestinal segment is brought out onto the skin to form the stoma. The stoma for the continent urostomy is usually flush to the skin and placed lower on the abdomen than the ileal conduit stoma.

Stoma assessment is an important postoperative consideration. The ileal conduit, colon conduit, and continent urostomy stomas should be edematous and a beefy-red color after surgery. Pallor or a gray color may indicate ischemia. Early complications after surgery include breakdown of the anastomosis in the gastrointestinal tract, leakage from the ureteroileal or ureterosigmoid anastomosis, paralytic ileus, obstruction of the ureters, wound infection, mucocutaneous separation, and stomal necrosis. Complications that may occur after hospitalization include stomal problems (retraction, stenosis, or hernia) and urinary infections.

The *orthotopic neobladder* is an alternative to urinary diversion for patients who have a competent sphincter without cancer in the urethra, trigone, or bladder neck. A reservoir is constructed and the patient's urethra is attached to the reservoir. This procedure produces good results, preserves the patient's ability to void, and eliminates the need of a stoma.[2,22]

Diet. No specific dietary modifications are necessary for the patient with bladder cancer. Anorexia and nausea are problems that need to be addressed. High-caloric supplements are encouraged to prevent wasting. Fluid intake of at least 2 L/day is recommended to avoid dehydration. Substances that irritate the bladder should be avoided, including alcohol, tea, spices, and smoking.

Activity. There are no specific activity restrictions related to treatment. Activity should be encouraged to promote the patient's well-being and return to ADLs.

Referrals. Care of the patient after radical cystectomy should be approached in a multidisciplinary manner. For diversions other than the orthotopic neobladder, an enterostomal therapist should be consulted to provide teaching on pouch and ostomy care. Home care is involved to provide supplies for pouch care. The American Cancer Society is a resource for all cancer patients and may provide supplies free of charge to patients. Another resource for patients is the United Ostomy Association, which has branches in most major cities.

NURSING MANAGEMENT OF PATIENT WITH URINARY DIVERSION SURGERY

PREOPERATIVE CARE

Any procedure for diversion of urine that results in an external stoma leads to a significant change in body image. Reactions may vary depending on the reason for the procedure, but virtually every person requires time and much nursing support while adapting to the altered means of urine elimination.

Assessment should include the patient's thoughts and feelings regarding urinary diversion. Information on the patient's lifestyle, occupation, and family roles helps the nurse plan appropriate interventions. The patient is prepared before surgery as for any other surgical procedure (see Chapter 16).

Counseling and Teaching

When the physician tells the person of the probable need for a urinary diversion, the first reaction is likely to be disbelief and disappointment. The reason for the surgery may influence the reaction. Time to grieve is essential, and the nurse can be a source of support during this time. Persons who have been well informed about the surgical procedure as well as the postoperative period and long-term management goals are generally better able to adjust to the entire experience than those who do not receive such preparation.

A person with a urinary diversion needs time to adjust to the change in body appearance, including the presence of an external pouch, internal reservoir, or the presence of a stoma. An opportunity should be provided for the patient to explore feelings and to begin to cope with all the changes.

The enterostomal therapy nurse specializes in the care of and instruction to persons who have or will have an ostomy. If possible, a preoperative meeting with the patient and enterostomal therapy nurse should be arranged. If time permits, a meeting with the patient and a representative from the United Ostomy Association can be arranged. The United Ostomy Association has trained volunteers who have coped well with an ostomy and are willing to visit patients and provide support, reassurance, and personal experiences. A postoperative or home visit can also be arranged.

The nurse's goals for preoperative teaching must reflect the patient's needs. However, certain basic information must be included. The patient should understand the surgical procedure and should know whether a pouch will have to be worn after surgery.

Preoperative instruction also involves preparing the person for the appearance of the stoma. The patient should be told that the stoma will be red, that the tissue is similar to the mucosal lining of the mouth, and that it will not be painful. Determination of the exact placement for the stoma should be made by the surgeon and/or the enterostomal therapy nurse. The stoma for the ileal conduit is usually constructed on the right side of the abdomen, below the waist, and within the rectus muscle. The continent urostomy stoma is placed lower on the right or left side of the abdomen because a flat surface for a pouch is not needed. Selection of the site is ideally made before surgery and should include evaluation of the proposed site when the patient is lying, sitting, and standing. Because smooth, even skin surrounding the stoma is important for optimal adherence of the pouch, it is important that the site selected is free of scars, skinfolds, and bony prominences.

Booklets designed for the person having a urinary diversion may be given to the patient before surgery. A simple drawing supplements and clarifies explanations of the surgical procedure. The patient should be given the definition of terms such as stoma, urostomy, and pouch. Some persons need this additional information to assist them in accepting the surgery. Others may be unable to review written materials until after surgery. The patient with an ileal or colon conduit is informed of the need to wear the pouch, the frequency of changing and emptying the pouch, and the function of the urinary stoma. Patients undergoing continent urostomy procedures are informed of the need to catheterize the stoma at regular intervals and to irrigate the internal reservoir to remove mucus. Assurance is given that the nurse will provide stoma care immediately after surgery and that the patient will be assisted to master self-care before discharge. Patients who have an orthoptic neobladder must be taught that urination will require increased pressure by abdominal straining and pelvic floor muscle relaxation. Because of the risk of inefficient voiding, patients should be taught to void when the bladder feels full or every 3 to 4 hours.

Guidelines for Safe Practice

The Patient After Urologic Surgery

1. Promote ventilation.
   a. Encourage breathing exercises.
   b. Encourage self-turning in bed frequently.
   c. Encourage ambulation.
2. Monitor patency and output of urinary catheters.
3. Prevent complications.
   a. Change wet dressings to protect skin.
   b. Restrict food and oral fluids if bowel sounds are absent.
   c. Encourage fluids to 3000 ml/day when permitted.
   d. Monitor for bright-red blood on dressings or in urine.
4. Administer analgesics to control pain.

Before urinary diversion surgery a complete cleansing of the bowel is required. Bowel preparation reduces the possibility of fecal contamination when the bowel is resected and used to form the conduit or internal reservoir. The cleansing routine consists of a low-residue diet for 2 days followed by a clear liquid diet for 24 hours before surgery and nothing by mouth after midnight the night before surgery. Large-volume oral bowel cleansing solutions (GoLYTELY or Colyte) or a special laxative and fluid program may be prescribed the day before surgery. Cleansing enemas may be ordered to supplement the clean-out procedure. Intestinal antibiotics such as erythromycin or neomycin may also be administered orally.

POSTOPERATIVE CARE

The basic needs of the patient requiring urologic surgery are the same as those of any other surgical patient (see Chapter 18). Special emphasis must be placed on promotion of ventilation and adequate urine output, prevention of distention and hemorrhage, and attention to drainage tubes and dressings (see Guidelines for Safe Practice box and Clinical Pathway). For persons who have had segmental resection, the decreased bladder size is of major importance in the postoperative period. The patient returns from surgery with catheters draining the bladder both from a cystostomy and from the urethra to avoid obstruction of drainage. The bladder would become distended rapidly if obstruction occurred, resulting in disruption of the bladder suture line.

As soon as the urethral catheter is removed, the patient becomes acutely aware of the small bladder capacity. Most patients need to void at least every 20 minutes and be reassured that the bladder capacity will gradually increase. Total fluid intake should be 3000 ml throughout the day. Large quantities of fluid should not be ingested at one time, and fluids should be limited for several hours before going out.

After an ileal or colon conduit procedure, stents are usually in place in the stoma for 1 week to 10 days to promote urinary drainage. The person with a continent urostomy usually has a catheter and/or stents in the stoma sutured in place to allow drainage from the reservoir. A drain tube is placed into the pelvic area for drainage of blood and surgical fluids. All tubes should be placed below the level of the kidney so that they can

clinical pathway *Cystectomy**

ATTENDING: POSTOP LOS 7 DAYS
MEDICAL DIAGNOSIS: ICD-9 CODE: 57.7x
Patient's/significant other's learning needs are identified and documented on PEP

	DATE: CLINIC DAY	INIT	DATE: PREOP DAY	INIT	DATE: DOS	INIT	DATE: POD 1 & 2	INIT
INTERDISCIPLINARY COMMUNICATION (CONSULTS)	Schedule PFTs if COPD/para (10.0) Schedule PAC if no preop day Smoking cessation reference PRN (10.0)		Anesthesia assmt Stomal marking (ET) (5.0) Home health (SW) (9.0) OR/blood consent Schedule OR PFT if indicated (10.0) Nutrition if hx pelvic radiation (7.0)		Notify HO or arrival Chaplain (8.0)		ET (5.0) SW discharge 9(.0) RT if unable to wean O_2 (10.0) PT PRN (6.0)	
ASSESSMENTS	High-risk screen (NSG) ET—discharge plan		Initiate database (RN) Physical assmt (RN) H&P (MD) Discharge assmt (SW/RN) Preprep weight (7.0)		VS q1hr × 4, q2hr × 4, then q4hr Urine output q4hr & notify HO if <30 ml/hr Pain (1.0) Epidural Gastric pH q6hr Protocols: Preop 1.56 OR care 1.115 PACU care 1.164		VS q4 with O_2 sat (10.0) Daily wt (7.0)	
DIAGNOSTICS (LABORATORY RADIOLOGY)			UA Electrolytes Type & screen CBC & PLT Chest x-ray ECG per anesthesia protocol				CBC & PLT Chem 7 AM	
MEDICATIONS	Home meds Multivitamin with iron 3 times/day		GoLYTELY PO 1100 obtain wt previously Erythromycin 1000 mg PO @ 1300, 1400, 2200 Neomycin 1000 mg PO @ 1300, 1400, 2200 D_5½NS IV @ 0000 150 ml/hr Protocol 1.40 Neomycin 1% enema @ 2200 Benadryl 50 mg PO HS if needed Home meds as ordered		Cefoxitin 1 gm IVPB q8hr × 7 doses Famotidine 20 mg IVPB q12hr PCA: MSO_4 1 mg q10min (max dose 6 mg) (1.2 acute pain) (1.79 IV opiates) Ketorolac 15 mg IVP q6hr × 9 doses Heparin flush 100 U IV q8hr PRN central line Heparin 5000 U SQ q8hr (2.0) Epidural–per APS 1.197 Epidural ⟶ Phenergan 12.5 mg IV q30min × 3 PRN (then q6hr PRN) Maalox 30 ml q4hr PRN for positive hem or pH <5 Benadryl 25 mg IVP QHS PRN Tylenol suppository 650 mg PR for temperature >38.5° C Cepstat Lozenges PRN		⟶ ⟶ ⟶ ⟶ ⟶ 2nd day change IV to D_5½NS with 20 KCl @ 100 ml/hr ⟶ ⟶ ⟶ ⟶	

Courtesy University of Virginia Medical Center.
*Times are given by 24-hour clock.
PEP, Patient education plan; *PFTs,* pulmonary function tests; *HO,* house officer; *SW,* social worker; *COPD,* chronic obstructive pulmonary disease; *para,* paraplegic; *RT,* respiratory therapy; *PT,* physical therapy; *PAC,* preadmissions center; *IVPB,* intravenous piggyback; *OBR,* orthopedic bowel routine; *PCA,* patient-controlled analgesia; *D5½NS,* 5% dextrose in 0.5 N saline solution; *APS,* acute pain service; *SP,* Jackson-Pratt drain.

DATE: POD 3	INIT	DATE: POD 4	INIT	DATE: POD 5	INIT	DATE: POD 6 & 7	INIT
		HHR development (9.0)		Solidify discharge plan: ET, SW & PT D/C needs identified (9.0) HHR done (9.0)			
VS q8hr or as indicated Continue to monitor sats q4hr × 2 after O_2 D/C (10.0) ——→ Wound assmt		——→ ——→		——→ Check BM (4.0) ——→			
		CBC & PLT Chem 7 AM				CBC Chem 7 AM	
——→ D/C Famotidine Nizatidine 150 mg PO q12hr ——→ ——→ ——→ D/C Maalox when NG out ——→ ——→ ——→		D/C PCA Percocet #2 PO q4hr PRN (1.0) ——→ D/C Epidural (1.0) ——→ ——→ ——→		OBR if no BM (4.0) ——→ Benadryl 50 mg PO q HS PRN ——→ Tylenol 650 mg PO q4hr PRN ——→		——→ ——→ ——→	

Continued

clinical pathway *Cystectomy—cont'd*

ATTENDING: POSTOP LOS 7 DAYS
MEDICAL DIAGNOSIS: ICD-9 CODE: 57.7x
Patient's/significant other's learning needs are identified and documented on PEP

	DATE: CLINIC DAY	INIT	DATE: PREOP DAY	INIT	DATE: DOS	INIT	DATE: POD 1 & 2	INIT
DRESSINGS, TUBES/DRAINS			Saline lock placed Protocol 1.40 Start fluids by 2100 TEDS: Apply thigh high at hs preop (2.0)		NG (1.43) to suction Check dressing with VS. reinforce PRN JP to bulb suction (1.41) If continent voiding diversion • stents to separate bag • irrigate Foley with 30 ml NS q3hr—start in PACU If catheterized continent diversion • irrigate Malecot 30 ml NS q3hr—start in PACU • stents to separate ostomy bags If ileal conduit • stents in ostomy bag		→ Dressing off with wound assmt (3.0) Ostomy supplies to room (5.0) →	
INTERVENTIONS/ TREATMENTS			Protocols: 1.5 Anxiety Cystectomy POC 2.122		Hibiclens 4% bath 0500 Turn cough and deep breathe q2hr (10.0) ICS while awake 10 × qhr (10.0) O_2 per cannula to keep sats >90 Protocol 1.48 (10.0)		→ Wean O_2 if sats >90 (10.0)	
ACTIVITY			As tolerated (6.0)		Bedrest Turn q2hr while in bed (6.0) 1.1 activity intolerance 1.103 ADL		OOB to chair for 20 min × 2 (2.0) (6.0) Walk into hallway POD 2 with assist (2.0) (6.0)	
NUTRITION	High-protein diet (7.0) until day of admission, then clear liquids		Encourage fluids until NPO after midnight (7.0)		NPO except hard candy (7.0)			
DISCHARGE PREPARATION	Discuss anticipated discharge plan with patient/family (include transportation		Assess home situation (SW, RN) with patient/family		Encourage open communication 1.5 Anxiety 1.210 Family coping		Home health inpt visit as indicated (9.0)	
EDUCATIONAL ACTIVITIES	Educational material Cystectomy information book given (8.0)		Preop teaching 3.9 Pain management teaching booklet Cystectomy educational plan		Postop ICS reinforcement (10.0) Review tubes with patient/family Review pain meds (1.0) PEPs 3.12 meds 3.21 anticoagulant therapy Urinary diversion Discuss operative outcome, preliminary plan with family (MD, RN) Protocol 1.210		Give discharge sheets Review teaching with patient/family	

DATE: POD 3	INIT	DATE: POD 4	INIT	DATE: POD 5	INIT	DATE: POD 6 & 7	INIT
D/C NG if + flatus (4.0) →		One JP out if drainage <5 ml/8 hr D/C central line as indicated Convert IV to heparin lock →		D/C heparin lock as indicated →		Staples out D/C JP day 6 Stents D/C day of discharge	
→ D/C O_2 (10.0)		→		→		→	
Walk in hallway with assist × 2 (2.0) (6.0)		Walk in hallway × 3 with assist (2.0) (6.0)		Walk in hallway × 3 with or without assist (2.0) (6.0)		Walk in hallway × 3 without assist (2.0) (6.0)	
IV fluids NPO 8 hr after NG removed Ice chip 30 ml max q1hr (7.0)		Clear liquids (7.0)		Reg diet (7.0)		Reg diet (7.0)	
Ostomy supply resource identified (SW, RN) (5.0)		HHR (NSG) (5.0)		All discharge orders in MIS (MD) Discharge plan complete, including patient transportation		Discharge plans validated/ implemented (9.0)	
Begin ostomy teaching (ET) (5.0)		Educational demonstration		Ostomy care with staff assist • Bag change • Empty bag • Night bag • Patient irrigate with assistance (5.0)		Patient/family member able to care for ostomy (5.0) MIS med information sheets reviewed (pharmacy, RN) Discharge teaching completed (RN) Patient irrigate with RN observation	

Continued

clinical pathway *Cystectomy—cont'd*

ATTENDING: POSTOP LOS 7 DAYS
MEDICAL DIAGNOSIS: ICD-9 CODE: 57.7x
Patient's/significant other's learning needs are identified and documented on PEP

	Process and discharge outcomes	
Concern	**Desired outcome**	**Data met/initials**
1.0 Pain management	Verbalizes successful postop pain management	
	Ability to describe and manage pain needs	
	On discharge verbalizes ability to manage level of pain	
	Aware of implications of increased level of pain and who to notify after discharge	
2.0 DVT	Free of all s/s of DVT	
	Aware of s/s of DVT and who to notify after discharge	
3.0 Infection	Free of all s/s of infection	
	Aware of s/s of infection and who to notify after discharge	
4.0 Bowel function	Bowel elimination maintained/restored to baseline	
5.0 Ostomy care	Patient/family member able to demonstrate care of ostomy/tubes/drains and equipment	
	Home health referral completed	
6.0 Mobility	Able to walk around unit 4 × with appropriate assistance on day 5	
7.0 Nutrition	Return to preop diet without GI distress	
	Able to describe high-protein foods	
	Able to describe maintaining intake of high-protein foods	
8.0 Support group	Support group contact made available	
9.0 Home health	Teaching communicated to home health agency in writing	
	Home health agency contacted	
10.0 Respiratory function	Free of s/s of respiratory complication	
	Contact with smoking cessation program	

drain by gravity. The newly created internal reservoir must be protected from distention to prevent leakage at the anastomosis.

A nasogastric tube with suction is used until effective intestinal peristalsis has returned and to administer medication. The nasogastric tube is maintained to prevent pressure on the intestinal anastomosis. The patient may have nothing by mouth until peristalsis returns. Intravenous fluids are given until adequate intake of oral liquids is tolerated. Once peristalsis resumes, clear liquids are started and the diet is advanced gradually.

Maintaining Skin Integrity

Skin care is an important consideration after urinary diversion surgery. Leakage of urine on surrounding skin can cause skin breakdown. For urinary diversions that exit to the skin's surface, care must be taken to prevent urine leakage onto the surrounding skin and abdominal incision. For the ileal or colon conduit, a transparent pouch is placed around the stoma in the operating room. The pouch allows visualization of the stoma, catheter or stents, and stoma sutures. The stoma should be bright pink or red. Any evidence of gray or black discoloration is reported to the surgeon, as this may indicate

ALTERED PATHWAY COURSE (note in progress notes)	
NOTE	DATE/SIGN

HOME EQUIPMENT/DISCHARGE	DATE/INITIAL
NEEDED:	PROVIDED:
Ostomy supplies	
If Malecot, irrigation setup	
Drain bag supplies	
If Foley, drain bag supplies	
Medication	

decreased circulation, which leads to necrosis of the stoma. Careful assessment of the stoma that is in contact with a catheter is imperative because improper positioning of a catheter may exert pressure on the stoma mucosa, leading to necrosis. The pouch is changed within 24 to 48 hours after surgery to allow for better visualization and assessment of the stoma and the peristomal skin. The abdominal incision is observed at least daily for healing of the suture line.

In the early postoperative period the pouch is positioned so that it drains to the side of the bed, facilitating drainage and emptying of the pouch. The urostomy pouch has a valve at the bottom that permits emptying. Drain tubing and a collection bag can be attached to the valve of the pouch to allow continuous drainage in the postoperative period (Figure 39-12). The procedure for changing the pouch is outlined in the Guidelines for Safe Practice box.

Monitoring Urine Output

After any type of urinary diversion, urine output is initially monitored every hour and output less than 30 ml/hr should be reported. Edema of the stoma or of the ureteral anastomosis site may prevent urine drainage, leading to hydronephrosis

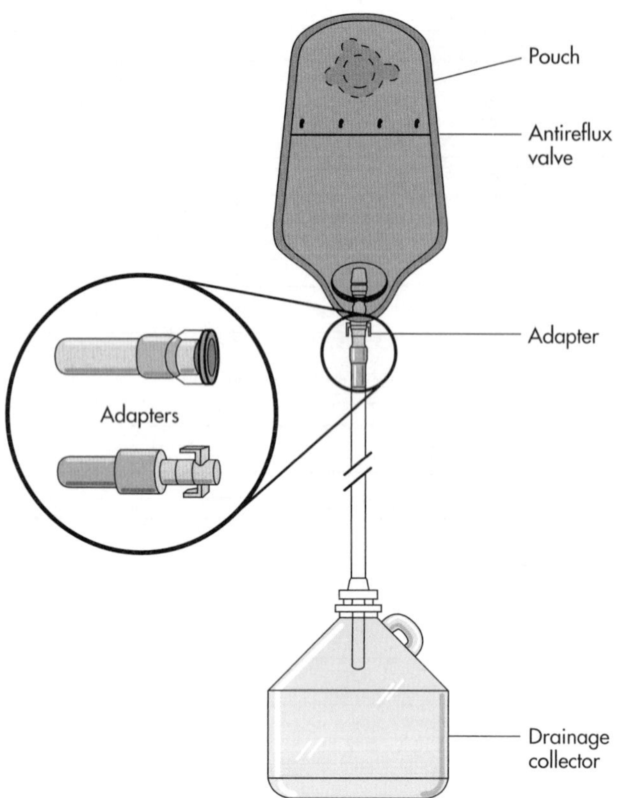

Figure 39-12 Urostomy pouch connected to continuous drainage.

Guidelines for Safe Practice

Changing a Urinary Pouch

1. Explain procedure to patient, being sure to include sensory information.
2. Assemble all supplies.
3. Empty the pouch and gently remove it from the skin.
4. Cleanse the peristomal skin with mild soap and water. Rinse and pat dry. Wash mucus secretions off the stoma gently.
5. Place a rolled piece of gauze or cotton balls over the stomal opening to absorb draining urine while caring for the skin.
6. Measure the diameter of the stoma and cut a corresponding opening in the skin barrier and the pouch or select the corresponding size of precut pouch.
7. Apply skin sealant around the stoma if desired. Allow the area to dry completely.
8. Attach the pouch to the skin barrier. The pouch and skin barrier may be applied to the skin separately or together. In the early postoperative period it is easier to attach the pouch to the skin barrier and then apply the system in one piece to the skin.
9. Apply the pouch and skin barrier around the stoma, keeping the adhesive area free of wrinkles or creases. Press gently but firmly into place. The valve at the bottom of the pouch must be closed or attached to drain tubing and a collection bag.

or a break in the anastomosis. Other complications that may first be detected by decreased urine output include dehydration, obstruction of the ureters, or compromised renal function. Decreased urine output is associated with symptoms of peritonitis (fever, abdominal distention, and pain). These symptoms should alert the nurse to the possibility of intraperitoneal leakage caused by a leak at either the intestinal or the ureterointestinal anastomosis. If this occurs, emergency surgery is required to repair the leak.

Urine is initially pink but should change to clear by the third postoperative day. Bright red blood and/or clots should be reported immediately, as it may indicate problems at the anastomosis or an infection. Mucus, a normal discharge from the intestinal segment, is usually secreted from an ileal or colon conduit or continent urostomy.

Epidural and parenteral opioids are given for the first 4 to 5 days after surgery. Opioids may be administered via patient-controlled analgesia (see Chapters 12 and 18). After the patient begins oral intake, oral analgesia can be used.

Patient/Family Education

Postoperative instruction is started as soon as the patient feels able to participate in urostomy care. During the active phases of teaching, the pouch is removed more often than is recommended after discharge. The patient (or caregiver) should learn how to manage the assembly and apply and empty the selected pouch.

After surgery the edema of the stoma begins to subside within 7 days, but the stoma continues to decrease gradually in size for the next 6 to 8 weeks. Therefore, before discharge the patient is taught how to measure the stoma and how to adjust the pouch size to accommodate the smaller stoma. Too large an opening can lead to skin problems for persons with an ileal or colon conduit. Too small an opening may restrict circulation or cause trauma to the stoma. The opening should be no more than 2 to 3 mm larger than the stoma.

Several types of pouches are available (Figures 39-13 and 39-14). All have two things in common: a pouch to collect the urine and an outlet or valve at the bottom for easy emptying every 3 to 4 hours. The basic types of pouches are (1) semidisposable pouches that fit onto a permanent disk or faceplate and (2) one-piece or two-piece disposable pouches. The pouches adhere to the body with a skin barrier to form a watertight seal. The type of pouch selected depends on the patient's preference, body build, and special needs, such as physical or visual impairment. The enterostomal therapy nurse can assist the patient in the assessment and selection of the appropriate pouch. Although most pouches can be worn for 5 to 7 days, reusable pouches are used less frequently because of the incidence of infection.

Health Promotion/Prevention. Because tobacco use accounts for a large majority of bladder cancer, teaching patients benefits and methods of smoking cessation is imperative. Smoking cessation programs should be encouraged for all tobacco users. Although most industries have rid the workplace of known carcinogens, patients should be questioned regarding occupational exposures, specifically in the rubber, manufacturing, textile, and printing industries.

GERONTOLOGIC CONSIDERATIONS

The older adult is at increased risk for developing cancer of the bladder. The disease is most common in the 60- to 90-year-old

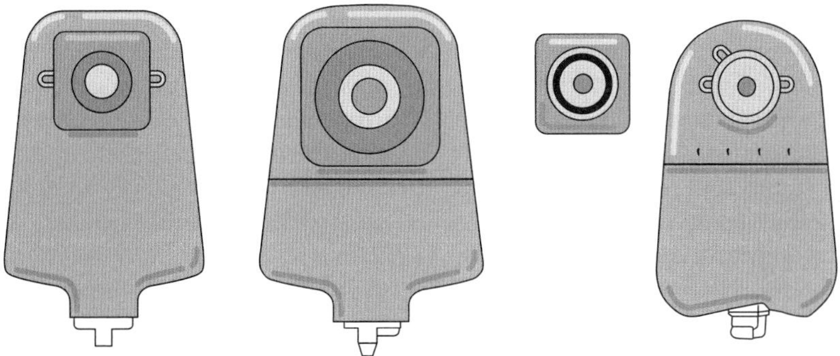

Figure 39-13 Disposable one- and two-piece pouches.

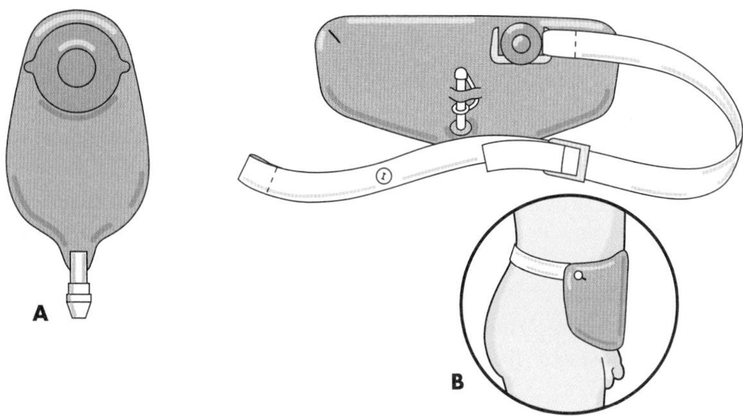

Figure 39-14 Reusable pouches. **A,** One-piece pouch. **B,** One-piece nonadhesive pouch.

age group. Radiation and chemotherapy may not be well tolerated by the elderly population. Modifications for stoma care and appliances may be necessary for older patients with decreased dexterity because of arthritis or sensory deficits. Home nursing care may be necessary to manage ostomy care. Because of age-related skin changes, fitting the pouch may be difficult and preventing skin breakdown may be a challenge.

SPECIAL ENVIRONMENTS FOR CARE

Community-Based Care

Before the patient is discharged from the hospital, the nurse must be certain that the individual can manage the urinary drainage system and can detect any deviations from normal. A return visit or an opportunity for telephone consultation with the primary nurse involved in the teaching or the enterostomal therapy nurse is extremely helpful. The majority of patients with bladder cancer undergoing urinary diversion requires home nursing care for stoma and pouch maintenance. Patients with a continent diversion should be informed that they will need a follow-up cystogram to assess the anatomic integrity of the reservoir.

COMPLICATIONS

The person with a urinary diversion is at greater risk for a UTI because of the shorter distance from the urinary diversion to the kidneys. The patient must be taught the signs and symptoms of a UTI (cloudy urine, blood in urine, strong odor to urine, flank pain, fever, and malaise). Urine cultures are obtained by catheter from the ileal or colon conduit stoma. A specimen taken from the pouch is likely to be contaminated. A pouch with an antireflux valve is recommended to reduce infection from bacteria found in the pouch.

Bowel segments used in continent reservoirs are subject to bacterial colonization leading to pouchitis and pyelonephritis. In addition, mucus, which can cause obstruction and be a source of infection, may be produced for about 1 year after surgery. Daily pouch irrigation with normal saline should be incorporated into care routines.

Problems with the peristomal skin include erythema and irritation from contact with urine, candidal infections, allergic dermatitis, and pseudoverrucous (wartlike) lesions.

Problems with the stoma include bleeding, stenosis, or hernia. A small amount of bleeding from the stomal mucosa may occur when the stoma is cleansed. Bleeding generally stops within a few seconds. If bleeding persists or is unusually severe, the physician is notified. Blood that originates from the urinary tract rather than the stoma may be related to complications such as infection or calculi.

Interaction of urine with the bowel epithelium causes altered transport of electrolytes. When the ileum or colon is used, the conduit mucosa resorbs chloride from the urine, and the patient may develop a metabolic hyperchloremic acidosis. A person with optimal renal function has no difficulty excreting the resorbed chloride. When renal function is compromised, the patient is more likely to develop electrolyte problems. This resorption can also occur in those with internal reservoirs because the urine is retained within the internal pouch until the stoma is catheterized and the urine drained. Follow-up urologic care visits and electrolyte studies are imperative. Early in the postoperative period as the suture lines heal, urine may leak into the peritoneal cavity causing peritonitis. Patients usually present with painful, rigid abdomen, fever, and absent bowel sounds.

Trauma to the Urinary Tract

Assessing the integrity of the urinary tract must be part of the evaluation of any person with traumatic injury to the lower trunk. Injuries particularly related to the urinary tract damage include penetrating and blunt trauma. The kidney is the most frequently injured urinary tract structure in trauma situations, followed by the bladder.

Etiology/Epidemiology

Blunt abdominal trauma from motor vehicle accidents, falls, and assaults account for the majority of renal and bladder trauma. Pelvic fractures may result in bladder perforation and urethral tearing. A sharp blow to the body, particularly to the lower back, may result in contusion, tearing, or rupture of a kidney. The mobility and anatomic location of the ureters make injuries from blunt trauma rare; most external ureteral injuries occur from gunshot wounds.

Pathophysiology

Renal injuries are classified into one of five grades based on radiographic and clinical history, ranging from contusion or hematoma to a shattered kidney[32] (Figure 39-15). Urine output may be scant or absent after trauma to the urinary tract. Although hematuria is present in trauma to the kidney, bladder, and urethra; hematuria is absent in approximately 40% of persons with renal vascular injuries.[4] However the amount of hematuria does not necessarily correlate to the amount of kidney trauma. The first symptoms of trauma to the kidney usually are hematuria and pain or tenderness of the upper abdominal quadrant and flank on the involved side. Persons with bladder injury may report abdominal pain and distention. The inability to urinate is common is persons with bladder and urethral trauma. Signs of shock may be present if hemorrhage is extensive.

Collaborative Care Management

Diagnostic Tests. Urine should be evaluated for hematuria and a complete blood count and chemistry profile should also be obtained. Urethral catheterization should never be attempted in persons with blood at the urinary meatus. A urology consult should be initiated.

A CT scan or MRI should be obtained to assess renal injuries. A cystography is the imaging test appropriate for bladder injuries. Ureteral injuries can be assessed by a CT scan or IVP. Retrograde urethrography is the diagnostic test used for males suspected of having urethral trauma and urethroscopy is indicated for females.

Treatment of injuries is focused on stabilizing the patient and surgically repairing any perforations or lacerations of the urinary tract. Initial treatment includes controlling bleeding, preventing shock, and promoting urinary drainage. A cystotomy may be performed to provide urinary drainage when injuries involve the bladder or urethra. Vital signs, fluid balance records, and hematocrit levels are monitored to assess bleeding. Reports of pain may indicate ureteral colic, signifying obstruction of the ureter by a clot. Surgery is required to control severe hemorrhage; otherwise the kidney is allowed to heal spontaneously. Bed rest is maintained until gross hematuria resolves; thereafter, activity progresses according to tolerance and absence of hematuria.

When urethral injuries are suspected, great care must be taken when inserting urinary catheters to prevent further urethral injury. A urologist may need to insert the catheter during a retrograde ureterogram or cystogram (see Chapter 38).

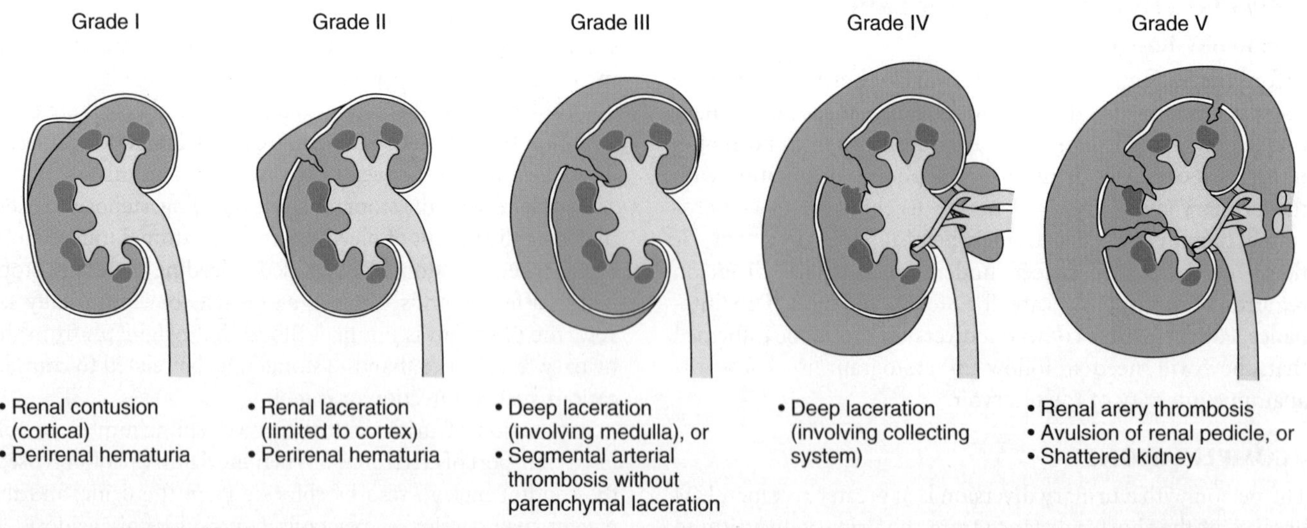

Figure 39-15 Severity of renal injury.

Nephrectomy may be indicated depending on the severity of the trauma. Adequate waste removal can be maintained by the remaining kidney or by less than half of one functioning kidney.

Patient/Family Education. Education for the patient with renal trauma focuses on treatment and surgical management. Much of the patient's concern depends on the type of surgery and cause of the trauma. Because the surgery temporarily or permanently alters urinary elimination, the person is concerned about the degree of change that will occur. Care of the person after nephrectomy is similar to that for persons with abdominal or urinary diversion procedures.

Because trauma to the kidney is often blunt, suffered as a result of motor vehicle accidents, contact sports, and falls, health promotion teaching is an important nursing intervention. Teaching should include preventive strategies such as wearing a seat belt when in an automobile, following safety rules when riding a bicycle or walking, and wearing protective equipment when participating in contact sports. Persons with one kidney should be cautioned regarding participation in contact sports.

Urinary Retention

Urinary retention is the inability to empty the bladder. The kidneys are producing sufficient urine, but the person is unable to expel the urine from the bladder.

Etiology

Causes of urinary retention are either mechanical or functional. Anatomic causes may be congenital or acquired and include anatomic blockage of urine flow in the lower urinary tract. Functional causes include impairment of urine flow in the absence of mechanical obstruction. Box 39-4 summarizes causes of urinary retention.

BOX 39-4 Causes of Urinary Retention

Mechanical

Congenital/Anatomic

Urethral stricture
Urinary tract malformation
Spinal cord malformation

Acquired

Renal calculi
Urinary tract infection
Trauma
Tumor
Pregnancy

Functional Causes

Neurogenic bladder dysfunction
Ureterovesical reflux
Decreased peristaltic activity of the ureter
Detrusor muscle atrophy
Atrophy (i.e., fear of pain after surgery)
Medications (i.e., anesthetics, opioids, sedatives, and antihistamines)

Epidemiology

The incidence of urinary retention increases with age, particularly in men.[34] Because of the multifactorial etiology of urinary retention, it is difficult to predict the frequency of occurrence. Urinary retention can be acute or chronic. Acute urinary retention, if unrelieved, may lead to acute kidney failure or bladder rupture. Chronic retention (>300 ml) is associated with a recurrent UTI, kidney stones, and hydronephrosis, which have been discussed previously.

Pathophysiology

Urinary retention may be related to bladder outlet obstruction, deficient detrusor muscle strength, or both. Acute urinary retention is often associated with a large volume of fluid intake and delayed urination, which causes distention of the detrusor muscle and impaired contractility. The end result and primary feature of urinary retention is the inability to void. The bladder becomes distended with urine and is sometimes displaced to either side of the midline. Percussion over a full bladder produces a "kettle drum" sound. Discomfort occurs from pressure of the bladder on other organs, and the person has an urge to urinate. Restlessness and diaphoresis also may occur with a full bladder.

Voiding 25 to 50 ml of urine at frequent intervals often indicates *retention with overflow.* The intravesicular (within the bladder) pressure increases as the bladder continues to fill with urine. As the bladder overfills, the restraining capability of the sphincter is taxed. A small amount of urine flows out of the bladder to reduce the intravesicular pressure to the level where the sphincter can control the flow of urine once again. The patient may state that the bladder continues to feel full. As the bladder fills again, the cycle is repeated. The urine specific gravity is normal or high in the presence of retention with overflow because the kidney's ability to produce urine is not impaired.

Collaborative Care Management

Urinary retention is a urologic emergency and, if untreated, can lead to kidney damage. Interventions for urinary retention are aimed at reestablishing urine flow.

Diagnostic Tests. The diagnosis of urinary retention is based on determining the amount of residual urine after voiding attempts. Urine yield of 250 to 300 ml on catheterization after voiding is indicative of retention. Postvoid residual should be less than 25% the person's total bladder capacity. If an attempt to pass an average-sized catheter (14F to 16F) fails, a urologist should be consulted. Cystoscopy may be indicated.

Medications. Medication use in urinary retention is determined by the etiology. Retention caused by sensory/neurologic problems may be treated with cholinergic medications. This group of medications stimulates bladder contraction and should not be used if obstruction is suspected. Bethanechol chloride (Urecholine) may be prescribed to initiate voiding by stimulating the detrusor muscle of the bladder. Urinary retention from prostate enlargement is discussed in Chapter 55.

Treatments

Direct Bladder Drainage: Cystostomy Tube. When obstruction occurs below the bladder, continuous drainage must be provided to prevent damage to the kidney. One means of providing drainage is the use of a cystostomy tube, which is placed directly into the bladder through a suprapubic incision. This method is usually used when the urethra is completely obstructed or when the prolonged use of a urethral catheter is contraindicated. During surgery, a cystostomy tube and a small urethral catheter are inserted to drain the bladder. Both catheters must be monitored for patency. Once patency is assured, it is not necessary to record the output from each catheter separately, as both tubes drain the bladder. The catheters do not necessarily drain equal amounts of urine. Securely anchoring these catheters is necessary to prevent them from slipping out of position.

Surgical Management

Drainage of Kidney, Pelvis, and Ureters. If a ureter becomes obstructed, a catheter must be placed directly into the renal pelvis. This prevents kidney damage that otherwise would occur as pressure increases because of continued urine formation. For a complete obstruction, a *nephrostomy* or *pyelostomy* tube may be inserted (surgically or under radiologic guidance) into the renal pelvis. The surgical incision is located laterally and posteriorly in the kidney region. An alternate form of drainage for a ureteral obstruction is the surgical placement of a ureterostomy tube passed through an incision in the upper outer quadrant of the abdomen into the ureter above the obstruction. The catheter is then passed through the ureter to the renal pelvis. If the ureter is unobstructed or partially obstructed, the renal pelvis may be drained by a ureteral catheter, which is passed up the ureter to the renal pelvis through a cystoscope.

All catheters must be firmly anchored to prevent accidental dislodging and trauma to the tissues. When a catheter is inserted during surgery, it is usually sutured in place and affixed to the skin. When not sutured in place, the tube should be anchored to the skin at two points using adhesive, with some slack in the tubing between the anchor points. Care must be taken to prevent kinking of the tubes while the patient is in the side-lying position in bed.

Unobstructed drainage of catheters leading to the renal pelvis is of the utmost importance. The normal renal pelvis has only a 5- to 8-ml capacity; if the catheter obstructs for even a few minutes, the resulting pressure can damage renal structures. In some patients, nephrostomy tubes may be left in place for several months, serving as a form of urinary diversion for long-term use. The person at home with a catheter draining the kidney pelvis must know how to obtain medical assistance quickly if the catheter becomes obstructed or dislodged.

Diet. No dietary modifications are necessary. Fluid intake should be encouraged. Optimally, 2 to 3 L of fluids per day should be consumed as prophylaxis for urinary tract infections.

Activity. No activity restrictions are indicated. Patients should be instructed not to obstruct the tubing if a nephrostomy is in place. Patients should also keep drainage bags empty during activity to avoid strain on the drainage tubes. Drainage bags should be kept below the level of the kidney or bladder (depending on location being drained) to prevent backflow of urine.

Referrals. Home health care support may be necessary for intermittent catheterization. Additionally, an enterostomal therapist may be needed to manage nephrostomy sites and to prevent skin breakdown. Community resources include the United Ostomy Association and the American Urological Association.

NURSING MANAGEMENT OF PATIENT WITH URINARY RETENTION

ASSESSMENT

Persons experiencing urinary retention may be unable to void any urine (retention) or may void small amounts of overflow urine but be unable to empty the bladder completely (retention with overflow). Urine remaining in the bladder is a good medium for bacterial growth, leading to a UTI.

Health History

Areas of the health history that need to be thoroughly explored when assessing the person with urinary retention are the patient's voiding pattern including the frequency of voiding and volume of each void; occurrence of pain or burning on urination (dysuria), which is indicative of a probable UTI; and presence of a sensation of need to void or bladder fullness immediately after voiding, which is indicative of retention with overflow. Fluid intake and output also need to be evaluated.

Physical Examination

Important aspects of the physical examination of the person with urinary retention include determination of the characteristics of the patient's urine (color, clarity, and odor) and palpation of bladder above the symphysis pubis after voiding.

NURSING DIAGNOSES

Nursing diagnoses are determined from analysis of patient data. Nursing diagnoses for the person with urinary retention may include but are not limited to:

Diagnostic Title	Possible Etiologic Factors
1. Urinary retention	Obstruction, position for voiding, immobility, inability to initiate stream
2. Risk for infection	Indwelling catheter, stasis of urine
3. Deficient knowledge	Lack of exposure/recall

EXPECTED PATIENT OUTCOMES

Expected patient outcomes for the person with urinary retention may include but are not limited to:

1a. Will void several times a day in adequate amounts
1b. Will state that bladder feels empty
1c. Will not have a palpable bladder after voiding
2a. Will be free from signs of a UTI

2b. Will perform self-catheterization correctly, using appropriate technique (if indicated)
2c. Will have unobstructed drainage of urine
3a. Will describe signs of retention or a UTI (for indwelling catheter)
3b. Will describe self-care, lifestyle adaptations, and need for follow-up care

INTERVENTIONS

1. Promoting Micturition

Before catheterization, noninvasive measures are attempted to stimulate voiding of urine. These measures may include assuming a position that facilitates voiding (positional stimuli: male standing upright; female sitting upright), running water (auditory stimuli), or pouring water over the perineum or placing the patient's hands in water (tactile stimuli). Sitting in lukewarm water may help relax the urinary sphincters. Providing privacy and encouraging use of the bathroom whenever possible also help to promote voiding. The patient can be taught to "double void" to promote complete bladder emptying. After voiding, the patient attempts a second void 5 minutes later to completely empty the bladder.

2. Preventing Infection

Urethral catheterization is the most common means of draining the bladder. The Foley catheter is most frequently used for this purpose. Because catheterization is the major cause of UTIs, strict asepsis must be practiced during insertion and in assembling the drainage equipment. The need for urethral catheterization must be carefully evaluated and should never be undertaken for nursing convenience.

If the nurse finds resistance or that a catheter is difficult to insert, the procedure is discontinued and the physician or health care provider is notified. Traumatic catheterization predisposes the patient to a UTI, formation of urethral strictures, and bleeding. In patients with urethral disorders, resistance may be encountered with a standard catheter; special equipment, such as catheter dilators or filiform catheters, may be needed. Catheterization after urologic surgery and the use of specialized catheter equipment are not nursing procedures.

The urethral catheter is changed when it is in danger of becoming obstructed by sediment within its lumen. Before discharge, the person going home with an indwelling urethral catheter needs to learn to change the catheter or have a family member demonstrate the ability to insert a catheter.

Urinary catheterization is used in a variety of clinical situations in both acute and chronic care. Major reasons for catheter drainage are to:

Relieve temporary anatomic or physiologic obstruction.
Permit healing of the urinary system after surgery.
Permit accurate measurement of urine output in severely ill patients.
Relieve inability to void.
Prevent retention of urine in persons with neurogenic bladder.
Permit irrigation to prevent obstruction or urine flow.

Reestablishing urine flow is an immediate treatment goal for obstruction. The type of catheter used to provide drainage in the presence of obstruction depends on location of the blockage. Table 39-6 summarizes the use of specific types of catheters.

Intermittent Catheter Drainage

Intermittent catheterization of the urinary bladder is used in the treatment of neurogenic bladder dysfunction secondary to spinal cord trauma, birth defects, urinary retention, and some chronic diseases.

Periodic complete emptying of the bladder eliminates residual urine (an excellent culture medium for bacteria) and maintains a good blood supply to the bladder wall by avoiding high pressures within the bladder.

Individuals are evaluated for the appropriateness of this form of management by the urologist. The potential for success should be evaluated, using input from the nurse, psychologist, social worker, and other involved health care professionals; however, teaching is generally a nursing responsibility. An individual catheterization regimen is planned using either clean or sterile technique as appropriate. The goals of intermittent catheterization are generally to prevent urinary retention and its sequelae (a UTI and kidney damage) and to achieve continence. The patient needs to know the expectations of the treatment plan to promote cooperation.

A size 14F catheter is generally used for an adult. A special silicone catheter without a balloon is used for intermittent catheterization. The volume of urine obtained with each catheterization is recorded so that the catheterization schedule can be adjusted as needed. The adult bladder should not be permitted to hold more than 300 to 500 ml at any time, as greater amounts lead to overdistention of the bladder and increased susceptibility to infection. The frequency of

TABLE 39-6 Types of Catheters

Type of Catheter	Description	Use
Whistle-tip	Open slant end	Hematuria or blood clots in urine
Robinson	Closed end, multiple lumen	Intermittent catheterization
Foley	Balloon (5 or 30 ml) to secure catheter in bladder	Constant drainage
Coudé	Tapered curved end	Suspected prostatic hypertrophy
Ureteral	4F to 6F size (urethral catheters are usually 14F to 16F)	Drain ureters
Malecot	Batwing-shaped tip	Drain renal pelvis, nephrostomy drainage
Pezzar	Mushroom-shaped tip	Drain renal pelvis, nephrostomy drainage

catheterization is determined by the amount of residual urine.

Even though the clean technique is suitable for home use,[11] sterile technique is necessary during hospitalization to decrease the possibility of nosocomial (hospital-acquired) infection. When hospitalized, the patient who customarily performs self-catheterization may continue to use clean technique, but preferably a sterile catheter will be used each time. Specimens for culture must be obtained by the usual sterile catheterization technique to avoid contamination of the specimen. The patient is informed why sterile technique is necessary in the hospital setting.

3. Patient/Family Education

The person needs to understand the rationale for intermittent catheter drainage and for regularity of bladder emptying (Patient Teaching box). Basic anatomy of the genitalia and urinary tract should be illustrated for the patient to alleviate fears of causing damage by incorrect placement of the catheter.

Most persons require much support during the actual teaching but usually become comfortable with the procedure. Initially a mirror is used to teach women catheter insertion. The woman should learn to catheterize while sitting on the commode, using palpation to locate the urethral meatus. Men may sit or stand for self-catheterization. It is important that men use generous amounts of lubricant to avoid urethral irritation; women generally do not require as much lubrication because of the shorter urethra. Family members may be taught catheterization if the patient is unable to perform self-catheterization. Clean technique has been shown to be effective in home use.

The tubing is disconnected at night to change from a leg bag to the overnight drainage bag and again in the morning to resume leg bag drainage. The drainage bag should hold at least 2000 ml for overnight collection. To lessen contamination, the caregiver is taught to wash the hands and then wipe the catheter and tubing with 70% alcohol before disconnection and reconnection. The disconnected ends of the drainage bags are protected with sterile gauze secured in place with a rubber band or protected with a connector cap. The drainage system should be kept as clean as possible by daily washing with soap and water. Teaching also includes the need to keep the drainage collection bag at a level lower than the cavity being drained to prevent urine reflux.

Persons requiring catheter drainage at home on a temporary or permanent basis must be able to safely maintain the urinary drainage system. A family member is instructed in all necessary care in case the patient is unable to perform care. Teaching includes care of the catheter and drainage system as previously described. A written list of needed specific supplies and where they can be obtained is helpful to avoid confusion.

The person needs to be well informed about adaptations that can be made with the urinary drainage system to allow a return to an optimal level of activity. A shower or tub bath with a catheter in place is generally permitted unless there is an unhealed surgical incision. The adhesive tape holding the catheter in place needs to be replaced after bathing. Leg bags are available in a variety of sizes and are concealed by clothing. Men or women do not need to remove an indwelling catheter before intercourse. This information should be included in all teaching because patients may hesitate to ask. The man can fold the indwelling catheter over the penis to facilitate insertion during intercourse.

The person with a urinary catheter of any type needs follow-up medical care. Instructions include the need to contact the physician if back pain, fever, or other urinary tract symptoms are present. Educating the patient about signs and symptoms of urinary retention, changes in the color and clarity of the urine, incontinence, and dysuria is undertaken when bladder drainage is discontinued. Often the first indicators of dysfunction are subjective comments from the patient. This information enhances detection of early recurrence of urinary drainage problems.

Patient Teaching
The Patient With Intermittent Catheterization

The patient or family can:

- Explain the need for adequate fluid intake, approximately 30 ml/kg of body weight.
- Explain the reason for the intermittent catheter drainage.
- State the need for regular, periodic, complete emptying of the bladder.
- Demonstrate self-catheterization using clean technique unless sterile technique is prescribed.
- Describe how to adapt the catheterization routine to the individual lifestyle.
- State how to obtain needed supplies.
- Describe symptoms of urinary tract infection requiring medical care.
- State plans for ongoing urologic care.

EVALUATION

To evaluate the effectiveness of nursing interventions, compare patient behaviors with those stated in the expected patient outcomes. Achievement of outcomes is successful if the patient with urinary retention:

1a. Voids several times a day in amounts of 150 to 400 ml/void.
1b. Has a bladder that is not palpable after voiding.
2a. Has no signs of UTI (fever, back pain, or increased serum white blood cell count).
2b. Correctly performs self-catheterization.
2c. Has a catheter that drains freely when in place.
3a. Lists signs of urinary retention or a UTI (for indwelling catheter) to be reported to physician.
3b. Describes self-care activities, lifestyle adaptations, and plans for follow-up care.

GERONTOLOGIC CONSIDERATIONS

Older patients are at increased risk for urinary retention because of decreased bladder tone and increased incidence of chronic disease. Structural changes in bladder muscle tone and prostatic enlargement in men play a key role. Although treatment options remain the same, the elderly patient must be fully evaluated regarding the ability to take part in treatment plans. Because of decreases in dexterity and sensory function, such as vision, catheterization and catheter care may be difficult.

SPECIAL ENVIRONMENTS FOR CARE

Community-Based Care

Clean (not sterile) catheterization technique is usually prescribed for home use. Hand washing is required before each catheterization, and the meatal area is cleansed with soap and water. After the catheter is inserted and the bladder is drained, the catheter is removed, washed with soap and water, and dried on a clean surface. Once dry, the catheter is stored in a closed container for the next use. The catheter is reused until it becomes either too soft or too hard to be directed properly.

If the hospital or outpatient teaching time is short, follow-up care may be required by a home health care nurse to help the person adapt the catheterization routine to life routines and to assist with any difficulties the patient may be having. Ongoing urologic care is essential, including periodic urine cultures.

COMPLICATIONS

Complications from treatment of urinary retention are related to catheterization. It is normal to note some dribbling of urine for a few hours after a urethral catheter has been removed because of dilation of the sphincter muscles by the catheter. Dribbling of urine that persists longer than a few hours should be reported to the physician; this symptom may indicate damage to the sphincters. In determining the type of intervention necessary to reestablish bladder control, information about the nature of the incontinence is gathered. Incontinence is described as complete (constant dribbling) or occurring only on urgency or stress. Assessment should include whether incontinence is present in all positions (lying, sitting, and standing). If muscular weakness of the sphincters is the major problem, incontinence is least likely to occur when the person is in a prone position and most likely to be a problem when the person is standing or walking. Perineal exercises may help to regain control of voiding.

Another problem that may arise after removal of a catheter is inability to void. The patient is encouraged to drink fluids and then attempt to void. The nurse carefully assesses the patient's bladder for distention. Efforts are made to provide comfortable positioning and privacy to facilitate voiding. A patient with adequate fluid intake should void within 8 hours. Patients with edema of the bladder neck may require temporary catheter reinsertion to facilitate urinary drainage.

Cystitis (inflammation of the bladder) may develop after catheter removal because of incomplete emptying of the bladder as muscle tone is being reestablished. Any abnormalities in color, odor, or sediment in the urine are reported.

Urinary Incontinence

Etiology

Urinary incontinence is the involuntary unpredictable expulsion of urine from the bladder and is encountered in several temporary and permanent conditions. There are several major types of incontinence: *urge* (the inability to suppress a sudden need to urinate), *stress* (intermittent leakage of urine resulting from a sudden strain, such as a cough or sneeze), *overflow* (characterized by dribbling, urgency, or frequency), and *functional* (inability to reach a toilet).

Epidemiology

Approximately 12 to 15 million Americans have urinary incontinence. The prevalence of incontinence is 1.5% to 5% in men and 10% to 25% in adult women under the age of 65 years. Urinary incontinence affects about 33% of women and 20% of men over age 60 who live in the community.[39] For persons who are institutionalized, the incidence increases to 50%. It is estimated that more than $15 billion a year are spent in managing patients with incontinence. Because of missed diagnoses and underreporting, the problem of urinary incontinence may be even more widespread. Risk factors related to urinary incontinence are found in the Risk Factors box.

Pathophysiology

Physiology of Urinary Continence. Most cases of incontinence are related to bladder and/or urethral dysfunction. As the bladder fills, the pressure within the bladder gradually increases. The detrusor muscle within the bladder wall responds by relaxing to accommodate the greater volume. When the bladder has filled to capacity, usually between 400 and 500 ml of urine, the parasympathetic stretch receptors located within the bladder wall are stimulated. The stimuli are transmitted through afferent fibers of the reflex arc for micturition. Impulses are then carried through the efferent fibers of the reflex arc to the bladder, causing contraction of the detrusor muscle. Completion of this reflex arc can be interrupted and voiding postponed through release of inhibitory impulses from the cortical center, which results in voluntary contraction of the

Risk Factors

Urinary Incontinence

TYPE	EXAMPLE
Stress	Loss of urethrovesicular junction in women
	Urethral irritation from infection or radiation after prostatectomy
	Obesity
	Sphincter incompetence
	Pelvic relaxation
	Multiple sclerosis
	Urinary tract infections
	Stroke
	Medications: hypnotics, tranquilizers, sedatives, diuretics
Overflow	Retention with bladder distention
	Fecal impaction
	Benign prostatic hyperplasia
Functional	Altered mental status
	Physical disabilities
	Physical barriers

external sphincter. If any part of this complex control system is interrupted, urinary incontinence results.

Urge incontinence is the involuntary loss of urine associated with an abrupt and strong desire to void (urgency). When active detrusor contractions overcome urethral resistance, urine leakage occurs. There are many potential causes for this type of incontinence including a UTI, obstruction, and neurologic diseases (multiple sclerosis or stroke). Urge incontinence can also be brought on by hearing running water, standing up after lying down, and rapid changes in temperature. Urge incontinence is more prevalent in elderly persons. The amount of urine lost can range from a few drops to the entire bladder contents.

Stress incontinence occurs as a result of dysfunction in the closure capabilities of the urethra or defective support structures.[17] The patient experiences a loss of 50 ml or less of urine as a result of increased abdominal pressure. Any activity leading to an increase in intraabdominal pressure on the bladder can result in urinary incontinence. These activities include lifting, exercising, coughing, sneezing, or laughing. Stress incontinence occurs primarily in women.

Increased distention of the bladder causes detrusor storage pressure to exceed urethral pressure, which results in *overflow incontinence.* Presenting symptoms include frequent or constant dribbling. Overflow incontinence can result from spinal cord injury, stroke, diabetic neuropathy, or radical pelvic surgery.

In *functional incontinence,* the urinary tract is normal but other factors contribute either to the inability to reach toileting facilities or the inability to perceive a full bladder. Lack of awareness of a full bladder is seen in those who are confused, demented, acutely ill, or sedated.

Last, incontinence may be caused by a disturbance of the urethrobladder reflex resulting from spinal cord lesions or damage to peripheral nerves of the bladder. Disturbances in urethrobladder reflex may be seen in persons with spinal cord malformations, injuries, or tumors and in those with compression of the spinal cord caused by fractures of the vertebrae, herniated disk, metastatic tumor, or postoperative edema of the spinal cord. The neurologic dysfunction results in detrusor inadequacy or *neurogenic bladder;* there are three types: reflex, spastic, and flaccid. The person with a neurogenic bladder has no control over bladder function.

Collaborative Care Management

Diagnostic Tests. Evaluation of the patient should begin with a voiding diary that includes voiding patterns and circumstances surrounding the episodes of incontinence. A urinalysis should be done to rule out a possible UTI as the cause of incontinence. Postvoid residual should be assessed because elevations may indicate an abnormality in bladder contraction and/or outlet resistance. Further diagnostic tests may be indicated if the cause of incontinence cannot be determined from these initial steps. A cystometrogram is a useful test especially for urge incontinence; it assesses the relationship between pressure and volume in the bladder primarily during the filling phase. There are many other urodynamic studies that can be used to determine the etiology of incontinence (uroflowmetry, electromyography, pressure flow studies). An ultrasound of the bladder, cystoscopy, and IVP may also be done to assess the structures and functioning of the urinary tract.

Medications. Medication management for the treatment of incontinence is based on the identified etiology of the incontinence. Box 39-5 lists common medications. These medications need to be used cautiously in older adults. Bladder outlet obstruction should be ruled out before use of medications.

Treatments. Treatment protocols and algorithms have been established by the U.S Department of Health and Human Services for the management of the incontinent adult. Treatments can be categorized as behavioral, pharmacologic, and surgical. A combination of therapies is often used. The type of therapy is guided by the type of incontinence (Table 39-7).

Behavioral therapy includes education about lifestyle changes and dietary modifications such as fluid restriction and avoidance of caffeine and other irritants. Behavioral techniques include bladder training, timed voiding, prompted voiding, and pelvic muscle exercises. Bladder training encompasses timed voiding (i.e., every 2 to 3 hours) in which the interval is gradually increased. Pelvic floor physiotherapy, often referred to as Kegel exercises, helps the patient suppress unwanted bladder contractions. These exercises involve the voluntary contraction and relaxation of the muscles that support the bladder and urethra. Although Kegel exercises have been part of incontinence therapy over the years, one recent study found pelvic floor exercises were effective in about 53% of the women studied.[7] The goal of pelvic floor physiotherapy is to

BOX 39-5 Medications Commonly Used for Urinary Incontinence

Urge

Anticholinergics

Over-the-counter cold/allergy formulations with antihistamines
Tricyclic antidepressants* (e.g., imipramine [Tofranil],* doxepin [Sinequan])*

Antispasmodics/anticholinergics

Oxybutinin, regular and sustained-release (Ditropan, Ditropan XL)
Tolterodine (Detrol)

*Estrogen**

Orally (opposed if uterus intact) or intravaginally

Stress

*Alpha-adrenergic stimulants**

Phenylpropanolamine, pseudoephedrine (over-the-counter cold/sinus formulations)

*Estrogen**

Orally (opposed if uterus intact) or intravaginally

From Rakel RE, Bope ET: *Conn's current therapy 2001,* Philadelphia, 2001, WB Saunders.
*Not FDA-approved for this indication.

increase the strength of the pelvic muscles, which prevents the downward rotation of the urethra and involuntary loss of urine. Because it is difficult for some women to isolate these muscles, a variety of methods have been used to help women exercise the correct muscles. These methods include the use of vaginal weights, vaginal electrical stimulation, and biofeedback. Vaginal weights, called vaginal cones, are inserted into the vagina and require contraction of the pelvic muscles to maintain their position. Biofeedback uses electromyography or vaginal pressure measurements that provide visual and/or auditory signals to an individual with respect to performance with pelvic floor muscle contraction.

The person with a brain tumor, meningitis, or traumatic injury to the brain that prevents adequate voluntary control of bladder function may benefit from a bladder retraining program. If the person's condition or response prohibits such a program, an internal or external drainage device should be used.

Persons with spinal cord injuries experience a transitory period of *spinal shock* in which urinary retention occurs (see Chapter 44). An indwelling catheter is placed to facilitate urinary drainage and prevent bladder distention. After the acute stage, management depends on the exact nature of any residual neurogenic bladder dysfunction. Persons with a lesion above the sacral segments and with an intact urethrobladder reflex may initiate voiding by pinching or stroking trigger areas of the thighs or suprapubic area. In persons with a lower motor neuron lesion, the use of *Credé's* method, which consists of exerting manual pressure over the bladder, may provide more complete bladder emptying. The appropriateness of this technique must be determined by the physician, based on the person's complete urologic status. Many individuals with neurogenic bladder dysfunction are taught intermittent self-catheterization using clean technique to prevent infection and to manage incontinence. Maintenance of a regular schedule for catheterization is stressed, and the frequency is determined on an individual basis.

Surgical Management. There are many surgical procedures to treat incontinence. The classic treatment has been surgical bladder neck suspension. The goal of this surgery is to return the bladder neck and urethra to their proper position. Treatment for a nonfunctioning sphincter includes a sling procedure, artificial urinary sphincter, and intraurethral bulking agents. Periurethral bulking is a relatively simple procedure performed under local anesthesia or sedation. This treatment involves injecting material around the urethra to increase urethral resistance. Other interventions include occlusive and supportive devices. Supportive devices improve continence by supporting the bladder neck. Tampons, traditional pessaries, contraceptive diaphragms, and intravaginal devices have been used for this purpose. Occlusive devices can occlude the urethra or bladder neck externally or internally via the urethra. For men, a clamp-type device is placed across the penile urethra. For women, occlusive devices may be inserted through the vagina or the urethra. An external occlusive device is a type of foam pad placed over the urethral meatus.[49] Finally, neuromodulation, modification of the sensory and/or motor function through electrical stimulation, can be tried when other conservative methods have failed. Although the precise mode of action is unclear, this method has been successful in inhibiting bladder activity.

Diet. Nutritional alterations for the patient with urinary incontinence involve the scheduling of fluid intake as well as avoidance of bladder stimulants such as alcohol, chocolate, and coffee. Fluid intake after dinner should be reduced or avoided.

Referrals. Patients with urinary incontinence should be referred to a urologist for management. Rehabilitation programs for bladder training are also useful for the patient with urinary incontinence. Community support programs are available in many areas. Companies marketing products used for incontinence management often sponsor these programs. Local hospital newsletters are a good source for programs related to incontinence management.

The U.S. Department of Health and Human Resources published Clinical Practice Guidelines for adults with incontinence. Publications are available for health care professionals and lay persons.

TABLE 39-7 Incontinence: Types, Causes, and Treatments

Type	Common Causes	Treatments
Stress	Pelvic floor muscular weakness; hypermobility of urethra	Behavioral therapy Kegel exercises Surgery: bladder neck suspension or sling alpha-adrenergic agonists
Urge	Detrusor overactivity related to urinary tract problems: UTI, kidney stones. Central nervous system problems: stroke, spinal cord injury	Behavioral therapy Bladder relaxants
Overflow	Obstruction: 1. Stricture, enlarged prostate 2. Neurogenic bladder (e.g., multiple sclerosis, certain spinal cord lesions)	1. Surgery 2. Catheterization (intermittent/chronic)
Functional	Dementia/immobility	Behavioral therapy Absorbent padding

NURSING MANAGEMENT OF PATIENT WITH URINARY INCONTINENCE

ASSESSMENT

Health History

Questions to ask the patient when assessing for urinary incontinence include these: What is the frequency of incontinence? What precipitates incontinence (stress, fear, coughing, sneezing, laughing, or exercise)? Is pain or burning present with incontinence? Is there an urge to void before incontinent episodes?

Physical Examination

Physical examination data to be collected to assess the person with urinary incontinence include volume of output; characteristics of the urine; and the patient's ability to follow directions, functional status, and ability to perform ADLs. The examination should also focus on identifying any physiologic reason for incontinence (e.g., spinal cord injury).

NURSING DIAGNOSES

Nursing diagnoses are determined from analysis of patient data. Several nursing diagnoses could be made for the incontinent patient for which the interventions are not specific to urinary incontinence and thus are not discussed in this section. These nursing diagnoses include skin integrity, impaired; body image disturbance; social isolation; self-care deficit; mobility, impaired physical; and coping, ineffective individual. Nursing diagnoses specific for the incontinent patient may include but are not limited to:

Diagnostic Title	Possible Etiologic Factors
1. Incontinence	Relaxed pelvic muscles, altered environment, sensory deficit, neurologic impairment, distention, decreased bladder capacity
2. Situational low self-esteem	Loss of urinary control
3. Deficient knowledge	Lack of exposure/recall

EXPECTED PATIENT OUTCOMES

Expected patient outcomes for the person with urinary incontinence may include but are not limited to:

1. Will achieve optimal urinary control

2a. Will verbalize feelings and concerns without self-deprecating statements

2b. Will socialize with others

3a. Will demonstrate perineal exercises (if appropriate)

3b. Will describe actions to control voiding (as appropriate), measures to maintain skin integrity, and plans for follow-up care

INTERVENTIONS

1. Assisting with Urinary Control

Bladder Retraining

When incontinence is caused by confusion or acute illness, control can usually be established if a persistent bladder retraining schedule is carried out. A voiding schedule is developed and strictly adhered to until the person gradually relearns to recognize and react appropriately to the urge to void. A successful program (Box 39-6), leading to complete rehabilitation or continence, requires mental competence of the individual. Otherwise, someone else must always remind the person to follow the schedule.

People ordinarily void on awakening, before retiring, and before or after meals. Consuming caffeinated beverages such as coffee creates a diuretic effect and the urge to void occurs in about 30 minutes. Using this knowledge, the nurse can begin to set up a schedule for placing the person on a bedpan or taking the person to the toilet. A record of involuntary voiding should be kept for a few days to determine the normal voiding pattern. If the schedule based on the pattern of incontinence is not successful, toileting every 1 to 2 hours should be carried out on a 24-hour basis.

When possible, toileting should be carried out in surroundings that remind the person of the voiding function; that is, the person should be taken to the bathroom to use the toilet. If this is not possible, a bedside commode can be an adequate substitute. Many men can void into a urinal more easily if allowed to stand at the bedside. The use of a bedpan is unfamiliar and distasteful to most persons, but in instances where women must remain in bed, voiding into a bedpan can be facilitated if the head of the bed is elevated as much as possible. This position is more consistent with the position normally assumed for voiding and facilitates complete bladder emptying. Few persons can void adequately in the supine position.

Providing adequate amounts of fluids, a minimum of 3000 ml/day, is necessary to ensure that adequate amounts of urine are produced and present in the bladder to stimulate the voiding reflex at the proper times. Fluids may be given at scheduled times, the largest portion being given during the day before 4 PM to decrease the frequency of voiding through the night. Persons with restricted fluid intake because of medical problems should receive the prescribed amount of fluid.

Catheterization

Occasionally the use of an indwelling catheter for the incontinent patient is justified. Reasons include the need to protect a surgical incision or to permit healing of a pressure ulcer in the area. Indwelling catheterization, however, presents

BOX 39-6 Bladder Retraining

- Establish patient's usual voiding patterns.
- Plan toileting based on the patient's usual pattern; assist patient as necessary.
- Plan toileting for every 1 to 2 hours (if no voiding pattern can be determined).
- Encourage patient to use normal toilet position.
- Encourage patient to empty bladder completely.
- Provide for a fluid intake of 3000 ml/day for adequate urine volume.
- Schedule majority of fluid intake before 4 PM.

many potential dangers, such as development of a UTI, urethritis, epididymitis, and urethral fistulae. All other means to manage the incontinence should be exhausted before resorting to catheterization.

External Urinary Drainage

For a man, external drainage can be accomplished with a condom catheter. Several commercial products are available. The following is an alternative method to purchasing external drainage devices. Select a condom of the correct size. Puncture a hole in the closed end of the condom with an applicator stick. Attach the punctured end of the condom to a firm rubber or plastic drainage tube with either a 3-mm ($\frac{1}{8}$-inch) piece of rubber tubing or a strip of adhesive tape (Figure 39-16). Before applying the condom, clean and dry the penis thoroughly and check for edema, skin breaks, or discoloration. Invert the condom and roll it onto the penis. There should be no roll at the top that could cause constriction. At least 2.5 cm (1 inch) of the condom should remain between the meatus and drainage tube to allow for penile erection, without allowing twisting and interference with drainage. Elastoplast is then applied over the condom and around the penis (never touching the skin) without causing constriction. Under no circumstances should adhesive tape be used.

The external catheter should be removed daily and the skin washed and inspected. Frequent assessment is necessary to determine whether edema or irritation is present and to ensure proper drainage. This is especially important in men with loss of sensation. The external device can be attached to either a leg bag or to straight drainage.

For persons who need external catheter drainage indefinitely, a rubber urinary appliance (sometimes called an incontinence urinal) may be used (Figure 39-17). Several models are available, and the one best suited to the person's needs is selected. Two appliances are recommended to allow for cleaning and drying of one device while using the other. They should be washed in mild soap, turned inside out, and thoroughly dried before application.

Most persons prefer to manage their own incontinence if they are at all able to do so. The nurse should support and encourage self-care, offering assistance as necessary and instruction in basic principles of skin care, equipment selection, and maintenance. The choice of management method should take into account the person's ability to manage as independently as possible.

Maintaining Skin Integrity

If none of the previous measures is appropriate or successful, nursing goals should focus on assisting the person to remain clean, free of odor, and free of skin breakdown. Incontinence leading to skin breakdown may lead to increased length of hospitalization, and increased costs.

Those who are unconscious or incapacitated by critical illness depend on the nursing staff to manage their incontinence by protective pads or pants or external catheter drainage. Others may be capable of some or all of their own management. Men and women may wear protective waterproof pants lined by disposable or washable absorbent pads. Adult briefs are available commercially, but they are quite bulky under clothing. Skin breakdown is a problem because of decreased air circulation. A resourceful person may be able to improvise equipment that is as comfortable and is less costly than commercially available pants. Zippers, Velcro, elastic, and a variety of waterproof materials may be used. Bedding and furniture can be protected with waterproof materials such as commercially available squares of absorbent cellucotton backed with light plastic.

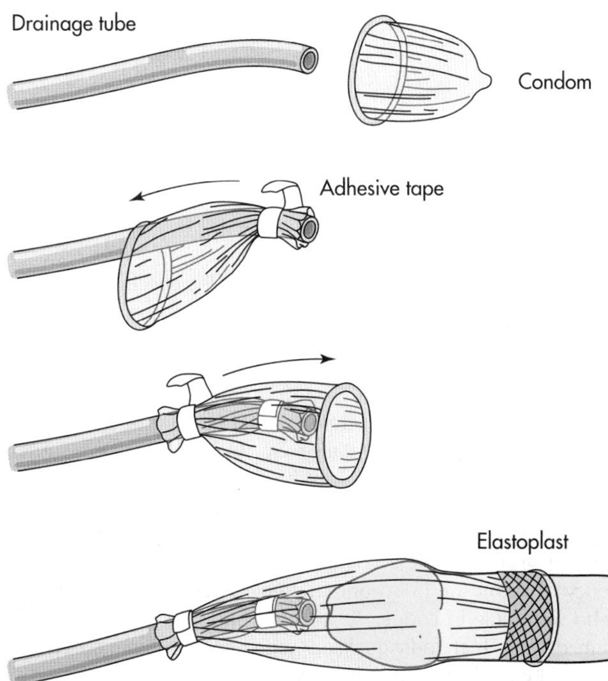

Figure 39-16 One method of making an external drainage apparatus.

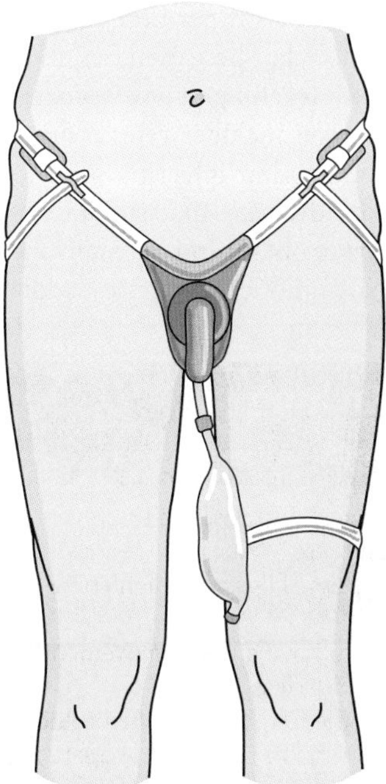

Figure 39-17 Rubber urinary appliance. Bag is emptied by drain valve at bottom of bag.

Whatever the type of padding, liners, or pants used, frequent changing is required for skin protection and comfort. The perineal and genital areas are thoroughly washed with soap and water and dried well at each changing. Periodic exposure of the perineal area to air is beneficial. A moisture barrier product (e.g., A&D ointment) helps protect the skin. Zinc oxide powder can be applied to lessen irritation. Excess amounts of powder are avoided, as this will cake on the skin and cause irritation.

2. Promoting Self-Esteem

Persons who are incontinent may feel isolated from their families and familiar surroundings. They may also have decreased self-esteem. These patients frequently respond well to mobilization in bladder retraining programs. When nurses believe that it is easier to change bed linen than to establish an appropriate bladder retraining program, a disservice is done to the individual and more work is actually created for the nurse. The person may have an increased risk of developing a UTI and skin breakdown, and feelings of worthlessness are increased. Urinary incontinence should not be considered inevitable in the elderly or institutionalized person.

3. Patient/Family Education

Teaching is an important aspect of care for the incontinent person. Patients and families are generally motivated to learn measures to manage incontinence. Explanation of the rationale for activities, such as the toileting schedule, mobility, and fluid requirements, increases the probability of the person following through with treatment plans.

Perineal exercises (Kegel exercises) may be helpful to control incontinence or to strengthen muscles after catheter removal. The exercises consist of tightening and relaxing perineal and gluteal muscles and can be performed in several ways (see Patient Teaching box). Stress incontinence in women can be prevented if perineal exercises are taught before and after childbirth. These exercises also may be included as part of the health teaching of any woman.

Additional teaching includes care of any drainage system, measures to maintain skin integrity, signs and symptoms of UTI (frequency or dysuria) that should be reported to the physician, and how to obtain and maintain any needed supplies and equipment (commode, protective padding, and drainage systems). The family or significant other should be included in the teaching.

Patient Teaching
Perineal Exercises

- Tighten the perineal muscles as if to prevent voiding; hold for 3 seconds, then relax.
- Inhale through pursed lips while tightening perineal muscles.
- Bear down as if to have a bowel movement. Relax, then tighten perineal muscles.
- Hold a pencil in the fold between the buttock and thigh.
- Sit on the toilet with knees held wide apart. Start and stop the urinary stream.

EVALUATION

To evaluate the effectiveness of nursing interventions, compare patient behaviors with those stated in the expected outcomes. Achievement of outcomes is successful if the patient with urinary incontinence:

1. Achieves urinary continence through bladder retraining (if appropriate) or uses a drainage system or padding.
2a. Describes self in positive terms.
2b. Socializes with others.
3a. Correctly demonstrates perineal exercises (if appropriate).
3b. Correctly describes measures to maintain skin integrity, signs and symptoms of a UTI, where to obtain needed supplies, and plans for follow-up care.

GERONTOLOGIC CONSIDERATIONS

Changes that occur with aging lead to decreased sensation and bladder muscle control, which may result in urinary incontinence. Because persons are often embarrassed about the loss of bladder control, they do not seek assistance and often become socially isolated.

Elderly patients, especially those with decreased ambulatory abilities, may not be able to reach the toilet in time to void. Older adults who are confused, disoriented, or receiving medications such as diuretics may also not reach the toilet in time to void. Portable commodes, urinals, and appropriate timing of medications will help manage functional incontinence. It is important to set realistic goals for the elderly patient to restore maximum efficiency of incontinence management. Prompted voiding and individualized toileting schedules may be an effective method of decreasing incontinence in older memory-impaired adults (see Evidence-Based Practice box).

Evidence-Based Practice

Reference: Jirovec MM, Templin T: Predicting success using individualized scheduled toileting for memory-impaired elders at home, *Res Nurs Health* 24(1):1, 2001.

The purpose of this study was to evaluate the effectiveness of an individualized scheduled toileting (IST) program on incontinent, memory-impaired elders being cared for at home. The sample consisted of 118 patients (69% women, mean age was 80, average length of incontinence was 30 months). The patients were randomly assigned to the experimental or control group. The caregivers in the experimental group were taught the IST program. Voiding records were kept by caregivers to determine the number of times persons were incontinent. Urinary incontinence significantly decreased in the experimental group, but not in the control group. Baseline cognitive ability, mobility, and consistency of using the IST program significantly predicted persons who were able to cooperate with toileting. The implications for nursing are that individualized scheduled toileting schedules should be implemented to improve incontinence.

SPECIAL ENVIRONMENTS FOR CARE

Community-Based Care

The incontinent patient may require supplies and equipment for home use. The home care nurse can evaluate the patient's home environment for ease of access to bathrooms, potential impediments to ambulation, and the need for supplemental equipment. The home nurse can also provide support for the family and reinforce patient teaching regarding incontinence.

COMPLICATIONS

The incontinent patient is at a high risk for developing skin breakdown. Any break in the integrity of the skin can greatly increase the risk of serious infection. Another complication of incontinence is depression related to social isolation.

Critical Thinking Questions

1. You are caring for a patient who had urinary diversion surgery. It is post-op day 3. You note blood clots in the tubing and urinary collection bag. Is this an expected finding after this type of surgery? What are appropriate nursing interventions?
2. You are caring for an 80-year-old man admitted after a fall. He is scheduled for repair of a hip fracture. You are preparing him for the OR. In the preop holding area, you insert a 14F Foley catheter, but do not obtain any urine. What should be done next?
3. You are planning the discharge for a 70-year-old woman with congestive heart failure. She is being discharged on a diuretic. She lives alone and has a history of arthritis and difficulty ambulating. She reports having problems with "dribbling" in the past. What other assessments need to be made? Devise a teaching plan for this patient. Are any referrals necessary?

References

1. American Cancer Society: website: http://www.cancer.org.
2. Blute ML, Gburek BM: Continent orthotopic urinary diversion in female patients: early Mayo Clinic experience, *Mayo Clin Proc* 73:501, 1998.
3. Brandes SB: Urethral stricture disease. In Hanno PM, Malkowicz SB, Wein AJ, editors: *Clinical manual of urology,* ed 3, New York, 2001, McGraw-Hill.
4. Brandes SB, Yu M: Urologic trauma. In Hanno PM, Malkowicz SB, Wein AJ, editors: *Clinical manual of urology,* ed 3, New York, 2001, McGraw-Hill.
5. Breschi LC: Urologic problems of the elderly. In Gallo JJ et al, editors: *Reichel's care of the elderly: clinical aspects of aging,* ed 3, Philadelphia, 1999, Lippincott Williams & Wilkins.
6. Cadeddu JA et al: Laparoscopic nephrectomy for renal cell cancer: evaluation of efficacy and safety: a multicenter experience, *Urology* 52(5):773, 1998.
7. Cammu H, Van Nylen M, Amy JJ: A 10-year follow-up after Kegel pelvic floor muscle exercises for genuine stress incontinence, *Br J Urol Int* 85:655, 2000.
8. Carroll PR: Urothelial carcinoma: cancers of the bladder, ureter and renal pelvis. In Tanagho EA, McAninch JW, editors: *Smith's general urology,* ed 15, New York, 2000, McGraw-Hill.
9. Carroll PR, Barbour S: Urinary diversion and bladder substitution. In Tanagho EA, McAninch JW, editors: *Smith's general urology,* ed 15, New York, 2000, McGraw-Hill.
10. Couser WG: Pathogenesis of damage in glomerulonephritis, 2001, website: http://uptodate.
11. Cravens DD, Zweig S: Urinary catheter management, *Am Fam Physician* 61(2):369, 2000.
12. Curhan GC: Dietary calcium, dietary protein, and kidney stone formation, *Mineral Electrolyte Metab* 23:261, 1997.
13. Curhan GC et al: A prospective study of dietary calcium and other nutrients and the risk of symptomatic kidney stones, *N Engl J Med* 328:833, 1993.
14. Dubose TD: Vascular disorders of the kidney. In Goldman L, Bennett JC, editors: *Cecil textbook of medicine,* Philadelphia, 2000, WB Saunders.
15. Dumyati G, Dolan JG: Pyelonephritis. In Rakel RE, Bope ET, editors: *Conn's current therapy,* Philadelphia, 2001, WB Saunders.
16. Falk RJ, Jennette JC, Nachman PH: Primary glomerular disease. In Brenner BM , Rector FC, editors: *Brenner's and Rector's: the kidney,* ed 6, Philadelphia, 2000, WB Saunders.
17. Foster HE: Female urology and incontinence. In Weiss RM, George NJR, O'Reilly PH, editors: *Comprehensive urology,* London, 2001, Mosby.
18. Gearhart JP, Baker LA: Congenital diseases of the lower urinary tract. In Weiss RM, George NJR, O'Reilly PH, editors: *Comprehensive urology,* London, 2001, Mosby.
19. Grantham, JJ: Cystic diseases of the kidney. In Goldman L, Bennett JC, editors: *Cecil textbook of medicine,* Philadelphia, 2000, WB Saunders.
20. Grantham JJ, Nair V, Winklhofer: Cystic diseases of the kidney. In Brenner, BM, editor: *Brenner's and Rector's: the kidney,* ed 6, Philadelphia, 2000, WB Saunders.
21. Hanno PM: Lower urinary tract infections in women. In Hanno PM, Malkowicz SB, Wein AJ, editors: *Clinical manual of urology,* ed 3, New York, 2001, McGraw-Hill.
22. Hautmann RE et al: Complications and functional results in 363 patients 11 years after follow-up, *J Urol* 161:422, 1999.
23. Irby PB: Renal calculi. In Rakel RE, Bope ET, editors. *Conn's current therapy,* Philadelphia, 2001, WB Saunders.
24. Kohn IJ, Weiss JP: Pylonephritis. In Hanno PM, Malkowicz SB, Wein AJ, editors: *Clinical manual of urology,* ed 3, New York, 2001, McGraw-Hill.
25. Kunin CM: Urinary tract infections and pyelonephritis. In Goldman L, Bennett JC, editors: *Cecil textbook of medicine,* Philadelphia, 2000, WB Saunders.
26. Nicolle LE: Bacterial urinary tract infections in women. In Rakel RE, Bope ET, editors: *Conn's current therapy,* Philadelphia, 2001, WB Saunders.
27. Lavine MA, Stein BS: Tumors of the kidney and urinary tract. In Brenner BM, editor: *Brenner's and Rector's: the kidney,* ed 6, Philadelphia, 2000, WB Saunders.
28. Maki DG, Tambyah PA: Engineering out the risk for infections with urinary catheters. *Emerg Infect Dis* 7(2):342, 2001.
29. Martin TV, Sosa RE: Shock wave lithotripsy. In Walsh PC et al, editors: *Campbell's urology,* ed 7, Philadelphia, 1998, WB Saunders.
30. Martini LA, Wood RJ: Should dietary calcium and protein be restricted in patients with nephrolithiaisis? *Nutr Rev* 58:111, 2000.
31. Malkowicz SB, Sanchez-Ortiz RF, Wein AJ: Adult genitourinary cancer. In Hanno PM, Malkowicz SB, Wein AJ, editors: *Clinical manual of urology,* ed 3, New York, 2001, McGraw-Hill.
32. McAninch JW, Safir MH: Genitourinary trauma. In Weiss RM, George NJR, O'Reilly PH, editors: *Comprehensive urology,* London, 2001, Mosby.
33. McRae SN, Dairiki Shortliffe LM: Bacterial infections of the urinary tract. In Tanagho EA, McAninch JW, editors: *Smith's general urology,* ed 15, New York, 2000, McGraw-Hill.
34. Mikel G: Urinary retention: management in the acute care setting, *AJN* 100:40, 2001.

35. Niaudet P: Treatment of idiopathic nephrotic syndrome in children, 2001, website: http://uptodate.
36. Nicolle LE: Urinary tract infection in long-term care facility residents, *Clin Infect Dis* 31:7757, 2000.
37. Nicolle LE: Bacterial infections in women. In Rakel RE, Bope ET, editors: *Conn's current therapy,* Philadelphia, 2001, WB Saunders.
38. Pahira JJ, Razack AA: Nephrolithiasis. In Hanno PM, Malkowicz SB, Wein AJ, editors: *Clinical manual of urology,* ed 3, New York, 2001, McGraw-Hill.
39. Peggs J: Urinary incontinence. In Rakel RE, Bope ET, editors: *Conn's current therapy,* Philadelphia, 2001, WB Saunders.
40. Raz R, Schiller D, Nicolle LE: Chronic indwelling catheter replacement before antimicrobial therapy for symptomatic urinary tract infection, *J Urol* 164(4):1254, 2000.
41. Redington J, Reller LB: The patients with urinary tract infection. In Schrier RW, editor: *Manual of nephrology,* ed 5, Philadelphia, 2000, Lippincott Williams & Wilkins.
42. Rose BR: Course of poststreptococcal glomerulonephritis, 2001, website: http://uptodate.
43. Safian RD, Textor SC: Renal-artery stenosis, *N Engl J Med* 344:431, 2001.
44. Schnaper HW, Ribson AM: Nephrotic syndrome: minimal change disease, focal glomerulosclerosis and related disorders. In Schrier RW, Gottschalk CW, editors: *Diseases of the kidney,* ed 6, Boston, 1997, Little, Brown.
45. Segura JW: Ureteral stones clinical guidelines panel summary report on the management of ureteral calculi, *J Urol* 158(5):1915, 1997.
46. Shinghal R, Payne CK: Emergency room urology. In Hanno PM, Malkowicz SB, Wein AJ, editors: *Clinical manual of urology,* ed 3, New York, 2001, McGraw-Hill.
47. Stapleton A, Stamm WE: Prevention of urinary tract infection, *Infect Dis Clin North Am* 11:719, 1997.
48. Textor SC, Wilcox CS: Renal artery stenosis: a common, treatable cause of renal failure? *Annu Rev Med* 52:421, 2001.
49. Wein AJ, Rovner ES: Voiding function and dysfunction. In Hanno PM, Malkowicz SB, Wein AJ, editors: *Clinical manual of urology,* ed 3, New York, 2001, McGraw-Hill.
50. Wilcox CS: Renovascular hypertension. In Massry SG, Glassock RJ: *Massry & Glassock's textbook of nephrology,* ed 4, Philadelphia, 2001, Lippincott Williams & Wilkins.
51. Zinman L: Urethral stricture disease. In Weiss RM, George NJR, O'Reilly PH, editors: *Comprehensive urology,* London, 2001, Mosby.

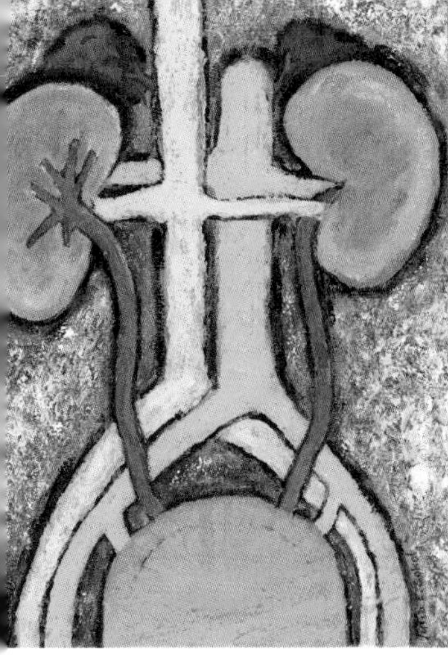

http://www.mosby.com/MERLIN/medsurg_phipps

Kidney Failure 40

Kelly A. Weigel, Cynthia Hollamon, Carol Genet Kelley

Objectives

After studying this chapter, the learner should be able to:

1. Analyze the pathophysiologic changes and clinical manifestations of acute and chronic kidney failure.
2. Differentiate the medical and nursing management of patients during the oliguric and diuretic phases of acute kidney failure.
3. Explain the benefits of continuous renal replacement therapy for patients with kidney failure.
4. Identify treatment goals for patients with chronic kidney failure.
5. Describe the physiologic principles of dialysis.
6. Compare the nursing assessment and management of patients undergoing hemodialysis, peritoneal dialysis, and kidney transplantation.

INTRODUCTION

Kidney failure is one of the most significant causes of death and disability throughout the world. Recent statistics from the United States Renal Data Systems (USRDS) report that more than 10 million persons in the United States alone are estimated to have chronic kidney disease.[10] The kidneys perform a large number of life-sustaining functions including filtration of waste from the blood, maintenance of acid-base balance, and regulation of blood pressure. Owing to the complexity of kidney function, kidney failure affects all body systems.

The kidneys have a tremendous ability to adapt to a decreasing number of functioning nephrons. With less than 25% of the original nephrons functioning, the kidneys are able to excrete waste products and maintain fluid and electrolyte balance. As kidney failure develops, laboratory tests reflect the changes in homeostasis, and the person appears clinically ill. The person in kidney failure cannot independently sustain life.

Kidney failure may be *acute* in onset (developing in hours to days) or *chronic* (developing slowly and progressively over a course of several years). When kidney failure occurs suddenly, as within a few days, biochemical changes are often dramatic, and the person has little time to adjust to these changes. The person becomes very ill and is frequently treated in a critical care area.

In chronic kidney failure (CKF), kidney function is progressively destroyed over the course of several months or years. The control of symptoms and preservation of function can be achievable goals. Kidney function may be preserved by medication and health promotion. Dietary adjustment may help delay the onset of symptoms of kidney failure. As function continues to deteriorate, dialysis or transplantation becomes necessary to maintain life.

Kidney insufficiency exists when a significant loss of kidney function occurs, but enough functioning remains to maintain an internal environment consistent with life. Kidney insufficiency generally refers to a decline in kidney function to approximately 25% of normal function or a glomerular filtration rate (GFR) of 25 to 30 ml/min. When kidney insufficiency exists, any additional physiologic stressor such as illness or a nephrotoxic drug can lead to failure. The individual experiencing kidney insufficiency may appear and feel well, even though laboratory data reflect deterioration in kidney function. Kidney insufficiency occurs as a phase in gradually but chronically progressive kidney disease.

Uremia is a syndrome of kidney failure characterized by elevated blood urea nitrogen (BUN) and creatinine levels. This syndrome (also referred to as *uremic syndrome*) is characterized by fatigue, anorexia, nausea, vomiting, pruritus, and neurologic manifestations.

Azotemia is defined as an increase in serum urea and creatinine levels. Azotemia and uremia are sometimes inappropriately used synonymously. Both terms refer to the buildup of nitrogenous waste products in the blood, but, unlike the person with uremia, the person with azotemia does not manifest symptoms of kidney failure.

ACUTE KIDNEY FAILURE

Etiology

Kidney failure refers to a significant loss of function; when only 10% of kidney function remains, the person is considered to have end-stage renal disease (ESRD).

Acute kidney failure (AKF) is an abrupt decline in kidney function as defined by increases in BUN and plasma creatinine levels. Urine output is generally less than 40 ml/hr (oliguria) but may be normal or even increased. Depending on cause, AKF is classified as *prerenal, intrarenal (intrinsic),* or *postrenal.* A total of 55% to 70% of the cases of AKF are due to prerenal factors such as intravascular volume depletion, decreased cardiac output, and vascular failure secondary to vasodilation or obstruction. Intrarenal causes account for 25% to 40% of cases of AKF . Intrarenal failure is caused by damage to the kidney tissues and structures and includes tubular necrosis, nephrotoxicity, and alterations in renal blood flow. Acute tubular necrosis (ATN) is the cause of approximately 90% of all cases of intrarenal AKF. Postrenal failure (approximately 5% of cases) is generally caused by obstruction of urine flow between the kidney and the urethral meatus. Box 40-1 summarizes the causes of acute kidney failure.

Epidemiology

Acute kidney failure is a common problem. It affects approximately 5% of all hospitalized patients and up to 30% of patients admitted to intensive care areas. The mortality rate for AKF approaches 50%, making it one of the leading causes of inpatient mortality.[3] Recovery from an episode of AKF depends on the underlying illness, the patient's condition, and management during the period of renal shutdown. Mortality associated with AKF approaches 50%. For those in whom AKF has been caused by glomerular disease or severe infection of the kidneys, return of kidney function is determined by the extent of scarring and obliteration of functional nephrons that occurred during the acute episode of kidney failure. Research indicates that the prognosis for these patients may not be as favorable as for those with AKF resulting from toxic or ischemic injury.

Pathophysiology

The kidneys receive approximately one fourth of the cardiac output; therefore they are very sensitive to alterations in perfusion. Thus an ischemic episode can rapidly result in nephron damage. Because a urinary output of at least 400 ml/day is necessary for adequate excretion of wastes, the resulting decrease in GFR that occurs in AKF is responsible for the increased BUN and serum creatinine levels.

The kidneys' response to hypoperfusion is the release of renin and an adaptive response to maintain perfusion to the glomerular bed. AKF develops when these adaptive responses are ineffective in maintaining normal kidney function.

The pathophysiology of AKF is not completely understood. Nephrotoxic factors and ischemia may be the cause.

Although a variety of conditions contribute to the development of AKF, ATN is the most common. ATN is classified as *postischemic* or *nephrotoxic.*

BOX 40-1 Causes of Acute Kidney Failure

Prerenal

Hypovolemia

Hemorrhage
Dehydration
Vomiting
Diabetes insipidus
Cirrhosis
Diarrhea
Inappropriate use of diuretics
Diaphoresis
Burns
Peritonitis
Pancreatitis

Decreased Cardiac Output

Congestive heart failure
Myocardial infarction
Tamponade
Dysrhythmias

Systemic Vasodilation

Sepsis
Acidosis
Vasodilating Medications
Anaphylaxis

Hypotension/Hypoperfusion

Cardiac failure
Shock

Intrarenal (Intrinsic)

Tubule/Nephron Damage

Acute tubular necrosis (most common cause)
Glomerulonephritis
Rhabdomyolosis

Vascular Changes

Coagulopathies
Malignant hypertension
Abdominal aortic aneurysm
Sclerosis
Renovascular disease
Abdominal aortic aneurysm

Nephrotoxins

Antibiotics (gentamicin, tobramycin, amphotericin B, polymyxin B, neomycin, kanamycin, vancomycin)
Chemicals (carbon tetrachloride, lead, ethylene glycol [antifreeze])
Heavy metals (arsenic, mercury)
Iodinated radiographic contrast media (IVP dye)
Drug-induced interstitial nephritis (nonsteroidal antiinflammatory agents, tetracyclines, furosemide, thiazides, phenytoin, penicillins, cyclosporine, tacrolimus, sulfonamides, cephalosporins)

Postrenal

Ureteral and Bladder Neck Obstruction

Calculi
Neurogenic bladder
Neoplasms
Prostatic hyperplasia

Ischemic events causing ATN occur most commonly after surgery (Box 40-1). Ischemia results in inflammation and causes cell swelling, injury, and necrosis along any part of the nephron. Necrosis associated with nephrotoxicity is generally limited to the proximal tubules.

There are three theories explaining the oliguria associated with ATN (Figure 40-1 and Table 40-1). Oliguria probably occurs as a result of a combination of all three mechanisms.

Phases. Acute kidney failure can be divided into four phases: onset, oliguric, diuretic, and recovery. The onset is the initial phase of injury to the kidney. Reversal or prevention of kidney dysfunction is possible at this stage by early intervention. The oliguric phase follows within 1 day of the onset. Major problems during the oliguric phase include inability to excrete fluid loads, regulate electrolytes, and excrete metabolic waste products. During the diuretic phase, large amounts of fluid (4 to 5 L/day) and electrolytes are lost. The recovery phase may last up to 12 months. Most patients are left with some residual renal dysfunction (Table 40-2).

With decreased kidney function, fluids are retained in the body, resulting in fluid overload and edema (see Chapter 13). When fluid overload is excessive, congestive heart failure and pulmonary edema may occur. Hypertension may accompany AKF when the person is hypervolemic.

Inability to excrete fluid leads to decreased urine output. Either oliguria or anuria (urine output less than 100 ml/day) may be present, although oliguria is more common.[6] Classically the patient in AKF shows a decrease in urine output to between 50 and 400 ml/day within 1 to 2 days. The urine specific gravity is low (1.010), and the osmolality of the urine approaches that of the person's serum (280 to 320 mOsm). Specific gravity and urine osmolality remain within this fixed range because the tubules have lost the ability to excrete sodium and water.[12]

Fluid and electrolyte imbalance occurs in the patient with AKF. The three major electrolyte problems are hyperkalemia, sodium imbalance, and metabolic acidosis.

Hyperkalemia. In the normal individual the potassium ion is exchanged in the distal convoluted tubule of the nephron for either a sodium or a hydrogen ion; healthy persons cannot conserve the potassium ion. However, in AKF with many tubular cells not functioning, no mechanism exists to remove potassium from the body. *Hyperkalemia* (the most sudden hazard in oliguric AKF) is said to exist when the serum concentration of this ion reaches a level of 5.5 mEq/L or higher. Serum concentrations of 7 to 10 mEq/L can be quickly reached in AKF and are incompatible with normal cardiac function and life.

The most reliable indicators of potassium toxicity are changes on the electrocardiogram such as widened QRS complexes and peaked T waves, and laboratory determinations of serum potassium. Occasionally neuromuscular symptoms such as paresthesias and paralysis (distal to proximal) are seen.[11] Changes in the patient's pulse are not indicators of the amount of potassium excess.

Sodium Imbalance. *Hyponatremia* in AKF most often develops with overhydration. The oliguric patient cannot excrete large volumes of urine; as the administration of sodium-free or low-sodium intravenous or oral fluids continues, the serum is diluted, and the serum concentration of sodium falls.

Hyponatremia is accompanied or caused by hypervolemia. In the acutely ill patient, the situation typically occurs when the person receives numerous drugs and fluids in an attempt to treat coexisting life-threatening problems. When the volume of drugs and fluids cannot be reduced to a safe level, dialysis is required to remove the excess fluid and restore sodium balance.

Signs and symptoms of hyponatremia include warm, moist, flushed skin; cerebral edema; and mental status changes such

TABLE 40-1 Pathophysiologic Theories of Oliguria of Acute Tubular Necrosis

Theory	Pathophysiology
Tubular obstruction	Tubular necrosis causes cell sloughing or ischemic edema, which results in tubular obstruction. The glomerular filtration rate (GFR) is decreased as a result of the obstruction.
Back leak	The GFR remains normal while tubular reabsorption of filtrate is increased. Ischemia is the underlying cause.
Alterations in renal blood flow	Exact mechanism is unknown. Ischemia may be responsible for changes in glomerular permeability and a decrease in the GFR. Arteriolar constriction may be associated with the release of angiotensin II.

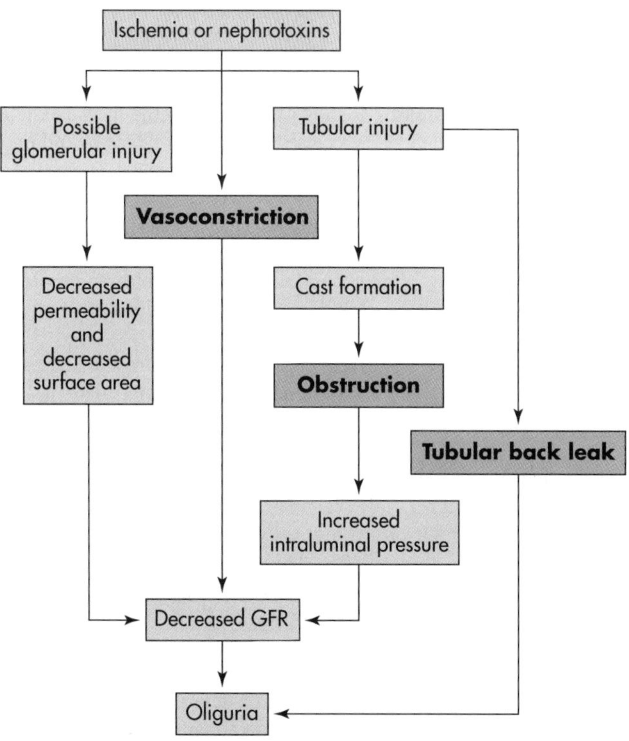

Figure 40-1 Pathogenesis of AKF.

as confusion, delirium, coma, and convulsions. Serum sodium concentrations are less than 130 mEq/L. The hematocrit and hemoglobin values fall suddenly in the absence of bleeding because of hemodilution.

Increases in the total body content of sodium also occur in AKF when the patient is receiving medications high in sodium content and excess sodium in the diet. Edema and increasing blood pressure indicate retention of sodium and water, even though the serum sodium concentration is normal or below normal.

Metabolic Acidosis. Acidosis develops when hydrogen ion secretion and bicarbonate ion production diminish in the tubules. The pH of the blood decreases, the carbon dioxide content decreases, and central nervous system symptoms of drowsiness progressing to stupor and coma may appear (see Chapter 13). Although the lungs cannot totally compensate for the increasing acid load, they help determine the rate at which acidosis develops and the frequency or need for dialysis. In compensating for increased metabolic acid loads, the lungs attempt to excrete more carbon dioxide by taking rapid breaths.

Inability To Excrete Metabolic Wastes. Decreased kidney function alters the body's ability to eliminate metabolic waste products, producing the typical signs and symptoms of uremia. BUN and serum creatinine values rise sharply. In the person who has already sustained illness and trauma, BUN values may increase at a rate of 30 mg/dl/day. Signs and symptoms include neurologic manifestations such as confusion, convulsions, coma, and asterixis.

Other pathologic changes also occur as a result of uremia. Gastrointestinal (GI) bleeding may result from a lesion such as an angiodysplasia (vascular dilation), which is associated with uremia and decreased platelet function.[25] Bruising and bleeding also result from changes in platelet function. Decreased cellular immunity causes an increased risk of infections. Pericarditis is thought to develop as a result of pericardial irritation from accumulated metabolic wastes. A pericardial friction rub may be present on auscultation.

The increased output associated with the diuretic phase indicates that the damaged nephrons are healing and are able to begin excreting urine. Daily urine volume increases slowly, although within 1 to 2 days, diuresis up to or exceeding 4 to 5 L/day may occur. Although fluid can be excreted, the kidneys are not yet healed. Often the person is unable to excrete proportional amounts of waste products, and the BUN and creatinine may rise or remain elevated as urine volume increases. At times, excessive excretion of sodium and potassium occurs during diuresis. Complete recovery of renal function is slow and requires weeks to months. Renal function is normal or near normal when the kidney can both concentrate and dilute urine, control serum electrolytes, and excrete nitrogenous wastes.

Collaborative Care Management

Diagnostic Tests. When altered kidney function is suspected, BUN, creatinine, and electrolyte levels are obtained. Urinalysis is done to determine specific gravity, osmolality, and urine sodium content. Additional studies include a com-

TABLE 40-2 Phases of Acute Kidney Failure

Phase	Physiologic Effect	Symptoms	Duration
Onset	Initial phase of injury; hypotension, ischemia, hypovolemia	Subtle	Hours to days
Oliguric (Urine output: <400 ml/24 hr)	Inability to excrete metabolic wastes: increased serum urea nitrogen and creatinine; BUN may increase 20 mg/dl/day	Nausea, vomiting; drowsiness, confusion; coma; gastrointestinal bleeding; asterixis; pericarditis	1-3 weeks, may extend to several weeks in older patients
or (Urine output: <30 ml/24 hr)	Inability to regulate electrolytes: hyperkalemia, hyponatremia, acidosis, hypocalcemia, hyperphosphatemia Inability to excrete fluid loads: fluid overload, hypervolemia Hematologic dysfunction: anemia, platelet dysfunction, leukopenia May still require dialysis	Nausea, vomiting; cardiac dysrhythmias, electrocardiogram changes; Kussmaul's breathing; drowsiness, confusion; coma; edema; congestive heart failure; pulmonary edema; neck vein distention; hypertension; fatigue; bleeding; infection	Duration also dependent on type of toxic injury and duration of ischemia
Diuretic (Urine output: >1000 ml/24 hr)	Increased production of urine (deficit in concentrating ability of tubules and osmotic diuretic effect of high BUN); slowly increasing excretion of metabolic wastes; hypovolemia; loss of sodium; loss of potassium; high BUN initially; BUN gradually returns to baseline	Urine output of up to 4-5 L/day; postural hypotension; tachycardia; improving mental alertness and activity; weight loss; thirst; dry mucous membranes; decreased skin turgor	2-6 weeks after onset of oliguria; duration varies
Recovery	Kidneys returning to normal functioning, some residual renal insufficiency; 30% of patients do not attain full recovery of GFR	Decreased energy levels	3-12 months

BUN, Blood urea nitrogen; *GFR,* glomerular filtration rate.

plete blood count (CBC), arterial blood gases, and urine protein. See Table 40-3 for laboratory values in AKF.

Radiographic examinations of the kidney and surrounding structures are used to help determine the cause of AKF, particularly in postrenal failure. Ultrasonography, computed tomography (CT), intravenous pyelography, and magnetic resonance imaging can be done to rule out obstructive causes of kidney failure. These procedures also determine the size and thickness of the kidneys. Enlarged kidneys may represent hydronephrosis. To visualize stones, a plain film of the abdomen or KUB (kidneys, ureters, and bladder) may be obtained. Cystoscopy may be performed to visualize obstructions. If the etiology of AKF is unknown, a renal biopsy may be done.

Medications. The use of medications in the treatment of AKF depends on the underlying cause and the presenting symptoms. Hypovolemia is treated with hypotonic solutions such as 0.45% saline. If hypovolemia is due to blood or plasma loss, packed red blood cells and isotonic saline are administered. Volume replacement rates must match volume losses on a 1:1 basis. Loop diuretics are used to manage altered electrolyte and fluid levels. Doses of up to 320 mg/day of furosemide may be required to produce adequate diuresis.

Kidney failure from nephrotoxins or ischemia is treated with agents that increase renal blood flow. These include mannitol and loop diuretics. Low-dose dopamine is still used extensively in the management of hospital acquired AKF, despite a lack of significant supporting data.[20] Inflammatory states as in acute glomerulonephritis are treated with glucocorticosteroids.

Patients with impaired renal function may have altered responses to therapeutic doses of many medications. Uremia alters the protein-binding sites, absorption, distribution, and metabolism of many drugs.[8] Nonsteroidal antiinflammatory drugs (NSAIDs) and angiotensin-converting enzyme inhibitors are contraindicated in patients with AKF.

Treatments. When conservative management is not effective, dialysis is required. Dialysis, the process by which waste products in the blood are filtered through a semipermeable membrane, is indicated when the patient with AKF is fluid overloaded and/or has rapidly progressive azotemia, hyperkalemia, and metabolic acidosis. Three methods of dialysis are used: hemodialysis, peritoneal dialysis, and continuous renal replacement therapy.

Continuous Renal Replacement Therapy. Continuous renal replacement therapy (CRRT) provides continuous (8 to 24 hours or more) ultrafiltration of extracellular fluid and clearance of uremic toxins. It must be administered in a critical care setting. This therapy may or may not necessitate the use of a hemodialysis machine and both arterial and venous access. CRRT that does not require a hemodialysis machine relies on the patient's own blood pressure to power the system and requires both arterial and venous vascular access usually via catheters placed in the femoral vessels. In most patients, a mean arterial blood pressure of 60 mm Hg is required to maintain adequate blood flow through this system. Whether or not a hemodialysis machine is used, success of CRRT depends on the maintenance of blood flow through the hemofilter, which is made up of a collection of hollow fibers. Blood flows through the inside of these hollow fibers, each of which serves as a semipermeable membrane. The ultrafiltration system is composed of outflow and return tubing, the hemofilter, and an ultrafiltration collection receptacle (Figure 40-2).

During CRRT, water, electrolytes, and other solutes are removed as the patient's blood passes through the hollow fibers of the hemofilter. The resulting ultrafiltrate is a protein-free fluid with solute and electrolyte concentrations similar to plasma. The plasma proteins and cellular components of the blood remain in the hemofilter circuit and return to the venous circulation. The ultrafiltrate is collected in a receptacle and discarded. The mass transfer of water and solutes across a semipermeable membrane is a result of *convection* and *diffusion.* The convection forces applied through the fibers of the hemofilter depend primarily on the blood pressure. The higher the blood pressure, the greater the hydrostatic pressure within the hemofilter. Diffusion is the process by which solutes are

TABLE 40-3 Laboratory Values in Acute Kidney Failure

Finding	Prerenal	Intrarenal	Postrenal
Blood value			
Blood urea nitrogen (BUN)	Increases	Increases	Increases
Creatinine	Normal	Increases	Increases
BUN/creatinine ratio	20:1 or greater (increased)	10:1 or less (not increased because both values elevated)	Normal to slightly increased
Urine Value			
Urea	Decreases	Decreases	Decreases
Creatinine	≈ normal	Decreases	Decreases
Specific gravity	1.020 or more (increased)	Fixed and may be high	Variable
Volume	Oliguria	Nonoliguria or oliguria	Oliguria/polyuria
Osmolality	400 mOsm or more (increases)	250-350 mOsm (low and fixed, similar to plasma osmolality)	Anuria Variable: increases or similar to plasma osmolality

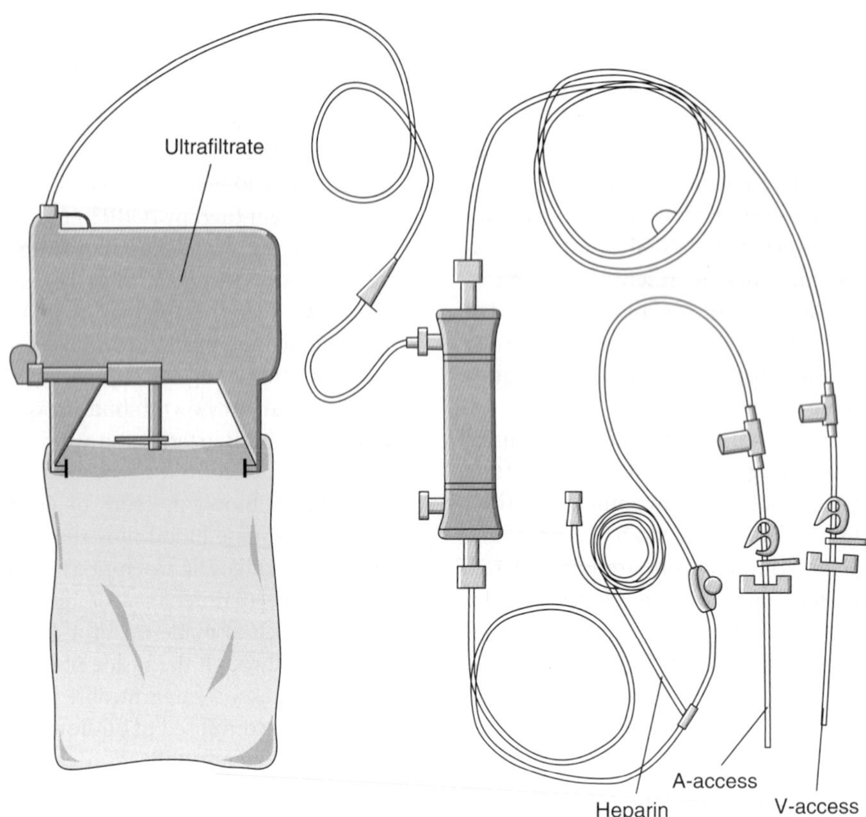

Figure 40-2 The ultrafiltration circuit.

passively transported across a semipermeable membrane. Diffusion depends on the presence of a concentration gradient across the membrane. In CRRT, a concentration gradient is established by infusing dialysate into the non–blood side of the hemofilter.

Removal of plasma water and electrolytes by CRRT is a gradual process that closely resembles the kidney's normal function. Because the process is gradual, rapid fluctuations in fluid and electrolyte status do not occur. Therefore CRRT is recommended for patients with AKF who are too hemodynamically unstable to tolerate hemodialysis or peritoneal dialysis. Patients who may benefit from CRRT are those with advanced cardiac disease, metabolic acidosis, abdominal wounds, cerebral edema, or sepsis.

Five variations of CRRT are in use: continuous venovenous hemofiltration, continuous arteriovenous hemofiltration, continuous venovenous hemodialysis, continuous arteriovenous hemodialysis, and slow continuous ultrafiltration. Each of these is designed to meet the renal replacement needs of a specific group of patients.

Continuous venovenous hemofiltration (CVVH) is favored by most clinicians.[12] Access to the patient's blood is obtained with a double-lumen catheter generally placed in a large central vessel. A significant benefit to this type of CRRT is that it does not require arterial access. Blood is pumped through a hemofilter by a specialized dialysis machine. This action of pumping generates hydraulic pressure for ultrafiltration. Control of fluid volume and electrolyte balance is achieved through pumped exchange of replacement fluids. Hourly ultrafiltrate loss is replaced by prescribed amounts of a sterile intravenous electrolyte solution. Systemic heparinization is usually instituted to prevent clotting; however, heparin requirements may be relatively low in patients with coagulopathy or thrombocytopenia.[12]

Continuous arteriovenous hemofiltration (CAVH) removes large amounts of plasma, water, and solutes at rates of 400 to 800 ml/hr. Patients with AKF, mild to moderate azotemia, and electrolyte disturbances can have CAVH as the primary method of dialysis while in the intensive care unit. This type of CRRT is less desirable because it requires the patient's own blood pressure to move the blood through the hemofilter and affords less reliable blood flow rates. This system also has the disadvantage of requiring arterial access. Because of heparinization required to prevent system thrombosis and the hemodynamic instability of the patient, cannulation of the arterial vessel puts the patient at increased risk for bleeding and blood loss. In addition, cannulation of the artery incurs a risk of distal atheroembolic or artery-occlusive complications.[12]

Continuous venovenous hemodialysis (CVVHD) is the most recently developed mode of CRRT. Like CVVH, the benefit of this mode is that it does not require arterial access. Sterile dialysate fluid is pumped into the ultrafiltration compartment of the hemofilter. The dialysate flows countercurrent to the blood flow, which increases diffusion of solutes from the blood to the ultrafiltration compartment.

Continuous arteriovenous hemodialysis (CAVHD) combines the convective transport of CAVH with diffusion dialysis. Like CAVH, this mode requires both arterial and venous blood access. Solute removal is much greater than in CAVH because as in CVVHD, sterile dialysate solution is pumped countercurrent to the blood flow, which increases the diffusion of solutes from the blood into the ultrafiltration compartment of the hemofilter. CAVHD can be used as primary dialysis therapy in a wide variety of critically ill patients, including patients with AKF who have severe azotemia, electrolyte imbalances, and acid-base disturbances.

Slow continuous ultrafiltration (SCUF), which is used to control fluid balance, slowly removes small amounts of plasma water and solutes at a rate of 150 to 300 ml/hr. SCUF is highly effective in patients with severe congestive heart failure (see Chapter 24) who do not respond to diuretic therapy. Fluid removal by ultrafiltration can achieve significant preload reduction in these patients. This method is unsuitable for patients with AKF who are azotemic or who have significant electrolyte abnormalities, because only small amounts of solutes are removed.

The goals of nursing management for patients undergoing CRRT are optimization of the patient's fluid volume and hemodynamic status, maintenance of ultrafiltration system patency, prevention of blood loss from line disconnection, and prevention of infection. Emotional support is important for the patient and family while in a critical care setting.

During the diuretic phase medical management centers on maintaining adequate fluid balance and regulating electrolytes. Even though the patient may be excreting large volumes of urine, dialysis may still be necessary to control electrolyte balance adequately. Protein restrictions are continued until BUN and serum creatinine levels decline.

Diet. Dietary management is important for patients with all types of kidney failure. Close collaboration between nurses, dietitians, and physicians is necessary to institute a diet that provides enough calories to avoid catabolism while preventing a surplus of nitrogen. Catabolism leads to an increased BUN level because of the breakdown of muscle for protein. Generally protein is restricted to 0.6 to 0.8 g/kg of body weight per day.[13] Carbohydrate intake should be maintained at around 100 g/day. Sodium and potassium are restricted, as is free water in patients for whom hyponatremia is an issue. Dietary supplements are usually prescribed. Patients who are unable to take in sufficient nutrients may be candidates for total parenteral nutrition and administration of fat emulsions, which provide a nonprotein source of calories.

Activity. The patient with AKF experiences fatigue and activity intolerance. Anemia may contribute to the fatigue. As the patient's energy level increases, walking should be encouraged as an aerobic exercise.

Referrals. A nutrition consultation is beneficial to establish the patient's caloric needs. Referrals to agencies that offer educational materials and resources for patients with kidney dysfunction are also helpful.*

*Such agencies include the National Kidney Foundation, 2 Park Ave, New York, NY 10006, and the American Kidney Fund, 7315 Wisconsin Ave, 203E, Bethesda, MD 20014.

NURSING MANAGEMENT OF PATIENT WITH ACUTE KIDNEY FAILURE

ASSESSMENT

Health History

When obtaining the health history of a person with AKF it is important to obtain information about:

- Voiding patterns, including any recent changes
- Weight gain (fluid retention)
- History of nausea or vomiting
- Presence of flank pain
- Presence of muscle weakness
- Mental status changes
- Patient and family history of renal disease or trauma
- Medication use (prescription and over the counter)
- Recent surgery, anesthesia, or trauma
- History of hypertension
- Exposure to nephrotoxins
- History of fatigue or lethargy
- Changes in bowel habits

Physical Examination

Objective data include:

- Amount of urine excreted in 24 hours
- Blood pressure, particularly postural changes
- Fluid status: presence of peripheral, periorbital, or sacral edema; lung sounds; skin turgor; daily weight
- Halitosis as a result of acidosis and/or ammonia secretion
- Mental status changes
- Pulse rate and rhythm
- Weight (compare to ideal body weight)
- Ecchymosis
- Pallor
- Muscle weakness
- Tachycardia

NURSING DIAGNOSES

Nursing diagnoses are determined from analysis of patient data. Nursing diagnoses for the person with AKF may include but are not limited to:

Diagnostic Title	Possible Etiologic Factors
1. Deficient/excess fluid volume	Abnormal fluid loss, compromised regulatory mechanism
2. Imbalanced nutrition: less than body requirements	Anorexia, nausea, restricted diet
3. Activity intolerance	Biochemical alterations
4. Risk for injury	Sensorimotor deficits, mental confusion
5. Risk for infection	Decreased nutrition, decreased immune response
6. Ineffective coping (individual)	Changes in health status
7. Deficient knowledge	Lack of exposure/recall

EXPECTED PATIENT OUTCOMES

Expected patient outcomes for the person with AKF during the oliguric phase may include but are not limited to:

1. Will maintain fluid volume, electrolytes, and waste products at a functional level as evidenced by:

1a. Will have absence of pulmonary edema; absence or control of peripheral edema

1b. Will have blood pressure readings between 135/80 and 100/60 mm Hg

1c. Will have balanced electrolytes: sodium 125 to 145 mEq/L, potassium 3.0 to 6.0 mEq/L, and bicarbonate greater than 14 mEq/L

1d. Will control protein catabolism: BUN less than 100 mg/dl, creatinine less than 12 mg/dl, and absence of skin breakdown

2. Will verbalize knowledge of a diet high in calories and fat and restricted in protein and potassium
3. Will report an increase in activity tolerance and decrease in fatigue
4. Will be free from injury
5. Will be free from infection
6. Will describe alternative ways of coping
7. Will verbalize knowledge of nature of illness, diet therapy, signs and symptoms to be reported to physician, and plans for follow-up care

INTERVENTIONS

Nursing care primarily focuses on (1) monitoring for signs of fluid overload, (2) monitoring for signs of electrolyte imbalance, and (3) the control of fluid intake (Guidelines for Safe Practice box).

1. Maintaining Fluid and Electrolyte Balance

Control of fluids is essential during the oliguric phase of AKF because of the deceased ability of the kidneys to excrete urine. All observations about the patient's state of hydration need to be recorded so that hour-to-hour and day-to-day comparisons can be made. Any finding indicating fluid retention is reported to the health care provider. Edema can first be noted in dependent areas such as the feet and legs, in the presacral area, and around the eyes (periorbital). It is important to remember, however, that edema may not be detected until the person has gained 5 to 10 pounds (2 to 5 kg) in fluid. The person is observed carefully for signs of pulmonary edema and congestive heart failure (see Chapter 24).

Central venous lines or arterial monitoring lines help provide data for short-term comparisons in managing the fluid balance of the critically ill person. Positioning and activity are determined daily based on assessment of the person's energy level and respiratory function.

All fluid (parenteral and oral) input must total only slightly more than daily output if severe overhydration is to be avoided. Devices that allow precise control of intravenous fluids help avoid fluid overload when giving parenteral fluids to anuric or oliguric patients. Accuracy in fluid balance records is essential.

2. Promoting Nutrition

Most patients with AKF are too ill to tolerate oral feedings. Oral intake can exacerbate nausea as a result of the altered biochemical environment and accompanying GI tract irritation. If the patient is able to tolerate oral feedings, dietary protein and potassium are restricted to modest amounts. The aim is to increase protein available for tissue building and the palatability of the diet without leading to metabolic waste buildup or hyperkalemia.

A high-carbohydrate, high-fat diet is encouraged. Calories in the form of carbohydrates and fats provide energy and spare body protein stores, thus decreasing nonprotein nitro-

Guidelines for Safe Practice

The Patient With Acute Kidney Failure

1. Maintaining fluid and electrolyte balance
   a. Maintain fluid restrictions.
   b. Monitor intravenous fluids carefully.
   c. Keep accurate records of intake and output.
   d. Weigh patient daily.
   e. Monitor vital signs frequently, including postural signs.
   f. Assess fluid status of patient frequently.
   g. Administer phosphate-binding medications as prescribed.
   h. Monitor serum electrolytes.
   i. During diuretic phase:
      (1) Assess for changes in mental status indicative of low serum levels.
      (2) Assess for presence of irregular apical pulse indicative of hypokalemia.
2. Maintaining nutrition
   a. Provide fluid in small amounts during oliguric phase; ginger ale and other effervescent soft drinks may be tolerated better than other fluids.
   b. Provide a diet:
      (1) Restricted in protein, as prescribed.
      (2) High in carbohydrates and fat during protein restriction.
      (3) Low in potassium during hyperkalemia and high in potassium during hypokalemia.
   c. Take measures to relieve nausea (antiemetics and comfort measures).
3. Preventing injury
   a. Assess orientation; reorient confused patient.
   b. When the patient is ambulatory, assess motor skills and monitor ambulation; assist patient as necessary.
   d. Assess patient for signs of bleeding.
   e. Protect patient from bleeding: instruct patient to use soft toothbrush; perform guaiac tests on stool, emesis, and nasogastric returns.
4. Preventing infection
   a. Avoid sources of infection.
   b. Assess for signs and symptoms of infection.
   c. Maintain asepsis for indwelling lines or catheters.
   d. Perform pulmonary hygiene.
   e. Turn weak or immobile patients every 2 hours and as needed.
   f. Provide meticulous skin care.
   g. Bathe patient with superfatted soap.
   h. Administer prescribed antipruritic agents.
5. Facilitating coping
   a. Encourage development of nurse-patient relationship to assist patient to express feelings as desired.
   b. Promote patient independence.
   c. Assist patient to explore alternative ways of coping.

gen production. The body recycles urea to synthesize amino acids for protein building so that some regeneration of tissues can occur even though protein intake is curtailed.

3. Promoting Rest/Activity Balance

The patient with AKF needs assistance with activities of daily living (ADL). As kidney function improves, progressive ambulation is indicated.

4. Preventing Injury

The patient with AKF is weak, may be confused, and may experience postural hypotension; thus the risk of falls may be increased. The amount of supervision required during daily care must be assessed continually and appropriate actions taken to prevent injury. The confused, agitated, or restless patient must be protected from injury; side rails may need to be elevated and padded. Meticulous skin care should be provided to prevent skin breakdown from edema.

Bleeding may occur from changes in platelet and endothelial function. Nursing interventions should include measures to prevent and detect bleeding. (Further information on protection from bleeding can be found in Chapter 27.)

5. Preventing Infection

Preventing infection is an important nursing intervention. Infection leads to tissue breakdown with production of metabolic wastes, which are difficult to eliminate for the patient with AKF. Aseptic technique must be maintained during all treatments, especially with invasive lines and catheters. Sources of infection should be avoided. Pruritus frequently occurs and may lead to skin lesions from scratching. Measures to relieve pruritus include bathing the patient with a superfatted soap and administering prescribed antipruritic medications as necessary.

To compensate for increased metabolic acid loads, the lungs attempt to excrete more carbon dioxide. Pulmonary hygiene measures should be carried out to maximize this pathway for acid excretion, to maintain maximal lung expansion, and to prevent atelectasis.

6. Promoting Coping

During the oliguric phase of illness, the biochemical alterations may affect both the patient's mental status and personality. Family members and occasionally the patient are aware of these changes, which include memory impairment or an inability to think clearly. Reassure the patient and family that mental capacities will return with recovery of kidney function. Structuring the patient's environment and activities may help with coping in the initial phase. The nurse can assist the patient/family to explore feelings concerning the nature of the illness and find effective ways of coping.

7. Patient/Family Education

Most of the patient teaching takes place after the acute phase of the illness is over; the patient is usually more receptive to teaching at this time. Items to include in the teaching plan are listed in the Patient Teaching box.

Patient Teaching
The Patient With Acute Kidney Failure

1. Cause of kidney failure and problems with recurrent failures
2. Identification of preventable environmental or health factors contributing to the illness, such as hypertension and nephrotoxic drugs
3. Prescribed medication regimen, including name of medication, dosage, reason for taking, desired and adverse effects
4. Prescribed dietary regimen
5. Explanation of risk of hypokalemia and reportable symptoms (muscle weakness, anorexia, nausea and vomiting, lethargy)
6. Signs and symptoms of returning kidney failure (decreased urine output without decreased fluid intake, signs of fluid retention, and increased weight)
7. Signs and symptoms of infection; methods to avoid infection
8. Need for ongoing follow-up care
9. Options for future; explanation of transplantation and dialysis if these are a possibility

Health Promotion/Prevention

Primary Prevention. The incidence of AKF can be reduced by the identification and control of environmental risk factors. A significant factor in preventive care is the control of nephrotoxic drugs, which is primarily a function of the Food and Drug Administration (FDA). Identification of nephrotoxic drugs and chemicals, enforced labeling of these substances, and drug dispensing only by prescription are examples of the FDA's attempts to promote public health. Proper labeling and storage of potentially toxic drugs and chemicals in the home can further reduce the number of accidental ingestions of nephrotoxic substances. Cleaners and solvents should be used in well-ventilated areas.

Secondary Prevention. Prevention of AKF includes increased medical supervision of persons with sore throats and upper respiratory infections and detection and treatment of individuals with bacteriuria and obstructive disease of the urinary system to monitor and prevent the development of glomerulonephritis associated with bacterial infections. The greatest incidence of AKF occurs in persons with major trauma, extensive burns, surgery of the heart or large blood vessels, massive blood loss, and severe myocardial infarction. Frequent monitoring of urinary output and detection of excessive losses of body fluid in these patients can help to identify instances of inadequate renal perfusion before kidney failure develops.

EVALUATION

To evaluate the effectiveness of nursing interventions, compare patient behaviors with those stated in the expected patient outcomes. Achievement of outcomes is successful if the patient with AKF:

1. Has a normal fluid balance with electrolytes and waste products at functional level.

1a. Shows no signs of respiratory distress, pulmonary, or peripheral edema.

1b. Has blood pressure ranges between 135/80 and 100/60.

1c. Has controlled serum electrolytes: sodium 125 to 145 mEq/L, potassium 3 to 6 mEq/L, and bicarbonate greater than 14 mEq/L.

1d. Has controlled protein catabolism: BUN less than 100 mg/dl, creatinine less than 12 mg/dl, and absence of skin breakdown.

2. Eats food high in calories and fat and restricted in protein and potassium.
3. Reports increased energy and rest.
4. Has no falls or bleeding; is free from injury.
5. Is free from infection.
6. Uses effective methods of coping; manages ADL to full extent of ability.
7. Verbalizes knowledge of AKF, diet therapy, signs and symptoms to be reported to physician, and plans for follow-up care.

GERONTOLOGIC CONSIDERATIONS

Mortality in AKF is greatest in the elderly population partially because of the prevalence of heart disease, hypertension, and diabetes in this population. Chronic illness and polypharmacy in the aging population can tax the kidneys. Early signs of AKF are vague and may be attributed to other causes. In the older person, signs of acute infection may be absent or diminished. Changes in mental status related to electrolyte imbalances may be attributed to early signs of dementia. In elderly men, decreased urine output, a sign of kidney failure, may be mistakenly attributed to benign prostatic hypertrophy.

Although the treatment for AKF remains the same regardless of the patient's age, treatment strategies are not tolerated easily in the older adult. Intravascular volume overload is particularly difficult to treat because of the increased risk of congestive heart failure. Older patients are much more likely to succumb to the severity of AKF because of an increased risk of complications such as pneumonia and sepsis.

SPECIAL ENVIRONMENTS FOR CARE

Critical Care

Most patients in the acute stages of AKF are cared for in the intensive care unit because of the need for constant monitoring of blood pressure, electrocardiogram, pulmonary status, and mental status. Many patients require mechanical ventilation and hemodynamic monitoring via a Swan-Ganz catheter to monitor intravascular fluid volume.

Patients who cannot tolerate hemodialysis because of hemodynamic instability may be treated with CRRT. These patients require one-to-one nursing care to continuously monitor blood pressure, administer and titrate medications, and maintain the patency of the system. The type of CRRT chosen is patient specific and is selected after careful assessment of hemodynamic status, fluid and electrolyte balance, and laboratory and clinical manifestations.

Community-Based Care

The home needs of the patient recovering from AKF vary, depending on the success of therapy. If progressing well through the recovery phase, the patient may be discharged from the hospital with instructions to follow up with his or her health care provider. Patients must be alert to early signs and symptoms of kidney failure. It may be necessary for a visiting nurse to monitor hemodynamic status. Mental status is also assessed to alert the nurse of early changes in electrolyte balance. If patients are discharged with a venous/arterial access device, assistance will be needed with dressing changes, care of the device, and monitoring for signs of infection.

COMPLICATIONS

The leading complication of AKF is the development of CKF. Approximately 50% of patients have some impairment of glomerular filtration. About 5% will never regain kidney function and require long-term hemodialysis or renal transplantation.[22] An additional 5% slowly develop CKF after initial recovery.[3]

CHRONIC KIDNEY FAILURE

Etiology

CKF exists when the kidneys are no longer capable of maintaining an internal environment that is consistent with life and damage to the kidneys is irreversible. For most individuals, the transition from health to a state of chronic or permanent illness is a slow process that may occur over a number of years. Recurrent infections and exacerbations of nephritis, obstruction of the urinary tract, systemic disease, and destruction of blood vessels from diabetes and long-standing hypertension all can lead to scarring in the kidney and progressive loss of function (Box 40-2). Some individuals, how-

BOX 40-2 Causes of Chronic Kidney Failure

Glomerular Dysfunction

Glomerulonephritis
Diabetic nephropathy
Hypertensive nephrosclerosis

Systemic Disease

Sickle cell anemia
Scleroderma
Polyarteritis nodosa
Systemic lupus erythematosus
Human immunodeficiency virus-associated nephropathy
Vasculitis

Urinary Tract Obstruction

Prostatic and bladder tumors
Lymphadenopathy
Ureteral obstruction
Calculi

Other

Chronic pyelonephritis
Nephrotic syndrome
Polycystic kidney disease
Kidney infarction
Cyclosporin nephrotoxicity
Multiple myeloma

ever, develop total irreversible loss of kidney function acutely. Such loss of function usually develops in a few hours or days and follows direct traumatic kidney insult. The leading causes of ESRD in order of occurrence are (1) diabetes mellitus 44%, (2) hypertension 16%, (3) glomerulonephritis 17%, and (4) other 23%.[23]

Epidemiology

Chronic kidney disease remains a significant health problem in the United States. More than 300,000 people have ESRD, and the number increases annually by 7%. The disease can affect persons of all ages, but the peak incidence is between 20 and 64 years old.

Until 1970 treatment for ESRD was cost-prohibitive to many patients. At the present time, private insurance as well as government programs subsidize most treatments for CKF.[2] Medicare benefits were extended to persons with ESRD by legislation passed in 1973.

Pathophysiology

CKF differs from AKF in that the damage to the kidneys is progressive and irreversible. Progression of CKF is through four stages: decreased kidney reserve, kidney insufficiency, kidney failure, and ESRD (Box 40-3). In practice, however, these stages are not sharply differentiated. Severe symptoms occur at the kidney failure stage. As many as 50% of nephrons are destroyed before renal deficits are apparent.

The specific pathophysiologic mechanisms depend on the underlying disease causing the destruction of the kidney. The following general pathophysiologic mechanism summarizes these changes. During CKF some of the nephrons, including the glomeruli and tubules, are thought to remain intact, whereas others are destroyed (*intact nephron hypothesis*). The intact nephrons hypertrophy and produce an increased volume of filtrate with increased tubular resorption despite a decreased GFR. This adaptive method permits the kidney to function until about three fourths of the nephrons are destroyed. The solute load then becomes greater than can be resorbed, producing an osmotic diuresis with polyuria and thirst. Eventually more nephrons are damaged, resulting in retention of waste products and oliguria.

Although the clinical course of CKF varies, some common features exist. Signs and symptoms result from disordered fluid and electrolyte balance, alterations in regulatory functions of the body, and retention of solutes. Anemia results from impaired red blood cell (RBC) production because of decreased secretion of erythropoietin by the kidney. Patients may report lethargy, dizziness, and fatigue. In addition, the life span of RBCs is shortened as a result of uremia and superimposed nutritional anemia resulting from dietary restrictions and poor GI absorption of iron. Azotemia and acidosis are present, and potassium and hydrogen ion excretion is impaired. Fluid and sodium balance is abnormal and may involve either abnormal retention or secretion of sodium and water; therefore urine volume can be increased, normal, or decreased.

Hyperuricemia is a common finding in ESRD, although the varied serum levels of uric acid do not seem to have a definite relationship with the level of kidney function. Increased levels of serum phosphate are characteristic, and calcium levels may be low or normal. These findings result from decreased kidney excretion of phosphate and a simultaneous reduction in ionized serum calcium. Through increased production of parathormone, the body may reestablish a normal serum calcium level, at the expense of the bone matrix.

Hypertension may or may not be present. As ESRD develops, blood pressure is elevated because of increased total body water, release of a vasopresser by the kidney, and inadequately secreted vasodepressors. Glucose intolerance may be seen, although usually not of sufficient severity to warrant treatment. The rising blood glucose level appears to be the result of an altered biochemical environment produced by the failing kidneys and does not signify the development of diabetes mellitus. As kidney failure progresses, the patient develops increased pigmentation of the skin; the skin becomes sallow or brownish in color. Uremic frost, though a rare occurrence, is a pale deposit of crystals on the skin caused by kidney failure and uremia. Metabolic waste products, unable to be excreted by the kidney, are instead excreted through the small capillaries of the skin. With more advanced and insufficiently treated kidney failure, the patient may develop muscular twitching, numbness in the feet and legs, pericarditis, and pleuritis.

BOX 40-3 Stages of Chronic Kidney Failure

Decreased Kidney Reserve (Kidney Impairment)

40%-75% loss of nephron function
GFR: 40%-50% of normal
BUN and serum creatinine levels normal
Patient asymptomatic

Kidney Insufficiency

75%-80% loss of nephron function
GFR: 20%-40% of normal
BUN and serum creatinine levels begin to rise
Mild anemia; mild azotemia, which worsens with physiologic stress
Nocturia, polyuria

Kidney Failure

GFR: 10%-20% of normal
BUN and serum creatinine levels increase
Anemia, azotemia, metabolic acidosis
Urine specific gravity low
Polyuria, nocturia
Symptoms of kidney failure

End-Stage Renal Disease

85% loss of nephron function
GFR: 10% of normal
BUN and serum creatinine at high levels
Anemia, azotemia, metabolic acidosis
Urine specific gravity fixed at 1.010
Oliguria
Symptoms of kidney failure

GFR, Glomerular filtration rate; *BUN,* blood urea nitrogen.

These signs usually resolve when the patient is treated with medication and/or dialysis.

The symptoms of uremia usually develop so slowly that the patient and family often cannot identify the time of onset. Symptoms of azotemia develop, which include lethargy, headaches, physical and mental fatigue, weight loss, irritability, and depression. Anorexia, persistent nausea and vomiting, shortness of breath, and pitting edema are symptomatic of severe loss of kidney function. Pruritus may be present. All body systems are affected by CKF (Table 40-4).

As ESRD develops, most women note changes in their menstrual cycle. Bleeding may occur at more widely spaced intervals, may be heavier or lighter in flow than normal, or may cease altogether. This obvious change in the reproductive cycle is usually accompanied by changes in fertility. Ovulation may occur normally or may occur only a few times a year. Pregnancy in uremic women is of much lower incidence than in the normal population. However, ESRD cannot be used as an effective method of birth control. In men, erectile dysfunction may occur as CKF progresses toward ESRD. Dialysis may be indicated to return or maximize reproductive function. It should be stressed that the sexual activity of some persons with CKF may remain quite normal even though changes occur in reproductive ability.

The point at which the patient becomes obviously symptomatic and displays signs typical of kidney failure occurs when approximately 80% to 90% of function has been lost (Figure 40-3). At this level of kidney function, creatinine clearance values fall to 10 ml/min or less.

Hypertriglyceridemia occurs in approximately 30% to 70% of persons with CRF. Atherosclerosis may develop as a result of an elevated ratio of high-density lipoproteins (HDL) to low-density lipoproteins (LDL). The production of HDL decreases because of decreased lipolytic activity caused by uremia.

Catabolism and proteinuria contribute to the negative nitrogen balance common in CRF. Muscle mass diminishes.

Collaborative Care Management

Diagnostic Tests. Because of the multisystemic effects of CKF, many serious abnormalities in laboratory values are characteristic of persons with CKF. Serum creatinine levels are essential in the evaluation of kidney function. Increased levels of creatinine are seen only when a significant number of nephrons are destroyed, resulting in impaired creatinine

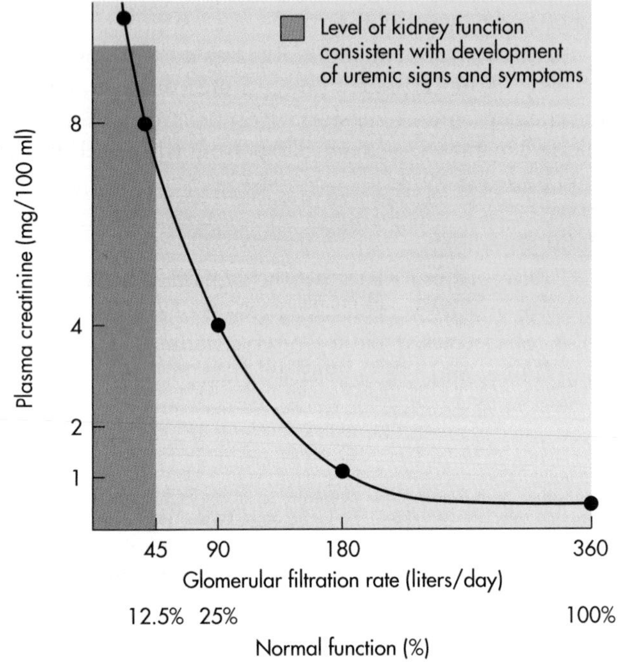

Figure 40-3 Glomerular filtration and plasma creatinine levels.

TABLE 40-4 Body System Manifestations in Chronic Kidney Failure

Causes	Signs/Symptoms	Assessment Parameters
Hematopoietic System		
Decreased erythropoietin by the kidney	Anemia	Hematocrit
Decreased survival time of RBCs	Fatigue	Hemoglobin
Bleeding	Defects in platelet function	Bleeding time
Blood loss during dialysis	Decreased hematocrit	Observe for bruising, hematemesis, or melena
Decreased activity of platelets and endothelin	Ecchymosis	
	Bleeding	
Cardiovascular System		
Fluid overload	Hypervolemia	Vital signs, body weight
Renin-angiotensin mechanism	Hypertension	Body weight, vital signs
Fluid overload, anemia	Tachycardia	Electrocardiogram
Chronic hypertension	Dysrhythmias	Heart sounds
Calcification of soft tissues	Congestive heart failure	Monitor electrolytes
Uremic toxins in pericardial fluid	Pericarditis	Assess for pain, pericardial friction rub
Fibrin formation on epicardium		

RBC, Red blood cell; *BUN,* blood urea nitrogen.

TABLE 40-4 Body System Manifestations in Chronic Kidney Failure—cont'd

Causes	Signs/Symptoms	Assessment Parameters
Respiratory System		
Compensatory mechanisms for metabolic acidosis Uremic toxins Fluid overload	Tachypnea Kussmaul's respirations Uremic fetor (or uremic halitosis) Tenacious sputum Pain with coughing Elevated temperature Hilar pneumonitis Pleural friction rub Pulmonary edema/frothy sputum	Respiratory assessment Arterial blood gas results Inspection of oral mucosa Vital signs Pulse oximetry
Gastrointestinal System		
Change in platelet activity Serum uremic toxins Electrolyte imbalances Urea converted to ammonia by saliva	Anorexia Abdominal distention Gastrointestinal bleeding Nausea and vomiting Diarrhea Constipation	Monitor intake and output Hematocrit Hemoglobin Guaiac test for all stools Assess quality of stools Assess for abdominal pain
Neurologic System		
Uremic toxins Electrolyte imbalances Cerebral swelling resulting from fluid shifting	Lethargy, confusion Convulsions Stupor, coma Sleep disturbances Unusual behavior Asterixis Muscle irritability	Level of orientation Level of consciousness Reflexes Electroencephalogram Electrolyte levels
Skeletal System		
Decreased calcium absorption Decreased phosphate excretion	Renal osteodystrophy Joint pain Retarded growth	Serum phosphorus Serum calcium Assess for joint pain Parathyroid hormone level
Skin		
Anemia Pigment retained Decreased size of sweat glands Decreased activity of oil glands Dry skin; phosphate deposits Excretion of metabolic waste products through the skin	Pallor Pigmentation Pruritus Ecchymosis Excoriation Uremic frost	Observe for bruising Assess color of skin Assess integrity of skin Observe for scratching
Genitourinary System		
Damaged nephrons	Decreased urine output Decreased urine specific gravity Proteinuria Casts and cells in urine Decreased urine sodium	Monitor intake and output Serum creatinine BUN Serum electrolytes Urine specific gravity Urine electrolytes
Reproductive System		
Hormonal abnormalities Anemia Hypertension Malnutrition Medications	Infertility Decreased libido Erectile dysfunction Amenorrhea Delayed puberty	Monitor intake and output Monitor vital signs Hematocrit Hemoglobin

excretion. A 12- or 24-hour urinary creatinine clearance test evaluates kidney function and determines the degree of dysfunction. This test is the most specific indicator of kidney function. The creatinine clearance rate is equal to the GFR. Measurements of serum and urinary creatinine levels and urine volume are necessary to complete the test. A creatinine clearance less than 10 ml/min is indicative of severe kidney impairment. Creatinine clearance is calculated based on 24-hour urine results (including serum and urinary levels) and data on body weight and height.

The BUN to creatinine ratio is also useful in evaluating kidney function. The creatinine level changes only in response to kidney dysfunction, while the BUN level changes in response to dehydration or protein breakdown.

Blood chemistry analysis, CBC, and urinalysis are performed to evaluate the degree of impairment in patients with CKF (Table 40-5). Because urinary output declines with the progression of kidney failure, urinalysis may not provide as much information as other laboratory tests.

Radiographic examinations are of little use in the evaluation of the patient with ESRD. A KUB film can evaluate kidney size, shape, and position. The patient with ESRD often has atrophic kidneys. Ultrasound or CT may be ordered to evaluate possible obstruction. CT is preferably performed without contrast because of the nephrotoxicity potential of the contrast agent.

Medications. Initial management of patients with CKF is focused on controlling symptoms, preventing complications, and delaying the progression of kidney failure (see Box 40-4 for treatment goals). Medications are used to control blood pressure, regulate electrolytes, and control intravascular fluid volume.

TABLE 40-5 Laboratory Findings in Chronic Kidney Failure

Test	Normal Values	Findings in Chronic Kidney Failure
Serum creatinine		
Male	0.6-1.5 mg/dl	Elevated
Female	0.5-1.1 mg/dl	> 4 mg/dl indicates significant renal impairment
Elderly	Decreased (due to decreased muscle mass)	May rise to 30 mg/dl before symptoms appear
BUN		
BUN	7-20 mg/dl	
Elderly	8-21 mg/dl	Values >100 mg/dl indicate severe kidney impairment*
Blood chemistry		
Sodium	135-145 mEq/L	Decreased
Potassium	3.5-5 mEq/L	Increased
Calcium		
Total	8.5-10.5 mg/dl	Decreased
Ionized	4.5-5.6 mg/dl	
Phosphorus	2.7-4.5 mg/dl	Increased
Magnesium	1.2-1.9 mEq/L	Increased
Serum pH	7.35-7.45	Decreased (metabolic acidosis) or normal
Serum bicarbonate	22-26 mEq/L	Decreased
Complete Blood Count		
Hemoglobin		
Male	10-17 g/dl	Decreased
Female	11.5-15.5 g/dl	
Elderly	Decreased	
Hematocrit		
Male	39%-49%	Decreased (may rise to near normal with epoetin therapy)
Female	33%-43%	
Elderly	Decreased	
Creatinine Clearance		
Male	70-150 ml/min	Decreased
Female	85-130 ml/min	Findings <10 ml/min indicative of kidney impairment
Elderly	Decreased up to 30% in absence of renal disease	Decrease reflects decreases in GFR
Uric Acid (Serum)		
Male	2.1-8.5 mg/dl	Increased
Female	2.0-6.8 mg/dl	Findings >12 mg/dl indicate serious kidney impairment
Elderly	3.5-8.5 mg/dl	

*Increased levels dependent on protein intake, liver disease, and hydration status.
BUN, Blood urea nitrogen; *GFR,* glomerular filtration rate.

Hypertension is controlled by the use of a variety of antihypertensive agents including angiotensive-converting enzyme inhibitors (ACEI), angiotensive II receptor antagonists, calcium channel antagonists, diuretics, and beta-blockers. If blood pressure cannot be controlled with a single agent, combination therapy may be instituted. Immunosuppressive therapy may be instituted in patients with glomerulonephritis. Intravascular fluid volume is also regulated by the use of diuretics.

Electrolyte imbalances are corrected by the use of sodium bicarbonate for metabolic acidosis. Hyperkalemia is treated with diuretic therapy or sodium polystyrene sulfonate (Kayexalate). In severe hyperkalemia insulin may be administered intravenously with dextrose to temporarily decrease the serum potassium level. Calcium and phosphorus levels are maintained by the use of phosphate-binding agents, calcium supplements, and vitamin D analogs.

Treatments

Fluid Control. Changes in the ability to regulate sodium and water excretion are often the first clinical signs of kidney failure. The ability to excrete sodium and water can vary considerably from one patient with CKF to the next. Although volume problems for most patients involve hypervolemia resulting from a marked inability to excrete sodium and water, some patients are unable to conserve these substances and hypovolemia results. With marked inability either to excrete or conserve body fluid, the patient can develop severe fluid imbalances in a relatively short time. Fluid imbalances are identified, and an intake of sodium and water equivalent to the amount of these substances excreted in a 24-hour period is prescribed. The desired effect is to maintain the person in a normotensive, normovolemic state.

BOX 40-4 Treatment Goals for the Patient with Chronic Kidney Failure

1. Stabilization of the internal environment as demonstrated by:
   a. Mental alertness, attention span, and appropriate interactions
   b. Absence or control of peripheral and pulmonary edema
   c. Control of electrolyte balance within the following limits:

Sodium	125 to 145 mEq/L
Potassium	3-6 mEq/L
Bicarbonate	>15 mEq/L
Calcium	9-11 mg/dl
Phosphate	3-5 mg/dl

   d. Serum albumin >2 g/dl
   e. Control of protein catabolism and protein metabolic wastes as indicated by the following parameters:

Urea nitrogen	<100 mg/dl
Creatinine	<10 mg/dl
Uric acid	<12 mg/dl

   f. Absence of joint inflammation and pain
   g. Control of anemia

Hematocrit	≥33%
Ferritin	>50-100 ng/ml
Iron saturation	>20%

2. Absence of infection
3. Absence of bleeding
4. Blood pressure controlled at 135/80 mm Hg sitting, <10 mm Hg postural change on standing
5. Control of coexisting disease including:
   a. Heart failure
   b. Anemia
   c. Dehydration
6. Absence of toxicity from inadequately excreted medications
7. Nutrient intake sufficient to maintain positive nitrogen balance
8. Anorexia and nausea controlled
9. Pruritus controlled

Electrolyte Control

Hyperkalemia. Hyperkalemia is defined as a plasma potassium (K^+) level greater than 5.5 mEq/L, although the level at which hyperkalemic complications occur may vary, depending on the steady-state value for a given patient. Potassium retention occurs in CKF because of a direct reduction in nephron excretory ability. Hyperkalemia can be controlled by decreasing dietary intake of foods high in potassium, such as citrus fruits, green leafy vegetables, and salt substitutes. Exchange resins, such as sodium polystyrene sulfonate, are also effective in removing K^+ from the body. The resin exchanges sodium ions for K^+ and calcium in the GI tract. Kayexalate can be given either as an oral preparation or by retention enema. It is usually given with sorbitol to enhance K^+ loss via the bowel. A 25-g dose removes approximately 12.5 to 25 mEq of K.[1] The use of a retention enema requires that the solution be retained in the colon for 30 to 60 minutes or longer.[11] In severe situations hemodialysis may be instituted.

Metabolic Acidosis. Metabolic acidosis occurs because the damaged kidneys are unable to excrete the normal load of acids generated by metabolism. When the GFR drops 30% to 40%, metabolic acidosis begins to develop primarily because of a reduced capacity of the distal tubules to produce ammonia and an impaired resorption of bicarbonate. Although there is continued hydrogen ion retention and bicarbonate loss, the plasma pH is maintained at a level compatible with life by other buffering mechanisms, particularly the bone salts.

Hypocalcemia/Hyperphosphatemia. When the kidneys fail, the ability to excrete phosphorus decreases, and a cycle of hypocalcemia/hyperphosphatemia results in significant bone demineralization. Several factors are responsible for these imbalances. In a state of acidosis there is dissolution of the alkaline salts of bone to serve as buffers because the kidney is no longer able to maintain acid-base balance. As a result, calcium and phosphorus are released into the bloodstream. Reduced glomerular filtration and excretion of inorganic phosphate lead to an elevation of plasma phosphate with a concomitant decrease in serum calcium. Decreased serum calcium concentrations stimulate the secretion of parathyroid hormone (PTH), which results in resorption of calcium from the bones. Normally PTH also inhibits tubular reabsorption of phosphates increasing their excretion, but the failing kidney is unable to excrete potassium so the level rises. The kidneys are also unable to complete the synthesis of vitamin D to its active form, 1,25-dihydroxycholecalciferol, which is necessary for absorption of calcium from the GI tract and deposition of calcium in the bones. This acquired resistance to vitamin D decreases calcium absorption, permits further retention of phosphorus, and contributes to secondary hyperparathyroidism. The result of these complex disturbances is growth arrest or retardation in children and bone pain and deformities known as *renal osteodystrophy* in adults. The aim of treatment is to decrease the serum phosphorus levels. This can be accomplished by restricting dietary phosphorus intake (eliminating dairy products and restricting protein) and using phosphate binders. The reduction of serum phosphorus toward normal is often associated with a small increase in serum calcium, a decline in serum PTH, and a reduced incidence of overt secondary hyperparathyroidism.

The goal of therapy with phosphate-binding agents is to reduce serum phosphorus to normal or near-normal levels. In dialysis patients predialysis serum phosphorus levels are ideally maintained between 4.5 and 6 mg/dl. To avoid GI upset, phosphate binders should be taken with meals and with snacks. The available agents for intestinal phosphate binding include calcium carbonate and calcium acetate. Another substance used for phosphate binding is sevelamer, a nonabsorbed, phosphate-binding polymer. Sevelamer (RenaGel) binds phosphate ions through a combination of ion exchange and hydrogen bonding without elevating serum calcium levels. Like other phosphate binders, it must be ingested during the meal. Historically phosphate binders containing aluminum were the mainstay of therapy. Because the kidney is the major route of aluminum excretion, prolonged ingestion of aluminum-containing phosphorus binders results in the accumulation of aluminum in kidney failure. Consequences of aluminum overload include dementia, myopathy, osteomalacia, and anemia.[5] Risks of calcium-containing phosphate binders include hypercalcemia and diarrhea. If the calcium carbonate is given with meals, less calcium is absorbed and the risk of hypercalcemia is reduced. It is critical that nurses adjust the medication times to coincide with meal delivery to enhance phosphate binding and to minimize calcium absorption.

Some patients may benefit from the administration of the active form of vitamin D (calcitriol 0.25 μg daily). Indications for use include inadequate control of serum phosphorus, hypocalcemia, bone pain, myopathy, and rising serum alkaline phosphatase concentration.[5]

Treatment of Concurrent Disorders

Anemia. Anemia universally accompanies chronic kidney disease. Hematocrit values of 16% to 22% were not uncommon in the days before epoetin alfa (EPO). When untreated, the anemia of chronic kidney disease is associated with a number of physiologic abnormalities, including decreased tissue oxygen delivery and use, increased cardiac output, cardiac enlargement, ventricular hypertrophy, angina, congestive heart failure, and decreased cognition and mental acuity.[15] The primary cause of anemia in these patients is insufficient production of erythropoietin by the diseased kidneys.[7] The introduction and subsequent clinical success of EPO, the recombinant form of human erythropoietin, have confirmed this hormone's primary role in regulating the erythropoietic cascade. Patients treated with this agent have an increase in hematocrit, a decrease in the need for blood transfusions, and improved energy levels. This increase in hematocrit enables the patient with CKF to carry out normal daily activities.

EPO is administered subcutaneously, three times a week, in a calculated dose of 50 U/kg of body weight. It is usually administered during a scheduled dialysis treatment. Patients who are in a predialysis state, receiving peritoneal dialysis, or receiving other home dialysis regimens learn to self-administer the drug.

Iron is a necessary component of erythropoiesis, and therapy with EPO is hindered if patients do not have adequate iron stores. Iron stores should be evaluated before and during therapy. Iron deficiency may occur with EPO as a result of an internal shift of iron from stores to RBCs during the acute correction of anemia. Iron deficiency is a major factor in the pathogenesis of anemia in patients with chronic kidney disease. A number of factors may contribute to the iron deficiency, including decreased dietary intake and GI absorption of iron, chronic GI bleeding, and chronic inflammatory responses associated with infection and/or autoimmune disease. In these conditions, iron stores may be adequate, but the availability of usable iron for the production of hemoglobin is reduced because iron is not released from the stores.[24] Because iron is necessary for continued RBC production, virtually all patients receiving EPO eventually require supplemental iron. Patients should be instructed that iron's adverse effects on the GI tract (nausea and constipation) can be avoided or minimized by taking iron on a full stomach and by adding a stool softener or laxative to the medication regimen. Furthermore, simultaneous ingestion of iron and phosphate binders should be avoided because phosphate binders impede the absorption of oral iron.

Folate and vitamin B_{12} are important cofactors in the production of RBCs and play a role in the formation and development of deoxyribonucleic acid (DNA). Shortages of these vitamins hinder the formation of DNA and thus RBCs. Folate can be taken orally at a dose of 1 mg/day, and vitamin B_{12} can be replaced with a monthly intramuscular injection of 100 to 1000 μg based on the vitamin B_{12} blood level.

Blood pressure may rise during EPO therapy, especially during the early stage of treatment when the hematocrit is rising. About 25% of patients experience this rise in blood pressure. Regulating a dialysis patient's blood pressure involves reevaluating dietary sodium intake, the dialysis prescription, and antihypertensive medications.

Gastrointestinal Disturbances. In patients with uremia, disturbances in fluid, electrolyte, and waste composition of body fluids produce changes in osmotic gradients in all cells. When these changes occur in the cells of the GI tract, anorexia, nausea, and vomiting result. Persons with uremia are subject to bleeding of the GI tract associated with lesions such as an angiodysplasia and decreased platelet function. Urea is broken down to ammonia by the action of intestinal bacteria. Because ammonia is a mucosal irritant, ulceration and bleeding can occur. Persons with chronic kidney disease also have decreased salivary flow. The smell and taste of ammonia resulting from urea breakdown increase anorexia. Treatment includes vinegar mouthwashes to neutralize ammonia and antacids every 2 to 4 hours to decrease GI irritation. Dietary control of uremia helps to control disturbances in fluid, electrolyte, and water composition of body fluids and thus helps to control nausea and vomiting.

Dialysis. Chronic intermittent hemodialysis was first used for the treatment of CKF in 1960. Before the early 1960s hemodialysis was reserved for the treatment of AKF. Once kidney failure was determined to be irreversible, hemodialysis was withdrawn. Many industrialized countries throughout the world continue to withdraw dialysis after irreversible kidney failure is confirmed.

In 1972 the U.S. Congress enacted legislation that provides some payment of health care costs for all U.S. citizens with ESRD. Under this legislation, any person with CRF is provided benefits under Medicare. As a result of this legislation, many persons are able to live longer by undergoing chronic hemodialysis.

Many technologic advances have been made in the treatment of persons with ESRD. Drastic changes in artificial kidneys allow for more efficient and comfortable hemodialysis treatments. Advances in the development of dialysis machines allow individuals the convenience of treatment in their own homes. Other developments in peritoneal dialysis permit patients to treat themselves with continuous peritoneal and intermittent peritoneal dialysis. Home dialysis provides persons with the opportunity to have more control over meeting their own health care needs.

Dialysis involves the movement of fluid and particles across a semipermeable membrane. It is a treatment that can help restore fluid and electrolyte balance, control acid-base balance, and remove waste and toxic material from the body. This treatment can sustain life successfully in both acute and chronic situations where substitution for or augmentation of normal kidney function is needed. Specifically, dialysis is used to remove excessive amounts of drugs and toxins in poisonings, to correct serious electrolyte and acid-base imbalances, to maintain kidney function when shutdown occurs as a result of transfusion reactions, to replace kidney function temporarily in persons with AKF, and to permanently substitute for the loss of kidney function in persons with ESRD.

Physiologic Principles of Dialysis. Dialysis is based on three principles: diffusion, osmosis, and ultrafiltration (Figure 40-4). *Diffusion* involves the movement of particles from an area of greater to an area of lesser concentration. In the body, this usually occurs across a semipermeable membrane. Diffusion is involved in the clearance of solute from the patient's body in both hemodialysis and peritoneal dialysis. Diffusion results in the movement of urea, creatinine, and uric acid from the patient's blood into the dialysate. This solution contains fewer particles of substances to be removed from the bloodstream and high concentrations of particles of substances to be added to the blood (Figure 40-5). Because the dialysate contains no protein waste products, concentration of these substances in the blood decreases because of random movement of the particles across the semipermeable membrane into the dialysate. The same principle applies to the movement of potassium ions. Although the concentration of RBCs and protein is high in blood, these molecules are quite large and do not diffuse through the membrane pores; thus they are not lost from the blood.

Osmosis involves the movement of water across a semipermeable membrane from an area of lesser to an area of greater concentration (osmolality) of particles. Osmosis is responsible for movement of extra fluid from the patient, particularly in peritoneal dialysis. Figure 40-5 shows that glucose has been added to the dialysate to make its particle concentration greater than that of the patient's blood. Fluid will then move through the pores of the membrane from the patient's blood to the dialysate.

Ultrafiltration involves the movement of fluid across a semipermeable membrane as a result of an artificially created

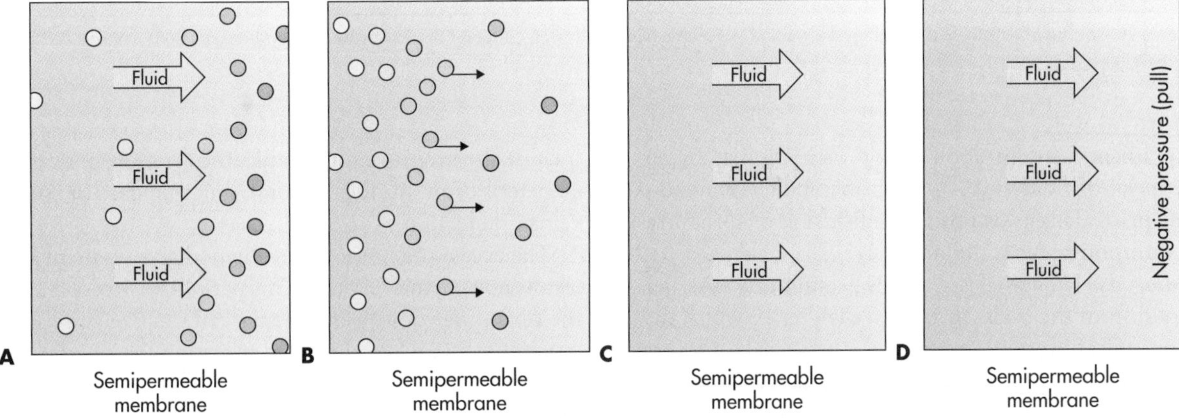

Figure 40-4 Dialysis is based on **A**, principles of osmosis, **B**, diffusion, and ultrafiltration. Ultrafiltration occurs when either **C**, positive pressure or **D**, negative pressure is placed on the system. Ultrafiltration can be maximized by simultaneously exerting both positive and negative pressure on the system.

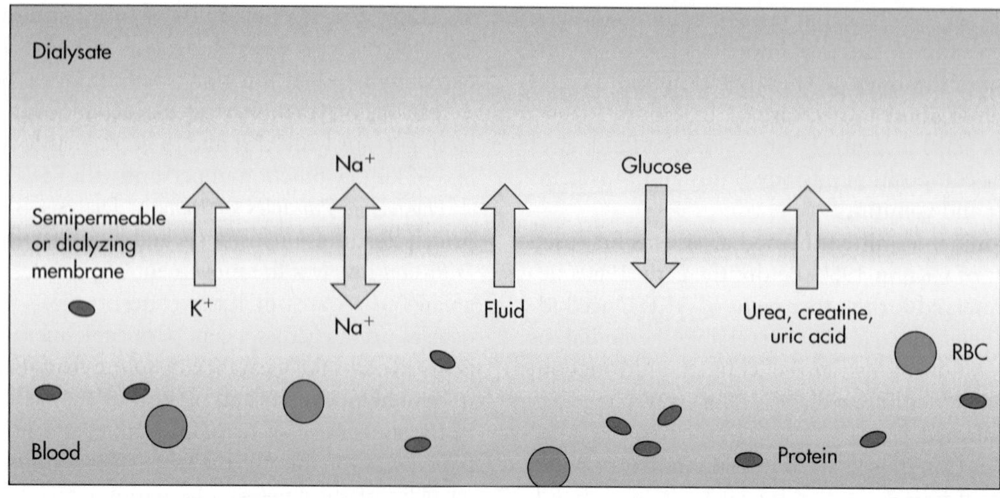

Figure 40-5 Osmosis and diffusion in dialysis. Net movement of major particles and fluid is illustrated.

TABLE 40-6 Dialysis Access

Type	Usable	Comments
Hemodialysis		
Central venous catheter (femoral/jugular/subclavian) Avoid subclavian where possible	Immediately	Usual maximum life of 2 weeks. Complications include venous stenosis, which may prevent subsequent fistula or graft from being successful (particularly with subclavian catheters)
Tunneled central venous catheter	Immediately	May last 1 year or more. Main complications are sepsis and catheter blockage.
Arteriovenous fistula	2-6 weeks	May last indefinitely. Requires adequate artery and vein: Doppler studies can be helpful in assessing patients with diabetes mellitus and peripheral vascular disease. Avoid cannulation of the veins of the forearm and wrist in those likely to require fistula formation.
Arteriovenous graft	1-2 weeks	More prone to thrombosis and infection than a fistula. Alternative for those whose vessels are inadequate for fistula formation.
Peritoneal Dialysis Access		
Hard cannula	Immediately	Usable for 1 week
Tenckhoff catheter	2 weeks	Can be placed by minilaparotomy, laparoscopy, or percutaneous technique. Risk of fluid leaks increased by using the catheter sooner than 2 weeks.

From Frasser D, Vinning M: Urologic nephrology. In Weiss RM, George N, O'Reilly PH, editors: *Comprehensive urology,* London, 2001, Mosby International Ltd.

pressure gradient. Ultrafiltration is more efficient than osmosis for removal of fluid and is used in hemodialysis for this purpose. During dialysis osmosis and diffusion or ultrafiltration and diffusion occur simultaneously.

Hemodialysis. Hemodialysis involves shunting the patient's blood from the body, through a dialyzer in which diffusion and ultrafiltration occur, and then back into the patient's circulation. Hemodialysis requires access to the patient's bloodstream, a mechanism to transport the blood to and from the dialyzer (area in which the exchange of fluid, electrolytes, and waste products occur), and a dialyzer. Currently the means of gaining access to the patient's bloodstream include the arteriovenous fistula, the arteriovenous graft, and catheterization of the femoral, interjugular, or subclavian veins (Table 40-6).

The access of choice for the hemodialysis patient is the arteriovenous fistula (AVF).[18] This peripheral access is created in the operating room using the patient's native vessels. The artery and vein are anastomosed, allowing the arterial blood to be diverted into the vein. The increased blood flow through the vein stimulates intimal hyperplasia of the vein with a thickening of the vein wall. The vein "matures" over 6 to 12 weeks and is then able to be cannulated by the dialysis needles. A well-matured AVF is able to provide the high blood flow re-

Guidelines for Safe Practice

Care of the Patient With an Arteriovenous Fistula

- Assess patency of fistula by palpating thrill or auscultating bruit.
- Instruct patient to avoid compression of fistula by tight clothing or when sleeping.
- Instruct patient to assess fistula for signs and symptoms of infection, including pain, redness, swelling, or excessive warmth.
- Instruct patient to monitor fistula patency by palpating the thrill daily.

quired for the dialysis procedure. If the fistula is cannulated before proper maturation, infiltration of the dialysis needle may occur. The patient may experience pain, edema, and hematoma. (See Guidelines for Safe Practice box above).

Many patients do not have blood vessels that will support the development of an adequate AVF. Because of possible vascular disease, patients with diabetes, long-term hypertension, or advanced age may not be candidates for a fistula. These patients are candidates for placement of the arteriovenous graft (AVG). The AVG is placed in the operating room by anastomosing a piece of tubular, synthetic material to an artery, tunneling the material through the soft tissue, and finally anastomosing the graft to the vein. As with the AVF, blood flow is diverted into the graft material with outflow through the vein. After about 3 weeks, the AVG becomes engrafted into the subcutaneous tissue and is ready for cannulation with dialysis needles. Over time, because of the increased blood flow, the venous outflow tract may become thickened, causing the AVG to be prone to thrombosis. Nursing implications for the patient with the AVG are the same as those for the patient with an AVF.

Dialysis catheters may also be used for hemodialysis access. These catheters may be placed in the femoral, internal jugular, or subclavian veins. In rare instances, the catheters may be placed in other large vessels such as the inferior vena cava. The vessel of choice for the dialysis catheter is the internal jugular vein.

Temporary dialysis catheters are devices placed at the patient's bedside or in a radiology suite for short-term dialysis use. These catheters are usually made of a firm plastic substance. This type of catheter is usually indicated for the patient with AKF or during the 3-week postoperative period after placement of an AVF or AVG.

The procedure for placing these catheters is the same as that for placing any central venous catheter. The temporary dialysis catheter is large, usually about 12 F. Two lumina are present, one for outflow to the dialysis machine and one for return of blood to the patient. Temporary dialysis catheters placed in the internal jugular vein may be left in place and used for up to 3 weeks. Temporary dialysis catheters placed in the femoral vein may be used for approximately 1 week.

Guidelines for Safe Practice

Care of the Patient With a Dialysis Catheter

- Maintain sterile technique when working with catheters or catheter exit site.
- Assess patient for bleeding at insertion site and tubing connections.
- Monitor patient for signs and symptoms of infection.

Tunneled, cuffed hemodialysis catheters may be placed for long-term dialysis use. These catheters are made of a soft, silicone-like substance and are placed in the operating room or radiology suite. If the catheter is placed in the internal jugular vein, a tunnel is made in the subcutaneous tissue. The exit site of the catheter is on the anterior chest wall. After about 4 weeks the cuff of the catheter becomes engrafted into the subcutaneous tissue. This anchors the catheter, preventing inadvertent removal, and acts as a barrier to the migration of bacteria. Like the temporary dialysis catheter, the tunneled, cuffed dialysis catheter has two ports. Regardless of the vessel placement, this type of catheter may be left in place for long-term dialysis of greater than 3 weeks' duration.

Once placed, dialysis catheters are ready for immediate use. At the end of dialysis, each port of the catheter is usually instilled with high-dose heparin to prevent thrombosis of the lumina. Access of the dialysis catheter should be performed by specially trained persons only. The dialysis catheter should not be used for routine intravenous procedures except in the dialysis unit. Functional complications associated with the dialysis catheter include thrombosis of the catheter and infections (see Table 40-6). See the Guidelines for Safe Practice box above for care of the patient with a dialysis catheter.

Many patients expect to leave the dialysis treatment with a feeling of well-being. Few persons feel this way; most experience some minor discomfort that diminishes within several hours after dialysis. The greatest feeling of well-being seems to occur the day after dialysis.

Immediately before dialysis the patient is weighed, vital signs are taken, and the patient's physical status is assessed. A sample of blood may be drawn to determine the level of serum electrolytes and waste products. Nursing care of the patient during hemodialysis centers around (1) monitoring physical status before and during dialysis for evidence of physiologic imbalance and change, (2) providing comfort and safety, and (3) helping the patient to understand and adjust to the care and changes in lifestyle. This latter objective involves educating the person as to the specifics of the treatment program (diet and medications in particular) and how these relate to altered kidney function. The person is encouraged to express concerns and feelings, and attempts must be made to help the individual work through these feelings. If dialysis is performed at home, the patient and dialysis partner must be able to institute all the care described (see Nursing Care Plan). Hemodialysis treatments last 2 to 4 hours.

Nursing Care Plan — *Patient With Kidney Failure Undergoing Dialysis*

DATA Mr. D. is a 52-year-old high school teacher with a 10-year history of chronic glomerulonephritis. He worked full time until 3 months ago, when his renal disease progressed to end-stage disease requiring hemodialysis. Mr. D. is married and has three adolescent children. Because of financial hardship, his wife has started to work full time as a sales clerk. Mr. D. finds his present situation depressing and confides that he seems to be losing control over his life.

Nursing assessment reveals that Mr. D.:
- Is scheduled for hemodialysis (which takes about 4 hours) three times weekly
- Has an arteriovenous fistula in his left arm
- Has a blood pressure ranging from 190/110 to 180/100 before dialysis and 120/70 to 100/64 after the second hour of treatment
- Often develops a headache during dialysis

NURSING DIAGNOSIS **Excess fluid volume related to fluid accumulation between dialysis treatments**
GOALS/OUTCOMES Will maintain fluid volume status within established parameters

NOC Suggested Outcomes
- Electrolyte and Acid-Base Balance (0600)
- Fluid Balance (0601)

NIC Suggested Interventions
- Hemodialysis Therapy (2100)
- Fluid and Electrolyte Management (2080)
- Acid-Base Management (1910)
- Hypervolemia Management (4170)

Nursing Interventions/Rationales
- Assess weight, lung sounds, and extremities for presence of edema. *To determine the fluid volume so that treatment parameters can be identified.*
- Monitor intake and output. *Some patients continue to urinate small amounts, but it is inadequate to clear all waste products. Intake is limited and must be monitored to prevent fluid volume overload.*
- Monitor laboratory data: blood urea nitrogen; serum creatinine, sodium, potassium, calcium, magnesium, and phosphorus levels; hemoglobin and hematocrit. *Nitrogenous waste and electrolytes accumulate between treatments. Anemia and blood losses associated with hemodialysis are complications associated with kidney failure.*
- Teach patient the need for maintaining fluid restrictions between treatments. *To prevent excess intake, which can lead to hypervolemia.*
- Teach patient the need for restricting sodium intake. *Sodium intake stimulates thirst, which can lead to excessive fluid intake and subsequent hypervolemia.*

Evaluation Parameters
1. Maintains fluid restrictions
2. Is free of peripheral edema
3. Clear lung sounds

NURSING DIAGNOSIS **Deficient fluid volume related to rapid fluid removal during dialysis and potential blood loss**
GOALS/OUTCOMES Will maintain fluid volume status within established standards

NOC Suggested Outcomes
- Electrolyte and Acid-Base Balance (0600)
- Fluid Balance (0601)

NIC Suggested Interventions
- Hemodialysis Therapy (2100)
- Fluid and Electrolyte Management (2080)
- Acid-Base Management (1910)
- Hypovolemia Management (2130)

Nursing Interventions/Rationales
- Monitor intake, output, and vital signs during dialysis. *To identify shifts in fluid balance.*
- Monitor effects of anticoagulant therapy every hour during dialysis. *Anticoagulant therapy is necessary to prevent clotting in the dialysis tubing; however, bleeding can occur.*
- Monitor blood-clotting time hourly during dialysis. *To identify and prevent excessive bleeding.*
- Minimize blood loss by returning all blood to patient at end of treatment and applying pressure to the access puncture site following needle removal. *Returning blood to the patient helps prevent anemia. Applying pressure to the puncture site prevents bleeding.*
- Monitor weight during dialysis. *To prevent weight loss greater than 3 to 4 kg during treatment, which can result in hypovolemia.*

Evaluation Parameters
1. Vital signs within normal parameters
2. Mucous membranes moist
3. Skin turgor good

Nursing Care Plan *Patient With Kidney Failure Undergoing Dialysis—cont'd*

NURSING DIAGNOSIS **Risk for infection related to frequent invasive procedure**
GOALS/OUTCOMES Will remain free of infection

NOC Suggested Outcomes
- Risk Control (1902)
- Immune Status (0702)

NIC Suggested Interventions
- Infection Protection (6550)
- Surveillance (6650)
- Hemodialysis Therapy (2100)

Nursing Interventions/Rationales
- Maintain Standard Precautions for exposure to blood and body fluids. *To protect both patient and nurse.*
- Maintain sterile technique when performing access site puncture and discontinuing hemodialysis. *To prevent site contamination with microorganisms.*
- Assess site for signs of localized infection (warmth, redness, swelling, tenderness). *To detect the presence of infection so that treatment can be initiated.*
- Monitor temperature and white blood cell (WBC) count. *To detect the presence of systemic infection so that treatment can be initiated.*
- Follow routine testing policies for hepatitis B and C and human immunodeficiency virus (HIV) antibodies. *To identify change in patient status. Patients are monitored monthly, and staff are monitored yearly.*

Evaluation Parameters
1. Absence of localized infection (redness, warmth, swelling, tenderness)
2. Absence of systemic infection (fever, elevated WBC count, lethargy, chills)

NURSING DIAGNOSIS **Risk for ineffective therapeutic regimen management related to change in life status and dependency on dialysis**
GOALS/OUTCOMES Will adhere to therapeutic regimen as prescribed

NOC Suggested Outcomes
- Family Normalization (0604)
- Knowledge: Treatment Regimen (1813)
- Health Beliefs: Perceived Control (1702)
- Health Beliefs: Perceived Resources (1703)

NIC Suggested Interventions
- Self-Modification Assistance (4470)
- Role Enhancement (5370)
- Family Support (7140)
- Financial Resource Assistance (7380)
- Mutual Goal Setting (4410)

Nursing Interventions/Rationales
- Monitor for indications of noncompliance with the treatment plan (abnormal laboratory data, missed appointments, excess fluid weight gain, verbalizations of noncompliance). *To determine if the patient is adhering to the prescribed treatment plan.*
- Determine factors that may interfere with patient's ability to adhere to the treatment plan. *To identify factors that may need to be addressed to assist the patient with treatment plan adherence.*
- Encourage patient to participate in decision making about his own care. *Allows the patient some control over his situation and increases the likelihood of adherence to the treatment plan.*
- Prepare patient and family for community dialysis center by reviewing the center's location and introducing them to a center representative who can review policies and procedures with them. *Preparing the patient and family in advance will give them time to work through their fears about the unknown, reduce anxiety, and increase the likelihood of compliance.*
- Acknowledge the impact that chronic kidney failure and hemodialysis has on the family. *The family is subjected to disruption, expenses, and considerable alterations in family routines to accommodate a patient with end-stage kidney failure on dialysis.*
- Explore with patient and family their perception of demands that the illness has made on them. *The family's perceptions and ability to cope affects patient outcomes both positively and negatively.*
- Support patient's and family's coping skills. *Previously successful coping skills are strengths to the family in new situations.*
- Refer to a support group as appropriate. *Group members often provide mutual support and share beneficial information with one another.*

Continued

Nursing Care Plan — Patient With Kidney Failure Undergoing Dialysis—cont'd

Evaluation Parameters

1. Attends all appointments for dialysis and follow-up care
2. Maintains fluid and dietary restrictions
3. Verbalizes ability to comply with therapeutic regimen
4. Takes active role in decision making

NURSING DIAGNOSIS **Situational low self-esteem related to chronic kidney failure requiring machine dependency and loss of family status**

GOALS/OUTCOMES Will maintain positive body image

NOC Suggested Outcomes

- Grief Resolution (1304)
- Self-Esteem (1205)
- HAcceptance: Health Status (1300)
- Body Image (1200)

NIC Suggested Interventions

- Self-Esteem Enhancement (5400)
- Body Image Enhancement (5220)
- Mutual Goal Setting (4410)
- Support Group (5430)

Nursing Interventions/Rationales

- Monitor patient's response to illness and treatments. *To determine the effect of health status changes so that appropriate interventions can be planned.*
- Allow patient to grieve over his losses. *Grieving is a necessary part of recovery.*
- Acknowledge patient's grief about being dependent on a machine. *Demonstrates empathy and validates the patient's feelings.*
- Support strengths, self-confidence, determination, and motivation to live. *Patients undergoing dialysis are not disabled in all aspects of life. Many live nearly normal lives while maintaining treatment schedules.*
- Help patient to develop or continue interests beyond dialysis and return to as near normal a life as possible. *Patients may tend to withdraw from social activities because of their new schedule and feelings of loss. Focusing on other interests will help the patient place less focus on his dependency.*
- Monitor for excessive expressed concerns about losses, depression, self-neglect, and noncompliance. *These may be indications of suicidal ideation, which needs to be identified and treated quickly.*
- Explore patient's feelings about changes in sexual functioning. *Kidney failure characteristically produces infertility and decreased libido and can interfere with the patient's marital and sexual life.*

Evaluation Parameters

1. Verbalizes positive feelings about self
2. Verbalizes acceptance of treatment regimen as part of lifestyle
3. Describes meaning of dependency on a machine for life (and loss of independence)
4. Grieves over perceived and actual losses

Peritoneal Dialysis

Peritoneal dialysis is used to treat acute and CKF in the hospital or at home.

In peritoneal dialysis the dialyzing fluid is instilled into the peritoneal cavity, and the peritoneum becomes the dialyzing membrane (Figure 40-6). Peritoneal dialysis can be continuous for up to 36 hours or done intermittently in the hospital setting. The procedure, once instituted, becomes largely a nursing responsibility.

The major advantages of peritoneal dialysis are:

- It provides a steady state of blood chemistry values.
- Patients can readily be taught the process.
- Patients can dialyze alone in any location without the need for machinery.
- Patients have few dietary restrictions; because of loss of protein in dialysate, patients usually consume a high-protein diet.
- Patients have much more control over daily life.
- Peritoneal dialysis can be used for patients who are hemodynamically unstable.

Procedure. Access to the peritoneum is gained through the introduction of a catheter into the peritoneal space. For acutely ill patients and those who are chronically ill and require sporadic dialysis, a sterile catheter is inserted for each dialysis procedure. For the chronically ill person treated on a routine basis, a Tenckhoff peritoneal catheter can be placed into the peritoneal space; the catheter remains in place until it malfunctions or until another treatment option, such as transplantation, is selected (see Table 40-6). Because these catheters present a continuous portal of entry for organisms into the peritoneum, each patient must be thoroughly instructed in the care of the catheter and the signs and symptoms indicative of local or peritoneal infection, which must be reported to the physician.

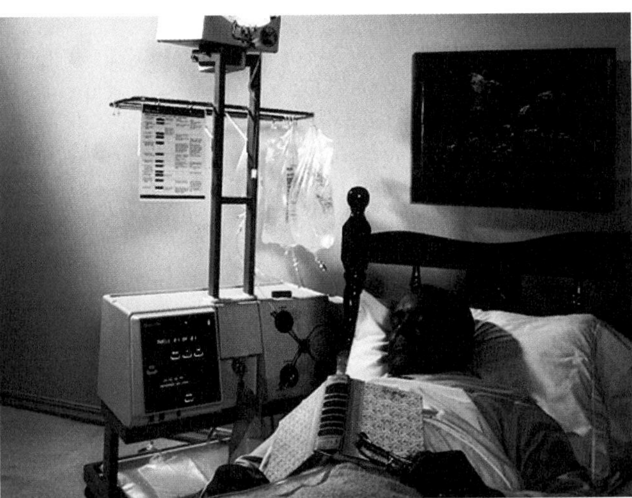

Figure 40-6 Automated peritoneal dialysis cycler, which is used while the patient is sleeping at night.

Guidelines for Safe Practice

Peritoneal Dialysis

1. Regulating fluid volume and drainage
   a. Assess vital signs.
   b. Monitor mental status.
   c. Record fluid balance after each cycle.
   d. Turn patient side to side to facilitate drainage.
   e. Elevate head of bed.
2. Promoting comfort
   a. Administer analgesics as ordered.
   b. Provide diversional activities.
   c. Encourage side to side movement.
   d. Assist with oral care and feeding.
3. Preventing complications
   a. Assess respiratory effort.
   b. Encourage frequent small meals.
   c. Use aseptic technique.
   d. Culture dialysate as directed.
   e. Monitor temperature.
   f. Observe for nausea, vomiting, abdominal tenderness, and cloudy outflow.

For all patients, weight, blood pressure, and pulse are recorded before the procedure is initiated. These values serve as baseline information against which to assess changes during treatment. For persons undergoing insertion of a peritoneal catheter before dialysis, assessment should be made of their knowledge of the procedure and their anxiety level. A mild sedative may help the severely anxious person to better tolerate the insertion of the catheter. It is important that patients void before catheter insertion to decompress the bladder and prevent accidental puncture during catheter placement.

To insert a peritoneal catheter, the physician cleanses the abdomen and anesthetizes a small area in the midline of the abdomen about 5 cm (2 inches) below the umbilicus. A small incision is made, and the multilumen nylon catheter is inserted into the peritoneal cavity. A dressing is placed around the protruding catheter.

Approximately 2 L of warm, sterile dialysate is attached by tubing to the catheter and allowed to run into the peritoneal cavity as rapidly as possible. This usually takes about 10 minutes. The tubing is then clamped. The maximal osmosis of fluid and diffusion of particles into the dialysate occurs in 20 to 30 minutes. At the end of the dwell time (amount of time the dialysate is left in the peritoneal cavity), the tubing is unclamped, and the fluid is allowed to flow by gravity from the abdomen. Fluid should drain in a steady stream. Drainage time should average about 10 to 15 minutes. The first drainage may be pink-tinged as a result of the trauma of catheter insertion; however, drainage should clear with the second or third cycle. At no time should fluid draining from the abdomen be grossly bloody. After fluid has drained from the abdomen, another cycle is started immediately. Dialysis is initiated for the person with a permanent catheter by carefully cleansing the catheter and surrounding skin with a bactericidal agent before the catheter is connected to the dialysate line. After the infusion of dialysate has been completed, the permanent catheter is again cleansed and a sterile cap is applied to the tip.

If the procedure is temporary, the catheter is removed, and the incision is covered with a dry, sterile dressing. The small abdominal wound from the catheter should heal completely in 1 to 2 days (see Guidelines for Safe Practice box).

Other Approaches to Peritoneal Dialysis. Several advances in the management of patients with ESRD have led to two variations of peritoneal dialysis. Continuous ambulatory peritoneal dialysis and continuous cyclic peritoneal dialysis are primarily for home and self-dialysis use.

Continuous ambulatory peritoneal dialysis (CAPD) is a method of self-dialysis that is practical, relatively inexpensive compared with hemodialysis, and promotes independence. CAPD involves continuous contact of dialysate with the peritoneal membrane. Approximately 2 L of dialysate is maintained in the peritoneal cavity and exchanged by the patient through a permanent peritoneal catheter four to five times each day. No special equipment is required for the exchanges, but patient education is imperative. CAPD allows the patient to lead a fairly normal life. Exchanges can take place at home or at work by connecting an empty bag to the catheter and opening a clamp to allow drainage. A full dialysate bag is then instilled, and the patient has completed an exchange.

The second method is *continuous cyclic peritoneal dialysis* (CCPD). CCPD differs from CAPD in that a machine known as a cycler is used to instill and drain dialysate from the patient (Figure 40-6). The machine has a series of time-controlled clamps. The timers open and close the clamps in sequence to allow for instillation and drainage of dialysate from the patient. The cycle times for patients with CKF generally allow for the patient to be dialyzed in 6 to 8 hours. Therefore a patient can connect to the cycler at bedtime, set the machine, and undergo dialysis while sleeping. Several alarms are built into the cycler to protect the patient from malfunctions such as dialysate that is too hot or cold, long or short dwell times, improper return of fluid, and changes in catheter pressures. The greatest advantage of CAPD and CCPD over other forms of dialysis is the unprecedented freedom the patient has in managing his or her own care.

Compliance is of utmost importance to the success of any CAPD/CCPD therapy for the dialysis patient. Conditions causing noncompliance in the peritoneal dialysis patients have not been adequately analyzed. From studies on compliance with chronic drug regimens, it is known that patients are more compliant when they are convinced about the appropriateness and beneficial effect of the prescribed treatment and that frequent reinforcement of the importance of the treatment is associated with better compliance. For the CAPD/CCPD patient, special emphasis should be placed on education about the importance and technique of the peritoneal dialysis prescription. Instructions should be repeated at least every 6 months, and patients should be monitored for signs of change in compliance.[17]

Evaluating Dialysis Effectiveness. Numerous outcome studies have demonstrated a correlation between the delivered dose of hemodialysis and patient mortality and morbidity.[16] Clinical signs and symptoms alone are not reliable indicators of hemodialysis adequacy. To ensure that ESRD patients treated with chronic hemodialysis receive a sufficient amount of dialysis, the delivered dose should be measured and monitored routinely.[15,16] *Kinetic modeling,* or prescription dialysis, is a tool developed by dialysis practitioners in the last decade to compute how much dialysis an individual needs. Kinetic modeling monitors the effectiveness of the delivered prescription. Hemodialysis is usually prescribed by nephrologists based on the mathematic formula Kt/V. This formulation includes individual patient parameters of dialyzer clearance (K), time of dialysis (t), and volume of urea distribution (V). In addition, the normalized protein catabolic rate of the individual patient must be determined and periodically reassessed. Using serum urea levels as the kinetic factor, practitioners are able to determine an expected outcome of treatment. If the patient's Kt/V is calculated to be inadequate, the patient's dialysis time or blood flow may be increased. A peritoneal dialysis patient may need to increase the number of dialysis exchanges.

Surgical Management

Kidney Transplantation. Kidney transplantation reverses many of the pathophysiologic changes associated with kidney failure. It also eliminates the dependence on dialysis and the need for dietary restrictions, provides the opportunity to return to normal life activities, and is more cost-effective than dialysis after the first year.

Although transplant procedures are expensive, the current success rates have made transplantation a cost-effective treatment option compared with traditional medical management. A patient undergoing chronic hemodialysis costs the federal government, through Medicare, about $50,000/year.[23] The cost of a kidney transplant is approximately $75,000 for the first year and $12,500/yr for follow-up care.[23] If the transplanted kidney functions for 5 years (the actual rate approaches 75%), the cost is $125,000 as opposed to $250,000 for 5-year chronic hemodialysis. Other financial factors that increase the cost-effectiveness of transplantation are the potential earning power of the transplant recipient and the discontinuation of disability benefits previously required. In short, transplantation can restore dignity and quality to the lives of patients and families dealing with ESRD and provide the potential for patients to become productive members of society again. (For a discussion of the methods of kidney transplantation and required care requirements, see Chapter 51.)

Diet. The goals of diet therapy are to (1) reduce the quantity of metabolic waste that requires excretion by the kidney, (2) provide sufficient calories and protein for growth and repair while limiting excretory demands on the kidney, (3) minimize metabolic bone disease, and (4) minimize fluid and electrolyte disturbances. The dietary protein restriction is calculated at 1 to 1.5 g/kg of ideal body weight. Adequate protein intake is reflected by a BUN/creatinine ratio of 10:1. Excessive intake of protein results in nausea and vomiting, apathy, weakness, and neurologic symptoms. Insufficient protein intake results in lowered serum albumin level, muscle wasting, edema, and weight loss. Two thirds of the total protein consumed should be protein of high biologic value, that is, containing the essential amino acids.

Ample calories are obtained from carbohydrates and fats because they do not require renal excretion of their metabolic by-products. This spares protein for growth and repair. Catabolism of existing protein stores liberates nitrogenous wastes. For this reason, sources of potential infection such as indwelling catheters are avoided. When infection is noted, it is immediately treated.

Activity. A patient undergoing hemodialysis must remain in a chair or in bed during dialysis because of the attachment to the machine. A patient with CAPD has more freedom during dialysis because the dialysate is in the abdominal cavity. However, the patient must cycle therapy over the 24-hour time frame; thus he or she must schedule the day around treatments. Apart from these considerations, there are no activity restrictions or recommendations for the patient with ESRD, and patients should be encouraged to continue with their normal activities. The Life Options Rehabilitation Advisory Council has suggested the five Es— encouragement, evaluation, employment, exercise, and education—for persons with ESRD.[9] Only 25% of Americans with ESRD are employed, in part because many persons with ESRD are older than 65 years of age.

Referrals. A patient with ESRD should be referred to a dietitian for education about meeting nutritional requirements and diet planning. ESRD patients may also need referrals to home health care to supervise treatments, provide dialysis supplies, and perform venipunctures. Social service referrals may be required to assist patients with financial concerns. Occupational and physical therapy is indicated to maximize independent functioning of the patient with ESRD.

NURSING MANAGEMENT OF PATIENT WITH CHRONIC KIDNEY FAILURE

ASSESSMENT

The nursing assessment of the patient with CKF is extremely complex. The assessment must include physical, psychologic, and social parameters. The basis of this assessment is the same as that described in Chapter 38 for the patient with suspected kidney problems. The initial nursing history and physical assessment must elicit adequate information to generate the appropriate nursing diagnoses. An example of a comprehensive nursing history is found in Figure 40-7 and an example of a physical assessment in Figure 40-8.

The extent and nature of subsequent assessments are determined by the medical regimen, nursing diagnoses, and patient condition. The frequency of assessment is a function of the medical regimen and stability of the patient. For example, the patient being managed conservatively may be able to go several months without follow-up assessments. On the other hand, the hemodialysis patient requires a thorough assessment with each treatment.

Health History

The history must be comprehensive and include not only information on physical symptoms but also on patient lifestyle. Health maintenance behaviors as well as the home environment should be explored to determine the consequences of various treatment options. The patient should report feelings of fatigue, nausea, pruritus, and lethargy.

Physical Examination

Data to be collected as part of the physical examination include vital signs, input and output, heart and lung sounds, mental status, and signs of pain. The skin should be assessed for increased pigmentation and signs of peripheral edema. Daily weight should also be part of the objective assessment.

NURSING DIAGNOSES

Nursing diagnoses are determined from analysis of patient data. Nursing diagnoses for the person with chronic kidney failure (CKF) may include but are not limited to:

Diagnostic Title	Possible Etiologic Factors
1. Excess fluid volume	Compromised regulatory mechanism
2. Imbalanced nutrition: less than body requirements	Anorexia, nausea, decreased salivary flow, bad taste, pain
3. Risk for infection	Compromised immune response
4. Risk for injury	Sensorimotor deficits, lack of awareness of environmental hazards, decreased level of consciousness
5. Fatigue	Uremia, anemia, insomnia
6. Acute pain	Sodium depletion, uremia, pruritus, ocular irritation, muscle cramping
7. Ineffective coping (individual)	Situational crisis
8. Situational low self-esteem	Changes in body appearance, change in social involvement
9. Deficient knowledge	Lack of exposure/recall

EXPECTED PATIENT OUTCOMES

Expected patient outcomes for the person with CKF vary, depending on the course of the disorder and the identified nursing diagnoses. Expected patient outcomes may include but are not limited to:

1. Will exhibit no signs of respiratory distress, peripheral edema, hypertension, or other signs and symptoms indicating fluid and electrolyte imbalance
2. Will explain dietary plan, including fluid, protein, potassium, and sodium restrictions
3. Will show no signs of infection; skin remains intact
4. Will be free from injury
5. Will report feeling more rested and less fatigued
6. Will be free of muscle cramping, itching, or ocular irritation
7. Will describe methods of effective coping; exhibits ability to perform ADLs and desired activities independently
8. Will affirm satisfaction with life and self
9. Will verbalize knowledge of nature of illness, treatment regimen, and plans for follow-up care

INTERVENTIONS

Because the condition of the person with CKF can vary, nursing care focuses on the specific identified nursing diagnoses. Most persons, however, require some help or teaching to maintain fluid and electrolyte balance; prevent infection or injury; promote comfort, rest, and sleep; and cope with the effects of kidney failure (see Guidelines for Safe Practice box).

Drug Therapy in Kidney Failure

Patients with either AKF or CKF typically receive multiple drugs to manage the associated complications. Currently, the drug approval process in the United States requires drug-dosing recommendations for patient with kidney failure as a part of the product labeling. In kidney failure, a number of factors can affect drug absorption: uremic gastroparesis, changes in gastric pH, gut wall edema, and alterations in first-pass metabolism.[1] As a result, many common doses for drug therapy must be adjusted for the patient with kidney failure. Clearance of drugs that are metabolized by the kidneys, such as insulin, meperidine, and numerous antibiotics, is greatly reduced in kidney failure.[1] The nurse should monitor patients closely for development of adverse reactions associated with drug overdose (Boxes 40-5 and 40-6).

1. Maintaining Fluid and Electrolyte Balance

The person with CKF must learn how to identify signs of imbalances, take fluids in the prescribed amounts, and eat within

Hemodialysis Nursing Notes Admission History (Inpatient)/Patient Notes (Outpatient)	

Date	Hour		
		I.	**Perception of Illness**
			Why, initially, did you come to the hospital?
			What does the doctor plan for you while you are here?
			What do you expect to happen to you when you start dialysis?
		II.	**History of Past Illness (Include dates and hospitalizations)**

Date	Hour	Medications	Dose	Frequency	Last Dose Taken	Reason for Taking

Date	Hour		
			Do you receive any special treatments or exercises?
		III.	**Activity**
			Do you have difficulty walking or getting in and out of a chair?
			Can you climb stairs?
			Are you employed?
			What are your usual daytime activities?
			What are your recreational interests?
		IV.	**Nutrition**
			Are you on a special diet?
			Do you have difficulty following a diet?
			How many meals do you eat a day?
		V.	**Sleep Habits**
			Do you sleep through the night at home?
			What helps in getting to sleep at night?
			What are your usual sleeping habits?

Figure 40-7 Hemodialysis nursing notes: admission history.

Date	Hour		
		VI. Elimination	
		How often do you urinate?	
		Do you have any difficulty with urination?	
		Frequency	Pain on urination
		Urgency	Other
		Have you ever had urinary tract infections?	
		24-hour urine output	cc/24 hr
		Color of urine?	
		What are your usual bowel habits?	
		Do you have difficulty with diarrhea or constipation?	
		How often do you use enemas or laxatives?	
		VII. Reproductive System	
		When was your most recent menses?	
		Have you recently had a change in menses?	
		Have you had any changes in sexual function recently?	
		Do you have any concerns about reproductive or sexual functions?	
		VIII. Social	
		Do you live with anyone?	
		Upon whom do you rely when you need help?	
		In what type of dwelling do you live?	
		Do you have to climb stairs?	
		Financial resources/insurance	

Admitting Nurse ______________________

Figure 40-7, cont'd Hemodialysis nursing notes: admission history.

(Inpatient)/Patient Notes (Outpatient)					
Date	Hour	A)	**Vital Signs**		
			Temperature		
			Pulses	Apical	
				Radial	
				Rhythm	
			Weight		
			Height		
		B)	**Cardiopulmonary**		
			Vascular access		
			Peripheral pulses:	Right	Left
			Radial		
			Femoral		
			Popliteal		
			Pedal		
			Peripheral edema?		
			Periorbital edema?		
			Friction rub?		
			Neck vein distention?		
			Cough?	Sputum?	Smoking habits?
			Adventitious breath sounds?		
			Shortness of breath?		
			Orthopnea		
		C)	**Neuromuscular**		
			Orientation		
			Level of alertness and responsiveness?		
			Muscle tone and strength, symmetry?		
			Weakness or loss of function of extremities?		
			Balance		
			Numbness, tingling, or tremors?		
			Patient experiencing difficulties with:		
			Sight		
			Speech		
			Touch		
			Taste/Smell		

Figure 40-8 Hemodialysis nursing notes: admission assessment.

Date	Hour	
		D) Skin
		Color
		Turgor
		Temperature
		Lesions
		Condition of nails
		E) General
		Presence of:
		Nausea
		Vomiting
		Headache
		Blurring of vision
		Ability to perform ADL

Admitting Nurse ____________________

Figure 40-8, cont'd Hemodialysis nursing notes: admission assessment.

the prescribed limits. This requires careful monitoring of intake and output.

Controlling sodium intake can be an extremely challenging problem for both the nurse and patient. Any sudden increase in weight indicates accumulating fluid, and the source of this fluid must be discussed with the patient. When the patient is not acutely ill and is responsible for diet restrictions, the problem can often be traced to excess sodium ingestion, which produces thirst. In helping to avoid this cycle of sodium-driven thirst leading to increased fluid ingestion and overhydration, the patient is taught about the amount of sodium and fluid allowed in the diet and restrictions to observe when purchasing prepared foods. The words *sodium* and *salt* should be checked on all food labels. All patients with CKF should avoid salt substitutes because these substitutes contain large amounts of potassium.

Sometimes the patient is unable to explain his or her increasing thirst and sodium ingestion. At this point the question of home self-medication is raised. The person may be taking over-the-counter antacids that are high in sodium. If the cause of the hypervolemia cannot be identified, the patient is asked to list all foods and fluids ingested over the previous 3 days. This list can be used to uncover dietary indiscretions, as well as serve as a teaching tool to reinforce the prescribed diet.

2. Facilitating Nutrition

Persons usually need help planning diets within the prescribed sodium, potassium, phosphorus, and protein limits. Modifying the diet to the individual's preferences can help to maintain intake of food. Dietary teaching and meal planning can be approached using an exchange system similar to that used for persons with diabetes.

Complying with a modified diet can be promoted through attempts to decrease emotional tension at the dinner table. Food that is attractively arranged and flavorful is also likely to promote the appetite. Herbs and other flavorings can add variety to foods that are prepared without sodium. When the GI tract is ulcerated, bland foods may be tried in an attempt to increase ingestion of food.

3,4. Preventing Infection and Injury

Tissue breakdown leads to infection. Extensive tissue damage can cause an elevation in serum potassium and must be avoided. Potassium is largely an intracellular cation, and extensive tissue damage can liberate a lethal amount of this ion into the system of the person with CKF. Edematous skin poses a high risk for skin breakdown; therefore, meticulous skin care is important. Patients with CKF should avoid others with infections and seek medical attention when symptoms of infections, GI bleeding, or other problems first appear.

The risk of constipation is also high in persons with CKF because of the fluid restrictions and required medication therapy. Stool softeners or laxatives may be needed.

Other important nursing activities include helping the patient to control blood loss. A soft toothbrush is recommended for oral care. The patient is instructed to observe for melena and to report this without delay to the physician. Aspirin should be avoided because it is normally excreted by the kidneys and may rapidly build to toxic levels and prolong bleeding time. Regular use of NSAIDs should also be avoided

Guidelines for Safe Practice

The Patient With Chronic Kidney Failure

1. Maintain fluid and electrolyte balance.
   a. Monitor for fluid and electrolyte excess.
      (1) Assess intake and output every 8 hours.
      (2) Weigh patient every day.
      (3) Assess presence and extent of edema.
      (4) Auscultate breath sounds.
      (5) Monitor cardiac rhythm and blood pressure every 8 hours.
      (6) Assess level of consciousness every 8 hours.
   b. Encourage patient to remain within prescribed fluid restrictions.
   c. Provide small quantities of fluid spaced over the day to stay within fluid restrictions.
   d. Encourage a diet high in carbohydrates and within the prescribed sodium, potassium, phosphorus, and protein limits.
   e. Administer phosphate-binding agents with meals as prescribed.
2. Prevent infection and injury.
   a. Promote meticulous skin care.
   b. Encourage activity within prescribed limits but avoid fatigue.
   c. Protect confused person from injury.
   d. Protect person from exposure to infectious agents.
   e. Maintain good medical/surgical asepsis during treatments and procedures.
   f. Avoid aspirin products.
   g. Encourage use of soft toothbrush.
3. Promote comfort.
   a. Medicate patient as needed for pain.
   b. Medicate with prescribed antipruritics, use emollient baths, keep skin moist, and control environmental temperature to modify pruritus.
   c. Encourage use of damp cloth to keep lips moist; give good oral hygiene.
   d. Encourage rest for fatigue; however, encourage self-care as tolerated.
   e. Provide calm, supportive atmosphere.
4. Assist with coping in lifestyle and self-concept.
   a. Promote hope.
   b. Provide opportunity for patient to express feelings about self.
   c. Identify available community resources.

because of increased risk of GI bleeding and prolonged bleeding time.

The buildup of osmotically active particles and fluid in the body that occurs with azotemia produces changes in the cells of the brain that may lead to confusion and impairment in decision-making ability. Fluid accumulation and hypertension can produce visual changes. The person's environment is assessed for potential for injury. At times the person may need help in limiting activities to a level commensurate with mental processes and level of awareness. For example, blurred vision and delayed reaction time contraindicate driving a motor vehicle.

BOX 40-5 Drugs That Require Very Different Prescriptions in the Dialysis Patient

Drug	Notes
Vancomycin	A large molecule poorly cleared by all forms of dialysis (but may be cleared to a greater degree by continuous hemofiltration techniques); dose of 1 g once weekly usually results in consistently therapeutic drug levels (usual dose 1 g twice daily)
Aminoglycosides, (e.g., netilmicin)	Cleared to a variable degree by both hemodialysis and peritoneal dialysis; dose likely to be greatly reduced (e.g., one third of usual daily dose every 2 days) and monitoring of plasma levels required; note that even if nephrotoxicity is no longer an issue, ototoxicity is still a serious complication of therapy
Morphine	Smaller doses are likely to be effective; accumulation of metabolites normally cleared by the kidney such as morphine-6 glucuronide can cause profound narcosis and respiratory depression; morphine-6 glucuronide is not cleared by dialysis, and clearance will take days to weeks in the anephric patient
Meperidine	Accumulation of normeperidine (a metabolite) can cause seizures; great care needed with use for longer than 24 hours
Digoxin	Reduced clearance; transient profound hypokalemia is common on hemodialysis, increasing the risk of arrhythmia with digoxin

From Frasser D, Vinning M: Urologic nephrology. In Weiss RM, George N, O'Reilly PH, editors: *Comprehensive urology,* London, 2001, Mosby International Ltd.

5,6. Promoting Comfort, Rest, and Sleep

The patient with CKF rarely has acute, sharp pain; however, these persons are subject to a wide variety of chronic discomforts including pruritus, muscle cramping, headaches, insomnia, and bone pain.

Most patients with ESRD develop pruritus and describe a sensation of deep itching. Itching is largely symptomatic, and measures that are effective in controlling it vary from person to person. Reducing levels of serum phosphorus with phosphate-binding preparations decreases itching for most patients. Medications such as diphenhydramine hydrochloride (Benadryl) and hydroxyzine hydrochloride (Atarax) may be effective for some patients. Keeping the skin moist and supple through use of lotions and bath oils, controlling the room temperature during sleep to prevent excessive warmth, and bathing with emollients or a vinegar solution are measures alone or in combination that may provide some relief from itching. The urge to scratch the skin is acute in some patients. Because scratching is often vigorous, injury to the skin with

BOX 40-6 Drugs To Be Used With Particular Caution in Those With Kidney Impairment

ACE inhibitors	Avoid in those with renal artery stenosis; renal blood flow is dependent on efferent arteriolar tone, and reduction of this by ACE inhibition may seriously damage renal function, sometimes irreversibly; risk of profound hypotension in patients with heart failure or volume depletion; these hazards are shared by angiotensin-receptor antagonists
Aminoglycosides	Very narrow therapeutic range and, with prolonged treatment, toxic within it; predominantly renal excretion; high risk of ototoxicity and nephrotoxicity in those with renal impairment; toxicity mainly relates to trough plasma concentration, so once-daily (or less frequent) dosing may be safer if their use is essential; netilmicin is probably the least nephrotoxic
NSAIDs	Risk of nephrotoxicity, partly from effect on prostaglandin-mediated renal vasoregulation; damage caused by other insults to the kidney (e.g., hypoxia, hypotension, or sepsis) is likely to be enhanced; increased risk of peptic ulceration in the uremic patient
Tetracyclines	Have an antianabolic effect, increasing blood urea, and should be avoided in those with renal impairment
X-ray contrast medium	Toxicity enhanced by kidney failure, particularly with diabetes mellitus, myeloma, dehydration, and low cardiac output states; even nonionized contrast can cause AKF; IVU relies on the excretion of the contrast by the kidney and so will not be helpful in the presence of advanced kidney failure

From Frasser D, Vinning M: Urologic nephrology. In Weiss RM, George N, O'Reilly PH, editors: *Comprehensive urology,* London, 2001, Mosby International Ltd.

subsequent infection can result. Fingernails should be trimmed closely. Instead of fingernails, a soft cloth should be used to scratch the skin.

Muscle cramping in the lower extremities and hands is common in kidney failure. Often, cramping can be correlated with sodium depletion. Primary treatment for muscle cramping involves controlling the state of uremia and fluid and electrolyte balance. Temporary measures of heat and massage are effective for some persons. Quinine sulfate, 325 mg, at bedtime often prevents cramping.

Insomnia and chronic daytime fatigue are common complaints of persons with CKF. This alteration of normal sleep patterns has been attributed to a variety of causes. These include (1) recurring preoccupation with thoughts concerning the disease state and resultant changes in lifestyle, (2) pruritus, and (3) the state of uremia itself. Reduction of high serum levels of urea nitrogen and creatinine through decreasing dietary intake of protein or dialysis may bring sleep patterns back to normal. When control of uremia fails to cure insomnia, mild central nervous system depressants may be prescribed.

The severely anemic person experiences extreme fatigue and shortness of breath. The lack of RBCs creates an inability to transport sufficient oxygen to cells for energy production. The anemic person with this extent of symptoms may require transfusion of packed RBCs. The anemic person may be unable to work or play without extended rest periods. Rest periods should be taken early enough in the day to prevent sleeplessness at night.

General comfort at bedtime is needed to induce sleep and is especially important when sleeping problems arise. Comfort measures include tepid baths, pursuing quiet activities an hour or two before bedtime, controlling itching, or relaxation techniques.

7,8. Facilitating Coping With Changes in Lifestyle and Feelings Regarding Self

The goals of therapy for patients with ESRD include not only the preservation of the patient's life in the presence of ESRD, but also restoration of optimal quality of life. There is broad agreement that patients' quality of life is related to their function in the physical/medical, ADL, psychologic, and social/occupational dimensions[14] (see Research box).

Optimal psychosocial care of patients with CKF requires careful and sophisticated psychosocial patient assessment. This assessment is accomplished as a collaborative effort by the physician, nurse, and social worker. Common psychologic problems include dysphoric moods (anxiety, depression, frustration, and anger), impaired body image (with a perceived loss of physical attractiveness), impaired self-esteem, and suicidal crises.

Noncompliance with the treatment regimen is a common behavioral problem; this may include treatment participation, diet and fluid restriction, and medication noncompliance, as well as noncompliance with other medical diagnostic and therapeutic procedures. Several factors contribute to noncompliance: the intrusive and demanding aspects of chronic dialysis regimen, strong feelings of frustration and depression, a strong desire to maintain control over one's life and deny the unpleasant personal reality of chronic illness, a need to indirectly express anger toward staff members, and attempts to balance health concerns with a short-term need for pleasure. Interventions that may effectively reverse significant patient noncompliance include (1) providing further information about the rationale for treatment procedures or restrictions, (2) helping the patient regain as much constructive control as possible over life's activities, (3) communicating with staff members to gather information and to design and implement a program to reward increased patient compliance, and (4) working with family members to educate them and enlist their support.

Social problems for patients with ESRD patients include strains in intimate relationships, loss of vocational function, and restriction of social and leisure activities. The introduction of a serious life-threatening illness such as ESRD is an added stress dimension to the already enormous demands placed on the contemporary family system. Role changes are common in families; spouses often take on the role responsibilities of the sick partner while maintaining their own roles. This leads to reduced rest and leisure for the spouse and lowers physical reserve. Major adjustments in thinking and living must be made, and at the same time, relationships must be maintained and nurtured. Nursing staff must be aware that additional social support for patients may need to be provided by professional caregivers, especially when family members take little responsibility for either physical and/or emotional support. These staff members may be viewed as important "significant others" for the patient with ESRD.

Vocational dysfunction is a result of decreased physical capacities, the time-intensive requirements of dialysis, depression and cognitive impairment, governmental policies about reimbursement for dialysis medical care, and the reluctance of employers to hire individuals with kidney disease. The problems of vocational function are quite complex, particularly for patients with limited skills and whose work previously involved manual labor. Implications for nursing and social work consist of identifying patients beginning dialysis and providing vocational counseling.

9. Patient/Family Education

The person with ESRD presents a unique opportunity for the nurse to promote optimal health through teaching and counseling. Important points to be included in patient teaching are listed in the Patient Teaching box.

Research

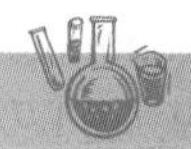

Reference: Kutner NG, Zhang R, McClellan WM: Patient-reported quality of life early in dialysis treatment: effects associated with usual exercise activity, *Nephrol Nurs J* 27(4):357-367, 2000.

The purpose of the study was to investigate factors associated with quality of life early in treatment in a cohort of newly diagnosed dialysis patients. This multicenter study investigated quality of life reported by patients on chronic hemodialysis and peritoneal dialysis at approximately 60 days after the start of treatment. Quality of life was assessed by the Medical Outcomes Study Short-Form 36 and by disease-targeted scales from the Kidney Disease Quality of Life. In univariate analyses, patients' quality of life scores were related to the following variables:

- Demographic (age, race, sex, educational level)
- Clinical (pre-dialysis blood urea nitrogen and creatinine, primary diagnosis of diabetes, cardiovascular comorbidity, average hematocrit and serum albumin)
- Dialysis (hemodialysis/peritoneal dialysis modality, dialysis adequacy, patient/staff ratio)
- Patient's level of usual exercise activity

The multivariate analyses showed that the most important independent quality of life predictor was patient's usual level of exercise activity. Continued study of patients outcomes in relation to adequacy of delivered dialysis, early versus late diagnosis of chronic kidney failure, and patient's usual exercise activity is important because these variables can be the focus of intervention strategies to prevent early deterioration in dialysis patients' functional health status.

The teaching plan for persons undergoing hemodialysis should include:

- The process of hemodialysis and relationship to body needs.
- Information necessary to care for vascular access devices including prevention of infection and clotting.
- Appropriate care of hemodialysis access.
- Common side effects of treatment, means of controlling mild symptoms, and means of obtaining medical attention for severe or persistent complications.
- Changes in medication schedule required before and after dialysis.
- A work and activity schedule as physical capabilities permit.

An example of a teaching care plan for the person receiving hemodialysis is illustrated in Box 40-7.

The teaching requirements for the patient undergoing peritoneal dialysis are consistent with the teaching plan for hemodialysis. However, the patient will need to be instructed in the specific details of the process of peritoneal dialysis. If the patient is to undergo continuous ambulatory dialysis, training should be accomplished in a home-training center that is equipped to assist the patient in dealing with home care.

The teaching plan should include:

Patient Teaching
The Patient With Chronic Kidney Failure

1. Relationships between symptoms and their causes
2. Relationships among diet, fluid restriction, medication, and blood chemistry values
3. Preventive health care measures: oral hygiene, prevention of infection, avoidance of bleeding
4. Dietary regimen, including fluid restrictions
   a. Prescribed sodium, potassium, phosphorus, and protein restrictions
   b. Label reading and identifying nutritional content of foods
   c. Use of small, frequent feedings to maintain nutrient intake when anorexic or nauseated
   d. Fluid prescription and sources of fluid in diet
   e. Avoidance of salt substitutes containing potassium
5. Monitoring for fluid excess
   a. Accurate measurement and recording of intake and output
   b. Monitoring for weight gain and edema
6. Medications
   a. Actions, doses, purpose, and side effects of prescribed medications
   b. Avoidance of over-the-counter drugs, especially aspirin, cold medications, and nonsteroidal antiinflammatory drugs
7. Measures to control pruritus
8. Planning for follow-up health care
   a. Symptoms requiring immediate medical attention: changes in urine output, edema, weight gain, dyspnea, infection, increased symptoms of uremia
   b. Need for continual medical follow-up

- The process of dialysis and how the dialysis relates to the patient's body needs.
- Signs and symptoms of infection of the peritoneal cavity or catheter site and where to obtain care if these occur.
- Appropriate care of the permanent peritoneal catheter.
- Common side effects of treatment, means of controlling mild symptoms, and means of obtaining medical attention for severe or persistent complications.
- Changes in medication schedule required before and after dialysis.

BOX 40-7 Example of a Teaching Plan for the Patient Undergoing Hemodialysis

Date	Hour	Teaching/learning	RN signature
		Chronic kidney failure being treated by hemodialysis	
Start	Stop	Plan	
		1. Introduce patient to hemodialysis unit using available printed material and a visit to unit when appropriate.	
		2. Explain normal kidney function.	
		3. Explain kidney failure specific to patient's pathophysiology:	
		a. Types	
		b. Causes	
		4. Explain and reinforce medication regimen:	
		a. Purpose of each prescribed medication	
		b. Common side effects	
		c. Dose and times of each medication	
		d. Prescription filling procedure	
		5. Reinforce dietary instruction:	
		a. Protein	
		b. Potassium	
		c. Sodium	
		d. Fluids	
		e. Calories	
		6. Instruct patient about need for and care of vascular access:	
		a. Procedure for assessing presence of thrill and bruit; who to notify if thrill or bruit is absent	
		b. Guarding against constriction of fistula, that is, sleeping on arm or wearing tight clothing	
		c. Hygiene and removing dressing after dialysis	
		d. Signs and symptoms of infection, that is, redness, swelling, or tenderness	
		e. Measures to control hemorrhage if it develops while away from dialysis unit	
		7. Instruct patient about process of hemodialysis:	
		a. Explain principles of dialysis in sufficient detail for learning level of patient.	
		b. Describe hemodialysis in full detail to patient.	
		c. Explain common sights and sounds of dialysis unit to patient.	
		d. Describe common complications of hemodialysis to patient as well as usual treatments:	
		(1) Hypotension	
		(2) Nausea	
		(3) Vomiting	
		(4) Cramping	
		8. Instruct patient in interpretation of laboratory data and effects of hemodialysis, diet, and medications on these values.	
		9. Introduce patient to alternative modes of treatment of end-stage renal disease:	
		a. Free-standing hemodialysis centers	
		b. Self-dialysis (home)	
		c. Peritoneal dialysis	
		d. Transplantation	

Continued

BOX 40-7 Example of a Teaching Plan for the Patient Undergoing Hemodialysis—cont'd

Date		Status of Problems at Discharge
Date		**Patient knowledge**
Date		**Follow-up plan**

RN signature ____________

- A work and activity schedule as physical capabilities permit.

Health Promotion/Prevention

Primary Prevention. Obstruction and infection of the urinary tract and hypertensive disease are common and often asymptomatic causes of kidney damage and failure. A significant reduction in the incidence of CKF can be effected through increasing attention to general health promotion. Yearly physical examinations in which blood pressure is measured, urinalysis is performed, and the person is questioned about dysuria or urinary tract pain assist in early detection of diseases that may lead to CKF. Meticulous blood glucose control in diabetic persons is critical to reducing kidney failure.

Secondary Prevention. General health maintenance can reduce the number of individuals who progress from kidney insufficiency to frank kidney failure. The aim of care is to adequately treat medical problems and closely supervise the person's health status in times of stress (e.g., infection or pregnancy).

Healthy People 2010. Healthy People 2010 has targeted chronic kidney disease as a focus area for specific improvement and several objectives have been developed. These objectives include reduction of the rate of new cases of ESRD, reduction of the death from cardiovascular disease in persons with CKF, and reduction of kidney failure resulting from diabetes. Other focus goals include increasing the proportion of treated patients with CKF who have received counseling on nutrition, treatment choices, and cardiovascular care 12 months before the start of renal replacement therapy from 45% to 60%; increasing the proportion of new hemodialysis patients who use arteriovenous fistula as the primary mode of vascular access from 29% to 50%; increasing the proportion of dialysis patients registered on the waiting list for transplantation from 20% to 66%; and increasing the proportion of patients with treated CKF who receive a transplant within 3 years of registration on the waiting list.[23]

Kidney Disease Outcomes Quality Initiative (K/DOQI). Although there have been significant improvements in dialysis technology, many opportunities for further improvement remain. The publication of the National Kidney Foundation-Dialysis Outcomes Quality Initiative (DOQI) Clinical Practice Guidelines in 1997 represented the first comprehensive effort to give evidence-based guidance to clinical care teams. These guidelines were developed to decrease variations in practice in more than 3100 dialysis facilities in the United States and to develop concrete plans to positively affect the quality of life for dialysis patients.

The initial four areas covered by the guidelines included hemodialysis adequacy, peritoneal dialysis adequacy, management of vascular access, and management of anemia. Each recommendation in the guidelines is accompanied by a rationale, enabling dialysis caregivers to make informed decisions about the proper care plan for each individual patient.

In 2000 these guidelines were revised and updated. Revisions included expanding the DOQI to encompass the spectrum of chronic kidney disease well before the need for dialysis. By prevention and early intervention, the need for dialysis may be delayed or avoided completely, and outcomes improved for patients with ESRD. To reflect this expansion, the initiative has become known as the Kidney Disease Outcomes Quality Initiative.[15]

EVALUATION

To evaluate the effectiveness of nursing interventions, compare patient behaviors with those stated in the expected patient outcomes. Achievement of outcomes is successful if the patient with CKF:

1. Is free of respiratory distress, peripheral edema, hypertension, or other signs of fluid and electrolyte imbalance.
2. Correctly explains dietary plan, including fluid, protein, potassium, and sodium restrictions.
3. Shows no signs of infection; skin remains intact.
4. Is free from injury.
5. Affirms feeling more rested and less fatigued.
6. States that no muscle cramping or itching is present.

7. Demonstrates effective coping and ability to perform ADL and desired activities independently.
8. States satisfaction with life and self.
9. Correctly describes nature of illness, treatment regimen, and plans for follow-up care.

GERONTOLOGIC CONSIDERATIONS

The elderly patient with ESRD is more likely to develop complications as a result of age-related stressors placed on the kidneys. The GFR decreases 10% every 10 years after the age of 50 years. The elderly patient is more likely to experience kidney insufficiency, predominantly related to atherosclerosis. Older adults often have multiple risk factors such as diabetes and hypertension, which increase the risk of kidney failure. Once faced with ESRD, all persons, particularly older adults, need to consider their overall health when choosing a treatment option.

The patient's home environment and resources must be evaluated to determine the best treatment options. Obstacles for elderly patients may be lack of transportation to a dialysis center. Lack of motor skills or a chronic illness such as osteoarthritis may prohibit elderly patients from performing home dialysis.

Options for the elderly patient include home health care or extended-care facilities. Agencies such as Help on Wheels offer transportation for patients free of charge to and from dialysis treatments. Complications are also more common among the elderly population.

SPECIAL ENVIRONMENTS FOR CARE

Critical Care Management

The patient with ESRD requires critical care management if severe complications develop from the disease or therapy for kidney failure. Treatment depends on clinical manifestations, and the patient may require ventilatory and circulatory support.

Community-Based Care

The home environment is a key issue when evaluating the feasibility of home care for the person with kidney failure. Home peritoneal dialysis requires space and can turn a home into a hospital clinic.

Safety and cleanliness must be of top priority. Patients receiving CAPD need to have dialysis equipment readily available. The cycler is currently being used in home CAPD. The cycler requires little hands-on manipulation and allows for dialysis to take place continuously during the night, which permits freedom from dialysis during the day. Because of the increased amount of equipment, the patient requires additional teaching about the use of the cycler, including troubleshooting guidelines. Home management of dialysis can be a strain on families and requires a high degree of commitment.

Hospice Care

Approximately 15% to 20% of dialysis patients voluntarily choose to discontinue dialysis.[9] Because patient autonomy in the United States is the overriding legal imperative to accepting treatment, patient wishes must be honored. If the burdens of a life with impaired quality are so great that continuation of therapy offers no benefit but only prolongs a miserable existence, then discontinuing dialysis is reasonable. This is not considered suicide by the major religious groups (Protestant, Catholic, Jewish, Muslim, and Buddhist). Patients are apprehensive about the process of dying; they fear pain and discomfort. Nurses can assure patients and families that death associated with complications of kidney failure, usually hyperkalemia, is generally quiet, peaceful, and without pain or discomfort. Hospice care is helpful for patients who wish to remain at home.

As the patient is dying, it is unreasonable to continue fluid and dietary restrictions. Many patients wish to enjoy favorite foods previously denied them; this wish should be honored. As the uremia progresses, patients will restrict their own intake. Fluid restriction may be maintained to assist patient comfort by decreasing the risk of pulmonary edema. The goals of nursing care are maintaining comfort and safety and providing the opportunity for patient and family to express their feelings and arrive at some degree of emotional comfort.

In providing physical comfort, frequent turning and repositioning are necessary to prevent skin excoriation and breakdown. Oral care is extremely important, because mouth sores, once developed, will not heal. Mineral oil is an acceptable protective lubricant for the alert patient; a water-soluble lubricant with a vegetable base (such as K-Y jelly) is preferable for the unresponsive patient. Hydrogen peroxide is helpful in removing blood from the mouth and nose. A vinegar mouthwash neutralizes the ammonia.

As death approaches and the patient's level of awareness and ability to control the environment decrease, it becomes the responsibility of the nursing staff to provide safety. (Chapter 42 describes the specific care required for the unconscious patient.)

Providing an opportunity for the patient and family to talk about their feelings is one of the more important aspects of nursing care. Thoughts concerning death and concern about treatments can produce considerable anxiety. The wishes of the patient and family regarding spiritual counseling should be determined. Through demonstrating interest in individual needs and providing comfort measures, the nurse can do much to help the patient and family through the process of dying. (For further information on loss, grief, and dying, see Chapter 6.)

COMPLICATIONS

Many of the complications of ESRD and its treatments have been discussed. Fluid and electrolyte imbalances, shock, sepsis, and bleeding have been described previously. Other complications include anemia, hypertension, hyperkalemia, congestive heart failure, pulmonary edema, pericarditis, atherosclerosis, peptic ulcer disease, osteodystrophy, peripheral neuropathy, and metabolic encephalopathy.

Treatment options for CKF place the patient at risk for developing other complications. Those treated with hemodialysis often require multiple hospital admissions for problems with vascular access devices.[21] Infection, clotting, and displacement lead to a need for additional surgical intervention, making proper care of these devices crucial.

The patient treated with CAPD is at risk for infection from improper technique, manipulation of the catheter, and from exit-site care of the dialysis catheter. Many patients have expressed concern over the need for education on proper site care.[4] Research does not support the effectiveness of a particular protocol over others. Peritonitis is an ever-present threat during peritoneal dialysis. Aseptic technique must be strictly maintained during insertion of the catheter and throughout the procedure. Care should be taken to avoid contaminating the solution or the tubing when dialysate solution is hung. Cultures of the dialysate fluid are performed routinely to rule out infection. The patient should be assessed for signs of peritonitis and be taught to recognize the symptoms at home. Signs of peritonitis include an elevated temperature, chills, abdominal pain or tenderness, nausea and vomiting, and cloudy outflow of solution. If these signs develop, the patient should contact the health care provider immediately.

Many drugs administered to dialysis patients are removed through the dialysis process. The nurse should be knowledgeable about each patient's medication regimen and set appropriate medication schedules for the dialysis patient.

Critical Thinking Questions

1. A 65-year-old man is seen at your clinic with complaints of voiding in small amounts and constant feelings of urgency despite having voided. He also complains of bouts of incontinence. His postvoid residual volume is 300 ml. Both BUN and creatinine levels are elevated. What are some risk factors that may contribute to this patient's problem? What diagnostic examinations might be ordered? He is admitted for kidney failure to a general medical unit. His blood pressure is stable. What nursing interventions are appropriate? What are treatment options?
2. A 50-year-old woman receiving CAPD enters the emergency room with complaints of severe abdominal pain and cramping. She is nauseated and febrile. Her CAPD catheter site is red and swollen. Her white blood cell count is elevated. What do you suspect her diagnosis to be? Will she receive her dialysis while she has these symptoms? If so, how will dialysis be accomplished?
3. A 39-year-old man is employed as an exterminator. He is admitted to the hospital for persistent flank pain and denies urinary frequency, urgency, or pain. He has had no recent illnesses or injuries except for a sore throat 3 weeks ago that subsided without treatment. His family history is positive for hypertension and diabetes. He is currently taking no medication. What risk factors does this patient have for developing disease?
4. A 57-year-old woman has a 10-year history of systemic lupus erythematosus. She has been treated intermittently with prednisone to control symptoms. Her disease has been slowly progressive but has not interfered with her ability to work. The patient is married with two adult daughters. She is 5 feet 4 inches tall and normally weighs 132 pounds. Does this patient have any significant risk factors for kidney failure? If so, what? Explain how lupus can affect her renal status.

References

1. Ateshkadi A: Principals of drug therapy in renal failure. In Greenberg A, editor: *Primer on kidney diseases,* ed 2, San Diego, 1998, Academic Press.
2. Blanford N: Renal transplantation: a case study of the ideal, *Crit Care Nurse* 13(1):40-55, 1993.
3. Brady HR, Brenner BM: Acute renal failure. In Fauci et al, editors: *Harrison's principles of internal medicine,* ed 14, New York, 1998, McGraw-Hill.
4. Chaing H, Liu H: An exploration of the factors influencing the needs for CAPD patient, an abstract *Nursing Res* 3(2):106-116, 1996.
5. Delmez J, Slatopolsky E: Renal osteodystrophy. In Brady HR, Wilcox CS, editors: *Therapy in nephrology and hypertension: a companion to Brenner's and Rector's the kidney,* Philadelphia, 1999, WB Saunders.
6. Denker DM, Brenner BM: Alterations in urinary function and electrolytes. In Fauci et al, editors: *Harrison's principles of internal medicine,* ed 14, New York, 1998, McGraw-Hill.
7. Eschbach JW: The anemia of chronic renal failure: pathophysiology and the effect of recombinant erythropoietin, *Kidney Int* 35:134-148, 1989.
8. Frasser D, Vinning M: Urologic nephrology. In Weiss RM, George N, O'Reilly PH editors: *Comprehensive urology,* London, 2001, Mosby International Ltd.
9. Foulks C: Ethical dilemmas in dialysis: to initiate or withdraw therapy. In Nissenson AR, Fine RN, editors: *Dialysis therapy,* St Louis, 1993, Mosby.
10. Jones CA et al: Serum creatinine levels in the US population: third National Health and Nutrition Examination Survey, *Am J Kidney Dis* 32:992-999, 1998.
11. Kamel K, Halperin M: Treatment of hypokalemia and hyperkalemia. In Brady HR, Wilcox CS, editors: *Therapy in nephrology and hypertension: a companion to Brenner's and Rector's the kidney,* Philadelphia, 1999, WB Saunders.
12. Kasiske BL, Keane WF: Laboratory assessment of renal disease: clearance, urinalysis and renal biopsy. In Brenner BM, editor: *Brenner and Rector's the kidney,* ed 6, Philadelphia, 2000, WB Saunders.
13. Kopple JD, Massry SG, editors: *Nutritional management of renal disease,* Baltimore, 1997, Williams & Wilkins.
14. Kutner NG, Zhang R, McClellan WM: Patient-reported quality of life early in dialysis treatment: effects associated with usual exercise activity, *Nephrol Nurs J* 27(4):357-367, 2000.
15. National Kidney Foundation: K/DOQI Clinical Practice Guidelines for Anemia of Chronic Kidney Disease, 2000, *Am J Kidney Dis* 37:S182-S238, 2001 (suppl 1).
16. National Kidney Foundation: K/DOQI Clinical Practice Guidelines for Hemodialysis Adequacy, 2000, *Am J Kidney Dis* 37:S5-S64, 2001 (suppl 1).
17. National Kidney Foundation: K/DOQI Clinical Practice Guidelines for Peritoneal Dialysis Adequacy, 2000, *Am J Kidney Dis* 37:S65-S136, 2001 (suppl 1).
18. National Kidney Foundation: K/DOQI Clinical Practice Guidelines for Vascular Access, 2000, *Am J Kidney Dis* 37(suppl 1):S137-S181, 2001.
19. Owen WF, Chertow G, Lazarus JM, Lowrie EG: The dose of hemodialysis: mortality responses by race and gender, *JAMA* 280:106, 1998.
20. Redden D, Szczech LA, Owen WF: Acute renal failure. In Rakel RE, Bope ET et al, editors: *Conn's current therapy,* Philadelphia, 2001, WB Saunders.
21. Stark J: Dialysis choice: turning the tide in acute renal failure, *Nursing 97* 27(2):41-46, 1997.

22. US Department of Health and Human Services: *Healthy People 2010: understanding and improving health,* Washington, DC, 2000, USDHHS.
23. US Renal Data System, USRDS 2000 Annual report: *Atlas of end-stage renal disease in the United States, National Institutes of Health, National Institute of Diabetes and Digestive and Kidney Diseases,* Bethesda, Md, 2000, USRDS.
24. Weiss G: Iron and anemia of chronic disease, *Kidney Int* 55(suppl):s12-s17, 1999 (suppl 69).
25. Wish JB, Weigel KA: Management of anemia in chronic kidney disease (predialysis) patients: nephrology nursing implications, *Nephrol Nurs J* 28(3):341-345, suppl, 2001.

http://www.mosby.com/MERLIN/medsurg_phipps

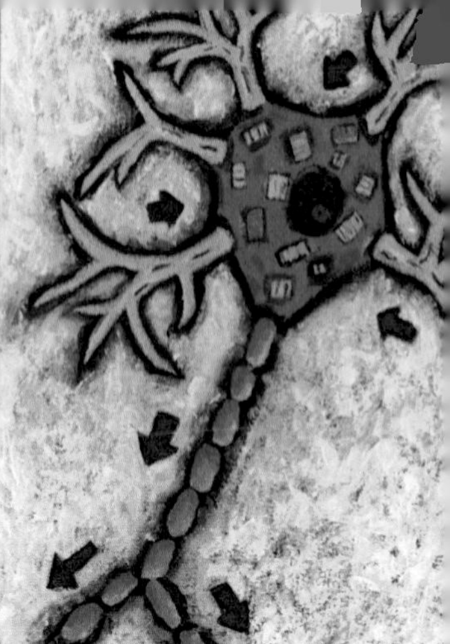

41 Assessment of the Nervous System

Shelley Yerger Huffstutler

Objectives

After studying this chapter, the learner should be able to:

1. State the four general functions of the nervous system.
2. Explain the normal anatomy and physiology of the nervous system.
3. Describe health history and physical examination data essential for assessment of the nervous system.
4. Analyze age-related physiologic changes that occur in the nervous system.
5. Explain the rationale for performing various diagnostic tests as a source of data collection in diagnosing neurologic diseases.
6. Describe the rationale for nursing interventions provided for patients experiencing various neurologic testing.

The ability to conduct an accurate neurologic assessment depends on the nurse's knowledge of neuroanatomy and neurophysiology along with skill in recognizing and interpreting subtle deviations from normal. This chapter contains an overview of neurologic anatomy and physiology, essential components of a neurologic assessment, and common neurologic diagnostic tests.

ANATOMY AND PHYSIOLOGY

The nervous system, like an electrical conduction system, coordinates and controls all activities of the body. It accomplishes this by means of four general functions:

1. Receiving stimuli or information from the internal and external environments over varied afferent, or sensory, pathways
2. Communicating information between distant parts of the body (periphery) and the central nervous system
3. Computing, or processing, information received at various reflex (spinal cord) and conscious (higher brain) levels to determine appropriate responses to existing situations
4. Transmitting information rapidly over varied efferent, or motor, pathways to effector organs for body action, control, or modification

Macroscopically the nervous system is divided into two major divisions: (1) the central nervous system (CNS) and (2) the peripheral nervous system (PNS). The CNS consists of the brain and spinal cord. The PNS includes the 12 pairs of cranial nerves, 31 pairs of spinal nerves, and the autonomic nervous system (ANS).

Neuron

The single neuron is the basic structural and functional unit of the nervous system. It shares all of the basic biologic and biochemical properties of other body cells and is highly specialized and differentiated. The single neuron acts as a miniature nervous system and has properties specialized for its electrical function.

Neuroglial cells serve as adjuncts to the neurons providing nourishment, support, and protection. They make up almost half of the microscopic structures of the brain and spinal cord. Four different types of neuroglial cells have been identified, each with different functions (Table 41-1). Neuroglial cells divide and multiply by mitosis and can be a source of tumors of the nervous system.

Microscopically the neuron consists of a cell body, or soma, and two extensions that project from it: a dendritic tree and an elongated cylindrical axon. The cell bodies are the primary components of the gray matter of the CNS. A cell membrane encloses the outer boundary of the soma, dendrites, and axon, thus separating the inside from the outside of the cell. This large surface area of cell membrane enables the neuron to receive a large number of synaptic contacts at one time (Figure 41-1). The axon is designed to transmit information along its extension away from the cell body to adjacent neurons; the dendrite or dendrites are designed to receive information from axon terminals at special sites called synapses and conduct impulses to the cell body. It should be noted that the word *axon* is used in various ways. It may be used to describe the extension of one cell or the extension of several cells making up a nerve. See Figure 41-2 for types of neurons.

Cell Membrane

Many of the most important functional properties of the neuron lie within the cell membrane itself. Structurally, the membrane is made up of lipids and proteins and has the ability to translocate materials across itself. The membrane exhibits differential permeability. For example, the membrane is permeable to oxygen, carbon dioxide, and certain inorganic ions, but impermeable to organic compounds (proteins) and other inorganic ions. This differential permeability results in a characteristic ion distribution. The inside of the neuron contains a high concentration of proteins and potassium (K^+), whereas the outside of the cell is high in sodium (Na^+). This unequal distribution, or gradient, of K^+ and Na^+ across the membrane is supported by the presence of an active sodium-potassium pump within the membrane. The pump requires metabolic energy for rapid movement of sodium and potassium across the membrane, and this produces an electrical potential difference, or charge, between the inside and the outside of the cell. The magnitude of the potential difference is a function of the ratio of charged particles on opposite sides of the membrane and is called the resting membrane potential (resting potential). Thus in the resting state all neurons possess a potential for action and are polarized. This resting potential is small, 260 mV, with the inside of the cell being electrically negative compared with the outside of the cell.

TABLE 41-1 Neuroglial Cells

Type of Cell	Function
Astrocyte	Maintain chemical environment for conduction and transmission of impulses
Ependyma	Produce cerebrospinal fluid
Microglia	Part of process of phagocytosis
Oligodendroglia	Produce lipid-protein complex that forms myelin

Excitability

The neuron also exhibits the property of "excitability," which means that the resting potential is unstable under certain conditions. For example, a neuronal membrane becomes unstable when subjected to stimulation, application of chemicals, or mechanical damage. This instability gives rise to the generation of action potentials (APs), which is a capacity unique to excitable cells. Action potentials transmit information within the nervous system and are, therefore, the basic phenomenon underlying all nervous system functions.

An AP occurs when a neuron is stimulated, resulting in a significant increase in membrane permeability to Na^+. Na^+

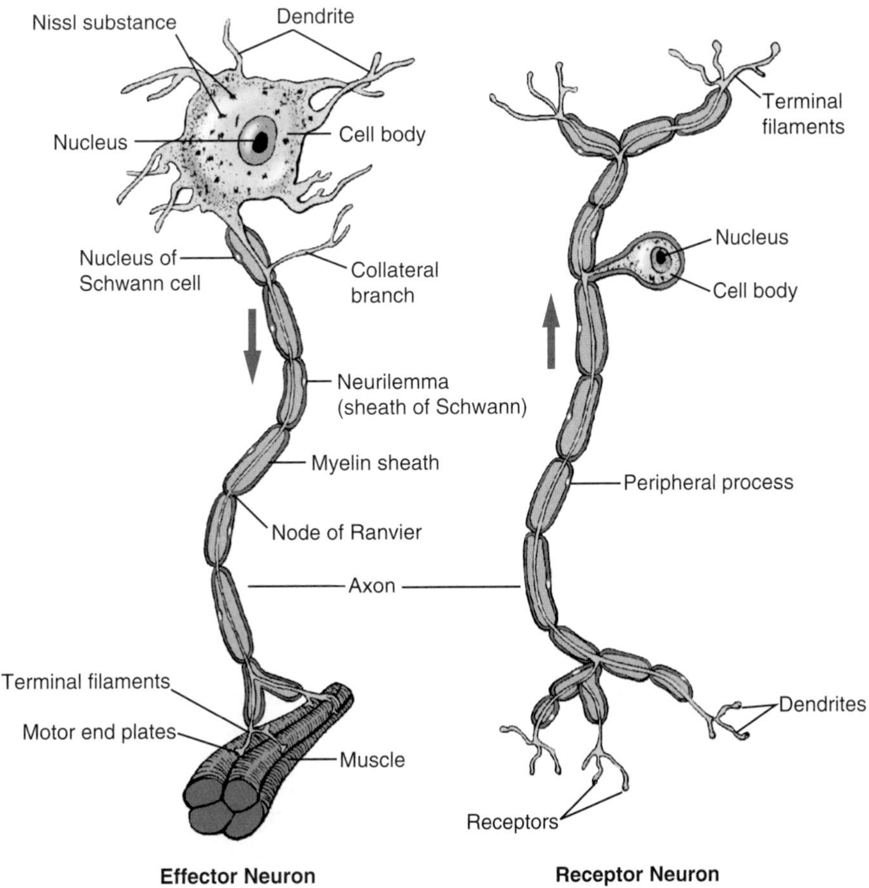

Figure 41-1 Diagram of a motor (effector) neuron and a sensory (receptor) neuron. Arrows indicate the direction of impulse conduction.

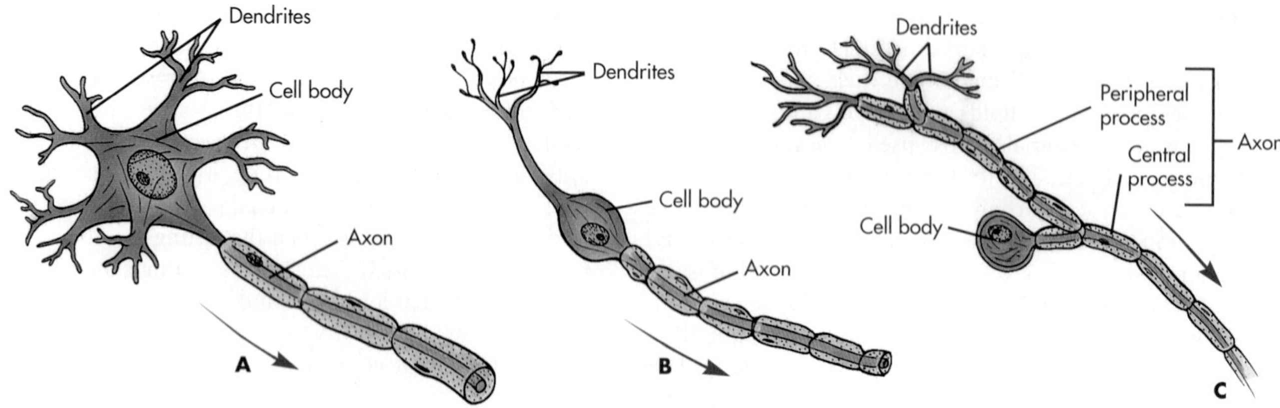

Figure 41-2 Structural classification of neurons. **A,** Multipolar neuron: neuron with multiple extensions from the cell body. **B,** Bipolar neuron: neuron with exactly two extensions from the cell body. **C,** Unipolar neuron: neuron with only one extension from the cell body. The central process is an axon; the peripheral process is a modified axon with branched dendrites at its extremity. The arrows show the direction of impulse travel.

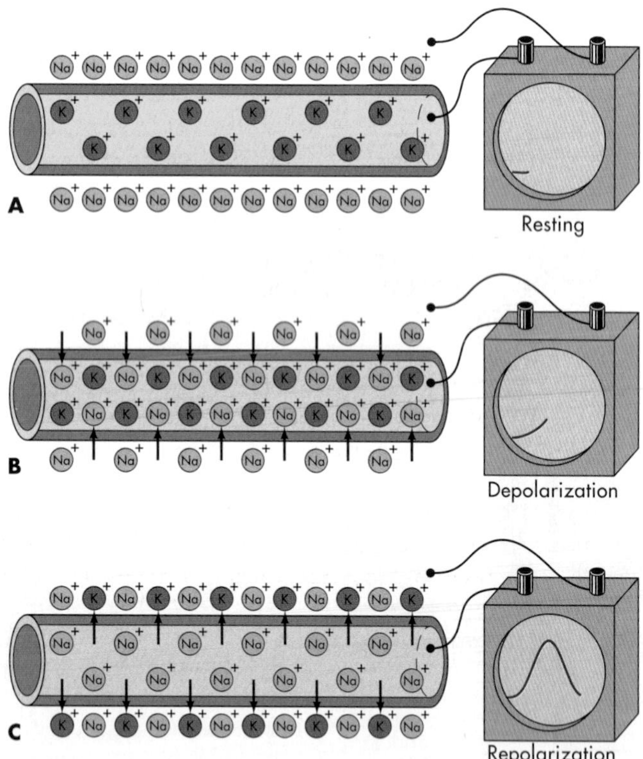

Figure 41-3 Depolarization and repolarization. **A,** Resting membrane potential (RMP) results from an excess of positive ions on the outer surface of the plasma membrane. More Na^+ ions are on the outside of the membrane than K^+ ions are on the inside of the membrane. **B,** Depolarization of a membrane occurs when Na^+ channels open, allowing Na^+ to move to an area of lower concentration (and more negative charge) *inside* the cell—reversing the polarity to an inside-positive state. **C,** Repolarization of a membrane occurs when K^+ channels then open, allowing K^+ to move to an area of lower concentration (and more negative charge) *outside* the cell—reversing the polarity back to an inside-negative state. Each voltmeter records the changing membrane potential as a red line.

quickly moves to the inside of the membrane through membrane pores or channels. These ions carry a sufficiently large positive charge to overwhelm the normal resting potential. A positive state develops within the cell and depolarization occurs (Figure 41-3).

Almost instantaneously the membrane pores return to being virtually impermeable to Na^+ while K^+ moves to the outside of the cell. Active transport then returns the Na^+ and K^+ back to their original state. These mechanisms result in the disappearance of the internal positive state and a return to the normal resting potential, a phase called repolarization. These two phases together form the AP. An entire AP occurs within 1 to 2 ms.

When an action potential is generated it proceeds automatically to completion, independent of the property of the stimulus that initiated the depolarization. In other words, a strong stimulus does not give rise to a larger AP; the AP proceeds to completion in an "all-or-none" fashion. The AP is also spread, or propagated, over the entire membrane without a decrease in its velocity. The propagation velocity is related to the size of the axon (the larger the diameter, the higher the velocity) and to the presence or absence of myelin.

Myelin

Myelin is an excellent insulator of axons and makes up the white matter of the CNS. The myelin sheath is deposited around the axons by Schwann cells, and this sheath may be as thick as the axon itself. Myelin prevents almost all ion flow across the axon and its membrane. However, at distances approximately 1 mm apart the sheath is interrupted by nodes of Ranvier. At these small, uninsulated areas, ions can flow easily between the extracellular fluid and the axon. The concept of conduction of nerve impulses from node of Ranvier to node of Ranvier is termed *saltatory conduction* (Figure 41-4).

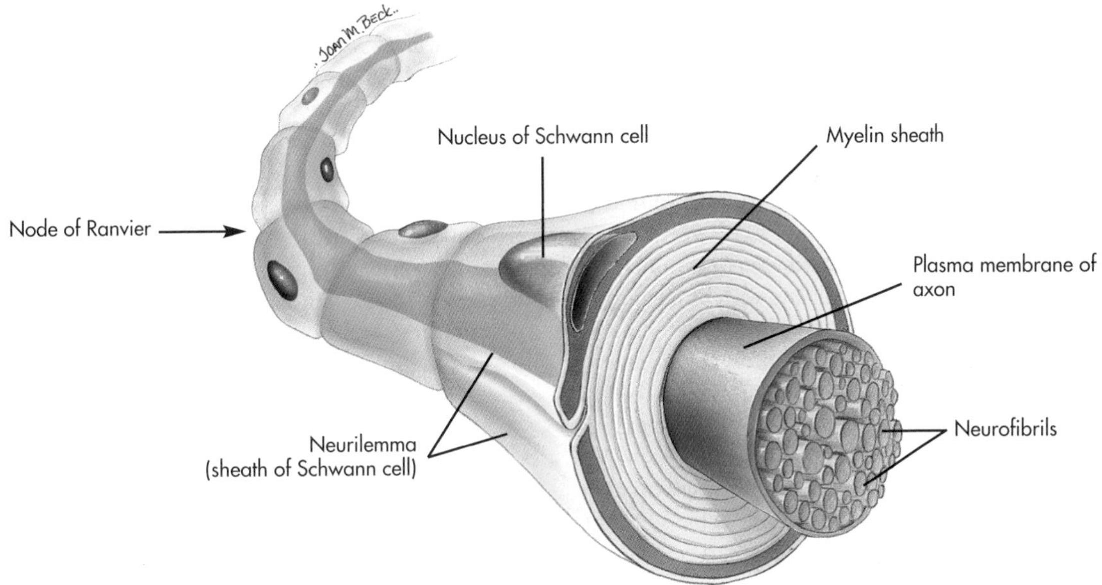

Figure 41-4 Diagram of a nerve fiber and its coverings. This myelinated axon is located outside the central nervous system. Myelin is produced in concentric layers by the Schwann cell. The neurilemma is the outer sheath of the Schwann cell and is indented by successive nodes of Ranvier.

The presence of myelin causes axons to be called large fibers; those without myelin are called small fibers. Large fibers have a greater conduction velocity because (1) the jumping effect allows depolarization to proceed quickly and (2) energy is conserved, because only the nodes depolarize. Large fibers appear white because of the myelin; the "white matter" of the nervous system is made up of myelinated fibers.

Many neuron APs originate in a receptor neuron where internal and external stimuli are normally received. A receptor is similar to a transducer in that it can change one form of energy into another form. A receptor, however, responds or depolarizes to only one type of stimulus. For example, the retina of the eye responds only to the stimulus of light. Therefore the receptor neuron may initiate depolarization but only in response to a specific stimulus. The receptor neuron obeys the all-or-none theory, although a strong stimulus makes the receptor neuron fire more action potentials per unit of time than does a weak stimulus.

Synapse

Neurons make functional contact with one another at specialized sites called synapses. Whenever an action potential is generated in a neuron synapse, a sequence of processes results in the action potential spreading to the second neuron. Transmission across a synapse is essentially a chemical process. The end of the axon contains a chemical substance located within its vesicles that is released when an AP reaches the vesicle. As the impulse travels down the axon, neurotransmitters are released at the terminal end and are taken up by the dendrites of the postsynaptic neuron. Excitatory neurotransmitters cause depolarization of the postsynaptic neuron.

Neuromuscular transmission occurs when the nerve impulse is transmitted from nerve to muscle at the neuromuscular junction. Acetylcholine is released as the nerve impulse travels down to the end of the axon. The acetylcholine travels across the synaptic cleft and binds with the postsynaptic receptor sites on the muscle. This increases permeability to sodium and potassium resulting in an action potential.

Synaptic transmission is both excitatory and inhibitory in nature. Inhibition means that the dendritic membrane becomes hyperpolarized because of the release of the specific neurotransmitter. The membrane potential shifts toward $K+$ equilibrium, thus stabilizing the membrane and taking the potential further from threshold. Each neuron acts only when its membrane is depolarized to threshold. Thus, a neuron fires based on the sum of excitatory and inhibitory inputs. Chemicals supporting excitatory transmission are acetylcholine, norepinephrine, dopamine, and serotonin. Those that inhibit transmission include gamma aminobutyric acid (GABA) in brain tissue and glycine in the spinal cord.

In summary, each single neuron contains all the structural and functional building elements of an electrical conduction system that also makes interconnections with adjacent neurons at synapses. Collectively, the neurons are organized into larger and larger units that serve to coordinate all the activities of the body.

Divisions of the Nervous System

Central Nervous System

The CNS is made up of collections of neurons and their connections organized within the brain and spinal cord. Specific areas of the brain and spinal cord can be distinguished where cell bodies are concentrated into nuclei, and groups of axons run in tracts that interconnect the parts. The connections determine the capabilities of each collection of neurons and are organized into circuits. Some circuits are simple and composed of relatively few neurons; others are highly complex. A single neuron may be a component of a number of different neuronal circuits and thus play a role in different functions.

Structurally the brain and spinal cord are continuous and are protectively housed within the skull and vertebral column. When injured, centrally located neuron cell bodies are unable to reproduce themselves. However, nerve endings can regenerate because of the presence of the neurolemma that covers all peripheral nerves and is believed to contain openings through which axonal regrowth occurs.

A blood-brain barrier exists in the nervous system that limits the free movement of substances from the blood to the brain tissue. The myelin sheath, as well as capillaries that have thickened basement membranes, slow the process of diffusion between the blood and the brain. The barrier is selective, allowing entry of fluid, gases, and small molecular substances, while preventing the entry of toxic substances, plasma proteins, and large molecules.

Meninges. The meninges are the coverings of the nervous tissue in the brain and spinal cord. The three coverings (dura mater, arachnoid, and pia mater) help support, protect, and nourish the brain and spinal cord (Figure 41-5). The outermost layer is the dura mater, a tough membrane consisting of two layers. This meningeal layer sends four processes deep into the cranium that form fibrous compartments for portions of the brain. These are the falx cerebri, the tentorium cerebelli, the falx cerebelli, and the diaphragm sellae.

The arachnoid, the delicate membrane lying beneath the dura, covers the brain more loosely. Projections called the arachnoid villi extend into the overlying dura. The pia mater, innermost of the meninges, is a vascular membrane having many small plexuses of blood vessels. The pia mater follows the course of the penetrating blood vessels as they dip into the substance of the brain. These three meningeal layers give rise to three potential spaces. The spaces are epidural, external to the dura; subdural, between the dura and arachnoid; and subarachnoid, between the arachnoid and pia mater.

These three meninges are also found in the spinal cord. The spinal cord arachnoid expands to surround the cauda equina; thus the subarachnoid space ends at S2 in the adult and is widest caudally. The spinal cord pia mater is thicker and less vascular than that of the cranium.

Brain. The brain (encephalon) is grossly divided rostrally to caudally into four main areas: the cerebrum, diencephalon (thalamus, hypothalamus), brainstem (midbrain, pons, and medulla), and cerebellum (Figure 41-6). Each area carries out unique functions.

Cerebrum. The cerebrum, or cerebral cortex, is composed of two frontal lobes, two parietal lobes, two temporal lobes, and two occipital lobes. Each cerebral lobe is named for its overlying cranial bones (Figure 41-7) and carries out one or more functions as listed in Table 41-2. The cerebral cortex is divided into right and left hemispheres, which have convoluted surfaces with many peaks, known as gyri (singular, gyrus), and valleys or indentations, known as sulci (sulcus). The hemispheres are connected at the bottom by the corpus callosum, a thick structure of nerve fibers that directly links corresponding areas of each hemisphere to one another.

Each of the hemispheres is further divided into the respective lobes by fissures or sulci. The frontal lobe is separated from the parietal lobe by the fissure of Rolando (also called the central sulcus) and from the temporal lobe by the sylvian fissure; the temporal lobe lies below the sylvian fissure. The parietooccipital fissure separates the frontal lobe from the occipital lobe.

The cortex of the cerebrum is approximately 0.25 inch thick. It controls more than 14 billion neurons, receives and analyzes all impulses, controls voluntary movement, and stores knowledge of all impulses received.

Speech is a function of the dominant hemisphere, which for all right-handed people and most left-handed people is the left side. The two identified speech centers are Broca's area and Wernicke's area (Figure 41-8). Broca's area is located in the lateral inferior portion of the frontal lobe adjacent to the motor cortex and its projections. This area appears to control verbal, expressive speech. Wernicke's area is located in the posterior

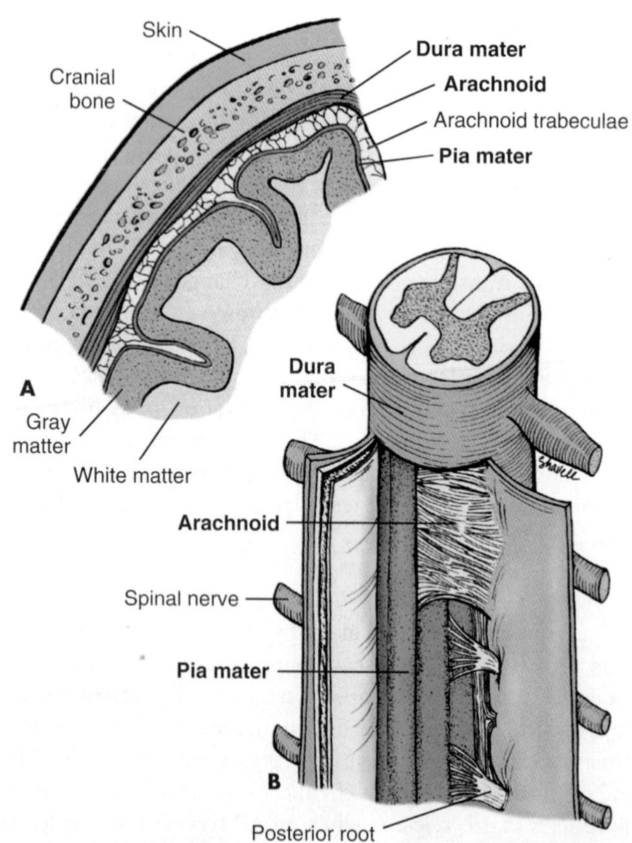

Figure 41-5 The three meninges, or membranes, that cover **A**, the brain and **B**, spinal cord. The dura mater is of leathery consistency and is the outermost of the three membranes. The arachnoid, which is loose, vascular, and like a spider web, is the middle membrane. The pia mater is thin, delicate, and closely adherent to the brain and spinal cord.

part of the superior temporal convolution and may extend to adjacent portions of the parietal lobe. This area is responsible for the reception and understanding of language. Other areas of the brain that are involved in speech include an area in the frontal lobe, which governs the ability to write, and an area in the occipital lobe, which governs the ability to understand written material (see Figure 41-8 for important cortical areas).

Deep within the cerebrum are structures called the basal ganglia. These masses of gray matter (cell bodies) include such structures as the caudate nucleus, putamen, and globus pallidus. In general, the basal ganglia function as part of the extrapyramidal system and are responsible for postural adjustments and gross volitional movements.

Diencephalon. The diencephalon consists of the hypothalamus, thalamus, subthalamus, and epithalamus. It surrounds and includes most of the third ventricle of the brain. The diencephalon often is called the interbrain because it lies directly beneath the cerebrum. The thalamus composes four fifths of the diencephalon and acts as a relay station for some sensory impulses while interpreting other sensory impulses. See Table 41-3 for a more detailed explanation of the structures and functions of the diencephalon.

Brainstem. The brainstem is located deep in the center of the hemispheres and is not visible when the intact brain is viewed. It includes a series of sections that make connections with the spinal cord at the level of the medulla, and it contains all nerve fibers passing from the hemispheres and the spinal cord. Twelve cranial nerves connect to the undersurface of the brain (Figure 41-9), mostly on the brainstem.

The brainstem is made up of several structures that include the midbrain, pons, and medulla oblongata. (See Table 41-3 for a more detailed explanation of the structures and functions of the brainstem.)

Of special importance is the core of tissue that extends throughout the entire brainstem called the reticular activating system (Figure 41-10). This interconnected network of cells

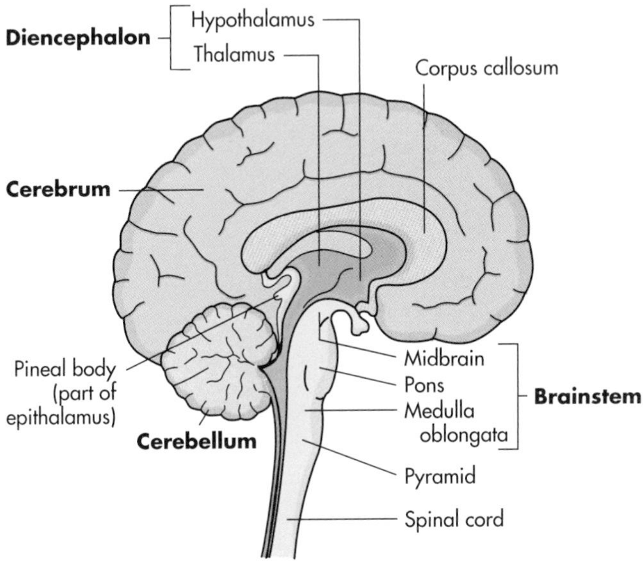

Figure 41-6 Major structures of the brain.

TABLE 41-2 Specific Functions of Cerebral Cortex

Lobe	Function
Frontal	Conceptualization Abstraction Motor ability Judgment formation Ability to write words
Parietal	Integrative and coordinating center for perception and interpretation of sensory information Ability to recognize body parts Left versus right
Temporal	Memory storage Integration of auditory stimuli
Occipital	Visual center Understanding of written material

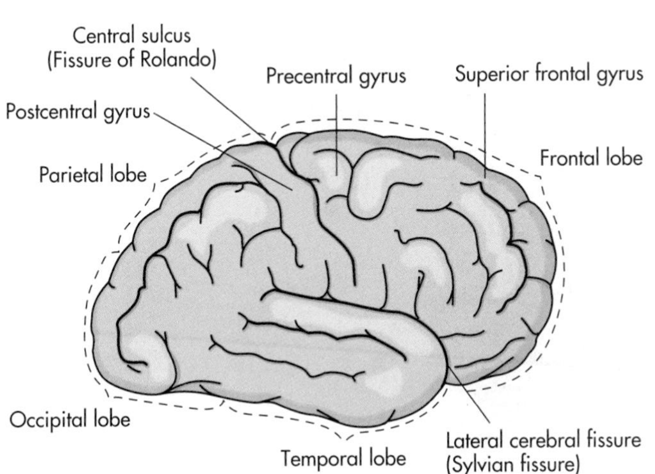

Figure 41-7 Lobes, sulci, and gyri of the brain.

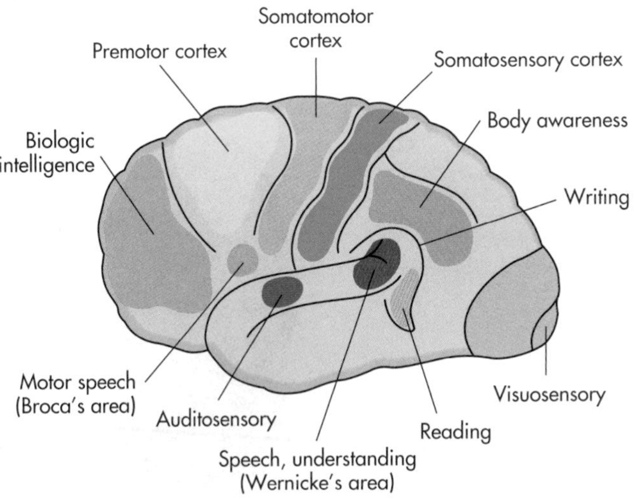

Figure 41-8 Lateral view of cerebral cortex with identification of major cortical areas.

TABLE 41-3 Diencephalon and Brainstem Structures and Functions

Structure	Function
Diencephalon	
Thalamus	All sensory fibers synapse for final relay to appropriate portion of sensory cortex General sensation perceived (meaning and locality imparted by cortex) Houses pain threshold
Epithalamus	Contains pineal body or epiphysis (thought to be endocrine gland whose secretion retards sexual development and growth)
Subthalamus	Receives fibers from globus pallidus, is part of efferent descending pathway
Hypothalamus	Contains cell bodies mediating most autonomic functions, endocrine functions, and emotional responses; regulates appetite, sexual arousal, sleep-wake cycle, and visceral-somatic activities; contains stalk of pituitary
Brainstem	
Midbrain	Relays impulses from cerebral cortex above and subcortical structures below Origin of righting and postural reflex located here
Pons	Connects medulla, midbrain, and cerebrum Contains pneumotaxic center—controls rhythmic quality of respirations
Medulla	Connects with central canal or spinal cord Vital centers of cardiac, respiratory, and vasomotor control, as well as swallowing and hiccoughing; gag and cough reflexes

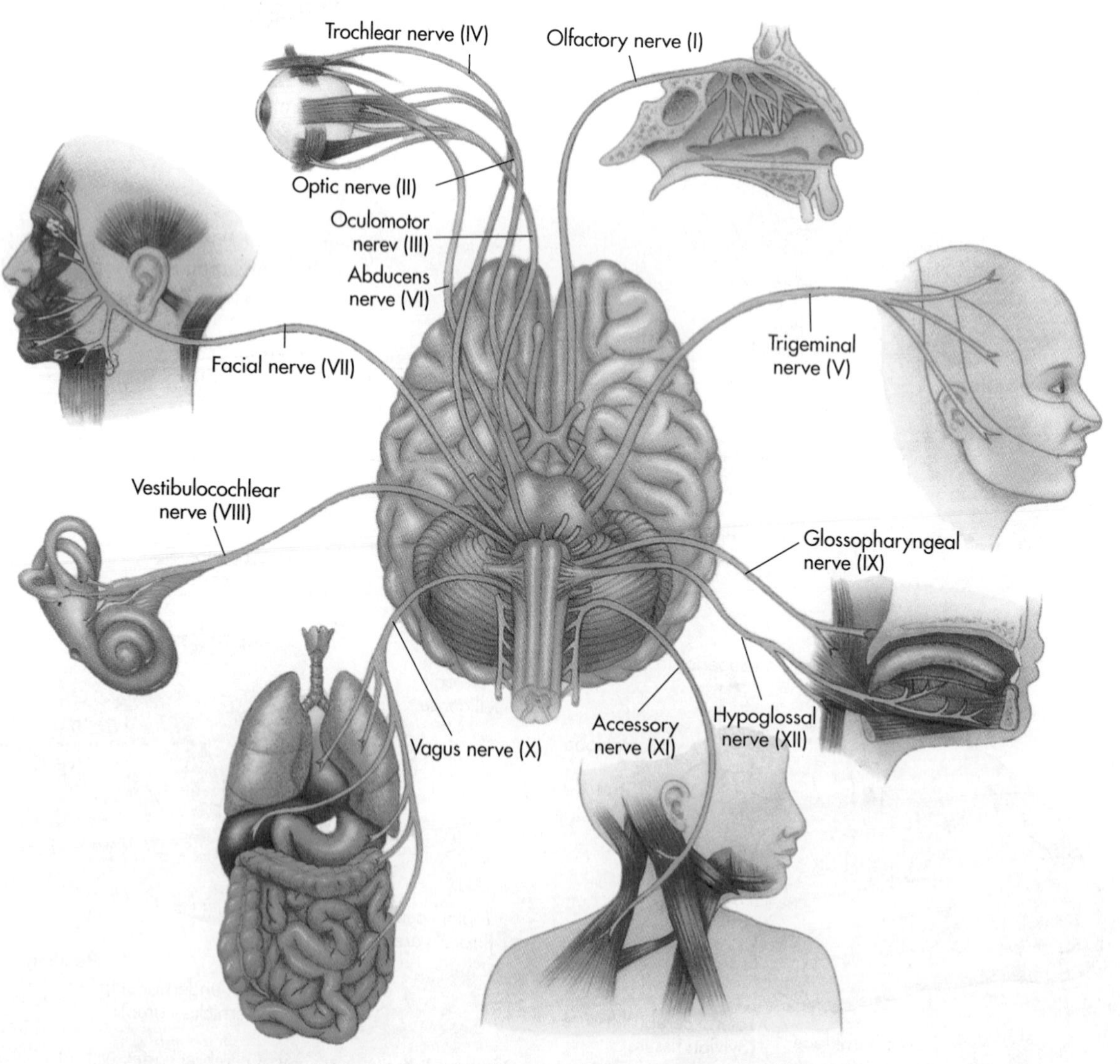

Figure 41-9 Cranial nerves. Ventral surface of the brain showing attachment of the cranial nerves.

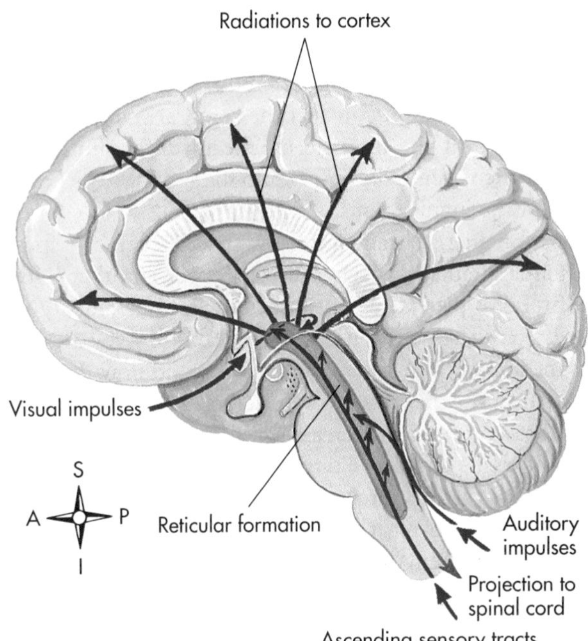

Figure 41-10 The reticular activating system consists of centers in the brainstem reticular formation plus fibers that conduct to the centers from below and fibers that conduct from the centers to widespread areas of the cerebral cortex. Functioning of the reticular activating system is essential for consciousness.

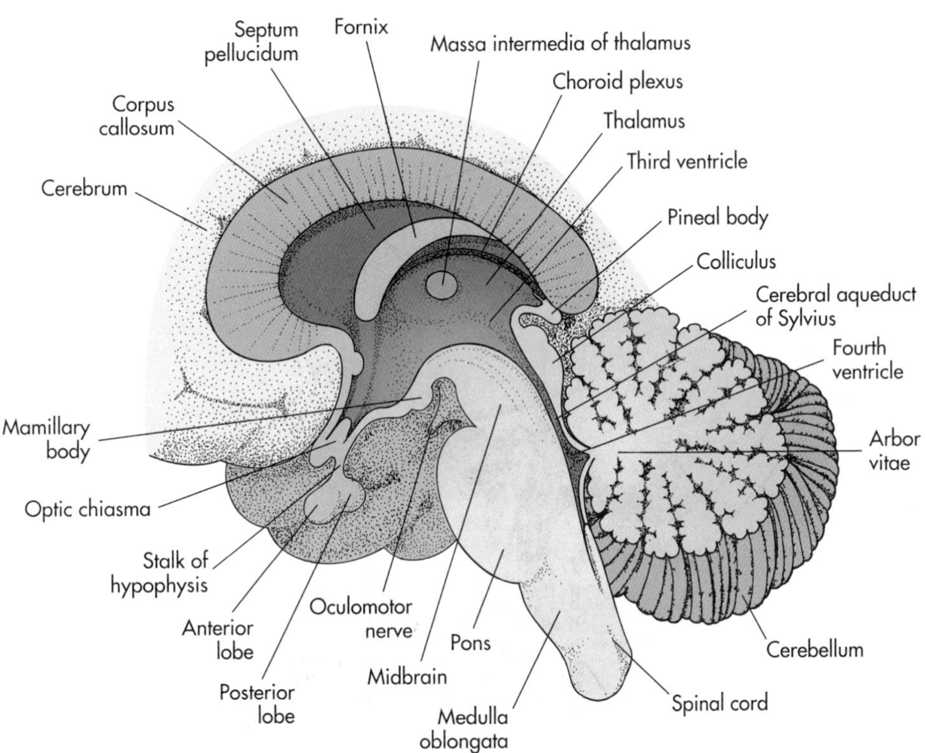

Figure 41-11 Sagittal section through midline of brain showing continuity of brain and spinal cord.

contains important integrating centers for respiration, cardiovascular function, afferent and motor systems, and state of consciousness. Increased stimulation leads to wakefulness, and decreased stimulation results in sleepiness.

Cerebellum. The cerebellum is located in the posterior cranial fossa, just below the posterior cerebrum, and contains short and long tracts. The short tracts act as connections between nuclei within the cerebellum; the long tracts enter and exit through three peduncles, the inferior, middle, and superior. The inferior peduncle connects the cerebellum with the medulla, the middle peduncle connects the cerebellum with the pons, and the superior peduncle connects the cerebellum with the midbrain (Figure 41-11).

The cerebellum has three main functions related to monitoring and making corrective adjustments of body movements:

1. Keeping the body oriented in space and maintaining truncal equilibrium
2. Controlling antigravity muscles
3. Checking or halting volitional movements

Circulation of the Brain and Spinal Cord. The blood supply for the brain derives from the aortic arch via the right innominate, left common carotid, and left subclavian arteries (Figure 41-12) and includes both conducting and penetrating vessels. The two conducting arteries are (1) the internal carotids, which supply most of the cerebral hemispheres, basal ganglia, and the upper two thirds of the diencephalon and (2) the vertebral arteries, which supply the brainstem, the lower one third of the diencephalon, the cerebellum, and the occipital lobes. These two systems anastomose at the circle of Willis, which is formed by the interconnection of the internal carotid, anterior cerebral, anterior communicating, and posterior communicating arteries as shown in Figure 41-13. The circle of Willis ensures equal circulation to both sides of the brain and helps compensate for alterations in blood flow and blood pressure. If blood flow via one side of the circle of Willis is inadequate, the other side supports blood flow to the area normally supplied by the damaged side (Figure 41-13). The parts of the brain supplied by each of these vessels are listed in Table 41-4.

The penetrating vessels enter the brain at right angles after branching off from the conducting vessels. These vessels supply nutrients to the neurons and brain tissue. The venous system of the brain is unique in that the cerebral veins have no valves. All veins of the brain terminate in dural sinuses or reservoirs, which eventually empty into the superior vena cava by means of the jugular veins.

Circulation in the brain possesses special characteristics. The systemic circulation favors the CNS over all other body parts. This helps provide a constant supply of nutrients (glucose and oxygen) to nervous tissue. The brain's vessels also possess the ability to maintain a constant blood flow through autoregulation. In the presence of increased blood pressure, cerebral vessels constrict, decreasing blood flow and preventing possible tissue damage. Conversely, in the presence of decreased blood pressure, cerebral vessels dilate to increase flow. Cerebral vessels also react to biochemical changes. Elevated carbon dioxide content causes notable vasodilation of cerebral vessels; hypoxia and elevated hydrogen ion concentration also cause vasodilation. These autoregulatory mechanisms become less responsive with increasing age and in the presence of arteriosclerosis.

The blood supply to the spinal cord comes from the spinal artery and two radicular arteries. The spinal artery arises from

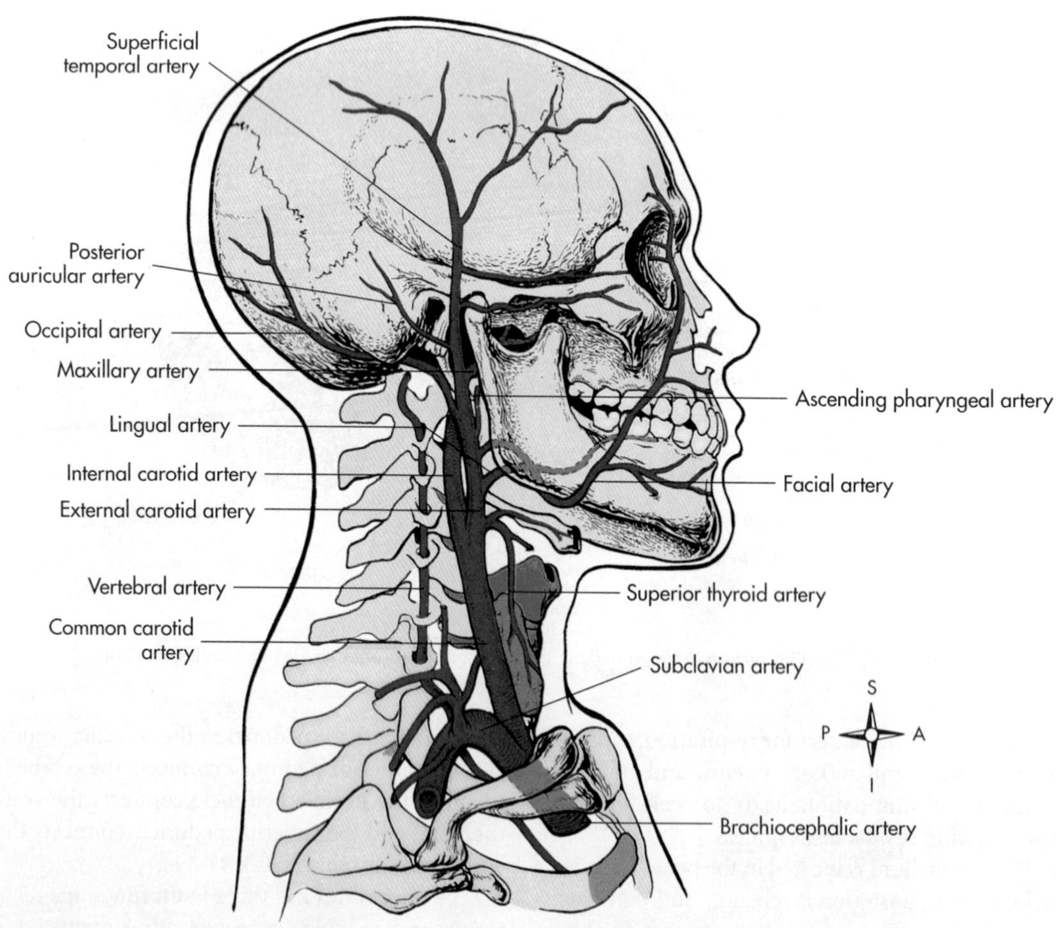

Figure 41-12 Major arteries of the head and neck.

the vertebral arteries, whereas the radicular arteries arise from the aorta.

Cerebrospinal Fluid. There are four fluid-filled spaces or ventricles in the brain. The two large lateral ventricles are located within each cerebral hemisphere. The third ventricle is a thin fluid pocket found below the lateral ventricles, and the small fourth ventricle is located where the cerebellum attaches to the back of the brainstem.

Cerebrospinal fluid (CSF) is a colorless, odorless fluid found in these ventricles as well as in the central canal of the spinal cord, and the subarachnoid space. The CSF serves four purposes. It acts as a fluid cushion for nervous tissue, supports the weight of the brain, carries nutrients to the brain, and removes metabolites. Normally, the total amount of CSF contained within the adult brain and spinal cord is 90 to 150 ml. Cerebrospinal fluid is continually formed by vessels of the choroid plexus at a rate of 18 ml/hr.

There is a constant circulation of CSF in the subarachnoid space around the brain and spinal cord. As the CSF returns to the brain, it is resorbed through the arachnoid villi and enters the venous system through the jugular veins to the superior vena cava (Figure 41-14).

Spinal Cord. The spinal cord is elliptical in shape and appears wider from side to side than from front to back. The spinal cord forms a continuous structure with the medulla oblongata extending 42 to 45 cm from the foramen magnum through the spinal foramina of the vertebral column to the upper border of the second lumbar vertebra. Cervical and lumbar enlargements are areas of nerve origin to the upper and lower limbs.

The spinal cord structurally includes H-shaped central gray matter (nerve cell bodies) surrounded by white matter that is divided into three columns or funiculi named according to their location (anterior [ventral], lateral, and posterior [dorsal] columns). Each column contains ascending and descending tracts that are described in more detail later in the chapter (Figure 41-15). These tracts connect different segments of the spinal cord to one another and connect the spinal cord with the brain. The names of the tracts usually indicate the point of origin by the first part of the name and the end point by the last part of the name (Table 41-5).

The spinal cord is also the site of reflex pathways. Reflexes are an example of the simplest neuronal circuit and do not require relay to the brain for action. A reflex consists of a

TABLE 41-4 Circulation of the Brain

Vessel	Part of Brain Supplied
Internal Carotid Arteries	
Anterior cerebral	Medial surface of the frontal and parietal lobes Basal ganglia Parts of the internal capsule and corpus callosum
Middle cerebral	Lateral surface of parietal, frontal, and temporal lobes Precentral (motor) gyri Postcentral (sensory) gyri
Vertebral Arteries	
Basilar	Brainstem Cerebellum
Posterior cerebral	Parts of temporal and occipital lobe Vestibular organs Cochlear apparatus

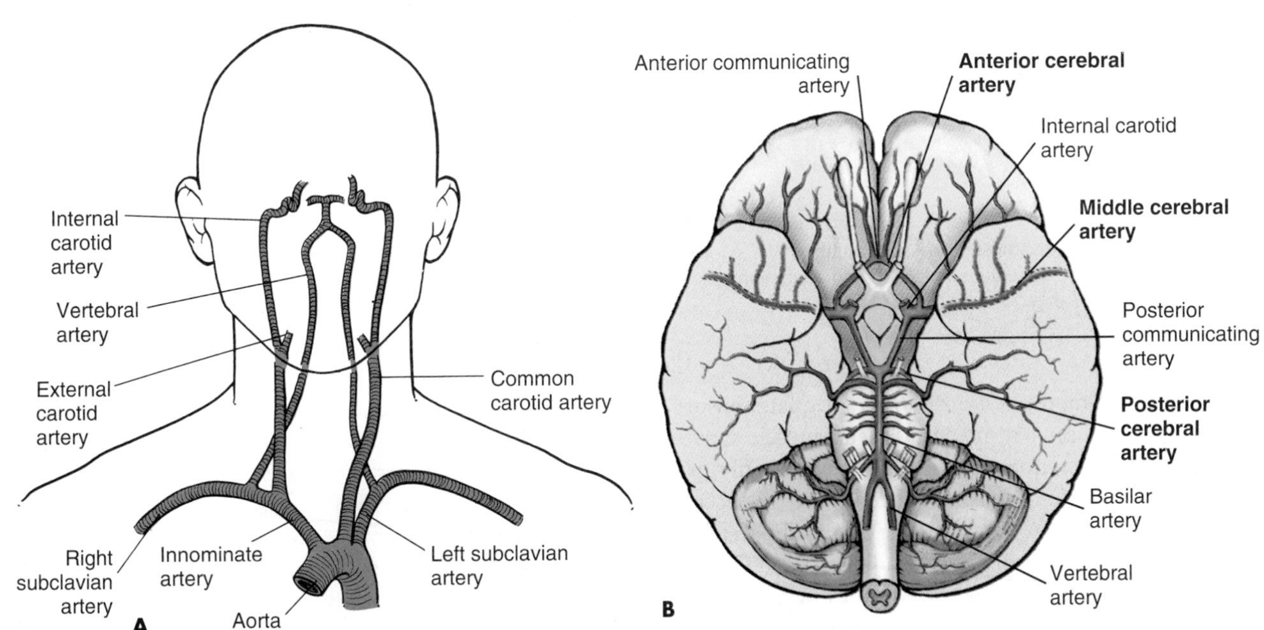

Figure 41-13 **A,** Major arteries supplying blood to the brain. **B,** The circle of Willis. Note the anterior, middle, and posterior cerebral arteries, which are the major pairs of arteries supplying the cerebrum.

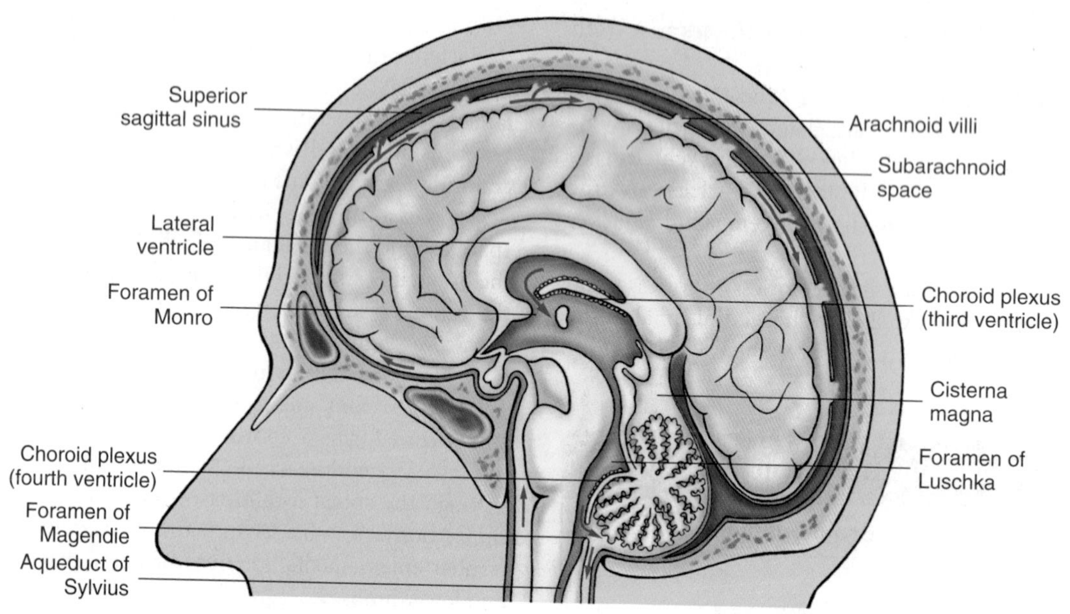

Figure 41-14 Cerebrospinal fluid circulation. Cerebrospinal fluid is produced by the choroid plexus in the lateral ventricles and flows around the brain and spinal cord until it reaches the arachnoid villi, from which it is absorbed into the venous circulation. Arrows indicate the major pathway of cerebrospinal fluid flow.

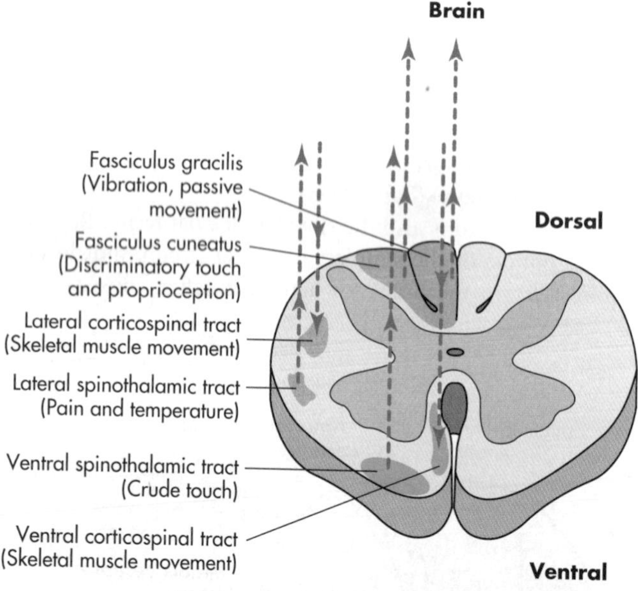

Figure 41-15 Nerve pathways arise from white matter of the spinal cord. Impulses travel to and from the spinal cord and brain along these pathways.

specific stereotyped motor response to an adequate sensory stimulus. The response may involve skeletal muscle movement or glandular secretion. A reflex may involve only two neurons as in the simple monosynaptic reflex arc that occurs with the knee-jerk reflex. A brisk tap over a partially stretched knee tendon stimulates sensory nerve endings within the tendons; subsequently, the stimulus travels over a sensory nerve fiber within a peripheral nerve toward the spinal cord where it synapses with a central motor neuron (anterior horn cell). The impulse is transmitted down the motor nerve (over the anterior nerve root of the spinal nerve or peripheral nerve) and across the neuromuscular junction to stimulate the muscle to contract. Figure 41-16 shows a reflex arc. A reflex may involve only one spinal cord level, as in the knee-jerk reflex; a few spinal cord levels (segmental reflexes); or structures in the brain that influence the spinal cord (supraspinal reflexes).

Peripheral Nervous System

The PNS is basically a set of communication channels located outside the CNS. Peripheral nerves are bundles of individual nerves that are sensory, motor, or mixed (having both sensory and motor fibers). Structurally, the PNS consists of 12 pairs of cranial nerves and 31 pairs of spinal nerves. The cranial nerves carry impulses to and from the brain. They originate mainly in the brainstem, except for the first nerve (olfactory), which arises in the olfactory bulb. (See Table 41-9, p. 1305, for an explanation of the functions of each cranial nerve.)

Spinal nerves are composed of a dorsal and ventral root. They correspond to the spinal cord segment from which they arise: 8 cervical, 12 thoracic, 5 lumbar, 5 sacral, and 1 coccygeal (the first pair of cervical spinal nerves come off the cord above C1). From L3 to S5, the spinal nerves branch out to form the cauda equina (Figure 41-17).

Peripheral nerves that transmit information toward the CNS are afferent, or sensory, in nature; peripheral nerves that transmit information away from the CNS are efferent, or motor, in nature. Peripherally the sensory and motor nerves usually travel together; however, they become separated centrally at the cord level into a posterior or sensory root and an anterior or motor root, respectively.

The PNS is divided into the somatic and autonomic nervous systems. The somatic nervous system innervates skeletal (striated) muscles. Its neuronal cell bodies lie in groups within

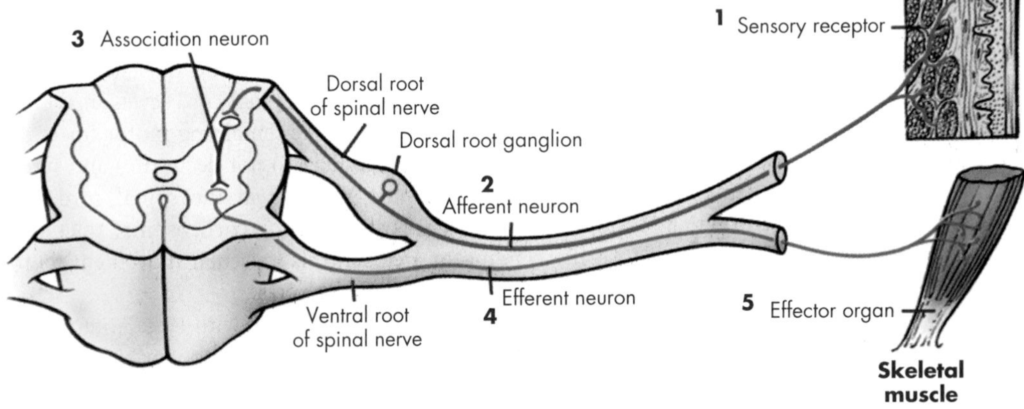

Figure 41-16 Basic diagram of a reflex arc, including the (1) sensory receptor, (2) afferent neuron, (3) association neuron, (4) efferent neuron, and (5) effector organ.

TABLE 41-5 Tracts of the Spinal Cord

Tract	Column	Direction	Function
Ventral corticospinal	Anterior	Descending	Voluntary motion
Vestibulospinal	Anterior	Descending	Balance reflex
Tectospinal	Anterior	Descending	Sight and vision reflex
Reticulospinal	Anterior	Descending	Muscle tone
Ventral spinothalamic	Anterior	Ascending	Light touch
Spinoolivary	Anterior	Ascending	Proprioception reflex
Lateral corticospinal	Lateral	Descending	Voluntary movements
Rubrospinal	Lateral	Descending	Synergy and muscle tone
Olivospinal	Lateral	Descending	Reflex
Dorsal spinocerebellar	Lateral	Ascending	Reflex proprioception
Ventral spinocerebellar	Lateral	Ascending	Reflex proprioception
Lateral spinothalamic	Lateral	Ascending	Pain and temperature
Spinotectal	Lateral	Ascending	Reflex
Fasciculus interfascicularis	Posterior	Descending	Integration and association
Septomarginal fascicularis	Posterior	Descending	Integration and association
Fasiculus gracilis	Posterior	Ascending	Vibration, passive movement, joint, and two-point movement
Fasiculus cuneatus	Posterior	Ascending	Vibration, passive movement, joint, and two-point movement

the CNS, and its axons exit the spinal cord at all levels. These fibers continue without synapse until they reach skeletal muscle cells. A small cleft exists between the nerve and the muscle. Vesicles containing acetylcholine are located at the end of the nerve terminal, and as the impulse moves down the nerve, the acetylcholine is released and crosses to the muscle, causing a muscle contraction. The muscle contraction is stopped by acetylcholinesterase, which is located in the muscle.

Sensory System Pathways. Sensation is initiated by stimulation of receptor neurons located throughout the body. Receptor neurons function to provide the brain with information about the condition and composition of both the internal environment (e.g., position [proprioception] and action [enteroception] of body parts) and the external environment (exteroception). The latter is achieved through the eyes, ears, nose, skin, and tongue. The general sensory system by which this information is conveyed includes (1) receptor neurons responsive to special stimuli from both the internal and external environments, (2) posterior roots of the peripheral or afferent sensory nerves carrying nerve impulses toward the central nervous system, (3) ascending or sensory tracts within the spinal cord and upper brain centers, and (4) sensory areas of the cerebral cortex where stimuli are perceived and localized.

From the receptor neuron, the sensory impulse travels to the spinal cord along the afferent fibers, enters the spinal cord through the posterior root, and proceeds along either the spinothalamic tracts or the posterior columns. The pathway followed is specific to the sensation. For example, nerve fibers conducting the sensations of pain and temperature pass into the posterior horn of the spinal cord, synapse with a secondary sensory neuron, cross immediately to the contralateral side of the cord, and continue upward as the lateral spinothalamic tract. These fibers arrive at the thalamus, synapse with a third sensory neuron, and terminate in the appropriate area of the sensory cortex.

Sensations for crude touch follow a similar pathway but ascend the spinal cord as the ventral spinothalamic tract. Impulses travel to the thalamus where they synapse with a third sensory neuron and terminate in the appropriate area of the sensory cortex. Sensations of fine touch, deep touch and pressure, vibration, and proprioception arrive at the spinal cord and are conducted by the posterior columns (fasciculus gracilis or fasciculus cuneatus) to the level of the medulla before synapsing with a second neuron, crossing over to the contralateral side, and continuing to the thalamus. At this location, they synapse with a third sensory neuron that terminates at the appropriate area of the sensory cortex (Figure 41-18).

Motor System Pathways. Motor impulses travel by one of three descending motor pathways. The pathways include the corticospinal (pyramidal) system, the extrapyramidal system, and the cerebellar system.

Corticospinal (Pyramidal) System. The corticospinal system is primarily concerned with skilled voluntary skeletal muscle movements of the distal extremities and, in particular, with the alpha and gamma motor neurons. Fibers that combine to form the corticospinal tracts arise from the upper motor neurons. Their cell bodies are located in the primary motor area of the cerebral cortex in the precentral gyrus of the frontal lobe and in the premotor cortex in the frontal lobe.

Motor fibers leave the cerebral cortex, descend through the internal capsule through the basilar portion of the pons, and then collect into discrete bundles within the medulla. The majority of the fibers cross over, or decussate, to the opposite side of the medulla and become the lateral corticospinal tract, which passes to all spinal cord levels in the lateral funiculus (Figure 41-19). The remaining motor fibers descend directly from the medulla (do not decussate) and synapse with alpha and gamma neurons in the spinal cord. This pathway is known as the anterior corticospinal tract. The left cerebral motor area controls muscular movement on the right side of the body and vice versa.

Motor fibers synapse with large anterior horn cells in the spinal cord. These cells are the lower motor neurons and are responsible for providing the final direct link or final common pathway with the muscles. Thus skeletal muscle activity is the result of the net influence of upper motor neurons on the alpha and gamma motor neurons through the anterior horn cells (lower motor neurons) in the spinal cord.

Extrapyramidal System. The extrapyramidal tracts are complex and provide separate pathways between the cortex, basal ganglia, brainstem, and spinal cord. Extrapyramidal (indicating that they do not pass through the medulla) tracts include all descending motor pathways other than the corticospinal tract. These tracts are named from point of origin to termination. The extrapyramidal tracts collectively assist in maintaining muscle tone and the control of gross automatic skeletal muscle movements. Some tracts facilitate extensor activity and inhibit flexor activity (lateral vestibulospinal tract

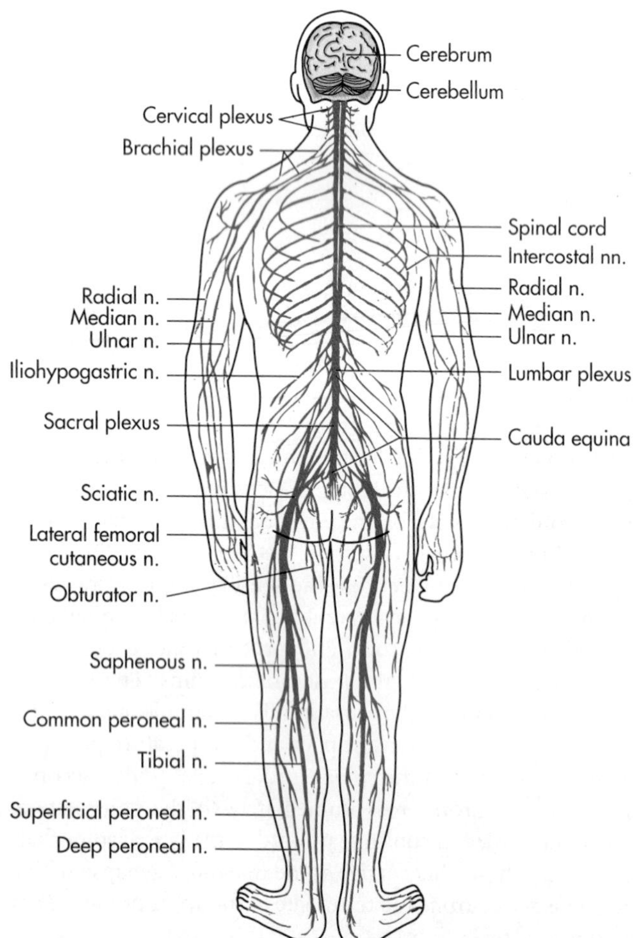

Figure 41-17 The central and peripheral divisions of the nervous system. The central nervous system consists of the brain and spinal cord. The peripheral nervous system is composed of the cranial and spinal nerves.

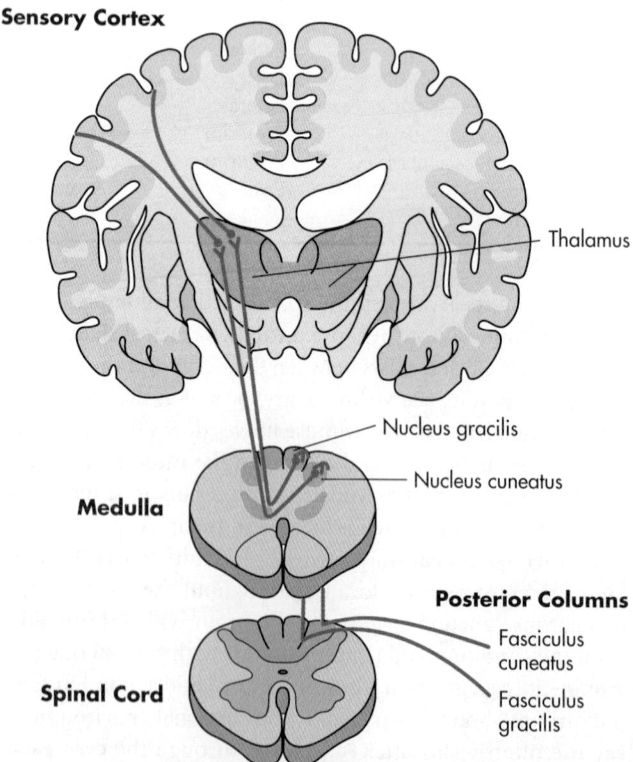

Figure 41-18 Pathways for fine touch, deep touch and pressure, vibration, and proprioception. Note how stimuli entering through the dorsal route (posterior) travel on the same side as posterior columns to the medulla where they cross to the opposite side, ascend to the thalamus, and end in the somasthetic area where perception occurs.

and pontine reticulospinal tract); others facilitate flexor activity and inhibit extensor activity (lateral corticospinal tract and rubrospinal tract).

Cerebellar System. The cerebellum coordinates the action of muscle groups and controls their contractions so that movements are performed smoothly and accurately. Voluntary movements can proceed without the cerebellum, but movements would be clumsy and uncoordinated (asynergia and cerebellar ataxia). The cerebellum receives tactile, auditory, and visual sensory stimuli and contains feedback circuits to all descending motor pathways. The functioning of the cerebellum allows nerve impulses to be returned to the same region from which they originated. The cerebellar cortex can detect any errors in muscle synergy and return the proper messages to adjust muscular control within the body.

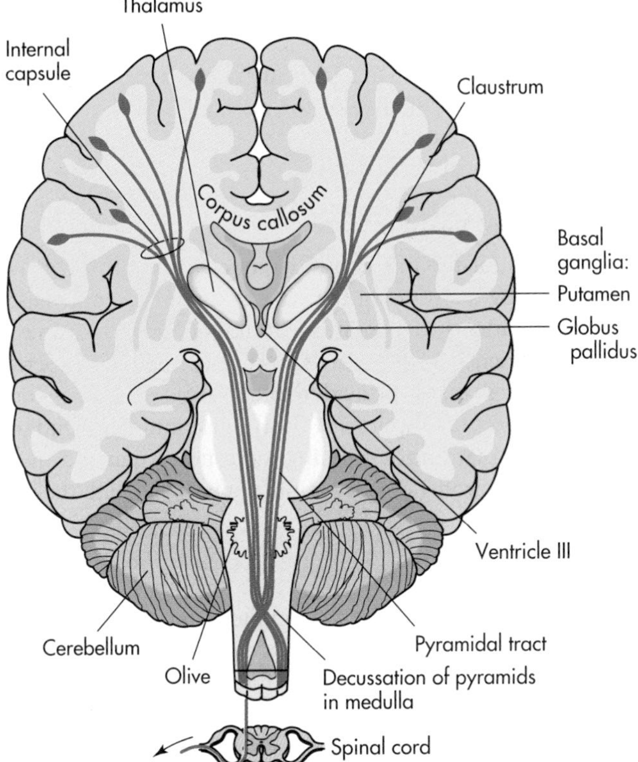

Figure 41-19 Crossed corticospinal (pyramidal) tracts. Axons that compose pyramidal tracts (corticospinal) come from neuron cell bodies in the cerebral cortex. After they descend through the internal capsule of the cerebrum and white matter of the brainstem, about three fourths of fibers decussate (cross over from one side to the other) in the medulla, as shown. Then they continue downward in the lateral corticospinal tract on the opposite side of cord. Each crossed corticospinal tract, therefore, conducts motor impulses from one side of the brain to interneurons or anterior horn motor neurons on the opposite side of the cord. Therefore impulses from one side of cerebrum cause movements of the opposite side of the body.

Visceral efferent motor pathways mediate the action of involuntary, or smooth, muscles located within the walls of tubes, hollow organs, the heart, and the glands. Most viscera are supplied by both excitatory and inhibitory fibers.

Effectors. Effectors may be considered as the cells of the body that "do something" by interacting with the internal and external environments and following the commands of the nervous system. The two classes of effectors are muscles and glands; both are transducers and capable of converting one form of energy into another. Effectors, like nerve tissue, are excitable tissues and are able to generate action potentials. The nervous system controls muscles and glands by directly turning them on or by altering their level of spontaneous activity through a neuron-to-effector chemical communication system.

Autonomic Nervous System. The autonomic nervous system regulates automatic body functions, usually in an effort to preserve homeostasis. Fibers of the autonomic nervous system synapse once after leaving the CNS and before arriving at the neuroeffector junction. The site of this synapse is called a ganglion, and its neurotransmitter is acetylcholine. The autonomic nervous system is further divided into the sympathetic nervous system (adrenergic), which functions to maintain homeostasis and to provide defense against stressors, and the parasympathetic nervous system (cholinergic), which is responsible for conserving and restoring vegetative functions (Table 41-6).

Fibers leaving the ganglia finally synapse at the effector organ. The neurotransmitter for the postganglionic synapse of the parasympathetic nervous system is acetylcholine; the neurotransmitter for the postganglionic synapse of the sympathetic nervous system is norepinephrine.

TABLE 41-6 Parasympathetic and Sympathetic Nervous System Influence

Organ System	Parasympathetic Influence	Sympathetic Influence
Heart	Decreases rate	Increases rate
Blood vessels	Dilates visceral and brain vessels	Constricts
Lungs	Constricts bronchi	Dilates bronchi
Gastrointestinal	Increases peristalsis	Decreases peristalsis
Gastric and salivary secretions	Increases	Decreases
Anal sphincter	Opens	Closes
Liver	Not applicable	Stimulates glycogen
Adrenal medulla	Not applicable	Stimulates production of epinephrine
Bladder	Contracts bladder	Relaxes bladder
	Opens sphincter	Closes sphincter
Eyes	Constricts pupil	Dilates pupil
	Accommodates for near vision	Accommodates for far vision
Skin	Not applicable	"Goose flesh"

Physiologic Changes With Aging

Changes in the nervous system occur with normal aging. However, it must be stressed that normal aging is not equated with senility or Alzheimer's disease. The healthy older person continues to function mentally at a high level into advanced age.

Changes in the nervous system associated with aging include the loss of brain cells with actual loss of brain weight. The nerve cell loss usually is diffuse and gradual. The gyri of the brain surface also atrophy, causing widening and deepening of the spaces between the gyri. Other changes include a decrease in blood flow to the brain. The ability of the brain to autoregulate its blood supply decreases with increased age.

The control of the autonomic nervous system over various functions of the body remains intact in the elderly but becomes more labile and unpredictable. In addition, the velocity of nerve impulses decreases, which slows sensory and motor conduction; sensory conduction decreases faster than motor. This change is more pronounced in peripheral nerves.

HEALTH HISTORY

Performing a nursing health history as part of a neurologic assessment is dependent on the condition of the patient and the urgency of the situation. The patient may be ambulatory, alert, and oriented, or may be experiencing an altered level of consciousness with neurologic deficits. The latter situation would necessitate that the nurse conduct the health history in phases over an extended time frame.[9] The interview not only provides a mechanism for gathering data or dispensing information but also serves as a tool for establishing a working relationship with both the patient and family. A patient and family history is explored along with the presence of classic neurologic symptoms such as headache, dizziness, vertigo, weakness, paresthesia, and pain.

Patient History

Patients often state that they are having difficulty performing usual activities but are unable to associate the change(s) with a neurologic disorder. The nurse always questions the patient about chronic diseases, use of both prescription and over-the-counter medications, and patterns of alcohol consumption, as these factors may contribute to the current problem and/or affect the patient's performance during the neurologic assessment. Important areas that are explored as part of the past medical history include previous trauma or injury to the CNS; diagnoses affecting the neuromuscular system such as strokes, seizures, multiple sclerosis, or Parkinson's disease; and neurosurgical procedures performed along with outcomes.

Family History

An accurate and thorough review of the patient's family history can help establish the diagnosis and affect the management of a patient experiencing a neurologic alteration. The patient is asked about relevant illnesses in the family. These include those of a neurologic origin, as well as diseases of other body systems that can affect neurologic status. Examples of the latter include hypertension, diabetes mellitus, renal disease, and peripheral vascular disease. Any history of a family member experiencing a stroke, seizure, CNS tumor, migraine headaches, and/or neuropathic disorders is thoroughly explored.

Headache

The nurse questions the patient about the occurrence of headaches that can be associated with a variety of conditions. Associated signs and symptoms such as nausea, vomiting, auras, tinnitus, lacrimation of the eyes, and vertigo are explored.[1] Transient headaches may occur after a diagnostic test such as a lumbar puncture.

Dizziness and Vertigo

It is essential for the nurse to differentiate between dizziness and vertigo by questioning the patient carefully about these symptoms. Patients who describe a feeling of light-headedness and/or experience a syncopal (fainting) episode are experiencing dizziness that is likely due to decreased cerebral blood flow. In contrast, descriptions of the room spinning around or the sensation that one is spinning indicates vertigo and may be related to neurologic dysfunction or a problem with the inner ear.

Weakness and Paresthesia

Any description of a sudden or gradual onset of weakness and/or paresthesia is also thoroughly explored. Weakness may be associated with a neuromuscular disorder such as myasthenia gravis or multiple sclerosis; however, the weakness may also be attributable to a nutritional deficiency or hematologic disorder such as an anemia. Paresthesias (abnormal sensations perceived as burning, tingling, prickling, etc.) may be associated with a diabetic neuropathy or other arterial insufficiency. The numbness and tingling may also be due to a PNS disorder such as a herniated disc or nerve impingement that can manifest itself in the upper or lower extremity.

Pain

Pain is a highly subjective symptom that nurses attempt to quantify using a pain scale of 0 to 10. Pain may be a symptom of a variety of disorders in other body systems such as angina, toothache, or a pleuritic-type pain. The pain could also indicate pressure on a sensory nerve such as with low back pain due to a trauma or injury. Individuals have different pain thresholds and nurses attempt to accurately record the pain experience from the patient's perspective[9] (see Chapter 12).

PHYSICAL EXAMINATION

The sequence of the neurologic examination varies with the examiner, but the nurse attempts to ensure completeness without exhausting the person being examined. The neurologic examination depends largely on inspection and palpation with occasional use of percussion. Auscultation may be used to detect related vascular abnormalities. Initially functions may be tested grossly, followed by definitive testing should an abnormality be identified. Equipment commonly used in a neurologic examination is listed in Box 41-1.

BOX 41-1 Equipment Needed to Perform a Neurologic Examination

- Cotton applicators
- Diagram of dermatomes
- Flashlight
- Miscellaneous items of varied shapes and sizes (coin, key, marble)
- Ophthalmoscope
- Otoscope
- Colored pencil
- Pins with sharp and blunt ends
- Printed page
- Reflex hammer
- Tape measure
- Tongue depressors
- Tuning fork
- Snellen chart
- Stoppered vials containing:
  - Peppermint, oil of cloves, coffee, soap (smell)
  - Sugar, salt, vinegar, quinine (taste)
  - Cold and hot water (temperature)
- Watch with second hand

Mental Status

Specific abnormalities of higher cerebral function are particularly significant in determining the presence of organic brain disease; therefore, clinical observation of mental function is important. Changes in level of consciousness (LOC) can be the most sensitive indicator of a person's level of neurologic function. The functional components of consciousness are arousal (alertness) and awareness (content) of self and environment. Arousal is mainly controlled by brainstem activity, including the reticular activating system (RAS). Awareness requires an intact cerebral cortex and association fibers. Thus the state of consciousness depends on the interactions between the brainstem and cerebral hemispheres.

Eye opening assesses arousal. A spontaneous opening of the eyes should occur when the examiner speaks to a person. A painful stimulus can be applied to determine whether the arousal mechanism is intact if eye opening does not occur with verbal and auditory stimuli (see p. 1304). Determining the patient's orientation to self and environment assesses awareness. Assessment of person, place, and time (day, month, year) is the most effective method to evaluate awareness.[5]

The assessment of mood and behavior is also included in a mental examination, because a particular mood may be associated with a specific disease. For example, emotional lability, where the mood shifts easily and quickly from one extreme to the other, often is seen in bilateral (diffuse) brain disease. The nurse determines whether the person's mood is appropriate to the topic of conversation. Personality changes with the appearance of violent temper and aggressive behavior may occur with destructive lesions of the inferior frontal parts of the limbic system. Family and friends can validate such behaviors.

The nurse tests the individual's knowledge and vocabulary by referring to current events. The ability to think abstractly may be tested by asking the person to explain the meaning of a proverb. The ability to serially subtract 7 from 100 tests calculation. Dyscalculia is the inability to solve simple problems. Recent memory loss is more common in brain disease than is remote memory loss. The findings of these gross tests may indicate the need for more definitive tests of mental function.

Language and Speech

Language ability is concentrated in a cortical field that includes parts of the temporal lobe, the temporoparietal-occipital junction, the frontal lobe of the dominant (usually the left) hemisphere, and the occipital lobe. Lesions in any of these areas produce some impairment of language ability.

To assess language and speech, it is important to distinguish between aphasia and dysarthria. Aphasia is the general term for impairment of language function; it represents a disorder of symbolic language. Dysarthria, on the other hand, causes indistinct word articulation or enunciation from interference with the peripheral speech mechanisms (e.g., the muscles of the tongue, palate, pharynx, or lips). Gross assessment of speech and language is made while the history is being taken.

Aphasia

Three different types of aphasia have been identified: (1) fluent, (2) nonfluent, and (3) global. Although one type often predominates, one or more of the other types is commonly present to some degree. See Table 41-7 for further information on the aphasias. Aphasic problems can be detected by assessing spontaneous speech and by asking the examinee to follow simple commands, written and oral; to read and interpret newspaper stories; or to write down thoughts.

Dysarthria

The nurse carefully assesses the person's ability to produce speech and observes for weakness or incoordination of the muscles used in articulating speech. Limitations may be observed during cranial nerve testing, particularly in cranial nerves V, VII, IX, X, and XII. Impairment of the motor component of these nerves may produce alterations in phonation, resonance, and articulation. The nurse asks the individual to produce different speech sounds to help localize the problem.

Dysarthrias are usually noticed during ordinary conversation or by having the person repeat a difficult phrase such as "Methodist Episcopal" or "third riding artillery brigade." Dysarthrias may be manifested by a single alteration or a variety of alterations, and there are characteristic changes that accompany particular diseases. For example, in cerebellar disease, speech is often thick with a prolongation of speech sounds occurring at intervals (scanning). In parkinsonism, speech is characterized by a decrease in loudness and a change in vocal emphasis patterns that makes sounds seem monotonous.

Perception

Sensation is integrated and interpreted in the sensory cortex, especially in the parietal lobe. It is important for the nurse to recognize perceptual problems, because they can be more difficult to deal with than changes in the patient's ability to move or sense. Disorders of perception commonly involve spatial-temporal relationships or the perception of self.

The ability to recognize objects through any of the special senses is known as gnosia. Lesions involving a specific association area of the cortex produce a specific type of agnosia (absence of this ability). One frequently tested ability is stereognosis, the ability to perceive an object's nature and form by touch. Asking the person to identify familiar objects that are placed in the hand one at a time with the eyes closed assesses stereognosis.

Apraxia is another common perceptual problem. This is the inability to perform skilled, purposeful movements in the absence of motor, sensory, or coordination losses. (See Table 41-8 for different types of apraxia.)

Sensory Status

Accurate assessment of sensory function depends on the person's cooperation, alertness, and responsiveness. The person should be relaxed and keep the eyes closed during all portions of the sensory examination to avoid receiving visual clues. Sensation is tested on both sides and distally to proximally.

Both superficial and deep sensation are tested on the trunk and extremities. Areas of sensory loss or abnormality are mapped out on a body diagram according to the distribution of the spinal dermatomes and peripheral nerves (Figure 41-17). A dermatome, or skin segment, may be thought of as the area of skin supplied by one dorsal root of a cutaneous nerve. An area in which sensation is absent (anesthesia) is differentiated from areas in which sensation is intensified (hyperesthesia) or lessened (hypesthesia or hypoesthesia). Paresthesia is an abnormal sensation that is perceived as burning, prickly, or itching.

Pain, Temperature, and Touch

The nurse assesses superficial pain perception by stimulating an area by pinprick and asking the person to report discomfort. Sharp and dull objects can be alternated for increased discrimination. Deep pain can be assessed by multi-

TABLE 41-7 Types of Aphasia

Type	Definition	Site of Lesion
Motor (Expressive)	Impairment of ability to speak and write; patient can understand written and spoken words	Insula and surrounding region, including Broca's motor area
Anomic	Inability to name objects, qualities, and conditions although speech is fluent	Area of angular gyrus
Fluent	Speech is well articulated and grammatically correct but is lacking in content and meaning	
Nonfluent	Problems in selecting, organizing, and initiating speech patterns May also affect writing	Motor cortex at Broca's area
Sensory (Receptive)	Impairment of ability to understand written or spoken language	Disease of auditory and visual word centers
Wernicke's	As above	Wernicke's area of left hemisphere
Mixed Aphasia	Combined expressive and receptive aphasia deficits	Damage to various speech and language areas
Global Aphasia	Total aphasia involving all functions that makes up speech and communication Few if any intact language skills	Severe damage to speech areas

TABLE 41-8 Apraxia

Type	Impairment Produced	Lesion Site
Constructional	Impairment in producing designs in two or three dimensions Involves copying, drawing, or constructing	Occipitoparietal lobe of either hemisphere
Dressing	Inability to dress oneself accurately Makes mistakes, as putting clothes on backwards, upside-down, inside-out, or putting both legs in the same pant leg	Occipital or parietal lobe usually in nondominant hemisphere
Motor	Loss of kinesthetic memory patterns, which results in patient's inability to perform a purposeful motor task although it is understood	Frontal lobe of either hemisphere, precentral gyrus
Idiomotor	Inability to imitate gestures or perform a purposeful motor task on command May be able to do task spontaneously	Parietal lobe of dominant hemisphere, supramarginal gyrus
Ideational	Inability to carry out activities automatically or on command because of inability to understand the concept of the act	Parietal lobe of dominant hemisphere or diffuse brain damage as in arteriosclerosis

ple means, some of which have the potential of causing tissue injury. It is necessary to assess deep pain only when the person has a decreased level of consciousness. Deep pain is assessed by applying pressure over the nail beds or supraorbitally. Pressure may also be applied over bony areas, such as the sternum. Figure 41-20 illustrates assessment of deep pain via nail bed pressure. Deep pain may also be elicited by squeezing the trapezius muscle. Pinching and pricking may damage tissues and are avoided whenever possible.

The nurse assesses crude touch by having the patient close his or her eyes and then touching an area with a cotton ball and requesting the person to indicate when the touch is felt. Temperature is assessed by touching areas of the body with warm to hot, and cool to cold, objects in a random fashion; the person states whenever a sensation is felt. Because pain and temperature sensations use the same nerve pathway (lateral spinothalamic), testing for temperature can be eliminated in the routine examination if the tests for pain perception are normal.[3]

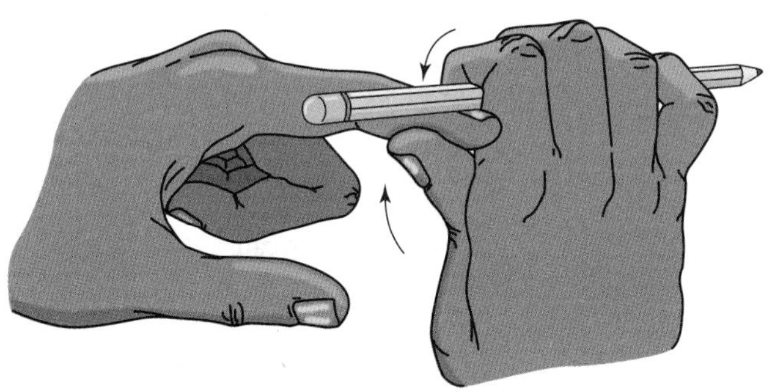

Figure 41-20 Nail bed pressure stimulation using pencil.

Motion and Position

Proprioceptive fibers (fasciculus gracilis and fasciculus cuneatus) transmit sensory impulses from muscles, tendons, ligaments, and joints. These impulses create an awareness of the position of one's limbs in space (kinesthetic sense). The nurse grasps the sides of the person's distal phalanx and moves it up and down to test proprioception. If proprioception is intact, the person reports correctly the direction in which the joint is being moved. Proprioceptive abilities can also be assessed by the Romberg test, in which the person is asked to stand erect with the feet together and eyes closed. A positive test occurs when the person loses balance; a positive test indicates the presence of a pathologic condition.

Vibration is assessed by placing the base of a low-frequency tuning fork on a distal bony prominence, such as the finger or toe, of one extremity at a time. The person indicates to the nurse when the vibration is initially felt and when it stops.

Cranial Nerves

The 12 cranial nerves are tested in either numbered sequence (Table 41-9). or by grouping cranial nerves with similar function, such as voluntary motor function, visceral motor function, and special sensory or general sensory functions. It is important to remember, however, that some cranial nerves have both motor and sensory functions.

TABLE 41-9 The Cranial Nerves and Their Functions

Cranial Nerves	Function
Olfactory (I)	Sensory: smell reception and interpretation
Optic (II)	Sensory: visual acuity and visual fields
Oculomotor (III)	Motor: raise eyelids, most extraocular movements Parasympathetic: pupillary constriction, change lens shape
Trochlear (IV)	Motor: downward, inward eye movement
Trigeminal (V)	Motor: jaw opening and clenching, chewing and mastication Sensory: sensation to cornea, iris, lacrimal glands, conjunctiva, eyelids, forehead, nose, nasal and mouth mucosa, teeth, tongue, ear, facial skin
Abducens (VI)	Motor: lateral eye movement
Facial (VII)	Motor: movement of facial expression muscles except jaw, close eyes, labial speech sounds (b, m, w, and rounded vowels) Sensory: taste—anterior two thirds of tongue, sensation to pharynx Parasympathetic: secretion of saliva and tears
Acoustic (VIII)	Sensory: hearing and equilibrium
Glossopharyngeal (IX)	Motor: voluntary muscles for swallowing and phonation Sensory: sensation of nasopharynx, gag reflex, taste—posterior one third of tongue Parasympathetic: secretion of salivary glands, carotid reflex
Vagus (X)	Motor: voluntary muscles of phonation (guttural speech sounds) and swallowing Sensory: sensation behind ear and part of external ear canal Parasympathetic: secretion of digestive enzymes; peristalsis; carotid reflex; involuntary action of heart, lungs, and digestive tract
Spinal accessory (XI)	Motor: turn head, shrug shoulders, some actions for phonation
Hypoglossal (XII)	Motor: tongue movement for speech sound articulation (l, t, n) and swallowing

From Seidel HM et al: *Mosby's guide to physical examination,* ed 4, St Louis, 1999, Mosby.

Cranial Nerve I (Olfactory)

The function of cranial nerve I is purely sensory, namely, smell. Special receptors located within the superior or uppermost part of each nasal chamber transmit neural impulses over the olfactory bulbs to the olfactory nerves in the area of the central cortex concerned with olfaction. When testing this cranial nerve the nurse asks if the patient smells an odor. If the answer is yes, the patient is asked to name the odor. Awareness of an odor must be differentiated from the ability to name a specific substance. Anosmia (absence of smell) or hyposmia (decreased sensitivity of the sense of smell) is often associated with complaints of lack of taste, even though tests may demonstrate that sense to be intact. Varied lesions involving any part of the olfactory pathways cause anosmia.

Cranial Nerve II (Optic)

The function of cranial nerve II is also purely sensory, (i.e., sight or vision). When the retina is stimulated, nerve impulses are transmitted over the optic nerves (extending from the optic disc to the chiasm), and the optic tracts with the radiations terminating in the visual cortex of the occipital lobes. As shown in Figure 41-21, the medial (nasal) fibers of each optic nerve cross at the chiasm to the opposite side of the brain, whereas the lateral (temporal) fibers remain uncrossed. Thus fibers of the left optic tract contain fibers from only the left half of each retina and carry impulses to the left occipital lobe; fibers of the right optic tract contain fibers from only the right half of each retina and carry impulses to the right occipital lobe. Optic nerve function is assessed in relation to visual acuity, visual fields, and the appearance of the fundus. Each eye is tested separately.

Visual Acuity. The cones of the retina mediate visual acuity. Reading newspaper print grossly tests central vision. Distance visual acuity is assessed through the use of the Snellen chart (see Chapter 57). Individuals with vision impairment are tested to determine light perception, hand movement, and finger count.

Visual Fields. Field of vision is defined as the range in which objects are visible when vision is fixed in one direction. The field of vision thus relates to peripheral vision, or indirect vision. Full visual fields depend on the intactness of all parts of the visual pathway of the eye. The visual fields are tested grossly by confrontation techniques where an object is moved into the periphery of each of the quadrants of the eye. The person is instructed to cover one eye, fix the other eye on a point straight ahead, and report when the moving object is first detected at the edge of each visual field. The nurse's finger may be used as the moving object. Visual fields may be altered in a variety of CNS diseases, such as neoplasia and vascular disease. Glaucoma is a major cause. Damage to one optic nerve anterior to the chiasm affects only the field of the involved eye. Lesions at the chiasm or posterior to it produce

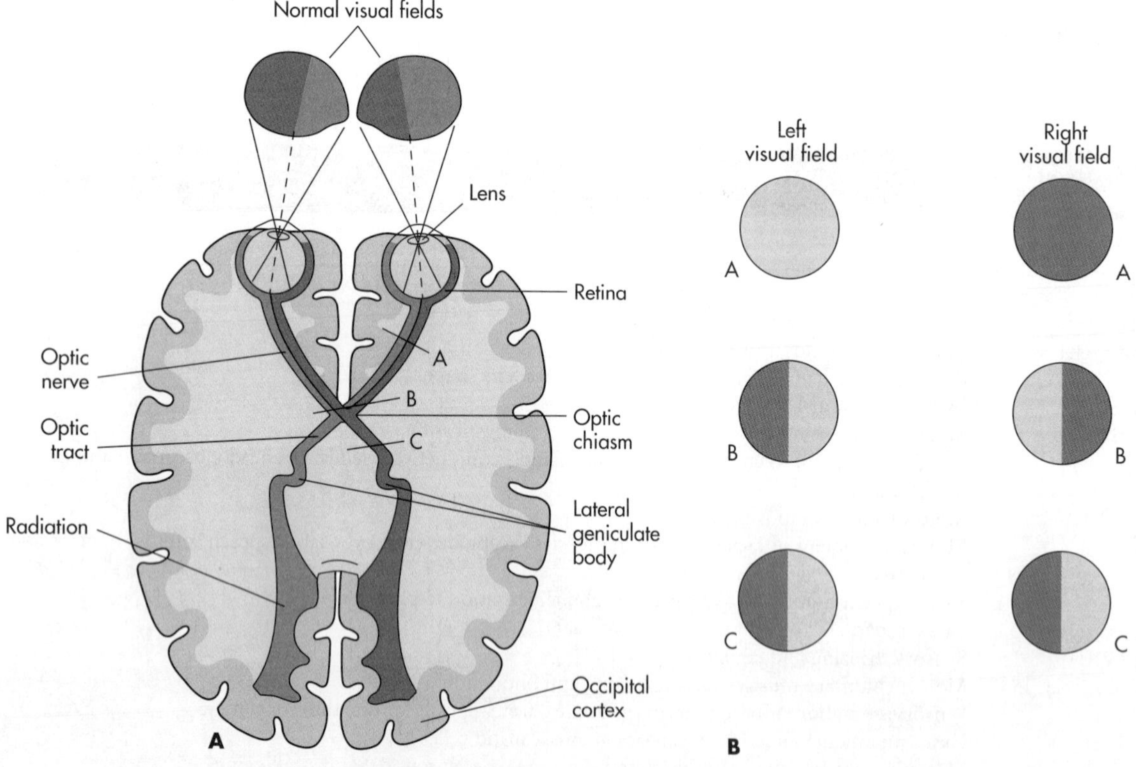

Figure 41-21 **A**, Visual pathways showing partial decussation of optic chiasm. Normal visual fields show reversal of light rays from the temporal and nasal sides to receptors in the retina. **B**, Abnormal visual fields. *A*, Normal left field of vision with loss of vision in right field as a result of complete lesion of right optic nerve. *B*, Loss of vision in temporal half of both fields as a result of lesion of optic chiasm (bitemporal hemianopia). *C*, Loss of vision in nasal field of right eye and temporal field of left eye caused by lesion of right optic tract (homonymous hemianopia).

a variety of bilateral visual fields defects as shown in Figure 41-21. For example, compression of the optic chiasm damages the crossing fibers from the nasal retina and causes bitemporal hemianopsia, or the loss of vision in the temporal halves of each eye. Loss of vision in the corresponding halves of both visual fields produces homonymous hemianopsia, which can be further designated as right or left.

Ocular Fundus. The ocular fundus is defined as that portion of the interior of the eyeball that lies posterior to the lens. It includes the optic disc, blood vessels, retina, and macula and is examined by means of an ophthalmoscope. The funduscopic examination begins with the optic disc (papilla), the area where the blood vessels and nerve fibers enter and exit the eyeball (Figure 41-22). The disc is normally the most prominent structure visible and is examined in detail to assess its size, shape, margins, and color. The normal characteristics of the optic disc are presented in Table 41-10. Either excessive pallor or redness may be present, as well as swelling, or papilledema, which can be caused by active inflammation or passive congestion. Papilledema that results from passive congestion or increased intracranial pressure is also called a choked disc. Optic atrophy indicates partial or complete destruction of the optic nerve and is associated with decreased visual acuity and a change in the color of the disc to a lighter pink or gray. The largest blood vessels visible in the fundus, the central retinal artery and central retinal vein, branch throughout the retina. The retina is the only site in the human body where the microcirculation can be viewed directly.

Cranial Nerve III (Oculomotor), Cranial Nerve IV (Trochlear), and Cranial Nerve VI (Abducens)

Cranial nerves III, IV, and VI are motor nerves that arise from the brainstem and innervate the six extraocular muscles attached to the eyeball. These muscles function as a group in providing the coordinated movement of each eyeball in the six cardinal fields of gaze, giving the eye both straight and rotary movement. The four straight, or rectus, muscles are the superior, inferior, lateral, and medial rectus muscles. The two slanting, or oblique, muscles are the superior and inferior (Figure 41-23).

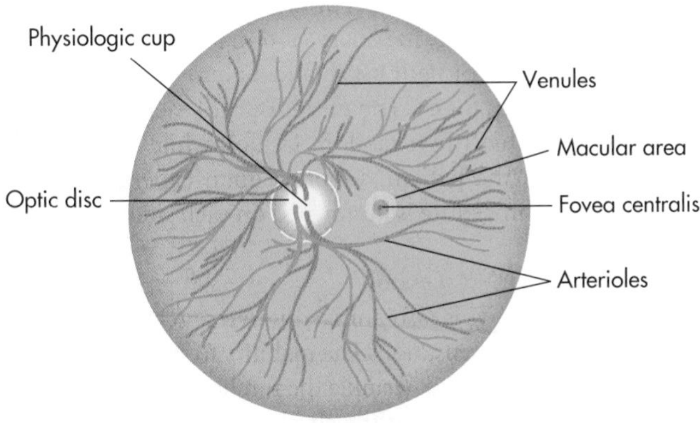

Figure 41-22 Structures of the left eye as visualized through the ophthalmoscope.

The action of each muscle is coordinated with one in the other eye, thus ensuring that the axes of the two eyes always remain parallel (conjugate movement). Parallel axes are important in a binocular system to present the brain with only one visual image. A single image is possible because the eyes move as a pair.

Extraocular Movements. Eye movements are tested by instructing the patient to cover one eye and follow the nurse's finger through all fields of gaze. Limitation of movement in any direction is noted, as well as actual paralysis (ophthalmoplegia). If one of the extraocular muscles is paralyzed, the eye is unable to move fully into the corresponding field of gaze.

Conjugate movements of the eyes also are tested by asking the person to look as far as possible to either side, then up and down, and then obliquely, as shown in Figure 41-23. The nurse observes for parallel movements of the eyes in each direction or any deviation from normal.

Double vision (diplopia), squint (strabismus), and involuntary rhythmic movements of the eyeballs (nystagmus) may be caused by deficits in the motor nerves that cause weakness in the extraocular muscles. Ptosis, or drooping of the upper eyelid over the eye, may be caused by damage to the oculomotor nerve. Normally, the upper lid minimally overlaps the iris as the person moves the eyes downward. The person with ptosis is unable to raise the lid voluntarily.

Pupils. Each pupil should be inspected first as to size and then as to shape and equality. Argyll Robertson pupils, for example, are constricted and do not react to light, although they exhibit accommodation in response to near objects. Pupil inequality, or anisocoria, may assist in the diagnosis of some neurologic diseases (Figure 41-24, *A*). The pupil is normally round, centrally placed, regular in outline, and equal in size to the other pupil. However, unequal pupils are found in approximately 25% of the normal population. Thus the briskness of the pupillary response is the more important part of the assessment.

Direct Light Reflex. The nurse darkens the room and focuses a small beam of light directly into each pupil. Normally the pupil constricts quickly when a light is focused on the retina. Constriction is reported to be especially brisk in young people and those with blue eyes. After a head injury, a dilated and fixed pupil may be observed on the side of the injury (Figure 41-24, *B*). A pupil is described as slow or sluggish if it contracts slowly or imperfectly and then relaxes immediately.

Consensual Light Reflex. When one pupil is directly stimulated by light, the pupil of the other eye also constricts. This consensual response is the result of the decussation (crossing)

TABLE 41-10 Normal Characteristics of the Optic Disc

Size	1.5 mm
Shape	Flat round or vertically oval
Margins	Sharply defined
Color	Creamy red with a small whitish depression in the center (physiologic cup)

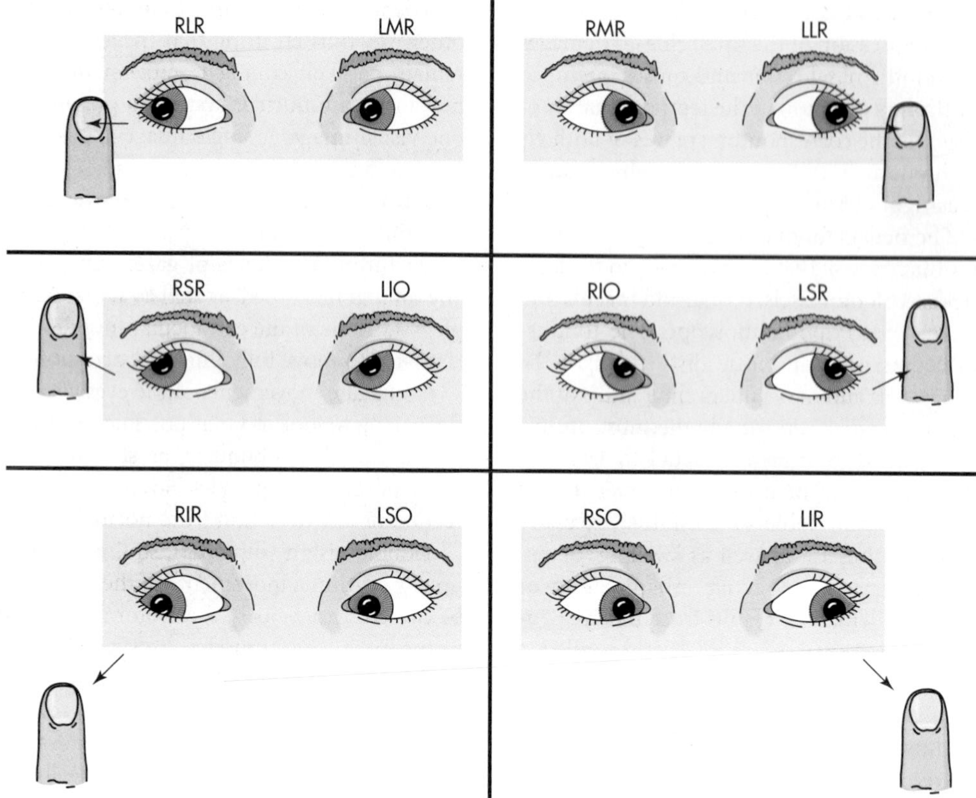

Figure 41-23 Examination of extraocular muscles. Note that two muscles are involved in each cardinal direction. *R,* right; *L,* left; *LR,* lateral rectus; *MR,* medial rectus; *SR,* superior rectus; *IO,* inferior oblique; *IR,* inferior rectus; *SO,* superior oblique.

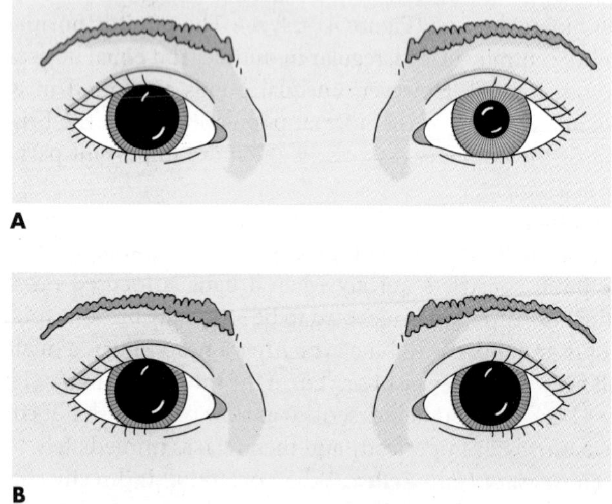

Figure 41-24 **A,** Unequal pupils, also called anisocoria. **B,** Dilated and fixed pupils, indicative of severe neurologic deficit.

of nerve fibers both in the optic chiasm and in the pretectal area, causing both the homolateral and contralateral pupil to react to light.

Cranial Nerve V (Trigeminal)

Cranial nerve V is a mixed nerve with both motor and sensory components and is the largest cranial nerve. The motor portion innervates the temporal and masseter muscles; the sensory part supplies the cornea, face, head, and the mucous membranes of the nose and mouth.

The motor portion of the nerve is tested through jaw movement. If muscle weakness is present the opened jaw tends to deviate to the side opposite the weakened muscles. The sensory components supplying the face are tested for touch, pain, and temperature. Bilateral corneal reflexes may also be assessed. Normally the person blinks bilaterally. This is an especially important reflex to assess in persons with a decreased LOC because the absence of the blink reflex can result in corneal damage.

Sensation of the face should be assessed for both light and deep touch. The three branches of the trigeminal nerve, which include the ophthalmic, maxillary, and mandibular, are tested using a cotton ball for light touch and a blunt object such as a paper clip for deep touch. The nurse touches each of the three areas with the object in a random fashion while the patient's eyes are closed; the patient responds upon experiencing the sensation. The procedure is performed on each side of the face.

Cranial Nerve VII (Facial)

Cranial nerve VII is also a mixed nerve concerned with facial movement and sensation. The inability to smile, close both eyes tightly, look upward, wrinkle the forehead, show the teeth, purse the lips, and blow out the cheeks demonstrate weakness or paralysis of the facial muscles innervated by this nerve. The nurse palpates the temporal and masseter muscles for strength and mass as the patient clenches his or her teeth. Special attention is given to asymmetry. Distinction must be made between central and peripheral neurologic involvement. Peripheral involvement is caused by compression of this cranial nerve and is a common type of lower motor neuron facial paralysis. Lesions affecting the facial nerve produce paralysis of half of the entire face, including the eyelids, forehead, and lips. Forehead function remains intact in central or upper motor neuron lesions and indicates that the lesion lies somewhere on the path from the cerebral cortex to the nucleus of the facial nerve.

Sensory branches of the facial nerve also supply the anterior two thirds of the tongue, and taste is assessed when the nurse suspects a facial nerve injury. The test is otherwise usually omitted from the assessment. A cotton applicator coated with a solution of sugar, salt, or lemon juice is applied to the tongue. The patient is then asked to identify the taste.

Cranial Nerve VIII (Acoustic)

Cranial nerve VIII is composed of a cochlear division related to hearing and a vestibular division related to equilibrium. The cochlear part is tested grossly by having the person listen and identify whispered words. A more complete examination, including bone and air conduction of sound, involves assessment with a tuning fork and audiometric testing (see Chapter 59). The Rinne test and Weber test are used most commonly (see Chapter 59). The vestibular function of the acoustic cranial nerve is evaluated by assessing balance through the Romberg test (discussed at right). A positive Romberg test suggests an inner ear or cerebellar problem.

Cranial Nerve IX (Glossopharyngeal) and Cranial Nerve X (Vagus)

Cranial nerves IX and X are tested together. The chief function of cranial nerve IX is to provide sensation to the pharynx and taste to the posterior third of the tongue. Both nerves supply the posterior pharyngeal wall, and normally when the wall is touched there is prompt contraction of these muscles on both sides, with or without gagging. This test is thus unreliable for evaluating either nerve alone. Because cranial nerve X is the chief motor nerve to the muscles of the soft palate, pharynx, and larynx , assessment includes testing voice and cough. In unilateral involvement of the motor portion of the vagus nerve the voice is harsh and nasal. When the person says "ah," the soft palate does not stay in the midline but deviates to the intact side. Bilateral involvement produces more severe speech problems; swallowing is difficult (dysphagia), and fluids regurgitate through the nose because of palatal and pharyngeal muscle impairment. Sensory function of the vagus usually is not tested.

Cranial Nerve XI (Spinal Accessory)

Cranial nerve XI is a motor nerve that supplies the sternocleidomastoid muscle and the upper part of the trapezius muscles. The muscles are assessed for weakness and paralysis.

Cranial Nerve XII (Hypoglossal)

Cranial nerve XII is a purely motor nerve and innervates the tongue. The person's tongue is first inspected at rest. Any asymmetry, unilaterality, decreased bulk, deviations, or fasciculations (fine twitching) are noted. When this nerve is impaired, the tongue deviates toward the side of the lesion. In an upper motor neuron lesion the tongue deviates toward the side opposite the lesion (contralateral). Atrophy of the tongue is shown through wrinkling and loss of substance on the affected side.

Motor Status

Function of the motor system is assessed through gait and stance, muscle strength, muscle tone, coordination, involuntary movements, and muscle stretch reflexes.

Gait and Stance

Gait and stance are complex activities that require muscle strength, coordination, balance, proprioception, and vision. Gait, or walking, and associated movements give considerable information about the person's motor status. Changes in gait may be characteristic of a specific neurologic disease. *Ataxia* is a general term meaning lack of coordination in performing a planned, purposeful movement such as walking. Ataxia can be caused by disturbance of position sense or by cerebellar or other diseases. To evaluate gait the person is asked to walk freely and naturally and then walk heel to toe in a straight-line, tandem walk, because this exaggerates any abnormalities. To evaluate stance, the person is asked to perform the Romberg test standing with the feet close together, first with eyes open and then with eyes closed. Patients with problems of proprioception have difficulty maintaining balance with their eyes closed; patients with cerebellar disease have difficulty even with their eyes open.

A variety of distinctive gaits characterize specific neurologic disorders. The hemiparetic gait seen in upper motor neuron disease is characterized by circumduction of the affected leg and inversion of the foot. Persons with Parkinson's disease walk with a slow, shuffling gait, and as they start walking, an increase in speed occurs until they are almost running (propulsive). They also have difficulty stopping, and deviation in the center of gravity can cause retropulsion or lateropulsion. In addition, loss of associated movements of the arms in walking is noticeable. Persons with cerebellar disease, on the other hand, walk with a wide-based, staggering gait.

Muscle strength, or power, is assessed systematically, including the trunk and extremity muscles. One common assessment of muscle strength involves asking the patient to grasp the nurse's hands and squeeze them simultaneously. The nurse compares the squeezing ability of one hand with the other. Assessment of muscle strength in the feet can be performed by plantar flexion and dorsiflexion. During manual testing of these and other muscle groups, the person attempts to resist the force applied by the nurse in moving the muscles. Identification of an impaired muscle requires the nurse to document the extent and degree of muscle weakness.

The person may also be tested for drift by asking them to hold the arms straight out for 20 to 30 seconds with palms up and eyes closed. Hemiparesis (weakness or incomplete paralysis) is suggested when there is pronation of one forearm or a downward drift of the arm.

Muscle Tone

Resting skeletal muscles have a certain number of fibers that are always partially contracted because of continuous stimulation of receptors of certain reflex arcs, especially the stretch reflex. The minimal degree of contraction exhibited by a muscle at rest is called muscle tone. When some of the lower motor neurons or afferent fibers innervating neuromuscular spindles are injured, there is a reduction in the stimulation of a muscle and a concomitant loss of tone referred to as hypotonia. In contrast, a muscle with increased tone is referred to as hypertonic.

To test muscle tone the nurse passively moves the person's limbs through a full range of motion. A skilled examiner can readily differentiate hypertonic from hypotonic muscles. Hypertonic extremities tend to stay in fixed positions and feel firm; hypotonic extremities assume a position governed by gravity. Overextension and overflexion are found in hypertonia; an initial resistance to passive movement may increase rapidly and then suddenly give way to spasticity, or clasp-knife rigidity. A steady, passive resistance throughout the full range of motion is characteristic of parkinsonian rigidity; the combination of passive resistance and parkinsonian tremor with small regular jerks is called cogwheel rigidity. In decorticate rigidity the upper limbs are flexed and pronated and the lower limbs are extended. In decerebrate rigidity, however, the upper limbs are extended.

Coordination

Coordination of muscle movements, or the ability to perform skilled motor acts, may be impaired at any level of the motor system. The cerebellum is primarily responsible for the coordination of movement, so that movements take place in a smooth and precise manner. Thus, disturbances in cerebellar function may result in ataxia, difficulty in controlling the range of muscular movement (dysmetria), and an inability to alternate rapid opposite and successive movements (adiadochokinesia). Simple motor activities are evaluated by asking the person to perform rapid rhythmic movements, such as the nose-finger-nose test, which requires the individual to alternately touch the nose and the tip of the nurse's finger, or the knee pat (pronation-supination).

Involuntary Movements

Involuntary movements are also assessed and described during the neurologic examination. It is important to observe the location of muscles involved, amplitude of movement, speed of onset, duration of contraction and relaxation, and rhythm. The effects of posture, rest, sleep, distraction, voluntary movements, and emotional stress on involuntary movements are determined. Emotional stress usually increases involuntary movements, and they may subside during sleep. Abnormal movements may be the result of organic disease or may be psychosomatic in origin.

Tremor consists of rhythmic to-and-fro movements, usually of small amplitude. These movements are the result of alternating contractions of opposing groups of muscles, are continuous while the patient is awake, and may or may not be present during sleep. Chorea refers to short, sharp, rapid, irregular movements, usually of small excursion, which occur in different parts of the body and persist during sleep. Hemiballismus is a variation of chorea in which movement is confined to one side of the body and affects the limbs to a great extent. Athetosis consists of slow, sinuous, and more sustained movements that may be of considerable amplitude; these movements occur in the neck and trunk, as well as the extremities. Myoclonus refers to irregular, abrupt, and arrhythmic contractions of a muscle or a group of muscles in the extremities, trunk, or face.

Reflexes

A reflex is a predictable response that results from a stimulus that initiates a reflex arc. The term *reflex* is typically used to describe involuntary responses. Although all muscles can be made to undergo reflex contraction, most are not tested clinically.

The stretch (myotatic) reflex is a two-neuron (monosynaptic) reflex arc. A well-known example is the knee-jerk reflex, or patellar reflex, which is produced by tapping the patellar tendon of the relaxed quadriceps femoris muscle (Figure 41-25). Such a reflex is described as ipsilateral because the response occurs on the same side of the body and spinal cord where the stimulus is received. Tapping on the patellar tendon elicits a stretching of the quadriceps tendon and its muscles along with some neuromuscular spindles within the muscle and generates nerve impulses. Afferent fibers convey these nerve impulses to the L2-L3 vertebral level of the spinal cord. The afferent neurons synapse with the lower motor neurons, which are large spinal neurons. Axons carry the impulse rapidly to the motor end plates of the quadriceps muscle, which stimulates contraction and extension of the lower leg.

Assessment of reflexes requires an experienced examiner, a reflex hammer, and a relaxed patient. The reflex is elicited by striking the hammer onto the muscle's insertion tendon. Comparison of right and left sides should reveal equal responses. Some of the more common diagnostic reflexes tested are listed in Table 41-11. The reflex response is graded on a subjective, four-point scale that requires clinical practice to use accurately (Table 41-12). If the reflex response fails to appear on the first attempt, the nurse encourages the person to relax by varying position or increases the strength of the hammer blow.

Any abnormal reflex response may indicate a disorder of the nervous system. For example, the Babinski or plantar reflex is abnormal and may indicate pyramidal tract disease. To test this reflex, the lateral aspect of the sole of the fool from the heel to the ball is stroked using the end of the handle on the reflex hammer. The expected finding is plantar flexion of all toes; however, a response of extension of the great toe along

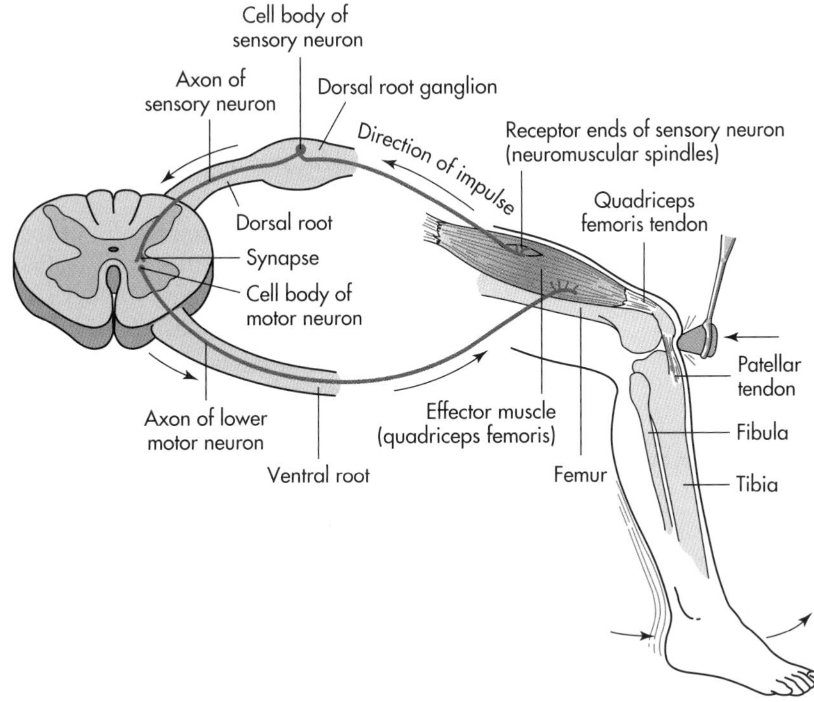

Figure 41-25 The two-neuron patellar reflex, or "knee jerk."

TABLE 41-11 Some Diagnostic Reflexes of the Central Nervous System

Reflex	Description	Indication
Abdominal reflex	Anterior stroking of the sides of lower torso causes contraction of abdominal muscles	Absence of reflex indicates lesions of peripheral nerves or in reflex centers in lower thoracic segments of spinal cord; may also indicate multiple sclerosis
Achilles reflex (ankle jerk)	Tapping of calcaneal (Achilles) tendon of soleus and gastrocnemius muscles causes both muscles to contract, producing plantar flexion of foot	Absence of reflex may indicate damage to nerves innervating posterior leg muscles or to lumbosacral neurons; may also indicate chronic diabetes, alcoholism, syphilis, subarachnoid hemorrhage
Biceps reflex	Tapping of biceps tendon in elbow produces contraction of brachialis and biceps muscles, producing flexion at elbow	Absence of reflex may indicate damage at the C5 or C6 vertebral level
Brudzinski's reflex	Forceful flexion of neck produces flexion of legs, thighs	Reflex indicates irritation of meninges
Kernig's reflex	Flexion of hip, with knee straight and patient lying on back, produces flexion of knee	Reflex indicates irritation of meninges or herniated intervertebral disk
Patellar reflex (knee jerk)	Tapping of patellar tendon causes contraction of quadriceps femoris muscle, producing upward jerk of leg	Absence of reflex may indicate damage at the L2, L3, or L4 vertebral level; may also indicate chronic diabetes, syphilis
Plantar reflex	Stroking of the lateral part of sole causes toes to curl down; if corticospinal damage, great toe flexes upward and other toes fan out (Babinski's sign)	Reflex indicates damage to upper motor neurons; normal in children less than 1 year old
Triceps reflex	Tapping of triceps tendon at elbow causes contraction of triceps muscle, producing extension at elbow	Absence of reflex may indicate damage at C6, C7, or C8 vertebral level

with fanning of the other toes is termed a Babinski response, which is abnormal. Hyporeflexia occurs when a reflex is less responsive than normal resulting from a lesion of the lower motor neurons; hyperreflexia, a reflex more responsive than normal, occurs from lesions in upper motor neuron pathways.

Assessment measures and variations in normal findings relevant to the care of older adults are presented in the Gerontologic Assessment box. Also identified are disorders common in older adults that may be responsible for abnormal assessment findings.

TABLE 41-12 Grading of Muscle Stretch Reflexes

Scale	Interpretation
0	Areflexia
1+	Hyporeflexia
2+	Normal
3+	Brisker than normal
4+	Hyperreflexia

Gerontologic Assessment

Reaction time increases with age.
Noticeable age-related effects on cognitive abilities include a slight and gradual decline in some intellectual abilities such as short-term memory.
Age-related changes in vision include a decrease in visual acuity, diminished peripheral vision, increased sensitivity to glare, and difficulty adapting to dark and light.
Hearing loss for high frequency sound is a common expectation.
Tactile sensation decreases; there is difficulty in temperature discrimination and performing fine motor tasks.
Both taste perception and olfactory sensation decline.
Deep tendon reflexes are less brisk. Ankle jerks are commonly lost; those in the upper extremities are usually present. Older adults often have difficulty relaxing their limbs; the examiner should always support the limb when eliciting reflexes.
Loss of the sensation of vibration at the ankle malleolus is common after age 65. Position sense in the big toe may be absent, but this is less common.
Gait may be slower and more deliberate. Also, the gait may deviate slightly from a midline path because of decreased coordination.
A decrease in muscle bulk often occurs and is most apparent in the hands. The hand muscles appear wasted; however, grip strength remains relatively good.
Senile tremors occasionally occur and are considered benign.
Common disorders in older adults include strokes, aneurysms, falls, Alzheimer's disease, and dementia.

DIAGNOSTIC TESTS

Relevant diagnostic tests provide an important source of data for diagnosing neurologic disease. A variety of laboratory, radiologic, and special tests are available to assist in the process.

Laboratory Tests

Blood

An important component of the neurologic assessment is blood screening. Screening usually includes electrolytes and a complete blood count. Serology screening is used to rule out syphilis, which in its tertiary form may cause neurologic symptoms. Arterial blood gases offer valuable information regarding oxygen and carbon dioxide levels. Additionally, drug levels may be drawn, which can provide information about the way a person metabolizes the drug and the person's adherence to the medication regimen. Abnormalities in any of the blood studies may be indicative of neurologic disease. See Table 41-13 for some specific abnormalities.

Urine

Urine output and electrolyte excretion are easily disturbed by cranial surgery and trauma. This is especially true if the pituitary gland is involved. Both diabetes insipidus and syndrome of inappropriate secretion of antidiuretic hormone are frequently encountered problems (see Chapter 42). See Table 41-14 for possible alterations in urinary results.

Cerebrospinal Fluid

CSF is a clear fluid that is formed in the third, fourth, and lateral ventricles of the brain. Samples are obtained through either a lumbar or cisternal puncture and examined for any increase or decrease in its normal constituents and for foreign substances such as pathogenic organisms and blood.

Spinal fluid normally is under slight positive pressure; 75 to 180 mm H_2O is considered normal. The pressure is measured with a manometer when a lumbar puncture is performed.

Normally each milliliter of spinal fluid contains up to eight lymphocytes. An increase in the number of lymphocytes can occur with both bacterial and viral infection. CSF can become

TABLE 41-13 Blood Abnormalities

Element	Abnormality Seen	Possible Reason
Potassium	Decreased	Poor dietary intake
White blood cells	Increased	Infection such as meningitis
		Common steroid effect
Po_2	Decreased	Increased intracranial pressure
Red blood cells	Increased	Dehydration
	Decreased	Anemia
Hematocrit and hemoglobin	Increased	Dehydration
	Decreased	Anemia
Anticonvulsant drug	Increased	Toxicity or patient overdose
	Decreased	Patient not taking drug
Plasma cortisol	Increased	Acute head injury
Sodium	Decreased	Inappropriate antidiuretic hormone

cloudy as a result of an increase in polymorphonuclear leukocytes from pyogenic infections. Bacterial infections can also alter the components of CSF. For example, tuberculosis and meningitis lower CSF glucose and chloride levels. Degenerative diseases and tumors usually cause an increased protein level in the CSF. See Table 41-15 for normal values of CSF.

Another test of CSF that is useful in diagnosing neurosyphilis or multiple sclerosis is the colloidal gold test. CSF is abnormal in about 90% of patients with multiple sclerosis, including CSF pleocytosis and abnormal gamma globulins as demonstrated by electrophoresis. A culture of CSF may be obtained to assist in organism identification in an ill patient. CSF testing for syphilis is important because serologic blood tests are often negative in the presence of neurologic involvement, whereas CSF tests are positive.[8]

Blood in the spinal fluid indicates bleeding into the ventricular system. It may be caused by a fracture at the base of the skull that has torn blood vessels or from the rupture of a blood vessel (e.g., with an aneurysm).[6] Occasionally the first specimen of CSF obtained contains blood from the trauma of the lumbar puncture. Therefore the specimens of CSF are numbered and the first vial is not used for the cell count.

Radiologic Tests

Multiple radiologic procedures of the brain and spinal cord may be performed, including plain radiographs, carotid Doppler studies, computed tomography, and special contrast studies of the ventricular system and the cerebral vessels.

Routine or Plain Radiographs

Plain radiographs of the skull and spinal column are commonly used diagnostic tests because they are safe and readily available. They can detect developmental, traumatic, or degenerative bone abnormalities.

TABLE 41-14 Urine Abnormalities

Element	Abnormality Seen	Possible Reason
Urinary output	Decreased amount Increased amount	Metabolic problem Kidney failure Diabetes insipidus
Specific gravity	Decreased Increased	Diabetes insipidus Dehydration
Glucose and acetone	Present	Steroid effect—possible chemical diabetes
Sodium	Increased amount	Inappropriate antidiuretic hormone Diabetes insipidus

TABLE 41-15 Normal Values of Cerebrospinal Fluid

Element	Normal Range
Pressure	75 to 180 mm H_2O
Glucose	50 to 80 mg/dl
Chloride	18 to 132 mEq/L
Protein	120 to 50 mg/dl
Gamma globulin	3% to 9%
Lymphocytes	0 to 5/ml

Carotid Doppler Studies

Carotid Doppler studies use a Doppler instrument that emits ultrasound waves to evaluate carotid arterial blood flow. Moving red blood cells reflect ultrasound waves back to the Doppler instrument; the velocity of the blood flow influences the reflection of the ultrasound waves. Velocity of blood flow is measured through an audible sound and a series of images for visualization. The test is noninvasive, painless, and accurate. No specific nursing care is required before or after the procedure. Stenosis or occlusion of the carotid arteries can be detected as the instrument is moved over the common carotid artery to the bifurcation of the internal and external carotid arteries.

Computed Tomography

Computed tomography (CT) scans can provide 100% more information than conventional radiographs, and they provide enhanced image detail. A series of x-rays studies are taken, with each image derived from a specific layer of brain tissue. The brain is thus scanned in successive layers by a narrow beam of x-rays.

Data are collected in x-ray and printout form, and information is also stored for future comparison. By comparing tissue densities found on the CT scan with norms, abnormalities can be detected. Tumor masses, infarctions, and displacements of bone and ventricles can be accurately detected. The CT scan is particularly efficient in detecting brain neoplasia and cerebrovascular lesions.[7]

No special physical preparation is required. The person is informed that the CT scan is painless except for insertion of an intravenous access before the procedure if a contrast medium is to be used, in which case patients are carefully assessed for allergies. The length of the procedure ranges from 30 to 60 minutes depending on whether a contrast medium is used. The person must be supine, with the head positioned in a rubber head holder.

After the completion of the CT scan, the nurse monitors the person for any signs of increased intracranial pressure (if dye was used). If the person becomes disoriented as a result of the test, reassurance is given and the person is protected from injury.

Brain Scan

The brain scan is a relatively safe and painless procedure that uses radioactive isotopes and a scanner to detect cerebral pathology. The patient is given an intravenous injection of a radionucleotide, and then the radioactivity is traced with a gamma scintillation camera or scanner, which converts the rays into images displayed on an oscilloscope screen. The underlying principle of the brain scan is that the radionucleotide can penetrate the brain only through a disruption in the blood-brain barrier and subsequently collects in abnormal brain tissue.

Nursing care is primarily focused on the educational needs of the patient who is informed that the injection of radioactive material causes burning at the insertion site, but no dangers are associated with its administration. The person is told that the scanner oscillates back and forth around the person's head during the scan and creates some loud noises. All jewelry and metal objects are removed before the procedure, which typically takes 45 minutes.

Myelography

Myelography is performed by introduction of either a gas or a radiopaque liquid into the spinal subarachnoid space following a lumbar or cisternal puncture. The flow of dye is monitored fluoroscopically as it moves through the subarachnoid space, and radiographs are taken to assist in the identification of lesions in the intradural or extradural compartments of the spinal canal.

A lumbar puncture is performed with the patient either in a side-lying position with the head and knees flexed, or sitting upright with the head flexed onto the chest. After the puncture, dye or air is injected into the spinal canal. Water-based dyes such as Amipaque are absorbed into the bloodstream and require no special considerations. Less frequently used oil-based dyes are removed at the completion of the test while the person remains upright to prevent the dye, which would cause meningeal irritation, from flowing above the level of the spine. Food and fluids are restricted for approximately 4 to 8 hours before the procedure. The nurse assesses for any history of allergies to iodine or dyes; the person is asked to sign a consent form and remove all jewelry and metal objects. A sedative may be given to relax the person immediately before the procedure.

After the procedure the person must lie supine for several hours if an oil-based dye was used. In contrast, the person assumes a semirecumbent position with the head elevated 30 to 60 degrees for 12 hours if a water-based dye was injected. These interventions attempt to decrease the incidence of headache, nausea and vomiting, and seizures in the posttest period. Complaints of neck stiffness or pain with neck flexion are immediately reported to the physician because these symptoms may indicate meningeal irritation. Other nursing interventions include monitoring vital signs and encouraging fluid consumption of 2400 to 3000 ml during the initial 24 hours. A normal diet can be resumed after 4 hours; however, phenothiazines are withheld for 48 hours after the procedure to decrease the risk of seizures.

Cerebral Angiography (Angiogram)

Cerebral angiography involves the injection of a contrast medium into the cerebral arterial circulation to assist in determining the etiology of strokes, seizures, headaches, and motor weakness. A catheter is inserted into the femoral artery (the most common entry site) and advanced to the carotid and cerebral vessels. Serial films are taken as the dye circulates throughout the cerebral circulation.

The nurse informs the person that the procedure takes 1 to 2 hours and that a feeling of warmth often occurs after dye injection. The nurse carefully assesses for any allergies to iodine, seafood, or contrast medium. The person is kept on nothing-by-mouth status for 6 to 10 hours before the procedure. Informed consent is required and jewelry, dentures, and hearing aids are removed before the angiogram. A sedative may be ordered before the test.

The person remains on bed rest for 12 to 24 hours; however, the duration of bed rest varies among institutions. Vital signs, distal pulses, intake and output, and hemostasis at the insertion site are monitored. The puncture site is immobilized for approximately 8 hours, and ice may be applied at the site to decrease the incidence of hemorrhage and edema.

Potential complications from cerebral angiography include allergic reaction to the radiopaque dye, vasospasm, hemorrhage, hematoma, embolism, or stroke. These complications usually manifest as motor, sensory, or language dysfunction.

Digital Subtraction Angiography

Digital subtraction angiography (DSA) is a method of radiographically studying blood vessels and is particularly useful when the area of study is blocked by bone. Intravenous DSA is often preferred over standard cerebral angiography because less radiation is used, the procedure is less expensive, and there is a lower incidence of serious complications. Images of target areas are taken before and after injection of the dye. Pictures are digitized, stored, and compared in a computer that subtracts anything common between the before (mask) and after (contrast) images.

The nurse addresses educational needs before the procedure. The person needs to lie completely still and is assessed carefully for potential allergy to the contrast medium. After the procedure fluids are encouraged, the insertion site is monitored for bleeding, and neurovascular checks are performed based on institution protocols.

Special Tests

Other tests can be important in determining the nature of neurologic symptoms. These include the lumbar puncture, electroencephalogram (EEG), electromyogram (EMG), and magnetic resonance imaging (MRI).

Lumbar Puncture

The lumbar puncture is performed to measure pressure and obtain CSF for examination. However, it is not typically performed in the presence of increased intracranial pressure or a suspected brain tumor because of the risk of brainstem herniation into the foramen magnum.

The needle is inserted below the level of the spinal cord at the L4-L5 or L5-S1 interspaces (Figure 41-26). After removal of the inner needle, CSF is collected and pressures are measured with a manometer. Queckenstedt's test is routinely performed to assess for subarachnoid blockage by compressing each jugular vein one at a time for approximately 10 seconds while monitoring for changes in spinal fluid pressures. Any pressure greater than 200 mm H_2O is considered to be abnormal.

No dietary or fluid restrictions are required before the test. A consent form is signed, and a sedative may be ordered. The person is encouraged to empty the bowel and bladder and is assisted either to assume a fetal position near the edge of the bed or to sit upright on the side of the bed with the chest and

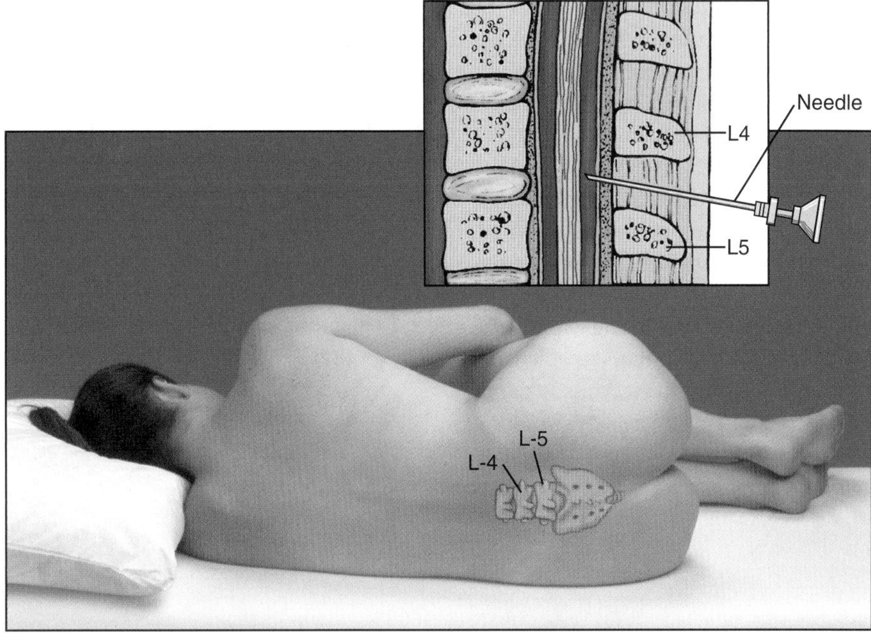

Figure 41-26 Lumbar puncture. With the patient in a flexed position to maximize the space between vertebrae, the lumbar puncture needle is inserted between L-4 and L-5 to gain entry to the subarachnoid space. During the actual procedure the patient would be gowned and draped to protect privacy.

head extended toward the knees. Local anesthesia is used but the patient may still experience sensations of pressure or brief pain as the spinal needle is inserted.

The person is encouraged to lie in a prone position with a pillow under the abdomen after the procedure to increase intraabdominal pressure and help seal the puncture site. A period of bed rest is encouraged but no specific duration is ordered. Nursing interventions include monitoring the insertion site for swelling, redness, and drainage. Signs of complications such as neck stiffness, irritability, and changes in LOC or vital signs are reported immediately to the physician. A postlumbar puncture headache can occur as a result of leakage of CSF at the puncture site and traction on the meninges. The headache may occur a few hours to several days after the procedure and is typically described as a throbbing in the frontal or occipital area.[2] The headache is not serious and is treated with analgesics along with bed rest in a quiet, darkened room.

Electroencephalography

The EEG amplifies and records the electrical activity of the brain (brain waves) transmitted by electrodes attached to the scalp. Any spikes, slowed activity, or asymmetric rhythms on the EEG are considered abnormal. Electroencephalography is indicated for all patients who experience unexplained confusion, LOC, or seizure activity. The EEG is also used to establish brain death.

The nurse reassures the patient that the test is painless and is not a form of shock therapy. Colas, teas, and coffees are avoided the morning of the EEG because consumption of these beverages produces a stimulating effect. The person's hair should be clean and free of hair sprays, gels, and lotions. The person is instructed to rest quietly and move minimally during the test; EEG recordings can be altered even by opening the eyes. Medications are usually not withheld before the test, but protocols vary.

Electromyography

The EMG measures the electrical activity of muscles and records the variations of electrical potential (voltage) detected by a needle electrode inserted into skeletal muscles. The electrical activity can be heard over a loudspeaker and simultaneously viewed on both an oscilloscope and a graph. No electrical activity can be detected in muscles at rest, but action potentials can be detected during movement. However, in motor disease abnormal electrical activity of various types appears in resting muscles. An EMG provides direct evidence of motor dysfunction and can be used to detect dysfunction in the motor neuron, the neuromuscular junction, or muscle fibers. This is particularly helpful in the detection of lower motor neuron disease, primary muscle disease, and defects in the transmission of electrical impulses at the neuromuscular junction.

The person is assured that there is no risk of electrocution from the needle but the sensation of needle insertion is painful and quite similar to an intramuscular injection. Informed consent is required. After the procedure the person may be encouraged to rest, and the nurse observes for any bleeding at the insertion sites.

Magnetic Resonance Imaging

MRI uses a powerful electromagnet to detect radio frequency pulses from the alignment of hydrogen protons in the magnetic field. Computers convert the electromagnetic echo into images. Because excellent visualization of tissue can be achieved without the use of contrast media, MRIs have become exceedingly popular. The MRI demonstrates an increased sensitivity to tissue variations and can often detect lesions such as brainstem tumors and brain abscesses that are not identifiable by CT scans.

The person is informed that the MRI is painless and requires no special preparation. A supine position is assumed, and the person is asked to lie still. The nurse prepares the patient for the narrow spaces, especially if there is any history of claustrophobia. The machine produces a "beating" noise, and earplugs are offered if the noise becomes bothersome. Jewelry is removed before the test; it is important to ascertain whether the person has surgical or orthopedic clips, heart valves, or a pacemaker because the MRI can cause displacement.

References

1. Bral EE: Migraine in children, *Am J Nurs* 99:35, 1999.
2. Connolly MA: Postdural puncture headache, *Am J Nurs* 99:48, 1999.
3. Jarvis C: *Physical examination and health assessment,* ed 3, Philadelphia, 2000, WB Saunders.
4. Lewis AM: Neurologic emergency, *Nursing* 29:54, 1999.
5. Messinger JA et al: Getting conscious sedation right, *Am J Nurs* 99:44, 1999.
6. Mower-Wade D, Cavanaugh M, Bush D: Protecting a patient with ruptured cerebral aneurysm, *Nursing* 31:52, 2001.
7. Reynolds PL: Which patients with minor head injury do not need computed tomography, *J Fam Pract* 49:886, 2000.
8. Sacher RA, McPherson RA: *Widman's clinical interpretation of laboratory tests,* ed 11, Philadelphia, 2000, FA Davis.
9. Victor K: Properly assessing pain in the elderly, *RN* 64(5):45, 2001.

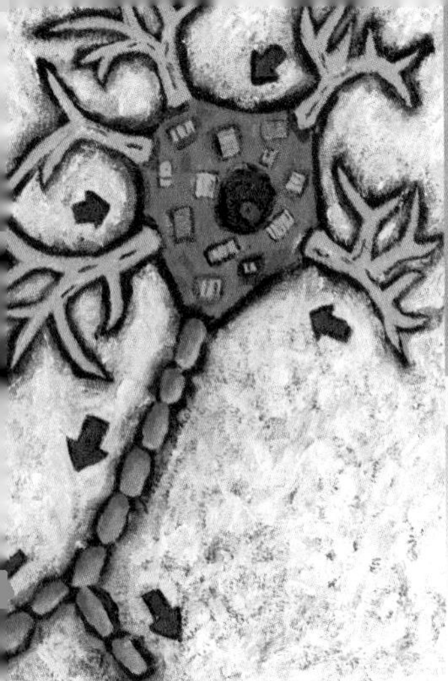

Traumatic and Neoplastic Problems of the Brain

42

Lisa Forsyth, Katherine Russell

Objectives

After studying this chapter, the learner should be able to:

1. Identify at least four causes of altered level of consciousness.
2. Describe three assessment parameters for the person with an altered level of consciousness.
3. Outline four nursing strategies to prevent increases in intracranial pressure.
4. Explain the significance of cerebral perfusion pressure in the patient with increased intracranial pressure.
5. Describe nursing assessment of the patient with a head injury.
6. Develop a plan of care for the patient with a severe head injury.
7. Outline preoperative and postoperative nursing care for the patient undergoing craniotomy for a brain tumor.
8. Differentiate among migraine, cluster, and tension headaches.
9. Differentiate between partial and generalized seizures.
10. Describe the emergent management of status epilepticus.
11. Design a plan of care for a patient with meningitis.

This chapter discusses the care of persons with traumatic, neoplastic, and related problems of the brain. The discussions of altered level of consciousness and increased intracranial pressure apply to the understanding and management of multiple neurologic conditions. The remaining sections present specific disease processes such as headache, epilepsy, intracranial tumors, craniocerebral trauma, and infections and inflammations of the nervous system.

ALTERED LEVEL OF CONSCIOUSNESS

Etiology

Consciousness and coma exist at opposite ends of a spectrum. Full consciousness is a state of awareness and ability to respond optimally to one's environment. Coma is the opposite, a state of total absence of awareness and ability to respond even when stimulated. A wide range of awareness and responsiveness exists between these two extremes (Figure 42-1). The labels used to identify the various points along the continuum are arbitrary and do not reflect any universal agreement as to the nature of consciousness. Terms such as *lethargy* or *stupor* may be interpreted differently by different health care professionals. Box 42-1 provides definitions for terms used to describe level of consciousness (LOC).

Consciousness has two primary components: arousal and content. Arousal is a function of the brainstem pathways that govern wakefulness, particularly the reticular activating system (RAS). Content is the sum of multiple interconnected cerebral hemisphere functions, including thought, behavior, language, and expression.[17] Disruptions in arousal, content, or both can alter the individual's LOC.

The two general types of causes underlying altered LOC are structural and metabolic. Structural causes include physical lesions interrupting neuronal pathways in the cortex or brainstem. Metabolic causes, such as hypoglycemia or hypoxia, involve alterations in the cellular environment that affect the function of neurons. Box 42-2 lists examples of both structural and metabolic causes of altered LOC.

The patient's LOC may fluctuate, and it is essential that there be clear communication and documentation of each assessment so that practitioners can recognize changes and trends in the patient's condition. Thorough documentation of a patient's LOC includes both the patient's response and the stimulation needed to obtain the response. This objective information about the patient's response to a specific stimulus allows other practitioners to reproduce the same results. For example, "Patient opens eyes and answers questions when his name is called" provides clearer and more useful information than simply documenting, "Patient is lethargic."

Three unique conditions of altered LOC demonstrate the complexity of the physiology of consciousness. A *persistent vegetative state* is a condition that can develop after a severe brain injury. Patients in this state demonstrate eye opening

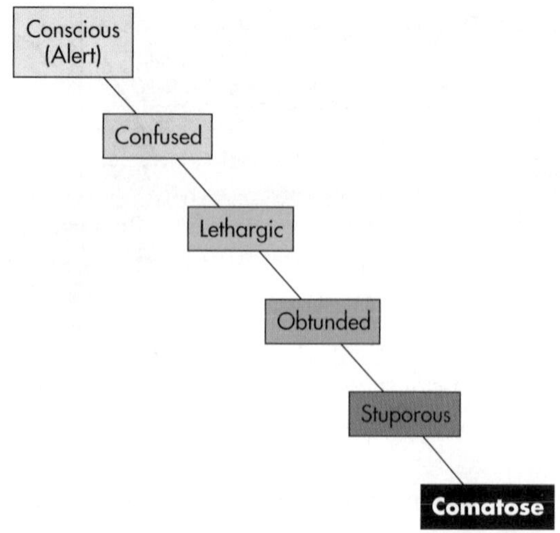

Figure 42-1 Continuum of consciousness.

BOX 42-1 Altered Level of Consciousness Terminology

Alert: attends to the environment; responds appropriately to commands and questions with minimal stimulation
Confused: disoriented to surroundings; may have impaired judgment; may need cues to respond to commands
Lethargic: drowsy, needs gentle verbal or touch stimulation to initiate a response
Obtunded: responds slowly to external stimulation; needs repeated stimulation to maintain attention and response to the environment
Stuporous: responds only minimally with vigorous stimulation; may only mutter or moan as a verbal response
Comatose: no observable response to any external stimuli

BOX 42-2 Possible Causes of Decreased Level of Consciousness

1. Structural causes
   a. Trauma (concussion, contusion, traumatic intracerebral hemorrhage, subdural hematoma, epidural hematoma, cerebral edema)
   b. Vascular disease (infarction, intracerebral hemorrhage, subarachnoid hemorrhage)
   c. Infections (meningitis, encephalitis, abscess)
   d. Neoplasms (primary brain tumors, metastatic tumors)
2. Metabolic causes
   a. Systemic metabolic derangements (hypoglycemia, diabetic ketoacidosis, hyperglycemic nonketotic hyperosmolar states, uremia, hepatic encephalopathy, hyponatremia, myxedema)
   b. Hypoxic encephalopathies (severe congestive heart failure, chronic obstructive pulmonary disease with exacerbation, severe anemia, prolonged hypertension)
   c. Toxicity (heavy metals, carbon monoxide, and drugs—especially opiates, barbiturates, and alcohol)
   d. Extremes of body temperature (heatstroke, hypothermia)
   e. Deficiency states (Wernicke's encephalopathy)
   f. Seizures

and sleep-wake cycles that indicate arousal, but they exhibit no cognitive function. In other words, these patients possess intact "vegetative" functions of the brainstem, such as respiratory drive, brainstem reflexes, and some functions of the RAS, but have no cognitive functions to enable them to interact voluntarily with their environment.

Locked-in syndrome is a condition in which the motor pathways in the brainstem are destroyed but the RAS and higher cognitive functions remain intact. In this state, patients are unable to move or speak because of destruction of the motor pathways that control those functions, but they are capable of interacting with their environment. The motor functions of blinking and extraocular movements are usually spared because those pathways lie above the level of the pons. Locked-in patients therefore can communicate with eye movements and are capable of full arousal and understanding.

Brain death is the third unique alteration in LOC with specific physiologic features. Severely brain-injured patients are considered brain dead when they meet strict criteria set forth by state law. The laws governing brain death may vary by state, but most include criteria such as a known cause of coma so that reversible causes, such as drug overdose or hypothermia, can be ruled out; unresponsiveness to external stimuli; absent brainstem reflexes; and absent respiratory effort in the presence of hypercapnea. These criteria are crucial because they do not include the classic layperson's criterion for death—an absent heartbeat. The definition of brain death becomes particularly important in situations involving tissue and organ donation (see Chapter 51).

Epidemiology

The number of people experiencing altered LOC is not known, but its multiple etiologies indicate that it is a commonly encountered problem in clinical practice. Patients of all ages may experience altered LOC—for brief periods of time or long term.

Pathophysiology

Full consciousness is a product of many delicate interactions within the nervous system. Arousal is a function of the RAS.[17] Fibers from the upper brainstem, thalamus, and hypothalamus receive input from sensory pathways in the brain and peripheral nervous system. The RAS fibers stimulate the cerebral hemispheres to initiate and maintain arousal. When a person is aroused, or awake, he or she is ready to respond to the environment. The cerebral cortex also provides feedback to the RAS to modulate and regulate the information sent to the cortex. See Chapter 41 for a further description of the function of the RAS.

The ability to consciously respond to the environment is a function of the cerebral hemispheres. The cerebral cortex, diencephalon, and upper brainstem act together to control voluntary motor functions, language, memory, and emotion. These higher-level cognitive functions represent the content portion of consciousness. A person needs both arousal, or wakefulness, and content to be considered fully conscious.

Disruptions to the nervous system controlling consciousness can be structural or metabolic. See Box 42-2 for examples. Structural lesions, such as a tumor or stroke, disrupt the pathways of nerve transmission and produce specific, localized neurologic deficits that reflect the location of the lesion. Metabolic causes, such as hypoglycemia or drug overdose, affect the biochemical environment of the brain and alter cellular function. Altered LOC resulting from metabolic changes usually produces more global, nonlocalized neurologic deficits.

Patients with selected sensory-perceptual alterations also may experience altered LOC. Patients experiencing hallucinations, agitation, and delirium are often found to have underlying metabolic problems such as hypoxia, infection, or medication interactions that disturb the metabolic environment of the brain. Classic clinical manifestations, including sensory-perceptual alterations, associated with altered LOC are presented in the Clinical Manifestations box.

Collaborative Care Management

Diagnostic Tests. Diagnostic evaluation of altered LOC includes searching for the structural or metabolic etiology of the changes. The workup includes a detailed history, extensive neurologic examination, radiologic examination, and laboratory testing.

In the emergency setting a rapid evaluation of life-threatening causes of reduced consciousness is carried out. Blood is drawn to assess electrolyte balance, glucose levels, and blood oxygen concentration. Since blood levels of opioids, sedatives, and other drugs cannot be immediately determined, a trial dose of naloxone (Narcan) may be administered to any patient in whom opioid overdose is suspected. A computed tomography (CT) scan of the head may be obtained to rule out the presence of space-occupying lesions that could be causing increased intracranial pressure (ICP). Interventions to protect the airway and support breathing and circulation are initiated while further diagnostic testing is done.

In the emergency setting, diagnostic tests can be subdivided into those tests that evaluate possible structural lesions and those that evaluate possible metabolic causes of altered LOC. Box 42-3 summarizes the range of diagnostic testing for alterations in LOC.

While diagnostic test results are pending or tests are being scheduled, the nurse completes a detailed history and performs a thorough physical examination. The health history is obtained from the patient when possible, but also from family, significant others, prehospital care providers, and home care providers, as appropriate.

A detailed neurologic examination is also performed that follows the standard neurologic assessment format of mental status, motor and sensory examination, and cranial nerve testing. The data from the neurologic examination are the most important part of diagnostic testing for alterations in LOC. (See Chapter 41 for details of a complete neurologic examination. The items discussed here are specific to the evaluation of altered states of consciousness.) The examination may be initially performed by a physician or advanced practice nurse and then repeated on an ongoing basis by the bedside nurse.

A mental status examination includes an overall assessment of consciousness and the patient's ability to remain awake and attentive and participate in the examination. Assessment of orientation, cognitive function, and language are included in the examination. Often, subtle changes in orientation are the first indications of altered LOC, and patients may be disoriented to varying degrees. Orientation to date is usually lost first as patients experience disruption of their usual routines and may not have access to newspapers, calendars, television, and radio. The nurse asks the patient about the day, month, and year. If a patient cannot name a specific date, the nurse asks about the season or recent holidays to obtain a

Clinical Manifestations

Altered Level of Consciousness

Decreased wakefulness
Decreased attention to surrounding environment
Confusion
Disorientation
Agitation
Poor memory
Decreased ability to carry out activities of daily living
Decreased mobility
Incontinence

SENSORY-PERCEPTUAL ALTERATIONS

Hallucinations: subjective sensory perceptions that occur in the absence of relevant external stimuli; may be auditory, visual, tactile, or somatic
Delusions: false, fixed, personal beliefs that are not shared by others
Illusions: misinterpretations of real external stimuli

BOX 42-3 Diagnostic Testing for Altered Level of Consciousness

Structural Tests

Skull x-ray films
Electroencephalography
Computerized tomography of the head
Cerebral angiogram
Magnetic resonance imaging
Evoked potentials

Metabolic Tests

Complete blood count
Urinalysis
Electrolytes (includes glucose, blood urea nitrogen, creatinine)
Calcium
Liver function studies
Cardiac enzymes
Serum osmolarity
Lumbar puncture
Arterial blood gases
Toxicology screens for drugs of abuse (opiates, alcohol, barbiturates, antidepressants)

more general response. Orientation to place may be lost, especially if the patient is in unfamiliar surroundings or has been transferred from one facility to another. If a patient cannot name the exact current location, the nurse asks the patient what kind of place he or she is in (for instance, a hospital, hotel, grocery store). If the patient can look around at medical equipment, staff uniforms, and hospital logos and still not be able to correctly answer a question about place, the patient is considered to be disoriented with an impaired ability to reason and use information. This may affect patient teaching and the patient's ability to participate in self-care.

Significant cognitive or language impairment is typically present when patients are unable to state or respond to their names. It is important to clarify what name the patient is used to responding to; this name should be used during interactions, and the appropriate name is shared with all staff. Some patients do not respond to their given name but do respond to a familiar nickname. It is important to remember that orientation is only a small part of the overall mental status examination. Patients may be able to guess or memorize the correct answers to basic orientation questions. Interaction with the patient during the rest of the neurologic examination provides important information about the patient's ability to think clearly, reason, and have insight into his or her illness.

Assessment of altered LOC includes attention, a component of mental status not often covered in the standard neurologic examination. The nurse assesses the patient's ability to focus, or concentrate, on the examination and evaluates his or her distractibility. Irritability, restlessness, and boredom are also considered, since these may all be signs of cerebral dysfunction.

The time frame associated with the altered LOC can be important in differentiating between delirium and dementia. Delirium develops over a short period, and its duration is usually brief. Because delirium is usually caused by an underlying organic disease process, the altered LOC often resolves when the disease is successfully treated. Dementia is not associated with reduced arousal or wakefulness, but it impairs intellectual functioning, memory, orientation, and the ability to care for self. Dementia develops slowly, is usually progressive, and is a chronic, irreversible state.

Motor examination is the next section of the neurologic examination as described in Chapter 41. The patient with reduced LOC is examined for strength and coordination, as well as the presence of reflexive or pathologic responses of the motor system. When patients have marked reductions in LOC, the nurse may need to use some degree of noxious stimuli to elicit a response. The nurse begins with verbal stimuli, such as calling the patient's name or asking the patient to follow some simple command. A slightly stronger stimulus would involve touching the patient's shoulder and gently tapping or shaking the patient while calling his or her name.

Some patients can respond only to a painful stimulus. Pressing on the sternum, pinching the trapezius muscle at the junction of the shoulder and neck, applying supraorbital ridge pressure, and applying pressure to the fingernail beds are examples of common painful stimuli. The nurse documents both the stimulus used and the patient's response so that the next nurse can duplicate the examination and accurately assess for changes in the patient's status.

The patient who reacts to a painful stimulus and attempts to push the nurse away is said to "localize to pain." If the patient grimaces or demonstrates nonpurposeful movement, he or she is said to "withdraw to pain."

Lesions in the cerebral hemispheres below the primary motor cortex can result in pathologic motor responses and cause abnormal flexor or extensor posturing. Abnormal flexion of the arms at the elbows, wrists, and hands with concurrent extension of the legs is called *decorticate posturing.* Lesions in the motor pathways of the midbrain or upper pons may cause abnormal extension of the arms with hyperpronation of the forearms, which is called *decerebrate posturing.* Abnormal motor postures are shown in Figure 42-2.

The sensory part of the neurologic examination may reveal deficits that affect a cognitively impaired patient's ability to function. Patients with a sensory-perceptual deficit after a stroke may neglect, or not attend to, the affected side of the body.

The last part of the neurologic examination is the cranial nerve examination. Several specific cranial nerve reflexes are particularly important in assessing altered LOC. Protective reflexes, including gag, corneal, and cough, are checked to assess the patient's ability to protect himself or herself from injury and aspiration (see Chapter 41).

The oculocephalic and oculovestibular reflexes are not part of a standard neurologic examination but are performed to assess the extent of brainstem pathology. The oculocephalic reflex (doll's eyes) is tested by holding the person's eyelids open and rotating the head quickly, first to one side and then to the opposite side. When the brainstem is intact, the eyes move in the opposite direction to the head turning. This is considered a positive or normal response (Figure 42-3). If a person has a brainstem lesion, the eyes passively follow the head movement. This is one of the tests used in determining brain death.

The oculovestibular reflex (calorics) is tested by stimulating the semicircular canals of the ear with ice water. The patient is positioned supine with the head of the bed elevated 30 degrees. The eyelids of the unresponsive patient are held open while the ear canals are irrigated with 50 ml of ice water. A normal response that indicates intact function of cranial nerves III, VI, and VIII is conjugate eye movements toward the side being irrigated, followed by rapid nystagmus to the opposite side (Figure 42-4). Absent or dysconjugate eye movement indicates brainstem damage. This test is also used in determining brain death.

A detailed neurologic examination provides the foundation for assessing patients with altered LOC, but health care providers also use a variety of standardized scales for the ongoing evaluation of a patient's functioning. Examples include the Glasgow Coma Scale (GCS), the Ranchos Los Amigos Levels of Cognitive Functioning, and the Mini-Mental State Examination. The GCS was developed specifically to evaluate head-injured patients, but it can be effectively used with a

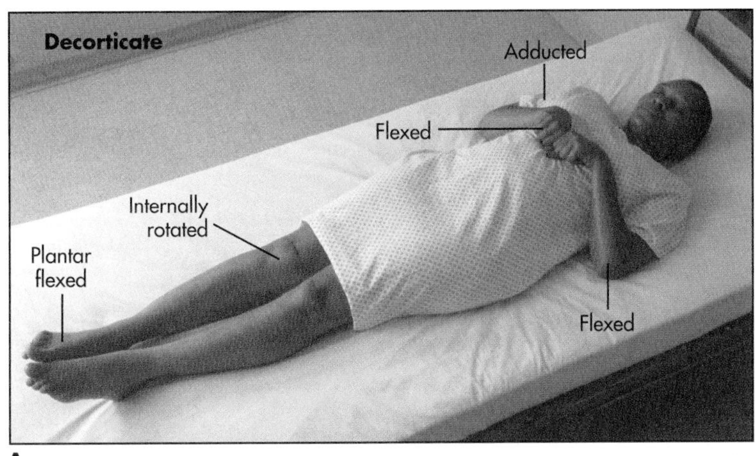

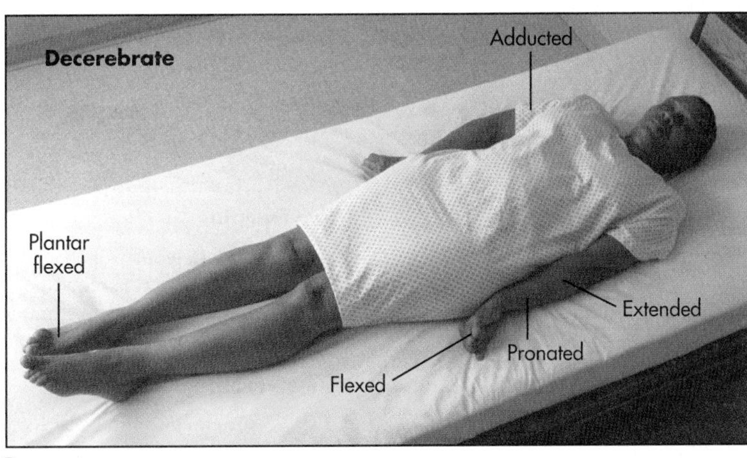

Figure 42-2 Types of posturing: decorticate and decerebrate.

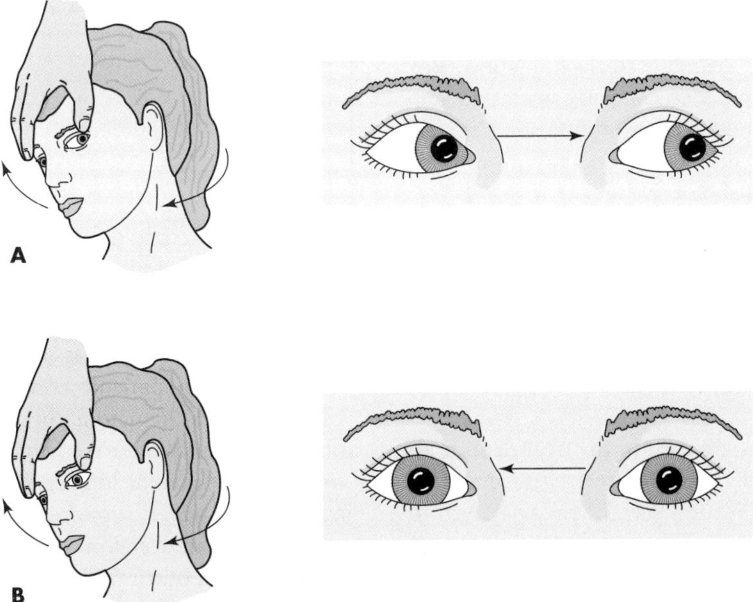

Figure 42-3 Oculocephalic reflex testing. **A,** Normal response: the eyes move to the left as the head is briskly rotated to the right. **B,** Abnormal response: the eyes do not move as the head is turned, but passively follow the head.

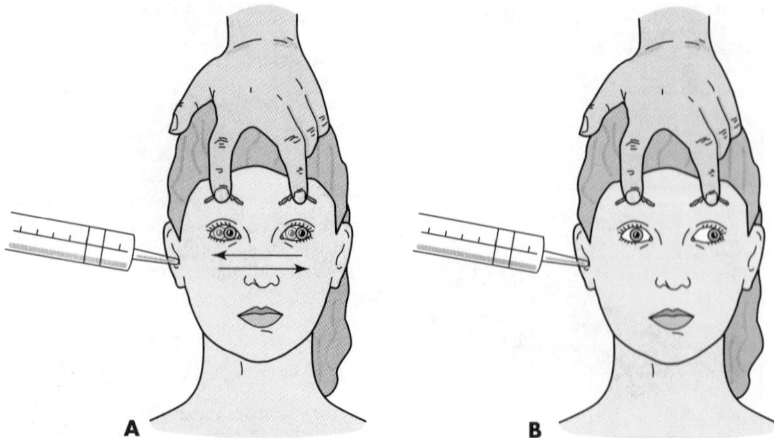

Figure 42-4 Test for oculovestibular reflex response (caloric ice water test). **A,** In the normal response, the individual's eyes slowly move toward the side being irrigated, followed by rapid conjugate eye movements to the opposite side as shown. **B,** Dysconjugate, or asymmetric, eye movements would be abnormal.

wide variety of other neurologic problems (Box 42-4).[24,26] The patient's total score is a sum of scores from three scales: eye opening, verbal response, and motor response. Numbers are assigned to the patient's best response in each area, and notations are made if a scale is not able to be evaluated, such as "eyes swollen shut" or "intubated; unable to test verbal score." The GCS does not take the place of a comprehensive neurologic examination, but the cumulative results can be graphed and used to identify trends in the patient's overall functioning and predict outcomes.

Another widely used scale is the Ranchos Los Amigos Levels of Cognitive Functioning. It was developed as a behavioral rating scale to aid in the assessment and treatment of brain-injured persons. It assesses the progressive recovery of cognitive abilities as demonstrated through behavioral change and is most commonly used in subacute and rehabilitation settings (Box 42-5).

A third tool is the Mini-Mental State Examination (Box 42-6). This classic brief examination assesses orientation, registration, attention, recall, and language and can also be used to follow trends in the patient's level of functioning. A total score below 24 is considered abnormal.[5]

Vital signs can also provide important information regarding a patient's altered LOC. Blood pressure and heart rate may reflect cardiac dysfunction affecting blood flow to the brain. The patient's respiratory rate and pattern can help to localize lesions in the central nervous system. Figure 42-5 provides examples of abnormal respiratory patterns that can result from neurologic problems.

Medications. Medications are used in the treatment of altered LOC to correct the underlying disease process or to control specific symptoms. Naloxone (Narcan) may be given to reverse the effects of opioid overdose. Flumazenil is a benzodiazepine antagonist, used to reverse the effects of overdoses of drugs such as diazepam (Valium) or lorazepam (Ativan). If seizures are the cause of decreased LOC, anticonvulsants are administered to treat actual seizures and prevent future ones. A variety of other medications (see p. 1332) may be administered to treat increased ICP, a common cause of altered LOC.

BOX 42-4 Glasgow Coma Scale

Eye Opening

4	Spontaneously open
3	Open to verbal request
2	Open with painful stimuli
1	No opening

Best Verbal Response

5	Oriented to time, place, person; converses appropriately
4	Converses, but confused
3	Words spoken, but conversation not sustained
2	Sounds made, no intelligible words
1	No response

Best Motor Response

6	Obeys commands
5	Localizes to painful stimulus
4	Withdraws to painful stimulus
3	Abnormal flexion to pain (decorticate posturing)
2	Abnormal extension to pain (decerebrate posturing)
1	No response

Treatments. Treatments for patients with altered LOC usually fall under the umbrella of nursing management. They are discussed in the section on nursing interventions.

Surgical Management. If the cause of the patient's altered LOC is a space-occupying lesion, surgical removal of the mass may improve the patient's condition. For example, a patient with a subdural hematoma becomes more alert and able to follow commands after the hematoma is evacuated. If the lesion has been present long enough to damage the surrounding tissue, however, some residual deficits may remain. See sections on craniocerebral trauma and brain tumors for further discussion of surgical management.

Diet. A patient's swallowing ability is carefully assessed before any decision is made about diet. Patients with decreased gag and cough reflexes, oral motor weaknesses, or decreased LOC may be candidates for placement of an enteral feeding tube to more safely deliver nutrients and medications.

BOX 42-5 Levels of Cognitive Functioning (Rancho Los Amigos Scale)

I. No Response

Patient is completely unresponsive to any stimuli.

II. Generalized Response

Patient reacts inconsistently and nonpurposefully to stimuli in nonspecific manner.

III. Localized Response

Patient reacts specifically but inconsistently to stimuli.

IV. Confused–Agitated

Patient is in heightened state of activity with severely decreased ability to process information.

V. Confused–Inappropriate

Patient appears alert and is able to respond to simple commands fairly consistently.

VI. Confused–Appropriate

Patient shows goal-directed behavior but depends on external input for direction.

VIII. Automatic–Appropriate

Patient appears appropriate and oriented within hospital and home setting, goes through daily routine automatically with minimal to absent confusion, and has shallow recall of actions.

VIII. Purposeful–Appropriate

Patient is alert and oriented, is able to recall and integrate past and recent events, and is aware of and responsive to culture.

From Malkmus D et al: *Rehabilitation of the head-injured adult: comprehensive cognitive management,* Downey, Calif, 1980, Professional Staff Association of Rancho Los Amigos Medical Center, Adult Brain Inquiry Service.

BOX 42-6 Mini-Mental State Examination

Possible Score	Actual Score	
		Orientation
5	________	What is the year? Season? Month? Day? Date?
5	________	Where are we (state, county, city, hospital, floor)?
		Registration
3	________	Name three objects: 1 second to say each. Ask patient to name all three after you have said them. (Give 1 point for each correct answer.) Repeat the objects until the patient has learned all three. Count trials, and record.
		Attention and Calculation
5	________	Serial 7s. Give 1 point for each correct answer. Ask patient to count backward from 100 by 7s. Stop after five answers. Alternative is to spell *world* backward.
		Recall
3	________	Ask for the three objects mentioned above. (Give 1 point for each correct answer.)
		Language
9	________	Display a pencil and a watch. Ask patient to identify them. (2 points)
	________	Repeat "No if's, and's, or but's." (1 point)
	________	Follow a three-stage command: "Take a paper in your right hand, fold it in half, and put it on the floor." (3 points)
	________	Read and obey: "Close your eyes." (1 point)
	________	Write a sentence. (1 point)
	________	Copy design as shown. (1 point)
30 total	________	**Total Score**

CLOSE YOUR EYES

Adapted from Folstein MF, Folstein SE, McHugh PR: Mini-Mental State: a practical method for grading the cognitive state of patients for the clinician, *J Psychiatr Res* 12(3):189, 1975.

Activity. Activity restrictions are rare for the patient with altered LOC unless precautions are in place to reduce ICP. Safety is the highest priority. Patients with altered LOC may easily become disoriented in unfamiliar surroundings and are at risk for both falls and wandering. Patients with decreased mobility require assistance with range-of-motion exercises, turning and bed mobility, and positioning.

Referrals. Nurses often coordinate referrals to other disciplines for patients with complex care needs, although discharge planning and counseling are performed by social workers in

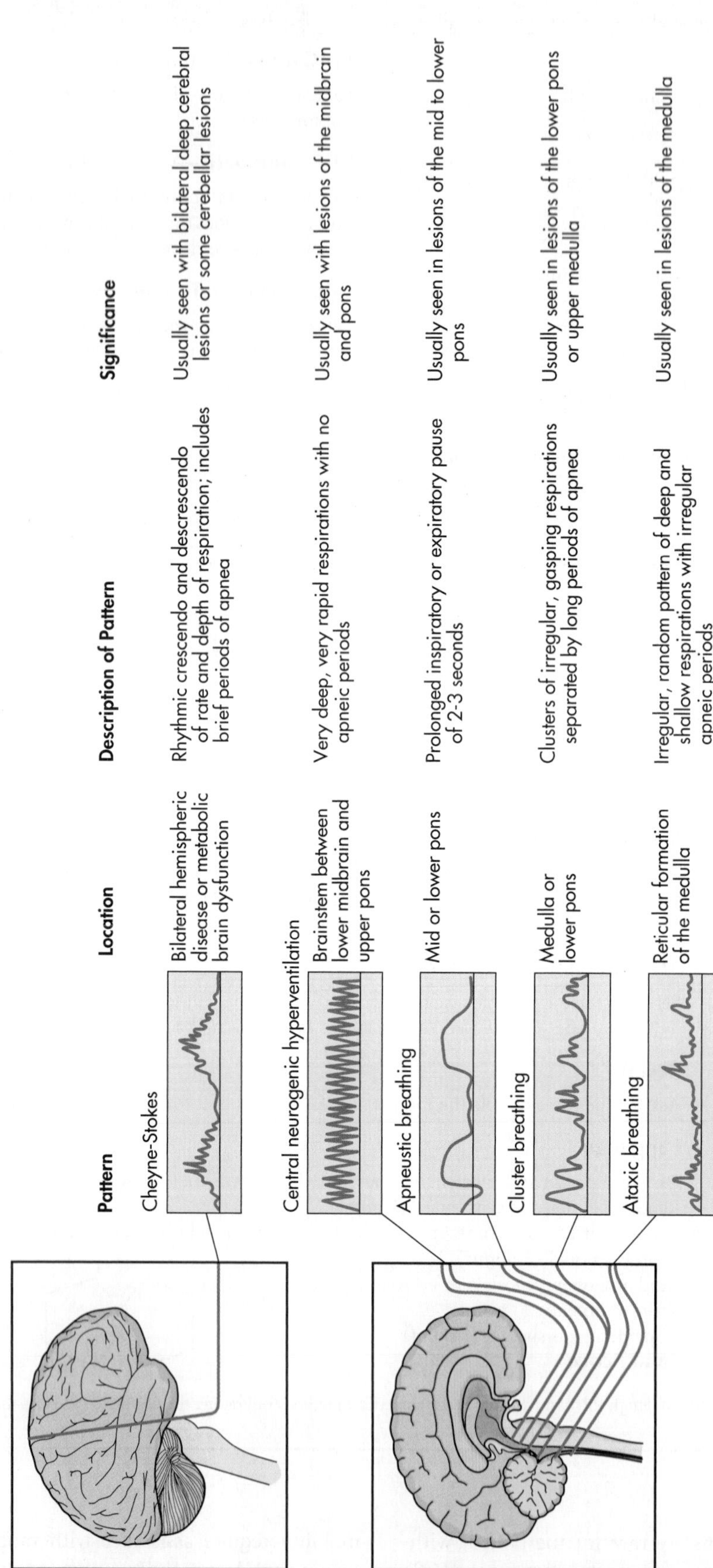

Figure 42-5 Abnormal respiratory patterns with corresponding level of central nervous system activity.

many inpatient settings. Specific patient needs determine the nature and extent of referrals. Physical and occupational therapists offer services to patients with motor, sensory, or self-care deficits. Speech therapists can assist the patient and family with communication and swallowing difficulties. Respiratory therapists collaborate with nursing and other disciplines to help protect the patient's airway and improve gas exchange. Nurses in outpatient or community settings use community resources and services to assist patients and families with home care needs.

NURSING MANAGEMENT OF PATIENT WITH ALTERED LEVEL OF CONSCIOUSNESS

ASSESSMENT

Health History

Obtaining a health history concerning a patient with altered LOC often involves using alternative data sources, such as family members and friends. Selected factors include:

- Date and type of onset
- When the change in LOC was first noticed
- Onset sudden or slowly progressive
- Patient's and family's awareness and understanding of the symptoms
- Recent history of falls, infection, or other trauma
- Medications in use—prescription and over-the-counter drugs; alcohol, nutritional supplements, herbal preparations
- Other comorbid health problems, treatment regimen

Physical Examination

- Ability to think, think abstractly, calculate, and make everyday decisions
- Motor status, presence of posturing
- Sensory status
- Visual changes
- Cranial nerve assessment, protective reflexes
- Breathing pattern
- Oxygenation status
- Other symptoms (pain, headache, fever, nausea)
- Laboratory results (electrolytes, hemoglobin, hematocrit, glucose, blood urea nitrogen [BUN], creatinine)
- Drug levels (opiates, sedatives, anticonvulsants)

NURSING DIAGNOSES

Nursing diagnoses are determined from analysis of patient data. Nursing diagnoses for the patient with altered LOC may include but are not limited to:

Diagnostic Title	Possible Etiologic Factors
1. Ineffective breathing pattern	Neuromuscular impairment, cognitive impairment
2. Ineffective tissue perfusion	Decreased or altered cerebral blood flow
3. Disturbed thought processes	Structural or metabolic imbalance
4. Ineffective thermoregulation	Impaired regulatory mechanisms
5. Risk for injury	Sensory/motor deficits, loss of integrative functions
6. Impaired physical mobility	Neuromuscular impairment
7. Imbalanced nutrition: less than body requirements	Decreased alertness, chewing/swallowing difficulties
8. Bowel incontinence	Perceptual or cognitive impairment
9. Impaired urinary elimination	Neuromuscular impairment
10. Risk for impaired skin integrity	Impaired mobility, nutrition, pressure or shearing forces
11. Ineffective health maintenance	Perceptual or cognitive impairment, loss of motor skills
12. Compromised family coping	Temporary family disorganization, crisis, role changes
13. Deficient knowledge: disorder, plan for treatment or rehabilitation	Lack of exposure, resources

EXPECTED PATIENT OUTCOMES

Expected patient outcomes for the patient with altered LOC may include but are not limited to:

1. Will maintain an effective breathing pattern
2. Will maintain adequate systemic blood pressure to perfuse the brain
3. Will maintain coherent thought processes; will not be confused
4. Will maintain body temperature within normal limits
5. Will not experience injury
6. Will maintain highest possible mobility with use of assistive devices and assistance of others
7. Will consume adequate balanced nutrients to maintain a stable body weight
8. Will maintain a regular pattern of bowel elimination without constipation, diarrhea, or incontinence
9. Will maintain urinary continence with or without an external continence device
10. Will maintain intact skin and have no evidence of redness or breakdown
11. Will participate in self-care to the maximum degree possible
12. Family will actively participate in all decision making and planning for the patient's care and will use coping strategies to adapt to family role changes
13. Patient and family will indicate understanding of the diagnosis and treatment plan

INTERVENTIONS

1. Supporting Effective Ventilation

The nurse closely monitors the breathing patterns of the patient with altered LOC. The patient may require assistance in keeping the airway clear, including the use of suctioning when warranted. The nurse positions the patient on either side and keeps the head of the bed elevated to at least 30 degrees to facilitate an open airway. Patients with swallowing difficulties may require additional precautions to prevent aspiration at mealtimes.

Patients with decreased LOC may not be able to turn themselves to mobilize pulmonary secretions or prevent atelectasis. The nurse helps patients to turn, encourages hourly deep breathing, and encourages the use of incentive spirometers. Patients with significant LOC reductions may hypoventilate and require supplemental oxygen or mechanical ventilation to maintain adequate oxygenation and prevent hypercapnea. The effectiveness of the patient's gas exchange can be evaluated with pulse oximetry and arterial blood gases. Pulse oximetry monitors oxygen saturation but cannot provide information about carbon dioxide exchange or blood pH, which require arterial blood gas sampling. The nurse checks breath sounds to evaluate the effectiveness of the patient's respiratory effort and pattern. The presence of decreased breath sounds indicates the potential for atelectasis and hypoventilation. Hypoxia or hypercapnea may result in increased ICP and further impair the patient's LOC. Changes in breathing pattern can also provide insight into the nature and extent of the patient's neurologic problems (see Figure 42-5).

2. Supporting Tissue Perfusion

Some patients with altered LOC have impaired cerebral tissue perfusion. Decreased perfusion may be a result of increased ICP (discussed later in this chapter) or decreased cardiac output and reduced systemic blood pressure. The nurse ensures that the patient receives adequate hydration to maintain blood volume and support blood pressure. The nurse works collaboratively with the physician to develop a medication plan that supports cardiac function and sustains the blood pressure at levels that ensure optimal peripheral and cerebral circulation.

Helping patients to change position at least every 2 hours enhances circulation and venous return. The nurse also ensures that clothing, bedclothes, and body position do not constrict circulation. Immobile patients develop impaired circulation at dependent sites. Passive or active range of motion is implemented to support blood flow and restore circulation to pressure-occluded or dependent sites. Intermittent compression sleeves may be applied to prevent venous pooling and thrombus formation in the legs.

3. Supporting Orientation

Patients with neurologic impairments may have a variety of sensory-perceptual problems that need to be taken into account when planning care. Patients with visual field deficits need to have objects placed within their functioning field of vision and learn to compensate for visual field losses. The nurse instructs patients to turn the head from side to side to maximize their functional range of vision. Alternating eye patches may be helpful for patients experiencing diplopia. Eye patches restore vision to a single image and allow the patient to read, reach for objects, and ambulate more safely.

Patients with hearing loss need adaptive devices or additional visual sources of information to participate in self-care. The nurse ensures that hearing aids work and are fitted properly. Notations are made on the chart to indicate that a patient is hard of hearing so that a lack of response to questions or instructions is not interpreted as disorientation or cognitive impairment. The nurse also ensures that the environment does not contain unnecessary background noise that can interfere with the patient's attempts to hear and communicate.

Patients with peripheral sensory losses such as hemiparesis may not attend to affected body parts, a condition termed *neglect.* The nurse helps the patient use the affected extremities during routine care and assists with positioning the limbs to prevent contractures, skin breakdown, or injury. Sensory loss on the face can affect the patient's ability to chew and swallow. Food or medications can unknowingly become pocketed in the cheek and later cause choking or aspiration. The nurse carefully checks the patient's mouth after meals and medication administration and removes any pocketed food.

Patients with sensory-perceptual alterations can easily misinterpret environmental stimuli, leading to confusion. The nurse gives special consideration to arranging the patient's environment to minimize confusion or altered thought processes. Large-print calendars and clocks within view can help maintain time orientation. Familiar pictures or objects from home provide a link to family and friends. Adequate lighting helps visually impaired patients see who is entering the room and may prevent the misinterpretation of shadows or unfamiliar objects. Lights should be kept to a minimum at night to promote sleep. The use of night-lights ensures sufficient light for the patient to find the call bell or get to the bathroom without falling while still promoting restful sleep. The need for a quiet, restful environment requires the nurse to carefully eliminate unnecessary noise. Some patients prefer to use background music to "drown out" other noise around them. The nurse carefully explains all of the unfamiliar elements in the environment that could be confusing to the patient, such as infusion pumps or beeps from monitoring equipment.

Communicating with a confused patient requires patience and consistency. The nurse speaks quietly and slowly, using simple sentences or phrases to explain all care. It is important to speak to patients before touching them and to request only one action at a time. If the patient can read, a schedule of activities can remind the patient of events that will occur during the day. Consistent caregivers allow the patient to recognize a few familiar faces.

A patient's altered LOC can be frightening to family members, who need to understand why the patient is behaving in a confused manner. The nurse encourages the family to participate in planning and delivering the patient's care. Family members are often helpful in explaining how the patient reacts to unfamiliar settings and in identifying strategies that are likely to be successful in reorienting the patient. Guidelines for care of the confused person are summarized in the Guidelines for Safe Practice box.

4. Maintaining Normal Body Temperature

Patients with severely reduced LOC are unable to communicate that they are too cold or too warm, and the nurse must

Guidelines for Safe Practice

The Patient With Confusion or Disorientation

1. Promote communication.
   a. Touch may be useful in establishing communication.
   b. Use a calm, quiet, and unhurried voice to talk to patient.
   c. Talk slowly and distinctly and use short sentences.
   d. Face patient when talking and stay within conversational range.
2. Promote orientation.
   a. Explain procedures in advance.
   b. Maintain a well-lighted environment.
   c. Keep large calendar and clock in view.
   d. Introduce self when caring for patient.
   e. Keep sensory stimulation to a minimum.
   f. Provide consistency in staff caring for patient.
   g. Keep decision making to a minimum.
3. Support family.

ensure that the patient maintains a stable body temperature. If the patient becomes febrile, the nurse initiates an assessment for potential sources of infection. Treatment for any fever includes treatment of infection, antipyretic medication, tepid baths, and lowering the room temperature. Patients with neurologic impairment can experience both fever and hypothermia as a result of damage of the hypothalamus. If a patient becomes hypothermic, the nurse carefully uses heat lamps, warmed blankets, and an increase in the room temperature to help restore the patient's temperature to the normal range.

5. Preventing Injury

Numerous nursing activities are geared toward providing a safe environment for the patient experiencing altered LOC. The nurse inspects the patient's environment for equipment that may present a hazard. Call bells should be left within reach, and the patient is instructed on how to use the device. Adaptive call bells are available for patients with limited motor abilities. When patients are unable to care for themselves, the nursing staff provides hygiene, eye care, and skin care to protect sensitive tissue. Seizure precautions may be appropriate for patients with a demonstrated history or suspected risk of seizures.

Patients with limited mobility also present safety risks. Some patients may need a "seat belt" or slide cushion to prevent them from slipping or falling out of chairs. Confused patients may attempt to climb out of bed or wander off, but physical restraints are used only as a last resort. Restraints have been consistently shown to increase patient agitation and actually increase the risk of injury.

The bed is kept in a low position. The nurse changes the patient's position frequently and provides regular opportunities for the patient to meet elimination needs. Assisting the patient in being out of bed as much as desired may prevent the patient from trying to get up on his or her own. This behavior cannot always be prevented but is sometimes a response to muscle aches, thirst, the need to urinate, or simple loneliness. Frequent visits and monitoring are essential. Simple reorienting and reassurance can be calming for agitated or confused patients. The nurse uses touch therapeutically with patients who respond positively to it. Electronic monitoring systems can be useful for patients who wander. These systems alert the staff when a patient moves outside the monitored area.

6. Promoting Mobility

The nurse positions patients who are unable to move themselves and performs range-of-motion exercise to prevent contractures and other musculoskeletal complications. Changes of position also help patients who are unable to move themselves to mobilize pulmonary secretions. Getting patients out of bed and assisting them with ambulation supports weight bearing on the long bones and slows the bone demineralization associated with bed rest. An upright posture also improves the patient's ability to interact with the environment. The physical therapist may recommend specific activities to promote mobility and supply adaptive equipment, such as walkers, canes, or wheelchairs, that can increase the patient's independence.

7. Supporting Nutrition

Decreased LOC makes it difficult for patients to meet their ongoing nutritional needs, particularly if they also have swallowing difficulties. Adequate nutrition is essential to prevent infection and protect tissue integrity. The nurse keeps records of the patient's food and fluid intake so that accurate assessments can be made. The nurse works with the dietitian to determine the best diet to meet patient needs. The patient may simply need reminders to take small bites and swallow carefully, but if the patient is unable to maintain an adequate oral intake without aspiration, enteral feedings may be started. Nasogastric tubes can be used for short-term feeding. If long-term nutritional support is anticipated, a gastrostomy, percutaneous endoscopic gastrostomy (PEG), or jejunostomy tube is placed (see Chapter 33). Daily or weekly weights are obtained to monitor the patient's status.

8. Promoting Bowel Elimination

Patients with altered LOC need to be started on a bowel program, especially if they are on bed rest, which increases the risk of constipation or impaction. The nurse uses preventive measures such as stool softeners, fiber added to tube feedings or diet, and additional hydration to prevent constipation. The patient is offered the bedpan or placed on a commode at times close to the patient's usual time for elimination, such as in the morning after breakfast. If constipation is suspected, the nurse checks the patient for impaction and gently removes the stool if needed. Mild laxatives or suppositories can also be used to treat constipation, but enemas are used only as a last resort because of their tendency to completely disrupt the normal elimination pattern.

The need for communication among the nursing staff about the patient's bowel function is especially important. Bowel movements are carefully recorded as to time, amount, and consistency to enable the nurse to make appropriate judgments about the need for timely intervention to support elimination.

9. Supporting Urinary Elimination

Indwelling catheters may be used in the acute care setting if frequent monitoring of urine output is required, but they are avoided for long-term management, if possible, because of the high risk of chronic infection. A condom catheter can be used for incontinent male patients, but female patients may require the ongoing use of an indwelling catheter. Some neurologic conditions cause urinary retention and necessitate the use of either an indwelling catheter or an intermittent catheterization program. When patients are able to communicate their needs, the nurse attempts to establish a regular schedule for bladder emptying that eliminates the need for catheters or diapers.

10. Maintaining Skin Integrity

Patients with altered LOC are prone to skin breakdown. Agitated patients may accidentally abrade their skin or bruise themselves if not protected. Immobilized patients need frequent position changes, and their skin must be kept clean and free of excess moisture but well lubricated to prevent dryness. Patients on prolonged bed rest or with actual skin breakdown are placed on special pressure relief mattresses. Adequate nutrition and hydration contribute greatly to the maintenance of skin integrity. The nurse carefully assesses the patient's skin during hygiene activities and protects the patient's skin from friction and shearing forces during position changes or when assisting the patient out of bed.

11. Facilitating Self-Care

Patients with altered LOC may be unable to meet their own self-care needs. Some patients may require simple assistance with activities of daily living (ADLs), such as supervision or verbal cueing during bathing or dressing. Others require the complete support of the nursing staff to complete hygiene activities. Engaging in self-care is an important part of rehabilitation. This may include bathing, hair shampooing, mouth care, eye care, and nail care. The nurse gives special attention to the skin in the axilla and perineal area and any skinfolds that might retain moisture, such as the skin under the breast. These areas are particularly vulnerable to breakdown and infection with yeast and other organisms.

12. Supporting the Family

Patients with altered LOC may be unaware of the severity of their situation, but the family is acutely aware. This awareness creates great anxiety and stress related to the crisis of a sudden illness or injury. The family may also need to make decisions about the patient's care, for which they may feel unprepared. The nurse listens carefully to family members' concerns and assesses their ability to cope. The nurse clarifies which family member usually helps the patient with health care decisions. The nurse then explores what information that person needs in order to make current decisions and asks if the patient has a living will or advance directive that can be used to guide decision making.

It is also important to find out what resources the family uses for support. Extended family, neighbors, and church friends are possible sources of support. The nurse ensures that the family is aware of other resources that are available, such as chaplains, social workers, and community groups appropriate to the patient's illness.

The nurse explains the hospital routines and surroundings to the patient and family to make the environment seem less foreign. The family is directed to a quiet place where they can sit, make phone calls, and wait while the patient is being cared for. When family members are in the patient's room, the nurse provides them with chairs and encourages them to touch and talk to the patient. Some institutions allow families to participate in care delivery. When the family leaves the hospital, they should be given a phone number that they can use to check on the patient's progress and talk to the nurse or the patient if he or she is able.

13. Patient/Family Education

Altered LOC may leave patients with deficits that profoundly affect many aspects of their lives and independence. Patients may not be able to resume their normal lifestyle because they have motor, sensory, or cognitive deficits that create safety concerns and interfere with their ability to be independent.

The patient's educational background and current cognitive abilities affect his or her ability to be involved in the education process. The patient and family need education about the diagnostic process and results, treatment options, and how the treatment plan will be carried out. As care is delivered, the nurse provides the patient and family with feedback about the progress of the treatments, as well as any changes that are made in the plan of care. Discharge planning involves identifying community resources and making appropriate referrals to ensure continuity of care. The nurse prepares a teaching plan to prepare the family for any care that the family will need to provide to the patient at home after discharge.

Health Promotion/Prevention

Specific disease processes that cause altered LOC cannot always be prevented. However, altered LOC resulting from medication side effects and other situational factors may be prevented by altering or eliminating the causative factor.

EVALUATION

Evaluation of care is an ongoing process. The current assessment is compared with the expected patient outcomes. Achievement of patient outcomes is successful if the patient:

1. Shows no evidence of aspiration; has strong cough, clear breath sounds, respiratory rate of 12 to 20 breaths/min, and pulse oximetry above 90%.
2. Has systemic blood pressure and cerebral perfusion pressure within normal ranges.
3. Is alert and oriented to the surroundings; shows no evidence of confusion.
4. Has body temperature within normal limits.
5. Shows no sign of physical injury; environment is uncluttered.

6. Uses assistive devices as needed to move about in the environment.
7. Takes a balanced oral diet; maintains stable body weight.
8. Uses diet, fluids, and stool softeners to maintain regular bowel elimination.
9. Follows a bladder training program to maintain continence.
10. Skin is intact without evidence of redness or breakdown.
11. Uses adaptive aids and assistive equipment to maintain self-care in ADLs.
12. Family uses coping strategies to plan effectively for patient's care.
13. Patient and family participate in planning for care after discharge.

GERONTOLOGIC CONSIDERATIONS

The healthy older adult should not experience memory loss, dementia, depression, or any decrease in LOC. All of these changes are considered unexpected and should be investigated and treated. Older adults do experience a reduction in the speed of their reflexes, and they are prone to decreases in vision and hearing that may affect their ability to interact with those around them. These sensory losses are usually treatable and need to be addressed so that the patient can continue to participate fully in education and self-care activities.

The older adult is more likely to experience comorbid medical problems and therefore is more likely to be taking multiple medications. Medication interactions or sensitivity to side effects may account for some alterations in cognition and awareness.

SPECIAL ENVIRONMENTS FOR CARE

Critical Care

The critical care environment can have serious effects on the patient with altered LOC. An emergent admission to a critical care unit can be frightening and confusing if the high-tech environment is not carefully explained to the patient and family. Sedation and pain medication may be given to help patients tolerate the discomfort of invasive lines, endotracheal tubes, and mechanical ventilation. Careful assessment must be ongoing to ensure that the patient receives sufficient medication to be comfortable but is not oversedated, masking changes in LOC. Other measures to increase comfort may be implemented, such as frequent repositioning, back rubs, or allowing the patient to choose soothing music or favorite TV shows.

For long-term patients in the intensive care unit (ICU), the noise and constant stimulation can lead to a type of altered LOC termed *ICU psychosis.* The patient becomes confused and agitated without discernible physiologic cause. Altering the patient's plan of care to include adequate periods of uninterrupted sleep at night and decreasing meaningless stimulation such as monitor alarms or intercom use may help alleviate this problem. Having the patient decide how and when some of his or her care is to be done and grouping care activities so that the patient may rest in between activities allows some control over care. Adequate pain control is also important.

Community-Based Care

The amount and complexity of care that is being delivered in the community setting continues to increase. Supplemental oxygen and respiratory therapy treatments, intravenous (IV) fluids and medications, and enteral or parenteral nutrition are all routinely provided to patients in their homes. When a patient with altered LOC needs ongoing nursing care at home, the nursing staff of the inpatient setting carefully assesses the patient's needs and the available resources in the community for care, family support, and respite care. If home care needs to be provided by the family, the nursing staff is also responsible for ensuring their knowledge and skill before discharge. Arranging needed services takes time, and the nurse needs to anticipate discharge to allow sufficient time for planning, teaching and referral.

COMPLICATIONS

Complications of altered LOC are discussed under the specific disease process causing the condition. Many complications are related to immobility or the failure to meet basic care needs. General guidelines for care of a patient with decreased LOC are summarized in the Guidelines for Safe Practice box.

INCREASED INTRACRANIAL PRESSURE

Etiology/Epidemiology

An increase in intracranial pressure (ICP) is a pathologic process common to many neurologic conditions. The intracranial volume is composed of brain tissue (85%), intracranial blood volume (5%), and cerebrospinal fluid (CSF) (10%). An increase in the volume of any of these contents, singly or in combination, results in an increase in ICP because the cranial vault is rigid and nonexpandable. Any lesion that increases one or more of the intracranial contents is considered a space-occupying lesion.[8] Common examples are listed in Box 42-7. Increased ICP is a common concern with a number of neurologic conditions, but no data are available concerning the incidence or distribution of this condition.

Pathophysiology

The cranial vault is a rigid, closed compartment. The intracranial contents of brain, blood, and CSF fully occupy the vault and exist in a dynamic equilibrium under normal conditions. The Monro-Kellie hypothesis states that conditions that increase one or more of the intracranial contents must cause a reciprocal change in the remaining contents or an increase in ICP will occur.[8] As the intracranial volume increases, compensatory mechanisms take place. CSF-filled spaces can be compressed and CSF redistributed to the lumbar cistern to reduce intracranial CSF volumes. Intracranial blood vessels, especially the veins, can be compressed by surrounding brain tissue and displace intracranial blood volume. These compensatory mechanisms initially are able to accommodate a growing intracranial volume without significant increases in ICP, but these mechanisms are quickly exhausted if the intracranial volume continues to increase.

Guidelines for Safe Practice

The Patient With Decreased Level of Consciousness or Coma

1. Protect airway and promote gas exchange.
   a. Turn side to side every 2 hours.
   b. Encourage coughing and deep breathing every hour while awake.
   c. Suction oral and pharyngeal airway as needed.
   d. Monitor oxygen saturation and blood gases.
2. Promote cerebral tissue perfusion.
   a. Maintain hydration; prevent hypovolemia.
   b. Monitor effects of antihypertensive, antidysrhythmic medications and promote adequate cardiac output and systemic blood pressure.
3. Promote tissue perfusion.
   a. Turn every 2 hours.
   b. Perform passive or active range of motion to enhance circulation at least once per shift.
   c. Apply elastic stockings or intermittent compression devices to prevent deep vein thrombosis.
4. Promote sensory-perceptual function.
   a. Provide meaningful stimuli.
   b. Speak to patient before touching.
   c. Orient patient to surroundings.
   d. Provide adequate lighting.
   e. Have calendar and clock within patient's view.
   f. Have familiar objects in patient's view.
5. Maintain normal body temperature.
   a. Hyperthermia
      (1) Remove excess bed coverings.
      (2) Maintain cool room temperature.
      (3) Administer antipyretic medications.
      (4) Provide tepid bath.
   b. Hypothermia
      (1) Apply warmed blankets.
      (2) Use heat lamps with caution.
      (3) Increase room temperature.
6. Prevent injury.
   a. Keep call bell within reach.
   b. Implement seizure precautions as needed.
   c. Provide eye care to prevent corneal damage at least once per shift.
   d. Apply restraints only as a last resort, with physician's order.
7. Promote mobility.
   a. Perform active or passive range of motion every shift.
   b. Assist patient with ambulation or position changes.
8. Maintain nutrition.
   a. Record intake to assess quantity and quality.
   b. Assist patient with feeding and swallowing safely, with instructions to take small bites and chew carefully.
   c. Administer enteral feedings at recommended rate for needs.
   d. Weigh patient daily or weekly to assess gain or loss.
9. Maintain regular bowel function.
   a. Provide adequate hydration.
   b. Ensure adequate fiber in diet or tube feedings.
   c. Administer stool softeners as needed.
10. Maintain bladder continence.
    a. Remove indwelling catheters as soon as possible.
    b. Provide regular toileting to prevent incontinence.
11. Maintain hygiene.
    a. Assist patient with activities of daily living as needed.
    b. If patient is unable to care for self, provide bath, mouth, eye, and skin care regularly.
    c. Shampoo patient's hair as needed.
12. Maintain skin integrity.
    a. Reposition patient at least every 2 hours.
    b. Use lotion or other skin moisturizers to prevent dry skin.
    c. Keep sheets dry and free of wrinkles.
    d. If skin breakdown is present or if patient is at high risk, use pressure relief device.
    e. Avoid shearing and friction when moving patient.
13. Support family coping.
    a. Assess family for usual coping skills and resources used.
    b. Introduce family to new resources available for support.
    c. Listen and address family concerns and provide needed information.
    d. Teach patient care skills needed for home care to family.

BOX 42-7 Space-Occupying Lesions

Edema caused by contusions or infarctions
Subdural hematoma
Epidural hematoma
Intracerebral hematoma
Tumors
Abscesses
Hydrocephalus

When the volume within the skull overwhelms the compensatory mechanisms, ICP begins to rise. The volume-pressure curve is illustrated in Figure 42-6. It shows that small changes in volume initially cause only small increases in pressure. However, as compensatory mechanisms fail, continued increases in volume cause dramatic increases in ICP. A normal ICP is between 0 and 15 mm Hg, and pressures over 20 mm Hg are considered "increased" ICP.

As pressure within the skull increases, the cerebral arteries and veins become increasingly compressed, causing a reduction in cerebral perfusion. Inadequate perfusion initiates a vicious cycle, causing the partial pressure of carbon dioxide (P_{CO_2}) to increase and the partial pressure of oxygen (P_{O_2}) and the pH to decrease. Cerebral arterioles have the ability to autoregulate, dilating or constricting as needed to maintain a constant blood supply to the brain. The increasing P_{CO_2} or decreasing pH associated with decreased perfusion causes vasodilation of the cerebral blood vessels and increases the intracranial blood volume, which contributes to further increases in ICP. Autoregulation is operative as long as the mean

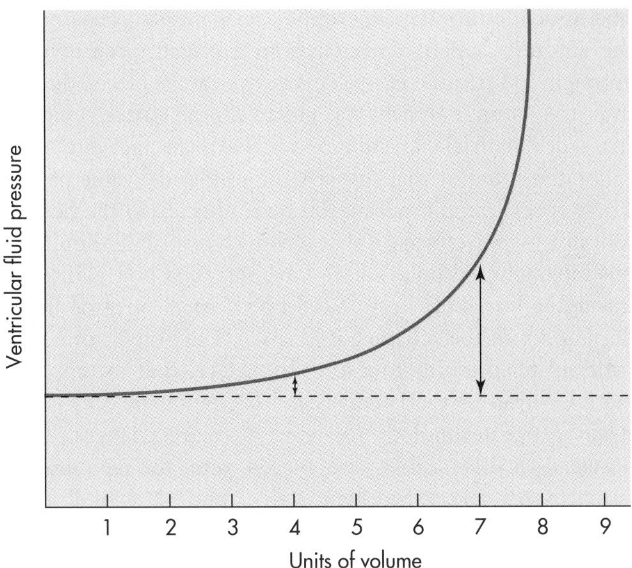

Figure 42-6 Intracranial volume-pressure curve. Note that for the addition of any given unit of volume (abscissa), a markedly different rise in pressure occurs, depending on the location (flat or steep portion) on the curve. Thus adding 1 U of volume at the second arrow results in nearly four times the increase in pressure from the same volume at the first arrow.

arterial pressure (MAP) is between 50 and 150 mm Hg and the metabolic environment of the brain is normal. Severe anoxia and hypotensive states cause a failure in autoregulation, subjecting the blood supply of the brain to the wide variations characteristic of systemic blood pressure.

Cerebral perfusion pressure (CPP) is a parameter used to monitor the adequacy of blood flow to the brain in the face of increased ICP. The systemic blood pressure needs to be high enough to overcome the ICP and deliver adequate amounts of oxygen and glucose to brain tissues. The CPP is measured by subtracting ICP from MAP:

$$CPP = MAP - ICP$$

The CPP is kept above 70 mm Hg to prevent cerebral ischemia. Autoregulation fails at high ICP ranges because the vessels cannot effectively dilate against the pressure of the surrounding brain tissues.

The actual brain structures can also be affected by increased ICP. The brain is surrounded and divided into compartments within the skull by the dura mater. The presence of edema or space-occupying lesions may cause brain tissue to shift or herniate. Subfalcial, or cingulate, herniation occurs when the brain is forced under the falx cerebri that separates the cerebral hemispheres. Uncal herniation occurs when the uncal portions of the temporal lobes shift over the edge of the tentorium cerebelli. Transforaminal herniation occurs when the brainstem is forced downward through the foramen magnum.

Increased ICP produces multiple signs and symptoms, but decreased LOC is the earliest and most sensitive sign. Altered blood flow and an altered cerebral metabolic environment reduce the brain's ability to respond to stimuli (see earlier discussion of altered LOC).

Pupillary responses are controlled by the oculomotor nerve (cranial nerve III), which carries the motor fibers for pupil constriction and eyelid opening. The oculomotor nerve becomes severely compressed when herniation of the uncal portion of the temporal lobe occurs. Dilation of the ipsilateral pupil occurs when the herniation is limited to one hemisphere. If ICP continues to rise and both hemispheres herniate, bilateral pupil dilation and fixation occur. If the nerve is only moderately compressed or stretched, pupil dilation with slowed constriction may be seen. A pupil that is fixed and dilated sometimes is referred to as a blown pupil.

The effect of ICP on blood pressure and pulse is variable. Ischemia in the vasomotor center excites vasoconstrictor fibers throughout the body, causing an increase in systolic blood pressure. The vasomotor center also sends parasympathetic impulses via the vagus nerve to slow the heart rate. A rising systolic blood pressure, widened pulse pressure, and slow heart rate are referred to as Cushing's response and are classic indicators of increased ICP. If the pressure on the brainstem is severe, the vasomotor center is no longer able to function. A drop in blood pressure and an increase in heart rate are seen as the patient's condition continues to deteriorate.[8]

Herniation also produces respiratory dysrhythmias that correspond to the level of brainstem compression (see Figure 42-5). An irregular respiratory pattern or periods of apnea are particularly significant. Cushing's triad adds the symptom of slowed respirations to the bradycardia and rising systolic blood pressure that are already present. Patients with decreasing LOC may have difficulty keeping the airway clear and exhibit shallow respirations that worsen the hypoxia or hypercarbia, which, in turn, worsen the cycle of vasodilation and increased ICP.

Failure of the thermoregulatory center is a late sign of increased ICP. The most common manifestation of this failure is a fever without a clearly identifiable source of infection. Hyperthermia, in turn, increases the metabolic needs of the already-compromised brain tissues and further increases ICP.

The rising pressure compresses the motor and sensory tracts between the primary motor and sensory areas in the frontal and parietal lobes and leads to contralateral loss of motor and sensory function. When disruptions to motor pathways become severe, the patient may exhibit posturing, described earlier in the section on altered LOC. Motor inhibitory fibers from the frontal lobes are blocked, resulting in hyperactive deep tendon reflexes. Damage to the corticospinal tracts also causes positive Babinski's reflexes.

The optic nerve attaches to the eye at the optic disc. The meninges surround both the optic nerve and its attachment to the eye. As ICP increases, the resulting pressure is transmitted to the eyes through the CSF in the subarachnoid space and to the optic disc, causing papilledema (choked disc). This may be a late sign of increased ICP. Other visual acuity changes are related to pressure on or shifting of optic pathways within the brain.

Headache is often an early nonspecific symptom of increased ICP. It is thought to result from tension on intracranial blood vessels. Vomiting may occur, but it is more common in children with increased ICP. A summary of common signs and symptoms of increased ICP is provided in the Clinical Manifestations box.

Collaborative Care Management

Patient outcomes for increased ICP are directly related to the nature of the underlying disease process. The collaborative care of the patient is aimed at controlling and reducing the increased ICP and preventing neurologic damage from herniation. The diagnosis of increased ICP is most accurately made when the pressure is measured by one of several available devices. However, the diagnosis can be made with careful neurologic examination and ongoing assessment when monitoring devices are not readily available.

A head CT scan can demonstrate the structural changes associated with increased ICP and locate space-occupying lesions and sites of edema or bleeding. A reduction in the size of the cisterns, CSF-filled spaces located at the base of the skull, indicates that CSF is being shunted out of the skull as a compensatory mechanism. Any herniation of brain tissue can also be readily identified on CT scans.[6]

Several methods have been developed to directly measure ICP. An intraventricular catheter, also known as a ventriculostomy, can be inserted through the brain and directly into one of the lateral ventricles by means of a small hole drilled into the skull. The catheter is connected to a sterile drainage system with a three-way stopcock that allows simultaneous monitoring of pressures via a transducer connected to a bedside monitor and drainage of CSF. Another approach uses a fiberoptic monitor. The fiberoptic device measures changes in the amount of light reflected from a pressure-sensitive diaphragm in the catheter tip. This device can be placed directly into the brain parenchyma, subarachnoid space, epidural space, or a ventricle. The fiberoptic cable is connected to a precalibrated monitor that displays the numerical value of ICP. These special monitors can also be connected to the bedside monitor for waveform display. A third type of ICP monitor is the subarachnoid bolt. The hollow, threaded bolt is inserted through a burr hole in the skull into a small opening in the dura and into the subarachnoid space. The bolt is connected via fluid-filled tubing to a transducer leveled at the approximate location of the lateral ventricles. A fourth device uses strain gauge technology to detect pressure changes. Thin, pressure-sensitive cables are placed into the epidural or parenchymal spaces. See Figures 42-7 and 42-8 for illustrations of various ICP monitors.

Medications used to treat increased ICP are selected on the basis of the underlying pathology. Osmotic diuretics such as IV mannitol (Osmitrol) or urea promote fluid removal from edematous brain tissue. Corticosteroids such as dexamethasone (Decadron) may be used to reduce the edema associated with tumors or abscesses. Anticonvulsant medication may also be prescribed to prevent seizures. Antibiotics may be prescribed if the patient has an ICP monitoring device in place.[10,19] Opioids and sedative medications are used cautiously because of their respiratory depressant effects. Opioids and sedatives may also alter the patient's ability to cooperate with an accurate neurologic examination.

Barbiturate coma is occasionally used for patients who do not respond to conventional management of elevated ICP. Large doses of barbiturates, usually pentobarbital, are given to slow the cerebral metabolic rate and minimize the damage caused by ICP-induced ischemia. The barbiturate coma is accompanied by numerous side effects, such as hypotension, that may require vasoactive drug treatment (e.g., dopamine infusion).[6] The high doses of barbiturate also obscure the accuracy of any neurologic assessment for the duration of the coma.

Surgical interventions are also designed to correct the underlying cause of the increase in ICP. Mass lesions such as tumors, abscesses, or hematomas are surgically removed if possible. Excess CSF can be removed with a surgically placed ventriculostomy. If hydrocephalus becomes a chronic problem, a shunt from the lateral ventricle to the peritoneum can be placed for long-term CSF drainage. On rare occasions a decompressive craniectomy may be performed to remove part of the skull and allow the edematous brain to expand. The bone can be replaced at a later date after the edema has resolved.[8]

Hyperventilation of the intubated patient decreases the $Paco_2$ and causes vasoconstriction of the cerebral blood vessels. This intervention is used commonly to temporarily help control ICP. However, if ongoing reductions in $Paco_2$ are needed, the vasoconstriction can lead to brain tissue ischemia (see Evidence-Based Practice box). A balance is sought that keeps the $Paco_2$ in the low-normal range of 30 to 35 mm Hg to prevent hypercapnea and subsequent vasodilation but does

Clinical Manifestations
Increased Intracranial Pressure

EARLY SIGNS

- Decreasing level of consciousness
  - Earliest and most sensitive sign
- Headache that increases in intensity with coughing, straining
- Pupillary changes
  - Dilation with slowed constriction
  - Visual disturbances such as diplopia
  - Ptosis
- Contralateral motor or sensory losses

LATE SIGNS

- Further decrease in level of consciousness
- Changes in vital signs
  - Rise in systolic blood pressure
  - Decrease in diastolic blood pressure
  - Widened pulse pressure
  - Slow pulse
- Respiratory dysrhythmias
  - Shallow, slowed respirations
  - Irregular patterns or periods of apnea
  - Hiccups
- Fever without a clear source of infection
- Vomiting (more common in children)
- Decerebrate or decorticate posturing

not reduce the Pa_{CO_2} to a level that results in vasoconstriction-induced brain ischemia.[2]

Control of activity plays an important role in the treatment of increased ICP. The pressure inside the skull is dynamic and changes in response to shifts in blood flow, CSF movement, and brain tissue edema. When the compensatory mechanisms are intact, transient increases in ICP are very brief and baseline normal values are rapidly restored. When compensatory mechanisms have been exhausted, however, the rise in ICP may be more dramatic and take much longer to return to

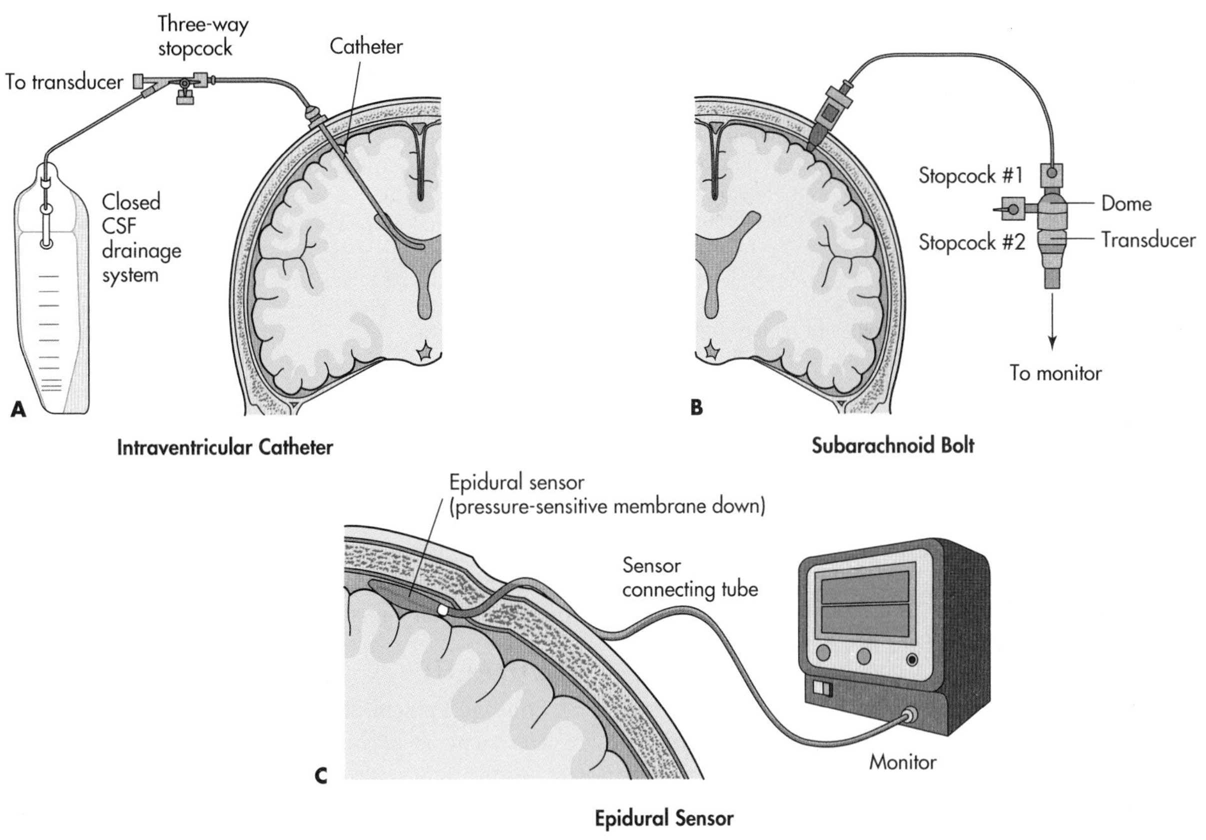

Figure 42-7 **A,** Intraventricular catheter monitoring system with a closed cerebrospinal fluid drainage system. **B,** Subarachnoid bolt monitoring system. **C,** Epidural monitoring system.

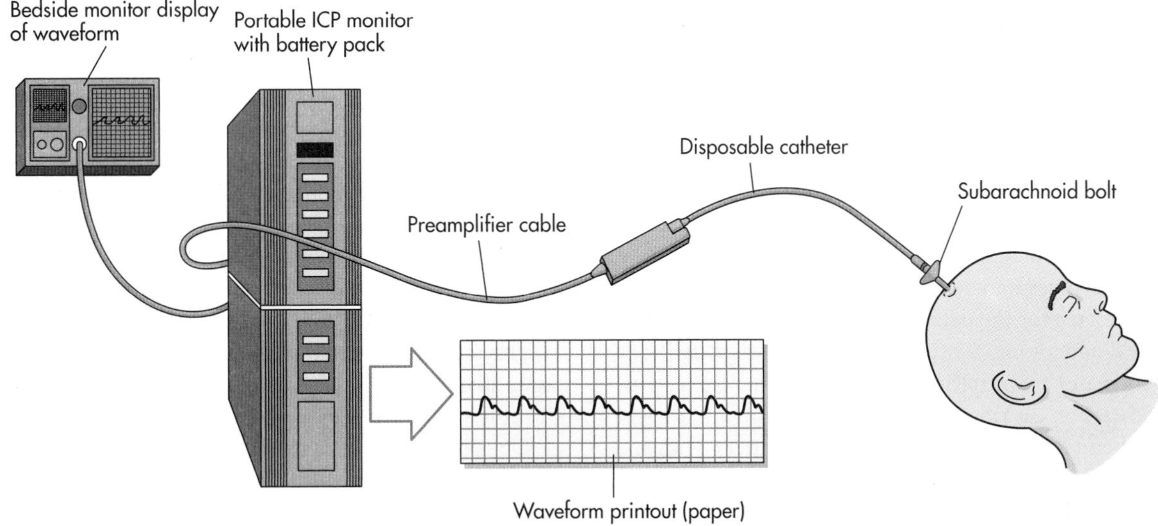

Figure 42-8 Fiberoptic monitoring system using the subarachnoid bolt *(patient),* disposable catheter connected to a preamplifier cable with continuous visual intracranial pressure (ICP) waveform display on the bedside monitor *(upper left),* and a continuous digital readout of ICP *(lower monitor)* with an ICP waveform printout.

Evidence-Based Practice

Reference: Brain Trauma Foundation; American Association of Neurological Surgeons: The joint section on neurotrauma and critical care: the role of steroids, *J Neurotrauma* 17(6/7):531-535, 2000.

The immediate administration of corticosteroids following spinal cord injury has made a significant impact on the severity of functional damage caused by the process of secondary injury. It was hoped that a similar intervention might have a positive impact on outcomes following traumatic head injury as well. This study reviewed the evidence of a decade of steroid administration following head injury and concluded that the administration of steroids to severely head-injured patients does not improve outcomes or lower intracranial pressure. It is acknowledged that an increased understanding of the complex variables associated with secondary brain injury may eventually uncover a role for steroids in the treatment of brain injury, but at the moment their routine use can no longer be recommended.

The study went on to evaluate the place of hyperventilation therapy in the treatment of traumatic brain injury. Although of proven effectiveness in lowering elevated intracranial pressure, hyperventilation was not associated with any clinical improvement and instead was potentially deleterious because it could contribute to cerebral ischemia. Prolonged hyperventilation therapy is therefore recommended for use only when documented elevations in intracranial pressure are present.

normal. The patient's ICP response to any and all activities and treatments is therefore monitored, and activities are restricted as needed.

The patient's neck is kept in proper alignment to promote venous drainage through the jugular veins (see Research box).[21] In some cases a cervical collar may be used to maintain the alignment. The head of the bed may also be elevated to promote venous drainage from the skull.[28] Activities that increase intrathoracic or intraabdominal pressure, such as coughing, straining to have a bowel movement, or moving in bed, may also increase ICP by interfering with venous drainage from the brain. These activities are prevented or avoided if possible.[8] Involuntary patient responses such as shivering, vomiting, agitation, or abnormal posturing also contribute to increased ICP. If increases in ICP become severe during these activities and do not promptly return to baseline, the patient may need to be sedated to decrease activity.

Nurses carefully time and coordinate the patient's care to prevent prolonged increases in ICP. Activities such as bathing and position changes may need to be alternated with rest periods to allow time for the patient's ICP to return to baseline.[8] Endotracheal suctioning contributes to increases in ICP because of increases in intrathoracic pressure and changes in oxygen and carbon dioxide levels. Preoxygenation and hyperventilation before suctioning the ventilated patient with increased ICP helps to minimize this problem (see Guidelines for Safe Practice box).

Patient/Family Education. The presence or risk of ICP creates a frightening and confusing situation for both patients and families. Patients are more likely to cooperate with the

Research

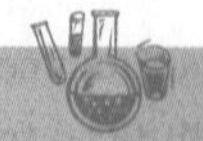

Reference: Sullivan J: Positioning of patients with severe traumatic brain injury: research-based practice, *J Neurosci Nurs* 32(4):204-209, 2000.

Traumatic brain injuries are the most common disabling injuries in the United States and account for over 40% of all trauma deaths. The primary injury is usually irreversible, and emergency interventions have focused on identifying interventions that can prevent or reduce the severity of the process of secondary brain injury. This study focused on the variable of head positioning in adults with traumatic brain injury. The analysis revealed that both intracranial pressure and cerebral perfusion pressure were important variables in determining outcomes, and that both variables needed to be monitored. Optimal outcomes for patients were associated with clinical decision making that avoided broad general rules and instead based positioning recommendations on the individual monitoring parameters of each patient.

need for frequent neurologic checks if the reason for them is explained. Patient and family education includes information about the underlying disease process and its relationship to increased ICP. As treatments and medications are introduced, the nurse explains their purpose to the patient and family. When patients are unable to care for themselves, the nurse includes the family in providing care and encourages them to touch and speak quietly with the patient.

HEADACHE

Etiology/Epidemiology

Headache is a common symptom of many neurologic conditions and is also a unique disease process. Headaches are classified by the International Headache Society as primary or secondary.[8] Primary headaches are not associated with any other known pathologic cause. Examples of primary headaches include migraine, tension, and cluster headaches. Secondary headaches are caused by a known pathologic condition such as meningitis, tumors, or subarachnoid hemorrhage. This section focuses on the care of the patient with a primary headache.

Migraines occur more often in women than in men and most commonly begin between adolescence and age 24. They demonstrate a strong hereditary pattern, but no specific genetic link has been identified.[12] Tension headaches can occur at any age and are typically associated with stress. No epidemiologic pattern has been identified for cluster headaches.

Pathophysiology

The pathophysiology of headache is not fully understood. Some structures of the head are incapable of sensing pain. The structures that are capable of feeling pain are the skin, muscles, periosteum of the skull, eyes, ears, nasal cavities and sinuses, meninges, cerebral blood vessels, and cranial nerves with sensory function. Pain is caused by traction, stretching, or movement of structures or by vasodilation of blood vessels. Serotonin is the primary neurotransmitter found in the pathways involved in headache, but its role is not fully understood.

Migraines are believed to be caused when cerebral blood vessels narrow and blood flow is reduced to some areas of the brain.[7] The initial vasoconstriction is followed by significant vasodilation and inflammation of the blood vessels, which triggers a release of serotonin and causes the headache.[12] Migraines vary in duration, frequency, and intensity from patient to patient and from episode to episode in the same patient.

Cluster headaches are thought to be similar to migraines, but the episodes are brief, usually lasting 45 minutes or less. They occur in "cluster" periods of weeks or months. Tension headaches are the result of stress-induced muscle tension over the neck, scalp, and face of the patient. These headaches are associated with the stresses of daily life. Table 42-1 compares the three major types of primary headaches.

Some headaches are preceded by prodromal signs and symptoms, or aurae. The aura occurs before the acute attack and may include visual field defects such as "flashing lights," photophobia, confusion, or paresthesias. Aurae typically last an hour or more. These symptoms are associated with the reduction in cerebral blood flow that precedes the vasodilation of the migraine.[12]

Collaborative Care Management

The diagnosis of headache is made from the patient's history. Careful questioning can help rule out secondary headaches caused by other illnesses. Headache caused by subarachnoid hemorrhage is sudden, severe, and generalized. Meningitis headaches are also generalized and severe and may radiate down the neck. Brain tumors can also cause headaches, usually as a result of increased ICP. These headaches may occur more often with straining, coughing, exertion, or sudden movement. Imaging studies such as CT and magnetic resonance imaging (MRI) are not usually performed unless symptoms suggestive of other neurologic processes are present.

Assessment parameters for headache are outlined in Box 42-8. The International Headache Society has developed specific criteria for the diagnosis of primary headache that include the presence or absence of an aura, presence or absence of nausea or vomiting, frequency, duration, location, aggravating factors such as exercise, severity of pain, and presence of photophobia.[12,22] Characteristic migraine symptoms include headaches that are preceded by an aura, are slow in onset, and build in intensity. Migraines are also often accompanied by other symptoms such as nausea and vomiting or photophobia.

The patient may be asked to keep a headache diary in which the events surrounding the occurrence of headache, such as food intake, sleep pattern, stressful events, stage of the menstrual cycle, and medication use, are recorded. By providing clues to headache triggers, the diary aids in the design of an individualized plan of care to prevent future attacks.

Medications for the treatment of headache fall into two broad categories: symptom relief and prevention. Symptomatic relief for mild, infrequent headache pain can usually be found with ibuprofen (Motrin), propoxyphene (Darvon), or codeine.

Guidelines for Safe Practice

The Patient With Increased Intracranial Pressure

1. Avoid hypotension (systolic blood pressure <90 mm Hg) and hypoxia (Pao_2 <60).
2. Elevate head of bed (check to see if spine films have been done and cleared for raising head of bed).
3. Avoid jugular venous outflow obstruction. (Keep neck midline, cervical collar or endotracheal tube tape not too tight; check collar frequently when edema is developing.)
4. Prevent or avoid coughing, Valsalva's maneuver, hip flexion, high levels of positive end-expiratory pressure.
5. Maintain normothermia. Work up and treat fever promptly.
6. Prevent seizures. Phenytoin is used to prevent early posttraumatic seizures. Fosphenytoin is a prodrug of phenytoin that causes fewer side effects when given intravenously and may be given in some circumstances.
7. Prevent or treat agitation. Search for causes of agitation, such as hypoxia or pain. Sedation with short-acting agents allows for neurologic monitoring. Pharmacologic paralysis may be used if sedation alone is inadequate in controlling agitation that contributes to increased intracranial pressure (ICP).
8. Monitor ICP to serve as an indicator of mass effect, to calculate cerebral perfusion pressure (CPP), and to assess effectiveness of interventions. Treatment for high ICP usually begins at 20 mm Hg. Ventriculostomies may be used if the patient has intraventricular blood or hydrocephalus.
9. CPP should be calculated if an ICP monitor is in use. (CPP = MAP − ICP.) The CPP should be kept above 70 mm Hg to prevent cerebral ischemia. Maintaining adequate CPP may be done with fluid resuscitation, by lowering the ICP, or by adding vasopressor support to the systemic blood pressure (BP).
10. Mannitol: osmotic diuretic used to treat cerebral edema. Usually given in bolus doses of 0.25 to 1.0 g/kg. Need to monitor for serum osmolarity of greater than 310 to 320 mOsm/L and effect of fluid and electrolyte shifts. Can contribute to dehydration and to decrease in BP and CPP.
11. Surgical intervention: surgical evacuation of hematomas or skull fracture repair. On some rare occasions a piece of skull may be removed and left off to allow the brain more room to swell (craniectomy).
12. Hyperventilation may be used initially in resuscitation when information about ICP is not readily available; may be used acutely for herniation. In general, ventilated patients will have their setting adjusted to keep Pco_2 between 30 and 35 mm Hg. Hyperventilating (and hyperoxygenating) patients before, during, and after endotracheal suctioning is still recommended to reduce the adverse effects of sudden rises in ICP with coughing and suctioning.
13. Barbiturates may be used but have significant complications. They work by reducing cerebral metabolic needs and cerebral blood flow. Monitoring of EEG burst suppression is suggested.

Adapted from Bullock MR, Povlishock JT: Guidelines for the management of severe head injury, *J Neurotrauma* 17(6/7):463-469, 2000.
MAP, Mean arterial pressure; *EEG*, electroencephalographic.

TABLE 42-1 Comparison of Migraine, Cluster, and Tension Headaches

Onset	Frequency/Duration	Pattern	Prodromal-Associated Symptoms	Treatment
Migraine Headaches				
Occur at any age Strongly hereditary More common in women than in men	Episodic; tend to occur with stress or life crisis Last hours to days	Occur slowly; pain becomes severe, with one side of head affected more than other	Prodromal: visual field defects, confusion, paresthesias Associated: nausea, vomiting, chills, fatigue, irritability, sweating, edema	Ergotamine tartrate Propranolol Nonopioid analgesics Relaxation techniques
Cluster Headaches				
Early adulthood; precipitated by alcohol or nitrate use More common in older men	Episodes clustered together in quick succession for a few days or weeks with remissions that last for months Last minutes to a few hours	Intense, throbbing, deep, often unilateral pain; begins in infraorbital region and spreads to head and neck	Prodromal: usually none Associated: flushing, tearing of eyes, nasal stuffiness, sweating, swelling of temporal vessels	Opioid analgesics during acute phase, often given intramuscularly
Tension Headaches				
Often in adolescence; related to tension or anxiety No family history	Episodic; vary with stress Duration is variable; can be constant	Dull, constant, aggravating pain; varies in intensity; usually bilateral and involves neck and shoulders; pain may be poorly defined	Prodromal: usually none Associated: sustained contraction of head and neck muscles Not aggravated by activity	Nonopioid analgesics Relaxation techniques Amitriptyline (Elavil)

BOX 42-8 Headache Assessment

- *Headache characteristics:* time of onset, location, frequency, severity, duration, quality (deep, superficial, steady, throbbing, stabbing, burning); situations or activities that make the headache better or worse
- *Presence of an aura:* duration, relation to onset of pain
- *Associated symptoms occurring before, during, or after a headache:* nausea, vomiting, photophobia, visual disturbances, dizziness, incoordination, redness of the eye, facial symptoms (sweating, paleness, flushing), fatigue or sleepiness, mood swings, weakness, paresthesia
- *Potential precipitating factors:* change in eating pattern, dietary substances (e.g., tyramine, nitrates), relationship to menstrual cycle, sexual intercourse, pregnancy, menopause, psychosocial stressors, change in sleep pattern, weather changes, hot or cold wind, altitude, lights, smog
- *Activities of daily living patterns:* eating, sleeping, exercise, relaxation
- *Drug history:* over-the-counter and prescribed headache medications, other medications (nitroglycerin, reserpine, birth control pills, vitamin A, indomethacin, hormone replacement), alcohol and drug use, smoking history
- *Medical history:* asthma; peptic ulcer; motion sickness; head injury; seizure disorder; sleepwalking; Raynaud's disease; irritable bowel syndrome; infertility; skin problems; pain in neck, head, or throat; abdominal distress; anxiety; depression; insomnia
- *Family history:* history of headache and other medical problems

NOTE: A headache daily diary must include a complete description of each headache, precipitating events, associated symptoms, and in women, the relationship to the menstrual cycle.

Adapted from Barker E: *Neuroscience nursing,* St Louis, 1994, Mosby.

Sumatriptan (Imitrex), a serotonin receptor agonist that causes vasoconstriction, is the first-line drug for treating a migraine headache. It can be given by mouth or subcutaneously and is administered at the first sign or symptom of the attack.[14] Ergot alkaloids, such as dihydroergotamine mesylate (D.H.E. 45) and ergotamine plus caffeine (Cafergot), are other drugs used to cause cerebral vasoconstriction and abort the attack. Opioids are rarely used for headache pain because of concerns over drug dependency. Antiemetics such as promethazine (Phenergan) or metoclopramide (Reglan) may be given to relieve associated symptoms of nausea and vomiting.

Other drugs are used to prevent migraines. Propranolol (Inderal) is a beta-blocker that inhibits vasodilation of cerebral blood vessels and inhibits the reuptake of serotonin. Amitripty-

TABLE 42-2 Common Medications for Headache

Drug	Action	Intervention
Symptomatic Treatment		
Ergot alkaloids	Causes cerebral vasoconstriction	Take as soon as migraine symptoms begin.
Ergotamine tartrate plus caffeine (Cafergot)	Decreases pulsation of cranial arteries	Nausea is a common side effect; patients may also need to use antiemetics.
Dihydroergotamine (D.H.E. 45)		Ergots have a cumulative effect; use sparingly and monitor for signs of ergotism—numbness and tingling, weakness, muscle pain.
Metoclopramide (Reglan)	Increases gastrointestinal motility to decrease incidence of nausea and vomiting	Patient should avoid driving or other hazardous activity after taking drug.
Sumatriptan (Imitrex)	Serotonin receptor agonist; causes vasoconstriction	Drug is contraindicated in pregnancy and coronary artery disease. Teach patient to take drug at first sign of a headache.
Prophylaxis		
Beta-blockers Propranolol (Inderal) Nadolol (Corgard) Atenolol (Tenormin) Timolol (Betimol) Metoprolol (Lopressor)	Inhibit vasodilation and serotonin uptake; propranolol is first drug of choice for prophylaxis of migraines	Drug may cause cardiac dysfunction; monitor for bradycardia, orthostatic hypotension, lethargy, depression.
Tricyclic antidepressants Amitriptyline (Elavil)	Block uptake of serotonin and catecholamines Most effective for migraine-associated tension headaches Alternative if beta-blockers are not tolerated	Drug may cause dry mouth, drowsiness, and urinary retention.
Methysergide (Sansert)	Used for migraine prophylaxis	Patient should avoid driving if drowsiness occurs and maintain a liberal fluid intake.

line (Elavil) is a tricyclic antidepressant used to block the uptake of catecholamines and serotonin.[25] Hydrochlorothiazide (HCTZ) or other diuretics may be given in low doses to prevent fluid retention, which can lead to migraines. Table 42-2 presents an overview of drugs commonly used to treat headache.

Other treatments for headache also attempt to prevent the attack or provide symptomatic relief. About one third of patients with migraine or tension headaches can be helped with biofeedback or relaxation techniques.[12] For patients who already have a headache, lying quietly in a darkened room and getting additional sleep offer some relief from pain. Chronic headache is a problem that is often self-treated using alternative and complementary therapies, and it is important for the nurse to carefully explore these practices during the patient assessment (see Complementary & Alternative Therapies box).

Once the patient has kept a headache diary, it may be possible for the nurse to assist the patient to identify specific foods that trigger headache and should be reduced or eliminated from the diet. Headache triggers can be confirmed by excluding them from the diet and monitoring the patient for the recurrence of symptoms. Foods that have been shown to cause cerebrovasodilation in migraine patients are nitrites, nitrates, tyramines, alcohol, monosodium glutamate, and caffeine. Eating small, frequent meals also helps to prevent fluctuations in glucose and serotonin levels. Fasting increases serotonin turnover in the brain, which can lead to vasodilation and trigger a headache. Nicotine has also been associated with an increased incidence of headache, and the nurse advises the patient to quit smoking, initiates referral to a smoking cessation program, and cautions the patient to avoid the use of nicotine gum or patches.[12] A high salt intake may lead to fluid retention, which is a problem for some women who

Complementary & Alternative Therapies
Chronic Headache

Alternative therapies have a long history of use in the treatment of selected neurologic disorders, and it is important for all health care professionals to be aware of the possible therapies that may be explored and their relative safety and efficacy for use in the management of selected disorders. Headaches and seizure disorders are two of the more common applications. Possible interventions include massage and relaxation therapy, biofeedback, energetic healing, aromatherapy, reiki, chakra balancing, yoga, and tai chi. Nurses need to incorporate these practices into their assessments of neurologic patients. This becomes even more important when patients are using herbal preparations that could negatively interact with prescription medications. All nurses need to be skilled in interviewing patients about their use of alternative medicine and encourage them to share all of this information with their primary care provider.

experience migraines around the time of their menstrual cycle. Oral contraceptives should not be used by migraine sufferers because of a recognized correlation between oral contraceptive use and an increase in migraine incidence.[12]

Vigorous activity has also been associated with triggering migraine headaches.[12] However, moderate exercise should not act as a trigger. Exercise is clearly associated with lowering stress and contributing to an overall sense of well-being. During the actual headache, patients benefit from rest until medication and other treatments take effect.

Patient/Family Education. The nurse may refer the patient to a dietitian if the patient needs guidance regarding dietary changes to prevent headache. Referrals may also be made for biofeedback or relaxation training to prevent stress-induced headache. In addition, there may be local support groups for headache sufferers. The National Headache Foundation is a good source of consumer health information for persons with headache.

Patients with headache commonly worry that their headache is a symptom of some other serious disease. The nurse encourages the patient to accurately report all signs and symptoms and provides education that helps the patient and family to satisfactorily prevent and treat headaches. Identification of triggers is just a first step. The patient must then make lifestyle changes to avoid these triggers. The nurse teaches the patient how to appropriately use all medications. Drugs prescribed to prevent migraine need to be taken on a regular schedule, without missing doses. Drugs prescribed to treat headache symptoms need to be available and taken as soon as the patient becomes aware of symptoms or the presence of an aura.

EPILEPSY

Etiology/Epidemiology

Epilepsy is a chronic disorder surrounded by many myths and misconceptions. Recent advances in the understanding and treatment of epilepsy have improved societal attitudes toward this condition, but the diagnosis still represents a social stigma for many patients. A seizure is an abnormal, paroxysmal electrical discharge from the cerebral cortex, and epilepsy is defined as recurrent, stereotypic seizures.[9] Seizures are clinically seen as alterations in sensation, behavior, movement, perception, or consciousness. Symptoms are related to the area of the cortex involved.

Any condition that causes cerebral irritation or alters the biochemical environment of the brain can result in seizures. The risk of having an isolated seizure during one's lifetime is thought to be about 10%.[15] Seizures can occur as a result of a wide range of metabolic derangements that affect the central nervous system, and if the underlying condition is corrected, the seizures do not recur. These seizures are not epilepsy. Genetics clearly plays a role in some forms of epilepsy.

An estimated 2 million people in the United States have epilepsy, and approximately 125,000 new cases are diagnosed each year. Thirty percent of newly diagnosed patients are under 18 years of age. The prevalence of epilepsy in persons over 65 years of age is 1%. When no identifiable cause for epilepsy can be found, the seizures are considered idiopathic, and idiopathic epilepsy accounts for 70% of all cases. The remaining 30% of cases are related to a known cause, such as central nervous system structural lesions. Risk factors for developing epilepsy in adulthood include lesions within the central nervous system (e.g., traumatic brain injury), meningitis or encephalitis, cerebral tumors, and stroke.[9] Initial seizures in children are often fever related. Common risk factors for seizures are listed in the Risk Factors box.

Pathophysiology

A seizure can be caused by any process that disrupts the cell membrane stability of a neuron. The point at which the cell membrane becomes destabilized and an uncontrolled electrical discharge begins is known as the seizure threshold. Some people have lower seizure thresholds than others and are therefore more prone to seizures.

In 1981 the International League Against Epilepsy proposed a revised classification for seizures (Table 42-3). The major categories are partial (focal) and generalized. Further subdivisions within the categories are based on the person's clinical behaviors during the ictal and interictal times. *Ictal* refers to the time during the seizure. *Interictal* refers to the time between seizure activity. *Postictal* refers to the time immediately after a seizure as the patient recovers.

Partial seizures do not always affect consciousness. Simple partial seizures have less motor, sensory, and consciousness involvement because they are limited to a smaller area of the brain. The wider the area of cerebral cortex affected, the more clinical symptoms are seen. With simple partial seizures a patient may experience uncontrolled movement of an extremity or a portion of the face. He or she is able to interact with others during the seizure and remembers the event afterward. Complex partial seizures affect consciousness. The patient may recall the presence of an aura, a warning sensation that occurs before the seizure. Patients having complex partial seizures often exhibit automatisms (automatic behaviors) such as lip smacking, chewing, rubbing, or picking at clothes. These

Risk Factors

Epilepsy

- Anoxia
- Cerebral palsy
- Perinatal problems (toxemia, difficult delivery, low birth weight, hypoxia)
- Congenital central nervous system defects
- Mental retardation
- Febrile conditions
- Family history of epilepsy
- Head trauma
- Central nervous system infections
- Central nervous system tumors
- Cerebrovascular disease
- Alcohol or drug abuse
- Metabolic disturbances
- Exposure to toxins
- Degenerative diseases (Alzheimer's disease)

behaviors are not voluntary, because consciousness is impaired. Some complex partial seizures spread to larger areas of the cortex and become generalized tonic-clonic seizures, but these are different from true tonic-clonic seizures, in which the initial seizure behavior is generalized.

Generalized seizures impair consciousness from the start. Absence seizures do not include motor signs and may last less than 1 minute, making them difficult to detect. These seizures are often seen in children and may initially be thought of as "daydreaming." There is no postictal state, and absence seizures can occur many times a day.

Tonic-clonic seizures have a tonic phase, during which the muscles become rigid, and then a clonic phase, which involves rhythmic muscle jerking. As the muscles of the trunk and diaphragm become rigid, the air moving past the vocal cords creates a "cry." Once the diaphragm is contracted, the patient is unable to breathe. If the seizure lasts long enough, the patient may become cyanotic. Bladder and bowel muscles are also affected, and the patient may experience incontinence.

Other generalized seizures include myoclonic and atonic types. Myoclonic seizures cause one or several muscles to jerk, often causing the patient to fall. Atonic seizures cause a brief loss of tone in one or more muscles, causing the patient to drop things or fall. They cause only a brief loss of consciousness and no postictal state. The patient is able to get up right away unless he or she is injured from the fall.

Postictal states represent periods of recovery from the seizure. The brain must recover from the intense burst of electrical activity. The length of the postictal period varies from patient to patient. Patients may have some degree of confusion, lethargy, or an inability to follow commands or speak clearly during this period. In some rare cases the patient may experience Todd's paralysis, which is a prolonged period of weakness involving one or more extremities. Although not permanent, the "paralysis" may persist beyond the postictal period of confusion or fatigue.

Status epilepticus is an episode of seizure activity lasting at least 30 minutes, or repeated seizures without full recovery between each seizure. Seizures cause a marked increase in cerebral metabolic activity and demands. These demands may outpace the delivery of oxygen and nutrients from the cerebral blood flow, and prolonged seizures can lead to cellular exhaustion and destruction, and even death, if not effectively interrupted.

Collaborative Care Management

The diagnosis of epilepsy is made from a health history that thoroughly explores the presence of risk factors such as those presented in the Risk Factors box. A thorough description of the seizure itself is also obtained, including:

- Description of the aura, if any (preseizure sensation or feeling)
- Precipitating factors, if any, such as lack of sleep, alcohol intake, emotional stress, excess caffeine, time of day, menses
- Description of the patient's behavior from the beginning of the seizure to the end, especially if the motor signs started in one part of the body and spread to another part (Jacksonian march)

TABLE 42-3 Classification of Seizures

Type of Seizure	Effect on Consciousness	Signs and Symptoms	Postictal State
Partial Seizures			
Simple partial (focal)	Not impaired	Focal twitching of extremity Speech arrest Special visual sensations (e.g., seeing lights), feeling of fear or doom	No
Complex partial (formerly psychomotor or temporal lobe seizures)	Impaired	May begin as simple partial and progress to complex Automatic behavior (e.g., lip smacking, chewing, or picking at clothes)	Yes
Complex partial generalizing to generalized tonic-clonic	Impaired	Begins as complex partial as above, then progresses to tonic-clonic as described below	Yes
Generalized Seizures			
Absence (formerly petit mal)	Impaired	Brief loss of consciousness, staring, unresponsive	No
Tonic-clonic (formerly grand mal)	Impaired	Tonic phase involves rigidity of all muscles, followed by clonic phase, which involves rhythmic jerking of muscles, and possibly tongue biting and urinary and fecal incontinence May be any combination of tonic and clonic movements	Yes
Atonic	Impaired for only a few seconds	Brief loss of muscle tone, which may cause patient to fall or drop something; referred to as drop attacks	No
Myoclonic	Impaired for only a few seconds or not at all	Brief jerking of a muscle group, which may cause the patient to fall	No

- Length of the seizure
- Length of the postictal recovery period and behavior during this phase
- Incidence of incontinence
- Frequency of the seizures (if more than one) and interval between them

A physical examination is performed to evaluate the patient for possible neurologic disease that could cause seizures and is supplemented by selected diagnostic tests such as a CT or MRI scan to check for structural lesions. Laboratory tests, including electrolytes, creatinine, BUN, arterial blood gases, and toxicology screens, are done to rule out metabolic causes for seizures.

An electroencephalogram (EEG) may be ordered to help identify the location, or foci, of the seizures and their pattern of spread, if any, over the cortex. The EEG may be recorded during a brief outpatient test, overnight, or after 12 to 24 hours of sleep deprivation. However, an EEG can only identify a seizure if one occurs during the test. A normal EEG does not rule out the possibility of a past or future seizure. In some cases patients may be monitored for several days as an inpatient.

Antiepileptic drugs (AEDs) are used to control seizures. These drugs are also referred to as anticonvulsants. See Table 42-4 for the most commonly used AEDs. Once the patient's regimen with the medication is established, drug levels are monitored to ensure that the patient has achieved and maintains a therapeutic level. While specific therapeutic ranges have been established for commonly used drugs, the appropriate dose for any patient is one that prevents seizures but does not cause excessive side effects or toxicity, even if the blood level is higher or lower than the established norm. In the past, patients were maintained on anticonvulsant therapy for life. Today the physician may attempt to wean the patient from the medication if the patient has remained seizure free for 1 to 2 years. A common side effect of most AEDs is drowsiness or other mental status changes. These side effects may in-

TABLE 42-4 Common Medications for Epilepsy

Drug	Action	Intervention
Hydantoins		
Phenytoin (Dilantin)	Blocks synaptic potentiation and propagation of electrical discharge in the motor cortex Blocks sodium transport and stabilizes membrane sensitivity Used alone or in combination to manage tonic-clonic, simple partial, and complex partial seizures Therapeutic range is 10-20 mg/L Takes at least 7-14 days to establish	Monitor for common side effects, including nystagmus, ataxia, fatigue, drowsiness, and cognitive impairment. Gastrointestinal symptoms (e.g., nausea, anorexia, vomiting) are common. Drug may be given with meals. Gingival hyperplasia is a common side effect. Patients are taught the importance of scrupulous oral hygiene. Regular follow-up for monitoring is encouraged.
Barbiturates		
Phenobarbital (Luminal)	Depresses postsynaptic excitatory discharge Used to manage tonic-clonic, simple partial, and complex partial seizures and status epilepticus	Monitor for side effects, which include sedation, drowsiness, and depression.
Succinimides		
Ethosuximide (Zarontin)	Depresses motor cortex and raises threshold to stimuli Used to manage absence seizures	Monitor for side effects (e.g., anorexia, nausea, vomiting, drowsiness). Caution patient to never abruptly discontinue the drug (doing so can precipitate status epilepticus).
Other		
Carbamazepine (Tegretol)	Believed to reduce polysynaptic responses and block synaptic potentiation Used to manage tonic-clonic, simple partial, and complex partial seizures	Monitor for side effects (e.g., drowsiness, dizziness, headache, anorexia, nausea, vomiting). Side effects tend to decrease in severity over time. Regular follow-up is encouraged because drug can cause rare but severe bone marrow toxicities.
Valproic acid (Depakene)	Increases levels of gamma-aminobutyric acid for membrane stabilization Used to manage absence seizures or in combination with other drugs for tonic-clonic and complex partial seizures	Monitor for side effects (e.g., anorexia, nausea, and vomiting). Teach patient to take drug with meals. Central nervous system side effects such as drowsiness, tremor, and ataxia. Regular follow-up is encouraged because drug may cause liver dysfunction and blood dyscrasias.

terfere with the patient's social life or work. Multiple changes in drug or dose may be needed to achieve the best seizure control with the fewest side effects.

Because of the emergent nature of status epilepticus, benzodiazepines are used to rapidly terminate the seizure activity while a loading dose of anticonvulsants is administered, since anticonvulsants take longer to achieve a therapeutic blood level (see Guidelines for Safe Practice box and the Nursing Care Plan).

The nurse institutes seizure precautions to protect the patient from injury if the patient's seizures are not well controlled or if the patient has a new illness or injury that predisposes him or her to a lower seizure threshold. In most hospitals, seizure precautions include keeping side rails up and padded if the patient has tonic-clonic seizures, ensuring that suction is available at the bedside, disabling the locks on bathroom and room doors, and avoiding taking oral temperatures with glass thermometers. Helmets may be used to prevent head injury in patients who are permitted to be up and walking.

Nurses need to be able to act quickly when a patient has a seizure. The nurse makes careful observations in order to

Guidelines for Safe Practice

The Patient in Status Epilepticus

1. Protect airway and provide oxygen. Position patient on side to prevent aspiration. Place an oral airway if the teeth are not clenched. Administer oxygen by mask. If respiratory depression occurs from seizures or medication used to control seizures, intubation may be necessary.
2. Establish intravenous access for medication delivery and fluids.
3. Draw blood for electrolytes, arterial blood gases, and toxicology to rule out metabolic causes for seizures.
4. Administer benzodiazepines, usually lorazepam (Ativan) 4 to 8 mg over 2 to 4 minutes or diazepam (Valium) 5 to 20 mg over 5 to 10 minutes to stop seizures. These drugs are fast acting and will control seizures until anticonvulsant drugs reach therapeutic levels.
5. Administer anticonvulsants, usually phenytoin (Dilantin) 15 to 20 mg/kg in normal saline at 50 mg/min maximum rate, at the same time as the benzodiazepines to begin establishing therapeutic levels. Dilantin can cause significant hypotension and cardiac dysrhythmias. Place patient on a monitor during loading doses.
6. Continue search for an underlying cause of seizures.

Nursing Care Plan — Patient With Status Epilepticus

DATA Mr. F. is a 29-year-old man with a history of seizures. He experiences complex partial seizures that occasionally generalize to tonic-clonic seizures. He takes phenytoin (Dilantin), 300 mg at bedtime, and carbamazepine (Tegretol), 200 mg three times a day, to control his seizures. Despite good compliance with medications, he has about four or five seizures a year.

This morning after mowing his lawn in very hot weather, Mr. F. was found having a tonic-clonic seizure by his wife, who turned him to his side. The seizure lasted 2 minutes. Five minutes later Mr. F. began to seize again, so his wife called for emergency assistance. By the time Mr. F. arrived at the emergency department, he had been seizing for 25 minutes without recovery between the seizures.

Oxygen was started by mask. An intravenous (IV) line was established, and an infusion of 0.9% saline was started. Blood was drawn for electrolytes, toxicology, and anticonvulsant levels. Lorazepam (Ativan), 2 mg was administered intravenously every 4 minutes for four doses for a total of 8 mg. Phenytoin, 1000 mg in saline, was infused over 1 hour. Following the fourth dose of lorazepam, the seizure stopped, but Mr. F.'s respiratory rate was 6 breaths/min and his oxygen saturation was 85%. His blood pressure was 85/50 mm Hg. He was electively intubated and ventilated and admitted to the intensive care unit (ICU).

It is now 1 hour after his admission to the ICU. He is localizing to pain stimuli but not following commands. His phenytoin bolus has infused, and his blood pressure has increased to 110/70; his respiratory rate is 8, with no breaths above the ventilator. Breaths sounds are clear bilaterally, and his oxygen saturation is 99% on 40% FiO_2.

NURSING DIAGNOSIS **Risk for injury related to seizure activity**
GOALS/OUTCOMES Will remain free of injury

NOC Suggested Outcomes
- Neurologic Status (0909)
- Risk Control (1902)
- Symptom Control (1608)

NIC Suggested Interventions
- Seizure Precautions (2690)
- Seizure Management (2680)
- Artificial Airway Management (3180)
- Surveillance: Safety (6654)

Nursing Interventions/Rationales
- Implement seizure precautions (side rails up and padded; bed in low position). *To minimize environmental risks when seizures occur.*
- Ensure rapid access to oxygen, suction, and other emergency treatment. *To ensure rapid access to emergency equipment to prevent respiratory compromise or arrest.*
- Administer antiseizures medication as prescribed. *Aggressive drug therapy is the key to halting seizures.*

Continued

Nursing Care Plan *Patient With Status Epilepticus–cont'd*

- Monitor patient's response to medications. *To determine the effectiveness of treatment or the need for more medication.*
- Insert nasogastric tube to administer carbamazepine if needed. *Carbamazepine cannot be administered intravenously and may be needed.*

Evaluation Parameters

1. Free of bruising, cuts
2. Rests quietly

NURSING DIAGNOSIS **Risk for deficient fluid volume related to altered mental status and sudden fluid losses**
GOALS/OUTCOMES Will maintain balanced intake and output

NOC Suggested Outcomes

- Fluid Balance (0601)
- Hydration (0602)

NIC Suggested Interventions

- Fluid Monitoring (4130)
- Fluid Management (4120)
- Intravenous (IV) Therapy (4200)
- Hypovolemia Management (2130)

Nursing Interventions/Rationales

- Assess and monitor for fluid volume deficiency (blood pressure, heart rate, urine output, skin turgor, mucous membranes). *The patient may be dehydrated from working in heat. The earlier fluid volume deficiency is identified, the more quickly fluid balance can be reestablished.*
- Allow patient nothing by mouth until fully awake. *To prevent aspiration. Aspiration is a risk until the patient is fully alert with protective reflexes intact.*
- Administer prescribed IV fluids. *To replace fluid losses and prevent hypovolemia.*
- Monitor vital signs every hour or more frequently if needed. *Phenytoin increases the risk of hypotension.*
- Monitor intake and output. *Intake should approximate output. Monitoring intake and output helps identify fluid deficits.*

Evaluation Parameters

1. Maintains blood pressure within normal limits
2. Intake equals output

document the seizure accurately. The patient is reassured that help is nearby if it is needed. If the seizure generalizes or begins as a generalized seizure, the nurse acts to protect the patient from injury. No attempt is made to restrain the patient, because this could cause injury. The nurse protects the patient from hitting his or her extremities or head on furniture or bed rails by moving them or padding obstructions. Nothing is forced into the patient's mouth. Patients having a tonic-clonic seizure will not have effective air exchange during the seizure, but a patient cannot "swallow" his or her own tongue. However, patients may occlude their airway by flexing their neck or clenching their jaw. After the seizure the nurse gently clears oral secretions, positions the patient to open the airway, and administers oxygen if needed. After securing the airway the nurse assesses the patient for injuries such as abrasions, bruises, or evidence of tongue biting that might have occurred during the seizure. The duration of the postictal phase is assessed and documented, including how much time elapses between the end of the seizure and when the patient can follow commands and answer questions. The nurse arranges for someone to remain with the patient until he or she becomes fully responsive to the surroundings.

There are no specific dietary restrictions for the patient with epilepsy. If the patient can identify certain foods that trigger seizures, these foods are eliminated from the diet. Examples include caffeine, chocolate, and alcohol. The intake of alcohol is known to lower the seizure threshold, and the nurse encourages the patient to use alcohol only in moderation if at all.

Most patients with epilepsy can achieve satisfactory control of their disease through the use of pharmacologic agents. More aggressive interventions may be necessary, however, if the patient's epilepsy remains unresponsive to standard treatment. Surgery may be performed to remove the epileptogenic focus in patients experiencing intractable epilepsy.

Patient/Family Education. Patients and their families must learn to cope with a chronic illness that greatly affects their everyday life and independence. The Epilepsy Foundation of America is a patient-focused organization providing education and support for patients and their families. Local chapters can provide information about services available in the local community, and the nurse encourages the patient to use this important resource.

Epilepsy was long believed to be of supernatural origin, and it has often been seen as a mark of the devil or evil. No

TABLE 42-5 Types of Brain Tumors Occurring in Adults

Type and Incidence	Pathology
Gliomas: Nonencapsulated, Tend to Infiltrate Brain Tissue	
Astrocytomas (grades I and II)—10% Glioblastoma multiforme (also called astrocytoma grades III and IV)—20% Oligodendroglioma (grades I to IV)—5% Ependymoma (grades I to IV)—6% Medulloblastoma—4%	Arise in any part of brain connective tissue; infiltrate primarily cerebral hemisphere tissue; not so well outlined as to be incised completely; grow rapidly—most persons live months to years; tumors assigned grade from I to IV, with IV being the most malignant
Tumors From Support Structures	
Meningiomas—15%	Arise from meningeal coverings of brain; usually benign but may undergo malignant changes; usually encapsulated, and surgical cure possible; recurrence possible
Neuromas (acoustic neuroma, schwannoma)—7%	Arise from Schwann cells inside auditory meatus on vestibular portion of third cranial nerve; usually benign but may undergo cellular change and become malignant; will regrow if not completely excised; surgical resection often difficult because of location
Pituitary adenoma—7%	Arise from various tissues; surgical approach usually successful; recurrence possible
Developmental (Congenital) Tumors	
Dermoid, epidermoid, craniopharyngioma—4%	Arise from embryonic tissue in various sites in the brain; success of surgical resection dependent on location and invasiveness
Angiomas—4%	Arise from vascular structures; usually difficult to resect
Metastatic Tumors–18%	Cancer cells spread to brain via circulatory system; surgical resection very difficult; even with treatment, prognosis is very poor; survival beyond 1 or 2 years is uncommon

disease has been more carefully concealed within families than epilepsy. Attitudes toward persons with epilepsy have been gradually changing, especially with the availability of effective treatment, but old prejudices persist.

Education regarding the causes of epilepsy can help to dispel the myth that persons with epilepsy are "possessed" or evil. With adequate pharmacologic control, the patient with epilepsy can lead a normal life, and the nurse helps the patient understand the importance of adhering to the medication regimen and avoiding precipitating factors for their seizures. Self-care is an ongoing challenge. Medications are prescribed and adjusted to achieve the best control of seizures without excessive side effects or toxicity. The timing of doses can be altered to fit the patient's lifestyle and prevent missed doses.

The nurse stresses the importance of carrying some form of identification with information about the seizure disorder and all prescribed medications in case strangers must provide first aid in the event of a seizure or accident. If the patient feels comfortable sharing the information, a colleague at work or school can be informed about the disease and instructed about what to do in the event of a seizure.

Safety is a primary consideration for the patient with epilepsy. Activity is not generally restricted unless it puts the patient at risk for injury should a seizure occur. However, a history of epilepsy does limit the patient's options in terms of employment, because employers must carefully consider their own liability in case of seizure activity on the job. Each state also has laws defining driver's licensing for persons with a seizure history. Driving may be permitted once a patient has been seizure free on medication for a period of time, often as much as 1 to 2 years.

INTRACRANIAL TUMORS

Etiology

Primary intracranial tumors arise from the support cells of brain tissues rather than from the neurons. These tumors invade or displace brain tissue as they grow, and lead to neurologic symptoms. They are therefore referred to as brain tumors. Brain tumors are generally believed to be the result of a change in the genetic control of cellular growth, leading to abnormal cell mutations and a loss of organized cell growth.[8] Both benign and malignant tumors occur, but this differentiation has less meaning for intracranial tumors than for other types of tissue. A histologically "benign" tumor can be surgically inaccessible, continue to grow, and cause increasing dysfunction ranging from increasing ICP to death.

Some intracranial tumors are graded from I to IV, reflecting the nature of the cellular changes. The more abnormal and anaplastic the tumor cells are, the higher the grade.[8] Highly malignant grades III and IV astrocytomas are the most common type of brain tumors, but a wide variety of tumors exist (Table 42-5).

Epidemiology

The annual incidence of primary brain tumors is about 17,500 cases.[1] An approximately equal number of secondary or metastatic tumors also occur each year.[1] Brain tumors affect people of all ages with two peak periods of incidence: early childhood and the fifth to seventh decades of life.

Children are primarily affected by infratentorial tumors of the posterior fossa such as medulloblastomas. Adults are most commonly affected by the various forms of gliomas. Gliomas and neuromas are more common in males, whereas meningiomas and pituitary adenomas are more common in females.

Pathophysiology

Brain tumors are named for the tissues from which they arise. The more common ones are gliomas, meningiomas, pituitary adenomas, and acoustic neuromas (see Table 42-5). Gliomas account for about 45% of all brain tumors and arise from the connective tissue, the glia cells, of the brain.[1] In adults gliomas primarily infiltrate the tissues of the cerebral hemisphere and are not encapsulated, making them difficult to excise. They grow rapidly, and most persons do not survive longer than a few years after diagnosis. The less malignant gliomas are low-grade astrocytomas and oligodendrogliomas. Ependymomas arise from cells lining the ventricular system. The most malignant and rapidly growing forms of gliomas are the glioblastoma mulitiforme and medulloblastoma. Gliomas may start as one grade and rapidly become more malignant, especially if left untreated.[20]

The meningiomas, which account for 15% of all primary brain tumors, arise from the meningeal coverings of the brain. They occur most commonly in the meninges over the cerebral hemispheres in the parasagittal region along the ridge of the sphenoid bone and in the anterior fossa near the olfactory groove or sella turcica. When located in the posterior fossa, they arise from the cerebellopontine angle, from the tentorium, or rarely from the region of the foramen magnum. Meningiomas are usually benign, but they may undergo malignant changes or be located in a place that makes surgery impossible without causing significant neurologic damage.

Acoustic neuromas constitute about 7% of all primary brain tumors. These tumors grow from the sheath covering the eighth cranial nerve, and the patient exhibits symptoms such as hearing loss or balance disturbance if the vestibular portion of the nerve is compressed. If the tumor becomes large, surrounding structures such as the trigeminal and facial nerves may also be involved, causing additional neurologic symptoms.

Pituitary adenomas make up about 7% of brain tumors. These tumors are considered benign but may be difficult to completely remove because of their location in the sella turcica and their close proximity to the pituitary gland. Symptoms include hormonal changes, such as acromegaly from increased growth hormone production. Visual symptoms may develop if the tumor expands beyond the sella turcica and compresses the optic chiasm, which crosses above the pituitary gland.

Metastatic tumors from primary sites in the lung, kidney, breast, colon, and other organs account for about 18% of all intracranial tumors. Primary brain tumors, conversely, rarely metastasize to other organs.

Brain tumors produce a wide range of neurologic symptoms depending on their size, location, and invasive qualities. Locally the tumor invades, displaces, and destroys brain tissue, producing symptoms related to the functions of that particular site (see Clinical Manifestations box). Brain tumors also exert direct pressure on nerve structures, causing degeneration and interference with local circulation. Local edema develops, which interferes with nerve transmission and exerts a mass effect.

An intracranial tumor of any type can cause an increase in ICP. The increased ICP is transmitted throughout the brain and ventricular system and can produce additional symptoms such as headache, confusion, and papilledema (see earlier discussion of ICP).

Some tumors can displace the structures of the ventricular system as they expand, leading to partial obstruction of the flow of CSF. The accumulation of CSF causes the ventricles to dilate and exert outward pressure on the brain. ICP rises, and hydrocephalus may result. One specific type of tumor, the ependymoma, originates in the ependymal cells that line the ventricular system.

Tumors occurring above the tentorium may disrupt brain function and lead to seizures. If the tumor is small and has not caused other symptoms, a seizure may be the first symptom that causes the person to seek medical attention.

Collaborative Care Management

Diagnostic Tests. The CT scan is the most commonly used test to diagnose and evaluate brain tumors and their effect on surrounding brain tissue. A cerebral angiogram may be per-

Clinical Manifestations

Intracranial Tumors

Symptoms can be generalized, as well as specific to the tumor location and the structures of the brain that are compressed:

- "Pressure" headaches (generalized or periorbital)
- Nausea and vomiting unrelated to food intake
- Symptoms of increased intracranial pressure
- Visual changes:
  - Blurred vision
  - Diplopia (with third, fourth, and sixth nerve compression)
  - Visual field alterations (with tumor compression of the optic chiasm or optic pathways)
  - Enlarged blind spot related to papilledema
- Seizures
- Weakness or hemiparesis (when tumor affects the motor cortex)
- Aphasia
  - Expressive (with frontal lobe tumor affecting the language area in the dominant hemisphere)
  - Receptive (with temporal lobe tumor)
- Alterations in level of consciousness (with a midbrain tumor)
- Personality changes from subtle to obvious psychosis (with frontal lobe tumors)
- Inappropriate affect (with frontal lobe tumors)
- Sensory-perceptual deficits (with parietal lobe tumors)

formed if the tumor is situated near major blood vessels, and information is needed regarding feeding vessels for the tumor. MRI is also used, particularly to help visualize tumors of the posterior fossa, where MRI can provide greater detail than CT.

Medications. Drug therapy is used in the management of brain tumors to both treat the tumor and manage symptoms. A wide variety of chemotherapeutic agents are used, typically in combination protocols. Chemotherapy can be delivered by the standard IV route, but the tight junctions of the blood-brain barrier make it difficult for therapeutic levels of the drugs to reach the brain tumor. Intrathecal administration delivers the drug directly into the central nervous system, but the distribution of the drug to the tumor is still uneven. The use of an Ommaya reservoir allows for the delivery of drugs directly into the lateral ventricle (Figure 42-9). Controlled-release polymer "wafers" allow the chemotherapy to diffuse directly into the tumor cavity. The wafers are implanted in the cavity when the tumor is resected and are left in place to gradually degrade after the drug has been delivered.[16,20]

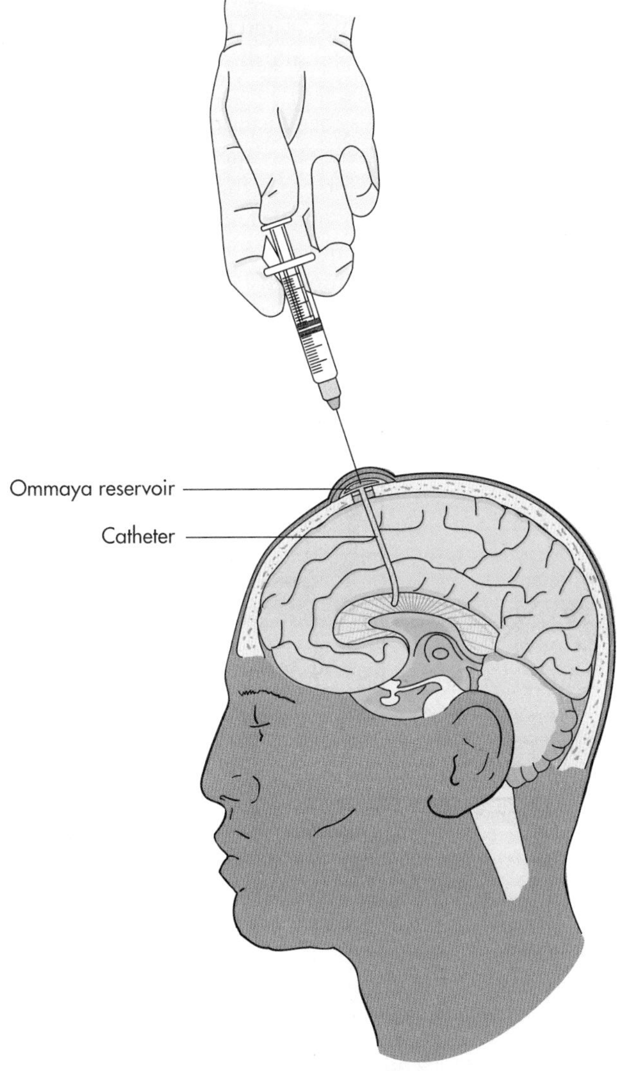

Figure 42-9 The Ommaya reservoir. The reservoir is a mushroom-shaped device with an attached catheter that is implanted into the lateral ventricle through a burr hole. A silicone injection dome rests over the burr hole under the scalp. Drugs can be injected directly into the reservoir with a syringe.

Drug therapy also plays a significant role in symptom management. Most patients receive a corticosteroid such as dexamethasone (Decadron) to help control cerebral edema around the tumor site. The effects are temporary, and steroids are usually tapered after about a month. A histamine receptor antagonist or proton pump inhibitor may be administered along with the steroid to decrease the risk of peptic ulcer formation. Anticonvulsant medications are also initiated to prevent the development of seizures. Phenytoin (Dilantin) is the drug of choice because carbamazepine (Tegretol) is known to cause bone marrow suppression.

Treatments. Radiation therapy is also used in the management of brain tumors. Radiation is usually administered after surgical resection of the tumor; however, it may be used as the primary therapy if the tumor is surgically inaccessible.[8] Metastatic lesions and medulloblastomas are the most responsive to radiation. Radiation is also used after surgery in the treatment of most gliomas because the infiltrative nature of these tumors makes them extremely difficult to completely remove.

Most patients respond well to radiotherapy, but some patients experience severe radiation-induced cerebral edema that is not controllable with steroids. These patients may exhibit symptoms of compromised brain function. Most brain tumors are invasive, and the radiation has to be administered to a large area of the brain, increasing the risk of collateral cell damage and necrosis in the surrounding brain tissue.

Stereotaxic radiation, or "gamma knife" therapy, is an alternative form of radiotherapy available at selected centers. It is used to noninvasively treat deep-seated tumors that are inaccessible to conventional surgery. Using a stereotaxic frame fixed to the patient's head, beams of radiation are concentrated and directed at small areas of brain tissue known to be malignant. This minimizes the radiation damage to surrounding normal brain tissue. The final effects of treatment are not known for several weeks because the irradiated area responds slowly to the treatment.[8]

Another adjunct to surgical treatment for brain tumors is the neuroradiologic procedure referred to as embolization. A cerebral angiogram is performed to identify the feeding blood vessels of a tumor, usually a meningioma. These vessels are then embolized by introducing a material that blocks blood flow through the vessel. Reduced blood flow to the meningioma enables the surgeon to resect the tumor with less blood loss.[20] Similar treatments are used in preparation for surgery to remove or repair aneurysms and arteriovenous malformations.[8]

Surgical Management. Surgery is the treatment of choice for most intracranial tumors. Surgery is used to establish the histologic tissue diagnosis and to either debulk or completely resect the tumor if possible. If the tumor is slow growing, the surgical procedure may keep the patient symptom free for years, even when complete resection is not possible. Surgery may also be used more emergently to deal with obstructions to the flow of CSF, which can cause increased ICP and hydrocephalus.

Surgical treatment of brain tumors typically involves a craniotomy, a surgical opening through the skull that allows access to brain tissue. The procedure is also used to repair the effects of trauma and to treat aneurysms and the effects of stroke. Preoperative preparation and postoperative care are virtually the same, regardless of the underlying condition.

The surgical site depends on the specific anatomic location of the lesion. The incision is usually made behind the hairline so that the scar will be hidden once the patient's hair grows back. A portion of the skull bone is removed, placed aside during the surgery, and replaced at the end of the procedure (Figure 42-10). On rare occasions the bone is not replaced, such as with depressed skull fractures or if the brain is severely swollen after trauma. If the bone is left off, the procedure is referred to as a craniectomy. If possible, the bone is saved, stored in a bone bank, and replaced at a later date. Repair of the cranial defect may be performed with stored bone or with substitute acrylic bonelike materials. Once the bone is off, the dura mater is opened, allowing access to the brain. At the end of the surgery the dura is carefully closed with sutures to prevent CSF from leaking while healing takes place.

Tumors involving the pituitary gland that do not extend outside the sella turcica may be removed by means of a transphenoidal approach. An incision is made beneath the nose under the upper lip, or sometimes through the nose, and access to the sella turcica is gained through an opening at the rear of the sphenoid sinus (see Figure 29-3 and the discussion in Chapter 29). After the surgery, packing is placed in the nose and a fat graft from the abdomen is used to close the defect in the dura.[20] Recovery is rapid, tissue damage in the brain is minimized, and the patient has no loss of hair or external visible incision.

The possibility of neurologic deficits after surgery must be considered, and the surgeon discusses this possibility with the patient and family. The location of the lesion and the overall health of the patient are important considerations in evaluating the patient's risks. A clear discussion of risks, presented in lay terms, is a necessary component of the process of informed consent.

Diet. No special diet is prescribed for the patient with a brain tumor. Rather, the patient's diet is modified as needed to reflect the patient's LOC and ability to swallow and protect the airway. A speech pathologist may be consulted if the patient is experiencing swallowing difficulties.

Activity. The patient is encouraged to remain as active as possible. The only contraindication to normal activity is the presence of increased ICP, which necessitates keeping the patient as quiet as possible. Physical and occupational therapists may be involved in planning and implementing an activity program for the patient.

Referrals. Nursing assessment determines the patient's and family's need for specific referrals. Patients who undergo surgery or other treatments for brain tumors may require the services of physical, occupational, and speech therapists as they recover and learn to compensate for residual deficits. Referrals for home care and community support help the patient

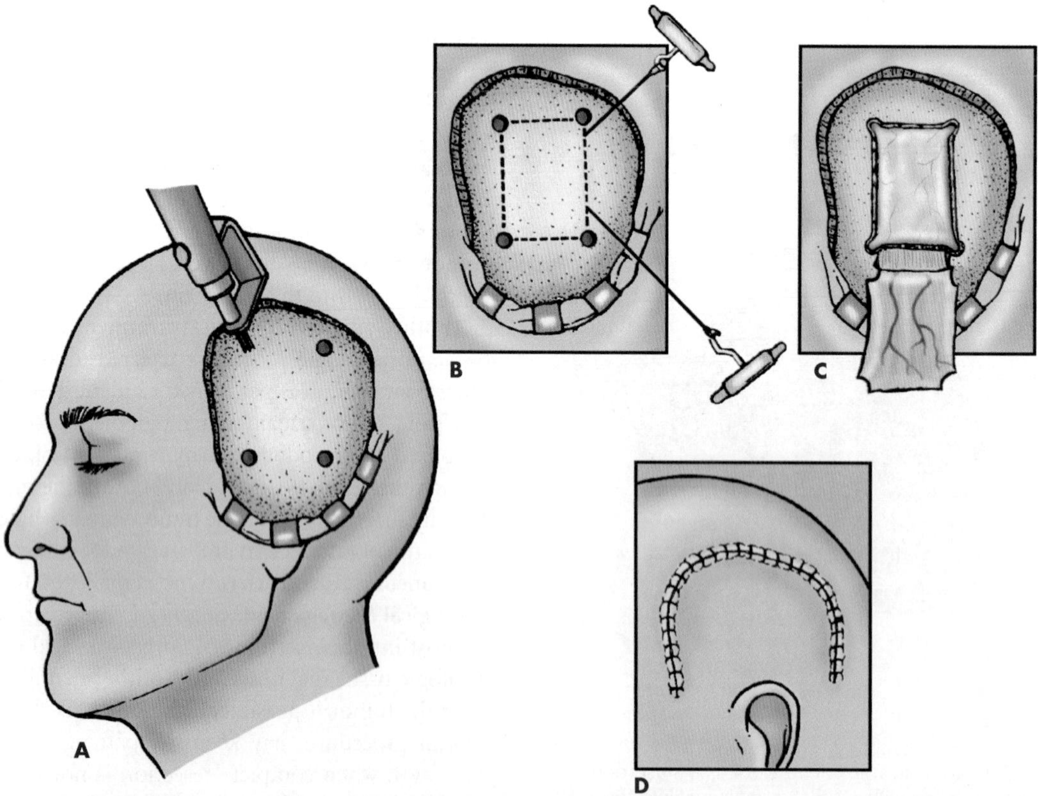

Figure 42-10 Craniotomy procedure. **A,** Burr holes are drilled into the skull. **B,** The skull is cut between the burr holes with a surgical saw. **C,** A bone flap is turned back to expose the cranial contents. **D,** After surgery, the bone flap is replaced and the wound is closed.

return home and continue with the therapy initiated in the hospital. The prognosis for patients with malignant brain tumors is guarded, and both the patient and the family need ongoing support to deal with both the psychologic and the physical complications of the illness and its treatment. Referral to the services of the American Cancer Society is always an appropriate first step.

NURSING MANAGEMENT OF PATIENT UNDERGOING INTRACRANIAL SURGERY

PREOPERATIVE CARE

A baseline neurologic assessment is performed and documented before surgery. The nurse involves both the patient and the family in all preoperative teaching because fears and concerns related to the surgery and postoperative care are normal and expected. Specific fears may relate to a permanent change in appearance or behavior, dependency, or death. Psychologic support for the patient and family is a priority nursing intervention. The nursing staff provides sufficient time for the family to ask questions and allay their fears. The patient or family may wish to see a spiritual counselor before surgery.

All treatments and procedures are carefully explained to the patient even if the person does not seem to fully understand. Shaving of the operative site is usually performed in the operating room. Long hair is saved in case the patient wishes to have a wig made. Some surgeons prefer to shave only the area directly around the surgical site; other surgeons shave the entire head. To avoid depressing the patient's LOC, preoperative sedatives and opioids are rarely administered.

Family members need to know where they may wait during surgery, approximately how long the surgery will take, and where the patient will be after surgery. If the patient is going to be in an ICU after surgery, the patient or family may want a brief tour of the unit to become familiar with the environment. Guidelines for preoperative care of the person undergoing intracranial surgery are summarized in the Guidelines for Safe Practice box.

POSTOPERATIVE CARE

Monitoring Vital Functions

In the immediate postoperative period frequent monitoring is performed to assess for subtle changes in the patient's neurologic status that might indicate complications requiring immediate management. The patient is assessed regularly for signs of increased ICP. The frequency of assessments depends on the patient's condition.

Any changes in the patient's vital signs, LOC, cranial nerve examination, or motor examination are reported at once to the physician. Subtle changes in behavior, such as restlessness, can indicate increased ICP or bleeding into the surgical site that might require further investigation or immediate corrective surgery.

An ICP monitor may be placed at the time of surgery. The monitor allows for direct monitoring of ICP and CPP (see p. 1332). Because the manipulation of brain tissue at the time of surgery can cause cerebral edema after surgery, precautions are taken to prevent activity-related changes in the patient's ICP. Coughing and vomiting are prevented, if possible, because they can dramatically increase ICP. If suctioning is permitted, it is performed in short, limited passes of the suction catheter to limit coughing and associated hypoxia. Deep breathing and incentive spirometry are encouraged but are not followed by forceful coughing.

Preventing Injury

Most patients are started on anticonvulsant therapy preoperatively to prevent postoperative seizures. Seizure precautions are maintained during the immediate postoperative period, and blood levels of the anticonvulsant are checked frequently. Care is taken to protect confused or agitated patients from injuring themselves by pulling at catheters, ICP monitors, or head dressings. Ventricular catheters can be taped securely and wrapped in bulky dressings, and a stockinette can be loosely tied under the patient's chin to keep a head dressing in place. As a last resort, and with a physician's order, restraints may be applied. The nurse attempts to use the least restrictive device possible because struggling against restraints increases the patient's ICP. Commercially available hand "mittens" prevent patients from using their fingers to pick at dressings or tubes but still allow arm movement and enable the nurse to adequately assess the patient's skin and circulation.

Caring for the Incision

Usually the craniotomy incision is covered with gauze dressings wrapped securely around the head. The head dressing is inspected regularly for the amount and type of drainage. Serosanguineous drainage on the dressing is measured and marked so that it can be accurately evaluated over time. Yellowish drainage is reported immediately to the physician because it might indicate a CSF leak. Individual surgeons usually have preferences about changing head dressings. It is not uncommon for the head dressing to be removed after 3 days and

Guidelines for Safe Practice

Preoperative Care of the Patient Undergoing Intracranial Surgery

1. Record baseline neurologic and physiologic data.
2. Encourage patient and family to verbalize fears.
3. Expalin all treatments and procedures fully, even if unsure whether patient understands.
4. If head is shaved, it usually is done in the operating room.
5. If hair is shaved, it is saved and given to patient or family.
6. An antiseptic shampoo may be ordered the night before surgery and repeated in the morning.
7. Prepare family for appearance of patient after surgery: head dressing; edema and ecchymosis of face common; possible decrease in mental status.

the incision left open to the air. Sutures or staples are removed after approximately 7 days. When the dressings are removed, the scalp can be gently cleansed with half-strength hydrogen peroxide and saline to remove any residual dried blood. A loose head covering, similar to the caps worn by operating room staff, may be used to protect the incision, to help remind the patient not to scratch the incision, and to improve the patient's appearance until his or her hair grows back. Head scarves or wigs are preferred by some patients and are available for both men and women. The patient who has had a piece of bone removed will have a depression in the scalp and is vulnerable to injury by bumping the head in this area. These patients are usually provided with a helmet to lessen the danger of inadvertent brain injury.

Promoting Nutrition

Fluid intake and output are accurately recorded. Fluids can be resumed as soon as the patient has active bowel sounds, is alert, and has adequate protective gag, swallow, and cough reflexes to drink without aspiration. IV fluids are used to supplement oral intake until the patient can drink 2000 to 2500 ml/day. An oral diet is resumed if the patient remains alert and does not experience nausea or vomiting.

Promoting Elimination

Urine output is usually monitored with an indwelling catheter for the first day or two postoperatively. The specific gravity of the urine is checked at least twice a day to rule out the presence of diabetes insipidus (DI). Although DI occurs most commonly after pituitary surgery, it can also occur after head trauma or other intracranial surgery (see discussion of DI in Chapter 29 and on p. 1350).

Stool softeners are given to prevent constipation and straining during defecation. Laxatives or suppositories may be used as needed to treat constipation.

Promoting Comfort

Patients often complain of headache after intracranial surgery because of manipulation of the coverings of the brain. Mild, nonopioid analgesics are administered to prevent central nervous system depression that might obscure the patient's neurologic examination. Other measures to promote comfort include treating nausea, keeping bright lights and loud noises to a minimum, and assisting the patient with hygiene, turning, and repositioning.

Promoting Mobility

The postcraniotomy patient may be allowed out of bed on the first postoperative day. If the patient has been on bed rest for more than a few days, some deconditioning is expected. The patient is helped to sit on the edge of the bed and dangle his or her legs. The nurse monitors the patient for postural hypotension or difficulty maintaining balance in the sitting position. Patients with motor or sensory deficits require additional support getting up to a chair or ambulating the first few times. Early mobility prevents the complications associated with bed rest and helps the patient return to normal activity before discharge. Guidelines for care of the person after intracranial surgery are summarized in the Guidelines for Safe Practice box.

GERONTOLOGIC CONSIDERATIONS

Older adults undergoing intracranial surgery have special needs, both before and after surgery. It is important to differentiate between deficits related to the brain tumor and those related to other disease processes. For example, the patient may have underlying weakness from a prior stroke or unrelated orthopedic problem. The elderly patient may have underlying cardiac or pulmonary dysfunction that requires special preparation before surgery and meticulous monitoring during the postoperative period. The patient with a significant medical history may spend more time in the ICU for close monitoring.

Elderly patients may be slower to recover after surgery. Patients with significant cerebrovascular disease are at greater risk for hemorrhage or ischemic stroke as a result of intracra-

Guidelines for Safe Practice

Care of the Patient After Intracranial Surgery

1. Perform monitoring.
   a. Assess neurologic status, including ability to move, level of orientation and alertness, and pupil checks.
   b. Assess degree and character of drainage.
      (1) Amount of drainage and bleeding should be minimal.
      (2) Initial head dressing can be reinforced as necessary.
      (3) Often incision is left open to air after first several days.
2. Promote mobility.
   a. Turning to either side is permitted.
   b. If supratentorial surgery was performed, the head of the bed is kept elevated at least 30 degrees.
   c. Early ambulation is encouraged to prevent complications of bed rest. Observe carefully for signs of postural hypotension; raise head of bed gradually; patient should always sit on edge of bed before standing.
3. Promote decreased intracranial pressure.
   a. Space nursing activities to allow patient to rest between them.
   b. Coughing and vomiting should be avoided.
   c. Suctioning should be performed only as necessary, and then gently and cautiously.
4. Protect safety of patient.
   a. Use soft hand restraints if restraints are necessary.
   b. Use mittens as alternative to restraints. Change mitt every 4 hours—provide range of motion to hand at this time.
   c. Keep side rails up at all times.
5. Promote electrolyte balance.
   a. Perform accurate intake and output with measurement of specific gravity. Do frequent testing for blood glucose.
   b. Have patient resume oral diet as soon as possible; assess for difficulty in swallowing or absence of gag reflex.
   c. Monitor electrolytes for evidence of abnormalities.
6. Promote comfort.
   a. Medicate for comfort with codeine sulfate or nonopioid analgesic.
   b. Ice cap for headache may be helpful.

nial vessel manipulation. Cerebrovascular disease can also compromise collateral circulation and cause ischemic damage during or after intracranial surgery. Slower postoperative recovery rates may necessitate planning for a short-term stay in a rehabilitation facility.

SPECIAL ENVIRONMENTS FOR CARE

Critical Care

Patients undergoing a craniotomy for tumor resection may spend a brief time in the ICU after surgery. The critical care environment allows for close monitoring of the hemodynamic changes that may result from extensive neurosurgery. Once the patient recovers from anesthesia and is breathing adequately without assistance, extubation will take place. When stable, usually within 24 hours, the patient is transferred to a regular patient unit.

Community-Based Care

In preparing the patient for discharge, the nurse assesses the patient's needs for ongoing care or assistance at home. In cooperation with the patient and family, the nurse helps to arrange any nursing or rehabilitation therapy needed after discharge. Short hospital stays increase the likelihood that patients are going to have continuing care needs after discharge. Rehabilitation after neurosurgery often takes months, and the nurse ensures that services have been arranged for the patient before discharge.

COMPLICATIONS

Hydrocephalus. Any obstruction of the normal flow of CSF can result in hydrocephalus. When the obstruction occurs between the ventricles, the CSF cannot flow out of the ventricular system and move through the brain and spinal cord. This is called *noncommunicating hydrocephalus.* When the obstruction prevents the CSF from being reabsorbed via the arachnoid granulations in the sagittal sinus, the resulting condition is called *communicating hydrocephalus.* The arachnoid granulations can become obstructed by blood or proteins produced by infection in the CSF.

Acute hydrocephalus may require immediate intervention via a ventriculostomy. A small catheter is placed into the lateral ventricle via a frontal opening in the skull, known as a burr hole. The catheter is connected to an external drainage system that monitors ICP and allows for drainage of CSF. The tubing and drainage system must be kept closed and sterile. If drainage appears to stop, the neurosurgeon is notified immediately. Ventriculostomies are left in place for only a few days to minimize the risk of infection. If the patient requires ongoing drainage of CSF, a shunt replaces the external drain (Figure 42-11). The different types of shunts are named for their points of origin and termination and include:

- Ventricular-peritoneal
- Lumbar-peritoneal
- Ventricular-jugular
- Cyst-peritoneal

When a shunt is placed, excessive CSF is diverted away from the central nervous system and into either the peritoneal cavity or, occasionally, the venous system, where it is reabsorbed. Shunts may include special valves or access reservoirs at the point where the catheter leaves the skull. These valves or reservoirs help control the volume and pressure of CSF leaving the ventricular system. Guidelines for care of the patient undergoing shunt placement are summarized in the Guidelines for Safe Practice box.

Respiratory Failure. Respiratory arrest may occur after posterior fossa surgery as a result of edema in the brainstem and the inability to protect the airway with the cough or gag reflex. Respiratory monitoring is one of the major reasons for temporary ICU placement after intracranial surgery. Any irregularity of respiration, reduction in pulse oximetry, or onset of dyspnea is reported at once. Equipment is kept ready to support ventilation, including intubation, if necessary.

Cerebrospinal Fluid Leak. Any opening into the dura, whether from trauma or surgery, predisposes the patient to a CSF leak. The nurse monitors the patient for clear fluid oozing from the suture line or clear drainage on the head dressing. If the patient had surgery via a transphenoidal approach, the nurse also checks for clear fluid draining from the nose. A dural leak allows CSF to escape and provides a pathway for bacteria to enter the brain, causing meningitis (see also Chapter 29).

CSF leaks usually heal spontaneously and do not require surgical intervention. The head of the bed is kept elevated to

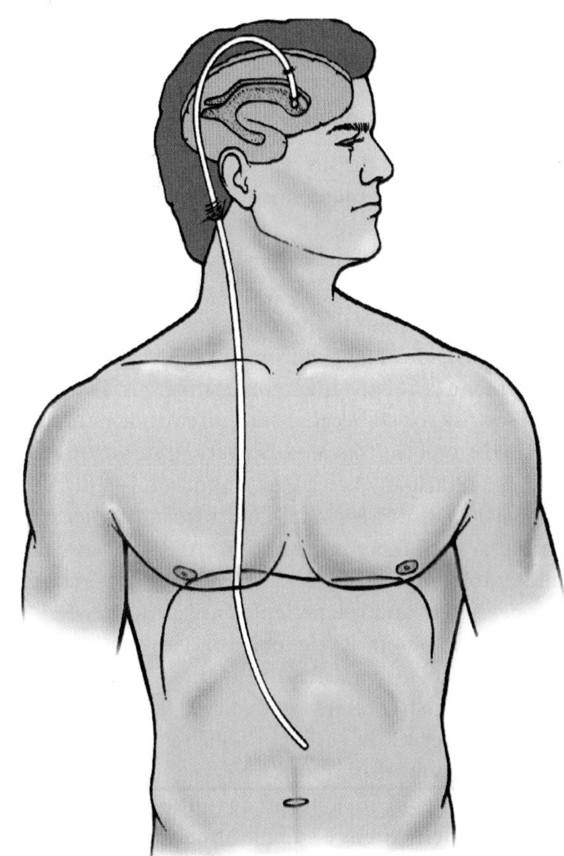

Figure 42-11 Ventriculoperitoneal internal shunt.

Guidelines for Safe Practice

The Patient Undergoing Shunt Placement

1. Perform monitoring.
   a. Assess neurologic status frequently for any decrease in mental status.
   b. Observe for symptoms of subdural hematoma, one of the possible side effects of the surgery.
   c. Monitor for symptoms of overdrainage, as evidenced by headache, especially when patient is sitting upright or standing.
   d. Assess degree and character of drainage.
      (1) Amount of drainage and bleeding should be minimal.
      (2) Reinforce dressing as needed.
      (3) Often incisional areas are left open to air after several days.
2. Maintain gastrointestinal status.
   a. Check frequently for signs of paralytic ileus; manipulation of the bowel that occurs with the placement of the shunt's peritoneal segment can predispose patient to ileus.
   b. Patient usually is given nothing by mouth for the first day, and then clear liquids are started.
   c. Regular diet is resumed as soon as good bowel sounds are present and patient tolerates liquids.
3. Maintain comfort.
   a. Patient may need frequent pain medication because of involvement of abdominal area.
   b. Keep pressure off incisional sites.
4. Promote mobility.
   a. Turning to either side is permitted.
   b. Raise head of bed gradually when mobilizing patient.
   c. Patient is encouraged to ambulate as much as possible to encourage adaptation to decreased intracranial pressure.

reduce CSF pressure at the site of the leak. Occasionally a lumbar drain is placed to remove small amounts of CSF and further reduce CSF pressure at the leak site. The patient is instructed not to blow his or her nose and to restrict activities that would increase ICP and force CSF out of the leak. Antibiotics are administered until the leak is resolved.

Diabetes Insipidus and Syndrome of Inappropriate Antidiuretic Hormone. Patients undergoing surgery in the pituitary region are at risk for DI because antidiuretic hormone (ADH) is made and stored in this area. Surgery, trauma, or cerebral edema from almost any neurologic condition can disrupt the delicate balance of this essential fluid regulatory mechanism.

DI occurs when there is insufficient ADH to cause the renal tubules to reabsorb water. Large quantities of very dilute urine are excreted, and the patient is at risk for severe dehydration. Serum sodium levels and osmolarity rise from the loss of fluid (Table 42-6). Treatment involves fluid replacement and administration of synthetic ADH in the form of desmopressin acetate (DDAVP) or aqueous vasopressin. The condition is usually self-limiting.

The syndrome of inappropriate antidiuretic hormone (SIADH) can also occur as a complication of intracranial surgery and is a direct contrast to DI. Patients with almost any central nervous system disorder, damage to the hypothalamus, bronchogenic carcinoma, or pulmonary disease may develop SIADH. In this syndrome too much ADH is secreted, causing the renal tubules to reabsorb excess amounts of water. The patient's urine output is low, generalized weight gain occurs, and the patient's serum sodium and osmolarity are low as a result of the dilutional effects of water retention (Table 42-6). The treatment for SIADH is fluid restriction, often to 1500 ml of fluid per day or less. If the patient is receiving IV fluids, normal saline is given to provide additional sodium. On rare occasions 3% hypertonic saline may be administered under close monitoring. The problem is usually self-limiting. In severe cases the drug demeclocycline (Declomycin) may be given to suppress the effects of ADH on the renal tubule.

Corneal Abrasions. Positioning of the patient during intracranial surgery may expose the patient to the risk of corneal abrasions. Trauma, dysfunction, or surgery in the area of the seventh cranial nerve, which controls the ability to close the eyes, also predisposes the patient to this complication. The nurse inspects the patient's eyes for redness and the ability to blink and keeps the eyes moist. If the corneal reflex is absent, lubricating eyedrops or eye ointment is used to keep the eyes moist. Patients may need teaching to continue this intervention after discharge. Preventive eye care is extremely important with patients experiencing severe impairments of LOC. Corneal abrasion is a serious complication that can rapidly progress to severe eye infection.

Gastric Ulceration. Neurosurgical procedures predispose the patient to gastric ulceration, commonly known as Cushing's ulcers. The underlying pathology is not well understood but is thought to represent a massive stress response. The use of steroids after surgery is also believed to increase gastric secretions and can contribute to gastric irritation and ulceration. Patients are usually placed on a histamine H_2 blocker or proton pump inhibitor as a preventive measure. If a nasogastric tube is in place, the pH of the gastric secretions can be monitored and antacids or sucralfate (Carafate) can be administered to protect the gastric mucosa. See Chapter 33 for a discussion of stress ulcer.

CRANIOCEREBRAL TRAUMA

Etiology

Craniocerebral trauma may result from injury to the scalp, skull, and/or brain tissues, either singly or collectively. Variables that influence the extent of the injury to the head include:

- Status of the head at the time of impact—moving or still
- Location and direction of the impact
- Rate of energy transfer
- Surface area involved in the energy transfer

Injuries vary from minor scalp wounds to concussions and open skull fractures with severe brain injury. The amount of obvious external damage does not necessarily reflect the seriousness of the injury. Serious craniocerebral damage can occur in the absence of visible external injury.

Contusions, abrasions, and lacerations of the scalp may occur (Table 42-7). Lacerations of the scalp bleed profusely because of the scalp's rich blood supply and the poor vasoconstrictive abilities of these vessels. Hematomas that form under the surface of

TABLE 42-6 Laboratory Parameters and Treatment of Diabetes Insipidus and Syndrome of Inappropriate Antidiuretic Hormone

Parameters	Diabetes Insipidus	Syndrome of Inappropriate Antidiuretic Hormone
Urine specific gravity	1.001 to 1.005	1.030 or more
Serum osmolarity	High	Low
Serum sodium	High	Low
Urine output	Very high	Low
Treatment	Fluid replacement Desmopressin 0.1-0.4 ml intranasally q12-24h Aqueous vasopressin 5-10 U SQ q3-6h	Fluid restriction Lasix for diuresis Demeclocyline 300 mg qid

TABLE 42-7 Damage of Brain Tissue Caused by Trauma

Characteristics	Structural Alteration	Effects
Concussion		
Characterized by immediate and transitory impairment of neurologic function caused by mechanical force	No	May be loss of consciousness that is instant or delayed; usually reversible
Contusion		
Likened to bruising with extravasation of blood cells	Yes	Injury may be at site of impact or at opposite side; often damage is to cortex
Laceration		
Tearing of tissues caused by sharp fragment or shearing force	Yes	Hemorrhage is serious complication

the scalp may obscure underlying skull fractures. The initial injury from head trauma is regarded as the primary trauma. Secondary trauma occurs from the body's response to the initial injury. Examples of secondary injuries are edema, hematoma formation, hydrocephalus, and infection.

Epidemiology

Craniocerebral trauma, or traumatic brain injury (TBI), causes death and serious disability in persons of all ages. Each year an estimated 1.5 million Americans sustain a TBI, and approximately 50,000 of these injuries result in death. An additional 230,000 people are hospitalized but survive, and approximately 80,000 to 90,000 people experience an injury that results in long-term disability.[6] Motor vehicle accidents are the cause of about 50% of TBIs, falls cause 21%, assaults and violence cause 12%, sports-related injuries make up 10%, and alcohol is implicated in a significant percentage of all injuries.[4] Both morbidity and mortality rates are higher in males. Head injury is the second most common cause of major neurologic deficits and the major cause of death in persons between ages 1 and 35 years.[26] In some states the repeal of laws requiring motorcyclists to wear helmets has resulted in an increase in death and injury from TBI sustained in motorcycle accidents. Motorcycle accidents pose an added risk for injury because of the body's total exposure to direct force injury.

Pathophysiology

Mechanisms of Injury. Head trauma results from three general types of injury: deformation, acceleration-deceleration, and rotation (Figure 42-12). Deformation results from the direct or indirect transmission of energy to the skull. If the force is sufficient, the skull is deformed or fractured. Acceleration-deceleration injuries typically occur when the accelerating skull, moving in a motor vehicle, suddenly decelerates when it hits an immobile object such as the steering wheel or windshield. The brain injury that results is often termed *coup–contra coup* because the brain first strikes the skull in the direction of movement and then rebounds and strikes the inner surface of the skull in the opposite direction. The damage from such injuries is highly variable and depends on the speed of acceleration and deceleration. Rotational forces also distort the brain and can cause tension, stretching, and diffuse shearing of brain tissues. Often the forces of acceleration-deceleration and rotation occur together, affecting both the brain and the spinal cord.

Skull Fractures. Skull fractures are a common form of primary craniocerebral trauma. Fractures of the skull may be linear, comminuted, depressed, or basilar (Figure 42-13). Linear skull fractures appear as a fine line on skull x-ray studies. If the fracture crosses the path of the meningeal artery, arterial bleeding above the dura can occur, creating a medical emergency. Comminuted or depressed skull fractures involve bone displacement, sometimes down into the brain tissue itself. If the dura is torn, a CSF leak may occur.

Basilar skull fractures are particularly serious because the vital respiratory and vasomotor centers, cranial nerves, and major nerve pathways may be permanently damaged. If the injury creates a direct communication between the cranial

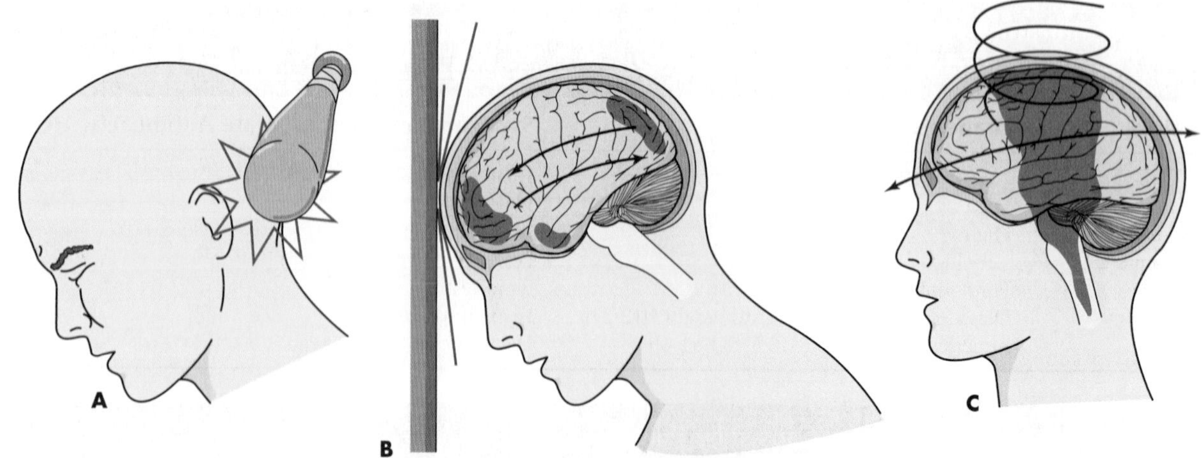

Figure 42-12 Mechanisms of injury. **A,** Deformation. **B,** Acceleration-deceleration. **C,** Rotation.

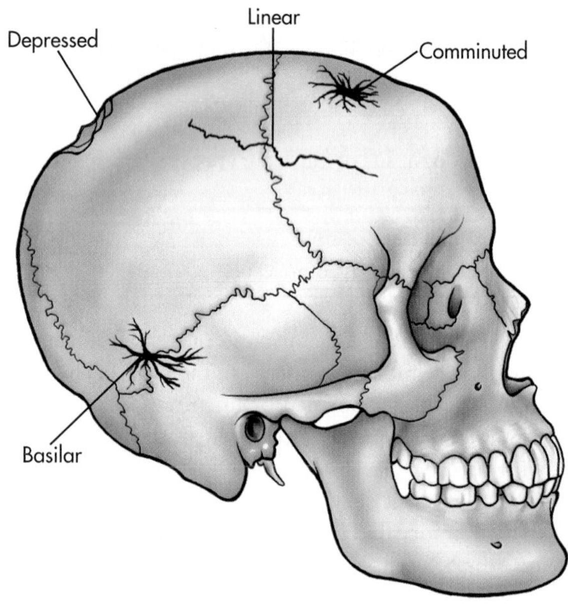

Figure 42-13 Types of skull fractures.

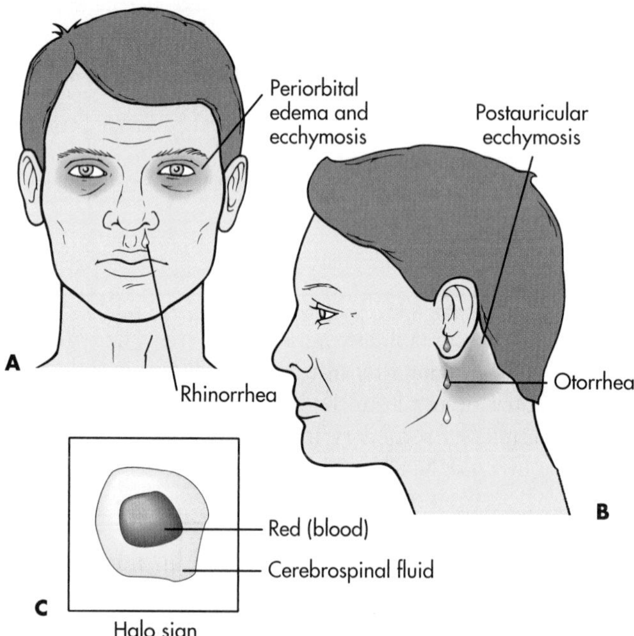

Figure 42-14 **A,** Racoon eyes and rhinorrhea. **B,** Battle's sign (postauricular ecchymosis) with otorrhea. **C,** Halo, or ring, sign. Drainage containing cerebrospinal fluid forms a ring, or halo, as it dries on a gauze pad.

cavity and the middle ear or the sinuses, meningitis or a brain abscess may develop. Bleeding from the nose and the ears suggests a basilar fracture. Serosanguineous drainage from the ears or nose may also contain CSF. Any drainage is routinely tested for the presence of glucose, and positive results are reported to the physician immediately. Drainage can also be blotted on a gauze pad. The presence of CSF causes it to form a ring, or halo, as it dries. Other signs suggestive of basilar skull fracture include hemotympanum (a hemorrhagic exudate into the middle ear), bruising over the mastoid process (Battle's sign), and periorbital ecchymosis (raccoon eyes) (Figure 42-14). The latter two signs may not be evident for the first 24 hours after injury.

Concussion and Contusion. Another primary brain injury is a concussion, which is characterized by an immediate and transient impairment of neurologic function induced by mechanical force. An instant or delayed loss of consciousness may occur, but the person usually recovers rapidly. A person who exhibits any alteration in consciousness after a blow to the head is closely observed after the injury, because the extent of the damage is not always immediately apparent. Postconcussion symptoms may develop and include headache, dizziness, fatigue, memory impairment, and impaired concentration. Although no structural neurologic changes are evident, current research indicates that there may be a correlation between the concussion of minor head injury and subsequent cognitive impairments.[13,26] Diffuse axonal injury is caused by rapid movement of the brain during which delicate axons are stretched and damaged. This damage interferes with nervous transmission and can cause extensive diffuse deficits.[11]

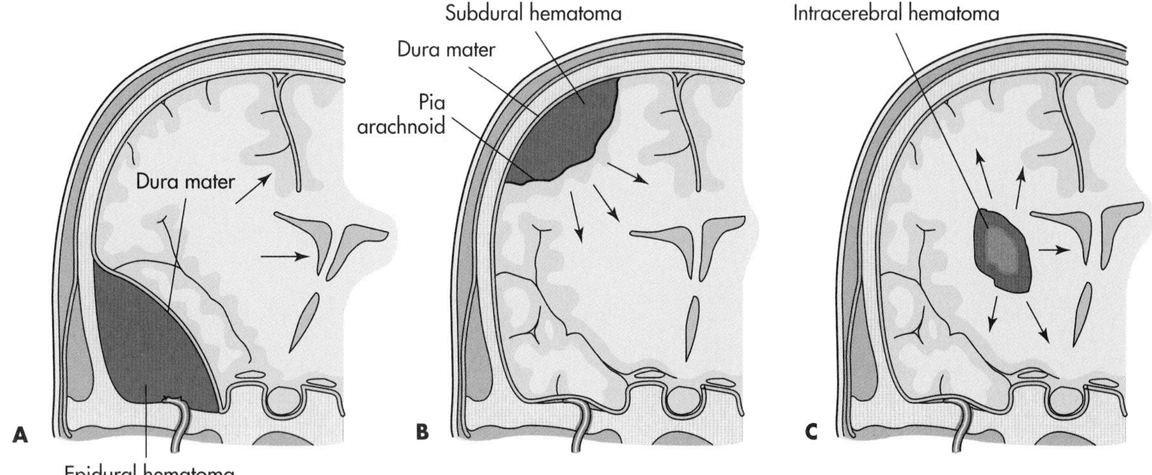

Figure 42-15 Cerebral hematomas. **A,** Epidural hematoma. **B,** Subdural hematoma. **C,** Intracerebral hematoma. Arrows indicate the direction of pressure generated by the hematoma.

A contusion is a structural alteration characterized by the extravasation of blood into the brain. It can be likened to bruising without tearing of tissues. The contusion may be at the site of impact or on the opposite side—a coup–contra coup type of injury. Contusions often damage the cerebral cortex. Laceration of the brain and its blood vessels can occur with severe contusions and may be caused by a sharp fragment or a shearing force. On CT scaning, small, petechial-like areas of bleeding are seen.

Secondary Injury. Secondary injury results from the body's response to the initial trauma and includes cerebral edema, increased ICP, and hematoma formation. The brain becomes edematous in response to local injury, bleeding, and disturbances in the circulation that result in hypoxia. Cell damage and hypoxia increase cell membrane permeability, leading to cytotoxic edema. The damaged capillaries also become more permeable and allow fluid to leak out into the interstitial space. The fluid leak creates a condition called vasogenic edema that contributes to increased ICP, as discussed earlier in the chapter. Most deaths from head injury occur from the effects of increased ICP rather than from the initial injury itself.

Hematoma formation is another form of secondary injury (Figure 42-15). An epidural hematoma forms as blood collects between the dura and the skull. Because bleeding in this area is usually caused by laceration of the middle meningeal artery, the hematoma forms rapidly. The bleeding must be controlled promptly and the blood evacuated, or life-threatening neurologic deterioration occurs. Epidural hematoma formation often accompanies basilar and temporal skull fractures. The nurse assesses frequently for signs of epidural hematoma when injuries occur in these sites.

A subdural hematoma forms when venous blood collects below the dural surface but above the brain. Because the bleeding is venous in nature, the hematoma forms relatively slowly. However, the accumulating clot puts pressure on the brain surface and eventually displaces brain tissue if it becomes large enough. Subdural hematomas are subdivided into acute, subacute, and chronic varieties. Acute subdural hematomas develop within 48 hours of injury and have an organized clot. Subacute subdural hematomas develop within 3 days to 2 weeks after injury. The clot may have already become more fluid as the body attempts to break it down and remove it. The chronic subdural hematoma can produce symptoms from about 3 weeks to several months after the injury. The damaged area is filled with fluid rather than an organized clot. Acute and subacute hematomas present a greater threat to neurologic function because of the rapidity of their development. Chronic subdural hematomas evolve over a longer period of time, and the symptoms are typically less acute.

A third type of hematoma is the intracerebral hematoma, which is common after a hemorrhagic stroke, or aneurysm rupture. The blood collects within the brain parenchyma itself, and the symptoms are related to the specific area of the brain where the clot forms.

Collaborative Care Management

Diagnostic Tests. Diagnostic procedures for head injury include CT scans, skull x-ray studies, and possibly cerebral angiography. The CT scan evaluates for hematomas, edema, or damage related to skull fractures. X-ray films reveal skull or facial fractures. Cerebral angiography may be used to assess for injury to blood vessels or to determine if blood found within the skull is the result of trauma or a stroke.

Laboratory tests performed on admission include arterial blood gases to evaluate oxygenation and detect hypoxia or hypercarbia. Blood alcohol levels and toxicology screens are routinely performed to rule out other potential metabolic causes for any altered LOC. Hemoglobin and hematocrit are used to establish a baseline for evaluating occult blood loss.

Medications. Medications for the patient with a head injury depend on the specific nature and severity of the patient's injury. Medications may include drugs to reduce ICP, prevent seizures, or provide analgesia.

Treatments. Treatments for the patient with a head injury depend on the presenting symptoms and the severity of the injury, as well as the presence of other systemic injuries.

Multiple injuries may be present. The patient may be intubated to protect the airway, undergo surgery to treat internal injuries, or be immobilized to treat concurrent musculoskeletal injuries.

Surgical Management. If the head injury causes hematoma formation, surgical intervention may be necessary. Craniotomies are performed to evacuate both epidural and subdural hematomas and repair the source of bleeding. If severe edema is present, the dura is closed surgically, but the overlying bone may be temporarily removed to allow room for anticipated brain expansion. The bone is replaced when the edema subsides. Patients with depressed skull and/or facial fractures also undergo surgery to repair the injury and relieve pressure on the brain or other structures.

Diet. No special diet is prescribed for the patient with a head injury. The diet is determined largely by the patient's condition. If, after several days, the patient is unable to take in sufficient nutrients by mouth, enteral or parenteral nutrition is initiated.

Activity. The patient's activity level is determined by his or her neurologic status. Safety is the primary concern. The patient with motor or sensory deficits or altered LOC needs supervision and assistance to prevent injury.

Referrals. In some settings the nurse assumes responsibility for making referrals to other services. For the patient with a head injury, this may include a dietitian, social worker, and physical and occupational therapists. The family is often aided by a referral to the local chapter of the Head Injury Foundation or another support group.

NURSING MANAGEMENT OF PATIENT WITH CRANIOCEREBRAL TRAUMA

ASSESSMENT

Health History

Data to be collected via the health history to assess a conscious head-injured patient include:

- Information about the nature of the injury—how it happened, treatment to date
- History of loss of consciousness, duration
- History of bleeding from the ears, nose, eyes, or mouth
- Patient's understanding of the injury and resulting pathologic consequences
- Patient's ability to understand
- Comorbid health conditions and current treatment regimen
- Medications in use: prescription, over the counter, and herbal
- Pattern of alcohol/drug use, type, and amount
- Living conditions, available family and social support

Physical Examination

Data to be collected during the physical examination include:

- Respiratory status (patency of the airway, ability to cough, need for intubation and mechanical ventilation)
  - Arterial blood gases
- Vital signs
  - Signs of increased ICP
- LOC, alertness, orientation
  - Presence of headache, nausea or vomiting
- Pupils: size, equality, reactivity
  - Presence of diplopia or other visual problems
- Motor status
- Sensory status, unusual sensations (paresthesias, ringing in the ears)
- Presence of bleeding
  - Battle's sign (ecchymosis behind the ears; indicates a basilar skull fracture)
  - Raccoon eyes (ecchymosis and swelling around the eyes; indicates a possible orbital fracture)
- Presence of discharge from the ears or nose
- Speech pattern abnormalities

NURSING DIAGNOSES

Nursing diagnoses are determined from analysis of patient data. Nursing diagnoses for the patient with a head injury may include but are not limited to:

Diagnostic Title	Possible Etiologic Factors
1. Ineffective breathing pattern	Central nervous system disturbance, trauma
2. Ineffective tissue perfusion	Decreased blood flow to brain; increased ICP
3. Ineffective thermoregulation	Trauma to vital control centers
4. Excess or deficient fluid volume	Hypersecretion or hyposecretion of ADH from pituitary
5. Risk for infection	Disruption of brain's dural protection, immobility
6. Activity intolerance	Sensory, motor deficits
7. Compromised family coping	Crisis of injury, uncertain outcomes
8. Deficient knowledge (knowledge of head injury)	Lack of exposure/recall to pathology, treatment plan

EXPECTED PATIENT OUTCOMES

Expected patient outcomes for the patient with a head injury may include but are not limited to:

1. Will maintain adequate ventilation as indicated by pulse oximetry readings above 90%, respiratory rate less than 20 breaths/min
2. Will maintain adequate cerebral perfusion and exhibit no signs or symptoms of increased ICP
3. Will maintain temperature within the range of 97.5° to 99.5° F
4. Will maintain urine output and specific gravity within normal limits
5. Will remain free of infection
6. Will return to preinjury activity level
7. Family members and/or significant other will verbalize adequate coping, use of support services
8. Patient and family members will be able to verbalize knowledge of head injury, treatment, and rehabilitation and resources available in the local community

INTERVENTIONS

1. Promoting Adequate Ventilation

Respiratory failure is a common complication of severe head injury, and cerebral anoxia, a common sequela of respiratory failure, is a leading cause of death in head-injured patients. The patient with respiratory failure may develop dyspnea, hypoxia, hypercapnia, and hypotension. Each of these problems results in adverse consequences for the injured brain, and intubation and mechanical ventilation are often necessary.

Arterial blood gases and pH are checked frequently to determine the adequacy of respiratory exchange. Pulse oximetry may be used as a less invasive means of monitoring the patient's oxygenation status. Alert patients are reminded to deep breathe frequently, but coughing is not encouraged because of the risk of increasing ICP. Suctioning is used only if absolutely necessary to ensure a patent airway, and the nurse carefully hyperventilates and hyperoxygenates the patient before suctioning to minimize the adverse effects on ICP.

2. Controlling Intracranial Pressure

Increased ICP is a major concern in patients with head injury, and bedside neurologic checks are performed frequently until the patient's condition stabilizes. Specific interventions to control increased ICP are discussed on p. 1332.

3. Maintaining Vital Signs and Temperature Control

Vital signs are assessed frequently until the patient's condition stabilizes. Patients with head injury are at immediate risk for increased ICP but may have also experienced trauma to other body systems and are at risk for shock. (See sections on altered LOC and ICP for specific changes in vital signs related to severe head trauma.) Patients who develop fever are immediately worked up to attempt to identify the specific source of infection. Once cultures are obtained, the patient may be treated with empiric antibiotics and antipyretics to increase comfort. Fever may reach life-threatening levels when the brain's thermoregulation completely fails, and tepid sponge baths or other more aggressive measures of reducing body temperature, such as cooling blankets, are used as a last resort.

4. Monitoring Fluid and Electrolyte Balance

Intake and output are carefully measured and recorded. The specific gravity of the urine is also tested and recorded if DI is suspected. These measurements may be performed hourly when the patient's condition is unstable.

Fluids are prescribed according to the patient's need for blood pressure support, for replacement of gastrointestinal losses from suctioning, or to balance urine output. Fluids are usually given parenterally but may be administered by feeding tube or by mouth, depending on the patient's condition. The nurse uses caution in administering fluids orally because the patient may have difficulty swallowing or may vomit and aspirate. The patient's urine output is also carefully monitored to assess the response to osmotic diuretics such as mannitol.

An indwelling catheter is inserted when mannitol is given because of the large amounts of urine produced and the need to measure output accurately. The presence of an indwelling catheter increases the risk of urinary tract infection, and the catheter is removed as soon as possible.

Careful monitoring of electrolytes is also necessary. Several types of sodium imbalances are known to occur after head injury. Natriuresis, or increased urinary excretion of sodium, is common. This is attributed to SIADH and an increased plasma level of ADH, serum hyponatremia, and hypoosmolarity, which aggravates cerebral edema. Hypernatremia, or sodium retention, also may occur and has negative consequences for cerebral function. No specific variations in potassium or chloride levels are associated with head injury, but serum levels of BUN, electrolytes, pH, and urinary electrolyte levels are checked frequently. Plasma cortisol levels also are elevated in acute head injury.

5. Preventing Infection

The patient's ears and nose are observed carefully for the presence of blood or serous drainage, which may indicate that the meninges have been torn (common in basal skull fractures) and that spinal fluid is escaping. Drainage from the nose can be tested for glucose to help differentiate CSF from mucus. Drainage can also be blotted on a gauze pad as CSF forms a halo on the gauze as it dries. No attempt should be made to clean the nose or ears or to block the drainage. Usually the leak of CSF subsides spontaneously, but there is a risk of meningitis whenever a tear in the dura allows communication between the nasal cavity, the ears, and the brain. Antibiotics are started immediately if a patient is believed to be at risk.

If a leak is suspected, the patient is instructed not to cough, sneeze, or blow the nose. These activities may, in addition to contributing to the development of meningitis, enable air to enter the cranial cavity and increase ICP.

Nasal suctioning is not used to remove secretions, and neither nasogastric nor nasotracheal tubes are used with any patient suspected of having a leak because of the risk of causing further damage or introducing infection.

6. Resuming Activities

The duration of convalescence following head injury depends entirely on how much damage has been done and how rapidly recovery progresses. Patients are usually encouraged to resume normal activities as soon as possible. Headache and occasional dizziness may be present for several months after a head injury but gradually resolve. Loss of memory and initiative may also be present.

Neuropsychologic testing can be used to identify subtle cognitive deficits and help guide rehabilitation.

Some persons require intensive physical rehabilitation, and others fail to make a satisfactory recovery and are left with serious functional deficits. Complete recovery from head injury is most likely to occur in persons younger than 20 years of age (see Research box). Persons between the ages of 20 and 50 years who remain in a coma longer than 2 weeks rarely recover.

7. Providing Emotional Support

The patient with a head injury may lose cognitive function and memory and develop behavioral problems associated

Research

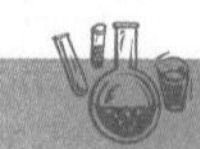

Reference: Gomez PA et al: Age and outcome after severe head injury, *Acta Neurochir* 142(4):373-383, 2000.

The study analyzed the records of over 800 patients admitted for treatment of a closed head injury in an attempt to determine if a relationship was present between age at the time of injury and the patient's final clinical status. A clear inverse relationship was found between age and final outcome, with clinical status becoming progressively worse with older patients. The odds of having an adverse outcome increase significantly after the age of 35 and then continue to worsen as the age increases. Individuals 65 years of age and older had a tenfold greater risk of adverse outcomes than those ages 12 to 25 years. The aspects of aging on brain function that contribute to these negative outcomes have not been adequately explained, but it is theorized that the older brain may have an impaired ability to recover after significant pathologic insult.

Patient Teaching

Monitoring the Patient With a Minor Head Injury

The patient should be awakened periodically through the first 24 hours to be sure he or she can wake up easily. Also, for the first 24 to 48 hours the family should watch carefully for the following warning signs:

1. Vomiting, often with force behind it
2. Unusual sleepiness, dizziness and loss of balance, or falling
3. Complaint of seeing two of everything or blurry objects; jerking movements of the eyes
4. Bleeding or discharge from nose or ears
5. A slight headache may be expected; however, if it worsens and the patient complains of feeling even worse when moving about, it should be reported
6. Seizures—any twitching or movements of arms or legs that the patient is not able to control
7. Any behavior or symptom that is not normal for the individual
8. Change in speech or ability to converse

Call a physician at once if any of these signs are observed. Call either your personal physician or emergency services.

with restlessness and a lack of judgment.[3] Emotional support is important for both the patient and family caregivers, because both are likely to experience significant frustration. Patients need firm but gentle care and specific guidelines for appropriate behavior.

The nurse encourages the patient and family to focus on short-term gains rather than long-term goals to avoid becoming discouraged with the slow pace of progress. Head injury support groups can be extremely helpful to the family as they learn to cope with the patient's behavior and deficits. The nurse also reinforces the importance of regular respite care for family caregivers.

8. Patient/Family Education

A patient with a head injury may be evaluated in the emergency department but not admitted to the hospital. The families of these patients need teaching about monitoring for complications. A sample set of instructions is presented in the Patient Teaching box.

Teaching for the head-injured patient who is left with deficits is targeted to the patient's and family's unique strengths and deficits. The rehabilitation principles used will be similar to those discussed in Chapters 43 and 44 for patients with stroke, spinal cord injury, or degenerative neurologic diseases.

Few illnesses challenge the physical and emotional resources of the patient's family as do neurologic problems. It is imperative that the family participate actively in all long-term planning for the patient. Family members may have severe emotional reactions to the patient's injury and need the assistance of a counselor to help them come to terms with the injury and its consequences. Both patients and families need time to work through their feelings. Sometimes neither the patient nor the family can grasp the enormity of the diagnosis and may need weeks or months to adjust to the reality of the patient's losses.

Even the person who has suffered a mild head injury can experience long-term effects. These most often include cognitive problems such as difficulty with concentration and loss of memory. Recovery of full intellectual functioning often is delayed, and the deficits may manifest in the inability to keep a job or manage the challenges of daily living.

If the patient with neurologic disease experiences severe personality changes, aphasia, or seizures, the family may even be afraid of the patient or may make tactless remarks in front of the patient. The nurse carefully assesses the family's response and reinforces teaching concerning head injury and its many possible consequences. The Guidelines for Safe Practice box summarizes the major elements involved in the care of a person who has experienced a head injury.

Health Promotion/Prevention

Traumatic head injuries can often be prevented. Primary prevention focuses on reducing the incidence of head injury through improved environmental safety and increased use of safety devices such as seatbelts and bicycle helmets (see Research box). These factors are reflected in the Healthy People 2010 objectives presented in the Healthy People 2010 box.[27] A variety of other strategies can also reduce the incidence of head injury in vulnerable populations. Public health and information campaigns focus on reducing risk through measures such as:

- Using seat belts, passive restraints, and air bags in automobiles
- Using helmets when riding motorcycles, snowmobiles, or bicycles
- Practicing firearm safety and gun control
- Avoiding excess consumption of alcohol and drugs
- Not driving after taking drugs or drinking alcohol
- Improving home environmental safety features (e.g., securing throw rugs, removing clutter on stairs, installing grab bars in bathrooms, and increasing lighting)

Nurses have multiple opportunities to participate in primary prevention efforts with professional and community or-

Guidelines for Safe Practice

The Patient With a Closed Head Injury

1. Promote rest.
   a. Provide quiet environment.
   b. Observe frequently.
   c. Administer anticonvulsants as ordered.
   d. Medicate for pain as necessary.
2. Maintain temperature.
   a. Give tepid sponge baths if hyperthermic.
   b. Administer antipyretics as ordered.
   c. Use hypothermia blanket if ordered.
   d. Reduce or increase temperature in patient's room as needed.
3. Promote adequate respiration.
   a. Suction only as necessary to provide adequate airway.
   b. Elevate head of bed to 30 degrees.
   c. Administer supplemental oxygen if ordered.
   d. Place patient in side-lying position.
4. Observe for drainage from ears or nose.
   a. Make no attempt to clean out orifice.
   b. Do not suction nose if drainage is present.
   c. Have patient avoid coughing, sneezing, or blowing nose.
   d. Test drainage for presence of cerebrospinal fluid and report immediately if present.
5. Control cerebral edema.
   a. Administer diuretics as ordered.
   b. Elevate head of bed to 30 degrees.
   c. Perform neurologic checks as ordered.
6. Maintain electrolyte balance.
   a. Observe for inappropriate antidiuretic hormone or diabetes insipidus.
   b. Monitor electrolytes.
7. Maintain elimination.
   a. Keep accurate intake and output record.
   b. Restrict fluid if ordered.
   c. Monitor output.
   d. Remove catheter as soon as possible.
8. Provide emotional support.
   a. Give specific guidelines for appropriate behaviors.
   b. Give positive feedback.
   c. Allow patient adequate time to complete tasks.

ganizations through the schools, senior centers, bike clubs, and civic groups.

EVALUATION

To evaluate the effectiveness of nursing interventions, compare patient behaviors with those stated in the expected patient outcomes. Achievement of patient outcomes is successful if the patient:

1. Has pulse oximetry readings above 90%, with regular and unlabored respirations.
2. Is free of signs and symptoms of increased ICP.
3. Maintains body temperature between 97.5° and 99.5° F.
4. Maintains a fluid intake of at least 1500 ml/day with balanced urine output, normal electrolyte and BUN values, and stable weight.
5. Remains free of infection.
6. Ambulates and performs transfers without assistance or moves independently via a wheelchair.
7. Has a family member or significant other who verbalizes understanding of and ability to cope with the injury of the loved one.
8. Has a family member or significant other who can correctly explain the pathologic process of head injury and rationale for associated care.

Research

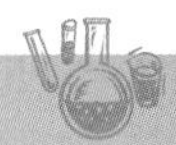

Reference: Attewell RG, Glase K, McFadden M: Bicycle helmet efficacy: a meta analysis, *Accid Anal Prev* 33(3):345-352, 2001.

This study analyzed the data related to bicycle helmet use and brain injury gathered from several countries over a decade between 1987 and 1998. The use of bicycle helmets was associated with a statistically significant reduction in brain injury, facial injury, and fatal injury associated with bicycle accidents. A subanalysis also revealed a connection between the use of older, heavier helmets and associated spinal cord injury that appeared to decrease as the lighter helmets came into widespread use. The authors make the case that the helmets remain less than optimally used and suggest the need for public education to make their use as uniformly accepted as the use of seat belts in automobiles.

Healthy People 2010

Goals and Objectives Related to Head Injury

1. Reduce hospitalization for nonfatal head injuries to 45 per 100,000 persons.
2. Reduce deaths caused by motor vehicle crashes to no more than 0.8 per 100 million vehicle miles traveled and 9.2 per 100,000 persons.
3. Increase the use of safety belts to 92% of the total population.
4. Reduce deaths from falls and fall-related injuries to no more than 3.0 per 100,000 persons.

From US Department of Health and Human Services: *Healthy People 2010: understanding and improving health,* Washington DC, 2000, USDHHS.

GERONTOLOGIC CONSIDERATIONS

The elderly patient may have preexisting conditions that contributed to the injury. Altered gait, balance, and reflexes make the elderly patient more prone to falls. Osteoporosis increases the risk, frequency, and severity of fractures of the skull and face. Syncope, hypotension, and cardiac dysrythmias can also lead to falls. Patients receiving anticoagulation therapy are more likely to develop hematomas after falls.

Elderly patients with significant medical histories, especially problems with hypertension or cerebrovascular disease, have less physiologic reserve to survive the acute period following a moderate to severe head injury.[18] The assessment of patients with a known degenerative disorder such as Alzheimer's disease is complicated by the need to differentiate between pretrauma abnormalities and those related to the trauma itself. Patients with sensory losses related to aging, such as vision or hearing losses, may have a more difficult time participating in therapy. An elderly patient who was barely independent before a nervous system trauma may not be able to regain independence even when the residual deficits are minor.

Nurses educate patients and families in ways to keep the older population safe from injuries that rob them of their independence and health. Environmental modifications to remove hazards, mobility aids, sensory enhancement aids, and structured exercise can help the elderly patient retain strength and mobility.

SPECIAL ENVIRONMENTS FOR CARE

Critical Care

The patient with a mild or moderate head injury does not usually require critical care. Patients with multisystem trauma, however, and those needing intubation and ventilation are admitted to a critical care setting. Initial management of the patient focuses on resuscitation and stabilization, as well as prompt identification of rising ICP and other complications. The full trauma evaluation is then completed to identify occult injuries. Effective ventilation is established, circulatory support is initiated to ensure perfusion to the injured brain, and frequent bedside monitoring is continued to identify subtle changes in the patient's status.

During the acute phase of recovery, the patient's ICP is monitored and treated as necessary. Ventilatory support is maintained and then gradually withdrawn as the patient recovers from his or her injuries. As the patient becomes more stable, less invasive monitoring is required and the patient is encouraged to participate more fully in ADLs. In rare instances the patient may need prolonged ventilatory support but is otherwise stable. In this case rehabilitation actually begins in the critical care setting.

The patient and family require a great deal of support during the critical care period. Trauma is unexpected, and families need to cope with sudden changes in their lives, as well as the threat of losing a loved one. Helping a family cope during the crisis phase is a major nursing responsibility in the ICU and is continued throughout the patient's recovery. Research has identified that the families of the critically ill list information about the patient's condition and access to the patient as their most important needs during this stressful time.[8]

Community-Based Care

Patients with moderate head injuries may be sent home to continue their rehabilitation on an outpatient basis. Hospital-based nurses assist families in identifying appropriate resources in the patient's local community. Resource selection is based on the patient's ability to perform self-care and the family's resources and supports for providing the needed care and support.

Patients with more severe head injuries may need long-term care either at a rehabilitation facility or at home. This care is often more supportive than restorative. The care needs of head-injured patients can be enormous because they include physical, psychologic, and cognitive challenges. Families need physical, social, and emotional support when providing this level of care long term.

COMPLICATIONS

A wide range of complications can occur following head injury. Complications related to immobility include atelectasis, pneumonia, cardiovascular deconditioning, skin breakdown, muscle atrophy, and constipation. Patients are also at risk for infection from breaks in the body's natural defenses. Invasive monitoring devices, IV lines, urinary catheters, and endotracheal tubes all breach the body's natural defenses and increase the risk of infection. If the patient has a skull fracture with a dural tear, meningitis is also a risk.

Head-injured patients are also at risk for complications specifically related to the neurologic injury. Some patients develop seizures and need lifelong anticonvulsant therapy. Other patients develop obstructions to CSF flow and need to be treated for hydrocephalus. Autonomic responses to the injury may increase stomach acid production and cause peptic ulcers. The nurse works collaboratively to identify possible complications and develop plans for prevention and treatment.

INFECTIONS AND INFLAMMATION

The nervous system may be attacked by a variety of bacteria and viruses that reach the nervous system by various routes. Chronic otitis media, sinusitis, mastoiditis, and fracture of any bone adjacent to the meninges can be a source of infection. Some organisms, such as the tubercle bacillus, reach the nervous system by means of the blood or lymph system. Infection can also occur as a complication of invasive procedures such as lumbar puncture. The exact route by which some infectious agents reach the central nervous system is not known. The infection may wall off and create an abscess, or the meninges and sometimes the brain itself may become involved. Two of the more common central nervous system infections—meningitis and encephalitis—are discussed next. Table 42-8 presents some of the common organisms that cause central nervous system infections.

Meningitis

Etiology/Epidemiology

Meningitis can be caused by both bacteria and viruses. Viral meningitis, also known as aseptic meningitis, is an inflammation of the meninges. Caused by viral or nonviral sources, the disease is usually self-limiting and does not require extensive treatment. Enteroviruses and mumps are the most common causative agents.

Bacterial meningitis affects the leptomeninges (the pia and arachnoid layers) and the CSF. The most common pathogens causing meningitis are *Haemophilus influenzae, Neisseria meningitidis,* and *Streptococcus pneumoniae.* The causative organisms vary significantly at different ages. *Haemophilus* is common in young children and often follows an upper respiratory or ear infection. *Neisseria* has its highest incidence in

TABLE 42-8 Organisms That Cause Central Nervous System Infections

Disease	Organism	Comments
Pneumococcal meningitis	*Streptococcus pneumoniae*	Gram-positive diplococci; most common type in adults, especially if history of pneumonia, sinus infection, trauma
Haemophilus influenzae meningitis	*H. influenzae*	Gram-negative cocci; most common in children, especially if history of upper respiratory infection or ear infection
Meningococcal meningitis	*Neisseria meningitidis*	Gram-negative diplococci; highest incidence in children or young adults; may have petechial rash; about 10% develop overwhelming septicemia
California encephalitis	Arbovirus of California, mosquito borne	Aseptic meningitis or encephalitis
St. Louis encephalitis	St. Louis encephalitis virus, mosquito borne	Encephalitis or aseptic meningitis

children and young adults and can cause an overwhelming septicemia. *S. pneumoniae* causes the pneumococcal form of meningitis, which is common in adults.

The incidence of meningitis is fairly constant throughout the year but typically declines slightly during the summer months. Certain forms of the disease are associated with serious adverse outcomes and complications.

Pathophysiology

The blood is the most common pathway for organisms to reach the nervous system. Bacteria in the nasopharynx can enter the bloodstream during an upper respiratory infection, and once organisms reach the brain, the CSF in the subarachnoid spaces and the pia-arachnoid membrane become infected. The infection then spreads rapidly throughout the meninges and eventually can invade the ventricles. Pathologic alterations include hyperemia of the meningeal blood vessels, edema of brain tissue, increased ICP, and a severe generalized inflammatory reaction that is accompanied by massive exudation of white blood cells into the subarachnoid spaces. Acute hydrocephalus may result when this exudate blocks the small passages between the ventricles.

Collaborative Care Management

The definitive diagnosis of meningitis requires culturing the CSF, which is obtained by lumbar puncture or from a ventriculostomy. A CT scan may also be performed to rule out other pathologic conditions.

Meningitis can present as a medical emergency. The onset is usually sudden and characterized by severe headache, stiff neck, fever, irritability, malaise, and restlessness. Nausea, vomiting, delirium, and complete disorientation may develop quickly. Kernig's sign (the inability of the patient to extend the legs when the knee is flexed at the hip) usually is present, and Brudzinski's sign (the hip and knee flex when the patient's neck is flexed) may also be present (Figure 42-16). The causative organism can usually be isolated from the spinal fluid, which is cloudy if a pyogenic organism is present. The CSF pressure is also usually elevated, as well as the protein level, whereas glucose content is usually decreased.

Treatment for bacterial infections consists of antibiotic therapy targeted at the specific causative organism. Parenteral antibiotics are given for at least 10 days and may be administered directly into the spinal canal (intrathecally). Respiratory isolation is required with meningococcal infections until the pathogen can no longer be cultured from the nasopharynx, usually after 24 hours of antibiotic therapy. Isolation is not needed with other forms of the disease. The use of hyperosmolar agents or steroids may be necessary to control cerebral edema. Anticonvulsants may be given to prevent or control seizures. If the patient develops hydrocephalus as a result of the meningitis, a shunt may need to be inserted to facilitate the flow of CSF.

General treatment measures include supportive care to control and reduce fever, balance fluids and electrolytes, and promote comfort. The headache can be severe, and the patient's fever may remain high throughout the illness. Acetaminophen (Tylenol) is typically given to reduce the fever and relieve the headache. Ice packs may increase the patient's comfort. Patients who are experiencing photophobia are more comfortable in a darkened room. Lights and noise are minimized as much as possible. The nurse monitors the patient frequently, avoiding unnecessary stimulation and touching. Seizure precautions are instituted, and tepid baths may be necessary to control the patient's fever.

Patient/Family Education. The patient and family are often extremely anxious and may have questions regarding how the disease started and the plan for treatment. The extent and severity of symptoms varies greatly from patient to patient. Some patients are only mildly affected and simply need supportive care. Others are severely affected and need critical care monitoring and support. The nurse keeps the family fully informed about the patient's status and prognosis and helps them to understand that the disease can cause permanent neurologic impairment and even occasionally prove fatal.

Encephalitis

Etiology/Epidemiology

Encephalitis is an acute infection of the brain parenchyma and meninges caused by bacteria, viruses, or fungi. Viral

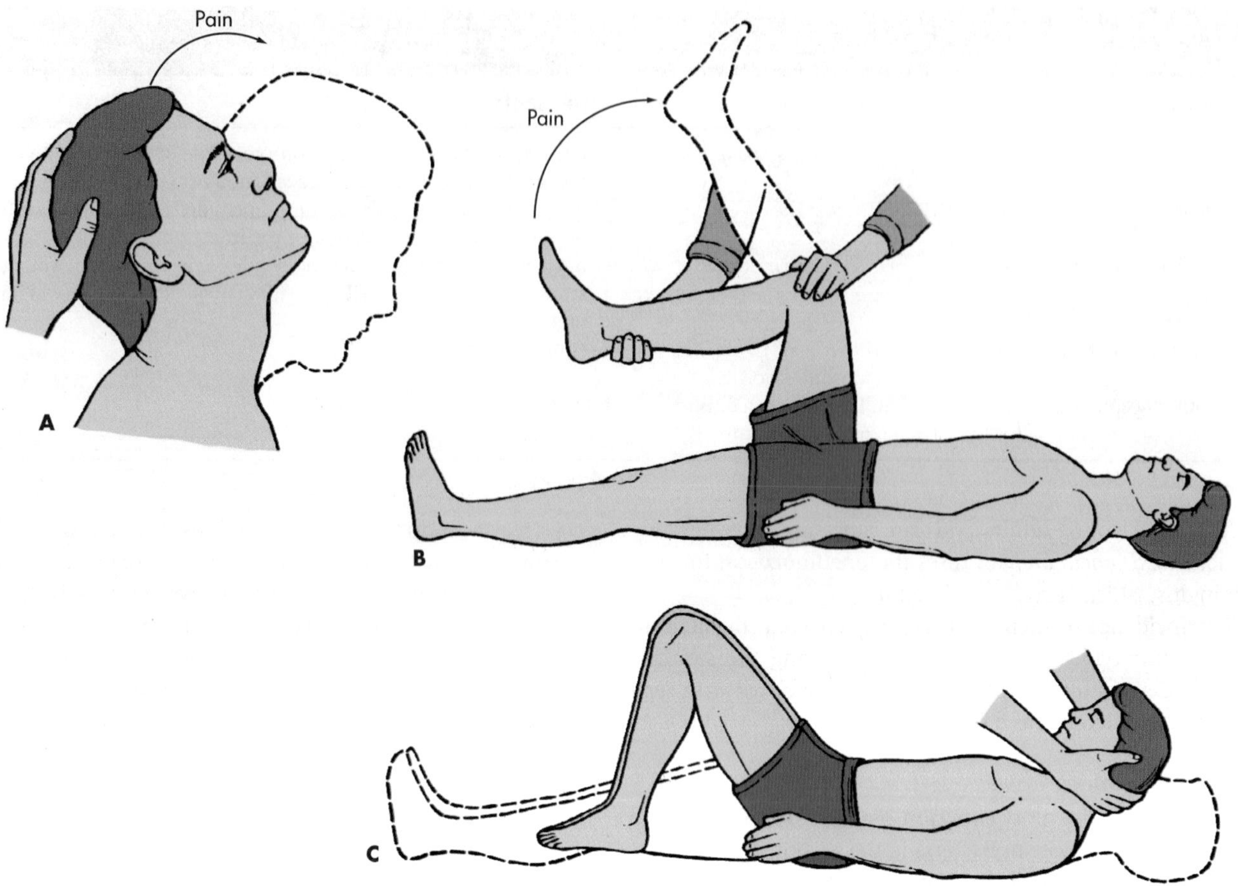

Figure 42-16 Signs of meningeal irritation. **A**, Nuchal rigidity. The neck is held extended and immobile. Attempts to flex the neck cause pain. **B**, Positive Kernig's sign: inability to extend the leg from a position of 90-degree flexion at the hip. Attempts to extend the leg cause pain and spasms in the hamstrings. **C**, Brudzinski's sign: passive flexion of the head and neck cause flexion of the thighs and legs.

infection is the most common and is typically caused by the arboviruses or herpes simplex. A wide variety of viruses, indigenous to various geographic areas, are capable of causing the disease if they gain access to the brain. Eastern equine encephalitis is the most serious, although least common, form. The most significant outbreak of encephalitis in the United States followed the influenza epidemic of 1918 and involved von Economo's disease. This particular form of encephalitis has not reappeared since 1926.

Pathophysiology

Encephalitis causes degenerative changes in the nerve cells of the brain and produces scattered areas of inflammation and necrosis. Some inflammation of the meninges is also typically present. The symptoms vary significantly, depending on the causative organism, but often include fever, headache, seizures, stiff neck, and a declining LOC that can progress from lethargy and restlessness to coma. A wide variety of local neurologic signs can also be present. The mortality rate for encephalitis also varies substantially with the causative organism, but most patients are left with some degree of residual deficit. Deficits include decreased cognitive functioning, personality changes, paralysis, and dementia. Patients can also be left deaf and blind.

Collaborative Care Management

Encephalitis is diagnosed primarily from the clinical picture, serology assays, and analysis of the CSF. Antiviral medications such as acyclovir are effective for some forms of the disease, but treatment is otherwise largely supportive and symptomatic. Prompt initiation of acyclovir therapy has reduced the mortality rate for herpesvirus infections from up to 80% to less than 28%.

Analgesics may be prescribed for the headache and neck pain that accompany the disease. Steroids are administered to suppress inflammation, and anticonvulsants are used to control seizures. In severe cases dramatic increases in ICP can result in brainstem herniation or cause widespread areas of cell necrosis.

Patient/Family Education. The needs of the patient and family for education and support are similar to those outlined for patients with meningitis, particularly when the patient is seriously ill. The fear associated with the disease and the uncertainty of the outcome necessitate frequent interventions and ongoing support from the nurse. It is essential that the nurse include the family in all decisions about the patient's care and keep them honestly apprised of the patient's status.

Critical Thinking Questions

1. A 34-year-old woman is admitted after having a tonic-clonic seizure. She has never experienced a seizure before. What would you assess during her postictal phase? Once she is completely alert, what areas would you explore as part of a detailed health history?
2. A 40-year-old patient with meningitis is admitted to your unit and started on a regimen of antibiotics. He complains of severe headache, stiff neck, and photophobia, and he is running a high fever. What comfort measures could you implement to address his symptoms?
3. Your assessment of a patient with a recent head injury reveals unequal pupils and decreased motor movement on the right side. An emergency CT scan shows an acute subdural hematoma on the left side. How would you explain the problem and its treatment to the patient and his family? How would you prepare him for surgery?
4. Does your state/community have helmet laws for motorcycle and bicycle riders? Prepare a teaching plan concerning the prevention of head injury to use with school-age children. How would the plan need to be modified to address adolescents? Older adults?

References

1. American Brain Tumor Association: *A primer of brain tumors,* Des Plaines, Ill, 1996, The Association.
2. Brain Trauma Foundation; American Association of Neurological Surgeons: The joint section on neurotrauma and critical care, *J Neurotrauma* 17(6/7):471-506, 2000.
3. Brewer T, Therrien B: Minor brain injury: new insights for early nursing care, *J Neurosci Nurs* 32(6):311-317, 2000.
4. Bullock MR, Povlishock JT: Guidelines for the management of severe head injury, *J Neurotrauma* 17(6/7):463-469, 2000.
5. Folstein MF, Folstein SE, McHugh PR: Mini-Mental State: a practical method for grading the cognitive state of patients for the clinician, *J Psychiatr Res* 12(3):189, 1975.
6. Ghajar J: Traumatic brain injury, *Lancet* 356(9233):923-929, 2000.
7. Goadsby PJ: Current concepts of the pathophysiology of migraine, *Neurol Clin* 15(1):27, 1997.
8. Hickey JV: *The clinical practice of neurological and neurosurgical nursing,* ed 4, Philadelphia, 1997, JB Lippincott.
9. Hilton G: Seizure disorders in adults: evaluation and management of new onset seizures, *Nurse Pract* 22(9):42, 1997.
10. Jacobs DG, Westerband A: Antibiotic prophylaxis for intracranial pressure monitors, *J Natl Med Assoc* 90(7):417-423, 1998.
11. King BS et al: The early assessment and intensive care unit management of patients with severe traumatic brain and spinal cord injuries, *Surg Clin North Am* 80(3):855-870, 2000.
12. Lin J: Overview of migraine, *J Neurosci Nurs* 33(1):6-13, 2001.
13. Marion DW: Management of traumatic brain injury: past, present and future, *Clin Neurosurg* 45:184-191, 1999.
14. Mathews NT: Serotonin 1D (5-HT) agonists and other agents in acute migraine, *Neurol Clin* 15(1):61, 1997.
15. McNew CD, Hunt S, Warner LS: How to help your patient with epilepsy, *Nursing* 27(9):57, 1997.
16. Nieder N, Nestle U: A review of current and future treatment strategies for malignant astrocytomas in adults, *Strahlenther Onkol* 176(6):251-258, 2000.
17. Plum F, Posner JB: *The diagnosis of stupor and coma,* ed 3, Philadelphia, 1982, FA Davis.
18. Rapoport MJ, Feinstein A: Outcome following traumatic brain injury in the elderly: a critical review, *Brain Injury* 14(8):749-761, 2000.
19. Rebuck JA et al: Infection related to intracranial pressure monitors in adults: analysis of risk factors and antibiotic prophylaxis, *J Neurol Neurosurg Psychiatry* 69(3):381-384, 2000.
20. Shapiro W: Current therapy for brain tumors: back to the future, *Arch Neurol* 56(4):429-432, 1999.
21. Simmons B: Management of intracranial hemodynamics in the adult: a research analysis of head positioning and recommendations for clinical practice and future research, *J Neurosci Nurs* 29(1):44-49, 1997.
22. Solomon S: Diagnosis of primary headache disorders: validity of the IHS criteria in clinical practice, *Neurol Clin* 15(1):15, 1997.
23. Sullivan J: Positioning of patients with severe traumatic brain injury: research-based practice, *J Neurosci Nurs* 32(4):204-209, 2000.
24. Teasdale G, Jennett B: Assessment of coma and impaired consciousness: a practical scale, *Lancet* 2(7872):81, 1974.
25. Tfelt-Hansen P: Prophylactic pharmacotherapy of migraine: some practical guidelines, *Neurol Clin* 15(1):153, 1997.
26. Thurman D et al: Traumatic brain injury in the United States: a public health perspective, *J Head Trauma* 14(6):602-615, 1999.
27. US Department of Health and Human Services, Public Health Service: *Healthy people 2010: national health promotion and disease prevention objectives,* DHHS Pub No (PHS) 91-50212, Washington, DC, 2000, US Government Printing Office.
28. Winkelman C: Effect of backrest position on intracranial and cerebral perfusion pressures in traumatically brain-injured adults, *Am J Crit Care* 9(6):373-382, 2000.

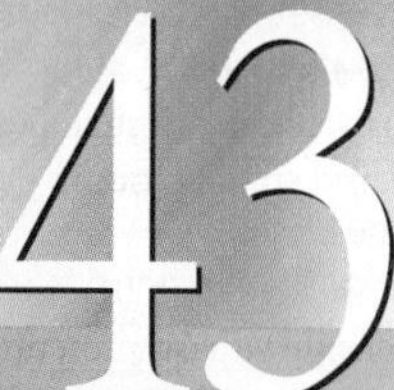

Vascular and Degenerative Problems of the Brain

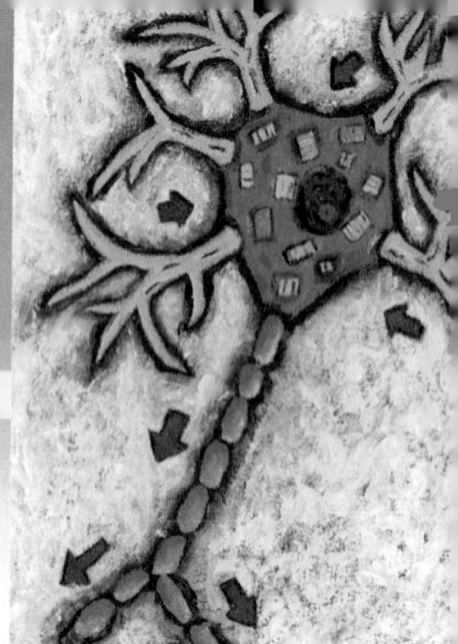

Lois Perry, Judith K. Sands

Objectives

After studying this chapter, the learner should be able to:

1. Identify the major risk factors for ischemic and hemorrhagic stroke.
2. Correlate stroke pathology with its major clinical manifestations.
3. Compare neurologic and behavioral findings associated with right versus left hemisphere strokes.
4. Develop specific assessment strategies for identifying the primary communication and sensory-perceptual deficits of stroke.
5. Discuss the rationale for antiplatelet therapy, reperfusion therapy, and carotid endarterectomy in the management of cerebrovascular disease and stroke.
6. Develop nursing interventions to assist patients in regaining self-care independence after stroke.
7. Describe nursing interventions to prevent the musculoskeletal and nutritional complications of stroke.
8. Develop a patient and family teaching plan to manage the communication, cognitive, behavioral, and emotional outcomes of stroke.
9. Compare the treatment options for aneurysms and arteriovenous malformations.
10. Compare the major degenerative and autoimmune neurologic disorders in terms of incidence, populations affected, and primary pathology.
11. Describe the pharmacologic management of myasthenia gravis and Parkinson's disease.
12. Compare the major nursing interventions used to manage mobility, self-care, nutrition, bowel and bladder elimination, and safety concerns for each of the major degenerative and autoimmune neurologic disorders.

This chapter presents the management of vascular, degenerative, and autoimmune disorders affecting the brain. Cerebrovascular accident is by far the most important of these disorders because of its incidence and its extensive residual deficits, which challenge patients, families, and health care providers. Numerous autoimmune and degenerative disorders could be included in the chapter discussion, but only the most common of these disorders are presented. All of them have complex associated care needs, but they all share the common goal of maximizing the patient's independence in self-care for as long as possible and supporting overall coping. These disorders are managed by a multidisciplinary team, but the nurse is commonly called on to serve as the case manager, coordinating needed services.

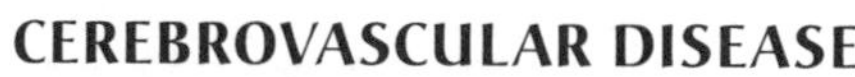

CEREBROVASCULAR DISEASE

The term *cerebrovascular disease* refers to any pathologic process involving the blood vessels of the brain. Cerebrovascular disease is the most common neurologic disorder in adults and is the third leading cause of death in the United States, after heart disease and cancer. The heterogeneous category of cerebrovascular disease encompasses two major types of disorders—ischemic and hemorrhagic—each of which can produce either temporary or permanent deficits in neurologic functioning. Major problems in either category create a syndrome of neurologic deficits that reflect impairment of oxygenation to a specific area of the brain. This syndrome is usually referred to as a cerebrovascular accident or stroke. Although strokes can have either an ischemic or a hemorrhagic origin, the following discussion is primarily directed toward the management of ischemic strokes, which are by far the most common form. Hemorrhagic strokes are discussed later in the chapter under Cerebral Aneurysm and Arteriovenous Malformation.

Cerebrovascular Accident/Stroke

Etiology

A cerebrovascular accident (CVA) is a neurologic deficit that has a sudden onset and lasts for more than 24 hours. Ischemic strokes account for an estimated 85% of the total, and this percentage can be further broken down into atherothrombotic strokes (61%) and embolic strokes (24%).[2] These categories are described in Box 43-1. Hemorrhagic strokes are typically classified by the location of the bleeding. Subarachnoid hemorrhagic strokes (about 7% of all strokes) occur from bleeding into the subarachnoid space, and intracerebral hemorrhagic strokes (about 10% of all strokes) occur from bleeding into the brain tissue itself.[2] Subarachnoid bleeding is usually the result of the rupture of a cerebral aneurysm or arteriovenous malformation, whereas intracerebral bleeds result from the rupture of a small artery, often a deep penetrating vessel, and are often related to poorly controlled hypertension.

Both modifiable and nonmodifiable risk factors are associated with stroke. The nonmodifiable risks of age, gender, sex, and race are discussed under Epidemiology and summarized in the Risk Factors box. In addition, hypertension, cardiac disease, diabetes mellitus, and blood lipid abnormalities can all increase the risk of stroke, particularly when they are present in combination. The presence of atherosclerosis elsewhere in the body is presumed to also involve the cerebral vessels. Patients who have preexisting heart disease have a clearly increased risk, as do patients with diabetes mellitus, which accelerates the processes of atherosclerosis and arteriosclerosis in the blood vessels. The reduction of modifiable risk factors such as hypertension, hyperlipidemia, tobacco use, and inactivity has been shown to reduce the incidence and recurrence of stroke.[13]

Epidemiology

Although a significant decrease in stroke incidence and mortality has occurred over the past two decades, stroke remains the third leading cause of death in the United States. An estimated 500,000 first-time strokes occur each year.[2] The mortality rate has declined about 15% since 1988,[2] but stroke leaves about 30% of its victims with mental or physical disabilities that require ongoing assistance with activities of daily living (ADLs).[32] This creates a pool of more than 1 million

BOX 43-1 Etiologies of Ischemic Strokes

Atherosclerotic

Atherosclerosis affects both the large extracranial and the intracranial arteries. The lumen of the vessel narrows and can be a target site for thrombus formation. Transient ischemic attacks occur in about half of patients before the stroke.

Small Penetrating Artery Thrombosis/Lacunar

Thrombosis of a small penetrating brain artery causes a small damaged area of tissue in the deep white matter structures of the brain, called a lacuna. Lacunae typically occur in the basal ganglia, internal capsule, pons, or thalamus.

Cardiogenic/Embolic

Most of these strokes are the result of emboli, usually of cardiac origin, that break off and travel in the arterial circulation until they reach a vessel that is too narrow to allow further passage. Atrial fibrillation is the most common cause of the emboli.

Other

Ischemic strokes can also result from vasospasm, inflammation, coagulation disorders, and the effects of drug abuse, particularly cocaine.

Idiopathic

No identifiable cause is established in up to 30% of all ischemic strokes.

Risk Factors

Stroke

AGE

From 60% to 75% of all strokes occur in persons over 65 years of age.

SEX

Men have a slightly increased incidence of stroke, possibly because of poorer control of hypertension and heart disease.

RACE

African-Americans are twice as likely to develop thrombotic strokes and three times more likely to develop hemorrhagic strokes. Whether this is truly a race-related risk is unknown.

HYPERTENSION

Hypertension is a major risk factor for stroke, particularly in combination with atherosclerosis. The improved diagnosis and treatment of hypertension have decreased the incidence and mortality of stroke over the past two decades.

HEART DISEASE

Heart disease is a major contributor to stroke, both from atherosclerosis and as a common source of emboli.

DIABETES

Diabetes is associated with an accelerated rate of microvascular and macrovascular changes that contribute to atherosclerosis.

OTHER

Cigarette smoking
Oral contraceptive use (especially if also a smoker)
Alcohol intake
Family history of transient ischemic attack or cerebrovascular accident
Obesity*
Sedentary lifestyle*
Elevated serum cholesterol and triglycerides*

*These factors are less well studied but are believed to contribute to stroke.

people who are currently partially or totally disabled from stroke, and this number is expected to rise as the population continues to age. The importance of stroke as a national health concern is reflected in the Healthy People 2010 goal "to reduce stroke deaths to no more than 48 per 100,000 people."[29]

Stroke has profound social and economic consequences for the person, family, and community. Direct and indirect costs for stroke management and ongoing care are estimated at 45 billion dollars.[2] The obvious economic impact of stroke is reflected in the rapid proliferation of clinical pathways for case management of stroke patients. These pathways attempt to clearly delineate the specifics of care to be provided at each stage of rehabilitation. The social and emotional tolls are more difficult to quantify but are readily apparent to anyone whose family has been touched by stroke.

About 72% of all strokes occur in persons over 65 years of age.[2] The remaining 28% affect younger persons. Strokes are slightly more common in men than in women. African-Americans are twice as likely to experience ischemic strokes and three times more likely to experience hemorrhagic strokes than Caucasians. It is unclear whether this increased incidence is directly related to racial factors or reflects generally poorer diagnosis and treatment of hypertension, heart disease, and diabetes in this population—particularly male African-Americans. Some variations in incidence and mortality have also been noted worldwide, particularly in Japan. The meaning of these differences is not clear.

Pathophysiology

The brain must receive a steady supply of nutrients from the blood because it has no capacity to store either oxygen or glucose. It is supplied with blood from two major pairs of arteries: the internal carotids and the vertebrals. The carotids supply the anterior portions of the brain, including most of the cerebral hemispheres except for the occipital lobes (Figure 43-1). The vertebrals join together to become the basilar artery and supply the posterior portions of the brain, including the cerebellum, brainstem, and occipital lobes. The Circle of Willis is the region of the brain in which the branches of the basilar and internal carotid arteries join, creating a circular network, which in theory allows blood to circulate from one hemisphere to the other and from the anterior to the posterior portions of the brain (Figure 43-2). Functionally, however, the circulations of the two hemispheres usually remain separate. The circle is composed of the middle cerebral arteries; the anterior cerebral arteries; the anterior communicating artery, which connects the anterior cerebrals; the posterior cerebral arteries; and the posterior communicating arteries, which connect the middle cerebrals with the posterior cerebrals, thus uniting the two systems. Figure 43-3 illustrates the major areas of the brain supplied by these cerebral vessels.

The complex processes of cerebral autoregulation maintain blood flow to the brain at a fairly constant rate of 750 ml/min. The cerebral vessels dilate and constrict in response to changes in blood pressure and carbon dioxide tension. Prolonged is-

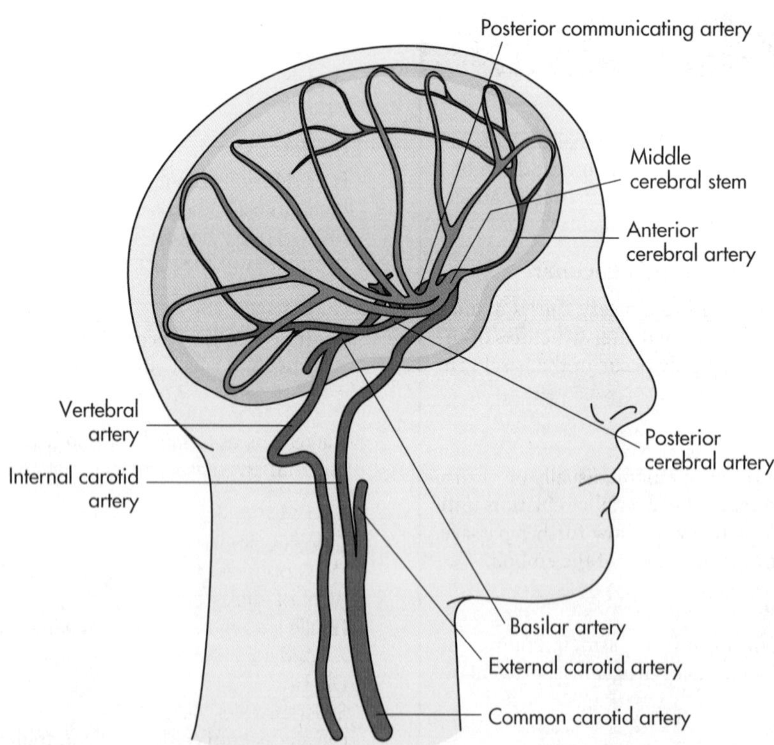

Figure 43-1 The major arteries that supply the brain. The internal carotids branch to supply the anterior portions of the brain. The vertebral arteries supply the posterior portions.

chemia can cause primary death of cerebral cells or cerebral infarction, which creates a core of necrotic tissue. The ischemia, in a process similar to that seen after myocardial infarction, also causes a second area of tissue damage in which cells are temporarily unable to function but may remain viable. A complex cascade of biochemical changes occurs in response to the ischemia, and this process is the target of intense current research.[12] When the components of the ischemic response can be accurately mapped, it may be possible to prevent or reverse its effects. Ischemia is known to cause the following disparate responses[12]:

- Impaired movement of calcium and potassium (High levels of calcium are believed to trigger the activation of enzymes that attack neuron cell membranes.)
- Accumulation of oxygen free radicals, which further disrupt calcium metabolism
- Enhanced lactate production from the presence of glucose in low perfusion areas, which worsens cellular damage and acidosis
- An influx of fluid-activated white blood cells and coagulation factors that further clog the microcirculation

The pathophysiology associated with hemorrhagic strokes is primarily related to an abrupt rise in intracranial pressure and ischemia followed by cerebral edema. With intracerebral bleeding, blood is forced into the adjacent brain tissue, where a hematoma forms. The compression of tissue then extends the ischemic damage and can even result in brain tissue displacement or herniation. The pathophysiologic process of elevated intracranial pressure is described in Chapter 42.

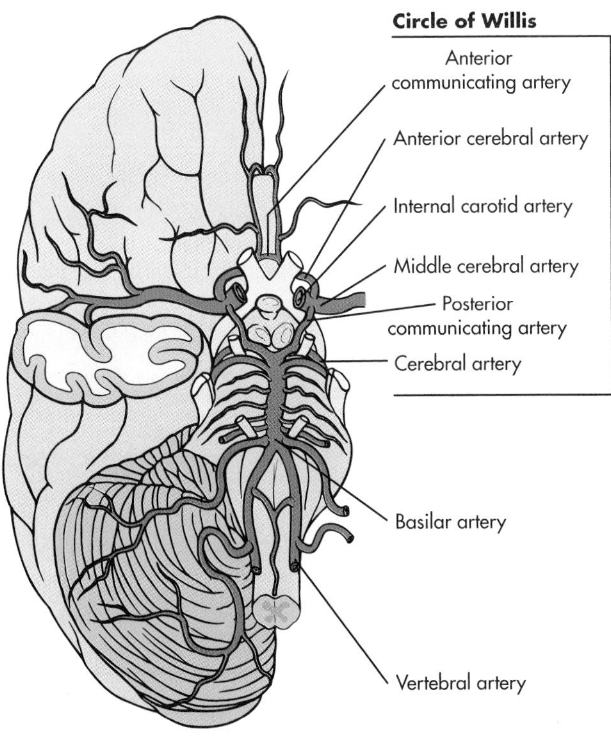

Figure 43-2 The Circle of Willis as seen from below the brain.

Transient Ischemic Attack. A transient ischemic attack (TIA) is a relatively brief episode of neurologic deficit that resolves without any residual effect. The episode may last for seconds, minutes, or hours, but the average duration is 10 minutes, and the vast majority resolve within an hour. By definition, the symptoms must resolve within 24 hours. The term *reversible ischemic neurologic deficit* may be used if the deficit persists beyond 24 hours but then resolves within 3 weeks with no permanent deficits.[21]

TIAs are generally thought to be warning signs of an impending ischemic problem and usually reflect advanced atherosclerotic disease. It is theorized that TIAs may be caused by microemboli that break off from atherosclerotic plaque lesions. However, TIAs can also be triggered by events that temporarily decrease blood flow to the affected area of the brain, such as vasospasm or hypotension.

An estimated one third of persons who experience a TIA will have future episodes, one third will have no future episodes, and about one third will have a stroke within 2 years. TIAs may also recur repetitively over days, weeks, and even years without progressing to stroke. The unique symptoms

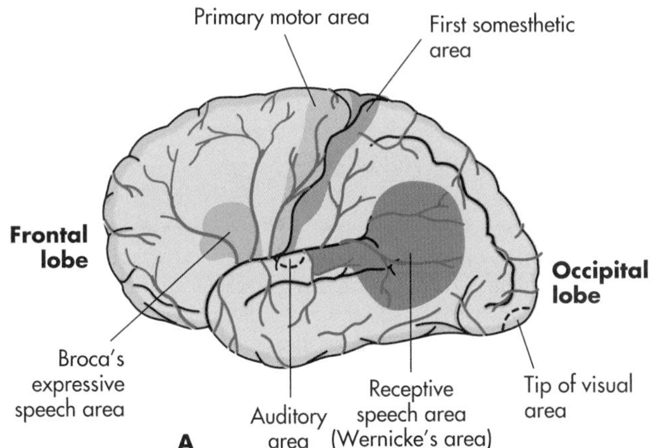

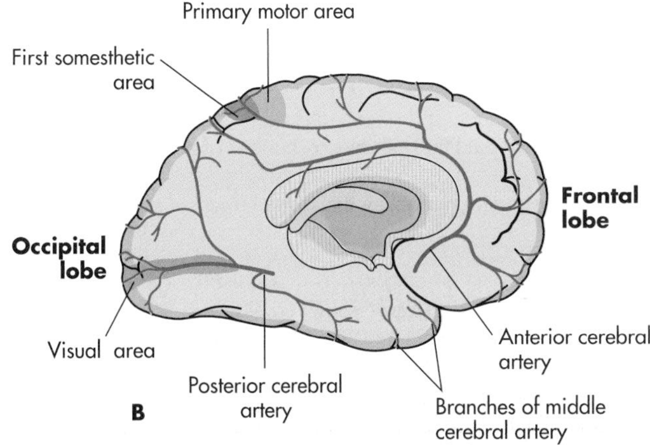

Figure 43-3 **A,** Distribution of the middle cerebral artery on the lateral surface of the brain. **B,** Distribution of the anterior and posterior cerebral arteries on the medial surface of the brain.

Clinical Manifestations

Transient Ischemic Attacks

SYMPTOMS RELATED TO CAROTID INVOLVEMENT

Visual disturbances
- Temporary blindness in one eye
- Blurred vision

Motor disturbances
- Hemiparesis
- Localized motor deficits in face or extremities

Sensory disturbances
- Hemianesthesia
- Sensory deficits in face or extremities

SYMPTOMS RELATED TO VERTEBRAL INVOLVEMENT

Motor disturbances
- Ataxia
- Dysarthria
- Dysphagia
- Unilateral or bilateral weakness

Visual disturbances
- Diplopia
- Bilateral blindness

Other
- Brief lapses in level of consciousness
- Sensory disturbance
- Dizziness, vertigo
- Tinnitus

NOTE: Clinical manifestations are brief in duration and reversible.

produced by the TIA are specific to the vessel involved and can usually be traced to involvement of the carotid supply or that of the vertebral arteries. There is tremendous variety in the range of possible symptoms. Common symptoms of TIAs are summarized in the Clinical Manifestations box.

Clinical Manifestations. The specific neurologic deficits that are produced by stroke reflect the location and severity of the ischemia and the adequacy of the collateral circulation in the region. The term *stroke* commonly evokes a classic mental picture of specific disabilities, but a wide variety of presentations can occur. Commonly encountered symptoms are summarized in the Clinical Manifestations box. Many of the features overlap with other forms of brain injury. A number of specific syndromes have been identified that reflect the involvement of specific vessels and the areas of the brain that they serve, but in clinical practice it is unusual to see these syndromes in their pure forms. Box 43-2 outlines a few of the major syndromes and their associated neurologic deficits. The two vessels affected most commonly are the middle cerebral artery and the internal carotid artery.

Each of the major types of stroke is associated with a fairly typical onset and course of symptoms. A stroke caused by a thrombus occurs during sleep or rest more than 60% of the time. This may be related to the decline in baseline blood pressure that occurs at rest or to increases in blood viscosity that develop during sleep periods. Symptoms may develop abruptly or progress over a period of hours, depending on

Clinical Manifestations

Stroke

NOTE: Specific symptoms will reflect the site and severity of ischemic damage. The following is a general listing of common deficits. See also Box 43-2 for specific deficits associated with ischemia in individual cerebral vessels.

MOTOR

Hemiparesis or hemiplegia of the side of the body opposite the site of ischemia
- Initially flaccid, progressing to spastic

Dysphagia
- Swallowing reflex may also be impaired

Dysarthria

BOWEL AND BLADDER

Frequency, urgency, and urinary incontinence
- Potential for bladder retraining is good if cognitively intact

Constipation
- Related more to immobility than to the physical effects of stroke

LANGUAGE

Nonfluent aphasia (also known as motor/expressive aphasia): difficulty or inability to express self verbally

Fluent aphasia (also known as sensory/receptive aphasia): difficulty or inability to comprehend speech

Alexia: inability to understand the written word

Agraphia: inability to express self in writing

SENSORY-PERCEPTUAL

Diminished response to superficial sensation
- Touch, pain, pressure, heat, and cold

Diminished proprioception
- Knowledge of position of body parts in the environment

Visual deficits
- Decreased acuity
- Diplopia
- Homonymous hemianopia (see Figure 43-4)

Perceptual (see Box 43-3)
- Unilateral neglect syndrome
- Distorted body image
- Apraxia: inability to carry out learned voluntary acts
- Agnosia: inability to recognize familiar objects through sight, sound, or touch
- Anosognosia: inability to recognize or denial of a physical deficit
- Possible deficits in:
  - Telling time
  - Judging distance
  - Right-left discrimination
  - Memory of locations, objects

COGNITIVE-EMOTIONAL

Emotional lability and unpredictability
- Behavior may be socially inappropriate (e.g., crying jags, swearing)

Depression

Memory loss

Short attention span, easy distractability

Loss of reasoning, judgment, and abstract thinking ability

BOX 43-2 Characteristics of Major Stroke Syndromes

Middle Cerebral Artery Syndrome (Most Common Occlusion)

If blockage of the main stem of the middle cerebral artery (MCA) occurs, the infarction can affect most of the hemisphere, because the MCA accounts for about 80% of the blood supply to the cerebral hemispheres.

- Contralateral hemiparesis or hemiplegia (arm affected more severely than the leg)
- Contralateral sensory impairment over same area affected by hemiplegia (proprioception, touch)
- Unilateral neglect or inattention (if nondominant hemisphere)
- Aphasia (if dominant hemisphere)
- Homonymous hemianopia

Internal Carotid Artery Syndrome

The symptoms of MCA and internal carotid artery strokes are almost identical, but if blockage of the main stem of the MCA occurs (see above), the deficits can be profound, because cerebral edema is usually extensive.

- Contralateral hemiparesis or hemiplegia
- Contralateral sensory losses
- Aphasia (if dominant hemisphere)

Vertebrobasilar Artery Syndromes

Occlusion of the vessels in this system creates unique symptoms that reflect the perfusion of the cerebellum and brainstem:

- Ataxia, clumsiness
- Dysphagia and dysarthria
- Dizziness and nystagmus
- Bilateral motor and sensory deficits
- Facial weakness and numbness

how much blood is able to move through the obstructed vessel lumen. The symptoms usually peak within 72 hours and then demonstrate some improvement as the cerebral edema resolves. Embolic and hemorrhagic strokes are more likely to develop suddenly and progress rapidly over minutes or hours. There is rarely any advance warning. Patients with embolic strokes usually remain conscious during the event, but a decreased level of alertness is expected during the first few days following any type of stroke.

The term *stroke in evolution* may be used to describe an ischemic stroke whose symptoms develop progressively over a period of hours or days. This pattern is most characteristic of a gradually enlarging thrombus. *Completed stroke* is a term used to describe a situation in which no further deterioration in function has occurred over a 2- to 3-day period. Active rehabilitation usually begins as soon as an ischemic stroke is considered complete.

Motor Deficits. Motor symptoms are the most widely recognized clinical manifestations of stroke. Compromise of the motor pathways can affect the initiation of movement, strength of movement, integration of movement, muscle tone, and reflex activity. The classic symptoms are hemiparesis or hemiplegia on the side of the body opposite the site of cerebral ischemia. Most patients are initially hyporeflexic and then progress to hyperreflexia and spasticity as recovery progresses. The upper and lower extremities may be affected to different degrees. Motor deficits also commonly impair swallowing and produce weakness in the muscles of speech.

Bowel and Bladder Deficits. Frequency, urgency, and incontinence are common problems in the initial days after stroke, but the reflex arc remains intact, as does at least a partial sensation of bladder filling. The stroke lesion usually affects only half of the motor and sensory control of the bladder, which makes effective continence rehabilitation a reasonable goal. The extent of motor deficits and the presence of cognitive deficits influence the degree of success. If extended indwelling catheterization can be avoided, there is a good chance of successful bladder retraining. The problems that develop with bowel elimination are more related to cognitive losses and immobility than to the physical effects of the stroke. Constipation is the most common problem.

Communication Deficits. The ability to communicate is a complex process that involves receiving and effectively processing the written or spoken word and being able to communicate appropriately both verbally and in writing. The left hemisphere is dominant for language in all right-handed and many left-handed individuals. Broca's area, which is located at the inferior gyrus of the frontal lobe, is critical for the motor control of speech. Wernicke's area, which is located in the temporal lobe on the superior temporal gyrus, is responsible for auditory association (see Figure 43-3). When the dominant hemisphere is affected, stroke can create aphasia, a language disorder that can be subdivided and classified in several ways. Nonfluent aphasia is an expressive, primarily motor disorder involving Broca's area. Patients have difficulty expressing thoughts because Broca's area contains the memory for motor patterns of speech. The deficits may range from difficulty finding the desired word to oral communication that is restricted to single-word responses. The ability to understand language usually remains intact, although many patients with aphasia have mixed patterns of abilities and disabilities. Agraphia, the inability to express ideas in writing, may or may not be present.

Fluent aphasia is a receptive, primarily sensory disorder involving Wernicke's area. The patient may speak fluently but be unable to comprehend speech. The patient's use of language is often full of errors, although automatic social responses such as *yes, no,* and *fine* are used appropriately. Either agraphia or alexia, the inability to understand the written word, may also be present. Global aphasia reflects damage to both regions of the brain and may result in the inability to either understand or use language. The presence of dysarthria can complicate the picture of aphasia.

Sensory-Perceptual Deficits. Perception is a complex process of recognizing and interpreting environmental stimuli. The right side of the brain (particularly the parietal lobe) plays a significant role in perception. Sensory-perceptual deficits are common following stroke and can take a variety of forms. Straightforward sensory losses manifest as a diminished response to superficial sensations such as touch, temperature, heat, and cold. These create a substantial risk for injury.

Visual deficits may complicate environmental management and commonly occur because the visual pathways pass through most of the cerebral hemispheres. These may manifest as decreased visual acuity or diplopia but more commonly present as some degree of homonymous hemianopia—loss of vision in a portion of the visual field of each eye. Figure 43-4 provides a comparison of the visual deficits created by ischemic damage at different portions of the visual pathway.

The more subtle perceptual problems that occur with stroke may initially be overlooked but can be profoundly disturbing to the family because of their more bizarre manifestations. Proprioceptive knowledge of the position of body parts in the environment may be affected, which contributes to the potential for injury. Distortions of body image, lack of ability to accurately judge spatial relationships, apparent denial of the physical effects of the stroke (anosognosia), and the loss of ability to identify or use familiar objects correctly (apraxia), particularly to complete tasks essential for self-care, can all be present to some degree. These deficits are outlined in Box 43-3.

Cognitive-Emotional Deficits. Patients commonly demonstrate a loss of control over their emotions following a stroke. Their emotional responses can be exaggerated, flattened, or inappropriate and are often unpredictable. Depression occurs in most patients and is compounded by frustration over the losses in functional abilities and communication. It is often difficult to distinguish between normal emotional responses and those related to emotional lability. Uncontrolled anger or tears can be frightening symptoms for families. Stress and fatigue may increase the unpredictability and severity of the patient's emotional responses.

Memory and judgment are also commonly compromised by stroke, although these losses may not be readily apparent in the early days of recovery. A short attention span with easy distractibility may be present, which interferes with self-care learning. The ability to reason and think abstractly may be significantly altered, which can deepen the depressive response to stroke, since patients must come to terms with the extent of their losses.

Effects of Laterality. As our understanding of the functions of each side of the brain continues to increase, some predictions about the effects of stroke injury to each hemisphere are possible. The effects of left hemisphere versus right hemisphere stroke for individuals who are left hemisphere dominant (all right-handed individuals and many left-handed persons) are summarized in Box 43-4.

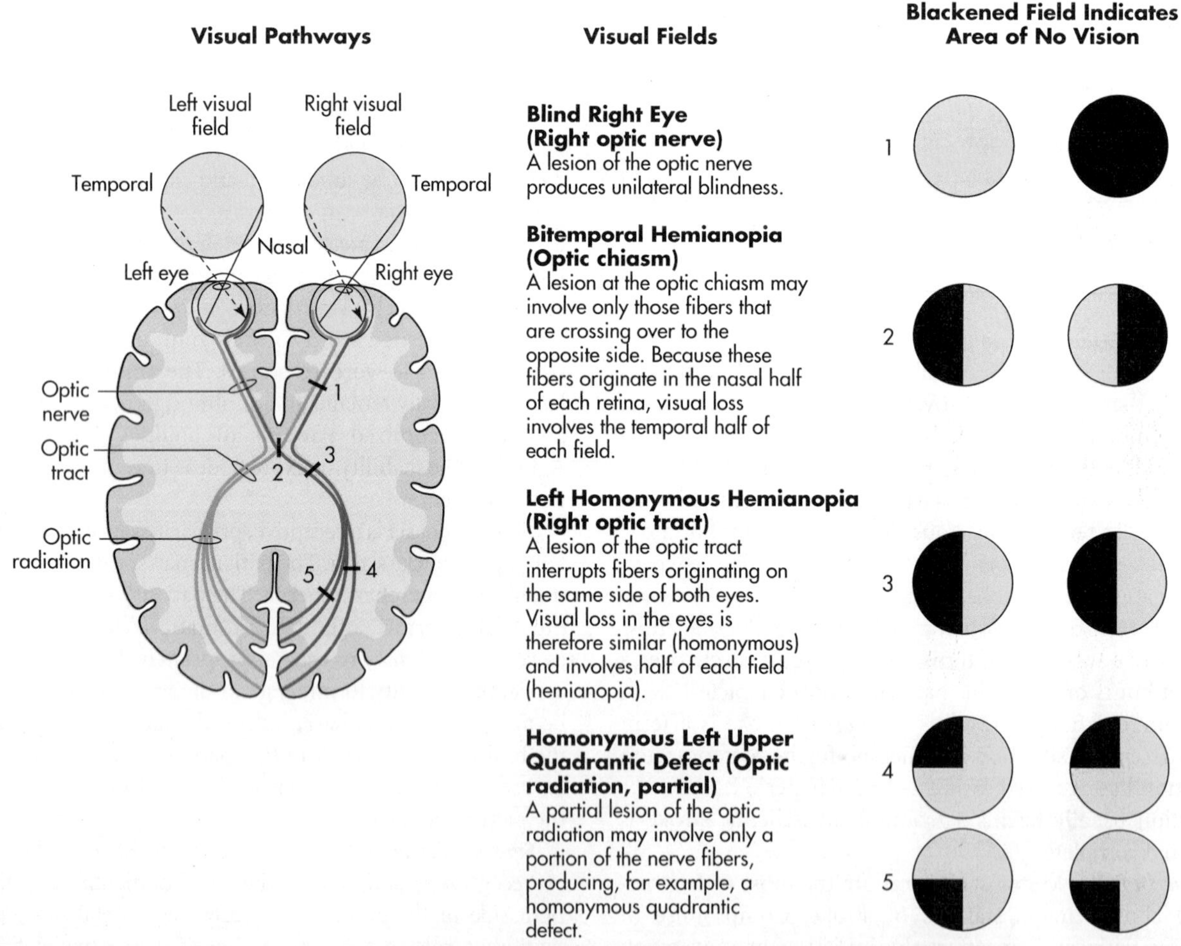

Figure 43-4 Visual field defects produced by selected lesions in the visual pathways.

Collaborative Care Management

Diagnostic Tests. A stroke is initially diagnosed by means of a careful history and physical examination. Aggressive early intervention to attempt reperfusion of the ischemic portions of the brain necessitates a rapid differentiation between ischemic and hemorrhagic etiologies, and this may be accomplished by either a computed tomography (CT) scan or magnetic resonance imaging (MRI).[8] A CT scan is used to rule out bleeding, but the extent of infarction will not be visible on CT scanning for about 48 hours. The MRI can demonstrate the ischemic zone within the first few hours following stroke, but its high cost and limited accessibility usually make MRI the second diagnostic option.

A variety of other tests may also be used to identify other problems that may have contributed to the stroke. These might include a cardiac workup to rule out the possibility of cardiogenic emboli. Carotid Doppler or ultrasonography may be performed to rule out or evaluate the degree of carotid stenosis. Angiography may be used to localize and evaluate a bleeding site if a hemorrhagic stroke has occurred, or to evaluate the extent of arterial occlusion. No laboratory tests confirm the presence of stroke, but routine blood work will be performed to assess the patient's baseline status and provide a framework for anticoagulation if needed.

Medications. Platelet aggregation inhibitor drugs are the mainstay of drug therapy for stroke. Aspirin, the most extensively used antiplatelet drug, has been proven to decrease platelet aggregation. It can be used in the management of TIAs and stroke in evolution, or following ischemic strokes. Aspirin has been shown to reduce recurrence after an initial stroke.[24] Even in low doses, however, some patients are unable to tolerate the long-term use of aspirin, and its use increases the risk of peptic ulcer disease. Several alternative antiplatelet drugs, including ticlopidine (Ticlid), clopidogrel (Plavix), and dipyridamole (Persantine), have been shown to be effective for secondary stroke prevention, but these agents are more costly than aspirin, and patients must be monitored for drug-specific side effects.[24]

Anticoagulants. Intravenous anticoagulation may be used during acute-stage management of a progressing ischemic or embolic stroke.[8] Authorities do not agree about the appropriateness of anticoagulant use in acute stroke management because of the significant risk of bleeding that may follow ischemic damage to brain tissue and because of the lack of conclusive evidence that acute anticoagulation therapy improves patient outcomes.[8]

Other. Patients with severe hypertension may require pharmacologic intervention, but moderate hypertension is usually not treated out of concern for reducing perfusion pressure in the brain. Blood pressure control is usually initiated for patients with hemorrhagic strokes, who also commonly require control of elevated intracranial pressure.

The evolving knowledge base about the mechanisms that contribute to the expansion of the ischemic zone of injury after stroke has opened a variety of new avenues for pharmacologic intervention. Calcium channel blockers, opiate antagonists, free radical scavengers (tirilazad), and lazeroids are all being used in research protocols.[20]

Treatments

Reperfusion Therapy. Reperfusion therapy with tissue plasminogen activator (t-PA) has been approved for use in selected stroke patients and represents one of the first major efforts to intervene and minimize the effects of ischemic damage. The risk of major bleeding is a serious concern, and only thrombotic and embolic strokes can be treated with t-PA. The risk of bleeding appears to be minimized if t-PA is administered within the first 3 hours following the onset of symptoms.[24] If t-PA is administered to necrotic tissue, the damage to the brain can worsen, so the window of opportunity is extremely narrow. Patients are carefully screened for risk factors because the risk of generalized bleeding from fibrinolysis is significant. Successful treatment with t-PA has

BOX 43-3 Perceptual Deficits Caused by Stroke

Unilateral Neglect Syndrome

A distortion in body image in which the patient ignores the affected side of the body

Anosognosia

Apparent unawareness or denial of any loss or deficit in physical functioning

Loss of Proprioceptive Skills

Lack of awareness of where various body parts are in relationship to each other and the environment

Agnosia

Inability to recognize a familiar object by use of the senses
- Visual agnosia
- Auditory agnosia
- Tactile agnosia

Apraxia

Loss of ability to carry out a learned sequence of movements or use objects correctly when paralysis is not present

Constructional: may not be able to sequence a planned act necessary for activities of daily living (e.g., dressing, brushing teeth, combing hair)

Spatial Relationships

Loss of ability to judge distance or size or localize objects in space

Impaired right-left discrimination

BOX 43-4 Left Hemisphere Versus Right Hemisphere Stroke

Left Hemisphere* Stroke

Motor deficits on right side
Language deficits
  Fluent, nonfluent, or global aphasia
  Agraphia or alexia
Right visual field deficits
Slow and cautious behavior
Severely anxious before attempting new skills
Intellectual impairment
High level of frustration, depression over losses

Right Hemisphere Stroke

Motor deficits on left side
Left visual field deficits
Spatial perceptual deficits
Denial or unawareness of deficits
Poor judgment, overestimates abilities
Impulsive, highly distractible
Appears unconcerned over losses

*Dominant hemisphere for most persons.

Future Watch

Stroke Treatment

In just the past several years, ischemic stroke treatment has been revolutionized with the development and growing use of tissue plasminogen activator (t-PA) a thrombotytic agent. New frontiers of stroke research are exploring the effects of ischemia on brain cells at the molecular level and are focusing on the development of treatments that can prevent or minimize the permanent damaging effects of ischemia on brain cells. A number of aggressive new treatments are already being evaluated (e.g., intraarterial clot lysis and the induction of mild hypothermia). A variety of other modalities are currently being developed:

- Recanalization and reperfusion: new antithrombotic, antiplatelet, and vasodilating drugs are being developed and tested.
- Prevention of inflammation: thrombolysis or spontaneous reopening of a blocked artery results in a cascade of responses that evokes an inflammatory response by the body. Drugs that can scavenge free radicals or that can suppress the inflammatory response in damaged brain tissue are being studied.
- Neuroprotective drugs: a number of drugs are being studied for their effects in blocking or interrupting the damaging intracellular processes that follow brain tissue ischemia.
- Hypothermia: experimental evidence suggests that mild hypothermia is protective after brain injury by means of lowering metabolism, thus reducing destructive cellular metabolic processes that follow ischemia.
- Hemicraniectomy: the damaging effects of the compression of a swelling brain against the skull can be reduced by the removal of cranial bone on one side of the head. Evidence suggests that this intervention substantially lowers the mortality rate in patients with malignant brain swelling.
- Facilitation of healing of surviving brain: brain recovery may be enhanced through measures such as environmental enrichment, use of human growth factors, and transplantation of fetal neural tissue or stem cells.

Reference: Lindsberg PJ et al: The future of stroke treatment, *Neurol Clin* 18(2):495, 2000.

been shown to significantly decrease the severity of the residual deficits of stroke[24] (see Future Watch box.).

Hypervolemic-Hyperdilution Therapy. Maintaining adequate and stable cerebral perfusion is an essential goal of early stroke management. As discussed previously, no effort is made to reduce moderate hypertension, and blood pressure stability is supported. Hypervolemia and hyperdilution can be achieved by the administration of saline and perhaps albumin. This treatment arguably supports a sustained blood pressure and promotes vasodilation of the cerebral vessels, theoretically maximizing perfusion to the brain.[20] Hypervolemic-hyperdilution therapy has been successfully used to treat vasospasm after subarachnoid hemorrhage, but its efficacy in acute ischemic stroke is unproven.[18]

Surgical Management. Carotid endarterectomy is the primary surgical intervention used in stroke management. It is targeted at stroke prevention primarily for patients with symptomatic carotid stenosis. Endarterectomy carefully removes the plaque after the artery has been clamped both above and below the obstruction (Figure 43-5). Circulation to the brain on the affected side is maintained through the vertebrobasilar arterial system with supplemental flow through a temporary bypass shunt. Despite these precautions, the greatest risks associated with the procedure relate to compromised cerebral blood flow, especially if carotid stenosis is present on both sides. Embolization of plaque and microthrombi resulting from the surgical manipulation increase the risk of additional strokes and are the primary postoperative concerns. Intervention is usually reserved for patients with greater than a 70% carotid blockage.[13]

Care in the postoperative period relates to blood pressure instability, which usually persists for about 12 to 24 hours and causes concern for the development of both hypertension and hypotension. The sudden restoration of blood flow through a significantly obstructed carotid artery can in itself result in hemorrhage, and the increased perfusion may initially overwhelm the brain's ability to effectively autoregulate. In appropriate surgical candidates, carotid endarterectomy significantly reduces the risk of stroke. The major nursing care considerations for patients undergoing carotid endarterectomy are listed in the Guidelines for Safe Practice box. A Clinical Pathway for a patient undergoing carotid endarterectomy is found on pp. 1372 to 1374.

Diet. The patient is usually placed on nothing-by-mouth (NPO) status on admission and is kept NPO until stabilization has occurred and a thorough evaluation of swallowing can be performed. Protecting the airway from aspiration of food, fluid, and secretions is the primary concern.[27] Intact gag and swallow reflexes are essential prerequisites for oral feedings, and their presence and strength are closely monitored. The process of swallowing is complex and requires the coor-

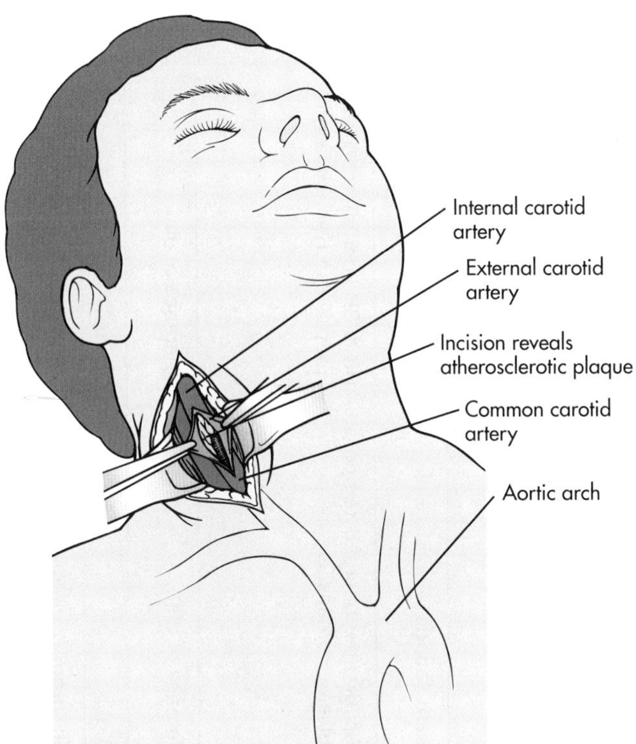

Figure 43-5 Carotid endarterectomy. Atherosclerotic plaque is removed from the internal carotid artery.

dination of several structures and muscle groups. If the patient is unable to ingest an oral diet, tube feedings may be initiated to prevent excessive catabolism and resultant malnutrition. A nasogastric route is initially used, and tube feedings may be either continuous or intermittent. The standard concerns related to formula hyperosmolality and problems with dehydration and diarrhea exist (see Chapter 33). A percutaneous gastrostomy may be needed for long-term nutrition management. Nutritional concerns are discussed further in the nursing management section.

Activity. Patients who have experienced an intracerebral hemorrhage require bed rest until the risk of rebleeding is minimized and intracranial pressure stabilizes. Patients who have experienced an ischemic stroke are mobilized into active rehabilitation as soon as the stroke has stabilized, usually within 48 hours.[22] A multidisciplinary team of physical and occupational therapy specialists and nurses then collaboratively plan the patient's self-care rehabilitation. Preventing immobility-associated problems (which can include pneumonia, urinary incontinence or urinary tract infection, pressure ulcers, deep vein thrombosis, and pulmonary embolus) is a major focus of collaborative in-hospital care.[3] Prophylactic measures against deep vein thrombosis, which occurs in up to 50% of hemiplegic stroke patients, may include the use of elastic hose, pneumatic compression stockings, or subcutaneous heparin injections.[28]

Referrals. Stroke rehabilitation is truly a multidisciplinary collaborative effort. A nursing case management approach can be extremely effective in ensuring that discharge planning is initiated in a timely fashion and that appropriate arrangements are made for assistance through home health care, short-term residential rehabilitation, or long-term care through a nursing facility. This process involves the direction of the physician; the coordination of the nurse case manager; and the active involvement of professionals from physical, occupational, and speech therapy, as well as social and dietary services.

Guidelines for Safe Practice
The Patient Undergoing Carotid Endarterectomy

Postoperative nursing care focuses on monitoring vital signs and the early identification of potential complications.

VITAL SIGNS

Monitor vital signs every 1 to 2 hours.
- Blood pressure instability is anticipated in the first 12 to 24 hours.
- Report incidence of blood pressure fluctuations above or below established parameters immediately.

MONITORING FOR COMPLICATIONS

Monitor neurologic status through frequent neurologic checks.
- Evaluate cranial nerves, particularly facial and vagus.

Monitor for dysrhythmias and assess for incidence of chest pain.
Monitor for signs of reperfusion injury, including:
- Worsening or recurring stroke symptoms
- Signs of increasing intracranial pressure

Monitor incision site for patency, drainage.

NURSING MANAGEMENT

ASSESSMENT

Health History

Assessment data to be collected as part of the health history of a patient with a stroke include:

- Baseline level of function
- History of hypertension and its management, coronary artery disease, diabetes, and history of TIA (symptoms, frequency, workup, and treatment, if any) and/or previous stroke
- Medications in use: prescription, over-the-counter drugs, herbal preparations
- Smoking history, and history of alcohol or other drug use
- Circumstances surrounding the stroke
- Onset, nature, severity, and duration of symptoms
- Presence of headache: nature and location
- Visual ability: acuity, diplopia, blurred vision, field cuts
- Ability to concentrate and follow commands, memory
- Emotional/affective response
- Family and social support network, current living situation, financial and insurance status

Physical Examination

Important aspects of the physical examination of a patient with a stroke include assessment of:

clinical pathway *Carotid Artery Endarterectomy*

	DAY 1 (OR)	DAY 2	DAY 3	DAY 4
Assessment				
Neurological/ Psychological:	Mental status • LOC/confusion • headache • vision • pupils (size, shape, reaction) • facial symmetry (smile/facial/eye ptosis) • ability to follow directions, speak (quality & tone of voice/hoarseness), & swallow • tongue movement • sensory loss • motor weakness (tingling, paralysis) • pain via pain scale (severity, quality, location, duration, radiation) • standard for recovery from anesthesia (local or general) • raise arms to horizontal position • risk for falls • explore anxiety/coping skills • begin assessment of health care problem & potential modifiable risk factors (smoking, diet, stress, exercise) • identify available & needed family/human/economic resources to resume independent self-care activities.	Mental status • LOC/confusion • headache • vision • pupils (size, shape, reaction) • facial symmetry (smile/facial/eye ptosis) • ability to follow directions, speak (quality & tone of voice/hoarseness), & swallow • tongue movement • sensory loss • motor weakness (tingling, paralysis) • pain via pain scale (severity, quality, location, duration, radiation) • raise arms to horizontal position • risk for falls • continue to explore anxiety/coping skills • continue assessment of health care problem & potential modifiable risk factors (smoking, diet, stress, exercise) • collaborate w/social services to identify available & needed family/human/economic resources to resume independent self-care activities.	Mental status • vision • pupils (size, shape, reaction) • facial symmetry (smile/facial/eye ptosis) • ability to follow directions, speak (quality & tone of voice/hoarseness), & swallow • tongue movement • raise arms to horizontal position • continue to explore anxiety/coping skills	Mental status • ability to follow directions
Pulmonary:	Breath sounds (atelectasis) • patent airway.	Breath sounds (atelectasis) • patent airway.	Breath sounds	Breath sounds
Cardiovascular:	VS per postop standard & then BP monitoring to continue q15min until stable • capillary refill • carotid bruits • peripheral pulses & temporal pulses • Homans' sign.	BP monitoring to continue q15min until stable • capillary refill • carotid bruits • peripheral pulses & temporal pulses • Homans' sign.	HR & BP • peripheral & temporal pulses • Homans' sign.	HR & BP • peripheral & temporal pulses • Homans' sign.
Gastrointestinal:	Ability to swallow • mucous membranes.	Ability to swallow • mucous membranes.	Tolerance of diet.	Tolerance of diet.
Genitourinary:	I & O • UO > 30 ml/h.	I & O • UO > 30 ml/h.	UO qs.	UO qs.
Integumentary:	Skin turgor, temp, color, & integrity • risk for pressure ulcers.	Skin turgor, temp, color, & integrity • risk for pressure ulcers.	Skin turgor & integrity.	Skin turgor & integrity.

Surgery Wound:	Dsg/incision line • amt & type of drainage • S & S of bleeding/ hematoma/edema/redness/heat • assess area under neck & shoulders for blood • neck swelling.	Dsg/incision line • amt & type of drainage • S & S of bleeding/ hematoma/edema/redness/heat • assess area under neck & shoulders for blood • neck swelling.	Dsg/incision line • amt & type of drainage • S & S of bleeding/ hematoma/edema/redness/ heat.	Dsg/incision line • amt & type of drainage • S & S of bleeding/hematoma/edema/redness/heat.
Focus	Hemodynamic stability • maintain airway • pain control.	Hemodynamic stability • pain control.	Improved PO fluid & food intake • teaching • initiate definitive treatment plan for therapeutic regimen for self-care.	Discharge • teaching • self-care.
Diagnostic Plan	Postop electrolytes & HCT @ 6 PM.	Repeat abnormal lab tests. *Consider:* repeat HCT.	Repeat abnormal lab test(s).	None.
Therapeutic Interventions	IV fluids to maintain BP systolic range of 100-160 mm/Hg & UO >30 ml/h • call physician if BP <100 mm/Hg systolic for 5 min & institute vasopressor-medicated infusion per standard • call physician if BP >160 mm Hg for 5 min & institute NTG or sodium nitroprusside-medicated infusion per standard • antibiotic • analgesic • use Doppler prn for temporal pulse assessment • NPO then progress to clear liquids (8 h postop) if swallowing intact • cough, deep breathe, & incentive spirometer q2-4h while awake • bedrest • assist w/turning q2h to maintain skin integrity unless BP labile • lotion to both heels & reapply heel protectors tid while in bed • encourage ankle dorsiflexion exercises q1-2h while awake • assist w/hygiene • elastic support stockings.	Continue IV therapy to maintain systolic BP within 100-160 range • continue w/ meds & treatments • progress diet to regular • encourage PO fluids & document plan for same • stool softener • OOB to chair tid unless BP labile.	Discontinue IV fluids • heplock line • independent w/ hygiene • progressive activity as tolerated • encourage participation in hygiene & wound care • OOB ad lib • walk in hall × 4.	Independent ADL • discharge.

From Birdsall C, Sperry S: *Clinical paths in medical-surgical practice,* St Louis, 1997, Mosby.

Continued

clinical pathway *Carotid Artery Endarterectomy—cont'd*

	DAY 1 (OR)	DAY 2	DAY 3	DAY 4
Patient/Family Teaching/ Discharge Planning	Teach use of pain scale & review meds available for pain & anxiety • reassure that responses (anxiety, etc.) are a normal reaction • initiate discharge plan • teach to cough, deep breathe, & use incentive spirometer & ankle dorsiflexion & extension exercises • discuss plan for daily review of plan of care w/patient/ family.	Teach adequate hydration to ensure UO >50 ml/h & to apply support stockings • identify learning needs & discuss potential lifestyle changes prn (smoking, diet, stress, weight, exercise) & document same • teach nutritional needs, carotid disease, & treatment plan.	Teach self-care strategies (no heavy lifting, no vigorous exercise, no prolonged sitting, no driving for 2 wk or as surgeon indicates) • teach S & S to report to physician (fever, drainage, redness, swelling, tenderness of back or calves) • review discharge plan & home care needs • clarify & confirm information given to date • allow time for verbalization of feelings • review meds & med/food interactions • review knowledge of health care problem & potential modifiable risk factors (smoking, diet, stress, exercise).	Review discharge plan, self-care strategies, S & S to report to physician, & to see physician in 3 wk • review appropriate health-seeking behaviors & need to modify lifestyle prn.
Expected Outcomes	Hemodynamically stable & UO >30 ml/h • assists w/ turning • verbalizes relief of pain w/ analgesia • acknowledges availability of analgesic/anxiolytic, plan of care, & need to communicate w/ nurse if S & S of anxiety & fear become overwhelming (subjective feelings, emotional lability, or inability to concentrate) • demonstrates coughing, deep breathing, & use of incentive spirometer.	Demonstrates how to cough, deep breathe, & use incentive spirometer effectively • demonstrates ankle dorsiflexion & extension exercises • BP stable within range w/ fluid support • verbalizes relief of pain w/ PO analgesia as evidenced by pain scale <3 (0-10) • acknowledges availability of analgesics/anxiolytics prn but denies anxiety • verbalizes appropriate anxiety & fears related to surgery • home care referral complete.	Voids independently & in qs • verbalizes meds & food/drug interactions • states will notify surgeon for S & S of infection/phlebitis • normal BM • uses fewer doses of prn meds as evidenced by pain scale <2 (0-10) • parenteral therapy discontinued • independent in ADL • acknowledges potential lifestyle changes & appropriate concerns & fears • social services screening documented • demonstrates applying support stockings.	Verbalizes self-care strategies & S & S to report to physician • states appointment date w/ physician • pain well controlled as evidenced by pain scale <2 (0-10) • social services referral to home care or outpatient follow-up documented • ambulates without assistance & independent in ADL • normal BM • verbalizes risk factors & health-seeking behaviors.
Trigger(s)	Hemodynamic instability • respiratory distress • neuro deficit (new).	Hemodynamic instability • neuro deficit • unable to get OOB.	Unable to tolerate fluids/food/ activity.	Unable to be independent in self-care.

Vital signs
Level of consciousness, orientation, and response to tactile stimuli
Motor strength: presence and severity of paresis or paralysis
Coordination: gait, balance
Ability to communicate (speak and understand speech)
Cranial nerve function, including gag and swallow reflexes, facial movement, tongue movement, eye blink, eye movement, and pupillary response
Bowel and bladder function

NURSING DIAGNOSES

Nursing diagnoses are determined from analysis of patient data. Nursing diagnoses for the patient with a stroke may include but are not limited to:

Diagnostic Title	Possible Etiologic Factors
1. Ineffective tissue perfusion	Interruption of arterial blood flow
2. Risk for disuse syndrome	Hemiparesis or hemiplegia, neglect, anosognosia
3. Self-care deficit: feeding, bathing/hygiene, toileting	Neuromuscular and sensory-perceptual impairments
4. Impaired swallowing	Oral and pharyngeal muscle weakness
5. Impaired verbal communication	Receptive, expressive, or global aphasia
6. Disturbed sensory perception (visual, tactile)	Altered sensory reception, transmission, and integration
7. Impaired urinary elimination	Altered neurologic stimulation, immobility
8. Impaired adjustment	Residual disability necessitating changes in lifestyle and independence; emotional effects of brain injury

EXPECTED PATIENT OUTCOMES

Expected patient outcomes for the patient with a stroke may include but are not limited to:

1. Will maintain cerebral perfusion as indicated by stable vital signs, stable or improving level of consciousness, stable or improving neurologic deficits, and the absence of signs of increased intracranial pressure
2a. Will transfer independently or with standby assistance from bed to chair/wheelchair
2b. Will remain free of the complications of disuse as evidenced by full range of motion and intact skin
3. Will use adapted equipment and strategies to regain independence in ADLs
4a. If able to tolerate food and fluid without choking or aspiration, will ingest sufficient nutrients to maintain a stable weight and meet the body's baseline nutritional needs
4b. If unable to take food and fluids by mouth, will tolerate tube feeding to meet nutritional needs
5. Will use alternative methods of communication to effectively communicate needs
6. Will compensate for visual and spatial perception impairments and remain free of injury
7. Will regain urinary continence
8. Will participate in appropriate social activities and make plans for the future

INTERVENTIONS

1. Monitoring Cerebral Perfusion

Immediately after the patient's admission, the focus of nursing care is on monitoring the patient's neurologic status and preventing complications while simultaneously assessing the severity of the stroke. Maintaining a patent airway is essential to support oxygenation and cerebral perfusion. The patient is placed on bed rest with the head of the bed elevated about 30 degrees and positioned to prevent the tongue from falling back and partially obstructing the airway. Supplemental oxygen may be administered. Vital signs and neurologic checks are performed frequently to monitor for stroke in evolution and to rule out the presence of increasing intracranial pressure. The environment is kept as quiet and restful as possible, and all activities that are known to increase intracranial pressure, such as coughing, straining, lying prone, isometric muscle contraction, emotional upset, and abrupt head or neck flexion, are avoided or minimized. See Chapter 42 for a more thorough discussion of the management of changes in intracranial pressure and Chapter 41 for a thorough review of neurologic assessment.

2. Preventing the Complications of Immobility and Disuse

Positioning

The mobility impairments associated with stroke place patients, especially elderly patients, at high risk for a variety of complications related to disuse. The rehabilitation plan incorporates active physical therapy, but the nurse also needs to incorporate a variety of interventions into the patient's daily care routines. Appropriate positioning is a key concern. Positioning is fundamental to preventing complications such as contractures and skin breakdown. The challenge of positioning is increased by the presence of sensory impairments, flaccidity or spasticity of muscle groups, and the need to minimize the time the patient spends lying on the paralyzed side. The patient is helped to change position every 2 hours and encouraged to move independently in bed as soon as possible. The affected arm is positioned with the hand elevated above the wrist and the wrist above the elbow to support venous return and minimize edema.

Special care must be taken to avoid excess pressure or pull on the affected shoulder joint, which is extremely vulnerable to joint subluxation and adduction contractures. The shoulder is positioned in a neutral position with support as needed from positioning devices. Pillows, rolled towels, and sandbags are used to support normal body alignment, with particular attention to preventing external rotation of the hip. The heels should be elevated off the mattress to avoid pressure injury, and foot-positioning aids such as boots and high-top sneakers may be used to decrease the incidence of footdrop. The use of a footboard to position the feet is no longer recommended because it is believed to stimulate plantar flexion. The same principles apply to the affected hand. Resting splints are often necessary to prevent contractures in the hand when spasticity is present, but rolled washcloths are avoided because they stimulate the grasp reflex. Firm hand splints are preferred. The supine position is also avoided for any patient who has a diminished or absent gag reflex in order to minimize the risk of aspiration. A side-lying position with the head of the bed elevated 10 to 20 degrees is preferred. Accomplishing these basic care goals is both labor intensive and time consuming for the nursing staff, but they must be recognized as high-priority interventions.

Skin care is another essential aspect of positioning. Pressure reduction devices such as 4-inch foam mattresses and elbow and heel protectors are standard, and the nurse assesses the patient for signs of pressure, shearing, or friction damage during each repositioning. Once the patient is out of bed, attention shifts to pressure reduction in chairs and preventing injury related to dragging and pulling on the affected extremities. Arm and shoulder supports are important when the patient is out of bed.

Exercise

The return of motor impulses is significant for the future use of the affected part, but it also presents new challenges. Most stroke patients are initially flaccid on the affected side (stage 1) but within a few days begin to exhibit signs of muscle spasticity (stage 2). If flaccidity persists, the chances of return of functioning decrease substantially.[10] Muscles that draw the limbs toward the midline become very active because the adductor and flexor muscles are stronger than opposing muscles. The arm may be held tightly adducted against the body, and the affected lower limb may be held inward and adducted to or beyond the midline. Without regular preventive exercise, the heel cord shortens, the heel may be lifted off the ground, and the knee becomes bent.[10] In the upper extremity the elbow flexes into a bent position, the wrist is flexed, and the fingers curl into palmar flexion. Contractures will develop rapidly if preventive measures are not instituted promptly and consistently. The use of resting splints may become necessary (Figure 43-6).

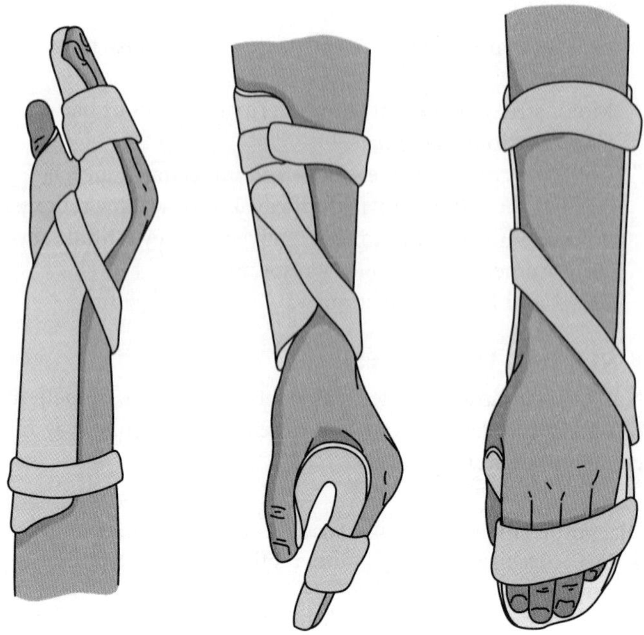

Figure 43-6 Volar resting splint provides support to the wrist, thumb, and fingers of a patient following a cerebrovascular accident, maintaining them in a position of extension.

Synergy, the third stage of recovery, develops after several weeks. In synergy the flexion of a single muscle group results in simultaneous flexion of a broader group of muscles such as the elbow, wrist, hand, and fingers. Over time, synergy can resolve into a nearly normal pattern of movement, although residual muscle weakness is almost always present. The patterns of recovery are unpredictable, however, and not uniform. The arm and hand recover sooner than the leg but rarely to the same extent. Recovery may also stop at any stage and progress no further.

Physical therapy is usually consulted to develop the overall exercise plan. Range-of-motion exercise for all joints is the foundation of the plan. The exercise is initially passive but will progress as soon as possible to active exercise of the unaffected side and assisted exercise of the affected side. Balance training is another important step. Patients may experience problems with proprioception, dizziness, and sensory-perceptual deficits that make it difficult to control movement even when they have adequate muscle strength and coordination. Voluntary muscles lose tone rapidly with bed rest, which makes fatigue an additional challenge during early rehabilitation. Patients need frequent reminders and assistance to sit straight and focus on maintaining a balanced posture.

Learning to make safe transfers to a chair or wheelchair is the next step. The chair is placed next to the patient's unaffected side. The patient stands and faces the chair and then turns and sits down after the unaffected arm has been placed on the distant chair arm. The nurse is positioned on the patient's affected side during transfers and can use a safety or transfer belt around the patient's waist to provide needed support and stability without ever needing to grasp or pull on the affected arm. If the patient's knees should buckle, the nurse can quickly move in front of the patient and block the unaffected knee so that it locks in position. The chair should provide firm support and have a high back and arms. A lapboard, pillow, or other device can provide additional support to the affected arm and shoulder. As strength and balance improve, the hemiplegic patient can be taught to transfer independently (Figure 43-7).

The same basic principles guide the gradual move to ambulation. Early ambulation promotes vasomotor tone and has strong positive psychologic effects on both the patient and the family. Correct walking patterns must be established early because incorrect patterns are difficult and sometimes impossible to change. A sideward shuffle should be prevented. A walker, crutch, or four-point cane may be helpful, and the affected arm can be placed in a sling for support during ambulation. Ambulation retraining begins between the parallel bars

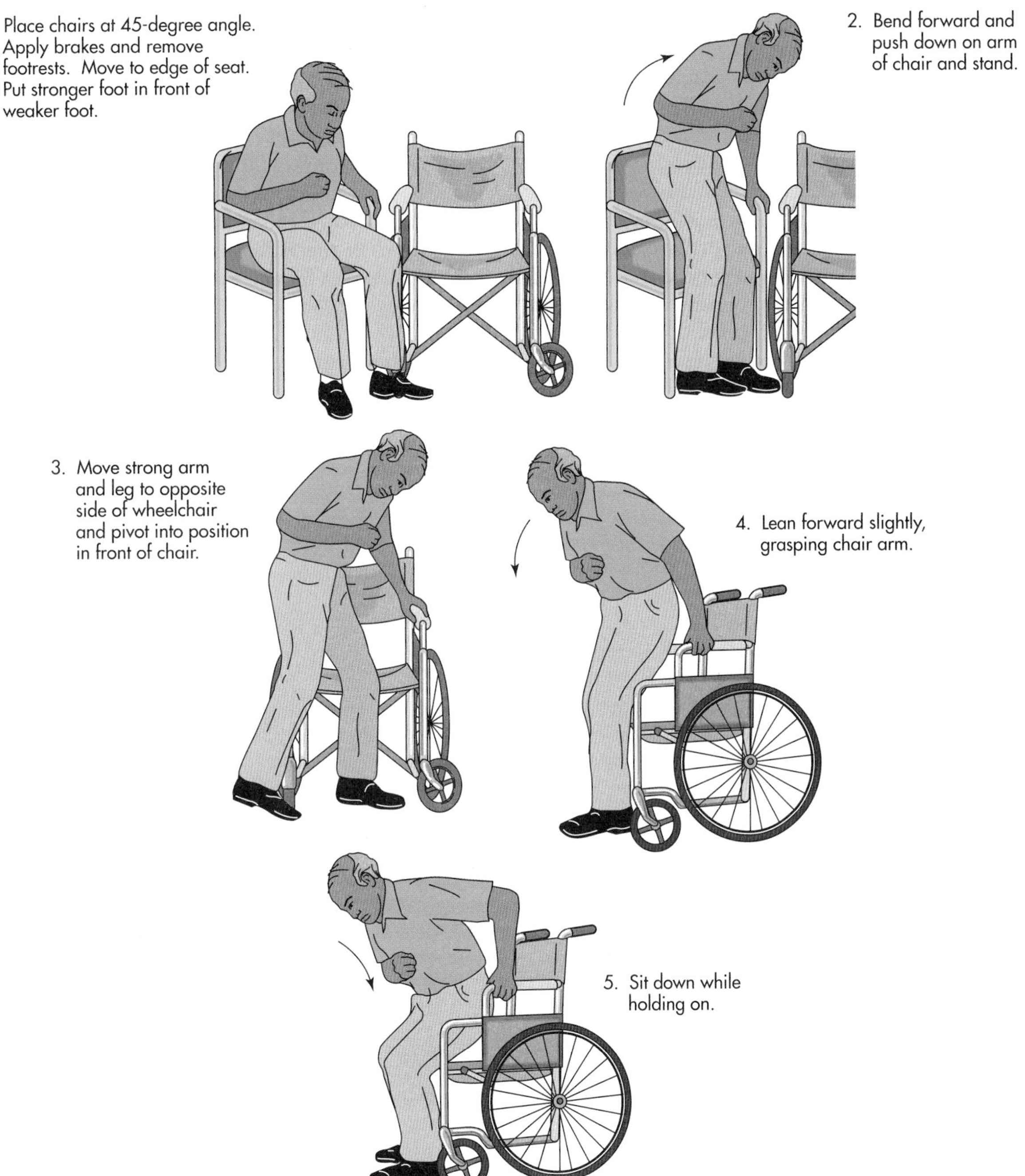

Figure 43-7 Doing a standing transfer from a chair to a wheelchair.

in physical therapy, but on-unit practice time provides essential reinforcement. The use of a safety belt can enable the nurse or therapist to provide additional support and stability.

In some rehabilitation settings the Bobath neurodevelopmental technique has been found to be useful in stroke rehabilitation. This approach seeks to normalize muscle tone, posture, and movement and promote bilateral functioning.[19] Therapy seeks to redirect short-term memory toward an appreciation of normal movement on the paralyzed side. When a Bobath approach is used, transfers are made to the affected and unaffected sides to promote bilateral functioning. Other principles of Bobath rehabilitation are presented in Box 43-5.

BOX 43-5 Application of Bobath Rehabilitation Principles

1. The use of both sides of the body is emphasized during activities of daily living and other activities.
2. Weight bearing on the affected side is encouraged during sitting and standing.
3. Movement toward the affected side is encouraged.
4. Positioning is accomplished in opposition to the patterns of spasticity.
5. The patient is consistently encouraged to straighten the trunk and neck to normalize body tone and posture.

3. Promoting Independence in Self-Care

Efforts to regain independence in self-care activities require the collaboration of the physical and occupational therapist, nurse, patient, and family. A rehabilitation plan is designed for the patient by the physical, occupational, and speech therapists, which is then implemented by the nursing staff and family. The plan is developed after thorough assessment of the patient's motor skills and deficits, as well as the cognitive and sensory-perceptual issues that will support or complicate rehabilitation. Rehabilitation seeks to help patients relearn lost skills and compensate for temporary or permanent losses.

Each new skill is demonstrated, and then the patient practices with ongoing support and encouragement from the nursing staff and family. Families need to be incorporated into all teaching so that they understand how to support independence rather than dependence. Providing extra time for activities is essential. Most motivated patients with moderate impairments can relearn the skills needed to complete basic ADLs.

Assistive devices play a major role in regaining self-care independence because accomplishing basic tasks with only one hand is both challenging and frustrating. A wide variety of devices exist to assist patients with eating and dressing, and the nurse can help the patient and family think of simple modifications that can promote independence, such as slip-on shoes, Velcro closures, loose pullover shirts, and elastic-waisted pants (Figure 43-8). Patients are encouraged to dress in simple workout-type clothes rather than pajamas and gowns as soon as active rehabilitation is started (Figure 43-9).

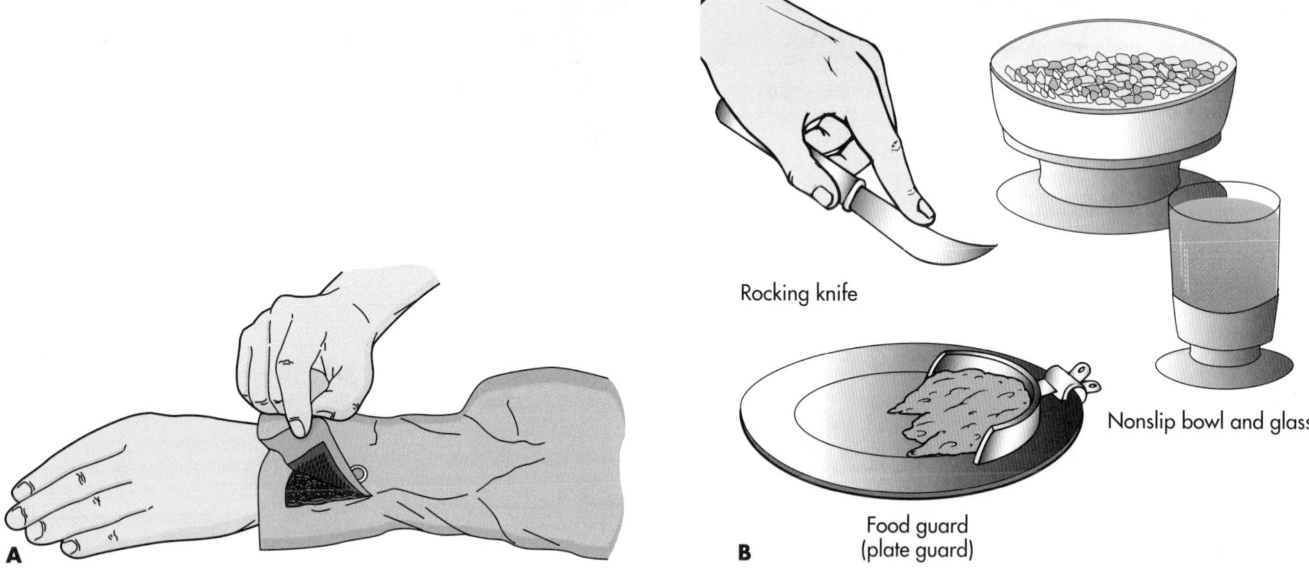

Figure 43-8 Assistive devices for self-care. **A**, Velcro closure on shirtsleeve. **B**, Assistive devices for eating.

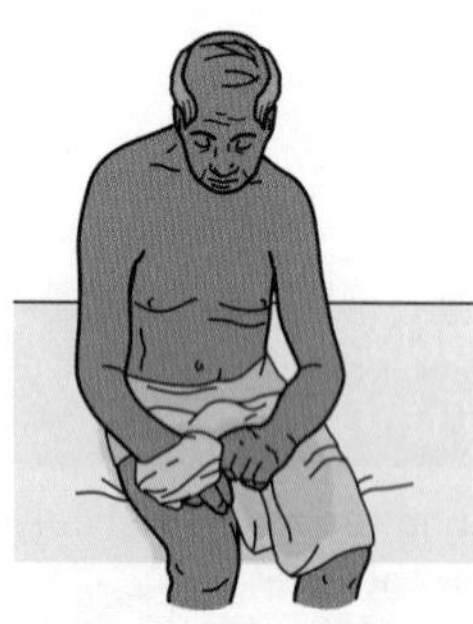

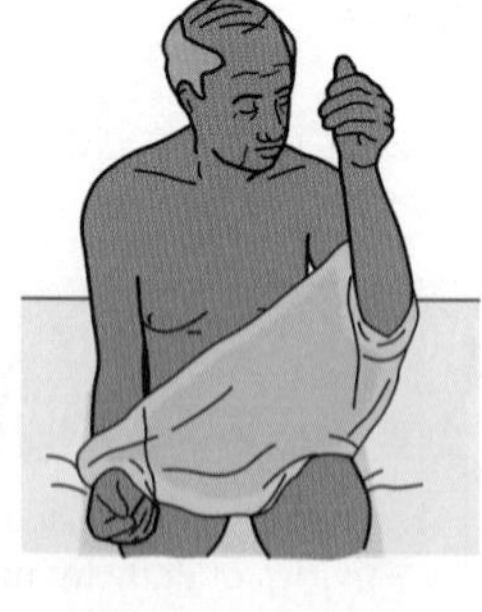

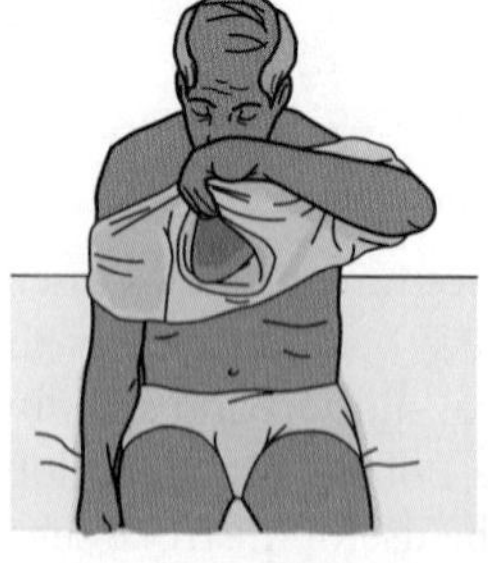

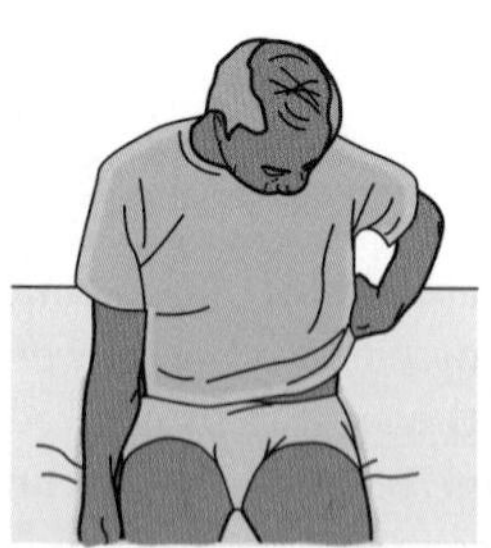

Figure 43-9 Putting on a pullover garment.

4. Promoting Safe Swallowing and Adequate Nutrition

The protective swallowing and gag reflexes usually return within a few days after the stroke, but the patient may have ongoing problems managing the complex act of swallowing. A number of cranial nerves are involved in this process. The presence of facial drooping or asymmetry, drooling, and a weak voice are strong indicators of swallowing difficulties. The gag and swallow reflexes are carefully assessed, and a speech therapist may be consulted to establish a management plan. At the bedside, the act of swallowing can be grossly assessed by placing the thumb and index finger on either side of the patient's larynx and feeling for symmetric elevation when the patient attempts to swallow. The nurse should never give anything by mouth to a patient whose swallowing has not been thoroughly evaluated because the patient can aspirate without the usual accompanying coughing or choking if protective reflexes are not intact.[9] It should be noted that up to 40% of stroke patients with dysphagia experience silent aspiration.[16] A modified barium swallow may be recommended to further assess swallowing function and the risk of aspiration. Even if swallowing is intact, the patient may still be at risk for aspiration because of easy distractibility. A quiet environment for eating where the patient can concentrate on effective swallowing is recommended. Specific strategies for approaching the problems of swallowing and nutrition in patients following stroke are presented in the Guidelines for Safe Practice box.

Guidelines for Safe Practice

The Patient With Impaired Swallowing

1. Place the patient upright in bed or preferably sitting in a chair for meals.
2. Offer mouth care before meals to stimulate saliva flow. Strong-tasting or salty liquids also stimulate saliva flow.
3. Position the patient's head and neck slightly forward with the chin tucked in to prevent premature movement of food to the back of the mouth before it is adequately chewed.
4. Experiment with food texture. Most patients tolerate a mechanically soft diet better than liquids. Avoid thin liquids. Consider adding a thickener to liquids if they are poorly tolerated.
5. Encourage the patient to take small bites and chew food thoroughly.
6. If hemiplegia is present, food should be placed in the unaffected side of the mouth. If "pocketing" of food occurs on the affected side, instruct the patient to sweep the affected side with a finger after each bite. Teach the patient to clean the affected side of the mouth with gauze wipes and perform mouth care after meals. Retained food causes mouth odors, infection, and tooth or gum disease.
7. Position foods within the patient's visual field if hemianopia is present (Figure 43-10).
8. Keep an accurate intake and output record until the patient is drinking sufficient liquids daily. Intravenous supplementation may initially be needed.
9. Monitor the patient's weight weekly. Add supplements to diet or liquids to increase caloric and nutrient intake.

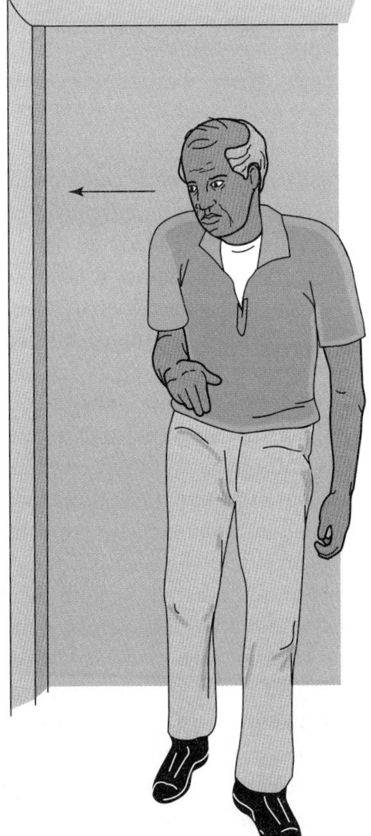

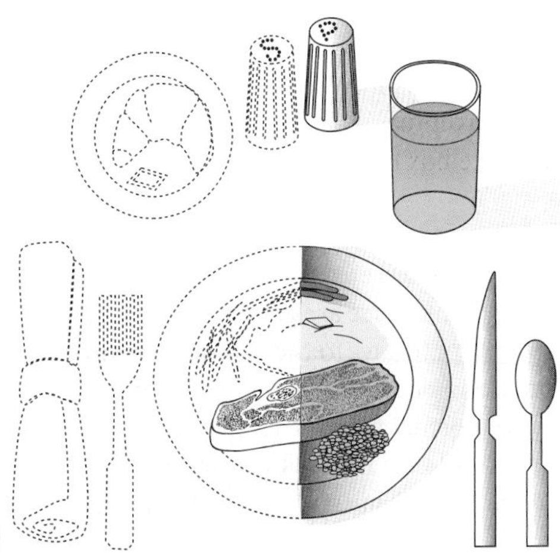

Figure 43-10 Spatial and perceptual deficits in stroke. **A**, The patient is instructed to look toward the affected side when walking to avoid bumping into things. **B**, With homonymous hemianopia, the patient is unable to see the left side of the tray and may ignore the items on that side.

5. Supporting Communication

Communication problems following stroke may include both aphasia and dysarthria. Each person reacts to language problems differently, but anger and frustration are common. Some patients become easily discouraged when they encounter problems and may quickly refuse to speak. This can progress to complete withdrawal from social interactions, even with family and close friends. Family members may be at a loss as to how to respond to the patient's problems and may even encourage the patient to avoid frustration by not trying to communicate. Embarrassment at the person's attempts at speech is common.

A speech therapist is an integral part of the patient's rehabilitation plan, but the nurse can reinforce that learning and help the family be an active part of the rehabilitation team. The patient needs frequent and meaningful communication and ample time to practice speaking in a nonstressful environment. Sitting down and spending time with the patient conveys interest and willingness to make communication a priority. Patients with fluent forms of aphasia may have baffling abilities to sing, recite poetry or Bible verses, or swear creatively. These actions can be extremely troubling to family members, who need to understand the organic basis of the behavior. Specific strategies for assisting patients with aphasia are summarized in the Guidelines for Safe Practice box.

6. Compensating for Sensory-Perceptual Deficits

A wide variety of sensory-perceptual deficits may be present following stroke, particularly strokes involving the right hemisphere. These deficits make it more difficult for patients to react appropriately to their environment. Deficits that involve proprioception, depth, and distance perception can present serious risks of injury as the patient becomes more active. These deficits are of particular concern when a patient also experiences denial of the stroke limitations and approaches activities with impulsive self-confidence. Until the exact nature and severity of the deficits are determined, the nursing staff provides increased supervision during all activities to ensure patient safety. The room should be kept as free of clutter as possible, but familiar personal objects from home can often help the patient remain oriented. Frequent verbal cueing can also help patients stay focused on the task at hand. Providing consistent caretakers improves ongoing assessment and evaluation and supports implementation of a consistent plan of care. Accurate documentation can be extremely valuable in evaluating outcomes and planning for future services. Specific interventions designed to address the major sensory-perceptual deficits are presented in the Guidelines for Safe Practice box on p. 1381.

7. Restoring Continence

Problems with urinary continence are common after stroke, but the chances for restoring continence are good because half of the innervation and control pathways to the bladder remain intact. The primary problem is poor bladder control. Efforts should be made to support normal bladder elimination and minimize the use of a Foley catheter if possible, even though this usually increases the amount of nursing care that the patient requires.[4] Long-term catheterization commonly results in urinary tract infection and makes regaining voluntary control more difficult. An adequate daily fluid intake is essential, although it may be necessary to restrict evening fluids to avoid nighttime incontinence. The patient is assisted to a commode every 2 hours and encouraged to empty the bladder. Efforts are made to keep the patient as dry as possible, and the skin is monitored frequently for signs of redness or irritation. The patient is verbally encouraged to maintain continence, and the family is enlisted in the total effort. Every effort is made to communicate to the patient the expectation that continence can and will be regained. The importance of continence cannot be overestimated because achieving continence is often the single most important variable in a family's decision about whether or not an elderly stroke patient can be successfully cared for at home (see Evidence-Based Practice box).

Constipation is the most common bowel problem after stroke. Regaining bowel continence is a reasonable expectation for most patients if a pattern of constipation, impaction, and laxative-induced diarrhea is prevented. The nurse needs to carefully monitor the patient's bowel elimination pattern

Guidelines for Safe Practice

The Patient With Aphasia

NONFLUENT EXPRESSIVE APHASIA

1. Allow the patient adequate time to respond. Establish a nonhurried atmosphere.
2. Be supportive and encouraging of the patient's efforts to communicate.
3. Use open-ended questions at intervals to assess spontaneous communication ability.
4. Involve the family or significant other in exercises to name objects used for routine self-care.
5. Express understanding and support for behavioral responses to frustration, such as tears or anger. Remind the patient that speech skills will improve.
6. If the aphasia is severe, a picture board or book may be necessary to communicate needs. Encourage the patient to communicate by whatever means are successful (e.g., pointing, pantomine). Anticipate the patient's needs when appropriate and verify your interpretation of the patient's meaning.

FLUENT SENSORY APHASIA

1. Face the patient and speak slowly and distinctly. Do not increase your volume; hearing is not the problem.
2. Break instructions into component parts and give them one at a time. Repeat as needed.
3. Use gestures appropriately to support your verbal messages.
4. Involve the family in planning and implementing all strategies.
5. Provide support and encouragement when the patient becomes frustrated.

GENERAL

1. Provide practice at times when the patient is rested and not fatigued.
2. Offer liberal praise and reinforcement for efforts. Remind the patient and family that small gains can still be made months into the rehabilitation process.

Guidelines for Safe Practice

The Patient With Sensory-Perceptual Deficits

HEMIANOPIA (LOSS OF VISION IN A PORTION OF THE VISUAL FIELD)

1. Approach the patient from the side of intact vision.
2. Position the patient in the room so that his or her intact visual field faces the door if possible.
3. Teach the patient to move the head from side to side (scan) to compensate for diminished visual fields. Scanning is also important with meals (see Figure 43-10).
4. Place objects needed for self-care within the patient's intact visual fields.

DENIAL/NEGLECT AND BODY IMAGE DISTORTIONS

1. Encourage the patient to look at and touch the affected side. Verbally remind the patient to check the position and safety of the affected side during activity.
2. Lightly touch and stimulate the affected side during care.
3. Provide gentle but consistent reminders to include the affected side in care (e.g., bathing, dressing).
4. Monitor the affected side for injuries when the patient is out of bed. A sling may be used to protect the affected side during ambulation.
5. Use a full-length mirror to assist the patient in reintegrating an intact body image and to assist with posture and balance.
6. Help the family to understand the nature of the patient's behavior.

AGNOSIA/APRAXIA

1. Encourage the patient to use all senses to compensate for problems in object recognition.
2. Practice the recognition and naming of commonly used objects and encourage the family to participate in the relearning process.
3. Encourage the patient to participate in self-care.
4. Correct the misuse of any object or task, guiding the patient's hand if necessary.
5. Continue to verbally cue the patient about the correct use of any objects or self-care tasks.
6. Be aware that memory deficits may make frequent reteaching necessary.
7. Explain the nature of all deficits to the family.

and ensure that the patient receives adequate daily fluid. A bowel program of stool softeners, fiber laxatives, and suppositories should be implemented on admission and modified as needed to support bowel regularity. Supporting the patient's normal daily pattern for elimination can also be helpful.

8. Promoting Effective Coping

The effects of stroke are usually life altering and can be devastating to the patient and family. Depression and despair are normal responses to stroke. In addition, the patient may experience significant difficulty in responding to situations with appropriate emotions. The patient's tolerance to stress is usually diminished, and significant emotional ability may be present. The patient may be extremely emotional and cry easily, and this behavior may be significantly different from the patient's prestroke baseline.

Evidence-Based Practice

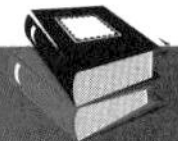

Reference: Chan H: Bladder management in acute care of stroke patients: a quality improvement project, *J Neurosci Nurs* 29(3):187, 1997.

Recognizing the importance of proactive nursing intervention in the return of continence after stroke, a group of nurses on a stroke care unit in Western Australia devised a study to demonstrate the effectiveness of their bladder retraining program. All nurses on the unit were trained in the use of a portable ultrasound bladder scanning device. The study sample comprised all stroke patients admitted to the unit for 13 weeks, with a total of 37 patients completing the study. Bladder function was assessed on admission for each patient, and a "bladder score" was assigned on the basis of the degree of continence. An individualized bladder management program was determined for each patient, consisting of a regimen of bladder scanning, intermittent catheterization (IMC), and/or determination of the patient's postvoid residual (PVR)), together with pelvic muscle exercise and/or pharmaceutical therapy. The IMC/PVR regimen was discontinued when a patient's PVR was found to be less than 100 ml for 3 consecutive days. At discharge, a bladder function score was again recorded.

Study results found that of the 37 patients enrolled in the study, 31 were continent at discharge from the hospital—a success rate of 84% in reestablishing continence. The remaining 6 patients were noted to have severe neurologic and self-care deficits that limited their ability to regain voluntary voiding control. The authors of this study recommend that given the substantial physical, economic, and social consequences of incontinence, a bladder management program that incorporates the monitoring of the patient's voiding pattern and consecutive assessment of the patient's PVR is indicated for all stroke patients who experience bladder dysfunction.

These emotional changes are distressing and commonly embarrassing to the spouse and family. Families need to be helped to understand that these emotional responses are outcomes of the stroke and are not volitional acts by the patient. Distraction and shifting the patient's attention can be successful strategies for assisting the patient in regaining control. The nurse teaches the family not to become sidetracked by attempting to explain or interpret the behavior and to avoid feeling responsible for causing it. Emotional responses typically become more stable with time. Problems with mood show potential for improvement with complementary therapies as discussed in the Complementary & Alternative Therapies box.[31]

Patient/Family Education

The greatest challenges for the patient and family occur after the patient has survived the initial acute stroke period (see Research box). Married couples often express the view that the stroke has happened to both of them because the threat to their established way of life is so profound. The patient and family need to be included in all explanations of interventions and procedures, as well as be provided with realistic appraisals of the patient's future status and deficits. Most people have a basic understanding of stroke and its classic manifestations, but this knowledge is rarely sufficient to understand the unique

Complementary & Alternative Therapies
Therapies in Long-Term Neurology Care

There is much current interest in alternative therapies, but to date, very little research is available regarding the effectiveness of these treatment modalities for neurologic patients. This pilot project involving a very small sample of just four patients was conducted to examine the effect of three complementary therapies—aromatherapy, relaxation, and reflexology—on the level of pain, mood, and physical health. Study participants were drawn from the patient population on a long-stay neurology unit, and each participant was randomly assigned to one of four treatment groups: relaxation only, aromatherapy only, reflexology only, or both aromatherapy and reflexology. Treatment was given once a week for 5 weeks. Data collection was by way of blinded interview (i.e., the interviewer did not know to which treatment group the patient had been assigned), with participants asked to report a perceived problem list (e.g., difficulty with mobility, eating, personal hygiene), perceived pain, and mood. Data were collected during the 2 weeks before the first treatment, and assessment interviews were conducted during treatment phases, as well as during "no treatment" phases of the study.

In general, the study found that patients' responses indicated that they experienced benefit from each of the four treatment modalities. Mood ratings were highest with the combination of aromatherapy and reflexology. Little change was found in ratings of perception of health, and although pain was reduced, the change was not significant. An inverse relationship between perceived problems and mood was found, with ratings of perceived problems lowest when mood ratings were elevated. Citing previous research regarding mood and functioning, which has provided evidence that an improved emotional state reduces disability, these researchers concluded that overall, this study found evidence for positive benefits of the use of these complementary therapies for this population of neurologic patients.

Reference: Walsh E, Wilson C: Complementary therapies in long-stay neurology in-patient settings, *Nurs Stand* 13(32):32, 1999.

Research

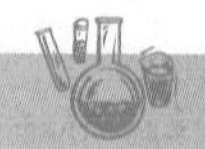

Reference: Johnson J et al: Stroke rehabilitation: assessing stroke survivors' long-term learning needs, *Rehabil Nurs* 22(5):243, 1997.

As a first step in the development of an educational program for stroke victims, this study was conducted as a needs assessment to examine the long-term self-identified learning needs and types of information desired by stroke survivors. It also examined the views of health care providers in the field of stroke rehabilitation regarding information needed by stroke survivors. A convenience sample of 258 participants was recruited: 68 stroke survivors, 37 family members, and 153 health care providers. Data were collected by means of questionnaires.

Study results found that although the stroke survivors and family members tended to articulate similar learning needs, differences were observed between the types of information desired by the patients and families and what the health care providers thought needed to be taught. For example, the providers believed that survivors needed to know more about the causes and mechanisms of stroke and about the emotional and social consequences of stroke, whereas the stroke survivors expressed a greater interest in learning about modalities such as massage, acupuncture, and vitamin supplements.

Results from this study also showed that learning needs of stroke survivors change over time, with recent stroke patients indicating concern with more immediate issues, such as learning about other problems stroke victims may face and how to deal with pain. The researchers used the information gleaned from this study to direct the development of an educational plan for stroke survivors and their families that uses a holistic approach to address the physical, social, and emotional impact of stroke.

challenges they face. The nurse uses every opportunity for teaching and encourages the family to be involved in the patient's actual care within the scope of their comfort level.

The acute care phase of stroke management is brief, and the family will need assistance to make decisions about the next phases of care for the patient. A social service referral is usually helpful. A lifetime of family dynamics and history complicate the efforts to make reasonable and rational decisions about bringing a patient home or seeking long-term nursing home placement. The financial consequences of either decision can be devastating. Ongoing and sometimes severe deficits are common after stroke, and most patients require some degree of supervision and assistance.[15] This support may be needed on a temporary or permanent basis. Stroke support groups and resources such as the American Heart Association and National Stroke Association can be useful sources of information and referral services.

Recent years have seen an increased emphasis on aggressive stroke rehabilitation, but this can increase the pressure on the family to attempt to manage the patient's care at home. Decision making about care is difficult, and the nurse attempts to support all parties, facilitate communication, and ensure that the family has all of the information they need. Involvement in the patient's daily care may help the family to have a more realistic picture of the patient's needs for assistance and their ability to provide such support at home. Chapter 10 provides additional information about the challenges of rehabilitation. The nurse may need to remind the family that regular respite for caregivers needs to be incorporated into the overall plan.

Health Promotion/Prevention. Increased attention to high blood pressure diagnosis and control has been successful in reducing the mortality and morbidity of stroke. Outreach efforts concerning hypertension control need to expand, especially for the African-American and Hispanic populations, and for the very old. Reducing cardiac risk factors, normalizing body weight, promoting smoking cessation, and controlling diabetes can all positively affect stroke statistics. High-risk patients are usually given antiplatelet agents, as are most patients who experience TIA. Compliance with these medication regimens can reduce stroke incidence. All patients who experience TIA are encouraged to undergo a workup to establish whether their symptoms are attributable to carotid stenosis that could possibly be surgically reversed. Current public health education efforts are teaching individuals to consider stroke as a form of "brain attack," viewed as a corollary of heart attack, in which early intervention can be critical in limiting the extent of ischemic damage and reducing poststroke disability.

EVALUATION

To evaluate the effectiveness of nursing interventions, compare patient behaviors with those stated in the expected patient outcomes. Achievement of patient outcomes is successful if the patient:

1. Maintains stable vital signs and has no signs of increased intracranial pressure.
2. Is able to move and transfer using adaptive equipment as needed; maintains an intact skin; shows no evidence of joint contractures.
3. Performs ADLs independently with the use of adaptive equipment.
4. Consumes a balanced oral diet without choking or aspiration, or tolerates tube feeding, and maintains a stable body weight.
5. Communicates effectively.
6. Uses techniques to compensate for perceptual deficits and remains free of injury.
7. Maintains bladder and bowel continence.
8. Participates with family in social interaction and planning for future care needs.

GERONTOLOGIC CONSIDERATIONS

The majority of all strokes affect the older population, and it is anticipated that the ongoing aging of the population will cause the incidence statistics to continue to increase. It is difficult to overestimate the impact of a stroke on an older adult's ability to maintain an independent lifestyle. The burdens for the spouse and family can be sudden and completely overwhelming. Even a mild stroke may require the complete restructuring of daily living patterns. In more severe strokes long-term institutionalization is commonly necessary. Even when the physical consequences are limited, the cognitive, emotional, and behavioral effects of stroke may still change the patient in small but significant ways.

The nature and scope of stroke rehabilitation are usually prescribed within the managed care framework. The nurse plays a crucial role in helping patients to gain access to needed services and move appropriately through the established care pathway. Stroke care for older adults necessitates multidisciplinary collaborative management and will continue to challenge the health care team to develop strategies to address the multiple areas of concern.

SPECIAL ENVIRONMENTS FOR CARE

Critical Care

Ischemic stroke management rarely necessitates admission to a critical care unit, although some institutions have specialized stroke units designed to increase the quality and intensity of patient monitoring. However, hemorrhagic strokes commonly create life-threatening situations that require management in critical care environments. This is particularly true for patients whose cerebral bleeding is the result of aneurysm rupture. These patients require aggressive management of increasing intracranial pressure to minimize extension of the damage. Older patients who have experienced nonaneurysmal intracerebral bleeding are usually transferred to general care as soon as CT scans confirm that the bleeding has stopped.

Community-Based Care

The challenges of reintegrating the stroke patient back into community and home care are substantial and have been previously discussed under each nursing diagnosis. The personal and financial costs and resource challenges for the patient and family, community services, and insurers can be enormous. Few diagnoses are as initially overwhelming as stroke or create as many challenges for ongoing care and support. The nurse usually serves as the patient's care coordinator, initiating discharge planning, helping the family to plan and implement necessary structural modifications in the home, and making referrals for the delivery of needed care in the home.

COMPLICATIONS

The list of possible complications of stroke is almost endless. Stroke may result in death or profound neurologic injury. With less severe strokes, the initial acute period may be complicated by respiratory problems related to aspiration and atelectasis. Other disuse-related complications include skin breakdown, deep vein thrombosis, muscle atrophy, and joint contractures. Urinary tract infections often result from the use of Foley catheters, and both constipation and impaction may result from immobility. Stroke patients are at high risk for environmental injury from a variety of physical and cognitive impairments, and the consequences of communication impairments can isolate the patient from full and active participation in the world. Furthermore, for each complication the patient experiences, there is the very real possibility that additional problems will develop for the family and support network. Prevention of these multiple complications is addressed in the collaborative care and nursing management sections.

Cerebral Aneurysm and Arteriovenous Malformation

Etiology/Epidemiology

A cerebral aneurysm is a thin-walled outpouching or dilation of an artery of the brain. Aneurysms typically develop at points of bifurcation of the blood vessels, and the vessels of the circle of Willis are affected most often. If the aneurysm ruptures, bleeding into the subarachnoid space usually ensues. This is termed *subarachnoid hemorrhage.* Aneurysms can be classified by both their shape and size.

Shape:

- Berry: berry-shaped with a neck or stem. These are the most common type.
- Saccular: any aneurysm that has a saccular outpouching
- Fusiform: an outpouching of the vessel wall without a stem
- Dissecting: the intimal layer of the artery pulls away from the medial layer, allowing blood to be forced between the layers

Size:
- Small: up to 15 mm
- Large: from 15 to 25 mm
- Giant: from 25 to 50 mm
- Supergiant: >50 mm

An estimated 10 to 15 million people in the United States have cerebral aneurysms, but most of these aneurysms are extremely small and remain asymptomatic throughout the person's life. Approximately 30,000 persons experience subarachnoid hemorrhage each year related to aneurysmal bleeding, and the outcome for these individuals remains poor.[12] From 20% to 40% die at the time of rupture. Subarachnoid hemorrhage primarily affects the 35- to 60-year-old age-group and is more common in women than in men by a ratio of 3:2.

A congenital developmental weakness in the artery has long been believed to play a major role in the etiology of aneurysms. Research also suggests that aneurysms develop as a result of degenerative vascular disease of the intima. Hypertension may predispose a person to aneurysm development; head trauma, bacterial and fungal infections, and atherosclerosis are all clearly implicated. Because multiple aneurysms are occasionally found in family groups, a genetic factor is being explored.

Arteriovenous malformations (AVMs) are also commonly diagnosed for the first time when the patient has signs of acute cerebral bleeding, but the nature of the problem is different. AVMs are among the more common developmental cerebrovascular malformations and are composed of a tangled mass of arteries and veins that lack a capillary network. Blood is directly shunted from the arteries to the veins. AVMs may form anywhere in the brain but are commonly found in the distribution of the middle cerebral artery. Most patients develop symptoms for the first time between the ages of 20 and 40 years. The annual incidence of AVMs is about 3 per 100,000, which represents 9% of all intracerebral hemorrhages and 1% of all strokes.[12]

Pathophysiology

When a cerebral aneurysm ruptures, blood at high pressure is forced out into the tissue, usually into the subarachnoid space. However, in some situations blood is forced into the brain substance itself, resulting in an intracerebral hemorrhage. The amount of blood lost is usually small because acute vasoconstriction occurs in adjacent vessels, and rising tissue pressure helps seal the bleeding site while fibrin and platelets initiate clot formation.

The pathology of AVM develops over time. The lack of a capillary network between the arteries and veins results in lower resistance in the arteries and the need for the veins to continually expand to handle the additional blood flow. Brain tissue within the AVM suffers degenerative changes. The patient may become steadily more symptomatic over time or have an active intracerebral hemorrhage.

Many patients are completely asymptomatic before the hemorrhage of either an aneurysm or AVM. The classic symptom is a sudden-onset violent headache, usually described as the "worst headache of my life." Immediate loss of consciousness may occur from the abrupt rise in intracranial pressure, and focal or widespread symptoms of an acute stroke develop. In addition, the blood itself irritates the blood vessels, meninges, and brain as it hemolyzes. Arterial spasms are triggered by the blood and the release of vasoactive substances, which can further decrease cerebral perfusion. AVMs also commonly manifest first as an acute hemorrhage, but some patients experience warning signs such as persistent unilateral headache or the onset of seizures.

Collaborative Care Management

The diagnosis of cerebral aneurysms and AVMs is usually made from the symptom pattern and the findings of CT scanning, which demonstrate bleeding. Once the diagnosis is made, cerebral angiography is used to visualize the major cerebral vessels, identify the specific characteristics of the aneurysm or AVM, and determine the presence and severity of vasospasm.

Surgical repair is the treatment of choice if anatomically and technically feasible. The surgery is performed as soon as possible after an initial period of stabilization and workup. Patients whose aneurysms are graded as I to III by an aneurysm classification system are the best candidates for early surgical intervention (Box 43-6).

The surgical approach depends on the location and size of the aneurysm. A berry aneurysm is usually clipped or ligated around the stem, whereas other types of aneurysms may be wrapped to support the weakened vessel and induce scarring around the wrapping (Figure 43-11). Balloon therapy involves the insertion and inflation of a small silicone catheter with a balloon to occlude either the aneurysm or the parent vessel. These latter procedures are still considered experimental.

Surgery for AVMs is extremely difficult from a technical perspective and may involve ligation or occlusion of feeder vessels. Surgery may be preceded by attempts to embolize feeder vessels with liquid polymerizing agents, Gelfoam particles, and microcoils. These treatment techniques progressively reduce the blood flow to the AVM. Gamma knife surgery may be used for certain inaccessible lesions (see Chapter 42).

BOX 43-6 Grading System for Symptoms and Neurologic Deficit after Subarachnoid Hemorrhage

Grade	Symptoms
Grade I: minimal bleed	Asymptomatic or minimal headache, slight nuchal rigidity
Grade II: mild bleed	Moderate to severe headache, nuchal rigidity, minimal neurologic deficits
Grade III: moderate bleed	Drowsiness, confusion, mild focal neurologic deficits
Grade IV: moderate to severe bleed	Stupor, moderate to severe hemiparesis, early decerebrate posturing
Grade V: severe bleed	Deep coma, decerebrate rigidity, disruption of vegetative functions

Rehabilitation aspects of care for patients with aneurysms and AVMs is similar to that previously discussed for ischemic stroke. However, initial management focuses on stabilizing the patient and minimizing the risk of rebleeding. The focus of medical management is on maintaining a stable cerebral perfusion pressure by sustaining systolic blood pressure in the 150 mm Hg range and intervening to prevent rebleeding and manage vasospasm.

Vasospasm complicates the course of significant numbers of persons who survive initial aneurysm hemorrhage. Symptomatic vasospasm occurs in about 30% of patients and peaks in incidence at 4 to 15 days postbleed.[1] Treatment is directed at increasing cerebral perfusion by administering crystalloid and colloid solutions to expand the intravascular volume and keep the vessels dilated. A calcium channel blocker is also routinely given to enhance collateral blood flow. Steroid use is widespread but remains controversial.

The focus of nursing care is careful patient monitoring and implementation of aneurysm bleeding precautions. The purpose of these precautions is to maintain a stable perfusion pressure. The rigor of aneurysm precautions has been decreased in recent years because concern has arisen over the development of sensory deprivation and related behavioral and cognitive impairments. Basic principles of care are outlined in the following Guidelines for Safe Practice box and are similar to those used for the management of increased intracranial pressure. Care after neurosurgery is described in Chapter 42.

Patient/Family Education. Aneurysm or AVM bleeding creates a sudden and potentially life-threatening crisis for the patient and family. The nurse plays an essential role in explaining all needed care routines, especially when a patient is in a critical care environment. Fear and anxiety can easily overwhelm the family's ability to learn and retain information. Participating in informed consent concerning high-risk surgical interventions can be particularly overwhelming. The nurse acts to bridge the gap between the neurosurgical team and the patient and family, providing concrete explanations and support as needed. The rationale for all treatments and restrictions is carefully explained, and the family is incorporated into the patient's care whenever it is safe and feasible to do so. Referral for social service and spiritual support may also be appropriate.

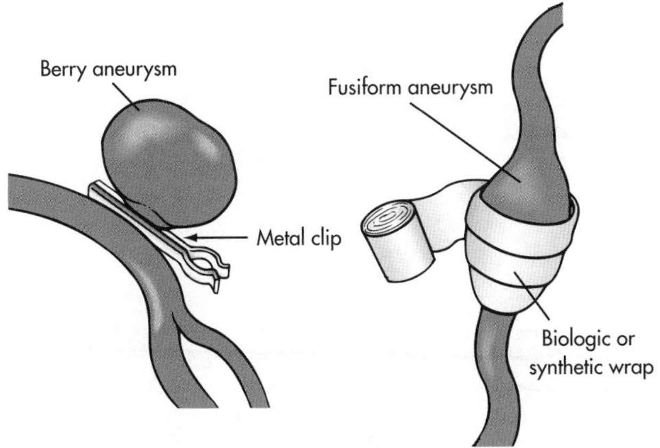

Figure 43-11 Clipping and wrapping of aneurysms.

DEGENERATIVE DISEASES

Degenerative neurologic disease includes a wide variety of neurologic disorders in which breakdown or progressive dysfunction of nerve cells exists. Only the most common of these disorders are discussed in this section. Alzheimer's disease is not included in the presentation because although it is an organic brain disorder, it is primarily seen and managed in nursing homes and long-term psychiatric care facilities. Conversely, a discussion of Guillain-Barré syndrome is included in the presentation even though it is not strictly a degenerative problem. It does, however, share many of the same care concerns as the other disorders presented.

Patients with degenerative neurologic diseases are primarily managed in the community setting. The focus of care is on achieving effective symptom management and supporting independence. This focus entails a multidisciplinary approach to care, with treatment decisions resting with the patient and family in close collaboration with medicine, nursing, physical therapy, occupational therapy, and social services.

Degenerative diseases typically cause a slowly progressive loss of independence. The patient must be helped to maintain a balance between the goal of independent self-care and acceptance of appropriate self-help aids and devices, or the need for direct assistance. Patients and families are forced to constantly adjust to changes in the patient's health status and cope with a future reality of declining abilities. The patient's and

Guidelines for Safe Practice

The Patient on Aneurysm Precautions

1. Place the patient in a quiet, private room without a telephone.
2. Maintain bed rest with the head of the bed elevated about 30 degrees. Some surgeons now permit bathroom privileges for selected patients. If the patient is allowed out of bed, stress the importance of not bending over (e.g., to pick up slippers or dropped objects).
3. Restrict visitors to close family or significant others and keep visits short. Prevent contact with visitors who upset or excite the patient.
4. Encourage quiet, restful activities such as reading or listening to quiet music. Television may be permitted if it does not excite the patient.
5. Keep the room slightly darkened and avoid bright, artificial light.
6. Use stool softeners to prevent straining at stool.
7. Discourage isometric contraction and use of Valsalva's maneuver (e.g., coughing, dragging self up in bed by the elbows, holding the breath during painful interventions such as venipuncture). Avoid the use of restraints.
8. provide gentle assistance with all needed care.
9. Administer analgesics as needed for headache.
10. Monitor the patient carefully for any changes in alertness or mental status.

family's psychosocial responses to these losses are often as important as the physical challenges of the disease process. The nurse's role is usually focused on ongoing patient education and support. Being knowledgeable about the disease process and treatment options allows the patient to effectively manage his or her environment and plan appropriately for the future. A major role for nurses is supporting the patient's and family's coping resources and remaining alert and sensitive to quality-of-life issues as they arise. Community support groups can be extremely helpful to patients and their families in dealing with both today's challenges and future crises.

Multiple Sclerosis

Etiology/Epidemiology

Multiple sclerosis (MS) is a chronic degenerative neuromuscular disease that is characterized by inflammation of the white matter of the central nervous system. The etiology of MS is unknown, although an underlying viral infection has been suggested as a cause. A slow viral infection is theorized to either directly cause the inflammation of the white matter or to trigger an autoimmune response that produces antibodies that result in the destruction of the myelin. Immunologic abnormalities are clearly part of the disease profile. Other autoimmune theories include the possibility that autosensitization occurs in response to an antigen on the myelin membrane or that a cell-mediated immune reaction triggers the demyelination process.

An estimated 250,000 to 350,000 persons in the United States have MS. The highest incidence is in young adults, and women are affected slightly more often than men.[23] Genetic makeup is implicated because the disease occurs 15 times more often in first-degree relatives of persons with MS than in the general population. Epidemiologic studies consistently demonstrate a higher incidence in colder northern latitudes.

MS is typically discussed as a single disease process, but it actually manifests in a variety of patterns, and in a significant minority of patients the disease causes little or no disability. Sclerotic lesions are even discovered on autopsy or by incidental scanning in individuals who are or were completely asymptomatic. Patients with more aggressive forms of the disease are obviously more likely to be hospitalized and have come to symbolize the disease for many health care professionals. MS is classified into two distinct disease courses[23]:

1. Relapsing/remitting disease (80% of all cases; female-male ratio, 2:1). Disease exacerbations occur over several days and then gradually resolve over several weeks, usually returning the patient to baseline or near-baseline functioning.
2. Primary progressive disease (20% of all cases, similar female-male ratio). This is a gradually progressive disease in which exacerbations occur but the patient does not return to baseline and is left with increasing amounts of residual disability.

Pathophysiology

MS causes scattered demyelination of the white matter of the central nervous system. Although the exact etiology remains unclear, research evidence suggests that viral infection initiates an autoimmune response that results in demyelination. The blood-brain barrier usually protects the brain from immune cell activity. In MS, however, this barrier is breached, and activated T cells, antibodies, and macrophages attack the fatty myelin sheath and the oligodendrocytes that produce it. The central nervous system damage is thought to be caused by a delayed type of hypersensitivity, a cell-mediated immune response.

The acute inflammation reduces the thickness of the myelin sheath that surrounds the axons and nerve fibers, and impulse conduction is slowed or blocked (Figure 43-12). Astrocytes or scavenger cells then remove the damaged myelin, and scar tissue forms over the affected areas. Natural healing may restore some of the function of the myelin, or the lesions may continue to interfere with nerve conduction. This partial healing accounts for the transitory nature of early disease symptoms. Eventually the nerve fibers may become permanently damaged, increasing the person's overt disabilities.

The course of MS is highly variable and unpredictable. Sites of inflammatory demyelination can occur virtually anywhere in the brain and spinal cord, and MS produces a wide range of signs and symptoms. Events that can precipitate a relapse of the disease include emotional stress, fatigue, infection,

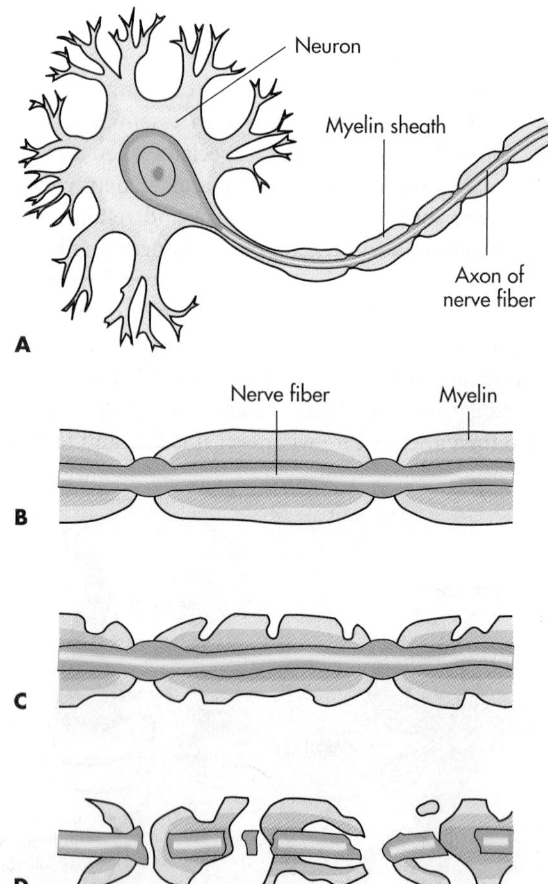

Figure 43-12 Process of demyelination. **A** and **B** depict a normal nerve cell and axon with myelin. **C** and **D** show the slow disintegration of myelin, resulting in a disruption in axon function.

fever, and hot and humid weather. Viral infections are again implicated in disease exacerbations. Early relapses may last just a day or two but typically become more prolonged as the disease progresses. A list of possible symptoms associated with MS is summarized in the Clinical Manifestations box. Classic symptom categories include sensory, motor, cerebellar, and neurobehavioral. Visual problems and fatigue are common early symptoms. Clinically silent relapses can also occur and are evident on MRI scans even in the absence of overt clinical symptoms.

Collaborative Care Management

The wide variety of initial symptoms and their transitory nature make the diagnosis of MS a challenge. There is no single reliable diagnostic test for the disease, and diagnosis often requires more than one episode of symptoms. MRI is extremely sensitive to white matter lesions and is useful in identifying specific sites of demyelination. When gadolinium is administered during the MRI, it is even possible to distinguish between old and new lesions. Nevertheless the diagnosis of MS remains a clinical one established by ruling out other neurologic causes of the symptoms.

Laboratory testing shows an increase in activated T4 lymphocytes and immune globulin G (IgG) content. Oligoclonal bands of IgG are commonly isolated from the cerebrospinal fluid (CSF). Myelin basic protein, which is found in the myelin sheath, is liberated during an acute attack and can be measured by radioimmunoassay. Finally, visual, auditory, and somatosensory evoked potentials are performed to assess nerve conduction.

Drug therapy is used in the management of MS to treat an acute attack, decrease the number and frequency of relapses, and support symptom management. The basic goal of all drug therapy is to decrease the inflammation and destruction of the myelin sheaths.[23] Some patients fail to respond to or respond poorly to drug therapy, and most approaches remain part of ongoing disease research studies. Drug therapy that is aimed at reducing the frequency and severity of relapses is summarized in Box 43-7. The development of recombinant forms of interferon-beta has offered patients with relapsing/remitting forms of MS a new drug therapy. Interferons have the ability to "interfere" with viral infections, but their mode of action in MS is not clear. Studies suggest that interferon-beta inhibits

Clinical Manifestations
Multiple Sclerosis

SENSORY SYMPTOMS

Numbness and tingling* on the face or extremities
Decreased proprioception
Paresthesias (burning, prickling)
Decreased sense of temperature, vibration, and depth

MOTOR SYMPTOMS

Weakness or a feeling of heaviness in the lower extremities
Paralysis
Spasticity and hyperreflexia
Diplopia
Bowel and **bladder** dysfunction (retention or urge incontinence)

CEREBELLAR SYMPTOMS

Spasticity and hyperreflexia
Incoordination, ataxia in lower extremities
Intentional tremor in upper extremities
Slurred speech, dysarthria
Scanning speech (slow, with pauses between syllables)
Nystagmus
Dysphagia

NEUROBEHAVIORAL SYMPTOMS

Emotional lability, euphoria, **depression** (occurs in 30% to 50% of patients)
Irritability
Apathy
Poor judgment, inability to problem solve effectively
Loss of short-term memory

OTHER

Optic neuritis (visual clouding, visual field deficits)
Impotence, sexual dysfunction
Fatigue (extremely common, ranges from mild to disabling)

*Commonly occurring symptoms are highlighted in **boldface**.

BOX 43-7 Principles of Drug Therapy for Multiple Sclerosis: Reducing the Frequency or Severity of Relapses

Acute Exacerbations

Short course of high-dose corticosteroids
- Methylprednisolone (Medrol) by IV infusion daily for 3 to 7 days with or without a follow-up taper of oral prednisone
- Oral prednisone tapered over 2 to 4 weeks
- Corticotropin (ACTH) by IV infusion or IM injection, gradually tapered over 2 to 4 weeks

Decreasing Relapses

- Interferon beta-lb (Betaseron) by SQ injection
- Interferon beta-1a (Avonex) by IM injection
- Glatiramer acetate (Copaxone; formerly known as copolymer 1), an injectable polymer that appears to have some effectiveness if started early in the disease
- Azathioprine (Imuran), an antiinflammatory and immunosuppressive agent; effectiveness is unproven

NOTE: Most drugs are effective for just one or two forms of multiple sclerosis.

Halting Disease Progression

Administration of selected immunosuppressive agents has shown some positive benefit in progressive disease. Drugs in use include:
- Cyclophosphamide (Cytoxan)
- Cyclosporine (Sandimmune)
- Cladribine (Leustatin)
- Oral myelin (currently in clinical trials)

Total lymphoid radiation may also be used.

ACTH, Adrenocorticotropic hormone; *IM*, intramuscular; *IV*, intravenous; *SQ*, subcutaneous.

the number of lymphocytes migrating to the central nervous system and suppresses production of macrophages.[5] These are the first drugs proven to decrease the frequency and severity of MS exacerbations. A wide variety of additional drugs may be used for symptom management. These include drugs to reduce tremor, spasticity, bladder dysfunction, and depression. Commonly used drugs are summarized in Box 43-8.

The goal of all collaborative interventions for MS is to keep the patient as independent as possible for as long as possible. Care is managed in the community and home setting except for short-term hospitalizations to treat disease exacerbations. A multidisciplinary team approach to care is essential, and the nurse commonly acts as the case manager. Physical therapy plays a crucial role. Range-of-motion and muscle-strengthening exercises are important in maintaining the function of uninvolved nerves.[25] Gait retraining is essential when spasticity or ataxia is present, and the patient may need to be fitted with assistive or supportive devices for safety. Stretching exercises are useful in compensating for mild spasticity. Range-of-motion exercise assumes greater importance as the need to prevent contractures develops.

BOX 43-8 Common Medications Used for Managing Symptoms of Multiple Sclerosis

Spasticity

Baclofen (Lioresal)
Dantrolene (Dantrium)
Diazepam (Valium)

Tremors

Hydroxyzine (Vistaril)
Isoniazid (INH)
Trihexyphenidyl (Artane)
Primidone (Mysoline)

Spastic Bladder and Urge Incontinence

Oxybutynin (Ditropan)
Imipramine (Tofranil)
Propantheline (Pro-Banthine)

Urinary Retention

Bethanechol chloride (Urecholine)

Antidepressants

Amitriptyline (Elavil)
Imipramine (Tofranil)
Trazodone (Desyrel)
Fluoxetine (Prozac)
Paroxetine (Paxil)
Sertraline (Zoloft)

Fatigue

Amantadine hydrochloride (Symmetrel)
Pemoline (Cylert)

Other

Stool softeners
Laxatives

Patient/Family Education. MS challenges patients and their families with its unpredictability and uncertainty. The threat of relapse and potential for loss of function are always present. These threats assume even greater magnitude for patients who may be in their young or middle adult years and at their height of productivity. Enormous pressure is placed on the patient to maintain normal daily activities, pursue a career, establish relationships, marry, and make responsible reproductive decisions. The uncertainty of the prognosis can be paralyzing to some patients and overwhelming to partners and families. Patient and family education plays a critical role in helping them to understand the disease process and how to prevent or minimize relapses if possible.

MS is a debilitating rather than a fatal disease process, and patients and families need to cope with disease challenges over many years. The nurse assumes major responsibility for coordinating patient education. The goal is to help the patient effectively manage self-care and minimize both recurrences and the need for hospitalization. The nurse encourages MS patients to maintain a general health-promoting lifestyle. This includes remaining active in normal daily activities to the limits of their energy tolerance and balancing activity with adequate rest to effectively manage fatigue.[25] The nurse stresses the use of energy conservation techniques, and an occupational therapist may be consulted about the use of appropriate self-help devices and aids. Chronic fatigue can be one of the disease's most debilitating features, and patients must become skilled at interpreting their body's responses and avoiding overexertion (see Research box).

The nurse instructs the patient on the importance of maintaining optimal nutrition. Patients with MS should eat a well-balanced diet that includes all major food groups. Natural fiber is encouraged to promote bowel regularity. Diets that limit the consumption of animal fat are recommended by some researchers because some polyunsaturated vegetable fatty acids are used by the body to produce myelin.

Patients with sensory losses need instruction about environmental safety. They need to compensate for their losses by using their eyes if possible to protect their extremities from trauma related to heat, cold, and pressure. Patients with diplopia often find that an eye patch is helpful. The nurse teaches the patient about the effect of heat, especially moist heat, on symptoms. When body temperature rises, the nerves may decrease or cease transmission, and disease symptoms can escalate dramatically. Hot baths, showers, hot tubs, steam baths, and saunas should all be avoided. Fever, stress, and infection can have the same effect. Chilling can also exacerbate symptoms. Female patients should be informed that pregnancy often exacerbates the disease, but they should be supported in their decision making about childbearing.

Bladder problems are extremely common in progressive disease. Drug therapy can be helpful in controlling symptoms, and the nurse instructs the patient about the effective use of prescribed medications. Urinary tract infection is a common cause of morbidity in MS and cannot always be prevented. A high daily fluid intake is important, and the nurse instructs the patient about the symptoms of infection that need to be reported to the health care provider. An intermittent catheterization program can be helpful for some patients with severe bladder problems. Bowel problems are best managed by the intake of adequate fluids and a high-fiber diet to establish a regular pattern of elimination.

If the patient progresses to permanent disabilities, a variety of additional interventions may be necessary. Referral to support groups such as the Multiple Sclerosis Association of America and the National Multiple Sclerosis Society can be helpful to both patients and families. Resources for coping will need to expand to adapt to the challenges posed by the steady loss of self-care abilities. Multiple changes may be required in family, occupational, and social roles. Changes in sexual patterns and abilities for couples should not be ignored. Families will also need ongoing support to deal with the cognitive and behavioral changes that may accompany MS. They need to understand that these symptoms, although often extremely troubling and frightening, are organic and disease related.

Parkinson's Disease

Etiology/Epidemiology

Parkinson's disease is a chronic degenerative disorder that primarily affects the neurons of the basal ganglia. First described in 1817 by James Parkinson, Parkinson's disease is currently one of the more common diseases of the nervous system. An estimated 100 to 150 persons per 100,000 population, or about 50,000 new cases, are diagnosed annually.[12] About 1 million persons are currently living with the disease in the United States.[17]

Parkinson's disease affects men and women about equally and usually occurs after the age of 50, with a median age of onset of about 55 years. A number of theories of causation for Parkinson's disease (including viral, vascular, metabolic, and environmental) are being tested, but the actual etiology remains unknown. The existence of a genetic component has been supported by recent research.[17] Primary Parkinson's disease is idiopathic, but a variety of other categories exist. Symptoms of Parkinson's disease may develop in response to the use of antipsychotic or neuroleptic agents; following an encephalitis infection; in response to brain trauma, tumors, hydrocephalus, or ischemia; in association with rare metabolic disorders; and in response to arteriosclerosis. Neurotoxins such as cyanide, manganese, and carbon monoxide have also been proposed as possible causes of the disease. Most cases are the primary idiopathic variety.

Research

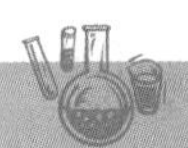

Reference: Stuifbergen AK: Physical activity and perceived health status in persons with multiple sclerosis, *J Neurosci Nurs* 29(4), 238, 1997.

This study examined the relationship of physical activity to overall health (social, mental, and physical) and perceived well-being in patients with multiple sclerosis (MS), a chronic and often debilitating illness. A convenience sample of 37 individuals with MS was recruited. Data about self-reported past and present types and levels of physical activity were obtained by means of questionnaires. Participants were also asked to complete a questionnaire regarding perceived health and well-being. A subset of four additional MS patients was recruited to participate in a 6-week twice-weekly swimming program. This group completed questionnaires at the start of the program, and at 6 weeks and 6 months later.

Although the researchers caution that it is not possible to make generalizations from a study with such a small sample, they offer the observation that participation in a program of regular exercise may lead to improvement in overall levels of activity and a perceived sense of well-being for MS patients. Study findings indicated that compared with the general population, MS patients have lower activity levels. Within this study group of MS patients, activity scores were found to be significantly correlated with the patients' overall health and level of physical activity. Those who reported regular physical activity had a higher sense of well-being than those who did not. Data from the subset of four patients who participated in the 6-week swimming program showed a 30% increase in perceived well-being from baseline at 6 weeks and, notably, a return to baseline 6 months after the end of the program. This suggests the importance of not only the encouragement of involvement in regular activity for MS patients, but also the continuation of activity over time.

Pathophysiology

The primary pathology of Parkinson's disease involves degenerative changes in the substantia nigra, which is an area within the basal ganglia. Destruction of the dopaminergic neurons in the substantia nigra significantly reduces the amount of available striatal dopamine.[12] Dopamine and acetylcholine are the primary neurotransmitters responsible for controlling and refining motor movements, and they have opposing effects. Dopamine produces inhibitory effects, and acetylcholine has excitatory effects. When the excitatory activity of acetylcholine is inadequately balanced by dopamine, an individual has difficulty controlling or initiating voluntary movements. Cellular degeneration in Parkinson's disease also leads to impairment of the extrapyramidal tracts that control semiautomatic and coordinated movements.

Clinical manifestations of Parkinson's disease do not usually occur until about 70% of the targeted neurons are destroyed. The disease begins insidiously and usually progresses so slowly that the person is seldom able to recall its onset. A faint tremor is a common early symptom that may be attributed to the aging process (Figure 43-13). The mnemonic TRAP, an acronym often used to describe the classic four major disease manifestations, stands for *t*remor, *r*igidity, *a*kinesia/bradykinesia, and *p*ostural instability. The disease is often categorized according to the nature and severity of the patient's symptoms. The major disease manifestations are described in more detail in the Clinical Manifestations box and are illustrated in Figure 43-14.

There are also numerous secondary disease manifestations. Patients usually experience generalized weakness and fatigue, difficulty with fine motor movements, loss of facial expression, difficulty chewing and swallowing, and voice changes. Many patients, particularly older adults, also experience memory loss, problem-solving difficulties, and visual-spatial deficits. There is no explanation for these cognitive losses at present, and many persons with Parkinson's disease remain

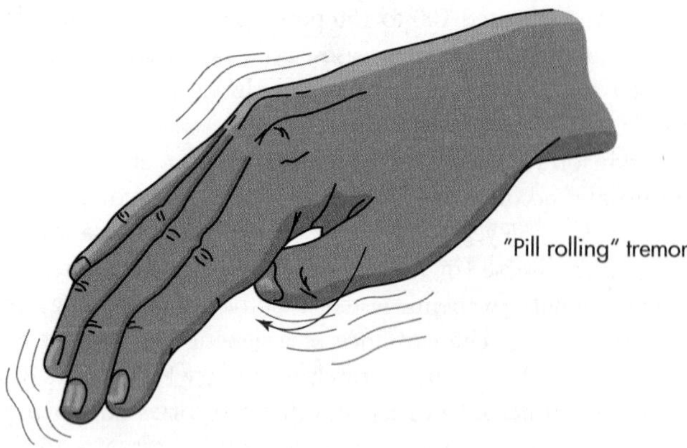

Figure 43-13 Classic tremor of Parkinson's disease. The movement of the thumb across the palm gives it a "pill rolling" appearance. The tremor is present at rest and may be relieved by movement.

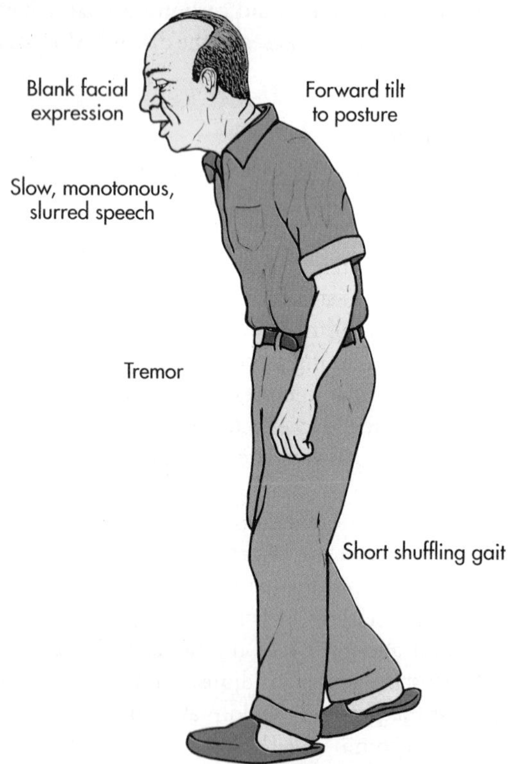

Figure 43-14 Characteristic appearance of a patient with Parkinson's disease.

Clinical Manifestations
Parkinson's Disease

TREMOR (see Figure 43-13)
Most recognized and least disabling symptom
Present in 75% of patients
Nonintentional, present at rest but usually not during sleep
Characterized by rhythmic movements of 4 or 5 cycles/sec
- Movement of the thumb across the palm gives a "pill-rolling" character
- Tremor also seen in limbs, jaw, lips, lower facial muscles, and head

RIGIDITY
Muscles feel stiff and require increased effort to move
Discomfort or pain may be perceived in muscle when rigidity is severe
"Cogwheel" rigidity refers to ratchetlike rhythmic contractions of the muscle that occur when the limbs are passively stretched

AKINESIA/BRADYKINESIA
Slowness of active movement
Difficulty initiating movement
Often the most disabling symptom; interferes with activities of daily living and predisposes patient to complications related to constipation, circulatory stasis, skin breakdown, and other related complications of immobility

POSTURAL INSTABILITY
Changes in gait
- Tendency to walk forward on the toes with small, shuffling steps
- Once initiated, movement may accelerate almost to a trot
- Festination may occur, which propels the patient either forward or backward propulsively until falling is almost inevitable

Changes in balance
- Stooped-over posture when erect (see Figure 43-14)
- Arms are semiflexed and do not swing with walking
- Difficulty maintaining balance and sitting erect
- Cannot "right" or brace self to prevent falling when balance is lost

cognitively intact despite major clinical manifestations of the disease. A decline in cognitive functioning is not universal.

Depression is seen in 20% to 43% of Parkinson's patients.[11] Many other signs and symptoms, primarily related to autonomic nervous system dysfunction, may also be present. The major secondary symptoms of Parkinson's disease are presented in Box 43-9. All symptoms typically worsen with stress and fatigue.

Collaborative Care Management

The diagnosis of Parkinson's disease is made clinically from the patient's history and symptoms. No definitive diagnostic test exists, and the diagnosis may be confirmed primarily from the patient's response to medication.

Parkinson's disease can neither be stopped nor cured, but developments in drug therapy over the past 40 years have resulted in enormous progress in the area of symptom control. In addition, general supportive care and education are provided to assist the patient in effectively managing disease manifestations in the home setting. Supportive care is primarily directed at supporting independence in self-care, developing coping resources, and ensuring safety. Multidisciplinary involvement of specialists such as physical, occupational, and speech therapists can help create a daily regimen that is effective in slowing the rate of disability.

Drug therapy for Parkinson's disease involves the potential use of six different classes of drugs (Table 43-1). Each patient's drug program is individually designed, taking into account the patient's age, type of symptoms, symptom severity, and

BOX 43-9 Secondary Manifestations of Parkinson's Disease

Facial Appearance

Expressionless
Eyes stare straight ahead
Blinking is much less frequent than normal

Speech Problems

Low volume
Slurred, muffled
Monotone
Difficulty with starting speech and word finding

Visual Problems

Blurred vision
Impaired upward gaze
Blepharospasm: involuntary, prolonged closing of the eyelids

Fine Motor Function

Micrographia: handwriting progressively decreases in size
Decreased manual dexterity
Clumsiness and decreased coordination
Decreased capacity to complete activities of daily living
Freezing: sudden, involuntary inability to initiate movement; can occur during movement or inactivity

Autonomic Disturbance

Constipation (hypomotility and prolonged gastric emptying)
Urinary frequency or hesitancy
Orthostatic hypotension (dizziness, fainting, syncope)
Dysphagia (neuromuscular incoordination)
Drooling (results from decreased swallowing)
Oily skin
Excessive perspiration

Cognitive/Behavioral

Depression occurs in about 40% of patients
Slowed responsiveness
Memory deficits
Visual-spatial deficits
Dementia

TABLE 43-1 Common Medications for Parkinson's Disease

Drug	Action	Intervention
Anticholinergics: trihexyphenidyl (Artane), benztropine (Cogentin), biperiden (Akineton)	Antagonize the transmission of acetylcholine in the central nervous system; most effective in decreasing rigidity; selective action but still have systemic anticholinergic effects	Monitor the incidence and severity of side effects: dry mouth, constipation, urinary retention, dysarthria, blurred vision, changes in memory, confusion.
Antivirals: amantadine (Symmetrel)	Block the reuptake and storage of catecholamines, allowing for the accumulation of dopamine	Positive effects may not last beyond 3 months. Monitor for effectiveness and severity of side effects (e.g., mental confusion, visual disturbances).
Levodopa: carbidopa-levodopa (Sinemet)	Restores deficient dopamine to the brain; carbidopa blocks peripheral conversion of levodopa	Monitor for side effects (e.g., nausea and vomiting, orthostatic hypotension, dry mouth, constipation, sleep disturbances, confusion, hallucinations). See teaching guidelines in the Patient Teaching box.
Dopamine agonists: bromocriptine (Parlodel), pergolide (Permax)	Directly stimulate dopamine receptors and increase the effect of levodopa; minimize fluctuations in drug response	Monitor for side effects, which are similar to those of levodopa. Mental dysfunction is common.
Monoamine oxidase B inhibitor: selegiline (Eldepryl)	Blocks the metabolism of dopamine; may slow the underlying disease process	Monitor for incidence of orthostatic hypotension. Do not exceed prescribed dose. May be given in combination with levodopa as the disease progresses.
COMT inhibitors: tolcapone (Tasmar)	Increase availability of levodopa by inhibiting COMT, thus increasing available CNS dopamine; may allow for decrease of levodopa dose	Monitor for side effects (e.g., orthostatic hypotension, diarrhea, nausea and vomiting, hepatic failure); monitor for elevated liver enzymes, electrolyte changes with diarrhea.

CNS, Central nervous system; *COMT,* catechol *O*-methyltransferase.

lifestyle. All treatment decisions are made collaboratively with the patient and family, who need to be carefully instructed about the advantages, disadvantages, and predicted side effects of each option. Drug categories include:

1. *Levodopa.* Levodopa is a precursor of dopamine that is able to cross the blood-brain barrier. Once present in the brain, it is converted to dopamine by the action of the enzyme dopa decarboxylase. This enzyme is also found outside of the central nervous system and acts on the levodopa wherever it is encountered. Most patients are therefore given Sinemet, which is a combination of levodopa and carbidopa. Carbidopa blocks the conversion

of levodopa in the peripheral tissues. This ensures that more levodopa reaches the brain and increases its effectiveness. Combining levodopa and carbidopa usually permits a reduction in the dose of levodopa, which helps control the multiple and sometimes disabling side effects of levodopa.

The effectiveness of levodopa gradually decreases over time, which may necessitate gradual increases in the dose to sustain its beneficial effects. Sensitivity to drug side effects also increases, however, which limits the ability to continue to increase the dose.[6] Some patients experience unpredictable responses to levodopa, including an "on-off" phenomenon. Motor function can fluctuate in a matter of minutes from active and ambulatory to severe motor freeze-ups. "Drug holidays" are recommended by some authorities for patients receiving prolonged levodopa therapy. Patients are admitted to the hospital and completely withdrawn from their medication. Although symptoms exacerbate dramatically, it is usually possible to restart the levodopa after about a week at a much lower dosage. Guidelines for the safe use of levodopa are summarized in the Patient Teaching box.

2. *Anticholinergics.* These drugs are typically used in conjunction with levodopa or for patients who cannot tolerate levodopa. They have been used in the treatment of Parkinson's disease for almost a century. They antagonize the excitatory effects of the cholinergic neurons, are most effective for treatment of tremor, and have some effect in relieving muscle rigidity. Although somewhat selective in action, they still produce widespread anticholinergic side effects and may not be well tolerated. Trihexyphenidyl (Artane) and benztropine mesylate (Cogentin) are two traditional drugs in this category.
3. *Antiviral agents.* Amantadine hydrochloride (Symmetrel) is an antiviral agent with known antiparkinsonian action. It blocks the reuptake of catecholamines, which allows dopamine to accumulate at synaptic sites. The drug's effectiveness is usually limited to about 3 months, and drug holidays do not prolong sensitivity to the drug's effects.
4. *Dopamine agonists.* Dopamine agonists stimulate dopamine receptors in the brain. They help prevent or minimize the fluctuations in motor response that occur in Parkinson's disease. Bromocriptine (Parlodel) and pergolide (Permax) are two forms in use.
5. *Monoamine oxidase B inhibitors.* Selegiline (Eldepryl) may be used in the early stages of Parkinson's disease. It blocks the metabolism of dopamine and often delays the need for levodopa therapy. This drug directly targets the disease process and not just its symptoms.
6. *Catechol O-methyltransferase inhibitors.* Tolcapone (Tasmar) is a relatively new drug that inhibits catechol O-methyltransferase (COMT), an enzyme that breaks down levodopa in the body. Given together with levodopa, COMT inhibitors can increase the availability of dopamine in the central nervous system. Because of the risk of significant side effects, including fatal liver dysfunction, it is recommended that the use of tolcapone be reserved for patients who have failed other drug therapy.[6]

A variety of experimental approaches have been or are being tried in the management of Parkinson's disease. Stereotactic surgery was used in the 1960s before levodopa became readily available. It is again being used in the management of severe tremor and rigidity. Thalamotomy and pallidotomy are procedures in which selected portions of the thalamus or basal ganglia are destroyed to relieve intractable tremors or dyskinesias. Case histories demonstrate positive outcomes in severe cases, but the risk of complications remains high.[33] Experimental treatment approaches also include autotransplantation of tissue from the adrenal medulla, where dopamine is produced peripherally. This therapy is based on the hope that the transplanted tissue will be able to produce dopamine in the brain. Experimental human and porcine embryonic tissue transfer has also been performed. The use of thalamic, or deep brain, stimulation to treat tremor has been approved by the Food and Drug Administration. In this procedure electrodes are implanted into the thalamus. These electrodes are connected to an external pulse generator, which is similar to a pacemaker, and is implanted under the skin of the chest. Clinical results of this surgery have been promising in patients with disabling tremor.[33]

Patient/Family Education. Parkinson's disease is primarily managed in the community and home setting, and the nurse's role is to educate the patient and family effectively for the

Patient Teaching

Guidelines for the Safe Use of Levodopa

1. Levodopa is best absorbed on an empty stomach. If nausea occurs, it can be taken with food.
2. Dry mouth is a common side effect. Chewing gum and hard candy can counter this effect.
3. Depression and mood swings may occur. Report these or other cognitive-behavioral changes such as insomnia, agitation, or confusion to the health care provider.
4. Avoid the use of alcohol or minimize alcohol intake. It is believed to antagonize the effects of levodopa.
5. Avoid protein ingestion near the times for medication administration. Some protein amino acids are believed to inhibit the absorption of levodopa. A pattern of a low-protein breakfast and lunch with a high-protein dinner has improved symptoms in selected patients.
6. Be alert to the possibility of orthostatic hypotension. Change positions slowly. Avoid steam baths, saunas, and hot tubs. Experiment with the use of support stockings to support venous return.
7. Avoid vitamin supplementation with products that contain vitamin B_6 (pyridoxine). Pyridoxine increases the conversion of levodopa in the liver, which decreases the amount available for conversion to dopamine in the brain.
8. Consult with the primary care provider and pharmacist about the use of all other drugs. Levodopa has multiple adverse drug interactions.

challenges of self-care. Patients and families need a thorough understanding of the disease process, appropriate self-care strategies, and signs that indicate medication failure or toxicity. The purpose of all interventions is to keep the patient as independent as possible in the face of a progressive decline in function. Teaching, support, and encouragement are needed throughout the course of the disease. A Nursing Care Plan for the patient with Parkinson's disease follows.

The nurse teaches the patient and family about the management of rigidity. Activity and exercise promote independence and reduce the risks of injury and complications. A physical therapist should be consulted to establish an initial

Nursing Care Plan *Patient With Parkinson's Disease*

DATA Mr. S. is a 75-year-old retired university professor who was diagnosed with Parkinson's disease 3 years ago. Over the past year he has developed tremors; a masklike appearance; slow, monotonous speech; difficulty swallowing; and a shuffling, unsteady gait. Mr. S. experienced two falls within the past month.

The nursing history reveals that Mr. S.:

- Lives with his wife in a two-story house
- Has a history of hypertension
- Underwent laparoscopic gallbladder surgery 8 months ago

Collaborative nursing actions include:

- Implementing aspiration precautions
- Implementing safety precautions to prevent falling
- Assessing for adverse reactions to medications

NURSING DIAGNOSIS **Ineffective airway clearance related to truncal muscle rigidity and resultant dysphagia, impaired cough mechanism, and decreased automatic swallowing**

GOALS/OUTCOMES Will maintain patent airway

NOC Suggested Outcomes

- Respiratory Status: Airway Patency (0410)
- Aspiration Control (1918)

NIC Suggested Interventions

- Airway Suctioning (3160)
- Aspiration Precautions (3200)
- Respiratory Monitoring (3350)

Nursing Interventions/Rationales

- Maintain elevation of head of bed (HOB) by at least 30 degrees. *An elevated position helps with gravitational flow of food and fluids into the stomach, decreasing the risk for aspiration.*
- Encourage swallowing of secretions if gag reflex is intact. *Increased salivation and decreased cough reflex increase the patient's risk of aspirating.*
- Remove excess secretions with tissue or by suctioning. *To remove excess secretions that cannot be swallowed or expectorated.*
- Encourage deep breathing and coughing every hour when sedentary. *Helps facilitate oxygenation and removal of secretions from the lungs.*
- Monitor respiratory status (lung sounds, respiratory rate and effort, altered level of consciousness). *To detect the flow of air and detect any adventitious sounds.*
- Assess ability to cough, gag, and swallow. *To determine existing deficits.*
- Avoid thin, warm liquids when cough and gag reflexes are intact. Thicken liquids as needed. *Thickened foods such as pudding are more easily swallowed than thin food because of their weight.*
- Institute aspiration precautions (check gag reflex before feeding; HOB elevated to 90 degrees; suction equipment at bedside). *Precautions are essential to prevent aspiration and respiratory compromise.*

Evaluation Parameters

1. Normal breath sounds
2. Nonlabored respiratory rate
3. Effective cough mechanism

NURSING DIAGNOSIS **Risk for injury related to decreased postural reflexes, orthostatic hypotension, rigidity, and retropulsive gait**

GOALS/OUTCOMES Will remain free of injury

NOC Suggested Outcomes

- Neurologic Status (0909)
- Risk Control (1902)
- Symptom Control (1608)

NIC Suggested Interventions

- Environmental Management: Safety (6486)
- Fall Prevention (6490)
- Surveillance: Safety (6654)

Continued

Nursing Care Plan — Patient With Parkinson's Disease—cont'd

Nursing Interventions/Rationales

- Assess blood pressure, pulse, and for dizziness immediately after changing to upright position. *To detect the presence of orthostatic hypotension in response to position change. Orthostatic hypotension can result in fainting and/or falling.*
- Change positions slowly when orthostatic hypotension is present. *Reduces orthostatic blood pressure changes.*
- Encourage patient to use sidebars in bathrooms, handrails in hallways, and chairs with back and arm rests.
- Use gait belt for assisted transfers. *Use of safety devices decreases the risk of falls and injury.*
- Encourage patient to choose a clear path for walking, avoiding crowds, narrow doorways, fast turns, uneven surfaces, and scatter rugs. *Environmental hazards can contribute to falls.*
- Encourage use of closed-heeled, supportive shoes or slippers. *Decreases the risk of the patient's shoes slipping from his feet and the patient falling.*
- Repeatedly remind patient to maintain upright position when ambulating. *Patients have a tendency to flex excessively at knees and hip, which increases the risk of falls.*
- Stop occasionally to slow walking speed (festinating gait). *To prevent falls.*
- Repeatedly remind patient to maintain wide-based gait (feet 12 to 15 inches apart). *Provides greater support and decreases the risk of falls.*
- Place chest restraint or loose bed sheet around patient's midriff while up in chair. *Prevents the patient from falling out of the chair. The patient must agree to use of restraint.*
- Place call light and telephone (and other such devices) within patient's reach. *To prevent leaning, which may result in falling.*

Evaluation Parameters

1. Patient and family express understanding of injury potential
2. Uses assistive devices correctly
3. Seeks assistance when needed

NURSING DIAGNOSIS **Impaired verbal communication related to micrographia and decreased ability to speak**
GOALS/OUTCOMES Will demonstrate effective communication of needs

NOC Suggested Outcomes

- Communication Ability (0902)
- Communication: Expressive Ability (0903)

NIC Suggested Interventions

- Active Listening (4920)
- Communication Enhancement: Speech Deficit (4976)

Nursing Interventions/Rationales

- Assess patient's ability to speak, read, and write. *Patients with Parkinson's disease have limited movement of facial muscles, tremors, and rigidity, which cause micrographia and decreased speech tone and volume.*
- Reduce environmental noise. *To reduce distractions that might interfere with communication.*
- Encourage patient to speak slowly and pause to breathe between words. *Assists the patient with articulation of words.*
- Watch patient's lips for clues and ask patient to repeat unclear words. *Aids the patient with communicating his needs accurately.*
- Teach patient to express ideas in short phrases or sentences. *Aids in articulation of words and communication of needs.*
- Teach patient to organize thoughts and plan what will be said. *Enhances articulation and communication of needs.*
- Teach patient to exaggerate pronunciation of words. *To aid articulation so that the caregiver can understand words.*
- Do not interrupt patient while trying to communicate. *Spontaneous speech may take time. Interrupting the patient increases anxiety and decreases the ability to articulate.*
- Encourage patient to use facial expressions when speaking. *This exercise aids with word articulation.*
- Encourage patient to talk or sing for 10 to 15 minutes each day. *To help maintain facial muscle tone to enhance the patient's ability to speak.*
- Encourage writing when antiparkinsonian medications are at their peak effectiveness. *Patient may experience less frustration by writing rather than trying to speak.*

Nursing Care Plan *Patient With Parkinson's Disease—cont'd*

- If speech cannot be understood, encourage patient to use alternative methods to communicate needs (communication board or list of words). *To enhance the patient's ability to communicate needs when speaking or writing is not possible.*

Evaluation Parameters

1. Makes known his needs
2. Uses alternative methods of communication
3. Is free of anxiety related to inability to speak

NURSING DIAGNOSIS **Risk for constipation related to decreased fluid intake, decreased peristalsis, and decreased mobility**

GOALS/OUTCOMES Will maintain normal pattern of bowel elimination

NOC Suggested Outcomes

- Bowel Elimination (0501)
- Hydration (0602)
- Mobility Level (0208)

NIC Suggested Interventions

- Bowel Management (0430)
- Fluid Management (4120)
- Exercise Promotion (0200)

Nursing Interventions/Rationales

- Assess patient's bowel regularity. *The patient's usual pattern of bowel elimination should be considered. A bowel movement every 2 to 3 days may be normal.*
- Increase fluid intake to 2 to 3 L/day if not contraindicated. *Adequate fluid is necessary to prevent hard, dry stool formation.*
- Encourage consumption of high-fiber foods. *Fiber coupled with adequate fluid stimulates peristalsis and elimination.*
- Encourage regular bowel elimination schedule. *A regular schedule aids with bowel elimination. The gastrocolic reflex may be helpful in stimulating bowel movement following meals.*
- Provide ample time for defecation. *Some patients take longer than others. Rushing the patient increases anxiety and prevents relaxation, which is necessary for normal elimination.*
- Use bathroom or bedside commode instead of a bedpan when possible. *Proper positioning allows gravity and abdominal muscles to promote stool elimination.*
- Implement bowel training program aided by suppositories. *May be necessary when regularity cannot be established through diet and exercise.*
- Avoid use of laxatives and enemas unless absolutely necessary. *The patient may become laxative or enema dependent and unable to establish normal bowel elimination patterns.*

Evaluation Parameters

1. Soft, formed stool
2. Daily bowel movement
3. No requests or need for laxatives or enemas

NURSING DIAGNOSIS **Imbalanced nutrition: less than body requirements related to decreased gag reflex, dysphagia, and difficulty chewing**

GOALS/OUTCOMES Will maintain weight within 5 pounds of baseline

NOC Suggested Outcomes

- Nutritional Status (1004)
- Nutritional Status: Food and Fluid Intake (1008)
- Nutritional Status: Nutrient Intake (1009)

NIC Suggested Interventions

- Nutrition Monitoring (1160)
- Nutrition Management (1100)
- Nutrition Therapy (1120)

Nursing Interventions/Rationales

- Provide small, frequent, high-calorie meals. *Patients who have difficulty chewing and swallowing become frustrated when they must eat large amounts of food. Small, frequent meals provide the same nutrients and are less tiring to consume.*
- Allow adequate time for eating. *Rushing the patient creates anxiety and frustration and may result in the patient's refusing to eat or not eating an adequate amount of food.*
- Provide thick, cold foods (ice cream, shakes, frozen liquid supplements). *These foods are easier to swallow than hot or thin foods.*

Continued

Nursing Care Plan Patient With Parkinson's Disease—cont'd

- Provide oral care before and after meals. *A clean mouth and pleasant taste stimulate eating. A bad taste can discourage eating.*
- Assess daily caloric intake. *To determine if the patient is consuming adequate calories to meet metabolic demands.*
- Record weight at least every third day. *To identify any pattern of weight gain, loss, or stability.*
- Schedule medications so that peak time coincides with meals. *Medications control symptoms that interfere with the patient's ability to self-feed and swallow.*
- Encourage family to bring patient's favorite meals from home. *Consumption of adequate nutrients is more likely to occur if the patient enjoys the foods that are served.*

Evaluation Parameters

1. Maintains balanced nutrient intake
2. Maintains stable weight
3. Is free of choking or aspiration
4. Maintains fluid intake >2000 ml/day

NURSING DIAGNOSIS **Self-care deficit (feeding, bathing, grooming) related to akinesia, decreased reflexes, and tremor**

GOALS/OUTCOMES Will independently perform self-care with use of self-help aids

NOC Suggested Outcomes

- Self-Care: Activities of Daily Living (0300)
- Self-Care: Bathing (0301)
- Self-Care: Dressing (0302)
- Self-Care: Eating (0303)
- Self-Care: Grooming (0304)

NIC Suggested Interventions

- Bathing (1610)
- Dressing (1630)
- Feeding (1050)
- Self-Care Assistance (1800)

Nursing Interventions/Rationales

- Obtain adaptive equipment for feeding (padded utensils and plate guards), bathing (sponge mitts), and dressing (Velcro straps), and teach patient correct use. *These devices aid the patient with completing self-care tasks, increase self-confidence, and allow some control over the situation.*
- Encourage use of chairs and commodes with elevated seats. *To aid the patient with sitting and prevent falls from loss of balance.*
- Provide unhurried atmosphere and allow time for completion of tasks. *Many patients can remain independent if they are allowed adequate time to complete tasks. Hurrying patients makes them frustrated and impedes their ability to function.*
- Foster independence and provide encouragement if problems arise. *Patients may become easily frustrated. Rewarding small successes provides encouragement for continued independence.*
- Perform active or passive range-of-motion exercises to all extremities. *Muscle rigidity can quickly progress to joint contractures.*
- Encourage patient to actively swing arms when ambulating. *Improves balance and decreases tremor, which facilitates movement.*
- If patient becomes "frozen" while ambulating, face patient and either hold patient's hands or have patient hold your shoulders or waist with both hands. Gently and slightly rock patient from side to side. *Bradykinesia is a classic sign of Parkinson's disease. Episodes of akinesia or freeze-up can occur wherein the patient cannot initiate movement. Gentle rocking helps unfreeze the patient so that he can continue walking.*

Evaluation Parameters

1. Uses self-help aids correctly
2. Completes self-care without assistance or frustration
3. Participates in daily exercises as prescribed

activity plan and teach the patient and family range-of-motion exercises. These exercises are performed several times each day to relieve stiffness and prevent joint contractures.

Massage and muscle stretching are also effective strategies for reducing rigidity. Strategies for managing gait problems and preventing injury during ambulation can also be taught. A wide-based stance helps maintain balance for ambulation. Holding the hands clasped behind the back when walking may help the patient keep the spine erect and counter the postural problems created by the arms hanging stiffly at the sides.

The nurse emphasizes the importance of correct posture. Lying on a firm bed without a pillow during rest periods may help prevent the spine from bending forward, and lying in the prone position at intervals is also helpful. The use of assistive devices to prevent injury and support mobility is also explored. Patients with severe resting tremor may find that holding an object or placing the hands firmly along the arms of a chair when sitting may reduce its severity.

Environmental safety is an ongoing concern. The nurse can help the patient and family to evaluate the home environment for fall risks posed by scatter rugs, clutter, or poor lighting. Simple home adaptations such as raised toilet seats and grab bars in the bathroom can significantly improve patient safety. Episodes of akinesia (freeze-ups) are more difficult to manage. The nurse reminds the patient to change positions frequently and avoid sitting in one position for extended periods. The use of firm, supportive chairs with arms and rocking movements to initiate large movements such as rising from a chair can be helpful for some patients.

Patients with Parkinson's disease may face a wide variety of other daily disease-related challenges. General teaching guidelines for patients with Parkinson's disease are summarized in the Patient Teaching box. Patients and families need ongoing support and encouragement because the burden of caregiving is heavy and will become steadily more severe as the patient's condition worsens. They may profit from referral to the National Parkinson Foundation or American Parkinson Disease Association. All persons involved with caring for an individual with Parkinson's disease should be aware of the possibility of cognitive changes and deterioration, as well as the frequency with which patients develop severe depression. Pharmacologic intervention to treat depression may be necessary, and information about this disease complication should be provided to the family.

Myasthenia Gravis

Etiology/Epidemiology

Myasthenia gravis (MG) is a rare, chronic disease that affects the myoneural junction. Although its exact etiology is unknown, MG is widely believed to result from an autoimmune response that destroys a variable number of acetylcholine receptors (AChRs) at the myoneural junction. This

Patient Teaching

Guidelines for Patients With Parkinson's Disease

ACTIVITY AND EXERCISE

Perform range-of-motion exercise to all joints three times daily.
Massage and stretch muscles to reduce stiffness.
Use a broad base of support when ambulating. Consciously lift and place the feet when ambulating.
Pay attention to posture. Try walking with the hands clasped behind the back.
Explore the use of assistive devices.
Avoid staying in one position for prolonged periods. Alter position regularly.

SAFETY

Examine the home environment for risks of injury.
Modify the environment to improve lighting and remove hazards.
Consider installing devices such as raised toilet seats and grab bars.
Change position slowly if orthostatic hypotension develops.
Be alert to the effects of heat, stress, and excitement on symptom severity.

NUTRITION

Monitor weight once a week.
Evaluate dysphagia and modify diet to increase ease of chewing and swallowing if appropriate.
Practice swallowing and take small bites.
Provide an unhurried atmosphere and allow additional time for meals.
Follow a plan of small, frequent meals if fatigue is a problem during meals.
Avoid eating high-protein meals at times of medication administration.
Do not use vitamin supplements containing pyridoxine (vitamin B_6).
Ensure adequate fiber and fluid intake to prevent constipation.
Manage drooling problems with soft cloths.

ELIMINATION

Monitor bowel elimination pattern.
Use diet, exercise, and fluids to ensure regularity if possible.
Use stool softeners if needed.
Keep a urinal or commode at the bedside.
Respond promptly to the urge to urinate, and be sure to empty the bladder at least every 2 to 4 hours. Bradykinesia can result in episodes of incontinence.

COGNITIVE/BEHAVIORAL

Monitor for depression. Report its presence to the health care provider.
Monitor for changes in sleep pattern, disordered thoughts, and the development of agitation, confusion, or hallucinations. Report these symptoms promptly.

COMMUNICATION

Exercise the voice regularly by singing or reading aloud.
Attempt to project the voice and alter volume and pitch.
Consult a speech therapist if vocal problems are severe.

results in the classic disease features of weakness and fatigue of selected voluntary muscles. It is estimated that the incidence of MG in the United States is 14:100,000.[7] MG can occur at any age, affecting men and women in equal numbers, although it tends to affect primarily women 20 to 40 years of age and men 60 to 80 years of age. Infants of affected mothers may exhibit symptoms at birth, but the symptoms generally disappear within a few weeks. The thymus gland has long been believed to play a role in the autoimmune process of MG, because thymic hyperplasia is seen in as many as 80% of MG patients and 15% have thymic tumors.[14] However, the exact role of the thymus gland in the disease is not understood.

Pathophysiology

Effective muscle contraction is contingent on adequate amounts of acetylcholine (ACh), a neuromuscular transmitter, being available at the postsynaptic membrane to generate an action potential that can spread along the length of the muscle and culminate in muscle contraction. Mitochondria in the motor nerve axons synthesize ACh, which is released when the nerve is stimulated. The ACh crosses the myoneural junction and binds with an acetylcholine receptor (AChR) on the postsynaptic membrane to initiate the action potential (Figure 43-15).

Acetylcholinesterase (AChE) is also released into the synaptic cleft. The AChE breaks down the ACh, which limits the duration of the muscle contraction. The number of AChR sites is significantly reduced in persons with MG as a result of the destructive effects of an antibody-mediated autoimmune attack that specifically targets the AChR sites. As a result, the stimuli may lack sufficient amplitude to trigger an effective action potential in some muscle fibers. The strength of muscle response is diminished, and with repeated stimuli the amount of ACh steadily decreases, resulting in profound muscle fatigue.

The severity of MG is directly related to the number of AChR sites involved.[14] Muscle biopsy can demonstrate the normal number of sites being reduced by as much as two thirds. The disease can be classified on the basis of either the severity of the clinical symptoms or the course of the disease (Box 43-10). The onset of MG is usually gradual, and the disease may elude diagnosis for a prolonged period if it is not considered a possible cause of the patient's symptoms. The course of the disease is also highly variable, as is commonly true with autoimmune disorders.

The classic symptoms of MG are muscle weakness and generalized fatigue, which occur in more than 80% of patients. Ptosis and diplopia are common early findings, and the disease is occasionally limited to the eye muscles (ocular myasthenia).[14] Muscles innervated by the cranial nerves are often affected, and it may be impossible for the patient to keep the mouth closed or to chew and swallow for extended periods. The mobility of the facial muscles is also affected, and the face may take on an expressionless appearance (Figure 43-16). Attempts to smile may result in the classic myasthenic "snarl." The patient's voice is often weak, and as fatigue sets in, it may even become difficult for the patient to swallow saliva effec-

BOX 43-10 Classification System for Myasthenia Gravis

Type 1: ocular myasthenia
Type 2A: mild
Type 2B: severe
Type 3: fulminating/acute
Type 4: chronic, late severe

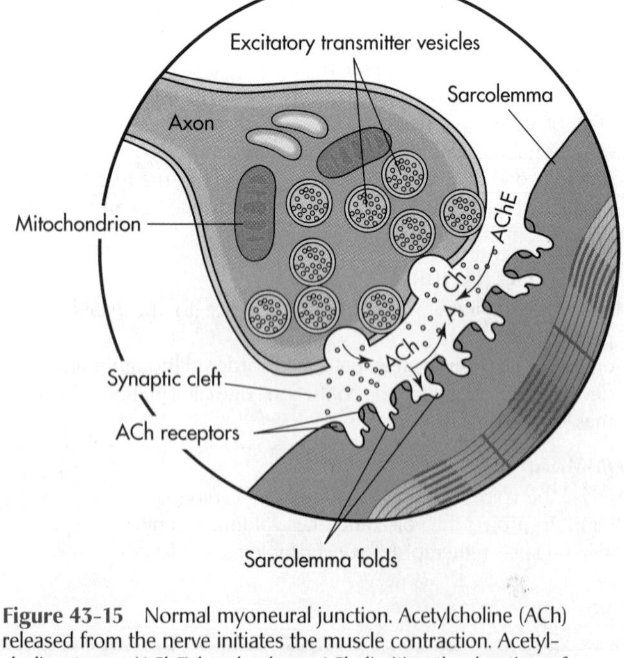

Figure 43-15 Normal myoneural junction. Acetylcholine (ACh) released from the nerve initiates the muscle contraction. Acetylcholinesterase (AChE) breaks down ACh, limiting the duration of contraction.

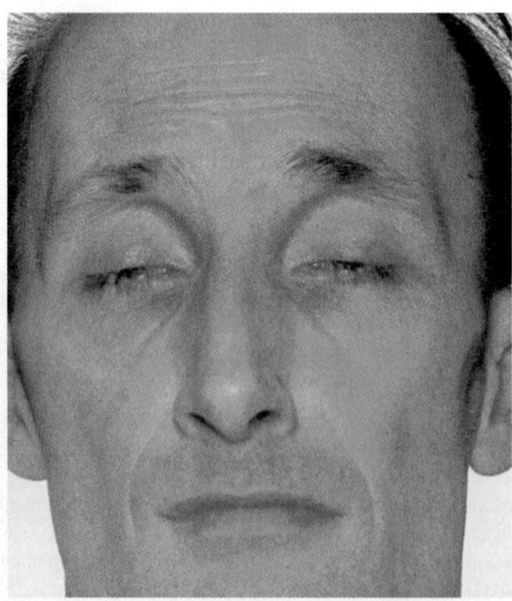

Figure 43-16 Facial appearance in myasthenia gravis. Note ptosis, lack of expression, and wrinkled brow.

tively. Weakness of the neck muscles tends to allow the head to fall forward.

Weakness of the arm and hand muscles may first become apparent during self-care activities such as shaving or combing the hair. Symptoms develop rapidly, but early in the course of the disease they are relieved easily with rest. As the disease progresses, fatigue becomes evident with less and less exertion. The muscles of the trunk and lower limbs may also become involved, creating difficulties with walking and even sitting.[14] The distal muscles are rarely affected as severely as the proximal muscles. During a disease exacerbation, muscle weakness of the intercostal muscles and diaphragm may become so severe that intubation and mechanical ventilation are necessary. Exacerbations of the disease can be triggered by upper respiratory infection, emotional stress, secondary illness, trauma, surgery, pregnancy, and even menstruation. There is no accompanying sensory loss in the affected areas.

Collaborative Care Management

The diagnosis of MG is first established presumptively from the patient's history and symptoms and is then confirmed through laboratory testing. A positive Tensilon test is considered diagnostic. In this test, edrophonium (Tensilon), a short-acting anticholinesterase, is administered intravenously. A patient with MG experiences a brief but significant increase in muscle strength in previously weakened muscles in response to the drug, and this response is considered a positive result.[7] AChR antibody titers are elevated in the vast majority of patients with MG, and electromyogram (EMG) results are believed to be 99% sensitive in diagnosing MG. The EMG can detect transmission delay or failure in muscle fibers that are repetitively stimulated. A thoracic MRI may be performed to evaluate thymus gland involvement.

There is no known cure for MG, but drug therapy is effective in managing symptoms in most patients. Individual responses vary tremendously, however, and an individualized treatment plan needs to be collaboratively developed for each patient. The management of MG primarily takes place in the community, and it is essential for patients to be well informed about self-care management of their disease. Patients may require hospitalization in rare circumstances to manage disease crises, but the bulk of care and treatment takes place in the home.

Drug therapy with AChE inhibitor agents is the cornerstone of MG treatment, but these drugs do not reverse the actual disease process. With the action of AChE being blocked in the myoneural junction, more ACh is kept available for receptor site binding.[7] Pyridostigmine (Mestinon) is the most commonly used drug. Its use is associated with multiple side effects (Box 43-11), and an individualized dosage schedule needs to be established that allows the patient to receive maximum benefit from the drug while keeping the side effects within tolerable limits. The drug effect peaks in about 2 hours, and its duration of effect is 3 to 6 hours, so its administration must be carefully timed to support specific muscle group activities such as chewing and swallowing at mealtimes. Atropine is the antidote for pyridostigmine and should be available to treat adverse side effects. The patient may be permitted to adjust the dosage and time of administration slightly within stated parameters to meet the fluctuating needs and demands of daily living.

Other treatment approaches for MG target the disease process itself. Long-term immunosuppression with corticosteroids, azathioprine, or cyclosporine may be prescribed for patients who do not respond well to cholinesterase inhibitors or develop disabling ocular or generalized MG. The potential benefits of this treatment must be carefully weighed against the risks of long-term immunosuppression. Prednisone is the drug of choice and produces improvement in 70% to 80% of patients, but it is often difficult to sustain these improvements when the drug is tapered. Azathioprine (Imuran) has been shown to reduce the number of circulating AChR antibodies, but improvement may not be noticed for months. Cyclosporine acts by decreasing T-cell function and also decreases circulating AChR antibodies. These drugs may also be used in conjunction with plasmapheresis to treat a serious disease exacerbation.

Plasmapheresis or intravenous immunoglobulin (IVIG) administration provides for short-term immunomodulation. During plasmapheresis the patient's plasma is removed and replaced with albumin or fresh frozen plasma. The AChR antibodies are removed in the process.[12] Improvements can be dramatic but are often temporary. IVIG is also used to treat disease exacerbations, and although its action is not understood, it has produced dramatic improvement in some MG patients. It is theorized that human immunoglobulins may react with antigens in the plasma and decrease the formation of the targeted antibodies.

The role of the thymus gland in MG has intrigued researchers for years. A thymectomy results in symptom remission in about 40% of patients. It appears to be most effective when performed in patients under 40 years of age who have had symptomatic MG for less than 5 years.

BOX 43-11 Side Effects of Pyridostigmine (Mestinon) Therapy

Muscarinic Effects (Effects on Smooth Muscle and Glands)

Gastrointestinal distress, heartburn
Nausea and vomiting
Increased peristalsis, abdominal cramping, diarrhea
Bradycardia
Increased bronchial secretions, bronchoconstriction/bronchospasm
Excess salivation
Sweating
Pupil miosis
Weakness

Nicotinic Effects (Effects on Skeletal Muscle)

Muscle twitching (fasciculations) and spasms
Profound muscle weakness

Myasthenic and Cholinergic Crises. Patients with MG are vulnerable to two crisis situations that may result in dramatic symptom exacerbation and the need for acute ventilatory support. A myasthenic crisis represents an acute exacerbation of the disease process and may occur in response to stress, trauma, or infection. Problems with breathing and swallowing can rapidly progress to life-threatening levels, and intubation is usually performed when the patient's vital capacity drops below 1 L. Mechanical ventilation is continued until the patient shows signs of return of muscle strength. Cholinesterase inhibitor drugs are gradually restarted in an effort to once again find an effective balance.

A cholinergic crisis represents a toxic response to medication. The muscarinic side effects develop slowly, but as toxic levels are reached, severe nicotinic effects can rapidly appear. The patient experiences profound weakness, copious respiratory secretions, and respiratory failure, which again may require intubation and mechanical ventilation. In this crisis the cholinesterase drug is temporarily stopped and then gradually restarted and retitrated. A Tensilon test can be used to differentiate between the two forms of crisis. If no improvement is seen with the administration of edrophonium (Tensilon), or if symptoms worsen, a cholinergic crisis can be assumed.

Acute care nurses are most likely to encounter patients with MG during an episode of disease exacerbation or crisis. Nursing care involves meticulous neurologic and respiratory monitoring and respiratory support. The nurse regularly monitors the severity of the patient's ptosis, the degree of swallowing impairment, hand strength, and voice quality. Respiratory rate and quality, the patient's ability to cough to clear the airway, and the use of accessory muscles are standard assessments. The patient's subjective assessment of breathlessness is also crucial, but decisions about intubation are generally made on the basis of vital capacity measurements. Patients who are weak enough to require intubation require total care and interventions to prevent the complications of immobility. Temporary placement in intensive care may be necessary. The experience of crisis is extremely frightening for the patient, who needs ongoing support and reassurance during the acute period. Patients and families dealing with any stage of the disease may profit from referral to the Myasthenia Gravis Foundation.

Patient/Family Education. Self-care is the foundation of care for MG, and education of the patient and family is its most critical component. Respiratory complications are the most serious disease threat, and knowledgeable self-care can positively affect their frequency and severity.[12] The medication regimen is also commonly adjusted by the patient within preset parameters, and the patient needs to be extremely knowledgeable about safe drug administration and the management of side effects. Box 43-11 outlines the major side effects associated with the use of pyridostigmine, and principles of patient teaching for MG are summarized in the Patient Teaching box.

Patient Teaching
Myasthenia Gravis

1. Use pyridostigmine (Mestinon) safely and appropriately.
   a. Take drug with food or fluid.
   b. Take drug before meals to permit maximum effect for chewing and swallowing.
   c. Adjust drug dosage and time of administration within set parameters in response to your individual pattern of weakness.
   d. Do not take any other medication, including over-the-counter products, without prior approval of the health care provider or pharmacist. Many drugs can compromise neuromuscular transmission and will worsen disease symptoms (e.g., local anesthetics, aminoglycosides, beta-blockers, and calcium channel blockers).
2. Modify diet as needed in response to swallowing problems.
   a. A soft diet is usually well tolerated.
   b. Eat slowly and take small bites.
3. Balance rest and activity throughout the day in response to weakness.
   a. Plan for additional rest periods.
   b. Seek out energy conservation strategies for routine activities.
4. Keep Medic-Alert identification with you at all times.
5. Know the symptoms of cholinergic and myasthenic crisis and contact physician promptly.
6. Be alert to disease response to periods of stress, infection, temperature extremes, and hormonal swings (e.g., menstruation or pregnancy).

Amyotrophic Lateral Sclerosis
Etiology/Epidemiology

Amyotrophic lateral sclerosis (ALS), or motor neuron disease, is a chronic and rapidly progressive disease that eventually weakens and paralyzes the respiratory muscles, resulting in death. It is also referred to as Lou Gehrig's disease after the New York Yankee baseball player who died from the disease.

ALS is a rare disease that occurs in 1 or 2 persons per 100,000 annually. Men have a higher incidence of ALS than women. The peak age at onset is from 55 to 75 years. The cause is unknown, but theories of causation include exposure to heavy metals, viral infection, and hydroxyl radicals.[30] ALS has also occurred in association with human immunodeficiency virus (HIV) infection.[12] Approximately 10% of ALS patients inherit an autosomal dominant gene that can result in the disease. Other theories of etiology include autoimmune destruction and neurotransmitter depletion.[12]

Pathophysiology

The term *amyotrophic* refers to the weakness and atrophy that occur from the degeneration of the alpha or lower motor neurons. Alpha motor neurons originate in the anterior horn of the spinal cord, and their axons connect the central nervous system with the voluntary muscles. They are essential for motor function and innervate the voluntary skeletal muscles. The term *lateral sclerosis* refers to the hardness of the spinal cord that is typically found in patients with the disorder. ALS involves degeneration of both cortical and alpha motor neurons of the final pathway. Cortical or upper motor neurons originate in the upper regions of the brain. The neurons of the brainstem are primarily affected by ALS. The axons of the upper motor neurons synapse in the descending corticospinal or pyramidal tract to the alpha or lower motor neurons.

ALS causes progressive degeneration of both the upper and lower motor neurons from demyelination and scar tissue formation. The disease gradually destroys motor pathways but leaves sensation and mental status intact. Lower motor neurons are usually affected first, resulting in muscle weakness and atrophy. The muscles of the upper body are affected much earlier than those of the legs. Patients may notice that they drop items or have a decreased ability to perform tasks that require fine motor skills. Other early symptoms include muscle atrophy, fasciculations and fibrillations of the muscles, and decreased tendon reflexes. Muscle cramping and generalized fatigue are also common. The disease is relentlessly progressive and eventually involves the upper motor neurons, which causes increased weakness and spasticity in affected muscles. Hyperactive reflexes, jaw clonus, tongue fasciculations, and a positive Babinski's reflex may be present. As the muscles of the neck, pharynx, and larynx become increasingly involved, slurring of the voice occurs, which gradually progresses to dysarthria and dysphagia. Paralysis is inevitable, and death usually results from pneumonia and respiratory failure within 5 years of diagnosis.

Collaborative Care Management

ALS is diagnosed by a process of elimination because no definitive diagnostic test exists. Muscle biopsies may be performed to determine the source of muscle weakness, and an EMG will show muscle denervation, fibrillation, and fasciculation, which are closely associated with ALS. Blood studies typically show elevations in the levels of creatine phosphokinase.

There is no cure for ALS, and treatment is primarily directed toward symptom relief. Riluzole (Rilutek) is the only drug currently approved for use in ALS treatment. Its action is unknown, but it is believed to have a neuroprotective effect and to extend the lives of ALS patients by several months.[30] Specific interventions are directed at managing complications as they arise. Nursing care focuses on supporting the self-care abilities of the patient and the coping resources of the entire family. General interventions are targeted at maintaining good general health, supporting nutrition, promoting adequate sleep, appropriately balancing activity and rest, and introducing the use of self-help devices as they become appropriate. Physical therapy targets both the muscle weakness and spasticity, and occupational therapy assesses the need for adapted equipment and assistive devices.

As ALS progresses, it is increasingly important to help the patient maintain a patent airway. Aspiration is a common concern and makes it increasingly difficult to meet the patient's nutritional needs with oral feedings. A gastrostomy may be created to support nutrition.

Patient/Family Education. Both the patient and the family need specific teaching concerning airway protection. The patient is taught to use a tucked-chin position while eating or drinking to encourage more effective swallowing and to always sit in an upright position for meals. If the patient's cough is weak, it may be necessary to keep suction equipment at the bedside during meals to assist in clearing the mouth. The patient is taught how to manage oral suctioning independently if possible.

Disease education is an important ongoing nursing responsibility. The reality of progressive physical deterioration can easily become overwhelming for both the patient and the family. Health care providers assist patients and families in making decisions about the types of interventions that will be used as the disease progresses. One of the most difficult decisions involves the use of a ventilator as respiratory muscles weaken. Death commonly results from aspiration, infection, or respiratory failure, and decision making in this area is essential. The issues need to be addressed before a respiratory crisis occurs, and the participants need to receive nonjudgmental support for whatever decision they make. Patients also need to be clearly aware that they can change their minds as the reality of their situation becomes apparent. The need for long-term ventilatory support may be accepted and incorporated into daily care or completely rejected. The inevitability of complete dependency is made clear. Referral to local or regional support groups for ALS patients and families may be helpful. The patient remains alert throughout the course of the disease, and most patients experience significant fear and anxiety over both the reality of today and the uncertainty of the future. Respite care for families who are caring for ALS patients at home needs to be addressed and legitimized, because the burden of caregiving can be overwhelming. Involvement with hospice services can be of tremendous aid to both patients and families. The nurse plays an important role in helping patients and families to deal with loss and grief (see Chapter 6).

Guillain-Barré Syndrome

Etiology/Epidemiology

Guillain-Barré syndrome (GBS) is an acute inflammatory polyneuropathy characterized by varying degrees of motor weakness or paralysis. It primarily affects the motor component of the cranial and spinal nerves and is known by a variety of other names, including acute inflammatory demyelinating polyradiculopathy, postinfectious polyneuritis, and idiopathic polyneuritis. It is a rare disorder with an incidence of 1 to 2 per 100,000 population.[12] GBS affects all races and age-groups, with peak incidence in the 50- to 74-year-old age-group.[26] The etiology of the disorder is unknown, but it is believed in most cases to be an autoimmune response triggered by a viral or bacterial infection. The onset of GBS usually occurs 1 to 3 weeks after an illness, infection, or immunization and commonly follows an upper respiratory or gastrointestinal infection.[26] The syndrome usually develops over days to weeks, is rapidly progressive, and can advance to full paralysis. Ninety percent of patients are weakest by the third week. The mortality rate is approximately 5%; the remaining 95% of GBS patients recover, and 80% recover completely within 1 year.[26] The mortality rate for GBS remains higher in elderly patients.

Pathophysiology

In GBS an immune-mediated response triggers destruction of the myelin sheath surrounding the peripheral nerves, nerve roots, root ganglia, and spinal cord. Collections of lymphocytes and macrophages are believed to be responsible for the myelin stripping. Demyelination occurs between the nodes of

Ranvier, which impairs or blocks the transmission of impulses from node to node. The nerve axons are generally spared, and recovery eventually takes place, although the process of remyelination occurs slowly.[26] In severe forms of the disease, wallerian degeneration occurs that involves the axons, making recovery slower and more difficult. In a small percentage of patients the disease does not resolve and becomes chronic or recurrent.

There are four major forms of GBS. Each reflects a different degree of peripheral nerve involvement.

1. Ascending GBS is the most common form. Weakness and numbness begin in the legs and progress upward. Fifty percent of patients experience respiratory insufficiency. Sensory involvement is also usually present.
2. Pure motor GBS is similar to the ascending form, but no sensory involvement is present. It is usually a milder form of the disease.
3. Descending GBS begins with weakness in the muscles controlled by the cranial nerves and then progresses downward. The respiratory system is quickly impaired. Sensory involvement is present.
4. Miller Fisher syndrome, a variant of GBS, is rare and primarily involves the eyes, loss of reflexes, and severe ataxia.

The patient with GBS has symmetric muscle weakness and flaccid motor paralysis. The paralysis usually starts in the lower extremities and ascends upward to include the thorax, upper extremities, and face. Cranial nerves may also be affected, and the fifth cranial nerve (facial nerve) is the most commonly involved. When the seventh, ninth, and tenth cranial nerves are involved, the patient may have difficulty swallowing, speaking, and breathing.[26] The vital centers in the medulla oblongata may also be affected, and involvement of the vagus nerve may explain the autonomic dysfunction that is commonly seen with the syndrome.

Pain and paresthesias are present when sensory nerves are involved. Tingling or a pins-and-needles sensation is common. Either numbness or a heightened sensitivity to touch may occur, and about 25% of patients experience pain.[26] The pain is usually experienced as a cramping in the extremities but can become severe enough to require analgesics.

Autonomic dysfunction is now recognized as a common problem with GBS and may include dysrhythmias, blood pressure instability, tachycardia or bradycardia, flushing, sweating, urinary retention, and paralytic ileus. GBS does not affect the patient's level of consciousness, alertness, or cognitive functioning.[26] The patient is alert and aware throughout the course of the disease and is acutely vulnerable to sensory deprivation problems from the decrease in environmental stimuli.

GBS generally progresses through three stages. The initial period lasts from 1 to 3 weeks and ends when no further physical deterioration occurs. A plateau period follows, which lasts from a few days to a few weeks. The recovery period can last from 6 months to well over 1 year. The remyelination of damaged nerves occurs during the recovery phase. Permanent deficits may remain, although complete recovery is the norm.

Collaborative Care Management

The diagnosis of GBS is made from the clinical presentation supported by a history of recent viral infection, elevations in the levels of protein in the CSF, and the results of EMG studies. Collaborative management of GBS is largely supportive and aimed at preventing complications until the recovery process can begin.[26] Respiratory support is always the priority intervention. Corticosteroid therapy is often used to attempt to reduce the autoimmune inflammation, but steroids have not been conclusively proven to be of benefit in GBS. Positive outcomes have been achieved with the use of plasmapheresis during the first 1 to 2 weeks after disease onset. With plasmapheresis, blood is removed and filtered of antibodies, immunoglobulins, fibrinogens, and other proteins. The filtered blood is then mixed with an isotonic solution or fresh frozen plasma and returned to the patient. IVIG is also used to treat GBS. IVIG is as expensive as plasmaphoresis, but it is easier to administer and is more readily available.[26]

Respiratory failure from neuromuscular weakness is common in GBS. Frequent monitoring of vital capacity, tidal volume, or minute volume is performed, and intubation with mechanical ventilation is generally initiated when the patient's vital capacity falls below a preset level, usually about 1.0 to 1.5 L for an average-size adult.[26] The need for long-term ventilatory support may necessitate a tracheostomy. Atelectasis and pneumonia are common complications. Intensive care placement may be necessary for weeks, and meticulous supportive care is needed. Rigorous assessment of motor, sensory, and cranial nerve status is ongoing.

Patients can lose weight rapidly with GBS, and nutritional support is a priority concern, especially for patients who will need to be weaned from mechanical ventilation. Complete immobility can cause a rapid loss of muscle mass.[12] Tube feedings may be used, but if the patient also experiences autonomic dysfunction and paralytic ileus, parenteral nutrition may need to be implemented.

Supportive care also addresses the range of concerns related to partial or total immobility and loss of self-care abilities. Interventions include standard measures for preventing skin breakdown and maintaining range of motion in all joints. The risk of deep vein thrombosis and pulmonary embolus is high, and low-dose anticoagulant therapy may be initiated.[26] A regular bowel program is established, and either indwelling or intermittent catheterization is implemented to address bladder dysfunction. A thorough rehabilitation plan is established as soon as the patient begins to recover.

It is critical to remember that the patient remains alert, aware, and cognitively intact throughout the course of GBS. Sleep disturbances are extremely common and can contribute to sensory deprivation or overload symptoms in patients who are cared for in intensive care unit settings for protracted periods of time. The patient needs meaningful stimulation and communication and should be included in care decisions as much as possible even if eyebrow raising or eye blinks are the full extent of the patient's ability to communicate. Family members are also encouraged to participate in care activities to their level of comfort.

Patient/Family Education. GBS is an alarming and unsettling disease process for the patient and family. It is often difficult to convince the patient and family that recovery from GBS is not just possible but expected. Teaching about the disease and its management is an important nursing responsibility. Reteaching of basic principles is commonly necessary. The nursing staff also need to encourage the patient and family to remain optimistic about the future. Each stage of GBS, particularly the need for intubation, increases the anxiety level of an alert patient. It is difficult for patients to communicate their needs for position changes, pain relief, and restful sleep. The slow pace of recovery may cause the patient and family to become discouraged about the future. Once patients are moved from the intensive care unit setting, they lose the constant support and care of the critical care nurses and may become extremely anxious about the ability of nurses on less acute units to adequately meet their needs. The patient's care manager needs to carefully coordinate all needed services to ensure that all transitions are as smooth and anxiety free as possible. Referral for community-based care and rehabilitation may also be needed.

Critical Thinking Questions

1. You are caring for a patient who was admitted 2 days ago with a left hemisphere ischemic stroke. You were told during report that the patient has "some aphasia." What kinds of assessment activities would you plan in order to thoroughly evaluate the nature and extent of the communication problems?
2. A patient has experienced a right hemisphere stroke, and you suspect that sensory-perceptual deficits may be present.
   a. *How would you assess the presence and severity of problems such as hemianopia, unilateral neglect, or agnosia?*
   b. *What effects might the right-sided stroke have on your plan for compensating for these deficits?*
3. The nursing diagnosis of risk for altered nutrition: less than daily requirements might apply to patients with Parkinson's disease and myasthenia gravis.
   a. *How would your nursing interventions related to nutrition be the same for patients with these two disorders?*
   b. *How would your interventions differ?*
4. A patient is admitted for an acute exacerbation of myasthenia gravis. You gave a dose of pyridostigmine (Mestinon) at 11:30 AM before lunch. It is now 1 PM, and the patient is reporting dramatically increased weakness, cramping, gastrointestinal upset, and difficulty swallowing saliva.
   a. *Is this likely to be a myasthenic or a cholinergic crisis? Support your answer.*
   b. *How could the two forms of crisis be differentiated?*

References

1. American Heart Association: *Guidelines for the management of aneurysmal subarachnoid hemorrhage,* 1998, website: http://www.americanheart.org/Scientific/statements/1994/119403.html.
2. American Heart Association: *2001 heart and stroke statistical update,* Dallas, 2000, The Association.
3. Brott T, Bogousslavsky J: Drug therapy: treatment of acute stroke, *N Engl J Med* 343(10):710, 2000.
4. Chan H: Bladder management in acute care of stroke patients: a quality improvement project, *J Neurosci Nurs* 29(3):187, 1997.
5. Clanet MG, Brassat D: The management of multiple sclerosis patients, *Curr Opin Neurol* 13(3):263, 2000.
6. Conley CC, Kirchner JT: Medical and surgical treatment of Parkinson's disease: strategies to slow symptom progression and improve quality of life, *Postgrad Med* 106(2):41, 1999.
7. Cunning S: When the dx is myasthenia gravis, *RN* 63(4):26, 2000.
8. Davenport R, Dennis M: Neurological emergencies: acute stroke, *Neurol Neurosurg Psychiatry* 68(3):277, 2000.
9. Galvan TJ: Dysphagia: going down and staying down, *Am J Nurs* 101:37, 2001.
10. Hayn AM, Fisher TR: Stroke rehab, *Nursing* 27(3):40, 1997.
11. Herndon CM et al: Parkinson's disease revisited, *J Neurosci Nurs* 32(4):216, 2000.
12. Hickey J: *The clinical practice of neurological and neurosurgical nursing,* ed 4, Philadelphia, 1997, Lippincott-Raven.
13. Hock HH: Brain attack: the stroke continuum, *Nurs Clin North Am* 34(3):689, 1999.
14. Hopkins LC: Clinical features of myasthenia gravis, *Neurol Clin* 12(2):243, 1994.
15. Johnson J et al: Stroke rehabilitation: assessing stroke survivor's long-term learning needs, *Rehabil Nurs* 22(5):243, 1997.
16. Kelly-Hayes M, Phipps MA: Preventive approach to poststroke rehabilitation in older people, *Clin Geriatr Med* 15(4):801, 1999.
17. Lang AE, Lozano AM: Medical progress: Parkinson's disease, part 1, *N Engl J Med* 339(15):1044, 1998.
18. Leira EC, Adams HP Jr: Management of acute ischemic stroke, *Clin Geriatr Med* 15(4):701, 1999.
19. Lennon S, Ashburn A: The Bobath Concept in stroke rehabilitation: a focus group study of the experienced physiotherapists' perspective, *Disabil Rehabil* 22(15):665, 2000.
20. Lindsberg PJ et al: The future of stroke treatment, *Neurol Clin* 18(2):495, 2000.
21. Love BB, Biller J: Neurovascular system. In Goetz CG, Pappert EJ, editors: *Textbook of clinical neurology,* Philadelphia, 1999, WB Saunders.
22. Mower DM: Brain attack—treating acute ischemic CVA, *Nursing* 27(3):35, 1997.
23. Noseworthy JH et al: Medical progress: multiple sclerosis, *N Engl J Med* 343(13):938, 2000.
24. Savitz SI et al: Antithrombotic and thrombolytic therapy for ischemic stroke, *Clin Geriatr Med* 17(1):149, 2001.
25. Stuifbergen AK: Physical activity and perceived health status in persons with multiple sclerosis, *J Neurosci Nurs* 29(4):238, 1997.
26. Sulton LL: A multidisciplinary care approach to Guillain-Barré syndrome, *Dimens Crit Care Nurs* 20(1):16, 2001.
27. Travers PL: Poststroke dysphagia: implications for nurses, *Rehabil Nurs* 24(2):69, 1999.
28. Treib J et al: Treatment of stroke on an intensive stroke unit: a novel concept, *Intensive Care Med* 26:1598, 2000.
29. US Department of Health and Human Services: *Healthy People 2010: understanding and improving health,* Washington, DC, 2000, USDHHS.
30. Walling AD: Amyotrophic lateral sclerosis, *Am Fam Physician* 59(6):1489, 1999.
31. Walsh E, Wilson C: Complementary therapies in long-stay neurology in-patient settings, *Nurs Stand* 13(32):32, 1999.
32. Warlow CP: Epidemiology of stroke, *Lancet* 352(suppl 3):1, 1998.
33. Young R: Update on Parkinson's disease, *Am Fam Physician* 59(8):2155, 1999.

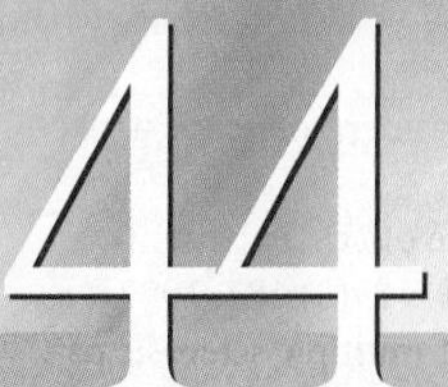

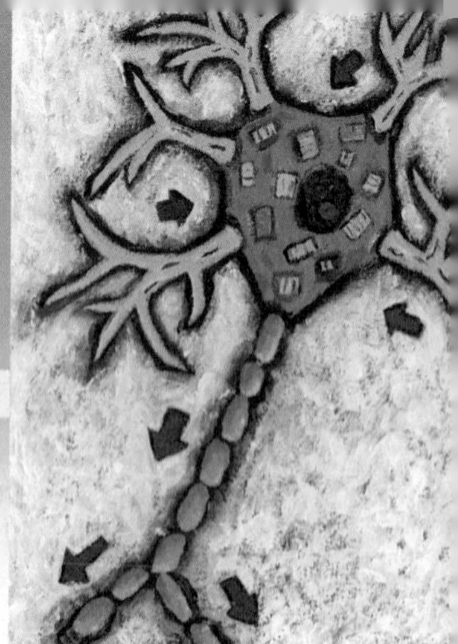

44 Spinal Cord and Peripheral Nerve Problems

Judith K. Sands

Objectives

After studying this chapter, the learner should be able to:

1. Discuss the demographics of spinal cord injury (SCI) and the major targets for prevention.
2. Describe how the process of secondary injury extends the damage that results from SCI.
3. Link the clinical manifestations of spinal shock and autonomic dysreflexia with the specific physiologic consequences of SCI.
4. Differentiate between the effects of upper motor neuron and lower motor neuron injury on muscle function, bowel and bladder function, and sexuality after SCI.
5. Discuss the options available for medical and surgical management of common spinal cord injuries, including compression, malalignment, and instability of the spine.
6. Describe the nursing management of the patient with SCI with a focus on skin care, bowel and bladder care, and patient and family teaching and support.
7. Outline a standard protocol for preventing and/or treating autonomic dysreflexia.
8. Contrast the care provided to patients with SCI with that required by patients with spinal tumors.
9. Compare the clinical manifestations and treatment of the patient with trigeminal neuralgia versus Bell's palsy.

This chapter presents an overview of the collaborative management of problems involving the spinal cord and peripheral nerves. The multidisciplinary challenges of spinal cord injury are the major focus. Spinal cord injury (SCI) is not a common problem, but its complexity and impact on the patient's life make it an enormous management concern in all phases of care. The pathophysiology of spinal cord and peripheral nerve injuries is complex, and the reader is referred to Chapter 41 for a review of neurologic anatomy and physiology.

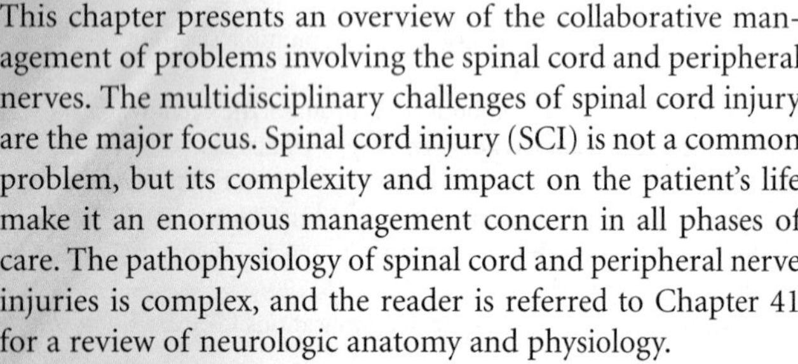

SPINAL CORD INJURY

Etiology

The spinal column is a circular bony structure that provides the spinal cord with excellent protection from most low-intensity injuries. Vertebrae, the individual bones of the column, are dense and have multiple articulations. These articulations allow a wide range of head and neck movement, but also create points of weakness that are vulnerable to a variety of types of injury. The close anatomic proximity of the spinal cord to the vertebrae, muscles, and ligaments increases the chance that injury to any of these supporting structures will also result in injury to the cord itself. Spinal injuries occur most commonly in the areas of maximum mobility in the lower cervical spine and the thoracolumbar junction.[24] Most injuries are the result of sudden and often violent external trauma, but persons who have chronic conditions that affect the vertebrae, such as stenosis, arthritis, or osteoporosis, are also at a high risk for injury.

Excessive force exerted on the spinal column can result in extreme flexion, hyperextension, compression, or rotation. Events that cause abrupt forceful acceleration and deceleration, frequently associated with vehicular accidents, are common initiating factors.

Injuries to the spinal cord can be classified in a variety of ways that take into account damage to both the vertebrae and the underlying spinal cord.

Mechanisms of Injury. Hyperflexion injuries (Figure 44-1) are frequently the result of sudden deceleration as might be experienced in a head-on collision or from a severe blow to the back of the head. The head and neck are forcibly hyperflexed and then may be snapped backward into forced hyperextension. These injuries are typically seen in the C5-6 area of the cervical spine. They may result in fracture of the vertebra, dislocation, and/or tearing of the posterior ligaments.

Hyperextension injuries (Figure 44-2) are frequently acceleration injuries such as those associated with rear-end collisions or falls in which the chin is forcibly struck. These injuries tend to cause significant damage because of the pronounced downward and backward arc of the head's movement. C4-5 is the area of the spine most commonly affected.

Compression injuries cause the vertebra to squash or burst (Figure 44-3). They usually involve high velocity and affect both the cervical and thoracolumbar regions of the spine. Blows to the top of the head and forceful landing on the feet or buttocks can result in compression injury.

Rotational injuries are caused by extreme lateral flexion or twisting of the head and neck (Figure 44-4). Tearing of ligaments can easily cause dislocation as well as fracture, resulting in a highly unstable spine. Soft tissue damage often complicates the primary injury. Many SCIs involve more than one type of directional force.

Box 44-1 describes the various types of damage that can affect the spinal cord itself. Spinal cord concussion, contusion, and laceration follow similar patterns to those described for head injury in Chapter 42. Complete transection, severing of the spinal cord, is a relatively rare initial outcome of spinal trauma because the protective layers of the cord are extremely tough. Complete transection usually results from secondary injury (see Pathophysiology), although penetrating injuries from knives or bullets may fracture the vertebra or directly enter the spinal cord. These injuries are most common in the thoracic and lumbar regions.

An SCI is termed complete when there is a total loss of motor and sensory function below the level of the injury. Complete injuries are more common in the thoracic spine because the spinal canal is quite narrow in that region. An incomplete lesion is one in which there is some preservation of motor and or sensory function below the level of the injury. Box 44-2

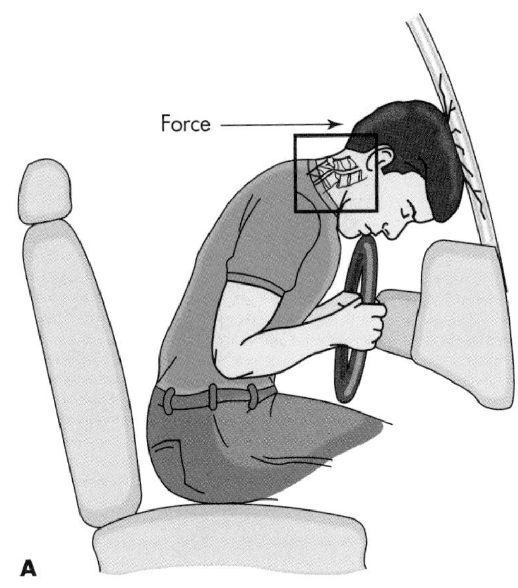

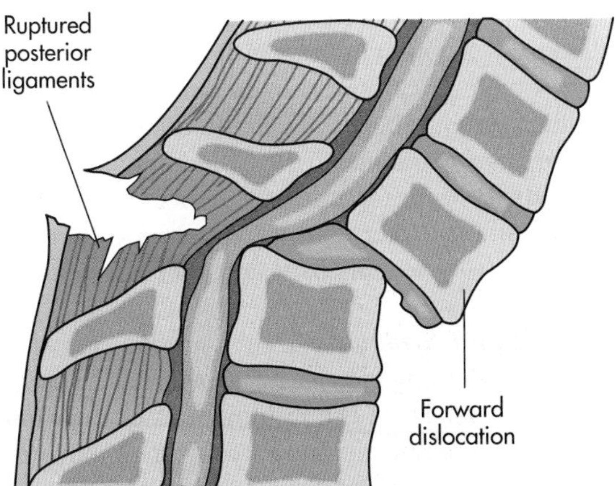

Figure 44-1 Hyperflexion injury. **A,** If hyperflexion occurs in the cervical spine, **B,** it can result in tearing or rupture of the posterior ligaments with resulting fracture or dislocation in the anterior spine.

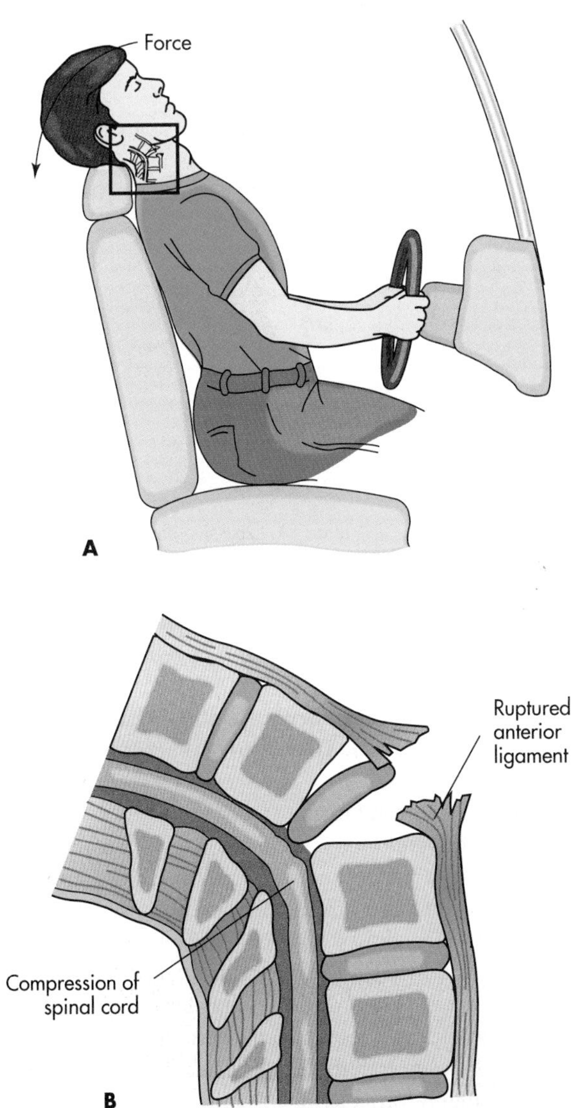

Figure 44-2 Hyperextension injury. **A,** If hyperextension occurs in the cervical spine, **B,** it can result in rupture or tearing of the anterior ligaments with dislocation or compression in the posterior spine.

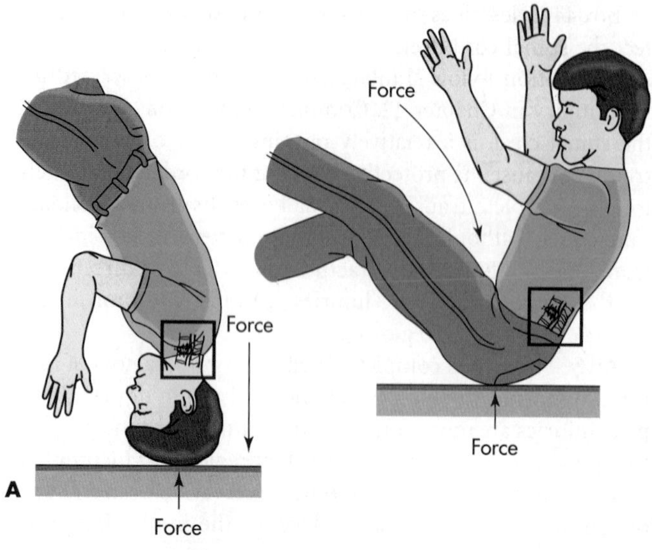

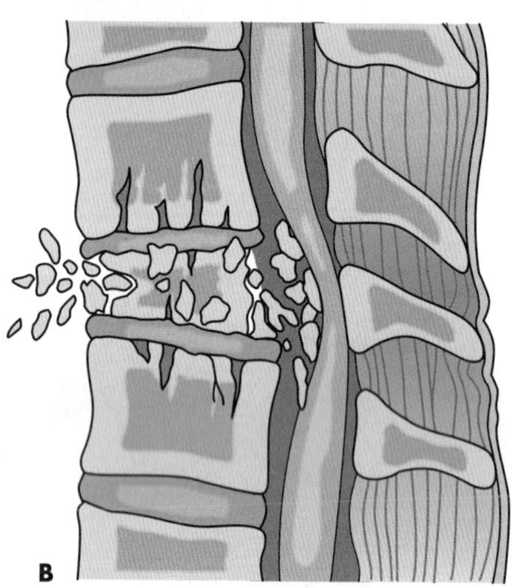

Figure 44-3 Compression injury. **A,** Excessive direct force to either the cervical or lumbar spine can **B,** result in shattering of the vertebra.

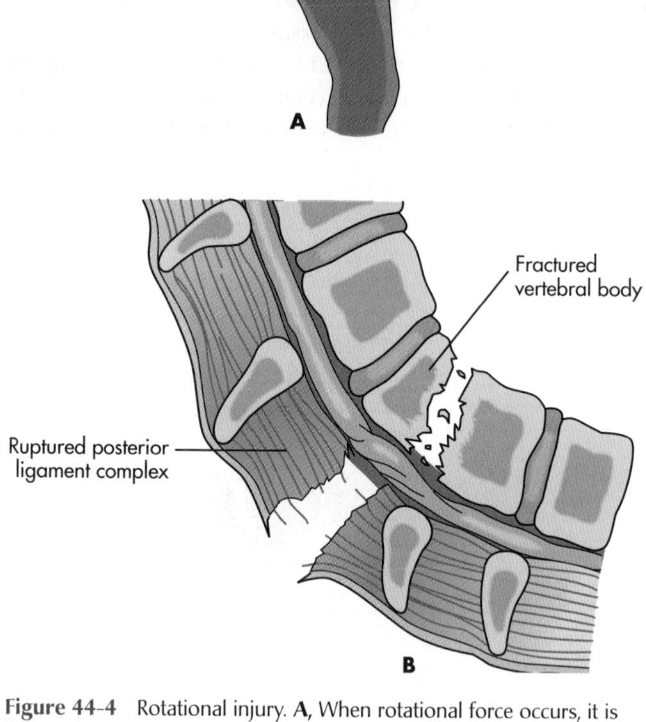

Figure 44-4 Rotational injury. **A,** When rotational force occurs, it is frequently accompanied by **B,** tearing and/or fracture of the ligaments.

outlines the SCI impairment scale developed by the American Spinal Injury Association.

Spinal Cord Syndromes. Several unique syndromes can occur after incomplete SCI. They represent specific types of localized damage, although it is unusual to see any of these syndromes in their pure form.

Central Cord Syndrome. This syndrome is caused by damage that primarily affects the central gray or white matter of the spinal cord (Figure 44-5). This fairly common syndrome usually occurs in older adults who experience a hyperextension injury in the cervical region. Hemorrhage and edema occur in the central part of the cord, causing bilateral upper extremity weakness and burning. Strength and sensation are usually preserved in the lower extremities.[3] The amount of sensory impairment is highly variable. Bowel and bladder function may or may not be affected. Improvement over time is expected.

Anterior Cord Syndrome. This syndrome typically results from injury or infarction involving the anterior spinal artery, which perfuses the anterior two thirds of the spinal cord (Figure 44-6). It can also result from tumors and acute disk herniation. Typically, the injury results in loss of strength and loss of pain and temperature sensation below the level of the injury. Position, vibration, and touch sensation remain intact.

Posterior Cord Syndrome. This is an extremely rare syndrome in which proprioreceptive sensation of position and vibration are lost due to damage to the posterior columns of the spinal cord while movement, pain, and temperature sensation remain intact.

Brown-Séquard Syndrome. This syndrome typically results from a penetrating injury that involves half of the spinal cord (Figure 44-7). There is a resulting loss of motor ability plus touch, pressure, and vibration sensation on the same side as the injury with a contralateral loss of pain and temperature sensation.

Conus Medullaris Syndrome. This syndrome results from damage to the sacral region of the spinal column and/or the

BOX 44-1 Types of Spinal Cord Damage

Cord Concussion

The cord is severely jarred or squeezed as is frequently seen with sports-related injuries (e.g., football). No identifiable pathologic changes are detectable in the cord, but a temporary loss of motor or sensory function, or both, can occur. The dysfunction usually resolves spontaneously within 24 to 48 hours.

Cord Contusion

This injury is frequently caused by compression. Bleeding into the cord results in bruising and edema. The extent of damage reflects the adequacy of the overall perfusion to the cord and the severity of the inflammatory response.

Cord Laceration

An actual tear occurs in the cord, which results in permanent injury because the neurons of the central nervous system do not regenerate. Contusion, edema, and compression will all usually be present and complicate the damage.

Cord Transection

A complete or incomplete severing of the spinal cord with loss of neurologic function below the level of the injury. The cord segment identified reflects the lowest cord segment in which neurologic function is preserved.

BOX 44-2 ASIA Impairment Scale

A—Complete injury: No motor function or sensation below the level of lesion

B—Incomplete injury: Selected sensation is preserved, but there is no evidence of motor function preservation below the level of injury

C—Incomplete: motor function is evident distal to the area of injury; however, key muscles are assessed at less than antigravity strength

D – Incomplete: Motor function is evident distal to the area of injury and key muscles are assessed at better than antigravity strength

E—Normal: Motor and sensory function assessed as normal

Source: American Spinal Injury Association: *International standards for neurological and functional classification of spinal cord injury,* Atlanta, 1994, ASIA.

lumbar nerve roots that comprise the cauda equina (Figure 44-8). It creates a lower motor neuron injury with flaccid paralysis of the bowel and bladder and loss of sexual function. Motor function in the legs and feet may be affected to various degrees, but sensory involvement is rarely present.[3]

Epidemiology

SCIs are catastrophic events whose incidence has remained fairly stable in recent years. Approximately 10,000 new injuries occur each year, roughly 3 per 100,000 population, and about 200,000 to 500,000 individuals are living with the

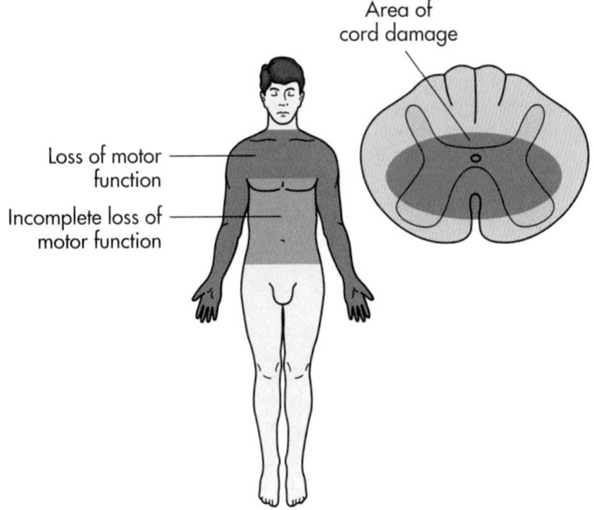

Figure 44-5 Central cord syndrome.

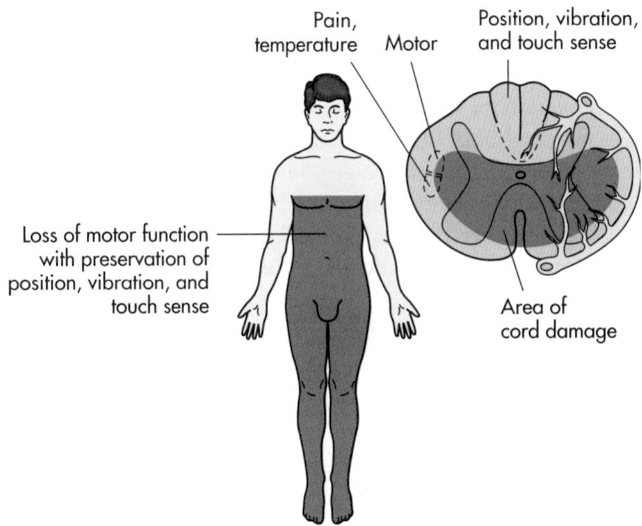

Figure 44-6 Anterior cord syndrome.

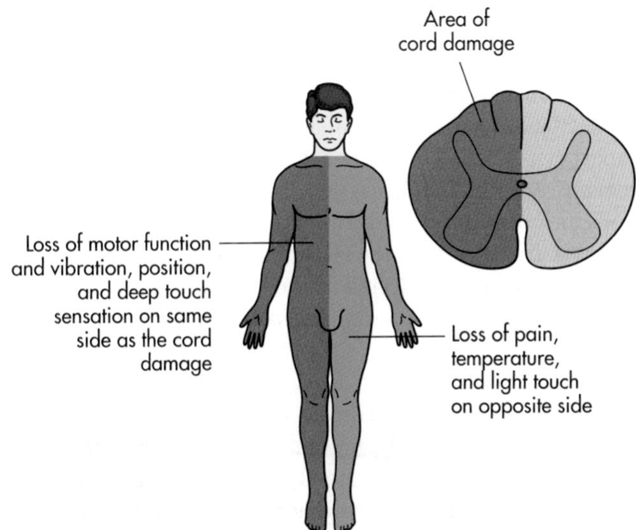

Figure 44-7 Brown-Séquard syndrome.

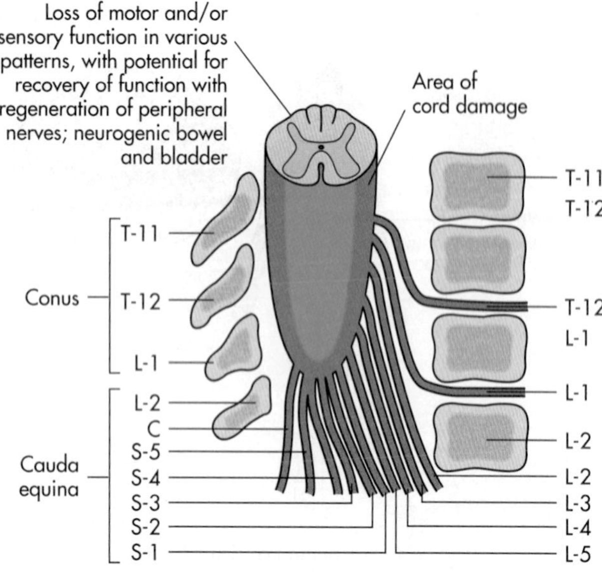

Figure 44-8 Conus medullaris and cauda equina syndrome.

> ## Healthy People 2010
> **Objective Related to Injury Reduction**
>
> Reduce hospitalizations for nonfatal spinal cord injuries from the baseline of 4.5 per 100,00 population to a target of 2.4 per 100,000 population.
>
> From US Department of Health and Human Services: *Healthy people 2010: understanding and improving health,* Washington, DC, 2000, USDHHS.

> ## *Risk Factors*
> **Spinal Cord Injury**
>
> AGE
>
> More than 60% of spinal cord injuries (SCIs) occur in persons 15-25 years of age
>
> Elderly persons experience the most fall-related injuries
>
> SEX
>
> Males are affected four times as often as females
>
> ALCOHOL/DRUG USE
>
> Substance abuse is present in the majority of motor vehicle accidents that result in SCI, as well as in many other accidents, diving incidents, and episodes of violent trauma

consequences of injury.[17] Age, sex, and race are the primary risk factors. About 80% of all SCIs occur in males, and more than 60% occur in young persons between 16 and 30 years old.[8] The incidence rate in young black males is almost double that of other groups.[2] Vehicular accidents are the most common cause (55%) and the injured person is usually the driver. Falls cause about 23% and penetrating injuries, which used to be extremely rare except during wartime, cause another 16%.[24] The remainder are caused by occupational and sports injuries.[2] Alcohol and/or drug use is present in the majority of "accidental" injuries, and failure to use safety equipment such as helmets and seatbelts significantly increases the risk of a fatal outcome. Falls are the most common cause of SCI in the elderly and are often related to osteoporosis.

Treatment and rehabilitation of persons with SCI are relatively recent phenomenon. SCI was long considered to be an untreatable injury, and the associated mortality was as high as 85% until the 1940s. The multitude of injuries produced by World War II stimulated a tremendous upsurge in research into SCI management. Today 94% of persons who experience a nonfatal SCI survive the initial hospitalization and their life expectancy is between 70% and 80% of normal.[2] However, SCI remains a multidisciplinary challenge of enormous proportions including direct costs for lifetime care that exceed $7 billion.[26] SCI is reflected in the Healthy People 2010 objectives for injury reduction as reflected in the Healthy People 2010 box. Risk factors for SCI are summarized in the Risk Factors box.

Pathophysiology

Trauma to the spinal cord causes both primary and secondary injuries. The primary damage results from the initial mechanical insult and is usually irreversible. Bruising and compression are the most common types of injury. The cord is rarely completely transected at the time of primary injury, but the initial impact initiates a complex self-destructive process that frequently results in a worsening of the injury. This multifactorial process is called secondary injury and is triggered by spinal cord ischemia.

The primary compression, stretching, jarring, or tearing of the spinal cord typically causes small hemorrhages in the gray matter of the cord, and the resultant edema causes the blood flow to the cord to slow in a matter of minutes.[20] Secondary injury mechanisms are triggered by the natural responses to tissue injury: ischemia, hypoxia, and edema. The body's natural responses to injury and inflammation have dramatic negative consequences for the spinal cord.[8] Capillary permeability increases in response to trauma, allowing fluid to move into the interstitial spaces. The resultant edema impairs the microcirculation and worsens the cord ischemia. The developing hypoxia stimulates the release of vasoactive substances such as catecholamines, histamines, and endorphins from the injured tissue, which further decrease blood flow in the microcirculation and may induce vasospasm.[20] Proteolytic and lipolytic enzymes, which can clog the microcirculation and worsen the edema and ischemia, are also released from the injured cells. The enzymes actively work to clear cellular debris, which includes removal of necrotic neural tissue that is incapable of regeneration. This secondary injury process can destroy the full thickness of the spinal cord at the level of injury and further extend its effects several cord segments above and below the original level of injury. The process of secondary injury is initiated within minutes after the original insult and progresses rapidly. Extensive research is attempting to identify all of the factors that are operational during secondary injury and determine which of these cellular processes can be slowed or interrupted. Inflammatory mediators, free radicals, and electrolyte imbalances are all believed to play important roles.[8] Blood flow to the injured spinal cord is further compromised by the onset of spinal shock.

Spinal Shock. Spinal shock represents a temporary but profound disruption of spinal cord function, which occurs immediately after injury, and is clinically evident within 30 to 60 minutes. It is a state of areflexia characterized by the loss of all neurologic function below the level of the injury. Spinal shock causes a complete loss of motor, sensory, reflex, and autonomic functioning. The severity of spinal shock varies depending on the extent and level of the primary injury, but injuries at T6 or above usually produce more severe forms.

Spinal shock is the direct result of the neuronal injury and is not preventable. Normal functioning of the spinal cord is dependent on a constant low-level axonal stimulation from the higher centers in the brain, which keeps the cord neurons in a state of excitability or readiness. Without this stimulation the resting excitability of the cord is dramatically reduced. Over time the spinal neurons gradually regain their excitability, which ends the period of spinal shock. The duration of spinal shock varies greatly, with an average of 1 to 6 weeks. The gradual reappearance of reflex activity signals the resolution of the spinal shock period. Clinical manifestations of spinal shock are summarized in the Clinical Manifestations box.

Injury above the thoracic outflow of the sympathetic nervous system (T6-7) disconnects the sympathetic nervous system from control by higher centers in the brainstem and results in a loss of autoregulatory contol of blood pressure.[3] Vasoconstrictive messages from the medulla cannot be transmitted, and sympathetic tone is lost. This lack of a functional sympathetic nervous system causes widespread venous pooling in the lower extremities and splanchnic circulation, which results in hypotension, that can be severe.[3] The unopposed parasympathetic stimulation of the vagus causes an extreme bradycardia. The presence of bradycardia helps to distinguish spinal neurogenic shock from hypovolemic shock, which is also commonly associated with trauma. The peripheral vasodilation causes the skin to feel warm and dry but also permits significant heat loss to occur. The body is unable to use either sweating or shivering as a means to control body temperature. These hemodynamic characteristics of neurogenic shock peak in the first 3 to 4 days and then gradually taper off and stabilize over 10 days to 2 weeks.[20] Orthostatic hypotension, however, may persist for months.

Clinical Manifestations. The clinical manifestations of SCI are dependent on the level of the injury and whether the injury is complete or incomplete. The terms *paraplegia* and *quadraplegia* (tetraplegia) are used to describe the functional consequences of SCI. Quadraplegia/tetraplegia involves the impairment or loss of motor and/or sensory function in cervical segments of the cord due to damage of neural elements within the spinal canal. The arms, trunk, legs, and pelvic organs are affected. Paraplegia refers to a similar impairment affecting the thoracic, lumbar, or sacral segments of the spinal cord.

Clinical Manifestations
Spinal Shock

Flaccid paralysis
- Affects all skeletal muscles below the level of injury

Loss of spinal reflex activity
- Paralytic ileus
- Loss of bowel and bladder tone

Sensory loss below the level of injury
- Pain, temperature, touch, pressure, and proprioreceptive senses
- Somatic and visceral sensation

Bradycardia (results from unopposed parasympathetic vagal slowing of the heart)

Hypotension (results from venous pooling in lower extremities and splanchnic circulation, related to loss of vasomotor tone)

Loss of temperature control
- Warm, dry skin
- Inability to shiver or perspire
- Poikilothermia: the body assumes temperature of external environment

The functional losses and residual functions that characterize injuries at specific spinal segments are summarized in Figure 44-9. The sensory dermatomes are illustrated in Figure 44-10. The sparing of even one spinal segment can have significant impact on the patient's future self-care potential, particularly when injuries affect the cervical spine.

Respiratory System Effects. The effects of SCI on respiratory function are of critical importance, particularly with cervical injuries. All ventilatory muscles receive their innervation from the spinal cord. Disturbance of respiratory function in injuries below T6 is minimal, but respiratory compromise becomes significant above this level.[18] The loss of the intercostal muscles (T1-7) interferes with expansion of the rib cage and decreases alveolar ventilation by as much as 60%.[18] Both the intercostal and abdominal muscles (T6-12) are essential for adequate and effective coughing.

Hypoventilation is the most dangerous immediate outcome of a cervical SCI.[27] The action of the diaphragm is controlled by the phrenic nerve and accounts for 50% to 60% of an individual's vital capacity. Phrenic nerve innervation occurs at C3-5, with the C4 root being most critical.[18] Therefore injury above C4 necessitates immediate intubation and mechanical ventilation. The accessory muscles are innervated from C2-8, and injuries in this area reduce their ability to assist in the effort of breathing.

Effects of Upper Motor Neuron or Lower Motor Neuron Injury. The effects of SCI are primarily determined by the level of injury, but injury to upper versus lower motor neurons is also an important consideration, particularly with the nerves that control bowel, bladder, and sexual function. Lower motor neurons (LMNs) (Figure 44-11) consist of the large anterior horn cells located in the anterior gray matter of the spinal cord or the motor cranial nuclei of the brainstem. Each anterior horn cell has a long axon that exits the cord via the anterior spinal root and extends out to a peripheral nerve (Chapter 41). When a lesion involves some part of the LMN,

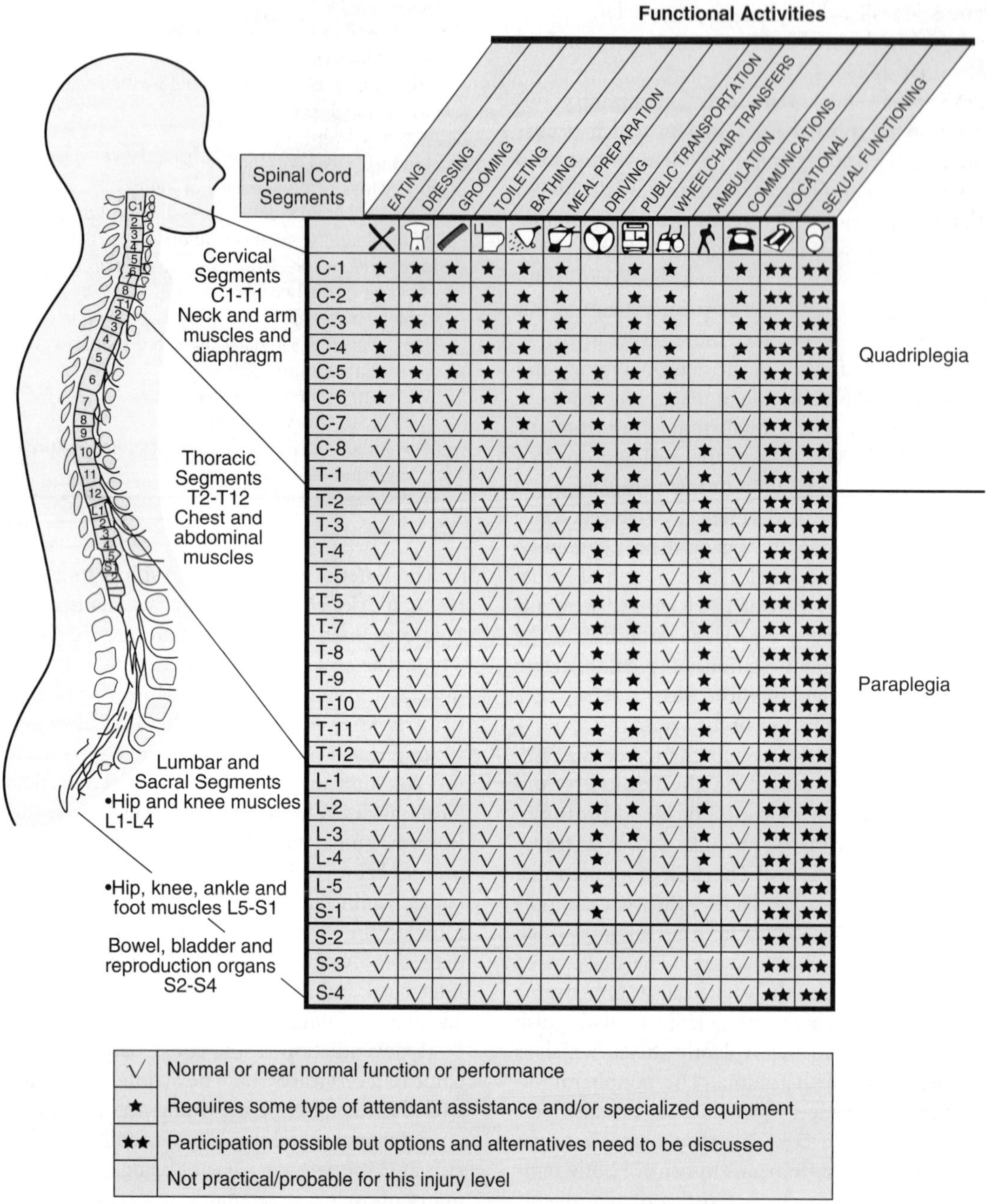

Spinal Cord Segments	Eating	Dressing	Grooming	Toileting	Bathing	Meal Preparation	Driving	Public Transportation	Wheelchair Transfers	Ambulation	Communications	Vocational	Sexual Functioning
C-1	★	★	★	★	★	★		★	★		★	★★	★★
C-2	★	★	★	★	★	★		★	★		★	★★	★★
C-3	★	★	★	★	★	★		★	★		★	★★	★★
C-4	★	★	★	★	★	★		★	★		★	★★	★★
C-5	★	★	★	★	★	★	★	★	★		★	★★	★★
C-6	★	★	√	★	★	★	★	★	★		√	★★	★★
C-7	√	√	√	★	★	√	★	★	√		√	★★	★★
C-8	√	√	√	√	√	√	★	★	√	★	√	★★	★★
T-1	√	√	√	√	√	√	★	★	√	★	√	★★	★★
T-2	√	√	√	√	√	√	★	★	√	★	√	★★	★★
T-3	√	√	√	√	√	√	★	★	√	★	√	★★	★★
T-4	√	√	√	√	√	√	★	★	√	★	√	★★	★★
T-5	√	√	√	√	√	√	★	★	√	★	√	★★	★★
T-5	√	√	√	√	√	√	★	★	√	★	√	★★	★★
T-7	√	√	√	√	√	√	★	★	√	★	√	★★	★★
T-8	√	√	√	√	√	√	★	★	√	★	√	★★	★★
T-9	√	√	√	√	√	√	★	★	√	★	√	★★	★★
T-10	√	√	√	√	√	√	★	★	√	★	√	★★	★★
T-11	√	√	√	√	√	√	★	★	√	★	√	★★	★★
T-12	√	√	√	√	√	√	★	★	√	★	√	★★	★★
L-1	√	√	√	√	√	√	★	★	√	★	√	★★	★★
L-2	√	√	√	√	√	√	★	★	√	★	√	★★	★★
L-3	√	√	√	√	√	√	★	★	√	★	√	★★	★★
L-4	√	√	√	√	√	√	★	√	√	★	√	★★	★★
L-5	√	√	√	√	√	√	★	√	√	★	√	★★	★★
S-1	√	√	√	√	√	√	★	√	√	√	√	★★	★★
S-2	√	√	√	√	√	√	√	√	√	√	√	★★	★★
S-3	√	√	√	√	√	√	√	√	√	√	√	★★	★★
S-4	√	√	√	√	√	√	√	√	√	√	√	★★	★★

Symbol	Meaning
√	Normal or near normal function or performance
★	Requires some type of attendant assistance and/or specialized equipment
★★	Participation possible but options and alternatives need to be discussed
	Not practical/probable for this injury level

Figure 44-9 Spinal cord injury functional activity chart.

it characteristically results in flaccid muscle weakness or paralysis, loss of reflex activity, and atrophy of the involved muscles.[11]

Upper motor neurons (UMNs) (Figure 44-11) originate in the motor strip of the cerebral cortex and in multiple brainstem nuclei, and they eventually synapse with LMNs in the spinal cord. Any lesion that destroys UMNs or interferes with their influence over LMNs is called an upper motor neuron injury.[11] Initially, the muscles affected by a UMN injury are flaccid (hypotonic) and hyporeflexic. This period of hypotonicity persists for a variable period of time, but gradually the reflex arcs become reactive in the absence of UMN modulation. Voluntary muscle function is lost, but hyperreflexia of all cord segments occurs with increased muscle tone and spasticity in response to muscle stretch, autonomic, or noxious stimuli.

The principles of upper and lower motor neuron injury apply to skeletal muscles below the level of SCI, but they are also important determinants of residual bowel, bladder, and sexual functioning. The micturition reflex center is located in the conus medullaris at S2-4 and is linked to the detrusor muscle of the bladder by sensory and motor fibers in the

C2
C3
C4
C5
T2
T3
T4
T5
T6
T7
T8
T9
T10
T11
T12
T1
C6
L1
S3
S4
S5
C8
C7
L2
L3
L4
L5
S1
S2
Coccyx

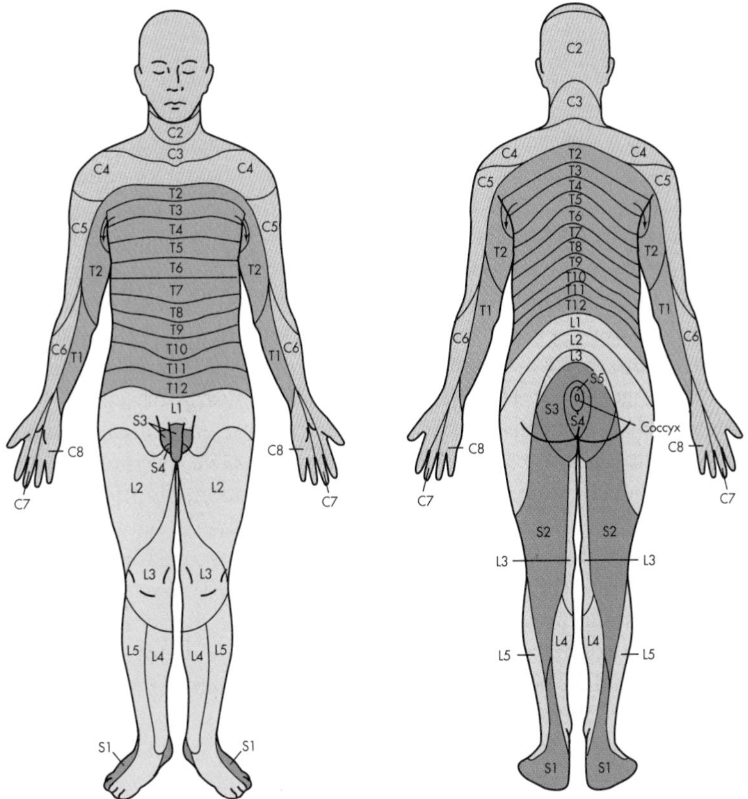

Figure 44-10 Sensory dermatomes.

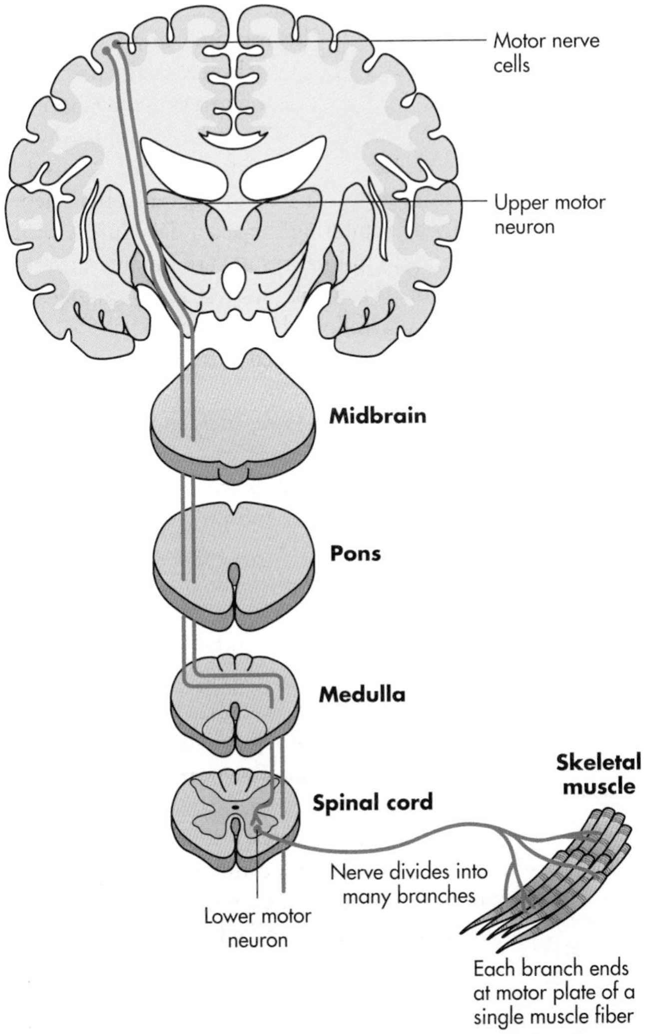

Motor nerve cells
Upper motor neuron
Midbrain
Pons
Medulla
Spinal cord
Skeletal muscle
Nerve divides into many branches
Lower motor neuron
Each branch ends at motor plate of a single muscle fiber

Figure 44-11 Upper and lower motor neurons.

pelvic nerves.[20] Injury above this level affects the UMN control of micturition. The micturition center remains functional, as does the internal sphincter, but they are no longer under voluntary control. The reflex arc is intact but the voluntary coordinated control of urination is lost. After the period of spinal shock, as spinal reflex activity resumes, a spastic automatic bladder develops. The person is unable to sense bladder fullness or an urge to void, but the bladder fills and empties spontaneously. An LMN injury below T12 directly affects the micturition center and results in an autonomous flaccid bladder. The reflex arc is no longer intact. The person is unaware of bladder distention, and the reflex center and both urinary sphincters are nonfunctional. The bladder can easily overdistend, and urinary retention, infection, and overflow incontinence are common.

The spinal defecation reflex center is also located at S2 through S4, and similar types of outcomes accompany injury to this area of the spinal cord. Injuries affecting the UMNs cause a loss of voluntary control over the external anal sphincter. The ascending impulses are blocked, and the person cannot feel rectal fullness nor the urge to defecate. The reflex center is intact, however, and continues to exert tone. This results in spastic bowel dysfunction, but the intact reflexes are capable of triggering regular evacuation of the bowel. Injuries below T12 affect the LMN and create flaccid bowel dysfunction. No tone exists, and incontinence can occur at any time. Peristalsis is not affected by SCI because the cell bodies that initiate peristalsis are found in nerve plexuses in the bowel wall, not in the spinal cord. This reflex activity remains intact.[19]

Similar principles govern the outcomes of spinal cord injury on sexual functioning. SCI at any level abolishes the communication between the genitals and higher brain centers, but the sexual reflex center, which controls erection in males and spontaneous lubrication in females, is affected differently by upper versus lower motor neuron injuries. The reflex center is located between S2 and S4. Psychologic sexual responses are not possible with injuries above T12, but reflex erections are usually possible, and the higher the level of injury the more likely a man is to be able to perform sexually. The reflex center is blocked when injuries occur below T12 and reflex erections do not occur.[20] Sex drive remains intact, but ejaculation is rare after any SCI. The experience of orgasm is possible, but men usually report it as being different from before the injury. Women with SCI can perform sexually, although again the experience of orgasm is usually altered. Fertility is decreased in males because of impaired temperature control in the scrotum, but remains intact in females once the menstrual cycle is reestablished.

Collaborative Care Management

Diagnostic Tests. SCI is initially diagnosed on the basis of the presenting clinical symptoms. Emergency services policies mandate that all trauma patients be treated as potentially spinal cord injured until this risk can be ruled out. Head trauma is frequently accompanied by SCI, and some of these patients present with no initial neurologic deficits. Standard x-rays can reveal the presence of fracture and/or dislocation of the vertebral bodies or spinal processes in the cervical region quite clearly, but they are less effective in identifying injuries to the thoracic spine.

Initial assessment roughly establishes the extent of injury and provides a baseline for evaluating symptoms related to secondary injury. Systematic assessment of the movement and strength of all major muscle groups is performed and documented. Baseline vital capacity is a critical value. A digital rectal examination is performed to determine whether the injury appears to be "complete." Any voluntary contraction of the perianal muscles or sensitivity to the examiner's finger indicates the presence of an incomplete injury and carries a much more favorable prognosis. A complete sensory evaluation of proprioception, pinprick, and response to light touch is performed and recorded for each dermatome.

Both computed tomography (CT) and magnetic resonance imaging (MRI) may be used to accurately evaluate the extent of injury. CT scans can reveal the exact anatomy of any bony injury and are useful in evaluating the patient who has neurologic symptoms or complaints of pain, but negative x-ray studies. MRI shows bone poorly but provides excellent visualization of the spinal cord and nerve roots. It can identify hemorrhage, contusion, or compression of the cord and appears to have some prognostic potential in being able to differentiate the effects of hemorrhage versus edema[8]; however, the patient's clinical status and restricted movement may make MRI scanning impractical in the acute period after injury.

Medications. Drug therapy is primarily targeted at delaying or suppressing the multiple physiologic processes that cause secondary injury. Each new factor that is revealed triggers a new wave of basic pharmacologic laboratory research. At present, only the administration of methylprednisolone has been validated by widespread clinical trials. Its use significantly improves neurologic recovery after incomplete SCI, primarily by inhibiting the secondary injury process of lipid peroxidation. Optimal results are obtained from prompt administration. Protocols suggest a 30 mg/kg bolus, ideally within 3 hours, followed by a 5.4 mg/kg infusion for 24 hours. A 48-hour infusion is used if treatment is delayed for 3 to 8 hours.[25]

Other drugs with a lower incidence of severe infection than is associated with the use of methylprednisolone are also showing promise. Lazeroids are a new group of drugs that inhibit lipid peroxidation without glucocorticoid activity.[25] The most promising agent in this class is tirilazad, which appears to have similar efficacy to methylprednisolone, with a significantly lower incidence of severe sepsis and pneumonia.

Gangliosides are glycolipids that are integrated into cell membranes in the central nervous system.

Although their mechanism of action is unknown ganglioside GM_1 has shown laboratory promise in fostering neurite outgrowth and regeneration of neurons (see Future Watch box).

The role of opioid antagonists such as naloxone in treatment remains controversial. It is known that endogenous opioid levels increase significantly after injury, but real benefit may need to wait until the specific opioid receptors related to secondary injury are identified.[25]

Future Watch
Spinal Cord Repair: Are We Getting Closer?

As recently as World War II, spinal cord injury was considered to be an untreatable injury. The intervening years have brought tremendous improvement to the care and rehabilitation of patients with spinal cord injuries, and most now achieve a near normal lifespan. As the processes of secondary injury continue to be unraveled, attention is now being directed toward attempting to minimize the consequences of injury and even repair damaged spinal cords.

High-profile sports and entertainment figures have directed the nation's attention to the problem of spinal cord injury and basic research is expanding exponentially. At the same time advances in cell manipulation and genetics make it possible to plan and carry out research that was impossible until recent years. Approaches under study include the use of embryonic stem cells to stimulate axon regeneration in the spinal cord, transplantation of glial cells to remyelinate damaged nerves, transplantation of gamma-aminobutyric acid inhibitory neurons to block chronic pain syndromes in patients with spinal cord injuries, and inhibition of the endogenous processes that result in secondary injury. All of these approaches show promise, but researchers caution that it could take years to successfully translate promising laboratory research into human applications. Rehabilitation will remain a key component of care for the foreseeable future.

Other drug therapies under intense investigation include antioxidants and free radical scavengers such as vitamins A, C, and E and selenium; platelet activating factor antagonists; ion (calcium) channel blockers; serotonin (5HT) receptor antagonists; and thyrotropin-releasing hormone analogs.[20,25]

The circulatory effects of spinal shock may also necessitate pharmacologic management with vasopressor agents, platelet inhibitors, and anticoagulants. A wide range of drugs may be used to manage specific problems such as muscle spasticity that occur during the rehabilitation period.

Treatments. Prehospital care at the site of injury has been a crucial aspect of SCI care since the late 1970s. The focus is on spine stabilization to prevent further damage and rapid transport to a specialty care center. A rigid cervical collar and long backboard are standard interventions before transport (Figure 44-12).[10,23] Highly trained rescue teams may initiate methyprednisolone protocols. The need for decompression and realignment can then be determined by diagnostic testing. The greatest concerns for spinal instability exist with injuries to the cervical spine, which is capable of extensive movement. Instability is also a concern with injuries from T11 to L2.

Decompression and stabilization procedures may need to take place on an emergency basis if the patient's neurologic status continues to deteriorate. Both surgical and nonsurgical approaches to stabilization are available. Surgical options are discussed later. In-line immobilization with a cervical collar is replaced by skeletal tongs or a halo ring with traction (Figure 44-13, see Figure 46-8). Once appropriate alignment has been achieved a halo vest may be used for stabilization.[7] The halo ring has the advantage of being compatible with both CT and MRI.[20] The halo device is applied with the patient under local anesthesia and consists of a metal ring that is attached to the skull by means of two anterior and two posterior pins. External vertical rods attach the halo to the body vest. The device provides for complete external immobilization of the head and neck without flexion, extension, or rotation movements. Patients with halos can be managed in standard hospital beds and be mobilized into active rehabilitation as soon as they are hemodynamically stable. Thus, length of stay in the acute care setting after SCI has been dramatically decreased. Care of the patient in a halo device is summarized in the Guidelines for Safe Practice box.

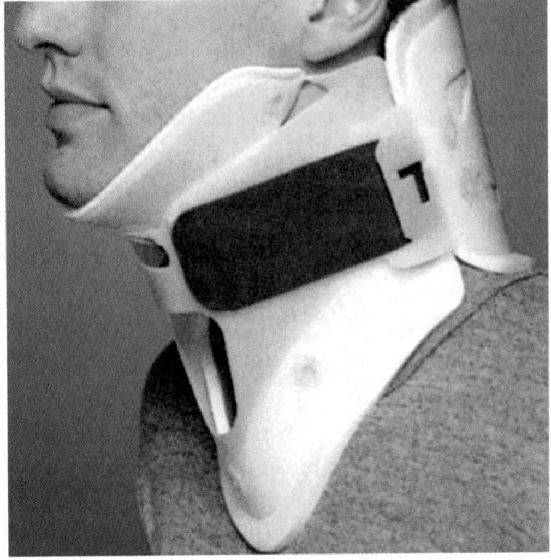

Figure 44-12 Rigid cervical collar.

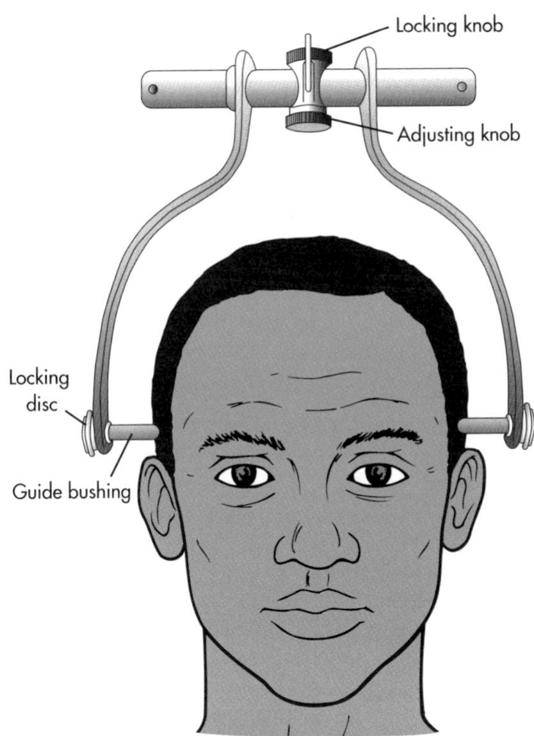

Figure 44-13 Vinke cervical tongs.

Bed rest alone may be sufficient to provide immobilization for lower thoracic and lumbar injuries. The thoracolumbar area cannot be stabilized with traction. Braces, corsets, or fiberglass shells may be used, but unstable fractures usually require surgical repair.

Numerous other treatments have been and are being investigated in the acute care management of SCI. Cord exposure and irrigation, cord cooling, and hyperbaric oxygen therapy are all being used experimentally (see Research box).

Managing Spinal Shock. Specific treatment for spinal shock is usually not necessary unless the patient is also experiencing hypovolemic shock from hemorrhage and associated trauma. An intravenous line is established and fluids are administered. Profound hypotension may require vigorous fluid resuscitation and the use of inotropic agents.[20] Mild vasomotor instability is managed by keeping the patient flat in bed and supporting venous return through the use of pneumatic compression devices, antiembolism compression stockings, or elastic bandages on the extremities, plus abdominal binders. Patients with high cervical injuries may also require intubation or a tracheostomy if their respiratory muscles are paralyzed or become excessively fatigued.

Surgical Management. Surgical intervention is used to relieve compression, correct alignment, and improve the stability of the spine. It may be performed immediately in an attempt to limit the extent of neurologic damage or after an initial stabilization period of medical management. Surgery may need to be delayed if the patient is not initially stable enough to tolerate the rigors of general anesthesia and spinal surgery. The MRI scan can help to determine the need for immediate surgical decompression. Early surgical intervention appears to be associated with improved outcomes and shorter hospital stays.[20]

Surgical options include laminectomy with fusion of the spinal elements via bone graft, intraspinous wiring, or the placement of rods. Harrington rods, which attach to the spinous processes by means of wires, have been used extensively over the last 30 years. The newer "CD" rods provide for multiple points of attachment with lamina hooks and screws. Rod systems are used primarily to stabilize thoracic and lumbar injuries. Anterior surgical techniques have been greatly improved in recent years, and cervical spine repair is now less risky and can be performed earlier during the hospital stay. An anterior approach is particularly effective for removing disk material or bone fragments from the injured area. Surgery on the cervical spine can be performed with the stabilizing halo device in place.

Diet. Ileus develops after SCI as part of the process of spinal shock and persists for a variable length of time. The patient is kept on a nothing-by-mouth status and a nasogastric (NG) tube is inserted to reduce abdominal distention and prevent aspiration. Decompression of the abdomen often improves ventilation.[24] The SCI triggers a profound metabolic stress response, which is often significantly greater than seems warranted by the severity of tissue damage. Energy needs are increased by as much as 50% and the patient with SCI may develop a severe catabolic state.[20] Glycogen stores are tapped to meet the body's immediate needs, but these reserves are typically exhausted within 24 hours. The body turns next to fats and proteins, which then are unavailable for tissue building and repair. A state of protein-calorie malnutrition that predisposes the patient to sepsis and other complications can develop within 3 to 5 days. A 7-kg weight loss is common in the early postinjury period.[20] Nutrition support is needed to meet nutritional needs that range from 30 to 35 Cal/kg per day with a protein need of 1.25 to 1.5 g/kg per day. Either enteral feedings or parenteral nutrition

Guidelines for Safe Practice

The Patient in a Halo With Vest

MANAGING THE HALO

Inspect the pins and pin sites each shift.
- Be sure that all pins are tight.
- Provide pin care if ordered.
- Inspect the margins of the vest for signs of skin irritation.
- Provide skin care to all areas affected by the halo and vest.
- Replace or add to vest padding as needed to prevent skin irritation.

Support the vest when the patient is in bed.

ENSURING PATIENT COMFORT

Keep rubber caps on the tips of the halo ring to minimize excessive sound magnification.

Provide mild analgesics for headache or discomfort at the pin insertion sites.

Turn and reposition the patient every 2 hours.

GENERAL CARE CONSIDERATIONS

Adjust the patient's diet to compensate for swallowing difficulties and discomfort.

Implement standard measures to minimize the complications of immobility:
- Bowel and bladder care
- Deep breathing and coughing
- Skin care
- Prevention of deep vein thrombosis

Research

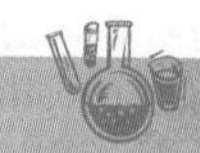

Reference: Asamoto S et al: Hyperbaric oxygen therapy for acute traumatic cervical spinal cord injury, *Spinal Cord* 38(9):538-540, 2000.

Thirty-four patients who experienced hyperextension injuries to the cervical spine were assigned at admission to two different treatment groups: with or without hyperbaric oxygen. The Neurological Cervical Spine Scale was used to evaluate the patients at admission and after initial treatment. Improvement rates ranged from 100% to 27% in the hyperbaric treatment group and from 100% to 25% in the nonhyperbaric treatment group. The mean response rates were significantly higher, however, in the patients treated with hyperbaric oxygen, indicating preliminary support that hyperbaric treatment demonstrates effectiveness in improving outcomes for traumatically injured patients with damage to the cervical spine.

may be used. Once the rehabilitation period is underway daily caloric intake is adjusted to maintain a stable body weight.

Development of stress ulcers is also a significant concern in the early days after SCI. The risk of overt hemorrhage is about 6% and is highest in patients with cervical injuries. H_2 blockers or proton pump inhibitors are administered, and the pH of all gastric secretions is carefully monitored. Antacids may be administered through the NG tube.

Activity. Most of the progress in the management of SCI over the last 40 years has come from treatment approaches that foster an early return to activity (e.g., halo devices). Flat bed rest is maintained in the initial spinal shock period, but patients are assisted out of bed and into aggressive multidisciplinary rehabilitation as soon as vasomotor status is stabilized and spinal alignment and stability are ensured. Early mobility helps to prevent the complications of disuse, improves mood, and facilitates patient involvement in intensive self-care rehabilitation.

Referrals. Management of patients with SCIs is truly a multidisciplinary effort. The nurse may serve as the case manager and coordinate the implementation of a critical pathway for care. At a minimum the patient's care necessitates the involvement of physical therapy, occupational therapy, and social work resources. Depending on the level and severity of the injury, the patient's care may also involve respiratory therapy, nutrition support, and spiritual counseling resources. Nurse specialists coordinate the family education efforts, but families are also referred to resources in their home communities for care, education, and support.

A clinical pathway for a patient with a traumatic SCI resulting in quadriplegia is presented below.

clinical pathway *Traumatic Spinal Cord Injury-Quadriplegia**

UNIT(s)	STABILIZATION PHASE DAY 0-3				
Day		INITIALS			
Date		0	1	2	3
Assessment	Nursing Assessment Trauma bath assessment when normothermic Vital signs and Neuro assessment every 1 hour for 24 hours, then every 2 hours Level of injury (motor/sensory) determined by neurosurgeon Respiratory assessment every 2 hours Review Lab results Skin Integrity Assessment and Risk Score day 0 and 3 Assessment for DVT daily				
Consults	Neurosurgery Service Physiatry to coordinate Rehabilitation Team Nutrition Services Social Work Services Psychiatry Liaison Services for Crisis Assessment/Intervention Plan Substance Abuse Consult for positive urine or serum screen Intensivist				
Labs					
Tests	Full spine series, CAT scan and/or MRI if not completed in E.D.				
Meds	Morphine 2-4 mgIV push q 1 hour prn Ativan 1-4 IV push q 2-4 hours prn Methylprednisolone __mg/hr x __ hours fluids Heparin 5,000 units S.Q. every 12 hours, begin after 24 hours Pepcid 20 mg IV every 12 hour x 48 hours If vasopressors needed, consider neosynephrine or norepinephrine Therevac daily for bowel training, begin after 48 hrs Multi-Vitamin with minerals daily or 1 ampule of MVI daily in IV Vitamin C 500 mg P.O. daily when taking P.O.				
IV	IV fluid as per orders				
Treatments	Pulse oximeter Traction and/or Rotorest bed prior to surgical stabilization Pin care every 8 hours wrench attached to halo vest, if applicable Mechanical ventilation if indicated Pulmonary Toilet prn Soft tissue injury repaired Suture line care Replace Salem Sump with smallest diameter Flexiflow after 24 hours of tolerating tube feedings Foley to gravity I & O Sequential Compression Device Consider IVC filter insertion Moisture barrier, prn if incontinent Rigid cervical collar post-op; check pressure points q shift				
Activity	Bedrest log roll until stabilized Turn and position every 2 hours, if in rotorest 60° continuous rotation Splints per PT/O.T. on/off every 2 hours				
Nutrition	NPO until surgical stabilization Post-op begin Propeptide trickle feedings, progress to Promote with fiber				
Teaching	Patient and family updated on tests, procedures, and plan of care SCI expectations Communication techniques Call Bell System				

Courtesy Allegheny General Hospital, Pittsburgh, Pa. Stabilization phase, days 0 to 3. Transition phase, days 4 to 7, follows as an example of changes in care.

Continued

clinical pathway *Traumatic Spinal Cord Injury-Quadriplegia–cont'd*

UNIT(s)	STABILIZATION PHASE DAY 0-3				
Day		INITIALS			
Date		0	1	2	3
Discharge	Formal multidisciplinary team meeting by Day 3 to establish plan				
Intermediate Outcomes	Hemodynamically stable Injuries identified and treated Neurologically stable Spine stabilized < 48 hours Level of functioning identified Pulse Oximeter >92% Nutritional needs met ≤ 72 hours Patient and family informed of plan of care Multidisciplinary plan established and goals identified Discharged destination options identified < 72 hours Pain is optimally managed				
Initials Signature Title					

000-000 Rev 10/01 The Clinical Pathway is only a guideline and may be modified at the discretion of the physician or caregiver, based on patient response.

UNIT(s)	TRANSITIONAL PHASE DAY 4 - 7				
Day		INITIALS			
Date		4	5	6	7
Assessment	Vital signs every 4 hours (Pulmonary Step Down) Neuro assessment every 4 hours Respiratory assessment every 4 hours Bowel assessment daily Bladder assessment daily Skin Integrity Assessment and Risk Score day 6 Assessment for DVT daily				
Consults	Physiatry to coordinate Rehabilitation Team: PT - conditioning, ROM and pressure relief BID O.T. - splints and ADL's BID S.T. - communication & swallowing evaluation BID Discharge referral - per patient/family decision				
Labs	PTT on day 7				
Tests					
Meds	Heparin 5,000 units S.Q. every 12 hours Multivitamin with mineral P.O. daily or 1 ampule of MVI in IV fluid daily Vitamin C 500 mg P.O. daily when taking P.O. Therevac daily for bowel training				
IV	INT				
Treatments	Mechanical ventilator if indicated Pulmonary Toilet prn Quad cough Consider trach day 3 - 7 Discontinue Foley on day 4 Straight cath every 4-6 hours to maintain urine ≤ 500 cc per cath I & O Sequential Compression Device Moisture barrier, prn if incontinent				
Activity	Sitting position bid Abdominal binder (not over hips) when in sitting position Evaluate for orthostatic hypotension: Check BP when in sitting position Weight shifts every 30 minutes when in sitting position PROM - AROM every 4 hours at bedside Splint on/off every 2 hours				
Nutrition	Promote with fiber, progress to Dysphagia diet once trached				
Teaching	SCI expectations Transition to Rehabilitation Institute				
Discharge	Multidisciplinary plan				
Intermediate Outcomes	Hemodynamically stable Pulse oximeter 92% Patient and family informed of plan of care Pain is optimally managed				

clinical pathway *Traumatic Spinal Cord Injury-Quadriplegia–cont'd*

000-000 Rev 10/01 The Clinical Pathway is only a guideline and may be modified at the discretion of the physician or caregiver, based on patient response.

UNIT(s)	TRANSITIONAL PHASE DAY 4 - 7					
Day			INITIALS			
Date			4	5	6	7
	Maintain intermittent cath schedule Transfer to Pulmonary step down					
Initials Signature Title						

NURSING MANAGEMENT

ASSESSMENT

Health History

Data to be collected during the health history include:

- Information about the nature of the injury and its circumstances
- History of loss of consciousness
- Patient's understanding of injury and the resulting deficits
- Other comorbid conditions, treatment, and medications
- Family and social resources
- Smoking history, substance abuse
- Preinjury weight, usual dietary pattern
- Time of last urination and defecation

Physical Examination

Data to be collected during the physical examination include:

- Level of consciousness
- Positioning and alignment of head, neck, and spine
- Baseline respiratory status
  - Rate and pattern, presence and severity of dyspnea
  - Tidal volume/vital capacity
  - Abdominal breathing, use of accessory muscle
- Baseline vital signs, apical pulse and blood pressure, temperature
- Baseline motor evaluation
  - Level of injury, motor strength, and movement
  - Presence/absence of spinal reflexes
  - Presence or absence of anal wink
- Baseline sensory evaluation
  - Dermatome assessment: pain, touch, temperature, pressure, proprioception
  - Presence of paresthesias, other abnormal sensation
- Baseline skin assessment
  - Signs of redness, pressure, or breakdown
- Presence and activity of bowel sounds
  - Presence of stool in rectum
- Presence and severity of bladder distention

NURSING DIAGNOSES

Nursing diagnoses are determined from analysis of patient data. Nursing diagnoses for the patient with a spinal cord injury may include but are not limited to:

Diagnostic Title	Possible Etiologic Factors
1. Ineffective breathing pattern	Neuromuscular weakness/ paralysis of intercostal muscles
2. Ineffective airway clearance	Paralysis of intercostal/ abdominal muscles
3. Decreased cardiac output	Decreased venous return with pooling of blood in the periphery
4. Ineffective thermoregulation	Autonomic dysfunction and loss of ability to shiver or perspire
5. Risk for disuse syndrome	Paralysis and treatment immobilization
6. Risk for impaired skin integrity	Sensory losses and physical immobilization
7. Urinary retention	Atonic flaccid bladder
8. Risk for constipation	Atonic bowel and immobility
9. Ineffective sexuality patterns	Physical effects of injury on sexual response
10. Interrupted family processes	Crisis of injury and loss of self-care capacity

EXPECTED PATIENT OUTCOMES

Expected patient outcomes for the patient with a spinal cord injury may include but are not limited to:

1. Will maintain a tidal volume of 7 to 10 ml/kg, respiratory rate of 25/min, and vital capacity of 15 to 20 ml/kg; will verbalize an absence of dyspnea
2. Will cough effectively; lungs will be clear to auscultation
3. Will be hemodynamically stable with a heart rate of 60/min; no occurrence of orthostatic hypotension
4. Will maintain a stable body temperature of 98° F (36.6° C)
5. Will maintain full range of motion in all joints; no objective sign of deep vein thrombosis (DVT) or pulmonary embolus

6. Will maintain intact skin
7. Will establish an intermittent catheterization program that ensures urine volumes of 400 ml/catheterization; will maintain a balanced intake and output
8. Will establish a regular pattern of bowel evacuation without incidence of impaction or incontinence
9. Will adapt sexual activity to limitations of residual sexual function
10. Will demonstrate the ability to use coping mechanisms effectively and to problem solve collaboratively with the family concerning present status and future care

INTERVENTIONS

1. Maintaining Adequate Ventilation

Respiratory complications are the leading cause of morbidity and mortality after acute SCI.[18,26,27] Adequate ventilation involves the coordinated functioning of the diaphragm, intercostal muscles, abdominal muscles, and accessory muscles. SCI can affect the innervation of any or all of these important muscle groups (Table 44-1). Any patient with a spinal cord injury at C4 or above can be expected to need short-term or permanent ventilatory support. Patients with lower cervical injuries may develop respiratory difficulties from the process of secondary injury or respiratory muscle fatigue. A baseline respiratory assessment is performed to establish parameters for ongoing monitoring.

Assessment is then performed hourly on unstable patients and at least every 4 hours on apparently stable patients. At a minimum, SCI can be expected to result in hypoventilation. Paradoxic respirations may also occur when the action of the intercostal muscles is lost. The thoracic cage collapses on inspiration as the diaphragm descends and expands when the diaphragm ascends. This reversed breathing pattern is extremely tiring for the patient and inefficient in meeting the body's needs.

The nurse closely monitors the patient's vital capacity, tidal volume, or both. A vital capacity less than 1000 ml indicates respiratory insufficiency and is associated with a higher risk of complications. A vital capacity less than 500 ml usually indicates a need to intubate,[20] particularly if the patient's respiratory rate is greater than 30/min, or if paradoxic breathing patterns are present. Earlier intubation may be indicated for patients with a history of smoking, pulmonary allergy, or chronic pulmonary disease that could further compromise the patient's respiratory reserve.

TABLE 44-1 Physical Effects and Functional Outcomes of Spinal Cord Injury

Level of Injury	Motor/Sensory Effects	Functional Potential
C1-C3	No voluntary movement or sensation below the level of the injury Diaphragm and intercostal muscles paralyzed	Ventilator-dependent
C4	As above but neck accessory muscle function intact plus potential for partial function of diaphragm	May be able to breathe without ventilator for intervals
C5	Phrenic nerve intact to diaphragm Deltoid and biceps function present which allows elbow flexion and good control of head and neck Full sensation to head, neck, chest, and upper arms	Independent breathing, but poor lung capacity Tidal volume 300 ml Self-feeding and dressing potential
C6-C8	Diaphragm and accessories can compensate for losses of intercostal and abdominal muscles and support normal breathing Hand grasp, sensation present	Potential for independent living; feeding, dressing, bathing, elimination, transfer, and wheelchair mobility
T1-T5	Full control of upper extremities Some intercostal and thoracic muscle function Sensation intact to arms and midchest/midback	Pulmonary function within acceptable norms; tidal volume 500-700 ml Independent in self-care; manual wheelchair Potential for full-time employment
T6-T10	Increasing control over abdominal and trunk muscles Sensation steadily increasing to level of umbilicus and midback	Full independence in care; manual wheelchair Employment reasonable expectation, can participate in sports activities
T11-L5	Increasing function of hip flexors, knee extension, knee flexion, and ankle dorsiflexion Sensation intact to lower abdomen, hips, anterior surface of legs, parts of posterior of legs No sensation present in groin, genitals, anus, or portions of buttocks	Independent in self-care Ambulation with long leg braces possible, but tires easily
S1-S5	Progressive return of full control to legs, ankles, and feet Progressive control of bowel, bladder, and sexual function; sensory function to groin, anus, and posterior aspects of legs and feet	Independent in self-care Independent ambulation; short braces may be used for support

Hypoxemia and hypercarbia can easily result from hypoventilation, and supplemental oxygen is routinely administered. The nurse monitors and records pulse oximetry and serial blood gas values. A Po_2 of less than 80 mm Hg or a Pco_2 greater than 45 mm Hg is a clear indicator of the need for intubation and mechanical ventilation. A tracheostomy may be performed to make patient management easier when extended ventilator support is anticipated. The use of fenestrated or "talking" tracheostomy tubes assist the patient to communicate. Deep breathing remains a critical intervention for patients who do not require intubation, and the nurse helps the patient use an incentive spirometer every 1 to 2 hours while awake to expand the alveoli and support adequate gas exchange.

2. Promoting Secretion Removal

Patients with SCI are at greatest risk for developing atelectasis and pneumonia 3 to 5 days after the injury.[18] Therefore, maintaining an open airway and effective secretion removal is a nursing care priority. Effective coughing ideally uses both the intercostal and abdominal muscles to build up sufficient pressure in the thorax so that air can be vigorously expelled. These muscles are typically affected by high thoracic and cervical injuries, and the patient loses the ability to effectively cough and clear the airway. Adequate humidity and hydration are provided to keep secretions thin, and chest physiotherapy is generally used to help the patient expel secretions. Frequent position changes are also important, but the positioning limitations of SCI make this extremely difficult in the early management period. To compensate for the inability to change positions, many centers use special beds such as the kinetic treatment table (Rotorest bed, which continually turn the patient through a maximal arc of about 120 degrees (Figure 44-14). Retrospective research studies indicate that continuous turning is effective in preventing mucus pooling in high-risk patients.[18]

The nurse performs endotracheal suctioning as needed, especially if the cough reflex is weak. A moist but unproductive cough clearly indicates the need for more aggressive airway clearance. Suctioning can trigger a vasovagal response in patients with SCIs and result in profound bradycardia. This could be life threatening, especially during the unstable period of spinal shock. The patient is attached to a cardiac monitor, and the nurse thoroughly hyperoxygenates the patient before suctioning. A variety of techniques have been used to remove secretions. The most effective appears to be a combination of positive pressure and assisted cough in a sitting position.[18] Assisted or "quad coughing" involves placing the nurse's hand between the patient's umbilicus and xyphoid and then pushing vigorously inward and upward as the patient exhales.

3. Supporting Cardiac Output

The patient with SCI is often hemodynamically unstable during the period of spinal shock. The bradycardia of spinal shock does not usually require treatment unless heart rate drops precipitously during movement or suctioning. Atropine may be given to block the vagal overactivity and correct bradycardia and dysrhythmia. Orthostatic hypotension can be severe. Patients are usually stable as long as they lie in a flat supine position, but they may develop severe blood pressure instability with position changes. The move from a supine to a vertical position quickly redistributes about 500 ml of blood and is associated with significant orthostasis in more than 73% of patients.[13] Severe orthostasis may significantly limit a patient's ability to become involved in active rehabilitation.

Initially the patient is kept in a flat supine position. Some combination of elastic bandages, antiembolism compression stockings, pneumatic compression devices, and abdominal binders are used to support venous return. The use of a kinetic movement bed also supports movement and circulation in the extremities. As spinal shock resolves, the patient is slowly moved toward an upright position in small increments. The angle of the head of the bed is increased just a few degrees at a time. The nurse carefully monitors the patient's response to each position change.

DVT is another common adverse outcome of the significant venous pooling associated with SCI. The risk of DVT is high, but the diagnosis is difficult to establish because the patient is unaware of calf pain or tenderness, and the clinical evaluation is unreliable as much as 50% of the time. The nurse monitors calf and thigh circumference at least daily and assesses the skin for discoloration or warmth each time the compression devices are removed for skin care.[24] Doppler ultrasound can also be used at the bedside to improve diagnostic accuracy. The nurse also performs range-of-motion exercise each shift and avoids putting the patient in any position that increases pressure behind the knee. Pulmonary emboli are a rare but serious complication of venous pooling, and low-dose heparin or low-molecular-weight heparin is frequently administered during the first postinjury weeks when the risk is highest. A sudden change in Po_2 or O_2 saturation is an important warning sign.

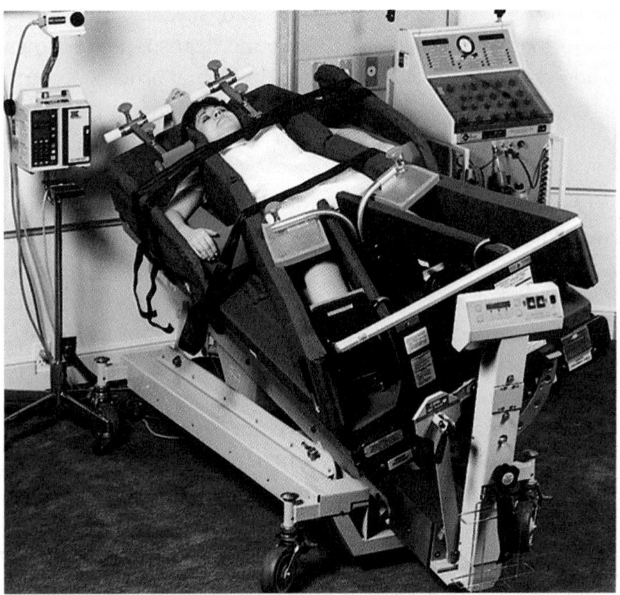

Figure 44-14 The Rotorest kinetic treatment table. This oscillating bed keeps the patient's spine in proper alignment yet slowly turns the patient through an arc of about 120 degrees every 1 to 2 hours.

4. Maintaining a Stable Body Temperature

The control of body temperature is significantly altered by SCI. Loss of sympathetic stimulation causes widespread vasodilation with an ongoing associated heat loss through the skin. Loss of upper motor neuron control by the thermoregulatory center of the brain means that the body can neither sweat nor shiver below the level of the injury to raise or lower body temperature. The nurse assesses the patient's temperature every 2 to 4 hours and ensures that minimal temperature variations occur in the care environment because the body gradually assumes the ambient temperature. The nurse uses extra blankets or environmental cooling as needed to keep the patient's temperature around 98° F. The patient and family are instructed about the risks of both chilling and serious overheating in hot weather.

5. Preventing the Complications of Disuse

Current approaches to the management of SCI emphasize early mobility and attempt to minimize the multiple problems associated with disuse. Early mobility is important regardless of the level of injury. Mobility initially involves active and passive range-of-motion exercise and position changes to prevent contractures and pressure damage to the skin. Mat and resistance exercises are initiated to increase strength and endurance in the muscles that remain under voluntary control. Rehabilitation gradually expands to include wheelchair activities, although orthostatic hypotension may initially limit the patient's ability to tolerate a sitting position. A tilt table is used in therapy, and a reclining wheelchair may be used until the patient is able to tolerate being upright.

Weight-bearing activities become extremely important in slowing down the osteoporotic changes associated with long-term immobility. As calcium leaves the bone matrix, the risk of pathologic fracture steadily increases. In all, 15% to 20% of patients experience excess bone deposits around the joints (heterotropic ossification), which can severely limit range of motion.[20] The cause of these bone deposits is unknown. In adolescents with SCI the bone remodeling process becomes so unbalanced that clinically significant hypercalcemia can develop along with its attendant risk of kidney stone formation.[12]

Disuse complications are a significant priority for nursing care. The nurse assesses joint range of motion every day and performs range-of-motion exercise at least twice daily. Range of motion becomes increasingly important because muscle spasticity develops over time, usually within the initial 6 months. Most joint deformities in a paralyzed person are preventable. The nurse carefully positions the limbs in their normal anatomic positions. Adaptive and functional splints are applied as needed to maintain functional position and prevent contracture. Knee flexion contractures and footdrop are serious complications that must be prevented. A flexion contracture in the knee joint interferes significantly with the patient's potential to bear weight in an upright position and accomplish transfers successfully. Patients with sufficient residual function will learn to accomplish transfers from bed to wheelchair and to propel a wheelchair independently (Figures 44-15 and 44-16). Instruction is initiated by the physical medicine team and practice is continued on the nursing unit. Wheelchair mobility is a major goal, but prolonged sitting can result in contractures of the hip. Positioning the patient in a prone position at intervals helps to prevent this problem.

The entire multidisciplinary team works collaboratively to assist the patient to compensate for the losses resulting from the SCI and restore a maximal level of self-care ability. Patients with high cervical cord injuries will need daily care for the rest of their lives, but patients with injuries as high as C7-8 have the potential for some degree of independent living. The rehabilitation process is arduous as the patient attempts to build strength in the remaining muscle groups. Occupational therapists facilitate the acquisition of appropriate assistive devices and teach the patient to use them appropriately to support independence.

6. Protecting the Skin

As the largest organ of the body, the skin is also the most vulnerable to damage related to SCI. The loss of sensory input and restricted mobility combine to create a lifelong threat of injury to the skin. Pressure ulcers are the second most common complication after SCI, and an estimated 12.3% of patients develop them.[1] Direct pressure-related skin injury is the primary concern, but shearing forces are also important. Skin protection will be a lifelong management problem.

Care for the skin begins immediately after injury. Microscopic tissue changes related to local ischemia can occur in less than 30 minutes. The significant venous pooling and inadequate tissue perfusion that characterize the hemodynamic instability of the spinal shock period further compromise the skin. Pressure injury is frequently initiated while the patient is strapped to a rigid backboard. It is important for the nurse to pad bony prominences if transport or diagnostic scanning must prolong the patient's time on the backboard.

The use of special beds such as the Rotorest decrease pressure-related concerns significantly during the acute phase. As the patient's condition stabilizes, a regular hospital bed may be used, but a minimum of a 4-inch foam antipressure mattress should be in place.

Inspection and pressure reduction are the two mainstays of preventive skin care. These strategies are initially implemented by the nurse, but the responsibility for skin protection is transferred to the patient as soon as possible. Frequent changes of position are essential throughout the day. They are especially important once the patient is out of bed in a sitting position. Pressure-relieving pads should always be used in wheelchairs. The nurse teaches the patient to perform weight shifts at frequent intervals.

Depending on the patient's mobility limitations, weight shifts may include wheelchair pushups to relieve pressure on the buttocks, leaning over the alternate sides of the wheelchair to shift weight, or brief rest periods with the wheelchair in a full reclining position. Weight is ideally shifted for 2 minutes every 15 minutes.[22] The importance of these routines cannot be overemphasized, as the development of open pressure ulcers creates serious management challenges. Pressure ulcers

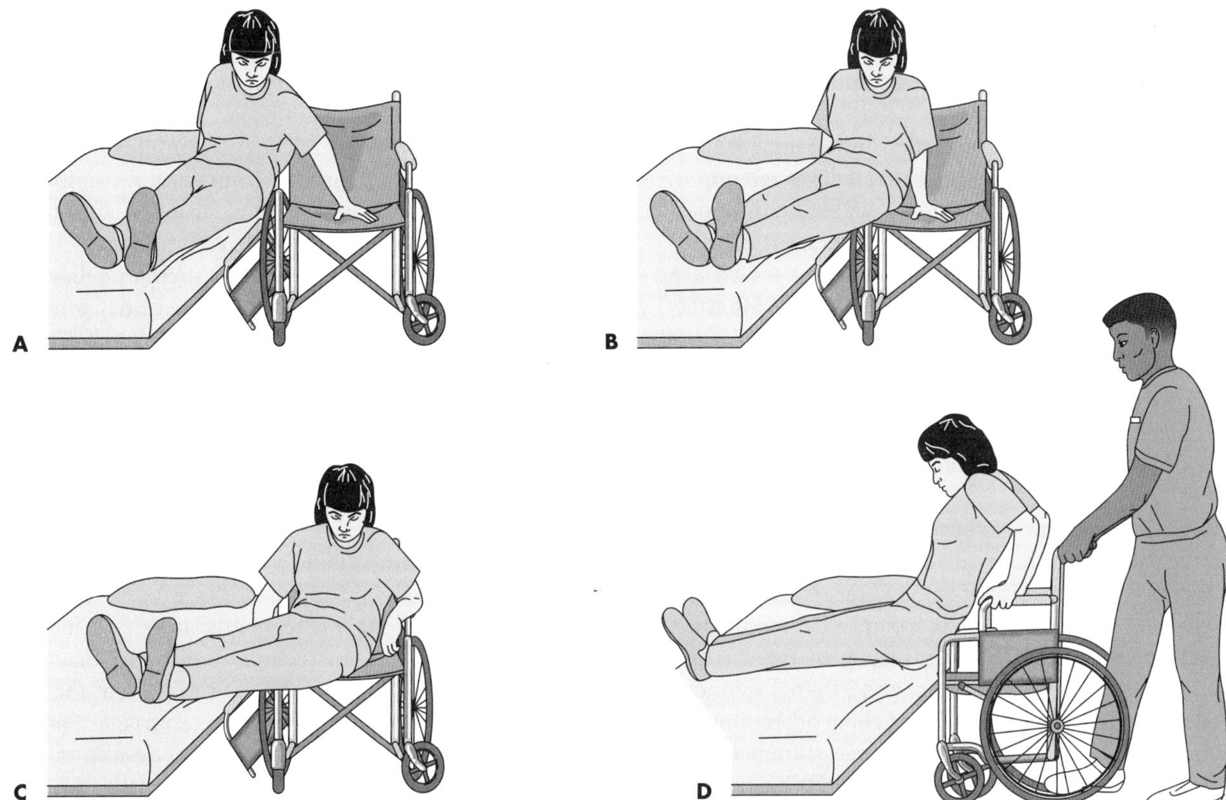

Figure 44-15 Two methods for patient with paraplegia and strong upper extremities to transfer from bed to chair. With one method: **A,** Patient moves sideways (note wheelchair, with right armrest removed, placed next to bed); **B,** then patient uses her arms to lift trunk into chair seat; and **C,** patient settles her hips comfortably into chair; she will then swing footrests into place and lift her legs from bed. **D,** Second method involves patient pushing backward off bed into chair.

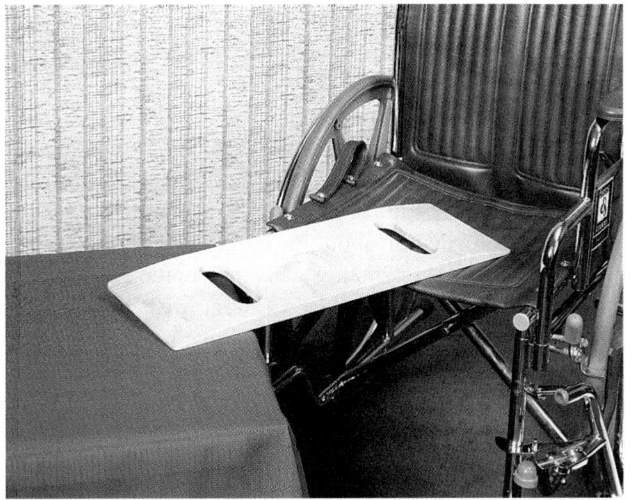

Figure 44-16 Patient with paraplegia whose upper extremity strength is not yet developed can use a sliding board to transfer from bed to chair. Board provides a firm surface on which to move, and trunk is supported by board through the move.

are extremely difficult to heal in patients with SCI and adversely affect the quality of the person's life.

Inspection is the second essential intervention. Pressure causes a period of sustained ischemia for the skin. Reddened areas that do not blanch within 20 to 30 minutes are serious warning signs of pressure damage. The nurse initiates routine skin inspection with each change of position and then teaches the patient to accomplish this task if possible with the use of mirrors or other devices.

The nurse avoids the use of incontinence pads that hold moisture close to the skin. The patient's skin is kept clean, but overdrying through frequent washing or the use of harsh soaps is avoided. The temperature of bath water is carefully monitored, and heating pads and hot water bottles are not used during care. If the patient's care regimen includes the use of braces or splints, a layer of thin cloth should always be worn between the brace and the skin. The nurse ensures that the patient and family receive specific instructions about the proper use and care of each piece of assistive equipment so that secondary injury does not occur. Adequate dietary intake with supplements of vitamin C and zinc help to maintain a positive nitrogen balance and keep the skin healthy.

7. Establishing a Regular Pattern of Urinary Elimination

Urinary tract infections and renal dysfunction are among the leading causes of long-term morbidity and mortality for patients with SCIs.[27] The incidence of UTIs is about 35%.[20] Therefore it is essential for the nurse to establish and maintain an effective regimen for managing urinary elimination. A Foley catheter is initially inserted to help assess the patient's fluid balance and monitor for shock-related complications during the first 3 to 4 days.

Most patients with SCIs have a reflex (autonomic or spastic) bladder. This occurs when the spinal reflexes remain intact, but the inhibiting controls from the higher brain centers are lost. An intermittent catheterization program is initiated in the rehabilitation period after spinal shock resolves. A schedule of catheterization every 3 to 4 hours is usually effective. The goal is to keep urine volumes below 500 ml, and this may require more frequent catheterization.[20] The patient is encouraged to drink at least 3000 ml of fluid daily, but the fluids need to be distributed throughout the day. No more than 600 to 800 ml should be consumed between catheterizations.

Strict aseptic technique is followed for the catheterizations, although the patient may be taught a clean technique to use at home. Patients with injuries at or below C8 are frequently able to manage their catheterizations independently. Stimulation of the bladder wall can lead to contraction of the detrusor muscle and relaxation of the internal and external sphincter with a reflex bladder. Stimuli such as touching or stroking the genitals, or lightly percussing the bladder may stimulate bladder emptying. This phenomenon is called "triggering" or "kicking off." Some patients are able to use this stimulation to induce voiding on command. Initially the amount of urine voided is small, leaving a large residual volume in the bladder. The residual volume can gradually drop to about 100 ml and may permit discontinuation of the catheterization regimen for some patients. Once the bladder is "triggering," the male patient may need to wear an external catheter device to catch urine when the bladder empties spontaneously. Female patients may need to wear disposable protective pads.

The nurse teaches the patient the correct technique for catheterization and instructs the patient to monitor for the presence of hematuria, clouding, increased sediment, or mucus in the urine. These are symptoms of urinary tract infection and need to be reported promptly to the physician. The classic sensory signs of urinary tract infection—burning and urgency—are not present. A urine acidifier such as vitamin C or methenamine hippurate (Hiprex) may be prescribed to help reduce the risk of urinary tract infection, but there is currently no research evidence to support their effectiveness.[20] Urinary antiseptics such as methenamine mandelate (Mandelamine) may also be used. A program of intermittent catheterization is also usually used with patients who have atonic bladders resulting from lower motor neuron damage.

8. Promoting Regular Bowel Elimination

The nurse is also responsible for developing an effective bowel elimination program. Bowel continence is a reasonable goal for many patients with SCI, but problems such as occasional incontinence, constipation, and the time-consuming nature of the regimen are serious causes of anxiety and depression. Bowel dysfunction adversely affects quality of life.[19] With most SCIs the neural innervation that is located in the bowel wall remains intact, although injuries above T6 eliminate the patient's ability to "bear down" using the abdominal muscles.

Planning for bowel evacuation should make use of the patient's normal body rhythms. The gastrocolic reflex, which is responsible for strong peristaltic contractions, is initiated by food and warm liquids and is often strongest after the first meal of the day. Planned bowel evacuation capitalizes on this factor. The nurse assesses the patient's preinjury elimination pattern and establishes an acceptable time of day for defecation. After breakfast is optimal for many people. The patient is positioned in a natural sitting position if possible, and pressure is applied with the hands across the lower abdomen to help compensate for the loss of the abdominal muscles. Stool softeners and suppositories are generally used, and a high-fiber diet is instituted if the patient can tolerate it. In the early phase of bowel training the nurse manually checks the patient's rectum daily for stool to prevent impaction.

Digital stimulation and suppositories are generally used to initiate defecation. The nurse gently inserts a lubricated gloved index finger into the rectum to dilate the anal sphincter. Anesthetic ointments may be used to prevent the spastic reflex responses that digital stimulation can trigger. Small volume enemas may also be used to stimulate defecation if digital stimulation and suppositories alone are ineffective.[19] Stool frequency and consistency are monitored and used to evaluate the effectiveness of the bowel program. Once a regular pattern of bowel elimination has been established, digital stimulation alone plus the ongoing management of diet and fluids may be sufficient to maintain regular bowel elimination. The bowel program needs to be acceptable and manageable for the patient to use at home after discharge. Many patients can achieve independence in bowel management, but ongoing assistance is required for patients with high cord injuries.

9. Supporting Sexual Function

SCI has profound effects on a person's ability to function sexually, and concerns about sexuality are a critical area for nursing intervention. The nurse provides the patient with accurate and specific information about the effects of the injury on sexual response and performance. This information needs to be provided to every patient with SCI along with written reference materials to supplement the teaching; research indicates that postdischarge support and education are also extremely important (see Research box). Generally, the higher the injury the more normal sexual functioning can be. Sacral injuries are the only SCIs that eliminate a man's ability to achieve any type of erection.

Effective nursing intervention in the area of sexuality requires far more than simple factual information. The nurse must explore each individual's sexual beliefs and practices and establish the parameters for acceptable sexual activity. Although most patients with an SCI are able to engage in satisfying sexual activity with a cooperative partner, clearly not all sexual alternatives are acceptable to every couple. The nurse also emphasizes to patients that sexuality encompasses far more than just intercourse.

Research

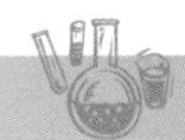

Reference: Byfield MG et al: Perception versus reality: inpatient sexual health needs of individuals with acute spinal cord injury, *SCI Psychosocial Process* 12(1):1, 4-8, 1999.

This study was designed to identify the perceived sexual health needs of patients with new spinal cord injuries. Forty-two patients were included in the study. Questionnaires were administered at several points in the treatment period. Analysis of the results indicated that patients tend to initially underestimate the impact of their injury on their ability to function sexually. They need to confront and cope with these realities in the postdischarge period when services are not as readily available. In-depth teaching and support services need to be targeted toward the postdischarge period and offered in the community setting for both patients and families.

Most men with SCIs are not able to experience psychogenic erections (those that occur in response to sexual thoughts), but they are usually capable of reflexogenic erections. Reflex erections occur from direct stimulation of the genitalia, but may also result from stroking the inner thigh, rectal stimulation, or manipulation of a urinary catheter. The ability to ejaculate is usually not present or may occur in a retrograde fashion; but orgasm, with a perceived release of tension, is possible. Patients often report that along with the extensive sensory loss associated with the injury, there is heightened sensitivity in the remaining intact tissue. The woman with a SCI is able to participate fully in sexual activity, but may not experience orgasm. Women also frequently require the application of a water-soluble lubricant to replace natural lubricating fluids.

The nurse stresses that spontaneous sexual activity is rarely possible or successful after SCI and that open communication between the partners is essential. Men with indwelling catheters can either remove the catheter just before sexual activity or fold it back on the penis and use the catheter to provide extra support for the erection. Women who have indwelling catheters can also leave them in place if desired. Both urinary catheterization and bowel emptying should be completed before intercourse to prevent the possibility of reflex emptying.

A variety of sexual resources are available for men whose reflex erections do not last long enough to engage in sexual activity. These include implants, injections, and vacuum pumps and are discussed more fully in Chapter 55. Nurses who are uncomfortable discussing sexual matters with patients should ensure that referrals are made to advanced practice nurses or other appropriate resources.

Most men with SCI experience infertility or low sperm counts, but this needs to be verified by laboratory analysis before sterility can be assumed. Sperm harvesting, artificial insemination, and in vitro fertilization offer couples the hope of successful pregnancy.[9] Women with SCIs typically retain their ability to conceive. The menstrual cycle is interrupted by the injury, but usually resumes after about 4 to 6 months, reestablishing fertility. Birth control counseling is therefore essential. Pregnancy can proceed safely after SCI, and infants can be successfully delivered vaginally, although there is an increased incidence of urinary tract infections and autonomic dysreflexia during both pregnancy and labor (see p. 1425).

10. Supporting Family Coping Resources

SCI has devastating effects on the patient and the entire family unit. Patients experience a wide range of emotional responses. Roles and relationships are abruptly and often permanently altered by the injury, and the family's sense of the future is shattered. The rapid pace and intensity of the initial rehabilitation period propel the patient and family at breakneck speed toward an unclear and often frightening future. The nurse needs to be aware of the range of possible responses to crisis and be skilled in assisting patients and families to progress toward effective coping.

Grieving is an essential task for both patient and family. The patient grieves the loss of functional abilities, and family members grieve the loss of the family unit as it was before the injury.[10] Each person moves through the stages of grief at a different pace. Family members are often so focused on being positive and supportive for the patient that they fail to acknowledge their own needs. SCI affects the entire family and may strain a marriage to the breaking point. The spouse is challenged to assume significant caregiving roles while frequently becoming the primary breadwinner. Both physical and emotional intimacy can be adversely affected.[9] The nurse plays a pivotal role in helping each family member deal openly and honestly with these complex feelings.

The nurse uses the principles of crisis theory to assist patients and families cope. Shock and disbelief dominate the first stage of care when the focus is on survival. As the physical crisis stabilizes, denial typically appears. The denial may center on the permanence of the situation or on some specific part of the injury such as the inability to walk. The nurse does not attempt to break the denial but attempts to focus the patient and family on the here and now and on actions and interventions that are necessary to meet the challenges of the present. As the reaction stage is entered, the full range of emotional responses may be encountered, but severe depression alternating with anger is an extremely common pattern.[9] Encouraging verbalization and providing consistent support are important nursing interventions. Multidisciplinary resources are used to ensure that the patient and family receive the support they need (see Research box).

In addition to the obvious psychologic challenges of SCI, the patient is also dealing with massive changes in the level of sensory input received from the body and the limited world that results from immobility. The patient is confronted with the helplessness and lack of control that result from being unable to perform self-care or possibly even change positions. The reality of total dependency can be overwhelming. The range of emotional responses is virtually unlimited but frequently includes intense anger, fear, and depression. Acting-out behaviors are expected at some point in the rehabilitation experience. Consistent caregivers are highly desirable, and the nurse must accept the patient's behavior

Research

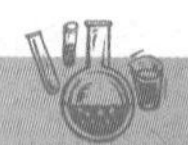

Reference: Kennedy P, Rogers BA: Anxiety and depression after spinal cord injury: a longitudinal analysis, *Arch Phys Med Rehabil* 81(7):932-937, 2000.

This study monitored a group of more than 100 patients who experienced traumatic spinal cord injury through the acute stage and for 2 years after discharge. Tools such as the Beck Depression Inventory, Beck Hopelessness Scale, State Anxiety Inventory, Social Support Questionnaire, and the functional independence measure were administered at intervals in the study period and the results analyzed for trends. Data revealed a consistent and striking pattern of heightened anxiety and depression across patient subcategories that were predictably highest during the acute care period but continued unabated long into the postdischarge period.

without being judgmental. Limit setting may become necessary. The physical, emotional, and financial impact of the patient's injury also becomes increasingly clear to the family, who may face an indefinite future of extensive caregiving responsibility. This can be particularly difficult when the injury affects a teenager or young adult and when alcohol, drug use, or other self-destructive behavior contributed to the injury.

Coping evolves over time, and it may take years to reach the stage of grief resolution. With support, the patient gradually becomes an active participant in care. The patient is then supported in making decisions and assuming some control in structuring the rehabilitation. Early mobility is a key strategy for effectively moving the patient past the stages of denial and reaction. The nurse reminds the patient and family that aggressive rehabilitation accomplishes solid functional outcomes after severe SCI, and almost 90% of SCI patients do return to their home settings.

EVALUATION

To evaluate the effectiveness of nursing interventions, compare patient behaviors with those stated in the expected patient outcomes. Achievement of patient outcomes is successful if the patient with an SCI:

1. Maintains spontaneous and adequate ventilation and experiences neither dyspnea nor hypoxia.
2. Uses quad-assisted coughing to adequately clear the airway.
3. Maintains stable vital signs without incidence of orthostatic hypotension.
4. Adjusts clothing and environmental conditions to maintain body temperature at 98° F (36.8° C).
5. Easily moves joints through their full range of motion; uses wheelchair and other assistive devices to support mobility.
6. Uses pressure-relieving devices and frequent weight shifts to maintain an intact skin.
7. Implements a spontaneous voiding or intermittent catheterization program to effectively empty the bladder and minimize episodes of incontinence.
8. Uses a bowel program to evacuate soft, formed stool daily or every other day without episodes of incontinence.
9. Speaks openly with partner about sexual effects of the SCI and refers to self as a sexual being.
10. Actively engages in the rehabilitation process and plans collaboratively with the family for the future.

GERONTOLOGIC CONSIDERATIONS

SCI is a devastating and life-altering process at any point in a person's life. Although most SCIs occur in young adults, about 20% occur in persons over 65 years old. These injuries are usually the result of falls and often reflect the weakening of vertebra related to osteoporosis. The challenges of SCI that have been outlined in the prior discussion can be even more overwhelming for the older person. Older adults experience an increased mortality related to respiratory failure, aspiration, and pneumonia; and they have more difficulty compensating for the other consequences of spinal shock.[28] The incidence of DVT and related pulmonary emboli is higher, and these complications are also more severe in older adults than in younger individuals.

The functional losses of SCI are also often more severe for older adults. Concurrent health problems contribute to increased complications and reduce self-care potential. The demands on families can be overwhelming and are compounded by distance, career, and nuclear family responsibilities. The dual challenges of dependency and depression can become insurmountable. Older adults with SCIs are less likely to achieve rehabilitation goals and are more likely to be placed in long-term custodial care.

SPECIAL ENVIRONMENTS FOR CARE

Critical Care

Critical care plays a significant role in the initial management of patients with SCIs, particularly injuries involving the cervical region of the cord. Motor vehicle accidents are the most common cause of SCIs, and these accidents frequently involve multiple trauma and head injury in addition to the SCI. Patients may be managed in surgical intensive care units or in specialized neurologic care areas.

Critical care monitoring and management are particularly vital in the treatment of unstable spinal injuries, especially if cervical traction is used to stabilize the spine. The use of specialized beds such as the kinetic treatment table requires constant nursing assessment and monitoring. Critical care expertise is essential in monitoring the patient's ongoing respiratory effort and appropriately timing the need for intubation and mechanical ventilation.

Critical care monitoring is also essential in the management of the complex hemodynamic instability that results when both hypovolemic and spinal shock occur. Hemodynamic monitoring is frequently required to adequately assess fluid balance and cardiac output (see Chapter 14). The presence of head trauma adds the additional challenge of intracranial pressure monitoring to this already complex situation.

Community-Based Care

The ultimate goal of aggressive multidisciplinary rehabilitation after SCI is to help the patient achieve the maximum self-care potential and return to the home environment. In the current world of managed care the patient's acute care hospital stay is likely to be quite brief. The patient is transferred to an acute rehabilitation setting as soon as he or she is hemodynamically stable and the problems of spinal instability and malalignment have been resolved. The patient is likely to be transferred to at least one or two additional facilities that focus on long-term SCI rehabilitation.

Case management is essential after SCI, and the nurse is the ideal professional to serve as a case manager for patients with SCIs. Social services and community resources need to be activated from the time of the patient's admission to allow adequate time for thoughtful planning about placements and the acquisition of needed equipment for patient care in the home or community. Social services are also essential to assist the family in dealing with the maze of financial costs and insurance coverage. Discharge planning must truly begin at admission even though the patient and family's shock and disbelief make it difficult for them to play an active role in the early planning.

Most patients require long-term rehabilitation. A total of 90% of patients with SCI eventually return to a home setting, but the path is neither straight nor easily traveled. The problems that accompany SCI are lifelong. Effective management focuses on long-term physical and psychosocial support to minimize the incidence and severity of complications.

COMPLICATIONS

The patient with an SCI is vulnerable to a wide range of complications, primarily related to immobility. Fecal impaction, pulmonary infections, contractures, skin breakdown, and urinary tract infection are all commonly occurring problems. Much of the patient's daily self-care routine is aimed at preventing the occurrence of these complications. Prevention strategies are discussed under nursing interventions. SCI patients are also vulnerable to several complications that are not routinely amenable to prevention, and these are discussed next.

Autonomic Dysreflexia. Autonomic dysreflexia is a unique complication of SCI that occurs in patients with cord injuries at T6 or above. The problem is most common in patients with cervical injuries. Autonomic dysreflexia is an exaggerated sympathetic response, which results in uncontrolled paroxysmal hypertension. The spinal nerves that innervate the preganglionic neurons of the sympathetic nervous system emerge from the thoracic and lumbar regions of the spine. The thoracic chain has primary control over vascular resistance. When injuries affect the upper cord, the sympathetic nervous system is shut off from the control of higher centers in the brain. During the period of spinal shock the sympathetic nervous system ceases to function below the level of the injury. As the hemodynamic instability gradually resolves, the sympathetic nervous system regains function but in an uncontrolled manner. When autonomic dysreflexia is triggered, a group of stimuli produce a massive sympathetic reflex discharge that causes profound vasoconstriction. The abrupt rise in blood pressure distends the baroreceptors in the carotid sinus and aortic arch. These baroreceptors stimulate the vagus nerve to slow the heart and induce vasodilation in the vessels above the level of the cord injury in an attempt to reduce the blood pressure. The intense sympathetic response continues below the level of the injury, however, because the inhibitive impulses from the higher centers are blocked. The majority of the blood vessels remain constricted, and extreme hypertension persists (Figure 44-17).

The clinical manifestations of autonomic dysreflexia are summarized in the Clinical Manifestations box. Paroxysmal hypertension is the classic defining feature, and the blood pressure can rapidly reach life-threatening levels. The hypertension is accompanied by a pounding headache, nausea, and blurred vision. Vasodilation above the injury level results in skin flushing and profuse perspiration in those areas. The continuing vasoconstriction in areas below the level of the injury causes cool pale skin and piloerection (goosebumps). The bradycardia produced by excess vagal stimulation can be severe. Patients experience variations in the symptom pattern but most patients are able to promptly recognize their own unique pattern of symptoms.

The abnormal stimuli that trigger autonomic dysreflexia arise from localized areas below the level of injury. Although a variety of stimuli can trigger the response (Box 44-3), the most common cause is some form of visceral stimulation—a distended bladder or stool in the rectum. A full bladder triggers 80% of all cases.[22]

Autonomic dysreflexia is a medical emergency that can result in stroke, blindness, or death. The major goal is to prevent episodes from occurring by maintaining effective regimens for bladder emptying and bowel evacuation to prevent overdistention. If the syndrome occurs, however, prompt treatment is essential. The patient is immediately placed in an upright position, which triggers orthostatic changes and helps to lower the blood pressure. Vital signs are monitored as frequently as every 5 minutes. Antiembolism compression stockings, elastic bandages, abdominal binders, and pneumatic compression stockings are all removed to promote venous pooling and reduce blood return to the heart.[3] If the patient has a urinary catheter, its patency is immediately checked. If the patient is using an intermittent catheterization routine, the bladder is immediately catheterized. If the dysreflexia does not resolve immediately, the nurse next checks the patient's rectum for the presence of stool. If it is necessary to remove stool from the rectum, dibucaine (Nupercaine) ointment or another anesthetic cream should be applied before inserting the finger. This prevents triggering another visceral stimulus and worsening the dysreflexia. If the triggering stimulus cannot be promptly identified and removed by these measures, most

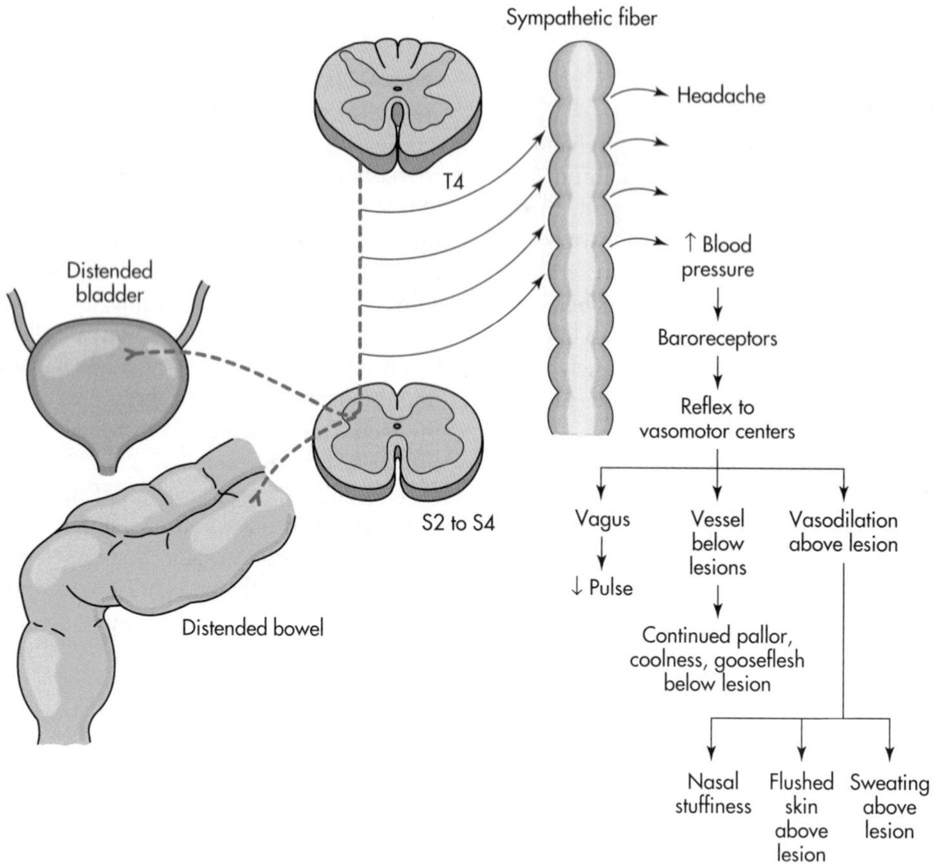

Figure 44-17 Pictorial diagram of causes of autonomic dysreflexia and results.

Clinical Manifestations

Autonomic Dysreflexia

Extreme hypertension
Pounding headache
Blurred vision, nausea
Bradycardia
Profuse sweating above the level of the injury
Flushed skin on the face and neck
Nasal congestion
Piloerection below the level of the injury
Cool, mottled skin below the level of the injury

BOX 44-3 Common Precipitating Factors for Autonomic Dysreflexia

Bladder distention (80% of all cases)
Distended bowel
Local pressure or irritation (especially to the penis, groin, or sacrum); pressure ulcers
Constrictive clothing
Catheterization of bladder; digital stimulation of rectum/anus
Exposure to hot or cold stimuli or drafts
Abdominal or pelvic distention or infection
- Menstruation
- Urinary tract infection
- Urinary calculi
- Sexual activity, ejaculation
- Gastritis, peptic ulcers, or gallstones
- Labor contractions

Muscle spasticity or pain

SCI unit protocols call for the prompt administration of emergency medications to lower the blood pressure (e.g., reserpine, hydralazine, guanethidine, nitroprusside, or diazoxide). Guidelines for safe practice with the patient experiencing autonomic dysreflexia are summarized in the accompanying Guidelines for Safe Practice box.

It is important to remember that patients become vulnerable to autonomic dysreflexia only after the period of spinal shock has been resolved. The two problems do not occur together. Once spinal reflexes begin to return, the risk of dysreflexia increases. Up to 80% of patients at risk develop dysreflexia within the first year after injury, although it has been known to occur for the first time several years after the initial injury. The incidence and severity of dysreflexia typically decrease over time.

Guidelines for Safe Practice

The Patient With Autonomic Dysreflexia

Elevate the head of the bed to a sitting position if possible.
Monitor the blood pressure and apical pulse every 2 to 5 minutes until the episode resolves.
Check the patency of the retention catheter if present.
- Ensure that it is not kinked or plugged. Insert new catheter as needed.
- Catheterize immediately if a retention catheter is not in place.

If dysreflexia persists, check for bowel impaction.
- If stool is present, apply an anesthetic agent to the rectum and anal area and monitor response.
- Stool can be gently removed once the blood pressure is lowered.

Initiate drug therapy as outlined in care protocols if blood pressure does not respond and notify the physician promptly.
If no cause can be identified:
- Change the patient's position.
- Send a urine specimen for culture and sensitivity.
- Assess the skin carefully for signs of irritation or breakdown.

Remain with the patient to provide support, reassurance, and needed explanations.

Spasticity. Spinal reflex activity begins to reappear with the resolution of spinal shock, and muscle spasticity can become a serious concern for patients whose spinal cord injuries affect the upper portions of the spinal cord. The appearance of spinal reflex activity is not an indication of returning function because the muscle movement is not under voluntary control, but it can represent false hope to patients who are experiencing extreme denial of the consequences of the SCI. The heightened muscle responsiveness does add resting tone to the flaccid muscles and may make it easier to move the patient and prevent muscle wasting. However, it also creates safety concerns and heightens the risk for contractures.[26] Flexor spasticity appears within the first 6 months and creates a risk for flexion contractures. Flexion contractures significantly limit a patient's rehabilitation and self-care potential and must be successfully prevented. Extensor spasticity develops later. Both sustained (tonic) and intermittent (clonic) spasticity can occur. Most patients experience a peak of spasticity within the first year after injury, which then stabilizes within about 2 years. The amount and severity of spasms may also be a reflection of other complications and need to be carefully evaluated.

Positioning and exercise are the two primary interventions for managing spasticity. The frequency of passive range-of-motion exercise is increased to at least four times a day as general muscle stiffness tends to worsen the spasticity. The nurse limits the amount of incidental tactile stimulation while providing care and handles the patient's limbs in a gentle yet firm manner. The patient's position is changed at least every 2 hours, and the joints are carefully positioned to prevent contracture. Splints may be needed to support optimal positioning in vulnerable joints such as the fingers. Physical and occupational therapists establish an appropriate exercise plan for the patient and design effective splinting devices. Noxious stimuli are avoided where possible, as spasticity is triggered by many of the same factors that cause autonomic dysreflexia. Spasticity that does not respond to these general measures may require the use of muscle relaxant medications such as baclofen (Lioresal), dantrolene (Dantrium), or diazepam (Valium). Long-term implantable delivery systems may be used if symptoms persist.[20] In severe cases surgical intervention with rhizotomy (section of the spinal nerve roots) or a similar procedure may be necessary.

Pain. The origins of pain following SCI are not completely understood, and there is no clear correlation between the pain and the level or completeness of the injury. Nevertheless pain can be an ongoing challenge for selected patients.[20] Pain in the early postinjury period is usually related to the fracture and soft tissue damage of the initial trauma. This pain usually responds well to traditional measures and decreases dramatically once the spine is decompressed, realigned, and stabilized.

Chronic pain syndromes can develop after SCI and become extremely difficult management issues. These syndromes are slightly more common with injuries that affect the lower portions of the spine, particularly the cauda equina, and seem to occur more frequently when the injury is incomplete. Most develop within the first 6 months after the injury. Management options vary with the nature and severity of the symptoms.

Radicular pain is produced by specific spinal nerve roots and causes an aching or shooting pain along the path of the nerve. Mild cases are often managed successfully with anticonvulsant drugs such as carbamazepine (Tegretol). Visceral pain is poorly localized and creates a burning or aching that diffuses throughout the abdomen or pelvis. Central pain is also diffuse and creates a general burning sensation that is aggravated by movement or touch. The latter two forms of chronic pain are theorized to occur from the abnormal firing of pain neurons, possibly because of the absence of normal sensory input that helps the nerves to maintain a steady state. These types of pain may be more responsive to interventions such as transcutaneous electrical nerve stimulation (TENS), or the use of tricyclic antidepressant medications such as imipramine (Tofranil) than to the use of more traditional analgesics. See Chapter 12 for a discussion of various forms of pain and their management. SCI pain is a complex problem, and patients can benefit from the involvement of an interdisciplinary pain management team. It is important to reassure the patient that caregivers accept the reality of the pain and will work collaboratively to find acceptable management strategies.

TUMORS OF THE SPINAL CORD

Etiology/Epidemiology

Both primary and secondary tumors affect the spinal cord. Primary tumors arise from the substance of the cord and meninges or from the surrounding bone or blood vessels. Primary spinal tumors are relatively rare and their

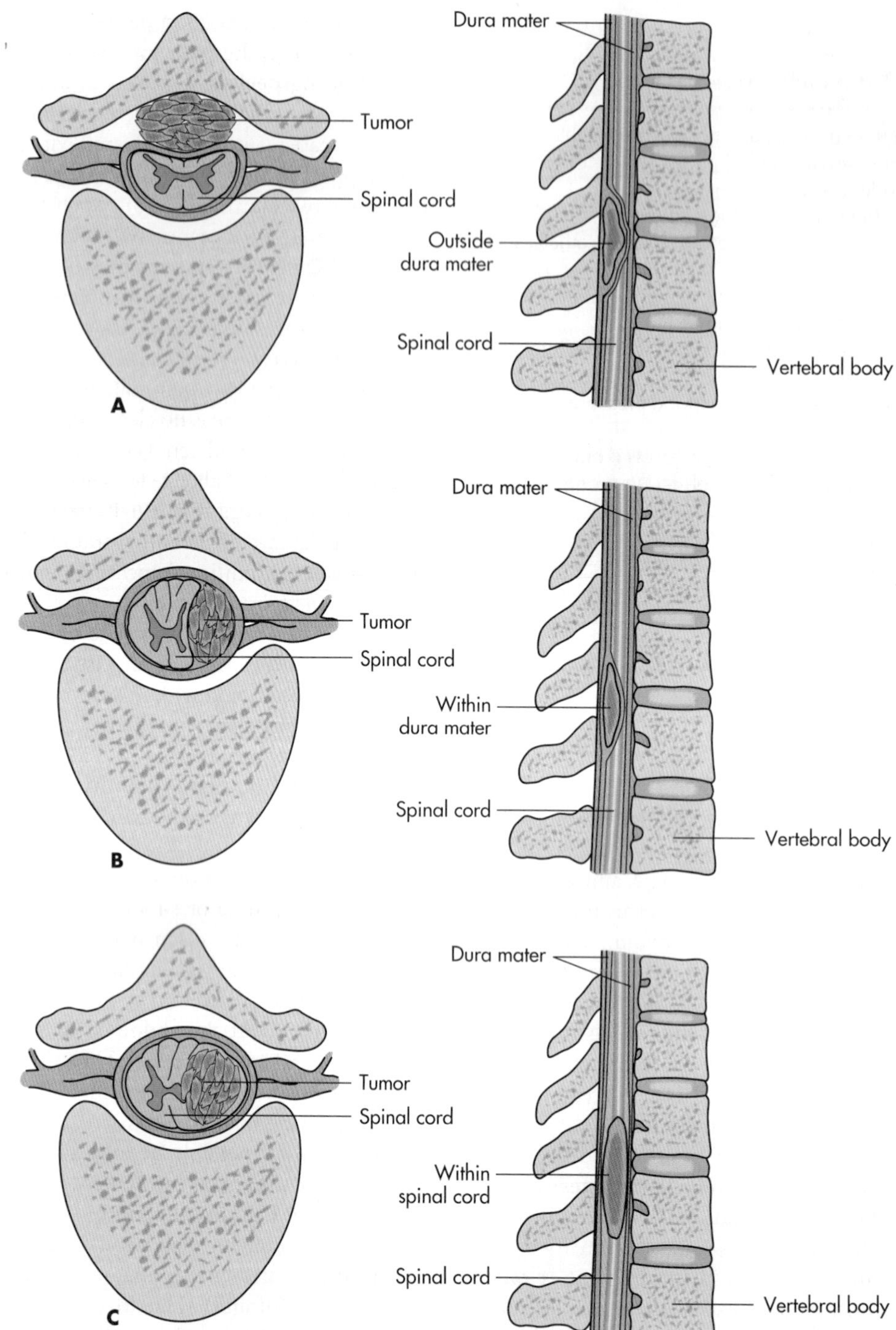

Figure 44-18 Spinal tumors. **A,** Extradural tumors–outside the dura mater. **B,** Subdural tumors–within the dura mater. **C,** Intramedullary tumors–within the spinal cord.

etiology is unknown.[3] A significant number of primary spinal tumors are benign, but the outcomes of spinal cord compression are just as serious as those caused by malignant neoplasms. The vast majority of primary spinal tumors are extramedullary, arising outside the substance of the spinal cord (Figure 44-18). Common examples include meningiomas and nerve sheath tumors. Primary spinal tumors affect both sexes and related risk factors are unknown. Spinal meningiomas affect women much more frequently than men (>80%) and the vast majority develop in the thoracic spine.[3] Men are affected much less often and their tumors appear equally in the cervical and thoracic spine. Most primary spinal tumors affect adults between 40 and 70 years old.

Secondary spinal cord tumors are metastatic and can be traced to primary tumors in other organs of the body.[3] They are three to four times as common as primary spinal tumors. Secondary tumors occur from primary sites in the lungs, breast, and prostate, and most of them are located in the epidural space in the lower thoracic spine and rarely infiltrate the spinal cord itself. The vast majority of metastatic tumors affect the richly vascular vertebral body or paravertebral tissue.

Pathophysiology

The pathologic consequences of both primary and secondary spinal tumors are primarily related to the effects of cord compression. Infiltration and invasion occur much less commonly. Pressure can irritate the spinal nerve roots, displace the cord, interrupt perfusion, cause ischemia and edema, and obstruct the flow of cerebrospinal fluid. The combined effects of pressure and edema cause the typical symptoms of pain, weakness, and motor and sensory loss.[3] The exact symptoms relate to the specific level of the spine affected by the tumor. The rate of tumor growth is important. Slow-growing tumors allow time for the spinal cord to initially adapt and may produce few symptoms until quite advanced. A rapidly growing tumor, particularly one composed of dense tissue, causes significant amounts of responsive edema.

Pain, with or without accompanying neurologic deficits, is the first symptom in 95% of patients with spinal tumors.[3] The pain may be localized or radiate along the path of the involved spinal nerve root. The pain varies in intensity from mild to severe. Sensory losses reflect the exact anatomic location of the compression within the cord and may be accompanied by weakness or paralysis in the same nerve distribution. Tumors are a common cause of anterior cord syndrome as discussed on p. 1406.

Collaborative Care Management

The diagnosis of a spinal cord tumor begins with a detailed history and neurologic examination. The diagnostic tests of choice are CT and enhanced MRI, although myelography may also be used. MRI clearly visualizes tumors in the vertebral bodies as well as those within the cord itself. Treatment is aimed at relieving pain and preserving neurologic function.

Surgical intervention is the treatment of choice for most primary spinal tumors. The surgery is often technically complex, especially when the blood supply is involved. Surgery is used less commonly in the management of secondary metastatic tumors and usually focuses on decompression of the spinal cord and debulking of the tumor to improve the patient's quality of life. Radiation therapy is the primary treatment approach for many secondary tumors and all tumors that exhibit invasive growth patterns that make complete surgical excision impossible. Radiation is an effective palliative strategy for relieving pain in patients with advanced disease. Administration of steroids is frequently combined with radiotherapy to minimize spinal cord edema. Chemotherapy has little documented effectiveness in the management of spinal tumors, although adjunctive hormonal treatment may be useful when the primary cancer site is the breast or prostate gland. Immobilization is a priority if the spine is unstable. Immobilization may involve simple bed rest with the patient in correct body alignment or the use of cervical collars, thoracic braces, and shells. Surgical stabilization may become necessary.

Patient/Family Education. Some of the nursing care priorities for patients with spinal tumors parallel those discussed under SCI. This is particularly true for the management of bowel and bladder problems. SCI, however, represents a single traumatic injury, and care is focused on restoring independence and limiting the incidence of complications. Patients with symptomatic spinal cord tumors are often in an advanced stage of a complex battle against cancer. The nurse plans holistically with the patient and family to clarify their goals and priorities for care. Ongoing meticulous assessment is critical to recognize subtle changes in the patient's status. Pain management may be an important issue requiring the input of a multidisciplinary pain team. Quality of life issues are a priority.

A major patient care goal is to return the patient to the home environment. To achieve this goal the family may need to learn transfer techniques, use of assistive equipment, a bowel and bladder regimen, positioning principles, pain management, and skin care. The nurse assesses the needs of both patient and family for community-based services and support and initiates appropriate referrals. A hospice referral may be appropriate. Both the patient and family require extensive teaching and support to adequately address each major area of concern.

CRANIAL NERVE DISEASES/DISORDERS

The three classic disorders affecting the cranial nerves are Meniere's disease, trigeminal neuralgia, and Bell's palsy. Meniere's disease is presented in Chapter 60 because of its primary effects on the auditory and vestibular systems. Trigeminal neuralgia and Bell's palsy are discussed here.

Trigeminal Neuralgia (Tic Douloureux)

Etiology/Epidemiology

Trigeminal neuralgia, a chronic condition affecting one or more branches of the fifth cranial nerve (trigeminal), causes intense paroxysmal pain along its pathway. No etiology has been clearly identified for the disorder, although a variety of associated factors are recognized. The most widely accepted theory of disease etiology involves injury or vascular compression of the nerve root resulting in irritation or even demyelination[14] (Figure 44-19). Trauma and infection in the teeth or jaw are often associated with the development of the pain syndrome. Other cases are believed to result from pressure on the trigeminal nerve as it exits the brainstem. The pressure can originate from an adjacent artery or the presence of an aneurysm or tumor.[4]

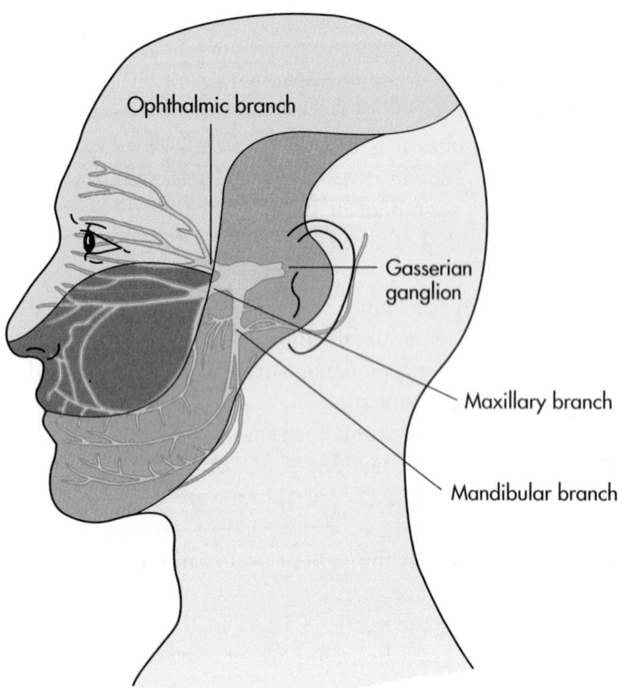

Figure 44-19 Pathway of trigeminal nerve and the facial areas innervated by each of its three main divisions.

Trigeminal neuralgia can occur at any age but is most common in middle-aged or older individuals. Women are affected more often than men.[21] The disease typically follows a pattern of exacerbation and remission, with the patient experiencing pain episodes over a period of weeks or months and then undergoing spontaneous remission of variable length. Trigeminal neuralgia is the most common facial neuralgia syndrome and is believed to be one of the most painful of all conditions.[14] The incidence and severity of the pain have a significant negative impact on the patient's quality of life and even on the ability to maintain self-care and adequate nutrition.

Pathophysiology

The trigeminal nerve exits the pons and merges into the gasserian ganglion before it separates into its three major branches (see Figure 44-19). The trigeminal nerve is the largest of the cranial nerves and has both motor and sensory fibers. The pain syndrome primarily affects the maxillary branch followed by the mandibular branch of the nerve. Involvement of the ophthalmic branch is rare. The pain typically affects the right side of the face for no known reason.[14] The pain occurs abruptly, lasts from a few seconds to a few minutes, and can recur at any time. Typically described as intense, piercing, burning, or "like a lightening bolt," the pain affects only one side of the face, and there are no identifiable motor or sensory deficits in the regions served by the nerve.

The classic pain pattern is the only diagnostic feature of trigeminal neuralgia, and the diagnosis is made by excluding other possible causes of facial pain. A head CT may be performed to rule out the presence of an intruding lesion, and an MRI can be useful in identifying the presence of demyelinating disease. Significant pathologic changes are frequently found in the myelin sheath of the nerve, which predisposes the nerve to erratic and hyperexcitable firing.[15] Most patients are able to identify specific trigger points along the course of the nerve where the slightest stimulus can initiate pain. Chewing, talking, smiling, brushing the teeth, cold liquids, and even a draft of air can trigger the pain.[4] Patients typically go to great lengths to avoid a triggering stimulus. It is not uncommon for patients to socially isolate themselves or neglect routine personal hygiene such as washing the face, brushing the teeth, or shaving in an effort to avoid pain. Significant weight loss can occur if chewing is a triggering stimulus.

Collaborative Care Management

Treatment options for trigeminal neuralgia include both medical and surgical options. Interventions seek to prevent or block the pain episodes in the most minimally invasive way and usually begin with drug therapy. In all, 80% of patients respond positively, at least initially, to treatment with anticonvulsants.[14] Carbamazepine (Tegretol) is the drug of choice. Carbamazepine is a sodium channel blocker that inhibits transmission of impulses that are perceived as pain. It is usually successful in lessening the frequency and duration of the pain episodes, but it may not be able to eliminate them. Phenytoin (Dilantin), gabapentin (Neurontin), clonazepam (Klonopin), or baclofen (Lioresal) may all be used if carbamazepine is ineffective.

In patients with refractory disease, alcohol or phenol injections, glycerol injections, cryotherapy, or thermocoagulation may be used to temporarily block specific branches of the nerve. Results are usually positive but rarely last beyond 12 to 18 months and may create an unacceptable degree of facial anesthesia.[4] Patients with uncontrolled pain often require surgery. The most common procedure involves percutaneous electrocoagulation of the nerve roots, which provides lasting pain relief with minimal destruction of the other sensory functions of the nerve. The procedure is performed with the patient under conscious sedation. Surgeons may also use a posterior fossa craniotomy to adequately visualize the trigeminal nerve and relieve any existing vascular compression. Block nerve rhizotomy is performed in intractable cases.

Patient/Family Education. The presence of trigeminal neuralgia can have devastating outcomes for the patient's daily lifestyle. The nurse assesses the patient's response to the disease process and ensures that both the patient and family have accurate information about the disease and the various treatment options. Medication teaching is particularly important, as anticonvulsants and muscle relaxants may affect the patient's alertness and safety during routine daily activities. Carbamazepine can cause myelosuppression and ongoing blood studies are important. The nurse assists the patient to explore ways to minimize triggering episodes and to modify the diet as needed to maintain a stable body weight. Alternatives for oral hygiene may also need to be explored if routine tooth brushing initiates pain.

Postoperative neurologic assessments help determine the presence and severity of any motor or sensory compromise. With lost or diminished pain sensation, the patient is instructed to avoid rubbing the eye on the affected side and to monitor the eye regularly for signs of irritation or infection. Regular dental care is also necessary when the protective pain warning sign is absent. A Nursing Care Plan for a patient with trigeminal neuralgia follows.

Bell's Palsy

Etiology/Epidemiology

Bell's palsy involves an acute paralysis of cranial nerve VII, the facial nerve, resulting in loss of motor, sensory, and parasympathetic function on one side of the face. The etiology of the disease is unknown, but it often follows a viral upper respiratory tract infection. The disease usually affects adults between 20 and 60 years old, and the incidence in men and

Nursing Care Plan — Patient With Trigeminal Neuralgia

DATA Mrs. P. is a 56-year-old teacher in whom trigeminal neuralgia was diagnosed 3 years ago. Her initial episodes were short and followed by an extended period of remission, but over the past year the attacks have been occurring more frequently and lasting longer each time. Mrs. P. is being managed through the neurologic service at a teaching hospital. Her physician has suggested surgery as the next logical step in her care. Mrs. P. is reluctant to agree to microsurgery despite the incapacitating nature of her pain episodes.

Nursing assessment reveals that Mrs. P.:

Has stable vital signs

Continues to lose weight from the difficulties she encounters while eating

Takes carbamazepine (Tegretol) faithfully but dislikes the drowsiness it causes

Has experienced no change in laboratory findings

Had to take disability retirement this year because of incapacitating pain

Is difficult to understand because her voice is low and she barely opens her mouth to speak

Has noticeably foul breath odor

Is generally unkempt in appearance (more unkempt than at last visit)

Rarely leaves her house except to keep her clinic appointments and keeps her phone unplugged

NURSING DIAGNOSIS **Chronic pain related to activation of trigger zones along the nerve pathway**
GOALS/OUTCOMES Will achieve pain-free status

NOC Suggested Outcomes
- Pain Level (2102)
- Pain Control (1605)
- Pain: Disruptive Effects (2101)

NIC Suggested Interventions
- Pain Management (1400)
- Analgesic Management (2210)
- Coping Enhancement (5230)

Nursing Interventions/Rationales
- Assess current pain management strategies and their effectiveness (pharmacologic and nonpharmacologic). *This is done to establish a baseline for measuring effectiveness of new pain control strategies.*
- Assess patient's knowledge of specific trigger activities for pain (chewing, talking, smiling/laughing, heat/cold, drafts, pressure, grooming, or mouth care). *This is done to identify factors that can be manipulated by pain control interventions.*
- Explore acceptability of cognitive and behavioral strategies to use in pain management (relaxation, imagery, distraction). *The patient must believe that nonpharmacologic strategies can be effective adjuncts to pain management.*
- Consult with physician, nurse practitioner, and pain management service regarding options for drug therapy. *Chronic pain necessitates a multidisciplinary approach to management.*
- Encourage patient to take medication at regular intervals and to use analgesics at the first sign of pain. *Steady blood levels increase drug effectiveness, and analgesics work more effectively if administered before pain reaches severe levels.*

Evaluation Parameters
1. Reports control of pain at acceptable level
2. No evidence of pain (facial grimace, withdrawn behavior, slowed speech)
3. Uses pain control methods consistently

Continued

Nursing Care Plan *Patient With Trigeminal Neuralgia—cont'd*

NURSING DIAGNOSIS **Imbalanced nutrition: less than body requirements related to fear of triggering pain with eating**
GOALS/OUTCOMES Will maintain weight within 5 pounds of baseline

NOC Suggested Outcomes
- Nutritional Status (1004)
- Nutritional Status: Nutrient Intake (1009)
- Pain Control (1605)

NIC Suggested Interventions
- Nutrition Monitoring (1160)
- Nutrition Management (1100)
- Pain Management (1400)

Nursing Interventions/Rationales
- Complete 24-hour recall assessment of dietary intake. *This provides objective data to determine adequacy of diet.*
- Explore dietary modifications to increase nutrient intake without exacerbating pain (consistency, texture, liquid supplements, adding skim milk or powders to foods). *An inadequate diet can be supplemented with powders and formulas to increase nutrient intake without substantially increasing volume.*
- Avoid empty calories. *Because eating triggers pain, all foods ingested should be nutritious and of sufficient value to meet metabolic needs.*
- Add liquid multivitamin supplement to food/fluid. *This is done to ensure adequate intake of vitamins in case of insufficient intake.*
- Ensure adequate fluid intake. *This is done to prevent dehydration, as the patient is reluctant to drink.*
- Assist patient in exploring ways to avoid pain while eating (mechanically soft foods, well-balanced liquid supplements). *Success in avoiding pain will allow the patient to consume more nutrients.*
- Place food in unaffected side of mouth. *This may reduce pain sensation, which will allow greater consumption of food.*
- Involve dietitian in planning. *Dietitians have expert knowledge about community access to appropriate supplements.*
- Teach patient to weigh self weekly and maintain weight record. *This helps track progress in meeting nutritional goals.*

Evaluation Parameters
1. Takes in adequate amount of food to maintain nutritional status
2. Is free of weight loss
3. Eats and drinks without triggering pain

NURSING DIAGNOSIS **Impaired oral mucous membranes related to inadequate oral hygiene secondary to fear of pain**
GOALS/OUTCOMES Will maintain health of teeth and gums without exacerbating pain

NOC Suggested Outcomes
- Oral Health (1100)

NIC Suggested Interventions
- Oral Health Promotion (1720)
- Oral Health Maintenance (1710)

Nursing Interventions/Rationales
- Inspect oral tissue on each visit. *This provides baseline for evaluation of progress or problems.*
- Assess patient's current practice for oral care and evaluate effectiveness. *This provides baseline for planning interventions.*
- Explore alternatives for oral care with patient (swabs, Water Pik, mouthwashes). *This provides patient with alternatives for achieving mouth care goals.*
- Encourage patient to carefully rinse mouth after eating. *This helps reduce mouth odor from retained food particles.*
- Encourage patient to perform thorough oral hygiene between pain episodes. *Patient should take advantage of pain-free intervals for performing more thorough mouth and teeth care.*
- Refer to dentist for regular assessment and care. *Infection in the mouth or teeth is a common trigger for increased pain episodes. Frequent dental assessments help identify early infections.*

Evaluation Parameters
1. Absence of foul breath odor
2. Performs daily mouth care
3. Teeth clean and free of debris

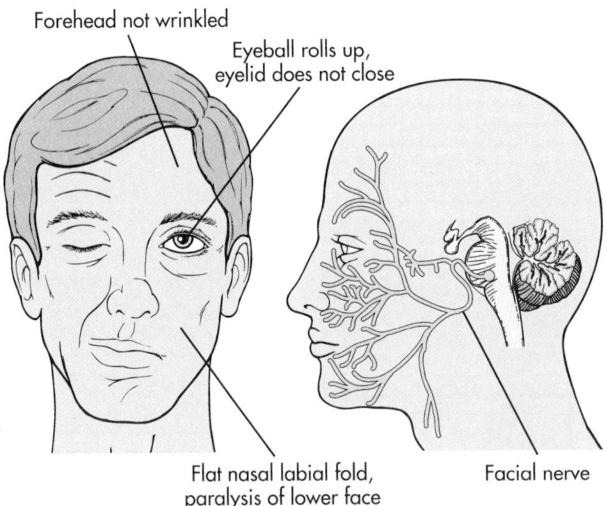

Figure 44-20 Bell's palsy.

women is about equal. More than 80% of patients recover over a period of a few weeks, although complete recovery may take 6 to 12 months.[6] Most patients experience no residual effects.

Pathophysiology

The facial nerve is primarily composed of motor nerves that innervate the muscles of expression on the face. The sensory branches supply the anterior two thirds of the tongue. Bell's palsy is characterized by a rapid weakening or paralysis of the facial muscles on one side of the face, which creates a masklike appearance. Symptoms are the result of rapid demyelination of the nerve, which completely interrupts its function. The eye on the affected side tears constantly, and the person may have difficulty swallowing (Figure 44-20). Symptoms typically develop over 24 to 36 hours but can also be fully present when the individual wakens from sleep. The diagnosis is one of exclusion and is established from the history and classic presenting symptoms.

Collaborative Care Management

There is no definitive treatment for Bell's palsy and most patients recover without intervention. The administration of steroids used to be standard but is now controversial.[6] Treatment is generally supportive, although heat, massage, and TENS therapy have all been used. Eye care is essential because the patient is unable to blink or close the eyelid on the affected side. Injury prevention and airway protection are other priorities for care.

Patient/Family Education. Most patients with Bell's palsy can be adequately managed in the community setting, and the nurse focuses on offering support and educating the patient and family about the disease process. The nurse teaches the patient the importance of protecting the affected eye from injury and infection. Artificial tears are recommended, and the eye should be patched or taped outdoors and at night to protect it from abrasion, wind, and light damage. The nurse recommends that the patient modify the diet as needed to support swallowing, and to eat and drink only in an upright position. Support and reassurance are critical as the patient copes with the sudden and frightening manifestations of the disease. As nerve function begins to return, the patient is instructed in facial exercises to help regain facial muscle tone.

PERIPHERAL NERVE TRAUMA

Etiology/Epidemiology

The peripheral nerves are vulnerable to injury from athletic injuries, vehicular accidents, mechanical and equipment injury, and acts of violence. Chronic nerve compression and entrapment can also result in nerve damage. Well-known syndromes such as carpal tunnel are described in Chapter 47. The mechanisms of injury in peripheral nerve trauma are similar to those discussed under SCI and include partial and complete transection, contusion, compression, ischemia, and stretch trauma. Peripheral nerves, however, possess the potential to regenerate after injury if conditions are favorable. Much has been learned about the process of repair, but clinical application has remained limited and recovery is frequently both slow and incomplete.[16] Specific epidemiologic data are not available concerning peripheral nerve injuries, but the median, ulnar, and radial nerves of the arm and the femoral, peroneal, and sciatic nerves of the legs are affected most commonly.

Pathophysiology

When a peripheral nerve is transected, several pathologic processes are initiated by injury. Edema in the axon fibers leads to demyelination and degeneration of the nerve fibers that progresses proximally back toward the nerve cell body. At the same time the distal nerve also degenerates and retracts (wallerian degeneration). The axon and its myelin sheath break down and the debris is cleared by an aggressive phagocytic process. A gap occurs in the nerve axon, and motor and sensory function are lost distal to the injury.[16] The body attempts to repair the damage through two major processes. Schwann cells in the neurolemma proliferate from both ends of the injury to form neurolemma cords, which act as guidewires for the regenerating axon (Figure 44-21). The axon cylinder generates multiple tiny buds or sprouts at its tip and if some of the sprouts are successful in using the neurolemma cords to cross the transected gap, they achieve union with the distal stump. Numerous sprouts develop at the axon tip, but they appear to preferentially grow toward the distal nerve segment by mechanisms that are not yet understood. A wide variety of trophic growth factors are released during the repair process that support the regeneration of the axon.[5] Nerve fibers regenerate at a rate of about 1 mm/day and major injuries require months to repair.[17] Successfully realigned nerves remyelinate and regrow to nearly their former size. The conduction velocity of regenerated nerves is typically about 80% of normal, and the chances for functional return are good.

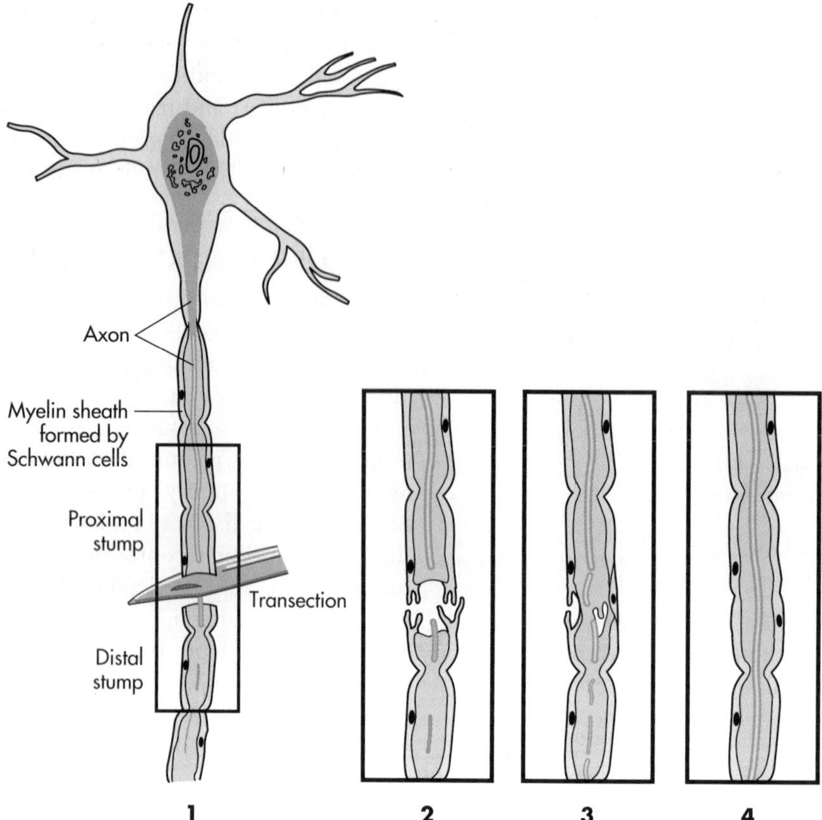

1 After nerve transection, degeneration and retraction of the distal stump occur within 24 hours.

2 Healing begins as Schwann cells of the neurolemma proliferate from both proximal and distal stumps, forming neurolemmal cords that will guide the regenerating axon.

3 Some unmyelinated axon sprouts that are generated from the proximal stump find their way to the distal stump, guided by the neurolemmal cords.

4 The axon regrows and remyelinates.

Figure 44-21 The process of repair and regeneration of a peripheral nerve.

The clinical manifestations of peripheral nerve injury depend on the exact location of the trauma and the specific function(s) of the involved nerve or nerves. Because peripheral nerves contain both sensory and motor components, deficits frequently exist in both areas distal to the site. Motor alterations include lower motor neuron signs such as flaccid paralysis and muscle wasting in the muscles innervated by the affected nerves. Autonomic changes may also be present after injury. Damage to sympathetic fibers creates an initial warm phase in which the affected area is dry and warm to the touch and flushed in appearance. A cold phase may follow in several weeks in which the extremity becomes cold and cyanotic.

Collaborative Care Management

Peripheral nerve injuries are diagnosed primarily from the injury history and presenting symptoms. Electromyography may be used to determine the presence and extent of any residual connection between the nerve and muscle. Microsurgical techniques now allow skilled surgeons to successfully explore the injury and perform decompression and repair. Early surgical intervention minimizes the extent of secondary injury and prevents extensive scar tissue formation at the nerve tips, but there is no consensus at present about the correct timing of surgical intervention. One of the many surgical challenges is that the severed portions of the nerve retract, and the remaining nerve is often shorter than desired. Nerve grafts may be used when the nerve segments are too short.

As more is learned about the biochemical processes taking place during repair, some surgeons are recommending bringing the severed nerve tips close to each other, but not attempting to repair the nerve. Instead, the tips are enclosed in a tube and the neurotropic factors accumulate around them.

A fibrin matrix is formed and the nerve segments rejoin and regenerate. Animal models are providing evidence that laser treatment, electromagnetic stimulation, and ultrasound all can be used to accelerate the natural process of regeneration and repair.[16]

A physical therapy program is initiated as soon as possible after the injury because the loss of nervous innervation causes the muscles to begin to atrophy, and a period of immobilization is frequently used to support healing. Physical therapy is critical and includes range of motion, resistive exercise, splints and braces to support proper positioning, and electrical nerve stimulation to the affected muscles to minimize atrophic changes. The flaccid muscles are unable to successfully balance their opposing muscles (i.e., flexors versus extensors), and the risk of contracture is high. Positioning in neutral or counter positions is essential to help prevent joint deformities. If the associated tendons are allowed to shorten, the contracture will be permanent.

Patient/Family Education. The rehabilitation process after peripheral nerve injury is prolonged and carries no guarantees. Distal nerve injuries appear to heal better than proximal injuries, and young persons heal more successfully than older persons. The nurse reinforces the rationale for all components of the treatment plan. Ongoing support and encouragement are essential, as the patient and family may become discouraged at the pace of progress and the cost of treatment. The nurse instructs the patient about safety measures to compensate for any sensory losses. Sensory nerve fiber healing is heralded by the return of pain and temperature sensation. Thorough visual assessment of all affected areas is essential. The nurse teaches the patient to carefully protect the affected areas from damage related to temperature extremes.

The nurse also emphasizes the importance of skin care to the affected areas. In the cold phase after injury the skin is fragile and vulnerable to injury. Daily inspection and gentle cleansing are critical. Lanolin creams or cocoa butter may be used to counteract dryness and scaling. Multiple adaptations in self-care skills may be necessary during the treatment and rehabilitation periods, and the nurse assists the patient to acquire and effectively use appropriate devices.

Critical Thinking Questions

1. A 19-year-old adolescent with a C8 spinal cord injury was injured 3 months ago and is in active rehabilitation. He has recently developed muscle spasticity, which is becoming increasingly severe. His family is optimistic that the spasms are an indication that he will eventually walk again. How would you respond to them? What nursing interventions can you implement to reduce the spasticity?
2. You are working on an acute spinal cord injury rehabilitation unit. Two of your patients are a 23-year-old man who suffered a T8 injury and a 32-year-old woman who suffered a C6 injury. In planning your day how will your priorities for these two patients be the same? How will they be different? Why?
3. A patient with an L2 spinal cord injury has been complaining of increasing levels of intense burning pain shooting through her legs and lower back. A fellow nursing student asks you whether you think that the patient really has pain, or whether she is just trying to get pain medication as a way of coping with her disability. "After all, spinal cord injury results in a loss of sensation below the level of the injury, doesn't it?" How would you respond to your friend? Support your answer.
4. What services exist in your community/region to care for patients with spinal cord injuries (SCIs)? Is there a specialty neurotrauma unit? Who offers acute specialty SCI rehabilitation? Do they accept patients without health insurance? If a family cannot provide care for a ventilator-dependent C_3 level injury, what choices are available for long-term care? Do any home health agencies offer services for this type of patient? What would this level of care cost per month?

References

1. American Injury Association: *International standards for neurological & functional classification of spinal cord injury,* Atlanta, 1994, American Injury Association.
2. Bracken MB et al: Administration of methylprednisolone for 24 or 48 hours or tirilazad mesylate for 48 hours in the treatment of acute spinal cord injury, *JAMA* 277(20):1597, 1997.
3. Burke DA et al: Incidence rates and populations at risk for spinal cord injury: a regional study, *Spinal Cord* 39:274, 2001.
4. Byrne TN, Benzel EC, Waxman SG: *Diseases of the spine and spinal cord,* New York, 2000, Oxford University Press.
5. Costa M: Trigeminal neuralgia, *Am J Nurs* 98(6):42, 1998.
6. Dahlin LB, Lundborg G: Use of tubes in peripheral nerve repair, *Neurosurg Clin North Am* 12(2):341, 2001.
7. Domanico S: Bell's palsy: a case study, *Internet J Adv Nurs Pract* 12(1):1, 1998.
8. Dorizzi A: Guidelines for management of spinal cord injury, *J Neurol Sci* 41(2):133-135, 1997.
9. Dubendorf P: Spinal cord injury pathophysiology, *Crit Care Nurs Q* 22(2):31,1999.
10. Gill M: Spinal cord injury, *Crit Care Nurs Q* 22(2):1, 1999.
11. Hauswald M et al: Out of hospital spinal immobilization: its effect on neurologic injury, *Acad Emerg Med* 5(3):214, 1998.
12. Hickey JV: *The clinical practice of neurological & neurosurgical nursing,* ed 4, Philadelphia, 1997, JB Lippincott.
13. Huston CJ: Cervical spine injury, *Am J Nurs* 98(6):33, 1998.
14. Illman A, Stiller K, Williams M: The prevalence of orthostatic hypotension during physiotherapy treatment in patients with an acute spinal cord injury, *Spinal Cord* 38:741, 2000.
15. Jackson EM et al: Trigeminal neuralgia: a diagnostic challenge, *Am J Emerg Med* 17(6):1, 1999.
16. Kish DL: Prehospital management of spinal trauma: an evolution, *Crit Care Nurs Q* 22(2):36, 1999.
17. Lazar DA et al: Acceleration of recovery after injury to the peripheral nervous system using ultrasound and other therapeutic modalities, *Neurosurg Clin North Am* 12(2):353, 2001.
18. Lipe AT, Lovasik D: Older patients with spinal cord injury, *Crit Care Nurs Q* 22(2):18, 1999.
19. Lucke KT: Pulmonary management following acute SCI, *J Neurosci Nurs* 30(2):91, 2000.
20. Lynch AC et al: Bowel dysfunction following spinal cord injury, *Spinal Cord* 39:193, 2001.
21. Mitcho K, Yanko JR: Acute care management of spinal cord injuries, *Crit Care Nurs Q* 22(2):61, 1999.

22. Mosiman W: Taking the sting out of trigeminal neuralgia, *Nursing* 31(3):86, 2001.
23. Murphy M: Traumatic spinal cord injury: an acute care rehabilitation perspective, *Crit Care Nurs Q* 22(2):51, 1999.
24. Orledge JD, Pepe PE: Out of hospital spinal immobilization: is it really necessary? *Acad Emerg Med* 5:203, 1998.
25. Prendergast V, Sullivan C: Acute spinal cord injury: nursing considerations for the first 72 hours, *Crit Care Nurs Clin North Am* 12(4):499, 2000.
26. Seidl EC: Promising pharmacological agents in the management of acute spinal cord injury, *Crit Care Nurs Q* 22(2):44, 1999.
27. Soden RJ et al: Causes of death after spinal cord injury, *Spinal Cord* 38:604, 2000.
28. Stewart-Amidei C, Kunkel JA: *AANN's neuroscience nursing: human responses to neurologic dysfunction,* ed 2, Philadelphia, 2001, WB Saunders.
29. Weitzenkamp DA et al: Aging with spinal cord injury: cross-sectional and longitudinal effects, *Spinal Cord* 39:301, 2001.

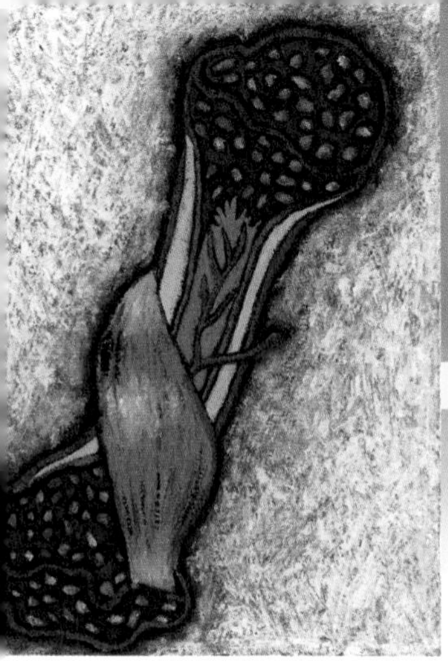

http://www.mosby.com/MERLIN/medsurg_phipps

Assessment of the Musculoskeletal System

45

Jane F. Marek

Objectives

After studying this chapter, the learner should be able to:

1. Describe the structure and function of the different tissues that compose the musculoskeletal system.
2. Analyze the interrelationship of the tissues of the musculoskeletal system with overall functioning of the system.
3. Discuss the physiologic changes that occur in the musculoskeletal system as a result of the aging process.
4. Explain the pathologic conditions that can occur within the musculoskeletal system.
5. Describe components of the nursing assessment of the musculoskeletal system, including the health history and physical examination.
6. Explain the diagnostic tests indicated for the person with a musculoskeletal problem, the rationale for each test, and appropriate nursing responsibilities associated with each test.
7. Synthesize a plan of care for a person with a musculoskeletal problem, using relevant subjective and objective data and results of diagnostic tests.

People often take the ability to move about freely in the environment for granted. Activities as simple as making a fist to movements as complex as a ballerina performing a cabriole depend on the structure, function, and integrity of the musculoskeletal system. The musculoskeletal system is one of the body's largest systems and accounts for over 50% of the body's weight. This dynamic system comprises bones, joints, muscles, and supporting structures. All the components of the system work together to produce movement and to supply structure and support to the body. Any disturbance in this well-integrated system results in musculoskeletal dysfunction. Problems can arise as a result of disease affecting the nerves, bones, muscles, or joints or as a result of trauma to these or surrounding structures. Problems arising outside of the musculoskeletal system, such as endocrine or neurologic diseases, may directly affect the system, resulting in some degree of disability.

Planning appropriate interventions for individuals with alterations in musculoskeletal functioning requires a careful and thorough assessment based on the nurse's knowledge and understanding of the anatomy and physiology of the musculoskeletal system. The patient's reaction to the disability and implications of the results of diagnostic studies must also be considered. This chapter discusses the anatomy and physiology of the musculoskeletal system, methods and rationale for collecting subjective and objective data from the patient and/or family, and the relevance of selected diagnostic studies.

ANATOMY AND PHYSIOLOGY

Bones

The human skeleton is made up of the axial and appendicular skeletons, which consist of 206 bones (Figure 45-1). The *axial* skeleton consists of 80 bones—the hyoid bone and those of the skull, vertebral column, and thorax. The remaining 126 bones make up the *appendicular* skeleton, which contains the bones of the upper and lower extremities, pectoral girdle, and pelvic girdle (os coxae). The skeleton makes up 14% of the weight of the adult body.

Types

Bones are divided into four types, according to their shape:

1. Long (femur, humerus)
2. Short (carpals): often cuboidal in shape
3. Flat (skull)
4. Irregular (vertebrae)

Each bone is composed of *cancellous* (spongy) and *cortical* (compact) bone. In the long bones the cancellous portions are found in the ends of the bones and cortical bone in the shaft. The short and irregular bones have an inner core of cancellous bone with an outer layer of cortical bone. Flat bones have two outer plates of cortical bone with an inner layer of cancellous bone. Cancellous bone is also found in the ends of long bones and in the iliac crests, tibiae, and sternum.

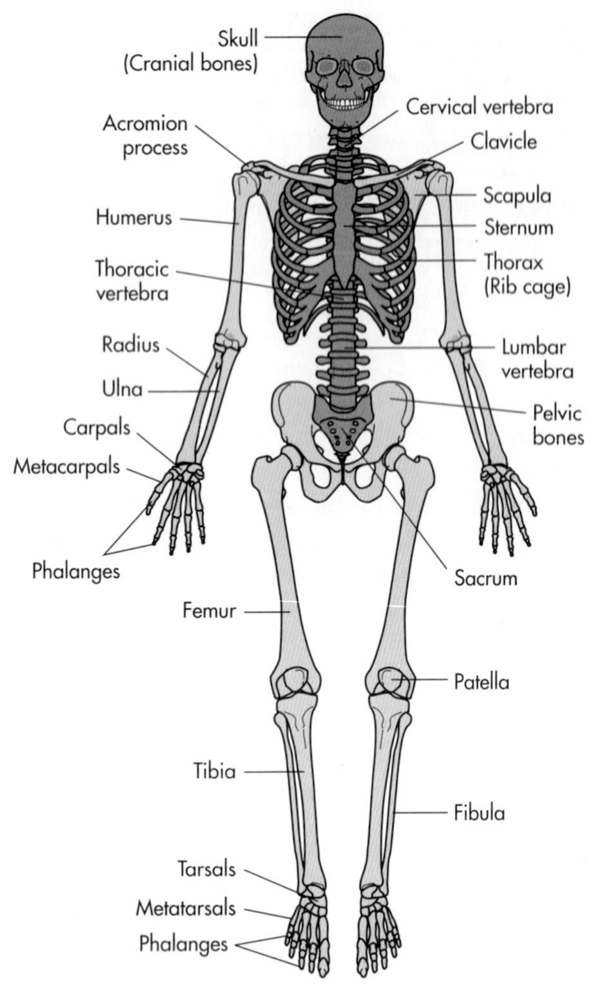

Figure 45-1 Axial and appendicular skeleton.

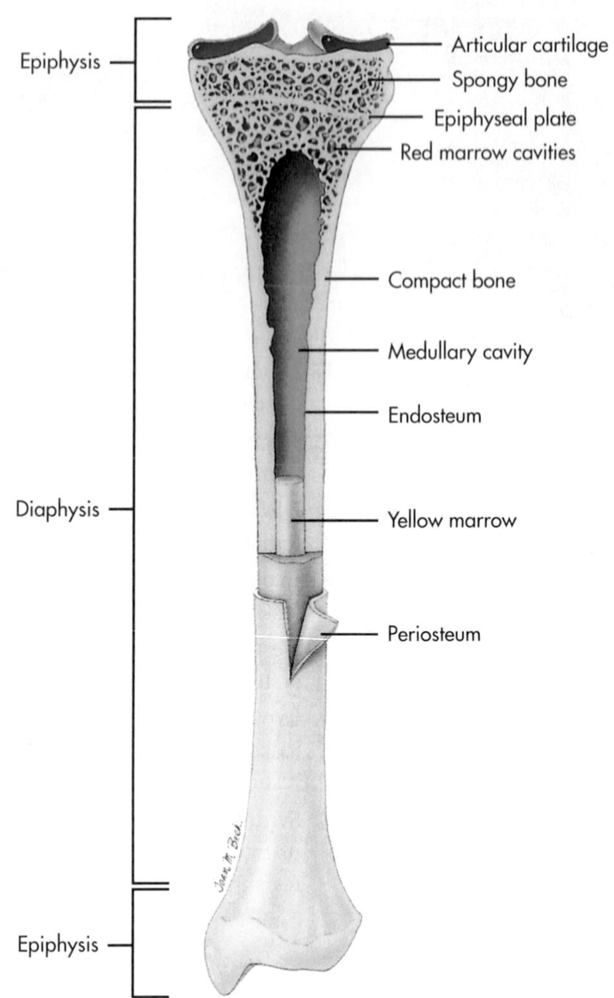

Figure 45-2 Cross section of a long bone.

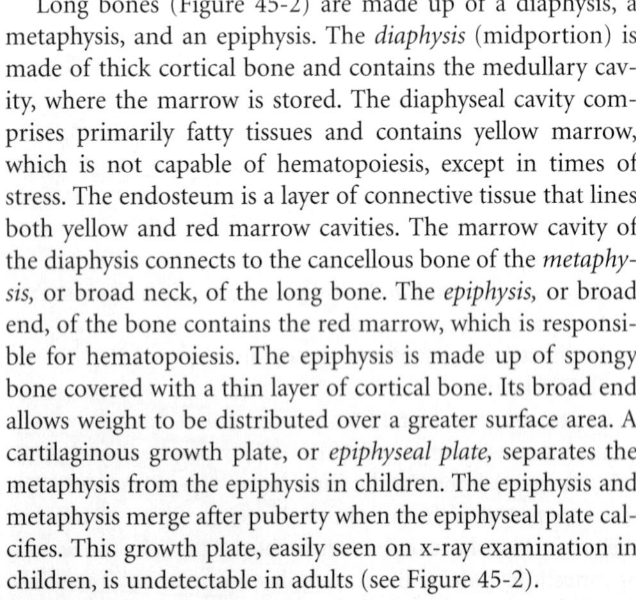

Long bones (Figure 45-2) are made up of a diaphysis, a metaphysis, and an epiphysis. The *diaphysis* (midportion) is made of thick cortical bone and contains the medullary cavity, where the marrow is stored. The diaphyseal cavity comprises primarily fatty tissues and contains yellow marrow, which is not capable of hematopoiesis, except in times of stress. The endosteum is a layer of connective tissue that lines both yellow and red marrow cavities. The marrow cavity of the diaphysis connects to the cancellous bone of the *metaphysis,* or broad neck, of the long bone. The *epiphysis,* or broad end, of the bone contains the red marrow, which is responsible for hematopoiesis. The epiphysis is made up of spongy bone covered with a thin layer of cortical bone. Its broad end allows weight to be distributed over a greater surface area. A cartilaginous growth plate, or *epiphyseal plate,* separates the metaphysis from the epiphysis in children. The epiphysis and metaphysis merge after puberty when the epiphyseal plate calcifies. This growth plate, easily seen on x-ray examination in children, is undetectable in adults (see Figure 45-2).

Structure

Bone, like other connective tissue, is made up of cells, fibers, and ground substance. In addition, unlike other connective tissue, bone contains crystallized minerals, which give it rigidity (Table 45-1).

Bone is a dynamic substance, continuously synthesizing and resorbing bone tissue. Bone cells allow growth, repair, and remodeling. Bone formation begins in the fetal stage as cartilage formation and continues throughout life. In the mature individual the first step in bone formation is the initiation of an organic matrix by the bone cells. Next, mineralization takes place as minerals are bound to collagen fibers, providing support and tensile strength to bone.

Three types of bone cells are found in the body. *Osteoblasts,* or bone-forming cells, are responsible for laying down new bone. They produce type I collagen and respond to changing levels of parathyroid hormone (PTH). New bone is formed as the osteoblasts produce osteoid and mineralize the bone matrix. Once this is accomplished, osteoblasts become *osteocytes* and are trapped in the mineralized bone matrix. Osteocytes maintain the mineral content and organic elements of bone. The third type of bone cell, *osteoclasts,* resorb bone during growth and repair. They are able to resorb bone by secreting citric and lactic acid and collagenases, which dissolve minerals and break down collagen.

TABLE 45-1 Structural Elements of Bone

Structural Element	Function
Bone Cells	
Osteoblasts	Synthesize collagen and proteoglycans; stimulate osteoclast resorptive activity
Osteocytes	Maintain bone matrix
Osteoclasts	Resorb bone; assist with mineral homeostasis
Bone Matrix	
Collagen fibers	Lend support and tensile strength
Proteoglycans	Control transport of ionized materials through matrix
Bone morphogenic proteins	Induce cartilage and bone formation
BMP-1	
BMP-2A	
BMP-3	
BMP-7	
Glycoproteins	
Sialoprotein	Promotes calcification
Osteocalcin	Inhibits calcium-phosphate precipitation; promotes bone resorption
Laminin	Stabilizes basement membranes in bones
Osteonectin	Binds calcium in bones
Albumin	Transports essential elements to matrix; maintains osmotic pressure of bone fluid
Alpha-glycoprotein	Promotes calcification
Minerals (elements)	
Calcium	Crystallizes to lend rigidity and compressive strength
Phosphate	Regulates vitamin D and thereby promotes mineralization

From McCance KL, Huether SE: *Pathophysiology: the biologic basis for disease in adults and children,* ed 4, St Louis, 2002, Mosby.

Bone is primarily composed of organic matrix and calcium salts. Collagen fibers account for 90% to 95% of the organic matrix; ground substance makes up the remainder. The collagen fibers extend along the lines of tensional force and give bone its great tensile strength. The ground substance functions as a medium for the diffusion of nutrients, oxygen, minerals, and wastes between bone tissue and blood vessels. Ground substance contains extracellular fluid and proteoglycans, particularly chondroitin sulfate and hyaluronic acid, which help control the deposition of calcium salts. The bone morphogenic proteins (BMPs), important substances responsible for inducing cartilage formation, are also found in the bone matrix. The glycoproteins found in the matrix play a role in the calcification, resorption, and metabolism of bone. The minerals contained in the matrix are primarily calcium and phosphate. Hydroxyapatite, the primary bone salt, is formed as a result of the mineralization and crystal formation of calcium and phosphate. Mineralization is the final step in the process of bone formation.

Both cancellous and cortical bone contain the same structural elements, but they differ in the organization of the bone matrix (Figure 45-3, *A* and *B*). Concentric layers of bone matrix are called lamellae.

The basic unit of cortical bone is the haversian system. At the center of this arrangement of concentric rings is the haversian canal, which runs through the long axes of bones. This canal contains blood vessels (capillaries, arterioles, or venules), nerve fibers, and lymphatics. Blood vessels in the canal communicate with blood vessels in the periosteum. Lacunae are small spaces between the rings of the lamellae and contain osteocytes. Canaliculi, very small canals that connect the lacunae and the haversian canal, run parallel to the long axis of the bone. This connection allows the osteocytes access to the nutrient supply. Haversian units (lamellae, haversian canal, lacunae, canaliculi) fit closely together in cortical bone. The hardness and density of cortical bone give it strength and rigidity.

In contrast, cancellous bone lacks haversian systems. The lamellae are arranged not in concentric layers but in connecting plates or bars called trabeculae, which form an irregular meshwork. The pattern of the trabecular bone depends on the direction of stress in the particular bone. Red marrow fills the spaces between the trabeculae. Lacunae, rich in osteocytes, are distributed among the trabeculae and connected by canaliculi. Capillaries flowing through the marrow provide nutrients to the osteocytes. The fine, thready structure of trabecular bone provides strength to cancellous bone while reducing its weight.

The outer, nonarticulating surfaces of long bones are covered with a white fibrous membrane called the periosteum. The outer layer of the periosteum contains blood vessels and nerves that reach the inner bones through Volkmann's canals. Nutrient arteries in the periosteum communicate with the haversian system. Collagenous fibers (Sharpey's fibers) anchor the inner layer of the periosteum to the bone.

The surfaces of bones contain grooves or ridges for nerves and blood vessels, prominences for muscular attachments,

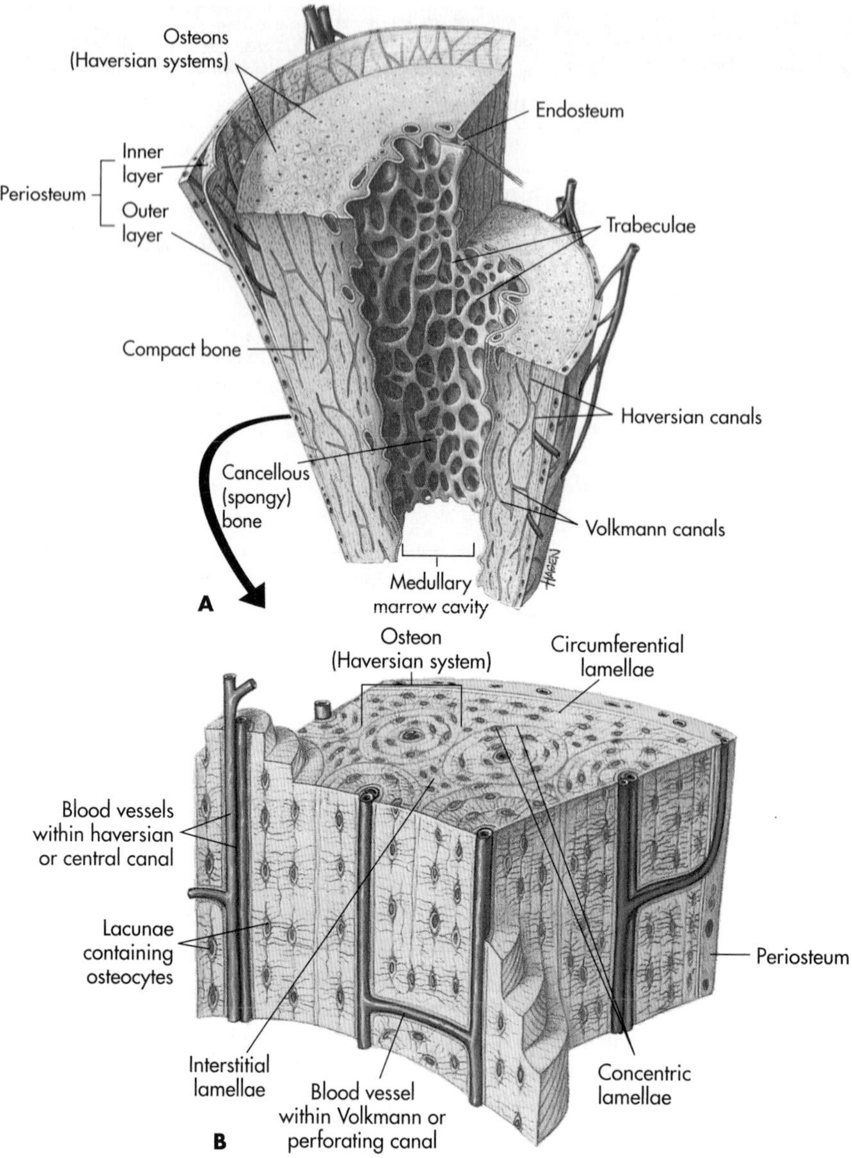

Figure 45-3 Structure of compact and cancellous bone. **A,** Longitudinal section of a long bone showing both cancellous and compact bone. **B,** Magnified view of compact bone.

and openings for blood vessels and muscles. Articulating surfaces are covered with hyaline cartilage (Figure 45-4).

Blood supply to bone is maintained through the haversian canals, periosteal vasculature, and vessels located in the marrow and ends of bones. Bones are supplied with sensory nerve endings in the periosteum that connect with the central nervous system.

Function

Bones have five functions:

1. *Support*—of body tissues as provided by the skeletal framework; they also give form and shape to the body.
2. *Protection*—of body organs; for example, the bony casing of the skull protects the brain, and the bones of the thorax and pelvis protect the heart, lungs, and reproductive organs.
3. *Movement*—by muscular attachments to bone and by joint movement.
4. *Hematopoiesis*—the marrow of some bones has a hematopoietic function. Normally after birth, red blood cell (RBC) production occurs only in the bone marrow (medullary hematopoiesis). Extramedullary hematopoiesis is usually a sign of disease. In adults the marrow in the bones of the skull, vertebrae, ribs, sternum, shoulders, and pelvis produces RBCs. The hematopoietic function of bone continues throughout life. Blood cells are produced to replace those lost through disease, bleeding, and cellular aging. An increase in RBC production can be triggered by anemia, hemorrhage, infection, stress, and other disorders that deplete their stores. Medullary hematopoiesis is accomplished by conversion of yellow marrow to red, increased differen-

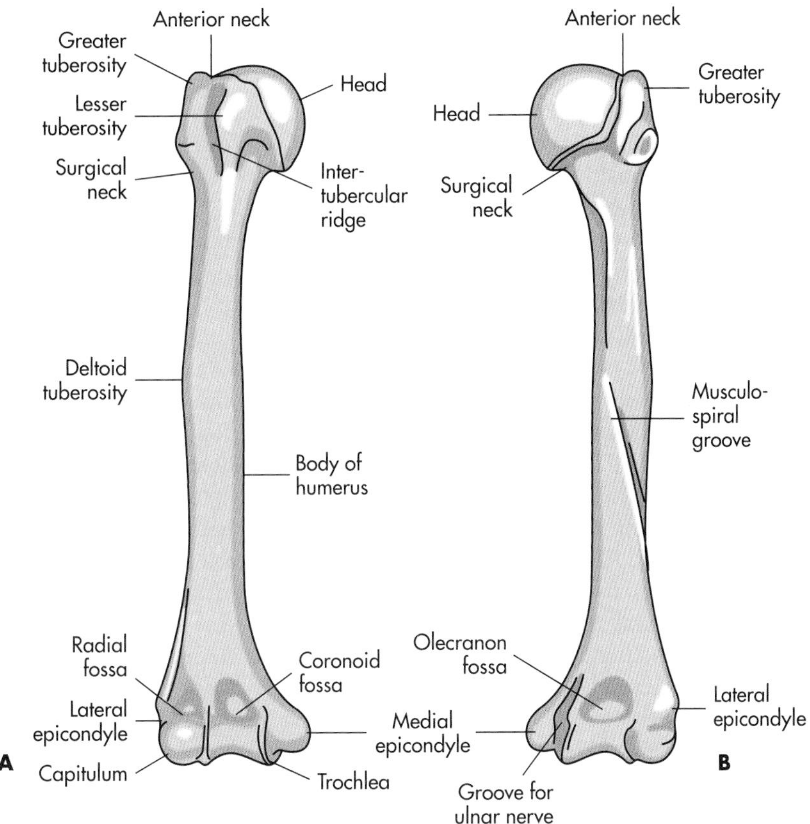

Figure 45-4 **A**, Anterior view of right humerus. **B**, Posterior view of right humerus. Note groove for ulnar nerve and tuberosities for muscular attachments.

tiation of daughter cells, and increased growth of stem cells.

5. *Mineral homeostasis*—bones store calcium, phosphate, carbonate, and magnesium, which are necessary for normal cellular function; approximately 99% of the body's calcium is stored in the skeleton.

Bone Growth and Remodeling

Longitudinal growth of the long bones emanates from the epiphyseal cartilage, which thickens because of rapid proliferation of the cartilage and undergoes ossification (endochondral ossification). Growth in the diameter of the bone is accomplished as osteoblasts in the periosteum produce new bone on the outside of the bone (membranous ossification). Bone reaches maturity after puberty.

Bone is continuously being deposited by osteoblasts and continuously being resorbed by active osteoclasts. In the adult, osteoblastic activity occurs on approximately 4% of all surfaces of living bone, resulting in a constant state of bone formation.[1] In contrast, osteoclastic activity is present on less than 1% of the bony surfaces of a normal adult.[1]

Except in growing bones, the rate of bone deposition equals the rate of bone destruction until approximately 35 years of age. Thus the total mass of bone remains constant. The value of the equilibrium between bone destruction and formation fulfills some physiologically important functions. Most important, bone responds to the amount of stress to which it is subjected; bone thickens and strengthens itself in response to a heavy load. Second, bone can also be reshaped in response to alterations in its mechanical function. These responses are in accordance with Wolff's law. Wolff was a German anatomist (1836-1902) who stated: "Every change in form and function of bones or their function alone is followed by definite changes in their external configuration in accordance with mathematical laws." Last, in old bone the organic matrix degenerates and the bone becomes weak and brittle; new organic matrix is necessary to maintain the strength and toughness of bone.

Remodeling is the process by which existing bone is resorbed and new bone replaces the old. In the first phase (activation), bone cell precursors form osteoclasts in response to a stressor or stimulus. In phase 2 (resorption), masses of osteoclasts form a cutting cone and begin to eat away at the bone for a period of approximately 3 weeks, creating a tunnel or cavity 0.2 to 1 mm in length.[1,3] In cancellous bone this tunnel is parallel to the trabeculae; in cortical bone it follows the longitudinal surface of the haversian system. In phase 3 (formation), the tunnel is then invaded by osteoblasts, and new bone (secondary bone) is laid down in lamellae on the inner surface of the tunnel until it is filled. New bone deposition is complete when the bone begins to encroach on the blood supply of the area. Subsequently, lamellae are formed until the tunnel is reduced to a haversian canal around a blood vessel. This process is responsible for the formation of new haversian systems and trabeculae. Areas of new bone are known as osteons. The entire process of remodeling takes place over a period of approximately 4 weeks.

Influencing Factors

Many factors influence the process of bone formation and resorption, including serum levels of calcium, phosphorus, and alkaline phosphatase (ALP); calcitonin; vitamin D levels; PTH; growth hormone (GH); glucocorticoids; sex hormones; infection and inflammation; and activity and weight bearing.

Approximately 99% of the body's calcium is found in bone. Calcium is necessary for bone formation and is an essential element in bone structure. Serum calcium levels are maintained in homeostasis by the actions of the small intestine, bones, and kidneys. These organs are regulated by PTH, calcitonin, and vitamin D_1, an inactive form of vitamin D. If serum calcium levels are low, the bone releases calcium into the vascular system in response to stimulation by PTH. Decreased serum levels of calcium delay bone formation.

Phosphorus and calcium have an inverse relationship. If serum levels of phosphorus are elevated, serum calcium levels are decreased. Phosphorus is found in bone and skeletal muscle and, like calcium, is controlled by PTH. Increases in PTH cause a decrease in serum phosphorus levels and increased excretion of phosphorus by the kidney. Bone resorption results in the release of phosphorus into the extracellular fluid.

The enzyme ALP is found in osteoblasts. It is excreted via the biliary tract and is necessary for the utilization of mineral salts and bone formation. Levels of ALP rise in response to increased osteoblastic activity in the bones (e.g., during fracture healing).

Calcitonin is a hormone produced and secreted primarily by the thyroid gland. Calcitonin inhibits bone resorption, inhibits calcium absorption from the gastrointestinal tract, and increases calcium and phosphorus excretion from the kidneys.

Vitamin D is derived from the action of ultraviolet light on provitamins found in the skin and from vitamin D–enriched foods. Vitamin D is activated in the liver and kidneys through the action of PTH. The activated form, calcitriol, is a hormone necessary for calcium absorption. Activated vitamin D elevates calcium and phosphate levels in the plasma by increasing intestinal absorption of calcium and phosphate and by increasing the release of calcium from bone into the blood. Vitamin D deficiencies can manifest themselves as rickets in children and osteomalacia in adults.

PTH, produced by the parathyroid gland, controls serum calcium and phosphorus levels. Decreased serum calcium levels are the stimulus for release of more PTH to keep the serum calcium levels normal. In conjunction with vitamin D, PTH works to stimulate absorption of calcium and phosphorus by the intestinal mucosa. It also causes mobilization of calcium from the bones by promoting osteoclastic activity and bone resorption.

GH is secreted by the anterior lobe of the pituitary gland and promotes the growth of bone and other tissue. Decreased levels of GH are manifested as dwarfism. Increased levels of GH in children result in gigantism; increased levels of GH in adults result in acromegaly (see Chapter 29).

Glucocorticoids (cortisol) regulate the metabolism of proteins. Increased levels cause a decrease in protein stores. Prolonged (longer than 6 months) increased levels may result in damage to the bone matrix, release of calcium from the bone, and eventually, osteoporosis.

Estrogen stimulates osteoblast activity and inhibits PTH. As estrogen levels decrease at menopause, women are at risk for decreased calcium levels, bone loss, and the development of osteoporosis. Androgens cause anabolism and increased bone mass. Infection and inflammation can cause lysis of bone and bone resorption.

Activity and weight bearing affect the structure of bone. Trabeculae within the bone develop and align themselves along lines of stress, and osteogenesis occurs along these lines. If the bone is not stressed, bone resorption occurs. The paraplegic or quadriplegic individual often experiences a reduction in bone mass (atrophy) as a result of inactivity and non–weight-bearing status (lack of stress) on the bone. Astronauts may experience a temporary loss of bone mass as a result of weightlessness in space. Conversely, a marathon runner or trained athlete may experience an increase in bony mass (hypertrophy) as a result of increased stress on bones. In older or inactive individuals, degeneration and resorption occur more rapidly than bone growth, which may lead to osteoporosis. Osteoporosis (see Chapter 47) is characterized by thin, weakened cortices and trabeculae, which render the bone more susceptible to fracture.

Physiology of Bone Healing

The process of bone healing is known as callus formation. Fractures and surgical disruption of bone both heal by the same process. Callus formation proceeds in five general stages (Figure 45-5):

1. *Hematoma formation.* Because bone is highly vascular, bleeding occurs at both ends of the fractured bone. Increased capillary permeability permits further extravasation of blood into the injured area. Blood collects in the periosteal sheath or adjacent tissues and fastens the broken ends together.
2. *Fibrin meshwork formation.* Fibroblasts invade the hematoma, forming a fibrin meshwork. White blood cells (WBCs) wall off the area, localizing the inflammation.
3. *Invasion by osteoblasts.* As osteoblasts invade the fibrous union to make it firm, blood vessels develop from capillary buds, thereby establishing a supply for nutrients to build collagen. Granulation tissue, or procallus, is formed. Collagen strands become longer and begin to incorporate calcium deposits, and cartilage begins to form. The bone morphogenic proteins, enzymes, and growth factors are active in this stage of bone healing.
4. *Callus formation.* Osteoblasts form woven bone, known as callus. Osteoblasts continue to lay the network for bone buildup as osteoclasts destroy dead bone and help synthesize new bone. Collagen strengthens and becomes further impregnated with calcium. Calcium and phosphate are deposited as mineral salts. Lamellar or trabecular bone continues to replace the callus.

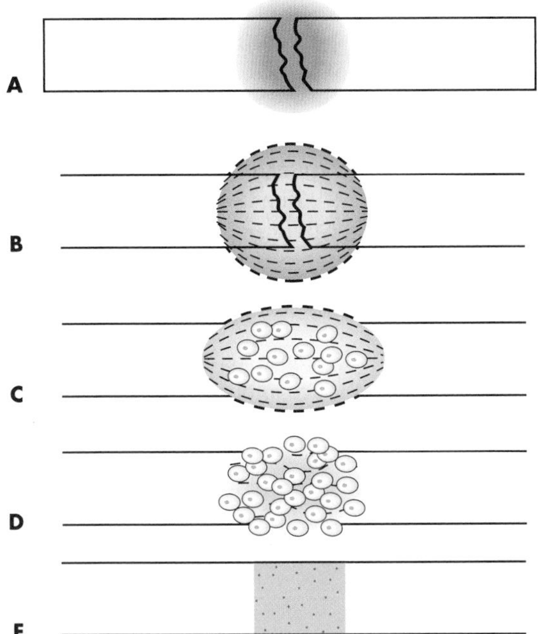

Figure 45-5 Bone healing (schematic representation). **A,** Bleeding at broken ends of the bone with subsequent hematoma formation. **B,** Organization of hematoma into fibrous network. **C,** Invasion of osteoblasts, lengthening of collagen strands, and deposition of calcium. **D,** Callus formation: new bone is built up as osteoclasts destroy dead bone. **E,** Remodeling is accomplished as excess callus is reabsorbed and trabecular bone is laid down.

5 *Remodeling.* Excess callus is reabsorbed, and trabecular bone is laid down along lines of stress in accordance with Wolff's law. Remodeling is an important stage because bone that has not undergone remodeling lacks the mechanical properties necessary for weight bearing.

Factors impeding callus formation include (1) inadequate reduction of the fracture; (2) excessive edema at the fracture site impeding the supply of nutrients to the area of injury; (3) excessive bone loss at the time of injury, which prevents sufficient bridging of the broken ends; (4) inefficient immobilization; (5) infection at the site of injury; (6) bone necrosis; (7) anemia or other systemic conditions; (8) endocrine imbalance; and (9) poor nutritional status. If callus formation does not occur normally and efficiently, the result is nonunion, or an ununited fracture (see Chapter 46).

Muscles

Types

There are three major types of muscle: visceral, cardiac, and skeletal. Visceral muscle, also known as smooth or involuntary muscle, is found in the blood vessels, stomach, and intestines. Visceral muscle is innervated by the autonomic nervous system and is not under voluntary control.

The cardiac muscle found in the myocardium has the properties of automaticity, rhythm, and conductivity. The cardiac conduction system and the autonomic nervous system exert control over cardiac muscle.

The primary focus of this chapter is skeletal muscle (Figures 45-6 and 45-7), also known as striated, voluntary, or extrafusal muscle. Skeletal muscle accounts for 45% to 50% of an average adult's body weight and contains 75% water, 20% protein, and 5% organic and inorganic compounds. Muscle contains 32% of all protein stores necessary for energy and metabolism.[3] Skeletal muscle is innervated by nerve fibers from the cerebrospinal system and can be controlled by will.

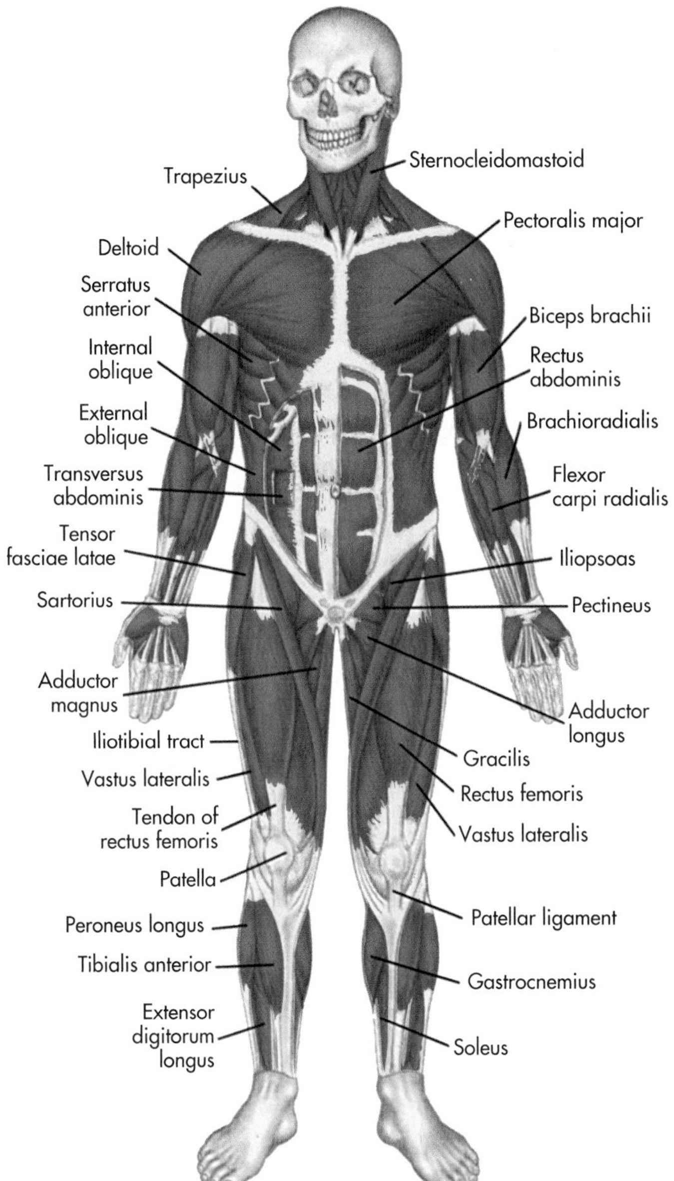

Figure 45-6 Skeletal muscles of body, anterior view.

The body has approximately 350 skeletal muscles, most in pairs. Muscle length varies greatly, from 2 to 60 cm. The function of a muscle determines its shape. Fusiform muscles are elongated and run from one joint to another (e.g., the quadriceps, which extends the knee). The deltoid is an example of a pennate muscle, which is characteristically broad and flat. The muscle fibers run obliquely to the muscle's long axis.

Structure

Each skeletal muscle is covered with a layered connective tissue called fascia. The epimysium, or outer layer, tapers at each end to form the tendon, which allows joint mobility. The middle layer, or perimysium, divides the muscle fibers into fascicles, or bundles of connective tissue. The endomysium, or inner layer, is the smallest unit of fibers and surrounds the fascicles (Figure 45-8).

Skeletal muscle fibers (cells) are contained within a membrane, the sarcolemma, which contains the sarcoplasm or cytoplasm. The sarcolemma transmits electrical impulses and plays a role in protein synthesis and nutrient supply. Sarcoplasm is similar to cytoplasm and contains proteins and enzymes necessary for the cell's energy production, protein synthesis, and oxygen storage. Small, closely packed fibers (called myofibrils) within the sarcoplasm alternate light and dark horizontal stripes and produce the striated appearance that lends this type of muscle its name. The myofibril is the functional unit of muscle contraction. The dark stripes are A bands, and the light stripes are I bands. Light bands crossing the middle of the dark stripes constitute the H zone, and dark lines crossing the middle of the light stripes are called Z lines. Myofibrils consist of several sections, called sarcomeres, that contain the contractile proteins actin and myosin. Each sarcomere is a section that extends from one Z line of a myofibril to the next (Figure 45-9). Bundles of muscle fibers (cells) make up the muscle itself. Glycogen is present in muscle as an energy source.

Function

Skeletal muscle provides controlled movement and maintains posture. Movement is accomplished by muscle contractions and work production. Muscular contraction is a complex process triggered by nerve impulses arriving at the muscle fiber. Calcium ions, released when the impulse is re-

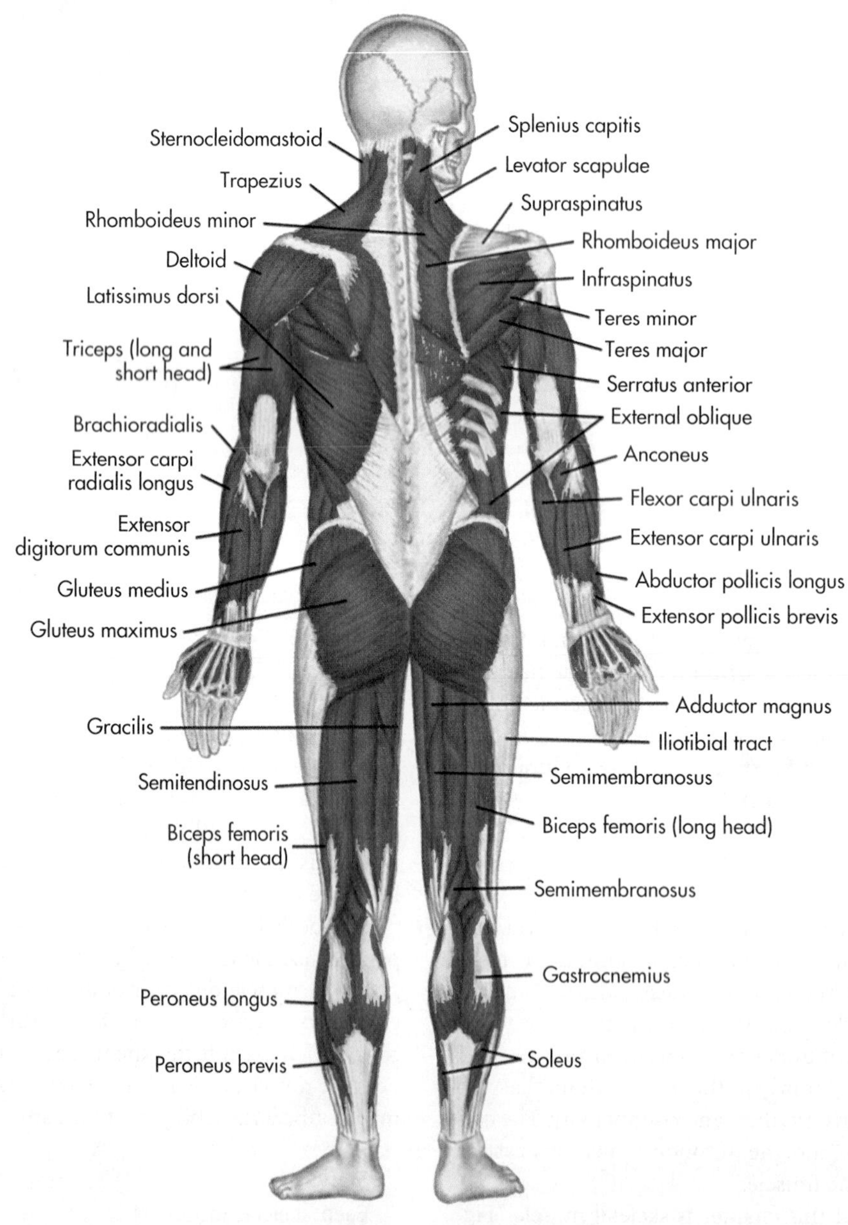

Figure 45-7 Skeletal muscles of body, posterior view.

ceived, bind to troponin (an inhibitor of the molecular myosin-actin interaction). Once troponin is bound, the myosin-actin interaction takes place and the sarcomeres of the myofibrils contract. This is known as the cross-bridge theory, which replaced the sliding filament theory described by Huxley.[5] The energy for muscle contraction is supplied by the breakdown of adenosine triphosphate (ATP), a substance that muscle cells produce by combining adenosine diphosphate with creatine phosphate. Relaxation of the muscle occurs when the calcium separates from the troponin (Figure 45-10).

Muscle cells obey the "all or none" law; that is, they contract fully or not at all. This does not mean that the entire muscle contracts fully. Only those individual cells that receive the nerve impulse contract. Adequately oxygenated muscle fibers contract more forcefully than those inadequately oxygenated.

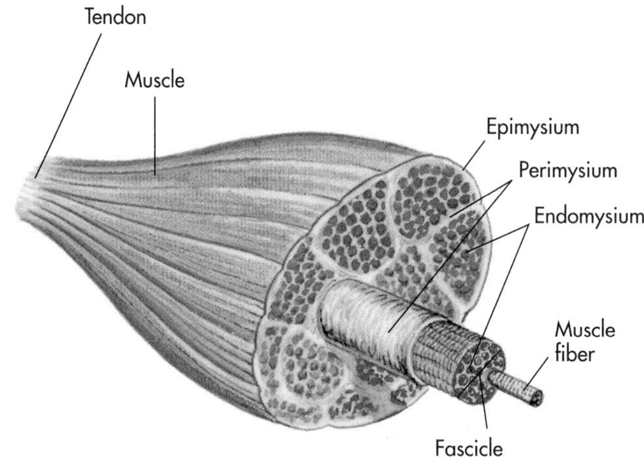

Figure 45-8 Cross section of skeletal muscle showing muscle fibers and their coverings.

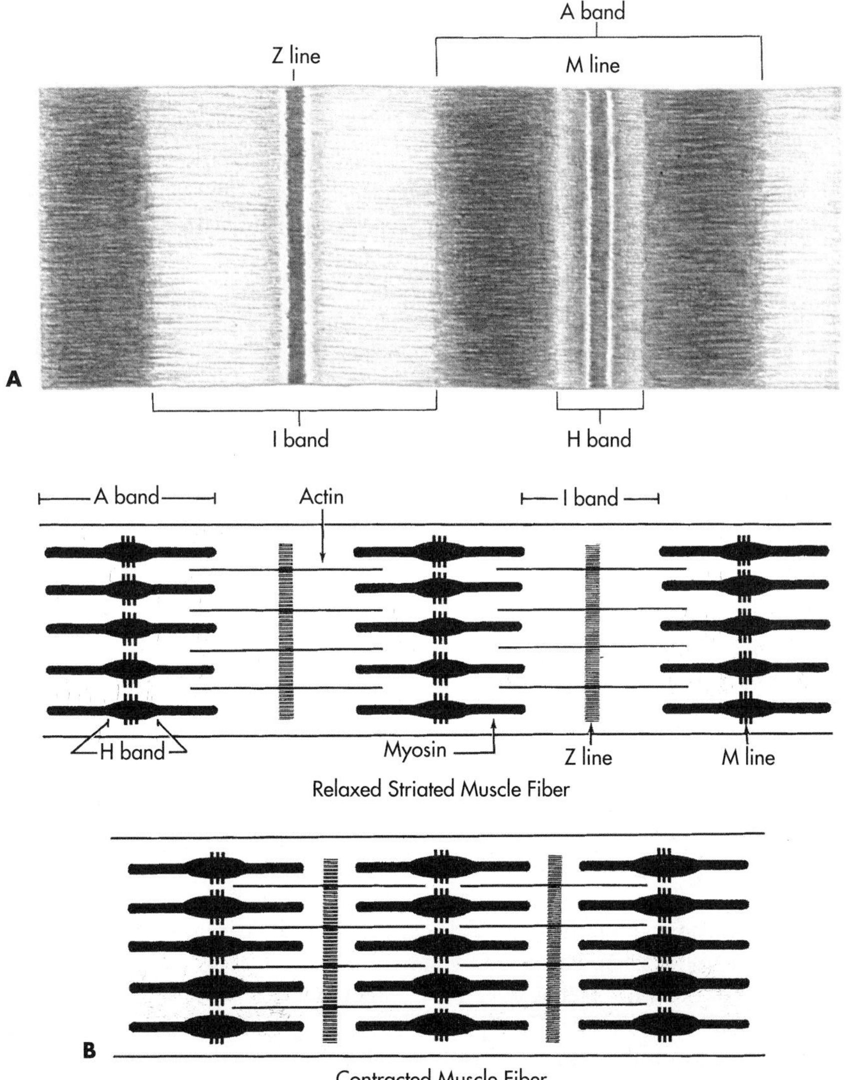

Figure 45-9 Muscle fibers. **A,** Lines and bands in striated muscle. **B,** Relationships of bands, actin, myosin, and lines in relaxed and contracted muscle fibers.

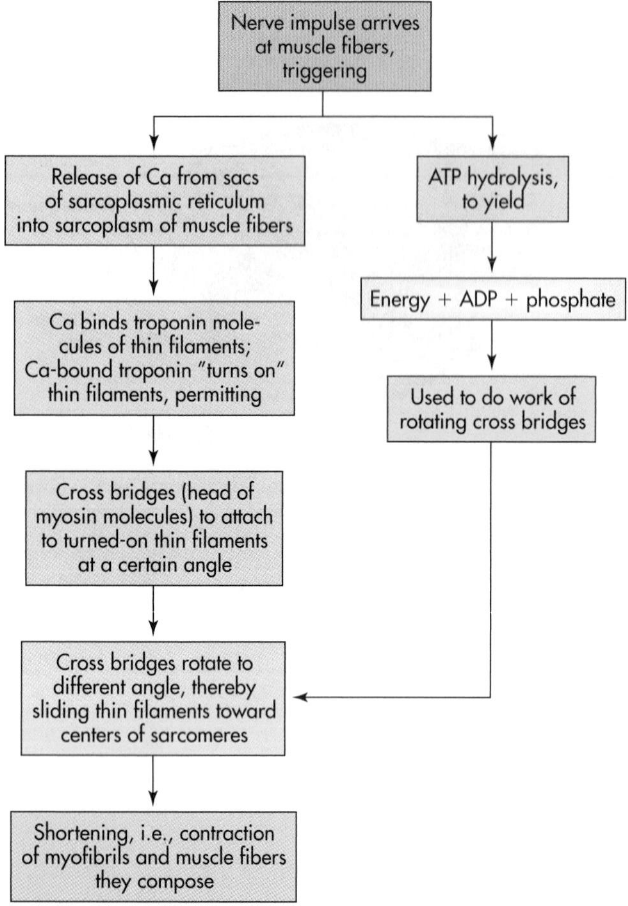

Figure 45-10 Mechanism of skeletal muscle contraction.

Types of Contractions

The arrangement of the fibers within the muscle determines the capacity of the forceful contraction of the muscle. Skeletal muscles contract only if they are stimulated. There are many types of contractions:

1. Tonic: a continual partial contraction that is vital in the maintenance of posture.
2. Isotonic: a contraction in which tension within the muscle is constant but the length of the muscle changes; it can either shorten (concentric contraction) or lengthen (eccentric). Examples of concentric contractions include lifting weights or climbing up stairs; going down stairs or putting down a weight are examples of eccentric contractions. Eccentric contraction uses less energy and results in pain and stiffness following unaccustomed exercise.
3. Isometric (static or holding): tension within the muscle increases, but the muscle does not shorten. Postoperative leg exercises are examples of isometric exercises.
4. Twitch: a jerky reaction to a single stimulus.
5. Tetanic: a more sustained contraction than the twitch, produced by a series of stimuli in rapid succession.
6. Spasm: an involuntary contraction caused by stimulation of an entire motor unit.
7. Treppe: stronger twitch contractions in response to regularly repeated, constant-strength stimuli.
8. Fibrillation: a synchronous contraction of individual fibers.
9. Convulsive: abnormal uncoordinated tetanic contractions occurring in varying groups of muscles.

Mechanism of Muscle Movement

Movements of the body are produced by muscles pulling on bones; the bones serve as levers, and the joints serve as fulcrums for the levers. Most movements depend on several muscles acting in a coordinated manner. To produce movement, a muscle acts as a prime mover, or agonist, as its reciprocal muscle, or antagonist, relaxes. Synergistic muscles contract at the same time as the prime movers, either to produce the movement or to stabilize a body part so that contraction of the prime movers is more efficient.

Muscle Metabolism

Energy for a muscle contraction can be generated both aerobically and anaerobically. The two anaerobic processes are the adenosine triphosphate—phosphocreatinine (ATP-PC) system and anaerobic glycolysis. The ATP-PC system is used for extremely short, explosive activities lasting no longer than 3 seconds. Anaerobic glycolysis is used at the beginning of sustained activity before the onset of aerobic metabolism and lasts for 2 to 3 minutes. During anaerobic glycolysis, lactic acid accumulates within the muscle. When 60 to 70 g of lactic acid has accumulated, the muscle reaches exhaustive levels. The rate of lactic acid accumulation is directly proportional to exercise intensity.

Anaerobic energy production is rapid and is valuable for quick bursts of energy to be used during intense activity. The aerobic method of energy production involves the burning of foodstuffs. Aerobic glycolysis depends on the presence of oxygen and relies on the production of ATP from the oxidation of carbohydrates, fats, and proteins. This method of energy production is used during prolonged activity.

Efficient muscle contraction depends on an adequate blood supply to and from the muscle fibers. Therefore skeletal muscle is highly vascular. Waste products resulting from the chemical changes that occur during muscle contraction must be transported to the liver to be resynthesized. When waste products are not adequately carried off, muscle fatigue and pain result. Conversely, oxygen must be transported to the muscle fibers to support the work of muscle contraction. Poor muscle work occurs when the oxygen supply is inadequate (e.g., in conditions such as anemia, in which the amount of oxygen-carrying hemoglobin is reduced, or trauma, in which circulation to the muscle fibers is interrupted).

Muscle Innervation

Adequate muscle contraction also depends on effective innervation. The cerebellum is primarily responsible for control of muscle movement. Every muscle cell is supplied with the axon of a nerve cell. Nerve cells that transmit impulses to skeletal muscles are known as somatic motor neurons. The neuron

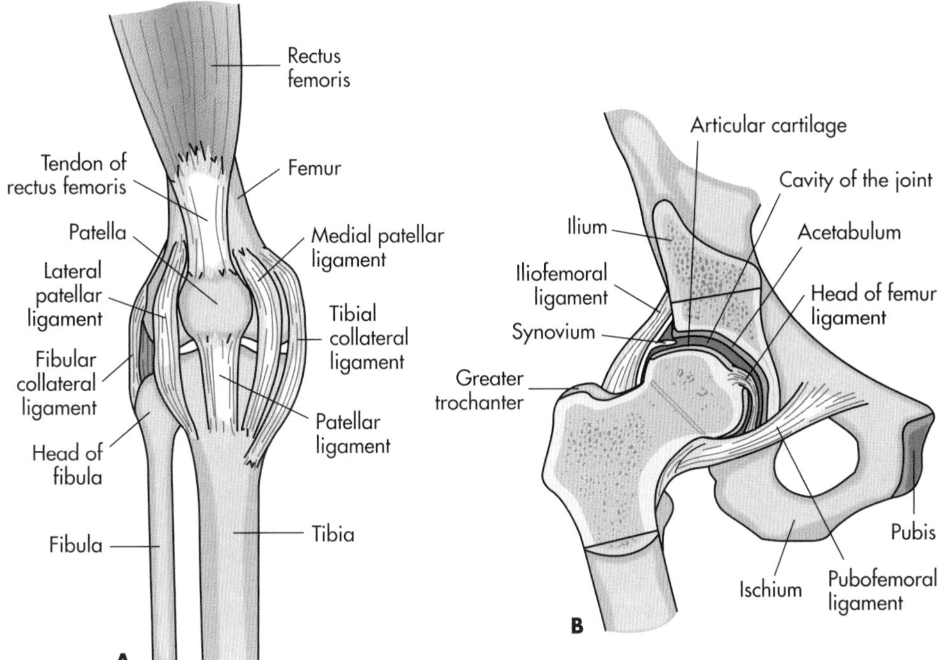

Figure 45-11 **A,** Ligaments of knee joint. **B,** Ligaments of hip joint.

and the muscle cell it activates are called a motor unit. The number of motor units per muscle varies significantly. The motor units, made up of lower motor neurons, extend to the skeletal muscle. The axon of one somatic motor neuron may be divided into any number of branches and therefore innervates a like number of muscle cells. The fewer muscle cells innervated, the more precise (or fine) are the resultant movements.

The actual contraction of the muscle is set off by the release of acetylcholine, a chemical contained in small vesicles in the axon terminal. When acetylcholine makes contact with the sarcolemma, it stimulates the contraction. This reaction takes place across a structure known as the motor end plate or neuromuscular junction, where the muscle and the nerve are in contact. Damage to the nervous system at the cerebrospinal level or at any point in the nerve's course through the local motor neuron level will result in muscular dysfunction.

Cartilage

Cartilage is composed of fibers embedded in a firm gel. Structurally cartilage is a strong but flexible material. Another important characteristic, particularly of articular cartilage, is its avascularity. Nutrients reach the cartilage cells by diffusion through the gel from capillaries located in the perichondrium (fibrous covering of the cartilage) or, in the case of articular cartilage, through the synovial fluid.

The number of collagenous fibers found in the cartilage determines its type: fibrous, hyaline, or elastic. Fibrous cartilage (or fibrocartilage) composes the intervertebral disks. The amount of fibrous cartilage increases with age; the transformation of hyaline cartilage into fibrous cartilage is a sign of aging. Hyaline, the most common type of cartilage, is composed of chondrocytes (cartilage cells), type II collagen fibers in the matrix, and protein polysaccharide complexes and water between the matrix and fibers. Its composition gives hyaline cartilage its spongy and elastic qualities, which are crucial to preventing injury to the bone during weight bearing. Articular cartilage is hyaline cartilage that covers the articulating surface on the ends of bone, reducing friction and evening weight distribution in the joint. The amount or thickness depends on the type of bone and amount of weight and shearing force to which the joint is subjected.

Articular cartilage contains 60% to 80% water and does not contain any blood vessels, lymph tissue, or nerves. As a result, it is insensitive to pain and does not easily repair itself following injury. Regeneration occurs at the junction of the synovial membrane and cartilage because of the adjacent blood supply and nutrients supplying the synovial membrane.

Yellow or elastic cartilage has the fewest fibers. Elastic cartilage may be found in areas such as the external ear and epiglottis.

Ligaments

Ligaments are parallel bands of flexible, dense fibrous connective tissue. Their primary function is to connect the articular ends of bones and provide stability. Ligaments permit movement in some directions but limit movement in others, preventing joint injury, as in the knee and hip joints (Figure 45-11). The medial and lateral collateral ligaments of the knee provide mediolateral stability to the knee joint; the anterior and posterior cruciate ligaments within the joint capsule of the knee provide anteroposterior stability. Ligaments may also attach to soft tissue to suspend structures (e.g., the suspensory ligament of the ovary that passes from the tubal end of the ovary to the peritoneum).

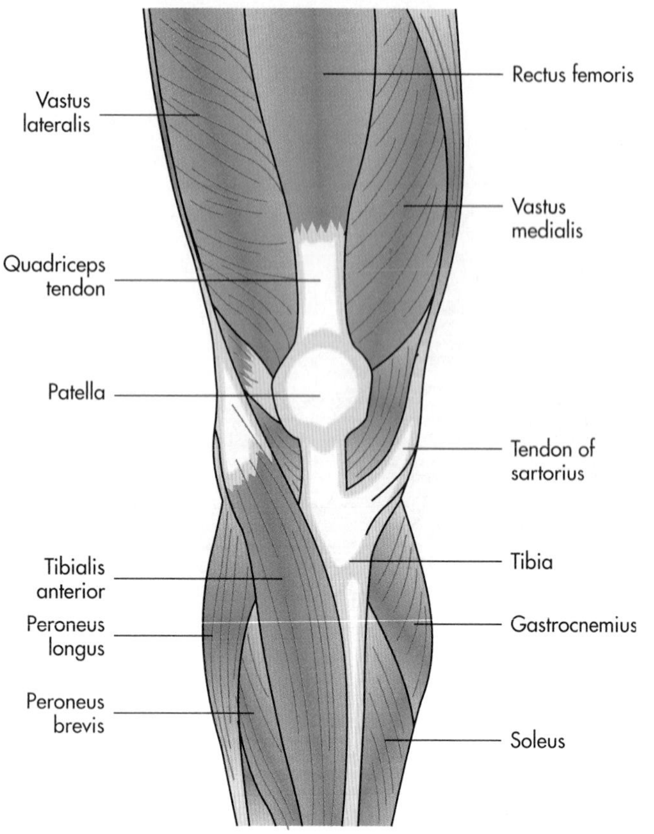

Figure 45-12 Anterior view of tendons around knee joint.

Tendons

Tendons are bands of dense fibrous tissue that form the origin and insertion of muscle to bone (Figure 45-12). The longitudinal arrangement of fibers provides tensile strength while preventing injury to the tendon. The tendon is an extension of the fibrous sheath that envelops each muscle and is continuous with the periosteum at its other end. Tendon sheaths are tubular structures of connective tissue that enclose certain tendons, especially in the wrist and ankle. These sheaths are lined with a synovial membrane, which provides lubrication (synovial fluid) for each movement of the tendon. Ligaments and tendons may add extra stability to the capsule. The synovial membrane, or synovium, lines the nonarticulating surfaces of the joint capsule. The synovium is capable of repair because of its rich blood and lymph supply. The synovial membrane secretes synovial fluid into the joint capsule for lubrication (Figure 45-13). Synovial fluid is plasma derived from blood vessels in the synovium. In addition to joint lubrication, synovial fluid provides nourishment to articular cartilage and contains leukocytes that have a phagocytic action on bacteria and debris in the joint. A decrease in synovial fluid can lead to destruction of the articular cartilage.

Fascia

Fascia is a sheet of loose connective tissue that may be found directly under the skin as superficial fascia or as a sheet of dense, fibrous connective tissue making up the sheath of muscles, nerves, and blood vessels. The latter is known as deep fascia.

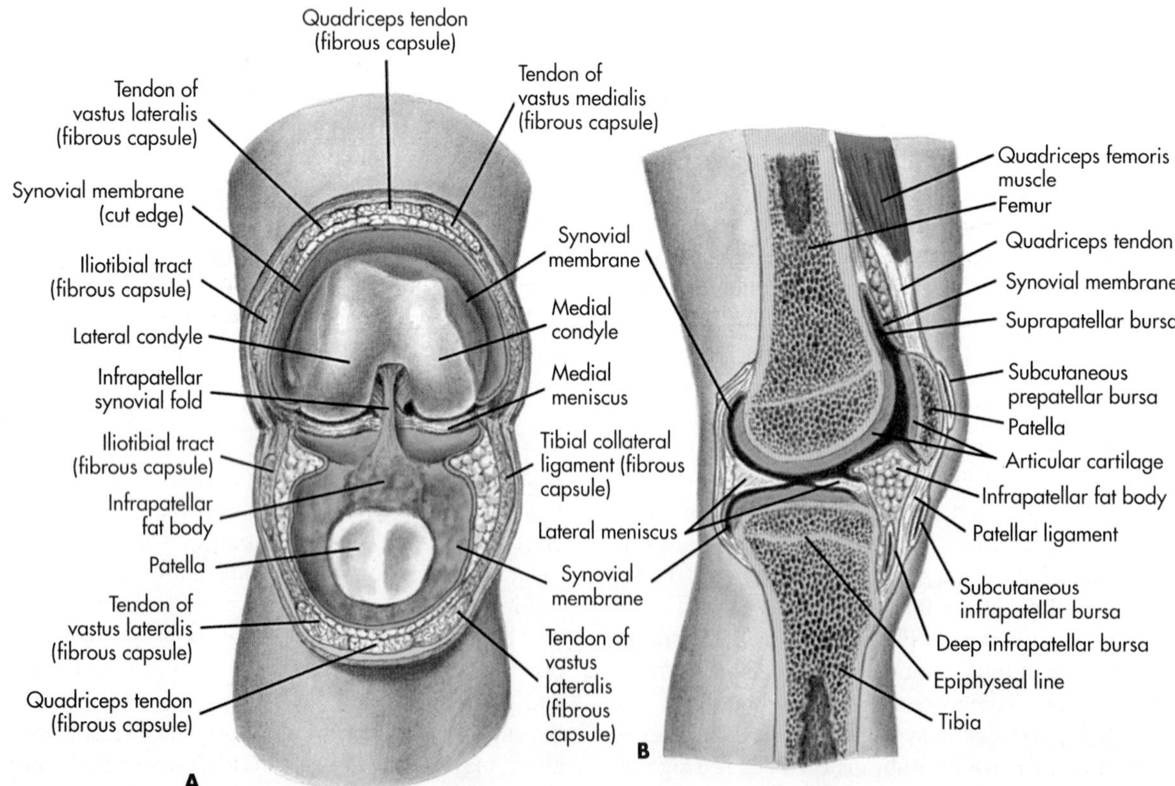

Figure 45-13 Knee joint (synovial joint). **A**, Frontal view. **B**, Lateral view.

Bursae

Bursae are small sacs of connective tissue located wherever pressure is exerted over moving parts. They may occur between skin and bone, between tendons and bone, or between muscles. Bursae are lined with synovial membrane and contain synovial fluid and serve as cushions between moving parts. One such bursa, the olecranon bursa, is located between the olecranon process and the skin. New bursae can develop as a result of prolonged or increased pressure or friction, often resulting in pain. The shoulder bursa (subacromial) is a common site of bursitis (Figure 45-14).

Joints

Movement would be impossible without flexibility within the skeletal framework. This flexibility is provided by the joints or places where the bones come together and articulate. The shape of the joint determines the amount and type of movement possible. Joints are classified by the amount of movement they allow and by the type of connective tissue that joins them.

Types

There are three major types of joints:

1. Synarthroses or fibrous: allow no movement and are exemplified by the sutures of the skull. Sutures bind bones tightly together with a thin layer of dense fibrous tissue.
2. Amphiarthroses or cartilaginous: allow little movement and are exemplified by the intervertebral joints and symphysis pubis. A syndesmosis is a type of amphiarthrosis joint that is joined by a ligament or membrane, such as the radioulnar joint and the tibiofibular joint.
3. Diarthroses or synovial: allow free movement and are exemplified by the hip, knee, shoulder, and elbow.

The synarthroses and amphiarthroses may be classified together as synarthroses, because both lack a joint cavity. Fibrous, cartilaginous, or osseous tissue grows between their articular surfaces. Because diarthroses are the joints that permit movement, they are discussed in the most detail.

Structure of Diarthrodial Joints

Each diarthrodial joint contains a small space, or joint cavity, between the articulating surfaces of the bones that make up the joint. Articular hyaline cartilage covers the articulating surfaces of both bones, allowing for the smooth, gliding motion of the joint. A joint capsule, or sleeve of fibrous tissue, encases the joint (see Figure 45-13).

Small pieces of dense cartilage may also be interposed between the articulating surfaces. These are crescent (or half-moon)–shaped structures (menisci) that provide additional cushioning of the joint. Examples include the medial and lateral menisci of the knee joint.

Function of Diarthrodial Joints

Joints provide the skeleton with both stability and mobility. In addition to the joint types already described, diarthrodial joints are further classified by the shape of their surface and the type of movement they permit. Examples include ball and socket (shoulder, hip), hinge (elbow, knee), pivot (atlas, axis), condyloid (wrist), saddle (first metacarpal, trapezium), and gliding (intervertebral disks).

Each joint has its own range and direction of movement. Diarthrodial joints permit one or more of the following

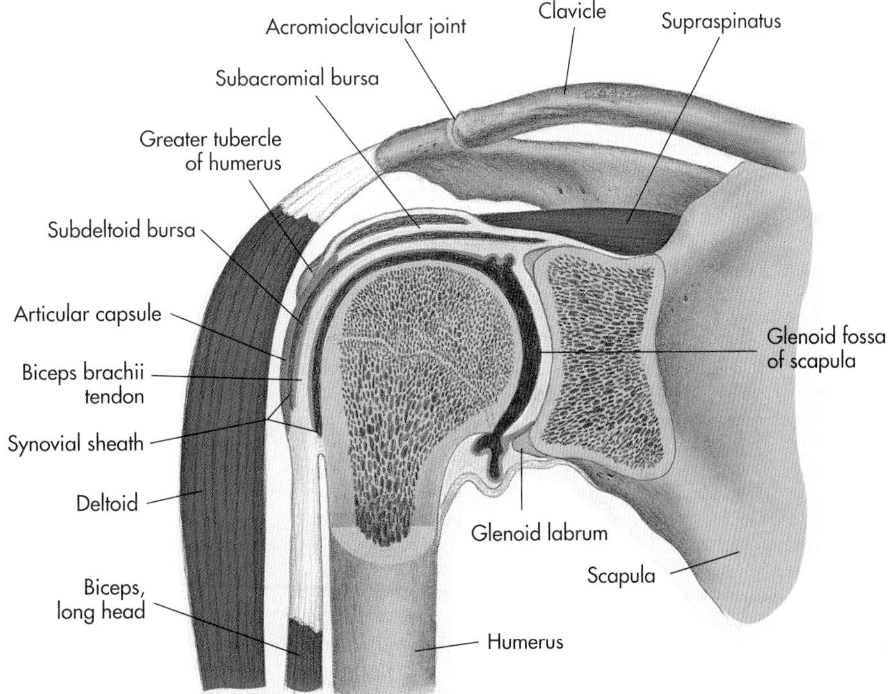

Figure 45-14 Shoulder joint bursae.

movements: flexion, extension, abduction, adduction, rotation, circumduction, supination, pronation, inversion, and eversion (Figures 45-15 to 45-17).

Physiologic Changes With Aging

Physiologic changes occur in the musculoskeletal system throughout a person's life span (Table 45-2). Childhood and adolescence are a time of rapid growth and development of the structures of the system. However, with maturity and aging, tissue strength and integrity begin to decline as the total number of body cells decreases. Connective tissues, particularly the articular cartilage of the joints and the intervertebral disks of the spine, lose some of their elasticity and resilience. Cartilage becomes more rigid because of increased cross-linking of collagen and elastin and decreased water content in the ground substance. As the amount of vigorous activity an individual engages in decreases, muscles lose bulk, tone, and strength.

Bone resorption takes place more rapidly than bone growth, and particularly in postmenopausal women, calcium is lost from the bone. A universal effect of aging is impaired osteoblastic activity. Women in particular experience loss of bone density and increased osteoclastic bone resorption with the aging process. By age 70 a woman has lost approximately 50% of her peripheral cortical bone mass.[2] In contrast, men experience bone loss later and at a slower rate than women. In addition, men initially have 30% more bone mass than women. African-Americans have denser bones than Caucasians, Asians, and Native Americans.

Muscle strength reaches a peak at 25 to 30 years, is maintained through the fifth decade, and then declines noticeably after 70 years of age. An estimated 30% to 40% of skeletal

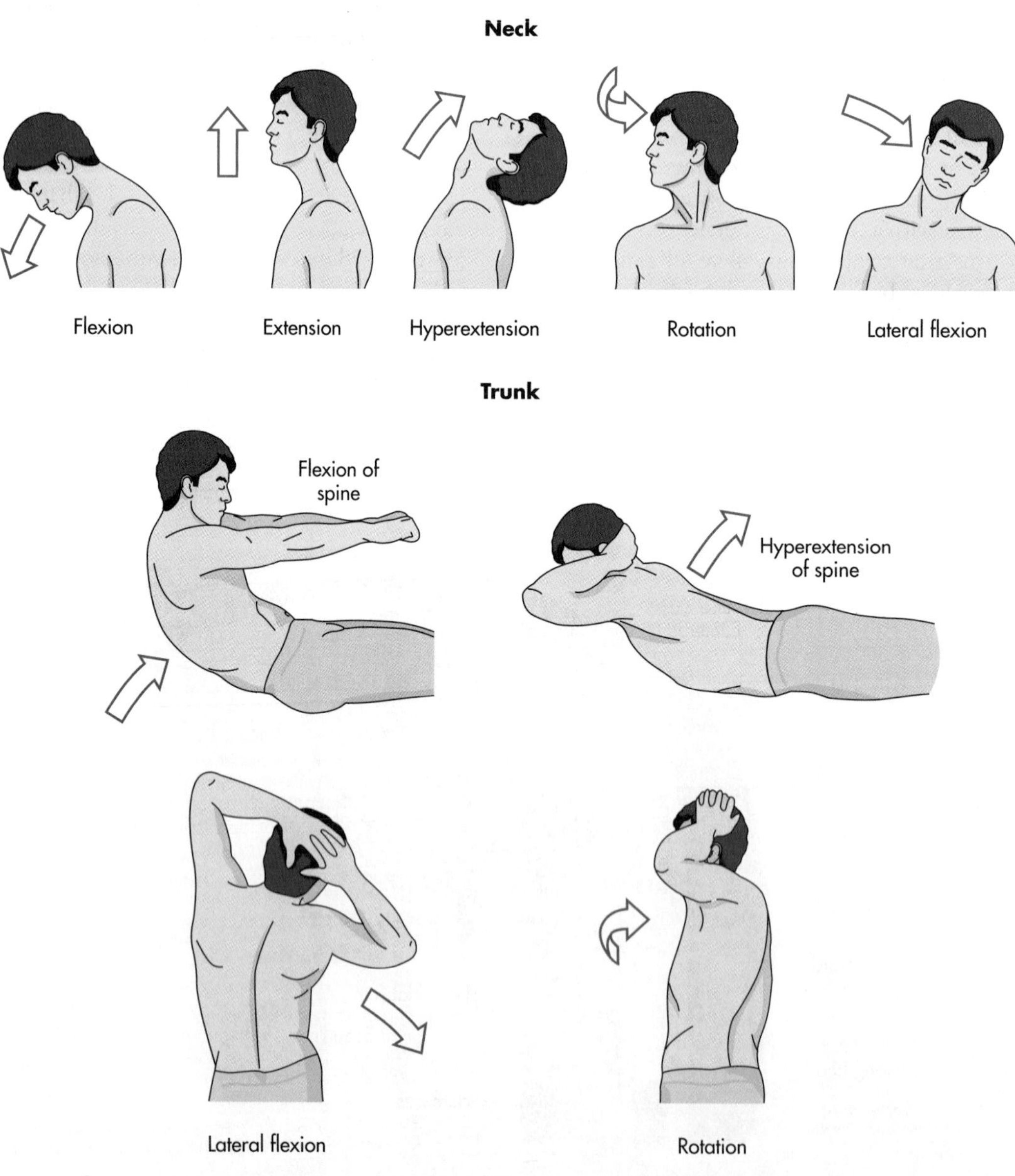

Figure 45-15 Range of motion for neck and trunk.

muscle mass is lost between the ages of 30 and 90 years.[2] The term *sarcopenia* refers to age-related skeletal muscle loss.

There are several age-related changes in the musculoskeletal system. With age, the shoulders may become stooped and narrowed. The knees and hips may be slightly flexed when standing or walking because of pain associated with joint degeneration. Posture becomes stooped as the body attempts to compensate for changes in the center of gravity caused by lower extremity joint flexion and forward thrusting of the head, neck, and shoulders. With these changes, height can

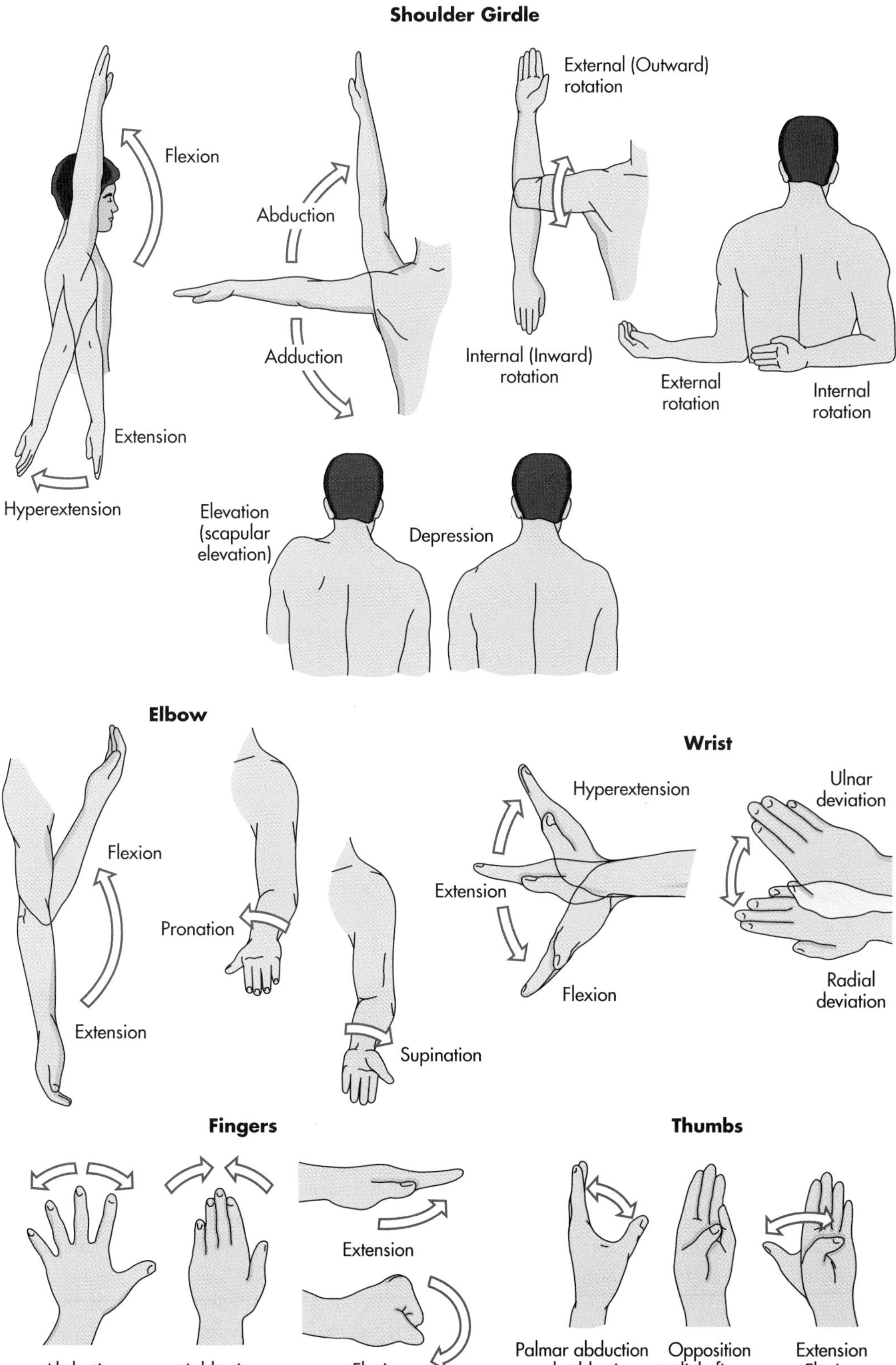

Figure 45-16 Range of joint motion for shoulder girdle, elbow, forearm, wrist, fingers, and thumbs.

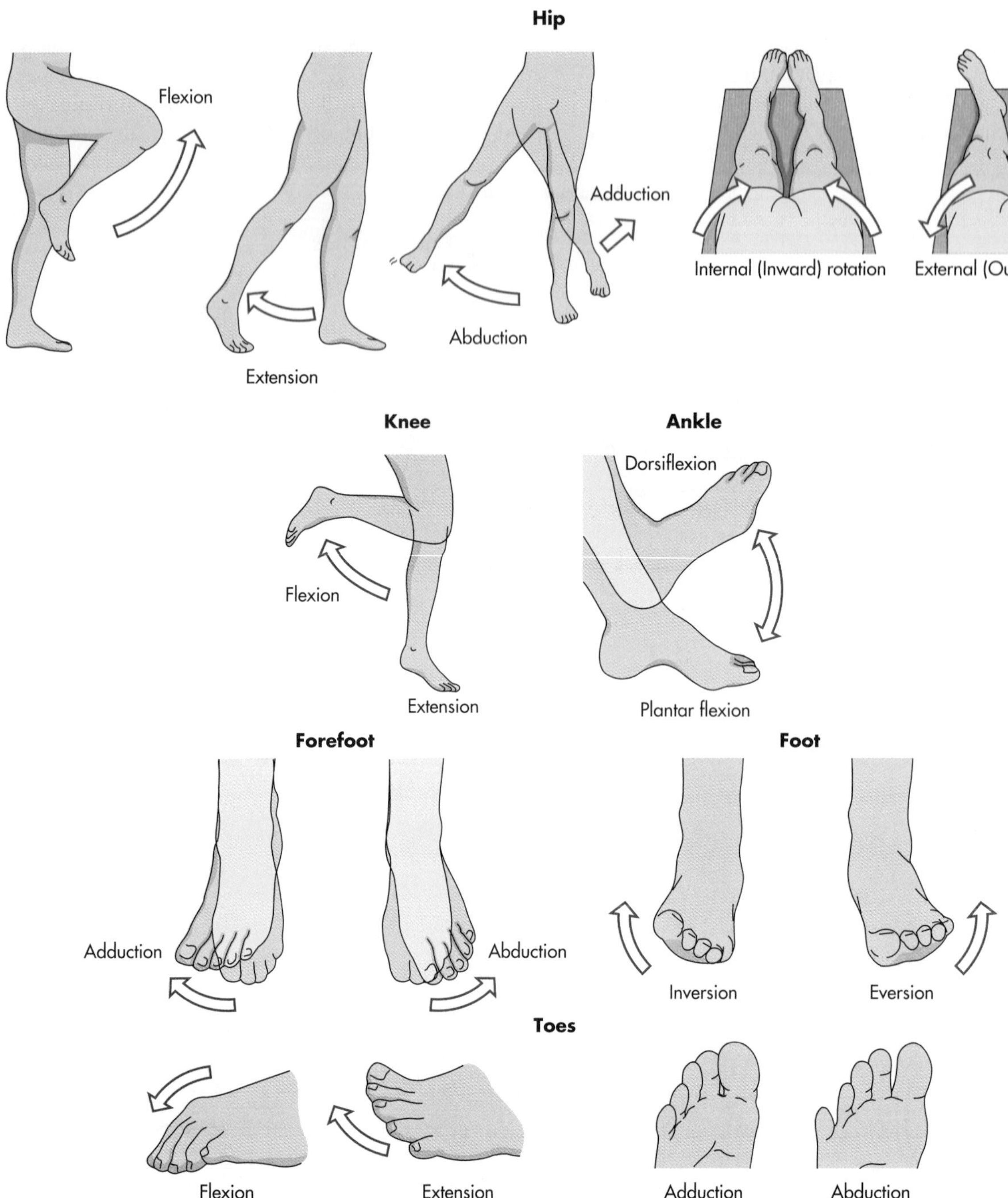

Figure 45-17 Range of joint motion for hip, knee, ankle, foot, and toes.

decrease by 6 to 10 cm. Gait may become unsteady because of loss of muscle strength and coordination, and the individual is more susceptible to falls. An estimated one third of persons 65 years of age and older experience falls annually.[2] Of this number, 2% are hospitalized as a result. Falls are common in nursing homes; an estimated 50% of nursing home residents fall each year. Assessment of fall risk and fall prevention are important nursing interventions, given that falls are the number one cause of accidental death in older adults.

Approximately 40% of community-dwelling older adults have arthritis, and 17% report chronic problems of the musculoskeletal system.[2] Independence and the ability to perform activities of daily living (ADLs) are commonly affected. Although diseases of the musculoskeletal system are not usually fatal, they do cause chronic pain and disability. However, complications arising as a result of a musculoskeletal problem can be fatal.

Programs of regular exercise (including weight-bearing activities) and resistive muscle strengthening can decrease or prevent some of the age-related changes in the musculoskeletal system. A nutritionally adequate diet is also beneficial.

TABLE 45-2 Physiologic Changes With Aging

Tissue	Change	Potential Problem
Bone	Decreased total bone mass Impaired osteoblastic activity Resorption exceeds growth Erosion of haversian systems Cortical bone changing to cancellous bone Porous cortical bone	Osteoporosis, pathologic fracture, delayed healing
Muscles	Decline in strength past 70 years Decline in number of muscle fibers Decrease in muscle mass Atrophy of muscle cells	Weakness, uncoordination, disuse atrophy, slow unsteady gait, poor posture, falls, contractures
Joints	Decreased elasticity of cartilage Increased susceptibility to tears in cartilage	Arthritis, decreased range of motion, contractures

ASSESSMENT

Health History

Plans for the care of any person with a musculoskeletal problem are based on a systematic assessment of needs, capabilities, and resources. A thorough assessment includes subjective data gathered from patient and family interviews. Information to be obtained and areas to be explored include:

- Age: age can be a predictor of common problems associated with a particular age-group. For example, older adults are susceptible to falls, older women have an increased risk for osteoporosis, and young men are at a higher risk for trauma.
- Height and weight: any changes? If so, were they intentional? What is the person's ideal weight and body mass index? Any loss of height, particularly in older adults?
- Nutrition: dietary intake of calcium, vitamin D, minerals, total calories, fad diets?
- Occupation (past, present): sedentary, standing, repetitive movements, safety factors, lifting, ergonomic environment?
- Exercise regimen: type, frequency, duration, weight-bearing activity, safety equipment, type of shoes, warm-up, cool-down activities?
- Ability to perform ADLs, noting type and amount of assistance required, use of assistive or adaptive devices.
- Transfer ability.
- Psychosocial factors such as marital status, support systems, methods and effectiveness of coping with stress, role changes, leisure activities, and cultural beliefs.
- Availability of transportation.
- Physical layout of home: steps, accessibility; assessment of risk for injury.
- Reliance on community services: past, present; usefulness of services.
- Exposure to environmental irritants, radiation.
- Allergies: record any reaction to iodine, shellfish.
- Medications: note use of aspirin, nonsteroidal antiinflammatory drugs, steroids, anticoagulants, hormones, vitamins, or analgesics. Include frequency, duration, indication, and effectiveness.
- Smoking, alcohol, and recreational drug use.
- Dominant hand.
- Childbearing history: nulliparity is a risk factor for osteoporosis.

Family History

- Genetic disorders, abnormalities
- Congenital abnormalities
- Arthritis, scoliosis, ankylosing spondylitis

Medical and Surgical History

- Developmental abnormalities
- Childhood diseases, illnesses, trauma
- Chronic illnesses, hospitalizations
- Past surgeries
- Age at menopause

Review of Systems

Obtain data regarding history of integumentary, ophthalmic, auditory, hematologic, immunologic, respiratory, cardiovascular, gastrointestinal, genitourinary, endocrine, neurologic, or psychologic problems that may have relevance to the presenting problem.

History of the Current Problem

- Onset of the problem
- Circumstances surrounding the onset of the problem: any precipitating or associated events or injuries?
- Duration of the problem
- Patient's perception of the problem
- Patient's perception of the impact the problem has had on his or her lifestyle, ability to carry out ADLs
- Any efforts to treat the problem and their effectiveness
- Adherence to treatment programs
- Trauma, mechanism of injury, sensations or sounds at the time of injury

TABLE 45-3 Physical Examination Data

Observations	Rationale
General Appearance	
Race Caucasian, Asian	Risk factor for osteoporosis
Posture	May be characteristic of a specific problem (e.g., scoliosis; kyphotic posture in ankylosing spondylitis; guarding of head, neck, and shoulders following whiplash)
Nutritional status	
Overweight	May indicate diminished ability to perform regular exercise or activity; excess weight causes increased stress on joints
Underweight	May indicate inability to secure or prepare nutritious meals or to carry out feeding activities adequately; women with thin build are at risk for osteoporosis
	May relate to specific systemic condition causing anorexia, nausea, vomiting, or malabsorption of food
Skin	
Turgor	Thin, papery skin may indicate aging, systemic connective tissue disease, or long-term steroid use; skin is easily broken
Texture	Thick, leathery patches over forearms, hands, chest, and face indicate scleroderma; ulcerates easily, especially over joints
Integrity Breaks in skin, ulcerations, reddened areas	Individuals with limited mobility are subject to skin breakdown and pressure ulcers from pressure over skin areas, which interferes with circulation; possibility of shearing forces against sheets, chair surfaces, bedpans, or other surfaces tearing or abrading skin
Temperature	Warmth, especially over painful joints, indicative of presence and degree of inflammatory or infectious process within joint
Erythema over joints	Indicates inflammation and the need to keep joint at rest
	May be present in systemic connective tissue disorders (psoriasis, scleroderma, dermatomyositis); initial observations provide useful baseline to determine effectiveness of treatment
Color change on exposure to cold	Change from white (resulting from arteriolar spasm) to blue (cyanosis caused by stagnation of blood) to red (warming and reactive vasodilation) present in some connective tissue disorders (Raynaud's phenomenon)
Bruising	Often present following trauma and consequent to long-term treatment of connective tissue disease with corticosteroids; anticoagulant use
Swelling of extremities or joints	In extremities, may denote prolonged dependent position, lack of activity, circulatory or renal impairment
	In joints, may indicate presence of effusion (serous, purulent, or bloody fluid in joint capsule); inflamed synovium (feels boggy): indication of need to rest joints involved
Bony enlargements	Indicative of disease process (e.g., Heberden's nodes, in osteoarthritis—hard, irregular swellings over distal interphalangeal joints of fingers—or Bouchard's nodes—cartilaginous or bony enlargement of proximal interphalangeal finger joints) (Figure 45-18)
Subcutaneous nodules	Indicative of rheumatoid arthritis: hard, mobile swellings commonly found in subolecranon area
Bursal swelling	Indicative of bursal inflammation: palpated as soft swelling over bursa
Synovial cyst	Indicative of hypertrophy of synovial tissue (e.g., Baker's cyst—swelling in popliteal area, often extending into calf)
Tophaceous deposits	Indicative of gout: hard translucent swellings over joints or in cartilage such as that of ear
Tenderness: may be elicited by direct pressure and graded by amount of pressure required to produce discomfort	Degree of tenderness is usually in direct proportion to severity of inflammation or trauma (e.g., in joint inflammation or injured soft tissue or overlying fracture)
General hygiene: evidence of uncleanliness of body, clothing	May indicate inability to adequately carry out hygienic requirements (because this may be embarrassing for the individual, plans must be made to introduce self-help devices or to provide assistance in ways that will not be demeaning)
Nails and Hair	
Poorly kept or diseased nails	May indicate lack of strength or inability to reach nails to care for them
	Change in nail structure may indicate presence of connective tissue disease
Poorly kept hair	May indicate inability to lift arms to comb hair
Alopecia, scaling of scalp	May indicate connective tissue disease, medications

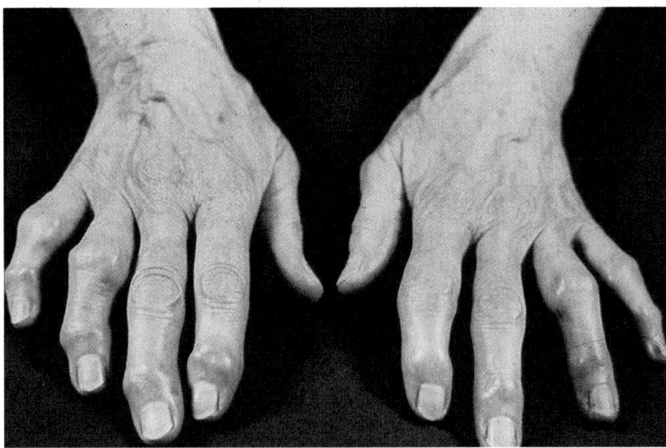

Figure 45-18 Heberden's nodes at distal interphalangeal joints and Bouchard's nodes at proximal interphalangeal joints.

- Any history of paresthesias, paralysis, swelling (location and timing), locking, "giving way"
- Unilateral or bilateral joint involvement
- Reasons for seeking and expectations of current treatment

Discomfort Associated With the Problem

Because pain or discomfort mark many musculoskeletal problems, questions should elicit the following information about the pain or discomfort:

- Nature
- Location
- Duration
- Radiating or referred pain
- Evaluation of pain, using pain-rating scale
- Measures the person has taken to alleviate pain or discomfort
- Effectiveness of measures taken
- Effect on daily or leisure activities
- Associated or precipitating events

Physical Examination

Observations are made regarding general appearance, skin, nails, and hair (Table 45-3). In addition, data are collected regarding deformities, strength and range of motion, ability to transfer and ambulate, and a complete functional assessment.

Inspection

Much information can be gathered even before the physical examination begins. The patient's gait as he or she enters the examining room is observed, and the person's ability to stand, sit, and rise from a chair is noted. If the patient uses assistive devices for ambulation or transferring, whether or not the devices are being used properly is observed. At the same time that patient privacy is ensured, the person's ability to dress and undress is assessed. These data are useful in determining the individual's functional status. The person's posture while standing erect is observed, and any abnormal curvatures of the spine are noted. A gentle lordotic (concave) curve in the lumbar spine is normal, and a gentle kyphotic (convex) curve in the thoracic spine is also normal (Figure 45-19). Any exaggeration of these normal curves, such as a lateral curvature or scoliotic curve of the spine, is considered abnormal.

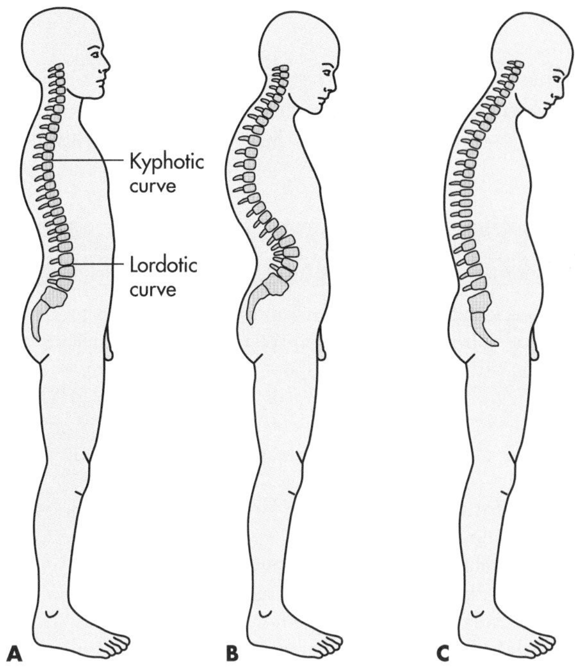

Figure 45-19 A, Curves of spine in good posture. B, Curves of spine in slumping posture. C, Obliteration of spinal curves, such as in early spondylitis.

BOX 45-1 Normal Gait Cycle

Stance phase	Begins with heel strike and ends with toe-off
Swing phase	Begins with toe-off and continues through heel strike
Double support	Brief period when both feet are on ground

A person's gait (Box 45-1) is his or her manner or style of walking. An altered gait pattern indicates a pathologic process. Having the patient walk 20 to 25 feet is usually adequate to make an accurate assessment of gait. During observation of ambulation, the presence and type of any limp, involved joints, the ability to bear weight, balance, and the degree of any deformity in the lower extremities are noted. Deformity of the lower extremities (e.g., genu varum, talipes varus) may not be as apparent when the joint is examined at rest as when weight-bearing forces are exerted across the joint. Furthermore, in persons with significant upper extremity involvement, some consideration must be given both to the amount of weight bearing that might be expected from the arms and hands and to the appropriate type of assistive device. For example, the individual with severe rheumatoid involvement of the hands might need a device that permits weight bearing on the forearms.

Other problems, such as cardiovascular disease, respiratory impairment, or anemia, may also affect ambulatory ability and must be considered during the assessment of ambulation. Assessment of transfer and ambulatory ability helps determine a suitable level of activity for the patient. All extremities must be observed for overall muscle mass, deformities, asymmetry, and masses. See Box 45-2 for a list of common musculoskeletal deformities.

BOX 45-2 Common Musculoskeletal Deformities

Swan neck deformity: flexion contracture of the metacarpophalangeal joints, hyperextension of the proximal interphalangeal joints, and flexion of the distal interphalangeal joints of the fingers (Figure 45-20), found in advanced rheumatoid arthritis

Ulnar deviation or drift: fingers deviate at the metacarpophalangeal joints toward the ulnar aspect of the hand (Figure 45-21)

Valgus deformities: distal arm of the angle of the joint points away from the midline of the body
- Hallux valgus: great toe turns toward the other toes
- Genu valgum: "knock-knees" (Figure 45-22)
- Talipes valgus: eversion of the foot

Varus deformities: distal arm of the angle of the joint points toward the midline of the body
- Genu varum: bowing of the knees
- Talipes varus: inversion of the foot

Scoliosis: lateral curvature of the spine

Kyphosis: thoracic spinal curvature, the convexity of the curve being posterior

Atrophy: reduction in size of an extremity or body part (e.g., wasting of muscles so that they appear to lack the bulk of normal muscle); can result from lack of use or disease process (e.g., polymyositis)

Hypertrophy: abnormal enlargement of an organ or body part; limitation of function may be associated with enlargement

Pes planus: flat feet (Figure 45-23, *A*)

Pes cavus: high instep (Figure 45-23, *B*)

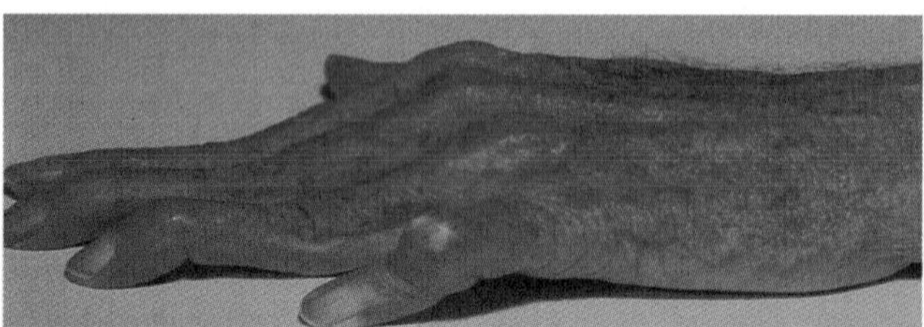

Figure 45-20 Swan neck deformities of fingers in rheumatoid arthritis.

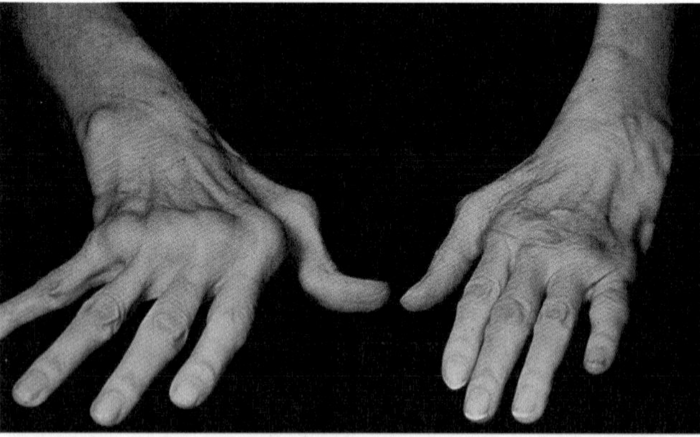

Figure 45-21 Ulnar deviation and subluxation of metacarpophalangeal joints.

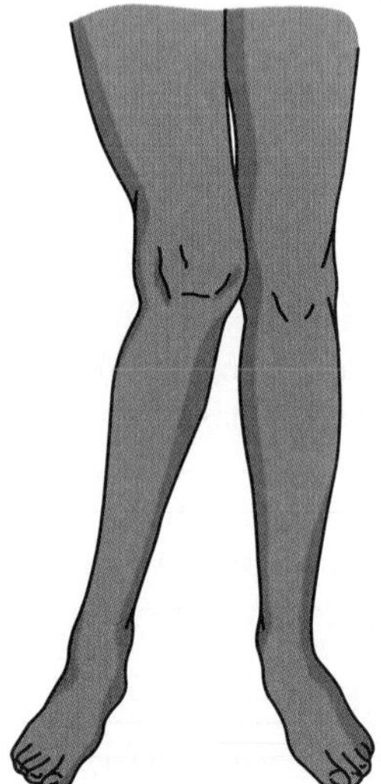

Figure 45-22 Valgus deformity of right knee.

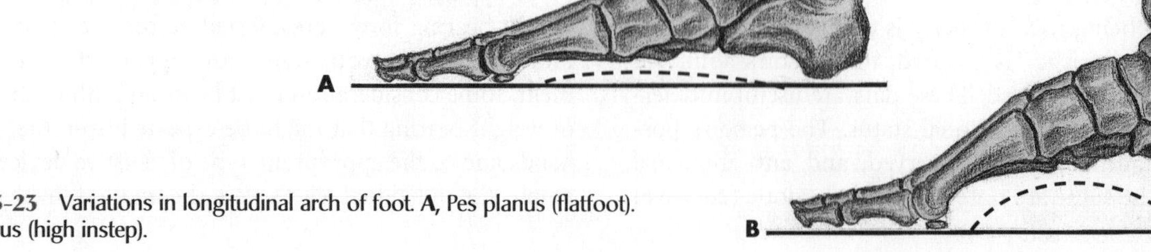

Figure 45-23 Variations in longitudinal arch of foot. **A,** Pes planus (flatfoot). **B,** Pes cavus (high instep).

Palpation

In a head-to-toe fashion, all bones, joints, and soft tissue are palpated for temperature, swelling, tenderness, pain, or masses. The spinous processes and intervertebral spaces are also palpated for tenderness.

Assessment of Sensory Function

To evaluate sensory innervation, the person's ability to discern light touch, gentle pressure, pain, and temperature is assessed. Each test is performed bilaterally, and results are compared. Sensation in the dermatomes is checked to detect abnormalities in spinal nerve innervation (Figure 45-24). The person's sense of proprioception (position sense) in the extremities is also evaluated.

Deep Tendon Reflex Activity

Absent reflexes may indicate neuropathy or a lower motor neuron lesion, whereas brisk reflexes indicate an upper motor neuron lesion. When reflexes are being checked, bilateral responses must be compared. Figure 45-25 shows the location of tendons and their corresponding spinal level, and Figure 45-26 illustrates the documentation of deep tendon response. The grading of responses is shown in Table 45-4.

Range of Motion

The term *range of motion* refers to the normal arc of movement provided for by the structure of a joint. Active range of motion is motion performed independently. Passive range of motion is accomplished with the assistance of someone else or with a mechanical device.

Before the muscle strength or range of motion of a joint is tested, some assessment of the position of the person's extremities must be made. Sudden changes from normal may indicate the presence of fractures, dislocations, or ruptures of supporting structures. Typical of this kind of sudden change is the marked external rotation and shortening of the leg following a hip fracture; the inability to extend a "dropped" finger following rupture of an extensor tendon in the hand; or postoperative "dropfoot," a complication that may occur following surgical procedures on the back, hip, or knee because of pressure on or stretching of the sciatic or peroneal nerve.

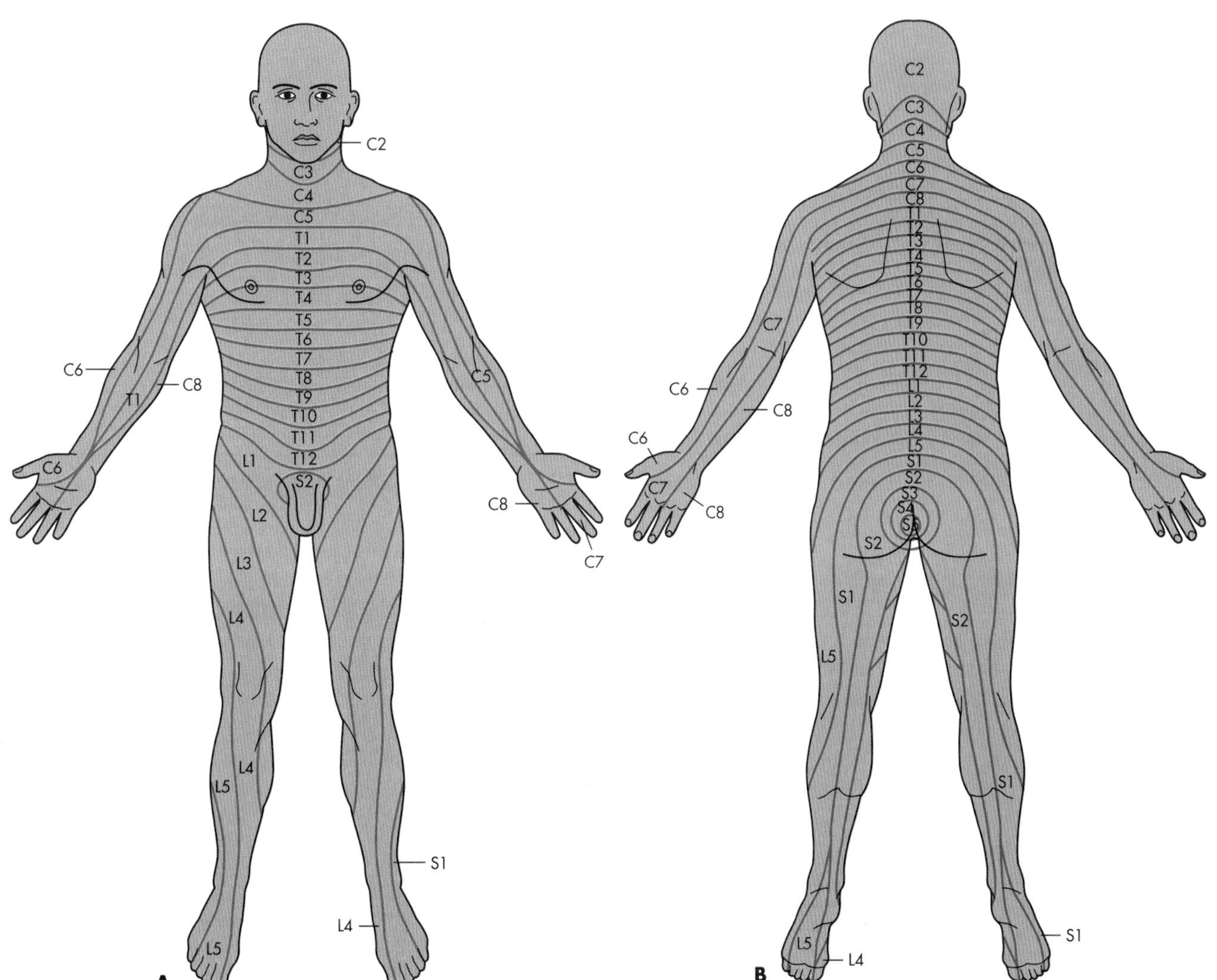

Figure 45-24 **A,** Dermatomes, anterior view. **B,** Dermatomes, posterior view.

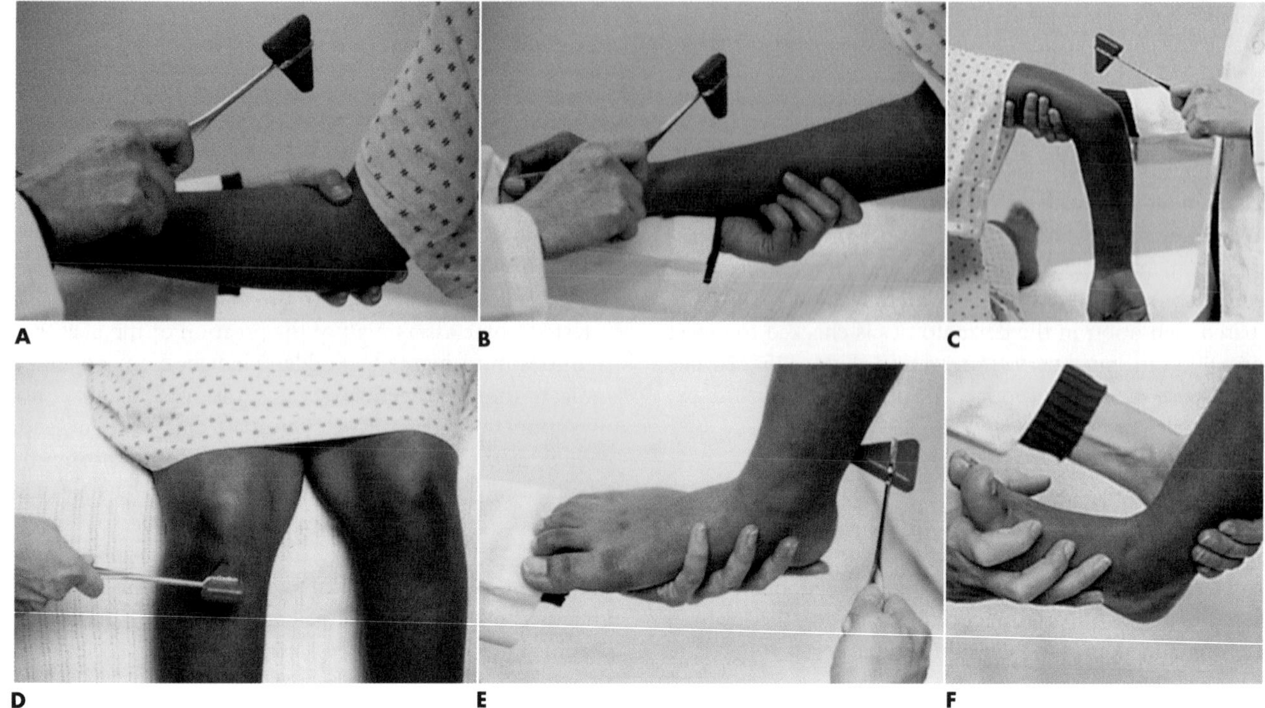

Figure 45-25 Location of tendons for evaluation of deep tendon reflexes. **A,** Biceps (C5, C6). **B,** Brachioradial (C5, C6). **C,** Triceps (C6, C7, C8). **D,** Patellar (L2, L3, L4). **E,** Achilles (S1, S2). **F,** Evaluation of ankle clonus.

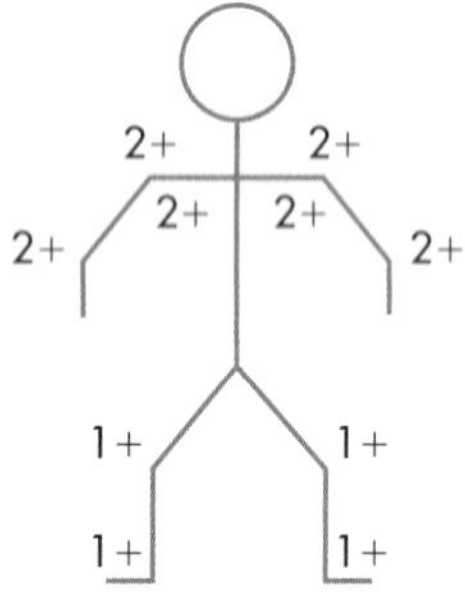

Figure 45-26 Documentation of deep tendon reflex response.

TABLE 45-4 Scale of Responses Used To Score Deep Tendon Reflexes

Grade	Deep Tendon Reflex Response
0	No response
1+	Sluggish or diminished
2+	Active or expected response
3+	More brisk than expected, slightly hyperactive
4+	Brisk, hyperactive, with intermittent or transient clonus

From Seidel HM et al: *Mosby's guide to physical examination,* ed 4, St Louis, 1999, Mosby.

Subluxation, or partial dislocation of a joint, should also be noted. This is often a chronic problem, as in the shoulder of the hemiplegic person or in the wrist of the arthritic person. Its presence is usually accompanied by some loss of function or need for support. Subluxation of the shoulder may be detected by examination; a space can be felt between the head of the humerus and the glenoid cavity of the scapula.

Loss of strength or limitation of joint motion results in some degree of loss of function. Loss of strength or joint range of motion may be the result of a neurologic, skeletal, muscular, or traumatic disorder.

Range of motion is tested by having the person actively perform the full range of motion of a particular joint (see Figures 45-15 to 45-17). In some instances, when the person cannot actively move a joint, as in the person with paresis (weakness) or paralysis, the joint may be moved passively. When passive range of motion is performed, support must be given proximal to the joint being moved (Figure 45-27).

Comparing the limitation of movement or instability present in one joint with its contralateral joint is helpful in differentiating normal from abnormal findings.

If a joint cannot be moved beyond a certain point in its normal arc of motion (e.g., a knee that does not extend beyond 130 degrees of flexion), a contracture is present. Contractures may exist because of soft tissue limitations (following immobilization for treatment of a fracture) or because of bony limitations (Figure 45-28). The location and nature of contractures can significantly limit function. For example, a person who can flex one knee only 15 degrees must climb stairs one at a time.

Crepitus, a crunching or grating sensation that is audible or palpable and elicited when the joint is actively or passively moved, is a significant indicator of a pathologic condition within the joint. This sensation can also be palpated or heard if the ends of a broken bone move against one another. In the presence of a possible fracture, no attempt should be made to elicit crepitus.

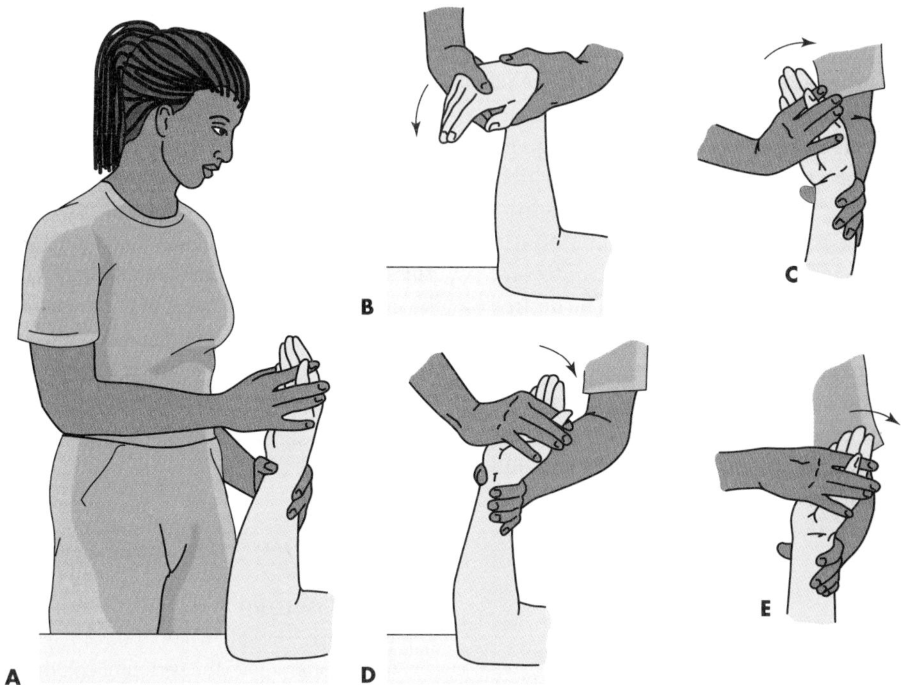

Figure 45-27 Techniques of passive range of motion. With patient in supine position, upper arm is supported on bed. **A,** Forearm is supported with nurse's hand; hand is supported with nurse's other hand. **B,** Wrist is flexed forward. **C,** Wrist is extended. **D,** Wrist is moved to ulnar side. **E,** Wrist is moved to radial side.

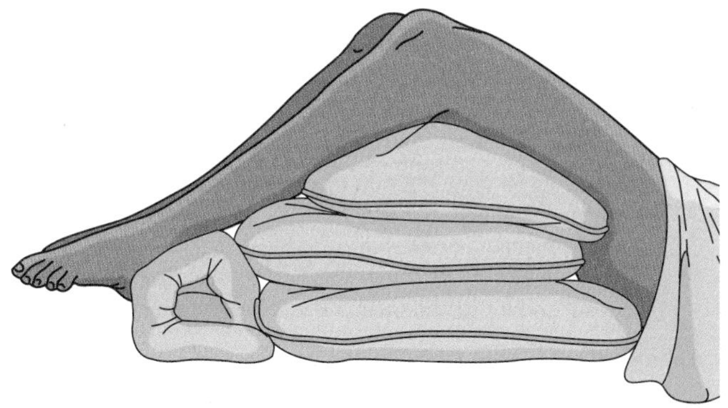

Figure 45-28 Contractures of hips and knees in patient with rheumatoid arthritis caused by continuous use of pillows to support knees in flexed position.

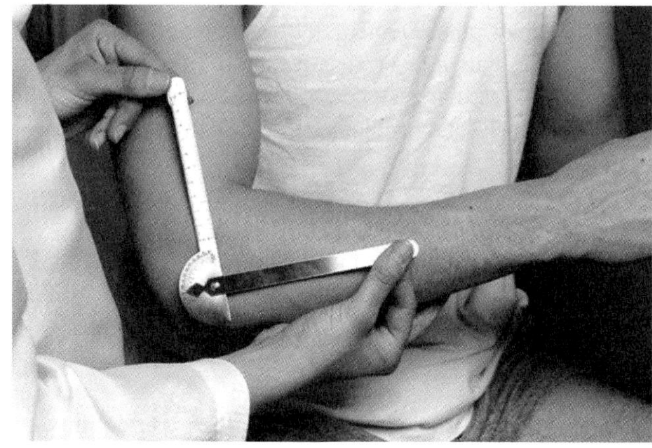

Figure 45-29 Measurement of joint motion with a goniometer.

A goniometer measures degrees of joint movement and allows comparison of findings with expected normal findings. A joint should not be forcefully moved if pain or resistance is encountered (Figure 45-29).

Muscle Strength

The manual muscle test (MMT) is performed to determine the degree of muscular weakness resulting from disease, injury, or lack of use. The MMT rates the strength of muscles by their performance in relation to gravity and manually applied resistance. Factors such as gravity, stabilization of the tested part, proper positioning, amounts of resistance, range of the joint, pain, and abnormal muscle tone may influence the objectivity of the MMT.

Muscle strength can be assessed by asking the person to contract a certain muscle group and resist while the examiner exerts an opposing force. Responses are compared bilaterally. If pain occurs, the joint is not forced past the point of pain. The presence of spasms is noted, and muscles are evaluated for flaccidity (lack of tone), hypotonicity (decreased tone), or hypertonicity (increased tone). Atrophy or hypertrophy of muscle mass is also noted. Findings are documented using a standard scale of measurement (Table 45-5).

The preceding tests of strength, dexterity, and range of motion are simple to perform; however, pain (rather than weakness, lack of coordination, or joint limitation) may limit the person's ability to perform the movement. It is often difficult to differentiate the cause of the deficit. Although the effect of pain is quantitatively the same as the effect of weakness or limitation (i.e., diminished function), pain is qualitatively different because treatment measures will be geared to pain relief rather than to muscle strengthening. The patient may have actual muscle weakness because of chronic pain and consequent lack of use of muscles. When these tests are being performed, it must be remembered that the person must not be moved beyond the point of pain. Pain indicates that something is wrong. Injudicious testing techniques can produce untoward results (e.g., the fracture of an osteoporotic bone). The desired result of diagnostic testing is the establishment of a baseline of strength, motion, and dexterity from which interventions to assist the person in gaining strength, regaining lost motion, and increasing functional capacity may be planned and evaluated. Many specialized physical examination techniques aid in the diagnosis of abnormalities of the musculoskeletal system. These are usually performed by advanced practice nurses, physician's assistants, or physicians. A summary of some of these techniques is found in Table 45-6. The reader is referred to a text on physical examination for a more in-depth description and illustration of these tests.

Assessment measures and variations in normal findings relevant to the care of older adults are presented in the Gerontologic Assessment box.

Diagnostic Tests

As with other illnesses, diagnostic test results offer data useful in diagnosing a patient's musculoskeletal illness and formulating a treatment plan. Elements of the patient's care may depend on the outcome of diagnostic studies. Some of the principal studies that may be performed on the person who has a musculoskeletal problem are described in the following sections.

Laboratory Tests

Laboratory tests consist of two major categories—serologic and urinary—as described in Tables 45-7 and 45-8, respectively.

Radiologic Tests

Bones and Joints. Radiologic tests of bones and joints are imperative for the identification and treatment of fractures. They are also helpful in determining the presence of disease (e.g., rheumatoid arthritis, spondylitis, avascular necrosis, and tumor), as well as the progress and effects of treatment on these disorders. Consult a specialized text for further discussion of specific radiologic tests.

Many patients are unable to lie on x-ray examination tables for long periods of time. In particular, persons with arthritis develop joint stiffness and pain if their ability to move is restricted. Because radiologic examinations for individuals with rheumatic diseases are often extensive, careful thought should be given to the scheduling of these examinations. Few of these patients can tolerate having all the required views of all the involved joints taken in a single session. Instead, 1 or 2 days of rest between shorter sessions may be required. Analgesics or

Gerontologic Assessment

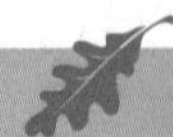

ASSESS POSTURE

In the older adult the trunk is short compared with the extremities; shortening of the vertebral column as a result of thinning of the intervertebral disks, decreased height of individual vertebrae from osteoporosis, and with advanced age, osteoporitic vertebral collapse results in loss of height.

Stooped posture (kyphosis) with a compensatory backward head tilt is common as a result of change in the center of gravity caused by lower extremity joint flexion.

ASSESS MUSCLE MASS AND STRENGTH

There is a decrease in total muscle mass with age because of a decrease in size of some muscles and atrophy of others.

Muscle contours become more evident and tendons are more distinct on palpation.

Muscle weakness is common as a result of decreased mass.

ASSESS GAIT AND BALANCE

Gait may be unsteady as a result of muscle weakness.

Loss of balance along with the need for assistive devices may be present secondary to changes in the center of gravity.

ASSESS BONES AND JOINTS

Flexion of the knees and hips accompanies joint degeneration.

Pain on palpation of spinous processes can indicate a compression fracture.

Enlarged, deformed joints occur with osteoarthritis and rheumatoid arthritis.

Tenderness and erythema of a joint is indicative of inflammation.

TABLE 45-5 Grading of Manual Muscle Test Scales

Muscle Functional Level	Grade	Percentage of Normal	Lovett Scale
No evidence of contractility	0	0	0 (zero)
Slight contractility, no movement	1	10	T (trace)
Full range of motion, gravity eliminated*	2	25	P (poor)
Full range of motion with gravity	3	50	F (fair)
Full range of motion against gravity, some resistance	4	75	G (good)
Full range of motion against gravity, full resistance	5	100	N (normal)

From Seidel HM et al: *Mosby's guide to physical examination,* ed 4, St Louis, 1999, Mosby.
*Passive movement.

local heat applications for relief of joint pain after x-ray examinations may be necessary.

Systemic Radiologic Studies. Systemic radiologic studies such as the barium enema, upper gastrointestinal series, and intravenous pyelogram are helpful in determining the extent of involvement of various internal organs (bowel, kidneys) in systemic rheumatic diseases. Discussion of these examinations can be found in Chapters 31 and 38.

Myelography. A myelogram is a radiologic examination of the spinal canal. Any portion of the spine (cervical, thoracic, or lumbar) can be examined. A radiopaque solution or, less commonly, air is injected into the subarachnoid space. Myelography is used to identify lesions such as herniated nucleus pulposus, nerve root involvement, spinal stenosis, tumor, or other lesions that may encroach on the spinal canal. Myelography has largely been replaced with magnetic resonance imaging (MRI) and computed tomography (CT) in the diagnosis of spinal disorders. However, myelograms may be used in conjunction with CT, particularly if the results of the CT scan are inconclusive. Other indications for myelography include obesity, postoperative spinal surgery, and inconclusive results with other studies.

The contrast medium used is either an oil- or a water-based solution. The viscosity of the oil-based solution (iophendylate [Pantopaque]) provides a good contrast medium for visualization of the spinal structures. However, its major disadvantage is that it must be removed as completely as possible after the examination or it may cause arachnoiditis, encephalopathy, or severe headaches.

Because of these limitations, water-soluble, nonionic solutions are primarily used. Metrizamide [Amipaque] and iohexol [Omnipaque] are commonly used contrast agents. Water-based

TABLE 45-6 Special Assessment Techniques for the Musculoskeletal System

Assessment Technique	Description	Abnormality Detected
Limb measurement	Measurement in centimeters of extremities from a major landmark	Asymmetric limb length may indicate pelvic obliquity or hip deformities; discrepancies in circumference may indicate atrophy or paresis of muscle groups; 1-cm discrepancy is normal in most people
Ballottement	Compression of suprapatellar pouch, which is normally snug against femur	Fluid wave indicates excess fluid in knee (effusion)
Bulge sign	Stroke medial aspect of knee, then tap lateral side of patella; if fluid is present, a fluid wave or bulge will appear	Effusion, excess fluid in suprapatellar pouch
McMurray's test	External rotation and valgus stress applied to knee while leg is held flexed at knee and hip (patient is lying supine); normally there is no pain or sound	"Click" or pain indicates meniscal tear
Drawer test (anteroposterior and mediolateral)	With patient supine and knee flexed, push forward and backward on tibia at joint line; with patient supine with knee extended, stabilize femur and ankle while attempting to abduct and adduct knee; normally there is little or no movement—assess symmetry of responses	Laxity or movement suggests instability of anterior or posterior cruciate ligaments or medial or lateral collateral ligaments of knee
Straight leg raising (LaSègue's) test	With patient supine, raise leg straight with knee extended; normally there is no pain	If maneuver reproduces sciatic pain, it is considered positive and suggests a herniated disk
Trendelenburg's test	While patient stands on one foot and then the other, both iliac crests should appear symmetric	Asymmetry suggests hip dislocation
Thomas test	With patient lying supine and one leg fully extended and the other flexed on chest, observe ability of patient to keep extended leg flat on table	Inability to keep leg extended suggests a hip flexion contracture in extended leg that may be masked by increased lumbar lordosis
Phalen's test	Flex both wrists together to 90 degrees and hold for 60 seconds; normally this produces no symptoms	Numbness, tingling, or burning in median nerve distribution suggests carpal tunnel syndrome
Tinel's sign	Tap over median nerve where it passes through carpal tunnel in wrist; normally this does not produce any symptoms	Tingling along median nerve distribution is associated with carpal tunnel syndrome
Drop arm test	Raise affected arm to 90 degrees of flexion, then have patient slowly adduct arm to side	Inability to lower the arm slowly or smoothly is associated with disruption of rotator cuff mechanism of shoulder
Scoliosis screening	"Forward bend" test; observe symmetry and height of scapulae, shoulders, iliac crests, rib cage	Asymmetry of scapulae or shoulder height, "winged" iliac crests, demonstrable curve of spine, rib hump indicates scoliosis

TABLE 45-7 Serologic Tests

Test	Rationale for Performing Test
Serum muscle enzymes	Enzymes can be elevated in presence of primary myopathic (muscle) diseases. Elevated levels may result from muscle fiber degeneration or from diffusion through a muscle membrane that has increased permeability.
Aspartate transaminase (AST; serum glutamatic-oxaloacetic transaminase [SGOT]) Aldolase Creatine phosphokinase (CPK) isoenzymes MM	Enzyme levels are an index of both progress of myopathic disorder and effectiveness of treatment. Aldolase levels are most commonly used to diagnose and monitor treatment of muscular dystrophy. NURSING PRECAUTION: Intramuscular injections should be avoided when these enzymes are being monitored. *Normal values:* AST 5 8-20 U/L Aldolase: 3-8.2 U/dl CPK-MM (muscle): percentage of total CK 90%-97%
Serologic test for syphilis (STS)	False-positive STS results occur in 10%-15% of persons with connective tissue diseases, so test may aid diagnosis.
Fluorescent treponemal antibody absorption (FTA-ABS)	FTA-ABS excludes presence of syphilis.
Rheumatoid factor or latex fixation (reaction of rheumatoid factor antibodies with IgG [7S] gamma globulin)	Rheumatoid factor antibodies are found in sera (50%-95%) of individuals with rheumatoid arthritis. Test is considered positive if rheumatoid factor is found in titrations of 1:40 or greater. May be positive in persons with systemic lupus erythematosus (SLE). CAUTION: Rheumatoid factor may be found in other conditions (e.g., aging, scleroderma, acute pulmonary tuberculosis, hepatitis).
Antinuclear antibodies (ANAs)	Circulating antibodies, which are composed of protein material and called antinuclear antibodies, react with cellular nuclei and various individual constituents of cellular nuclei, and can be identified by fluorescent techniques using antihuman gamma globulin labeled with fluorescein. Positive tests are used in diagnosing Sjögren's syndrome, scleroderma, and SLE. Pattern of nuclear staining varies with different diseases. Poor positive predictive value for SLE and other rheumatic diseases.
Serum complement	Protein substances that are found in serum and synovial fluid and are associated with immune and inflammatory mechanisms; low levels often occur in SLE and rheumatoid arthritis.
Erythrocyte sedimentation rate (ESR)	Increased rate of settling of erythrocytes is an important index of presence of inflammation. *Normal values:* men, <15 mm/hr; women, <20 mm/hr
Hematocrit	Individuals with systemic connective tissue disease often have normocytic (normal red blood cell [RBC] count), normochromic (normal amount of iron carried by RBCs) anemia in absence of any abnormal bleeding. Individuals who suffer trauma or undergo major surgery to musculoskeletal system sustain significant blood loss. Symptoms of anemia (e.g., extreme tiredness, fatigue, weakness) are experienced when hematocrit drops quickly; acute symptoms may be absent if anemia develops gradually or is chronic. Individuals with acute anemia should not be physically stressed. *Normal values:* men, 45-50 vol/dl; women, 40-45 vol/dl
Calcium	Immobility and bone demineralization (bone cancers, multiple myeloma) will show an increase in serum levels. Rickets, vitamin D deficiency, will show a decrease in levels. Malnutrition also results in decreased levels. *Normal values:* total 9-10.5 mg/dl; ionized 4.5-5.6 mg/dl
Alkaline phosphatase (ALP)	Bone tumor and infections, fractures, Paget's disease, rickets, and other conditions that cause an increase in osteoblastic activity will cause an increase in ALP levels. Also used to monitor response to treatment for osteoporosis. In hypophosphatasia (characterized by a defect in bone formation), levels are decreased. *Normal value:* 30-85 ImU/ml; slightly higher in older adults
Phosphorus	Together with calcium, plays a vital role in bone metabolism. Conditions that cause an increase in calcium levels will cause a decrease in serum phosphates. *Normal value:* 2.5-4.5 mg/dl
Anti-DNA antibody	Used in diagnosis of SLE or to monitor response to treatment. Antibodies to DNA are present in serum of 60%-80% of persons with SLE.
C-reactive protein	Used as a nonspecific indicator of infection and inflammation. Commonly used to aid in diagnosis of rheumatoid arthritis. May also be used to monitor responses to antibiotics or antiinflammatory medication.
LE prep	Used in diagnosis and treatment of SLE. Antinuclear factor in SLE is LE factor; LE test detects antinuclear antibodies, but many patients with SLE have negative results.

TABLE 45-8 Urinary Tests

Diagnostic Test	Rationale for Test
24-hour urine for creatine-creatinine ratio	In presence of muscle disease, ability of muscle to convert creatine is decreased, amount of creatine excreted by kidneys increases, and ratio of urinary creatine to creatinine increases. Periodic studies are helpful in diagnosis and evaluation of progress of treatment of primary myopathies.
Urinary uric acid levels (24-hour collection)*	Helpful in diagnosis and decisions regarding treatment modalities for gout. *Normal value:* should not exceed 900-mg uric acid excretion per day
Urine for deoxypyridinoline (first or second morning void) routine collection	Deoxypyridinoline (Dpd) crosslinks assay provides a quantitative measurement of Dpd, which is excreted unmetabolized in urine during bone resorption.

*NOTE: 24-hour urine collections must be accurate to facilitate proper diagnosis and treatment.

dyes are less viscous and fill the canal and narrow spaces easily, allowing good visualization of the structures. They are absorbed into the cerebrospinal fluid (CSF) and excreted by the kidneys, and need not be removed after the procedure. Major adverse effects are seizures, nausea, headache, and vomiting after the procedure. Iohexol has a lower risk of neurotoxicity and seizures than metrizamide. Emergency medications and equipment should be immediately available in case of allergic response to the contrast medium. Informed consent is necessary before the procedure.

Patient education is vital before the procedure. A thorough explanation of events before, during, and after the procedure may help allay fears and clarify any misconceptions regarding myelography.

Myelography is an outpatient procedure done in the radiology department by a radiologist with the assistance of a radiology technician. The patient is admitted to the hospital the morning of the procedure. The patient should be instructed to fast, usually for 4 hours before the procedure. A careful history should be taken, noting any previous allergic reactions to other contrast agents, iodine, or shellfish. If a water-based solution is being used, the patient may not take amphetamines, phenothiazides, or tricyclic antidepressants for 12 hours before the procedure because these drugs lower the seizure threshold.

If necessary, a sedative may be prescribed before the procedure. In the radiology department the patient is transferred to the x-ray table. The patient is placed in either a lateral or a sitting position for the lumbar puncture. Local anesthetic is injected before the lumbar puncture (see Chapter 41). The myelogram is performed with the patient in the prone position. Approximately 10 ml of CSF is withdrawn and sent to the laboratory for analysis. The contrast medium is then injected, and the x-ray table is moved and tilted, allowing the dye to fill the canal as films are taken. The procedure may take up to 1 hour. Commonly a CT scan follows the myelography.

After a myelography, fluids are encouraged to replace the removed CSF and to aid in the excretion of the contrast medium. If an oil-based dye was used, the patient is kept flat in bed for approximately 8 hours. If a water-soluble dye was used, bed rest is maintained, with the head of the bed elevated 30 degrees for 6 to 8 hours. If air was used, the head of the bed should be kept lower than the trunk for up to 48 hours.

Contrast material has a diuretic effect. Output should be monitored for at least 8 hours after the test. The patient's diet is resumed as tolerated, and fluids are encouraged, regardless of the dye used. The patient should be observed for any reactions to the contrast agent. Headaches, nausea, and vomiting are the most common side effects. Neurologic checks are performed hourly. The lumbar puncture site is covered with a small adhesive strip and should be observed for any bleeding. The patient can be discharged the afternoon of the procedure. Patients should continue with bed rest at home and then gradually resume normal activities. Lifting or strenuous activity should be avoided for 24 hours.

The patient should be taught to check the puncture site for any drainage, swelling, or signs of infection. Anticonvulsants or other medications withheld before the procedure may be resumed in 48 hours. The patient should be instructed to contact the physician if persistent nausea or vomiting develops.

Myelography is contraindicated for persons with multiple sclerosis. Allergy to contrast material or renal impairment affects the choice of contrast medium.

Bone Densitometry. Bone densitometry measures bone density to aid in the diagnosis of osteoporosis, predict fracture risk, and monitor the effectiveness of treatment protocols. The most widely used method is dual x-ray absorptiometry (DEXA or DXA scan). This noninvasive radiologic test measures bone mass and density in the lumbar spine, proximal femur, and wrist. A digital imaging device that scans the fingers is also available. The two types of scanners are the pencil-beam and the fan-beam. The fan-beam produces images with better resolution in less time. Both emit low-dose radiation, approximately 1 to 3 mrem as compared with 20 to 50 mrem for a chest x-ray film. The duration of the procedures varies from 30 seconds per site to 4 minutes per site. No special preparation or aftercare for this test is needed. A certified x-ray technologist performs the tests. The patient's results are compared with the bone density expected for someone of the same age, sex, and race and with the peak bone density of a healthy adult of the same age, sex, and race. These scores are known as "young normal" or T scores and as "age-matched" or Z scores. Densities 1 standard deviation (SD) below the "normals" represent a reduction in bone mass of about 12% and an increased risk for fracture.

Treatment is generally initiated for persons with bone mineral density (BMD) results 2.5 SD below the T score. The American Association of Clinical Endocrinologists recommends that all women 65 years and older have screening BMD; women under 65 years should have BMD performed if they are at risk for osteoporosis.[4] BMD should be reassessed every 2 years for most persons.

Arthrography. Arthrography permits visualization of structures within the joint that are not normally seen on routine radiographic films. An arthrogram is usually performed on the knee or shoulder for evaluation of persistent pain or preoperative assessment. Although the knee and shoulder are the most common joints evaluated, the elbow, wrist, hip, and temporomandibular joints may also be visualized.

The joint cavity is injected with radiopaque dye, air, or both. When both are used, the test is referred to as a double-contrast arthrogram. The dye or air serves as a contrast medium against which the outlines of soft tissue components of the joint may be seen. Tears of the menisci and internal derangement of the joint such as ligament disruption and synovial cysts can be diagnosed with the aid of arthrograms.

Before the examination the patient should be checked for allergies to iodine or seafood. Patients may experience pain while the joint is expanded by the dye or air, and local anesthetic may be injected before the examination. Analgesics are prescribed after the examination. The patient should be instructed to watch for redness, edema, or unusual pain in the joint after the procedure.

Radioisotope Bone Scans. Radioisotope bone scans are performed primarily to demonstrate the presence of metastatic disease, tumors, infection (osteomyelitis), and other conditions with increased bone activity. This nuclear scanning test can also be used to diagnose the cause of undetermined bone pain and assess the healing of fractures. Intravenously injected sodium pertechnetate technetium-99m (^{99m}Tc) is the isotope most commonly used in this study. The ^{99m}Tc concentrates in areas of osteoblastic activity involved in the exchange of calcium.

Technetium, a bone-seeking radioisotope, is taken up by the bone in areas of adequate blood supply and metabolic activity. "Hot spots" on the scan indicate areas of increased bone turnover, as in the case of fractures, bone healing, and inflammatory responses. "Cold spots," or areas of decalcified bone, indicate no bone activity, as in lytic lesions. Lesions may be visualized on bone scans as early as 3 to 6 months before the lesions are evident on routine x-ray films. Bone scans are commonly used to rule out bony metastases from the prostate, breast, and lung.

Technetium scans are also of some use in determining the degree of parotid gland involvement in Sjögren's syndrome. The uptake, concentration, and excretion of the isotope by the major salivary glands are measured by a technique known as sequential scintiphotography.

Persons being prepared for these procedures should know that the procedures are not painful and that the isotopes will not harm them. However, the patient may have to remain quietly in one position for 1 hour or more. The radioisotope is injected intravenously about 2 hours before scanning. The patient is assessed for iodine or seafood allergies and is encouraged to drink fluids before the examination. The bladder should be emptied just before the scan to avoid interference with visualization of the pelvis. Procedures using barium or iodine are not scheduled before the bone scan, because these substances interfere with scanning. The kidneys excrete the radioisotope in the urine within 6 to 24 hours. Fluids should be encouraged after the scan to aid in excretion of the isotope.

Computed Tomography. Tomography is an x-ray technique by which detailed images of "slices" of tissue are obtained by focusing x-ray beams at predetermined planes or depths of the tissue being studied. Detailed images of the structures at that level are produced, and details of structures surrounding that level are blurred or eliminated. Computed tomography (CT) scanning is tomography employing a computer to compose a picture of the tissue being studied. A series of x-ray beams is rotated, 1 degree at a time, around the specific area being examined. With each rotation a picture is generated that depicts the difference in tissue density. These pictures are extremely clear and detailed. CT may be used in conjunction with intravenous or oral contrast media to allow better visualization of structures.

The scan picks up disruptions in normal structures. The procedure can be used in diagnosing spinal pathologic conditions and tumors and in evaluating the hip before custom joint replacement. The procedure is noninvasive and does not require repositioning of the patient, as does conventional tomography. Disadvantages of CT include poor depiction of intraspinal processes and poor differentiation between disk herniation and postoperative scar tissue. CT is commonly done after myelography in diagnosing spinal pathologic conditions. Patients who are claustrophobic may have difficulty tolerating the procedure because they must lie in a cylindric metal scanner for up to 1 hour.

Magnetic Resonance Imaging. Magnetic resonance imaging (MRI) is a scanning technique that produces tomographic images by using magnetic forces rather than x-ray beams. The patient lies on a nonmagnetic scanning table that slides, head first, into a large cylindric magnet. The magnet causes the body's atomic protons to line up and spin in the same direction. A radio frequency signal is beamed into the magnetic field, causing the protons to move out of alignment. When the signal stops, the protons move back into alignment and release energy. A receiver coil measures the energy released by the movement of the protons and the time it takes for the protons to return to their aligned position. These measurements provide information regarding the type of tissue in which the protons lie, as well as the condition of the tissue. A computer uses this information to construct an image on a television screen, showing the distribution of protons of hydrogen atoms; the television image may also be recorded on film or magnetic tape. The images produced by MRI are more accurate than those produced by CT or myelography.

Patients being prepared for MRI should know that the procedure is painless and requires no special preparation. However, because a magnetic field is used, the patient will be asked to remove any metallic objects, such as jewelry, hairpins, credit cards, and nonpermanent dentures. Patients who have cardiac pacemakers or intracranial vascular aneurysm clips are excluded from MRI. Persons who have metal implants cannot have that area scanned.

As with CT scanning, patients who are claustrophobic may have difficulty being placed in the scanner. Sometimes medication such as diazepam (Valium) is prescribed to help the patient relax. "Open-air" MRI scanners allow the patient to feel less confined but still obtain quality images. These scanners are an option for some patients. During the scan the patient hears the hum of the machine, a loud thump when the radio waves are turned on and off, and other machinelike noises. The thumping can be particularly annoying to patients, and many persons are frightened if they are not told what will happen. Scanning time is usually 30 to 90 minutes. Many facilities offer earplugs to reduce outside noise while in the scanner.

Contrast media may be used with MRI to enhance the quality of the images. Gadolinium-DPTA, an intravenous contrast agent often used with MRI to enhance imaging, differentiates recurrent disk herniation from epidural scarring.

Diskography. A diskogram is a radiologic procedure that uses a contrast medium to evaluate the integrity of the intervertebral disks. Diskography is performed on an outpatient basis in the operating room or radiology department with the use of fluoroscopy. The patient is placed in the prone position, and local anesthetic is administered. The patient may require additional sedation, because the procedure can be quite uncomfortable. Needle position is confirmed by fluoroscopy; contrast medium and saline are then injected into the disk space. If a pathologic condition is present, injection of the saline reproduces the patient's back or leg pain. Despite the accuracy of myelography, CT, and MRI, the diskogram is still a useful diagnostic tool because the ability to reproduce the patient's symptoms may aid the surgeon in differential diagnosis, especially when several vertebral levels are involved. However, this technique is less specific than myelography.

Special Tests

Electromyography. Electromyography measures the electrical activity of muscles; an electromyogram (EMG) is a recording of the variations of electrical potentials (voltage) detected by a needle electrode inserted into skeletal muscle. An EMG, an electrophysiologic test, differentiates between myopathies (muscle diseases) and neuropathies (nerve diseases). The electrical activity can be heard over a loudspeaker and viewed on an oscilloscope and graph at the same time. No electrical activity can be detected in normal muscles at rest, but during volitional movement, action potentials can be detected. In both primary myopathic and neuropathic disorders, specific variations exist in the size of individual motor unit potentials. In neurogenic atrophy, fibrillations may be present in the resting muscle. An EMG provides direct evidence of motor dysfunction and can be used to some extent to detect a dysfunction located in the motor neuron, the neuromuscular junction, or the muscle fibers. Thus it is particularly helpful in the diagnosis of lower motor neuron disease, primary muscle disease, and defects in the transmission of electrical impulses at the neuromuscular junction, such as occurs in myasthenia gravis. However, electromyography cannot be used to differentiate specific disease entities in either the myopathic or neuropathic categories.

No special preparation is required for this procedure. The patient may fear that insertion of electrode needles will be painful or that electrical stimulation of the needles will cause severe shock. Although the patient may be reassured that the procedure is not dangerous, some individuals do experience mild to moderate discomfort. Therefore nurses preparing patients for this test should not refer to the test as "painless."

Biopsy. Biopsies of tissue from a variety of organs are helpful in the diagnosis of disease or disorders affecting the musculoskeletal system. Table 45-9 lists the tissues that may be biopsied, the tests performed, the significance of results, and general nursing considerations for patients undergoing biopsy.

Joint Aspiration. Joint aspiration (arthrocentesis) is performed to obtain a sample of synovial fluid from within the joint cavity. This procedure (performed by introducing a needle into the joint cavity and withdrawing fluid) helps determine the presence of an aseptic inflammatory process such as rheumatoid arthritis or a septic process such as bacterial arthritis. Samples of synovial fluid are cultured and examined both microscopically and chemically.

The synovial fluid is normally straw colored and clear; the viscosity resembles that of clean motor oil. In the presence of inflammation, the fluid becomes turbid and watery. The mucin clot test is performed by mixing synovial fluid with glacial acetic acid. Normal synovial fluid forms a white, ropy mucin clot. When inflammation is present, the clot breaks apart easily and becomes flaky (flocculent). The degree of flocculence increases with the degree of inflammation. Also, when inflammation is present, the WBC count, the protein content, and the number of polymorphonuclear cells in the synovial fluid are increased and the glucose content is decreased.

A local anesthetic is usually administered before the procedure. Strict asepsis is observed during the procedure. After the procedure the joint is often wrapped in a small compression (elastic) dressing. The joint may be rested for 8 to 24 hours.

Endoscopy

Arthroscopy. Arthroscopy (visualization of a joint) is a procedure performed in the operating room, usually in an ambulatory surgical center, with the patient under local or regional anesthesia. A specially designed endoscope (arthroscope) is inserted through a small incision into the joint cavity, enabling the physician to visualize the structure and contents of the joint (Figure 45-30). Most arthroscopic procedures are performed on the knee, although the wrist, ankle, hip, shoulder, and temporomandibular joint are also examined and treated using this technique.

The procedure is used to diagnose and treat such conditions as chondromalacia of the knee, ligamentous disruption, meniscal tears, carpal tunnel syndrome, osteoarthritis, rheumatoid arthritis, and impingement syndrome. Endoscopy is also used to perform lumbar and thoracic diskectomy.

TABLE 45-9 Types of Biopsies

Organ Test(s)	Performed	Positive Results	Nursing Considerations
Skin (punch biopsy)	Immunofluorescent staining—tissue is washed with solution of fluorescein-labeled antihuman gamma globulin antibody	Band of immunofluorescence at epidermal-dermal junction, indicating presence of rheumatic disease (i.e., scleroderma, systemic lupus erythematosus, psoriatic arthritis)	Biopsy site kept clean and dry with small adhesive bandage until scab develops; only very mild discomfort experienced by patient
Muscle (operative procedure)	Histochemical staining	Tissue reveals features of lower motor neuron disease, degeneration, inflammatory reaction as in polymyositis, or involvement of specific fibers indicating primary myopathic disease	Patient instructed and prepared for surgery; patient monitored per postanesthesia routine (local or general); mild to moderate pain and stiffness in biopsy area; routine activity encouraged within 24 hours to avoid undue stiffness; dressings changed as necessary
Synovium (closed—performed with needle; open—performed in surgery)	Histologic examination—synovial fluid obtained at same time; may be cultured to determine presence of infection	Differentiates various forms of arthritis	Patient instructed about procedure; patient may require postanesthesia monitoring; strict asepsis observed throughout procedure and in caring for wound; small compression dressing applied to joint, and joint rested for 24 hours to prevent hemorrhage or effusion
Buccal mucosa (punch biopsy)	Histologic examination of tissue from inside lower lip	Helpful in diagnosing Sjögren's syndrome	Patient instructed about procedure; generally minor discomfort experienced; diet altered to avoid rough and very hot foods (they will irritate surgical site)
Bone (operative procedure)	Microscopic analysis	Can confirm presence of infection or neoplasm	Patient instructed and prepared for surgery; patient monitored per postanesthesia routine; mild to severe discomfort may be experienced; activity restrictions dependent on location and extent of surgical procedure; dressings changed as necessary

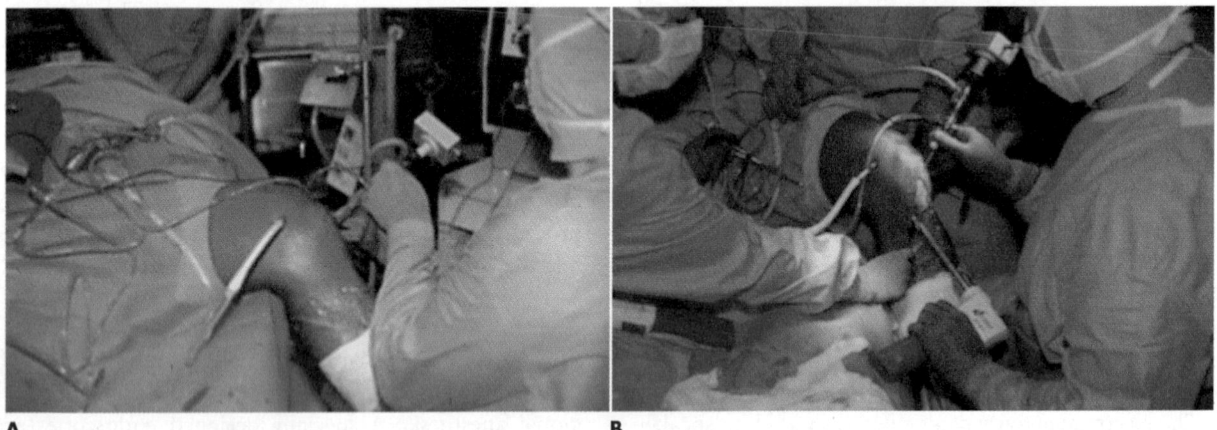

Figure 45-30 **A,** Arthroscopy of knee. **B,** Arthroscopically aided reconstruction of anterior cruciate ligament.

Analgesics are prescribed after surgery. The patient is taught to observe the operative site for swelling and signs of infection. The period of time the joint is rested and the use of any immobilizing device are determined by the location and extent of the procedure. The surgeon should be consulted regarding the activity the patient is permitted after the procedure so that damage to the joint may be avoided.

References

1. Guyton AC, Hall JE: *Textbook of medical physiology,* ed 10, Philadelphia, 2000, WB Saunders.
2. Lueckenotte AG: *Gerontologic nursing,* ed 2, St Louis, 2000, Mosby.
3. McCance KL, Huether SE: *Pathophysiology: the biologic basis for disease in adults and children,* ed 4, St Louis, 2002, Mosby.
4. Morgan A: The basics of bone density testing, *Clin Adv* 44(4):76, 2002.
5. Thibodeau GA, Patton KT: *Anatomy and physiology,* ed 4, St Louis, 1999, Mosby.

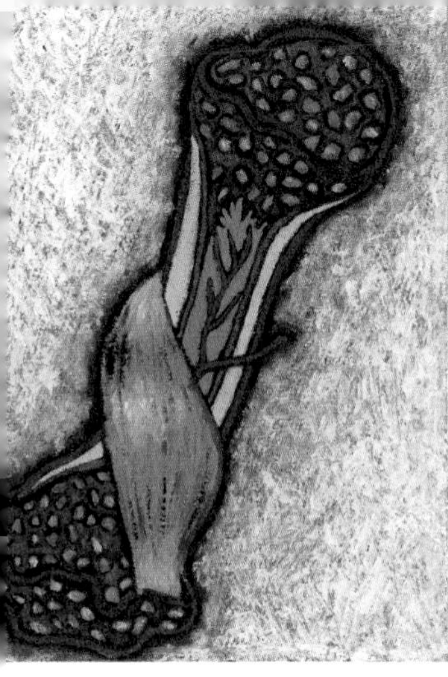

Trauma to the Musculoskeletal System

46

Jane F. Marek

Objectives

After studying this chapter, the learner should be able to:

1. Relate appropriate measures to prevent the causes of bone fractures.
2. Explain various treatment modalities for fracture healing.
3. Correlate complications of fractures with the available treatment regimens.
4. Describe the components of the nursing assessment of the person who has had a fracture.
5. Explain the nursing role in the management of fractures and prevention of complications.
6. Develop a nursing care plan for a person who has undergone surgical repair of a hip fracture.
7. Compare the nursing care required for a person with a prosthetic implant for a hip fracture with that required for a person who has received an internal fixation device.
8. Delineate the special nursing considerations in caring for the patient with a spinal fracture.
9. Analyze the various types of soft tissue trauma and joint injuries.
10. Discuss the nursing care of patients who have sustained soft tissue trauma and joint injuries.
11. Discuss the special care considerations of the patient who has sustained multiple injuries.

The person with musculoskeletal trauma has sustained an interruption in the integrity of one or more components of the system. Musculoskeletal trauma is most commonly manifested as a bone fracture, but it may also include injury to soft tissue or to a muscle, ligament, meniscus, tendon, or joint.

The National Center for Health Statistics estimates that annually an average of 1 in 10 persons suffers acute injury to the musculoskeletal system. The most common injuries are fractures, dislocations, and sprains.

TRAUMA TO BONE

FRACTURE

Etiology

A fracture is a disruption in the continuity of a bone and usually is a result of a blow to the body, a fall, or another accident. The amount of force or stress required to cause a break in the bone is dependent on several factors, including the size and density of the bone involved, the type and amount of stress applied, and the age of the patient. A fracture results when the bone is unable to absorb the stress. Although most fractures occur as a result of an accident or injury, stress fractures occur as a result of normal activity or after minimal injury. There are two types of stress fractures: fatigue and insufficiency related. *Fatigue* fractures are more common in younger, healthy persons and occur as a result of repeated stress and impact, usually from sports-related activities. The fracture begins as a small area of cortical infarct and progresses with continued stress.[15] *Insufficiency-related* fractures occur as a result of normal weight bearing or minimal activity; the bone is unable to absorb the stress and recover. These types of fractures typically occur to bones weakened by disease, such as primary or metastatic cancer, metabolic disorders, or osteoporosis. This type of fracture is also referred to as a pathologic fracture. Another type of fracture, avulsion fracture, occurs when a strong ligamentous or tendinous attachment pulls a fragment of bone away from the rest of the bone.

Epidemiology

Fractures occur in all age-groups, but the highest incidence is in young men, 15 to 24 years of age, and in older adults, particularly women, 65 years of age and older. Tibial fractures are the most common long bone fracture and are usually a result of motor vehicle accidents. Neuromuscular instability is an important contributing factor to the risk of falls, which commonly precede a fracture in the elderly population. Wrist, hip, and vertebral fractures are most common in older adults. The incidence of fatigue stress fractures is 4% to 15% generally and 0.12% in athletes.[15] The higher incidence of stress fractures in female athletes with menstrual irregularities is thought to be a result of decreased estrogen levels, which cause decreased bone density.[15] Persons in high-risk occupations (e.g., steelworkers and race car drivers) and persons with chronic degenerative or neoplastic diseases are also at higher risk for injury. In this section, fractures in general are discussed. Later in the chapter, complications of fractures and hip and spinal fractures are discussed.

Pathophysiology

Types of Fractures. A fracture is a complete or partial interruption of osseous tissue. *Complete* fractures penetrate both cortices, producing two bone fragments; only one cortex is broken in *incomplete* fractures. The part of the bone nearest the center of the body is referred to as the proximal fragment; the part more distant from the center is called the distal fragment. The proximal fragment is also called the uncontrollable fragment, because its location and muscular attachments prevent it from being moved or manipulated in an attempt to bring the separate fragments into alignment. The distal fragment is called the controllable fragment because it can usually be moved to bring it into correct relationship to the proximal fragment. Fractures in long bones are designated as being in the proximal, middle, or distal third of the bone.

If the skin over the fracture is intact, the fracture is classified as *simple* or *closed*. A fracture is classified as compound or open when there is direct communication between a skin wound and the fracture site. An open or compound fracture has a high risk of contamination, which is an important factor in treatment. Open fractures can be classified into three categories based on the severity of the fracture and the degree of soft tissue involvement. Type 3 fractures are the most severe and are further subdivided into three subtypes (Box 46-1).[13] When the two bone fragments are in proper alignment with no change from normal position despite the break in continuity of bone, the fracture is referred to as a *nondisplaced fracture*. If the bone fragments have separated at the point of fracture, the fracture is referred to as a *displaced* fracture. The degree of displacement varies with the type of injury and the condition of the bone and soft tissues. The position of the bone fragments depends on the mechanism of injury. The type, direction, and strength of the force and pull of the attached muscles determine the position of the bone fragments. Bone fragments that slide over each other are referred to as overriding fragments.

The line of fracture as revealed by x-ray film or fluoroscopy is usually classified according to type. It may be a *greenstick* fracture, with splintering on one side of the bone (this occurs most often in older adults and in young children); *transverse*, with the break being straight across the bone; *oblique*, with the line of the fracture at an oblique angle to the bone shaft; or *spiral*, with the fracture lines partially encircling the bone. The fracture may be referred to as *telescoped* or *impacted* if the distal fragment is forcibly pushed against and into the proximal fragment. This occurs most often with compression and force applied to the distal fragment. If there are several bone fragments, the fracture is referred to as *comminuted* (Figure 46-1 and Box 46-2).

Because bones are more rigid than their surrounding structures, any injury severe enough to cause a bone fracture may also cause injury to adjacent muscles, nerves, connective tissue, and blood vessels. The force that causes the fracture is dissipated through the surrounding soft tissue, and small fragments of bone may become embedded in muscle, blood vessels, or nerves.

Healing of Fractures. A fracture disrupts the cortex, periosteum, and adjacent soft tissues. Bleeding occurs at the broken ends of the bone and surrounding soft tissues. Important considerations in fracture healing are the blood supply to the fracture site and adequate immobilization. Once immobilization is accomplished, the bone heals by the process of callus formation (see Chapter 45). Immobilization of the fracture is vital for proper healing and may be accomplished in any of the following three ways:

1. Physiologic splinting, a naturally occurring phenomenon related to pain in the affected area that causes guarding, muscle spasm, and avoidance of use, as well as a desire to rest the whole body until some repair has occurred
2. External orthopedic splinting with devices such as casts, plaster splints, and braces

BOX 46-1 Classifications of Open Fractures

Type 1

Length of wound <1 cm
Low-energy injury

Type 2

Length of wound >1 cm
More energy absorbed during fracture

Type 3

Length of wound >10 cm
Comminuted fracture with extensive soft tissue damage
High-energy injury typically from gunshot wounds, motor vehicle accidents, farming accidents

Type 3A

Do not require major reconstructive surgery for closure

Type 3B

Major soft tissue defects requiring reconstructive surgery for closure

Type 3C

Vascular and neural compromise
Require major reconstructive procedures

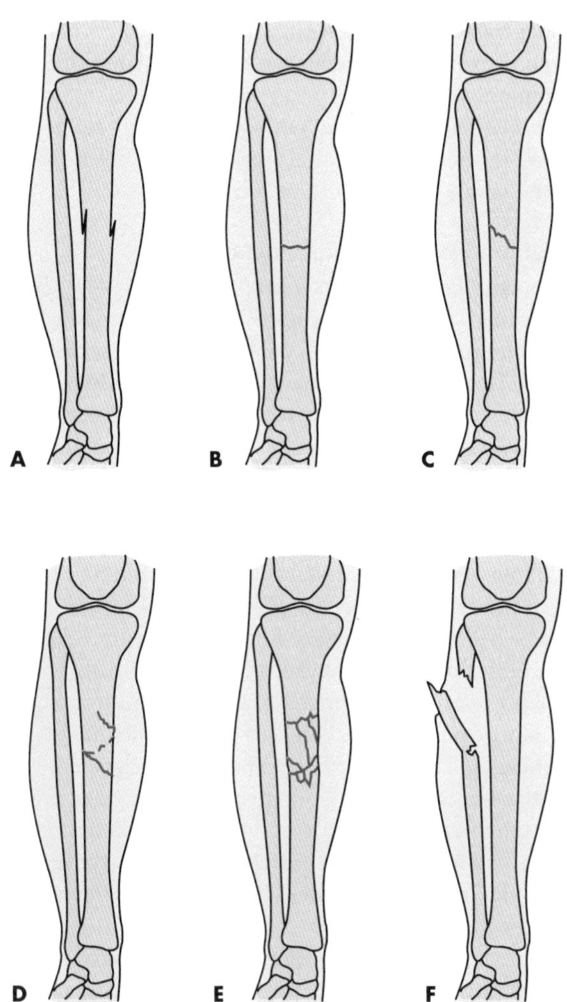

Figure 46-1 Types of fractures. **A,** Greenstick. **B,** Transverse. **C,** Oblique. **D,** Spiral. **E,** Comminuted. **F,** Open.

3. Internal fixation with screws, plates, or rods to hold the opposing ends of the fracture in place

The clinical manifestations of fractures differ, depending on the location and type of fracture and associated soft tissue injuries (see Clinical Manifestations box). Characteristics of most fractures include pain, impairment or loss of function, deformity, abnormal or excessive motion, swelling, altered sensation, and radiologic evidence of fracture. The immediate pain associated with a fracture is usually severe. Attempts at movement increase the pain. Factors contributing to the pain are associated soft tissue injuries, muscle spasms, and overriding of fracture fragments. Alterations in sensation are caused by pressure, pinching, or severing of nerves from the trauma, or by bone fragments.

Fracture healing begins with hematoma formation 24 to 72 hours after the injury. The healing time required for fractures depends on many factors. The age of the patient and type of bone fractured are important considerations. Adults require a longer healing time than children. Age is not a significant consideration in the rate of healing in adults after age 20, unless a metabolic disorder such as osteoporosis is present.[15] Osteoporotic bone, commonly found in older adults, requires additional healing time.

BOX 46-2 Types of Fractures

Typical Complete Fractures

Closed (simple) fracture: noncommunicating wound between bone and skin
Open (compound) fracture: communicating wound between bone and skin
Comminuted fracture: multiple bone fragments
Linear fracture: fracture line parallel to long axis of bone
Oblique fracture: fracture line at 45-degree angle to long axis of bone
Spiral fracture: fracture line encircling bone
Transverse fracture: fracture line perpendicular to long axis of bone
Impacted fracture: fracture fragments pushed into each other
Pathologic fracture: fracture at a point in the bone weakened by disease (e.g., by tumor or osteoporosis)
Avulsion fracture: fracture in which a fragment of bone connected to a ligament breaks off from the main bone
Extracapsular fracture: fracture close to the joint but outside the joint capsule
Intracapsular fracture: fracture within the joint capsule

Typical Incomplete Fractures

Greenstick fracture: break on one cortex of bone with splintering of inner bone surface
Torus fracture: buckling of cortex
Bowing fracture: bending of the bone
Stress fracture: microfracture
Transchondral fracture: separation of cartilaginous joint surface (articular cartilage) from main shaft of bone

Source: McCance KL, Huether SE: *Pathophysiology: the biologic basis for disease in adults and children,* ed 4, St Louis, 2002, Mosby.

Clinical Manifestations

Fractures

1. Pain (caused by swelling at site, muscle spasm, damage to periosteum)
   a. Immediate
   b. Severe
   c. Aggravated by pressure at site of injury
   d. Aggravated by attempted motion
2. Loss of normal function (injured part incapable of voluntary movement)
3. Obvious deformity resulting from loss of bone continuity
4. Excessive motion at site (i.e., motion where motion does not usually occur)
5. Crepitus* or grating sound if limb is moved gently
6. Soft tissue edema in area of injury resulting from extravasation of blood and tissue fluid
7. Warmth over injured area resulting from increased blood flow to the area
8. Ecchymosis of skin surrounding injured area (may not be apparent for several days)
9. Impairment or loss of sensation or paralysis distal to injury resulting from nerve entrapment or damage
10. Signs of shock related to severe tissue injury, blood loss, or intense pain
11. Evidence of fracture on x-ray film

*No attempt should be made to elicit this sign when a fracture is suspected, because it may cause further damage and increase pain.

The objective of healing is to restore the normal anatomy and function of the fractured bone. A fracture is considered united when radiographic evidence demonstrates a bony bridge at the fracture site. Other evidence that supports healing includes lack of motion at the fracture site, a nontender fracture site, the ability to resume normal function, and pain-free weight bearing (in lower extremity fractures).

In general, fractures of cancellous bone heal faster than cortical bone fractures because of the rich blood supply, especially when fracture fragments remain in direct contact. Midshaft fractures of the humerus, ulna, and tibia usually heal slowly because of the poor blood supply. An adequate blood supply enables the bone to bleed with the injury, allowing adequate hematoma formation, which is the first stage of bone healing. A greenstick fracture takes only a few weeks to heal, in contrast to an open, comminuted fracture, which may take up to 2 years for complete healing. Articular fractures are technically difficult to treat and are slower to heal; the fibrinolysin in synovial fluid is thought to slow the first stage of healing.[13] Factors conducive to fracture healing include close approximation of fracture fragments, an adequate blood supply, a surrounding muscular envelope, absence of infection, and adequate immobilization. Once immobilization is achieved, weight bearing stimulates healing and bone repair. Factors that impede bone healing include inadequate reduction, immobilization, and/or blood supply; systemic disease; and infection (Table 46-1).

Failure of a fracture to consolidate in the time usually required is termed *delayed union,* and failure to form a stable union after 6 months is termed *nonunion.* The incidence of nonunion in tibial fractures is higher than the incidence in other long bones, especially when the fracture occurs as a result of a high-energy injury, such as a motor vehicle accident. Certain bones are more likely to result in nonunion, regardless of proper fracture management. The distal tibia, carpal navicular, and proximal fifth metatarsal have the highest incidence of nonunion.[18]

Malunion refers to healing with angulation or deformity. If a fracture is nonunited, there is excessive mobility at the fracture site, creating a false joint, or *pseudoarthrosis.*

Collaborative Care Management

Diagnostic Tests. Diagnosis is confirmed by x-ray examination. Other studies, including CT and MRI, may be indicated if multiple injuries or complex fractures have been sustained. Healing progress may be documented by x-ray examination; stress films may be needed in some cases.

Medications. A fracture results in pain. Pain is managed by opioid and nonopioid analgesics and adjuvant drugs. Skeletal muscle relaxants may be prescribed in addition to analgesics. Antibiotics are given when an open fracture has occurred or surgical intervention is necessary. Tetanus toxoid may be necessary in the case of an open fracture. If prolonged immobilization or bed rest is necessary for treatment, anticoagulants may be prescribed as prophylaxis for deep vein thrombosis (DVT) and pulmonary embolism. Vitamin and iron supplements may be prescribed to prevent or treat anemia.

Treatments. The primary objectives of management are to reduce the fracture by realigning the fracture fragments, to maintain the fragments in correct alignment through immobilization, and to restore function and prevent excessive loss of joint mobility and muscle tone. Thus immediate treatment of the injury consists of:

1. Maintaining the airway and assessing for signs of shock
2. Splinting the fracture to prevent movement of the fracture fragments and further injury to the soft tissues by bony fragments (Splinting and immobilization also decrease pain.)

TABLE 46-1 Major Factors That Impede Bone Healing

Factor	Effect on Bone
Inadequate immobilization	Movement of fragments
Poor approximation of fracture fragments	Inaccurate reduction or malalignment of fracture fragments Excessive bone loss at time of fracture, preventing sufficient bridging of broken ends Excessive fragmentation of bone, allowing soft tissue to be interposed between bone ends Inability of patient to comply with restrictions imposed by immobilizing/fixation device(s), resulting in movement of fragments
Compromised blood supply	Damage to nutrient vessels Periosteal or muscular injury Severe comminution Avascularity (type of fracture, result of internal fixation device)
Excessive edema at fracture site	Tissue swelling impedes supply of nutrients to area of fracture
Bone necrosis	Injury to blood vessels impedes supply of nutrients to involved bone
Infection at fracture site	Infection disrupts normal callus formation
Metabolic disorders or diseases (cancer, diabetes, malnutrition, immunodeficiency, Paget's disease)	Retard osteogenesis
Soft tissue injury	Disruption of blood supply
Medication use (e.g., steroids, anticoagulants)	Steroids can cause osteoporosis, avascular necrosis; long-term use of heparin may cause osteoporosis

3. Preserving correct body alignment
4. Elevating the injured body part to decrease edema
5. Applying cold packs (during the first 24 hours) to reduce hemorrhage, edema, and pain
6. Observing for changes in color, sensation, circulation, movement, or temperature of the injured part

Subsequently, simple fractures are reduced (replacing bone fragments in their correct anatomic position) and immobilized. Reduction of simple fractures can be through manual manipulation (also known as closed reduction) in which bone fragments are moved into position by applying manual traction and pressure to the distal fragment; through the use of traction; or through open reduction, which is a surgical intervention that may incorporate the use of an internal fixation device.

The secondary management of compound fractures includes surgical debridement; irrigation of the wound to remove dirt, foreign material, devitalized tissue, and necrotic bone; and wound culture. The wound is packed and observed for signs of osteomyelitis, tetanus, and gas gangrene. The wound is closed when there is no sign of infection. The fracture is reduced and immobilized. In some cases of nonunion, bone growth stimulators that use low-voltage electrical impulses are used to enhance healing.

The purpose of immobilization is to hold the broken bone fragments in contact with each other (or in very close approximation) until healing takes place. Immobilization can be accomplished externally with external fixation devices (cast, splint, brace, cast brace), traction, or external fixators, or internally with metal plates, pins, screws, and nails, alone or in combination with bone grafts or prosthetic implants. Combinations of both external and internal methods can be used. The appropriate period of immobilization must be maintained to prevent nonunion or malunion.

Methods of External Fixation

Casts. The most common external fixation device is the cast. Materials used for casts include plaster of paris, fiberglass, and plastic. All of these materials are available as rolled bandages and are applied over the body part to be immobilized in much the same manner as an elastic bandage. Plaster, which has to be moistened before application, dries very slowly, is heavy, and loses its strength and integrity if it becomes wet after the initial drying. If a plaster cast requires revision, it usually must be removed and a new one applied. However, plaster is less expensive than fiberglass or plastic. Fiberglass and plastic dry quickly, are lightweight, and may be immersed in water without losing their strength. Plastic casts may be reheated and remolded if revision is necessary. Some types of fiberglass require drying under special ultraviolet lights, and persons wearing fiberglass or plastic casts may suffer maceration of the skin unless they dry the skin thoroughly with a warm air dryer after bathing or showering. Specific advantages or disadvantages of various cast materials are discussed in orthopedic texts.

A cast may enclose (1) all or part of an extremity (Figure 46-2), (2) all or part of the trunk and cervical area, or (3) all or part of the trunk with all or a portion of one or more extremities. The latter type of cast is called a spica cast (Figure 46-3). Splints are made from cast material, but they may be thought of as half-casts because they do not wholly enclose a body part. They can be applied anteriorly, posteriorly, medially, or laterally and are wrapped in place with an elastic bandage. Cast braces are made of two separate casts, applied above and below the involved joint and joined by metal or heavy polyethylene hinges incorporated into the cast material. Cast braces permit the patient joint mobility below the fracture while still providing immobilization for the fracture fragments.

Casts are applied over skin that has been cleansed and assessed for potential areas of infection or breakdown. Skin lesions should be treated before cast application. Before the cast is applied, the skin may be treated with tincture of benzoin and wrapped with cotton padding or stockinette. Bony prominences are padded with sheet wadding or felt to prevent pressure points. For specific techniques of cast application, consult specialized texts.

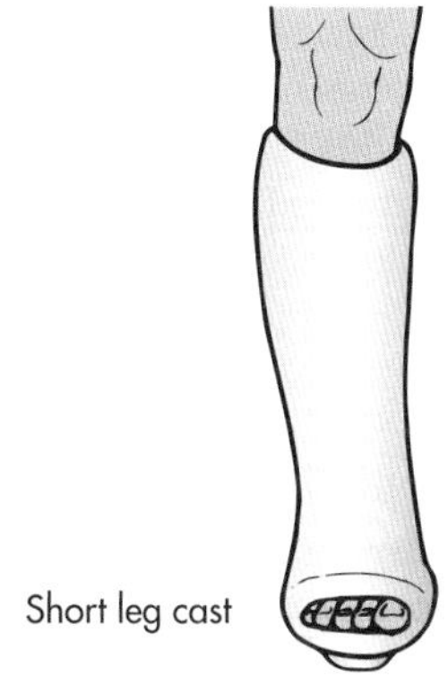

Figure 46-2 Short leg walking cast.

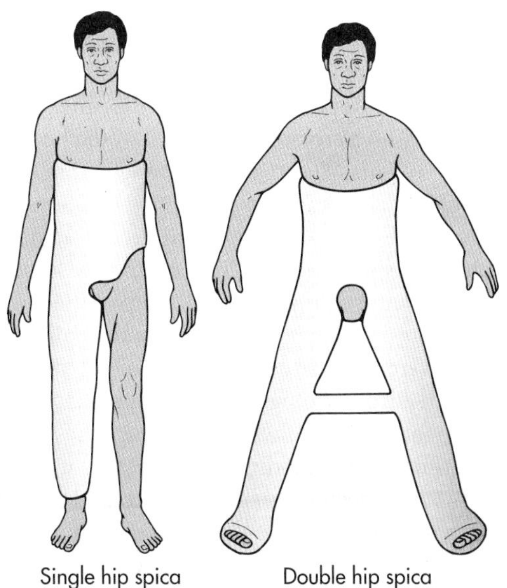

Figure 46-3 Hip spica casts.

Traction. Traction is the mechanism by which a steady pull is exerted on a part or parts of the body. Traction may be used to:

- Reduce a fracture.
- Maintain correct alignment of bone fragments during healing.
- Immobilize a limb while soft tissue healing takes place.
- Overcome muscle spasm.
- Stretch adhesions.
- Correct deformities.

Countertraction is a force that counteracts the pull of traction. The patient's body may be the countertraction, in which case the patient's feet should not rest on the foot of the bed. Buck's traction is an example of traction in which the patient's body is used as countertraction.

Suspension is the use of traction equipment, such as frames, splints, ropes, pulleys, and weights, to suspend but not exert a "pull" on a body part. To suspend the part correctly and continuously, the suspension must be balanced by weights. Suspension is often referred to as balanced suspension. Balanced suspension is often used in conjunction with traction to allow the patient to move about more freely and easily in bed.

Two types of traction are used: skin traction and skeletal traction. Skin traction is achieved by applying wide bands of moleskin, adhesive, or commercially available devices directly to the skin and attaching weights. The pull of the weights is transmitted indirectly to the involved bone or other connective tissue. Buck's extension and Russell's traction are the two most common forms of skin traction for injury to the lower extremities.

Buck's extension is the simplest form of skin traction and provides for straight pull on the affected extremity (Figure 46-4). It is often used to relieve muscle spasm and to immobilize a limb temporarily (e.g., to treat a hip fracture before open reduction and internal fixation [ORIF]). If adhesive substances are to be used, the leg is shaved and tincture of benzoin is applied to protect the skin. Adhesive tape or moleskin is then placed on the lateral and medial aspects of the leg and secured with a circular gauze or elastic bandage. The adhesive material should not cover the malleoli because of the risk of skin breakdown over these bony prominences. The tapes are attached to a spreader bar wide enough to pull the tapes away from the malleoli. Rope is attached to the spreader, passed through a pulley on a crossbar at the foot of the bed, and suspended with weights. The maximum weight that should be applied by skin traction is 2 to 4 kg (5 to 10 pounds); more weight can cause skin damage. Commercial foam rubber Buck's extension splints are widely used and are applied with Velcro straps. Contraindications to placing a patient in Buck's extension are stasis dermatitis, arteriosclerosis, allergy to adhesive tape, severe varicosities or varicose ulcers, diabetic gangrene, or marked overriding of bone fragments that would require more than 3.6 kg of weight to reduce the fracture.

Russell's traction is sometimes used because it permits the patient to move somewhat freely in the bed and permits flexion of the knee joint (Figure 46-5). It requires an overhead frame attached to the bed and preparation of the leg as for Buck's extension. A footplate with pulley attachments is used instead of a spreader bar. The knee is suspended in a sling to which a rope is attached. The rope is directed up to a pulley that has been placed on the overhead frame directly above the tibial tubercle of the affected extremity. The rope is then passed down through a pulley on a crossbar at the foot of the bed, back through a pulley on the footplate, back again to another pulley on the crossbar, and then suspended with weights. This arrangement places a double pull from the crossbar to the footplate, so the traction is approximately double the amount of weight used. Usually the foot of the bed is elevated on blocks (or the bed is put in Trendelenburg's position) to provide countertraction.

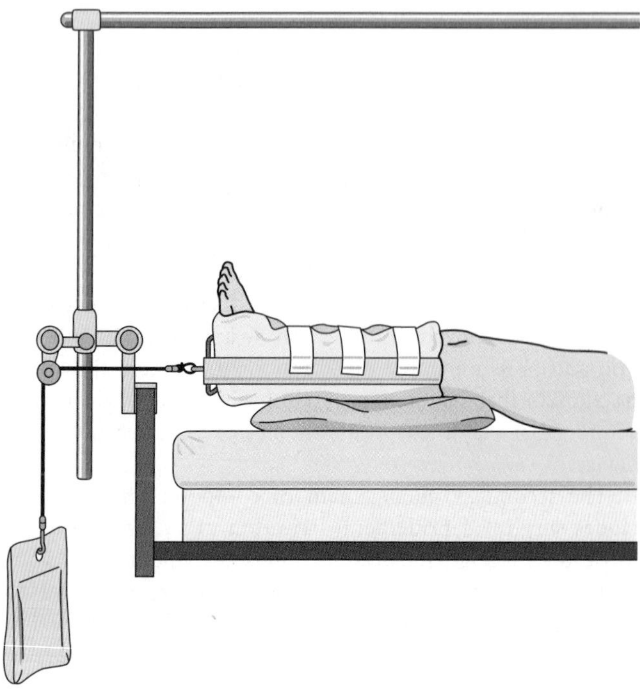

Figure 46-4 Buck's extension. The heel is supported off the bed to prevent pressure on the heel; the weight hangs free of the bed, and the foot is well away from the footboard of the bed. The limb should lie parallel to the bed unless prevented, as in this case, by a slight knee flexion contracture.

Russell's traction is used in the treatment of an intertrochanteric fracture of the femur when surgery is contraindicated. Either bilateral Russell's traction or Buck's extension may be used to treat back pain, because both partially immobilize the patient and reduce muscle spasm.

Skeletal traction is traction applied directly to bone. With the patient under local or general anesthesia, a Kirschner wire or Steinmann pin is inserted through bone distal to the fracture; the site of insertion varies with the type of fracture. The pin protrudes through the skin on both sides of the extremity, and the ends of the pin are covered with cork or metal protectors. Small sterile dressings are usually placed over the entry and exit sites of the pin, or pin sites may be left uncovered for easier observation. A U-shaped metal spreader or bow is attached to the pin, and the rope on which the traction weights are hung is tied onto the spreader. Skeletal traction can be used for fractures of the tibia, femur, humerus, and cervical spine. Skeletal traction applied to the cervical spine is achieved through the use of tongs applied to the skull (Figure 46-6).

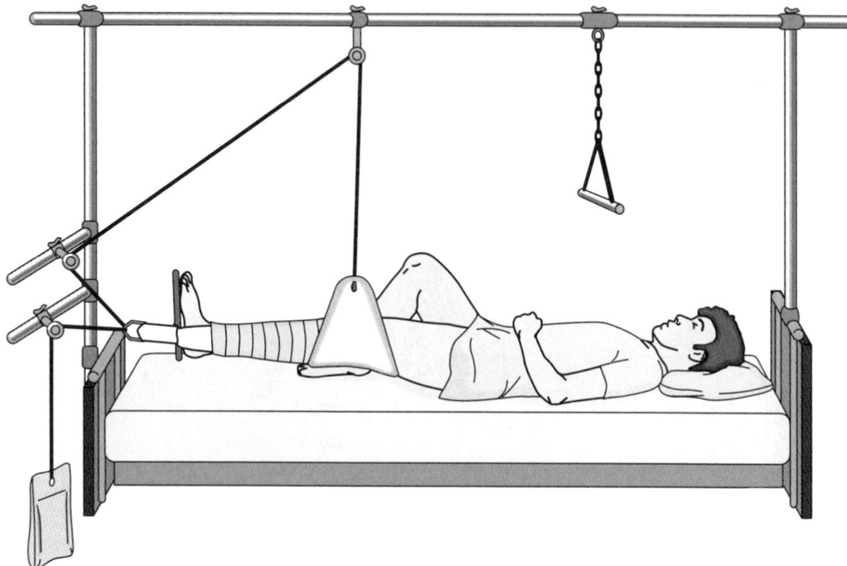

Figure 46-5 Russell's traction. The hip is slightly flexed. Pillows may be used under the lower leg to provide support and keep the heel free of the bed.

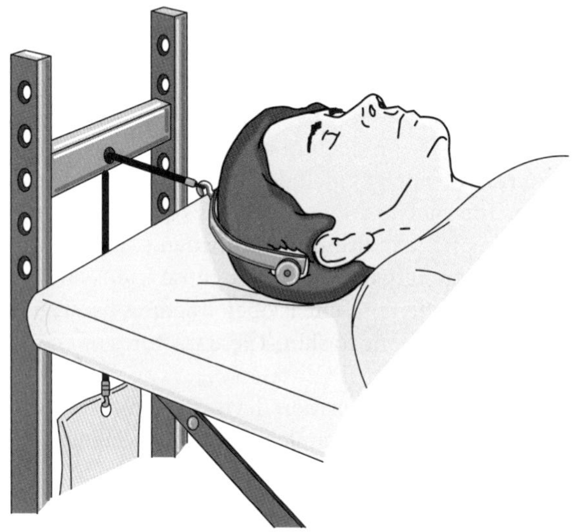

Figure 46-6 Traction to the cervical spine can be maintained through the use of Crutchfield tongs inserted into the skull.

When a balanced suspension apparatus is used in conjunction with skin or skeletal traction, the patient is able to move about in bed more freely without disturbing the line of pull of the traction. A full- or half-ring Thomas or Hodgen splint is commonly used for suspension of the lower extremity (Figure 46-7). Straps of canvas, muslin, or synthetic lamb's wool are placed over the splint and secured to provide a support for the leg. The areas under the popliteal space and heel are left open to prevent pressure. If knee flexion or movement of the lower leg is desirable, a Pearson attachment is clamped or fixed to the Thomas splint at the level of the knee.

Other Types of External Immobilization. Other devices for external immobilization of fractures include:

- Braces made of rigid plastic material
- Plaster or plastic braces that incorporate metal struts attached to pins inserted into bone, such as a halo brace (Figure 46-8)

Surgical Management. A variety of procedures and materials exist for operative fracture fixation. The materials selected and type of procedure performed depend on the individual patient, the surgeon, and the type of fracture. Materials selected for internal fixation must be strong and flexible. Two common materials are titanium alloy and stainless steel. Both of these materials provide adequate strength and fatigue resistance to allow healing of the fracture. Both may be contoured to fit irregularities in bone surfaces.

One method of fracture fixation is the *external fixator,* which consists of metal struts attached to pins inserted into bone (Figure 46-9). Advantages of external fixators include access to soft tissue injuries, management of complex comminuted fractures, alignment of fracture fragments, and early mobilization. External fixators such as the Hoffman or Synthes device may be used alone or in conjunction with plaster. All of these devices provide extremely rigid fixation while allowing the patient some degree of mobility. The patient with an external fixator on the lower leg can be out of bed in a wheelchair and can ambulate without bearing weight on the affected leg. As healing progresses, progressive weight bearing is allowed. The potential for infection is a major concern with the use of external fixators. In cases of severely comminuted fractures, bone grafting may be needed to promote healing.

The Ilizarov external fixator was developed in the Soviet Union in 1951 (Figure 46-10). It can be used to treat fractures, nonunions, osteomyelitis, deformities, and bony defects (caused by resection of malignancies) and to lengthen limbs. The basic principle of the Ilizarov technique is to achieve new bone growth by performing *corticotomies* (osteotomies through the cortex)

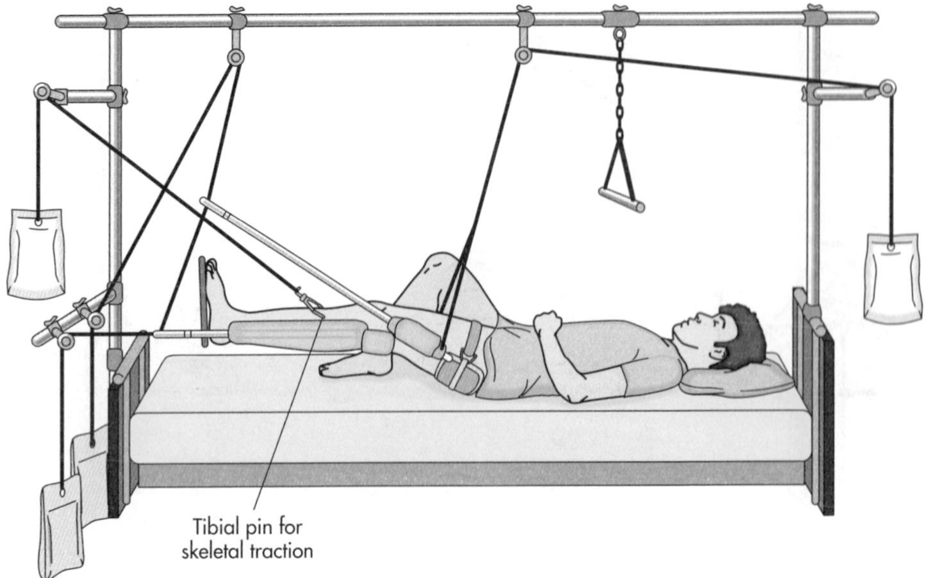

Figure 46-7 Balanced suspension with a Thomas splint and Pearson attachment. This apparatus can be used alone or, as in this case, with skeletal traction.

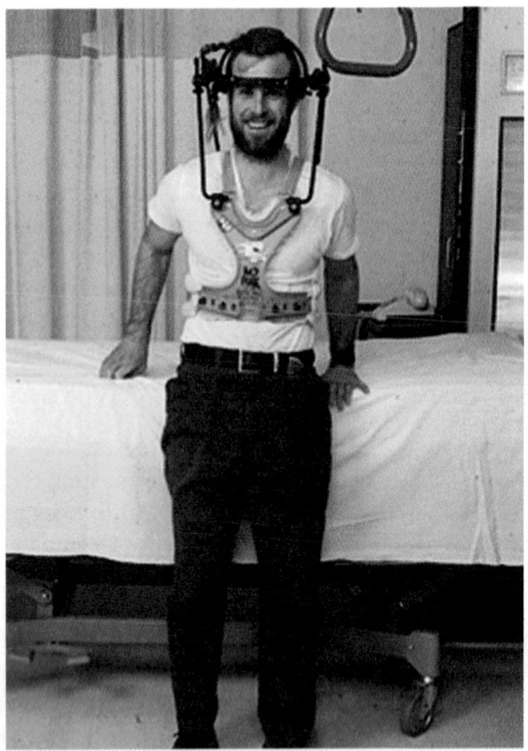

Figure 46-8 Halo vest. Note the rigid shoulder straps and encompassing vest. Various vest sizes are available prefabricated. The halo ring, superstructure, and vest are magnetic resonance imaging compatible.

and through the application of distraction. The corticotomy creates a "pseudo" growth plate without disrupting the medullary cavity, thereby preserving blood supply and allowing new bone to fill in the distraction gap. The application of gentle traction on the bone stimulates growth. Weight bearing, which also stimulates new bone growth, is usually encouraged.

Open surgical reduction of fractures has the advantage of allowing visualization of the fracture and surrounding tissues. ORIF is indicated for unstable or open fractures and those with significant soft tissue injuries. Other indications include failed closed reduction and displaced or intraarticular fractures. Advantages include solid fixation and early mobilization. Internal fixation is carried out under the most vigorous aseptic conditions, and patients may receive a course of perioperative prophylactic intravenous antibiotics. Tibial fractures often present as open fractures because of the close proximity of bone to skin. These fractures often require ORIF.

A variety of internal fixation devices are available, including plates and nails, intramedullary rods (Figure 46-11), transfixion screws (Figure 46-12), and prosthetic implants (Figure 46-13). Hip implants are indicated for fractures through or immediately below the femoral head, when blood supply to the femoral head is threatened. Fixation with internal devices does not preclude additional fixation with external devices (casts, braces, or traction), particularly in cases of highly complicated fractures or multiple trauma.

Rigid internal fixation with hardware is often used in conjunction with bone grafting, particularly when there has been excessive bone loss at the fracture site. *Autogenous* bone grafting (the patient's own bone) achieves the best results. The bone can be harvested from a variety of sites, commonly the iliac crest. Disadvantages include increased blood loss, the potential for infection, and increased pain at the donor site. Alternatives to autogenous grafting include *allograft* (human donor bone) and bone "substitutes." Allograft is bone derived from living or cadaver donors. During total hip arthroplasty (see Chapter 47), if suitable, the femoral head can be harvested and processed for future grafting.

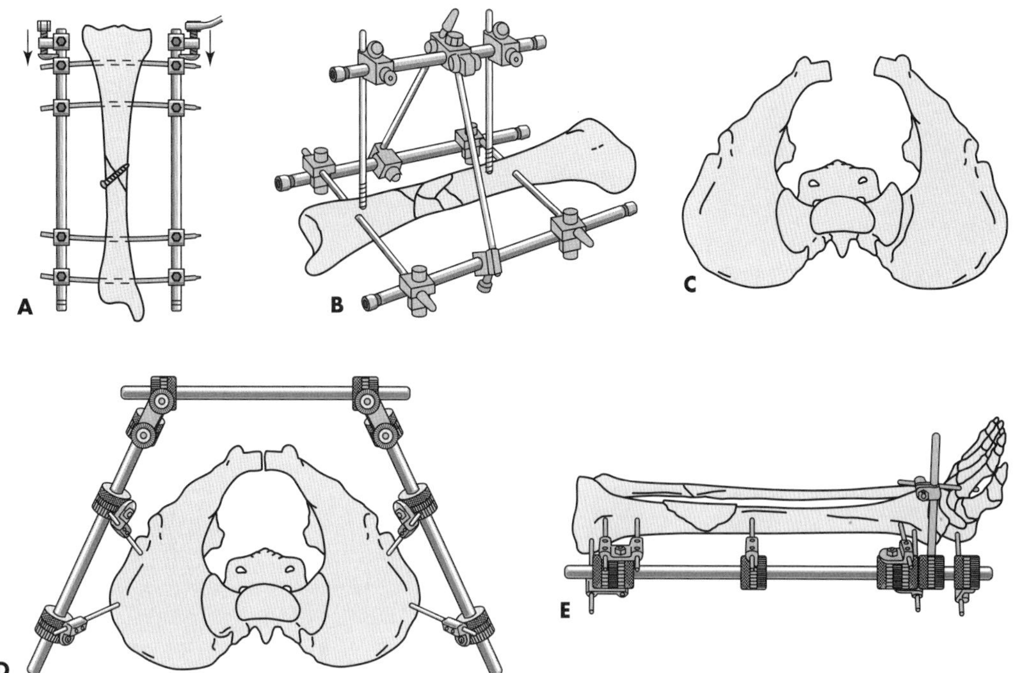

Figure 46-9 External fixators. A, Tibial fracture with simple AO external fixation with lag screw at fracture site. B, AO (Synthes) external fixator with three-dimensional or triangular fixation of comminuted fracture of tibia. C, Pelvic diastasis (dislocation). D, Hex-Fix external fixator in place, showing reduction of pelvic fracture. E, Hex-Fix external fixator used to treat tibial fracture. Immobilization of ankle and foot allows soft tissue healing.

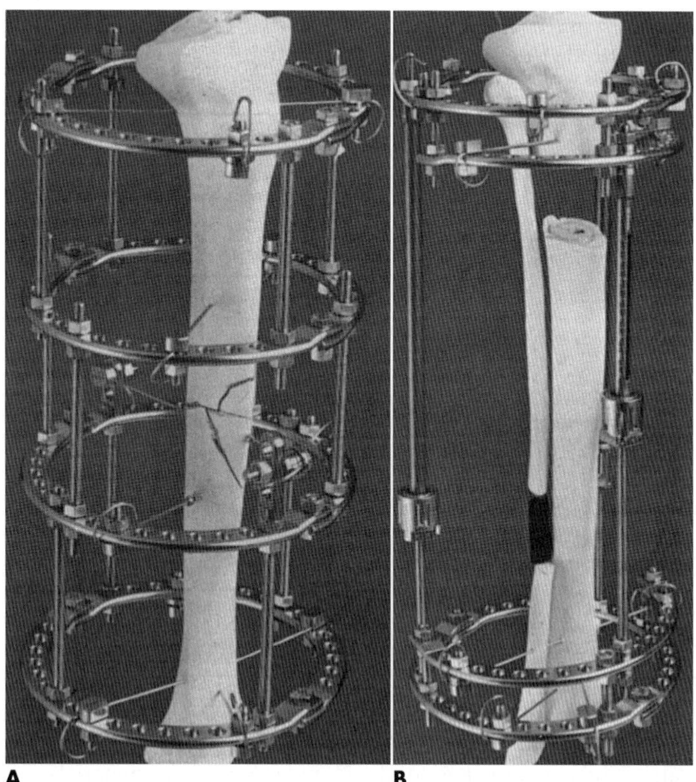

Figure 46-10 A, Ilizarov device in place to treat comminuted fracture. B, Ilizarov device assembly for lengthening of tibia.

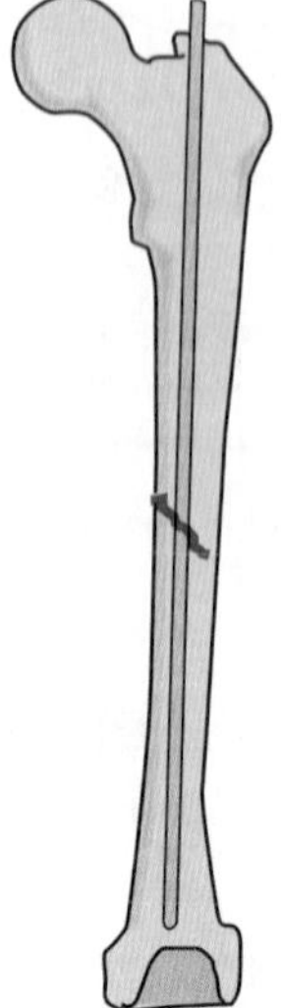

Figure 46-11 Intramedullary rod used to repair midshaft femoral fractures.

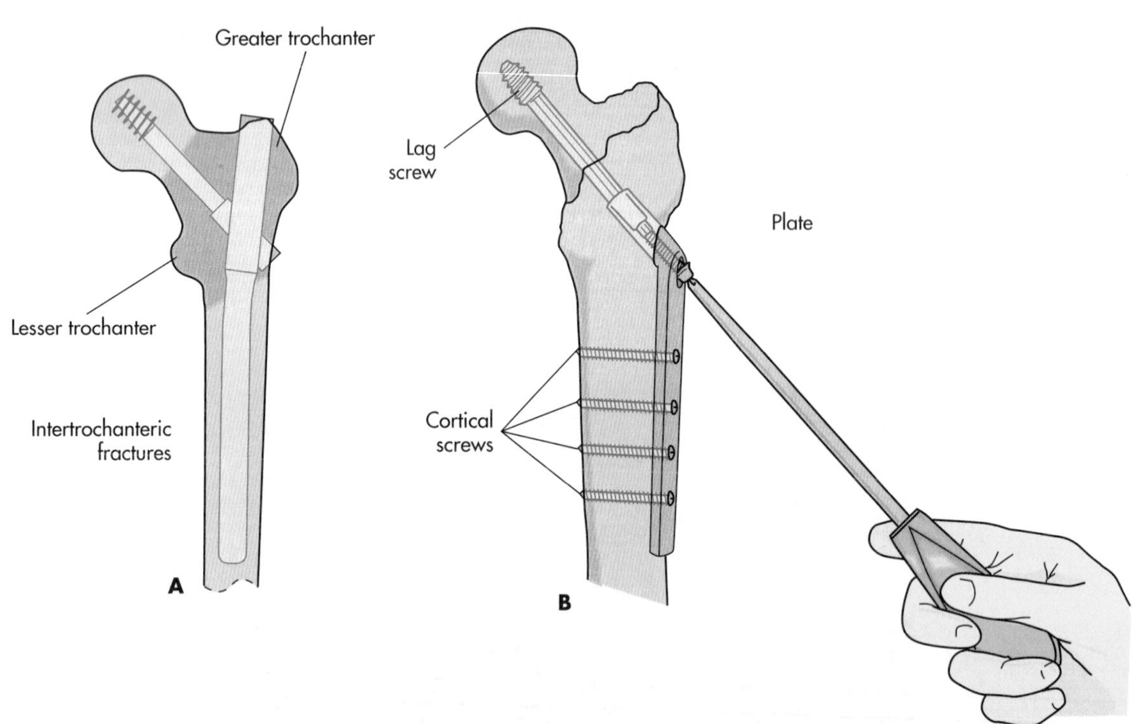

Figure 46-12 **A**, Richards intramedullary hip screw used for proximal femur fractures. Shown here for management of intratrochanteric fracture *(shaded area)*. The device consists of an intramedullary nail, lag screw, compression screw, centering sleeve, and set screw. **B**, Richards compression screw and plate for hip fractures. The compression screw *(shown at end of screwdriver)* threads into the distal end of the lag screw and draws the fracture fragments together. The sliding feature of the nail and plate assembly reduces the risk of acetabular penetration and allows weight-bearing forces to be transferred to the bone, rather than to the device.

The use of allograft bone carries the risk of transmission of blood and tissue-borne disease. Before use, bone bank bone must undergo processing. Methods of processing the bone differ. Immunogenicity, sterility, mechanical properties, and bone stimulation potential depend on the method of collection and processing. Bone that carries the highest risk of viral and bacterial contamination is cadaveric bone collected by sterile technique and used without further processing. However, cadaveric bone also contains the most bone growth factors, and thus it has the greatest potential to stimulate new bone formation. Ethylene oxide, a sterilizing agent, is not able to penetrate large pieces of allograft; therefore large grafts must be secondarily sterilized with gamma radiation.

Another alternative for grafting is the use of hydroxyapatite and other similar materials. Hydroxyapatite, a material derived from coral, is useful for filling bone defects but does not stimulate bone growth. Other materials, including synthetics and combinations of collagen, tricalcium phosphate, and hydroxy-

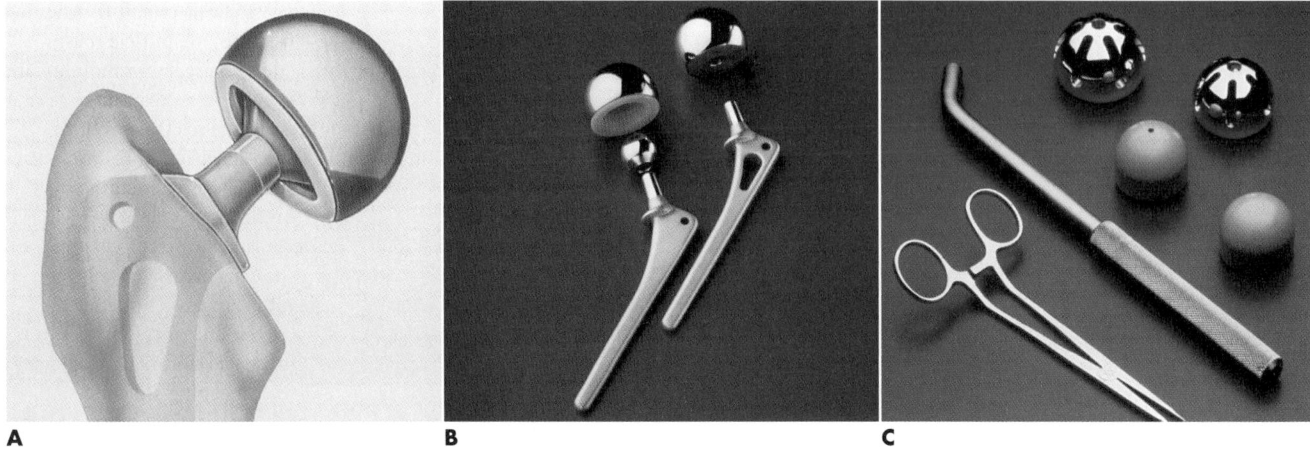

Figure 46-13 A, Bipolar modular prosthesis commonly used to replace the femoral head and neck in hip fractures when the vascular supply to the femoral head may be compromised. **B**, Bipolar *(left)* and unipolar *(right)* hip prostheses for hip fractures. In unipolar prostheses the femoral head attaches directly to the femoral stem. In bipolar prostheses the femoral head consists of two components. **C**, Instrumentation used for hip prostheses. Trial components used for sizing actual implant.

apatite, also require autogenous bone grafting to stimulate bone growth. The biomechanical and structural properties of these bone substitutes differ greatly from those of bone. In general, their structural properties are inferior to those of human bone. Augmenting bone substitutes with a human bone graft may improve their structural properties, particularly elasticity.[22] These bone "pastes" can be injected directly into the fracture site and harden in about 10 minutes. Twelve hours later, they are as strong as normal human bone. Ideally, as with a human bone graft, the body eventually resorbs the graft material and transforms it into bone mineral.

In general, the major objective of care is to protect the fixation until healing takes place. Metal, which can fatigue and break, cannot be expected to substitute for intact bone. If the fixation device breaks, healing of the fracture is disrupted. However, mobilization of patients who have had internal fixation is usually much faster than that for patients who have had external fixation.

Special consideration must be given to prevent infection in open fractures. Antibiotics and/or wound debridement may be necessary before open reduction. Severe open fractures can be treated with antibiotic "beads" placed directly in the wound. Antibiotic-impregnated (usually tobramycin) beads of bone cement (polymethylmethacrylate) are placed temporarily in the wound, and the wound is covered with a porous, transparent dressing. This method, first used in total hip arthroplasty, is effective in reducing infection.

Diet. The essentials of a nutritious diet, including fruits, vegetables, proteins, and vitamins, are especially important for the individual after a fracture. If mobility is restricted, catabolic activity is accelerated, producing a rapid breakdown of cellular materials, leading to protein deficiency and a negative nitrogen balance. In addition, metabolic needs are increased during healing. Decalcification and demineralization of bone take place during immobility, regardless of the quantity of calcium intake. Therefore increasing dietary calcium above normal requirements is not recommended, because the excess calcium cannot be used. However, a diet high in protein (150 to 300 g daily) is indicated to overcome protein deficiency and to return the body to a state of positive nitrogen balance. Patients who have had fractures have increased needs for iron, protein, and vitamins if bone repair is to progress normally.

Patients with fractures, particularly if immobilized, are at risk for developing bladder infections and renal stones. Dietary interventions to decrease the risk of bladder infections and renal calculi include increasing fluid intake and decreasing intake of calcium and citrus fruits and juices. Adequate fluid intake also aids in preventing urinary stasis, which contributes to the development of urinary tract infection.

Weight gain or loss is to be avoided, especially if the patient is in a cast or molded brace, because it affects the proper fit of the device. Excess body weight also increases stress on joints. Constipation is a complication of immobility. Fluids (2000 to 3000 ml daily) and fiber should be encouraged to promote bowel elimination.

Activity. Activity is limited, depending on the individual patient, the type and location of the fracture, and the method of reduction. The physician determines the amount of ambulation, activity, and weight bearing and prescribes specific exercises. In many institutions physical and occupational therapists do much of this teaching. However, the nurse needs to reinforce the teaching and supervise the patient in performing exercises and the correct use of crutches, walkers, and other devices. Range-of-motion (ROM) and isometric exercises should be performed while in bed to promote circulation and prevent muscle atrophy. The patient should be encouraged to be as active as possible within prescribed limitations to prevent the complications associated with immobility.

Referrals. Common referrals for persons with fractures include physical therapy and occupational therapy for instructions regarding exercises and proper use of assistive and adaptive devices. Placement in a rehabilitation facility or home care may be necessary for some persons with multiple injuries or complicated fractures.

NURSING MANAGEMENT

ASSESSMENT

Health History

A complete health history should be obtained (see Chapter 45), focusing on:

- Mechanism of injury and events leading up to injury
- Pain
- Loss of sensation or movement of the affected part
- Medication history
- Ability to perform activities of daily living (ADLs); amount of assistance required
- Past medical and surgical history (The presence of chronic diseases may affect the healing process.)
- Previous musculoskeletal injuries and surgical procedures
- Nutritional history (The patient's nutritional status will affect the healing process.)
- Support of family/significant others; coping skills
- Expectations of treatment

Physical Examination

Physical examination focuses on assessment of/for:

- Warmth, edema, or ecchymosis over and surrounding the injured part
- Obvious deformity; changes in normal alignment
- Crepitus
- Loss of normal function in the injured part
- Status of the immobilization device
- Neurovascular status (Table 46-2)
- Skin condition
- Indicators of pain, anxiety

NURSING DIAGNOSES

Nursing diagnoses are determined from analysis of patient data. Various methods of treatment, including surgical repair and immobilization by cast, traction, or external devices, are considered in the discussion of nursing diagnoses and interventions. (Refer to Chapters 16 and 18 for general preoperative and postoperative care.) Prevention of infection is an important nursing intervention, particularly for patients with open fractures or those who have undergone ORIF of the fracture. If injuries are extensive or prolonged immobilization or bed rest is required for treatment, disuse syndrome is an appropriate diagnostic choice. This comprehensive diagnosis guides the nurse in planning care to prevent multisystem complications associated with immobility. Nursing diagnoses for the patient with a fracture may include but are not limited to:

Nursing Diagnoses	Possible Etiologic Factors
1. Impaired physical mobility	Musculoskeletal impairment, prescribed weight-bearing limitations or activity restrictions, decreased strength and endurance, pain
2. Acute pain	Injury to bone or soft tissue at fracture site, muscle spasm, edema, surgery, immobility, improper pressure points
3. Risk for peripheral neurovascular dysfunction	Pressure, restrictive envelope, mechanical compression, trauma, casts, traction, immobility
4. Risk for impaired skin integrity	Decreased mobility, pressure, shearing forces
5. Powerlessness	Health care environment, decreased mobility, changes in role, level of functioning, ineffective coping strategies
6. Impaired home maintenance	Surgery, altered mobility, activity restrictions
7. Deficient knowledge	Lack of experience with a fracture, hospitalization, treatment protocols

EXPECTED PATIENT OUTCOMES

Expected patient outcomes for the patient with a fracture may include but are not limited to:

1a. Will demonstrate maximal mobility within prescribed activity and weight-bearing limits
1b. Will demonstrate proper use of adaptive/assistive devices
1c. Will participate in a program of progressive activity
2. Will state that pain is decreased; will rate pain at 4 or below using a scale of 0 to 10 (0 = no pain; 10 = most severe pain imaginable)
3. Will maintain intact peripheral neurovascular status in all extremities
4. Will maintain skin integrity
5a. Will verbalize a sense of power and control of the situation
5b. Will participate in the plan of care and treatment decisions; will demonstrate effective coping strategies; will report having an adequate support system
6a. Will demonstrate ability to meet role expectations
6b. Will adapt the home environment to meet his or her needs: will remove scatter rugs and obstacles to avoid injury when ambulating with a walker or crutches; will use safety devices in the bathroom (grab bars, elevated toilet seat, tub rails)
7. Will demonstrate knowledge of the disease and treatment essential to self-care management
7a. Nature of injury and course of treatment that must be followed to prevent injury or infection and to achieve the desired result
7b. Preoperative and postoperative routines and treatment protocols if surgical repair of the fracture is indicated
7c. Type and duration of weight-bearing and activity restrictions
7d. How to perform or modify ADLs within prescribed limitations of activity and motion; correct use of adaptive devices

TABLE 46-2 Signs and Symptoms of Neurovascular Impairment*

Signs and Symptoms	Interpretation
Pallor	Decreased arterial blood supply
Cyanosis	Venous stasis and poorly oxygenated tissue
Prolonged capillary refill	Decreased arterial blood supply
Edema	Fluid accumulating in tissues; poor venous return
Tissue cold or cool to touch	Decreased arterial blood supply
Patient unable to move parts distal to injury or external fixation device; paralysis or paresis	Pressure on nerves innervating parts distal to injury or underlying external fixation device
Patient report of extreme pain unrelieved by elevation, analgesic, or repositioning	Pressure on nerves innervating parts distal to injury or underlying external fixation device; ischemia
Patient report of heightened or decreased sensation or paresthesia in part distal to injury or underlying external fixation device	Pressure on nerves innervating parts distal to injury or underlying external fixation device
Diminished or absent pulses	Arterial injury; vascular compromise secondary to tissue edema

*Comparison of tissue should be made with uninvolved limb to determine the extent of the deviation from normal.

7e. Care for the cast, pins, or other immobilization devices, if applicable
7f. Safe use of an ambulatory or other ADL assistive device, if necessary
7g. Proper technique for wound care, if necessary
7h. Techniques appropriate to prevent skin breakdown, swelling, and neurovascular impairment
7i. Pain management techniques
7j. Appropriate use of prescribed medications
7k. Plans for follow-up care
7l. Methods to prevent further fracture or injury

INTERVENTIONS

1. Maintaining Strength and Mobility/Promoting Activity

One objective in the care of the patient who has sustained a fracture is to prevent loss of mobility and muscle tone. This is true for the fractured part, as well as for the rest of the body. The patient should move about to the greatest extent possible within the restrictions of the fracture reduction and the immobilizing devices. When permissible, weight bearing is encouraged, since it stimulates bone healing.

An initial assessment of the patient's strength, ROM, transfer ability, and functional status is useful in planning outcomes and measuring progress. Before beginning physical activity, the patient's response to and tolerance of activity should be assessed, since prolonged immobilization may result in physical deconditioning. Management of pain is another important consideration before beginning activity; untreated pain may result in reluctance to move or exacerbation of pain.

The patient should be encouraged to perform ROM and isometric exercises at least twice daily to prevent contractures, maintain joint mobility, and increase circulation and muscle tone. Another benefit of exercise is that it promotes a sense of well-being. The nurse should perform passive ROM exercises for immobile patients. A physical therapy consult may be initiated for specific exercises, weight training, and progressive ambulation. If appropriate, the use of walkers, crutches, walking belts, and/or wheelchairs should be encouraged to increase mobility. The patient should be encouraged to be as independent as possible in self-care activities. Occupational therapy can provide assistive devices to aid in self-care. An overhead trapeze can increase the patient's mobility in bed and increase upper body muscle tone.

2. Promoting Comfort

The person with a fracture often has severe pain at the fracture site, pressure from edema in the damaged soft tissues adjacent to the fracture, and spasm of the muscles in the fracture area. If the fracture is repaired by ORIF, the patient also has operative pain. Continued pain and muscle spasm can put undue stress on the fracture fragments and retard efforts both to reduce and to maintain reduction of the fracture. Patients who are in severe pain may resist efforts to help them carry out measures designed to prevent complications.

Effective pain management requires a team approach and the involvement of the patient in the treatment plan. Both pharmacologic and nonpharmacologic methods are used in treating pain. Depending on the severity of pain, opioids and/or nonopioid analgesics are prescribed. The patient's self-report is the most reliable indicator of pain. Adjuvant drugs may be added, including muscle relaxants or anxiolytics.

Methods of administration include around-the-clock dosing, as-needed dosing, and patient-controlled analgesia. If opioids are used, the patient's level of consciousness, respiratory status, sedation level, and pain intensity should be assessed at least every 4 hours. The patient and family should receive instructions regarding the pain management plan. The effectiveness of the treatment should be evaluated at regular intervals. As pain subsides, reduction in the strength or frequency of analgesic administration should be negotiated with the patient.

In addition to pharmacologic methods, nonpharmacologic interventions are effective in managing pain. The patient's previous experiences with these methods, including guided

Guidelines for Safe Practice

The Patient in Traction

1. Patient education
   a. Explain traction in relation to the fracture and the physician's plan of treatment.
   b. Explain the amount of movement permitted and how to achieve it (e.g., how the trapeze can be used to assist with movement).
   c. Explain correct body positioning. Maintain proper body alignment.
2. Maintain continuous traction, unless indicated otherwise
   a. Inspect the traction apparatus frequently to ensure that the ropes are running straight and through the middle of the pulleys, that the weights are hanging free, and that nothing impinges on the traction apparatus.
   b. Check ropes frequently to be sure they are not frayed.
   c. Avoid releasing weights or altering the line of pull of the traction.
   d. Avoid adding weight to the traction.
   e. Check the position of the Thomas splint frequently; if the ring slides away from the groin, readjust the splint to its proper position without releasing traction.
   f. Avoid bumping into or jarring the bed or traction equipment.
   g. Be sure weights are securely fastened to their ropes.
   h. Avoid manipulation of pins.
3. Maintain countertraction
4. Skin care
   a. Encourage the patient to turn slightly from side to side and to lift up on the trapeze to relieve pressure on the skin of the sacrum and scapulae; have the patient lift up for routine skin care to prevent friction and shearing forces.
   b. Avoid padding the ring of the Thomas splint, because this will create dampness next to the skin. Bathe the skin beneath the ring, dry it thoroughly, and powder the skin lightly.
   c. Inspect the skin frequently to be sure it is not being rubbed, contused, or macerated by traction equipment; readjust splints or the extremity in the splint to free the skin from pressure.
   d. Keep skin areas around pin sites clean and dry. Data are inconclusive to support the best practice for pin site care (see Evidence-Based Practice box). Use institutional protocol or physician order regarding pin care frequency and method.
5. Toileting
   a. Use a fracture pan with a blanket roll or padding as support under the small of the back.
   b. Protect the ring of the Thomas splint with waterproof material.
6. Prevention of neurovascular problems
   a. Perform neurovascular checks every hour for the first 24 to 48 hours; notify the physician of changes from baseline status.
   b. Monitor for signs of deep vein thrombosis, pulmonary embolism, and fat embolism syndrome (if applicable).

Evidence-Based Practice

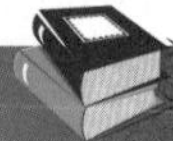

Reference: McKenzie LL: In search of a standard for pin site care, *Orthop Nurs* 8(2):73-78, 1999.

Although often encountered in clinical practice, there has been no standard of care for the care of skeletal pin sites. Care has been based on clinicians' preferences rather than research. Practices include the use of saline, hydrogen peroxide, alcohol, povidone-iodine solution and/or ointment, antibiotic ointment, and soap and water. Frequency of care varies. The author conducted a review of the medical and nursing literature regarding pin care practices; there was a paucity of data to support a best technique for pin site care. On the basis of the pathophysiology of pin site infections and current literature, the author developed a protocol for care. Recommendations include using normal saline as a cleansing agent, no use of ointments after cleansing the sites, removing any crusted drainage, and applying a dressing to the pin sites. Pin care should be performed three times a day if there is drainage present, or once daily if the sites are clear. Sterile technique should be used while the patient is hospitalized; clean technique can be used once the patient is discharged to home.

imagery, distraction, and relaxation, should be assessed. Also, application of ice decreases pain by reducing swelling.

The patient must be repositioned frequently within the prescribed position or activity limitations to avoid prolonged pressure over bony prominences and to prevent stiffness. Positioning is a measure that promotes comfort, provides for adequate ventilation and mobilization of pulmonary secretions, enhances circulation, and relieves pressure on vulnerable skin areas. To safely reposition a patient, the nurse must know the location and type of fracture, reduction techniques used, and any special activity or positioning restrictions.

The nurse should use the following guidelines for positioning the patient with a fracture:

Maintain the alignment of the fracture.

Maintain the direction of pull of traction (see Guidelines for Safe Practice box for the patient in traction).

Maintain the integrity of the cast (see Guidelines for Safe Practice box for the patient in a cast).

Maintain positioning, activity, and weight-bearing restrictions of an internal fixation device (see Guidelines for Safe Practice box for the patient with an internal fixation device).

Generally, nurses should avoid changing the position of patients with unreduced, unsplinted fractures. Manipulation of fracture fragments, particularly long bones, may cause release of fat into the vasculature (see discussion under Fat Embolism Syndrome). Once the parameters for safe positioning are defined, the nurse should assist the patient in changing position at least every 2 hours until the patient can do so independently.

Guidelines for Safe Practice

The Patient in a Cast

1. Patient education
   a. Before cast application, explain why and how the cast will be applied.
   b. Advise the patient that the plaster cast will feel warm as it dries.
   c. Explain the extent to which the patient will be immobilized.
   d. Following cast application, explain care of the cast and expectations after discharge.
   e. Instruct the patient not to insert sharp objects (coat hangers or pencils) under the cast, because these may abrade the skin and lead to infection.
   f. Cast removal: explain that the saw used for removal is noisy; the saw will not harm the skin.
2. Handling the new cast
   a. Support the wet cast with the flat of the hands or on pillows to avoid indentations that will cause pressure on the underlying skin.
   b. Place cotton blankets or other absorbent material under the cast to aid the drying process.
   c. Expose the cast to air as much as possible to aid the drying process.
   d. Turn the patient frequently to aid the drying process.
   e. Use a fan to circulate air over the cast.
   f. Instruct the patient not to apply anything to the cast; plaster is a porous material that allows air to circulate to the skin.
3. Skin care and prevention of infection
   a. Inspect the skin at the edges of the cast and underlying the cast for redness or irritation; apply petal-shaped strips of adhesive tape or moleskin around the rough edges of the cast.
   b. Instruct the patient to report any drainage, foul odor, or increased pain, which may indicate infection, bleeding, or skin irritation. Circle existing drainage with a marker to detect increases.
   c. Remove plaster crumbs from the skin with a washcloth moistened with warm water.
   d. Use creams and lotions sparingly, because they may soften the skin and cause the cast to stick to the skin.
   e. Apply waterproof material around the perineal area to prevent skin irritation and soiling of and damage to the cast.
   f. Attend to the patient's report of pain under the cast, particularly over bony prominences, because this may indicate pressure on the skin. If discomfort is not relieved by repositioning, report to the physician. Cast pressure may need to be relieved by windowing or bivalving (cutting the cast in half).
   g. Following cast removal, provide skin care to remove built-up exudate of secretions and dead skin. Mineral oil and warm water soaks are helpful.
4. Turning
   a. Turning to any position is generally permitted, as long as the integrity of the cast is not compromised and the patient is comfortable.
5. Toileting (for a long leg or hip spica cast)
   a. Use a fracture pan with a blanket roll or padding as support under the small of the back.
   b. Elevate the head of the bed if permitted, or place the bed in reverse Trendelenburg's position.
6. Abdominal discomfort
   a. Spica cast may be "windowed" (cut an opening into cast) to provide relief of abdominal distention or as a port for checking bladder distention.
7. Mobilization
   a. The amount of weight bearing permitted will be prescribed by the physician.
   b. A cast shoe or a walking heel incorporated into a lower extremity cast will permit weight bearing without damaging the cast.
8. Prevention of neurovascular problems
   a. Perform neurovascular checks every hour for at least 24 hours after cast application to detect difficulty from swelling or pressure of the cast on nerves or vessels. Notify the physician of changes in color, changes in pulse quality, or alterations in sensation or motion unrelieved by position change; the cast may need to be bivalved to relieve pressure.
   b. Elevate the affected extremity on pillows until the danger of swelling is over (usually 24 to 48 hours).
   c. After mobilization of the patient with a lower extremity or upper extremity cast, avoid keeping the extremity in a dependent position for prolonged periods.
   d. After a lower extremity cast is removed, encourage the patient to wear an elastic stocking and elevate the affected leg at rest until full mobility is regained. Isometric exercises should be encouraged to prevent circulatory complications.

3. Maintaining Neurovascular Status and Tissue Perfusion

Monitoring for neurovascular compromise must be carried out every hour in the initial stages of a fracture. Damage to blood vessels or nerves may occur at the time of the fracture or following reduction. Some swelling of a fractured extremity may be expected and is often well controlled by elevating the extremity. However, unrelieved swelling of an extremity that is confined in a cast or compression dressing causes undue pressure on vessels and nerves and can result in circulatory or neurologic impairment or skin breakdown. The affected extremity should be evaluated frequently for signs of compression. Evidence of impaired circulation or sensation must be reported to the physician immediately. The frequency of neurovascular checks can usually be reduced if there is no evidence of compromise within 48 hours of the fracture or reduction (see Table 46-2). Observations of the involved extremity should be compared with observations of the uninvolved extremity to validate deviations from the patient's "normal."

Monitoring neurovascular status of the injured part includes:

- Palpating for warmth
- Observing color
- Assessing capillary refill time
- Questioning the patient about pain and paresthesias in the injured part

Guidelines for Safe Practice

The Patient With an Internal Fixation Device

1. Patient education
   a. Prepare the patient for anesthesia.
   b. Explain the surgical procedure and general perioperative care.
   c. After surgery explain the limits of motion and weight bearing to the affected part.
2. Promoting mobility
   a. Consult with the physician regarding activity, range-of-motion, and weight-bearing limits.
   b. Instruct and help the patient to turn, transfer, and ambulate within the prescribed limits (mobilization may begin as early as the day of surgery).
   c. Instruct and help the patient to use an appropriate ambulatory aid if lower extremity fracture.
3. Prevention of neurovascular problems
   a. Perform neurovascular checks every hour for the first 24 to 48 hours; notify the physician of any change from preoperative status, because this may indicate pressure from swelling, constricting bandages, or damage to nerves or vessels during surgery.
   b. Keep the affected extremity elevated.
   c. Monitor for signs of deep vein thrombosis, pulmonary embolism, and fat embolism syndrome, if applicable.
4. Maintenance of immobilization of fracture (Considerations for care would be the same as for patients in cast/traction if those devices are used.)

Assessing the patient's ability to discriminate sensation
Observing the patient's ability to voluntarily move the body part distal to the fracture

Immobility is a risk factor for the development of DVT. Ambulation should begin as soon as possible to help prevent clot formation. Isometric leg exercises help promote venous return and decrease venous stasis. Other interventions that have proved to be effective in decreasing the development of DVT include the use of graduated compression elastic stockings, intermittent compression devices, and prophylactic anticoagulants. The patient should be monitored frequently for signs of DVT, which include redness, swelling, tenderness, pain, and a palpable cord in the involved leg. Homans' sign is not a reliable indicator for the presence of DVT. The most common presentation is pain and swelling in the affected extremity. Calf and thigh circumferences should be measured daily; differences greater than 2 cm should be reported to the physician. The affected extremity should be elevated for the first 48 hours; thereafter the extremity should be elevated when the patient is at rest.

4. Maintaining Skin Integrity

When determining interventions to maintain skin integrity, the nurse must consider ways to prevent skin breakdown, as well as ways to promote wound healing. A risk assessment tool such as the Braden Scale can be used on admission and at regular intervals thereafter. The skin should be monitored at least daily for signs of pressure, which include color changes (redness or pallor), warmth or coolness, induration, and nonblanchable areas. Bony prominences (heels, sacrum, elbows, scapulae, ischial tuberosities) are at increased risk for breakdown. Skin over bony prominences should not be massaged, because massage can traumatize the underlying deep tissues. Patients with sensory deficits are at increased risk for skin breakdown.

Because moisture contributes to the development of skin breakdown, the patient should be assisted with keeping the skin clean and dry, especially under casts, slings, and traction apparatus. Skin care should be performed after toileting. If the patient is incontinent, exposure to urine and feces should be minimized to prevent breakdown. Skin areas in contact with cast edges or traction apparatus should be assessed frequently, and measures taken to eliminate moisture, chafing, or pressure in those areas.

If permissible, the patient should be turned every 2 hours, using a turn sheet to reduce friction and shearing forces. During transferring or positioning of the patient, friction and shearing forces should be eliminated or reduced. Foam wedges, pressure-relieving devices, sheepskin, pillows, and heel and elbow pads can be used to relieve pressure. In some instances a special bed or mattress or a turning frame may be required. When sitting in a chair, the patient should be taught to perform weight shifts at least every 2 hours.

5. Promoting Autonomy and a Sense of Control

An unexpected event such as an injury disrupts the normal routine and lifestyle of the patient and his or her family, and all need support to cope effectively and resolve the crisis. Developing a therapeutic relationship helps establish trust. Allowing adequate time for questions allows the patient some control over the situation. Factors contributing to feelings of powerlessness include hospitalization, immobility, prognosis, role changes, and misinformation. A frank discussion of what is under the patient's control is beneficial in establishing realistic goals. Assessing family dynamics, support systems, and coping strategies can help the nurse develop a plan of care with the patient. The patient's locus of control (external versus internal) should be considered and incorporated into the care plan. Providing explanations of the treatment plan and supporting the patient's and family's decisions help increase feelings of control and autonomy. The patient should be allowed to make as many choices regarding daily care and treatment routines as possible. Allowing the patient time to verbalize feelings of frustration also can help decrease feelings of frustration and accept limits of the situation. The patient should be encouraged to pursue activities that provide relaxation and distraction.

6. Promoting Self-Care and a Safe Home Environment

As healing progresses and pain diminishes, patients are more receptive to learning what activities are necessary for a safe return home. The easiest and most effective way to teach patients self-care is to have them function as independently as possible within their prescribed limitations, using the appropriate assistive devices, while they are in the hospital. Assessing the probable level of functioning at the time of discharge allows the health care team to determine the type of assistance and equipment that is needed. As necessary, referrals are made to the home care team, community health nurse, or other agencies that will meet with the patient and family to determine what help (aide, homemaker) may be needed. This is especially important for persons who live alone or who will be alone for long periods of time while family members are at work.

An assessment of the home environment and the availability of caregivers should be done as soon as possible. If the family plans to care for the patient at home, relief for caregivers should be explored. Before discharge, arrangements should be made to obtain any necessary assistive or adaptive devices for the home (elevated toilet seat, walkers, safety bars, etc.). The patient should be able to demonstrate safe and proper use of these devices before discharge. Instructions should be given regarding the use of any immobilization devices.

7. Patient/Family Education

Treatment of the acute fracture is usually carried out in the hospital's emergency department or in the operating room before the patient is admitted to the general hospital unit. Patients may have little or no opportunity to become oriented to the hospital or to the care they will be receiving. In addition, they are probably frightened or overwhelmed by what has happened to them, may be experiencing pain, and possibly may be groggy from pain medication or anesthesia. Careful and often-repeated explanation and direction is necessary. Patients must be given time to adjust to their situations before they can begin to understand how they can cooperate in their care. Instructions should include information regarding the nature and course of treatment, including follow-up care, skin and wound care, pain management, activity and weight-bearing restrictions, the use of prescribed medications, and signs of complications.

Health Promotion/Prevention

Because most fractures occur as a result of accidents or injuries, a key intervention is prevention. Interventions should be targeted at high-risk groups. These include children, young men ages 15 to 24 years, and older adults. Young men ages 15 to 24 years have the highest incidence of motor vehicle–related deaths, and persons older than 75 years of age have the second highest incidence of motor vehicle–related deaths.[4] Each day more than 400 persons in the United States die as a result of motor vehicle accidents, guns, falls, and other injuries.[5] Nurses can be instrumental in providing education to prevent accidents and fractures.

Public education regarding prevention should include the following information:

- The dangers of driving while impaired
- Use of seat belts and air bags in motor vehicles; adhering to speed limits
- Attending to safety precautions when climbing ladders and using power tools or heavy equipment
- Wearing recommended protective clothing (e.g., steel-toed shoes and hard hats for hazardous work at home or on the job)
- Wearing proper protective clothing while engaging in sports (e.g., protective padding, helmets, and proper-fitting running shoes)

Safety measures and fall prevention are important for older adults. Ensuring a safe home environment can be an effective prevention against falls and fractures. Grab bars, handrails, nonskid floor and tub surfaces, night lights, and an obstacle-free environment can help prevent falls and injury. Individuals who must use ambulatory devices and wheelchairs should be instructed on how to use them properly. Knowledge of the patient's medication history, with attention to drugs that may cause dizziness, sedation, or orthostatic hypotension, may alert the family and/or caregivers to the risk of falls. A third approach to prevention is education regarding prevention of osteoporosis (see Chapter 47).

Healthy People 2010

Injury and violence are the leading health indicators related to fracture; objectives include reducing deaths caused by motor vehicle crashes. Other Healthy People 2010 objectives related to osteoporosis are discussed in Chapter 47 in the section on osteoporosis.

EVALUATION

To evaluate the effectiveness of nursing interventions, compare patient behaviors with those stated in the expected patient outcomes. Achievement of patient outcomes is successful if the patient:

1a. Participates in activities to maximum potential, adhering to prescribed restrictions.
1b. Ambulates safely using a cane, walker, or crutches.
1c. Participates in a program of progressive exercise; attends physical therapy sessions as indicated to practice prescribed exercises.
2. Controls pain effectively.
2a. Rates pain as less than 4 on a scale of 1 to 10.
2b. States correct use of prescribed analgesics.
2c. Uses ice packs for 20 minutes after exercising.
3. Maintains intact peripheral neurovascular status in all extremities.
3a. Pulses are palpable, strong, and symmetric in both extremities.
3b. Extremities are warm and pink.
3c. Sensation and motor function are intact.
3d. Capillary refill is less than 3 seconds bilaterally.
4. Has intact skin that is free from pressure.
5a. Verbalizes a feeling of being in control of the situation.
5b. Participates in the treatment plan and decisions regarding care; uses effective coping strategies; has an adequate support system.
6a. Assumes some aspects of usual role.
6b. Adapts the home environment to individual safety needs and uses appropriate safety devices.

7. Demonstrates knowledge of the disease and treatment essential to self-care management.
7a. Describes the nature of the injury and course of treatment.
7b. Describes perioperative routines and treatment protocols if surgical repair is indicated.
7c. Explains the limitations and duration of motion and activity restrictions.
7d. Explains how to perform ADLs using assistive devices; walks with a cane or other ambulatory aid without assistance; is able to ascend, descend stairs safely.
7e. Describes how to care for cast, pins, or other immobilization devices.
7f. Demonstrates the correct way to walk with a cane, walker, or crutches.
7g. Explains proper technique for wound and skin care.
7h. Explains how to prevent skin breakdown, swelling, and neurovascular impairment.
7i. Explains appropriate use of pain management techniques.
7j. Explains correct use of prescribed medications.
7k. Describes plans for follow-up care.
7l. Describes methods of preventing further fracture or injury.

GERONTOLOGIC CONSIDERATIONS

Older persons who sustain fractures often incur some loss of functional ability. Older adults are prone to fractures for many reasons, including osteoporosis, neoplasms, sensorimotor deficits, and falls. Falls are the most common cause of fractures in the elderly. Bones most commonly fractured are the proximal femur (hip), distal radius (Colles' fracture), vertebrae, and clavicle. Colles' fractures usually occur as a result of placing an outreached hand to break a fall, most commonly in a woman with osteoporosis. Treatment usually consists of closed reduction and immobilization. The majority of clavicular fractures in older adults are sustained in a manner similar to that with a Colles' fracture. The fracture usually occurs in the medial third of the clavicle. The patient exhibits swelling, point tenderness, local deformity, and crepitus. Treatment consists of closed reduction and immobilization with a sling or cast. Vertebral fractures are usually pathologic and are a result of osteoporosis. The fracture is usually a compression fracture of the vertebral body.

SPECIAL ENVIRONMENTS FOR CARE

Critical Care

The person who has sustained a fracture does not usually require critical care nursing management. Exceptions include a patient with fat embolism and the victim of multiple trauma. The patient with a fat embolus is at risk of developing pulmonary edema and acute respiratory distress syndrome (ARDS). Treatment includes oxygen therapy, mechanical ventilation, positive end-expiratory pressure, fluid replacement, and administration of steroids (their use is controversial). See Chapter 21 for a full discussion of ARDS.

Community-Based Care

The home should be assessed for environmental hazards, including scatter rugs, highly waxed floors, electrical cords, and other potential hazards. Safety equipment such as grab bars, nonskid mats in the bathroom and tub, secure handrails, an elevated toilet seat, an elevated chair with arms, and nightlights should be rented or installed in the home if possible.

A home health aide may be required for assistance with ADLs. Meals-on-Wheels is an excellent resource for those who are unable to purchase or prepare their own meals. If dressing changes or intravenous medications are to be continued at home, a home care agency must be consulted for nursing visits. The patient may be transferred to a rehabilitation facility before going home if extensive therapy is needed.

COMPLICATIONS OF FRACTURES

Complications can arise as a result of the initial trauma, treatment, or the resulting loss of mobility. Systemic complications usually are a result of immobility or surgical intervention (see Chapter 18) and include cardiovascular, respiratory, gastrointestinal, and urinary complications.

Complications of fractures affect the patient's recovery and functional outcome. Early recognition and treatment of complications is extremely important. In this section, fracture blisters, fat embolism syndrome, and compartment syndrome are discussed. DVT and pulmonary embolism are also complications of fracture and are discussed in Chapters 18, 21, and 25.

Impaired fracture healing may result in nonunion, malunion, or pseudoarthrosis. These complications are generally treated with revision of the reduction. Posttraumatic arthritis and refracture may also occur. Posttraumatic arthritis occurs mainly in weight-bearing joints; severe cases may require joint replacement surgery. Of persons with tibial fractures, 5% to 40% have complications, including osteomyelitis, nonunion, compartment syndrome, and delayed union.[13]

Infection, which is the leading cause of delayed union and nonunion, occurs primarily in open or compound fractures. Most symptoms of infection occur within 4 weeks of the injury. Pain is the primary symptom, followed by erythema and edema. Infections following open fractures commonly result in osteomyelitis (infection of the bone), which is discussed in Chapter 47.

Heterotopic bone formation occurs as a result of trauma in approximately 10% of cases and may cause pain and restricted joint motion. Evidence of heterotopic ossification is detectable by x-ray examination as early as 1 to 2 months after injury. Persons with head injuries are more prone to heterotopic bone formation. Treatment consists of surgical resection and, in some cases, low-dose radiation.

Two types of complex regional pain syndrome (CRPS) can occur as complications following a fracture. These pain syndromes are progressive and potentially disabling chronic conditions. Both are recognized by the International Association for the Study of Pain.[14] Although they typically occur in a distal extremity, symptoms are systemic. CRPS I, or reflex sympathetic dystrophy, occurs in 5% to 30% of persons with fractures or bone or soft tissue injury. This condition is characterized by pain, hyperalgesia, edema, sweating, weakness, flushing or pallor (thought to be a result of sympathetic nervous system dysfunction), and skin changes.[13] Anxiety may exacerbate the symptoms.

The precipitating event for CRPS II is injury to a nerve. CRPS II, or causalgia, has symptoms similar to those of CRPS I. Symptoms are progressive and include severe, burning pain; restricted joint motion; osteopenia; muscle atrophy; and joint fibrosis. Treatment goals are preservation of limb function and pain relief. Modalities include gabapentin and/or adjuvant medications, physical therapy, nerve blocks, electrical stimulation, and physical therapy.[14]

Fracture Blisters

Etiology/Epidemiology

Fracture blisters are skin bullae and blisters representing areas of epidermal necrosis with separation of the stratified squamous cell layer by edema fluid. They are associated with fractures, twisting types of injuries, and joint trauma. Fracture blisters may also develop as a result of compartment syndrome, as the body attempts to relieve rising tissue pressures. Other factors influence the development of blisters, including the interval between the occurrence of the fracture and immobilization. The presence of fracture blisters predisposes the patient to infection, delays in treatment, nonunion, impaired healing, and ultimately a longer hospital stay and increased costs. Wound complications can result in serious infection. Delaying surgery for up to 2 weeks until swelling has lessened may decrease the development of wound infection.[19] Early surgical reduction results in a lesser incidence of blistering.[19] The highest incidence of fracture blisters occurs in the ankle, elbow, distal tibia, and foot, which are anatomic areas with tight skin constraints and little muscle or surrounding fascia, both of which contribute favorably to the formation of fracture blisters.

Pathophysiology

After the acute injury, severe tissue edema and swelling develop as a result of damage to bone, ligaments, tendons, and surrounding soft tissues. The vasculature and lymphatic drainage are disrupted, which causes the epidermis to separate from the dermis. Detachment of the epidermis results in disruption of its blood supply, causing necrosis of the epidermal layers. The edema and venous stasis that occur after the injury cause collapse and thrombosis of the affected blood and lymph vessels, which increase circulatory problems. Blisters may result from the local tissue hypoxia. Deep tissue damage may result, necessitating later full-thickness skin grafting. The time period for reepithelialization is an estimated 4 to 21 days.

Collaborative Care Management

Preventive nursing measures include identifying persons at risk and early and frequent assessment of the skin. In addition to fractures associated with a greater incidence of blisters, other risk factors include the presence of diabetes, hypertension, peripheral vascular disease, smoking history, alcohol use, and lymphatic obstruction. Initial treatment measures that may decrease the development of blisters include early immobilization and elevation to limit edema formation, both of which help maintain normal blood and lymphatic circulation. If the patient develops a fracture blister, a dry dressing is recommended for protection. "Popping" the blister is not recommended, because the blister covering provides a biologic dressing.[19] A ruptured blister provides an excellent environment for infection; it is moist, provides nutrients (serum), lacks initial phagocytic activity, and has few coexisting microorganisms. If blister rupture occurs, a hydrocolloid dressing is helpful to maintain a moist wound environment. Despite treatment, a ruptured blister may result in a full-thickness loss. Intravenous antibiotics are recommended if the wound culture reveals *Staphylococcus aureus*. Anticoagulants such as low-dose heparin or warfarin are prescribed to prevent thrombus formation.

Patient/Family Education. Persons with high-risk fractures should be taught the etiology of blisters and treatment protocols. This is especially important for patients who are treated in the emergency department or urgent care center and discharged home. The patient and family should be taught the importance of proper wound care, signs and symptoms of infection, dressing techniques, and signs and symptoms of potential complications such as compartment syndrome. Other interventions include teaching the patient and family about the significance of fracture blisters, their effect on healing, and the rationale for delaying fracture fixation if blisters develop. They should be given the name and number of the appropriate person to contact if symptoms develop.

Fat Embolism Syndrome

Etiology/Epidemiology

Fat embolism syndrome (FES) is a potentially fatal complication associated with fractures, multiple crush injuries, total hip arthroplasty, and total knee arthroplasty. Fat embolism was first described in 1862 following an autopsy of a railroad worker who had suffered a crush injury.[10] Fat emboli may lead to ARDS, with an associated mortality rate of 50%, especially if the onset is more than 5 days after trauma.

FES is most common after fractures of the pelvis, femur, and tibia. Persons with total hip and knee arthroplasties are at risk for FES because of surgical reaming of the intramedullary canal to allow seating of the prosthesis and pressurizing of the medullary canal during sizing and cementing of the prosthesis, which may cause fat to enter the venous system. Cerebral microemboli have occurred during total hip arthroplasty, with both cemented and uncemented prostheses.[6,8,16] The incidence of FES after long bone fractures is reported to be 0.5% to 2.2% and increases with pelvic fractures and multiple trauma.[10] Increased serum glucose and beta-lipoprotein levels may increase the incidence of FES. FES usually occurs within 24 hours of injury in 46% of patients and within 72 hours of injury in 91% of patients.[10] The average time of onset of symptoms is 12 to 24 hours after injury. Morbidity, although difficult to determine, is estimated at 12% to 87%.[10]

Pathophysiology

On autopsy, fat globules have been found in the lungs of a number of patients with long bone fractures. After a fracture, fat globules and tissue thromboplastin are released from the bone marrow and local tissue into the circulation, increasing clotting and blood viscosity. The fat molecules enter the venous circulation, travel to the lungs, and embolize the small capillaries and arterioles. Lipase is produced to break down fat molecules into fatty acids. These chemical changes irritate pulmonary tissue and result in deterioration of lung surfactant, increased permeability of the alveolocapillary membrane, interstitial hemorrhage, edema, and atelectasis. Eventually, hypoxemia and ARDS may develop. Fatty acids attract red blood cells and platelets, forming an aggregate, which can lead to disseminated intravascular coagulation and emboli to the brain and other vital organs. Retinopathy as a result of FES has developed in almost 50% of patients.[10] Other serious complications include pneumonia, coma, kidney failure, and congestive heart failure.

Symptoms of FES include hypoxemia, tachypnea, tachycardia, petechiae, fever, lipuria, chest pain, and altered mental status. Alteration in mental status and changes in arterial blood gas readings (primarily hypoxemia) are early clinical indicators of FES. Approximately 75% of persons with FES develop significant neurologic symptoms, which may manifest as restlessness, confusion, lethargy, or coma. Petechiae, considered a "classic" symptom of FES, occur in only 50% to 60% of persons with FES. They usually occur 24 to 48 hours after the injury. They are usually found on the conjunctivae, axillae, chest, and neck and are thought to be caused by capillary occlusion with fat and fibrin. Other causative factors include capillary fragility and platelet defects. The rash does not blanch with pressure but usually disappears within 48 hours of onset. The presence of unexplained fever, especially when accompanied by a change in mental status and petechiae, should alert the caregiver to the possibility of FES. This is a medical emergency, and the physician should be notified immediately.

TABLE 46-3 Comparison of Fat Embolism and Pulmonary Embolism

Fat Embolism	Pulmonary Embolism
Pathophysiology	
Fat globules released from marrow following fracture(s) enter bloodstream and obstruct pulmonary circulation	Deep vein thrombus dislodges and obstructs pulmonary circulation
Onset of Symptoms	
Usually 1-4 days after injury	Usually 4-10 days after trauma or development of thrombophlebitis but can occur much later
Signs and Symptoms	
Altered mental status Dyspnea Tachypnea Tachycardia Petechial rash Fever Restlessness Agitation	Dyspnea Chest pain Apprehension Anxiety Cough Hemoptysis Tachypnea Tachycardia Fever
Risk Factors	
Hypovolemia Shock Delayed immobilization of fracture Multiple fractures	Venous stasis Immobility Obesity Trauma Major surgery History of heart disease Age >40 years History of deep vein thrombosis, pulmonary embolism

Collaborative Care Management

Diagnosis is confirmed by a decrease in arterial PO_2, an increase in systemic PCO_2, infiltrates on chest x-ray films, petechiae, and mental confusion in persons at risk. A drop in the hemoglobin level due to sequestration of red blood cells in fat and a platelet count of less than 150,000/ml is considered diagnostic of FES.[10] Thrombocytopenia occurs as a result of hemodilution, the clotting process, and platelet attraction to fat globules. The platelet count usually returns to normal within 1 week. Prothrombin and partial thromboplastin times increase. Pathologic examination of the lungs reveals fat globules diffusely distributed throughout the pulmonary vasculature.

Arterial blood gases are obtained to determine the amount of hypoxemia. Fat may be found in the blood and urine. However, lipuria is a normal finding after a fracture and therefore is not of clinical significance in the diagnosis of FES. Chest x-ray films detect changes related to a fat embolus in only one third of patients. If ARDS develops, chest films will show areas of consolidation. A lung scan (ventilation-perfusion [V/Q] scan) may be used to rule out a pulmonary embolus (Table 46-3).

The most important nursing interventions are the recognition of patients who are at risk for developing FES and careful monitoring for early detection of clinical indicators of FES. Careful handling of the fractured extremity, especially when turning and positioning the patient, decreases manipulation of the fracture site, thus decreasing the risk of fat emboli.

As stated earlier, medical management is the same as for a person with ARDS (see Chapter 21). Adequate hydration to prevent kidney failure and to flush out fatty acids is an important intervention. The use of corticosteroids has been effective in reducing morbidity but must be used cautiously because of side effects. Steroids are beneficial in reducing cerebral edema, restoring capillary permeability, and decreasing capillary leakage. Hemodynamic monitoring is usually indicated. Other treatments include packed red blood cells to restore volume and decrease hypoxemia and low-dose dopamine to increase cardiac output and renal perfusion. Preventive measures include early stabilization (within 24 hours of injury) of patients with long bone fractures. Patients who undergo early stabilization of fractures experience shorter hospital stays and less incidence of respiratory complications than those with late stabilization (more than 48 hours after injury) of fractures.

Early recognition of symptoms, including respiratory insufficiency, decreased oxygenation, mental status changes, unexplained drop in hemoglobin, thrombocytopenia, and the presence of fat in the urine or sputum, should alert the caregiver to the possibility of a fat embolus.

Patient/Family Education. The patient and family require much emotional support and information regarding treatment regimens. Because the onset of FES is abrupt, the patient and family may not be prepared to deal with the severity of the situation. Early teaching regarding the risk for developing complications and signs and symptoms may help prepare them if the situation occurs. Early recognition of discrete mental status changes is often best recognized by family or friends. If FES develops, education regarding the rationales for treatment and emotional support while the patient is in the critical care environment are essential. If complications develop, the patient and family will require long-term support.

Compartment Syndrome

Compartment syndrome is a complication of trauma in which increased pressure within a limited anatomic space compromises the circulation, viability, and function of the tissues within that space. Compartment syndrome was first recognized more than 100 years ago. In 1881 Volkmann described an upper extremity contracture that he attributed to trauma, swelling, and restrictive dressings. This phenomenon was later termed *compartment syndrome* (Figure 46-14). If unrecognized, compartment syndrome can lead to loss of function, deformity, and possibly amputation. Failure to recognize compartment syndrome is one of the most common causes of medical litigation in the United States.

Compartment syndrome can be either acute or chronic. Acute compartment syndrome is usually a complication of trauma. Chronic compartment syndrome commonly occurs in persons who are active in sports such as long-distance running, cycling, dancing, and cross-country skiing. Symptoms usually resolve with rest and rarely result in tissue damage. *Crush syndrome* (rhabdomyolysis) is also a form of compartment syndrome. Trauma from extensive soft tissue and muscle damage results in multisystemic effects. Protein breakdown from the damaged cells results in myoglobinuria, release of potassium from the cells, and an inflammatory reaction; third-space fluid loss, kidney failure, acidosis, and shock may ensue. The following sections pertain to acute compartment syndrome.

Etiology/Epidemiology

For compartment syndrome to occur, there must be a space-limiting sleeve surrounding the tissue and increased tissue pressure. The space-limiting sleeve can be a restrictive dressing, a splint, a cast, fascia, or epimysium. Increased pressure within the compartment results from anything that either increases the contents of the compartment or decreases its size. Compartments consist of muscles, nerves, and blood vessels surrounded by a nonelastic covering. The body contains 46 compartments, 38 of which are in the extremities. These compartments are the most vulnerable to the development of compartment syndrome. The most common sites are the four compartments of the lower leg (deep posterior, superficial posterior, lateral, and anterior) (Figure 46-15), the dorsal and volar compartments of the forearm, and the interosseous compartments of the hand. Persons with tibial shaft fractures are at increased risk for developing compartment syndrome. Older adults may have a lower risk of developing compartment syndrome, because of increased tolerance for higher tissue pressures as a result of relatively higher blood pressures; smaller muscle mass may also be a factor.[11]

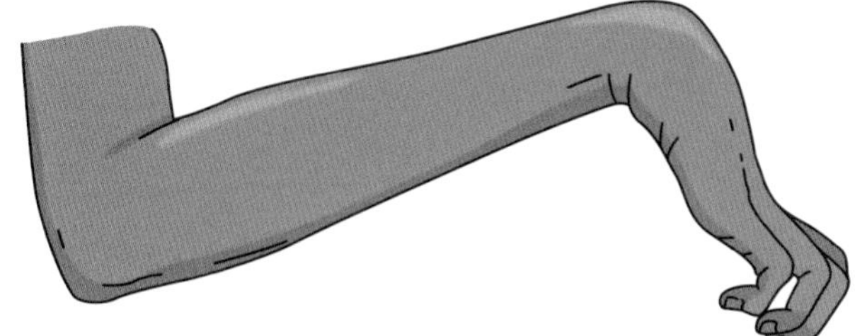

Figure 46-14 Volkmann's ischemic contracture.

Although compartment syndrome usually occurs as a result of trauma, there are several other causes (Box 46-3). Fracture blisters may be an early warning sign of increased intracompartmental pressure.[11] Shock can also increase the risk of compartment syndrome.

Pathophysiology

Following trauma, fluid accumulates in the compartment, and fascia cannot expand to accommodate the excess fluid, causing compartmental pressure to rise. Increases in tissue and venous pressures result in a decreased arteriovenous gradient. The end result is decreased blood supply and tissue hypoxia. In an attempt to correct the hypoxia, histamine is released, causing vasodilation and increased capillary permeability, which causes compartmental pressure to continue to rise. Rising pressures lead to tissue ischemia and eventually to necrosis. Peripheral muscle tissue undergoes ischemic changes within 6 hours of injury. Necrotic muscle cannot regenerate and is eventually replaced by dense, fibrous scar tissue. Peripheral neuropathy can develop within 24 hours, and contracture (ischemic paralysis) development begins within 4 to 12 hours of ischemia. If extensive ischemic muscle damage occurs, myoglobinuria may occur, leading to systemic complications that include kidney failure, metabolic acidosis, hyperkalemia, and sepsis. Normal tissue compartmental pressure is 0 to 10 mm Hg; pressure in excess of 20 mm Hg is abnormal. Sustained pressure readings of 30 to 40 mm Hg usually require prompt treatment with fasciotomy, but this varies with the individual patient.

Early recognition of symptoms and prompt treatment may preserve the function of the limb. Pain is the most common symptom of compartment syndrome. The patient may report

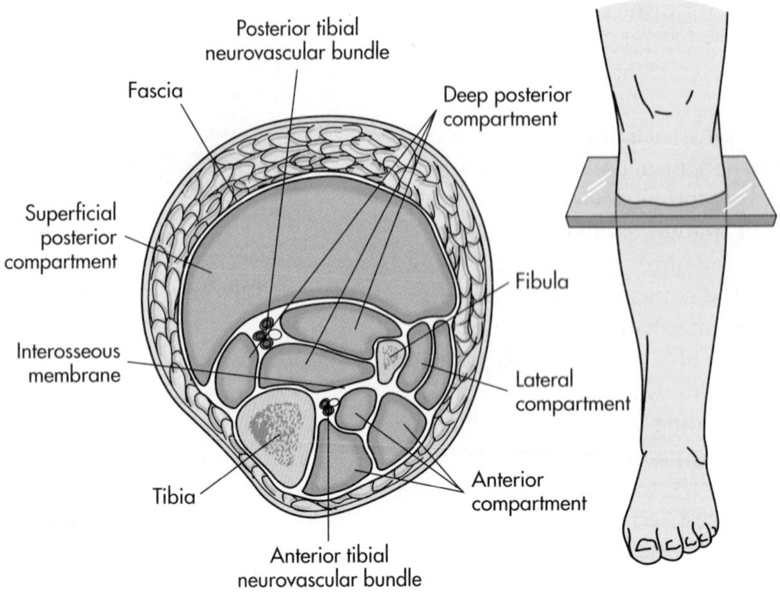

Figure 46-15 Compartments of lower leg.

BOX 46-3 Causes of Compartment Syndrome

Bleeding
Vascular injury
Coagulation defect (hemophilia, anticoagulant therapy)

Nephrotic Syndrome

Excessive Muscle Use
Exercise
Seizures
Tetany
Eclampsia

Trauma
Fractures
Crush injuries
Hypothermia, frostbite
Burns
Snake or spider bites

Infiltrated Infusions

Surgery

External Pressure
Positioning (lying on limb)
Surgical tourniquets
Military antishock trousers (MAST)
Circumferential restrictive dressings
Tight cast
Splints

Decreased Compartment Size
Excessive traction
Closure of fascial defects

severe, unrelenting pain, unrelieved by analgesia and increased by elevation of the extremity. The intensity of the pain is usually greater than that expected for the extent of the injury. As pressures increases, so does the intensity of the pain. Passive movement or stretching of the digits increases pain. It is important to note that epidural analgesia may mask the onset of compartment syndrome.

Motor and sensory function is also affected. Hypoesthesia, paresthesia, and muscular weakness or paralysis are common. It may be helpful to remember the six *P*'s: *p*ulselessness, *p*aresthesia, *p*ain, *p*ressure, *p*allor, and *p*aralysis. Skin color, temperature, capillary refill, and the quality of peripheral pulses are not reliable early clinical indicators for the presence of compartment syndrome. If pallor, coolness, slow capillary refill, and diminished or absent pulses are present, extensive and potentially irreversible damage has probably already occurred.

Laboratory data supporting the diagnosis of compartment syndrome include an elevated white blood cell count and erythrocyte sedimentation rate as a result of the inflammatory response; hyperkalemia due to cell damage; myoglobinuria; elevated creatine phosphokinase, lactate dehydrogenase, and aspartate aminotransferase levels, indicative of muscle damage; and a decreased serum pH. An elevated temperature may occur as a result of ischemia or infection.

Collaborative Care Management

Goals of treatment include (1) decreasing tissue pressure, (2) restoring blood flow, and (3) preserving function of the limb. Removal of external compression devices by splitting dressings or bivalving casts may alleviate early compartment syndrome. If conservative measures fail, surgical intervention

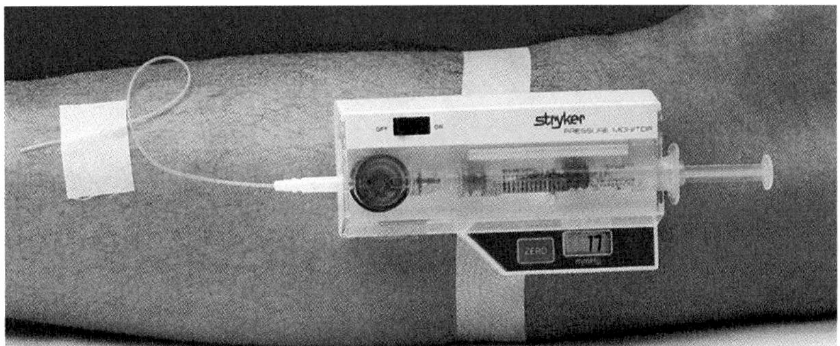

Figure 46-16 Compartmental pressure monitor.

may be indicated. Decompressive fasciotomy is performed along the complete length of the compartment to open the affected compartments, decrease the pressure, and restore normal perfusion. Epimysiotomy, in which the outermost sheath of connective tissue is removed from the skeletal muscle, also may be necessary. Necrotic tissue is debrided to prevent infection. Postoperatively the wound is covered with wet saline dressings, and the extremity is splinted in a position that avoids stretching of the tissues (functional position). Further debridement may be necessary until secondary closure is possible. If extensive damage or infection occurs, amputation of the affected limb may be necessary.

If contractures develop, splints and physical and occupational therapy may be indicated. In some cases additional surgery such as joint fusion, tenotomy, or tendon transfers may be performed.

As mentioned earlier, recognition of early signs and symptoms may lead to prompt diagnosis and treatment. In an unconscious patient or if sensory deficits are present, pain and changes in neurovascular status may be difficult to assess. Therefore if compartment syndrome is suspected, invasive measurement of compartmental pressures can be performed. A variety of systems are available either for one-time use or for continuous monitoring (Figure 46-16). Compartmental pressure readings should always be evaluated in relation to the clinical picture. The patient's blood pressure must be considered when evaluating compartmental pressures. To maintain compartmental perfusion, the diastolic pressure minus the compartmental pressure must be at least 30 mm Hg. Maintaining adequate compartmental perfusion may eliminate the necessity of surgical decompression.[10]

Segmental limb blood pressures and Doppler-derived ankle-brachial indices are sometimes used to evaluate compartment syndrome. Nerve conduction studies may be performed to evaluate nerve function. Venograms or arteriograms may be ordered to rule out DVT or vascular injury.

Nursing management of the patient with or at risk for developing compartment syndrome focuses on maintaining neurovascular integrity of the extremities. Careful monitoring of the neurovascular status of the extremities is crucial in the detection and prevention of compartment syndrome. Baseline and ongoing assessments are made on both extremities; it is important to compare the findings.

Knowledge of the innervation to the extremities is useful when assessing for deficits. Hourly assessments should be performed and recorded, noting any reports of increased pain, pain that occurs with passive stretching, and alterations in sensory or motor function. The patient with upper extremity involvement should be assessed for the ability to extend, flex, abduct, adduct, and oppose the fingers and thumbs and flex the wrist. If the lower extremities are involved, the ability to extend and flex the toes, perform plantar flexion and dorsiflexion, and invert and evert the foot should be assessed.

If compartment syndrome is suspected, the physician is notified and restrictive dressings are loosened. To reduce edema, the extremity should be elevated to, but not above, heart level because elevation above heart level compromises arterial flow.[10] If ice packs are being used, they are removed because the application of cold and elevation of the limb may further impair the circulation.

Dressings, splints, and casts are checked for excessive pressure, and compartmental pressures are monitored and recorded. Any significant changes are reported to the physician. Reports of pain are monitored, and the effectiveness of pain relief measures is assessed.

Patient/Family Education. Persons at risk should be taught to recognize the signs of compartmental pressure and to report them immediately. Clear instructions regarding pain management, treatment, and prognosis should be given to the patient and family. ROM exercises to other extremities are performed, and/or the patient is ambulated if possible. Isometric exercises are taught and encouraged. ROM exercises are continued throughout rehabilitation. The patient may need instructions about wound care, crutch use, and splint care. The family and patient should be knowledgeable about the symptoms of recurring compartment syndrome and infection. If extensive damage has occurred or amputation is necessary, rehabilitative care will be necessary. Return to normal activities is gradual and depends on the type of injury.

HIP FRACTURE

Etiology/Epidemiology

Hip fractures are a leading cause of morbidity and mortality in the elderly population. The incidence of hip fracture increases with age; an estimated one of every five women older than 80 years of age will suffer a hip fracture. Currently more than

250,000 hip fractures occur annually, and the associated health care costs are estimated at 7 to 10 billion dollars.[12] As a result of the aging population, the number of hip fractures worldwide will increase six times to 6.26 million fractures annually by 2050.[12,23] Repair of a hip fracture is probably the most common surgical procedure for persons older than 85 years of age.

Risk factors commonly associated with hip fractures include osteoporosis (see Chapter 47), advanced age, being female and Caucasian, decreased estrogen levels (because of postmenopausal changes or bilateral oophorectomy), prior hip fractures, Alzheimer's dementia, institutional residence, and sedentary lifestyle. Other risk factors include an inadequate dietary intake of calcium and vitamin D, excessive dietary protein, caffeine intake, smoking, alcohol use, and use of psychotropic drugs. Although the incidence of hip fracture is most commonly associated with women, the risk of hip fractures in elderly men has increased as well. African-Americans older than 45 years of age are less likely to experience hip fractures than Caucasians because of increased mineral content and increased bone mass.

The hospital stay of elderly patients with hip fractures is often complicated and prolonged and may result in chronic disability, transfer to an extended care facility, or death. The older the individual, the lower the chance of regaining prefracture functional status. Factors that negatively influence recovery and increase the risk of mortality following a hip fracture include being male, preexisting medical problems, cognitive impairment, and the development of postoperative complications.

Pathophysiology

A hip fracture is a fracture of the proximal femur and may be classified as follows (Figure 46-17):

1. Intracapsular (femoral neck): within the hip joint and capsule
   a. Subcapital
   b. Transcervical
   c. Basal neck
2. Extracapsular or intertrochanteric: outside the hip joint and capsule to an area 5 cm (2 inches) below the lesser trochanter
3. Subtrochanteric: below the lesser trochanter

The location of the fracture is an important consideration in predicting healing. Intracapsular fractures, especially displaced fractures, can disrupt the blood supply to the femoral head (Figure 46-18). They are associated with an increased incidence of nonunion and avascular necrosis of the femoral head. Intertrochanteric fractures occur in the well-nourished vascular metaphyseal region of the hip and do not generally interfere with the blood supply of the proximal femur. Complications associated with intertrochanteric fractures include malunion and shortening of the affected extremity. Intertrochanteric and femoral neck fractures account for approximately 90% of all hip fractures, and subtrochanteric fractures account for approximately 10%.

Signs and symptoms of a hip fracture are severe pain at the fracture site, inability to move the leg voluntarily, shortening and external rotation of the leg, and other signs and symptoms consistent with those of any fracture.

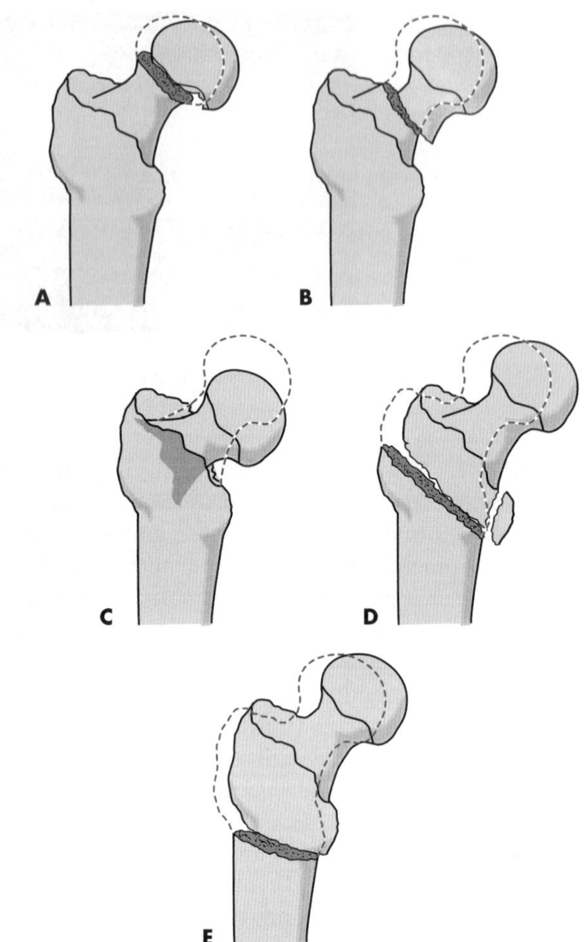

Figure 46-17 Fractures of the hip. **A**, Subcapital fracture. **B**, Transcervical fracture. **C**, Impacted basal neck fracture. **D**, Intertrochanteric fracture. **E**, Subtrochanteric fracture.

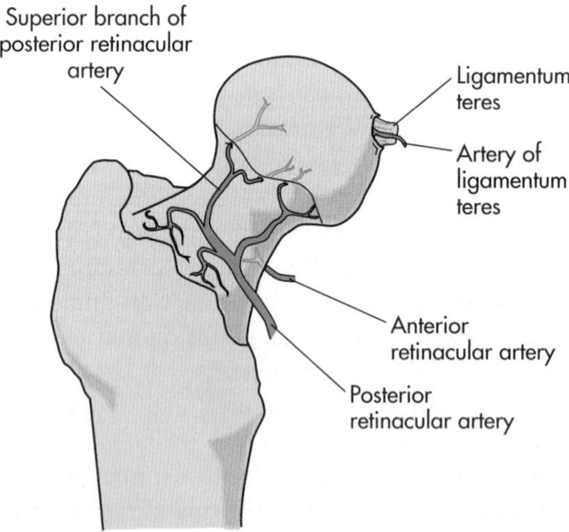

Figure 46-18 Posterior view of blood supply to head of femur.

Collaborative Care Management

Surgical intervention is the standard of care unless the patient's general medical condition precludes that option. Conservative management (Buck's traction) involves prolonged immobility with the associated complications, including DVT, pulmonary embolism, pneumonia, and skin breakdown. The goals of management are to return the patient to prefracture functional ability and to prevent any further disability.

Surgery involves reduction and stabilization of the fracture and insertion of an internal fixation device. The choice of fixation device depends on the location of the fracture, the potential for avascular necrosis of the femoral head, and the individual patient. An impacted intracapsular fracture without displacement may be treated only with bed rest. Other surgical options include a compression screw and plate, a fixed or sliding nail and plate, percutaneous pinning, and a prosthetic implant. A hemiarthroplasty (usually a bipolar prosthesis), which replaces only the femoral head, or a total hip arthroplasty (see Chapter 47) (replacement of both articular surfaces of the joint) is also an option. The amount of weight-bearing limitation (up to 2 months) and positioning restrictions vary with the type of implant used and the type of fixation. Cemented prostheses often allow immediate full weight bearing, which may make compliance easier for older adults, especially those with impaired cognition.

Improving the general medical condition of the elderly patient before surgery, which includes the stabilization of preexisting medical problems and the correction of fluid and electrolyte imbalances, increases the chances for functional recovery. Nursing interventions include those to prevent the most common postoperative complications, such as thromboembolism, pneumonia, alterations in skin integrity, and voiding dysfunction (see Chapter 18 and the Nursing Care Plan).

Nursing management includes those interventions already noted for general care of patients with fractures, with specific attention given to interventions for persons with internal fixation. Positioning and weight-bearing limitations after

Nursing Care Plan *Patient With an Intracapsular Hip Fracture*

DATA Mrs. W. is an 81-year-old widowed, Caucasian, retired secretary. She tripped and fell on an icy step when leaving her niece's home. She complained of immediate, severe pain in her left hip and was unable to move her leg. Emergency personnel were summoned, and Mrs. W. was taken to the emergency department of the local hospital. Initial assessment revealed that Mrs. W.'s left leg was shorter than her right and externally rotated. Her vital signs were stable, and the neurovascular status of the left leg was intact. An x-ray examination revealed an intracapsular femoral neck fracture. Intravenous fluids were initiated. An electrocardiogram, urinalysis, complete blood count, and serum electrolytes were obtained. Mrs. W. was transferred to the orthopedic unit with physician's orders for morphine sulfate via a patient-controlled analgesia (PCA) pump, bed rest, pneumatic compression devices bilaterally, and diet as tolerated. Five pounds of Buck's traction was applied to the left leg. Informed consent was obtained for surgical repair of the fracture. A hemiarthroplasty (prosthetic replacement of the femoral head and neck) is scheduled to take place the next morning.

The nursing history reveals that Mrs. W.:

- Lives alone in her own apartment in a senior citizen complex
- Has no children but does have nieces and nephews in the area who see her regularly and assist with shopping and other errands
- Would like to return to her own apartment after being discharged from the hospital but is worried that she may need help at home (Her family is considering hiring a home health aide.)
- Takes no medications other than aspirin for occasional "stiffness" on awakening
- Has never been hospitalized and last saw a physician 2 years ago for the flu

Collaborative nursing actions include monitoring:

- For pressure areas and wound healing
- Lung sounds for atelectasis/respiratory infection
- Urine output for retention or stasis
- Bowel status for constipation
- Fluid and electrolyte status for hydration and electrolyte balance
- For signs of deep vein thrombosis

NURSING DIAGNOSIS **Deficient knowledge related to lack of exposure to surgery and treatment protocols**
GOALS/OUTCOMES Will express decreased anxiety regarding impending surgery; will verbalize understanding of injury, impending surgery, and need for continued follow-up care; will participate in postoperative rehabilitation care and exercises

NOC Suggested Outcomes
- Knowledge: Disease Process (1803)
- Knowledge: Health Resources (1806)
- Knowledge: Infection Control (1807)
- Knowledge: Medications (1808)
- Knowledge: Prescribed Activity (1811)

NIC Suggested Interventions
- Teaching: Disease Process (5602)
- Teaching: Individual (5606)
- Teaching: Preoperative (5610)
- Teaching: Prescribed Activity/Exercise (5612)
- Teaching: Prescribed Medication (5616)

Nursing Interventions/Rationales
- Assess need for instruction and provide as needed. *Teaching needs vary among patients. Assessment helps individualize teaching to specific patient needs.*
- Provide written materials if available. *Patients often want to review material later or may not remember specifics.*

Continued

Nursing Care Plan — Patient With an Intracapsular Hip Fracture—cont'd

- Review perioperative care with patient and family before the surgery; provide examples of prostheses if available. *Understanding the surgical procedure and postoperative care lessens anxiety and promotes participation in postoperative routines.*
- Evaluate patient's understanding of information taught and reinforce learning as needed. *To determine the need for further teaching. Reinforcement of information previously taught improves retention.*
- Keep patient and family informed of the plan of care and rationales for treatment. *Encourages family support and participation in care routines while the patient is hospitalized and following discharge.*
- Perform neurovascular checks every 2 hours for the first 24 to 48 hours and notify physician of changes from preoperative status. *To detect signs of neurovascular compromise as quickly as possible so that correct interventions can be initiated.*
- Encourage performance of active dorsiflexion, plantar flexion, isometric quadriceps and gluteal exercises, and active range of motion of unaffected limbs every 12 hours until ambulatory. *Exercising promotes venous return, prevents thrombus formation, and helps maintain muscle tone.*
- Administer anticoagulants as prescribed and educate patient about their use and potential side effects. *Bleeding and thrombocytopenia are side effects of some anticoagulants.*
- Monitor coagulation studies. *To monitor drug effectiveness and to prevent excessive anticoagulation, since the patient takes aspirin, which can potentiate anticoagulation.*
- Provide information and rationales for discharge restrictions and activities. *Understanding the rationale for activities and restrictions may promote compliance and avoidance of complications.*
- Assess patient's ability to ambulate independently on level surface and stairs with appropriate ambulatory aid before discharge. *To determine patient's ability to ambulate and potential risk for falls.*
- Teach patient the importance of follow-up examinations. *To determine effectiveness of the treatment plan and detect problems for early intervention.*

Evaluation Parameters

1. Explains preoperative and general postoperative care
2. Reports decreased anxiety
3. Actively participates in plan of care
4. Performs prescribed exercises every 12 hours until ambulatory
5. Verbalizes understanding of prescribed home medications

NURSING DIAGNOSIS **Acute pain related to surgical procedure**
GOALS/OUTCOMES Will report decrease or absence of pain following use of pain relief measures

NOC Suggested Outcomes
- Pain Control (1605)
- Pain Level (2102)

NIC Suggested Interventions
- Pain Management (1400)
- Analgesic Administration (2210)

Nursing Interventions/Rationales

- Assess patient's pain before and after comfort interventions. *To determine the degree of postoperative pain and effectiveness of pain relief measures.*
- Apply ice to operative hip for 48 hours after surgery. *Ice reduces swelling, which contributes to pain.*
- Encourage use of PCA before pain becomes severe. *Milder pain is more readily controlled than severe pain.*
- Monitor use and effectiveness of PCA. *PCA avoids peaks and valleys associated with intermittent use of analgesics. It also allows the patient greater control over her pain and its elimination.*
- Encourage use of nonpharmacologic pain relief measures if acceptable to patient. *Relaxation, repositioning, and distraction are helpful for reducing and controlling pain. However, the patient must believe that they will be beneficial.*

Evaluation Parameters

1. Reports pain relief within 30 minutes of prescribed analgesics
2. Reports satisfaction with pain relief measures
3. Decreased use of pain medications before discharge

NURSING DIAGNOSIS **Impaired physical mobility related to pain secondary to surgical repair and placement of prosthesis**

GOALS/OUTCOMES Will regain mobility within prescribed limitations by discharge

NOC Suggested Outcomes
- Pain Control (1605)
- Pain Level (2102)

NIC Suggested Interventions
- Pain Management (1400)
- Analgesic Administration (2210)

Nursing Interventions/Rationales
- Maintain prescribed limits of motion and weight bearing. *Positioning restrictions are designed to prevent dislocation of the prosthesis.*
- Turn patient from back to nonoperated side every 2 hours and as needed. Avoid positioning patient on operative side and observe flexion restrictions when elevating the head of the bed. *Frequent turning and repositioning promotes circulation, respiratory effort, and muscle activity. Maintaining prescribed positioning restrictions prevents dislocation of the prosthesis.*
- When turning patient, hold opposite leg in abduction and use pillows to maintain 30-degree abduction. *Prevents adduction of the leg and dislocation of the prosthesis.*
- Help patient to walk using appropriate ambulatory aid. Begin walking on the second postoperative day and increase the frequency and distance of ambulation as tolerated. *Hastens recovery and prevents postoperative complications related to immobility.*
- Encourage sitting when patient demonstrates sufficient control of affected leg to sit within flexion restrictions. *Prepares patient for discharge while ensuring that patient functions safely within prescribed flexion limits.*
- Elevated sitting surface with pillows to keep angle of hip within prescribed limits. *To prevent hip flexion beyond 90 degrees.*
- Reinforce use of assistive devices provided by physical or occupational therapy. *Assistive devices aid with mobility while helping to prevent injuries.*
- Teach patient/family that for the first 2 to 3 months hip flexion is limited to <90 degrees, adduction beyond midline and extreme internal or external rotation are prohibited, and partial weight bearing with the aid of a walker is maintained. *To aid with healing and prevent dislocation of the prosthesis.*

Evaluation Parameters
1. Uses assistive devices correctly to aid with mobility
2. Remains free of complications of immobility
3. Performs prescribed exercises
4. Maintains prescribed limitations

NURSING DIAGNOSIS **Risk for impaired home maintenance related to age and prolonged recovery**

GOALS/OUTCOMES Patient and family will express satisfaction with arrangements made for rehabilitation facility or self-care management at home

NOC Suggested Outcomes
- Compliance Behavior (1601)
- Participation: Health Care Decisions (1606)

NIC Suggested Interventions
- Discharge Planning (7370)
- Home Maintenance Assistance (7180)
- Family Support (7140)
- Mutual Goal Setting (4410)

Nursing Interventions/Rationales
- Assess patient's/family's perception of problems that may occur with management of self-care at home. *To identify actual or perceived needs and obstacles to the patient's caring for herself at home.*
- Determine the type of equipment needed (e.g., crutches, walker, elevated toilet seat) and obtain any needed equipment. *To facilitate the patient's/family's ability to successfully care for the patient at home.*
- Assess the home environment for needed changes (e.g., stairs, proximity of bathroom to bedroom). *To facilitate the patient's recovery at home and the patient's/family's ability to provide that care.*
- Encourage patient to participate in decisions about rehabilitation and self-care at home. *Involving the patient in decision making increases the likelihood of compliance with the prescribed treatment/rehabilitation plan.*

Evaluation Parameters
1. Verbalizes understanding of prescribed medications
2. Accurately describes bleeding precautions and side effects of anticoagulant therapy
3. Correctly self-administers prescribed medications
4. Verbalizes need for keeping follow-up appointments

hemiarthroplasty or total arthroplasty generally require the patient to:

- Avoid hip flexion beyond 60 degrees for up to 10 days.
- Avoid hip flexion beyond 90 degrees from day 10 to 2 months.
- Avoid adduction of the affected leg beyond midline for 2 months.
- Maintain partial weight-bearing status for approximately 2 months (varies with the type of prosthesis and method of implantation [cement versus bony ingrowth]).

The patient must be carefully instructed on the limits of motion to be observed, and nursing care must be provided within these constraints. Generally, positioning the patient on the operative side is avoided, although this can vary, depending on the surgeon's preference. The patient is helped to maintain hip abduction using an A-shaped abduction pillow or bed pillows as shown in Figures 46-19 and 46-20. Maintaining hip abduction requires that the patient's position during transferring be carefully monitored. A chair with armrests and a firm, nonreclining seat should be provided; the sitting surface is elevated as necessary with pillows or foam cushions to keep the angle of the hip within the prescribed limits when the patient is sitting. In general, patients who have had any kind of internal fixation for a fractured hip should avoid elevation of the operative leg when sitting in a chair because this puts excessive strain on the fixation device.

Patient/Family Education. Most patients are discharged to a rehabilitation facility. The patient and family should be reminded that complete recovery might take as long as 6 months. Recovery is generally measured by the patient's ability to regain prefracture functional status. The patient and family need reassurance that the process of healing and recovery is gradual. Discharge instructions include medication instruction, positioning and weight-bearing restrictions, ambulation techniques with assistive devices, signs and symptoms of complications, and prevention of further injury.

Adaptive equipment for the home includes an elevated toilet seat, grab bars for the bath, long-handled reachers, and an elevated chair with armrests. Many patients are prescribed anticoagulants for as long as 3 months postoperatively. DVT may occur in as many as 70% of patients after a hip fracture. The patient and family should be familiar with medication administration (the patient may be prescribed subcutaneous injections of low-molecular-weight heparin), side effects, and the potential for periodic laboratory assessment of coagulation times.

Instructions regarding the prevention of falls (see Research box), which is a major cause of hip fractures, should also be given. Because osteoporosis is a significant contributing factor to hip fractures, primary prevention should focus on the education of persons at risk for osteoporosis (see Chapter 47). Adequate dietary intake of calcium decreases bone loss and helps prevent fractures. Weight-bearing exercise is required to

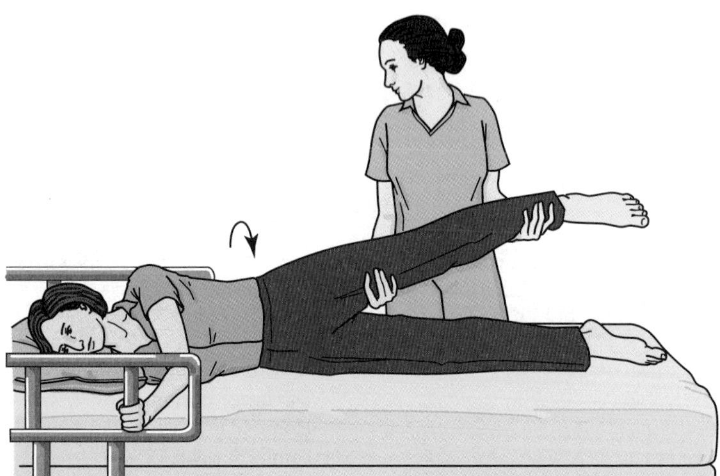

Figure 46-19 Assisting patient with turning while maintaining abduction of the hip. The leg is supported at the thigh and just above the ankle to avoid putting undue stress on the hip. An abduction pillow may also be used.

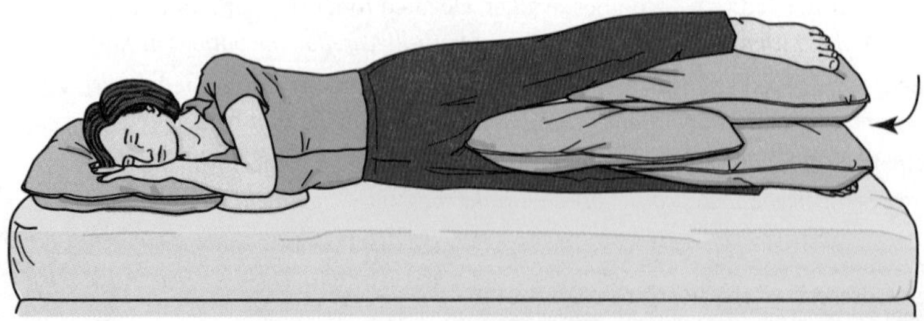

Figure 46-20 Pillows are staggered in a wedge-shaped arrangement to maintain abduction of the hip.

maintain bone mass; studies indicate that regular exercise decreases the risk of hip fractures by 50%.[12] Thirty minutes of exercise daily is recommended. Exercise has the added benefit of reducing the risk of falling in older adults (see Complementary & Alternative Therapies box).

Secondary prevention includes early detection of the disease process and methods to decrease the severity of the disorder. Much emphasis has been placed on women as a high-risk group for hip fractures, but because of the rising incidence of fractures in older men, education also needs to be directed toward this previously overlooked group.

FRACTURE OF THE SPINE

Etiology/Epidemiology

Spinal or vertebral fractures occur as a result of falls, motor vehicle or diving accidents, or blows to the head or body by heavy objects. With increasing frequency, fractures of the spine are also occurring as a result of osteoporosis (see Chapter 47) and metastatic lesions of the spine. A spinal fracture can occur at any age.

Pathophysiology

A vertebral fracture may occur with or without displacement. Displaced fracture fragments may place pressure on spinal nerves or injure the spinal cord itself. Such pressure results in partial or complete dysfunction of the body parts innervated by nerves at the level of injury. Depending on the extent of injury to the nervous system, dysfunction may be permanent or temporary.

A fracture can occur at any level of the spine, from the occiput through the sacrum. Signs and symptoms of a vertebral fracture include pain at the site of injury, partial or complete loss of mobility or sensation below the level of injury, and evidence of a fracture or fracture dislocation on routine x-ray examination, myelography, a computed tomography scan, or a magnetic resonance imaging (MRI) scan.

Collaborative Care Management

Long-term goals of treatment are stabilization and reduction of the fracture and decompression (i.e., removal of pressure from spinal nerves or the spinal cord). Immediate management objectives are (1) immobilization of the patient with a backboard and cervical collar and (2) immediate transport to a hospital.

Objectives of surgical management are:

- Decompression of nerve structures through laminectomy (see Chapter 47) or appropriate reduction of the fracture and removal of fracture fragments
- Reduction of the fracture through operative procedures or, in some cases, traction (e.g., cervical traction through application of tongs to the skull)
- Stabilization of the fracture with bone grafting or internal fixation devices such as pedicle screws and plates or rods
- Maintenance of stabilization with external fixation devices such as casts, corsets, or braces as necessary

Nondisplaced compression fractures without neurologic compromise may be treated with bed rest until the patient's pain subsides. The patient is then gradually mobilized, sometimes with stabilization by a corset or brace.

Many of the nursing interventions required by the patient with a spinal fracture are identical to those outlined for the patient with spinal cord injury in Chapter 44. Of special concern are interventions designed to (1) maintain the stability of the fracture fixation; (2) prevent neurovascular problems; and (3) promote psychologic comfort. To maintain stability of the fracture fixation, the head of the bed should not be elevated beyond the prescribed level, which is usually only 30 degrees. In the absence of an elevation order, the bed is maintained in a flat position. When the patient is in a side-lying position, pillows are placed between the patient's legs and behind the back to prevent back strain. Changes of position are best accomplished with the use of special beds that rotate 45 degrees from side to side, because the literature indicates that when the spine is unstable, logrolling and the use of turning frames are contraindicated

Research

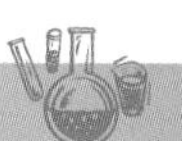

Reference: Kannus P et al: External hip protectors for the elderly, *N Engl J Med* 343(21):1506-1513, 2000.

Falls are a common cause of hip fractures. The mechanism of injury is usually a sideways fall, with the force of impact directly on the greater trochanter. This study, conducted in Finland, evaluated the effectiveness of an external hip protector in reducing the severity of falls among elderly persons.

The sample consisted of 1801 community-dwelling elders. All were at risk for hip fractures as a result of a previous fall or fracture; impaired vision; poor balance; or alterations in cognition, mobility, or nutrition. The hip protector device was an undergarment made of stretch fabric with padded protectors to redirect the force of impact from the fall to the soft tissues anterior, posterior, and superior to the proximal femur. Results were statistically significant. In the experimental group 1404 falls occurred, 74% while the garment was worn; researchers noted an 80% reduction in fracture risk from falls. The control group experienced 67 fractures, the experimental group 13 (4 with the garment). Further research is needed to evaluate the effectiveness of this garment.

Complementary & Alternative Therapies

T'ai Chi May Reduce the Risk of Falling in Older Adults

Falls are a major cause of hip fracture in the elderly. T'ai chi, an ancient Chinese exercise form, may be an effective intervention to reduce the risk of falls in this population. This review of 31 controlled experimental studies and clinical trials examined the physiologic responses and effects on general health and fitness of t'ai chi on 2216 elderly men and women. T'ai chi is considered moderate exercise and does not demand more than 55% of maximum oxygen intake. Data analysis revealed that T'ai chi has positive effects on cardiorespiratory, immune, and musculoskeletal functioning. In addition to reducing the incidence of falls in the elderly, T'ai chi improved the flexibility, balance, posture, and mental control of the study participants.

Source: Li JX, Hong Y, Chan KM: Tai chi: Physiological characteristics and beneficial effects on health, *Br J Sports Med* 35(3):148-156, 2001.

because they can stress the fracture site. When logrolling is done, strict attention must be paid to avoid twisting the spine and placing stress at the fracture site. If a corset or brace is ordered, it should be applied before getting the patient out of bed.

To prevent neurovascular problems, neurovascular checks are done every hour for the first 24 to 48 hours postoperatively. Any decrease in neuromotor function must be reported to the physician, because this may indicate displacement or pressure at the fracture site. Passive ROM to involved extremities is performed at least three times daily to maintain joint motion, and the patient is encouraged to perform active ROM to noninvolved extremities hourly to maintain joint motion and promote circulation.

Promotion of psychologic comfort begins with recognizing that the patient may have feelings of powerlessness, anger, or fear about the situation, particularly if there is sensorimotor deficit. The patient must be encouraged to express his or her feelings, and the services of a counselor should be offered if indicated. The patient also is prepared for long-term care in a rehabilitative facility if needed.

Other nursing interventions are similar to those for any patient who has a fracture, including interventions for individuals in casts or traction, which are discussed earlier in this chapter.

Patient/Family Education. The patient should be taught proper body mechanics and lifting techniques to avoid strain on the spine. If permissible, exercises may be prescribed to strengthen back and abdominal muscles. If a brace or corset is to be worn, instructions are needed regarding skin care and care of the brace. If the fracture was a result of trauma, teaching should focus on prevention of further injury. Persons with a spinal fracture should be extremely cautious when engaging in contact sports.

TRAUMA TO SOFT TISSUE STRUCTURES

TRAUMA TO LIGAMENTS AND TENDONS

Etiology/Epidemiology

Trauma to ligaments and tendons is usually seen in connection with injury to a joint caused by a blow, twisting, or severe stretching. The most common site of ligament damage is the knee, often resulting from a sports injury, because of the anatomy, location, and complex motions of the joint. The Achilles tendon is susceptible to partial or complete tears, usually caused by a sports injury. Shoulder and ankle injuries are common, particularly sports injuries. Ankle sprains are the most common injury seen in emergency departments.[21] Sports-related injuries account for 500,000 visits to health care providers annually.[21] Many of these injuries are to the musculoskeletal system (Table 46-4).

This section contains a general discussion of ligamentous and tendon injuries. A more detailed discussion of anterior cruciate ligament trauma and rotator cuff trauma follows.

Pathophysiology

The most common ligamentous or tendon injuries are partial or complete tears. Injury to the knee may include damage to the medial, lateral, and posterior ligaments and to the anterior and posterior cruciate ligaments (see Clinical Manifestations box). Injuries may be classified as mild, moderate, or severe:

- Mild (class I) injuries: stretching of ligament without obvious tear
- Moderate (class II) injuries: several ligament fibers torn with a partial loss of function; partial tear
- Severe (class III) injuries: severe or complete disruption of the ligament with resulting instability

Signs and symptoms of class I injuries are mild pain and swelling. Class II injuries are associated with moderate pain and swelling, and persons with class III injuries typically report severe pain, swelling, joint instability, and disability or loss of function.

Collaborative Care Management

Immediate first-aid measures for soft tissue injuries of the musculoskeletal system can be easily remembered by the mnemonic RICE (rest, ice, compression, elevation):

- Rest of the injured part
- Ice for at least 48 to 72 hours to decrease bleeding and edema
- Compression with elastic bandages, splints, or casts (Be sure to monitor for signs of compartment syndrome.)
- Elevation of the extremity to slightly above the level of the heart to increase venous return and decrease edema

Diagnosis is based on evaluation of the patient history and physical examination, including specialized tests to detect ligamentous instability. It is especially important to elicit a complete history of the specific mechanism of injury, which aids in differential diagnosis. X-ray films are used to rule out a fracture. Arthrography and arthroscopy may be performed to visualize the extent of the injury.

Treatment. Treatment varies with the extent of injury. For mild injuries, rest and a compression dressing are used. Moderate injuries are also treated with rest but may require aspiration of excess fluid. A compression dressing is used to control swelling and further effusion, and support is provided with a splint or a brace. Strengthening exercises are needed.

In cases of severe injury, surgical repair to prevent disability and instability, via arthroscope, open, or arthroscopically aided procedures, is needed. A modified compression dressing is applied to prevent effusion, and the joint is immobilized for a prescribed time. Joint remobilization may include a continuous passive motion machine and physical therapy for strengthening exercises. The use of crutches is necessary for lower extremity injuries.

Medications used for pain relief depend on the severity of discomfort. Choices include opioids and nonopioids. Skeletal muscle relaxants may be used to relieve pain and spasm. Relaxation of hypertonic muscles promotes healing and decreases pain.[2]

TABLE 46-4 Common Soft Tissue Injuries

Mechanism of Injury	Symptoms	Treatment
Meniscal		
Medial and lateral tears usually occur with rotary or extension/flexion injuries of knee	Joint pain Swelling "Locking"	Splint, bracing, or cast Surgical treatment by meniscectomy via arthroscopy or arthrotomy
Anterior Cruciate Ligament (ACL)		
Valgus stress applied to knee while in hyperextension and external rotation Associated with deceleration and changes in direction	Audible "pop" or "snap" Pain Joint effusion Hemarthrosis Joint deformity Joint instability "Giving way" of knee Positive Anterior Drawer test	Treatment depends on age and lifestyle of patient Conservative treatment: quadriceps and hamstring strengthening, bracing, and avoidance of high-risk activities Surgical reconstruction of ACL, either open or arthroscopically aided, using autologous or synthetic graft followed by extensive rehabilitation program
Rotator Cuff		
Strain or tear of rotator cuff muscles or tendons of shoulder (supraspinatus, infraspinatus, teres minor, subscapularis) Usually results from falling on an outstretched hand, throwing objects (baseball pitchers), or chronic or excessive use	Severe pain with loss of ability to flex and abduct shoulder Positive drop arm test	Rest, sling and swath for immobilization, physical therapy, NSAIDs Surgical repair for complete rupture, disability, or chronic pain; followed by physical therapy
Ankle Sprain		
Approximately 75% of all ankle injuries are sprains; 25% of injuries occur in running and jumping sports Higher incidence in sports—basketball, soccer; also can occur while walking on uneven surfaces; lateral ligaments more susceptible to injury Usually injury results from an inversion and plantar flexion force on ankle (95% as a result of inversion) Position of foot, type of sport, directional changes, joint laxity, and magnitude of force affect severity of injury	Swelling Tenderness Reluctance to bear full weight, perform full range of motion Deformities Ecchymoses	Rest, ice, elastic compression, elevation for grades I, II sprains Grade II sprains—immobilization by cast or bracing, gradual resumption of activity Aggressive treatment may include primary surgical repair or ankle stabilization procedure

NSAIDs, Nonsteroidal antiinflammatory drugs.

Postoperative nursing interventions for the patient with a ligamentous or tendon tear include the same considerations as for the partially immobilized patient after fracture reduction and application of an external fixation device.

Patient/Family Education. Patient teaching is particularly important. If surgery was performed, general perioperative instructions are given. Instructions include information regarding the correct use and application of the immobilization device (brace, cast, splint), activity or weight-bearing restrictions, medication use, symptoms of complications, and the plan for follow-up care.

Methods to prevent future injury are stressed. Patients need to understand that repetitive injuries may result in

Clinical Manifestations

Knee Trauma

- Tenderness
- Swelling, effusion (usually within 2 to 4 hours of injury)
- Pain
- Hematoma
- Disability; "knee gives way"
- Abnormal motion at joint
- Audible pop

posttraumatic degenerative arthritis and that safety equipment, proper footwear, and warm-up and cool-down exercises should be a part of any sports activity.

TRAUMA TO THE ANTERIOR CRUCIATE LIGAMENT

Etiology/Epidemiology

Trauma to the anterior cruciate ligament (ACL) is the most common ligamentous injury to the knee; more than 100,000 injuries are diagnosed annually.[1,21] It is also the knee injury most often treated surgically. Ninety percent of all injuries occur in the middle third of the ligament. The highest incidence is in persons 15 to 25 years of age who participate in pivoting sports; the incidence is also higher in women than in men.[9] As mentioned earlier, the anatomy and function of the knee make it vulnerable to injury because of the stresses of motion and load bearing on the joint. Injury usually occurs in instances when the knee is hyperextended and the femur is externally rotated on a fixed tibia. Injuries commonly occur during soccer, football, skiing, and basketball, with the affected leg firmly planted on the ground. The patient usually sustains a twisting type of injury and typically reports a "pop" as the injury occurs.

Pathophysiology

The ACL provides support to the knee joint. It is paired with the posterior cruciate ligament to stabilize the knee joint. The ligament originates from the posterior medial aspect of the lateral femoral condyle and crosses (origin of the name *cruciate*) the knee joint obliquely. The insertion is on the anteromedial aspect of the tibial plateau. The ACL functions primarily to prevent anterior displacement of the tibia, hyperextension, and excessive internal rotation of the knee. Lesser functions include decreasing varus and valgus stresses to the knee while in flexion.

The patient usually reports the knee "giving way" and severe swelling and pain. Effusion usually occurs 2 to 4 hours after the injury. Ruptured blood vessels are the cause of hemarthrosis, which is particularly indicative of ACL injury. Examination of the patient is often difficult because of the pain.

Chronic injury occurs as a result of a missed diagnosis, failure to seek treatment, or unsuccessful conservative treatment of an acute injury. The knee becomes increasingly unstable anteriorly and "gives way" more frequently. Muscle weakness and decreased activity are common.

Collaborative Care Management

Diagnosis is made on the basis of the history and physical examination. The drawer test and Lachman's test are both done to determine the degree of anterior displacement of the tibia and the amount of laxity of the knee (see Chapter 45). The pivot shift maneuver also detects anterolateral stability of the knee. It is important to evaluate both knees for comparison. Radiographs and MRI scans are performed to confirm the diagnosis. Although x-ray films are not useful in diagnosing ACL tears, they are essential to rule out a fracture or avulsion of the ACL from its insertion site.

The patient's age, activity level, type of job and leisure activities, and general medical condition are factors to be considered before determining the type of treatment. If meniscal damage is also present, surgical treatment is highly recommended because the resultant degenerative arthritis is difficult to treat. Options are physical therapy and rehabilitation or surgical intervention and rehabilitation. The goals of treatment are to prevent further damage to the knee (traumatic arthritis and meniscal tears) and allow the patient to return to his or her former level of functioning.

Conservative management usually consists of nonsteroidal antiinflammatory drugs (NSAIDs); application of ice and heat; electrical stimulation; rest and immobilization for a few days, followed by physical therapy to restore muscle strength; ROM; and weight bearing as quickly as possible. A brace and activity modification to avoid further injury are recommended. If the patient is not willing to modify activity, surgical repair should be considered.

The goal of surgical reconstruction is elimination of anterior subluxation of the tibia. Surgical options include repair with or without augmentation of the ligament and reconstruction using various types of grafts. The procedure is often performed with the aid of arthroscopy, limiting the need to open the joint surgically. A popular reconstructive technique involves the use of a patellar tendon graft with a bone block at both ends; the graft is passed through to the original origin and insertion sites of the ligament. Hamstring tendons and the Achilles tendon may be substituted. Both autograft and allograft can be used for the patellar tendon, although autograft is preferable.

Controversy surrounds the ideal time between injury and surgical repair. Patients undergoing reconstruction of a chronic ACL tear may actually attain more joint ROM than those who have had acute injuries repaired. Early reconstruction is indicated for high-performance athletes and those persons who wish to remain active in vigorous sports.

The surgical procedure is generally performed on an outpatient basis. The degree of pain control is usually the main determinant of the hospital length of stay. Newer techniques are aimed at minimizing the amount of postoperative pain control and facilitating early discharge. Intraarticular injection of bupivacaine in the operating room provides pain relief for up to 4 hours. Intraarticular morphine also shows promise as an effective method of reducing postoperative knee pain for as long as 3 to 6 hours after injection. Cryotherapy, or the use of cooling pads, is another method of controlling pain, as well as swelling, which contributes to pain.

Postoperative complications include nausea, infection, DVT, pulmonary embolism, graft failure, and recurrent laxity.[1] Depending on protocol, the patient may be seen in the office the next day for a dressing change and evaluation of the knee for hemarthrosis. Approximately 10% of patients require joint aspiration for hemarthrosis.[1]

Patient/Family Education. If surgical repair is performed, patient education focuses on postoperative activity restrictions, exercises, weight-bearing limits, brace instruction, crutch walking, and recognition of signs and symptoms of complications.

The goals of rehabilitation are to protect the graft, restore ROM, promote early weight bearing, and return to preinjury activity levels. The amount of permissible weight bearing depends on the surgeon's protocols. Generally, touching down or weight bearing as tolerated is prescribed after surgery. Physical therapy sessions usually begin 1 to 4 weeks after surgery. The rehabilitation process can take as long as 1 year. Ankle pumps, quadriceps and hamstring isometrics, and straight leg raises are taught before discharge. The patient is cautioned against overdoing exercising too early in the rehabilitation process. The graft often takes up to 12 months to revascularize and up to 24 months to attain preinjury strength.[1] The patient and family are instructed to call the physician if the patient experiences fever, chills, increased swelling, increased wound drainage, or pain unrelieved by analgesics. The patient and family are also instructed regarding the appropriate use of prescription pain medication.

OVERUSE AND TRAUMATIC INJURIES OF THE SHOULDER

Etiology/Epidemiology

The shoulder is the third most commonly injured joint, after the knee and ankle. Injury commonly occurs during athletic activities. Sports injuries are associated with direct trauma and overuse (as with throwing motions), which causes overloading of the shoulder's supporting structures. Overhead arm motion can stress the soft tissues surrounding the glenohumeral joint, causing injury over a period of time. The large head of the humerus and the comparatively shallow glenoid fossa allow the shoulder to be the most mobile joint in the body. Because of the mobility of the shoulder joint, there are fewer structural restraints to prevent potentially damaging movements. Chronic overuse is insidious in onset and usually results in impingement syndrome. Acute trauma may result in a partial or complete tear of the rotator cuff, dislocation, subluxation, separation, or fracture. Acromioclavicular separation is one of the most common shoulder injuries. Injuries to the rotator cuff usually occur as a result of chronic impingement in persons over the age of 40.

Pathophysiology

The rotator cuff is composed of subscapularis, supraspinatus, infraspinatus, and teres minor muscles and tendons. The rotator cuff functions to stabilize the humeral head in the glenoid while the arm is raised. Primary movements of these muscles are abduction, external rotation, joint stabilization, and to a lesser extent, internal rotation. The term *impingement syndrome* refers to the impingement of the rotator cuff by the acromion, coracoacromial ligament, and acromioclavicular joint. The syndrome occurs as the arm is abducted past 90 degrees and the greater tuberosity of the humerus impinges the rotator cuff against the acromion. The impingement causes microtrauma to the cuff, edema, hemorrhage, and cuff shortening. A poor blood supply to the tendons results in decreased potential for healing. Fibrosis, tendinitis, bony changes, a rotator cuff tear, or a biceps tendon rupture may progressively result. Symptoms of impingement are limited movement, increased pain on external rotation and abduction, weakness on manual muscle testing, muscle atrophy, and point tenderness over the insertion of the rotator cuff. Differentiating the pain occurring from impingement from the pain that occurs as a result of a rotator cuff tear is difficult.

Collaborative Care Management

Treatment is based on the following principles: decrease the inflammatory response by administering an NSAID or applying ice, alleviate pain, immobilize the joint or provide limitation of motion, and rehabilitate the patient to achieve maximal functional outcome. Rehabilitation begins with isometrics, passive ROM progressing to active ROM, and exercises to promote strengthening of the rotator cuff and the surrounding muscles. Subacromial cortisone injections, activity modifications to avoid repetitive overhead motions, heat, and electrical stimulation are also prescribed to decrease inflammation and promote healing. The use of cortisone injections should be limited because repeated injections into the cuff may weaken the cuff and predispose the tissues to tearing.

Surgical intervention is indicated if conservative methods fail to improve functioning within 6 months to 1 year. Extremely active persons or athletes may opt for immediate surgical treatment, without a trial of conservative therapy. Most procedures can be performed arthroscopically. Arthroscopic procedures offer the advantage of less discomfort, less chance of infection, and quicker return to overhead activities, usually within 6 to 8 weeks. Laser surgery can also be used for rotator cuff repair and relief of impingement. Rehabilitative exercises are prescribed after surgery, in the same progression as described earlier (Figure 46-21).

Patient/Family Education. Surgical repair of shoulder injuries is performed on an outpatient basis or requires a short hospitalization. Discharge instructions focus on wound care, hygiene methods, medication instruction, signs of infection, and activity restrictions. The patient should be familiar with the proper application of any immobilization devices (slings, splints) and how to inspect the skin for signs of irritation. Passive ROM techniques should be taught in addition to prescribed exercises. A physical therapist provides the initial instruction, which is then reinforced by the nurse. The amount of active ROM and shoulder movement permitted varies, depending on the type of injury and treatment. The patient and family should understand the signs of potential complications, such as decreased sensation in the affected arm, increased pain, unusual swelling, increased drainage from the wound (if applicable), and coolness of the extremity.

CUMULATIVE TRAUMA DISORDERS

Cumulative trauma disorder (CTD) and *repetitive strain injury* are relatively new terms for a group of upper extremity soft tissue musculoskeletal disorders. However, written reports of use-related complaints date back centuries. Less commonly used terms are *work-related upper extremity disorder* and *occupational overuse syndrome.* As these names imply, these disorders are caused by cumulative trauma and overuse of the neck and upper extremities in the workplace. The widespread use

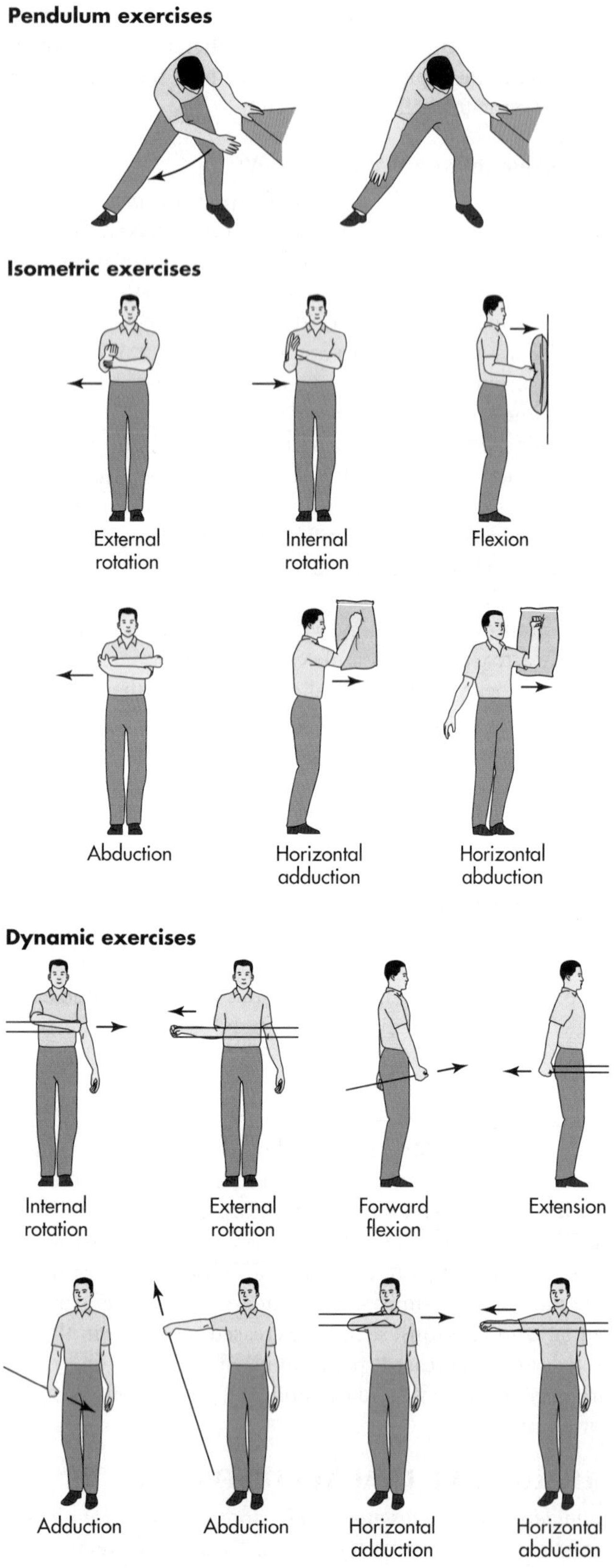

Pendulum exercises

Isometric exercises

External rotation

Internal rotation

Flexion

Abduction

Horizontal adduction

Horizontal abduction

Dynamic exercises

Internal rotation

External rotation

Forward flexion

Extension

Adduction

Abduction

Horizontal adduction

Horizontal abduction

Figure 46-21 Rehabilitative exercises of the shoulder.

of computers in the home and workplace for both recreational and occupational purposes has been cited as a significant factor in the development of CTD.

The impact of CTD on society is significant. CTD claims are more costly than the average traumatic injury claim and are the basis of a large number of lawsuits filed against employers by data processors, telephone operators, and keyboard operators. More time is lost from work because of CTD than because of any other musculoskeletal disorder, including lower back pain. The National Institute for Occupational Safety and Health (NIOSH) has named occupational musculoskeletal disorders, including CTD, as one of the top 10 priority work-related conditions.[7] The goal of NIOSH is to promote a better understanding of the incidence, presentation, prevention, treatment, and rehabilitation of these common disorders. The Occupational Safety and Health Administration has proposed ergonomic standards to address work-related disorders. Adoption of such standards would require employers to make efforts to reduce workplace exposure to CTD. Healthy People 2010 has also addressed repetitive motion disorders (see Healthy People 2010 box).

CTD can occur in any muscle group that is used repeatedly for long, uninterrupted periods with the body in a relatively fixed posture. Women are affected twice as often as men. Most sources cite repetitive motion as the predominant risk factor for the development of a CTD. Other risk factors include obesity; excessive, forceful movements; poor tool design; ergonomic factors in the workplace; vibration exposure; extremes of flexion or extension; and static positioning. The most common CTDs include carpal tunnel syndrome, medial and lateral epicondylitis, thoracic outlet syndrome, and de Quervain's tenosynovitis (Table 46-5). Symptoms are primarily those of entrapment neuropathies, including pain and paresthesias.

Carpal Tunnel Syndrome

Etiology

Carpal tunnel syndrome (CTS), which was first described in 1854, is caused by pressure exerted on the median nerve of the wrist. The condition occurs most commonly in women 30

Healthy People 2010

Objective Related to Repetitive Motion Disorders

Objective 20-3: Reduce the rate of injury and illness cases involving days away from work due to overexertion or repetitive motion.

Target: 338 injuries per 100,000 full-time workers

Baseline: 675 injuries per 10,000 full-time workers due to overexertion or repetitive motion were reported in 1997.

Target setting method: 50% improvement

Data source: Annual Survey of Occupational Injuries and Illnesses

From US Department of Health and Human Services: *Healthy People 2010: understanding and improving health,* Washington, DC, 2000, USDHHS.

to 50 years of age and usually affects the dominant hand. Many conditions can cause an increase in pressure in the carpal tunnel, thereby producing symptoms of median nerve compression. Symptoms are usually consistent, regardless of etiology. CTS is considered a CTD because the etiology is often repetitive hand or wrist motions. CTS is closely related to computer use. It should be stressed that as with all other CTDs, the etiology is not always repetitive motion.

Epidemiology

Inflammatory processes such as rheumatoid arthritis, flexor tenosynovitis, and gout can cause thickening of the flexor synovium, which leads to elevated pressure in the carpal tunnel. Patients receiving long-term hemodialysis for chronic kidney failure may be at risk for developing CTS because of synovial edema and amyloid deposits.

Previous trauma may contribute to the development of CTS. Burns, fractures, and dislocations of the wrist can constrict the tunnel by the formation of contractures, scarring, or bony deformities.

Repetitive motion of the wrist may also contribute to the development of CTS. Work-related CTS is a CTD caused by job-related tasks that involve certain motions or actions:

- Forceful grasping or pinching of objects (e.g., tools)
- Awkward positions
- Direct pressure over the carpal tunnel
- Repetitive motions
- Use of vibrating handheld tools

Other conditions that contribute to the development of CTS include diabetes; myxedema; pregnancy; abnormalities of the median artery and flexor muscles, ganglions, and lipomas. Alcoholism has also been associated with the development of CTS. Certain occupations put workers (typists, computer operators, assembly line workers, and truck drivers) at risk for developing the syndrome.

Pathophysiology

The median nerve passes through a tunnel bounded by the carpal bones on the dorsal surface and by the transverse carpal ligament on the volar surface (Figure 46-22). Through this "tunnel" pass nine flexor tendons and the median nerve. The median nerve provides sensation to the radial aspect of the palm and volar surfaces of the thumb, index finger, middle finger, and radial half of the ring finger. The median nerve also innervates the muscles of the anterior forearm and thenar muscles of the thumb and supplies sensation to the skin of the thumb, index finger, middle finger, and half of the ring finger. Any narrowing within this canal leads to compression of the medial nerve and CTS.

Initially pressure on the median nerve causes temporary blockage of the myelinated nerve fibers, which results in numbness of and pressure on the hand and fingers. Continued pressure

TABLE 46-5 Common Types of Cumulative Trauma Disorders

Disorder	Manifestations	Etiology	Treatment
de Quervain's tenosynovitis	Pain with thumb and wrist movement; pain radiating to forearm; aching over dorsal thumb surface; swelling; decreased pinch-grip strength	Inflammation of abductor pollicis longus and extensor pollicis brevis tendons in first dorsal compartment of wrist, at base of thumb; first described in 1895 as "washerwoman's strain" from wringing clothes; workers at risk include operating room personnel, housekeepers, musicians, and butchers (repetitive pinching and forearm rotation)	Wrist and thumb spica splint, gentle active range-of-motion exercises, joint protection, and ergonomically designed workplace and tools; surgical treatment (release of first dorsal compartment) only if conservative measures fail
Thoracic outlet syndrome	Pain; paresthesias; swelling; temperature changes; weakness of the forearm, shoulder, arm	Compression of brachial plexus, subclavian artery, and subclavian vein; mechanical compression; posture of head, neck, shoulders; cervical rib; overhead activities	Physical therapy; patient education about posture, workstation dynamics, ergonomics, physical activity; surgical resection if compression is due to cervical rib
Lateral epicondylitis (tennis elbow)	Microscopic tears in extensor carpi radialis brevis tendon, which originates at lateral epicondyle of elbow; repetitive activities	Pain over lateral epicondyle and extensor muscle mass; increased pain with elbow extension and forceful grip; persons at risk include construction workers, assembly line workers, tennis players (only 5% of identified cases), swimmers, golfers, and carpenters (hammering)	Reduce elbow extension; splinting; cold compresses followed by stretching; electrical stimulation, heat, and ultrasound; patient education about avoidance of aggravating movements or postures, tool or handle modification; surgical intervention to lengthen and repair tendon if conservative measures fail

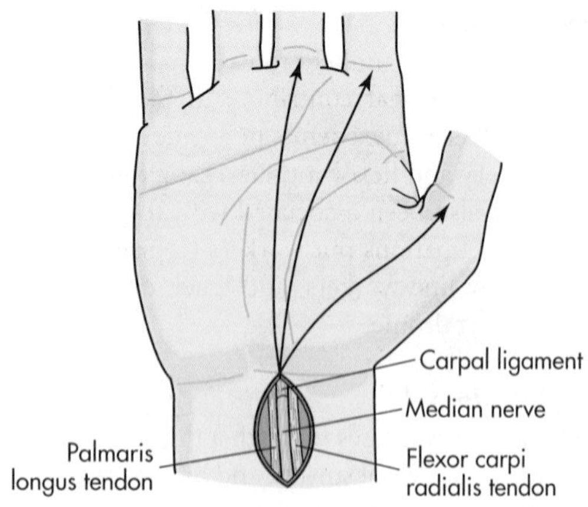

Figure 46-22 Carpal tunnel syndrome. Volar aspect of wrist retracted to demonstrate position of median nerve. Distribution of median nerve is to thumb and first two fingers.

causes ischemia, resulting in axonal death, muscular atrophy, and pain. The severity of symptoms varies. Mild manifestations include intermittent paresthesias, tingling, and pain in the median nerve distribution. The pain may awaken the patient at night; symptoms persist and increase if the condition is not treated. More severe cases of CTS include symptoms of hypoesthesia, awkwardness, and loss of dexterity and pinch strength. The patient may complain of dropping things or changes in handwriting. Symptoms may be worse at night, perhaps as a result of sleeping with the wrists in a flexed position. Complaints usually increase when there has been forced flexion of the wrist for long periods, as with knitting or typing. The patient may describe the hand as "swollen" and may complain of clumsiness. Pain referred to the upper extremity and base of the neck is common. Long-standing CTS may manifest with pronounced thenar atrophy (the padded area of the palm below the base of the thumb), chronic pain, and major functional impairment secondary to axonal death. The prognosis at this stage is poor, regardless of treatment.

Collaborative Care Management

Diagnosis is based on the patient history, physical examination, and evaluation of diagnostic tests. Other conditions with similar symptoms must be eliminated, including cervical radiculopathy, brachial plexopathy, de Quervain's tenosynovitis, arthritis, and thoracic outlet syndrome. Symptoms can be reproduced by tapping the median nerve at the wrist (positive Tinel's sign). Phalen's test is also used to diagnose CTS. The examiner holds the wrists in acute flexion for 60 seconds; if symptoms are reproduced or increased, the test is considered positive. Direct compression of the median nerve at the wrist for 30 seconds will also reproduce or increase symptoms in the presence of CTS. Nerve conduction studies and electromyography are also used to evaluate nerve function and muscle abnormalities.

Medical management of the patient with CTS begins with rest and splinting to maintain the wrist in a neutral position. Splinting is most effective if begun within 3 months of the onset of symptoms. NSAIDs are used for pain relief. Short-term use of diuretics may be prescribed to reduce fluid volume in the carpal tunnel, and oral vitamin B_6 may be prescribed because pyridoxine deficiency has been noted in some persons with CTS. If inflammation is prominent, local steroid injections may be given. Surgical decompression of the median nerve is done if conservative treatment fails or in the presence of long-standing symptoms. This surgery involves open or endoscopic release and decompression. Endoscopic release is associated with decreased postoperative pain, reduced scarring, and decreased recovery time. This approach is contraindicated in patients with rheumatoid arthritis and flexor synovitis.

Nursing care of patients having a surgical decompression procedure includes teaching regarding rest and splinting of the wrist, as well as general preoperative instructions (see Chapter 16). An occupational history should be obtained and referrals made for job counseling/retraining if occupational factors such as wrist flexing and repetitive tasks contributed to development of the condition.

Postoperative care focuses on promotion of circulation, comfort, and the prevention of complications. The affected hand and arm are elevated for 24 hours, and ice is used to reduce swelling and pain. The fingers are checked for circulation, sensation, and movement every 1 to 2 hours for 24 hours. Active thumb and finger motion is encouraged within the limits imposed by the dressing. Analgesics are administered as prescribed, and their effectiveness is assessed.

Discharge instructions include directions for recognizing and reporting symptoms of neurovascular compromise and directions for care of the splint, which usually is maintained for 2 to 3 weeks after surgery. The patient is also scheduled for follow-up wound assessment and a dressing change in the physician's office within 1 week. The need for this follow-up care and for lifestyle modification if repetitive motions (workplace or leisure) contributed to the disease process is explained. Referral to physical therapy for ROM and strengthening exercises is initiated.

Patient/Family Education. Because of the increasing incidence of cumulative trauma–related injuries in the workplace, it is important for nurses to recognize persons at risk and to teach preventive measures. As a result of the number of lawsuits against employers filed by employees, many businesses have initiated programs to decrease the development of CTD. These programs include redesign of the workplace with the focus on ergonomics, stress reduction techniques, and classes to teach proper mechanics and body awareness and reduce computer stress. Nurses are in an ideal position to promote wellness and reduce the risks associated with the development of CTS and other CTDs.

Depending on the work environment and type of job the patient has, it may be possible to reorganize the work structure to avoid long periods of repetitive motions. The patient should be taught to organize the day in an efficient but diverse schedule. The patient should be instructed to take frequent short breaks and to get out of the office chair and move around, exercising the neck, shoulders, and upper extremities. Simple ROM exercises can be performed at the desk if moving around is not an option. The work space should be redesigned to reduce fatigue and stress while increasing efficiency.

Instructions regarding body mechanics during computer use are beneficial to both the patient and the family. The position of the computer and the person's posture while working are important factors in reducing CTS risk. The patient should be taught to sit erect and lean slightly forward while using the keyboard. The arms should be elevated with the wrists straight to reduce pressure on the nerves, tendons, and muscles of the arms and hands. The forearms and palms should be angled toward each other while typing to reduce fatigue.[13] The keyboard height should be modified to avoid placing the wrists into hyperextension, which stretches the muscles and ligaments. Foam pads on which to rest the wrists while typing are available commercially. When keystroking, the patient should understand that rapid, prolonged movements of the fingers can cause pain. Patients who use the keyboard frequently should be instructed to avoid long fingernails, which cause awkward positioning of the fingers and wrists during keystroking. In addition, general health teaching should be done, including education regarding the benefits of a healthy diet and regular exercise.

TRAUMA TO JOINTS AND JOINT STRUCTURES

Injuries to joints and joint structures may occur as a sprain (tearing of the capsule or ligaments surrounding a joint, including disruption of the synovial membrane), meniscal tear, joint dislocation, or joint subluxation.

Trauma to ligaments and tendons and principles of patient management are discussed earlier in the chapter. Joint dislocation is discussed in this section. The shoulder is susceptible to traumatic dislocation. Closed reduction, followed by rehabilitative exercises, is the first choice of treatment. Chronic instability may necessitate surgical stabilization.

TRAUMATIC HIP DISLOCATION

Etiology/Epidemiology

Traumatic hip dislocation usually occurs as a result of a motor vehicle accident, especially if a frontal impact is sustained. This type of force can drive the victim's knees into the dashboard, forcibly dislocating the hip. Traumatic dislocation of the hip is considered an orthopedic emergency because of the risk of avascular necrosis of the femoral head. Prompt treatment is critical; reduction within 6 hours of injury decreases the risk of persistent pain, decreased ROM, and avascular necrosis. Traumatic dislocations occur most commonly in persons under 50 years of age unless an underlying disease is present, such as a neuromuscular disease or rheumatoid arthritis.

Pathophysiology

As the hip is forcibly dislocated, the blood supply to the femoral head can be disrupted (see Figure 46-18). Damage to the sciatic nerve is also possible and can result in partial to complete motor and sensory loss in the affected extremity (see Clinical Manifestations box). Sciatic nerve injury is present in 10% to 20% of persons with a posterior dislocation. Another potential problem is fracture of the femoral head, acetabulum, or pelvis. The articular surface of the femoral head may be eroded by bone fragments. Most dislocations of the femoral head occur posteriorly with the thigh in flexion. The femoral head cannot be completely displaced from the acetabulum unless the ligamentum teres is torn or ruptured. Anterior dislocations occur with the hip in extension and external rotation. The femoral head may be palpable anteriorly below the inguinal area. Complications of dislocation include avascular necrosis, infection, malunion, posttraumatic arthritis, and sciatic nerve injury. Avascular necrosis may occur as late as 2 years after the injury. Residual neuropathy occurs in approximately 20% of persons in whom sciatic nerve damage has been sustained.

Clinical Manifestations

Traumatic Hip Dislocation

- Pain
- Deformity
- Decreased range of motion
- Decreased sensation
- Diminished or absent pulses
- Anterior dislocation: hip in extension and external rotation; palpable femoral head
- Posterior dislocation: hip in flexion and internal rotation; shortening; may be a visible leg length discrepancy when compared with unaffected leg

Collaborative Care Management

Diagnosis is made on the basis of the history, physical examination, and evidence of dislocation on x-ray films. If possible, the hip is reduced immediately. The patient is given intravenous sedation, and the physician uses manual traction to relocate the hip (closed reduction). If closed reduction is not feasible, or in the presence of an acetabular or pelvic fracture, skeletal traction may be used to reduce the hip until surgery is possible. If there is no fracture, open reduction is accomplished by opening the hip capsule and relocating the head. For pelvic and acetabular fractures, internal fixation devices are usually used; a pelvic external fixator may also be used. If avascular necrosis results, prosthetic replacement of the hip is required.

Nursing management of the patient with a traumatic hip dislocation is the same as that for the patient with a hip fracture. The major emphasis is on keeping the limb in alignment by proper positioning. In addition, some patients have a brace applied either in surgery (if an orthotist is available) or the next day.

Patient/Family Education. The patient is taught active and passive exercises. Teaching also includes prevention of further injury and the use of assistive devices. The use of crutches or a walker is usually required until the patient has progressed to full weight bearing, generally in 4 to 6 weeks.

MULTIPLE TRAUMA

Etiology/Epidemiology

The leading cause of death in the United States for persons under the age of 45 is trauma. Causes of trauma include falls, crush injuries, vehicular (including airplane) accidents, and gunshot wounds. The nature of the injuries sustained in trauma is often extensive, involving multiple organ systems and multiple sites of injury. Approximately 50% of trauma deaths occur at the scene of injury, before medical help can arrive. Death usually results from brainstem trauma, spinal cord injury, hemorrhage, or major organ injuries. The second peak of trauma deaths occurs within 2 hours of injury, as a result of hemorrhage or head, chest, or abdominal injuries. Death during the third peak occurs within days to weeks of the initial injury, usually because of sepsis or multisystem failure.

More than 60 million persons survive following major trauma.[17] Survival rates are related to care at the accident scene, quick methods of transport to hospitals, and advances in the field of emergency medicine and nursing. Regional trauma centers allow transfer of patients to facilities equipped to manage complex care needs of the victim of polytrauma. Personnel in any hospital may be confronted with a multiply injured patient and should be prepared to treat the patient. Often the patient is stabilized and then airlifted to a trauma center.

The most common orthopedic injuries that occur as a result of multiple trauma are pelvic fractures and crush injuries. Approximately 30% of persons with multiple injuries sustain a pelvic fracture. Fractures of the pelvis usually occur as a result of motor vehicle accidents, falls, and crush injuries. Depending on the type of fracture and coexisting injuries, closed pelvic fractures have an associated mortality rate of 8% to 15%, and open pelvic fractures have an associated mortality rate of 30% to 50%.[17] Hemorrhage is usually the cause of death. Shearing forces from the impact of trauma cause rupture of blood vessels surrounding the pelvic ring, causing hemorrhage and hypotension. Damage to internal organs, especially urogenital injuries, can occur from shearing forces, bone fragments, and compression. The retroperitoneal space can accommodate up to 4 L of blood before tamponade results. Coagulopathy is a significant problem because of loss of clotting factors and because of continued bleeding at the fracture site. Pelvic fractures are classified by the mechanism of injury and degree of instability.

Crush injuries (see discussion under Compartment syndrome) may result from falls, motor vehicle accidents, and blunt trauma, such as being trapped under heavy fallen objects. Multiple fractures and internal bleeding may result, with hemorrhage being the usual cause of death. Crush syndrome was first described during World War II. Crush syndrome follows crush injury and is characterized by muscle necrosis, hypovolemia, compartment syndrome, rhabdomyolysis, fluid and electrolyte imbalance, coagulopathy, and kidney failure. The development of kidney failure increases the mortality rate. Fluid and electrolyte imbalances commonly seen in crush syndrome include hypocalcemia, hyperphosphatemia, hyperkalemia, edema, and third spacing.

Collaborative Care Management

Treatment of victims of multiple trauma is based on the ABCs of *a*irway management with cervical spine control, *b*reathing, and *c*irculation (see Chapters 7 and 8). The pelvis and abdomen must be evaluated for fractures and hemorrhage (Box 46-4). Rib fractures and spinal fractures may cause life-threatening neurologic and cardiovascular injuries.

Obvious fractures are immobilized and splinted, and sterile dressings are applied to open fractures until surgical reduction is feasible. The goals of management are to correct or stabilize any life-threatening problems (e.g., obstructed airway, pneumothorax, bleeding) and then to reestablish the continuity of injured tissues. Musculoskeletal injury may require reduction of fractures and repair of related soft tissue injuries. Because life-threatening problems must be addressed first, musculoskeletal injuries are usually not repaired until the patient has been stabilized. However, sites of fractures or potential fractures must be splinted or otherwise protected until reduction can be effected.

The principles of nursing management are:

1. Before reduction, all actual or potential sites of fractures must be protected by maintaining splints, traction, or positioning precautions; manipulation of fracture frag-

BOX 46-4 Pelvic Fractures

Signs and Symptoms

Pain with compression of iliac crests
Asymmetry of iliac crests
Abnormal rotation of femurs
Leg length discrepancy
Lacerations of perineum, vagina, or rectum
Hematuria
Neurologic deficits
Hypotension

Diagnostic Tests

X-ray study
Computed tomography scan*
Peritoneal lavage to determine presence of intraabdominal bleeding*
Arteriogram: intravenous pyelogram may be done (if patient is stable) to determine extent of internal injury

Management

Pelvic sling
Skeletal traction
Spica cast
Open reduction and internal fixation
External fixators are the treatment of choice

Associated Injuries

Vascular
Genitourinary
Abdominal
Intestinal and rectal

*Controversial.

ments must be avoided; and the patient must be monitored for hemorrhage and other complications.
2. After reduction, all of the previously discussed principles of nursing management of the patient with a fracture must be observed.

The challenge for the nurse is to devise a plan of care that takes into account the demands of the variety of fixation techniques, fracture sites, and mobilization or immobilization requirements for that patient. The psychosocial needs and the rehabilitation requirements for individuals who have sustained multiple injuries are often long term and extensive. Consideration of rehabilitation requirements must occur early in the patient's hospital course and be reviewed frequently (see Chapter 5).

Patient/Family Education. Nurses can play a role in the prevention of multiple trauma by promoting safety awareness among all persons, especially those at risk. Promoting safety in the work environment may prevent industrial or on-the-job accidents. Public awareness of the dangers of driving while intoxicated and the importance of wearing seat belts may help decrease the number of motor vehicle accidents and the injuries sustained in them.

Persons who have sustained multiple injuries may have residual deficits and require an extensive rehabilitative process. Teaching focuses on adaptive techniques and measures to prevent further disability.

Critical Thinking Questions

1. Compare the nursing care for a patient undergoing an open reduction of a fracture with that for a person undergoing a closed reduction. What would you include in discharge instructions for each patient?
2. Discuss nursing interventions and rationales for the care of a patient following open reduction of a midshaft femoral fracture. What are potential complications? Discuss the essential assessment parameters used by the nurse to detect systemic complications of a bone fracture.
3. Develop a health promotion plan for a group of office workers to prevent the development of a repetitive motion disorder.
4. Describe nursing interventions for a 24-year-old man who suffered a pelvic and femoral fracture in a motor vehicle accident. What are potential complications of his injury? What preventive nursing measures are indicated?
5. What information would be included in the home-going instructions for a person who has undergone an anterior cruciate ligament reconstruction in an ambulatory surgery center?

References

1. Bach BR, Boonos CL: Anterior cruciate ligament reconstruction, *AORN J* 74(2):152-164, 2001.
2. Barnett R et al: A patient oriented approach to the management of musculoskeletal injury, *Ther Bull Suppl Clin News* 6(2):1-8, 2002.
3. Barry ME: Ankle sprains, *Am J Nurs* 101(10):40-42, 2001.
4. Burggraf V, Barry RJ: Healthy people 2010: protecting the health of older individuals, *J Gerontol Nurs* 12:16-22, 2000.
5. Doheny MO, Deucher MJ: Healthy people 2010: implications for orthopaedic nurses, *Orthop Nurs* 20(4):59-65, 2001.
6. Edmonds CR et al: Intraoperative cerebral arterial embolization during total hip arthroplasty, *Anesthesiology* 93(2):315-318, 2000.
7. Eliff B: Work injuries: circumstances for orthopaedic case management, *Orthop Nurs* 17(2 suppl):20-30, 1998.
8. Gelinas JJ, Cherry R, MacDonald SJ: Fat embolism syndrome after cementless total hip arthroplasty, *J Arthroplasty* 15(6):809-813, 2000.
9. Griffin LY et al: Noncontact anterior cruciate ligament injuries: risk factors and prevention strategies, *J Acad Orthop Surg* 8(3):141-150, 2000.
10. Hager CA, Brncick N: Fat embolism syndrome: a complication of orthopedic trauma, *Orthop Nurs* 17(2):41-46, 1998.
11. Harvey C: Compartment syndrome: when it is least expected, *Orthop Nurs* 20(3):15-25, 2001.
12. Lappe JM: Prevention of hip fractures: a nursing imperative, *Orthop Nurs* 17(3):15-26, 1998.
13. Maher AB, Salmond SW, Pellino TA: *Orthopaedic nursing,* ed 3, St Louis, 2002, Mosby.
14. McCaffery M, Pasero C: *Pain: clinical manual,* ed 2, St Louis, 1999, Mosby.
15. Morrison C: A practical approach to stress fractures, *Orthop Nurs* 19(6):23-34, 2000.
16. Ott MC et al: Cerebral embolization presenting as delayed, severe obtundation in the postanesthesia care unit after total hip arthroplasty, *Mayo Clin Proc* 75(11):1209-1213, 2000.
17. Parsons LC, Krau SD, Ward KS: Orthopedic trauma: managing secondary medical problems, *Crit Care Clin North Am* 13(3):433-442, 2001.
18. Skinner HB: *Current diagnosis and treatment in orthopedics,* ed 2, Norwalk, Conn, 2000, Appleton & Lange.
19. Thordarson DB: Complications after treatment of tibial pilon fractures: prevention and management, *J Am Acad Orthop Surg* 8(4):253-265, 2000.
20. Unger J, Selfridge-Thomas J: Common sports injuries. Part 1: Ankle injuries. In *Nursing contact hours for nurse practitioners,* Atlanta, 2001, American Health Consultants, pp 45-50.
21. Unger J, Selfridge-Thomas J: Common sports injuries. Part 2: Knee and shoulder injuries. In *Nursing contact hours for nurse practitioners,* Atlanta, 2001, American Health Consultants, pp 51-60.
22. Verdonschot N et al: Time dependent mechanical properties of HA/TCP particles in relation to morsellized bone grafts for use in impaction grafting, *J Biomed Mater Res* 58(5):599-604, 2001.
23. Yarnold BD: Hip fracture: caring for a fragile population, *Am J Nurs* 99(2):36-41, 1999.

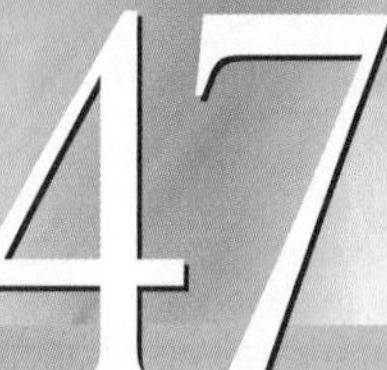

47 Degenerative Disorders

Jane F. Marek

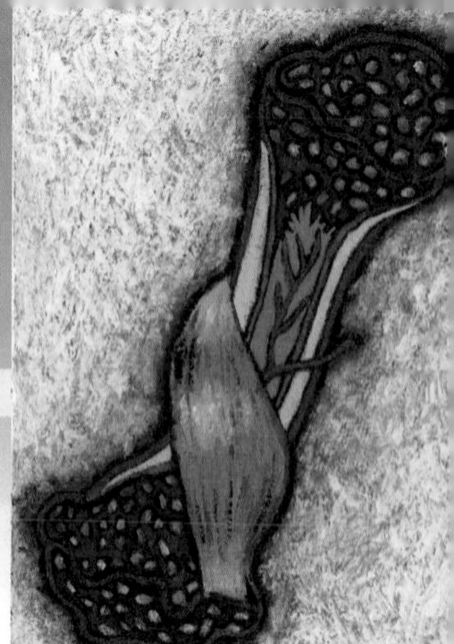

Objectives

After studying this chapter, the learner should be able to:

1. Differentiate the etiology/epidemiology, pathophysiology, and clinical manifestations of rheumatoid arthritis and osteoarthritis.
2. Compare the collaborative care management of rheumatoid arthritis and degenerative joint disease.
3. Correlate the pathophysiology with the collaborative care management for persons with inflammatory and degenerative disorders affecting the joints.
4. Develop a plan of care for a person undergoing joint replacement surgery.
5. Compare the pathophysiology and collaborative care management of the different types of degenerative and inflammatory processes affecting bones.
6. Discuss the incidence, pathophysiology, and clinical manifestations of osteoporosis.
7. Describe the collaborative care management of persons with osteoporosis.
8. Develop a teaching plan for persons at risk for osteoporosis, including preventive measures to reduce the risk of osteoporosis.
9. Relate the pathophysiology and clinical manifestations to the collaborative care management of persons with a degenerative disease of the spine.
10. Correlate the pathophysiology with management strategies for persons with scoliosis.
11. Describe the etiology, pathophysiology, and treatment for common tumors of the musculoskeletal system.
12. Explain the medical, surgical, and nursing management for persons with osteosarcoma.
13. Compare potential complications after limb salvage surgery with those following amputation.
14. Discuss the etiology/epidemiology, pathophysiology, and clinical manifestations of disorders affecting the soft tissues of the musculoskeletal system.
15. Explain the medical and nursing interventions used in the care of persons with soft tissue disorders of the musculoskeletal system.

The essence of nursing care for individuals with musculoskeletal problems lies in helping them make the physiologic and psychosocial adaptations necessary to cope with a temporary or permanent disability. Inflammatory and degenerative processes can affect all structures in the musculoskeletal system and are often chronic and disabling. Pain and impaired mobility are major problems that must be considered when planning nursing care. Nursing interventions are focused on helping the patient to maximize independent functioning and teaching methods of joint protection, energy conservation, and prevention of further disability.

DISORDERS AFFECTING THE JOINTS

Arthritis (inflammation of a joint) is a common disorder of the musculoskeletal system that causes joint pain and stiffness. Although there are more than 100 arthritic conditions, rheumatoid arthritis and osteoarthritis are the two main types. Found worldwide, arthritis affects 1% of the world's population and is the major cause of disability in the United States.[48] The number of persons in the United States affected by arthritis continues to increase; it is estimated that 20% of the population, or one in five persons, will have arthritis by the year 2020.[71]

RHEUMATOID ARTHRITIS

Etiology

Rheumatoid arthritis (RA) is a chronic systemic inflammatory disease affecting primarily the diarthrodial joints and surrounding soft tissues. The disease process is characterized by inflammation of the connective tissues throughout the body. Systemic manifestations include pulmonary, cardiac, vascular, ophthalmologic, dermatologic, and hematologic effects. Mortality is associated with the extraarticular manifestations of RA and may shorten the individual's life expectancy by 3 to 18 years.

The etiology of RA is not known. However, several theories have been postulated regarding the pathogenesis of RA. The stimulus that triggers the inflammatory process remains unknown. RA is thought to be an autoimmune process, specifically the interaction of immunoglobulin (Ig) G with rheumatoid factor, which appears to perpetuate the rheumatoid inflammation. A genetic predisposition has also been identified in relation to certain human leukocyte antigens (HLAs). Another theory postulates that the disease occurs as an altered immune response to an unknown antigen. Possible causative antigens include the Epstein-Barr virus, human T-lymphotrophic virus type 1, parvovirus B19, bacteria, and mycoplasma.[38] Environmental factors have also been thought to trigger the inflammatory response. Prolonged exposure to the antigen causes normal antibodies (Ig) to become autoantibodies and attack host tissues (self-antigen). These autoantibodies, called *rheumatoid factors,* bind with self-antigens in the blood and synovial membrane to form immune complexes (Figure 47-1).

Epidemiology

RA affects 1% to 2% of the U.S. population, with health care costs exceeding $8.7 billion annually. In addition to the physical and psychologic costs associated with a chronic disabling disease, the estimated direct cost of medical care per patient is $4798 per year.[48] Women are two to three times more likely to be affected by RA than men. More than 1.5 million American women have RA.[42] The age of onset is between 20 and 50 years, with women usually diagnosed in later childbearing years. The incidence in persons under 35 years of age is less than 0.3% but increases to more than 10% for those over 65 years of age.[48]

Pathophysiology

Key pathologic features of RA are proliferation of the synovial membrane and erosion of articular cartilage and subchondral bone. These processes result in destruction of intraarticular and periarticular structures and joint deformity.

The stimulus that triggers the inflammatory process is unknown. The disease begins in the synovial membrane within the joint. Edema, vascular congestion, fibrin exudate, and cellular infiltrate occur as a result of the inflammatory process. Activated T cells, not present in normal joints, are found in joints affected by RA. Macrophages and monocytes are also found in rheumatoid joints and produce cytokines, which affect immune responses and inflammatory reactions. The cytokines, including interleukins, tumor necrosis factor (TNF)–alpha, granulocyte-macrophage colony-stimulating factors, and other growth factors cause cartilage destruction and increase inflammation.

White blood cells (WBCs) release chemicals (including superoxide radicals and hydrogen peroxide) that destroy both the bacteria and normal cells. Prostaglandins (chemicals that mediate inflammation), leukotrienes (producers of inflammation), and digestive enzymes are released. Particularly damaging to joint tissue is the enzyme collagenase, because it breaks down collagen, the main structural protein of connective tissue. The presence of these substances within the joint attracts more WBCs, and in RA the process becomes chronic. Continued inflammation leads to thickening of the synovium, particularly where it joins the articular cartilage. At these junctures fibrin develops into a granulation tissue, known as *pannus,* that covers the surface of the cartilage. The pannus also invades subchondral bone and interferes with the normal nutrition of the articular cartilage, causing necrosis. Pannus formation leads to adhesions between the joint surfaces, and a fibrous or bony union *(ankylosis)* develops. Destruction of cartilage and bone, in addition to some weakening of tendons and ligaments, may lead to subluxation, or dislocation, of joints. Invasion of the subchondral bone may cause eventual regional osteoporosis (Table 47-1).

Pain occurs as a result of cartilage degeneration. Areas of exposed bone due to erosion of cartilage may develop fissures or bone cysts. These cysts, caused by an excessive amount of inflammatory exudate, may develop into draining fistulas, communicating with the skin. Bone spurs and osteophytes (outgrowth of bone) may also occur, decreasing joint mobility and increasing pain.

Constitutional symptoms and new onset of joint pain are early manifestations of RA. The patient may report lymphadenopathy, malaise, depression, fever, weight loss, fatigue, and generalized aching. Early-morning stiffness lasting more than an hour is characteristic. Morning stiffness is thought to occur as a result of synovitis. The person may describe the location of aching and stiffness in general terms as opposed to naming specific joints. This kind of discomfort, commonly referred to as *fibrositis,* is poorly localized. Such discomfort may be the patient's earliest report. These symptoms may be present for some period of time before they are replaced by more specific, or localized, problems (i.e., frank articular inflammation with joint swelling, pain, redness, warmth, and tenderness). In other persons fibrositis and joint inflammation occur together at the onset (see Clinical Manifestations box).

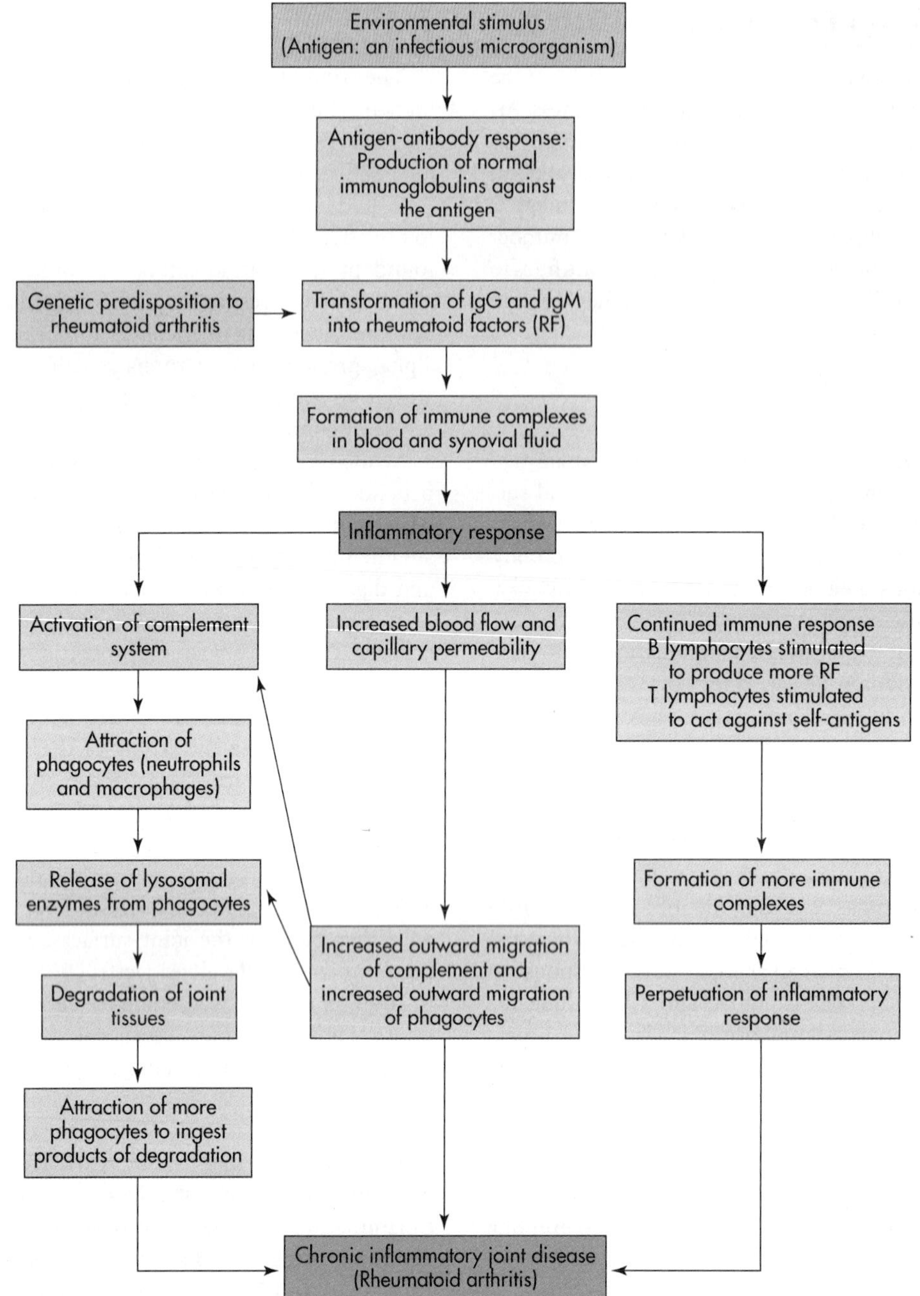

Figure 47-1 Probable pathogenesis of rheumatoid arthritis.

The proximal interphalangeal (PIP) and metacarpophalangeal (MCP) joints of the hands and fingers are often affected early. As the disease progresses, the fingers develop a characteristic tapering (fusiform) appearance with a classic ulnar deviation of the hand (Figure 47-2). Virtually all joints can become involved, but the ones most commonly involved are those of the hands, wrists, ankles, elbows, and knees. Shoulder and hip involvement occurs later. Joint involvement most often occurs in a bilaterally symmetric pattern.

Joint swelling is caused by inflammation of the synovial membrane, new bone formation, and tissue hyperplasia. The joint feels warm and boggy on palpation and may be erythematous.

Eventually all joints may be affected by RA. Involvement of the temporomandibular joint (TMJ) may limit the person's ability to open the mouth. Spinal involvement is usually limited to the cervical spine, particularly the first and second vertebrae. Subluxation or dislocation of the cervical vertebrae may result in death or paralysis. Both TMJ and cervical spine pathologic conditions should be assessed before the use of general anesthesia.

Inflammation of the tendon sheaths, particularly in the wrist, may occur. Muscle spasms contribute to the deformity of involved joints. Muscle atrophy may occur as a result of disuse secondary to pain. *Rheumatoid nodules* are an aggregate of inflammatory cells around a center of cellular debris and may

TABLE 47-1 Normal Function, Primary Pathophysiology, and Clinical Manifestations of Rheumatoid Arthritis

Normal Function	Pathophysiology	Clinical Manifestations
Synovial tissue secretes synovial fluid, which contains leukocytes, mucin, fat, albumin, and electrolytes. Provides joint lubrication and nourishment to articular cartilage.	Proliferation of synovium: inflammation causes edema, vascular congestion, fibrin exudate, and cellular infiltrate to build up around synovium. White blood cells move into synovium, releasing superoxide radicals, H_2O_2, prostaglandins, leukotrienes, and collagenase.	Synovium thickens, particularly at articular junctions. Symptoms of inflammation occur within and overlying joint (pain, swelling, erythema, warmth). Joint mobility is limited by pain.
Articular (hyaline) cartilage covers ends of articulating bones to reduce joint friction and to distribute weight-bearing forces in joint.	Pannus forms at junctions of synovial tissue and articular cartilage, interfering with nutrition of cartilage and resulting in scar tissue formation. Pannus invades subchondral bone and supporting soft tissue structures (ligaments, tendons), causing fibrous ankylosis.	Joint pain increases at rest and with movement. Destruction of soft tissue structures (ligaments, tendons) causes joint to sublux or dislocate. Fibrous tissue becomes calcified, and bony ankylosis occurs. Depending on amount of articular cartilage destroyed, adhesions can develop and joints can fuse, prohibiting joint motion. Atrophy of soft tissues adjacent to involved joint may result.

Clinical Manifestations

Rheumatoid Arthritis

EARLY SYMPTOMS

Fatigue
Weight loss
Fever
Malaise
Morning stiffness
Pain at rest and with movement, night pain
Edematous, erythematous, "boggy" joint

LATE SYMPTOMS

Pallor
Anemia
Color changes of digits (bluish, rubor, pallor)
Muscle weakness, atrophy
Joint deformities
Paresthesias
Decreased joint mobility
Contractures (usually flexion)
Subluxation
Dislocation
Increasing pain

develop near joints, over body prominences, or along extensor surfaces in the subcutaneous tissues. Twenty percent of persons with RA develop rheumatoid nodules.[11]

RA may also affect other body systems, and rheumatoid nodules may form in the heart, lungs, and spleen (Table 47-2). Glaucoma may result from rheumatoid nodule formation on the sclerae. Other manifestations of the multisystem involvement of RA include pleuritis, pulmonary fibrosis, pericarditis, aortic valve disease, lymphadenopathy, and splenomegaly. Acute necrotizing vasculitis, also common in other autoimmune disorders, may result in myocardial infarction, cerebrovascular accident, kidney damage, or Raynaud's phenomenon.

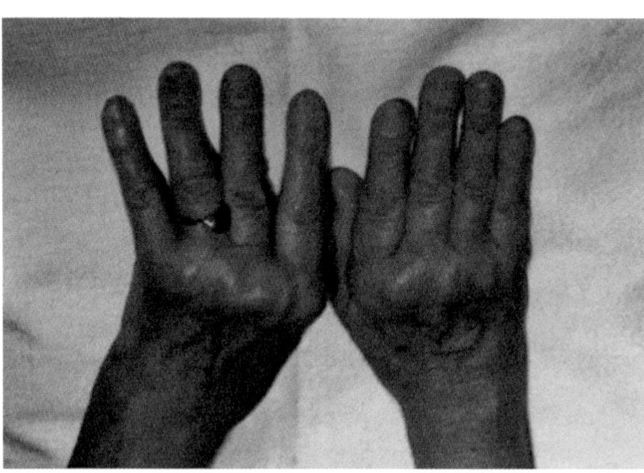

Figure 47-2 Rheumatoid arthritis of hands.

The course and severity of RA is unpredictable and is marked by periods of exacerbation and remission. However, in most patients narrowing of the joint space and bony erosion progress most rapidly during the first 2 years of disease.[38] Individuals with seropositive rheumatoid disease (positive rheumatoid factor) tend to have a chronic progressive pattern of disease. In a small number of individuals, the disease may be rapidly progressive, marked by unremitting joint destruction and diffuse vasculitis. This form of the disease is referred to as malignant rheumatoid disease.

The length of time between exacerbations varies with individuals. Physiologic and psychologic stress can contribute to exacerbations of the disease.

Increased morbidity and mortality are associated with more severe active cases of the disease. Remission is unlikely after 3 years of sustained disease activity. If untreated, RA tends to relapse and recur in a more severe form. Even with careful management, approximately 10% of patients with RA develop a severe, crippling form of the disease.

TABLE 47-2 Systemic Manifestations of Rheumatoid Arthritis

Body System	Clinical Manifestations
Cardiovascular	Pericarditis, valvular lesions, myocarditis, vasculitis, Raynaud's phenomenon
Pulmonary	Pleurisy, rheumatoid nodules on lungs, pneumoconiosis (Caplan's syndrome), interstitial pneumonitis, pulmonary fibrosis, pulmonary hypertension
Neurologic	Compression neuropathy, peripheral neuropathy, cervical myelopathy
Hematologic	Anemia, leukopenia (Felty's syndrome when accompanied by hepatosplenomegaly)
Renal	Rheumatoid nodules on kidney
Dermatologic	Rheumatoid nodules, brown lesions on skin due to ischemia, ulcers, draining fistulas
Ophthalmologic	Scleritis, sicca syndrome (keratoconjunctivitis); Sjögren's syndrome (keratoconjunctivitis, xerostomia, vaginal dryness), glaucoma, scleromalacia
Other	Fever, malaise, weakness

BOX 47-1 Diagnostic Criteria for Rheumatoid Arthritis

1. Morning stiffness >1 hour and at least 6-week duration
2. Soft tissue swelling of three or more joints for at least 6 weeks
3. Swelling of wrist, metacarpophalangeal, or proximal interphalangeal joints for at least 6 weeks
4. Symmetric soft tissue swelling
5. Rheumatoid nodules
6. Positive serum rheumatoid factor test
7. Radiographic changes (bone erosion or decalcification) in hand or wrist joints

BOX 47-2 Diagnostic Criteria for Remission of Rheumatoid Arthritis

1. Duration of joint stiffness less than 15 minutes
2. Absence of fatigue
3. No joint pain (per history) and no joint pain or tenderness with motion
4. Absence of soft tissue swelling in joints or tendon sheaths
5. Erythrocyte sedimentation rate less than 30 mm/hr in women; less than 20 mm/hr in men

Collaborative Care Management

Diagnostic Tests. The American Rheumatism Association has devised a system for the diagnosis of RA; the presence of four of the seven criteria is necessary for the diagnosis of RA. (Box 47-1).[2,38]

Criteria defining remission of disease have been proposed by the American College of Rheumatology; the criteria must be present for at least 2 consecutive months (Box 47-2).[2]

Diagnostic tests results usually include:

- Elevated erythrocyte sedimentation rate (ESR)
- Positive C-reactive protein test during acute phases
- Positive antinuclear antibody test, present in 30% to 40% of cases
- Mild leukocytosis or normal WBC count; possibility of eosinophilia in persons with severe disease
- Anemia (hypochromic, normocytic in the range of 30% to 35%); low serum iron and iron-binding capacity
- Positive rheumatoid factor or latex fixation test (present in 50% to 90% of patients, depending on disease duration and severity)
- Narrowing of the joint space and erosion of articular surfaces on roentgenographic examination; subluxation, dislocation of joints; radiographic changes are proportional to the degree of inflammation and disease activity; in persons with early RA, magnetic resonance imaging (MRI) may show focal bone changes undetectable by plain x-ray films.
- Inflammatory changes in synovial tissue obtained by biopsy
- Synovial fluid analysis: poor mucin clot test, elevated WBC count, immune complexes present, increased turbidity and decreased viscosity of fluid

Medications. The purposes of pharmacologic therapy are relief of pain, control of inflammation, and prevention of bone erosion (Table 47-3). Minimization of drug side effects is also desirable. Early aggressive drug therapy is recommended to prevent irreversible changes in articular cartilage that typically occur within 2 years of disease onset.[2,38]

The use of nonsteroidal antiinflammatory drugs (NSAIDs) has traditionally been the first line of treatment. Cyclooxygenase-2 (COX-2) inhibitors, newer NSAIDs, have demonstrated less platelet and gastrointestinal (GI) dysfunction than other NSAIDs, but like all NSAIDs they have the potential for renal toxicity. The use of NSAIDs is contraindicated in persons with poor renal function.

Research indicates that the use of disease-modifying antirheumatic drugs (DMARDs) or slow-acting antirheumatic drugs may be more effective in suppressing symptoms of RA in some persons. The use of DMARDs has been shown to result in less functional disability, less pain, less joint tenderness and swelling, and lower ESRs than in persons using NSAIDs, although NSAIDs are still considered first-line therapy by some practitioners. Persons with minimal joint involvement and absence of radiologic changes are well suited to initial treatment with NSAIDs. NSAIDs, including salicylates, modify the inflammatory process by inhibiting prostaglandin synthesis but do nothing to prevent bony erosion and alone are usually ineffective in the management of RA. Many agents are available, and patients respond differently to different agents; a 2- to 3-week trial is necessary to judge the effectiveness of therapy. The American College of Rheumatology recommends that before initiation of therapy with NSAIDs, baseline values be obtained for the following: complete blood count (CBC); blood urea nitrogen, creatinine, liver enzymes, and potassium levels; and urinalysis.[2] Monitoring should be done again in 1 to 3 months,

TABLE 47-3 Common Medications for Rheumatoid Arthritis

Drug	Action	Intervention
NSAIDs, Salicylates		
Aspirin	Modify inflammatory process by inhibiting prostaglandin synthetase; analgesic, antipyretic	Larger dose required, usually 3-6 g daily. Monitor for toxic levels and signs of toxicity (tinnitus, hearing loss, GI upset). Buffered or enteric coating recommended.
Diclofenac (Voltaren, Cataflam) Diflunisal (Dolobid) Etodolac (Lodine) Fenoprofen (Nalfon) Ibuprofen (Motrin) Indomethacin (Indocin) Naproxen (Naprosyn) Oxaprozin (Daypro) Piroxicam (Feldene) Sulindac (Clinoril) Tolmetin (Tolectin)	Do not modify disease progression	Monitor patient for dyspepsia, gastritis, hemorrhage, renal and hepatic function, platelet dysfunction, headache, confusion. Administer with food (check individual drug; food may interfere with absorption). Avoid concomitant use of salicylates and NSAIDs.
Celecoxib (Celebrex)		Contraindicated for persons with allergies to sulfonamides
Diclofenac sodium and misoprostol (Arthrotec)	Reduces risk of gastric ulcers	
Corticosteroids		
Prednisone (oral) Hydrocortisone (intraarticular)	Antiinflammatory	Long-term use only for persons with aggressive joint disease unresponsive to other agents; use smallest dose possible (prednisone 5-10 mg every other day) when necessary. Take with food or milk. Do not abruptly discontinue medication. Monitor patient for fluid and electrolyte balance, glucose levels, hypertension, skin lesions (purpura), decreased healing potential, cataract formation. Encourage adequate calcium and vitamin D intake to retard osteoporosis. Teach patient to avoid sources of infection. Systemic effects are rare with intraarticular use; avoid more than three injections per joint per year.
DMARDs		
Methotrexate (Rheumatrex), oral or intramuscular	Rapid onset of action inhibits degradation of folic acid, which inhibits DNA synthesis of inflammatory cells; effective for long-term therapy; concomitant use with folic acid 1 mg/day decreases toxicity without decreasing effectiveness	Evaluate renal function before therapy; monitor patient for hepatic and pulmonary toxicity, leukopenia, thrombocytopenia, anemia. Explain to patient that nausea, diarrhea, and stomatitis are common. Advise patient to use birth control while taking medication. Check for drug interactions that may increase toxicity risk.
Hydroxychloroquine (Plaquenil)	Mechanism of action unclear; acts on DNA synthesis, anti-inflammatory	Inform patient of need for eye examination before therapy and every 6 months thereafter (retinal edema may result in blindness). Monitor patient for hematologic toxicity, GI irritation, and hypertension; evaluate renal function.
Sulfasalazine (Azulfidine)	Unknown, antiinflammatory	Monitor patient for neurologic and GI toxicity, leukopenia, anemia, and Stevens-Johnson syndrome. Educate patient about need for CBC and liver function tests throughout therapy.
Gold salts (Myochrysine, Ridaura, Solganal), oral and intramuscular	Antiinflammatory mechanism unclear; effect not noted until several months of therapy	Monitor patient for renal and hepatic damage, dermatitis, and mouth ulcerations. Inform patient of need for CBC and urinalysis before and at intervals throughout therapy. Stress the need for oral hygiene; therapy may cause metallic taste in mouth. Oral gold has fewer side effects.
Azathioprine (Imuran)	Unknown, immune suppressant	Monitor patient for blood dyscrasias, hepatitis, and pancreatitis. CBC necessary as baseline and throughout treatment.
D-Penicillamine (Depen, Cuprimine)	Unknown	Monitor patient for fever, rash, GI upset, blood dyscrasias, and delayed wound healing; assess for penicillin allergy. Inform patient of potential for dysgeusia (taste alteration). Food interferes with absorption. Rare side effects include polymyositis and Goodpas-

CBC, Complete blood count; *DMARDs*, disease-modifying antirheumatic drugs; *NSAIDs*, nonsteroidal antiinflammatory drugs; *DNA*, deoxyribonucleic acid; *GI*, gastrointestinal; *TNF-alpha*, tumor necrosis factor–alpha.

Continued

TABLE 47-3 Common Medications for Rheumatoid Arthritis—cont'd

Drug	Action	Intervention
DMARDs–cont'd		
D-Penicillamine—cont'd		ture's syndrome. Urinalysis and CBC required before and at intervals during therapy.
Leflunomide (Arava)	Pyrimidine antagonist, immunomodulator, antiinflammatory; inhibits activated T lymphocytes	Begin with loading dose followed by maintenance dose. Use caution with renal or hepatic disease. Few toxic effects; monitor liver function. Doses >25 mg/day associated with increased incidence of side effects, including alopecia, weight loss, and elevated liver enzymes. Educate patient regarding use of contraception while taking medication.
Immunosuppressant		
Cyclophosphamide (Cytoxan)	Suppresses synovitis; retards bony erosions	Monitor patient for toxic effects, including GI distress, bone marrow suppression, alopecia, and hemorrhagic cystitis. Inform patient of possible long-term effects, including bladder fibrosis and cancer, infections, sterility, and hematologic malignancies. Inform patient of need for monitoring CBC and urinalysis during therapy. Teach patient to increase fluid intake to ensure frequent bladder emptying.
Biologic Response Modifiers (Kineret)		
Anakira	Recombinent human interleukin-1 (IL-1) receptor antagonist.; counteracts the effects of IL-1, decreasing inflammation, bone erosion, and cartilage destruction; also relieves pain; given alone or in combination with other DMARDs; contraindicated for use with ethanercept and infliximab	Administered daily by subcutaneous injection. Daily dosing provides greater relief of symptoms than by weekly or thrice-weekly dosing.[31a] The most common adverse effect is pain at injection site (rotating sites is recommended). Other adverse effects are rare and include neutropenia, neoplasia, and infection. Medication must be refrigerated and protected from light.
Etanercept (Enbrel)	Recombinant TNF-alpha antagonist; originally developed for use with methotrexate, now used as monotherapy	For use in patients with severe disease unreceptive to other disease-modifying agents. Cost is high, and biweekly subcutaneous injections are required. There are no data regarding long-term use; it is contraindicated in pregnancy, lactation, malignancy, and sepsis. Avoid vaccinations (particularly live) while taking drug. Side effects include pain at injection site, respiratory infections.
Infliximab (Remicade)	TNF-alpha moclonal antibody and immunoglobulin G1 antibody that neutralizes TNF-alpha; administered intravenously; commonly used with methotrexate; approval as monotherapy pending	Side effects include headache, rash, respiratory and urinary infections, and local infusion site reactions.

then at 3- to 12-month intervals thereafter. GI side effects can be controlled with the addition of an H_2 blocker, proton pump inhibitor, or sucralfate. Misoprostol has been shown to be effective for reducing the incidence of gastric ulcers and hemorrhage and should be considered in high-risk persons (those with a history of ulcers, older adults, smokers, and those who are receiving concomitant steroid therapy).

Persons with polyarthritic involvement, persistent inflammation, elevated ESRs or positive rheumatoid factor tests, and radiologic evidence of bone erosion are usually treated with second-line agents or DMARDs. Patients often receive NSAIDs and DMARDs simultaneously.

Formerly used later in the course of RA, DMARDs are now introduced early in the disease to preserve joint function and improve outcomes. DMARDs "modify" the disease by preventing erosions. Therapy with DMARDs is usually begun if a 2- to 3-month trial of NSAIDs has been ineffective. Most persons with moderate or severe RA are started on a regimen of methotrexate. Long-term studies have demonstrated the safety and effectiveness of methotrexate, especially when prescribed with folic acid.

The effectiveness of DMARDs may not be evident until after weeks to months of therapy. Disadvantages of DMARD therapy include the high cost, toxic effects, and long onset of action. DMARDs are continued at low dosages even after disease control is achieved because of the risk of a rebound effect after drug discontinuation. Careful monitoring is required to prevent the development of toxic effects. Most adverse effects are reversible

TABLE 47-4 Types and Functions of Splints and Braces

Type	Function
Spring-loaded braces	Oppose the action of unparalyzed muscles and act as partial functional substitutes for paralyzed muscles (Figure 47-3)
Resting splints	Maintain a limb or joint in a functional position while permitting the muscles around the joint to relax (Figure 47-4)
Functional splints	Maintain the joint or limb in a usable position to enable the body part to be used correctly
Dynamic splints	Permit assisted exercise to joints, particularly following surgery to finger joints (Figure 47-5)

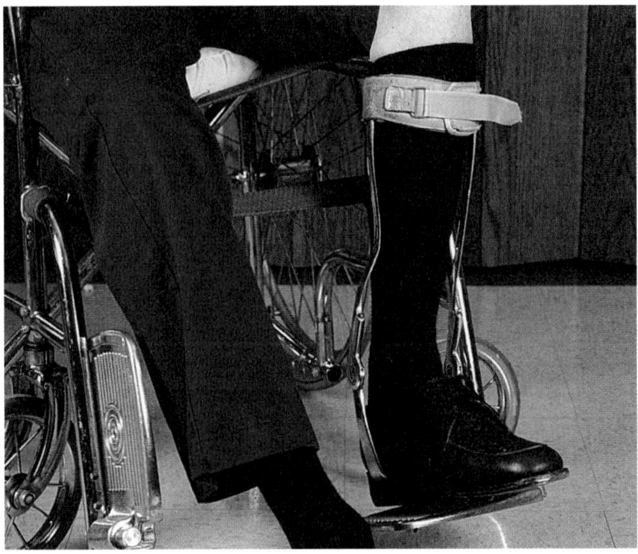

Figure 47-3 Leg brace.

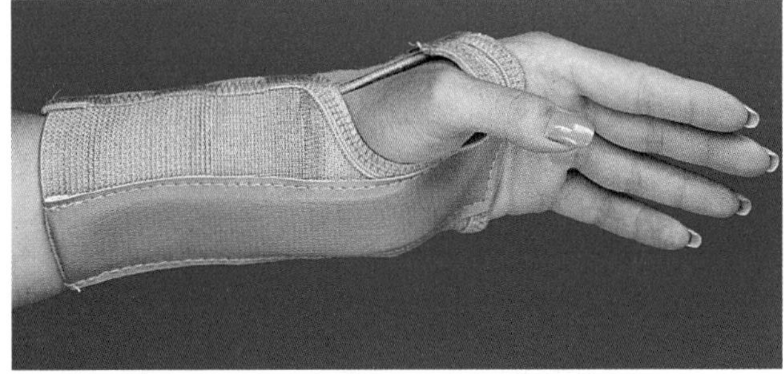

Figure 47-4 Wrist splint.

after the drug is discontinued. Many physicians prescribe two or more DMARDs in combination. Failure to respond to multiple DMARDs is associated with a poor prognosis.

Steroid therapy, oral and intraarticular, is also used in the management of RA. The many side effects associated with steroid use rarely occur with intraarticular injections. More than three injections in the same joint per year is not recommended. The use of low-dose (5 to 7.5 mg) prednisone can significantly reduce the incidence of side effects. This regimen is often effective in controlling inflammation, particularly in elderly patients at risk for NSAID toxicity. Supplemental calcium (1200 to 1500 mg/day) and vitamin D can be prescribed to reduce steroid-induced osteoporosis.

Newer agents include TNF-alpha antagonists, which have been shown to retard radiographic progression of disease. Disadvantages include the high cost and paucity of data regarding safety and efficacy of long-term use. Because of cost, most insurance companies require proof that other agents have been ineffective in retarding disease progression before approving the use of these agents. Anakira, the newest agent approved by the U.S. Food and Drug Administration (FDA), blocks interleukin-1, a protein present in excess in persons with RA. The use of anakira is recommended for persons unresponsive to other DMARDs.

Other pharmacologic therapies used to treat RA include cytokines, cytokine agonists, cyclosporine, antibiotics (minocycline, tetracycline), and monoclonal antibodies. These therapies are experimental and are reserved for use in persons who do not respond to conventional therapy.

Adjuvant drugs to control chronic pain and to improve sleep quality are also used in the treatment of RA. Tricyclic antidepressants are commonly prescribed; patients should be monitored for side effects, including sedation and dry mouth.

Treatments. The goals of therapy for persons with RA are to relieve symptoms, prevent joint destruction, maintain joint and muscle function, and promote independence and quality of life. In addition to pharmacologic therapy, occupational therapy (OT) and physical therapy (PT) are mainstays of treatment to preserve joint mobility and promote independence. An exercise program, designed with the physical therapist, is important for maintaining mobility and preventing muscle atrophy. There is ample evidence to support the fact that exercise can improve the individual's sense of well being, which is beneficial to an individual trying to cope with a chronic, disabling disease.

Splints and orthoses (braces) are prescribed by the physician and fitted by a physical therapist, occupational therapist, or orthotist. The purposes of splints and braces are to:

- Stabilize or support a joint.
- Protect a joint or body part from external trauma.
- Mechanically correct a dysfunction such as footdrop by supporting the joint in its functional position.
- Assist patients in exercising specific joints.

Splints and braces (Table 47-4) are designed to be as lightweight and cosmetically acceptable as possible. Many splints are made of plastic (Figure 47-6), which can be molded to fit. In many instances plastic has replaced metal and leather braces that are often obvious, even though worn under loose-fitting clothing. Shoes may be modified or corrective shoes may be prescribed to provide special support for the feet. Braces can be fitted to the patient's own shoes (see Figure 47-3).

Many assistive devices are available for individuals who have impaired upper and/or lower extremity function (Box 47-3). These devices are obtained by referring the patient to an occupational therapist.

Supportive devices or ambulatory aids (walkers, canes, and crutches) are usually recommended for persons who cannot bear weight on one or more joints of the lower extremities. Other indications for use include instability, loss of balance, or pain on weight bearing. The physical therapist evaluates the patient to determine the specific device that matches the patient's needs and abilities.

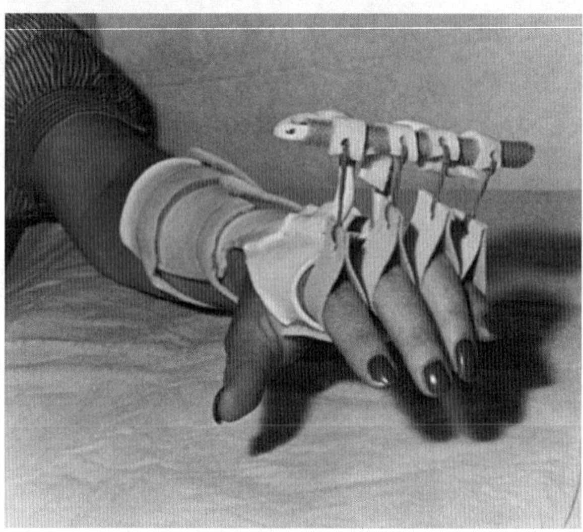

Figure 47-5 Dynamic hand splint.

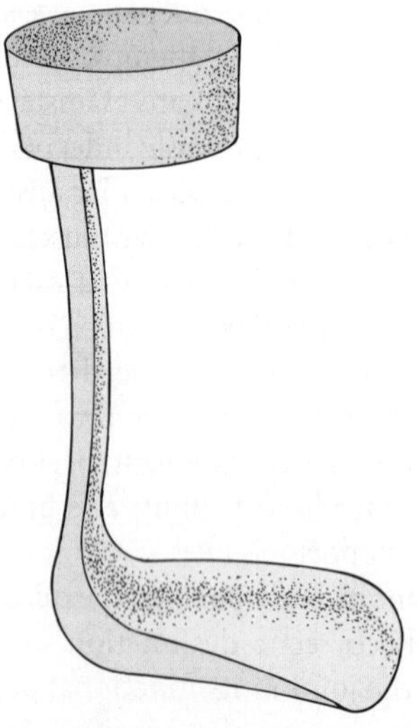

Figure 47-6 Ankle-foot orthosis.

Nurses are expected to supervise patients in their use of these devices and encourage patients to use their walking aids correctly. Advantages and disadvantages of different aids and the techniques of walking with each are presented in Table 47-5.

Other treatment modalities for the person with RA include the application of hot and cold packs to the affected joint(s). Heat may be applied by means of:

- Hydrocollator packs (packs containing chemical filler that expands in water and retains heat; may be heated in a pot of water or special machines that maintain a constant temperature of 80° C [174° F])
- Paraffin baths
- Electric heating pads that are approved for use with moist towels
- Electric heating pads that produce moisture
- Warm soaks, tub soaks, or showers

Application of cold or ice packs is helpful in reducing or preventing swelling (especially after trauma), reducing pain, and relieving stiffness. Cold packs may take the form of plastic bags containing ice, commercially available gel packs that can be refrozen and reused, or large bags of frozen vegetables (especially for home use).

BOX 47-3 Assistive Devices for Persons With Motor Impairments

Assistive Device	Patient Limitation
Utensil with built-up handle (Figure 47-7)	Cannot adequately close hand
Utensil with cuffed handle	Loss of opposition of thumb
Combination knife-fork	Loss of only one hand
Mug with special handle (Figure 47-8)	Unable to grasp regular cup handle
Long-handled shoehorn (Figure 47-9)	Unable to bend to reach feet; hip flexion limitation
Long-handled reacher (to reach for or pick up objects) (Figure 47-10)	Unable to stoop or reach; hip flexion limitation
Stocking guide (Figure 47-11)	Unable to reach feet; hip flexion limitation

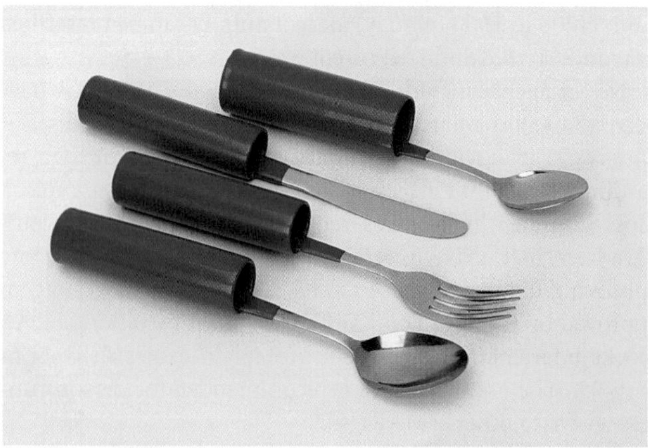

Figure 47-7 Utensils with special handles.

Heat or cold should be left on for 15 to 20 minutes to achieve maximum effect. Cold packs and moist heat packs should be wrapped in protective towels to prevent burns to the skin, and the skin should be checked 5 minutes after application for any evidence of tissue damage. Heat or cold should be applied with caution to any individual with decreased sensation, because of the risk of injury.

Persons with RA and other chronic diseases are particularly susceptible to claims of "cures" and nontraditional therapies. The patient should be educated to carefully evaluate risks and benefits before trying any of these remedies (see Complementary & Alternative Therapies box). For management of systemic manifestations of RA, the reader is referred to the appropriate section of the text.

Surgical Management. Referral to an orthopedic surgeon is indicated if conservative therapies are ineffective. Surgery is indicated for the prevention or correction of deformity, relief from pain, and restoration or maintenance of function.

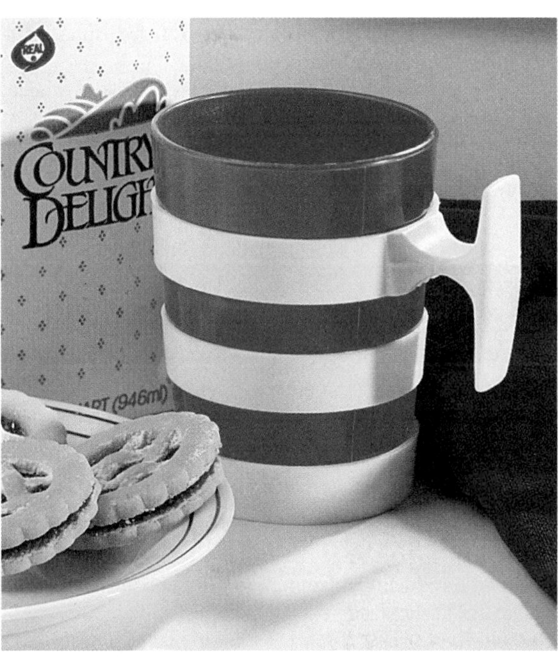

Figure 47-8 Cup with special handle.

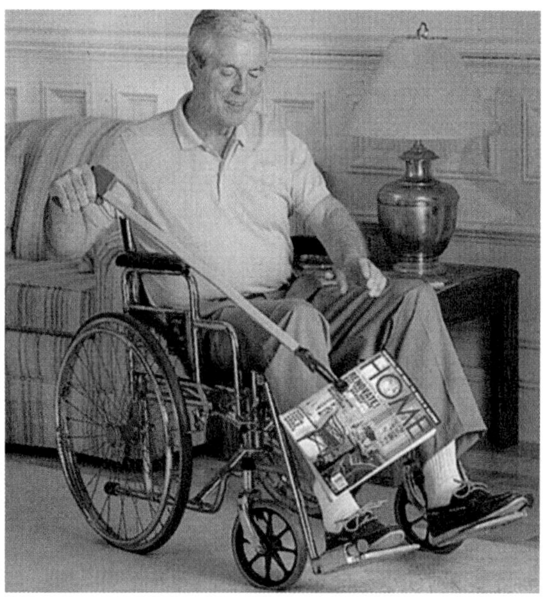

Figure 47-10 Long-handled reachers.

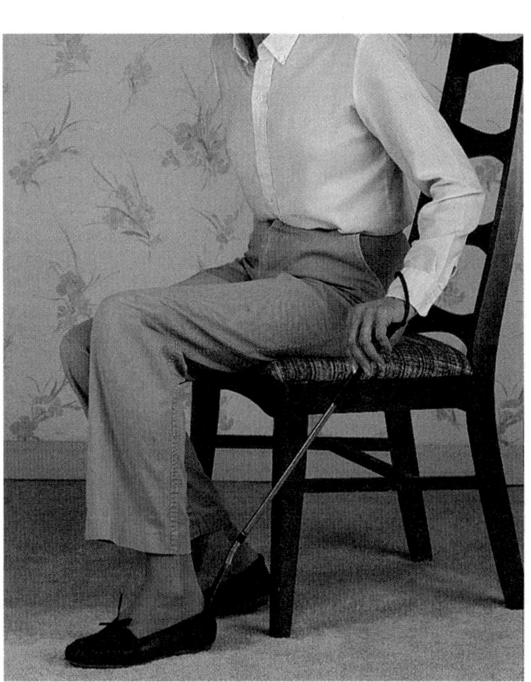

Figure 47-9 Long-handled shoehorn.

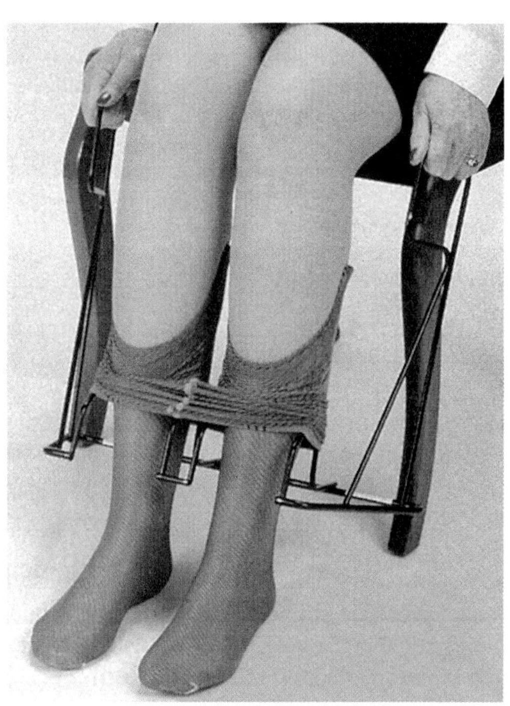

Figure 47-11 Stocking helper.

TABLE 47-5 Comparison of Ambulatory Aids

Device	Advantages/Disadvantages	Gait*
Single-support device: cane, quad cane, single crutch	Less cumbersome than crutches or walkers Less effective in unloading weight as a double support	Device is held in hand opposite involved leg Device and involved leg are advanced first, followed by uninvolved leg
Double-support device Walker	Provides solid support Can be used by individuals with loss of balance Limits speed of ambulation Hazardous on stairs or uneven ground	Walker is advanced first, then involved extremity, then uninvolved extremity
Crutches	Require dexterity and a good sense of balance Permit faster ambulation than a walker Can be used on stairs	3-point gait—same as walker gait 4-point gait—crutch, opposite leg, opposite crutch, other leg 2-point gait—both crutches, both legs (one leg may be non–weight bearing)

*SPECIAL NOTE: Climbing stairs is accomplished by moving the uninvolved leg first, then the device and the involved leg; to descend stairs, the involved leg and the device are moved first, then the uninvolved leg. The device and the involved leg always move together.

Complementary & Alternative Therapies

Rheumatoid Arthritis

There are a myriad of supplements available claiming to provide relief from pain and inflammation and other symptoms associated with rheumatoid arthritis (RA). Pharmacologic treatment often causes adverse side effects, and as a result, many patients may be tempted to try "natural remedies." Nurses caring for patients with RA should be familiar with the most common products so that they can provide patients with information necessary to make an informed decision regarding their use. The Arthritis Foundation has identified the following supplements as potentially beneficial for persons with RA. Before trying these products, the patient should discuss their safety and efficacy with his or her health care provider.

- *Dehydroepiandrosterone (DHEA)* is a naturally occurring hormone compound; when used as a supplement, it is derived from chemically treated yams. It claims to relieve pain and inflammation and reduce fatigue; it may increase bone density. DHEA is currently under review by the U.S. Food and Drug Administration (FDA) as a treatment for lupus. Because it is a hormone, there are potentially serious side effects, including acne, abdominal pain, hypertension, hair growth, and menstrual irregularities. This supplement should be used only under medical supervision.
- *Fish oil* derived from cold-water fishes contains omega-3 fatty acids that have been shown to decrease the inflammation and pain associated with RA. It may increase the blood-thinning effects of anticoagulants and nonsteroidal antiinflammatory drugs (NSAIDs). Fish oil may be taken as a supplement or by eating cold-water fish two to three times weekly.
- *Flaxseed (Linum usitassimum)* is derived from meal or oil of the flax plant. It is available as a pill, meal, flour, or oil. Flaxseed is also a source of omega-3 fatty acids, which are effective in reducing inflammation. Flaxseed is also a laxative, so gastrointestinal side effects may occur.
- *Gamma-linoleic acid (GLA)* is found in black currants, borage oil, and evening primrose oil. It is available as a capsule or oil. Claims include relief from inflammation and stiffness and symptoms of Sjögren's syndrome and Raynaud's phenomenon. There are some studies supporting its efficacy in reducing pain and inflammation, but none to support topical use for aching joints. Side effects include increased action of anticoagulants and, with evening primrose oil use, gastrointestinal symptoms.
- *Green tea (Camellia sinensis)* supposedly relieves pain and inflammation, but there are no human studies to support this claim. Green tea contains polyphenols, which are antioxidant compounds that may relieve inflammation. Green tea has been used medicinally in Asia for years; when taken as a beverage in moderate amounts, it is considered safe.

Reference: Horstman J: *Arthritis Today's* supplement guide, *Arthritis Today,* pp 34-49, July-Aug 2001.

If loss of function or permanent deformity is not preventable, the patient's powers of compensation and adaptation must be developed.

Before performing surgery, the orthopedist considers the procedure best suited to achieve the desired objectives for the individual patient. It is important that those caring for the patient know and understand what the expected outcomes are so that care may be adapted to achieving them.

A description of commonly performed surgical procedures is found in Table 47-6. Synovectomy is performed early in the disease to decrease pain and retard the degenerative changes in the joint. Osteotomy and joint arthroplasty are performed in advanced disease.

Diet. There is evidence to suggest that ingestion of fish oil (a type of n-3 polyunsaturated fat) as a dietary fat is beneficial to persons with RA. Benefits include a decrease in the number of swollen joints, decrease in the duration of morning stiffness, and overall improvement in function.[48] How fish oil produces a therapeutic effect is unknown, but it does suppress inflammatory mediator (prostaglandins, leukotrienes, and cy-

TABLE 47-6 Surgical Management of Rheumatoid Arthritis

Procedure	Indication
Arthroscopy	
Endoscopic examination of a joint	Diagnosis Synovectomy Chondroplasty Removal of bone spurs, osteophytes, and "joint mice"
Arthrotomy	
Opening of a joint	Exploration of joint Drainage of joint Removal of damaged tissue
Arthroplasty	
Reconstruction of a joint	Restore motion Relieve pain Correct deformity Avascular necrosis
Interposition	
Replacement of part of a joint with a prosthesis or with soft tissue	
Hemiarthroplasty	
Replacement of one articulating surface	
Replacement (Total Joint)	
Replacement of both articulating surfaces of a joint with prosthetic implants	
Synovectomy	
Removal of part or all of the synovial membrane	Delay the progress of rheumatoid arthritis
Osteotomy	
Cutting a bone to change its alignment	Correct deformity (varus or valgus) Alter weight-bearing surface of diseased joint to relieve pain
Arthrodesis	
Surgical fusion of a joint by removal of articular hyaline cartilage, introduction of bone grafts, and stabilization with internal or external fixation devices	Stabilize joint Relieve pain
Tendon Transplants	
Moving a tendon from its anatomic position	Substitute one tendon for another that is not working Realign tendon function (e.g., for stability)

tokines) production. More research is needed to determine the optimal effectiveness of fish oil in the diet.

Persons with RA often have anemia. A diet containing iron-rich foods (liver, oysters, clams, organ meat, lean meat, whole grains, legumes, and leafy green vegetables) is recommended to decrease anemia. Calcium and vitamin D supplements can reduce bone resorption.

Fatigue and malaise are common in persons with RA. A diet containing adequate calories and balanced nutrition is necessary to prevent fatigue and increase energy. Malnourishment also increases susceptibility to infection, which can exacerbate symptoms. If the patient is being treated with an immunosuppressant, the risk for infection is intensified. If the patient is overweight, a weight reduction diet, combined with exercise, is recommended to decrease the strain on weight-bearing joints.

Activity. Rest is often used as therapy for persons with RA. Rest is beneficial in reducing fatigue and decreasing the systemic inflammatory response. Resting specific joints or immobilization may also be prescribed.

Activity must be balanced with adequate rest. Individuals who have pain and stiffness with or after certain activities must learn to recognize their tolerances and adapt their activities of daily living (ADLs) accordingly. This does not mean stopping all activity; it means modifying activity.

Exercise is prescribed to:

- Preserve joint mobility (active and passive range of motion [ROM]).

- Maintain muscle tone (active ROM and isometrics).
- Strengthen selected muscle groups (resistive exercises performed against resistance provided by another person or by weights).

Exercise may be facilitated by the application of heat or cold or the administration of an analgesic before the exercise period. Exercise is contraindicated in the presence of acute joint or muscle inflammation until the inflammatory process subsides. Patients may benefit from an aquatic exercise program, which reduces stress on joints.

Exercise programs should be tailored to the patient's specific needs and capabilities. Nurses need to be aware of the specific exercise program the patient is following and be prepared to provide support and assistance in performing the exercises as needed and reinforcing the purpose, technique, frequency, and duration of the exercises.

Referrals. Common referrals for persons with RA include PT and OT. A social service consultation may be initiated to assist the patient with discharge needs. The patient and family may benefit from a referral to the Arthritis Foundation.* The Arthritis Foundation sponsors support groups, self-help classes, and exercise programs.

NURSING MANAGEMENT OF PATIENT WITH RHEUMATOID ARTHRITIS

ASSESSMENT

Health History

A complete health history, including a functional assessment, is important in persons with RA. Early in the disease, the patient may report chronic fatigue, generalized aching and stiffness in the extremities, and weight loss. As the disease progresses, the patient will report specific joints that are painful, loss of strength, decreased mobility, early-morning stiffness, and fatigue. Generally, pain interferes with normal ADLs. The patient will also note that affected joints are changing in appearance. Many patients express fear or despair over loss of function and independence.

Physical Examination

The nurse performs a complete head-to-toe examination, focusing on:

Inspection and palpation of the same joints on both sides of the body for symmetry, skin color, size, shape, tenderness, heat, and swelling
Assessment of limitation of active joint ROM
Evidence of pain with active ROM
Evidence of atrophy or loss of tone or tenderness in muscles associated with involved joints
Transfer ability and ability to perform ADLs

*1314 Spring Street NW, Atlanta, GA 30309; (800) 283-7800 or (404) 872-7100; website: www.arthritis.org.

NURSING DIAGNOSES

Nursing diagnoses are determined from analysis of patient data. Possible nursing diagnoses for the person with RA may include but are not limited to:

Diagnostic Title	Possible Etiologic Factors
1. Chronic pain	Inflammation and swelling in joints
2. Self-care deficit (related to bathing/hygiene, dressing/grooming, feeding, toileting)	Pain and musculoskeletal impairment
3. Fatigue	Chronic systemic disease
4. Situational low self-esteem	Change in body appearance, functioning
5. Risk for injury	Loss of muscle strength and joint motion
6. Deficient knowledge (related to arthritis)	Lack of exposure to information

EXPECTED PATIENT OUTCOMES

Expected patient outcomes for the person with RA may include but are not limited to:

1. Will state that pain is decreased and verbalizes ways to control pain
2. Will demonstrate improved ability to perform self-care activities and participate in usual activities to fullest extent possible
3. Will state factors that lead to fatigue and how fatigue might be avoided
4. Will verbalize a more positive self-concept
5. Will maintain active joint ROM within limits of disease to strengthen muscles and prevent injuries; will be free of injury
6. Will explain the disease process, the applicability of treatment measures, and plans for follow-up care

INTERVENTIONS

1. Promoting Comfort

A complete pain assessment (see Chapter 12) is performed. Patients with RA have both chronic and acute pain. The challenge to the nurse caring for the person with RA is managing pain control while promoting mobility. Exercise and movement are difficult when a person is in pain; weight bearing increases stress on inflamed joints, possibly causing more pain. Both pharmacologic and nonpharmacologic methods should be used to manage the pain associated with RA.

Medications are used to decrease the pain and inflammation associated with exacerbations of symptoms. The nurse should provide the patient with information regarding prescribed medications, adverse and therapeutic effects, dosage, and administration. Additional interventions to control pain include the application of heat/cold, relaxation techniques, proper body alignment, joint protection and rest, and ROM to decrease stiffness. A warm shower or tub bath may be effective in reducing pain and stiffness, whereas cold can reduce pain and decrease swelling. Transcutaneous electrical nerve stimulation (TENS) may be prescribed as an adjunct for pain relief.

2. Promoting Independence and Self-Care

Most people want to be able to live their lives independently. However, persons with musculoskeletal problems may be unable to manage one or more activities for themselves. Assistive devices (e.g., button hook or Velcro closures) are available to increase independence in ADLs. An OT referral may be necessary to evaluate the patient for appropriate assistive devices. Overhead trapezes, handrails, tub rails or shower chairs, grooming aids, elevated toilet seats, and shoes with Velcro fasteners may assist the patient in performing self-care. The patient should allow extra time for completing ADLs; frequent rest periods may be needed because of pain or fatigue.

3. Reducing Fatigue

Persons with RA commonly report fatigue; the patient may experience an overwhelming feeling of exhaustion and an inability to complete his or her usual activities. The nurse can use an intensity scale (0 to 10) to evaluate the severity of fatigue and to establish a baseline assessment. Inadequate nutrition and poor quality or amount of sleep can contribute to fatigue. Dietary counseling and methods to enhance sleep and rest may help decrease fatigue. The patient should be encouraged to discuss factors that cause fatigue and identify times of greatest fatigue and structure activities accordingly. Rest is often prescribed to decrease feelings of fatigue; the patient should be helped to set small, attainable goals and to use energy conservation techniques (Box 47-4). Daily routines may need to be modified to accommodate decreased abilities. Some tasks may be delegated to family or friends, and the patient may need to temporarily limit social and/or work responsibilities. Referral to a support group can help the individual deal with body and role changes. A regular aerobic exercise program, if permitted by the physician, may reduce fatigue.

4. Promoting a Positive Self-Concept

A major problem faced by many individuals who have musculoskeletal problems is that the disorder may be disfiguring in addition to being disabling. Not only must they adapt to functional disability, but also they may have to adapt to "looking different" from other people. Loss or alteration of function or the need to use an assistive device or prosthesis can also cause patients to view themselves as different from others. Depending on the nature and strength of pressures from family, social, or work situations or the individual's degree of self-esteem, the individual may attempt to cover up the disability so as not to lose support, esteem, or a livelihood. If the disability cannot be concealed, some persons may withdraw or limit their contact with others. Feelings of loneliness or social isolation may result.

Nursing interventions to enhance self-esteem include establishing a trusting relationship with the patient and family members, encouraging expression of feelings regarding the disease process and personal appearance, supporting positive coping mechanisms, and conveying respect and nonjudgmental acceptance. Positive feedback should be provided, and the patient helped to perform a self-appraisal, identifying strengths and weaknesses and a realistic approach to achieving desired goals. If necessary, referral to self-help groups, support groups, or counseling services is made.

BOX 47-4 Joint Protection and Energy Conservation Techniques

- Maintain good standing and sitting posture and proper body alignment.
- Avoid keeping joints in flexion for prolonged periods of time.
- Avoid twisting motions with small joints, such as turning a jar lid.
- Change positions frequently.
- Use the strongest joints and muscles when performing activities.
- When working at a desk, stand up and walk about for a few minutes every half hour.
- Use the knees, not the back, when lifting heavy objects.
- Push a door open with the shoulder, not the wrist.
- Use a shoulder strap, not a handheld strap, to carry a heavy bag or purse.
- Avoid reaching or bending when another approach would work as well.
- Work at a comfortable height.
- Avoid trying to accomplish difficult tasks in a single time period.
- Take breaks during work periods.
- Slide rather than lift objects.
- Use a wheeled cart to move objects from one place to another.

5. Promoting Mobility and Preventing Injury

Safety devices can be used by the patient to enhance function and prevent accidents when normal function, balance, or dexterity is compromised. Examples of safety devices include safety arms around toilets, grab bars mounted at tubs or showers, elevated toilet seats, adhesive strips on tub or shower floors, handrails along staircases, and nonskid wax applied to floors. Nurses need to be familiar with the various devices available and help patients learn to use them.

Optimal joint mobility and muscle strength help reduce accidents and falls. A regular exercise program helps to build muscle tone and increases strength and coordination. Interventions to promote joint mobility include a baseline assessment of functional abilities and joint motion. Active and, if necessary, passive ROM exercises should be encouraged at least twice daily. Controversy exists regarding performing ROM exercises during exacerbations of acute inflammation; periods of joint rest may be prescribed. Complete bed rest should be avoided because of the significant risk of complications associated with immobility. Activity should be balanced with rest.

Splints may be prescribed to provide joint rest or proper alignment. Positions that may lead to contractures must be avoided. For example, pillows should not be placed under knees when the patient is supine or under the head, forcing the neck into forward flexion. It is important that the patient wear properly fitted footwear with nonskid soles for safety. Ways to improve the safety of the home environment to prevent falls and injury should be discussed with the family or caregivers.

6. Patient/Family Education

As with any chronic illness, patient teaching is perhaps the most important aspect of nursing care of patients with RA. The patient has to evaluate the response to and effectiveness of the prescribed therapy.

It is estimated that hundreds of millions of dollars are spent each year on gadgets, programs, and "medicines" that allegedly are able to "cure" arthritis. In some instances the disease and associated disability may progress despite all efforts to control the disease process; this is extremely discouraging for the patient, family, and members of the health care team. However, many persons are able to live reasonably normal, productive lives while managing their arthritis. Their ability to do so partially depends on their knowledge of the disease and its treatment.

Nurses teaching persons about RA (and other rheumatic diseases) may find it helpful to use some of the teaching material prepared by the Arthritis Foundation. The Arthritis Foundation is an important resource for both health care professionals and patients. Local chapters holds classes and exercise programs.

Patient teaching should include information about the following: balance of rest and activity, joint protection and energy conservation methods, medication use, exercise programs, proper use of walking aids or assistive devices, proper care of splints or braces, safety measures, and follow-up care. The patient should be referred to the orthotist for problems with fitting orthoses.

Health Promotion/Prevention

Several objectives in Healthy People 2010 are related to arthritis treatment strategies and the effect of a chronic disease on daily functioning (see Healthy People 2010 box).

EVALUATION

To evaluate the effectiveness of nursing interventions, compare the patient's behaviors with those stated in the expected patient outcomes. Achievement of patient outcomes is successful if the patient:

1a. Verbalizes that pain is reduced or tolerable; demonstrates effective pain relief measures.
1b. Demonstrates adequate sleep and rest; sleep is not disturbed by pain.
2. Performs own ADLs to the fullest extent possible.
3a. Lists factors that cause fatigue.
3b. Describes measures to prevent or reduce fatigue; plans for adequate rest periods and techniques for energy conservation to increase activity level as tolerated.
4. Demonstrates behaviors to promote positive self-esteem; identifies feelings and underlying issues of negative self-perception.
5a. Demonstrates active ROM exercises and strengthening exercises such as straight leg raises and quadriceps sets; achieves maximum mobility of extremities; is injury free.
5b. Describes plan for balancing rest and exercise and use of cold or heat after exercising.
6. Verbalizes understanding of disease process of RA and rationales for treatment.

Healthy People 2010
Goals Related to Chronic Joint Symptoms

Decrease:
- The number of days with severe pain
- Limitation in activities of daily living and other activity because of arthritis symptoms

Increase:
- The number of persons who seek help in coping with psychosocial problems associated with arthritis
- The employment rate among working-age adults
- The number of persons seeking health care for joint problems
- The proportion of persons receiving evidence-based education for arthritis management

Eliminate racial disparities in the rate of total knee replacement surgeries

From US Department of Health and Human Services: *Healthy people 2010: understanding and improving health,* Washington, DC, 2000, USDHHS.

GERONTOLOGIC CONSIDERATIONS

Early manifestations of RA, such as fatigue and myalgia, are vague and can also be attributed to a number of other conditions. The elderly patient with rheumatic disease probably has at least one other comorbid condition. Fatigue and myalgia can be symptoms of hypothyroidism, a common condition in the elderly population. Care must be taken to be sure that the arthritic symptoms are not a result of a comorbid condition. The elderly patient may not exhibit the typical symptoms associated with RA. In contrast to the usual presentation, the larger joints are usually affected in the older adult, and the onset is usually acute.[37]

An important factor when considering treatment of RA in older adults is the choice of drug therapy. It is well known that altered drug metabolism is a physiologic event of aging, and the dosage of many drugs needs to be decreased in the elderly patient. The older adult is more sensitive to the toxic and therapeutic effects of analgesics. Even with reduced dosages, drug toxicity occurs more often and is more serious in the elderly patient.

The use of NSAIDs is a particular concern with older adults. Side effects include GI complications, platelet dysfunction, and renal toxicity. Renal function may already be impaired in the older adult, and drug dosage should depend on age and renal function. The risk of GI side effects occurs most often in the first 90 days of treatment with NSAIDs.[43] Concomitant use of misoprostol and lower NSAID dosages have been effective in reducing the incidence of GI side effects. If long-term NSAID therapy is prescribed, a CBC and liver and renal function studies should be done every 6 to 12 months.

Acetaminophen may be an alternative to the use of NSAIDs in older adults with RA. Acetaminophen does not cause GI side effects or platelet dysfunction; however, it lacks antiinflammatory properties. When used as analgesia in a dosage of 4 g/day, acetaminophen was as effective as ibuprofen in providing pain relief.[43] Long-term use of acetaminophen is contraindicated in persons with hepatic or renal impairment.

Even medications such as methotrexate and steroids, which are associated with serious adverse effects, may be safer and more effective than the use of NSAIDs in treating RA in elderly patients. Methotrexate, started in dosages of 5 to 7.5 mg once weekly, then increased to 15 to 20 mg weekly, is well tolerated in older adults. Low doses of prednisone (5 to 7.5 mg/day) take up to 10 years to produce osteoporosis and may be an alternative therapy for older adults, particularly those at risk for developing side effects from NSAIDs. Gold salts are another alternative.

Another factor relevant to treatment of RA in older adults is the need for modification of the home environment to meet the needs of the individual. Mobility impairments induced by RA, coupled with changes associated with aging (hearing loss, decreased vision, loss of balance, and loss of muscle mass), are potential obstacles to preserving independence and function. Raised toilet seats, support bars in the bathroom, handrails, avoidance of scatter rugs, and other modifications to prevent injury may allow the person to remain at home and avoid relocation to an extended care or assisted living facility. Prevention of falls is an important intervention for the older person with RA to avoid fractures and the possible associated complications. Coping with a chronic and potentially disabling condition, in addition to pain and alterations in body image and role performance, may result in depression in the older adult. Nurses are in an ideal position to provide support and counseling to patients. If depression is suspected, a referral for evaluation is indicated.

SPECIAL ENVIRONMENTS FOR CARE

Community-Based Care

In addition to the adaptive and assistive devices previously mentioned, adaptations to the home environment may be necessary. Elevated toilet seats and safety equipment for the bathroom can be installed in the home. Doorways should be wide enough to accommodate a walker or wheelchair if necessary. A ramp can be added for access to the front door if there are stairs. Countertops and cupboards can be lowered to accommodate the person who is wheelchair bound. These modifications may be costly. Patients with severe RA are quite disabled and may need the assistance of a family member or friend to complete ADLs; if that is not feasible, a home health aide may be needed. The patient should continue in a regular exercise program, eat a nutritious, balanced diet, take medications as prescribed, and participate in follow-up care. Meals on Wheels may help provide nutritious meals for those unable to independently prepare meals. Maintenance of social supports and continued participation in social and recreational activities are necessary to prevent social isolation and depression.

COMPLICATIONS

Complications associated with RA are usually a result of systemic manifestations. Pericarditis occurs in approximately 40% of patients with RA.[38] Pulmonary complications are usually asymptomatic but may manifest as infiltrates, nodules, or interstitial pneumonitis. Pulmonary complications may also result from treatment of RA with methotrexate and gold.

Compression neuropathy may develop in the form of carpal and tarsal tunnel syndrome and ulnar nerve palsy. Atlantoaxial (C1 and C2) subluxation is a potentially fatal complication in persons with RA. Cervical subluxation occurs in approximately 15% of persons with RA within 3 years of the onset of disease; patients with RA should be carefully screened for cervical subluxation, particularly if they are undergoing general anesthesia. Any patient with a new onset of neck pain or myelopathy should be evaluated for cervical subluxation.

Rheumatoid vasculitis, inflammation and blockage of small blood vessels, is another potentially severe complication of RA. The extremities are most commonly affected, but involvement of the heart, abdominal organs, muscle, and nerves is possible. Treatment for internal organ involvement is usually high-dose corticosteroids and cyclophosphamide. The initial manifestation of vasculitis may be 1- to 3-mm brown spots on the fingers and fingernails, resulting from small areas of skin infarction. Eventually skin ulcers may form, which may be difficult to heal. Concomitant treatment with corticosteroids or other immunosuppressants may compound the problem.

DEGENERATIVE JOINT DISEASE

Etiology

Degenerative joint disease (DJD), also known as osteoarthritis (OA), hypertrophic arthritis, osteoarthrosis, or senescent arthritis, is an extremely common disease that is probably as old as civilization. Almost everyone older than 40 years of age has hypertrophic changes in the joints. Although symptomatic DJD is usually seen in the 50- to 70-year age-group, it has been observed as early as 20 years of age.

OA results from a series of cellular, biochemical, and biomechanical factors affecting cartilage, subchondral bone, and soft tissues of diarthrodial joints. The cause of primary OA is unknown, but several genetic and acquired risk factors have been identified. The quantity and quality of proteoglycans decrease with the aging process and predispose the cartilage to break down and degenerate. Genetic factors suggest a mutation of the gene that directs the formation of type II collagen.

Epidemiology

OA is the most common form of arthritis; by age 65, over 80% of the population have radiographic evidence of the disease, and 5% to 10% have clinical symptoms. It is estimated that by the year 2020 the incidence of OA in the United States will be greater than 18%, affecting more than 59 million persons.

The pattern of joint involvement is affected by age, gender, and occupation. The incidence of OA increases with age; men usually develop symptoms before 45 years of age; women usually do not develop symptoms until after age 55. Before age

55 there is little difference in joint involvement by gender. Older women usually develop OA in the hands (particularly PIP joints and thumbs) (Figure 47-12) and knees, whereas men typically develop OA in the hips, knees, and spine. Heberden's nodes are more likely to develop in women than in men; a familial tendency has also been noted. Racial background also influences the development of OA; African-American women have a higher incidence of OA of the knee than do Caucasian American women, but a lower incidence of Heberden's nodes. There is a relatively low incidence of hip OA in Asia and among black Africans and Jamaicans.[4,60]

An important modifiable risk factor for developing OA is weight. Studies have shown that obesity contributes 21% to the risk of knee OA.[67] This is an important consideration, in view of the fact that more than 50% of Americans are overweight (as defined as body mass index >25).

The joints most commonly affected by OA are the PIP and distal interphalangeal joints, first carpometacarpal joint, hips, knees, and cervical and lumbar spine. The two forms of OA are primary (idiopathic) and secondary.

Primary joint disease is the most common type of noninflammatory joint disease. Primary DJD is distributed throughout the central and peripheral joints of the body, usually affecting the joints of the hand, wrist, neck, lumbar spine, hip, knee, and ankle.

Secondary joint disease is caused by any condition that damages cartilage, subjects the joints to chronic stress, or causes joint instability. Causes of secondary joint disease include previous joint infection, inflammation, trauma, surgery, and certain occupations or activities. Other causes include endocrine disorders (acromegaly or hyperparathyroidism); neurologic disorders (pain and proprioceptive responses are altered, thereby increasing the risk of abnormal movement or weight bearing); skeletal deformities; and hemophilia (bleeding into the joints). Regular moderate exercise does not appear to cause or increase existing DJD in normal joints.[60,67] Injury to the joint is a significant risk factor for later development of OA.[21]

Pathophysiology

Despite the name osteoarthritis, there is not a significant inflammatory component associated with the disorder. A small amount of low-grade inflammation is observed, and mechanical abnormalities in the joints irritate surrounding soft tissues and can cause inflammation. OA is generally termed noninflammatory to distinguish it from RA (Table 47-7). Both primary and secondary DJDs affect the articular cartilage. Characteristic pathologic changes include:

- Erosion of articular cartilage
- Thickening of subchondral bone
- Formation of osteophytes or bone spurs

Normal articular cartilage is white, translucent, and smooth. When affected by DJD, it becomes yellow and opaque. Areas of cartilage soften, and the surface becomes rough, frayed, and cracked. This process is thought to occur as a result of digestion of the cartilage by enzymes and alteration of the nutrition of the cartilage. Eventually the cartilage is destroyed, and the underlying subchondral bone goes through a remodeling process. Osteophytes, or bone spurs, appear at the joint margins and at the sites of attachment of supporting structures. These may break off and appear in the joint cavity as "joint mice."

Symptoms vary, depending on the joints involved and degree of pathology (see Clinical Manifestations box). Pain is the primary feature and is usually described as a deep aching in the joint. Weather changes and increased activity tend to increase the pain; rest usually provides relief. In contrast to RA, joint stiffness typically lasts less than 1 hour. Decreased joint motion may be caused by the loss of articular cartilage, muscle spasms, shortening of ligaments, and osteophytes; loss of articular cartilage and subchondral bone can lead to joint subluxation and deformity. As the joint degenerates, the person may report decreased mobility and the sensation of grinding and catching. Joint laxity may also develop as a result of effusion and remodeling of tendinous and ligamentous insertions.

Arthritic changes in the hip cause an antalgic gait, and pain is usually felt on the outer aspect of the hip and in the groin, buttocks, inner thigh, and knee. Patients with OA of the knee are most likely to report pain with motion, stiffness after inactivity, and decreased flexion. A varus deformity is common (Figure 47-13 and Box 47-5). OA of the spine is the most common cause of low back pain. Patients may report pain, stiffness, and occasionally neurologic symptoms. Neurologic symptoms can be caused by osteophytes, foraminal stenosis, disk protrusion, or subluxation.

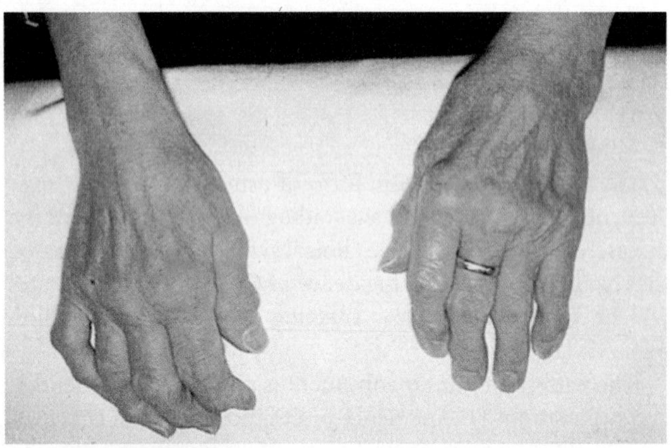

Figure 47-12 Osteoarthritis of hands.

Collaborative Care Management

Objectives in management include relief of pain, restoration of joint function, and prevention of disability or further progression of the disease.

Diagnostic Tests. Diagnosis is based on evaluation of the patient history and physical assessment and the results of radiologic studies. Serologic and synovial fluid examinations are essentially normal. Synovial fluid is pale yellow or clear with a low leukocyte count—500 to 2000 cells/mm^3. Leukocyte counts in excess of 2000 to 3000 are indicative of inflammation; a workup for RA, gout, lupus, and other inflammatory arthropathies should follow. Bloody effusions are usually the result of trauma, fractures of osteophytes or subchondral bone, or synovial or ligamentous tears. Arthroscopy is not

TABLE 47-7 Distinguishing Features of Osteoarthritis and Rheumatoid Arthritis

	Osteoarthritis	Rheumatoid Arthritis
Etiology	Primary: unknown, genetic component Secondary: mechanical stress, trauma, hormonal	Unknown Theories: overstimulation of inflammatory process; autoimmune, genetic, antigen-antibody reaction, viral
Onset	45 to 55 years Insidious	After age 30 Average age 55 years Insidious or acute
Pathophysiology	Disease of articular cartilage Biochemical changes leading to deterioration and loss of cartilage Reactive new bone formation Changes in articular surface Areas of exposed bone may occur Formation of osteophytes No systemic manifestations	Inflammatory disease of joints, connective tissue with systemic manifestations Inflammatory process destroying joint components Formation of pannus Cartilage erosion Soft tissue changes causing joint subluxation and dislocation Formation of rheumatoid nodules
Joint involvement	Asymmetric, monoarticular, or polyarticular DIP joints (Heberden's nodes) PIP joints (Bouchard's nodes) First CMC, first MTP Hips, knees, lumbar and cervical spine	Symmetric, polyarticular PIP joints MCP joints MTP joints Cervical spine Large joints (hip, knee; more common in older adults)
Clinical manifestations	Joint enlargement Crepitus Pain increased with weight bearing, relieved with rest Limitation of joint motion Noninflammatory joint effusion Morning stiffness <1 hour Joint stiffness or laxity	Fever Weight loss Fatigue Night pain Pain with rest Morning stiffness >1 hour Joint "boggy" with palpation, tender, erythematous Inflammatory joint effusion Subluxation, dislocation Rheumatoid nodules
Diagnostic data	No laboratory abnormalities Radiographic evidence of joint space narrowing, osteophytes, bony sclerosis	Rheumatoid factor positive in 75%-80% of patients; elderly onset positive in 90% of persons[48] Elevated ESR Radiographic evidence of joint space narrowing, bone erosion, osteopenia

CMC, Carpometacarpal; *DIP*, distal interphalangeal; *ESR*, erythrocyte sedimentation rate; *PIP*, proximal interphalangeal; *MCP*, metacarpophalangeal; *MTP*, metatarsophalangeal.

necessary for diagnosis of OA, but it is helpful because it allows direct visualization of articular surfaces and early disease may be detected. X-ray films reveal narrowing of the joint space, osteophyte formation, and eburnation (sclerosis) of subchondral bone. Almost 50% of patients with evidence of OA on x-ray studies are asymptomatic.

Medications. Analgesics, NSAIDs, and intraarticular corticosteroids are the mainstays of pharmacologic treatment of OA (Table 47-8). The objective of treatment is symptomatic relief of pain; benefits such as improved mobility and functioning have not been established.

Acetaminophen is a first-line agent for treatment. Doses up to 4 g/day may be given in the absence of hepatic or renal disease. Liver function studies must be done at regular intervals while the patient is receiving therapy. Constant pain is best relieved by dosing at regular intervals; intermittent pain may be relieved by "as needed" dosing. The effectiveness of acetaminophen is similar to that of NSAIDs. Moderate to severe pain

Clinical Manifestations

Degenerative Joint Disease

Pain	Worse with weight bearing; improves with rest; may be accompanied by paresthesias
Swelling and joint enlargement	May be from inflammatory exudate or blood entering joint capsule, causing an increase in synovial fluid, or from fragments of osteophytes entering synovial cavity
Decreased range of motion	Depends on amount of destroyed cartilage
Muscular atrophy	From disuse, joint instability, and deformity
Crepitus	May be present on movement
Joint stiffness	Worse in morning (morning stiffness <1 hour) and after a period of rest or disuse

BOX 47-5 Characteristic Changes or Symptoms in Certain Joints

- Knee involvement: varus (Figure 47-13), valgus (knocked knees), flexion deformity; crepitus; limited range of motion
- Heberden's nodes: bony protuberances occurring on the dorsal surface of the distal interphalangeal joints of the fingers (Figure 47-14)
- Bouchard's nodes: bony protuberances occurring on the proximal interphalangeal joints of the fingers (Figure 47-14)
- Coxarthrosis (degenerative joint disease of the hip): pain in the hip on weight bearing, with pain progressing to include groin and medial knee pain and limited range of motion

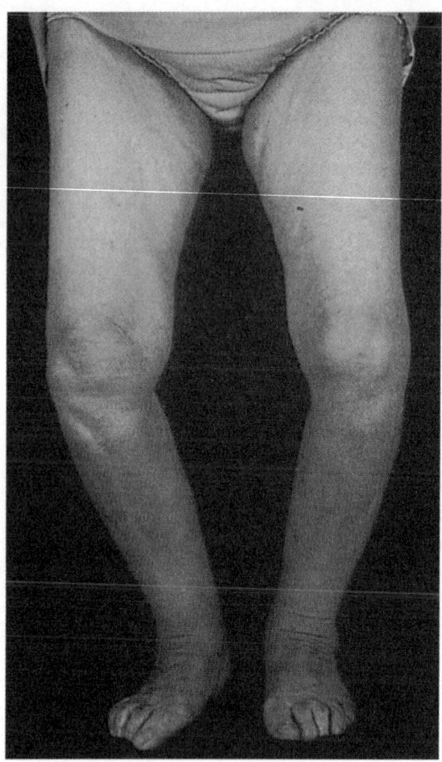

Figure 47-13 Typical varus deformity of knee osteoarthritis.

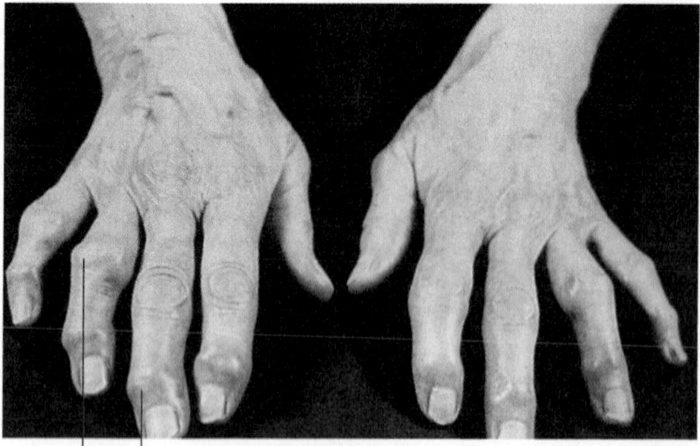

Figure 47-14 Heberden's and Bouchard's nodes.

can also be managed by opioids or adjuvant drugs if nonopioids and NSAIDs are ineffective.

If acetaminophen is contraindicated because of liver or renal disease, NSAIDs are the next choice for therapy. As mentioned earlier, a small degree of inflammation may be present; thus NSAIDs have the advantage of having an antiinflammatory effect. There is no convincing evidence to support the hypothesis that NSAIDs retard articular cartilage degeneration or alter the course of the disease.

NSAIDs act by preventing the formation of prostaglandins, which play a major role in pain and inflammation; most inhibit both COX-1 and COX-2 enzyme formation. Inhibition of COX-1 formation can lead to serious adverse effects, including bleeding and GI ulceration. Newer selective COX-2 inhibitors have a lesser incidence of GI side effects and are the NSAID of choice in OA therapy; however, these drugs are more expensive than older COX-1 inhibitors.

All NSAIDs have the potential for renal and hepatic dysfunction; kidney and liver function studies should be monitored for persons receiving long-term therapy. Studies show that NSAIDs have increased blood pressure by 5 mm Hg in normotensive and hypertensive persons.[67a] Hypertensive effects are increased in persons taking angiotensive-converting enzyme inhibitors, diuretics, and beta blockers. More research is necessary to determine the cardiovascular effects of the COX-2 inhibitors. The risk of developing side effects is increased with a history of ulcers, GI bleeding, congestive heart failure, cirrhosis, diabetes, and NSAID intolerance; with concomitant use of steroids or anticoagulants; in the elderly; and in persons in poor general health.[4,18] Certain NSAIDs are available in cream or gel form for topical application.

Intraarticular injection of steroids may be needed if analgesics and NSAIDs are ineffective or as an adjunct to therapy. Unstable or infected joints should never be injected. Steroid injections are effective in controlling pain and improving function. However, repeated injections may actually accelerate joint degeneration. To prevent articular cartilage damage, a joint should not be injected more than three to four times per year. Other complications include infection and cutaneous atrophy.

Viscosupplementation, developed in the 1960s, is based on the fact that synovial fluid in persons with OA is less elastic and less viscous than normal synovial fluid. The objective of treatment is to restore the normal elasticity and viscosity of the synovial fluid and restore the normal balance of hyaluronan within the fluid. Hyaluronan (hyaluronic acid) is a glycosamine polysaccharide and is found in high concentrations in normal synovial fluid. In persons with OA, the concentration of hyaluronan is decreased, and the amount of synovial fluid is increased. Viscosupplementation may be used in combination with other medications for treatment of OA.

Treatments. Treatment early in the course of DJD can make a significant improvement in the person's quality of life

TABLE 47-8 Common Medications for Osteoarthritis

Medication	Action	Intervention
Acetaminophen (dosage 1-4 g/day)	Analgesic for mild to moderate pain; first-line treatment for patients with minimal inflammation	Low cost, good safety profile. Monitor liver function at beginning of therapy and every 6-12 months while taking medication; contraindicated in persons with liver disease or regular high intake of alcohol because of risk of liver toxicity. Teach patient not to exceed 4 g/day, to carefully read over-the-counter (OTC) medication labels, since many contain acetaminophen. Nausea most common side effect.
NSAIDs (nonselective)	Analgesic and antiinflammatory; prevent formation of prostaglandins	Studies show NSAIDs do not provide superior pain relief to acetaminophen.[4,18,71] Prescribe with caution because of incidence of side effects (nausea, heartburn, GI bleeding, platelet dysfunction, renal and liver dysfunction, congestive heart failure). Prescribe in lowest effective dose and with prophylactic gastroprotective drug. Monitor blood pressure, renal and liver function, and signs of GI bleeding while patient is receiving therapy. Avoid concomitant use of other NSAIDs, steroids, anticoagulants, and alcohol.
NSAIDs (COX-2 selective inhibitors) Celecoxib (Celebrex) Rofecoxib (Vioxx) Meloxicam (Mobic)	Analgesic and antiinflammatory; selectively inhibits prostaglandin synthesis by inhibiting cyclooxygenase-2 (COX-2); gastroprotective prophylaxis may be beneficial in high-risk patients	Contraindicated in persons with allergies to aspirin, other NSAIDs, sulfonamides (with celecoxib); renal and hepatic dysfunction; asthma; and in pregnancy. Monitor for renal and hepatic function, signs of bleeding. Use cautiously in persons with congestive heart failure or hypertension; peripheral edema may occur.
Opioid analgesics Tramadol (Ultram) Codeine Oxycodone (may be combined with acetaminophen [Percocet] or aspirin [Percodan]) Propoxyphene (Darvon) may be combined with acetaminophen (Darvocet)	Bind with receptors in central nervous system to produce analgesia; relief of moderate to severe pain when acetaminophen or NSAIDs are ineffective in relieving pain	Causes central nervous system depression, respiratory depression; side effects include nausea, dizziness, constipation, sedation. Use cautiously in persons with renal or hepatic disease. Monitor for signs of toxicity. Teach patient to avoid hazardous activity when taking medication; institute safety precautions. Monitor bowel function; may take stool softener to prevent constipation. Potential for drug dependence and tolerance.
Intraarticular steroid injection (triamincinolone [Kenalog], methylprednisolone [Depo-Medrol])	Antiinflammatory; used in cases of inflammation or knee infusion	Potential adverse effects on connective tissue; limit injections to two to three per year per joint.
Intraarticular hyaluronan hylan G-250 (Synvisc) Sodium hyaluronate (Hyalgan)	Glycosaminoglycan; simulates synovial fluid; mode of action poorly understood; substitutes for naturally produced hyaluronic acid, which lubricates joint and acts as shock absorber	Require a series of injections; expensive ($500 per series). Pain relief begins 5-9 weeks after completing injections and may last up to 6 months.[71] Pain may occur at injection site; risk of infection; few local reactions; no systemic reactions. Rate of response less in persons with advanced disease; may benefit those awaiting joint replacement. Hyaluronan hylan G-250 is made from chicken combs and is contraindicated in persons with poultry allergy.
Topical agents Capsaicin NSAIDs (salicylate, benzydamine, diclofenac, ibuprofen) OTC preparations (Icy Hot, Aspercreme)	Provide pain relief and/or antiinflammatory action; capsaicin, derived from pepper plant, acts as substance P inhibitor; others may contain local anesthetics	Relatively safe and inexpensive; fewer side effects with short-term use of topical agents than with systemic NSAIDs. Avoid contact with mucous membranes.

GI, Gastrointestinal; *NSAIDs*, nonsteroidal antiinflammatory drugs; *OTC*, over-the-counter.

and may alter the course of the disease. Three foci of therapy are relief of pain, joint protection, and PT to stabilize joints and prevent deformity. Joint protection techniques may include weight reduction and the use of canes or splints.

Exercise is indicated to maintain and restore function. Maintenance of muscle strength can be attained by engaging in regular exercise. An appropriate warm-up and cool-down program is essential to prevent muscle strain and damage. ROM exercises should be performed daily. Isometric and isotonic exercises, which do not stress the joint, are an excellent starting point. As strength and endurance increase, progressive, resistive exercises can be added to the regimen. Low-impact aerobic exercise improves cardiovascular functioning, increases well-being, and helps with weight reduction if needed. Swimming and water exercises, which decrease stress on joints, are good choices. In general, persons with OA should avoid high-impact activities and exercises, which can increase symptoms, especially if weight-bearing joints are involved. The Arthritis Foundation offers exercise classes at many community centers for persons with arthritis.

Heat applied before exercise can be helpful in relaxing the muscles, increasing blood flow to the region, and decreasing pain. Moist heat is generally preferred. Application of cold after exercise or during periods of acute inflammation decreases pain and swelling. For the patient with decreased function due to DJD, adaptive aids, PT, and pain relief medications can be prescribed. Adaptive devices may be beneficial for completing ADLs for persons with DJD of the hands. (See section on treatments for RA for information on assistive and adaptive devices and joint protection techniques.) Persons with advanced DJD, severe pain, or severe limitations in function or mobility may be candidates for surgical management of their disease.

Surgical Management. Surgical management of the person with OA is indicated to relieve pain, improve function, or correct deformity. Surgical procedures include those that preserve or restore articular cartilage and those that realign, fuse, or replace joints. Surgical management usually provides the patient with excellent results; however, the patient is at risk for developing surgical complications, including infection, nerve and blood vessel injury, deep vein thrombosis, and pulmonary or fat embolism. Surgery is performed when medications and PT have failed. However, surgery should be performed before severe deformity, joint instability, contracture, or severe muscle atrophy develop, all of which can seriously compromise the outcome and place the patient at a higher risk for developing complications.

Procedures to restore or preserve articular cartilage include joint debridement (via arthroscopy), abrasion chondroplasty (abrasion of subchondral bone to stimulate growth of cartilage), and replacement of articular cartilage with grafts. These procedures are not indicated for patients with advanced DJD, because they usually produce only short-term results. An alternative therapy is the transplantation of healthy cartilage (autologous cartilage implantation) cells into the knees of persons with traumatic arthritis or other cartilage defects. Chondrocytes are harvested, cultured in the laboratory, and injected into the knee.[49] Young persons with small areas of damaged cartilage are the ideal candidates for cartilage transplantation; the patient must be committed to a 12-month rehabilitation program.

An osteotomy is a surgical incision through a bone. Osteotomy may be thought of as a surgical or intentional fracture. The purpose of osteotomy is to realign a joint or bone or to redistribute the load-bearing surface of a joint to a region that has more articular cartilage (Figure 47-15). Osteotomy is useful for correcting angulation or rotational deformities. The patient is treated similarly to a patient who has suffered a fracture. Persons with stable joints, functional ROM, adequate musculature, and some remaining articular cartilage benefit the most from osteotomy.

Arthrodesis, or joint fusion, is performed to relieve pain and to restore stability and alignment. Joint fusion, as the term implies, results in lost motion; hence this procedure has limited application. The fusion of one joint increases the load bearing of adjacent joints, which may accelerate degeneration of those joints. Arthrodesis is most commonly performed on the cervical and lumbar spine, interphalangeal joints, first metatarsal joints, and the wrist and ankle.

Joint replacement, or arthroplasty, has been a mainstay of treatment for OA since the 1960s. Sir John Charnley, a pioneer in arthroplasty surgery, first described his success with hip arthroplasty in 1961. The hip was the first joint to be successfully replaced and continues to be replaced in many persons with OA. More than 200,000 total hip replacements are performed annually in the United States.[56] Although arthroplasty procedures of the hip and knee are the most common (Figures 47-16 and 47-17), the procedure can also be performed on the shoulder, elbow, ankle, and finger joints.

Materials for prosthetic implants are metal (titanium or cobalt-chrome alloy), high-density polyethylene, ceramic (low friction and longer wear), and other synthetic materials (Figure 47-18). Replacement prostheses may be implanted with polymethylmethacrylate, may be uncemented, or may be a combination of both (hybrid). Uncemented prostheses are

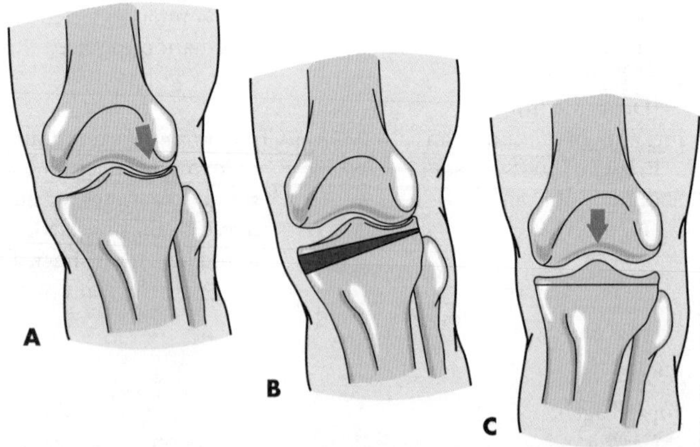

Figure 47-15 Osteotomy of tibia for genu valgum (valgus deformity); anterior view of left knee. **A**, Weight-bearing force is concentrated on one compartment of the knee. **B**, A wedge of bone is removed from the tibia. The amount of bone removed is determined by how much correction in angulation is necessary. **C**, The distal portion of the tibia is swung to the proximal portion. The correction of angulation obtained allows weight-bearing forces to be more evenly distributed through both compartments of the knee.

treated with a porous coating that promotes bony ingrowth (see Figure 47-18). New, minimally invasive techniques for hip replacement (traditionally performed as an open procedure) are being developed that could significantly reduce postoperative pain and recovery time (see Future Watch box); robotically aided surgery is also being developed for joint replacements.

The decision whether or not to use cement depends on such factors as the individual patient, including his or her bone stock, age, and ability to comply with weight-bearing restrictions after surgery. Uncemented components are thought to last longer, since the bony growth lessens the likelihood of the prosthesis loosening, which is a consideration with cemented joints. Loosening of the components may lead to implant failure. In addition, uncemented joints are usually easier to replace and revise than cemented joints.

Total knee (medial and lateral femorotibial) arthroplasty is a technically more difficult procedure than total hip replacement, because of the complex movements of the knee joint. The patella may or may not be replaced in total knee surgery. A unicompartmental or unicondylar knee arthroplasty replaces the medial or lateral compartment of the femorotibial joint.

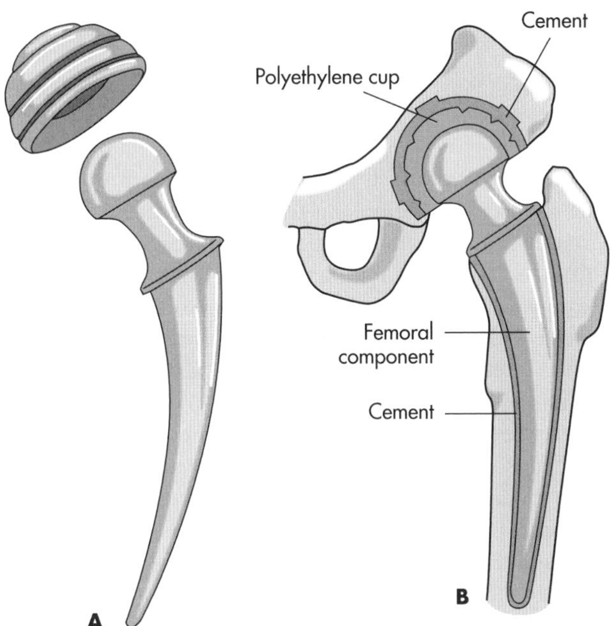

Figure 47-16 **A,** Acetabular and femoral components of total hip prosthesis. **B,** Total hip prosthesis in place.

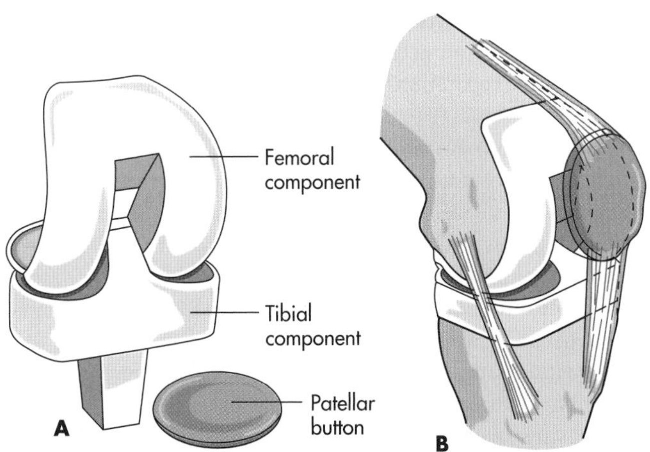

Figure 47-17 **A,** Tibial and femoral components of total knee prosthesis. A patellar button, made of polyethylene, protects the posterior surface of the patella from friction against the femoral component when the knee is moved through flexion and extension. **B,** Total knee prosthesis in place.

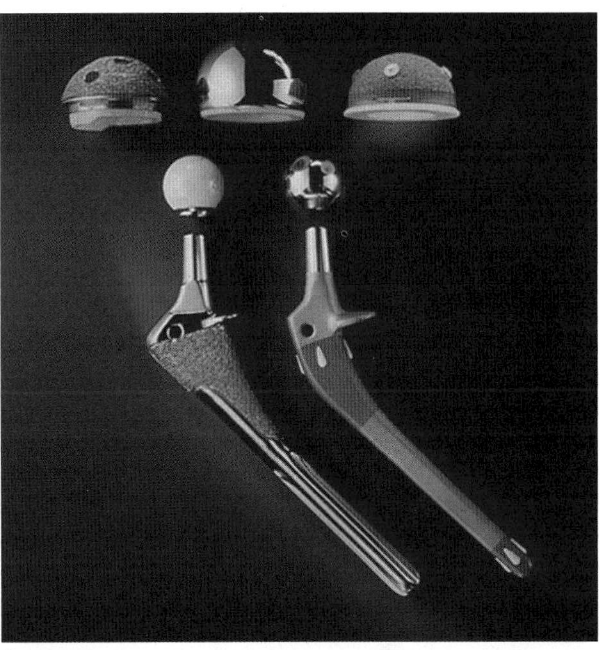

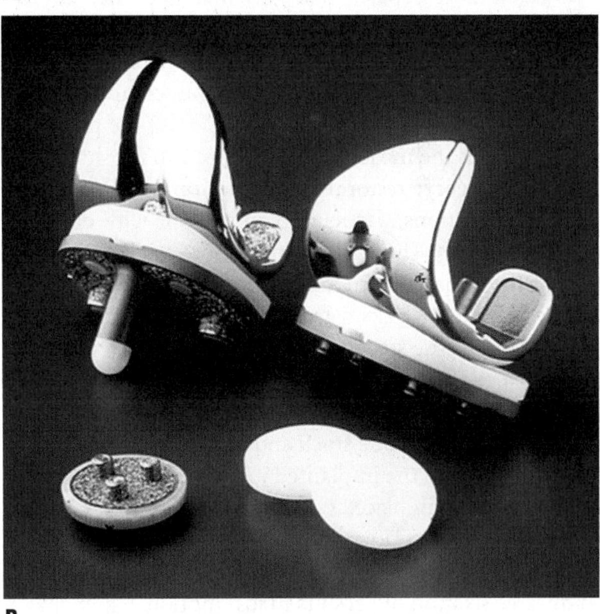

Figure 47-18 **A,** Hip prostheses. *Left:* Porous ingrowth acetabular cup and femoral stem, ceramic femoral head. *Middle:* Bipolar head for hemiarthroplasty (component fits on top of femoral head component). Used with either cemented or uncemented femoral stems. *Right:* Cemented femoral stem and cemented acetabular cup. **B, K**nee prostheses. *Left:* Porous ingrowth femoral and tibial components; porous ingrowth patellar button. *Right:* Hybrid: cemented femoral component and patellar button; porous ingrowth tibial component.

Future Watch
Minimally Invasive Hip Replacement Surgery

Orthopedic surgeons are developing a minimally invasive approach for hip replacement surgery. Instead of the traditional 12- to 18-inch posterolateral hip incision, the procedure is performed through two 1-inch incisions and with smaller instruments. The same types of joint components are used as in open procedures. The less invasive approach involves less blood loss and less soft tissue dissection, with resultant decreased pain after surgery. A study of 120 patients is underway to evaluate long-term effectiveness of this new procedure.

Reference: Minimally invasive hip surgery eases pain and reduces recovery time, *The Cutting Edge News for the OR Professional,* July 30, 2001, website: http://www.orsoftware.com/newsletter/2001_0730/.

All joint components have a finite life span. When originally developed in the 1970s, joint prostheses were expected to last about 10 years; then revision surgery was indicated. Today approximately 85% of joint implants will last 20 years.[30] Advances in prosthetic components, surgical technique, bearing surfaces, and methods of fixation have resulted in increased implant survival rates. The prosthetic implants are subject to fatigue, wear, breakage, and failure. A particular risk associated with total joint arthroplasty is infection, which usually necessitates removal of the prosthesis. Most revisions are done because of component loosening; infection and implant failure are other reasons for revision. Revision surgery typically lasts longer, involves more blood loss, and results in less joint function than the primary procedure.

Total shoulder replacement was first described in 1893, long before the first hip replacement. Since the 1970s, replacement of the shoulder joint has become more common; both total arthroplasty (glenoid and humeral component) and hemiarthroplasty (humeral component only) are performed. Relief of pain is the most common indication for shoulder replacement surgery; restoration of motion and strength are lesser considerations, particularly in persons with damage to the rotator cuff.[56] The surgical procedure is challenging because of the dynamic structure and movements of the joint. The shoulder joint lacks a true socket and depends on surrounding soft tissue structures for its stability.

Total elbow replacements are primarily performed to relieve the pain and disability associated with RA. The patient must have adequate bone stock and ligamentous structures to provide stability to the implanted joint. Both components are usually cemented in place.

Ankle fusion has traditionally been the procedure of choice for surgical treatment of ankle OA. Fusion provides pain relief and durable fixation but results in lost motion, which may result in arthritis of the hindfoot. Joint replacement offers the benefit of pain relief and ankle motion. Disadvantages of ankle arthroplasty include problems with wound healing, loosening of components, and higher complication rates.[10] The ankle joint is formed by the tibia, talus, and fibula; the joint space is called the ankle mortise. Both two- and three-component prostheses are available; currently all are bony ingrowth.

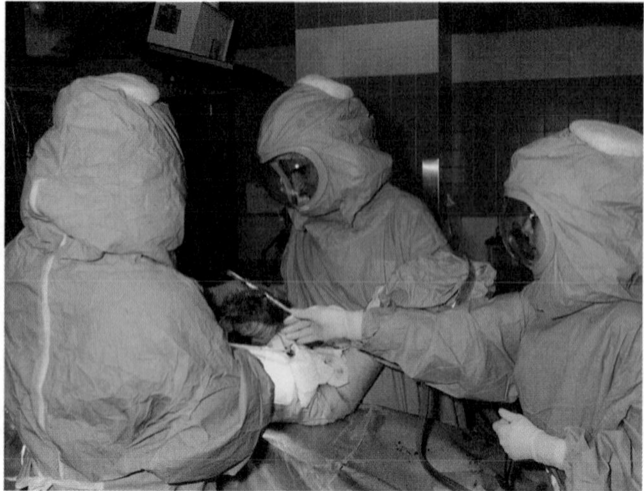

Figure 47-19 Body exhaust system during total joint replacement surgery.

Wound healing has historically been a major problem with ankle replacement; more long-term data are needed to evaluate newer prostheses and surgical techniques.[10]

Another type of joint replacement is the interposition arthroplasty, in which the joint surface on one or both sides is replaced with metal, inert material (polyethylene), fascia, or tendon. Interposition arthroplasty is usually performed on the wrist or MCP joints of the fingers.

Preventing infection is a priority of care with all joint replacement surgery. Revision surgery carries a higher risk of infection because of the longer operating time. Sources of infection in the operating room include direct contamination of the wound and contamination of the sterile field or personnel. The rate of infection in patients with total hip replacements is approximately 1%; the rate is 2% in total knee replacement and 5% to 10% in ankle replacement.[1,14] An estimated 50% to 80% of infections originate in the operating room by direct wound contamination.[1] Measures taken to prevent surgically acquired infection include the use of laminar airflow systems; body exhaust systems for scrubbed and circulating personnel; limited traffic in the operating room and use of an "outside circulating nurse," skin preparation, and strict adherence to sterile technique (Figure 47-19). Other techniques include antibiotic-impregnated cement and prophylactic perioperative antibiotics.

Diet. Appropriate nutritional intake is encouraged to maintain ideal body weight and avoid weight gain. Weight gain places an unnecessary stress on joints, particularly the hips and knees. Nutritional supplements are also used in combination with medications and other treatments (see Complementary & Alternative Therapies box).

Activity. As described earlier, exercise is a cornerstone of treatment for persons with DJD. Emphasis is placed on unloading the stress on painful weight-bearing joints through the use of canes, walkers, or crutches; ROM exercises to prevent deformities and contractures; and muscle-strengthening exercises to increase or maintain muscle tone and strength.

Exercise is also beneficial in reducing fatigue, a common complaint in persons with chronic disease. In persons with

Complementary & Alternative Therapies
Osteoarthritis

Both glucosamine and chondroitin are classified as nutritional supplements and are not approved by the U.S. Food and Drug Administration (FDA) for the treatment of osteoarthritis (OA). Both products are available over the counter and are widely used to relieve mild pain and stiffness associated with OA. Glucosamine has been used successfully in Europe for over 25 years.[51]

Glucosamine (glucosamine hydrochloride and sulfate) occurs naturally in the body and when taken as a supplement is derived from chitin in the shells of shrimp, crab, and lobster. It is available as a tablet, cream, or beverage and has been shown to be effective in reducing pain and possibly in improving the health of cartilage by contributing to cartilage repair.[4,18] Most studies demonstrating the effectiveness of glucosamine have involved glucosamine sulfate; there are less data to support the effectiveness of glucosamine hydrochloride. Known side effects are few. They include nausea, rash, and possible allergic reactions in persons with shellfish allergy. Glucose metabolism, particularly in persons with diabetes, should be monitored, since glucosamine is a derivative of glucose. The usual dose is 1500 mg daily (2000 mg/day for persons weighing over 200 pounds); at least 2 months of therapy is necessary to determine effectiveness.

Chondroitin sulfite is a component of human cartilage; when taken as a supplement, it is derived from the trachea of cattle. The recommended dose is 1200 mg/day in two divided doses. It is available in pills, capsules, lotion, or liquid and is often sold in combination with glucosamine. Studies have shown chondroitin to be effective in relieving pain and stiffness associated with OA, with few or no adverse effects. There is no evidence to support topical use of chondroitin. Persons taking warfarin should not use chondroitin, since it interferes with warfarin levels. As with glucosamine, it may take 2 months or longer to determine effectiveness of therapy. Monthly costs for both substances average $30 to $45.

The American College of Rheumatology believes that more studies are indicated to prove the efficacy of these agents in the treatment of OA. The National Institute of Arthritis and Musculoskeletal and Skin Diseases, the National Institutes of Health, and the National Center for Complementary and Alternative Medicine are conducting studies to evaluate the effectiveness of both these substances.[51] Nurses should be prepared to discuss the benefits and precautions regarding the use of these nutritional supplements for treatment of OA.

advanced disease, exercise may exacerbate symptoms. Rest relieves most joint pain but should be avoided for prolonged periods, because immobility promotes joint stiffness. Persons with DJD of the lower extremities should also avoid prolonged standing or kneeling.

Referrals. Common referrals for persons with DJD include PT and OT. As described earlier, the Arthritis Foundation is an excellent resource and offers the "Arthritis Self-Help" course to help individuals manage pain, fatigue, and stress and to develop individualized exercise programs. The Arthritis Foundation is a nonprofit organization; it also publishes the magazine *Arthritis Today.*

NURSING MANAGEMENT OF PATIENT UNDERGOING JOINT REPLACEMENT SURGERY

A Nursing Care Plan for a patient undergoing joint replacement is found on pp. 1530 to 1532.

PREOPERATIVE CARE

As described in Chapter 16, preoperative data are usually gathered at a preadmission appointment or surgeon's office. Many institutions have joint replacement classes, brochures, videos, and other teaching aids to enhance preoperative instruction and decrease anxiety. The patient is assessed for risk factors (see Chapter 16) that may influence perioperative care. Nursing interventions should focus on providing accurate information on the perioperative experience.

The presence of infection is a contraindication to joint replacement surgery. Infection causes loosening of the prosthetic components and may progress to osteomyelitis. The presence of respiratory conditions may delay surgery. Persons with severe chronic obstructive pulmonary disease or those with pneumonia are at particular risk perioperatively, since methylmethacrylate (bone cement) is excreted through the lungs, which may cause pneumonitis or worsen a preexisting respiratory condition.

The patient and family require teaching about potential complications and preventive measures after joint replacement surgery. Persons having knee or hip joints replaced are at risk for the development of deep vein thrombosis (DVT) and pulmonary or fat embolism. A history of previous DVT or bilateral knee or hip replacement surgery places the patient at an increased risk. Without prophylactic anticoagulation, the frequency of DVT in persons undergoing hip replacement surgery is as high as 50% to 60% and up to 80% in persons undergoing knee replacement surgery.[56,65] Persons with recurrent embolism or in whom anticoagulant therapy is contraindicated may require a more invasive approach to prevention of thromboembolism, including placement of an inferior vena cava filter.[56] The high incidence of DVT in patients with a hip replacement may be related to occlusion of the femoral vein, which occurs during the operative procedure. The femoral vein may become twisted, damaging the endothelium during disarticulation of the femoral head from the acetabulum. These factors, in addition to postoperative immobility and hypercoagulability, place the patient at a significant risk for the development of DVT.[24,65] Length of surgery in excess of 30 minutes is the most documented risk factor for DVT. Any joint replacement surgery takes longer than 30 minutes; revision surgery may last as long as 4 or more hours. Proximal DVTs are more likely to occur because of the surgical technique. Persons undergoing a total knee replacement are at an increased risk for DVT because of surgical technique. Intraoperatively, the extremity is wrapped in an elastic bandage and a pneumatic tourniquet is inflated to reduce blood loss. The use of the tourniquet and elastic wrap may damage the endothelial lining of the vein, attracting platelets and causing aggregation and possibly thrombus. In addition, the use of bone cement, which produces release of heat, may

Nursing Care Plan — Patient With a Total Knee Replacement

DATA Mr. C. is a 59-year-old married office manager with osteoarthritis of the left knee. Over the past 8 months he has experienced increased pain with only minimal relief from nonsteroidal antiinflammatory drugs (NSAIDs). He now ambulates with a cane when his pain is severe. Because of pain and limited mobility, he is no longer able to participate in many activities he once enjoyed. On the advice of his physician, he has elected to undergo total knee replacement.

The nursing history reveals that Mr. C.:

- And his wife reside in a two-story house with the bedroom upstairs
- Plans to return home after his hospitalization, where he will remain during his 6-month leave from work
- Has no other preexisting medical problems and takes only NSAIDs
- Was last hospitalized 18 years ago for a cholecystectomy
- Attended a total knee replacement class 2 weeks before his admission as part of his preadmission screening
- Discontinued taking NSAIDs 1 week before his scheduled surgery

Collaborative nursing actions include monitoring for:

- Neurovascular compromise
- Bleeding
- Fluid and electrolyte imbalance
- Elimination problems
- Impaired skin integrity and/or delayed wound healing

NURSING DIAGNOSIS **Deficient knowledge related to lack of exposure to total knee replacement surgery**
GOALS/OUTCOMES Will verbalize understanding of impending surgery and need for continued follow-up care; will participate in postoperative rehabilitation care and exercises

NOC Suggested Outcomes

- Knowledge: Disease Process (1803)
- Knowledge: Health Resources (1806)
- Knowledge: Infection Control (1807)
- Knowledge: Medications (1808)
- Knowledge: Prescribed Activity (1811)

NIC Suggested Interventions

- Teaching: Disease Process (5602)
- Teaching: Individual (5606)
- Teaching: Preoperative (5610)
- Teaching: Prescribed Activity/Exercise (5612)
- Teaching: Prescribed Medication (5616)

Nursing Interventions/Rationales

- Assess need for instruction and provide as needed. *Teaching needs vary among patients. Assessment helps individualize teaching to specific patient needs.*
- Review preoperative instructions with patient and wife. Provide written materials, videos, anatomic model of knee, and sample knee prostheses if available. *To help the patient and wife understand the surgical procedure, decrease anxiety, and increase the likelihood of postoperative compliance with the treatment plan. Written materials reinforce verbal teaching. Models or videos demonstrate the procedure better than oral descriptions.*
- Evaluate patient's understanding of information taught and reinforce learning as needed. *To determine the need for further teaching. Reinforcement of information previously taught improves retention.*
- Keep patient and family informed of plan of care and rationales for treatment. *Encourages family support and participation in care routines while the patient is hospitalized and following discharge.*
- Have patient demonstrate independent transfer and ambulation with appropriate ambulatory aid before discharge. *To assess the patient's ability to ambulate and determine the need for further teaching or assistance.*
- Have patient demonstrate exercises to be performed at home (straight leg raises and active flexion). *To determine the need for further teaching or assistance.*
- Have patient verbalize the need for maintaining activity restrictions for 2 months or until follow-up appointment with surgeon. *Kneeling and jarring activities are to be avoided to prevent dislocation of the prosthesis.*
- Provide information and rationales for discharge restrictions and activities. *Understanding the rationale for activities and restrictions may promote compliance and avoidance of complications.*
- Assess the wife's ability to assist with home care. *To determine if the need for further support exists.*
- Assess layout of home, number of stairs, proximity of bathroom to bedroom, and potential safety hazards. *The home environment may need to be arranged to increase the patient's independence and decrease the risk for injury.*
- Teach patient the importance of follow-up examinations. *To determine effectiveness of the treatment plan and detect problems for early intervention.*

Evaluation Parameters

1. Explains preoperative and general postoperative care
2. Reports decreased anxiety
3. Actively participates in plan of care
4. Performs prescribed exercises and maintains activity restrictions
5. Verbalizes understanding of prescribed home medications

Nursing Care Plan — *Patient With a Total Knee Replacement—cont'd*

NURSING DIAGNOSIS **Acute pain related to knee replacement surgery**
GOALS/OUTCOMES Will report decrease in or absence of pain following use of pain relief measures

NOC Suggested Outcomes
- Pain Control (1605)
- Pain Level (2102)

NIC Suggested Interventions
- Pain Management (1400)
- Analgesic Administration (2210)

Nursing Interventions/Rationales
- Assess patient's pain before and after comfort interventions. *To determine the degree of postoperative pain and effectiveness of pain relief measures.*
- Apply ice or a cooling pad to operative site for 48 hours after surgery as prescribed. *Ice reduces swelling, which contributes to pain.*
- Encourage use of patient-controlled analgesia (PCA) before pain becomes severe. *Milder pain is more readily controlled than severe pain.*
- Encourage use of PCA before exercise periods. *The patient can perform exercises better if pain is manageable.*
- Monitor use and effectiveness of PCA. *PCA avoids peaks and valleys associated with intermittent use of analgesics. It also allows the patient greater control over his pain and its elimination.*
- Encourage use of nonpharmacologic pain relief measures if acceptable to patient. *Relaxation, repositioning, and distraction are helpful for reducing and controlling pain; however, for these measures to be beneficial, the patient must believe that they will help.*

Evaluation Parameters
1. Reports pain relief within 30 minutes of prescribed analgesics
2. Reports satisfaction with pain relief measures
3. Decreased use of pain medications before discharge

NURSING DIAGNOSIS **Impaired physical mobility related to pain secondary to total knee replacement**
GOALS/OUTCOMES Will regain mobility within prescribed limitations by discharge

NOC Suggested Outcomes
- Pain Control (1605)
- Pain Level (2102)

NIC Suggested Interventions
- Pain Management (1400)
- Analgesic Administration (2210)

Nursing Interventions/Rationales
- Turn patient from side to back to side every 2 hours and as necessary while on bed rest. *Frequent turning and repositioning promotes circulation, respiratory effort, and muscle activity.*
- Elevate operative leg on pillows when in bed and up in chair for first 24 to 48 hours, avoiding passive flexion of knee. *Elevating the leg enhances venous return. Avoiding flexion prevents flexion contracture.*
- Assist patient with transfer out of bed on the first postoperative day, allowing weight bearing on operative leg with assistive device only. *To prevent complications of immobility. Weight-bearing restrictions are dependent on the method used to implant the prosthesis.*
- Encourage patient to perform active dorsiplantar flexion, isometric quadriceps setting exercises, and straight leg raises (after drain is removed) every 2 hours until fully ambulatory, then four times a day. *Exercising the lower extremities prevents venous stasis and promotes muscle strengthening.*
- Help patient to walk using the appropriate ambulatory aide, increasing the distance walked each day. *Hastens recovery and prevents postoperative complications related to immobility.*
- Encourage patient to sit up in chair as tolerated, especially for meals. *To encourage movement to prevent complications from immobility.*
- If continuous passive motion machine is used, patient's leg should be in the machine a minimum of 8 to 12 hours/day up to 22 hours/day if tolerated. *To prevent excessive swelling and bruising at the site of surgery and to promote even healing of the involved joint tissues.*
- Begin active flexion exercise of the knee on the second postoperative day and encourage flexion four times a day. *Promotes return of function. It is desirable that the patient achieve approximately 90 degrees of active flexion before discharge from the hospital.*
- Encourage use of knee exerciser. *Promotes return of function.*
- Advise patient that a knee immobilizer may be worn at night as a resting splint. *Helps prevent painful muscle spasms by supporting the knee at rest.*

Continued

Nursing Care Plan Patient With a Total Knee Replacement—cont'd

Evaluation Parameters
1. Uses assistive devices correctly to aid with mobility
2. Remains free of complications of immobility
3. Performs prescribed exercises
4. Maintains prescribed limitations

NURSING DIAGNOSIS **Risk for ineffective therapeutic regimen management related to lack of knowledge and altered ability to care for self**

GOALS/OUTCOMES Will assume responsibility for self-care at home

NOC Suggested Outcomes
- Compliance Behavior (1601)
- Participation: Health Care Decisions (1606)

NIC Suggested Interventions
- Discharge Planning (7370)
- Home Maintenance Assistance (7180)
- Family Support (7140)
- Mutual Goal Setting (4410)

Nursing Interventions/Rationales
- Assess patient's/wife's perception of problems that may occur with management of self-care at home. *To identify actual or perceived needs and obstacles to the patient caring for himself at home.*
- Determine the type of equipment needed (e.g., crutches, walker, elevated toilet seat) and obtain any needed equipment. *To facilitate the patient's/wife's ability to successfully care for the patient at home.*
- Assess the home environment for needed changes (e.g., arranging for first-floor sleeping arrangements). *To facilitate the patient's recovery at home and the patient's/wife's ability to provide that care.*
- Encourage patient to participate in decisions about rehabilitation and self-care at home. *Involving the patient in decision making increases the likelihood of compliance with the prescribed treatment/rehabilitation plan.*

Evaluation Parameters
1. Correctly self-administers prescribed medications
2. Verbalizes the need for keeping follow-up appointments
3. Participates in decision making about home care

cause local venous damage and an increased risk of DVT.[65] Reaming of the intramedullary canal and seating of the femoral component may result in a fat embolus.

Prophylaxis for DVT may begin preoperatively or intraoperatively using low-molecular-weight heparin (LMWH), heparin, or warfarin. Other protocols begin anticoagulation postoperatively. Using institutional or surgeon protocol, the patient should be advised to discontinue any NSAIDs, aspirin, anticoagulants, or steroids at the prescribed interval before surgery. Steroid therapy needs to be tapered and may take several weeks to discontinue; aspirin and NSAIDs are generally discontinued 7 to 10 days before surgery. Results of coagulation studies should be within the normal range before surgery. Despite the use of prophylaxis, the incidence of DVT in elective orthopedic surgery is estimated to be 20%.[46]

Persons undergoing major orthopedic surgery often have significant perioperative blood loss; persons undergoing total hip replacement may lose 1000 to 2000 ml.[19] Depending on the procedure performed and expected blood loss, either type and screen or type and cross-matching is ordered. Autologous donation (see Chapter 16) is another alternative. The patient should be informed about autologous donation of blood in sufficient time to allow donation. Preoperative autologous donation decreases the patient's hemoglobin and hematocrit levels before surgery and can exacerbate anemia.[19] An iron supplement is usually prescribed if the patient opts for autologous donation.

Erythropoietin-alfa given before surgery is effective in stimulating erythropoiesis and reducing the need for allogenic transfusion by 50%.[19] Candidates for erythropoietin therapy include persons scheduled for major elective hip or knee surgery with baseline hemoglobin values between 10 and 13 g/dl.[21]

In cases where anticipated blood loss is significant, intraoperative and postoperative blood salvage techniques may be used to allow for reinfusion either intraoperatively or after surgery. A pneumatic tourniquet is used intraoperatively during knee replacement surgery to reduce blood loss.

Preoperative diagnostics depend on the patient's age and medical condition (see Chapter 16). The results of the examinations and laboratory testing should be evaluated before the patient's admission to the hospital, in case additional studies are needed or abnormal results require medical intervention. Objective data to be gathered regarding the musculoskeletal system include the following: joint ROM; presence of deformities such as varus, valgus, or flexion; leg length discrepancies; condition of joints, enlargement, erythema, crepitus, and asymmetry; gait; and ability to perform ADLs.

The patient is also instructed about the perioperative routine, including respiratory and leg exercises (see Chapter 16). The patient may have a PT evaluation before surgery and be measured for crutches, a walker, or a cane. Persons with arthritis involving the joints of the upper extremity may be fitted with a platform walker, in which most of the upper body weight is distributed on the forearms during ambulation. Platform walkers are particularly beneficial to persons with RA, who typically have wrist and finger joint involvement. The patient should be informed about what adaptive equipment will be needed on discharge. Postoperative pain control is usually achieved with the use of patient-controlled analgesia (PCA) pumps. Both epidural and intravenous pain control are used for patients with joint replacement surgery. The patient should be shown the pump and given instructions regarding its use at the preoperative interview.

The patient is instructed to take nothing by mouth after midnight on the day preceding surgery and is admitted to the hospital on the day of surgery. Intravenous antibiotics are begun at least 30 minutes before the incision time to establish a therapeutic level; antibiotics are usually continued for 24 to 48 hours after surgery. The lowest rate of infection occurs when antibiotics are given no more than 2 hours before incision time.[20]

Discharge planning is also begun at the preadmission interview. The length of hospital stay varies with the joint replaced and the individual patient's condition. Most patients admitted for hip or knee replacement are discharged after 4 days, usually to a rehabilitative facility or subacute division for continued therapy. The patient's and family's resources and preferences should be assessed at the preadmission interview to begin planning for transfer after discharge.

POSTOPERATIVE CARE

Routine postoperative nursing care for the patient recovering from total joint replacement surgery includes monitoring vital signs and level of consciousness, assisting with coughing and deep breathing, monitoring and recording intake and output (including suction drains at the operative site), providing adequate nutrition and hydration, managing pain, assessing the surgical site for drainage and signs of infection, maintaining the position of the operative extremity to prevent dislocation of prostheses, performing frequent neurovascular checks, providing skin care, encouraging progressive ambulation, preventing infection, teaching, and monitoring the patient for signs of complications. See Chapter 18 for general postoperative care.

Priorities of care include interventions to prevent the complications associated with immobility, including constipation, urinary retention, respiratory complications, altered skin integrity, and venous stasis. Nursing interventions specific to the joint replaced are discussed separately following this section.

DVT is a common complication after both hip and knee replacement. Measures to prevent DVT include the administration of anticoagulants, use of intermittent pneumatic compression devices and antiembolism hose, and leg exercises performed by the patient. As mentioned earlier, the threat of DVT and pulmonary embolism continues 4 to 6 weeks after surgery. Proximal DVT is most often associated with pulmonary embolism. Depending on the individual patient and surgeon preference, patients are given heparin, low-dose heparin, LMWH (enoxaparin or dalteparin), or warfarin for prophylactic anticoagulation. LMWH has a longer half-life than standard heparin and does not require laboratory testing for twice-daily dosing. LMWH has been shown to be more effective than standard heparin in reducing the incidence of proximal DVT but showed no difference in preventing distal DVT.[54] LMWH is usually administered subcutaneously twice daily for a period of 7 to 14 days and is highly effective in reducing the incidence of proximal and distal DVT after total hip and knee replacement. Low doses of warfarin can be administered daily on the basis of the patient's daily prothrombin time or INR results. The goal is to maintain a prothrombin time of 15 seconds and a control of 1.5 seconds.

Generally, a combination of treatments is implemented to reduce the incidence of DVT, including prophylactic anticoagulation, graduated elastic stockings, leg exercises, pneumatic compression devices, and early mobilization. In many institutions pneumatic compression devices are applied intraoperatively and are continued until the patient is fully ambulatory.

The venous foot pump is an alternative method of decreasing venous stasis and thus the risk of DVT. This device has been shown to be as effective as natural weight bearing in producing adequate pumping action to increase venous return. Nurses should encourage the patient to perform isometric leg exercises every 1 to 2 hours, with 10 repetitions per session. The use of antiembolism hose should be continued until the patient is fully ambulatory. Some institutions include ultrasound or other diagnostic testing to rule out DVT as part of the postoperative protocol.

Early ambulation is a safe and inexpensive method of preventing venous stasis. Most patients are assisted out of bed on the first postoperative day, with progressive ambulation and PT sessions daily to follow. Activity and weight-bearing restrictions vary, depending on the joint replaced, whether or not cement was used, and surgeon protocol. The nurse should help and encourage the patient to perform active and passive ROM exercises, isometrics, and other exercises prescribed by the physical therapist to increase muscle strength and decrease the complications of mobility.

While the patient is receiving anticoagulants, the nurse is responsible for monitoring the patient for signs of bleeding. The stool, urine, and sputum should be monitored for blood; a soft-bristled toothbrush should be used; dental floss should be avoided; electric razors should be used in place of razor blades; and needle punctures should be kept to a minimum. The suction drain and dressing should be assessed for excessive drainage, and the patient's coagulation studies and CBC should be monitored daily.

Closed wound drainage systems are surgically placed at the time of closing of the incision to prevent hematoma formation and are left in place 24 to 48 hours after surgery. Because of intraoperative blood loss, the patient may require a transfusion after surgery. An alternative is an autotransfusion drain, a closed drainage system that collects and filters the blood, which can then be reinfused intravenously into the patient. Used alone, postoperative salvage and reinfusion have been shown to be effective in reducing the amount of autologous blood needed postoperatively. The blood obtained through intraoperative and postoperative salvage methods has several advantages over homologous banked blood. Platelets and clotting factors remain intact in the salvaged blood, the pH of the blood is identical to the patient's, red blood cells are viable, reinfused blood has a greater affinity for oxygen, and the risk of transfusion reaction or transmission of bloodborne diseases is less.[19]

In addition to monitoring of the drain and dressing site for signs of excessive bleeding, the patient's hemoglobin and hematocrit must be monitored daily. Persons undergoing bilateral knee replacement surgery experience an average 5.42 g/dl drop in hemoglobin values in the perioperative period.[19] Output from the surgical drain is generally less than 300 ml per shift. Patients are often given an iron supplement postoperatively to increase blood counts.

Preventing infection is a nursing priority for any patient who has undergone total joint replacement. A postoperative wound infection can lead to prolonged hospitalization with significant cost increase, permanent disability, and removal of the prosthesis with a decreased chance for success in subsequent replacements. Infection rates for persons receiving total hip replacements are 0.1% to 1%; the risk increases with revision surgery because of the longer operative time. Infection rates for persons undergoing elbow replacement surgery are significantly higher because of the superficiality of the joint and poor skin coverage for closure.

Gram-positive organisms are responsible for 60% to 65% of all joint infections; *Staphylococcus aureus* and *Staphylococcus epidermidis* are the most often cultured organisms from hip and knee wounds.[1] The patient's skin has been identified as the major source of infection; airborne bacteria in the operating room are another major source of pathogens. Bone and joint infections are particularly difficult to treat because of the multiple channels in bone that may harbor organisms for long periods of time. The use of prophylactic antibiotics in the perioperative period has been effective in reducing the incidence of postoperative infection in patients undergoing hip or knee replacement. Antibiotics should be given as prescribed to maintain therapeutic blood levels.

The patient should be monitored for any signs of infection, including elevated temperature, elevated WBC count, and erythema, edema, or drainage from the wound. Dressing changes should be performed using aseptic technique. A report of a dull aching pain or unusual or persistent pain may be an indication of joint infection and should be reported to the physician for further evaluation. The patient and family should be taught to recognize the signs and symptoms of infection. Discharge instructions should include methods of avoiding sources of infection, including the necessity for prophylactic antibiotics when undergoing dental or genitourinary procedures or other invasive procedures and for instances of systemic bacterial infections. Many institutions provide patients with wallet-sized cards with antibiotic prophylaxis information.

Pain management is an important aspect of nursing care for patients after total joint replacement. Many patients with arthritis have endured years of chronic pain as a result of degenerative changes in the joint. Total joint replacement may offer relief from that pain. However, postoperative pain is different from that associated with arthritis. Many institutions use intravenous or epidural PCA with opioid analgesics (morphine, fentanyl, hydromorphone) as a method of pain control. The PCA pump is usually continued for up to 48 hours postoperatively; then oral analgesics are ordered as needed. The patient should be monitored for bowel function because of the side effects of the medication and immobility after surgery. Ice is applied to the incision area for the first 48 hours to prevent swelling and to decrease pain. Ice also helps alleviate pain after PT sessions. The nurse should consider the patient's PT schedule and make sure the patient is adequately medicated before going to therapy.

Total Hip Arthroplasty

In addition to general postoperative care, there are some important considerations for care after total hip arthroplasty (see Guidelines for Safe Practice box). Positioning restrictions protect the prosthesis and depend on the surgical approach and technique and type of prosthesis. The positioning restrictions outlined pertain to the posterolateral approach to the hip, which is commonly used. Patients undergoing an anterolateral approach are able to tolerate sitting upright with 90 degrees of flexion and should avoid active abduction, external rotation, and extension of the operative leg. After total hip arthroplasty, dislocation of the prosthesis is a serious complication that may require additional surgery or anesthesia to relocate the prosthesis. Signs of possible dislocation include a sudden onset of pain unrelieved by medication, a "popping" sensation associated with movement, loss of movement, leg length discrepancy, and deformity. The affected extremity may be either externally or internally rotated, depending on the direction of the dislocation, and the head of the femoral prosthesis may be palpable.

Extremes of flexion, adduction, or rotation should be avoided because these motions may cause dislocation (Figure 47-20). Flexion is generally limited to 60 degrees for 6 to 7 days and then to 90 degrees for 2 to 3 months. When the patient is supine or lying on the side, the legs should be kept in abduction; pillows or an abduction splint can be used (Figure 47-21). Positioning the patient on the operative side is usually avoided to prevent adduction of the operative limb. Positioning restrictions are maintained until the hip capsule is well healed and the risk of dislocation has passed. Bone growth around the prosthesis begins in approximately 10 days.

Most patients have some restriction in weight bearing, which limits the distraction force on the prosthesis. The surgeon prescribes the amount of weight bearing allowed. Patients with cemented prostheses are usually allowed weight bearing as tolerated. With the help of physical therapists, the

Guidelines for Safe Practice

Postoperative Care of the Patient With Total Hip Replacement

1. Positioning
   a. Positioning will depend on the surgical approach and technique, method of implantation (cemented or bony ingrowth prosthesis), and prosthesis design.
   b. Restrictions to avoid dislocation of the prosthesis usually include:
      (1) Flexion is limited to 60 degrees for 6 to 7 days, then to 90 degrees for 2 to 3 months.
      (2) No adduction is permitted beyond midline for 2 to 3 months; therefore no side lying on the operative side unless ordered by the surgeon. The leg is maintained in abduction when the patient is lying supine or on the unoperative side (see Figure 47-21).
      (3) No extreme internal or external rotation is permitted (see Figure 47-20).
2. Wound care
   a. Drains are inserted in the wound to prevent formation of a hematoma and left in place for 24 to 48 hours.
   b. Maintain constant suction through a self-contained suction device.
   c. Note amount and type of drainage.
   d. Use aseptic technique.
   e. Following the initial dressing change, change dressing once daily and as needed, using aseptic technique. Observe incision line for signs of infection. The wound may be left open to air if there is no drainage. Staples/sutures are removed 7 to 10 days after surgery.
3. Activity
   a. Observe flexion restrictions when elevating the head of the bed.
   b. Encourage periodic elevation and lowering of the head of the bed to provide motion at the hip.
   c. Instruct patient in use of the overhead trapeze to shift weight and lift for the bedpan and change of linen.
   d. Encourage active dorsiflexion/plantar flexion exercise of the ankles and quadriceps and gluteal setting exercises to promote venous return, prevent thrombus formation, and maintain muscle tone (see Chapter 18). Gluteal sets also help strengthen the muscle around the hip joint capsule, which will help decrease the risk of dislocation.
   e. The patient may be turned to the unoperative side with the operative leg maintained in abduction and extension.
   f. Begin ambulation as early as the first postoperative day, if tolerated. Physical therapy consult is initiated.
      (1) Observe flexion and adduction restrictions.
      (2) Observe weight-bearing restrictions prescribed by the surgeon (usually partial weight bearing assisted with a walker or crutches).
      (3) Increase amount of walking each day according to the patient's tolerance.
   g. Begin sitting when the patient demonstrates sufficient leg control to sit within flexion restrictions (usually requires elevation of sitting surfaces, including use of a raised toilet seat).
4. Medications
   a. Prophylactic anticoagulant drugs are usually prescribed to decrease the risk of thrombus formation. Monitor patient for signs of deep vein thrombosis, pulmonary embolism, and fat embolism syndrome.
   b. Initially control pain with positioning and opioid analgesics (usually patient-controlled analgesia), transition to oral opioids, nonsteroidal antiinflammatory drugs (NSAIDs), or nonopioid analgesics according to the patient's tolerance.
5. Discharge instructions
   a. The patient must use an ambulatory aid, avoid adduction, and limit hip flexion to 90 degrees for about 2 to 3 months.
   b. A raised toilet seat is to be obtained and used at home until flexion restrictions are removed.
   c. The patient may need a long-handled shoehorn and reacher to facilitate activities of daily living within flexion restriction.
   d. The patient must be made aware of the lifelong need for antibiotic prophylaxis when undergoing invasive procedures or dental work to protect the prosthesis from bacteremic infection.
   e. Inform patient that the implant may activate metal detector alarms. Provide a wallet identification/information card if available.

goal is for the patient to accomplish safe transfer from bed to chair and toilet, perform prescribed exercises independently, and ambulate with the appropriate weight-bearing restrictions using a walker, cane, or crutches. The patient should also be taught to ascend and descend stairs safely.

Assistive devices to aid the patient in completing ADLs are usually obtained through the OT department. The patient is given instructions about the use of an elevated toilet seat, which prevents extreme hip flexion; long-handled reachers; and devices that aid in donning shoes and stockings; these items will be used after discharge as well.

Total Knee Arthroplasty

Postoperative management of persons with total knee replacement may include the use of a continuous passive motion (CPM) machine (Figure 47-22). The CPM machine supports the operative extremity while passively moving it within preset limits of flexion and extension. Use of the CPM machine reduces postoperative swelling, prevents adhesions, decreases pain, and facilitates early mobility. The CPM is usually applied in the operating room or postanesthesia care unit, and patients are encouraged to use the machine while in bed as tolerated (up to 22 hours/day). Increases in the amount of knee flexion are ordered by the physician; the goal is usually 90 degrees. If the CPM is not used, a knee immobilizer is often placed over the bulky dressing and is kept in place until the dressing is reduced. Other surgical protocols call for the use of a knee exerciser, which is attached to the overhead frame of the bed and allows the patient to exercise the knee while in bed. The physician determines when active flexion exercises may begin. There are no real positioning restrictions, although the patient should adhere to the physician's orders

Do
Do Not
Do not cross your operated leg past the midline of the body or turn your kneecap in toward your body.
Do not sit in low chairs or cross your legs.
To sit: Use a high chair with arms or add pillows to elevate the seat.
Avoid flexing your hips past 90 degrees.
To bend: Keep the operative leg behind you or as instructed by your therapist.
To reach: Use long-handled grabbers or as therapist advises.
Use an elevated toilet.
Sleep with a pillow between the legs.

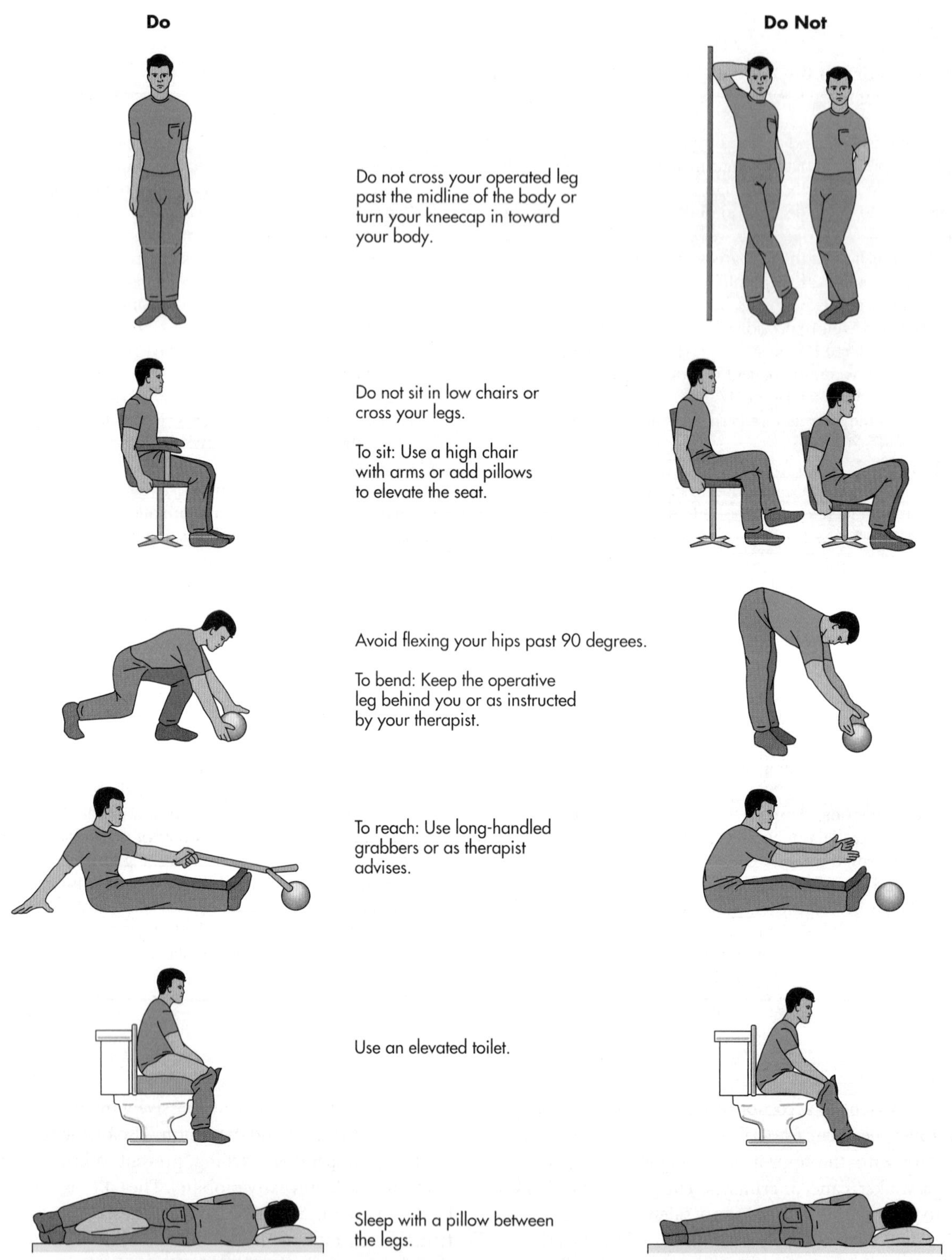

Figure 47-20 Home-going instructions illustrating *do's* and *do not's* for patients with a total hip replacement. Patients are to avoid extreme flexion (past 90 degrees), adduction, and internal rotation of the operated hip—any of which may cause dislocation of the prosthesis.

regarding the amount of weight bearing and knee flexion permitted. Kneeling is usually discouraged. Flexion is increased at intervals. While in bed, the patient is cautioned against having a pillow under the knee, which may cause the knee to remain in a flexed position (see Guidelines for Safe Practice box).

Total Shoulder Arthroplasty

Priorities of care for the patient following total shoulder arthroplasty are pain management, assessment of neurovascular status, promotion of self-care and mobility, and prevention of complications. Nerve damage is uncommon, but the brachial

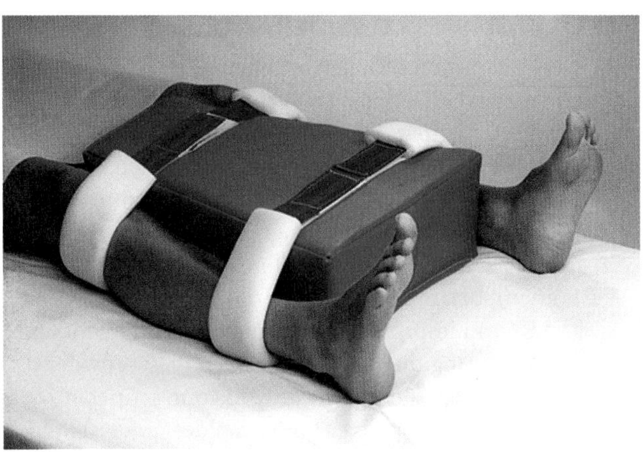

Figure 47-21 Abduction splint for postoperative hip arthroplasty.

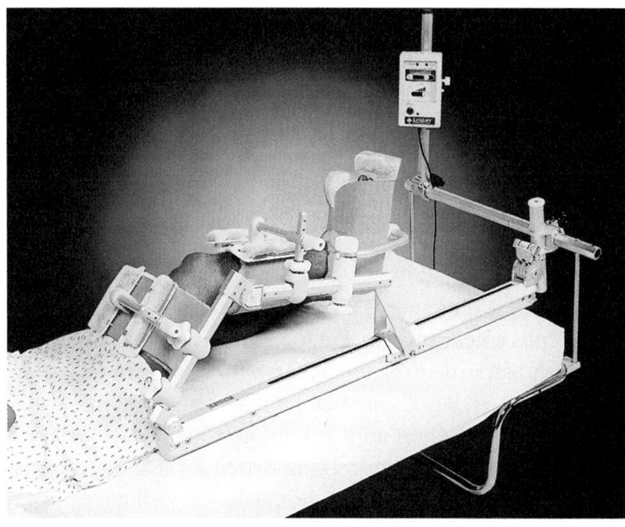

Figure 47-22 Example of continuous passive motion machine.

Guidelines for Safe Practice

Postoperative Care of the Patient With Total Knee Replacement

1. Positioning
   a. The operative leg(s) is elevated on pillows to enhance venous return for the first 48 hours. Pillows are placed with caution not to flex the knee(s). It is becoming more common for patients to have bilateral total knee replacements done at one surgery.
   b. The patient may be turned from side to back to side.
2. Wound care
   a. Care of drains is as for total hip replacement.
   b. The patient is assessed for systemic evidence of loss of blood (hypotension, tachycardia) if a bulky compression dressing is used, since it may hold large quantities of drainage before drainage is visible.
   c. Bulky dressings are removed before the patient begins active flexion.
   d. Assess wound for healing and signs of infection. Perform a dry sterile dressing change once the bulky dressing is discontinued. Leave incision open to air if there is no drainage.
3. Activity
   a. Passive flexion is provided in a continuous passive motion (CPM) machine within prescribed flexion-extension limits. The patient's leg may remain in the CPM machine as much as tolerated (up to 22 hours/day) to facilitate even healing of tissue.
   b. The patient is encouraged to perform active dorsiflexion/plantar flexion of the ankles, gluteal and quadriceps setting, and after drain(s) are removed, straight leg raising exercises.
   c. The patient begins active flexion exercises three to four times per day on about the second to third postoperative day. The time when active flexion is permitted varies.
   d. Partial weight bearing with an assistive device may be started as early as the first postoperative day and increased as the patient tolerates. Physical therapy consult initiated.
   e. Sitting in a chair with the leg(s) elevated may be started on the first postoperative day.
   f. The patient may be encouraged to wear a resting knee extension splint (immobilizer) on the operative extremity until able to demonstrate quadriceps control (independent straight leg raising).
4. Medications
   a. Prophylactic anticoagulants are usually prescribed to decrease the risk of thrombus formation. Monitor the patient for signs of deep vein thrombosis, pulmonary embolism, and FES.
   b. Initial control of pain is with opioid analgesics (usually patient-controlled analgesia [PCA]) and positioning; after PCA is discontinued, oral opioids, nonsteroidal antiinflammatory drugs (NSAIDs), or nonopioids are given as needed.
   c. Ice is usually prescribed to be applied to the knee to reduce swelling and pain.
   d. The patient is encouraged to apply ice to the knee(s) for 20 to 30 minutes before and after active flexion exercise.
5. Discharge instructions
   a. The patient must observe partial weight-bearing restrictions and use an ambulatory aid for approximately 2 months after discharge. Kneeling should be avoided indefinitely.
   b. The patient should continue active flexion and straight leg raising exercises at home.
   c. The patient must be made aware of the lifelong need for antibiotic prophylaxis before invasive procedures or dental work.
   d. Inform patient that the implant may activate metal detector alarms. Provide a wallet identification/information card if available.

plexus may have been injured intraoperatively or as a result of positioning. Motor, sensory, and vascular assessment of the operative extremity should be done every 4 hours, and the findings compared with the patient's preoperative baseline. After total shoulder replacement, the operative extremity is placed in an immobilizer, which is kept in place for 1 to 2 days (Figure 47-23). The sling is then worn at night and for comfort during the day. Passive exercises are initiated immediately after surgery, and pendulum exercises are begun 1 to 10 days after surgery (see Chapter 46). Shoulder CPM machines may be used for passive ROM exercises. Isometric exercises are started the second week. The patient is cautioned to limit the amount of external rotation. Patients undergoing total shoulder replacement may require only overnight hospitalization. Lifelong precautions include prevention of infection and avoidance of contact or load-bearing activities. Joint instability accounts for 38% of complications following shoulder replacement surgery.[56]

Total Elbow Arthroplasty

Damage to the ulnar nerve is a possible complication following elbow replacement surgery. Frequent neurovascular checks, focusing on assessment of ulnar nerve function, are important interventions. Edema and hematoma formation may cause alterations in sensation and/or motion. Knowledge of the patient's preoperative function is important for making comparisons. The surgeon should be notified of any changes in the patient's neurovascular status.

After total elbow replacement the operative extremity is placed in a plaster splint and bulky dressing (Figure 47-24). The splint may be flexed up to 90 degrees. The arm should be elevated, and ice applied. Active ROM of the fingers is encouraged to maintain mobility and decrease edema. The drain is removed within 24 to 36 hours, and the bulky dressing is reduced. Elbow flexion and extension exercises are begun after the dressing is removed. Activity restrictions include limiting lifting to no more than 1 pound for 3 months and less than 5 pounds long term. The patient should avoid contact sports for life.

Total Ankle Arthroplasty

Total ankle replacement is performed most often for patients with RA. Neurovascular assessment is important to evaluate intraoperative damage to the neurovascular bundle. A drain is placed to decrease hematoma formation; elevation helps reduce swelling.

After surgery the extremity is placed in a soft compression dressing and plaster splint. The operative extremity should be kept elevated, with ice applied. The dressing is removed, and a short leg walking cast is applied for 2 to 3 weeks. Nursing care is similar to care for the person with a fracture (see Chapter 46). PT and exercises are begun after cast removal. Preventing infection and promoting wound healing are key interventions to avoid serious complications with skin closure and healing.

GERONTOLOGIC CONSIDERATIONS

Arthritis is a common problem among the elderly population and may affect their ability to perform ADLs and to enjoy usual leisure activities. OA is the most common form of arthritis in the older adult. Over 40% of women older than age 60 have OA. Joint involvement is typically symmetric, and the onset of pain is insidious, progressing to more persistent pain, unrelieved by rest (see Guidelines for Safe Practice box).

PT is an important treatment for older adults with OA. Exercise and PT can improve the quality of life and maintain independence. Resting the affected joint typically provides pain relief but can contribute significantly to contractures, atrophy of disuse, and osteoporosis. Thus the older adult should be advised to maintain a constant level of physical activity, even in the presence of active arthritis. Passive and active exercises should be performed to maintain ROM and muscle tone. Swimming and walking are good choices for regular exercise.

Assistive and adaptive devices can improve the quality of life and allow the patient independence in ADLs. Orthoses and special shoes for foot problems can help maintain alignment and provide support for diseased joints.

Medications to treat OA should be chosen carefully when elderly patients are being treated. The health care provider should be aware of any other medications the patient is taking because of the possibility of drug interactions. Hepatic and renal function should be evaluated before a pharmacologic regimen is prescribed. Acetaminophen in doses up to 4 g is a good choice for elderly patients without renal or hepatic disease. A dose of 4 g of acetaminophen has been shown to be as effective as 2.4 g of ibuprofen in the treatment of OA.[4] If NSAIDs are prescribed, a CBC, urinalysis, and liver and kidney function tests should be performed before treatment and at 1- to 3-month intervals thereafter. Increased age has been identified as a significant risk factor for the development of side effects associated with NSAIDs.[4,71] All NSAIDs should be used with cau-

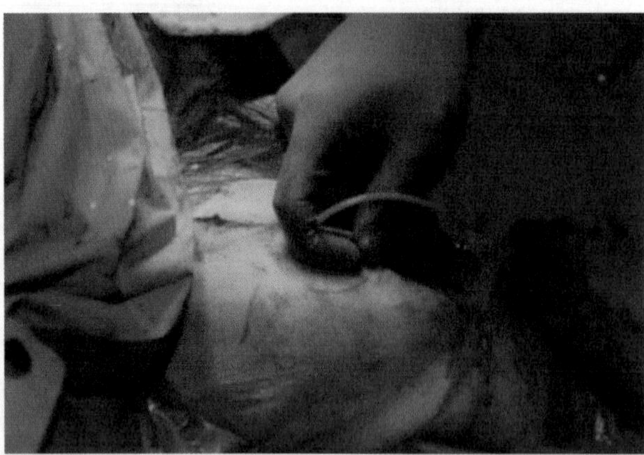

Figure 47-23 Total shoulder arthroplasty with postoperative immobilization. Note Hemovac drain.

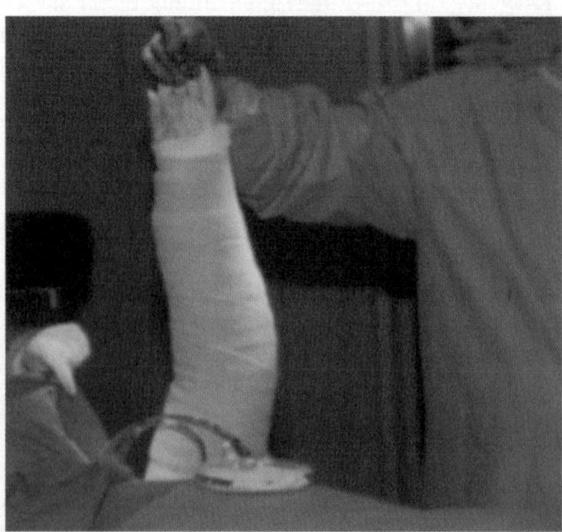

Figure 47-24 Total elbow arthroplasty with postoperative splint and dressing. The elbow is in full extension.

tion in older adults; piroxicam should be avoided because of its long half-life.[43] A chronic pain management program should include nonpharmacologic modalities as well. Some forms of exercise may benefit chronic pain (see Research box).

Many elderly patients with OA require or elect surgical intervention to relieve pain or to improve mobility. Any coexisting disease such as heart disease, hypertension, diabetes, or kidney problems must be stabilized before elective surgery. See Chapters 16 to 20 for perioperative considerations for the elderly patient.

After surgical intervention the elderly patient may be discharged to a rehabilitative facility to continue with PT and to attain independence in ADLs, transfers, and ambulation. If the patient is transferred directly to home, a family member, friend, or home health care referral will be necessary to assist in care.

SPECIAL ENVIRONMENTS FOR CARE

Community-Based Care

Patients and their families should be informed that the rehabilitative phase after joint replacement lasts at least 1 year. At 1 year most patients have achieved approximately 90% of functional return. Patients and families should be reminded that cooperation in the rehabilitative process is necessary for success. Daily exercise is an important component of the recovery process.

Because of the shortened length of stay (4 to 5 days for total hip replacement), most patients are discharged to a subacute facility or rehabilitative center for PT. Some patients do opt to be discharged directly to home. Patients who are discharged to home need a referral for home PT or need to make arrangements for outpatient PT. A home health nurse visit should be scheduled for suture or staple removal.

The follow-up appointment with the orthopedic surgeon is usually at 6 weeks after surgery. After 6 weeks patients are allowed a little more flexibility in activity and can usually resume sexual activity. When it is safe to resume sexual activity is a topic that nurses need to address, preferably at the preoperative visit, but certainly before discharge. Generally, 6 to 8 weeks is the recommended time for refraining from sexual intercourse. Persons with joint revisions may need additional time. Once intercourse is resumed, appropriate positioning of the affected extremity is a key consideration. Persons with hip replacements should continue to follow positioning guidelines to avoid dislocating the prosthesis.

The patient should be cautioned against driving without consulting the surgeon. Patients with total hip replacements generally have sufficient muscle strength to resume driving a car with an automatic transmission at 6 to 8 weeks; driving while using pain medication is contraindicated.

When the patient has regained maximal strength, he or she may resume low-impact activities such as walking, swimming, golfing, biking, bowling, and tennis. High-impact activities and

Guidelines for Safe Practice

The Elderly Patient With Arthritis

ASSESSMENT

- Assess all older adults for muscle strength and tone, gait, sensory deficits, painful joints or muscles, contractures, deformities, and foot problems that may interfere with ambulation and activities of daily living (ADLs).
- Assess availability, condition, and use of assistive aids, such as walkers, canes, or crutches.
- Assess environmental factors conducive to falls because older adults are at high risk for falls.

INTERVENTION

- Order assistive aids to foster independence and to increase ambulation, such as a walker, cane, lift, and bedside commode.
- Encourage an exercise program to maintain baseline muscle and joint function.
- Perform active and passive range of motion for elderly patients needing bed rest.
- Obtain orders for progressive ambulation as early in hospitalization as possible.
- Position extremities in proper body alignment to prevent contractures.
- Teach good foot care and the importance of well-fitted shoes.
- Request physical therapy for patients with gait or mobility problems.
- Request occupational therapy for problems with ADLs and fine-motor coordination.
- Teach elderly patients how to transfer and ambulate safely.
- Initiate a fall prevention program that identifies risk factors and promotes an individualized plan for each patient, depending on his or her ability and tendency to fall.
- Be sure the environment is free of clutter, the bed is kept in lowest position, and a night-light illuminates the floor.

Research

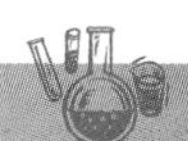

Reference: Adler P et al: The effects of tai chi on older adults with chronic arthritis pain, *J Nurs Sch* 32(4):377, 2000.

Tai chi has been used in China for hundreds of years to decrease pain in older adults. Tai chi combines meditation and movement and is a safe exercise for persons with arthritis. Benefits include improved flexibility, muscle strengthening, and aerobic exercise, but little is known about its effects on general health and pain relief.

This study examined the effects of T'ai chi on the pain intensity of older adults with chronic arthritis pain. Exclusion criteria were activity limitations, orthostatic hypotension, history of falls, and Meniere's disease. Participants were community-dwelling adults ages 68 to 87 years. The experimental group participated in 10 weekly, 1-hour T'ai chi classes; the control group maintained their usual level of activity. Pain intensity was scored using a numerical scale (0 to 10); pretest and posttest measurements of pain and health were scored using the Short-Form McGill Pain Questionnaire and the Rand Health Survey. Participants rated their pain intensity, analgesic use, and activity weekly. There were no significant differences in analgesic use, activity, or health between the two groups. The experimental group's ratings of pain intensity decreased after the 10-week session. Because of the small sample size ($n = 16$) and other effects of pain measurement, the change in pain intensity as a result of T'ai chi was not statistically significant. Further studies with a larger sample are needed to evaluate T'ai chi as an effective intervention in chronic pain management of older adults.

exercises that place an increased load on the joints are not recommended, since they decrease the longevity of hip prostheses.

Teaching includes information about home-going medications, particularly anticoagulants. The patient and family should be aware of the purpose, side effects, dosage, and method of administration of prescribed medications. The patient and family should be knowledgeable about the signs and symptoms of complications, such as prosthesis dislocation, infection, DVT, fat embolism, and pulmonary embolism.

Temporary rearrangement of the home environment may be necessary, especially if the patient returns directly home. It may be more convenient if the bathroom and bedroom are on the same floor; a bedside commode or urinal can be used temporarily. The bed should be arranged so that the patient can exit the bed on the opposite side of the operative leg. The floors and doorways should be free of any obstructions. Throw rugs should be removed. A firm chair with armrests is necessary for persons recovering from total hip or knee surgery. Adding pillows can raise the height of the seat. The room can be arranged with commonly used items within close reach of the patient. A tote bag can be attached to the patient's walker to carry the phone, reachers, or other necessary items. A raised toilet seat is needed for persons with total knee and hip replacements. For bathing, a long-handled sponge will allow the patient to wash his or her legs. A walk-in shower is best, and a chair can be added for safety. If the patient has a tub, a sponge bath may be easier for the first few weeks. If the patient has pets, a friend or family member may be needed to help care for them. Small dogs or cats may easily trip a person using a walker, cane, or crutches. The patient should be instructed to wear comfortable, well-fitting, nonskid, walking shoes. Regular follow-up appointments are continued for the first year and as necessary thereafter.

COMPLICATIONS

Complications associated with total joint replacement include the following: wound infection (superficial or deep), thrombophlebitis or DVT, pulmonary embolism, fat embolism, dislocation of the prosthesis, and mechanical failure of the components. Other complications associated with the surgical procedure include urinary tract infection (if an indwelling catheter is used) and pneumonia. It should be stressed that infection is a potentially severe complication after joint replacement. Deep infection may necessitate removal of the prosthesis.

More than 50% of hip infections occur more than 3 months after surgery. Infections that develop within the first 3 postoperative months are usually superficial or suprafascial infections (stage I). Deep or subfascial infections are commonly seen within 3 to 24 months after surgery (stage II). Infections occurring later than 24 months after surgery are usually attributed to hematogenous spreading from other locations in the body (stage III).[1]

Stage II infections are attributed to direct contamination of the wound in the operating room (50% to 80% cases).[1] Symptoms associated with mechanical loosening of the prosthesis resemble those of stage II infections; however, loosening rarely occurs in the first year after replacement. A patient's report of new pain in the operative site should be immediately investigated. Conditions such as diverticulitis, cellulitis, abscesses, or seeding resulting from dental procedures, GI procedures, or any surgery can be a source of stage III infections.

Once an infection occurs, there are several treatment options. The patient's condition and the causative organism are major determinants of treatment. Surgical debridement, resection arthroplasty, arthrodesis, amputation, antibiotic therapy, and reimplantation are all options for treating persons with infected total joints. If infection necessitates removal of the prosthesis, first the area is debrided and then the appropriate antibiotics are administered on the basis of culture and sensitivity results. Reimplantation of the joint is done between 6 weeks and 1 year, depending on the causative organism and the condition of the patient. Antibiotics are continued for several weeks. Intraoperatively, antibiotic-treated cement can be used for susceptible organisms during reimplantation. If it is not possible to replace the prosthesis in a patient with a total hip replacement, a "girdlestone" hip results. Fibrous scar tissue replaces the hip joint, but the patient can still ambulate. In the case of a total knee replacement that cannot be replaced, the patient can undergo an arthrodesis, resulting in an immobile knee joint. Patients with severe systemic infection, intractable pain, or extensive bone loss may eventually require an amputation.

Persons with RA are more likely to develop major wound complications as a result of immunosuppressive medications used to treat RA. Patients with diabetes are also at an increased risk for developing infections after total joint replacement.

In addition, DVT, pulmonary embolism, and fat embolism are potentially fatal complications occurring after total knee or hip replacement. The rate of DVT and fatal pulmonary embolism in patients with hip or knee replacements who do not receive prophylactic anticoagulation is as high as 40%.[53] With prophylaxis, 2% of patients develop pulmonary embolism.[54]

Dislocation of the prosthesis is a particular concern for persons with hip replacements. Dislocation can result in significant morbidity and possibly an additional surgical procedure. Dislocation often occurs during transfers. Safety precautions and education of patients and personnel are necessary during the rehabilitation process and during the acute care phase. See Box 47-6 for other complications of total joint arthroplasty.

GOUT

Etiology/Epidemiology

Podagra, or foot pain, was first described in the fourth century BC. Gout was considered a disease of the wealthy and was associated with rich food and wine. Gout is a clinical syndrome resulting from the deposition of urate crystals in the synovial fluid, joints, or articular cartilage. Most cases are idiopathic; genetic defects in purine metabolism have been identified. Considered a metabolic disorder, gouty arthritis develops as a result of prolonged hyperuricemia (elevated serum uric acid) caused by problems in the synthesis of purines or by poor renal excretion of uric acid.

Gout must be distinguished from pseudogout, which occurs as a result of calcium pyrophosphate dihydrate (CPPD) crystals.

BOX 47-6 Complications of Total Joint Arthroplasty

Hip

Dislocation
Infection
Deep vein thrombosis (DVT)
Pulmonary embolism (PE)
Fat embolism
Leg length discrepancy
Altered gait
Pneumonia
Footdrop (secondary to nerve damage)

Knee

Infection
DVT
PE
Fat embolism
Acute compartment syndrome
Instability
Loosening of prosthesis
Patellar fracture
Poor patellar tracking
Vascular injury (intraoperative) and hemorrhage
Reflex sympathetic dystrophy
Nerve damage

Shoulder

Infection
Loosening of the prosthesis
Glenohumeral instability
Dislocation, subluxation
Intraoperative fracture
Rotator cuff tears
Deltoid dysfunction
Nerve damage
Impingement syndrome
PE

Elbow

Infection
Dislocation
DVT
PE
Loosening of prosthesis
Delayed healing of wound

Ankle

Infection
Problems with wound healing or skin closure
Residual pain
Impingement
Loosening of prosthesis

Pseudogout resembles gout with intraarticular calcium deposits and CPPD crystals in synovial fluid and affects primarily older adults. Articular cartilage, menisci, and adjacent tendinous or ligamentous structures are affected by pseudogout. Persons with previous joint trauma or a history of meniscectomy are prone to developing pseudogout. Both disorders resemble RA.

BOX 47-7 Causes of Secondary Gout

Overproduction of Uric Acid

Paget's disease
Cancer
Polycythemia vera
Multiple myeloma
Chronic myelocytic and lymphocytic leukemia
Hemolytic anemias
Cytotoxic drugs

Underexcretion of Uric Acid

Chronic renal insufficiency
Ketoacidosis
Lactic acidosis
Drug ingestion (diuretics, cyclosporine, levodopa, pyrazinamide, low-dose salicylates)

Unknown Etiology

Hyperparathyroidism
Hypoparathyroidism
Hypothyroidism
Adrenal insufficiency

Gout primarily affects adult men; less often it occurs in postmenopausal women. Risk factors associated with the development of gout include familial history, male gender, obesity, excessive alcohol use, hyperlipidemia, hypertension, renal insufficiency, diuretic use, and lead exposure.[64] Persons who have received organ transplants have a higher incidence of gout, secondary to the use of diuretics and cyclosporine.[64]

Pathophysiology

Hyperuricemia is not necessary for the diagnosis of gout. Uric acid levels are controlled by diet, purine metabolism, and renal clearance. Gout is classified as primary or secondary. Underexcretion of uric acid is caused by decreased tubular secretion, increased tubular resorption, or a combination of both. Approximately 75% of patients develop primary gout as a result of undersecretion of uric acid. The remaining 25% of persons develop primary gout as a result of overproduction of uric acid.

Secondary gout results from an overproduction of uric acid secondary to increased purine catabolism or impaired excretion of uric acid. Secondary gout usually occurs in the acute care setting (Box 47-7).

Urate crystals form in the synovial tissue, causing severe inflammation. The inflammatory process is extremely rapid, occurring over a few hours. Acute symptoms are extreme pain, swelling, and erythema of the involved joints. Typically, the first metatarsophalangeal joint of the great toe is involved (50% of patients), but other joints, such as the ankle, heel, knee, or wrist, may also be affected. Pain is so severe that the patient may not tolerate even the weight of a sheet over the joint. Renal damage may occur, especially if recurrent uric acid stones have been present. Between attacks of gout, the patient may be asymptomatic, but repeated attacks can occur with gradually increasing frequency if the disease is untreated. Patients with gouty symptoms may develop *tophi,* or deposits of monosodium urate, in their tissues. These consist of a core of monosodium urate with a surrounding inflammatory reaction. Patients with tophaceous deposits (Figure 47-25) tend to have more frequent and more severe episodes of gouty arthritis.

Collaborative Care Management

Laboratory studies indicate an elevated serum uric acid level and a normal or increased urinary uric acid level over a 24-hour period, as well as the presence of monosodium urate monohydrate crystals in the synovial fluid and in the tophi. Treatment is focused on control of acute attacks, prevention of recurrent attacks, and long-term uricosuric therapy to prevent the formation of tophi. Results are best when therapy is initiated shortly after the onset of symptoms.

Colchicine, once considered the mainstay of treatment, is used less often for management of acute attacks because of the distressing side effect of diarrhea. The ability to inhibit phagocytosis of urate crystals by neutrophils is the key to colchicine's effectiveness. Colchicine is not effective once an attack has been present for several days. However, in persons who are able to recognize the symptoms of an acute attack, one or two 0.6-mg tablets of colchicine may be taken to thwart the attack. Colchicine 0.6 mg. is given orally every 1 to 2 hours until diarrhea develops (to a maximum of 10 mg).[7,64] Joint inflammation usually subsides within 48 hours in most patients.

For persons with adequate renal function and no other contraindications, NSAIDs are a good choice for therapy. Although any NSAID may be prescribed, indomethacin has been successful in the treatment of gout. Long-term use of NSAIDs can help prevent acute attacks.

For persons in whom NSAIDs are contraindicated, the administration of corticosteroids is effective. Intraarticular injections or systemic therapy can be used for treatment of acute attacks.

Future attacks of acute gout can be prevented by the administration of colchicine or NSAIDs. Pharmacologic prophylaxis should be initiated before uric acid levels are corrected. Prophylaxis with colchicine decreases the number of acute attacks, regardless of the serum uric acid level. Medications that lower uric acid levels, such as allopurinol, may precipitate an acute attack; these drugs should be started after resolution of acute symptoms. Controversy exists regarding the duration of prophylactic therapy. Treatment is usually maintained until the patient has normal urate levels and has been asymptomatic for at least 6 months.[71]

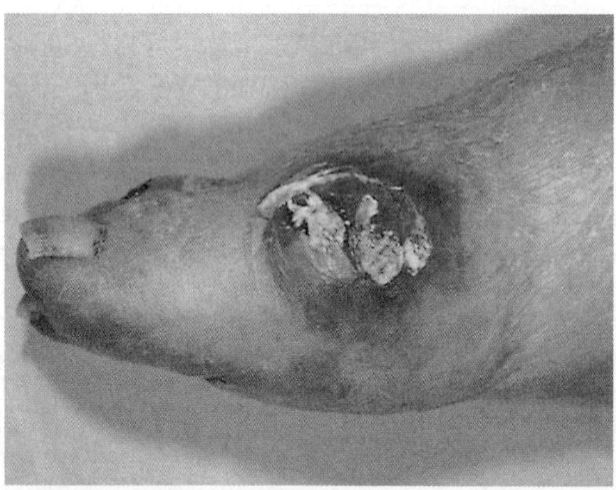

Figure 47-25 Gouty tophus on right foot.

Identifying and correcting the cause of hyperuricemia can accomplish prevention of gouty attacks. Medications can be given that inhibit the synthesis of urate or increase its secretion. Some causes of hyperuricemia may require lifelong medication to decrease serum levels. Attention should be focused on factors that increase uric acid levels. The factors that contribute to increased urate production are regular alcohol consumption, obesity, and a high-purine diet. Alcohol should be avoided because it not only increases production of uric acid but also prevents its excretion.

Rest and joint immobilization are recommended until the acute attack subsides. Local application of cold can relieve pain. Application of heat should be avoided, since it will increase the inflammatory process.

Patient/Family Education. Most persons with gout are cared for at home; patient education should focus on prevention of further attacks and complications. Instructions should include information regarding medication use and possible side effects. Dietary instructions include reducing or eliminating alcohol intake and avoiding excessive intake of purines (sweetbreads, yeast, heart, herring, herring roe, and sardines). In the absence of renal or cardiac disease, the patient should be encouraged to drink 2 to 3L/day to eliminate uric acid and prevent renal calculi. Skin care is another important consideration, including daily assessment for tophi formation, use of emollients for softening, and positioning for comfort. Properly fitting shoes decrease skin irritation and increase comfort. Ice or heat may be used for pain relief. During acute attacks, pain management is important; immobilizing the affected joint may decrease pain until inflammation subsides.

BACTERIAL OR SEPTIC ARTHRITIS

Etiology/Epidemiology

Bacterial arthritis is the result of invasion of the synovial membrane by microorganisms, most often *Neisseria gonorrhoeae,* meningococci, streptococci, *Staphylococcus aureus,* coliform bacteria, *Salmonella,* and *Haemophilus influenzae.* Bacteria can enter the joint by hematogenous spread, direct inoculation, or extension from an adjacent infection. Hematogenous infection is the most common cause of bacterial arthritis.

Persons with an underlying medical illness are at greatest risk. Immunodeficiency, chronic disease, intravenous drug abuse, local joint surgery or trauma, intraarticular injections, and RA also place the person at risk for bacterial arthritis.

Pathophysiology

Synovial tissues respond to bacterial invasion by becoming inflamed. The joint cavity may become involved, and pus develops in the synovial membrane and the synovial fluid. If allowed to progress, the infection causes abscesses in the synovium and subchondral bone, eventually destroying cartilage. Ankylosis of the joint may result. The patient reports pain, swelling, and tenderness of the joint.

Collaborative Care Management

Joint aspiration is performed to identify the causative organism and determine treatment. Strict aseptic technique must be followed to avoid introducing additional bacteria into the joint. WBC counts are high, and the glucose content of synovial fluid may be reduced. X-ray films taken days to weeks after the onset of infection may reveal loss of joint space and lytic changes in bones.

Treatment should begin immediately. Medical management begins with appropriate antibiotic therapy and rest or immobilization of the joint. If infection does not respond to antibiotic therapy, or if osteomyelitis is present, surgical drainage by needle aspiration, arthroscopy, or arthrotomy is done. Needle aspiration of purulent exudate may be required daily until drainage ceases. Infections of the hip joint must be drained immediately to prevent necrosis of the femoral head. When infection subsides and motion can be tolerated, active ROM is resumed.

Nursing management focuses on promoting rest of the affected joint; administering antibiotics on time and as prescribed to maintain blood levels; and administering prescribed pain medication as necessary. The nurse also encourages the patient to participate in self-care to the extent possible within restrictions of prescribed rest for the joint.

Patient/Family Education. The results of treatment depend on the infecting organism, duration of infection before treatment, and host defenses. The patient should be educated about signs and symptoms of bacterial arthritis and to seek prompt treatment if symptoms recur. Prompt diagnosis and treatment can save the joint from destruction. The immunodeficient patient should be taught how to avoid sources of infection.

Antibiotic therapy may be prescribed for prolonged periods of time; the patient should be encouraged to comply with treatment to ensure eradication of infection. Other teaching includes cast or splint care, exercise and ROM, the use of crutches or assistive devices, antibiotic therapy, and follow-up care.

LYME DISEASE

Etiology/Epidemiology

Lyme disease (LD) is caused by the tickborne spirochete *Borrelia burgdorferi.* The disease was discovered in Lyme, Connecticut, in 1976 and declared a nationally notifiable disease by the Centers for Disease Control and Prevention (CDC) in 1991; between 1982 and 1996 more than 99,000 were reported to the CDC.[16] For surveillance purposes, the presence of an erythematous migrans rash 0.5 cm in diameter or laboratory documentation of infection with evidence of musculoskeletal, neurologic, or cardiovascular disease confirms the diagnosis of LD.[68] LD is transmitted by ticks, present most commonly on deer, mice, dogs, cats, raccoons, cows, and horses. Deer ticks are responsible for 95% of cases of LD. Birds help spread infected ticks by their migratory flights. The tick bite is usually painless, and the patient may not remember being bitten.

The disease has been reported in most European countries, throughout Asia, and in 49 states and the District of Columbia in the United States. LD is the number one vectorborne disease in the United States. The disease is prevalent in the northeastern, north-central, and mid-Atlantic regions of the United States. LD affects all ages, although the highest incidence is in children under 15 years of age and in adults over 29 years of age; those living in endemic areas with outdoor exposure are at risk. The peak months for early clinical manifestations of the disease are June through October. Increased public awareness, increasing deer populations, and the trend in the United States toward utilization of farmlands and forest increases the contact between humans and vectors and is responsible for the increasing rates of the disease.[68] Humans can be exposed to the ticks in wooded areas and in well-landscaped areas in endemic regions. Transmission of the disease from the tick to humans requires some time. Attachment of the tick for less than 24 hours rarely transmits the disease; attachment for at least 72 hours or more almost certainly transmits the disease. The incubation period from exposure to the onset of symptoms is from 3 to 32 days.[16]

Pathophysiology

LD has been called the "great imitator" because it mimics other diseases such as influenza, RA, multiple sclerosis, chronic fatigue syndrome, amyotrophic lateral sclerosis, fibromyalgia, lupus erythematosus, and Alzheimer's disease. Infection with *B. burgdorferi* stimulates inflammatory cytokines and autoimmune mechanisms, which results in Lyme arthritis. Primarily an extracellular organism, *B. burgdorferi* is thought to invade some cells and cross the blood-brain barrier, resulting in the neurologic manifestations of LD.

Infection with *B. burgdorferi* can be divided into three stages. Not all patients develop all stages. The early manifestations of the disease are usually self-limiting, and the late manifestations can become chronic (see Clinical Manifestations box). The arthritis associated with LD is either monoarticular or oligoarticular, affecting the knee and other large joints. Inflammation is a result of immune complex deposition in the synovium. Chronic and recurrent arthritis develops, possibly as a result of genetic factors or an autoimmune process.[16]

Collaborative Care Management

The varied signs and symptoms, coupled with the fact that most persons do not remember the tick bite, make diagnosis difficult. Laboratory testing should be done to confirm a clinical diagnosis. Serologic tests used to diagnose LD include enzyme-linked immunosorbent assay (ELISA), Western blot, and indirect immunofluorescence assay. Less than 50% of persons with stage I disease have detectable antibodies; in stage II disease the percentage rises to 70% to 90%. Both serum and cerebrospinal fluid should be tested to diagnose LD. Synovial fluid may be sampled if arthritic symptoms are present. An electrocardiogram should be done for patients with cardiac symptoms.

Treatment of LD is usually successful if therapy is initiated early with penicillins, cephalosporins, macrolides, or tetracyclines.[68] Patients in stage I disease should be treated with amoxicillin or doxycycline to prevent the development of further symptoms. During stages II and III, intravenous therapy is indicated, usually ceftriaxone (crosses the blood-brain barrier), cefotaxime, or penicillin.

The patient should be monitored for the development of cardiac and neurologic sequelae. Persons with musculoskeletal symptoms resulting in impaired mobility may require PT

Clinical Manifestations

Lyme Disease

STAGE I (EARLY LOCALIZED INFECTION)

Symptoms appear days to 16 weeks after tick bite
Erythema migrans appears in 50% to 70% of patients; resolves spontaneously in a few weeks
Fatigue
Headache
Lethargy
Myalgia, arthralgia
Lymphadenopathy

STAGE II (EARLY DISSEMINATED INFECTION)

Symptoms occur weeks to months after tick bite

Cardiac Symptoms

Carditis
Dysrhythmias
Heart failure
Pericarditis
Palpitations
Dyspnea

Neurologic Symptoms

Meningitis
Encephalitis
Cranial and peripheral neuropathy
Myelitis

Musculoskeletal Symptoms

Arthralgia, myalgia
Fibromyalgia

Other Symptoms

Conjunctivitis, optic neuropathy
Hepatomegaly, hepatitis
Generalized lymphadenopathy

STAGE III (LATE INFECTION)

Symptoms occur months to years after tick bite
Monoarticular or oligoarticular arthritis
Chronic arthritis
Acrodermatitis chronica atrophicans (bluish red, doughy lesions)
Lyme encephalitis, encephalomyelitis
Ataxia
Spastic paresis
Periventricular lesions
Memory loss
Behavioral changes

and OT, as well as analgesics to relieve joint pain. Nursing care would be similar to interventions for patients with RA.

Patient/Family Education. A vaccine for LD (LYMErix) was approved by the FDA in 1998. One year is required for optimal immunity, and the need for booster shots has not been determined. The vaccine is for persons ages 15 to 70 years. There have been no studies of the use of the vaccine in pregnant women, persons over 70 years of age, and those with chronic disease.[3,16,68] Persons with a history of LD may benefit from vaccination; previous infection does not guarantee immunity.[16] The vaccine is administered intramuscularly in a three-shot series over 12 months. Once the series is completed, the vaccine provides 79% immunity; after two injections it is only 50% effective. LYMErix does not treat LD, nor does it provide immunity against other tickborne diseases.[16] The cost of the vaccine is about $240; side effects include redness, swelling, and flulike symptoms. There are no known drug interactions, but the vaccination causes a false-positive ELISA and Western blot assay. The CDC recommends that the vaccine not be given to persons with Lyme arthritis that is resistant to antibiotic treatment, because of the possible relationship between the vaccine and developing chronic arthritis.[3,16,68] However, because of decreased consumer demand, the drug manufacturer is considering removing LYMErix from the market.[15a]

Patient Teaching

Lyme Disease Prevention

- Avoid tick-infested areas and sitting directly on the ground. Stay on paths while hiking.
- When outdoors in high-risk areas, wear long sleeves and long pants in light colors (to easily see ticks). Tuck shirt into pants and pants into shoes or socks.
- Wear closed shoes when hiking.
- Use Environmental Protection Agency (EPA)–approved tick repellents on skin and clothing. Wash off repellent thoroughly when returning inside. Avoid spraying repellents directly on the skin of small children.
- Check frequently for ticks; pets should be checked also.
- Have pets wear tick collars; do not allow outdoor pets on furniture or bedding.
- If a tick is found, use fine-pointed tweezers to grasp the tick at the point of attachment; gently pull the tick straight out. Place the tick in a sealed jar, and have it tested by a local veterinarian or health department. Do not squeeze the tick; doing so may release infected fluids.
- Wash the tick site thoroughly with soap and warm water, apply antiseptic, and disinfect the tweezers. Wash hands. Wash clothes thoroughly.
- Ticks are susceptible to dehydration. Reduce humidity by pruning trees, clearing brush, and mowing the lawn on your property.
- Do not have bird feeders or birdbaths in your yard; these attract animals that may have ticks.
- Keep woodpiles away from the house.
- Keep children's play areas away from wooded areas.
- See a physician or nurse practitioner if flulike symptoms or a rash develops.
- Discuss vaccination with the primary care provider, especially for persons at risk for contracting Lyme disease.

Education is the best prevention against LD (see Patient Teaching box). For persons with the disease, education about the signs and symptoms and complications of later disease is necessary. Patients and families need to learn about joint protection and energy conservation techniques.

Healthy People 2010 has named prevention of LD as a priority. Goals include decreasing the overall incidence of LD by 40% in endemic regions.[16] Nurses can provide community education to prevent the disease, especially in areas where the disease is prevalent. Education about the signs and symptoms of the disease is important to ensure early recognition and treatment of persons with LD. If LD is untreated, severe neurologic, cardiac, and musculoskeletal manifestations may occur. If the disease is diagnosed, cases should be reported to community health officials. Patients can be referred to the Lyme Disease Foundation.*

SERONEGATIVE ARTHROPATHIES

The term *seronegative arthropathies* is used to describe a group of diseases characterized by arthritis (arthropathy) in which the rheumatoid factor is not present in the serum. Another commonality is the absence of rheumatoid nodules. Approximately 2 million persons in the United States have seronegative arthropathies. Diseases included in this category are Reiter's syndrome, psoriatic arthritis, enteropathic arthritis, and ankylosing spondylitis (Table 47-9). In many instances symptoms overlap and do not meet the diagnostic criteria, so these patients are often diagnosed with the disease given the more general term *spondyloarthropathy.*[13,29] The majority of persons with ankylosing spondylitis and Reiter's syndrome have a specific gene, HLA-B27, which is found in 8% of North American Caucasians.[13]

These diseases are also known as *spondylarthritides* and have several characteristics in common, including:

- Axial arthritis (sacroiliitis and spondylitis [inflammation of the vertebrae characterized by stiffness and pain])
- Peripheral inflammatory arthritis, usually asymmetric and oligoarticular
- Enthesitis (inflammation at tendon attachment sites to bone)
- Presence of the cell marker HLA-B27
- Extraarticular manifestations, including ocular inflammation (conjunctivitis, uveitis), skin and nail lesions, aortitis, and ulceration of the GI and genitourinary tracts

*1 Financial Plaza, 18th Floor, Hartford, CT 06103; (860) 525-2000 or National Hotline (800) 886-LYME; e-mail: lymefnd@aol.com; website: www.lyme.org.

TABLE 47-9 Seronegative Arthropathies

Disorder	Etiology	Signs and Symptoms	Collaborative Management
Reiter's syndrome (reactive arthritis)	Sexually transmitted organisms or intestinal bacteria Precipitating event commonly urethritis Common organisms: *Chlamydia, Salmonella, Shigella*	Classic triad: arthritis, urethritis, and conjunctivitis (present in 33% of patients)[13] Acute onset of monoarthropathy or oligoarthropathy Fatigue, fever, generalized aching, joint stiffness, and back pain Arthritis usually affecting knees, ankles, feet, or toes; upper extremity involvement (sausage digits) with long-term disease Oral or genitourinary lesions; cutaneous lesions on soles and palms	Goals: alleviate pain, maintain joint mobility, and relieve systemic symptoms Medications: antibiotics for underlying infection, NSAIDs, sulfasalazine, methotrexate, ocular or topical steroids PT referral may be indicated; application of heat or cold for comfort Patient education regarding the disease No cure; exacerbations in one third of persons
Psoriatic arthritis	Complication of psoriasis Occurs in 7% of persons with psoriasis Possible genetic predisposition May result from abnormal immune response to *Streptococcus* that collects in psoriatic skin lesions	Distal interphalangeal joints of fingers, toes (sausage digits) Spondyloarthropathy similar to ankylosing spondylitis Sacroiliac joint involvement Skin lesions Nail changes (see Chapter 62)	Similar to treatment for rheumatoid arthritis
Enteropathic arthritis	Develops in 9%-20% of persons with inflammatory bowel disease, specifically ulcerative colitis and Crohn's disease (see Chapter 34) May result from an immune response to intestinal bacteria	Arthritis in multiple joints, particularly the knees, ankles, and wrists Spine, hips, and shoulders also affected Occurs during exacerbations of bowel disease and disappears when bowel symptoms subside In persons with spondylitis, symptoms not correlated with bowel symptoms	Similar to treatment for rheumatoid arthritis

NSAIDs, Nonsteroidal antiinflammatory drugs; *PT,* physical therapy.

Ankylosing Spondylitis

Etiology/Epidemiology

Ankylosing spondylitis (AS) (Marie-Strümpell disease) is a chronic inflammatory disorder of the axial skeleton, affecting primarily the sacroiliac joints and spine. The etiology is unknown. The course of the disease is marked by remissions and exacerbations.

The incidence of AS in the Caucasian population ranges from 0.02% to 23%, affecting men more than women by a 3:1 ratio.[13,29] The disease may be underdiagnosed in women because of milder symptoms and delayed onset.[13] The onset of disease is usually early adulthood. The genetic marker HLA-B27 is present in 95% of persons with AS; it is questionable whether bacterial infection triggers the disease.[29]

Pathophysiology

Spondylitis means inflammation of the spine. As a result of inflammation, the bones of the spine grow together and ankylose (fuse). The primary site of pathologic findings is the enthesis, where ligaments, tendons, and the joint capsule insert into bone. In AS, fibrous ossification and eventually fusion of the joint occur. The joint capsule, articular cartilage, and periosteum are invaded by inflammatory cells that trigger the development of fibrous scar tissue and growth of new bone. The bony growth changes the contour of the vertebrae and forms a new enthesis, or syndesmophyte, on top of the old one. As the spinal ligaments continue to undergo progressive calcification, the vertebral bodies lose their original contour and appear square, which gives the spine the classic bamboo appearance of AS. Inflammation usually begins around the sacroiliac joints and progresses up the spine, eventually resulting in fusion of the entire spine. As the inflammatory process involves the costosternal and costovertebral cartilage, it causes chest pain, which is worse on inspiration.

Initial symptoms may include low back pain or aching; pain and swelling of the hips, knees, or shoulders; mild fever; loss of appetite; and fatigue. Low back pain flares and subsides intermittently. Over time, pain subsides and motion of the back becomes restricted. Fusion of the sacroiliac joints and spine up through the cervical vertebrae may occur over a period of 10 to 20 years. As a result of rigidity, fractures may develop at multiple sites. The spine loses its normal lordotic curve, and the patient may have either a "poker back" deformity or a kyphosis at the cervicodorsal junction (Figure 47-26). The knees are flexed as the person attempts to move the head upright.

Extraarticular manifestations include iritis, uveitis, pulmonary fibrosis, and aortic insufficiency. One third of persons develop uveitis, which can cause tearing, photosensitivity, and ocular pain. Involvement is typically unilateral.

Collaborative Care Management

Differential diagnosis should include other causes of low back pain. Diagnosis is made primarily by the patient history and radiographic findings. The ESR is usually elevated, but this is not specific for diagnosis. X-ray films show the presence of syndesmophytes and "bamboo" spine. Ankylosis of peripheral joints may be seen. Computed tomography (CT) scans and MRI may show changes before they are visible on plain films. Testing for HLA-B27 is not useful for diagnosis.

Goals of treatment are to relieve pain and stiffness, achieve and maintain the best possible alignment of the spine, strengthen the paraspinal muscles, and prevent complications. Antiinflammatory medications (aspirin or NSAIDs) are given to control pain and inflammation, but they do not retard disease progression. NSAIDs shown to be beneficial in treating AS include indomethacin, diclofenac, naproxen, piroxicam, meloxicam, and celecoxib.[29] Systemic steroids are not recommended, although intraarticular or periarticular injections may be beneficial. The use of DMARDs for persons unresponsive to NSAID therapy is being studied.[29] If pain is unrelieved, additional analgesia should be added to the regimen (acetaminophen, opioids, and/or adjuvants).

Exercise is an important component of treatment. Swimming in a warm pool is a good choice for exercise. Rest should be discouraged unless a fracture is present. PT is recommended to maintain mobility and reduce the severity of deformity; for example, ROM exercises and lying prone (extension) may be done three to four times per day for 15 to 30 minutes, and deep breathing exercises may be performed to promote maximal chest expansion (rib cage mobility is decreased) (Figure 47-27). Surgery is indicated for persons with unrelieved pain and mobility problems. Procedures may include spinal osteotomy (usually cervical) and fusion and hip replacement.

Patient/Family Education. Patient teaching focuses on the nature and course of the disease, therapy regimen, appropriate use of prescribed medications, pain management, signs and symptoms of complications, and plans for follow-up care. Maintaining mobility and reducing the severity of deformity are important considerations. Stretching and extension exercises for the spine are beneficial in maintaining flexibility and mobility. Heat and hydrotherapy can help with stiffness and pain relief as an adjunct to exercise. Regular deep breathing and chest expansion exercises should be included in the regimen to optimize respiratory function. If respiratory complications occur, promoting adequate oxygenation is a priority of care. Adequate rest and pacing of activities is necessary to decrease dyspnea and activity intolerance. The patient should be advised of the risks associated with smoking.

Maintaining proper sitting and standing posture to decrease spinal flexion are important in the workplace and at home. Ergonomic modifications to the individual's work area can increase comfort and decrease stiffness. The individual should be encouraged to change positions frequently. For sleep, the patient should be encouraged to use a firm mattress or a bed board. Lying with the head flat helps maintain spine extension; sleeping with pillows causes cervical extension.

The patient is encouraged to participate in ADLs and usual activities to the fullest extent possible. The occupational therapist can provide assistive devices for persons with decreased mobility. Support and acceptance for persons with changes in appearance and body image are essential. Clothing may be difficult to fit if significant spinal deformity is present.

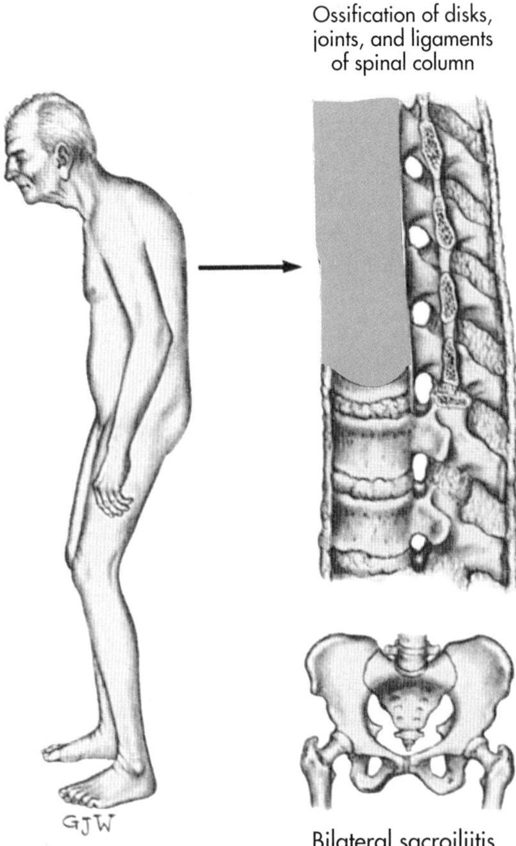

Figure 46-26 Characteristic posture and sites of ankylosing spondylitis.

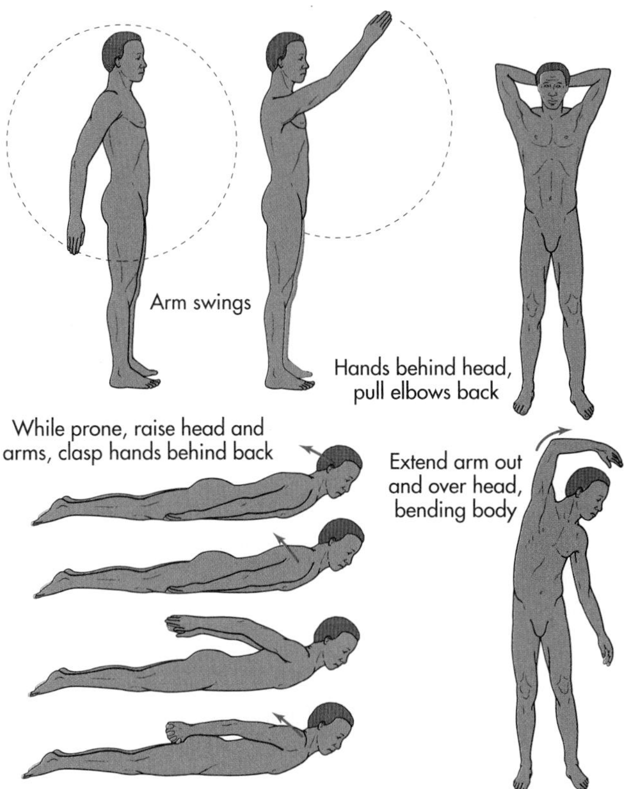

Figure 47-27 Typical chest cage stretching and deep chest breathing exercises for ankylosing spondylitis.

AUTOIMMUNE CONNECTIVE TISSUE DISEASES

Several autoimmune disorders affect the joints. These diseases are of unknown etiology and are similar to RA, affecting the skin and other organs. These disorders include systemic lupus erythematosus, scleroderma, CREST syndrome (*c*alcinosis cutis, *R*aynaud's phenomenon, *e*sophageal motility disorder, *s*clerodactyly, and *t*elangiectasia), and Sjögren's syndrome (Table 47-10). Although rare, Sjögren's syndrome is the most common autoimmune disorder among women; 95% of affected persons are female.[35] Nursing care for the person with musculoskeletal symptoms is similar to the care for the person with RA. Lupus is discussed in the following section.

SYSTEMIC LUPUS ERYTHEMATOSUS

Etiology/Epidemiology

Lupus was described as early as the time of Hippocrates. Today, lupus is classified as discoid (see Chapter 62), systemic, or drug induced. Systemic lupus erythematosus (SLE), which means "red wolf," refers to a chronic inflammatory disease of autoimmune origin that affects primarily the skin, joints, and kidneys, although the disease may affect virtually every organ of the body. The disease was named after the characteristic erythematous butterfly rash over the nose and cheeks, which resembles a wolf's snout.

Although the etiology is unknown, genetic, hormonal (disturbances in estrogen metabolism), and immune factors have been identified. Drugs, including procainamide, isoniazid, and hydralazine, are known to induce lupuslike syndromes. Persons with drug-induced lupus usually do not develop renal and neurologic disease. The symptoms usually resolve after the drug is discontinued.

SLE affects women, particularly of childbearing years. The incidence is estimated to be 40 to 50 per 100,000 women and is higher in African-American women.[40,61] The incidence is higher among Native Americans, Asians in Hawaii, and Chinese persons. Lupus has been seen in some men with Klinefelter's syndrome.[61] Menses and pregnancy can cause an exacerbation of the disease. The risk for developing SLE drops significantly after menopause in women but remains constant throughout the life span in men. Although there is no cure, the course of SLE can usually be controlled. Although potentially fatal, 85% of persons with SLE survive 15 years or longer.[40] Mortality is usually a result of lesions affecting major organs or from secondary infections.

Pathophysiology

The exact mechanism of pathogenesis is unknown. However, several alterations in the immune system are associated with SLE. Numerous cellular antibodies have been identified in persons with the disorder. Antinuclear antibodies, antibodies to deoxyribonucleic acid (DNA), antihistones, and antibodies to ribonucleoprotein (Smith antigen) are all strongly associated with SLE.

TABLE 47-10 Autoimmune Connective Diseases

Disorder	Pathophysiology	Clinical Manifestations	Treatment
Scleroderma (systemic sclerosis)	Most common in middle-aged women Causes microvascular damage and fibrous degeneration of tissue in skin, GI tract, heart, lung, and kidneys; excess collagen causes fibrosis and malfunction of involved organ	Raynaud's phenomenon GI: dysphagia, gastroesophageal reflux disease (GERD), diarrhea, and malabsorption Renal: hematuria, proteinuria, renal crisis, hypertension Cardiopulmonary: pericarditis, dysrhythmias, pulmonary hypertension, fibrosis Dermatologic: hardening, tightening, and thickening of skin; edema, pallor, and deepened pigmentation Musculoskeletal: muscle atrophy, rheumatoid arthritis, tightening of tendons, flexion contractures	Arthralgia, myalgia Dependent on amount of organ involvement Avoidance of cold; protective clothing Skin care for ulcers Doppler evaluation of palmar circulation; thrombolytics if needed Thoracic sympathectomy for Raynaud's phenomenon Metoclopramide, proton pump inhibitors, and esophageal dilation for GI symptoms ACE inhibitors for renal symptoms Cyclophosphamide for alveolitis; calcium channel blockers or epoprostenol for pulmonary hypertension; lung transplant for persons with end-stage lung disease NSAIDs, PT, OT, exercises to maintain joint mobility Splints for contractures and deformities Heat and cold as needed
CREST syndrome (limited cutaneous scleroderma)	Variant of scleroderma, classified by extent of skin thickening More favorable prognosis and less organ involvement	Calcinosis (result of chronic vascular insufficiency) Intracutaneous or subcutaneous calcifications on digital pads, periarticular tissues, extensor surfaces of forearms, olecranon, and prepatellar bursae Raynaud's phenomenon Esophageal dysmotility Sclerodactyly Telangiectasia Pulmonary involvement in many patients	As for scleroderma Surgical removal of calcium deposits
Sjögren's syndrome	Inflammation and dysfunction of exocrine glands, particularly lacrimal and salivary glands, which results in dryness of mouth, eyes, and mucous membranes Lymph nodes, bone marrow, and organ involvement Rheumatoid arthritis in 50% of patients	Xerostomia, xerophthalmia; (dry mouth and dry eye, known as sicca syndrome) Oral candidiasis (complication of xerostomia) Dyspareunia Decreased tearing Gritty sensation in eyes Dysphagia Dental caries Cough Enlarged parotid glands Rheumatoid and antinuclear antibody factors positive in most patients Anemia	Artificial tears Vaginal lubrication or estrogen creams Surgical punctal occlusion Saliva substitutes; pilocarpine to promote salivary and lacrimal flow[25,35] Increased fluid intake, especially with meals Good dental and oral hygiene, especially after meals Avoidance of respiratory infections and smoking Increased humidity in home and work environment Antimalarials NSAIDs for arthritic symptoms Steroids, immunosuppressants for renal, lung symptoms

ACE, Angiotensin-converting enzyme; *GI,* gastrointestinal; *NSAIDs,* nonsteroidal antiinflammatory drugs; *OT,* occupational therapy; *PT,* physical therapy.

Abnormalities in both B cells and T cells also have been identified in persons with the disease. The appearance of B cells is thought to cause an increase in the production of antibodies to self and nonself antigen. These antibodies are responsible for the tissue injury seen in SLE. Most visceral lesions are mediated by type III hypersensitivity, and antibodies against red blood cells are mediated by type II hypersensitivity. An acute necrotizing vasculitis can occur in any tissue. Most lesions are found in the blood vessels, kidney, connective tissues, and skin.

TABLE 47-11 American College of Rheumatology: Criteria for Classification of Systemic Lupus Erythematosus*

Criterion	Definition
1. Malar rash	Fixed erythema, flat or raised, over the malar eminences, tending to spare the nasolabial folds
2. Discoid rash	Erythematous raised patches with adherent keratotic scaling and follicular plugging; atrophic scarring may occur in older lesions
3. Photosensitivity	Skin rash as a result of unusual reaction to sunlight, by patient history or physician observation
4. Oral ulcers	Oral or nasopharyngeal ulceration, usually painless, observed by a physician
5. Arthritis	Nonerosive arthritis involving two or more peripheral joints, characterized by tenderness, swelling, or effusion
6. Serositis	a. Pleuritis—convincing history of pleuritic pain or rub heard by a physician or evidence of pleural effusion, or b. Pericarditis—documented by electrocardiogram or rub or evidence of pericardial effusion
7. Renal disorder	a. Persistent proteinuria greater than 0.5 g/dl or greater than 3+ if quantitation not performed, or b. Cellular casts—may be red blood cell, hemoglobin, granular, tubular, or mixed
8. Neurologic disorder	a. Seizures—in the absence of offending drugs or known metabolic derangements (e.g., uremia, ketoacidosis, or electrolyte imbalance) or b. Psychosis—in the absence of offending drugs or known metabolic derangements (e.g., uremia, ketoacidosis, or electrolyte imbalance)
9. Hematologic disorder	a. Hemolytic anemia—with reticulocytosis, or b. Leukopenia—less than 4.0×10^9/L (4000/mm^3) total on two or more occasions, or c. Lymphopenia—less than 1.5×10^9/L (1500/mm^3) on two or more occasions, or d. Thrombocytopenia—less than 100×10^9/L (100×10^3/mm^3) in the absence of offending drugs
10. Immunologic disorder	a. Positive lupus erythematosus cell preparation, or b. Anti-DNA antibody to native DNA in abnormal titer, or c. Anti-Sm—presence of antibody to Sm nuclear antigen, or d. False-positive serologic test for syphilis known to be positive for at least 6 months and confirmed by negative *Treponema pallidum* immobilization or fluorescent treponemal antibody absorption test
11. Antinuclear antibody	An abnormal titer of antinuclear antibody by immunofluorescence of an equivalent assay at any point in time and in the absence of drugs known to be associated with drug-induced lupus syndrome

Data from Tan EM et al: The revised criteria for the classification of systemic lupus erythematosus, *Arthritis Rheum* 25:1271, 1982.
*The classification is based on 11 criteria. For the purpose of identifying patients in clinical studies, a person shall be said to have systemic lupus erythematosus if any 4 or more of the 11 criteria are present, serially or simultaneously, during any interval of observation.

Because of the multisystem involvement and characteristic remissions and exacerbations, the clinical manifestations of SLE can be overwhelming. The American College of Rheumatology has developed criteria for the diagnosis of SLE (Table 47-11). The initial manifestation of SLE is often arthritis, typically a nonerosive synovitis without deformity. Ninety-five percent of persons with SLE develop arthritis. Joint deformity occurs without bony erosion and resembles that of persons with RA. Contractures may also develop. In many instances the joint symptoms are transient and respond to treatment. Weakness, fatigue, and weight loss may be present. The patient may report photosensitivity, development of a rash, and at times fever or arthritis on exposure to sunlight. Erythema, usually in a butterfly pattern, appears over the cheeks and bridge of the nose. The margins of these lesions are bright red, and the lesions may extend beyond the hairline with partial alopecia above the ears. Lesions may also occur on the exposed part of the neck. Lesions spread slowly to the mucous membranes and other tissues of the body, or they may originate there. These lesions do not ulcerate but cause degeneration and atrophy of tissues.

Depending on the organs involved, glomerulonephritis, splenomegaly, hepatomegaly, pleuritis, pericarditis, lymphadenopathy, peritonitis, neuritis, or anemia may be present. Renal and neurologic manifestations are among the more serious complications of the disease.

Collaborative Care Management

Diagnosis is made after evaluation of the patient history and physical examination and results of laboratory tests. See Table 47-11 for selected laboratory findings.

The immunofluorescence test for antinuclear antibodies (ANA) is positive in more than 95% of patients with SLE; the higher the titer, the more likely the diagnosis of SLE. However, the diagnosis of SLE cannot be made solely on the basis of a positive ANA result, because it is also positive in many other autoimmune disorders, such as systemic sclerosis (both CREST syndrome and diffuse sclerosis), Sjögren's syndrome, and polymyositis. Positive results are also found among older adults and pregnant women, and secondary to many prescription medications.[33] As mentioned earlier, antibodies against double-stranded DNA and anti-Smith antigen are positive in 20% to 60% of patients with SLE. The LE cell test is positive in 70% of patients with SLE. The LE cell is any phagocytic leukocyte that has engulfed the nucleus of an injured cell.

Kidney failure is the most common cause of death in persons with lupus. Cyclophosphamide, either orally or by intravenous pulse therapy, is effective in treating lupus nephritis but is associated with significant toxicity. Dexamethasone and ondansetron can be given to improve tolerance of side effects. Treatment with azathioprine is an alternative to cyclophosphamide, especially for those who wish to preserve reproductive function. Renal symptoms are often silent; urinalysis and renal function tests should be done at regular intervals. Renal biopsy may be indicated to evaluate the condition of the parenchyma.[58] Dialysis or a transplant may be indicated for patients with uncontrolled lupus nephritis.

Arthritis and arthralgia are the most common presenting symptoms of SLE; avascular necrosis may develop as a result of the disease or steroid therapy. Orthopedic surgery may be required for persons with severe arthritic manifestations of SLE. Pharmacologic management of arthritic symptoms is similar to treatment for RA. NSAIDs are first-line treatment, but patients with SLE are prone to developing NSAID-induced hepatitis and should be monitored carefully. Renal function should be monitored regularly; NSAIDs are contraindicated with renal impairment. Hydroxychloroquine sulfate to suppress synovitis is indicated for those unresponsive to NSAIDs. Corticosteroids and methotrexate are used if other medications are ineffective in controlling symptoms. If methotrexate is used, folic acid should be given to decrease side effects and blood and liver function studies should be monitored.

Antimalarials are also effective in treating skin lesions, serositis, fever, and fatigue. Topical corticosteroids are prescribed for less extensive skin lesions. Corticosteroids are also effective in treating neurologic, cardiac, or hematologic effects. Because of the side effects associated with systemic steroids, their use should be limited to persons with severe, life-threatening complications (severe hemolytic anemia, thrombocytopenia, pulmonary hemorrhage) or those unresponsive to other, less toxic therapies.[33]

During exacerbations, persons with SLE are acutely ill, and nursing care depends on the symptoms manifested. The patient should be monitored for the effects of medications and the possibility of renal dysfunction. The patient's neurologic status must be assessed frequently for the development of cognitive dysfunction. Seizures may occur in 15% to 20% of persons with SLE; psychosis may develop as a result of steroid therapy or the disease process.[58]

Patient/Family Education. Instructions for joint protection, pain management, energy conservation techniques, and self-care are similar to those for the patient with RA. In addition, the patient should be instructed to avoid sun exposure and to apply sunscreen (sun protection factor [SPF] 15 or higher) liberally when outdoors. Sun exposure exacerbates skin and systemic manifestations. When skin manifestations are present, the patient should be taught to keep the lesions clean and to avoid secondary sources of infection. Any cosmetics used on the face should be hypoallergenic. Wigs may be used to mask hair loss.

The patient and family may need help in coping with a chronic systemic disease with an unpredictable course. Compliance may be an issue, particularly because strict adherence to the treatment regimen does not necessarily prevent exacerbation.

Because most persons affected with SLE are women in childbearing years, pregnancy should be addressed. The incidence of exacerbation during pregnancy ranges from 22% to 58%.[40] Pregnancy should be planned in consultation with the patient's physician, usually an obstetrician who treats high-risk patients. The safety during pregnancy of medications used for treatment must be considered carefully.

Factors such as fatigue, sun, stress, and infection can exacerbate SLE. The patient and family should be taught measures to deal with stress. Physical changes, such as the rash, alopecia, or joint deformities, may cause problems with body image or social isolation. Nursing interventions can assist the patient in accepting changes and coping with a chronic disease.

INFLAMMATORY MYOPATHIES

Polymyositis and dermatomyositis are considered to be both rheumatic connective tissue diseases and idiopathic inflammatory myopathies. Both may occur alone or in combination with other rheumatic diseases, most notably scleroderma, SLE, and Sjögren's syndrome.

Polymyositis/Dermatomyositis

Etiology/Epidemiology

Polymyositis (PM) is a chronic acquired inflammatory disorder of skeletal muscle. When a characteristic skin rash is present, the disorder is referred to as dermatomyositis (DM). The etiology of both disorders is unknown, but abnormal reactions of the immune system have been implicated, perhaps triggered by a virus. Autoantibodies are found in the serum of affected individuals. The incidence of both disorders is estimated to be 1 per 1,000,000 population; PM and DM are the most common inflammatory muscle diseases.[5] PM occurs two times more often in women than in men.

Pathophysiology

Both PM and DM are characterized by inflammation of muscle fibers and connective tissue, resulting in extensive tissue necrosis and destruction of muscle fibers. Both cell-mediated and humoral immune mechanisms are associated with the diseases. Inflammatory cells found at the perimysial and perivascular sites contain B cells and helper T cells in DM. Less vascular involvement occurs in PM, and B and T cells are found surrounding the muscle fibers and fascicles.

Results of histologic studies of muscle biopsy are variable, but the pathologic alterations found, in order of their frequency, are:

- Primary degeneration of muscle fibers, either focal or extensive
- Basophilia of some fibers with central migration of the sarcolemmal nuclei
- Necrosis of parts or entire groups of muscle fibers
- Inflammation of blood vessels supplying the muscles
- Interstitial fibrosis varying in severity with the duration and, to some extent, the type of the disease
- Variation in the cross-sectional diameter of fibers

The initial symptoms of both disorders are similar to those associated with any inflammatory response: fever, swelling, malaise, and fatigue. The diseases, which run a course of exacerbations and remissions, are usually first noted in proximal muscles, in particular the pelvic and shoulder girdles. The weakness is symmetric. Climbing stairs, rising from a chair, and other activities that involve lifting the body become increasingly difficult or impossible. Lifting the arms becomes progressively more difficult, and hair combing may be impossible. Other muscles such as the neck flexors and the muscles of swallowing may also become involved. Muscle pain or tenderness is present in some instances in the early stages.

Clinical manifestations common to both PM and DM include dysphagia, dyspnea, decreased esophageal motility, cardiomyopathy, and Raynaud's phenomenon. A dusky red lesion may be found in the periorbital region (heliotrope rash), along with periorbital edema in persons with DM. This dusky red rash may extend over the face, forehead, neck, upper shoulders, chest, and upper back. Scaly lesions on the arms and legs commonly affect the extensor surfaces. Erythema occurs over the MCP and PIP joints (Gottron's sign). Calcinosis can also occur in DM.

The weakness of myositis, if it persists, can lead to contractures and atrophy. Older adults with DM seem to have a greater chance of malignancy than the population at large, although the frequency ranges from 6% to 45%. The most common sites of cancer are the lungs, breasts, ovaries, and GI tract, as well as myeloproliferative disorders.[5]

Collaborative Care Management

Diagnosis is based on:

- The patient history and physical examination, including manual muscle tests to delineate weakness in specific muscles
- An electromyogram to delineate a specific pattern of findings to differentiate PM from other types of muscle disease
- Muscle biopsy to define specific pathologic changes in muscle
- Serum enzyme levels (creatine phosphokinase, lactate dehydrogenase, and aldolase), which are elevated in the presence of active disease
- A 24-hour urine test to determine an abnormal creatine-creatinine ratio

High-dose corticosteroid therapy (prednisone up to 60 mg daily) is used for patients with PM or DM. Serial muscle testing helps document response to treatment. With clinical improvement, steroid dosage should be tapered to 10 to 20 mg daily and continued for 1 year. With exacerbations, high-dose steroid therapy is resumed. If steroids are contraindicated or ineffective, an immunosuppressant such as methotrexate is prescribed. Blood counts and liver enzymes should be monitored while the patient is receiving therapy. Cyclosporine has been used effectively in some patients, and hydroxychloroquine may improve the rash in persons with DM.

Nursing interventions focus on maintaining the patient's strength, ROM, and level of functioning. Measures to prevent falls from muscle weakness include the use of assistive devices for ambulation, strengthening exercises, and evaluating the home and work environment for safety. Osteoporosis may develop as a result of steroid therapy; prevention of falls and fractures is an important intervention. ROM exercises should be performed regularly to prevent contractures. Sitting surfaces may need to be elevated to facilitate transfer—a chair with a firm surface with back and arm rests is best; an elevated toilet seat and handrails can be added to the commode.

Patient/Family Education. The patient's and family's knowledge of the disease process and treatment plan is assessed. The patient should be aware of the need for serial laboratory and clinical examinations. The patient is instructed in the use of selected ADL devices to enhance function (e.g., a long-handled comb). Home health services may be required during acute phases of illness because of muscle weakness. Family and caregiver support is needed. Medication instruction focuses on the side effects associated with long-term steroid therapy (see Chapter 29). The importance of following the medication regimen and not altering dosages or frequency should be stressed. Patients should wear a Medic-Alert bracelet or identification card indicating that they are receiving steroid therapy.

Fibromyalgia Syndrome

Although fibromyalgia syndrome (FMS) is considered to be a generalized pain syndrome, it is discussed here because of its association with RA, SLE, PM, and Sjögren's syndrome.

Etiology/Epidemiology

After OA and RA, FMS is the most commonly diagnosed rheumatologic disorder in the United States. An estimated 3 to 6 million persons in the United States are affected by this disorder, as well as 2% to 10% of the population in industrialized countries.[9,69] The typical age of onset is between 29 and 37 years.[27] FMS has been described since antiquity; however, some practitioners are reluctant to recognize this syndrome as a legitimate diagnosis, perhaps because of the nonspecific pain and unknown mechanism of disease.[9,47] This disabling disease is characterized by widespread pain and tenderness to palpation at anatomically defined tender points.

The etiology is unknown, but there is an association between sleep disturbance, lack of exercise, and fibromyalgia. Fibromyalgia-like symptoms have occurred in persons deprived of sleep and/or exercise; specific exercise prescriptions effectively treat symptoms. Other theories include a low pain threshold and malfunction in supraspinal processing of external stimuli and hypoactivity of the autonomic nervous system and hypothalamic-pituitary-adrenal axis.[9] Possible triggers include stress, viral infection (parvovirus, Epstein-Barr), hormonal alterations, hypothyroidism, and Lyme disease. A familial pattern of disease prevalence has been identified.

Pathophysiology

Fibromyalgia may appear with RA or SLE or other pain syndromes and is considered in the differential diagnosis of RA, SLE, polymyalgia rheumatica, myositis, neuropathies, and hypoparathyroidism. The pathophysiology of FMS is not completely understood. Several abnormalities in muscle have been documented in persons with FMS, including lower adenosine triphosphate and adenosine diphosphate levels, higher levels of adenosine monophosphate, and changes in the number of capillaries and fiber area. A general hypothesis is that increased muscle tenderness is the result of generalized pain intolerance, perhaps as a result of central nervous system

(CNS) abnormalities (Figure 47-28). Decreased levels of serotonin and tryptophan and low levels of growth hormone may be responsible for the sleep dysfunction and weight gain experienced by many persons with FMS.

Collaborative Care Management

The American College of Rheumatology defined diagnostic criteria for FMS in 1990 (Box 47-8 and Figure 47-29). Palpation of the tender points should reproduce pain, not tenderness or pressure. A pressure threshold meter can be used for objectivity. Excessive or inadequate pressure can lead to false-positive or false-negative results. Tender points must be present bilaterally, above and below the waist, and in the midline.

BOX 47-8 Diagnostic Criteria for Fibromyalgia Syndrome

Patient history of chronic (lasting longer than 3 months) widespread pain in all four quadrants of the body

Pain in 11 of 18 specific tender point sites when palpated is significant for diagnosis;

4 kg of palpation pressure used for examination

Bilateral tender point sites are:

- Occiput
- Cervical
- Trapezius
- Scapular
- Second rib
- Epicondyle
- Gluteal
- Trochanter
- Medial knee

Sources: Clauw DJ: Elusive syndromes: treating the biologic basis of fibromyalgia and related syndromes, *Cleve Clin J Med* 68(10):830-839, 2001; Mortensen SE: Bursitis, tendinitis, myofascial pain, and fibromyalgia. In Rakel RE, Bope ET, editors: *Conn's current therapy,* Philadelphia, 2002, WB Saunders.

The characteristic symptom of fibromyalgia is a generalized chronic pain, which may be described as "burning or gnawing." Common symptoms include chronic aching, nonrestorative sleep, morning stiffness, and fatigue. Patients with FMS demonstrate loss of functional abilities similar to that in patients with RA, yet no radiographic changes in articular structures are found in persons with FMS. Depression is a common finding in persons with FMS. Headaches, sensitivity to extreme temperatures, abdominal pain, paresthesias, menstrual irregularities, irritable bowel, and difficulty concentrating may be reported. There are no visible signs of FMS.

There is no cure for FMS. Goals of therapy are to restore sleep and reduce pain. A multidisciplinary approach to managing the person with FMS is most effective. Medications used to treat FMS include tricyclic antidepressants to increase non-REM sleep (amitriptyline or nortriptyline); cyclobenzaprine (has both antidepressant and muscle relaxant qualities) and selective serotonin reuptake inhibitors (SSRIs) are also used effectively. A combination of a tricyclic given at bedtime and an SSRI taken in the morning may be effective in restoring adequate sleep and reducing fatigue. Tramadol and gabapentin have been used successfully for pain control. NSAIDs also may be used for pain control.

Exercise is an important treatment modality for persons with FMS. Stretching exercises, PT, and massage can aid in relaxation, reducing fatigue, and improving overall condition-

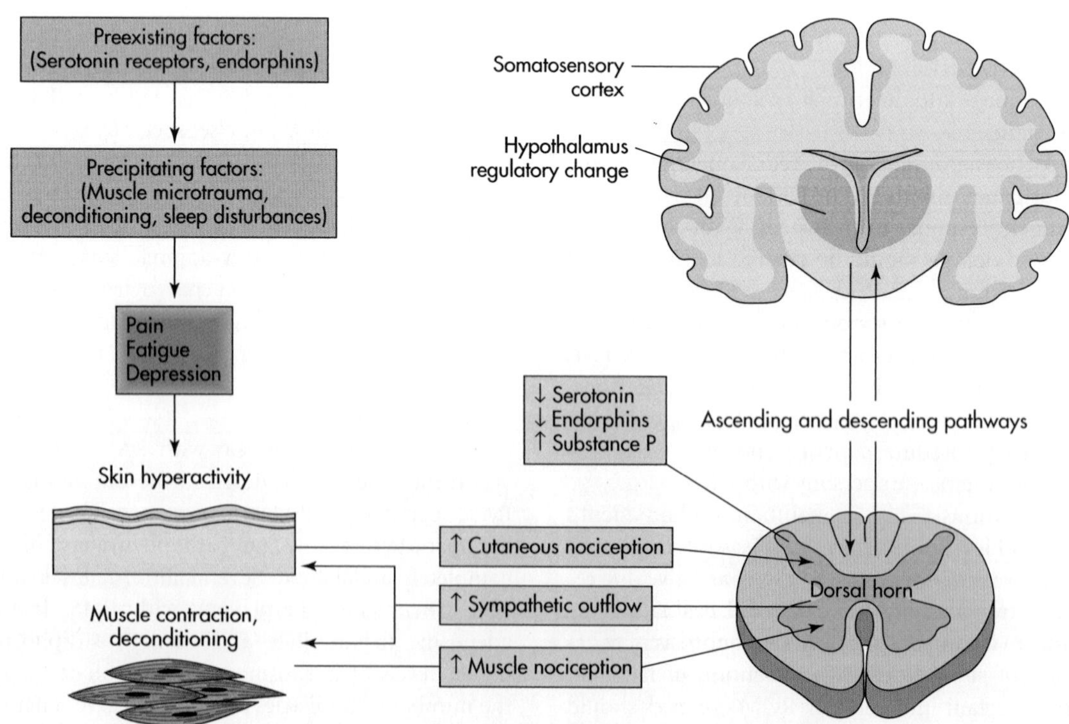

Figure 47-28 Theoretic pathophysiologic model of fibromyalgia.

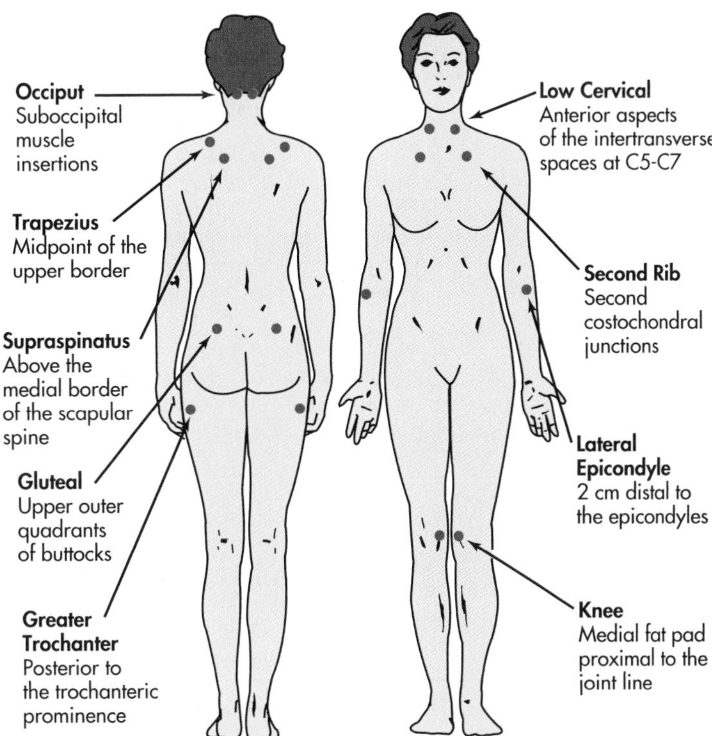

Figure 47-29 Location of specific tender points for diagnostic classification of fibromyalgia.

ing. Other relaxation techniques such as biofeedback, deep breathing, and meditation can be useful adjuncts to pharmacologic therapies. Stress management techniques should be included in treatment. Other treatments that may be effective include heat in the form of whirlpools, moist packs, or a hot shower; acupuncture; and acupressure.

Patient/Family Education. Support of the patient and family is an important nursing responsibility. FMS affects not only the patient but also the entire family. The patient may have considerable anxiety, especially if diagnosis of the disorder was difficult; the patient may need assurance that she or he is not "crazy." Because of the lack of objective signs of illness, others may doubt the reality of the illness. Psychologic counseling may be necessary for some patients. Reassurance and validation of the patient's reports of symptoms are important. The patient and family should be encouraged to discuss their feelings openly. Stress can cause exacerbations of the disorder, so stress management and reduction techniques are important.

Teaching should include information about the disease and the rationales for treatment. The patient should be taught the relationship between exercise and sleep and other factors that may disturb sleep (alcohol, stress, noise, and pain). Making a lifetime commitment to regular exercise can decrease symptoms and improve well-being.

Nurses can provide support to individuals trying to cope with chronic disease. The principles of therapeutic communication are important when listening to patients' reports of illness and coping strategies. Support groups are available for patients with FMS. The Arthritis Foundation may be helpful as a resource for exercise programs in the community. Other resources are the Fibromyalgia Network* and the American Fibromyalgia Syndrome Association, Inc.†

Other generalized pain syndromes affecting the musculoskeletal system include polymyalgia rheumatica, which can be accompanied by a destructive, inflammatory arthritis and which often occurs with giant cell arteritis (Table 47-12).

DISORDERS AFFECTING THE BONES

METABOLIC BONE DISEASES

Metabolic bone diseases affect the normal homeostatic functioning of the skeletal system. The etiology of metabolic bone diseases includes hormonal, genetic, and dietary factors. Paget's disease and osteoporosis are discussed in the following sections.

Paget's Disease

Etiology/Epidemiology

Sir James Paget, an English surgeon first described Paget's disease, also referred to as osteitis deformans, in 1876. Characterized by an excess of bone destruction and unorganized bone formation and repair, Paget's disease is the second most common bone disorder in the United States following osteoporosis. The etiology of Paget's disease is unknown; a genetic predisposition has been identified in 10% of patients, most probably as an autosomal-dominant pattern of inheritance.[28]

*5700 Stockdale Highway, Suite 100, Bakersfield, CA 93309; (805) 631-1950.
†Website: http://www.afsafund.org.

TABLE 47-12 Polymyalgia Rheumatica

Epidemiology	Etiology	Clinical Manifestations	Treatment
Peak incidence: Caucasians older than age 50 years; average age at onset 70 years Twice as many women as men 10% of persons with PR develop GCA; 50% of persons with GCA have PR[26]	Unknown etiology Theories include trauma to cell-mediated response, immune process; normal aging process; genetic predisposition or environmental influences such as infectious agents, drugs, and toxins Studies suggest single causative agent for PR and GCA	ESR 50 mm/hr Anemia Elevated C-reactive protein and elevated alkaline phosphatase Creatine kinase normal and rheumatoid factor negative Acute or insidious onset of symptoms Morning stiffness lasting >30 minutes classic symptom Bilateral aching in the shoulders, neck, and pelvic girdle Knees, elbows, wrists, and metatarsophalangeal joints also affected No radiologic evidence of bone erosion Fever, anorexia, night sweats, apathy, depression, weight loss, and malaise Diagnosis of GCA confirmed by temporal artery biopsy	Steroid therapy, typically prednisone, in lowest dose to control symptoms for shortest period of time (PR: 10-20 mg/day, then tapered; GCA: 40-60 mg/day, then tapered); NSAIDs for discomfort after steroids discontinued Possibility of disease recurrence within 18 months of cessation of prednisone Patient teaching about signs and symptoms of disease and medications Encourage adequate rest and regular exercise

ESR, Erythrocyte sedimentation rate; *GCA*, giant cell arteritis; *NSAIDs*, nonsteroidal antiinflammatory drugs; *PR*, polymyalgia rheumatica.

Research suggests that a slow viral infection of the osteoclasts triggers the disease in genetically predisposed individuals. Other causative theories include autoimmune dysfunction, vascular disorders, vitamin D deficiency in childhood, and mechanical stressors to bone.

Paget's disease is a common disorder in Northern Europe, North America, Australia, and New Zealand but is relatively uncommon in other parts of the world. It is commonly found in the United Kingdom, where the incidence is 5% of the population older than 55 years of age.[28] The average age at diagnosis is 50 to 60 years of age; the incidence of symptomatic disease increases with age.

Paget's disease usually affects the axial skeleton, particularly the vertebrae and skull, although the pelvis, femur, and tibia are other common sites of disease. Most persons are asymptomatic, and diagnosis is incidental.

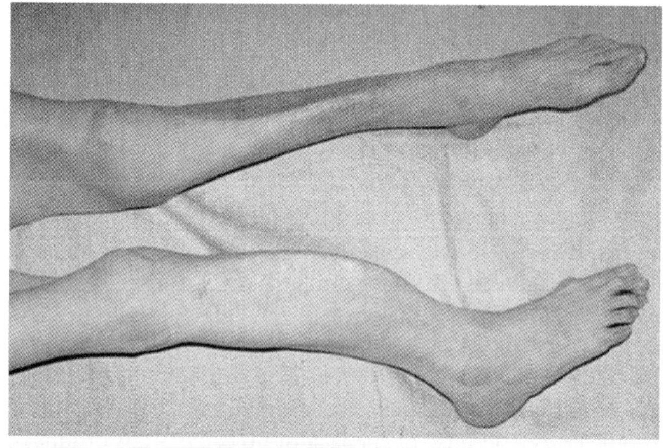

Figure 47-30 Paget's disease with bilateral tibial deformities.

Pathophysiology

Initial changes in Paget's disease involve an increase in osteoclast-mediated resorption of cancellous bone, along with an increase in osteoblast-mediated bone formation. Bone resorption and formation are increased, resulting in a mosaic-like mix of abnormal woven and normal lamellar bone. Mineralization may encroach into the marrow, and excessive bone formation usually occurs around partially resorbed trabeculae, causing thickening and hypertrophy. Vascularity is increased in affected portions of the skeleton. Lesions may occur in one or more bones, but the disease does not spread from bone to bone.

Deformities and bony enlargement often occur. Bowing of the limbs and spinal curvature may occur in persons with advanced disease. Bone pain is the most common symptom of Paget's disease. Degenerative arthritis may occur at adjacent joints. Microfractures, cortical swelling, and lytic bone lesions contribute to the pain. Pain is usually worse with ambulation or activity but may also occur at rest. Involved bones may feel spongy and warm as a result of the increased vascularity. Weight-bearing bones such as the tibia and femur may become deformed, and the person's gait is affected (Figure 47-30).

Skull pain is usually accompanied by headache, warmth, tenderness, and enlargement of the head. Flattening of the base of the skull *(platybasia)* may result in serious complications of obstructive hydrocephalus or brainstem compression. Facial bone involvement may cause deformity or, less often, affect the airway. Conductive and/or sensorineural hearing loss and vertigo may develop secondary to otosclerosis or neurologic abnormalities. With extensive skeletal involvement, cardiac involvement may develop as a result of increased vascularity and increased cardiac output.

Pathologic fractures are a problem for persons with Paget's disease. Because of the increased vascularity of the involved bone, bleeding is a potential danger. Long bones with lytic lesions are the most susceptible to fracture. Long-standing disease may lead to malignant transformation, usually osteosarcoma. Symptoms include increased pain and swelling of affected bones. The most common sites for malignancy are the pelvis, femur, and humerus.

Alkaline phosphatase levels are usually markedly elevated as a result of osteoblast activity. Serum calcium levels are usually normal except with generalized disease or immobilization. The development of kidney stones is a potential complication if immobility is prolonged. Calcium deposits may also occur in the joint spaces. There is the risk of developing secondary hyperparathyroidism in persons with normal serum calcium levels and increased levels of serum alkaline phosphatase. Gout and hyperuricemia may develop as a result of increased bone activity, which causes an increase in nucleic acid catabolism.

Collaborative Care Management

Radiographs of individuals with Paget's disease reveal radiolucent areas in the bone, typical of increased bone resorption. Deformities and fractures may also be present. A bone scan is indicated at the time of diagnosis to determine the extent of disease. A CT scan may be indicated if malignancy or neural compression is suspected. Urinary pyridinoline cross-links (see Chapter 45), a marker of bone turnover, can be followed to determine the effectiveness of treatment.

Goals of treatment are to relieve pain and prevent fracture and deformity. Asymptomatic patients generally do not require treatment.

Pharmacologic agents are used to suppress osteoclastic activity. Medications include the bisphosphonates and calcitonin. The bisphosphonates and calcitonin are effective agents to decrease bone pain and bone warmth and may also relieve neural compression, joint pain, and lytic lesions. Deformity or hearing loss does not improve with pharmacologic treatment. Gallium nitrate, a bone metabolism regulator, although not approved for treatment, is also used for therapy.

Plicamycin is not approved for treatment of Paget's disease but has been used parenterally to treat persons with severe disease or neurologic symptoms. Dexamethasone may be used in combination with plicamycin in the case of spinal cord compression. Some individuals may require surgical decompression.

Other treatments include the use of analgesics and NSAIDs. Assistive devices, including canes and walkers, may be needed. A shoe lift may be required for persons with deformities resulting in leg length discrepancy. Deformities may also be corrected by surgical intervention (osteotomy). Open reduction and internal fixation may be necessary for fractures. In some cases total joint arthroplasty may be indicated for severe degenerative arthritis.

The patient may benefit from a PT referral. Local application of ice or heat may help alleviate pain. However, application of heat may increase the warmth associated with increased vascularity, which some patients find uncomfortable. Massage may be effective in some patients.

Patient/Family Education. The patient and family should receive information regarding the course of disease, complications, and treatments. Instructions for taking medications should be included. The patient should understand the need for follow-up medical care and monitoring for complications.

A regular exercise program should be maintained; walking is best. Patients should avoid extended periods of immobility to avoid hypercalcemia. A nutritionally adequate diet is recommended. Because of the pathologic fractures, safety precautions are very important to avoid falls or other injuries. The patient may need assistance in learning to use canes or other ambulatory aids. If deformities are present, the patient may need support in dealing with changes in body image. The Arthritis Foundation and the Paget Foundation* are useful resources for patients and their families.

Risk Factors
Osteoporosis

Aging
Female
Caucasian or Asian race
Nulliparity
Family history
Postmenopausal–surgical or natural
Chronic calcium deficiency
Vitamin D deficiency
Sedentary lifestyle
Small frame, low body weight
Smoking
Diet high in protein and fat
Chronic alcohol use
Excessive caffeine intake

Osteoporosis

Etiology

Osteoporosis is the most common bone disorder in the Western world and is second only to arthritis as a cause of musculoskeletal morbidity in the elderly population. The initial definition of *osteoporosis,* which means "porous bone," was "too little bone in the bone" and was provided by Albright.[65] Although the exact etiology of osteoporosis is unknown, several risk factors have been identified (see Risk Factors box). Important risk factors are a low peak bone mass at skeletal maturity, aging, and accelerated postmenopausal bone loss. The gene controlling bone density has been identified by researchers and may have significant implications for the prevention of osteoporosis.[63]

Osteoporosis was initially categorized as postmenopausal (women up to age 65 years), senile (any sex over 65 years), or

*120 Wall Street, Suite 1602, New York, NY 10005; (800) 237-2438 or (212) 509-5335.

idiopathic. Subsequently it was redefined as consisting of type I and type II forms (Table 47-13). In some persons the two types of osteoporosis overlap.

Osteoporosis can also be further classified as primary or secondary. Primary osteoporosis, the more common form, has no underlying pathologic condition. Secondary osteoporosis results from another cause or medical condition, such as glucocorticoid-induced osteoporosis (Box 47-9). The focus of treatment of secondary osteoporosis is removal of the underlying cause.

Low bone mass is a critical element in the diagnosis of osteoporosis. The World Health Organization has established the following classifications of bone mass[34,66]:

- *Normal skeletal status:* bone mineral density (BMD) values of no more than 1 standard deviation (SD) below the young adult woman (30 to 40 years of age) mean value (T-score above −1)
- *Osteopenia* (low bone mass): BMD values between 1 and 2.5 SDs below the young adult mean value (T-score between −1 and −2.5)
- *Osteoporosis:* BMD values 2.5 or more SDs below the young adult mean value (T-score at or below −2.5)
- *Severe osteoporosis:* BMD values 2.5 or more SDs below the young adult mean value and the presence of one or more pathologic (fragility) fractures

These definitions are used in reference to BMD values determined by dual-energy x-ray absorptiometry (DXA) of the hip or spine. They are not applicable to bone density measurements at all sites or with all types of measuring devices. Another disadvantage is that the young adult "normal" refer-

TABLE 47-13 Types of Osteoporosis

	Type I: Postmenopausal	Type II: Senile
Age	Postmenopausal women (natural or surgically induced) Age of onset 55-75 years	Women >70 years Men >80 years
Sex	F:M 6:1	F:M 2:1
Pathology	Osteoclast mediated Increased resorption	Osteoblast mediated Decreased bone formation
Rate of bone loss	Rapid	Slow
Type of bone lost	Predominantly trabecular Associated with vertebral (compression-type) and distal radial fractures; hip fracture possible	Cortical and trabecular Associated with vertebral (wedge), proximal humerus, tibia, and hip fractures
Bone density	>2 SD below normal	Low normal

BOX 47-9 Causes of Secondary Osteoporosis

Endocrine Disorders

Diabetes
Cushing's syndrome
Hyperparathyroidism
Parathyroidism
Hypogonadism
Prolactinoma

Rheumatoid Arthritis

Drug Induced

Glucocorticoids
Heparin
Chronic use of phosphate-binding antacids
Loop diuretics
Anticonvulsants
Barbiturates
Thyroid medication
Lithium
Chemotherapy
Cyclosporine

Disuse

Prolonged immobilization (prolonged bed rest, immobilization of limb by casting or splinting)
Paraplegia
Quadriplegia
Lower motor neuron disease

Chronic Illness

Sarcoidosis
Cirrhosis
Renal tubular acidosis

Cancer

Multiple myeloma
Lymphoma
Leukemia

Malabsorption Syndrome

Anorexia Nervosa

Prolonged Parenteral Nutrition

Alterations in Gastrointestinal and Hepatobiliary Function

Amenorrhea in Premenopausal Women

ence range used for comparison are Caucasian women's scores; criteria are needed for men and women of diverse racial backgrounds.[34]

Decreased bone mass and susceptibility to fracture with little or no trauma are hallmarks of the disease. At age 50, the lifetime risk of hip, spine, and forearm fracture is 40% in Caucasian women and 13% in Caucasian men.[12,52,55] The mortality risk for osteoporotic fracture in women is 2.8%, or equal to that for breast cancer.[52] BMD decreases with aging and may decrease as rapidly as 5% every 5 years after age 65.[52] As bone density decreases by 1 SD, the risk of fracture increases 2.6 times.[52] Osteoporosis is usually an asymptomatic condition until fracture occurs. With the advent of bone densitometry, the ability to safely and easily measure the amount of bone density allows persons at risk for fracture to be identified before fracture occurs (see Chapter 45). Early intervention can prevent or decrease further bone loss and decrease the risk of fractures.

Bones are constantly undergoing remodeling. The remodeling process is a complex and highly integrated activity that strategically balances the forces of resorption with the process of bone formation. The osteoblastic forces predominate throughout childhood and young adulthood, until peak bone mass is reached at about age 35. After a variable period of relative balance, the resorptive breakdown forces begin to predominate. High rates of bone turnover and progressive loss persist throughout aging. In osteoporosis, the bone is essentially normal, but there is not enough of it to withstand mechanical stresses. Simple bone mass is the major determinant of bone strength and accounts for about 75% to 85% of its variance.

Other factors associated with the development of osteoporosis are related to hormonal balance. The loss of natural estrogen at menopause appears to dramatically increase the process of bony resorption, although the exact mechanism is not well understood. Chronic calcium deficiency is a common problem in the aging population, and adequate calcium is essential for bone production. The mechanism of intestinal absorption of calcium becomes less efficient with advancing age, increasing the demand for calcium. Diets high in fat appear to decrease calcium absorption, and excess protein ingestion—particularly animal protein—increases the excretion of calcium by the kidney. Alcohol may be toxic to osteoblast cells, and chronic use usually results in malnutrition. Alcohol and possibly caffeine also increase calcium excretion. Both a history of smoking and current smoking affect bone remodeling and appear to both lower body estrogen levels and block calcium absorption. Current smokers have a 4.3% lower BMD than nonsmokers; BMD scores for persons with a history of smoking are 1.7% lower than those of nonsmokers.[52]

Lack of exercise is another causative factor. In accordance with Wolff's law (see Chapter 45), bone is a dynamic substance that responds to stressors and weight-bearing forces. Chronic immobility is accompanied by well-documented increases in bone resorption. In normal daily lifestyles, this translates into an increased risk of osteoporosis for individuals with small frames, low body weight, and a sedentary activity pattern.

The use of steroids for treatment of persons with chronic illness is widespread. However successful it is in controlling conditions such as RA or asthma, steroid use is associated with many side effects. Osteoporosis is one of these side effects. Glucocorticoids interfere with calcium metabolism, reduce the synthesis of proteins by osteoblasts in the bone matrix, and may interfere with calcium absorption in the gut and renal tubule.[32] A reduction in serum sex hormone levels has also been noted, particularly in men and postmenopausal women. The rate of bone loss is greatest during the first few months of steroid therapy. The amount of bone lost during the first year of therapy has been reported to be as high as 20%.[32] Studies show fracture risk increases significantly with steroid use: the risk for hip fracture in persons receiving prednisone increases 77% to 127%. Higher risk is associated with higher daily doses.[12]

Epidemiology

Characterized by decreased bone mass and increased susceptibility to fracture, osteoporosis has become a major health problem. The prolonged longevity of the American population is expected to increase the number of persons affected by osteoporosis.

Ten million persons (8 million women) in the United States are affected by osteoporosis, and more than 3 million others are at risk of developing the disease.[12] An additional 18 million persons have osteopenia.[8] One in eight men is affected by osterporosis, and half of all women.[13a] The lifetime risk for osteoporosis-related fracture women is one in two.[59] More than 1.5 million fractures occur annually as a result of osteoporosis, with more than 250,000 of those being hip fractures.[59] Hip fracture and its sequelae are of major concern. Proximal hip fractures are associated with a significant mortality rate; as many as 70% of persons suffer functional losses as a result of fracture. Of persons with hip fracture, 25% die within 1 year; 50% are unable to return to independent living.[59]

The racial distribution of osteoporosis is influenced by differences in bone mass, rather than rates of bone loss. African-Americans have approximately 10% greater bone mass than do Caucasians and consequently are at less risk of developing osteoporosis. Asians and persons of northern European or Scandinavian ancestry are at greatest risk of developing osteoporosis.

Considered primarily a women's disease, attention is now being focused on the development of osteoporosis in men. More than 5 million men in the United States have or are at risk for developing osteoporosis (see Risk Factors box).[70] The age-related increase in fractures begins about 10 years later in men than in women; the mortality rate following hip fracture is greater in men than in women. BMD of the hip in men decreases by 1% each year, regardless of hormonal status.[45] Interventions to prevent or decrease bone loss in both sexes is well warranted.

Pathophysiology

In the process of normal bone remodeling, bone formation equals bone resorption. An osteoporotic state develops if bone resorption exceeds bone formation. Trabecular bone accounts

Risk Factors
Osteoporosis in Men

Hypogonadism (majority prostate cancer)[45]
Alcoholism
Smoking history
Liver disease
Renal tubular acidosis
Hypercalciuria
Hyperparathyroidism
Hyperthyroidism
Mastocytosis
Hyperprolactinemia
Vitamin D deficiency
Gastrointestinal disease (postgastrectomy)[70]
Glucocorticoid therapy

for approximately 20% of the skeletal mass; cortical bone accounts for the remaining 80%. Age-related bone loss begins in both sexes at approximately age 40 years. In women the most significant bone loss begins after menopause as a result of decreased levels of estrogen. Once menses cease, the rate of bone loss increases by 7.[17] During the first 5 to 10 years of menopause, women can lose up to 15% of cortical bone and 30% of trabecular bone.[17] This loss can be prevented by estrogen therapy.[17] The skeleton continues to lose bone mass in the hip and appendicular skeleton, even after the age of 80 years.

Two processes of bone loss have been identified: rapid bone loss and gradual bone loss. Rapid bone loss occurs during menopause and is osteoclast mediated, whereas gradual bone loss is osteoblast mediated and occurs after menopause. The time required to complete one cycle of bone remodeling in a healthy adult is about 4 months; that time is increased to almost 2 years for individuals with osteoporosis.

The remodeling process consists of the following steps: clusters of bone precursor cells respond to a stimulus (drug, hormone, or physical stressor) to activate the remodeling process and form osteoclasts. Osteoclasts form a cutting cone and begin to resorb bone, leaving a resorption cavity. In cortical bone, osteoblasts line the cavity and begin laying down layers (lamellae) of new bone until a haversian canal results (see Chapter 45). Trabeculae are formed in cancellous bone. If this process of remodeling is disrupted, osteoporosis may result. A decrease in the number of bone precursor cells or in the rate of bone formation, an increase in the rate of bone resorption, or an increase in the number of stimuli that activate the process can all result in osteoporosis. Osteoporosis also occurs if the whole process is not completed in entirety. Interference in the bone's vascular system results in a decreased number of bone precursor cells, which may also cause osteoporosis.

Cortical thinning begins at age 40 years, increases with age, and almost ceases late in life. Following menopause women lose cortical bone at a rate of 2% to 4% per year, returning to normal levels approximately 10 years after menopause.[17] The rate of trabecular bone loss differs. Trabecular bone loss begins earlier in both sexes and is lost in greater amounts. Following menopause the rate of trabecular bone loss is as high as 8% annually.[17] There are fewer and smaller trabeculae, with large spaces between them, decreasing the bone density. The compressive strength of trabecular bone is related to its density; as the density decreases, so does its compressive force and ability to withstand mechanical stressors. The bones most susceptible to fracture are those rich in trabecular bone, particularly the vertebrae, proximal femur, and distal radius. Cortical bone undergoes osteoporotic changes as well, becoming thin and porous and thus susceptible to fracture. Collapse and deformity may occur as a result of the bone's decreased density.

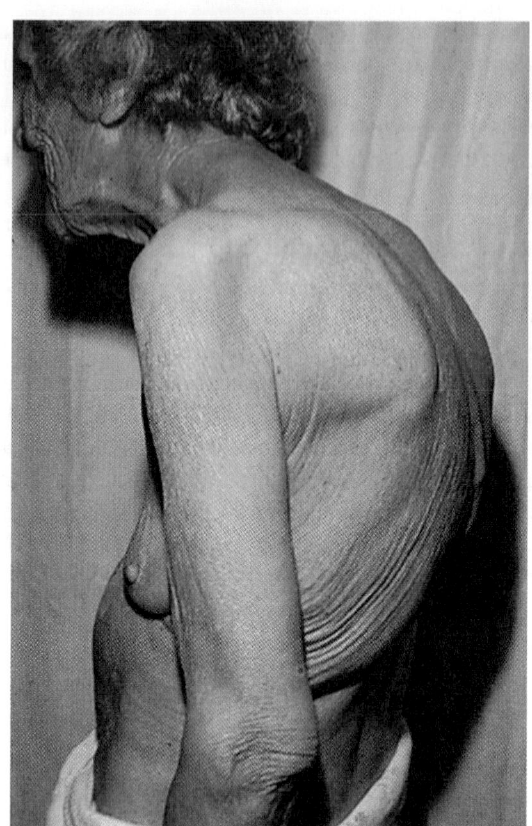

Figure 47-31 Kyphosis. This elderly woman's condition was caused by a combination of spinal osteoporotic vertebral collapse and chronic degenerative changes in the vertebral column.

Osteoporosis has been called the "silent thief" and "the silent disease" because most persons affected have no outward manifestations of disease. Previously the disease was not diagnosed unless fracture occurred. Many fractures related to osteoporosis occur without the patient's knowledge, although some are associated with excruciating pain. The earliest manifestation of osteoporosis may be an acute onset of back pain in the mid to low thoracic region as a result of vertebral fracture, occurring at rest or with minimal activity. Vertebral fracture can involve the entire vertebrae (compression) or a portion, usually the anterior section (wedge). Motion of the spine is restricted, especially forward flexion. Anterior compression fractures of the thoracic vertebrae may cause a "dowager's hump," or thoracic kyphosis (Figure 47-31). Loss of height and a protruding abdomen (due to pressure on abdominal viscera) are

TABLE 47-14 Methods of Measuring Bone Mineral Density

Method	Site	Advantages and Disadvantages
Single-photon and x-ray absorptiometry (SPA, SXA)	Radius, calcaneus	Inexpensive, easy to use Lengthy time required for results First technique developed to measure bone mineral density
Dual-photon absorptiometry (DPA)	Lumbar spine, proximal femur, total body	Reasonably precise, inexpensive Lengthy examination times; largely replaced by DXA
Dual-energy x-ray absorptiometry (DXA or DEXA)	Lumbar spine, proximal femur, proximal radius, distal radius, calcaneus, whole body	Accurate, gold standard; DXA most widely used; allows precise measurement of hip and spine with low radiation exposure
Quantitative CT (QCT)	Spine, radius (both cortical and trabecular)	Rapid results, widely available, able to assess trabecular content of spine Higher exposure to radiation than other methods; expensive
Quantitative ultrasound (QUS)	Calcaneus, tibia	Inexpensive, portable, no radiation exposure, questionable value in predicting fracture risk[17]; persons identified at risk should be referred for DXA

associated with this condition. Eventually the lower rib cage may rest on the iliac crests. Paravertebral muscle spasm often occurs, but neurologic deficits are rare with spontaneous vertebral compression fractures. These postural changes may affect exercise tolerance and food tolerance. The patient reports early satiety. The patient's body image may also be affected as a result of the spinal deformity.

Distal radial fractures (Colles' fractures) usually occur after a fall on a outstretched hand. Fractures of the proximal femur are associated with considerable morbidity and mortality (see Chapter 46). Osteoporotic hip fracture often occurs after little or no trauma. Intracapsular hip fracture is caused by bone loss, and intertrochanteric fracture is caused by both cortical and trabecular bone loss.

Collaborative Care Management

Diagnostic Tests. The risk for fracture can be assessed by identifying the patient's risk factors and history and measured precisely with noninvasive diagnostic tools. Measurement of BMD and biochemical markers of bone resorption are the basic tools for diagnosis of osteoporosis. Diagnostic techniques can assess the extent of disease, effects of treatment, progression of disease, and perhaps most important, risk of fracture. There are a variety of techniques used to measure bone density at various parts of the skeleton (Table 47-14), and the accuracy of predicting fracture risk measuring the BMD of the finger is being studied.[12] Once the diagnosis of osteoporosis is established, BMD studies should be performed every 1 to 2 years to determine response to treatment.

Biochemical markers of bone turnover (bone formation [bone alkaline phosphatase, serum osteocalcin] bone resorption [urine deoxypyridinolines, urine pyridinium cross-links]) are easily assessed by either a blood or a urine sample, and their effectiveness in predicting fracture risk and in monitoring therapy continue to be tested.[17] These studies are most often used in conjunction with BMD and may be helpful in monitoring response to treatment.

Guidelines for screening are controversial. Medicare provides reimbursement for BMD testing for women over 65 years of age who are at clinical risk for osteoporosis. The National Osteoporosis Foundation recommends BMD screening for persons under 65 years of age who have one or more risk factors for osteoporosis (in addition to menopause) and for all women over 65 years of age, regardless of associated risk factors. The U.S. Preventive Services Task Force concluded that there is insufficient evidence to warrant routine BMD testing of postmenopausal women.[66]

DXA scanning of the proximal femur or spine is usually done. Using the proximal femur for BMD testing is recommended as the best predictor of hip fracture and is preferred in older persons because degenerative changes in the spine may mask decreases in bone density of the vertebral bodies if measurements are taken of the spine.

Medications. The goal of pharmacologic therapy for persons with osteoporosis is to prevent further bone loss and to decrease the risk of fracture. Relieving symptoms associated with skeletal deformity and fracture and maximizing functional capacity are other goals of treatment. Medications used to treat osteoporosis either decrease bone resorption or increase bone formation and are summarized in Table 47-15. Alendronate has been approved to treat osteoporosis in men; androgen replacement may be beneficial in treating androgen-deficient men with osteoporosis but is associated with significant adverse effects.[45] Combination therapy using estrogen and bisphosphonates results in a greater increase in BMD than either therapy alone.[45] Other drugs used to treat osteoporosis, including fluorides, growth factors, calcitonin, anabolic steroids, and parathyroid hormone analogs, are under investigation (see Future Watch box). Mild analgesics are used to relieve pain associated with muscular aches and spasms.

Treatments. Osteoporosis is easier to prevent than to treat. Diet, medications, exercise, and prevention of falls and fractures are the foundations of therapy. There are no specific treatments for persons with osteoporosis. Treatments for

TABLE 47-15 Common Medications for Osteoporosis

Drug	Action	Intervention
Calcium	Necessary for bone formation High calcium intake may retard bone loss; insufficient alone to prevent or treat osteoporosis	Daily recommended dose for adults over age 65 is 1500 mg taken in divided doses of 500 mg/day or 600 mg bid for maximum absorption. Observe for signs of hypercalcemia. Calcium is contraindicated with severe renal disease.
Vitamin D: calcitriol, calcifediol	Necessary for bone formation and calcium absorption from gastrointestinal (GI) tract Improves calcium balance	Effectiveness of therapy depends on adequate calcium intake. Monitor for effects of hypercalcemia.
Estrogen replacement therapy (ERT): conjugated estrogen, estropipate, estradiol oral, transdermal patch	Inhibits osteoclastic bone resorption; positive effect on calcium balance; protects against postmenopausal osteoporosis Prevents cortical and trabecular bone loss Increases bone mineral density (BMD) and reduces fracture risk	Inform patients of risks/benefits. Side effects include breast tenderness, vaginal bleeding, hypertension, and deep vein thrombosis. Protective effect shown for coronary artery disease. Relationship between use and breast cancer uncertain; long-term use (over 15 years) associated with increased risk of breast cancer in postmenopausal women. When given without progestin, increases risk of endometrial cancer. Encourage women to have regular gynecologic (Papanicolaou smears and uterine biopsy if indicated) and breast examinations and mammograms during therapy; contraindicated in women with history of endometrial and breast cancer.
Selective estrogen receptor modulators (SERMs) antiestrogens, "designer estrogens": raloxifene (Evista)	Mimics effects of estrogen in some, but not all, tissues Blocks estrogen's cancer-promoting effects in other tissues Reduces rate of bone resorption and decreases rate of overall bone turnover Increases bone density, lowers blood lipid levels, does not increase high-density liproprotein (HDL) level Does not adversely affect breast, uterine tissue; studies being done to determine effect on breast cancer risk in younger women FDA approved for prevention of osteoporosis in postmenopausal women Inconclusive data regarding decreasing fracture risk; has been shown to decrease vertebral fracture risk in older women with postmenopausal osteoporosis	Risk of venous thromboembolic events, similar to risks associated with HRT. Avoid use in women with history of blood clots. Inform patient of side effects, including hot flashes and leg cramps. Smoking should be avoided while taking SERMs. Caution women of childbearing potential to avoid pregnancy.
Hormone replacement therapy (HRT): estrogen in combination with progestin	Increases BMD, decreases fracture risk Adding progestin reduces risk of endometrial cancer Increases bone mass in women older than age 65 years	Initiation of therapy is recommended early in postmenopausal period.
Bisphosphonates: etidronate, pamidronate, alendronate (Fosamax), risedronate, tiludronate	Inhibit osteoclast-mediated bone resorption Also used in treatment of Paget's disease Increase bone resorption, increase BMD, and prevent fractures in postmenopausal women with osteoporosis (alendronate) Protect against bone loss during long-term steroid therapy (risedronate)	Use is alternative for ERT or HRT. Administer on an empty stomach (before any food or medications) with full glass of water because of poor absorption. Alendronate: poorly absorbed with food; fast evening before and 30 minutes after administration. To decrease risk of esophagitis and GI side effects, patient should remain standing or upright for 30 minutes after administration. Take with at least 8 ounces of water; do not take within 2 hours of calcium-containing foods, beverages, or medications. Alendronate: Convenience of once-weekly dosing. Etidronate: for maximum absorption, patients should not eat or drink 2 hours before and after administration.

TABLE 47-15 Common Medications for Osteoporosis—cont'd

Drug	Action	Intervention
Calcitonin (human or salmon): intranasal (Miacalcin)	Opposes effect of parathyroid hormone on bone and kidneys Inhibits bone resorption; decreases fracture risk Increases bone mass in persons with steroid-induced osteoporosis Analgesic effect with osteoporotic fractures	Use is limited to parenteral or intranasal administration; side effects with subcutaneous injection include nausea, flushing, and local inflammatory reaction; administering dose at bedtime may decrease adverse effects. Monitor for hypocalcemia. Assess for allergy. Teach importance of reading labels; many over-the-counter products contain calcium. Few systemic effects with intranasal use.

Future Watch

Thiazide Diuretic Therapy for Osteoporosis

Thiazide diuretics, widely used in the treatment of hypertension, are known to decrease the urinary excretion of calcium. Studies show that thiazide therapy is associated with a decreased risk for hip fracture. In this study 320 normotensive adults received either 12.5 mg or 25 mg of hydrochlorothiazide (HCTZ) daily for 3 years; the control group received placebo. The participants ranged in age from 60 to 79 years and had normal bone mineral density (BMD). At the conclusion of the study, BMD of the hip decreased 0.3% in the control group and increased 0.5% in the 12.5 mg/day experimental group and 0.6% in the 25 mg/day group. There were no significant differences in BMD of the spine and total body in any group. The mean urinary calcium of the participants receiving HCTZ decreased. Potassium supplementation was necessary in the higher-dose group; only one subject required supplemental potassium in the lower-dose group. Further studies are needed to determine if thiazide diuretic therapy is beneficial for persons with osteoporosis.

Reference: LaCroix AZ et al: Low-dose hydrochlorothiazide and preservation of bone mineral density in older adults, *Ann Intern Med* 133(7):516-526, 2000.

persons with fractures are discussed in Chapter 46. Wrist fractures are usually treated by closed reduction and immobilization. Treatment for acute vertebral fractures is bed rest for 1 to 2 days and analgesics. Persons who have sustained a vertebral fracture as a result of osteoporosis may benefit from a corset (fitted by an orthotist) to provide support. Rigid bracing should be avoided, since complete immobilization results in bone loss. Pain usually subsides after 6 to 12 weeks as the fracture heals. Activity is essential during the healing period to avoid chronic back symptoms. Calcitonin has been effective in relieving the pain after vertebral fracture. Ultrasound, massage, and local application of heat or cold may alleviate pain and muscle spasms. Assistive or adaptive devices may be needed in the home or work environment. Persons who have had one fracture are at risk for subsequent fractures.

Surgical Management. Surgical intervention is necessary to repair some fractures. However, vertebral fractures without neurologic deficits usually do not require surgical intervention. Severe kyphotic deformities and vertebral fracture can be treated with kyphoplasty and percutaneous vertebroplasty—relatively new, minimally invasive procedures. Both procedures are performed with fluoroscopy to identify the fracture site. Kyphoplasty is preformed for vertebral compression fractures; methylmethacrylate is injected into the vertebrae for stabilization and relief of pain. Both procedures reduce deformities and relieve pain. Kyphoplasty also restores vertebral height.[13a] Wrist fractures may need open reduction for the person to achieve maximum functional results. Almost all hip fractures are managed surgically (see Chapter 46 and section on hip arthroplasty). The choice of procedure and fixation depends on the individual patient, the location of the fracture, and the vascular supply to the femoral head. As with all types of fractures, the principles of management are to mobilize the patient as quickly as possible to prevent the complications of immobility and to restore the patient to his or her maximum level of functioning.

BOX 47-10 Recommendations for Daily Calcium Intake

Age	Daily Recommendation	Servings*
1 to 3 years	500 mg	2
4 to 8 years	800 mg	3
9 to 18 years	1300 mg	4
19 to 50 years	1000 mg	3
51+ years	1200 mg	4

*1 serving is equal to:
- 1 cup whole, reduced-fat, fat-free, or flavored milk
- 1 cup yogurt
- $1\frac{1}{2}$ ounces natural cheese
- 1 cup pudding made with milk

Diet. Adequate nutrition is essential throughout life for a healthy skeleton. Calcium and vitamin D intake should be adequate from childhood through maturity to develop peak bone mass before menopause, thus protecting against osteoporosis later in life. The importance of adequate calcium intake increases with aging. Vitamin D and calcium absorption is gradually impaired as a result of the aging process. The daily recommended intake of calcium for adults older than 51 years of age is 1200 mg (Box 47-10).[15] Persons with osteoporosis should have a daily intake of calcium of 1500 mg. If the person is unable to take in adequate calcium in the form of dairy products, supplements are needed. Single doses of calcium should not exceed 600 mg per dose. Calcium-enriched juices and breads, which contain approximately 300 mg of calcium, equal to the calcium content of one glass of milk, are available. Foods rich in calcium include dairy products, green vegetables, and tofu (Table 47-16).

Vitamin D is necessary for calcium absorption and stimulates bone formation. Deficiencies of vitamin D are common in persons with osteoporosis, strict vegetarians, and those living in northern latitudes with restricted sunlight exposure. The recommended daily allowance of vitamin D is 400 IU. Persons with vitamin D deficiencies may require supplements, but persons with sun exposure throughout the year usually do not. Foods rich in vitamin D include milk, fish, and eggs.

TABLE 47-16 Major Dietary Sources of Calcium

Food	Quantity	Calcium (mg)
Milk	1 cup (240 ml)	
Skim		302
1%		300
2%		297
Ice Cream	1 cup	
Hard		176
Soft		236
Ice Milk (Vanilla)	1 cup	
Hard		176
Soft		274
Cheese		
Cheddar	1 oz	204
Swiss	1 oz	272
American	1 oz	150
Cottage	1 cup	155
Beans		
Pinto (cooked)	1 cup	86
Soy (cooked)	1 cup	131
Navy (cooked)	1 cup	95
Green (cooked)	1 cup	80
Vegetables		
Turnip greens (cooked)	1 cup	249
Broccoli (cooked)	1 cup	90
Tofu	4 oz	108
Fish and Shellfish		
Oysters (raw)	1 cup	226
Salmon (canned)	3 oz	167
Yogurt		
Plain (low fat)	8 oz	415
Fruit (low fat)	8 oz	343
Frozen (fruit)	8 oz	240
Frozen (chocolate)	8 oz	160

Another dietary recommendation for persons with osteoporosis is avoidance of excessive intake of alcohol and caffeine, both of which are risk factors associated with the development of osteoporosis. For persons with fractures, a diet adequate in proteins and vitamin C is necessary to promote wound and tissue healing.

Activity. Exercise is an often-prescribed, but not completely understood, intervention for the prevention and treatment of osteoporosis. Benefits of exercise include increased muscle tone and muscle mass, which may improve balance and flexibility and thus prevent falls. In addition to the benefits of overall well-being and cardiovascular effects, impact-loading exercise seems to be effective in maintaining bone mass. Regular weight bearing or bone stressing (weight training and resistance exercises) is necessary to maintain bone mass in both children and adults. The effects of exercise on peak bone mass are most significant during the years of skeletal growth and have less significance in older adults. Premenopausal women who exercise regularly and have regular menstrual cycles have the greatest bone mass; amenorrhea leads to bone loss.

The ideal amount and type of exercise needed to maintain bone mass have not been determined. Research has shown positive effects of exercise on BMD in postmenopausal women. Weight-bearing or weight-training exercise appears to be beneficial in maintaining and, in some cases, increasing BMD.[23]

Recommendations for all adults should include a daily (or at least five times per week) program of weight-bearing and mild weight-training exercises. Brisk walking or low-impact aerobics are good choices for the older adult. Extension exercises of the spine are beneficial for posture and flexibility, but flexion exercises may contribute to fracture. Jogging may also precipitate vertebral fracture. Walking outdoors has the added benefit of sunlight exposure, essential for vitamin D formation. Swimming or water exercises have no direct effect on bones but are good choices for an aerobic workout.

Referrals. Referrals for PT and OT may be necessary for exercise regimens and assistive and adaptive devices. A nutritionist can assist the elderly patient in meal planning to include adequate calcium and vitamin D. National organizations and support groups for patients and families are excellent resources for information about osteoporosis. An example is the Osteoporosis and Related Bone Diseases–National Resource Center, National Osteoporosis Foundation.*

NURSING MANAGEMENT OF PATIENT WITH OSTEOPOROSIS

The nursing management section pertains to persons with osteoporosis, but without fractures. The nursing management of persons with fractures is discussed in Chapter 46.

*1150 17th Street NW, Suite 500, Washington, DC 20036-4603; (202) 223-2226 or (800) 624-BONE; TTY: (202) 466-4315; fax: (202) 223-2237; website: http://www.nof.org.

ASSESSMENT

Health History

The patient should be assessed for the presence of risk factors for osteoporosis. The patient's diet, exercise habits, amount of caffeine and alcohol consumption, and amount and frequency of sunlight exposure are all relevant data. Medication use and coexisting medical conditions may be contributing factors to osteoporosis. The medication list should also include over-the-counter preparations. Any family history of osteoporosis should be noted. Female patients should have a gynecologic history taken. The regularity of menstrual cycles, pregnancies, time of menopause, and medications are important factors in the development of osteoporosis.

If the patient has an established diagnosis of osteoporosis, the nurse asks what treatments or therapies have been prescribed and whether the patient noted any changes in height or posture. In addition, the nurse should question the patient regarding his or her expectations of treatment. A complete assessment of the patient's level of pain should be included in the history. The patient's previous methods of pain control may be beneficial in planning interventions for pain relief.

A history of falls or previous fractures, especially occurring after minimal trauma, is important for planning care. The nurse should assess the patient's home environment for fall hazards and injury potential. Information to be obtained includes whether the patient needs to climb stairs, whether the bedroom and bathroom are on the same floor, and whether the home is carpeted.

Psychosocial assessment should include noting any disturbances in self-esteem due to loss of independence or functional ability. Pain or limited mobility may impair the patient's ability to pursue necessary and leisure activities, leading to anxiety, social isolation, and depression. Depression is a common finding in older persons. The amount of family support can influence the patient's coping abilities, especially with a chronic degenerative disease.

Physical Examination

A complete physical examination focusing on the musculoskeletal and neurologic system should be performed. The patient's gait, balance, coordination, and sensory ability should be assessed to determine the risk for falls and injury. The patient's baseline level of functioning should be assessed, including the ability to perform ADLs.

The physical examination should include an assessment of all joints and extremities. Areas prone to pathologic fracture should be thoroughly and carefully assessed. The presence of kyphosis is common in older women. When kyphosis is present, a complete respiratory and GI assessment should be performed, since decreased respiratory excursion, respiratory compromise, abdominal distention, ileus, and constipation may occur as a result of the deformity. Tenderness with palpation over the intervertebral disk spaces may indicate a vertebral fracture, so the spine should be palpated gently. Loss of height may be attributed to osteoporosis and vertebral fractures. Loss of motion, particularly flexion, may also occur.

NURSING DIAGNOSES

Nursing diagnoses are determined from analysis of patient data. Nursing diagnoses for the patient with osteoporosis may include but are not limited to:

Diagnostic Title	Possible Etiologic Factors
1. Risk for injury	Altered mobility, minimal trauma, falls, advanced age, previous fall
2. Impaired physical mobility	Decreased bone mass, decreased strength, musculoskeletal impairment, pain
3. Situational low self-esteem	Chronic illness, anxiety, loss of usual role, body changes, limitation in mobility, chronic pain, loss of independence

EXPECTED PATIENT OUTCOMES

Expected patient outcomes for the patient with osteoporosis may include but are not limited to:

- **1a.** Will experience no injuries, falls, or fractures
- **1b.** Will identify factors that contribute to potential injury and steps to correct the situation or modify the environment
- 2. Will maintain maximum level of mobility and functioning
- 3. Will have positive self-esteem and participate in desired activities at fullest level

INTERVENTIONS

1. Preventing Injury

Pathologic fracture can result from minor trauma in the individual with osteoporosis. Falls commonly result in hip fracture, a significant cause of mortality in the older adult. The environment should be modified to protect the patient from accidental harm or injury.

The patient should be monitored for level of consciousness, ability to make judgments, motor strength, coordination, balance, and sensory deficits. Many medications may cause weakness, drowsiness, or dizziness, which pose an additional risk for injury. If adverse effects are occurring, the physician should be consulted for alternatives. Electrolyte imbalances are common in older adults and may manifest as mental status changes or weakness. Blood chemistry results should be evaluated for abnormalities.

Instructions should be given about the proper technique for transferring from bed to chair, bending, and lifting. Proper body mechanics can protect the patient from back injuries (Figure 47-32). Excessive flexion of the spine may contribute to compression fracture of the vertebrae. Kyphosis may alter the patient's center of gravity and diminish vision. The patient should be encouraged to maintain an upright posture to improve ambulatory ability and also to enhance respiration. Assistive devices and ambulatory aids may be necessary for some persons. A PT referral may be needed to teach the patient the proper technique for using a walker or cane. Walkers and canes provide support, decreasing the risk for falls.

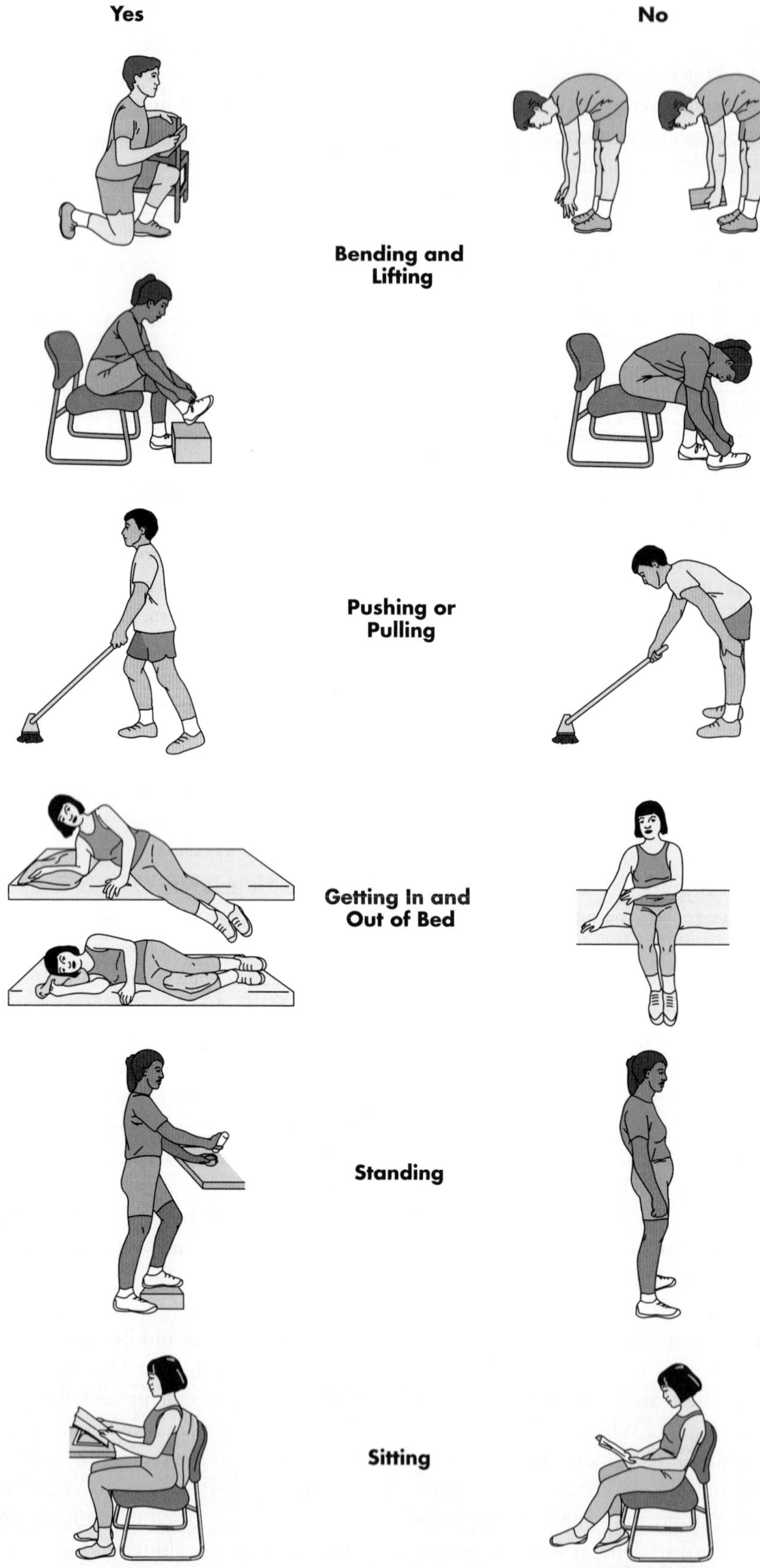

Figure 47-32 Proper body mechanics.

The environment should be kept as hazard free as possible while the patient is hospitalized. The bed should be kept in low position, and the need for side rails should be assessed. Confused persons or those receiving sedation should have the side rails elevated. However, careful monitoring of the patient is crucial, since some persons may attempt to climb over the rails and sustain a fall. The call light should be within reach, and the patient should be instructed in its use. Nonskid shoes or slippers can also help prevent falls. Environmental hazards such as equipment, electrical cords, and slippery floors should be eliminated. The home environment should also be assessed for safety hazards (see Patient Teaching box).

Exercise is an important intervention for preventing falls. Regular exercise increases energy, muscle tone, strength, flexibility, and coordination, which may help in fall prevention. ROM exercises should be included in the program to maintain joint mobility. Weight-bearing, regular exercise for 30 minutes five times per week should be recommended to persons with osteoporosis.

2. Promoting Mobility

The patient's ROM and muscle strength should be monitored, and limitations in mobility should be documented. The level of the patient's pain should also be monitored, because unrelieved pain may interfere with mobility. Analgesics should be given as needed, especially before planned activities, such as PT. Active ROM should be encouraged daily; if the patient is unable to perform active ROM, passive ROM should be performed by the nurse.

If the patient has a vertebral fracture, a corset may be prescribed to provide support and increase mobility while fracture healing occurs. Encouraging maximal mobility while the fracture heals is recommended to avoid bone loss from immobility. Again, weight-bearing exercises are recommended to maintain bone mass. In addition, strengthening exercises increase circulation to both bone and muscle. A PT referral is an option for teaching weight-bearing and resistive exercises. OT can provide the patient with adaptive devices to complete ADLs. Participation in ADLs should be encouraged to maintain independence, allowing the patient adequate time to complete self-care.

Affected parts of the body can be supported with slings or pillows as needed, especially during periods of rest. Uninterrupted periods of rest should be ensured to increase energy and prevent fatigue throughout the day. Fatigue is common among persons with musculoskeletal impairments. The

Patient Teaching

Home Safety and Fall Prevention

Unintentional injury is the third leading cause of death and disability for persons older than 65 years of age. The disability that may result from an injury may end the independence of an older person living at home. Falls are the leading cause of injury for the older adult. Because the bones in the body may become more brittle with aging, a fall may potentially cause a serious injury. A hip fracture secondary to a fall may be a catastrophic event for an older person. Most falls in the older adult occur because of an environmental hazard, loss of muscle strength and coordination, an impaired sense of balance, and slowing reaction time. To ensure the safety of an older person, and to help prevent falls and other injuries, it is important to make the person's living space safe and free of hazards.

ENVIRONMENTAL SAFETY

- Steps should be highly visible and have good lighting, nonskid treads, and handrails.
- A strong banister running along all indoor and outdoor steps is essential.
- Clearly mark and light the top and bottom steps.
- Use bright lighting in the living space.
- Remove all floor clutter in the walkways.
- Remove slippery floor coverings such as polished linoleum, small mats, and area or throw rugs.
- Use nonskid floor wax, wall-to-wall carpeting, or rubber-backed rugs. Tack down the corners of area rugs.
- Install nonskid mats and handrails in the bathtub and near the toilet and bed.
- A bedside lamp or low-wattage night-light should be available in the bedroom.
- Secure electrical cords along the walls or baseboards.
- Store frequently used dishes, clothes, and other items within easy reach; climbing on a stool or chair should be avoided.
- Set the temperature on the hot water heater to no hotter than 130° F or have a mixing valve installed on the bathtub faucet to prevent burns.

PERSONAL SAFETY ACTIVITIES

- If you need glasses, wear them, but never walk around with glasses that are meant only for reading. Take them off before moving around.
- If you are even slightly unsteady on your feet, use a cane. Do not hesitate to use a walker either inside the house or outdoors.
- Always turn lights on and use adequate-wattage lightbulbs to brighten the room.
- Wear wide-based, low-heeled shoes with corrugated soles to help prevent slips and falls.
- Do not wear flimsy or slippery-soled shoes or slippers.
- When getting up at night, first sit on the edge of the bed to make sure you are awake and steady, then turn on a light before walking to the bathroom or around the room.
- Don't ever smoke in bed. If you are sleepy, don't light up a cigarette regardless of where you are sitting.
- Always wear clothing with short sleeves when you are cooking. Never reach over a hot burner on the stove.
- If you live alone, have a safety plan to call for help or to get assistance.
- If you take a medication that makes you dizzy or weak, discuss these symptoms with your health care provider. Being dizzy or weak when you get up to walk or go down stairs may increase your risk of falling.

From *Mosby's patient teaching guides: update 3*, St Louis, 1997, Mosby.

patient's family and friends should be encouraged to participate in care, since they can assist the patient in managing problems associated with immobility.

3. Promoting a Positive Self-Image

Osteoporosis, in addition to the effects on musculoskeletal functioning, also significantly affects an individual's social and emotional functioning. Changes in the body and body functioning may cause anxiety. Deformities such as kyphosis, the onset of menopause, or decreased mobility as a result of musculoskeletal disease may be difficult changes for the patient to assimilate. With spinal curvature and changes in body contours, finding attractive clothing to fit, particularly without requiring alterations, may be problematic. This may compound changes in body image. Depression is not an uncommon reaction to an altered body image and functional limitations. Kyphosis can result in height loss, spinal deformity, and difficulty wearing one's usual clothing. Dissatisfaction with appearance may cause a patient to avoid going out and pursuing social activities. Patients who experienced previous falls often fear falling again. Explaining the process of aging, menopause, and the effects on bone can help reassure patients that aging and menopause are normal events of life. Knowledge of the treatment and preventive strategies for protecting bone mass can alleviate patients' fears. Nurses can provide support and help patients adapt to change and maintain a positive outlook.

Women with chronic illnesses such as osteoporosis often have to modify their roles as a result of the limitations imposed by disease. These changes often have negative effects, creating feelings of dependency and isolation. Changes in physical appearance may have similar effects.

Changes in appearance and level of functioning, as well as fear of falling and fracture, may limit a person's willingness to go out and pursue necessary or social activities. Interventions are needed to assist women in adapting to physical changes and to assist them in devising methods to avoid injury and lessen fears.

As a result of the negative feelings associated with osteoporosis, the social support of family and friends is essential for assisting a patient in dealing with dependency as a result of pain, disability, and physical deformities. Spouses, friends, or family can assist the patient with household tasks. Social contacts should continue, and outings that do not pose hazards to the person with osteoporosis can be arranged. Walking with friends outdoors or in a mall during bad weather can foster social support and fulfill the need for exercise. The woman with osteoporosis can continue to perform as many aspects of her usual role as possible, perhaps with some adaptations. Clothing can be purchased or altered to decrease the prominence of back deformities, thus decreasing feelings of embarrassment or negative self-image. Explanations about treatments and medications can allay fears.

Patient/Family Education

Teaching the family and patient with osteoporosis should include instructions about the disease process, medications, body mechanics, exercise, and prevention of falls (see Patient Teaching box and Figure 47-33; see also Figure 47-32).

The patient and family also need information about diet, including foods rich in calcium and vitamin D. Patients should be instructed to read the labels of over-the-counter medications, particularly for calcium content.

Health Promotion/Prevention. Teaching should include health promotion techniques, especially for persons at risk of developing osteoporosis. To decrease the risk of osteoporosis in all persons, a diet adequate in calcium and vitamin D and regular weight-bearing exercise, beginning in childhood, should be advocated to accumulate peak bone mass at skeletal maturity. Education pertaining to bone health should begin in

Patient Teaching

What Is Osteoporosis?

Osteoporosis is the most common metabolic bone disease. It results from the loss of calcium in the bones, causing the bones to become brittle and susceptible to breaking. The term *osteoporosis* means "porous bone." The disease is usually not diagnosed until the person suffers a fracture or broken bone.

WHY ARE WOMEN AFFECTED MORE OFTEN?

One out of four women and half the women older than 65 years of age have osteoporosis to some extent. Most are Caucasian women who have gone through menopause. Generally, African-Americans have greater bone mass than Caucasians, and men have greater bone mass than women. Petite women with small bones and thin bodies have very small bone masses. Thus women are at greater risk of developing osteoporosis if they are Caucasian, Asian, or petite.

Osteoporosis is also caused by low estrogen levels that occur in women after menopause. Although the role of estrogen is not clear, it is linked to the processes of bone formation and resorption. Estrogen is thought to reduce bone resorption, to reduce calcium loss through the kidneys, and to increase calcium absorption in the digestive tract. Estrogen protects women who have had an inadequate intake of calcium in their growing years. However, when estrogen levels drop after menopause, bone resorption in women increases greatly.

WHAT ARE THE RISK FACTORS?

Two major risk factors for osteoporosis are lack of exercise and inadequate intake of calcium, vitamin D, and protein. Osteoporosis caused by calcium and vitamin D deficiencies affects men and women 70 to 85 years of age. Other risk factors contributing to the disease are:

- A family history of osteoporosis
- Smoking and consuming too much alcohol and caffeine, which interfere with the absorption of calcium
- Prolonged use of drugs or medications such as steroids, magnesium-based antacids such as Maalox, and heparin
- Diseases and hormonal disorders such as rheumatoid arthritis, liver disease, certain cancers, and an overactive thyroid gland
- Poor calcium absorption in the intestines

Although osteoporosis primarily affects middle-aged or older adults, it can occur in young adults. Injuries that result in paralysis or long periods of immobility can lead to osteoporosis.

From *Mosby's patient teaching guides: update 3*, St Louis, 1997, Mosby.

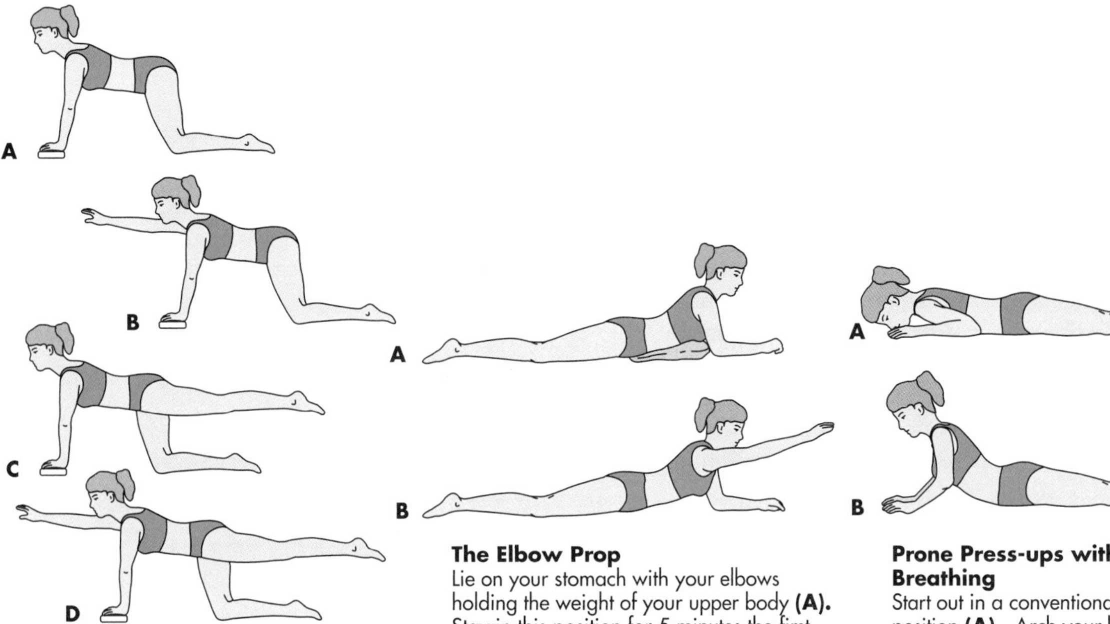

All Fours Arm/Leg Lifts
Position yourself on your hands and knees, with your hands directly under your shoulders and your knees directly under your hips **(A).** Your back should be flat or slightly arched. Lift one arm and hold for 3 seconds **(B).** Repeat with the other arm. Then lift one leg and hold for 3 seconds **(C).** Repeat with the other leg. If you can do these exercises comfortably, try lifting your right arm and left leg simultaneously **(D),** and then your left arm and right leg.

The Elbow Prop
Lie on your stomach with your elbows holding the weight of your upper body **(A).** Stay in this position for 5 minutes the first day; gradually increase the time to half an hour. You may be more comfortable if you put a pillow under your stomach. The elbow prop position helps reverse the effects of bad posture by passively decompressing the vertebrae and disks. To exercise the back as well, reach the right arm forward **(B),** then the left, and repeat.

Prone Press-ups with Deep Breathing
Start out in a conventional "push-up" position **(A).** Arch your back, pinching your shoulder blades together **(B).** As you push up, inhale; as you lie down, exhale. Keep elbows partially bent to protect the back. Make sure you don't lift your pelvis.

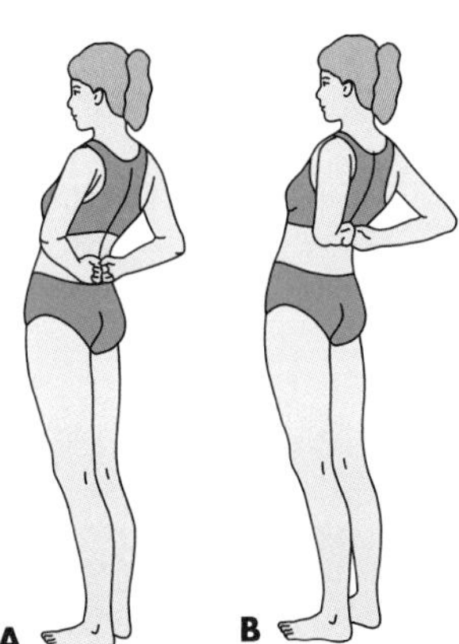

Standing Back Bend
Put your fists on your lower back. Arch backwards slowly while taking a deep breath **(A).** Relax and put your arms down, then repeat, this time with the fists on the middle back **(B).**

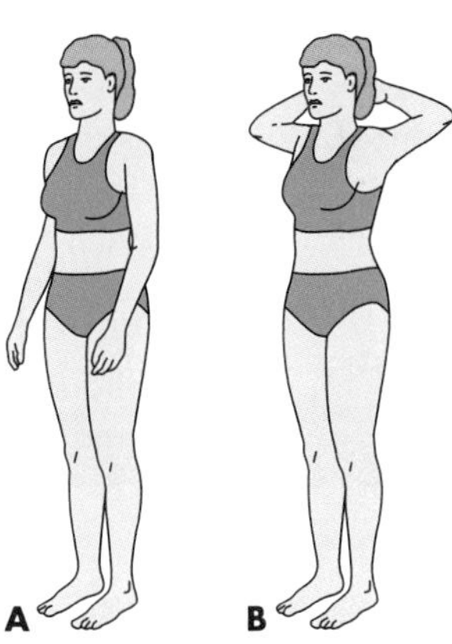

Isometric Posture Correction
Stand as tall as you can, with your chin in, not up **(A).** Place your palms against the back of your head. Simultaneously push your hands against your head while pinching your shoulder blades together **(B).** Hold for 3 seconds, then relax for 3 seconds. Maintain an erect posture throughout the exercise.

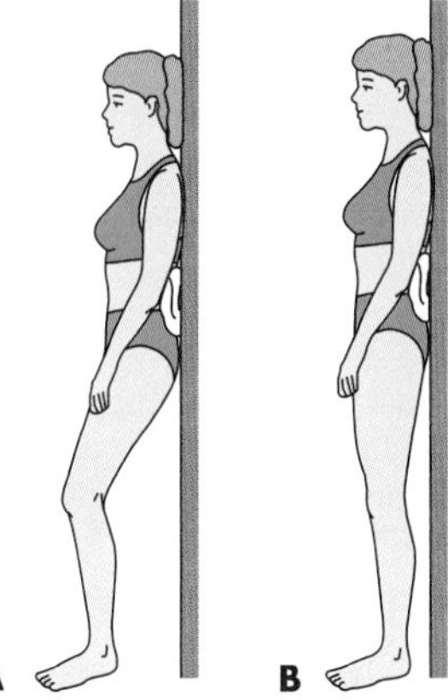

Standing and Pelvic Tilt
Stand with your feet about a foot from the wall, with your knees slightly bent and your back straight **(A).** Use a towel to support your lower back. Slide up and down, keeping the back straight and the stomach muscles contracted. You should be able to plant your feet closer to the wall as you improve **(B).**

Figure 47-33 Exercises for prevention of osteoporosis.

childhood and adolescence. Older adults, including older men (see Research box), are another at-risk target population. Premenopausal women benefit from an explanation of the effects of estrogen on bone mass and strategies to prevent osteoporosis before the need arises. Osteoporosis is one of the targeted initiatives for Healthy People 2010 (see Healthy People 2010 box). Screening for BMD should be done for persons at risk of developing osteoporosis or before beginning treatment to determine baseline levels to monitor the effectiveness of treatment.

The National Osteoporosis Foundation is an excellent resource for information about osteoporosis. A newsletter is published quarterly regarding advances in treatments for osteoporosis. Boning Up on Osteoporosis is an excellent guide to the treatment and prevention of osteoporosis and is available from the National Osteoporosis Foundation. National Osteoporosis Week is usually held in May each year.

Complementary and Alternative Therapy. Complementary therapies for osteoporosis include tai chi and yoga to improve muscle strength and flexibility. Isoflavones, plant chemicals found in soybeans, are similar in structure to estrogen and may play a role in improving bone density. Tofu is a good source of isoflavones. Collard greens, rich in vitamin K, may have protective effect for bone and reduce risk of fracture.

Research

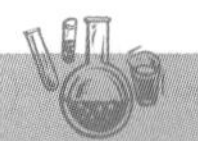

Reference: Sedlak CA, Doheny MO, Estok PJ: Osteoporosis and older men: knowledge and health beliefs, *Orthop Nurs* 19(3):38-46, 2000.

Osteoporosis has primarily been considered a women's health problem, although it affects more than 2 million men in the United States. Osteoporosis is a debilitating disease and is commonly associated with fractures of the hip, spine, and radius. Bone loss in men is associated with decreased levels of testosterone and decreased ability to absorb calcium. More than 80,000 men sustain hip fractures annually, and more than one third of these men die of complications within 1 year. However, little is known about elderly men's understanding of osteoporosis.

The purpose of this study was to describe elderly men's knowledge, health beliefs, and prevention strategies regarding osteoporosis. The sample consisted of 138 community-dwelling men age 65 and older. Participants completed several questionnaires that evaluated their knowledge of osteoporosis, perceived susceptibility to the disease, and performance of preventive behaviors. The Osteoporosis Health Belief Scale was used to evaluate susceptibility, seriousness, benefits and barriers regarding exercise and calcium intake, and self-efficacy. Osteoporosis-preventing behaviors included ensuring adequate calcium intake, performing weight-bearing exercise, and limiting the amount of smoking and alcohol intake. Results indicated that the men had a poor knowledge of osteoporosis and did not perceive themselves as susceptible to developing the disease. Very few men engaged in osteoporosis-preventing behaviors, although 98% of the sample were nonsmokers.

This study validates the need for education regarding osteoporosis targeted to men, including information regarding risk factors, the disease process, and methods of prevention. More studies using a more diverse sample are needed. Participants were all Caucasian and similar in demographics. Targeting education to younger men may enable them to incorporate health-promoting behaviors into their lifestyle.

EVALUATION

To evaluate the effectiveness of nursing interventions, compare patient behaviors with those stated in the expected outcomes. Achievement of patient outcomes is successful if the patient:

1a. Has had no falls or fractures.
1b. Verbalizes knowledge of safety measures, exercises, and strategies to prevent falls, injuries, and fractures.
2. Demonstrates maximum degree of mobility and functioning.
3. Has positive self-esteem, participates in usual roles to fullest extent, and engages in social activities as desired.

SPECIAL ENVIRONMENTS FOR CARE

Community-Based Care

Many of the home care considerations for persons with osteoporosis pertain to modification of the home environment to prevent falls or fractures. In addition, a home health care referral may be needed if the patient is unable to complete ADLs independently. Homemaking services may also be required. Meals on Wheels is an option for patients who are unable to prepare their meals independently. Assistive and adaptive devices may need to be purchased for the home. If the patient does not have the necessary resources, several community agencies may offer assistance. These items may also be rented. If patients are severely disabled or lack family support for care, transfer to an assisted living or nursing facility may be necessary.

COMPLICATIONS

Complications of osteoporosis are primarily fractures. Fractures and complications of fractures are discussed in Chapter 46.

Healthy People 2010

Goals Related to Osteoporosis

- Reduce the number of adults with osteoporosis.
- Increase the number of culturally competent community health prevention programs.
- Increase the number of persons who meet dietary requirements for calcium intake.
- Increase the number of adults who engage in regular, moderate physical activity for at least 30 minutes/day.
- Increase the number of adults who engage in physical activities that promote flexibility, muscular strength, and endurance.
- Reduce the number of adults hospitalized for osteoporosis-related vertebral fractures.

From US Department of Health and Human Services: *Healthy People 2010: understanding and improving health,* Washington, DC, 2000, USDHHS.

INFECTIOUS BONE DISEASE

Osteomyelitis

Etiology/Epidemiology

Although the development of osteomyelitis is often precipitated by a traumatic event or is a complication of trauma, it is included with the degenerative disorders because of its chronic and debilitating aspects. Osteomyelitis is an infection of the bone, most often of the cortex or medullary portion. It is most commonly caused by bacteria but can also be caused by fungi, parasites, and viruses.

The two types of osteomyelitis are classified by the mode of entry of the pathogen. *Contiguous focus* or *exogenous osteomyelitis* is caused by a pathogen from outside the body or by the spread of infection from adjacent soft tissues. The most common offending organism is *Staphylococcus aureus.* Examples include pathogens from an open fracture or surgical procedure, particularly a joint replacement or procedure involving instrumentation. *Staphylococcus epidermis* is associated with implant-related infection. The infection can also be caused by human or animal bites and by fist blows to the mouth. The most common organism found in human bites is *S. aureus;* the most common organism found in animal bites is *Pasteurella multocida.* The infection spreads from the soft tissues to the bone. Risk factors for developing exogenous osteomyelitis are chronic illness or diabetes, alcohol or drug abuse, and immunosuppression. In persons with diabetes or vascular disease, osteomyelitis occurs most often in the feet. Pain may be absent as a result of neuropathy. The onset is insidious: initially cellulitis progressing to the underlying bone.

Hematogenous osteomyelitis is caused by bloodborne pathogens originating from infectious sites within the body. Examples include sinus, ear, dental, respiratory, and genitourinary infections. In hematogenous osteomyelitis the infection spreads from the bone to the soft tissues and can eventually break through the skin, becoming a draining fistula. This type of osteomyelitis is more common in infants, children, and older adults. In the older adult age-group men are more commonly affected. Again, *S. aureus* is the most common causative organism. Other responsible organisms include streptococcus B, *Haemophilus influenzae, Salmonella,* and gram-negative bacteria. *Salmonella* is linked with sickle cell anemia, and gram-negative organisms are associated with infections occurring in older and immunocompromised individuals. Acute osteomyelitis left untreated or unresolved after 10 days is considered chronic osteomyelitis. Osteomyelitis of long bones can also be categorized by the stages of infection (Box 47-11).[41]

Pathophysiology

Pathologic mechanisms of osteomyelitis are inflammation and destruction of bone, bone necrosis, and formation of new bone. Necrotic bone is the distinguishing feature of chronic osteomyelitis. In hematogenous osteomyelitis the organisms reach the bone through the circulatory and lymphatic systems. The bacteria lodge in the small vessels of the bone, triggering an inflammatory response. Blockage of the vessel causes thrombosis, ischemia, and necrosis of the bone. The femur, tibia, humerus, and radius are commonly affected. Infections of the pelvic organs often spread to the pelvis and vertebrae. The pathophysiology of osteomyelitis is similar to that of infectious processes in any other body tissue.

Bone inflammation is marked by edema, increased vasculature, and leukocyte activity. Exudate seals the bone's canaliculi, extends into the metaphysis and marrow cavity, and finally reaches the cortex. New bone, laid down over the infected bone by osteoblasts, is referred to as *involucrum.* Openings in the involucrum allow infected material to escape into soft tissues. The infectious process weakens the cortex, thereby increasing the risk of pathologic fracture. *Brodie's abscesses* are characteristic of chronic osteomyelitis. These are isolated, encapsulated pockets of microorganisms surrounded by bone matrix, usually found in long bones. These pockets of virulent organisms are capable of reinfection at any time. The microscopic channels found in bone allow bacteria to proliferate without being affected by the body's defenses.

In patients with exogenous osteomyelitis the infection begins in the soft tissues, disrupting muscle and connective tissue, and eventually forming abscesses. Signs and symptoms associated with soft tissue infection are most common.

Chronic osteomyelitis is difficult to treat. Recurrent infection, areas of dead bone *(sequestrum),* and scar tissue are contributing factors to its resistance to treatment. Complications of chronic osteomyelitis include sepsis, nonunion, draining fistulas, shortening of the affected extremity, and eventually amputation.

The clinical manifestations of osteomyelitis vary with the individual, type of responsible organism, precipitating event, and type of infection (acute or chronic). The patient may report fever, malaise, anorexia, and headache. The affected body part may be erythematous, tender, and edematous. There may be a fistula draining purulent material.

Collaborative Care Management

Blood tests reveal an increase in WBCs, ESRs, and C-reactive protein levels. A culture and sensitivity test of the drainage reveals the causative organisms, allowing identification of appropriate antibiotic therapy. Blood cultures

BOX 47-11 Classification of Long Bone Osteomyelitis by Cierny-Mader System

Stage 1: Medullary

Necrosis limited to medullary canal and endosteal surfaces

Stage 2: Superficial

Bone necrosis only at exposed surface

Stage 3: Localized

Bone stable; sequestrum through one cortex; well-marginated infection

Stage 4: Diffuse

Unstable bone, infection all around bone, through both cortices determine the presence or absence of septicemia. MRI and a radionuclide bone scan may be performed. Pathologic changes are visible after the infection has been present for 7 to 10 days.

Treatment is difficult and costly. The goals of treatment are:

- Complete removal of dead bone and affected soft tissue
- Control of infection
- Elimination of dead space (after removal of necrotic bone)

Treatment depends on the area of bone involved, causative organism, ability to maintain a functional limb, duration of treatment, and expected outcomes. Other considerations include ensuring adequate soft tissue coverage and restoration of the blood supply. Debridement surgery to remove necrotic tissue is the foundation of management of persons with osteomyelitis. Debridement involves removal of sequestrum and surrounding granulation tissue. Surgical excision of the bone must be adequate to ensure eradication of the causative organism. Debridement often results in a bony defect or dead space. Techniques to fill the dead space include flaps, antibiotic beads, and bone grafts. The goal is to replace necrotic bone and scar tissue with vascularized tissue. Closure of the wound is done whenever possible; healing by secondary intention is to be avoided because of the risk of decreased vascular supply to scar tissue.[41] Irrigation and drainage systems, once popular for management, are not recommended because of the high incidence of nosocomial infection.[41]

Temporary placement of polymethylmethacrylate antibiotic beads in the wound can be used to stabilize and temporarily maintain dead space.[41] Agents commonly used include vancomycin, tobramycin, and gentamicin. An implantable pump can also be used to deliver antibiotics directly to the wound. Placement of antibiotic beads offers higher drug levels at the infection site than occur with systemic administration. The wound is closed and covered; the beads are usually removed after 2 to 4 weeks, and then reconstruction is performed. Soft tissue defects can be repaired with a split-thickness skin graft; larger defects may require flaps and vascularized muscle flaps.

Other options include the use of allograft bone and stabilization by external or internal fixation. The Ilizarov technique (see Chapter 46) can be used for difficult cases, nonunion, and large bone defects. Prevention of infection is crucial. The Papineau technique was introduced in the 1970s as a means of treating osteomyelitis occurring in the diaphysis of long bones. It consists of removal of infected and necrotic bone, immobilization (usually achieved by an external fixator [see Chapter 46]), delayed cancellous bone grafts, and finally, soft tissue closure. This technique has been shown to be highly successful in the treatment of chronic osteomyelitis.

Revascularization procedures, including local pedicle flaps and myocutaneous flaps, are commonly performed for recurrent osteomyelitis. Hyperbaric oxygen treatments have been used for gas gangrene and chronic osteomyelitis and should be an adjunct to surgical and antibiotic therapy.[41]

The choice of antibiotic therapy depends on the causative organism, which is verified by culture and sensitivity. Most treatment involves 2 to 4 weeks of intravenous therapy, followed by 4 weeks of oral medication.

Essential to the nursing management of the patient with osteomyelitis is the use of aseptic technique during dressing changes. The patient is observed for signs and symptoms of systemic infection, and antibiotics are administered on time and as prescribed. Prescribed analgesics and/or antipyretics are administered, and the patient is monitored for their effectiveness. Rest of the affected joint or limb is promoted, and the affected extremity is handled carefully to avoid pathologic fracture. Splints are often used for immobilization.

ROM exercises are encouraged to prevent contractures and flexion deformities, and participation in ADLs to the fullest extent possible is encouraged. The patient is instructed in the correct use of assistive devices as needed.

Patient/Family Education. If home-going therapy is prescribed, the proper administration of antibiotics should be taught. A peripherally inserted central catheter or central line allows for long-term venous access. Instructions for care of the insertion site and catheter should be given to the patient and family. A discussion of drug side effects should be included. Long-term antibiotic therapy can be performed at home with the help of a home health nurse. The patient and family can also administer antibiotics with periodic visits by the nurse. Dressing changes may also be performed at home. The patient and family can be taught aseptic technique.

Persons with total joint implants need instruction regarding the signs and symptoms of infection and avoiding sources of infection. The patient with an acute infection should be instructed to avoid the use of heat and exercise, which increase circulation and may spread infection. Information regarding follow-up care should be provided.

If surgery is performed, perioperative instructions are necessary. Persons with radical resections, flaps, external fixators, or amputations need emotional support in accepting body image changes and decreased mobility and independence. The patient and family need much support in coping with a chronic illness. Depression may occur in response to a chronic illness. The patient and family may need support and referrals for financial assistance, particularly if they lack insurance or have insufficient coverage.

DISORDERS AFFECTING THE SPINE

LOW BACK PAIN

Etiology/Epidemiology

Low back pain (LBP) is one the most common conditions a nurse encounters in any practice setting. Although a common disorder, LBP is also a challenge to health care professionals. Worldwide, it is estimated that up to 80% of the population experience LBP at some time during the life span.[44] Second only to the respiratory problems in the number of primary care office visits and time lost from work, LBP is also a major cause of permanent work disability.[50]

LBP is a challenge to the health care professional because it is a symptom that is not usually attributable to a specific cause or disease. Eighty percent of cases of LBP are idiopathic. Indeed, in approximately 80% of persons with LBP without neurologic symptoms, the pain resolves within 4 to 6 weeks without specific treatment.[44] Some patients develop chronic pain conditions, and approximately 15% have LBP attributable to specific causes, including a herniated disk, spinal stenosis, compression fracture, systemic disease related to the spine, and systemic disease unrelated to the spine.[44]

Common systemic conditions related to LBP include malignancy and infection. Persons in whom a systemic cause of LBP should be suspected include those younger than 20 years of age or older than 50 years of age and those with a history of cancer, symptoms of fever or chills, and unexplained weight loss. Other symptoms that require immediate attention include severe pain, significant neurologic deficit, sensory loss in the saddle area, abdominal pain, and trauma.

LBP affects the area below the ribs and gluteal muscles, often radiating to the thigh, and can be acute or chronic. The most common cause is a lumbar strain after lifting or twisting. More men than women are affected by back pain; postmenopausal women have a higher incidence than premenopausal women.[43] Risk factors associated with LBP include occupational hazards (repetitive motions, prolonged exposure to vibrations, and forward bending and twisting motions of the spine), smoking, osteoporosis, and hyperthyroidism.

Pathophysiology

The pathophysiology of common causes of back pain, including herniated disk, spinal stenosis, and spondylolisthesis, is discussed in the following sections. If disk herniation is the cause of back pain, the pain comes from the irritated dura and spinal nerves, since the nucleus pulposus lacks intrinsic innervation. Pain can arise from the joint capsule, ligaments, or muscles in the lumbar spine. The ligamentous structures of the lumbar spine are richly supplied with pain receptors and are susceptible to tears, sprains, and fracture. Muscle sprains and strains are also common causes of back pain. See Chapter 12 for a discussion of the theories of pain.

Collaborative Care Management

A detailed history and complete physical examination are required for accurate diagnosis and treatment of the person with LBP. The patient should be asked about any associated symptoms, any neurologic deficits, and any loss of bowel or bladder control. The presence of bowel or bladder symptoms should alert the health care provider to the possibility of *cauda equina syndrome,* which requires emergency surgical intervention. Cauda equina syndrome is compression of the caudal sac by herniated disk material. The presence of abdominal pain may suggest the presence of abdominal aortic aneurysm.

The physical examination should include neurologic assessment, ROM, and muscle testing. The lower extremities should be evaluated for any asymmetry in neurologic function. Measurements of calf and thigh circumference should be done; inequality may indicate muscle atrophy due to neurologic deficit. Limits in forward flexion are commonly found, with localized pain in the lumbosacral area. Screening for malignancy should also be done. Specialized tests, including straight leg raising (see Chapter 45) and crossed leg raising, should be incorporated into the examination. A complete assessment of the pain should be done. The patient's descriptors of the pain are important in determining the effect the pain has had on the person's lifestyle.

Routine laboratory examinations are not indicated. Controversy exists regarding the appropriateness of ordering x-rays at the first visit. Federal guidelines recommend a conservative approach. Many cases of back pain resolve; hence delaying diagnostics may avoid unnecessary expense and radiation exposure. Plain films are recommended only for persons over age 50, those with symptoms suspicious of systemic disease, and persons with radiculopathy.[50] CT scans and MRI are indicated for persons with neurologic compromise and for surgical candidates.

Most persons with LBP respond well to conservative therapy. Only 1% to 2% of patients require surgical intervention.[43] A multidisciplinary approach is necessary. Patients benefit from an early return to work and physical activity. Prolonged bed rest and missed work are actually harmful, reinforcing the concept of illness and disability. Bed rest is limited to 2 to 3 days for patients with radiculopathy. For those without neurologic symptoms bed rest is not recommended, or at most is recommended for 1 to 2 days.[50] Management strategies using the least amount of analgesics and fewest activity restrictions have been shown to have the best outcomes.[44]

Back exercises to strengthen lumbar musculature are indicated for treatment of LBP. Stretching and extension exercises have shown positive results, whereas flexion exercises are of little benefit. A PT referral is beneficial to instruct patients in the proper method to perform exercises.

The application of heat or cold applied within 48 hours of the onset of symptoms or heat for symptoms persisting over 48 hours is effective in reducing pain. Massage therapy has provided some patients with temporary relief. Traction, TENS, and ultrasound have not been proved to be effective.[50] Other treatments include trigger-point therapy and spinal manipulation. Chiropractic treatment is contraindicated for patients with radiculopathy. See Chapter 12 for other nonpharmacologic methods of pain control.

Pharmacologic treatments include NSAIDs, analgesics, and adjuvants. Topical medications for local pain relief may be effective for some persons. Steroid injections have also been used with some success. Implantable pumps to deliver intrathecal or epidural opioids have been used for persons with chronic pain, but their use is controversial.[72]

Interventions addressing psychosocial needs are important in the management of persons with LBP. Depression and substance abuse are common in persons with LBP. Secondary gain may be a motive in some persons, making treatment difficult. Persons whose pain has persisted for longer than 3 months may need referral for management of chronic pain.

Patient/Family Education. The patient and family need education about the pathogenesis of back pain, particularly if no specific cause is found. Reassurance that most persons with back pain respond favorably to conservative treatment and are able to return to work and leisure activities can help decrease anxiety about long-term effects of the pain on lifestyle. If appropriate, information about lifestyle changes such as cessation of smoking, weight loss, and institution of a regular exercise program should be given. Body weight should be maintained within 10% of the ideal body weight. If environmental conditions such as occupational hazards are contributing to the LBP, perhaps a modification in the work environment can be made. In some cases employment retraining may be indicated. Ergonomics should be incorporated into the design of the worksite.

Persons with depression or substance abusers should be referred to a psychologist or counselor for additional therapy. Cognitive coping strategies have been used effectively in helping patients cope with chronic pain. Patients' positive perceptions of their self-efficacy may assist them in implementing strategies to relieve pain and cope with a chronic pain condition. Self-efficacy theory states that a person's perceived ability to carry out a behavior necessary for a desired outcome positively influences the probability that the person will perform the behavior.[64] Nurses can assist patients in learning these behaviors.

Providing information about proper body mechanics and methods to avoid back injury is very important. The proper way to sit, stand, bend, and lift objects should be demonstrated to all patients with LBP (see Figure 47-32). When seated, the feet should rest flat on the floor or stool. The knees should be higher than the hips with the arms supported. When lifting, the knees, not the back, should be bent, and objects should not be lifted higher than the level of the elbows. While sleeping supine, a pillow should be placed under the knees. A firm mattress or bed board is beneficial for adequate support. Giving the patient information to prevent further episodes of back pain allows the patient responsibility for management of the condition and some sense of control. Many back pain clinics have a "Back School" where patients are referred and taught principles of body mechanics, posture, and exercises. Regular aerobic exercise in addition to back-strengthening exercises (Figure 47-34) should be done for at least 30 minutes five times per week. Walking and swimming are good choices for persons with LBP. Some persons may believe that exercise will do further harm to the back; they need reassurance and encouragement to participate in a regular exercise program.

Support groups may help the individual with LBP. Exercising at community centers may provide the person with companionship. For persons with chronic pain, a referral to a pain support group may be indicated. Information can be obtained from the American Pain Society.*

*4700 West Lake Avenue, Glenview, IL 60025; (847) 375-4715; website: info@ampainsoc.org.

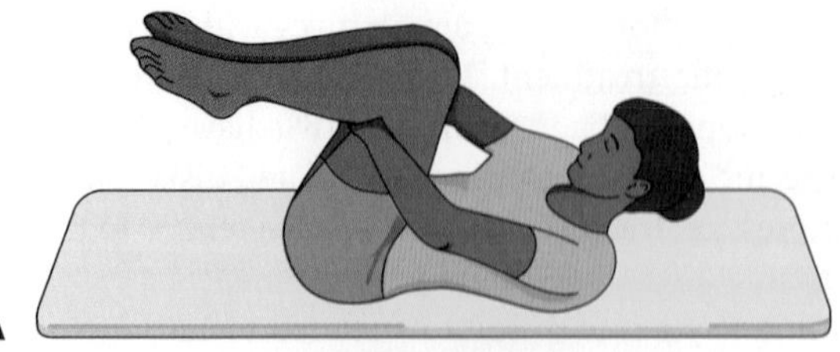

Back Roll

The back roll stretches your back, buttocks, and neck muscles. Lie on your back on the floor, relax, and bring your knees to your chest. Clasp your hands behind your knee and rock back and forth, from your buttocks to your neck. Slowly return to the starting position. Repeat 5 to 10 times.

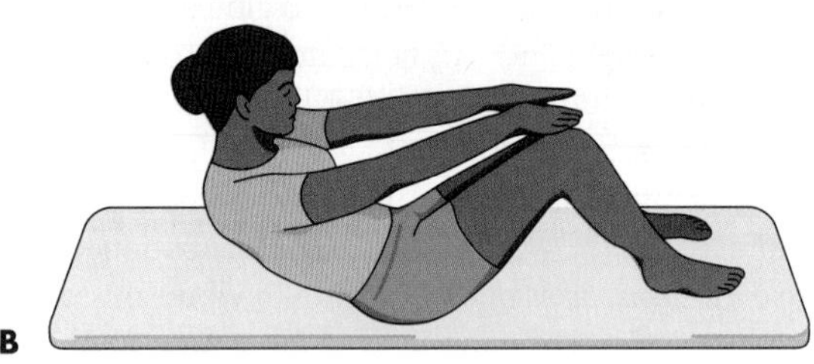

Partial Sit-ups

Partial sit-ups strengthen your abdominal muscles. Lie flat on your back on the floor with your knees bent and feet flat on the floor. Tuck in your chin and tighten your abdomen. Slowly raise your head and neck while reaching out with your hands to touch your knees. Hold your knees for a count of five and slowly return to the starting position. Repeat 5 to 10 times.

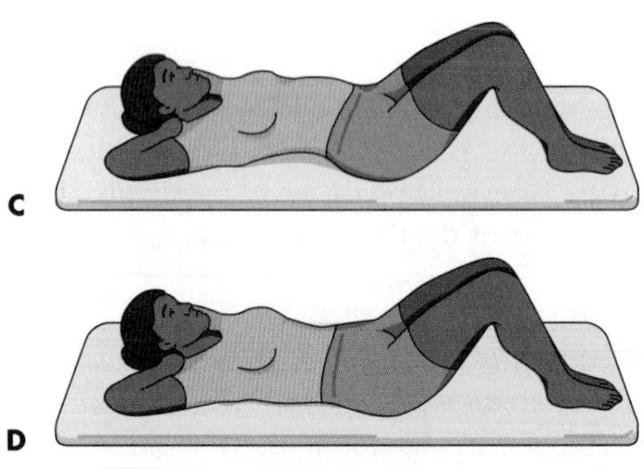

Pelvic Tilt

The pelvic tilt strengthens your abdominal and back muscles. Lie flat on your back on the floor with your knees bent and feet flat on the floor. Join your hands behind your head. Firmly tighten your buttock and abdominal muscles, pressing your lower back flat against the floor. Hold for a count of five and relax muscles. Repeat 5 to 10 times.

Figure 47-34 Exercises for lower back pain. **A**, Back roll. **B**, Partial sit-ups. **C** and **D**, Pelvic tilt.

DEGENERATIVE DISORDERS OF THE SPINE

A number of degenerative disorders that affect the cervical, thoracic, and lumbar portions of the spine are treated by surgical intervention. The collaborative care and nursing management sections pertain to persons with any of these disorders.

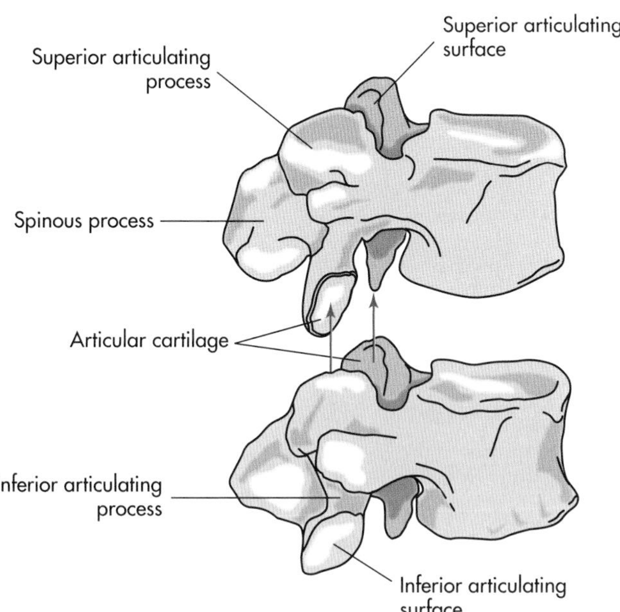

Figure 47-35 Posterior facet joints of lumbar vertebrae. Each vertebra has four surfaces by which it articulates with its adjacent vertebrae: two on its superior aspect and two on the inferior. Superior articulating surfaces are medially located; inferior articulating surfaces are laterally located. These joints are diarthrotic, having a joint capsule with a synovial lining.

Etiology

Degenerative disease of the spine is a common but difficult problem. The spine has 23 intervertebral disk joints and 46 posterior facet joints (Figure 47-35), all of which are subjected to stresses and strains in holding the human body upright and moving it about. The vertebrae in the spinal column are articulated in a series of "couplets" that are able to move through an intervertebral disk joint and two posterior facet joints. The intervertebral disks are composed of an outer layer of cartilage called the annulus fibrosus and an inner layer called the nucleus pulposus. Several common problems arise with these structures in degenerative disease of the spine. These include degenerative disk disease, herniated intervertebral disk, spinal stenosis, spondylolisthesis, and spondylosis.

Degenerative disk disease develops as a result of biochemical and biomechanical changes in the intervertebral disks. The gelatinous mucoid material of the nucleus pulposus is replaced with fibrocartilage as a result of aging. The water content of the disk also decreases with aging.

Spinal stenosis occurs as a result of aging, degenerative disk disease, spondylosis, osteophyte formation, or a congenital condition. The disk space is narrowed and less resilient and may be unstable at the affected levels. Smoking is a risk factor for the development of disk degeneration and herniation. Other identified risk factors include a sedentary lifestyle and extensive motor vehicle driving.

Spondylosis is degeneration of the vertebrae; it may occur in the cervical, thoracic, or lumbar spine. It is often accompanied by arthritic changes, including osteophyte formation, ligamentous disruption, and subluxation.

Epidemiology

Degenerative disorders of the spine develop most commonly in persons over 50 years of age. Cervical spondylosis is generally found in persons over 55 years of age.[60] Disk herniation is seen in persons of all ages, but the peak incidence is between 35 and 45 years of age.

Pathophysiology

Pathophysiologic changes associated with degenerative disk disease include spinal stenosis (narrowing of the spinal canal), spondylosis (degeneration and stiffness of the vertebral joints), subluxation, and vertebral degeneration. Initial disk changes are followed by facet arthropathy, osteophyte formation, and ligamentous instability. Myelopathy and radiculopathy (disease involving a spinal nerve root) may follow. The degenerative process usually involves synovitis, which causes cartilage erosion, leading to the formation of osteophytes.

Herniated intervertebral disk is a protrusion of the nucleus pulposus through a tear or rupture in the annulus. Herniation can occur anteriorly, posteriorly, or laterally. Extrusion of the disk material may impinge on a nerve root or on the spinal cord (Figure 47-36). Herniation may occur as a result of trauma, a sharp or sudden movement, or degeneration. In the cervical spine, herniation usually occurs at the more mobile segments—C5-6, C6-7, and C4-5. Most lumbar herniations occur at the L5-S1 and L4-5 levels.[65] Herniation of thoracic disks is less common. Symptoms may develop immediately or take years to manifest themselves. The location and size of the herniation determines the signs and symptoms associated with the herniation (see Clinical Manifestations box). Pain associated with disk herniation may be caused by direct pressure of disk fragments on the nerve root, by breakdown products from a degenerated nucleus pulposus, or by an autoimmune reaction. The nurse's knowledge of dermatomes and spinal nerve innervation aids in the assessment of a patient with a herniated intervertebral disk (Table 47-17). Another consideration is the size of the patient's spinal canal. A slight herniation may cause significant symptoms in an individual with a congenitally narrow canal.

Spinal stenosis is a narrowing of the spinal canal or intervertebral foramina at any level, creating pressure on the involved nerve root(s), resulting in neurologic symptoms. Spinal stenosis results from hyperplasia and cartilaginous changes in the ligamentum flavum, laminae, and facet joints. Anatomic abnormalities may also contribute to spinal stenosis. The condition can be congenital or acquired. Osteophyte formation may cause neuroforaminal stenosis, resulting in joint instability and subluxation.

Spondylolisthesis is an anterior or posterior slippage of one vertebral body on another. Spondylolisthesis can be a congenital abnormality or be caused by degenerative changes, trauma, or bone disease. Spondylolysis or a structural defect in the lamina is often the cause. The pars interarticularis (between the superior and inferior articular facets) is usually the site of the defect. The degree of spondylolisthesis is graded on a scale of 1 to 4, depending on the percentage of slip that is

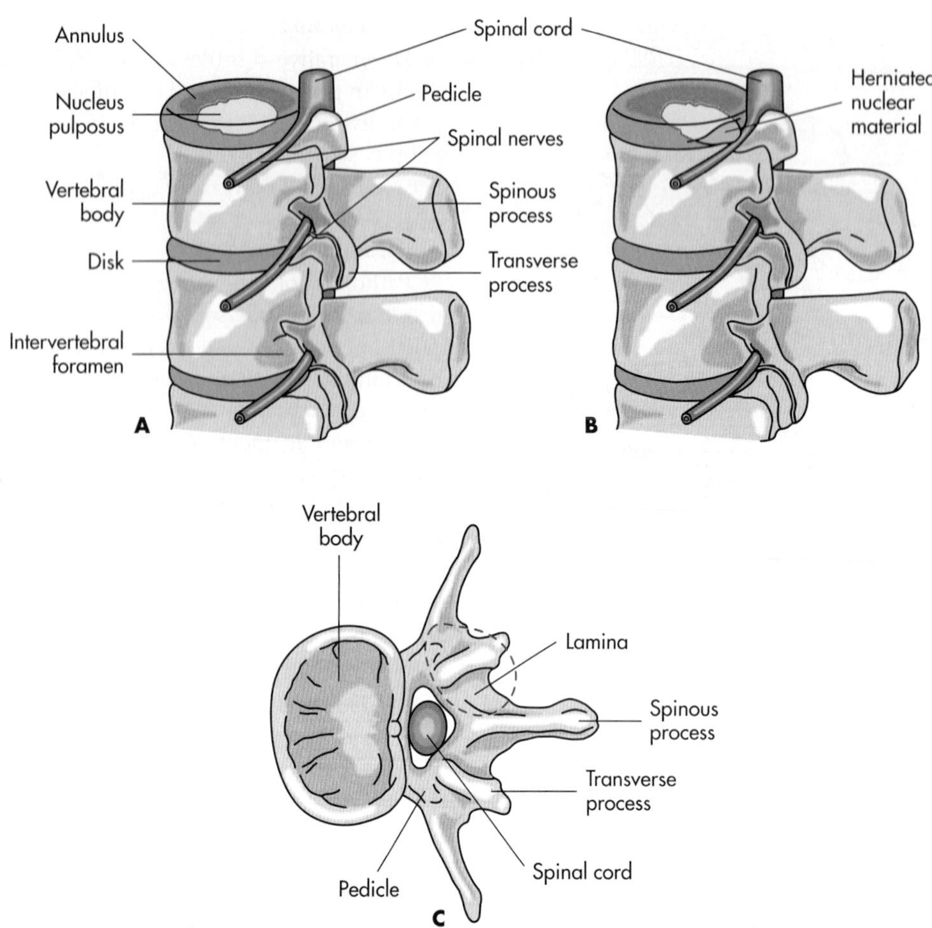

Figure 47-36 Compression of spinal cord and nerve root. **A,** Disks, composed of a cartilaginous outer layer (anulus fibrosus) and a gel-like inner layer (nucleus pulposus), lie between vertebral bodies. Spinal nerves exit the spinal cord laterally just above the pedicle. **B,** Laminae compose posterior portions of vertebrae. Each pedicle joins with a lamina; the transverse and spinous processes project from laminae. **C,** When nucleus pulposus herniates posteriorly through its fibrous covering and the posterior longitudinal ligament, it may compress the spinal cord and trap the nerve root. The surgical approach to relieve this compression is through lamina *(dotted line)*, posterior to the transverse process.

Clinical Manifestations

Herniated Intervertebral Disk

CERVICAL

Decreased range of motion of cervical spine
Paresthesias of upper extremities, depending on nerve root involved
Weakness or atrophy of upper extremity musculature, depending on level involved
Pain in affected nerve root distribution
Abdominal reflex activity
May have motor or sensory disturbances in lower extremities

LUMBAR

Sciatica in 40% of persons
Tenderness or pain with palpation of disk spaces and sciatic notch
Painful and/or decreased range of motion of lumbar spine
Motor and sensory impairment in affected nerve root distribution (may note discrepancies in calf circumference, weakness in lower extremity muscle groups, pain and numbness in dermatomal distribution)
Decreased or absent reflexes
Bowel or bladder impairment
Positive straight leg raising (Lasegue's test): straight leg raising with opposite leg flat will produce leg pain or radicular symptoms
Pain radiating down leg in dermatomal distribution
Pain relieved by lying down

TABLE 47-17 Lumbar Disk Herniation

Level of Herniation	Nerve Root	Reflex	Sensation	Muscle Testing
L3-4	L4	Patellar	Medial aspects of leg and foot	Inversion of foot (tibialis anterior)
L4-5	L5	—	Lateral aspect of leg and dorsal surface of foot	Extension of toes (extensor hallucis longus)
L5-S1	S1	Achilles	Lateral aspect of foot	Eversion of foot (peroneus longus, brevis)

shown on x-ray films of the spine. Grades 3 and 4 are usually treated surgically. Spondylolisthesis usually occurs at L5-S1. The forward slip of the vertebra can cause nerve impingement, manifested by motor and sensory deficits at the level(s) involved, such as pain, weakness, and/or bowel and bladder involvement. The slip may be detected when the spinous processes are palpated.

Cauda equina ("horse's tail") syndrome may occur after trauma, spinal stenosis, fracture, tumor, or disk herniation. Pressure on the cauda equina nerve roots causes neurologic deficits, varying in intensity, depending on the degree of compression.

Collaborative Care Management

Diagnostic Tests. Diagnostic tests to determine defects in the spine include x-ray films, myelography, CT scanning, and MRI. See Chapter 45 for more information.

Medications. Conservative management of degenerative problems of the spine includes the use of antiinflammatory agents (usually NSAIDs). Concomitant use of alcohol or aspirin may increase GI irritation and bleeding tendencies and therefore should be avoided. Pain relief is usually noted after 1 week of therapy. If pain relief is not effective, opioids should be prescribed. Oral corticosteroids are useful for treating pain for short periods of time; long-term use is not recommended. Steroids may also be prescribed for acute symptoms of cauda equina syndrome. Antiinflammatory medications or local anesthetics may be injected directly into the affected joint or structure (epidural space to relieve nerve root pain). The use of steroid injections should be limited because of adverse effects on tissue healing.

Skeletal muscle relaxants may also be prescribed. The patient should be cautioned against driving or engaging in potentially hazardous activities because of drowsiness, a frequent side effect of muscle relaxants. The patient should be informed that the use of alcohol or other CNS depressants will increase the effects of the muscle relaxant. Muscle relaxants often cause dry mouth, and the nurse can instruct the patient in measures to counteract this side effect.

Treatments. Conservative treatment is implemented initially (see discussion under Low Back Pain). Pain control and return to functioning are the goals of treatment. Conservative management is given a trial before surgical intervention is considered, unless neurologic deficits are present. Corsets or braces are sometimes prescribed to provide external support to the spine, especially during physical activity. Braces and corsets are fitted by an orthotist.

BOX 47-12 Types of Spinal Surgery

Laminectomy: removal of a portion of the lamina, the posterior arch of the vertebra, to gain access to the disk and spinal canal

Discectomy: removal of all or part of a herniated intervertebral disk

Foraminotomy: widening of the intervertebral foramen to allow free passage of the spinal nerve

Spinal fusion: stabilization of two or more vertebrae by insertion of bone grafts with or without the addition of hardware (rods, plates, screws, cages, or disk prostheses) to achieve vertebral stability

Decompression: release of pressure or impingement on spinal nerve roots by removal of osteophytes, bone, or soft tissues

Surgical Management. Most spinal disorders are treated conservatively. Surgery is indicated when conservative modalities fail or for the following reasons: neurologic deficits, such as loss of bowel or bladder control or loss of motor function; severe, intractable pain; bony instability; and progressive deformity with resultant loss of function.

Spinal surgery is also performed for fractures and tumors. A variety of procedures are performed on the cervical, thoracic, and lumbar spine. Surgical approaches to the spine include anterior, transthoracic, retroperitoneal, and posterior approaches. Box 47-12 gives examples of commonly performed types of spinal surgery. Anterior approaches to the lumbar spine allow direct visualization of the disk space; a general surgeon often opens and makes the exposure. The transthoracic approach involves thoracotomy.

Spinal surgery may involve the use of instrumentation. A number of different implants are available. Instrumentation is used to maintain correction of deformity, stabilize the spine, prevent neurologic damage, enhance bony fusion, avoid external immobilization, and allow for early mobilization, thereby facilitating rehabilitation. The type of instrumentation used depends on the pathologic condition, individual patient, and surgeon preference. Table 47-18 gives examples of spinal instrumentation.

Some types of spinal surgery involve the use of bone grafts. Bone grafts function as a form of scaffolding into which osteogenic cells grow and/or as a means of mechanical support. Autograft, allograft, or bone substitute may be used for grafting. The success of the bone graft depends partially on the type of fixation of the graft and the site and condition of the host recipient.

TABLE 47-18 Common Types of Spinal Instrumentation

Indications	Approach	Components	Advantages and Disadvantages
Cotrel-Dubousset (CD) (Horizon)			
Idiopathic scoliosis, kyphosis, trauma	Posterior	Parallel rods Hooks Screws C-rings Cross-link plate	*Advantages:* ability to correct rib hump deformity; early mobilization; bracing not necessary *Disadvantages:* time-consuming, difficult technique; difficult to revise; hook shift; expensive
Harrington			
Thoracolumbar fracture scoliosis	Posterior	Rods Hooks Screws	*Advantages:* rigid fixation; uncomplicated technique *Disadvantages:* increased immobility postoperatively; instrument failure, breakage; loss of correction; inability to control rod; loss of lumbar lordosis; need to fuse above and below level of pathologic condition, resulting in immobile spine; requires bracing
Kaneda			
Thoracolumbar fracture Kyphosis Compromised spinal canal	Anterior (transthoracic retroperitoneal)	Threaded rods Staples Vertebral body screws Nuts	*Advantages:* rigid fixation *Disadvantages:* possible damage to vascular structures
Luque			
Scoliosis Kyphosis Thoracolumbar fracture	Posterior	L-shaped rods Sublaminar wires	*Advantages:* rigid stabilization; ability to contour rod *Disadvantages:* risk of neural damage associated with sublaminar wiring
Pedicle Screw-and-Plate Systems (Roy Camille, AO, Steffee, Danek)			
Spinal instability Spinal stenosis Thoracolumbar fracture Pseudoarthrosis Failed instrumentation Tumor Spondylosis Spondylolisthesis	Posterior	Screws Plates Rods Cables	*Advantages:* reduces deformity, restores alignment, and achieves stability while fusing fewer levels; rigid fixation; early, less painful mobility postoperatively *Disadvantages:* screw breakage, failure; pseudoarthrosis; loosening of hardware; lengthy procedure; proximity of pin, screw to neural elements
TSRH (Texas Scottish Rite Hospital) (Pedicle Screw and Plate)			
Scoliosis Spinal fracture Tumor Kyphosis	Anterior or posterior	Parallel rods Cross-link plates Hooks	*Advantages:* easily revised; can be adapted for anterior use; easily contoured rods; early ambulation *Disadvantages:* pseudoarthrosis; hardware failure
Unit			
Neuromuscular scoliosis	Posterior	Precontoured, continuous rod Sublaminar wiring	*Advantages:* ends of rods able to be implanted in pelvis; stability: little rod migration; good correction of rotational deformities; correction of pelvic obliquity *Disadvantages:* risk to neural elements associated with sublaminar wiring
Fusion Cages (Moss, BAK)			
Spinal stenosis Tumor Interbody fusion Spinal instability	Anterior Posterior Endoscopic	Metal cage Screws with bone graft or bone substitute	*Advantages:* immediate stabilization; allows bony in-growth from superior and inferior vertebral bodies into matrix of bone graft; can be used in a variety of approaches, particularly endoscopic; uncomplicated technique; high success rate *Disadvantages:* long-term results unknown
Z Plate			
Instability Corpectomy Fusion	Anterior	Z-shaped plates and screws	*Advantages:* rigid stabilization *Disadvantages:* hardware failure; pseudoarthrosis

Both cortical and cancellous bone can serve as graft material. Allogeneic and autogenic cortical grafts both initially act as weight-bearing struts to provide support until the host bone has incorporated and remodeled the graft and is able to bear weight. Freshly implanted autografts are capable of osteogenesis, the process of bone synthesis by graft or host cells. Cancellous bone, because of its larger surface area, has greater potential for osteogenesis than does cortical bone. Host bone is produced by osteoconduction, a process in which mesenchymal cells of the host differentiate into osteoblasts.

Initially all types of bone graft are partially resorbed. Incorporation of the bone graft takes place in overlapping stages. It begins by creeping substitution (gradual resorption of the graft) and finally results in replacement of the graft by new bone. Both autografts and allografts produce an acute inflammatory response within the first week, followed by the formation of fibrous granulation tissue and an increase in osteoclastic activity. This is followed by osteoinduction, which is probably regulated by bone morphogenic protein, which promotes new bone production by the host. Bone morphogenic protein is present in fresh autografts and in modified allografts, but autoclaving for sterilization destroys bone morphogenic protein. Osteoinduction is followed by osteoconduction, characterized by capillary growth and infiltration of the graft by perivascular tissue and osteoprogenitor cells of the host. This process may last for several months in cancellous autografts and for years in cortical autografts or allografts. Cancellous grafts are eventually completely replaced, whereas cortical grafts remain a mixture of necrotic graft bone and viable host bone. As remodeling takes place, the graft is resorbed and replaced by living bone, subject to Wolff's law.

Advantages of autografts are tissue compatibility and low cost. Disadvantages include a limited supply of bone, a weakened donor site with a potential for fracture, and an added surgical site that can cause considerable pain. The most common sites for graft harvesting are the iliac crests and the fibulae.

Advantages of allografts are fewer surgical sites and thus less pain. Allografts also come in a variety of sizes and shapes. Disadvantages include a limited and costly supply and a high graft failure rate. Allografts trigger local and systemic immune responses that may affect their failure rate. Freezing and freeze-drying implants have decreased rejection rates.

Surgical techniques have evolved to replace the traditional open approach to spinal surgery and instrumentation. Microdiskectomy involves a surgical incision, but one that is much smaller than that with the open approach. The use of MRI and other imaging techniques allows direct access to the disk through a very small incision. Decompression and disk removal can be accomplished with less exposure and thus less pain and a shorter hospital stay. The surgeon must have considerable experience to perform the procedure with limited exposure. The success rates for open diskectomy and microdiskectomy are equal.

An alternative to microsurgery is another, less invasive method of accessing the spinal structures. Endoscopic approaches to the spine allow the surgeon to perform diskectomy, decompression, and fusion through endoscopic portals. These procedures are most commonly preformed on the thoracic or lumbar spine. Procedures performed without fusion can usually be performed as an outpatient procedure. Patients undergoing endoscopic fusions can expect a 2- to 4-day hospital stay. Persons with multilevel disease or previous spinal surgery may not be candidates for these techniques.

Diet. Although a special diet is not indicated for the treatment of degenerative disorders of the spine, weight reduction may be advised in the case of an overweight individual. Every effort should be made to attain or maintain ideal body weight to decrease the mechanical stressors on the back, as well as other joints.

Activity. The physical therapist will instruct the patient in a program to strengthen the muscles of the back and abdomen, which will increase support of the vertebral column. Exercises to increase flexibility, which will enable the person to bend and move with less chance of injury, are also prescribed. Aerobic exercises, such as swimming, may be prescribed to improve overall conditioning and to maintain or reduce weight, without placing stress on the back. The patient should be taught to avoid lifting heavy objects (generally heavier than 10 pounds), participating in contact sports, and extreme twisting or bending of the spine. Logrolling and maintaining proper body alignment are important to decrease muscle strain and injury.

Referrals. A referral to a back school or occupational therapist may be initiated to assist the patient and family in functioning effectively within the confines of the patient's disability. Emphasis is placed on body mechanics and modifications of daily routines to decrease the possibility of further injury. Job retraining may be indicated. Sometimes a referral to a pain management center is initiated, especially in the case of an individual having difficulty coping with chronic pain. If back or leg pain persists longer than 6 weeks, or if a psychologic component of pain is suspected, a psychologic referral may be indicated.

NURSING MANAGEMENT OF PATIENT UNDERGOING SPINAL SURGERY

PREOPERATIVE CARE

Preoperative nursing care that is relevant to persons undergoing all types of spinal surgery is discussed. Persons undergoing elective spinal surgery are admitted on the morning of their surgery. Preoperative teaching and testing are completed and evaluated before admission. Depending on the patient's condition, preoperative evaluation may include the following: complete history and physical examination; laboratory work, including CBC; urinalysis; blood chemistry; prothrombin time and partial thromboplastin time; type and screen or cross-matching of blood; chest x-ray films; electrocardiogram; and diagnostic tests related to the spine, such as x-ray films, myelography, CT scans, and MRI. If significant blood loss is expected, autologous donation should be discussed with the patient.

If postoperative bracing is required, the patient is fitted for the brace and given instructions for its use preoperatively. An orthotist measures and fabricates the brace. Many types of braces are available, depending on the type of procedure performed. Some examples are cervical four-poster braces, a thoracic lumbar sacral orthosis (TLSO), and soft corsets.

General preoperative teaching should be given to the patient and family (see Chapter 16). Many patients are curious about the types of implants to be used. If a sample of the instrumentation is available, it may be helpful to show it to the patient. The patient should also be informed about the location and extent of the surgical incision(s). If a spinal fusion with autologous graft is planned, an explanation of the donor site location and degree of postoperative pain is beneficial. The patient should also be informed if allograft bone is to be used.

The patient should be given instructions in performing logrolling technique, isometric exercises, incentive spirometry, and coughing and deep breathing. Instructions are also given regarding general postoperative care, such as postanesthesia care, care of intravenous lines and catheters, vital sign routines, and pain management.

POSTOPERATIVE CARE

Postoperative care of the patient recovering from spinal surgery includes interventions to prevent or minimize complications (Chapter 18). If an anterior or lateral approach was used, general care of the patient is as described in Chapters 21 and 34.

Prevention of DVT and PE is an important nursing intervention after surgery. The use of elastic stockings and pneumatic sleeves applied in the operating room is continued after surgery. Patients are instructed to perform isometric exercises hourly while awake. Anticoagulants are prescribed after surgery as prophylaxis against DVT and pulmonary embolism. Ambulation is encouraged as soon as possible. The patient is evaluated daily for signs of DVT.

Monitoring of hemoglobin and hematocrit levels is important, especially if the patient has experienced an extensive blood loss during surgery. The surgical site and dressing should be assessed for signs of infection and hemorrhage. Clear drainage may indicate leakage of cerebrospinal fluid and should be reported to the surgeon.

With any spinal procedure, careful monitoring of neurologic function is critical. Knowledge of the patient's baseline functioning is vital when monitoring for changesafter surgery. Neurovascular checks to the extremities are performed hourly in the immediate postoperative period and less frequently thereafter. The patient's ability to detect touch and discern sharp from dull is tested. Motor strength in the extremities is evaluated, and any changes are reported to the surgeon. Neurologic changes can occur up to 72 hours after surgery. If neurologic deficits were present before surgery, improvement in sensation may not be immediately evident after surgery. Careful assessment to monitor sensation and motor function is essential to detect changes from baseline. Drainage from surgical drains should be assessed and measured. Drains are usually removed after 24 to 36 hours. If a fusion has been done, the donor site should be assessed for bleeding.

Urinary retention is common after spinal surgery. If the patient does not have an indwelling catheter, he or she should be assessed for the ability to void. Lying flat in bed can make voiding difficult, particularly for male patients. Patients who have not undergone fusion are usually allowed out of bed the evening of surgery, which may facilitate the ability to void. The physician may order that the patient be catheterized if the patient is unable to void after 8 hours.

Correct positioning of the patient after spinal surgery is important. When turning, patients should be logrolled to keep the spinal column straight. If bracing is required postoperatively, the patient may be in bed without the brace, but it must be worn while ambulating. A straight-backed chair should be used for sitting to avoid twisting the back.

Discharge planning focuses on teaching and performing ADLs. Assistive devices such as long-handled brushes, shoehorns, and grabbers may be necessary to avoid extreme bending or reaching. If bracing is used, the patient and family should be able to demonstrate the proper technique of applying and removing the brace. The patient should be taught to assess the skin for evidence of pressure or breakdown, and the patient or family member should be instructed about how to inspect the wound for any signs of infection.

Lumbar Spine Surgery

The length of stay for persons undergoing lumbar spine surgery varies. Patients undergoing endoscopic disk removal may go home the same day; persons underoing fusions may be hospitalized for up to 4 days (see Guidelines for Safe Practice box, p. 1578, top). Note the differences in care for patients undergoing lumbar spine surgery with and without fusion in the Clinical Pathways on pp. 1580 to 1585.

Cervical Spine Surgery

Persons undergoing cervical spine surgery may require tongs or halo traction (see Chapter 46) or a halo brace. Edema of the throat is present in the early postoperative period, requiring careful assessment of the airway and ability to swallow (see Guidelines for Safe Practice box, p. 1578, bottom). The estimated length of stay for persons undergoing procedures on the cervical spine is 1 to 3 days. A Clinical Pathway for a patient undergoing cervical fusion is found on pp. 1587 and 1588.

Thoracic Spine Surgery

Mobility restrictions are more prolonged than with lumbar surgery, because the thoracic spine is more mobile; consequently, there is a greater risk of dislodging grafts through improper motion (see Guidelines for Safe Practice box on p. 1586).

GERONTOLOGIC CONSIDERATIONS

As stated earlier, degenerative changes occur as the skeleton ages. Degenerative disk disease and spinal stenosis primarily affect the elderly population.

Disk degeneration causes the facet joints and posterior ligamentum flavum to hypertrophy in an attempt to stabilize the posterior elements of the spine. These anatomic changes result in a narrowed spinal canal. Consequently, nerve roots may

Text continued on p. 1586

Guidelines for Safe Practice

Postoperative Care of the Patient Who Has Undergone Lumbar Spine Surgery

1. Positioning
   a. The patient is encouraged to logroll to change position from side to back to side.
   b. Use of a turning sheet is advised until the patient can assist with turning.
2. Neurovascular checks to assess circulatory status and motor and sensory function
   a. Monitor the patient for signs of neurologic deficit, deep vein thrombosis, and pulmonary embolism. Prophylactic anticoagulants may be prescribed.
3. Wound care (drains placed in wound to prevent hematoma formation, if necessary)
   a. Maintain constant suction through drains as required.
   b. Maintain drains free of contamination.
   c. Monitor for excessive output from drains. Output ranges from 20 to 250 ml/8 hours for the first 24 hours, tapers for 12 hours postoperatively, and usually is removed 24 to 36 hours postoperatively. Drains that allow reinfusion of serous drainage may be used.
   d. Inspect surgical area frequently for evidence of excess drainage or hematoma formation (bulging of tissues surrounding the surgical site).
   e. If a spinal fusion with autologous graft has been done, inspect donor site (usually iliac crest) for drainage, hematoma.
4. Promoting comfort
   a. Reposition patient frequently.
   b. Administer opioids; change from intravenous route to oral route as tolerated, transition to nonopiods as patient tolerates. Monitor respiratory status and effectiveness of pain management.
   c. Monitor use and effectiveness of the patient-controlled analgesia pump, if ordered.
   d. Use a fracture bedpan.
5. Promoting mobility
   a. Activity out of bed varies depending on whether fusion was done. Bed rest may be ordered if there was damage to the dura intraoperatively.
   b. Transfer patient out of bed with as little time spent in the sitting position as possible.
      (1) Start the transfer with the patient in a side-lying position at the edge of the bed.
      (2) Have patient push off the bed with the upper hand and the lower elbow.
      (3) One person assists by guiding the patient's trunk, and another assists the patient's legs over the side of the bed.
      (4) Reverse the process for return to bed.
   c. The patient may be permitted to walk as much as tolerated, with an assistive aid if necessary.
   d. Braces or corsets, if prescribed, are applied before the patient gets out of bed.
   e. Encourage patient to participate in activities of daily living within prescribed limits of mobility.
6. Discharge instructions
   a. Do not lift or carry anything heavier than 2.25 kg (5 pounds).
   b. Do not drive a car until permitted by the surgeon.
   c. Avoid twisting motions of the trunk.
   d. Report any signs of infection or neurologic deficit to surgeon.

Guidelines for Safe Practice

Postoperative Care of the Patient Who Has Undergone Cervical Spine Surgery

1. Positioning
   a. Keep head of bed elevated 30 to 45 degrees, particularly if an anterior surgical approach was used, to decrease swelling in the throat and facilitate respiration.
   b. If the patient is in a cervical brace, position is not restricted except by the patient's tolerance.
   c. If the patient is in cervical traction, the patient may be turned side to back to side to the patient's tolerance.
2. Promoting safety
   a. Assess the airway and respiratory function frequently. Swelling may compromise the airway.
   b. Provide suction equipment and a tracheotomy set in the patient's room until swelling in the throat subsides and the patient is swallowing and breathing normally.
   c. Check adjustment screws and straps frequently to ensure that there is no loosening of the brace.
   d. Advise physician or orthotist of loosening of the brace consequent to a decrease in edema so that the brace can be readjusted.
3. Wound care
   a. Inspect surgical area, including the iliac crest donor site, frequently for evidence of excess drainage or formation of a hematoma. Apply an ice bag to the donor site for comfort.
   b. If a tong or halo traction is being used, pin care may be required (see Chapter 46).
4. Promoting comfort and relieving pain
   a. Provide ice chips to soothe sore throat.
   b. Make progressive diet changes slowly; the patient will have difficulty swallowing and will be afraid of choking. Full liquids or semisolids (ice cream, custards, gelatin, nectars) are often better tolerated than clear juice or broth; however, milk products may increase mucus production.
   c. Administer analgesics as for any patient undergoing spinal surgery. The donor site often causes more discomfort than the neck incision.
   d. The patient may require aerosol treatments or humidification of air to loosen mucus secretions or make breathing more comfortable.
5. Promoting mobility
   a. If the patient is in traction, encourage patient to perform ankle dorsiflexion/plantar flexion exercises and quadriceps setting on a regular basis to promote circulation and maintain leg strength. Monitor the patient for signs of deep vein thrombosis and pulmonary embolism.
   b. If the patient is in a brace, out-of-bed activity, including walking, may begin as soon as the patient tolerates.
   c. Provide for temporary use of a walker if the donor site pain restricts mobility.
   d. Encourage patient to participate in activities of daily living to the greatest extent possible.
6. Discharge instructions
   a. Wear the brace at all times.
   b. Report any difficulty with the brace to the physician immediately.
   c. Do not drive a car during the period that the brace must be worn.
   d. Report symptoms of graft dislodgment (dysphagia and a feeling of "fullness" in the throat), infection, or neurologic deficit.

clinical pathway *Lumbar Laminectomy Fusion Risk Factors*

Directions:
1. Review CCT approximately every 8°.
2. Appropriate and completed interventions need no additional documentation.
3. Cross through any interventions which are not applicable.
4. Circle any intervention not completed.
5. The plan of care—nursing interventions and outcome evaluation statements—may be added to the CCT as necessary.

DRG 215 Expected LOS 4
Physician(s) ____
Admit Date ____
Discharge Date ____
Surgery/Procedure ____
____
Date of Surgery/Procedure ____

Discharge Plan:
☐ Homecare ____
____
☐ Rehab/Subacute ____
____

Comorbid Conditions:
☐ CHF
☐ IDDM
☐ Angina
☐ Atrial fib/flutter

Imprint/Label

Complications during this admission:
☐ DVT
☐ PE
☐ Infection
☐ Continued wound drainage
☐ Mental status change
☐ Cardiac
☐ Urinary retention
☐ Ileus
☐ Stroke

Risk Factors:
☐ Obesity ☐ ETOH/Substance Abuse ☐ Smoking ☐

DATE	PROBLEM LIST	DISCHARGE CRITERIA	DATE INITIALLY MET	MET ON DISCHARGE	
				YES	NO
	1. Patient education knowledge deficit 2. Pain 3. Impaired mobility 4. Impaired skin (potential) 5. Impaired gas exchange (potential) 6. Altered tissue perfusion (potential) 7. Constipation (potential)	1. Vital signs baseline. 2. Pain controlled by po pain meds. 3. Incision well approximated/no signs of infection. 4. Patient ambulates independently or with assistive device. 5. Patient appropriately utilizes brace if required. 6. Patient/caregiver has knowledge, resources & ability to safely provide care outside the hospital environment.			
		Explain any discharge criteria not met:			

Courtesy The Cleveland Clinic Foundation, Cleveland, Ohio, 12/21/2000. This is a general guideline to *assist* in the management of patients. This guideline is not designated to replace clinical judgment or individual patient needs.

clinical pathway *Lumbar Laminectomy Fusion Risk Factors—cont'd*

PLAN	DISCHARGE PLANNING RECORD TEAM MEMBERS (INCLUDE BEEPER #)		HOMEGOING EQUIPMENT/SUPPLIES	HAS @ HOME	ORDERED	PATIENT EDUCATION (INITIATED IN HOSPITAL)
Anticipated date of discharge: ________________ To: ☐ Home ☐ Home Care ☐ Rehab ☐ SNF ☐ Intermediate care ☐ Hospital transfer ☐ Subacute Services ☐ Other APEX FORM COMPLETED AS APPROPRIATE: ________________ (date/initials of ASC) Person assisting with care at home ________	Clinical Resource Manager: __________ Social Worker: __________ Alternate Site Coordinator(s): __________ __________ __________ Nutrition Service: __________ Pastoral Care: __________	Physical Therapist: __________ Occupational Therapist: __________ Respiratory Therapist: __________ Speech Therapist: __________ Other: __________ __________ __________	Wheelchair Bedside Commode Walker Crutches Hospital Bed Dressing Supplies BP kit Pharmacy Supplies Ventilator Oxygen Other:	☐ ☐ ☐ ☐ ☐ ☐ ☐ ☐ ☐ ☐	☐ ☐ ☐ ☐ ☐ ☐ ☐ ☐ ☐ ☐	☐ Medication ☐ Discharge needs ☐ Nutrition Diet ________ ☐

OUTSTANDING ISSUES:

Continued

clinical pathway *Lumbar Laminectomy Fusion Risk Factors—cont'd*

TIME FRAME LOCATION	HOSPITAL DAY POD DAY OF SURGERY DATE UNIT	HOSPITAL DAY POD# 1 DATE UNIT	HOSPITAL DAY POD# 2 DATE UNIT	HOSPITAL DAY POD# 3 DATE UNIT
Patient Satisfaction	What can we do to enhance your stay with us?	What can we do to enhance your stay with us?	What can we do to enhance your stay with us?	What can we do to enhance your stay with us?
Discharge Planning	Identify primary caregiver If pt lives alone consult ASC (44663) for possible subacute placement; Social Work (46552) prn	ASC for home care, rehab, or subacute	Visit from nurse clinician	D/C to home ASC finalize homecare Visit from nurse clinician
Patient Education	Orient to room Review IS, PCA Review importance of logrolling	Transfer techniques No sitting >30 min. Importance of logrolling	Reinforce transfer techniques No sitting >30"; log rolling "Do's & Don'ts (nurse clinician) Applications/removal of brace by orthotist prn	Review transfer techniques; limitations/precautions; "Do's and Don'ts"; S/S infection; pain control/ scripts; brace care if applicable Dressing changes
Tests/Procedures/ Consults		Orthotics and prosthetics prn Assess need for PT/consult Consult PT if pt. requiring Assistance ambulating		
Allied Health Interventions		PT-gait training prn, precautions, transfers, stairs OT-if brace required	PT gait training prn, stairs OT for ADL's if brace, application	PT for gait training OT for ADL's if necessary
Nursing/Medical Interventions	PCA pump assess q4 hr Bedrest logroll q2 hrs Assess drsg, skin-protect heels IS as ordered; O_2 via N/C prn, O_2 sat >92% Lung sounds qs IVF as ordered; I/O qs & drains PAS stockings bilat LE's Foley CL diet; po stool softener Neuro/CMS ✓'s qs	Assess PCA pump q4 hrs OOB to chair TI; 30 min or less Ambulate in room; assess skin; protect heels IS as ordered; O_2 via N/C prn, Maintain O_2 sat >92%; lung sounds qs IVF as ordered PAS stockings bilat LE's Neuro/CMS ✓s CL/select diet D/C foley Monitor voiding pattern, ISC Q6 hr prn if no void Po stool softeners Assess drsg, reduce or wait for drain D/C if applicable	DC PCA pump; assess PO pain analgesics q4 hrs Ambulate to bathroom; no bedpan Assess skin; protect heels IS as ordered-D/C O_2, PO_2 sat >92% roomair Lung sounds qs; d/c IV; monitor I/O qs Pas stockings bilat LE Neurovascular checks qs Select diet D/C foley Monitor void pattern; ISC Q6hr prn PO stool softener bid △ dressing qd/prn; d/c drains per MD	PO pain meds Continue ambulation; no bedpans Dressing change Diet as tolerated Assess voiding qs Verify BM-enema after d/c if no BM
Outcome Criteria	Pt moves arms/legs freely with full sensation; oriented × 3 VS stable, lungs clear UO >240cc/shift Pain controlled with analgesics Pt compliant with logrolling Incision/dressing with scant drainage Patient/Family Satisfaction addressed	Pt moves arms/legs freely with full sensation; oriented 3 3 Pain controlled with PCAs Patient begins to learn transfer techniques in/out of bed Patient OOB × 3 to chair with assist <30 min Voids independently after foley removed Patient/Family Satisfaction addressed	Tolerates gait training in PT Ambulates in room to bathroom with assist Pain controlled with no analgesics Tolerates diet; baseline bladder fx Understands "Do's/Don'ts" Demonstrates braced donning/doffing Patient/Family Satisfaction addressed	Patient understands d/c instruction (see d/c criteria) Ambulates independently with/without assistive device Pain controlled Dons/duffs brace if needed Understands transfer techniques; do's/don'ts; SS of infection Patient/caregiver performs dressing changes if ordered Patient/Family Satisfaction addressed

clinical pathway *Lumbar Discectomy*

<table>
<tr>
<td>Directions:
1. Review CCT approximately every 8°.
2. Appropriate and completed interventions need no additional documentation.
3. Cross through any interventions which are not applicable.
4. Circle any intervention not completed.
5. The plan of care—nursing interventions and outcome evaluation statements—may be added to the CCT as necessary.</td>
<td>DRG __215__ Expected LOS __1__
Physician(s) ____________
____
____
Admit Date ______ M60 ______
Discharge Date ____________

Surgery/Procedure
____
____
Date of Surgery/Procedure ________
____________</td>
<td>Comorbid Conditions:
☐ CHF
☐ IDDM
☐ Angina
☐ COPD ☐ UTI
☐ Malignant HTN
☐ Dehydration</td>
<td>Imprint/Label

Complications during this admission:
☐ DVT ☐ Ileus
☐ PE ☐ Stroke
☐ Infection ☐ Mental status change
☐ Continued wound drainage ☐ Cardiac (dysrhythmia)
☐ Urinary retention Other</td>
</tr>
<tr>
<td colspan="2"></td>
<td colspan="2">Risk Factors:
☐ Obesity ☐ ETOH/Substance Abuse ☐ Smoking ☐</td>
</tr>
</table>

<table>
<tr><th rowspan="2">DATE</th><th rowspan="2">PROBLEM LIST</th><th rowspan="2">DISCHARGE CRITERIA</th><th rowspan="2">DATE INITIALLY MET</th><th colspan="2">MET ON DISCHARGE</th></tr>
<tr><th>YES</th><th>NO</th></tr>
<tr><td rowspan="2"></td><td rowspan="2">1. Knowledge deficit
2. Pain
3. Impaired mobility
4. Impaired skin (potential)
5. Impaired gas exchange (potential)
6. Altered tissue perfusion (potential)
7. Constipation (potential)</td><td>1. Vital signs baseline.
2. Pain controlled by po pain meds.
3. Incision well approximated/no signs of infection.
4. Patient ambulates independently.
5. Patient/caregiver has knowledge, resources & ability to safely provide care outside the hospital environment.</td><td></td><td></td><td></td></tr>
<tr><td colspan="4">Explain any discharge criteria not met:</td></tr>
</table>

Courtesy The Cleveland Clinic Foundation, Cleveland, Ohio, 12/21/2000. This is a general guideline to *assist* in the management of patients. This guideline is not designated to replace clinical judgment or individual patient needs.

Continued

clinical pathway *Lumbar Discectomy—cont'd*

PLAN	TEAM MEMBERS (INCLUDE BEEPER #)		HOMEGOING EQUIPMENT/SUPPLIES	HAS @ HOME	ORDERED	PATIENT EDUCATION (INITIATED IN HOSPITAL)
Anticipated date of discharge: __________ To: ☐ Home ☐ Home Care ☐ Rehab ☐ SNF ☐ Intermediate care ☐ Hospital transfer ☐ Subacute Services ☐ Other APEX FORM COMPLETED AS APPROPRIATE: __________ (date/initials of ASC) Person assisting with care at home __________ __________	Clinical Resource Manager: __________ Social Worker: __________ Alternate Site Coordinator(s): __________ __________ __________ Nutrition Service: __________ Pastoral Care: __________	Physical Therapist: __________ Occupational Therapist: __________ Respiratory Therapist: __________ Speech Therapist: __________ Other: __________ __________ __________	Wheelchair Bedside Commode Walker Crutches Hospital Bed Dressing Supplies BP kit Pharmacy Supplies Ventilator Oxygen Other:	☐ ☐ ☐ ☐ ☐ ☐ ☐ ☐ ☐ ☐	☐ ☐ ☐ ☐ ☐ ☐ ☐ ☐ ☐ ☐	☐ Medication ☐ Discharge needs ☐ Nutrition Diet __________ ☐

OUTSTANDING ISSUES:

clinical pathway *Lumbar Discectomy—cont'd*

TIME FRAME LOCATION	HOSPITAL DAY POD DAY OF SURGERY DATE UNIT		HOSPITAL DAY POD# 1 DATE UNIT		HOSPITAL DAY POD DATE UNIT
Patient Satisfaction	What can we do to enhance your stay with us?		What can we do to enhance your stay with us?		
Discharge Planning	Identify primary caregiver ____________________ If pt lives alone consult ASC (44663) for home care Consult SS (46552) as needed		Visit from nurse clinician and ASC for home care		
Patient Education	Orient to room Review IS, PCA Review importance of logrolling		Transfer techniques No sitting >30 min. Importance of logrolling "Do's & Don'ts" (nurse clinician) Anticipate D/C in a.m. D/C instruction: -review transfer technique -"Do's & don'ts, pain control S/S infection -Review dressing △ if needed		
Tests/Procedures/ Consults			Assess need for PT/consult Consult PT if pt. requiring assistance with ambulating		
Allied Health Interventions			PT-gait training prn OT ADL's, Do's/Don'ts, brace application if ordered		
Nursing/Medical Interventions	PCA pump assess pain level q4 hr Assess drag/skin—protect heels Lung sounds qs PAS stockings bilat LE's Monitor voiding patterns	Bedrest logroll q2 hrs IS as ordered; O_2 via N/C prn IVF as ordered; monitor I/O Neuro vascular checks qs CL liquid/regular diet	D/C pump by p.m. (dinner time) Begin po pain meds-assess 4 hrs OOB to chair, no sitting >30 min No bed pans-ambulate to BR by pm Assess dressing; skin-protect heels IS as ordered; O_2 via N/C prn D/C IV by p.m.; continue to monitor I/O PAS stockings bilat LE's Assess neuro status Select diet △ drag qd/PRN Continue independent ambulation DC O_2 if O_2 >92% room air	Lung sounds qs Neuro checks qs	
Outcome Criteria	Moves arms/legs freely with full sensation Orientation × 3 VS stable, lungs clear UO >240cc/shift Pain controlled with analgesics Pt compliant with logrolling Incision/dressing with scant drainage Patient/Family Satisfaction addressed		Ambulates with assistance in room Pain controlled on po meds by p.m. Tolerates diet Baseline bladder Pt understands "Do's, Don'ts" Verbalizes understanding of D/C instructions Meets D/C criteria Ambulates independently in room Pain controlled with po meds Verbalizes understanding of limitations/ precautions/Do's, Don'ts Patient states S/S of infection Pt/SO performs dressing △ if needed Patient/Family Satisfaction addressed		

Guidelines for Safe Practice

Postoperative Care of the Patient Who Has Undergone Thoracic Spine Surgery

Same as for lumbar surgery with the following additions and exceptions:

1. Positioning
   a. The head of the bed may often be elevated to 30 degrees.
2. Wound care
   a. If the pleural cavity is entered, a chest tube will be inserted and must be managed postoperatively (see Chapter 21).
3. Promoting comfort
   a. Help patient to splint the chest while coughing.
4. Promoting mobility
   a. Encourage and assist patient in performing vigorous pulmonary hygiene measures.
   b. Encourage dorsiflexion/plantar flexion, gluteal and quadriceps exercises hourly while awake. Monitor the patient for signs of deep vein thrombosis and pulmonary embolism. Prophylactic anticoagulants may be prescribed.
   c. Keep spine in alignment; help patient to logroll.
   d. A brace is routinely prescribed and must be applied before the patient is allowed out of bed.
   e. Permit patient to perform whatever activities are comfortable within the limitations of the brace.
   f. Encourage patient to participate in activities of daily living within prescribed limits of mobility.
5. Discharge instructions
   a. Apply and remove the brace before getting out of bed.
   b. Wear the brace whenever out of bed; assess the skin under the brace.
   c. Use proper body mechanics; avoid lifting over 5 to 10 lbs.
   d. Report symptoms of infection or neurologic deficit to surgeon.

not receive an adequate blood supply and nutrition, depending on the diameter of the person's spinal canal. The onset of spinal stenosis is usually insidious, and physical symptoms may take years to manifest. Care must be taken to differentiate spinal stenosis from peripheral vascular disease, since the claudication (leg pain and weakness after walking) symptoms are similar. In persons with spinal stenosis, the pain in the legs is reproduced by walking and relieved by resting. Back pain often accompanies the leg pain, probably as a result of facet arthritis and degenerative disk disease.

SPECIAL ENVIRONMENTS FOR CARE

Community-Based Care

Because of shortened lengths of stay, considerable recovery from spinal surgery takes place at home. The patient and family should understand the indications for the prescribed medications. If opioid analgesics are prescribed, the patient should understand the precautions associated with administration.

A follow-up appointment with the surgeon (usually 6 weeks after surgery) is necessary to evaluate progress. Before that, a home care nurse may visit to remove any sutures or staples (7 to 10 days) used for skin closure. The patient or family member should evaluate the incision for signs of infection and healing. Dressing changes should be done daily or as needed until the wound is free of drainage; then the incision may remain open to air. Any excessive or purulent drainage should be reported to the physician. A nutritionally adequate diet should be recommended to promote wound healing. The patient may require some assistance with meal preparation until energy reserves are restored. Cigarette smoking is not recommended and actually delays bone healing.

Depending on the degree of mobility restrictions, the patient may require assistance with ADLs. Clothing should be loose fitting, especially if worn under a brace. The patient may benefit from long-handled reachers and sponges if back flexion is limited. The occupational therapist can supply these and other assistive devices before discharge. An elevated toilet seat should be obtained. Bathing may be easier if a shower chair is used. If the patient does not have a shower, a sponge bath is best until activity restrictions are lifted. Special attention should be given to the skin if a brace is worn. A cotton T-shirt should be worn under the brace. Sensible low-heeled walking shoes with a nonskid sole are a good choice for footwear.

An exercise program should be recommended once healing is progressing. Walking is a safe and effective exercise for patients recovering from back surgery. Activities should be resumed gradually, allowing adequate time for rest and sleep. Driving is usually not permitted until cleared by the surgeon at the 6-week appointment. If a cervical collar is needed, the patient may not drive until the collar is removed. Driving with a halo vest is illegal in most states. When riding in a car as a passenger, the patient should be encouraged to comply with seat belt laws. To avoid injury, proper body mechanics are required for getting in and out of an automobile. The patient should be encouraged to comply with recommendations for activity and mobility restrictions to prevent dislodgment of the graft if a fusion was performed. Physical activities that involve bending, twisting, and lifting should be avoided until cleared by the surgeon. Lifting is generally restricted to objects lighter than 10 pounds. For reference, a gallon of milk weighs about 9 pounds. Parents with small children may require assistance with child care in the early postoperative period.

Symptoms to report immediately to the surgeon include increased temperature, new onset of neurologic deficit, bleeding from the incision(s), or new onset of pain. The patient should be reminded that numbness and tingling present before surgery do not always abate immediately after surgery. Months or years may be needed for resolution of symptoms, and occasionally symptoms never completely resolve.

Most persons can return to work after 6 weeks. The work environment should be modified to include proper body mechanics and ergonomic design. The patient should avoid staying in one position for prolonged periods of time. Frequent breaks to get up and move about should be taken if possible. If the patient's job involves heavy manual labor, vocational retraining may be an option.

Modification of the home environment should be considered if potential hazards exist. Safety is a key concern for the patient recovering from spinal surgery. Falls and injury can cause neurologic injury or graft displacement.

clinical pathway *Cervical Fusion: Orthopaedics*

	PREADMISSION	DAY OF SURGERY DAY 1	POD #1 DAY 2	POD #2 DAY 3	POD #3 DAY 4
Outcomes: Medical/Health Status	Potential problems identified	1. Surgery completed 2. Medically stable 3. Neurologically intact 4. Acceptable level of pain	1. Medically stable 2. Neurologically intact 3. Incision(s) healing well with minimal drainage 4. Acceptable level of pain	1. Medically stable 2. Neurologically intact 3. Bone graft position satisfactory 4. Incision(s) healing well with minimal drainage 5. Acceptable level of pain	1. Medically stable 2. Neurologically intact 3. Incision(s) clean & dry 4. Acceptable level of pain
Tests	PAT protocol	HCT	HCT	HCT AP and lateral x-ray of neck	
Treatment		I/O × 48 hr. NV q 2 hr. × 24 hr. VS q 4 hr. × 24 hr. Foley → CD 1.8. q 1 hr. W/A Teds/SCD's Tonsil suction set up at bedside Trach set at bedside Maintain 2-poster brace Inspect incision(s) q shift Check scalp pressure points q shift Check brace pressure points q shift Phili Collar at bedside	I/O q shift NV q 8 hr. VS q 4 hr. → q 8 hr. Foley → CD I.S. q 2hr. W/A Teds/SCD's Tonsil suction set up at bedside Maintain 2-poster brace Inspect incision(s) q shift Check scalp pressure points q shift Check brace pressure points q shift Initial dressing change done per MD Phili Collar at bedside	VS q 8 hr. I/O q shift D/C if po >400 cc q shift I.S. q2-4 hr. W/A NV q 8 hr. Teds D/C SCD's D/C Foley Tonsil suction & trach set at bedside Maintain 2-poster brace Inspect incision(s) q shift Dressing change p.r.n. Check scalp pressure points q shift Check brace pressure points q shift Phili Collar at bedside	Teds Maintain 2-poster brace Inspect incision(s) D/C I.I.P. if applicable Outplacement pre-scriptions:
Medications/ IV Fluids	Assess for use of NSAIDS + Discontinue	PCA-Morphine/Demerol IM analgesics PO analgesics Intra-op antibiotics Post-op antibiotics IV fluids	Maintain PCA - or change to PO after assessing pain status Continue post-op antibiotics IV fluids	D/C PCA - convert to oral pain medications I.I.P. if need to finish IV antibiotics	PO analgesics Colace FeSO4 Muscle relaxants
Nutrition		NPO, few ice chips	Progress diet as tolerated		Regular diet

Courtesy The Cleveland Clinic Foundation, Cleveland, Ohio.

Continued

clinical pathway *Cervical Fusion: Orthopaedics—cont'd*

	PREADMISSION	DAY OF SURGERY DAY 1	POD #1 DAY 2	POD #2 DAY 3	POD #3 DAY 4
Consults	Initial nursing evaluation PST Care Management Orthotic Specialties		Physical therapy Occupational therapy if indicated Orthotic Specialties for brace adjustments		
Outcomes: Functional Status	Fitted for 2-poster brace	Dangle at bedside post-op night HOB ↑ 20-30 degrees Ankle pumps q 2 hr. W/A and with VS at night	Progressive ambulation Up chair ADL's	Continue ambulation Up chair ADL's	Ambulates with/without assistive device Transfers independently Stairs with/without assistance Independent with ADL's
Outcomes: Educational	Patient verbalizes understanding of surgical routine, exercises, precautions, equipment Review pathway Cervical fusion homecare booklet given	Education complete re: I.S./C & DB Activity level PCA/PO meds Tonsil suction IV therapy	Teach patient how to wash hair, apply clothes. Show patient/family cervical fusion book. Instruction given on walker/cane if needed. OT-instruction initiated on use of adaptive equipment if needed.	Teaching completed	Verify cervical fusion homebook given Teaching completed
Outcomes: Community Re-entry	Discharge plans completed	Discharge plans verified after surgery	Verify equipment ordered Adjustments made on brace if necessary.		Discharge plans implemented
Discharge Targets	1. Incision(s) clean and dry, healing well 2. Neurologically intact 3. Medically stable 4. Independent with ambulation/ADL's 5. Patient to be discharged before hospital day 4 (POD #3) 6. Acceptable level of pain				

COMPLICATIONS

Complications associated with general anesthesia are important considerations after surgery. These include complications such as atelectasis, paralytic ileus, and urinary retention. Infection is a complication associated with the operative procedure. When instrumentation is used, the risk for infection increases. There is also a risk for hardware failure.

Posterior approaches to the spine are performed with the patient in the prone position, using a variety of frames and positioning devices. Complications can arise from positioning techniques and lengthy procedures. Potential complications include pooling of blood in the lower extremities; pressure areas on the knees, forehead, chest, and other bony prominences; and neuropathies as a result of local ischemia caused by prolonged pressure.

Complications of the procedure and the postoperative period include dural tear and cerebrospinal fluid leakage, blood loss, hypovolemia and decreased cardiac output, hematoma formation, infection, instrumentation or graft failure, pseudoarthrosis, loss of correction of deformity, persistence of pain and/or deficits, neurologic impairment or loss, DVT, pulmonary embolism, fluid volume overload, and fat embolism. Monitoring of sensory evoked potentials is often used as a method of reducing injury to the neural elements intraoperatively. Before surgery begins, electrodes are placed on the patient's scalp and extremities. Baseline data are collected, and impulse transmissions through the posterior columns of the spinal cord are monitored throughout the procedure. Any changes indicate possible injury, and the patient is given a "wake-up test." The level of anesthesia is lightened sufficiently to allow the patient to follow commands to move the extremities. Inability to do these tasks is considered indicative of neurologic impairment. This monitoring technique allows the surgeon an opportunity to explore, ascertain, and possibly correct the cause of neurologic loss before closing the incision.

A complication often occurring in the postoperative period of patients undergoing spinal fusion is the syndrome of inappropriate antidiuretic hormone (SIADH). Contributing factors include decreased blood volume, the use of anesthetic agents and analgesics, and physical and emotional stressors. Postoperative monitoring of spinal fusion patients should include accurate measurement of intake and output. SIADH should be suspected if the patient has decreased hemoglobin and hematocrit values (which should be normal 2 to 4 days postoperatively) and the blood pressure and pulse remain within the patient's normal range.

Complications associated with approaches to the cervical spine include vascular injury and injury to the laryngeal nerve because of the proximity of these structures to the surgical site. Complications associated with surgical correction of thoracic spine disorders also include those associated with thoracic surgery (see Chapter 21), because the thoracic cavity is entered through an anterior approach to the thoracic spine.

When fusions are performed, complications include graft failure, infection, and pseudoarthrosis. The use of hardware is associated with potential complications, including hardware failure or loosening, infection, damage to neurovascular structures, and adverse reactions to implant materials.

Endoscopic procedures, although less invasive, are also associated with complications. Complications include visceral injury; bleeding, instrument breakage or failure; oxygen retention in the abdomen, chest, or vasculature; hypoxia to local tissues; infection; carbon dioxide absorption; and scar tissue formation.[31]

SCOLIOSIS

Etiology/Epidemiology

Scoliosis, or lateral curvature of the spine, can be classified as nonstructural or structural. Nonstructural scoliosis is also described as postural or functional and is caused by posture, pain, leg length inequality, and other factors. This form of scoliosis is usually easily corrected, either by exercise or by removing the underlying cause. An important distinction is the absence of vertebral rotation. However, untreated nonstructural scoliosis can progress to structural scoliosis.

Structural scoliosis involves a rotational deformity of the vertebrae. It is further divided into three major categories:

1. *Congenital* scoliosis (present at birth) occurs as a result of vertebral malformations in fetal life and accounts for 15% of structural scoliosis cases.
2. *Neuromuscular* scoliosis results as a consequence of several diseases and represents approximately 15% of cases. Curves generally appear early and progress rapidly.
3. *Idiopathic* scoliosis has an unknown cause, but genetic factors have been linked to the development of disease. It accounts for approximately 65% to 80% of cases and affects about 1% of all children, mostly preadolescents and adolescents.[57] Idiopathic scoliosis is further divided into three groups, depending on the age of onset (Box 47-13). Girls and boys are affected equally; however, curvatures in girls are usually more progressive.[57]

BOX 47-13 Classification of Scoliosis

Congenital

Neuromuscular Causes

Cerebral palsy
Charcot-Marie-Tooth disease
Syringomyelia
Spinal cord injury
Poliomyelitis
Myelomeningocele
Muscular dystrophy
Neurofibromatosis
Marfan's syndrome

Idiopathic

Infantile: 0 to 3 years of age
Juvenile: 3 to 10 years of age
Adolescent: older than 10 years of age

Pathophysiology

Scoliosis may develop in localized areas of the spinal column or involve the whole spinal column. Curvatures may be S shaped or C shaped (Figure 47-37).

The earliest pathologic changes begin in the soft tissues. Muscles and ligaments shorten on the concave side of the curve, progressing to deformities of the vertebrae and ribs. In skeletally immature persons, vertebral deformation occurs as asymmetric forces are applied to the epiphysis by the shortened and tight soft tissue structures on the concave side of the curve. The Scoliosis Research Society has devised a method of classifying curves. Deformities are classified by magnitude, direction, location, and etiology. Curve direction is designated by the convex side of the curve.

The degree of rotation of the curve is important because it determines the amount of impingement on the rib cage. The amount of vertebral compression and twisting depends on the position of the vertebrae in the curve. The forces of compression are greatest on the apical vertebrae, which become the most deformed. Deformity progresses quickly during skeletal growth and slows later in life, but the greatest increase in curvature may occur in adult life. Gravity and an increase in upper body weight may increase the deformity in adulthood. Curves greater than 60 degrees have a significant effect on pulmonary function.

Initially the individual may have slight, mild, or severe deformity. Early deformity may not be obvious except on specific examination. In the early stages individuals may note that clothing does not fit correctly or hang evenly, because the height of the shoulders is uneven. Pain is not usually an accompanying factor. Persons affected with structural scoliosis may exhibit asymmetry of hip height; pelvic obliquity (tilting of the pelvis from the normal horizontal position); inequalities of shoulder height; scapular prominence; rib prominence; and rib humps, which is a posterior, unilateral prominence of the rib cage visible on forward bending. In severe cases cardiopulmonary and digestive function may be affected because of compression or displacement of internal organs. Total lung capacity, vital capacity, and maximum voluntary ventilation may be decreased in persons with scoliosis. Cardiac output may also be compromised. Significant deviations in balance of the curve may also affect gait patterns.

Right thoracic, right thoracic and left lumbar, and right thoracolumbar curves are most common in idiopathic scoliosis. A compensatory curve may develop, allowing the head to be centered over the pelvis. In general, compensatory curves are of a lesser degree, are more flexible, and are less rotated.

Collaborative Care Management

A complete radiologic examination of the spine is performed. Curve angles, flexibility, and the degree of vertebral rotation are calculated. Radiographs may also be done to determine skeletal maturity. In patients with severe thoracic scoliosis, pulmonary function studies may be completed to evaluate the degree of restrictive lung disease.

Treatment depends on the individual patient and the degree of lateral curvature. Early or postural scoliosis may be amenable to postural exercise or exercise combined with traction. Cottrell's traction, which is a combination of a cervical head halter with 5 to 7 pounds and pelvic traction with 10 to 20 pounds, may be used. When the curve is flexible (less than 40 degrees) and the patient is cooperative, bracing, in combination with exercise, may be sufficient to correct the deformity (e.g., Milwaukee brace [Figure 47-38], Risser cast, or halofemoral or helopelvic traction). Maintaining ideal weight is a consideration in reducing the stress on the spine. The patient should be advised against weight gain, especially if bracing is prescribed, because the brace is specifically fitted and contoured to the individual. The brace can usually accommodate a 10-pound gain or loss. Transcutaneous electrical muscle stimulation may be used to stimulate the muscles on the convex side of the curve. Repeated stimulation strengthens the muscles and pulls the spine into alignment. The patient usually uses the stimulator at night.

Surgery is indicated for patients when conservative management has failed to halt curve progression; for those with se-

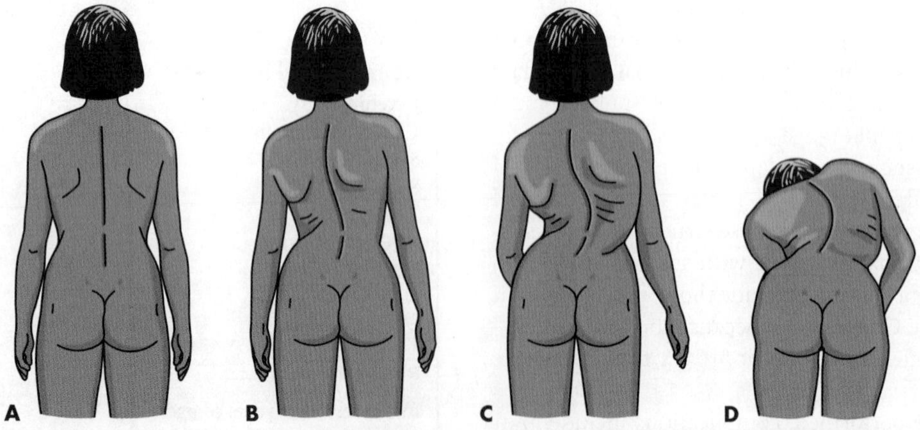

Figure 47-37 Normal spinal alignment and abnormal spinal curvatures associated with scoliosis. **A**, Normal. **B**, Mild. **C**, Severe. **D**, Rotation and curvature of scoliosis.

vere, progressing curves, intractable pain, or compromised pulmonary function; or for cosmesis. Many individuals with neuromuscular scoliosis are unable to walk. Surgical correction is sometimes performed in these patients to facilitate the ability to transfer or to increase sitting ability or tolerance.

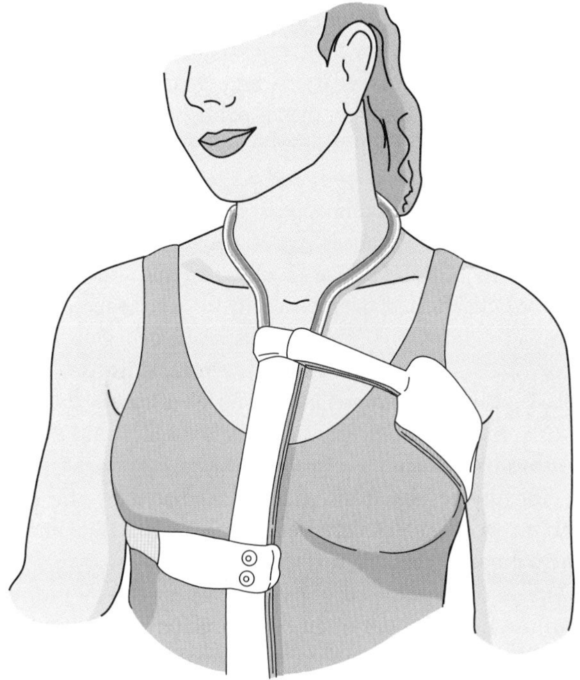

Figure 47-38 Milwaukee brace.

Surgical correction is usually performed when curves are greater than 45 degrees[57] (Figure 47-39).

Surgical correction usually involves a posterior approach to the spine with instrumentation and bony fusion. Patients with severe, rigid curves and pelvic obliquity often require a staged procedure. A transthoracic or retroperitoneal approach to the spine is performed first, followed by a posterior procedure in 1 to 2 weeks. Many types and combinations of types of instrumentation are available. The type used is based on the individual patient and surgeon preference. Refer to Table 47-17 for examples of commonly used implants and see also Figure 47-39. Complications of scoliosis fusion are similar to those described under Nursing Management of Patient Undergoing Spinal Surgery.

Nursing management of the patient undergoing surgery of the spine is discussed in the preceding section. This nursing care is also applicable to the patient with a scoliosis fusion. Particular attention should be paid to assessment of respiratory function, management of pain, and acceptance of changes in body image.

Patient/Family Education. When conservative interventions are being used, patient instruction is most important for achieving the desired outcomes. Patients need to be instructed about the disease process and rationales for treatment. The patient's and family's expectations of treatment need to be clarified, and the patient instructed and supervised in the performance of prescribed exercises and use of traction equipment. The patient is advised that wearing a brace need not restrict normal or desired activities and is instructed in how to

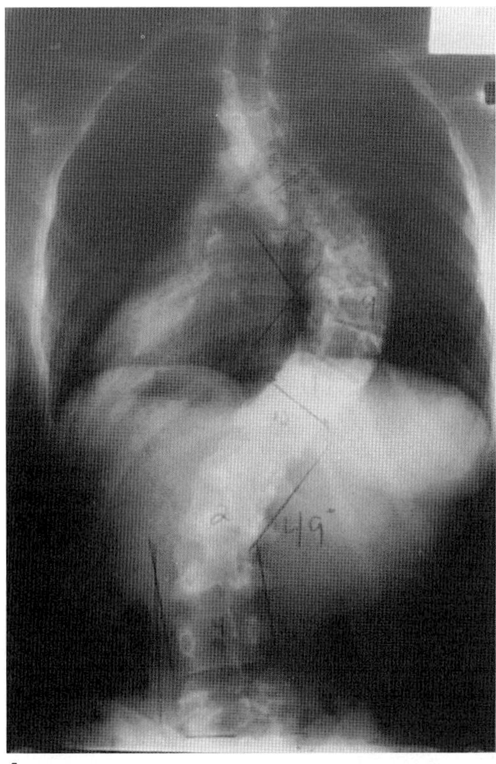

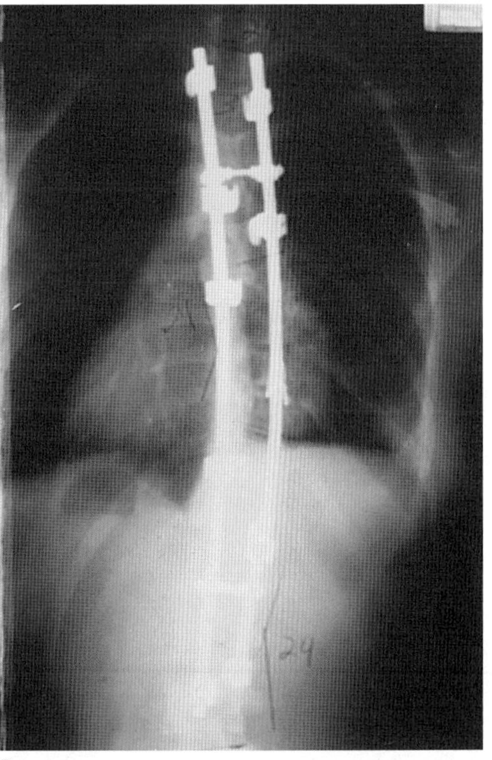

A **B**

Figure 47-39 **A,** Preoperative radiograph of adult with idiopathic scoliosis. **B,** Postoperative film showing correction of curve with Cotrel-Dubousset instrumentation in place.

apply, remove, and care for the brace. The patient is also instructed and supervised in methods of inspecting the skin. The patient is advised to select loose-fitting but attractive clothing that conceals the brace (particularly important for women and adolescents) and is informed about patient and family support groups.

Persons who have undergone spinal fusion need teaching as described in the section on spinal surgery. In addition, the patient and family must be knowledgeable regarding brace care and application (Figure 47-40).

There are no specific measures to prevent scoliosis. However, attention to proper posture may be effective in preventing some types of nonstructural scoliosis in both children and adults.

The Scoliosis Research Society recommends annual screening of all children ages 10 to 14 years. Scoliosis screening is mandated by law in some states; others have voluntary screening programs. The U.S. Preventive Services Task Force has insufficient evidence to recommend either for or against routine screening of asymptomatic adolescents.

Interested patients and families can be referred to the following support groups: the Scoliosis Association, Inc.,* and the National Scoliosis Foundation.†

*PO Box 811705, Boca Raton, FL 33481-1705; (800) 800-0669.
†72 Mount Auburn Street, Watertown, MA 02172; (617) 926-0397.

DISORDERS AFFECTING THE HANDS AND FEET

DUPUYTREN'S CONTRACTURE

Etiology /Epidemiology

Dupuytren's contracture, first described in the early 1800s by a French surgeon, is a progressive condition marked by hypertrophic hyperplasia of the palmar fascia that results in a flexion deformity of the distal palm and fingers (Figure 47-41). The cause of Dupuytren's contracture is unknown. A familial tendency has been noted.

Dupuytren's contracture appears most commonly in persons of Northern European ancestry, between 40 and 60 years of age. Caucasian men, middle aged or older, are more frequently affected. When affected, women seem to experience only mild deformity. Dupuytren's deformity is associated with diabetes, epilepsy, alcoholism, penile lesions (Peyronie's disease), and hyperplasia of the plantar fascia (Lederhose's disease).

Pathophysiology

Deformity results from changes mediated by the myofibroblasts, which is not completely understood. The anatomy of the palmar fascia is distorted.

Dupuytren's contracture may take up to 20 years to reach maximum deformity. It often occurs bilaterally and symmetrically. Hyperplasia and progressive fibrosis of the palmar fascia on the ulnar side of the band cause progressive shortening of the pretendinous bands of the ring and small fingers. The bands shorten, and the MCP joints are drawn into flexion

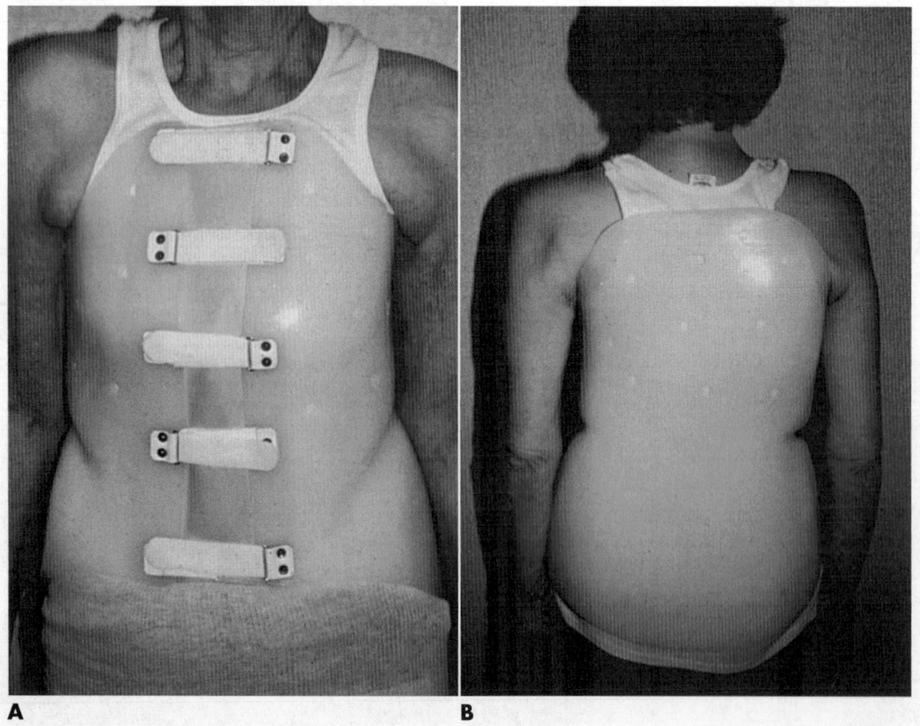

Figure 47-40 **A,** Anterior view of thoracolumbar sacral orthosis (TLSO). **B,** Posterior view of TLSO. Note cotton shirt worn under brace.

contractures. Web space contractures and scissoring of the fingers develop from ligamentous contracture. The PIP joint may also be involved. The skin of the palm is drawn down, forming tight puckers and nodules.

Depending on the severity of the deformity and hand dominance, the patient may experience difficulty in grasping objects. Burning pain may accompany attempts at grasping. Usually, the main complaints are deformity and mild interference with hand function.

Collaborative Care Management

Surgery is the preferred method of treatment. Persons with fixed flexion contractures of 30 degrees or more at the MCP or PIP joints are candidates for surgical intervention. Surgical repair involves regional fasciectomy or subtotal palmar fasciectomy to allow the patient full motion. Recurrence of disease is common. Patients with more advanced cases may require joint fusion or amputation if neurovascular structures are involved. Splints worn at night may decrease residual flexion contractures of the digits. Referrals to PT and OT are necessary after surgery for exercises to regain ROM and splinting.

Surgical repair is performed as an outpatient procedure. The most common postoperative complications are hematoma and inadequate skin closure. Nursing management focuses on postoperative care, including pain management, neurovascular assessment of the fingers, care of the dressing or splint, and promotion of self-care.

Patient/Family Education. The patient and family need instruction about care of the dressing and splint. The hand should be elevated for comfort and to decrease swelling. A sling may be worn. The patient should be instructed to contact the surgeon if the fingers become cool, pale, or painful, or if paresthesias, increased pain, or decreased movement is experienced. The splint should be maintained until the follow-up visit. Analgesics are prescribed as needed. If the patient's dominant hand is affected, assistance in ADLs may be needed. The patient can generally return to work in a few days. A PT referral is indicated for postoperative ROM exercises. The patient and family should understand the signs and symptoms of recurrent disease.

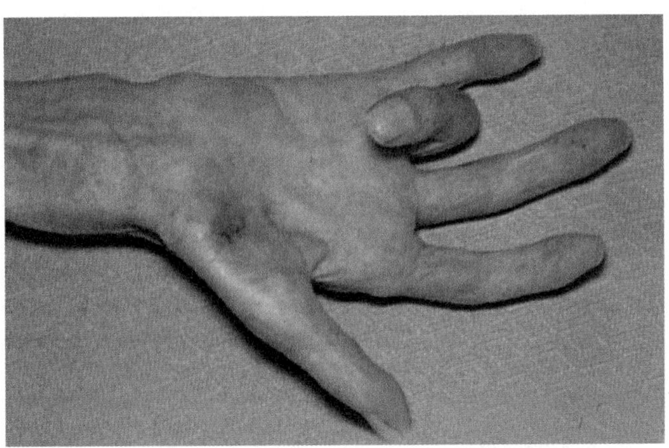

Figure 47-41 Dupuytren's contracture.

HALLUX VALGUS

Etiology/Epidemiology

Foot problems are a significant source of pain, deformity, and disability. Hallux valgus is the lateral angulation of the proximal phalanx on the metatarsal head of the great toe. This common foot problem is often bilateral (Figure 47-42). Depending on the degree of angulation, prominence of the medial eminence may occur, resulting in bunion deformity (Figure 47-43).

Women develop hallux valgus deformity 10 times more often than men. There is a familial tendency. The type of shoes worn also contributes to the development or worsening of the deformity; pointed-toe shoes that cause crowding and angulation of the toes are associated with the development of hallux valgus and bunions. Other associated factors include pes planus (flat foot), chronic tightening of the Achilles tendon, spasticity, and rheumatoid arthritis.

Pathophysiology

Lateral deviation of the proximal phalanx causes pressure on the medial metatarsal head and attenuation and contracture of

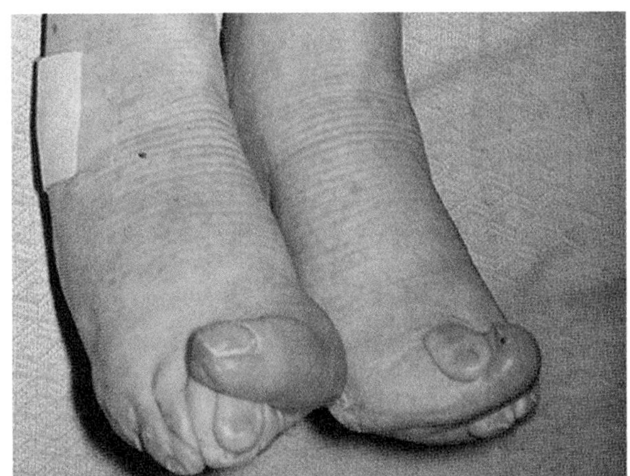

Figure 47-42 Bilateral hallux valgus.

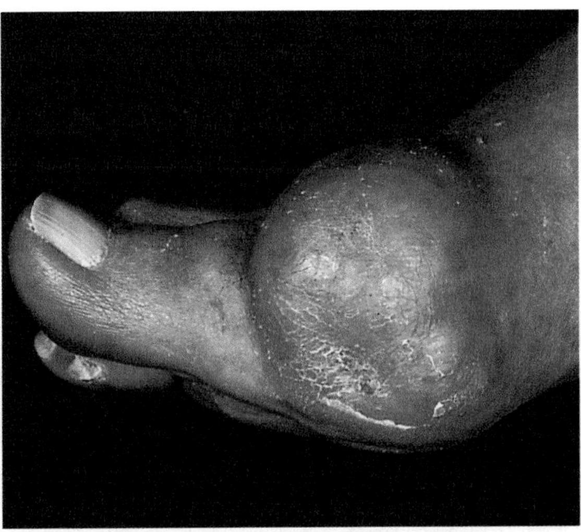

Figure 47-43 Bunion.

the joint capsule. The adjacent sesamoid bones, anchored by the adductor tendon and transverse metatarsal ligament, become subluxed. The flexor and extensor hallicus longus, which insert at the base of the distal phalanx, also deviate laterally, increasing the deformity. The medial eminence of the metatarsal head becomes prominent, and a protective bursa forms as it rubs against the shoe. The great toe may cause crowding and deformity of the second toe.

Collaborative Care Management

Diagnosis is made by the patient history and physical examination. The type of shoes worn, occupation, and amount of exercise are important points to include in the history. The gait and neurovascular status of the feet are important points of the objective examination. Corns and callus may also be present, and the patient may have flat feet. Radiographs confirm the diagnosis and define the severity of the deformity.

Conservative treatment includes encouraging the patient to wear properly fitting shoes of the correct size and shape to allow room for the toes; this alone may alleviate the problem. Shoes should be wide enough to accommodate the medial eminence. A protective pad can be taped under the metatarsal head to change the weight-bearing pressure. Insoles can be purchased to cushion the foot in shoes. A pad can be placed over the corn or bunion to decrease pain and pressure. Medications such as NSAIDs or acetaminophen can be prescribed for pain relief.

If conservative treatment fails or the patient is reluctant to change footwear, surgical intervention may be indicated. There are several surgical procedures to correct hallux valgus and bunions (Figure 47-44), including osteotomy and fusion. Pain relief, correction of deformity, and a functional foot are goals of surgical correction.

Before consenting to surgery, the patient should be completely informed of the risks and benefits of the procedure. After bunion surgery, it is not always possible to wear whatever type of shoes is desired. The surgical procedure is not indicated for cosmesis, but to correct a structural deformity.

After surgery the foot is wrapped in a soft, bulky dressing, and in some patients a splint or cast is applied. The patient wears a postoperative cast shoe and ambulates with crutches or a walker until full weight bearing is permitted.

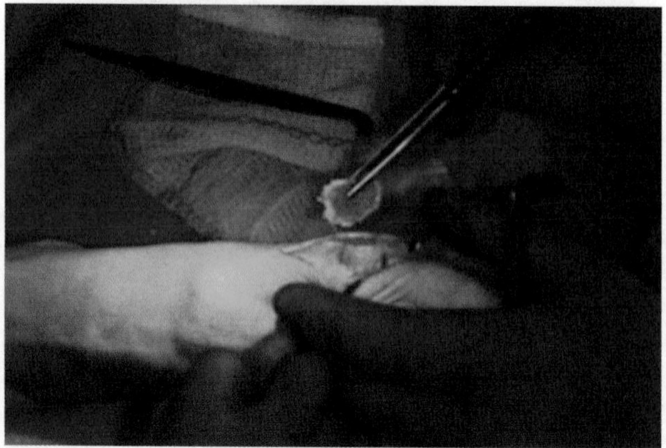

Figure 47-44 Surgical correction of bunion and hallux valgus. Medial eminence is removed.

Patient/Family Education. Bunion surgery is performed as an outpatient procedure, and the patient and family will need discharge instructions. The cast shoe is worn for approximately 2 weeks or until the splint or cast is removed. Activity and weight bearing should be limited during this time. Two to 4 weeks after surgery, round-toed, lacing shoes or sandals can be worn. A bunion splint is worn at night for approximately 6 weeks. At 6 weeks full activity can be resumed. The patient also needs teaching about wearing properly fitting shoes and avoiding pointed-toe shoes. High-heeled shoes, which alter the weight-bearing pressure on the feet, should be avoided. A PT referral may be required for some patients. A podiatry consult for custom shoes may be required for patients with severe deformity. Teaching should be done regarding proper foot care (see Patient Teaching box).

The patient may need support in accepting body image changes associated with the appearance of the feet. Because bunions often occur bilaterally, the patient should be taught to

Patient Teaching

Foot Care

In addition to recognizing common problems, there are many things that you can do to promote healthy feet and prevent problems. Follow these guidelines:

- Walk regularly. This will improve circulation, increase flexibility, and encourage bone and muscle development. Walking is very important for maintaining overall foot health.
- Always wear comfortable shoes that provide proper support. The shoes should be sufficiently wide and have low enough heels so that you feel no leg fatigue, leg or foot cramps, or pain.
- Massage your feet to improve circulation and promote relaxation of the feet at least daily.
- If you have bunions, wear shoes that are extra long or wide. This will help ease pressure on your toes. In addition, use donut-shaped bunion cushions or moleskin to take pressure off of the joints.
- Wear heel pads or cushions in the bottom of your shoes to protect your heels if you walk on hard surfaces for long times.
- Wash your feet every day in warm water. Dry them by blotting with a towel, rather than rubbing.
- If your feet perspire a lot, dust your feet with talc or a hygienic foot powder. You may also sprinkle some powder into your shoes. Do not use cornstarch powder because it may lead to a fungal infection.
- Trim your nails shortly after you have taken a bath or shower, while they are soft. Cut the nails straight across with a toenail clipper.
- Do not go barefoot outdoors, especially if you are in an area that is not your own yard. A foreign body may cut or puncture your foot.
- Inspect your feet every day for cuts, blisters, and scratches. Provide care as needed and observe for proper healing.

From *Mosby's patient teaching guides: update 3*, St Louis, 1997, Mosby.

assess the other foot for signs of beginning deformity. Finally, the patient should be educated about the signs and symptoms of infection and any medications that may be prescribed.

TUMORS OF THE MUSCULOSKELETAL SYSTEM

Etiology

Tumors may arise from any of the structures of the musculoskeletal system (Tables 47-19 and 47-20). The type of tumor is determined and classified by the tissue of origin (Figure 47-45). Tumors can be benign or malignant and can affect both adults and children. Musculoskeletal tumors constitute 3% of all malignant tumors.

Generally malignant tumors tend to cause more bone destruction, invasion of the surrounding tissues, and metastasis. Benign bone tumors tend to be less destructive to normal bone, do not invade soft tissues, and are not capable of metastasis. The cause of bone tumors is unknown. A tumor can be defined as a new growth or hyperplasia of cells. This growth may be in response to inflammation or trauma. Other tumors are a result of a spontaneous, rapid, poorly differentiated proliferation of cells.

Epidemiology

The incidence of bone tumors varies with age. Adults 30 to 35 years of age have a low incidence of bone tumors. Adolescents and adults older than the age of 60 years have the highest incidence of bone tumors; the higher incidence in the older adult is related to metastatic tumors. Osteosarcoma is the most common type of primary bone tumor, representing 20% of all cases.[22,62]

Other factors are associated with the development of bone tumors. A history of Paget's disease or radiation therapy increases the risk of development of a bone tumor. Bone tumors can also occur as a result of metastases from other primary sites of neoplasia. Cancers of the breast, prostate, kidney, thyroid, and lungs often metastasize to bone. Common sites for metastases include the spine, ribs, pelvis, hip, and proximal long bones. Survival rates for those with metastatic disease depend on the primary tumor site.

Pathophysiology

The pathophysiology of neoplasms is found in Chapter 15. Bone tumors commonly cause bone destruction and erosion of the cortex. Benign bone tumors have a controlled growth rate, normally compressing and displacing rather than invading normal bone tissue. This eventually leads to weakening of the normal bone. Other types of tumors destroy normal bone by either resorption or disruption of the blood supply to the bone. Three patterns of bone destruction have been identified[65]:

1. *Geographic:* characterized by slow-growing tumors. There is an identifiable margin between the normal and abnormal bone.
2. *Moth-eaten:* margins are less defined. This type of destruction characterizes rapidly proliferating tumors and malignancies.
3. *Permeative:* tumor and normal bone are meshed with no perceivable margins.

A staging system has been developed for bone tumors. Malignancies are classified according to their growth patterns and sites of metastases (Table 47-21). Common tumors of the musculoskeletal system, their characteristics, and treatment are described in Table 47-22.

TABLE 47-19 Common Tumors of the Musculoskeletal System*

Benign	Malignant
Bone	
Osteoma	Osteosarcoma
Cartilage	
Osteochondroma Enchondroma Periosteal Chondroblastoma	Chondrosarcoma
Fibrous	
Fibroma	Fibrosarcoma
Bone Marrow	
Giant cell	Ewing sarcoma Myeloma
Uncertain Cell	
Unicameral bone cyst Aneurysmal bone cyst	

*See also Table 47-20.

TABLE 47-20 Muscle Tumors

Characteristics	Treatment
Leiomyoma	
Affects smooth muscle, usually uterus Palpable mass Tenderness	Surgical excision
Rhabdomyoma	
Affects striated muscle Rare Tenderness	Surgical excision
Leiomyosarcoma	
Affects smooth muscle, usually uterus, stomach, or small bowel Radical growth	Surgical excision with wide margins Radiation Chemotherapy
Rhabdomyosarcoma	
Affects striated muscle, usually in inguinal, popliteal, or gluteal areas Slow-growing mass Tenderness	Radiation Surgical excision Chemotherapy

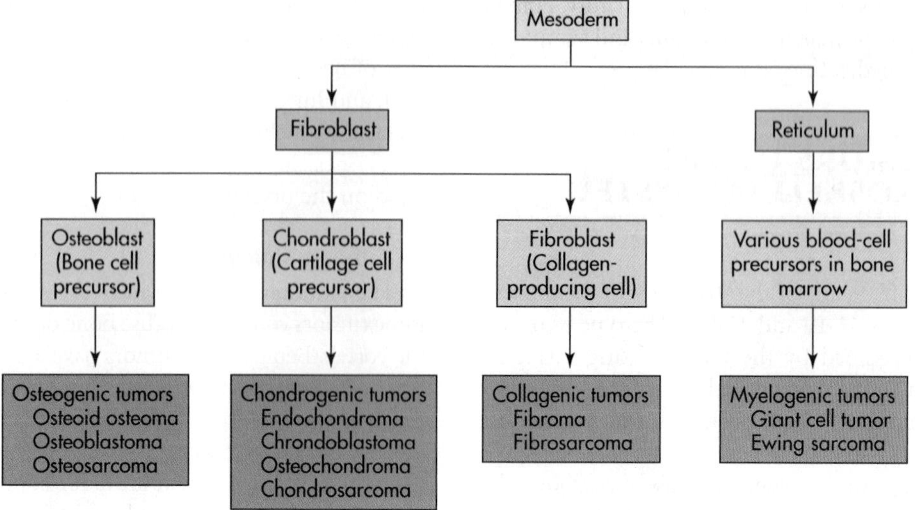

Figure 47-45 Derivation of bone tumors.

TABLE 47-21 Surgical Staging System for Bone Tumors

Stage	Grade	Site (T)	Metastasis (M)
IA	Low (G_1)	Intracompartmental (T_1)	None (M_0)
IB	Low (G_1)	Extracompartmental (T_2)	None (M_0)
IIA	High (G_2)	Intracompartmental (T_1)	None (M_0)
IIB	High (G_2)	Extracompartmental (T_2)	None (M_0)
IIIA	Low (G_1)	Intracompartmental or extracompartmental (T_1 or T_2)	Regional or distant (M_1)
IIIB	High (G_2)	Intracompartmental or extracompartmental (T_1 or T_2)	Regional or distant (M_1)

Data from Simon SR, editor: *Orthopaedic basic science,* Chicago, 1994, American Academy of Orthopaedic Surgeons.

TABLE 47-22 Other Common Tumors of the Musculoskeletal System

Characteristics	Treatment
Osteochondroma	
Compromise of cancellous bone with cartilaginous cap	Surgical excision
Develops during growth periods at metaphysis of bone	
Also appears in tendons	
May limit joint motion	
May recur	
Enchondroma	
Destroys cancellous bone	Surgical excision with wide margins
Usually occurs in humerus or finger	Amputation
Can cause pathologic fractures	
May become malignant, especially in long bones or pelvis	
Chondrosarcoma	
Usually affects persons 50-70 years old	Surgical excision
Accounts for 20% of all bone tumors	Amputation
Affects males more than females	
Chondrosarcoma—cont'd	
Slow growing, insidious onset	
Most common in humerus, femur, pelvis	
Local pain, swelling	
May have palpable mass	
Severe, persistent pain	
May infiltrate joint space and soft tissue	
May metastasize to lung tissue	
May recur	
Fibrosarcoma	
Usually affects persons 30-50 years old	Wide surgical excision
Affects females more than males	Amputation
Occurs in bony fibrous tissue of femur and tibia	
Accounts for 4% of primary malignant bone tumors	
May result from radiation therapy, Paget's disease, or chronic osteomyelitis	
Night pain, swelling, possible palpable mass	

TABLE 47-22 Other Common Tumors of the Musculoskeletal System—cont'd

Characteristics	Treatment
Fibrosarcoma—cont'd	
May cause pathologic fractures May metastasize to lungs	
Giant Cell Tumor (Figure 47-46)	
Usually affects ages 20-40 years Affects females more than males Accounts for 4%-5% of all benign bone tumors Appears in epiphyseal area; destroys bone matrix; can invade soft tissues Commonly found in femur, tibia, or humerus Dull, aching night pain Limitation of motion Swelling High incidence of recurrence	Wide excision May require bone graft Amputation
Myeloma, Multiple Myeloma (Multifocal)	
Poor prognosis Common in persons >40 years old Affects males more than females Accounts for 27% of bone tumors Higher incidence in African-Americans Neoplastic proliferation of plasma cells Causes cortical and medullary bone lysis and infiltrates bone marrow Aching, intermittent pain in spine, pelvis, ribs, or sternum Pain increased with weight bearing May complain of weight loss, malaise, or anorexia Causes pathologic fractures	Palliative treatment Radiation Chemotherapy
Osteoma	
Usually affects persons 10-20 years old Accounts for 20% of benign bone tumors Slow growth	Treatment only if symptomatic, then excision

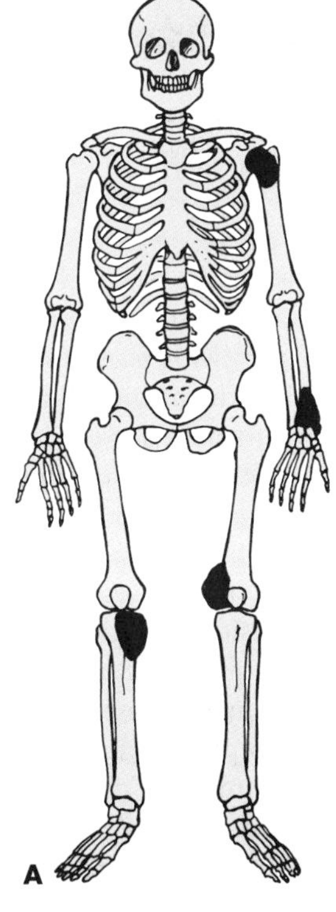

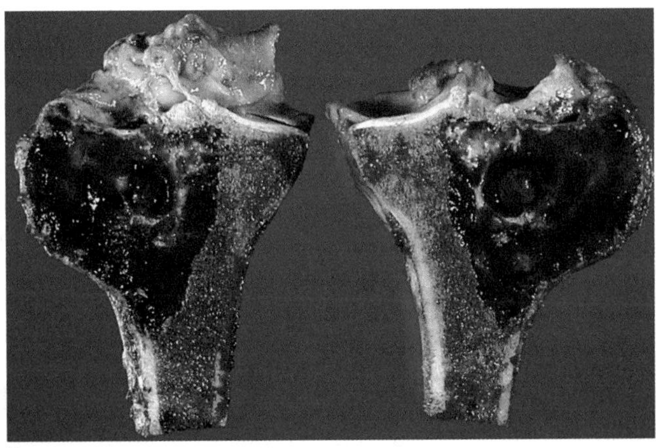

Figure 47-46 Giant cell tumor. **A**, Common skeletal locations. **B**, Gross picture of cell tumor on bone (epimetaphysis).

The rest of this section refers only to osteosarcoma.

Osteosarcoma. Osteosarcoma exhibits a moth-eaten pattern of bone destruction with poorly defined margins (Figure 47-47). Osteoid and callus produced by the tumor invade and resorb normal cortical bone. The tumor erodes through the cortex and periosteum and eventually invades soft tissues. Metastasis to the lungs is common.

Ninety percent of osteosarcomas occur in the metaphyses of long bones, especially the distal femur and proximal tibia.[22] Pain and swelling are often reported. The initial complaint of

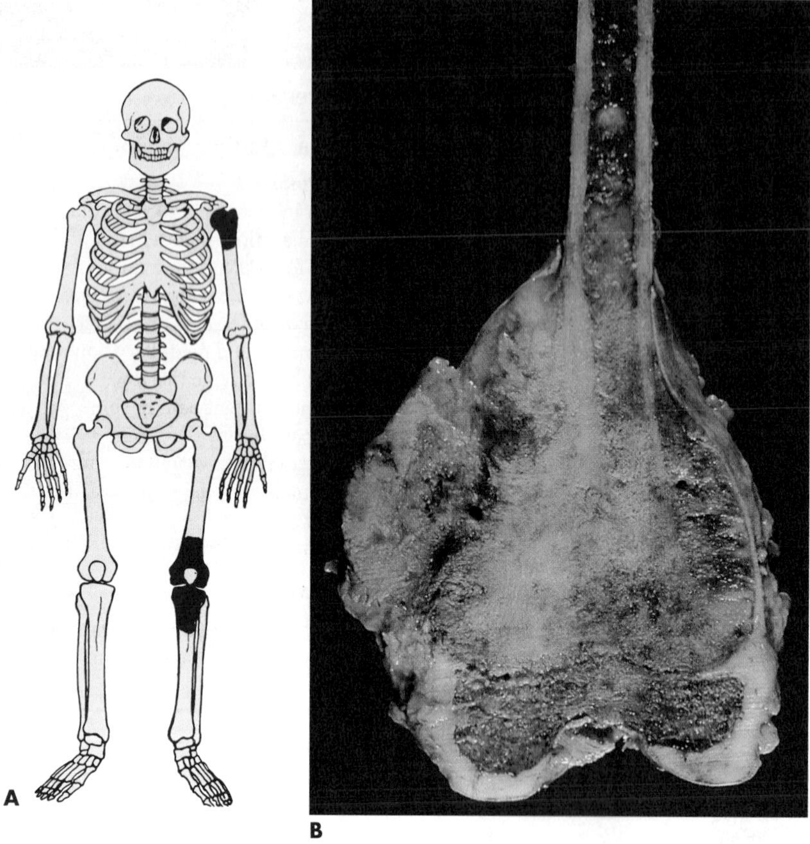

Figure 47-47 Osteosarcoma. **A**, Common locations of osteosarcoma. **B**, The femur has a large mass involving the metaphysis of the bone; the tumor has destroyed the cortex, forming a soft tissue component.

pain is often described as dull, aching, and intermittent, but the pain rapidly increases in intensity and duration. Night pain is common. Other frequent complaints include generalized malaise, anorexia, and weight loss.

Two types of lesions are seen with metastatic tumors. Bone destruction exceeds bone formation in lytic lesions, which are commonly seen in lung metastases. Tumors in which bone formation exceeds bone destruction, as seen in prostate metastases, are called blastic lesions. Bone lysis generally occurs with metastatic disease and hypercalcemia. Another potential problem of persons with metastatic disease is pathologic fracture. Pathologic fractures can occur with any activity and pose a significant risk to persons with metastatic bone lesions.

Collaborative Care Management

Bone biopsy is used to confirm the diagnosis. Because of the rapid growth rate of osteosarcomas, the prognosis is poor. Death, usually from pulmonary complications as a result of metastases, may occur within 2 years of diagnosis if the tumor is left untreated.

X-ray films, CT scans, MRI, and bone scans show tumor location and size. X-ray films have limited use, since 50% of trabecular bone must be destroyed before lesions are visible. Blood tests reveal an elevated serum alkaline phosphatase level. Chest x-ray films confirm the presence of metastases.

Treatment options for the patient with metastatic disease include radiation, hormonal therapy, chemotherapy, surgical excision, surgical repair (with prostheses or hardware), and palliative measures. Treatment modalities may be combined to improve outcomes. Radiation is effective in relieving pain, especially from fracture and nerve compression. Treatment for primary lesions depends on the size and location of the tumor; the presence of metastases; and the patient's age, general health, lifestyle, and preferences. Surgical management includes excision of the lesion, resection, amputation, and limb salvage procedures (Figures 47-48 and 47-49). The extent of the procedure varies from wide resection to more radical procedures, including hemipelvectomy and hip disarticulation.

Historically, the treatment of choice for high-grade bone sarcomas has been amputation. Advances in chemotherapy, diagnostic techniques, and surgical techniques led to the development of a less radical treatment option—limb salvage surgery (LSS). Disease-free survival rates after LSS are similar to those following amputation. With current adjuvant chemotherapy protocols, the disease-free survival rate for osteosarcoma is 40% to 70%.[22,62] LSS has no adverse effects on survival rates. With tumor recurrence, amputation is usually indicated (in the absence of metastases).

There are no histologic contraindications to LSS. In addition to treatment of osteosarcoma, LSS is used to treat patients with Ewing's sarcoma, chondrosarcoma, giant cell tumor, and

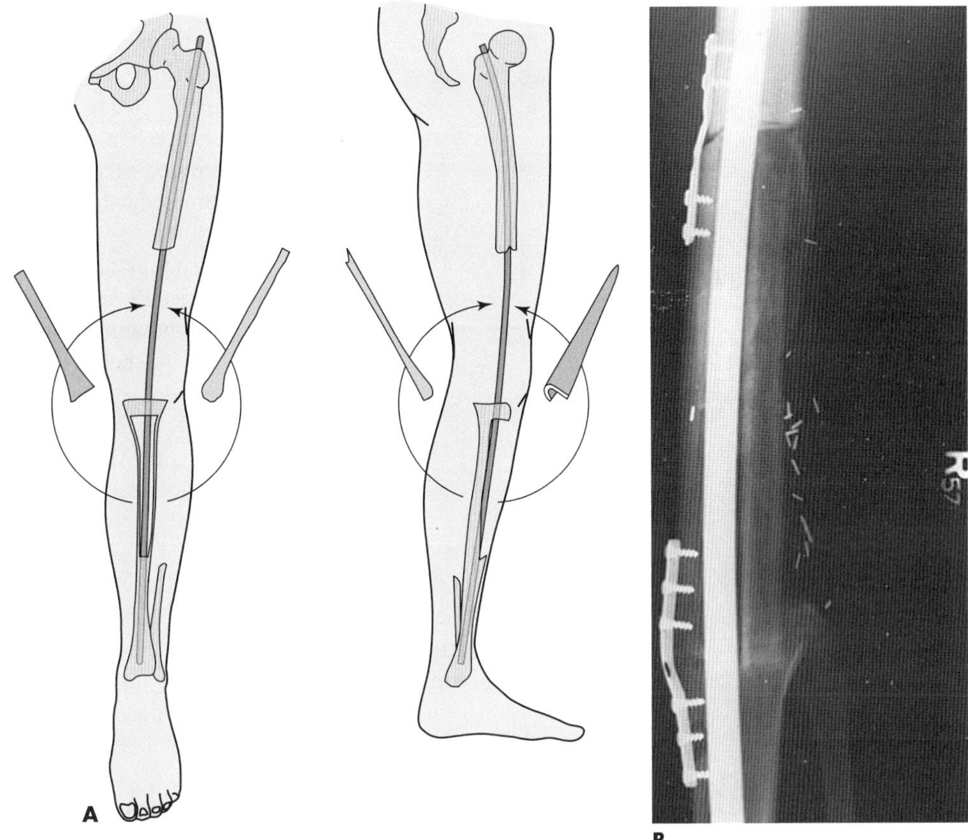

Figure 47-48 **A,** When the distal femur has been resected and arthrodesis is desired, the anterior one third of the tibia and proximal fibula may be used to span the defect. The extremity is stabilized with a long, fluted intramedullary rod. When the proximal tibia is resected, the anterior one third of the distal femur and a segment of the fibula are used to span the defect. An iliac bone graft is added to improve the strength of the reconstruction. Allograft segments also have proved to be successful in filling defects. **B,** Postoperative radiograph of a patient who had resection arthrodesis for stage IIB tumor in the distal femur. He uses no external aids and is fully active.

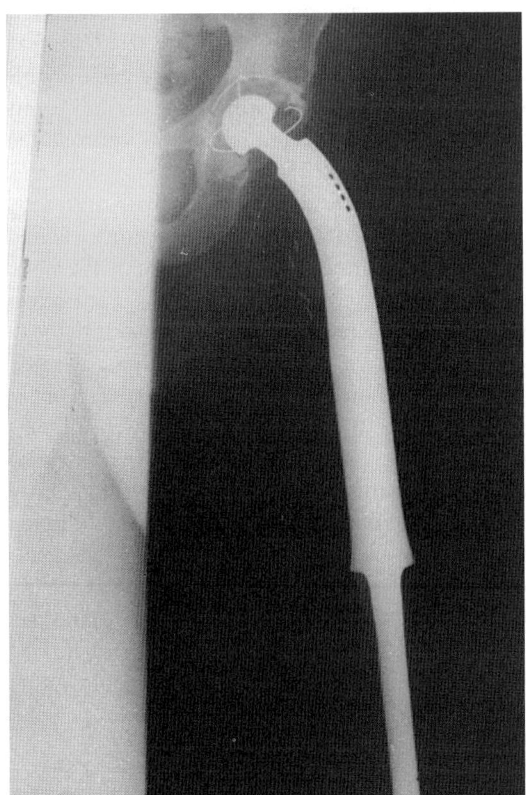

Figure 47-49 This custom-made total hip was used to replace the proximal femur and hip joint of a 50-year-old woman with a chondrosarcoma. She has had no recurrence of tumor and walks with a modest limp while using a cane, but has no active abduction of the hip.

BOX 47-14 Complications of Limb Salvage Surgery and Amputation

Limb Salvage Surgery

Local recurrence of tumor
Wound and skin necrosis (The procedure may necessitate extensive soft tissue flaps.)
Deep infection (Risk may be increased by the immunosuppressant action of chemotherapy.)
Neurovascular complications
Deep vein thrombosis
Nonunion
Hemorrhage
Implant and/or graft failure
Arthritis (long term)

Amputation

Infection
Wound necrosis
Phantom limb pain
Contractures
Skin breakdown

other tumors. Preoperative chemotherapy has allowed more persons to be considered for LSS. Contraindications to LLS include a large invasive tumor, involvement of the neurovascular bundle, inability to achieve tumor-free margins, or a technically difficult surgical approach, such as a tumor in the distal tibia. Complications of amputation and LSS are summarized in Box 47-14.

Patient/Family Education. Nursing care for the patient with cancer is discussed in Chapter 15. Nursing care for the patient undergoing tumor resection surgery is challenging. The patient and family, who may still be trying to cope with the diagnosis of cancer, are now faced with difficult decisions regarding treatment options. Nursing interventions focus on education, support, and clarification of information. The nurse should validate that the patient and family are fully informed regarding expected treatment outcomes and the risks and benefits. A full explanation of the possible side effects associated with chemotherapy and radiation therapy, as well as interventions to reduce their incidence, is important. Depending on the type of surgical resection, alterations in body image and functioning may result. Providing support and promoting acceptance of body image and role changes are important nursing interventions. Referrals to support groups or community services may help the patient and family cope with the diagnosis of cancer and changes in functioning.

DISORDERS AFFECTING THE MUSCLES

MUSCULAR DYSTROPHY

Etiology/Epidemiology

The muscular dystrophies are a group of familial disorders characterized by varying degrees of skeletal muscle weakness and degeneration, leading to disability and deformity. Classification has traditionally been by phenotype, mode of inheritance, rate of progression, and distribution of involvement. At least 10 types of muscular dystrophy (MD) have been identified; of these, 5 types are commonly seen in adults (Table 47-23).

Duchenne's MD, discovered in 1868, is the most common type, affecting 1 in 3500 male births.[6] Becker's MD is also an X-linked recessive disease but is less common than Duchenne's. Other types of MD seen in adults can occur in either sex. Children with MD rarely live past 25 years of age. The mechanism of the genetic defects is unknown. Theories include defects in muscle cell membranes and biochemical abnormality.

Pathophysiology

The genetic abnormality in MD causes a defect in the intracellular metabolism of the muscle fibers. Defects in creatine metabolism and intracellular enzymes in the glycolytic system have been identified. Muscle cells exhibit phagocytosis and necrosis, with dissolution of myofilaments. The striation of the fibers is altered, and the fibers are either hypertrophied or atrophied. Eventually, muscle fibers are replaced with fat and connective tissue, causing fatty infiltration and fibrosis. There is no pattern of the involved muscle fibers. Mental retardation occurs in some types of MD.

Collaborative Care Management

Diagnosis is made by the patient history and physical examination. Laboratory and diagnostic data include muscle biopsy, electromyography, and serum muscle enzyme levels. Ninety-percent of persons with Duchenne's MD have abnormal electrocardiograms. Creatine kinase levels are elevated during infancy and before the onset of weakness. There is no cure for any of the muscular dystrophies. Treatment varies with the type of disorder (Table 47-24). Genetic counseling is important. Steroids and immunosuppressants have been used with some success in treating persons with MD.

Patient/Family Education. Nursing care of the person with MD is supportive. Because of the severity of the disability and the multiple manifestations, a multidisciplinary approach is necessary. Referrals to PT and OT can assist the patient and family in dealing with ADLs and problems with mobility. Monitoring for cardiac and other system involvement is important. The patient and family should be aware of the signs and symptoms and possible complications of MD. Prevention of the complications associated with immobility is vital. Medication teaching is necessary if the patient is receiving steroids or immunosuppressants. Emotional support is vital, especially for parents of children with MD. The family may need help dealing with feelings such as grief and guilt about disease transmission. Genetic counseling should be offered to appropriate individuals. Encouraging ambulation and mobility to the fullest extent should be balanced with ensuring adequate rest and sleep to prevent fatigue. Family members need instruction about transfer techniques for wheelchair-bound patients. A lift may be necessary if the family members are unable to assist with transfers. The Muscular Dystrophy Association is a good resource for patients and families of persons with MD. All states have local chapters.

TABLE 47-23 Common Types of Muscular Dystrophy

Dystrophy	Genetics	Onset	Progression	Muscular Distribution
Duchenne's	X-linked recessive Only males affected	18 months to 3 years	Rapid, death from cardiac or respiratory failure by third decade	Symmetric shoulder and hip involvement Cardiac involvement and mental retardation common
Becker's	X-linked recessive Only males affected	5-25 years	Gradual, normal life span, inability to walk ~25 years after onset of disease	Pelvic and shoulder muscle atrophy
Limb-girdle	Autosomal-dominant or autosomal-recessive Either sex affected	Variable, second or third decade	Variable, shortened life span, severe disability by 15-20 years after onset of disease	Pelvic and shoulder girdle, neck muscles
Facioscapulohumeral (Landouzy-Dejerine)	X-linked autosomal-dominant Either sex affected	Usually second decade	Moderate, normal life span	Facial, neck, shoulder girdle, and pelvic muscles
Myotonic (Steinert's disease)	Autosomal-dominant Either sex affected	Birth to fourth decade	Gradual, if adult onset	Muscle atrophy Delayed muscle relaxation, eyelids, facial, neck muscles Cataract development Dysphagia Hypersomnolence

TABLE 47-24 Treatment for Common Types of Muscular Dystrophy

Type	Treatment
Duchenne's	Function of unaffected muscles maintained; muscle fiber breakdown hastened by strenuous exercise Physical therapy (PT) for range of motion (ROM) Orthoses, braces, use of wheelchair Surgical release of contractures Spinal fusion Respiratory exercises
Becker's	Surgical release of contractures, tenotomies Ambulation maintained as long as possible Monitor for cardiac complications
Limb-girdle	PT for ROM; contracture development rare; patient usually ambulatory up to 20 years after diagnosis
Facioscapulohumeral	PT for exercises Orthoses Preserve ambulation Wheelchair for distance Surgical stabilization to prevent winged scapulae Arthrodesis of scapulae to ribs
Myotonic	Monitor for cardiac and endocrine disorders Aspiration precautions for dysphagia Decreased esophageal motility; feeding tube may be necessary Cataract surgery Pemoline or methylphenidate for somnolence

Critical Thinking Questions

1. A patient is admitted to the hospital with systemic manifestations of rheumatoid arthritis. The patient remarks, "I thought I just had arthritis. How did this happen?" Develop a teaching plan for this patient.
2. A 70-year-old patient is admitted 6 months after a right knee replacement with right knee pain, an elevated temperature, and general malaise. What are probable causes for his symptoms? What treatment might you expect? Develop a discharge teaching plan for this patient.
3. You are asked to speak to a group of perimenopausal women at a local community center. The topic is "healthy bones." Describe essential components of your presentation.
4. A 45-year-old woman is admitted for surgery to correct scoliosis. She has decreased respiratory function as a result of the severity of the spinal curvature. What preoperative assessments are necessary to plan her care? Describe priority interventions for postoperative care.
5. A 73-year-old woman has undergone left hip revision arthroplasty. She has a history of dislocation. Devise a teaching plan for her to prevent further dislocation of the prosthesis.

References

1. Anderson LP, Dale KG: Infections in total joint replacements, *Orthop Nurs* 17(1):7-11, 1998.
2. Arnett FA: Rheumatoid arthritis. In Goldman L, Bennett JC, editors: *Cecil textbook of medicine,* ed 21, Philadelphia, 2000, WB Saunders.
3. Aucott JN, Sigal LH, Smith RP: Lyme disease: the debate continues, *Patient Care Nurse Pract* 26(6):38-54, 2001.
4. Baird C: First-line treatment for osteoarthritis, *Orthop Nurs* 20(5):17-26, 2001.
5. Barohn RJ: Inflammatory and other myopathies. In Goldman L, Bennett JC, editors: *Cecil textbook of medicine,* ed 21, Philadelphia, 2000, WB Saunders.
6. Barohn RJ: Muscular dystrophies. In Goldman L, Bennett JC, editors: *Cecil textbook of medicine,* ed 21, Philadelphia, 2000, WB Saunders.
7. Blumenthal DE: Hyperuricemia and gout. In Rakel RE, Bope ET, editors: *Conn's current therapy,* Philadelphia, 2002, WB Saunders.
8. Burke S: Boning up on osteoporosis, *Nursing 2001* 31(10):36-43, 2001.
9. Clauw DJ: Elusive syndromes: treating the biologic basis of fibromyalgia and related syndromes, *Cleve Clin J Med* 68(10):830-839, 2001.
10. Cook RA, O'Malley MJ: Total ankle arthroplasty, *Orthop Nurs* 4:(21):30-37, 2001.
11. Crowther CL, Mourad LA: Alterations of musculoskeletal function. In McCance Kl, Huether SE, editors: *Pathophysiology: the biologic basis for disease in adults and children,* ed 4, St Louis, 2002, Mosby.
12. Curry LC, Hogstel MO: Osteoporosis, *Am J Nurs* 102(1):26-33, 2002.
13. Cush JJ, Lipsky PE: The spondyloarthropathies. In Goldman L, Bennett JC, editors: *Cecil textbook of medicine,* ed 21, Philadelphia, 2000, WB Saunders.

13a. Davidson M, DeSimone ME: Osteoporosis update, *Clin Rev* 12(4):76-82, 2002.

14. DeBaun BJ: Prevention of infection in the orthopedic surgery patient, *Nurs Clin North Am* 33(4):671-681, 1998.
15. Dowd R: Role of calcium, vitamin D, and other essential nutrients in the prevention and treatment of osteoporosis, *Nurs Clin North Am* 36(3):417-429, 2001.

15a. Drug News: LYMErix: lack of demand kills lyme disease vaccine, *Nursing 2002* 32(5):18, 2002.

16. Fell E: An update on Lyme disease and other tick-borne illnesses, *Nurse Pract* 25(10):38-57, 2000.
17. Finkelstein JS: Osteoporosis. In Goldman L, Bennett JC, editors: *Cecil textbook of medicine,* ed 21, Philadelphia, 2000, WB Saunders.
18. Freeman S: Diagnosis and management of osteoarthritis, *Am J Nurse Pract* 5(8):9-24, 2001.
19. Geier K: Perioperative blood loss, *Orthop Nurs* 17(1 suppl):6-36, 1998.
20. Geier K: Management approaches for improved patient outcomes, *Orthop Nurs* 19(3 suppl):10-21, 2000.
21. Gelber AC et al: Joint injury in young adults and risk for subsequent knee and hip arthritis, *Ann Intern Med* 133(5):321-328, 2000.
22. Gibs CP, Weber K, Scarborough MT: Malignant bone tumors, *J Bone Joint Surg Am* 83A(11):1727-1745, 2001.
23. Hertel KL, Trahiotis MG: Exercise in the prevention and treatment of osteoporosis, *Nurs Clin North Am* 36(3):441-450, 2001.
24. Hill N, Davis P: Nursing care of total joint replacement, *J Orthop Nurs* 4(1):41-45, 2000.
25. Hochberg MC: Sjögren's syndrome. In Goldman L, Bennett JC, editors: *Cecil textbook of medicine,* ed 21, Philadelphia, 2000, WB Saunders.
26. Hunder GG: Polymyalgia rheumatica and giant cell arteritis. In Goldman L, Bennett JC, editors: *Cecil textbook of medicine,* ed 21, Philadelphia, 2000, WB Saunders.
27. Jones A: Getting past the pain of fibromyalgia, *Nursing 2001* 31(4):62-64, 2001.
28. Kanis JA: Paget's disease of bone. In Goldman L, Bennett JC, editors: *Cecil textbook of medicine,* ed 21, Philadelphia, 2000, WB Saunders.
29. Koehler L, Zeidler H: Ankylosing spondylitis and other spondylarthritides. In Rakel RE, Bope ET, editors: *Conn's current therapy,* Philadelphia, 2002, WB Saunders.
30. Krebs VE: *Total joint replacements: an overview for the orthopaedic nurse.* Presented at the symposium on Orthopaedic Nursing: Excellence through Education, Cleveland Clinic Foundation, April 27, 2001.
31. Kuklo TR, Lenke LG: Thoracoscopic spine surgery: current indications and techniques, *Orthop Nurs* 19(6):15-21, 2000.

31a. Kupecz D, Berardinelli C: Using anakira for adult rheumatoid arthritis, *Nurse Pract* 27(4):62-65, 2002.

32. Lacasey B: Corticosteroid-induced osteoporosis, *Nurs Clin North Am* 36(3):455-464, 2001.
33. Lahita RG, Pisetsky DS, Wallace DJ: Lupus: high stakes Dx; broad treatment options, *Patient Care Nurse Pract* 23(4):19-29, 1998.
34. Lappe JM: Pathophysiology of osteoporosis and fracture, *Nurs Clin North Am* 36(3):393-398, 2001.
35. Lash AA: Sjögren's syndrome: pathogenesis, diagnosis, and treatment, *Nurse Pract* 26(8):50-58, 2001.
36. Reference deleted in proofs.
37. Leukenotte AG: *Gerontologic nursing,* ed 2, St Louis, 2000, Mosby.
38. Lohr KM: Rheumatoid arthritis. In Rakel RE, Bope ET, editors: *Conn's current therapy,* Philadelphia, 2002, WB Saunders.
39. Reference deleted in proofs.
40. MacDonald PA: Autoimmune and inflammatory disorders. In Maher AB, Salmond SW, Pellino TA, editors: *Orthopaedic nursing,* ed 3, Philadelphia, 2002, WB Saunders.
41. Mader JT, Shirtliff ME: Osteomyelitis. In Rakel RE, Bope ET, editors: *Conn's current therapy,* Philadelphia, 2002, WB Saunders.
42. Mahat G: Rheumatoid arthritis, *Am J Nurs* 98(12):42, 1998.

43. McCaffery M, Pasero C: *Pain: clinical manual,* ed 2, St Louis, 1999, Mosby.
44. McCann MT: Low back pain. In Rakel RE, Bope ET, editors: *Conn's current therapy,* Philadelphia, 2002, WB Saunders.
45. Miller PD: Osteoporosis. In Rakel RE, Bope ET, editors: *Conn's current therapy,* Philadelphia, 2002, WB Saunders.
46. Morris BA, Colwell CW, Hardwick ME: The use of low molecular weight heparins in the prevention of venous thromboembolic disease, *Orthop Nurs* 17(6):23-31, 77, 1998.
47. Mortensen SE: Bursitis, tendinitis, myofascial pain, and fibromyalgia. In Rakel RE, Bope ET, editors: *Conn's current therapy,* Philadelphia, 2002, WB Saunders.
48. Nash BA: Arthritis: rheumatoid and osteoarthritis, *Ohio Nurses Rev* 74(5):5-6, 14-16, 1999.
49. Ocleus SM: Autologous cultured chondrocytes for the treatment of knee cartilage injury, *Orthop Nurs* 19(4):19-27, 2000.
50. O'Grady ET: Low back pain: an evidence-based approach, *Adv Nurse Pract* 7(8):55-58, 80, 1999.
51. O'Rourke M: Determining the effectiveness of glucosamine and chondroitin for osteoarthritis, *Nurse Pract* 26(6):44-52, 2001.
52. Paduchi-Hyde L: Assessment of risk factors for osteoporosis and fracture, *Nurs Clin North Am* 36(3):401-406, 2001.
53. Pellino TA et al: Complications of orthopedic disorders and orthopaedic surgery. In Maher AB, Salmond SW, Pellino TA, editors: *Orthopaedic nursing,* ed 3, Philadelphia, 2002, WB Saunders.
54. Rice KL, Walsh E: Minimizing venous thromboembolic complications in the orthopaedic patient, *Orthop Nurs* 20(6):21-27, 2000.
55. Rizzoli R, Schaad MA, Uebelhart B: Osteoporosis in men, *Nurs Clin North Am* 36(3):467-477, 2001.
56. Roberts D: Degenerative disorders. In Maher AB, Salmond SW, Pellino TA, editors: *Orthopaedic nursing,* ed 3, Philadelphia, 2002, WB Saunders.
57. Rodts MF: Disorders of the spine. In Maher AB, Salmond SW, Pellino TA, editors: *Orthopaedic nursing,* ed 3, Philadelphia, 2002, WB Saunders.
58. Rus V, Via CS: Connective tissue disorders. In Rakel RE, Bope ET, editors: *Conn's current therapy,* Philadelphia, 2002, WB Saunders.
59. Schmitt M: Osteoporosis: focus on fractures, *Patient Care Nurse Pract* 25(2):61-71, 2000.
60. Schnitzer TJ: Osteoarthritis (degenerative joint disease). In Goldman L, Bennett JC, editors: *Cecil textbook of medicine,* ed 21, Philadelphia, 2000, WB Saunders.
61. Schur PH: Systemic lupus erythematosus. In Goldman L, Bennett JC, editors: *Cecil textbook of medicine,* ed 21, Philadelphia, 2000, WB Saunders.
62. Scully SP et al: Pathologic fracture in osteosarcoma: prognostic importance and treatment implications, *J Bone Joint Surg Am* 84A(1):49-57, 2002.
63. Searle T, Baughn P, editors: Researchers find bone-density gene, *Campus News* (Case Western Reserve University) 13(31):1, 4, 2001.
64. Sedlak CA, O'Doheny MO: Metabolic conditions. In Maher AB, Salmond SW, Pellino TA, editors: *Orthopaedic nursing,* ed 3, Philadelphia, 2002, WB Saunders.
65. Skinner HB: *Current diagnosis and treatment in orthopedics,* ed 2, Norwalk, Conn, 2000, Appleton & Lange.
66. Taft LB, Looker PA, Cella D: Osteoporosis: a disease management opportunity, *Orthop Nurs* 19(2):67-76, 2000.
67. Taylor G, Stein CM: Osteoarthritis. In Rakel RE, Bope ET, editors: *Conn's current therapy,* Philadelphia, 2002, WB Saunders.
67a. Unger J, Selfirdge-Thomas J: *The role of COX-2 inhibitors in inflammatory arthritis and common pain syndromes,* Atlanta, Ga, 2001, Nursing Contact Hours for Nurse Practitioners.
68. Wade CF: Keeping Lyme disease at bay, *Am J Nurs* 100(7):26-32, 2000.
69. Wassem R, Beckham N, Dudley W: Test of a nursing intervention to promote adjustment to fibromyalgia, *Orthop Nurs* 20(3):33-43, 2001.
70. Wildauer JM: Men and osteoporosis, *Adv Nurse Pract* 9(4):31-35, 2001.
71. Wright W: Arthritis update: new treatments for an old problem, *Adv Nurse Pract* 8(2):44-50, 2000.
72. York M, Paice JA: Treatment of low back pain with intraspinal opioids delivered via implanted pumps, *Orthop Nurs* 17(3):61-69, 1998.

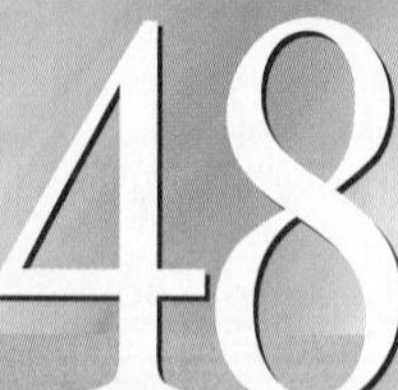

48 Assessment of the Immune System

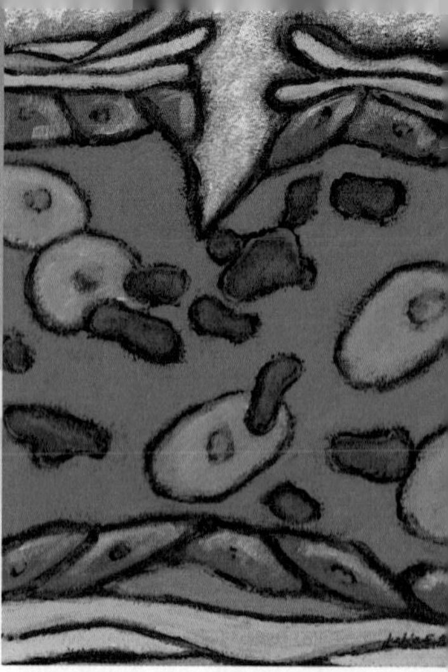

Carol J. Green

Objectives

After studying this chapter, the learner should be able to:

1. Recall the structure and function of the immune system.
2. Differentiate between natural and acquired immunity.
3. Discuss changes that occur within the immune system as a result of normal aging.
4. Identify assessment data relative to actual or potential alterations in immune functioning.
5. Describe common diagnostic tests used to identify immune alterations.
6. Explain the nursing implications of immune-related diagnostic tests.

This chapter provides a review of the structure and function of the immune system, essential components of natural and acquired immunity, related assessment data, and diagnostic tests for immune function. The inflammatory response as a clinical phenomenon is discussed in Chapter 11 along with clinical concepts of infection and infection control. Immune disorders are presented in Chapters 49 and 50.

ANATOMY AND PHYSIOLOGY

The Immune System

The immune system is a unique network of specialized cells, tissues, and organs that protect the body from invading microorganisms, destroy malignant cells, neutralize foreign substances, and dispose of cellular debris. The immune system performs these functions by distinguishing "self" cells from "nonself" cells. It does this on the basis of proteins unique to each individual organism, which protrude through the membrane surrounding each cell. Substances that are identified as nonself because they do not carry these self markers are destroyed. Nonself cells and proteins include all foreign particles and microorganisms, infected or weakened body cells, or self cells that have undergone malignant transformation. Any nonself substance capable of eliciting an immune response is known as an *antigen.* Microorganisms, pollens, foods, drugs, transplanted organs or tissues, and venoms are a few examples of antigenic nonself cells.

The immune system has two levels of defense: natural and acquired immunity. These basic responses are meshed together to give individuals their own unique immunologic reaction to antigens. Variations in immunologic response occur because each person has a different genetic background, is exposed to different environmental conditions, and responds differently to antigenic stimulation.

Specialized cells and organs that make up the immune system are located throughout the body. Immune organs are also called lymphoid organs because they are involved with the growth, development, and function of lymphocytes (white blood cells). The primary lymphoid organs are the bone marrow and thymus gland where lymphocytes mature and become *immunocompetent* cells capable of producing an immune response. Lymphocytes maturing in the bone marrow are called B lymphocytes. Those that migrate and mature in the thymus gland are called T lymphocytes.

The thymus gland is believed to regulate the overall immune system. Its activity reaches its peak in childhood and the gland begins to shrink in size after puberty. Animal research has shown that if the thymus is removed (thymectomy) very early in life, a severe state of immunodeficiency is induced and T-cell-mediated immunity never develops.

The lymph nodes, spleen, tonsils and adenoids, appendix, and patches of specialized lymphoid tissues that lie beneath the mucous membrane layer of the respiratory, gastrointestinal (GI), and genitourinary tracts are the secondary lymphoid organs (Figure 48-1). Within these secondary lymphoid organs, mature immune cells are concentrated.

Lymph nodes are small, bean-shaped structures that occur along lymphatic vessels. They consist of an inner medullary and paracortical region made up primarily of T cells and an outer cortex composed of clusters, or germinal centers, of B cells known as follicles. Lymph nodes (Figure 48-2) filter foreign substances from lymph. When stimulated, macrophages and B cells in the lymph nodes can rapidly proliferate and differentiate into immunoglobulin-producing cells and may be evidenced by palpably enlarged lymph nodes (lymphadenopathy).

The spleen lies inferiorly and posteriorly to the stomach in the upper left quadrant of the abdomen. The spleen is a

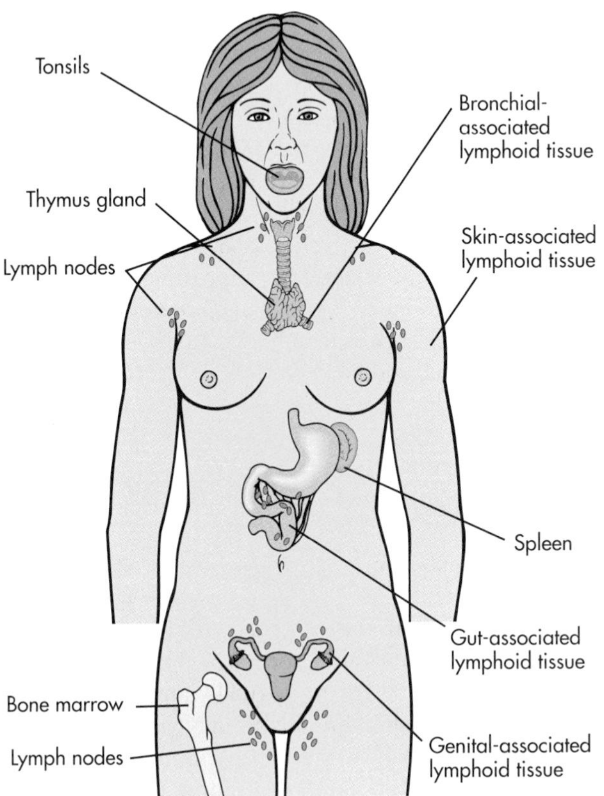

Figure 48-1 Structures of the immune system.

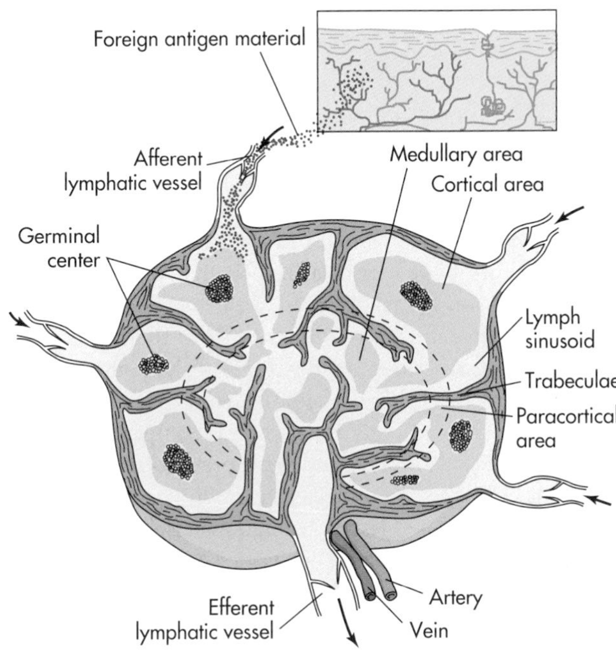

Figure 48-2 Structure of a lymph node. Lymph nodes are organized into three main areas: the outer cortex, where B cells proliferate and mature; the deeper paracortex, populated mainly by macrophages and T cells; and the inner medulla, containing both B cells and T cells. Macrophages, B cells, and T cells interact with each other, often in the presence of antigen percolating through the node, resulting in the inductive phase of the immune response.

major storage depot for macrophages and lymphocytes, both of which can launch an immune response when stimulated by bloodborne antigens. The spleen is composed of two types of tissues: white pulp and red pulp. White pulp primarily contains B lymphocytes, which support immune surveillance and lymphocyte proliferation.

Mucosa-associated lymphoid tissues are patches of specialized cells, called Peyer's patches, similar to those found in the spleen. They block submucosal entry of antigens into the area where they are located (e.g., the respiratory, GI, and genitourinary tracts and skin). Collectively, the tonsils, Peyer's patches, and appendix are known as gut-associated lymphoid tissues. The tonsils filter out airborne and ingested antigens. The appendix and Peyer's patches specifically protect against alimentary antigens. Collectively, the lymphoid cells and organs act in concert to protect skin surfaces, mucous membranes, blood, lymph, and internal organs from foreign invasion.

Natural and Acquired Immunity

Natural immunity is nonspecific, present at birth, and does not require exposure to an antigen for its development. It consists of anatomic and chemical barriers that recognize and respond to damaged self cells or nonself, foreign antigens. Because natural immunity is nonspecific it is always the same except for the degree of response. Acquired immunity begins after birth as the result of the immune system's response to repeated antigenic stimulation. It is specific in that it is initiated by and targeted against particular antigens. It is this immunity that results in lifelong protection against many diseases.

Natural Immunity

External Nonspecific Defenses. The skin, mucous membranes, protective secretions, enzymes, phagocytic cells, and protective proteins provide the body with its nonspecific natural immunity. The most basic of these defenses is the external barrier protection, which derives from the structures and functions of the skin, and mucous membranes, which act to prevent entry of harmful agents into the body. The intact skin serves as an extremely efficient physical barrier to harmful agents and environmental forces such as heat, cold, and trauma. The keratinized surface cells of the skin provide a tough, dense, waterproof covering. Some of the fatty acids released to the skin surface by the sebaceous glands have antimicrobial activity and inhibit the growth of selected microorganisms. Also, the acetic acid and salt concentration of perspiration is toxic to many pathogenic microorganisms. Microbial antagonism, the competition between resident and transient flora, further assists in preventing invasion by pathogenic microorganisms. The normal or resident flora compete for nutrients and space with transient, potential pathogens and some release antimicrobial substances that retard the growth of transient organisms seeking to colonize the same site.

Mucous membranes protect the eye and line all body tracts that have external openings. When intact, the mucous membranes, like the skin, are basically impervious to foreign materials and microorganisms. A viscous secretion that tends to trap and inactivate microorganisms covers the surfaces. A specific class of immunoglobulins (antibodies) known as immunoglobulin A (IgA) are found in this mucosal secretion and, in high concentration, within the secretory mucosal cells of the respiratory and intestinal tracts. IgA antibodies are secreted from the mucosal cells and have antibacterial, antiviral, and antitoxic properties. These antibodies prevent microbial adherence and colonization of the tracts by pathogens.

The mucous membrane of the respiratory tract is further protected by the surface activity of the ciliated epithelial cells, which sweep foreign material out of the tract. The mucous membranes are highly vascularized so that the internal defense mechanisms are readily available to attack any microorganisms that do gain access to the surface of these cells.

Many other structures and functions of the body also contribute to external defense. The nasal hairs have a unique filtration action that serves to trap particles and microorganisms. The flushing action of saliva and urine prevents the buildup of organisms. The eyes are protected from dirt particles and organisms by the lids and lashes. Foreign material that does gain entrance to the eye tends to be washed out by tears. In the stomach, the acidity (approximately pH 2) of the gastric juice kills many organisms and detoxifies certain potentially toxic substances. For this reason, when gastric pH is increased, special precautions must be taken to avoid introduction of organisms through the nose and mouth. A higher gastric pH is characteristic in neonates; therefore special care should be taken in feeding and handling babies to prevent exposure to pathogens by the oral route. The action of bile and proteolytic enzymes generally keeps the upper intestine free of organisms. The constant movement of foods through the stomach and intestines also works to prevent the buildup of organisms and toxic waste products. Even vomiting and the watery stools of diarrhea are active modes of removal of harmful products from the GI tract.

In the vagina, secretions support the colonization of lactobacilli, which are harmless, acid-producing bacteria. This colonization results in an acid environment and reduces the chance of pathogens colonizing the vagina. When either the amount or the acidity of the vaginal secretions is reduced, the risk of vaginal infection increases. Because vaginal secretions are not present before puberty and are greatly reduced after menopause, both young girls and older women are more prone to vaginitis. The use of certain types of oral contraceptives may cause a shift in the composition and pH of the vaginal secretions, which increases the possibility of colonization of the vagina, especially by the causative agent of gonorrhea, *Neisseria gonorrhoeae*.

The bactericidal enzyme called lysozyme also plays a significant role in external defense. It is capable of lysing (splitting) the bacterial cell wall of many gram-positive organisms and causing their destruction. The enzyme is present in mucus, tears, saliva, and skin secretions. Lysozyme is also found in many of the internal fluids and cells of the body where it tends to work in combination with complement and other blood factors to destroy bacteria directly. Thus lysozyme plays a role in both external and internal nonspecific defense.

If antigens are successful in penetrating these external protective barriers, an even more complex array of internal defense mechanisms come into play. These internal defenses, which involve the cells and molecules of the mononuclear phagocyte system, blood, complement, and interferons, underlie the inflammatory response (see Chapter 11).

Internal Nonspecific Defenses

Mononuclear Phagocyte System. The mononuclear phagocyte system, formerly known as the reticuloendothelial system, is a widespread system of phagocytic cells located in the blood and various body tissues. In the blood, these phagocytic cells are referred to as monocytes. After approximately 24 hours of life, the monocytes move into tissue and become fixed. Once anchored in tissues such as lymphoid tissue, liver, spleen, bone marrow, lungs, and blood vessels, these monocytes mature into macrophages. Macrophages have been given unique names, dependent on their specific tissue location within the body (Table 48-1). The function of the macrophages is to capture and destroy foreign materials found in the fluids of their environment.

Other cells making up the phagocytic network are not stationary and are called *wandering macrophages*. The wandering macrophages carry out the important role of final cleanup of a damaged site in preparation for repair. These cells have the capacity to engulf and destroy virtually any type of foreign material or debris within the body. Both types of macrophages play an important role in the nonspecific inflammatory response and the specific immune response discussed later in this chapter.

Blood. Blood is one of the primary sources of elements designed to provide protection against injurious agents. The important cellular components of blood in the nonspecific response include granulocytes, lymphocytes, monocytes, and thrombocytes (platelets). The granulocytes, also referred to as polymorphonuclear leukocytes (PMNs), and the monocytes are the most important because of their phagocytic activity.

One of the chief internal nonspecific defense mechanisms is the ingestion of microorganisms and other particulate matter by phagocytic white blood cells (WBCs). The phagocytes carry out the process of phagocytosis in several discrete steps (Figure 48-3). Most infecting microbes are quickly and efficiently destroyed by phagocytosis; however, some pathogens can escape this destruction. Some bacteria, such as strains of streptococci and staphylococci and *Bacillus anthracis* (an-

TABLE 48-1 Distribution and Names of Macrophages in Various Tissue Sites

Tissue	Name
Peripheral blood	Monocyte
Loose connective tissue	Histiocyte
Liver	Kupffer cells
Spleen, MPS	Wandering or fixed macrophage
Lung	Alveolar macrophage or dust cell
Granulomatous tissue	Epithelioid and giant cells
Peritoneal cavity, pleural cavity, bone	Macrophages

thrax), actually produce factors that kill the phagocyte. Other organisms resist ingestion or digestion. Some organisms may survive within the phagocytes and multiply there. This may lead to the transport of the organism to other sites in the body or may serve as a chronic focus of continued infection.

The granulocytes can be divided on the basis of their structure and function into neutrophils, eosinophils, and basophils. The "granules" found within these cells represent discrete packets of degradative enzymes used to digest the ingested materials. The neutrophils are the most numerous in circulation and are the most efficient and responsive phagocytic cells involved in the inflammatory process. Provided there is adequate blood supply to a region, the neutrophils are constantly available to move from the blood vessels to the site of injury or infection. The neutrophils and monocytes are actually attracted to the scene by chemicals released during infection or injury. This cellular response to chemical attractants is known as chemotaxis, and the substances released are called chemotactic substances.

Eosinophils constitute about 4% of the total WBC count. They are known to destroy parasitic organisms and play a major role in allergic reactions.

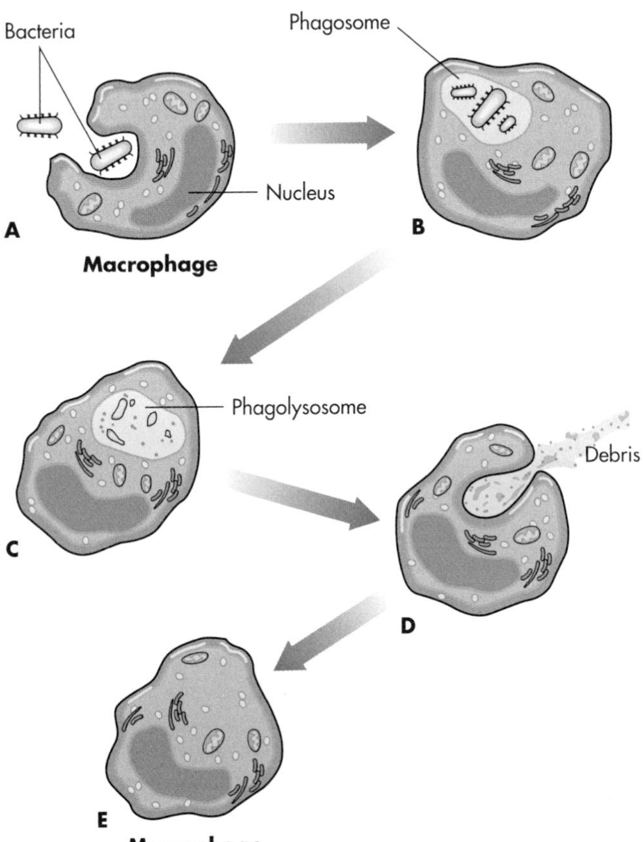

Figure 48-3 Phagocytosis sketched in macrophage. **A,** Opsonized bacteria engulfed by phagocyte (macrophage). **B,** Phagosome formed. **C,** Phagosome becomes phagolysosome; bacteria digested. (To this point the process of phagocytosis is comparable to either macrophage or neutrophil, not shown. **D,** Debris is egested. (Neutrophil would succumb here.) **E,** Macrophage returns to resting state.

Basophils make up less than 1% of the total WBC count. They play an important role in the inflammatory process by their actions on blood vessels. They release histamines and other chemicals that act on smooth muscle and blood vessel walls. The histamine that is released narrows the lumens of the respiratory system and restricts breathing. Histamine also works to decrease blood flow through veins through vasoconstriction, thereby increasing blood in the small arteries and capillaries, and enhancing capillary permeability. This increased capillary permeability is thought to enhance the antimicrobial properties of the blood at sites of inflammation and infection.

The fluid portion of uncoagulated blood is called plasma. Immunoglobulins, which are produced as part of the acquired specific immune response to antigen stimulation and which bind and coat specific antigens, are transported throughout the body by the plasma. The immunoglobulin-bound antigen can be recognized by receptors on the surface of the phagocytic cells, thereby greatly enhancing the ability of these cells to engulf antigen. This process of enhanced phagocytosis is known as opsonization. Through this process the specific immune response mechanism contributes to the nonspecific mechanism and makes it significantly more efficient.

Another plasma constituent, fibrin, participates in the inflammatory process by creating a meshwork around the injured area and sealing it off. Microorganisms become trapped within this meshwork, where the phagocytic cells can more easily capture them.

Complement. One of the most important constituents of plasma is a complex series of proteins known by the singular name of complement. There are as many as 20 different protein components, with 11 designated as major components in the complement cascade. The liver is the primary site of synthesis of the components of complement. The primary role of complement is to provide specific lysis (rupturing) of cell membranes. The initiation of the complement cascade most often is triggered by the binding of the first complement protein to complement-binding immunoglobulins that have already bound to their antigens. Thus complement serves to accentuate or complete the action of an immunoglobulin. The immunoglobulin by itself cannot produce cell lysis, but with the recruitment of complement in the reaction, the cell may be ruptured. However, other nonimmune substances also can activate complement. Complement is considered a nonspecific component of the plasma because it is not increased by immunization. In addition to its cytolytic effects, complement is involved in leukocyte chemotaxis, release of histamines, enhancement of phagocytosis by PMNs, viral neutralization, and bactericidal activity.

The classic activities ascribed to complement depend on the sequential interaction of nine protein subunits (C1 to C9), the first component of which consists of three subfractions termed C1q, C1r, and C1s (thereby accounting for the 11 separate proteins). The C1q, C1r, and C1s components constitute the recognition unit, inasmuch as this unit is capable of recognizing the antibody and fixing it. When an antigen-antibody complex on the surface of a cell binds the first component, C1, it acquires the enzymatic ability to activate many molecules of the next components in the sequence, C4 and C2, to form an active C42 complex (Figure 48-4). (Unfortunately, the numbering system of the complement components reflects their order of discovery and not their sequential additive pattern.) Each of the activated C42 complexes (the activation units) is then able to act on multiple molecules of the next components and so on, producing a cascade effect and a greatly amplified reaction. As each component is added, new enzymatic activity is created to initiate the next step similar to what occurs in the clotting process. The final component, C5b6789, has the ability to create a lesion in the cell membrane and, if enough lesions are created on the membrane, cell death results. This complex is sometimes called the *membrane attack unit.* The intermediate stages in the complement sequence also give rise to complexes and fragments with other significant biologic activities that include the following:

1. *Histamine release.* Histamines cause an extreme increase in vascular permeability and contraction of smooth muscle. A fragment (C3a) split off during the activation of C3 and another fragment (C5a) created by the activation of C5 are released into the surrounding tissues, where they cause the release of histamine from mast cells. The histamines in turn exert their physiologic effects on the smooth muscle tissues and vascular system.
2. *Enhanced phagocytosis.* Neutrophils and macrophages have receptors for C3b on their cell surfaces, which add to the opsonization effect. Complement activation at the site of infection labels foreign materials with the C3b fragments and makes them more subject to phagocytosis. The contribution of the process to protection is most apparent in persons with a genetic deficiency in the synthesis of the C3 protein. Such individuals suffer from recurrent bacterial infections and septicemia.
3. *Chemotactic substance formation.* Several of the fragments and intermediate factors serve as chemotactic substances to attract phagocytes to the site of the reaction.

All these activities are central to the inflammatory response as described in Chapter 11.

Interferons. Interferons comprise a group of proteins produced by various human cells, usually in response to a viral infection of the cell. When a virus infects a cell, the infected cell begins to make interferon almost immediately (Figure 48-5). The interferon is released into its surrounding environment, where it induces uninfected cells to produce alterations that protect those cells from viral multiplication. This antiviral action is exerted before the synthesis of immunoglobulins specific for the virus reach protective levels. The elaboration of interferons from virally infected cells continues for a few hours (up to about 24 hours) after infection, thereby playing a significant role in isolating the infective foci in many, but not all, viral infections.

Although viruses seem to be the most potent agents for the induction of interferon, other intracellular parasites such as rickettsia, bacteria, and parasites may also trigger its formation. Even bacterial and fungal extracts, as well as materials such as double-stranded ribonucleic acid (RNA), synthetic polymers, and plant extracts, may serve as signals.

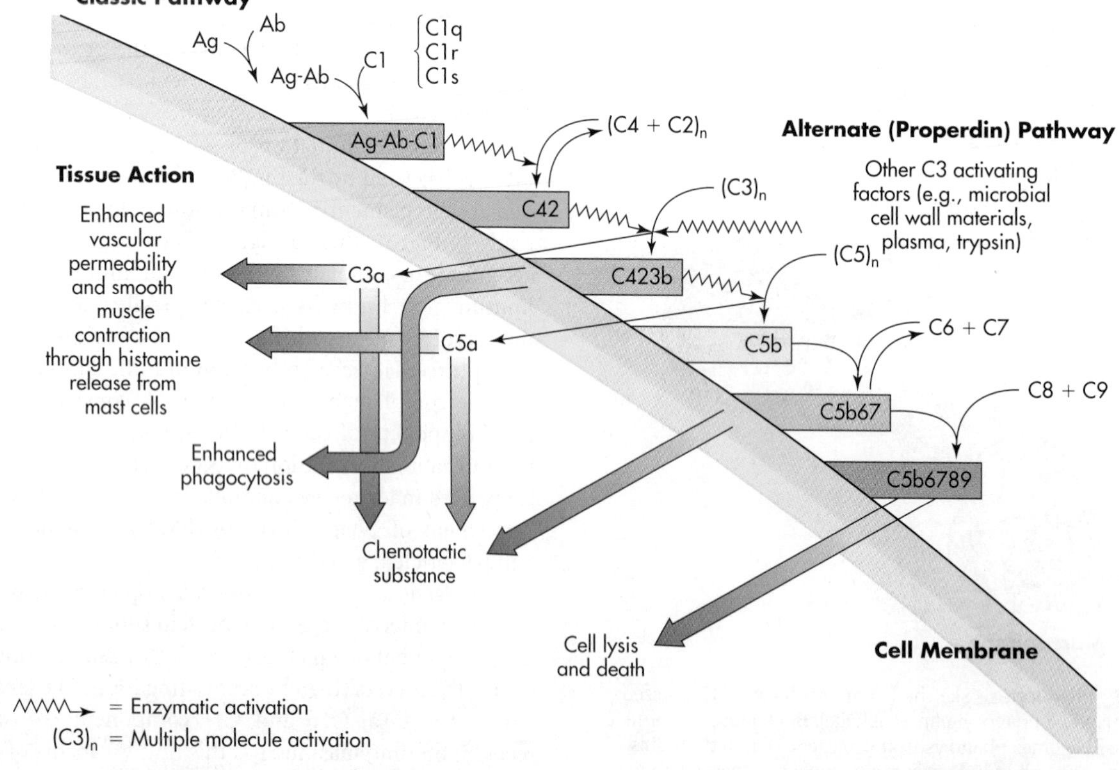

Figure 48-4 Classic and alternate complement cascade. Sequence of complement activation generates multiple biologically active intermediate molecules, which are active in the inflammatory response.

Different cell types in the human body produce three distinct types of interferons, and each type seems to exert different protective effects. Alpha-interferon is produced by lymphocytes and seems to have antiviral activity. Fibroblasts, epithelial cells, and macrophages form beta-interferon, which is definitely antiviral. Gamma-interferon is produced by T lymphocytes of the specific immune response system and has an immunoregulatory effect. In addition to their antiviral activities, the interferons are capable of inhibiting cell growth; therefore they are being used widely in clinical trials as antitumor agents. Interferons slow down cell replication and enhance natural killer (NK) cell activity, thereby acting as anticancer agents.

Acquired Immunity

Acquired immunity is specific immunity against a particular microorganism or molecular entity. It follows exposure to antigens or transfer of antibodies from one individual to another. An antigen is a substance that, in the body, is recognized as nonself and elicits the formation of antibodies (reactive proteins), and/or specifically sensitized cells called cytotoxic lymphocytes. Most antigens are naturally occurring proteins of at least 10,000 molecular weight. However other substances, such as polysaccharides, nucleoproteins, lipoproteins, and glycoproteins, can also be antigenic. Some molecules, because of their small size, cannot induce the formation of antibodies unless they are coupled with a high-molecular-weight carrier. These molecules are known as incomplete antigens or haptens.

The *antigenic determinant* is the part of an antigen molecule that can be recognized by immune cells and hence elicit the formation and proliferation of *antibodies* and *cytotoxic* lymphocytes. These antibodies and lymphocytes subsequently bind to the antigenic determinant. This binding can have direct beneficial effects such as detoxification of toxins, inactivation of viruses, or, coupled with complement, the direct lysis of cells. However, in most cases the antigen-antibody combination initiates and facilitates the nonspecific defense mechanisms such as phagocytosis, complement, and the inflammatory response (see Chapter 11). The specific type of immune response—that is, synthesis of antibodies, development of antigen reactive lymphocytes, or a combination of the two—varies with the characteristics of the antigen.

Acquired immunity possesses memory, which allows the system to remember prior contact with antigenic material. It takes days to weeks for the immune system to produce a sufficient response to be protective after first exposure to the antigen. However, the immune system is able to respond faster and more vigorously to subsequent encounters with the same antigen.

Immunity acquired from exposure to antigens such as measles is *active* immunity. It is active because the host's immune system recognizes the antigen and responds against the specific antigen. Acquired immunity that is transferred from one person to another is *passive* immunity. It is passive because the host's immune system is not involved in production of the protective antibodies. Infants receive antibodies from their mother while in utero and through breast milk. Other forms of passive immunity include gamma globulin, antiserum, and immune serum, all of which are administered by injection. Passive immunity provides short-term, temporary protection against diseases such as tetanus or rabies as well as snake bites.

Acquired immunity consists of two functional components. One is a cell-mediated system that provides cytotoxic lymphocytes. The other is a humoral-mediated system that provides circulating antibodies. Cells of both components are derived from undifferentiated stem cells of the bone marrow. The primary cells of the immune response system develop from the lymphocytic cell population (Figure 48-6). One population of lymphocytic cells undergoes differentiation under the influence of the thymus gland and become thymus-dependent lymphocytes, or T cells. These cells become responsible for facilitating the cell-mediated immune response. Another population of

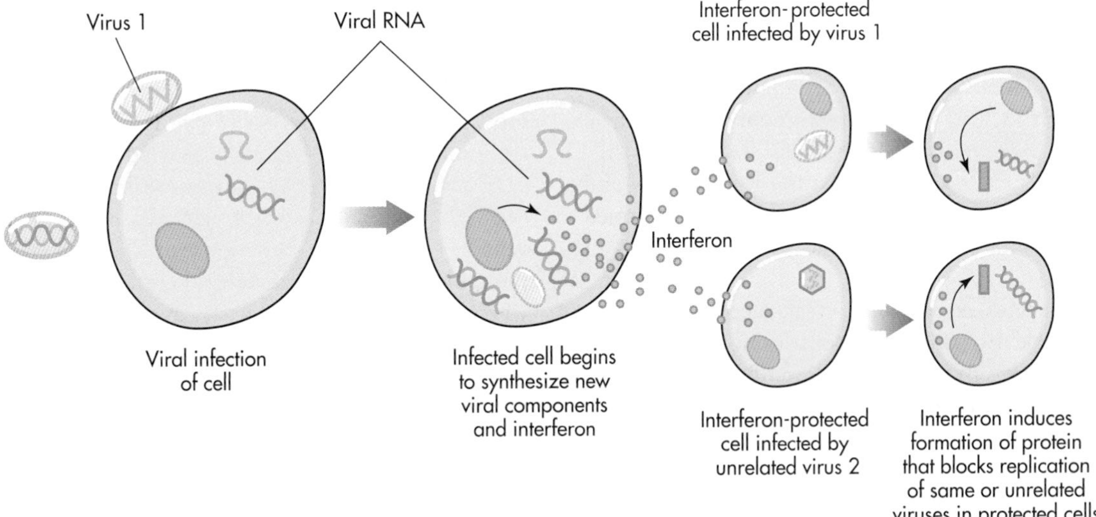

Figure 48-5 Mechanism of interferon action.

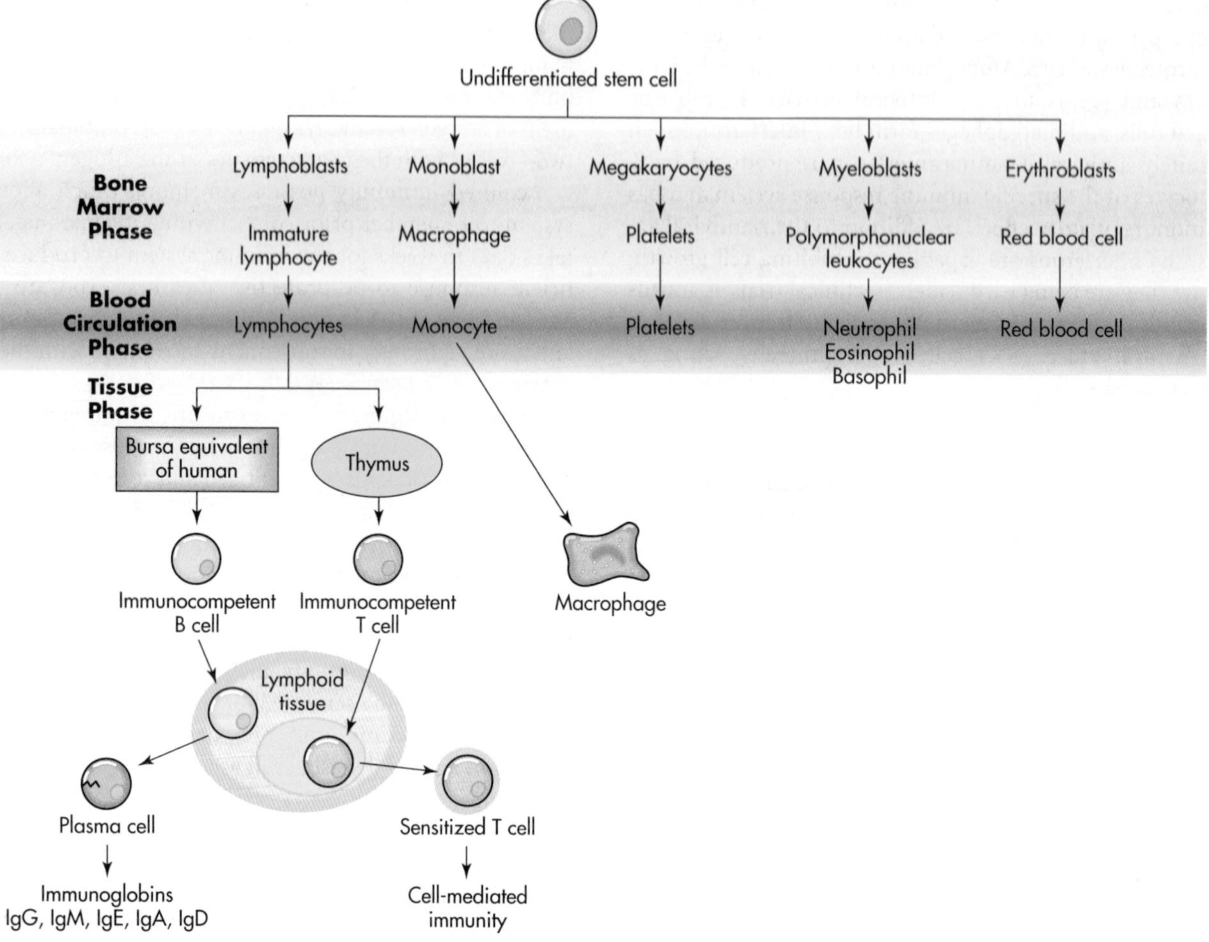

Figure 48-6 Development of B and T lymphocytes.

lymphocytes matures in a site other than the thymus and is known as thymus-independent lymphocytes, or B cells. The B cells are responsible for production of the immunoglobulins and provision of the humoral immune response. B and T lymphocytes can be differentiated from each other on the basis of specific markers (membrane-bound proteins) on their surface.

Cell-Mediated Acquired Immunity. The cell-mediated system offers protection from (1) chronic bacterial infections (e.g., syphilis, tuberculosis, leprosy), (2) many viral infections (e.g., measles, herpesvirus infections, chickenpox), (3) fungal infections (e.g., candidiasis, histoplasmosis, cryptococcosis), (4) parasitic infections (e.g., leishmaniasis, toxoplasmosis, and *Pneumocystis carinii*), and (5) transplanted or transformed cells (e.g., tissue transplants and some transformed cells of cancer).

T-cell lymphocytes, responsible for cell-mediated or cellular immunity, make two important contributions to immune defense. They are vital to the coordination of cellular and humoral immunity and they directly attack antigens. T lymphocytes are produced in the bone marrow and mature in the thymus gland. From the thymus gland they migrate to regional lymph nodes and the spleen where they populate the medullary regions. Each mature immunosensitive T-cell lymphocyte is capable of responding to a specific antigen. Upon exposure to its specific antigen, the T cell proliferates. Cells are shed into the circulation where they are transported throughout the body (Figure 48-7).

Several T-cell lymphocyte subsets act to regulate T-cell function and augment production of antibodies by B cells. Helper/inducer T cells (also called TH, T4, or CD4) are essential for activating other T-lymphocyte cells, B-lymphocyte cells, NK cells, and macrophages. Without the helper T cell, B cells are unable to make sufficient antibody against most invading antigens. Cytotoxic T cells (Tc) attack and destroy antigen or antigenically labeled cells on site. Specifically they attack infected, tumor, and foreign graft cells.[7] T cells known as suppressor T cells (Ts or T8) operate to prevent or modify the functions of the two systems. It is thought that they may turn off the specific immune reaction when it is no longer needed. Delayed cells (Td) are involved in delayed hypersensitivity involving fungi and mycobacteria allergic responses.[2] The last subset of T lymphocytes is the memory T cell. They are named for their ability to remember contact with specific antigens and immediately respond on subsequent exposure.

T lymphocyte cells work primarily by secreting potent chemical messengers known as cytokines, or specifically lymphokines. Lymphokines are soluble substances that recruit

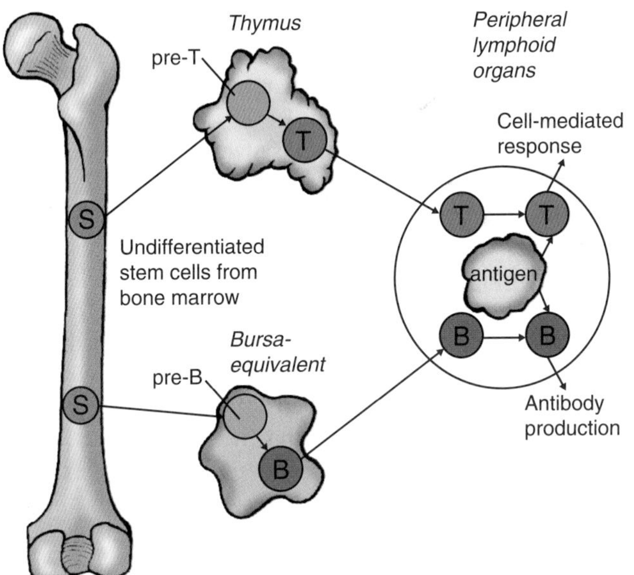

Figure 48-7 Undifferentiated stem cells move from the bone marrow to either the thymus gland or the bursa-equivalent, where they are transformed into T cells or B cells. They then move to one of the secondary lymphoid organs, where they may contact an antigen and become activated.

and activate nonspecifically reactive phagocytes, including components of the inflammatory response and lymphokine-activated killer cells.[2] T-helper cells produce a lymphokine known as interleukin-2 (IL-2), which stimulates the production of NK cells that target tumor cells and virally infected cells. NK cells are similar to the cytotoxic T-cell subset, but do not need to recognize a specific antigen to attack. Once activated by IL-2, NK cells release potent chemicals that kill on contact.[5] Table 48-2 summarizes the functions of the various T lymphocytes.

Humorally Mediated Immunity. The humorally mediated system provides major immunity against (1) bacteria that produce acute infection (such as *Staphylococcus, Streptococcus,* and *Haemophilus* organisms), (2) bacterial exotoxins (diphtheria, botulinus, and tetanus toxins), (3) viruses that must enter the bloodstream to reach their target tissues (e.g., poliomyelitis and hepatitis virus), and (4) organisms that enter the body from the mucosal tissues (e.g., cold viruses, enteroviruses, and influenza viruses). Even though circulating antibodies may be produced against other organisms (such as tuberculosis, human immunodeficiency virus [HIV], and fungi), these antibodies do not protect the body from infection.

B-cell lymphocytes, the lymphocytes providing the humorally mediated immune response, are produced and are believed to primarily mature in the bone marrow after which they migrate to the spleen and lymphoid tissues located along the gut, bronchus, and tonsils (Figure 48-7). These are all strategic locations that are continuously exposed to antigens.[7]

The immunosensitive B cells are programmed to respond to a single antigen. When the antigen is present, the B cell begins to proliferate and differentiate into a plasma cell. A plasma cell is designed to synthesize and release large amounts

TABLE 48-2 Functions of Various T Cell Subsets

T Cell Subsets	Function(s)
T helper cell (T_4, T_H CD_4)	Release lymphokines that: Regulate antibody production by B cells Activate other T cells Activate macrophages Activate natural killer cells
T suppressor cell (T_8, T_S)	Prevent or modify the functions of T cells and B cells May suppress the immune reaction when no longer needed
Cytotoxic (T_c) cell	Kill virus infected cells, tumor cells, and foreign graft cells
Delayed (T_d) cell	Delayed hypersensitivity Inflammatory response
T memory cell (T_M)	Induce secondary immune response

of immunoglobulin (antibody) that will combine with the antigen that caused its production. These antibody molecules are released into the circulation where they become part of the gamma-globulin fraction of the serum. The B cells producing the immunoglobulin remain in the lymphoid tissue and continue to synthesize additional molecules of the specific antibody. This process is different from the T-cell response where cytotoxic T cells are released; in this case the B cells remain, and their product is released. Thus the level of active specific antibodies begins to rise in the serum fraction (antibody titer), as well as in the level of the gamma-globulin fraction in general. Antibodies bind to their specific antigen after being carried by the blood and other body fluids to the site where needed. On binding, the antibody may inactivate the antigen, precipitate it, or activate other antigen-damaging processes, such as the complement cascade, to remove it.

The immunoglobulins are subdivided into different classes on the basis of molecular structure and function. The generic symbol for immunoglobulins is Ig, and each class is designated by a letter of the alphabet: IgG, IgM, IgA, IgE, and IgD. The basic structural pattern for all immunoglobulins is four-peptide chains arranged in a Y shape (Figure 48-8). The two chains of higher molecular weight are called heavy (H) chains and the two of lower molecular weight are called light (L) chains. At the ends of the two arms of the Y are the sites where antigen is bound (variable region). Both the H and L chains participate in the formation of these antigen-binding sites. The two arms of the Y are designated the Fab regions (for fragment, antigen-binding). The base of the Y is called the Fc region (for fragment, crystallizable). The Fc fragment binds to complement and to white blood cells, including macrophages.

The predominant class of immunoglobulins in normal adult serum is IgG, which makes up about 75% to 85% of the immunoglobulin fraction. IgG, which is capable of crossing the placenta to provide the newborn with temporary natural passive immunity to those diseases against which the mother has circulating antibodies, is also found in extravascular fluids.

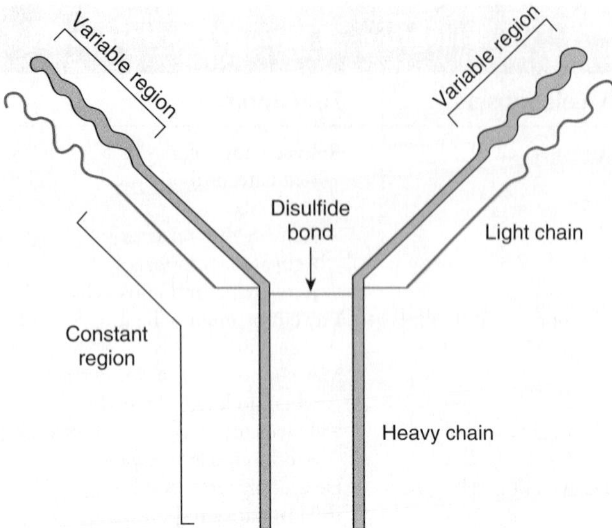

Figure 48-8 The basic antibody molecule is a Y-shaped unit composed of two heavy chains and two light chains. Each chain has a constant region and a variable region that contains the specific antigen-binding site.

Its primary functions are to neutralize toxins and inactivate viruses and bacteria. It also forms antigen-antibody complement immune complexes that are associated with certain types of hypersensitivity (see Chapter 49). IgG is the immunoglobulin class primarily responsible for the rise in serum antibodies during a secondary (booster) response to an antigen.

IgM is primarily found in intravascular fluids and constitutes about 7% of the immunoglobulins in serum. Also called macroglobulin because of its molecular size, IgM, like IgG, is capable of binding the C1 component of complement and initiating the complement cascade. In each antigenic stimulation, IgM antibodies are the first to appear, but they neither reach the levels of IgG nor exhibit a booster response on subsequent antigen contact. The chief function of IgM is to protect against viral and bacterial invaders in the blood. IgM is also involved in certain immune complex hypersensitivities and autoimmune diseases, such as rheumatoid arthritis, as a result of its ability to bind complement.

About 10% of the total immunoglobulin in serum is IgA. IgA is termed the secretory immunoglobulin because it is found in the exocrine secretions of the body (milk, mucin, saliva, and tears). IgA specifically protects of the mucosal surfaces of the respiratory, digestive, and genital tracts from pathogenic invasion by preventing the attachment of bacteria to epithelial surfaces.

IgD, whose function is unknown, makes up only about 1% of the immunoglobulin fraction of serum. Because most IgD is found on the surface of lymphocytes, it is thought to play a role in activating or suppressing their function.

IgE is present in the serum in extremely small amounts (0.002%), as it selectively attaches to the surface of mast cells and basophils. When bound to the surface of these cells, which are rich in the potent, physiologically active substances histamine, kinins, and serotonin, IgE mediates hypersensitivity reactions such as hay fever, allergic asthma, and anaphylactic shock (see Chapter 49). The protective role of this immunoglobulin is unclear.

Table 48-3 summarizes the characteristics and clinical significance of immunoglobulins.

The humorally mediated B cell system is similar to the T-cell system in that it is controlled by T-helper and T-suppressor cells, produces memory (BM) cells, and is rendered self-tolerant by the same mechanisms. See Figure 48-9 for a depiction of the relationships and functions of macrophages, T cells, and B cells.

Either the cell-mediated or the humorally mediated system or both can be immunodeficient (see Chapter 50). When one system is not functioning properly, the person becomes susceptible to infection or encroachment by the agents against which that system provided primary protection. For example, infection with HIV reduces the protection afforded by the cell-mediated system, making the individual susceptible to fungal infections (candidiasis), protozoan infections *(P. carinii* pneumonia), viral infections (herpesvirus infection), and cancers (Kaposi's sarcoma or lymphoma). Alternatively, the loss of the humorally mediated system that occurs in Bruton's agammaglobulinemia is accompanied by increased incidence of acute bacterial infections, respiratory tract infections, and GI tract problems. If both systems are lost or compromised, the individual is fully susceptible to infectious agents and cannot survive in an unprotected, nonsterile environment.

Immune Response Sequence

Antigen Challenge

When an antigen is introduced into the body (an antigenic challenge), it can trigger a wide or narrow spectrum of response mechanisms. The specific pattern of response depends on (1) the type of antigen introduced, (2) the site of introduction, and (3) the amount of antigen introduced.

Highly invasive antigens (e.g., bacteria such as *S. aureus* or *S. pyogenes*) or those introduced directly into the bloodstream by blood transfusion, intravenous catheterization, or injection can immediately establish a systemic type of immune response. This is why extreme care must be exercised in the use of any type of medical procedure that would allow the introduction of antigens into the general circulation.

Small amounts of noninvasive, large, particulate antigens introduced at a single body site are quickly and efficiently handled with little or no systemic involvement beyond the local lymph node and the immune response may go unnoticed. Small, soluble antigens, however, are more difficult for the lymph nodes to clear from the circulation and hence are more likely to induce a wider spread response. Similarly large amounts of any antigen can overwhelm and escape the local defenses. An excessively large, sustained antigen dose can exhaust not only the local site but the entire system. This greatly reduces the body's ability to respond to even minor invasive challenges and renders the host vulnerable to secondary infections.

When an antigenic substance is introduced into the body, either it is carried directly by lymphocytic circulation to a regional lymphoid tissue, where it is engulfed by an antigen processing cell (APC), or an APC engulfs the antigen at the site of

TABLE 48-3 Characteristics of Immunoglobulins

Class	Relative Serum Concentration (%)	Location	Characteristics
IgG	76	Plasma, interstitial fluid	Is only immunoglobulin that crosses placenta Fixes complement Is responsible for secondary immune response
IgA	15	Body secretions, including tears, saliva, breast milk, colostrum	Lines mucous membranes and protects body surfaces
IgM	8	Plasma	Fixes complement Is responsible for primary immune response Provides specific antitoxin action when combined with IgG Forms antibodies to ABO blood antigens
IgD	1	Plasma	Is present on lymphocyte surface Assists in the differentiation of B lymphocytes
IgE	0.002	Plasma, interstitial fluids, exocrine secretions	Causes symptoms of allergic reactions Fixes to mast cells and basophils Assists in defense against parasitic infections

From Lewis SM, Heitkemper MM, Dirksen SR: *Medical-surgical nursing: assessment and management of clinical problems,* ed 5, St Louis, 2000, Mosby.

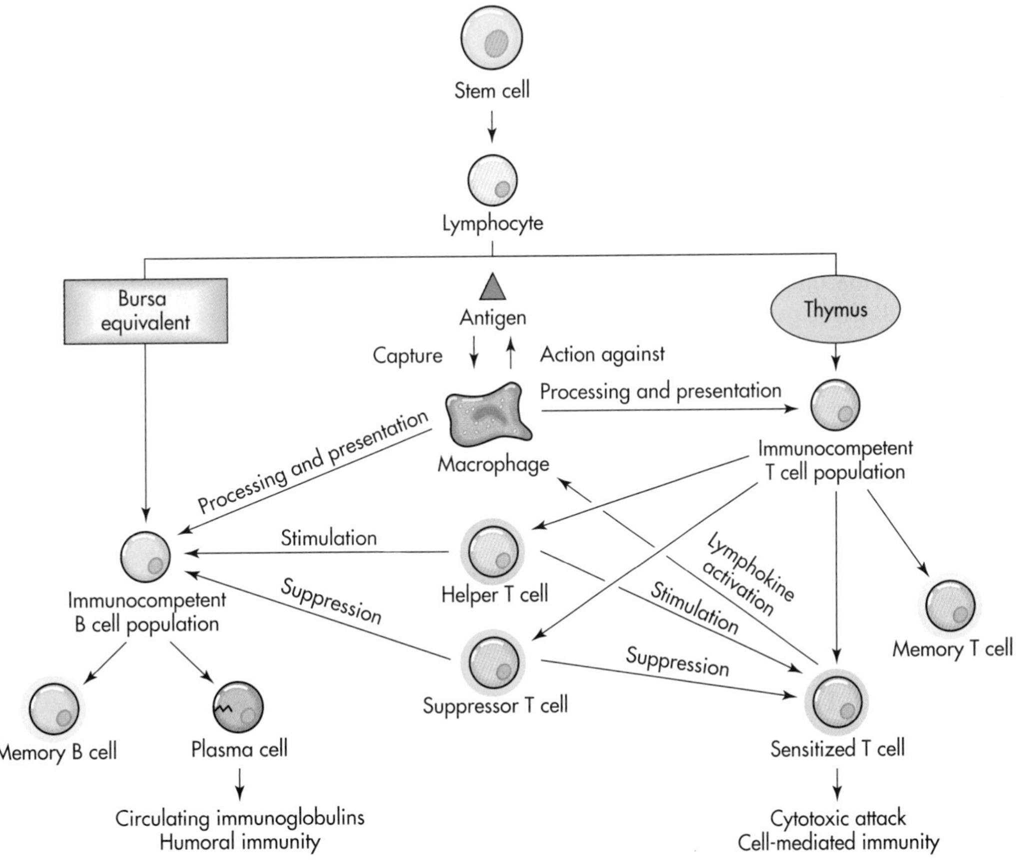

Figure 48-9 Combined response of B and T cell systems.

introduction and carries the antigen to the lymphoid tissues. In the APC the complex antigen is degraded, and the antigenic determinants are attached to one of the cell membrane proteins on the APC known as a major histocompatibility complex (MHC) antigen on its surface. These same MHC antigens are the markers on the surface of the cell that allow recognition of self versus nonself cells. The APC, with the concentrated antigenic determinants, then presents the antigenic signal to specifically reactive B or T cells in the regional lymph node. This is accomplished by a cell-to-cell contact. With this interaction the specific B or T cell is stimulated to undergo proliferation (cell division) and differentiation (change in structure and function). A soluble material known as interleukin 1 (IL-1) released from the APC signals the lymphocyte to divide and differentiate.

The progeny of the stimulated cell increases in number within the lymph node, forming clones of specifically adapted lymphocytes. If a B cell is stimulated each new generation of lymphocytes becomes more differentiated toward a cell population ideally suited for the synthesis and release of immunoglobulin. These cells are known as plasma cells.

With the development of the plasma-cell population in the lymph node (several days after the introduction of the antigen), antibodies can be detected in the lymph node. It is not until about 7 days after the antigenic challenge, however, that detectable levels of specific antibodies appear in the serum. The plasma cell population of the lymph node and the levels of antibody in the blood continue to increase for another 2 to 3 weeks, and then both begin to retreat. Some of the lymphocytes of the activated clone become "memory cells," which are much more responsive, both in time of reaction and efficiency of antibody synthesis, to subsequent contact with the antigen (Figure 48-10).

If a T cell is stimulated by an antigen it is referred to as a sensitized T-cell lymphocyte.

Proliferation occurs and sensitized lymphocytes are released into the circulation. These cells migrate to the site of the antigen's entrance into the body, where the invading agent or residual antigen is found. These activated lymphocytes, along with macrophages, infiltrate the regions of the tissue and begin a direct attack on the antigen or tissue cells labeled with the antigen. The T cells participating in this direct attack are known as cytotoxic T cells.

To amplify the site reaction further, the sensitized lymphocytes activate the nonspecific phagocytotic cells (macrophages, PMNs, and null cells) in the region of the antigen. This is accomplished through the release of the soluble cytokines, which marshal this additional cellular involvement to attack the antigenic materials.

The observable results of this attack of antigen-labeled tissues are classically illustrated by a positive tuberculin test reaction. In this case the inflammation (erythema, induration) observed at the site of the intradermal injection of a small amount of cell wall extract of *Mycobacterium tuberculosis* represents a T-cell attack on the antigen-labeled cells. The positive test result is actually mediated by a secondary immune response (see following discussion) produced by prior exposure to *M. tuberculosis.* With the introduction of the antigen, it is engulfed, processed, and presented by the APC to responsive clones of T cells in the regional lymph node. That clone of cells is stimulated to undergo proliferation, and activated T cells are released into circulation. The activated T cells seek out the antigen (at the site of injection) and begin to accumulate at the site, where they release cytokines (lymphokines) that stimulate null cells and macrophages to attack the tissues at the focal site. The lag time (24 to 48 hours) required for the development of the inflammation at the site is consistent with the time needed to trigger the release of the responsive cells from the regional lymph node and to accumulate at the site of the antigen-labeled tissues.

Control of Immune Response

Cytokines are soluble protein mediators that induce and regulate various aspects of immunity. They act as hormones and are synthesized by a variety of cells: macrophages, neutrophils, eosinophils, monocytes, and T lymphocytes. These protein mediators have been called by various names, as in-

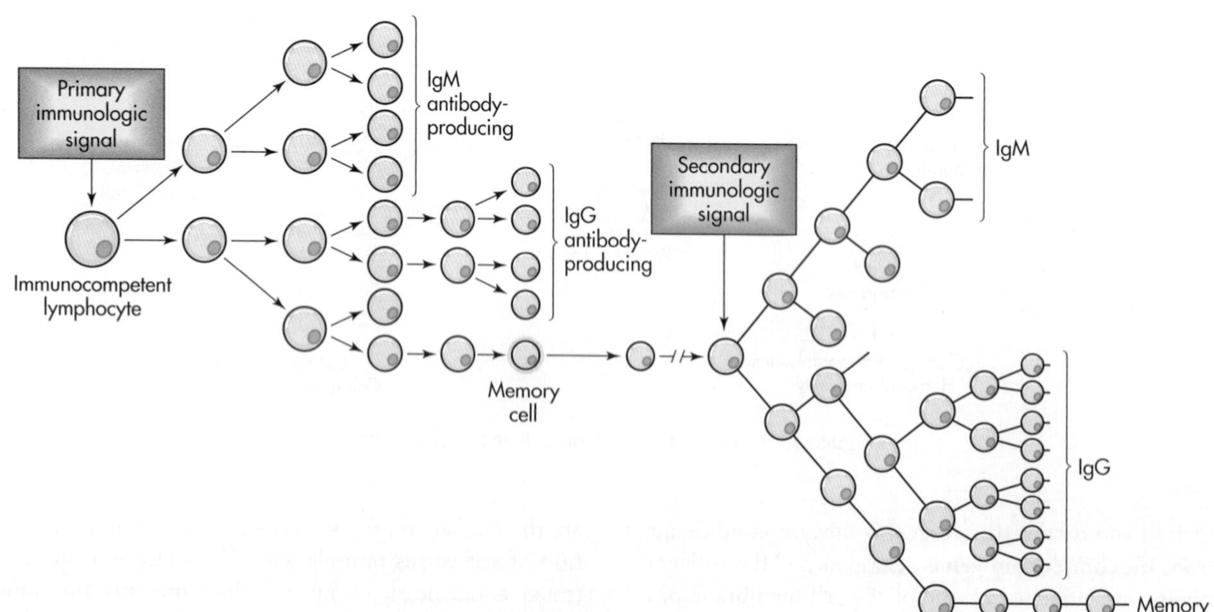

Figure 48-10 Response of memory cells to antigen signal.

formation about them was uncovered. Initially they were termed lymphokines when it was recognized that many of them were produced by activated T lymphocytes. When it was generally acknowledged that other cells secreted them as well, they were termed cytokines. An even more specific name, interleukins, recognizes that the major function of many of the cytokines is communication among various leukocytes. As many as 14 interleukins have been recognized, each with specific functions and structures.

IL-1 is produced by macrophages when they come into contact with bacterial products, the helper T cell, or tumor necrosis factor. IL-1 is an endogenous pyrogen; it increases the proliferation of helper T cells, stimulates growth and differentiation of B lymphocytes, and induces the secretion of other interleukins. Interleukin 2 (IL-2) is produced by helper T cells; it increases the growth and differentiation of T lymphocytes and also stimulates increased production of more IL-2 from activated lymphocytes. In addition, it increases nonspecific cytotoxic functions in NK cells (lymphokine-activated killer cells). Interleukin 3 (IL-3), produced by helper T cells, stimulates production of immature bone marrow stem cells in the presence of infection. Interleukin 4 (IL-4) and interleukin 5 (IL-5) also are produced by helper T cells; IL-4 stimulates growth and proliferation of B lymphocytes, whereas IL-5 stimulates their differentiation into actively producing antibody cells. Interleukin 6 (IL-6), made by both macrophages and T cells, is thought to have antiviral and possibly antitumor effects. IL-6 stimulates the growth of activated B lymphocytes.

Some of these interleukins are called colony-stimulating factors (CSFs) because of their role in stimulating the growth and differentiation of myeloid precursors, including a subset of pluripotent stem cells in the bone marrow. Among the known CSFs are IL-1 (for B lymphocytes), IL-2 (for T lymphocytes), IL-3 (for pluripotent bone marrow cell), IL-4, IL-5, and IL-6 (for B lymphocytes), granulocyte macrophage CSF (for granulocytes and macrophages), granulocyte CSF (for granulocytes), and monocyte macrophage CSF (for mononuclear phagocytes). Table 48-4 summarizes the major cytokines.

A second type of control is a nonspecific mechanism known as antibody feedback, in which the increasing level of circulating antibodies serves as a negative force on the further synthesis of antibodies. In other words, if circulating antibody levels are elevated, it is more difficult to stimulate antibody production with further antigenic challenge. This has clinical significance in the case of abnormal antibody production by persons with gammopathies, such as multiple myeloma or macroglobulinemia (see Chapter 49). These diseases are marked by significant elevation of the gamma-globulin fraction of the blood and a seemingly paradoxic increased susceptibility to infection. The high levels of nonspecific gamma-globulin exert an immunosuppressive effect on further specific antibody synthesis when the host is challenged by a pathogen.

The immune response system also is controlled by the presence of the helper T cells (TH or T4), which cooperate with the B cells and T cells to allow the full expression of a B-cell or T-cell response. If a B-cell clone requires the aid of a helper T-cell clone that is missing, the B-cell clone will not undergo proliferation and differentiation to form plasma cells that produce the specific immunoglobulin. On the other hand, the presence of suppressor T-cell clones (designated TS or T8 cells) prevents or suppresses the full development of the immunoresponsive clones (Figure 48-9).

If the normal balance between immunoresponsive T or B cells and TS and TH cells is disrupted, control over proper immune response reactions may be lost. The classic example of this problem is acquired immunodeficiency syndrome (AIDS), in which a disproportionate ratio occurs in the number of TS (T8) cells compared with TH (T4) cells in peripheral circulation; this results from destruction of the TH cells caused by HIV infection. In other conditions, such as some autoimmune diseases, the loss of certain TS clones may allow the production of antibodies against self-antigens.

In addition to these "in system" controls, immune cells are influenced by and in turn influence other regulatory systems in the body, specifically, the endocrine and neural systems. The immune response cells have receptors on their surfaces to receive modifying input from hormones, such as insulin, growth hormone, glucocorticoids, estrogen, and testosterone. Some of these hormone signals (glucocorticosteroids, testosterone, estrogen, and progesterone) have been shown to depress immune function. Other hormones (growth hormone, thyroxine, and insulin) tend to improve immune function. Other neurotransmitters and hormones found in lower doses in the body also influence immune response cell function. The negative effects of the corticosteroids are so great that they are

TABLE 48-4 Cytokines Liberated in the Immune Response

Cytokine	Function
Interferon	Inhibits viral replication Activates macrophages and neutrophils Activates natural killer cells
GM-CSF	Stimulates growth and differentiation of myeloid stem cells
M-CSF	Stimulates production of monocytes and macrophages
G-CSF	Stimulates production of neutrophils
Interleukin 1	Pyrogenic; stimulates helper T cells and B lymphocytes
Interleukin 2	Stimulates production of T lymphocytes
Interleukin 3	Stimulates production of bone marrow stem cells
Interleukin 4	Stimulates growth of B lymphocytes
Interleukin 5	Stimulates growth of eosinophils and function of plasma cells
Interleukin 6	Stimulates growth of B lymphocytes and stem cell production
Tumor necrosis factor	Pyrogenic; stimulates secretion of CSFs and some interleukins

GM-CSF, Granulocyte macrophage colony-stimulating factor; *M,* monocyte; *G,* granulocyte.

widely used as pharmacologic agents to suppress immune function (see Chapters 49 and 51).

Primary and Secondary Immune Response

The first contact between the immune response system and an antigen leads to the primary response in which there is significant lag time to the appearance of antibodies in the circulation (Figure 48-11). Immunoglobulins of the IgM class are the first to appear, but they maintain protective levels for only a short period. Specific IgG antibodies follow and reach protective levels within 12 to 14 days, but they also fall off fairly quickly with only this initial exposure. When the "primed" immune response system encounters the antigen again, a secondary response ensues, which is more rapid, of greater intensity, and longer lasting than the primary response. This secondary response is termed an anamnestic response. This "remembered" response is a characteristic of both the B- and T-cell systems. The prior contact with the antigen is stored in special memory cells of both cell lines. As illustrated in Figure 48-10, the memory cells respond immediately to the antigenic signal, so the lag time between exposure to the antigen and production of protective antibody levels is greatly reduced. This phenomenon provides the basis for active immunization and "booster" doses to maintain the protective levels of immunity. In an immunized person the memory cells elicit the rapid response in time for the immune system to overwhelm the pathogen or toxin before it can produce its damage. These memory cells are long-living lymphocytes, surviving and able to respond for years after their development.

Immune Tolerance

Immune tolerance is the state of immunologic nonresponsiveness. Normally the body is immune tolerant of self while maintaining responsiveness to foreign materials. Research has established that self-tolerance is acquired primarily during embryonic development though the exact mechanism is unclear.

Physiologic Changes With Aging

The extent of immunologic change that occurs with aging varies among individuals, depending on multiple factors such as genetics, nutritional status, and the presence of disorders that deplete the immune system. In general, however, the thymus gland atrophies and aspects of the immune response decrease. There is a decline in T-cell responsiveness and proliferation, even though the number of T cells are not reduced overall. T-helper and T-suppressor proportions are decreased, which results in increased numbers of circulating autoantibodies. Leukocyte migration ability slows and there are decreased numbers of cytoxic (killer) T cells, which diminishes antigen specific cytotoxicity. T-helper cells produce less IL-2, which further diminishes stimulation of T lymphocytes and NK cells. T cells respond more slowly to certain viral antigens, allografts (transplants from other persons), and tumor cells. B cell function is thought to remain relatively stable, even though autoantibody production is increased.[4]

Other physiologic changes affect older adults' immune competence and place them at increased risk for infection. Decreased epidermal and dermal skin thickness and decreased elasticity ("give" of the skin) make older adults more vulnerable to trauma and environmental injuries. Once the skin is broken, the healing process occurs more slowly because of decreased vascularity.[6]

Chemical barriers within many organs decrease, increasing older adults' susceptibility to pathogenic invasion. Estrogen loss in females, urinary retention, bladder muscle weakness, and prostatic disease place older adults at increased risk for urinary tract infections. Decreased ciliary action of the respiratory tract and decreased cough reflex can lead to aspiration or pneumonia. Decreased gastric acid and emptying predis-

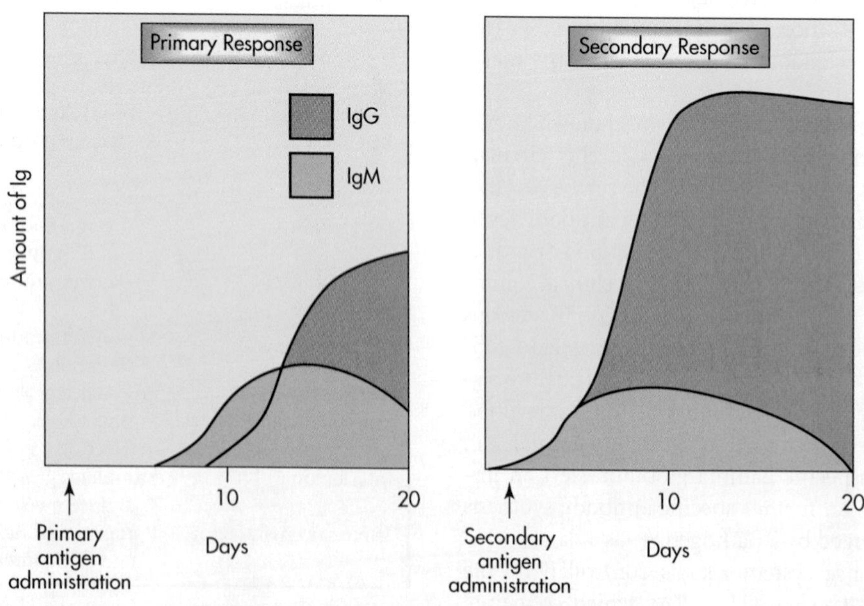

Figure 48-11 Primary and secondary humoral responses.

pose older adults to gastroenteritis or diarrhea. These changes in biologic processes can cause poor removal of organisms and an increase in microbe flora.

Older adults experience multiple chronic illnesses, are hospitalized more frequently than younger persons, and undergo treatments that put them at risk for infection. Chronic illness may cause older adults to be less mobile, and immobility coupled with altered immune responses increases the risk of complications such as pneumonia and skin breakdown.[4]

The end result of immune system changes in older adults is an increased risk for and incidence of infections, increased number of tumors, and an increased incidence of autoimmune disorders. Common infections tend to be more severe, with slower recovery and less probability of developing effective immunity after an infection. Older adults are not, however, immune compromised to the same degree or in the same manner as a person with AIDS or those receiving immunosuppressive drugs.

HEALTH HISTORY

Persons at increased risk for infection (children, older adults, immunosuppressed, or immunodeficient) need to be identified so that preventive measures can be taken and early treatment initiated. Consequently an accurate health history is essential. The health history should include recent and/or recurrent infections, known allergies, history of autoimmune disorders, diet, and any therapy or environmental factors that may affect the immune system.

Infection History

Recurrent infections can be good indicators that the immune system is compromised. Patients need to be asked about the number and type of infections they have experienced, when the infections occurred, and if the patient has any insight into what might be causing the infections. This information provides a guide to physical examination as well as to needed teaching.

Fever may be due to an inflammatory response, an impaired immune system, or from rapid proliferation of WBCs. The pattern of the fever often provides clues to the type of infective process involved; therefore the onset, range and duration of the fever, and the presence of night sweats or chills are important data to collect. High fevers may be associated with viral or bacterial infections or serum sickness, whereas low-grade fevers may indicate allergies or autoimmune processes. Fever may also be a sign of transplant rejection.

Enlarged lymph nodes (lymphadenopathy) usually accompany inflammation but may also be seen with Hodgkin's disease or non-Hodgkin's lymphoma, or they may be a sign of transplant rejection. Location of the enlarged nodes provides data about the source of the inflammation or infection.

Allergy History

Allergic symptoms are triggered by a variety of allergens; therefore data are collected regarding allergens such as food, contrast media, medications, or other substances. The reactions to particular allergens can vary from a slight rash to life-threatening anaphylactic shock. The most common signs and symptoms of allergic reactions are skin rash, difficulty hearing from obstruction of eustachian tubes, watery eyes, nasal discharge, coughing or wheezing, and gastrointestinal problems such as diarrhea or colic.[2]

An environmental assessment is useful for patients with allergies, as it can help identify factors in the patient's environment that might be causing the allergies. Common home allergens include animal dander, house dust, mold, and mites. Chemicals or other items used at work, home, or with hobbies may be associated with allergies. Data about potential allergens help to identify sources that can be eliminated or controlled.

Other Data

A person's immune system can be adversely affected by medical problems and associated treatments. For example, patients with autoimmune disorders are often treated with steroids or immunosuppressant drugs, such as azathioprine (Imuran) to control the autoimmune process. Patients with cancer undergo treatments with radiation or chemotherapy, which may cause bone marrow destruction and further immune deficiency. Patients with diabetes mellitus or renal failure may undergo systemic changes that depress the immune response. Medical treatments, such as surgery, or diagnostic tests can interrupt the integrity of immune defense mechanisms. Because all of these conditions place the patient at increased risk for infection, it is important to collect data about their presence and any prescribed, alternative, or over-the-counter treatments or medications.

The patient's nutrition and psychosocial status are two aspects of lifestyle that can greatly influence the immune system. Malnutrition is a common cause of immune deficiency (defects in cell-mediated immunity, phagocytosis, and the complement system) therefore, it is important to collect data about nutritional habits. Patients' usual eating habits and present appetite need to be investigated.

Stress, which increases the production of cortisol, can compromise immune function. If the patient has experienced recent stressors, it is important to examine this aspect more completely and determine how the patient is coping with the stressor and how it has changed the patient's relationships with others.

Risk factors for HIV infection (blood transfusions, illicit drug use, high-risk occupations such as nursing and medical technology, homosexuality, unprotected sexual intercourse, or multiple sexual partners) need to identified during the assessment.

PHYSICAL EXAMINATION

Disorders of the immune system are more difficult to assess objectively because of less obvious physical markers. However, observations of the patient's general behavior, as well as the skin, lymph nodes, lungs, ears, eyes, nose, throat, and other body systems, may provide clues about immune dysfunction.

Patient Behavior

Immune disorders such as AIDS and systemic lupus erythematosus (SLE) may produce dementia from inflammation and cellular destruction. Patients with multiple sclerosis often experience personality changes, varying from inappropriate euphoria to severe depression, which can alter behavioral patterns. Cognitive dysfunction, disorientation, or confusion need to be investigated as they may indicate an immune alteration.

Skin, Hair, and Nails

The skin is inspected carefully for color, skin turgor, texture, temperature, and moisture. Skin changes provide information about altered immune processes. For example, jaundice of the skin may indicate an autoimmune disorder such as hemolytic anemia. Systemic sclerosis (scleroderma) is associated with thick, smooth, taut, shiny skin, whereas patients with Sjögren's syndrome have scaly skin and experience decreased sweating. Increased skin temperature may indicate the presence of inflammation, whereas coldness suggests arterial insufficiency as seen with Raynaud's disease (see Chapter 25).

Various skin lesions are often associated with immune alterations. People with allergic reactions often have a maculopapular rash at the site where they were exposed to the allergen or over the whole body if the allergy is systemic. Persons with SLE have a characteristic erythemic rash across the bridge of the nose and cheek in a butterfly pattern. Patients with AIDS often have malignant skin lesions called Kaposi's sarcoma, which are typically maculopapular and range in color from pink to bluish-purple (see Chapter 50). Patients with rheumatoid arthritis experience bony spurs located primarily over the knuckles and finger joints (see Chapter 47). Some autoimmune processes will cause notable patches of alopecia (patchy hair loss) or dry, brittle, and broken hair. The nails may show changes in color and configuration, or brittleness.

Ears, Eyes, Nose, and Throat

Assessment of patients with allergies may reveal serous otitis media with retracted tympanic membranes, which indicates obstruction of the eustachian tubes and fluid collection within the ear. The patient may repeat questions many times because of difficulty with hearing.

Patients with autoimmune disorders or hypersensitivity reactions may have periorbital edema. Dark circles may be noted under the eyes of patients with allergy because of chronic nasal obstruction that results in venous stasis.[3] Autoimmune disorders may cause changes in the conjunctiva, such as discoloration and vascular hemorrhage.

Nasal obstruction may cause the patient to breathe through the mouth, and the voice will have a nasal tone. Examination of the mouth and throat will identify any lesions in the mucous membrane or changes in mucosal color. Many autoimmune disorders cause oral lesions, and immunosuppressed or immunodeficient patients may experience thrush, a white exudate that occurs over the tongue and mucous membranes.

Lymph Nodes

Assessment of the lymph nodes includes inspection, as well as palpation, beginning at the neck and extending to the entire body. The location, size, surface characteristics, consistency, symmetry, mobility, and discomfort with palpation of the lymph nodes are documented. Inflamed, tender, or fixed nodes indicate the need for further investigation. The location of enlarged lymph nodes helps with the identification of possible sources of infection by the pattern of node involvement and usual drainage route (Figure 48-12).

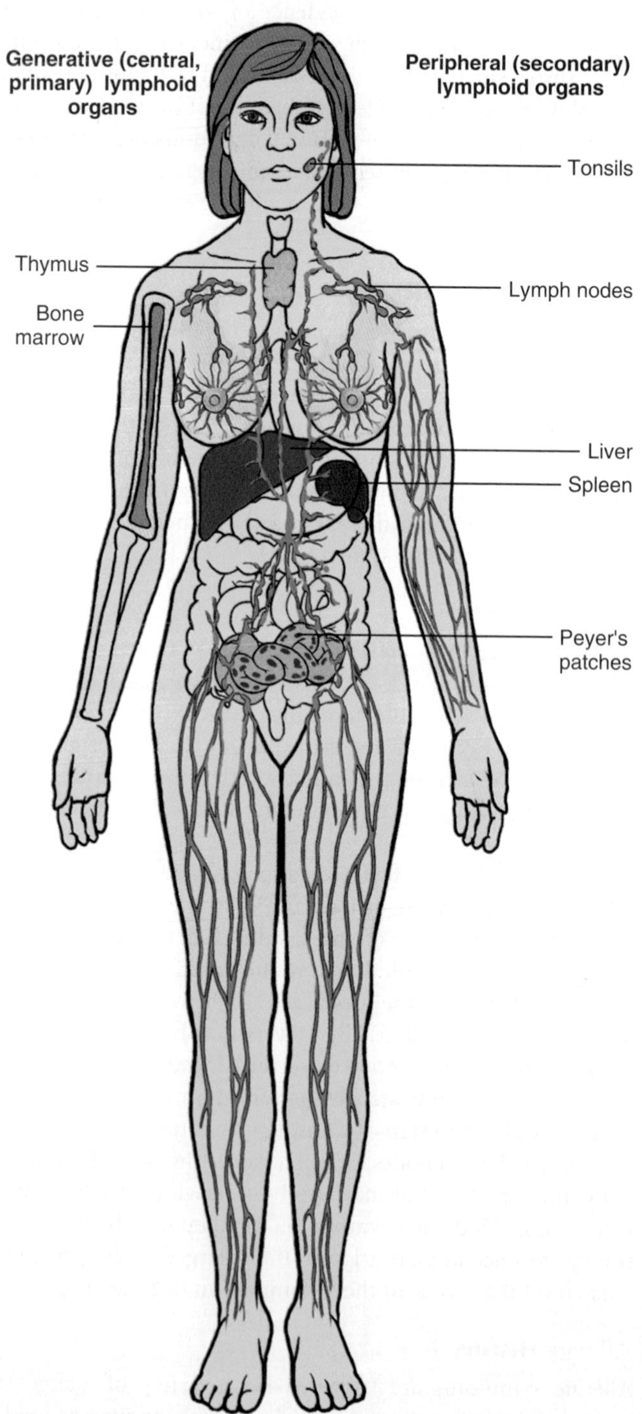

Figure 48-12 Major primary and secondary lymphoid organs and tissues.

Gerontologic Assessment

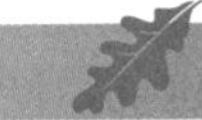

Assess for decreased skin thickness, elasticity, and neurosensory function.
- Decreased awareness of injury makes aging skin more vulnerable to trauma.
- Torn skin provides a portal of entry for microorganisms.

Assess for signs of infection (fever, increased heart rate, increased respirations, fatigue) and for decreased breath sounds or crackles, which may indicate pneumonia.
- Increased risk for respiratory infections because of decreased ciliary action, reduced respiratory muscle strength, and decreased gag and cough reflexes, which reduces the ability to expel inhaled microorganisms.

Assess skin for evidence of adequate circulation.
- Increased risk for altered circulation because of decreased cardiac output and increased peripheral resistance. Altered circulation delays inflammation and increases the risk for ischemic injury.

Assess for indigestion, nausea.
- Decreased gastric emptying, secretion of hydrochloric acid, and selected dietary enzymes, which results in less efficient digestion and decreased production of serum proteins.

Assess for signs of infection.
- Increased risk for infection because of decreased number and size of lymph nodes, decline in T-cell.
- Responsiveness, and proliferation and decreased number of circulating antibodies.

Respiratory System

Because persons with allergies typically show respiratory symptoms and immunosuppressed patients are particularly prone to pneumonias, it is critical that a complete respiratory assessment be performed. Cough pattern, sputum color, skin color, the work of breathing, and lung sounds need to be given special attention. Patients with pneumonia will display tachypnea and thick yellow or green sputum. They will use accessory muscles for breathing. Allergic patients will typically wheeze and cough, but experience little or no dyspnea. An allergic cough is characteristically hacking and nonproductive.

Assessment measures and variations in normal findings relevant to the care of older adults are presented in the Gerontologic Assessment box.

DIAGNOSTIC TESTS

Laboratory tests, skin tests, and biopsies are the main sources of diagnostic evaluation of the immune system.

Laboratory Tests

Laboratory tests are used to assess the patient's immune status, identify offending antigens, and monitor the effectiveness of treatments. The WBC count with differential, erythrocyte sedimentation rate (ESR), C-reactive protein, total complement activity test, and phagocytic cell function tests measure the natural, nonspecific inflammatory response and phagocytosis. Protein electrophoresis, immunoelectrophoresis, autoantibody tests, and antigen tests measure specific, acquired immune processes.

White Blood Cell Count With Differential

The WBC count with differential provides information about the type of infection and the body's response to it. Normally a healthy adult will have a WBC count between 5000 and 10,000/cm^3; the healthy older adult range is typically 3000 to 9000/cm^3. Leukopenia, a WBC count less than 5000, often signifies a compromised inflammatory response or a viral infection. Leukocytosis, a WBC count greater than 10,000, indicates an inflammatory response to a pathogen or a disease process.[8]

If the WBC count is elevated, the differential count is examined to determine which specific group of WBCs (neutrophils, basophils, eosinophils, lymphocytes, or monocytes) is increased or decreased. The differential is listed in such a way that the percentages of cells total 100%. This means that if the bone marrow proliferates one type of cell, it will increase the percentage of this cell and conversely decrease the percentage of the other cell types. Neutrophils are among the first cells to migrate to the site of a bacterial infection, so an increase in the total neutrophil percentage greater than 70% usually indicates the presence of bacterial infections. The phrase *shift to the left* refers to the decrease in number of mature neutrophils (segmented neutrophils) and corresponding increase in number of immature neutrophils (bands or stabs) that occurs during acute bacterial infections (Table 48-5).

Lymphocytes are some of the first cells to respond to viral infections. Lymphocytes are the second most commonly occurring white blood cell. An elevated lymphoycte count is generally associated with viral infections, mononucleosis, tuberculosis or some tumors. Increased eosinophil counts are associated with allergic reactions and parasitic infestations.[8]

Erythrocyte Sedimentation Rate

The ESR or sed rate is the rate at which red blood cells (RBCs) settle and is expressed in millimeters/hour. An increased ESR indicates that there are increased globulins, fibrinogen, or other substances in the blood, which make it clump faster than normal, usually because of infection, malignancy, or collagen vascular disease.[8] The ESR is frequently higher in healthy older adults.

C-Reactive Protein

C-Reactive protein (CRP) measures an abnormal protein found 18 to 24 hours after certain inflammatory processes. It is commonly used to distinguish inflammatory from noninflammatory diseases, such as osteoarthritis from rheumatoid arthritis. A positive test result indicates the presence of an acute inflammatory reaction. CRP is frequently monitored in patients with acute inflammatory disorders to determine the best treatments.

Total Complement

Total complement (CH50) is a group of nine major protein components and some inhibitor proteins that assist with the inflammatory and immune responses. Once activated, complement facilitates chemotaxis, phagocytosis, and immune destruction of antigen. In healthy adults the CH50 ranges from

TABLE 48-5 Comparison of Normal and Abnormal White Blood Cell Count and Differential

	Bands (Stabs) %	Neutrophils (segs) %	Eosinophils %	Basophils %	Lymphocytes %	Monocytes %
Normal WBC Differential 5000	1	49	1	1	38	10
Bacterial Infection 23,000 (with "shift to the left")	15	65	2	1	13	4

A comparison of a normal and abnormal WBC and differential with a "shift to the left" demonstrating a shift from mature to immature neutrophils, called stabs or bands. The absolute neutrophil count has increased from 2500 to 18,400 (which is derived from multiplying the total WBC count by the combined percentage of bands and segmented neutrophils).

75 to 160 U/ml. During active antibody/antigen reactions or acute inflammation, complement is consumed and serum levels fall. As these conditions are treated and reversed, complement levels return to normal. Similar to the CRP, complement levels are monitored in patients with acute inflammatory conditions such as SLE to determine the effectiveness of treatment. Low serum complement levels are associated with autoimmune diseases, glomerulonephritis, renal transplant rejection, and serum sickness. Elevated total complement levels are associated with acute rheumatic fever. Older adults typically show higher values for these proteins than younger adults, because they have a higher incidence of inflammatory conditions.

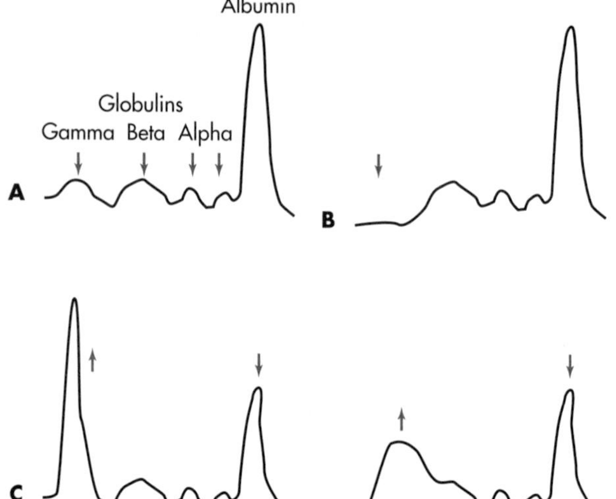

Figure 48-13 Electrophoretic patterns. **A,** Normal. **B,** Hypogammaglobulinemia. **C,** Monoclonal gammopathy. **D,** Polyclonal gammopathy.

Phagocytic Cell Function Tests

Tests can be performed to evaluate the phagocytic ability of PMNs and macrophages. One method is observing the absolute and relative numbers of monocytes and PMNs on the WBC count. The neutrophil functional assay is a primary test to evaluate the motility, recognition and adhesion, ingestion, degranulation, and killing ability of the leukocytes and macrophages.

Protein Electrophoresis

This test analyzes blood for protein content, specifically albumin and the globulins (alpha-globulin, beta-globulin, and gamma-globulin. These measurements are helpful in assessing immune function and in identifying various disease states such as hypogammaglobulinemias, macroglobulinemia, inflammatory disorders, neoplastic disorders, and dysproteinemia.[8] Figure 48-13 illustrates typical patterns seen with normal, increased, and decreased immunoglobulin levels. Immunoglobulins can be either increased or decreased, depending on the specific immune disorder present.

Immunoglobulin Electrophoresis

Immunoglobulin electrophoresis separates serum immunoglobulins from one another based on their quantity and electrical charge. The separated immunoglobulins are compared with specific antisera to determine which immunoglobulins are present. The test shows relative but imprecise quantities of immunoglobulins. Normal adult IgG levels are 600 to 1800 mg/dl, IgA levels are 100 to 400 mg/dl, and IgM levels are 60 to 150 mg/dl. Serum electrophoresis is used to detect and monitor hypersensitivity disorders, autoimmune disorders, chronic viral infections, immune deficiency diseases, multiple myeloma, and intrauterine infections.[8]

Nephelometry is a rapid yet accurate quantitative measurement of IgG, IgM, and IgA. The specific antibody is introduced into a fluid containing the specific antigen. The interaction of the antigen and antibody makes the fluid turbid; the degree of turbidity is measured by a photometric instrument. IgD and IgE are generally present in amounts too small to measure. Table 48-6 presents a summary of the clinical significance of altered levels of immunoglobulins.

Radioallergosorbent Test

The radioallergosorbent test (RAST) measures minute quantities of IgE contained in the serum. RAST is useful for detecting allergies and correlates well with skin test results. RAST testing is expensive, but is useful in testing patients for allergies who are taking antihistamines that suppress skin reactions.

Antibody Screening Tests

Numerous tests are available to detect antibodies formed against specific bacteria, viruses, fungi, or parasites Antibody screening tests confirm the presence of antibodies toward a

TABLE 48-6 Summary of the Clinical Significance of Altered Levels of Immunoglobulin

Class of Immunoglobulin	Increased Level	Decreased Level
IgG	IgG myeloma bacterial infections, hepatitis A, glomerulonephritis, rheumatoid arthritis, SLE, AIDS	Agammaglobulinemia, IgA myeloma, IgA deficiency, chronic lymphocytic leukemia, type I dysgammaglobulinemia, lymphoid aplasia, combined immunodeficiency, common variable immunodeficiency, X-linked hypogammaglobulinemia
IgM	Hepatitis A and B, Waldenström's macroglobulinemia, trypanosomiasis, chronic infections, type I dysgammaglobulinemia, hepatitis, SLE, rheumatoid arthritis, Sjögren's syndrome, AIDS	Lymphoid aplasia, hypogammaglobulinemia, chronic lymphocytic leukemia, IgG myeloma, IgA myeloma, agammaglobulinemia
IgA	SLE, rheumatoid arthritis, IgA myeloma, glomerulonephritis, chronic liver disease	Ataxia, telangiectasia, hypogammaglobulinemia, acute and chronic lymphocytic leukemia, IgA deficiency, combined immunodeficiency, common variable immunodeficiency, X-linked hypogammaglobulinemia, agammaglobulinemia, IgG myeloma, chronic infections (especially upper respiratory type)
IgE	Atopic disorders: allergic rhinitis, allergic asthma, atopic dermatitis, Wiskott-Aldrich syndrome with eczema, parasitic infestation, hyperimmunoglobulin E	Associated with IgA deficiency, intrinsic (nonallergic) asthma
IgD	Eczema, skin disorders	Unknown

From Mudge-Grout CL: *Immunologic disorders,* St Louis, 1983, Mosby.

particular antigenic source but do not necessarily mean that the person has the disease. Medications, infections, or chronic diseases can influence test results.

Autoantibody Tests

Abnormal antibodies that the body produces against itself are termed autoantibodies. Autoantibodies injure self-tissues and produce the symptoms associated with autoimmune conditions. Several tests are useful in confirming the presence of autoantibodies. Rheumatoid factor (RF) is an abnormal protein consisting of IgM antibodies found in the serum of persons with rheumatoid arthritis and other autoimmune diseases. Antinuclear antibodies (ANAs) or anti-DNA antibodies are gamma-globulins formed against properties of the cell nucleus. Tests for ANAs are positive in a large number of patients with autoimmune disorders such as SLE or systemic sclerosis. Healthy elders have increased antibodies (ANAs and RF), but the clinical relevance of these increases is unclear.[4]

Antigen Tests

Laboratory tests are useful for isolating and identifying specific invading antigens. For example, a positive result for HBSAG indicates the presence of the hepatitis B surface antigen, a specific antigenic determinant of the hepatitis B virus. Other tests isolate the antigenic properties of the antibodies toward RBCs. The indirect Coombs' test indicates serum antibodies to RBCs, which are not connected to the cell. It can be used to identify a patient's Rh factor. ABO and Rh typing are used to help determine blood type compatibility and thereby reduce the possibility of transfusion reactions. The direct Coombs' test detects antibodies coating the RBCs that are not detected by ABO typing. A positive test facilitates diagnosing hemolytic disease and autoimmune disorders.[1]

The lupus erythematosus (LE) cell test is used to help confirm the diagnosis of systemic LE (SLE), a classic autoimmune disorder. LE cells are neutrophils that contain large groups of abnormal DNA in their cytoplasms. Such cells are seen in 70% to 80% of patients with SLE. Cryoglobulins are abnormal serum globulin proteins found in the blood of patients with various diseases. Cryoglobulins can precipitate within blood vessels of the fingers when exposed to low temperatures. This produces arthralgia or Raynaud's phenomenon (coldness, pain, cyanosis).[8]

Certain subsets of T-lymphocyte cells called clusters of differentiation (CD) provide the clinician with information about the extent of immunodeficiency present in patients with AIDS. When the CD4 levels fall below certain parameters, therapy is initiated to help restore immune function. Infection and autoimmune disorders can also result in reduced CD4 levels. Other T-cell subsets are used to detect T-cell leukemias, T-cell lymphoma, or B-cell tumors.[8]

Human Immunodeficiency Virus Tests

The enzyme-linked immunosorbent assay (ELISA) and Western blot tests are used to detect the presence of HIV antibodies. The ELISA is positive when blood or body fluid reacts with the surface antigen of a killed HIV virus. The test is highly sensitive and is the primary test used for mass screening for HIV infection. The Western blot, another immune assay test, is used to confirm the presence of HIV antibodies in persons who test positive on the ELISA test. It identifies very specific HIV protein antigen-specific antibodies. When used in combination, the specificity of these tests for HIV antibodies is greater than 99.9%.[1]

The absolute CD4 cell count is used to test the progressive depletion of CD4 T lymphocytes in persons with HIV infection. The risk for disease progression and development of opportunistic infections increases as the number of CD4 T lymphocytes decline. Another test that predicts HIV disease progression is the plasma viral load. This test measures the amount or concentration of HIV in the circulation and is a reflection of viral replication. As viral load increases, the risk for disease progression increases. Both of these tests are used to determine the need for more or less aggressive HIV therapy and to monitor treatment effectiveness.

Special Tests

Biopsy

A lymph node biopsy may be performed in patients with enlarged lymph nodes (lymphadenopathy) to determine if inflammation or malignancy is present. A synovial biopsy may be performed to obtain synovial fluid from a joint to differentiate among various types of arthritis or bone malignancies.

The nurse's role in biopsy procedures includes teaching the patient about the procedure and assisting the physician. Most biopsies are completed under local anesthetic in an ambulatory setting. After anesthesia is effective, the patient should perceive only a pressure sensation; pain generally indicates insufficient anesthesia. After biopsy, the area is covered with a sterile bandage, and the patient is instructed to monitor for bleeding and infection. Postbiopsy discomfort can be relieved by analgesics.

Skin Tests

Skin tests are a simple, relatively painless, and inexpensive means to diagnose particular IgE-mediated allergies. The suspected allergen is delivered by intradermal injection, or a scratch, prick, or puncture of the skin. Skin tests are influenced by skin reactivity to the allergen, amount of allergen administered, and degree of host mast cell sensitivity. Elderly persons tend to have a poorer response to skin testing owing to changes in their mast cell reactivity. Although intradermal skin tests are the most sensitive, they can also produce systemic reactions, anaphylaxis, or false-positive results. The scratch test is difficult to standardize and has the highest probability of producing a systemic reaction, anaphylaxis, or a false-positive result. The prick test enables more substances to be tested at one time, but bleeding can cause false-positive results. Closely placed sites can also interfere with accurate interpretation of results. The puncture method is used more than the other skin testing methods because of greater reliability, safer administration, and ease of use with children.

Anergy Tests

Skin testing is used to screen patients for T-cell immunodeficiency. Specific antigens, including purified protein derivative, candida, mumps antigen, streptokinase-streptodornase, coccidiodin, histoplasmin, and trichophyton, are injected intradermally. Reactions are read at 24-, 48-, and 72-hour intervals. The reactions determine hypersensitivity to the antigen, not the presence of disease. More than 90% of healthy persons will show a response to one of these antigens within 48 hours. Areas of induration are carefully measured. An induration of 5 mm or greater indicates a positive result. A person who does not react to any of these antigens is said to be anergic. Anergy is associated with immunodeficiency disorders.

Nurses frequently administer skin tests. The correct amount of allergen must be administered by the correct method to ensure patient safety and test reliability. Emergency equipment should be available before skin tests are administered because of the risk of anaphylaxis, and the patient should be monitored for at least 30 minutes after allergen administration.

Nursing Implications for Laboratory Testing

Many of the tests presented in this chapter require little patient preparation or nursing intervention other than teaching. In addition, they require little or no observation after the test. Even so, a clear understanding of the various tests will allow the nurse to conduct routine teaching, answer patient questions accurately, and recognize abnormal data that need to be monitored and reported.

References

1. Copstead LC, Banasik JL: *Pathophysiology: biological and behavioral perspective,* ed 2, Philadelphia, 2000, WB Saunders.
2. Huether SE, McCance KL: *Understanding pathophysiology,* ed 2, St Louis, 2000, Mosby.
3. Jarvis C: *Physical examination and health assessment,* ed 3, Philadelphia, 2000, WB Saunders.
4. Lueckenotte A: *Gerontologic nursing,* ed 2, St Louis, 2000, Mosby.
5. McCance KL, Huether SE: *Pathophysiology: the biologic basis for disease in adults and children,* ed 3, St Louis, 1998, Mosby.
6. Maas M et al: *Nursing care of older adults: diagnoses, outcomes, and interventions,* St Louis, 2001, Mosby.
7. National Cancer Institute (NCI), 2001, Internet document: *Understanding the immune system,* website: http://rex.nci.nih.gov/behindthenews/uis/uisframe.htm.
8. Pagana KD, Pagana TJ: *Mosby's diagnostic and laboratory test reference,* ed 4, St Louis, 2001, Mosby.

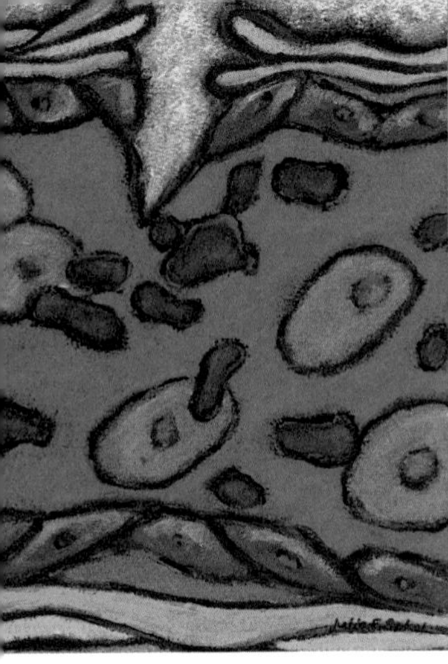

Immunologic Problems 49

Carol J. Green

Objectives

After studying this chapter, the learner should be able to:

1. Compare primary and secondary immunodeficiency disorders.
2. Develop a nursing care plan for the patient with an immunodeficiency disorder, addressing physical, psychosocial, and educational needs.
3. Describe the pathophysiologic changes that occur with monoclonal and polyclonal gammopathies.
4. Discuss nursing problems and interventions necessary for a patient experiencing multiple myeloma.
5. Examine the differences in immunologic reactions that occur between the four classifications of hypersensitivity disorders.
6. Delineate the nursing interventions that are imperative to prevent a hypersensitivity reaction.
7. Formulate a nursing care plan that includes discharge teaching for a patient with a type I hypersensitivity disorder.
8. Explain the pathophysiologic factors involved in immunologic blood reactions.
9. Describe the role of the nurse caring for patients with serum sickness.
10. List three examples of type IV hypersensitivity reactions.
11. Outline the possible etiologies of autoimmune disease.
12. Describe nursing management for the person with chronic fatigue syndrome.

In the normal healthy individual the immune response is a protective one; however, that protection depends on an intact immune system. Four primary aberrations in immunity can lead to disease: (1) a deficiency of one or more immune components (immunodeficiency), (2) an abnormal production of antibodies (gammopathy), (3) an exaggerated or inappropriate immune response (hypersensitivity), and (4) immunologic attacks on host cells (autoimmunity). These disorders are the basis of organization for this chapter.

IMMUNODEFICIENCIES

The four components of the immune system—antibody-mediated (B cell) immunity, cell-mediated (T cell) immunity, phagocytosis, and complement—act together and independently to protect the individual from infection and disease. Both primary (congenital) and secondary (acquired) immunodeficiencies produce chronic or recurrent infections that can lead to death.

Etiology/Epidemiology

Primary immunodeficiencies are disorders that occur from intrinsic, inherited defects in the immune system. There are many primary immunodeficiencies, and they are usually seen in infants and young children. The World Health Organization (WHO) recognizes 70 primary immunodeficiencies including, but not limited to agammaglobulinemia, common variable immune deficiency (hypogammaglobulinemia), selective immunoglobulin A (IgA) deficiency or low levels of IgA antibody, and severe combined immunodeficiency disease (SCID).[2] They are grouped according to the immune system component that is defective or lacking.

Primary immunodeficiency disorders are not common. Agammaglobulinemia occurs in 1:50,000 people, but severe combined immunodeficiency disorders are rare, occurring in 1:100,000 to 1:500,000 persons. Selective immunoblobulin (Ig)A deficiency occurs more commonly that other immunodeficiencies and may affect as many as 1 in 500 to 1000 individuals.[15]

Primary immunodeficiencies usually manifest themselves within the first year of life and have a familial pattern. Chromosomal abnormalities have been noted in some primary immunodeficiency disorders, but despite modern medical advances in understanding the immune system, the biologic errors of most primary immunodeficiencies remain unknown.

The most common immunodeficiencies are secondary or acquired. Any factor that interferes with the normal growth or expression of the immune system can lead to a secondary immunodeficiency. Immunosuppressive agents, malignancies, and chronic diseases such as diabetes mellitus are common causes of secondary immunodeficiency. Prolonged physical and psychosocial stress stimulates the production of corticosteroids, which suppress immunity and increase the risk for infections and tumors. T and B cells are reduced for up to a month after surgery, most likely related to stress. Malnutrition and subsequent protein and calorie deficiencies result in reduced T-cell numbers. The immune systems of older adults are less efficient, with decreased T-cell function, variable ability to respond to antigenic stimulation, and decreased proliferation of immune cells.[5] Human immunodeficiency virus causes a serious secondary immunodeficiency, acquired immune deficiency syndrome (AIDS) (discussed in detail in Chapter 50). Specific conditions that can suppress immunity are presented in Table 49-1.

Pathophysiology

Primary immunodeficiency disorders are characterized by intrinsic defects in immunologic cell development or function that results in B-cell (antibody), T-cell, complement, or phagocytic cell deficiency (Figure 49-1). Recurrent infections or repeated infection treatment failures generally prompt the clinician to suspect the presence of immunodeficiency. Without treatment, most individuals suffering from these deficiencies will die of overwhelming infections early in life.[14]

B lymphocytes produce proteins known as *antibodies* that recognize and mark foreign antigens such as bacteria and viruses, so that other immune components will react and destroy the antigen. X-linked agammaglobulinemia is an example of an inherited, B-cell immunodeficiency that results from failure of pre-B cells to differentiate into mature B cells. This disorder occurs exclusively in males and is usually diagnosed within the first three years of life.[17] Individuals with agammaglobulinemia are particularly susceptible to infections from pyrogenic bacteria such as streptococci, staphylococci, *Pseudomonas,* and *Haemophilus influenzae;* infections that affect the eyes, sinuses, ears, nose, and lungs; and viruses such as hepatitis and polio.[15]

Selective IgA deficiency is the most common primary immunodeficiency and has both autosomal dominant and recessive inheritance traits. The exact defect that leads to low serum immunoglobulin IgA levels is unknown, but may be related to impaired B-lymphocyte differentiation and subsequent loss of

TABLE 49-1 Conditions That Can Suppress Immunity

Condition	Effect on Immune System
Nephrotic syndrome	Loss of serum protein
Burns	
Protein-losing enteropathy	
Severe liver disease	Decreased protein synthesis
Cancer	Severe malnutrition; decreased protein synthesis
Alcoholism	
Malabsorption	
Uremia	Decreased T-cell function
Diabetes mellitus	
Infections (especially viral)	
Autoimmune disorders	
Lymphomas	Alterations in B-cell and T-cell numbers and function
Leukemias	

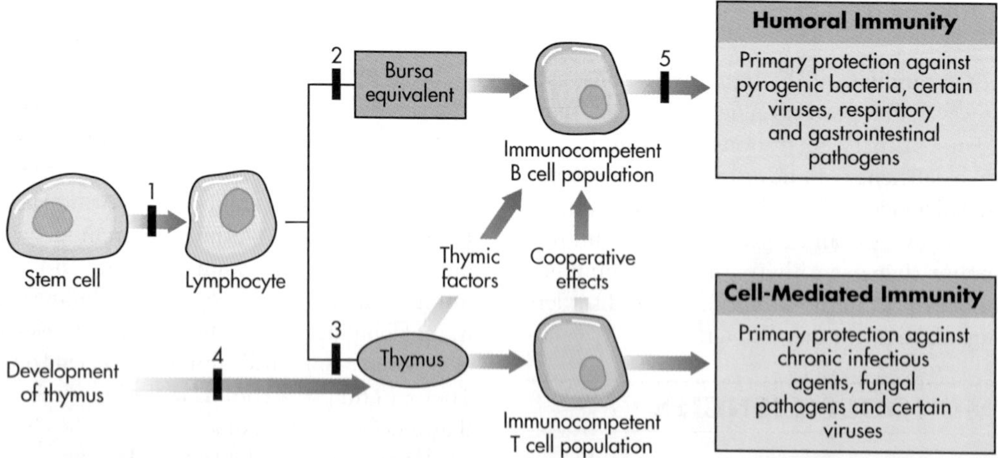

Figure 49-1 Causes of immunodeficiencies. Abnormalities at *1* result in combined humoral and cell-mediated immunodeficiency. Blockage at *2* produces agammaglobulinemia. Blockage at *3* or *4* results in drastic reduction in T-cell-mediated function and, because of cooperative effects on B cell system, some reduction in humoral response. Abnormalities in synthesis of specific immunoglobulin classes are reflected by blockage at *5*. Some blockages result in complete deficiency; others show up as reduction in response.

immunoglobulin-secreting ability. The disorder is associated with increased incidence of infections, autoimmunity, allergies, gastrointestinal disorders, and cancer.[17]

Thymic hypoplasia (DiGeorge syndrome) is a developmental disorder in which the thymus gland is unable to assist in the maturation of T cells, resulting in T-cell deficiency. Even though B cells are normal, children with total loss of thymus function are at increased risk for infection and rarely live more than 5 or 6 years without treatment.[5]

SCID refers to the complete absence of both T-cell (cellular) and B-cell (humoral) immunity. There are many variants of this disorder. In the most severe form, reticular dysgenesis, the common stem cell for white blood cells is absent resulting in subsequent loss of B cells, T cells, and phagocytic cells. Infants with reticular dysgenesis generally die in utero or soon after birth. A less severe form of SCID results from impaired stem cell maturation, which impedes T- and B-cell lymphocyte development. T and B lymphocytes are significantly reduced or absent even though other white blood cells are present in normal numbers.[11] People with SCID are at high risk for developing nearly every type of infection resulting from pancytopenia.

Phagocytes (neutrophils and macrophages) are white blood cells that engulf and destroy antibody-coated antigens. Phagocyte defects may affect their ability to move to the site of an infection or destroy pathogens. Chronic granulomatous disease is the most severe form of phagocytic cell deficiency. It involves a deficiency in the molecules needed by neutrophils to destroy foreign antigens.[15] Individuals with phagocytic disorders are at risk for developing mild to severe bacterial infections, whereas those with complement deficits have problems that range from recurrent infections to autoimmune diseases. Signs and symptoms depend on the site of infection and type of infecting organism.

The complement system is composed of proteins that attach themselves to antibody-coated antigens to facilitate destruction of the antigen. Persons with complement deficiency have a diminished ability to destroy invading pathogens and are at increased risk for infection. A common complement deficiency, C2 deficiency, is associated with an increased incidence of autoimmune disease and severe infection such as meningitis.[15] Table 49-2 presents a summary of selected primary immunodeficiencies.

TABLE 49-2 Selected Primary Immunodeficiencies

Disorder	Basis of Deficiency
B Cell Deficiencies	
Bruton's agammaglobulinemia	Sex-linked depression of all immunoglobulin classes; failure of prelymphocytes to mature into B lymphocytes; all serum immunoglobulins decreased
Common variable immunodeficiency	Variable degree of ability to synthesize primarily IgA or IgM in adults; high concentrations of autoantibodies and abnormal immunoglobulins
Selective IgA deficiency	Total absence or severe deficiency of IgA; the B lymphocytes that normally produce IgA are unable to convert to IgA-producing plasma cells
T-Cell Deficiencies	
DiGeorge syndrome (thymic hypoplasia)	Nongenetic failure of thymic development related to abnormal embryonic development of head and neck tissues and cells; normal or increased serum immunoglobulins; decreased T cells
Mixed T-Cell and B-Cell Deficiencies	
Severe combined immunodeficiency disease	Defect in stem cell differentiation and maturation of T and B cells; T and B cells decreased or absent
Wiskott-Aldrich syndrome	Sex-linked IgM and T-cell deficiency in males; tendency toward bleeding because of low numbers of platelets
Ataxia-telangiectasia	Autosomal-recessive deficit in IgA and IgE; decreased or normal T cells
Nezelof syndrome	Congenital failure of embryonic thymic development; normal or increased serum immunoglobulins; lymphopenia
Phagocytic Cell Deficiencies	
Chronic granulomatous disease	Sex-linked genetic disease in males that results in failure to destroy phagocytized organisms and particles
Chédiak-Higashi syndrome	Autosomal-recessive disorder with abnormal granule formation, neutrophil chemotactic response, and intracellular killing of microorganisms
Complement Deficiencies	
C1, C3, and C4	Develop bacterial infections; more prone to autoimmune processes (systemic lupus erythematosus, glomerulonephritis, Sjögren's syndrome)
Hereditary angioedema	Autosomal-dominant disorder associated with C1 inhibitor deficiency; results in large amount of vasoactive peptides and increased vascular permeability

Secondary immunodeficiencies result from numerous factors. Generalized *immunosuppression* is often induced therapeutically to decrease unwanted immune reactions, such as hypersensitivity reactions, autoimmune diseases, neoplasia, or organ rejection. Corticosteroids have both antiinflammatory and immunosuppressive properties. They inhibit movement of leukocytes and alter cellular and humoral immunity. When infection is present in a person receiving corticosteroids, the severity of the infection may increase despite the induced minimization of symptoms. Cyclosporine, a primary immunosuppressant drug used after organ transplantation, acts by inhibiting helper T cells and facilitating development of suppressor T cells.

Cytotoxic drugs and other cancer chemotherapeutic agents (alkylating agents, antifolates, and antimetabolites) destroy replicating cells. Consequently, they produce immunosuppression by destroying rapidly dividing immunologically stimulated cells. They also interfere with basic cellular metabolic processes in which B- and T-cell numbers are reduced.

Specific immunosuppression may be induced in people with hypersensitivities by administration of antigens in small amounts over time. This antigenic stimulation forms circulating IgG antibodies (immunoglobulins) that combine with the offending antigen to block contact with immunocompetent cells or IgE-coated mast cells, thus suppressing the immune response and preventing hypersensitivity reactions. Allergists use an adaptation of this method to desensitize persons who are allergic to antigens such as pollens or dust mites. A slightly different method of immunosuppression involves administration of a specific antibody, which then combines with the antigen to block contact with the immunocompetent cell. This method is used successfully in obstetrics to prevent the sensitive Rh-negative mother from reacting to an Rh-positive fetus during pregnancy.

Antilymphocytic globulin and antithymocytic globulin are antisera prepared by isolating the active globulin fraction from the serum of horses, goats, or rabbits that have been immunized with human lymphocytes or thymocytes. These antisera produce immunosuppression by decreasing all lymphocytes, although T cells are more affected than B cells. Because these globulins are xenogeneic (from another species), serum sickness may occur, and this limits their use to short-term therapy.

Monoclonal antibodies (MoAbs) are also used to suppress immunity. Because they are derived from a single cell line (monoclonal), they are very specific and can be targeted against subpopulations of lymphocytes, such as helper T cells.[17] Monoclonal antibodies are useful in treating cancers, (see Chapter 15), autoimmune disorders, and renal allograft rejection (see Chapter 51). Drugs commonly used for immunosuppression are described in Table 49-3.

TABLE 49-3 Major Immunosuppressive Drug Categories

Immunologic Action	Indications for Use
Corticosteroids (e.g., Prednisone)	
Inhibit T-cell proliferation Decrease interleukin-2 production Decrease macrophage and neutrophil function Inhibit T-helper and T-suppressor cell activity	Disease in which immune disorder is unknown Autoimmune diseases (e.g., systemic lupus erythematosus) Allergic disorders (e.g., asthma) Transplant rejection (e.g., kidney transplant)
Cytotoxic Drugs	
Alkylating Agents (e.g., Cyclophosphamide)	
Interfere with DNA, RNA, and protein synthesis Lymphocytolytic Depress B-cell, macrophage, and monocyte function	Autoimmune diseases (e.g., systemic sclerosis) Lymphomas Leukemias Granulomatous diseases (e.g., thyroiditis)
Antimetabolites (e.g., Azathioprine)	
Interfere with RNA, DNA, and protein synthesis Depress bone marrow and antibody production Depress T-cell function	Autoimmune disease (e.g., multiple sclerosis, systemic lupus erythematosus) Organ transplantation Pemphigus (e.g., skin disease) Neoplasia (e.g., cancers)
Antifolates (e.g., Methotrexate)	
Cause deficiency of folate coenzymes preventing synthesis of thymine and purines	Autoimmune disease (e.g., rheumatoid arthritis) Neoplasia (e.g., cancers)
Transplant Immunosuppressants	
(e.g., Cyclosporine, Sandimmune)	
Inhibits helper T-cell, lymphokine, and interleukin-2 production Facilitates suppressor T-cell development	Allograft rejection Graft-versus-host disease

Many chemicals have immunosuppressive effects in exposed humans. T lymphocytes seem to be affected more severely than other immune cells. Examples of potentially damaging environmental chemicals are asbestos, dioxin, insecticides, and heavy metals. Irradiation also suppresses immunity by suppressing both primary and secondary immune responses, although primary suppression is more effective. Irradiation destroys lymphocytes either directly or through depletion of precursor stem cells.

Collaborative Care Management

The primary goals of collaborative management for patients with suspected immunodeficiency disorders are to (1) identify those at risk for the disorder, (2) prevent infection or effectively treat existing infections, and (3) replace missing humoral or cellular immunologic factors.

Diagnostic tests for immunodeficiencies include complete blood count with differential, immunoglobulin assays and titers, absolute neutrophil counts, total lymphoycte counts, qualitative B-cell and T-cell studies, antinuclear antibody studies, and CH50. Fetoscopy and chromosome analysis aid in the early detection of some of the primary immunodeficiencies. See Chapter 48 for a more detailed discussion of diagnostic tests for immune function.

Research has led to improved therapy for patients with immunodeficiencies. Immunoglobulin replacement therapy, which contains primarily IgG and small amounts of other antibodies is accepted treatment for patients with antibody deficiencies (hypogammaglobulinemia). The optimal dose of IgG, which is usually between 400 and 500 mg/dl, is maintained by monitoring the trough levels of IgG in the blood. Immunoglobulins are usually given intramuscularly or intravenously on a monthly basis. Reactions to immunoglobulins can include back or abdominal pain, nausea and vomiting, chills and fever, headache, myalgia, or fatigue. Fortunately, anaphylactic reactions to immunoglobulins are rare. Immunoglobulin therapy is extremely expensive; the annual cost of therapy for a 70-kg adult starts at approximately $25,000 per year.

Bone marrow transplantation may be used for patients with T-cell deficiencies. The major risk of this therapy is graft-versus-host disease (GVHD). Bone marrow cells from a family member with identical human leukocyte antigens (HLA) has been used successfully in treating patients with combined immunodeficiencies.[15] Immune system modulators such as interferon gamma has been shown to improve the function of white blood cells (WBCs) (neutrophils) in patients with chronic granulomatous disease.

Antimicrobial agents to prevent and treat infections is a key aspect of treatment for both primary and secondary immunodeficiencies. Patients who are immunodeficient or immunosuppressed are particularly susceptible to viral and fungal pathogens and must be protected from infection. Protective isolation to prevent exposure to pathogens may be necessary if the person must undergo hospitalization. A private room is warranted for patients with severe leukopenia and laminar flow unit or hepa filtered room is indicated for those who are severely immunodeficient. Good hand washing for anyone coming in contact with the patient is essential to decrease the patient's risk for infection. All equipment and supplies are sterilized before being taken into the patient's room. As an additional precaution, the number of persons entering the controlled environment is kept to a minimum and staff and visitors are screened for colds and infections. If severe neutropenia is present (<500), fresh fruits, vegetables, and flowers are avoided because they could harbor bacteria.

Patients with immunodeficienies or undergoing induced immunosuppression are consistently monitored for indications of systemic infection, such as fever, changes in vital sign pattern, irritability, fatigue, or cough (see Chapter 11). Meticulous skin and perineal care and a clean environment reduce the patient's potential for infection. Adequate nutrition and hydration help support the immune system. Injections are avoided and invasive lines are kept to a minimum whenever possible. When invasive lines are necessary, insertion sites are carefully monitored. Suspicious drainage is cultured. Laboratory data are monitored to detect new infections and to determine the effectiveness of medications and other treatments. No live immunizations or oral polio vaccines are administered to immune-compromised patients because of the risk of viral infections contracted via the immunizations.

Patient/Family Education. Immunodeficient or immunosuppressed patients and their families need to know the nature of the immunodeficiency and how to avoid infection. Many patients do not require hospitalization, but they do need to be taught about infection control measures to follow at home. The nurse educates family members about signs and symptoms of infection and what symptoms need to be reported to the health care clinician. People who have infections such as colds or chickenpox should be requested not to visit. Teaching includes information about the use of protective strategies such as hand washing, dietary precautions (e.g., thorough cooking of meat products), and washing of fruits and vegetables. Careful attention should be given to older adults because of their increased risk for infection due to a decline in T-cell function and immune response efficiency[5] (see Patient Teaching and Evidence-Based Practice boxes).

A balanced, nutritious diet is an important part of treatment for persons with immunodeficiency diseases. The diet should include all food groups, with adequate calories and protein to support tissue building. There are no specific activity restrictions; however, the nurse cautions patients about becoming overly tired. Patients with immunodeficiency disorders need to understand the importance of ongoing follow-up care. Referrals to community or home health nurses for continued assessment and treatment of infections may be necessary. Hospice care may be appropriate for patients with terminal primary or secondary immunodeficiency disorders (see Complementary & Alternative Therapy box).

Patient Teaching
The Patient With Immunodeficiency

1. Explain the nature of the immunodeficiency (the inability of the body to adequately fight infection).
2. Teach measures to prevent infections.
   a. Avoid persons with infections (especially colds).
   b. Inspect skin daily for lesions or breaks.
   c. Avoid bumping, breaking, or tearing skin.
   d. Eat a well-balanced diet with sufficient calories to maintain ideal weight.
   e. Drink at least six glasses of fluid daily.
   f. Avoid becoming overly fatigued.
   g. Try to get sufficient sleep every night.
   h. Decrease environmental contaminants.
      (1) Avoid stagnant water (vases) to prevent bacterial growth.
      (2) Keep indoor pets clean by bathing frequently.
      (3) Avoid cold-mist humidifiers that can harbor bacteria.
   i. Take prophylactic antibiotics before any manipulative or invasive procedures (dental procedures, biopsies, endoscopies, arteriograms).
   j. Keep scheduled follow-up appointments with health care provider.
3. Report signs of infection immediately (increased temperature, redness or swelling of skin or mucous membranes, change in color of sputum, unusual drainage, diarrhea).

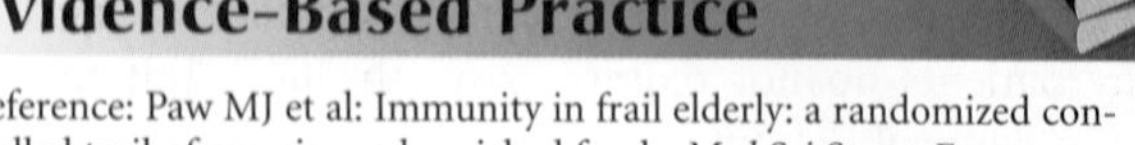

Evidence-Based Practice

Reference: Paw MJ et al: Immunity in frail elderly: a randomized controlled trail of exercise and enriched foods, *Med Sci Sports Exerc* 32(12):2005, 2000.

The study examined the effect of a progressive exercise program and an enriched diet on the cellular immune response of 112 independently living, frail older adults. The control group received the identical, but nonenriched foods and no exercise program. After 17 weeks nonexercising subjects had a larger decline in cellular immunity than exercising subjects. The study demonstrated that microenriched foods had no effect, but exercise may prevent or slow the age-related decline in immune response.

Complementary & Alternative Therapies
Garlic

Garlic is a well-known culinary and medicinal herb *(Allium sativum)*. It has been used since the days of the Egyptians to treat wounds, infections, tumors, and intestinal parasites. The herb contains sulfur compounds, which give it its pungent, spicy aroma, and are responsible for many of its healing properties.

Studies indicate that garlic enhances the immune system by stimulating the activity of macrophages and white blood cells, and increasing the activity of T-helper cells. Garlic's immune properties seem to be effective against viruses, bacteria, and yeast. It is particularly useful for respiratory viral infections since it clears mucus from the lungs.

Garlic also inhibits the growth of parasites in the intestine, such as amebas that cause dysentery. Currently it is being studied as a possible treatment for cryptosporidium infection in patients with AIDS.

Garlic may be consumed raw, although it does leave its potent, characteristic aroma. Dried garlic is an alternative, more acceptable choice, as it contains the important sulfur compound without leaving an unpleasant odor.

Reference: Holladay S: Garlic: the great protector. Botanical.com, website: http://www.botanical.com/botanical/article/garlic.html, 2001.

GAMMOPATHIES

Gammopathies, also termed hypergammaglobulinemias, are elevated levels of gamma globulin in serum resulting from overproduction. The blood normally contains a large number of different proteins collectively called plasma proteins. One type of protein, gamma globulin, combines to make varying types of antibodies for fighting different infections. When the majority of protein produced is an identical type of gamma globulin, the abnormally produced protein is called monoclonal gammopathy or plasma cell dyscrasia. Multiple myeloma and macroglobulinemia are plasma cell dyscrasias that have distinctive clinical patterns.

When a monoclonal gammopathy occurs in the absence of disease such as myeloma or lymphoma, the disorder is called monoclonal gammopathy of unknown significance (MGUS). About 2% of people aged 65 years or older have MGUS in the United States. The clinical importance of MGUS is not yet well understood. The majority of patients with MGUS have a low level of monoclonal proteins, remain symptom free, and lead a normal life. Of patients with MGUS, 20% to 25% will develop multiple myeloma or related lymphoproliferative disorder.[3]

Polyclonal gammopathies involve the overproduction of virtually all classes of immunoglobulins in response to inappropriate antigenic stimulation. High levels of dysfunctional immunoglobulins depress the synthesis of normal immunoglobulins, leaving the patient susceptible to infection. IgG and IgM are the most commonly involved immunoglobulins. The immunoglobulin levels reflect the severity of disease produced. Polyclonal gammopathies are associated with chronic bacterial infections and connective tissue diseases such as lupus erythematosus and rheumatoid arthritis. The polyclonal gammopathies are summarized in Table 49-4.

Multiple Myeloma

Etiology/Epidemiology

Multiple myeloma is the most serious and prevalent of the monoclonal gammopathies. It affects approximately 2 to 3 per 100,000 people in the United States, with 13,000 to 15,000 new cases appearing each year.[3] The male/female ratio is 1.6:1 and most patients are over the age of 40.[1] African-Americans are affected twice as often as Caucasians (see Evidence-Based Practice box). The origin of multiple myeloma is unknown, but studies have shown associations with agricultural occupations and radiation and benzene exposure.[3]

Pathophysiology

Multiple myeloma is a cancer of the bone marrow, which occurs from uncontrolled growth of plasma cells. Normally the

TABLE 49-4 Polyclonal Gammopathies (Hypergammaglobulinemia)

Etiologies	Characteristics
Infectious diseases Chronic bacterial infections (lung abscess and osteomyelitis)	Diffuse increase in antibody synthesis as a result of inappropriate antigen stimulation IgG and IgM most commonly involved immunoglobulins
Connective tissue disease Systemic lupus erythematosus Rheumatoid arthritis Chronic active liver disease	The immunoglobulin levels correlate the severity of disease High levels of dysfunctional immunoglobulins depress the synthesis of normal immunoglobulins, leaving the person susceptible to infection

Evidence-Based Practice

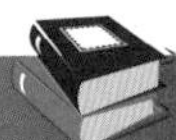

Reference: Baris D et al: Socioeconomic status and multiple myeloma among U.S. Blacks and Whites, *Am J Public Health*, 90(8):1277, 2000.

This study examined the relationship between socioeconomic status and risk for multiple myeloma among African-American and Caucasian populations in the United States. Information on occupation, income, and education was obtained from study subjects. Risks for multiple myeloma were significantly elevated for subjects in the lowest categories of occupation, income, and education, with low education and low income accounting for 17% and 28%, respectively, of excess incidence in African-Americans. The study concluded that socioeconomic factors do account for a substantial degree of the differential between African-Americans and Caucasians in the incidence of multiple myeloma.

bone marrow contains less than 5% plasma cells. Patients with multiple myeloma have bone marrow that contains between 10% and 90% plasma cells. Because of their numbers, the plasma cells are readily visible on microscopic examination of bone marrow specimens. The malignant plasma cells are most often monoclonal, originating from one single defective cell.[9]

The disease is often associated with multiple osteolytic lesions, hypercalcemia, anemia, renal damage, and increased susceptibility to bacterial infections.[1] The onset is slow and insidious, so symptoms may not develop until late in the disease. By the time of diagnosis, bone lesions are typically present in the skull, spine, and pelvis.

Diagnosis is based on computed tomography scans and radiography that show a "punched-out" type of bone lesion or generalized osteoporosis of the axial skeleton. Normal immunoglobulins are decreased and anemia, leukopenia, and thrombocytopenia may be present depending on the degree of bone marrow involvement and coexisting vitamin B_{12} or folate deficiencies.[4] Bone demineralization may result in increased serum calcium levels and protein breakdown may result in elevated serum uric acid levels. Twenty percent of patients have impaired renal function as a result of hypercalcemia and hyperuricemia. The estimated myeloma cell mass estimates tumor burden. Less than 0.6 trillion cells per square meter indicates low burden; greater than 1.2 trillion cells per square meter indicates high burden and advanced disease.[18] The clinical manifestations of multiple myeloma are summarized in the Clinical Manifestations box.

Clinical Manifestations
Multiple Myeloma

- Frequent recurrent infections (especially respiratory)
- Anemia, leukopenia, thrombocytopenia; abnormal immunoglobulin formation, depressed normal immunoglobulin formation
- Skull, spine, and pelvis fractures
- Spinal cord compression–paraplegia, quadraplegia
- Hypercalcemia, hyperuricemia, renal insufficiency, renal failure

Collaborative Care Management

Collaborative management of multiple myeloma is directed at reducing tumor cell burden and reversing complications. Chemotherapy prolongs the survival for patients with stage I disease for 40 to 46 months, stage II disease for 35 to 40 months, and stage III disease for 24 to 30 months. Oral melphalan combined with prednisone is the treatment of choice to reduce tumor load. Other chemotherapy agents such as vincristine sulfate and doxorubicin are used for patients with resistant tumors.[19]

Maintenance interferon alpha therapy has been shown to prolong the duration of initial remission. Glucocorticoids and calcitonin are used to reduce the lytic bone destruction and hypercalcemia. Intensive chemotherapy supported with bone marrow transplant has resulted in increased remission rates and improved disease-free 5-year survival rates from 12% to 52%. However, relapses continue to occur at a constant rate.[19]

When a patient has a solitary skeletal lytic lesion of plasma cells, is otherwise asymptomatic, and has fewer than 5% of plasma cells in bone marrow collected from an uninvolved site, isolated plasmacytoma exists. This condition responds well to local radiation therapy and has survival rates of over 50% at 10 years.[19] If the bone damage to the spine is extensive, orthopedic fixation devices may be used for stabilization and to prevent cord compression. If the patient has renal failure, dialysis may be necessary to correct the severe azotemia, hypercalcemia, and fluid overload.

Patient/Family Education. The major problems encountered by the patient with multiple myeloma are pathologic fractures, fluid overload caused by kidney failure, and infection. Nursing interventions, therefore, are focused around three areas: safety during mobility, fluid balance, and infection prevention.

Patients with multiple myeloma have extremely fragile bones owing to plasmacytosis and subsequent bone destruction. Ambulation is encouraged to prevent further bone demineralization associated with immobility. Safety is of vital importance because of the risk of fractures; a fall can have disastrous outcomes. Skeletal pain may be a deterrent to ambulation; therefore a lightweight spinal brace, analgesics, and local radiotherapy are used to control the pain. The nurse encourages the family to remove throw rugs from the home to eliminate a potential source of falls. If the patient is completely immobile, careful turning is important. In late stages, even a tug on the arm or a turn toward the bed rail can cause a fracture. A lift sheet and the assistance of several people are necessary to facilitate moving the patient gently and safely.

Patients and families are taught that adequate hydration is necessary to prevent renal complications from the increased amounts of urates and calcium being excreted in the urine. Fluid intake needs to be sufficient to ensure a minimum urinary output of 1500 ml/24 hr. If the patient is unable to maintain adequate fluid intake orally or requires nothing-by-mouth status for diagnostic or surgical procedures, intravenous fluids are administered. The patient is weighed daily to assess for fluid retention. The patient's blood urea nitrogen and serum creatinine levels are monitored frequently to evaluate renal function.

The nurse instructs the patient and family about measures to prevent infection, including avoiding persons with infections; maintaining skin integrity; avoiding fresh fruits, vegetables, and flowers; and following meticulous hand washing routines. The patient is reminded to seek medical attention for any signs of impending infection. Frequent turning and deep breathing exercises are encouraged to prevent atelectasis and pneumonia. A Nursing Care Plan for a patient with multiple myeloma is found below.

Nursing Care Plan — *Patient With Multiple Myeloma*

DATA Mr. T. is a married, 66-year-old African-American farmer admitted for primary treatment of multiple myeloma. Mr. T. has worked on his family farm his entire adult life. He was in excellent health until 2 years ago, when he began experiencing a series of bacterial infections. The multiple myeloma was diagnosed during a recent episode of pneumonia. He was immediately started on high-dose corticosteroid treatment, but his disease is believed to be fairly advanced and he has consented to aggressive treatment with chemotherapy plus radiotherapy to reduce the mass of the multiple bone tumors.

The nursing history reveals:

- Mr. T.'s wife is in failing health, and with no children in the area the couple is extremely concerned about losing the farm.
- Mr. T. has been experiencing severe fatigue over the past 9 months but has been reluctant to discuss this symptom with anyone. When directly asked, he admits to chronic bone pain in his lower back and pelvis.
- Mr. T. neither smokes nor drinks alcohol, and he and his wife have a strong religious faith, believing that "nothing happens without good reason."
- Mr. T. believes himself to be a strong person and is confident that he can regain his health and strength after treatment.

Admission diagnostic data include:

- Hemoglobin, 9.6 g; hematocrit, 28%; white blood cell (WBC) count, 6000
- Chemistry: serum calcium, 12.1 mg/dl; creatinine, 2.1 mg/dl; uric acid, 10.0 mg/dl
- Computed tomography scan and radiographic studies confirm the presence of multiple bone tumors and "punched-out" lesions plus evidence of widespread osteoporosis

NURSING DIAGNOSIS **Chronic pain related to presence of bony tumors and osteoporosis**

GOALS/OUTCOMES Will state that pain is controlled at manageable levels with pharmacologic and nonpharmacologic interventions

NOC Suggested Outcomes

- Comfort Level (2100)
- Pain Control (1605)
- Pain: Disruptive Effects (2101)
- Pain Level (2102)

NIC Suggested Interventions

- Pain Management (1400)
- Analgesic Administration (2210)
- Medication Management (2380)
- Progressive Muscle Relaxation (1460)
- Heat/Cold Application (1380)

Nursing Interventions/Rationales

- Obtain a thorough pain history, including (1) rating of pain severity, duration, and frequency; (2) factors that exacerbate and relieve pain; (3) pain control strategies used at home; (4) effects of pain on daily activities, appetite, sleep, mood, and general coping; and (5) knowledge of physiologic basis for pain. *To establish a baseline regarding pain and pain control methods. Chronic pain is a complex challenge and usually requires a multifocal management plan. It is essential to fully understand the patient's situation before planning any interventions.*
- Initiate referral to pain management team. *Chronic pain is best managed by a multidisciplinary team of specialists who can explore the entire scope of management options for the patient.*

Nursing Care Plan Patient With Multiple Myeloma–cont'd

- Administer nonsteroidal antiinflammatory drugs as ordered and encourage patient to use the medication on a consistent basis. *Management of chronic pain is best achieved by maintaining constant blood levels of analgesics rather than peaks and valleys. Medicating before pain becomes severe provides better pain control.*
- Explore patient's preferences in terms of pharmacologic pain management strategies and encourage him to begin incorporating those strategies into his daily routines. *Nonpharmacologic strategies work most effectively when patients are receptive to them. Such strategies often require practice before they become fully effective.*
- Explore effectiveness of heat/cold and relaxation for pain relief. *Heat increases circulation to the affected area. Cold reduces swelling and inflammation. Muscle relaxation may augment the effectiveness of other pain control methods and analgesics.*

Evaluation Parameters
1. Reports pain reduced and/or controlled
2. No facial grimace or expression of pain
3. Demonstrates use of nonpharmacologic pain measures
4. Reports satisfaction with nonpharmacologic pain measures
5. Self-administers prescribed analgesics accurately

NURSING DIAGNOSIS **Risk for injury to self related to bone demineralization**

GOALS/OUTCOMES Will identify injury risks in home environment and modifications that can be made to reduce those risks; will accurately verbalize the physiologic nature of his disease-related risk for injury; will maintain high daily fluid intake to prevent renal stone formation

NOC Suggested Outcomes
- Knowledge: Personal Safety (1809)
- Risk Control (1902)
- Safety Behavior: Home Physical Environment (1910)

NIC Suggested Interventions
- Environmental Management: Safety (6486)
- Fall Prevention (6490)
- Teaching: Disease Process (5602)
- Medication Management (2380)

Nursing Interventions/Rationales
- Ensure patient safety in hospital environment by maintaining adequate lighting and keeping the floor free of clutter. *An unfamiliar environment increases the risk of falls and injury, especially when equipment or unnecessary clutter impedes ambulation.*
- Encourage patient to change positions slowly and to avoid sudden, jarring movements. *Pathologic fractures can result from sudden movements when bone matrix is fragile, as occurs with bone tumors and osteoporosis.*
- Equip bed with firm mattress. *A firm mattress supports the skeleton and maintains vertebrae and joints in optimal position.*
- Explore home safety concerns with patient and wife, including equipment, rugs, and polished floors. *The majority of falls occur at home. Most homes contain numerous hazards that can be prevented or decreased with minor adaptations, such as removing scatter rugs or avoiding highly polished and slick floors.*
- Explore use of light braces or other assistive devices. Consider adding nonslip pads and hand grips, particularly in the bathroom. *The use of supports can allow the patient to remain active yet provide a sense of security and reduce the risk for injury.*
- Encourage a daily fluid intake sufficient to ensure at least 1500 ml of urine output daily. As much as 3000 ml may be necessary. *Bone demineralization creates severe hypercalcemia. Adequate fluid intake is the best strategy for preventing the development of renal calculi.*

Evaluation Parameters
1. Absence of injury
2. Reports methods to reduce home environmental hazards
3. Absence of renal calculi
4. Demonstrates correct use of assistive devices
5. Maintains fluid intake sufficient for 1500 ml of urine output
6. Accurately describes disease process

Continued

Nursing Care Plan Patient With Multiple Myeloma—cont'd

NURSING DIAGNOSIS **Risk for infection related to impaired internal defenses secondary to disease process, chemotherapy, and radiotherapy**

GOALS/OUTCOMES Will verbalize understanding of risk factors for infection; will implement risk control practices to prevent infection

NOC Suggested Outcomes
- Immune Status (0702)
- Knowledge: Infection Control (1807)
- Nutritional Status (1004)

NIC Suggested Interventions
- Infection Protection (6550)
- Nutrition Management (1100)
- Surveillance (6650)
- Teaching: Disease Process (5602)

Nursing Interventions/Rationales
- Teach patient/wife the importance of thorough, frequent hand washing. *Hand washing remains one of the most effective strategies for preventing infection.*
- Limit visitors if needed; avoid contact with persons who have active infections. *The patient may need assistance with limiting visitors and explaining the need for limited visitors while undergoing chemotherapy and radiotherapy. Visitors may unintentionally expose the patient to infections.*
- Monitor vital signs. *Clinical manifestations of infection generally include fever, chills, lethargy, and an increased WBC count. Immunosuppressive agents or immunocompromising diseases may mask overt manifestations of infection.*
- Teach patient the signs of infection and encourage him to report the development of any signs indicating infection. *The patient may be the first to recognize signs of infection. Early detection of infection is essential to institute early treatment.*
- Encourage frequent deep breathing, position changes, and routine hygiene. *Immobility coupled with shallow breathing can quickly progress to respiratory infection. Routine hygiene reduces the presence of microorganisms and enhances patient comfort.*
- Encourage patient to limit contact with fresh plants and soil and to wash fresh fruits and vegetables thoroughly. Explore implications for home routines on the farm. *Normal pathogens in soil and on foods can be sources of infection in the immunocompromised patient. Farmers are at particular risk for such infections.*

Evaluation Parameters
1. Absence of infection
2. Vital signs within normal limits
3. WBC count within normal limits
4. Demonstrates deep breathing exercises
5. Verbalizes understanding of infection control measures
6. Limits visitors

NURSING DIAGNOSIS **Activity intolerance related to fatigue secondary to altered tissue perfusion**

GOALS/OUTCOMES Will establish priorities for daily activities; will balance activity and rest effectively to complete desired daily activities

NOC Suggested Outcomes
- Activity Tolerance (0005)
- Knowledge: Energy Conservation (1804)
- Nutritional Status: Energy (1007)

NIC Suggested Interventions
- Energy Management (0180)
- Nutrition Management (1100)
- Sleep Enhancement (1850)

Nursing Interventions/Rationales
- Assess severity of fatigue and patient's understanding of the physiologic cause. *The patient is reluctant to admit his fatigue. Patients often consider fatigue to be a sign of weakness. A baseline assessment of the patient's fatigue is essential for later comparisons.*
- Encourage patient to prioritize daily activities and let go of unessential tasks. *Fatigue compromises one's ability to participate in daily activities. It is important that the patient's available energy be used to complete priority activities.*
- Explore strategies to (1) modify existing activities, conserving energy when possible; (2) seek assistance or delegate activities; (3) pace activities throughout the day to allow a balance between activity and rest. *Many daily activities can be modified to consume less energy, but this requires the patient's willingness to*

Nursing Care Plan Patient With Multiple Myeloma—cont'd

think about routine activities in a different way. Accepting the reality of fatigue may allow the patient to consider ways of seeking assistance or delegating activities that would not usually be considered acceptable.

- Encourage patient to obtain at least 8 hours of uninterrupted sleep at night. *Effective nighttime sleep patterns may decrease daytime fatigue.*

Evaluation Parameters

1. Balances activity with rest
2. Explains physiologic reason for fatigue
3. Performs only essential activities
4. Reports obtaining adequate nighttime sleep

HYPERSENSITIVITIES

The immune system is always ready to respond to foreign antigens. Under certain circumstances, however, this response may harm as well as protect. Occasionally, reexposure of a previously sensitized person to a specific antigen results in an exaggerated or inappropriate immune response that produces injury to local tissues or a dramatic systemic effect that can cause death. Such reactions are called hypersensitivity reactions, or allergies. The antigen producing the hypersensitivity reaction is referred to as an *allergen.* Whether an allergic response occurs and to what degree depend on a combination of interrelated factors that are summarized in Box 49-1.

Hypersensitivities are broadly divided into two categories based on the components of the immune system involved in mediating the hypersensitivity reaction: humoral response (B-cell mediated) or cellular response (T-cell mediated). This basic division corresponds with the clinical symptom division of immediate and delayed, which describes the timing of appearance of clinical symptoms and the speed of skin test reactions when a host is challenged with various allergens.

Hypersensitivity reactions are more narrowly classified into four types, as shown in Table 49-5. Reaction types I, II, and III are mediated by the humoral system (B cell), whereas type IV reactions are cell mediated (B cell). Because the first three types of hypersensitivities result from interactions involving circulating antibodies, they can be serum transferred from a sensitized to a nonsensitized host. Type IV sensitivities can be transferred only by lymphocyte exchange.

BOX 49-1 Factors That Determine an Allergic Response

1. *Responsiveness of the host to the allergen.* If the host is highly sensitive to the antigen, a greater than normal chance exists that a tissue-damaging reaction will occur.
2. *Amount of allergen.* Generally, the greater the amount of allergen contacted, the more severe the reaction.
3. *Nature of the allergen.* Any foreign protein or protein-containing component can serve as an allergen when coupled with a normal tissue protein carrier. Examples include pollens, foods, animal dander, house dust, and feathers.
4. *Route of entrance of the allergen.* Allergens may gain host entry via the respiratory tract, through epidermal or mucosal surfaces, by injection, or through the digestive tract.
5. *Timing of exposure to the allergen.* If the host's contacts with the allergen are widely separated by time, the immunologic mediators may be so dilute that there is little response. Conversely, if frequent contact is made with the allergen, reactions are more likely to occur.
6. *Site of the allergen–immune mediator reaction.* A reaction can occur in the tissues with little consequence; however, the same reaction occurring in the bloodstream can lead to a severe reaction.
7. *Host's threshold of reactivity.* The host's immune system can be changed by factors such as stress, fatigue, or infection, all of which can decrease the responsiveness of the immune system to potential allergens.

TYPE I HYPERSENSITIVITIES

Type I hypersensitivity (anaphylactic) reactions include a wide variety of conditions. All of these diseases are characterized by a rapid and exaggerated response directed by IgE antibodies toward an external substance serving as the allergen.

Etiology/Epidemiology

The tendency to become hypersensitive and produce IgE antibodies in response to inhaled or ingested substances is inherited as a dominant trait and referred to as *atopy.* If both parents are atopic, there is a high probability their children will be atopic. What an individual becomes hypersensitive to, however, is determined by the allergens to which that individual is exposed. A person does not inherit a specific allergy, only the predisposition to develop allergies. Allergic rhinitis, hay fever, asthma, atopic eczema (atopic dermatitis), venom hyperreactivity, and food allergy are examples of atopic diseases, which are often divided into two categories: seasonal and perennial. Seasonal allergens include pollens from trees, grasses, and weeds. Symptoms are produced when the person reacts to a brief tree season, followed by the grass and then weed season. Perennial allergens such as house dust, mites, molds, food, venom, latex, and animal dander are present throughout the year, and the sensitized person can experience symptoms at any time.

TABLE 49-5 Summary of Hypersensitivity Reactions

	Immune System Mediators	Allergens	Response to Intradermal Skin Test	Pathophysiologic Effects	Examples
Humoral (Immediate)					
I-Anaphylactic	IgE bound to mast cells	Exogenous antigens	Wheal and flare within 30 min, edema	Release of histamines, kinins, chemotactic factors, and active products of arachidonic acid metabolism (leukotrienes, prostaglandins, and thromboxanes) from mast cells, which affect smooth muscle, mucous glands	Systemic anaphylaxis, atopic allergies, hayfever, insect sting reactions
II-Cytotoxic	IgG or IgM (plus complement)	Foreign cells or alteration of cell surface antigens	Not done	Direct cytotoxic destruction of cells	Hemolytic disease of the newborn (Rh), transfusion reactions
III-Immune complex	IgG or IgM (plus complement)	Soluble antigens	Erythema and edema within 3-8 hr	Acute inflammatory reaction; primarily polymorphonuclear neutrophil leukocytes	Serum sickness, Arthus reaction, glomerulonephritis
Cellular (Delayed)					
IV-Cell mediated	T cells, macrophages	Infectious agent, contact allergens, foreign tissues, cancer cells	Erythema and induration within 24-48 hr	Tissue destruction, primarily lymphocytes and macrophages	Tuberculin reaction, skin graft rejection, poison ivy

There are nonatopic disorders that are also mediated by IgE (e.g., urticaria/angioedema and systemic anaphylaxis). These disorders lack the genetic link or specific organ hyperresponsiveness displayed by atopic disease. The allergic form of urticaria is usually caused by foods, especially eggs, fish, and nuts, or by drugs such as penicillins, sulfonamides, cephalosporins, aspirin, and other nonsteroidal antiinflammatory drugs. Angioedema is a form of urticaria, but it involves the subcutaneous tissue rather than the skin.

A more severe form of nonatopic reaction in humans is systemic anaphylaxis. Anaphylaxis is most often associated with drugs such as penicillin, streptokinase, or amphotericin B; insect or snake venoms; or foods, although almost any antigen to which a person is hypersensitive and previously sensitized has the potential for producing anaphylaxis. Latex hypersensitivity, which has a high potential for producing anaphylaxis, has become a universal concern among health care workers as evidenced by the 1987 precautions implemented by the Centers for Disease Control and Prevention. Numerous medical products contain latex, including gloves, catheters, and tubes. Studies have shown the prevalence rate for latex hypersensitivity among health care workers to be between 3.8% and 17% in the United States and between 2.8% and 12.1% worldwide.[20]

The onset of allergic diseases most commonly occurs between the ages of 2 and 15 years, although they can begin at any age. Skin test studies support the presence of allergies in more than 50 million people in the United States, with atopic disorders being the most common. Pollen allergies affect approximately 26 million people, or 10% of the American population. Allergic rhinitis accounts for about 9.2 million primary care provider office visits annually, and researchers estimate that between 2% and 4% of children have food allergies. Anaphylaxis (life-threatening hypersensitivity) occurs far less frequently, affecting approximately 0.4 cases per million a year in the general population. Allergic reactions to drugs such as penicillin or cephalosporine occur in about 2% to 3% of hospitalized patients, and insect stings produce anaphylaxis in 3.3% of the U.S. population.[17] No association has been found between gender, race, or geographic area and an increased risk of developing anaphylaxis.

Pathophysiology

Type I hypersensitivities are mediated by the IgE class of immunoglobulins. In genetically predisposed people, initial exposure to an allergen prompts B lymphocytes to produce IgE antibodies, which sensitize the person to the allergen. This initial contact with the allergen is known as the sensitizing dose. In some cases it may take several sensitizing doses of allergen before the person's immune system is fully ready to react. Once the person is fully sensitized, subsequent exposure (termed the

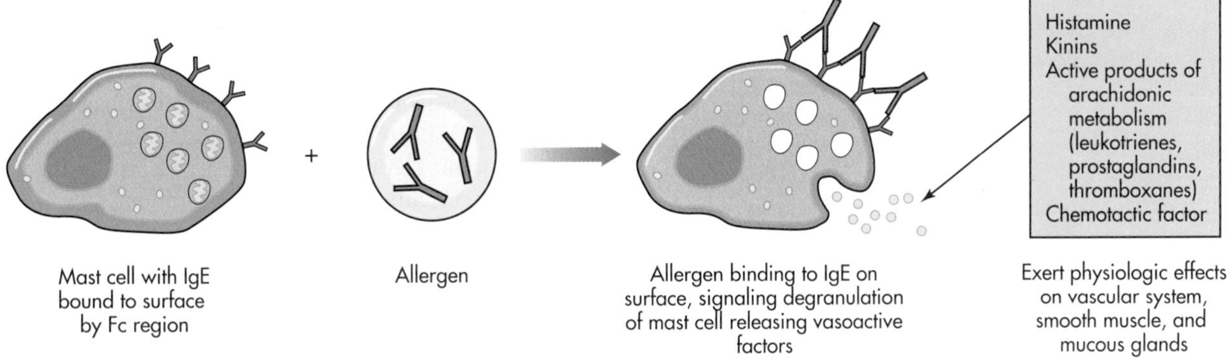

Figure 49-2 Mediators of type I hypersensitivity.

> ## *Future Watch*
> ### A New Hypoallergic Rubber on the Horizon?
>
> There is a growing incidence of hypersensitivities, including type 1 immediate hypersensitivity reactions, among users of natural rubber latex products throughout the world. These reactions are not only elicited through skin contact, but from inhaling airborne particles.
>
> Researchers in the Polymer Science Department at the University of Akron have developed a process to render natural rubber hypoallergenic. Most rubber products are made from Brazilian tropical trees, but these researchers are testing the process on rubber from the guayule shrub, which is native to North America. The scientists treated the rubber by a new process that removes essentially all of the proteins that serve as antigens in the previously sensitized host. The altered rubber products were tested on mice, and no hypersensitivity reactions occurred.
>
> The researchers claim that the rubber products from this new procedure are ideally suited for medical products and industrial and consumer products such as foam rubber, bandages, adhesives, garment elastic, and dipped goods such as gloves, condoms, tubing, and balloons.
>
> Reference: Schloman W: Polymer Homepage, University of Akron, website: http://www.polymer.uakron.edu/tech/286.html

shocking dose or challenging dose) results in the allergen combining with specific IgE antibodies that are bound to receptor sites on tissue mast cells and blood basophils. This antigen-antibody reaction results in a rapid release of potent vasoactive mediators such as histamine, kinins, chemotactic factors, and active products of arachidonic acid metabolism (leukotrienes, prostaglandins, and thromboxanes)[12] (Figure 49-2). Latex hypersensitivity reactions include the classic type 1 immediate hypersensitivity, which is IgE antibody mediated as well as the T cell mediated delayed hypersensitivity reaction. There is no cure for latex hypersensitivity, and avoidance is the only option for sensitized individuals (see Future Watch box).

Vasoactive mediators produce the clinical manifestations associated with type 1 hypersensitivity, which includes smooth muscle contraction, increased vascular permeability, and increased mucous gland secretion. Repeated cycles of exposure to allergens and type I responses can lead to chronic diseases.

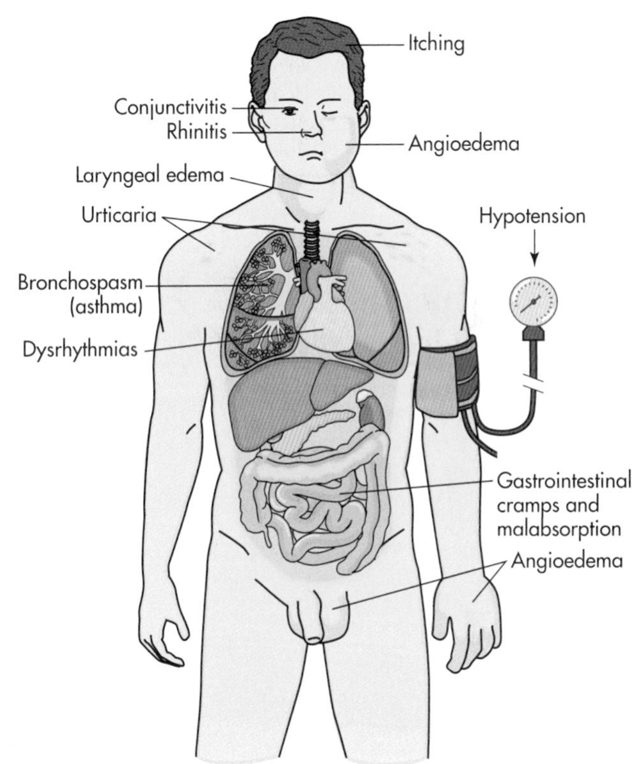

Figure 49-3 Clinical manifestations of type I hypersensitivity reactions.

The clinical manifestations of type I hypersensitivity reactions reflect changes in a wide variety of organs, because the reactions do not occur at the site of the antigen-antibody reaction. Rather, they occur in the organs where the pharmacologically active mediators exert their actions. If the mediators remain confined to a local area, the tissue reactions remain localized. This is known as local anaphylaxis. If the mediators are released systemically, the response is known as systemic anaphylaxis (Figure 49-3).

Atopic diseases are rarely life threatening, but the symptoms can be uncomfortable and may cause the individual to miss school or work. The local hypersensitivity that most people demonstrate in response to a mosquito bite is a classic example of this type of reaction; the intradermal injection of the mosquito anticoagulants produces a wheal-flare type of reaction within a matter of minutes. The clinical manifestations

Clinical Manifestations
Type I Atopic Hypersensitivity

RESPIRATORY
Rhinorrhea
Watery, itching eyes
Obstruction of eustachian tubes
Sneezing
Sinusitis
Headache
Facial pain
Bronchospasm
Dyspnea
Stridor
Tachypnea
Wheezing
Cyanosis
Use of accessory muscles for breathing
Flaring of nares

DERMAL
Hives
Rash
Angioedema

ABDOMINAL
Nausea
Vomiting
Cramping
Diarrhea

GENERAL
Fever
Diaphoresis
Malaise
Joint pain
Hematopoietic suppression
Anxiety
Anaphylaxis

Clinical Manifestations
Type I Nonatopic Hypersensitivity

LOCALIZED REACTION
Hives
Angioedema

SYSTEMIC ANAPHYLAXIS
Apprehension
Edema of the face, hands, or other parts of body
Wheezing
Dyspnea
Respiratory collapse
Vascular collapse with shock
- Rapid, weak pulse
- Falling blood pressure
- Cyanosis

Death

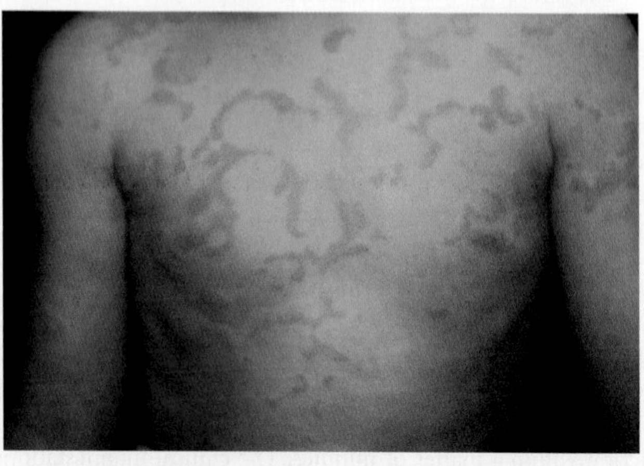

Figure 49-4 Urticaria.

associated with type 1 atopic hypersensitivity are summarized in the Clinical Manifestations box.

Nonatopic diseases can range from a local reaction such as hives or angioedema to a systemic reaction such as anaphylactic shock. Hives (urticaria) are pruritic lesions characterized by a pale pink elevated edge (wheal) on an erythematous background (Figure 49-4). Urticaria are generally transient and may reappear in different areas of the body. Skin exposed to latex, such as latex gloves, can precipitate contact urticaria. Chronic urticaria that occurs in response to heat, cold, or various light waves is not an IgE-mediated hypersensitivity. Cholinergic urticaria can occur in response to stress or physical exertion. Angioedema is a form of urticaria that involves the subcutaneous tissue rather than the skin. It can involve an entire anatomical part, such as the eyelid, thumb, or lip. Swelling is present, but not pruritus.

Apprehension and sneezing are two of the earliest symptoms of systemic anaphylaxis. Edema and itching occur at the site when injected drugs or venoms are the allergens. Signs of latex allergy depend largely upon the route of exposure. When latex particles are aerosolized, wheezing, rhinitis, and conjunctivitis may occur. Mucosal exposure frequently results in angioedema. These mild reactions are rapidly followed, sometimes in a matter of seconds or minutes, by severe manifestations that lead to vascular collapse, shock, or death unless rapid action is taken. The clinical manifestations associated with type I nonatopic hypersensitivity are summarized in the Clinical Manifestations box.

Collaborative Care Management

Diagnostic Tests. The health history, including an environmental assessment, is one of the most valuable diagnostic tools for the health care provider evaluating the patient for type I hypersensitivities. Skin testing and the radioallergosorbent test (RAST) may be helpful in determining therapy for persons with atopic allergies (Figure 49-5). Test results must

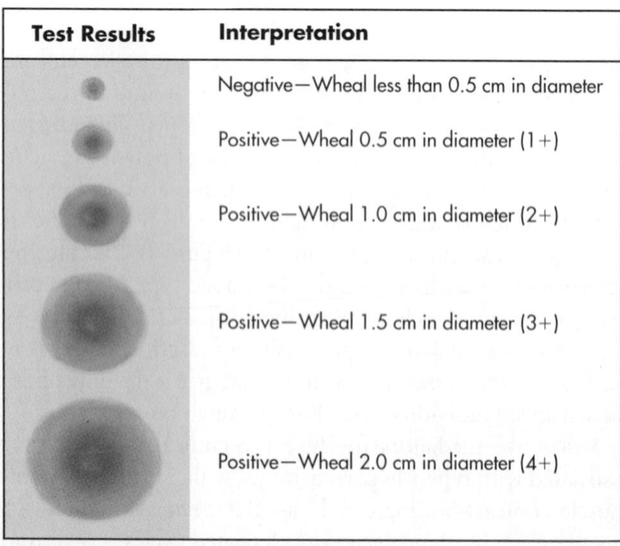

Figure 49-5 Interpretation of intradermal allergy test results based on the size of the wheal after 15 to 30 minutes.

be correlated with the patient's history, however, to accurately identify the cause of the allergic reaction. Eosinophilia (increased eosinophil count) is associated with antigen-antibody reactions and occurs in persons with allergies, hay fever, and drug hypersensitivity. IgE levels are elevated during exacerbations of atopic dermatitis, however, they are not diagnostically useful in atopic asthma and allergic rhinitis.[2]

Medications. Symptom relief is the primary aim of drug therapy for atopic allergies. Urticaria and angioedema are usually self-limiting; therefore treatment is not often required. Anaphylaxis is treated with epinephrine to shorten its duration and prevent relapse. Antihistamines, such as diphrenhydramine (Benadryl) may be given to prevent the actions of histamine. Short term corticosteroid therapy may be useful for decreasing the inflammation associated with allergic responses (Table 49-6).

Treatments. Avoidance therapy, in which the patient is taught to reduce exposure to triggering antigens, is the most effective treatment to decrease allergic attacks. This therapy appears to be most effective with food, drug, and allergens such as animal dander, but it can also be useful in treating seasonal allergies. For instance, limiting outdoor activities and staying in air-conditioned settings when the pollen counts are high decrease seasonal allergy symptoms.

Immunotherapy is often useful in reducing symptoms in patients who cannot avoid antigens such as dust mites or pollen. An extract of the allergen is injected subcutaneously starting with the dose at which the person was found to be

TABLE 49-6 Common Medications for Type I Hypersensitivities

Drug	Action	Intervention/Implication
Antihistamines		
Diphenhydramine (Benadryl) Chlorpheniramine (Chlor-Trimeton) Brompheniramine (Dimetane) Astemizole (Hismanal) Loratadine (Claritin) Clemastine (Tavist) Fexofenadine hydrochloride (Allegra)	Antihistamine; compete with histamine for effector cell H_1 receptor sites, thus preventing the action of histamine	May produce significant drowsiness (Benadryl) or central nervous system stimulation (Chlor-Trimeton); causes dry mouth; may produce blurred vision Contraindicated in hypersensitivity, narrow-angle glaucoma, pregnancy, breastfeeding, lower respiratory tract disease, acute asthma attacks, or within 14 days of taking monoamine oxidase inhibitors Advise to take 1 hour before or 1 hour after meals to facilitate drug absorption
Decongestants		
Phenylephrine (Neo-Synephrine) Pseudoephedrine (Sudafed)	Stimulate alpha-adrenergic receptors to shrink respiratory mucous membranes	May produce nausea, vomiting, headache, anxiety, tremors, dizziness, seizures, tachycardia, hypertension, dysrhythmias, mucous membrane irritation, or dry mouth Monitor blood pressure and pulse; give several hours before bedtime if drug produces sleeplessness Contraindicated in patients with hypertension Teach patient to stop drug if tremors or restlessness occur
Mast Cell Degranulator Inhibitor		
Cromolyn sodium inhaler (Intal) Cromolyn sodium nasal spray (Nasalcrom)	Inhibit mast cell release of histamine and slow-reacting substance of anaphylaxis, thus preventing an allergic response	For prophylactic use only May produce nasal irritation and burning, sneezing, cough, or throat irritation; dry mouth; nausea and vomiting; angioedema or bronchospasm Do not give in hypersensitivity, acute asthma, or to patients with a history of coronary artery disease or dysrhythmias Teach effective use of inhaler for accurate dosing
Corticosteroids		
Prednisone Methylprednisone Decadron phosphate Vancenase Beconase Nasalide	Suppress migration of polymorphonuclear leukocytes and fibroblasts, thereby reducing inflammation	Contraindicated in patients with hypersensitivity, psychoses, fungal infections, AIDS, tuberculosis Monitor for thrombocytopenia, increased intraocular pressure, poor wound healing, nausea, diarrhea, headache, and mood changes Monitor daily weight, serum potassium levels, blood glucose levels, blood pressure, signs of infection, mood changes Give with food or milk to decrease gastrointestinal irritation Caution patient not to stop taking drug abruptly and to notify health care provider if infection develops

Continued

TABLE 49-6 Common Medications for Type I Hypersensitivities—cont'd

Drug	Action	Intervention/Implication
Adrenalin		
Epinephrine	Opposes the action of histamine through vasoconstriction to raise blood pressure; promotes bronchiole relaxation to facilitate breathing; stimulates both alpha and beta receptors to reproduce effects of sympathetic nervous system	Temporary relief from anaphylaxis, hypersensitivity reactions, bronchospasm, and acute asthma attacks Contraindicated in hypersensitivity, narrow-angle glaucoma, dysrhythmias Monitor for anxiety, tremors, palpitations, tachydysrhythmias, hypertension, pulmonary edema
Aminophylline		
Theophylline (Theo-Dur)	Xanthine blocks phosphodiesterase, thus increasing cyclic adenosine monophosphate, which alters intracellular calcium and ion movement; produces respiratory tract relaxation and bronchodilation and increases pulmonary blood flow	Monitor for central nervous system stimulation, dizziness, anxiety, restlessness, seizures, tachycardia, dysrhythmias, nausea, vomiting, insomnia Contraindicated in hypersensitivity to xanthine and in patients with history of tachydysrhythmias Avoid intake of stimulant foods such as coffee, tea, and colas Monitor theophylline blood levels Avoid smoking because it interferes with absorption

sensitive by skin testing. Over time, serum IgE specific antibody levels fall, IgG blocking antibodies increase, and lymphocyte responsiveness to the antigen is reduced. Increasing amounts of allergen are injected at weekly intervals. If large local reactions occur during therapy, the dose is repeated or lowered until better tolerated (see Clinical Manifestations box).

Systemic reactions, although uncommon, may occur within 30 minutes of injection of the allergen extract. Treatment includes placing the person in a supine position and administering epinephrine. If signs and symptoms of systemic anaphylactic shock are noted, oxygen is administered and intravenous fluids are infused rapidly to support blood pressure (see Chapter 14 for treatment of shock). Because of its potential for anaphylaxis and death, the patient and primary caregiver must be sure that the symptoms warrant the risk, expense, and inconvenience of immunotherapy.

The future of atopic disease treatment appears to lie in learning how to more effectively modulate the immune response. Possible therapies include manipulating IgE response by using IgE-specific suppressor T cells; using antibodies against IgE idiotopes; or using cytokines to suppress IgE synthesis.

Diet. The diet may be altered in patients with food allergies to avoid those foods causing allergy. Common foods that cause allergies are milk, nuts, fish, egg, soy, wheat, corn, and chocolate.

Activity. Patients with allergies have no activity restrictions. Persons with atopic allergies are encouraged to avoid activities when environmental allergens or pollutant levels are high. Pollen counts are usually the highest between the hours of 12 midnight and 8 AM and on dry, windy days.

Referrals. Individuals with atopic allergies who have not achieved control of their symptoms by avoiding allergens or using symptom-treating drugs may be referred to allergists for testing and possible immunotherapy.

Clinical Manifestations
Immunotherapy Reactions

LOCAL	SYSTEMIC
Redness	Nasal stuffiness
Edema	Sneezing
Pruritus	Reddening of conjunctiva
Tenderness	Chest tightness
	Wheezing
	Fainting
	Apprehension
	Anaphylactic shock

NURSING MANAGEMENT

ASSESSMENT

Health History

Assessment data to be collected as part of the health history of a patient with allergy includes:

- History of allergic reactions in the past (e.g., type, frequency, or perceived causes)
- Familial history of allergies
- Recent exposure to sensitizing substances (chemicals, drugs)
- Changes in living, working, or environmental conditions
- Characteristics of present environment (house, clothing, plants, trees, or animals)

Increased stress in recent past (stress aggravates asthmatic response)
Types of symptoms experienced: respiratory, dermal, gastrointestinal, or general
Alleviating factors, either prescribed, herbal, or over-the-counter
All patients should be questioned about allergies and sensitivities to drugs before any drug therapy is initiated. If there is a positive history, the physician is consulted before a new drug is given; when a new drug is given, the patient is monitored closely for allergic responses.

Physical Examination:

Important aspects of the physical examination of the patient with allergy include inspection and observation for:
Rashes (location, color)
Mouth breathing (nasal obstruction)
Flaring nares
Difficulty hearing (plugged eustachian tubes)
Pale bluish turbinates that are edematous with clear secretions
Tearing
Dark areas under eyes (venous dilation of skin)
Scleral or conjunctival infections
Increased respiratory rate
Audible wheezing
Use of accessory muscles for breathing
Anxious expression

NURSING DIAGNOSES

Nursing diagnoses for the patient with allergies and/or anaphylaxis may include, but are not limited to:

Atopy

Diagnostic Title	Possible Etiologic Factors
1. Risk for ineffective health maintenance	Effects of allergy on preferred lifestyle
2. Deficient knowledge of environmental and lifestyle modifications to control allergies	Inadequate information about allergy control and treatments

Anaphylaxis

1. Ineffective airway clearance	Excess secretion production and bronchoconstriction
2. Decreased cardiac output	Inadequate venous return to heart, peripheral vasodilation
3. Deficient knowledge	Inadequate information about allergy control and treatments

EXPECTED PATIENT OUTCOMES

Expected outcomes for the person with a type I hypersensitivity may include but are not limited to:

Atopy

1. Will maintain health status by verbalizing:
1a. Understanding of the disease process
1b. Understanding of the substances that are allergenic and approaches for avoidance
1c. Will plan to alter habits or environment to reduce exposure to allergens
2. Will demonstrate knowledge of treatments by verbalizing:
2a. Will understand rationale for immunotherapy (if applicable)
2b. Will understand need for avoiding allergens when feasible
2c. Will understand prescribed, alternative and over-the-counter drugs used to relieve symptoms

Anaphylaxis

1. Will maintain patent airway
1a. Will demonstrate use of anaphylaxis emergency equipment
1b. Will verbalize need for having anaphylaxis emergency equipment constantly available
2. Will remain free of clinical manifestations of shock
3. Will demonstrate knowledge of risk for latex allergy by verbalizing:
3a. Will understand latex allergy and products that contain latex
3b. Will understand the need to avoid all latex products (gloves, condoms, tubing)
3c. Will verbalize the need to inform all health care providers regarding latex sensitivity

INTERVENTIONS—ATOPY

1. Health Maintenance

An important aspect of nursing care for the patient with allergies is helping the patient identify and adjust to lifestyle changes that may be necessary to reduce exposure to allergens and maintain health. In many cases this may involve few lifestyle changes, and the patient and family readily adjust. In other cases, lifestyle changes may involve adjusting to a complex medication schedule, giving up a beloved pet, or moving to another climate. Patients may have to change employment to avoid allergens such as chemicals, molds, or fibers. These changes may place emotional or financial burdens on the patient and family, especially if the job market or patient's skills are limited. The nurse's role is to help the patient explore alternative solutions and make the best choices possible to maintain health.

2. Deficient Knowledge

Teaching the patient and family about the nature of the disorder and the methods that can be used to avoid the allergen is another important nursing intervention for the patient with allergies. Results of allergy testing, assessment findings, and patient history are reviewed with the patient and family so they understand which allergens need to be controlled or avoided. Patients are taught the importance of controlling their living and working environments to reduce exposure to antigens and hence, the risk of reactions. If animal dander is a source of allergy and removal of a family pet is unacceptable to the patient or family, the nurse can explore ways to decrease the impact of the pet on the allergic patient, such as keeping pet outdoors, or in a room separate from where the patient sleeps or spends large amounts of time. The need for total avoidance of latex is emphasized to those patients who are latex sensitive. The nurse explains all prescribed medications, including desired actions, dosage schedules, and potential side effects. The importance of maintaining drug schedules for prophylactic drugs, such as cromolyn, is stressed, and the patient and family are reminded that these drugs are of no value during an acute allergic attack.

INTERVENTIONS—ANAPHYLAXIS

Anaphylaxis can occur following exposure to offending antigens or from immunotherapy, consequently, the patient and family need to be taught about such reactions and how to deal with them. The nurse instructs both the patient and family about signs and symptoms that need to be reported, potential reactions that can result in the need for emergency measures, and use of emergency care kits. If immunotherapy is elected as a treatment choice, the risks and benefits, schedules, and costs of such therapy are discussed. The patient is informed that immunotherapy can be reinstituted if symptoms recur.

1. Airway Clearance

Death from anaphylaxis occurs from asphyxiation because of upper airway edema and congestion, irreversible shock, or a combination of these factors (see the section on clinical manifestations of type I nonatopic anaphylaxis). The primary concern of the nurse during an anaphylactic reaction is making certain that the patient's airway is patent. The patient is positioned in high Fowler's position to maximize ventilation; an oral airway is inserted if necessary, and secretions are removed by suction or by encouraging the patient to cough. Oxygen therapy may be given according to health care provider's orders or facility protocols. The nurse encourages slow, deep breathing. The administration of epinephrine or bronchodilators such as aminophylline may be necessary to decrease bronchospasm. In severe cases, tracheostomy may be necessary to maintain a patent airway. The patient is monitored closely both during and after anaphylaxis, since recurrence is possible.

2. Cardiac Output

Respiratory compromise quickly leads to decreased cardiac output that can produce death within a matter of minutes. The nurse is alert for clinical manifestations that indicate anaphylactic shock and is prepared to address the problem should it occur. At the first sign of anaphylaxis, the patient is given epinephrine 1:1000 solution 0.3 to 0.5 ml subcutaneously or intramuscularly. If shock continues, albuterol (Ventolin) or epinephrine administered through aerosol treatments may be administered. Vasopressors such as dopamine or metaraminol bitartrate (Aramine) may be prescribed for severe shock to assist in increasing blood pressure and cardiac output.

3. Risk for Allergy Response

Because persons with a history of allergies are more likely to develop anaphylactic reactions to drugs than those without such a history, all patients are questioned about allergies and drug sensitivities before drug therapy is initiated. High-risk persons are instructed to wear an identification bracelet or tag at all times that indicates the known allergy. Such tags may be obtained from Medic Alert or other commercial sources.

Allergic individuals are advised to alert health care workers of their allergies when animal sera, allergenic extracts, or contrast media containing iodide need to be given for any reason, so that epinephrine can be readily available. The patient is then monitored for at least 30 minutes after administration of such substances. Any reaction that occurs within a few minutes forewarns of an impending emergency.

Nurses need to recognize the potential for drug cross sensitivity when administering alternative drugs to allergic patients. For example, cephalosporins are frequently administered to patients who are sensitive to penicillin. A small percent of patients will, however, be sensitive to the cephalosporin due to its cross sensitivity with penicillin. The yellow dye contained in some tablets cross sensitizes with aspirin and may cause anaphylaxis in aspirin sensitive patients.

Patient/Family Education. Patient and family education is a major component of care for the patient with type 1 hypersensitivity reactions. In addition to the teaching described previously under Deficient Knowledge, the rationale, risks, and benefits of immunotherapy are explored if this option is being considered by the patient (see Patient Teaching box).

Patient Teaching
The Patient With Atopic Allergy

The nurse instructs the patient to:

1. Avoid allergen, if possible.
   a. Animal dander
      (1) Avoid fur-bearing pets, if possible, or keep pets outdoors.
      (2) Avoid furniture stuffed with horsehair or feathers.
   b. Pollen spores
      (1) Use air conditioning if possible; keep windows closed at night; if using air conditioner in car, start car, roll down windows, and allow air conditioner to run for 10 to 15 minutes before entering car.
      (2) Limit time outdoors between sunset and sunrise, especially when windy.
      (3) Do not hang wash outside to dry. (Pollen and molds stick to wet wash.)
      (4) Avoid gardening, raking leaves, mowing lawn, or being near freshly cut grass.
      (5) Keep car windows closed when driving.
      (6) Minimize number of indoor plants.
      (7) Vacation in selected geographic areas, such as beach or sea, that are free of specific allergen during seasonal height, if possible.
   c. House dust
      (1) Use synthetic materials; avoid wool and cotton.
      (2) Use a minimum of lint-producing articles.
      (3) Put away articles that are difficult to dust.
      (4) Dust with damp cloth daily.
      (5) Use air conditioner, if possible.
      (6) Change furnace filter every month when in use.
2. Use all medications as prescribed and report the incidence of side effects.

EVALUATION

1,2,3. To evaluate the effectiveness of nursing interventions, compare patient behaviors with those stated in the expected patient outcomes. Achievement of outcomes is successful if patients with allergy understand the information that has been provided to them, the choices that need to be made, and the benefits and risks of various therapies. Patients at increased risk for anaphylaxis to latex or other allergens need to verbalize understanding of the importance of the condition and the need for immediate intervention, and be able to demonstrate use of home emergency kits. Patients need to verbalize understanding of the expected effects, dosages, side effects, and potential interactions of prescribed and over-the-counter medications. Persons who are sensitive to latex need to verbalize understanding of the need to avoid contact with latex or latex-containing products or the inhalation of latex particles or powders that contain latex.

GERONTOLOGIC CONSIDERATIONS

Older adults undergo changes in their patterns of immunologic response that leave them with a decreased ability to respond to immunologic events, including allergens. Even so, between 27% and 38% of adults with a history of childhood allergic asthma have a recurrence of the disease in later life. Because there are no conclusive data to support that older adults have fewer hypersensitivities than younger adults, they are assessed for allergies and taught the same emergency interventions as younger adults. If older adults are unable to care for themselves, it is particularly important that the nurse teach the family or caregiver how to deal with potential and actual hypersensitivities.

SPECIAL ENVIRONMENTS FOR CARE

Critical Care Management

Critical care management does not play a role in the routine management of atopic allergy, but it may be essential for the patient experiencing anaphylactic shock. Persons experiencing anaphylaxis and anaphylactic shock require hospitalization until they are free of respiratory distress. Tracheostomy may be required when airway compromise is severe. Anaphylaxis has a propensity to recur as emergency medications are excreted from the body; therefore patients are likely to remain hospitalized until the likelihood of recurrence has passed.

Home Care Management

Except in the case of anaphylaxis, people with atopic hypersensitivities are cared for at home and seen as necessary in the primary caregiver's office or outpatient clinic. The home environment should be altered to decrease the risk of exposure to allergens (see earlier discussion regarding home maintenance).

Persons with type I hypersensitivities should be aware of situations in which their allergens may be present. Persons with insect sting sensitivity need know how to use an insect sting emergency kit. Kits are available commercially and should be readily available. Both the patient and family are taught how to use the self-injecting syringe to administer epinephrine. If the patient is unable to use the syringe or give the injection, an inhalation high-dose epinephrine may be taken from a metered-dose aerosol, which is found in some emergency kits (see Patient Teaching box).

Patient Teaching

The Patient With Type I Hypersensitivity: Sting

The nurse instructs the patient and family concerning the following:

1. Emergency care for the specific allergy
2. Availability and use of commercially prepared emergency kit
3. Concentration and route of emergency use epinephrine (1:1000 epinephrine injection)
4. Use of self-injecting syringe of epinephrine supplied with kit (spring loaded; can be given through clothing)
5. Emergency procedure if sting occurs
   a. Immediately swallow the uncoated antihistamine tablet
   b. Inject the epinephrine
   c. If unable to self-inject, inhale high-dose epinephrine from metered-dose aerosol* (if included in kit)

*Epinephrine is rapidly absorbed through respiratory tract and will help relieve bronchoconstriction and bronchospasms; not recommended as primary treatment because it does not correct hypotension.

TABLE 49-7 ABO Blood Groups

A—antigen A is present on cell; anti-B antibodies in serum
B—antigen B is present on cell; anti-A antibodies in serum
AB—antigens A and B are present on cell; no antibodies in serum
O—neither antigen A nor B is present on cell; anti-A and anti-B antibodies in serum

COMPLICATIONS

The primary complication of type I hypersensitivities is anaphylactic shock, which can lead to death within minutes without emergency treatment. This complication was previously discussed, and a detailed discussion of shock can be found in Chapter 14.

TYPE II HYPERSENSITIVITIES

A classic example of a type II hypersensitivity reaction, also known as cytotoxic hypersensitivity, occurs with the infusion of mismatched blood. Other examples include hemolytic disease of the newborn, hyperacute graft rejection, autoimmune hemolytic anemia, myasthenia gravis, and thyroiditis.[5]

Etiology/Epidemiology

ABO System. Four major blood groups are found in humans: A, B, AB, and O (Table 49-7). Inherited erythrocyte antigens provide humans with their blood types. Within 3 months of birth, a person has formed antibodies against the other types of major erythrocyte antigens. The exact cause of this antibody formation is not clear, but is suspected to occur through natural contact with antigenically similar agents that stimulate antibody formation. For example a person with type A blood possesses anti-B antibodies and can cross-react with either the A or B antigen on the surface of other ABO types. People with type O blood are considered universal donors because everyone is tolerant of the O antigen within the ABO system.[18] People with type O, however, cannot receive other types of blood without experiencing a reaction. People with type AB blood can receive blood from any other blood type because they have both A and B antigens (Figure 49-6).

Acute hemolytic transfusion reaction (ABO incompatability) is the most serious adverse reaction to blood transfusions and results in 1 death per 100,000 units of blood infused. The reaction occurs within the first 30 minutes of blood administration. Studies of hemolytic reactions have shown that mistakes in specimen collection and labeling or inadequate patient identification are the primary errors that lead to hemolytic reactions.[10]

Rh System. When the mother is sensitized to antigens on the infant's erythrocytes and makes antibodies against those antigens, hemolytic disease of the newborn (HDNB) occurs. The Rhesus D (RhD) antigen is the most commonly involved antigen of the 27 known antigens within this system. The term *Rh positive* means that the antigen Rh-D is present; the term *Rh negative* means that the Rh-D antigen is absent. Approximately 85% of the population has Rh-positive blood.

When the Rh-negative person is first exposed to Rh- positive blood, Rh antibodies are formed. On subsequent exposures to Rh-positive blood, the Rh antibody binds to its corresponding antigen on the surface of the erythrocyte containing the Rh antigen. The Rh antibodies do not usually fix complement; therefore there is no immediate hemolysis as occurs in the ABO system. Instead, the Rh-antigen erythrocytes are rapidly broken down by macrophages in the spleen, with conversion of hemoglobin to bilirubin, resulting in jaundice. Between 10% and 15% of Caucasian infants and approximately 5% of African-American infants experience Rh incompatability.[11]

HLA System. Another system that has clinical significance in blood transfusion is the HLA system. Human leukocyte antigens are found on many types of tissue cells and on blood leukocytes and platelets. The system is more complex than the erythrocyte antigen system, and thousands of combinations of antigens may occur. Sensitization can occur through pregnancy or through exposure to platelets and WBCs during transfusions. Repeated transfusions of blood cells may lead to transfusion reactions. These reactions occur in only about 3% to 4% of all transfusions.[10]

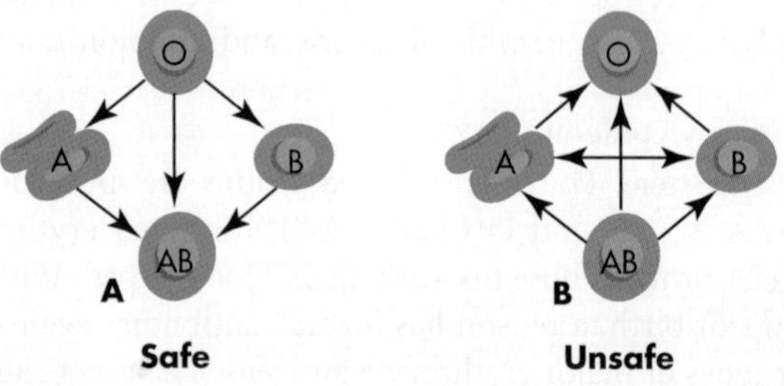

Figure 49-6 Blood groups and their donor/recipient relationships. **A**, Safe. **B**, Unsafe.

Pathophysiology

The underlying mechanism of type II hypersensitivities involves the direct binding of IgG or IgM immunoglobulins to an antigen on the surface of a cell. Once binding occurs, the cell is destroyed by phagocytic attack, nonspecific lymphocytic attack, or lysis of the cell through the activation of the full complement cascade (see Chapter 48). Figure 49-7 illustrates the mechanism of type II hypersensitivity reactions.

Transfusion Reactions. Transfusion reactions can be broadly grouped into immunologic and nonimmunologic types. Table 49-8 presents an overview of each of the major immunologic transfusion reactions along with their associated clinical manifestations and management.

Immunologic Transfusion Reactions. *Acute hemolytic reactions* are caused by antigen-antibody complexes on the erythrocyte membrane. These complexes activate the Hageman factor (coagulation factor XII) and the complement cascade. The Hageman factor initiates the kinin system, causing increased capillary permeability, arteriole vasodilation, and hypotension. The activated complement system initiates intravascular hemolysis, as well as histamine and serotonin release from the mast cells. Hageman factor and free incompatible erythrocyte stroma (covering) activate the intrinsic clotting cascade causing disseminated intravascular coagulation (DIC).

Febrile nonhemolytic reactions are among the most common transfusion reactions. They occur because the recipient becomes sensitized to the donor's WBCs, platelets, or plasma.

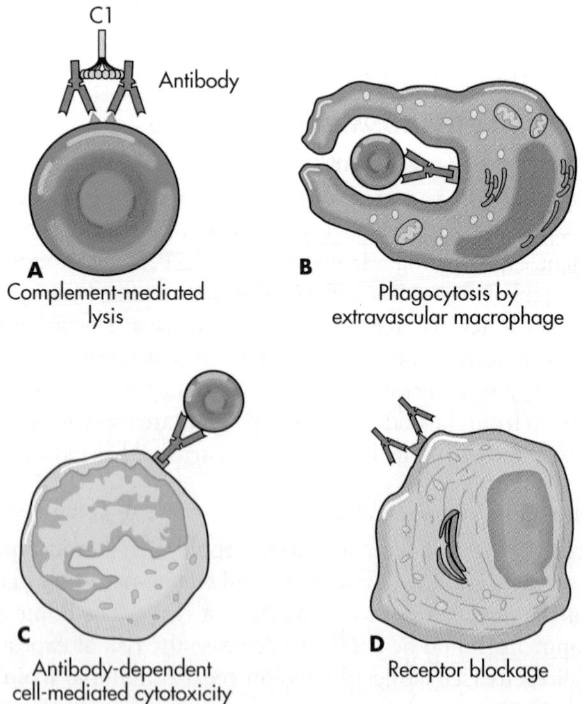

Figure 49-7 Mechanisms of type II, tissue-specific reactions. Antigens on the target cell bind with antibody and are destroyed or prevented from functioning by **A**, complement-mediated lysis; **B**, clearance by macrophages in tissues; **C**, antibody-dependent cell-mediated cytotoxicity (ADCC); or **D**, the modulation or blockage of receptors on the target cell.

Symptoms usually begin 30 minutes after the start of the infusion. Although this reaction is not usually serious, it is uncomfortable for the patient.

Allergic transfusion reactions are caused by sensitivity of the recipient to foreign plasma proteins. Common symptoms include hives, rash, and urticaria. If the symptoms are mild, the patient is treated with antihistamines and the transfusion is restarted slowly. A more severe allergic reaction (anaphylaxis) with symptoms of bronchospasm, respiratory distress, and shock can occur but is rare.

TABLE 49-8 Immunologic Reactions to Blood Transfusion

Reaction	Clinical Manifestations	Management	Prevention
Acute hemolytic*	Chills, fever, low back pain, flushing, tachycardia, tachypnea, hypotension, vascular collapse, hemoglobinuria, hemoglobinemia, bleeding, acute renal failure, shock, cardiac arrest, death	Treat shock. Draw blood samples for serological testing. To avoid hemolysis from the procedure, use a new venipuncture (not an existing central line) and avoid small-gauge needles. Send urine specimen to the laboratory. Maintain blood pressure with intravenous (IV) colloid solutions. Give diuretics as prescribed to maintain urine flow. Insert indwelling catheter or measure voided amounts to monitor hourly urine output. Dialysis may be required if renal failure occurs. Do not transfuse additional red blood cell–containing components until the transfusion service has provided newly cross-matched units.	Meticulously verify and document patient identification from sample collection to component infusion. Transfuse blood slowly for first 15-20 minutes with nurse at patient's side.
Febrile, nonhemolytic (most common)*	Sudden chills and fever (rise in temperature of greater than 1° C [2° F], headache, flushing, anxiety, muscle pain	Give antipyretics as prescribed. Do not give aspirin to thrombocytopenic patients. *Do not restart transfusion.*	Consider leukocyte-poor blood products (filtered, washed, or frozen).
Mild allergic*	Flushing, itching, urticaria (hives)	Give antihistamines as directed. If symptoms are mild and transient, restart transfusion slowly. Do not restart transfusion if fever or pulmonary symptoms develop.	Treat prophylactically with glucocorticosteroids or antihistamines (Decadron, Benadryl) given 30-60 min before transfusion.
Anaphylactic*	Anxiety, urticaria, wheezing, tightness and pain in chest, difficulty swallowing, progressing to cyanosis, shock, and possible cardiac arrest	Initiate cardiopulmonary resuscitation if indicated. Have epinephrine ready for injection (0.4 ml of a 1:1000 solution subcutaneously or 0.1 ml of 1:1000 solution diluted to 10 ml with saline for IV use). *Do not restart transfusion.*	Transfuse extensively washed red blood cell products from which all plasma has been removed. Alternatively, use blood from IgA-deficient donor.
Delayed hemolytic	Fever, chills, back pain, jaundice, anemia, hemoglobinuria	Monitor adequacy of urinary output and degree of anemia. Treat fever with Tylenol. May need further blood transfusion.	Do more specific type and cross-match when giving patient blood.
Posttransfusion graft-versus-host disease	Anorexia, nausea, diarrhea, high fever, rash, stomatitis, liver dysfunction	No effective treatment. Administer steroids.	Give irradiated blood products.
Noncardiac pulmonary edema	Fever, chills, hypotension, cough, orthopnea, cyanosis, shock	Stop transfusion. Continue IV saline. Give oxygen prn. Administer steroids as directed. Give furosemide (Lasix) and epinephrine as ordered.	

*Modified from *National blood resource education program's transfusion therapy guidelines for nurses,* NIH Pub No 90-2668, 1990.

Delayed hemolytic reactions occur 7 to 14 days after the transfusion and are thought to be the result of sensitization of the recipient's immune system to the transfused erythrocyte antigens. The recipient may also have been previously sensitized but have antibody titers that are undetectable at the time of the transfusion.

Posttransfusion graft-versus-host disease, which was once relatively rare, is occurring more frequently because of increased use of purposeful immunosuppression as treatment (e.g., bone marrow transplantation). The donor lymphocytes begin to reject the patient's host cells 4 to 30 days after the infusion of blood.

Noncardiac pulmonary edema is thought to be caused by a high titer of leukocyte antibodies in either the donor or recipient plasma. These antibody-to-granulocyte reactions cause granulocyte aggregates that are filtered out by the lung. The antibodies attached to the granulocytes initiate the complement cascade and promote histamine release, causing an influx of inflammatory cells into the lung.

Nonimmunologic Transfusion Reactions. Blood transfusion can result in reactions that are not immunologic in nature. These include circulatory overload, sepsis, and transmission of disease. These reactions are summarized in Box 49-2. Clinical manifestations associated with nonimmunologic transfusion reactions are presented in the Clinical Manifestations box.

Collaborative Care Management. Prevention is the key to management of transfusion reactions. Accurate prescreening of potential donors, meticulous laboratory testing, and close patient monitoring are all essential components of care. Blood received from volunteer donors through the American Red Cross Blood Service or hospital blood banks is preferred to that of paid donors, because paid donors may be less likely to report past or present diseases that may be transmitted to the recipient. Common screening guidelines for blood donation are outlined in Box 49-3.

BOX 49-2 Major Nonimmunologic Transfusion Reactions

Circulatory Overload

Can occur when blood is given too rapidly or in large quantities. The elderly are particularly vulnerable. Patients develop signs of fluid overload and pulmonary congestion. The transfusion is stopped and oxygen and diuretics may be administered.

Sepsis

Bacterial contamination may occur at any time during the collection or handling of blood. Signs of sepsis begin almost immediately. The transfusion is stopped, and the patient receives antibiotics and treatment for shock if it occurs.

Disease Transmission

Hepatitis, cytomegalovirus, and human immunodeficiency virus are the most common diseases transmitted by blood transfusions. Hepatitis A and B are effectively identified with current screening capabilities, but hepatitis C is still readily transmissible.

One method for preventing immunologic blood transfusion reactions and disease transmission is planned autologous transfusion, which involves using the person's own blood for replacement. Blood is collected at regular intervals before anticipated use, such as forthcoming surgery. The blood is then stored or frozen until needed. This method is especially useful for persons with rare blood types, for those whose religious beliefs preclude receiving donor blood, or when several units of blood are expected to be necessary during surgery (e.g., selected heart surgeries or joint replacements).

Autotransfusion, which consists of collecting, filtering, and immediately reinfusing the person's own blood, may be performed in the emergency department, the operating room suite during surgery, the postanesthesia care unit, or the criti-

Clinical Manifestations
Nonimmunologic Transfusion Reactions

CIRCULATORY OVERLOAD	SEPSIS
Dyspnea	Fever >40° C
Chest tightness	Abdominal cramps
Headache	Nausea
Hypertension	Vomiting
Tachypnea	Diarrhea
Cough	Septic shock
Cyanosis	
Peripheral edema	
Jugular vein distention	
Crackles (rales)	
Abnormal heart sounds	
Hypertension	

BOX 49-3 Screening Guidelines for Blood Donors

Persons with any of the following are not permitted to donate blood:

1. History of infectious diseases such as hepatitis, HIV infection and AIDS, tuberculosis, syphilis, or malaria
2. Malignant diseases
3. Allergies or asthma
4. Polycythemia vera
5. Abnormal bleeding tendencies
6. Hypotension (current)
7. Anemia (current)
8. Recent pregnancy or major surgery
9. Men with at least one homosexual or bisexual contact since 1975 (concern for AIDS)
10. International travel to malarial areas or high-risk countries (concern for AIDS)
11. Blood transfusion during last 6 months
12. History of jaundice
13. Diseases of the heart, lung, or liver
14. Immunizations or vaccinations with attenuated viral vaccine rubella or rabies vaccine
15. Hgb level below 13.5 g/dl for men or 12.4 g/dl for women
16. Abnormalities in vital signs, particularly fever
17. History of residence for greater then 6 months in the United Kingdom between 1980-1996.

cal care unit. The blood is suctioned into a bag and passes through a filter to remove microaggregates. When the bag is full, it is disconnected from the system and the blood is infused into the patient with an administration set, using a standard or microembolic filter.

Blood components, as opposed to whole blood, are being increasingly administered. Blood can be fractionated into red blood cells (RBCs), platelets, and plasma (Table 49-9) either by centrifuge or automated cell separators. Blood can also be withdrawn from a donor, a portion separated out, and the

TABLE 49-9 Types of Blood Components

Blood Component	Description	Usage	Comments
Red Blood Cells (RBCs)			
Packed RBC (PRBCs)	RBCs separated from plasma and platelets	Anemia Moderate blood loss	Decreased risk of fluid overload as compared with whole blood
Autologous PRBCs	Same as packed RBC	Elective surgery for which blood replacement is expected	Units may be stored for up to 35 days
Washed RBCs	RBCs washed with sterile isotonic saline before transfusion	Previous allergic reactions to transfusions	Increased removal of immunoglobulins and protein
Frozen RBCs	RBCs frozen in a glycerol solution; cells washed after thawing to remove the glycerol	Storage of rare type blood Storage of autologous blood for future use	Relatively free of leukocytes and microemboli Expensive
Leukocyte-poor RBCs	RBCs from which most leukocytes have been removed	Previous sensitivity to leukocyte antigens from prior transfusions or from pregnancy	Fewer RBC than packed RBC; washed leukocyte-poor RBC units have more RBC than nonwashed
Neocytes	RBC units with high number of reticulocytes (young RBCs)	Transfusion-dependent anemias	Fewer problems with iron overload Expensive
Other Cellular Components			
Platelets			
Random donor packs	Platelets separated from RBCs by centrifuge; given in 50 ml of plasma	Thrombocytopenia Disseminated intravascular coagulation	Plasma base is rich in coagulation factors Platelet preparations can also be packed, washed, or made leukocyte poor
Pheresis packs	Platelets from an HLA-matched donor, separated by apheresis	Allosensitized persons with thrombocytopenia	Requires specialized techniques
Granulocytes	Granular leukocytes separated by apheresis	Granulocytopenia from malignancy or chemotherapy	Allergen sensitization may occur with chills and fever
Plasma Components			
Fresh frozen plasma (FFP)	Freezing of plasma within 4 hr of collection	Clotting deficiencies Liver disease Hemophilia Defibrination	Preserves factors V, VII, VIII, IX, and X and prothrombin Minimizes hepatitis risk Administered through a filter
Factor concentrates VIII and IX	Prepared from large donor pools Heated to inactivate HIV	VIII: hemophilia A IX: hemophilia B	Increased risk of hepatitis (VIII, IX) and thromboembolism (IX) Given in small volumes
Cryoprecipitate	Precipitated material obtained from FFP when thawed	Hemophilia A Infection of burns Hypofibrinogenemia Uremic bleeding	Contains factors VIII, XIII, and fibrinogen
Serum albumin Normal serum albumin Plasma protein fraction (PPF)	Albumin chemically processed from pooled plasma	Hypovolemic shock Hypoalbuminemia Burns Hemorrhagic shock	No risk of hepatitis Does not require ABO compatibility Lacks clotting factors Hypotension may occur if PPF is given faster than 10 ml/min
Immune serum globulin	Obtained from plasma of preselected donors with specific antibodies	Hypogammaglobulinemia Prophylaxis for hepatitis A, tetanus	Given intramuscularly

remainder returned to the donor (apheresis). Using blood components rather than whole blood is a more efficient use of a scarce commodity for an increased number of recipients, prevents fluid overload, and decreases the risk for adverse effects.

Most of the serious reactions that occur during transfusions are the result of human error. Typing, screening, and cross-matching of blood in the laboratory must be accurate. Typing is confirmed by testing the recipient's serum against commercial A and B cells to detect isoagglutinins. The recipient's serum is then screened for all antibodies that were not found in the typing. The goal of cross-matching is to ensure that the recipient's blood does not contain antibodies that will attack and destroy the transfused erythrocytes. When mismatched blood cells are transfused, antibodies immediately agglutinate the incompatible erythrocytes and activate complement. This reaction produces cell lysis and subsequent intavascular hemolysis.

Blood transfusions are carefully monitored and follow strict institutional protocols. Care of the person receiving a blood transfusion is outlined in the Guidelines for Safe Practice box. If a patient reports any of the symptoms associated with transfusion reaction, the nurse immediately stops the transfusion and maintains patency of the vein by administering normal saline. The primary care provider is notified immediately. Patients who exhibit any sign of anaphylaxis or hemolytic reaction receive frequent vital sign monitoring and are assessed for signs of impending shock, renal failure, or DIC. The blood and tubing are returned to the laboratory for analysis, and a first-voided urine specimen is collected to analyze for signs of hemolysis. The patient's hemoglobin and hematocrit levels are carefully monitored to determine the extent of the reaction. Patients who experience mild allergic reactions to blood may receive premedication with an antihistamine if they should need transfusion in the future. A Clinical Pathway for a patient receiving a blood transfusion can be found on p. 1647.

Patient/Family Education. Informed consent is necessary before the administration of blood; therefore the patient and family are queried about their understanding of the procedure, and permission for the transfusion is secured. The nurse answers questions and clarifies misunderstandings about blood transfusions. The prospect of receiving blood is frightening to many individuals because of concerns about contracting AIDS. The nurse reassures patients and families that blood is carefully screened and tested for disease before being prepared for transfusion.

Teaching includes information regarding how the blood or blood component will be administered, approximately how long the transfusion will take, and signs and symptoms associated with transfusion reactions. Patients are encouraged to promptly report any unusual sensations experienced during the transfusion. They are also informed that their vital signs will be frequently monitored throughout the procedure, and that this is normal protocol and does not mean that a reaction is actually occurring.

Guidelines for Safe Practice

The Patient Receiving a Blood Transfusion

1. Carefully check all of the following:
   a. Identity of patient to receive transfusion
   b. The label of the unit of blood for the name of the person for whom it is intended; make certain that it matches the patient's wristband before administering the blood
   c. Expiration date of the blood
   d. Color and consistency of blood (if the bag appears to have clots, gas, or a dark purple color, it could be contaminated and should not be infused)
2. Obtain baseline vital signs and check again at frequent intervals throughout the procedure.
3. Administer all blood products through micron mesh filters.
4. Assess patient for any unusual sensations felt throughout the transfusion. (This information may help with early identification of any reactions that occur.)
5. Infuse blood within 4 hours after it is taken from the blood bank (to prevent bacterial growth).
6. If blood cannot be infused within 4 hours, return it to the blood bank for proper refrigeration.
7. Follow facility guidelines for proper disposal of empty blood bag and tubing.
8. Record patient's response to the infusion.
9. Report any adverse effect to the primary care provider immediately.
10. Return the blood bag and tubing to the laboratory for testing if a reaction occurs.

TYPE III HYPERSENSITIVITIES

Type III hypersensitivities are due to the formation or deposition of antigen-antibody complexes in various tissues, which results in complement activation and inflammation. These reactions are not immediate and generally occur over several hours after exposure to the antigen. Examples of the more common type III hypersensitivities include systemic lupus erythematosus (see Chapter 47), immune complex glomerulonephritis (see Chapter 39), and serum sickness.

Serum Sickness

Etiology/Epidemiology

Serum sickness develops within 1 to 3 weeks after administration of foreign serum, such as horse or rabbit serum. It may also occur after administration of certain drugs (e.g., antimicrobials such as penicillin and sulfonamides). Classic serum sickness is rarely encountered today because large doses of foreign sera are rarely administered.

Pathophysiology

The pathogenesis of serum sickness lies in the union of soluble antigens (foreign serum proteins) and immunoglobulins of the IgM and IgG classes. The complexes formed in these interactions are not properly cleared by the reticuloendothelial system because of their small size, which tends to defy phagocytosis. The complexes can then bind

clinical pathway *Blood Transfusion*

PROBLEM LIST AND OUTCOMES	DATE UNIT 1		DATE UNIT 2	DATE UNIT 3	DATE UNIT 4	DATE UNIT 5
Knowledge deficit R/T need for transfusion	Verbalizes understanding of procedure and symptoms to report to nurse	☐	---> ☐	---> ☐	---> ☐	---> ☐
Potential for adverse physical effects R/T administration of blood component therapy	Demonstrates no adverse physical effects (see symptoms of reaction)	☐☐	---> ☐☐	---> ☐☐	---> ☐☐	---> ☐☐
Tests	H&H post infusion as ordered	☐	☐	☐	☐	☐
Treatments	Check Nsg H&P for previous transfusion history	☐	--->	--->	--->	--->
	Have pt review and sign blood consent	☐	--->	--->	--->	--->
	Establish adequate IV access	☐	--->	--->	--->	--->
IMPORTANT	VS: prior to getting unit from bloodbank, 15min & 1hr after start of infusion	☐☐	---> ☐☐	---> ☐☐	---> ☐☐	---> ☐☐
Do not remove any attached identification from the unit of blood until the transfusion is completed.	Temperature elevation prior to starting blood is reported to physician for pre-treatment	☐	---> ☐	---> ☐	---> ☐	---> ☐
	Blood started within 30 minutes of pickup	☐	--->	---> ☐	---> ☐	---> ☐
	Infuse unit in 4 hours or less as ordered	☐	---> ☐	---> ☐	---> ☐	---> ☐
Blood tubing is used for 1 unit of blood and hangs no longer than 4 hrs.	Check VS immediately & 1 hr after infusion is complete	☐☐	---> ☐☐	---> ☐☐	---> ☐☐	---> ☐☐
	Transfusion form completed and returned to blood bank within 8 hours.	☐	---> ☐	---> ☐	---> ☐	---> ☐
	If symptoms occur: Stop infusion, notify MD & Blood Bank, KVO IV w/ normal saline, assist pt. to collect specimens, send bag, tubing, & saline to lab, complete suspected transfusion reaction form.	☐☐	---> ☐☐	---> ☐☐	---> ☐☐	---> ☐☐
	Benign urticaria (hives with no other symptoms): Notify physician, notify Blood Bank, treat symptoms, no workup required					
Teaching	Instruct pt. & family on rationale, procedure symptoms to report of reaction	☐☐	Reinforce teaching ☐	---> ☐	---> ☐	---> ☐
<u>Symptoms of Reaction:</u> BLDTRANS.WK1 11/00	Fever (1.5 degree F rise), Chills, Shock, Excessive bleeding, BP change, chest pain Back pain, Flushing, Oliguria, Dyspnea, Hemoglobinuria, Urticaria (Hives) with other symptoms, Jaundice, Itching, Rash					

Courtesy Columbia Overland Park Regional Medical Center (Health Midwest, Inc.) Overland Park, KS.

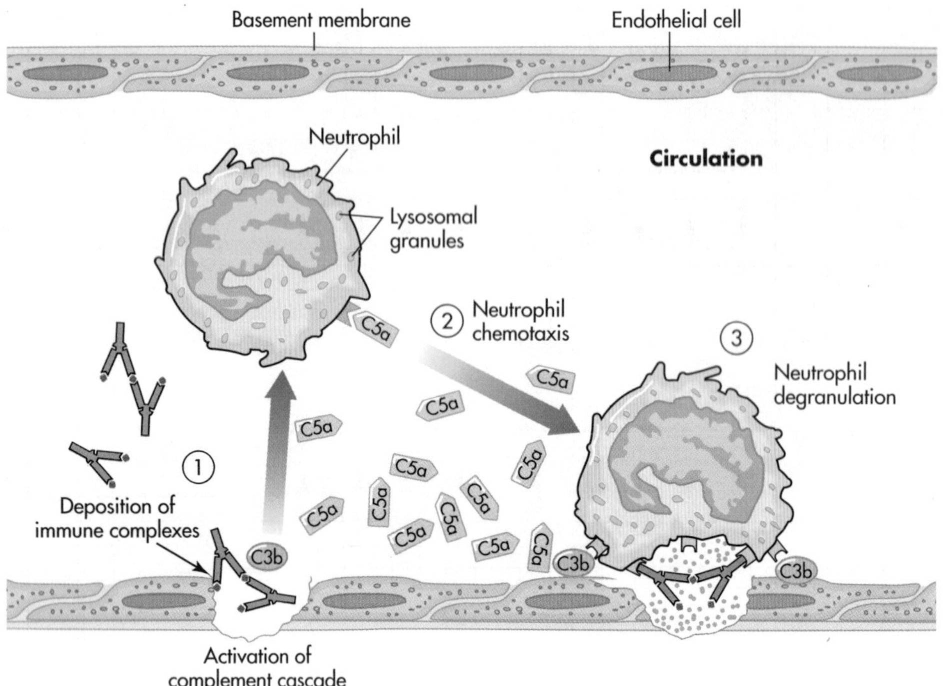

Figure 49-8 Mechanism of type III, immune complex-mediated reactions. Immune complexes are deposited in the vessels of other healthy tissue, where they activate the complement cascade and generate complement fragments including C5a (*1*). C5a is chemotactic for neutrophils, which migrate into the inflamed area (*2*) and attach to the IgG and C3b in the immune complexes. The neutrophils degranulate a variety of degradative enzymes that destroy healthy tissues (*3*).

complement, initiating the complement cascade and resulting in chemotaxis, vasodilation, and cell lysis. The chemotactic factors released by the complement cascade lead to an influx of phagocytes, which tend to intensify the inflammatory response (Figure 49-8).

The antigen-antibody reactions of serum sickness occur in many organs, but the kidneys, choroid plexus, joints, skin, and lungs are primarily affected. Itching and discomfort at the injection site are usually the first symptoms noted. These are followed by lymphadenopathy, fever, urticaria or erythematous rash, angioedema of the face, and joint pain. Splenomegaly, abdominal pain, headache, nausea, and vomiting may also occur.

Collaborative Care Management

Treatment of type III hypersensitivities depends on the cause. Serum sickness is a self-limiting disease. Mild symptoms respond well to antihistamines and salicylates. More severe symptoms are treated with steroids such as prednisone, and relief of symptoms is often obtained within hours. Epinephrine is given if an anaphylactic reaction occurs.

Patient/Family Education. Patients who develop serum sickness are concerned about the cause of this unusual disorder and how it is treated. They are taught that serum sickness is a reaction to foreign protein, that symptoms can be controlled, and that it is a self-limiting condition. Persons who develop serum sickness are encouraged to inform future health care providers of their tendency toward hypersensitivity.

TYPE IV HYPERSENSITIVITIES

Type IV hypersensitivity, also known as delayed hypersensitivity, is cell mediated as opposed to antibody mediated. Graft rejection, contact dermatitis, and hypersensitivity induced by chronic infection (e.g., tuberculosis) are examples of type IV hypersensitivity reactions.

Etiology/Epidemiology

Type IV hypersensitivities generally occur within 12 to 72 hours after a sensitized individual comes in contact with the offending antigen. The reaction that occurs from an inactivated or purified protein derivative tuberculin test is a classic example of type IV hypersensitivity. People who have undergone sufficient exposure to *Mycobacterium tuberculosis* to be sensitized to the organism, whether or not they have the disease, develop redness and induration in response to the injection within 8 to 12 hours.

Allergic contact dermatitis is an inflammatory response confined to the skin that results from repeated exposure of a sensitized person to an allergen. Environmental substances such as cosmetics, hair dyes, or detergents; poison ivy or oak; or latex may serve as the offending antigen in type IV hypersensitivity.

Another important type IV hypersensitivity reaction occurs when organs or tissues are transferred from one person to another. Transplantation has been done for many years, but has been limited because of the rejection process resulting from type IV hypersensitivity.

Pathophysiology

Type IV hypersensitivities are cell mediated and do not involve antibodies such as IgE. Macrophages pick up antigens identified as "foreign" to the body. These macrophages take pieces of the antigen and present them to the T lymphocytes, which become sensitized to the specific antigen. The next time the person comes in contact with the antigen, the sensitized lymphocyte forms cytotoxic T cells or activates nonspecific phagocytic cells. The cytotoxic T lymphocytes destroy the antigen directly by breaking down the cell membrane, causing lysis and cell death. The sensitized T lymphocyte can also activate nonspecific phagocytic cells (macrophages and polymorphonuclear leukocytes) through release of lymphokines.

Allergic contact dermatitis is one of the most commonly encountered types of allergic disease. Usually, both the route of sensitization and the clinical manifestations are produced by direct dermal contact. The allergen attaches to skin proteins, which function as haptens to stimulate the proliferation of a T-cell population sensitized to the allergen. After sensitization, subsequent contact with the contact allergen leads to formation of an erythematous, vesiculated (blistered) lesion. The inflamed area is red, swollen, and warm and may itch, burn, or sting. The location of the lesions often provides data about the causative allergic agent.

The tubercle bacillus *(M. tuberculosis)* itself is not directly toxic to human cells or tissues. The organism invades the tissues of a nonsensitized host and establishes residence in the host tissues, causing virtually no damage. However, in the course of time, as the organism sheds antigenic material, the cell-mediated immune response is triggered. The sensitized lymphocytes and the activated macrophages attack not only the organism but also the tissues surrounding the organism. This process is aimed at destroying the foreign organism; however, in the course of the attack, tissue destruction may result. The lesions associated with tuberculosis (such as caseation necrosis cavitation) and general toxemia are results of the hypersensitivity. After the initial sensitization with the infectious organism, subsequent contact with the tuberculosis organism or an extract of a purified protein from the organism will elicit a hypersensitivity reaction. This is the basis of the Mantoux tuberculin skin test. The skin rashes of smallpox and measles and the lesions of herpes simplex virus are all examples of an infectious type IV hypersensitivity.

In transplantation the foreign tissue or organ serves as the allergen against which the cell-mediated response is directed. Cytotoxic T lymphocytes attack and destroy the tissues directly, resulting in destruction of transplanted tissues.[5] A discussion of organ transplantation can be found in Chapter 51.

Collaborative Care Management

Treatment for contact dermatitis includes elimination of known allergens, decreased exposure, or both. Topical antiinflammatory agents such as corticosteroid creams may be useful in reducing the discomfort associated with itching and decreasing healing time. For severe reactions, systemic corticosteroids and antihistamines may be necessary.

There is no specific treatment, other than treatment of the underlying infection, for hypersensitivity reactions to infective agents. If secondary infection develops as a result of the patient scratching the area, antibiotics may be prescribed. Immunosuppression therapy is used to control transplant rejection.

Patient/Family Education. The nurse provides the patient and family with information about the hypersensitivity reaction and how it manifests. Specific antigens are identified and strategies are planned to reduce exposure. Patients with contact dermatitis are cautioned to avoid scratching lesions, because scratching may further spread the lesion or infect the site. Patients are also taught how to use topical corticosteroids. Patients on systemic corticosteroids are cautioned to never abruptly stop taking their medication. For care of the person with contact dermatitis, see Chapter 62.

AUTOIMMUNE DISEASES

Etiology/Epidemiology

Autoimmunity is influenced by genetic, hormonal, viral, and environmental factors. Autoimmune disorders run in families but are not passed on by simple mendelian inheritance. Human leukocyte antigens and non-HLA antigens have a well-documented association with certain autoimmune diseases. Many individuals with these same gene markings, however, do not have the disease, so there is not a direct relationship between the genetic predisposition and disease.

The role of sex hormones is not clearly understood, but autoimmune diseases are far more common in females than in males. Interactions of the host with certain environmental agents such as bacteria, viruses, drugs, and toxins have been shown to initiate autoimmune disease.

Pathophysiology

Autoimmunity, the formation of antibodies against self-tissues, is a natural phenomenon that occurs when the body looses some of its tolerance to self and is no longer able to fully distinguish self from non-self cells. Autoimmunity may involve either T or B cells or both. Antibodies produced against one's own cells are referred to as *autoantibodies.* When produced against DNA, they are called anti-DNA antibodies. These self-reactive immunoglobulins are often associated with pathologic states in the body; however, they can also be isolated from the serum of disease-free individuals and are present in about half of adults over the age of 70 years.

The exact mechanism of autoimmunity is not known, although several theories have been proposed:

- *Release of sequestered antigens.* If an antigen does not come into contact with the immune system during fetal development when self-tolerance normally develops, the antigen remains antigenic. Later, as a result of trauma or infection, the antigen may be exposed to the immune system, eliciting an autoimmune response (e.g., autoantibodies against heart muscle after acute myocardial infarction).
- *Defective T suppressor cells.* Suppressor T cell function may be lost or altered so that autoantibodies are allowed to proliferate.

- *Synthesis of cross-reactive antibodies.* Antibodies synthesized in response to certain foreign antigens may have cross-reactivity with similar antigenic components within human tissues. Contact with antigens called heterophile antigens may trigger the production of autoantibodies. This process is theorized to account for the damage of rheumatic heart disease.
- *Alteration of self-antigens.* Normal body proteins may be altered by chemicals, infectious organisms, or therapeutic drugs and present new antigenically active groups to the immune system. Autoimmune hemolytic anemia may result from alteration of the Rh antigens of the RBC, rendering it antigenic. Certain antibiotics can have a similar effect.

Autoimmune disorders are grouped into categories according to the part of the body involved. Autoimmune diseases that are organ specific produce chronic inflammatory changes in a specific organ. Nonorgan-specific autoimmune disorders are characterized by chronic inflammatory changes in many different organs and tissues throughout the body. Box 49-4 presents a listing of selected autoimmune disorders.

BOX 49-4 Classification of Autoimmune Disorders

Organ Specific

Blood

Autoimmune hemolytic anemia
Idiopathic thrombocytopenic purpura

Heart

Rheumatic fever

Central Nervous System

Multiple sclerosis
Guillain-Barré syndrome

Muscles

Myasthenia gravis

Endocrine System

Addison's disease
Autoimmune thyroiditis (Hashimoto's disease)
Graves' disease
Hypothyroidism

Eye

Uveitis

Gastrointestinal System

Pernicious anemia
Ulcerative colitis

Kidneys

Glomerulonephritis
Goodpasture's syndrome

Skin

Pemphigus vulgaris

Nonorgan Specific

Systemic lupus erythematosus
Rheumatoid arthritis
Progressive systemic sclerosis

Collaborative Care Management

Treatment for many autoimmune disorders is suppression of cell-mediated immunity and control of clinical manifestations, primarily achieved through treatment with systemic corticosteroid therapy. Initial doses of 60 mg of oral prednisone often bring about a noticeable decrease in symptoms. Once symptoms are controlled, dosages are slowly decreased and then discontinued until the next exacerbation occurs. Cytotoxic drugs such as cyclosphosphamide, azathioprine, and methotrexate, are sometimes prescribed for patients with severe or persistent manifestations. Treatment of specific autoimmune disorders is discussed elsewhere in this textbook.

Patient/Family Education. Emotional support and patient teaching are important aspects of care for the person with an autoimmune disorder. Patients are taught about their illness, symptoms that warn of exacerbation, and any measures that may reduce the chances for exacerbation. Teaching includes manifestations that need to be reported immediately versus those that can be managed at home.

The nurse encourages patients to eat a well-balanced diet, maintain daily exercise patterns that do not result in fatigue, and get plenty of rest and sleep. The nurse also explains the anticipated benefit of prescribed medications, dosage schedules, and adverse effects, especially when the patient is taking corticosteroids or other immunosuppressive drugs. The patient is cautioned against abruptly withdrawing steroid medications, because abrupt cessation can result in adrenal insufficiency or crisis. The nurse stresses the importance of close follow-up care. The patient and family are referred to available local support groups.

CHRONIC FATIGUE SYNDROME

Chronic fatigue syndrome (CFS) is a condition of unexplained fatigue that lasts 6 months or longer and eventually becomes debilitating. CFS may follow a cold, influenza, bronchitis, or mononucleosis. In other instances, CFS develops gradually, with no clear initiating event.[13] Accompanying manifestations, such as muscle and joint discomfort, headache, loss of concentration, weakness, and tender lymph nodes, may go unnoticed because they are similar to the flu. Unlike the flu, however, the fatigue and other symptoms remain or reappear frequently.

Etiology/Epidemiology

The exact cause of CFS remains unknown despite intensive decade-long research into possible causative factors. Genetic and environmental factors, viruses, bacterium, toxins, and psychologic factors have been considered. Currently, anemia, hypoglycemia, environmental allergy and body-wide yeast infection is being investigated as causative or contributing factors.[6]

BOX 49-5 Diagnostic Criteria for Chronic Fatigue Syndrome

Major Criteria

- New, debilitating, persistent, or relapsing fatigue that does not improve with rest and that has impaired daily activities by 50% for 6 months or longer
- Absence of other conditions that produce similar symptoms (autoimmune diseases, cardiac disease, cancer, HIV, AIDS, gastrointestinal dysfunction, hepatic problems, endocrine dysfunction, neuromuscular complaints, psychiatric problems, etc.)

Minor Criteria

- Four or more of the 11 symptoms must be present

Symptoms

Symptoms must have started after fatigue onset and persisted or recurred for 6 months or longer.

- Low-grade fever
- Sore throat
- Cervical or axillary adenopathy
- Generalized muscular weakness
- Myalgia
- Prolonged fatigue (≥24 hours) after exercise that was previously tolerated
- New onset of generalized headache
- Noninflammatory arthritis
- Complaints of one or more of the following: photophobia, transient visual scotomata, forgetfulness, excessive irritability, confusion, difficulty thinking, inability to concentrate, or depression
- Insomnia or hypersomnia
- Onset of symptoms over a few hours to a few days

Signs

Must be documented by a physician on two occasions at least 1 month apart.

- Low-grade fever
- Nonexudative pharyngitis
- Palpable/tender cervical or axillary lymph nodes of 2 cm or less

Modified from Holmes GP et al: *Ann Intern Med* 108(3):387, 1998.

Chronic fatigue syndrome affects as many as 800,000 people in the United States. One four-city study by the Centers for Disease Control and Prevention (CDC) found that 98% of patients with CFS were Caucasian and 85% were female, with an average age of onset of 30 years. More than 80% of the women in this study were well educated and from upper income families, which may be one reason why CFS was mislabeled as "yuppie flu." CFS is now recognized in people of all ages, races, and socioeconomic groups.[13]

The CDC published the first case definition of CFS and a set of diagnostic criteria in 1988. A revised set of diagnostic criteria and clinical manifestations is presented in Box 49-5. The primary clinical manifestation of CFS is prolonged, debilitating fatigue accompanied by any or all of the symptoms listed in the diagnostic criteria for CFS.

Evidence-Based Practice

Reference: Cleare AJ et al: Low-dose hydrocortisone in chronic fatigue syndrome: a randomized crossover trial, *Lancet* 353:455, 1999.

The purpose of the study was to determine if patients with chronic fatigue syndrome could benefit from low-dose hydrocortisone therapy. A total of 32 study subjects received 5 or 10 mg of hydrocortisone daily and control subjects received a placebo. Nine of the subjects who received the hydrocortisone therapy reported short-term improvement in their fatigue, but 10% of those nine experienced side effects. The study concluded that any benefit derived from hydrocortisone therapy was short lived and associated with adverse effects.

Pathophysiology

The clinical course of CFS varies considerably among patients and is difficult to diagnose because the same symptoms occur with many other conditions and diseases. CFS often follows a cyclical course, alternating between illness and relatively symptom-free intervals, which is similar to that of autoimmune disorders such as lupus erythematosus or multiple sclerosis. About 50% of patients recover within the first 5 years after onset. No characteristics of the disease or persons with the disease have been identified that make one person more likely to achieve recovery than another.[13]

Collaborative Care Management

Treatments for CFS have included antiviral agents, antidepressants, and immune modulators, but none have proven to be effective (see Evidence-Based Practice box). Consequently, treatments are aimed at controlling symptoms. Nonsteroidal antiinflammatory drugs may be beneficial in reducing body aches or fever, and nonsedating antihistamines have been useful for relieving allergic symptoms. There is no cure for this disease at this time.

Patient/Family Education. Education for the patient with CFS focuses on how to manage fatigue to improve functioning and quality of life. The nurse carefully assesses the extent of the patient's symptoms and physical limitations and helps the patient identify potential triggers of fatigue. The patient is encouraged to avoid situations or activities that adversely affect energy levels. Periods of activity are scheduled at times when the patient feels better and are alternated with rest periods. Exercise may seem contradictory in the presence of fatigue, but exercise improves conditioning and can restore energy. The nurse assists the patient with developing an individualized exercise program that incorporates a gradual increase in intensity and duration. Exercise needs to be incorporated in a manner that does not exacerbate fatigue, yet promotes regular participation.

A well-balanced diet is essential to promote adequate energy stores and is therefore another important part of patient/family education. Nighttime sleep should be as free of interruption as possible, and daytime naps are avoided if they interfere with nighttime rest. The patient may also benefit from relaxation, meditation, massage, imagery, touch, music, or biofeedback.

Chronic fatigue syndrome is a disease with overwhelming subjective symptoms, and patients experiencing persistent debilitating fatigue are commonly treated with overt skepticism if not direct accusations of malingering by health care providers. Symptoms of CFS may be attributed to life stress, unhappiness, female hormone imbalances, or simply labeled as psychosomatic. The nurse plays an important role in reassuring the patient about both the validity and severity of the symptoms. The nurse also includes the family in all discussions and teaching sessions about disease etiology and management. Family support is critical to the patient because many occupational and family roles may have to be reduced or eliminated in the face of overwhelming fatigue. The nurse encourages the patient and family to contact local or national CFS support groups to establish a network of information and support for dealing with this debilitating chronic disease.

Critical Thinking Questions

1. You are caring for two patients. One has a primary immune deficiency disease, and the other has a secondary immune deficiency. How will the care of these two patients be similar? How will it be different?
2. A patient resided in a warm and humid climate for 30 years. After moving to another climate, she developed an upper respiratory infection for which her physician gave her an injection of penicillin. She stated that she had never been given penicillin, and that she had no known allergies. Within 20 minutes after receiving the penicillin, she developed symptoms of anaphylaxis. What explanation can be given for her reaction?
3. A woman was recently diagnosed with seasonal allergies to pollens and grasses. She cleans houses 3 days each week, and she lives in a house near a large open field. What additional data, if any, do you need to collect from her, and what do you need to include in her teaching plan?
4. What aspects of care are similar for any patient with autoimmune disease, regardless of cause?

References

1. Beers MH, Berkow R, editors: Plasma cell disorders. *Merck manual of diagnosis and therapy,* ed 17, Whitehouse Station, NJ, 1999, Merck Co.
2. Beers MH, Berkow R, editors: Disorders with type 1 hypersensitivity reactions, *Merck manual of diagnosis and therapy,* ed 17, Whitehouse Station, NJ, 1999, Merck Co.
3. Cleveland Clinic: Multiple myeloma and plasma cell dyscrasia, website: http://www.clevelandclinic.org/myeloma/mm%2Dpt.htm, 2001.
4. Cleveland Clinic: Diagnosis and treatment of multiple myeloma and other plasma cell disorders, website: http://www.clevelandclinic.org/myeloma/mm%2Dpt.htm, 2001.
5. Copstead LC, Banasik JL: *Pathophysiology: biological and behavioral perspective,* ed 2, Philadelphia, 2000, WB Saunders.
6. Chronic Fatigue Syndrome Association of America (CFIDS): Chronic fatigue syndrome fact sheet, http:www.cfids.org/news/factsht.html, 2001.
7. Huether SE, McCance KL: *Understanding pathophysiology,* ed 2, St Louis, 2000, Mosby.
8. Immune Deficiency Foundation: Overview of primary immune deficiency diseases, website: http://www.primaryimmune.org, 2000.
9. International Myeloma Foundation: Multiple myeloma, *Myeloma Today* 1(6), 2001.
10. Kardon E: Transfusion reactions, website: http://www.emedicine.com/emerg/topic603.htm, 2001.
11. Loudermilk DL, Perry SE, Bobak IM: *Maternity and women's health care,* ed 7, St Louis, 2000, Mosby.
12. McCance KL, Huether SE: *Pathophysiology: the biologic basis for disease in adults and children,* ed 3, St Louis, 1998, Mosby.
13. National Center for Infectious Diseases: Chronic fatigue syndrome: demographics, Center for Disease Control and Prevention, website: http://www.cdc.gov/ncidod/diseases/cfs/demographics.htm, 2000.
14. National Institute of Allergy and Infectious Diseases, National Institutes of Health: Improved therapy means a better and longer life, website: http://www.niaid.nih.gob/publications/pid/what.htm, 1998.
15. National Institute of Allergy and Infectious Diseases, National Institutes of Health: the 10 warning signs of primary immunodeficiency disease, website: http://www.niaid.nih.gob/publications/pid/what.htm, 1998.
16. National Institute of Allergy and Infectious Diseases, National Institutes of Health: What are primary immunodeficiency diseases? website: http://www.niaid.nih.gov/publications/pid/what.htm, 1998.
17. National Institute of Allergy and Infectious Diseases, National Institutes of Health: Asthma and allergy statistics, *Fact Sheet,* U.S. Department of Health and Human Services, 2000.
18. Roitt I, Brostoff J, Male D: *Immunology,* ed 5, St Louis, 1998, Mosby.
19. University of Pennsylvania Cancer Center: Multiple myeloma and other plasma cell neoplasms, website: http://cancer.med.upenn.edu/pdq_html/1/engl/110392-3.html, 2000.
20. Zak HN: Health-care workers and latex allergy, *Arch Environ Health* 9:43, 2000.

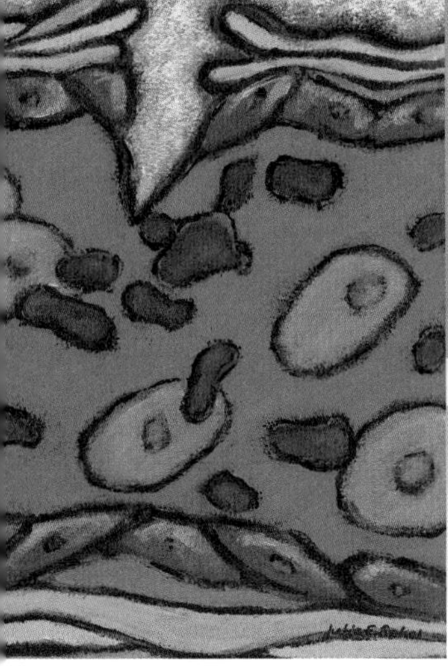

http://www.mosby.com/MERLIN/medsurg_phipps

HIV Infection and AIDS 50

Carol J. Green

Objectives

After studying this chapter, the learner should be able to:

1. Describe the epidemiology of HIV infection.
2. Identify the causative agent of HIV infection.
3. Discuss the infection and replication process of HIV.
4. Distinguish between primary, secondary, and tertiary prevention measures for HIV infection.
5. Describe the continuum of HIV infection.
6. Describe the clinical manifestations and collaborative management of the common opportunistic infections that occur with AIDS.
7. Compare nursing care for the person with HIV infection and AIDS.

HUMAN IMMUNODEFICIENCY VIRUS INFECTION

Human immunodeficiency virus (HIV) infection is an acquired infection in which the HIV integrates itself into CD4 (T4 helper) cells, causing severe immune dysfunction. HIV infection renders the person unusually susceptible to other life-threatening infections and malignancies. In its most serious form it results in the HIV syndrome known as acquired immunodeficiency syndrome (AIDS).

Etiology

The origin of HIV is still largely unknown. Evidence appears to support the hypothesis of an African origin, since an AIDS-like illness in central Africa has been known to exist since the early 1960s. It is further hypothesized that the most likely source of human infection was from nonhuman primates.

The causative agent of HIV infection and AIDS is the human immune deficiency virus, a retrovirus that belongs to the lentivirus subfamily. Several human retroviruses have been identified. Two of them, HIV-1 and HIV-2, are associated with T4-helper-cell depletion and subsequent loss of cellular immunity. HIV-1 is the predominant cause of HIV infections in both developed and developing countries, accounting for more than 80% of AIDS cases worldwide. HIV-2 seems to be limited in geographic distribution and is most prevalent in West Africa.[12] Although there has been scientific and clinical progress and development of new treatments and comprehensive models of care, HIV disease remains an incurable disease.

Epidemiology

In December 2000 the Centers for Disease Control and Prevention (CDC) estimated that there were between 800,000 and 900,000 people living with HIV and approximately 40,000 new HIV infections occurring every year in the United States. By gender, approximately 70% of new HIV infections are among men, although the incidence among women has been steadily increasing. By race, African-Americans and Hispanics are disproportionately affected by HIV in the U.S. population. More than half (54%) of the new HIV infections occur among African-Americans, and 12% occur among Hispanics, even though these groups represent 13% and 12% of the population, respectively[5] (Figure 50-1).

Early in the U.S. epidemic more than 80% of those infected with HIV were men who have sex with men (MSM). Currently about 42% of infections occur in this group. Persons now at greatest risk for acquiring HIV infection in the United States include heterosexual women and their children and intravenous (IV) drug users[5] (Figure 50-2).

As of June 2000, 753,907 cases of AIDS had been reported in the United States, 43% of which were among Caucasian, 37% among African-Americans, and 20% among Hispanics. A total of 438,795 deaths from AIDS had been reported, which included 374,422 men and 64,373 women. Of these, 203,695 were Caucasian, 154,695 were African-American, and 75,966 were Hispanic. Advances in HIV treatments in the mid to late 1990s led to dramatic declines in AIDS deaths in the United States and slowed the progression of HIV to AIDS. In recent years, however, the annual number of AIDS cases is leveling, although the number of AIDS deaths continues to decline[5] (Figure 50-3).

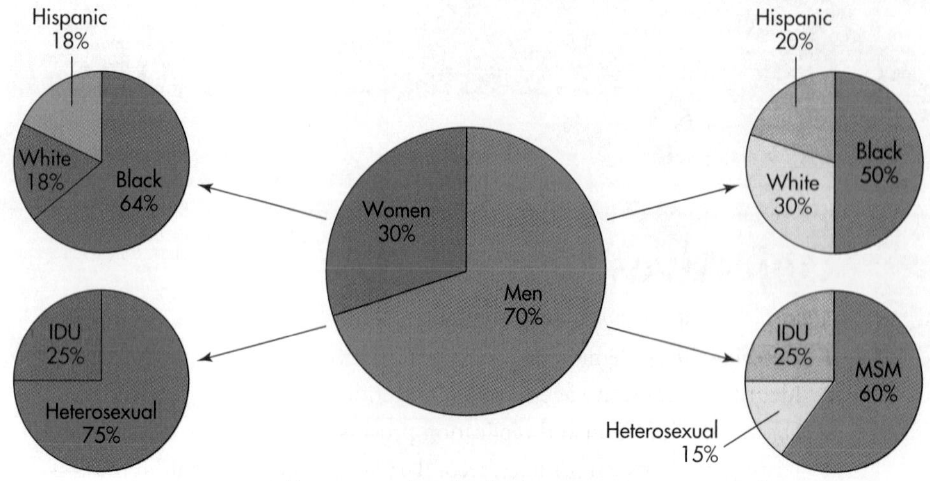

Figure 50-1 National estimates of annual new HIV infections among men and women by race/ethnicity and risk, 2000. *IDU,* Infection drug users; *MSM,* men who have sex with men.

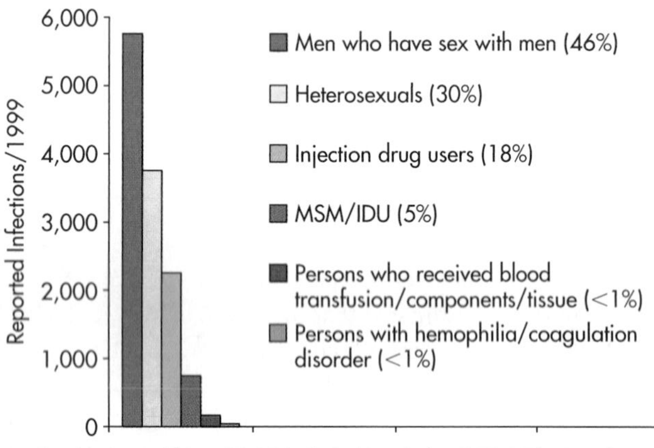

Figure 50-2 Adult and adolescent HIV infections by known risk, 1999.

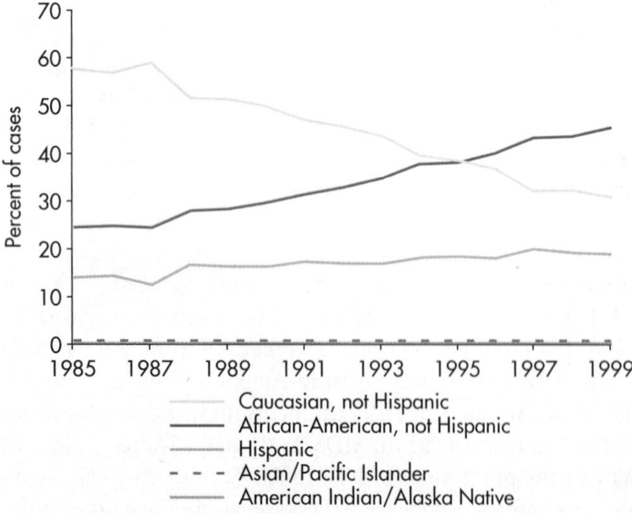

Figure 50-3 Proportion of AIDS cases by race/ethnicity and year of report, 1985-1999, United States.

By the end of 1999, the World Health Organization (WHO) estimated that 34.3 million people were infected with HIV/AIDS worldwide, with 95% of those individuals living in developing countries. WHO further estimated that in 1999 alone 5.4 million people became infected, averaging 15,000 new infections per day. WHO reported that 85% of the total global HIV/AIDS cases occur in sub-Saharan Africa, where more women are infected than men, even though only one tenth of the world's population lives there.[21] Other areas of concern are India, Southeast Asia, Latin American, and the Caribbean because the cost of new pharmacologic treatments is beyond the reach of these populations.

The routes for transmission of HIV are well documented: (1) directly from person to person by sexual contact; (2) direct inoculation with contaminated blood products, needles, or syringes; and (3) from infected mother to her fetus or newborn. HIV has been cultured from a variety of body fluids, including blood, semen, vaginal secretions, cerebrospinal fluid (CSF), saliva, tears, and breast milk. However, blood, semen, and vaginal secretions are the primary transmitters of infection. Epidemiologic studies indicate that transmission through body fluids such as saliva, tears, and breast milk is inefficient and unlikely to produce infection.

HIV is a bloodborne, sexually transmitted disease. Sexual practices, including vaginal or anal penetration without a condom and oral sexual practices, are associated with a high risk for infection. The use of contaminated needles for subcutaneous, intramuscular, or IV injection represents another serious risk for HIV infection. Women who are HIV infected may pass the virus on to their newborns via three potential routes: during gestation, during delivery, and rarely via breast milk.[7] HIV is not transmitted by casual contact, including sneezing, coughing, spitting, handshakes, and contact with potential secretions on toilet seats, bathtubs, showers, swimming pools, utensils, dishes, or linens used by infected persons. HIV is not transmitted by biting or bloodsucking insects.[3]

Blood transfusions are not a significant source of HIV infection today. In the United States each unit of donated blood

Risk Factors

HIV

Sexual practices*
- Unprotected sex
- Multiple sexual partners
- Anal or oral sexual activity
- Improper condom use or condom breakage
- Open sore, lesions, or irritation in the genital area

Contaminated blood

Contaminated needles

Occupational exposure
- All health care workers—acute care, long-term care, and home care
- Dental workers
- Corrections officers and law enforcement personnel

Perinatal exposure (during pregnancy, birth, or breast feeding)

NOTE: Approximately 25% of children of HIV-positive mothers are infected with the virus.

*An individual's sexual practices, not sexual preferences, create the HIV risk. The only true "safe sex" involves two seronegative partners in a monogamous relationship.

is tested for HIV infection, as well as several other bloodborne infections, such as hepatitis B. HIV screening of blood products has been conducted since 1985; only recipients of transfusions before that time were at significant risk for infection via the blood supply. It is possible for a contaminated unit of blood to test negative for HIV if the donor has not yet formed antibodies to the virus at the time of donation. As a result the risk of exposure to HIV via the US blood supply is estimated to be 1 in 400,000 units of blood.[3]

Risk factors for HIV infection are summarized in the Risk Factors box. The risk of HIV transmission to health care workers prompted the development and implementation of Universal Precautions by the Centers for Disease Control and Prevention. Recently, Universal Precautions were expanded to include all patients regardless of their medical diagnosis and are now referred to as Standard Precautions. The new precautions acknowledge that recognized and unrecognized microorganisms can exist in any body fluid and aim to reduce the risk of transmission within the hospital environment. These principles, which are summarized in Box 50-1, are to be used in the care of all patients at all times regardless of their HIV status (see Future Watch box).

BOX 50-1 Standard Precautions

Standard Precautions are designed to reduce the risk of transmission of microorganisms from both recognized and unrecognized sources of infection in the hospital. *Standard Precautions apply to all patients, regardless of their diagnosis.* Standard Precautions expand the coverage of Universal Precautions by recognizing that any body fluid may contain contagious microorganisms.

Standard Precautions are implemented when contact with blood, all body fluids (secretions and excretions except sweat, regardless of whether they contain visible blood), nonintact skin, and mucous membranes.

1. Hands are washed:
   a. After touching blood, body fluids, secretions, excretions, and contaminated items, whether or not gloves are worn.
   b. After removing gloves
   c. Between patient contacts
2. Gloves are worn (changed or removed):
   a. Before touching body fluids, secretions, excretions, nonintact skin, and contaminated items
   b. When performing veinpuncture and other vascular procedures
   c. Change gloves when changing tasks and procedures on the same patient
   d. Remove gloves before touching non-contaminated items and before going to another patient.
3. Gowns are worn if soiling with blood or body fluid is likely to occur.
4. Masks, eye protection, or face shields are worn if splashes or sprays of blood or body fluids are likely during care activities.
5. All sharp instruments and needles are discarded in a puncture-resistant container. Needles are disposed of uncapped.
6. Contaminated linens are placed in leak-proof bags for disposal.

NOTE: Additional precautions may be necessary to decrease the risk of infection with specific organisms. These precautions are instituted on a per patient basis and include airborne precautions, droplet precautions, and contact precautions. They are not needed for care of the HIV-positive patient unless a specific opportunistic infection such as tuberculosis is also present.

Adapted from Hospital Infection Control Practices Advisory Committee: *Guideline for Isolation Precautions in Hospitals,* Atlanta, Georgia, January 1996, Centers for Disease Control and Prevention, Public Health Service, US Department of Health and Human Services.

Pathophysiology

The natural history of HIV infection is associated with an unpredictable course of disease progression. Patients may undergo a prolonged period of clinically silent infection, often lasting more than 10 years. Although the virus is consistently detectable throughout this time, patients may exhibit only subtle immunologic alterations. Once the patient becomes symptomatic, however, decreases in the number of T4 helper cells can be detected and viral replication increases.

The life cycle of HIV is similar to that of the other retroviruses. Mature virons interact with specific host receptors and then use the host cell for viral replication. HIV interacts with the CD4 glycoprotein, which occurs on the membrane of specific cells, primarily the CD4 (T4) helper lymphocytes. The CD4 protein may also be found on the surface of several other cells, including some monocytes, macrophages, glial cells, and gastrointestinal (GI) cells. Presence of the CD4 glycoprotein allows the virus to fuse to the host cell. The viral core is subsequently injected into the cell cytoplasm, where the viral ribonucleic acid (RNA) genome is translated into deoxyribonucleic acid (DNA) by a retroviral enzyme called reverse transcriptase. Infection and subsequent viral replication eventually deplete the host's T4 helper cells, resulting in a dramatic loss of the protective immune response against invading microorganisms (Figure 50-4).

Several potential cofactors, which may be viral, host, or environmental, are thought to directly influence the replication of HIV or the severity of its pathogenic effects. Viral cofactors

Future Watch

AIDS Vaccine

The National Institutes of Health reports that more than 60 trials of vaccines against HIV have been conducted worldwide. Although many of the vaccines were safe and immunogenic in diverse populations, they failed to induce adequate cytotoxic T-cell lymphocytes or neutralize isolates of the HIV virus.

Currently, research is taking place to identify a vaccine that induces broadly neutralizing antibody against HIV, cytotoxic T-cell responses in a vast majority of recipients, and strong mucosal immune responses. Many barriers exist to the development of an effective vaccine; however, more is known about HIV than other pathogens for which vaccines were successfully developed.

The National Institute of Allergy and Infectious Disease has established a number of resources to facilitate private sector involvement and public-private collaborations in HIV vaccine research and development, including but not limited to, grant programs, training of investigators from developing countries in vaccine research and development, evaluation of possible vaccines, and doubling funding for HIV/AIDS research within the United States. Multiple organizations, including Walter Reed Army Institute of Research, The Centers for Disease Control and Prevention, the International AIDS Vaccine Initiative, and WHO/UNAIDS vaccine program are devoting time, effort, and funding to the development of an effective vaccine against HIV infection.

Reference: National Institute of Allergy and Infectious Disease: HIV vaccine development status report, National Institutes of Health, website: http://www.niaid,nih.gov/daids/vaccine/whsummarystatus.htm, 2000.

that may influence the progression of the disease include herpes simplex virus, cytomegalovirus (CMV), and Epstein-Barr virus (EBV). Host cofactors may include a variety of cytokines and intracellular mediators. Environmental cofactors may include repeated exposure to HIV, which may induce hyperactivation of the immune system, resulting in an expansion of the pool of HIV-replicating cells. As viral replication increases, depleting the body of T4 lymphocytes, the body's defense mechanisms are progressively weakened. Infections that were once disarmed by the healthy immune system are eventually able to cause serious and potentially life-threatening disease.

The spectrum of HIV infection ranges from asymptomatic infection to potentially life-threatening opportunistic infections. Early in the AIDS epidemic, it was believed that HIV infection could be divided into four separate processes: acute HIV infection, latent infection, AIDS-related complex, and AIDS. It is now known that the infection is one continuous disease process with three stages: acute retroviral infection, asymptomatic disease, and symptomatic disease (AIDS) (Figure 50-5). The CDC uses a Case Definition for AIDS surveillance and reporting, which has evolved over time and incorporates both laboratory and clinical stages[4] (Box 50-2). However, it is more useful to discuss the disease in terms of staging.

Acute Retroviral Infection. Symptoms generally occur within 1 to 3 weeks following HIV infection although they may occur up to 4 or 5 months after infection, and last for a week or two. Symptoms are similar to the flu or mononucleosis, consisting of fever, sore throat, fatigue, nausea, vomiting, headache, rash, or lymphadenopathy. Most of these manifestations go away without intervention, however, the lymphadenopathy usually persists throughout the course of the disease. It is during this time that the person converts to seropositive HIV status.

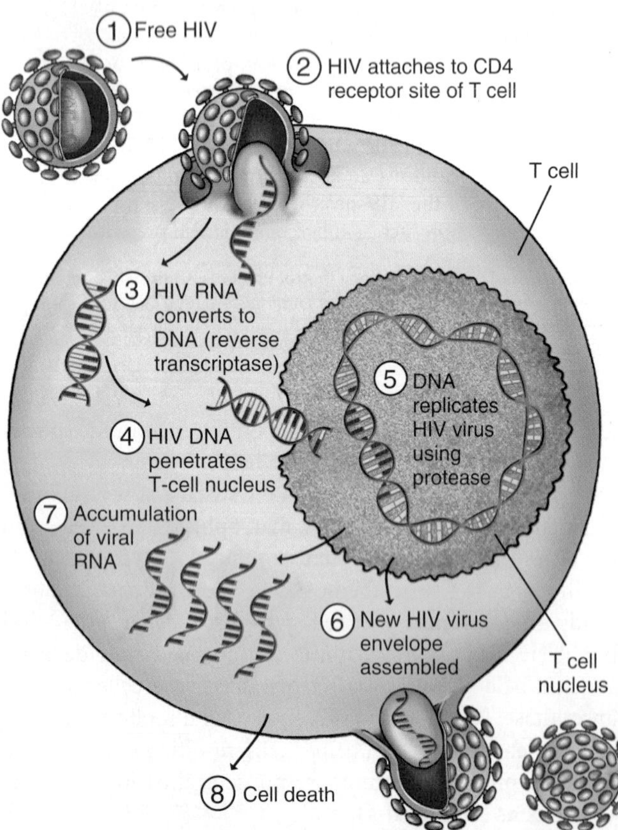

Figure 50-4 Life cycle of HIV.

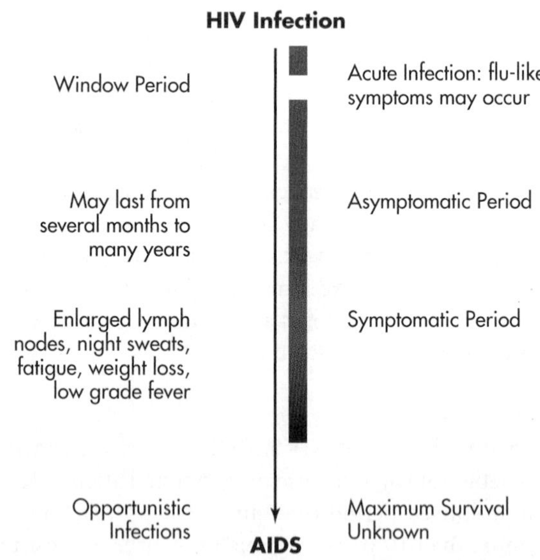

Figure 50-5 Spectrum of HIV infection. The initial phase of infection may be followed by a period of latency that may last from several months to several years. During this time the person may be completely asymptomatic or experience only mild symptoms. AIDS is said to exist when opportunistic infections are present and CD4 cell counts drop.

BOX 50-2 CDC Surveillance Case Definition for AIDS

I. HIV status of patient is unknown or inconclusive
If laboratory tests for HIV infection were not performed or gave inconclusive results and the patient had no other cause of immunodeficiency listed in IA (see below), a definitive diagnosis of any disease listed in IB (see below) indicates AIDS.
   A. Causes of immunodeficiency that disqualify a disease as an indication of AIDS in the absence of laboratory evidence of HIV infection
      1. The use of high-dose or long-term systemic corticosteroid therapy or other immunosuppressive/cytotoxic therapy within 3 months before the onset of the indicator disease
      2. A diagnosis of any of the following diseases within 3 months after diagnosis of the indicator disease: Hodgkin's disease, non-Hodgkin's lymphoma (other than primary brain lymphoma), lymphocytic leukemia, multiple myeloma, any other cancer of lymphoreticular or histiocytic tissue, or angioimmunoblastic lymphadenopathy
      3. A genetic (congenital) immunodeficiency syndrome or an acquired immunodeficiency syndrome that is atypical of HIV infection, such as one involving hypogammaglobulinemia
   B. Diseases that indicate AIDS (requires, definitive diagnosis)
      1. Candidiasis of the esophagus, trachea, bronchi, or lungs
      2. Cryptococcosis, extrapulmonary
      3. Cryptosporidiosis with diarrhea persisting for more than 1 month
      4. Cytomegalovirus disease of an organ other than the liver, spleen, or lymph nodes in a patient older than 1 month
      5. Herpes simplex virus infection causing a mucocutaneous ulcer that persists longer than 1 month; or herpes simplex virus infection causing bronchitis, pneumonitis, or esophagitis for any duration in a patient older than 1 month
      6. Kaposi's sarcoma in a patient younger than 60 years
      7. Lymphoid interstitial pneumonia or pulmonary lymphoid hyperplasia (LIP/PLH complex) in a patient younger than 13 years
      8. Lymphoma of the brain (primary) affecting a patient younger than 60 years
      9. *Mycobacterium avium* complex or *M. kansasii* disease, disseminated (at a site other than or in addition to the lungs, skin, or cervical or hilar lymph nodes)
      10. *Pneumocystis carinii* pneumonia
      11. Progressive multifocal leukoencephalopathy
      12. Toxoplasmosis of the brain in a patient older than 1 month

II. Patient is HIV positive
Regardless of the presence of other causes of immunodeficiency (see IA, above), in the presence of laboratory evidence of HIV infection, any disease listed in IB (see above) or in IIA or IIB (see below) indicates a diagnosis of AIDS. In addition, beginning in 1993, all HIV-positive adults and adolescents with $CD4^+$ T-cell counts less than 200/mm^3 or with pulmonary tuberculosis, recurrent pneumonia, or invasive cervical carcinoma should also be included in the AIDS case definition.
   A. Diseases that indicate AIDS (requires definitive diagnosis)
      1. Bacterial infections, multiple or recurrent (any combination of at least two within a 2- to 4-year period), of the following types in a patient younger than 13 years: septicemia, pneumonia, meningitis, bone or joint infection, or abscess of an internal organ or body cavity (excluding otitis media or superficial skin or mucosal abscesses) caused by *Haemophilus, Streptococcus* (including pneumococcus), or other pyogenic bacteria
      2. Coccidioidomycosis, disseminated (at a site other than or in addition to the lungs or cervical or hilar lymph nodes)
      3. Histoplasmosis, disseminated (at a site other than or in addition to the lungs or cervical or hilar lymph nodes)
      4. HIV encephalopathy
      5. HIV wasting syndrome
      6. Isosporiasis with diarrhea persisting for more than 1 month
      7. Kaposi's sarcoma at any age
      8. Lymphoma of the brain (primary) at any age
      9. *M. tuberculosis* disease, extrapulmonary (involving at least one site outside the lungs, regardless of whether there is concurrent pulmonary involvement)
      10. Mycobacterial disease caused by mycobacteria other than *M. tuberculosis,* disseminated (at a site other than or in addition to the lungs, skin, or cervical or hilar lymph nodes)
      11. Non-Hodgkin's lymphoma of B-cell or unknown immunologic phenotype and the following histologic types: small noncleaved lymphoma (Burkitt's or non-Burkitt's) or immunoblastic sarcoma
      12. *Salmonella* (nontyphoidal) septicemia, recurrent
   B. Diseases that indicate AIDS (presumptive diagnosis)
      1. Candidiasis of the esophagus
      2. Cytomegalovirus retinitis, with loss of vision
      3. Kaposi's sarcoma
      4. Lymphoid interstitial pneumonia or pulmonary lymphoid hyperplasia (LIP/PLH complex) in a patient younger than 13 years
      5. Mycobacterial disease (acid-fast bacilli with species not identified by culture), disseminated (involving at least one site other than or in addition to the lungs, skin, or cervical or hilar lymph nodes)
      6. *P. carinii* pneumonia
      7. Toxoplasmosis of the brain in a patient older than 1 month

III. Patient is HIV negative
With laboratory test results negative for HIV infection, a diagnosis of AIDS for surveillance purposes is ruled out unless
   A. All the other causes of immunodeficiency listed in IA (see above) are excluded; and
   B. The patient has had either of the following:
      1. *P. carinii* pneumonia diagnosed by a definitive method
      2. A definitive diagnosis of any of the other diseases indicative of AIDS listed in IB (see above) and a $CD4^+$ helper-inducer T-cell count of less than 400/mm^3

AIDS, acquired immunodeficiency syndrome; *CDC,* Centers for Disease Control and Prevention; *HIV,* human immunodeficiency virus.

Asymptomatic HIV Disease. The initial phase of infection may be followed by a period of latency that may last from several months to 10 years or more. During this time the person may be completely asymptomatic or experience only mild symptoms such as fatigue, headache, or lymphadenopathy.

During this stage $CD4^+$ cell counts gradually decline. The actual rate of decline varies among individuals and can be altered by antiretroviral therapy.

Clinical Manifestations

HIV/AIDS

Chills and fever	Malaise
Night sweats	Fatigue
Dry productive cough	Oral lesions
Dyspnea	Skin rash
Lethargy	Abdominal discomfort
Confusion	Diarrhea
Stiff neck	Weight loss
Seizures	Lymphadenopathy
Headache	Progressive generalized edema

Symptomatic HIV Disease. As the immune system becomes further compromised, the symptoms of AIDS develop. Clinical manifestations associated with AIDS are primarily those of opportunistic infections. Common symptoms are summarized in the Clinical Manifestations box. Symptoms of specific opportunistic infections are presented later in this chapter. Figure 50-6 illustrates the scope of HIV infection in the body and the range of organs and tissues that can be affected.

AIDS and its associated opportunistic infections can affect every organ and body system. Pulmonary infection from a variety of organisms is a constant threat to the person with HIV and is often the first manifestation of HIV infection. Pulmonary infections can very rapidly lead to severe hypoxemia. Compromised respiratory function can also result from pulmonary infiltration by a lymphoma.

Numerous GI problems associated with opportunistic infections or chemotherapy may plague the person with HIV infection. Common problems include granulomatous hepatitis, drug toxicity hepatitis, or coinfection with a hepatitis virus; masses or lesions from lymphomas and Kaposi's sarcoma; cholangitis or cholestasis; and pancreatic lesions. Patients may have difficulty eating or swallowing or may experience dys-

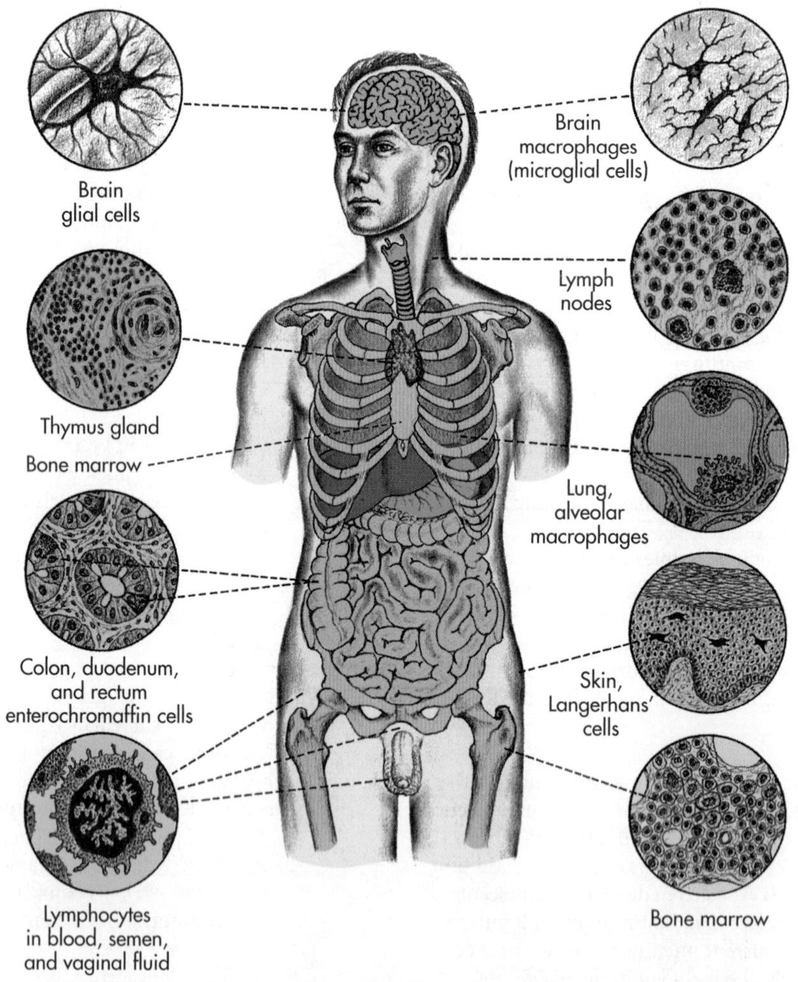

Figure 50-6 Distribution of tissues that can be infected by HIV. Infection is closely linked to the presence of CD4 receptors on host tissue, with the possible exceptions of glial cells in the brain and chromaffin cells in the colon, duodenum, and rectum.

pepsia, diarrhea, and weight loss. Loss of lean muscle mass is common.

HIV is able to cross the blood-brain and blood-CSF barriers and infect microglia and possibly other cells, resulting in encephalopathy. This process results in loss of cognitive and motor function. Many of the opportunistic infections can affect the central nervous system. Peripheral neuropathy with loss of motor function often occurs.

Macular roseola skin eruptions may be present during the initial infection with HIV. Later, seborrheic dermatitis, psoriasis, and Kaposi's sarcoma lesions can occur, along with cutaneous infections.

HIV infection causes the eyes to be vulnerable to invasion by CMV, which can result in blurring of vision and decreased acuity. The lesions are progressive and may lead to total blindness unless treated early and aggressively.

Thrombocytopenia, anemia, and neutropenia may be present with HIV. The causes of these problems are not precisely known, but it is thought that HIV decreases red blood cell production. Drug side effects also impact the hematologic system and can cause impaired production and increased destruction of blood cells.

Opportunistic infections can affect the heart, by producing pericarditis or myocarditis. Severe pulmonary hypertension associated with multiple episodes of *Pneumocystis carinii* pneumonia can cause right ventricular failure.

Although not as common as other system dysfunctions, all endocrine glands can be infiltrated with HIV. The adrenal gland is most commonly affected. Adrenal insufficiency may result from invasion by infective organisms, tumor growth, or drug therapy.

Musculoskeletal manifestations of HIV are common and may be mild or severe. Arthralgia is seen with acute infection and may also result from drug therapy. Myalgia, weakness, and wasting may also occur secondary to decreased appetite.

Fluid and electrolyte and acid-base imbalances occur from a variety of causes, including renal, GI, endocrine changes, or drug therapy. Renal dysfunction may occur from acute kidney failure secondary to hypovolemia, interstitial nephritis due to invasion of renal tissue by tumors or infective organisms, or glomerulosclerosis from HIV-associated nephropathy.

Collaborative Care Management

Diagnostic Tests. The most commonly used screening test for HIV infection is the enzyme-linked immunosorbent assay (ELISA), a highly specific test for HIV antibodies that has a sensitivity of 93.4% to 99.6%. A positive ELISA must be confirmed by the Western blot technique. Both the ELISA and the Western blot depend on antibody formation. Approximately 90% of the population form antibodies in response to HIV exposure within 6 weeks to 3 months after exposure, although this period may be as long as 6 months. A negative antibody test may occur in the "window phase" between the dates of actual exposure leading to infection and development of detectable serum antibodies. Because newborns maintain maternal antibodies for as long as 18 months, antibody testing is unreliable until the infant is 18 months of age.

Plasma HIV RNA levels measure the amount of virus in the person's serum, which is a reflection of active viral replication, or viral load. The steeper the rate of increase in plasma HIV RNA, the greater the risk of disease progression. A plasma HIV RNA level of less than 10,000 copies/ml is considered low risk for development of AIDS. Levels between 10,000 and 100,000 copies/ml double the risk for developing AIDS, and greater than 100,000 copies/ml indicates a high risk for developing AIDS.[6,8]

HIV RNA levels are measured periodically to determine the risk for disease progression and to monitor the effectiveness of antiretroviral therapy. Therapy is aimed at reducing plasma HIV RNA levels to below the limit of detection by the sensitive assay. For accuracy, two HIV RNA assays are completed within 1 to 2 weeks of each another, and both values are used to establish a baseline for the infected person. It is important for nurses to understand that suppression of HIV RNA levels to below the limits of detection does not mean that HIV infection has been eliminated or that viral replication has been halted completely. It simply means that HIV levels have been reduced to such a degree that they cannot be measured by present methods. Tests that can detect viral loads of between 20 and 100 copies/ml are being developed, which will improve the practitioner's ability to predict HIV disease progression.

CD4 + T cell counts are used to measure the extent of immune damage that has occurred as a result of HIV infection and its complications, and to monitor the immunologic benefit of antiretroviral therapy. CD4 refers to the particular protein expressed on the surface of the T4 helper lymphocyte. CD4 + T cell counts should be obtained on all newly diagnosed persons, and once every 6 months as long as the counts are above 500 cells/ml. When the counts decrease to less than 500 cells/ml, the assessments should occur every 3 months. Should the cell count fall below 200, more frequent monitoring is advisable.[15] Figure 50-7 illustrates the relationship among HIV viral load, CD4 lymphocyte counts, and HIV antibody levels at various points along the HIV continuum.

Medications. Recent drug developments have significantly improved the outlook for many HIV-infected persons. In 1995 the U.S. Food and Drug Administration approved a class of drugs named protease inhibitors. When a protease inhibitor was combined with two other drugs (reverse transcriptase inhibitors) a highly active antiretroviral therapy (HAART) "cocktail" was created that reduced HIV viral load to undetectable levels.[17]

The drug combination works by disrupting HIV at different stages during its replication process.

AZT, ddl, d4T, 3TC, and ddC are nucleoside reverse transcriptase inhibitors (NRTIs). NRTIs become incorporated into the growing DNA chains by viral reverse transcriptase, thereby interfering with the early stages of HIV viral replication.[3] Protease inhibitors (PIs) such as indinavir, ritonavir, saquinavir, and nelfinavir prevent HIV from making the long protein molecules necessary to create new viruses, thus halting replication toward the end of viral replication. Nevirapine and delavirdine are nonnucleoside reverse transcriptase inhibitors (NNRTIs, or nucleoside analogs), the newest group of drugs that block HIV replication by protecting non–HIV infected cells. The goal of treatment with combination therapy is to suppress plasma HIV RNA levels to below detectable levels on assay and elevate CD4$^+$ T cell counts for as long as possible.[3] New drugs are undergoing constant development and clinical trials. Table 50-1 summarizes the medications commonly used to treat HIV infection and AIDS.

In 2001 the CDC released revised guidelines for use of antiretroviral agents in HIV-infected adults and adolescents. The guidelines include recommendations for initiating

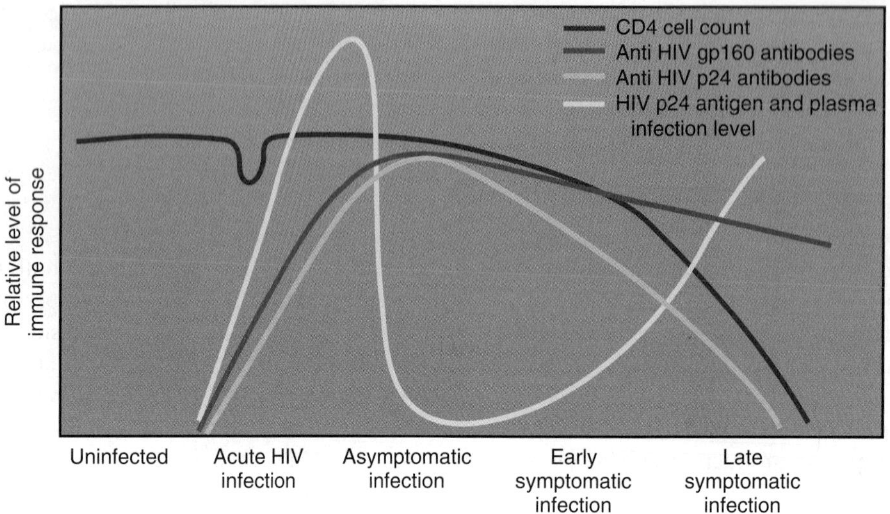

Figure 50-7 Relative levels of immune response to HIV infection.

TABLE 50-1 Common Medications for HIV/AIDS

Medication	Action	Intervention
Nucleoside Reverse Transcriptase Inhibitors (NRTIs)		
Zidovudine (AZT, ZDV) (Retrovir)	Nucleoside analog. Prevents the initial step in which HIV turns its RNA into DNA and integrates itself into human genes. Drug acts as decoy preventing replication of HIV.	Monitor for bone marrow suppression: anemia or neutropenia. Monitor for gastrointestinal (GI) intolerance, headache, insomnia, asthenia. Monitor for drug effectiveness. Teach patient/significant other regarding drug dose, schedule, and possible adverse effects.
Didanosine (ddl) (Videx)	Nucleoside analog. Prevents replication of HIV.	Monitor for drug-associated pancreatitis, peripheral neuropathy, nausea, diarrhea. Monitor CD4$^+$ cell counts for drug effectiveness. Teach patient/significant other regarding drug dose, schedule, and possible adverse effects.
Zalcitabine (ddC) (Hivid)	Nucleoside analog. Prevents replication of HIV.	Monitor for peripheral neuropathy, stomatitis. Monitor for drug effectiveness. Teach patient/significant other regarding drug dose, schedule, and possible adverse effects.
Stavudine (d4T) (Zerit)	Nucleoside analog. Prevents replication of HIV.	Monitor for peripheral neuropathy. Monitor for drug effectiveness. Teach patient/significant other regarding drug dose, schedule, and possible adverse effects.
Lamivudine (3TC) (Epivir)	Nucleoside analog. Prevents replication of HIV.	Minimal toxicity noted. Monitor for drug effectiveness. Teach patient/significant other regarding drug dose, schedule and possible adverse effects.
Abacavir (ABC) (Ziagen)	Nucleoside analog. Prevents replication of HIV	Monitor for drug effectiveness, toxicity, and side effects (hypersensitivity, fever, rash, nausea, vomiting, malaise, loss of appetite). Hypersensitivity and lactic acidosis may be life threatening. Drug should not be restarted when hypersensitivity is suspected. Numerous drug interactions.

Adapted from Guidelines for the use of antiretroviral agents in HIV-infected adults and adolescents, Panel on Clinical Practices for Treatment of HIV Infection, Department of Health and Human Services and the Henry J. Kaiser Foundation, 2000.

TABLE 50-1 Common Medications for HIV/AIDS—cont'd

Medication	Action	Intervention
Nonnucleoside Reverse Transcriptase Inhibitors (NNRTIS)		
Nevirapine (Viramune)	Blocks HIV replication by protecting non–HIV-infected cells.	Monitor for rash. Monitor drug effectiveness. Drug interactions: rifampin, rifabutin, oral contraceptives, protease inhibitors.
Delavirdine (Rescriptor)	Blocks HIV replication.	Monitor for rash. Do not administer within 1 hour of antacids.
Efavirez (Sustiva)	Blocks HIV replication.	Drug interactions: terfenadine, astemizole, alprazolam, midazolam, cisapride, rifabutin, rifampin. Drugs that decrease drug effectiveness: phenytoin, carbamazepine, phenobarbital. Increases drug levels of clarithromycin, dapsone, rifabutin, ergot alkaloids, dihydropyridines, quinidine, warfarin, indinavir, saquinavir. Monitor for adverse effects: rash, CNS symptoms, increased transaminase levels. Numerous drug interactions.
Protease Inhibitors		
Indinavir (Crixivan)	Protease inhibitors interfere with the step of HIV replication in which the virus makes the long protein chains necessary to reproduce itself from DNA. The long protein chains must be cut by a protease enzyme to turn the proteins into the correct length to create HIV. Protease inhibitors prevent this action and render the virus noninfectious.	Monitor $CD4^+$ cells and viral load for drug effectiveness. Teach patient/significant other about drug dose, schedule, and potential side effects. Monitor for nephrolithiasis, GI intolerance, headache, asthenia, blurred vision, dizziness, rash, metallic taste, thrombocytopenia. Drug interactions: rifampin, terfenadine, astemizole, cisapride, triazolam, ergot alkaloids, ketoconazole, rifabutin, midazolam.
Ritonavir (Norvir)	Protease inhibitor	Monitor $CD4^+$ cells and viral load for drug effectiveness. Teach patient/significant other about drug dose, schedule, and potential side effects. Monitor for GI intolerance, nausea, vomiting, diarrhea. Must be kept refrigerated. Drug interactions: meperidine, piroxicam, flecainide, quinidine, rifampin, bepridil, terfenadine, cisapride, bupropion, clozapine, diazepam, alprazolam, dihydroergotamine, ergotamine.
Saquinavir (Invirase)	Protease inhibitor	Monitor $CD4^+$ cells and viral load for drug effectiveness. Teach patient/significant other about drug dose, schedule, and potential side effects. Monitor for GI intolerance, nausea, diarrhea, headache, elevated transaminase enzymes. Drug interactions: rifampin, rifabutin, astemizole, terfenadine, cisapride.
Nelfinavir (Viracept)	Protease inhibitor	Monitor for diarrhea. Monitor $CD4^+$ cells and viral load for drug effectiveness. Teach patient/significant other about drug dose, schedule, and potential side effects. Drug interactions: rifampin, astemizole, terfenadine, cisapride, midazolam, triazolam.
Amprenavir (Agenerase)	Protease inhibitor	High-fat meal can decrease effectiveness. Adverse effects: GI intolerance, rash, oral paresthesias, hyperglycemia, fat redistribution. Alters liver function tests. Numerous drug interactions.
Iopinavir and ritonavir (Kaletra)	Protease inhibitors	Adverse effects: GI intolerance, nausea, vomiting, asthenia, elevated transaminase enzymes, hyperglycemia, fat redistribution, increased bleeding in hemophilia. Numerous drug interactions.

TABLE 50-2 Indications for Initiation of Antiretrovial Therapy in HIV-Infected Persons

Clinical Category	CD4 + T-Cell Count	HIV RNA Count	Recommendations
Asymptomatic	CD4 + T cells > 350/mm³	<30,000 (bDNA)	Many clinicians defer treatment recognizing the 3-year risk of developing AIDS is <15% in untreated patients.
Asymptomatic	CD4 + T cells > 350/mm³	>30,000 (bDNA)	Some clinicians initiate therapy; others do not. The 3-year risk for developing AIDS is >30% in untreated patients.
Asymptomatic	CD4 + T cells > 200 but <350/mm³	Any value bDNA	Treatment is generally offered.
Symptomatic (AIDS)	Any value CD4 + T cells	Any value bDNA	Treat.

Adapted from Guidelines for use of antiretroviral agents in HIV-infected adults and adolescents. Panel on Clinical Practice for Treatment of HIV Infection. U.S. Department of Health and Human Services, HIV/AIDS Treatment Information Service, Feb. 2, 2002, p. 44.

TABLE 50-3 Risks and Benefits of Delayed and Early Therapy in Asymptomatic HIV-Infected Persons

	Risks	Benefits
Early therapy	Reduced quality of life due to drug side effects Greater cumulative drug-related adverse effects Earlier development of drug resistance (if viral suppression is suboptimal) Limited future antiretroviral treatment options	Control of viral replication easier to achieve and maintain Delay or prevention of immune system compromise Lower risk of resistance with complete viral suppression Possible decreased risk of HIV transmission
Late therapy	Possible risk of irreversible immune system depletion Possible greater difficulty with suppressing viral replication Possible increased risk of HIV transmission	Avoid negative effects on quality of life (side effects and inconvenience) Avoid drug-related adverse effects Delay in development of drug resistance Preserve maximum number of available future treatment options

antiretroviral therapy in persons who are asymptomatic as well as those with established disease. The recommendations were derived from studies designed to identify the risks versus benefits of treatment. Clinical trials indicated that patients whose CD4+ T cell counts fell below 200 cells/mm³ were at significantly increased risk for opportunistic infections and should be offered antiretroviral therapy.[16] See Table 50-2 for indications for initiation of antiretroviral therapy (see Evidence-Based Practice box).

No optimal time for the initiation of antiretroviral therapy was established for HIV infected patients with CD4 + T cell counts greater than 200 cells/mm³ who are asymptomatic. The drug regimens currently available are potent, complex, and pose a challenge for adherence. Thus the decision to initiate therapy for this group of patients must be a joint decision between the patient and practitioner. Patients are likely to experience drug toxicity and numerous side effects, must be compliant with large pill burdens and tightly prescribed administration regimens, be able to financially withstand the cost of therapy, and be prepared for the possibility of drug resistance, which may limit future therapy options. Drug resistance can develop if viral replication is not sufficiently suppressed or the person is already infected with a resistant strain of HIV. On the other hand, patients who delay therapy run the risk of permanent immune system damage, inability to effectively inhibit viral replication at a later stage in the disease, and increased risk of HIV transmission. Table 50-3 presents a summary of risks versus benefits of early and delayed retroviral therapy for asymptomatic HIV-infected persons.[9]

Treatments. There are no special treatments in the early stages of HIV infection. Respiratory treatments may become necessary as the patient's disease progresses. Standard Precau-

Evidence-Based Practice

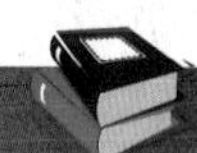

Reference: Kaplan J et al: *Late initiation of antiretroviral therapy is associated with increased risk of death,* Atlanta, February 2000, Centers for Disease Control and Prevention.

Teams of researchers led by the CDC have found new evidence suggesting that delaying the initiation of antiretroviral treatment in patients with T-helper cell counts below 200 increases their risk of death. Specifically, the study found that about 95% of the 5000 patients included in the study who began antiretroviral treatment at a CD4+ level of 200 or higher survived for at least 2 years. Survival rates declined significantly for those who started treatment after CD4+ levels fell below 200.

The study also indicated that delaying treatment for patients with CD4+ levels below 500 but above 200 had little impact on survival rates of HIV infected persons. These findings add to the growing body of research that suggests delaying treatment until CD4+ levels fall well below 500 can reduce side effects and drug resistance and potentially improve dug adherence.

tions are necessary when the patient is hospitalized or being treated at home. Treatments associated with maintenance and improvement of nutritional status usually become necessary. Specific treatments related to opportunistic infections are discussed later in this chapter.

Surgical Management. Surgery does not play a role in the standard management of HIV. Patients may undergo surgical biopsy of skin lesions, surgical treatment of internal Kaposi's sarcoma lesions that do not respond to chemotherapy, or drainage of abscesses or other sites of infection. These all represent management of AIDS complications, however, and are not primary therapies for HIV disease.

Diet. No special diet is indicated for persons with HIV, even though nutritional deficits commonly develop from both the disease itself and the opportunistic infections associated with the disease. Anorexia, nausea, and diarrhea are commonly associated with antiretroviral therapy, further contributing to nutritional alterations. Many persons with AIDS develop wasting syndrome, especially toward the later stages of the disease. Wasting syndrome occurs when non-voluntary weight loss occurs in excess of 10% to 15% of normal baseline weight. It is related to decreased nutrient intake, decreased nutrient absorption, and metabolic disturbances.[15]

Each patient must be carefully monitored to evaluate the adequacy of intake, any food intolerances, and ways to promote a high-calorie, high-protein diet. In the later stages of disease when infections and muscle wasting prevent adequate food intake, intravenous nutritional support may be necessary.

Activity. There are no activity restrictions for the person with HIV infection. A pattern of rest and activity should be encouraged to help maintain lean body mass and prevent deconditioning. More frequent rest periods are necessary for individuals with AIDS because fatigue is a common complaint. During acute infections, activity may need to be restricted. Increasing the amount of sleep and reducing sleep interruptions may be effective in increasing the adequacy of sleep and combating fatigue (see Evidence-Based Practice box).

Referrals. Most HIV-infected individuals are managed on an outpatient basis. The goal of management is to reduce the number of hospitalizations by providing needed services. Consequently a thorough assessment of the HIV- infected person should be undertaken to determine whether referrals need to be made. In some settings the nurse assumes responsibility for making referrals. In other settings, a multidisciplinary approach is taken whereby referrals are made by various health care professionals.

Social services should always be consulted, whether the HIV-infected person is being cared for at home or hospitalized. This department can verify that the individual is covered by insurance or has completed the application process for Medicare/Medicaid and associated programs. Social services can also facilitate contact with a variety of services, including food pantries, housing assistance, community AIDS services, and support groups. For hospitalized persons, social services can assist with discharge planning and facilitating home care.

Evidence-Based Practice

Reference: Mustafa T et al: Association between exercise and HIV disease progression in a cohort of homosexual men, *Ann Epidemiol* 9(2):127, 1999.

The purpose of this study was to determine the relationship between exercise and human immunodeficiency virus (HIV) disease progression. Exercise (defined as self-report of exercising three to four times a week or daily) and CD4 cell counts were monitored in 415 cohort subjects. The study showed that exercise was associated with slower progression to death and increased CD4 cell counts. Exercising three to four times a week had a more protective effect than daily exercise. Researchers concluded that moderate physical activity may slow the progression of HIV disease.

Referrals are commonly made to physical and occupational therapists. Some HIV-infected individuals have difficulty with exercise tolerance related to acute infections, fever, fatigue, and nutritional deficits. Physical and occupational therapy may assist HIV-infected persons to return to their usual state of activity and improve their ability to perform activities of daily living (ADLs).

Psychiatry, counseling, or spiritual referrals may be desired or requested by HIV-infected individuals. The nurse must assess each individual and family for need and interest in such referrals.

NURSING MANAGEMENT

ASSESSMENT

Health assessment of all patients should include an appraisal of potential risk factors for HIV infection. Obtaining a complete, accurate sexual history, including past and present sexual activities, requires skillful interviewing techniques and a professional relationship based on trust. Nurses need to be able to explain the need for information on intimate sexual activities and phrase questions in appropriate but comprehensive terms. The sexual history, in addition to identifying individuals at risk for possible HIV infection, may also provide an opportunity for health education concerning risk reduction and disease prevention. A discussion on taking a sexual history can be found in Chapter 52.

The standard admission database may not include all the information necessary for the person with AIDS and opportunistic infections since it will be used to determine the type and level of nursing care required. In addition to information about the patient's physical status, which includes clinical manifestations, allergies, medications and alternative remedies, the nurse needs to assess for family or other support systems, advanced directives, and HIV-specific data that may influence the patient's care.

Assessment may be difficult due to the clinical diversity of HIV infection and disease.

Health History

Assessment data to be collected as part of the health history of a patient with AIDS include:

Symptoms experienced (e.g., weakness, fatigue, headache)
Factors that exacerbate or relieve symptoms
Ability to perform ADLs
Current drug therapy (prescribed, over-the-counter, and alternative) (see Alternative & Complementary Therapy boxes)
Risk factors (unprotected sex, exposure to blood or blood products, needle exposure, use of mood-altering drugs)
Other concurrent medical problems
Surgical history

Physical Examination

Important aspects of the physical examination of a patient with AIDS include:
Nutritional status, height, weight
Vital signs
Skin and mucous membranes (turgor, temperature, integrity, lesions)
Respiratory status (cough, dyspnea, crackles, wheezing)
Gastrointestinal status (presence of diarrhea)
Urinary status (urine color, quality, and quantity)
Mental status (alertness, orientation)

NURSING DIAGNOSES

Nursing diagnoses are derived from analysis of data collected from the interview and physical examination. Nursing diagnoses for the person with HIV disease may include but are not limited to:

Diagnostic Title	Possible Etiologic Factors
1. Risk for infection	Compromised host defenses
2. Imbalanced nutrition: less than body requirements	Anorexia, nausea, drug side effects, and chronic diarrhea
3. Fatigue	Chronic inflammatory process and side effects of drug therapy
4. Risk for (or actual) ineffective individual coping	Uncertainty about the future
5. Risk for (or actual) ineffective individual	Lack of experience with complex treatment (or family) therapeutic regimen management regimen, disease, or its sequelae.

EXPECTED OUTCOMES

Expected outcomes for the person with HIV disease may include but are not limited to:

1. Will report absence of infection
1a. Will be free of fever, chilling and malaise
1b. Will have white blood cell count within normal limits
2. Will maintain present weight or weight returns to within 0.5 kg. of preillness weight
2a. Will verbalize need to increase caloric intake
2b. Will increase intake to 3000 calories daily as tolerated
2c. Will maintain fluid hydration
3. Will report independence in performance of ADLs
3a. Will engage in daily routines without experiencing fatigue

Complementary & Alternative Therapies
Goldenseal *(Hydrastis canadensis)*

Goldenseal, also known as yellow root, orange root, or turmeric root, may be effective in preventing and treating some infections. Because of its antimicrobial activity, goldenseal has a long history of use by Native Americans for infectious diarrhea, upper respiratory tract infections, and vaginal infections. It may be beneficial in preventing colds and flu.

The alkaloids hydrastine and berberine are the active ingredients in goldenseal that have been most extensively researched. These ingredients appear to have a wide spectrum of antibiotic activity against pathogens, such as *Chlamydia* species, *E. coli*, *Salmonella typhi*, and *Entamoeba histolytica*.

Goldenseal may be taken in capsule, tablet, or liquid form. The dried root dose ranges between 1.5 and 3 g daily for adults and is taken in three divided doses. For liquid herbal extracts, 4 to 6 ml is taken daily. The capsule dose ranges between 250 and 500 mg/day in divided doses. Goldenseal should not be taken continuously for more than 3 weeks.

Goldenseal can be associated with central nervous system stimulation, jaundice, nausea, vomiting, or shortness of breath. It can interfere with the anticoagulants and antihypertensive agents. Patients on prescription medications should inform their health care practitioner of their intended or actual use of goldenseal.

Reference: Mother Nature.com, website:
http://www.mothernature.com/ency/Herb/Goldenseal.asp.

Complementary & Alternative Therapies
Echinacea *(Echinacea purpurea)*

Echinacea, commonly known as purple cornflower, is a wildflower native to North America. Echinacea has been used by the American Indians for a variety of conditions, including venomous bites and other external wounds. In the late 1800s it was used for infections such as colds and syphilis. In the 1830s the Germans began researching the antiinfective properties of Echinacea.

Research has demonstrated Echinacea's effect on the immune system. It increases the production and activity of white blood cells, lymphocytes (T cells), and macrophages and increases production of interferon and cytokines. Echinacea has been shown to have antibacterial, antiviral, and antiinflammatory properties.

As an immune system stimulant, Echinacea is taken three to four times a day for 10 to 14 days; 3 to 4 ml of liquid extract or 300 mg capsules are taken three times a day. Regardless of the type of Echinacea used, therapy is followed by a "rest" period so that it does not lose its effectiveness.

Echinacea can cause dizziness, fatigue, headache, vomiting, or allergic reactions. It may interact with immunosuppressant agents, anabolic steroids, or ketoconazole. Patients on prescribed medications should consult their health care provider before taking Echinacea.

Reference: Mother Nature.com, website:
http://www.mothernature.com/ency/Herb/echinacea.asp.
Davis Drug Guide: website: http://www.drugguide.com/documents/mongraphs/herbals/echinacea.htm.

3b. Will demonstrate usual strength and activity tolerance
4. Will engage in communication that leads to sharing of feelings, decision making, and problem resolution as pertinent and appropriate.
5. Will report ability to manage and adhere to prescribed treatment regimen
5a. Will develop and follow a plan to achieve treatment regimen
5b. Will avoid risk-taking behaviors
5c. Will recognize and report changes in disease status

INTERVENTIONS

The HIV epidemic in the United States has brought social stigmatization, public fear, and a growing number of legal and ethical concerns. Nurses providing care in a variety of settings face many of these issues, which may jeopardize the quality of patient care. In addition, nurses face many personal stresses, including fear of personal contamination and burnout related to caring for terminally ill patients. The professional commitment needed by nurses who provide care to HIV-infected patients requires clarification of personal values and renewed dedication to service.

1. Preventing Infection

Infection is a major complication of HIV disease. The already compromised AIDS patient, in particular, must be protected from further infectious insults. The nurse monitors vital signs, skin integrity, mucous membranes, respiratory status, GI function, and mental status routinely for signs of possible infection. White blood cell levels are monitored when signs of infection are present.[7]

A diet free of foods that may be contaminated or harbor bacteria (raw fruits, vegetables, fish, or seafood) is recommended for patients with absolute neutrophil counts less than 500 cells/cm^3. The nurse educates significant others about signs and symptoms of infection and when to report them to the clinician. Visitors can be requested to wear a mask during their visit to the home if the patient's condition warrants it. People who have infections such as colds or chickenpox should be requested not to visit until they are well.

The nurse reinforces the importance of protective strategies, including hand washing, scrupulous personal hygiene, dietary precautions such as thorough cooking of meat products and washing of fruits and vegetables, removing fresh plants and flowers from the patient's bedroom, and keeping inside pets clean. Meticulous asepsis of all invasive lines is essential.

The need for control of infections does not mean that the person with HIV disease should be socially isolated. It is important that patients maintain their usual social relationships to prevent feelings of social isolation. Many communities have support groups with volunteers who are willing to make routine visits or become the patient's "buddy" or "ally." This can be of particular benefit to those who have no nearby relatives or significant others.

2. Promoting Nutrition

The nutritional status of patients with HIV disease may range from normal early in the disease process to extreme cachexia and wasting syndrome with progressive disease. Therefore the nurse monitors the nutritional status of all patients and promotes food intake necessary to maintain maximal health and functioning. Current dietary intake, likes and dislikes, dietary restrictions, food tolerances and intolerances, and height and weight are all identified. The nurse monitors the patient for signs of altered nutrition or factors that may alter nutritional status, such as decreased weight, decreased muscle strength and tone, decreased energy levels, anorexia, nausea, stomatitis, impaired swallowing, or self-care deficits. Teaching includes the side effects of drug therapy that may affect nutritional status. Eating toast or dry crackers and drinking beverages 30 minutes before meals may be effective in reducing nausea.

Antiemetics may be necessary for severe nausea and vomiting. Oral analgesics and topical anesthetics can often aid in reducing mouth pain. The nurse encourages the patient to perform mouth care before meals, sit in a chair to eat, eat with others, and take meals in pleasant surroundings. These measures can be successful in promoting an adequate oral intake.

A high-calorie, high-protein diet divided into six small meals per day is recommended. Specific food likes and dislikes are incorporated into meal planning to enhance intake. If the patient is losing weight, the nurse keeps a calorie and protein count or food diary for 1 week to determine the presence of deficits. Teaching includes normal nutrient requirements, calories required to maintain or gain weight, and the distribution of nutrients and calories in food. The nurse assists the patient with feeding and encourages the use of adaptive equipment if needed. Impaired swallowing is reported promptly to the physician. Family members, friends, or community agencies can be an important source of support and can be contacted to provide meals, visit during mealtimes, or assist with feeding.

3. Controlling Fatigue

Fatigue is a primary complaint of persons with HIV infection or disease; therefore energy management is important. The nurse assesses the person's ability to perform ADLs, including weakness, gait, endurance, strength, and motor and sensory deficits. The importance of balancing activities with rest periods in order to maintain normal or near-normal activity levels is stressed. The nurse encourages the person to respect the signs and symptoms of fatigue and reduce activities when required. The use of assistive devices, such as wheelchairs, canes, or walkers, can help conserve energy[7] (see Evidence-Based Practice box).

The environment is arranged so that items of necessity are within easy reach. Items used on a daily basis need to be conveniently located and readily accessible. The nurse and patient may have to be creative in finding ways to help the person conserve energy in a home environment that may be less than optimal. Attention is given to conditions that may jeopardize patient safety, such as stairs, use of small scatter rugs, or lack of handrails on bathtubs. The support of family members or

Evidence-Based Practice

Reference: Crystal S et al: Physical and role functioning among persons with HIV: results from a nationally representative survey, *Medical Care* 38(12):1210, 2000.

The purpose of this study was to determine the physical and role-functioning abilities of HIV-infected individuals. The researchers assessed the physical and role limitations of 2836 HIV-infected people; 51% of HIV-infected persons experienced difficulty in carrying out their roles at least part of the time. The study concluded that limitations are more common for energy-demanding activities (climbing stairs) than self-care tasks. People who were older, less educated, had more advanced disease, or had a higher symptom load experienced greater role and function difficulties. Symptoms most significantly associated with decreased function included nausea, cough, and diarrhea.

significant others can be solicited to assist with home maintenance tasks to prevent or relieve the patient's fatigue.

Environmental stimuli can be adjusted so that a restful night's sleep can be achieved. At least 6 to 8 hours of sleep per night are recommended. Visits from a home health aide or community support group can be arranged to assist the patient with physical care when necessary.

4. Supporting Individual Coping

HIV-infected persons have many fears and concerns, including fear of losing their jobs and independence, fear of becoming debilitated, fear of bodily changes, and fear of death. Fear produces anxiety, which can result in ineffective coping patterns. The recognition of fear is often the first step in alleviating it. The nurse assesses the patient's psychological response to the situation and availability of support systems and helps the patient identify additional sources of financial and physical support. Patients are encouraged to talk about their concerns and assisted with identifying means for dealing with those concerns. The nurse encourages patients to maintain social and community activities with persons who have common interests and goals and use available support groups because they offer a safe place for individuals to express themselves.[7] Uncontrolled fear may interfere with care. In this case a counseling referral should be considered. A Nursing Care Plan for a person with HIV/AIDS can be found on pp. 1667 to 1670.

5. Promoting Effective Therapeutic Regimen Management

Caring for the person with HIV disease at home places heavy physical, psychologic, and financial burdens on both the patient and caregiver. The nurse assesses the patient for functional abilities, disabilities, and extent of illness, as well as the caregiver's ability and willingness to assist with or perform needed care. The patient is encouraged to maintain self-care to the extent possible, without incurring injury. Activity is not only physiologically important, but it provides a sense of control for the individual. It is important for the nurse to educate the person in safety measures and the importance of calling for assistance when needed. Diet, activities, self-monitoring needs, prevention of infection, stress reduction (see Chapter

Evidence-Based Practice

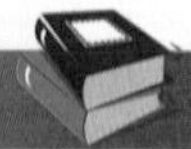

Reference: Standish L et al: Alternative medicine use in HIV-positive mean and women: demographics, utilization patterns and health status, *AIDS Care* 13(2):197, 2001.

A team of researchers at Bastyr University AIDS Research Center in Kenmore, Washington, DC, collected information from 1675 HIV-positive men and women from 48 states to determine their use of conventional and CAM (complementary and alternative medicine) therapies. Participants of the study reported using more than 1600 different types of CAM for treating their HIV/AIDS: 63% of participants reported using antiretroviral drug therapy and 37% used alternative therapies 6 months before the study, although the majority of subjects reported using both conventional and CAM therapies at some point in their illness. The most frequently reported CAM substances used by participants included vitamin C, multiple vitamin and mineral supplements, and garlic. CAM providers most commonly consulted included massage therapist, acupuncturists, nutritionists, and psychotherapists. CAM activities most commonly used were aerobic exercise, prayer, massage, and meditation. Few study participants reported that their conventional and CAM providers worked as a team.

6), and follow-up monitoring needs are all discussed. The nurse reviews treatment protocols, particularly drug regimens, and teaches the patient about drug dosages, administration schedules, and side effects. The patient is encouraged to anticipate unpleasant drug side effects and plan strategies for addressing them, such as using a cool cloth to the head or napping to relieve nausea. Patients are encouraged to report their use of complementary or alternative medications (CAM) so that drug interactions can be avoided (see Evidence-Based Practice box).

The nurse encourages the patient to consider the consequences of disease progression and the potential for further physical and mental deterioration. The patient-caregiver relationship is assessed, and the nurse attempts to anticipate how the stressors of disease progression may affect that relationship. A therapeutic nursing relationship built with empathy, acceptance, and support is essential. HIV-infected people often feel stigmatized by their disease. An empathetic nurse can do much to support individuals simply by taking time to talk to them at times other than when providing physical care. The nurse encourages the patient and caregiver to explore and express their feelings and fears and helps them identify past and current coping strategies, as well as effective and ineffective components of their relationship. The use of effective coping strategies is reinforced.

The early success of drug cocktail protocols has added new uncertainties to the lives of persons with HIV. Dramatic successes have been widely reported, with some patients experiencing a drop in their viral load to undetectable levels. It may be difficult for patients to know how to use this newly found well being, especially if their lives have been fully consumed with disease management. Even if returning to work is not a possibility due to ongoing fatigue, the person may no longer be overtly sick. This creates new and unexpected challenges

Nursing Care Plan Patient With HIV/AIDS

DATA Ms. B. is a 41-year-old Caucasian hair stylist who lives with her 70-year-old mother, her primary caregiver. Eight years ago Ms. B. was diagnosed as being HIV positive. Three years before her diagnosis Ms. B. was involved in an automobile accident. She received several blood transfusions for multiple traumas. Ms. B. has been divorced for 14 years and has one adult son who lives in another state. Her current medications include a protease inhibitor combined with two nucleoside reverse transcriptase inhibitors. She has been able to work full time until recently. During the past 3 months she has experienced increased fatigue and a 10-pound weight loss. Ms. B. has been admitted to the hospital with complaints of fever, night sweats, myalgia, malaise, chest discomfort, dry nonproductive cough, abdominal discomfort, and diarrhea. Her CD4+ helper count is 200/mm^3, and her HIV RNA count is 18,000 (bDNA).

Physical examination reveals:

- Bilaterally diminished lung sounds with coarse crackles
- Axillary adenopathy
- Vital signs: oral temperature, 101.8° F; heart rate, 92 and regular; respiratory rate, 28 and mildly labored
- Clear sensorium, oriented times 3
- Abdomen firm and tender with the presence of hyperactive bowel sounds

Physician orders include:

- Oxygen by nasal cannula, 4 L/min
- Bed rest with bathroom privileges
- Diet as tolerated
- Lactated Ringer's solution at 125 ml/hr

The nursing history also reveals that Ms. B.:

- Is concerned about her condition and fears that she will be unable to return to work full time
- Is concerned about the health of her mother, who has diabetes mellitus and arthritis
- Has not told her son that she is HIV positive
- Has a boyfriend, is sexually active, and consistently uses safe sexual practices

Following diagnostic bronchoscopy and stool specimen examination, Ms. B. is diagnosed with *Pneumocystis carinii* pneumonia and *Cryptosporidium* infection.

Collaborative nursing actions include:

- Monitoring for other opportunistic infections (e.g., *Candida,* cytomegalovirus, *Mycobacterium avium* complex)
- Monitoring vital signs for changes denoting improvement or nonimprovement
- Maintaining intravenous fluids and prescribed antibiotics on schedule
- Monitoring intake and output
- Maintaining Standard Precautions

NURSING DIAGNOSIS **Risk for impaired gas exchange related to opportunistic infection *(Pneumocystis carinii)***
GOALS/OUTCOMES Lungs will remain clear

NOC Suggested Outcomes

- Respiratory Status: Ventilation (0403)
- Respiratory Status: Gas Exchange (0402)
- Respiratory Status: Airway Patency (0410)
- Vital Signs Status (0802)

NIC Suggested Interventions

- Respiratory Monitoring (3350)
- Airway Management (3140)
- Cough Enhancement (3250)
- Vital Signs Monitoring (6680)
- Chest Physiotherapy (3230)

Nursing Interventions/Rationales

- Monitor respiratory rate, rhythm, and effort. *To detect respiratory compromise and determine effectiveness of treatment.*
- Monitor lung sounds. *To detect breathing pattern abnormalities and determine effectiveness of treatment.*
- Encourage slow, deep breathing. *To alleviate dyspnea while allowing for maximum oxygenation.*
- Teach patient how to cough effectively. *To prevent stasis of secretions without expending excessive respiratory energy.*
- Encourage increased fluid intake. *To promote liquefaction of secretions for easy expectoration.*
- Administer prescribed supplemental oxygen. *To enhance oxygenation and prevent hypoxia.*

Evaluation Parameters

1. Absence of cough
2. Oxygen saturations above 95%
3. Absence of cyanosis and/or dyspnea
4. Arterial blood gases within normal limits
5. Demonstrates effective cough technique

Continued

Nursing Care Plan — Patient With HIV/AIDS—cont'd

NURSING DIAGNOSIS **Risk for infection: opportunistic (in addition to those present) related to HIV infection and subsequent immunodeficiency**

GOALS/OUTCOMES Will remain free of other opportunistic infections; health care workers will not become infected with HIV

NOC Suggested Outcomes
- Immune Status (0702)
- Knowledge Deficit: Infection Control (1807)
- Risk Control (1902)
- Risk Detection (1908)

NIC Suggested Interventions
- Infection Protection (6550)
- Infection Control (6540)
- Medication Management (2380)
- Teaching: Disease Process (5602)

Nursing Interventions/Rationales
- Monitor for signs and symptoms of infection (fever, chills, dyspnea, fatigue, oral lesions, dysuria). *To identify new infections so that treatment can be instituted early. Frequent and/or prolonged infections contribute to the wasting syndrome that occurs with HIV infection.*
- Monitor laboratory data (white blood cell [WBC] count, differential), CD4 cell count, and viral load. *To detect new infections and monitor effectiveness of treatment. Infections are more likely to occur when CD4 cell counts are below 500 mm^3 and viral load is above 10,000 (bDNA).*
- Teach patient to report signs and symptoms of infection. *To assist with early detection of infections.*
- Screen all visitors for communicable diseases. *To protect the immunocompromised patient from sources of new infections.*
- Culture wound drainage, mouth lesions, sputum, blood, stool, or urine as needed. *To identify the pathogenic organism so that appropriate treatment methods can be initiated.*
- Administer prescribed antimicrobial medications on time. *To maintain blood levels of antimicrobial agents for maximum effectiveness.*
- Teach patient ways to reduce exposure to infections, such as practicing good hand-washing technique, avoiding the handling of pet wastes, cleaning household surfaces with disinfectant solutions, maintaining personal hygiene, and thoroughly cooking meats, eggs, and vegetables. *To decrease exposure to new infections and prevent exposing others to HIV infection.*
- Ensure aseptic handing of all intravenous lines and invasive procedures, such as catheterizations or injections. *To decrease exposure to new, hospital-acquired infections.*

Evaluation Parameters
1. Vital signs return to normal
2. WBC count returns to normal
3. Health care workers implement and maintain Standard Precautions

NURSING DIAGNOSIS **Imbalanced nutrition: less than body requirements related to diarrhea secondary to opportunistic infection**

GOALS/OUTCOMES Will cease to lose weight; will describe meal plan with adequate calories and fluids; will maintain electrolyte balance

NOC Suggested Outcomes
- Nutritional Status: Food and Fluid Intake (1008)
- Nutritional Status: Nutrient Intake (1009)
- Weight Control (1612)

NIC Suggested Interventions
- Fluid Monitoring (4130)
- Nutrition Monitoring (1160)
- Fluid Management (4120)
- Nutrition Management (1100)
- Fluid and Electrolyte Management (2080)
- Weight Management (1260)

Nursing Interventions/Rationales
- Monitor intake and output. *To determine if fluid output is excessive when compared with fluid intake so that fluid deficits can be avoided or treated early.*
- Monitor hydration status (skin turgor, mucous membranes). *To determine adequacy of fluid intake and to initiate fluid replacement early if needed.*
- Obtain daily weights and monitor trends. *Weight is a clinical indicator of adequate nutrition and fluid balance. Weight loss indicates the need for nutritional supplements or total parenteral nutrition.*

Nursing Care Plan — Patient With HIV/AIDS–cont'd

- Monitor laboratory data (blood urea nitrogen, serum protein, hemoglobin, hematocrit, transferrin levels). *Provides objective data regarding nutritional status so that corrective actions can be initiated early.*
- Encourage six small meals, excluding dairy products and raw fruits and vegetables. *Small meals prevent gastric distention and nausea. Lactose in dairy products may enhance diarrhea. Raw foods contain naturally occurring microorganisms that may cause infection in the immunocompromised host.*
- Administer intravenous fluids as prescribed. *To prevent fluid volume deficits, hypovolemia, and cellular dehydration.*
- Teach patient to increase intake of high-calorie, protein-rich, carbohydrate foods. *To provide calories, aid healing, and prevent wasting.*
- Assess and monitor for factors that impede intake (oral lesions, pain). *To prevent nutritional deficits due to inability to intake food or fluids.*

Evaluation Parameters

1. Begins to gain weight, and weight moves to within 5 pounds of baseline
2. Verbalizes nutritional needs accurately
3. Appetite and food intake increase

NURSING DIAGNOSIS **Risk for deficient fluid volume related to diarrhea secondary to cryptosporidiosis**
GOALS/OUTCOMES Will maintain fluid volume balance

NOC Suggested Outcomes

- Immune Status (0702)
- Knowledge Deficit: Infection Control (1807)
- Risk Control (1902)
- Risk Detection (1908)

NIC Suggested Interventions

- Infection Protection (6550)
- Infection Control (6540)
- Medication Management (2380)
- Teaching: Disease Process (5602)

Nursing Interventions/Rationales

- Monitor skin turgor and mucous membranes. *Poor skin turgor and sticky mucous membranes are indications of fluid deficit.*
- Monitor weight daily. *Weight is a good indicator of hydration status. Rapid changes in weight are usually due to changes in fluid volume.*
- Monitor consistency and amount of stools. *Fluid lost in stool must be replaced, since diarrhea is a significant source of fluid loss.*
- Monitor vital signs. *To detect changes associated with fluid deficit. Tachycardia, hypotension, and low-grade fever are associated with fluid volume deficit.*
- Monitor intake and output. *To determine if imbalance between intake and output exists and to determine fluid deficiency effect on renal function.*
- Encourage fluid intake when tolerated. *To replace fluid losses.*
- Administer prescribed intravenous fluids. *To replace fluid losses.*
- Administer prescribed antidiarrheal medications. *To correct the cause of the fluid loss.*

Evaluation Parameters

1. Good skin turgor
2. Moist mucous membranes
3. Weight remains within 5 pounds of baseline
4. Urine output >30 ml/hr

NURSING DIAGNOSIS **Activity intolerance related to decreased oxygen transport and reduced energy reserves secondary to opportunistic infection**
GOALS/OUTCOMES Will perform daily activities without dyspnea

NOC Suggested Outcomes

- Activity Tolerance (0005)
- Endurance (0001)
- Energy Conservation (0002)

NIC Suggested Interventions

- Energy Management (0180)
- Teaching: Prescribed Activity/Exercise (5612)
- Sleep Enhancement (1850)

Continued

Nursing Interventions/Rationales

- Assess severity of fatigue and patient's understanding of the physiologic cause. *To establish a baseline for later comparisons and to determine effectiveness of treatment.*
- Encourage patient to prioritize daily activities and let go of unessential tasks. *Fatigue compromises one's ability to participate in daily activities. It is important that the patient's available energy be used to complete priority activities.*
- Explore strategies to (1) modify existing activities, conserving energy when possible; (2) seek assistance or delegate activities; and (3) pace activities throughout the day to allow a balance between activity and rest. *Many daily activities can be modified to consume less energy. Accepting the reality of fatigue may allow the patient to consider ways of seeking assistance or delegating activities that would not usually be considered acceptable.*
- Encourage patient to obtain at least 8 hours of uninterrupted sleep at night. *Effective nighttime sleep patterns may decrease daytime fatigue.*
- Encourage intake of well-balanced diet. *To supply adequate nutrients to meet energy needs.*

Evaluation Parameters

1. Participates in daily care activities without experiencing dyspnea or fatigue
2. Reports feeling rested and having increased energy

NURSING DIAGNOSIS **Anxiety related to fear of losing independence, job, and income**
GOALS/OUTCOMES Will report decreased anxiety regarding outcome of illness

NOC Suggested Outcomes

- Anxiety Control (1402)
- Fear Control (1404)
- Coping (1302)

NIC Suggested Interventions

- Anxiety Reduction (5820)
- Calming Technique (5880)
- Coping Enhancement (5230)

Nursing Interventions/Rationales

- Explain all care and procedures. *Decreases anxiety that often occurs when unfamiliar procedures are scheduled.*
- Encourage verbalization of fears and concerns. *Venting of feelings often allows the patient to put fears into perspective and may decrease anxiety.*
- Discourage decision making while under extreme stress. *Stress inhibits the ability to problem solve and approach decisions in a rational manner.*
- Discourage decision making until outcomes are known. *Decisions based on inadequate information may cause greater stress in the future.*
- Explore past effective coping strategies that were successful. *Patterns of past successful coping are indicators of present resources and strengths.*

Evaluation Parameters

1. Identifies previous effective coping strategies for stress
2. Verbalizes sources of fear
3. Verbalizes decreased anxiety and fear

NURSING DIAGNOSIS **Risk for impaired skin integrity related to frequent diarrhea**
GOALS/OUTCOMES Will maintain intact skin

NOC Suggested Outcomes

- Tissue Integrity: Skin and Mucous Membranes (1101)
- Fluid Balance (0601)
- Nutritional Status (1004)
- Bowel Elimination (0501)

NIC Suggested Interventions

- Skin Surveillance (3590)
- Perineal Care (1750)
- Diarrhea Management (0460)
- Fluid Management (4120)

Nursing Interventions/Rationales

- Monitor skin for signs of breakdown (redness, excoriation). *To detect skin deterioration so that treatment can be implemented as early as possible.*
- Inspect skin turgor and mucous membranes daily. *Dry mucous membranes and poor skin turgor indicate fluid deficit, which predisposes the patient to skin breakdown.*
- Keep rectal area clean and dry. *Prevents secondary infections and spread of existing microorganisms.*
- Apply topical protective cream to reddened areas as prescribed. *To protect skin from wetness and acidic stool and prevent breakdown while increasing comfort.*

Evaluation Parameters

1. Skin free of redness, excoriation
2. Decreased number of diarrheal stools

for patients and caregivers, who must find new ways to relate and effectively use this gift of time.

The persistent threat of disease recurrence is consistently present and can easily create a state of chronic anxiety in which the present is difficult to enjoy because of pervasive worries over how long the respite will last.

A wide range of knowledge, skills, and resources may be needed to provide care at home and manage a complex treatment regimen during various stages of HIV and AIDS, and the nurse needs to carefully explore the availability and adequacy of those resources. Family members, friends, clergy, and community support groups available to assist the patient and caregiver are thoroughly explored. The services of such resources can be enlisted to provide rest periods or time away from home for the caregiver. Referrals to home health agencies, social workers, AIDS support groups, respite care, spiritual counselors, and other community resources are initiated as available.

Some individuals with AIDS may be able to continue to work as their disease progresses, whereas others find it necessary to quit because they can no longer meet the physical requirements of their job. Inadequate health insurance coverage forces some patients to stop working prematurely and seek disability to qualify for medical assistance to cover the costs of drug therapy. This step makes it nearly impossible for patients to then return to work at some point in the future even if their health status allows it. Loss of work generally means loss of income and eventual loss of independence. The impact of lost income and the psychologic impact of inability to work both need to be explored. Information about how and where to apply for financial assistance and medical care should be provided before it becomes a crisis, to reduce the burden on both patient and caregiver. The nurse needs to use all available multidisciplinary resources, including social services, clergy, public and private mental health resources, and special funding initiatives such as the Ryan White Fund, to assist patients in their efforts to effectively self-manage HIV infection or AIDS in their home environment.

Patient/Family Education

Because HIV is a multifaceted national and international problem, the first priority of care is to halt the spread of infection. To achieve this goal, the U.S. Department of Health and Human Services, Public Health Service, has developed Healthy People 2010 objectives related to HIV infection (see Healthy People 2010 box).[16] Prevention efforts must include accurate, reliable, and clear information about risk factors for HIV disease and ways to decrease these risks by limiting exposure to infected blood, semen, or vaginal secretions.

Persons identified with HIV infection have numerous knowledge needs, including but not limited to prevention of transmission, treatment options, legal and medical rights, and community resource availability. The nurse begins by assessing the patient's current knowledge base. The patient's family or significant other is included in teaching sessions. The importance of collaborative planning for future care is stressed. Depending on the extent of the patient's knowledge, teaching involves all aspects of the disease and its treatment.

Healthy People 2010

Objectives Related to HIV/AIDS

- Reduce the prevalence of HIV infection to no more than 1 new case per 100,000 people.
- Reduce the number of new cases of HIV infection among men who have sex with men to no more than 13,385 cases per year.
- Reduce the number of new AIDS cases among women and men who inject drugs to no more than 9075 cases per year.
- Reduce the number of new cases of HIV infection among men who have sex with men and inject drugs to no more than 1592 per year.
- Increase to 85% the proportion of adults with tuberculosis who have been tested for HIV.
- Increase to 50% the proportion of sexually active persons who use condoms.
- Increase the proportion of adults in publicly funded HIV counseling and testing sites who are screened for common bacterial sexually transmitted diseases (chlamydia, gonorrhea, and syphilis) and are immunized against hepatitis B virus.
- Increase the proportion of HIV-infected adolescents and adults who receive testing, treatment, and prophylaxis consistent with current Public Health Service treatment guidelines.
- Increase the number of HIV-positive persons who know their serostatus.
- Increase by 70% the proportion of substance abuse treatment facilities that offer HIV/AIDS education, counseling, and support.
- Increase the number of state prison systems that provide comprehensive HIV/AIDS, sexually transmitted diseases, and tuberculosis education.
- Increase the proportion of inmates in state prison systems who receive voluntary HIV counseling and testing during incarceration.
- Reduce deaths from HIV infected to no more than 0.7 deaths per 100,000 persons.
- Extend the interval of time between an initial diagnosis of HIV infection and AIDS diagnosis to increase years of life of an individual infected with HIV.
- Increase years of life of an HIV-infected person by extending the interval of time between an AIDS diagnosis and death.
- Reduce new cases of perinatally acquired HIV infection.
- Reduce HIV infections in adolescent and young adult women aged 13 to 24 years that are associated with heterosexual contact.
- Increase the proportion of pregnant women screened for sexually transmitted diseases (including HIV infection and bacterial vaginosis) during prenatal health care visits, according to recognized standards.

From US Department of Health and Human Services, *Healthy People 2010: Understanding and improving health,* Washington, DC, 2000, USDHHS.

The patient and caregiver are assisted with organizing information so that it is readily available and easy to understand. Emergency phone numbers and community resources need to be readily accessible. The nurse reviews the patient's plan of care and current treatment protocols and answers questions as needed to clarify information. The importance of physician visits and follow-up care is stressed. During the later stages of disease, education may shift from providing specific information about the disease to keeping patients informed and discussing their wishes in regard to their own care.

EVALUATION

1,2,3,4,5. To evaluate the effectiveness of nursing interventions, patient behaviors are compared with those stated in the expected outcomes. Successful achievement of outcomes for the person with HIV disease may include freedom from opportunistic infections; reduced fatigue and increased ability to provide self care and manage the prescribed treatment regimen; regaining lost weight or maintaining desired body weight; eating a nutritious and well balance diet; seeking assistance as needed; maintaining social interactions and freely verbalizing fears and concerns.

Evidence-Based Practice

Reference: Kalachman SC et al: Depression and thoughts of suicide among middle-aged and older persons living with HIV-AIDS, *Psychiatric Service* 51(7):903, 2000.

This study examined the prevalence and characteristics of suicidal ideation among middle-aged and older persons who have HIV infection or AIDS. A total of 113 subjects over the age of 45 who had HIV/AIDS completed questionnaires covering suicidal ideation, emotional distress, quality of life, coping, and social support. The study concluded that people with HIV/AIDS experience significant emotional distress and thoughts of suicide. The data suggest a need for planning interventions that address mental health and prevent suicide.

GERONTOLOGIC CONSIDERATIONS

As of 2001 approximately 11% of people with AIDS in the United States were 50 years of age or older.[5] This percentage is expected to rise steadily as adults being treated with HAART live longer. Recognition of HIV infection in older adults may be difficult for several reasons. A diagnosis of AIDS may be missed since this group commonly experiences symptoms such as pneumonia, dementia, shortness of breath, weakness, fatigue, poor nutritional intake, and weight loss. In addition, caregivers may fail to evaluate thoroughly such risk factors as IV drug use or unprotected sex in this age-group.[1]

Care and counseling of the older adult with HIV infection or HIV disease are similar to that of the younger adult, except that age-related changes need to be incorporated into the plan of care. Older adults with compromised immune functions or chronic illnesses often have little reserve to resist or fight the multiple infections that accompany the HIV infection. In general, this age group exhibits more side effects from aggressive antibiotic therapy used to fight infections of any kind, which makes them particularly susceptible to the side effects associated with aggressive HIV drug therapy.

Because older adults are not generally targeted as an at-risk group for HIV infection, they are often neglected when it comes to AIDS outreach and teaching. Nurses must keep in mind that older adults are sexually active and be prepared to provide health teaching about HIV infection and transmission when appropriate.

SPECIAL ENVIRONMENTS FOR CARE

Critical Care Management

The majority of individuals with HIV disease are cared for at home and are followed on an outpatient basis. However, the occasion may arise when it is necessary to hospitalize the person for induction therapy or to treat severe physical compromise related to opportunistic infections. Critical care management of overwhelming infections may include aggressive intravenous antibiotic therapy or respiratory support. All medical and nursing efforts are directed at controlling or eliminating symptoms and the underlying infection when possible and desirable.

The decision to treat infections aggressively depends on the patient's and family's wishes and the extent of physical deterioration present. It is important for the nurse to understand and support the patient's wishes in this regard. Persons with early HIV disease are likely to request aggressive treatment, whereas persons who have experienced repeated infections and HIV wasting syndrome may not desire aggressive therapy.

Home Care Management

The majority of HIV-infected and AIDS patients are cared for at home by family or friends. Diagnostic testing and monitoring are performed in the outpatient setting. With improvements in antiretroviral therapy and treatments for opportunistic infections, continuing therapy can now be accomplished at home.

A vital resource for the person with HIV disease is the assistance and support of a competent and dependable caregiver. That person may be a spouse, partner, friend, or relative. During the early stages of disease, the patient may rely on the caregiver to help diminish mood fluctuations, provide encouragement, foster motivation, and assist with some aspects of daily care. As the condition of the person with HIV deteriorates, however, the caregiver's role is significantly increased to include physical, psychologic, and financial support. Consequently, caregiver burden can become an important issue. It is important to assist caregivers with finding suitable outlets for their own emotions. They are encouraged to maintain adequate rest and nutrition so that they will have the physical stamina to meet the demands placed on them. Use of community resources, family members, or friends is encouraged to provide time periods away from the physically ill individual for the purpose of shopping, work, or recreation.

Persons with HIV disease who do not have a dependable support system are at a considerable disadvantage. Not only do they require earlier referrals for home care and other community services, but they do not have the day-to-day comfort and encouragement offered by a close personal companion. Patients without support systems are at risk for suicide (see Evidence-Based Practice box). In many cases, it is the nurse who has to fill part of the void by being a compassionate listener, offering encouragement, and fostering hope.

COMPLICATIONS

The complications of HIV disease present a complex picture of opportunistic infections, neoplasms, or other conditions related to immunodeficiency. When CD4 cell counts fall below 500/mm^3, signs and symptoms of immune deficiency are likely to be noted; when counts fall below 200/mm^3, oppor-

TABLE 50-4 Prophylactic Treatment of Common Opportunistic Infections

Infection	Prophylactic Interventions	Comments
Pneumococcal pneumonia	Pneumococcal vaccine	Provide as soon as possible during course of infection; antibody response is optimal when CD4+ cells are >350/μl
Hepatitis B virus (HBV)	Hepatitis B vaccine series; screen and vaccinate those who show no evidence of previous HBV infection	Provide as soon as possible during course of infection; encourage vaccine in injecting drug users, sexually active gay men, and sex partners or household contacts of HBV-infected individuals
Herpes simplex virus (HSV) 1 and 2	Low-dose acyclovir therapy may be initiated if prompt treatment of outbreaks is not sufficient for control	Provide ongoing assessment and intervention
Pulmonary tuberculosis	Treat if PPD is >5 mm reactive or if patient is anergic or at risk; INH for 12 mo; consider directly observed therapy (clinical disease requires treatment with four or more drugs)	Rule out active or extrapulmonary disease, which requires multidrug therapy; remember that a negative PPD in the presence of HIV does not exclude a diagnosis of tuberculosis; provide ongoing assessment and intervention
Pneumocystis carinii pneumonia (PCP)	Trimethoprim-sulfamethoxazole (TMP-SMX) (drug of choice) or dapsone or pentamidine per inhalation	Initiate when CD4+ cells go below 200/μl; offer TMP-SMX to any patient with a history of PCP, regardless of CD4+ cell count; oral drugs that provide systemic effect are preferred
Mycobacterium avium complex (MAC)	Rifabutin	Initiate when CD4+ cells go below 100/μl; rifabutin has caused dose-related uveitis (above 600 mg/day), which is reversible with drug withdrawal or dose reduction;
Toxoplasmosis	Trimethoprim-sulfamethoxazole (TMP-SMX) or dapsone with pyrimethamine and folinic acid	Initiate when CD4+ cells go below 100/μl

Adapted from USPHS/IDSA: Guidelines for the Prevention of Opportunistic Infections in Persons Infected with Human Immunodeficiency Virus, *MMWR*, 1999.

tunistic infections and neoplasms are encountered.[10] Bacterial, fungal, protozoan, and viral infections are the four categories of opportunistic infections seen in immunodeficient individuals. Kaposi's sarcoma is the most commonly seen neoplasm associated with HIV disease, but non-Hodgkin's lymphoma and cervical cancers can also occur.

The infections associated with HIV disease are called opportunistic because the organisms producing infection are not ordinarily pathogenic. The organisms are found throughout the environment but are rendered harmless by the intact immune system. In patients with HIV infection, however, the organisms multiply, thrive, and produce disease because the immune regulators are severely compromised. Opportunistic infections are not limited to persons with HIV disease, but may affect any person who is immunodeficient or immunosuppressed as a result of chronic illness or chemotherapy.

Persons with HIV disease may experience one or more infections at the same time, producing numerous problems that present a challenge for both the physician and the nurse. The patient may be on several antibiotics for extended periods of time, causing an increased incidence of side effects and the potential for the development of drug resistance. It is not uncommon for opportunistic infections to return when antibiotics are reduced or discontinued.

In 1999 the U.S. Public Health Service (USPHS) and the Infectious Diseases Society of America (IDSA) revised their earlier guidelines for preventing opportunistic infections in persons infected with human immunodeficiency virus, which are summarized in Table 50-4. HAART is the most effective means of preventing opportunistic infections in HIV-infected people. However, there are patients who are not ready or able to take HAART, or have tried HAART regimens without success. These patients benefit from prophylaxis against opportunistic infections. Prophylaxis from opportunistic infections has been shown to provide survival benefits even among persons who are receiving HAART.[10] The goal of treatment is to prevent infection or reduce its incidence and severity. This section reviews common opportunistic infections and other complications associated with HIV disease.

AIDS-RELATED OPPORTUNISTIC INFECTIONS

BACTERIAL INFECTIONS

Mycobacterium avium complex

Etiology/Epidemiology

Mycobacterium avium and *Mycobacterium intracellulare* are closely related nontuberculous or atypical mycobacteria that are usually grouped together as *M. avium* complex (MAC). These organisms are widespread in the environment, with high concentrations found in water, soil, unpasteurized dairy products, and aerosol droplets. There is a low incidence of clinical disease in the normal host because of the low pathogenicity of the organism, but MAC is the most common bacterial infection in AIDS, occurring in up to 50% of patients late in the course of HIV infection.

Pathophysiology

M. avium complex is generally manifested as a tuberculosis-like pulmonary process. The majority of people who are colonized with MAC but do not have HIV infection are asymptomatic. It is unusual to find an HIV-infected person with MAC who is asymptomatic. Persistent fevers as high as 104° F (40° C), night sweats, fatigue, anorexia, weight loss, abdominal pain and diarrhea are the most commonly occurring clinical manifestations of MAC. *M. avium* complex is most often disseminated and may be found in every organ. Physical examination may reveal lymphadenopathy or hepatosplenomegaly. It is thought to be a major contributing factor to the development of wasting syndrome.

Collaborative Care Management

Most people with MAC have high-grade bacteremia; consequently, a single blood culture is usually sufficient for diagnosis. Diagnosis can also be confirmed by culture of MAC from other normally sterile body sites such as the liver, bone, or lymph nodes. The most common laboratory abnormality associated with MAC is anemia. A sudden fall in hematocrit or the need for repeat transfusions may be associated with disseminated MAC. An elevated alkaline phosphatase level may indicate direct liver involvement.

Disseminated MAC is associated with significant morbidity and mortality, therefore, preventing it is a rational part of therapy for patients at risk. The preferred prophylactic agents for HIV infected adults with CD4+ T-lymphocyte count of less than 50 cells/μl are clarithromycin or azithromycin, which are similar drugs. Use of drugs to prevent MAC are particularly advantageous because they also confer protection against other respiratory bacterial infections.[10]

The most useful drugs for treating disseminated MAC are azithromycin or clarithromycin combined with ethambutol, clofazimine, or rifabutin. Combining drugs may prevent the development of drug resistance but is also associated with increased incidence of drug side effects. Table 50-5 lists medications used to treat MAC. Persons who have been diagnosed with MAC infection are continued on full therapeutic doses of antimycobacterial agents for life.[10]

Patient/Family Education. Teaching for the person with MAC is similar to teaching for HIV disease in general. No special diet is required; however, weight loss is a common problem, and oral, enteral, or parenteral supplementation may be necessary. There are no specific activities or activity restrictions. Fatigue is usually present and may be a limiting factor in activity levels. Patients are encouraged to stay as active as possible. Supplemental oxygen may be necessary to prevent hypoxia, in which case the patient and family are instructed about how and when to use oxygen. The nurse educates patients and families about drug therapy and side effects, symptoms that should be reported to the physician,

TABLE 50-5 Common Medications for *Mycobacterium avium* Complex

Drug	Action	Intervention
Rifampin (Rifadin)	Bacteriostatic and bactericidal; inhibits DNA-dependent polymerase activity, thereby decreasing replication	Monitor for rash, hepatotoxicity, neutropenia Assess skin integrity Monitor liver function studies, CBC Institute neutropenic precautions if necessary May turn urine orange
Clarithromycin (Biaxin)	Inhibits protein synthesis by binding to the 50S ribosomal subunit of susceptible bacteria	Monitor for nausea, abdominal pain, diarrhea, hepatotoxicity Assess nutritional status Monitor intake and output Monitor liver function studies
Azithromycin (Zithromax)	Same as clarithromycin	Monitor for nausea, abdominal pain, diarrhea, hepatotoxicity Same as clarithromycin
Amikacin (Amikin)	Bactericidal; inhibits protein synthesis in susceptible organisms	Monitor for ototoxicity, nephrotoxicity Obtain peak and trough as ordered Monitor renal studies
Streptomycin (Streptomycin)	Bactericidal; interferes with bacterial protein synthesis	Monitor for ototoxicity, nephrotoxicity Same as amikacin
Ciprofloxacin (Cipro)	Bactericidal; interferes with conversion of intermediate DNA into high-molecular DNA	Monitor for nausea, abdominal pain, diarrhea, rash Monitor nutritional status Assess hydration status Assess skin integrity
Ethambutol (Myambutol)	Inhibits RNA synthesis, decreasing organism replication	Monitor for nausea, abdominal pain, changes in visual acuity Monitor nutritional status Assess visual acuity and monitor for changes
Clofazimime (Lamprene)	Binds to mycobacterial DNA, inhibiting growth of organism	Monitor for nausea, abdominal pain Assess and monitor nutritional status Educate patient that drug may cause hyperpigmentation

and the need for continuing drug therapy for the rest of their lives.

Because most people with MAC are likely to have end-stage HIV disease and significant immune compromise, the patient and family should be informed about the availability of community resources. In particular, a respiratory therapist may be able to provide valuable insights into managing respiratory difficulties.

Mycobacterium tuberculosis

Mycobacterium tuberculosis is affecting increasing numbers of immunodeficient or immunosuppressed individuals. HIV is thought to be one of the most important factors responsible for the increased incidence of *M. tuberculosis* in the United States. USPHS guidelines recommend that all HIV-positive persons be skin tested annually for tuberculosis, and those with positive results placed on prophylactic isoniazid daily (or twice weekly) for 9 months, or either rifampin or pyrazinamide therapy for 2 months. This respiratory disease represents a complex community health illness that is discussed in detail in Chapter 32.

All HIV-infected persons who have a positive tuberculin skin test (>5 mm induration) should be suspected of having active tuberculosis and should undergo diagnostic evaluation. HIV-infected persons who are symptomatic should undergo diagnosis even if their TST is negative.[10] Definitive diagnosis of tuberculosis is made when acid-fast *M. tuberculosis* bacilli are identified in sputum or tissue samples.

Five primary drugs are used to treat tuberculosis: isoniazid, rifampin, pyrazinamide, streptomycin, and ethambutol. HIV-infected persons with active tuberculosis are placed on a multidrug treatment regimen and kept on respiratory isolation while chemotherapy is initiated and until sputum specimens are free of the bacillus. Chronic suppressive therapy for the HIV-infected person who has completed chemotherapy for active tuberculosis is not necessary or recommended. HIV-infected persons who are in close contact with people who have active, infectious tuberculosis are started on prophylactic therapy regardless of their tuberculin skin test result, age, or prior courses of chemotherapy after active tuberculosis has been ruled out.[10]

FUNGAL INFECTIONS

Fungal infections are a common problem among HIV-infected patients. The three most commonly encountered fungal diseases are candidiasis, cryptococcosis, and histoplasmosis.

Candidiasis

Etiology/Epidemiology

Thrush (candidiasis), caused by *Candida albicans,* may be one of the earliest signs of HIV infection. It is normally found in the mouth, GI tract (throat, esophagus, stomach, or bowel), vagina, and skin. Not usually pathogenic, *Candida* can become pathogenic when the immune system is altered by disease, diabetes, cancer, or immune-suppressing drugs. In HIV-infected people, mucocutaneous Candida infections of the mouth are most common, followed by infections of the esophagus, skin, rectum, and vagina. Although annoying, oral or vaginal candidiasis presents no significant risk of mortality. Disseminated infections, although rare, can be associated with significant morbidity and mortality. There are no known measures to reduce exposure to this fungus.[19]

Pathophysiology

C. albicans is characterized by the formation of white, curd-like patches, erythema, and ulcers on mucous membranes. The patches are painful and often bleed when disturbed or removed. Oral lesions occur as thrush. Esophageal lesions produce irritation and dysphagia. Vaginal infections are associated with itching, irritation, and discharge (often described as thick and cheesy). Rectal lesions also produce itching and irritation. Disseminated infections are characterized by high fever, chills, and hypotension.

Candida infections are generally diagnosed by their characteristic appearance of glistening white patches on the tongue or oral mucosal surfaces or creamy white vaginal discharge. Scrapings of the lesions and examination under a microscope allow identification of the yeast organism. Candida infections can progress to other mucocutaneous sites as well. Oral infections, when left untreated, can progress into the esophagus and stomach. Diagnostic scraping of these lesions may then require an endoscopic procedure to obtain the sample and assess the extent of infection.

Collaborative Care Management

The current recommended treatment and maintenance therapy for mouth and esophageal candidiasis is oral fluconazole or ketoconazole. However, fluconazole-resistant strains of *C. albicans* are emerging. Alternative treatments include ketoconazole, itraconazole, clotrimazole, and nystatin.[19] Vaginal yeast infections may be treated with nystatin cream, ointments, or suppositories. For persistent or systemic infections, amphotericin may be required. Table 50-6 presents an overview of these medications.

Although candidiasis is a common complication of HIV infection, primary prophylactic drug therapy is not recommended because the mortality rate is low and therapy for acute infections is highly effective. Persons with repeated episodes of esophageal candidiasis, however, are considered candidates for chronic suppression therapy with fluconazole.[19]

Patient/Family Education. There are no dietary restrictions, and patients may eat whatever they can tolerate. Oral candida lesions do, however, make it difficult for patients to tolerate temperature extremes and spicy foods. Soft foods may be better tolerated. Use of a soft-bristled toothbrush for oral hygiene will decrease the risk of pain and bleeding. Referral to a dietitian may be necessary for patients having difficulty maintaining their nutrition because of pain from oral lesions.

Patients with disseminated disease require amphotericin therapy and are likely to be acutely ill. Many patients receiving this drug experience fatigue, which may greatly reduce activity tolerance. Patients may need assistance in establishing an activity regimen they can tolerate. A gynecological referral is initiated for women who have recurrent vaginal yeast infections.

TABLE 50-6 Common Medications for *Candida* Infections

Drug	Action	Intervention
Fluconazole (Diflucan)	Fungistatic; fungicidal; inhibits ergosterol biosynthesis, producing damage to fungal cell wall	Monitor for headache, nausea, vomiting, hepatotoxicity, gynecomastia Monitor liver function studies, CBC Monitor nutritional status
Ketoconazole (Nizoral)	Fungistatic; fungicidal; inhibits fungal enzymes; alters cell membrane; prevents fungal metabolism	Same as fluconazole
Clotrimazole (Mycelex)	Fungistatic; fungicidal; changes integrity of cell membrane, allowing leakage of cell nutrients and halting fungal replication	Monitor for nausea and vomiting Monitor liver function studies Monitor nutritional status
Nystatin (Mycostatin)	Fungistatic; fungicidal; same as clotrimazole	Monitor for nausea, vomiting, epigastric pain, diarrhea Assess nutritional status Educate patient about swish-and-swallow procedure
Amphotericin (Fungizone)	Fungistatic; increases cell membrane permeability, thus inhibiting replication; decreases potassium, sodium, and nutrients in fungal cell	Monitor for fever with shaking chills, headache, anorexia, malaise, generalized pain Treat symptoms of discomfort during therapy

A dermatologist may be consulted regarding lesions that do not resolve.

Cryptococcosis

Etiology/Epidemiology

Cryptococcus neoformans is a yeastlike fungus that is ubiquitous and occurs worldwide. The organism is found in pigeon droppings and can be contracted from nesting places, soil, fruit, and fruit juices. *C. neoformans* can remain viable for up to 2 years even in desiccated pigeon feces. Neither person-to-person nor animal-to-person transmission has been documented. The disease is naturally acquired from the environment, where the organism is aerosolized and inhaled. In patients with prolonged, severe immunodeficiency caused by HIV, the immune system may not be competent against *C. neoformans,* and cryptococcosis can develop. Cryptococcal infection usually manifests as meningitis in HIV-infected patients.

Pathophysiology

Cryptococcus primarily affects the central nervous system and lungs, but it can also affect the skin, mouth, bones, liver, and kidneys. Pulmonary cryptococcal infection is generally asymptomatic, but may cause dyspnea, cough, and chest discomfort. Central nervous system findings include low-grade fever, headache, blurred vision, dizziness, memory changes, irritability, nausea or vomiting, lassitude, fatigue, and convulsions. If untreated, coma and death can occur as a result of cerebral edema or hydrocephalus. Cryptococcal skin lesions are painless, red papules that may be similar in appearance to Kaposi's sarcoma.

Collaborative Care Management

Diagnosis of *Cryptococcus* is achieved by identification of the fungus in the CSF. The organism may also be detected by antigen testing in urine or serum. Cryptococcal antigen titers and cultures of blood or CSF are the most reliable diagnostic measures. Computed tomography (CT) of the head may be performed to rule out hydrocephalus and to look for focal lesions. Chest radiographs are helpful if cryptococcal pneumonia is suspected.

Central nervous system infection can be fatal if appropriate therapy is not instituted in a timely manner. The primary drug used to treat an initial cryptococcal infection is amphotericin B; however, studies have shown that fluconazole and itraconazole can also reduce the frequency of cryptococcal infections in HIV-infected persons. HIV-infected patients with CD4 + T lymphocyte counts less than 50 cells/ml may be considered for prophylactic treatment with fluconazole. Patients who have had an episode of Cryptococcus infection are generally placed on lifelong suppressive therapy.[19] In addition to the usual IV infusion of amphotericin B, intrathecal administration has been used in patients failing to respond to IV infusion.

Other medications used include flucytosine and fluconazole. Flucytosine is an oral agent and is given in combination with amphotericin B. Fluconazole is less toxic than amphotericin and is better tolerated but may not be as efficacious in certain patients. The side effects and nursing implications of drug therapies for cryptococcosis are summarized in Table 50-7.

As with many of the opportunistic infections associated with HIV disease, the successful treatment of the initial acute infection does not cure the patient. Long-term suppressive therapy is necessary to prevent recurrence. Primary prophylaxis (instituted before the patient ever develops an initial infection) and long-term suppressive therapy may be accomplished with oral fluconazole therapy.

Patient/Family Education. There are no special dietary considerations for this infection. Patients need to be encouraged to maintain a healthy, well-balanced diet. Activity restrictions are as needed based on the degree of fatigue. Patients with meningitis may experience somnolence or confusion; consequently, activity restrictions may be necessary to protect the patient from injury. Patients and families are educated and

TABLE 50-7 Common Medications for *Cryptococcosis*

Drug	Action	Intervention
Flucytosine	Antiinfective; antibiotic; antifungal; converted to fluorouracil within fungal cell, inhibiting fungal cell metabolism	Monitor for anemia, jaundice, skin rash, itching, sore throat, fever, unusual bleeding/bruising, confusion, diarrhea, nausea, vomiting, headache, light-headedness, drowsiness Assess for signs of unusual bleeding Monitor nutritional status
Fluconazole (Diflucan)	Fungistatic; fungicidal; inhibits ergosterol biosynthesis, producing damage to fungal cell wall	Monitor for headache, nausea, vomiting, hepatotoxicity, gynecomastia Monitor liver function studies, CBC Monitor nutritional status
Amphotericin (Fungizone)	Fungistatic; increases cell membrane permeability, thus inhibiting replication; decreases potassium, sodium, and nutrients in fungal cell	Monitor for fever with shaking chills, headache, anorexia, malaise, generalized pain Treat symptoms of discomfort during therapy

counseled about the modes of transmission of *Cryptococcus* and cautioned about contact with infected animals, human or animal feces, soil, and sexual practices that may result in oral exposure to feces.

As with other serious opportunistic infections that occur in late-stage disease, patients with cryptococcal infections may require multiple referrals. Social services, home nursing services, physical or occupational therapy, and psychiatry or counseling may be appropriate.

Histoplasmosis

Histoplasma capsulatum causes the common, usually benign fungal infection, histoplasmosis that occurs primarily in the lungs. Histoplasmosis in HIV-infected persons may manifest as acute pulmonary infection or, more often, as disseminated disease. Because chest radiographs are unreliable and are normal in up to 30% of individuals with disseminated histoplasmosis, bone marrow biopsy and cultures, examination and culture of pulmonary tissue and secretions, as well as blood cultures are the most common means of establishing a diagnosis in HIV-positive patients.

Disseminated histoplasmosis in AIDS is invariably fatal if not treated aggressively with antifungal therapy. Amphotericin B and fluconazole are the drugs of choice in induction therapy for acute infection. Candida patients who have been diagnosed with histoplasmosis will require lifelong suppressive treatment with itraconazole. HIV-infected individuals with CD4 + T lymphocyte counts less than 100 cells/*m*l are considered for prophylactic therapy with itraconazole; however, concerns over drug toxicities, interactions, drug resistance, and cost may delay prophylactic treatment.[19]

Patients placed on prophylactic therapy are taught the signs and symptoms of drug toxicity and informed about potential drug interactions. As with other serious opportunistic infections that occur in late-stage disease, patients with histoplasmosis may require multiple referrals. Dietary services, social services, home nursing services, physical or occupational therapy, and psychiatry or counseling may be appropriate.

PROTOZOAL INFECTIONS

Protozoal infections are caused by a variety of organisms, many of which are parasitic. *Cryptosporidium, P. carinii,* and *Toxoplasma gondii* are commonly encountered opportunistic infections in HIV-infected individuals.

Cryptosporidium

Etiology/Epidemiology

Cryptosporidium is a parasite present in a variety of animal species, including birds, reptiles, fish, cattle, sheep, and humans. It is a well-recognized pathogen in both immunologically intact individuals and immunocompromised hosts, such as persons with HIV disease. In addition to animal-to-human transmission, person-to-person transmission has also been documented among day care centers, household contacts, hospitalized patients, and health care workers. Water-borne transmission has also been documented. Chlorination of water does not kill *Cryptosporidium.*

Pathophysiology

The most common site of *Cryptosporidium* infection is the small intestine. It is a self-limiting disease in immune-competent individuals; however, it is extremely pathogenic in immunocompromised persons. It can affect the entire GI tract, producing fever, nausea, vomiting, abdominal pain and cramping, and severe watery diarrhea. Death from profound malabsorption, electrolyte imbalances, malnutrition, and dehydration can occur.

Collaborative Care Management

Diagnosis is made by identifying *Cryptosporidium* oocytes in fresh or formalin-preserved stool specimens. No effective anticryptosporidial therapy currently exists for either treatment or prevention.[19] The drugs paromomycin and azithromycin may help suppress the infection in some people, but it is not always effective. Octreotide may be used to reduce the volume of stool. Otherwise therapy is aimed at controlling pain and decreasing peristalsis.

Patient/Family Education. Education of the HIV-infected person emphasizes modes of transmission and ways to avoid contact with the organism. Patients and families are advised to avoid contact with infected animals, contaminated drinking water, lake water, diaper-age infants and children, and human and animal feces.

Patients with *Cryptosporidium* require intravenous therapy for fluid replacement and may require nutritional supplements or total parenteral nutrition (TPN) to replace fluids, calories, and nutrients lost through the massive volumes of diarrhea. Reducing bulk in the diet may reduce stool volume. If octreotide is prescribed, patient education about the drug is essential. Side effects may include hyperglycemia, hypoglycemia, abdominal pain, nausea, vomiting, pain at the injection site, headache, fatigue, dizziness, edema, facial flushing, and hepatic dysfunction. The patient is taught how to self-monitor stool volume to assess the drug's effectiveness.

Frequent perineal care is essential for patients experiencing *Cryptosporidium* diarrhea. Patients are instructed to use nondrying soaps and to keep the skin clean and dry. Protective topical creams or lotions are applied to prevent skin cracking and excretion.

Pneumocystis carinii

Etiology/Epidemiology

P. carinii pneumonia (PCP) is a very common severe opportunistic infection affecting HIV-infected patients. *P. carinii* is a ubiquitous organism with worldwide distribution. It is found in the air, on food, and in water, although most transmission appears to be via airborne routes. Most healthy children have acquired *P. carinii* infection by 4 years of age. It is not highly virulent, and infection in a normal host is usually asymptomatic. In the immunocompromised host, however, *P. carinii* can cause fulminant disease. PCP occurs in 90% of HIV-infected persons in the United States and is the leading cause of death.[20]

Pathophysiology

P. carinii is generally confined to the lungs, although extrapulmonary *Pneumocystis* can occur. The infection causes increased permeability of alveolar capillary membranes, degenerative lung cell changes, and diffuse alveolar injury, resulting in impaired gas exchange and altered lung compliance. Without treatment, the infection leads to respiratory insufficiency and death. Clinical manifestations include dyspnea, nonproductive cough, intermittent fever, fatigue, anorexia, weight loss, and tachypnea. Persons with advanced disease may exhibit crackles, decreased breath sounds, and cyanosis.

Collaborative Care Management

Bronchoalveolar and transbronchial biopsies are usually performed to identify *P. carinii* in patients with pneumonia. If unsuccessful, an open lung biopsy via thoracotomy may be performed as a last resort. Chest radiograph may reveal pneumonia, although 5% to 10% of chest radiographs in AIDS patients with PCP appear normal. Pulmonary function studies usually reveal decreased vital capacity, decreased total lung capacity, and decreased single-breath diffusing capacity of carbon monoxide. Arterial blood gas studies may reveal hypoxemia, hypocarbia, and an increase in the alveolar-arterial oxygen gradient, particularly with exercise.

Presumptive diagnosis of PCP may be made according to the CDC guidelines: (1) history of dyspnea on exertion or nonproductive cough of recent onset; (2) chest radiographic evidence of diffuse bilateral interstitial infiltrates or gallium scan evidence of diffuse bilateral pulmonary disease; (3) arterial blood gas analysis showing an arterial oxygen tension of less than 70 mm Hg, a low respiratory diffusing capacity, or an increase in the alveolar-arterial oxygen tension gradient; and (4) no evidence of bacterial pneumonia.[19]

The most effective treatments for PCP are IV pentamidine isethionate or either IV or oral co-trimoxazole (trimethoprim and sulfamethoxazole). Co-trimoxazole is the preferred therapy because it is better tolerated. However, many patients are sensitive to sulfa drugs such as co-trimoxazole, which may limit the medication options. Other therapies that may be used include aerosolized pentamidine, trimetrexate, clindamycin, primaquine, or atovaquone. Table 50-8 summarizes information about pentamidine and co-trimoxazole.

Prophylactic therapy is recommended for patients who have not yet developed PCP but have $CD4^+$ T lymphocyte counts less than 200 cells/*ml*, exhibit unexplained fever for 2 weeks or longer, or have a history of oropharyngeal candidiasis. Significant progress has been made in controlling PCP.

Trimethoprim-sulfamethoxazole (TMP-SMZ) is the recommended prophylactic agent. One double-strength tablet per day is preferred if it can be tolerated, otherwise one single-strength tablet is administered. If TMP-SMZ cannot be tolerated, dapsone, dapsone plus pyrimethamine plus leucovorin, aerosolized pentamidine, or atovaquone are alternative drugs. An advantage of dapsone is that it also protects against toxoplasmosis. Secondary prophylaxis is recommended after the first episode of PCP.[19] The use of prophylactic therapy has significantly reduced the number of PCP recurrences, ultimately reducing the mortality rate.

Patient/Family Education. Drug therapy for PCP may produce severe adverse effects in immunodeficient individuals, including bone marrow suppression, fever, nausea, vomiting, and hepatotoxicity. Patients are encouraged to seek follow-up care and report signs of adverse or toxic drug effects. The nurse assesses the patient's drug administration technique to ensure that inhaled drugs reach the lung bases. Supplemental oxygen may be necessary to enhance oxygenation when dyspnea is severe. Mechanical ventilation may improve the chance of survival for persons with advanced disease who develop respiratory failure.

There are no special diet or activity recommendations for the person with PCP. A well-balanced, nutritional diet with adequate fluid intake is encouraged. Activity depends on the person's degree of illness. Dyspnea often results in fatigue; therefore activities should be alternated with rest periods. As with other serious opportunistic infections, the person with *Pneumocystis* infection may require multiple referrals. A respiratory therapy referral for airway management is essential. A

TABLE 50-8 Common Medications for *Pneumocystis carinii* Pneumonia

Drug	Action	Intervention
Pentamidine isethionate (Pentam 300)	Interferes with protozoan DNA and RNA synthesis, thus interfering with parasite reproduction	
Intravenous		Monitor for blood dyscrasias, rapid irregular pulse, hyperglycemia, hypoglycemia, diabetes mellitus, skin rash, hypotension, pain at injection site Monitor blood and renal studies Rotate injection sites
Inhalation		Implement respiratory therapy precautions Administer bronchodilators as indicated Monitor for chest pain, congestion, cough, dyspnea, pharyngitis, wheezing, skin rash, metallic taste, pneumothorax
Co-trimoxazole (Bactrim, Septra) (sulfamethoxazole and trimethoprim)	Trimethoprim: antiinfective and folic acid antagonist; interferes with bacterial cell growth Sulfamethoxazole bacteriostatic sulfonamide; halts the multiplication of bacteria	Monitor for hemolytic, megaloblastic, or aplastic anemia; agranulocytosis, skin rash, Stevens-Johnson syndrome, dysphagia, nausea, vomiting, stomatitis, headache, convulsions Contraindicated in hypersensitivity to sulfa agents Give oral preparation with full glass of water Monitor intake and output

sample Clinical Pathway for an immunocompromised patient with pneumonia is presented on p. 1680.

Toxoplasma gondii

Etiology/Epidemiology

T. gondii is a protozoan that occurs worldwide and infects both humans and domestic animals. The definitive hosts are members of the cat family, although not all cats are infected, and toxoplasmosis has been documented in locales without cats. Transmission of *Toxoplasma* in humans is primarily through ingestion of meats and vegetables containing oocysts. The prevalence of *Toxoplasma* tissue cysts in meat consumed by humans may be as high as 25%. Cockroaches, earthworms, snails, and slugs may serve as transport hosts for the oocysts. It is estimated that 5% to 10% of young adults in the United States are seropositive for toxoplasma, and this rate rises to 50% by 50 years of age.[14] Human-to-human transmission is from mother to fetus, by blood transfusion, or by organ transplantation.

Pathophysiology

Toxoplasmosis infection does not generally cause significant illness in healthy hosts. It is, however, a major cause of encephalitis in persons with AIDS. Toxoplasmosis produces localized and disseminated infections. Localized infections may be mild and are manifested by symptoms similar to mononucleosis. Disseminated infections are serious and include manifestations such as headache, confusion or delirium, fever, encephalitis, vomiting, hemiparesis, seizures, and loss of vision.

Collaborative Care Management

Persons newly diagnosed with HIV infection are tested for toxoplasma antibodies to detect latent toxoplasmosis infection.[19]

Because *Toxoplasma* causes encephalitis, definitive diagnosis generally requires brain biopsy. Presumptive diagnosis is most often accomplished by (1) brain-imaging evidence of a lesion with a mass effect, (2) recent onset of focal neurological abnormality, (3) serum antibody to toxoplasmosis, or (4) successful response to therapy for toxoplasmosis.

HIV-infected persons who are seropositive for toxoplasmosis and who have CD4 + T cell counts of less than 100/*ml* are started on prophylactic drug therapy with TMP-SMZ. Dapsone with pyrimethamine is alternate therapy for patients who are unable to tolerate TMP-SMZ. HIV-infected persons who have been diagnosed with toxoplasmosis are placed on suppressive drug therapy for the remainder of their lives.

The primary therapy for toxoplasmosis in persons with AIDS is a combination of sulfadiazine and pyrimethamine (Table 50-9). Adjunctive therapy include dexamethasone (Decadron) for cerebral inflammation associated with abscesses and phenytoin (Dilantin) for infection induced seizures. Approximately 40% to 60% of patients may have severe adverse reactions during the initial treatment phase, and alternative regimens, including cessation of sulfadiazine or addition of clindamycin, may be required.[19]

Patient/Family Education. The nurse warns HIV-infected persons against eating raw or undercooked meat, advises them to wash their hands after contact with raw meat or contact with soil and to wash raw fruit and vegetables before eating them, and recommends that they avoid changing cat litter if they own a cat. If the patient must change cat litter, thorough hand washing afterwards is essential.

There are no specific dietary or activity restrictions for the person with toxoplasmosis. Patients with mental status changes or seizures may require safety precautions. Because drug therapy can cause blood dyscrasias, teaching includes signs and symptoms of drug toxicity and the importance of follow-up

clinical pathway *Pneumonia With Immunocompromise*

Expected LOS: 5 days
Developed by Team

	DAY/HOUR/VISIT ADMISSION	1	2	3
Consults	Dietician			
Tests	Chem 18 with LDH CBC CXR Blood cultures × 2, AFB × 1, Fungal × 1 RC: ABG RC: Sputum C&S & GM stain Silver Stain (order on misc. requisition)	Lab as Ordered Monitor reports Alert MD to any microscopic evidence of organisms Sputum results called	→ Consider line placement (PICC, Midline) if antibiotics to be prolonged →	→ →
Medication	Antibiotics IV *Antibiotics started within 1 hr of admission PO meds as ordered	Continue until DC'd →	→ →	→ →
Treatment	IV Fluids RC: treatments as ordered O_2: titrate O_2 to 95% & notify MD NSG: Advanced Directive in chart Report abnormal labs Nsg Assessment q shift resp rate & rhythm, lung aeration, abnorm. gas exchange Functional level assessed based on Karnofsky scale (see page 2)	Continue until DC'd → Continue until DC'd →	→ RC TX or MDI → → Reassess functional level based on Karnofsky scale (see page 2) Reassess appropriateness of Advanced Directive	S.L. → → →
Diet	Advera/Ensure supplement TID	Food intake recorded 24 hr Calorie Count NPO p MN if bronch in AM Advera/Ensure supplement TID	NPO p MN if bronch in AM Advera/Ensure supplement TID	Advera/Ensure supplement TID
Activity	As ordered, encourage activity Assist to chg position q2h from sitting to lying as tolerated NSG: If ADL rating 3-4, order for PT/OT/TR assessment obtained	Chair (for meals) →	Chair (for meals) (× 3 for _____ min) Ambulate with assist Reassess for need for PT/OT evaluation	→ (3 × for _____ min.) Ambulate ad lib
Teaching	Orient to room and routines Review intended effect of therapy and CCP & goals RC: Instruct on treatment plans and O_2 safety (if applicable)	Reinforce teaching Discuss changes in diet, activity, medications if appropriate	Reinforce teaching Discuss possibility of move to SNU or home with Home Health if appropriate	→
Discharge Planning	Assess for barriers to discharge NSG: If from LTC facility, VNA, home O_2, financial issues, notify Social Services	NSG: Notify Resource Nurse of any changes in discharge plans	SS/NSG: Discuss with physician if pt is candidate for move to SNU ie., IV therapy, IM injection, rehabilitative nsg procedures, or PT/OT needed	If candidate for SNU prepare for discharge RC: If going home on O_2, make home arrangements

Team Problem Identification		Intermediate Goals		
Anxiety R/T hospitalization	NSG: Pt. /family verbalizes concerns	→	→	→
Knowledge deficit R/T tests/ procedures disease process	NSG: Verbalizes understanding of tests/procedures	→	→	→
	NSG: Verbalizes understanding of information on the teaching pathway & goals/CCP			
	NSG: Pt/family verbalize agreement with Advance Directive/Living Will status			
	RC: Verbalizes understanding of O_2 therapy and aerosol TX	→	RC: Verbalizes understanding of correct method to use MDI	RC: Demonstrates independence in use of MDI
Home maintenance management impaired R/T disease process	NSG: Verbalize beginning knowledge of home care needs	→	Verbalizes agreement with current discharge plans	
	NSG: Verbalizes understanding of safety measures	Demonstrates compliance with safety measures	No injury	→
Potential for injury R/T unfamiliar environment	RC: Verbalize understanding of safety R/T oxygen therapy			
Ineffective breathing pattern R/T disease process	NSG: Demonstrates comfortable breathing pattern	→	→	→
	RC: Adequate ventilation/respiration per ABG results. PaO_2 >60 (PaO_2 = to pre disease with or without O_2, and SpO_2 >90.)	RC: Verbalizes a sense of improvement from respiratory treatments	→	→
Potential alteration in nutrition R/T disease process	NSG: Verbalizes understanding of need for adequate nutritional intake	NSG: Demonstrates tolerance of nutritional regimen	→	→
Potential alteration in self care R/T disease process	NSG: Demonstrates tolerance of activity levels without respiratory distress	NSG: Demonstrates able to sit up in the chair for 30 min	→	NSG: Demonstrates returning to pre-illness care abilities

Courtesy Columbia Overland Park Regional Medical Center, Overland Park, KS.

Continued

clinical pathway *Pneumonia With Immunocompromise*

Expected LOS: 5 days
Developed by Team

DAY/HOUR/VISIT				
	ADMISSION	**1**	**2**	**3**
Team Problem Identification		Intermediate Goals		
Signatures: NSG	7-3	7-3	7-3	7-3
	3-11	3-11	3-11	3-11
RC (Respiratory Care)	11-7	11-7	11-7	11-7
	7-3	7-3	7-3	7-3
	3-11	3-11	3-11	3-11
	11-7	11-7	11-7	11-7
SS				
Baseline Data:				

DISCHARGE DAY*********** 4	
Nursing Diagnosis	
Anxiety R/T hospitalization	NSG: Pt./family demonstrate appropriate coping mechanisms
Knowledge deficit R/T tests/procedures disease process	NSG: Verbalizes understanding of tests/procedures
Home maintenance management impaired R/T disease process	NSG: Verbalize understanding of discharge plans/instructions
Potential for injury R/T unfamiliar environment	NSG: No injury
Ineffective breathing pattern R/T disease process	NSG: Demonstrates optimal ventilation with measures taken RC: Verbalizes a sense of improvement from resp. treatments
Potential alteration in nutrition R/T disease process	NSG: Demonstrates tolerance of nutritional regimen
Potential alteration in self care R/T disease process	NSG: Demonstrates pre-illness self care abilities
Signatures: NSG	
	7-3
	3-11
RC	11-7
	7-3
	3-11
SS	11-7

TABLE 50-9 Common Medications for *Toxoplasmosis*

Drug	Action	Intervention
Sulfadiazine PO	Bacteriostatic sulfonamide; halts the multiplication of bacteria but does not fully kill the mature microorganism	Maintain fluid intake of 1500 ml/day. Educate patient about the importance of maintaining drug dosage and schedules Monitor for fever, blood dyscrasias Monitor liver and renal studies
Pyrimethamine PO	Inhibits folic acid metabolism in organism; stops growth of fertilized gametes to inhibit parasitic transmission	Contraindicated if hypersensitivity exists Monitor for CNS stimulation, convulsions, tremors, fatigue, nausea, vomiting, anorexia, diarrhea, gastritis, thrombocytopenia, leukopenia, megaloblastic anemia, agranulocytosis Monitor liver and renal studies
Clindamycin PO, (Cleocin) IM, IV	Antibacterial agent that suppresses protein synthesis; binds to 50S subunit of bacterial ribosomes	Monitor for rash, urticaria, nausea, vomiting, diarrhea, pseudomembraneous colitis, vaginitis, leukopenia, eosinophilia, agranulocytosis Monitor liver studies Contraindicated if hypersensitivity exists Competes with chloramphenicol and erythromycin

monitoring. As with other opportunistic infections, patients with toxoplasmosis may require multiple referrals.

Viral Infections

Cytomegalovirus (CMV) and herpes simplex virus (HSV) types 1 and 2, which are widespread in the general population, are viruses that can significantly affect HIV-infected individuals.

Etiology/Epidemiology

CMV infection is caused by CMV, a virus belonging to the herpesvirus family. Seroprevalence of CMV ranges from 30% to 100% in the United States. It is found in breast milk, saliva, cervical secretions, semen, feces, urine, and blood.[19]

Herpes simplex virus is caused by *Herpesvirus hominis.* Type 1 HSV is transmitted via oral and respiratory secretions. Type 2 HSV is transmitted by sexual contact. Both CMV and HSV remain dormant in tissues after initial infection and are reactivated in the presence of HIV and immunodeficiency.

Pathophysiology

CMV is thought to spread throughout the body via lymphocytes or mononuclear cells. The infection is usually asymptomatic in the immune-competent host and can exist as a latent or chronic infection. In the immune-compromised host, CMV is pathogenic and produces symptoms. Disseminated infection can produce inflammatory reactions in the lungs, GI tract, liver, central nervous system, and eyes, leading to chorioretinitis, pneumonitis, encephalitis, adrenalitis, colitis, esophagitis, cholangitis, and hepatitis. CMV is a significant cause of blindness in persons with HIV disease.[2]

HSV type 1 affects the skin and mucous membranes, producing painful vesicular lesions. Similar lesions are produced by HSV type 2, but they occur in the genital or perianal regions. Disseminated herpes infections affect the brain, liver, and lungs, producing blindness, seizures, deafness, and death.

Collaborative Care Management

CMV and HSV types 1 and 2 are diagnosed by identification of antibodies in the serum. Parenteral or oral ganciclovir, parenteral foscarnet, and parenteral cidofovir are the drugs of choice for both treatment and prophylaxis of CMV infections. Prophylaxis with oral ganciclovir may be considered for HIV-infected adults with CD4+ T-lymphocyte count of less than 50 cells/μl. It is not always recommended, however, because of costs, limited effectiveness, and side effects. Chronic suppressive therapy or maintenance therapy is recommended for persons with recurrent disease.[19]

HSV is treated effectively with acyclovir. Prophylaxis is not generally recommended because acyclovir is an effective treatment for acute episodes. Persons who tend to have chronic herpes lesions are candidates for daily suppressive therapy with acyclovir. Intravenous foscarnet and cidofovir are alternative drugs that can be used when acyclovir is not effective.[2]

Patient/Family Education. HIV-infected persons are advised that CMV is shed in saliva, semen, and cervical secretions and that HSV is spread by oral and sexual contact. Latex condoms must be used during sexual contact to reduce the risk of viral transmission. Use of good hygienic practices, such as hand washing, can significantly reduce the risk of infection.

There are no specific dietary or activity restrictions for the person with CMV or HSV. Teaching regarding antiviral therapy should include signs and symptoms of drug toxicity and the importance of follow-up monitoring. All HIV-positive individuals are provided with home screening tools for identifying early CMV-related visual changes and are encouraged to have regular professional eye screening. CMV retinitis rapidly progresses toward blindness. As with other opportunistic infections, patients with viral infections may require multiple referrals.

HIV-Related Cancer

Etiology/Epidemiology

Kaposi's sarcoma is by far the most common neoplasm found in patients with HIV infection. Kaposi's sarcoma is a rare cancer that may occur in aged non–HIV infected persons. It has commonly been associated with HIV but may affect any person who is immunosuppressed or immunodeficient. The incidence of unexplained cases of Kaposi's sarcoma was one of the initial manifestations that led to the identification of HIV infection in this country.

Pathophysiology

The exact cause of Kaposi's sarcoma is unknown. The lesions may appear on the skin, mucous membranes, mouth, tongue, tonsils, sclera, or conjunctiva and may also affect the internal organs. Lesions extend from the mid dermis upward into the epidermis and appear as dark blue, purple, or red papules (Figure 50-8). They may ulcerate and are associated with pain and itching. Systemic manifestations include lymphatic obstruction with resulting edema, dyspnea or respiratory distress when the lungs are affected, and digestive problems when the GI tract is involved.

Collaborative Care Management

Kaposi's sarcoma is diagnosed by skin biopsy, but high suspicion exists when persons with lesions are immunocompromised. Local lesions can be surgically removed, but systemic lesions are treated with radiation or chemotherapy.[19] Doxorubicin, vinblastine, vincristine, and etoposide are agents of choice for treatment of Kaposi's sarcoma. Kaposi's sarcoma is not a major cause of death in persons with HIV disease; however, systemic disease can result in the need for medical or surgical intervention.

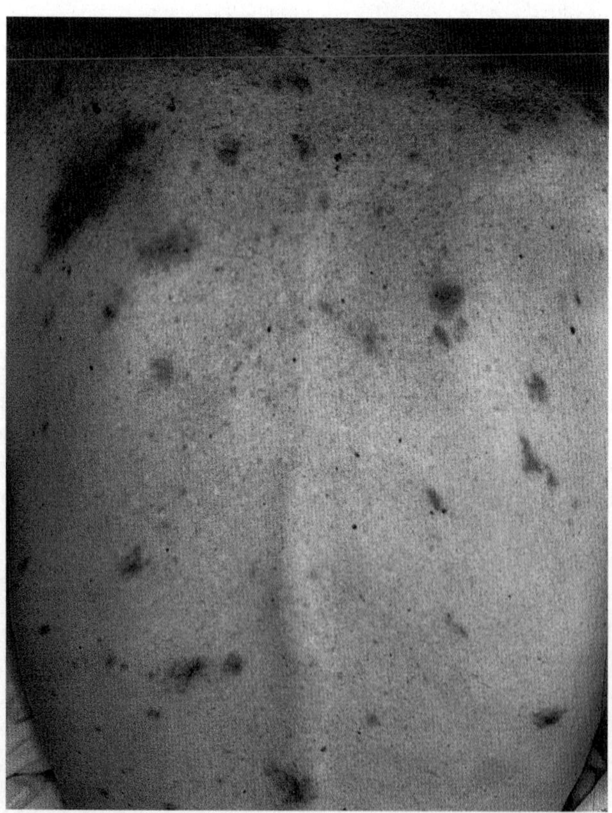

Figure 50-8 Kaposi's sarcoma.

Patient/Family Education. There are no known measures to prevent Kaposi's sarcoma; consequently, patients need information regarding what to expect and how to care for lesions. The nurse explains infection prevention methods such as keeping draining lesions covered, avoiding scratching or picking at lesions, and keeping lesions clean and dry. Skin care protocols are implemented for ulcerated areas. Patients are encouraged to express their feelings about the changes in appearance produced by Kaposi's sarcoma. If chemotherapy is elected, education must include an explanation of medications, potential side effects, drug interactions, and signs and symptoms that need to be reported to the physician.

Critical Thinking Questions

1. A woman engaged in unprotected sex 2 weeks ago. Concerned, she decided to have her blood drawn to determine her HIV status. Four days later she learns that her ELISA is negative. What conclusions can be drawn about her ELISA findings at this time?
2. You have been asked to talk to a group of high school freshmen about HIV infection and AIDS. What information will be most relevant to this group? What information is irrelevant or not appropriate for this age-group?
3. Your co-worker confides in you that he thinks his assigned patient, who has AIDS, deserves the disease because he is gay. Discuss the ramifications of your co-worker's attitude toward his patient with AIDS. How should you respond? Should the patient be assigned to another nurse? Why or why not?
4. Your patient, who is HIV infected, has a $CD4^+$ T helper lymphocyte cell count of 250 cells/μl. She asks your advice about initiating antiretroviral therapy. How will you respond?
5. Your AIDS patient has several opportunistic infections, one of which is Kaposi's sarcoma. No treatment has been ordered for the problem. Given your understanding of Kaposi's sarcoma, explain why the disease is not being medically treated.

References

1. Burke M, Walsh M: *Gerontologic nursing: wholistic care of the older adult,* ed 2, St Louis, 1997, Mosby.
2. Calvert W: Preventing and treating major opportunistic infections in AIDS, *Postgrad Med* 102(4):89, 1997.
3. Centers for Disease Control and Prevention (CDC): HIV and its transmission, website: http://www.cdc.gov/hiv/pubs/facts/transmission.htm.
4. Centers for Disease Control and Prevention (CDC). Revised surveillance case definition for HIV Infection, *MMWR* 48(13):29, 1999.
5. Centers for Disease Control and Prevention (CDC): A glance at the HIV epidemic, *Update* 12:1, 2000.
6. Kirton, C, Talotta, D, Zwolski K: *Handbook of HIV/AIDS nursing,* St Louis, 2001, Mosby.
7. McCloskey J, Bulechek G: *Nursing interventions classifications (NIC),* ed 3, St Louis, 2000, Mosby.
8. Mellors J et al: Prognosis in HIV-1 infection predicted by quantity of virus in plasma, *Science* 272:1167, 1997.

9. Office of AIDS Research and the National Institutes of Health: Report of the NIH panel to define principles of therapy of HIV infection, Washington, DC, 1997, U.S. Government Printing Office.
10. Panel on Clinical Practices and Treatment of HIV Infection: *Guidelines for the use of antiretroviral agents in HIV-infected adults and adolescents,* Rockville, Md, February, 2001, U.S. Department of Health and Human Services and the Henry J. Kaiser Family Foundation.
11. Reference deleted in proofs.
12. Roitt, I, Brostoff J, Male D: *Immunology,* ed 5, St Louis, 1998, Mosby.
13. Reference deleted in proofs.
14. The Body: OI update: toxoplasmosis, website: http://www.thebody.com/hivnews/newsline/aug99/advances.html.
15. Ungvarski P, Flaskerud J: *HIV/AIDS: a guide to primary care management,* ed 4, St Louis, 1999, Mosby.
16. U.S. Department of Health and Human Services, Public Health Service: *Healthy people 2010,* Washington, DC, 2001, U.S. Government Printing Office.
17. U.S. Food and Drug Administration: Attacking AIDS with a "cocktail" therapy, 1999, website: http://www.fda.gov/fdac/features/1999/499_aids.html.
18. U.S. Food and Drug Administration. Antiretroviral drugs approved by FDA for HIV, February 14, 2001, website: http://www.fda.gov/oashi/aids/virals.html.
19. U.S. Public Health Service and Infectious Diseases Society of America: UPHS/IDSA guidelines for the prevention of opportunistic infections in persons infected with human immunodeficiency virus, *MMWR* 48(10):1, 1999.
20. Wilkin A, Feinberg J: *Pneumocystis carinii* pneumonia: a clinical overview, *Am Fam Physician* 60:1699, 1999.
21. World Health Organization: Programme for surveillance of HIV/AIDS/and sexually transmitted infections, 2000, website: http://www.who.int/emc/diseases/hiv/index.html.

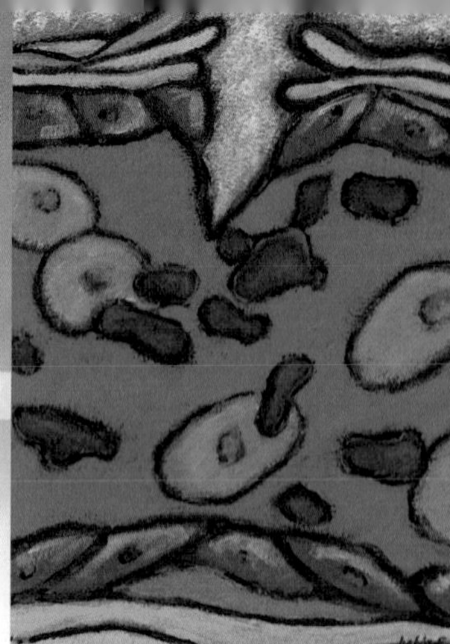

51 Organ Transplantation

Carol J. Green

Objectives

After studying this chapter, the learner should be able to:

1. Describe the criteria used to select candidates for transplantation.
2. List the general organ and tissue donor criteria.
3. List the steps of the donor evaluation process.
4. Examine the influences of current and past legislative initiatives on organ donation and transplantation.
5. Construct a plan of care for the organ donor family.
6. Differentiate among hyperacute, acute, and chronic rejection.
7. Discuss the histocompatibility testing and matching required for transplantation.
8. Compare mode of action, indications for use, dosage, administration, side effects, and nursing interventions for the commonly used immunosuppressive agents.
9. Describe the major infections for which the immunosuppressed transplant recipient is at high risk.
10. Describe the general nursing diagnoses and care needs of the transplant recipient before and after transplantation.
11. Design care plans that address the common needs and interventions for persons with corneal, kidney, liver, pancreas, heart, lung, or bone marrow transplantations.

OVERVIEW OF TRANSPLANTATION

Organ transplantation has evolved from being a medical experiment to a major therapeutic intervention for selected patients. Advances in organ procurement and preservation, surgical technique, tissue typing and matching, management of the immune system, and the prevention and treatment of rejection have dramatically increased the demand for organs and tissues for transplantation. Unfortunately, organ donation has not kept pace with organ/tissue demand, which is expected to continue as more and more diseases can be treated by transplantation. Nurses play a pivotal role in addressing the shortage of organs/tissues because they care for potential donors and closely interact with donor families.

Although many types of organ/tissue transplants are performed, this chapter focuses on allograft transplantation (transplantation of organs/tissues from one member of a species to another member of the same species) of solid organs (kidney, liver, heart, pancreas, and lung), corneas, and bone marrow.

Etiology/Epidemiology

In 2000, 40,000 cornea,[18] 13,290 kidney, 4934 liver, 2197 heart, 436 pancreas, 956 lung, and 48 heart-lung transplants were performed in the United States.[26] In all, 450,000 people received tissue transplants, which included bone, heart valve, artery, vein, tendon, and cartilage allografts. Donated skin was used on about 100,000 patients.[24] Table 51-1 provides a summary of tissues that can be transplanted. Transplantation offers new life to individuals dying of liver, heart, and lung failure. It restores lost body function and improves quality of life for individuals with kidney failure, diabetes, blindness, heart disease, bone disease, and eye disease.

Conservative medical management of patients with end-stage kidney, liver, heart, or lung disease is costly. Although transplantation procedures are expensive, the current success rates have made transplantation a cost-effective treatment option compared with traditional medical management. For example, Medicare expenditures for one individual undergoing chronic hemodialysis costs between $60,000 and $70,000 a year. The cost of a kidney transplantation is approximately $111,400 for the initial hospitalization and first year of follow-up care and immunosuppressive medications.[20] Because about 90% of transplants function for 5 years, the cost for transplantation is $191,400, as opposed to $300,000 to $350,000 for 5 years of chronic hemodialysis. Likewise, patients with end-stage liver,

TABLE 51-1 Summary of Tissues That Can Be Transplanted

General Criteria for Donation of Tissues:

No history of significant disease processes affecting tissues.
No sepsis/transmissible disease
Known cause of death

Eye	Bone	Heart	Ear	Other
Cornea	Ilium	Heart valves	StapesSkin	Dura mater
	Radius		Incus	Fascia lata
	Ulna		Malleus	Cartilage
	Femur		Tympanic membrane	
	Humerus		Tendons	
	Tibia		Ligaments	
	Fibula			
	Ribs			
	Mandible			

Source: UNOS, website: http://www.unos.org.

TABLE 51-2 Estimated Average Cost for First Year of Organ Transplantation

Organ	Estimated Cost
Kidney	$111,400
Heart	$303,400
Heart-Lung	$301,200
Liver	$244,600
Lung	$257,700
Pancreas	$113,700
Kidney-Pancreas	$136,300

Adapted from Milliman USA: Cost implications of human organ and tissue transplantation, an update, 1999, website: www.milliman.com.

TABLE 51-3 Number of Transplants and Transplant Programs in the United States

Organ	Number of Transplants	Number of Programs
Kidney	22,423	246
Kidney/Pancreas	1806	96
Pancreas	415	96
Heart	4012	142
Lung	1646	77
Heart/Lung	94	83
Liver	7161	121

Source: *Transplant Patient Data Source:* February 16, 2000, Richmond, Va: United Network for Organ Sharing. Retrieved [date of retrieval, e.g., February 16, 2000], website: http://207.239.150.13/tpd/.

heart, or lung disease have multiple costly hospital admissions for conservative management of their disease before death occurs (Table 51-2).

Other financial factors that increase the cost-effectiveness of transplantation include the potential earning power of the transplant recipient and the discontinuation of existing disability benefits. Transplantation can restore dignity and quality to the lives of patients and families dealing with end-stage organ disease and allow patients to once again become productive members of society.

Availability of Donor Organs

The United Network for Organ Sharing (UNOS) reported that in 2000, there were 11,589 donors, many of whom provided more than one organ, and that 22,423 solid organ transplants took place (Table 51-3). As of May 2001, the national patient waiting list included 76,617 registrants. If donor recoveries do not increase, an organ shortage as high as 65% could occur. UNOS estimates that a new patient is added to the national patient waiting list for organ transplantation every 20 minutes and that seven people die every day while waiting for organ transplants.[25]

The shortage of organs reflects both organ accessibility and availability. Only an estimated 40% of organs from people who die meeting donor eligibility criteria are actually donated each year.[30] Despite extensive public awareness campaigns and the existence of laws mandating that all families be given the opportunity to donate the organs of a loved one who dies, the ratio of potential to actual donors has not been affected. Some of the important reasons why people do not donate are that (1) they fear they are compromising their religious beliefs, (2) they find the subject distasteful, (3) they are not approached about donation in a respectful manner, or (4) they feel the system is unfair.[4]

Another difficulty of the organ procurement process relates to the definition and declaration of death. Both the medical profession and lay public agree that the absence of a heartbeat and respirations are acceptable criteria for a declaration of death. However, advances in life-support technology enable health care professionals to maintain respiration and circulation in individuals whose brain function is minimal or absent and have created uncertainty about what constitutes death.

Although the 1981 Uniform Definition of Death Act includes the cessation of all functions of the brain as a criterion for death, many health care professionals feel uncertainty over implementing this criterion.[9] People are strongly conditioned to view a breathing body with a beating heart as alive, even when those functions result only from life-support systems.

Organ Sources

Because of the disparity between the supply and demand for organs, there is ongoing interest in increasing the potential organ donor pool with the use of living donors, non–heart-beating donors (NHBDs), marginal donors, and animals.

Living Donors. Living donors have been used in kidney transplantation since 1954. In the past, donors were restricted to blood relatives (i.e., parents, children, siblings). More recently, unrelated donors have been added to the donor pool. These donors are not blood relatives, but have an emotional relationship with the potential recipient (e.g., spouse, stepparent, stepchild, friend). The advantages of a live donor include (1) improved patient and graft survival rates, (2) immediate availability of an organ, (3) the ability to schedule the surgery when the recipient is in the best possible medical condition, and (4) immediate functioning of the organ because there is minimal preservation time. In 2001, 5227 live donor kidney transplants were performed in the United States, accounting for 39% of the total.[26]

Living donors are becoming sources for livers, pancreases, lungs, and hearts. The concept of living donor liver transplantation grew out of the need for appropriately sized livers for patients weighing less than 15 kg. The initial work with reduced-size and split-liver transplants established the feasibility of using a portion of an adult liver in a child. Live donors are also being used for pancreas transplantation. The donor gives up a part of the tail of the pancreas but is left with enough islet cells to produce adequate amounts of insulin to prevent diabetes.[5] Living donor lung transplantation was first performed in 1990 when a child received a right upper lobe from the mother.[13]

There are ethical concerns that arise when people donate organs or portions of organs. These relate to the risk of surgical complications for the healthy donor, loss of income if the donor is a primary wage earner, uncertain outcomes for the recipient, and guilt experienced by the donor if the recipient dies. The concerns of the donor must be weighed against the recipient's risk of dying while awaiting a cadaver donor of the right match. Respect for autonomy supports the right of the donor to assume these risks if the donor's decision is informed, free from coercion, and truly autonomous (see Evidence-Based Practice box).

Patients who have been declared dead by traditional cardiopulmonary criteria rather than brain death criteria are another source of transplantable organs. These are NHBDs because organ procurement takes place after the heart has stopped beating. Before the institution of brain death criteria, these donors were the major source of transplantable kidneys, but problems with extended ischemia and resultant cellular and tissue damage limited their usefulness. Now, organs are procured from NHBDs by in situ organ preservation immediately after cardiopulmonary arrest, and from patients who die after choosing to forego life-sustaining treatment.[2]

In situ organ preservation involves the infusion of cooled preservation solution through a catheter inserted into the abdominal aorta immediately after death has been declared. This process must be instituted immediately after asystole. Unfortunately, obtaining family consent for the procedure is difficult, because the family does not have time to adjust to the news of their loved one's death before having to make a decision about organ donation.

The alternative method, allowing patients and families the option of donating organs after they have decided to forego life-sustaining treatment, has two advantages. First, the decision to donate is made by the patient and family before death; therefore there is time for them to discuss, reflect, and give informed consent before the initiation of any invasive procedure. Second, the time and place of death are controlled to minimize warm ischemia time. The patient is taken to the operating room, where a surgical team begins organ removal and preservation within minutes of the declaration of death. It is estimated that use of NHBDs could increase the potential donor pool by 20% to 25%; however, less than 3% of organ donors in the United States are currently NHBDs.[7]

Cadaver Donors. The criteria for cadaver donors have been liberalized to include increasing age (up to 72 years), diabetes, hypertension, some infections, high-risk social history but negative human immunodeficiency virus (HIV) test, some hemodynamic instability, some chemical imbalances, and increased organ preservation time. These expanded criteria could add 25% to 39% to the cadaver donor supply.[25] A careful evaluation, including histologic assessment of the recovered organs, is made before transplantation; and careful, long-term follow-up is provided to ensure that patient and graft survival rates are comparable to those obtained with traditional cadaver donors. The decision to transplant a marginal donor organ requires not only a thorough anatomic and physiologic evaluation of the organ but also a similar evaluation of the recipient, including age, comorbid conditions, and immunologic compatibility.[2]

Xenografts. Xenografting is the transplantation of animal organs into humans. The major obstacle to success is hyperacute rejection, which occurs when the human recipient pro-

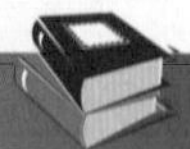

Evidence-Based Practice

Reference: Corley MC et al: Attitude, self-image, and quality of life of living kidney donors, *Nephrol Nur J* 27(1):43, 2000.

The purpose of the study was to assess the attitude, self-image, and quality of life of living kidney donors. Several instruments, including social desirability, quality of life, donor attitudes, and self-image, were used to assess 55 living donors. The study concluded that men were more ambivalent about donating organs than women; African-Americans, donors with higher levels of education, and those who donated organs recently had higher predicted levels of self-esteem and independence; and that quality of life of donors is high and similar to other healthy persons.

duces xenoreactive antibodies that destroy the organ. The transmission of viral diseases from animal to human is another concern. Potential advantages of xenografting include a readily available organ supply, fewer patient deaths on the waiting list, lower organ procurement costs, a more elective surgical procedure, and size matching for donor and recipient. Research in this area is continuing, although substantial resistance is occurring from various organizations such as the Campaign for Responsible Transplantation.[3]

NURSING ROLE IN THE DONATION PROCESS

Nurses are commonly the first health care professionals to identify a potential organ donor and make the appropriate referral to the local organ procurement organization (OPO). Nurses are in the best position to provide compassionate support to families and are well prepared both educationally and through experience to help the family through this crisis. Studies indicate that 87% of the general public is knowledgeable about transplantation and willing to donate organs at the time of death.[4] In an emergency situation, however, the family cannot be expected to initiate the idea of donation. The nurse provides both sufficient factual information and the emotional support needed for the next of kin to arrive at a decision about organ/tissue donation.

A common concern that arises in the minds of caregivers relates to whether organ donation and transplantation are supported by their religious group. Although the specific standards and positions about transplantation vary both within and among various faiths and denominations, the major religious groups in the United States all support donation and transplantation. Many groups (e.g., Roman Catholics, Amish, Moslems, and Jews) view donation as an act of charity, fraternal love, and self-sacrifice. Hindus, Jehovah's Witnesses, and various Protestant groups express the belief that donation is a matter of individual conscience.

Requests for organ/tissue donation must be carefully timed and sensitive to the needs of the family. The donation process is initiated only after the physician has communicated to the family the hopelessness of the clinical situation and the family has had time to assimilate this information. Once the next of kin have been informed of their family member's death, the physician, nurse, procurement coordinator, or hospital designee can offer the family the opportunity to donate organs/tissues. The discussion takes place in a comfortable, private area, conducive to the family's expression of grief. The success of the request usually reflects the attitude exhibited by the caregivers during this sensitive period. The request for donation is handled as part of the natural support provided to a family at the time of a loved one's death. It is the death that is the most important event, not the donation. The family is approached, not to acquire organs, but to show compassion and offer assistance and support during their bereavement (see Guidelines for Safe Practice box). The discussion begins with an expression of sympathy and allows the family time to express their feelings. It is important that the caregivers verify the family's understanding of the loved one's condition, and reexplain, if necessary, why the patient is considered to be dead.

Initiating a request for organ/tissue donation before the family has had time to assimilate the news of their loved one's death results in a high rate of denied consent. Separating the explanation of the certainty of death of a loved one and the request for donation allows for a period of acceptance and results in greater likelihood of consent.

The organ procurement team responds to commonly expressed family concerns such as pain experienced by the donor, payment, disfigurement of the body, funeral delays, and confidentiality. A brief reexplanation of brain death can allay fears related to pain during the organ/tissue procurement surgery. The team informs the family that the procurement agency pays all costs associated with the procurement of the organ/tissue and care of the donor, including laboratory tests, operating room costs, surgeon fees, and intravenous (IV) fluids and medications. The family remains financially responsible for all health care costs incurred up to the pronouncement of death. Families are often concerned about whether donation interferes with an open-casket funeral. Assurance can be given that the donor will appear normal, and donation does not preclude use of an open casket. Funeral

Guidelines for Safe Practice

Talking With Families About Organ and Tissue Donation

1. Potential donor identified by nurse/physician/health care team.
2. Death declared and discussed with family. Make certain the family understands that brain death is irreversible.
3. Allow time for family to assimilate information.
4. Notify local organ procurement organization to determine suitability for organ/tissue donation.
5. Attempt to determine the beliefs of the potential donor (donor card or driver's license signed).
6. Identify legal next of kin and other family members who need to be included in the discussion.
7. Provide a comfortable, private place for discussions between health care providers, procurement coordinator, and family.
8. Respect cultural beliefs and differences.
9. Acknowledge the family's pain; speak slowly and with compassion.
10. Provide adequate, accurate information on the options available for discontinuing life support.
11. Provide adequate, accurate information about organ/tissue donation, including informed consent and required evaluations.
12. Ensure that the family understands that there is no cost to the donor family, and that donation will not interfere with the timing of the funeral service or open casket service.
13. Provide time for the family to discuss the request and make their decision.
14. Request written consent only after the family has had time to make their decision and have given an affirmative response.
15. Respect the family's decision. Avoid being judgmental or condescending if the family chooses not to donate.

delays usually are not necessary unless procurement teams are coming from various parts of the country. After procurement, the body is released to the funeral home. Gifts of organs or tissues are confidential. No one who receives a transplant is told the identity of the donor, and donor families are told only the age and sex of the various recipients and how they are doing after transplantation.[27]

Health care professionals often fear that asking grieving families for organ/tissue donation adds to the family's grief. Studies have consistently shown, however, that the strongest advocates of donation are donor families, who view donation as the highest form of charity, giving the ultimate gift, life, to another person.

ORGAN DONATION AND ALLOCATION

Organ procurement organizations are responsible for organ recovery in the United States. These organizations have offices in major cities and provide services on a local, state, and regional basis. Organ procurement organizations provide 24-hour assistance to evaluate potential donors, discuss donation with the next of kin, and assist with physical assessment and hemodynamic monitoring to maintain organ function until surgical removal. They also implement organ recovery and placement through the UNOS allocation policies. Additionally, they provide follow-up bereavement support for donor families, relay information regarding the outcome of the donation, and provide feedback to the donor hospital regarding transplant outcomes.

UNOS is a nonprofit corporation whose members include all U.S. transplant centers, OPOs, histocompatability laboratories, voluntary health organizations that promote organ donation, professional scientific organizations with an interest in transplantation, and members of the general public. UNOS, operating under the auspices of the U.S. Department of Health and Human Services, maintains the national waiting list of persons needing transplants, matches potential recipients with donor organs, and allocates each type of organ. Because of the size of the country and the need to avoid prolonged organ ischemia, organs are offered locally first, then regionally, and finally nationally. If the organ is a kidney, pancreas, liver, or intestine and cannot be used locally, it is allocated within the UNOS region from which it was procured. Thoracic organs that cannot be placed locally are allocated within successive concentric 500-mile radius circles from the OPO to avoid unacceptable ischemia.[15]

Because a major obstacle to organ/tissue donation is failure to identify potential donors early in the process, it is essential that nurses become knowledgeable about donor eligibility criteria and understand how to activate the organ procurement process. Organ donors are previously healthy individuals who have suffered an irreversible brain injury. The most common causes of injury are cerebral trauma from motor vehicle accidents or gunshot wounds, intracerebral or subarachnoid hemorrhage, and anoxic brain damage resulting from a drug overdose or cardiac arrest. The brain-dead donor must have effective cardiovascular function and receive ventilator support to preserve organ function. The age range for most suitable donors is newborn to 70 years. The age of the donor is generally less important than the quality of organ function. The donor must be free of malignancy, sepsis, and communicable diseases, including HIV, hepatitis B and C, syphilis, and tuberculosis, and have no history of IV drug abuse. Unlike organ donors, tissue donors (e.g., donors of eyes, bone, skin, heart valves) do not need to have a beating heart. Death is pronounced, and tissue may be recovered hours after the heart has stopped beating.

Recipient Selection

Appropriate recipient selection is important for both a successful outcome and the best use of this scarce resource. Candidacy is determined by a wide variety of medical and psychosocial factors that vary among transplant centers. These factors include disease status, therapeutic benefits of transplantation, age, functional ability, and presence of family support. A careful evaluation is completed before transplantation to attempt to identify and minimize potential complications after transplantation. Contraindications for transplantation include disseminated malignancies, chronic infections (except hepatitis B and C), and ongoing psychosocial problems such as noncompliance with medical regimens and chemical dependency.

Payment for Transplantation

Reimbursement for transplantation occurs through private insurance, self-payment, Medicare, and Medicaid. Private insurance and managed care companies currently reimburse at a fixed rate, and reimbursement may not equal the actual charges. The recipient may be responsible for the difference.

Medicare is the primary payer for kidney transplants and certain heart, liver, and bone marrow transplants, but restrictions for coverage include the length and extent of the patient's disability, age of the recipient, underlying disease requiring transplantation, and the transplant center that will perform the procedure. Medicare not only covers the transplantation procedure and hospitalization, but 80% of the cost of immunosuppressive medications for 36 months from the day of hospital discharge. After 3 years, the recipient either pays out of pocket or purchases a supplemental insurance policy that covers the medications.[10]

Immunology and Transplantation

Successful transplantation of allografts requires manipulation of the recipient's immune response. All cells and tissues in the body have markers or antigens on the cell membrane surface. These antigens allow cells to be recognized by other cells as either *self* or *nonself* (see Chapter 48). The antigens distributed on the surface of the cells of any one person are unique for that person, except for identical twins, and are controlled by genes. These cell markers are important in protecting the body from invasion by foreign substances. Because transplanted tissues and organs have markers different from the host, they are recognized as nonself by the immune system. Once recognition takes place, B and T lymphocytes are activated, differentiate, proliferate, and attack and destroy the transplanted organ or tissue.

The ability of immune cells to recognize foreign substances is the result of genetic factors on chromosome 6. This region of the chromosome is called the major histocompatibility complex. It codes for human leukocyte antigens (HLA), which initiate the process of rejection and serve as the targets for immunologic attack against the transplanted organ. The entire HLA genetic complex encodes cell membrane markers or antigens on almost every cell in the body. It contains two groups. Class I HLAs (A, B, C) are expressed by almost all cells, including leukocytes, platelets, and solid organ cells. Class II HLAs (D) are expressed on many of the immune system cells including B and some T lymphocytes, macrophages, monocytes, and vascular endothelium.

In all, 100 antigens have been identified in the HLA system. Because of the millions of possible combinations of antigens, the chance of two unrelated persons having an identical combination of histocompatibility genes is less than 1 in 20 million. Any cell surface protein configuration that is different from a person's own is an antigen capable of provoking the immunologic defense response.[21]

The other antigen system important to the acceptance of transplant tissue is the ABO blood typing system. ABO antigens are on red blood cells (RBCs) and other tissues. Some minor RBC antigens, particularly the Lewis system, are important to transplantation rejection or acceptance and are assessed in recipients and donors. The RHO antigen system is not thought to have a role in the survival or rejection of transplanted tissue or organs.

Tissue Typing and Matching Procedures

In preparation for transplantation, some tissue typing and leukocyte cross-matching may be performed. See Box 51-1 for a description of the major tests that may be used to establish compatibility between the donor and recipient. The number and types of tests vary depending on the organ being transplanted. Several reasons exist for this variability. All antigens play some role in allowing self-cells to be differentiated from non-self cells; however, the individual locations of the HLA and RBC antigens are not equally important in transplant graft rejection. Matching at the HLA-D locus seems to be the most critical for graft acceptance. The immunogenicity of transplanted organs also varies from most allogeneic to least allogeneic as follows: bone marrow, skin, islets of Langerhans, heart, kidney, and liver. Additionally, the preservation time of many organs is too short to allow all these various tests to be completed before transplantation.

Histocompatibility Testing for Different Types of Transplants

Transplantation of organs from live donors is associated with maximal histocompatibility testing, the purpose of which is to enhance the probability of graft acceptance. Transplantation of a kidney from a live donor, for example, requires the establishment of ABO compatibility, HLA matching by means of microlymphocytotoxicity testing, and mixed leukocyte (or lymphocyte) culture. White blood cell (WBC) cross-match and mixed lymphocyte cross-match are also conducted.[10,21]

BOX 51-1 Tests Used for Tissue Typing and Matching

ABO Compatibility

Tests surface antigens on red blood cells (RBCs) and other tissues; compatibility is same as for blood transfusions; recipient would have antibodies to any ABO antigens present on donor cells and not on recipient cells.

Minor RBC Antigen Testing

Tests surface antigens on RBCs; transplant recipients who have had multiple transfusions may have antibodies to known minor RBC antigens.

Microlymphocytotoxicity Testing

Detects class I HLA antigens (A, B, C) and matches these antigens between recipient and donor.

Mixed Leukocyte Culture or Mixed Lymphocyte Culture

Lymphocytes of the potential donor are treated to prevent them from responding. In this way an estimate of the response of a potential recipient (living cells) to a potential donor (treated cells) can be made. The mixed lymphocyte culture is primarily the result of HLA-D differences between donor and recipient. A low response of the recipient's cells to the donor's cells is predictive of a successful transplant. This test is helpful in live donor transplants. Because the test takes approximately 7 days to complete, it cannot be used for cadaver transplants.

T Cell Crossmatch

A positive crossmatch occurs when the recipient has demonstrable circulating antibodies against the donor's T cell antigens. These circulating cytotoxic antibodies are detected by incubating donor lymphoid cells in recipient serum in the presence of complement. After a period of incubation, a marker of cell death is added to the suspension, and the proportion of dead cells is counted. The presence of significant numbers of dead cells indicates a positive crossmatch and predicts a poor outcome after transplantation (i.e., hyperacute rejection).

Panel Reactive Antibody

A blood test using lymphocytotoxic antibodies to determine the presence of preformed antibodies to HLA antigens. The results range from 0% to 100% and reflect the percentage of antigens on the test panel against which the potential recipient has preformed antibodies. If a potential recipient is found to have antibodies against specific HLA antigens, an organ donor carrying those antigens would not be suitable for that recipient because of the increased risk of rejection. A high panel reactive antibody means that a potential transplant recipient has antibodies against many HLA antigens, and finding a suitable donor will be more difficult.

Because of the short preservation times of the heart, liver, lung, and pancreas, only minimal histocompatibility testing is possible. With a heart transplant, ABO compatibility is established and a mixed lymphocyte cross-match is carried out. In liver transplants, the ideal transplant comes from an identical ABO donor. However, incompatible matches are acceptable in emergency situations.[2] HLA typing and matching and mixed leukocyte culture (MLC) testing are not thought to be as clinically important in liver transplantation as in other types of transplants.

Successful allograft bone marrow transplantation requires maximal compatibility between donor and recipient. This compatibility is identified by microlymphocytotoxicity testing for class I HLAs and by MLC testing for class II HLAs. However, ABO and Rh compatibility is not necessary. If a transplant with ABO-incompatible bone marrow is planned, the recipient must undergo plasma exchange to eliminate antibodies against the ABO group of the donor.[6,10]

Research is ongoing to improve histocompatibility testing and identify the most important antigens for matching to prevent rejection of transplants. As new information and technology accumulate, tissue-matching procedures for transplants may change to decrease the incidence of rejection.

COMPLICATIONS OF TRANSPLANTATION

Rejection

The major reason for transplant failure is rejection. There are three types of rejection: hyperacute, acute, and chronic. A special type of rejection that occurs in recipients of allogeneic bone marrow transplants is graft-versus-host disease (GVHD)[23] (see Future Watch box).

Hyperacute Rejection

Hyperacute rejection occurs at the time of transplantation or within 48 hours after transplantation. It is mediated by the humoral immune system. Preformed circulating cytotoxic antibodies to incompatible ABO blood group antigens, antigens on the vascular endothelium, or histocompatability antigens are responsible for the hyperacute rejection. The combination of the preformed antibody with the antigen causes activation of complement, entrapment of formed blood elements and clotting factors, massive intravascular coagulation, and necrosis of the graft from decreased perfusion. The degranulation of phagocytic cells causes the release of hydrolytic enzymes that also cause tissue destruction.[11]

Hyperacute rejections are rare as a result of careful cross-matching and tend to be isolated to kidney transplants.

A special type of hyperacute rejection is accelerated rejection. This type of rejection occurs over 3 to 5 days and may be reversed if detected early.

Acute Rejection

Acute rejection usually occurs from 1 week to 3 months after the transplantation and recurs at any time after the first incident. Acute rejection is mediated by both humoral and cellular immunity. In acute rejection, transplanted antigens are trapped by macrophages. This macrophage-antigen interaction stimulates differentiation and maturation of various B-cell and T-cell subsets, which cause destruction of the transplanted tissue directly or indirectly through activation of other immune cells. Acute rejection is treated by pharmacologic interventions consisting of increased doses of steroids, the use of monoclonal antibodies (e.g., OKT3), or polyclonal antibodies such as ATG or ALG.

> ***Future Watch***
>
> **Leukemia Drug Effective Treatment for Graft-versus-Host Disease?**
>
> Nipent, a drug that is currently approved by the U.S. Food Drug Administration for the treatment of hairy cell leukemia, is undergoing investigation into its effectiveness as a treatment for graft-versus-host-disease (GVHD). The drug was administered to 12 steroid-refractory GVHD patients as "salvage thearapy" because each had failed all other treatments. Nipent was well tolerated by all. A 75% success rate was achieved, with five patients undergoing a complete response and four others undergoing a partial response. No significant drug toxicity was reported. The drug's manufacturer SuperGen is conducting further studies to determine Nipent's effectiveness as a GVHD drug choice.
>
> Reference: Presentation to the December 2000 42nd Annual Meeting of the American Society of Hematology. CenterWatch Database of Study Results, website: http://www.centerwatch.com/patient/results/details.asp?I=3457.

Chronic Rejection

Chronic rejection occurs 3 months or longer after transplantation. It is mediated by both the cellular and humoral immunity and results in slow, progressive loss of graft function. Chronic rejection remains the major unresolved problem in transplantation, because it is less responsive to immunosuppressive therapies.[6]

Hypertension

Hypertension occurs in approximately 70% of kidney transplant recipients and up to 90% of recipients of other solid organs such as heart, liver, lung, and pancreas. Hypertension has been associated with several antirejection drugs such as prednisone, cyclosporine, and tacrolimus.[16]

Infection

Infection remains a major cause of morbidity and mortality after transplantation. The transplant recipient is at risk for infection resulting from alteration of the body's normal defense mechanisms by surgery, immunosuppressive medications, and the effects of end-stage organ disease. Advancing age plus the presence of other illnesses such as diabetes mellitus, lupus erythematosus, and malnutrition further impair the immune response. Signs and symptoms of infection can be subtle, and prompt diagnosis and treatment are important.

The most common infections observed in the first month after transplantation are similar to those acquired by any postoperative patient, including wound and IV line infections, pneumonia, and urinary tract infections.[12] Viral infections, especially cytomegalovirus (CMV), Epstein-Barr virus, herpes simplex virus, and varicella-zoster virus, may occur as primary or reactivated infections. Reactivation of dormant viruses can

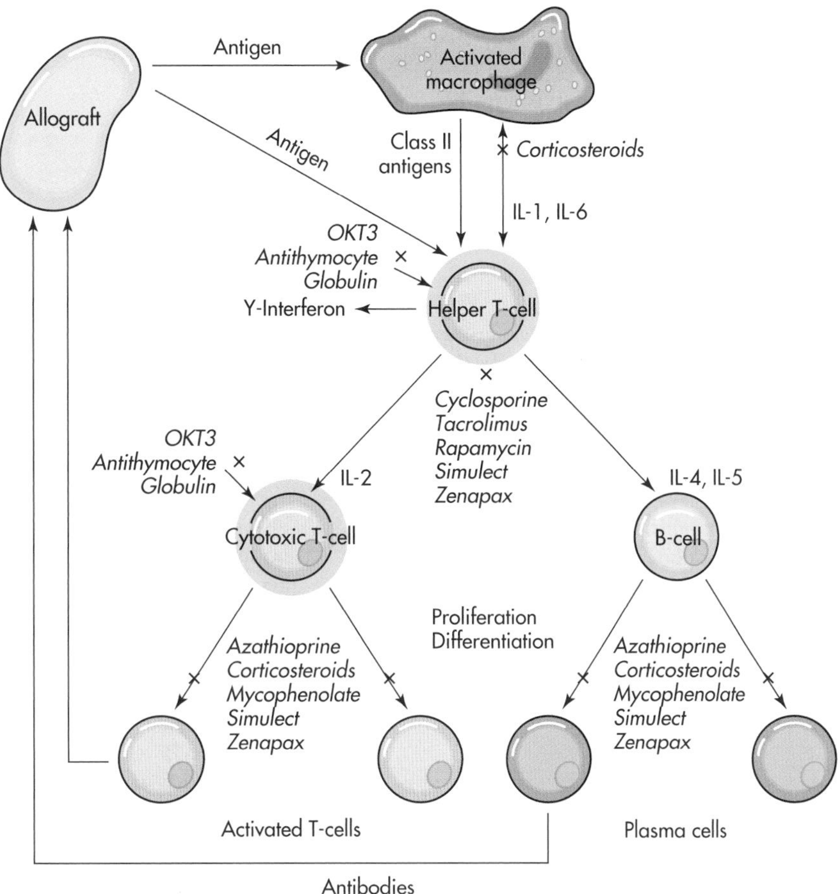

Figure 51-1 Sites of action for immunosuppressive agents.

BOX 51-2 Organisms Responsible for Infections in Transplant Recipients

Bacterial Infections

Gram-negative organisms, including *Pseudomonas aeruginosa, Serratia marcescens, Proteus rettgeri, Enterobacter cloacae, Legionella pneumophila,* and various *Nocardia* species

Viral Infections

Herpesviruses, including herpes simplex viruses 1 and 2, varicella-zoster virus, cytomegalovirus, and Epstein-Barr virus

Fungal Infections

Candidal species (most often *C. albicans*) and other fungi, including *Aspergillus fumigatus, Cryptococcus neoformans, Coccidioides immitis,* and *Histoplasma capsulatum*

Parasitic Infections

Include *Pneumocystis carinii* and *Toxoplasma gondii*

occur from pharmacologic immunosuppression. Primary infections that occur after transplantation can often be traced to an exogenous source such as the donated organ or blood transfusion. Matching the CMV status of the donor and recipient is not considered to be practical because of the shortage of donor organs and the high incidence (70%) of previous exposure to CMV in the normal population. The risk of acquiring CMV disease from the donor has been significantly reduced by the use of prophylaxis with anti-CMV hyperimmune globulin in high-risk patients. Common organisms responsible for infection in transplant recipients are presented in Box 51-2.

Malignancies

The incidence of malignancies is approximately 5% in transplant recipients, a rate 100 times greater than that in the general population. The increased incidence is related to an altered immune system caused by chronic immunosuppressive therapy. Common malignancies include cancer of the skin, lips, cervix, as well as lymphomas.

DRUG THERAPY TO PREVENT REJECTION

In the absence of immunosuppression, transplanted organs are rejected within about 2 weeks.[17] Thus, the goal of immunosuppressive drug therapy is to adequately suppress the immune response to prevent rejection of the transplanted organ while maintaining sufficient immunity to prevent overwhelming infection. By using a combination of medications that work during different phases of the immune response, effective immunosuppression can be achieved with lower doses of each drug, thereby minimizing side effects (Figure 51-1). Immunosuppressive protocols used at different transplant centers vary significantly in the different combinations of medications used. Table 51-4 provides an overview of the major agents used for transplantation immune suppression.

TABLE 51-4 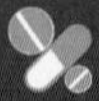 **Common Medications for Prevention of Rejection After Organ Transplantation**

Nursing Interventions for all Immunosuppressive Agents

Institute infection control measures
Assess for signs/symptoms of infection
Inspect oral mucous membranes
Maintain good oral hygiene including flossing
Monitor for drug side effects

Calcineurin Inhibitors	Action	Intervention/Implication
Cyclosporine (Sandimmune, Neoral)	Inhibits T-cell interleukin-2 production Inhibits maturation of T-cytotoxic lymphocyte precursors	Monitor for drug side effects: acute and chronic nephrotoxicity, hypertension, dyslipidemia Monitor trough concentrations, serum creatinine, blood urea nitrogen, potassium, liver enzymes, and coagulation factors
Tacrolimus (Prograf)	Prevents production and release of interleukin-2 Inhibits maturation of T-cytotoxic lymphocyte precursors cyclosporine	Monitor for edema, hypertension, jaundice, and neurologic status (tremors, paresthesias, headache, confusion, seizures) Tacrolimus: Monitor GI status (anorexia, nausea, vomiting, diarrhea, weight loss)
Sirolimus (rapamycin, Rapamune)	Suppresses lymphocyte proliferation Inhibits B cells from synthesizing antibody	Monitor daily weight, intake and output, blood glucose Teach patient regarding: Drug side effects being dose related Use of a depilatory if hirsutism develops Need for dental cleaning every 6 months if gingival hyperplasia develops Decrease dose as prescribed Administer diuretics and hypertensive agents as prescribed Tacrolimus: Monitor blood glucose levels and administer prescribed insulin or oral hypoglycemic agent Sirolimus: Administer via central line over 4-6 hours
Antiproliferative Agents		
Azathioprine (Imuran)	Suppresses proliferation of rapidly dividing cells, including sensitized B and T cells Alkylating agent that interferes with DNA, RNA, and protein synthesis	Monitor hematocrit, white blood cell count, platelet count, liver enzymes, coagulation factors Monitor for infection, bleeding, jaundice, nausea, vomiting, abdominal pain, hematuria, and hair loss Administer prescribed oral antifungal agent
Cyclophosphamide (Cytoxin)		Reduce dose as prescribed Encourage increased fluid intake, especially water
Corticosteroids Prednisone	Suppresses inflammatory response, prevents proliferation of T-cytotoxic lymphocytes	Monitor daily weight, blood glucose, wound healing Monitor for blood in stool or emesis, complaints of acid indigestion, esophageal or gastric burning, changes in muscle strength Encourage low sodium intake, low-fat, low-cholesterol diet (especially in presence of high serum cholesterol levels) Administer antacids, H_2 receptor blockers as prescribed Administer with food to decrease gastric irritation Administer oral antifungal agent if prescribed Teach patient regarding: Need for controlling intake to maintain ideal weight Need for consistent exercise to counteract muscle weakness Hyperglycemic effect of corticosteroids Avoid skin trauma and use of adhesive tape
Monoclonal Antibodies	Monoclonal antibody that removes circulating T lymphocytes	Administer prescribed acetaminophen, diphenhydramine, and hydrocortisone at time of IV infusion
Muromonab-CD3 (Orthoclone OKT3)	Monoclonal antibody against IL-2 receptor Blocks T-cell activation and proliferation	Monitor daily weight, lung sounds, GI status (nausea, vomiting, diarrhea), intake and output, temperature

TABLE 51-4 Common Medications for Prevention of Rejection After Organ Transplantation—cont'd

Monoclonal Antibodies–cont'd		
Chimeric anti-IL-2 Receptor Antibody (Simulect)		Monitor for peripheral edema, complaints of headache, photophobia
Dacliximab (Humanized anti-TAC, Zenapax)	Polyclonal antibody directed against lymphocytes	Monitor platelet count and report if below <100,000
		Administer prescribed diuretics
Antilymphocyte globulin (ALG)	Reduces circulating lymphocytes	Arrange for outpatient infusion to complete course of therapy after discharge
Antithymocyte globulin (ATG)	Decreases lymphocyte proliferation	
Purine Synthesis Inhibitor	Inhibits purine synthesis	Monitor daily weight, GI status (nausea, vomiting, diarrhea, abdominal cramping, dyspepsia), intake and output, white blood cell count
Mycophenolate mofetil (CellCept)	Suppresses T-cytotoxic lymphocyte proliferation	Administer antiemetics and antidiarrheals as ordered

TABLE 51-5 Transplant Recipient and Graft Survival Rates

Organ	Transplants	1 Year Graft Survival	1 Year Patient Survival	3-Year Graft Survival	3-Year Patient Survival
Kidney	22,423	22,423	22,341	20,791	20,680
Kidney/Pancreas	1806	1806	1806	1754	1754
Pancreas	415	415	410	258	253
Heart	4012	4012	4000	4117	4100
Lung	1646	1646	1637	1535	1525
Heart/Lung	94	94	93	85	85
Liver	7161	7161	6755	6724	6283

Source: *Transplant Patient DataSource.* (2000, February 16). Richmond, Va: United Network for Organ Sharing. Retrieved [date of retrieval, e.g., February 16, 2000], website: http://207.239.150.13/tpd/.

Allergic reactions to foreign proteins contained in immunosuppressive agents are common but usually are not severe enough to preclude use. Fever, arthralgias, and tachycardia commonly occur. These reactions can be attenuated by administering the preparation slowly, over 4 to 6 hours, and premedicating patients with acetaminophen (Tylenol) and diphenhydramine hydrochloride (Benadryl). Patients may develop antibodies against antisera type drugs. This problem limits the drugs' effectiveness during subsequent courses of treatment. The main toxicities of antisera are lymphopenia and thrombocytopenia caused by antibody contaminants that are not completely removed during preparation of antisera.

Monoclonal antibodies are usually used for treating acute rejection episodes, but they can be used for induction to prevent acute rejection after transplantation. OKT3 was the first of these monoclonal antibodies to be used. OKT3 is a mouse monoclonal antibody that reacts with the T3 antigen found on the surface of human thymocytes and mature T cells. Thus OKT3 is an antiantigen receptor antibody that interferes with the function of the T lymphocyte, the pivotal cell in the response to graft rejection. This agent reverses 95% of acute rejection episodes.[11,14]

Vasoactive substances released from the T3 cells cause a flulike syndrome that lasts through the first few days of treatment. All patients receive Tylenol, Benadryl, and corticosteroids at the time of IV infusion to reduce the severity of the symptoms. Severe pulmonary reactions manifested by dyspnea, wheezing, or acute respiratory failure have occurred in some patients. The side effects associated with OKT3 virtually mandate hospital admission during treatment. However, all of the side effects tend to subside within 3 to 5 days, making a switch to outpatient administration feasible.

Overall survival rates for transplant recipients continue to improve as advancements are made in immunosuppressive therapies. The 1-year patient survival rates for kidney and pancreas transplant recipients lead the way at 94.3% and 91.1%, respectively. Three-year survival rates range from 90% for kidney, heart, pancreas, and liver; 81.2% for heart-lung; and 75.9% for lung transplant recipients. These patient survival rates indicate that patients who survive their first year after organ transplantation have excellent long-term prospects[31] (Table 51-5).

KIDNEY TRANSPLANTATION

Etiology

Kidney transplantation is used primarily to treat patients experiencing end-stage renal disease resulting from glomerular diseases, diabetes mellitus, polycystic kidney, and hypertension.[25] The advantages of kidney transplantation include the reversal of many of the pathophysiologic changes associated with renal failure as normal kidney function is restored. However, hypertension, which is a common complication of kidney failure, is rarely cured. Transplantation also eliminates the patient's dependence on dialysis and its accompanying dietary restrictions, provides the opportunity to return to normal life activities (including employment), and is less expensive than dialysis after the first year. Some patients who are approaching end-stage renal disease may be transplanted before they require dialysis if a kidney becomes available. This approach is most advantageous for children, whose physical and mental development is significantly impaired by renal failure, and for patients with diabetes, who have a much higher mortality rate on dialysis than nondiabetic patients.

Epidemiology

Kidney transplantation is the oldest and most common type of transplant procedure. The first kidney transplantation was performed in the early 1950s, and the procedure is now well established as a viable and desirable alternative to dialysis as a treatment for end-stage renal disease. Currently, more than 100,000 persons in the United States have received kidney transplants, and between 13,000 and 14,000 new transplants are performed each year. However, more than 160,000 people are being maintained on dialysis, and the lack of available organs is significant. Currently, about 49,000 people are on the transplant waiting list for kidneys.[26]

Collaborative Care Management

Diagnostic Tests. Kidney transplantations involve maximal histocompatibility testing, especially in situations involving a live donor. ABO compatibility, HLA matching, WBC cross-match, and mixed lymphocyte cross-match are all performed. Other routine laboratory tests include complete blood count, renal panel, liver panel, partial thomboplastin time, prothrombin time, viral titers, and creatinine clearance. Potential recipients are also screened for the presence of HIV, CMV, and Epstein-Barr virus, which are contraindications to renal transplantation[11] (see Evidence-Based Practice box).

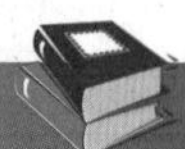

Evidence-Based Practice

Reference: Couchoud C: Cytomegalovirus prophylaxis and antiviral agents for solid organ transplantation, *The Cochrane Library,* Issue 1, 2001, website: www.update_software.com.

The objective of the study was to assess the efficacy of antiviral agents in the prevention of cytomeglovirus (CMV) infection and symptomatic CMV disease in adult and child recipients of solid organs (liver, heart, kidney, pancreas, lung). A second objective was to assess the efficacy of antiviral agents in decreasing the incidence of acute organ rejection, graft loss, and death. Study results demonstrated that prophylactic treatment with antiviral agents (acyclovir or ganciclovir) were associated with a significant decrease in CMV disease compared with placebo or no treatment. Prophylactic antiviral treatment was also associated with a significant decrease in graft loss, acute rejection, and death. The study supports the use of antiviral agents for preventing CMV infection and disease in patients who receive solid organ transplants.

Medications. Patients undergoing kidney transplantation will be started and maintained on a full regimen of immunosuppressive therapy. Immunosuppressive therapy is maintained for life to preserve the transplanted kidney.

Treatments. Patients awaiting kidney transplantation continue on their regular schedule of dialysis right up to the time of transplantation. Dialysis is conducted as close to the surgery as possible to ensure that the patient is in the best possible metabolic condition to withstand the rigors of surgery. Living donor kidneys usually begin to function immediately after surgery. Cadaver kidneys may experience a delay in functioning, and the patient might need to have dialysis resumed after surgery to maintain physiologic homeostasis.

Surgical Management. The donor kidney is carefully dissected free with its renal artery and vein intact. The ureter is also dissected with great care to preserve the periureteral vascular supply. The kidney is removed, flushed with a chilled, sterile electrolyte solution, and prepared for transplantation into the recipient. The procedure takes about 2 hours.

The transplanted kidney is placed extraperitoneally in the iliac fossa (Figure 51-2). Generally the peritoneal cavity is not entered. The patient's own kidneys are not removed unless they are infected or are causing significant hypertension in order to maintain erythropoietin production, blood pressure control, and prostaglandin synthesis and metabolism. Efficient revascularization is critical to prevent ischemic injury to the kidney.

The donor ureter is used to the extent possible. If long enough, the donor ureter is tunneled through the bladder submucosa and sutured in place. This allows the bladder to clamp down on the ureter as it contracts for micturition, thereby preventing reflux of urine up the ureter into the transplanted kidney. The entire transplantation procedure takes about 3 hours.

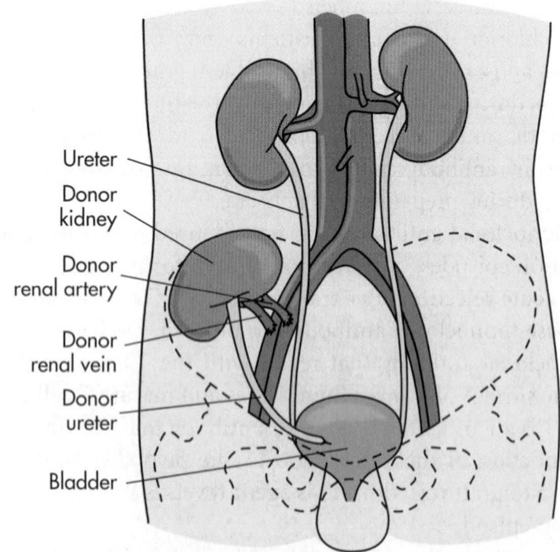

Figure 51-2 Location of a transplanted kidney showing the anastomosis of the renal artery, renal vein, and ureter.

Diet. Before surgery the patient with end-stage renal disease continues on the renal failure diet that has been prescribed. One of the major benefits of successful kidney transplantation is the ability to eat a more normal diet without the extensive restrictions of protein, fluid, sodium, and potassium that are characteristic of the management of end-stage renal disease. However, the patient will need to continue to control sodium and calorie content after transplant to manage the side effects of high-dose steroid administration that is required for immunosuppression.

Activity. Activity restrictions are not necessary after successful kidney transplantation. The patient typically experiences significant improvement in energy level and mood and is able to gradually resume a more active role in family and social activities. The ultimate goal is to support the patient's return to gainful employment.

Referrals. Various referrals may be needed for patients undergoing kidney transplantation. During the first year, transplant centers monitor patients regularly to detect early signs of rejection or adverse drug reactions.[14] The services of a dietitian may be helpful as the patient attempts to understand the differences in dietary restrictions that are in place after transplantation. The patient may need assistance understanding and managing the complex medication regimen and usually profits from involvement with a support group. The psychologic and emotional responses to transplantation are highly unpredictable, but can be profound, especially when a kidney has been donated by a family member.

A Clinical Pathway that outlines the care for a patient undergoing kidney transplantation is found on pp. 1698 to 1702.

NURSING MANAGEMENT

PREOPERATIVE CARE

Nursing care of the patient in the preoperative phase includes emotional and physical preparation for surgery. Because the patient and family may have been waiting 2 to 3 years for the transplant, a review of the operative procedure and what can be expected in the immediate postoperative recovery period is important. The nurse informs the patient that there is a 20% chance the kidney will not function immediately, and dialysis may be required for the first few weeks. In addition, the rationale for the immunosuppressive therapy and the importance of preventing infection after surgery are stressed.

To ensure that the patient is in optimal physical condition for surgery, an electrocardiogram, chest x-ray study, and laboratory studies are performed. Dialysis is often required to achieve optimal fluid, electrolyte, and acid-base balance, as well as to remove excess nitrogenous wastes. Because dialysis may be required after transplantation, the patency of the vascular access must be maintained. The extremity containing the vascular access is wrapped in Kerlix and labeled "dialysis access." This identification reminds all caregivers to avoid using the affected extremity for blood pressure measurement, phlebotomy, or IV infusions.

POSTOPERATIVE CARE

Care of the Donor

The postoperative care of a live donor is similar to that provided after a nephrectomy (see Chapter 39). The donor can easily become a forgotten person in the transplantation process because most of the attention is focused on the recipient. The pain of a nephrectomy is significant, and adequate analgesia is essential to ensure comfort, promote ambulation, and prevent atelectasis and possible pulmonary complications. Most donors are discharged within 3 to 5 days and can usually return to work in 1 month.

The majority of kidney donors feel good about the donation because of the improved health of their family member or significant other. Nurses caring for live donors need to acknowledge the precious gift they have given. Care of the cadaver donor is outlined in the Nursing Care Plan on p. 1703.

Care of the Recipient

Maintaining Fluid and Electrolyte Balance

The first priority of care for the recipient is maintenance of fluid and electrolyte balance. Kidney transplant recipients often spend the first 24 hours after surgery in the intensive care unit because of the close monitoring required. Rapid diuresis may take place soon after the blood supply to the kidney is reestablished, especially in live donor transplants. This diuresis is related to the kidney's ability to filter blood urea nitrogen (BUN), which acts as an osmotic diuretic; the abundance of fluids administered intravenously during the operation; and renal tubular dysfunction, which inhibits the kidney from concentrating urine normally. Urine output during this phase may be as high as 1 L/hr, but decreases when BUN and serum creatinine levels return toward normal. The patient's urine output is measured and replaced with IV fluids hourly for the first 12 to 24 hours. Central venous pressure readings are essential for monitoring the patient's postoperative fluid status. Dehydration is avoided to prevent renal hypoperfusion and further tubular damage. The patient's electrolyte levels are closely monitored to detect hypokalemia, which is often associated with rapid diuresis and/or the kidney tubules' inability to concentrate. Delayed graft function occurs in 20% of patients receiving cadaver kidneys that have been preserved for longer than 24 hours. The ischemic damage from prolonged preservation results in acute tubular necrosis (ATN), which can last anywhere from several days to weeks, followed by gradually improving kidney function. Dialysis may be necessary initially, but is discontinued when the patient's urine output increases and serum creatinine and BUN levels normalize. Some patients develop high-output ATN—that is, they are able to excrete fluid but unable to excrete metabolic wastes or regulate electrolytes. Other patients experience oliguric or anuric ATN. These patients are at risk for fluid overload in the immediate postoperative period.[14]

A sudden decrease in urine output in the early postoperative period may be caused by dehydration, rejection, a technical complication such as vascular thrombosis, or an obstruction that impedes urine flow. Any decrease in output is thoroughly

Text continued on p. 1706.

clinical pathway *Kidney Transplantation*

UNIVERSITY HOSPITALS
of Cleveland

CARE PATH NAME: KIDNEY TRANSPLANT
DRG: ELOS: 7 days
Expected Disposition: Home
Surgery Date: ___/___/___
Pre-op Dry Weight: ___ Kg

Collaborative Problem List
1. Impaired Home Maintenance Management
2. Potential for Infection
3. Knowledge Deficit
4. Fluid and Electrolyte Imbalance
5. Pain Management
6.
7.

FOCUS	PRE-OP DATE: ___/___/___	DAY OF SURGERY DATE: ___/___/___	POST-OP DAY 1 DATE: ___/___/___	POST-OP DAY 2 DATE: ___/___/___	POST-OP DAY 3 DATE: ___/___/___	POST-OP DAY 4 DATE: ___/___/___
Laboratory/ Tests/ Procedures	• Chem 23 • CBC + Diff • PT/PTT • Urine C&S • T&C 2 U PRBC • Check CMV status • Chemstick if diabetic • CMV IgG quantitative	• Immediately Post-op: Chem 7, CBC • 8 hours post-op: Chem 7, CBC • CXR on arrival to PACU	• CBC + Diff • Chem 23 • CD3 level if on OKT3 • CXR • Ultrasound as indicated per protocol	• Chem 7 → • Urine for bacteria/ fungus • CBC (Diff if on OKT3) → • CD3 level if on OKT3 → • CYA level starting day 2 of therapy →	→	• Chem 23
Consults/ Referrals			• Consider PT Consult • Dietary screen and evaluation			
Physical Assessment	• VS q4h • Weight • Baseline skin assessment • Renal assessment regarding need for dialysis	• BP, AP, Rq 1/2 h until stable then q2h-q4h then q4h prn • Temp. immediately and q2h × 16 h then q4h • CVP q2-4 × 16 h then q 4 h • Pulse ox baseline and prn → • Urine output q1h × 24 h then q4h × 24 then qs	• VS q4h with CVP • Urine output q4h weight • Bowel sounds	• VS q4h • I&O q shift → • Weight → • Pulse ox × 2	• VS q shift →	→
Activity	• Up ad lib	• Bed rest	• Out of bed → chair			
Treatments	• Fleet enemas × 2 • Hibiclens shower • SCDs with patient to OR • Apply Teds pre-op	• O_2 per order, wean as tolerated • CVP dressing • JP dressing → • Incision dressing • Incentive spirometry q1h W/A → • Foley care → • Guaiac stools → • SCDs and Teds →	• D/C O_2 if RA pulse ox > 92% • Incision care	• Up with assistance • CVP dressing • D/C JP if output <30 cc → • Remove incision dressing	• Out of bed ad lib → • Incentive spirometry q2h W/A →	• CVP dressing • D/C Foley

Diet	• NPO	• NPO, ice chips • Advance as tolerated	• Diabetic/or any other diet restrictions as indicated →	→	→	→
Medications	• On call to OR: Antibiotic, Solumedrol 250 mg IV, Imuran 5 mg/kg IV maximum dose—500 mg • Induction Options: OKT3, ATG, Cyclosporine, MMF, Neoral	• Solumedrol 60 mg q6h IV → • Antibiotic • Fluid replacements	→ • Imuran or Mycophenolate • OKT3, ATG, Cyclosporine, Neoral • Gancyclovir 2.5 mg/kg qd if CMV (+) or CMV (−) receiving (+) organ • MSO4 prn	• Solumedrol 60 mg IV q8h • OKT3, ATG, Cyclosporine, Neoral → • Gancyclovir → • Bactrim ss or Trimethoprim qd → • Colace → • Clotrimazole → • Acyclovir → • Zantac →	• Solumedrol 60 mg IV q12h → • Tylenol #3 • Cytogam if donor CMV (+) and recipient (−)	→ • Prednisone 1 mg/kg/day • OKT3, CYA or ATG • Tylenol or Darvon
Patient/ Family Teaching	• View pre-op transplant video • Orient to Tower 9		• Give teaching materials to patient • Renal transplant booklet • Preprinted cards • I&O sheet • Outcome criteria form	• Review of meds and teaching material with patient/family →	→	• Continued review and if ready, take test
Discharge Planning		• Social Worker review notes from information appointments	• Review chart, interview RN and patient → • Collect psychosocial data (insurance, financial issues, discharge needs) →	→ • Psychosocial assessment, support and education/ information →	→ • Initial note in chart • Discuss prescription plan	• Arrange financial applications • Begin arranging prescription plans • Meet/talk with family prn • Consult/refer to other disciplines prn • For patients using mail order program, arrange forms with physicians

University Hospitals' carepaths have been developed to assist clinicians in patient management and clinical decision-making. The carepaths are intended to meet the needs of patients in most circumstances. They are not intended to replace a clinician's judgment or establish a protocol for all patients with this diagnosis.

SP-9601 (01/05/96)

SCDs, Sequential compression devices; *AP,* apical pulse; *JP,* Jackson-Pratt.

Continued

clinical pathway *Kidney Transplantation—cont'd*

FOCUS	PRE-OP DATE: ___/___/___	DAY OF SURGERY DATE: ___/___/___	POST-OP DAY 1 DATE: ___/___/___	POST-OP DAY 2 DATE: ___/___/___	POST-OP DAY 3 DATE: ___/___/___	POST-OP DAY 4 DATE: ___/___/___
Intermediate Outcomes	1. Viewed video 2. Negative cross-match	1. Hemodynamically stable 2. CVP 10-12 3. Euvolemic with fluid replacements 4. Vital signs returned to baseline 5. K + <6.0 6. Equal and clear breath sounds 7. Pain controlled	1. Hemodynamically stable 2. CVP 10-12 3. Euvolemic with or without fluid replacements 4. Vital signs at baseline 5. Decrease in BUN and Cr from pre-op 6. Equal and clear breath sounds 7. Pain controlled 8. Teaching material given to patient/ family 9. Immunosuppression dosages adjusted	1. Hemodynamically stable 2. Euvolemic without fluid replacements 3. Decrease in BUN and Cr 4. Electrolytes WNL 5. Equal and clear breath sounds 6. Pain controlled 7. Ambulating 8. Tolerating oral meds and diet 9. Teaching begun 10. JP removed if drainage is <30 cc for 24 h 11. Immunosuppression dosages adjusted 12. Wound dry and approximated	1. Hemodynamically stable 2. Euvolemic 3. Decrease in BUN and Cr 4. Electrolytes WNL 5. Equal and clear breath sounds 6. Pain controlled 7. Actively participates in ADLs 8. Ambulates at baseline 9. Has bowel movement 10. Initial Social Worker note in chart 11. Teaching continues 12. JP removed if drainage is <30 cc for 24 h 13. Immunosuppression dosages adjusted 14. Wound dry and approximated	1. Hemodynamically stable 2. Euvolemic 3. Decrease in BUN and Cr 4. Electrolytes WNL 5. Equal and clear breath sounds 6. Actively participates in ADL 7. Pain controlled 8. Ambulates at baseline 9. Has bowel movement 10. Teaching continues 11. Foley discontinued 12. JP removed if drainage is <30 cc for 24 h 13. Immunosuppression dosages adjusted 14. Wound dry and approximated 15. Financial and prescription arrangements made
Intermediate Outcomes RN Signature Days	☐ Met ☐ Not Met (see notes) #s not met ______ Signature ______	☐ Met ☐ Not Met (see notes) #s not met ______ Signature ______	☐ Met ☐ Not Met (see notes) #s not met ______ Signature ______	☐ Met ☐ Not Met (see notes) #s not met ______ Signature ______	☐ Met ☐ Not Met (see notes) #s not met ______ Signature ______	☐ Met ☐ Not Met (see notes) #s not met ______ Signature ______
Intermediate Outcomes RN Signature Evenings	☐ Met ☐ Not Met (see notes) #s not met ______ Signature ______	☐ Met ☐ Not Met (see notes) #s not met ______ Signature ______	☐ Met ☐ Not Met (see notes) #s not met ______ Signature ______	☐ Met ☐ Not Met (see notes) #s not met ______ Signature ______	☐ Met ☐ Not Met (see notes) #s not met ______ Signature ______	☐ Met ☐ Not Met (see notes) #s not met ______ Signature ______
Intermediate Outcomes RN Signature Nights	☐ Met ☐ Not Met (see notes) #s not met ______ Signature ______	☐ Met ☐ Not Met (see notes) #s not met ______ Signature ______	☐ Met ☐ Not Met (see notes) #s not met ______ Signature ______	☐ Met ☐ Not Met (see notes) #s not met ______ Signature ______	☐ Met ☐ Not Met (see notes) #s not met ______ Signature ______	☐ Met ☐ Not Met (see notes) #s not met ______ Signature ______

Laboratory/ Tests/ Procedures	• CBC (Diff if on OKT3) → • Chem 7 → • CD 3 level if on OKT3 → • CYA level →	→	→
Consults/ Referrals	• Consider Home Team referral		
Physical Assessment	• VS qs → • I&O qs → • Weight →	→	→
Activity	• OOB ad lib →	→	→
Treatments	• Guaiac stools → • Incentive spirometry q2h W/A	→ • CVP dressing	→ • D/C central line
Diet	• Diabetic or any other diet restriction as indicated →	→	→
Medications	• Prednisone—taper as indicated → • Imuran or Mycophenolate → • OKT3, ATG, Neoral or Cyclosporine → • Gancyclovir → • Bactrim → • Colace → • Clotrimazole → • Acyclovir → • T3 or Darvon → • Zantac →	→	• D/C Gancylovir • Acyclovir **SrCr** — **Dosage** <1.4 — 800 mg PO q6h 1.5-2.5 — 800 mg PO q8h 2.6-4.5 — 800 mg PO q12h >4.5 — 800 mg PO q24h HD — 800 mg PO q48h

Continued

clinical pathway *Kidney Transplantation—cont'd*

FOCUS	POST-OP DAY 5 DATE: __/__/__	POST-OP DAY 6 DATE: __/__/__	POST-OP DAY 7 DATE: __/__/__
Patient/ Family Teaching	• Take test • Diet teaching prn	• Review material as needed and retake test if needed	• Review homegoing med dosages, clinic and lab test follow-up appointments
Discharge Planning	• Arrange financial applications • Arrange prescription plans • Meet/talk with family prn • Other D/C plans • Psychosocial assessment, support, and education/information	• Transportation arrangements prn → • Other D/C plans carried out prn → • Final note in chart with D/C plan Psychosocial assessment, support, and education/information →	→
Homegoing Medications	• Mail order prescription forms completed and faxed by 2:00 PM. (If weekend/holiday D/C anticipated must do this by 2:00 PM, Friday).	• Delivery of medications prn →	→
Intermediate Outcomes	1. Hemodynamically stable → 2. Euvolemic → 3. Electrolytes WNL → 4. Independent in ADL and ambulation → 5. Has bowel movement → 6. Test taken and passed with 90% or continue med review 7. Scale and thermometer arranged for home 8. JP removed if drainage is <30 cc for 24 hr 9. Immunosuppression dosage assessed → 10. Financial and prescription plans arranged 11. Cyclosporine levels assessed and adjusted	→	1. D/C to home with written instructions 2. Medications available to take at home 3. Refer to discharge order form
Intermediate Outcomes RN Signature Days	☐ Met ☐ Not Met (see notes) #s not met ______ Signature ______	☐ Met ☐ Not Met (see notes) #s not met ______ Signature ______	☐ Met ☐ Not Met (see notes) #s not met ______ Signature ______
Intermediate Outcomes RN Signature Nights	☐ Met ☐ Not Met (see notes) #s not met ______ Signature ______	☐ Met ☐ Not Met (see notes) #s not met ______ Signature ______	☐ Met ☐ Not Met (see notes) #s not met ______ Signature ______

Nursing Care Plan — *Patient Who Is an Organ Donor*

DATA Mr. G., a 31-year-old married man and the father of three young children, was involved in a serious automobile accident in which he sustained multiple traumas, including a severe head injury. Despite aggressive initial management, Mr. G. did not respond to treatment and has since met the criteria for brain death.

His wife has been informed of his status and approached about organ donation. Despite Mrs. G.'s shock and grief, she believes that donation is something her husband would have wanted and has signed permission. The organ procurement process has been initiated.

Collaborative care interventions for Mr. G. include:

- Frequent monitoring of vital signs, intake and output, central venous pressure (CVP), pulmonary wedge pressure, and electrocardiogram
- Vasopressor administration to support blood pressure within established parameters
- Mechanical ventilation
- Use of heating/cooling blankets to maintain normothermia

NURSING DIAGNOSIS **Decreased cardiac output related to central nervous system dysfunction (loss of vasomotor control) and hypovolemia**

GOALS/OUTCOMES Cardiac output will remain within normal limits

NOC Suggested Outcomes

- Cardiac Pump Effectiveness (0400)
- Thermoregulation (0800)
- Tissue Perfusion: Abdominal Organs (0404)
- Tissue Perfusion: Cardiac (0405)
- Vital Signs Status (0802)

NIC Suggested Interventions

- Temperature Regulation (3900)
- Fluid and Electrolyte Management (2080)
- Hemodynamic Regulation (4150)
- Hypovolemic Management (4180)
- Invasive Hemodynamic Monitoring (4210)

Nursing Interventions/Rationales

- Monitor hourly heart rate and blood pressure. *To determine effectiveness of life support measures in maintaining adequate cardiac output and tissue perfusion.*
- Maintain continuous electrocardiographic monitoring. *To identify cardiac dysrhythmias and monitor effectiveness of life support measures.*
- Monitor hourly central venous or pulmonary artery pressures. *To determine fluid volume status and arterial pressures and to evaluate effectiveness of cardiac support measures.*
- Monitor hourly fluid intake and output. *Adequate urine output indicates adequate tissue perfusion. Urine output should approximate fluid intake.*
- Administer intravenous fluids as prescribed. *To maintain fluid volume and support blood pressure.*
- Administer vasopressors as ordered and monitor for untoward effects. *To sustain organ and tissue perfusion before organ harvest.*
- Obtain serum cardiac enzyme levels as prescribed. *To determine injury to the cardiac muscle related to decreased cardiac perfusion.*

Evaluation Parameters

1. Systolic blood pressure remains greater than 100 mm Hg
2. Heart rate within normal limits
3. CVP greater than 10 cm H_2O or 7 mm Hg

NURSING DIAGNOSIS **Ineffective tissue perfusion related to central nervous system dysfunction, hypovolemia**

GOALS/OUTCOMES Adequate tissue perfusion will be maintained

NOC Suggested Outcomes

- Tissue Perfusion: Abdominal Organs (0404)
- Tissue Perfusion: Cardiac (0405)
- Tissue Perfusion: Peripheral (0407)
- Tissue Perfusion: Pulmonary (0408)

NIC Suggested Interventions

- Hemodynamic Regulation (4150)
- Hypovolemia Management (4180)

Nursing Interventions/Rationales

- Monitor hourly heart rate, blood pressure, CVP, or pulmonary artery pressure. *Provides insight into status of peripheral perfusion.*
- Monitor quality of peripheral pulses. *Peripheral pulses reflect the status of tissue perfusion.*
- Monitor capillary refill in fingertips and nail beds and lips for cyanosis. *To detect changes or inadequacy of tissue perfusion.*

Continued

Nursing Care Plan — Patient Who Is an Organ Donor–cont'd

- Obtain arterial blood gases as indicated. *Provides direct measure of effectiveness of life support measures in maintaining tissue perfusion.*
- Obtain serum electrolytes, blood urea nitrogen (BUN), and serum creatinine. *To monitor electrolyte balance and renal function.*
- Administer vasopressors as ordered, and document changes in blood pressure and urine output after administration. *To sustain organ and tissue perfusion before organ harvest.*

Evaluation Parameters

1. Systolic blood pressure >100 mg Hg
2. CVP >10 cm H_2O or 7 mm Hg
3. Urine output >2 to 3 ml/kg/hr
4. Peripheral pulses present
5. Absence of cyanosis
6. Blood pH within normal limits
7. BUN and serum creatinine within normal limits

NURSING DIAGNOSIS **Impaired gas exchange related to central nervous system dysfunction (loss of respiratory drive and mechanics) and neurogenic pulmonary edema**

GOALS/OUTCOMES Adequate ventilation and gas exchange will be maintained

NOC Suggested Outcomes

- Respiratory Status: Gas Exchange (0402)
- Respiratory Status: Ventilation (0403)
- Tissue Perfusion: Pulmonary (0408)
- Electrolyte and Acid-Base Balance (0600)

NIC Suggested Interventions

- Acid-Base Management: Respiratory Acidosis (1913)
- Mechanical Ventilation (3300)
- Respiratory Monitoring (3350)

Nursing Interventions/Rationales

- Monitor mechanical ventilation. *Patients who experience brain death lack any ventilatory drive and must be mechanically ventilated.*
- Auscultate breath sounds bilaterally. *To determine adequacy of gas exchange.*
- Obtain arterial blood gases every 4 to 6 hours and after ventilator changes. *To determine adequacy of gas exchange and the need for ventilator adjustments.*
- Observe tracheobronchial secretions for amount, color, consistency, and odor. *To determine the presence of infection.*
- Maintain patent airway with sterile suctioning to remove tracheobronchial secretions. *To help mobilize secretions and prevent stasis.*
- Turn every 2 hours and administer chest physiotherapy. *To prevent mobilization of secretions and to prevent stasis.*

Evaluation Parameters

1. PaO_2 between 80 and 120 mm Hg with normal breath sounds bilaterally
2. Oxyhemoglobin saturation above 90%
3. $PaCO_2$ between 35 and 45 mm Hg
4. IMV rate between 8 and 14 breaths/min
5. Tidal volume, 12 to 15 ml/kg
6. pH, 7.35 to 7.45
7. Hemoglobin, 12% to 18%

NURSING DIAGNOSIS **Risk for deficient fluid volume related to diabetes insipidus**

GOALS/OUTCOMES Adequate fluid balance will be maintained

NOC Suggested Outcomes

- Fluid Balance (0601)
- Hydration (0602)
- Electrolyte and Acid-Base Balance (0600)

NIC Suggested Interventions

- Fluid Monitoring (4130)
- Fluid Management (4120)
- Hypovolemia Management (4170)

Nursing Care Plan Patient Who Is an Organ Donor—cont'd

Nursing Interventions/Rationales

- Monitor hourly intake and output. *To determine fluid balance. Intake should approximate output when fluid balance is maintained.*
- Obtain daily weight. *Changes in weight reflect subtle and dramatic shifts in fluid balance.*
- Monitor urine specific gravity every 2 hours. *To assess effectiveness of measures to maintain fluid balance.*
- Administer intravenous maintenance and replacement fluids. *To replace heavy fluid losses in urine due to altered pituitary secretion of antidiuretic hormone.*
- Administer aqueous vasopressin as prescribed and document changes in urine output following administration. *Vasopressin replaces antidiuretic hormone effect and helps reduce fluid losses.*

Evaluation Parameters

1. Stable vital signs
2. Urine output >2 to 3 ml/kg/hr
3. Stable weight
4. Normal serum and urine electrolytes

NURSING DIAGNOSIS **Ineffective thermoregulation related to central nervous system dysfunction**
GOALS/OUTCOMES Normal body temperature will be maintained

NOC Suggested Outcomes

- Thermoregulation (0800)
- Vital Signs Status (0802)

NIC Suggested Interventions

- Temperature Regulation (3900)
- Fever Treatment (3740)
- Hypothermia Treatment (3800)

Nursing Interventions/Rationales

- Monitor body temperature for hyperthermia or hypothermia. *The patient's temperature can fluctuate out of control because of loss of adequate central temperature regulation.*
- Restore normal body temperature with use of heating/cooling blankets as needed. *To restore body temperature to normal.*
- Warm intravenous fluids before administration if hypothermia is present. *To prevent hypothermia related to fluid infusion.*

Evaluation Parameters

1. Absence of body temperature fluctuations
2. Body temperature between 36.1 and 37.7° C (97° and 100° F)

NURSING DIAGNOSIS **Risk for infection related to presence of indwelling catheters and endotracheal tube**
GOALS/OUTCOMES Will remain free of infection

NOC Suggested Outcomes

- Risk Control (1902)
- Infection Status (0703)

NIC Suggested Interventions

- Infection Protection (6550)
- Wound Care (3660)
- Surveillance (6550)

Nursing Interventions/Rationales

- Maintain careful hand washing. *General asepsis is the best preventive measure against infection.*
- Obtain complete blood count with differential. *To determine changes denoting the presence of infection.*
- Maintain aseptic care of indwelling urinary catheter, observing urine color and consistency. *To prevent urinary tract infection. Cloudiness, sediment, and odor indicate the presence of infection.*
- Monitor wounds, incisions, and puncture sites for signs of infection. *Erythema, warmth, swelling, and drainage indicate the presence of infection.*
- Culture secretions, urine, and blood as indicated. *To determine the causative organism of the infection so that appropriate antibiotics can be administered.*
- Administer antibiotics as prescribed. *Prophylactic antibiotics may be administered to prevent sepsis.*

Evaluation Parameters

1. White blood cell count within normal limits
2. Absence of fever
3. Absence of purulent respiratory or wound drainage

Continued

Nursing Care Plan — Patient Who Is an Organ Donor–cont'd

NURSING DIAGNOSIS **Anticipatory grieving (wife/family) related to imminent death of a loved one**
GOALS/OUTCOMES Will be able to make decisions about anticipated loss; will discuss feelings about loss of loved one

NOC Suggested Outcomes
- Grief Resolution (1304)
- Coping (1302)
- Family Coping (2600)

NIC Suggested Interventions
- Grief Work Facilitation (5290)
- Emotional Support (5270)
- Organ Procurement (6260)

Nursing Interventions/Rationales
- Assess and evaluate accuracy of family's perceptions of loved one's condition. *Brain death is a difficult concept to understand because the patient's heart is beating. Misconceptions about the loved one's prognosis need to be corrected.*
- Listen attentively and with empathy to accounts of circumstances leading up to the trauma. *Coping with traumatic loss is fostered by the wife/family reliving and processing the circumstances. This includes talking about the patient's life and qualities.*
- Encourage family to talk about loved one. *Helps the family to process their loss and facilitates movement through the grief process.*
- Allow family to visit any time and participate in care if they so desire. *Quiet time at the bedside can facilitate movement through the grief process.*
- Explain the variety of thoughts, feelings, behaviors, and physical sensations the family may experience as a normal part of healthy grieving. *Brief discussion of grief can help the wife understand the nature of her physical and emotional responses.*
- Evaluate support systems (e.g., other family members, friends, clergy). *Support systems are an essential coping resource, and bereavement therapy may help the wife to cope with this traumatic event.*
- Refer to bereavement therapy if appropriate. *To provide additional support and guidance to help the family cope with their loss.*
- Reinforce altruism and benefit of the gift of organ donation. *Organ donation is a gift of life from sudden death. This is a comfort to many survivors.*

Evaluation Parameters
1. Family is able to discuss feelings about loss of a loved one
2. Family is able to identify thoughts, feelings, behaviors, and physical sensations they experience as a result of their loss
3. Support system (other family members, friends, clergy, or counselor) available to assist family in beginning their grief work

investigated. A blood clot in the Foley catheter is a common cause of early obstruction. Because the catheter remains in the bladder for 3 to 5 days after surgery to allow the bladder anastomosis to heal, its patency must be ensured. The physician may order careful sterile catheter irrigation to dislodge the occluding clots.

Most patients undergo ultrasonography within 24 hours of transplantation to assess the kidney's vascular supply and look for any fluid collections, such as hematoma, lymphocele, or urine leak. The presence of hydronephrosis, with or without a dilated ureter, may indicate obstruction.

Once the patient has sufficiently recovered from the operative procedure, nursing care involves ongoing assessment, diagnosis, intervention, and evaluation of the patient's response to the transplant. This includes the prevention or treatment of allograft rejection, monitoring for the complications of surgery and immunosuppression, and prevention of and monitoring for infection. Some institutions still use protective isolation, but scrupulous patient hygiene and thorough staff hand washing are two of the most effective interventions to prevent infection. Environmental cleanliness is also carefully assessed and ensured and all insertion sites of invasive lines and devices are monitored for signs of infection. People with active infections should not visit or care for the patient (see Evidence-Based Practice box).

Patient/Family Education

Patient/family education is an integral part of a smooth transition from hospital to home. The first priority for discharge preparation is medication teaching. Patients and their families must be able to explain the action, dosage, and potential adverse effects of all medications. A written list of discharge medications with the administration schedule is supplied for the patient to use as a home resource.[19]

Patients should be able to describe clinical manifestations associated with rejection and infection, and explain when and

Evidence-Based Practice

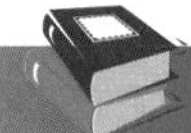

Reference: Starzomski R, Hilton A: Patient and family adjustment to kidney transplantation with or without an interim period of dialysis, *Nephrol Nurs J* 27(1):17, 2000.

This study examined the process of patient and family adjustment to kidney transplantation and compared differences between those who did versus those who did not receive dialysis pretreatment. A longitudinal study of 20 patients with end-stage renal disease and their partners was conducted. Data were obtained during the assessment phase before kidney transplantation and at 3- and 6-month intervals after organ transplantation. A total of 47 patients and their partners composed the cross-sectional sample. A series of self-report questionnaires on family functioning, support and resources, uncertainty, sickness impact, and sense of coherence were administered. The study found that patients and their partners experienced considerable stress related to the transplantation process, which included illness, family strain, and financial strain. Uncertainty decreased over time from the period of pretransplant to posttransplant. The study concluded that education and support programs are needed during both the pretransplant and posttransplant periods to help patients and their partners adjust to kidney transplantation.

how to contact the transplant office if symptoms occur (see Clinical Manifestations box). A follow-up appointment is scheduled, along with instructions for any routine laboratory testing. Careful timing of immunosuppressive medication administration is essential if 12-hour trough level testing is scheduled.

The nurse discusses postdischarge activity limitations, sexuality issues, and dietary recommendations. Most patients can return to work in 6 to 12 weeks. Heavy lifting (more than 20 pounds) is avoided for the first 6 weeks, until the incision completely heals. Regular exercise is encouraged to counteract the proximal muscle weakness associated with steroid administration.

Patients can resume sexual intercourse after 4 to 6 weeks. Women of childbearing age are encouraged to postpone pregnancy for at least 1 year after transplantation to ensure stable renal function and allow for lower doses of immunosuppressive drugs. Barrier contraceptive methods such as condoms, diaphragms, and foam are recommended. Oral contraceptives and intrauterine devices are not recommended because of the risks of thrombophlebitis and infection. Some women prefer to use contraceptive injections because they are easier and are more reliable in protecting against pregnancy.

The dietitian is an excellent resource for educating patients and families about good eating habits. Steroids commonly stimulate appetite, and the dietitian can offer suggestions for low-calorie snacks to minimize weight gain. The dietitian also provides teaching about cholesterol restriction because of the risk of hyperlipidemia associated with the use of steroids and cyclosporine. Although most renal patients are accustomed to following a low-sodium diet, a review of foods to avoid and hidden sources of sodium in fast food and convenience foods may help the patient minimize the salt- and water-retaining effects of steroids.

Clinical Manifestations

Renal Transplant Rejection

- Fever greater than 37.7 ° C (100 ° F); may be masked by steroid therapy
- Pain or tenderness over grafted kidney
- Sudden weight gain (2 to 3 pounds in 24 hours)
- Edema
- Hypertension
- General malaise
- Elevated serum creatinine and blood urea nitrogen
- Decreased creatinine clearance
- Ultrasound or biopsy evidence of rejection

GERONTOLOGIC CONSIDERATIONS

The incidence of end-stage renal disease is increasing most rapidly in the older adult population, which makes issues related to kidney transplantation particularly relevant for this group. Almost one third of all new cases of end-stage renal disease are diagnosed in persons over 65 years old. Age itself is not an absolute contraindication for kidney transplantation, and transplants are successfully performed in healthy older adults. However, a higher incidence of concurrent health problems and systemic disorders may contraindicate transplantation for any particular person. Arteriosclerosis and atherosclerosis are more common in this population and may be a factor in the transplant decision.

Older adults typically experience a decline in immune system function, and the immunosuppressive regimen may leave the individual extremely vulnerable to infection. The accelerated incidence of malignancy related to immunosuppression is also a concern, because cancer is already much more common within this age group. Many older adults undergoing transplantation have type 2 diabetes mellitus, and the need for high-dose corticosteroid therapy may seriously compromise their regimen for glucose control as well as impair wound healing.

SPECIAL ENVIRONMENTS FOR CARE

Critical Care

Patients undergoing solid organ transplantation are typically cared for in a critical care environment during the early postoperative period. Meticulous monitoring of all cardiovascular, fluid and electrolyte, and hemodynamic parameters is critical. If the patient stabilizes promptly, the stay in the critical care area is usually brief.

Community-Based Care

Hospitalization for successful kidney transplantation is typically brief, and patients are discharged to their home environments quickly. Discharge teaching is initiated as soon as the patient is able to focus and attend to it. Written materials prepared at an appropriate reading level for the patient's understanding supplement all teaching.

Preventing infection and adhering to the immunosuppressive regimen are two major areas of emphasis. The nurse stresses the importance of meticulous personal hygiene, frequent mouth care, and a liberal intake of fluids to prevent urinary stasis. Infections, besides occurring more frequently, also tend to generalize more rapidly in patients after transplantation and can quickly result in sepsis.

Adherence to a complex immunosuppressive drug regimen is difficult and cannot be assumed. The nurse lays the groundwork for successful regimen management and ensures that all necessary appointments have been made to initiate appropriate follow-up monitoring. Patients with ongoing needs for wound care management are referred for home health supervision.

HEART TRANSPLANT

Etiology/Epidemiology

The first heart transplant was performed in 1967. The procedure has evolved into a viable treatment option for patients with terminal cardiac disease. End-stage cardiomyopathy is the most common reason for cardiac transplant (50%) followed by inoperable coronary artery disease (CAD).

Donor availability is a serious problem with cardiac transplant, and the waiting period may be prolonged. As the patient's condition deteriorates, extended hospitalization may be required until a suitable donor is found. These patients are usually physiologically unstable and may require intensive treatment in a critical care setting because of the need for complex drug therapy, intraaortic balloon pump therapy, or the placement of a ventricular assist device.

Potential candidates for heart transplant are usually less than 60 years old and free of systemic illnesses or diseases in other organ systems that would limit their chances for long-term survival. Donor matching includes ABO blood group compatibility, negative lymphocyte cross-match, and avoidance of a CMV-positive donor if the recipient is CMV negative. HLA screening is not usually performed and has no proven benefit in light of the scarcity of donors.

Collaborative Care Management

Heart transplant surgery consists of the removal of the diseased heart (leaving the posterior walls of the recipient's atria to spare the sinoatrial node), followed by anastomosis of the atria, aorta, and pulmonary arteries.[25] Figure 51-3 shows the recipient's atrial cuffs and great vessels after cardiectomy, at the beginning of the left atrial suture line, and after completed cardiac transplant.

The patient who undergoes heart transplantation receives care similar to that of any patient having open heart surgery (see Chapter 24). A clinical pathway may be used to specifically guide the patient's postoperative care. A healthy donor heart usually functions well and the patient's cardiac output stabilizes.

Dysrhythmias are common in the initial postoperative period, and hypervolemia can result from fluid replacement and high-dose corticosteroid therapy. These complications are managed with the same treatments used for other cardiac patients. Critical care placement is usually maintained until the patient's condition stabilizes.

> ***Clinical Manifestations***
> **Heart Transplant Rejection**
>
> Fluid retention (peripheral edema, crackles, jugular vein distention, S_3 gallop)
> Fever
> Weakness or malaise
> Heart failure (decreased cardiac output)
> Cardiac enlargement
> Dysrhythmias
> Hypotension
> Dyspnea

Either acute or chronic rejection of the transplanted heart can occur. Endometrial biopsy is performed to confirm the presence of rejection. Biopsies are used routinely to monitor the patient's progress because the classic signs of rejection may or may not be present.

The patient showing signs of rejection (see Clinical Manifestations box) may be treated with increasing doses of immunosuppressive agents. In addition, methylprednisolone boluses, lymphocytic immune globulin, or OKT3 may be given. The patient needs considerable support during rejection episodes because of the potentially life-threatening nature of rejection and the anxiety associated with the threat of losing the new heart.

Chronic rejection is insidious and is characterized by graft atherosclerosis, which can result in myocardial ischemia, myocardial infarction, or cardiac failure. Ischemia and infarction may not be associated with pain because the transplanted heart is denervated. No effective treatment exists to stop the chronic rejection process or the associated atherosclerosis. Treatment focuses on interventions to improve cardiac function until another heart becomes available.

Patient/Family Education. Preparation for discharge involves the same teaching as discussed for the kidney transplant recipient. Health care measures to improve cardiac fitness, particularly exercise, are reviewed. Patients who have had long waits for donor hearts may have become virtually immobilized before surgery, and they need to very gradually increase their activity and fitness. The patient and family must understand the plan for repeat cardiac catheterization with biopsies and the timing intervals for these monitoring tests.

LIVER TRANSPLANT

Etiology/Epidemiology

The first liver transplantation was performed in 1963. It is now a therapeutic option for both adults and children with liver failure. Liver transplantation is used to treat biliary atresia, fulminant hepatic failure, cirrhosis, hepatitis, metabolic disorders, and primary hepatic malignancy. Cirrhosis of the liver is the major pathology in adult patients seeking transplantation, and the importance of abstinence from alcohol creates unique dilemmas in the selection procedures for liver transplant recipients. The use of transplantation to treat liver

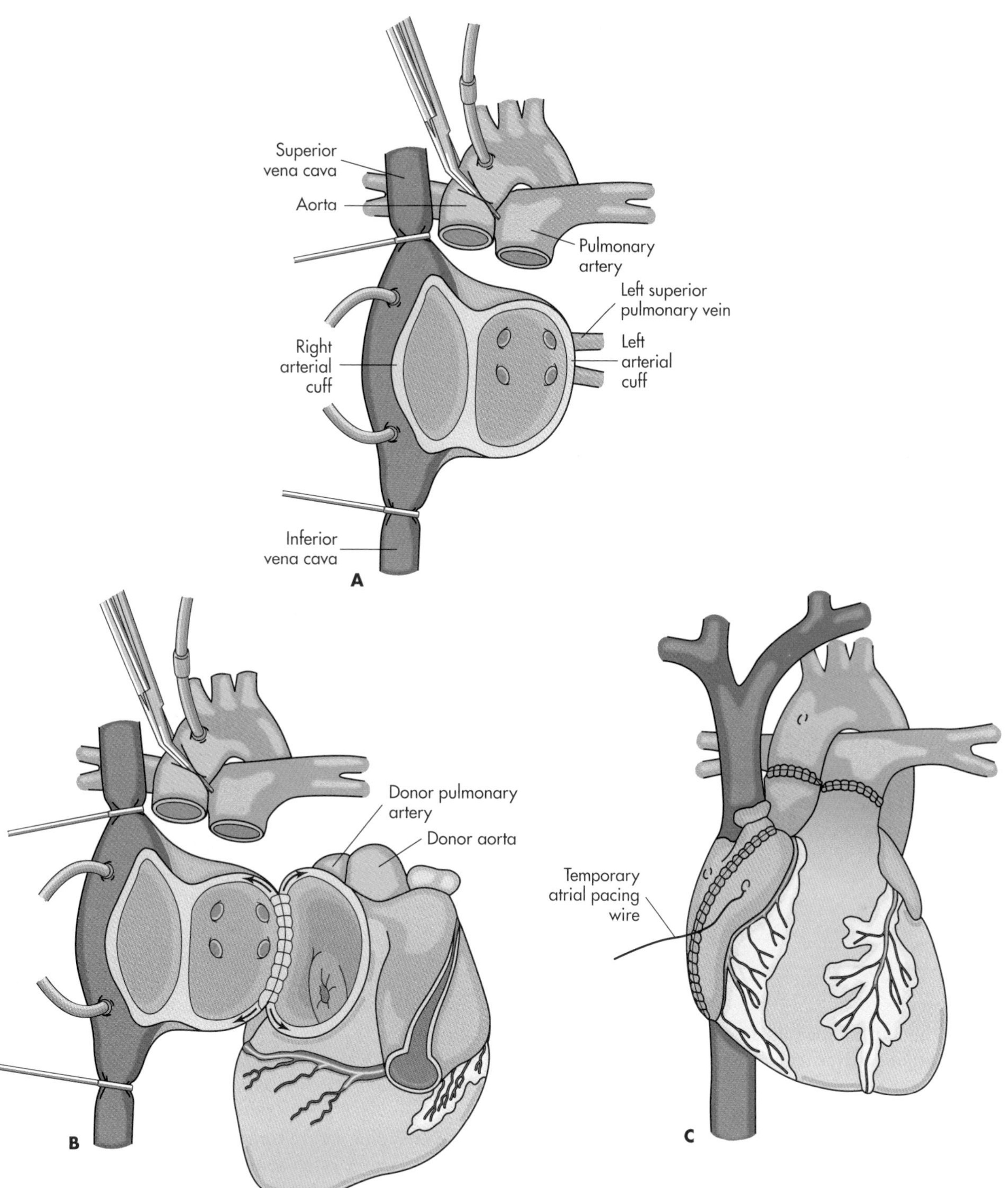

Figure 51-3 **A**, Recipient arterial cuffs and great vessels after cardiectomy. **B**, Beginning of left atrial suture line. Arrows indicate direction of suture line. **C**, Completed cardiac transplant.

cancer is controversial because of the high rate of recurrence, even when there is no evidence of disseminated disease.

Bilirubin concentrations greater than 10 mg/dl, serum albumin concentrations less than 2.5 mg/dl, and prothrombin times greater than 5 seconds beyond the control value are clinical features predictive of the need for liver transplantation. Other criteria include incapacitating encephalopathy, recurrent variceal bleeding not controlled by sclerotherapy, intractable ascites that does not respond to diuretic therapy or paracentesis, and recurrent spontaneous bacterial peritonitis.[11]

Collaborative Care Management

A liver transplant takes 8 to 12 hours and involves the removal of the recipient's diseased liver followed by implantation of the donor liver allograft.[29] The diseased liver is removed en bloc. A venovenous bypass system may be used to

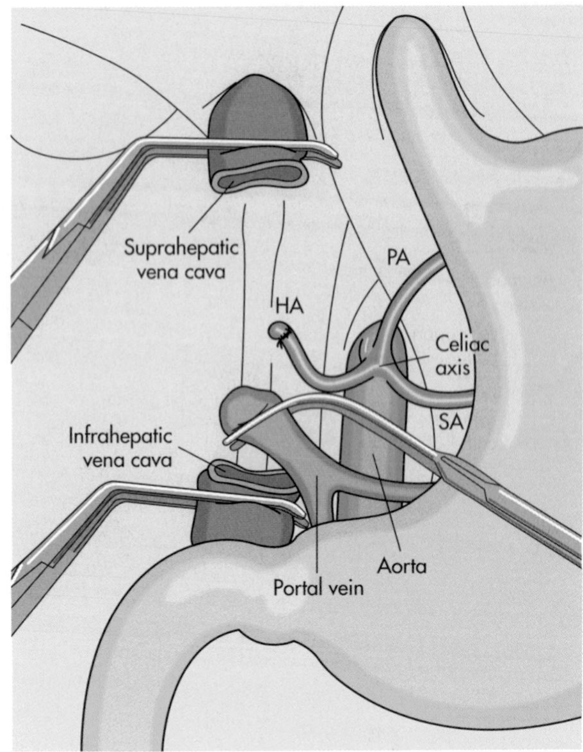

Figure 51-4 Vascular anastomoses of liver transplant.

Clinical Manifestations
Liver Transplant Rejection

Fever
Flulike symptoms
Jaundice
Itching
Abdominal or back pain
Elevated liver enzymes

allow normal hemodynamic values to be maintained while the recipient is without a liver. This bypass system helps prevent venous hypertension, circulatory instability, and excessive bleeding. The liver transplant procedure is the most technically complex of the solid organs because of the intricate vascular and biliary anastomoses that are required (Figures 51-4 and 51-5).

The major postoperative complications include rejection, infection, and occlusion of vessels. The liver is less susceptible to acute rejection than the kidneys, but adequate immunosuppressive therapy is still a priority concern.[28] The extensive nature of the surgery combined with the presence of preoperative liver failure significantly increases the patient's risk for postoperative complications (see Clinical Manifestations box).

Initial care of the liver transplant recipient is challenging and complex; therefore the postoperative patient is admitted to an intensive care setting. Constant monitoring of the patient's hemodynamic status and liver function is critical. Bed rest is maintained for several days. The patient's liver function

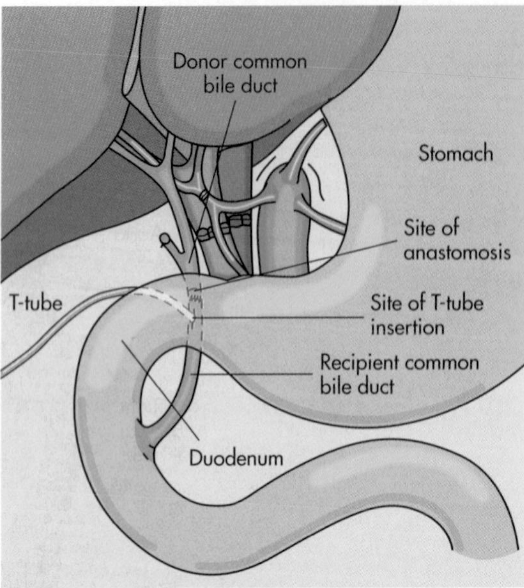

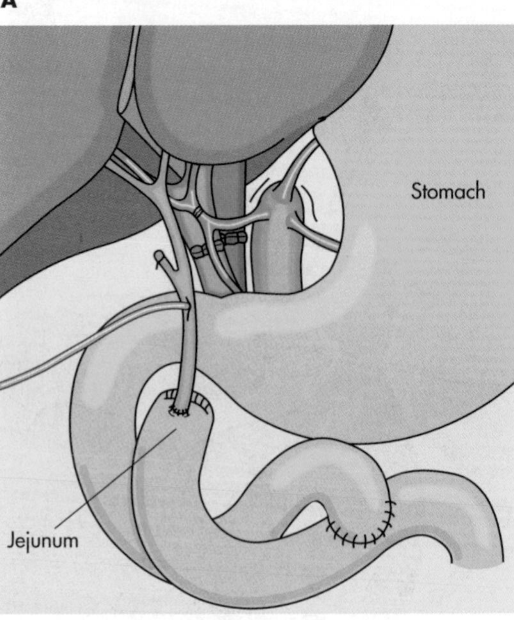

Figure 51-5 Biliary anastomoses of liver transplant. **A,** Choledochocholedochostomy. **B,** Choledochojejunostomy.

tests, including serum transaminases, bilirubin, albumin, and clotting factors, often show improvement within 24 hours if complications do not occur. Immunosuppressive therapy is started before surgery and continued on a regular schedule after the procedure. Worsening liver function, fever, swelling, and tenderness of the liver are all warning signs of a complication.[11] Infection is a crucial concern and can be bacterial, viral, or fungal in nature. The risk of infection is greatest during the first 3 months after surgery.

Patient/Family Education. Preparation for discharge involves the same teaching discussed for the kidney transplant recipient. In addition, the patient with alcoholic cirrhosis is counseled that the ongoing involvement with a chemical dependency program is an essential strategy to prevent disease recurrence from relapse.

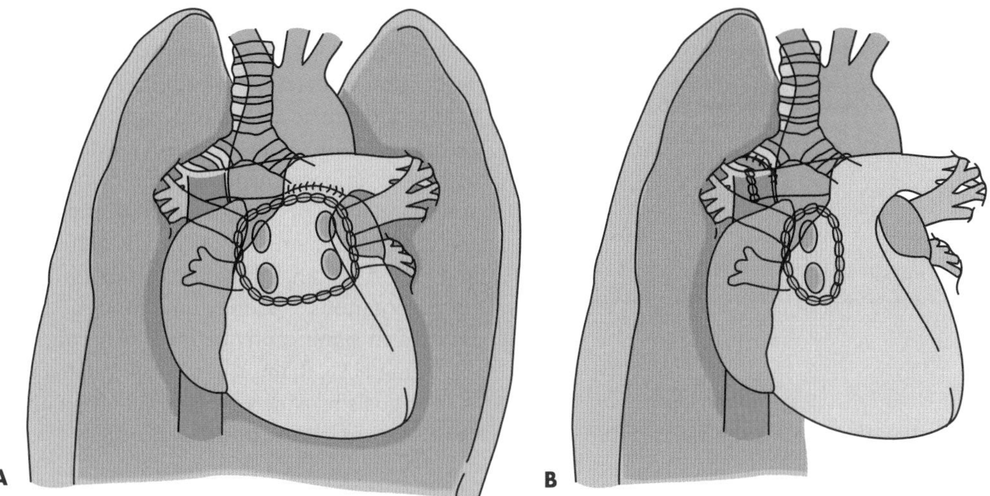

Figure 51-6 Anastomoses for **A**, double-lung and **B**, single-lung transplantation.

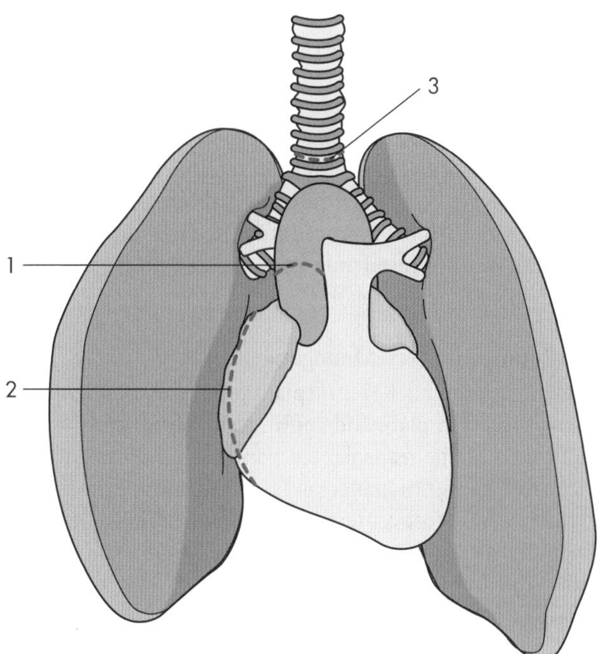

Figure 51-7 Anastomotic sites in heart-lung transplant. *1*, Aorta; *2*, Right atria; and *3*, Trachea.

LUNG TRANSPLANT

Etiology/Epidemiology

Successful transplantation of the lungs became a reality in the 1980s. Lung transplants may involve a single lung, two lungs, or a lobe of a lung. Advances in surgical technique and immunosuppressive therapy have raised the 1- and 2-year survival rates for lung transplants to about 75%. The procedure is used with patients less than 60 years old who are not active smokers and who suffer from advanced pulmonary diseases such as pulmonary hypertension, emphysema, cystic fibrosis, and sarcoidosis.

Single lung transplantation is used for restrictive lung disease, because the decreased compliance and increased pulmonary resistance of the recipient's remaining lung result in preferential ventilation and perfusion of the transplanted lung. Double lung transplants are typically used in persons with emphysema or cystic fibrosis. Most lobe transplants are for cystic fibrosis patients.[25]

Collaborative Care Management

Single lung transplants are performed through an anterolateral thoracotomy (Figure 51-6). Some patients require cardiopulmonary bypass, especially those patients with primary pulmonary hypertension. The double lung transplant procedure has been modified to a bilateral single lung transplant procedure with individual bronchial anastomoses (Figure 51-7). Cardiopulmonary bypass is required in the double lung procedure.

When heart-lung procedures are performed with the use of cardiopulmonary bypass, the recipient's heart is first removed and the phrenic nerves are isolated. Enough left atrium is removed to allow the donor's right lung to fit into the right pleural space. The lungs are then removed individually and the donor's heart-lung bloc is placed into the recipient's chest. Tracheal anastomosis completes the surgical process.

The patient is cared for in an intensive care setting after surgery. The most important aspects of care are promoting adequate airway clearance and gas exchange and instituting measures to prevent major complications associated with lung transplant. Poor gas exchange is a common complication and may be caused by reperfusion edema of the lung, impaired cough, infection, or rejection. Appropriate immunosuppressive therapy is initiated, and the patient is monitored closely for signs of rejection.

One difference in the immunosuppressive regimen for lung transplants is that corticosteroids are not used for the first 7 to 14 days after the transplant procedure. Corticosteroids jeopardize the healing of the tracheal and bronchial anastomoses; therefore OKT3 is used instead.[6] Once healing has occurred, immunosuppressive therapy with corticosteroids is initiated (see Clinical Manifestations box).

Aggressive respiratory care is critical. It is difficult for the patient to clear the airway because the transplanted lung (or

Clinical Manifestations

Lung Transplant Rejection

- Fever
- Dyspnea
- Nonproductive cough
- Malaise
- Decreased oxygen saturations
- Abnormal pulmonary function tests

lungs) is denervated below the level of the trachea and mucociliary clearance is decreased. Care includes frequent position changes and deep breathing along with postural drainage and coughing. Supplemental oxygen is necessary. Patients with lung transplants are prone to cardiovascular complications from hypervolemia or hypovolemia, myocardial irritability, or decreased contractility. Hemodynamic status is carefully managed to maintain adequate cardiac output without fluid overload that can lead to pulmonary edema and elevated pulmonary vascular resistance. Patients are at risk for dysrhythmias because of the use of cardiopulmonary bypass.

The use of anticoagulants with cardiopulmonary bypass or excessive replacement of blood products puts patients at risk for bleeding from coagulopathy. Careful monitoring of coagulation studies and blood loss from mediastinal tubes is imperative. Administration of platelets or fresh frozen plasma may be necessary. Additional care needs include nutritional support, comfort measures, and promotion of adequate sleep.

It is common for the patient undergoing lung transplantation to experience two or three episodes of acute rejection during the first 6 weeks after transplantation. Clinical manifestations of lung rejection include pulmonary infiltrates, poor arterial blood gases, dyspnea, low-grade fever, and elevated WBC count. Transbronchial biopsies can provide valuable information by helping differentiate among infection, rejection, and lung injury.[14] As with other solid organ transplants, treatment of rejection involves enhancement of immunosuppression.

Patient/Family Education. Preparation for discharge involves the same teaching discussed for the kidney transplant recipient. The importance of adherence to the regimen and regular follow-up monitoring is stressed. Infection is a risk for any transplant recipient but is of particular concern for lung transplant recipients. Obliterative bronchiolitis causes severe deterioration of lung function in as many as 50% of lung transplant recipients after the first year. It is mostly irreversible, and the only viable treatment option is retransplantation. The cause of this complication has not been determined. Possibilities include chronic rejection, viral infection, cyclosporine toxicity, long-term denervation of the lung, the lack of lymphatics, and the loss of bronchial blood supply. Patients experience a cough and progressive dyspnea. Obliterative bronchiolitis is diagnosed with fiberoptic bronchoscopy and transbronchial lung biopsy.

PANCREAS TRANSPLANT

Etiology/Epidemiology

Because diabetes is the leading cause of end-stage renal disease in the United States, pancreas transplants are being performed with increasing frequency with patients experiencing a marked improvement in overall outcomes. Simultaneous transplantation of both the kidney and pancreas (KP) from the same donor into a patient with type 1 diabetes mellitus and end-stage renal disease accounts for 85% of all pancreas transplantations.[26] Kidney and pancreas transplantation has resulted in significantly better 1-year pancreas graft survival, exceeding 80%, than pancreas transplantation alone.

The goals of pancreas transplantation are to eliminate the need for exogenous insulin and dietary restrictions and to prevent or stabilize the microvascular and neuropathic complications of diabetes. The recipient eligibility criteria for KP transplantation are similar to those for kidney transplantation except that the age range is more restricted at 18 to 45 years, and cardiovascular clearance must be obtained from a cardiologist. Some centers do not consider diabetics with secondary complications such as blindness or severe peripheral vascular disease as acceptable candidates for KP transplantation. Generally, pancreas transplantation is offered to a select group of patients who are at low to moderate cardiac risk, highly motivated, and well informed about the benefits and risk associated with the procedure. The risks include greater morbidity, an increased rate of acute rejection, and an increased risk of cardiac death.[22]

Collaborative Care Management

In the combined KP transplantation, the recipient's own pancreas is left in place and continues to perform its exocrine function while the transplanted pancreas provides endocrine function. The donor pancreas is placed intraperitoneally in the pubic area. Most centers use a bladder drainage technique to handle the exocrine juices from the donor pancreas. The head of the donor pancreas is anastomosed to the dome of the recipient's bladder with a segment of the donor's duodenum. The donor kidney is placed in the iliac fossa as described earlier (Figure 51-8).

The KP transplant recipient has nursing care needs similar to those of any patient after extensive abdominal surgery. Blood glucose levels are monitored closely during the immediate postoperative period. Increasing glucose levels may indicate decreased graft perfusion as a result of thrombosis. Metabolic acidosis can occur from the loss of bicarbonate in the exocrine pancreatic secretions that are eliminated in the urine. Supplemental sodium bicarbonate may be added to the patient's IV infusions or may be administered orally.

The extra digestive secretions and fluids that are excreted in the urine account for an additional 1000 to 1500 ml of fluid output daily. Consequently, fluid replacement must be adjusted to compensate for these additional losses. The KP recipient may need to drink more than 5 L of fluid daily to prevent fluid deficits.

The diagnosis of pancreas rejection is difficult because many clinical manifestations are late indicators of rejection.

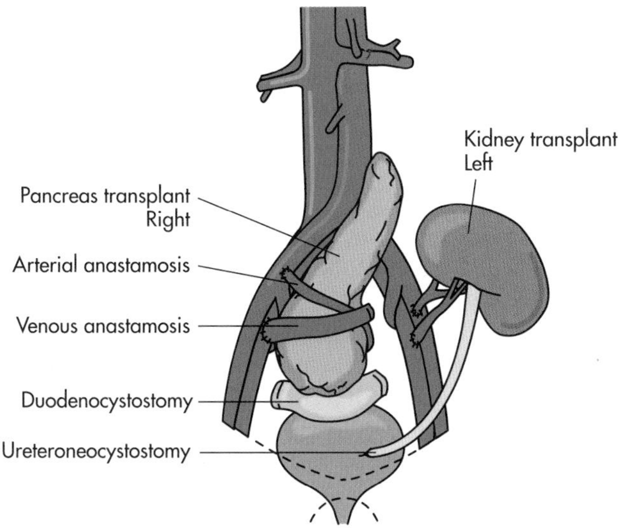

Figure 51-8 Diagram of the combined kidney-pancreas transplant.

Clinical Manifestations

Pancreas Transplant Rejection

Fever
Tenderness over graft site
Decreased serum amylase (if pancreas attached to urinary bladder)
Hyperglycemia (late sign)

Hyperglycemia becomes apparent only after 90% of the pancreas is damaged. A major advantage of urinary drainage is the ability to monitor amylase and bicarbonate levels in the urine and detect a rejection episode before hyperglycemia occurs. The exocrine pancreas typically malfunctions approximately 3 days before the endocrine pancreas; therefore decreases in urine amylase and urine pH can be early indicators of pancreatic rejection. Changes in kidney function also precede signs of pancreas rejection, and an increase in serum creatinine is an important warning sign. Reversal of kidney rejection is almost always associated with preservation of pancreas graft function as well (see Clinical Manifestations box).

Patient/Family Education. Many patients find it difficult to maintain an adequate oral fluid intake because they are so accustomed to the fluid restrictions of dialysis, and they do not have a normal response to thirst. Some patients are discharged from the hospital with a venous access device in place for home IV fluid administration. A total of 1 to 2 L of fluid can be administered at night to ensure an adequate fluid balance. In most patients, the exocrine secretions produced by the pancreas and excreted in the urine significantly decrease after the first 2 months. The patient can then discontinue IV supplementation and maintain fluid balance with oral intake alone. Before discharge, it is critical that KP transplant recipients be instructed in the signs and symptoms of dehydration, including decreased weight, dizziness (especially with position changes), increased pulse rate, and generalized weakness. All KP transplant recipients must be alert for signs and symptoms of metabolic acidosis, including weakness, anorexia, nausea, and vomiting.

If a bladder drainage procedure is used, the patient is instructed to monitor the urine pH with a dipstick to detect early signs of pancreas rejection. If the patient's vision is impaired, a family member or significant other is taught how to perform the test.

BONE MARROW TRANSPLANT

Etiology/Epidemiology

Bone marrow transplant (BMT) is used to treat a wide variety of malignant and nonmalignant disorders. The malignant diseases amenable to BMT are the leukemias, lymphoma, and selected solid tumors. The 5-year disease-free survival rate average 50%. Nonmalignant diseases requiring BMT include immunologic deficiency disease, aplastic anemia, and thalassemia. The 5-year disease-free survival rate for these conditions average 80%.[11]

There are three types of bone marrow donors: allogeneic, the use of marrow from an HLA-matched donor, most often a sibling; syngeneic, from an identical twin; or autologous bone marrow transplant, in which patients serve as their own donors. With the hope of making BMT more accessible to patients who lack an HLA-matched sibling, many centers are exploring the use of partially matched or unrelated donors. Advances in histocompatibility testing have enabled researchers to more clearly define disparity between the recipient and the donor. In general, as the disparity between the donor and recipient increases, the incidence and severity of GVHD and the risk of graft failure increase, and the survival rate decreases. Donor registries have been established in the United States and abroad to assist in the search for HLA-matched unrelated donors. The National Marrow Donor Program has a registry of more than 200,000 donors.

The type and extent of disease are the primary determinants of a patient's eligibility for BMT. The risk of relapse after transplantation is reduced if BMT is performed in patients whose disease is in complete remission or those who have minimal residual disease at the time of transplantation. Additional eligibility criteria include age, lack of preexisting organ toxicity or comorbid conditions, and availability of a suitable marrow donor.

Collaborative Care Management

In preparation for BMT, the recipient undergoes intensive chemoradiotherapy to eradicate residual disease, make space in the recipient's marrow for donor cell engraftment, and establish immunosuppression to prevent the rejection of donor marrow in allogeneic transplants.

Bone marrow stem cells capable of engraftment can be obtained from peripheral blood, fetal liver tissue, fetal umbilical cord blood, cadavers, or the sternum or pelvis of a live donor. Most autologous or allogeneic bone marrow is obtained by multiple needle aspirations from the posterior iliac crests with the donor under general or spinal anesthesia. The amount of

Clinical Manifestations

Bone Marrow Rejection (Graft-versus-Host Disease)

Fine, maculopapular, erythematous rash of the hand palms and soles of feet
Generalized erythroderma
Right upper quadrant pain
Hepatomegaly
Jaundice
Green, watery diarrhea
Abdominal cramping
Nausea, vomiting
Ileus

marrow extracted ranges from 600 to 2500 ml. Complications of bone marrow donation include bruising, bleeding, pain at aspiration sites, infection, transient neuropathies, and hypotension secondary to volume loss.[8]

After processing, the marrow is given to the recipient intravenously, frozen at −140° C (−284° F), or cryopreserved at −196° C (−384.8° F) and kept for 3 years or more. The bone marrow reinfusion process is technically similar to blood transfusion and takes 2 to 4 hours. The recipient is hydrated with IV fluids containing sodium bicarbonate before and after marrow infusion. This ensures adequate renal perfusion and urine alkalinization if red cell hemolysis occurs as a result of incompatibility or trauma. All BMT recipients can expect a red tinge to their urine for up to 12 hours after marrow infusion because of mild intravascular red cell lysis.[8]

The recipient is closely monitored during reinfusion. Many of the common problems seen after transplantation result from the conditioning regimen of radiation and chemotherapy required before transplantation. Gastrointestinal complications are the most common problems and include anorexia, nausea, vomiting, diarrhea, stomatitis, and mucositis. Bone marrow suppression can result in bleeding and infection.

Graft-versus-Host Disease

Persons who receive allogeneic bone marrow are at risk for GVHD, depending on the degree to which the donor and recipient are HLA incompatible. Irradiation and chemotherapy are used before allogeneic transplantation to destroy the recipient's immunocompetent cells. The donor's immunocompetent cells, once they engraft in the recipient, recognize other cells of the recipient as foreign and attack them. The tissue and organs most often affected are the skin, liver, and gastrointestinal tract[23] (see Clinical Manifestations box). GVHD can occur as an acute or a chronic process. Histocompatibility testing and effective immune suppression are used to prevent or minimize GVHD.

Patient/Family Education. Patients can be discharged after BMT when they are afebrile, are able to maintain an adequate oral intake, and have met or exceeded specific blood count criteria, including a platelet count greater than 15,000, a granulocyte count greater than 500, and a hematocrit above 30%. Important components of discharge teaching are similar to those discussed for the kidney transplant recipient. Preventing infection is a priority concern. In addition, BMT recipients must be knowledgeable about bleeding precautions and the signs and symptoms of GVHD.

CORNEA TRANSPLANT

Etiology/Epidemiology

Although cornea transplantation is not a lifesaving procedure, it has great potential for enhancing quality of life. The number of Americans, young and old, with impaired vision resulting from corneal damage underscores the importance of this technology. Defective corneas cause blindness in more than 40,000 Americans each year.[1] The leading causes of corneal damage requiring transplantation are keratoconus, Fuchs' dystrophy, herpes simplex keratitis, pseudophakic bullous keratopathy, and chemical burns.[18] Corneal transplants are successful in 95% of patients, but the degree of visual acuity restored can be highly variable. It is not unusual for patients to require eyeglasses or contact lenses to correct refractive error.

Patients considering a cornea transplant must be evaluated for other ocular conditions that can affect visual acuity after transplant, such as strabismus, amblyopia, retinal disease, glaucoma, and previous cataract surgery. A complete examination of all ocular structures is performed to determine existing conditions that can affect graft survival. The eye is carefully assessed for infection since corneal transplantation cannot be performed in the presence of infection.

Collaborative Care Management

The ideal corneal donor is under the age of 65 years and has undergone enucleation within 6 hours of death. Beyond 6 hours, the supply of glucose in the aqueous humor and endothelium is exhausted and necrosis occurs. In addition, the risk of contamination by bacteria and fungi increases as the interval between death and enucleation lengthens. Donor corneas are usually transplanted within 24 hours, but new preservation methods can extend preservation up to 35 days without significant loss of endothelial cells and ultrastructural integrity.

The type of corneal graft used depends on the depth and size of the damaged area (Figure 51-9). Corneal transplants or grafts may involve the entire thickness of the cornea (total penetrating), only part of the depth of the cornea (lamellar), or a combination of these, in which a small part of the graft involves the entire thickness of the cornea (partial penetrating). Penetrating grafts establish least well.

Patients are permitted out of bed after recovery from the anesthetic. Discharge takes place within 2 to 4 days. The eye is covered with a sterile eye pad, and a metal or plastic shield is placed over the pad for extra protection. The patient continues to wear the shield at night for several weeks. Cornea grafts heal very slowly because of the lack of blood vessels in the cornea and require 3 to 6 months for complete healing.[18]

Patient/Family Education. Patient teaching includes instruction about medications and assessment for graft rejection (see Clinical Manifestations box). Patients are usually

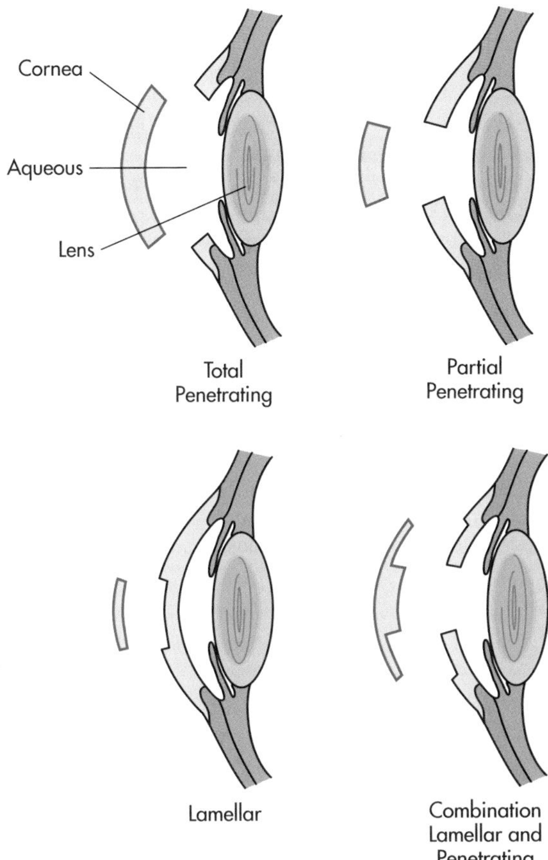

Figure 51-9 Types of corneal grafts currently in use. Note that the lamellar graft does not penetrate the entire thickness of the cornea.

Clinical Manifestations
Cornea Transplant Rejection

Abrupt or sudden change in visual clarity
Unusual redness of the eye
Increased sensitivity to light
Eye pain

discharged on cycloplegic, steroid, and sulfa eye drops. Because the cornea is normally avascular, the recipient's immune cells are not exposed to the cornea; thus immunosuppressive therapy is not required. However, patients are instructed to check for graft rejection daily for the rest of their lives. The eye is checked at the same time each day for new or increased redness, irritation, or discomfort; or decrease in vision. Any symptoms that persist or increase in severity in a 24-hour period should be reported to the surgeon.

Often patients expect to have their vision restored immediately after the graft. However, vision is generally blurred for the first few weeks, but it progressively clears. Sutures are left in place while the wound heals, which is a slow process. After 2 or 3 months part of the sutures are removed and vision usually improves. It may take 6 months to 1 year before all sutures are removed and full vision is achieved. Patients are evaluated monthly during this time period.

Critical Thinking Questions

1. The following patients are awaiting liver transplantation:
   a. *Patient A is a 46-year-old patient with alcoholic cirrhosis and liver failure who first entered an alcohol treatment program when he was placed on the transplant list 2 months ago. His condition is deteriorating rapidly, but he is not hospitalized.*
   b. *Patient B is a 22-year-old woman in liver failure related to an acetaminophen overdose. She has just been placed on the transplant list but is in full liver failure.*
   c. *Patient C is a 65-year-old man with idiopathic cirrhosis hospitalized and fading in and out of hepatic coma. He has been on the transplant list for 3 years. A liver has just become available in Patient B's home state. The liver is an excellent ABO and HLA match for Patient A, who lives halfway across the country. Who should get the transplant? What criteria did you use to make your decision?*
2. Kidney and pancreas transplantation may allow a patient with type 1 diabetes mellitus to stop taking insulin and relax dietary restrictions. Given the cost of the procedure and its associated rejection and complication rates, should health insurance plans be required to cover it for anyone seeking it? Why or why not?
3. Compatible Asian/Pacific Islander bone marrow donors are in extremely short supply nationwide. You live in an urban area with a dense population of this ethnic group. Design a community outreach program targeted at getting Asian/Pacific Islander ethnic group members typed as potential bone marrow donors.
4. A 32-year-old father of three has been pronounced brain dead after a motorcycle accident. Outline a plan for approaching his young wife about organ donation.

References

1. American Association of Tissue Banks: *Tissue bank statistics,* Washington, DC, 1997, American Association of Tissue Banks.
2. Briceno J et al: Impact of marginal quality donors on the outcome of liver transplantation, *Transplant Proc* 29(1-2):477, 1997.
3. Campaign for Responsible Transplantation, website: http://www.crt-online.org/.
4. Caplan A: *Due considerations: controversy in the age of medical miracles,* New York, 1998, Wiley.
5. Cole MR: Trends in living donor transplantation, *Nurs Spectrum* 11A(17):1, 1999.
6. Committee on Non-Beating Transplantation II: *Non-heart-beating transplantation practice and protocols.* Division of Health Care Services, Institute of Medicine, Washington, DC, 2000, National Academy Press.
7. Denton MD: Immunosuppressive strategies in transplantation, *Lancet* 357:342, 1999.
8. Division of Hematologic Malignancies: *Bone marrow transplantation program: the transplant process,* Baltimore, 2001, Johns Hopkins Oncology Center.
9. DuBois JM: Ethical assessments of brain death and organ procurement policies: a survey of transplant personnel in the United States, *J Transplant Coordination* 9(4):210, 1999.
10. Expanded Medicare coverage for transplant recipients, website: http://www.organdonor.gov/expanded.htm.
11. Ginns LC, Cosimi AB, Morris PJ, editors: *Transplantation,* New York, 1999, Blackwell Science.
12. Giuliano K, Sims T: Transplant issues: Infections and immunosuppressant drugs, *Dimens Crit Care Nurs* 18(2):16, 1999.

13. Goldsmith MF: Mother to child: first living donor lung trasplant, *JAMA* 264(21):2724, 1990.
14. Good EW: Caring for patients with donor organs, *Nursing 2000* 30(6):34, 2000.
15. Graham WK: *Organ transplantation in the United States,* Richmond, Va, 2001, United Network for Organ Sharing.
16. Halloran PF: Sirolimus and cyclosporin for renal transplantation, *Lancet* 356(9225):179, 2000.
17. McCance KL, Huether SE: *Pathophysiology: the biologic basis for disease in adults and children,* ed 3, St Louis, 1998, Mosby.
18. Midwest Eye Banks and Transplant Center: *Fun facts: Cornea transplants,* Ann Arbor, Mich, 2000, website: www.mebtc.org/who12.htm.
19. Milliman USA: Cost implications of human organ and tissue transplantation, an update, 1999, Milliman USA, 2001, website: www.milliman.com.
20. Ohler L: Educating patients and families about solid organ transplantation, *Prog Transplantation* 10(3):138, 2000.
21. Roitt I, Brostoff J, Male D: *Immunology,* ed 5, St Louis, 1998, Mosby.
22. Steen DC: The current state of pancreas transplantation. *AACN Clinical Issues Advanced Practice Acute Critical Care* 10(2):164, 1999.
23. The John Hopkins Oncology Center: More information about GVDH, website: http://www.med.jhu.edu/cancerctr/hematol/moregvh.htm.
24. Transplant Resource Center of Maryland: Tissues donation, website: http://www.mdtransplant.org/tissuea.htm.
25. United Network for Organ Sharing: *Transplant patient DataSource.* Richmond, Va, January, 2001, website: http://207.239.150.13/tpd/.
26. United Network for Organ Sharing: Critical data: U.S. Facts about transplantation, Richmond, 2001, UNOS.
27. United Network for Organ Sharing: *The organ donation process,* Richmond, 2001, UNOS.
28. USC Liver Transplant Program and Center for Liver Disease: *A patient's guide to liver transplant surgery: medications and complications,* Los Angeles, 2001, USC.
29. USC Liver Transplant Program and Center for Liver Disease: *A patient's guide to liver transplant surgery: the organ donation process.* Los Angeles, 2001, USC.
30. U.S. Department of Health and Human Services: *Improving the nation's organ transplantation system,* Washington, DC, 1999, HRSA Press.
31. U.S. Department of Health and Human Services: Organ transplant recipients' survival rates improve nationwide, website: http://www.hrsa.gov/NEWS-PA/Unos_csr.htm.

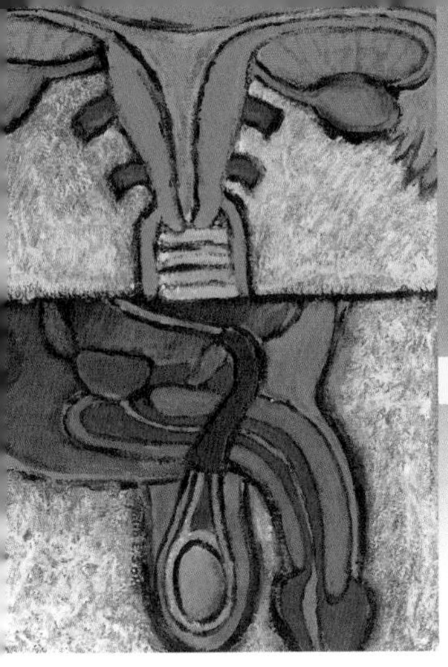

Assessment of the Reproductive System

52

Kathleen Barta

Objectives

After studying this chapter, the learner should be able to:

1. Describe the structures and functions of the female and male reproductive systems.
2. Explain the functions of the major hormones that control the reproductive systems.
3. Describe age-related changes in the reproductive systems.
4. Identify data related to the reproductive system and sexuality that should be obtained from a patient history.
5. Discuss patient preparation and related nursing interventions for diagnostic and laboratory tests used in identifying reproductive tract problems.

Conditions affecting healthful functioning of the reproductive systems of men and women take a high toll in loss of life and acute and chronic physical and emotional stress. The nurse assists in general health education, refers patients for appropriate health care, and uses knowledge of the usual treatments available and nursing care needed when disease develops. A basic knowledge of the structure and function of the reproductive system is important for accurate assessment and planning.

ANATOMY AND PHYSIOLOGY

Pelvis

The pelvis is the weight-bearing structure of the upper body and trunk. The pelvic bones consist of the innominate bones, the sacrum, and the coccyx. Each of the two innominate bones is made up of the pubic bone, ilium, and ischium. Anteriorly, the pubic bones join at the symphysis pubis. The inferior borders of the pubic bones and symphysis form an inverted V, called the pubic arch. The sacrum and coccyx come together at the sacrococcygeal joint, which is movable. The bones of the pelvis are shown in Figure 52-1.

The pelvis is divided into the true and the false pelvis by a bony ridge called the pelvic brim (Figure 52-2). The false pelvis is the broad, expanded portion above the pelvic brim. The narrow part below the pelvic brim is the true pelvis. The true pelvis has an inlet and an outlet. The inlet is located at the pelvic brim, and the outlet is at the base of the pelvis. The iliac spines mark the midpoint between the inlet and the outlet. The distances between the bones of the true pelvis have special significance during childbirth, since it is through this bony canal that the baby must pass to be born.

There are four basic pelvic types: gynecoid, anthropoid, android, and platypelloid. The gynecoid, or typical female pelvis, occurs in the majority of women. It is wide and shallow and especially well-suited for childbirth. The android, or typical male pelvis, is heart shaped and characterized by a narrow subpubic angle and straight sacrum. These pelvic types vary by age, race, and gender. True pelvic types are rare; most pelves are a combination of two types, for example, gynecoid and android. The major differences between the pelves of men and women are in the contour of the pelvis and thickness of the bones.

Female Genital System

External Structures

The external genitalia, known collectively as the vulva or pudendum, consist of the mons pubis (mons veneris), labia majora, labia minora, clitoris, prepuce, frenulum, vestibule, urethral meatus, Skene's (paraurethral) glands, vaginal orifice, hymen, fossa navicularis, Bartholin's (vulvovaginal) glands, fourchette, perineum, and escutcheon. The escutcheon is the triangular pubic hair pattern from the upper portion of the pubic bone to the lateral areas of the labia majora. The mons pubis is the rounded area in front of the symphysis pubis. It consists of a collection of fatty tissue beneath the skin and is covered with hair after puberty. Figure 52-3 shows the external female genitalia.

The labia majora are two prominent, longitudinal folds of tissue extending from the mons pubis. The labia are thicker in front, gradually become thinner as they extend back, and appear to flatten out as they merge with the adjacent tissues in the area of the perineum. The labia majora have two surfaces. The outer surface is covered by a thin layer of skin containing hair follicles and sebaceous and sweat glands. The inner surfaces are smooth, lack hair, and are supplied with many sebaceous

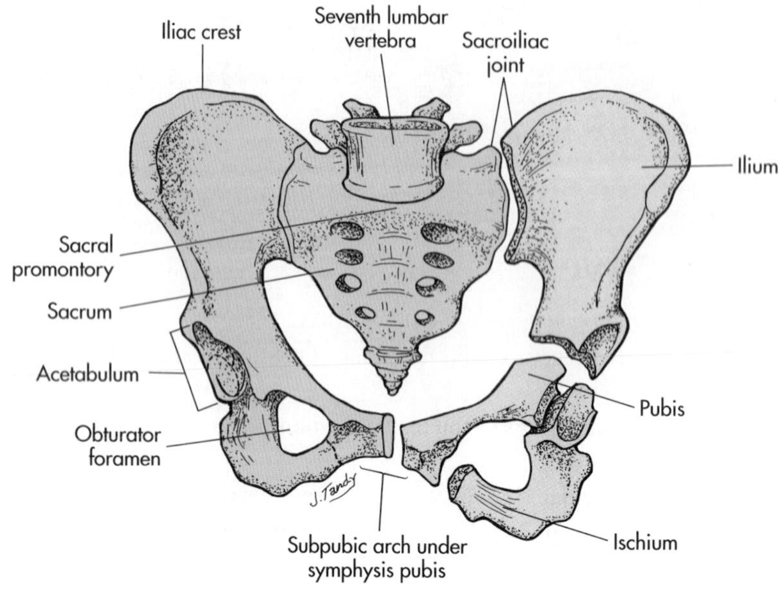

Figure 52-1 Adult female pelvis.

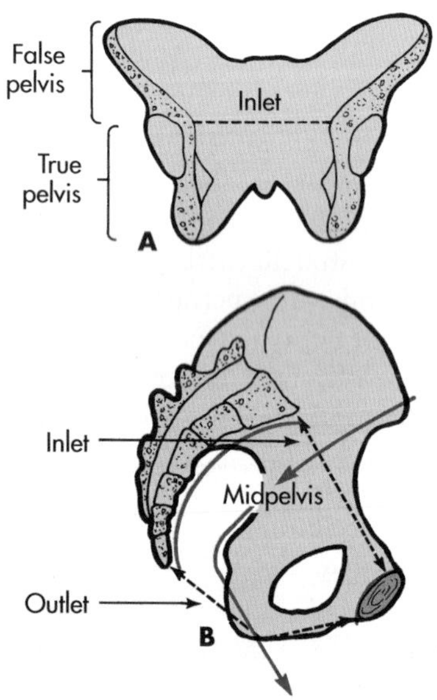

Figure 52-2 Female pelvis. **A,** Cavity of the false pelvis is a shallow basin above the inlet; the true pelvis is a deeper cavity below the inlet which is completely surrounded by bone. **B,** Cavity of the true pelvis is an irregularly curved canal *(arrows).*

follicles. The labia are homologous to the male scrotum and serve as protection for the inner structures of the vulva.

The labia minora are two smaller folds of tissue inside and parallel to the labia majora. In sexually active women and in women who have borne children, the labia minora may project beyond the labia majora. The labia minora join near the prepuce, which covers the clitoris, extend backward to enclose the urethral and vaginal orifices, and merge with the labia majora in the perineum. The labia minora are made up of connective and elastic tissue and contain little fatty tissue. Sweat glands and hair follicles are absent from the labia minora, but sebaceous glands are present. The labia minora increase in size and deepen in color in response to sexual stimulation.

The clitoris is situated near the anterior folds of the labia minora. The glans of the clitoris is a small, rounded area consisting of erectile tissue enclosed in a layer of fibrous membrane. The physiologic functions of the clitoris are the initiation and elevation of sexual tension levels. Sexual stimulation initiates a process whereby the clitoris becomes enlarged, erect, and very sensitive to stimuli. Female orgasm can occur from stimulation of the clitoris as well as from stimulation of other sites sensitive to touch.

The vestibule is a boat-shaped fossa formed between the labia minora, clitoris, and fourchette. The fossa navicularis is a small depression between the fourchette and hymen. The vaginal and urethral orifices can be seen inside the labia minora.

The hymen is a thin membrane that partially covers the vaginal orifice or introitus. It can be broken or avulsed by coitus, digital examination, tampon use, vigorous exercise, or surgery. Remnants of the hymen called caruncles remain after avulsion and form an irregular border around the vaginal orifice.

The paraurethral or Skene's glands are located on either side of the urethral meatus and drain the multiple urethral glands. The Bartholin's glands are located near the vaginal orifice on either side of the labia and secrete a lubricating mucus needed for intercourse. The Skene's and Bartholin's glands are usually not visible or palpable unless infected. If infected, the glands are enlarged, erythematous, and painful.

The perineum is the area between the vagina and anus. It is composed of muscles and subdermal and dermal tissue. It is the site for an episiotomy incision that is sometimes needed during labor and delivery.

Appearance of the external genitalia varies with age and development and can be quantified using the five stage Tanner scale. Before puberty, there is no pubic hair, and the labia minora are larger than the labia majora. Sexual maturation in

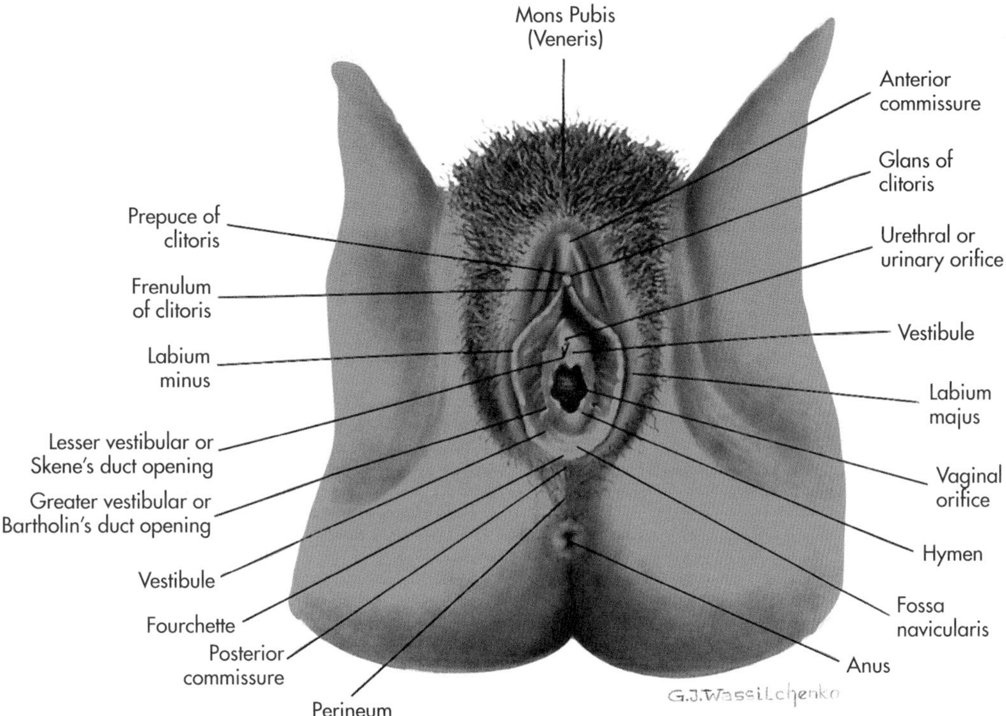

Figure 52-3 External female genitals.

girls usually begins between 8½ and 13 years of age. Physical changes include development of the breasts and pubic hair until adult proportions and distribution are established. With the onset of menopause and gradual withdrawal of hormones, the external genitalia atrophy, and the pubic hair begins to thin. In elderly women, the mons pubis is thinner secondary to the loss of the fat pad, and the clitoris and labia become smaller. See p. 1728 for reproductive physical changes related to aging.

Internal Structures

The female internal reproductive organs are shown in Figures 52-4 and 52-5. The internal reproductive organs are located in the true pelvis and remain there unless altered by a disease process, pregnancy, or sexual stimulation.

Vagina. The vagina is a soft, tubular structure that extends upward and back from the vaginal orifice to connect the vulva with the cervix and uterus. Located between the rectum and urethra, the vagina permits discharge of the menstrual flow, accommodates the penis during intercourse, contracts during orgasm, and is the passageway for childbirth. The length of the vaginal canal varies, and the posterior wall is longer (8 to 9 cm) than the anterior wall (6 to 8 cm).

The vagina is lined with pink mucous membrane arranged in transverse folds called rugae. The rugae make it possible for the vagina to distend and stretch during coitus and childbirth. The rugated appearance of the vaginal canal is prominent during adolescence and tends to disappear with multiparity and menopause. The length of the vagina shortens after menopause, and the vaginal mucosa becomes thin and dry because of the decrease in estrogen.

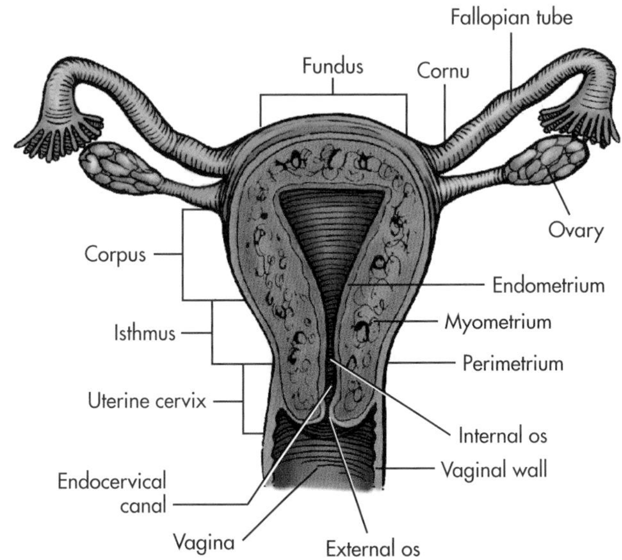

Figure 52-4 Lateral view of the internal female genitals.

The external os of the cervix projects into the upper vagina, creating a cup shape, and the vaginal walls end in a blind pouch around it called the fornix. The vaginal epithelium is continuous with the epithelium of the cervix. The cervix has the same pink color as the vaginal epithelium, but is smoother in texture. The position of the cervix varies somewhat and can be influenced by the position of the uterus.

The vagina is lubricated by transudation from its own cells and by secretions from the cervix and Bartholin's glands. Before puberty, the vaginal pH tends to be neutral (7.0). With the

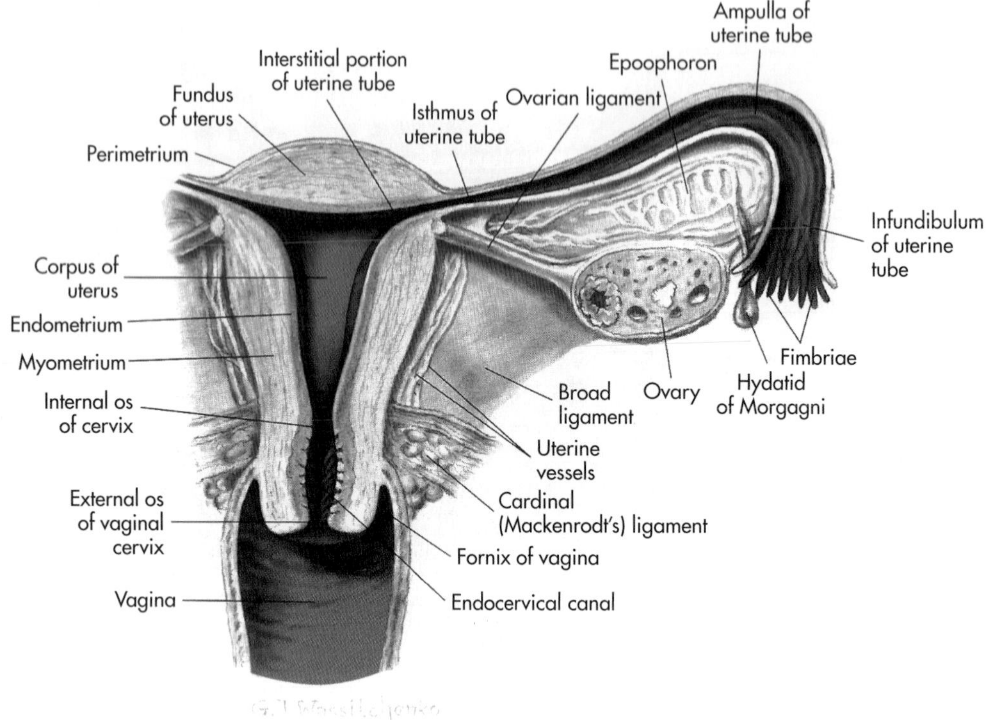

Figure 52-5 Cross section of uterus, adnexa, and upper vagina.

TABLE 52-1 Reproductive System Physical Changes That Occur at Puberty and Menopause

	Puberty	Menopause*
Breasts	Tissue increases	Tissue decreases, less elastic
Nipple and areola	More pronounced	Smaller, flatter
Mons pubis	More prominent, fat deposits	Thinner, loss of fat deposits
Pubic hair	Increases in texture and amount	Sparse, gray
Clitoris	More erectile	Smaller
Labia majora	Enlarges, thickens	Smaller
Labia minora	Enlarges	Thinner
Vaginal opening	1 cm	Smaller
Vaginal epithelial	Layers thicken	Thin, pale, fragile
Vaginal secretions	More acidic, increase	Less acidic, decrease
Vagina	Lengthens	Shortens
Uterus	Increases in size	Decreases in size
Endometrial lining	Thickens	Thins
Ovaries	Increase in size	Shrink to 1-2 cm, no longer palpable

*Changes may be influenced by hormone replacement therapy.

onset of puberty, the pH drops to 4.0 to 5.0. The vaginal secretions remain acidic throughout the reproductive years and become even more strongly acidic during pregnancy. Neutral or alkaline values are normally found in postmenopausal women. Acidity is strongly influenced by the estrogen concentration, which controls the glycogen levels of the cells. The normal vaginal flora, Döderlein's bacilli, interact with the secreted glycogen to produce lactic acid and maintain an acid pH.

The vaginal pH can be influenced by personal hygiene measures such as douches, deodorant tampons, and bubble baths or by pathogenic bacteria. Any increase in vaginal pH lessens the natural vaginal defenses and increases the risk of infection. See Table 52-1 for additional physical changes that occur at puberty and at menopause.

Uterus. The uterus is a hollow, muscular organ located between the urinary bladder and rectum. Its three sections are the fundus, corpus (body), and cervix. The fundus is the thick muscular region above the insertion of the fallopian tubes. The corpus is the main portion of the uterus joined to the cervix by an isthmus of constricted tissue. The cervix is the narrow lower segment. The external os extends into the vagina. The size of the uterus decreases from the fundus to the cervix, creating a triangular, pear-shaped appearance. The size of the uterus varies among women, ranging from 5.5 to 9 cm long, 3.5 to 6

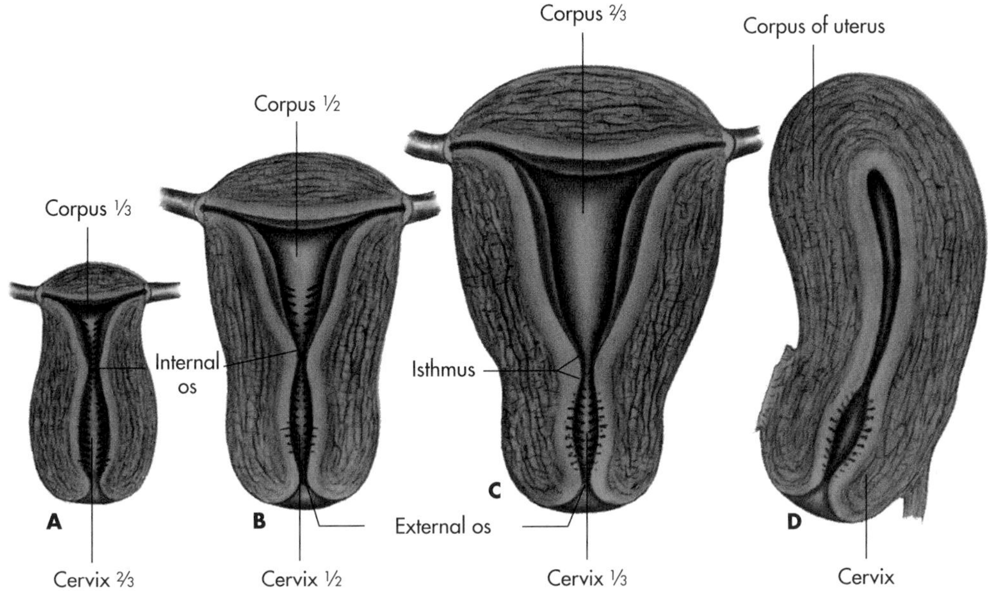

Figure 52-6 Comparative sizes of uteri at various stages of development. **A**, Prepubertal. **B**, Adult nulliparous. **C**, Adult multiparous. **D**, Lateral view, adult multiparous. The fractions give the relative proportion of the size of the corpus and the cervix.

cm wide, and 2 to 4 cm thick in nonparous women. All dimensions may be 2 to 3 cm larger in multiparous women (Figure 52-6).

The position of the uterus is subject to considerable variation. The uterus is usually anteverted and slightly anteflexed, although it may be retroverted, retroflexed, or in midposition. The body of the uterus is positioned over the bladder so that the fundus is behind the symphysis pubis. The uterus is in direct contact with the bladder and may also touch the rectum, sigmoid colon, and small intestines. The cervix curves forward. With sexual excitation, the uterus elevates into the false pelvis and contracts during orgasm. During pregnancy, the uterus changes in size, shape, structure, and position and then returns to its prepregnancy state within 6 to 8 weeks after delivery.

The outer surface of the uterus is covered by peritoneum, which is reflected from the abdominal wall. The anterior and posterior reflections of the peritoneum join at the sides to enclose the fallopian tubes and ovaries. Reflection of the peritoneum over the top of the pelvic organs creates spaces between the uterus and bladder anteriorly and the uterus and rectum posteriorly. The posterior space of the pelvic cavity is known as the cul-de-sac of Douglas and is a common entry site for culdoscopy, culpotomy, and surgical drainage.

The uterus has three functional layers. The perimetrium is the peritoneal and fascial outer layer that supports the uterus within the pelvis. The myometrium is the middle muscular layer which prevents the backflow of menstrual fluids, supports the developing fetus, and during labor, moves the term fetus toward the cervix. The endometrium is the inner lining of the uterus and responds to cyclic levels of estrogen and progesterone. The cavity of the uterus is continuous with the cervical canal and has an average fluid capacity of 3 to 8 ml. Near the fundus, the uterus opens into the lumen of the fallopian tubes. Thus a direct route exists from the vagina through the cervix, uterus, and fallopian tubes to the peritoneum.

The cervix is firm, smooth, and round. It is primarily made up of elastic and fibrous connective tissue and smooth muscle. The external os is located in the center of the vaginal portion of the cervix. Extending upward from the external os is the cervical canal, which averages 2 to 3 cm long. The cervical canal terminates as it joins the corpus. The junction of the cervical canal and the corpus is termed the internal cervical os. The cervix provides a channel for discharge of the menstrual flow, secretes mucus to facilitate the transport of sperm, and dilates during labor for the passage of the fetus.

Fallopian Tubes. The term adnexa refers to the fallopian tubes, ovaries, and supporting tissues. The fallopian tubes are two narrow, muscular canals ranging from 8 to 14 cm long. They function as the site for fertilization and transport of the ovum to the uterus. The fallopian tubes extend outward from the corpus near the fundus and are enclosed in the folds of the broad ligaments. The tubes are divided into four sections. The interstitial section lies within the myometrium. The isthmus is the narrow section extending from the fundus. The ampulla is the longer, middle section where fertilization usually occurs. The distal section is the infundibulum, which terminates in the fimbriae (Figure 52-5). The wavelike motion of the fimbriae encourages the ovum to enter the infundibulum. The walls of the fallopian tubes contain smooth muscles that possess peristaltic properties and are lined with a mucous membrane that contains cilia. At the time of ovulation, both peristaltic and ciliary actions increase and facilitate ovum transport.

Ovaries. The ovaries are endocrine glands as well as reproductive organs. The ovaries store primordial follicles, produce mature ova, and produce and secrete estrogen, progesterone, and androgens. The two almond-shaped ovaries, which are 3 to 4 cm long, 2 cm wide, and 1 to 2 cm thick, lie near the fimbriae of the fallopian tubes. They are partly enclosed by the broad ligaments. The innermost portion of the ovary is the medulla, which contains nerves and blood vessels.

The cortex, which is the outer layer of the ovary, is where primordial follicles are stored. Each follicle contains an undeveloped ovum that has the capacity to respond to stimulation by pituitary hormones. Each ovary contains an estimated 500,000 primordial follicles at birth. Unlike sperm, which are produced constantly, only one ovum normally matures at a time, and the process of ovum maturation requires an average of 28 days. When the ovum reaches maturity, it leaves the ovary by the process of ovulation. Many primordial follicles disintegrate before puberty, and the process of disintegration continues throughout the childbearing years. Few if any primordial follicles are found in the ovaries after menopause.

The ovaries undergo physical changes in position, size, and shape during the life span. At birth the ovaries are very small and are located in the false pelvis. Between infancy and puberty, the ovaries increase in size and descend into the true pelvis. During the childbearing years the ovaries appear long and flat and have a nodular surface caused by the presence of follicles. During pregnancy, the ovaries are lifted out of the pelvis by the enlarging uterus, but they descend back into the pelvis after childbirth. After menopause, the ovaries undergo rapid regressive changes, decrease in size, and become wrinkled. In most postmenopausal women, the ovaries are so small that they cannot be palpated during vaginal examination.

Pelvic Ligaments and Muscles

The internal and external reproductive structures are maintained in their positions by groups of ligaments and muscles. In the female, the broad, round, cardinal, ovarian, infundibulopelvic, pubocervical, and uterosacral ligaments support the uterus, ovaries, cervix, and vagina (Figure 52-5).

The levator ani and external anal sphincter muscles comprise the pelvic diaphragm or pelvic floor. The muscles of the perineum, located between the anus and vagina, commonly called the perineal body, reinforce the support provided by the levator ani muscles.

Blood, Lymph, and Nerve Supply

In males and females the organs of reproduction are supplied with blood from the aorta as it branches and divides into the internal iliac (hypogastric) artery with branches to the uterus and genitalia. The ovarian arteries branch off the aorta to furnish the ovaries with blood. The venous drainage empties into the vena cava. In both males and females, lymphatic drainage of the external and internal organs of reproduction is extensive, structurally follows much of the blood supply network, and includes the inguinal area.

Nerve supply is derived from both sympathetic and parasympathetic fibers of the autonomic nervous system. In the female, the pudendal nerve and its branches supply the majority of the motor and sensory fibers of the muscles and skin of the vulvar region. The pudendal nerve arises from the second, third, and fourth sacral roots. In the male, the motor segment of the pudendal nerve innervates the urinary sphincter, and the sensory portion supplies the glans penis and urethra.

Breasts

The paired female breasts or mammary glands, are accessory structures of the reproductive system meant to nourish the infant after birth (Figure 52-7). They are located between the second and sixth ribs, the edge of the sternum, and the midaxillary line. They develop in response to hormonal stimulation from the hypothalamus, pituitary gland, and ovaries.

The tissue of the breast has three primary components: an interconnected network of glandular and ductal tissue, fibrous tissue, and fat. The proportion of each tissue is a reflection of the individual woman's genetic make-up, age, obstetric history, and weight. The breast is supported by the suspensory ligaments of Cooper, which attach to the underlying muscles.

The nipple is the primary external structure of the breast and arises from the center of the pigmented areola and consists of erectile tissue responsive to sexual stimulation. Montgomery's glands are sebaceous glands that appear as small, round elevations on the areola. They are believed to secrete a fatty substance that offers some protection to the nipple during breastfeeding.

Internally each mature breast is composed of 15 to 25 lobes arranged radially around the breast and separated from each other by fatty tissue. Each lobe is composed of several lobules, which in turn are composed of numerous alveoli. Each alveolus is connected by a duct to a larger lactiferous duct from the lobule, which join to form one duct from each lobe and then converge at the nipple. Just before the nipple, the ducts expand into sinuses, which serve as reservoirs. The epithelial linings of the alveoli synthesize and secrete the components of breast milk in response to stimulation by prolactin from the pituitary.

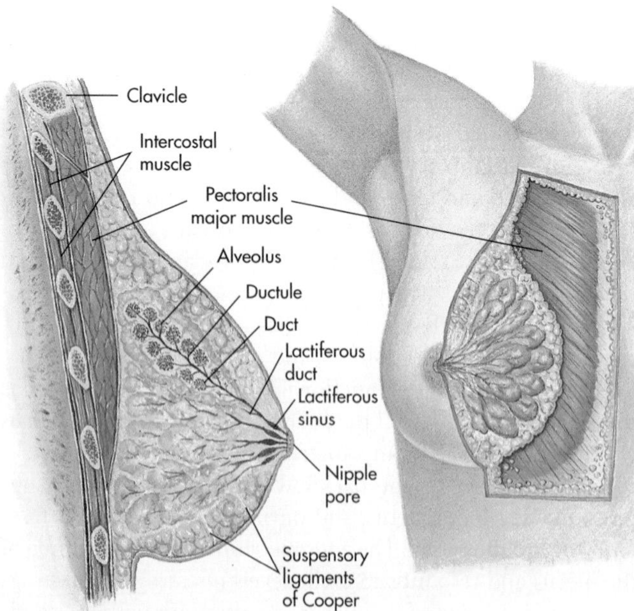

Figure 52-7 Anatomy of the breast, showing position and major structures.

The breasts receive an abundant blood supply from the internal mammary and lateral thoracic arteries. Their venous drainage connects to the superior vena cava. They contain an extensive lymph drainage network originating within the breast and draining radially into the axillary and subclavian nodal system. Drainage from the axillary region empties into the jugular and subclavian veins. This short and direct route assumes significance in the metastasis of breast cancer (Figure 52-8).

Many women experience noticeable changes in their breasts in response to the menstrual cycle. The breasts may enlarge and become tender or nodular in the premenstrual period in response to the increasing levels of estrogen and progesterone. The cellular growth regresses after menstruation, and water retention is relieved. See Table 52-1 for changes in the female reproductive system at puberty and at menopause.

Male Genital System

The male reproductive organs and associated structures are shown in Figure 52-9. The male reproductive organs produce sperm, suspend the sperm in a liquid, and deliver the

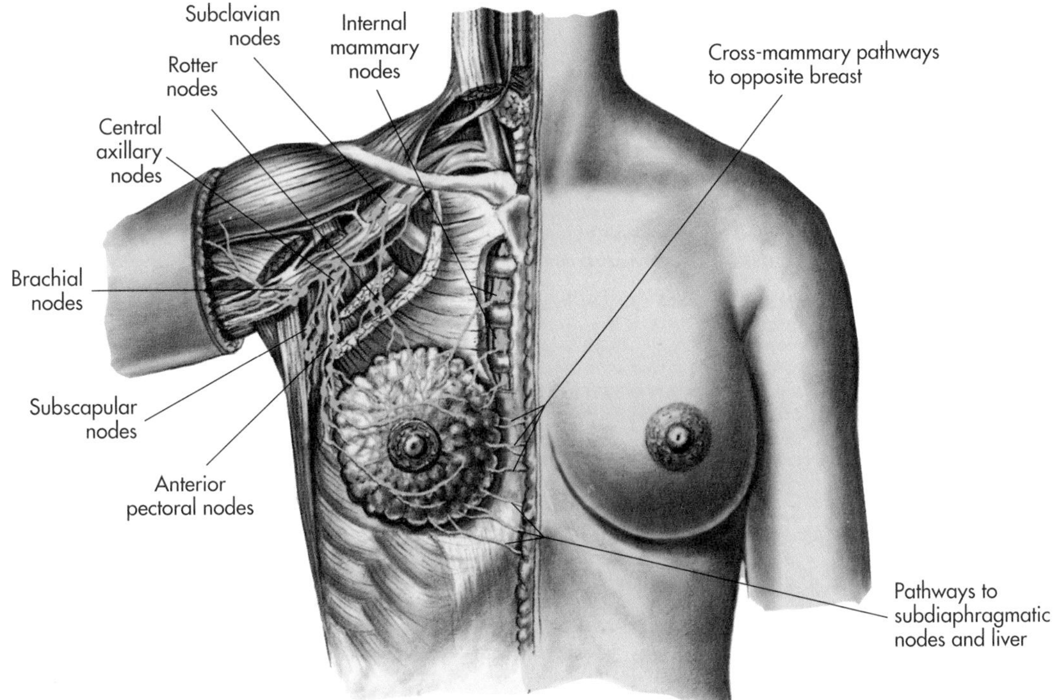

Figure 52-8 Lymphatic drainage of breast.

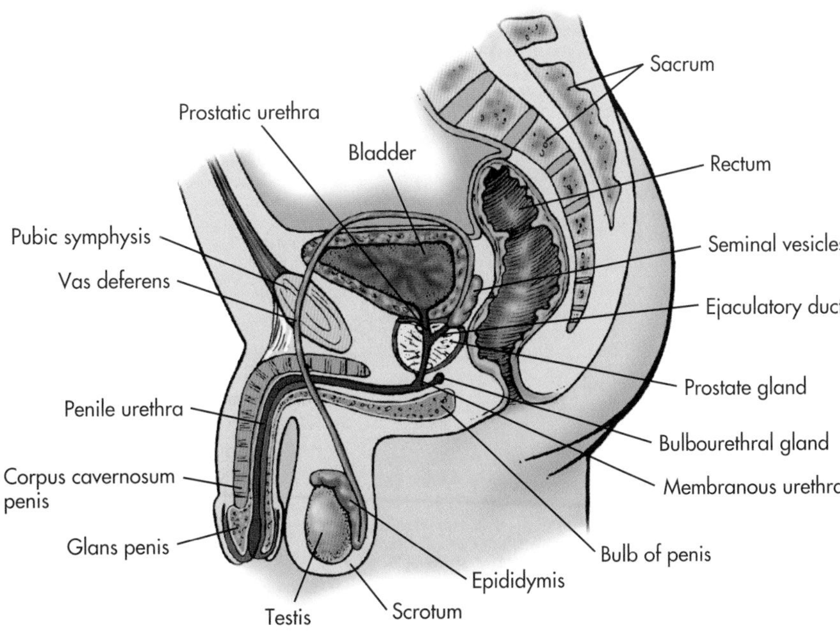

Figure 52-9 Male reproductive system: internal and external genitals.

sperm into the vagina to fertilize an ovum. They also secrete male hormones, the androgens. The male genitalia include the penis, scrotum, testes, epididymis, vas deferens, spermatic cord, seminal vesicles, prostate gland, and Cowper's glands.

External Structures

Penis. The penis is a conduit for elimination of ejaculate and urine through the urethral orifice. It includes the pendulous portion or corpus, and the perineal portion or radix (root). The penis consists of three erectile columns of cavernous tissue. The two corpora cavernosa form the dorsum and sides of the penis. The corpus spongiosum forms the ventral side. In the root of the penis, the spongiosum is bulbous and is called the bulb of the penis. The corpus spongiosum continues distally and expands at the end of the penis to the glands or balanus. The urethra is encircled by the corpus spongiosum, with a meatus at the distal end.

The glans covers the distal third of the corpus of the penis. The dorsum and lateral sides of the glans are called the corona. The dorsal surface of the glans meets the corpus in the neck of the penis or (retroglandular) sulcus.

The corpus of the penis is covered with a thin skin that contains no fat, is darker than body skin, and has redundant tissue, which allows for erection. In an uncircumcised male, the skin at the glans is folded over on itself to form the prepuce or foreskin.

Under the skin of the penis, the body of the penis is covered with the dartos layer, which is continuous with the fascia of the anterior abdominal wall, the scrotum, and the perineum. Contained within this layer are the superficial dorsal veins. The deep fascia of the penis, or Buck's fascia, contain the neurovascular bundle.

The root of the penis is attached to the abdominal wall through a thickening and extension of the dartos and Buck's fascia. In addition, the root is covered by the bulbocavernous muscle. This muscle also contains the perineal artery, vein, and nerve, and the pudendal artery, vein, and nerve.

The venous and arterial blood supply to the penis is complex. Several pairs of arteries supply blood (Figure 52-10), but the main arterial source is the internal pudendal artery, which branches to form the cavernous, bulbar, urethral, and dorsal arteries. These arteries continue to branch to form the vascular complex of the corpora cavernosa.

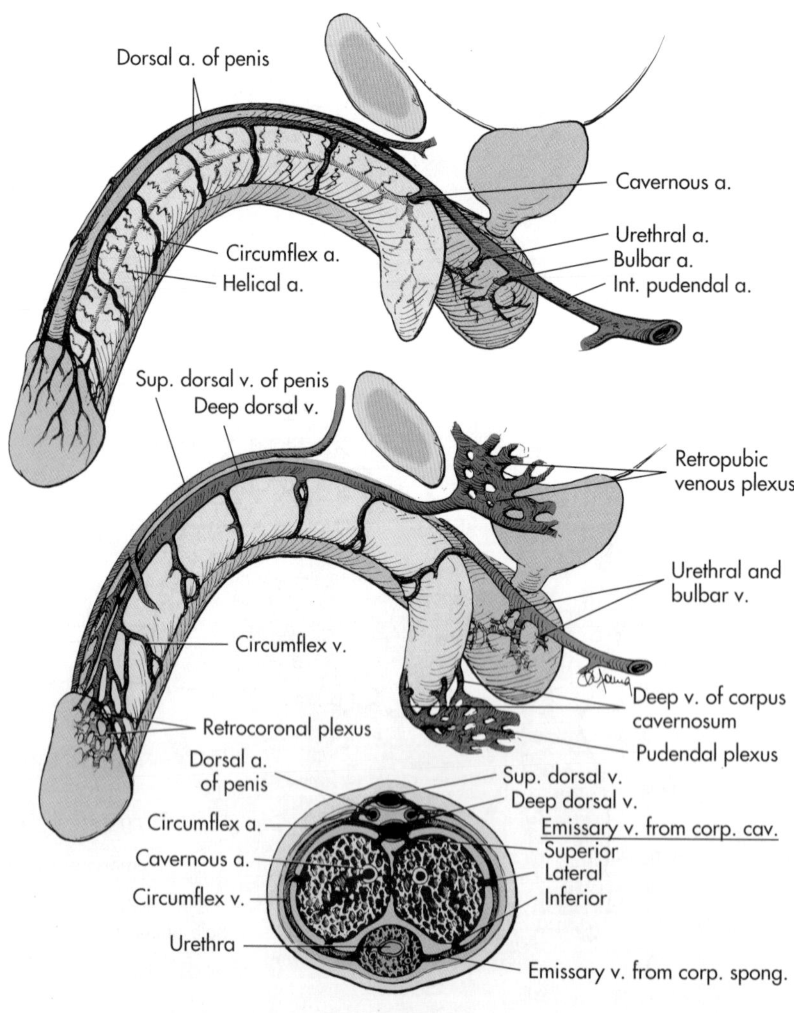

Figure 52-10 Illustration of vasculature of penis. *a*, artery; *v*, vein.

The venous drainage includes the superficial dorsal veins in the dartos tunic, the deep dorsal vein under Buck's fascia, and the deep or cavernous veins of the corpus cavernosum. The deep dorsal vein branches to form multiple circumflex veins. The corpus spongiosum is drained via the emissary veins through the urethral and bulbar veins, and the corpora cavernosa drain through the deep dorsal vein or cavernous veins.

For the penis to deposit sperm into the vagina, an erection must occur. The two types of erections are reflexogenic and psychogenic. Reflexogenic erections follow local stimulation, while psychogenic erections follow stimulation of erotic centers in the brain. Erection and ejaculation are mediated by the sympathetic nervous system, but the exact mechanism is unknown. During erection, the corpora cavernosa and the corpus spongiosum vascular spaces fill with blood, which transforms the penis into a firm organ permitting entry into the vagina.

Ejaculation is a two-part process: emission and ejaculation. In the first phase, secretions from the periurethral glands, seminal vesicle, and prostate move into the posterior urethra. Through peristalsis, sperm from the vas deferens is also moved into the posterior urethra.

During ejaculation, the internal sphincter of the bladder closes, the external urethral sphincter relaxes, and ejaculate is expelled by contraction of the perineal and bulbourethral muscles. The typical emission is 3 to 4 ml and contains fluid from the prostate and seminal vesicles and 200 to 400 million spermatozoa. After ejaculation, the penis returns to a flaccid state in 1 to 2 minutes.

Scrotum. The scrotum is a cutaneous pouch that covers and protects the testes and spermatic cords (Figure 52-11). Because the testes are surrounded by serous membrane and are suspended in the cavity of the scrotum, the testes are capable of being moved about readily. The ease of movement within the scrotum protects the testes against injury.

The skin of the scrotum is thin, brownish, and very elastic because it contains rugae. Because of the rugae, the scrotum distends readily and may become greatly enlarged when edema is present. The scrotal skin is covered by thinly scattered hair and contains sebaceous follicles. The surface of the scrotum is divided into two halves by a ridge (raphe) that extends anteriorly to the undersurface of the penis and posteriorly along the midline of the perineum to the anus. Internally, a septum divides the scrotum into two halves, each containing a testis and its epididymis and portion of spermatic cord. The left side of the scrotum normally hangs lower than the right side because the left spermatic cord is longer.

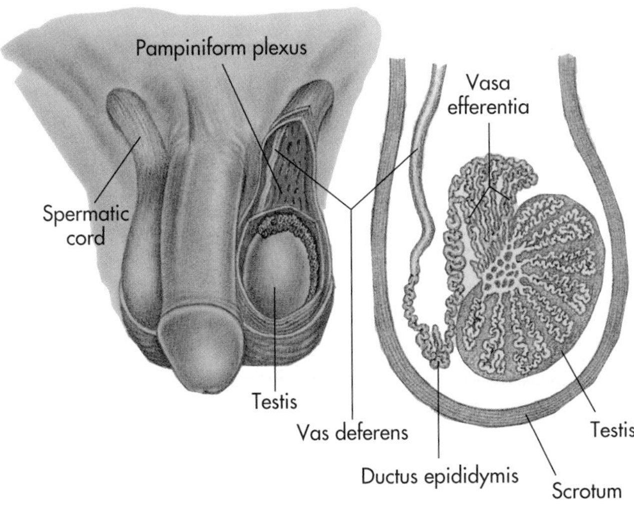

Figure 52-11 Scrotum and its contents.

The external appearance of the scrotum varies under different conditions. In warm temperatures and in older or debilitated men, the scrotum becomes elongated and flat. In young, healthy men and in cool temperatures, the scrotum appears short and more wrinkled.

Internal Structures

Testes. The oval-shaped testis is the essential organ of reproduction in the male. During fetal life, the testes are located in the abdominal cavity behind the peritoneum. Two to 3 months before birth the testes descend through the inguinal canals and inguinal rings into the scrotum and are suspended in position by the spermatic cords, which are attached to the posterior borders of the testes. This process is stimulated by the increased secretion of testosterone by the testes. At the lateral edge of each spermatic cord is the epididymis, which appears as a narrow flattened structure (Figure 52-11).

The testes are composed of glandular tissue covered by fibrous tissue. The glandular tissue is composed of many lobules differing in size according to their location. Each lobule consists of 600 to 1200 small, convoluted structures, the seminiferous tubules that produce the sperm, and spermatozoa in different stages of development can be seen along the cells of the tubules.

After puberty, the lining of the seminiferous tubules forms sperm continually. In a young man sperm are produced at a rate of 120 million/day. Each mature sperm has a whiplike tail that makes free movement possible, but the sperm are passive within the testes. The fluids produced within the seminal vesicles and prostate gland suspend the sperm and cause them to become active and motile.

In addition to producing sperm, the testes function as an endocrine gland. Production of androgens by the testes is stimulated by gonadotropin-releasing hormone (GnRH) from the hypothalamus. GnRH stimulates the anterior pituitary gland to secrete luteinizing hormone (LH) and follicle-stimulating hormone (FSH). LH stimulates testosterone production in the testes. FSH stimulates sperm development. The testes produce testosterone, dihydrotestosterone, and androstenedione. Testosterone is produced in much greater amounts than the other hormones and is therefore considered the most important testicular hormone.

Increased testosterone production at puberty causes several changes in the male body. These include an increase in the size of the penis and scrotum, hair growth on the pubis and face, and a deepening of the voice. The five-stage Tanner scale is used to quantify changes in secondary sex characteristics. See Box 52-1 for physical changes in males related to testosterone.

BOX 52-1 Physical Changes in Males Related to Testosterone

- Eightfold increase in the size of penis, scrotum, and testes
- Enlargement of larynx and deepening of voice
- Increased skin thickness
- Increased secretion of sebaceous glands, may cause acne
- 50% increase in muscle mass
- Thickening of bones
- Narrowing of pelvis, with greater strength
- 10% increase in basal metabolic rate
- Increase in red blood cells

Epididymis/Vas Deferens. The comma-shaped epididymis is located at the lateral edge of the posterior segment of the testes where it creates a bulge (see Figure 52-11). Newly formed sperm enter into the epididymis, which in turn empties into the vas deferens. The vas deferens serves as the excretory duct of the testes, is a constituent of the spermatic cord, and separates from the spermatic cord at the inguinal ring. Although the testes form the sperm, only a small number are stored in the epididymis. The majority of sperm are stored in the acidic environment of vas deferens, and although inactive, they stay viable for about 1 month. After taking a complex path through the pelvis, the vas deferens descends, enters the base of the prostate gland, becomes greatly narrowed, and joins the ducts of the seminal vesicles to form the ejaculatory duct.

Spermatic Cords. The spermatic cords extend from the deep inguinal rings and consist of arteries, veins, lymphatics, nerves, and the excretory duct of the testes held together by the spermatic fascia (see Figure 52-11). At the deep inguinal rings the structures of the spermatic cords converge with the structures of the testes, pass through the inguinal canals, emerge through the superficial inguinal rings, and pass downward into the scrotum.

Seminal Vesicles. The seminal vesicles are two lobulated, membranous pouches, 5 to 10 cm long, located between the bladder and the rectum (see Figure 52-9). They secrete fluid that is added to the secretions of the testes. This alkaline fluid contains fructose, citric acid, prostaglandins, and fibrinogen, which add to the bulk of the ejaculate. The fructose provides nutrients to the ejaculated sperm; the prostaglandins react with cervical mucus in the female to make it more receptive and probably help to propel the sperm to the fallopian tubes.

The lower end of each seminal vesicle becomes constricted into a straight duct and joins the vas deferens to form the ejaculatory duct. The ejaculatory duct begins at the base of the prostate gland, runs posteriorly and downward, and enters the prostate gland in the midline. In the prostate gland, the ejaculatory duct opens into the prostatic portion of the urethra.

Prostate Gland. The prostate gland is located below the internal urethral orifice, behind the symphysis pubis, and close to the rectal wall, extending around the beginning of the urethra (see Figure 52-9). Enveloped in a firm adherent capsule, the prostate gland grows to the size and shape of a walnut during puberty and weighs about 20 g. Internally, the prostate gland is partly muscular and partly glandular. The glandular substance consists of numerous follicular pouches that open into long canals and join to form 12 to 20 small excretory ducts. Prostatic ducts open into the prostatic portion of the urethra, thus adding the prostatic secretion to the seminal fluid. The prostatic secretion is a thin, white fluid that helps raise the pH of the fluid from the vas deferens and enhance motility and fertility of the sperm. Another substance secreted by the prostate gland is acid phosphatase.

Cowper's (Bulbourethral) Glands. Cowper's (bulbourethral) glands are two small, round bodies located at the sides and to the back of the membranous portion of the urethra (Figure 52-9). Each gland has an excretory duct that opens into the urethra. The main excretory duct of a Cowper's gland represents the joining of many ducts from its internal glandular tissue. Cowper's glands secrete an alkaline substance into the semen to counteract vaginal and urethral acidity.

Endocrine Functions

Male Hormones

In males andrenarche refers to the increased secretion of the androgenic hormones at puberty, which results in the appearance of secondary sex characteristics and production of mature sperm. Testosterone is the androgen most closely related to reproduction, because it specifically stimulates maturation of sperm and is responsible for maintaining the reproductive organs in a functional state. Testosterone secretion is closely related to pituitary gland function. The rate of secretion of testosterone is determined by levels of LH in the blood. Testosterone levels show temporary elevations during the fetal and neonatal periods with peak levels seen during adolescence.

Female Hormones

The major hormones produced by the ovaries are estrogen and progesterone. The ovaries produce three different forms of estrogen. Estriol is produced during pregnancy. Estradiol is produced in the ovulatory follicle and is the primary estrogen of premenopausal women. The third form, estrone, is a byproduct of the metabolism of estradiol and is also produced and held in adipose tissue. Estrogen is responsible for the development of secondary sex characteristics at puberty. After puberty estrogen primarily causes development of the endometrium in preparation for implantation of a fertilized ovum. Progesterone enhances the action of estrogen on the endometrium. The ovaries depend on stimulation from the pituitary hormones FSH and LH to fulfill their functions.

Menstruation

Menarche is the term used to designate the onset of menstruation, and it reflects the time when reproduction is first possible. The onset of menarche varies with age, heredity, general health, weight, and nutritional status and cannot be accurately predicted. The average age at menarche has decreased significantly over the past 100 years and is now 12.5 years, with a normal range from 10.5 to 14.5 years. It is believed that a percentage of body fat (17%) must be attained for the average girl to reach menarche.

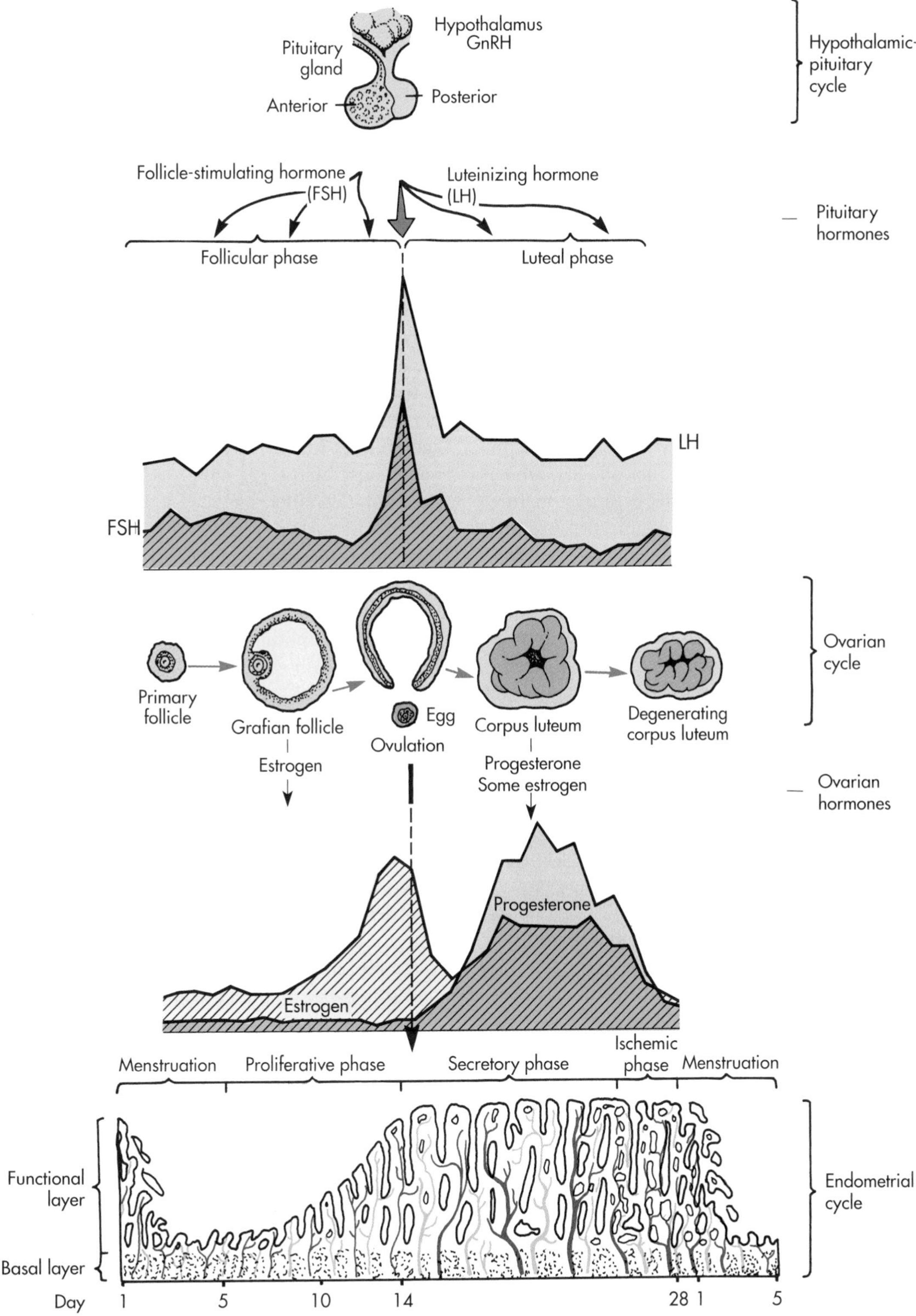

Figure 52-12 Menstrual cycle: hypothalamic-pituitary, ovarian, and endometrial.

Menstrual Cycle. The menstrual cycle includes a complex series of uterine and ovarian changes that result in menstruation. The uterine cycle includes the menstrual, proliferative, and secretory phases that correspond to specific phases of the ovarian cycle as illustrated in Figure 52-12. Both cycles require an average of 28 days. The first day of menstrual flow is considered to be the first day of the menstrual cycle. Normal variation exists in the intervals between menstrual periods, but most cycles occur within a range of 26 to 36 days and last for 3 to 7 days. The greatest variance typically occurs during the perimenarchal and perimenopausal years. The smooth functioning of the menstrual cycle depends on complex relationships among the hypothalamus in the central nervous system, anterior pituitary, ovaries, and uterus.

Menstrual Phase. During the menstrual phase of the cycle, the endometrium breaks down and is shed. The production of estrogen and progesterone stops before the onset of menstrual flow, which results in rupture of uterine capillaries and necrosis of endometrial tissue. The menstrual phase of the cycle lasts an average of 4 days. Menstrual fluid does not clot unless it is retained in the uterus or vagina for a prolonged time. It is believed that the endometrium produces an anticoagulant that prevents the clotting of blood in the uterus.

Proliferative Phase. When menstruation ceases, the proliferative phase begins, extends over the next 14 days, and ends with ovulation. During the proliferative (ovarian follicular) phase, the hypothalamus releases GnRH, which signals the pituitary gland to secrete increasing amounts of FSH, which stimulates a primordial follicle to develop into a mature graafian follicle containing a mature ovum. Because the graafian follicle produces estrogen, FSH is essential for estrogen production. While increasing in size, the graafian follicle moves toward the surface of the ovary, where it appears as a blisterlike structure. Finally, the graafian follicle ruptures (ovulation), allowing the ovum to enter the fallopian tube and be carried in the direction of the uterus.

As the graafian follicle matures, it secretes increasing amounts of estrogen. Estrogen causes the endometrium to become thicker and softer as it prepares for implantation of a fertilized ovum. Estrogen also causes the cervical mucus to increase in quantity and attain a clear, elastic state that permits sperm to enter the cervix more readily. The high level of estrogen also suppresses pituitary release of FSH and triggers release of LH. A sharp rise in LH levels occurs 12 to 24 hours before ovulation, followed by a peak level about 8 hours after ovulation.

On the day of ovulation, about 25% of women experience pain in the lower abdomen on the side of ovulation. This pain is referred to as mittelschmerz and is probably a result of peritoneal irritation from follicular fluid or blood released from the ovary with the ovum.

Secretory Phase. The proliferative phase ends with ovulation and the secretory phase begins, lasting for approximately 10 to 14 days. The secretory (ovarian luteal) phase is the least variable part of the menstrual cycle. Irregular menstrual cycles are usually related to variations in the menstrual or proliferative phases.

Under the influence of LH, the corpus luteum forms in the ovary at the site of the ruptured graafian follicle and produces progesterone. Progesterone further alters the endometrium by stimulating growth of cells and circulation of blood to the uterus. With these additional endometrial changes, the uterine environment is prepared for implantation of a fertilized ovum.

If pregnancy occurs, the corpus luteum remains secretory by the action of human chorionic gonadotropin, which the placental cells produce within 1 week of conception. By 6 to 8 weeks after conception, the placenta is developed and assumes the function of secreting progesterone to maintain the endometrium. If pregnancy does not occur, the corpus luteum degenerates in about 10 days, progesterone secretion drops significantly, and the endometrium degenerates; menstruation results, and the cycle begins again.

Menopause. The medical term menopause refers to a single, specific physical event in a woman's life—the occurrence of the final menstrual period; however, research has expanded to include the entire perimenopausal period, which may extend from age 35 to as old as 60 years of age. This is the period in which physical changes can be clearly linked to altered levels of hormones. Natural menopause may occur in women between the ages of 35 and 60 years of age. The average age is 49 to 51 years in Western societies. This average has remained quite stable over time, despite fairly significant changes in the average age of onset for menstruation: 25% of all women experience menopause before age 45, 50% between 45 and 50 years of age, and 25% after age 50. Factors influencing the onset of menopause include genetic differences in the estrogen receptors and current smoking status. Menopause may be artificially induced by surgical removal or irradiation of the ovaries, severe infections, and the effects of alkylating chemotherapeutic agents. The removal of the uterus, hysterectomy, results in a cessation of menses but does not itself result in menopause, as long as the ovaries are left intact.

Changes during the perimenopausal period are primarily related to a gradual decline in ovarian production of estrogen. Over a period of years, the menses become more scanty and may become irregular or spaced further apart until they eventually stop. Estrone is the primary postmenopausal estrogen and has a potency of only one-tenth that of estradiol. Cellular estrogen receptors are found in organs throughout the body, so a decline in estrogen triggers a wide variety of potential symptoms. The intensity of symptoms is thought to be related to the rapidity of changes in estrogen level and may be mediated somewhat by the fat content of the body. Women with higher fat stores in their bodies retain a storage pool of estrogen to buffer them through the early transition period. Commonly reported symptoms of the perimenopausal period are summarized in Box 52-2.

Physiologic Changes With Aging

The major physiologic changes that occur in the female reproductive tract with aging are related to the process of menopause. When ovulation ceases the production of progesterone is halted, and estrogen levels decrease. These two primary hormone changes are responsible for most aging-related changes in the uterus, ovaries, and vagina. The ovaries begin to atrophy around age 40 and become nonpalpable within 3 to 5 years of menopause. The uterus decreases in size. The vagina decreases in width and length, and the entrance narrows. The mucosal lining becomes thinner, and vaginal secretions are diminished. Externally the mons pubis decreases in fullness and the labia majora and minora decrease in size. Pubic hair becomes thinner and turns gray or white. Muscle weakness in the pelvis can lead to cystocele, rectocele, or uterine prolapse and may cause problems related to stress incontinence.

BOX 52-2 Common Perimenopausal Symptoms

Vasomotor

Hot flashes
Hot flushes
Perspiration
Palpitations

Vaginal

Dryness
Vulvar itching or burning
Dyspareunia

Menstrual

Irregular uterine bleeding
Shorter or longer cycles
Missed periods

Urinary

Frequency or urgency
Stress incontinence
Urinary tract infections

Psychologic

Sleep disorders/insomnia
Irritability
Mood swings
Depression
Anxiety

Other

Weight gain
Skin changes
Sensory changes
Osteoporosis
Joint pain
Headache

The woman's capacity for sexual response, however, remains intact.

The primary changes in the male reproductive tract during the climacteric are also related to variations in hormone level. After peaking in adolescence, testosterone levels decline throughout adulthood and appear to level off around age 60. This causes a decrease in the size and firmness of the penis and testes. The scrotum is more pendulous in appearance and has fewer rugae. Although some spermatogenesis continues throughout life, the seminal fluid decreases in amount and force of ejaculation decreases. The prostate gland typically hypertrophies and creates problems with urinary retention. The pelvic muscles decrease in strength and the pubic hair thins and turns gray or white. The capacity for sexual response remains intact in healthy men and fertility, although diminished, does continue.

HEALTH HISTORY

Information about the patient's sexuality, sexual activity, and genitourinary functioning may be gathered as a part of a complete health history or during an episodic examination. Assessment of the reproductive system can be uncomfortable for both the nurse and patient. It is important to examine one's own attitudes about the various ways people express their sexuality so that personal prejudices do not interfere with patient care. As with any nursing history, questions should be asked in a nonjudgmental manner, using open-ended and focused questions. Attention to supportive nonverbal communication is also important. The interview should take place before the patient undresses for the physical examination.

Chief Complaint

Information may be organized through a review of systems or by a history of the chief complaint with a system review. For example, a sexually transmitted disease (STD) can mimic a urinary tract infection; therefore information about both the urinary and reproductive systems is important. Begin the interview with open questions. Record the chief complaint in the patient's own words. Follow-up with focused questions to assess the critical characteristics of the symptoms including onset, duration, location, character/quality, quantity/severity, timing, setting, aggravating or relieving factors, associated factors, and the patient's perception of the problem.

BOX 52-3 Sample Abuse Screening

1. Have you ever experienced unwanted touching or sexual experiences in childhood?
   Yes ☐
   No ☐
2. Have you ever been forced or pressured to have sex when you did not want to?
   Yes ☐
   No ☐
3. Have you ever been hit, kicked, slapped, pushed, or shoved by your boyfriend, husband, or partner?
   Yes ☐
   No ☐

Sexuality and Sexual Activity

It is best to incorporate questions about intimate relationships and sexual activity as part of the genitourinary and gynecologic portions of an annual health assessment or during evaluation of specific complaints in these areas. Open-ended questions that can be helpful include: "What concerns do you have about your sexual functioning?" and "What changes have you experienced in your sexual relationships in the past 6 months?" and, if appropriate, "How has your illness affected your sexual relationship?" Sexual preference can be determined by asking, "What is your sexual preference?" Satisfaction with intimate relationships can also be assessed with a focused question such as the following: "How satisfied are you with your sexual relationships?" Determine if a patient is currently sexually active, practices safer sex behaviors, or has recently changed sexual partners. Record the number of current and past sexual partners to determine risk status for STDs. Although the risk of exposure to STDs certainly increases with the number of partners, sexual activity with one partner in a nonmonogamous relationship also carries risk.

Screening for childhood or adult sexual abuse or sexual assault needs to be a routine part of the health history, as the incidence is estimated to range from 12% to 40%. Screening questions/tools should be a part of all documentation systems. Survivors of childhood sexual abuse can present with a variety of symptoms related to the reproductive system including chronic pelvic pain and sexual dysfunction such as dyspareunia, nonspecific vaginitis, vaginismus, fear of intimacy, lack of enjoyment, and compulsive promiscuity. Having a vaginal, pelvic, or prostate examination may be especially traumatic for adult survivors of sexual abuse. Including questions that address issues of abuse in assessment tools ensures that these issues are not excluded or missed. See Box 52-3 for sample abuse assessment questions that can be adapted for use with male patients. Document any areas of injury on a body map in the patient record.

Female Genitourinary Assessment

Genitourinary health histories for women generally include data about the urinary system, menstruation, sexual activity, contraceptive use, pregnancies, and history of gynecologic problems or surgeries. Although not part of the reproductive system, breast health is usually assessed during a routine gynecologic visit. The assessment interview must be tailored to the patient's age. For example, middle-aged women can be questioned about perimenopausal symptoms, whereas older women should be screened for postmenopausal bleeding and incontinence.

Screening for proper use of contraceptives can be easily accomplished during the assessment. The method of contraception used and the patient's satisfaction with the method need to be assessed. Screening for common complications or serious side effects is also possible. The following outline summarizes the interview items, symptoms, and health promotion activities to be included in the assessment.

Female Breast and Genitourinary History

- Current breast health
- Problems with breasts
  - Pain/tenderness
  - Lumps
  - Skin dimpling
  - Lesions or changes in the skin
  - Discharge from the nipples
- Current genitourinary health
- Urinary symptoms including infections and voiding dysfunction
  - Dysuria
  - Frequency
  - Urgency
  - Hematuria
  - Nocturia
  - True incontinence (loss of urine without warning)
  - Stress incontinence (loss of urine with cough or sneeze)
- Menstrual history
  - Age at menarche (first menses)
  - Last menstrual period
  - Interval or frequency; regular or irregular
  - Duration
  - Menstrual flow: light, medium, or heavy (number of pads or tampons used in a specified time period)
  - Menorrhagia (increased amount or duration of flow)
  - Dysmenorrhea (pain with menstruation): frequency and severity
  - Bleeding between periods
  - Postcoital bleeding (bleeding after intercourse)
  - Postmenopausal bleeding: essential to assess for any bleeding since menopause to screen for endometrial cancer
  - Premenstrual syndrome symptoms: irritability, depression, weight gain, headaches, breast tenderness, and breast swelling
- Obstetric history
  - Number of pregnancies (gravida)
  - Pregnancy outcomes
    - Term: number of births between 37 and 42 weeks of pregnancy
    - Premature: number of births before 37 weeks of pregnancy
    - Abortions: spontaneous or elective
    - Living: number of living children
  - Types of deliveries: vaginal, forceps, vacuum, or cesarean
  - Complications of pregnancies
- Perimenopausal symptoms
  - Hot flashes/flushes
  - Headaches
  - Night sweats
  - Vaginal dryness
  - Mood swings
  - Numbness and tingling
- Vulvovaginal problems
  - Discharge: color, amount, and odor
  - Vaginal itching
  - Lesions or lumps
  - Dyspareunia (pain with intercourse)
  - Vaginismus (spasms of muscles around vagina)
  - History of STDs
- Sexual health
  - Sexually active: monogamous versus multiple partners, male/female/both
  - Types of sexual activity
  - Satisfaction with or problems related to sexual activity
  - Changes in ability to engage in sex: vaginal dryness, loss of libido, female sexual arousal disorder, inhibited orgasm, or pain with intercourse
- Health promotion practices
  - Contraceptive choice, barrier protection, proper use of method, satisfaction, and side effects
  - Pelvic examinations: date of last Pap smear and results
  - Breast self-examination (technique and frequency)
  - Vulva self-examination
  - Date of last mammogram and results
  - Nutritional patterns, intake of folic acid
  - Personal hygiene: douche, bubble baths, use of tampons, and feminine sprays
  - Smoking cessation efforts
  - Use of complementary and alternative products or practices
  - Immunization status
- Family history
  - Breast cancer
  - Cervical, ovarian, or endometrial cancer
  - History of exposure to diethylstilbestrol (DES)

Male Genitourinary Assessment

A male genitourinary history includes current health status as well as past medical history. Depending on the age of the patient, the interview can be tailored to screen for specific age-related problems. For example, prostate enlargement occurs in older men, and therefore it is necessary to screen for factors such as urinary retention, straining, and hesitancy. Data can be collected about the bladder, kidney function, the penis and testes, possible hernias, sexual health, and health promotion activities. The following outline summarizes symptoms and health-promotion behaviors to be included in the assessment.

Male Genitourinary History

- Current genitourinary health status
- Urinary symptoms relating to infections, voiding dysfunction, or prostate problems
  - Dysuria (pain with urination)
  - Frequency
  - Urgency
  - Hematuria
  - Nocturia
  - Urinary retention
  - Straining
  - Hesitancy
  - Change in force/caliber of stream
  - Dribbling
  - History of prostate problems
  - History of urinary tract infections
- Incontinence
  - True (loss of urine without warning)
  - Stress (loss of urine with cough/sneeze)
- Problems with the penis such as skin lesions, cancer, or STDs
  - Pain
  - Lesions or sores
  - Discharge
  - History of STDs
- Problems with testes such as torsion, cancer, or infection and problems with the scrotum such as hydrocele, hernia, or varicocele
  - Lump or swelling in testes
  - Bulge or swelling in scrotum
  - Change in size of scrotum
  - History of hernia
- Sexual health
  - Sexually active: monogamous versus multiple partners, male/female/both
  - Types of sexual activity
  - Satisfaction with or problems related to sexual activity
  - Changes in ability to engage in sex: erectile dysfunction, premature ejaculation, loss of libido
- Health-promotion practices
  - Contraceptive choice, barrier protection, proper use of method, satisfaction, and side effects
  - Prostate examination: date of last examination and results
  - Testicular self-examination (technique and frequency)
  - Smoking cessation efforts
  - Use of complementary and alternative products or practices
  - Immunization status

PHYSICAL EXAMINATION

Physical examination of the breasts or genitourinary system may cause embarrassment for the patient. Before the examination it is important to inquire if the patient has previously had an examination of this nature. The procedure is explained, and any questions answered before the patient is undressed and on the examination table. If this is the first breast, pelvic, testicular, or prostate examination, ignorance about the process may also cause fear. Take the time to explain the process, review normal anatomy, and teach self-examination of the breasts or testes. Pictures, three-dimensional anatomic models, and examples of equipment such as a speculum aid in the educational process. Models of the pelvic organs and pamphlets assist with the presentation of information about the purpose of the pelvic or prostate examination, what is done, and what to expect.

Breast Examination

Female Breast

In a menstruating female, the ideal time to examine the breasts is several days after menstruation when they are less tender and nodular. In nonmenstruating females the timing of the examination is less important. Examination of the breasts begins with inspection of the skin and areola. The examination should be performed in both the sitting and supine position. See Figure 52-13 for patient positions during breast examination.

With the woman's hands at her sides, inspect the breasts for symmetry and the skin for dimpling, puckering, scaling, scars, or discharge from the nipples. A dimple, pucker, or retraction in breast tissue may indicate an underlying chest wall lesion. Scaly skin or nipple tissue can be seen in eczema of the breast or Paget's disease. While the woman slowly raises her hands over her head, observe for signs of retractions. Ask the woman to put her hands on her waist and flex her shoulders and elbows. Observe for puckering or retractions and for symmetric movement. Women with large breasts should lean forward. The breast should move smoothly without signs of adhesions to the chest wall.

The breasts and axilla can be palpated in both sitting and supine positions. Bimanual palpation of large breasts is easily accomplished while the patient is sitting. It should be repeated in a supine position. Before the patient lies down, palpate the supraclavicular and axillary lymph nodes for size, shape, mobility, or tenderness. The majority of the breast lymphatics drain toward the axilla.

When the patient is supine, place a small pillow or towel under the shoulder of the breast to be examined. Ask the woman to raise her arm over her head, as this helps flatten the breast tissue. The breast can be palpated in a circular, spokes of a wheel, vertical, or horizontal pattern (Figure 52-14). The breast tissue is systematically palpated at three different depths using the pads of three fingers. It is important to palpate the entire breast, including the tail of Spence in the upper outer quadrant near the axilla. The consistency of the breast tissue and the presence of any tenderness, lumps, or nodules are noted. If a nodule is identified, its location, size in centimeters, shape, and consistency are noted. After the examination, instruct the woman in breast self-examination.

The nipple is palpated for underlying masses or tumors, and is gently squeezed to check for masses or discharge. A milky discharge may be related to pregnancy, lactation, hormones, or

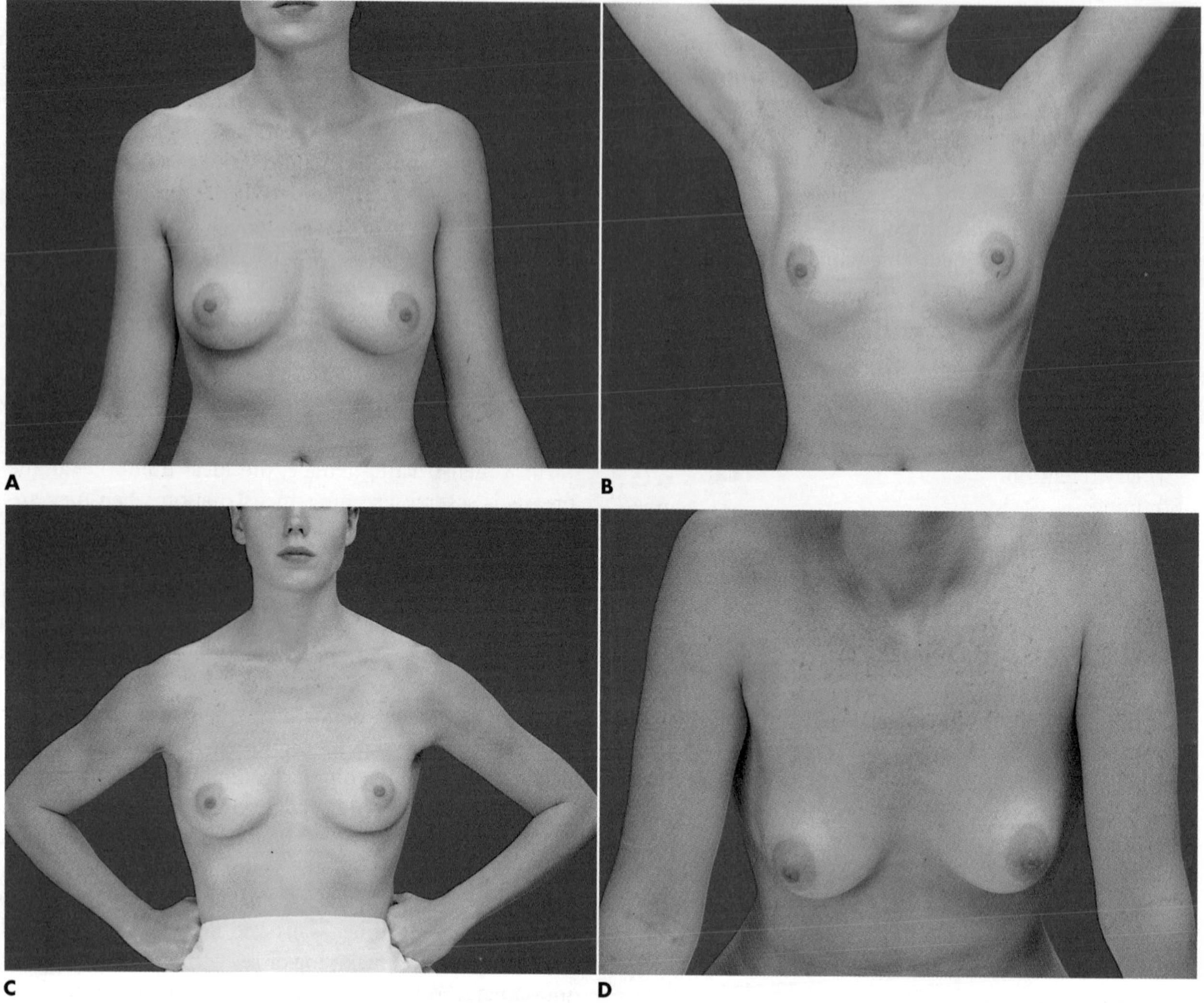

Figure 52-13 Patient positions during breast self-examination. Note the distribution of breast tissue in the different positions. **A,** Patient position at start of examination: sitting with arms at sides. **B,** Arms over the head position. **C,** Patient with arms lowered and hands pressed against hips. **D,** Forward leaning position, typically used for patient with large, pendulous breasts.

drugs. A nonmilky discharge may indicate a pathologic condition. The process is then repeated on the opposite breast.

Male Breast

The male breast can be easily and quickly examined during a routine physical examination. Although rare, breast cancer does occur in males, most frequently in the areolar area. The examination is initiated with inspection of the skin and areolae. The presence of any swelling, retractions, or lesions is noted. The breast, areola, and axilla are then palpated for masses.

Abdominal Examination

Physical assessment of the reproductive organs includes a standard assessment of the lower abdomen (see Chapter 31). Any localized areas of prominence are noted, as these may indicate enlargement of the reproductive organs or adjacent structures. The skin of the abdomen and pubic area is inspected for amount, distribution, and character of hair; abnormal pigmentation; and lesions. Abdominal muscle tone is assessed by having the patient cough or raise the head.

Auscultation of the abdomen for bowel sounds and bruits should precede palpation. After auscultation, percussion of the abdomen is completed to identify any enlarged organ, tumor, or masses. A tumor, such as an ovarian cyst or uterine myoma, produces a dull, flat, tone. Because the reproductive organs in the female are normally situated in the pelvic cavity, they are usually not palpable through the abdominal wall unless enlarged with pregnancy. Abdominal palpation is performed to rule out or discover abnormalities. If an abdominal mass is felt, its position, size, shape, consistency, contour, tenderness, movability, and relationship to any pelvic or abdominal organ are described.

Enlargement of the uterus is detected by palpating in the midline of the lower abdomen. Palpation is started just below the umbilicus and continued in the direction of the symphysis pubis. In contrast with a full bladder, which feels soft, an enlarged uterus feels firm and may be round or asymmetric. A firm, isolated area of enlargement may be caused by the presence of a tumor of the uterus.

Enlargement of the fallopian tubes and ovaries may be detected by palpation of the right and left lower quadrants. Even

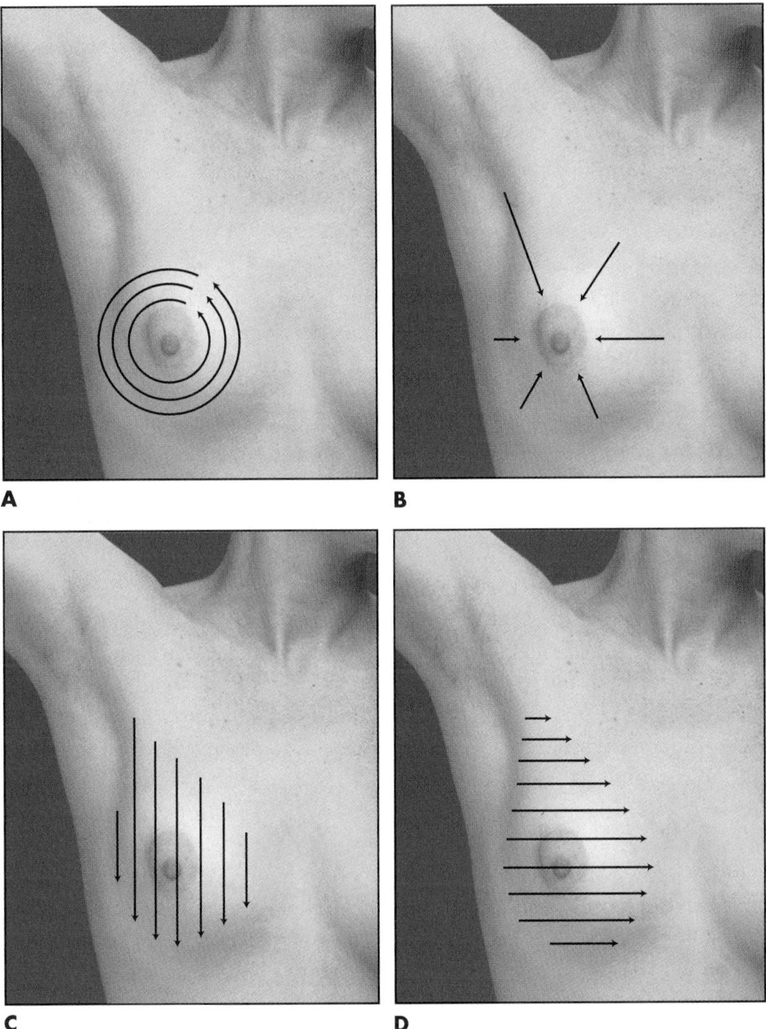

Figure 52-14 Different patterns used in palpation of the breasts. **A**, Spiral. **B**, Spokes of a wheel. **C**, Vertical lines. **D**, Horizontal lines.

when enlarged, these organs are not always palpable through the abdominal wall. However enlargement is often associated with pain or tenderness on palpation of the lower quadrants.

Physical Examination of the Female External Genitalia

The external genitalia are examined before performing the internal examination. Self-examination of the vulva can be simultaneously explained to the patient with the use of a mirror and good lighting. Before each step of the examination, remind the patient of what you plan to do. For example, "First I am going to examine the vulva. You will feel me touching the labia (or skin) around the vagina." The mons, pubis, labia, and perineum are inspected for nits, lesions, swelling, inflammation, altered pigmentation, or discharge. Small painful vesicular lesions may indicate genital herpes, whereas condylomata acuminata appear as warty lesions. The labia are gently separated and the clitoris, urethral orifice, and vagina are inspected. Next Bartholin's glands are palpated between the index finger and thumb if swelling is seen. Note and culture any discharge from the glands. If urethritis or inflammation of the Skene's glands is suspected, the urethra is milked by inserting a finger into the vagina and gently stroking the urethra in a downward motion. Note and culture any discharge.

Pelvic Examination

The pelvic examination is frequently a stressful event for the patient. The nurse can help the woman overcome pain, embarrassment, and anxiety by establishing a relaxed, positive atmosphere and addressing the woman's questions and concerns. Women who are scheduled for pelvic examination should be advised to avoid douching, sexual intercourse, using tampons, and applying any vaginal preparations (medicinal or deodorant) for at least 48 hours before examination. A Pap smear should not be performed if there is significant menstrual bleeding, as this makes interpretation of the test difficult. Patients should void and defecate, if needed, immediately before examination because an empty bladder and lower bowel make palpation of the pelvic organs easier, decrease patient discomfort, eliminate possible distortion of the position of pelvic organs caused by a full bladder, and obviate the risk of incontinence during examination.

Positioning

The most common position used for the pelvic examination is the lithotomy position. This position may need to be modified for a woman with poor mobility or arthritis (Figure 52-15). Assist the older woman to a position of comfort for pelvic examination if lithotomy position is not possible. The stirrups can be adjusted depending on the age of the woman. The head of the examination table can be raised for comfort, and so that the woman can see the examiner. The woman may or may not prefer to be draped with a sheet. In addition, a mirror can be offered to the woman if she is interested in watching the examination. Encourage the older woman to change positions slowly after pelvic examination as orthostatic hypotension may occur.

Inspection of the Vagina and Cervix

Before insertion of the speculum, the labia majora and minora are separated with the nondominant gloved hand. The appropriately sized speculum is gently inserted into the vagina at an oblique angle along the natural plane of the vagina. The speculum is rotated to a horizontal plane, and the blades are opened (Figure 52-16). The cervix is visualized at the tip of the speculum. Note the cervical color, location of the os, and characteristics such as lesions, nodules, or discharge.

Vaginal samples for pH and wet mount are obtained first, followed by the Pap test. The best cervical specimen can be obtained by first using a plastic ectocervical spatula followed by an endocervical brush (Figure 52-17). Some facilities use a cotton-tipped swab for the endocervical sample, which should be moistened with sterile saline before specimen collection to avoid cell trapping.

With the long end of the spatula in the os, the spatula is rotated circumferentially around the entire cervical os. The endocervical brush is inserted into the endocervical os and just rotated 180 degrees to limit bleeding. The specimen should be obtained from the entire transformational zone of the cervix, as the majority of cervical cancers develop at the junction of the squamous epithelium and the columnar epithelium of the endocervix. The presence of endocervical cells on the Pap smear is considered the gold standard for an adequate Pap test. The specimens are then "unrolled" onto a glass slide and fixed immediately with a spray or alcohol solution. A new method, approved by the U.S. Food and Drug Administration, of transporting cervical cells in liquid suspension may eventually replace the conventional glass slide method. With this technology the sample is immediately placed in the liquid preservative after each collection. It is important to swirl the spatula or brush several times to release the maximum number of cervical cells into the preservative.[4] After transport to the laboratory, cells are filtered and plated in a thin layer on a slide. After collection of the cervical sample, cultures for chlamydia and gonorrhea are collected with the appropriate swabs.

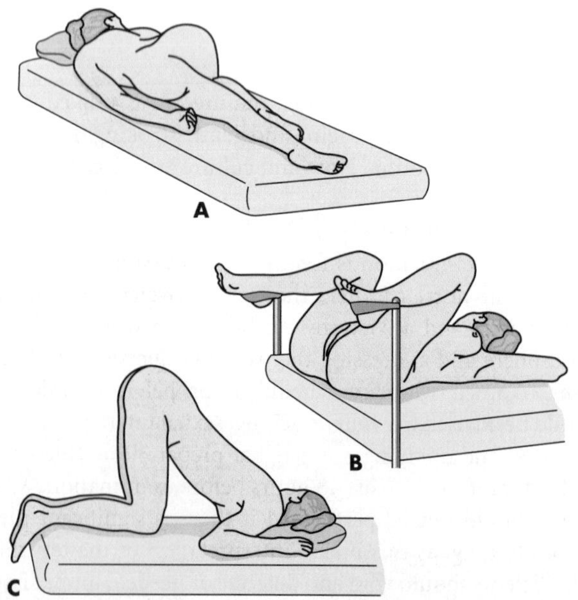

Figure 52-15 Various positions that can be assumed for examination of rectum and vagina. **A**, Sims' (lateral) position. Note position of left arm and right leg. **B**, Lithotomy position. Note position of buttocks on edge of examining table and support of feet. **C**, Knee-chest (genupectoral) position. Note placement of shoulders and head.

Bimanual examination follows the Pap test. The ovaries are normally slightly tender to palpation and are not always palpable, especially in obese women. When palpable, healthy ovaries feel smooth and oval in shape. Any irregular, firm palpable mass in the area of the fallopian tubes and ovaries indicates a possible deviation from normal. Because the ovaries atrophy during menopause, any mass felt in the areas of the ovaries in postmenopausal women is usually a sign of a problem.

The rectovaginal examination is performed to confirm uterine position, reassess the adnexal areas, follow-up on complaints of pain or bleeding, and determine rectal sphincter tone. The woman is told that it may be uncomfortable, and she may feel as though she has to have a bowel movement. Hemorrhoids, fistulas, and fissures can be observed. Stool for occult blood is obtained.

After the pelvic examination, a woman may need assistance removing lubricating jelly or discharge from her genitalia, removing her legs from the stirrups, and getting down from the table. If a bloody discharge is present, a sanitary pad is provided. Older women merit careful assistance after pelvic examination because positions such as the knee-chest and lithotomy positions may alter the normal circulation of blood sufficiently to cause blood pressure changes or faintness.

Physical Examination of the Male Genitalia

Physical examination of the male genitalia includes inspection, auscultation, and palpation of the lower abdomen; inspection and palpation of the external genitalia; and palpation of the prostate gland by rectal examination.

Positioning

Depending on the patient's age, the external genitalia can be examined after the abdominal examination with the patient in the supine or standing position. However, the patient should be in a standing position to evaluate hernias. The inguinal and femoral areas are inspected for any bulges or masses, and the patient is asked to bear down as the area is reinspected. A bulge while straining may indicate a femoral

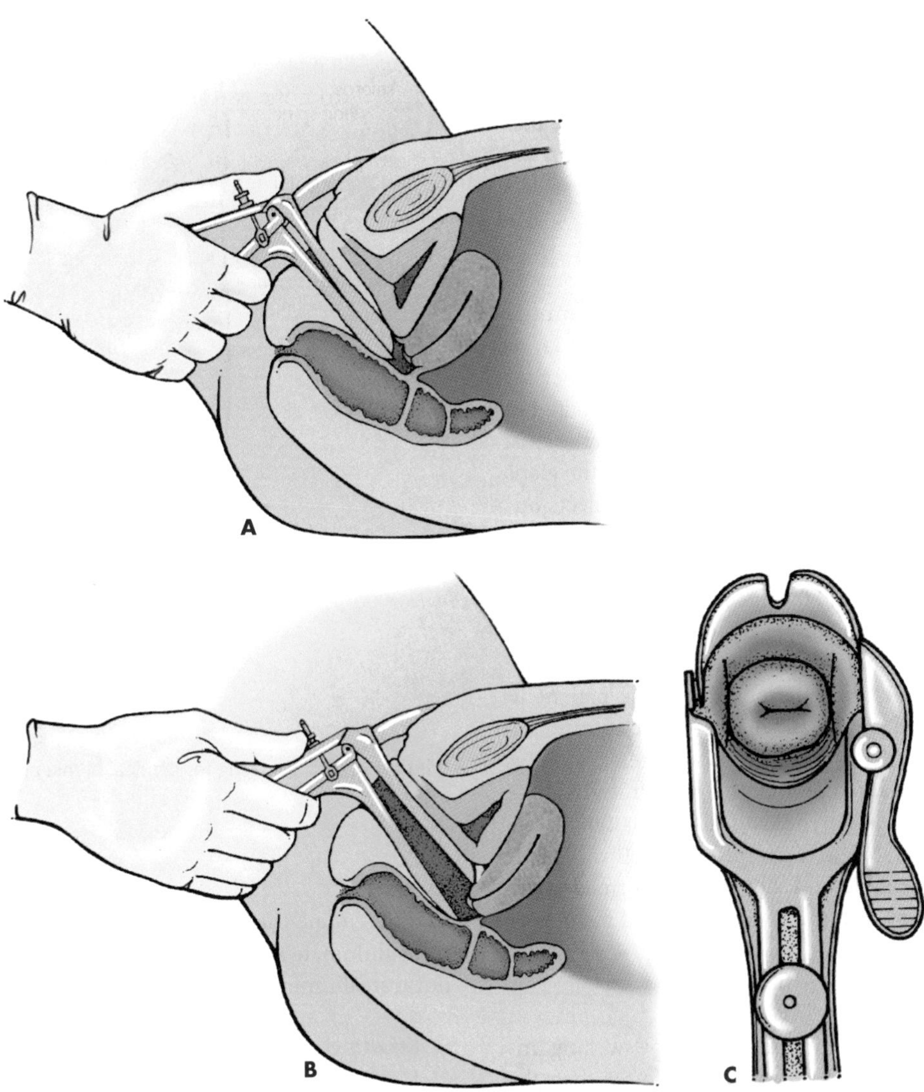

Figure 52-16 Speculum examination of the cervix. **A**, Insertion of a speculum. **B**, Open speculum within the vagina. **C**, Examiner's view of the cervix through an open speculum.

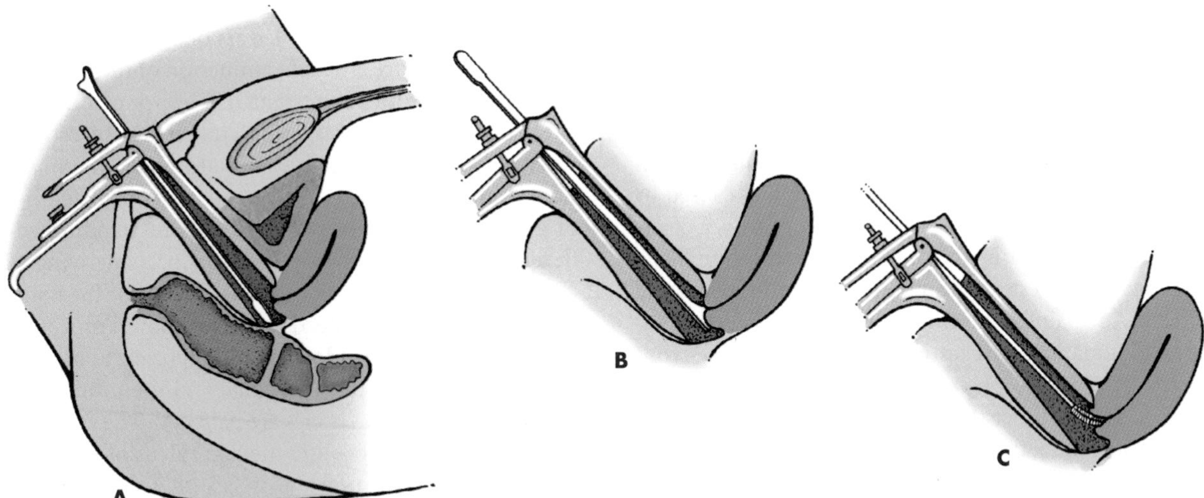

Figure 52-17 Method of obtaining specimen for a Pap test. **A**, Blunt end of an Ayre spatula used to scrape the specimen from the posterior fornix. **B**, Most pointed tip of the bifid end of an Ayre spatula inserted into the cervical os and rotated 360 degrees to obtain a specimen from the squamocolumnar junction. **C**, Cytobrush inserted into cervical os and rotated 360 degrees to collect a specimen from the endocervix. A glass pipette or cotton swab may also be used.

hernia. Straining is preferred over coughing as a method of assessment, as it causes more sustained pressure in the lower abdomen. After auscultation of the abdomen and palpation of the upper abdomen, the inguinal and femoral areas are palpated for enlarged lymph nodes and hernias. Once again the patient is asked to bear down and the inguinal region is palpated. A bulge will be felt with a direct hernia.

Penis

The skin of the penis is inspected for swelling, inflammation, or lesions caused by chancres, genital warts, herpes, or penile cancer. Pubic hair should be inspected for nits, lice, or scabies. In an uncircumcised male, the patient is instructed to retract the foreskin while the glans is inspected for lesions. Normally the foreskin or prepuce retracts easily and the glans is smooth. Smegma, a cheesy white substance that collects under the prepuce, is a normal finding.

The location and color of any discharge from the urethral meatus are noted. The urethral meatus is usually centrally located on the glans. Congenital displacement of the meatus can occur on either the ventral surface (hypospadius) or on the dorsal surface (epispadius) of the penis. Ask the patient to compress the glans and collect any discharge for culture and smear. If the patient has complained of discharge but none is seen, the patient can be asked to milk the penis from the base to the glans. Cultures for gonorrhea and chlamydia can be collected by inserting a swab 2 to 4 cm into the urethra. This is an uncomfortable procedure and should be performed at the end of the examination. Last, the penis is palpated for masses and tenderness.

Scrotum and Testes

The scrotum is inspected for size, symmetry, swelling, inflammation, and/or lesions. The left testis is lower than the right, which causes the scrotum to appear asymmetric under normal conditions. Scrotal size is also determined by room temperature and age. In warm temperatures the dartos muscles relax, and the testes are more pendulous. Likewise, with age the dartos muscles atrophy, which also causes a pendulous appearance. Marked asymmetry can be caused by an undescended testicle, indirect hernia, hydrocele, tumor, or edema.

Palpation of the scrotum is necessary to distinguish between enlargement caused by a mass and swelling caused by the collection of fluid. The size, shape, and consistency of the testes are noted by palpating the testes between the thumb and first two fingers. The testes feel smooth and firm, are oval, and move freely. Any painless hard nodule should be further investigated, as it may indicate testicular cancer. The epididymis and spermatic cord are palpated from the testes to the inguinal ring. At this time, the examination for hernia is repeated by invaginating the scrotal skin with the index finger to the external inguinal ring (Figure 52-18). The patient is asked to strain; the presence of a hernia will produce a bulge or tap. A load test can be done at this time if the hernia is not palpated despite complaints of hernia symptoms. Finally, transillumination of the scrotum with a flashlight may be attempted to differentiate the cause of scrotal swelling. Serous fluid will transilluminate and produce a red glow. Tissue and blood will not transilluminate.

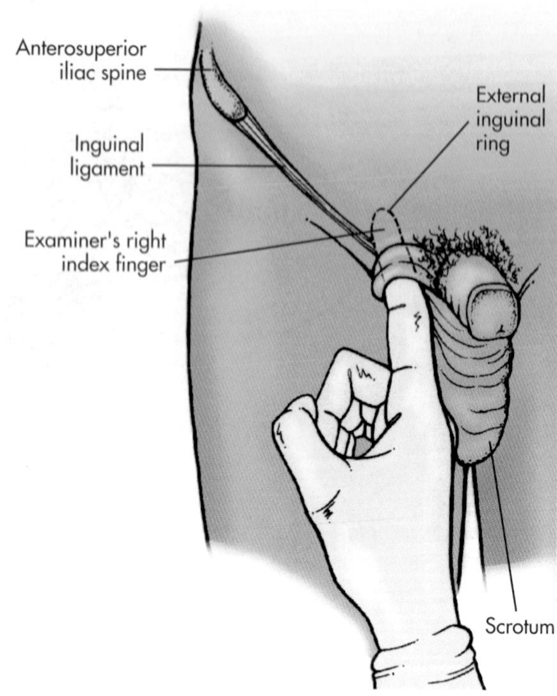

Figure 52-18 Palpating for inguinal hernia at the right inguinal ring.

Prostate

Rectal examination is the most important step in the diagnosis of prostatic disease, especially carcinoma. Cancer of the prostate gland may start as a localized, hard nodule, which is palpable by rectal examination, before proceeding to an advanced stage. For this reason, it is recommended that all men, especially those older than 50 years of age, have a rectal examination at least once a year. Examination of the prostate can be a stressful event for the patient. The nurse can help the man overcome pain, embarrassment, and anxiety by establishing a relaxed, positive atmosphere and addressing the man's questions and concerns. The prostate gland is palpated by means of a rectal examination with the patient standing with hips flexed over an examination table or in a side-lying position (Figure 52-19). Before the examination advise the man that he may feel as though he needs to have a bowel movement. The patient is asked to bear down while a lubricated index finger is gently inserted into the anal canal and then the rectum. The prostate and seminal vesicles are palpated. The size, shape, and consistency of the lobes and median sulcus of the prostate are noted. The normal prostate is 2.5 × 4 cm, smooth, heart shaped, rubbery, and nontender.

Assessment measures and variations in normal findings relevant to the care of older adults are presented in the Gerontologic Assessment box. Also identified are disorders common

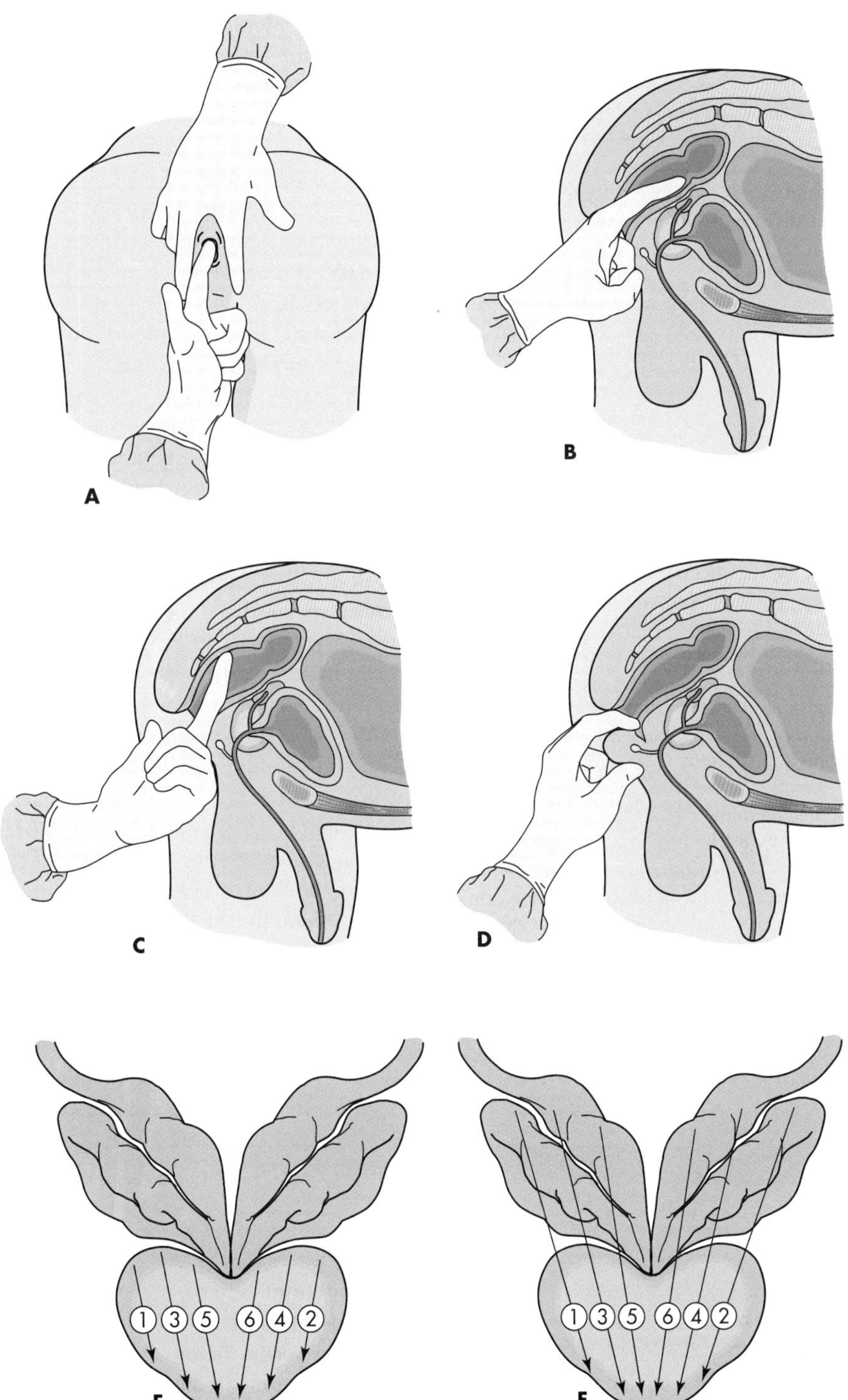

Figure 52-19 Rectal examination. **A**, Introduction of protected, well-lubricated finger. **B**, Palpation of prostate gland and seminal vesicles, lateral view. **C**, Palpation of anterior surface of sacrum and coccyx. **D**, Palpation of Cowper's glands. **E**, Massage of prostate gland for specimen collection or treatment; order of strokes is indicated by gradually working toward center (verumontanum). **F**, Massage of seminal vesicles and prostate gland.

Gerontologic Assessment

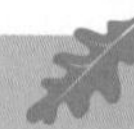

ASSESSMENT

Determine meaning of sexuality to patient and level of sexual satisfaction and assess for problems engaging in sexual intercourse.
- Personal beliefs and social mores influence attitudes toward sexuality. Disability or disease can interfere with sexual satisfaction.

Inquire about the use of complementary or alternative therapies.
- Complementary or alternative therapies, which are in common use today, can interact positively or negatively with conventional therapies and must be considered when planning care.

For women:
- Determine frequency of regular gynecologic examinations, mammography, and breast self-examination.
- Some women are not aware that these examinations should be continued after menopause.

Assess for signs of vaginitis (vaginal pruritus and discharge).
- Older women are at risk for vaginitis because of changes in hormone levels and the resulting thinning of the vaginal epithelium and rise in vaginal pH.

Assess for signs of cystocele or rectocele (urinary incontinence and low back pain).
- Cystocele and/or rectocele are common findings in older women as a result of long-standing childbirth injuries and decline in muscle tone and strength.

For men:

Inquire directly about problems urinating.
- Benign prostatic hypertrophy (BPH) is common in older men and the classic symptoms are frequency, nocturia, hesitancy, dribbling, and a feeling of being unable to empty the bladder. Dysuria and hematuria present if cystitis develops.

Assess knowledge and understanding of common prostate problems.
- Prostatitis, BPH, and prostatic cancer affect large numbers of older men and are responsible for significant morbidity/mortality. Early diagnosis and effective treatment depend on understanding of the problem and the need for screening and/or intervention.

COMMON REPRODUCTIVE DISORDERS IN OLDER ADULTS

Vaginitis
Uterine prolapse
Cystocele, rectocele
Erectile dysfunction
Hernias
Cancer of cervix, uterus, breast, prostate

in older adults, which may be responsible for abnormal assessment findings.

DIAGNOSTIC TESTS

Many diagnostic tests are useful in providing data about the reproductive system. They include blood tests, urine tests, cytologic tests, radiologic tests, biopsies, and endoscopic procedures.

Laboratory Tests

Blood Tests

Endocrine Testing. Because the endocrine system is so closely related to reproductive function, almost any study of endocrine function may be ordered, including determination of estrogen levels and thyroid hormones in women and 24-hour urine collections for ketosteroids and pituitary gonadotropins in both sexes. Endocrine system tests are presented in Chapter 28.

Coagulation Studies. Women who present with menorrhagia may be evaluated for underlying coagulation disorders. Tests could include activated partial thromboplastin time, platelet count, factor levels and ristocetin-induced platelet agglutination assay, which are discussed in Chapter 26.

HIV Testing. Assessment of HIV status is presented in Chapter 50.

Prostate-Specific Antigen. Prostate-specific antigen (PSA) is a glycoprotein that is specific to the prostate gland but not to prostate cancer. PSA serum levels are currently used to identify men at risk for prostate cancer. Other conditions such as benign prostatic hyperplasia or inflammation can also cause an elevated PSA level. Conversely, a man with prostate cancer can have a normal PSA level. PSA levels should be 4.0 or less. The American Cancer Society and the American Urological Association currently recommend annual PSA testing for all men older than 50. African-American men and those with a positive family history should begin annual examinations in their early forties.

The PSA is most valuable when evaluated in conjunction with the patient's symptoms, a family history of prostate cancer, and the findings of the digital rectal examination. Men who are believed to be at risk for prostate cancer are further evaluated by transrectal ultrasound or biopsy. The PSA is also valuable in evaluating the efficacy of treatment and in the detection of recurrence of prostate cancer. Contrary to previous belief, blood for the PSA test does not have to be drawn before the rectal examination. PSA levels can be increased after recent ejaculation, cycling, infection, and prostate massage, needle biopsy, or ultrasound.[6]

Prostatic Acid Phosphatase. Another glycoprotein used in the evaluation of prostate cancer is prostatic acid phosphatase (PAP). PAP is found in the epithelium of the prostate, and persistently elevated levels may indicate metastasis, although metastasis can also be present with a normal PAP level. Although useful in following the course of prostate cancer, the test is not a practical screening test because of the high rate of false-positive results. An elevated PAP level can occur after a rectal examination or with either prostatitis or benign prostatic hyperplasia.

Other Serum Tumor Markers. Alkaline phosphatase is followed in men with metastatic prostate cancer. Alpha-fetoprotein and human chorionic gonadotropin can be elevated in metastatic testicular cancer.

Genetic Testing

Genetic testing for the general population is not recommended; however, the American Society of Clinical Oncology does recommend that women who are found to have an increased risk of breast and/or ovarian cancer be offered genetic testing for mutations in the tumor suppressor genes BRCA1 and BRCA2. Such women include those with three or more first- or second-degree relatives who develop the disease, cancer diagnosis before age 45, family members with known

BRCA1 or BRCA2 mutations, family history of ovarian cancer, multiple breast cancers, breast cancer in male relative, Ashkenazi Jewish descent and breast or ovarian cancer history.[3] Genetic testing should be conducted only within the context of a pretesting and posttesting counseling program. Women with the BRCA1 or BRCA2 gene mutations should be screened earlier than the recommendations for low-risk women and may consider other options such as prophylactic surgery or chemoprevention.[1]

Syphilis Studies. Serologic testing can also be used to detect syphilis because two identifiable antibodies appear in the blood 1 to 4 months after syphilis is contracted. Two types of tests, treponemal and nontreponemal, are presently available. The tests differ in the type of antibody measured and in the antigen used to detect antibodies.

The nontreponemal tests, typically called serologic tests for syphilis (STS), measure an antibody-like substance called reagin. Blood samples are obtained by venipuncture. The Venereal Disease Research Laboratory (VDRL) and the rapid plasma reagin (RPR) screening tests are the most common syphilis tests and are typically used for routine premarital and prenatal screening. The RPR screening test has replaced the VDRL in many institutions.

Syphilitic reagin is thought to form from tissue breakdown products resulting from the interaction of the organism and body tissues. STS are usually reported as nonreactive, weakly reactive, or reactive. If any degree of reactivity is found, a quantitative test is also performed. Quantitative reactions are reported in ratios and reflect the highest dilution at which the serum reacts.

Reactive STS are confirmed by alternate serologic tests because hypersensitivity reactions, acute bacterial and viral infections, and chronic systemic diseases such as tuberculosis or collagen disease can all trigger reactivity without exposure to syphilis. It is important, therefore, not to tell patients they have syphilis based on STS alone. The microhemagglutination-*Treponema pallidum* (MHA-TP) assay has replaced the fluorescent treponemal antibody absorption (FTA-ABS) test as the most often used serologic test to confirm reactive STS. A positive MHA-TP or FTA-ABS assay must be obtained before the diagnosis of syphilis can be confirmed.

The serologic tests in use today do not always indicate an active syphilitic infection and only detect the presence of antibodies. There is an urgent need for a specific, rapid method of detecting infection caused by syphilis, and until new tests are developed, the patient's history, clinical symptoms, and serologic testing are the best available tools for the diagnosis.

Scrapings, Cultures, Smears, Urine Tests

Screening for STDs can be done by obtaining a culture of any discharge from the male and female reproductive tract. STDs can be asymptomatic or produce only mild symptoms. Routine periodic screening for STDs among sexually active persons is essential in identifying asymptomatic infected persons to prevent long-term problems (e.g., the sequelae of untreated chlamydia can include pelvic inflammatory disease and infertility).

Syphilis. During the primary stage of syphilis a painless chancre develops within 1 to 3 weeks at the site of initial exposure to the *Treponema pallidum* organism, usually on the genitals, mouth, or lips. Dark field examination of the chancre scrapings may reveal the *T. pallidum* spirochete. A negative scraping does not necessarily rule out syphilis, however, as the specimen may have been inadequate.

Chlamydia and Gonorrhea. *Chlamydia trachomatis* infection is the most common STD in the United States; gonorrhea is the second most common. Both gonorrhea and chlamydia produce similar symptoms and often occur simultaneously. Infected men complain of urethral discharge and dysuria. Women may note postcoital bleeding or an increase in vaginal discharge or have mucopurulent cervicitis. Testing for *C. trachomatis* has evolved in recent years to include direct antigen detection and nucleic acid amplification techniques using either polymerase or ligase chain reactions, as well as cultures, which used to be the gold standard.

Nonculture testing for chlamydia is not as specific as the culture method, but is cheaper and easier to complete. Direct fluorescent antibody detection uses visualization of chlamydia elementary bodies, whereas enzyme immunoassay uses spectrophotometry to identify color changes in the elementary bodies. These tests require a cervical specimen and have a sensitivity of about 60% and a specificity of about 96% to 99%.[3] The sensitivity reflects the ability of the test to identify someone who has the disease, and the specificity reflects the ability of the test to identify someone who does not have the disease.

The direct DNA probe test screens for both *C. trachomatis* and *Neisseria gonorrhoeae* with one culture. In women, a swab is inserted 1 to 1.5 cm into the endocervical canal for 30 seconds and rotated several times before removal. A smaller urethral swab is used to obtain a culture in men. The male patient is advised not to urinate for at least 2 hours before the culture. The swab is inserted 2 to 4 cm into the urethra and rotated gently for 2 to 3 seconds.

New nucleic acid amplification tests for detecting chlamydia only require a first-voided urine sample (FVU). These techniques include polymerase chain reaction, ligase chain reaction, strand displacement assay, hybrid capture system, and transcription-mediated amplification of RNA all with specificity and sensitivity ranging from 82% to 100%. FVU samples are easier to collect than cervical and urethral swabs and can be easily used for screening. The Centers for Disease Control and Prevention[3] offers clinicians a software program called SOCRATES (Screening Optimally for Chlamydia: Resource Allocation, Testing and Evaluation Software) to guide decision making regarding the most appropriate tests to use to screen for chlamydia.

Herpes Simplex Virus. Genital herpes is a sexually transmitted disease most frequently caused by herpes simplex virus type 2 (HSV-2), although it can also be caused by herpes simplex virus type 1 (HSV-1), previously thought to cause only cold sores. Primary genital HSV is characterized by multiple, painful genital blisters and flulike symptoms. Diagnosis can be confirmed by physical examination, culture for herpes virus, Pap smear, and serology testing for HSV antibodies. A culture is obtained by rubbing a suspicious lesion with a cotton- or Dacron-tipped swab and then inserting it into a transport medium. A final culture report may take 7 days.

Wet Mounts. Vaginal discharge can be easily examined microscopically for the presence of *Gardnerella vaginalis, Trichomonas,* and *Candida.* During a pelvic examination vaginal discharge is collected with a cotton swab and mixed with saline on a clear slide. The specimen is covered with a cover slip and examined under a microscope for bacteria, white blood cells, "clue" cells (stippled epithelial cells), and trichomonads. Several drops of 10% potassium hydroxide are then added to the slide, and it is reexamined for a positive whiff test and *Candida.* Potassium hydroxide causes the epithelial cells to lyse and in cases of yeast infections release hyphae. In bacterial vaginosis, vaginal discharge that is mixed with potassium hydroxide produces a fishy smell or positive whiff test. See Table 52-2 for interpretation of wet mounts.

Prostatic Smear. For a prostatic smear the prostate is first massaged during a digital rectal examination and any discharge from the penis is collected. If no discharge is expressed, the first urine sample after the examination is collected. Although some cases of tuberculosis and cancer can be detected by this method, the use of the prostatic smear has declined in recent years. Findings from the digital rectal examination, PSA levels, and biopsy are used to diagnose prostate cancer.

Cytology

Pap Smear. The Pap smear is a screening test for abnormal cervical cells including cancer. It is designed to determine who needs further evaluation and the type of evaluation needed. Pap smears can also identify vaginal infections such as *Trichomonas* and human papillomavirus, as well as evaluate hormone status.

The accuracy of the Pap test depends on the quality of the sample and the reliability of the laboratory interpreting the test. Results of 10% to 40% of tests are estimated to be reported as false negative partly as a result of inadequate specimens or misdiagnosis on the part of the cytologist. Several new systems have been developed to improve the reliability of Pap smear samples and thereby reduce the incidence of false-negative results. The speculoscopy has been shown to improve the identification of abnormal cervical lesions during a pelvic examination. In speculoscopy, a chemiluminescent light is attached to the blade of a speculum. Once the Pap smear is obtained, the cervix and vagina are washed with 5% acetic acid. Using 4003 magnification, the cervix is examined for areas of distinct acetowhite areas, which indicate cervical pathologic changes.[7] The use of speculoscopy, combined with Pap smears, identifies more cervical lesions than Pap smears alone.

The preparation of the Pap smear slide or specimen can also lead to false-negative results. Traditionally, Pap smear samples are rolled or scraped across a slide and sprayed with a fixative. The thin-layer preparation* is a new slide preparation method developed to reduce the effects of air-drying distortion, excessive blood or mucus, or a thick layer of cells.[5] After the Pap smear sample is obtained, the collection device is rinsed in a bottle of preservative solution. A slide is prepared from the suspended cells and screened by a cytologist in a conventional manner. The ThinPrep slides produce an evenly distributed sample without obscuring artifacts, which is easier to interpret. The ThinPrep method is associated with an increase in the number of cervical lesions identified as well as better Pap samples.

A new system has also been developed to rescreen Pap smears initially reported as negative or normal. The AutoPap 300 QC computer is a high-speed image processing computer with the ability to analyze the specimen for size, shape, density, and color of cells. Any Pap smear with abnormalities is reexamined by a cytologist. The misinterpretation of Pap smears should decline with this process.

The American Cancer Society recommends that all women who are, or have been, sexually active or who are at least 18 years of age have an annual Pap smear for 3 consecutive years

*ThinPrep, Cytic Corp.

TABLE 52-2 Wet Mount Interpretations

	Normal	Bacterial Vaginosis	Candida	Trichomonas	Atrophic
Symptoms	None	Thin, gray discharge; malodorous, pruritus can be present	Thick, white, curdlike discharge; pruritus	Increased, thin, frothy, yellow discharge; prutitus	Vulvar and vaginal dryness
pH	3.5-4.1	5-6	3.5-4.5	6-7	7.0
Microscopic findings	Lactobacilli	Clue cells, bacteria	Budding yeast	Increased white blood cells (WBCs), trichomonads	Increased WBCs, parabasal and intermediate cells
KOH	No findings	Positive whiff test, fishy odor	Budding yeast, pseudohyphae	No findings	No findings

KOH, Potassium hydroxide.

and then every 3 years until middle age. A woman should not douche, take a tub bath, use vaginal medications or deodorants, or have sexual intercourse for at least 24 hours before the test. Some physicians request a 48-hour delay before the test. Pap smears are preferably obtained 5 to 6 days after menstruation, as menses makes interpretation difficult and may camouflage atypical cells. Infections can also interfere with hormonal cytology. Pap smears should be delayed for at least 1 month after use of topical antibiotics, which produce rapid, heavy shedding of cells. Many women experience slight vaginal bleeding after a Pap smear has been taken. They should be advised that this is expected, but that any bleeding in excess of spotting should be reported to the health care provider.

The results of Pap smears are reported using the Bethesda System. The Bethesda System evaluates the adequacy of the sample, for example, satisfactory or not satisfactory for interpretation, and provides a general classification of normal or abnormal and a descriptive diagnosis of the Pap smear. The descriptive diagnosis indicates whether the cells were atypical squamous cells of undetermined significance, low-grade squamous intraepithelial lesions, high-grade squamous intraepithelial lesions, or glandular cells. It is important to monitor Pap smears and ensure proper follow-up including treatment of vaginal infections and colposcopy if necessary (see Evidence-Based Practice box).

Radiologic Tests

Diagnostic radiographic studies including computed tomography (CT), magnetic resonance imaging (MRI), ultrasonography of the male and female reproductive system, and mammography/xerography are used to identify soft tissue and bony abnormalities, to diagnose tumors and masses, and to diagnose infertility problems. Patient preparation and aftercare associated with the use of CT and MRI tests are similar to those described for other body systems and are not repeated here.

Ultrasonography

Ultrasonography (ultrasound) has become a useful diagnostic tool for persons with reproductive system problems. It can be used to locate pelvic masses, intrauterine devices, ectopic pregnancies, and prostatic neoplasms. Abdominal ultrasounds require the patient to have a full bladder. Transvaginal ultrasonography provides improved picture clarity of the immediate area compared with transabdominal sonography. Transvaginal sonography is currently being used to inspect and assess the uterus, ovaries, fallopian tubes, and extragenital structures (Box 52-4). The patient is asked to void before the procedure and then assisted into the lithotomy position. A female staff member should be available to provide emotional support for the woman during the procedure. Vaginal probes are lubricated with coupling gel and inserted into a condom or latex glove before insertion. The clinician uses one hand on the patient's abdomen to assess organ mobility. Additional assessments of pain and size of masses are obtained. The transvaginal probe is also used to guide procedures involving needle puncture, such as ova retrieval for in vitro fertilization. Transvaginal color Doppler sonography (TV-CDS) adds information on the quality of blood flow for the assessment of pelvic masses.

Transrectal Ultrasonography

Transrectal ultrasonography (TRUS) may be used as part of a workup for benign prostatic enlargement or prostate cancer. The procedure is preceded by a rectal examination and possibly an enema. A transrectal probe is inserted 8 to 9 cm into the rectum. TRUS is valuable in evaluating the size of the prostate, determining the response of a prostate tumor to treatment, and guiding placement of needles for biopsy. However, TRUS is not sensitive enough to be used alone for the diagnosis of cancer because the numbers of false-negative and false-positive results are too high.

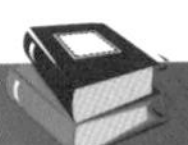

Evidence-Based Practice

Reference: Abercrombi PD: Improving adherence to abnormal Pap smear follow-up, *J Obstet Gynecol Neonatal Nurs* 30(1):80-97, 2000.

The purpose of this study was to critically review research studies that examined factors related to adherence to follow-up evaluation for abnormal Pap smears and interventions designed to increase adherence to follow-up care. Early detection of cervical cancer can lead to longer survival rates for women. Characteristics of women who do not seek follow-up care for abnormal Pap smears include ethnic minority, younger age, and lower socioeconomic status. Women with stronger social support and more severe Pap results were more likely to seek follow-up care. Interventions that improved adherence to follow-up care included telephone counseling and appointment reminders, reminder letters, and brochures. The researchers encouraged nurses to individualize their follow-up interventions and include clear information, emotional support, and reminder procedures.

BOX 52-4 Uses of Transvaginal Sonography

Uterus

Size, position
Inspection of myometrium and endometrial lining
Detection of malformations
Identification of small fibroids
Early pregnancy determination
Early fetal heartbeats

Ovaries

Size, texture, location
Monitoring follicular growth
Evaluation of ovulation
Identification of corpus luteum
Identification of tumors and structural deformities
Follicular aspiration

Fallopian Tubes

Diagnosis of tubal pathologic changes
Detection of tuboovarian abscess
Early recognition of tubal pregnancy

Extragenital Structures

Evaluation of free pelvic fluid
Detection of pelvic blood clots

Hysterosalpingography

Hysterosalpingography involves radiographic visualization of the uterine cavity and fallopian tubes after the injection of contrast material through the cervix. The test is useful in the evaluation of uterine tumors, tubal obstructions, and abnormalities. The procedure is usually performed in the radiology department, and the patient is placed in a lithotomy position on a fluoroscopy table. A plastic speculum is inserted into the vagina rather than a metal one, to allow for better visualization. A cannula is filled with a water-soluble contrast material, which is injected slowly under direct fluoroscopy. The hysterosalpingogram has largely replaced the older Rubin test, which was associated with numerous false-negative and false-positive results. The patient is assessed for allergy to iodine dye or shellfish, although allergic reactions are rare, as the contrast material is not injected intravenously. The bowel may be cleansed with laxatives, suppositories, or enemas before the test, but no food or fluid restrictions are needed. The patient may be given a sedative or antispasmodic agent before the test. The patient is advised that she may feel menstrual-type cramping and that she may experience shoulder pain caused by subphrenic irritation from the dye as it leaks into the peritoneal cavity.

After the procedure the nurse assesses the patient for nausea, faintness, and discomfort. Analgesics may be prescribed. The patient is instructed to apply a perineal pad, as vaginal drainage may be present for 1 to 2 days after the test, and the radiopaque dye may stain clothing. The patient should report any signs of infection such as fever, increased pulse rate, or pain to the health care provider.

Mammography/Xeromammography

Mammography is a radiologic study of the breast used to evaluate differences in the density of tissue, particularly small or poorly defined masses or nodules. It is capable of detecting many breast cancers that are too small to be palpated on physical examination. Mammograms are most effective in older women who have a higher percentage of fatty tissue in their breasts, which creates a greater contrast density on x-ray film. The density of benign cysts and malignant tumors may be similar, but their appearance is usually quite different. Suspicious lesions may be referred for needle aspiration or biopsy.

Recommendations for mammography screening are under constant evaluation and revision. Currently it is recommended that a woman have a single baseline mammogram taken between ages 35 and 40. Routine screening is then undertaken at the advice of the physician, considering all known and suspected risk factors for breast cancer (see Chapter 54). Recommendations from various groups are contradictory and reflect political and economic pressures as well as research outcomes. Some sources believe that low-risk women can delay further screening until age 50. Others recommend mammography every 1 to 2 years for women in their forties. General consensus does exist that annual screening after age 50 is appropriate.

No special preparation is required before a mammogram, but the woman should be instructed to avoid using deodorant, cream, or powder, which can mimic calcium clusters on x-ray film. Pretest teaching about the test is critical, as most women are highly anxious about the examination and the possibility of breast cancer. The woman is positioned standing next to the x-ray machine, and one breast at a time is placed between the platform and film plate. Most women experience some degree of discomfort from the breast compression. At least two views of each breast are taken.

Aftercare involves providing clear information concerning how and when the results of the test will be communicated to the patient. Most centers use this opportunity to reinforce skill and understanding of the purpose, technique, and timing of breast self-examination as well.

The xeromammogram provides an x-ray image with a much lower dose of radiation than that required for a traditional mammogram. The images are recorded on paper rather than film. The technique has become increasingly popular because the high contrast result is easier to read and may be more accurate.

Special Tests

Pregnancy Tests

Most of the frequently used pregnancy tests are based on the fact that human chorionic gonadotropin (hCG) is present in the blood and urine of pregnant women. Results are obtained within minutes to 2 hours. The newer tests can detect as little as 25 mIU/ml of hCG as early as 3 to 4 days after implantation. First morning urine specimens provide the best sample. Do-it-yourself pregnancy tests are available to women over the counter. These tests are sensitive and easy to perform.

The radioreceptor assay test for pregnancy is rapid and reliable. It is extremely accurate, and serial blood samples may be used to determine the viability of the pregnancy or identify molar or ectopic pregnancies. Serum hCG levels double approximately every 2 days until the 10th week of pregnancy. In men and nonpregnant women the normal hCG level is less than 5 mIU/ml. At 2 weeks' gestation the value is 50 to 500 mIU/ml. In ectopic pregnancies the level increases at a slower rate.

Schiller's Test

Schiller's test is a simple test that reveals the presence of atypical cervical cells. A solution of 3.5% iodine or Lugol's solution is applied to the cervix. Atypical cells, both malignant and benign, do not contain glycogen and will fail to stain. Early cancerous lesions and benign lesions, such as cervicitis, may appear as glistening areas of a lighter color than surrounding tissue. Biopsies can then be obtained from these targeted areas. The test is used infrequently because colposcopy is a more accurate method of obtaining the same information.

Biopsies

Cervical Biopsy

A cervical biopsy is performed to obtain a tissue specimen for pathologic examination. It is almost always performed with colposcopic direction. Although bleeding is minimal, the biopsy is ideally performed shortly after the menses when the cervix is less vascular. A punch biopsy can be safely performed as an office procedure without the use of anesthesia because the cervix has few pain receptors. The woman is instructed to leave the packing or tampon in place for 8 to 24 hours and report the incidence of excessive bleeding.

Conization of Cervix

Conization of the cervix may be performed as a diagnostic or therapeutic measure. It is typically performed in an outpatient setting with the woman under local anesthesia. A cone-shaped portion of the cervix containing the suspected malignant or infected tissue is removed. Bleeding from the site of conization is greater than that occurring from punch biopsy. If the bleeding is excessive or if hemorrhage seems likely, the cervix is sutured to control blood loss. Oozing is controlled by packing, which is kept in place for 24 to 48 hours. The patient is instructed to rest and avoid heavy lifting for at least 3 days. She should be informed that her next two or three menstrual periods may be heavy and prolonged.

Endometrial Biopsy

Although an ideal method for screening for endometrial cancer has not been developed, a variety of methods are now in use. Less than one half of women with uterine cancer have an abnormal Pap test at diagnosis. Cells rarely exfoliate from the endometrium in the early stages of the cancer, making this an unsatisfactory method of screening and diagnosis. The best results are obtained when cervical aspiration is performed as part of the Pap test. It is important to make sure the woman is not pregnant before performing the procedure. A paracervical block or local anesthetic may be used.

Endometrial cells obtained by aspiration smear show malignant changes 75% to 90% of the time when uterine cancer exists. A small cannula is inserted through the cervix into the uterine cavity, and suction is applied by means of a syringe attached to the cannula. The specimen obtained is prepared as for a Pap smear.

Endometrial biopsy can be used to diagnose cancer; evaluate bleeding, polyps, or inflammatory conditions; and determine whether ovulation has occurred by assessing the effects of estrogen or progesterone on the endometrium. It is performed by introducing a small curette into the uterus and obtaining several strips of endometrial tissue. The specimens are taken from several sites in the uterine cavity to increase the chances of obtaining malignant cells. The biopsy method is considered to be about 90% accurate in diagnosing endometrial cancer.

Complications include perforation of the uterus, uterine bleeding, interference with early pregnancy, and infection. Any temperature elevation after the biopsy should be reported to the physician because this procedure may activate pelvic inflammatory disease. The patient is advised to wear a pad after the procedure because some vaginal bleeding is expected. If excessive bleeding occurs, the physician should be notified. The patient is advised that douching and intercourse should be avoided for 72 hours after the biopsy. The patient is encouraged to rest during the next 24 hours and avoid heavy lifting to prevent uterine hemorrhage.

Breast Biopsy

It is widely accepted that most breast masses need to be evaluated for cancer. Biopsy can differentiate fibrocystic lesions, fibroadenomas, and intraductal papillomas. Three major approaches are in use. An excisional biopsy removes the mass for pathologic evaluation. An incisional biopsy samples some of the tissue from the mass, and an aspiration biopsy involves the removal of fluid or tissue from the mass through a large-bore needle. The aspiration method is in widespread use. Bloody fluid aspirated from the mass indicates the possibility of cancer. If nothing can be aspirated, the mass is considered to be solid and needs to be evaluated via the incisional route. Breast biopsies are usually performed in ambulatory settings with the patient under local anesthesia. It is crucial that the woman clearly understand what procedure is planned, the anesthesia to be used, and the sensations she may experience during the procedure. Aftercare is straightforward. The incision site is assessed for bleeding, edema, or infection. Mild analgesics are provided for discomfort. Numbness at the biopsy site may persist for months.

Needle Biopsy of Prostate

A needle aspiration biopsy of the prostate is performed to retrieve cells for histologic study. The procedure is usually performed at the same time as cystoscopy but can also be done as an office procedure with the patient under local anesthesia. Either a transrectal or a transperineal approach is used.

A transrectal approach uses guided ultrasound to identify biopsy sites (Figure 52-20). Before the procedure a digital rectal examination is performed to locate the suspicious lesions. A condom-covered ultrasound transducer is inserted into the rectum, and tissue samples are collected from suspicious lesions and other areas of the prostate.

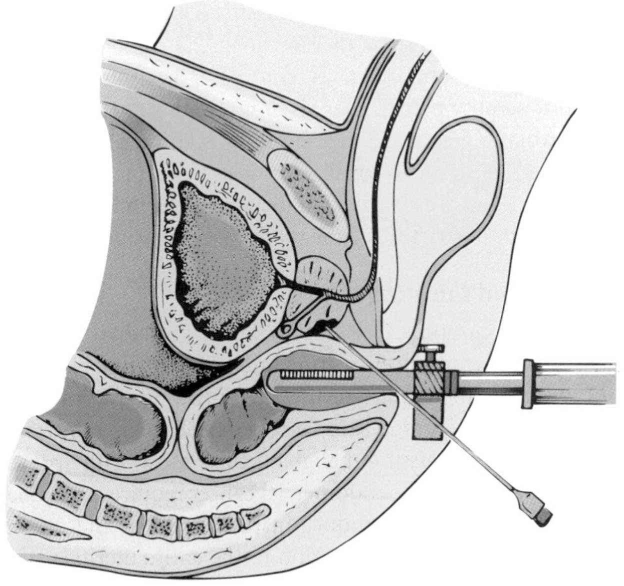

Figure 52-20 Diagram demonstrating transrectal biopsy with transrectal ultrasound.

Aspiration may be repeated several times in different locations to sample the tissue adequately. This method is thought to be slightly more accurate than the transperineal approach, which involves insertion of the needle through the perineum into the prostate using the examiner's finger, which is placed in the rectum, as a guide.

Patient preparation for prostatic biopsy may include bowel cleansing if a rectal approach is used. Sepsis is a rare but potentially life-threatening complication. Prophylactic antibiotics are usually prescribed before and after the procedure. The patient may also experience transient hematuria and rectal bleeding. The patient should be advised to promptly report a temperature of greater than 100° F (37.7° C), chills, or difficulty voiding.

Open Perineal Biopsy

To obtain a specimen of tissue by open perineal biopsy, a small incision is made in the perineum between the anus and scrotum. This technique gives the greatest accuracy because the suspect lesion can be clearly identified, and multiple specimens can be taken from the prostate gland. The procedure requires regional or general anesthesia.

A dressing is applied to the biopsy site and can be held in place for about 24 hours with a two-tailed binder. The patient is instructed to wipe from front to back after defecation so as not to contaminate the incision. Perineal irrigation is sometimes advised for both cleanliness and comfort. Unless the physician prescribes a solution, warm water poured from front to back over the incision can be used. After the sutures are removed, sitz baths may be used and add much to the patient's general comfort. The man is instructed to promptly report any signs of infection to the physician.

Testicular Biopsy

Smears or biopsy specimens from the testes can be obtained by the needle method or by an incision made through the scrotum. Most often an incision is used. After a local anesthetic has been administered, a small incision about 2.5 cm long is made, and a small piece of the testis is removed. A dressing is applied, and postoperative management is similar to that after open perineal prostatic biopsy. Testicular biopsy specimens are sometimes used to evaluate fertility. If sperm are present in the biopsy tissue but are absent from the semen, the infertility is often the result of stricture of the tubal system beyond the testes.

Dilation and Curettage

Dilation and curettage (D&C) may be performed for a variety of purposes, including evaluating infertility, treating bleeding, and inducing abortion. Because the entire uterine cavity is "scraped," a large tissue sample is obtained. This minimizes the likelihood of missing malignant cells. Most of the procedures used to diagnose endometrial cancer require some dilation of the cervix to introduce instruments into the uterus. Vacuum curettage applies suction to the entire uterine cavity to obtain tissue specimens.

For a D&C, metal dilators of graduated sizes are inserted into the cervical canal. Once the cervix is dilated, sharp curettes are used to remove endometrial tissue. The major complications of a D&C are hemorrhage and perforation of the uterus. Postoperative care is summarized in the Guidelines for Safe Practice box. Most women are discharged on the day of the procedure. Normal daily activities can be resumed, but vigorous exercise is discouraged. Sexual intercourse may be resumed when the woman feels comfortable. The menstrual cycle usually is not disturbed by a D&C, and all vaginal bleeding should disappear in a week to 10 days. Women are advised to report the recurrence of bright-red blood or the development of a vaginal discharge with an unpleasant odor.

Infertility Tests

The purposes of an infertility evaluation are to establish the cause of infertility, give a prognosis for future fertility, provide a basis for medical or surgical treatment, and assist the couple to accept their diagnosis, treatment, and future options. The assessment and intervention can be physically painful as well as emotionally and economically stressful.

A full description of an infertility workup is beyond the scope of this discussion. Both the man and woman undergo a thorough physical examination to rule out any undetected medical problems. Specific diagnostic studies used in infertility evaluation include determination of ovulation status of the woman using a basal temperature assessment, luteinizing hormone assessment, and serum progesterone. A biopsy of the endometrium may be done to see assess barriers to implantation. A hysterosalpingogram can determine if the fallopian tubes are scarred or blocked. The man's semen is examined to determine adequacy of sperm counts.

Endoscopy

The pelvic organs and surrounding tissues can be visualized directly by endoscopy. The procedures by which this can be accomplished are colposcopy, culdoscopy, laparoscopy (peritoneoscopy), hysteroscopy, and falloposcopy (Box 52-5). Most of the procedures can be performed on an outpatient basis even if general anesthesia is used. Culposcopy is used to

Guidelines for Safe Practice

After Dilation and Curretage

1. Apply a perineal pad to absorb the expected drainage.
2. Take vital signs every 15 minutes until stable.
3. Monitor bleeding every 15 minutes for 2 hours; if active bleeding continues, monitor every hour for about 8 hours.
4. Record each pad change and amount of blood loss in estimated milliliters (60 ml saturates a perineal pad).
5. Monitor urine output.
6. Give mild analgesics as prescribed; report immediately any abdominal pain that is continuous, sharp, and not relieved by analgesics (may indicate perforation of uterus).
7. Encourage ambulation when patient is awake and vital signs are stable.

BOX 52-5 Procedures for Visualization of Pelvic Organs

Colposcopy

Visualization of vagina and cervix under low-power magnification

Culdoscopy

Insertion of culdoscope through posterior fornix into cul-de-sac of Douglas for visualization of fallopian tubes and ovaries (Figure 52-21)

Falloposcopy

Transcervical endoscopic examination of fallopian tubes

Hysteroscopy

Insertion of hysteroscope through cervix for visualization of inside of uterus

Laparoscopy

Insertion of laparoscope (patient under local or general anesthesia) through small incision in abdominal wall (inferior margin of umbilicus), which is insufflated with carbon dioxide; permits visualization of all pelvic organs (Figure 52-22)

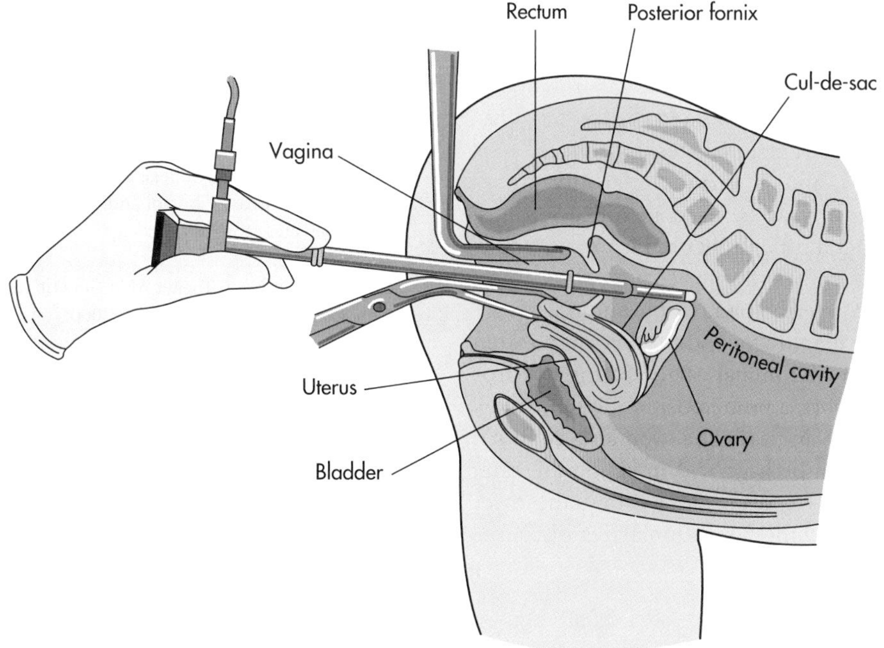

Figure 52-21 With patient in knee-chest position, culdoscope is inserted through posterior fornix of vagina into cul-de-sac of Douglas. Note that ovaries can be seen.

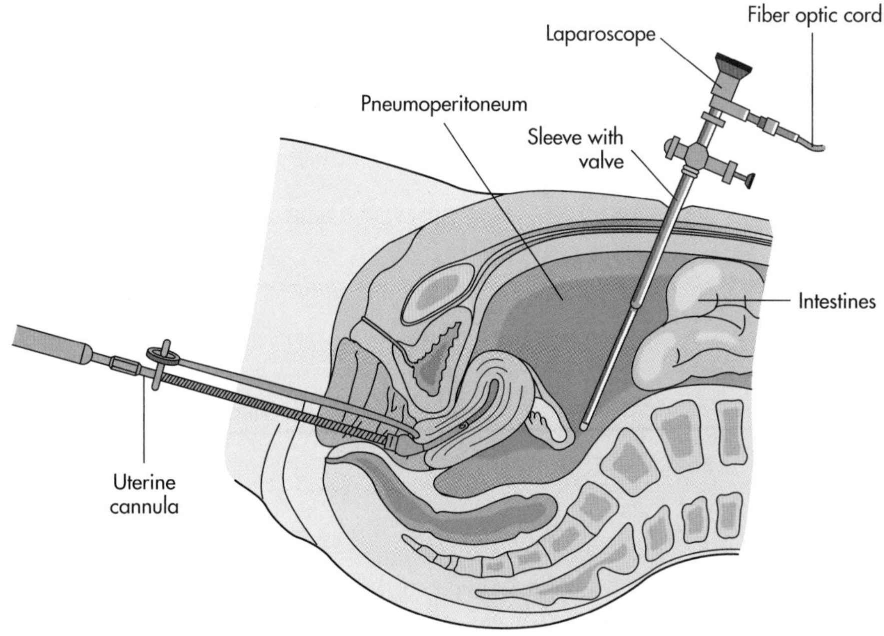

Figure 52-22 Scheme of gynecologic laparoscopy.

augment a detailed examination of the vagina and cervix or to guide cervical biopsy. The associated care is the same as that for other types of cervical biopsy. The use of culdoscopy (Figure 52-21) is declining because laparoscopy has become a standard diagnostic and treatment intervention. Hysteroscopy is routinely performed as part of a D&C to allow the physician to inspect the inside of the uterus before scraping or treatment. In the male, cystoscopic examination allows the physician to inspect the condition of the urethra and bladder mucosa and to detect prostatic encroachment on the urethra (see Chapter 38).

Laparoscopy (pelvic endoscopy or peritoneoscopy) may be used to inspect the outer surface of the uterus, fallopian tubes, and ovaries (Figure 52-22). A laparoscope is inserted through the abdominal wall through a small incision in the subumbilical area. The peritoneal cavity is filled with 3 to 4 L of carbon dioxide to separate the abdominal wall from the viscera and increase visualization. The laparoscope is then inserted to conduct the planned procedure. Laparoscopy may also be used for tubal sterilization, for lysis of adhesions, for biopsy, and in various infertility procedures. Conscious sedation may be used in office settings; however, general anesthesia is typically used for more extensive procedures. At the end of the procedure, the carbon dioxide is removed, but referred pain to the shoulder from gaseous irritation of the diaphragm and phrenic nerve often occurs. Air may enter the abdominal cavity during the procedure and cause discomfort; a prone position with a pillow under the abdomen may increase the woman's comfort. Complications such as hemorrhage and infection are rare, but women are cautioned to report fever or pain in the lower abdomen. The Patient Teaching box summarizes discharge instructions.

Patient Teaching

Discharge Instructions After Routine Laparoscopy

1. Rest for 24 hours before resuming normal activities.
2. Avoid sexual intercourse until after postoperative visit with physician.
3. Discomfort may be experienced in shoulder and upper abdominal area. Take oral pain medications as prescribed.
4. Call the physician if abdominal pain increases, if temperature elevates, if abnormal vaginal bleeding occurs, or if there is increased redness, swelling, soreness, or foul drainage at wound sites before first postoperative visit.
5. Wound dressings may be removed in 24 hours, and showering is permitted.
6. Resume regular diet and drink plenty of fluids.

References

1. American College of Obstetricians and Gynecologists: *Breast-ovarian cancer screening*, ACOG Committee Opinion, No 239, Washington, DC, 2000, American College of Obstetricians and Gynecologists.
2. Centers for Disease Control and Prevention: SOCRATES software, 2001, website: http://www.cdc.gov/nchstp/dstd/Software/Socrates.htm.
3. Clark RA, Garber J, Tucker MA: Genetic testing for cancer, *Patient Care for the Nurs Pract* 3(2):46, 2000.
4. Huff BC: Screening for cervical cancer, *AWHONN* 4:53, 2000.
5. Lee KR et al: Comparison of conventional Papanicolaou smears and a fluid-based, thin-layer system for cervical cancer screening, *Obstet Gynecol* 90(2):278, 1997.
6. Marks SHF: Prostate-specific antigen testing: an essential guide to its use and meaning, *ADV Nurse Pract* 9(4):38-44, 2001.
7. Wertlake PT et al: Effectiveness of the Papanicolaou smear and speculoscopy as compared with the Pap smear alone: a community based clinical trial, *Obstet Gynecol 90*(3):421, 1997.

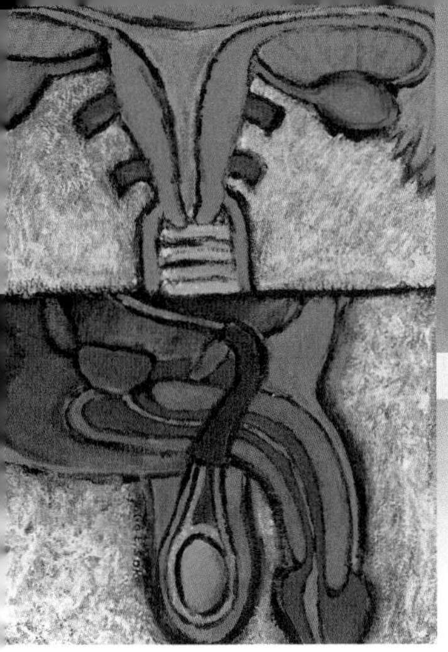

Female Reproductive Problems

53

Kathleen Barta

Objectives

After studying this chapter, the learner should be able to:

1. Discuss the collaborative management of common infectious diseases of the female reproductive tract.
2. Discuss the management of various disorders of menstruation.
3. Adapt preoperative and postoperative care for women undergoing hysterectomy.
4. Discuss nursing management for women undergoing intracavitary radiotherapy to the female reproductive tract.
5. Discuss options for couples considering sterilization or experiencing problems with fertility.
6. Identify anticipatory guidance for promoting reproductive health in women.

Diseases and disorders of the female reproductive system impair the physical and emotional health of millions of women each year. Infectious processes and disorders of menstruation are common and pervasive problems. Malignant neoplasms destroy childbearing potential and end numerous lives each year. Disorders affecting the female reproductive system are important national health concerns and are reflected in the Healthy People 2010 goals as summarized in the Healthy People 2010 box.

INFECTIOUS PROCESSES

VAGINITIS

Etiology/Epidemiology

Although the vulva and vagina are relatively resistant to infection, vaginitis is one of the most common problems for which women seek medical care. The most commonly involved organisms are *Candida albicans, Trichomonas vaginalis,* and *Gardnerella vaginalis.*

Bacterial vaginosis is the most common cause of vaginal discharge and occurs from an overgrowth of normal flora in the vagina, usually *G. vaginalis,* primarily in women who are sexually active.

Pathophysiology

Disturbances in the flora of the normally acidic vaginal environment result in a variety of symptoms, including vaginal discharge, vulvar pruritus, tissue irritation and inflammation, and burning. Different organisms are associated with specific types of discharge and symptom patterns, but pruritus is an extremely common symptom, regardless of the cause, and commonly is severe.

If the pH of the vaginal mucosa is altered or the woman's resistance is decreased by aging-related changes, stress, or disease, her risk of vaginitis increases. Specific factors that increase this risk include the use of antibiotics, which destroy the normal protective flora of the vagina; diseases causing immunocompromise, such as human immunodeficiency virus (HIV) infection; diseases altering carbohydrate metabolism, such as diabetes mellitus[2]; the use of steroids or other medications that suppress the immune response; and tissue injury from mechanical irritation by foreign objects such as tampons or by chemical irritation from douches, which makes tissues more susceptible to invasion by organisms. Because many organisms proliferate in a more alkaline environment, postmenopausal women are at increased risk for vaginitis because of the decrease in normal vaginal secretions and a rise in vaginal pH caused by a decline in estrogen levels. Risk factors for vaginitis are listed in the Risk Factors box.

Collaborative Care Management

The diagnosis of vaginitis is based on the history, physical examination, and laboratory testing. Abnormal vaginal discharge is evaluated using a wet preparation, potassium hydroxide (KOH) test (whiff test), and pH analysis. Serologic testing and urine culture may also be used. The management of vaginitis is primarily pharmacologic. Antifungal oral and topical agents are used for candidiasis; antianaerobic oral and intravaginal preparations are used for bacterial vaginitis (Table 53-1). Many of these drugs are available as over-the-counter preparations, but women are advised to seek diagnosis from

TABLE 53-1 Common Causes, Signs and Symptoms, and Treatment of Vaginitis

Cause	Signs and Symptoms	Treatment
Bacterial vaginosis *(Gardnerella vaginalis)*	Pruritus Thin, "fishy" vaginal discharge pH <4.5, clue cells, positive potassium hydroxide (KOH) test	Antibiotics with anaerobic activity (oral or intravaginal) Metronidazole Clindamycin
Fungal infections *(Candida albicans)*	Pruritus Vulvar burning Thick white drainage Presence of yeast buds on wet-mount preparation	Antifungal agents (oral or intravaginal) Clotrimazole Miconazole Fluconazole
Protozan infections *(Trichomonas vaginalis)*	Copious, foul-smelling discharge pH >4.5, leukocytes and flagellated organisms on wet-mount preparation "Strawberry cervix"	Antibiotics (oral) Metronidazole
Estrogen deficiency	Dryness and burning	Estrogen (oral or topical)

Healthy People 2010

Goals Related to Female Reproductive Problems

CERVICAL CANCER DEATHS

Reduce the death rate from cancer of the uterine cervix to 2 per 100,000 women.

PAP TESTS

Increase to at least 97% the proportion of women age 18 and older who have ever received a Pap test and to at least 90% of those who received a Pap test within the preceding 3 years.

CHLAMYDIAL INFECTION

Increase the proportion of sexually active women age 25 and younger who are screened annually for genital *Chlamydia trachomatis* infection.

Reduce the proportion of adolescents and young adults with *C. trachomatis* infection to 3% of those attending family planning and sexually transmitted disease (STD) clinics.

PELVIC INFLAMMATORY DISEASE (PID)

Reduce the proportion of women who have ever required treatment for PID to 5%.

FERTILITY PROBLEMS

Reduce the proportion of childless women with fertility problems who have had an STD or who have required treatment for PID to 15%.

SMOKING CESSATION BY ADULTS

Reduce cigarette smoking by adults to 12%.
Increase smoking cessation attempts by adult smokers to 75%.

From US Department of Health and Human Services: *Healthy People 2010: understanding and improving health,* Washington DC, 2000, USDHHS.

Risk Factors

Infections of the Vulva and Vagina

- Pregnancy
- Age–premenarche and postmenopause
- Low estrogen levels
- Dermatologic allergies
- Diabetes mellitus
- Oral contraceptive use
- Inadequate hygiene
- Douching
- Treatment with broad-spectrum antibiotics
- Use of vaginal contraceptives–foams, inserts
- Sexual intercourse with infected partner
- Frequent sexual intercourse with multiple partners
- Tight, nonabsorbent, and heat-retaining clothing

their primary health care provider for an initial episode of vaginitis if symptoms do not subside after one course of over-the-counter treatment.

The drugs may be administered orally or by ointment, cream, or suppository. Women are informed that the use of metronidazole (Flagyl) causes urine to turn a dark reddish brown. It also causes numerous gastrointestinal (GI) side effects that may be reduced by taking the drug with meals. The use of alcohol can trigger a disulfiram (Antabuse)–like reaction of severe nausea, vomiting, and abdominal distress and should be avoided during treatment and for 48 hours after completing the medication. Probiotics, the use of microbial foodstuffs, is under investigation as a way to restore normal vaginal flora and reduce the recurrence of candidal infections and bacterial vaginosis (see Complementary & Alternative Therapies box).

Patient/Family Education. Women have self-managed vaginitis for generations, and a number of alternative treatments are in common use. The nurse explores the woman's use of alternative therapies, ensures that the treatment is not contraindicated for the specific causative organism, and provides the woman with specific instructions about the safe and appropriate use of soaks, irrigations, and douches in vaginitis treatment. Women may benefit from including cultured food products such as yogurt or kefir in their diet.

Complementary & Alternative Therapies
Probiotics

Probiotics are beneficial bacteria contained in food that provide protection against invasive organisms. Examples include yogurt, milk with added probiotic bacteria, and kefir. Beneficial effects have been shown in adults and children with acute diarrhea and other intestinal disorders, lactose intolerance, and allergies. Research studies in women with candidal infections and bacterial vaginosis showed a decrease in the recurrence rate when they were treated with probiotics. Theories about the mechanisms of protection include (1) direct action against harmful bacteria, (2) decrease in pH through the production of lactic acid, (3) competition with harmful bacteria for receptor sites and nutrients, (4) increased immunity, and (5) production of lactase. The U.S. Food and Drug Administration (FDA) allows the addition of such organisms as *Lactobacillus acidophilus* in milk products, although the exact amount is not mandated. Studies indicate that fermented products have increased amounts of folic acid, a critical nutrient for women of childbearing age because of its protection against neural tube disorders in the developing fetus. Fermented products also improve the digestibility of lactose in dairy products, which are an important source of calcium, critical in the prevention of osteoporosis in women. With so many benefits to health, women should be encouraged to include some source of fermented milk product in their daily diets. As research into the health effects of probiotics continues, we will likely see a refinement in our ability to control the dose and target the organism for particular conditions.

Reference: Kopp-Hoolihan L: Prophylactic and therapeutic uses of probiotics: a review, *J Am Diet Assoc* 101(2):229-38, 2001.

Patient Teaching
Preventing Vaginal Infections

1. Cleanse genital area thoroughly with mild soap and water daily.
   a. Wipe genital area from front to back after bowel movements.
   b. Avoid use of vaginal irritants (e.g., harsh deodorant and perfumed soap, deodorant sprays, douches).
   c. Avoid routine douching, which can alter the vaginal pH.
2. Use underwear with a cotton crotch and change panties daily; avoid use of any clothing that is tight in the crotch or thighs. Avoid wearing underpants while sleeping.
3. Assess sexual partners for any sign of infection (e.g., discharge, lesions, reddened areas on genitals).
   a. Use a barrier method of contraception.
   b. Avoid any sexual practice that is painful or abrasive.
   c. Avoid anal-genital intercourse.
   d. Cleanse genital area of self and partner and void before and after sexual intercourse.
4. Change tampons or napkins frequently during menstruation.
5. Treat athlete's foot and "jock itch" with over-the-counter antifungals.
6. Consider using vitamin C 500 mg orally twice a day to increase the acidity of vaginal secretions.
7. Recognize the signs of infection and respond promptly.

Nursing management focuses primarily on the appropriate use of prescribed therapy and measures to prevent reinfection. The hands should be washed carefully before and after treatment. The nurse instructs the woman to cleanse the genital area thoroughly with soap and water and dry well before applying any medication. The nurse advises the woman to remain recumbent for 30 minutes after insertion of a suppository or cream to facilitate absorption and prevent loss from the vagina. Tampons should be avoided during treatment. If vaginal drainage is present, the woman is encouraged to wear a minipad. Sitz baths can be comforting. The woman is instructed to refrain from sexual intercourse while the infection is being treated, and the male partner should use a condom until all symptoms of inflammation have resolved.

Prevention of reinfection is an important consideration because vaginitis can easily become a recurrent problem. The nurse discusses the various lifestyle modifications that can be made to reduce the incidence of vaginal infection as presented in the Patient Teaching box.

CERVICITIS

Etiology/Epidemiology

The term *cervicitis* is used for a number of conditions characterized by inflammation and infection of the cervix. Risk factors include early initiation of sexual intercourse, oral contraceptive use, and multiple partners.[28] When cervicitis is associated with human papillomavirus (HPV), there is an increased risk of cervical cancer.

Pathophysiology

Chlamydia trachomatis is the most common offending organism, along with *Neisseria gonorrheae*, herpes simplex virus, and HPV.[28] Leukorrhea is the most common sign, but the amount may not be significant. On examination, the cervix is grossly erythematous and edematous with or without erosion. There is usually a mucoid purulent discharge, but the amount may be so small that the patient does not notice it. The woman commonly has no subjective signs but may report backache, lower abdominal pain, or painful sexual intercourse. Urinary frequency and urgency may also be present. It is important to rule out the presence of a cancerous lesion.[23]

Collaborative Care Management

The cervix is cultured, and appropriate pharmacologic therapy is initiated. See Chapter 56 for a more thorough discussion of the treatment of sexually transmitted diseases (STDs). If the woman's cervicitis does not respond to antibiotics or if she has significant cervical erosion, cryosurgery, electocauterization/loop electrosurgical excision procedure (LEEP), or laser therapy may be necessary.[28]

Patient/Family Education. The prevention of cervicitis includes those measures outlined in the Patient Teaching box, because many cases of cervicitis develop from vaginal infection. If surgical intervention is needed, it is generally performed as an outpatient procedure, and women are instructed accordingly. Women are told that a watery discharge is common, especially after cryosurgery, but that it resolves in several weeks. Healing is usually complete within 6 weeks. Women are also told that they may experience mild to moderate cramping during the procedure.[28]

BARTHOLINITIS (BARTHOLIN'S CYSTS)

Etiology/Epidemiology

Bartholin's cysts are one of the most common disorders of the vulva. They result from obstruction of a duct and may become infected. Thickened mucus, stenosis, or mechanical trauma may initiate the process.

Pathophysiology

The infection usually is unilateral but can be bilateral. *N. gonorrhoeae* is the most common infecting organism. The secretory function of the gland continues, and the duct fills up with fluid, producing severe inflammation, enlargement of the gland, and tissue edema. The area becomes tender, and even walking may be difficult. The pain is constant, and dyspareunia can be severe. The abscess may rupture, resulting in temporary symptom relief, but it usually re-forms. Occasionally, the acute inflammation resolves, leaving scar tissue that can form a cyst. The cyst usually is nontender but may interfere with ambulation or sexual intercourse.

Collaborative Care Management

Cultures are taken, and the woman is treated for any underlying infectious process with broad-spectrum antibiotics. If the cysts are symptomatic, incision and drainage may be performed. The cysts tend to recur, and a permanent opening for drainage of the gland may need to be constructed by placing a tiny catheter through a stab wound into the cyst cavity. The catheter remains in the cyst for 4 to 6 weeks until healing has occurred and a new duct has formed. The catheter is assessed weekly. Bathing is permitted for hygiene and comfort.[28]

Patient/Family Education. Nursing interventions focus on comfort. Mild analgesics and sitz baths help relieve pain. Because most procedures are performed on an outpatient basis, the nurse instructs the woman on home care and reinforces the need to report any signs of infection.

PELVIC INFLAMMATORY DISEASE

Etiology/Epidemiology

Pelvic inflammatory disease (PID) is a general term that refers to acute, subacute, recurrent, or chronic infection of the reproductive organs, pelvic peritoneum, veins, or connective tissue. The infection may be confined to just one structure or be widespread.

Sexually active adolescents are at greatly increased risk of contracting PID, which is the cause of a significant number of hospitalizations for women. PID occurs in women using intrauterine devices (IUDs) more often than in women using other forms of contraception.

The risk factors for PID are the same as those for STDs. These risk factors include low socioeconomic status, early onset of sexual activity, multiple sex partners, vaginal douching, lower educational level, and ethnicity. Chlamydial infection and gonorrhea are frequent causes; therefore sexually active women should be screened for the organisms causing these infections in an effort to prevent PID.[24] Surgery on the reproductive organs, childbearing, and abortion all lower the woman's resistance to infection and provide portals of entry for pathogens.

Pathophysiology

The routes of pelvic infection are illustrated in Figure 53-1. Pathogenic organisms usually are introduced from outside the body and pass up the cervical canal into the uterus. Common causative organisms include gonococci, *Chlamydia, Haemophilus,* and streptococci. The causative organisms invade the pelvis by way of the fallopian tubes or through the uterine veins or lymphatics. Many of the pathogens lodge in the fallopian tubes and create an acute or chronic inflammatory reaction. Purulent material collects in the tubes, adhesions and strictures form, and sterility, which is one of the most serious consequences of PID, may occur. Partial obstruction of the tubes may predispose a woman to ectopic pregnancy because the fertilized ovum cannot reach the uterus. Inflammatory adhesions become so severe that surgi-

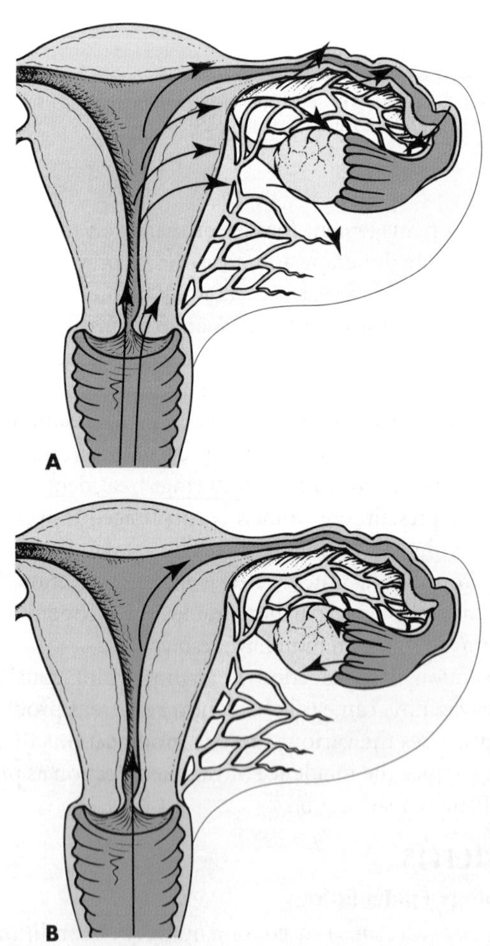

Figure 53-1 Common routes of spread of pelvic inflammatory disease. **A,** Direct spread of bacterial infection other than *Neisseria gonorrhoeae.* **B,** Direct spread of *N. gonorrhoeae.*

cal removal of the uterus, tubes, and ovaries may be necessary. The infection usually remains localized in the lower abdomen and pelvis, although abscesses may form.

Clinical manifestations of acute PID include severe abdominal pain, lower abdominal cramping, intermenstrual bleeding, dyspareunia, fever and chills, malaise, nausea, and vomiting. A sensation of pelvic pressure and back pain may also be present, as well as a foul-smelling, purulent vaginal discharge. The vaginal discharge is copious and commonly purulent and may cause pruritus and excoriation. Abdominal palpation reveals pain and tenderness in the lower quadrants of the abdomen, which is confirmed on pelvic examination. Masses may be felt, indicating enlargement of the fallopian tubes or ovaries or the presence of an abscess. In contrast, some women with PID may have no symptoms.

Collaborative Care Management

Diagnostic studies include white blood cell counts, C-reactive protein, erythrocyte sedimentation rate, and culture of any purulent secretions. Laparoscopy may be ordered to visualize pelvic structures and accomplish drainage of abscesses and lysis of obstructing adhesions. Transvaginal sonography may be used to evaluate masses and structural thickening.[24]

Treatment is aimed at eradicating the infection and preventing complications. Hospitalization may be necessary if the woman is acutely ill. Broad-spectrum antibiotics are used until drug sensitivities are determined. If the woman has an IUD, it is removed.

Nursing interventions are largely supportive. Bed rest in a semi-Fowler's position is recommended to assist with pelvic drainage. Heat applied to the abdomen may be comforting, but tub or sitz baths should be avoided during the period of active infection. Naproxen can be used for pain management. Adequate oral fluids are encouraged. Other nursing measures include managing fever, monitoring vital signs, monitoring intake and output, and providing emotional support.

Patient/Family Education. The nurse instructs the woman to cleanse the perineal region every 3 to 4 hours and maintain scrupulous hygiene after urination and defecation. Tampons should not be used, and drainage pads should be changed frequently. A minimum of 2000 ml of fluids daily is recommended.[24] Women treated as outpatients are reminded of the importance of completing the antibiotic regimen and seeking appropriate follow-up, because PID can have serious lifelong consequences for fertility. Sexual activity should be avoided until the infection is adequately treated. Partner notification, treatment, and counseling should be done. The importance of using condoms to prevent reinfection or future infections is stressed.

TOXIC SHOCK SYNDROME

Etiology/Epidemiology

Toxic shock syndrome (TSS) is a severe disease caused by strains of staphylococci that produce a unique epidermal toxin. It can occur in any situation in which staphylococcal organisms can be harbored, but it is most clearly associated with women during menstruation, particularly women who use tampons. TSS has occurred in infants, children, and men and has been associated with a variety of surgical procedures, including gynecologic, urologic, and orthopedic procedures. Women at increased risk include those who use superabsorbent tampons, insert tampons with their fingers, or have chronic vaginal infections or herpes genitalis. The overall incidence has decreased dramatically with the awareness of appropriate use of tampons.

Pathophysiology

The exact mechanism by which staphylococcal toxins gain access to the circulatory system is unknown. The role of tampons also remains unclear. They may cause mucosal damage, but it is theorized that superabsorbent tampons obstruct the vagina and cause retrograde menstruation with peritoneal absorption of bacteria or toxins. The use of a diaphragm during menstruation creates a similar risk. Tampons may also cause an increase in aerobic bacteria from oxygen trapped in the interfibrous spaces. The longer a tampon is left in place, the greater the risk for TSS. The mortality rate is 4% to 5%.[24]

The onset of symptoms is usually abrupt, with fever, vomiting, watery diarrhea, headache, and myalgia. The patient appears acutely ill, with a fever near 39° C or higher, and the syndrome can progress to hypotensive shock within hours. An erythematous, sunburnlike rash develops over the face, proximal extremities, and trunk, and both the conjunctivae and the pharynx become erythematous. Muscle and abdominal tenderness commonly are present. Signs of central nervous system irritation may be present. Prompt diagnosis is critical, and these symptoms occurring in a menstruating woman using tampons are thoroughly explored. If the woman is wearing a tampon, it is removed immediately.

Collaborative Care Management

Diagnostic tests for TSS include a complete blood screen and cultures of the blood, throat, urine, vaginal secretions, and possibly cerebrospinal fluid. Vaginal cultures usually show penicillinase-producing *Staphylococcus aureus.* The cornerstone of medical care is beta-lactamase–resistant antibiotics such as nafcillin, methicillin, and oxacillin.[24] Penicillinase-resistant agents, antistaphylococcal agents, and corticosteroids may all be used. Aggressive fluid and electrolyte management is indicated if the patient shows signs of shock. Mechanical ventilation may be necessary if acute respiratory distress syndrome develops. The management of shock is discussed in detail in Chapter 14. Nursing care revolves around careful monitoring and supportive care similar to that provided for any critically ill patient (see Chapter 8).

Patient/Family Education. Approximately 30% of women who develop TSS experience recurrences. The greatest risk for recurrence is during the first three menstrual periods after treatment. Recurrent episodes are usually less severe than the initial one. Women can almost entirely eliminate the risk of TSS by avoiding tampon use. In addition to providing this information, the nurse instructs women about the importance of careful perineal hygiene, avoiding douching, and limiting the use of a contraceptive diaphragm to no more than 24 hours at one time. The continued use of tampons requires thorough handwashing before insertion. This is essential, especially for health care workers in hospital settings.

DISORDERS OF MENSTRUATION

Almost all women experience a problem with their menstrual cycle at some point in their reproductive years. Problems produce a variety of symptoms that may be related directly or indirectly to the pelvic organs. Most problems are self-managed and are rarely brought to a physician's attention unless they become severe or persistent.

DYSMENORRHEA

Etiology/Epidemiology

Dysmenorrhea involves uterine pain with menstruation and is commonly known as menstrual cramps. Primary dysmenorrhea is not associated with pelvic pathology and occurs in the absence of any organic disease. Its severity usually declines after pregnancy or by age 30. Secondary dysmenorrhea occurs in response to organic disease such as PID, endometriosis, leiomyomas (uterine fibroids), and IUD use.

Primary dysmenorrhea affects about 60% to 95% of menstruating young women, with 5% to 18% reporting severe symptoms. It is associated with earlier age of menarche, longer duration of menses, and cigarette smoking.[27]

Pathophysiology

Dysmenorrhea is related to the high levels of prostaglandins during the second phase of the menstrual cycle. The exact mechanism by which prostaglandins cause dysmenorrhea is not understood. What causes some women to have excess prostaglandins or increased sensitivity to them also remains in question, but women with dysmenorrhea have been found to have concentrations up to four times higher than those in women without pain.

The pain of primary dysmenorrhea typically occurs on the first or second day of the menses. It is usually described as colicky, cramping pain in the lower abdomen that may be perceived as minor, controllable with mild analgesics, or incapacitating. Backache and other systemic symptoms, particularly involving the GI tract, may also occur.

Collaborative Care Management

Primary dysmenorrhea is treated with prostaglandin inhibitors, which block prostaglandin synthesis and metabolism. Nonsteroidal antiinflammatory drugs (NSAIDs) such as ibuprofen and naproxen are more effective than aspirin in providing pain relief. (Women did report more adverse reactions from naproxen than from ibuprofen.) Other treatments demonstrated to be more effective than placebo include high-frequency transcutaneous electrical nerve stimulation, acupuncture, and vitamin B_1 (thiamine).[27]

Treatment of secondary dysmenorrhea is aimed at correcting the underlying organic cause. Options include both pharmacologic and surgical interventions.

Patient/Family Education. Women rarely seek professional help for mild primary dysmenorrhea. However, women who are consistently unable to engage in normal activities because of menstrual pain should be encouraged to seek medical care. The nurse instructs the patient that NSAIDs are most effective when taken at the onset of the menses before pain becomes severe, and can be buffered with food or antacid if GI irritation occurs. The nurse also encourages the woman to ensure adequate rest, nutrition, and exercise. Constipation should be avoided. If pain occurs, the nurse can suggest that the woman (1) use local heat, which helps dilate the blood vessels and relieve ischemia, and (2) use progressive relaxation strategies, although there is insufficient evidence of their effectiveness.[27]

AMENORRHEA

Etiology/Epidemiology

Amenorrhea is the absence of menstruation. Primary amenorrhea exists if the first menses has not occurred by age 16. Secondary amenorrhea exists when a previously menstruating woman ceases to menstruate for more than 3 to 6 months (3 months in a woman with a history of regular menstrual cycles). Skipping an occasional single period is normal. Pregnancy is the most common cause of secondary amenorrhea. Amenorrhea can result from anatomic abnormalities, genetic conditions, hypothalamic or pituitary dysfunction, or ovarian failure.[23]

Pathophysiology

Prolonged secondary amenorrhea is common among certain groups of conditioned athletes on aggressive training schedules, because of decreased body fat percentages. A weight loss of 10% to 15% of total body weight can also result in amenorrhea.

The consequences of prolonged amenorrhea are not fully known, but strong evidence indicates that it is detrimental to bone density and can hasten the development of osteoporosis. A woman who does not ovulate may also develop endometrial cancer, breast disease, or dysfunctional uterine bleeding and is infertile.

Collaborative Care Management

The diagnostic workup for amenorrhea includes a detailed history and careful examination of the reproductive system. Laboratory analysis of levels of follicle-stimulating hormone, prolactin, thyroid-stimulating hormone, cortisol, calcium, and autoantibodies, as well as assessment of karotype, may be indicated.[23] Pregnancy should be ruled out as a possible cause. The treatment depends on the cause. An organic problem is corrected, if possible, through surgery or hormone replacement.

Patient/Family Education. The nurse teaches the woman about the problem, its causes, and the diagnostic studies planned. Teaching may include information about weight gain, stress reduction, and reducing the energy drain of strenuous exercise. Women may need counseling and support to deal with feelings of threat to their self-concept and concerns over fertility that may be caused by the amenorrhea.

PREMENSTRUAL SYNDROME

Etiology/Epidemiology

The term *premenstrual syndrome (PMS)* has been given to a cluster of distressing physical and behavioral symptoms that occur in the second half of the menstrual cycle and are followed by a symptom-free period. About 10% of women experience severe symptoms and seek medical assistance. The peak prevalence for PMS occurs in the thirties, with a slight decline noted in the forties.

The etiology of PMS is unknown. A disturbance in serotonin regulation is the most recent theory supported by research.[5]

Pathophysiology

Symptoms of PMS are many and varied and range in severity from mild to severe. The symptoms are not well defined and involve multiple body systems. The lack of a proven etiology makes it difficult to track a cause-and-effect relationship for physiologic changes and observed or reported symptoms. The symptoms appear only in the luteal phase of the menstrual cycle and disappear completely with menopause. Symptoms include affective and somatic complaints, including depression, irritability, anger, confusion, anxiety, social withdrawal, breast tenderness, abdominal bloating, headache, and swelling.[5]

Collaborative Care Management

No objective means of diagnosing PMS exists, and the diagnosis is primarily established by exclusion. A careful clinical history is critical. The woman is asked to keep an accurate diary during her menstrual periods of the occurrence, nature, and severity of symptoms. A woman is considered to have PMS if her symptoms interfere with activities of daily living. Symptoms that occur in the 5 days preceding menses for two consecutive cycles confirm the diagnosis.

Numerous treatments have been suggested, including both pharmacologic and nonpharmacologic strategies, but no treatment has proved to be effective in all cases. The American College of Obstetricians and Gynecologists recommends a step approach in the treatment of women with PMS. The first step includes supportive therapy, particularly relaxation therapy; dietary modification to increase complex carbohydrate intake; use of calcium, magnesium, and vitamin E supplements; aerobic exercise; and spironolactone. Second-step therapy includes the use of selective serotonin reuptake inhibitors or an anxiolytic for nonresponders. Third-step therapy involves the use of hormonal ovulation suppression with oral contraceptives or gonadotropin-releasing hormone (GnRH) agonists.[5]

Patient/Family Education. The nurse helps the woman and her family understand the possible causes of the syndrome and the rationale for any planned treatments. Simple lifestyle modifications can reduce symptoms and improve the woman's overall well-being. Regular aerobic exercise is strongly recommended, because exercise results in a release of endorphins, which can elevate the mood. The nurse encourages the woman to avoid fatigue, because it exaggerates the symptoms of PMS. This is particularly important in the premenstrual period. Stress management techniques are also recommended. The Patient Teaching box summarizes patient teaching related to PMS. The nurse can refer interested patients and families to the National Women's Health Information Center (NWHIC) (website: www.4woman.gov) or the National PMS Society.*

DYSFUNCTIONAL UTERINE BLEEDING

Etiology/Epidemiology

Dysfunctional uterine bleeding (DUB) is excessive or irregular uterine bleeding with no demonstrable cause. It can take many forms, including excessive flow, prolonged duration of menses, and intermenstrual bleeding.

DUB may be caused by a variety of factors. Pregnancy must be ruled out. Table 53-2 lists and defines various types of DUB and their associated etiologies. Some systemic diseases can cause DUB. Liver disease may interfere with estrogen metabolism, and blood dyscrasias can produce spontaneous bleeding. DUB related to the menstrual cycle is usually anovulatory and painless and generally occurs at the extremes of menstrual life, when disturbances of ovarian function are common. In perimenopausal and postmenopausal women DUB is commonly associated with uterine cancer.

Pathophysiology

DUB may occur between or during the menstrual periods. When menorrhagia is present, the woman may soak a tampon or pad every 1 to 2 hours for a week or more. The exact cause of the anovulatory episode is not understood, but it may represent a dysfunction of the hypothalamic-pituitary-ovarian axis that results in continuing estrogen stimulation of the endometrium. The endometrium outgrows its blood supply, partially breaks down, and is sloughed in an irregular manner. Anovulation may also result from other endocrine abnormalities.[23]

*PO Box 11467, Durham, NC 27703.

Patient Teaching
The Patient With Premenstrual Syndrome

1. Teach about the possible causes of the condition and its treatment.
2. Teach relaxation techniques.
3. Teach patient to:
   a. Avoid stressful activities during the premenstrual period.
   b. Ensure adequate rest, especially during the premenstrual period. Fatigue exaggerates symptoms.
   c. Take medications as prescribed (explain rationale).
   d. Reduce or eliminate smoking and alcohol consumption.
   e. Follow a regular exercise program.
   f. Eat a well-balanced diet with complex carbohydrates and a reduced intake of salt and refined sugars.
   g. Incorporate stress-reducing strategies into daily lifestyle.

TABLE 53-2 Causes of Dysfunctional Uterine Bleeding During Childbearing and Postmenopausal Years

Type	Cause
Menorrhagia: prolonged profuse menstrual flow during regular period	Submucous myomas, pregnancy complications, adenomyosis, endometrial hyperplasias, malignant tumors, hypothyroidism, von Willebrand's disease
Metrorrhagia: bleeding between periods	Endometrial polyps, endometrial and cervical cancer, exogenous estrogen administration
Polymenorrhea: increased frequency of menstruation	Anovulation, shortened luteal phase
Cryptomenorrhea: unusually light menstrual flow	Hymenal or cervical stenosis, Asherman's syndrome (uterine synechiae), oral contraceptives
Menometrorrhagia: bleeding at irregular intervals	Any condition causing intermenstrual bleeding; sudden onset is indication of malignant tumors or complications of pregnancy
Oligomenorrhea: menstrual periods more than 35 days apart	Anovulation from endocrine causes (pregnancy, menopause) or systemic causes (excessive weight loss); estrogen-secreting tumors
Dysfunctional uterine bleeding: abnormal bleeding without known organic cause	Unknown

Collaborative Care Management

The diagnostic workup for DUB begins with a thorough history of the frequency, amount, and duration of bleeding. Pelvic examination is done to detect gross abnormalities, which are further evaluated by pelvic or transvaginal ultrasound, hysteroscopy, or endometrial biopsy. Laboratory tests may include blood counts to estimate blood loss, pregnancy tests, endocrine studies, ovulation tests, and coagulation studies.

The cause of the bleeding guides medical care. In the absence of an organic cause, the preferred treatment is usually conservative. Pharmacologic options to stop heavy bleeding or reduce future blood loss in subsequent menstrual cycles include the use of estrogens, progestins, NSAIDs, antifibrinolytic agents, and GnRH agonists such as danazol. Endometrial ablation or hysterectomy may be necessary for those women whose bleeding cannot be controlled with hormones.[23]

Patient/Family Education. Because most care for DUB is provided in the outpatient setting, the nursing role is largely educational. The impact of chronic excessive bleeding on a woman's lifestyle can be profound. The nurse teaches the woman to accurately assess the amount of bleeding in terms of number of pads or tampons, type of pad or tampon, and degree of saturation. The nurse helps the woman set up and maintain an accurate record of the bleeding in the form of a diary. The nurse also encourages the woman to express her concerns and fears. Anxiety related to infertility or fear of cancer can be intense but remain unexpressed.

ENDOMETRIOSIS

Etiology/Epidemiology

Endometriosis is a condition in which endometrial cells that normally line the uterus are seeded throughout the pelvis. Endometriosis typically affects women during their childbearing years. Although the age-specific prevalence is unknown, it is estimated that the incidence is 2% to 22% in the general female population. The incidence in women with dysmenorrhea is 40% to 60%.[8]

The etiology of endometriosis remains unknown. The condition may be hereditary, because it occurs more often in women whose mothers had the disorder. Theories include the congenital presence of endometrial cells out of their normal location, the transfer of endometrial cells by means of the blood or lymph system, reflux of menstrual fluid containing endometrial cells up the fallopian tubes and into the pelvic cavity, and ineffectiveness of the cellular immune response.[23]

Pathophysiology

With each menstrual period the seeded endometrial cells are stimulated by ovarian hormones and bleed into the surrounding tissues, causing an inflammatory response. Encased blood may lead to palpable masses known as chocolate cysts. Occasionally the cysts rupture and spread endometrial cells deeper into the pelvis. Repeated inflammation and healing may create adhesions severe enough to fuse pelvic organs or cause bowel or bladder strictures.

The ovaries are the most common site of involvement, and the process is usually bilateral (Figure 53-2). The pelvic peritoneum; the anterior and posterior cul-de-sac; and the uterosacral, round, and broad ligaments are other common sites.

Endometriosis progresses gradually and usually does not produce symptoms until the woman is 30 to 40 years of age. The classic feature is menstrual pain or discomfort that becomes progressively worse. Other possible symptoms include abdominal pain, dyspareunia, irregular menses, bowel problems, and urinary dysfunction. Pelvic examination often reveals a fixed, retroverted uterus that is enlarged, tender, and nodular. Occasionally, the disease is far advanced but causes no symptoms, and it may first be diagnosed as part of a workup for infertility.

Collaborative Care Management

Laparoscopy is the only definitive method of diagnosing endometriosis. The endoscopy is used to carefully map and

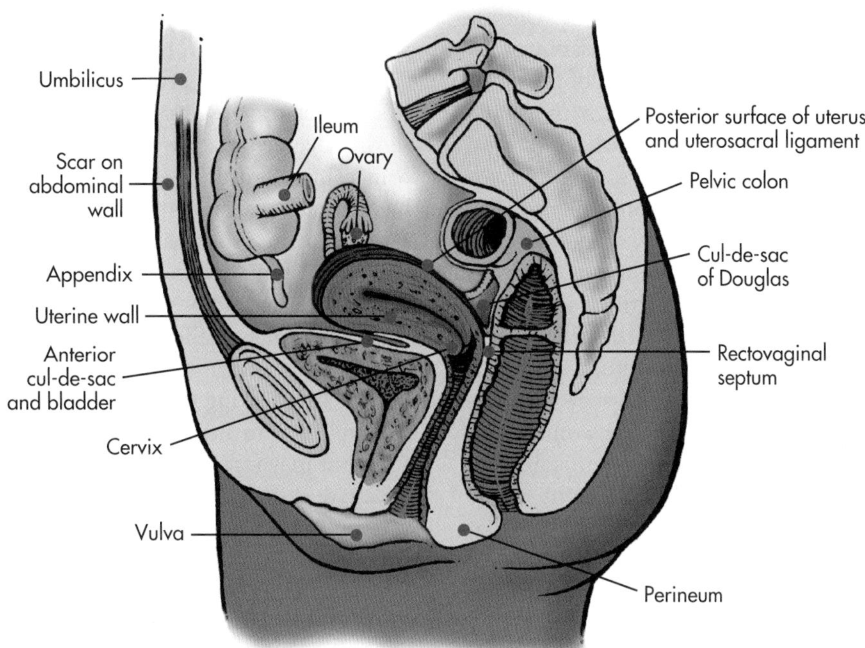

Figure 53-2 Common locations for endometriosis.

describe the extent of disease involvement, and biopsies of suspicious tissue can be obtained during the procedure.

Because the cause of endometriosis is not understood, treatment is highly individualized. In rare cases endometriosis disappears spontaneously. Pregnancy appears to slow the progression of the condition because menstruation is halted during pregnancy and lactation. Some women remain asymptomatic after pregnancy. A couple may be encouraged to attempt pregnancy if children are desired, because the fertility rate is low and continues to deteriorate with time. Mild cases may be managed with NSAIDs and regular monitoring.

Hormonal treatment with agents such as danazol, medroxyprogesterone, gestrinone, oral contraceptives, and GnRH agonists has been effective in reducing the pain of endometriosis.[27] Oral contraceptives with minimal estrogen and high levels of progestins may be used to produce endometrial atrophy. Disadvantages to this approach include irregular bleeding and symptoms such as nausea, fatigue, and depression. Drugs with antigonadotropic action, such as danazol, may be used to suppress ovarian activity. Danazol stops endometrial proliferation, prevents ovulation, and produces atrophy of the ectopic endometrial tissue.

The major drawbacks to the treatment are its high cost and the occurrence of common side effects such as hot flashes, depression, and weight gain. GnRH agonists are an even more expensive approach to treatment. These drugs induce a hypoestrogenic state and result in amenorrhea. Side effects mimic the symptoms of menopause. A steady loss in bone density limits the duration of possible treatment.

Surgical intervention may be necessary if the disorder does not respond to drug therapy. Conservative approaches that attempt to preserve the woman's fertility include lysis of adhesions and destruction of pockets of implanted endometrial tissue by means of laparoscopic laser surgery. More radical surgery involves the removal of the uterus, tubes, and possibly the ovaries. Ovarian function is preserved if at all possible. The onset of menopause halts the disorder.

Patient/Family Education. Because most care for women with endometriosis is delivered in the community, the nurse's role is largely educational and supportive. The nurse reassures the woman that endometriosis can be treated. The nurse teaches about the prescribed drugs and the management of side effects. Strategies to manage chronic pain are particularly important. The importance of ongoing care and follow-up is reinforced. Referral to support groups may be beneficial. This is particularly important if infertility related to the endometriosis is diagnosed. Two excellent organizations are the Endometriosis Association* and Resolve Incorporated.†

STRUCTURAL PROBLEMS

UTERINE DISPLACEMENT/PROLAPSE

Etiology/Epidemiology

The uterus may undergo minor displacement in ways that are considered to be normal variations with little or no clinical effect (Figure 53-3). Retroversion is the most common variation and occurs in about 20% of women. Uterine prolapse represents a severe uterine problem in which the uterus protrudes through the pelvic floor aperture or genital hiatus.

*8585 North 76th Place, Milwaukee, WI 53223.
†5 Water St., Arlington, MA 02174.

It is usually associated with a cystocele or rectocele. Uterine prolapse occurs most often in multiparous Caucasian women as a response to injuries to the muscles and fascia of the pelvis incurred during childbirth. Systemic conditions, such as obesity and chronic pulmonary disease, and local conditions, such as ascites and uterine or ovarian tumors, are other potential causes. Chronic coughing can also contribute to prolapse.[23] Prolapse usually develops gradually, suggesting that the effects of aging play a major role. As the uterus begins to drop, the vaginal walls become relaxed and the bladder may herniate into the vagina (cystocele), or the rectal wall may herniate into the vagina (rectocele). These structural problems are illustrated in Figure 53-3. Both conditions may occur simultaneously. Cystoceles are common, and the woman may remain completely asymptomatic until after menopause. Estrogen helps maintain adequate blood flow and tone of the paravaginal tissues, and its loss results in atrophic changes that render the tissues more subject to prolapse.

Pathophysiology

Variations in the normal position of the uterus or prolapse can result from congenital or acquired abnormalities of the pelvic support structures. Acquired weaknesses occur after childbirth, surgery, and closely spaced pregnancies and in response to obesity and the loss of tissue elasticity with aging. The severity of the prolapse is designated by degree. In a first-degree prolapse the cervix is still within the vagina. In a second-degree prolapse the cervix protrudes from the vaginal orifice. In a third-degree prolapse the entire uterus, suspended by its stretched ligaments, hangs below the vaginal orifice. Before menopause the uterus hypertrophies and is engorged and flabby. The vaginal mucosa thickens, and stasis ulcers may develop. Anterior and posterior vaginal wall relaxation often accompany prolapse, allowing for the development of cystocele or rectocele. Older women may have these conditions for years before seeking medical attention.

Patients with first-degree prolapse experience few symptoms but may report sensations of heaviness or fullness and a feeling that something is falling out of the vagina. In more severe prolapse, when the cervix protrudes at the introitus, the patient may complain of feeling like she is sitting on a ball. With severe prolapse the woman is clearly aware of the mass. Leukorrhea or menometrorrhagia may develop in premenopausal women with prolapse as a result of uterine engorgement. After menopause, discharge and bleeding with prolapse usually result from infection and ulceration.

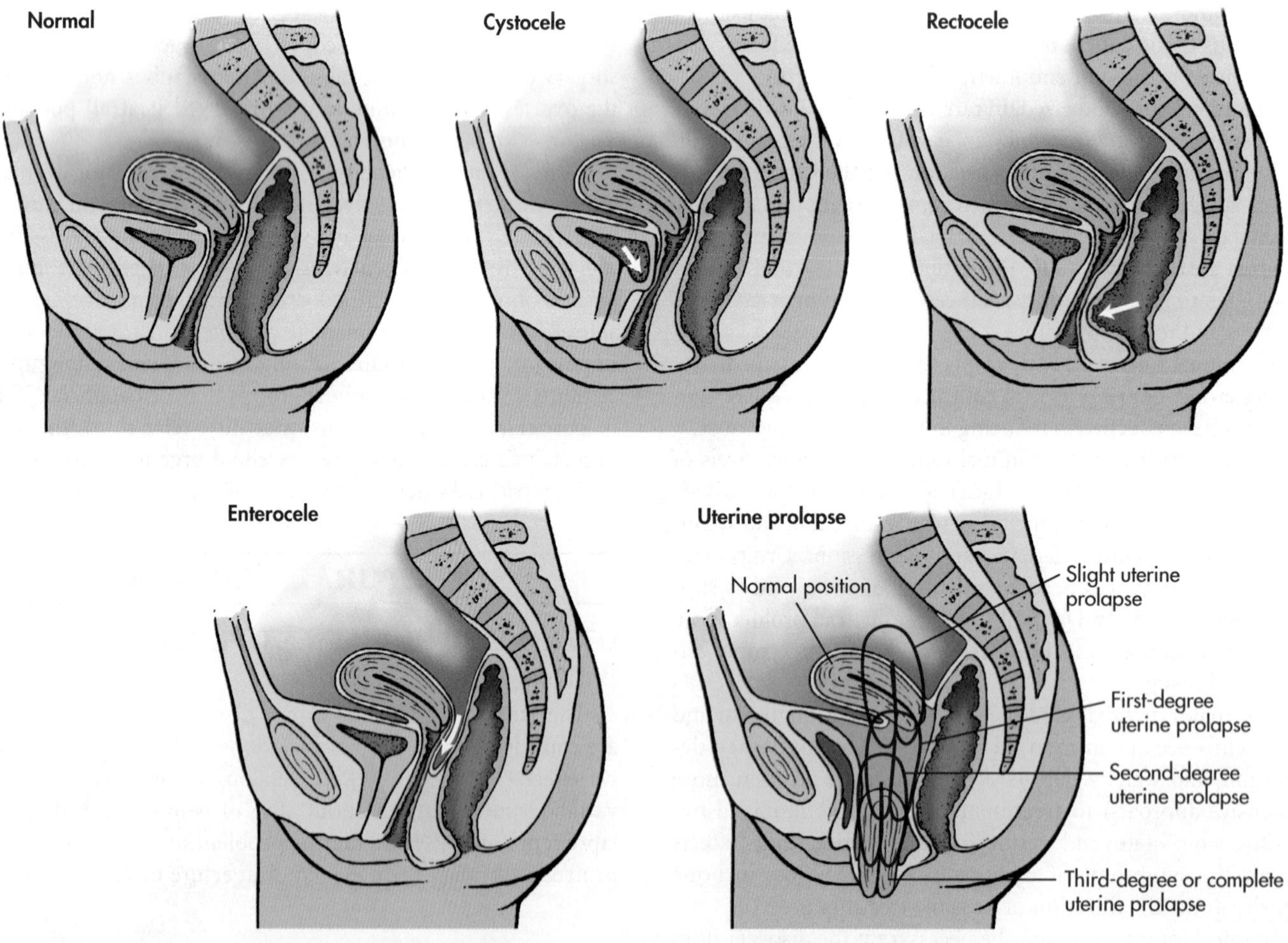

Figure 53-3 Types of uterine prolapse.

The woman with a cystocele may complain of urinary incontinence accompanying any activity that increases intraabdominal pressure, such as coughing, laughing, or lifting. She may also experience frequent urinary tract infections. The patient with a rectocele may complain of chronic constipation and develop hemorrhoids.

Collaborative Care Management

Uterine prolapse can be readily identified on pelvic examination. If a cystocele is present, the vaginal outlet is relaxed with a thin-walled, smooth, bulging mass present in the anterior vaginal wall below the cervix. The mass descends when the patient is asked to bear down. If a rectocele is present, palpation of the vaginal area reveals a thin-walled rectovaginal septum projecting into the vagina. Many women are found to have both a cystocele and a rectocele.

A first-degree prolapse in a postmenopausal woman is treated with estrogen therapy to maintain the tone and integrity of the pelvic floor muscles. Exercise therapy is suggested for all women. (Exercises for the pelvic floor are discussed under Patient/Family Education.) If pain or bleeding occurs, the uterus may be manually repositioned and supported by the insertion of a vaginal pessary (Figure 53-4). Pessaries are devices made of hard rubber or plastic that maintain the uterus in a forward position by exerting pressure on the ligaments attached to the posterior wall of the cervix.

Conservative treatment with estrogen, exercise, and a pessary may also be employed for a cystocele or rectocele if the woman experiences only mild symptoms. Surgery to repair cystoceles, rectoceles, and more advanced prolapses is undertaken when symptoms significantly interfere with the patient's lifestyle or threaten other organ function, such as the kidney if repeated urinary track infections are present. The procedures designed to tighten the vaginal wall are referred to as anterior and posterior colporrhaphy. They are often combined with hysterectomy. Cystocele repair may be done abdominally and combined with a urethrovesical suspension procedure, called a Marshall-Marchetti-Krantz procedure, to correct stress incontinence.

Patient/Family Education. Exercise teaching is an important nursing intervention for any patient with a uterine displacement or prolapse. Kegel perineal exercises are the mainstay. The woman is instructed to tighten the muscles of the perineum as if to stop the flow of urine, maintain the tension for 5 seconds at a time, and repeat the exercise in sets of 10. The exercise is repeated 10 to 12 times daily. Knee-chest exercises are used less often but may be ordered to stretch or strengthen the pelvic ligaments. Corrective exercises for poor posture may also be prescribed.

The nurse encourages obese patients to lose weight to reduce intraabdominal pressure. Chronic cough and chronic constipation are also corrected, because these conditions contribute to weakness of the muscular wall.

Women fitted with a pessary need to be taught how to insert it and withdraw it if the device becomes displaced or uncomfortable. Pessaries are removed and cleaned once every few weeks or months as recommended by the physician. If the pessary is neglected, it can cause infection or fistula. Women who undergo anterior colporrhaphy are instructed to refrain from heavy lifting, straining, and strenuous exercise for 3 months. Sexual intercourse may be resumed after about 3 weeks. See Guidelines for Safe Practice box on p. 1758.

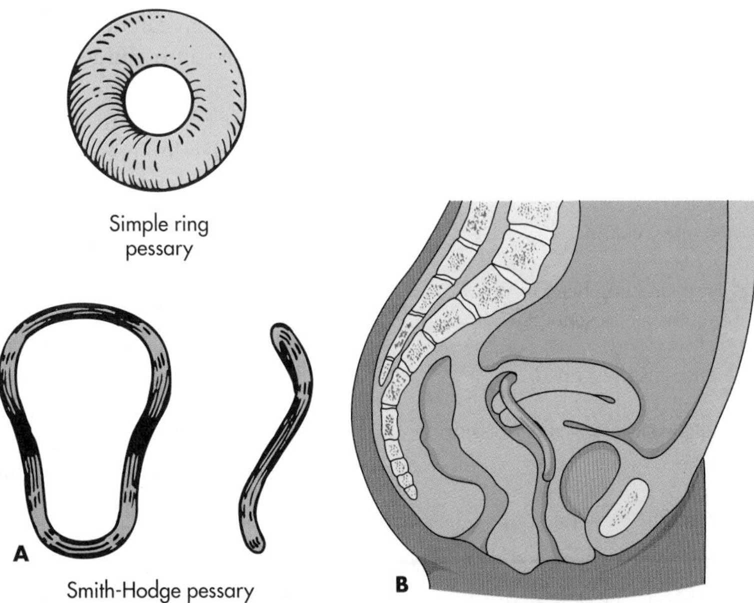

Figure 53-4 **A,** Examples of pessaries (simple ring, Smith-Hodge). **B,** Pessary in place to hold posterior vaginal fornix and, with it, attached cervix wall backward and upward in pelvis.

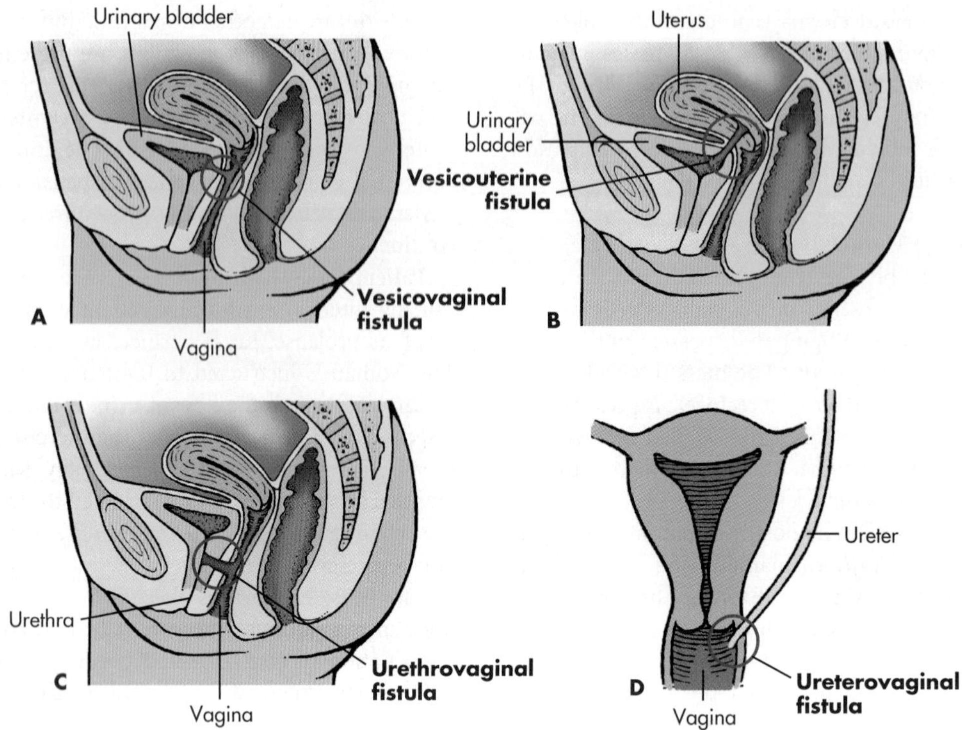

Figure 53-5 Types of genitourinary fistulas. **A,** Vesicovaginal (bladder to vagina). **B,** Vesicouterine (bladder to uterus). **C,** Urethrovaginal (urethra to vagina). **D,** Ureterovaginal (ureter to vagina). Fistulas range in size from tiny and difficult to locate to large, disfiguring the base of the bladder. The primary symptom of a genitourinary fistula is leakage of urine into the vagina, which can be a source of embarrassment for the woman. The fistula may be seen during a vaginal examination with the patient in the knee-chest position and confirmed by an intravenous pyelogram. If healing does not occur within 6 months, surgical closure is used.

Guidelines for Safe Practice

The Patient Undergoing Vaginal Surgery

1. Provide perineal care after each voiding or defecation.
   a. Pour sterile normal saline over vulva and perineum.
   b. Cleanse perineum as needed with sterile cotton balls; cleanse away from vagina toward rectum.
   c. Dry perineum as needed with sterile cotton balls.
2. Encourage sitz baths after sutures are removed.
3. If douches are ordered during immediate postoperative period:
   a. Use sterile equipment and sterile solution.
   b. Insert douche nozzle very gently.
4. Prepare patient for discharge by instructing her to:
   a. Take daily douches and tub baths as prescribed.
   b. Avoid straining at stool.
   c. Use stool softeners and laxatives as prescribed.
   d. Avoid lifting for 6 weeks.
   e. Avoid sexual intercourse until physician gives permission (usually about 6 weeks).
   f. Avoid jarring activities.
   g. Avoid prolonged standing, walking, or sitting.
   h. Continue leg exercises for 6 weeks.
   i. Recognize that vaginal sensation may be lost for several months postoperatively, but sensation will return.
   j. Eat a high-fiber diet and drink 3000 ml of fluids daily.

FISTULAS

Etiology/Epidemiology

A fistula is an abnormal tunnel-like opening between hollow internal organs or between an organ and the exterior of the body. Fistulas can develop from a variety of causes but are usually the result of surgery, childbirth, trauma, or radiation therapy.

The name of the fistula indicates the connecting structures. Fistulas can develop between the vagina and the rectum (rectovaginal), bladder (vesicovaginal), or urethra (urethrovaginal). They are illustrated in Figure 53-5. Vesicovaginal fistulas are the most common, followed by rectovaginal fistulas.

Pathophysiology

Conditions that cause fistulas to form typically compromise the blood supply and cause tissue damage. A passageway between the vagina and the bladder and/or rectum results in a constant leak of urine or escape of flatus and fecal material through the vagina. This is highly distressing to the patient and creates an offensive odor. The drainage excoriates and irritates the vaginal and vulvar tissue.

Collaborative Care Management

Fistulas are diagnosed primarily through pelvic examination. A fistulogram, which involves the injection of dye into the vagina, may be used to assess the exact location and severity of the fistula. Small fistulas may heal spontaneously if the tissue is allowed to rest. Surgery is otherwise necessary to close the fistula tract. Tissue inflammation and edema must be treated first, and this can take months. Either anterior or posterior colporrhaphy may be done. It may be necessary to temporarily divert the urinary or fecal stream in complex situations. A Foley, ureteral, or nephrostomy catheter is used to keep the area well drained and is left in place for weeks in some patients.

Postoperative care focuses on tissue healing. A small amount of serosanguinous drainage is expected, but the patient is carefully monitored for evidence of continued fecal or urinary drainage. Douches may be ordered, and the nurse administers them gently and at low pressure to protect healing tissue. Bed rest is often enforced for several days.

If the fistula is being conservatively managed, nursing intervention focuses on comfort and the prevention of infection. Sitz baths and careful cleansing with mild soap and water are helpful. Although protective pads may be worn, the nurse stresses that cleansing must be repeated at regular intervals to prevent skin breakdown and odor.

Surgical repair is not always successful, and repeat procedures may be needed. The risk of infection is constantly present, and the nurse anticipates that the patient may become anxious and depressed about her situation. The nurse encourages the patient to verbalize her concerns and seek support from family and friends.

BENIGN AND MALIGNANT NEOPLASMS OF THE FEMALE REPRODUCTIVE TRACT

NEOPLASMS OF THE CERVIX

Cervical Polyps

Etiology/Epidemiology

Cervical polyps are relatively common. The two main types are (1) endocervical from the canal in the opening of the cervix and (2) ectocervical from the lower portion of the cervix that protrudes into the vagina. Endocervical polyps tend to occur in middle-aged multiparous women. Ectocervical polyps are found most often in postmenopausal women. Polyps are thought to arise from hyperplasia, possibly in response to chronic inflammation, abnormal responses to hormonal stimulation, or localized vascular congestion. Hyperestrinism is thought to play a major role. Although most cervical polyps are benign, some cervical cancers manifest as a polypoid mass.

Pathophysiology

Most polyps are asymptomatic and discovered on routine pelvic examination. Endocervical polyps are usually reddish purple to cherry red, smooth, soft growths that may vary in size from a few millimeters to 2 or 3 cm in diameter and length. They are usually attached to the mucosa by a narrow pedicle and may be single or multiple in number. Ectocervical polyps are pale or flesh colored, round or elongated, and often attach with a broad pedicle. Polyps are usually very vascular.[23] The classic symptom is intermenstrual bleeding, particularly after sexual intercourse or douching. Leukorrhea may be present. The chronic irritation and bleeding can lead to cervicitis, endometritis, or even salpingitis.

Collaborative Care Management

Cervical polyps are usually diagnosed by direct inspection and can be removed safely in a physician's office through clamping or incision.[23] The procedure causes minimal bleeding, but if bleeding should occur, it can be controlled by electrical or chemical cautery. All of the excised tissue is sent for pathologic examination.

Patient/Family Education. The nurse encourages the woman to rest and avoid strenuous activity after polyp removal. A perineal pad can be provided to absorb drainage. The nurse instructs the woman to report any significant bleeding or signs of infection. The nurse also instructs the woman to avoid tampon use, douches, and sexual intercourse for about a week while healing takes place.

Cancer of the Cervix

Etiology

Although the cause of carcinoma of the cervix remains unknown, a close association exists between early and frequent sexual contact with multiple partners and cervical viral infection, particularly with HPV. HPV has been isolated in the vast majority of precancerous and cancerous changes of the cervix. A vaccine for HPV may reduce the incidence of cervical cancer.[17] Risk factors for cervical cancer include multiple sexual partners, a history of HPV infection, first sexual intercourse before age 16, cigarette smoking, environmental tobacco smoke exposure, prolonged use of oral contraceptives for more than 5 years, and ethnicity.[13]

Immunosuppression also increases the risk of cervical cancer, and studies indicate that women positive for HIV are at high risk for cervical cancer and have a poorer disease prognosis. STDs are also linked with atypical cell transformation. Dietary factors include deficiencies of vitamins A and C and derangement in folic acid metabolism.

Epidemiology

Cervical cancer is the sixth most common type of solid cancer in women following breast, colorectal, lung, endometrial, and ovarian cancers.[23] Papanicolaou (Pap) smear screening has significantly reduced the mortality rate associated with cervical cancer in the United States, but 4800 women still die annually of cervical cancer in the United States. Cancer of the cervix is the leading cause of cancer deaths among women in underdeveloped countries with inadequate cervical cancer screening programs.

There has been a general decline in the incidence of cervical cancer in the United States, although the overall incidence of Pap smear abnormalities has risen rapidly over the past 2 decades. Cervical carcinoma in situ, a precancerous noninvasive stage, is now the most common form diagnosed and peaks in incidence between the ages of 25 and 35. Preinvasive lesions seem to occur in some populations at a very early age, perhaps related to the sexual practices of teenagers. The incidence of invasive cervical cancer increases with age. The risk factors for cervical cancer are summarized in the Risk Factors box. Women need to be informed of and supported in their efforts to reduce their modifiable risk factors for cervical cancer. Patient teaching relative to the prevention of cervical cancer is presented in the Patient Teaching box.

Pathophysiology

Ninety-five percent of all cervical cancers are squamous cell, arising from the epidermal layer of the cervix. Cell dysplasia indicates the presence of a precursor lesion, typically called cervical intraepithelial neoplasia (CIN), which has been divided into the following three stages:

CIN I: mild to moderate dysplasia
CIN II: moderate to severe dysplasia
CIN III: severe dysplasia to carcinoma in situ

Women diagnosed with dysplasia may experience disease regression, persistence, or a progression to carcinoma. There are usually no signs or symptoms of dysplasia, and the diagnosis is based on cytologic findings. Early detection is important to ensure positive outcomes. Routine Pap screening begins once a woman engages in regular sexual intercourse or turns 18 years old. Increased frequency of screening reduces deaths from cervical cancer; however, optimal frequency has not been established (see Evidence-Based Practice box). Undertested groups, including ethnic minorities and older women, need special encouragement to have routine Pap screening. Abnormal smears should be followed up with colposcopy and biopsy to further investigate cellular change.[23]

Cervical cancer spreads through the blood, by direct extension, and by lymph invasion. As the lymph nodes grow larger, venous flow is obstructed, and leg edema, ureteral obstruction, or hydronephrosis may occur. Distant organ metastasis to the lung, liver, or bone can occur in the advanced stage.[23] Prognosis is based on the stage of the disease, depth of invasion, and vascular involvement of the tumor (Table 53-3).

Risk Factors

Cervical Cancer

RISK FACTORS

- Human papillomavirus infection
- Cigarette smoking
- Low socioeconomic status
- Early age at first coitus
- Multiple sexual partners
- History of sexually transmitted diseases
- High-risk male partner
- Compromised immunity, including human immunodeficiency virus (HIV) infection
- Early age at first pregnancy
- Multiparity, especially for African-Americans, Mexican-Americans, and Native Americans
- Prostitution

POTENTIAL RISK FACTORS

- Heavy use of talc
- Use of oral contraceptives
- Deficiencies of vitamins A and C
- Derangement of folic acid metabolism
- Intrauterine exposure to diethylstilbestrol (DES)
- Diabetes
- Nulliparity
- Frequent douching

Patient Teaching

Prevention of Cervical Cancer

1. Reinforce importance of condom use during sexual intercourse to limit transmission of sexually transmitted diseases (STDs) and genital viruses.
2. Encourage adolescent girls to delay the onset of sexual activity and limit the number of their sex partners.
3. Teach importance of prompt and effective treatment of vaginal or cervical infections.
4. Stress importance of following American Cancer Society Guidelines for Pap screening.
   a. Annually for sexually active women age 18 and older and at intervals recommended by health care provider once a pattern of three annual negative tests is established
   b. Annually throughout life for women who are considered to be at high risk
5. Implement Agency for Healthcare Research and Quality (AHRQ) guidelines on tobacco cessation. Ask about smoking status and exposure to environmental sources. Advise about quitting; ask if woman is ready to set quit date. Support smoking cessation efforts and plan follow-up support.

Evidence-Based Practice

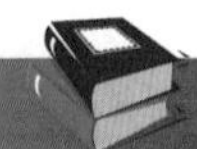

The Institute for Clinical Systems Improvement publishes clinical practice guidelines for a variety of health-related conditions, including cervical cancer screening. The guidelines include algorithms supported by a range of evidence, from randomized clinical trials and cross-sectional studies to meta-analyses and expert opinion. Published guidelines are reviewed on a rotational basis approximately every 18 months. Use of the cervical cancer screening guideline should contribute to achievement of the Healthy People 2010 goals related to increasing the number of women who receive Pap smears and ultimately decreasing the number of deaths from cervical cancer. The guideline indicates that there is strong research support, including clinical trials for time spent on prescreening educational and counseling activities, to increase the number of women who are up-to-date on cervical screening. The guideline also states that the ideal time to initiate cervical cancer screening is after the start of sexual activity, which for many adolescents is before age 18. Women who have had three consecutive normal Pap smears and no dysplasia can reduce the screening frequency to every 3 years.

Cervical cancer is asymptomatic in the early stages. As the disease progresses, the woman may experience a slight watery vaginal discharge and occasional bloody spotting, especially after sexual intercourse. With advanced disease, a foul-smelling discharge may develop from sloughing of the epithelial tissue. Pain is usually a late sign and can involve the pelvis, flank, lower back, and abdomen. The growing tumor may place pressure on the rectum and bladder, causing irritation and discharge. Hemorrhage is possible with advanced infiltrative tumors, which may also erode the walls of adjacent organs and create fistulas. The signs and symptoms of cervical cancer are summarized in the Clinical Manifestations box.

Collaborative Care Management

Diagnostic Tests. Women with CIN are followed closely with repeat Pap tests. Colposcopy is used to examine cervical lesions and to direct cervical biopsies.[23] Cervical conization can also be used therapeutically to remove the entire lesion and remains a valuable tool for preserving a woman's fertility. Cone biopsy is illustrated in Figure 53-6.

Clinical Manifestations

Cervical Cancer

EARLY SYMPTOMS

Thin, watery vaginal discharge
Bloody spotting after coitus or douching
Metrorrhagia
Postmenopausal bleeding
Polymenorrhea

LATE SYMPTOMS

Dark, foul-smelling vaginal discharge
Pelvic, abdominal, or back pain
Flank pain
Weight loss
Anorexia
Anemia
Leg edema
Dysuria
Rectal bleeding

TABLE 53-3 Clinical Stages in Carcinoma of the Cervix Uteri (FIGO System)

Stage	Involvement
Stage 0	Carcinoma in situ, cervical intraepithelial neoplasm (CIN)
Stage I	Carcinoma strictly confined to cervix (extension to corpus should be disregarded)
Stage Ia	Preclinical carcinoma of cervix diagnosed only by microscopy
Stage Ia1	Stroma invasion of 3 × 7 mm
Stage Ia2	Stroma invasion of 5 × 7 mm
Stage Ib	Lesions of cervix or preclinical lesions larger than Ia
Stage II	Involvement of vagina but not lower third, or infiltration beyond cervix but not into wall
Stage IIa	Involvement of up to upper two thirds of vagina but no evidence of parametrial involvement
Stage IIb	Infiltration of parametrium but not out to sidewall
Stage III	Involvement of lower third of vagina or extension to pelvic sidewall; includes all cases with a hydronephrosis or nonfunctioning kidney, unless they are known to be attributable to other cause
Stage IIIa	Involvement of lower third of vagina but not out to pelvic sidewalls
Stage IIIb	Extension onto pelvic sidewall or hydronephrosis or nonfunctional kidney
Stage IV	Extension outside reproductive tract
Stage IVa	Involvement of mucosa of bladder or rectum
Stage IVb	Distant metastasis or disease outside true pelvis

Source: National Cancer Institute: Screening for cervical cancer, *PDQ summary,* website: www.nci.gov, 2001.
FIGO, International Federation of Gynecology and Obstetrics.

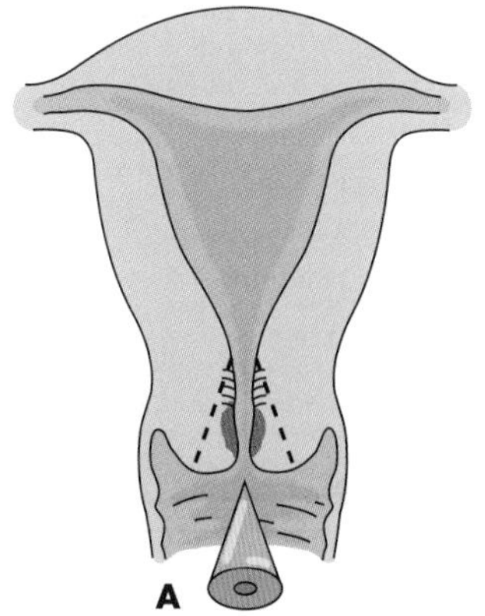

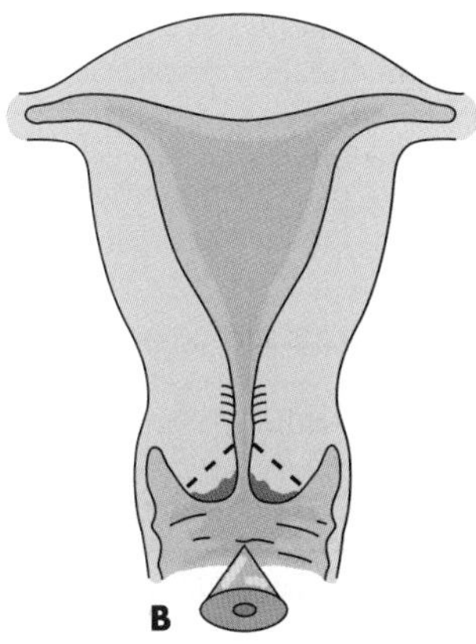

Figure 53-6 **A,** Cone biopsy for endocervical disease. Limits of lesion were not seen on colposcopy. **B,** Cone biopsy for cervical intraepithelial neoplasia of exocervix. Limits of lesion were identified on colposcopy.

Chest x-ray films, intravenous pyelography, skeletal x-ray films, and barium studies of the lower GI tract are used to stage the cancer. Additional procedures used in staging include cystoscopy, proctoscopy, and endocervical curettage. During the staging workup the nurse ensures that the woman has all the information necessary to understand the tests and their rationale. Anxiety is typically high until the extent and invasiveness of the cancer can be determined.

Medications. Chemotherapy has not played a significant role in the management of most cervical cancer. Squamous cell cancers tend to be relatively unresponsive to drug treatment. Recurrent cancers tend to reappear in areas previously irradiated where the tissue is fibrotic and relatively avascular, making it difficult to obtain high tissue concentrations of the drugs. For more advanced stages of cervical cancer, cisplatin-based chemotherapy treatment combined with radiation appears to improve survival.[20] Nursing care related to chemotherapy is discussed in Chapter 15.

Treatments. Cervical cancer is treated according to the stage of the disease. Figure 53-7 illustrates the extent of anatomic involvement represented by each stage. Carcinoma in situ may be treated by excisional conization, LEEP, cryosurgery, or laser surgery, particularly if the woman wants to have more children. Hysterectomy may be chosen if fertility is not an issue. More invasive cancer is treated with increasingly extensive surgical procedures or radiotherapy. Table 53-4 summarizes the major treatment options for various stages of cervical cancer and their associated long-term survival projections.

Radiotherapy. When radiotherapy is used in the treatment of cervical cancer, it may consist of external pelvic irradiation or intracavitary implants (Figure 53-8). Intracavitary implants are usually left in place for 24 to 72 hours. The use of radiotherapy as a cancer treatment is discussed in detail in Chapter 15.

During treatment with an intracavitary implant, it is important that all untreated tissues remain in their normal positions and not come in close contact with the radioactive substance. The bowel is cleansed before therapy, and the woman is maintained on a low-residue diet during treatment to prevent bowel distention with feces. A Foley catheter is typically inserted to keep the bladder small and decompressed. Gauze packing may be used in the vagina to support the rectum and bladder away from the treatment field. The woman is kept flat in bed during treatment to prevent dislodgment of the radioactive substance. The exact position of the implants can be verified by x-ray film.

The presence of the implant in the cervix may stimulate uterine contractions that may become severe. A foul-smelling vaginal discharge develops from the destruction and sloughing of cells. The woman may also develop symptoms of radiation syndrome, with nausea, vomiting, anorexia, and malaise. Local reactions include cystitis, proctitis, and acute

TABLE 53-4 Summary of Treatment Options for Cervical Cancer

Clinical Stage	Treatment Options	5-Year Survival (%)
Stage 0 (CIN)	Loop electrosurgical excision procedure (LEEP), cryosurgery, conization, laser surgery, hysterectomy for postreproductive women	Nearly 100
Stage Ia	Total hysterectomy Conization Radical hysterectomy Intracavitary radiation alone	95-100
Stage Ib	Radiation therapy Radical hysterectomy and bilateral pelvic lymphadenectomy Postoperative total pelvic irradiation plus chemotherapy with subsequent radical hysterectomy and bilateral pelvic lymphadenectomy Radiation therapy and cisplatin-based chemotherapy	85-95
Stage IIa	Radiation therapy Radical hysterectomy and bilateral pelvic lymphadenectomy Postoperative total pelvic irradiation plus chemotherapy with subsequent radical hysterectomy and bilateral pelvic lymphadenectomy	75-80
	Radiation therapy and cisplatin-based chemotherapy	60
Stage IIb	Radiation therapy and cisplatin-based chemotherapy	45
Stage III	Radiation therapy and cisplatin-based chemotherapy	18
Stage IVa	Radiation therapy and cisplatin-based chemotherapy	Palliation
Stage IVb	Radiation, chemotherapy clinical trials of other agents such as paclitaxel, ifosfamide, and irinotecan	
Recurrent cervical cancer	Radiation with chemotherapy (flurouracil with or without mitomycin)	40-50
	Pelvic exenteration	
	Palliative chemotherapy	32-62

Source: National Cancer Institute: Cervical cancer treatment, *PDQ summary,* website: www.nci.gov, 2001.
CIN, Carcinoma in situ.

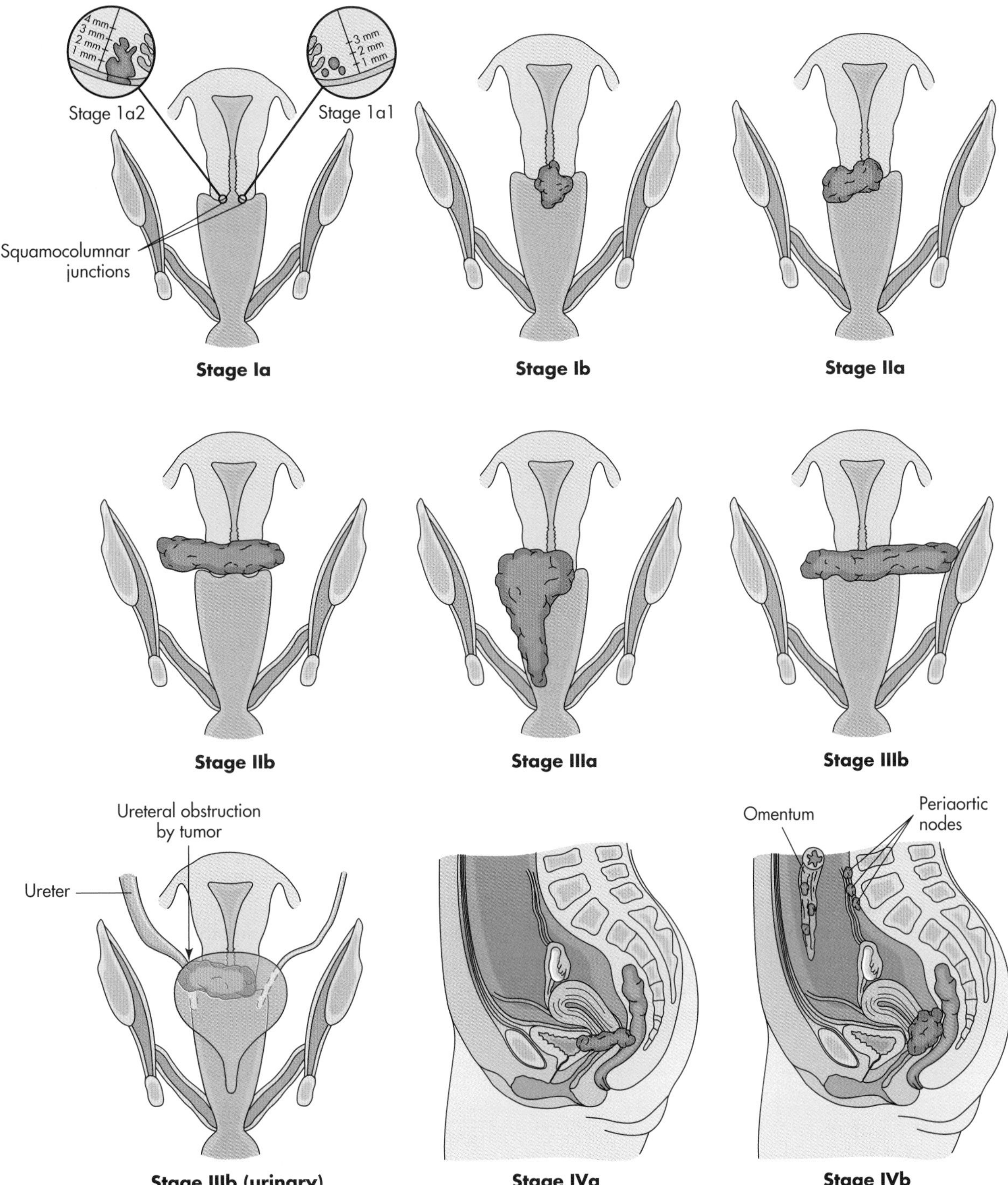

Figure 53-7 International Federation of Gynecology and Obstetrics staging and classification of cancer of cervix.

radiation enteritis. After treatment, the catheter is removed, and an enema may be administered to restore bowel function. The vaginal discharge persists for weeks, and the woman may need to douche regularly at home to control odor. Slight vaginal bleeding may occur for 1 to 3 months after treatment. The woman can usually be discharged within 1 day after removal of the applicators.

External pelvic radiation treatments are usually given over a course of 5 to 6 weeks. General care for the patient receiving external radiotherapy is presented in Chapter 15; the nursing care of patients receiving intracavitary implants is discussed on p. 1770.

Chemotherapy. Both the National Cancer Institute and the American College of Obstetricians and Gynecologists now

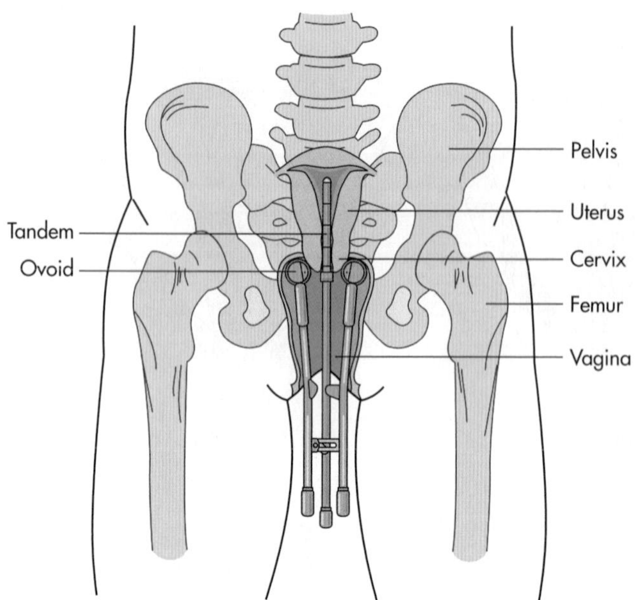

Figure 53-8 Placement of tandem and colpostats before vaginal packing.

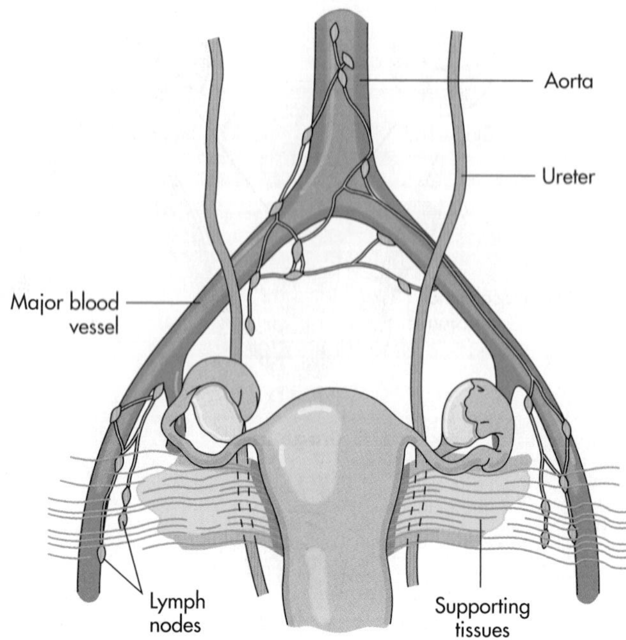

Figure 53-9 Radical hysterectomy includes removal of the uterus, nearby supporting tissues, uppermost part of the vagina, and pelvic lymph nodes.

recommend the concurrent administration of cisplatin chemotherapy for women with cervical cancer who require radiation therapy to treat their disease. The use of concurrent chemoradiation resulted in a reduced death risk of 30% to 50%.[4]

Surgical Management. Simple or radical hysterectomy is the most commonly recommended surgical procedure for treating stage I and stage II cervical cancer. A radical hysterectomy removes the uterus, supporting tissues, distal vagina, and pelvic lymph nodes (Figure 53-9). In some patients the cancer may be locally advanced but still confined to the pelvis. In these situations a pelvic exenteration procedure may be considered (Figure 53-10). The surgery is controversial, but it can be lifesaving in certain malignancies, particularly advanced or recurrent cervical cancer.[20] The procedure involves removal of all the pelvic viscera, including the bladder, rectosigmoid colon, and all reproductive organs. Five-year survival rates after this radical surgery range from 20% to 62%. The procedure is contraindicated if the disease has spread beyond the pelvis. Improved operative techniques support the possibility of reconstructive surgery to create a neovagina. This can be done at the time of surgery or as a second surgery later. Figure 53-11 illustrates an approach to vaginal reconstruction.

Nursing care of the patient undergoing hysterectomy is presented on p. 1775. Women undergoing exenteration receive this standard care but also receive care for an abdominal-perineal resection of the bowel and an ileoconduit or a continent urinary diversion. The extensive nature of the surgery usually necessitates at least a short stay in a critical care unit. Clear and honest teaching is a prerequisite for this surgery. Women need to be fully aware of the nature and consequences of the procedure in terms of both body appearance and function. Complications are numerous, occurring in 25% to 50% of all patients, and usually involve the urinary and GI systems. Fistula formation is a common problem.

Diet. No special diet is required for a patient who has cancer of the cervix. Any change in diet is usually made in response to the side effects of radiation, chemotherapy, or surgical interventions.

Activity. No activity restrictions are required by the diagnosis. Sexual activity may be restricted temporarily after biopsy, radiation treatment, or surgery. General activity restrictions are made in response to the short-term requirements of specific treatments.

Referrals. In some settings the nurse assumes responsibility for making referrals to other services. The nurse may need to initiate a referral to an enterostomal therapist for stomal care if the patient undergoes pelvic exenteration. Sexual dysfunction as a result of disease or treatment may necessitate a psychiatric or sexual counseling referral.

NURSING MANAGEMENT OF PATIENT WITH CERVICAL CANCER

ASSESSMENT

Health History

Aspects of the health history that have particular relevance to the diagnosis of cervical cancer, and hence need to be thoroughly explored, relate to vaginal discharge or abnormal bleeding, pain, and elimination. Vaginal discharge that begins as thin and watery and advances to dark and foul smelling; spotting or intermittent metrorrhagia; or increased amount or duration of menstrual flow are all signs that can indicate cervical cancer. Pain may be generalized or limited to the pelvis, back, flank, or leg. Some patients may report only abdominal discomfort or

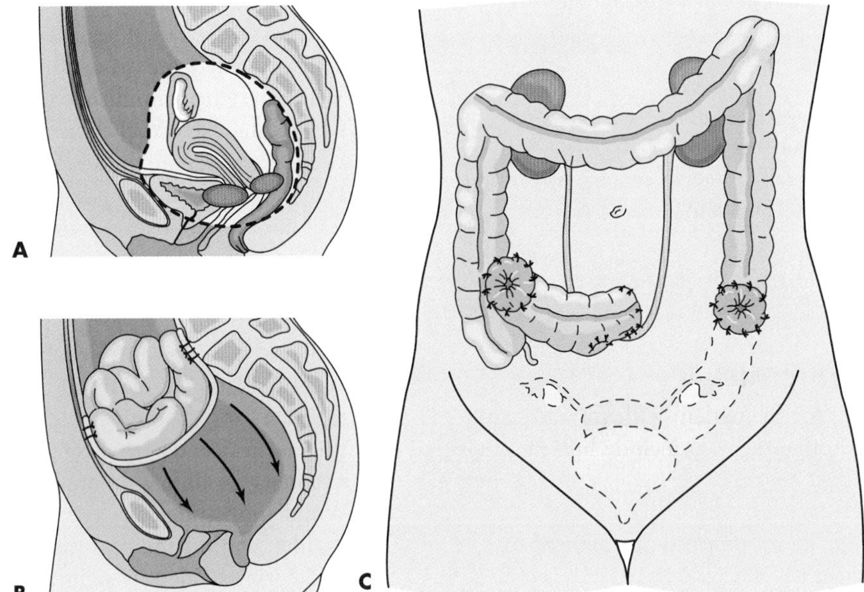

Figure 53-10 A, Lateral view of recurrent cancer involving cervix and upper vagina with extension into bladder and rectum. Stippled area is tissue to be removed by exenteration. B, Lateral view after pelvic viscera have been removed. An omental "carpet" is used to keep the intestines out of the pelvis during the immediate postoperative period. With time, the omental "carpet" descends into the pelvis and adheres to the pelvic floor. C, Urinary conduit and colostomy diversion after exenteration. Dotted areas of sigmoid colon, bladder, and internal genitalia have been removed.

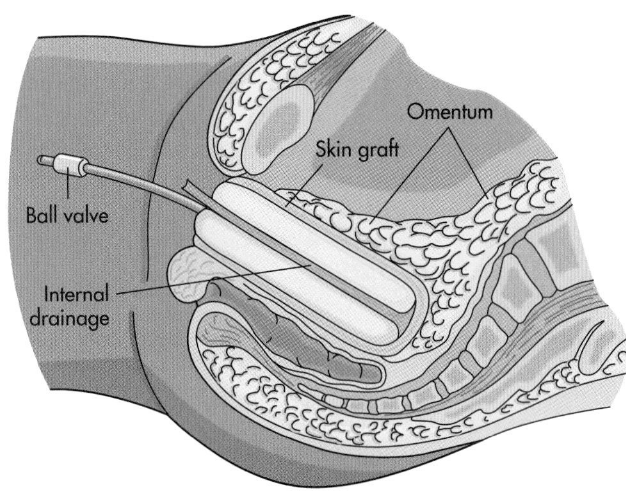

Figure 53-11 Vaginal reconstruction with skin graft. Omentum is placed in the pelvis and sutured to the rectum posteriorly and to the sigmoid colon laterally to create a "pocket" for the neovagina. Two split-thickness skin grafts are harvested, sutured together over a Heyer-Schulte stent, and inserted into the newly created pelvic space.

pain with sexual intercourse. Dysuria or constipation are common. Information also needs to be obtained about any general complaints such as anorexia, weight loss, or fatigue.

Physical Examination

A primary focus of the physical examination is the condition of the cervix. Foul-smelling discharge may be evident, and the cervix may be enlarged or barrel shaped with a smooth surface. Its consistency may be hard on palpation. Colposcopic examination may demonstrate erosion of epithelium and an obvious lesion. Muscle guarding or rigidity may be found on examination of the abdomen. A rectal examination is done to check for rectal bleeding and any palpable lesion. The legs are examined for edema due to lymphatic obstruction. Edema may be present along the entire length of the leg, making one leg larger than the other.

These assessments pertain to any patient with cancer of the cervix. Other pertinent assessments relate to the specific type of treatment the patient is receiving, as do nursing diagnoses, expected patient outcomes, and interventions. These factors as they pertain to the patient being treated with internal radiotherapy are discussed here. Those pertaining to the patient having a hysterectomy are found in the Nursing Care Plan on pp. 1766 to 1769. Care of the patient receiving chemotherapy or external radiation is found in Chapter 15.

NURSING DIAGNOSES

Nursing diagnoses for the patient with cervical cancer being treated with internal radiotherapy may include but are not limited to:

Diagnostic Title	Possible Etiologic Factors
1. Anxiety	Diagnosis of cancer; uncertainty of outcome
2. Self-care deficit: bathing/hygiene, toileting	Activity restrictions during treatment

3. Risk for loneliness	Isolation and safety precautions necessitated by implant
4. Impaired urinary elimination	Inflammation
5. Diarrhea	Cell wall necrosis secondary to irradiation
6. Fatigue	Decreased metabolic energy production
7. Effective therapeutic regimen management (individual)	Treatment program
8. Sexual dysfunction	Vaginal changes secondary to radiation

EXPECTED PATIENT OUTCOMES

Expected patient outcomes for the patient with cervical cancer being treated with radiotherapy may include but are not limited to:

1. Will control anxiety
1a. Will verbalize rationales for precautions followed by both staff and visitors
1b. Will communicate feelings about diagnosis and treatment
1c. Will express less anxiety about treatment and future outcomes
2. Will understand self-care bathing/hygiene and toileting restrictions; will adapt self-care tasks to activity restrictions and accept assistance as needed
3. Will control loneliness and boredom
3a. Will interact with staff and visitors within the established safety guidelines
3b. Will engage in appropriate diversional activities
4. Will maintain urinary elimination
4a. Will have adequate fluid intake
4b. Will have adequate urine output
4c. Will experience diminished burning and frequency
5. Will reestablish bowel elimination
5a. Will have adequate fluid intake
5b. Will have normal skin integrity
5c. Will have usual bowel pattern
6. Will conserve energy
6a. Will adjust activities of daily living to reduced energy levels
6b. Will use social support network
7. Will understand and comply with treatment regimen
7a. Will accurately describe components of home care and need for follow-up monitoring
7b. Will demonstrate competency in care skills such as vaginal dilation and perineal cleansing
7c. Will correctly identify signs and symptoms of complications
8. Will maintain sexuality
8a. Will openly communicate with partner
8b. Will use alternative methods of sexual expression
8c. Will have knowledge of referral resources

INTERVENTIONS

1. Reducing Anxiety

A cancer diagnosis can produce a barrage of negative feelings in the patient that commonly escalate during the overwhelming diagnostic and staging period. The nurse establishes a

Nursing Care Plan — Patient After Hysterectomy for Cervical Cancer

DATA Mrs. C., age 42, saw her gynecologist 2 weeks ago because of bleeding between periods and occasional postcoital bleeding. Her last Papanicolaou (Pap) smear was 5 years ago and negative. This Pap smear was positive, and a cervical biopsy confirmed cancer of the cervix, stage I. She was admitted yesterday for a total abdominal hysterectomy.

Admission notes indicate that Mrs. C. is married and has two teenage children. Her husband was with her on admission and appears to be supportive. Her preoperative concerns centered on the total removal of the cancer and whether or not a hysterectomy would affect her sex life. She stated that she felt like she was being "neutered." The nurse explored Mrs. C.'s knowledge of the surgery and explained that the surgery would not physically affect sexual functioning.

Mrs. C. has returned from postanesthesia recovery alert with an intravenous line infusing and vital signs stable. Her dressing is dry and intact. She is receiving morphine sulfate per a patient-controlled analgesia (PCA) pump at 1 mg/hr and a bolus of 1 mg available every 8 minutes.

Nursing assessment includes monitoring:

- Vital signs
- Breath sounds
- Urine output
- Fluid intake
- Respiratory rate
- Pain status

NURSING DIAGNOSIS **Acute pain related to abdominal incision**
GOALS/OUTCOMES Will achieve pain-free status

NOC Suggested Outcomes
- Pain Level (2102)
- Pain Control (1605)

NIC Suggested Interventions
- Pain Management (1400)
- Progressive Muscle Relaxation (1460)

Nursing Care Plan — Patient After Hysterectomy for Cervical Cancer—cont'd

Nursing Interventions/Rationales

- Assess duration and intensity of pain. *To monitor effectiveness of pain control measures.*
- Maintain analgesic infusion so that medication is delivered on a regular basis for the first 24 hours. *Provides more effective pain control because it prevents severe pain, which is harder to control.*
- Encourage frequent changes of position in bed and early ambulation. *Activity decreases pain by increasing circulation and reducing muscle tension. Ambulation encourages peristalsis, decreasing the intensity of gas pains.*
- Assess adequacy of pain relief every 2 to 4 hours. *To determine if the drug is effective or if a change in analgesia is needed.*
- Encourage use of PCA bolus to maintain comfort. *Allows the patient control over her pain and prevents pain from becoming severe, which is more difficult to control.*
- Encourage use of nonpharmacologic pain relief measures (massage, relaxation, music, distraction). *May work with analgesics to provide better pain control.*

Evaluation Parameters

1. Verbalizes feeling comfortable within 1 to 2 hours following comfort measures
2. Decreased use of PCA pump

NURSING DIAGNOSIS **Risk for situational low self-esteem related to loss of uterus and concern about sexuality**
GOALS/OUTCOMES Will actively plan for assuming usual role

NOC Suggested Outcomes

- Identity (1202)
- Self-Esteem (1205)
- Body Image (1200)

NIC Suggested Interventions

- Body Image Enhancement (5220)
- Role Enhancement (5370)
- Self-Esteem Enhancement (5400)

Nursing Interventions/Rationales

- Provide patient the opportunity to express feelings and concerns about loss of uterus. *The patient may feel free to talk about her concerns if the opportunity is provided. Identification of the patient's feelings helps direct the plan of care.*
- Assess significant others' concerns and perceptions of body changes. *Helps the patient and significant others to ventilate doubts and resolve concerns. Provides an opportunity to correct misconceptions.*
- Provide factual information regarding anticipated bodily changes; include significant other if possible. *Provides accurate information and corrects misconceptions.*
- Be empathetic about patient's feelings, which may include grief, guilt, shame, or remorse. *Feelings associated with many emotions may be expressed when grieving over the loss of a body part. Expression of feelings helps the patient progress through the grief process.*
- Encourage patient to continue activities associated with femininity, such as fixing her hair, wearing her own apparel, and applying makeup. *Feelings of femininity will emphasize "feminine" rather than "neuter" and that she herself is not changed.*
- Help patient make plans for resumption of former activities. *If her life patterns are reestablished, her thoughts about her body changes may diminish.*

Evaluation Parameters

1. Verbalizes fears and concerns
2. Makes positive statements about self
3. Talks about resuming usual role

NURSING DIAGNOSIS **Risk for constipation related to surgical manipulation of bowel and pain medications**
GOALS/OUTCOMES Will be free of constipation

NOC Suggested Outcomes

- Bowel Elimination (0501)
- Hydration (0602)

NIC Suggested Interventions

- Bowel Management (0430)
- Constipation/Impaction Management (0450)

Nursing Interventions/Rationales

- Monitor stool characteristics and frequency. *To identify the need for a treatment plan and evaluate the effectiveness of that plan.*
- Encourage ambulation every 4 hours. *Ambulation promotes peristalsis, which facilitates bowel movements.*

Continued

Nursing Care Plan — Patient After Hysterectomy for Cervical Cancer—cont'd

- Assess abdomen for presence and quality of bowel sounds. *Peristalsis may be decreased from the handling of pelvic viscera; helps determine flatus buildup.*
- Encourage oral fluids when permitted. *Adequate hydration promotes soft stool formation and prevents constipation and impaction.*
- Teach patient to avoid straining at stool. *Increases abdominal pain and can induce postoperative bleeding.*

Evaluation Parameters

1. Passage of soft, formed stools
2. Absence of complaints about constipation

NURSING DIAGNOSIS **Impaired urinary elimination related to loss of bladder tone, pain with muscle contraction, and discomfort from urinating position**

GOALS/OUTCOMES Will void spontaneously and empty bladder completely

NOC Suggested Outcomes

- Urinary Elimination (0503)

NIC Suggested Interventions

- Urinary Elimination Management (0890)
- Urinary Retention Care (0620)
- Urinary Catheterization: Intermittent (0582)

Nursing Interventions/Rationales

- Monitor urine output until patient reestablishes her normal voiding pattern. *Urinary retention can occur from the handling of the bladder during surgery, which decreases bladder tone postoperatively.*
- Encourage patient to void every 2 hours. *Promotes optimal bladder tone and prevents distention.*
- Monitor for urinary bladder distention above symphysis pubis and for lower abdominal discomfort other than incisional pain every 2 hours. *Detects bladder distention and the degree of bladder fullness.*
- Provide privacy during attempts to urinate. *Allows the patient to relax, which facilitates urination.*
- Catheterize for residual urine as ordered. *Residual urine in the bladder provides a good medium for bacterial growth and infection.*
- Teach patient good perineal care. *Helps prevent the development of urinary tract infection.*

Evaluation Parameters

1. Is free of urinary bladder distention
2. Voids without hesitancy
3. Denies feeling of bladder fullness or abdominal pain (other than incisional pain)

NURSING DIAGNOSIS **Risk for ineffective tissue perfusion related to pelvic venous stasis from surgery**

GOALS/OUTCOMES Will maintain normal circulation

NOC Suggested Outcomes

- Tissue Perfusion: Peripheral (0407)
- Circulation Status: 0401)

NIC Suggested Interventions

- Circulatory Care: Venous Insufficiency (4066)
- Embolus Precautions (4110)

Nursing Interventions/Rationales

- Monitor for discomfort in legs/thighs, sudden dyspnea, Homans' sign, and color, warmth, and blanching of lower extremities every 8 hours. *To detect abnormalities in tissue perfusion to ensure early treatment.*
- Encourage patient to lie completely flat in bed for short periods every 4 hours for 24 hours or until ambulating well. *To help promote blood return from pelvic veins.*
- Encourage leg exercises and frequent turning in bed until ambulating well. *Exercise promotes venous return via muscle pumps.*
- Avoid elevating knees or placing pillows under knees. Encourage patient to keep knees flat when lying in bed, and minimize use of high Fowler's position. *Pressure on the popliteal veins or sharp knee flexion may increase venous stasis.*
- Provide antiembolism stockings or apply intermittent pneumatic compression stockings. *To help prevent venous stasis. Patients with varicose veins are at increased risk for phlebothrombosis.*
- Encourage ambulation. *Promotes venous return by contracting muscles to compress veins.*

Evaluation Parameters

1. Absence of thrombus, emboli, or leg/thigh pain
2. Negative Homans' sign
3. Extremities remain warm and pink (or normal color)
4. Performs leg exercises as taught

Nursing Care Plan — Patient After Hysterectomy for Cervical Cancer—cont'd

NURSING DIAGNOSIS **Risk for ineffective therapeutic regimen management related to lack of knowledge concerning postoperative self-care following discharge from hospital**

GOALS/OUTCOMES Will assume independent performance of self-care

NOC Suggested Outcomes
- Adherence Behavior (1600)
- Knowledge: Treatment Regimen (1813)
- Participation: Health Care Decisions (1606)

NIC Suggested Interventions
- Teaching: Individual (5606)
- Family Support (7140)
- Mutual Goal Setting (4410)

Nursing Interventions/Rationales
- Teach patient when activities can be resumed (see text). *Activities are resumed gradually to permit healing; heavy lifting and strenuous activities are avoided for 6 to 8 weeks postoperatively.*
- Teach patient the signs of phlebothrombosis to be monitored and reported. *Phlebothrombosis may occur 7 to 10 days postoperatively after the patient goes home.*
- Teach patient the signs of vaginal bleeding to be reported. *Excessive or persistent bleeding indicates impaired healing.*
- Teach patient that bathing and light activity are permitted after hospital discharge. *Bathing maintains hygiene, and light activities prevent complications related to immobility.*
- Teach patient to avoid driving a car, especially one with a standard shift, for 2 to 4 weeks. *The patient may be too fatigued to shift or handle turns while driving.*
- Teach patient the importance of follow-up care. *Follow-up care is essential to evaluate the patient's progress or lack thereof.*
- Include significant other in teaching when possible. *Promotes compliance with discharge teaching.*
- Reinforce preoperative explanations of the surgery and its effect on sexual functioning, including significant other when possible. *Preoperative anxiety may have decreased the patient's awareness. Hysterectomy does not interfere with satisfactory sexual functioning.*

Evaluation Parameters
1. Describes self-care accurately
2. Increasingly participates in self-care
3. Complies with prescribed treatment plan, restrictions, and follow-up recommendations

trusting relationship and encourages the woman to talk about her feelings and concerns. The nurse supports the need to ventilate emotions through anger or crying. As anxiety is controlled, effective teaching can begin concerning the condition, treatment options, and expected side effects. The nurse should assess the meaning of the diagnosis to the patient and her significant others, clarify misconceptions, and provide reliable information to enhance their understanding. Both patient and spouse or significant other need to understand the grief response and how it may affect the woman's responses during treatment and recovery.

Careful teaching takes place before the insertion of the implant so that the woman understands the sensations she will experience. The woman and her family need to understand the rationale for all restrictions and safety measures (see Guidelines for Safe Practice box). It is particularly important to review the precautions related to the implant itself, which are summarized in Box 53-1. The cesium implant is a source of high-dose ionizing radiation to all who come into its range, and these risks must be minimized to the fullest extent possible. The radiation hazard is clearly marked on the door to the room, and a radiation safety officer is available in the institution to deal with questions and concerns.

2. Assisting With Self-Care: Bathing/Hygiene and Toileting

The activity restrictions outlined in the Guidelines for Safe Practice box on p. 1770 must be followed carefully during the treatment period to prevent accidental dislodgment of the device or movement of the implant that endangers normal tissue. To promote adherence to the treatment plan, it is critical that the woman understand the rationale for all restrictions. The nurse provides bed rest care and ensures that all needed articles are kept within easy reach, but assistance may be necessary because the woman must remain supine. Hourly turning is encouraged, and back rubs may help relieve some of the discomforts of bed rest. The foul-smelling vaginal discharge may be both physically irritating and embarrassing. The nurse assists with frequent perineal hygiene and provides a room deodorizer.

Guidelines for Safe Practice

The Patient Undergoing Internal Radiotherapy

PREIMPLANTATION

Care before the insertion of the radioactive implant usually includes the following:

1. Provide cleansing enema to empty the bowel.
2. Insert Foley catheter to keep the bladder empty and small during treatment.
3. Provide povodine-iodine (Betadine) douche and shave pubic area if ordered.

IMPLANTATION PERIOD

Care during the 24 to 72 hours of treatment includes the following:

1. Maintain strict bed rest.
2. Elevate head of bed no more than 20 degrees. Keep patient as flat as possible.
3. Assist patient in turning from side to side as needed for comfort.
4. Provide low-residue diet and possibly antimotility agents to prevent bowel distention.
5. Administer analgesics as needed for uterine cramping, which can be severe.
6. Perform routine perineal cleansing if drainage is present; provide room deodorizer if discharge is foul smelling.
7. Ensure a minimum fluid intake of 2500 ml daily.
8. Visit patient frequently from the room doorway for emotional support.
9. Provide diversional activities appropriate to activity restrictions.
10. Monitor implant for proper placement; keep long-handled forceps and lead-lined container in the room in case of dislodgment.
11. Monitor for complications.
    a. Infection: increased vaginal redness or swelling; increasingly dark, foul-smelling drainage; cloudy urine; fever
    b. Thrombophlebitis: painful leg swelling; positive Homans' sign

Thrombophlebitis is another concern during bed rest; therefore embolus precautions are instituted. The nurse also teaches the woman range-of-motion and isometric exercises that support venous return and encourages her to perform them 10 times each hour. Elastic or compression stockings are applied and removed for 15 to 20 minutes every 8 hours.

3. Providing Diversion and Social Interaction

The woman receiving intracavitary radiation often feels alienated and depressed. The nurse spends time talking with the patient but must remain at a safe distance and observe the time restrictions for safety. Family members are also encouraged to visit, following the same guidelines. Alternative communication methods for children or pregnant women should be used, since visitation is contraindicated for them. Strict bed rest rapidly creates a boring and uncomfortable situation for the patient. The nursing staff should maintain frequent contact with the patient, checking on her at least hourly, and ensuring that her call bell is within easy reach. The nurse

BOX 53-1 Radiation Precautions for Internal Radiotherapy

- Time at the bedside is limited—each contact should last no more than 30 minutes.
- Children and pregnant women/staff should not visit during treatment.
- Staff members should wear a dosimeter during every patient contact to monitor radiation exposure.
- A lead shield may be installed at the side and foot of the bed.
- Staff should use the principles of distance, time, and shielding in all contacts with the patient.
- The implant is always handled by means of long-handled forceps, never with the hands. A lead-lined container should be present in the room for use if the implant dislodges.
- A sign that clearly identifies the radiation hazard is posted on the room door.
- A contact number for the radiation safety officer of the institution should be posted on the warning sign.

attempts to create a pleasant, odor-free environment. Diversional activities, such as reading materials, music, telephone, and television, are provided for the patient.

4,5. Supporting Elimination

Urinary catheterization is necessary during the treatment and is followed by urinary elimination management before discharge. Patients may develop symptoms of radiation syndrome that may alter nutrition and elimination. Uterine cramping can become severe. Diarrhea management, including the use of antidiarrheal agents as needed, may be necessary. An adequate fluid intake is essential to maintain fluid and electrolyte balance and prevent irritation of the bladder. The nurse encourages the patient to maintain a fluid intake of 2500 to 3000 ml daily, even in the face of anorexia and nausea, and administers antiemetics as needed.

6,7. Teaching

The hospitalization period for intracavitary radiotherapy is short, and the patient is discharged soon after the removal of the implant. The woman must learn several self-care skills for home management and be aware of the signs and symptoms of potential complications. Radiotherapy causes fatigue, vaginal stenosis, loss of vaginal lubrication, and induced menopause. Energy management strategies are discussed that allow the woman to reduce fatigue and build endurance.

The vaginal discharge often continues for weeks, and the woman may need to douche at least twice daily as long as discharge and odor persist. The nurse cannot assume that the woman has experience with douching and reviews the technique and precautions in detail. Some vaginal bleeding may also persist for a few months after treatment, and the woman should receive information from her physician about acceptable amounts of bleeding. Local application of estrogen cream may prevent bleeding. Medication management of hormone replacement therapy may be necessary.

The cesium implant causes vaginal narrowing and fibrosis. Regular vaginal dilation is essential to minimize these effects. If the woman has a spouse or sexual partner, regular sexual intercourse, usually at least three times per week, is one method of minimizing stenosis. The woman may prefer to use a manual obturator to dilate the vagina. The importance of this intervention is also explained to women who are not sexually active. Even routine pelvic examination can become difficult or almost impossible if the vagina becomes severely stenosed. Dilation should be performed at least three times a week for 1 year after treatment. The obturator is lubricated before use and washed carefully with soap and water after each use. A vinegar-and-water douche may be ordered after treatment. The nurse informs the woman that slight bleeding may occur after dilation for up to a year.

Other self-care teaching focuses on gradually increasing activity, maintaining a liberal fluid intake to prevent urologic problems, and adjusting the diet to prevent bowel problems. Either constipation or diarrhea may occur in response to the radiation, and these problems may persist for months after treatment. The nurse also teaches the woman about symptoms that indicate complications. The woman should promptly report unusually heavy discharge, foul-smelling urine, low-grade fever, persistent bowel problems, or pain. Radiotherapy can cause fistulas in the pelvis, both in the early posttreatment period and in the future. Written materials can be helpful resources for the woman at home. The importance of follow-up care and monitoring is emphasized.

8. Supporting Sexuality

Sexual intercourse may be resumed about 3 weeks after discharge, but the woman is instructed to use a water-soluble lubricant for comfort because vaginal secretions will be decreased or absent. The woman's partner is included in all discussions about sexual activity if the woman is comfortable with her partner's presence. Alternative forms of expressing affection and relating sexually should be considered, especially during the initial recovery period. The woman and her partner need to be informed of referral sources for sexual counseling in the community, such as support groups and counselors who specialize in assisting couples with illness-related sexuality issues.

EVALUATION

To evaluate the effectiveness of nursing interventions, compare patient behaviors with those stated in the expected patient outcomes. Achievement of patient outcomes is successful if the patient:

- **1a.** Correctly explains rationales for all radiation and activity restrictions.
- **1b.** Communicates feelings to partner, family, or staff.
- **1c.** States that anxiety is minimal or absent.
- **2.** Performs self-care activities independently or with appropriate assistance.
- **3a.** Regularly interacts with family, friends, and staff using alternative means of communication when necessary.
- **3b.** Uses selected diversional activities to reduce social isolation.
- **4a.** Drinks a variety of oral fluids (2500 to 3000 ml/day) to promote urine elimination.
- **4b.** Voids a minimum of 50 ml/hr.
- **4c.** On follow-up visits, reports diminished burning and frequency.
- **5a.** Drinks a variety of oral fluids (2500 to 3000 ml/day) to promote bowel elimination.
- **5b.** Reports intact perineal skin.
- **5c.** On follow-up visits, reports reestablishment of usual bowel function.
- **6a.** Reports adjustment of activities of daily living with frequent rest periods.
- **6b.** Uses social support network to help maintain activities of daily living.
- **7a.** Correctly describes treatment regimen and planned pattern for follow-up care.
- **7b.** Correctly demonstrates perineal care and use of an obturator for dilation.
- **7c.** Correctly describes signs of complications that need to be reported.
- **8a.** Reports open communication with partner.
- **8b.** Uses alternative methods of sexual expression during recovery period.
- **8c.** Uses referral resources if necessary.

GERONTOLOGIC CONSIDERATIONS

Cancer of the cervix occurs in women of all ages. Early diagnosis is critical and is an ongoing challenge in older women. After the childbearing years many women stop having routine gynecologic examinations. Pap smear screening for elderly women remains controversial, and current screening guidelines reflect no upper age limit. Symptoms are often discounted or attributed to the multiple effects of aging on the reproductive system. Therefore it is less likely that cervical cancer will be detected in the early and curable stages. Elderly women are less able to withstand the rigors of radical surgery, are more prone to complications of treatment, and often experience exaggerated tissue responses to radiotherapy. It is critical that teaching and outreach be provided to this population about the ongoing importance of Pap smear screening for cancer because the incidence and mortality rates for cervical cancer in the United States are highest among elderly women.

SPECIAL ENVIRONMENTS FOR CARE

Critical Care Management

Women undergoing treatment for cancer of the cervix do not usually need critical care support except if undergoing radical surgery. Total pelvic exenteration is a complex assault on the body and involves extensive urinary and bowel diversion procedures. Short-term postoperative critical care monitoring is usually indicated, particularly for older patients and women who have concurrent major organ system diseases.

Community-Based Care

Much of the diagnostic and conservative treatment for cervical cancer takes place in an outpatient environment. Even hospitalization for radiotherapy extends only for the duration of the implant placement. It is therefore critical that the woman be an informed partner in her own care. Extensive teaching needs to be provided, with full understanding that the anxiety associated with the diagnosis of cancer and its treatment will make it difficult for the woman to hear and process much of the information. Repeat sessions and written reference materials are critical. The woman's partner is included in teaching sessions if possible, because the disease and treatment have significant potential impact on the couple's sexual activities, at least in the short term. The nurse ensures that the woman has the name and phone number of all appropriate support groups and services available in her home community.

COMPLICATIONS

Recurrence and metastasis of the cancer are the primary concerns. The diagnosis can compromise the woman's body image, sexuality, and fertility. Implant therapy results in radiation-induced menopause, which adds to the challenge of keeping the vagina dilated, supple, and lubricated for sexual intercourse. The presence of prolonged vaginal discharge does not promote the resumption of sexual activity, and the couple's relationship can deteriorate as a result of communication problems and mixed messages between the partners. The woman must also cope with odor and drainage that can compromise her image of herself as a desirable sexual being. Physical complications such as fistula formation, tissue fibrosis, and inflammatory bowel problems are addressed in the discharge teaching, but the woman typically finds herself alone at home, dealing with the reality of all the changes. The nurse again stresses the importance of social support.

NEOPLASMS OF THE UTERUS

Uterine Leiomyomas (Fibroids)

Etiology

Leiomyomas (myomas) are benign tumors of muscle cell origin that contain varying amounts of fibrous tissue. The etiology of leiomyomas is not completely understood. The stimulus for growth is unclear but is thought to be related to estrogen, because leiomyomas are rare before menarche and often decrease in size after menopause. The tumors often enlarge during pregnancy and with the use of oral contraceptives. Women who smoke tend to be relatively estrogen deficient and have been found to have a lower incidence of leiomyomas. The tumors can reach enormous proportions, weighing as much as 50 pounds. Malignant transformation is rare.

Epidemiology

Leiomyomas are the most common type of pelvic tumor, developing in 30% of women.[1] Leiomyomas occur more often in African-American women and account for more than 50% of hysterectomies.[1] Leiomyomas are more common in women who are obese and who do not smoke.[23] The frequency increases during the perimenopausal period.

Pathophysiology

Leiomyomas originate in the myometrium and are classified by their anatomic location (Figure 53-12). The tumor is the result of overgrowth of a single muscle cell influenced by estrogen and progesterone-stimulated growth factors.[23] Submucous myomas lie just beneath the endometrium and compress it as they grow. They can develop a pedicle and protrude into the uterine cavity or even through the cervical canal. Intramural myomas lie within the uterine muscle, and subserosal tumors lie at the serosal surface of the uterus or may bulge outward from the myometrium. These external tumors also tend to become pedunculated. They occasionally are found in the fallopian tubes or round ligament, and approximately 5% originate from the cervix.

Most leiomyomas are asymptomatic and may go undetected. The development of symptoms depends on the location, size, and condition of the tumor. Menorrhagia is the most common symptom. Bleeding can result from distortion and congestion of surrounding vessels or from ulceration of the overlying endometrium. Bleeding usually takes the form of premenstrual spotting or prolonged light bleeding after the menses. Metrorrhagia is associated with venous thrombosis or necrosis on the surface of the tumor, particularly if it extrudes through the cervix.

Pain is not a characteristic symptom, although it can result from tumor degeneration or occur with myometrial contractions that attempt to expel the myoma from the uterus. If the

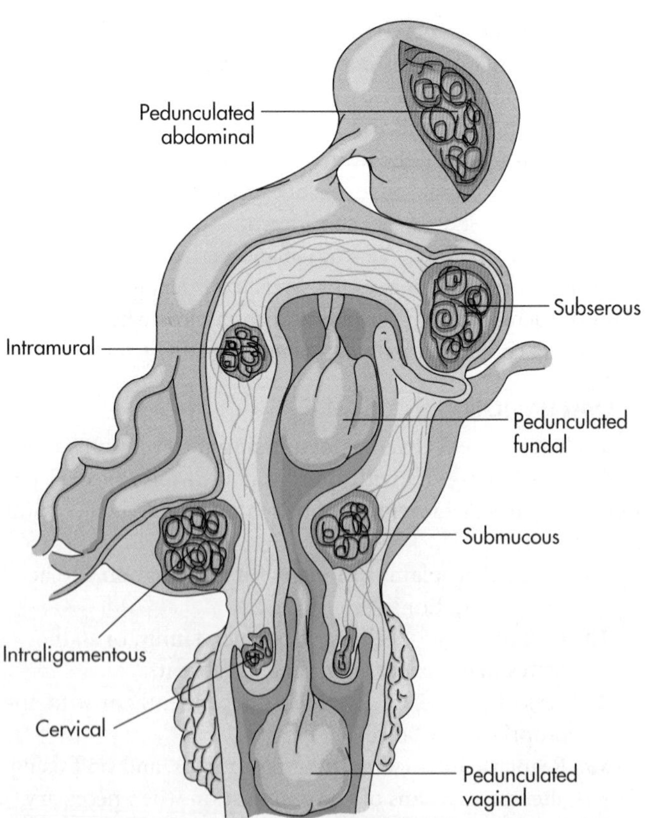

Figure 53-12 Myomas of uterus.

pedicle stalk becomes twisted, it can cause sudden, severe pain. Women often report a sensation of pressure in the pelvis or a "bearing down" feeling, especially with large tumors. The tumor may cause pelvic circulatory congestion and create backache, constipation, or dysmenorrhea. The woman may even notice an increase in abdominal girth.

Leiomyomas interfere with fertility by blocking the opening of the fallopian tubes, inducing spontaneous abortion, or obstructing the cervical canal, making delivery hazardous. Sudden growth of a myoma after menopause is considered to be a classic sign of leiomyosarcoma, which necessitates hysterectomy.

Leiomyomas increase the risk of complications during pregnancy, including placental abruption and malpresentation.[23] Anemia is associated with chronic blood loss, but women may also exhibit polycythemia secondary to erythropoietin produced by the myometrium.[23] The signs and symptoms of leiomyomas are summarized in the Clinical Manifestations box.

Collaborative Care Management

Diagnostic Tests. Myomas often can be detected by routine pelvic examination when the uterus is displaced and irregular nodules are felt on the uterine surface. Diagnosis is confirmed through the use of magnetic resonance imaging (MRI), computed tomography (CT) scanning, pelvic sonography, and hysterography or hysteroscopy. These tests are used to determine the size and placement of the tumor(s) and to evaluate the degree of urologic compression.

Clinical Manifestations

Leiomyomas

Abnormal bleeding
Abdominal mass
Pressure in the pelvis
Iron deficiency anemia
Sudden-onset pain indicates a complication
NOTE: Most leiomyomas are asymptomatic.

Medications. GnRH agonists may be used to reduce the level of circulating estrogens and shrink the tumor. The GnRH agonists are able to reduce tumor size by as much as 90%, but their effect is temporary. These drugs may be used in perimenopausal women to avoid the need for surgery because the tumors are known to regress after menopause. The GnRH agonists are also prescribed preoperatively to reduce the incidence and severity of postoperative bleeding. Reducing the tumor size also may permit the use of a vaginal, rather than an abdominal, approach for the hysterectomy and decrease recovery time. Antiprogestins such as RU-486 are under study for possible use in both treatment and prevention.[23]

Treatments. Small, asymptomatic myomas are simply monitored. The myomas tend to shrink as estrogen levels begin to decline. If a patient is experiencing bleeding, an endometrial biopsy may be performed to verify the diagnosis and rule out cancer. Submucous myomas may be resected via the cervical canal using the hysteroscope and laser therapy as an outpatient procedure.

Surgical Management. Leiomyomas are the most common indication for hysterectomy.[1] The decision to undergo surgery depends on the woman's age, symptom severity, and desire to preserve her childbearing ability. Asymptomatic leiomyomas are not treated with a hysterectomy until the uterus reaches the size of a 12-week pregnancy.[1] Myomectomy can be performed if the tumor is near the outer wall of the uterus, leaving the muscular walls of the uterus relatively intact. Abdominal and vaginal hysterectomies are illustrated in Figure 53-13. Various gynecologic surgical procedures are defined in Box 53-2.

Diet. Diet therapy does not play a role in the management of leiomyomas.

Activity. A woman's usual pattern of activity does not need to be altered by the presence of leiomyoma. The development of anemia often causes fatigue and activity intolerance. Women who experience pelvic heaviness or backache may curtail their activities in response to their symptoms.

Referrals. Unless the situation becomes complex, a patient with leiomyoma generally does not need multidisciplinary referral.

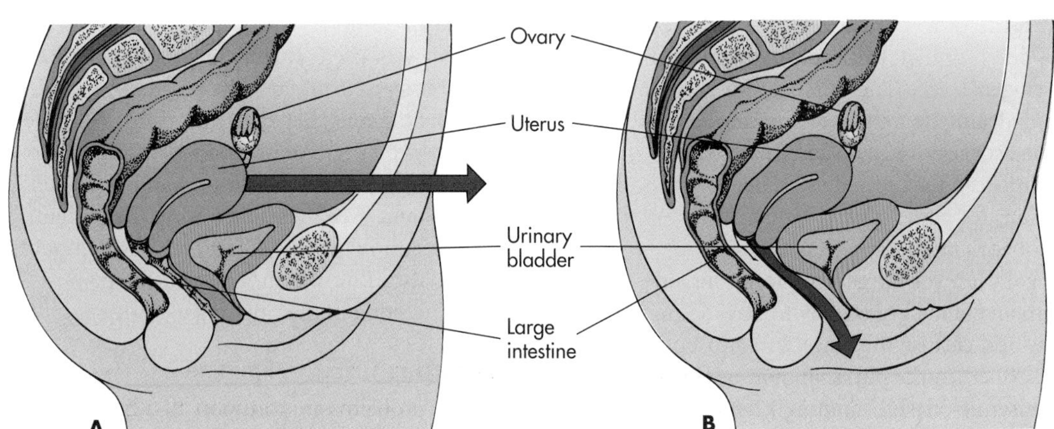

Figure 53-13 **A,** Abdominal hysterectomy. The uterus is removed through an abdominal incision. **B,** Vaginal hysterectomy. The uterus is removed through the vagina, and there is no abdominal incision.

BOX 53-2 Surgeries of the Female Reproductive System

Oophorectomy: removal of an ovary
Salpingectomy: removal of a fallopian tube
Bilateral salpingo-oophorectomy (BSO or Bil S&O): removal of both ovaries and fallopian tubes
Total hysterectomy: removal of the entire uterus, including the cervix; may be referred to as a total abdominal hysterectomy (TAH); the procedure can be done vaginally or abdominally
Subtotal hysterectomy: removal of the uterus except for the cervix; rarely done today
Hystero-oophorectomy: removal of the uterus and an ovary
Hysterosalpingectomy: removal of the uterus and a fallopian tube
Total abdominal hysterectomy and bilateral salpingo-oophorectomy (TAH-BSO): removal of the entire uterus and both fallopian tubes and ovaries; the term *panhysterectomy* has been used previously to refer to this type of surgery
Radical hysterectomy (Wertheim procedure): TAH-BSO, partial vaginectomy, and dissection of the lymph nodes in the pelvis

Research

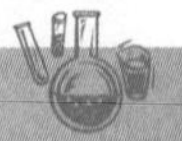

Reference: Wade J et al: Hysterectomy: what do women need and want to know? *J Obstet Gynecol Neonatal Nurs* 29:33-42, 2000.

Hysterectomy is a common treatment for many gynecologic problems. Women's experiences of the procedure are both physical and psychologic. The researchers used a qualitative survey design to examine women's experience of having a hysterectomy. Responses from 102 women were examined for themes. The average time since surgery was 1 year. Positive aspects of the experience included relief of physical symptoms and improved quality of life. Women commented on the value of information received from their providers, the importance of support, and the need to be involved in decision making. Fears included concerns about hormone replacement therapy and potential secondary cancers. Insufficient information was a problem for a third of the women. A fourth of the women expressed sexual concerns and a lack of information about what to expect. Some women described surprise at the mood changes they experienced following surgery and their lack of preparation for the changes. A few women expressed grief at the loss of childbearing, although the average age of respondents was 43. The researchers stressed the need for more anticipatory guidance, especially in the areas of sexuality and mood. Nurses' holistic approach to patient care puts them in a strong position to develop and implement such supports.

NURSING MANAGEMENT OF PATIENT UNDERGOING HYSTERECTOMY FOR LEIOMYOMA

PREOPERATIVE CARE

Hysterectomy is used as a treatment for a variety of reproductive tract problems in addition to leiomyoma, including cancer of the cervix, uterus, and ovaries, as well as structural problems such as severe prolapse. Vaginal, abdominal, and laparoscopic approaches are used. Women report that knowledge of their treatment choices and participation in decision making are important to them[26] (see Research box). Women desire information on their options, including differences in symptom relief, length of stay, cost, and quality of life.[10]

Preoperative teaching is essential and usually is initiated in the physician's office or by the preadmissions team. Women who smoke should receive counseling and support for smoking cessation before surgery and at discharge.[7] Most women are familiar with the term *fibroid* but have little real understanding of the development, treatment, or relationship of fibroids with estrogen levels. The nurse verifies that teaching has been provided and that the woman can accurately describe the planned surgery and associated care. The nurse then clarifies and reinforces that teaching as needed, thoroughly discussing the plans for pain management and the importance of early and frequent ambulation.

Physical preparation for surgery typically includes bowel preparation with an enema or laxative the day before the procedure to empty and cleanse the bowel. An antiseptic douche may also be prescribed, or the physician may order the woman to insert an antiseptic-soaked tampon 12 hours before the surgery. Ferrous sulfate therapy may be prescribed several weeks before surgery if the woman is anemic from chronic blood loss.

POSTOPERATIVE CARE

Much of the postoperative care provided after hysterectomy is similar to that provided after any major surgery and includes assessment for hemorrhage and pulmonary embolism (see Chapter 18). Unique aspects of care are addressed here.

Promoting Activity

Ambulation begins on the day of surgery or the first postoperative day, and the nurse encourages regular brief periods of ambulation throughout the day. Ambulation supports oxygenation through natural deep breathing, assists in the prompt elimination of residual anesthetic, stimulates the return of peristalsis, and supports venous return. Venous pooling and pelvic congestion are common complications after hysterectomy because of the inflammatory response to the trauma of surgery. This is particularly true if the lithotomy position was used during surgery. The risk of thromboembolism is significant, and the physician may order prophylactic subcutaneous heparin injections. Routine interventions include applying compression stockings or external devices, encouraging leg and foot flexion and extension exercises every 2 hours, and avoiding positioning the patient with the knees bent. Elevating the legs at intervals throughout the day may be helpful also. Routine monitoring for pain or swelling in the calf is included in the ongoing assessment.

Supporting Urinary Elimination

Urinary problems are common after hysterectomy. The woman who undergoes vaginal hysterectomy may have a catheter left in place for 24 hours to allow for resolution of edema around the urethra. The catheter is typically removed on the first postoperative day, but many women experience some difficulty in voiding spontaneously or emptying the bladder completely. Careful assessment during the postoperative period for return of normal function is essential, since the delicate structures of the urinary tract may be injured during surgery.

Supporting Return of Peristalsis

Peristalsis is typically suppressed after hysterectomy, particularly if an abdominal approach with extensive handling of the GI organs was used. Gaseous distention is one of the most common and troublesome postoperative complaints. The woman typically receives nothing by mouth until bowel sounds return, and intravenous fluids are continued until she is taking oral fluids well. If problems do not occur, the patient moves quickly from a liquid to a regular diet. When paralytic ileus is severe, a nasogastric tube may be placed to relieve gaseous pressure. Frequent ambulation is encouraged as the most reliable means of stimulating peristaltic activity. The woman's potassium level is monitored to ensure that hypokalemia does not contribute to the ileus.

Promoting Sleep

Sleep pattern disturbance is commonly reported by women following hysterectomy and may be related to the surgical procedure and hospital environment. Efforts to promote normal sleep-wake patterns need to be balanced with the need for frequent monitoring.[10]

Providing Emotional Support

Hysterectomy may be accompanied by emotional upset and ambivalence concerning the loss of reproductive ability, but this is not always the case. Many women are equally concerned about the effects of the surgery on femininity and sexuality. After surgery almost all women experience some degree of depression for several days and may be inexplicably tearful. Grieving for losses is both appropriate and important, and the nurse encourages the woman to deal honestly with her emotions. Family members need to be informed about these expected responses, and partners may need to be encouraged to offer the patient specific reassurance and understanding during this time. Depression resulting from hormonal changes may respond to postoperative hormone replacement therapy in women who also undergo oophorectomy.[10] Women are instructed to avoid sexual intercourse until the vaginal vault is satisfactorily healed. This usually takes about 6 weeks. Satisfactory sexual relations can then be reestablished and often are improved.[22] Women need to adjust to changes in the nature of pelvic sensations and stimuli during sex. Open communication between the woman and her partner is essential. Alternative methods of expressing affection can be encouraged during the postoperative period.

Managing Fatigue

Persistent fatigue related to pain and sleep pattern disturbance is a frequent complaint of women following hysterectomy.[10] Women should be encouraged to use social support to free up time for rest periods throughout the day. A gradual return to preoperative responsibilities will be needed.

Guidelines for Safe Practice

The Patient Undergoing Hysterectomy

PREOPERATIVE CARE

1. Verify patient understanding of the procedure and anticipated care.
2. Administer prescribed enemas, laxatives, and douches.
3. Verify completion of prescribed skin preparation.
4. Promote circulation and oxygenation.
   a. Apply antiembolic stockings.
   b. Teach deep breathing, effective coughing, use of incentive spirometer, how to splint abdomen, and how to change positions.
   c. Teach leg and foot exercises.
5. Teach how to use patient-controlled analgesia (PCA) for pain control.
6. Encourage expression of feelings and concerns.

POSTOPERATIVE CARE

1. Promote comfort.
   a. Administer analgesics and encourage PCA use.
   b. Administer antiemetics as needed.
2. Promote circulation and oxygenation.
   a. Encourage turning, deep breathing, coughing, and use of incentive spirometer.
   b. Encourage leg and foot exercises every hour while in bed.
   c. Maintain use of antiembolic stockings as ordered.
   d. Encourage frequent ambulation.
   e. Monitor for signs of thromboembolism.
3. Accurately record all output and drainage.
4. Promote elimination.
   a. Monitor effectiveness of bladder emptying after catheter removal. Catheterize for residual if ordered.
   b. Monitor for signs of returning peristalsis.
   c. Encourage frequent ambulation and a liberal fluid intake.
   d. Teach diet modifications to prevent constipation.
5. Provide discharge teaching regarding medications and therapeutic regimens.
   a. Reinforce importance of and support for continued smoking cessation in those women who smoked before surgery.
   b. Teach signs of urinary tract infection.
   c. Provide teaching regarding incision care.
   d. Instruct patient to avoid heavy lifting, prolonged sitting, and long car rides.
   e. Tell patient to refrain from coitus for about 6 weeks and not to douche unless prescribed by her physician. Vaginal bleeding or discharge may persist for up to 6 weeks.
   f. Help patient anticipate the occurrence of mood swings and emotional lability during healing.

The nursing care for the hysterectomy patient is summarized in the Guidelines for Safe Practice box. A Clinical Pathway for a patient undergoing total abdominal hysterectomy is on pp. 1776 to 1777.

GERONTOLOGIC CONSIDERATIONS

Leiomyomas typically develop in middle-aged women and are rarely a significant problem in postmenopausal women. However, estrogen replacement therapy (ERT) will continue to

clinical pathway *Total Abdominal Hysterectomy* *Doe, Jane*

DAY DATE	1 06/13/02	2 06/14/02	3 06/15/02	4 06/16/02
Diet	06/13. NPO to ice chips.	06/14. CLEAR LIQUIDS advance as tolerated	06/15. REGULAR DIET as tolerated	------→
Vital Signs/Frequency	06/13. TPR/BP q4 hrs.	------→	------→	TPR/BP q8 hrs.
Intake & Output	06/13. I & O Call MD if urine output < 30 cc/hr	06/14. Discontinue I & O when IV discontinued and adequate PO intake.		
Weights	06/13. Weight obtained on admission.			
Elimination	06/13. Foley catheter	06/14. Foley to be D/Ced at ________		
Hygiene/ADL assistance	06/13. Assisted ADL's	------→	06/15. Independent ADL's	------→
Nursing Treatments	06/13. Abdominal binder applied 06/13. Venodyne boots as ordered	------→	06/15. D/C Venodyne boots	
Safety	06/13. Assess for fall prevention			
Safety	06/13. High risk skin assessment performed			
Activity	06/13. Bedrest; dangle at bedside	06/14. OOB: with assistance	06/15. OOB ad lib	------→
Respiratory treatments	06/13. Incentive spirometer: q 1 hr when awake	------→	06/15. Incentive spirometer: PRN	------→
ORDERS	**(MEDS/IVs/LABS/DIAGNOSTICS)**			
Lab tests		06/14. CBC as ordered, routine		
PLANS	INTERDISCIPLINARY PLANS OF CARE (Pharmacy, Nutrition Services, OT, PT, RT, Speech Therapy			
Case management: Pt/SO demonstrated knowledge of follow-up/community resources upon D/C		06/14. Medical record reviewed		
LOS: Pt. safely discharged on day 4	------→	------→	------→	Day of discharge ------→
OUTCOMES	Documentation of Nursing Assessments, Interventions, Expected outcomes			
Safety: Pt remained free of injury. Safety awareness maintained.	06/13. Oriented to environment. Evaluated for Fall Prevention. Maintained safe environment. Side rails up, bed in lowest position, call light handy as per policy.	06/14-06/15. Maintained safe environment. Side rails up, bed in lowest position, call light handy as per policy. Safety measures reinforced. Pt. compliant with and verbalized knowledge of safety measures.		06/16. Reinforced safety measures. Pt. compliant w/safety measures. No injury noted. Pt. demonstrated good safety awareness.

Psych: Pt. demonstrated adaptive coping skills. Affect appropriate. No s/s neglect or abuse. Characteristics of appearance/ verbalizations/behaviors approp. to situation.	06/13. Coping skills assessed as normal. Support system assessed as adequate. Emotional support provided prn. Tests, treatments, & procedures explained.	06/14. Pt. verbalized issues of self-care management. Pt. demonstrated knowledge of tests and treatments. Assessed coping skills related to outcome of surgery and female sexuality issues. Verbalized feelings related to surgery and body image changes.	---------→	06/16. Pt. demonstrated adequate coping skills. Expressed feelings openly concerning outcome of surgery. Support systems, community resources available discussed and secured.
PT/SO EDUCATION: Pt./SO demonstrated knowledge of diet, meds, food/drug interactions, safety, use of med equipment, community resources, smoking cessation support (if needed) & self care management.	06/13. Pt./SO verbalized reason for surgery. Pt. oriented to room, call light, safety measures. Instructed in diet progression, bowel and urinary function, activity level, pain medication, comfort measures, and respiratory care. Demonstrated cooperation in post-op teaching.	06/14. Pt./SO instructed on safe transfer method, mobility/ activity expectations and limitations, signs and symptoms to report to MD. Reinforced S&S of wound infection. Pt./SO return demonstrated understanding of material and present treatment plan.	06/15. Pt./SO verbalized knowledge of S&S of wound infection. Medications reviewed; new medications taught. Discharge teaching incisional care, bleeding, activity level, F/U MD visits, estrogen replacement therapy (if applicable). Verbalized content of post-op discharge teaching. Instructed Pt./SO on appropriate diet & food/drug interactions.	06/16. Pt./SO verbalized knowledge of S&S of wound infection. Pt./SO verbalized acceptance of discharge instructions.
COMFORT: Pt. verbalized minimal discomfort. Required prn medication only.	06/13. Pt. pain assessed q3-4 hrs. & prn. Pain reduction techniques taught and pt. was able to return demonstrate. Abdominal binder applied. Pt. demonstrated knowledge of analgesia method used (PCA/Epidural/IM). Medicated for pain prn. Pt. verbalized pain relief obtained.	06/14. Pt. pain assessed q3-4 hrs. & prn. Pain reduction techniques taught and pt. was able to return demonstrate. Pt. demonstrated knowledge of analgesia method used (Epidural/IM). Medicated for pain prn. Pt. verbalized pain relief obtained.	06-15. Pt. pain assessed q3-4 hrs. & prn. Pain reduction techniques taught and pt. was able to return demonstrate. Pt. demonstrated knowledge of analgesia method used (IM/PO). Medicated for pain prn. Pt. verbalized pain relief obtained.	06/16. Pt. pain assessed q3-4 hrs. & prn. Pain reduction techniques taught and pt. was able to return demonstrate. Pt. demonstrated knowledge of analgesia method used (PO). Medicated for pain prn. Tolerated PO analgesia. Pt. verbalized pain relief obtained.
RESPIRATORY: Respirations WNL. No wheezing, coughing, orthopnea. Bilateral breath sounds equal & clear.	06/13. C&DB encouraged. Instructed pt. in use of incentive spirometer and splinting of incision. Pt. return demonstrated.	06/14. C&DB encouraged. Reinforced use of incentive spirometer and pt. used as directed.	06/15. C&DB encouraged. Pt. independently used incentive spirometer as directed.	---------→
06/16. GI/ELIM: No distention. Bowel sounds active. Abd. soft.	06/13. Assessed for return of bowel function.	06/14. (+) bowel sounds and flatus.	06/15. Passing flatus and/or BM.	---------→
GU/ELIM: Bladder not distended after voiding. Urine yellow & clear.	06/13. Assessed for bladder distention.	06/14. Assessed for bladder distention and awareness of bladder sensation. Return to normal function.	---------→	---------→
SURG. WOUND SITE: Incision site free from redness, swelling, and drainage.	06/13. Assessed incision & dressing q 4 hrs. Dressing dry & intact. Wound care performed per MD orders.	06/14. Assessed incision & dressing q 8 hrs. Dressing dry & intact. Wound care performed per MD orders.	---------→	---------→
SIGNATURES	06/13.	06/14.	06/15.	06/16.

Modified from Bridgeport Hospital, 267 Grant Street, Bridgeport, CT 06610.

stimulate the growth of a myoma. There are no major differences in treatment approaches for older women, and most older women tolerate hysterectomy extremely well. Older patients need to be carefully monitored because complications are more common in this age-group, especially after abdominal surgery.

SPECIAL ENVIRONMENTS FOR CARE

Critical Care Management

Critical care management would rarely be indicated in the standard treatment of leiomyomas unless a woman developed severe and unexpected complications or had severe concurrent health problems in other major organ systems.

Home Care Management

Patients are rapidly discharged to their home environments, especially following vaginal hysterectomy. They rarely need home health support unless complications develop. The nurse provides thorough teaching about care of the incision and the signs of wound infection. Ileus can be an ongoing problem, and patients are instructed to contact their physician if abdominal distention, nausea, or vomiting develops. Stool softeners, liberal fluids, and diet modifications are used until a normal bowel pattern is reestablished. Discussion of strategies for managing fatigue and mood changes, promoting sleep, and resuming life patterns is essential.

COMPLICATIONS

The complications of hysterectomy are typically those associated with any major surgery and the use of general anesthesia. These include hemorrhage, pulmonary embolism, thrombophlebitis, infection, and ileus.

Cancer of the Endometrium

Etiology/Epidemiology

Cancer of the endometrium (uterine corpus) is the most common form of gynecologic cancer. It is highly curable and primarily affects women over 50 years of age. Endometrial cancer is twice as common as ovarian cancer and three times more common than cervical cancer.

Multiple risk factors have been identified in addition to age. These include obesity, diabetes, nulliparity, late menopause (after age 52), use of ERT, and use of tamoxifen for breast cancer. The risk of endometrial cancer among women taking ERT appears to be limited to unopposed estrogen products.[18] Adding progesterone to the therapy appears to eliminate the risk, and women receiving combined estrogen-progesterone products actually have a lower total risk of endometrial cancer than do women who are not receiving ERT.

Pathophysiology

Uterine hyperplasia is somewhat analogous to dysplasia of the cervix. Some lesions revert to normal, some persist as hyperplasia, and a few progress to endometrial adenocarcinoma. Unfortunately, unlike cervical dysplasia, no reliable, widely available screening method for endometrial hyperplasia exists. Most women with this condition are diagnosed when they seek medical care for abnormal uterine bleeding. The diagnosis of endometrial hyperplasia can be made only by pathologic examination of uterine tissue.

Endometrial cancer is an excellent example of an estrogen-dependent lesion. The underlying pathologic process involves overgrowth of the uterine endometrium in response to an estrogen-dominant hormonal environment. Abnormal vaginal bleeding is the most common symptom. Occasionally women have a purulent, blood-tinged discharge.

Collaborative Care Management

Cancer of the endometrium is a slow-growing form of cancer and is very responsive to treatment if detected early. High-risk women may have endometrial tissue samples taken periodically. Tissue samples may be acquired in a variety of ways, as outlined in Table 53-5.

Endometrial cancer is treated according to its stage. Table 53-6 outlines the staging criteria. The most common treatment is total abdominal hysterectomy with bilateral salpingo-oophorectomy. Radiation and surgery often are combined to treat early-stage disease. In high-risk stage I disease, patients may receive vaginal cuff brachytherapy to prevent local recurrence.[14] Lymphadenectomy is added for stage II tumors. Radiotherapy is used as a primary modality if the woman is a poor risk for surgery or refuses surgery.

Hormonal therapy and chemotherapy are often added for stage III or IV disease. Progestational agents have been successfully used for years. Chemotherapy with doxorubicin has shown some positive results. Women with stage IV disease should be encouraged to consider relevant clinical trials of chemotherapy agents.[14]

Patient/Family Education. The nursing care associated with hysterectomy and radiotherapy has been discussed previously. Nurses play a major role in health teaching about the impor-

TABLE 53-5 Methods of Detection of Endometrial Cancer

Method	Effectiveness (%)
Endometrial aspiration	70-80
Endometrial washings	80-90
Dilation and curettage (fractional)	85-90
Pap smear	45-50
Combination of above	90

TABLE 53-6 Stages of Cancer of the Endometrium

Stage	Involvement
I	Confined to corpus
II	Involves corpus and cervix
III	Extends outside corpus but not outside pelvis (vaginal wall but not bladder or rectum)
IV	Involves bladder, rectum, or outside pelvis

tance of careful evaluation of all abnormal uterine bleeding in the postmenopausal population. This single factor is the most important strategy for reducing the death rate by identifying endometrial cancer in a treatable stage.

Gestational Trophoblastic Neoplasia

Etiology/Epidemiology

Gestational trophoblastic neoplasia (GTN) is the term used to describe choriocarcinoma and related diseases such as hydatidiform mole and invasive mole. The etiology of GTN is not thoroughly understood. The hydatidiform mole often precedes malignant diseases.

The risk of hydatidiform mole varies significantly in different regions of the world, being more prevalent in the Far East than in the United States. Deficiencies of protein and carotene may contribute to the development of hydatidiform mole.[23]

Pathophysiology

GTN is an abnormal pregnancy characterized by a degeneration, or abnormal growth, of the trophoblastic tissue of the placenta, usually in the absence of an intact fetus. It produces a serum marker, human chorionic gonadotropin (hCG), whose levels are directly related to the number of tumor cells.

Early stages of GTN may be similar to normal pregnancy. As the disease progresses, most women experience uterine bleeding. Rapid uterine growth occurs, often accompanied by nausea and vomiting.

Collaborative Care Management

The diagnosis of GTN usually involves pelvic examination, blood chemistries, ultrasound, chest x-ray films, and analysis of hCG levels. Suction curettage is the most common method used for evacuation of a molar pregnancy. Hysterectomy may be considered for women who have completed childbearing. Weekly hCG levels are monitored in all women until normal levels are maintained for 6 months.[23] Women are advised to use a reliable contraceptive method and avoid pregnancy. Should hCG levels rise in the absence of pregnancy, prophylactic chemotherapy with methotrexate or dactinomycin is added, usually with excellent results.[23] Women with malignant GTN are evaluated for the extent of disease and treated with chemotherapy and possibly surgery and radiation.[23]

Patient/Family Education. Patient and family teaching includes an overview of this rather strange disease process, implications for future pregnancies, the effect of chemotherapy on future children, and the need for effective contraception during the first year after diagnosis.

NEOPLASMS OF THE OVARIES

Ovarian Cysts

Etiology/Epidemiology

Many types of benign tumors affect the ovaries; 80% are classified in the epithelial group, which includes serous, mucinous, endometrial, and mesonephroid lesions. Epithelial tumors are composed of supporting connective tissue and ovarian stroma but have the capacity to alter the woman's hormonal status. Other types of ovarian neoplasms include simple cysts and nonneoplastic cysts originating in the graafian follicle. Nearly 80% of ovarian tumors are discovered during routine pelvic examination and are asymptomatic. Women between ages 45 and 60 years are at greatest risk. Each of the various tumor types tends to affect a different age-group and behave in a different way.

Pathophysiology

Benign cysts and tumors develop from a variety of physiologic imbalances. Elevated levels of luteinizing hormone may cause hyperstimulation of the ovaries. Follicular cysts depend on gonadotropins for growth and generally occur during the menstrual years and resolve spontaneously. Simple cysts occur commonly during menopause. Box 53-3 summarizes the characteristics of various common types of ovarian cysts and tumors.

Most ovarian tumors are asymptomatic for long periods or produce only nonspecific symptoms. Menstrual irregularities may be present when hormonal imbalance exists. Dull, unilateral, lower quadrant pain may occur, especially as the cyst grows in size, but overt pain is an unusual symptom. Fatigue or a sense of heaviness in the pelvis also may occur. Ascites and increasing abdominal girth have been reported in slender women. Large tumors may cause symptoms of pelvic pressure, such as urinary frequency and constipation.

Collaborative Care Management

Palpation of the reproductive organs during pelvic examination commonly reveals the presence of any mass or enlargement of the ovary (Figure 53-14). Any mass palpated in a postmenopausal woman requires further investigation because the ovaries normally atrophy after menopause.

Ultrasonography may be used to distinguish functional from neoplastic cysts. A CT scan is capable of distinguishing solid tumors, cysts, and ascites, but laparoscopy may be performed to confirm the diagnosis.

Many ovarian cysts resolve spontaneously. If the cyst does not decrease in size, oral contraceptives may be prescribed to shrink it. Surgery is usually recommended only when the cyst is larger than 8 cm or occurs after menopause or before puberty. A cystectomy rather than oophorectomy will be performed if possible.

Patient/Family Education. The woman is reminded of the importance of follow-up care to continue to monitor the tumor's size. Most women are extremely anxious concerning the effects of the tumor on fertility and should be reassured that even oophorectomy does not reduce childbearing potential as long as the second ovary is healthy. If both ovaries are removed, the woman undergoes surgical menopause and needs to receive information concerning ERT.

Cancer of the Ovary

Etiology/Epidemiology

Malignant neoplasms of the ovaries occur at all ages, including infancy and childhood. Cancer of the ovary is the fifth most common cancer in women in the United States and has the highest mortality rate of the gynecologic cancers. More

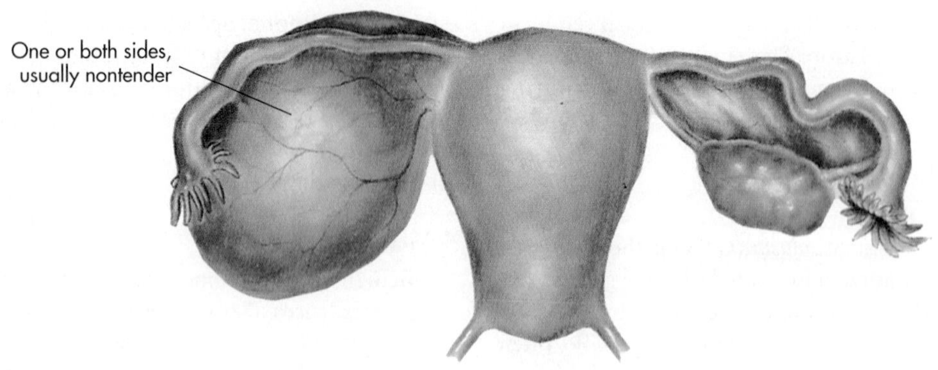

Figure 53-14 Ovarian cyst.

BOX 53-3 Characteristics of Various Types of Benign Ovarian Cysts and Tumors

Cysts

Follicular Cysts

Most common form of cysts
Often multiple; range in size from a few millimeters to as large as 15 cm in diameter
Depend on gonadotropin for growth
Occur during menstrual years and usually resolve spontaneously
May cause menstrual irregularities if blood estrogen elevated

Corpus Luteum Cysts

Less common variety
Associated with normal ovarian function or elevated progesterone
Average diameter 4 cm
May appear purplish red from bleeding within corpus luteum
May cause delayed menstrual bleeding from progesterone secretion; menorrhagia common

Theca Lutein Cysts

Least common variety
Usually bilateral and produce significant ovarian enlargement, up to 30 cm in diameter
Develop from prolonged or excessive stimulation by gonadotropins
Associated with hydatidiform mole 50% of the time and with choriocarcinomas 10% of the time

Epithelial Tumors

Serous Tumors

Found in all age-groups
Can be extremely large, filling pelvis or abdomen

Mucinous Tumors

Occur in second to third decade of life
May be bilateral
Can reach spectacular size; largest form

Endometroid Tumors

Small lesions, purplish blue in color
Large tumors called "chocolate cysts" because they contain brownish fluid
Very low malignancy potential

Mesonephroid Tumors

Usually multifocal
Involve peritoneal surfaces and may cause intestinal or urinary tract complications
Characterized by papillary proliferations without mitotic activity

than 23,000 new cases are expected each year, with a 5-year survival rate of less than 50%, making ovarian cancer one of the deadliest cancers for women.[19]

The etiology of ovarian cancer is not understood, but several factors appear to be associated with its incidence. Family history is the most important risk factor.[19] Increasing age, nulliparity, early menarche, late menopause, use of hormone replacement therapy, and a history of breast cancer add to the risk of ovarian cancer.[19] Protective effects include long-term use of oral contraceptives; completing at least one pregnancy; breastfeeding; having a tubal ligation, hysterectomy or oophorectomy; and, avoiding agents such as talc, fertility drugs, and a high-fat diet.[19] The survival rate is highest when the disease is diagnosed and treated early but decreases dramatically for advanced forms of the disease.

Recent genetic linkage studies reveal an association between the risk of ovarian cancer and the presence of mutations of the tumor suppressor genes BRCA1 and BRCA2. Approximately 16% of women with mutations of these genes are expected to develop ovarian cancer.[15] The American College of Obstetricians and Gynecologists does not recommend widespread genetic testing for ovarian cancer risk.[3]

Pathophysiology

Ovarian cancer is a broad term, and ovarian neoplasms can be divided into many categories, depending on the cell type of origin. The major histologic types occur in distinctive age ranges. The four main types are described in Table 53-7. Malignant epithelial cell tumors are the most common and are seen in women over age 50. Malignant germ cell tumors

TABLE 53-7 Classification of Ovarian Neoplasms

Neoplasm	Examples
Epithelium	Serous, mucinous, endometrioid
Germ cell	Teratoma (mature and immature), dysgerminoma
Gonadal stroma	Granulosa (theca, Sertoli's, Leydig's cells)
Mesenchyme	Fibroma, lymphoma, sarcoma

TABLE 53-8 Stages of Cancer of the Ovary

Stage	Involvement
I	Limited to ovaries
II	Involving one or both ovaries with pelvic extention
III	Involving one or both ovaries with intraperitoneal metastasis outside pelvis or positive lymph nodes
IV	Involving one or both ovaries with distant metastasis (e.g., liver, lungs)

are more uncommon and are seen primarily in women under age 20.[16]

The clinical manifestations of advancing disease include pelvic discomfort, low back pain, weight change, abdominal pain, nausea and vomiting, constipation, and urinary frequency. Any ovarian enlargement should be evaluated for malignancy. Palpable ovaries in premenarchal or postmenopausal women are abnormal physical findings.

Collaborative Care Management

The early diagnosis of an ovarian neoplasm usually occurs by chance rather than successful screening. No useful screening test exists at present for widespread use. Even ultrasonography, CT scanning, and MRI are not sufficiently specific to distinguish between benign and malignant tumors. Although the use of transvaginal ultrasonography improves the recognition of early malignancies, both abdominal and transvaginal ultrasound are usually inadequate to confirm the diagnosis. CA-125, a tumor marker produced by ovarian cancer cells, is not specific enough to be diagnostic, although it is used to monitor response to chemotherapy.[12] A variety of other tests may be used in the search for metastasis.

Laparotomy is the primary tool for both diagnosis and staging. Table 53-8 presents the staging system. Surgery is also the primary therapeutic approach and usually involves total abdominal hysterectomy with bilateral salpingectomy-oophorectomy. Ascitic fluid or washings are submitted for cytology. All of the tissue of the pelvis is carefully assessed, and biopsy specimens of any suspicious tissue are sent for analysis.

Adjuvant therapy is often employed, depending on the stage of the disease. Chemotherapy is typically used for stage I disease, and various combinations of agents are under investigation. Patients with stage II disease may be treated with instillation of radioactive phosphorus (^{32}P) into the peritoneum, external irradiation, or combined chemotherapy. Patients with stage III or IV disease undergo surgical attempts to remove as much tumor as possible. This intervention appears to be directly related to survival. Surgery is followed by aggressive combination chemotherapy with such agents as cisplatin, paclitaxel, and cyclophosphamide. Patients may also want to consider participation in one of the many clinical trials underway for epithelial cancer (see Future Watch box).

Patient/Family Education. Patient teaching concerning diagnosis, surgery, and adjuvant therapy for ovarian cancer is an integral aspect of nursing care. Support and education are offered to the patient and family throughout each aspect of diagnosis and treatment. Genetic testing may involve several members of the family. Cancer of the ovary carries a poor prognosis, and the woman and her family will need ongoing support.

Future Watch

Clinical Trials Investigate the Use of Angiogenesis Inhibitor Agents in Ovarian Cancer

Angiogenesis inhibitors are chemicals that signal the body to stop making new blood vessels. The National Cancer Institute (NCI) is currently investigating the potential use of angiogenesis inhibitors for possible antitumor effects. Angiogenesis inhibitors could potentially "starve" the tumor and reduce its size. An example of a phase II clinical trial is a study of the effects of carboplatin and squalamine lactate in patients with recurrent or refractory stage III or IV ovarian cancer. The trial is a combination of a standard intravenous cisplatin agent with squalamine lactate, an angiogenesis inhibitor agent. The therapy repeats every 3 weeks for six courses. In a phase II trial the primary focus is on response rate, time to progression, and safety of the regimen. Consequently, participants are women for whom standard therapies have not worked. The NCI is expanding its use of clinical trials. Health care providers should have discussions with women regarding their interest in participating in clinical trials. A listing of NCI-sponsored clinical trials is also provided on the NCI's website: http://cancertrials.nci.nih.gov. The Institute for Clinical Systems Improvement, a national information and education network, can be reached by the following toll-free phone number: (800) 4-CANCER ([800] 422-6237).

Reference: Institute for Clinical Systems Improvement: *Health care guideline—cervical cancer screening,* March 2001, website: www.icsi.org.

NEOPLASMS OF THE VULVA

Cancer of the Vulva

Etiology/Epidemiology

Vulvar cancer is rare, with invasive disease accounting for just 5% of malignancies of the female genital tract. It is a disease that primarily affects older women. Preinvasive disease (vulvar carcinoma in situ) is occurring more commonly in younger women, possibly because of factors such as exposure to HPV and HIV. Three times as many Caucasians are affected as African-Americans. Parity does not seem to play a role in the incidence. Survival rates are high with early detection of noninvasive disease but drop to 50% when lymph nodes are positive.[21]

The exact etiology of cancer of the vulva is still unknown. Etiologic factors are believed to include STDs involving the vulva and the use of tight-fitting apparel or nylon undergarments, perineal deodorants, smoking, and trauma. Herpes, syphilis, and genital warts have all been associated with the development of carcinoma.

Pathophysiology

Most cancers of the vulva are squamous in origin (90%). The initial lesion often arises from an area of intraepithelial neoplasia, which can eventually form a firm nodule and ulcerate. The diagnosis of vulvar cancer can be made only by biopsy and histologic tissue examination. The lesion can develop anywhere on the vulva, but 70% of lesions arise on the labia. The lesion is usually localized and well demarcated. Common clinical manifestations include vulvar itching and burning.

Collaborative Care Management

Treatment of carcinoma of the vulva varies significantly, depending on the location and extent of the disease. Preinvasive disease is usually treated surgically, with laser therapy, or with skinning vulvectomy. Carcinoma in situ may also be treated nonsurgically with topical 5-fluorouracil (1% Efudex) applied daily; the response rate is 50% to 60%.[21] The standard treatment for invasive carcinoma has been radical vulvectomy, although the procedure has been modified for women with certain types of lesions to make it less mutilating. Radical vulvectomy involves excision of the mons pubis, terminal portion of the urethra, and vagina; excision of portions of the round ligaments and saphenous veins; and selected lymph node dissection (Figure 53-15). Radical surgery achieves an 80% to 90% 5-year survival rate for stage II lesions.[21] Radiation treatment following surgery is used in stage III disease. Chemotherapy is used for recurrent disease.[21]

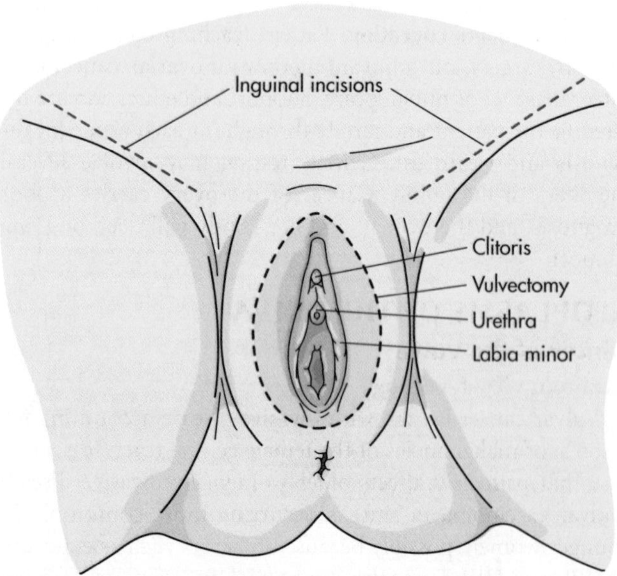

Figure 47-15 Vulvectomy with operative incision lines shown. Note groin incisions.

Complications related to radical vulvectomy include wound infection and disruption because the wounds are typically left open to heal by secondary intention. Delayed complications include stenosis of the vagina from scar tissue formation, pelvic muscle relaxation leading to stress incontinence, and swelling of the legs from obstructive lymphangitis.

Postoperative care focuses initially on comfort. Because of the widespread tissue destruction, the inguinal suture line is very tight and extremely uncomfortable. The woman needs frequent assistance to achieve a comfortable position. Wound breakdown is often a problem. The vulvar wound is usually left open, and sitz baths, whirlpool therapy, and topical agents may be used to support healing.

Patient/Family Education. The nurse teaches the patient that despite meticulous care, the wounds heal very slowly and complications may occur. The nurse encourages the woman to express her feelings concerning this difficult and disfiguring surgery. The woman is reassured that sexual intercourse usually can be resumed after complete wound healing has occurred—usually at least 6 weeks. Lymphedema in the legs is treated with compression stockings for at least 6 months after surgery. The warning signs of other complications are discussed with the woman before discharge. The Guidelines for Safe Practice box summarizes nursing care for patients experiencing radical vulvectomy.

STERILIZATION

Etiology/Epidemiology

Voluntary sterilization is the most commonly used method of fertility control for married couples over 30 years of age and is the most widely used contraceptive method worldwide. In the United States about 1 million sterilization procedures are performed annually.[23] The primary reasons given are the desire to limit family size and the desire to be free of the risk of pregnancy with advancing age.

About 1% of sterilized women subsequently request reversal. Successful reversal is more likely in those cases where a higher failure rate method was originally used.[23] Microsurgical techniques are used and typically involve an end-to-end anastomosis of the ligated tubes.

Pathophysiology

Tubal sterilization terminates a woman's ability to bear children but does not alter ovarian hormone secretion or menstrual functioning. Artificial menopause is not induced, and the ability to enjoy sexual intercourse should not be impaired. Women appear to have little regret after the surgery if they understand what to expect during and after the procedure and are able to express their feelings and have their questions answered before surgery. Occasionally, however, women who are ambivalent about the choice or have preexisting self-esteem issues develop psychologic problems after sterilization.

Collaborative Care Management

Tubal sterilization was first performed in 1823, and since that time more than 200 different techniques for the procedure have been developed. Most methods involve the mechanical removal of a part of the female reproductive system so that the sperm and ovum cannot unite. Table 53-9 summarizes available methods of sterilization. Minilaparotomy and laparoscopy are by far the most common methods.

In minilaparotomy a small (2- to 3-cm) transverse abdominal incision is made about 3 cm above the pubis, and the peritoneal cavity is entered. The fallopian tubes are located, and a portion of each tube is elevated and ligated at the base. The free ends may be tied off or cauterized. Minilaparotomy is an ambulatory procedure performed with the patient under local anesthesia.

Laparoscopic tubal sterilization is more common and requires only a small subumbilical incision for insertion of the laparoscope. A segment of each tube is coagulated by application of an electric current. Clips or rings may also be applied to the tube. The procedure is brief and safe and is performed with the patient under local anesthesia.

The laws governing sterilization vary from state to state and have undergone many changes over the years. In general, the surgery may be performed if written, informed consent is given by a woman capable of giving permission. Patients using federal funds for payment must be at least 21 years of age, and there may be a prescribed waiting period for patients using Medicaid funds.

Patient/Family Education. Patient teaching is the foundation of nursing care. The discussion of sterilization methods

Guidelines for Safe Practice

The Patient Undergoing Radical Vulvectomy

PREOPERATIVE CARE

1. Explain treatment and plan of care.
2. Administer enemas and douches as prescribed.
3. Provide emotional support.
4. Teach deep breathing exercises and leg exercises.

POSTOPERATIVE CARE

1. Maintain bed rest for 72 hours in semi-Fowler's position.
   a. Support legs with pillows.
   b. Turn every 2 hours.
   c. Encourage frequent deep breathing and use of incentive spirometer.
   d. Encourage leg exercises.
   e. Avoid stress on suture lines.
   f. Assess for signs of complications—atelectasis, deep vein thrombosis.
2. Assess discomfort level and ensure adequate analgesia. Use a patient-controlled analgesia pump, if possible, to allow patient to control dosage.
3. Monitor wound healing.
   a. Provide perineal hygiene and give sitz baths when ordered; keep perineum dry.
   b. Cleanse wound twice a day and after defecation.
4. Maintain patency of the Foley catheter.
5. Provide a low-residue diet.
6. Provide diversional activities.
7. Encourage expression of feelings.

DISCHARGE TEACHING

1. Use support hose for 6 months; elevate legs frequently.
2. Can resume sexual activity in 4 to 6 weeks.
3. Discuss possible need for lubrication and position changes with coitus; genital numbness may be present.
4. Avoid straining with defecation.
5. Discuss signs and symptoms of complications to report to physician.
6. Note the possible altered directional flow of urine.

TABLE 53-9 Methods of Tubal Sterilization for Women

Description	Comments
Abdominal	
Minilaparotomy: ligation or cutting of fallopian tubes under direct vision through small abdominal incision or near umbilicus	Complications: wound infection, hematoma, bladder injury Advantages: good chance for sterility reversal
Laparoscopy: electrocoagulation of segment of fallopian tubes by laparoscopy through small abdominal incision near umbilicus	Local anesthesia Advantages: minimal discomfort, short procedure
Vaginal	
Culpotomy: ligation or cutting of fallopian tube through small incision in cul-de-sac of Douglas	Local, spinal, or general anesthesia Higher complication rate than with laparoscopy (infection, hemorrhage)
Culdoscopy: electrocoagulation of segment of fallopian tubes by culdoscope through small incision in cul-de-sac of Douglas	Local anesthesia Higher complication rate than with laparoscopy Local or general anesthesia

BOX 53-4 Informed Consent Guidelines (Federal) Relating to Sterilization

1. Choice is made by patient. No pressures are placed on choice (e.g., loss of welfare benefits, wrath of health care provider).
2. Benefits and risks of sterilization are described.
   a. Benefits: permanent, no further costs or decision making
   b. Risks: usual surgical risks, possibility of future pregnancy (i.e., not 100% effective)
3. Alternative contraceptive methods are described.
4. Patient is encouraged to ask questions.
5. Patient may withdraw from using the method without penalty.
6. Explanations are given about the entire sterilization procedure, costs, and possible side effects (effects of hormones, weight changes, menstrual changes, sexual response).
7. Written instructions and risk factors are given to patient.
8. A written consent to the procedure is signed by patient and witnessed.

BOX 53-5 Causes of Infertility

Female

- Developmental: uterine abnormalities
- Endocrine: pituitary, thyroid, and adrenal dysfunctions; ovarian dysfunctions (inhibit maturation and release of ova)
- Diseases: Pelvic inflammatory disease (especially from gonococcus); fallopian tube obstructions; diseases of cervix and uterus that inhibit passage of active sperm
- Other: malnutrition, severe anemia, anxiety

Male

- Developmental: undescended testes, other congenital anomalies (inhibit development of sperm)
- Endocrine: hormonal deficiencies (pituitary, thyroid, adrenal) (inhibit development of sperm)
- Diseases: testicular destruction from disease, orchitis from mumps, prostatitis
- Other: excessive smoking, fatigue, alcohol, excessive heat (hot baths), marijuana use

Both Female and Male

- Diseases: sexually transmitted diseases (STDs), cancer with obstructions (inhibit transport of ovum or sperm)
- Other: immunologic incompatibility (inhibit sperm penetration of ovum), marital problems
- Diethylstilbestrol exposure in utero (suggested but not proved as a cause of male infertility)

should be based on the federal government's informed consent guidelines (Box 53-4). The nurse confirms that the woman understands the nature and consequences of the surgical procedure. The facts concerning reversibility, including current success rates, are discussed. Many people equate sterilization with a loss of femininity, and even women who know the difference may appreciate reassurance.

After surgery the woman is instructed to rest for 24 to 48 hours and avoid all heavy lifting and strenuous exercise for 1 week. The nurse instructs the woman to abstain from sexual intercourse until the wound is completely healed and to report any signs of fever, incisional bleeding, or persistent abdominal pain to the physician. Care of the woman after a laparoscopic procedure is discussed in Chapter 52.

INFERTILITY

The term *infertility* refers to the inability to achieve a pregnancy within a stipulated period of time, usually 1 year. The problem may be considered primary if the couple has never conceived or secondary if conception was successfully achieved in the past.

Etiology/Epidemiology

An estimated 10% to 15% of all couples in the United States are infertile. Infertility is most often attributed to women, but about 30% of cases result from male infertility and 20% from both partners.[28] More couples today are seeking infertility treatment, despite its high costs. The majority of couples who undergo assessment and treatment for infertility successfully conceive.[23]

From 80% to 90% of all women become pregnant within 1 year when they practice unprotected sexual intercourse. Fertility in women is low during the early teenage years, peaks in the mid-twenties, and declines after age 30. Approximately 33% of women who delay pregnancy until after age 35 experience problems with infertility. This rate increases to 60% after age 40. Fertility in men also reaches its peak in the mid-twenties and subsequently declines, but the decrease is much less significant than in women. The frequency of coitus is another recognized variable in fertility, because increased frequency appears to enhance sperm motility. Other risk factors for infertility include increased age, a history of STDs, and occupational and environmental hazard exposure.[28]

Pathophysiology

Three basic categories of infertility account for most reproductive dysfunction: anovulation, anatomic defects of the female genital tract, and abnormal sperm production. Common causes of infertility in men and women are presented in Box 53-5. No cause can be found in 10% to 20% of cases.

Ovulatory dysfunction is a leading cause of infertility. It can result from a malfunction at any point in the hormonal feedback system. Fallopian tube obstruction is a common structural defect. Acute salpingitis from gonorrhea or chlamydial infection is the most common cause of this obstruction. Pelvic infections, use of IUDs, and endometriosis can also cause fallopian tube obstruction.

Infection may destroy the glands that secrete the thin, watery mucus essential for sperm survival and migration. Estrogen deficiency may decrease the volume and quality of the cervical mucus. Anomalies of the uterus, including the presence of leiomyomas, may interfere with successful implantation.

A number of studies suggest that tobacco may be a causal factor in infertility. Nicotine appears to adversely affect tubal transport and implantation. *Mycoplasma*, which causes cervici-

TABLE 53-10 Diagnostic Testing for Infertility

Gender	Tests	Purpose
Male	Semen analysis	Determine presence, number, and motility of sperm
	Testicular biopsy if sperm count low or absent	Check for presence of sperm, which indicates obstruction of vas deferens
Female	Basal body temperature chart	Determine that ovulation is occurring
	Postcoital test of cervical secretions	Measure ability of sperm to penetrate cervical mucus and remain active; determine quality of mucus
	Endometrial biopsy	Determine whether ovulation is occurring (if in question)
	Laparoscopy	Examine pelvis and determine patency of fallopian tubes
	Hysterosalpingography (x-ray film after insertion of contrast media)	Determine patency of uterus and fallopian tubes
Male/female	Hormonal tests	Determine whether problem is hormonal

tis, may contribute to infertility, and the role of other infectious agents is under investigation. Dietary deficiencies are known to adversely affect secretion of pituitary gonadotropins, and strenuous exercise, such as running more than 10 miles per week, has been implicated in infertility, either through its caloric demands or the effects of endorphins on the pituitary gland.

Infertility can produce profound psychologic effects. When couples find themselves unable to have children, the trauma can affect every aspect of their lives and marriage. The experience of diagnosis and treatment can be an emotional roller-coaster of raised expectations and dashed hopes.

Collaborative Care Management

The purposes of an infertility evaluation are to establish the cause of infertility and provide a basis for determining medical or surgical treatment options. The process can be physically painful, as well as emotionally and economically stressful. The various diagnostic tests used in the diagnosis of infertility are discussed in Chapter 52 and summarized in Table 53-10.

Artificial insemination is a simple, safe, inexpensive, and highly successful infertility treatment when male infertility is the cause. Semen may be deposited by a cervical-vaginal, intracervical, or intrauterine route. A few drops of semen are injected as close to the time of ovulation as possible. Treatment may use the partner's semen (homologous) or donor semen (heterologous). The fertility of donors is carefully determined, and the sperm are screened for HIV. This can be an emotional topic for some couples and may induce strong reactions.[9]

In the past decade a virtual explosion of reproductive technology has occurred. These procedures, known as assisted reproductive technologies, are expensive and raise ethical issues regarding parenting. There is a movement to mandate insurance coverage for nonexperimental methods of treating infertility; however, only about 25% of U.S. companies provide any form of coverage.[6] Box 53-6 summarizes other, less commonly employed approaches to infertility.

The correction of structural problems is undertaken first if feasible. Transcervical balloon tuboplasty may be performed to correct blocked or scarred fallopian tubes. A modified cardiovascular balloon is passed into the fallopian tube and inflated to clear the occlusion.

BOX 53-6 Alternative Approaches to Fertility Management

In Vitro Fertilization and Embryo Transfer

One or more ova are recovered from the ovarian follicles and fertilized with the partner's sperm in a Petri dish. Oocyte retrieval is performed by means of ultrasound-guided needle aspiration. The cleaved ova are placed in the patient's uterus through a small catheter about 48 hours after retrieval. Pregnancy rates are related to the number of embryos placed and vary from 18% to 30%.

Gamete Intrafallopian Transfer (GIFT)

Oocytes aspirated from follicles are mixed with washed sperm and placed in the uterine tube via laparoscopy. This approach appears to achieve a higher pregnancy rate than in vitro fertilization. The preembryo travels toward the uterus, following the natural timetable for implantation in 4 days.

Zygote Intrafallopian Transfer (ZIFT) and Tubal Embryo Transfer (TET)

These procedures are similar to GIFT, except transfer to the fallopian tubes occurs at the zygote stage, about 16 to 18 hours after oocyte insemination. TET involves transfer of embryos into the fallopian tube around 40 to 48 hours after oocyte insemination.

Surrogate Mothers

Surrogate mothers are women who contract to conceive by artificial insemination and give the baby to the semen donor after delivery. Many social and legal implications with the process have received recent attention through some extremely public lawsuits over custody of the child.

Ovum Transfer

A donor provides the ovum, which is fertilized with the partner's sperm. The embryo is transferred to the infertile woman's uterus after about 5 days via a small catheter. Pregnancy rates have been as high as 25% to 50%.

A variety of drugs can be used to induce or support ovulation. Clomiphene citrate (Clomid, Serophene) is used for women with intact pituitary function. Follicle-stimulating and leutinizing hormones, such as mentropin (Pergonal), are used when patients have pituitary dysfunction. Recombinant deoxyribonucleic acid (DNA)–origin gonadotropins, such as follitropin-beta (Follistim) and follitropin-alfa (gonal F), are also used. hCG may be given to trigger the release of mature follicles, and progesterone preparations may be used for luteal phase support. The drugs may also be used in combination.

Multiple births can occur with ovulatory induction therapy. The onset of low abdominal pain can indicate the development of an ovarian cyst or cyst rupture. The woman is informed of the multiple-drug side effects, which include hot flashes, emotional lability and depression, fatigue, nausea, and bloating.

Problems of sperm production are addressed by first eliminating alterations of thermoregulation. Optimal sperm production occurs at temperatures approximately 1° to 3° F below body temperature. The man is instructed to avoid sitting for long periods of time in hot tubs, wearing tight clothes that pull the testicles against the body, and sitting for long periods of time with poor heat dispersion. Medications (clomiphene citrate, hCG, menotropin, and a GnRH pump) can also be used to treat male infertility.[28]

Traditional drug therapy may be combined with intrauterine insemination. This approach has achieved a success rate comparable with that of in vitro fertilization—approximately 20%.

Patient/Family Education. Infertility can produce profound psychologic effects. The nurse is challenged to help couples to be active participants in the entire infertility workup and treatment plan, carefully exploring their own feelings about the limits they wish to set on the attempt to become pregnant. Sexual dysfunction often occurs, because this formerly pleasurable and spontaneous private activity becomes a public process to be dissected and often used as a measure of their success or failure concerning pregnancy. The nurse encourages the honest expression of feelings and provides time for dealing with the couple's intense feelings during treatment. Anticipatory guidance regarding side effects of medications is provided to improve tolerance.[11]

Nurses also play an important role in promoting fertility. Patient teaching aimed at preventing infection of the pelvic organs, particularly gonorrhea and chlamydial infection, is critical. Salpingitis is often the first overt sign of gonorrhea and can result in obstruction of the fallopian tubes. Early diagnosis and effective treatment of all vaginal and cervical infections is critical. The nurse encourages the use of barrier contraceptives, which help reduce the risk of infection, and encourages the woman to limit the number of her sexual partners. Women with ovarian and hormonal problems commonly experience symptoms such as menstrual irregularities. Many of these problems can be successfully managed with hormone therapy if identified early, before problems with infertility develop.

Critical Thinking Questions

1. You have been asked to speak to a group of high school students about women's health issues. Outline how you would address the relationships among the development of pelvic inflammatory disease, cervical cancer, and infertility.
2. A 21-year-old woman completes a symptom diary to determine the severity of her premenstrual syndrome. What teaching is relevant in the initial management of documented premenstrual syndrome?
3. A 45-year-old woman is 2 days postoperative following a total abdominal hysterectomy and bilateral salpingo-oophorectomy to treat severe leiomyomas. What are the discharge teaching priorities for her?
4. A patient is completing intracavitary radiation treatment for early cervical cancer. You are beginning her discharge teaching related to vaginal fibrosis when she breaks into tears. She says, "How will we ever resume sexual intercourse? I stink, this drainage is disgusting, and my husband will never find me attractive again." How will you respond?
5. Describe the following methods of assisted reproductive technologies: in vitro fertilization and embryo transfer, gamete intrafallopian transfer (GIFT), zygote intrafallopian transfer (ZIFT), tubal embryo transfer (TET), surrogate mothers, and ovum transfer.

References

1. Agency for Health Care Policy and Research: *Management of uterine fibroids,* Summary, Evidence Report/Technology Assessment No 34, AHRQ Pub No 01-E052, Rockville, Md, 2001, website: http://www.ahrq.gov/clinic/utersumm.htm.
2. American College of Obstetricians and Gynecologists: *Vaginitis,* ACOG Technical Bulletin No 226, Washington, DC, 1996, ACOG.
3. American College of Obstetricians and Gynecologists: *Breast-ovarian cancer screening,* ACOG Committee Opinion No 239, Washington, DC, 2000, ACOG.
4. American College of Obstetricians and Gynecologists: *Concurrent chemoradiation in the treatment of cervical cancer,* ACOG Committee Opinion No 242, Washington, DC, 2000, ACOG.
5. American College of Obstetricians and Gynecologists: *Premenstrual syndrome,* ACOG Practice Bulletin No 15, Washington, DC, 2000, ACOG.
6. Association of Women's Health, Obstetric and Neonatal Nurses: *Infertility treatment as a covered health insurance benefit,* AWHONN Position Statement, 2000, website: www.awhonn.org.
7. Department of Health and Human Services, Public Health Service: *Treating tobacco use and dependence,* Washington, DC, 2000, USDHHS.
8. Farquhar C: Endometriosis, *Clin Evidence* 5:1267-1275, 2001.
9. Holzman G: *Precis: an update in obstetrics and gynecology,* 1998, American College of Obstetricians and Gynecologists.
10. Kim KH, Lee KA: Symptom experience in women after hysterectomy, *J Obstet Gynecol Neonatal Nurs* 30:472-480, 2001.
11. Leibowitz D, Hoffman J: Fertility drug therapies: past, present, and future, *J Obstet Gynecol Neonatal Nurs* 29:201-210, 2000.
12. National Cancer Institute: Cancer facts: tumor markers, *PDQ summary,* website: www.nci.gov, 1998.
13. National Cancer Institute: Cervical cancer treatment, *PDQ summary,* website: www.nci.gov, 2001.
14. National Cancer Institute: Endometrial cancer treatment, *PDQ summary,* website: www.nci.gov, 2001.
15. National Cancer Institute: Genetics of breast and ovarian cancer, *PDQ summary,* website: www.nci.gov, 2001.
16. National Cancer Institute: Ovarian germ cell tumor treatment. *PDQ summary,* website: www.nci.gov, 2001.
17. National Cancer Institute: Prevention of cervical cancer, *PDQ summary,* website: www.nci.gov, 2001.

18. National Cancer Institute: Prevention of endometrial cancer, *PDQ summary,* website: www.nci.gov, 2001.
19. National Cancer Institute: Prevention of ovarian cancer, *PDQ summary,* website: www.nci.gov, 2001.
20. National Cancer Institute: Screening for cervical cancer, *PDQ summary,* website: www.nci.gov, 2001.
21. National Cancer Institute: Vulvar cancer treatment, *PDQ summary,* www.nci.gov, 2001.
22. Rhodes JC et al: Hysterectomy and sexual functioning, *JAMA* 282:1934-1941, 1999.
23. Scott JR et al, editors: *Danforth's obstetrics and gynecology,* ed 8, Philadelphia, 1999, Lippincott Williams & Wilkins.
24. Scott LD, Hasik KJ: The similarities and differences of endometritis and pelvic inflammatory disease, *J Obstet Gynecol Neonatal Nurs* 30:332-341, 2001.
25. Stovall TG, Ling FW, editors: *Gynecology for the primary care physician,* Philadelphia, 1999, Current Medicine.
26. Wade J et al: Hysterectomy: what do women need and want to know? *J Obstet Gynecol Neonatal Nurs* 29:33-42, 2000.
27. Wilson M, Farquhar C: Dysmenorrhoea, *Clin Evidence* 5:1254-1266, 2001.
28. Youngkin EQ, Davis MS: *Women's health: a primary care clinical guide,* Stamford, Conn, 1998, Appleton & Lange.

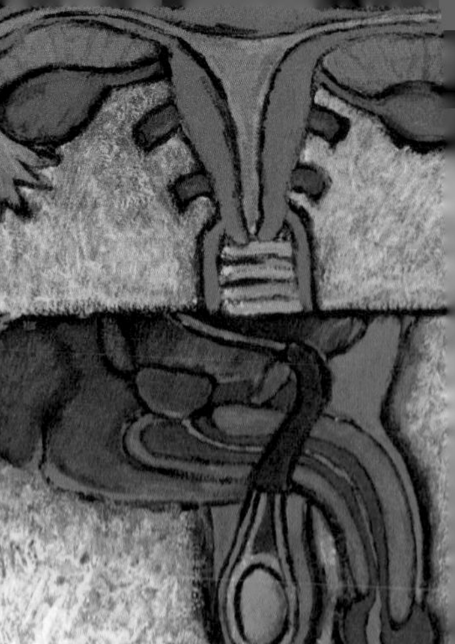

54 Problems of the Breast

Angela Sammarco

Objectives

After studying this chapter, the learner should be able to:

1. Describe the differences between benign and malignant breast conditions.
2. Identify the risk factors for developing breast cancer.
3. Describe early detection methods and diagnostic tests for breast evaluation.
4. Discuss the advantages and disadvantages of surgery, chemotherapy, radiotherapy, and hormonal therapy in the treatment of breast cancer.
5. Describe the types of breast preservation and reconstruction procedures available.
6. Demonstrate how to correctly perform postmastectomy exercises.
7. Discuss the management and prevention of lymphedema in patients treated for breast cancer.
8. Discuss the aspects of psychosocial adjustment to breast cancer.
9. Compare the treatments for common benign breast conditions.

This chapter discusses the collaborative management of both breast cancer and other cystic and inflammatory breast conditions. Breast cancer is by far the most important of these disorders, and it is presented first. The nonmalignant conditions are discussed later in the chapter, followed by problems that affect the male breast.

MALIGNANT CONDITIONS OF THE BREAST

Etiology

Breast cancer is the most common cancer among women. The incidence of breast cancer continues to increase, partly as a result of the steady aging of the population, and partly because of improved diagnostic technology. The mortality rates associated with breast cancer were relatively stable between 1950 and the late 1980s. Beginning in 1989, the rate of breast cancer mortality has declined annually. This reduction in mortality has been attributed to improvements in breast cancer treatments and the benefits of mammography screening.[3] The underlying cause of breast cancer is still unknown, but a number of risk factors have been identified.

Age and Gender. Breast cancer is almost exclusively a disease affecting women. Only 1500 of the 192,200 new cases of breast cancer anticipated in 2001 are predicted to involve men.[17] Women today have a 1 in 8 chance of developing breast cancer in their lifetime. As is the case with most malignant conditions, the incidence of breast cancer increases with age.[3]

Breast cancer is diagnosed most frequently in women older than 50 years. One reason for this age-related finding may be an increased probability of mutagenic changes occurring over a longer life span. Another is that older women are at greater risk, and they outnumber younger women in the present population.

Heredity. Inherited breast cancer accounts for up to 10% of all breast cancer cases in Western countries. The presence of inherited breast cancer is demonstrated by the incidence in first-degree relatives, which include mother, daughter, or sister. A woman's risk of breast cancer is two or more times greater if a first-degree relative developed the disease before the age of 50, and the younger the first-degree relative at the time of breast cancer development, the greater the risk.[34] Additional hereditary risk factors include a family history of bilateral breast cancer, a combination of breast cancer and another epithelial cancer, and male breast cancer[34,40] and an Ashkenazi Jewish heritage. Most breast cancers that occur before age 65 are attributed to a genetic mutation.[34]

An important breakthrough in understanding breast cancer risk factors occurred with the discovery of mutations in the BRCA1 and BRCA2 genes in high-risk families. These genes are located on the long arms of chromosomes 17 and 13, respectively, and are transmitted through an autosomal dominant pattern of inheritance. This means that the abnormal gene can be inherited through either sex and that some family members may transmit the abnormal gene without developing cancer themselves.[34] It is thought that mutations in BRCA1 and BRCA2 genes play a role in approximately 30% to 70% of all inherited breast cancer cases and may account for 5% to 10% of all ovarian cancers.[40] Ongoing genetic research on BRCA1 and BRCA2 will provide more definitive data on inherited breast cancer and how to treat and counsel families about this most sensitive and serious health problem. The characteristics of inherited breast cancer are listed in Box 54-1.

The development of noninherited breast cancer is considered to be a two-step process. The first step involves a change in cell structure or function, followed by a second event that promotes another change in the cell and causes it to become malignant. In hereditary breast cancer the inherited cell may already be in an altered state (first step) and require only one event to change it to a cancer cell.

Menstrual and Reproductive History. The risk of breast cancer is increased when menstruation begins before age 12 and extends to a late menopause after age 55. Women who have a natural menopause after the age of 55 have twice the risk of developing breast cancer than women who experience menopause before the age of 45.[40] The probability of mutagenic changes taking place from an intermediate phase to a malignant phase is more likely when the menstrual cycle spans more than 30 years.

Women who have never been pregnant (nulliparity) or who have their first child after the age of 30 are at an increased risk of breast cancer. Women ages 30 to 35 years in their first full-term pregnancy are at greater risk for breast cancer than women who deliver for the first time at 18 years of age or younger. The implication is that a full-term pregnancy at an early age promotes changes in breast development that protect the breast from cancer. However, studies have suggested that an induced abortion may adversely affect a woman's subsequent risk of breast cancer and that an interrupted pregnancy does not impart the protective effects of full-term pregnancy against breast cancer.[8]

Hormones and Oral Contraception. Postmenopausal hormone replacement therapy has become controversial because of the increased risk of breast cancer associated with prolonged estrogen exposure. Postmenopausal women who are exposed to hormone replacement therapy exhibit an increase in breast cancer risk, although not all studies support these findings.[19] Overall the incremental risk is small, but evidence suggests breast cancer risk increases with long-term use.[33]

BOX 54-1 Characteristics of Inherited Breast Cancer

- Occurs at an early age (premenopausal)
- Incidence of bilateral disease increased
- First-degree relative (mother, daughter, sister) with breast and ovarian cancer
- Ashkenazi Jewish heritage
- Family history of male breast cancer

Adapted from Nogueria S, Appling S: Breast cancer genetics, risks, and strategies, *Nurs Clin North Am* 35(3):663, 2000.

Breast cancers diagnosed in women taking hormone replacement therapy were found to be less advanced clinically as compared to those found in women who have not used hormone replacement therapy. In addition, current research findings suggest that hormone replacement therapy does not increase breast cancer mortality.[34]

Current findings indicate that, during the time women are taking oral contraceptives and for 10 years after, there exists a small increase in the risk of developing breast cancer. The effect of factors such as age at first use, duration of use, dose, and type of hormone in the contraceptive agent and their effects on breast cancer risk[34,50] is unclear, as different studies have had conflicting findings. Research findings also indicate that women who begin use of oral contraceptives before the age of 20 appear to have a higher risk of breast cancer than women who begin taking oral contraceptives at an older age.[34]

Diet and Body Weight. Research on the relationship between a high-fat diet and breast cancer has produced conflicting and controversial results. Evidence suggesting that high dietary fat contributes to an increased risk of breast cancer became questionable because of study bias, discrepant data, and inherent difficulties with study designs and data collection.[8,33] Nevertheless, there is evidence of a lower incidence of breast cancer in countries in which a diet low in fat is the norm.[40] Although a high-fat diet is not thought to cause breast cancer, dietary fat intake may indirectly support increased serum estrogen levels.[40]

Among postmenopausal women the risk of breast cancer appears to rise as body mass index increases. A possible explanation for this finding is that in the postmenopausal woman, androgens in adipose tissue can be converted to estrogen and become a source for stimulating cancer growth and spread.[8,33] A number of other studies have found a reduced risk of breast cancer in former college athletes and ballet dancers. This suggests that physical activity and reduced body weight around menarche, early adolescence, or throughout life may be important factors associated with decreased risk.[8] Until further research can support the association between fat intake, obesity, and breast cancer, women should be advised to limit dietary fat intake and maintain optimum body weight.

Benign Breast Disease. The risk of breast cancer is four to five times higher in women with severe atypical hyperplasia (increased cellular proliferation) compared with women who have no proliferative changes in their breasts. Women with atypical hyperplasia and a first-degree relative with breast cancer have a ninefold increase in risk. The presence of palpable cysts, complex fibroadenomas, ductal papillomas, sclerosis adenosis, and moderate or florid epithelial hyperplasia present a slightly higher risk of breast cancer compared with women without these changes. This increase is not considered clinically significant.[34]

Ionizing Radiation. Ionizing radiation has been shown to significantly increase the risk of breast cancer. A very high incidence of breast cancer has been found among women who survived the atomic bomb explosions in Japan during World War II. Particularly high risk of breast cancer is associated with exposure of the breast to radiation around menarche. It is postulated that breast tissue is especially vulnerable to the effects of ionizing radiation during adolescence, which is a period of rapid breast development. In addition, women who have had repeated fluoroscopic examinations of the chest, mantle radiation for Hodgkin's lymphoma, or radiation as a treatment for mastitis have demonstrated a markedly increased risk of breast cancer later in life.[8,33,34] Risk factors associated with breast cancer are summarized in the Risk Factors box.

Epidemiology

A comparison of the estimated cancer incidence and death rate figures reveal that breast cancer accounts for about one third (31%) of all cancers detected in women and 15% of all cancer-related deaths.[17] The mortality rate for women with breast cancer has decreased an average of 2.2% per year between 1990 and 1997, with most notable decreases observed among Caucasian women and among younger women. It is estimated that as more breast cancers are detected in situ or at earlier stages of invasive disease, the mortality rate should continue to decline.[3] The cancer death rates in females by site are shown in Figure 54-1.

Incidence and mortality rates for breast cancer are highest in the United States and Western Europe. The reason for this is debatable. One theory is that these countries are highly industrialized and therefore more economically and socially advantaged than some of the developing countries. As a consequence of this affluence, prevailing dietary patterns and lack of exercise promote obesity, which may be a contributing factor (see preceding discussion of diet and obesity).

Although this theory is merely speculative, it is known that when women emigrate from developing countries and the Far East to the United States and other Western countries, their rate of breast cancer incidence rises, possibly because of changes in eating patterns.

In the United States Caucasian women have an overall higher incidence of breast cancer than do African-American women. However, African-American women younger than 50 years old are more likely to develop breast cancer than are Caucasian women of the same age,[3] and at almost every age

Risk Factors

Breast Cancer

Female gender	Increased	99% of all breast cancers occur in women and 1% in men.
History of a previous breast cancer	Increased	The risk of developing a cancer in the opposite breast is five times greater than for the average population at risk.
Age >40	Increased	Incidence increases with age and peaks in the fifth decade.
Menstrual history		
Early menarche or late menopause or both	Increased	The risk of breast cancer rises as the interval between menarche and menopause increases; shortening the interval by oophorectomy reduces the risk, especially if performed in women younger than 35 years old.
Reproductive history		
Nulliparity First child born after age 30 years	Increased	Childless women have an increased risk as do women who bear their first child near or after age 30 years.
Family history		
Mother or sister or both	Increased	Risk increases two to three times if a mother or sister has had breast cancer and is further increased if the relative was diagnosed during the premenopausal state and if the cancer was bilateral.
Diet	Controversial	Animal data and descriptive epidemiology of breast cancer incidence strongly suggest an association of dietary factors, specifically a high-fat diet, with an increased risk of breast cancer. The National Academy of Sciences recommends decreasing total fat intake to 30% of available calories.
Alcohol	Unknown	A suggested small increase in risk with moderate alcohol consumption has been reported, although limitations in methodology have been cited, and results require confirmation.
Obesity	Controversial	Obesity and increased body mass index have been reported to be associated with an increased risk of breast cancer.
Ionizing radiation	Increased	Women who received ionizing radiation exposure, particularly during adolescence, demonstrated a markedly increased breast cancer risk.
Benign breast disease	None	Fibrocystic breast disease is not associated with breast cancer. However, biopsy-proven atypical hyperplasia is associated with an increased risk.
Oral contraceptives	None	There is no evidence yet to suggest a causal relationship between oral contraceptives and incidence of and survival from breast cancer.
Exogenous hormones	Controversial	Several studies report no link with replacement hormones and breast cancer, and those that do appear to identify only subsets of patients at risk: those who have taken replacement estrogens for very long periods and those who have taken large cumulative doses.

Adapted from Boyle P, Maisonneuve P, Autier P: Update on cancer control in women, *Int J Gynecol Obstet* 70:263-303, 2000; McPherson K, Steel CM, Dixon JM: ABC of breast diseases: breast cancer-epidemiology, risk factors, and genetics, *Br Med J* 321(9):624-628, 2000.

African-American women have a higher mortality rate from breast cancer than do Caucasian women[23,25] (Figure 54-2). African-American women are more likely to present with advanced stages of breast cancer, have poorer survival within each stage category, are less likely to have estrogen/progesterone receptor- (ER/PR) positive tumors, and have more aggressive tumor biology compared with Caucasian women.[25] In other racial/ethnic subgroups in the United States, breast cancer incidence rates vary widely. A high rate of breast cancer incidence has been observed among Native Hawaiian women, as well as a more advanced stage at diagnosis. A more advanced stage at diagnosis has also been observed in Hispanic, American-Indian, and Filipino-American women. The lowest incidence rates have been found among Korean-American, American-Indian of New Mexico, Vietnamese-American, and Chinese-American women.[4] Incidence rates intermediate to these groups have been found among Japanese-American, Alaska native, Filipino-American, and Hispanic women.[23]

In 2000 the federal government proposed health care-related objectives for the nation in Healthy People 2010, which is an initiative to improve health for the first decade of the twenty-first century. The single, overarching purpose of Healthy People 2010 is that of promoting health, and preventing illness, disability, and premature death.[52] Objectives from this initiative that specifically relate to breast cancer are found in the Healthy People 2010 box.

Prognostic Factors

Overall prognosis at the time of diagnosis of breast cancer is based on several factors. These include whether the tumor is invasive or noninvasive, grade, lymph node involvement,

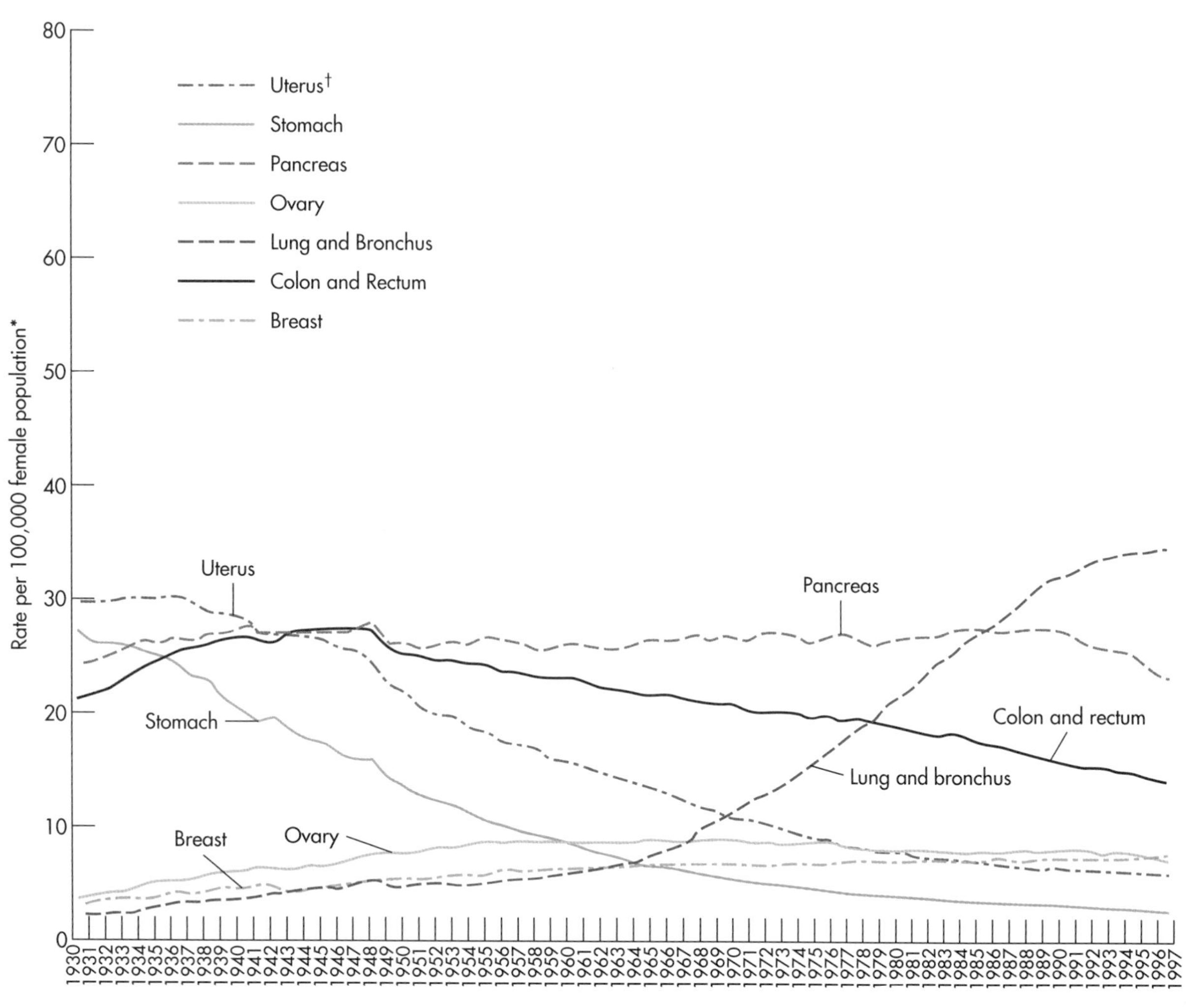

Figure 54-1 Age-adjusted cancer death rates: females by site, United States, 1930-1997. (*Rates are per 100,000 and are age-adjusted to the 1970 US standard population. †Uterus cancer death rates are for uterine cervix and uterine corpus combined. Note: As a result of changes in ICD coding, numerator information has changed over time. Rates for cancers of the uterus, ovary, lung, and bronchus, and colon and rectum are affected by these coding changes.

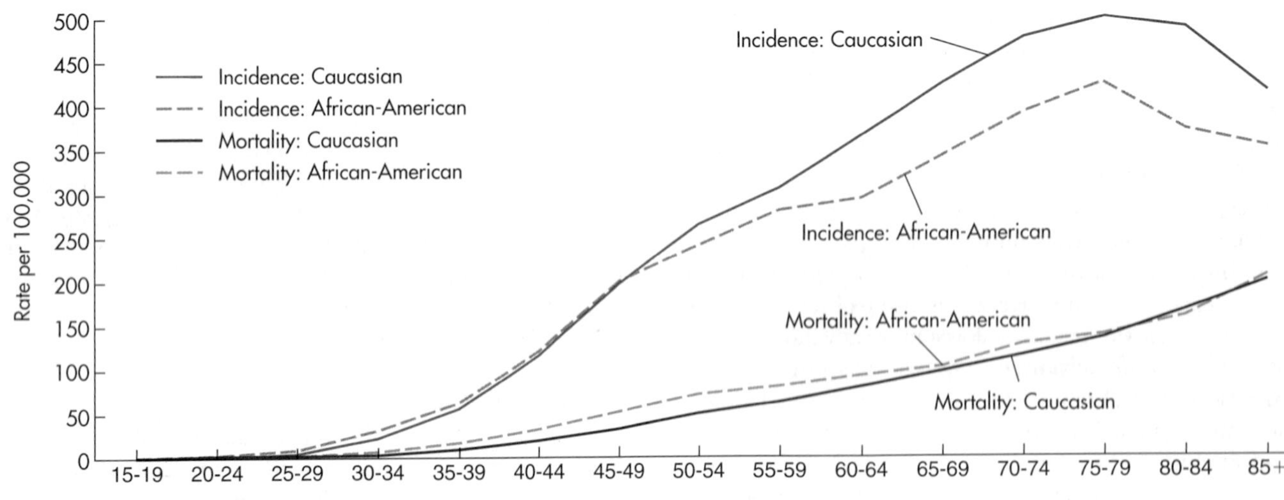

Figure 54-2 Female breast cancer mortality trends by age and race, United States, 1992-1996.

Healthy People 2010

Objectives To Reduce Breast Cancer Mortality

1. Reduce breast cancer deaths to no more than 22.3 per 100,000 women by the year 2010.
2. Increase, to at least 70%, the proportion of women 40 years old and older who have received a mammogram within the preceding 2 years.

From US Department of Health and Human Services: *Healthy People 2010: understanding and improving health,* Washington DC, 2000, USDHHS.

tumor size, tumor proliferation/DNA analysis, estrogen/progesterone markers, and genetic influence.

Invasive versus Noninvasive. Breast cancer may be categorized as noninvasive or invasive. Noninvasive cancers include ductal carcinoma in situ and lobular carcinoma in situ. These cancers are completely contained in the ductal and lobular systems of the breast and unable to reach the bloodstream or invade adjacent tissues and organs. They are considered rarely life threatening and have excellent prognoses.[45] The majority of primary invasive cancers are adenocarcinomas, of which infiltrating ductal carcinoma is a variant.

Grade. An indicator of a tumor's invasive or metastatic potential can be found in its histologic differentiation or similarity to normal breast tissue. Differentiation or grade is determined by using the Scarff-Bloom-Richardson system, which grades tumors based on the cellular factors of tubule formation, nuclear features, and mitotic index. Tumors graded with low numbers are considered well differentiated, whereas higher numbers indicate poorer differentiation.[45]

Lymph Node Involvement. The presence of cancer cells in axillary lymph nodes is considered the most important prognostic factor, and the number of positive lymph nodes present is directly proportional to the risk of breast cancer recurrence.[47] Nodal involvement is found in approximately 40% of women diagnosed with breast cancer. Those patients who have histologically negative lymph nodes have a 70% to 80% chance of remaining disease free. There are four categories of lymph node status: 0 lymph nodes or negative involvement, 1 to 3 positive nodes, 4 to 9 positive nodes, and 10 or more positive nodes. Progressively greater nodal involvement implies worsening survival.[45]

Tumor Size. The size of the tumor is also directly related to the risk of breast cancer recurrence. For node-negative patients with tumors less than 1 cm, the recurrence rate is approximately 1% to 10%. For node-negative patients with tumors measuring 1 to 3 cm, the recurrence rate is approximately 30%. For node-negative patients with tumors larger than 3 cm, the recurrence rate is more than 50%.[47] Tumor size is obtained by a three-way measurement of the gross tumor, with the largest dimension used for staging determination. When tumors display mixed invasive and noninvasive components, only the invasive component is measured to obtain a more accurate prognostic indicator.[45]

Tumor Proliferation/DNA Analysis. Flow cytometry is used to measure tumor proliferation through determination of the fraction of tumor cells in the synthesis (S) phase of cell division. S-phase is a sign of DNA activity. Designating the DNA activity provides information regarding the ability of breast cancer to proliferate.[45] A high S-phase is associated with a fast-growing tumor and a short disease-free survival time. Ploidy status refers to the amount of DNA contained in tumor cells. Diploid tumors have the normal amount of DNA as found in normal cells. Aneuploid tumors have more than the 46 normal chromosomes. Shorter survival is associated with aneuploid tumors.[45] (See Chapter 15 for a more detailed discussion on cell kinetics.)

Estrogen/Progesterone Markers. ER and PR are well-recognized predictors of long-term survival in women with breast cancer. These receptors are proteins present in and on the surface of cancer cells that bind with estrogen and progesterone and subsequently influence DNA activity and cell growth. A tumor that contains receptors that bind with estrogen or progesterone is ER-positive or PR-positive, respectively. Approximately 60%

of all breast cancers are ER-positive.[45] Tumors that are hormone receptor positive are more responsive to endocrine therapy than tumors that are negative for hormone receptors. A major advantage of an ER-positive or PR-positive tumor lies in the ability to use hormonal management as first-line treatment in advanced breast cancer.[53]

Genetic Influence. Approximately 30% of breast and ovarian cancers are associated with overexpression of the proto-oncogene, c-erB-2/HER-2/neu. In breast cancer this overexpression and gene amplification is directly related to early metastasis and poor prognosis. Women with overexpression of this gene are noted to have aggressive breast cancers that are resistant to standard therapy regimens.[51]

Staging of Breast Cancer

Staging of breast cancer incorporates the primary tumor, regional nodes, and metastasis. This TNM classification is shown in Box 54-2. Treatment decisions are based on the stage of the breast cancer, as well as on those factors already discussed.

Pathophysiology

Tumors of the breast arise in the epithelial cells of either ductal or lobular tissue and are referred to as carcinomas. The breast is divided into four quadrants, as shown in Figure 54-3. Most breast tumors are located in the upper outer quadrant, but they can occur in any area of the breast. When the tumor is confined within a duct or a lobule and has not invaded surrounding tissue, it is considered localized or in situ carcinoma of the breast. Infiltrative ductal or lobular carcinomas are tumors that have spread directly into surrounding tissue and may have distant metastases if they have penetrated the axillary or internal mammary nodes or the systemic circulation. Of the invasive breast tumors, infiltrating ductal carcinoma is the most prevalent histologic cell type, followed by infiltrating lobular carcinomas. Subtypes of each of these histologic cell types comprise the remainder of breast tumors. Table 54-1 reviews selected histologic types of breast cancer.

The breast is served by an extensive lymphatic drainage system: central axillary, pectoral (anterior), subscapular (posterior), and lateral nodes. The ipsilateral axillary nodes drain up to 75% of lymph from the breast. Additional drainage flows upward to the infraclavicular and supraclavicular lymph nodes. The normal lymphatic system and directional flow are shown in Figure 54-4.

Paget's disease is an eczema-like inflammatory process affecting the nipple and areola. It may progress from an epidermal condition to an intraductal carcinoma of the breast. It may be accompanied by burning, itching, discharge, and a palpable lump.

Clinical Manifestations. Early-stage cancer of the breast is symptomless and can be detected only on physical examination of the breast or by mammogram. It is difficult to differentiate from benign tumors. With more advanced tumors a variety of signs and symptoms are helpful in differentiating a benign tumor from a malignant tumor. Benign tumors generally have well-defined edges, are encapsulated, and are freely movable. The shape of a malignant tumor is more difficult to define and is less mobile on palpation, usually the result of the tumor becoming "fixed" and adhering to the chest wall. As the tumor infiltrates into surrounding tissue, it can cause retraction of the overlying skin and create what is referred to as dimpling. The nipple also may be retracted or deviated at an odd angle from the same growth pattern. A peau d'orange

BOX 54-2 Staging of Breast Cancer

T—Primary Tumor Size

TX	Primary tumor cannot be assessed
T0	No evidence of primary tumor
Tis	Carcinoma in situ: intraductal carcinoma, lobular carcinoma in situ, or Paget's disease of the nipple with node
T1	Tumor 2 cm or less in greatest dimension
T2	Tumor more than 2 cm but not more than 5 cm in greatest dimension
T3	Tumor more than 5 cm in greatest dimension
T4	Tumor of any size with direct extension to chest wall or skin

NOTE: Paget's disease associated with a tumor is classified according to the size of the tumor

N—Regional Lymph Nodes

NX	Regional lymph nodes cannot be assessed (e.g., previously removed)
N0	No regional lymph node metastasis
N1	Metastasis to movable ipsilateral axillary lymph node(s)
N2	Metastasis to ipsilateral axillary lymph node(s) fixed to one another or to other structures
N3	Metastasis to ipsilateral internal mammary lymph node(s)

M—Distant Metastasis

MX	Presence of distant metastasis cannot be assessed
M0	No distant metastasis
M1	Distant metastasis (includes metastasis to ipsilateral, supraclavicular lymph node[s])

Stage Grouping

Stage 0	Tis	N0	M0
Stage I	T1	N0	M0
Stage IIa	T0	N0	M0
	T1	N1	M0
	T2	N0	M0
Stage IIB	T2	N1	M0
	T3	N0	M0
Stage IIIA	T0	N2	M0
	T1	N2	M0
	T2	N2	M0
	T3	N1	M0
	T3	N2	M0
Stage IIIB	T4	Any N	M0
	Any T	N3	M0
Stage IV	Any T	Any N	M1

From American Joint Committee on Cancer: *Manual for staging of cancer,* ed 5, Philadelphia, 1997, Lippincott-Raven.

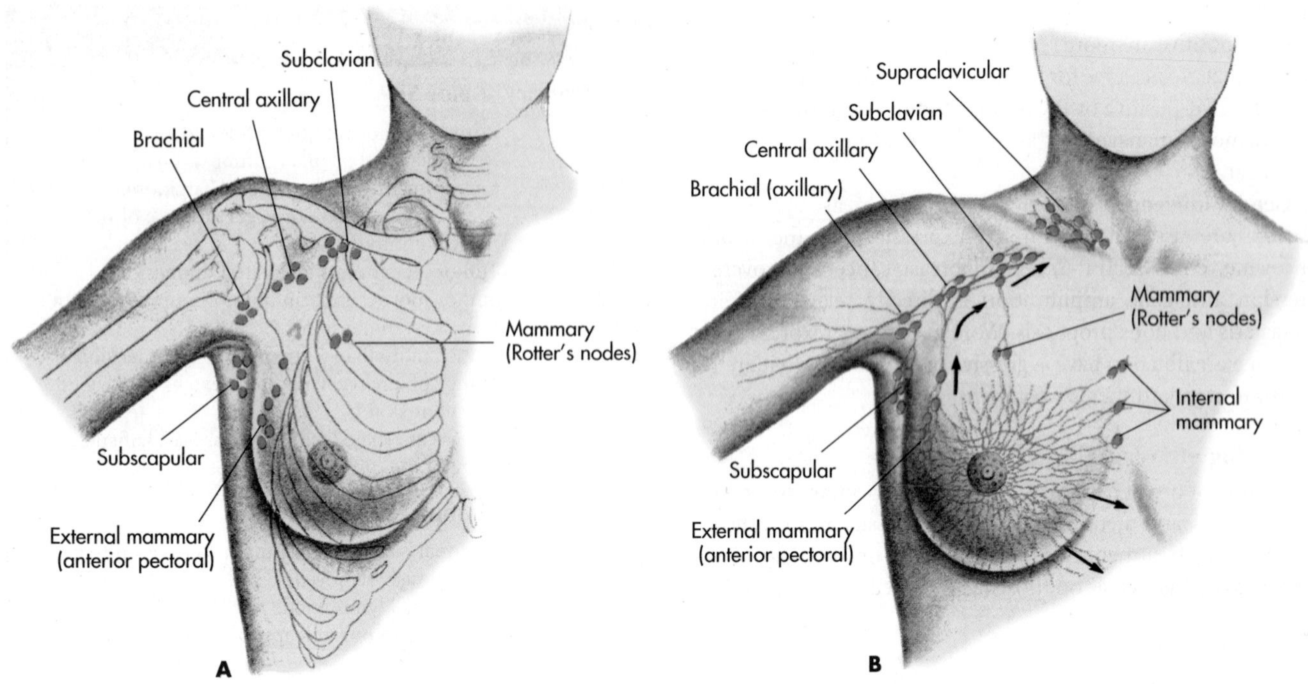

Figure 54-3 **A,** Lymph nodes of the axilla. **B,** Lymphatic drainage of the breast.

TABLE 54-1 Selected Histologic Types of Breast Cancer

Type	Incidence (%)	Characteristics	Prognosis
Infiltrating ductal carcinoma	70-80	Solid mass; hard and firm on palpation	Poor; common involvement of axillary nodes
Medullary carcinoma	6	Characterized by a prominent lymphocyte infiltrate, frequently seen in younger patients, can reach large size	Favorable
Mucinous, or colloid, carcinoma	3	Slow growing; mucus producing	Good if tumor is predominately mucinous
Invasive lobular carcinoma	5-10	Multicentricity common; may involve both breasts, tumors have ill-defined margins	Similar to ductal types
Paget's disease	Rare	Scaly, eczematoid nipple with burning, itching, discharge; usually unable to palpate mass beneath nipple	Related to histologic type of underlying tumor
Inflammatory breast cancer	1-2	Diffuse edema, skin and breast redness, firmness of underlying tissue, tenderness, pain, nipple retraction	Poor
Carcinoma in situ (ductal-DCIS, lobular-LCIS)	2-3	Proliferation of malignant cells within ducts and lobules, without invasion into surrounding tissue. DCIS appears as clustered microcalcifications on mammography	Good, depends on histologic subtypes

Adapted from Liu L: Histologic classification of breast cancer. University of Pennsylvania, 1999. Available from www.oncolink.upenn.edu/disease/breast/screen/breast_type.html, and Dow KH: Breast cancer. In Varricchio C, editor: *A cancer sourcebook for nurses,* ed 7, Sudbury, Mass, 1997, Jones and Bartlett International.

breast sign in which the breast resembles an orange peel with large prominent pores, indicates lymphatic obstruction from tumor growth with resulting edema. These signs are more ominous and usually reflect advanced disease. The clinical manifestations of breast cancer are found in the Clinical Manifestations box.

Collaborative Care Management

Management of breast cancer is both complex and controversial. Treatment options are ever changing and influenced by new and better surgical techniques, new cytotoxic drug combinations, and more accurate knowledge of breast cancer growth and dissemination.

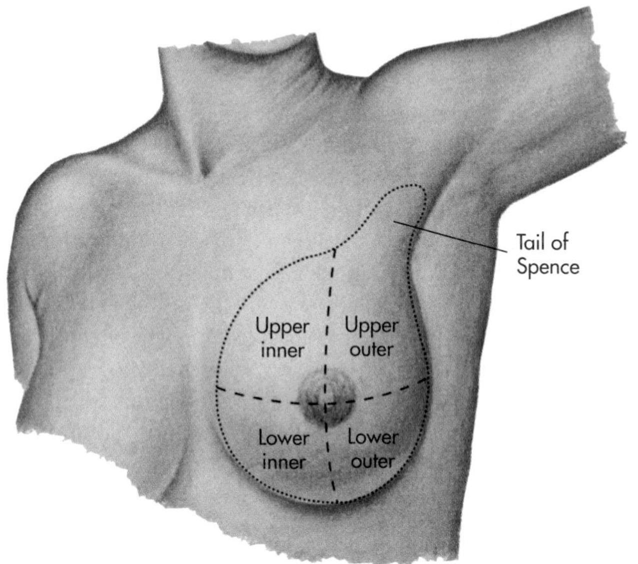

Figure 54-4 Quadrants of left breast and axillary tail of Spence. Most tumors develop in the upper outer quadrant.

Clinical Manifestations

Breast Cancer

Lump that is:
- Irregular, star-shaped
- Firm to hard in consistency
- Fixed, not mobile
- Poorly defined or demarcated
- Usually not tender, but can occasionally cause discomfort
- Single

Presence of skin or nipple retraction
Nipple discharge
Peau d'orange appearance of the skin
NOTE: Most breast tumors identified by mammography are completely without discernible symptoms.

Diagnostic Tests. When a breast lump has been found, the exact nature of the lesion must be determined. The presence of a benign lesion, such as a fibroadenoma, cyst, or fibrocystic breast disease, must be ruled out. Most breast lesions are benign; however, only histologic examination of tissue from the lesion can determine the true nature of the disease process.

Noninvasive Diagnostic Tests. Monthly breast self-examination (BSE) is recommended by the American Cancer Society as an early detection method. Although its true value in detecting breast cancer at an early stage and decreasing breast cancer mortality has not been fully determined, studies have found that women whose tumors were discovered during purposeful BSE had significantly smaller tumors, had less nodal involvement, and had smaller lesions in involved nodes.[29] Even though 80% to 95% of all breast lesions initially are detected by women themselves,[29] the promotion of BSE has not resulted in more women performing the examination on a regular schedule. Furthermore, statistics reveal that approximately 21% to 50% of women over the age of 40 do not perform monthly BSE.[28] Barriers that deter women from regular practice of BSE include anxiety, forgetfulness, lack of skill, fear of finding breast cancer, embarrassment, being unaware of their personal breast cancer risk, having large breasts, and uneven texture.[28,29] Educating women about the importance of regular monthly self-examination and teaching the proper technique are essential to early detection and intervention (see Chapter 15).

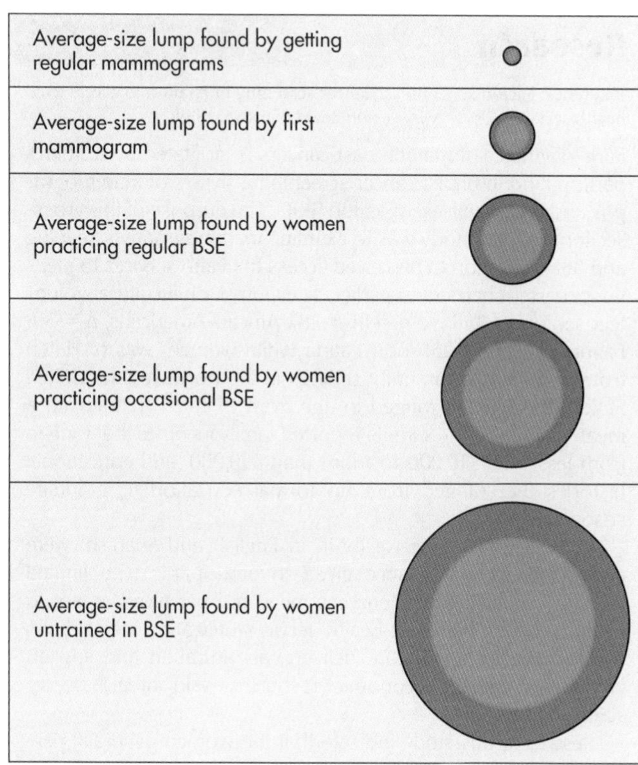

Figure 54-5 Relative sizes of tumors detected by various detection methods, as reported by the Breast Health Program of New York.

At the present time mammography is the best diagnostic tool available to detect breast tumors, especially for older women. Mammography may have limitations for those with dense breast tissue or women using hormone replacement.[11] Nevertheless, a mammogram can detect breast lesions before they become palpable on physical examination (1 cm) or before they can be seen on conventional roentgenogram. Figure 54-5 compares the average size of a lesion discovered by a woman on BSE and one capable of being detected on mammogram.

The recent increase in breast cancer incidence has been at least partially attributed to the increased use of mammography and its detection of cancer in an earlier, localized stage. Many women, however, are still reluctant to undergo mammographic examination (see Research box). The most frequent barriers cited for not complying with health care provider recommended examinations or for nonparticipation in screening programs are cost of the examination (no insurance coverage or only partial coverage), fear of radiation exposure or pain during the procedure, lack of knowledge of

Research

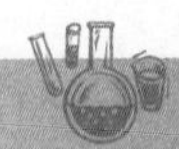

Reference: Facione NC: Breast cancer screening in relation to access to health services, *Oncol Nurs Forum* 26(4):689-696, 1999.

Early diagnosis of many breast cancers is facilitated by women's participation in breast cancer screening activities of mammography and breast self-examination (BSE). The purpose of this cross-sectional survey study was to examine mammography screening and BSE in relation to perceived access to health services to identify persistent barriers to earlier detection. A multicultural volunteer sample of 838 women (n = 287 African-Americans, n = 316 Latinas, and n = 235 non-Latina white women) was recruited from work and community settings in the northwestern United States. The women ranged in age from 19 to 99 years, with a mean age of 46. The sample reported family incomes that ranged from less than $10,000 to more than $90,000, and educational histories that ranged from no formal education to graduate school.

Surveys and interviews (both in English and Spanish) were conducted, with assistance given to participants with limited reading capabilities. The surveys measured perceived access to health services, habits of health services utilization, perceptions of prejudice in health care delivery, acculturation and spoken language, available economic resources, and breast cancer screening behaviors.

Results of this study indicate that the women generally perceived that they had access to health care services. Those who perceived a relative lack of access were more likely to have less-developed habits of health care use for health promotion and treatment of illness. Moreover, those who perceived lack of access were more likely to be Spanish-speaking and perceive that health care providers treat them with prejudice because of their race, age, income, or sexual orientation. In addition, those who perceived lack of access had lower annual income, were uninsured, and had little available money to spend on health care.

These findings underscore the importance of providing true economic access to breast cancer screening, which will help improve participation and early detection. Implications of these findings include supporting legislation that makes mammography screening economically available to all women, as well as the treatment inevitably needed by those whose mammograms detect cancer. Also inclusive is the implementation of strategies designed to increase adherence to breast cancer screening guidelines, such as reminder postcards, personal contact, and media campaigns. Tolerance and culturally sensitive service delivery are vital to eliminate prejudice as a barrier to breast cancer screening services.

---

recommended guidelines, and belief that mammography is unnecessary in the absence of symptoms.[20,39]

For a mammogram to be accurate, two views of sufficiently compressed breast tissue are needed. Compression is required to decrease breast thickness, separate mammary structures, and eliminate motion, thus resulting in a more accurate image with less radiation scatter.[39] When accurately performed and read by an experienced radiologist, a mammogram can detect the presence of a lesion 2 to 4 years before it is large enough to be detected by conventional x-ray film or palpated on physical examination.[2] The major limitation of mammography is its inability to differentiate between malignant and benign lesions. Figure 54-6 shows a mammogram with a malignant lesion.

Digital mammography is currently under investigation. This procedure uses a detector that emits an electronic signal in response to an x-ray exposure. This signal can be stored and processed on a computer for use later on film or display on a monitor. Digital mammography shows promise in improving the quality of the breast image and in enhancing accuracy in distinguishing between malignant and benign tumors.[11] Ultrasound is a noninvasive test that can be used to determine the size of a lesion and differentiate a fluid-filled cyst from a solid lesion. In women with dense breast tissue, it may also help to detect cancer at an earlier, more curable stage. The effectiveness of ultrasound used in combination with mammography for women with dense breasts is currently under investigation.[24]

Invasive Diagnostic Tests. Most breast tumors are not malignant; however, an accurate diagnosis cannot be made until tissue from the tumor is examined for histologic cell type. Therefore, when a tumor mass is discovered, whether on physical examination or mammogram, an invasive procedure such as needle biopsy or excisional or incisional biopsy is required.

Fine-needle aspiration can differentiate cysts from other solid tumor masses. The contents of a cyst range from clear aspirate to bloody or even black fluid. The fluid generally is sent for cytologic examination and may be helpful in the identification of histologic cell type.

A wide-needle biopsy is a procedure used to obtain a small piece of tissue from a breast mass. This tissue sample undergoes cytologic examination for the presence of cancer cells. Needle biopsies are performed using local anesthetics and can be done in an outpatient setting. If the needle biopsy shows cancer cells, a surgical biopsy is done to remove tissue for examination. A cytologic examination is never used alone as a diagnostic tool for cancer because of the chance of both false-positive and false-negative reports.

Technologic advances in breast biopsy systems now enable the removal of mammographic densities with or without calcifications that measure up to 20 mm. These innovative techniques, which combine digital stereotactic imaging and a minimally invasive biopsy system, locate and remove tissue specimens for diagnostic purposes. These systems are rapidly becoming established as the preferred method for removing indeterminate breast lesions.[7]

Excisional or incisional biopsies can be performed with the patient under local anesthesia in an outpatient department or a physician's office. Biopsies of deep lesions in a large breast are better performed in an operating suite. A needle-wire localization procedure done under mammographic, sonographic, or stereotactic visualization may be performed before the excisional biopsy to locate suspicious but nonpalpable areas of the breast tissue.

Tissue specimens obtained from excisional or incisional biopsies are examined for cell type. If the lesion is malignant, the estrogen and progesterone receptor status should be determined at the same time. This information is important because the ER and PR status helps determine treatment choices.

Other Diagnostic Tests. Breast cancer has a predilection to metastasize to bones; therefore, a bone scan and bone marrow biopsy may be ordered. Positive findings on these tests indicate

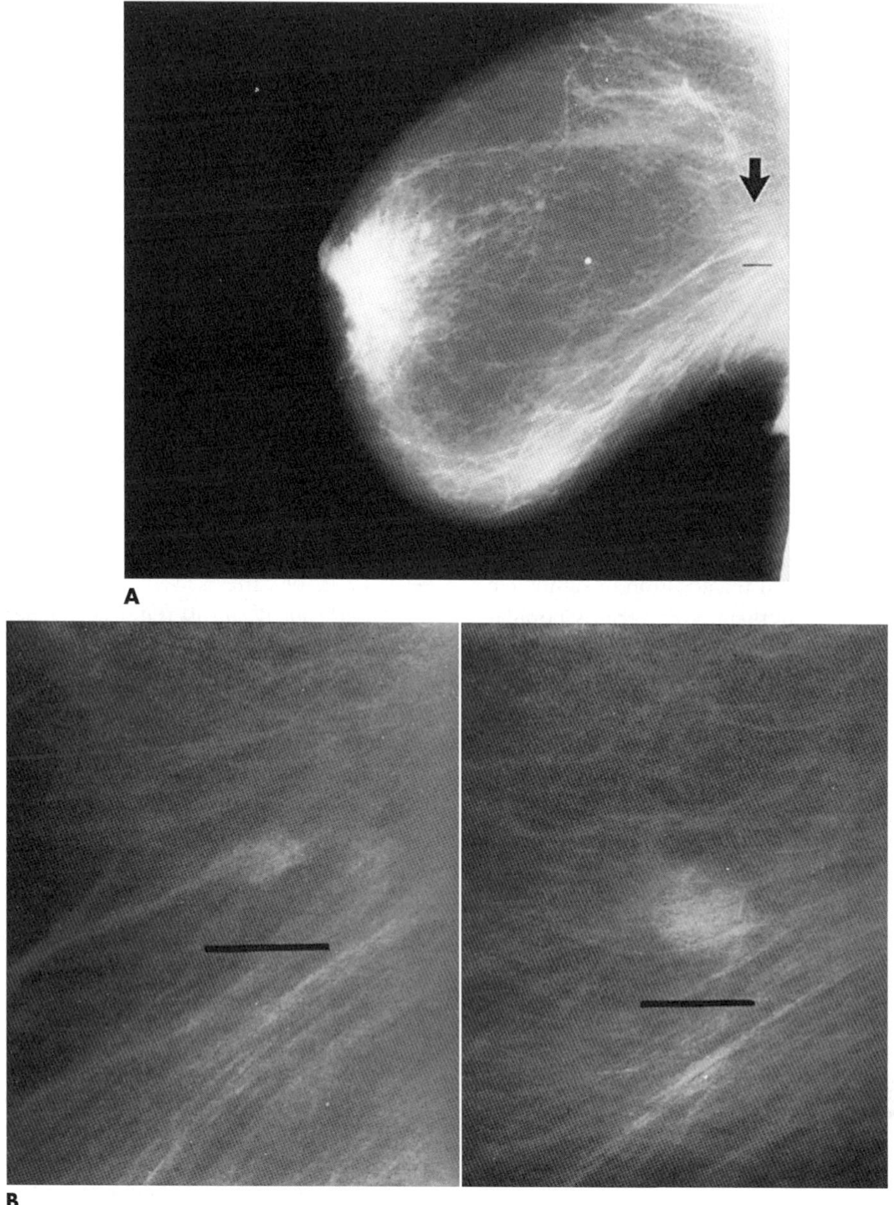

Figure 54-6 Mammogram of patient with area of density indicating carcinoma. A small nodule *(arrow)* in a large fatty breast (**A**) was oval in shape with ill-defined margins (**B**). The nodule increased in size over a 12-month interval. Black line represents 10-mm measure.

the presence of widespread disease and a poorer prognosis. A liver scan may be indicated when results of liver function tests are abnormal. A chest x-ray film reveals lung status before any surgical intervention and also shows the presence of metastasis.

Medications. The role of systemic drug therapy in the treatment of breast cancer (chemotherapy and endocrine therapy) is to either eradicate or impede the growth of micrometastatic disease.

Chemotherapy

Stages I and II Disease (Localized). As a result of improved diagnostic tests, breast cancer is being discovered earlier and in a more localized stage, frequently without nodal involvement. It is estimated that more than 90% of women with tumors 1 cm or less and without nodal involvement can be expected to achieve long-term disease-free survival.[41] However, because the tumor cells of breast cancer are heterogeneous in nature—that is, there is no uniformity of cells and the cells are subject to changes with each cell generation—even localized, node-negative tumors can and frequently do recur. The presence of micrometastasis may be undetected at the time of initial treatment. When micrometastasis is present, changes (mutations) can occur in the tumor cells, making them resistant to the effects of chemotherapeutic agents even though tumor sensitivity to drug therapy is greatest when the tumor burden is small. Thus it is not always possible to predict with confidence that all tumors 1 cm or less without node involvement are "cured" with initial local or regional treatment. Therefore early introduction of systemic adjuvant therapy, as determined by the estimated risk of tumor recurrence in certain subsets of women with node-negative disease, is advocated. Moreover, research findings suggest that adjuvant chemotherapy effectively reduces the risks for recurrence and mortality in patients with node-positive disease.[47] Box 54-3 provides a list of chemotherapy agents and drug regimens most commonly used in the treatment of node-positive and node-negative breast cancer.

Administering preoperative chemotherapy to patients with operable stage I and stage II breast cancer has many potential benefits. Preoperative use of chemotherapy may decrease drug resistance arising from ongoing cellular mutation. Additionally, preoperative use of chemotherapy can enhance prevention of micrometastasis that can occur with primary tumor removal. Preoperative chemotherapy also can render larger inoperable tumors more amenable to surgical removal, and has the potential advantage of permitting an increased rate of breast conservation.[47]

The National Cancer Institute issued a clinical alert in 1989 that advocated systemic adjuvant therapy in certain subsets of women with node-negative disease. Numerous clinical trials ensued since then that investigated the addition of tamoxifen alone and tamoxifen with chemotherapy in various populations of patients with node-negative disease. Research findings showed significant improvement in survival and mortality with the use of adjuvant chemotherapy. Although research results supported the recommendation that adjuvant chemotherapy can be justified in all patients with stage I and II breast cancer, regardless of age, hormone-receptor status, and nodal status, additional follow-up time is needed for these patients before any definite conclusions can be drawn regarding their optimal management.[47]

BOX 54-3 Chemotherapy Agents and Regimens Effective for Treating Breast Cancer

Cyclophosphamide
Methotrexate
Fluoroucil
Doxorubicin*
Paclitaxel/Docetaxel†

Regimens Currently Used in Node-Positive and Node-Negative Disease

CMF	Cyclophosphamide, methotrexate, 5-fluorouracil
CAF	Cyclophosphamide, doxorubicin, 5-fluorouracil
CMF/VP	Cyclophosphamide, methotrexate, 5-fluorouracil, vincristine, prednisone
AC	Doxorubicin, cyclophosphamide
A'CMF	Doxorubicin followed by CMF
AC'T	Doxorubicin, cyclophosphamide followed by a taxane
AT	Doxorubicin and a taxane

*Anthracyclines. Doxorubicin is the most effective agent in the treatment of advanced breast cancer.
†Taxanes. Research suggests an increase in survival benefit when used sequentially with standard chemotherapy in node-positive breast cancer.
Adapted from: Shuster TD, Girshovich L, Whitney TM, Hughes KS: Multidisciplinary care for patients with breast cancer, *Surg Clin North Am* 80(2):505, 2000.

At present there are few new chemotherapeutic agents useful in the treatment of breast cancer. Therefore treatment approaches that use established agents in new ways are being investigated. Alternating drug combinations may be more effective in treating breast cancer than using a single drug protocol. Also the use of various combinations of drugs (Box 54-3) may prove beneficial in improving tumor cell sensitivity to drug therapy by reducing drug resistance. Another current approach is to administer the prescribed chemotherapeutic agents at their maximal safe dosage levels while providing a "rescue" for the bone marrow. Most chemotherapeutic drugs have an adverse effect on the bone marrow's ability to produce vital cellular components (white blood cells, red blood cells, and platelets). Therefore hematopoietic growth factors such as granulocyte colony-stimulating factors and granulocyte-macrophage colony-stimulating factors are given, or bone marrow transplant is performed, to stimulate bone marrow recovery after high-dose therapy.[6] See Chapter 15 for a more detailed discussion of chemotherapy and related nursing care.

Stages III and IV Disease (Advanced). Chemotherapy with multiple drug combinations has been used in the treatment of recurrent and advanced breast cancer for many years with positive results. Many of the modalities used to treat localized breast cancer are being used to treat recurrent and advanced disease as well.

Paclitaxel (Taxol) and docetaxel (Taxotere, a semisynthetic toxoid) comprise first-line therapy for patients with locally advanced or metastatic breast cancer in whom anthracycline-based therapy (doxorubicin) has failed or who have a recurrence during anthracycline-based therapy. Capecitabine (Xeloda), an oral chemical precursor of 5-fluorouracil, has been approved as a treatment for metastatic breast cancer refractory to paclitaxel and an anthracycline-containing regimen, or to cancer resistant to paclitaxel and for whom further anthracycline therapy is contraindicated.[36] Another drug developed for use in advanced breast cancer is the recombinant, humanized monoclonal antibody Herceptin. Herceptin is used in situations in which advanced tumors demonstrate overexpression of the c-erB-2 gene.[16] These cytotoxic agents give patients with metastatic breast cancer other treatment options.

The use of chemotherapy continues to generate many unanswered questions, such as optimal drug combinations, optimal dosage, and length of treatment. These are just a few of the concerns currently being addressed in clinical trials.

Hormonal Therapy

Stages I and II Disease. Hormonal therapy has been a useful treatment modality for breast cancer for many decades. Whereas chemotherapy acts on rapidly dividing cells to achieve its effects, hormonal therapy targets cells that are dependent on estrogen for growth. The underlying reason for the success of hormonal therapy was not known until the development of bioassay methods that revealed the presence of estrogen receptors on the tumor cell surface. Before this discovery it was known only that surgical removal of the ovaries interfered in some way with breast cancer growth. Research revealed that tumors that are ER rich (>10) grow in response to stimulation by estrogen and are classified as ER positive. It was theorized that if the level of circulating estrogen was removed or decreased, the growth of ER positive tumors could be impeded and disease-free interval and survival time increased. However, estrogen ablation through oophorectomy also induced menopause, as the primary source of estrogen is the ovaries. Hot flashes, vaginal dryness, a rise in plasma lipids, atherosclerosis, and osteoporosis resulted. To counteract these menopausal effects, antiestrogen drug research led to the development of the antiestrogen drug tamoxifen, and more recently, raloxifene. Tamoxifen is a nonsteroidal drug that competes for the estradiol-binding site on the ER-positive cell, thus removing the stimulus (estrogen) for tumor growth. Although tamoxifen is most effective in ER-positive breast cancer, it also affects (but to a lesser degree) ER-negative tumors as well. Tamoxifen is considered the hormonal therapy of choice for both premenopausal and postmenopausal women.[42] Tamoxifen is also used in early-stage breast cancers in women with both node-negative and node-positive tumors. The greatest benefits are seen in women 50 years of age and older with ER-positive tumors.[42]

Stages III and IV Disease. Hormonal therapy is a mainstay of treatment for advanced breast cancer. The therapy is well tolerated and offers the possibility of temporary tumor remission or inhibition of tumor growth. Ideal candidates for endocrine therapy include women with advanced disease with ER-positive tumors, who had a long prior disease-free interval, had a prior response to hormonal treatment, or lack rapidly progressing disease. Findings from clinical trials have demonstrated response rates with tamoxifen for treatment of metastatic disease range from 15% to 53%. Tamoxifen has been used alone or in combination with chemotherapeutic agents. Chemotherapy combined with tamoxifen therapy has been shown to significantly reduce recurrence and mortality in women more than 50 years old.[42]

Analysis of data from the National Surgical Adjuvant Breast and Bowel Project found that tamoxifen increased the risk of development of endometrial cancer twofold to threefold in women receiving it compared with women with breast cancer not treated with tamoxifen.[14] Other side effects of therapy include symptoms similar to those of menopause (hot flashes, irregular menstrual periods, nausea, fluid retention, and vaginal discharge).

The usefulness of tamoxifen as a breast cancer prevention agent in high-risk women is under investigation. Preliminary results indicate that patients receiving tamoxifen were 45% less likely to develop breast cancer than those receiving placebo. These findings provide compelling evidence of the usefulness of tamoxifen for the reduction of breast cancer risk in the short term for women at risk for developing the disease. Approval for such usage of tamoxifen has been granted by the U.S. Food and Drug Administration (FDA).[16]

Until more data become available and standard treatment protocols can be agreed on for both chemotherapy and hormonal manipulation, the patient and her physician need to discuss each modality for its known advantages and disadvantages and select the one that meets each woman's individual needs and concerns.

Treatments

Radiation Therapy

Stages I and II Disease. Radiation to the breast after preservation surgery (lumpectomy) is a standard therapy for early stage breast cancer. Radiation to the breast eradicates tumor cells left behind after manipulation and handling of the tumor during surgery. The total recommended radiation dose is 4500 to 5000 cGy over 6 to 7 weeks. A booster dose of up to 1000 cGy may be prescribed with the use of either implants or external beam irradiation (Figure 54-7). The risk of local recurrence is minimal after this protocol. Tumors of less than 1 cm generally are not treated with radiation after breast preservation surgery because the risk of metastasis is minimal, and prognosis is considered excellent (see discussion under Medications on early-stage breast cancer). Although radiation after conservative surgery is widely used, some large breast tumors may be irradiated before surgery to facilitate easier surgical removal. Close medical follow-up care is important after conservative surgery and radiation. Recommended guidelines include a breast physical examination every 4 to 6 months for 2 years, twice a year for 3 years, and then yearly. A mammogram is recommended 6 months after radiation and then annually.[37]

When the breast is irradiated, the side effects include skin reactions (redness, dryness, and itching), edema, mild tenderness, and fatigue. Fatigue is the result of bone marrow suppression from radiation to the thorax, as the adult sternum, ribs, and thoracic vertebrae contain more than one third of the total body bone marrow (sternum 3%, ribs 16%, and thoracic vertebrae 16%). Patient instruction for managing the side effects of anemia and increased vulnerability to infection is vital to achieve patient compliance in completing treatment with the total prescribed radiation dose.

Local Recurrence. Local recurrence of breast cancer usually occurs within 2 to 8 years after the initial diagnosis and treatment. Approximately 80% occur within 3 years. Generally the earlier the recurrence, the graver the prognosis. When recurrence follows conservative surgery and radiation therapy,

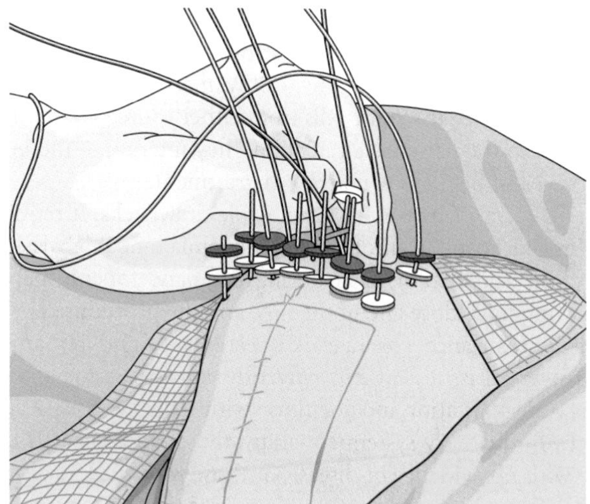

Figure 54-7 Interstitial "booster" radiation therapy for breast cancer using iridium needles.

mastectomy alone or with adjuvant systemic therapy is recommended.

Tissue subjected to radiation therapy given at a dose intended for a "cure" does not respond well to repeated radiation exposure. This is because of the changes that occur in the vascular bed after initial radiation treatment, which results in a reduced blood and oxygen supply to the irradiated tissue. Radiation therapy works best on tissue with a good blood supply and high oxygen saturation content.

Complications of repeated radiation therapy include fibrotic changes to the lung, tissue necrosis, and rib fractures.

Stages III and IV Disease. The role of radiation therapy in advanced breast cancer usually is palliative. Breast cancer has the propensity to metastasize to bone, which is a major source of pain. Bone involvement can result in pathologic fractures of the spinal vertebrae, causing compression of nerve roots and the spinal cord. Radiation therapy can help to alleviate the discomfort from these complications. Metastasis from breast cancer often causes lymphatic obstruction and may result in pleural effusion. In addition, metastasis frequently involves other vital organ systems such as the lung and liver. Radiation therapy frequently is used to treat these metastatic lesions. When radiation is prescribed, the patient requires information and instruction on the rationale for the therapy and any specific care measures that will be necessary during treatment. It is important that the patient be aware that the radiation treatments will not cure the disease but can provide pain relief and improve quality of life. (See Chapter 15 for a more thorough discussion of radiation therapy in the treatment of cancer.)

Bone Marrow Transplantation. The use of bone marrow transplantation (BMT), a therapy developed for treatment of hematologic cancers, is an increasingly used treatment modality for breast cancer. Two sources of marrow cells that are used in this procedure are the patient's own marrow (autologous BMT) and the patient's circulating blood stem cells (peripheral blood stem cell transplantation [PBSCT]). BMT and PBSCT are able to "rescue" the breast cancer patient's bone marrow after ablation by high-dose chemotherapy or radiation therapy.[1] High-dose chemotherapy is administered to kill all tumor cells, and then the destroyed bone marrow is rescued with the patient's own healthy marrow or peripheral stem cells. Once the stem cells from either source are reintroduced into the patient's circulation, they migrate to the bone marrow and begin new marrow engraftment.

This form of treatment has notable drawbacks. It requires prolonged hospitalization, there is anemia, and high risk of infection and hemorrhage during the pancytopenic period following high-dose chemotherapy, and the procedure is very costly.[31] Insurance coverage is questionable and remains a controversial issue. Patients currently considered for autologous transplantation include those with stage IV disease after successful primary systemic therapy, those with stage III disease with no evidence of disease, or those with stage II disease with a poor prognosis (10 or more positive axillary lymph nodes) following standard, multidrug adjuvant regimens.[15] Early clinical trials have demonstrated a 54% to 73% response rate in stage IV breast cancer. More recent studies have shown improved long-term survival and disease-free intervals.[1] Although current data are extremely encouraging, more research is needed to further determine the true value of these therapies in breast cancer. (See Chapter 51 for further discussion of bone marrow transplantation.)

Surgical Management

Stages I and II (Local Disease). Surgery is the initial treatment of early stage breast cancer, especially when the disease is localized without distant metastasis. The surgical removal of breast cancer has evolved over the past 100 years from the mutilating radical mastectomy to the more conservative surgical approaches in use today. Halsted introduced the radical procedure (removal of the entire breast, skin, chest wall muscles, and axillary lymph nodes) in the mistaken belief that as a breast tumor grows, it will spread in an orderly manner from the tumor core outward to all adjacent tissue and lymph nodes in its path. This surgical procedure became the standard form of treatment up until the early 1970s. Today, after years of clinical trials, surgery using less extensive tissue removal is now the rule.

When primary, localized breast cancer (less than 2 to 4 cm and no metastasis) is diagnosed, two surgical options may be offered: modified radical mastectomy, with or without breast reconstruction, or breast-sparing (lumpectomy) procedures. The goal of both modified radical mastectomy and lumpectomy is to control local/regional disease, to accurately stage the disease so that patients at high risk for recurrence are identified, and to provide the best chance for long-term survival, in addition to achieving the best cosmetic result. The overall long-term survival rates for the two surgical methods are approximately the same.[47]

Modified radical mastectomy is the standard form of mastectomy surgery. This procedure involves the removal of the whole breast, some fatty tissue, and dissection of the axillary lymph nodes. The pectoral muscles and surrounding nerves are left intact. The cosmetic result avoids the devastating chest wall defects, shoulder and arm limitations, and skin graft requirements that accompanied the more radical procedure. However, the modified surgery is significantly more extensive than the breast-sparing procedures.

Breast-sparing procedures, known as partial mastectomy, wedge resection, or lumpectomy, involve the least removal of breast tissue and, therefore, have the best cosmesis. The tumor is removed, including a margin of normal tissue. The pathologist usually examines the specimen immediately to be sure that the margins around the tumor are cancer free. If not, a wider excision is required. A separate incision is used to determine axillary node involvement. Breast-sparing treatment for local disease is followed in 2 to 4 weeks by radiation therapy when wound healing is complete. Breast-sparing surgery is not advised for all stage I and II disease. Contraindications are listed in Box 54-4.

Both modified radical mastectomy and lumpectomy include axillary lymph-node dissection because metastatic dissemination takes place primarily through these nodes. Axillary node status is a significant prognostic indicator in breast can-

BOX 54-4 Contraindications for Use of Breast-Sparing Procedures

Pregnancy: first and second trimesters preclude the use of radiation therapy
Locally advanced or inflammatory breast cancer
Multiple lesions located in separate quadrants of the breast or diffuse malignant or indeterminate-appearing microcalcifications
Prior irradiation of the breast
History of collagen-vascular disease, which is recognized as having poor tolerance to the effects of radiation therapy
Tumor size: large tumor in a small breast, which will not allow adequate resection of tumor
Breast size: large pendulous breasts, which are difficult to irradiate; small breasts, which may result in an unacceptable cosmetic outcome

Source: Schuster TD et al: Multidisciplinary care for patients with breast cancer, *Surg Clin North Am* 80(2):505, 2000.

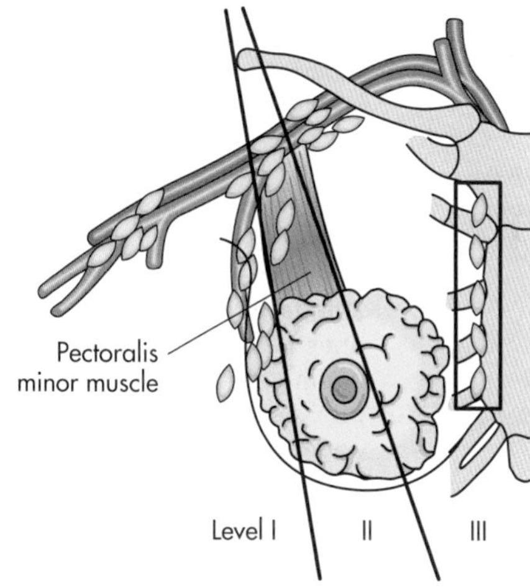

Figure 54-8 Regional axillary lymph nodes demonstrating levels I, II, and III node dissection.

cer and provides valuable information towards determination of adjuvant therapy.[54] Low axillary dissection (level I) is the removal of an entire bloc of nodes in the area from the latissimus dorsi muscle laterally to the medial pectoralis muscle. Levels II and III dissection remove en bloc nodes from the middle to the entire axillary node chain, respectively (Figure 54-8). Approximately 80% of axillary nodes are found within a level I to II dissection, with the remainder in level III. When axillary nodes are negative for cancer, a level I to II dissection is adequate. If nodes are positive for disease, a complete level III dissection is advised.

Sentinel lymph node dissection (SLND) is a promising technique currently under investigation that may help to identify axillary node involvement before axillary dissection.[47] This procedure is based on the concept that a certain anatomic region renders all of its lymphatic drainage into one or two lymph nodes in the regional nodal basin. The sentinel node can reflect the tumor status of the entire nodal basin and thus reduce the number of unnecessary lymph node dissections in negative patients.[22]

On the day of surgery, a radioisotope is injected around the tumor site or biopsy cavity. Then a lymphoscintigram is obtained to identify the pathways of lymphatic drainage and the approximate location of the sentinel node. After this, isosulfan blue dye is injected around the tumor or biopsy cavity. The dye is expected to travel via the lymphatics and become trapped in the sentinel node. After an axillary incision is made, a gamma probe is used to help locate the sentinel nodes, which are identified by the blue dye. After excision of all identifiable sentinel nodes, the axilla is examined for residual radioactivity that may indicate additional sentinel nodes remaining, thus requiring further exploration. All sentinel nodes are sent for frozen section analysis, during which time the surgeon proceeds with any additional surgery that may be required in the breast (e.g., lumpectomy or mastectomy). If the sentinel node is positive for metastatic cells, the surgeon performs a standard axillary lymph node dissection. If the sentinel node is negative for metastatic cells, the lymph node dissection is omitted.[5] When performed by an experienced surgeon according to exacting standards, SLND can be successfully done in more than 90% of eligible breast cancer patients. In addition, the tumor status of the sentinel node can accurately predict the tumor status of all axillary nodes in more than 95% of cases.[22]

Stages III and IV Disease. Surgery for advanced breast cancer includes mastectomy in combination with systemic chemotherapy or hormonal therapy. A Clinical Pathway for a patient undergoing mastectomy for breast cancer is found on pp. 1802 and 1803.

Breast Reconstruction. The goal of breast reconstruction is to create a symmetric breast mound that approximates the appearance of the opposite breast.[38] Two types of procedures are available for breast reconstruction: implants and autogenous tissue flaps. Implants, in their simplest form, are soft sacs filled with saline or silicone gel that are placed in a pocket beneath the pectoralis major muscle and held in place by the pectoralis major, anterior serratus, and upper rectus abdominis muscles. The size and shape of the implant are matched to the size of the remaining breast. Some surgeons prefer to first use a tissue expander. This expandable implant is placed in the manner just described and progressively filled with sterile saline over a period of weeks or months to stretch the skin until the desired size of breast is reached. The sterile saline is added to the expander sac through a needle inserted into a subcutaneous access port. The expander is then replaced by a permanent implant, either saline or silicone gel–filled, during a second operation.[27] No activity restrictions are necessary during the expansion period, and pain and discomfort are usually easily controlled.

The use of implants is not without complications or controversy. Complications include fibrous capsular contractions around the implant causing pain, tenderness, and fixation of the implant to the chest wall. Infection is a rare cause for implant removal. As a result of questions and concerns about the

clinical pathway *Mastectomy*

	DAY 1 (OR)	DAY 2	DAY 3
Assessment			
Neurologic/ Psychologic	Mental status; pain via pain scale (severity, quality, location, duration, radiation); standard for recovery from anesthesia; explore anxiety/ coping skills (patient/spouse); begin assessment of knowledge of health care problem; identify available and needed family/human/economic resources to resume independent self-care activities	Mental status; pain via pain scale (severity, quality, location, duration, radiation); continue to explore anxiety/coping skills (patient/spouse); continue assessment of knowledge of health care problem; collaborate with social services to identify available and needed family/human/economic resources to resume independent self-care activities	Mental status; pain via pain scale; continue to explore anxiety/coping skills (patient/spouse)
Pulmonary	Breath sounds	Breath sounds	Breath sounds
Cardiovascular	VS per postop standard; capillary refill; pulses; Homans' sign.	CR; BP; pulses; Homans' sign	CR; BP; pulses; Homans' sign
Gastrointestinal	Mucous membranes; nausea; vomiting; bowel sounds	Mucous membranes; stool	Mucous membranes; stool
Genitourinary	I&O; UO qs	UO qs	UO qs
Integumentary	Skin turgor, temperature, color, integrity	Skin turgor and integrity	Skin turgor and integrity
Surgical Wound	Surgical drain (Jackson-Pratt/Hemovac) to self-suction; dsg/incision line; amount and type of drainage; S&S of bleeding/hematoma/edema/ redness/heat	Surgical drain (Jackson-Pratt/Hemovac) to self-suction; dsg/incision line; amount and type of drainage; dsg; S&S of bleeding/hematoma/edema/ redness/heat	Surgical drain (Jackson-Pratt/Hemovac) to self-suction; dsg/incision line; amount and type of drainage; dsg; S&S of bleeding/hematoma/edema/ redness/heat
Musculoskeletal	Measure circumference of affected arm above elbow and compare with preop baseline	Measure circumference of affected arm above elbow and compare with preop baseline	Measure circumference of affected arm above elbow and compare with preop baseline
Focus	Hemodynamic stability; pain control	Self-care; pain control	Discharge
Diagnostic Plan	Postop Hct @ 6 PM	Repeat Hct	None
Therapeutic Interventions	Full fluid diet as tolerated this evening, then progress diet to regular; force fluids to 1500 ml by 10 PM; keep affected arm and hand elevated on pillow with elbow higher than shoulder; notify surgeon if arm circumference increases or S&S of lymphedema appear; cough, deep breathe, and use incentive spirometer q2-4h while awake; elastic support stockings; assist with getting up the first time; OOB to chair this evening and ambulate with assistance around room; assist with hygiene; *Consider:* arm sling.	After surgical dsg debulked, cleanse and cover wound with DSD daily; initiate hand and elbow exercises; full regular diet; OOB and ambulate in hall; reapply support stockings bid; social services to coordinate Reach to Recovery volunteer visit	Independent ADL; discharge

From Birdsall C, Sperry SP: *Clinical paths in medical surgical practice,* St Louis, 1997, Mosby.

Continued

clinical pathway *Mastectomy*

	DAY 1 (OR)	DAY 2	DAY 3
Patient/Family Teaching/ Discharge Planning	Teach use of pain scale and review meds available for pain and anxiety; reassure that responses (anxiety/fear, etc.) are a normal reaction; begin to explore threats to femininity/ self-esteem if patient appears ready to discuss same; teach to use incentive spirometer, to limit movement of affected arm and shoulder for 24 hr, to keep arm and shoulder elevated on pillows to facilitate drainage, to empty and measure surgical drain reservoir; review treatment plan; initiate discharge plan; discuss plan for daily review of plan of care with patient/family	Remove surgical dsg and encourage patient to look at wound (allow time in an attempt to have patient share concerns of self-image/ femininity before discharge); review how to empty and measure surgical drain reservoir and teach wound care (cleanse per standard and apply DSD); teach to apply support stockings and to do hand and elbow exercises (squeeze ball, open and close fist, flex and extend wrist and elbow) 10 × q2h while awake; introduce Reach to Recovery program, verify that volunteer will arrange a visit and leave patient pamphlet about exercise at bedside; review discharge plan and home care needs; review, clarify, and confirm information given to date	Review discharge plan; teach wound self-care (empty and record drain volume, cleanse and apply DSD, keep incision and drain dry until drain removed (7-10 days postop); teach that nerve-related numbness/tingling of arm and breast will gradually disappear; teach strategies to protect arm (no BP, injections, or blood tests; no constricting clothes, jewelry, wristwatch; no stretching, straining, or lifting packages/ pocketbook; do not allow arm to be dependent); to prevent a frozen shoulder, explain that a long-term, vigorous outpatient exercise program will be initiated; tell to notify physician if drainage changes (increase in volume/odor) and S&S of bleeding/hematoma/lymphedema/ redness/heat appear
Expected Outcomes	Hemodynamic stability with no signs of hematoma formation; verbalizes relief of pain with analgesia; acknowledges availability of analgesic/anxiolytic, plan of care, and need to communicate with nurse if S&S of anxiety and fear become overwhelming (subjective feelings, emotional lability, or inability to concentrate); demonstrates use of incentive spirometer; participates in self-care	Voids qs; normal stool; needs fewer doses of prn meds as evidenced by pain scale <3 (0-10); demonstrates correct arm position to facilitate drainage; ambulates freely; verbalizes discharge plan, meds, and drug/food interactions; verbalizes appropriate anxiety and fears related to surgery; demonstrates how to empty and measure surgical drain reservoir	Demonstrates self-care of wound and drain; verbalizes planned exercises per teaching plan; states appointment date with physician; pain well controlled as evidenced by pain scale <3 (0-10); verbalizes health-seeking behaviors (nutrition, fluids, daily exercise, monthly breast self-exam, and annual mammogram); verbalizes community resources and support groups available
Trigger(s)	Hemodynamic instability from bleeding; hematoma formation	Reluctance to participate in self-care activities, especially wound care	Unable to be independent in ADL

Consults for Consideration: (Date and initial when completed) Social Services ________ Dietary Dept. ________
Oncology CNS ________ Reach to Recovery ________ Home Care ________

safety of silicone implants, the FDA has restricted the use of these implants to women undergoing breast reconstruction for cancer under strictly controlled clinical trials. This restriction has been in place since 1992, awaiting more definitive data on the safety of silicone implants. Research in this area is ongoing.[27]

Nipple reconstruction, using tissue obtained from the opposite nipple-areola complex or skin from the upper part of the inner thigh, requires another surgical procedure about 3 to 6 months after breast reconstruction. The use of a dermal tattoo that can match normal breast pigment is an alternative method of nipple formation.

The use of autogenous tissue flaps is a second means of breast reconstruction that can be performed at the time of mastectomy or at a later date. Tissue flaps eliminate the need for an implant unless insufficient tissue is available to form a breast of dimensions equal to the remaining normal breast. Performing immediate breast reconstruction avoids the cost of a second hospitalization and surgery and loss of time from normal activities. Flaps used include latissimus dorsi musculocutaneous tissue from the upper portion of the back to create a breast or transverse rectus abdominis myocutaneous (TRAM) tissue from the lower portion of the abdomen. The latissimus dorsi flap leaves a scar on the upper back that may be visible with certain types of clothing. A TRAM flap uses tissue that is similar in elasticity to normal breast tissue and is available in sufficient quantity to construct a new breast of equal size and shape of the uninvolved breast. The scar from a TRAM flap on the lower abdomen is easily concealed beneath clothing.[27] Nipple reconstruction is performed in the same manner as already described. Figure 54-9 shows the three types of breast-reconstruction methods.

The patient's desire to have breast reconstruction surgery and whether it is to be performed immediately or at a later date depend on various factors. These factors may include the type of tumor, need for radiation or chemotherapy, and the patient's wishes. When chosen, immediate reconstruction can lessen feelings of loss and disfigurement.[13] Delayed reconstruction gives the woman more time to consider all options, and some surgeons believe that a wait of 3 to 6 months is beneficial before reconstruction surgery. This delay permits sufficient recovery of tissue integrity.[38]

When mastectomy without breast reconstruction is chosen as the option, a breast prosthesis is necessary. For some women this may not be viewed as a problem. Others find the need for prostheses an uncomfortable nuisance and a constant reminder of their breast cancer experience. Some women describe feeling "out of balance" when wearing the prosthesis compared with the weight of the opposite normal breast. They also may feel confined in their choice of clothing or participation in physical activities. These kinds of concerns may prompt women to undergo breast reconstruction many months or years after selecting mastectomy alone.

Diet. Maintenance of good nutrition is essential for all patients with cancer. Dietary requirements include an increase in calories, carbohydrate (CHO), and protein. Body energy demands are known to increase with cancer, and more energy is

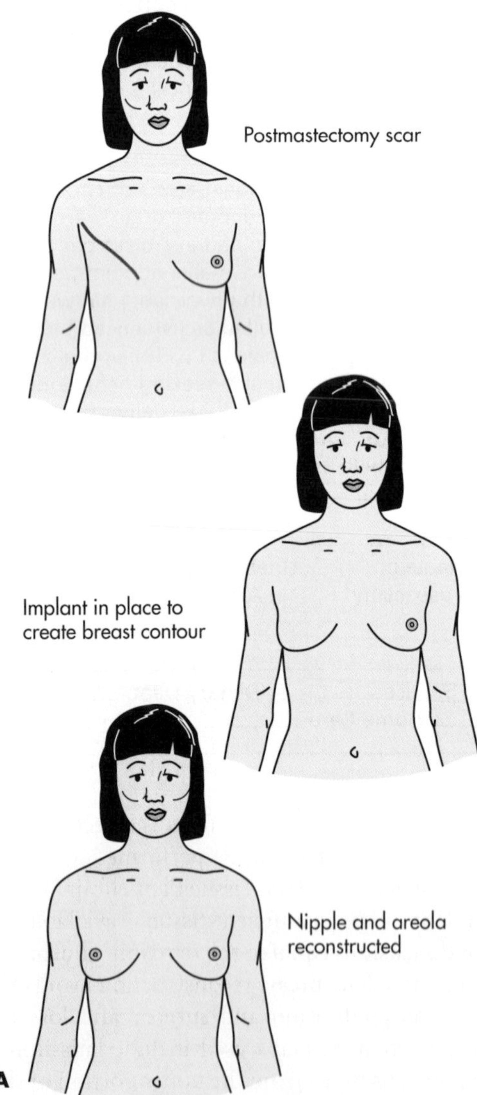

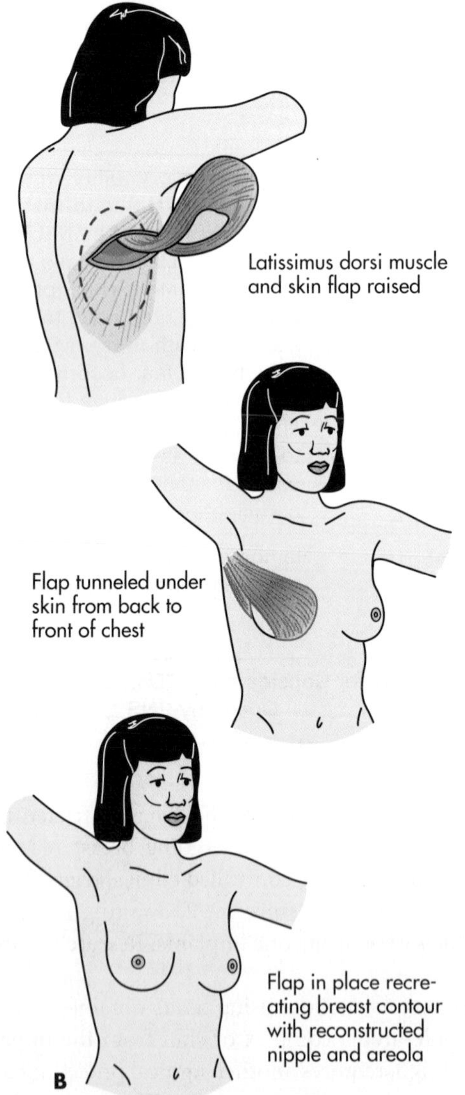

Figure 54-9 Three types of breast reconstruction procedures. **A,** Simple implant placement. **B,** Latissimus dorsi reconstruction.

Continued

necessary to withstand the potentially debilitating side effects of treatment. A diet high in calories and CHO spares body protein, necessary for tissue and wound repair, from being broken down for energy needs.

Good dietary management and patient education are especially important for the person with breast cancer. This diagnosis can evoke great emotional stress, and its treatment can affect appetite and nutrition in many ways. Additionally, all of the prescribed treatment options—surgery, radiation therapy, chemotherapy, and hormonal therapy, as well as adjunct medication and activity restrictions—affect body nutritional needs and maintenance to some degree. Table 54-2 provides an overview of nutritional problems generated by various cancer treatment options and the interventions commonly used to treat them.

Activity. The activity level of the patient with breast cancer depends on several factors: extent of the disease process, type of treatment used, phase within the treatment modality, and state of physical and emotional adjustment. The patient is encouraged to engage in any activity that she finds enjoyable and for which she feels able. At least 8 hours of sleep each night and incorporation of rest periods throughout the day are advisable, especially in the immediate postoperative period and during chemotherapy or radiation therapy. Sexual activity is not contraindicated and can be resumed as desired.

Referrals. During the period of diagnosis and treatment, the patient's primary physician may refer her to breast cancer specialists: surgeons and medical or radiation oncologists. The rationale for the referrals should be thoroughly discussed with the woman and her family. If breast reconstruction is to be performed at the time of mastectomy, a plastic surgeon will evaluate the patient to determine which procedure can be most easily performed and will best meet her needs. When radiation therapy or chemotherapy is to be part of the treatment plan, a re-

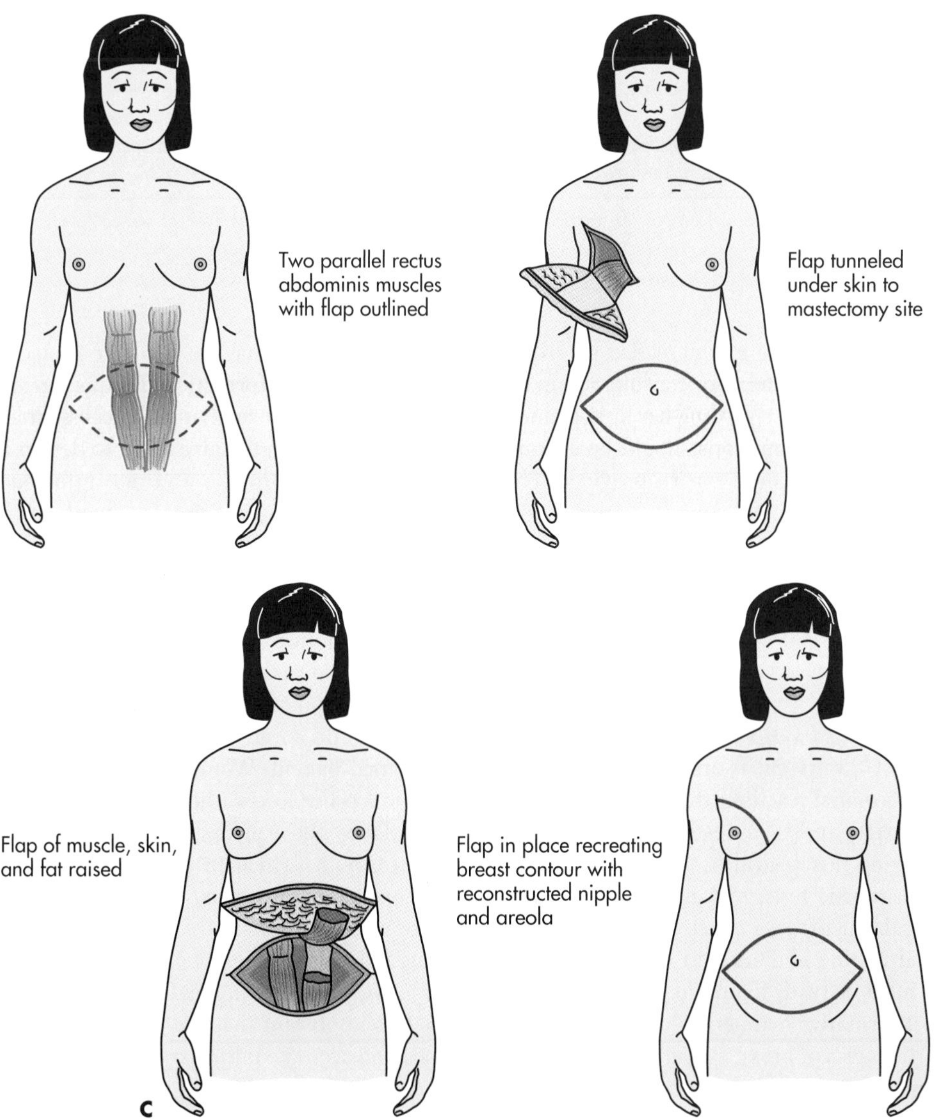

Figure 54-9, cont'd Three types of breast reconstruction procedures. **C,** Rectus abdominis reconstruction.

TABLE 54-2 Plan of Care for Treatment-Induced Nutritional Problems

Nutritional Problem Generated	Treatment Options Involved and Stress-Related Factor	Intervention
Oral		
Stomatitis (mouth sores)	Chemotherapy, radiation therapy	Eliminate acidic, salty, and spicy foods; abstain from alcohol and tobacco; use good oral hygiene.
Anorexia	Chemotherapy, radiation therapy, emotional distress	Provide small, frequent high-caloric meals; make meal time an enjoyable occasion; avoid noxious odors.
Xerostomia (dry mouth)	Chemotherapy, radiation therapy, medications; mouth breathing	Ensure adequate fluid intake; suck on hard candies; use artificial saliva; moisten mouth with water, using a dropper or syringe if necessary.
Abnormal taste	Chemotherapy, radiation therapy, medications	Avoid offensive foods (red meat); mask bad taste by adding wine/beer to soups and sauces; marinate meats; use more and stronger seasonings; serve cold or room-temperature food; drink more liquids; add tartness with lemon juice or vinegar; remedy dental problems.
Nausea and vomiting	Chemotherapy, surgery, radiation therapy, narcotics; behavioral factors (anticipatory vomiting)	Use antiemetics as needed; withhold food before chemotherapy or radiation treatment: eliminate offensive foods; avoid noxious odors; avoid food preparation if possible.
Dysphagia (difficult swallowing), odynophagia (painful swallowing)	Chemotherapy, radiation therapy; neuromuscular defects	Eat soft foods or foods processed in a blender; avoid spicy or highly seasoned foods.
Constipation	Chemotherapy, medications; inactivity	Increase fluid intake (prune juice, water, coffee); increase bulk in diet; use bran cereal, increase activity level.
Diarrhea	Chemotherapy, medications, radiation therapy; infection	Chemotherapy, medications, radiation therapy; infection

Modified from Wilkes GM, Yemma T: Nutritional support. In Varricchio C et al, editors: *A cancer source book for nurses,* ed 7, New York, 1997, American Cancer Society.

ferral to an expert in these areas is common practice. Often it is the woman herself who initiates a referral or consultation in the effort to obtain a "second opinion" regarding her breast cancer diagnosis and treatment. Second opinions should be encouraged and names of appropriate medical experts provided. This ensures the patient "peace of mind" and confidence that the diagnosis and prescribed treatment are in fact appropriate.

NURSING MANAGEMENT

PREOPERATIVE CARE

Assisting With Treatment Decisions

The discovery of a breast "lump" elicits one of the most powerful and distressing emotional reactions that a woman of any age can experience. Anxiety and stress levels are high. Nurses caring for patients during this critical time (discovering the tumor, undergoing diagnostic tests, making treatment decisions) need to be cognizant of the impact these events have on a woman's normal coping abilities and decision-making processes. The nurse must be ready to provide emotional support in a caring and informative manner.

Once a definitive diagnosis of breast cancer has been established, a complete explanation of treatment options must follow. Most patients come to this situation with some prior knowledge about breast cancer, either from media exposure or through friends or relatives who have had breast cancer. Their knowledge base may be accurate or laden with misconceptions and false information. Because treatment of breast cancer is constantly evolving, it is essential for the nurse, in conjunction with the physician, to determine what the patient knows and to provide accurate information so that an informed treatment choice can be made. Inclusion of family and especially the spouse or partner in all discussions about treatment is vital to a successful outcome.

The physician will discuss the stage of the disease and the treatment options in detail so that the patient is aware of the advantages and disadvantages of each, as well as the immediate and long-term outcome expectations. The information is often complex and confusing even to the most intelligent and well-informed patient. Women are no longer pressured to select a surgical procedure without knowledge of the final biopsy report. Delay between breast biopsy and definitive treatment provides time in which to consider the options and choose the option that is most personally suitable. The nurse should plan to be present, if possible, when treatment options are presented. This allows assessment of patient and family understanding and time to clarify misinformation and misconceptions.

It is important that the physician and nurse provide unbiased and accurate information on each option. Studies have revealed that the manner in which information is presented can influence the patient's final decision. Even when physician treatment preference is not indicated or solicited, the patient may perceive that one exists and make her choice accordingly.[10,48,49]

Contrary to past reports, patients who choose mastectomy do so not because they were uninformed about breast-sparing surgery but because they may not wish to go through an additional 6 to 7 weeks of radiation therapy. Radiation may be perceived as decreasing quality of life. Mastectomy surgery allows the patient to have definitive surgery, recover, and return more readily to previous activities and lifestyle.

Financial concerns also can influence treatment decisions. If the patient has health insurance, generally she can be assured that costs for both mastectomy and breast reconstruction surgery are covered. It is important to note that concern for treatment-related problems and out-of-pocket costs might lead some women to choose less intense treatment regimens.[49]

Assisting With the Grieving Process

The diagnosis of breast cancer is extremely traumatic, but contrary to common belief, most women cope well with surgery and the loss of a breast. Most women state that they are not concerned about body image or sexuality when deciding on a surgical procedure (lumpectomy versus mastectomy). Their most immediate concern is to have the cancer eradicated from the body. It may not be until after the mastectomy surgery that issues related to body image and sexuality arise. Therefore during the presurgical phase of treatment, it is essential for the nurse and physician to determine what impact breast cancer and total or partial loss of a breast will have on the patient's self-esteem and perceived sexuality. The loss of a breast can engender feelings similar to those caused by limb amputation. Reactions include anger, depression, denial, and withdrawal. Grieving for the lost body part is normal, and the patient should be permitted time to work through her grief. The nurse should offer reassurance that the expression of grief is accepted and understood by staff members and is therapeutic for the patient. It is important that family members be made aware of the grieving process and encouraged to provide emotional support to the woman for as long as it is needed. Patients with problems regarding intimate relationships and sexuality should be referred for counseling. Characteristics of women at higher risk for self-esteem problems and poor sexual adjustment after mastectomy are listed in Box 54-5. Women without partners may benefit from referral to a support group of women similar to themselves. Advancing age does not exempt a woman from concerns over self-esteem and sexuality, and older adults should be included in all interventions and referrals for assistance. The spouse or partner should be present, if at all possible, during all discussion about sexual concerns so that his anxieties can be addressed as well.

Referral to the Reach to Recovery program of the American Cancer Society (ACS) provides another means of assisting the patient to work through her grief and anxieties after breast cancer surgery. A Reach to Recovery volunteer is a woman who has had breast cancer and has undergone successful surgery and rehabilitation. These volunteers have personal knowledge of the problems and fears faced by the patient. If possible, the volunteer is matched to the patient by age and type of surgery undergone. The volunteer is able to answer questions about rehabilitation, as well as types of prostheses and brassieres (Figure 54-10) and where these items can be purchased. If the patient has not undergone breast reconstruction surgery, the volunteer provides the patient with a temporary breast prosthesis and demonstrates its use. In addition, the volunteer provides pamphlets that illustrate the prescribed rehabilitative exercises, as well as a rope and ball used for some of these activities.

BOX 54-5 Women at Risk for Sexual and Self-Esteem Problems After Loss of Breast

1. Reported lack of support from a loving spouse or partner
2. Existence of an unhappy, unstable, intimate relationship
3. Desire to conceive more children if still in the childbearing years
4. Past sexual problems
5. History of sexual abuse such as rape or incest

From Schover LR: The impact of breast cancer on sexuality, body image, and intimate relationships, *CA Cancer J Clin* 41(12):112, 1991.

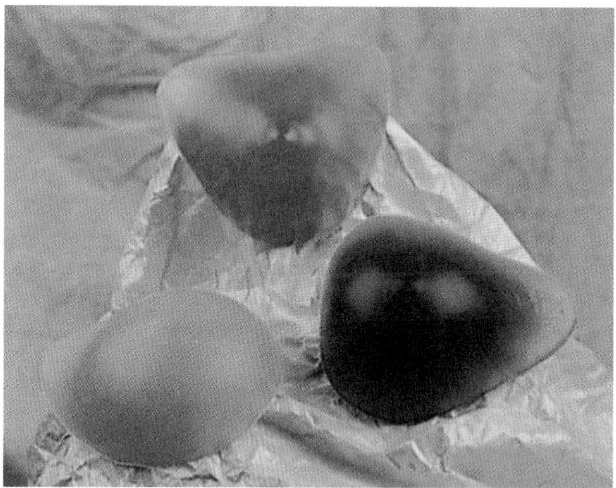

Figure 54-10 Examples of common silicone breast prostheses.

The impact of breast cancer and its treatment on the quality of life of breast cancer survivors and their families is an area of ongoing concern. Breast cancer can cause not only physical and psychologic difficulties but social and spiritual problems as well, which can extend well into survivorship (see Research box). Quality of life issues should be explored with patients and their families and strategies developed to assist each family member in coping with the disease.

Promoting Patient Participation in the Treatment Plan

The focus of nursing during the preoperative period is to provide teaching in regard to what the patient can expect after surgery. Instruction for the patient undergoing mastectomy and lymph node dissection includes a review of the expected incision line and the type of dressing, drains, and drainage collection device anticipated. If breast reconstruction is to be performed immediately, the location of the donor tissue is indicated (upper back area or lower abdomen). The use of pictures or diagrams similar to those shown in Figure 54-9, *A* to *C*,

Research

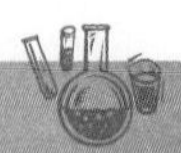

Reference: Ferrell BR et al: Quality of life in breast cancer survivors: implications for developing support services, *Oncol Nurs Forum* 25(5):887-895, 1998.

As advances in treatment extend the period of survivorship for women with breast cancer, quality of life has become an important issue. The purpose of this study was to provide a description of the unique multidimensional quality of life concerns of breast cancer survivors. The sample consisted of 298 randomly selected breast cancer survivors who were stratified to include three age groups: younger than 40 (n = 80), 40-60 (n = 128), older than 60 (n = 89). About 73% of the women were Caucasian, with the remainder of the sample representing other ethnic groups. Most women had undergone surgery as primary treatment for breast cancer. Approximately half of the women had adjuvant chemotherapy, and half had adjuvant radiation therapy. Annual income ranged from less than $10,000 to more than $50,000. About 39% of the sample was employed outside the home, with the remainder of the sample either unemployed, retired, or disabled. The mean time since diagnosis was 107 months.

The mailed survey method was used. The survey measured the quality of life of breast cancer survivors according to the domains of physical well-being, psychologic well-being, social well-being, and spiritual well-being. Another survey measured pain associated with breast cancer. Results of the study indicate that the physical demands of breast cancer, including fatigue and pain, as well as psychologic burdens related to fear of recurrence and anxiety, continue well into survivorship. The social domain illustrated that the greatest areas of concern were for female relatives and family distress. The spiritual domain illustrated disruption related to uncertainty about the future.

The findings of this study identified breast cancer survivors' various areas of concern across the domains of quality of life. This information offers direction for nurses in planning and implementing supportive-care services intended to improve the quality of life of breast cancer survivors.

will facilitate patient understanding. If an implant is to be inserted, the nurse clarifies position and placement guidelines. The patient is informed that movement of the arm and shoulder on the affected side will be limited for the first 24 hours and that the arm and hand will be elevated on a pillow to facilitate lymphatic and venous drainage. A return demonstration of breathing exercises and turning techniques prepares the patient to actively participate in postoperative recovery.

POSTOPERATIVE CARE

The focus of postoperative care after breast surgery is to provide physical comfort, maintain nutritional support, prevent complications, and prepare the patient for discharge and successful home management. Adequate information must be provided so that the patient has full understanding of each intervention and the degree of participation required of her to make a successful transition from hospital to home management.

Managing Pain

Surgical pain after mastectomy results from the transverse incision that usually extends from the sternum to the axilla. In addition, discomfort may result from either trauma to or transection of thoracic and intercostal nerves and from fluid collection in the chest wall or at the site of the lymph node dissection. If the patient has had immediate breast reconstruction using the TRAM flap procedure, abdominal pain is another factor to consider in pain management.

Pain relief is managed after mastectomy surgery by the administration of prescribed analgesics and comfort measures. The amount of discomfort experienced varies with the individual patient and her degree of pain tolerance. Most patients are relatively pain free by the time of discharge, requiring only a mild analgesic. Thorough assessment of the patient's pain level and prompt administration of analgesics ensure both pain relief and adequate sleep and rest. Patient-controlled analgesia can be an effective intervention. Maintaining physical comfort also helps diminish the high stress level seen in the immediate postoperative period. Medicating the patient before activities such as turning or getting out of bed for the first time is advisable.

Instructing the patient to get out of bed from the unaffected side lessens pain and tension on the operative site. Providing support to the affected side for the first few days after surgery is necessary because movement of the affected arm and shoulder is restricted for at least 24 hours. The patient is informed that she may feel "out of balance" initially because of the weight of the dressing and the presence of the drainage collection apparatus. Temporary use of a sling on the affected arm during ambulation, if approved by the physician, provides comfort and support by lessening strain on the shoulder and prevents dependent lymphatic and venous stasis.

Abdominal pain after a TRAM flap procedure is managed using patient-controlled analgesia (PCA). Oral analgesics are started by the third postoperative day as tolerated.[35] Maintaining a semi-Fowler's position with the knees flexed and elevated also reduces pressure on the abdomen. An abdominal binder may be ordered to provide added support during ambulation.[35] Abdominal drainage devices are checked at least every 1 to 2 hours for proper function and for the amount and type of drainage. Excessive bright red drainage may indicate hemorrhage, whereas little to no return may indicate obstruction of the drain or drainage apparatus. The occurrence of either is promptly reported to the physician.

When nerves are cut or traumatized within the operative field, the patient may experience sensory changes such as numbness, tingling, changes in skin sensitivity of the chest wall, and even phantom breast sensations. The patient is informed that these changes are common and expected outcomes after surgery. The nurse can assure the patient that nerve-related discomforts gradually decrease and usually cease within a few months.

Preventing Infection

Fluid collection in the chest wall or at the axillary node dissection site can be a source of infection. The build-up of lymphedema can be a secondary source. Lymphedema usually is a transitory event until collateral lymph channels are formed. When measures are not implemented to increase lymphatic flow, fibrosis can occur within the system, and lymphedema becomes an irreversible condition. The chronic collection of fluid and any subsequent injury to the involved extremity can result in infection.[43]

After the initial dressing change by the physician, the nurse performs wound care and dressing changes as needed, noting the condition of the wound and observing for signs of infection (redness, swelling, drainage, odor, increased discomfort, and fever). Proper placement of drains and drainage collection devices can prevent fluid collection and stasis. The nurse assesses the devices (Hemovac, Jackson-Pratt) for placement and for the amount and type of drainage. When the drain and drainage-collection device are functioning properly, the amount of fluid around the incision is minimal. The patient is instructed to avoid touching the dressing and drainage device, unless she is changing the dressing or measuring output.

When immediate breast reconstruction is performed, the hospital stay is between 2 and 7 days depending on the extent of reconstruction (simple implant, tissue expander, or autologous tissue reconstruction).[35] If reconstruction involves the use of a tissue flap, such as a TRAM flap, it is important to observe for tissue perfusion, flap color, temperature, and capillary refill for the first 3 days after surgery.[35]

When breast reconstruction is performed by the placement of a tissue expander, the patient will probably experience pulling and stretching sensations of the overlying muscles. This discomfort is caused when the expander pouch is filled with 100 to 300 ml of saline solution during surgery. Discomfort gradually subsides as the muscles adjust to their new length.

Promoting Mobility of the Arm and Shoulder

One of the priority nursing interventions after mastectomy surgery is to maintain elevation of the affected arm and hand on pillows so that they are higher than the elbow and the elbow is higher than the shoulder. This strategy must be performed while the patient is in bed or sitting in a chair so that venous and lymphatic pooling are prevented. The nurse monitors for lymphatic and venous stasis by measuring the circumference of the affected arm 6 inches above and below the elbow and comparing results with a preoperative baseline measurement and with the unaffected arm. The affected arm is kept relatively immobile for 24 hours to decrease any strain on the incision line. Hand exercises may be started, consisting of squeezing a ball, opening and closing the fist, and flexing and extending the wrist and elbow several times each hour. These exercises help facilitate lymphatic flow. More rigorous range-of-motion exercises for the arm and shoulder are initiated at the discretion of the physician. Some exercises are delayed 7 to 10 days until the sutures and drains have been removed. Figure 54-11 presents an overview of exercises prescribed after mastectomy surgery (Box 54-6).

Patient Teaching
Discharge Instructions After Breast Cancer Surgery

DRESSINGS

Incision

There will be a dry gauze dressing over the incision when you leave the hospital. It is not necessary to change this dressing until you return to see the doctor.

Drain Site

A small dry dressing will be around the site where the drain is placed. Often there is some leakage of fluid around the drain. Check the gauze dressing for drainage and change if soiled. Some leakage is normal, but if the dressing becomes soaked more than once a day, call your doctor.

Drains

Your nurse has shown you how to empty the reservoir from your drain and how to measure the volume of drainage. You should empty the drain twice a day and record the measurements.

Drains are generally removed when drainage is about 30 ml in 24 hours.

Drains are often removed at the same time as the stitches, generally 7 to 10 days after surgery.

BATHING

Sponge baths or tub baths, making certain that the area of the drain and incision stay dry, are permitted. You may shower after the stitches and drains are removed.

HAND AND ARM CARE

You can begin using your arm for normal activities such as eating or combing your hair. Exercises involving the wrist, hand, and elbow such as flexing your fingers, circular wrist motions, and touching hand to shoulder are very good. More strenuous exercises can usually be resumed after the drains have been removed.

COMFORT

Some discomfort or mild pain is expected after surgery. Within 4 to 5 days most women have no need for medication or require something only at bedtime.

Numbness in the area of the surgery and along the inner side of the arm from the armpit to the elbow occurs in virtually all patients. It is a result of injury to the nerves that provide sensation to the skin in those areas. Women have described sensations such as heaviness, pain, tingling, burning, and "pins and needles." These sensations change over the months and usually resolve by 1 year.

SUPPORT AND INFORMATION

Pamphlets on exercises, hand and arm care, and general facts about breast cancer are available from your nurse or volunteer visitor. The American Cancer Society has volunteers who have had surgery similar to yours and are available to visit you.

Adapted from McCorkle R et al: *Cancer nursing: a comprehensive textbook,* Philadelphia, 1996, WB Saunders.

Patient/Family Education

Before discharge, the patient is instructed about wound care management, exercise guidelines and sensory change precautions, assessment and management of lymphedema, and prevention of trauma and infection. The Patient Teaching box provides an overview of some general discharge instructions.

Teaching Wound Care Management

Having the patient perform wound care before discharge is a major nursing goal. Instruction focuses on aseptic technique, care of drains, the signs and symptoms of infection, and frequency of dressing change. Because hospital stay is limited and is generally a time of high stress and anxiety, all verbal teaching

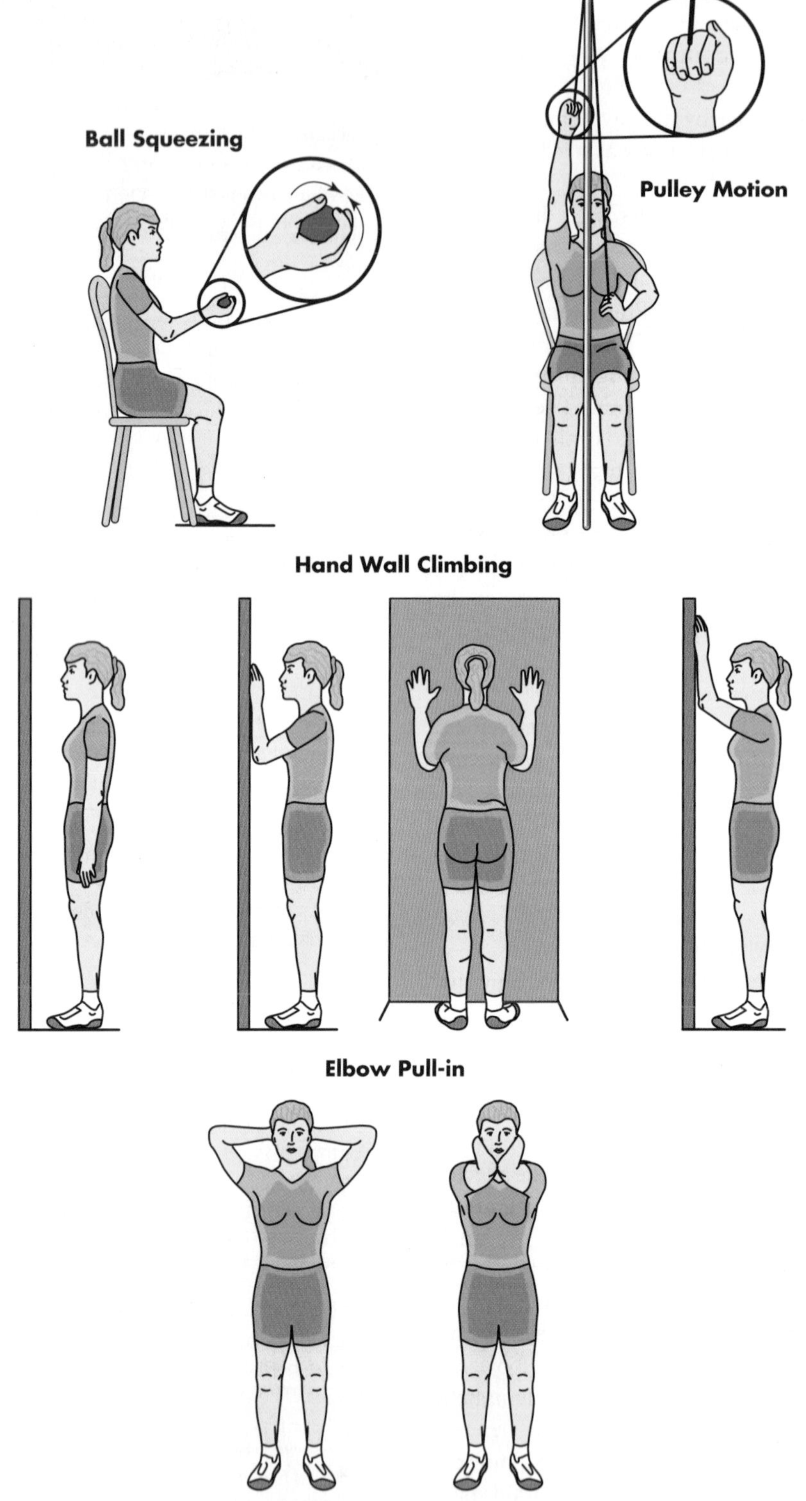

Figure 54-11 Arm and shoulder exercises commonly prescribed for patients after mastectomy surgery.

Continued

should be accompanied by simple, clearly written instructions. At least one return demonstration of the care ensures that the patient understands the procedure and performs it correctly. Dressing change is necessary at least once a day to examine the incision site for signs of infection and to ensure that the drainage device is working satisfactorily. The wound should be kept dry inasmuch as infection is more likely to develop in a warm, moist environment. The patient is instructed that once the sutures and drains are removed, usually in 7 to 10 days, the physician will indicate whether the incision requires any further dressing.

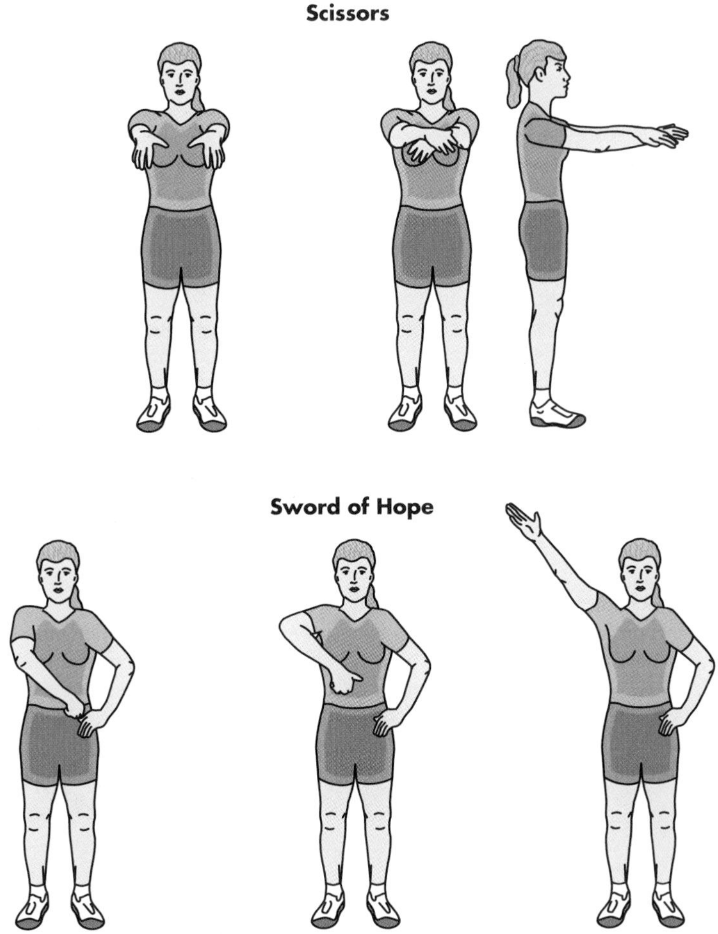

Figure 54-11, cont'd Arm and shoulder exercises commonly prescribed for patients after mastectomy surgery.

Teaching Arm/Shoulder Exercises

At the time of discharge the patient will still have restrictions on the type and amount of exercise permitted for the affected arm and shoulder. Squeezing a ball and bending and flexing the wrist and elbow of the affected arm are continued at home. The more rigorous exercises meant to restore full range of motion to the shoulder are delayed until the drain and sutures are removed. The physician will then prescribe a gradual increase in the amount and type of exercises to be performed (such as wall climbing or combing hair). Some of these exercises are described in Box 54-6. Performing these exercises several times daily helps to restore full range of motion to the arm and shoulder, thus preventing a "frozen shoulder" from lack of normal movement. The exercises also facilitate the development of collateral lymphatic channels and help prevent lymphedema.

If the patient has had breast reconstruction surgery, she is cautioned to avoid heavy lifting (more than 5 lb) for 6 weeks. This time frame ensures that complete healing has occurred and strain on the incision line is minimal.[35] A well-fitted brassiere provides support and normal alignment of the newly formed breast. When the patient has sensory changes because of transection or trauma to nerves at the time of surgery, some side effects may persist well after discharge. Although most sensory problems resolve within 1 year, some may persist and can cause atrophy of muscles that move the shoulder on the affected side. The patient should be alert to any signs and symptoms of impaired shoulder mobility and report them immediately.

Assessing and Managing Lymphedema

Instructions on how to assess for the presence of lymphedema and how to avoid its occurrence are important. Patients should be taught to observe for signs of numbness, tightness, stiffness, pain, and redness. Decreased strength and infection may also indicate the presence of lymphedema.[46] The nurse stresses the importance of the prescribed rehabilitative exercises and teaches the patient to avoid placing the affected extremity in a dependent position for extended periods. Compliance with these instructions helps to prevent the chronic form of lymphedema, which can occur soon after discharge or many months afterward. Some edema may be present at discharge, especially if lymph node dissection was performed. The greater the number of nodes removed, the greater the chance of edema. As the wound heals and the prescribed exercises are performed, the edema usually subsides.

BOX 54-6 Postmastectomy Arm Exercises

Ball Squeezing

1. Standing, sitting, or lying in bed, hold a rubber ball in your hand on the operated side. Keep your arm bent, with your palm toward the ceiling, while lifting your hand higher than your heart.
2. First squeeze and then relax the ball. Repeat.
3. Do this exercise as often as recommended by your doctor.
4. If it is uncomfortable to hold your arm straight out, support the arm using several pillows or the back of a chair.

Pulley Motion

1. Place knots at each end of the rope.
2. Toss the rope over the top of the door with the unoperated arm.
3. Sit with legs hugging both sides of the door and keep feet firmly planted on the floor.
4. Hold the ends of the rope in each hand with knots between your second (middle) and third (ring) fingers.
5. Slowly raise arm on operated side as far as comfortable by pulling down on the rope with arm on unoperated side; keep the raised arm close to your head. Reverse the motion to raise opposite arm. Rest and repeat.

Hand Wall Climbing

1. Start in standard position, with toes 4 to 6 inches from and facing the wall.
2. Bend elbows and stand with arms, from elbow to wrist, against the wall and your hands at eye level.
3. Work both hands up the wall trying to keep them parallel to each other until incisional pulling or pain occurs. Mark the spot you reach so progress can be checked.
4. Work hands down to shoulder level. Move feet and body closer to wall as comfort allows and reach requires.
5. Return to standard position. Rest and repeat. (It will relax you a bit if you rest your head against the wall.)
6. Once you reach your goal, push your fingers against the wall.

Elbow Pull-In

1. While sitting or standing, clasp fingers in front of you with elbows straight.
2. Raise your arms slowly over your head, keeping your arms straight. At first you may not be able to raise your arms over your head, but keep trying.
3. Bend elbows and bring hands behind your neck, keeping your fingers clasped together. Try to push your elbows backward so they are in a horizontal line with your shoulders.
4. Pull elbows in toward each other until they touch at chin level. It is OK to unclasp fingers to let your elbows touch.
5. Release elbows back to position in step 3.
6. Lift your arms back over your head to position in step 2 with arms straight.
7. Lower your arms in front of you to the starting position. Rest and repeat.

Crossed Arm

1. Stand with elbows flexed and raised to shoulder level.
2. Cross one arm on top of the other arm so your fingers are over the opposite elbow.
3. Push elbows backward while attempting to squeeze your shoulder blades (scapula) together. You will feel a slight pulling in the chest. Be sure to keep elbows at shoulder level as you do this exercise.
4. Return arms to crossed position but place opposite hand on top this time. Rest and repeat.

Scissors

1. Keep your arms straight, with palms toward the floor, while lifting them in front of you to shoulder height.
2. Cross hand over hand (left over right) while keeping arms straight. Uncross and recross same position.
3. Return to beginning position.
4. Cross over with opposite hand on top—right over left. Uncross and recross same position. Return to starting position. Rest and repeat.
5. Repeat the above exercise, except start with palms facing up. This change will work different muscles.
   (This exercise may be more difficult to do at first because of lack of support of the extended arm. It may be better to do the CROSSED ARM exercise in the beginning.)

Sword of Hope

1. Place the hand of your unoperated side on your hip. Make a fist with your hand on the operated side. Place your fist on the opposite hip with the thumb touching the hip. Raise your elbow slightly.
2. Lift your hand in a diagonal line from your hip to the breast area on the opposite side while keeping your elbow flexed.
3. Open your hand, palm up, as you straighten your arm over your head continuing the diagonal line.
4. Reverse the movements from position in step 3, step 2, step 1. Rest and repeat.
   (It may be recommended to do this exercise with the arm of the unoperated side for the first week before starting with the arm of the operated side.)

From Reach to Recovery, exercises after breast surgery, no 4668-PS, Atlanta, 1996. Reprinted by permission of the American Cancer Society, Inc.

Demonstration of the proper technique to measure arm circumference and a method to record arm measurements enables the patient to quickly recognize the presence of a problem and report it immediately. Although there is no standard degree of enlargement that constitutes lymphedema, the most common definition is a 2-cm difference in arm circumference between the affected and unaffected arm.[43] When edema is present, the patient is instructed to keep the affected extremity elevated as much as possible. If edema persists or increases, the physician should be notified. Treatment regimens may include application of a compression garment, extremity elevation, exercise regimens, skin care, manual decompression, and external compression.[9]

Strategies to Prevent Trauma and Infection

The patient who has had breast surgery with a level II or III lymph node dissection must be vigilant in avoiding trauma and infection to the affected arm. Protecting the arm and hand is essential because lymphatic circulation has been compromised by the removal of axillary lymph nodes. Radiation therapy is also known to interfere with the ability of the lymph nodes to remove foreign substances and destroy bacteria. Thus node dissection and radiation therapy can both lead to lymphatic dysfunction. Infectious agents can easily enter the lymphatic system from cuts, scratches, or burns. Special instructions to avoid these complications are listed in the Guidelines for Safe Practice box, top right. The patient must understand that these precautions need to be followed for the rest of her life.

Health Promotion/Prevention

The ultimate goal of primary prevention is to prevent a disease from occurring. Although many risk factors for breast cancer have been identified (see Risk Factors box, p. 1790) the specific cause is unknown. Women, even with knowledge of their own personal risk factors, cannot control risks such as age, gender, family, and menstrual or reproductive history. The risk of breast cancer may be reduced, however, through diet control, weight reduction, and avoidance of prolonged use of oral contraceptives and/or exogenous hormones.

Secondary prevention is used to detect a disease process in its early stage so that it can be successfully treated or cured. Important measures to detect breast cancer in an early localized stage include monthly BSE, and mammographic examination as directed by a physician or as part of a mammography screening program. The ACS has designated physical examination of the breast and use of mammography as the approved basic detection methods for breast cancer at right. The criteria are listed in the Guidelines for Safe Practice box.

Breast cancer centers have been established across the United States to provide care for women with breast problems, whether benign or malignant. Major goals of breast cancer centers include educating the public about risk-factor reduction; providing of breast examinations; instructing women in BSE techniques; initiating referrals for screening, diagnosis, and treatment; and increasing the detection of breast cancer in its early localized stage. The empowerment and education of women to take an active role in promoting their own personal breast health care is a positive outgrowth of breast cancer centers.

A Nursing Care Plan for a patient with breast cancer undergoing mastectomy and immediate breast reconstruction with a TRAM flap can be found on pp. 1814 to 1816.

GERONTOLOGIC CONSIDERATIONS

Nearly half of all breast cancers occur in women more than 65 years old. Advanced-stage breast cancer is more often detected in elderly women than in their younger counterparts. One reason for this occurrence may be that elderly women tend to receive less instruction on BSE technique and less encouragement to perform it on a regular schedule.[26,30] Many older women are reluctant to touch and examine their breasts even with appropriate teaching. In addition, older women may not be aware of their increased vulnerability to cancer, especially breast cancer, nor know the suspicious signs and symptoms that they should report to the physician.

Changes occurring in the breast as a result of aging—such as fibrosis, calcification, shrinkage, and loss of subcutaneous fat—may cause confusion regarding changes that are normal for aging and those that may indicate a possible malignant condition. Women with arthritis may have difficulty performing BSE and may discontinue the practice altogether.

Other factors that affect early diagnosis of cancer and successful treatment may be related to the socioeconomic status of older adults. Retirement with reduced financial resources and the lack of health insurance beyond Medicare/Medicaid may deter older women from seeking medical care for a breast

Guidelines for Safe Practice

Arm Precautions After Mastectomy

- Ensure that the affected arm is never used for blood pressure, injections, or venipunctures.
- Wear no constricting clothing or jewelry, including wrist watch, on affected arm.
- Do not carry heavy objects (pocketbook, packages) in affected arm.
- Wear rubber gloves when washing dishes.
- Use unaffected arm when removing items from hot oven, or protect by wearing a padded glove pot holder.
- Use a thimble when sewing; wash needle pricks and cover as necessary.
- Take care when trimming fingernails and cuticles; avoid using scissors for this task.
- Use softening lotions or creams to keep skin in soft; supple condition.
- Outdoor activities:
  - Wear gloves when gardening.
  - Avoid sunburn—wear protective clothing or use sunscreen liberally.
  - Use insect repellent when in an area where biting or stinging insects may be located.
  - Tend to cuts and scratches immediately by washing and applying protective covering.

Adapted from Rockson SG: Precipitating factors in lymphedema: myths and realities, *Cancer* 83:2814, 1998.

Guidelines for Safe Practice

Breast Cancer Screening in Asymptomatic Patients

TEST OR EXAMINATION	AGE	RECOMMENDATION
Breast self-examination	20 and older	Monthly
Breast physical	20-39	Every 3 years
Mammogram	40+	Annually

Adapted from American Cancer Society: *1999-2000 breast cancer facts and figures*, New York, 1999, The American Cancer Society.

Nursing Care Plan *Patient With Breast Cancer Undergoing Mastectomy and Immediate Breast Reconstruction With a TRAM Flap*

DATA Mrs. J. is a widowed 53-year-old Caucasian woman who has been admitted to the surgical unit with the diagnosis of cancer of the left breast. Mrs. J. had her annual mammogram 1 week before admission, at which time a 2-cm lesion was revealed. Tissue reports following needle biopsy confirmed the presence of infiltrative ductal carcinoma. Treatment options were discussed. Since the lesion was small and in a localized stage (stage I to II), Mrs. J. elected to undergo mastectomy and immediate reconstruction using the transverse rectus abdominis muscle (TRAM) flap procedure. Construction of a new areola and nipple are planned to take place after surgical healing has been achieved.

Routine preoperative orders included a complete blood count, urinalysis, electrocardiogram, chest x-ray study, bowel preparation, and nothing by mouth (NPO) status after midnight. Nursing orders included assessing Mrs. J.'s understanding of the impending surgical procedure; assessing any concerns or fears not previously discussed; preoperative teaching regarding turning and breathing techniques; teaching regarding the need for a nasogastric tube (optional), an indwelling urinary catheter, incentive spirometry, and antiembolism stockings; and teaching regarding the method of pain control (patient-controlled analgesia [PCA] pump), nutrition plan (NPO status to clear liquids to regular food as tolerated), positioning and mobility postoperatively, and Mrs. J.'s expected involvement in her postoperative recovery. The nurse also initiated a referral to Reach to Recovery for a visit by a volunteer who had undergone TRAM flap reconstruction.

The nursing history reveals that Mrs. J.:

- Performs monthly breast self-examination (BSE) and has a yearly mammogram
- Has no known family history of breast cancer in first-degree relatives (mother, sister)
- Has excellent family support available and employer health insurance that provides complete coverage for surgical reconstruction
- Is in good general health, does not smoke, and only drinks alcohol socially
- Has two pints of her own blood reserved to be administered as needed during or after the surgical procedure

Collaborative nursing actions include monitoring for:

- Signs of infection: redness, swelling, purulent drainage, pain at site, and elevated temperature
- Signs of neurovascular changes in the TRAM flap: decreased capillary refill, warmth, increased swelling, and loss of sensation

NURSING DIAGNOSIS **Deficient knowledge related to lack of exposure to physical and cosmetic changes after mastectomy and TRAM flap reconstruction**

GOALS/OUTCOMES Will verbalize understanding of surgery, recovery, and rehabilitation

NOC Suggested Outcomes

- Knowledge: Infection Control (1807)
- Knowledge: Prescribed Activity (1811)
- Knowledge: Treatment Procedures (1814)
- Knowledge: Treatment Regimen (1813)

NIC Suggested Interventions

- Teaching: Individual (5606)
- Teaching: Prescribed Activity/Exercise (5612)
- Teaching: Prescribed Procedure/Treatment (5618)

Nursing Interventions/Rationales

- Clarify location of TRAM flap from site of lower abdomen; also explain that removal of muscle flap will result in some abdominal weakness and an abdominal scar. *Provides a knowledge base to enable a full understanding of the procedure so that the patient will not be surprised or frightened.*
- Reinforce that surgery will take about 7 hours to complete, hospitalization will be 6 to 7 days, and employment can be resumed in about 6 weeks. Explain that a second surgery will be required to reconstruct an areola and nipple. *To prepare the patient for the need to continue therapy on an outpatient basis following discharge from the hospital.*
- Show pictures of reconstructed breast mounds. Indicate that the mound will have feelings of sensation and pressure. Explain that reconstructed breast will be similar in size to original breast if adequate abdominal tissue is available. *Provides realistic expectation of appearance and feel of reconstructed breast.*
- Instruct patient to gradually increase activities and exercise over a 3-month period. *Activities and exercises are increased as strength and endurance return.*
- Initiate referral to American Cancer Society Reach to Recovery Program for a visit from a volunteer who has undergone mastectomy with TRAM flap reconstruction. *Provides support from a woman with the same diagnosis, surgical reconstruction, and concerns.*

Evaluation Parameters

1. Accurately discusses location of donor site and aftereffects, length of recovery, and rehabilitation
2. Accurately describes appearance of new breast mound
3. Maintains activity/mobility restrictions
4. Receptive to visit from Reach to Recovery volunteer

Nursing Care Plan — *Patient With Breast Cancer Undergoing Mastectomy and Immediate Breast Reconstruction With a TRAM Flap—cont'd*

NURSING DIAGNOSIS **Ineffective tissue perfusion to affected arm related to compromised circulation and lymphatic drainage following TRAM flap breast reconstruction**
GOALS/OUTCOMES Will remain free of circulatory compromise or lymphatic stasis

NOC Suggested Outcomes
- Risk Control (1902)
- Tissue Integrity: Skin and Mucous Membranes (1101)
- Tissue Perfusion: Peripheral (0407)

NIC Suggested Interventions
- Skin Surveillance (3590)
- Positioning (0840)
- Neurologic Monitoring (2620)

Nursing Interventions/Rationales
- Assess flap every hour for 24 hours, then every 2 to 4 hours, for capillary refill, color, warmth, edema, and decreased sensation. Use Doppler if necessary. *To monitor viability of flap and adequacy of blood supply.*
- Perform neurovascular checks in affected arm every hour for 24 hours, then every 2 to 4 hours. Teach patient how to perform checks when able to participate. *Lymphedema may be present with axillary node dissection. Lymphedema causes pressure on peripheral nerves, leading to a cool, pale extremity, diminished pulse, and poor movement.*
- Check drainage devices at TRAM flap and axillary area for patency, amount, color, and consistency each shift. Document changes and report to physician. *Increased drainage may indicate that the drain is improperly placed or obstructed, leading to lymphedema or impaired circulation at the flap.*

Evaluation Parameters
1. Good capillary refill in affected limb
2. Maintains full sensation in affected limb
3. Drainage devices patent
4. No evidence of decreased tissue perfusion

NURSING DIAGNOSIS **Acute pain related to surgical procedure (graft and mastectomy)**
GOALS/OUTCOMES Will achieve pain-free status

NOC Suggested Outcomes
- Pain Level (2102)
- Pain Control (1605)

NIC Suggested Interventions
- Pain Management (1400)
- Progressive Muscle Relaxation (1460)
- Positioning (0840)

Nursing Interventions/Rationales
- Assess duration and intensity of pain. *To monitor effectiveness of pain control measures.*
- Administer prescribed analgesics to provide maximum level of comfort. If using PCA pump, assess ability to use correctly. *Freedom from pain promotes patient cooperation and compliance with the plan of care. A PCA pump provides the patient with some control in pain management.*
- Elevate affected arm on pillow as directed. Position in semi-Fowler's position with knees flexed and elevated on a pillow when in bed. *Promotes lymphatic and venous return and helps prevent lymphedema, which increases pain.*
- Use abdominal binder if ordered. *Reduces strain on the abdominal incision and promotes healing and competency of abdominal muscles necessary in the performance of daily activities.*
- Assist with turning and ambulation. *To promote mobility without increasing pain.*
- Restrict upper extremity exercise/activity until permitted by physician. *Reduces strain on incision and helps prevent lymphedema.*
- Secure drainage devices properly (two at breast and two in abdominal wound). Check function every 2 hours. *Prevents hematoma or seroma formation, pressure on incision line, and risk of infection. Drainage becomes clear as healing progresses.*

Evaluation Parameters
1. Decreased complaints of pain
2. Decreased use of analgesics
3. Voices satisfaction with pain control methods

Continued

Nursing Care Plan — *Patient With Breast Cancer Undergoing Mastectomy and Immediate Breast Reconstruction With a TRAM Flap–cont'd*

NURSING DIAGNOSIS **Risk for infection related to mastectomy, axillary node dissection, abdominal wound, and invasive equipment (intravenous [IV] lines, catheter, drains)**

GOALS/OUTCOMES Will remain free of infection

NOC Suggested Outcomes
- Risk Control (1902)
- Infection Status (0703)
- Immune Status (0702)

NIC Suggested Interventions
- Infection Protection (6550)
- Wound Care (3660)
- Surveillance (6550)

Nursing Interventions/Rationales
- Assist with performing deep breathing, turning every 2 hours, and incentive spirometry. Splint abdomen for coughing. Encourage early ambulation as permitted. *To prevent inadequate respiratory efforts and pooling of secretions that cause respiratory infection.*
- Assess for signs and symptoms of infection (elevation of temperature, redness, swelling, pain, and purulent drainage). *Provides for early recognition and treatment.*
- Teach patient signs and symptoms of infection. *So the patient can recognize and report infection to ensure early treatment.*
- Perform drain care using sterile technique. Teach patient how to perform drain care before discharge and the need for good hand-washing technique. *Promotes patient involvement and self-care before discharge. Decreases the risk for infection.*
- Monitor invasive equipment as a cause of infection. Document and report findings. *Provides for early detection and treatment if needed.*
- Post sign in room alerting staff not to use affected arm for blood pressure measurements, injections, venipuncture, or IV lines. Inform patient of guidelines to follow to protect herself from infection. *Lymph node dissection disrupts lymphatic function. An inflated blood pressure cuff can obstruct lymph flow through channels and increase damage. Injections and venipunctures cause breaks in skin and provide a source for infection.*

Evaluation Parameters
1. Accurately lists signs and symptoms of infection
2. Absence of fever
3. Absence of wound redness, warmth, swelling, tenderness, and purulent drainage
4. White blood cell count within normal limits

NURSING DIAGNOSIS **Ineffective therapeutic regimen management related to lack of knowledge regarding long-term recovery and rehabilitation**

GOALS/OUTCOMES Will assume self-care and carry out therapeutic regimen as prescribed

NOC Suggested Outcomes
- Adherence Behavior (1600)
- Knowledge: Treatment Regimen (1813)
- Participation: Health Care Decisions (1606)

NIC Suggested Interventions
- Teaching: Individual (5606)
- Family Support (7140)
- Mutual Goal Setting (4410)

Nursing Interventions/Rationales
- Teach wound care and care of drainage devices following discharge, and have patient return demonstration. *Demonstration and return demonstration along with written instructions give the patient/family confidence in their ability to carry out the therapeutic regimen accurately.*
- Teach patient activity limitations (see text) and the need to protect the reconstructed breast from pressure until healed. *To prevent complications from occurring and to ensure full recovery and rehabilitation.*
- Reinforce BSE technique and compliment patient's past adherence. Discuss the need to continue BSE and mammograms with new and remaining breast. *Provides a means of detecting recurrence of breast cancer. Complimenting the patient's past adherence to BSE increases self-confidence and reinforces future adherence.*

Evaluation Parameters
1. Accurately describes exercise, wound care, and activity limits
2. Adheres to therapeutic regimen
3. Progressively assumes self-care without difficulty
4. Participates in care planning and goal setting

lump. Financial concerns about ability to pay for long-term chemotherapy or radiation therapy may cause them to terminate treatment. Becoming a burden, both physically and financially, on their families is frequently a concern of the elderly patient with cancer.[10,49]

Older women may also be offered fewer breast cancer treatment options. Mastectomy, rather than the conservative surgical lumpectomy procedure, is frequently the only surgical treatment advised for older women, even those with early, localized disease and negative nodes.[48]

The nurse must encourage the older woman to participate in cancer screening and detection programs, have a yearly mammogram, and perform monthly BSE. The nurse should also act as a patient advocate when treatment options are being presented and advised.

SPECIAL ENVIRONMENTS FOR CARE

Critical Care Management

The critical care setting is seldom used for the care of early-stage breast cancer patients. An exception may be a patient with a comorbid condition, such as diabetes or emphysema, that could complicate normal recovery and require more intensive nursing care. The older patient is more likely to have a chronic or acute comorbid condition that would benefit from close nursing and medical management.

Home Care Management

For most women the home has become the setting in which recovery and rehabilitation after breast cancer treatment take place. Women who will receive additional treatment with radiation or chemotherapy should be provided with information about when and where treatment will begin and why it is necessary to keep all follow-up appointments. If a tissue expander was used for breast reconstruction, the nurse provides the patient with information about the timing of subsequent injections of saline solution into the implant. The nurse advises the woman that the procedure is uncomfortable because the muscle overlying the expander is stretched immediately after each injection. Once the muscle has been stretched to the desired size, the expander may be removed or left in place over the implant. If an autogenous tissue flap was created, nipple reconstruction may be planned after the operative site has healed.

Unfortunately, breast cancer can recur or develop in the remaining breast. Therefore the nurse determines the patient's knowledge and skill in the performance of BSE. If necessary, the proper procedure should be demonstrated and a pamphlet on BSE provided. Because breast cancer has a tendency to recur at the incision line, the nurse teaches the patient how to assess this area. Follow-up mammograms and clinical breast examinations are an integral part of long-term care. The necessity for these examinations cannot be overstressed.

The ACS is an important resource for all cancer patients. Reach to Recovery volunteers are available to meet with patients after discharge to answer questions and address concerns. Some will make home visits, accompany the patient in purchasing a permanent prosthesis and brassiere, and talk about breast-reconstruction issues. Other ACS volunteer groups, such as I Can Cope, are helpful to persons who need support in coping with life after cancer. Family members frequently find needed support from this group as well.

COMPLICATIONS

The woman who has undergone treatment for breast cancer will always live with the fear of recurrent disease even when the cancer was found and treated in an early, localized stage. Recurrent disease can develop within months of initial treatment or many years later. It is important that all women, regardless of age or stage of disease, be reminded to report the presence of symptoms such as bone pain or changes at the incision site, which could indicate disease recurrence or the presence of distant metastasis.

In addition to recurrence, the development of lymphedema is a dreaded complication of breast cancer treatment. Along with deformity, disability and discomfort are experienced, and recurrent episodes of lymphangitis and cellulitis may be expected.[43] Lymphedema is a serious problem that requires a physician's evaluation for the institution of a proper treatment regimen. It is important for patients with lymphedema to be treated by a physician or clinic that can offer therapeutic treatment for this condition. Presently, there are not enough centers available or clinicians with specialized training in management of severe lymphedema to provide a comprehensive treatment program for women. Nurses can assist women with finding treatment centers through contacting the National Lymphedema Network and the American Cancer Society.

The threat of trauma and infection after mastectomy and node dissection is ever present and requires that the woman comply with the aforementioned arm precautions. If signs and symptoms of trauma or infection occur, the woman is advised to inform her physician immediately so that appropriate measures can be instituted.

NONMALIGNANT CONDITIONS OF THE BREAST

Benign breast disease is common and accounts for about 90% of all breast problems. Because there is no universally accepted classification system for benign disorders, the term fibrocystic disease has been used as an umbrella category into which most benign disorders are placed. This has resulted in confusion in diagnosing and treating patients with benign conditions.

CYSTIC BREAST DISEASE

Etiology/Epidemiology

The underlying cause of cystic breast disease is not fully known. Changes in the breast are cyclic and thought to be caused by hormonal imbalance or the exaggerated response of breast tissue to ovarian hormones. Breast tenderness is more pronounced during or before menstruation. Cystic breast disease is most common in nulliparous women between the ages of 40 and 50 years but can occur at any age. Occurrence is least frequent after menopause.

Pathophysiology

A number of commonalities are seen in cystic disease, regardless of the diagnostic name used. Changes once thought to be abnormal such as microcysts, apocrine change, adenosis, fibrosis, and varying degrees of hyperplasia are now recognized as part of the involutional process of the breast. These changes include the presence of lumps of varying size, nipple discharge, and breast pain (mastodynia). Cystic lesions are soft, well demarcated, and freely movable. The process is almost always bilateral, with most lesions located in the left breast. The cysts may contain clear, milky, straw-colored, or yellow to dark brown fluid. Occasionally the contents may be blood-tinged. The common clinical manifestations of fibroadenomas and fibrocystic disease of the breast are compared in Table 54-3.

Collaborative Care Management

The woman who discovers a mass or masses in her breast should seek the advice of a health care provider who will decide whether aspiration or biopsy should be performed. A needle aspiration generally confirms the presence of a cyst. Because the presence of nodular tissue in the breast makes the early detection of malignant lesions more difficult, some physicians suggest periodic mammograms to detect any changes. There is no evidence to suggest that cystic disease predisposes women to the development of a malignant lesion, but these women are at more risk than those without cystic disease.

The traditional treatment of fibrocystic disease consists of diuretics and restrictions in fluid and salt intake. The limitation or exclusion of methylxanthines (a class of chemicals found in coffee, tea, cola, and chocolate) is frequently recommended as a means of controlling cystic disease, but there is no research evidence that methylxanthines is associated with benign breast disease.[32]

Vitamin therapy, especially vitamin E, may have some anticancer properties, but again, no conclusive evidence exists that vitamin E therapy reduces the risk of cancer or relieves the distress of cystic breast disease. Danazol and bromocriptine have been tried for symptom relief but ineffectiveness and unpleasant side effects have precluded their use.[32] Studies of tamoxifen are ongoing. Some women with cystic disease have reported results that range from some regression of lesions to the complete disappearance of breast pain with tamoxifen use, but its appropriateness for cystic breast disease has not been established.

Patient/Family Education. The role of the nurse in the care of patients with benign breast disorders is primarily that of educator and facilitator. The nurse should be knowledgeable about benign conditions, understand their medical management, provide and clarify information, and support the patient, emotionally and physically, through diagnosis and treatment.

Hospitalization is seldom required for the treatment of cystic breast disease. The nurse teaches BSE to those women who are not familiar with it and stresses its use every month. Women should be taught to recognize through touch their normal breast tissue and the location and size of any lesions present. They should report significant changes that differ from the normal cyclic fluctuations or that appear at a different time in the menstrual cycle. The use of a mild analgesic and wearing a firm supportive brassiere may provide comfort and reduce pain on movement. The use of warm, moist heat also may be beneficial to relieve aching pain. Eliminating caffeine consumption and decreasing salt content before menstruation to relieve bloating and weight gain can be recommended. The woman is advised to consult her health care provider before using vitamin E as a therapeutic intervention, so its beneficial effects, if any, can be professionally monitored. Side effects of vitamin E use are few.

FIBROADENOMA

Etiology/Epidemiology

Fibroadenomas, or adenofibromas, are the most common benign breast neoplasms. The tumors occur most often in women younger than 25 years old; some lesions become evident by age 15. Fibroadenomas usually are firm, rubbery, round, freely movable, nontender, and encapsulated; they may be multiple and bilateral. Tumor size ranges from 1 to 3 cm. A "giant" fibroma is the most common lesion seen in the adolescent breast.

TABLE 54-3 Clinical Manifestations of Fibroadenomas and Fibrocystic Disease of the Breast

	Fibroadenoma	Fibrocystic Disease
Likely age	15-20, can occur up to 55	30-55, decreases after menopause
Shape	Round, lobular	Round, lobular
Consistency	Usually firm, can be soft	Firm to soft, rubbery
Demarcation	Well demarcated, clear margins	Well demarcated
Number	Usually single	Multiple usually, may be single
Mobility	Very mobile, slippery	Mobile
Tenderness	Usually none	Tender, increases before menses
Skin retraction	None	None
Pattern of growth	Grows quickly and constantly	Size may increase or decrease rapidly
Risk to health	None: benign; must diagnose by biopsy	Benign, although general lumpiness may mask other cancerous lumps

From Jarvis C: *Physical examination and health assessment,* ed 3, Philadelphia, 2000, WB Saunders.

Pathophysiology

Fibroadenomas are estrogen-dependent tumors of fibroblastic and epithelial origin, and usually associated with menstrual irregularities. Fibroadenomas are slow growing and often are stimulated by pregnancy and lactation. Regression may occur after delivery. At menopause, they tend to regress and become hyalinized. "Giant" fibroadenomas grow rapidly to 10 to 12 cm in diameter but are not more prone to malignant change than smaller lesions. Dimpling or nipple retraction is not associated with fibroadenomas.

Collaborative Care Management

Surgical removal is the standard treatment for fibroadenomas. Many can be removed under local anesthesia in an outpatient setting. Although the tumor is examined for definitive pathologic characteristics, the association between fibroadenomas and cancer is weak.

Patient/Family Education. When the woman discovers a breast mass, her primary concern is always a diagnosis of cancer. Reassurance that most breast lesions are not malignant should be avoided. Only the final pathology report will provide this reassurance. Before the surgical removal of the fibroadenoma, the nurse prepares the woman for the type of surgery to be performed, what to expect during the procedure, and how to care for the incision afterward. Practice of BSE should be encouraged, as well as the reporting of any unusual changes found during the examination.

INFLAMMATORY LESIONS

Mammary Duct Ectasia

Etiology/Epidemiology

Mammary duct ectasia, also referred to as plasma cell mastitis, is a benign condition of unknown etiology. Some investigators believe an anaerobic bacteria may be implicated. Another causative factor may be bacterial infection that results from stasis of fluid in the large ducts of the breast. Age is the primary risk factor for duct ectasia, with a mean age ranging from 45 to 55 years. Breast pain and a palpable mass are typical symptoms in premenopausal women, nipple discharge predominates in perimenopausal women, and nipple retractions secondary to periductal fibrosis are more often noted in postmenopausal women.

Pathophysiology

Mammary duct ectasia involves inflammation of the ducts behind the nipple, duct enlargement, and a collection of cellular debris and fluid in the involved ducts. As the inflammatory response resolves, the ducts become fibrotic and dilated. Nipple discharge usually is bilateral and ranges from serous to thick, sticky, or pastelike. Drainage may be green, greenish brown, or blood stained. Nipple itching, suggestive of Paget's disease, may accompany transient pain in the subareolar and inner quadrants of the breast. On palpation the areolar area may feel wormlike; the nipple may be red and swollen or flat and retracted. The condition is not associated with breastfeeding.

Collaborative Care Management

Treatment varies, depending on the severity of the problem. Because of the chronic nature of this problem, most women are monitored with routine physical examination of the breast. The symptoms of mammary duct ectasia may engender the fear of malignant disease in the patient. Once the benign nature of this chronic condition is affirmed, fears generally are dispelled, and most women are able to deal with their symptoms. Although there is no cure for mammary duct ectasia, antibiotics are prescribed for acute inflammatory episodes, such as the development of an abscess. If the chronic discharge can no longer be tolerated, surgical excision of the retroareolar ducts is performed.

Patient/Family Education. The nurse must be cognizant of the chronic yet benign nature of this condition and offer support and understanding care. The woman is taught how to cleanse the breast to minimize the risk of infection. Good hand washing and personal hygiene measures are stressed. Wearing a supportive yet nonconfining brassiere padded with sterile gauze and changing the brassiere daily or as necessary helps prevent abscess formation. The nurse teaches the woman the signs and symptoms indicative of abscess that should be reported immediately.

Acute Mastitis and Abscess

Etiology/Epidemiology

There are two forms of mastitis: acute and chronic. The acute form is a rare condition almost always found in breastfeeding mothers during the first 4 months of lactation. It occurs most frequently from *Staphylococcus aureus* or *Staphylococcus epidermidis* infection that spreads from a break in the skin surface of the nipple to underlying breast tissue. It may be confined to only one quadrant of the breast. Symptoms include a fissured nipple, fever, chill, localized tenderness, and erythema. Purulent discharge from the nipple is usually not observed.

The chronic form of mastitis can follow acute mastitis or have a slow and insidious onset. Both acute and chronic mastitis are caused by the same bacterial agents. The chronic form occurs more often in older women, and the symptoms can mimic inflammatory breast cancer. The infection usually arises in the sweat or sebaceous glands and spreads to the breast. Symptoms of chronic mastitis include a painful breast mass that involves the nipple and areola and a low-grade fever.

Pathophysiology

In both acute and chronic mastitis there is edema and congestion of the periductal and interlobular stomata. The ducts are distended from the accumulation of neutrophils and retained secretions. If an abscess forms, its central core may be necrotic and contain creamy, yellow exudate. Fibrosis of the involved tissue can develop after treatment. Both the acute and chronic forms of mastitis should be investigated for inflammatory breast carcinoma, but recent lactation usually excludes the acute form from the need for further evaluation.

Collaborative Care Management

Acute mastitis is easy to diagnose in a nursing mother. Treatment with antibiotics resolves the infectious process. In older women, because the condition has similarities to inflammatory breast carcinoma, incision and drainage of the inflammatory exudate are performed to determine the cause. Antibiotics can then be prescribed. In cases where the condition is unresponsive to antibiotics, a complete ductal excision may be performed.[32]

Patient/Family Education. When acute mastitis is the result of an infection during lactation, most women immediately stop breastfeeding. Women should be informed that discontinuing breastfeeding is not always necessary or advisable. The infant is not affected by sucking on the involved breasts and symptoms are usually relieved within 48 hours of antibiotic treatment.[32] Continued breastfeeding is believed to reduce the pain and lessen the volume of milk that can be a source for bacterial growth. If breastfeeding is discontinued, the woman is instructed to keep her breasts as empty as possible by pumping. If the breast is not emptied, it becomes engorged, and pain increases. The woman is instructed to complete the entire course of antibiotics and not discontinue them when symptoms are relieved. Because the infection generally does not originate in the breast, teaching about personal hygiene measures is important. The older woman with mastitis may be anxious about a diagnosis of cancer. Emotional support and frank discussion of her concerns are provided until the aspiration biopsy results are known.

Both acute and chronic mastitis resolve with antibiotic therapy, rest, and the application of local heat. Discomfort generally is relieved by analgesics.

MALE BREAST PROBLEMS

GYNECOMASTIA

Etiology/Epidemiology

Gynecomastia is a common disorder of the male breast. This condition is estimated to occur in up to 70% of pubertal boys during the time of rapid testicular growth between the ages of 12 and 15 years. Symptoms include a firm, circular, disklike, circumscribed, tender mass beneath the areola, usually bilateral at onset. In adolescent boys the condition is transient and lasts for approximately 12 to 24 months. Gynecomastia is seen again in men ages 45 years and older, with 40% of elderly men having some degree of the condition.[44] Gynecomastia is seen in obese men because obesity increases the rate of conversion of androgens to estrogen and in patients with cirrhosis of the liver, because of the incomplete hepatic clearance of estrogen. Gynecomastia may develop in men who are receiving drugs such as estrogen, cimetidine, certain antibiotics (isoniazid), antihypertensive agents (reserpine and methyldopa), calcium channel blockers, and digoxin.[18]

Pathophysiology

Gynecomastia is caused by hormonal imbalance. As a result of the large estrogen secretion, hyperplasia (overdevelopment) of the stomata and ducts in the mammary glands occurs. The primary cause of gynecomastia in the older man is the aging process. As men age, the plasma testosterone concentration declines at the same time that the plasma testosterone-estrogen level increases. Thus less free testosterone is available.

Collaborative Care Management

When gynecomastia occurs and the condition cannot be attributed to rapid testicular growth (teenaged boys), treatment with estrogen therapy (middle-aged men), or hepatic dysfunction, a human chorionic gonadotropin-beta subunit (hCG-*b*) level should be obtained. This finding assists in ruling out a malignant testicular germ cell condition, which can manifest with gynecomastia and an elevated hCG-*b* level. Chest and mediastinal roentgenograms and a careful testes examination are also included in the evaluation. In older men the physician may suggest obtaining a breast biopsy specimen because this age group is more prone to male breast cancer. Surgery is used for cosmesis only when the gynecomastia persists over a long time and is not associated with an underlying disease process.

Patient/Family Education. The nurse who cares for men with gynecomastia must offer sympathetic understanding. Most men are intensely embarrassed about the condition because enlarged breasts constitute a serious assault on the male self-image. The condition is visible whenever the man removes his shirt for work or recreation and frequently results in taunts and jokes. Similar problems exist for the man who undergoes mastectomy for breast cancer and is visibly asymmetric. The problems and needs of these patients have not been fully recognized.

Patients who are treated with hormonal therapy for prostate cancer should be warned that gynecomastia is one of the side effects of treatment. Treatment of cancer takes priority over breast enlargement, but it may still constitute a psychologic stress for the man. Elderly men should be informed that with normal aging, breast enlargement may occur. If the man is obese and elderly, the enlargement may be more pronounced. The nurse should be aware of the variety of drugs, other than hormones, that can increase male breast size. Men should be forewarned of this side effect.

MALE BREAST CANCER

Etiology/Epidemiology

Male breast cancer is a rare disease and often presents late with a poor prognosis. It accounts for approximately 1% of breast cancer incidence and mortality.[3] The epidemiology and clinical features of the disease generally parallel those of female breast cancer. Men with breast cancer tend to be older and have subareolar tumors, and their disease is found in more advanced stages as compared to women with breast cancer.[12] A family history places men at increased risk for breast cancer, as does prior exposure to radiation, exogenous estrogen therapy, and Klinefelter's syndrome. Gynecomastia is a controversial risk factor, with several studies reporting conflicting correlations with breast cancer.[21]

Pathophysiology

Approximately 75% to 100% of breast cancers in men are ER positive, with ductal infiltrating carcinoma being the predominant histologic cell type.[21] Bioassay for the presence of ER and PR is performed at the time of biopsy. Tumor staging is based on the TNM system.

Physical examination, mammography, fine-needle aspiration, and incisional or excisional biopsy are standard diagnostic procedures. The presence of advanced disease at the time of initial diagnosis is common, largely because of delays in seeking medical evaluation that average 12 to 24 months.[21]

Gynecomastia caused by drug, alcohol, or hormone ingestion can be differentiated from a malignant lesion by both physical examination and mammogram. Fine-needle aspiration of the lesion may also be used to differentiate gynecomastia from a malignancy. Gynecomastia generally is bilateral, whereas a malignant lesion generally occurs in a single breast.

The symptoms commonly seen at the time of diagnosis include a firm mass directly beneath the nipple in the subareolar area, most frequently in the left breast. A lesion in the upper outer quadrant is the next most frequent location for tumor growth. Bloody nipple discharge with nipple inversion is common. Evidence of Paget's disease of the nipple (eczema), itching, ulceration, and local tenderness also may be present. Metastasis may occur to bone, the lungs, and the liver.

Collaborative Care Management

Treatment for a primary localized tumor is modified radical mastectomy with node dissection. Breast-sparing procedures are not often used because of the belief that men do not have the psychologic need for this body image-sparing procedure. In addition, the typical location of the lesion in the subareolar area requires that the nipple be removed along with a tumor-free margin of tissue. Thus breast-preservation procedures cannot be safely used. Radiation therapy may be prescribed before or after surgery for control of micrometastasis or to prevent local recurrence, but radiation has not been shown to significantly increase long-term disease-free survival time.[21] When axillary nodes are involved in the disease process, systemic adjuvant therapy (chemotherapy or hormonal) is advised.

Recurrent or advanced disease is highly amenable to palliative therapy with hormonal manipulation inasmuch as most tumors are ER positive. Tamoxifen is the treatment of choice for metastatic disease. Additional hormonal agents that may be used include progestins, LHRH agonists, and aminoglutethimide.[1] Chemotherapy protocols such as cyclophosphamide, methotrexate, and 5-fluorouracil (CMF), and 5-fluorouracil, Adriamycin (doxorubicin), and cyclophosphamide (FAC) may be prescribed.

Patient/Family Education. Nursing management of the man with breast cancer reflects the basic principles outlined earlier in the chapter. However, a man in whom breast cancer is diagnosed faces unique psychosocial stressors that the nurse needs to address on an individual basis. The long delays in diagnosis may reflect in part a basic disbelief that this "female problem" can be occurring. A subtheme of embarrassment needs to be identified, if present, and acknowledged. The threats of cancer remain present, however, and the treatment is aggressive. The use of tamoxifen has reduced the need for palliative surgeries such as orchiectomy, with their accompanying assault on male self-concept and body image. The male patient treated for breast cancer is an uncommon occurrence; however, the nurse will need to be sensitive to his unique needs and tailor the standard surgical care routines to the individual situation.

Critical Thinking Questions

1. A 78-year-old widow is recovering from a modified radical mastectomy for stage II ductal carcinoma. She has a history of osteoarthritis and hypertension. She is undergoing chemotherapy and tamoxifen therapy. Discuss the issues that may impact on the quality of life of this patient as a result of her age, diagnosis, treatment regimen, and psychosocial needs. What interventions should you plan for her?
2. A 39-year-old woman underwent a modified radical mastectomy and has been receiving weekly chemotherapy treatments, which have left her fatigued and weak. She tells you that she has decided to quit chemotherapy because, "I have four children to look after, my husband already works two jobs, and he can't be expected to manage the house also. I can't be much of a wife to him since this surgery anyway—the least I can do is meet my responsibilities as a mother." You know that 6 more months of chemotherapy have been planned. What major concerns do you have for her and what interventions would you plan to help her?
3. Use the research information presented in the chapter to discuss the importance of BSE and mammography as diagnostic tools for breast cancer. What nursing strategies would be helpful in overcoming barriers to earlier breast cancer detection?

References

1. Anderson-Reitz L, Mechling B, Hertz SL: High dose therapy for treatment of breast cancer, *Nurse Pract Forum* 10(3):154, 1999.
2. Andolina VF, Lille SL, Willison KM: *Mammographic imaging: a practical guide*, Philadelphia, 1992, JB Lippincott.
3. American Cancer Society: *1999-2000 breast cancer facts and figures*, New York, 1999, The American Cancer Society.
4. Baquet CR, Commiskey P: Socioeconomic factors and breast carcinoma in multicultural women, *Cancer Suppl* 88(5):1256, 2000.
5. Baron R: Sentinel lymph node biopsy in breast cancer and the role of the oncology nurse, *Clin J Oncol Nurs* 3(1):17, 1999.
6. Berman AJ: Supporting the home care client receiving chemotherapy, *Home Care Provid* 4(2):81, 1999.
7. Boshaw DL: New instrumentation allows for removal of nonpalpable breast lesions, *AORN J* 66(2):296, 1997.
8. Boyle P, Maisonneuve P, Autier P: Update on cancer control in women, *Int J Gynecol Obstet* 70:263, 2000.
9. Brennan MJ, Miller LT: Overview of treatment options and review of the current role and use of compression garments, intermittent pumps, and exercise in the management of lymphedema, *Cancer* 83:2821, 1998.
10. Cameron S, Horsburgh ME: Comparing issues faced by younger and older women with breast cancer, *Can Oncol Nurs J* 8:40, 1998.
11. Cole CF, Coleman C: Breast imaging today and tomorrow, *Nurse Pract Forum* 10(3):129, 1999.

12. Donegan WL: Cancer of the male breast, *J Gend Specif Med* 3(4):55, 2000.
13. Dow KH: Breast cancer. In Varricchio C, editor: *A cancer sourcebook for nurses,* ed 7, Sudbury, Mass, 1997, Jones and Bartlett International.
14. Fisher B et al: Endometrial cancer in tamoxifen treated breast cancer patients: findings from the National Surgical Adjuvant Breast and Bowel Project (NSABP) B-14, *J Natl Cancer Inst* 86(7):527, 1994.
15. Foelber R: Autologous stem cell transplant plus interleukin-2 for breast cancer: review and nursing management, *Oncol Nurs Forum* 25(3):563, 1998.
16. Goldhirsch A, Coates AS, Castiglione-Gertsch M, Gelber RD: New treatments for breast cancer: breakthroughs for patient care or just steps in the right direction? *Ann Oncol* 9:973, 1998.
17. Greenlee RT, Hill-Harmon MB, Murphy T, Thun M: Cancer statistics, 2001, *CA Cancer J Clin* 51(1):15, 2001.
18. Harris JR et al, editors: *Breast diseases,* ed 2, Philadelphia, 1999, Lippincott, Williams & Wilkins.
19. Hilakivi-Clarke L: Estrogens, BRCA1, and breast cancer, *Cancer Res* 60:4993, 2000.
20. Holm CJ, Frank DI, Curtin J: Health beliefs, health locus of control, and women's mammography behavior, *Cancer Nurs* 22(2):149, 1999.
21. Hsi A: Male breast cancer, University of Pennsylvania, 1997, website: www.oncolink.upenn.edu/disease/breast/mbc.html.
22. Hsueh EC, Hansen N, Giuliano AE: Intraoperative lymph node mapping and sentinel lymph node dissection in breast cancer, *CA Cancer J Clin* 50(5):279, 2000.
23. Hunter CP: Epidemiology, stage at diagnosis, and tumor biology of breast carcinoma in multiracial and multiethnic populations, *Cancer Suppl* 88(5):1193, 2000.
24. Jefferson TC: Ultrasound may markedly improve cancer detection in dense breasts, *JAMA* 281(4):311, 1999.
25. Joslyn SA, West MM: Racial differences in breast cancer survival, *Cancer* 88(1):114, 2000.
26. Kimmick G, Muss H: Breast cancer in older women, *Clin Geriatr Med* 13(2):265, 1997.
27. LaRossa D: Breast reconstructive surgery options, University of Pennsylvania, 1997, website: www.oncolink.upenn.edu/disease/breast/treat/recon/.
28. Lauver DR et al: Engagement in breast cancer screening behaviors, *Oncol Nurs Forum* 26(3):545, 1999.
29. Leslie N, Roche BG: The effectiveness of the breast self-examination facilitation shield, *Oncol Nurs Forum* 24(10):1759, 1997.
30. Lickley L: Primary breast cancer in the elderly, *Can J Surg* 40(5):341, 1997.
31. MacRae K, Humphreys A, Lind M: Home care for stem cell transplantation patients, *Prof Nurse* 15(2):87, 1999.
32. Marchant DJ: Controversies in benign breast disease, *Surg Oncol Clin North Am* 7(2):285, 1998.
33. Martin AM, Weber BL: Genetic and hormonal risk factors in breast cancer, *J Natl Cancer Inst* 92(14):1126, 2000.
34. McPherson K, Steel CM, Dixon JM: ABC of breast diseases: breast cancer-epidemiology, risk factors, and genetics, *Br Med J* 321(9):624, 2000.
35. Moran SL, Herceg S, Kurtelawicz K, Serletti JM: TRAM flap breast reconstruction with expanders and implants, *AORN J* 71(2):354, 2000.
36. Mrozek-Orlowski ME, Frye DK, Sanborn HM: Capecitabine: nursing implications of a new oral chemotherapeutic agent, *Oncol Nurs Forum* 26(4):753, 1999.
37. National Comprehensive Cancer Network: *Breast cancer treatment guidelines for patients,* Atlanta, 2000, American Cancer Society.
38. Neill KM, Briefs BA: Factors that influence plastic surgeons' advice about reconstruction to women with breast cancer, *Plast Surg Nurs* 17(2):61, 1997.
39. Newman J: Early detection techniques in breast cancer management, *Radiol Technol* 68(4):309, 1997.
40. Nogueria SM, Appling SE: Breast cancer genetics, risks, and strategies, *Nurs Clin North Am* 35(3):663, 2000.
41. Overmayer BA: Chemotherapy in the management of breast cancer, *Cleve Clin J Med* 62(1):36, 1995.
42. Pasacreta JV, McCorkle R: Providing accurate information to women about tamoxifen therapy for breast cancer: current indications, effects, and controversies, *Oncol Nurs Forum* 25(9):1577, 1998.
43. Petrek JA, Heelan MC: Incidence of breast carcinoma related lymphedema, *Cancer* 83:2776, 1998.
44. Powell DE, Stellilag CB, editors: *The diagnosis and detection of breast disease,* St Louis, 1994, Mosby.
45. Rosenzweig MQ, Rust D, Hoss J: Prognostic information in breast cancer care: helping patients utilize important information, *Clin J Oncol Nurs* 4(6):271, 2000.
46. Runowicz CD: Lymphedema: patient and provider education: current status and future trends, *Cancer* 83:2874, 1998.
47. Shuster TD, Girshovich L, Whitney TM, Hughes KS: Multidisciplinary care for patients with breast cancer, *Surg Clin North Am* 80(2):505, 2000.
48. Silliman R, Dukes K, Sullivan L, Kaplan S: Breast cancer in older women, *Cancer* 83(4):706, 1998.
49. Silliman R et al: The impact of age, marital status, and physician-patient interactions on the care of older women with breast carcinoma, *Cancer* 80(7):1326, 1997.
50. Snyder GM, Sielsch EC, Reville B: The controversy of hormone replacement therapy in breast cancer survivors, *Oncol Nurs Forum* 25(4):699, 1998.
51. Strauss B: Best hope or last hope: access to phase III clinical trials of HER-2/neu for advanced stage breast cancer patients, *J Adv Nurs* 31(2):259, 2000.
52. U.S. Department of Health and Human Services: *Healthy People 2010: understanding and improving health,* Washington, DC, 2000, USDHHS.
53. Wasaff B: Current status of hormonal treatments for metastatic breast cancer in postmenopausal women, *Oncol Nurs Forum* 24(9):1515, 1997.
54. Welykholowa NL: Lymphatic mapping and sentinal node biopsy: new technology for women's health, *Can Oper Room Nurs J* 16(3):18, 1998.

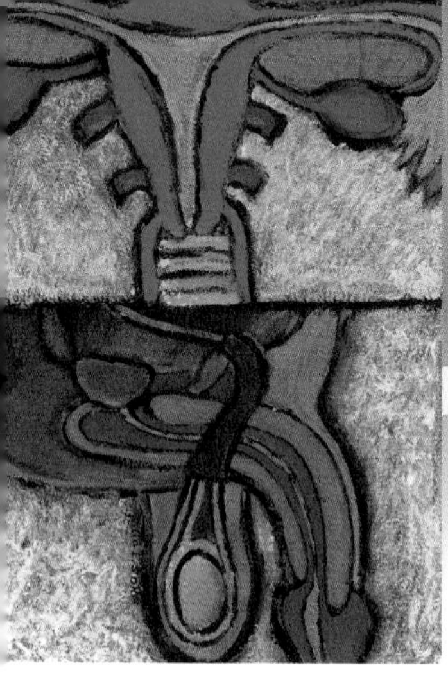

Male Reproductive Problems

55

Carolyn Eddins

Objectives

After studying this chapter, the learner should be able to:

1. Describe the process of infectious diseases specific to men's reproductive health.
2. Compare the nursing care associated with benign and malignant neoplasms that are specific to men's reproductive health.
3. Describe expected patient outcomes for each condition discussed.
4. Identify teaching needs for various treatments of male reproductive problems.
5. Compare the common causes of impotence, both physical and psychologic.
6. Discuss nursing interventions related to the structural and infectious problems presented in the chapter.
7. Identify the common complications related to the different problems of the male reproductive system.

Men's reproductive health care is one dimension of an emerging specialty area of nursing practice, men's health. Traditionally problems of the male reproductive system have been viewed only as problems related to aging or lifestyle choices. Often the complexity of the male reproductive system and the multiple psychosocial needs of the patient have been minimized by the health care system. Consequently, men often do not seek medical care until symptoms are well advanced. Also, myths and knowledge deficits related to the specifics of sexual function are common in the male population. It is important to provide health care that is sensitive, accurate, and timely for this population that often limits health care visits. The information in this chapter is divided into sections according to specific organ structures and functions of the male reproductive system. The focus is on the most common health problems of the male reproductive system. Particular emphasis is placed on common infections, problems of the prostate gland, and impotence. Sexually transmitted diseases are presented in Chapter 56. Figure 55-1 illustrates the male reproductive organs and associated structures.

PROBLEMS OF THE TESTES AND RELATED STRUCTURES

The scrotal sac contains the testes, epididymis, and part of the spermatic cord as well as other associated structures that include nerve, lymphatic, and vascular networks (Figure 55-2). These structures are responsible for the production and storage of sperm and provide the pathway for ejaculation. The testes are also involved in the production of hormones, primarily testosterone. Consequently, any disorders related to these structures have the potential to affect male fertility adversely, as well as interfere with testosterone production.

Pathologies of these structures include problems with swelling, twisting of cords, trauma, and carcinomas. The testes are particularly sensitive to changes in scrotal environment. Fluctuations in temperature and blood flow often have a negative affect on fertility. Infection is also a common problem. Accurately differentiating between pathologies related to infection versus structural problems or neoplasms can facilitate timely therapy and positively affect the patient's prognosis.

Epididymitis

Etiology/Epidemiology

The epididymis is a convoluted tubular structure within the scrotal sac that acts as a reservoir for sperm. While in this structure, sperm mature and become fertile and mobile. Epididymitis is an acute inflammatory process within the epididymis and is one of the most common intrascrotal inflammations in adult males. In the United States epididymitis accounts for more than 600,000 visits per year to health care providers.[24] This inflammation is rarely seen in children and occurs infrequently in the elderly adult male. The average age for patients presenting with epididymitis is 20 years.[24]

Inflammation of the epididymis most often is caused by an ascending infection via the ejaculatory duct through the vas deferens into the epididymis. Such infections can occur in three ways. First, infection may be introduced when surgical or diagnostic procedures are performed. This occurs more frequently among boys less than 15 years old and in men over

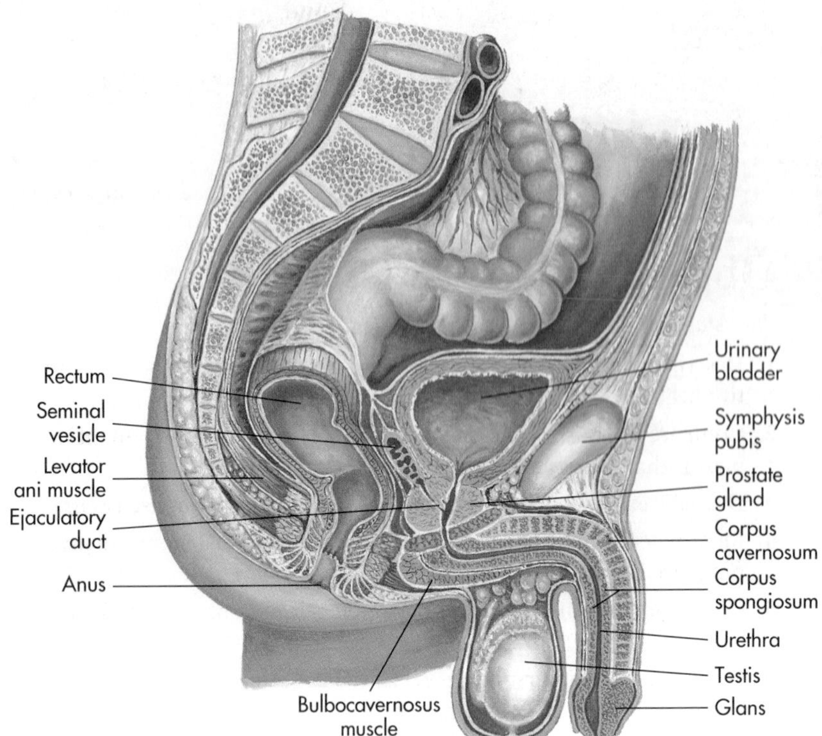

Figure 55-1 Male reproductive organs and associated structures.

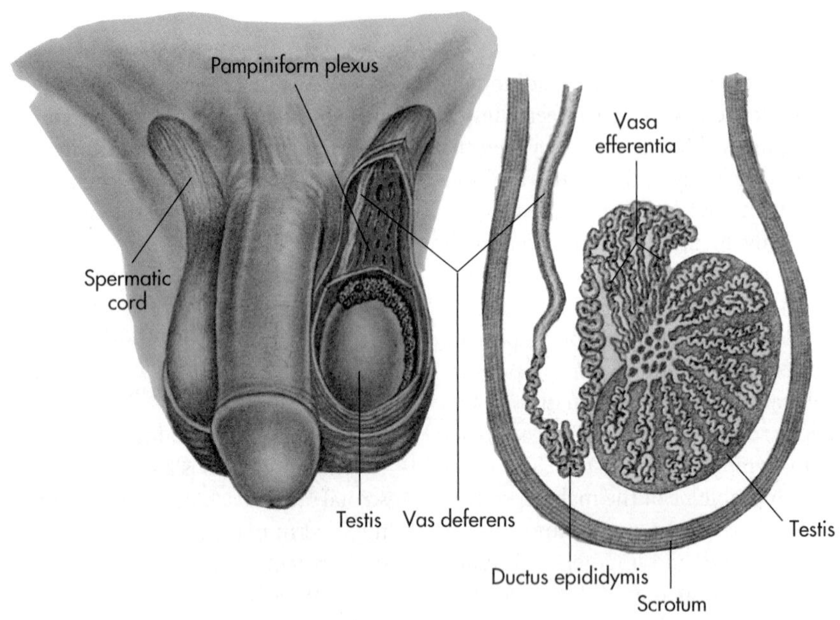

Figure 55-2 The scrotum and its contents.

45 years old. The most common organism of contamination in these age-groups is *Escherichia coli.* Second, structural malformations or developmental structural insufficiencies in the child may contribute to problems of urinary reflux. Reflux of infected urine can cause infection; reflux of sterile urine causes a chemical irritation in the epididymis and is another common cause of inflammation.

Finally, in the adult male between the ages of 19 and 35, sexual transmission is the most common means of infection. The pathogens most likely to cause epididymitis in heterosexual men are *Chlamydia trachomatis* and *Neisseria gonorrhoeae.*[8] In homosexual men, the most common pathogens are the ones that would be found in the anal canal, *E. coli* and *Haemophilus influenzae.*

Pathophysiology

Epididymitis results from inflammation of the epididymis and scrotal sac. Fluid accumulates in the scrotal sac as an inflammatory response to the infectious process. Excess fluid loss into the interstitial space of the scrotal sac can lead to diminished blood flow, nerve damage, and resultant pain and swelling. Inflammatory fluids also can form pockets of pus called abscesses. Heat generated from the inflammatory process can negatively affect the testicular function of spermatogenesis. Consequently, complications of epididymitis include testicular infarction, chronic pain from nerve damage, abscess formation, and infertility.

The most common clinical manifestations are severe tenderness, pain in the scrotal area, and noticeable swelling of one or both sides of the scrotum. The onset of pain is usually gradual, increasing over hours or days. Scrotal swelling can cause pain on ambulation and discomfort that is exacerbated by wearing restrictive clothing. Men with epididymitis often walk with a type of "waddle" to help spare the scrotum from rubbing up against the thighs or clothing. Elevation of the scrotum reduces pain in approximately 50% of patients (Prehn's sign).[15,24,27] Other symptoms include an increase in temperature of the scrotum and sometimes a systemic rise in temperature. A urethral discharge may also be present,[15] with the color and consistency varying according to the type of causative organism. Urethritis is often associated with epididymitis, and the associated symptoms include burning on urination, frequency, urgency, and general malaise.

Collaborative Care Management

Assessment of the patient with symptoms of epididymitis should include a sexual history. For young children, it should include questions to determine possible sexual abuse and any history of recent urinary examinations or instrumentation. In older men questions focus on history or symptoms of urinary obstruction or recent urinary examinations.

Prompt diagnosis is essential to decrease the risk of complications. Urinalysis is used to differentiate epididymitis from emergency conditions such as testicular torsion (see later discussion). If epididymitis is present, the urinalysis usually shows an increased white blood cell (WBC) count and the presence of bacteria. Urine and urethral cultures are used to determine the specific causative organism and its sensitivity to various antibiotics, as well as to provide information for needed drug therapies.

Other diagnostic tests to detect epididymitis focus on changes in blood flow to the inflamed scrotum. An initial increase in blood flow to the area would indicate inflammation and/or infection, whereas other conditions resulting in swelling might impede blood flow. Scrotal ultrasound is a noninvasive diagnostic measure used on adults when urinalysis and cultures are not conclusive. Ultrasound for this condition is usually done serially, and if possible, by comparing the nonaffected scrotum to the affected side. Any indication of reduced blood flow to the affected side usually indicates a more serious condition or a complication of epididymitis. Radionuclide scanning can also be performed when the diagnosis is questionable. These scans are more sensitive than ultrasound and generally show increased blood perfusion to the affected side of the scrotum if epididymitis is present.

The nature of the patient's pain is assessed; whether the pain is bilateral or unilateral, and if the pain is of sudden onset or has developed over hours or days. The nurse also notes whether the pain is relieved by elevating the scrotum. Any symptoms of dysuria are documented, such as burning, frequency, urgency, fever, and general malaise. A recent history of urethral discharge or change in the discharge is important to help determine the possible type of causative organism. The color, consistency, and amount of any discharge are documented.

The patient is also observed for the classic "waddle," or a somewhat rolling gait, indicating that the patient is attempting to protect his scrotum. Swelling of the scrotum is documented, as well as whether it is on the left, right, or both sides. Palpation of the scrotum at this time is generally deferred to avoid causing severe pain. The nurse instructs the patient to obtain a urine sample using the *first* voiding (not midstream) to help differentiate urinary contamination from the urethra, rather than the bladder.

Treatment of epididymitis usually consists of pain management, medications to treat the infection, and supportive care. Nonsteroidal antiinflammatory drugs (NSAIDs) such as ibuprofen may be used to decrease the inflammation and relieve the discomfort and swelling. Narcotic analgesics may be prescribed if the pain is severe. Stool softeners are given to prevent constipation and reduce straining on defecation, which may cause severe pain in the inflamed scrotum.

Eradication of the infection generally is accomplished by giving oral antibiotics. Most antibiotics prescribed are broad spectrum. Oral quinolones or cefazolin are frequently the antibiotics of choice.[8] These antibiotics may be prescribed for a course of 14 to 30 days depending on the patient's history of chronicity. The nurse instructs the patient that it is important to take these medications for the entire time they are prescribed to avoid recurrence of the disease. If sexually transmitted diseases (STDs) are present, antibiotics are prescribed to eradicate the STD. The patient's sexual partners also should be treated at the same time.

Unless high fever and the potential for complications are present, most men with epididymitis can be treated as outpatients. Frequent return appointments are indicated if swelling does not resolve in a few weeks. Because this condition can be associated with other pathologies of the scrotum, a more comprehensive palpation of scrotal structures is performed after the swelling has resolved. The examination incorporates such diagnostic tests as ultrasound, magnetic resonance imaging (MRI), and aspiration of fluid from the scrotum.

Patient/Family Education. Patient education initially focuses on measures to reduce the swelling of the scrotum. Bed rest with the scrotum elevated on a towel, application of ice packs, and the use of scrotal supports when the swelling is less severe decrease the discomfort caused by the heavy sensation resulting from the enlarged scrotum (Figure 55-3). Also these measures prevent traction on the spermatic cord and improve venous drainage. Bed rest is helpful until the patient is pain

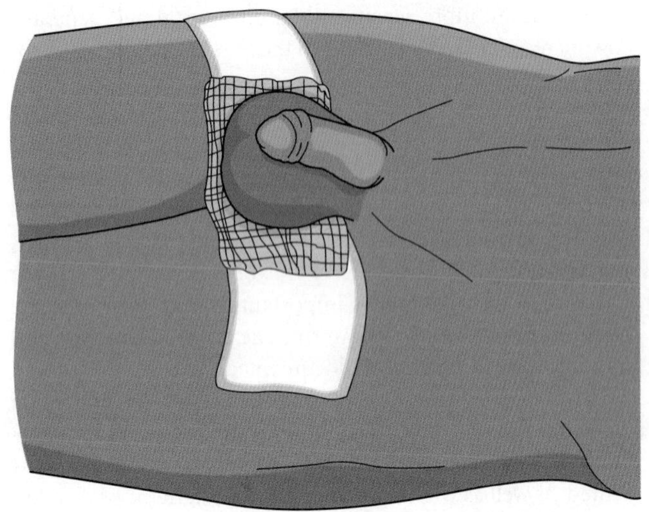

Figure 55-3 A simple scrotal support.

free, then a scrotal support is worn for approximately 6 weeks. The patient is instructed to avoid work and sexual arousal that would strain the lower abdomen and scrotal area.

Because STDs are the most common causes of epididymitis, it is important for the patient to be educated about prevention. The importance of using condoms and maintaining good hygiene are stressed in patient teaching. (Methods of preventing STDs are discussed more completely in Chapter 56.)

Orchitis

Etiology/Epidemiology

Inflammation or infection of the testicle is known as orchitis. Orchitis may be caused by pyogenic bacteria, gonococci, tubercle bacilli, or viruses (e.g., paramyxovirus, the agent responsible for mumps), or it may follow any septicemia. Orchitis often occurs after epididymitis. Orchitis occurs as a complication of mumps in approximately 20% of all cases contracted after puberty. Symptoms may develop 4 to 6 days after the onset of parotitis. If the case of mumps is mild, there may be no symptoms until the onset of orchitis.

Pathophysiology

Inflammatory fluid seeps from the testicle into the serous membrane lining the epididymis and the testicle to create unilateral or bilateral swelling. Hydrocele (a collection of fluid within the tunica vaginalis testis) is frequently associated with orchitis. The signs and symptoms of orchitis are the same as those of epididymitis. However, because orchitis is caused by a systemic infectious process rather than a localized infection, more systemic symptoms are present. These include nausea, vomiting, and pain radiating to the inguinal canal.

As a result of inflammation and fibrosis, some degree of testicular atrophy occurs in 20% to 50% of patients. Atrophy of the testes may lead to sterility in 20% of cases. Unless both testes are severely involved, however, infertility is rare.[16]

Collaborative Care Management

Any postpubertal boy or man who is exposed to mumps may be given gamma globulin immediately unless he has already had mumps or been vaccinated for the disease. Gamma globulin may not prevent mumps, but the disease is usually less severe and less likely to cause complications. Bacterial orchitis is treated with broad-spectrum antibiotics. Antiinflammatory medication is given to help reduce pain and swelling.

Patient/Family Education. Patient education focuses on measures to reduce discomfort from gonadal swelling and alleviate systemic symptoms. During the acute phase of gonadal swelling, the scrotum may be supported as described for the patient with epididymitis. Warm or cold compresses may be applied to help reduce swelling and increase comfort. Rest and an increased fluid intake are encouraged for all patients.

Testicular Torsion

Etiology/Epidemiology

Testicular torsion is a condition in which testicular circulation is acutely impaired by the twisting of the spermatic cord. Torsion may follow activities that put a sudden pull on the cremasteric muscle, such as jumping into cold water, blunt trauma, or bicycle riding. It may also occur at night when there is less gravitational pull from the testes on the cord, allowing more movement and consequent twisting. The congenital defect known as "bell clapper" deformity is a major risk factor for torsion. The testicle and spermatocord are not properly supported causing the testicle to be tilted, which results in greater risk for twisting. There is a genetic predisposition for "bell clapper" deformity, but not every male that has this deformity has resultant torsion.

Approximately 1 in 4000 males under age 25 years experiences torsion. Peak incidence of testicular torsion is around 1 year and then between ages 12 and 18 years, but it can occur at any age. Of the cases reported, 40% occur spontaneously, awakening the male at night.[27]

Pathophysiology

Torsion interrupts the blood supply to the testes, leading to ischemia and severe unrelieved pain that may be aggravated by manual elevation of the affected side. The scrotum is swollen, tender, and red. The affected side is usually elevated because the twisting and shortening of the cord pull up the testicle. The cremasteric reflex, elicited by stroking the inner aspect of the thigh to cause reflex retraction of the testicle, is usually absent on the side of the suspected torsion. Although the scrotum appears infected because of the swelling and redness, both urinalysis and blood tests are typically normal. Fever is rarely present. Absence of pain after a time may indicate infarction and necrosis. Gangrene may be a serious sequela.

Testicular viability after torsion is directly related to the duration of the torsion episode. If torsion has occurred for less than 4 hours, there is an 80% salvage rate for the testicle. If more than 12 hours have elapsed, the salvage rate is 20%. Early recognition and treatment are imperative if the testicle is to be preserved.[24,27] Table 55-1 lists assessment criteria to help differentiate torsion from epididymitis.

TABLE 55-1 A Comparison of Testicular Torsion and Epididymitis

Torsion	Epididymitis
Age	
First year through adolescence; most common age, 12-18 years	Adolescence and later
Onset	
Acute	May be gradual
Signs and Symptoms	
Pain	
Localized to testis and radiates to groin and lower abdomen; severe in nature; similar episodes of self-limiting pain not unusual	Usually localized to epididymis and testis, sometimes to groin; increasing severity of pain; similar episodes of self-limiting pain rare
Fever	
Rare	Common
Vomiting	
Common	Rare
Dysuria	
Rare	Common
Physical Examination	
Testis may be in elevated position with abnormal lie; testis will be swollen and tender; epididymis also may be tender	Epididymis will be firm, tender, and swollen; testis may be normal or tender
Cremasteric Reflex	
Usually negative	Usually positive
Prehn's Sign	
Pain constant	Pain decreased
Urethral Discharge	
Not found	Common with sexually acquired infections
Urinalysis	
Usually normal	Pyuria common

Collaborative Care Management

Diagnostic studies for testicular torsion may include color Doppler ultrasound. Doppler studies help to identify reduced blood flow diagnostic of torsion. Doppler ultrasound also helps in the imaging of the structures that can help determine risk factors such as "bell clapper" deformity or rule out associated problems such as trauma.

Detorsion (a process of untwisting the spermatic cord) can be attempted manually. If detorsion is unsuccessful, surgical intervention is imperative within 6 to 12 hours to maintain viability of the testis. Even so, the testis may atrophy. Unless gangrenous, the testis is not excised, as it may still produce hormones, even if spermatogenesis is destroyed. The testis is fixed surgically to the scrotal wall (orchiopexy) to prevent recurrence. The contralateral testis is usually fixed prophylactically at the same time.

If the testicle is gangrenous or found to be nonviable after surgical detorsion, an orchiectomy (removal of the testicle) is carried out. If orchiectomy is performed, a testicular prosthesis is usually inserted. Hyperbaric oxygen treatments may be ordered to enhance oxygenation of the oxygen-deprived testicle.[24]

Nursing care after orchiopexy and orchiectomy is similar. Ice bags and scrotal elevation may be ordered to reduce swelling. The nurse continues to monitor the patient for signs of testicular necrosis and fever in the case of orchiopexy. A small Penrose drain may be placed in the scrotum, which will necessitate dressing changes.

Patient/Family Education. After scrotal surgery, the patient should be instructed to limit stair climbing to two flights and not to lift or carry heavy objects for 4 weeks. He is instructed to refrain from sexual activity for 6 weeks. The use of a scrotal support for at least 3 weeks is recommended to control edema. Sitz baths may help relieve any discomfort.

Body image disturbances may result from castration and involve fears of loss of masculinity, and issues relating to sterility and impotence. The nurse provides specific information about the physiologic changes resulting from testicular atrophy or surgical removal of the testicle. The patient is still able to have an erection after trauma or surgery to the testicles. Fertility may or may not be affected if there is still a remaining healthy testicle. If necessary, counseling on alternative means of conception may be suggested. The patient is reminded that the appearance of the scrotum will not be altered if a testicular prosthesis is inserted after orchiectomy.

Testicular Cancer

Etiology/Epidemiology

The causes of testicular cancer are still unknown. A wide range of genetic and environmental causes are being explored. Chemical carcinogens, trauma, and orchitis all are theorized to initiate malignant changes. Because there is a greater incidence of testicular cancer in men who live in rural areas, environmental triggers are also suspected. Possible congenital etiologies include familial predisposition, gonadal dysgenesis (developmental abnormality), and cryptorchidism (failure of the testis to descend at birth). There is a 40% greater risk of testicular cancer in men who have a history of cryptorchidism.[2]

Cancer of the testis is the leading cause of death from cancer in the 15- to 35-year-old age-group. Two to three men per 100,000 have testicular cancer, but the number is increasing. The age-groups that are most prone to testicular cancer are infants, men between 20 and 40 years, and men over age 60. Testicular cancer is more common in Caucasian than in African-American males. If detected and treated early, there is a 90% to 100% chance of cure. Unfortunately, approximately half the cases are found in advanced stages. Common areas of metastasis are the spine, peritoneum, and lung. If testicular cancer remains untreated, death often occurs within 2 to 3 years.[2]

Pathophysiology

Testicular neoplasms are divided into two classifications: germinal and nongerminal. Germinal cancers make up 90% to 95% of all testicular neoplasms and are further divided into two groups: seminomatous (50%) and nonseminomatous (NSGCT) (50%) tumors. In addition, tumors with mixed cell types can occur.[2]

The determination of cell type helps to focus treatment. The diagnostic workup includes chest x-ray studies, computed tomography (CT), intravenous pyelogram, skeletal surveys if the patient's alkaline phosphatase is elevated, and lymphangiography. Biopsy of the testis is contraindicated because of the highly metastatic character of testicular carcinoma. Manipulation and invasion of the cancer could cause it to seed to other areas. Laboratory tests include evaluation of alpha-fetoprotein (AFP), the beta subunit of human chorionic gonadotropin (beta-hCG), and lactate dehydrogenase (LDH). AFP is considered a marker that indicates the presence of nonseminomatous disease, although a small number of men (less than 10%) with diagnosed seminoma also have elevations in this marker hormone. LDH is elevated in 60% of patients with metastatic NSGCT and 80% of patients with metastatic seminoma.[16] No one combination of elevated and normal markers specifically indicates testicular neoplasm. However, changes that occur in the laboratory values of these markers help to monitor the effectiveness of therapeutic interventions. The markers are monitored throughout the course of therapy.

Clinical manifestations of testicular cancer are often subtle and go unnoticed by the male until he notices a feeling of heaviness or dragging in the lower abdomen and groin area. A lump or swelling may be present, which is usually nontender and painless. Other symptoms are nonspecific, such as back pain, weight loss, and fatigue. Testicular tumors are often rapidly growing. Some complex tumors have been reported to double in size in a few days.[24]

Collaborative Care Management

In any suspected case of testicular cancer, the testis is usually removed immediately. Men who are at higher risk for testicular cancer as a result of cryptorchidism may be encouraged to undergo orchiectomy as a prophylactic measure. Orchiectomy consists of excision of the spermatic cord, the contents of the inguinal canal, and the testis with the tunicae attached. The adjacent area is explored for metastases. The specimens are then examined to determine the cancer cell type. If NSGCT is found then a nerve-sparing retroperitoneal lymph node dissection is usually done at the time of orchiectomy. Staging of the disease (Box 55-1), as well as pathologic findings, determines the course of treatment.

Of the two major types of testicular cancer, seminoma is highly responsive to radiation therapy. For stage I seminoma, irradiation is administered to the retroperitoneal nodes. In stage II, irradiation of the mediastinal and supraclavicular nodes may be added. Chemotherapy may be done for both stage II and III.[2] If tumor markers are present or elevated after irradiation, nonseminomatous involvement must be suspected. Seminoma can metastasize into a different type of cancer. A second primary lesion can develop in the remaining testis. The prognosis in that case is the same as if it were the first lesion.

Nonseminomatous neoplasms are radioresistant. Therefore retroperitoneal lymphadenectomy or radical node dissection is performed at the time of orchiectomy. Chemotherapy is given for clinical, radiologic, or tumor marker evidence of metastasis. If the lymph node dissection is positive, the patient has stage II disease. Cyclic combination chemotherapy is administered for stages II and III. Drugs used in combination chemotherapy include cisplatin, vinblastine, and bleomycin.

Nongerminal testicular tumors are rare. Treatment consists of various combinations of the four modes of treatment (orchiectomy, radiation, lymphadenectomy, chemotherapy) used in germinal neoplasms. Table 55-2 lists treatments for testicular cancer based on tumor type.

Seminoma has the best prognosis of any of the germinal neoplasms. Five-year survival rates are 95% to 100% for stage

BOX 55-1 Staging of Testicular Neoplasia

Stage I	No metastasis; confined to testis
Stage II	Metastasis to retroperitoneal lymph nodes or other subdiaphragmatic areas
Stage III	Metastasis to mediastinal and supraclavicular nodes or other areas above diaphragm

I, 70% to 90% for stage II, and 50% to 70% for stage III. Relapses are more common in patients with advanced stage cancer, and thus chemotherapy with radiation is used to achieve a higher rate of sustained remission. For nonseminomatous neoplasms (NSGCT), 5-year survival rates are 90% for stage I, 60% to 85% for stage II, and 30% to 40% for stage III.[2]

Patient/Family Education. Patient teaching focuses on the planned treatment and its expected side effects. Radiotherapy and chemotherapy are discussed in Chapter 15. Low-dose radiation is used for the seminomatous tumors and has a lower incidence of side effects than the dose given for NSGCT. Although the normal testis is shielded during external radiation, it is exposed to radiation scattered from the abdomen and thighs. The nurse explains to the patient that a period of 70 days is required to determine if spermatogenesis has been affected. Spermatogenesis may be decreased for 7 months to 5 years or more. The patient is encouraged to seek genetic counseling related to questions about the effects of radiation on sperm and consequently the possibility of genetic defects. Sperm banking before treatment is often recommended.

The nurse explains the effects of orchiectomy on fertility. Orchiectomy alone does not result in infertility if the contralateral testis is normal. The remaining testis undergoes hyperplasia, producing sufficient testosterone to maintain sexual function, drive, and sexual characteristics.

After a radical node dissection, there is danger of hemorrhage. Vigorous movement may be contraindicated, as nodes may have been resected from around many large abdominal vessels. The patient should not do any lifting or driving for 10 to 14 days after surgery. Pain and swelling of the scrotum are treated with pain medications, elevation of the scrotum when the patient is supine, and scrotal support when the patient is ambulating. Application of a warm or cool compress may also provide comfort and decrease swelling.

Even though prosthetic testes are used to lessen the change in the physical appearance of the scrotum, the patient is usually aware of the loss of a sexual organ. The nurse needs to explore the emotional effect that this loss has on the patient and provide support and possible referral for counseling.

After a retroperitoneal lymphadenectomy, 90% of patients experience decreased ejaculatory ability. Decreased ejaculation results from a disruption of the sympathetic nervous system pathways. The nurse informs the patient that ejaculation is independent of other sexual functions and that erection and orgasm is still possible. The sexual partner should also be invited to learn about these changes in function.

Follow-up visits are often scheduled monthly for the first year after surgery to have serum tumor markers drawn, chest x-ray films, and possibly a CT scan. The interval between visits increases to 2 months for 2 more years to continue monitoring for signs of cancer recurrence.

The nurse also teaches the patient how to perform monthly testicular self-examination. Testicular self-examination should be performed by all males starting at puberty. Because men are at greatest risk for testicular cancer between the ages of 18 and 38 years, teaching needs to be targeted to this age group. Men should be taught to examine each testicle and spermatic cord monthly. Any lump should be reported to a physician. Figure 55-4 illustrates the testicular self-examination.

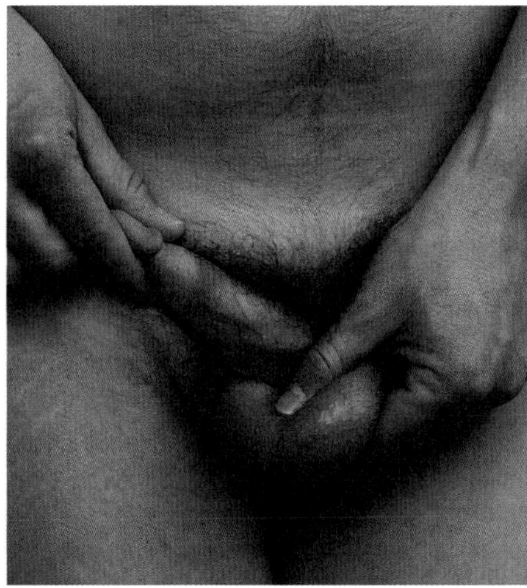

Figure 55-4 Testicular self-examination. Examination is performed after a shower when the testicles are relaxed, descended, and easier to palpate. The man thoroughly palpates each testicle. Lumps are usually painless and circumscribed.

TABLE 55-2 Treatment of Testicular Cancer Based on Tumor Type

Stage	Tumor Type	Treatment
0	Benign	Surveillance
I	Seminomatous	Orchiectomy Radiation therapy
	Nonseminomatous	Orchiectomy Modified retroperitoneal lymph node dissection Radiation therapy
II	Seminomatous	Orchiectomy Radiation
	Nonseminomatous	Orchiectomy Radiation therapy/ modified or full retroperitoneal lymph node dissection
III	Seminomatous	Combination chemotherapy/full retroperitoneal lymph node dissection
	Nonseminomatous	Combination chemotherapy/full retroperitoneal lymph node dissection

PROBLEMS OF THE PROSTATE

The prostate is a chestnut-sized gland that is located below the bladder and surrounds the urethra. The gland is composed of cells that depend on male hormone to maintain its growth and size. The gland provides fluid that supports the viability and motility of sperm and modifies the pH of the vagina to help protect the sperm.

The most common disorders of the prostate gland are prostatitis (inflammation of the prostate), benign prostatic hypertrophy (benign enlargement of the prostate), and cancer of the prostate.

Prostatitis

Etiology/Epidemiology

Prostatitis is one of the more common inflammations of the male reproductive system. It is most often seen in young and middle-aged men. The two types of prostatitis are bacterial and nonbacterial. Nonbacterial prostatitis is the most common type. Chlamydia trachomatis has been suspected as the cause in many cases of nonbacterial prostatitis[7,11] but frequently the infective organism cannot be identified. In other cases nonbacterial inflammations may be attributed to allergic or antibody-antigen reactions. Chemical irritation from urate in noninfected urine can reflux into the prostate also causing inflammation.

Bacterial prostatitis can be acute or chronic. It is often caused by the same bacteria that cause urinary tract infections (UTIs), such as *E. coli* and *Pseudomonas.* Ascending UTIs or reflux of infected urine may be the route of bacterial contamination. Urethral instrumentation is another source of bacterial infection as are sexually transmitted organisms.

Pathophysiology

The prostate gland becomes swollen, inflamed, and painful because of either a bacterial infection or other inflammatory process. The prostate surrounds the urethra and, when it becomes swollen, can compress the urethra and cause urinary obstruction. Prostatic abscess may also form in severe cases. Men with prostatitis typically complain of changes in voiding patterns, such as difficulty starting the stream or the need to strain on urination. Low back pain, pelvic pain, and perineal pain are other common symptoms. Pain during or after ejaculation may also be experienced. In addition, the patient with bacterial prostatitis frequently complains of symptoms of UTIs that can include urgency, frequency, painful urination, and hematuria. Bacterial infection of the prostate typically causes fever, chills, and general fatigue. Symptoms of acute bacterial prostatitis are often severe, whereas symptoms of nonbacterial prostatitis are usually more vague.

Collaborative Care Management

Urine cultures are usually obtained to determine the organism causing bacterial prostatitis. Cultures of prostatic secretions can verify a diagnosis of bacterial infection. Patients with nonbacterial prostatitis usually have negative urine cultures, but prostatic secretions can show an increased number of leukocytes and fat-containing macrophages.[7]

Treatment is conservative and consists of antibiotics for 30 days to prevent chronic infection, forced fluids, physical rest, stool softeners to decrease irritation of the prostate from hard feces, and local application of heat by sitz baths. Prompt treatment of prostatitis may prevent edema and resultant urinary obstruction. Urethral straight or indwelling catheterization is avoided if possible because of the risk of epididymitis. Suprapubic drainage is established if necessary. Prostatic massage may be used to eliminate residual pus pockets, but it is contraindicated during the acute phase because of the risk of bacteremia.

Recurrent episodes of acute prostatitis may cause fibrotic tissue to form. The fibrosis causes a hardening of the prostate, which may initially be confused with carcinoma. In the granulomatous form of prostatitis, the enlargement may take 3 to 6 months to resolve.

Inadequate treatment of acute infection can result in chronic prostatitis. A subacute infection may also develop into a chronic prostatitis that remains asymptomatic. Therefore prostatic secretions should be examined routinely to detect infection and to prevent complications such as acute or chronic cystitis, pyelonephritis, or epididymitis. It is believed that inflammation permits entry of antibiotics that normally do not diffuse into the prostatic fluid. They can be used during an acute infection but are ineffective in a chronic condition. Antibiotics that may diffuse into the prostatic fluid and be helpful include trimethoprim/sulfamethoxazole, carbenicillin, and ciprofloxacin.[7] Occasionally prostatic abscesses complicate the clinical course and may have to be drained surgically. If prostate calculi are present, they also may be infected. Antibiotics are ineffective against infected calculi, and surgical excision is required. Prostatectomy may be necessary to eradicate the infection.

Patient/Family Education. Patient teaching focuses on how to reduce the effects of swelling of the prostate. The patient is taught how to take warm sitz baths, use anti-inflammatory medications, and avoid foods causing irritation that may exacerbate the inflammation.

The patient should refrain from sexual activity until the antibiotic has started to work, approximately 2 weeks into therapy. After 2 weeks regular ejaculation is encouraged to promote "flushing" of the prostate gland. The antibiotic must be taken for the entire prescribed time, even if the symptoms have been relieved sooner. Avoiding the use of alcohol and over-the-counter drugs (e.g., decongestants) can help prevent exacerbation of the symptoms of urinary obstruction. The continued use of stool softeners can decrease irritation to the inflamed prostate during defecation.

Benign Prostatic Hypertrophy (Hyperplasia)

Etiology

Benign prostatic hypertrophy (hyperplasia, BPH) is an enlargement and change in the tissue consistency of portions of the prostate. Parts of the gland may atrophy, whereas other parts become large and nodular. These changes usually occur in the transitional zone of the prostate, which is near the inner core that surrounds the urethra. The changes that take place can eventually cause problems with urination and compromise the function of the kidneys. During puberty, the prostate grows rapidly. After puberty, growth tapers off by age 30 years. Changes in the size and firmness of the gland next occur after age 50. Consequently, signs and symptoms of BPH are common in men over age 50.[18]

The changes in the size and shape of the prostate are associated with increased androgen levels, increased estrogen and decreased free testosterone. There is also an elevation of the enzyme 5-alpha-reductase. This enzyme converts testosterone to dihydrotestosterone, which stimulates the prostate cells to grow. There is a greater concentration of dihydrotestosterone in males with BPH.[19,23] Studies have shown that BPH does not occur in males castrated before puberty and that BPH does not progress after castration. Males without the enzyme 5-alpha-reductase cannot convert testosterone to dihydrotestosterone and also do not develop BPH.[19,23]

Epidemiology

BPH is the most common problem of the male reproductive system. It occurs in at least 50% of all men over 50 years old and 75% of men over 70 years. Symptomatic disease typically occurs in men in their mid 60s, although not all men with enlarged prostates develop symptoms, and symptomatic disease can occur as early as age 30. Symptoms appear slightly earlier in African-American men.[21] An estimated 30% of men with symptomatic disease eventually need surgery. The presence of benign prostatic hypertrophy does not appear to predispose a man to the development of cancer in the gland. BPH most often develops in the inner portions of the gland, whereas cancer typically arises in the outer portions.

Pathophysiology

The changes that occur in the prostate gland of older men can create a number of problems with the associated urinary system. When the enlarged nodular tissue in the transitional zone of the prostate impinges on the urethra, the urethra elongates and compresses, causing obstruction of urinary flow. This can result in a compensatory hypertrophy of the bands of bladder muscles. This in turn increases the trabeculation (contouring) of the bladder wall, providing pockets for urinary retention. These trabeculated areas show up on ultrasound. Because of the muscular thickening, the bladder has less capacity and is less compliant leading to increased pressure in the bladder during filling. Prolonged exposure to high bladder pressures can adversely affect the upper urinary tract, causing hydronephrosis and kidney atrophy. Bladder muscle tone can diminish over time. Consequently, the bladder cannot empty completely at each voiding (residual urine); the urine becomes alkaline from stasis and is a fertile medium for bacterial growth.

These urethral and bladder changes can result in symptoms of urinary obstruction and irritation. Often the symptoms of obstruction are gradual and characterized by exacerbations and remissions. Consequently the symptoms are often not noticed by the male until acute urinary retention occurs. Symptoms of gradual obstruction include a decrease in the urinary stream with less force on urination and often dribbling at the end of voiding. Other related symptoms include hesitancy, a difficulty in starting the stream, intermittency, and inability to maintain a constant stream. The patient may also complain of a sense of incomplete emptying of the bladder. Straining and urinary retention are the symptoms that often convince the patient to seek medical attention.

Symptoms of irritation often accompany the obstructive problems. Nocturia from incomplete emptying is common. Dysuria, urgency, and urge incontinence are symptoms associated with loss of muscle tone in the bladder and changes in the angle of the bladder neck. The patient also may have symptoms of UTI because of incomplete emptying and the increased risk of infection. As the prostate enlarges, so do the blood vessels, and when straining takes place, these vessels may break and cause hematuria. Urinalysis and culture and sensitivity tests are routinely done to screen for blood and possible UTIs. The typical signs and symptoms of BPH are summarized in the Clinical Manifestations box.

Common complications are kidney disorders caused by pressure and backflow of urine. Urinary retention can lead to UTIs, pyelonephritis, and sepsis. Anemia may also occur if blood loss is severe or as a result of secondary renal insufficiency.

Collaborative Care Management

Diagnostic Tests. Diagnostic tests for BPH include tests of renal function. These include blood and urine tests, monitoring changes in blood urea nitrogen (BUN), creatinine, proteinuria, specific gravity, hematuria, and increases in WBC. Other diseases that result in outflow obstruction need to be ruled out. Prostate cancer, bladder neck contracture, urethral stricture, bladder calculi, bladder cancer, inflammatory prostatitis, and neurogenic bladder are all problems that have similar symptoms. Prostate specific antigen (PSA), a blood test, is often performed on men 50 years and older. It provides a rough estimate of the volume of the prostate. The PSA blood test is divided into free PSA and combined PSA, resulting in the total PSA score. Men who have 25% or greater free PSA are more likely to have BPH than prostate cancer[18] (see further discussion under Cancer of the Prostate later in this chapter).

Clinical Manifestations

Benign Prostatic Hypertrophy

- Prostate gland enlarges, becomes more nodular
- Straining on urination
- Hesitancy in starting urine flow
- Decreased urine stream
- Postvoid dribbling
- Nocturia
- Dysuria
- Blood in urine
- Urgency

Besides the urinary and blood tests already mentioned, cystoscopic procedures may be performed. Cystourethroscopy is used to assess for outflow obstruction, measure the length of the urethra, and visualize the extent of bladder involvement. Uroflowmetry is a noninvasive procedure that can evaluate bladder emptying. Urodynamics is a computerized test that measures bladder pressures and can diagnose obstruction and bladder decompensation. An intravenous pyelogram (IVP) can be performed to outline the urinary tract. Sequential x-ray films are taken to assess the anatomy of the upper urinary tract, check for calculi (stones), and evaluate the degree of bladder emptying. IVPs are not routinely ordered for evaluation of BPH unless hematuria is present. Measuring postvoid residual urine using a catheter is an easy but invasive technique that can also assess bladder emptying. Use of a bladder ultrasound is a noninvasive method of estimating postvoid residuals.

Medications. Medications used to treat BPH are aimed at either reducing the size of the prostate gland or relaxing the bladder neck to open the internal urethral sphincter. Finasteride (Proscar) inhibits the activity of 5-alpha-reductase so that it cannot turn testosterone into dihydrotestosterone, and consequently Proscar can reduce the prostate size.[23] Often the therapeutic effects of finasteride are not noticed for several months because of the time required to demonstrate an appreciable difference in the size of the prostate. Even though this drug actually changes the size of the prostate, it may not always help the symptoms of urinary retention. The urethra may remain compressed because the nodular growth in that immediate area may not shrink sufficiently to affect the flow of urine positively. It seems to be most effective in the treatment of large prostates. Adverse drug effects include decreased libido, impotence, and ejaculation disorders. Finastride can interfere with PSA monitoring by lowering the PSA levels by 50%.

Other drugs are used to relax muscles and reduce straining on urination. These drugs tend to be effective in treating prostate glands of any size. Drugs include selective or nonselective alpha-blockers. Alpha-receptors are found in the bladder neck and when stimulated help store urine. Blocking these receptors promotes voiding. The most selective alpha-blocker for the bladder is tamsulosin (Flomax). This drug has fewer side effects and does not need to be titrated like other alpha-blockers. Other less selective blockers are prazosin (Minipress), doxazosin (Cardura), and terazosin (Hytrin). Nonselective alpha-blockers such as phenoxybenzamine (Dibenzyline) tend to have more severe side effects. The main side effects of most of these drugs are orthostatic hypotension and fatigue. They are usually taken in the evening to reduce side effects. Alternative medicine approaches are also being used to both prevent and treat BPH. Dietary supplements such as lycopene and the use of botanicals such as saw palmetto are reported to reduce prostate size and decrease the symptoms of BPH. Research is ongoing.

Certain medications can exacerbate the symptoms of urinary retention because of their effects on the muscles of the bladder and urethral sphincter and should be avoided. Drugs that affect muscle function include anticholinergics such as decongestants, tranquilizers, and antidepressants.

Treatments. No specific treatment exists for mild BPH besides medication and some dietary restrictions, namely, limitation of alcohol consumption and decreased fat intake. Patients are routinely monitored for signs of subtle changes in kidney function, which may initially be diagnosed by the use of blood tests. The phrase "watchful waiting" often is used to describe the monitoring of the condition with regular checkups.

For patients who do not have large prostates and who are not candidates for conventional prostatectomy because of complicating medical problems such as bleeding disorders, heat therapies may be an option. These include microwave therapy and laser therapy. The microwave and laser techniques burn the area of the prostate adjacent to the urethra and the tissue sloughs, creating a larger lumen in the urethra. These procedures result in less postprocedural bleeding and take much less time than conventional surgical approaches. Postoperative care for laser and microwave therapy is similar to that for transurethral resection of the prostate (TURP) except that microwave and laser procedures rarely require bladder irrigation, but may require a Foley catheter to stay in place for 3 weeks instead of the few days. Microwave may be done as a same day surgery, or the patient is admitted for an overnight stay in the hospital.

There are potential complications to both these heat therapies. If the heat probes are not positioned exactly in the right place burning and sloughing of tissues in adjacent organs may take place, causing rectal fistulas, erosion of the penis, and bladder scaring. Also they may not be as effective as conventional surgery and the patient may need a repeat procedure in a few years.[22,26]

Surgical Management. For patients with recurrent and obstructive problems caused by BPH, surgery is often the treatment of choice. The decision for surgery is based on the severity of urinary symptoms, persistent UTIs, and the degree of physiologic change. Surgery removes the nodular gland tissue but leaves the capsule of the prostate gland intact. Men who undergo this treatment are typically symptom free for at least 8 years, after which there is a 5% to 15% retreatment rate.[29]

Transurethral Prostatectomy. TURP is performed when the major glandular enlargement exists in the medial lobe that directly surrounds the urethra. There must be a relatively small amount of tissue requiring resection so that excess bleeding will not occur and the time required to complete the surgery will not be prolonged. A TURP may be performed with the patient under general or spinal anesthesia.

A resectoscope (an instrument similar to a cystoscope but equipped with a cutting and cauterization loop attached to an electric current) is passed through the urethra. The bladder and urethra are continuously irrigated during the procedure. Tiny pieces of tissue are cut away, and the bleeding points are sealed by cauterization (Figure 55-5).

After a resectoscope TURP, a large three-way Foley catheter is inserted into the bladder if a significant amount of bleeding is expected after the procedure. A large-size catheter is used to facilitate removal of clots from the bladder. After the retention

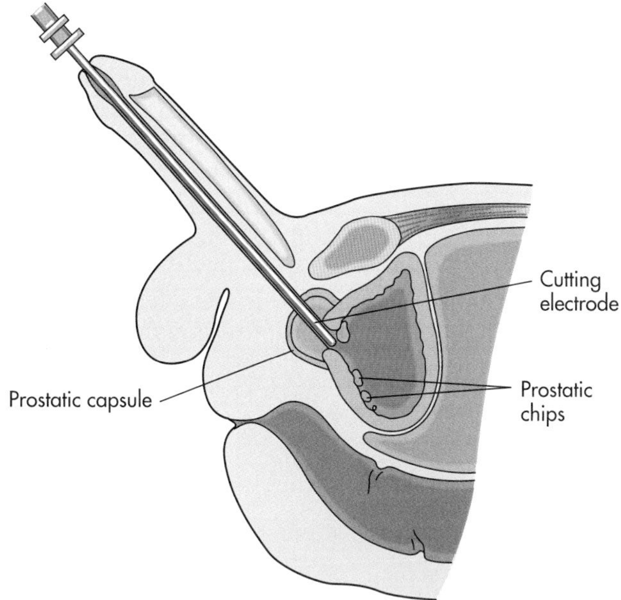

Figure 55-5 Transurethral resection of prostate gland by means of resectoscope. Note enlarged prostate gland surrounding urethra and tiny pieces of prostatic tissue that have been cut away.

balloon of the catheter is inflated, the catheter is pulled down so that the balloon rests in the prostatic fossa and supports hemostasis. Traction may be applied to the Foley catheter to increase pressure on the operative area to control bleeding and prevent hemorrhage. Because the catheter balloon exerts pressure on the internal sphincter of the bladder, the patient may continually feel the urge to void. If the catheter is draining properly, the strongest of these sensations usually passes momentarily. Attempting to void around the catheter causes the bladder muscles to contract and results in a painful "bladder spasm." As the nerve endings become fatigued, the frequency and severity of spasms decrease. This usually occurs within 24 to 48 hours.

A constant bladder irrigation may be used to prevent excessive clotting or clot retention. This irrigation is usually performed via a three-way Foley and intravenous drip apparatus and uses a GU irrigating solution. Constant bladder irrigation after resectoscope TURP usually is discontinued within 24 to 48 hours if no clots are draining from the bladder.

Patients can develop water intoxication, formerly known as transurethral resection (TUR) syndrome, as a result of excessive irrigating solution being absorbed during surgery. Cerebral edema may result, which creates a medical emergency. Confusion and agitation may be the first signs of this condition. Inability to void after removal of the catheter may also be a problem because of urethral edema. When this occurs, the catheter may need to be reinserted. Continence is carefully assessed because the internal and external sphincters lie above and below the prostate, close to the operative area, and may have been damaged during surgery.

About 2 weeks after TURP, when desiccated tissue is sloughed out, a secondary hemorrhage can occur. The patient, who is home at this time, must contact the physician immediately if bleeding occurs.

Persistent bladder discomfort, bladder spasms, or failure of a catheter to drain properly usually signifies one of the following serious complications, which requires immediate medical attention: (1) hemorrhage and clot retention, (2) displacement of the catheter, or (3) unsuspected perforation of the bladder during surgery.

Long-term complications of TURP occur in approximately 18% of patients. These complications include problems with potency and a "change" in orgasms. Fertility can be affected because of retrograde ejaculation, which affects sperm viability and turns the urine cloudy. Other problems include chronic incontinence, which occurs in about 3% of all patients, and urethral strictures, which are rare.[21]

Diet. Alcohol can exacerbate urinary retention and overflow incontinence and should be avoided. Dietary supplements of zinc and vitamin E are sometimes recommended if the patient has deficiencies. These nutritional supplements are thought to help reduce nocturnal urinary symptoms. Saw palmetto, a palm extract that inhibits the effect of dihydrotestosterone on the prostate gland, is being researched as an herbal approach to reducing the size of the prostate. It is given in a pill form and at present is considered an over-the-counter dietary supplement.

Activity. The man with BPH does not need to restrict his normal activity in any way. Frequent emptying of the bladder and avoiding bladder distention are important to prevent hypertrophy of the bladder. Avoiding straining and lifting heavy weights help prevent hemorrhage resulting from strain on the increased vasculature in the prostate.

Referrals. In some settings the nurse assumes responsibility for making referrals to other services. Referrals for persons with BPH are rarely needed because of the temporary nature of any complications associated with the therapies.

NURSING MANAGEMENT OF PATIENT UNDERGOING TURP

PREOPERATIVE CARE

A thorough preoperative assessment of the patient undergoing TURP enables the nurse to anticipate problems that put the patient at risk for complications. A baseline description of the patient's presurgical symptoms is documented. This information is used to compare the symptoms presurgical and postsurgical intervention, as well as to follow long-term improvement of the patient. See Table 55-3 for a standardized format for collecting important assessment information.

Medication information is of particular importance in the assessment of the patient undergoing surgery on the vascular prostate gland, as bleeding is a common postoperative problem. Information on the patient's use of over-the-counter medications that impair clotting, such as acetylsalicylic acid and NSAIDs, is documented as is the use of prescription NSAIDs and anticoagulants, such as warfarin (Coumadin). The nurse also carefully assesses the patient for a history of problems such as anemias that can affect clotting times.

Bowel elimination also is assessed before surgery. Constipation and hard stool can significantly increase the patient's discomfort in the postoperative period, and straining during defecation can cause pressure and pain to the prostate gland and as well as exacerbate bleeding. If the patient is laxative dependent before surgery, he will need some form of stool softener or laxative to prevent constipation after surgery.

The nurse assesses the patient's knowledge of the purpose of surgery and its effects on urinary elimination, sexual functioning, and fertility. Teaching about the effects of local or general anesthesia is provided before surgery (see Chapter 17). In addition the nurse informs the patient about the three-way Foley catheter and bladder irrigation system that may be used after surgery. The patient is informed that his urine may appear red or pink for several days after the procedure, and that this is a normal result of the manipulation of the prostate. Pain management is always a concern with surgical patients, and the nurse instructs the patient about the discomfort associated with bladder spasms and the presence of a large catheter and how this discomfort will be managed. Without an external incision of any kind, the TURP procedure is not associated with any significant incisional discomfort.

TABLE 55-3 American Urological Association (AUA) Symptom Index

	AUA Symptom Score (Circle One Number on Each Line)					
Questions to Be Answered	**Not at All**	**Less Than One Time in Five**	**Less Than Half the Time**	**About Half the Time**	**More Than Half the Time**	**Almost Always**
Over the past month, how often have you had a sensation of not emptying your bladder completely after you finished urinating?	0	1	2	3	4	5
Over the past month, how often have you had to urinate again less than 2 hours after you finished urinating?	0	1	2	3	4	5
Over the past month, how often have you found you stopped and started again several times when you urinated?	0	1	2	3	4	5
Over the past month, how often have you found it difficult to postpone urination?	0	1	2	3	4	5
Over the past month, how often have you had a weak urinary stream?	0	1	2	3	4	5
Over the past month, how often have you had to push or strain to begin urination?	0	1	2	3	4	5
Over the past month, how many times did you most typically get up to urinate from the time you went to bed at night until the time you got up in the morning?	0	1	2	3	4	5
Sum of seven circled numbers (AUA Symptom Score):________						

Adapted from Benign prostatic hyperplasia: diagnosis and treatment, Rockville, Md, 1994, Department of Health and Human Services, AHCPR Pub No 94-0582.
Mild, 0 to 7; moderate, 8 to 19; severe, 20 to 35.

POSTOPERATIVE CARE

Nursing management of the patient following traditional resectoscope surgery is discussed next. A Nursing Care Plan follows.

Promoting Adequate Urine Elimination

The first 24 to 48 hours after prostatectomy surgery are critical in maintaining patency of the catheter or restoring spontaneous voiding. The chance of blood clots forming and interfering with the flow of urine is greatest at this time. If bladder irrigation is being used, the flow rate of the irrigation must be set so that the urine remains free from clots and remains a light red to pink color. If a dark-red color is noted, the flow of the fluid needs to be increased. The nurse is responsible for regulating the flow of the irrigation in response to the color and consistency of the urine output. If bleeding persists

Nursing Care Plan — *Patient After TURP for Benign Prostatic Hypertrophy*

DATA Mr. J. is a 67-year-old married, retired automobile mechanic who has been diagnosed with benign prostatic hypertrophy. Although Mr. J. has undergone medical examinations on an outpatient basis, this is his first admission to a hospital for any reason. Physical examination findings are unremarkable except for slight obesity and a blood pressure of 140/90. Mr. J. has denied any history of hypertension and takes only over-the-counter Tylenol for headaches. He had a transurethral prostatic resection (TURP) performed this morning to relieve urinary retention.

Collaborative nursing activities include monitoring for:

- Postoperative bleeding
- Infection
- Urinary retention

NURSING DIAGNOSIS **Impaired urinary elimination related to surgery**
GOALS/OUTCOMES Will maintain urine output greater than 50 ml/hr

NOC Suggested Outcomes

- Urinary Elimination (0503)

NIC Suggested Interventions

- Bladder Irrigation (0550)
- Urinary Elimination Management (0590)
- Urinary Retention Care (0620)

Nursing Interventions/Rationales

- Monitor urine output and characteristics. *To determine adequacy of urinary elimination and detect complications such as bleeding or infection.*
- Maintain constant bladder irrigation (CBI) as prescribed during the first 24 hours. *To ensure urinary drainage and prevent the formation of clots.*
- Maintain patency of indwelling urinary catheter. *To ensure bladder emptying. Clots may obstruct urinary flow and must be detected early.*
- Encourage high fluid intake (2500 to 3000 ml/day). *To promote increased urine flow.*
- After catheter is removed, monitor for signs of retention and/or infection. *Initiation of the urinary stream may be difficult because of swelling following catheter removal. Fever, chills, and pain on urination coupled with retention or frequency may indicate infection.*

Evaluation Parameters

1. Absence of urinary bladder distention
2. No complaints of urinary frequency, urgency, or pain
3. Consistent urine output in relation to intake

NURSING DIAGNOSIS **Acute pain related to bladder spasms**
GOALS/OUTCOMES Will achieve pain-free status

NOC Suggested Outcomes

- Pain Level (2102)
- Pain Control (1605)
- Hydration (0602)

NIC Suggested Interventions

- Pain Management (2210)
- Analgesic Administration (2210)
- Fluid Management (4120)

Nursing Interventions/Rationales

- Maintain patency of urinary catheter. *Bladder distention from inadequate emptying may exacerbate bladder spasms.*
- Encourage patient to avoid trying to urinate around the catheter. *Forced voiding encourages bladder spasms.*
- Monitor patient's pain status at regular intervals for 48 hours after surgery. *To identify early signs of bladder spasms so that pain relief can be implemented early.*

Continued

Nursing Care Plan — Patient After TURP for Benign Prostatic Hypertrophy–cont'd

- Administer prescribed analgesics and antispasmodics. *Antispasmodics may offer best relief by reducing or eliminating painful spasms.*
- Reassure patient that spasms will decrease in intensity and frequency within 24 to 48 hours. *May reduce the patient's anxiety about long-term effects of urinary surgery.*

Evaluation Parameters

1. Decreased number of requests for and use of pain medication
2. Expresses satisfaction with pain control measures

NURSING DIAGNOSIS **Risk for excess fluid volume related to absorption of irrigating fluid**
GOALS/OUTCOMES Will maintain normal fluid balance

NOC Suggested Outcomes

- Fluid Balance (0601)

NIC Suggested Interventions

- Bladder Irrigation (0550)
- Fluid Monitoring (4130)
- Fluid Management (4120)

Nursing Interventions/Rationales

- Monitor patient for signs of water intoxication during the first 24 hours following surgery or until CBI is discontinued. *Irrigation fluid may be reabsorbed through the bladder wall, resulting in water intoxication. Signs and symptoms of water intoxication include confusion, agitation, warm moist skin, anorexia, nausea, vomiting, and a low serum sodium level.*
- Monitor fluid intake (oral, intravenous, CBI) and output. *To detect shifts in fluid balance so that early treatment can be instituted.*

Evaluation Parameters

1. Urine output approximates fluid intake
2. Absence of signs of water intoxication

NURSING DIAGNOSIS **Risk for infection related to surgical removal of prostate gland**
GOALS/OUTCOMES Will remain free of infection

NOC Suggested Outcomes

- Immune Status (0702)
- Risk Control (1902)

NIC Suggested Interventions

- Infection Protection (6550)
- Surveillance (3590)

Nursing Interventions/Rationales

- Monitor vital signs and report signs of infection. *Fever, chills, and excessive lethargy are associated with infection.*
- Monitor appearance of urine. *Cloudy, frothy urine with a foul odor is associated with infection. Persistent bright red color is associated with active bleeding.*
- Maintain strict asepsis of urinary drainage system and irrigate catheter only when essential. *To prevent introduction of microorganisms into urethra and urinary bladder.*
- Encourage high–fluid volume intake. *Flushing the urinary bladder prevents excessive growth of bacteria.*
- Teach patient to avoid Valsalva's maneuver and avoid rectal temperatures, rectal examinations, and enemas for at least 1 week. *To prevent prostatic bleeding, which makes the patient more susceptible to infection.*

Evaluation Parameters

1. Body temperature within normal limits
2. White blood cell count within normal limits
3. Progressive clearing of urine from blood tinged to clear yellow

NURSING DIAGNOSIS **Risk for stress (or urge) urinary incontinence related to catheter use and prostatic surgery**
GOALS/OUTCOMES Will achieve urinary continence

NOC Suggested Outcomes

- Urinary Continence (0502)
- Urinary Elimination (0503)

NIC Suggested Interventions

- Urinary Elimination Management (0590)
- Urinary Incontinence Care (0610)
- Pelvic Muscle Exercise (0560)

Nursing Interventions/Rationales

- Assess patient for dribbling after catheter is removed. *Dribbling may occur after TURP as a result of trauma and the use of a catheter but should resolve quickly. Continued dribbling indicates the need for further interventions to reestablish continence.*
- Reassure patient that dribbling is common and continence is possible. *To relieve the patient's anxiety about loss of continence.*
- Teach patient how to perform perineal exercises and encourage their use. *Perineal exercises strengthen sphincter tone and enhance continence.*
- Explain use of devices and pads for temporary incontinence. *To protect the patient from embarrassment and possible skin breakdown associated with incontinence.*

Evaluation Parameters

1. Absence of urinary dribbling or incontinence when coughing, laughing, or sneezing
2. Absence of complaints about involuntary loss of urine

NURSING DIAGNOSIS **Anxiety related to fear of sexual dysfunction following prostate surgery**
GOALS/OUTCOMES Will report decreased anxiety and fear

NOC Suggested Outcomes

- Sexual Functioning (0119)
- Body Image (1200)
- Anxiety Control (1402)
- Coping (1302)

NIC Suggested Interventions

- Anxiety Reduction (5820)
- Sexual Counseling (5248)
- Coping Enhancement (5230)
- Body Image Enhancement (5220)

Nursing Interventions/Rationales

- Provide opportunities for patient to discuss feelings about possible effects of prostatectomy on sexual functioning. *Patients often need to be encouraged to discuss their concerns regarding sexuality, which is a very private issue. Identifying fears and concerns is necessary for planning appropriate interventions.*
- Reassure patient that the majority of patients eventually return to their former level of sexual functioning. *To reassure the patient that impotence is most likely temporary, which may reduce his anxiety.*
- Explain retrograde ejaculation to the patient and that it may occur the first few times he experiences an ejaculation. *So that the patient will not be alarmed if his first voiding after intercourse has a milky appearance.*
- Teach patient the need for avoiding sexual intercourse for 3 to 4 weeks following surgery. *To prevent bleeding or infection.*

Evaluation Parameters

1. Discusses fears and concerns about loss of sexual functioning
2. Identifies anxiety-reducing strategies that have been effective in the past

NURSING DIAGNOSIS **Deficient knowledge regarding activity restriction, prevention of complications related to lack of prior exposure**
GOALS/OUTCOMES Will accurately describe and participate in self-care

NOC Suggested Outcomes

- Knowledge: Health Promotion (1823)
- Knowledge: Prescribed Activity (1811)
- Knowledge: Treatment Regimen (1813)

NIC Suggested Interventions

- Teaching: Individual (5606)
- Teaching: Prescribed Activity/Exercise (5612)

Nursing Interventions/Rationales

- Teach patient to avoid heavy activities for 3 to 4 weeks. *To prevent postoperative bleeding.*
- Encourage use of stool softeners or laxative, if needed, for 4 to 6 weeks after surgery. *To prevent straining during defecation, which can stimulate postoperative bleeding.*
- Encourage increased intake of fluids. *Drinking 10 or more 8-ounce glasses of fluid per day decreases the risk of constipation and straining at stool.*
- Maintain prescribed activity restriction. *To prevent fatigue, bleeding, and other postoperative complications.*
- Teach patient to be alert for possible postoperative bleeding occurring about 2 weeks after surgery. *Tissue sloughing occurs about 2 weeks after surgery, which increases the risk for bleeding.*
- Teach patient to report bleeding immediately should it occur. *So that treatment can be immediately implemented to prevent hemorrhagic shock and possible urinary obstruction from blood clots.*

Evaluation Parameters

1. Describes activity restrictions and need for follow-up care
2. Reads written resources
3. Verbalizes understanding of self-care and signs and symptoms that need to be reported

despite the increased rate of irrigation, the physician is notified promptly.

The intake and output record documents the urine output compared with the flow of the irrigation solution. The output should be at least 50 ml/hr greater than the hourly flow of the irrigation. Less urine output indicates a possible obstruction. All tubing is first checked for patency, and if no equipment problem can be determined, manual irrigations using a 50-ml syringe may be ordered to help clear the catheter of clots.

Because irrigation solutions may be used in large quantities, there is a potential risk for water intoxication. The patient may absorb excess amounts of the irrigation fluid, and problems of hyponatremia, and other electrolyte imbalances may occur. The nurse assesses the patient for symptoms of elevated blood pressure, decreased pulse rate, confusion, and nausea. The nurse treats the hyponatremia as ordered by the physician. This often includes infusions of hypertonic saline and the use of diuretics such as furosemide (Lasix).

Controlling Discomfort from Bladder Spasms and Straining

Narcotics may be given to lessen the pain sensation of bladder spasms, but they are frequently unnecessary. Belladonna and opium suppositories are most often prescribed to reduce bladder spasm. These soft suppositories do not cause pain or damage to the fragile tissue around the rectum, which may have been involved in the surgical procedure. Encouraging fluids, at least 8 to 10 full glasses of fluid per day, helps to flush the system and reduce irritation that causes spasms. Frequent voiding after the catheter has been removed also decreases irritation that causes spasms.

To prevent straining during defecation, which can put pressure on the recently traumatized tissues of the perineum, the patient is encouraged to use stool softeners or take mild laxatives and maintain a well-hydrated state to promote painless defecation.

Preventing Infection

Intravenous antibiotics or oral antibiotics often are administered in the first few days after surgery. The patient is again encouraged to increase his fluid intake to promote flushing of the system and help prevent urinary stasis and decrease the chances of infection. The nurse reviews the symptoms of UTI, which the patient should report to his physician.

Relieving Anxiety

The patient is told that most men have some temporary difficulty with continence after any type of prostatectomy. The man should understand that this is normal but will improve. Teaching perineal exercises such as Kegel exercises (see Chapter 53) can be helpful in controlling voiding. Frequent voiding can help reduce problems of dribbling. The nurse provides specific suggestions about absorptive devices and specialty underwear products that can be used for the temporary control of incontinence as needed.

Surgical procedures used to treat BPH do not usually affect a man's ability to have an erection. The patient needs to be reassured that there is a difference between infertility and impotence. Depending on the amount of prostate removed, fertility can be minimally or greatly reduced. Also, if the patient has continued retrograde emission of prostatic fluid even after several months, fertility will remain diminished.

The nurse must not assume that because men with BPH routinely are older, fertility is not an issue. Even if the man is not planning to have children, fertility is often closely associated with sexuality. The nurse may need to provide opportunities for the patient to express these concerns. Reminding the patient that the ability to have an erection is unchanged is often helpful. The ability to experience orgasm is also intact. The patient is cautioned that he may still be fertile, and use of birth control may still be necessary to prevent unwanted pregnancies.

■ GERONTOLOGIC CONSIDERATIONS

Benign prostatic hypertrophy rarely affects men before late middle age. Therefore all of the preceding discussion clearly relates to an older population. Older patients withstand surgical intervention very well and do not have a significantly increased rate of problems postoperatively if they are in good general health. New developments in treatment, which have decreased the invasiveness and length of the procedures, have also clearly benefited older patients.

■ SPECIAL ENVIRONMENTS FOR CARE

Critical Care Management

TURP surgery is on the verge of becoming a 1-day outpatient procedure. Critical care management is therefore clearly not an expected part of the management plan for any patient. It would be used only if the patient experienced a catastrophic response to the surgical experience, perhaps an acute hemorrhage.

Home Care Management

After any prostatectomy surgery, the patient is instructed to avoid heavy lifting and climbing more than two flights of stairs. The patient should avoid sexual activity for at least 3 weeks and should not drive for 2 weeks.

The patient is instructed to watch for and report any sign of infection. The patient should also watch for blood or clots in the urine and any change in the urine stream. The patient rarely leaves the hospital with a Foley catheter, but if the catheter must remain in place after discharge, the nurse provides instructions for Foley care. (See the discussion under Cancer of the Prostate later in this chapter.) Mild analgesics, antibiotics, and stool softeners are often prescribed, and information on their use and side effects is provided.

The nurse teaches the patient to avoid the use of alcohol and over-the-counter medications such as antihistamines that increase the risk of urinary retention. The patient is reminded to void at regular intervals and avoid straining and physical activities that create excessive abdominal or perineal pressure. See the Research box for implications for postoperative nursing care derived from a study of patients who had a transurethral resection of the prostate.

■ COMPLICATIONS

The major complications of TURP surgery already have been presented in the overview of surgical management. They can

Research

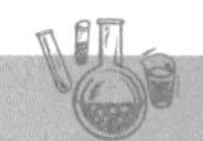

Reference: Pateman B et al: Men's lived experience following transurethral prostatectomy for benign prostatic hypertrophy, *J Adv Nurs* 31(1):51-58, 2000.

Most of the literature related nursing interventions related to posttransurethral resection of the prostate (TURP) focuses on the immediate postoperative period. There is little literature on the longer-term side effects or complications and possible need for nursing intervention. The research that has been done relates more to when and if complications developed or if the patient was ultimately satisfied with the outcome of his surgery. There is a need to determine if the patient would benefit from nursing interventions to help the patient prevent, cope with, or manage these side effects or complications.

Access to study participants was obtained by patient permission via a Urology clinic patient list. Men that had a TURP in the last 3 to 6 months were included in the study. Informal semi-structured interviews were used to elicit information related to the men's feelings, concerns, and questions after the TURP. The interviews were taped, transcribed, and reviewed for recurrent themes. The themes were used to compile a description of the experiences and validated with the patient for accuracy.

Three themes immerged from the interviews. The patients had "put-up" with very problematic symptoms before the TURP, and the symptoms now experienced could be more easily tolerated. A female nurse often does the postprocedural care, and this is embarrassing to the patient. Last, there is a communication gap between hospital and home. The patients thought they had no one to talk to once they left the hospital.

Nursing implications from this study include the need for nurses to anticipate patient problems. Nurses should provide information on how to cope with side effects before discharge. Same-gender care needs to be considered as much for male patients as it is now for female patients, and follow-up phone interviews or earlier clinic visits may need to be considered for these patients.

include problems with bleeding, sexuality, fertility, and incontinence. Most patients, however, tolerate the surgery extremely well and are able to resume their normal lifestyle without ongoing difficulties.

Cancer of the Prostate

Etiology

Cancer of the prostate is the most common cancer in adult American men, but its etiology remains basically unknown. Tumors typically arise in areas of the gland that are atrophic rather than hyperplastic, but the process is not fully understood.

Factors that may affect the development of prostate cancer include hormonal changes and viral infections. Hormonal influences have been proved clinically to be a cancer risk factor, as men castrated before puberty do not develop prostate cancer. Hormonal changes during aging are the reason that prostate cancer is seen almost exclusively in men over age 40. A direct viral etiology has not been proved, but a strain of cytomegalovirus isolated from the prostate gland can produce malignant transformation in prostate tissue in the laboratory setting.[9] In addition, positive antibody titers to herpes simplex and cytomegalovirus have been found in men with prostate cancer.

Environmental influences may increase the risk for prostate cancer. Immigrants from countries with a low incidence of prostate cancer have demonstrated an increased incidence after living in a country with a high incidence of prostate cancer.[25] Other risk factors include a history of multiple sexual partners, episodes of STDs, the presence of cervical cancer in sexual partners, high-fat diets, and industrial exposure to cadmium.

Epidemiology

Prostate cancer has the highest incidence rate and second highest mortality rate of all cancers affecting men in the United States. Prostate cancer accounts for approximately 11% of male cancer-related deaths in the United States. According to the American Cancer Society, almost 200,000 new cases of prostate cancer have been diagnosed in the last year. One man in six will be diagnosed with prostate cancer in his lifetime, but only 1 of 30 men will die of prostate cancer.[28] Prostate cancer rarely occurs before age 40, the incidence increases sharply with age, and there is a clear familial risk. African- Americans have the highest incidence of prostate cancer in the world. Although Caucasian men in the United States have a lower incidence than African-American men; they have a rate higher than men in other parts of the world. Ninety-three percent of all men, regardless of severity of the prostate cancer survive at least 5 years. If the prostate cancer is localized to the gland (not spread to other organs) the 5-year survival rate is nearly 100%.[9,12]

Pathophysiology

Cancer of the prostate, which is most often an adenosarcoma, typically starts as a discrete, localized hard nodule in an area of senile atrophy. In all, 75% of prostate cancers arise in the peripheral zone (outer area of gland, contiguous with the capsule), 20% in the transitional zone (midportion of gland), and 10% in the central zone surrounding the urethra. Because the growth is generally on the outer portion of the gland, compression of the urethra and subsequent voiding symptoms are not common until late in the disease. Nonurinary symptoms, if present, are often so ambiguous that the disease is not diagnosed until it is well advanced.

The cancer readily can spread outside of the capsule boundaries and be disseminated through the lymphatic and vascular systems. The most common sites of metastasis are the bones of the pelvis, lumbar and thoracic spine, femur, and ribs. Involvement of organs such as lung, liver, and kidneys usually is not seen until the late stages of the disease.

Because the posterior of the prostate gland is adjacent to the rectal wall, the tumor may be detected by rectal examination before symptoms appear. On physical examination prostate cancer may present as a discrete or diffuse area of increased firmness. Unfortunately, up to 40% of cancers arise anterior to the midline of the prostate gland and consequently cannot be felt on rectal examination.[25]

Blood screening for prostate specific antigen (PSA) measures the elevation of a glycoprotein secreted by the prostate, and is used to help identify possible cancers. Factors that can influence PSA levels are identified in Box 55-2. Epithelial cells in the ductal system of the prostate gland also secrete acid phosphatase. Elevated serum acid phosphatase usually indicates that prostatic cancer has spread beyond the capsule of the gland.

Prostate cancer can spread slowly or aggressively. The biologic aggressiveness of malignant tumors depends at least in part on the degree of differentiation of the cells. Most prostatic malignancies are defined as adenocarcinomas or sarcomas. It is frequently difficult to determine the severity or extent of the tumor because multiple tumor sites may be present with varying degrees of cell differentiation.

Clinical manifestations of prostate cancer may include complaints of stiffness, back pain, hip pain, and occasionally pathologic fractures. Symptoms may also mimic those of BPH, with urinary outflow obstruction or severe bladder irritation with no signs of infection. Often there are no symptoms in the initial stages of prostate cancer (see Clinical Manifestations box).

Collaborative Care Management

Diagnostic Tests. Because symptoms are often ambiguous, regular screening for prostate cancer is important. A combination of diagnostic tests is now used to improve the accuracy of prostate cancer detection. Blood screens, rectal examination, and ultrasound techniques all help in early detection (Box 55-3). High-risk patients, with histories of multiple sexual partners, STDs, and certain viral infections, should be given special attention in screening routines.[11]

It is recommended that all men over the age of 40 have an annual rectal examination (see Research box). Hard nodular areas felt on the prostate at the time of the digital rectal examination are often indicative of cancer.

Even before disease is noted on the rectal examination, the blood screening test for PSA may show that there is a possible prostatic cancer. Blood screening is often done serially because a rise in PSA or a consistently high PSA is more reliable than a

BOX 55-2 Factors That Affect PSA Levels

Race: African-Americans have higher PSA levels.
Age: Older adults have increased PSA levels.
BPH: Prostatic hypertrophy increases the gland volume and the PSA level.
Manipulation of the prostate (e.g., instrumentation) elevates PSA level
Sexual orgasm within 24 hours elevates PSA level.
Flomax and *saw palmetto* lower PSA by 50%.

Clinical Manifestations

Prostate Cancer

- Often no symptoms if cancer is confined to the gland
- Symptoms of urinary obstruction
- Symptoms of urinary tract infection
- Low back pain, malaise, aching in legs, and hip pain if cancer has metastasized

BOX 55-3 Diagnosis and Staging Tests

Examinations and Visualizations

Digital Rectal Examination (DRE)

A procedure in which a physician inserts a gloved, lubricated finger into the rectum to feel the prostate

Chest X-ray

An image that can show whether cancer has spread to the lungs or other structures such as the ribs

Bone Scan

A picture that can show whether cancer has spread to the bone

Transrectal Ultrasonography (TRUS)

A procedure in which an instrument is inserted into the rectum and produces sound waves directed at the prostate; from these sound waves, a picture is created.

Computed Tomography (CT)

A picture produced by a computer from x-rays, showing the prostate and other nearby parts of the body

Intravenous Pyelogram (IVP)

An x-ray of the kidneys, *ureters,* and bladder that is taken after the patient has been injected with a special dye

Magnetic Resonance Imaging (MRI)

A picture produced by a computer and a high-powered magnet that shows the prostate and other nearby parts of the body

Blood Tests

Prostate-Specific Antigen (PSA)

A test useful both in diagnosis and follow-up of prostate cancer that detects a blood substance that often increases in cases of prostate cancer and other prostate diseases

Percent Free-PSA Ratio

A newer type of PSA test that measures how much PSA is unbound and how much is bound to other proteins in the blood; a low percent-free PSA ratio combined with a borderline PSA can help confirm a diagnosis of prostate cancer

Tissue Samples

Prostate Biopsy

The removal and microscopic examination of a small sample of the prostate to determine whether it contains cancer cells

Pelvic Node Dissection (Also Called Lymphadenectomy)

A procedure used to help determine whether prostate cancer has spread—typically done during surgery to remove the prostate single assay. Because PSA levels can rise with inflammation, benign hypertrophy, or irritation as well as in response to cancer, PSA screening is performed in conjunction with other diagnostic procedures. Knowledge of prostate size, along with PSA levels, provides a more definitive diagnosis than PSA alone. Blood for PSA levels is now routinely drawn starting at age 50 as part of physical examinations, and before and after biopsies or surgery on the prostate gland. Serial levels can be followed after the test or treatment to detect recurrence of the cancer. Laboratory parameters for significant PSA levels are somewhat age dependent: the younger the male the more significant a small rise in PSA. The PSA test can be divided into two scores: a bound PSA and a free PSA. If the patient has a high percentage of free PSA, this tends to indicate BPH rather than prostate cancer. A total PSA value above 4 with a low percent of free PSA indicates a higher probability of prostate cancer.[4,5]

Transrectal ultrasound (TRUS) aids in the screening of nonpalpable tumors. It may also be used to help direct the physician in biopsy of palpable tumors so that these tumors can be graded and staged. TRUS allows greater accuracy in tumor localization and needle placement than using digital rectal examinations to help guide the biopsy.[20] Biopsy of any firm or nodular area is necessary to confirm the diagnosis of prostate cancer. The biopsy procedure may be done in a office setting or minor surgery operating rooms. The biopsy can be done with the patient under local anesthesia or light general anesthesia. If combined with ultrasound, a probe is placed in the rectum; otherwise, the surgeon uses a digital technique to guide the procedure. The needle biopsy can be performed by either a transperineal or transrectal route, depending on the physician's choice.

Patient preparation for prostate biopsy focuses on providing an optimal environment for visualization, preventing complications, and baseline data gathering for follow-up care. Rectal cleansing by enema or oral laxative is often done before the procedure as a means of preventing potential infection. Preprocedural antibiotics are used and may be continued for several days after the procedure. The patient may be on a nothing-by-mouth regimen or permitted to eat a light breakfast before the biopsy. The extreme vascularity of the prostate gland increases the risk of bleeding, and coagulation profiles usually are drawn before the procedure. Patients are taken off any anticoagulants and drugs such as aspirin at least 48 hours before the test.

Staging. A common system of staging prostate cancer is the TNM (tumor-nodes-metastasis) system. This documents the location of the *T*umor, whether it has spread to the lymph *N*odes, and if there is evidence of *M*etastasis. The extent of tumor spread is assigned a number (0-4) and a letter (A-D) For example a tumor that is confined to the prostate gland, spread to a single lymph node, but with no evidence that the cancer has metastasized to distance areas would be staged as: T2aN1M0 (Box 55-4). Stages confined to within the prostatic capsule have a good prognosis. Stages with higher numeric values and/or with additional higher letter values of C or D attached to the numbers, have a poorer prognosis. Staging helps determine prognosis and provides the basis for treatment recommendations.

Treatment decisions are based on both the results of the staging and the Gleason grading scale. The Gleason grading scale is used to rank the correlation between the extent of tissue differentiation and the patient's prognosis. This grading of the tissue type helps determine the aggressiveness of the cancer. The Gleason system of grading has total scores ranging from 2 to 10. Two biopsy sites are used in testing, and the scores of each (which range from 1 to 5) are added together to obtain the total score of 2 to 10. The lower the score, the less aggressive the cancer and the better the prognosis.

Medications

Hormone Therapy. When cancer of the prostate is inoperable, or when signs of metastasis occur after surgery, pharmacologic treatment is given. Some patients experience dramatic improvement with hormonal therapy that may last for 10 years or more. Usually the response is quite good for about 1 year, and then the patient's condition begins to deteriorate. Because a large portion of the growth in prostate cancer is testosterone dependent, medication is used to block the production or action of this hormone. The testicles produce testosterone when stimulated by the release of hormones from the pituitary gland. Therefore drugs that inhibit the release of these pituitary hormones are often first-choice therapies. Hormone analogs such as leuprolide (Lupron) and goserelin (Zoladex) are given every 1 to 3 months, depending on the preparation, by intramuscular injection.

Research

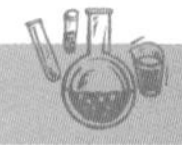

Reference: Weinrich SP et al: Barriers to prostate cancer screening, *Cancer Nurs* 41(2):117-121, 2000

Getting men to participate in prostate screening has always been difficult. Even though the African-American male is at greater risk for prostate cancer, he is less likely to participate in prostate screening programs than Caucasian American males. This study used univariate and multivariate logistic regression models to evaluate barriers to prostate cancer screening. African-American men for this study were recruited from 11 counties in South Carolina. Sampling sites included churches, meal sites, barber shops, and work sites. An instrument was developed to measure perceived barriers to prostate screening and used in two pilot studies to establish content validity. This 15-item questionnaire was then administered, and the men asked to check the items that would make it difficult for them to be screened. Analysis of the data found that cost and lack of knowledge were major barriers to prostate screening.

This study found that, even with the institution of free prostate screening and programs on the reason for prostate screening, barriers still remained. A follow-up phone survey was done to determine reasons African-American males still did not participate in screening, even when free screening was offered in the area and educational programs provided. Lack of knowledge related to specific sites for screening, and transportation or the ability to "take off work" for screening purposes were the specific barriers found. The nursing implication of this study is that education needs to be individualized. It is important for the nurse to provide information that includes addresses, directions, and office hours to help promote participation in health screening programs.

BOX 55-4 Prostate Cancer Staging

The TNM (tumor-nodes-metastasis) system is also used by doctors to stage prostate cancer. This system focuses on tumor anatomy by looking at first the tumor itself, then at the regional lymph nodes, and finally at the metastasis.

T *The primary tumor:* Evaluates whether or not the cancer has spread.

TX Tumor cannot be assessed
T0 No evidence of tumor
T1 Tumor is not clinically apparent, is not palpable, cannot be visualized with imagining devices
T2 Tumor is confined to the prostate
T3 Tumor has broken through the prostatic capsule
T4 Tumor has invaded or affixed itself to adjacent tissue (other than the seminal vesicles)

N *The lymph nodes:* Evaluates whether or not the cancer has begun to spread to the local lymph glands.

NX Cannot be assessed
N0 No evidence of spread to regional lymph nodes
N1 Spread to a single lymph node
N2 Larger spread to a single lymph node, or to more than one node
N3 Larger spread to a regional lymph node

M *The metastasis:* Evaluates whether or not the cancer has spread to distant parts of the body.

MX Cannot be assessed
M0 No evidence of spread to distant areas
M1 Spread to distant areas

Source: http://www.prostate90.com/book/p12.html

In conjunction with drugs that inhibit the production of testosterone, antiandrogenic drugs may be given to inhibit the action of testosterone produced by the adrenal glands. These regimens of combination hormonal therapy are called "maximal androgen blockade" (MAB or combined androgen blockade, CAB). Examples of antiandrogen drugs include flutamide (Eulexin) and bicalutamide (Casodex). Side effects of both of these classes of drugs can include impotence, hot flashes, nausea, vomiting, chemical hepatitis, and diarrhea.

Treatments

Radiation Therapy. Radiation can be used to treat localized tumors confined to the inside of the prostate capsule. It is also used if a patient cannot tolerate or chooses not to undergo surgery. Radiation may be delivered by external beam or by implant (brachytherapy). The testes are shielded during external radiation. The external beam radiation is usually given in short sessions, once a day for several weeks. Internal retropubic prostatic implantation may be used initially or after failure of external radiation therapy. Brachytherapy is often done as an overnight or same day surgery. Very small radioactive seeds are inserted into the prostate and remain in the patient. The patient gives off minimal radiation immediately adjacent to the prostate gland and then is not "radioactive" after the seeds have encapsulated into the gland (approximately 1 week) because the area of radiation from the seeds is confined to the prostate. The patient is asked to refrain from ejaculation for a week until the seeds can encapsulate into the gland. Complications of seed implantation include blood loss from multiple needle punctures during implantation, deep vein thrombosis, pulmonary emboli, hematomas, and abscesses.[6] Impotence from radiation develops over time as a result of scar tissue formation. There is a greater risk of complications if radioactive implants are used after external beam radiation. Irritability of the bladder caused by radioactive implants can produce urinary symptoms of frequency, urgency, and nocturia.

Surgical Management. A radical resection of the prostate gland usually is curative for patients with low-grade and confined prostate cancer. The entire prostate gland, including the capsule and the adjacent tissue, is removed. The remaining urethra then is anastomosed to the bladder neck. The surgery is accomplished by using a suprapubic, retropubic, or perineal approach. The suprapubic and retropubic approaches use a low midline incision, and the perineal approach uses a perineal incision. The patient has a Foley catheter in place for a period of days to several weeks, depending on the approach used by the physician, and whether or not the patient is at risk for delayed healing because of previous radiation therapy. Table 55-4 compares the different surgical methods, and Figure 55-6 illustrates the placement of drains and incisions.

Suprapubic Prostatectomy. In the suprapubic resection, the prostate gland is removed from the urethra by way of the bladder; this type of resection is performed when a large mass of tissue must be resected. Some type of hemostatic agent is placed in the prostatic fossa, and urine is drained by Foley catheter, cystotomy tube, or both.

Hemorrhage is a possible complication, and the precautions are the same as those taken after TURP. Since some oozing of blood from the prostatic fossa occurs, continuous bladder irrigations may be ordered for the first 24 hours.

Cystotomy tubes are usually removed 3 to 4 days after surgery; urethral catheters generally remain until the suprapubic wound is well healed. After the urethral catheter has been removed, the nursing care of the patient is similar to that for the patient undergoing TURP. If the suprapubic wound should reopen and drain, a urethral catheter is usually reinserted.

Retropubic Prostatectomy. In a retropubic prostatectomy, a low abdominal incision similar to that used for suprapubic prostatectomy is made, but the bladder is not opened. The bladder is retracted, and the prostatic tissue removed through an incision in the anterior prostatic capsule. A large-diameter Foley catheter is inserted. Hemorrhage and infection are potential complications, but the sphincter muscles are not damaged, and the patient rarely has difficulty voiding. Nerve-sparing surgeries are the treatment of choice if the patient has less invasive cancer.[30]

Perineal Prostatectomy. The perineal approach results in a draining incision in the perineal area. Often a Penrose drain is placed to help direct the serous drainage from the wound site. The bladder remains intact during this surgery. Nerves that control urinary continence and penile erection may be damaged with this surgical approach. Also muscles and nerves around the rectal sheath can be traumatized. Consequently these patients may have difficulty with bladder and bowel continence as well as impotence. Nerve-sparing approaches

TABLE 55-4 Comparison of Types of Prostate Surgery

Reason for Surgery	Location of Incision	Drainage Tubes	Bladder Spasms	Dressing	Complications
Transurethral Resection					
Enlargement of medial lobe surrounding urethra—benign prostatic hypertrophy	No incision; removal by way of urethra	Three-way Foley catheter with 30 ml balloon in urethra; constant irrigation 1-24 hr	Yes	None	Hemorrhage; water intoxication; incontinence; obstruction
Suprapubic Resection					
Extremely large mass of obstructing tissue—prostate cancer	Low midline abdominal incision through bladder to prostate gland	Cystotomy tube or drain through incision; Foley catheter with 30 ml balloon in urethra	Yes	Abdominal dressing easily soaked with urinary drainage	Hemorrhage; obstruction; wound infection; impotence; sterility
Retropubic Resection					
Large mass located high in pelvic area—prostate cancer	Low midline abdominal incision into prostate gland (bladder not incised)	Foley catheter with 30 ml balloon in urethra, constant irrigation for 24 hr	Few	Abdominal dressing; no urinary drainage	Hemorrhage; obstruction; wound infection; impotence; sterility
Perineal Resection					
Large mass located low in pelvic area—prostate cancer	Incision between scrotum and rectum	Foley catheter with 30 ml balloon in urethra; perineal drain	Few	Perineal dressing; no urinary drainage	Hemorrhage; obstruction; wound infection; impotence; sterility; incontinence
Radical Perineal Resection					
Mass extends beyond the capsule; includes lymph node dissection—prostate cancer	Large perineal incision between scrotum and rectum	Foley catheter with 30 ml balloon in urethra; drain in incision	Few	Perineal dressing; no urinary drainage	Urinary incontinence; wound infection; impotence; sterility

are being successfully used with perineal approaches as well, but the surgery is technically difficult.

Orchiectomy. When testosterone suppression is necessary, one of the methods to decrease testosterone production is a bilateral orchiectomy (castration). This procedure is technically minor and is often performed using local anesthesia, but it may cause the patient considerable emotional distress. The man's permission for sterilization must be obtained. If he is married, he is usually urged to discuss the procedure with his wife. This surgery eliminates the testicular source of male hormones and seems to cause regression of the cancer or at least slow its growth. Very seldom, a hypophysectomy (removal of the pituitary gland, which secretes a testosterone-stimulating hormone) may be performed to further reduce hormonal stimulation.

Diet. No therapeutic diet exists for patients with prostate cancer. A high-fiber, low-fat diet is recommended because men from countries that routinely eat this type of diet have a lower incidence of prostate cancer. There is now clinical evidence that diet can play a role in preventing or slowing the growth of prostate cancer. A diet high in lycopene (a substance found in tomatoes), vitamin E, and selenium can reduce the risk of prostate cancer.[3] Diets are routinely modified if the patient is to have surgery. Increasing fluid intake after prostate surgery helps to prevent problems with constipation.

Activity. If the patient has undergone radiation therapy or prostatic surgery, he should limit heavy lifting or straining. The patient should not drive a vehicle for 2 weeks after surgery. If the Foley catheter has been left in place at the time of discharge, the patient is cautioned not to engage in any activity that could pull or put strain on the catheter.

Referrals. Because many of the therapeutic interventions affect the patient's fertility and ability to have an erection, a specialist in sexual therapy or counseling may be helpful to the patient. Sometimes patients are also interested in family-planning counseling for alternative means of conceiving children. If persistent urinary incontinence is a problem, nurses specializing in the care of incontinent patients (WOC/enterostomal therapy nurses) may be consulted. The American Cancer Society can help the patient deal with the emotional issues related to the diagnosis of cancer, as well as provide information on a variety of helpful resources. Support groups such as

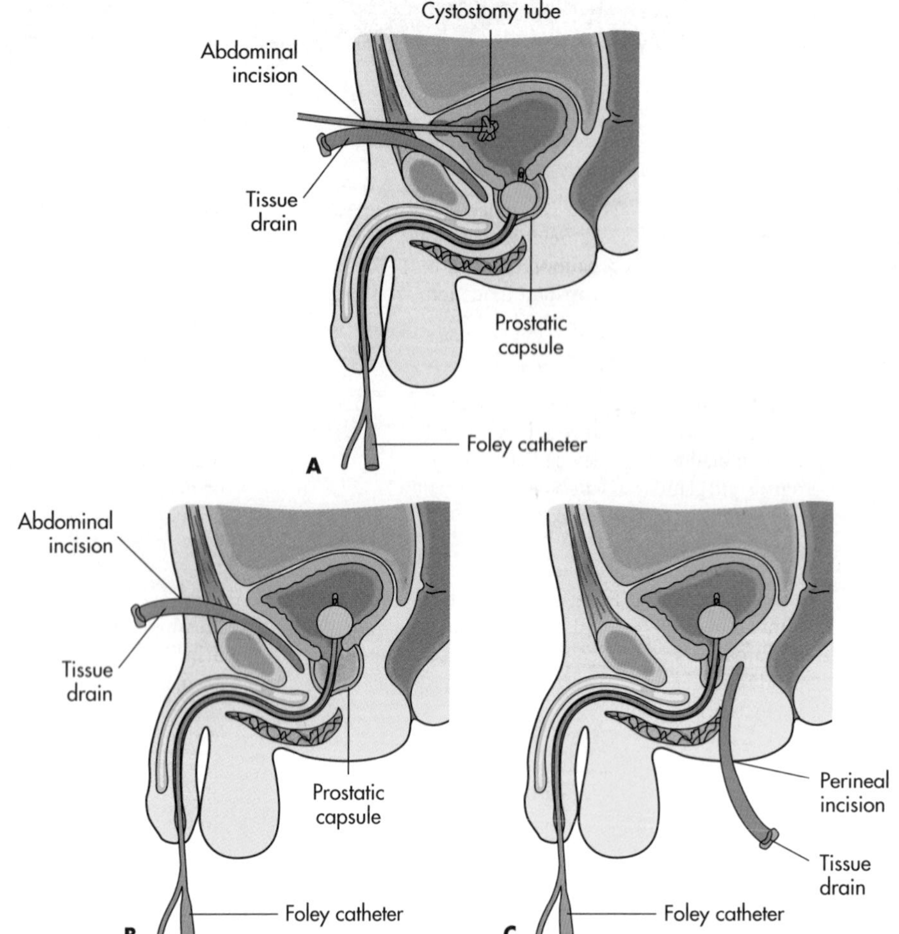

Figure 55-6 Three types of prostatectomies. **A**, Suprapubic: note placement of inflated Foley catheter in prostatic fossa. **B**, Retropubic. **C**, Radical perineal: note tissue drain placed in incision between scrotum and rectum.

"US TOO" and "MAN to MAN" are specifically for the patients with a diagnosis of/or who have been treated for prostate cancer.

NURSING MANAGEMENT OF PATIENT WITH PROSTATE CANCER UNDERGOING PERINEAL PROSTATECTOMY

PREOPERATIVE CARE

If the patient is to have a perineal approach in surgery, he is given a bowel preparation, which may include enemas, cathartics, and sulfasalazine (Azulfidine) or neomycin before surgery and only clear fluids the day before surgery to prevent fecal contamination of the operative site. The remainder of the preoperative care is similar to that described under benign prostatic hyperplasia.

POSTOPERATIVE CARE

Caring for the Perineal Wound

Care of the perineal wound consists of monitoring for possible urine leaks, hemorrhage, and signs of infection. Drains may be placed in the incision, and the wound may be left partially open to heal by secondary intention. Often the patient wears a Fuller shield or briefs-type underwear to support the dressing on the perineal incision. Open wounds may drain copious amounts and frequent dressing changes are usually necessary. The use of a "donut" or "Life Saver" cushion may be used to relieve pressure on the incision site while sitting. The use of rectal thermometers, rectal tubes, and suppositories is avoided to prevent injury to the fragile perineal area.

When solid food is permitted, a low-residue diet may be given until wound healing is well advanced. Diphenoxylate hydrochloride with atropine sulfate (Lomotil) may be prescribed to inhibit bowel action in the first postoperative week to prevent contamination of the incision.

Restoring Urinary and Bowel Continence

A large amount of urinary drainage on the perineal dressing for a number of hours is not unusual. This can be managed by the use of an ostomy bag around the dressing. The urinary drainage should decrease rapidly. The amount of bleeding in the urine should not be the same as after suprapubic prostatic surgery. Because the catheter is not being used for hemostasis, the patient usually experiences less bladder spasm. The catheter is used both for urinary drainage and as a splint for the urethral anastomosis;

therefore, care should be taken that it does not become dislodged or blocked. Clinically, the risk of blockage from clots is greatest during the first hour. The catheter may be irrigated intermittently or continuously as ordered by the physician. The catheter is usually left in the bladder for at least 2 to 3 weeks.

Temporary urinary incontinence is usually a problem with patients who have had any type of radical prostatectomy. The patient needs to be encouraged, and provisions should be made to keep him dry so that he will feel able to be up and to socialize with others without fear of incontinence.

Because perineal surgery causes relaxation of the perineal musculature, the patient may also have problems with fecal incontinence. It is disturbing to the patient, and sometimes can be avoided by starting perineal (Kegel) exercises within a day or two after surgery. Control of the rectal sphincter usually returns readily. Perineal exercises should be continued even after rectal sphincter control returns, as the exercises also strengthen the bladder sphincters, and unless the bladder sphincters have been permanently damaged, the patient will regain urinary control more readily on removal of the catheter.

Promoting Sexual Function

Total prostatectomy that includes bilateral pelvic lymphadenectomy can result in physiologic sexual dysfunction as a result of disruption of genital innervation. The patient may be impotent for several months even after a nerve-sparing prostatectomy. In all, 95% of patients who undergo the nerve-sparing prostatectomy regain potency within 1 year.[30] The patient needs to know that return of erectile capability may be delayed and that alternative sexual interactions may be used until function returns (see the following section on impotence).

The patient and his spouse/partner should understand the sexual consequences of prostatectomy surgery. The nurse teaches both partners if the patient is comfortable having his partner present. The nurse clarifies that the man is no longer fertile after any radical prostatectomy and that the loss of the prostate gland interrupts the flow of semen and he will not ejaculate. However, the ability to have an erection will gradually return, and he can still experience orgasm.

Dealing With Grief

Patients who have low-grade and low-stage prostate cancer have an excellent survival rate. It is important to remind patients that prostate cancer is very different from many other forms of cancer, as even men with higher grades of prostate cancer often have a long survival rate. Prostate cancer is usually slow growing, and many older men do not die of their prostate cancer but from other causes. The fear of cancer must be acknowledged, however, and the patient needs time and encouragement to express these fears. If surgery has resulted in impotence, the patient needs to be supported through his grief over the loss of sexuality. For more information on the grieving process related to cancer, see Chapter 15.

GERONTOLOGIC CONSIDERATIONS

Because prostatic cancer is often slow growing, treatment options for older patients may be more palliative in nature. Radical prostatectomies do not necessarily prolong life for these patients. Consequently, radiation or measures to decrease the size of the prostate (e.g., TUR) to relieve symptoms of urinary obstruction may be the treatment of choice rather than radical prostatectomy.

If surgery is performed, healing times may be prolonged. The perineal muscles of the older patient are weaker, and problems of urinary incontinence and bowel incontinence may take longer to resolve. Perineal muscle exercises may be started before surgery to help the older patient regain muscle tone sooner.

SPECIAL ENVIRONMENTS FOR CARE

Critical Care Management

Despite the radical nature of the surgical approaches that may be used to treat prostate cancer, critical care management would not be a planned part of the treatment approach. If older patients have multiple concurrent health problems that would significantly increase the risks associated with surgery, a less invasive type of treatment is usually selected, negating the need for critical care management.

Home Care Management

If the patient has a radical perineal prostatectomy, the perineal wound may still be open when the patient is discharged from the hospital. Cleansing the wound after defecation should consist of simple cleansing with water and possible use of a spray bottle to provide low-pressure irrigation to the area. Many physicians allow showers within the first week of surgery. The dressing to the incision site is held in place with the use of briefs-type underpants, just as in the hospital. The dressing should remain dry, and the patient should be encouraged to change the dressing whenever the drainage becomes irritating, often twice a day or more.

The patient is taught how to use a urinary leg bag and how to connect and disconnect the Foley catheter from the bedside drainage bag into the leg bag. Signs of UTI are taught to the patient, and he is told to notify his physician if any signs of infection occur. The catheter insertion site at the penis should be washed once a day with water and/or a mild soap if desired. The catheter needs to remain securely anchored to the thigh or abdomen to avoid pulling. Perineal exercises to promote the return of urinary continence when the catheter is removed should be practiced on a regular basis at home.

Reminding the patient that bowel incontinence may still be a problem for a few days when he returns home is important. The patient should have easy access to a bathroom. Instructing the patient to use the toilet a few hours after meals may help to promote bowel continence. Postoperative care for patients undergoing any type of prostatectomy is summarized in the Guidelines for Safe Practice box.

COMPLICATIONS

Complications of radical prostatectomy for prostate cancer include, but are not limited to, hemorrhage, urinary and bowel incontinence, infertility, impotence, and leakage at the anastomotic site of the urethra and bladder. Prostate cancer

Guidelines for Safe Practice

Postoperative Care for the Patient Undergoing Prostatic Surgery

1. Maintain patency of catheter system.
2. Monitor appearance of urine: red to light pink (24 hours) to amber (3 days).
3. Monitor patient for signs of water intoxication after TURP (confusion, agitation, warm moist skin, anorexia, nausea, vomiting).
4. Instruct patient not to try to void around catheter; explain feeling of needing to void from pressure of catheter.
5. Avoid use of enemas and rectal thermometers.
6. Give prescribed medications (analgesics, antispasmodics) as needed; tell patient spasms will decrease in intensity and severity within 24 to 48 hours.
7. After catheter removal:
   a. Monitor for signs of urinary retention.
   b. Monitor for continence; teach perineal exercises if dribbling occurs.
   c. Encourage increased fluids and frequent voiding.
8. Change dressings frequently around suprapubic wounds after suprapubic prostatectomy to prevent skin maceration.
9. Give patient opportunities to discuss feelings about sexuality and possible incontinence.
10. Teach patient to:
    a. Avoid vigorous exercise, heavy lifting (over 20 pounds), and sexual intercourse for at least 3 weeks.
    b. Avoid driving for 2 weeks.
    c. Avoid straining with defecation; use stool softeners or mild laxatives if needed.
    d. Drink at least 2500 ml of fluids per day to prevent urinary stasis and infection and to keep stools soft.
    e. Notify physician if urinary stream diminishes or if bleeding occurs.

may metastasize to local organs such as the lymph nodes, bowel, bladder and bony areas such as the pelvis and spine. Sites of distant metastasis include the liver and lungs.

PROBLEMS OF THE PENIS

Structural problems of the penis typically involve the head of the penis or the foreskin. The head of the penis is susceptible to problems caused by irritation, cancer, and trauma. The foreskin is the source of structural difficulties that can affect urination, cause pain, and interfere with blood flow to the penis. Functional problems of the penis primarily involve disorders of erection. Impotence is discussed later in the chapter. The anatomy of the penis is illustrated in Figure 55-7.

Phimosis and Paraphimosis

Etiology/Epidemiology

Phimosis is a condition in which the opening of the prepuce or foreskin is unable to be retracted behind the glans. The condition may be congenital or acquired as a result of inflammation or infection.

Paraphimosis, conversely, is a condition in which the prepuce is retracted over the glans and forms a constriction at the base of the glans (Figure 55-8). This is usually a result of manipulation of the foreskin over the glans and failure to return it to cover the glans. This condition is most often seen in children or in men with changes in mental status that predispose them to memory loss or with decreased sensation in the penis.

Pathophysiology

The inability to retract the foreskin may interfere with adequate hygiene. Consequently, urine and smegma (mucuslike drainage) may be trapped in the preputial sac, resulting in irritation and predisposing the glans to infection. Chronic irritation may be a cause of penile carcinoma. Healing of the irritation or infection causes scar tissue formation, which can worsen the acquired phimosis. If the constriction of the foreskin at the head of the penis is severe enough, it causes urinary obstruction and painful urination.

Constriction is also a major problem with paraphimosis. The constriction at the base of the glans usually results in swelling of the glans. If the swelling is not reduced, blood vessels to the glans are compressed, reducing flow. Inadequate blood flow can result in necrosis of the glans.

Collaborative Care Management

Treatment for severe cases of phimosis may consist of incisions in the foreskin to reduce the contracture and widen the opening. Congenital phimosis may be successfully treated by gentle repeated stretching of the foreskin over the glans. Circumcision may be performed if the prepuce cannot be satisfactorily retracted.

Circumcision is done to prevent recurrence of paraphimosis. When the penis is circumcised, the wound is covered with gauze generously impregnated with petrolatum. Bleeding usually is controlled by applying a pressure dressing that may be bulky and must be removed before the patient can void. It is removed cautiously and replaced after voiding with a fresh petrolatum dressing.

Patient/Family Education. Patient education focuses on strategies to reduce the inflammation. Hot soaks and oral antibiotics are often used to treat the swelling and infection that can result from phimosis. Cool compresses are used for paraphimosis. The cool compress is applied to the penis, and the penis is elevated for a short period before a gentle attempt is made to reduce the prepuce.

If circumcision has been necessary, the nurse teaches the patient how to change the petrolatum dressing and observe for signs of infection. The nurse also instructs the patient to be alert for signs of bleeding. If severe bleeding occurs, a firm dressing should be applied to the penis, and the patient should be taken to the physician's office or the emergency room. If bleeding persists it may be necessary to resuture the wound. An estrogen preparation may be prescribed for the adult patient for several days after surgery to prevent painful erections.

Cancer of the Penis

Etiology/Epidemiology

In America penile cancer accounts for 0.5% to 1.5% of all male malignancies. Although most common between ages 50 and 70, it can occur in younger men and has been reported in

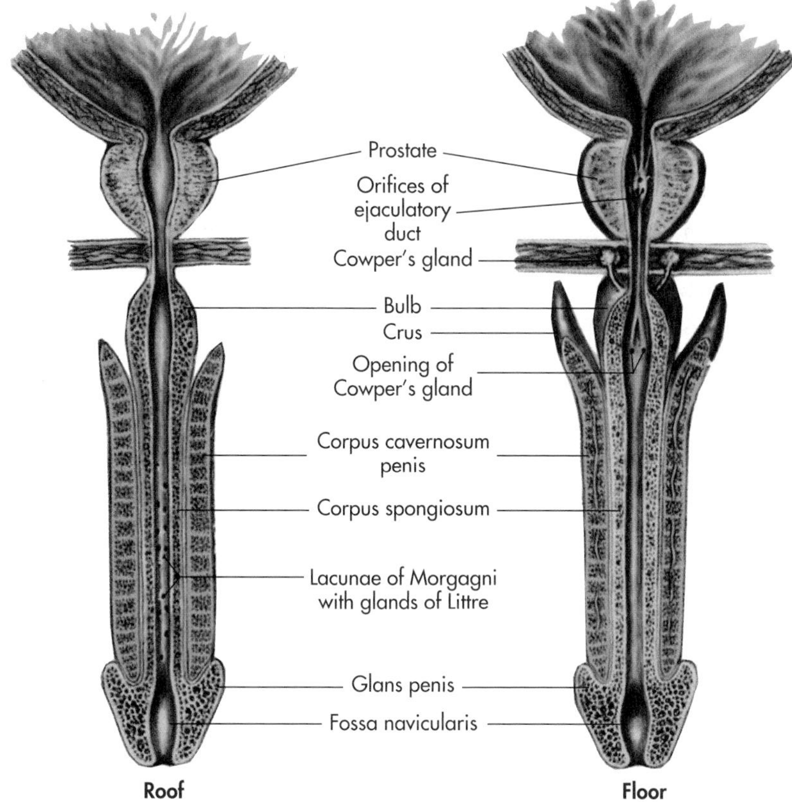

Figure 55-7 Anatomy of the penis.

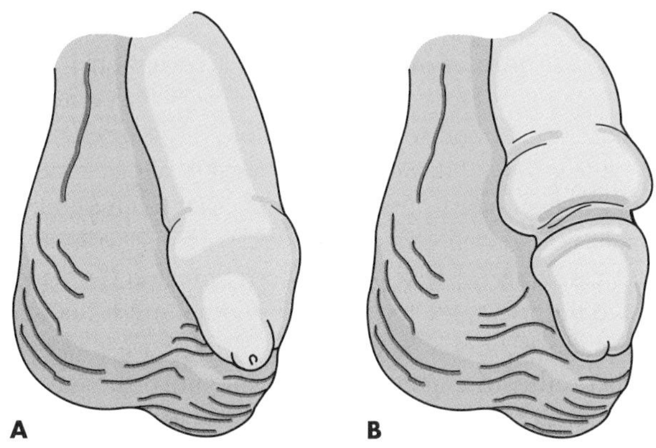

Figure 55-8 **A**, Phimosis: note pinpoint opening of foreskin. **B**, Paraphimosis: note foreskin is retracted but has become constricting band around penis.

children.[10] There is a higher incidence in African-Americans than Caucasians, possibly because of a lower incidence of circumcision. Penile cancer accounts for 10% to 20% of all malignancies among African-American and Asian-American men.[10]

The incidence of penile cancer depends greatly on hygienic standards and cultural and religious practices. It almost never occurs in a male who was circumcised at birth. Circumcision after puberty does not decrease the risk of cancer when compared with the incidence among uncircumcised males. Circumcision removes the prepuce, or foreskin, which provides a haven for bacteria. The bacteria act on desquamated cells, producing smegma, which is irritating to the tissue of the glans penis and the prepuce. This chronic irritation is considered to be carcinogenic. Therefore adequate hygiene theoretically is sufficient prophylaxis against penile cancer, making circumcision unnecessary. Trauma and STDs are thought to be coincidental to penile cancer rather than causative. Box 55-5 lists the stages of penile cancer.

BOX 55-5 Stages of Penile Cancer

Stage A	Lesions confined to glans or foreskin
Stage B	Shaft or corpora cavernosa invaded by tumor
Stage C	Shaft involvement; lymph nodes involved but operable
Stage D	Shaft involvement; lymph nodes inoperable; metastases to distant sites

Pathophysiology

Penile cancer starts as a small lesion usually on or under the prepuce and extends until the entire glans and shaft are involved. The initial lesion may assume a variety of forms. It may appear as a small bump, resemble a pimple or wart, or occur as a nonhealing ulcer with the edges rolled inward. The latter is associated with earlier metastases and a poorer 5-year survival.

The most common (95%) type of malignancy is squamous cell carcinoma. Phimosis, which is present in 25% to 75% of patients with penile cancer, may obscure the lesion. The lesion may then cause erosion through the prepuce, resulting in a foul odor and discharge. Bleeding may or may not be present. Urethral and bladder involvement are rare. Eventually the disease can become autoamputative. If left untreated, death occurs in 2 to 3 years.

Clinical manifestations of penile cancer include weakness, fatigue, malaise, and weight loss. Men may complain of itching and burning under the prepuce and an occasional foul discharge. A 1-year delay before seeking treatment occurs in 15% to 50% of cases. Biopsy is performed to establish the diagnosis; however, benign penile lesions occur infrequently.

Metastasis usually occurs at the regional femoral and iliac nodes and is associated with a significantly worse prognosis. Five-year survival with inguinal node involvement is 20% to 25%.[10]

Collaborative Care Management

Treatment is usually surgical. Radiation therapy is indicated only in patients who have small superficial lesions and strongly desire to preserve sexual function.

If the lesion is confined to the prepuce, circumcision may be adequate. If the lesion is on the glans, partial penectomy or amputation of the penis is required. If the shaft of the penis is involved, total amputation may be necessary. The decision is based on the amount of penis remaining after excision with an adequate tumor-free margin. The remaining penis must be long enough for the patient to void in a standing position and direct the urinary stream. If this is possible, sexual function will probably be retained. If total amputation is required, a perineal urethrostomy is performed, in which the urethra is redirected to an opening between the scrotum and the anus. With spread of the cancer to the scrotum, radical removal is required, either hemipelvectomy or hemicorporectomy.

Approximately one third of men with penile cancer have metastatic nodal disease at the time of initial diagnosis. Radiation therapy is used as adjuvant therapy at all stages. Lymphadenectomy is indicated for lymph node involvement. Accurate detection of metastases is difficult, as enlarged lymph nodes may be free of cancerous tissue, whereas normal-size lymph nodes may contain metastatic lesions.

Chemotherapeutic agents have been used with some success, particularly in patients with stages A and B (low-grade) disease. Agents include high-dose methotrexate, bleomycin, and cisplatin. Because of the rarity of the disease, large-scale clinical studies to evaluate chemotherapeutic agents are lacking. Methotrexate has been somewhat successful. If the disease is confined to the penis, 5-year survival is 80% to 85% with amputation. With metastasis to the lymph nodes, it is only 20%.

Patient/Family Education. The nurse teaches the patient about the potential side effects of radiation in the perineal area. Radiation in this location can cause the skin to become dry, itchy, and sensitive. Special gels that are safe to use during radiation may be applied to the affected area.

Urethral strictures can develop several months to years after radiation therapy. The nurse informs the patient of symptoms of urethral stricture, which include difficulty starting or stopping the urine flow, frequent UTIs, and nocturia. Bowel patterns may change during radiation therapy and for up to several weeks. Effects of chemotherapy and nursing interventions are discussed in Chapter 15.

The emotional devastation of a diagnosis of penile cancer is difficult to overestimate. The proposed surgery may be unthinkable to the patient, who is frequently in a state of shock. The scope of support and sexual counseling needed by this patient is beyond the expertise of most nurses. The patient is referred for sexual counseling with experts who can clearly explain his options. Some patients with a urethrostomy have experienced orgasm and ejaculation after stimulation of the perineal, scrotal, and testicular regions.

Impotence/Erectile Dysfunction

Etiology

Impotence is the inability of a man to have an erection firm enough or sustain an erection long enough for satisfactory intercourse. The term satisfactory is defined by the couple involved and may vary from couple to couple. The ability to have an erection depends not only on a healthy psychologic state, but also on adequately functioning neurologic, vascular, and hormonal systems. The brain is the controlling organ for sexual arousal. The brain perceives sexual stimuli and controls the physiologic changes that occur during arousal. The two fundamental causes of impotence are physical and psychologic.

Physical causes include changes in blood flow to the penis and neurogenic dysfunctions. Diseases such as diabetes, lupus, and rheumatoid arthritis can damage blood vessels and cause obstruction of blood flow in the penis. Anemia and dehydration can cause insufficient blood volumes to maintain an erection. Cardiac diseases and antihypertensive drugs can interfere with the capillary blood pressure.[17] Trauma to the peritoneum can cause scaring and reduce blood flow.

A wide variety of disorders that affect neurologic functioning (e.g., spinal cord injury, diabetes, renal failure, multiple sclerosis, and Parkinson's disease) can interfere with erectile function. Changes in testosterone levels can affect the male sex drive. Aging affects the level of testosterone, and sexual function usually declines somewhat with advancing age.

Other causes of impotence include surgical procedures that interfere with both blood engorgement and neurogenic innervation of the penis, and prescription drugs that produce the side effect of impotence.

Psychologic impotence can be attributed to many factors, such as long-term stressors, fears, anxiety, anger, and frustrations. "Performance anxiety," a fear of not performing well during sexual intercourse, is common. Fatigue also influences the ability to have an erection (see Risk Factors box).

Epidemiology

Most men occasionally experience impotence. Short-term impotence can be caused by fatigue, stress, anxiety, or the use of alcohol or other drugs. Until recently, psychologic problems were considered to be the cause of 90% of impotence cases. Now, physical causes have been found in 85% of cases. One in every 10 males in the United States has continuing or chronic impotence.[16] The tremendous anxiety produced by

Risk Factors
Impotence

Stress
Fatigue
Drug effects (e.g., antihypertensive agents, beta-blockers, or alcohol)
Diabetes mellitus
Vascular disease (e.g., hypertension or peripheral vascular disease)
Neurologic disorders (e.g., multiple sclerosis or spinal cord injury)
Effects of colorectal, cystectomy, or selected prostatectomy procedures
Trauma to the perineal area
Psychologic factors

BOX 55-6 Priapism

Priapism is a painful condition, characterized by prolonged erection (>4 to 6 hours). Penile ischemia can result, causing permanent impotence or necrosis of the penis.

Etiology

- Caused by either prolonged venous occlusion or arterial blood engorgement
- Possible side effect of some impotence therapies

Treatment

- Treatment is directed at the specific cause.
- Options include administration of alpha-agonists directly into the corpora cavernosa, and IV therapy to reestablish acid-base balance.
- Pain management is a high priority.

occasional or chronic impotence worsens the problem, even when the underlying disorder is physical in nature.

Pathophysiology

Inability of the brain to respond to sexual stimuli can interrupt the signals to the parasympathetic nervous system that release a transmitter substance causing the small arteries in the penis to dilate. The result is insufficient blood flow to fill the network of sinusoids inside the corpora cavernosa (erectile chambers) that cause the penis to enlarge and become firm. When the blood volume in the erectile chambers is inadequate, they cannot create enough pressure to block blood return. Blood drains from the penis and an erection cannot be maintained.

The sympathetic nervous system controls both orgasm and ejaculation. These two functions therefore can occur without an erection. After ejaculation, or when sexual stimulation diminishes, the arteries in the penis constrict, reducing blood flow, and the veins expand to allow disengorgement.

Collaborative Care Management

Diagnostic Tests. Diagnostic tests for impotence include complete blood count, urinalysis, BUN, creatinine, and fasting blood sugars. These tests help rule out entities such as anemia, renal disease, and diabetes as possible causative factors. Other blood tests include cholesterol levels and hormonal studies.

Nocturnal monitoring of penile tumescence is also performed. This test involves the man wearing a device around the penis at night that can gauge normal nocturnal engorgement of the penis. Results indicate the ability of the penis to enlarge and become firm.

Invasive studies are ordered only when other testing measures are inconclusive. Arteriograms and cavernosometry, which measures pressures and blood vessel responses in the erectile chambers, are sometimes performed.

Psychologic testing is also performed, which ideally also includes the man's partner.

Medications. A phosphodiesterase inhibitor, Viagra promotes local vasodilation and has demonstrated 50% to 70% effectiveness during clinical trials. All oral agents still require sexual stimulation for the patient to achieve an erection. Viagra can lower the blood pressure significantly and has resulted in cardiac arrest in a few cases when taken in combination with nitrates. Other side effects include headache and gastrointestinal disturbances.

Topical agents are occasionally used to enhance venous congestion of the penis. These drugs can support an erection over a period of hours. Nitroglycerin ointment is an example of a topical vasodilator. Topical and oral agents are often combined with other therapies to treat impotence.

Hormonal therapy is prescribed for the 2% of the impotent population who have a low serum testosterone or an elevated serum prolactin level. Testosterone is given either intramuscularly or transdermally to avoid the hepatotoxicity of the oral preparations. Testosterone can stimulate growth of normal prostatic tissue, promote metastasis of prostatic cancer, stop sperm production, and cause fluid retention and therefore must be used cautiously.

Vasodilators can induce penile erections by means of increased arterial blood flow, sinusoidal relaxation, and increased venous resistance. The drugs generally used are a papaverine and phentolamine combination injected by the patient into the corpus cavernosum of the penis, or inserted into the tip of the penis via suppository. Drug combinations may include prostaglandin E (PGE). Once the drug is injected or inserted, the penis becomes turgid within 5 to 10 minutes, and the erection may last up to 2 hours. Response rate is about 100% for those with neurogenic impotence and 60% to 70% for those with vascular problems.[17] Test doses are given initially to determine the appropriate drug dosage for each patient. Dosages range from .05 to 1.5 ml of the combination drug. Side effects include dizziness, facial flushing, hypotension, and priapism (an erection that lasts longer than 4 to 6 hours; Box 55-6).

Many medications have side effects that inhibit erectile function. Modifying the dosage, changing the brand, or trying an alternative medication can be helpful for many patients.

Treatments. External vacuum devices are sometimes used to achieve an erection for a short time. These devices are cylinders

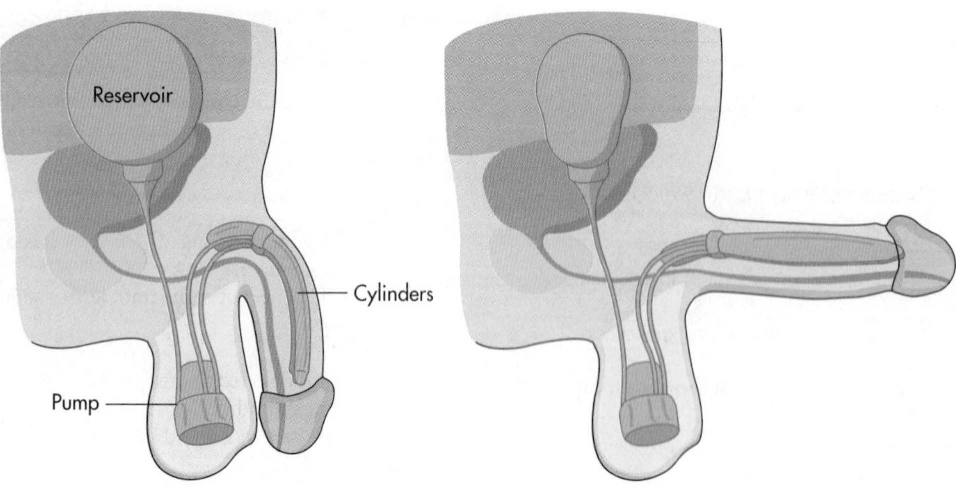

Figure 55-9 The Scott Inflatable Prosthesis has both erect and flaccid positions designed to mimic normal erectile function.

that fit over the penis and use a suction pump to pull blood into the penis. A band is applied to the proximal aspect of the penis when an erection is achieved to impede the venous return. The erection may be maintained for approximately 30 minutes. The devices can be used daily and have minimal side effects if used properly. These devices are contraindicated for patients with bleeding disorders, sickle cell anemia, and severe circulatory compromise.

Counseling and sexual therapy classes may be suggested for patients who have identified psychologic impotence. They may also be suggested for men dealing with the problem of impotence and the need to find alternative measures for sexual fulfillment.

Surgical Management. Vascular reconstructive surgery may be helpful for the approximately 5% of impotent men who have problems with venous leakage. Venous leakage is defined as the inability to maintain an erection for more than about 2 minutes. The surgery may include the microscopic reconstruction of arterial vessels or removal of some veins to slow the draining of blood from the penis. These surgeries have a limited success rate of only 30% to 50%.[17] There is also a high rate of relapse because of arteriosclerosis and the continued development of incompetent veins. Complications of vascular surgery include numbness of the penile skin, shortened length, curvature, and hematoma formation.

A penile prosthesis may be implanted to treat organic erectile dysfunction. There are two types of penile prostheses. One type consists of two sponge-filled silicone rods, which are implanted in the corpora cavernosa. They support the penis in a constant semierect position. Another method, which more closely simulates an actual erection, is the inflatable penile prosthesis (Figure 55-9). This consists of two inflatable rods inserted into either side of the penis. The rods are connected to a reservoir that allows fluid to flow in or out of them when the man presses on a pump device inserted in the thigh or scrotum.

Both types of prostheses are implanted surgically and do not interfere with normal urinary elimination. The silicone implants are inserted through perineal or penile incisions and the inflatable prostheses through perineal and abdominal incisions. Penile edema is minimal, but scrotal edema may occur with the inflatable type. Pain may be severe during the first week, and mild pain may continue for several weeks after surgery. As with any prosthetic device, the man needs to integrate the device successfully into his body image and sexual relationship.[1] Table 55-5 compares treatment options for erectile dysfunction.

Diet. A well-balanced diet is recommended for men with impotence. No studies have proved that any vitamin or mineral supplements specifically enhance a man's ability to have an erection. However, some foods are considered to be aphrodisiacs in various cultures, including oysters, avocados, and bull testicles. Obesity can interfere with erectile functioning. Low-fat reducing diets are recommended for patients who are overweight.

Activity. Men who are in better physical condition often have more endurance and may fatigue less quickly when engaging in sexual activity. However, no specific exercise plan is known to have any positive effect on erectile function.

Referrals. In some settings the nurse assumes responsibility for making referrals to other services. Common referrals for a man with impotence include certified sex therapists, social workers, and family counselors.

NURSING MANAGEMENT OF PATIENT WITH IMPOTENCE

ASSESSMENT

Data to be collected to assess the patient with impotence include:

- History of sexual dysfunction
- Partner's view of sexual history
- Ability to have an erection: type, length of time penis remains engorged
- Length of time sexual functioning has been a concern

TABLE 55-5 Treatment Options for Male Sexual Dysfunction

Advantages	Disadvantages
Nonsurgical	
Oral Medications (sildenafil [Viagra], alprostadil)	
Increases libido Inexpensive Minimal side effects Can be used with other options	Newly released and still in trials, 50%-70% effective Side effects include headache, diarrhea Contraindicated for concurrent use with nitrates
Hormonal Therapy (Testosterone)	
Increases libido Inexpensive Does not interfere with other treatment options Widely available	Limited effectiveness (10% to 15%) Contraindicated with prostate cancer Must be taken on long-term basis Side effects include fluid retention, liver damage
External Vacuum Devices	
Easy to understand Inexpensive Safe, reversible Can be used with other treatment options	Requires preparation Long-term effects not known Side effects include bruising, pain Requires manual dexterity
Sexual Devices	
Inexpensive Easy to understand May enhance foreplay/orgasm	Does not produce satisfactory erection May not fit into value system Inaccessiblity
Counseling	
Involves partner Can be used with other treatment options May improve other psychosocial issues	Limited effectiveness Long-standing problems may be difficult to treat
Penile Injections/Suppositories	
Use only when desired Produces rapid, natural-appearing erections Can be used with other treatments Minimal pain	Requires close monitoring Moderately expensive Not effective with severe blood flow problems Side effects include priapism, fibrosis Patient may have aversion to needles/insertion device

Advantages	Disadvantages
Surgical	
Vascular Reconstructive Surgery	
Possibility of restoration to normal function Natural appearance	Expensive Technically difficult surgery Low long-term success rate (30%-50%) High relapse rate
Inflatable Prosthesis	
Natural-looking erection No preparation time Use as desired Increases girth of penis No concealment problem	Device failure Requires manual dexterity May require removal/reimplant Expensive Risk of infection, erosion
Self-contained Inflatable Prosthesis	
Natural-looking erection No preparation time Use as desired No concealment problem Simpler surgery than that for full inflatable prosthesis	Device failure Requires manual dexterity May require removal/reimplant Expensive Risk of infection, erosion Does not increase girth
Semirigid/Malleable Prosthesis	
Simple surgery No moving parts Least expensive implant Use as desired	May be difficult to conceal Does not increase girth of penis Expensive Risk of infection/erosion May require removal/reimplant

Presence of psychosocial stressors

History of physical diseases; especially vascular and neurogenic

History of surgeries; especially TURP, prostatectomy, cystectomy

Treatment approaches tried to alleviate the problem

Sensory/motor deficits: manual dexterity and visual acuity needed for many treatment options

General assessment of sexual organs to note any obvious deformity or structural defects

NURSING DIAGNOSES

Nursing diagnoses are determined from analysis of patient data. Nursing diagnoses for the patient with impotence may include but are not limited to:

Diagnostic Title	Possible Etiologic Factors
1. Sexual dysfunction (impotence)	Difficulty in attaining or maintaining an erection
2. Anxiety	Sexual performance

EXPECTED PATIENT OUTCOMES

Expected patient outcomes for the patient with impotence may include but are not limited to:

1a. Will identify alternative methods of sexual intimacy that will provide a positive sexual interaction
1b. Will demonstrate the effective use of devices to obtain an erection
2. Will demonstrate a relaxed positive attitude about sexual performance

INTERVENTIONS

1a, b. Identifying Alternatives

Helping the patient choose sexual therapy options by providing accurate and up-to-date information is an important part of nursing care for the patient with impotence. Myths and erroneous information are common obstacles in sexual rehabilitation. The patient is informed of the physiologic and psychologic aspects of erectile function. The use of external devices and medications is reviewed, including their modes of action, side effects, and contraindications. Early referral to advanced practice nurses and other specialists is usually appropriate.

Penile Injections

The nurse may be responsible for teaching the patient to administer penile injections. These patients need to be evaluated in an office or clinic on a regular basis. Systemic complications of the injections include orthostatic hypotension and dizziness. Local complications include pain, hematoma, edema, decreased glandular sensation, fibrosis, and priapism. Priapism may be reversed by application of ice, manual masturbation, injection of epinephrine, or the use of antihistamines. If priapism persists longer than 4 to 6 hours, the patient should notify his physician.

Injection sites are to the lateral sides of the penis and should be rotated, and injection into the urethra should be avoided. Applying pressure to the injection site can help decrease the possibility of fibrosis. The patient is instructed not to use injections more than twice a week. Liver enzyme levels should be monitored about every 3 months. If liver function studies are elevated or fibrosis is noted on the penis, it usually is recommended that the injections be discontinued. The drug should be kept in the refrigerator to avoid degeneration of the solution. Dosages can be altered if initial results are not satisfactory.

External Vacuum Devices

Vacuum devices come in one size with ring seals at the end that are different diameters to accommodate individual erection size. The patient is taught to use the device and make sure that the seals are the appropriate size to ensure sufficient vacuum to the penis. The vascular ring is applied once the penis is engorged and should be left on only for approximately 30 minutes to prevent possible vascular damage. The nurse involves both partners in the teaching session if possible. Couples need to discuss in advance how sexual activity may be modified comfortably with the use of the device.

The vacuum device may be used every day if desired. Complications include pulling of scrotal tissue, hematoma, inability to achieve or maintain the erection, and discomfort with the vascular ring. These complications can usually be managed by adjusting the procedure or switching to a different product. Blocked or retrograde ejaculation may also occur. Orgasm should not be affected. The patient is encouraged to schedule ongoing medical support to help him cope with this altered sexual pattern.

Penile Implants

Infection rates are generally low with penile implant surgery. Antibiotics may be administered a few days before surgery and for a week after surgery to prevent infection. The patient also may be told to perform a Hibiclens prewash before surgery, to decrease the chance of infection. The nurse instructs the patient to take all antibiotics and report any symptoms of infection, such as unusual swelling, redness, excessive pain, or drainage around the incision sites.

To prevent the device from eroding through the penile skin, the patient is instructed to avoid sexual intercourse for at least 6 to 8 weeks after surgery. When sexual activity resumes, the patient is instructed to use a water-soluble lubricant. The patient needs to avoid wearing tight-fitting clothing and sitting with the legs crossed or in other positions that put pressure or cause friction to the penis.

The nurse explains to the patient that his erections will not necessarily be any larger than before surgery, that the implant will not affect sex drive or interfere with penile sensation, and that he should be able to have an orgasm and ejaculate with the implant in place. Patients with inflatable implants need to be instructed on how to inflate and deflate the prosthesis. The patient's partner is included in teaching sessions if possible.

2. Reducing Performance-Related Anxiety

Sexual counseling usually is offered in conjunction with other forms of treatment for the impotent patient. The nurse is often the person to encourage patients to avail themselves of counseling opportunities. The nurse helps the patient understand his needs and explains the general nature of sexual counseling, as patients often have misconceptions concerning the treatment. The nurse provides some specific examples of exercises used during sexual counseling and explains how partner communication can be enhanced.

EVALUATION

To evaluate the effectiveness of nursing interventions, compare patient behaviors with those stated in the expected patient outcomes. Achievement of outcomes is successful if the patient with impotence:

1a. Engages in gratifying sexual intimacy with a significant other.
1b. Uses devices to obtain an erection correctly and safely.
2. States he feels more relaxed and positive about sexual performance.

GERONTOLOGIC CONSIDERATIONS

The nurse should not assume that older adults do not have sexual needs. Impotence in the older patient is often caused by narrowing of the blood vessels and consequently decreased blood flow to the penis. Most healthy males can obtain an erection even at an advanced age. Often the elderly male needs more and prolonged stimulation than his younger counterpart to have an erection. The nurse can inform patients and their partners of the need for longer "foreplay" with the older man.

SPECIAL ENVIRONMENTS FOR CARE

Critical Care Management

Critical care does not play a role in the management of impotence. Treatment is largely based in the outpatient setting and surgery would not be recommended for any man who was not in good general health.

Home Care Management

If the patient had surgical treatment for impotence, any signs of infection or erosion of the penile implant should be immediately reported to the physician. Often, when the patient uses the penile erectile devices for the first few times at home, questions arise. Patients need to be discharged with explicit instructions about whom to contact with concerns and phone numbers for resource persons.

COMPLICATIONS

Complications of penile implant surgery include malfunction of the device, infection, and erosion of the prosthesis through the penis. Complications of injections and mechanical erectile devices include possible priapism and circulatory occlusions to the penis, causing tissue necrosis.

VASECTOMY: MALE STERILIZATION

Etiology/Epidemiology

Voluntary sterilization has become increasingly acceptable to both men and women as a method of preventing pregnancy. It is the most frequently used method of fertility control for married couples over 30 years old and is the most widely used contraceptive method worldwide, protecting approximately 100 million couples. It has been estimated that more than 13.7 million adults have been sterilized in the United States and 100 million worldwide. Each year, 500,000 to 1 million American men have vasectomies.[13]

The primary reason given by both men and women for wishing sterilization is a desire to limit family size. More frequently than women, men give as an important reason for sterilization their wish for an effective contraceptive that does not interfere with sexual pleasure. Also, men express concern over the health of their sex partners. Some men believe that the "pill" is actually or potentially harmful to the woman.

Laws governing sterilization vary from state to state and have undergone many changes. In general, if the surgery does not violate specific state provisions and if written informed consent is given by a man or woman legally capable of giving permission, the surgery can be performed. Because sterilization is a permanent method of contraception, informed consent is absolutely necessary before the procedure.

Pathophysiology

Bilateral vasectomy is the surgical procedure used for male sterilization. Vasectomy interrupts the continuity of the vas deferens, and sperm are prevented from being ejaculated with other components of the semen. However, sperm still are produced, and the ejaculate is not noticeably diminished in amount. Residual fertility may be present for a variable period because of existing sperm in the semen beyond the point of occlusion of the vas deferens. Sperm gradually disappear from the ejaculate; thus conception is possible in the immediate postoperative period.

After vasectomy, antibodies to sperm develop in about 50% to 66% of men. No relationship has been found in humans between the presence of sperm antibodies and any systemic pathologic condition. It is hypothesized that antisperm antibodies may result in circulating immune complexes that exacerbate atherosclerosis, but this has not been proven in human studies.

Collaborative Care Management

At least 11 different techniques for vasectomy exist. Bilateral partial vasectomy is the surgical method used most often. Because of its safety and simplicity, the procedure can be performed on an outpatient basis using a local anesthetic. A small incision is made in the scrotum to expose the sheath of the vas deferens. The sheath is opened, and a 0.63 to 1.27 cm segment of the vas deferens is removed. The severed ends of the vas deferens are then ligated or coagulated to ensure sterility. The incision is then sutured closed.

Complications after vasectomy are rare and usually minor. Bruising, mild edema, and mild discomfort are common and usually subside without treatment. Infection of the wound occurs in about 3% of patients. Hematoma, epididymitis, and granuloma formation can occur. The incidence of failure as a result of recanalization (reanastomosis) is reported to be 0% to 6%. The cause of spontaneous recanalization is unknown, but duplication of the vas deferens has occasionally occurred. A preoperative specimen of semen is examined to serve as a baseline for monitoring sperm disappearance after surgery.

Research is ongoing concerning techniques to reverse vasectomy and restore fertility. A vasovasostomy attempts to rejoin the severed ends of the vas deferens. Success is measured by the presence of sperm in semen specimens after reconstruction. Reports of success in restoring fertility range from 29% to 85%.[13]

Patient/Family Education. Patient education focuses on ensuring that the patient has made a careful and informed decision concerning sterilization. Teaching is based on the federal government's informed consent guidelines (see Chapter 18). The nature and consequences of the surgery are explained to the patient. It is important to emphasize that the sterilization procedure does nothing to increase or decrease sexual performance or enjoyment, but simply removes the risk of pregnancy. Visual aids and models can be of great value in explaining the surgery to patients.

Every effort is made to ensure that the decision for sterilization is not based on a lack of knowledge concerning other options for contraception. Most patients are satisfied with the results of vasectomy, but emotional difficulties can be experienced, as sterilization affects both partners.

The facts concerning reversibility, including current success rates, are discussed. In the case of vasectomy, the chance of recanalization and return of fertility should be pointed out. The man or couple must also be informed that sterility occurs progressively rather than immediately after vasectomy, and alternate methods of contraception need to be used until sterility is achieved. Men are taught to expect slight swelling of the scrotum, minor pain, and a small amount of bleeding after surgery. Ice to the scrotal area, sitz baths, and rest will ameliorate these discomforts. Any signs of infection should be reported promptly to the physician for evaluation and treatment.

It is important for the man to schedule follow-up semen analysis. A sperm count usually is taken 4 weeks after vasectomy. Two consecutive sperm-free specimens are necessary before the man can be considered sterile. Reanastomosis of the vas deferens is suspected if sperm fail to disappear from the ejaculate, if there is an increase in sperm in the semen after two successive sperm counts, or if motile sperm are found in the semen 3 months after vasectomy.

Critical Thinking Questions

1. A 40-year-old patient is postorchiectomy and radical node dissection for a nonseminomatous neoplasm. The nurse identifies hemorrhage, atelectasis, thrombosis, and paralytic ileus as potential complications of the surgery. Discuss preventive nursing measures for these potential complications specifically with regard to activity.
2. As a community health nurse in an industrial company, you are designing a program to teach men in the company about reproductive health. Develop an outline depicting the priority diseases and preventive measures to teach.
3. A 59-year-old man is admitted to the hospital complaining of difficulty urinating. The emergency room physician orders routine urinalysis, complete blood count, and chemistry profile. Outline questions designed to help differentiate the cause of these symptoms.

References

1. Backmann GA et al: Patients with sexual dysfunction, *Patient Care* 2:4, 1999.
2. Carroll PR, Presti JC: Testes cancer, *Urol Clin North Am* 3:25, 1998.
3. Catalona WJ et al: Treating early prostate cancer: difficult decisions abound, *Patient Care* 2:10, 1999.
4. Cookson MS, Smith JA: PSA testing: update on diagnostic tools, *Consultant* 4:40, 2000.
5. Critz FA et al: Prostate specific antigen bounce after radioactive seed implantation followed by external beam radiation for prostate cancer, *J Urol* 163(4):1085-1089, 2000.
6. Davis DL: Prostate cancer treatment with radioactive seed implantation, *AORN J* 1:68, 1998.
7. Donovan DA, Nicholas PK: Prostatitis: diagnosis and treatment in primary care, *Nurse Pract* 22(4):144, 1997.
8. DuFour JL: Short communications: assessing and treating epididymitis, *Nurse Pract* 26(3):23, 2001.
9. Goolsby MJ: Screening, diagnosis, and management of prostate cancer: improving primary care outcomes, *Nurse Pract* 3:23, 1998.
10. Gordon SI et al: When the diagnosis is penile cancer, *RN* 60(3):41-44, 1997.
11. Gray M: Urinary retention, *Am J Nurs* 7(100):40, 2000.
12. Greifzer SP: Oncology today: prostate cancer, *RN* 6:63, 2000.
13. Hans JM, Butta PG, Giruin S: A comprehensive and efficient process for counseling patients desiring sterilization, *Nurse Pract* 22(6):52, 1997.
14. Reference deleted in proofs.
15. Kolon TF, Albertsen PC: Diagnosis and treatment of scrotal abnormalities, *Clin Advisor* 5:3, 2000.
16. Leasia MS, Monahan FD: *A practical guide to health assessment,* ed 2, Philadelphia, 2000, WB Saunders.
17. Lue TF: Erective dysfunction, *Urol Clin North Am* 2:28, 2001.
18. Mosier WA, Scheymanski TJ, Walgren KD: Benign prostatic hyperplasia, *Clin Rev* 7:8, 1998.
19. National Kidney and Urologic Diseases Information Clearinghouse: *Prostate enlargement: benign prostatic hyperplasia,* National Institute of Diabetes and Digestive and Kidney Diseases (NIDDK), Washington, DC, 1998, National Institutes of Health, USDHHS.
20. Pagana KD, Pagana TJ: *Mosby's diagnostic and laboratory test reference,* ed 4, St Louis, 1999, Mosby.
21. Pateman B, Johnson M: Men's lived experiences following transurethral prostatectomy for benign prostatic hypertrophy, *J Adv Nurs* 1:31, 2000.
22. Peacock P: A new procedure for prostate patients, *RN* 12:61, 1998.
23. Reznicek S: Common urologic problems in the elderly, *Postgrad Med* 1:107, 2000.
24. Tamkin G: Evaluating acute scrotal pain, *Emerg Med* 32(5):20, 2000.
25. Vetrosky DT et al: Prostate cancer: pathology, diagnosis, and management, *Clin Rev* 5:7, 1997.
26. Wareing M et al: Piloting day case surgery for prostate resection, *Professional Nurse* 11:14, 1999.
27. Zitkus BS, Dumas MA: Testicular discomfort, *Am J Nurse Pract* 7:4, 2000.
28. website: http://www.cancernet.nci.nih.gov
29. website: http://www.mayohealth.org/home?id=5.1.1.2.8
30. http://www.prostateinfo.com

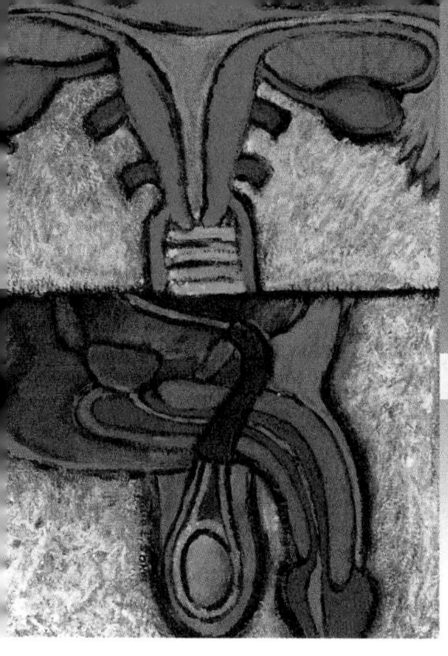

http://www.mosby.com/MERLIN/medsurg_phipps

56 Sexually Transmitted Diseases

Gretchen G. Mettler, Wilma J. Phipps

Objectives

After studying this chapter, the learner should be able to:

1. Define sexually transmitted diseases (STDs).
2. Describe the transmission, prevention, and control of STDs and urovaginal infections.
3. List the causative agent, incubation period, signs and symptoms, medical therapy, and long-term effects of gonorrhea, chlamydia, syphilis, herpes genitalis, and human papillomavirus infections.
4. Identify the information to be collected from a person suspected of having any STD or urovaginal infections.
5. Write a teaching plan for a unit on the prevention of STDs for a sexuality education course for adolescents.

Etiology

Sexually transmitted diseases (STDs) are diseases that usually are or can be transmitted from one person to another with heterosexual or homosexual intercourse or intimate contact with the genitalia, mouth, or rectum. Because the causative organisms survive only briefly outside a warm, moist environment, there is almost no way to contract STDs from toilet seats, towels, or bed linens. Although STDs are not usually transmitted in public restrooms, conditions caused by fungi, bacteria, and lice can possibly be transmitted from water in unclean toilet bowls. Women using a conventional toilet expose the vaginal and anal area to pathogens that can be introduced by the backsplash of contaminated toilet water.

There are some notable exceptions to sexual transmission. If a mother has syphilis during pregnancy, the fetus may become infected in utero by placental transmission, and the neonate may acquire congenital syphilis or be stillborn. Infants of mothers with gonorrhea or chlamydia may contract an infection of the eyes (ophthalmia neonatorum) during birth, and unless treated, the infection can lead to permanent blindness. *Chlamydia* present at birth is a common cause of subacute, afebrile pneumonia occurring in the infant between 1 and 3 months old.

Since the 1980s, several diseases have been added to the list of STDs. Originally syphilis, gonorrhea, chancroid, lymphogranuloma venereum, and granuloma inguinale were identified. Now the list includes *Chlamydia trachomatis*, genital herpes, human papillomavirus (HPV), genital mycoplasmas, cytomegalovirus, hepatitis B, enteric infections, and ectoparasitic disease. Early in the 1980s the human immunodeficiency virus (HIV) was identified, and acquired immunodeficiency syndrome (AIDS) emerged as a major STD.[21] Because of the profound effect of AIDS on the immune system, Chapter 50 is devoted to its discussion.

The diseases classified as STDs and urogenital infections and their causative organisms are listed in Table 56-1. Many of the newly recognized STDs have become epidemic or hyperendemic as a consequence of changing sexual behavioral patterns. In addition to this increase in many STDs, the sexually transmitted proportion of infections by agents with multiple modes of transmission (e.g., hepatitis B virus, enteric pathogens) has increased. All states require that each case of syphilis, gonorrhea, and AIDS be reported to the state or local health officer.[6] Most states also require the reporting of chlamydia, chancroid, granuloma inguinale, hepatitis A, B, and C, and lymphogranuloma venereum. Herpes genitalis does not need to be reported in any state. The true incidence of STDs is not known because of variable reporting requirements and because many cases are not reported by the clinicians who treat them. STDs not only have immediate consequences but have the recognized effects on maternal and infant morbidity, as well as on human reproduction and fertility.

Epidemiology

In the United States almost 12 million cases of STDs occur yearly, 86% of them in persons between 15 and 29 years old. By the age of 21 years, approximately one of every five young persons has received treatment for an STD. Because only some teenagers are sexually active, this amounts to an effective case rate of at least 25% among those who are sexually active.[8]

Most STDs exhibit "biologic sexism" because their serious complications have the greatest impact on women and children. These complications are pelvic inflammatory disease (PID), sterility, ectopic pregnancy, blindness, cancer associated

TABLE 56-1 Sexually Transmitted Diseases/ Urovaginal Infections

Type of Organism	Disease
Bacteria	Gonorrhea, chancroid, granuloma inguinale, bacterial vaginosis
Spirochete	Syphilis
Chlamydia	Nongonococcal urethritis, epididymitis, cervicitis, pelvic inflammatory disease, lymphogranuloma venereum
Virus	Herpes genitalis, hepatitis B, cytomegalovirus, human immunodeficiency virus/acquired immune deficiency syndrone, human papillomavirus (condylomata acuminata), molluscum contagiosum
Protozoa	Trichomoniasis
Fungi	Candidiasis
Parasites	Pediculosis pubis, scabies

with the HPV, fetal and infant deaths, birth defects, and mental retardation. The populations most affected are medically underserved persons, poor persons, and racial and ethnic minorities. The direct and indirect societal costs of STDs total $17 billion annually, with the cost of PID and PID-associated ectopic pregnancy and infertility alone exceeding $2.6 billion.[8]

In explaining the trends of reported cases of STDs in the United States, societal changes occurring since the 1960s are often cited in the literature. The first of these relates to the use of antibiotics and resultant changes in the antibiotic susceptibility of pathogenic organisms. The widespread, perhaps indiscriminate, use of penicillin and other antibiotics in the late 1940s and early 1950s parallels the decline in both syphilis and gonorrhea. It is postulated that the organisms developed a greater resistance to antibiotics over that time and hence are now less effective. No firm evidence indicates a decrease in effectiveness of penicillin against syphilis. The gonococcus clearly tends to develop resistance even to newer generations of. antibiotics.

Another explanation concerns sexual behavior patterns and includes permissiveness. Concern has been expressed particularly about the prevalence of gonorrhea among adolescents and young adults. Rates for gonorrhea show that young adults 20 to 24 years old accounted for 40% of reported cases of gonorrhea, whereas persons 15 to 19 years old accounted for 25% of cases. The highest morbidity rate for men was in the 20- to 24-year age-group; for women it was in the 15- to 19-year age-group.

The preceding discussion makes an assumption of relaxed social values and behaviors and, in doing so, requires acknowledgment of advances in contraceptive technology since the development of "the pill." These social changes are often referred to as the three Ps (permissiveness, promiscuity, and the pill). The underlying idea is that, with the advent of antibiotics and the pill, people began to lose fear of untreated venereal disease and pregnancy and that the number of lifetime partners increased significantly, leading to greater exposure to infection. According to Hatcher and associates,[14] the type of contraception chosen has a direct impact on STD risk.

Most unmarried persons admit to practicing "serial monogamy," which is a mutually faithful sexual relationship with one person for a period of time, rather than reporting multiple sexual partners. In the past, prostitution was a major force in the transmission of STDs. Today, the practice of serial monogamy increases the number of lifetime sexual partners, thereby increasing the risk for contracting STDs.[14]

For example, currently, most persons with gonorrhea are single, under 25 years old, and report being in a monogamous relationship.

Before 1960 homosexuals were rarely mentioned in the literature as carriers of STDs. With the development of the AIDS epidemic in the early 1980s, much more attention has been given to the risk of STDs among homosexual and bisexual men. Homosexual men also carry pathogens in the rectum and colon, including gonococcus, *Giardia*, ameba, *Shigella*, and *Campylobacter*. Although lesbians are considered to be at low risk for contracting STDs and gay males are at higher risk, it is important to note that sexual orientation does not determine individual forms of sexual behavior.

Before the advent of oral contraceptives, condoms were the main method of contraception followed by diaphragms. Use of the condom is believed to have prevented the spread of STDs by providing a mechanical barrier to the organisms. The pill revolutionized contraceptive practices, unlinking contraception from the sexual act. In addition estrogen, a component of oral contraceptives, alters the vaginal and cervical ecology, predisposing it to infection.

Two events during the 1980s and 1990s bear mentioning:

1. The designation of AIDS as an STD put other STDs in competition with it for attention and resources.[19]
2. Studies of the sociodemographic and geographic distribution of gonorrhea clearly indicate that the transmission of gonorrhea is predicated on the existence of small groups of persons who share common sociodemographic, behavioral and geographic characteristics of a so-called core group. This concept was verified empirically in such diverse locations as New York State; Colorado Springs, Colorado; Dade County, Florida; and Liverpool, England. With the understanding of a core group pattern comes the opportunity to design intervention programs tailored to the group at risk.[19]

Pathophysiology

Although many persons with STDs are clinically asymptomatic, others commonly have genital lesions, genital itching or burning, changes in vaginal discharge, lower abdominal pain, penile discharge, or pain with intercourse.

Collaborative Care Management

Diagnostic Tests. Specific diagnostic tests are used to establish the diagnosis of each of these diseases. Diagnostic tests are discussed under the specific disease later in this chapter.

Medications. Treatment depends on the causative organisms identified through the history, physical examination, and

TABLE 56-2 Selected Sexually Transmitted Diseases

Incubation Period	Signs and Symptoms	Medical Therapy
Gonorrhea		
Men: 3-30 days Women: 3 days to an indefinite period	Men: purulent urethral discharge, dysuria, epididymitis, prostatitis Women: asymptomatic in early stages: cervicitis with purulent discharge, bartholinitis, salpingitis	Ceftriaxone, 125 mg IM in a single dose, or cefixime, 400 mg PO in a single dose, or ciprofloxacin, 500 mg PO in a single dose, or ofloxacin, 400 mg PO in a single dose, plus azithromycin,1 g PO in a single dose or doxycycline, 100 mg PO bid, for 7 days (individuals with gonorrhea are concurrently treated for chlamydia)
Syphilis		
3 weeks (9 days to 3 mo)	Positive serologic tests, chancre in primary; condyloma lata in secondary	Benzathine penicillin G, 2.4 million U IM
Herpes Genitalis		
3-14 days	Vesicles that rupture and form ulcerations, pain, inguinal lymph node enlargement, dysuria, flulike symptoms	Herpes primary occurrence: acyclovir, 400 mg PO tid, for 7-10 days, or 200 mg PO five times a day for 7-10 days, or famciclovir, 250 mg PO tid, for 7-10 days, or valacyclovir, 1 g PO bid, for 7-10 days; recurrence: acyclovir, 400 mg PO tid, for 5 days; suppression: acyclovir, 400 mg PO bid, for 1 year, or famciclovir, 250 mg PO QD Diet: Usually no dietary modifications or restrictions during the treatment of STDs Activity: No standard activity limitations Referrals: Pregnant women with STDs may be referred to obstetricians/CNMs for treatment; persons with resistant strains of STDs may be referred to public health officials or infectious disease specialists
Chlamydia		
5-10 days or longer	Women: painful or difficult urination, abnormal vaginal discharge or bleeding, pain or bleeding with coitus, irregular menses; one third are asymptomatic Men: testicular pain, nonspecific urethritis or epididymitis	Azithromycin, 1 g PO in a single dose, or doxycycline, 100 mg PO bid, for 7 days
HPV/Genital Warts (Condylomata Acuminata)		
1-6 mo	Horny papules on vulva, vagina, cervix, perineum, anal canal, urethra, glans penis	Patient-applied: podofilox, 0.5% solution bid for 3 days, then 4 days of no therapy, repeat up to four cycles; or Imiquimod, 5% cream qhs, three times a week for up to 16 weeks. Provider applied: 80%-90% trichloroacetic/bichloroacetic acid; intralesional interferon; surgical treatment: laser, cryotherapy, electrocautery, or loop electrosurgical excision procedure

HPV, human papilloma virus; *STD*, sexually transmitted disease.

diagnostic tests and is discussed in the following pages. It is not unusual for an individual to harbor two or more organisms simultaneously. See Table 56-2 for standard treatment modalities for gonorrhea, chlamydia, syphilis, HPV (condylomata acuminata), and genital herpes.

NURSING MANAGEMENT

ASSESSMENT

Health History

Data to be collected to assess the patient suspected of having any STD include:

- Exposure to STD contact, including HIV
- Prior STD history, treatment
- Sexual orientation: "Have you been having sex with men, women, or both?"
- Relationship of onset of symptoms to last sexual intercourse
- Number of sexual partners in the past 6 months

Women are questioned about last menstrual period, vaginal discharge (color, odor, amount), vulvar itching, dysuria, urinary urgency, lower abdominal pain, rectal symptoms, sore throat, genital lesions, skin rashes or itching, and menstrual periods.

Men are questioned about urethral discharge, dysuria, genital lesions, skin rashes, itching, testicular pain, and sore throat.

Gay and bisexual men are also asked about rectal symptoms such as pain, bleeding, discharge, and diarrhea.

If hepatitis is also suspected, the person is questioned about dark-colored urine, clay-colored stools, fatigue, and jaundice.

Physical Examination

Essential components of the physical examination of the patient suspected of having any STD include inspection and palpation of the integumentary system, reproductive system, and anorectal area.

Examination for women includes:
Inspection of skin of lower abdomen, inguinal area, hands, palms, and forearms
Inspection of pubic hair for lice and mites
Inspection and palpation of external genitalia, including perineum and anus
Speculum examination of vagina and cervix
Bimanual examination of the uterus and adnexa
Palpation for inguinal and femoral lymphadenopathy
Inspection of mouth and throat, including tonsils
Pregnancy test for all women of childbearing age
Examination of men includes:
Inspection of the skin and pubic hair
Inspection of the penis, including the meatus, with retraction of the foreskin and "milking" of the urethra
Palpation of the scrotum
Inspection of the mouth, throat, and tonsils
Examination of homosexual or bisexual men also includes:
Inspection of the anorectal area
Anoscopic examination if there are rectal symptoms

NURSING DIAGNOSES

Nursing diagnoses are determined from analysis of patient data. Nursing diagnoses for the person with any STD may include but are not limited to:

Diagnostic Title	Possible Etiologic Factors
1. Deficient knowledge	Lack of exposure/recall, information misinterpretation, lack of familiarity with information sources about STDs
2. Ineffective health maintenance	Lack of knowledge, cultural practices, lack of material resources

EXPECTED PATIENT OUTCOMES

Expected patient outcomes for the person with any STD may include but are not limited to:

1a. Person and partner will be able to explain the etiology and factors contributing to the STD.
1b. Person and partner will be able to state the name, dosage, and schedule of administration of drug therapy, as well as its possible side effects.
1c. Person and partner will be able to explain the need for adherence to the entire treatment regimen.
1d. Person and partner will be able to state the reasons for abstaining from sexual activity during the infectious stages of the STD.
1e. Person and partner will be able to state effects of the STD on the reproductive system of oneself and one's partner.
1f. Person and partner will be able to state indications for seeking immediate health care if signs and symptoms reappear.
1g. Person and partner will be able to explain necessity for treatment of sexual partner or partners.
1h. Person and partner will be able to accept the occurrence of the STD.
1i. Person and partner will be able to explain how to prevent the transmission of STDs by using safer sex practices, including the type of condom to use, when and how to apply it, and how to remove it.[14] Recommendations on the proper use of condoms to prevent transmission of STDs can be found in Box 56-1.

BOX 56-1 Recommendations from the CDC for the Use of Condoms

The following recommendations for proper use of condoms to reduce the transmission of STDs are based on current information:

1. Latex condoms should be used, because they offer greater protection against viral STDs than natural membrane condoms.
2. Condoms should be stored in a cool, dry place out of direct sunlight.
3. Condoms in damaged packages or those that show obvious signs of age (e.g., those that are brittle, sticky, or discolored) should not be used. They cannot be relied on to prevent infection.
4. Condoms should be handled with care to prevent puncture.
5. The condom should be put on the erect penis (either partner can do this) before the penis comes into contact with the woman's genitals to prevent exposure to fluids that may contain infectious agents. Hold the tip of the condom and unroll it onto the erect penis, leaving 1 to 2 inches of space at the tip to collect semen, yet ensuring that no air is trapped in the tip of the condom.
6. Adequate lubrication should be used. If exogenous lubrication is needed, only water-based lubricants should be used. Petroleum- or oil-based lubricants (e.g., petroleum jelly, cooking oils, shortening, and lotions) should not be used, because they weaken the latex of the condom.
7. Use of condoms containing spermicides may provide some additional protection against STDs. However, vaginal use of spermicides along with condoms is likely to provide greater protection.
8. If a condom breaks, it should be replaced immediately. If ejaculation occurs after condom breaks, the immediate use of a vaginal spermicide has been suggested. However, the protective value of postejaculation application of spermicide in reducing the risk of STD transmission is unknown.
9. After ejaculation, care should be taken so that the condom does not slip off the penis before withdrawal; the base of the condom should be held while withdrawing. The penis should be withdrawn while still erect.
10. Condoms should never be reused.

Modified from Hatcher PA et al: *Contraceptive technology,* ed 16, New York, 1994, Irvington.

2a. Person and partner will describe resources necessary to achieve health.

2b. Person and partner will recognize personal strengths and weaknesses.

2c. Person and partner will participate actively in health maintenance activities.

INTERVENTIONS

The following interventions apply to the person with any STD.

1. Patient/Family Education

The nurse's first responsibility in STD control is to educate persons who have a sexually transmitted infection or may develop one in a nonjudgmental manner. Nurses must be knowledgeable about the most prevalent diseases, the signs and symptoms, methods used in diagnosis, treatments used, and where individuals can obtain help and information. They also can influence the knowledge and attitudes of their colleagues and peers toward STD and its control. Nurses can exert influence in the community by taking an active role in education programs. The best way to reduce the risk of STD is for every person who is sexually active to limit his or her number of sexual partners. Sexual activity with different partners increases the risk of infection. Using a condom is recommended but is no guarantee against passing on or acquiring an STD.

Before nurses can be effective in working with persons who have STDs, they must confront their own feelings and attitudes about STDs. The person with an STD is often young, fearful of pain, and unaccustomed to surroundings in a clinic or physician's office. Young people especially fear that their families and friends may learn they have an STD.

Once the diagnosis, tentative or conclusive, is made, focus is placed on obtaining a cure and preventing complications and reinfection. Because some of the diseases respond to penicillin or other antibiotics, many people believe that all genital infections can be cured easily, but this is not so. Some people believe that antibiotics not only cure an infection but also produce immunity against reinfection. Persons receiving an antibiotic or other medications for STDs are informed of the action of the drug, its duration of effectiveness, side effects, chances of cure, and the need for follow-up care. They need to be advised that treatment failures do occur and that reinfection rates are high. Return visits for follow-up care are encouraged when necessary.

Many persons focus on how the diseases are spread rather than on the consequences of having an infection. For adolescents, contracting an STD and securing help means they must admit to sexual activity, which may cause feelings of guilt. People with STDs may feel their self-esteem is threatened by what has happened to them. They may express feelings of anger. Persons with an STD have not only physical and social problems but perhaps economic problems (paying for the treatment), and an emotional problem dealing with the diagnosis. They need constructive and comprehensive help. The nurse who is successful in working with persons who have an STD is one who can create an atmosphere of trust in which the person feels free to discuss all aspects of the problem.

Persons who seek help recognize that they have a problem; they want to get better and stay well. Because of this they are highly motivated to do what is necessary, receptive to information and advice, and attentive when advice is given. Nurses can take advantage of the patient's readiness to learn and motivation to improve and maintain health.

Persons treated for STDs need information about self-care. To understand their therapy and to responsibly engage in self-care, they must be informed about the sexual nature of the infection, how it is transmitted, and the possibility of reinfection and infection of their sexual partner or partners. The person needs to know that it is important for sexual partners to be checked for signs of infection, to be advised of what the signs are, and to be tested for asymptomatic infection. The person should be advised to abstain from intercourse until he/she and the partner is cured. The use of condoms must be stressed to prevent infection or reinfection if persons persist in engaging in intercourse even when advised not to do so.

Teaching about hygiene and personal health practices is beneficial in reducing the chances of secondary infection, recurrence, and various types of infections in the future. Frequent bathing and hand washing are indicated. Soap and water destroy many of the organisms causing STDs. For women, douching is contraindicated. All women should be informed that douching at any time is not advisable, because this may disturb the vaginal and cervical environments and predispose the woman to infection.

If the lesions are present on body surfaces, the person should be instructed in their care. Unless contraindicated, a hot bath (sitz bath) is taken two or three times a day, and lesions are kept as dry as possible between baths. Both men and women should be advised to wear cotton underwear, and women should be advised to avoid wearing pantyhose, because they tend to trap moisture and prevent circulation of air to the genitalia. Unless lotions, creams, or ointments are specifically prescribed as local medications, the patient should not apply them to any of the lesions associated with an STD.

Genital self-examination is important for sexually active persons. Inspecting skin, mouth, genitalia, and perianal areas for lesions and discharges is recommended. Self-inspection helps the person become educated about the signs and symptoms of STDs and how to look for them. In addition, people can learn to casually inspect their partners during the initial period of lovemaking to identify any signs of STDs. Urinating after sexual activity can be helpful in cleansing the urethra of organisms.

Opportunities for promoting healthy attitudes about sexual activity and STDs frequently arise. These topics are approached tactfully and with consideration of the person's feelings. Adolescents especially require an approach that indicates understanding balanced with the ability to help them set limits. They need to understand that they are responsible for their own bodies, and they do not have to give in to sexual pressures. It is well documented, however, that the strongest influence on teenagers comes from their peer group. For this reason, discussion with groups of teenagers about their sexual responsibilities may be helpful. In the climate of the twenty-first century there should be no doubt that abstinence is the only absolute way to prevent STD. If a teen elects to be sexually active he or she needs to understand that the consequences of unprotected sex may include unwanted pregnancy, or an STD, and possibly cervical cancer. Monogamous relationships and the proper use of condoms should be stressed for those who are sexually active.

As mentioned earlier, a problem among sexually active teenagers and unmarried adults is serial monogamy. When questioned about their sexual activities, most of them consider themselves to be monogamous, but the monogamy lasts for only a few weeks or months. Thus they are not having sex with more than one person in a time span, but are going from one short-term relationship to another without concern about their partners' sexual histories.

2. Health Promotion/Prevention

Prevention and control measures for STDs include three levels of prevention. Primary prevention is directed at preventing the disease. This includes educating uninfected persons so that they can take responsibility for their own health and not expose themselves to an infected person; identification and treatment of exposed persons who are asymptomatic; interviewing persons with infection for identification of contacts, examination, and preventive treatment of contacts; educational programs for the public; and active involvement of professionals in programs of control. The goal of these efforts includes eradication of the reservoir of disease in the population. Secondary prevention is directed toward screening, early diagnosis, and treatment. Tertiary prevention focuses on prevention of complications, supporting and counseling infected persons to receive treatment, and asking infected persons to notify their sexual partners so that they can be examined and treated if infected.

In the prevention and control of STDs, young people often fear that their parents and the parents of the sexual partner(s) will find out about their infection. Minors need to know that they can probably obtain treatment without parental consent. Presently most states permit health care providers to treat minors for STDs without obtaining parental consent, and several states are proposing changes in existing legislation that restricts treatment of minors.

The patient is interviewed about his or her contacts at the time of the initial visit in the event that the patient does not return for follow-up care. It is probably best that this interview take place after the patient is examined, the type of infection is determined, and the treatment is prescribed. If assessment is accompanied by information giving, the person should be better informed about STDs and how they are treated and be more willing and able to give information about sexual contacts. People may perceive reporting of STDs as a threat from an official agency and may hesitate to name their contacts out of a sense of protection if they do not know that no punishment is involved.

Healthy People 2010

Goals Related to the Reduction of STDs

1. Reduce the proportion of adolescents and young adults with *Chlamydia trachomatis* infections.
2. Reduce gonorrhea.
3. Eliminate sustained domestic transmission of primary and secondary syphilis.
4. Reduce the proportion of adults with genital herpes infection.
5. Reduce the proportion of persons with human papillomavirus (HPV) infection.
6. Reduce the proportion of females who have ever required treatment for pelvic inflammatory disease (PID).
7. Reduce the proportion of childless females with fertility problems who have had a sexually transmitted disease or who have required treatment for PID.
8. Increase the proportion of adolescents who abstain from sexual intercourse or use condoms if currently sexually active.
9. Increase the number of positive messages related to responsible sexual behavior during weekday and nightly prime-time television programming.

From US Department of Health and Human Services: *Healthy People 2010: understanding and improving health,* Washington, DC, 2000, USDHHS.

Because one focus of STD control is increasing self-referrals, the patient is asked to inform her or his sexual partner(s) (partner notification) to come in for examination and treatment. Confidentiality is stressed. Because of the understandable reluctance of many people to name their sexual partner(s), the patient may be given the responsibility of informing the contacts and advising them of their need for treatment. Local health departments cooperate in locating, examining, and treating contacts when necessary.

Whenever possible, the sexual partners of the infected person are advised to have an examination and tests as soon as possible. If the sexual partner or partners do not have symptoms of infection at the time of the first examination, treatment is still instituted. Giving preventive treatment to contacts who have no clinical evidence of infection is common practice in the United States; this same approach is used in management of patients with "minor" STDs.

Healthy People 2010 follows up on the goals attained by Healthy People 2000, and establishes several goals related to the reduction of STDs to be achieved by the year 2010. These goals are listed in the Healthy People 2010 box.

The special population targets for objective 1 appear in Table 56-3. To support the achievement of these important goals, Leading Health Indicators have been identified. Those for the area of STDs are responsible adolescent sexual behavior and condom use by adults.[23]

■ EVALUATION

Evaluation of care is achieved by comparing the patient's responses to interventions with the expected outcomes. Achieve-

TABLE 56-3 Healthy People 2010 Goals to Reduce Sexually Transmitted Diseases

Disease	Population	Baseline	Goal
Chlamydia trachomatis	Females 15-24 years attending family planning clinics	5.0% (1997)	Expand Healthy People 2000 and tracks percent positivity among women ages 15 to 24 who attend STD clinics in addition to family planning clinics
	Females 15-24 years attending STD clinics	12.2% (1997)	
	Males 15-24 years attending STD clinics	15.7% (1997)	Expand Healthy People 2000 to include men ages 15-24 years who attended STD clinics with positive results
Gonorrhea		123 cases per 100,000 (1997)	Reduce gonorrhea Targets not yet specified
Syphilis (primary and secondary)		3.2 cases per 100,000 (1997)	Eliminate sustained domestic transmission of primary and secondary syphilis
Genital herpes	Adults 20-29 years	17% (1988-1994)	Modify Healthy People 2000 to track the proportion of person with a positive laboratory test for herpes simplex virus, type 2
HPV	15-44 years	Operational definition does not yet exist	Propose reducing the number of HPV cases to minimize the prevalence of subtypes 16 and 18 and other subtypes associated with cervical cancer

HPV, Human papillomavirus; *STD,* sexually transmitted disease.

ment of outcomes is successful if the patient and his or her partner:

1a. State the factors that contributed to the present infection with STD (multiple/serial sexual partners, not using a condom).
1b. State the drug therapy to be followed, including name of drug, dosage, schedule of administration, and side effects.
1c. Explain why the therapy must be taken without interruption (to prevent resistant strains of organisms from developing).
1d. State why he or she should not engage in sexual activity while the STD is infectious.
1e. State effects of STDs that may develop in the reproductive system of either partner.
1f. State signs and symptoms (fever, pain, discharge) that indicate the need for immediate health care.
1g. Verbalize understanding of the necessity of treatment for his or her sexual partner or partners.
1h. Verbalize that she or he has an STD, and identify ways to prevent further STD infections.
1i. Explain what is meant by practicing "safer sex," including what type of condom to use, when and how to apply it, and how to remove it.
1j. Describe resources necessary to achieve health.
1k. Recognize personal strengths and weaknesses.
2. Participate actively in health maintenance activities.

GONORRHEA

Etiology/Epidemiology

Gonorrhea, sometimes referred to as GC or the clap by lay people, is caused by *Neisseria gonorrhoeae.* Gonorrhea is of great concern, because persons with it often have another STD such as chlamydia or HIV. There is a possibility for a high reinfection rate and serious residual effects. The incubation period is 3 to 30 days in men and 3 days to an indefinite period in women.

The incidence of gonorrhea in the United States declined rapidly from 1985 to 1996, but between 1997 and 1999 gonorrhea rates increased. (Figures 56-1 to 56-4). In men the rate increased from 124.9 per 100,000 to 136 per 100,000. In women the rate increased from 119 per 100,000 in 1994 to 129.9 per 100,000. These rates are still lower than rates of the mid-1990s, but the concern is with the alarming rise in gonorrhea among gay and bisexual men.[8]

Southern states continue to have the highest gonorrhea rates of any region. Gonorrhea mainly affects teens and young adults. The rates are highest among females between 15 and 19 years and males between 20 and 24 years, regardless or race or ethnicity. Reported rates of gonorrhea among African-Americans increased from 802.4 to 848.8 cases per 100,000 people, more than 30 times higher than for Caucasians and more than 11 times higher than for Hispanics. Among adolescents, gonorrhea increased 13% between 1997 and 1999. Young African-American women and men remain at extremely high risk.[8]

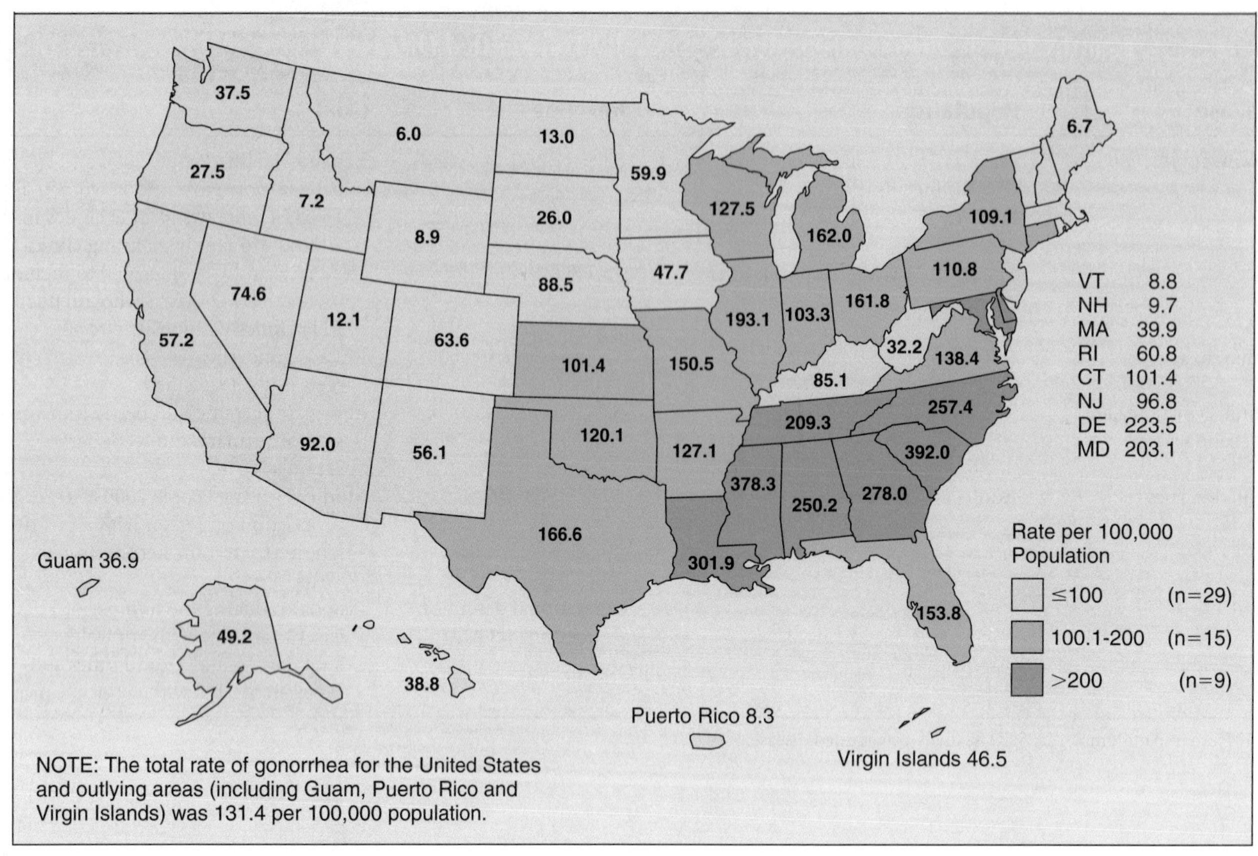

Figure 56-1 Reported cases of gonorrhea per 100,000 population, United States and outlying areas, 1999.

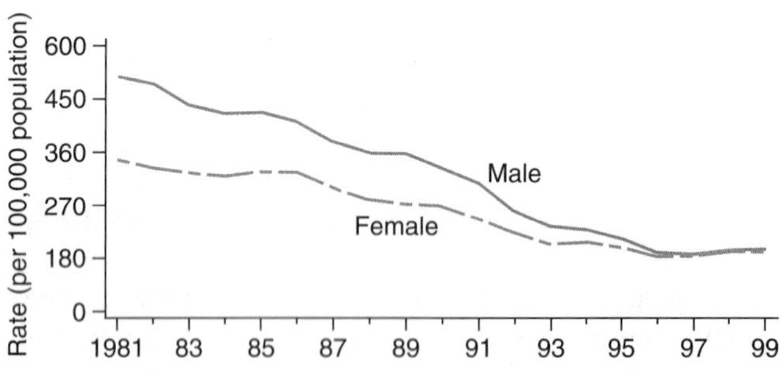

Figure 56-2 Reported cases of gonorrhea per 100,000 population by gender, United States, 1981-1999.

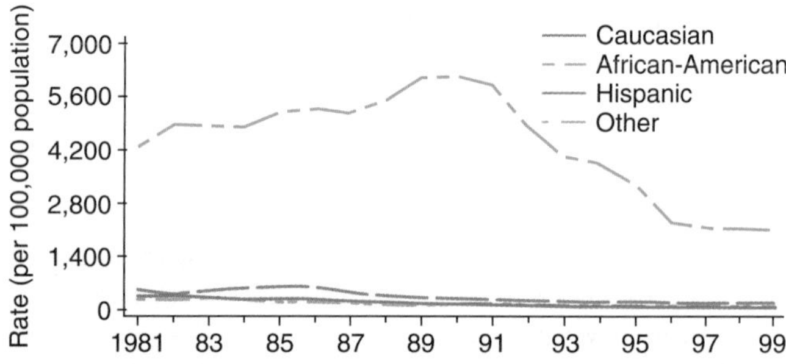

Figure 56-4 Reported rate for 15- to 19-year-old males by race/ethnicity: United States, 1981-1999.

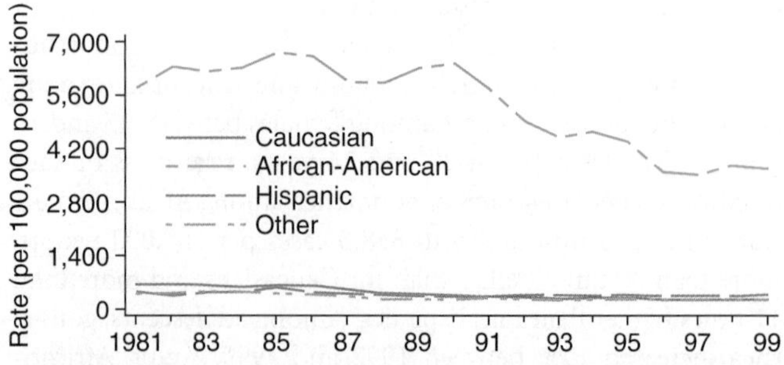

Figure 56-3 Reported cases of gonorrhea for 15- to 19-year-old females by race/ethnicity: United States, 1981-1999.

An estimated 650,00 cases of gonorrhea occur each year in the United States. The incidence of gonorrhea is believed to be much higher than reported, because it is known that the cases of many patients treated by private physicians are never reported to public health authorities and therefore are not reflected in the statistics. It is generally accepted that only 50% of cases treated by private physicians are reported. In addition, women have few if any signs or symptoms of gonorrhea and thus are often not diagnosed. For this reason it is commonly believed that the actual number of cases per year in the United States is probably more than 1.5 million.[7]

Asymptomatic persons are an important reservoir for infection because they usually remain untreated. Women are more likely to be asymptomatic than men, but suffer more severe complications from unrecognized early infections. Among men rectal infections result from penetration by an infected penis and are followed by symptomatic proctitis in half of cases. Rectal infection is found in 5% to 10% of women with cervical infections.[16]

It is estimated that the total cost of gonorrhea in the United States is several billion dollars yearly. Women and their offspring suffer the major physical, emotional, and economic burden. Pelvic inflammatory disease occurs in 10% to 20% of women with gonorrhea. Even when treated, these women are likely to suffer from recurrent salpingitis, ectopic pregnancy, infertility, and menstrual abnormalities and may face surgical removal of the pelvic organs, as well as fetal loss.

Pathophysiology

The most common signs and symptoms of gonorrhea are listed in the Clinical Manifestations box. In men the gonococcus is introduced into the anterior urethra during sexual activity. Because most men are diagnosed and treated early, complications and residual effects of gonorrhea are uncommon among men. Sterility from orchitis or epididymitis can occur as a rare residual effect.

The incidence of asymptomatic gonorrhea in men is believed to be low; however, men with asymptomatic infection are an important factor in the transmission of gonorrhea. Some men have been found to have no symptoms of infection despite positive tests for gonorrhea 2 weeks after exposure.

Gonorrhea in women most often begins as asymptomatic cervicitis. The infection can be present for extended periods without causing noticeable signs; hence there is a high number of infected, asymptomatic women. These women do not receive treatment unless gonorrhea is diagnosed through screening or unless the woman is identified by a sexual partner and presents herself for treatment. Complications are commonly the first indicators of gonorrhea in women. In cases of untreated gonorrhea, the residual effects of chronic PID, infertility, and ectopic pregnancy are well known. Other complications of untreated gonorrhea in both men and women include dermatitis, carditis, meningitis, and arthritis. The incidence of these complications is higher among women because of the prolonged period of infection without symptoms.

Collaborative Care Management

Although fluroquinolones are the treatment of choice (Table 56-2), some *N. gonorrhoeae* strains resistant to fluoroquinolones have been reported sporadically and are more widespread in parts of Asia. Quinolone-resistant N. gonorrhoeae (QRNG) occurs rarely in the United States; in 1997 the rate was <0.05%. As long as QRNG strains are <1% of all *N. gonorrhoeae* strains isolated in 26 target cities, fluoroquinolones can be used with confidence. However, the prevalence of QRNG could increase in the United States causing the discontinuation of fluoroquinolone treatment.[4,16]

There is no clinical difference in the infections caused by resistant strains of N. gonorrhoeae and those caused by sensitive strains. Culture and sensitivity testing is performed when there is apparent treatment failure after recommended therapy. These failures are reported to the local health department. When a high number of resistant strains are present in a community, there is more likely to be an increase in sequelae of acute gonococcal infections such as PID, gonococcal ophthalmia, and disseminated gonococcal infection.[4]

Patient/Family Education. Prevention of gonorrhea and its complications can be achieved in three stages. The first and most crucial stage, *primary prevention,* is prevention of the disease. The second stage, *secondary prevention,* involves prevention of complications of the disease such as PID. The third stage, *tertiary prevention,* is reversal of the damage caused by the disease, such as by tubal reconstruction.

Early treatment of infected persons is the most effective method to prevent new infection of sexual partners. Treatment of choice is ciprofloxacin, 500 mg orally in a single dose, or ceftriaxone, 125 mg IM in a single dose. Mechanical barrier methods such as condoms used with spermicides may reduce but not guarantee 100% prevention of gonorrhea. Education to acquaint people with the symptoms of gonorrhea, the efficacy of condoms, and the availability of diagnostic and treatment resources is important. Early detection through partner notification and screening can reduce serious complications of gonorrhea, especially in women.

Most health care providers recommend that all persons with gonorrhea should be treated for chlamydia even though there are no signs or symptoms of it because it may inhibit the development of antibiotic-resistant gonococcal strains, and because it may treat unrecognized syphilis.[16] All patients with gonorrhea should be offered testing and counseling for HIV and other STDs.

Clinical Manifestations

Signs and Symptoms of Gonorrhea

HETEROSEXUAL MEN

1. Urethritis—often first symptom
2. Severe dysuria—especially with first voiding in morning
3. Purulent discharge from urethra
4. Swelling of the penis and balanitis—rare symptoms

HOMOSEXUAL AND BISEXUAL MEN

1. Proctitis (rectal gonorrhea)—50% asymptomatic; diagnosed by rectal culture
2. Pharyngeal gonorrhea—usually asymptomatic

WOMEN

Women rarely have early, distressing symptoms such as men have. When symptoms are present, they include the following:

1. Slight purulent vaginal discharge
2. Vague feeling of fullness in pelvis
3. Discomfort or aching in abdomen
4. If bladder is involved—burning, frequency, and urgency, which usually cause the woman to seek medical attention

The first three symptoms are so slight that they may be ignored by the woman.

SYPHILIS

Etiology/Epidemiology

Syphilis is caused by a spirochete, *Treponema pallidum*, that gains entry into the body through either the mucous membrane or skin during intercourse. The organism is readily destroyed by physical and chemical agents, including heat, drying, and soap and water. This disease is curable, but progresses in stages if untreated leading to cardiovascular and neurologic diseases and blindness.

The incubation period for syphilis is usually 3 weeks. However, symptoms can appear as early as 9 days or as long as 3 months after exposure. The genital ulcers of primary syphilis increase the likelihood of sexual HIV transmission twofold to fivefold.[8,18]

Since the 1940s when penicillin became available and a national STD control program began, the initial near elimination of syphilis in 1957 has been followed by cyclic national epidemics every 7 to 10 years. The most recent epidemic peaked in 1990 at 20.3 per 100,000 people. Since 1990, syphilis rates have declined to 2.5 cases per 100,000 people, or 6657 cases reported to the Centers for Disease Control and Prevention (CDC) in 1999 (Figure 56-5).[8] Reported cases to the CDC are believed to represent about 80% of all recently acquired cases.[4]

The trends for congenital syphilis—infants acquiring infection from their mothers during pregnancy or birth—have paralleled the trends for primary and secondary syphilis among women. Peaks in congenital syphilis usually occur 1 year after peaks in primary and secondary syphilis in women. The congenital syphilis rate in the United States peaked in 1991 at 107.3 cases per 100,000 live births and declined to 14.3 cases per 100,000 live births, or 556 cases, in 1999.[8]

Pathophysiology

The signs and symptoms of the four stages of syphilis are listed in Table 56-4. If syphilis is adequately diagnosed and treated during the primary stage, the other stages can be prevented.

Collaborative Care Management

As with gonorrhea, three levels of prevention are important. *Primary prevention* is prevention of the initial infection by finding and treating those with the disease so that they cannot spread it to others. Treatment of choice for syphilis is penicillin G benzathine (2.4 million units IM). *Secondary pre-*

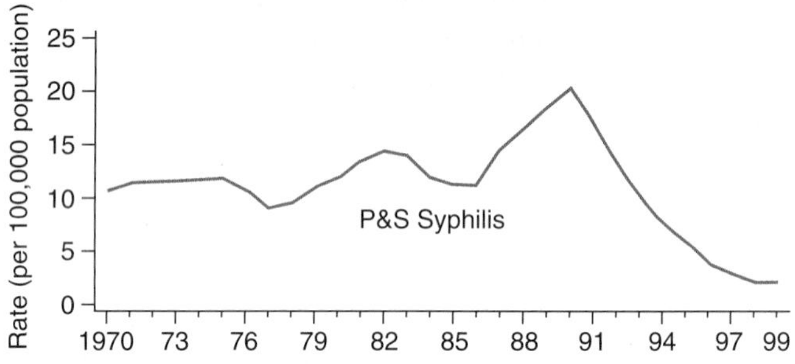

Figure 56-5 Primary and secondary syphilis rates per 100,000 population by year, United States, 1970-1999.

TABLE 56-4 Stages of Syphilis

Primary	Secondary	Latent	Late
Duration			
2-8 wk	Appears 2-4 wk after chancre appears; extends over 2-4 yr	5-20 yr	Terminal if not treated
Signs and Symptoms			
Hard sore or pimple on vulva or penis that breaks and forms painless, draining chancre; may be a single chancre or groups of more than one; may be present also on lips, tongue, hands, rectum, vagina, cervix, or nipples; chancre heals, leaving almost invisible scar	Depends on site; low-grade fever, headache, anorexia, weight loss, anemia, sore throat, hoarseness, reddened and sore eyes, jaundice with or without hepatitis, aching of joints, muscles, long bones; sores on body or generalized fine rash; condylomata lata on rectum or genitalia	No clinical signs	Tumorlike mass (gumma) on any area of body; damage to heart valves and blood vessels; meningitis; paralysis; lack of coordination; paresis; insomnia; confusion; delusions; impaired judgment; slurred speech
Communicability			
Exudates from lesions and chancre are highly contagious	Exudates from lesions highly contagious; blood contains organisms	Contagious for about 2 yr; not contagious to others after that; blood contains organisms; may be transmitted placenta to fetus	Noncontagious; spinal fluid may contain organisms

vention is directed at early treatment of cases to prevent late syphilis or congenital syphilis. In *tertiary prevention* efforts are made to treat the complications of syphilis when they occur. Contact investigation is necessary as for all STDs and HIV testing is mandated for anyone with syphilis because of the high coprevalence.[18]

HERPES GENITALIS

Etiology/Epidemiology

Herpes genitalis (genital herpes, HSV-2) is caused by infection with herpesvirus hominis type 2 (HSV-2). Its chronicity and frequent recurrences distinguish it from other STDs. It can be treated but not cured. It is estimated that more than one in five Americans are infected with genital herpes and that as many as 1 million people become infected each year.[8] Its peak incidence parallels the young age-groups affected by other STDs. Once acquired, herpes genitalis is a *lifelong disease* and carries with it not only recurrent discomfort, but also anxieties about future childbearing, and sexual and marital function. Women with a primary infection in pregnancy may rarely have transplacental infection of the fetus resulting in congenital infection. The disease is potentially fatal in newborns, so if labor begins during a herpetic outbreak cesarean delivery is necessary. Pregnant women can be offered suppression therapy from 36 weeks to decrease the likelihood of an outbreak near delivery.[5]

Pathophysiology

The incubation period for genital herpes is 3 to 7 days. The primary lesion appears as a vesicle on the external genitalia in men; often in the rectum in homosexual men; and on the vagina, cervix, or external genitalia in women. Following primary herpes, the virus persists in a latent or unrecognized form. It is believed that the latent virus is localized in the ganglia of sensory nerves to the genitalia. When the host factors favor it, the latent infection becomes clinically apparent as recurrent herpes.

Common signs and symptoms of primary herpetic infection are local inflammation; pain; enlargement of inguinal lymph nodes; generalized signs of infection such as photophobia, headache, and flulike symptoms of chills, fever, and malaise; dysuria; and urinary retention.

Primary herpetic lesions begin as single or multiple reddish painful papules, which then develop into clear, fluid-filled vesicles. These lesions often ulcerate, especially when located on moist surfaces. Once they rupture ulcers form that may fuse with other lesions to form large ulcerated areas. The disease tends to be more extensive in women than in men. Cervical infection can accompany external lesions, and often it may be the only infected site. In a primary infection, genital lesions often worsen during the first 10 to 15 days but usually heal within 3 to 4 weeks. These symptoms usually lead the individual to seek medical attention.

Vaginal discharge is common among women with primary or recurrent infections, and discharge from the urethra is usual in men who have primary infections. Urinary tract involvement may occur and is reflected in symptoms of dysuria or urinary retention. The lesions can cause severe pain, requiring hospitalization for parenteral analgesia or urinary catheterization. Most people with herpes have no symptoms and are unaware of their infection. In a national household survey, less than 10% of people who tested positive with herpes knew they were infected.

A majority of persons with herpes genitalis have at least one recurrence. Fortunately, recurrent infections are usually milder and of shorter duration than primary infections and usually produce a local rather than systemic reaction. The patient experiencing a recurrent infection often has a prodromal paresthesia (an abnormal sensation or itching) and burning of a localized genital area where the lesion will erupt. Factors that may predispose to recurrent infection include fever, emotional upsets, premenstrual states, and overexposure to heat and sunshine. Although the mode of recurrent infection is not clear, it has been theorized that during primary infection the virus ascends sensory nerve sheaths, localizing in corresponding nerve ganglia, and that when the environment becomes favorable, the virus is reactivated. Lesions of recurrent infections usually occur at the site of the primary infection. Herpes encephalitis is rare, but possible.

Collaborative Care Management

Treatment for herpes genitalis consists of acyclovir or other antiviral agent as specified in Table 56-2 and symptomatic care. Use of antiviral agents for initial outbreaks does not prevent recurrences.

Patient/Family Education. Persons with herpes should abstain from sexual contact from the onset of prodromal signs to complete healing of lesions. Risk of transmission during asymptomatic periods exists; therefore, the person is advised to always use condoms to prevent transmission of the disease. A person presenting with a primary infection should be screened for other STDs, especially HIV.

Because herpes genitalis is a recurrent disease with no cure, persons infected with the virus require considerable emotional support. Some infected persons withdraw from an active social life rather than face the possibility of making a commitment that will require them to share knowledge of their disease with another person. For this reason, in some communities support groups have been formed for persons who have herpes genitalis.

CHLAMYDIAL INFECTION

Etiology/Epidemiology

Chlamydia trachomatis is caused by the gram-negative obligate *C. trachomatis.* Chlamydial infection is recognized as the most prevalent of the STDs in the United States (Figure 56-6). Because it is not a reportable disease, the actual number of cases is unknown. It is estimated, however, that each year more than 3 million Americans experience epidemic chlamydial infections. Age, number of sex partners, socioeconomic status, and sexual orientation are predictors of infection with *C. trachomatis.*[7]

Age. A total of 40% of chlamydia cases are reported among people 15 to 19 years old. Prevalence among sexually active

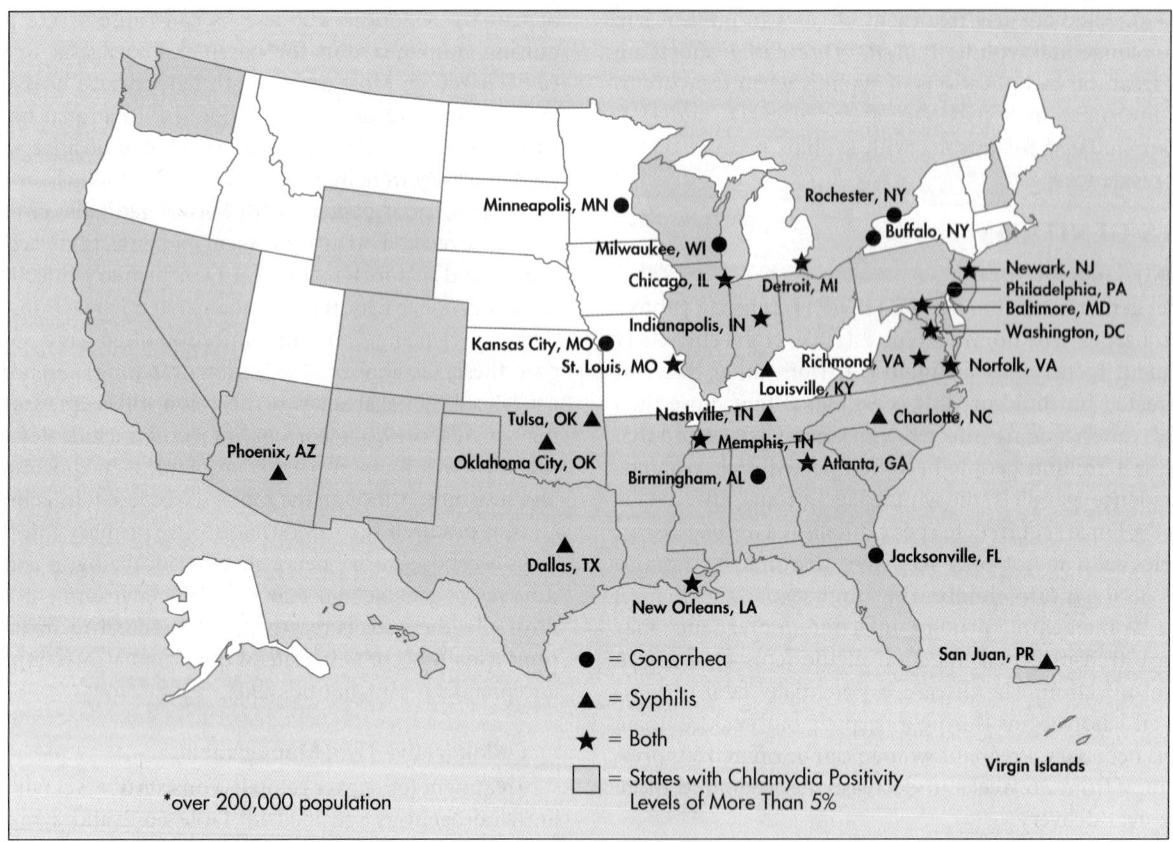

Figure 56-6 Cities on the top 20 list for rates of gonorrhea and syphilis, and states with *Chlamydia* positivity Levels of more than 5% among 15- to 24-year-old women tested in family planning clinics, United States, 1999.

teenage girls exceeds 10%. The reported rate for adolescent boys is lower, probably because programs to screen and treat are directed at women. True rates are probably similar to those of girls. One program that screened high-risk youth in the field found a 12% rate among the young men.[8]

Number of Sex Partners. Persons with several sex partners are at higher risk of infection.

Socioeconomic Status. Some studies have shown that persons of lower socioeconomic status are at increased risk for infection with *C. trachomatis.* The highest rates for infection in the United States are in areas without longstanding screening and treatment programs.[8]

Sexual Preference. The prevalence of urethral chlamydial infection among homosexual men is one third of the rate of heterosexual men. However, 4% to 8% of homosexual men seen in STD clinics have rectal chlamydia infection.

Chlamydial infections are responsible for about 20% to 30% of PID cases. It is estimated that up to 40% of women with untreated chlamydial infections will develop PID. One in five of those will become infertile, and an estimated 36,000 will have ectopic pregnancies as a result of this organism.[8] Chlamydial infections can be transmitted to infants during delivery, causing conjunctivitis and pneumonia in many.

C. trachomatis is the leading cause of pneumonia in infants under 6 months old. The rate of infection with pneumonia is 3 to 10 per 1000 live births and may go as high as 50 to 60 per 1000 in areas where *C. trachomatis* is epidemic. The organism has superseded *N. gonorrhoeae* as a cause of neonatal conjunctivitis.[14]

The overall decline in *Chlamydia* infections in the United States is probably due to increased efforts to screen and treat women for chlamydial infections. Further reduction in the level of *Chlamydia* will require not only continuing expansion of screening and treatment among women, but also increased effort to screen and teach men. Young people will need to be educated about how to reduce their risk of infection through safer sexual behaviors.[8]

Pathophysiology

C. trachomatis is an intracellular parasite that has specific requirements for adenosine triphosphate and amino acids. There are two stages in the life cycle of the organism. In stage 1, the infective stage, the elementary body attaches to the host cell and is ingested by phagocytosis. In stage 2 the elementary body undergoes metamorphosis to become a reticulate or initial body. This is the metabolic phase of the life cycle. The ini-

TABLE 56-5 *Chlamydia trachomatis* **Infections**

Males	Females	Infants
Transmission		
Males ⟷	Females ⟶	Infants
Infections		
Urethritis	Cervicitis	Conjunctivitis
Postgonococcal urethritis	Urethritis	Pneumonia
Proctitis	Proctitis	Asymptomatic pharyngeal carriage
Conjunctivitis	Conjunctivitis	Asymptomatic gastrointestinal carriage
Pharyngitis	Pharyngitis	
Subclinical lymphogranuloma venereum	Subclinical lymphogranuloma venereum	
Complications		
Epididymitis	Salpingitis	
Prostatitis	Endometritis	
Reiter's syndrome	Perihepatitis	
Sterility	Ectopic pregnancy	
Rectal strictures*	Infertility	
	Vulvar/rectal carcinoma*	
	Rectal strictures*	

From Centers for Disease Control and Prevention: *Chlamydia trachomatis* infections, policy guidelines for prevention and control, *MMWR* 35(suppl):54, 1985.
*Associated with lymphogranuloma venereum.

tial body duplicates by binary fission and changes into the elementary body. The host cell, which contains the elementary bodies, undergoes lysis, liberating infectious organisms that are capable of reinfecting new cells.[24]

Serotypes D through K cause chlamydial infections. It is estimated that between 20% and 40% of sexually active women have been exposed to the bacterium and have antibody titers to *C. trachomatis.*[24] Table 56-5 shows how the infection can be transmitted between male and female sexual partners and from women to infants. It also lists the various ways the disease is manifested in men, women, and infants.

Collaborative Care Management

The treatment of choice for chlamydial infections is azithromycin, 1 g orally in a single dose, or doxycycline, 500 mg twice a day for 7 days.[10]

Patient/Family Education. It is important that the patient encourage sexual partner(s) to seek care as soon as possible to avoid reinfection of the patient and complications in the partner. Patients who are sexually active should be advised to always wear condoms and use spermicides to reduce reinfection. Social and emotional support of these patients is important, as it is with any person with a STD. HIV testing and screening for other STDs should be offered.

LYMPHOGRANULOMA VENEREUM

Etiology/Epidemiology

Lymphogranuloma venereum is a systemic STD caused by serotypes L1, L2, and L3 of *C. trachomatis.* Other species of *Chlamydia* are the causative organisms of trachoma and psittacosis. The disease is contracted by vaginal, anal, or oral intercourse; primary inoculation with the organism may occur at any site involved in close contact. The incubation period is 3 to 30 days. Lymphadenitis of regional lymph nodes draining the site of primary infection occurs, and the disease spreads by way of the lymphatic system.

Lymphogranuloma venereum is most prevalent in the tropics. It is endemic in parts of Africa, Southeast Asia, India, the Caribbean, and South America.[12] It is very rare in the United States, about 200 cases per year, and is mainly found in the southern states.[19] It may be underreported because the initial symptoms resolve spontaneously.

Pathophysiology

The three clinical phases of infection in lymphogranuloma venereum are (1) inoculation and appearance of the primary lesions, (2) lymphatic spread and generalized symptoms, and (3) late complications. In individual cases any one of the phases may be absent or go unnoticed.

The primary lesion, which is *transient, appears as a papule, small erosion, or vesicle.* The most common sites of the primary lesion are the prepuce and glans in men and the vagina and cervix in women. Because it is painless, the primary lesion may go unnoticed, especially in women. Localized edema may be present. If the rectum is infected, a bloody discharge is followed by a mucopurulent discharge, diarrhea, and cramping.

Involvement of the lymphatics occurs 2 to 6 weeks after the vesicular lesions have healed. The superficial inguinal lymph nodes or the deep iliac and anorectal lymph nodes are involved. Inguinal lymphadenopathy leads to *buboes* that appear firm and lobular and contain the organism. The skin over the superficial nodes is bluish red and adheres to the nodes.

The first indication of infection in most patients is a feeling of stiffness and aching in the groin followed by swelling in the inguinal area, usually unilateral. Symptoms of nongonococcal urethritis may be present (mucopurulent or purulent discharge from the urethra and burning during urination). Constitutional symptoms of infection may or may not appear at this time. Untreated, the involved lymph nodes may suppurate, causing extensive scarring and obstruction of the lymphatics, leading to chronic edema and ulceration. Lymphatic spread of the infection is accompanied by generalized symptoms of mild to high fever, malaise, nausea, and vomiting. Abdominal pain, symptoms of cystitis, and urinary retention are common when pelvic lymph nodes are involved. Acute proctocolitis is common in homosexual men.

Late complications of untreated lymphogranuloma venereum include perianal abscesses, rectovaginal or rectovesical fistulas, and rectal strictures.[12] In the last clinical phase, generalized infection is indicated by blood values showing anemia, leukocytosis, and an elevated sedimentation rate.

Collaborative Care Management

Lymphogranuloma is treated with doxycycline, 100 mg orally twice a day for 21 days, or erythromycin base, 500 mg orally four times a day for 21 days.

Patient/Family Education. These patients may require much counseling and teaching as they deal with their disease. Because the fluctuant lymph nodes may be disturbing to the patient's self-image, social and emotional support is extremely important.

CHANCROID

Etiology/Epidemiology

Chancroid is an STD caused by a gram-negative bacillus, *Haemophilus ducreyi.* The peak incidence of chancroid occurred in 1987 when 5035 cases were reported to the CDC. The number of cases has declined steadily since then, with 143 cases reported in 1999.[8]

Although it is found worldwide, chancroid is most prevalent in tropical and semitropical areas in Asia, the West Indies, and North Africa. In areas where it is endemic, chancroid is transmitted primarily by prostitutes, but the outbreak in the 1980s was associated with crack cocaine abuse and sexual activity.[15] Many women have minimal symptoms and usually present only with dysparunia or dysuria.[1] However, men usually develop severe symptoms and seek treatment because of pain and the appearance of an ulcer that causes them to cease sexual activity.

The disease occurs more often in men, more often among non-Caucasians, and more often in people over 35 years old. Chancroid is probably substantially underdiagnosed and underreported. The incubation period varies from 2 to 10 days.[8]

Chancroid is a cofactor for HIV transmission. A high rate of HIV infection among people with chancroid has been reported in the United States and other countries. As many as 10% of people with chancroid may be coinfected with *T. pallidum* or HSV.[15]

Pathophysiology

The initial lesions are acutely tender genital ulcers. The ulcers found in chancroid are typically ragged and irregular. They are highly infectious and autoinfection may occur, resulting in multiple lesions. The ulcers appear excavated; have a granulating, purulent surface and are painful. Often, edema of the surrounding tissues is present.

Lymphadenopathy and tender buboes appear about 1 to 2 weeks after the primary lesion. Involvement of the inguinal lymph nodes occurs in about 50% of all cases. The buboes are most often unilateral, painful, and spheric in shape; the skin over the buboes is inflamed. The buboes may suppurate and lead to abscesses. These abscesses in turn may suppurate and rupture, further spreading the infection. Generalized symptoms of infection usually appear when inguinal abscesses form.

In women the lesions of chancroid are most often found on the labia, anus, clitoris, vagina, and cervix. A few women do not have any lesions but may report dyspareunia or dysuria. In men the lesions appear on the prepuce, glans, or shaft of the penis.

Collaborative Care Management

Chancroid is treated with azithromycin, 1 g orally in a single dose, or ceftriaxone, 250 mg IM in a single dose, or ciprofloxacin 500 mg orally twice a day for 3 days, or erythromycin base, 500 mg orally four times a day for 7 days.

Successful treatment for chancroid cures the infection, resolves the clinical symptoms, and prevents transmission to others. Follow-up evaluation is essential. If treatment is successful, ulcers improve symptomatically within 3 days. If treatment failure occurs reasons need to be explored.

Patient/Family Education. The individual is taught to report any signs or symptoms that persist or worsen during treatment and to abstain from sexual activity until all lesions are healed. The individual needs to be screened for HIV. Proper use of a condom should also be stressed (Box 56-1).

GRANULOMA INGUINALE (DONOVANOSIS)

Etiology/Epidemiology

Granuloma inguinale, or granuloma venereum, is believed to be most often transmitted by sexual contact, although nonsexual transmission has been reported. The infection is caused by a gram-negative bacillus, *Calymmatobacterium (Donovania) granulomatis,* widely referred to as *Donovan bacillus.* The organism is related to *Klebsiella.*

Donovanosis is common in tropical and subtropical areas of Papua New Guinea, the Caribbean, and parts of Africa and Southeast Asia; it rarely occurs in the United States. The disease is mildly contagious and probably requires repeated exposures for spread of infection. Predisposing factors are poorly understood. The disease is more common in men than in women and is especially common among homosexual men. The incubation period varies from several days to months.[11]

Pathophysiology

Lesions appear on the genitalia and in the perianal area. The infection first appears with development of red subcutaneous nodules. These elevated areas eventually ulcerate, producing sharply defined, painless lesions. The ulcers enlarge slowly and bleed on contact. With ulceration, the infection tends to spread along the pubic region. Involvement of the lymph nodes is uncommon but can occur and produce occlusion of the lymphatics, resulting in elephantiasis.

Collaborative Care Management

Granuloma inguinale is treated with trimethoprim-sulfamethoxazole (Bactrim DS) orally twice a day for a minimum of 3 weeks or doxycycline, 100 mg orally twice a day, for a minimum of 3 weeks. Therapy should be continued until all lesions have healed completely.

Patient/Family Education. Clinician follow-up care of anyone diagnosed with granuloma inguinale is extremely important, because of the possibility of treatment failure. All persons should be advised to abstain from sexual activity until all sexual partners complete a course of treatment, and all lesions are healed.

HUMAN PAPILLOMAVIRUS

Etiology/Epidemiology

The most commonly recognized clinical signs of genital HPV infections are genital warts. However in many cases HPV infects people without causing noticeable symptoms. Genital warts caused by HPV are the most commonly diagnosed viral disease in both the United States and the United Kingdom. Epidemiologic and molecular biologic evidence demonstrate that some types of HPV cause cervical cancer.[3,22]

An estimated 5.5 million people acquire a genital HPV infection every year. It is estimated that 20 million people in the United States have genital HPV infections that can be transmitted. Between 500,000 and 1 million cases of genital warts occur per year in the United States. They are the leading cause of office visits.[8]

Pathophysiology

There are 30 distinct types of HPV that can infect the genital area; more than 70 types of HPV have been identified in all. Of these, types 6 and 11 are most commonly found in genital warts. Types 6 and 11 can cause cervical dysplasia, but are not found in cancer of the cervix.[2] Genital warts occur in or around the vulva, vagina, cervix, perineum, anal canal, urethra, and glans penis. People who have visible genital warts can be infected simultaneously with multiple HPV types. They can enlarge during pregnancy and may cause difficulty with birth. Most HPV infections appear to be temporary and probably are cleared by the body's immune system. However, reactivation is possible after a period of up to decades. Reinfection is also possible.[8]

Types 16, 18, 31, 33, and 35 are strongly associated with cervical dysplasia. These types are occasionally found in visible genital warts and have been associated with vaginal, anal, and cervical intraepithelial dysplasia and squamous cell carcinoma. Types 16 and 18 are especially likely to progress to high-grade lesions and cancer if left untreated. People infected with these types usually do not have any apparent visible lesions.[22] About 40% of untreated cervical dysplasia cases progress to invasive cancer over an average of 10 years.[20] Multiple cofactors are necessary for progression from dysplasia to invasive cervical cancer with the HPV infection.[13]

Collaborative Care Management

Multiple treatment modalities exist for HPV depending on the location and extent of the infection. The primary goal of treating visible genital warts is to remove the symptomatic warts. Treatment should be guided by patient preference, available resources, and experience of the health care provider. No available treatment is superior to other treatments and no single treatment is ideal for all persons with HPV.

Patient/Family Education. Because a diagnosis of HPV has been linked to an increased risk for cervical cancer, the woman is advised to have an annual Pap smear. More frequent Pap smears are recommended when abnormal Pap smears develop. Malignant changes may not develop for 5 or more years.

After visible genital warts have cleared, follow-up care is not mandatory; however, the patient should be advised to watch for recurrences. Recurrences occur most frequently in the first 3 months after treatment. People with HPV infections need to understand that they might remain infectious even though the warts are gone. The use of condoms may reduce, but does not eliminate, the risk of transmission.[6] As with all STDs, HIV and other STD testing should be offered.

Prevention of HPV should be stressed. It includes (1) abstaining from intercourse, (2) avoiding sexual relationships with persons in known high-risk groups, (3) using latex condoms for sexual intercourse, and (4) avoiding anal intercourse.

The CDC does not recommend a cesarean birth to prevent transmission of HPV to newborns. Cesarean delivery may be indicated for warts obstructing the pelvic outlet or if a vaginal birth would cause excessive bleeding of the warts.

TRICHOMONIASIS

Etiology/Epidemiology

A protozoa, *Trichomonas vaginalis,* causes trichomoniasis. Evidence suggests that the incubation period ranges between 4 and 28 days. There are an estimated 5 million cases of trichomoniasis annually in the United States.[5] *T. vaginalis* organisms are found in 3% to 15% of women under the care of private physicians, 13% to 23% of women attending gynecologic clinics, and 50% of women who have gonorrhea. It is transmitted most easily by the sexual route, but laboratory conditions have demonstrated transmission by fomites such as towels and toilet seats. The parasite commonly exists in vaginal and cervical secretions and in seminal fluid. It is estimated that one in five women will have a trichomonas infection during her lifetime.

Pathophysiology

Trichomoniasis presents as a malodorous copious, frothy, thick or thin, white to yellow-green/gray discharge. The vagina may be inflamed. About 90% of patients with trichomoniasis have cervical erosions and leukorrhea with subsequent cervical bleeding. Trichomoniasis results in urethritis and causes prostatitis in men 40% of the time. Reversible sterility can occur as a result of inhibition of sperm motility by toxins produced by the organism

Trichomoniasis is commonly viewed as an innocuous infection, yet there are serious implications for health. In pregnant women, trichomoniasis may cause prematurity or low birth weights. During the postpartum period, the rate of persistent fever, prolonged vaginal discharge, and endometritis is twice as high as in women who do not harbor the organism. Trichomoniasis may increase the risk of HIV infection.[8]

Collaborative Care Management

Trichomoniasis is usually treated with metronidazole, 2 g orally in a single dose taken with food. Alternatively the person may take metronidazole, 500 mg twice a day for 7 days.

Patient/Family Education. The CDC recommends that both partners be treated simultaneously with oral metronidazole to prevent reinfection. The partners should be cautioned against drinking alcohol while taking the drug. The drug is known to cross the placental barrier, but does not cause teratogenic effects; therefore it is deemed safe to give in the first trimester, a recent treatment change. Condom use is advised. HIV and all other STD testing should be offered.[5]

BACTERIAL VAGINOSIS

Etiology/Epidemiology

Bacterial vaginosis (BV) is the most common vaginal infection among women of childbearing age. In the United States as many as 16% of pregnant women have BV.[5] It is characterized by an overgrowth of normal flora resulting from the introduction of other flora and altered vaginal pH related to sexual activity or poor hygienic practices such as douching or incorrect wiping after bowel movements. Women who have never been sexually active are rarely affected. Recent studies have linked BV with preterm labor, infection of amniotic fluid, postpartum uterine infections, and PID.[8,17]

Pathophysiology

Bacterial vaginosis infection is characterized by a small amount of homogeneous gray or grayish white discharge. The discharge usually has a disagreeable odor, and because it is less irritating than discharges caused by other organisms, pruritus is mild or absent. On inspection the vaginal walls are slightly reddened, and the discharge appears to adhere to the mucosal lining.

Collaborative Care Management

Bacterial vaginosis can be treated with metronidazole, 500 mg orally twice a day for 7 days, or with clindamycin cream 2%, one applicatorful at bedtime for 7 days, or with metronidazole gel 0.75% (Metrogel), one full applicator vaginally at bedtime for 7 days.

Patient/Family Education. The goal of therapy for BV is to relieve vaginal symptoms and signs of infection. The woman can take metronidazole orally or as a vaginal gel, or she may be prescribed clindamycin cream for vaginal use. Self-care measures should be emphasized.[5] These include use of condoms for 4 to 6 weeks after diagnosis, eliminating douching, and wiping from front to back after voiding.

HEPATITIS B VIRUS

Etiology/Epidemiology

Hepatitis B virus (HBV) is a DNA virus that causes acute hepatitis and is a major cause of chronic liver disease, which may cause cirrhosis, and hepatocellular cancer, leading to death. There are more than 300 million persons infected worldwide. In the United States an estimated 200,000 new infections occur each year. About 5000 to 6000 deaths occur each year from chronic hepatitis B–related liver disease. Infants and children have the highest risk of developing chronic HBV infection.[8] The chronic carrier rate in the United States is 0.1% to 0.5% of the population. The rate is considerably higher in other parts of the world.

In the United States transmission of HBV is primarily through blood or intimate contact (usually sexual). About 120,000 of new infections are acquired through sexual transmission, usually by young adults.[8] Hepatitis B virus is transmitted sexually, and risk factors include multiple sexual partners, a history of STD, and receptive anal intercourse. HBV is transmitted parenterally[9] by drug abusers sharing needles or by health care workers by accidental needle sticks. Since blood screening programs were implemented in the 1980s it is not transmitted by blood transfusion. Transmission from mother to neonates occurs in 70% to 90% of mothers positive for hepatitis B e antigen (HBeAg). HBeAg-negative mothers have a 10% to 40% risk of infecting their neonates. Other transmission risk factors include patients on hemodialysis and those who are institutionalized.[5] Between 30% and 40% of patients with HBV infection in the United States deny any of the risk factors, and the source of their infection may never be known.

Pathophysiology

The hepatitis caused by HBV results in the same symptoms seen in other types of hepatitis. The liver is inflamed, and the patient may have jaundice, anorexia, slight fever, and gastrointestinal upset. For more information see Chapter 37.

Collaborative Care Management

Treatment of HBV is described in Chapter 37.

The CDC recommends vaccination for persons identified as being at high risk, including residents of correctional or long-term care facilities, persons seeking treatment for an STD, teens and young adults, health care workers, prostitutes, homosexuals, and anyone living with someone with HBV. The CDC also recommends that all children regardless of their exposure risk be vaccinated against HBV. The vaccine is given at birth, 1 month, and 6 months. If serum HBsAg is not detected after 5 to 7 years, a booster dose of the vaccine should be considered. Vaccination is recommended for all health care workers because of the possibility of needle sticks and blood exposure.[5]

The CDC recommends that postexposure prophylactic treatment with hepatitis B immune globulin (HBIG) should be considered in the following situations: sexual contact with a person who has active hepatitis B or who contracts hepatitis B and sexual contact with a hepatitis B carrier (blood test positive for HBsAg). The prophylactic treatment should be given within 14 days of sexual contact. The HBIG is also given to unvaccinated health care workers who suffer a needlestick.[5]

All pregnant women should be screened during their first obstetric visit for the presence of HBsAg. If they are HBsAg positive, their newborns should be given HBIG and hepatitis B vaccine within 12 hours of birth and subsequent follow-up immunizations with hepatitis B vaccine.[5] For more information about hepatitis see Chapter 37.

OTHER SEXUALLY TRANSMITTED DISEASES

In addition to the diseases already discussed, pediculosis pubis, molluscum contagiosum, and scabies are considered to be STDs.

Pediculosis pubis, also known as "crabs," is caused by pubic lice. Although lice can be transmitted by bedding or clothing, they are often transmitted during sexual contact. They produce erythematous, itchy papules. The lice adhere to hair around the pubic area, anus, abdomen, and thighs. Diagnosis is made by observation of lice or microscopic observation of nits found on the pubic hairs. Recommended treatment is 1% Kwell lotion or shampoo. One treatment per episode is necessary, but itching may persist.

Molluscum contagiosum is a viral infection manifested by papular lesions on the abdomen, thighs, and genitals. Although molluscum contagiosum may be transmitted via fomites, its transmission in adults is primarily sexual. Diagnosis is often made on sight of the characteristic lesion. A punch biopsy may be used for diagnostic evaluation if visual diagnosis is uncertain. There is no effective medical treatment. Most often patients are advised to allow the lesions to resolve spontaneously. If only a few lesions are present the core of the lesions may by surgically excised. Multiple lesions may be treated with cryotherapy.

Scabies, caused by mites known as *Sarcoptes scabiei,* is transmitted by close body contact, bedding, and clothing. Diagnosis is made from linear burrows, often characterized by a reddened papule containing the mite. Common sites are finger webs, wrists, elbows, ankles, and the penis. Nocturnal itching is common. A one-time use of 1% Kwell shampoo is recommended. Family, household, and sexual contacts should also be treated.

Critical Thinking Questions

1. You have been requested to give a presentation on STDs to several health education classes at a local high school. What information should you be prepared to discuss? If you are limited to 45 minutes, what information do you think is most important to cover and why?
2. Explain why the incidence of STDs is high among American teens. How might the care of a teenager who has an STD differ from that of an adult with the same disease?
3. Discuss the social and economic factors that affect the spread of STDs.
4. What social interventions may be needed to facilitate a decrease in the incidence and prevalence of STDs?

References

1. Abbuhl S: Chancroid, *EMedicine J* 2(5):1, 2001, website: http://www.emedicine.com/EMERG/topic95.html, 2001
2. Birley HD: Continuing medical ignorance: modern myths in the management of genital warts, *Int J STD AIDS* 12(2):71, 2001.
3. Bonn D, Bradbury J: The warts and all approach to tackling cervical cancer, *Lancet* 351(9105):8, 1998.
4. Cates W et al: Estimates of the incidence and prevalence of sexually transmitted diseases in the United States, *Sex Transm Dis* 26(suppl): S2, 1996.
5. Centers for Disease Control and Prevention (CDC): Guidelines for treatment of sexually transmitted diseases, *MMWR*(RR-1):1-29, 1998.
6. Centers for Disease Control and Prevention (CDC): National Center for Health Statistics, Sexually transmitted disease, website: http://www.cdc.gov/nchs/fastats/stds.htm. retrieved 8/13/01.
7. Centers for Disease Control and Prevention (CDC): Recommendations for prevention and management of *Chlamydia trachomatis* infections, *MMWR* 41:1, 1993.
8. Centers for Disease Control and Prevention (CDC): Tracking the hidden epidemics, Trends in STDs in the United States 2000, corrected April 6, 2001, website: http://www.cdc.gov/nchstp/dstd/dstdp.html
9. Cooksley WG: Acute and chronic viral hepatitis. In Rakel RE, editor: *Conn's current therapy 1999,* Philadelphia, 1999, WB Saunders.
10. Faro S: *Chlamydia trachomatis* infection. In Rakel RE, editor: *Conn's current therapy 1999,* Philadelphia, 1999, WB Saunders.
11. Felman YH: Granuloma inguinale (Donovanosis). In Rakel RE, editor: *Conn's current therapy* 1999, Philadelphia, 1999, WB Saunders.
12. Felman YH: Lymphogranuloma venereum. In Rakel RE, editor: *Conn's current therapy 1999,* Philadelphia, 1999, WB Saunders.
13. Goodman A: Role of routine human papillomavirus subtyping in cervical screening, *Curr Opin Obstet Gynecol* 12(1):11, 2000.
14. Hatcher RA et al: *Contraceptive technology,* ed 16, New York, 1994, Irvington.
15. Martin DH: Chancroid. In Rakel RE, editor: *Conn's current therapy 1999,* Philadelphia, 1999, WB Saunders.
16. Moran JS: Gonorrhea. In Rakel RE, editor: *Conn's current therapy 1999,* Philadelphia, 1999, WB Saunders.
17. Reed BD: Vulvovaginitis. In Rakel RE, editor: *Conn's current therapy 1996,* Philadelphia, 1996, WB Saunders.
18. Rein, MF: Syphilis. In Rakel RE, editor: *Conn's current therapy 1999,* Philadelphia, 1999, WB Saunders.
19. Roberts RB: Lymphogranuloma venereum (LGV)—*Chlamydia trachomatis* website: http://edcenter.med.cornell.edu/Pathophysiology_Cases/STDs/STDs_08.html, retreived 8/16/01.
20. Sawaya GF, Brown AD, Washington AE, Garber AM: Current approaches to cervical-cancer screening, *N Engl J Med* 344(21):1603, 2001.
21. Those other STDs, *Am J Public Health* 81(10):1250, 1991 (editorial).
22. Trofatter KF: Diagnosis of human papillomavirus genital tract infection, *Am J Med* 102(5A):21, 1997.
23. U.S. Department of Health and Human Services: *Healthy People 2010: understanding and improving health,* Washington, DC, 2000, USDHHS.
24. Workowski KA: *Chlamydia trachomatis* infection. In Rakel RE, editor: *Conn's current therapy 1996,* Philadelphia, 1996, WB Saunders.

57 Assessment of the Visual System

Sarah C. Smith

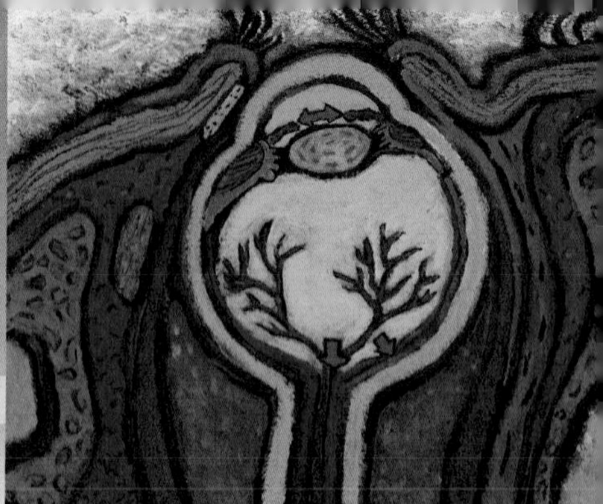

Objectives

After studying this chapter, the learner should be able to:

1. Describe the structure and function of the eye.
2. Identify the normal physiologic and anatomic ocular changes that occur with aging.
3. Identify the subjective and objective data that should be obtained when assessing the eye.
4. Discuss the nursing interventions and patient teaching associated with common ocular diagnostic tests.

Orientation to our world is primarily visual. We learn much about our environment and ourselves through our eyes. Practically every behavior is affected by the visual sense. One hears a noise and looks in the direction from which it came. Something touches our body, and we look to see what it was. Vision contributes meaning and pleasure to the human experience.

Assessment of the visual system is an integral part of the nurse's role. Visual screening is conducted with persons of all ages and in all settings, and most eye disorders are identified by nurses and physicians in schools, industry, outpatient clinics, or ophthalmologists' offices. Admission to the hospital is usually limited to medical or surgical treatment that cannot routinely be accomplished on an outpatient basis.

Because persons with eye problems usually are managed on an outpatient basis, visual impairment is usually not the major diagnosis of persons for whom the nurse is providing care. However, visual impairment is frequently present and may be undiagnosed. Therefore nurses should routinely assess visual ability, especially in persons who have systemic diseases that affect vision or who are taking medications with known visual side effects.

ANATOMY AND PHYSIOLOGY OF THE EYE

Layers of the Eye

The eyeball has three main coats or layers (Figure 57-1). The tough outer layer consists of the opaque sclera (white) and the transparent cornea. These structures are joined at the corneoscleral sulcus or limbus. The middle vascular layer or uvea is composed of three parts: the choroid, the ciliary body, and the iris, which contains an opening in its center called the pupil.

The retina, the third and innermost layer of the eye, is composed of two parts: a sensory portion and a layer of pigmented epithelium. The sensory portion contains the photoreceptors (rods and cones). These photoreceptors synapse in the retina with bipolar neurons and then with ganglion neurons, and these become the fibers of the optic nerve that pass visual information to the brain.

The cones, which are less numerous than the rods, are mainly concentrated near the center of the retina in an area termed the macula (Figure 57-2). They are considered to be the receptors for bright daylight and color vision and allow us to see sharp images. The rods, which are found mostly in the periphery of the retina, are receptors for dim or night vision. Rods contain rhodopsin, a photosensitive protein that rapidly becomes depleted in bright light. The slow regeneration of rhodopsin, which depends on the presence of vitamin A, explains the time needed to adjust from a bright to a dim light.

Chambers of the Eye

The interior of the eyeball is divided into two segments (anterior and posterior). The anterior segment includes the space from the back of the cornea to the lens, and the posterior compartment is the space from the posterior surface of the lens to the retina.

The anterior segment is further subdivided into an anterior chamber (between the cornea and the iris) and a posterior chamber (between the iris and the lens). This segment is filled with a clear liquid called aqueous humor, whose purpose is to nourish and bathe the lens and cornea. Produced by the ciliary body in the posterior chamber, aqueous humor flows through the pupil into the anterior chamber and leaves the eye through the filtration structures at the junction of the iris and cornea (anterior chamber angle). The filtration structures consist of the trabecular meshwork and an encircling tubular channel into which the aqueous humor drains (Schlemm's canal).

Schlemm's canal has several exit channels that empty into the scleral and episcleral veins. Aqueous humor passes through these exit channels and eventually is absorbed into general circulation (Figure 57-3).

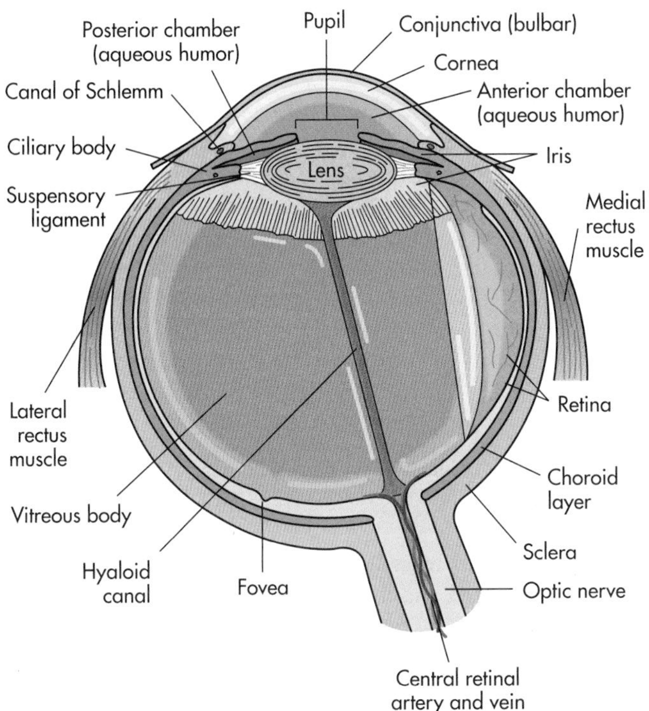

Figure 57-1 Horizontal section through the left eye.

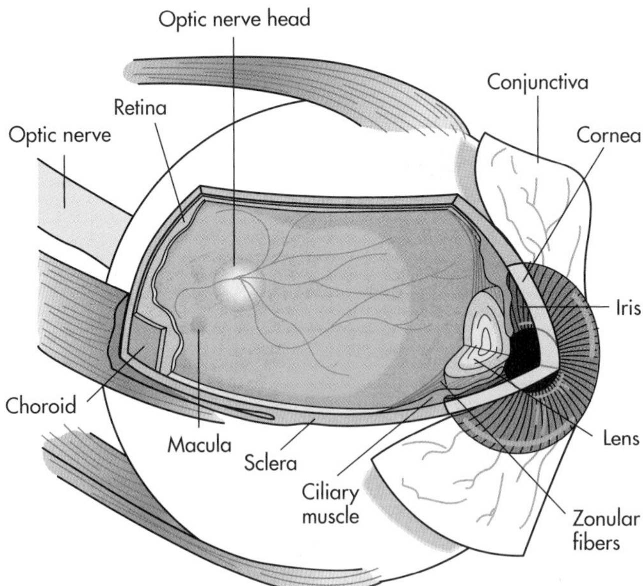

Figure 57-2 Cutaway section of the eye.

The posterior segment is the larger of the two segments and is filled with a clear gel-like substance called the vitreous humor. The structure of the vitreous humor can be pictured as fine collagen fibers crossing one another to form a scaffolding that helps to maintain the shape of the eyeball. This fibrous network becomes more dense toward the outermost portion of the vitreous humor, particularly in the areas of strong attachment between the vitreous humor and retina. These attachments occur at the anterior edge of the retina, the optic disc, the equator of the eye, and the macula. The vitreous humor is clear, thus allowing transmission of light posteriorly to the retina.

Lens

The lens is a transparent biconvex structure located directly behind the iris and pupil. It is enclosed in a clear capsule and attached to the ciliary body by multiple suspensory ligaments called zonules. The lens is the fine-focusing mechanism for the eye. It bends light rays entering the eye so that they focus on the retina producing a clear image.

Eye Muscles

There are two types of eye muscles: extrinsic and intrinsic. The six extraocular muscles are extrinsic voluntary muscles that control the extraocular movements of each eye (Table 57-1 and Figure 57-4). The lateral and medial rectus muscles control outturning (abduction) and inturning (adduction), respectively, with the remaining four muscles. The rectus muscles move the eye up and down and toward the nose while the oblique muscles also control up and down movement plus movement toward the ear. The simultaneous actions of the muscles of each eye are integrated by the brain.

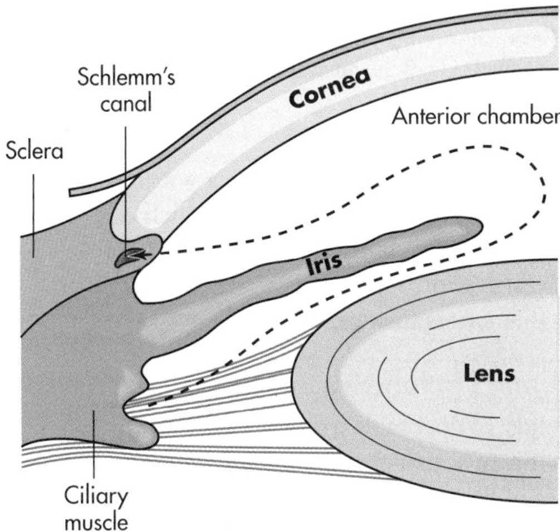

Figure 57-3 Flow of aqueous humor. Aqueous humor is largely produced by the ciliary processes in the posterior chamber; it flows into the anterior chamber and leaves the eye through Schlemm's canal.

TABLE 57-1 Extrinsic Muscles

Name	Function
Superior rectus	Rotates eye upward and toward the nose
Inferior rectus	Rotates eye downward and toward the nose
Lateral rectus	Moves eye toward the temporal side
Medial rectus	Moves eye toward the nose
Inferior oblique	Rotates eye upward and toward the temporal side
Superior oblique	Rotates eye downward and toward the temporal side

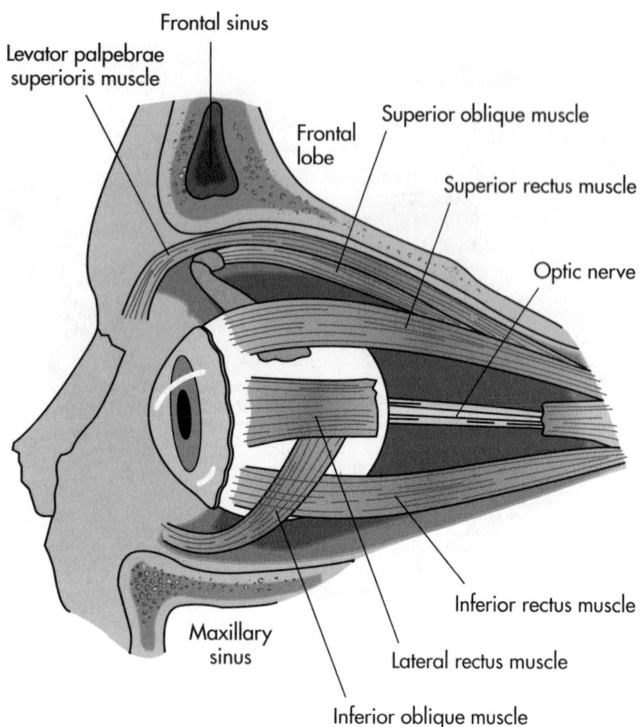

Figure 57-4 Extrinsic muscles of the eye. Both oblique muscles insert behind the equator of the globe. The inferior oblique muscle passes inferiorly to the body of the inferior rectus muscle but beneath the lateral rectus muscle.

The intrinsic involuntary muscles within the eye are the ciliary muscles (in the ciliary body), which control the shape of the lens, and the sphincter and dilator pupillae muscles in the iris, which control pupil size and consequently the amount of light that enters the eye.

Eyelids and Conjunctiva

The eyelids (palpebrae) are made up of thin layers of skin, muscle, fibrous tissue, and mucous membrane. The main purposes of the eyelids are to protect the eye from external irritation, spread tears over the front of the eye, and interrupt and restrict the amount of light entering the eye. The conjunctiva, the mucous membrane lining of the eyelid (palpebral conjunctiva) that extends over the anterior sclera (bulbar conjunctiva), is of particular significance. This membrane and its blood vessels provide nutrients, antibodies, and leukocytes to the avascular cornea. The conjunctiva and glands within the eyelid secrete mucus and oil, which help keep the cornea moist and clear and decrease friction when the lids close.

Lacrimal System

The lacrimal system consists of the lacrimal gland and a tear drainage system (Figure 57-5). The lacrimal gland produces the tears that flow across the eye and enter the drainage system nasally. Each time the eyelids blink, the tears are pumped by the blinking action and flow across the surface of the eyes. The tears flow through small holes in the eyelids (puncti) and ducts (canaliculi) to the lacrimal sac. They then drain into the nasolacrimal duct through the opening of the inferior meatus of the nasal cavity. Tears keep the surface of the eye and conjunctiva moistened and lubricated. Tears also contain an enzyme that functions as an antibacterial agent.

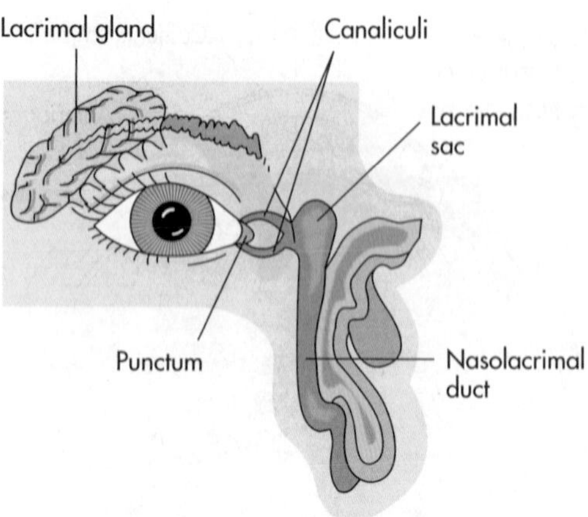

Figure 57-5 Lacrimal system.

Orbit

The eye rests within the confines of the bony orbit. This orbit is a cone-shaped cavity formed by the union of cranial and facial bones. The eyeball itself occupies only about one fifth of the space of the orbit. The remainder is filled with the lacrimal gland, muscles, blood vessels, nerves, and fatty tissue. This fatty tissue serves as a protective cushion for the eye. The optic nerve exits the orbit posteriorly, transmitting visual information from the eye to the brain.

Physiology of Vision

Light rays entering the eye are bent (refracted) as they pass over the curved surfaces of the cornea and through the various (more posterior) structures of the eye (aqueous humor, lens, and vitreous humor) to focus on the retina. The cornea provides the major refractive change for light entering the eye, with the lens providing the fine focus for light transmitted posteriorly to the retina.

The eye can adjust (accommodation) to seeing objects at various distances by the flattening or thickening of the lens. Near vision requires contraction of the ciliary muscles in the ciliary body. This contraction allows the ciliary muscle to move forward and relaxes the zonules attached to the lens. The lens then bulges to bend the light rays more acutely so the rays focus on the retina. Accommodation also is facilitated by changing the size of the pupil. With near vision, the iris constricts the pupil to force light rays to pass through the shortened but thicker lens. The pupils also constrict with bright lights to protect the retina from intense stimulation.

Light rays are absorbed by photoreceptors on the retina, changed to electrical activity, and transmitted via the optic nerve to the visual cortex areas of the brain for processing. The fibers of the optic nerve (cranial nerve II; see Chapter 41) divide at the optic chiasm; the medial portion of each nerve crosses to the opposite side, and the impulses are then transmitted to the visual cortex. In this way, visual information received by each eye is transmitted simultaneously to both sides of the brain. Binocular vision creates depth perception.

Physiologic Changes With Aging

Aging affects many aspects of visual function, both physiologic and anatomic.[9] Decreased flexibility and elasticity of the lens lead to one of the first noted signs of aging—the decreased ability of the eye to focus (accommodate) for near and detailed work (presbyopia).

With the aging process an older person's color vision declines and contributes to impaired depth perception.[6] This decline in color vision causes greater difficulty in distinguishing among colors at the blue end of the spectrum, whereas warm colors are easier to differentiate. A smaller pupil (senile miosis) adds to this distortion of color. It also affects the amount of light that reaches the peripheral retina and the ability of the person to adapt to dim light and darkness. As a result, the older person has impaired night vision. Persons older than 60 years of age need about twice as much light to see as they did when they were 20.

This increase in the amount of light needed for close work can also create problems with glare. Glare, a veil-like luminance superimposed on the retinal image, masks and reduces the brightness of objects in the visual field.[9] Glare is related to increased light scatter in the eye caused by corneal, scleral, lens, and vitreal changes.

The field of vision also begins to decrease with age, affecting the breadth of vision.[3] It is uncertain whether this decrease is caused by retinal changes, decreased pupil size, or loss of lens transparency.

The decrease in lens transparency, which begins to appear in the fifth decade of life, is not fully understood. The compression of lens fibers, yellowing of the lens, and efficiency of aqueous humor circulation may all play a part in the increased opaqueness of the lens, leading to cataract formation. Cumulative lifetime exposure to ultraviolet B radiation is associated with lens opacities, supporting the practice of wearing sunglasses.[12]

Aqueous humor production drops off sharply in the sixth decade. This compensates for the reduced drainage and shallowness of the anterior chamber and enables the eye to maintain a relatively stable intraocular pressure.[8]

The quantity and quality of tears also decrease with age, and the tears tend to evaporate more readily. The eyes take on a duller appearance, and there is a feeling of tightness, scratchiness, or dryness. The drainage of tears also is less efficient.

One of the more common eye changes that occurs with aging is arcus senilis. This hazy gray ring around the periphery of the cornea is a result of fat deposits. Another important change in the cornea is its change in shape. It tends to flatten, resulting in an irregular curvature in the corneal surface. As a result light entering the eye tends to be refracted at varying angles, leading to a distorted and blurred image (astigmatism).

HEALTH HISTORY

A complete visual assessment consists of a careful patient history combined with a physical examination of the eye structures. General areas explored during the history include the patient's assessment of his or her vision and any recent changes in visual acuity, whether glasses or contacts are used, and the date of the last professional eye examination. The presence and severity of common eye symptoms such as blurred vision, floaters (tiny particles in the vitreous humor seen by the patient as black specks or moving spots in the visual field), dry scratchy eyes, burning, or chronic headache are explored. The history also allows the nurse to explore the person's health promotion and risk reduction practices such as the use of protective eyewear and care of contact lenses if worn. Any history of head trauma, loss of consciousness, or direct eye trauma or infection is important to explore.

Because many eye disorders are inherited, a family history is essential. Questions specifically address any family history of cataracts, glaucoma, diabetes, hypertension, poor vision that could not be corrected with glasses, or blindness. A personal medical history is also obtained, with particular attention to all medications in current use.

PHYSICAL EXAMINATION

The tissues of the eye are for the most part transparent, making abnormalities easily detectable. Ocular manifestations of systemic disease also can be identified. In addition, the vascular system (retinal vascular system) and cranial nerve (optic nerve) of the eye can be visualized on examination. Physical examination includes inspection of the external structures and gross measures of visual acuity. More complete eye examinations, such as electrophysiologic studies of the retina and other fundus examinations, are performed by physicians in conjunction with specially trained nurses or technicians. A basic assessment of the eye and vision is summarized in Table 57-2.

Inspection of External Structures

The nurse first inspects the general appearance of the face and eyes of the patient. The presence of an abnormal protrusion or bulging of an eye is called exophthalmia or exophthalmos. In older adults the eyes tend to sink into the orbit (enophthalmos) primarily as a result of the loss of orbital fat.

The eyelids are assessed for color, texture, mobility, and position. The lids should be able to close completely to prevent drying of the conjunctiva and cornea. Any swelling, redness, or discharge is noted. If one upper lid seems to be lower than the other, or "droops," ptosis of the eyelid may be present. If ptosis is present in both eyes, the upper lid is noted to be in an abnormally low position, covering the upper portion or more of the iris. Ptosis may be the result of extreme debility or neuromuscular disease. Extreme ptosis can interfere with vision by covering the pupil.

As the person ages, the eyelids become thinner and less elastic and positional defects may occur. In addition to ptosis, ectropion, entropion, and dermatochalasis may be present. Ectropion is eversion of the lower lid. It is usually bilateral, and symptoms include tearing and irritation. Entropion is the turning in of the eyelids. The person experiences a foreign body sensation caused by the eyelashes rubbing against the cornea. Dermatochalasis is a redundancy of upper or lower lid

TABLE 57-2 Basic Assessment of the Eye and Vision

Facial and ocular expression	Prominence of eyes; alert or dull expression
Eyelids and conjunctiva	Symmetry, presence of edema, ptosis, itching, redness, discharges, blinking, equality, growths
Lacrimal system	Tears, swelling, growths
Sclera	Color
Cornea	Clarity
Anterior chamber	Depth, presence of blood/pus
Iris and pupils	Irregularities in color, shape, size
Pupillary reflex	
Light	Constriction of pupil in response to light in that eye (direct light reaction); equal amount of constriction in the other eye (consensual light reaction)
Accommodation	Convergence of eyes and constriction of pupil as gaze shifts from far to near object
Lens	Transparent or opaque
Peripheral vision	Ability to see movements and objects well on both sides of field of vision
Acuity with and without glasses	Ability to read newsprint, clocks on wall, and name tags and to recognize faces at bedside and at door
Supportive aids	Glasses, contact lenses, prosthesis

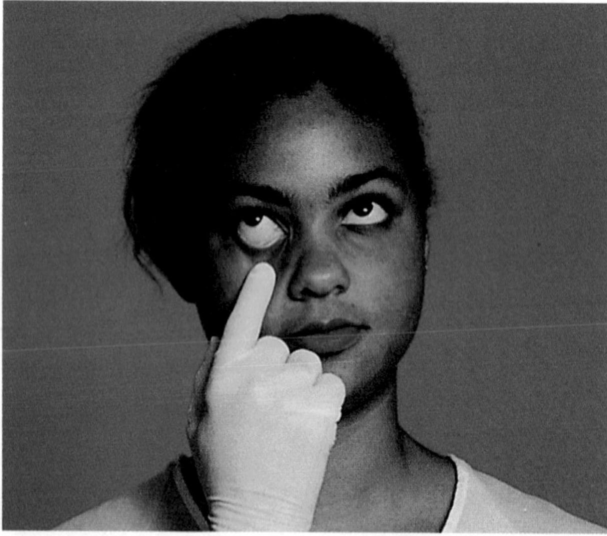

Figure 57-6 Eversion of lower eyelid by drawing margin downward as subject looks upward.

tissues. This usually occurs from loss of elasticity and results in wrinkles and drooping folds.

The conjunctiva of the lower lid is examined by pulling downward on the lid as the person looks upward (Figure 57-6). To examine the conjunctiva of the upper lid, the lid must be everted (Figure 57-7).

The lacrimal gland normally is not observable. Enlargement of the gland may occur in certain disorders that cause inflammation of the eye. This may be most evident when the upper lid is everted.

Small blood vessels normally are visible in the conjunctiva. The sclera shows through the conjunctiva and has a shiny porcelain-like appearance. Dilation of blood vessels of the conjunctiva may indicate disease of the cornea or disease within the eye. Spontaneous small hemorrhages may occur beneath the conjunctiva in the normal eye. A yellow discoloration of the sclera indicates jaundice but must be distinguished from the normal yellow tinge that may be present in dark-skinned individuals.

The cornea, which is normally visible except for surface reflections, must be smooth and transparent for good vision. It should look shiny and bright when examined with a penlight. Moving the light and directing it from the side, the nurse looks for abrasions and opacities. If the cornea is clear, the iris and pupils should be clearly visible.

Defects in the epithelium of the cornea may be demonstrated with the use of topical dyes. Contact lenses should be removed before dye instillation because the dye tends to stain soft lenses. The dye is put on the conjunctiva by drops or by touching the conjunctiva with a moistened strip of filter paper that has been impregnated with the dye. Injured tissue absorbs the dye allowing visualization of foreign bodies, abrasions, and inflammation of the cornea. After the test, the nurse cleans the dye from the patient's face with a moist tissue.

Occasionally the nurse performs a tear test (Schirmer test). This test is performed to verify abnormal tear production (dry eyes). The nurse explains the procedure to patients and informs them that the test may be uncomfortable but is not painful. The quantity of tears is measured with a strip of filter paper, folded and hooked over the lower lid, and left in place for approximately 5 minutes. The extent to which the filter paper is soaked with tears is then measured.

Next the anterior chamber is inspected. The anterior chamber of the eye, that segment between the cornea and the iris, can be inspected with the aid of a penlight and the "naked" eye or with the use of magnification, such as an ophthalmoscope and/or ophthalmic slit lamp. The fluid in the anterior chamber, aqueous humor, should be clear/transparent. If some of the fluid is reddish, quite possibly blood is present. If the fluid appears hazy to opaque, there are likely white cells present, and this is termed a hypopion (pus pocket).

The iris of each eye is compared for color, pattern, and shape. When looking through the pupillary opening with an ophthalmoscope, the nurse should be able to visualize the red pigment of the retinal fundus. If the nurse looks nasally (to-

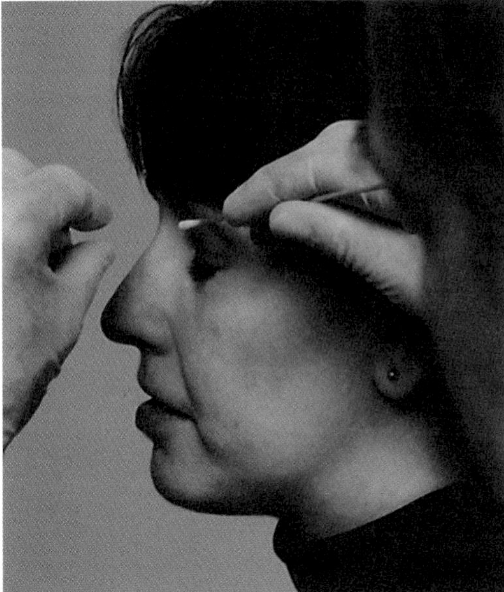

A

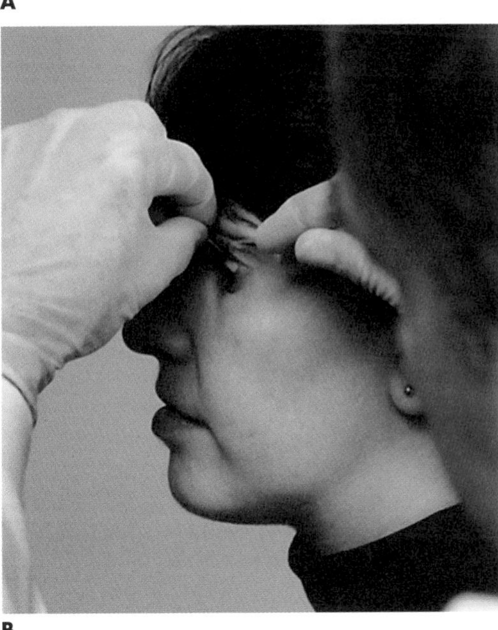

B

Figure 57-7 Eversion of upper eyelid. Patient is instructed to look downward, and lashes of upper eyelid are grasped between thumb and index finger. **A,** Cotton-tipped applicator is placed at level of tarsal fold. **B,** Eyelid is folded back on applicator while patient continues to look downward.

ward the patient's nose) with the ophthalmoscope or has the patient look outward the optic nerve head (optic disc) should be seen. If the interior of the eye cannot be visualized it may be due to opacification of the normally transparent lens. An opaque lens is termed a cataract.

Pupillary Reflexes

The pupils normally are equal and round and react to light and accommodation (PERRLA).[5] When assessing the pupillary reflexes, the nurse approaches from the side and quickly shines a light into one eye, causing constriction of the pupil in that eye (direct light reaction). The pupil of the other eye also should constrict the same amount (consensual light reaction). The other eye is then tested in the same manner.

A light shining into a blind eye will not produce a pupillary response; however, a light shining into a normal eye will produce a pupillary response in the blind eye by consensual reaction if the oculomotor nerve is intact.[2]

The pupillary reflex can also be tested by having the person focus on an object that is moved directly toward the nose. When the person focuses on the near object, the pupils of both eyes should constrict (near reaction, reaction in accommodation). The nurse looks for the presence of a response and notes whether the response is equal in both eyes. Loss of pupillary reflexes when sight is present is caused by neurologic disease.

Assessment of Vision

Visual acuity means acuteness or sharpness of vision and includes measurement of distance and near vision. Visual acuity can vary with attention, intelligence, and physical conditions such as lighting.[11]

Distance Vision

Distance vision usually is determined by the use of a Snellen chart (Figure 57-8, *A*), with the person positioned 20 feet (6 m) from the chart. The chart consists of rows of letters, numbers, or other characters arranged with the larger ones at the top and the smaller ones at the bottom. The uppermost letter on the chart is scaled so that it can be read by the normal eye at 200 feet, and the successive rows are scaled so that they can be read at 100, 70, 50, 40, 30, 20, 15, and 10 feet, respectively. Visual acuity is expressed as a fraction, and a reading of 20/20 is considered normal. The upper figure refers to the distance of the person from the chart, and the lower figure indicates the distance at which a normal eye can read the line. Each eye is tested separately, using a piece of stiff paper or a plastic occluder to cover the eye not being tested. The person is tested with and without distance lenses, and the results are recorded.

For preschool children, illiterate adults, and others unable to read the English alphabet, a modified Snellen chart may be used (Figure 57-8, *B*). A block E is shown in varying positions, and the person is asked to indicate in which direction the "legs" or "fingers" of the E point (Figure 57-8, *B*).

Near Vision

Near vision can be tested with the use of a Jaeger chart or newsprint. The Jaeger chart is a card containing varying sizes of print that is held 14 inches (35 cm) from the eye. The score obtained can be expressed in Jaeger or Snellen equivalent. For example, J1 is equal to Snellen 20/25; J2 = Snellen 20/30, J16 = Snellen 20/200.

For persons without sufficient vision to read letters, visual acuity can be assessed by asking them to count the number of the nurse's fingers that they can see held in front of their eyes. Some persons may not be able to count fingers but can see hand movement. Still others may be able to tell only the direction from which light is coming (light projection) or just respond to light flashed in their eyes (light perception).[7] Table 57-3 presents examples of visual acuity measurements and their meanings. Any person with vision less than 20/30 OD

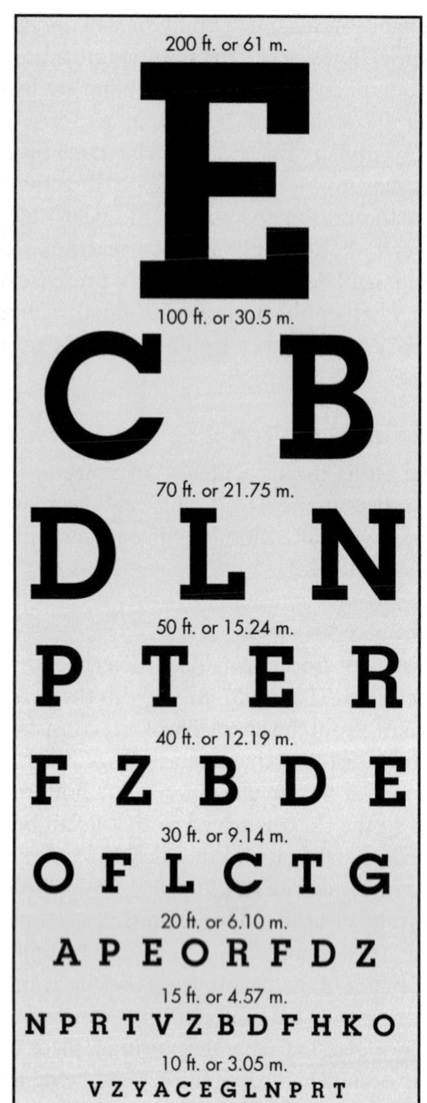

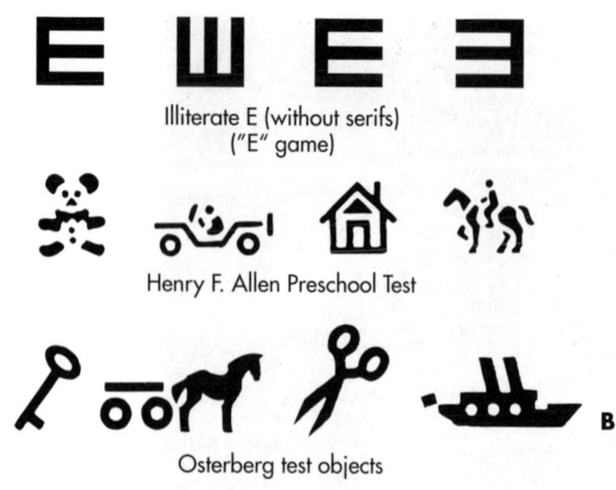

Figure 57-8 **A,** Snellen chart used in vision screening. **B,** Modified Snellen chart used in testing distance vision in children and illiterate adults.

TABLE 57-3 Examples of Visual Acuity Measurement

Measurement	Meaning
20/20	Normal
20/40-2	Missed two letters of the 20/40 line
10/400	At 10 ft, reads line that normal eye sees at 400 ft
CF/2 ft	Counts fingers at 2 ft
HM/3 ft	Sees hand movement at 3 ft
LP/Proj.	Light perception with projection
NLP	No light perception

(right eye) or OS (left eye) or with a two-line difference between eyes should be referred to an ophthalmologist for further testing and treatment, as the Snellen, block E, and Jaegar chart examinations provide only basic screening test data.

Refraction

A ray of light entering the eye passes through the various transparent refractive media and is bent (refracted) to focus on the retina. The bending of the light rays and the location of the image depend on the shape and condition of the eye. If the anteroposterior dimension of the eye is abnormally long, the light rays will focus in front of the retina (myopia) (Figure 57-9, *A*). Conversely, if the anteroposterior dimension is abnormally short, the rays will focus behind the retina (hyperopia) (Figure 57-9, *B*). When the lens becomes less elastic and responds less to the need for accommodation, blurring of near objects (presbyopia) results. The curvature of the cornea also may be asymmetric or irregular so that rays in the horizontal and vertical planes do not focus at the same point (astigmatism).

When the image is not clearly focused on the retina, refractive error is present (Box 57-1). Refractive errors account for the largest number of impairments of good vision.

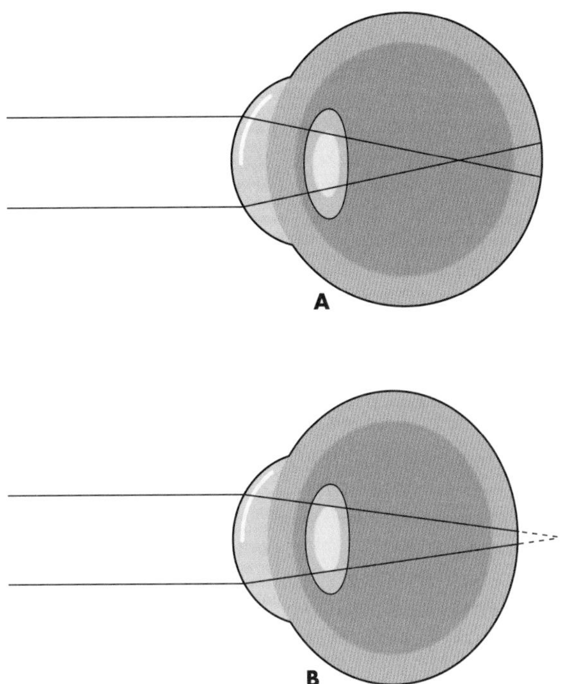

Figure 57-9 Two major types of refractive errors. **A**, Myopia. Parallel light rays come to a focus in front of the retina. **B**, Hyperopia. Parallel light rays come to a focus behind the retina.

To obtain a more definitive refractive error measurement, a cycloplegic drug often is instilled before the examination. A cycloplegic drug temporarily dilates the pupil and paralyzes the ciliary muscle (placing it at rest), thus paralyzing accommodation. This is called a cycloplegic refraction. Cyclopentolate (Cyclogyl), 1% or 2%, usually is used because it is effective in 30 minutes, and the effect generally wears off completely after 6 hours. Common medications used for eye examinations are summarized in Table 57-4. The nurse informs the patient that blurred vision will be present after the examination, and driving or reading will not be possible until the effect of the drug subsides.

Visual Fields

The visual field is that portion of the world that the eye can perceive. Lesions of the retina, optic pathways, and central nervous system affect sections of the field of vision. The location of visual field loss indicates the location of the lesion. For instance, glaucoma decreases peripheral vision, indicating damage to the optic nerve at its head or the optic disc. A rough measurement of the visual fields can be made with the confrontation test (see Chapter 41). If there appears to be any abnormality in the field of vision, more precise testing is performed by an ophthalmologist or a specially trained nurse or technician. The patient's peripheral vision can be precisely plotted using the perimeter, an instrument that measures the visual fields in degrees of arc. The tangent screen is the simplest perimeter, in which peripheral vision is plotted as a test object is moved against a black screen. Several automated and computer-assisted perimeters are also used to measure visual fields.

BOX 57-1 Terms Describing Refraction

Accommodation	Ability to adjust between far and near objects
Emmetropia	Normal eye; light rays focus on retina
Ametropia	Refractive error; light rays do not focus on retina
Myopia	Nearsightedness; light rays focus in front of retina
Hyperopia	Farsightedness; light rays focus behind retina
Presbyopia	Hyperopia from loss of lens elasticity because of aging
Astigmatism	Irregular curvature of cornea; light rays do not focus at same point

The central portion of the visual field can also be measured with the Amsler grid, a 20-cm square divided into 5-mm squares with a dot in the center (Figure 57-10). The grid is used to detect and follow a central area of blindness (scotoma). It most commonly is used at home by the patient to detect progression of macular disease.

With glasses on and one eye closed, the person holds the grid at the customary reading distance (12 inches). While fixating on the central dot, the person describes and outlines any area of distortion or absence of the grid. Distortions or "blind spots" are abnormal and imply dysfunction of the central retina (macula) or diseases of the optic nerve.

Color Vision Testing

Color vision testing is not always part of the normal eye examination. It is used most frequently to test for color blindness in persons seeking motor vehicle licenses or jobs for which color discrimination is important. Color vision deficiencies occur as a hereditary defect in both men (7%) and women (0.5%). Nutritional deficiencies, drug toxicities, and various disorders of the optic nerve and fovea centralis also can alter color perception.

There are both gross and sensitive measures of color vision. A common test consists of color plates on which numbers are outlined in primary colors and surrounded by confusion colors. The person with a color vision problem is unable to recognize the figure. The more sensitive tests involve hue discrimination. One such test consists of 84 chips of color that are matched in terms of increasing hue.

Assessment of Ocular Movements

Ocular movements are evaluated to determine whether the eyes are moving in a synchronous manner. Muscle imbalances and cranial nerve damage also can be detected.

To test ocular muscles the nurse and patient sit facing each other. The patient looks straight ahead, and a penlight is shone on the cornea. The corneal light reflex should be in exactly the same position on each pupil. The nurse then covers one of the person's eyes while the person looks at the light. When the cover is quickly removed, the nurse notes whether that eye moves to regain fixation on the light. Movement may

TABLE 57-4 Common Eye Medications Used for Diagnostic Purposes

Drug	Action	Intervention
Mydriatics (eyedrops): phenylephrine hydrochloride (Neo-Synephrine, Mydrin)	Pupil dilation by blocking the responses to the sphincter muscle of the iris from cholinergic stimulation	Evaluate the effectiveness (dark-eyed individuals usually require more drops to achieve the dilation required). Use is contraindicated in patients with a history of narrow or closed anterior chamber angles as may precipitate an increase intraocular pressure or angle closure attack. Monitor for temporary blurred vision— caution patients about driving or operating machinery until vision improves. Monitor for photophobia, and instruct patient to wear dark glasses in the sunlight or brightly lit rooms as needed.
Cycloplegics (eyedrops): atropine sulfate, cyclopentolate hydrochloride, homatropine hydrobromide, topicamide	Pupil dilation, but also blocks accommodation by paralyzing the ciliary muscles	Same as for mydriatics

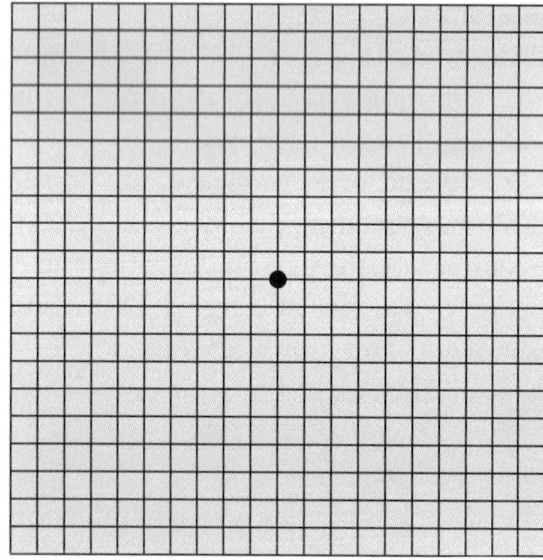

Figure 57-10 The Amsler grid.

indicate a drift of the eye behind the cover, which can indicate muscle imbalances.

To evaluate possible weaknesses of individual extraocular muscles, muscle testing can be performed in six cardinal fields of gaze, as well as straight ahead. More detailed information about assessment of ocular movements is presented in Chapter 41.

Inspection of Internal Structures

Ophthalmoscopy

The fundus of the eye is examined with a handheld instrument called an ophthalmoscope, which magnifies the view of the back of the eye so that the optic nerve, retina, blood vessels, and macula can be seen through the pupil (Figure 57-11). The examiner may use either the direct (Figure 57-12) or the indirect (Figure 57-13) method of ophthalmoscopic examination. The indirect ophthalmoscope allows the examiner to view the retina stereoscopically, thus allowing a wide-angle, three-dimensional view. This method provides visualization of the ocular fundus as far as the ora serrata (anterior margin of the retina). The indirect method, which requires a great degree of skill, normally is performed by an ophthalmologist. Nurses trained to perform an ophthalmoscopic examination use the direct method, the more commonly used approach. Because the entire retina cannot be visualized at one time, the examiner moves the ophthalmoscope until the entire fundus is visualized.

Difficulty in visualizing the fundus may be caused by interference with the light penetrating the eye as a result of intraocular inflammation, corneal scarring, or cataract. Data obtained from visualization of the fundus may indicate eye disease (cupping of the disc in glaucoma) or systemic disease (arteriosclerosis or hypertension). Hemorrhages in deep retinal layers occur in advanced hypertension, severe renal disease, certain collagen diseases, advanced diabetes, and blood dyscrasias.

Slit-Lamp Examination of the Fundus

The anterior segment of the eye can be examined with a slit-lamp, an instrument that combines a microscope and a light source. By adjusting the lens, the examiner can test for such problems as corneal ulcerations, lens changes, foreign bodies in the vitreous, or retinal changes.

Estimation of Intraocular Pressure

An instrument known as a tonometer is used to measure ocular tension and is helpful in detecting early glaucoma. The most common tonometer in general use worldwide is that of Schiøtz. The procedure is performed with the patient lying down or in the chair with the head back and looking upward at some fixed point. The eye may be anesthetized, after which the tonometer is placed on the cornea (Figure 57-14). While the weight of the tonometer is supported by the cornea, the amount of indentation that the instrument makes in the cornea is measured on the attached scale. This reading is used to determine the pressure within the eye. Readings over 24 mm Hg (Schiøtz) suggest glaucoma, but tests usually are repeated because temporary increases sometimes are caused by occurrences such as emotional stress. The applanation tonometer

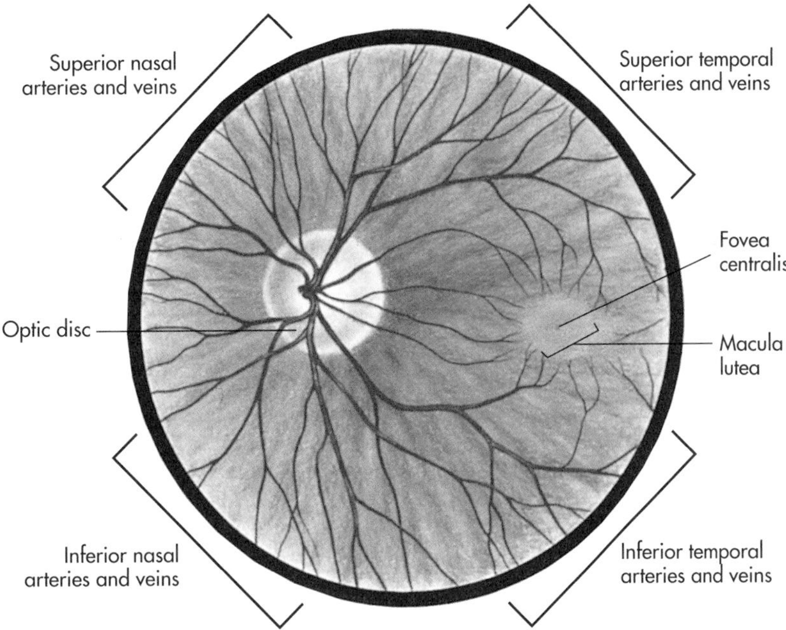

Figure 57-11 A normal right fundus as seen through a direct ophthalmoscope.

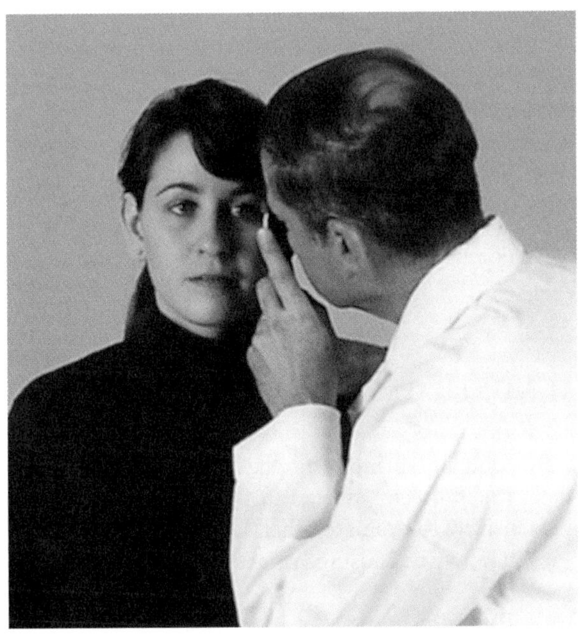

Figure 57-12 Direct method of ophthalmoscopic examination.

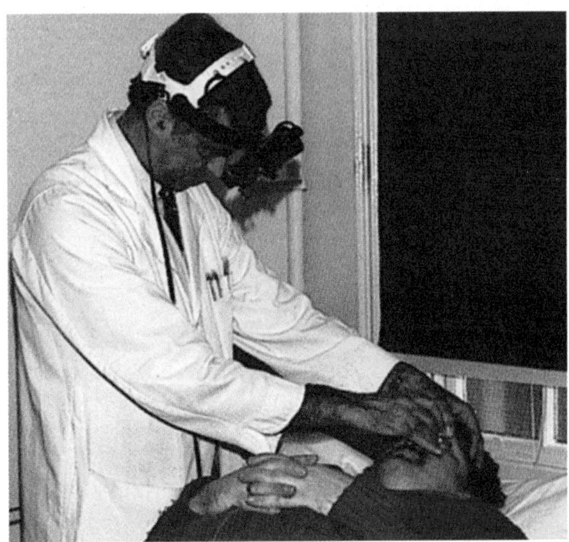

Figure 57-13 Indirect method of ophthalmoscopic examination.

(Goldmann) is more accurate in estimating intraocular pressure and is frequently attached to the slit-lamp (Figure 57-15). Instead of indenting the eye, a small area of the cornea is flattened to counterbalance a spring-loaded measuring device, and the pressure is measured directly.

A relatively new tonometer, the Tono-Pen (Figure 57-16) is widely replacing the Schiøtz in the Western World. The instrument is handheld in a perpendicular position to the cornea. Gentle tapping over the central cornea enables several readings to be taken and averaged. A digital LED screen displays the final reading.

Assessment measures and variations in normal findings relevant to the care of older adults are presented in the Gerontologic Assessment box. Also identified are disorders common in older adults, which may be responsible for abnormal assessment findings.

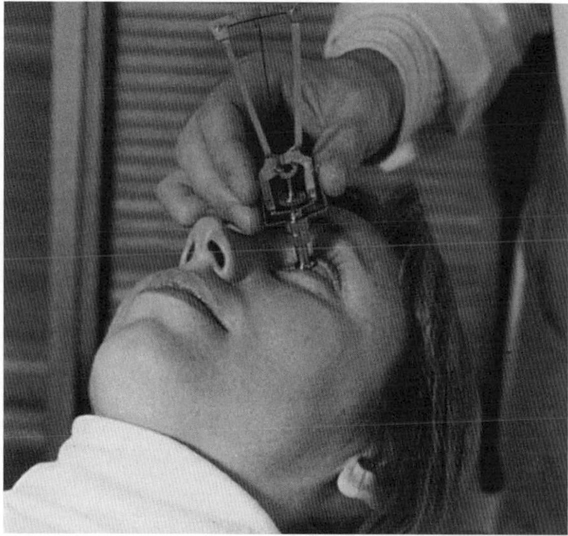

Figure 57-14 Measurement of intraocular pressure with Schiøtz tonometer.

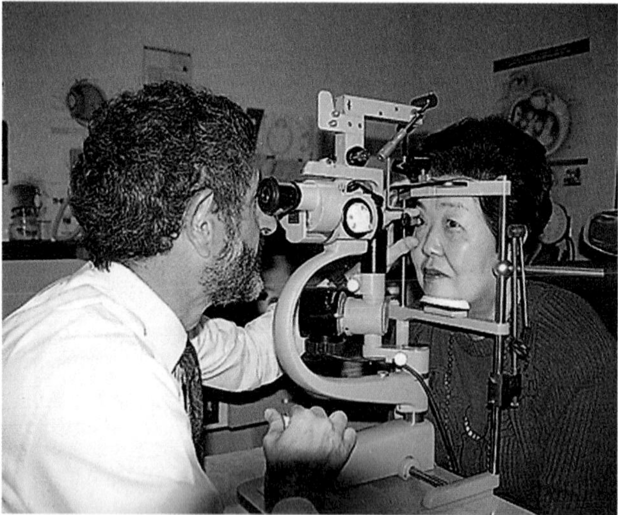

Figure 57-15 Measurement of intraocular pressure with applanation tonometer.

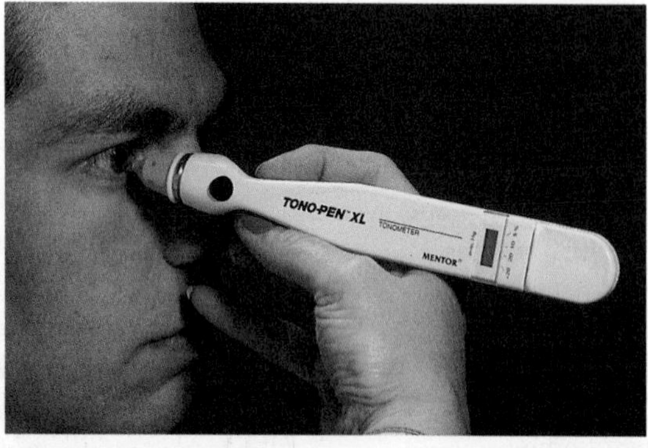

Figure 57-16 Tono-Pen tonometer.

Gerontologic Assessment

Inspect the general appearance of the face and eyes.
- Loss of orbital fat and decreased muscle tone may cause the eyes to sink into the orbit.

Examine the upper and lower eyelids.
- Loss of elasticity creates wrinkles and folds; redundant lid tissue is called dermatochalasis.
- Muscle relaxation may impair the ability to look up.

Examine the cornea.
- Irritation and scratchy and itchy sensations may result from decreased tear production.
- Fat deposits may create a hazy gray ring around the periphery (arcus senilis).
- Corneal dystrophy creates clouding of the central cornea.

Examine the size of the pupil.
- Pupillary size typically decreases with age.

Examine the lens.
- Yellow discoloration may be present, which can progress to cataract formation.

Examine the retina with an ophthalmoscope.
- The effects of diabetes, hypertension, and macular degeneration are often evident in hemorrhages, exudates, and abnormal areas of pigmentation.

Perform vision screening.
- Normal aging is associated with refractory changes, senile miosis, and decreased visual acuity.

Explore the impact of any change in vision or color perception on the patient's ability to perform activities of daily living and engage in desired pursuits.

COMMON DISORDERS IN ELDERS

Corneal dystrophy
Glaucoma
Cataract
Diabetic retinopathy
Macular degeneration/macular hole

DIAGNOSTIC TESTS

Laboratory Tests

Neither blood nor urine tests play a significant role in the evaluation of problems related to the eye, although they are used extensively to evaluate other systemic disorders such as diabetes that may be causing visual symptoms.

Radiologic Tests

Several radiologic procedures are used to aid in the diagnosis of eye conditions. These include plain x-ray films, computed tomography (CT) scans, and magnetic resonance imaging (MRI).

Plain X-Ray Films

Plain x-ray films of the orbit are used to assist in the diagnosis of orbital fractures and tumors. Right and left oblique views and a lateral view of the affected side usually provide the needed information.

Computed Tomography Scan

The CT scan is a rapid, safe, and noninvasive technique for the investigation of serial sections of the orbit and eye. The globe, lens, vitreous humor, optic nerve, extraocular muscles, visual pathway, and brain can all be evaluated. The CT scan is valuable in the diagnosis of orbital disease, retrobulbar tumors, intraocular eye masses, and intracranial disease and can be augmented by the injection of contrast material that increases the density of inflammatory or vascular lesions.[11] The nurse's primary responsibilities relate to careful pretest patient teaching.

Magnetic Resonance Imaging

MRI is a noninvasive technique that uses a high magnetic field to evaluate the brain, orbit, and eye. MRI provides better definition of tissues and fluids in the brain and eye than can be achieved with a CT scan. It is particularly helpful in identifying edema.[13] The nurse explains the procedure and carefully prepares the patient for the noises and sensations experienced during the test.

Special Tests

Ultrasonography

Ultrasonography is a noninvasive test that uses high-frequency sound waves to outline and detect intraocular and orbital structures and measure the distance between them.[10] Various abnormalities, such as retinal masses and detachments, intraocular foreign bodies, and changes in the orbit, can be easily delineated by this test. Two types of ultrasonography, A-scan and B-scan, are used in ophthalmology. The A-scan is useful in differentiating between benign and malignant tumors and measuring the axial length of the eyeball, a value that is needed to calculate the power of an intraocular lens for implantation after a cataract extraction. The B-scan provides a two-dimensional image that helps visualize tumors, retinal detachments, swollen muscles, or inflamed tissue. In both scans, a probe is placed on the front of the eye (or on the closed eyelid), sound waves are delivered, and measurements are recorded on the screen of the oscilloscope. The test is not uncomfortable although anesthetic drops may be instilled if the probe is applied directly to the eye. The nurse gives the patient information about the procedure itself and any sensory effects.

Fluorescein Angiography

Fluorescein angiography is a specialized procedure used in the diagnosis, monitoring, and treatment of eye diseases. After the pupil is dilated, fluorescein dye is injected into a vein in the antecubital fossa of the patient's arm. The retinal and ciliary arteries transmit the dye into the eyes, and the retinal arteriovenous circulation is visualized. The dye reaches the retinal arteries 10 to 16 seconds after the injection, and the veins are filled within 25 seconds. To provide a permanent record of this circulation, photographs are taken with a specially designed camera called a fundus camera. The camera is equipped with an optical system for viewing the retina and a light flash system for illumination and is mounted on a stand similar to that for a slit-lamp. The patient sits in a chair with the chin placed in the chin rest and the forehead against a bar while a rapid series of photographs are taken to capture the movement of the dye through the retinal arteriovenous circulation. This test may take as long as 1 hour to complete. When the photographs are assessed, they provide definitive information about any avascular obstruction, the growth of new vessels (neovascularization), microaneurysms, abnormal capillary permeability, and defects in the pigmented layer of the retina.

Fluorescein angiography is a relatively safe procedure with few untoward effects. The patient is assessed for any allergies or previous reaction to dye. Those with a history of hay fever or asthma may be given a small test dose before the entire dose is injected.[1] Although rare, a severe allergic reaction can occur.

The nurse explains the procedure, obtains an informed consent, and explains the need to keep the head still during the test. The nurse warns the patient that a dazzle effect may occur from the frequent camera flashes. Mydriatic eye drops are instilled to dilate the pupils, facilitating visualization of the fundus. Some patients experience transient nausea or vomiting as the dye is injected.

Patients are informed that it may require several minutes for the dazzle effect to resolve after the test. The nurse also informs the patient that yellowing of the skin, especially in persons with fair complexions, and a fluorescent orange or green discoloration of the urine usually is present for 24 hours. Patients are encouraged to drink increased amounts of fluids to promote excretion of the dye. The pupils remain dilated for a few hours, and the patient should avoid bright light and wear sunglasses when outdoors until the pupils return to normal.

Electrophysiology Examinations

There are four electrophysiology examinations performed in ophthalmology: electroretinogram (ERG), electrooculogram (EOG), dark adaptometry, and visual-evoked potential (VEP). The main purpose of these examinations is to assess the function of the visual pathway from the photoreceptors of the retina to the visual cortex of the brain. Electrophysiologic testing is useful in diagnosing retinal vascular occlusions, toxic drug exposure, inherited retinal diseases, and intraocular foreign bodies.[4]

Electroretinogram. ERG is a process of graphing the electrical response from the retina that occurs as a consequence of light stimulation. In this test the pupil is dilated, a topical anesthetic is applied, and a corneal electrode is placed on the cornea using a contact lens. A grounding electrode is placed on the ear. Lights at various intensities and intervals are then flashed and the nervous response graphed.

ERG tests the function of the rods and cones and is helpful in evaluating widespread retinal disease such as retinitis pigmentosa. The visual potential of an eye that has a dense cataract or other opacification also can be assessed with ERG. However, normal results do not rule out the presence of macular or optic nerve disease. The patient is told the nature of the test and the steps of the procedure. A demonstration of the flashing lights often is helpful. The test does not require any special follow-up care.

Electrooculogram. EOG measures the difference in the electrical potential between the front and back of the eye (retina) in response to periods of dark and light. The preparation of the patient requires that skin electrodes be placed on the lateral and medial canthi of both eyes. Corneal contact lenses are not required.

Dark Adaptometry. Dark adaptometry measures the universal phenomenon of dark adaptation. Normally, when a person is placed in a room and the lights are suddenly turned out, the eyes gradually become more sensitive and vision in the darkness improves over time. For this test, the patient is placed in a totally darkened room with a dark adaptometer machine. The patient is then exposed to a standardized level of light for a specified period of time. The light is gradually dimmed until total darkness is restored. Patients respond to the various intensities of light to which they are exposed by pushing a button on the machine.

Visual-Evoked Potential. VEP is a measurement of visual function monitored at the level of the occipital cortex with scalp electrodes that evaluate the integrity of the visual pathways from the optic nerve to the occipital cortex. Stimulation of the retina with light changes the electrical activity of the cortex. Through various computer processes, the electrical activity associated with this stimulation of the retina is summed and shown as a measurable electrical wave. Optic neuritis, demyelinating disease, and optic atrophy can alter this wave. For these electrophysiologic tests, the nurse explains the procedures, indicating that they are pain free and require no special follow-up care.

References

1. Anand R: Fluorescein angiography. I. Technique and normal study, *J Ophthalmol Nurs Technol* 8:48, 1989.
2. Bickley LS et al: *Bates' guide to physical examination and history taking,* ed 7, Philadelphia, 1999, Lippincott, Williams & Wilkins.
3. Ebersole P, Hess P: *Toward healthy aging: human needs and nursing response,* ed 5, St Louis, 1998, Mosby.
4. Follmer BA, Smith SC: Electrophysiology testing and the ophthalmic registered nurse, *Insight* 19(4):12, 1994.
5. Hunt L: Ophthalmic nursing assessment, *Insight* 17(3):9, 1992.
6. Elfervig LS: Normal aging eye, *Insight* 22(4):125, 1997.
7. Leasia S, Monahan FD: *A practical guide to health assessment,* ed 2, Philadelphia, 2002, WB Saunders.
8. Smith SC: Aging, physiology and vision, *Nurse Pract Forum* 9(1):19, 1998.
9. Kelly JS: Visual impairment among older people, *Br J Nurs* 2(2):110, 1993.
10. Mrochuk J: Introduction to diagnostic ophthalmic ultrasound for nurses in ophthalmology, *J Ophthalmol Nurs Technol* 9:234, 1990.
11. Newell F: *Ophthalmology: principles and concepts,* ed 8, St Louis, 1996, Mosby.
12. West S: Ultraviolet B exposure and lens opacities: a review, *J Epidemiol* 9(suppl 6):97, 1999.
13. Wirtschafter JD, Berman EL, McDonald CS: *Magnetic resonance imaging and computed tomography: clinical neuro-orbital anatomy,* San Francisco, 1992, American Academy of Ophthalmology.

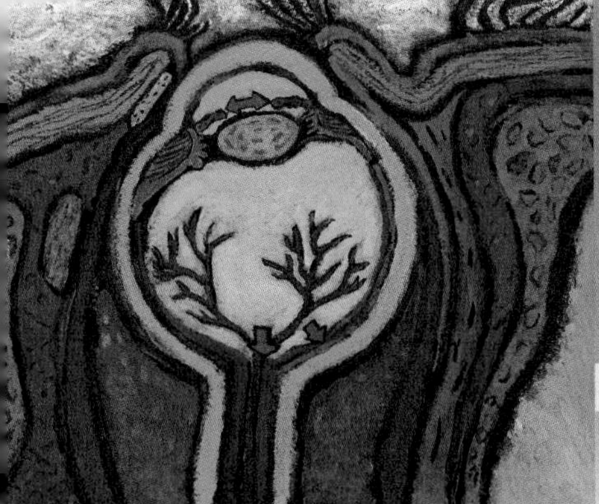

Problems of the Eye 58

Sarah C. Smith

Objectives

After studying this chapter, the learner should be able to:

1. Discuss the etiology and management of common forms of visual impairment.
2. Compare the pathophysiology of common eye inflammations and infections.
3. Describe the emergency treatment of eye injury.
4. Discuss the collaborative management of glaucoma.
5. Compare the preoperative and postoperative care of patients undergoing surgery for cataracts and retinal detachment.
6. Outline the effects of diabetes, hypertension, and human immunodeficiency virus (HIV) infection on the eye.

Eye disease and blindness affect millions of people throughout the world. In the United States nearly 11.5 million persons have some degree of visual impairment, and approximately 1.5 million persons do not have useful vision in one or both eyes. This chapter discusses the major causes of visual impairment, common eye infections and injuries, and the management of major eye disorders such as glaucoma and cataracts. The nurse plays a significant role in the collaborative care of patients experiencing eye disorders and also has an important role in educating the general public about primary and secondary prevention strategies to maintain eye health.

VISUAL IMPAIRMENT

Etiology/Epidemiology

Visual impairment ranges in severity from diminished visual acuity to total blindness. Legal blindness is defined in the United States as (1) a visual acuity, with maximal correction, of 20/200 or less and/or (2) a visual field reduction to a range of 20 degrees (compared with a normal range of about 180 degrees). This is an arbitrary definition that was established early in the century to identify individuals who would need public assistance to function in society. The definition is not accepted or used worldwide.

An estimated 1 million persons in the United States are legally blind, and most of these persons are older than 65 years of age. Almost 80 million Americans have a disorder of one or both eyes, and this figure does not include the additional millions of persons with straightforward refractive errors who require the use of corrective lenses to participate fully in daily activities. These figures make visual impairment one of the most common disorders affecting adults in this country. Uncorrected vision problems have a negative impact on school and work performance and contribute to injury. Loss of vision limits the individual's interaction with the environment and reduces the range and variety of experiences available. Personal care, home maintenance, social interaction, and interpersonal communication are all affected.

Visual impairment has numerous causes, and preventable blindness is a major worldwide health problem. Refractive errors are by far the most common problem, but numerous other nutritional, infectious, metabolic, and systemic disorders adversely affect the function of the eye. Nutritional deficiencies are a major global health concern. A lack of adequate vitamin A and B complex can cause changes within the retina, cornea, and conjunctiva. Night blindness is a classic outcome of vitamin A deficiency, and optic neuritis can result from deficits of vitamin B, especially in persons with alcoholism. Infection (e.g., trachoma) is another common cause of visual impairment and causes blindness in millions of persons in developing countries. Macular degeneration, a disease of the aging retina, is the leading cause of blindness in older adults.[2] Twenty to thirty percent of persons between 75 and 85 years of age are affected. The leading causes of visual impairment/blindness in the United States include glaucoma, cataracts, diabetic retinopathy, and macular degeneration.

The eye can also be adversely affected by a variety of systemic diseases (Table 58-1). The exophthalmos associated with Graves' disease is one of the most visible examples, and visual field problems are common outcomes of cerebrovascular accidents. The demyelination associated with multiple sclerosis also commonly affects the eye. Retinopathy is a complication of vascular disease, particularly uncontrolled hypertension, and is often both progressive and irreversible. Cytomegalovirus retinopathy has become a serious complication associated with

TABLE 58-1 Eye Manifestations of Systemic Diseases

Disorder	Effect on the Eyes
Vascular Disorders	
Hypertension	Persistent uncontrolled hypertension can cause hemorrhage, edema, and exudates in retina. Retinal arteries narrow, causing degenerative changes.
Cerebrovascular accident	Depending on location of stroke, patient may experience hemianopsia or blindness.
Sickle cell disease	This can cause neovascularization, arterial occlusions, or retinal hemorrhage.
Neurologic Disorders	
Multiple sclerosis	Demyelination can result in optic neuritis, diplopia, and nystagmus.
Endocrine Disorders	
Graves' disease	Accumulation of fat and fluid in the retroocular tissue can produce exophthalmos (protrusion of eye) and lid retraction.
Diabetic retinopathy	Retinal capillary walls thicken and develop microaneurysms. Retinal veins widen and become tortuous (Figure 58-1). Small hemorrhages occur, which leave scars that decrease vision. As disease worsens, neovascularization occurs, and new vessels grow into vitreous humor. These vessels are vulnerable to both obstruction and rupture. Vision decreases, and "floaters" are perceived in eye.
Connective Tissue Disorders	
Rheumatoid arthritis, systemic lupus erythematosus	Neovascularization, inflammation of cornea, sclera, or uveal tract occur.
AIDS-Related Disorders	
Herpes zoster ophthalmicus	Herpes can invade the cornea and create ulceration that is potentially blinding.
Cytomegalovirus (CMV)	CMV affects an estimated 20% of AIDS patients. It spreads rapidly through cells of the retina and blood vessels and can totally destroy the retina (Figure 58-2).
Kaposi's sarcoma	Lesions of Kaposi's sarcoma can affect skin of eyelids and conjunctiva or orbit itself.

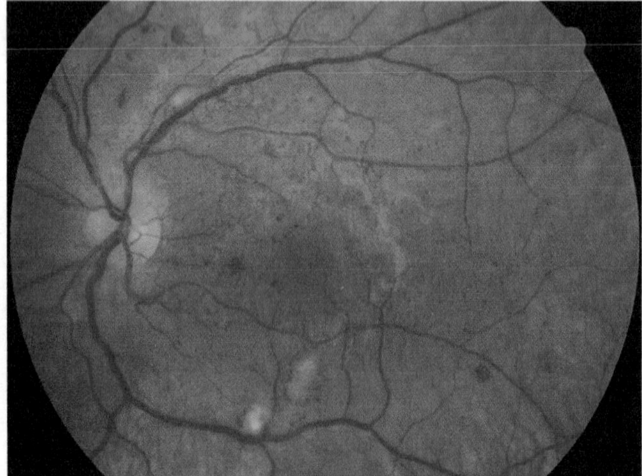

Figure 58-1 Diabetic retinopathy with cotton wool spots (exudates) below macula.

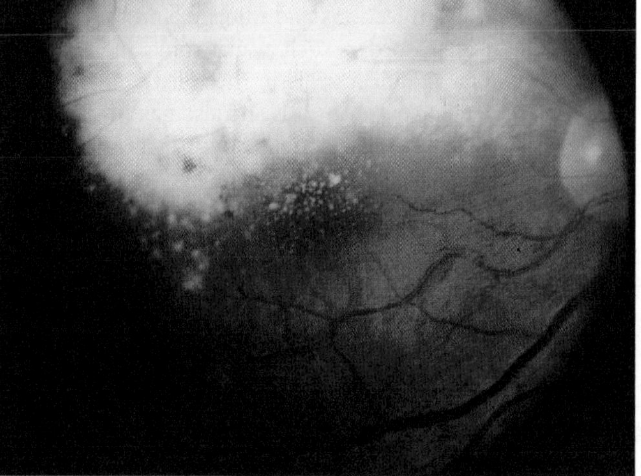

Figure 58-2 Cytomegalovirus retinitis infiltrating superior retina.

the severe immunocompromise of acquired immunodeficiency syndrome (AIDS). Diabetic retinopathy, despite laser treatment, which is effective in its early stages, commonly results in a steady progression toward blindness in diabetic patients with uncontrolled or brittle disease (see Chapter 30).

Pathophysiology

Refractive Disorders. Refractive disorders include irregularities of the corneal curvature, length, and shape of the eye, as well as the focusing ability of the lens. There are three main types of refractive disorders (Figure 58-3). The major symptoms of all three disorders include blurred vision and headache.

Myopia, or nearsightedness, occurs when parallel rays of light focus in front of the retina as the person looks at a distant object. Hyperopia, or farsightedness, occurs when light rays focus in back of the retina as the individual looks at a near object. A shortened eyeball may contribute to the problem.

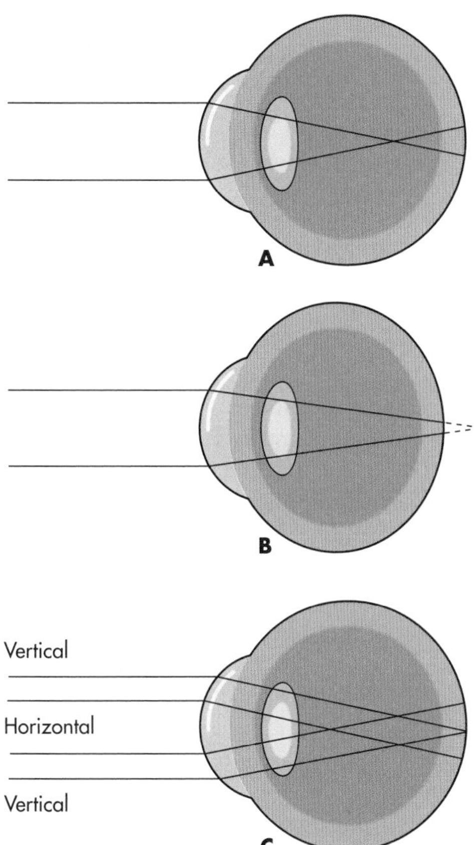

Figure 58-3 Three types of refractive errors. **A**, Myopic eye. Parallel rays of light are brought to a focus in front of the retina. **B**, Hyperopic eye. Parallel rays of light come to a focus behind the retina in the unaccommodative eye. **C**, Simple myopic astigmatism. The vertical bundle of rays is focused on the retina; the horizontal rays are focused in front of the retina.

Astigmatism is caused by an unequal curvature of the cornea. Light rays are bent unevenly and do not focus on a single spot on the retina. Presbyopia is a common problem associated with aging. The lens loses elasticity, making it more difficult to focus on near objects.

Macular Degeneration. Degenerative changes occur in the thin layer of blood vessels that arise in the retina and extend into the choroid and their membrane cover. Both neovascular (exudative or wet) and nonneovascular (nonexudative or dry) forms occur. In neovascular degeneration there is a sudden proliferation of new, fragile blood vessels in the macular area that tend to leak and damage the macula. Scarring occurs, and functional losses progress rapidly. The neovascular form of macular degeneration occurs in only 5% to 10% of all patients, but it is responsible for about 80% of the severe loss of vision attributed to the disease. The nonneovascular form of macular degeneration is more common. Degeneration occurs from the deposit of waste products and slow atrophy of the choroid, retina, and pigment epithelium.

Macular degeneration causes a variety of symptoms, including visual blurring and distortion, and usually causes some degree of central vision loss and a decreased ability to distinguish colors. Early signs and progression of the disease can be readily detected with the use of the Amsler grid (see Chapter 57). The individual perceives dark spots, missing areas, and distorted wavy lines. Intravenous fluorescein angiography may be used to visualize or confirm the extent of neovascularization if vessel leakage is suspected.

Collaborative Care Management

Corrective Lenses. Visual impairments caused by refractive errors are usually diagnosed as part of a routine eye examination. The person may initiate the diagnostic process in response to chronic headache or an awareness of blurred or failing vision. Eyeglasses and contact lenses are widely used to correct common refractive errors and restore visual acuity. Federal law requires that all prescription glasses be made with impact-resistant lenses. Plastic lenses are lightweight but scratch easily. Hardened and safety lenses have been tempered to make them extremely resistant to breakage.

Contact lenses are made of various types of thin plastic that fit over the cornea. Their popularity is primarily cosmetic, but some people do achieve better vision correction with contact lenses than with glasses.

Contact lenses may be rigid or soft. In addition to standard hard and soft lenses, the rigid category includes gas permeable lenses, and the soft category includes extended-wear and disposable lenses. Rigid (hard) lenses are easy to care for, are relatively inexpensive, and correct vision efficiently. However, rigid lenses that are not gas permeable are generally uncomfortable and require a prolonged period of adaptation. Wearing time generally does not exceed 12 hours. Gas-permeable lenses have the optical quality of other hard lenses but are permeable to oxygen and other gases and are generally more comfortable for the wearer.

Soft lenses are very flexible and can often be used successfully by persons who cannot tolerate hard lenses. They are higher in cost and require frequent replacement. Extended-wear soft contact lenses can be left in place for as long as a month, but their use is generally limited to 1 week, at which time they are removed for cleaning and disinfection.

Disposable soft contact lenses are similar to standard soft contact lenses, but they can be inexpensively manufactured and are discarded after 1 week, thus eliminating cleaning and disinfecting. There is concern that use of any extended-wear contact lens increases the risk of ulcerative keratitis (inflammation of the cornea). Extended-wear contact lens users were found to have a 10 to 15 times higher risk of developing ulcerative keratitis than wearers who removed and cleaned their lenses every day.

All contact lenses can cause problems, and careful attention to recommended regimens for cleaning and disinfection are important for the overall success of the wearer.

Refractive Surgery. Refractive surgery, defined as any operative procedure performed for the purpose of eliminating a refraction error, has become an increasingly viable alternative to glasses and contact lenses for persons with visual impairment related to refraction errors. The most common procedure (Figure 58-4), photorefractive keratotomy, uses an excimer laser to reshape the surface of the cornea and has become increasingly

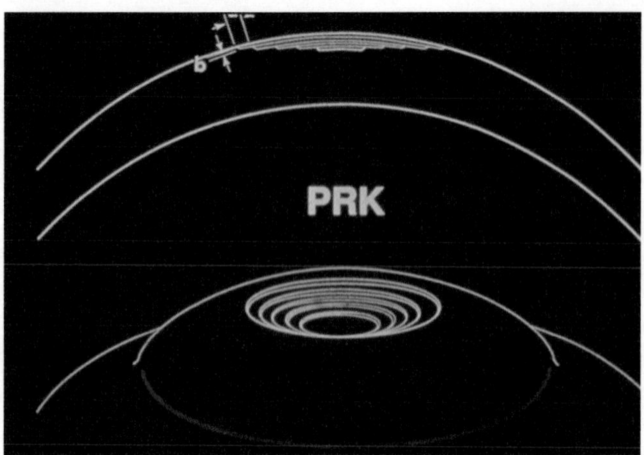

Figure 58-4 Photorefractive keratectomy showing raised flap of corneal epithelium with stromal layer to be ablated with eximer laser.

popular. Thin sections of outer cornea can also be removed to correct higher degrees of myopia. Recent advances have added the ability to correct hyperopia and the age-related condition, presbyopia. The most recent innovation in refractive procedures is the implantation of two semicircular plastic rings called Intacs. Intacs are placed within the layers of the cornea but do not involve the optical center. They may be removed, if necessary, which reverses the effect. They are currently available only to treat low levels of nearsightedness (myopia). All of these procedures are performed in ambulatory surgery centers. Careful preoperative teaching about the goals and limitations of the surgery, as well as the expected postoperative course, is essential. Patients are permitted to gradually resume activities and usually experience a slow improvement of vision over a period of weeks or months. The nurse administers analgesics as needed to keep the patient comfortable and administers antibiotics to decrease the incidence of infection.

Macular Degeneration. There is no adequate treatment currently available for the nonneovascular (dry) form of macular degeneration. A small percentage of patients with neovascular (wet) degeneration may benefit from laser therapy to coagulate the abnormal vessels, or from photodynamic therapy (PDT) with intravenously injected verteporfin (Visudyne). PDT uses low-level laser light to activate the drug within the abnormal blood vessels, rendering them inactive and subsequently temporarily stabilizing central vision. Patients usually require multiple treatments spaced at least 90 days apart to obtain the desired result. Vision is not improved with either type of laser intervention; however, additional loss of central vision is often spared. The Age-Related Eye Disease Study and the Carotenoids and Age-Related Eye Disease Study are two randomized, multicenter clinical trials funded by the National Eye Institute that are looking at variables related to age and diet, specifically the effects of carotenoids and their possible effects of reducing and/or preventing Age-Related Macular Degeneration.[1]

Patient/Family Education. Some forms of visual impairment are preventable, and most forms can be slowed or treated with early diagnosis and appropriate therapy. Regular eye examinations by a competent professional are an important health promotion measure throughout life, especially as a person ages. Early identification of eye disorders such as glaucoma is essential to prevent loss of vision. Appropriate intervention for cataracts can restore useful vision, and the rigorous control of systemic diseases such as diabetes and hypertension can minimize the adverse visual consequences.

Multiple opportunities exist for education and intervention with patients and families regarding preserving visual function and promoting eye health. The importance of this area is reflected in the Healthy People 2010 goals, one goal of which is to improve the visual health of the nation through prevention, early detection, treatment, and rehabilitation.[9]

Maintaining eye health is an important teaching intervention for all patients, not just those experiencing eye problems. The eye is a remarkably resilient organ. It cleans itself through the constant production and excretion of tears and the secretions from the conjunctivae, which also are protective. As a consequence, normal healthy eyes do not need special care or cleaning. Care should be taken not to irritate the eyes or introduce bacteria into the eyes by rubbing them.

Adequate nutrition is as important for eye health as it is for maintaining other body functions. Vitamin deficiencies can cause night blindness (vitamin A), corneal damage (vitamin A), optic neuritis (vitamin B), and other disorders. Although a sufficient vitamin intake is necessary, an excessive amount is wasted and may actually do more harm than good.

It is difficult to predict the course of any progressive visual impairment, and patients rightly fear becoming blind. The nurse ensures that the patient has accurate information about the specific disease, type of vision loss, and prognosis. Opportunities to express fears and frustrations related to declining vision can be helpful to the patient and family. Social support is a key factor in the adjustment of patients to visual impairment. The nurse can also provide referrals for the patient to the numerous community agencies that provide services and support to visually impaired persons as they attempt to incorporate their changing vision status into their daily lives. Integration of declining vision or blindness into one's self-concept can take a long time. A social stigma related to blindness still exists, and patients need ongoing support and understanding.

Visual impairment requires a major life adjustment. Persons need to adjust to both the initial impact of the loss and the subsequent changes that will occur in their life because of the loss of vision. Over time most patients learn new ways or adapt their present ways of doing things to carry out their normal activities. Most recognize that there are some things that they will never be able to do again or that they can do only with help.

The nurse ensures that the patient has any and all visual aids that may be useful to him or her, including magnifying glasses and high-intensity reading lights. Patients with progressive macular degeneration need to learn how to optimize their peripheral vision as their central vision deteriorates.

Adjustment is an ongoing process, and time is a key variable. Time is needed to grieve for the lost sight and to recognize and come to terms with the implications of the loss. Time is also needed to master many of the difficult tasks and the work associated with adjustment to a visual impairment.

The dependence on others and the need to ask for help are two of the most difficult things to which these persons must

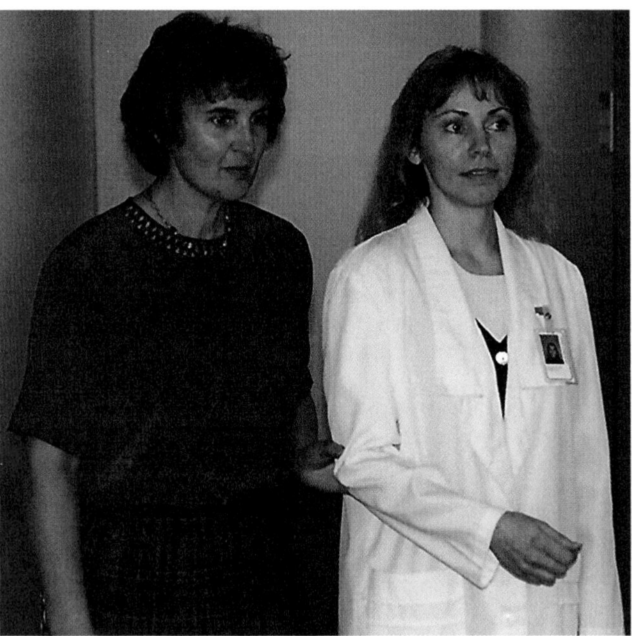

Figure 58-5 Helping a visually impaired person to ambulate. Note that the woman is holding the nurse's arm and is led without being held.

Guidelines for Safe Practice

Facilitating Independence in Activities of Daily Living for Visually Impaired Patients

1. Place clothing in specific and consistent locations in drawers and closets.
2. Place food and cooking utensils in specific and consistent locations in cupboards and/or the refrigerator.
3. Encourage use of a cane when walking.
4. Keep furniture and household objects in specific and consistent places.
5. When walking with a blind person, let the person take your arm (see Figure 58-5).
6. Provide descriptions of food on the plate using clock placement of food; for example, put the peas at "7 o'clock." Cut food as appropriate.
7. Always permit blind persons to pull out their own chairs and seat themselves.

adjust. Fluctuating vision leads to frustration and difficulties in planning or implementing tasks.

Figure 58-5 and the Guidelines for Safe Practice boxes provide useful strategies for assisting the visually impaired person.

INFECTIONS AND INFLAMMATION

Infections and inflammation can occur in any of the eye structures and may be caused by microorganisms, mechanical irritation, or sensitivity to some substance. Inflammation of the eye is the most common acute condition affecting the eye. Conjunctivitis represents about two thirds of the total cases of inflammation. Table 58-2 summarizes the common eye infections/inflammations and their management. Conjunctivitis is discussed in the following section. Box 58-1 summarizes ophthalmic drugs used to treat inflammation and infection.

Guidelines for Safe Practice

Communicating With the Visually Impaired Patient

1. Talk in a normal tone of voice.
2. Do *not* try to avoid common phrases in speech, such as "See what I mean?"
3. Introduce yourself with each contact (unless well known to the patient). If in a hospital, knock on the door before entering.
4. Explain any activity occurring in the room or what you will be doing.
5. Announce when you are leaving the room so that the patient is not put in the position of talking to someone who is no longer there.

Conjunctivitis

Etiology/Epidemiology

Conjunctivitis (inflammation of the conjunctiva) is a common infection that can occur from a variety of causes. It may result from mechanical trauma, sunburn, or infection with organisms such as staphylococci, streptococci, or *Haemophilus influenzae.* Two sexually transmitted agents that cause conjunctivitis are *Chlamydia trachomatis* and *Neisseria gonorrhoeae.* Inflammation is often caused by allergic reactions within the body or by external irritants (e.g., poison ivy or cosmetics). Viral agents that cause conjunctivitis include most human adenovirus strains and the herpes simplex viruses.

Acute mucopurulent bacterial conjunctivitis (often called pinkeye) is the most common form of conjunctivitis. It is prevalent in school-age children but can occur at any age. It is highly infectious, especially in crowded environments such as schools and nursing homes. It is usually self-limited and causes no permanent damage.

Pathophysiology

The symptoms of conjunctivitis vary in severity. Hyperemia and burning are common initial symptoms that progress rapidly to a mucopurulent exudate, which crusts on the base of the eyelashes and is easily transferred to the uninfected eye. Viral infections produce minimal exudate. The conjunctivae are grossly reddened and inflamed. Invasion of the cornea can result in ulceration and even perforation, usually in response to virulent organisms such as *N. gonorrhoeae.* Involvement of the cornea, although rare, is extremely serious and can even result in loss of the eye. The corneal ulcer is usually identified on slit-lamp examination and may be outlined with the use of sterile fluorescein dye.

Collaborative Care Management

Treatment of conjunctivitis includes careful cleansing of the eyelids and lashes and the use of topical antibiotics. Warm, moist compresses may be used to gently remove firm, adherent crusts from the eyes, especially in the morning. The procedure for applying warm compresses is outlined in the Guidelines for Safe Practice box. Because the drainage material is infectious, it should be disposed of carefully.

Common ophthalmic antibiotics include polymixin B, bacitracin, and gentamicin in ointment or eyedrop form (see

TABLE 58-2 Eye Infection/Inflammation

Disorder	Description	Collaborative Management
Hordeolum (stye)	Common infection of small glands of lid margins, caused by staphylococcus; creates a tender, swollen pustule that gradually resolves or ruptures	Application of warm compresses three to four times per day; antibiotic ointment if severe; incision of pustule if it does not resolve spontaneously
Chalazion	Sterile cyst located in connective tissue in free edges of eyelid; lump is small, hard, and nontender, but may put pressure on eye and affect vision	May disappear spontaneously, become infected, or require local excision if impairing vision
Trachoma	Chronic infectious form of conjunctivitis believed to be caused by *Chlamydia trachomatis;* common in Africa and Asia; one of leading causes of blindness worldwide	Can be effectively treated early in disease with antibiotics; hard to eradicate once chronic
Keratitis	Inflammation of cornea; can be superficial or deep, acute or chronic; *Staphylococcus* and *Streptococcus* bacteria and herpes simplex viruses are common causes; pain, photophobia, and blepharospasm are common; can result in loss of vision	Steroids to control inflammation; antibiotics; cycloplegics to rest the eye; corneal transplant may be necessary
Uveitis	Acute inflammation of uvea from infection, allergy, toxic agents, and systemic disorders; causes eye pain, swelling, photophobia, and visual impairment	May be self-limiting; treatment of underlying cause plus cycloplegics to rest the eye; warm, moist compresses to reduce inflammation and increase comfort
Blepharitis	Inflammation of eyelids; often begins in childhood and recurs, causing redness and scaling of upper and lower lid at lash borders	Daily facial cleansing and shampoo to remove scales; local antibiotics may be helpful
Corneal ulcer	Infection of cornea is not common, but can readily lead to ulceration; ulcers typically cause pain, tearing, and spasms of eyelid; grayish white corneal opacity seen with fluorescein evaluation	Minor abrasions heal spontaneously and without scarring; comfort measures are critical, since pain can be severe; possible need for antibiotics and corticosteroids

BOX 58-1 Ophthalmic Drugs Used to Treat Infection/Inflammation

Antibiotics and Antiviral Drugs

Polymyxin B, bacitracin (Polysporin)
Polymyxin B, neomycin, bacitracin (Neosporin)
Bacitracin
Gentamicin, chloramphenicol, ciprofloxacin hydrochloride, erythromycin, norfloxacin, ofloxacin, tobramycin
Idoxuridine (IDU)

Steroids

Prednisone
Prednisolone acetate
Methylprednisolone (Depo-Medrol)
Triamcinolone (Aristocort)
Dexamethasone (Decadron, Maxidex)
Fluorometholone (FML)

Cycloplegic and Mydriatic Action

Atropine sulfate (Atropisol, Isopto Atropine)
Cyclopentolate hydrochloride (Cyclogyl)
Homatropine hydrobromide (Isopto Homatropine)
Scopolamine hydrobromide (Isopto Hyoscine)
Tropicamide (Mydriacyl)

Box 58-1). Ophthalmic ointments remain in contact with the eye much longer, providing a prolonged effect. There is also less absorption into the lacrimal passages than with eyedrops. Eye ointments can, however. produce a film in front of the eye that may blur vision.

Guidelines for Safe Practice

Applying Warm, Moist Compresses

1. Use sterile technique when infection or ulceration is present; clean technique may be used for allergic reactions.
2. Use separate equipment for bilateral eye infections.
3. Wash hands before treating each eye.
4. The temperature of the compress should not exceed 49° C (120° F).
5. Change compresses frequently—every 5 minutes or as ordered. Always wash hands first.
6. Do not exert pressure on the eyeball.
7. Sterile petrolatum may be used on the skin around the eyes, if desired, to protect the skin.
8. If sterility is not required, moist heat may be applied by means of a clean facecloth.

Patient/Family Education. The nurse teaches the patient about the disease and its treatment. The infectiousness of the disorder is emphasized, and the patient is encouraged to avoid crowded environments and to keep the hands away from the face. Frequent hand washing is critical, especially before and after the use of warm compresses or the instillation of eye medications.

The nurse instructs the patient about how to correctly instill the ophthalmic ointment. The procedure is similar to that used for eyedrops. The ointment is gently placed directly onto the exposed conjunctiva from the inner to the outer canthus, being careful to avoid the eyelashes or any part of the eye that would

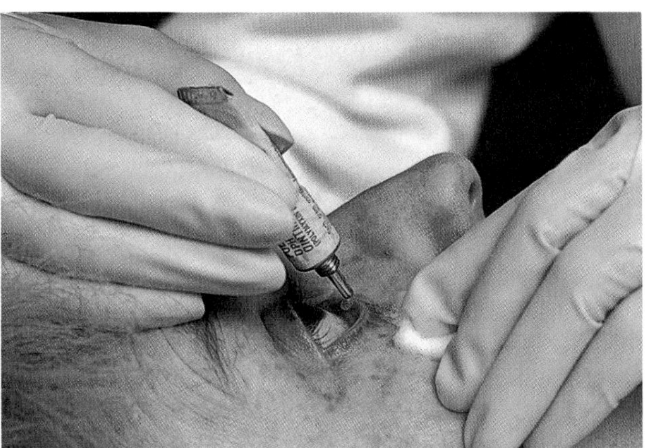

Figure 58-6 Ophthalmic ointment is squeezed onto the conjunctiva of the lower lid.

contaminate the tip of the tube (Figure 58-6). The nurse warns the patient about the possible blurring of vision. If both eyedrops and ointments are to be used, the ointment is applied last. Treatment at bedtime minimizes the adverse effects of blurred vision caused by the instillation of the ointment.

EYE TRAUMA AND INJURY

Etiology/Epidemiology

Each year in the United States, 2 to 3 million persons sustain an injury to their eyes. Of these, 4000 will have permanent blindness as a result. Most of these injuries are considered preventable.

The two major categories of injury are burns and mechanical trauma. Chemical burns can occur in the home, school, and industrial setting and may involve either an acid or an alkali substance. Prompt treatment is essential to prevent permanent eye damage. Ultraviolet burns are also a concern and may occur from excess sun exposure (skiing, outdoor work, or sunbathing) or the use of heat lamps and tanning beds. Thermal burns are less common but may destroy the eyelids and necessitate skin grafting.

Mechanical trauma can include lacerations of the eyelids, as well as direct injury to the eye itself. Contusions can cause bleeding into the anterior chamber (hyphema). Corneal injuries present unique problems because they are extremely painful and resistance to infection is low. Scarring on the cornea can impair vision. Foreign bodies on the surface of the cornea are estimated to account for about 25% of all eye injuries.

Pathophysiology

Although the eye is vulnerable to trauma, its natural protective mechanisms both prevent and minimize minor eye injury. The heavy orbital bone protects the eye from most blunt mechanical injuries. The eye's natural lubricating system is augmented by tears to help flush away chemicals and other foreign bodies, and the blink reflex protects the eye from most low-impact forces.

Acid causes coagulation in the cornea, which, although it produces significant local trauma, actually prevents the substance from penetrating and damaging the deeper structures of the eye. Alkaline substances, however, penetrate the corneal epithelium and release proteases and collagenases that can cause corneal necrosis and perforation.

Penetrating injuries or retained foreign bodies can result in sympathetic ophthalmia, a serious inflammation of the ciliary body, iris, and choroid that occurs in the uninjured eye. The cause of the acute inflammation is unknown, but it is believed to be some type of autoimmune response. The inflammation can spread rapidly from the uvea to the optic nerve. The uninjured eye becomes inflamed, painful, and photophobic with a decline in visual acuity. Prompt aggressive treatment of eye injuries has decreased the incidence of this rare disorder that can result in loss of the "good" eye.

Guidelines for Safe Practice

Eye Irrigations

PURPOSE

1. Remove chemical irritants, foreign bodies, and secretions.
2. Cleanse.

PROCEDURE

1. Prepare solution. Physiologic solutions of sodium chloride or lactated Ringer's solution are most commonly used.
2. Position patient comfortably toward one side so that fluid cannot flow into the other eye.
3. Use appropriate means (e.g., kidney basin, large towel) to catch irrigating fluid.
4. Use appropriate amounts of solution.
   a. If small amounts are needed (to cleanse the eye postoperatively), sterile cotton balls moistened with solution can be used.
   b. If moderate amounts of fluid are needed (i.e., for removing secretions), a plastic squeeze bottle is used to direct irrigating fluid along the conjunctiva and over the eyeball from the inner to the outer canthus.
   c. If copious amounts of fluid are needed (i.e., for removing chemical irritants), bags of solution such as intravenous bags along with tubing to direct the flow into the eye can be used.
5. Avoid directing a forceful stream into the eye.
6. Avoid touching any eye structures with the irrigating equipment.
7. If there is drainage, wrap a piece of gauze around the index finger to raise the lid and ensure thorough cleansing.

Collaborative Care Management

Prompt professional evaluation and care are perhaps the most important aspects of management of eye injuries and may protect the eye from serious visual impairment. First aid measures for eye injury should be widely taught and posted clearly in all settings in which eye injury is a significant risk. Chemical burns are immediately treated with copious flushing of the eye with water (see Guidelines for Safe Practice box and Figure 58-7). A litmus paper may be applied to the conjunctiva to determine the pH if the substance is unknown. Irrigation is continued for at least 15 minutes before the patient is transferred for further evaluation and treatment. This simple measure may preserve eye function. Further treatment may include topical antibiotics, steroids, and antiglaucoma

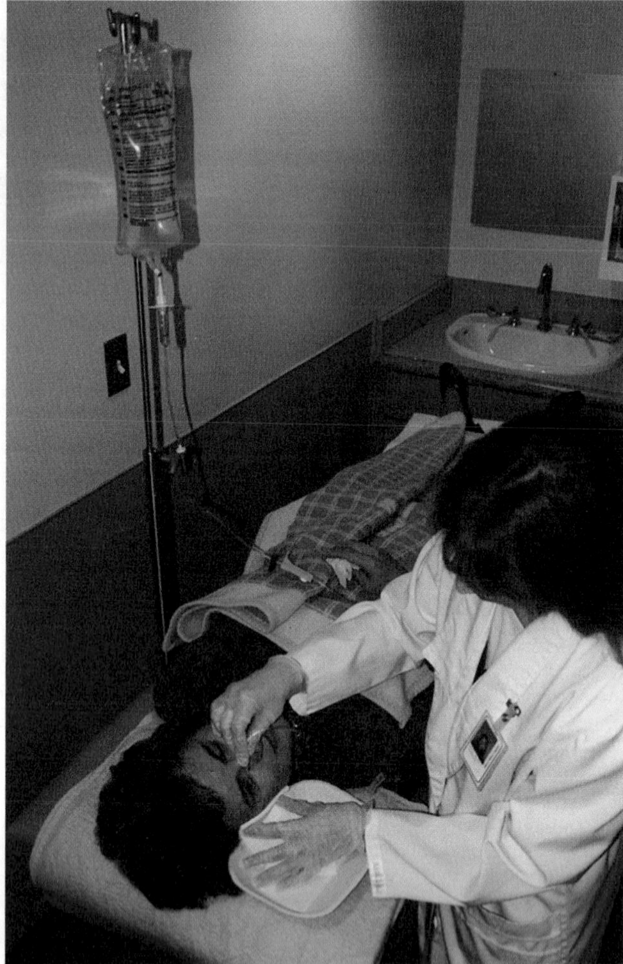

A

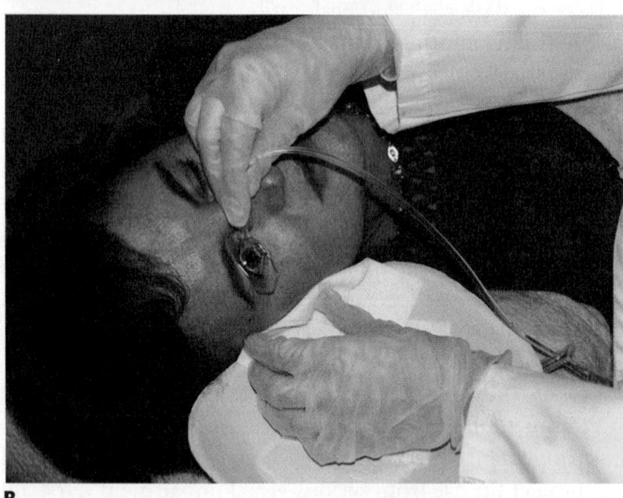

B

Figure 58-7 **A,** Eye irrigation using an intravenous bag and tubing. **B,** Note lid speculum in place.

agents to reduce intraocular pressure (IOP). Ultraviolet burns are treated with cool compresses, analgesics, and anesthetics.

Mechanical trauma also requires prompt professional care and evaluation, since there is risk of both infection and losing the eye. Antibiotics, wound suturing, cycloplegic agents, and cold compresses are all possible interventions, depending on the exact nature of the injury.[5] Table 58-3 outlines the basic first aid for common eye injuries. Significant damage can be done by well-intentioned efforts to remove a foreign body from the eye. The eye may be kept closed and loosely covered during transport to prevent further injury and until definitive treatment can be provided. Sterile fluorescein solution may be distilled to help outline the foreign body for removal. Antibiotic drops may be used to reduce the risk of infection and support healing.

TABLE 58-3 First Aid for Eye Injuries

Injury	Intervention
Burns: chemical, flame	Flush eye immediately for 15 minutes with cool water or any available nontoxic liquid. Seek medical assistance.
Loose substance on conjunctiva: dirt, insects	Lift upper lid over lower lid to dislodge substance, produce tearing. Irrigate eye with water if necessary; do not rub eye. Obtain medical assistance if above interventions fail.
Contact injury: contusion, ecchymosis, laceration	Apply cold compresses if no laceration present; cover eye if laceration present. Seek medical assistance.
Penetrating objects	Do not remove object. Place protective shield over eye (e.g., paper cup); cover uninjured eye to prevent excess movement of injured eye. Seek medical assistance.

Extensive or penetrating injuries to the eye can result in blindness or loss of the eye. Repair is surgically performed if possible. Contusions are treated with rest and the application of cold compresses to reduce swelling. When penetrating injuries occur, no attempt is made to remove the object or to clean the eye. Professional management is essential.

Patient/Family Education. The nurse may be responsible for community education efforts concerning eye safety and first aid for eye injuries.[4] The body's natural eye defenses can be appropriately augmented by the use of goggles, shields, and safety lenses for sports and high-risk activities. Children need to be taught about the risks associated with BB guns, slingshots, and even rubber bands. The use of protective sunglasses may also be important, depending on the patient's occupational and leisure time sun exposure. General guidelines for eye safety are summarized in Box 58-2.

GLAUCOMA

Etiology

Glaucoma is an eye disease characterized by progressive optic nerve atrophy and loss of vision. Elevated IOP is the most important risk factor for developing glaucoma. In primary open-angle glaucoma many persons have elevated IOP, but some have normal IOP. Because of this, elevated IOP is no

BOX 58-2 Rules of Eye Safety

1. Spray aerosols away from eyes.
2. Wear protective glasses during active sports such as racquetball.
3. Slowly release steam from ovens, pots, pressure cookers, and microwave popcorn bags.
4. Gaze at solar eclipses only through adequate filters.
5. Wear safety goggles whenever you are doing hazardous work or if you are in a workplace area where such hazards exist.
6. Fit all machinery with safeguards.
7. Keep dangerous items and chemicals away from children.
8. Store sharp objects safely.
9. Pick up rocks and stones rather than going over them with a lawn mower.

longer a defining characteristic of glaucoma. The term *glaucoma* actually refers to a group of disorders, as shown in Table 58-4. The two major forms of glaucoma are open-angle glaucoma and angle-closure (formerly referred to as closed-angle) glaucoma. The disease is primary when its etiology is unknown and secondary when it results from another eye disorder, such as a forward shift of the iris, pupillary blockage, or contracture of the fibromuscular membrane in the anterior chamber.

Epidemiology

Glaucoma is the third leading cause of blindness in the general U.S. population and the leading cause among African-Americans.[7] The prevalence rate among African-Americans is 15 times higher than that of Caucasians. About 2% of the population older than age 40 has glaucoma, and an estimated 1 million additional persons have undiagnosed disease. The incidence is expected to continue to rise as the population ages. Age, race, myopia, and a family history of glaucoma are the only identified risk factors. Angle-closure glaucoma is more prevalent in Asians. Glaucoma is a major cause of visual impairment and blindness worldwide.

Pathophysiology

The normal balance of production and drainage of aqueous humor allows the IOP to remain relatively constant within the normal range of 10 to 21 mm Hg with a mean pressure of 16 mm Hg. Normal diurnal variations are limited to about 5 mm Hg. Obstruction in any part of the outflow channels for aqueous humor results in a backup of fluid and an increase in IOP (Figure 58-8). A sustained elevation gradually damages the optic nerve and impairs vision. In primary open-angle glaucoma, which represents 90% of all cases, the changes occur slowly, and the damage is insidious. The process can also occur more rapidly in response to injury or infection or as a complication of surgery. Signs and symptoms of glaucoma are summarized in the Clinical Manifestations box. Figure 58-9 shows the progressive loss of peripheral vision that can occur with glaucoma.

TABLE 58-4 Types of Glaucoma

Type	Description
Primary open-angle (chronic, simple)	Most common type (90%) Usually caused by obstruction in trabecular meshwork
Secondary open-angle	Can occur from abnormality in trabecular meshwork or increase in venous pressure
Primary angle-closure (narrow angle, acute)	Outflow impaired as result of narrowing or closing of angle between iris and cornea Intermittent attacks—pressure normal when angle open; if persistent, acute ocular emergency
Secondary angle-closure	Can result from ocular inflammation, blood vessel changes, trauma
Congenital	Abnormal development of filtration angle; can occur secondary to other systemic eye disorders Rare (0.05%)

Collaborative Care Management

Diagnostic Tests. Several diagnostic tests are used to diagnose and monitor glaucoma. These include:

- Tonometry: measurement of IOP
- Tonography: estimation of the resistance in the outflow channels by continuously recording the IOP over 2 to 4 minutes
- Ophthalmoscopy: evaluation of the color and configuration of the optic cup
- Perimetry: measurement of visual function in the central field of vision
- Gonioscopy: examination of the angle structures of the eye, where the iris, ciliary body, and cornea meet[8]

Medications. Drug therapy is the foundation of treatment for most forms of glaucoma. The goal of treatment is to lower the individual's IOP and keep it at a level that prevents loss of vision. Drug therapy is administered topically or systemically to lower the IOP by either increasing the outflow of aqueous humor or decreasing the production of aqueous humor. Drug options include:

- Miotic agents that constrict the pupil and increase the drainage of aqueous humor
- Prostaglandin agonists that increase the uveoscleral outflow of aqueous humor
- Beta-adrenergic blockers and carbonic anhydrase inhibitors that decrease aqueous humor formation

Table 58-5 presents the medications commonly used in the treatment of glaucoma. Once initiated, drug therapy is continued for the rest of the patient's life.

Angle-closure glaucoma usually requires more aggressive management because it represents an emergency situation with the threat of permanent loss of vision if the pressure is not controlled promptly. Intravenous carbonic anhydrase inhibitors may be given in combination with osmotic agents

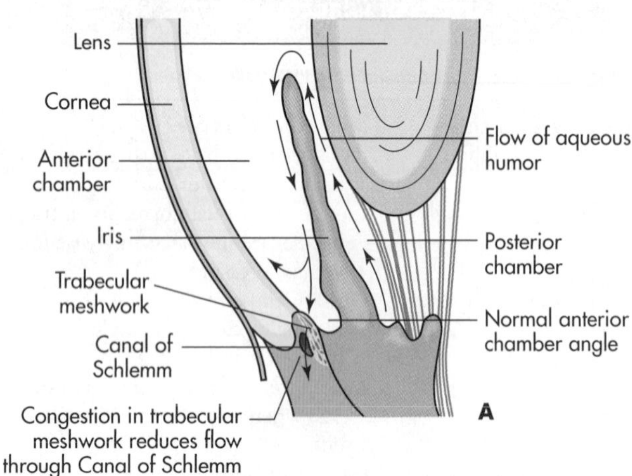

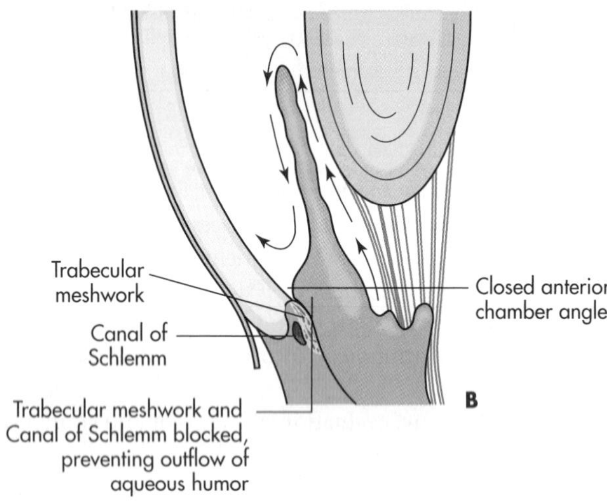

Figure 58-8 **A,** Chronic open-angle glaucoma. Congestion in the trabecular meshwork reduces the outflow of aqueous humor. **B,** Acute angle-closure glaucoma. The angle between the iris and the anterior chamber narrows, obstructing the outflow of aqueous humor.

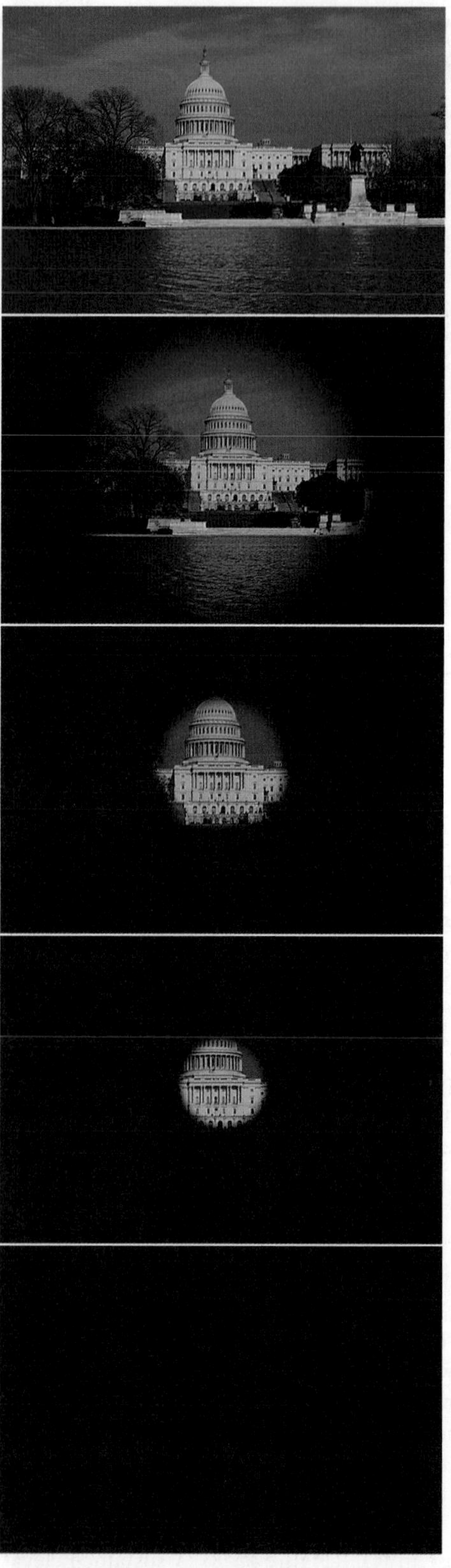

Figure 58-9 Glaucoma causes a progressive loss of peripheral vision. The changes may be so insidious that extensive irreversible damage occurs before the problem is recognized.

that draw fluid from the intraocular spaces, and with topical beta-blockers and miotics. Topical steroids may also be given in an attempt to minimize damage to the iris and the trabecular network. Regular ophthalmic care often permits identification of patients with narrow angles and the potential for angle-closure glaucoma. Prophylactic laser peripheral iridotomies may be performed to avoid an angle-closure glaucoma crisis.

Treatments. Cyclodestructive procedures such as cyclocryotherapy and YAG (yttrium, aluminum, and garnet) or diode laser thermal procedures attempt to lower the IOP by permanently damaging the ciliary body. The results of these procedures are unpredictable, and repeat treatment may be necessary to achieve the desired effect. Patients require close follow-up because they have an increased risk of retinal detachment, hemorrhage, and severe inflammation in the treated eye.

Surgical Management. Surgical intervention is indicated when conservative treatment fails to control the IOP. Two of the common procedures are argon laser trabeculoplasty (ALT) and trabeculectomy. ALT uses a laser beam to produce a nonpenetrating thermal burn on the trabecular meshwork that changes the configuration of the meshwork, increases tension in the meshwork, and leads to increased outflow of aqueous

Clinical Manifestations

Glaucoma

OPEN-ANGLE GLAUCOMA

Often no signs or symptoms in early stages
Intraocular pressure (IOP) typically elevated >24 mm Hg
Slow loss of vision
Peripheral vision lost before central vision (see Figure 58-9)
Tunnel vision
Persistent dull eye pain
Difficulty adjusting to darkness
Failure to detect color changes

ANGLE-CLOSURE GLAUCOMA

Acute: severe ocular pain, decreased vision, pupil enlarged and fixed, colored halos around lights, eye red, steamy cornea, may cause nausea and vomiting
IOP usually dramatically elevated; may exceed 50 mm Hg
Permanent blindness if marked increase in IOP for 24 to 48 hours

CONGENITAL GLAUCOMA

Enlargement of eye, lacrimation, photophobia, blepharospasm

TABLE 58-5 Common Medications for Glaucoma

Drug	Action	Intervention
Miotics		
Cholinergics Pilocarpine hydrochloride (Pilocar, Isopto Carpine) Carbachol (Isosopto Carbachol)	Contrict pupil (miosis) by directly stimulating sphincter muscle Increase outflow of aqueous humor by ciliary muscle pull on trabecular meshwork	Evaluate effectiveness. Monitor frequency of use. Inform patient that blurred vision and poor night vision may occur because of a small pupil. Other side effects include eye, brow, or lid discomfort, or burning sensation with drop instillation.
Cholinesterase Inhibitors		
Physostigmine (Eserine) Isoflurophate (Floropryl) Demecarium bromide (Humorsol) Ecothiophate iodide (Phospholine Iodide)	Constrict ciliary muscle and iris sphincter; iris is pulled away from anterior chamber angle, allowing drainage of aqueous humor and lowering of intraocular pressure (IOP)	Avoid use of isoflurophate, demecarium during pregnancy. Inform patient that blurred vision, watering eyes, brow ache, and change in vision may occur.
Beta-Adrenergic Antagonists		
Timolol maleate (Timoptic) Betaxolol (Betoptic) Levobunolol (Betagen) Carteolol hydrochloride (Ocupress) Metipranolol (OptiPranolol)	Decrease aqueous humor production and increase outflow, thereby decreasing IOP	Evaluate effectiveness. Use caution when administering nonselective beta-blockers to patients who have pulmonary or cardiac disease—can cause bronchospasm.
Carbonic Anhydrase Inhibitors		
Acetazolamide (Diamox) Ethoxzolamide (Cardrase) Dichlorphenamide (Daranide) Methazolamide (Neptazane) Dorzolamide (Trusopt)	Decrease aqueous humor production by inhibiting carbonic anhydrase in ciliary processes (an enzyme necessary to produce aqueous humor)	Evaluate effectiveness. Monitor for tingling sensation in extremities, tinnitus, gastric upset, or hearing dysfunction. Monitor for signs of hypokalemia.
Adrenergic Agents		
Epinephryl borate (Eppy/N, Epinal) Epinephrine hydrochloride (Glaucon) Epinephrine bitartrate (Epitrate) Dipivefrin (Propine) Apraclonidine (Lopidine)	Reduce aqueous humor formation and increase outflow	Evaluate effectiveness. Monitor for side effects: headache; brow ache; blurred vision; tachycardia; pigment deposits in cornea, conjunctiva, lids.
Osmotic Agents		
Glycerin (Osmoglyn) Mannitol (Osmitrol) Isosorbide (Ismotic)	Move water from intraocular structures, resulting in a marked ocular hypotonic effect, thereby decreasing IOP	Evaluate effectiveness. Monitor electrolytes for depletion. Monitor glucose levels in patients with type 1 diabetes. Drugs can cause hyperglycemia.
Prostaglandin Agonist		
Latanoprost (Xalatan)	Increase outflow of aqueous humor; used primarily with patients intolerant to or unresponsive to other glaucoma agents	Monitor renal and hepatic function during treatment. Teach patient about adverse side effects (e.g., burning on administration, blurred vision, itching, photophobia).

humor. Trabeculectomy creates an opening, or fistula, at the limbus under a partial-thickness scleral flap. The new opening circumvents the obstruction, and aqueous humor flows into the subconjunctival spaces. Fibrosis can occur at the site of the scleral flap and interfere with drainage, causing the IOP to rise again. Antimetabolites such as 5-fluorouracil and mitomycin C may be given to inhibit fibrosis. Releasable sutures and laser suture-lysis can also be used to support drainage at the site. ALT can usually be performed on an outpatient basis, whereas trabeculectomy typically requires an overnight hospital stay.

IOP control is achieved in about 85% of all patients, but most (75%) continue to require medications to treat glaucoma. Nursing care for the person after trabeculectomy is summarized in the Guidelines for Safe Practice box.

Molteno implants and other seton implants (e.g., Schoket, Krupin, and Ahmed implants) provide an alternative for patients with glaucoma that is resistant to other forms of surgery. In implant surgery a polymethylmethacrylate plate is implanted against the sclera. A tube is then surgically implanted directly into the anterior chamber. The aqueous humor drains out of the eye through the tube and collects under the plate posteriorly. The plate is designed to block scar tissue formation that could affect aqueous reabsorption or physically block the outflow tube. Overdrainage of aqueous humor is a potential complication that can increase the risk of retinal detachment and choroidal and vitreous hemorrhage.

Acute angle-closure glaucoma is treated with either a laser peripheral iridotomy (YAG or argon) or a surgical peripheral iridectomy, which penetrates the iris and permanently connects the anterior and posterior chambers of the eye. This prevents the iris from occluding the anterior chamber.

Diet. Diet does not play a role in the management of glaucoma. Patients experiencing acute angle-closure glaucoma may develop nausea and vomiting from the acute eye pain.

Activity. Activity does not need to be restricted for the treatment of open-angle glaucoma, but the patient is instructed to avoid heavy lifting, isometric exercises, and constipation that would cause straining.[10] The loss of peripheral vision that can result from the disease and the blurred vision and loss of night vision that are common side effects of several of the medications do create safety risks that may need to be addressed through a modification in activity, particularly driving.

Referrals. Referrals are not routinely needed in the treatment of glaucoma, but patients with acute angle-closure glaucoma need immediate treatment by an ophthalmic surgeon. Patients with loss of vision may benefit from referrals to the National Federation of the Blind,* and the National Eye Care Project.†

Guidelines for Safe Practice

The Patient Undergoing Trabeculectomy

Nursing care for the patient after trabeculectomy includes:

1. Routine postanesthesia care
2. Protection of the operative eye with a patch or shield, positioning the patient on back or unoperative side, and safety measures
3. Maintaining comfort in the operative eye
4. Assessment, as appropriate, of the intraocular pressure, appearance of the bleb, and anterior chamber depth
5. Administration of medications such as a cycloplegic, a mydriatic, and a combination antibiotic and steroid

NURSING MANAGEMENT OF PATIENT WITH GLAUCOMA

ASSESSMENT

Patients with open-angle glaucoma are typically asymptomatic in the early stages of the disease and may remain asymptomatic if they receive adequate treatment.

Acute angle-closure glaucoma causes an abrupt rise in IOP and can produce a variety of symptoms. Nausea and vomiting are often so severe in some persons with acute angle-closure glaucoma that an acute abdomen is mistakenly diagnosed. A popular misconception is that symptoms of headache, halos around lights, blurred vision, and eye pain are seen in persons with primary open-angle glaucoma.

Health History

Assessment data to be collected as part of the health history of patients with glaucoma include:

- Symptoms: onset; duration; severity; precipitating, aggravating, and alleviating factors; other characteristics
  - Sudden onset of severe pain in the eye
  - Acute blurring of vision
  - Halos around lights
  - Nausea and vomiting
  - Excessive tearing

Physical Examination

Important aspects of the physical examination of the patient with glaucoma include examining for:

- Pupil dilation, which is usually mild
- Hazy, bluish appearance of the cornea
- Sharp elevation in IOP (may be >50 mm Hg)
- Impaired visual fields indicative of central involvement late in the disease process
- Enlarged optic disc cup and disc pallor seen on ophthalmoscopic examination

NURSING DIAGNOSES

Nursing diagnoses are determined from analysis of patient data. Nursing diagnoses for the patient with open-angle or angle-closure glaucoma may include but are not limited to:

*1800 Johnson Street, Baltimore, MD, 21230; (410) 659-9314.
†Toll-free helpline (8 AM to 4 PM Pacific time): (800) 222-3937.

Diagnostic Title	Possible Etiologic Factors
1. Acute pain	Increased IOP
2. Deficient knowledge:	Lack of exposure/recall of information or misinterpretation of treatment/ disease process information
3. Ineffective health maintenance	Impairment in vision

EXPECTED PATIENT OUTCOMES

Expected patient outcomes for the patient with glaucoma may include but are not limited to:

1. Will experience a decrease in eye pain
2. Will accurately describe the nature of the disease process, components of the treatment plan, and the need for lifelong treatment
3. Will adapt lifestyle and self-care activities to accommodate losses in vision

INTERVENTIONS

1. Relieving Pain

Aggressive pharmacologic intervention is required to control the IOP and reduce the patient's pain. The nurse carefully explains all interventions and assesses the patient's pain level frequently. The nurse administers analgesics as needed to control the pain and carefully evaluates their effectiveness. The nurse modifies the patient's environment by controlling light levels, visitors, and stimulation and offers cool eye compresses to augment comfort. The nurse assists the patient in using relaxation strategies to help control disabling anxiety.

2. Patient/Family Education

Glaucoma is a chronic condition, and teaching focuses on the essential knowledge and skills for self-management. The nurse teaches the patient and family about the disease and its treatment and emphasizes that the disease can be controlled through lifelong management but that there is no cure. Vision that has been lost to elevated IOP cannot be restored, but further loss of vision can be prevented with careful adherence to the pharmacologic regimen and ongoing follow-up. A normal lifestyle is possible with minimal restrictions or modifications.

The nurse instructs the patient about all prescribed medications and their side effects and teaches the patient how to correctly administer topical eyedrops. Eyedrops are quickly eliminated from the eye and may need to be administered several times a day. Guidelines for administering eyedrops are summarized in the Guidelines for Safe Practice box. The nurse recommends that the patient keep a reserve bottle of the medication available, if possible, in case the drug is lost or spilled. The medication should always be carried in a pocket or purse when traveling and never packed in luggage. A Medic-Alert or other information card indicating that the patient has glaucoma and takes a specific medication can be an important safety precaution in case the patient is involved in an accident.

3. Supporting Self-Care

The use of miotic drugs causes pupil constriction and may adversely affect the patient's night vision and adaptation to dark places. The nurse assists the patient in planning for any adaptations in home or daily activities to ensure safety. Extra lighting in the home and reducing clutter can be helpful. The nurse cautions the person to carefully evaluate his or her ability to drive at night. The nurse also frankly discusses the adverse side effects of the drugs, including temporary blurred vision after administration and a stinging or burning sensation. Patients need both professional and family support to adhere to the treatment regimen, especially when an absence of disease symptoms makes the disease process seem tenuous, since the treatment can certainly seem worse than the disease. Honesty is an important tool for the nurse to use in all patient education efforts.

Health Promotion/Prevention

Early diagnosis and treatment of glaucoma is essential to prevent permanent destruction of fibers on the optic disc. All persons with a family history of glaucoma should have their eyes examined, including measurement of IOP, every 2 years after the age of 40. Mass screening programs are important for detecting glaucoma in persons who do not have periodic medical eye examinations, because the permanent loss of vision it causes is usually preventable.

Once the diagnosis has been made, regular medical follow-up is essential to evaluate the effectiveness of treatment. Follow-up every 2 to 3 months may be necessary initially until it is clear that the patient's IOP is under control. Adherence to treatment and regular monitoring are the best means available to prevent loss of vision from progressive disease activity.

EVALUATION

To evaluate the effectiveness of nursing interventions, compare patient behaviors with those stated in the expected patient outcomes. Achievement of patient outcomes is successful if the patient:

Guidelines for Safe Practice

Self-Administration of Eyedrops

1. Wash hands thoroughly before administering the medication.
2. Tilt head back and look up toward the ceiling.
3. Pull lower lid gently down and out to expose the conjunctiva and create a sac.
4. Bring dropper from the side and apply the eyedrops. Avoid touching the eyelashes, conjunctiva, or surface of the eye with the dropper. Resting the thumb on the forehead can help to stabilize the hand.
5. Close both eyes gently. Do not squeeze them tightly, or the medication will be expelled.
6. Apply slight pressure at the inner canthus of the eye to decrease systemic absorption of the medication.
7. If more than 1 drop is to be administered, wait 2 to 5 minutes before administering the second drop.

1a. Reports no eye pain or headache.
1b. Has IOP within target range.
2a. Has an appointment for follow-up monitoring and care.
2b. States commitment to lifelong therapy of the disease.
3. Makes needed alterations in home environment and activities to ensure safety despite impaired night vision or compromised peripheral vision.

GERONTOLOGIC CONSIDERATIONS

The incidence of glaucoma increases with aging, and the entire discussion of the disease and its management applies primarily to the older adult. Screening initiatives for glaucoma need to be particularly targeted to this population, because the disease is often not diagnosed until irreversible loss of vision has already occurred. Adherence issues are particularly challenging in this population. Fixed incomes can make the purchase of any medications difficult. The fact that most patients with glaucoma are asymptomatic can make it difficult for the patient to accept these medication purchases as essential. Compliance with a regimen that does not make you feel better and even compromises your night vision skills can be difficult to achieve. Often it is more difficult for patients with any degree of mobility or dexterity impairment, such as with arthritis or other problems, to learn to correctly self-administer eyedrops. In addition, most older adults are already dealing with some degree of visual impairment, and these impairments often have an impact on their ability to drive. Blurred vision and impaired visual acuity for night driving can create significant safety risks for individuals who are already struggling to remain independent. The issues for elders are real and challenging, and the nurse can neither solve nor eliminate them. Honest acknowledgment can be helpful, however, as the nurse attempts to assist the patient to anticipate areas of difficulty and develop strategies for addressing these problems.

SPECIAL ENVIRONMENTS FOR CARE

Critical Care Management

Critical care would not be used in the management of glaucoma. Angle-closure glaucoma can represent a real and emergent threat to the patient's vision, but the intense invasive monitoring and supervision inherent in the critical care environment does not add any benefits to management.

Home Care Management

Glaucoma is a community-based problem. Patients are typically diagnosed in the community and manage their disease process independently in their own homes. Hospitalization is rarely necessary unless the glaucoma does not respond to standard pharmacologic treatment and surgery is indicated. Even in these situations, the surgery is typically performed in an ambulatory center or as an overnight procedure. All of the nurse's interventions related to teaching and self-care must be targeted toward the reality of the patient's home situation and the supports available.

COMPLICATIONS

Loss of vision is the primary complication of glaucoma, and preventing vision loss and blindness is the ultimate goal of all therapy. Most patients with glaucoma can be successfully managed with routine pharmacologic therapy. Selected patients may require surgical intervention, and in rare instances the disease cannot be successfully controlled and severe visual impairment or blindness results. Glaucoma-related blindness remains a major international health concern.

CATARACT

Etiology

A cataract is a clouding or opacity of the lens that leads to gradual painless blurring and eventual loss of vision (Figure 58-10). Cataracts are generally classified as senile (associated with aging), traumatic (associated with injury), congenital (present at birth), or secondary (occurring after other eye/systemic diseases).

Senile cataracts are associated with the aging process and are not preventable. There is some evidence that exposure to ultraviolet radiation may significantly contribute to cataract formation, but a cause-and-effect relationship has not been proved. Speculation exists that antioxidant use, such as the combined intake of vitamins A, C, and E, may reduce the risk of senile cataracts, but this also is not proved.

Eye injury is the next most common identifiable cause of cataracts. The transparency of the lens may be destroyed by either a penetrating wound or a contusion. Cataracts may result from the ingestion of injurious substances such as dinitrophenol or naphthalene. Some researchers report that cataracts may result from systemic absorption of hair dye. The incidence of most traumatic cataracts is preventable through adherence to standard eye safety precautions (see Box 58-2).

Cataracts may also occur secondary to eye diseases, such as uveitis, or with systemic diseases, such as diabetes mellitus, galactosemia, or sarcoidosis.

Epidemiology

Cataracts are the third leading cause of preventable blindness in the United States, and their incidence increases steadily

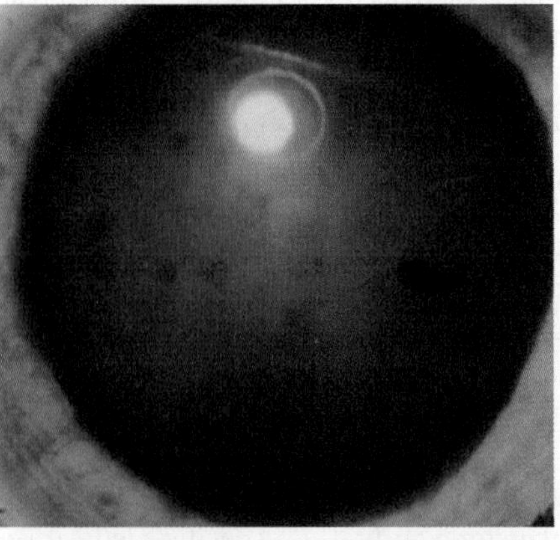

Figure 58-10 Mature senile cataract viewed through dilated pupil.

with age. Visible lens changes are present in 42% of the 52- to 64-year-old population, and 5% of this group demonstrate some degree of visual impairment related to the cataract. Of the population older than 65 years of age, 60% to 90% have visible lens changes, and between 25% and 45% have some degree of related visual impairment. A higher incidence of cataracts is found among people residing in warm, sunny climates. Risk factors for cataract formation are summarized in the Risk Factors box.

Pathophysiology

Senile cataracts occur because of a decrease in protein, an accumulation of water, and an increase in sodium content that disrupts the normal fibers of the lens. The cause of these pathologic changes is unknown. Cataracts usually develop bilaterally, but at different rates.

The primary symptom of cataracts is a progressive loss of vision. The degree of loss depends on the location and extent of the opacity. Persons with an opacity in the center portion of the lens can generally see better in dim light when the pupil is dilated. The person with presbyopia may find that reading without glasses is possible in the early stage of cataract formation because the greater convexity of the lens creates an artificial myopia.

Signs and symptoms of a cataract are summarized in the Clinical Manifestations box.

Collaborative Care Management

Diagnostic Tests. There are no particular diagnostic tests for a cataract. The diagnosis is made by direct inspection of the lens with an ophthalmoscope after pupil dilation. The progression of the cataract is monitored over time. Before surgery A-scan ultrasonography, keratometry, B-scan ultrasonography, endothelial cell counts, and potential acuity meter (PAM) tests may be performed. The A-scan measures the length of the eye and is done to help estimate the power of the intraocular lens (IOL) that will be needed. Keratometry measures the curvature of the cornea and is also used to determine the power of the IOL. A B-scan may be performed to evaluate the health of the retina if a dense cataract obscures visualization through an ophthalmoscope. Endothelial cell counts evaluate the health of the cornea and its ability to withstand surgery. The PAM test enables the surgeon to ensure that cataract surgery will be beneficial in increasing the patient's visual acuity by preoperatively measuring functional retinal response.

Medications. Medications do not play a role in the management of cataracts. Anesthetics, antiinflammatory agents, and antibiotics are all used after surgery to facilitate the healing process and promote patient comfort.

Treatments. Surgery is the treatment of choice for cataracts and can be used with virtually all patients. Various types of lenses are used after surgery to restore the person's vision, as discussed under surgical management.

Surgical Management. Surgery is the definitive treatment for cataracts, and it can be used safely and effectively with older adults. The success rate is between 90% and 95%. It was previously believed that a cataract had to "ripen," or mature, before it could be successfully removed. Currently, cataracts are removed when the visual impairment interferes with the individual's daily activities. The person's general health is the most important variable.

Cataract removal is performed with the patient under local anesthesia. The anesthetic is injected behind the eye and in and around the eyelids. The most popular method of cataract removal is the extracapsular cataract extraction (Figure 58-11). In this procedure only the anterior portion of the lens capsule and the capsule contents are removed, using techniques such as irrigation and aspiration or phacoemulsification (ultrasonic vibration to break up the lens).

Phacoemulsification is performed in about 80% of all cataract patients in North America. This procedure uses a smaller (⅛ inch) incision that promotes healing and decreases postoperative inflammation. Other surgical innovations include making the incision on the sclera rather than the cornea and using a single stitch to close the incision, or even no stitch. These innovations are all attempts to facilitate healing and decrease the incidence of postoperative astigmatism.

Extracapsular extraction leaves the posterior lens capsule intact, which avoids disruption of the vitreous humor and facilitates the placement of a lens implant (see Figure 58-11). Cataracts can also be removed with intracapsular extraction,

Risk Factors

Cataract

Age (The incidence increases dramatically after age 65.)
Sex (Cataracts are slightly more common in women.)
Ultraviolet light exposure
- More common in persons living in warm, sunny climates
- More common in persons who have worked outdoors extensively

High-dose radiation exposure
Drug effects from use of corticosteroids, phenothiazines, and selected chemotherapeutic agents
Poorly controlled diabetes mellitus resulting in accumulation of sorbitol (by-product of glucose)
Trauma to the eye

Clinical Manifestations

Cataract

Gradual, painless blurring and loss of vision
Peripheral vision may be affected first
Near vision may initially improve
Glare at night and in bright light
Halos around lights
Loss of ability to discriminate between hues
Cloudy white opacity on pupil

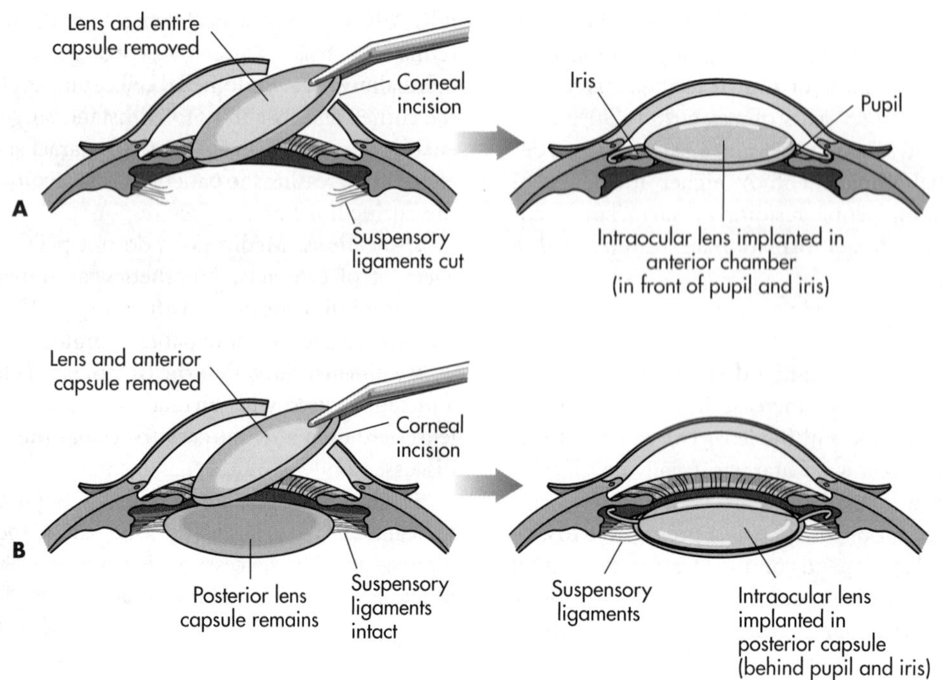

Figure 58-11 **A,** Intracapsular cataract extraction with removal of entire lens and capsule. **B,** Extracapsular cataract extraction leaving posterior lens capsule intact.

which involves the removal of the entire lens and its surrounding capsule using a freezing probe that adheres to the surface of the lens. This technique was popular at one time but is rarely used anymore.

An IOL implant is the preferred method for replacing the focusing power of the lens. A posterior chamber lens made of polymethylmethacrylate is placed behind the iris at the time of surgery and is supported by the posterior portion of the lens capsule that was left in place (see Figure 58-11). This type of implant is not dependent on the pupil or iris for support and rarely moves out of position. It is the most commonly used type of lens implant, because it is believed that the lens position most closely approximates the natural lens, and magnification is minimized.

Vision can be restored to near 20/20. The field of implants is rapidly evolving. Currently multifocal, bifocal, and even foldable implants are available. Foldable implants can be folded for insertion into the eye and allow the surgical incision to be even smaller.

If an IOL is not inserted during surgery, the person must wear an external lens. Cataract glasses are the least desirable option but are used if the person cannot tolerate contact lenses. Cataract glasses tend to magnify objects about 25%, making them appear closer than they actually are. The person's field of vision is also narrowed, and a circular blind area (ring scotoma) may occur at the edge of the glasses because the glasses bend the light rays so much that they do not enter the eye. Objects tend to "pop" in and out of the person's visual field as the eyes are moved away from the center of the glasses. An accurate prescription cannot be made for several months until the person's vision stabilizes after surgery.

Contact lenses correct some of the problems encountered with cataract glasses, but not all of them. The extended-wear soft contact lens is commonly used. Interruption of the nerve supply to the cornea from surgery usually facilitates the wearing of a contact lens, but persons with rheumatoid arthritis or any other form of impaired mobility may be unable to insert and maintain contact lenses.

Diet. Diet does not play a role in the management of cataracts, but it is important that the individual use diet modification and stool softeners or laxatives as necessary after surgery to prevent constipation. Straining during defecation can significantly increase the patient's IOP.

Activity. Activity used to be severely curtailed after cataract surgery, but the newer surgical techniques have allowed the restrictions to be significantly eased. Most of the positioning and activity restrictions are focused on preventing increases in the patient's IOP. These are discussed under Nursing Management of Patient Undergoing Cataract Surgery.

Referrals. Referrals are not generally necessary after cataract surgery unless the older adult lives alone and is not able to manage self-care safely during the first few days after surgery. A referral for home health supervision or assistance may be appropriate, especially for dressing changes and eyedrop administration.

Research

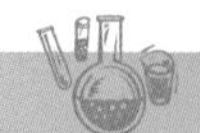

Reference: Morrel G: Effects of structured preoperative teaching on anxiety levels of patients scheduled for cataract surgery, *Insight* 26(1):4-9, 2001.

Structured preoperative instruction has clinical significance on anxiety levels and blood pressures. A significant difference was found between the state anxiety scores of the control group and those of the experimental group after preoperative teaching. A positive correlation was also evident between blood pressure and structured preoperative teaching.

Guidelines for Safe Practice

The Patient After Cataract Surgery

1. Position patient on the back or unoperative side to prevent pressure on the operative eye.
2. Keep side rails up as necessary for protection.
3. Place bedside table on the side of the unoperative eye (the patient then turns toward the unoperative side).
4. Place call light within reach.
5. Stress avoidance of actions that increase intraocular pressure (e.g., sneezing, coughing, vomiting, straining, or sudden bending over with the head below the waist).

NURSING MANAGEMENT OF PATIENT UNDERGOING CATARACT SURGERY

PREOPERATIVE CARE

Most cataract surgery is performed in ambulatory surgery centers; few patients require hospitalization. Routines for preoperative care vary with the setting and the eye surgeon. Inclusion of structured preoperative teaching can significantly decrease patients' anxiety level (see Research box above).

The patient may be asked to perform a face scrub before admission, and the eyelashes may be cut. The pupil of the operative eye is dilated and paralyzed before surgery, and sedation may be initiated. The nurse ensures that the patient has understood all explanations about the surgery and expected postoperative care and restrictions. The nurse also ensures that plans are in place for someone to transport the patient home and hopefully to assist with the patient's care during the first few postoperative days.

POSTOPERATIVE CARE

Most patients are discharged within a few hours. Immediate care considerations are summarized in the Guidelines for Safe Practice box. Because of the steady advances in surgical technique, patients do not need to restrict their activities in any substantive way, and they are encouraged to resume normal self-care activities as soon as they feel able.

Protecting the Eye

After any cataract operation, a dressing is applied to the eye and covered with a metal shield to protect the eye from injury.

Research

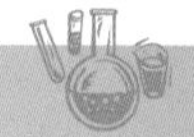

Reference: Morlet N, Kelly M: Improving drop administration by patients, *J Ophthalmol Nurs Technol* 15(2):60-64, 1996.

Twenty-three patients who underwent cataract surgery were observed during eyedrop administration to identify problems in their technique. The teaching of the next group of 10 patients was modified to address the problems identified. The performance of this group was then compared with the performance of a group of patients whose drops were administered by a caregiver. The performance of both groups was found to be equal, and the mean number of drops used was similar in each group. Patients who self-administered drops were found to be most effective when they stabilized the bottle by placing the thumb of their hand against their forehead to administer the drops.

The dressing is usually removed the day of or a day after surgery, but a metal eye shield is worn at night for a few weeks until the eye is healed to avoid accidental bumping of the eye during sleep. The patient is cautioned not to sleep on the operative side for 3 to 4 weeks to prevent pressure on the operative eye. Depending on the technique used to implant the lens, patients may be cautioned not to bend over with the head lower than the waist for about 2 weeks. Other patients have no restrictions on bending. The nurse instructing the patient clarifies with the surgeon what restrictions are necessary, if any.

The use of stool softeners is recommended to prevent constipation and straining. The nurse instructs the patient to avoid rubbing the eye and to continue using the eye shield as instructed.

Patient/Family Education

The nurse instructs the patient to be careful to prevent soap or water from entering the operative eye during face or hair washing. The nurse also instructs the patient to avoid heavy lifting, active exercise, isometric exercise, or straining during defecation until cleared by the surgeon to prevent abrupt fluctuations in IOP. The nurse reviews plans for follow-up care and ensures that appointments have been made and confirmed.

Most patients receive postoperative medications to relieve inflammation and facilitate healing. Antiinflammatory agents,[3] antibiotics, analgesics, cycloplegics, and mydriatics may all be used. Dilating the pupil alleviates discomfort and prevents the iris from adhering to the lens implant. Pupil dilation necessitates the use of sunglasses, since the eye is not able to respond naturally to light. Beta-blockers or carbonic anhydrase inhibitors may be administered to reduce aqueous humor formation and prevent postoperative increases in IOP (see Table 58-5).

The nurse ensures that the patient and the caregiver understand the purpose of all prescribed medications and can administer them correctly. Eyedrop solutions are commonly prescribed. If the patient is receiving multiple topical solutions or ointments, the nurse reminds the patient to wait 2 to 5 minutes between the administration of each drop and to administer the ointment last (see Research box above and

Guidelines for Safe Practice box on p. 1897). The nurse ensures that all discharge instructions are provided to the patient and family in writing for easy reference and that they have a phone number to call if questions or problems arise.

The nurse reviews safety precautions and reminds the patient that depth perception is initially compromised after surgery and that the risk of injury is increased. Special care is taken with any stairs, and driving is prohibited until cleared by the physician.

GERONTOLOGIC CONSIDERATIONS

Since cataracts are a problem that primarily affects older adults, the entire discussion is directed to that population. It is particularly important for the nurse to perform a careful assessment of the patient's support system for care after discharge, physical dexterity to be able to perform dressing changes and medication administration, and understanding of the important components of home care. If a patient needs cataract glasses, additional teaching is given for safety precautions to be followed at home. Objects appear larger, and both peripheral vision and depth perception can be seriously compromised after surgery. Extra care must be taken in ambulation, particularly when the patient attempts to go up and down stairs or curbs.

SPECIAL ENVIRONMENTS FOR CARE

Critical Care Management

Critical care does not play a role in the treatment of a cataract. The surgery is performed in an ambulatory surgery center, and even extremely aged individuals are successfully discharged back to their home environments the same day.

Home Care Management

The patient is likely to need assistance during the first days after surgery, and if family or friends are not available, the nurse ensures that referral for home health supervision is initiated. The acuity of vision in the unoperative eye may influence the person's ability to perform activities of daily living and administer medications safely.

Anticipatory planning can reduce the patient's dependence on others. Items needed for self-care can be temporarily relocated for easy access without bending over at the waist (e.g., slippers and pet supplies). The patient's hair is washed before surgery to delay the need to wash it in the postoperative period. Meals can be prepared ahead and frozen for easy access. Frail elderly patients without strong family or social supports may need a brief admission to an assisted living facility.

COMPLICATIONS

Infection, bleeding, and elevated IOP are the major complications of cataract surgery. The patient is instructed to promptly report the incidence of drainage, excessive tearing, bleeding, or a decline in visual acuity. Irritation and discomfort are expected after surgery, but acute pain would indicate a complication and should be reported immediately. When severe pain occurs, it often indicates that the position of the iris has been disrupted, causing an acute rise in IOP. This may require surgical correction to preserve the patient's vision.

RETINAL DETACHMENT

Etiology/Epidemiology

Retinal detachment occurs when the outer pigmented layer and the inner sensory layer of the retina separate (Figure 58-12). Inflammation and bleeding are common contributors to the detachment. Myopic degeneration and trauma are the most common causes of detachment, but it is also a common complication in eyes that are aphakic (without a lens). In many cases no apparent cause can be found.

Pathophysiology

The retina is a smooth, unbroken, multilayered surface. Degenerative holes or tears in the retina can allow vitreous humor to pass through and initiate a detachment (rhegamatogenous detachment). The presence of an inflammatory mass, blood clot, or tumor can also separate the retinal layers (exudative detachment). The vitreous also undergoes some deterioration with aging and can fall forward, exerting a traction pull on the inner lining of the retina, causing detachment (traction detachment).

Retinal detachment may occur suddenly or develop slowly. Symptoms include floating spots or opacities before the eyes, flashes of light, and progressive loss of vision in one area. The floating spots are blood and retinal cells that are freed at the time of the tear; they cast shadows on the retina as they drift about the eye. The flashes of light are caused by vitreous traction on the retina. The area of vision loss depends entirely on the location of the detachment.

If the detachment extends to include the macula, blindness results. When the detachment is extensive and occurs quickly, the patient may have the sensation that a curtain has been drawn before the eyes, but there is no pain associated with the detachment.

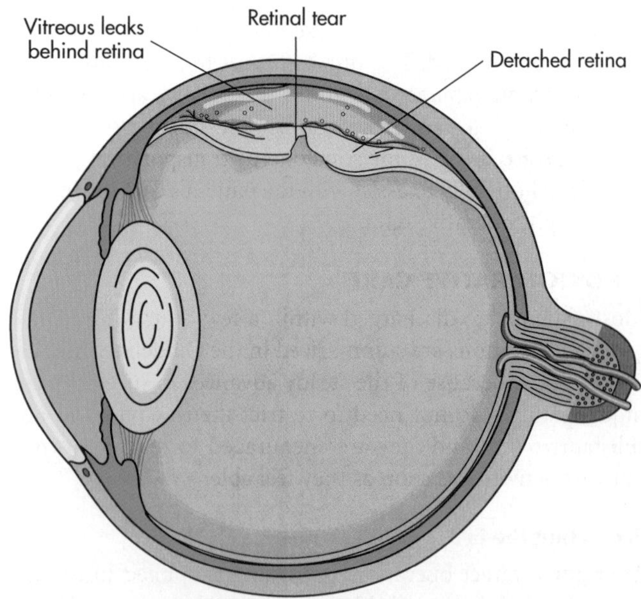

Figure 58-12 Retinal detachment.

Collaborative Care Management

The diagnosis of retinal separation is established by ophthalmoscopic examination of the retina to identify the location and extent of the retinal tear. B-scan ultrasonography may be used to improve the accuracy of the diagnosis, particularly if the vitreous is opaque. Minor tears and retinal holes are often identified as part of a routine eye examination, but if the individual is asymptomatic, no intervention is necessary.

Detachments that compromise vision are repaired surgically if possible. Surgery has a 90% success rate in reattaching the retina. Several different surgical techniques may be used. Fluid is usually first drained from the subretinal space to return the retina to its normal position. The tear is then sealed by producing an inflammatory reaction that causes adhesions to form between the margins of the break and the choroid (chorioretinitis). Diathermy can be used for small tears of recent origin. Needlepoint electrodes are applied to stimulate the inflammatory process. Laser photocoagulation can also provide the energy source to trigger the chorioretinitis. In cryopexy or cryotherapy, subfreezing nitrous oxide or carbon dioxide is applied to the sclera in the area of the tear or hole to produce the inflammatory reaction.

Cryopexy is a commonly used procedure that is often combined with a scleral buckling procedure in which the sclera and choroid are indented (buckled) toward the break by placing various sizes and shapes of silicone in the region of the break. An encircling band of silicone can also be placed around the eye (Figure 58-13) .These procedures ensure that the choroid remains in contact with the tear during healing and reduce the traction pull of any vitreous adhesions. The hole is thereby closed, and a watertight intraretinal space is reestablished.

Pneumatic retinopexy may also be used to repair a detachment, particularly small holes on the superior portion of the retina. The instillation of an expandable gas, such as sulfur hexafluoride (SF6) or perfluoropropane (C3F8), or silicone oil provides internal tamponade and supports the healing retina.

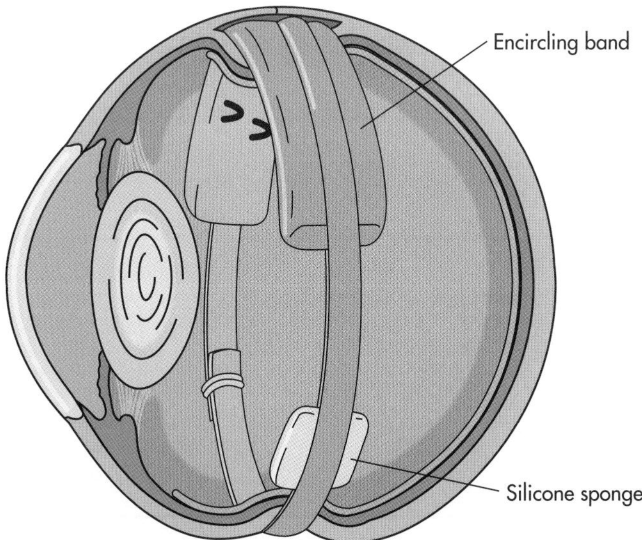

Figure 58-13 A band of silicone is placed around the eye to ensure that the choroid and retina remain in close contact during healing. A sponge is placed directly over the tear to depress the sclera.

The gas is gradually absorbed and replaced with vitreous. Silicone oil may remain in the eye and can only be removed surgically, and only if necessary. Laser demarcation is performed 1 to 2 days later to provide additional support to the retina.

The location and severity of the retinal detachment guide the patient's preoperative care. With small tears the patient may be permitted to continue with normal activities. When the detachment is large, however, or the macula is threatened, the patient needs quiet bed rest and may have both eyes patched to minimize eye movement and prevent extension of the detachment if possible. This is an extremely stressful time for the patient who needs careful teaching about the planned procedure and postoperative care. Patients with eye patches require thoughtful supportive care and frequent monitoring to remain oriented in a strange and frightening environment. The nurse also needs to assist the patient with all routine care.

Eye patching may be continued in the postoperative period, depending on the preference of the surgeon. The nurse continues to orient the patient to the environment and ensures patient safety through the use of side rails, assistance with self-care activities, close supervision when the patient is out of bed, and placement of the call bell securely within easy reach. The nurse provides ongoing support and encouragement to the patient and family while the eye patches are in place and while the success of the surgery is in question, reinforcing the 90% success rate. The threat of permanent blindness can be extremely frightening for both the patient and the family.

The exact location and severity of the detachment also govern the patient's specific activity restrictions in the postoperative period. If a gas bubble has been injected into the eye to reinforce the repair, the patient is positioned so that the gas rises in the eye and presses against the repair. This usually necessitates positioning the patient face down or angled toward the unoperative side. This position can be extremely difficult for patients to maintain, especially older adults, and the nurse assists the patient in achieving as much comfort as possible through the use of support pillows and head supports. Positioning restrictions may be in place for as long as 4 to 30 days. The patient is permitted out of bed for brief periods but is encouraged to keep the head parallel with the floor as much as possible. The nurse works to ensure both the patient's safety and relative comfort. The nurse encourages the patient to practice deep breathing every hour to decrease the risk of respiratory infection. Prone positioning significantly compromises respiratory excursion. Coughing is contraindicated because of the risk of elevating the IOP.

The nurse attempts to increase the patient's physical and emotional comfort. Eye pain is expected to be moderate, and the nurse administers analgesics as needed and evaluates their effectiveness. Cycloplegic agents may be administered to rest the eye, and corticosteroid drops are given to reduce inflammation. The combined effects of the medications and surgery may cause acute photophobia, and the nurse adjusts the room light to increase the patient's comfort. Vision is initially blurred because accommodation has been paralyzed. Care of the patient after repair of a retinal detachment is presented in the Nursing Care Plan on pp. 1904 to 1906.

Nursing Care Plan — Patient With Retinal Detachment

DATA Mr. A. is a 56-year-old warehouse clerk with a complaint of decreasing vision in his left eye over the past few days. He stated that he began to notice spots floating in front of his eye, as well as flashes of light out of the corner of his eye, about 2 weeks ago. He did not feel concerned because he thought his symptoms were due to his age. He visited his physician when it began to feel like a curtain was draped over his eye. His physician sent him to the hospital immediately.

The nursing history reveals that Mr. A.:

- Has never experienced eye problems except for nearsightedness, which is corrected by glasses
- Is generally healthy except for high blood pressure, which is well controlled by medication and diet
- Does not recall any accidents or injuries to his eye
- Swims and jogs regularly to feel his best

Examination of his left eye revealed a superior retinal detachment with inferior vision loss. His visual acuity was 20/80. Mr. A. underwent emergency scleral buckling (retinal reattachment surgery). Postoperatively, he has a patch over his left eye and is restricted to bed rest. He is experiencing eye discomfort, which he rates as a 5 on a scale of 1 to 10. Both he and his wife have little understanding of what happened to his eye or the surgery that repaired it. They are concerned about whether Mr. A. will regain his vision in that eye and if the same thing will happen to the right eye.

NURSING DIAGNOSIS **Acute pain related to inflammation and increased intraocular pressure (IOP) secondary to retinal detachment and scleral buckling**

GOALS/OUTCOMES Will achieve pain-free status

NOC Suggested Outcomes
- Pain Level (2102)
- Pain Control (1605)

NIC Suggested Interventions
- Pain Management (2210)
- Analgesic Administration (2210)

Nursing Interventions/Rationales
- Assess patient's level of discomfort, including the duration and quality. *Postoperative discomfort is expected, but severe pain suggests increased IOP or hemorrhage.*
- Apply cool, moist compresses to left eye. *Reduces swelling and promotes comfort.*
- Administer prescribed analgesics as prescribed. *Pain medication may be needed to decrease pain so that the patient can comply with prescribed activity restrictions.*
- Teach patient to avoid rapid head movements and bending the head below the waist (when ambulatory). *Prevents pain and avoids increasing IOP.*

Evaluation Parameters
1. Decreasing complaints of pain
2. Verbalizes satisfaction with comfort measures

NURSING DIAGNOSIS **Anxiety related to fear of unknown outcome of surgical procedure**

GOALS/OUTCOMES Will verbalize decreased anxiety related to surgical outcome

NOC Suggested Outcomes
- Anxiety Control (1402)
- Coping (1302)

NIC Suggested Interventions
- Anxiety Reduction (5820)
- Coping Enhancement (5230)

Nursing Interventions/Rationales
- Provide patient and wife an opportunity to explore concerns about possible loss of vision in left eye. *Identification of specific fears will direct the plan of action. Talking about one's fears often relieves anxiety.*
- Answer all questions honestly. *Information decreases uncertainty and helps the person gain control and feel less anxious.*
- Encourage realistic hope about maintaining vision. *Helps relieve anxiety.*
- Explore patient's understanding of the disorder and therapy. *To correct misunderstandings that may be contributing to the patient's fears and anxiety.*

Evaluation Parameters
1. Absence of physical signs of anxiety (tachycardia, restlessness, increased blood pressure)
2. Verbalizes fears and feelings of anxiety
3. Identifies past successful strategies for coping with anxiety

Nursing Care Plan *Patient With Retinal Detachment—cont'd*

NURSING DIAGNOSIS **Risk for injury related to sensory deficit and anxiety**
GOALS/OUTCOMES Will remain free of injury

NOC Suggested Outcomes
- Risk Control: Visual Impairment (1916)
- Safety Behavior: Fall Prevention (1909)

NIC Suggested Interventions
- Environmental Management: Safety (6486)
- Fall Prevention (6490)
- Surveillance (6650)

Nursing Interventions/Rationales
- Orient patient to physical surroundings. *Increases the patient's awareness of potential hazards.*
- Keep bed in lowest position and side rails up on left side. *To ensure the patient's safety while the eye is patched and vision is reduced.*
- Assist patient when initially ambulating after surgery. *To ensure safety. The patient may experience dizziness or altered proprioception from having one or both eyes patched.*
- Instruct patient to avoid sneezing, coughing, and vomiting. Administer cough medication or antiemetic if required. *To avoid increasing IOP.*
- Instruct patient to wear eye shield at night, or when taking a nap, for 2 weeks after surgery. *To prevent accidental bumping of the eye while resting or sleeping.*
- Teach the importance of maintaining prescribed activity and position restrictions. *Restricted eye movement helps increase adherence of the scleral buckle and decreases the risk of another detachment.*
- Place bedside table within patient's reach without need to turn head. *To decrease head movement, since gravity helps keeps the retina in its proper position.*
- Assist with activities of daily living (ADLs) as necessary. *To prevent excessive head movement while allowing the patient to assume his usual routine as much as possible.*
- Approach patient from unaffected side and place bed so that patient is facing away from the wall. *Allows the patient to see who is approaching, offsets isolation, and aids with orientation to a new environment.*
- Encourage diversional activities such as radio and conversation. *Provides sensory input and encourages feelings of normalcy.*

Evaluation Parameters
1. Asks for assistance when ambulating
2. Adheres to activity restrictions as prescribed

NURSING DIAGNOSIS **Risk for infection related to surgical repair of retina**
GOALS/OUTCOMES Will remain free of infection

NOC Suggested Outcomes
- Immune Status (0702)
- Infection Status (0703)

NIC Suggested Interventions
- Surveillance (6650)
- Infection Protection (6550)

Nursing Interventions/Rationales
- Assess for signs and symptoms of infection (purulent drainage, increased eye pain, swelling, warmth, increased white blood cell count, fever). *To identify infection early so that treatment can be initiated during the early stages.*
- Use sterile technique when performing eye care and changing dressings. *To prevent the introduction of microorganisms that can cause infection.*
- Administer antibiotic eyedrops as prescribed. *To prevent infection or treat existing infection.*

Evaluation Parameters
1. Absence of fever
2. Absence of purulent drainage, swelling, or increased pain of eye
3. White blood cell count within normal limits

Continued

Nursing Care Plan — Patient With Retinal Detachment–cont'd

NURSING DIAGNOSIS **Deficient knowledge related to lack of previous exposure to condition, surgery, postoperative care, and self-care**

GOALS/OUTCOMES Will accurately describe and participate in self-care as prescribed

NOC Suggested Outcomes
- Knowledge: Treatment Regimen (1813)
- Knowledge: Prescribed Activity (1811)
- Knowledge: Disease Process (1803)

NIC Suggested Interventions
- Teaching: Disease Process (5602)
- Teaching: Individual (5606)
- Teaching: Prescribed Activity/Exercise (5612)
- Teaching: Psychomotor Skill (5620)

Nursing Interventions/Rationales
- Teach about the eye and the role of the retina in vision. Explain symptoms associated with detaching retina. *To increase understanding of the disease process and promote cooperation with postoperative routines and the treatment regimen.*
- Explain importance of following prescribed postoperative activities. *To prevent increased IOP or precipitating another detachment.*
- Teach patient that he may engage in activities as long as they do not precipitate eye pain (climbing stairs, watching TV, reading, ADLs). *To allow increased freedom of activities without increasing the risk of increased IOP or another detachment.*
- Encourage patient to avoid driving, heavy house or yard work, or sports activities until released by physician to do so. *To prevent increased IOP or another detachment.*
- Suggest ways the patient can make himself comfortable if he must maintain a specific position (e.g., face down). *If a gas bubble is injected to cover the retinal hole, a specific position will be required to ensure its success (usually prone).*
- Demonstrate and have patient return demonstrate correct technique for hand washing and cleansing his eye from inner to outer canthus using a clean cotton ball for each wipe. *To reduce the risk of introducing microorganisms into the operative eye.*
- Demonstrate and have patient return demonstrate correct technique for self-administering eyedrops and ointments and applying an eye shield. *To ensure that the patient receives the prescribed dose of medication without increasing the risk of contamination of the eye.*
- Instruct patient to notify physician immediately if he experiences new flashing lights, floaters or shadows, severe or persistent eye pain, increased redness of the eye or lid, or increased quantity or change in color of eye drainage. *May indicate increased IOP or infection, which necessitates immediate intervention.*

Evaluation Parameters
1. Accurately describes retinal detachment and corrective surgery
2. Accurately describes activity restrictions and need for keeping follow-up appointments
3. Participates in self-care within prescribed restrictions

Patient/Family Education. The patient is discharged within a few days. The nurse ensures that the patient or family caregiver can correctly administer all medications and eyedrops. The nurse reinforces the need to limit activity, avoid bending over below the level of the waist, and avoid constipation and straining. Activities that require close vision, such as reading, needlework, or writing, are limited because they require rapid eye movements and accommodation. Watching television and walking are appropriate, although patients with gas bubbles may still have restrictions on positioning their heads. An eyeshield is worn during sleep for about 2 weeks. The nurse instructs the patient to contact the surgeon immediately if acute eye pain develops, eye discharge increases or turns yellow-green, or symptoms of detachment recur.

STRABISMUS

Etiology/Epidemiology

Strabismus is an ocular misalignment that results from an imbalance in the intraocular muscles. The eyes may be misaligned in any direction (e.g., esotropia [turning in], exotropia [turning out], hypertropia [turning up[, or hypotropia [turning down]). Strabismus is usually associated with childhood, but it can also be a lifelong disorder. Adult strabismus is also associated with brain tumor, head trauma, stroke, and thyroid ophthalmopathy. An estimated 2% to 3% of the general population have some degree of strabismus.

Pathophysiology

The ability to move the eyes in all directions and fixate on an object is the function of the six pairs of extraocular muscles (see Chapter 57). Strabismus interferes with the ability to use binocular vision and focus both eyes on an object, often causing double vision. Children with strabismus are often able to compensate for the confused images and avoid diplopia. Adults with new-onset strabismus are rarely able to compensate.

Collaborative Care Management

Strabismus is diagnosed through a standard visual field assessment. A variety of treatment options exist. Glasses with prisms may successfully realign the eyes and restore binocular vision. Eye exercises have been widely prescribed for patients with strabismus to "strengthen" the weak muscles, but there is little evidence of their effectiveness. Surgical correction is the standard treatment. The extraocular muscles are selectively weakened (recession), tightened (resection), or physically shifted (transposition) to achieve balanced eye movement. Adjustable sutures can be used to achieve an even more accurate alignment. A slip knot is attached during surgery. Once the anesthetic has worn off, the patient's ocular alignment is checked, and minor corrections can be made by tightening or loosening the knot.

Drug therapy with botulinum neurotoxin A (Botox) may eliminate the need for surgery or be used in conjunction with surgery. Botox is injected into the extraocular muscle and interferes with the release of acetylcholine at the neuromuscular junction. The toxin appears to strengthen the antagonist muscle and weaken the injected muscle over a period of weeks to months.

Patient/Family Education. Most strabismus surgery is performed on an outpatient basis with the patient under either local or general anesthesia. Postoperative care focuses on careful monitoring and preparation of the patient for self-care at home. The eyes may be patched initially for protection, especially if an adjustable suture was used. Patients are instructed to avoid strenuous exercise and heavy lifting until approved by the surgeon. Slight redness, swelling, and irritation are expected, and the nurse instructs the patient to use cold compresses for comfort. Dust and heavy pollen can irritate the eye and should be avoided. The nurse instructs the patient to monitor the eye for healing and to promptly report any sign of infection.

EYE TUMORS

Both benign and malignant tumors may affect the eye and related structures. They may originate within the eye or metastasize from another primary site. Benign neoplasms include lymphomas, hemangiomas, and mucoceles from the sinuses. Malignant tumors threaten both the patient's vision and life, since extension commonly involves vital structures within the brain. The eyelids are vulnerable to any of the standard tumors that affect the skin, including nevi and xanthelasma (lipid deposits near the corner of the eye). Positive outcomes often require early diagnosis and prompt treatment. Treatment usually involves surgical excision but may also include various forms of radiotherapy.

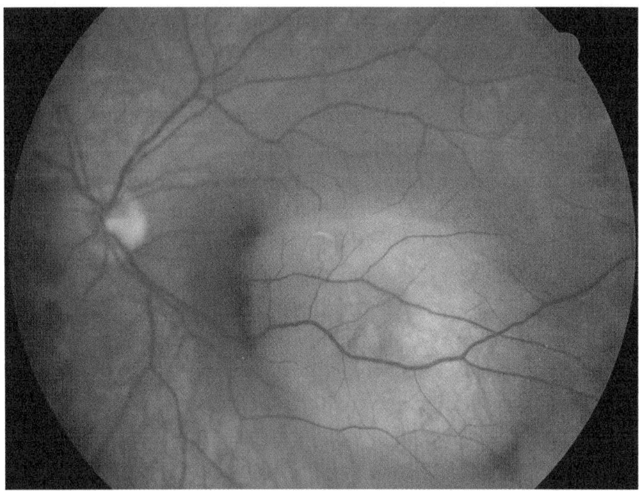

Fig 58-14 Large choroidal melanoma.

MALIGNANT MELANOMA

Etiology/Epidemiology

A melanoma involving the eye is rare, but it is the most common form of intraocular tumor in adults. Retinoblastoma is the most common form of eye tumor, but it is congenital and is typically diagnosed in childhood. Melanomas usually occur unilaterally. See Chapter 62 for a more complete discussion of melanoma.

Pathophysiology

Malignant melanomas occur in the choroid (Figure 58-14), ciliary body, and iris. They are slow growing, but they metastasize early because of the vascularity of the choroid. Vision may not be affected until the tumor becomes large or affects the macula.

Collaborative Care Management

Intraocular malignant melanomas are often diagnosed with an ophthalmoscopic examination. Ultrasonography and fundus photography may be useful in documenting the size and placement of the tumor. Fluorescein angiography may be used to document the vascular involvement of the tumor.

Surgery is the primary treatment for an intraocular melanoma. Treatment is based on the exact size, shape, and location of the tumor. Every effort is made to preserve the patient's vision if possible. Small tumors that involve the iris may be successfully treated with iridectomy, often with removal of the ciliary body as well. Large melanomas of the choroid are usually treated with enucleation of the eye, which involves surgical removal of the entire eye, including the sclera. Evisceration is removal of the contents of the eye with retention of the sclera. Exenteration involves removal of the entire eye and all other soft tissues in the bony orbit.

Nonsurgical treatments include radiation therapy, photocoagulation, and brachytherapy, in which radioactive plaques are sutured into the sclera.

If feasible, the eyeball alone is removed, leaving the surrounding layers of fascia (Tenon's capsule) and the muscle attachments. A silicone, plastic, or tantalum implant is inserted into the eye socket, the cut ends of the muscle attachment are overlapped and sutured around it, and the Tenon's capsule and the conjunctiva are closed. This procedure supplies both support and motion for an artificial eye.

A newer implant called hydroxyapatite, which has the same consistency as bone, may provide better movement of an ocular prosthesis.[20] The ball-shaped implant is left in place permanently. A plastic conformer is placed in the socket until edema subsides and an artificial eye (prosthesis) can be inserted, because the extraocular muscles strongly anchor to it. This provides superior motion and improved cosmetic appearance.

Pressure dressings are used for 1 or 2 days to help control possible hemorrhage. Headaches or pain on the operative side could indicate a venous thrombosis or the onset of meningitis. Infection is a dangerous complication of eye surgery, and most patients receive prophylactic antibiotics.

A custom-made prosthetic eye can be used as soon as healing is complete and edema has disappeared. Healing is usually complete 4 to 8 weeks after surgery, although many patients begin to wear a temporary prosthetic eye after only 2 to 3 weeks. Today artificial eyes are made of plastic instead of glass and can be made in shades that closely match the normal eye.

Patient/Family Education. The diagnosis of eye malignancy, along with the need to undergo enucleation, creates a crisis situation for the patient and family. The virulence of the malignancy may necessitate immediate surgery with little time to prepare for the loss of the eye either physically or emotionally. The nurse plays an important role in providing support and counseling to the patient during this difficult time. Both the patient and the family need to be encouraged to talk about their feelings and concerns and to be helped to adjust their lives when confronted by this serious situation.

When a person has lost one eye, the preservation of sight in the other eye becomes crucial. Wearing impact-resistant glasses provides some protection from injury. Because binocular vision is gone when there is only one functioning eye, depth perception is affected. The nurse teaches the person about the adjustments necessary to carry out normal activities with one eye and about potential safety hazards. For example, driving a car is potentially dangerous because of the alteration in depth perception. With patience and practice, however, almost all normal activities are possible.[6]

Care of the prosthetic eye is relatively simple. Frequent removal and cleaning are no longer recommended. Patients are referred for follow-up to an ocularist, who will clean and polish the eye to remove salt and protein buildups. This may be done just one or two times per year.

Critical Thinking Questions

1. How would you teach a visually impaired person who is using three different types of eyedrops to identify the correct drops?
2. What approaches might you consider for a person with glaucoma who refuses to administer eyedrops four times a day as prescribed by the physician?
3. A 20-year-old woman has a foreign object floating on the surface of her left eye. The nurse has her lie on her right side and begins irrigating the left eye with a syringe filled with normal saline. She directs the fluid from the outer to the inner canthus. Critique this irrigation procedure.

References

1. Age-Related Eye Disease Study Research Group: The risk factors associated with age-related macular degeneration (AMD): a case-control study in the Age-Related Eye Disease Study, Age-Related Eye Disease Report No 3, *Ophthalmology* 107(12):2224-2232, 2000.
2. Bressler SB: *Age-related macular degeneration,* San Francisco, 2000, American Academy of Ophthalmology.
3. Brown RM, Roberts CW: Preoperative and postoperative use of nonsteroidal antiinflammatory drugs in cataract surgery, *Insight* 21(1):13-16, 1996.
4. Burlew JA: Preventing eye injuries—the nurse's role, *Insight* 16(6):24-28, 1991.
5. Buttaraboli P, Stein T: *Minor emergencies: splinters to fractures,* St Louis, 2000, Mosby.
6. Hill JE, editor: *Ophthalmic procedures—a nursing perspective,* San Francisco, 2000, American Society of Ophthalmic Registered Nurses.
7. Newell FW: *Ophthalmology: principles and concepts,* ed 8, St Louis, 1996, Mosby.
8. Stein HA, Slatt BJ, Stein RM: *The ophthalmic assistant: a guide for ophthalmic medical personnel,* ed 7, St Louis, 2000, Mosby.
9. US Department of Health and Human Services, Public Health Service: *Healthy people 2000: midcourse review and 1995 revisions,* Washington, DC, 1995, US Government Printing Office.
10. Whitaker RJ et al: Glaucoma: what the ophthalmic nurse should know, *Insight* 24(3):86-90, 1999.

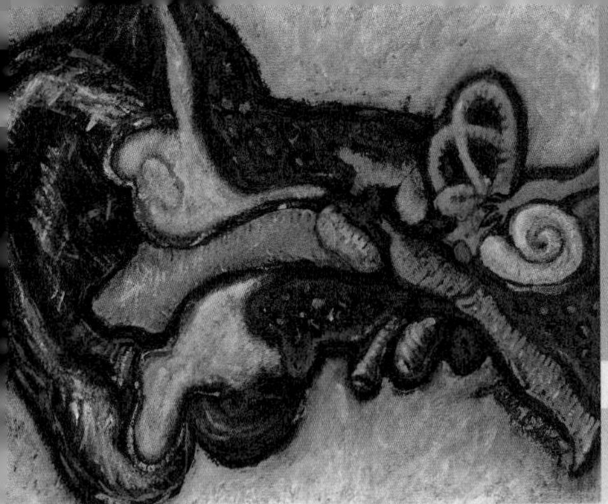

http://www.mosby.com/MERLIN/medsurg_phipps

Assessment of the Auditory System 59

Carol Meadows

Objectives

After studying this chapter, the learner should be able to:

1. Describe the basic structure and function of the temporal bone and ear.
2. Use behavioral cues to detect loss of hearing and balance.
3. Describe anatomic and physiologic age-related changes in the auditory and vestibular systems.
4. Recognize normal assessment findings related to the ear and its functions.
5. Identify specific diagnostic tests for hearing and balance and their associated nursing interventions.

The two major functions of the ear relate to hearing and balance, both of which play an important role in the activities of daily living. Hearing helps us interact with the environment. It is essential for the normal development and maintenance of speech, provides warning of danger, and adds a dimension of aesthetic pleasure to life. The organs of balance contained within the ear relay information about the body's position to the brain and thus are critical to the ability to function within the environment.

Nurses are involved in all aspects of patient care related to auditory and vestibular problems: prevention, detection, and treatment. In fact, the nurse is frequently the first member of the health care team to be approached by patients regarding problems with hearing and balance. Thus every nurse needs to be skillful in examining the outer ear and grossly assessing the patient's hearing and equilibrium.

ANATOMY AND PHYSIOLOGY

The ears are a pair of complex sensory organs located in the middle of both sides of the head at approximately eye level (Figure 59-1). The position of the ears is important because the use of both ears simultaneously produces binaural hearing, allowing a person to detect the direction of sound and aiding in maintaining equilibrium. A person detects the direction from which a sound comes by the time lag between the sound entry into one ear compared with the sound entry into the other ear and by the intensity of sound in each ear.

The ears are housed in the "temporal" bones of the skull, which are part of both the base and the lateral wall of the skull. The temporal bones are the hardest bones in the human body and provide adequate protection for the organs of hearing and balance.

Each ear is divided into three parts: the external ear, the middle ear, and the inner ear.

The External Ear

The external ear consists of the pinna or auricle and the external auditory canal. The pinna is primarily composed of cartilage covered by skin and is attached to the side of the head at approximately a 10-degree angle. The parts of the pinna are illustrated in Figure 59-2. The external auditory canal extends from the concha, which is the deepest part of the pinna, to the tympanic membrane or eardrum, in an inward, forward, and downward path in an adult. The canal is irregular and constricts about midway and again near the eardrum. Skin lines the canal and covers the eardrum. The supporting wall of the first half of the ear canal is cartilaginous and the second half is osseous. The skin lining this bony portion of the canal is thin and highly sensitive and contains fine hairs and sebaceous glands.

Ceruminous glands, which are modified sweat glands found in the external auditory canal, produce cerumen or ear wax. Cerumen has a protective function in that its sticky consistency, along with the fine hairs of the ears, help to cleanse the auditory canal of foreign matter.

The funnel shape of the external ear collects sound and channels it toward the tympanic membrane, which is a thin, semitransparent membrane, that protects the middle ear and conducts sound vibrations from the external ear to the ossicles. The tympanic membrane is approximately 9 mm in diameter, nearly oval in shape, obliquely directed downward and inward, and is pearly gray in color.

Distinguishing landmarks of the normal eardrum include the annulus, which is the thickened border that attaches the

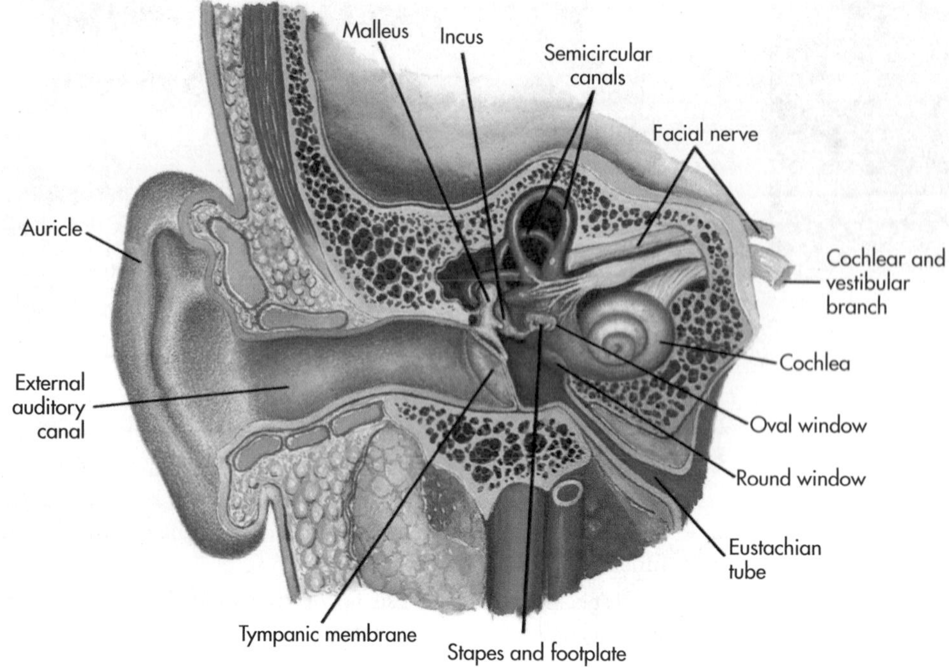

Figure 59-1 Structures of the ear.

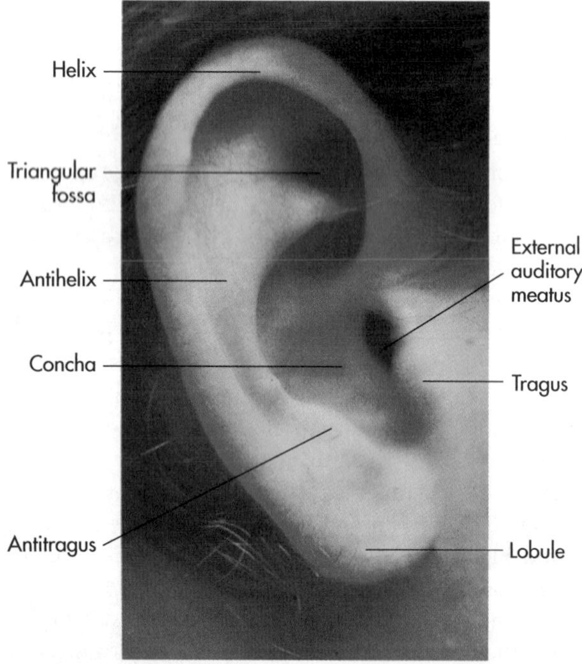

Figure 59-2 Anatomic structures of the pinna. The helix is the prominent outer rim, whereas the antihelix is the area parallel and anterior to the helix. The concha is the deep cavity containing the auditory canal meatus. The tragus is the protuberance lying anterior to the auditory canal meatus, and the antitragus is the protuberance on the antihelix opposite the tragus. The lobule is the soft lobe on the bottom of the auricle.

eardrum to the temporal bone; the umbo, the most depressed point where the first ossicle attaches to the eardrum; the pars flaccida, a small triangular area above the short process of the malleus; and the largest portion, the pars tensa (Figure 59-3).

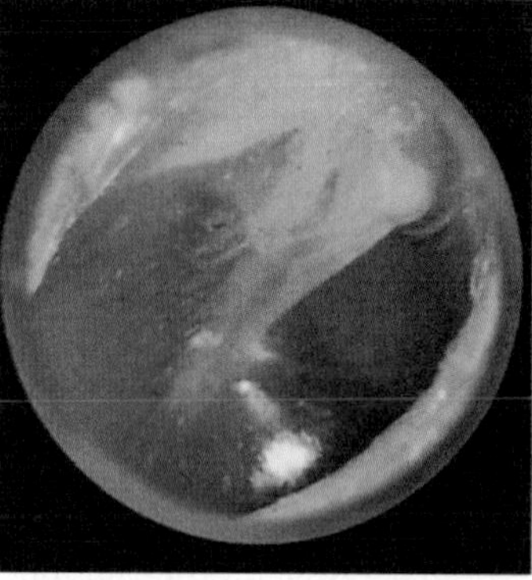

Figure 59-3 Structural landmarks of the tympanic membrane.

The tympanic membrane is composed of three layers: an outer skin layer continuous with the skin of the external ear canal, a fibrous middle layer, and an inner mucosal layer continuous with the lining of the middle ear.[1] The pars flaccida is composed of only two layers. The absence of the fibrous middle layer makes the pars flaccida more vulnerable to negative pressure and resulting disorders.

The Middle Ear

The middle ear consists of an air-filled cavity and its contents: the ossicles, the oval and round windows, and the opening of the eustachian tube.

The ossicles—the malleus (hammer), the incus (anvil), and the stapes (stirrup)—are the three smallest bones in the body. The ossicles have been given these common names because of their appearance. The ossicles joined together in a movable chain, connect the tympanic membrane to the labyrinth. They are held in place by muscles, ligaments, and joints. The ossicles function to mechanically transmit sound vibrations and

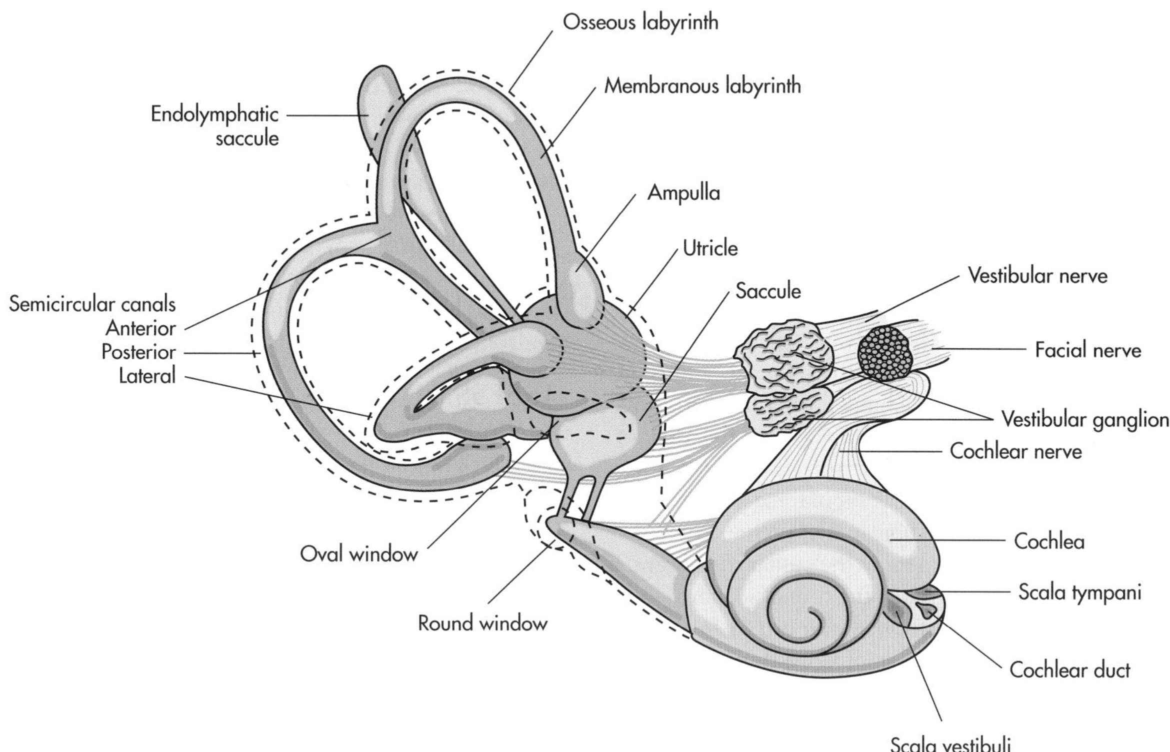

Figure 59-4 Structures of the inner ear.

also protect the inner ear from loud sounds by means of a dampening mechanism. The ossicles provide an efficient means by which the moving air molecules of sound in the external ear can be transferred to the fluid molecules that circulate in the inner ear. Liquids offer more resistance than air and need more force to produce movement; the ossicular chain produces this force against the inner ear fluids.[1]

The oval window, which is covered by the footplate of the stapes, is the opening into the inner ear where sound vibrations enter. The round window is a true window and provides an exit for sound vibrations from the inner ear.

The eustachian tube is a channel approximately 35 mm (1½ in) long that connects the middle ear with the nasopharynx. The tube is composed of bone, cartilage, and fibrous tissue lined with mucous membrane. The eustachian tube allows air to enter and leave the middle ear and is responsible for both ventilation and pressure regulation, which are necessary for normal hearing.

Only a small segment of the eustachian tube remains open permanently; otherwise the walls are in direct contact with each other. This prevents the sound of normal nasal respiration and one's own voice from passing up the eustachian tube into the middle ear. The tube can be forcibly opened by increasing nasopharyngeal pressure ("popping the ears").

The mastoid includes the mastoid bone (part of the temporal bone); the mastoid process, which can be felt as a bony protuberance behind the lower portion of the pinna; the mastoid cavity, a large cavity that is continuous with the middle ear; and the mastoid air cells that branch off the mastoid cavity. The cavity and system of air-filled cells contained within the mastoid bone aid the middle ear in adjusting to changes in pressure and lighten the weight of this protective bony structure.

The Inner Ear

The inner ear is a complex system of intercommunicating chambers and connecting tubes located in the petrous part of the temporal bone (Figure 59-4). The two major structures of the inner ear are the bony labyrinth and the membranous labyrinth. The membranous labyrinth lies within, but does not completely fill, the bony labyrinth. The bony labyrinth consists of three semicircular canals (the superior, the lateral or horizontal, and the posterior), the vestibule, and the cochlea.

The vestibule connects the semicircular canals and the cochlea. The cochlea looks like a snail shell and has two compartments. The upper compartment is called the scala vestibuli and leads from the oval window to the apex of the cochlea. The lower compartment is called the scala tympani and continues from the apex of the cochlea to the round window. This system allows sound vibrations to enter at the oval window and exit at the round window. The membranous labyrinth consists of the utricle, saccule, three semicircular ducts, the cochlear duct, and the organ of Corti. The organ of Corti, the end organ for hearing, is located on the basilar membrane and stretches from the base to the apex of the cochlea.

The membranous labyrinth contains a fluid called endolymph and is continuously bathed in another fluid, called perilymph.

The three semicircular canals, the utricle, and the saccule are the sense organs responsible for position and balance. The semicircular canals are arranged to sense rotational movement, whereas the utricle and saccule are involved with linear movements.

Sound Transmission

Sound is transmitted from the external ear to the inner ear by two routes, air conduction and bone conduction. Air conduction transmits sound vibration through the middle ear to the inner ear, whereas bone conduction transmits sound vibrations through the skull to the inner ear.

In air conduction the tympanic membrane conducts sound vibrations to the ossicles and then through the oval window into the perilymph. The pressure exerted by the vibrations on the stapes in the oval window is 22 times greater than the pressure exerted on the tympanic membrane because the force of the sound vibrations increases with transmission from a larger area to a smaller area. From the perilymph, these amplified vibrations travel through the vestibular membrane, enter the cochlear duct, and cause movement of the basilar membrane.[2] They then exit the inner ear through the round window.

Sound energy must be transformed into neural energy for transmission to the brain. The organ of Corti transforms mechanical sound vibrations into neural activity for transmission to the brain. It also separates sound into different frequencies. Nerve impulses are transmitted between the ear and the brain by the eighth cranial nerve, the acoustic (vestibulocochlear) nerve, which has two branches. The cochlear branch of the vestibulocochlear nerve innervates the acoustic portion of the ear while the vestibular branch of the nerve innervates the vestibular portion of the ear. Electrochemical impulses travel via the acoustic nerve to the temporal cortex of the brain and are interpreted as meaningful sound. In a similar way, the inner ears send impulses to the brain via the vestibular portion of the nerve that are decoded to maintain normal balance.[2]

Physiologic Changes With Aging

A variety of changes occur in the ear as a result of normal aging. The auricle enlarges and loses its elasticity; the lobe also enlarges and becomes pendulous. At the entrance to the external auditory canal, a tuft of wiry hair frequently develops. Within the canal, cilia become coarse and stiff; production of keratin in the skin increases; and the apocrine glands atrophy and secrete decreased amounts of cerumen. As a result cerumen is drier. It also tends to harden and accumulate, as it is not efficiently moved outward by the cilia. Ultimately impaction and decreased hearing acuity can occur. The tympanic membrane atrophies and may become sclerotic. It appears dull white or cloudy, and opaque. Landmarks are more prominent because of retraction. Within the middle ear muscles and ligaments stiffen and calcification of the ossicles may cause fixation of the foot of the stapes in the oval window. These changes in the tympanic membrane and the ossicles contribute to a conductive hearing loss. In the inner ear, hair cells in the organ of Corti usually begin to degenerate after 50 years of age. In addition, cochlear capillaries atrophy with age, the basilar membrane becomes less flexible, and neurons and endolymph diminish. A sensorineural hearing loss known as presbycusis results. This is the most common type of hearing loss in elderly persons and is characterized by decreased perception of high frequency sounds (S, Sh, Ph, K). Decreased perception of consonants (Z, T, F, G) also occurs. Tinnitus, a sensation of buzzing, ringing, or other noise in one or both ears, accompanies most sensorineural hearing loss and thus is common in older adults.

Generalized degenerative changes in the labyrinth cause presbyastasis or presbyvertigo, which is a balance disorder of aging. Also contributing to the imbalance are decreased visual acuity and compromised proprioception. Presbyastasis can be controlled but not cured.[4]

ASSESSMENT

Health History

Before beginning the health history, the nurse obtains a general impression of the patient's hearing ability by observing for behavioral clues. Specific behavioral clues that suggest the presence of hearing loss are presented in Box 59-1. The individual may also focus on the speaker's face and lips, rather than making eye contact. If the patient has a hearing loss, it is important for the nurse to face the patient directly and speak clearly. If the patient wears a hearing aid, the nurse ensures that it is in use and functioning properly.

The nurse asks the patient about the presence or history of earache (otalgia), drainage (otorrhea), tinnitus, or vertigo. An environmental and work history is also obtained, as previous or current occupational exposure to loud noise or living in a noise polluted area may result in hearing loss. Any history of old trauma, such as a blow to the ears or a foreign body, is explored, as these can result in hearing loss later in life.

The nurse completes a thorough medication history to identify use of potentially ototoxic drugs (Table 59-1).[6] Ototoxic agents either directly affect the eighth cranial nerve or the organs of hearing and balance, causing symptoms such as tinnitus, headache, dizziness, vertigo, nausea, ataxia, nystagmus, or a discernible change in hearing.

BOX 59-1 Behavioral Cues Suggesting Loss of Hearing

Any adult with a loss of hearing may exhibit one or more of the following traits:

- Is irritable, hostile, or hypersensitive in interpersonal relations
- Has difficulty hearing upper frequency consonants
- Complains about people mumbling
- Turns up volume on television
- Asks for frequent repetition or misunderstands
- Answers questions inappropriately
- Loses sense of humor; becomes grim
- Leans forward to hear better; face looks serious and strained
- Shuns large- and small-group audience situations
- Appears aloof and "stuck up"
- Complains of ringing in the ears
- Has an unusually soft or loud voice
- Has garbled speech

The patient is questioned regarding self-care of the ears: frequency of hearing tests and the method and frequency of cleaning. This information helps the nurse plan appropriate health teaching. Incorrect methods of cleaning the ears, such as the use of cotton-tipped applicators, can lead to impacted cerumen and hearing loss. The nurse also asks the patient about any history of ear infections and the method of treatment. A history of chronic ear infections alerts the nurse to the possibility of sequelae.

Dizziness and/or hearing loss can have devastating effects on the patient's quality of life. The nurse carefully explores the extent of disruption of the patient's lifestyle caused by the symptoms and evaluates the patient's emotional response to it. If the ability to communicate is impaired, the patient may feel socially isolated. The nurse assesses the nature and effectiveness of the patient's coping mechanisms. When either balance or hearing is affected, the patient's risk for injury increases, and use of appropriate safety measures is carefully explored.

Physical Examination

External Ear

The external ear is inspected for size, configuration, and angle of attachment to the head. The configuration of the pinna is observed for gross deformity. Whether the ears protrude and the degree of protrusion, the color of the skin of the ear, and whether any additional skin tags are present are noted. The skin of the ear should be smooth and without breaks or inflammation, especially behind the ear in the crevice. The presence of any lumps or skin lesions is documented by approximate size and location. The nurse also assesses all pierced ear holes for irritation or infection.

The pinna is palpated for the presence of tenderness or nodules. Palpation in the mastoid area may produce pain or discomfort that could indicate inflammation or infection. A normal mastoid bone is smooth, hard, and nontender, and the two sides are not always equal in size. For direct observation of the ear canal, the adult is asked to tip the head slightly to the opposite side while the nurse pulls the pinna up, back, and out. A penlight is used to inspect the ear canal for any abnormalities such as extreme narrowing, excessive wax, redness, scaliness, swelling, drainage, cysts, or foreign objects.

Tympanic Membrane

An otoscope is used to examine the tympanic membrane. An otoscope consists of a handle, a light source, a magnifying lens, and an attachment for visualizing the ear canal and eardrum. Some otoscopes have a pneumatic device for injecting

TABLE 59-1 Common Potentially Ototoxic Medications

Drug	Effect on the Auditory/Vestibular System
Aminoglycosides	Affect auditory and vestibular functions, usually related to persistently high drug levels; elderly patients, persons taking other ototoxic drugs, and persons with preexisting auditory loss most susceptible; damage may be reversible if detected early and drug discontinued; however, may be permanent
Gentamicin Tobramycin Streptomycin	Primarily affect vestibular function
Amikacin Neomycin Kanamycin	Primarily affect auditory function
Vancomycin	Elderly and those with hearing loss most susceptible; ototoxicity more common with high serum levels
Loop Diuretics	Rapid parenteral administration may cause hearing loss, deafness, or tinnitus
Furosemide Torsemide Bumetanide Ethacrynate sodium Ethacrynate acid	
Erythromycin	Hearing loss associated with IV administration of high doses, especially with patients with kidney failure
Salicylates	
Aspirin	Tinnitus, hearing loss, audiometric testing indicated before and/or after long-term therapy; elderly most susceptible; effects generally reversible
Nonsteroidal Antiinflammatory Drugs	Auditory function monitored before and during therapy to prevent ototoxicity; elderly most susceptible
Cisplatin	Tinnitus, high-frequency hearing loss
Quinine Sulfate	Tinnitus, impaired hearing; serum concentrations $\geq$10 mg/ml may confirm toxicity as cause of tinnitus or hearing loss

air into the ear canal to test the mobility and integrity of the eardrum.

The diameter of the meatus and the length of the ear canal vary; thus the speculum with the largest diameter that fits comfortably into the ear canal is chosen.

The otoscope is held with the dominant hand, which is braced lightly against the patient's head to decrease the risk of damage to the external canal if the patient moves suddenly. With the patient's head gently tilted away, the nurse uses the nondominant hand to pull the pinna up, back, and out to straighten the ear canal while slowly and carefully inserting the speculum into the ear canal (Figure 59-5). The otoscope is moved in a circular fashion to allow for visualization of the entire ear canal.[3] It should not touch the bony walls of the auditory canal as this will be painful. The cartilaginous portion of the canal is normally not tender.

Any abnormalities such as extreme narrowing of the ear canal, nodules, redness, scaliness, swelling, drainage, cysts, foreign objects, or excessive wax are noted.[3] Color and consistency of cerumen, which are genetically determined, are also noted. Dark sticky cerumen is common in Caucasians and African-Americans, whereas flaky, dry cerumen that is light brown to gray is commonly found in Asian-Americans and Native-Americans. Sometimes the ear canal must be cleaned of wax, dead skin, and other debris before the eardrum can be visualized. Hearing remains normal even when 90% to 95% of the ear canal is blocked with cerumen. Total occlusion creates a sudden hearing loss or feeling of fullness in the ear.

The normal eardrum is slightly conical, shiny and smooth, and pearly gray in color. The position of the drumhead is oblique to the ear canal. In the presence of disease the color of the eardrum changes, and other abnormalities such as retraction, bulging, perforation, or a white plaque in the eardrum may be present.[7] The entire eardrum is carefully inspected, including the border or the annulus. The umbo and the long and short process of the malleus should be easily visible through the eardrum.

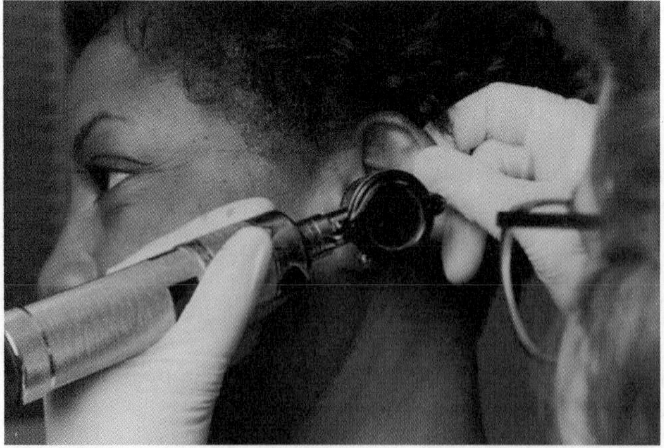

Figure 59-5 Otoscopic examination. The external auditory canal is straightened by pulling the auricle up and back to examine the ear with the otoscope.

The mobility of the eardrum is tested by injecting a small puff of air into the ear canal with the pneumatic device on the otoscope. Gentle movement of the eardrum should occur.

Middle Ear

Assessment of the middle ear involves evaluating hearing and inspecting the middle ear through the tympanic membrane with the otoscope. Gross assessment of hearing can be accomplished through general conversation and whisper tests that compare one ear to the other. Tuning forks are also used to assess hearing. Typical tuning fork tests are the Weber and Rinne tests (see Special Tests and Figures 59-7 and 59-8).

Inner Ear

The inner ears are not accessible to direct examination. However, some inferences about their condition can be made based on auditory and vestibular function. Thus the physical examination should include not only a gross assessment of the patient's hearing as discussed in previous paragraphs, but also balance testing, which assesses the vestibular function of the inner ear.

DIAGNOSTIC TESTS

Assessment of Balance

Balance and equilibrium depend on four systems being intact: the vestibular (the labyrinth or inner ear), the proprioceptive (somatosensors of joints and muscles), the visual (the eye), and the cerebellar (coordination). Sensations transmitted from the muscles and joints and the inner ears are integrated in the brainstem and cerebellum and perceived in the cerebral cortex. Dizziness is most likely to occur when two or more systems are impaired simultaneously or when they transmit sensory information that is contradictory.

Balance is assessed by observation of gait, the gaze test for nystagmus, and the Romberg test.

Gait is tested by asking the patient to walk away from the nurse and then turn and walk back. Posture, balance, swinging of the arms, and movement of the legs are all observed. To test for nystagmus, which is the involuntary, rhythmic oscillation of the eyes associated with vestibular dysfunction, the finger of the examiner is placed directly in front of the patient at eye level, and the patient is asked to follow the finger without moving the head. The finger is moved slowly from the midline toward the ear in each direction and the eyes are observed for any jerking movements.

For a Romberg test, the patient stands with feet together and the arms at the sides first with the eyes open and then with the eyes closed (Figure 59-6). The ability to maintain an upright posture with eyes closed is assessed. Normally only a minimal amount of swaying occurs. A loss of balance (positive Romberg test) may indicate an inner ear problem (vestibular problem) or cerebellar ataxia. Assessment of gait, nystagmus, and the Romberg test is discussed in more detail in Chapter 41.

Assessment measures and variations in normal findings relevant to the care of older adults are presented in the Gerontologic Assessment box. Also identified are disorders common in older adults, which may be responsible for abnormal assessment findings.

Laboratory Tests

Routine blood and urine tests rarely provide significant information related to disease of the ears. An elevated white blood cell count indicates an infection but is not diagnostic of ear disease. Drainage from the ear canal can be cultured to identify specific organisms causing infection. Cultures are important for treatment of acute infections, but are less helpful with long-term drainage because gram-negative bacilli cover up the original pathogen.

When clear fluid is found in the ear, it is important to rule out the presence of cerebrospinal fluid. Fistulas, skull fractures, and other head injuries can cause leakage of cerebrospinal fluid with the accompanying risk of meningitis. Cerebrospinal fluid tests positive for glucose on a reagent strip and feels "slippery" to the touch.

Radiologic Tests

Computed Tomography

Computed tomography (CT) scanning can be used to evaluate the temporal bone in thin sections or slices producing more and smaller components than a plain film x-ray. The CT scan can also be done with a contrast medium to improve the imaging of vascular lesions and to increase the clarity of the images. The person is carefully assessed for any allergy to iodine, shellfish, or contrast media, and the nurse prepares the patient for what to expect during the test.

Magnetic Resonance Imaging

Magnetic resonance imaging (MRI) uses a large magnet rather than ionizing radiation to emit energy. MRI effectively details soft tissues. Therefore the membranous organs, nerves, and blood vessels of the temporal bone can be examined. The nurse carefully prepares the patient for the expected sensory experiences associated with MRI, including loud pounding noises and often some sense of claustrophobia. Newer MRI machines make less noise, which makes them more comfortable for the patient.

Arteriography and Venography

Adjuncts to radiography are arteriography and venography in which contrast medium is injected into blood vessels. These studies are especially useful for diagnosing vascular abnormalities in the temporal bone. Compression of the vessels can be recognized, and tumors of the temporal bone and related structures can be recognized in greater detail.[9]

Special Tests

Auditory Acuity Tests

Whispered Voice Test. The patient occludes one ear with a finger and the nurse softly whispers two-syllable words toward the unoccluded ear. The patient is then asked to repeat the words. The intensity of the nurse's voice can be increased from a soft, medium, or loud whisper to a soft, medium, or loud

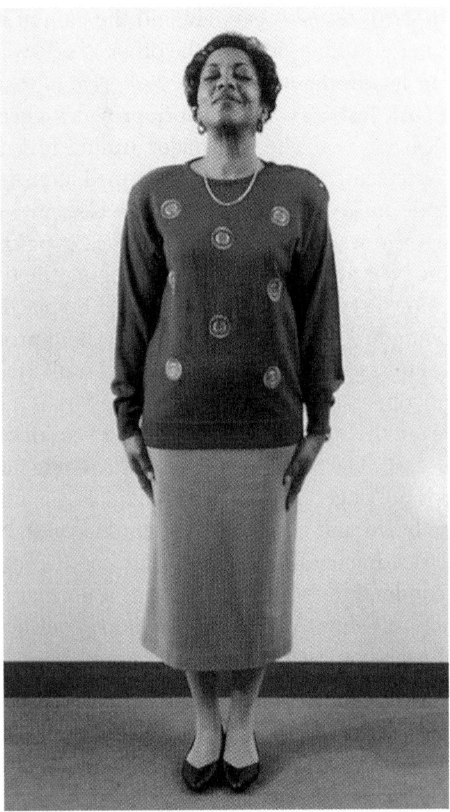

Figure 59-6 Evaluation of balance with the Romberg test. Person maintains balance with eyes closed.

Gerontologic Assessment

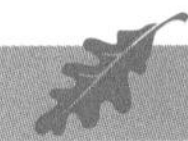

Assess the patient's level of functional hearing before beginning the health history and determine if any compensatory actions are needed (e.g., modulation of tone or speed of diction, adjustment of a hearing aid, involvement of a family member).
- Close to one third of people over age 65 have some type of hearing loss.

Inspect the external ear.
- The auricle may be enlarged and lack elasticity, earlobes may be pendulous, and a tuft of wiry hair may be present at the entrance to the external auditory canal.

Examine the external auditory canal and tympanic membrane with an otoscope.
- Impacted cerumen may be present because of decreased secretion, increased amounts of keratin, and stiff, coarse cilia, which result in cerumen that is harder and more easily impacted.
- Because of atrophy and retraction, the tympanic membrane may appear dull white or cloudy, and opaque with prominent landmarks.

COMMON DISORDERS IN ELDERS

Presbycusis
Impacted cerumen
Tinnitus
Presbyastasis
Conductive hearing loss
Sensorineural hearing loss

voice. Each ear is tested separately, and the patient is asked if hearing is better in one ear than the other. A soft whisper can normally be heard in both ears.

Tuning Fork Tests. The tuning fork provides a general estimate of hearing loss. The two major tuning fork tests date from the nineteenth century and are named after their originators: Rinne and Weber. The tuning fork is set into vibration by striking the tines on the examiner's knuckles or knee, holding only the base of the fork without touching the tines.

Rinne Test. The Rinne test is performed by placing the vibrating tuning fork against the patient's mastoid process (Figure 59-7, *A)* to assess bone conduction (BC) until the vibrating sound is no longer heard. The still vibrating fork is then placed 1 to 2 cm from the auditory canal to assess air conduction (AC) (Figure 59-7, *B)*. The patient is asked to inform the nurse when the sound is no longer heard. The nurse times the intervals the sounds are heard and compares the number of seconds. The results are documented using AC for air conduction and BC for bone conduction. AC>BC represents a normal finding of air conduction being twice as long as bone conduction. The test is performed on each ear.

The Rinne test is useful in differentiating between conductive and sensorineural hearing losses. When normal conduction pathways are blocked, transmission through the mastoid may be able to bypass the obstruction. Bone conduction therefore lasts longer than air conduction in these situations (BC>AC).

Weber Test. The vibrating tuning fork is placed on the patient's head or teeth (Figure 59-8). Placement on the teeth (even if the patient has false teeth) is generally more reliable. The patient is asked whether the tone is heard equally in both ears or is stronger in the right or left ear. Normally the sound should be heard equally in both ears. Lateralization, an abnormal finding, indicates the sound is heard better in one ear. The Weber test is useful in identifying patients with unilateral hearing loss. Table 59-2 presents the results of Weber and Rinne tests with normal hearing and with conductive and sensorineural hearing loss.

Pneumatoscopy

Pneumatoscopy tests the ability of the eardrum to respond to changes in air pressure introduced into the ear canal and the middle ear. A pneumatic otoscope is used to introduce air into the ear and to assess mobility of the tympanic membrane. The air causes the tympanic membrane to move in an out if it is intact. The membrane does not move if a perforation is present or if there is fluid in the middle ear space.[8]

Audiometric Hearing Tests

Audiometric hearing tests are conducted in a soundproof booth by an audiologist or trained technician. Hearing is measured in decibels, a logarithmic function of sound intensity. The sound is presented through an audiometer. The patient wears earphones and signals the audiologist when a tone

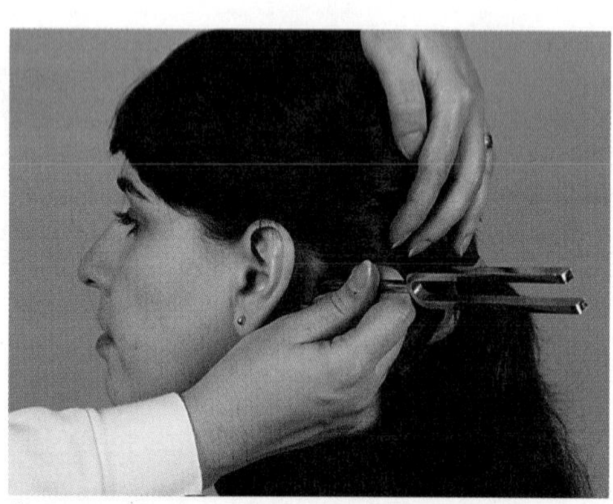

A

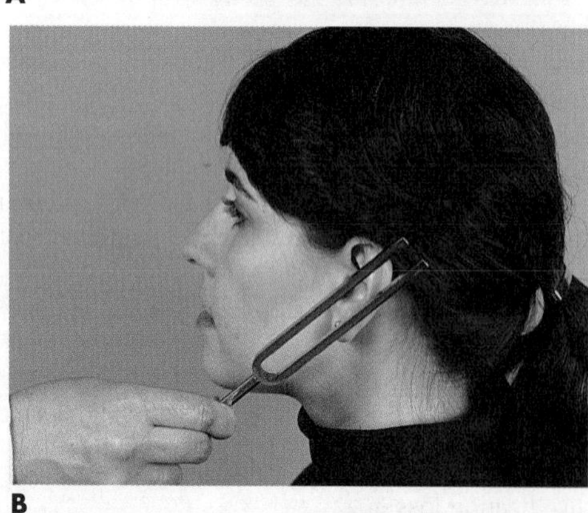

B

Figure 59-7 Rinne test. **A,** The vibrating tuning fork is placed on the mastoid bone for bone conduction. **B,** The vibrating tuning fork is placed in front of the ear for air conduction.

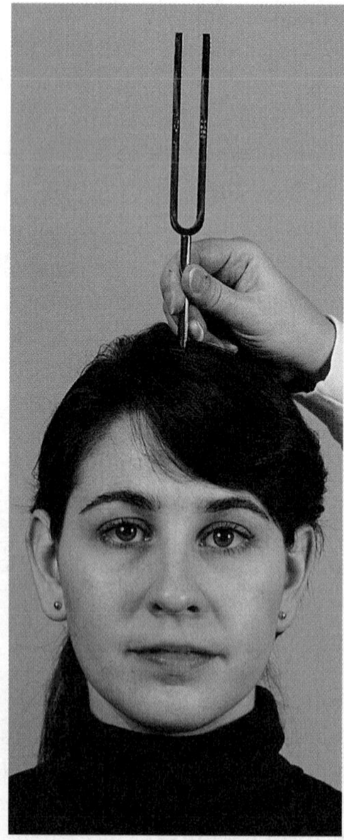

Figure 59-8 Weber test. The vibrating tuning fork is placed on the midline of the skull.

is heard by raising a hand or pushing a button. Responses are plotted on a graph called the audiogram.

Pure-tone audiometry is the standard measure of hearing acuity. To test air conduction, pure tones within the range of 250 to 8000 Hz are presented at varying intensities to one ear at a time, beginning with the better-hearing ear. For bone-conduction testing, tones are delivered through a bone conduction oscillator placed against the forehead or mastoid process while masking noise is presented to the untested ear by an earphone to prevent it from participating in the test of the opposite ear. By presenting the sound in this way, the middle ear structures are bypassed, and a bone conduction level is established. The bone conduction level represents the level at which the cochlea can hear and is commonly referred to as the nerve hearing level. A person with normal hearing would have the same air conduction as bone conduction hearing levels. A difference in air and bone conduction levels is indicative of conductive hearing loss. If air and bone conduction levels are equal but not within the normal range, a sensorineural nerve hearing loss is present. It is quite common for a patient to have both conductive and sensorineural hearing loss, a condition called a mixed hearing loss. The speech audiometry/speech reception threshold test determines the lowest intensity at which the patient can hear and correctly repeat 50% of a list of two-syllable words presented through earphones. The result usually corresponds closely to the air-conduction threshold.

In the Speech Discrimination Test, a list of 50 monosyllabic words is presented through earphones to the patient. The score indicates the percentage of words that the patient can hear and repeat correctly.

Impedance Audiometry. Impedance audiometry or tympanometry can be used for differentiating problems in the middle ear. The test applies pressure to the tympanic membrane and measures the result, creating a distinctive tracing on a graph called a tympanogram. Abnormalities of the tympanogram indicate problems of the middle ear, eustachian tube, or the ossicles. Tympanometry can also be used to measure the stapedial muscle reflex and the status of the acoustic nerve.[5] With pathologic conditions of the cochlea, acoustic reflexes often occur at less intense stimulation levels. With a retrocochlear lesion, the reflex thresholds are elevated or even absent. With conductive hearing loss, the reflex thresholds may be elevated but usually are absent. The nurse thoroughly explains all aspects of the test before its start.

Auditory Brainstem Response. Brainstem auditory evoked potential testing assesses dysfunction of the auditory nervous system at the level of the eighth cranial nerve (acoustic nerve), pons, or midbrain. Evoked potentials measure and record changes in brain electrical activity that occur in response to auditory sensory stimulation. The test involves placing electrodes on the vertex, mastoid process, or earlobes while the patient is seated in a comfortable chair. Test data are fed into a computer. Abnormal findings suggest dysfunctions at the various levels in the auditory nervous system, for example, a lesion of the acoustic nerve or brainstem.

Seventh cranial nerve (facial nerve) testing may also be performed. Tests of the seventh cranial nerve are related to audiometric tests because the facial and acoustic nerves share the internal acoustic canal. The facial nerve is tested in the same way as other motor nerves with nerve conduction tests and muscle excitability tests. The auxiliary functions of the facial nerve (taste and tearing) can also be measured. The facial and acoustic nerves are usually both involved when lesions involve the temporal bone.

Balance Testing

Electronystagmography. Electrophysiologic tests can be used to test balance and the status of the vestibular system in assessing the causes of dizziness, vertigo, and tinnitus. They can suggest the presence and location of central or peripheral lesions.

In some settings the tests are performed by audiologists, because of the close physical proximity of the vestibular and cochlear systems in the labyrinth. Although the physical assessment of balance is important, the most common objective measurement of balance is accomplished by electronystagmography, which measures nystagmus in response to stimulation of the vestibular system. The patient is tested at rest, and electrodes are placed on the head. The patient is tested in different positions and with different temperatures (Caloric Test) in the ear canals, thus stimulating the semicircular canals. The test results create an electronystagmogram that reflects the status of each labyrinth.

TABLE 59-2 Tuning Fork Tests for Auditory Acuity

Site of Problem	Weber Test	Rinne Test
Normal Hearing		
No problem	Tone heard in center of head	Air conduction lasts twice as long as bone conduction
Conductive Loss		
External or middle ear	Tone heard in poorer ear because ear not distracted by room noise	Bone conduction lasts longer than air conduction
Sensorineural Loss		
Inner ear	Tone heard in better ear because inner ear less able to receive vibrations	Air conduction lasts longer than bone conduction

The patient is instructed to discontinue any vestibular sedatives or tranquilizers and to avoid alcohol use for at least 24 hours before the test. Patients are also cautioned to avoid a heavy meal before the test because vertigo and nausea may be stimulated. Because the electrodes are placed with conduction paste, the patient is assisted in washing his or her hair after the procedure.

Platform Posturography. Platform posturography is a computerized test performed while the person is standing on a platform surrounded by a screen. Postural control is evaluated under six conditions such as both platform and screen moving, both stationary, and platform moving with screen stationary etc. The platform test helps to identify, quantify, and localize the source of balance disorders by separating the balance problem into inner ear, visual, and muscle stretch origins. The nurse explains the procedure and the sensations the patient can expect. Although painless, the test can cause vertigo and nausea. Sedatives, tranquilizers, and alcohol can alter the test results and should be restricted before the procedure.

References

1. Bailey BJ: *Head and neck surgery in otolaryngology,* ed 2, vol 2, 1903-1910, Philadelphia, 1998, JB Lippincott.
2. Bennett JC, Plumb F: *Cecil textbook of medicine,* ed 20, vol 2, Philadelphia, 1996, WB Saunders.
3. Bickley LS: *Bates' guide to physical examination and history taking,* ed 7, Philadelphia, 1999, JB Lippincott.
4. Fook L, Morgan R: Hearing impairment in older people: a review, *Postgrad Med J* 76(899):537, 2000.
5. Lilley LL, Aucker RS: *Pharmacology and the nursing process,* ed 2, St Louis, 1999, Mosby.
6. Pelton SI: Otoscopy for the diagnosis of otitis media, *J Pediatr Infect Dis* 17:540, 1998.
7. Preston K: Pneumatic otoscopy: a review of the literature, *Iss Comp Pediatr Nurs* 21(2):117, 1998.
8. Weissman JL, Hirsch BE: Imaging of tinnitus: a review, *Radiology* 216(2):342, 2000.
9. Wilson SF, Giddens JF: *Health assessment for nursing practice,* ed 2, St Louis, 2001, Mosby.

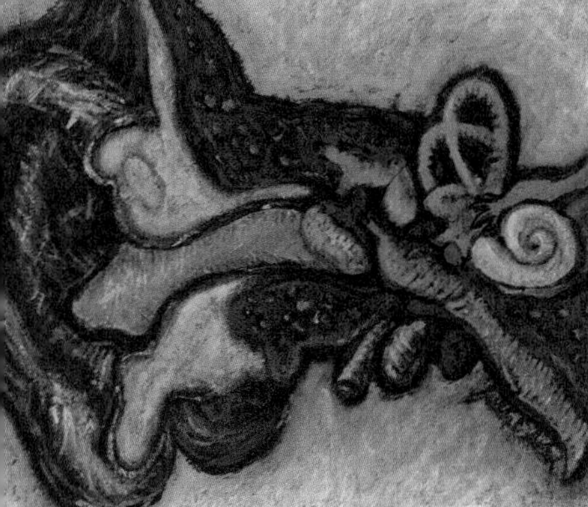

Problems of the Ear 60

Carol Meadows, Frances D. Monahan

Objectives

After studying this chapter, the learner should be able to:

1. Identify three measures that are important in preventing hearing loss.
2. Compare the etiologies and assessment features of conductive and sensorineural hearing loss.
3. Contrast the pathophysiology and nursing care of patients with external and middle ear infections.
4. Discuss the preoperative and postoperative care of the patient undergoing ear surgery.
5. Relate the signs and symptoms of Meniere's disease to its underlying pathology.
6. Develop strategies for communicating with a hearing-impaired person.
7. Describe common clinical manifestations of ear dysfunction.

A wide range of disorders can affect the ear. These include infections, tumors, and trauma. However, hearing loss is by far the most common and important ear problem affecting adults. Any problem with the ear threatens its function and acuity and hence, the ability of the individual to interact effectively with the environment. Selected ear disorders can also create problems with an individual's sense of balance.

HEARING LOSS

Etiology/Epidemiology

Hearing loss has become the nation's number one disability, affecting more than 10 million Americans.[7] Hearing impairment ranges from difficulty in understanding words or hearing certain sounds to total deafness.

Hearing impairment can hinder communication with others, limit social activities, and negatively impact employment. Hearing loss diminishes the individual's aesthetic enjoyment of major aspects of daily living and can adversely affect quality of life.[9]

Hearing loss is a symptom rather than a specific disease or disorder and can be the result of mechanical, sensory, or neural problems. The major types of hearing loss are:

Conductive Hearing Loss: Loss of hearing from a mechanical problem in the outer or middle ear that interferes with conduction of sound waves

Sensorineural Hearing Loss: Loss of hearing involving the cochlea and auditory nerve

Neural Hearing Loss: A sensorineural hearing loss originating in the nerve or brainstem

Fluctuating Hearing Loss: A sensorineural hearing loss that varies with time

Sensory Hearing Loss: A sensorineural hearing loss originating in the cochlea and involving the hair cells and nerve endings

Sudden Hearing Loss: A sensorineural hearing loss with a sudden onset

Central Hearing Loss: Loss of hearing from damage to the brain's auditory pathways or auditory center

Mixed Hearing Loss: Elements of both conductive and sensorineural hearing loss

Functional Hearing Loss: Loss of hearing for which no organic lesion can be found

Figure 60-1 illustrates the relationship between the anatomic location of the causative problem and the type of hearing loss that results. Some problems causing conductive hearing loss can be treated with medicine or surgery to either restore hearing or to minimize permanent hearing loss. However, the vast majority of persons with a hearing impairment cannot be treated effectively because 80% of all hearing impairments are caused by nerve deafness for which, at present, there is no known cure.

Hearing loss can also be classified according to severity. The decibel (dB) is a measure of the loudness or intensity of sound. A hearing loss of 15 to 50 dB is a mild to moderate loss and the person with a hearing loss in this range is said to be hearing impaired. A loss of 50 to 80 dB is a severe hearing loss. A loss of more than 80 dB in both ears is a profound hearing loss, and the patient may be referred to as deaf.

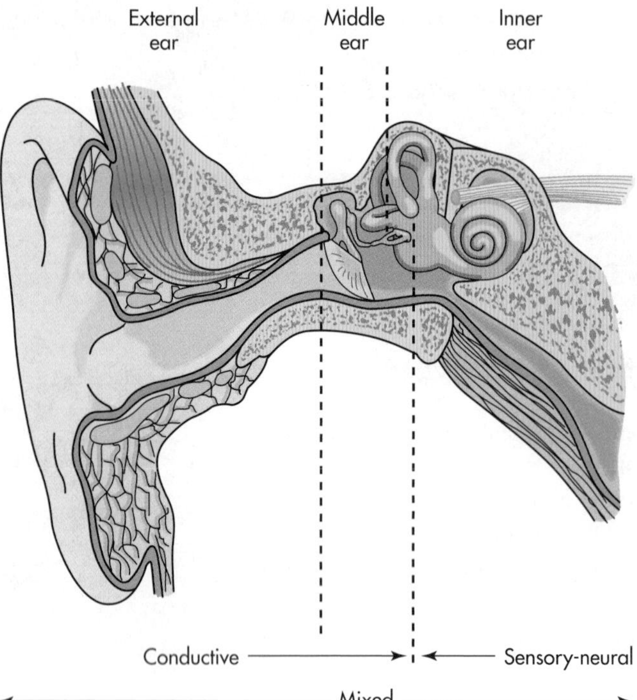

Figure 60-1 Three types of hearing loss. Conductive loss results from interference with conduction in the external and middle ear, sensorineural loss results from interference with conduction in the inner ear, and missed hearing loss results from interference with conduction.

Pathophysiology

Conductive hearing loss results from interference with the conduction of sound impulses through the external auditory canal, the tympanic membrane, or the ossicles of the middle ear. Conductive hearing loss may be caused by anything that blocks the external ear such as wax, infection, or a foreign body. It may also be caused by thickening, retraction, scarring, or perforation of the tympanic membrane or any pathophysiologic change in the middle ear that affects or fixes one or more of the ossicles. Examples of the latter include tumors, scar tissue from previous surgery, and otosclerosis.

Sensorineural hearing loss results from disease or trauma to the inner ear, neural structures, or nerve pathways leading to the brainstem. Disease that results in sensorineural hearing loss may be systemic or local, and in some cases may be drug induced. Systemic diseases, which can cause sensorineural hearing loss, include diabetes mellitus, arteriosclerosis, and infectious disease such as measles, mumps, and meningitis. Local disorders that can cause sensorineural deafness include neuromas of cranial nerve VIII, otospongiosis (form of progressive deafness caused by the formation of new abnormal spongy bone in the labyrinth), trauma to the head or ear, or degeneration of the organ of Corti, which occurs most commonly with advancing age.

A rare form of sensorineural hearing loss is central deafness, also known as central auditory dysfunction. In this disorder hearing ability remains intact, but the patient is deaf because the central nervous system is unable to interpret normal auditory stimuli. Central deafness can result from tumors or a cerebrovascular accident.

Hearing loss as a result of exposure to noise accounts for the major proportion of hearing impairment among people between the ages of 35 and 65. If hearing loss results from a single exposure to a sudden loud noise or blast, it is referred to as acoustic trauma. More commonly, hearing loss occurs over time from repeated injury from noise[8] in which case it is referred to as *noise-induced hearing loss.*

Occupational noise is a primary cause of noise-induced hearing loss in Western society. Other causes of noise-induced hearing loss include the use of firearms and high-intensity music. Noise from rock bands can exceed 120 dB, and hearing losses have been measured in some members of these bands. In the United States, the Occupational Safety and Health Administration (OSHA) has established acceptable noise levels for work environments. In general, exposure to noise levels in excess of 90 dB over an 8-hour day is considered excessive and should be avoided. Ordinary speech is about 50 dB and heavy traffic about 70 dB; above 80 dB, noise becomes uncomfortable to the human ear. Exposure to levels greater than 85 to 90 dB for months or years can cause cochlear damage. Whatever the cause, noise-induced hearing loss is characterized by a greater loss in the higher frequencies with the ability to distinguish sounds such as "s," "sh," "f," "th," and "ch" impaired first. The sensory cells in the ear are progressively destroyed, and the problem cannot be medically or surgically repaired. The only treatment is to prevent the injury by avoiding noise or by wearing ear protection. OSHA regulations require that workers exposed to noise above the designated limits must wear ear protection to decrease the risk of noise-induced hearing loss.

Presbycusis is a hearing loss associated with aging that becomes more common after age 50. Changes in the delicate labyrinthine structures over the decades cause a hearing loss predominantly in the higher frequencies. The incidence of presbycusis increases with age, and the disorder affects almost 50% of persons age 85 years and older.[3] In some persons the amount of hearing loss warrants the use of a hearing aid. Presbycusis cannot be cured.

Tinnitus, which is defined as a ringing or other noise in the ear, accompanies most sensorineural hearing losses and is often a warning of impending or worsening hearing loss[4] (see Research box). Persistent tinnitus is extremely annoying. The only cure for tinnitus is to correct the underlying condition.

Collaborative Care Management

A hearing loss in one ear is more difficult to detect than bilateral loss. Unilateral hearing loss may be noticed only when using a telephone or when having difficulty determining the direction of sounds. Often, hearing loss first is detected by a family member rather than by the affected person. Behavioral cues suggesting loss of hearing are found in Box 60-1, and assessment questions related to hearing status are found in the accompanying section on obtaining a health history. Because the auditory nerve does not regain function, early detection and evaluation of any hearing loss are important. Routine

Research

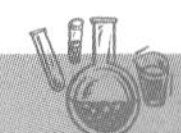

Reference: Griest SE, Bishop, PM: Tinnitus as an early indicator of permanent hearing loss, *AAOHN J* 45(7):325-329, 1998.

This longitudinal, retrospective study was designed to evaluate tinnitus (ringing or other sounds in the ears or head) as a potential early indicator of permanent hearing loss in a population of workers exposed to noise. Data were examined from 91 male employees working in environments with noise levels ranging from 8 hour time weighted averages of 85 to 101 dB over 15 years. Results of annual audiometric testing were obtained as part of an ongoing hearing conservation program conducted since 1971 by ESCO Corporation, a steel foundry located in the Portland, Oregon metropolitan area. Results indicated the prevalence of tinnitus increases more than 2.5 times for workers experiencing maximum threshold shifts greater or equal to 15 dB in hearing level. Results also provide evidence that reports of tinnitus at the time of annual audiometric testing may be useful in identifying workers at greater risk for developing significant shifts in hearing thresholds.

hearing assessment should be a part of the annual physical examination of all persons over age 40 because aging is associated with degenerative changes in the ear. When indicated additional diagnostic testing is done as described in Chapter 59. Because a variety of diseases and disorders affect the ear and the majority of persons with ear problems experience some degree of hearing loss, any disease that causes prolonged ear symptoms such as pain, swelling, drainage, a "plugged" feeling, or decreased hearing should be promptly assessed by a health care provider. Many chronic problems such as perforations and necrotic ossicles can be prevented with prompt and adequate medical attention.

Hearing aids offer assistance to many individuals with hearing impairments. Hearing aids amplify sound in a controlled manner and are used by both hard-of-hearing and deaf persons. While hearing aids make sound louder, they do not improve the ability to hear. As a result, amplification of background noise can create confusion, especially in crowded settings. Persons with decreased discrimination (ability to understand what is spoken) have limited benefit from the use of a hearing aid.

The evolution in hearing aid development has led to smaller and more effective aids. Hearing aids currently are available that fit into the ear canal, fit within the ear concha, or fit behind the ear. Special hearing aids can transmit sound by radio waves to the opposite ear or by vibration to the inner ear through the skull. Regardless of the type, the hearing aid consists of the following parts:

1. Microphone to receive sound waves from the air and change sounds into electrical signals
2. Amplifier to increase the strength of the electrical signals
3. Battery to provide the electrical energy needed to operate the hearing aid
4. Receiver (loudspeaker) to change the electrical signals back into sound waves

Figure 60-2 illustrates several common types of hearing aids.

BOX 60-1 Questions to Assess Vertigo

When did the dizziness first occur?
Did the dizziness start suddenly or gradually?
Is the dizziness constant, or does it come in "attacks"?
How often do the attacks occur?
How long do the attacks last?
List anything that stops an attack of dizziness or makes it better.
Overall, has the dizziness gotten better or worse since starting?
List anything that brings on an attack of dizziness or makes it worse.
Does the dizziness occur only in certain positions?
Do any other symptoms occur simultaneously with the dizziness such as nausea, vomiting, or ear pressure?
Does stress have any relationship to the dizziness?
Have you ever fallen because of the dizziness?
Do you get dizzy after heavy lifting, straining, exertion, or overwork?
Do you get dizzy if you have not eaten for a long time?
For women: Is your dizziness connected with your menstrual cycle?
How has the dizziness affected the quality of your life?

Adapted from Sigler BA, Schuring L: *Ear, nose, and throat disorders*, St Louis, 1993, Mosby.

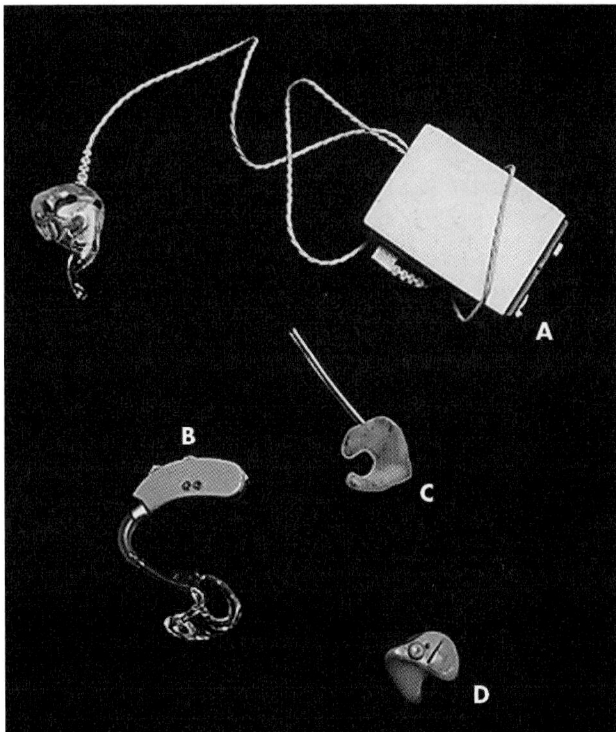

Figure 60-2 Types of hearing aids. **A,** Older aid with a battery pack worn on the body and a wire connected to the ear mold. **B,** Behind-the-ear battery with ear mold. **C,** Small ear canal mold with battery. **D,** Newer, smaller mold worn in the ear canal.

Implantable Hearing Devices. There are three types of implanted hearing devices: cochlear implants, bone conduction devices, and fully or semiimplantable hearing aids.[2]

Cochlear implant devices directly stimulate the auditory nerve and are used to provide sound awareness for persons with sensorineural hearing loss originating in the organ of Corti. The device does not allow the person to hear speech but creates an awareness of environmental sounds such as door bells or telephones and also provides auditory clues that facilitate lip reading. Cochlear implant devices have both internal and external components. The internal components include one or more electrodes implanted into or onto the cochlear, and a receiver implanted behind the auricle. The external components include a small microphone, a speech processor, and a transmitter coil with a magnet that holds it in place over the implanted receiver. Sound is picked up by the microphone and is sent to the processor, which converts it into electrical impulses. These impulses go on to the transmitter and then to the internal receiver, where further processing occurs. Finally they travel to the electrodes in the cochlea (Figure 60-3). The external components are put in place 4 to 6 weeks after surgery when the wound is healed so no change occurs in the patient's hearing until this time. Once in place, settings on the device must be calibrated to the individual patient's needs and a rehabilitation program completed. Typically the rehabilitation program includes care of the unit, simple auditory training, and speech reading practice with the added sounds from the implant. Length of rehabilitation varies but is usually 40 hours or more. Subsequently regular follow-up visits are needed for several years.[2]

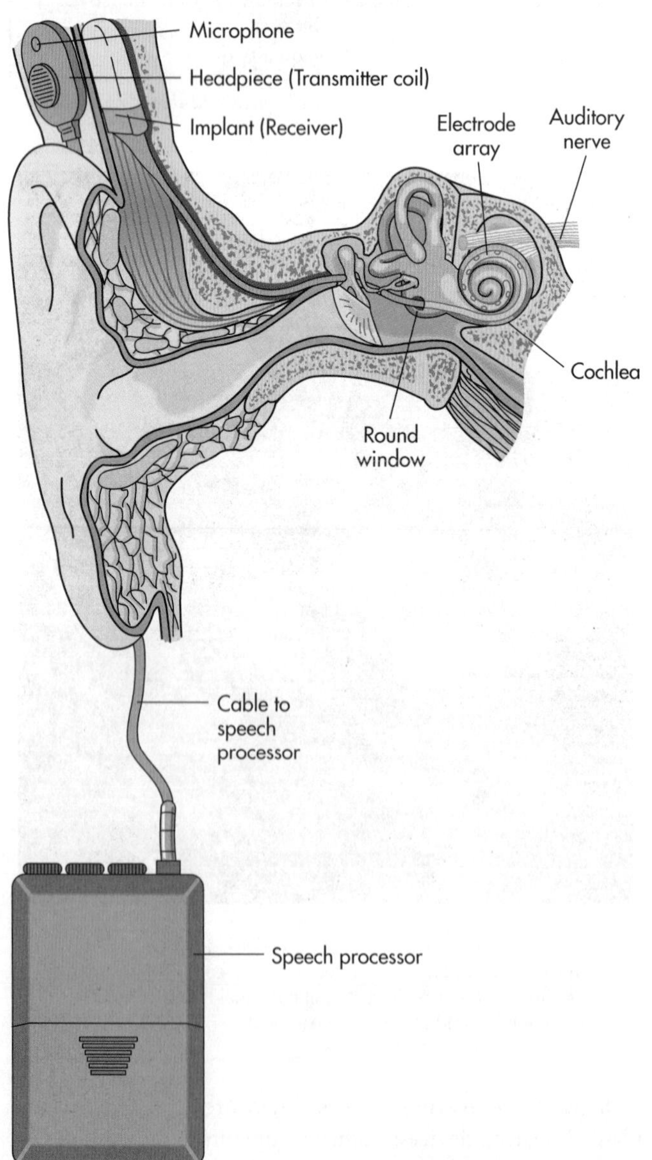

Figure 60-3 Cochlear implant is placed transmastoid through round window into the cochlea.

The best cochlear implants use multiple channels and are able to return about half the patient's hearing and understanding.

Bone conduction devices (Bone-anchored hearing aid [BAHA]) transmit sound through the skull to the inner ear.[2] One such device uses an orthopedic screw implanted under the skin into the skull. The external device transmits the sound through the skin and is worn above the ear and not in the ear canal. Patients who already use a hearing aid gain the most from the implantable device.

If hearing loss is irreversible and not amenable to surgical correction or if the person elects not to have surgery, aural rehabilitation may be recommended. Aural rehabilitation includes auditory training, speech reading, and speech training and is designed to maximize the hearing-impaired person's communication skills. Auditory training attempts to increase the hearing-impaired person's listening skills by fine tuning the person's ability to discriminate between similar sounds. Speech reading, formerly called lip reading, is a difficult skill to master but can be an important means of communication. Speech training focuses on the preservation of speech skills (pitch, clarity, and rate) to prevent deterioration as auditory feedback diminishes. Guidelines for communicating with hearing-impaired persons are summarized in the Guidelines for Safe Practice box.

Patient/Family Education. Hearing loss is a major health concern in the United States, and nurses play a major preventive role in interactions with all patients and families. Healthy People 2010 national health objectives related to hearing loss are to:

- Reduce to no more than 15% the proportion of workers exposed to average daily noise levels that exceed 85 dB.
- Reduce significant hearing impairment to a prevalence of no more than 82 per 1000 people, as measured by self-reported hearing impairment.

Individuals 45 years old and older are identified as special target populations.[10]

Prevention through education is key to achieving these goals. Patient education begins with an exploration of the patient's understanding of the role of noise in hearing loss. Explanation of the relationship between noise and hearing loss is provided as needed, and the use of protective ear covers in noisy environments is strongly recommended. The importance of maintaining moderate sound levels when listening to music, especially when using headphones, is stressed.

Patients should be taught to avoid inserting hard articles into the ear canal, obstructing the ear canal with any object, inserting unclean articles or solutions into the ear, and swimming in polluted water. Patients also should be taught that wax should not be cleaned out of the ear routinely. It should be explained that the ear canal is generally "self-cleaning." Wax is to the ears what tears are to the eyes; it serves as a protective mechanism. Earwax lubricates the skin and traps foreign material that enters the canal. The external ear may be washed with soap and water daily while bathing or showering, but cotton-tipped applicators or other objects should not be used to clean the ear. The ear canal and eardrum can be easily damaged, and the applicator may push accumulated wax against the eardrum.

The person with a hearing aid needs to be taught how to care for the aid and what to do if the aid does not work. The nurse must also have a basic knowledge of the hearing aid to assist the person who is unable or unwilling to do this when ill. The person is encouraged to use the hearing aid and to store it safely in its case when it is not in use. The Guidelines for Safe Practice box at right presents key points of hearing aid care and trouble-shooting suggestions.

Patients taking drugs that are ototoxic (see Table 59-1) (i.e., that damage the cochlea, the vestibule of the ear, the labyrinth, or the eighth cranial nerve) need to know that symptoms such as dizziness, decreased hearing acuity, and/or tinnitus should be promptly reported.

Guidelines for Safe Practice

Communicating With the Hearing-Impaired Patient

1. Get the person's attention by touching him or her lightly, flickering the room lights, or raising an arm or hand.
2. Stand facing the patient with the light on your face; this will help the person speech (lip) read.
3. Speak slowly and clearly, but do not overaccentuate words.
4. Speak in a normal tone; do not shout. Shouting overuses normal speaking movements and may cause distortion. If the person has a conductive loss, making the voice louder without shouting may be helpful.
5. Alert the person to the topic before beginning the discussion to enable use of contextual clues.
6. If the person does not seem to understand what is said, express it differently. Some words are difficult to "see" in speech reading, such as white and red.
7. Do not smile, chew gum, or cover the mouth when talking to a person with limited hearing.
8. Use phrases to convey meaning rather than one-word answers. Supplement words with body language.
9. Do not show annoyance by careless facial expression. Persons who are hard of hearing depend more on visual clues.
10. Write out proper names or any statement that you are not sure was understood.
11. Encourage the use of a hearing aid if the person has one; allow him or her to adjust it before speaking.
12. Avoid the use of the intercom when communicating with the patient.
13. Do not avoid conversation with a person who has hearing loss.
14. Post a note at the bedside and nurses station alerting personnel that the person is hard of hearing.

PROBLEMS OF THE EXTERNAL EAR

The external ear may be affected by masses, trauma, wax impaction, and infection. External ear infection is by far the most common disorder and is discussed next. The other problems are summarized in Table 60-1.

External Ear Infection (External Otitis)

Etiology/Epidemiology

External otitis is an inflammation or infection of the external auditory canal or the auricle. It occurs more frequently in summer than in winter, and is usually bacterial or fungal in origin. Cultures indicate that the most common infecting bacteria are *Staphylococcus aureus, Escherichia coli, Proteus vulgaris,* and *Pseudomonas aeruginosa;* the most common infecting fungi are *Candida albicans* and the *Aspergillus* organisms. A localized form of this infection, which begins in the skin lining the ear canal, is a furuncle or abscess. In the presence of a systemic disease such as diabetes, external otitis can spread wildly through cartilage and bone and is then termed malignant external otitis. The most common forms of external otitis are (1) swimmer's ear, so called because it tends to occur when water remains in the ear canal, and (2) opportunistic fungal infection, which is most prevalent in warm, moist climates. Occasionally, infection involves only the cartilage of the auricle and is then called perichondritis. Necrosis of the cartilage and loss of the distinctive shape of the auricle occur if perichondritis is not treated quickly.

Pathophysiology

Local trauma such as picking the ear, contamination, or ongoing exposure to moisture produces an environment conducive to the overgrowth of normal flora. Pain (otalgia) in the

Guidelines for Safe Practice

Care of a Hearing Aid

1. Turn the hearing aid off when not in use.
2. Open the battery compartment at night to avoid accidental drainage of the battery.
3. Keep an extra battery available at all times.
4. Wash the earmold frequently (daily if necessary) with mild soap and warm water and use a pipe cleaner to cleanse the cannula.
5. Do not wear the hearing aid if an ear infection is present.

WHAT TO DO IF A HEARING AID FAILS TO WORK

1. Check the on-off switch.
2. Inspect the earmold for cleanliness.
3. Examine the battery for correct insertion.
4. Examine the cord plug for correct insertion.
5. Examine the cord for breaks.
6. Replace the battery, cord, or both, if necessary. The life of batteries varies according to amount of use and power requirements of the aid. Batteries last from 2 to 14 days.
7. Check the position of the earmold in the ear. If the hearing aid "whistles," the earmold is probably not inserted properly into the ear canal, or the person needs to have a new earmold made.

TABLE 60-1 Disorders of the External Ear

Disorder	Etiology	Collaborative Management
Masses Cysts Exostosis (bony protrusions) Infectious polyps Malignant tumors	Most cysts arise from sebaceous glands. Polyps typically arise from the middle ear or tympanic membrane. Malignant tumors are usually basal cell carcinomas on the pinna and squamous cell carcinomas in the canal.	Masses of all types are fairly rare, and, if treatment is indicated, surgical excision is performed. Squamous cell carcinomas can invade the underlying tissue and spread throughout the temporal bone.
Trauma	Both sharp and blunt force injuries are common. Penetrating injury can damage hearing, but infection and cosmetic appearance are more common concerns.	Supportive care and protection from infection are indicated. Cosmetic surgery may be needed.
Foreign bodies	Many options exist. Insects and cotton pieces are the most common.	Remove carefully aided by microscopic visualization. Insects are removed by filling the canal with mineral oil.
Pruritis	This frequent complaint in elders results from sebaceous gland atrophy and dry epithelium. Dry cerumen worsens the itching.	Daily application of glycerin or mineral oil drops decreases dryness and softens cerumen.
Impacted cerumen	This may result from use of cotton-tipped applicator or other object to clean the ear. Age-related drying of cerumen increases incidence.	Impacted wax is softened and loosened with alternating instillation of glycerine to soften and hydrogen peroxide to loosen the cerumen for removal by warm water irrigation.

Guidelines for Safe Practice

Performing an Ear Irrigation

Ear irrigations or washes are used to remove excess cerumen[4] or a foreign body from the ear (Figure 60-4).

1. Wash hands before and after the procedure.
2. Fill a 2- to 3-ounce ear syringe with the solution (water or a saline solution), warmed to body temperature (between 90° F and 100° F).
3. Position the patient lying on his or her side with the affected ear up or in a sitting position with an ear basin under the ear.
4. Gently pull the pinna back and up while placing the tip of the syringe gently into the ear canal. Do not be afraid to insert it into the ear.
5. Instill the solution from the syringe back semiforcefully into the ear. The fluid must actively move in the ear canal to be effective.
6. The patient may experience dizziness with movement; however, if procedure is painful, stop the ear wash.
7. Apply eardrops if instructed.
8. Continue to use the ear wash solution as instructed for about 2 weeks or until the ear is dry and without drainage.

NOTE: If not done by a health care provider, the procedure should be performed by a family member or significant other if possible. It cannot be performed effectively by the patient alone.

external ear is the most common symptom. Pain can be significant especially when palpating the ear because of the close proximity of bone (a hard surface). A clue to early external otitis is pain or tenderness when gently pulling on the pinna or putting pressure on the tragus. A forerunner of pain in external otitis is itching in the ear canal. Inflammation is easily identified with an otoscope. Early in the infection, drainage from the ear may be clear; later it may be serosanguinous or

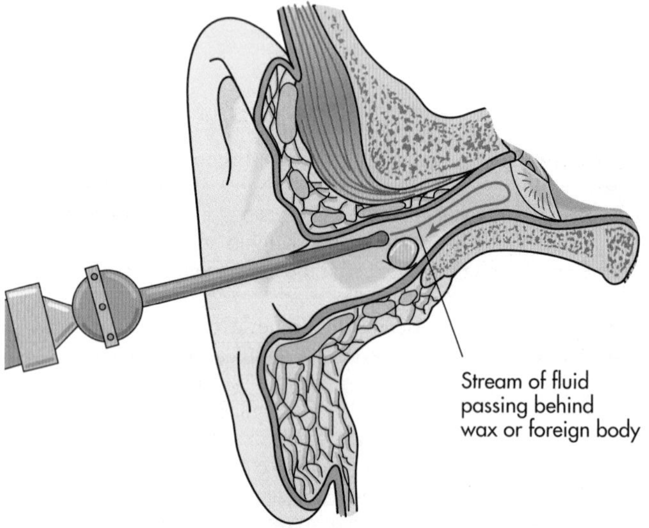

Figure 60-4 Ear irrigation.

purulent. Hearing may be impaired from swelling and accumulated debris in the canal. Dizziness also may occur.

Collaborative Care Management

Treatment for external otitis depends on the cause and extent of the infection. Local/topical antibiotics are the mainstay of treatment.[6] Systemic antibiotics may also be prescribed if the infection extends beyond the ear canal. If the ear canal is swollen shut, a "wick" made of a 1-inch length of $\frac{1}{4}$-inch wide gauze may be inserted to allow the antibiotic drops to penetrate the canal. Irrigations may be performed to remove infective debris (see Guidelines for Safe Practice box). Comfort measures such as mild analgesics and warm soaks are pro-

TABLE 60-2 Disorders of the Middle Ear and Mastoid

Disorder	Etiology	Collaborative Management
Perforated tympanic membrane	Perforations may occur acutely after trauma or as the result of chronic infection. Damage may extend to the ossicles and worsen the hearing loss.	Acute perforation may heal spontaneously. Infection is treated with appropriate local and/or systemic antibiotics. Surgical correction of the perforation may be performed: myringoplasty for the membrane or tympanoplasty if repair includes the middle ear structures. Grafts may be taken from the muscle fascia, a vein, or perichondrium. Success rate is high.
Otosclerosis (hardening of the ear)	Problem involves the stapes. Sclerotic bone forms on the stapes limiting its movement and resulting in conductive hearing loss. Underlying cause is unknown.	A hearing aid may be initially prescribed. Advanced disease is treated surgically through stapedectomy in which a prosthesis replaces the otosclerotic footplate. The success rate is high (Figure 60-5).
Mastoiditis	Chronic otitis media can result in the extension of the infection into the mastoid cavity. The volume of drainage from the middle ear increases.	Antibiotic therapy is the foundation of care, possibly supplemented by irrigations. Aggressive treatment is appropriate to prevent serious complications. Surgical mastoidectomy may be necessary in rare situations.

Guidelines for Safe Practice

Administering Ear Drops

1. Wash hands before and after the procedure.
2. Warm the ear drops to body temperature before administration. Dizziness may occur from insertion of drops that are too warm or too cold.
3. Instruct the patient to tilt the head so that the ear to be treated is up.
4. Straighten the ear canal by pulling the external ear up and back.
5. Instill prescribed number of drops to run along ear canal.
6. Press gently several times on the tragus of the ear to ensure proper instillation, or hold the head in position for 2 to 3 minutes.
7. Wipe the external ear with a cotton ball or tissue to prevent skin irritation.
8. A cotton ball may be placed in the ear but is not necessary.

vided to control the symptoms. Abscesses and perichondritis may require excision and drainage.

Patient/Family Education. The nurse instructs the patient/family in the safe administration of ear drops (see Guidelines for Safe Practice box). If an ointment is prescribed to control itching or inflammation, the patient is instructed to apply it using a cotton-tipped applicator, being certain not to insert the applicator any deeper into the ear than the cotton end. The need to use a new applicator each time is stressed.

The nurse also instructs the patient to avoid getting water in the ear by using earplugs or by placing cotton with Vaseline on it in the auditory meatus. If earplugs are used, thorough cleansing with alcohol or a mild detergent between uses is recommended to prevent reinfection. The patient should not swim during this time.

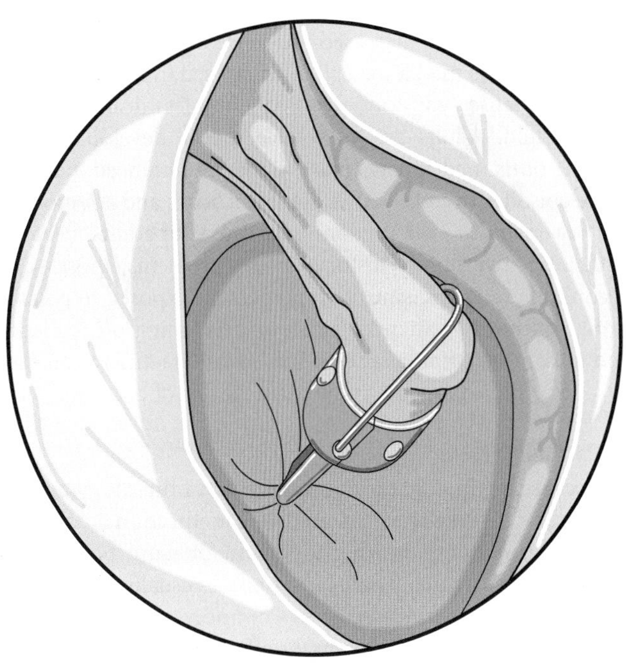

Figure 60-5 Stapedectomy with Robinson stainless steel prosthesis in place.

PROBLEMS OF THE MIDDLE EAR

Infection with its associated complications is the most common disorder of the middle ear, but masses, trauma, and other conditions may occur. The less common disorders of the middle ear are summarized in Table 60-2.

Middle Ear Infection (Otitis Media)

Etiology

Otitis media is a general term that refers to inflammation of the mucous membranes of the middle ear, eustachian tube, and mastoid. These mucous membranes are continuous with those of the respiratory tract, and thus infection can easily ascend to the ear. Otitis media is most often caused by various types of bacteria, although viral cases can occur.

There are three distinct types of otitis media: acute, chronic, and serous. Acute otitis media develops suddenly and is usually of short duration. Chronic otitis media is the result of recurrent or untreated infection and is usually characterized by drainage and perforation of the tympanic membrane. Serous otitis media is characterized by a collection of noninfectious fluid in the middle ear as a result of incomplete resolution of an acute infection, an allergic reaction, or an obstruction of the eustachian tube. If fluid is present within the ear for a protracted period of time, the tympanic membrane retracts, and adhesive otitis media may develop. Likewise, any long-term blockage of the eustachian tube can lead to adhesive otitis media and result in hearing loss.

Epidemiology

Otitis media is classically considered to be a childhood disorder associated with upper respiratory infection. The vast majority of cases occur in children from infancy to school age. The incidence is clearly increased during the colder months in association with the increased incidence of upper respiratory infection. Otitis media may go undiagnosed in the adult population because symptoms are frequently less dramatic than in the child. Adults are vulnerable to the development of chronic otitis media, particularly if they experienced multiple acute episodes in their youth. Staphylococcus and streptococcus organisms are the predominant causes in adults. Persons with a positive family history for ear problems, those with chronic allergies and sinusitis, and persons exposed to passive smoke all have an increased risk of developing otitis media and its complications as adults. Inadequate treatment can easily lead to the emergence of resistant strains of bacteria.

Pathophysiology

Because the middle ear transmits sound from the tympanic membrane to the inner ear, middle ear infection frequently causes a conductive hearing loss from pressure behind the tympanic membrane. The hearing loss is usually correctable with resolution of the infection. Common additional symptoms include throbbing pain in the affected ear, inflammation, fever, and drainage and bulging of the eardrum with possible perforation. Blood, pus, and other material may be present when perforation occurs. A thick yellow purulent discharge is a common finding with chronic otitis media. Tympanosclerosis, a deposit of collagen and calcium within the middle ear, can also result from repeated infection. The deposit can harden around the ossicles and contribute to a worsening of any conductive hearing loss. Because of the anatomy of the temporal bone, middle ear infection can, in rare cases, lead to a life-threatening brain abscess. Common symptoms of otitis media are summarized in the Clinical Manifestations box.

Collaborative Care Management

The diagnosis of otitis media is made based on the patient's symptoms and otoscopic examination of the ear, which readily reveals a bulging tympanic membrane and perforation or drainage if present.

Clinical Manifestations
Otitis Media

Throbbing pain in infected ear
Fever
Drainage: clear, bloody, or purulent
Bulging of the eardrum
Conductive hearing loss, usually reversible with effective treatment

Research

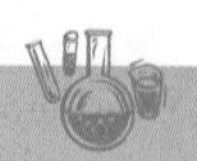

Reference: Tigges BB: Acute otitis media and pneumococcal resistance: making judicious management decisions, *Nurse Practitioner* 25(1):69, 73-80.

Based on a study of recent literature, the author concluded that the emergence of drug-resistant *Streptococcus pneumoniae* (DRSP) has implications for the primary care provider who treats acute otitis media (AOM) in children. AOM must be carefully distinguished from otitis media with effusion (OME). Antibiotic treatment for AOM is recommended because of the low rate of spontaneous resolution of *S. pneumoniae* infection and the risk of suppurative complications. Amoxicillin continues to be the first drug of choice. When the first course of antibiotics fails, the patient should be treated with amoxicillin-clavulanate, cefuroxime axetil, or ceftriaxone. Trimethoprim-sulfamethoxazole, the macrolides, and most of the cephalosporins have limited effectiveness against DRSP and should no longer have a major role in AOM treatment. OME need not be treated with antibiotics unless the effusion has been present for 3 to 4 months. Tympanostomy tubes are an effective treatment for both chronic OME and recurrent AOM.

Medications. Antibiotic therapy is the key to treatment of otitis media. Broad-spectrum antibiotics are used unless drainage is present that allows for culture of the organism and sensitivity testing (see Research box). Chronic infections frequently do not respond to the usual antibiotics and may require local treatment with irrigations and antibiotic ear drops. Drugs commonly used to treat otitis media are summarized in Table 60-3.

Treatments. An ear wash may be prescribed, particularly if chronic drainage is present that is irritating to the tissue of the ear canal. The most common solution used is boric acid and alcohol, which is obtained by prescription. The solution cleanses the ear of debris and infection and provides a drying agent. When the eustachian tube is chronically obstructed, it may be necessary to remove fluid from the middle ear. Myringotomies, with or without tubes, are performed to regain normal middle ear and eustachian tube function. Myringotomy involves making a tiny incision in the tympanic membrane through which the fluid can be suctioned out. To keep the incision open and prevent a reaccumulation of fluid, various types of transtympanic tubes can be inserted into the incision (Figure 60-6). These tubes fall out by themselves in 3 to 12 months and rarely have to be removed.

TABLE 60-3 Common Medications for Treatment of Otitis Media

Drug	Action	Intervention
Antibiotics: amoxicillin, trimethoprim sulfamethoxazole, amoxicillin-clavulanate, cefaclor	Inhibits cell wall synthesis, bacteriocidal	1. Assess for allergies or sensitivities. 2. Instruct patient to take medication around the clock, not to miss any doses, and to finish prescription completely. 3. Assess for superinfection.
Analgesic/antipyretic or narcotic analgesics: acetaminophen with codeine	Central nervous system (CNS) depressant, analgesic, antipyretic, antiinflammatory	1. Assess vital signs, especially temperature. 2. Caution patient not to drive or operate machinery if taking codeine; also not to take other CNS depressants, including alcohol, while taking medication. 3. Teach patient to increase fluid and roughage intake to avoid constipation. 4. Take medication with meals to decrease possible nausea. 5. Do not increase dose; assess effectiveness of pain relief.
	H_1-receptor antagonist, antiemetic, antitussive, anticholinergic, and local anesthetic actions	1. Monitor blood pressure (BP) in hypertensive patients. 2. Avoid driving a car or operating machinery until drug effects are determined. 3. Caution against alcohol use, which may cause an additive effect or drowsiness.
Decongestants: pseudoephedrine	Sympathomimetic, acts directly on smooth muscle, produces little congestive rebound that occurs with nasal sprays	1. Monitor heart rate and BP, especially in patient with cardiac history. 2. Teach patient not to take medication before bedtime because of stimulant effect. 3. Withhold medication if restlessness or tachycardia occurs. 4. Teach patient to avoid other over-the-counter medications, which may contain ephedrine.

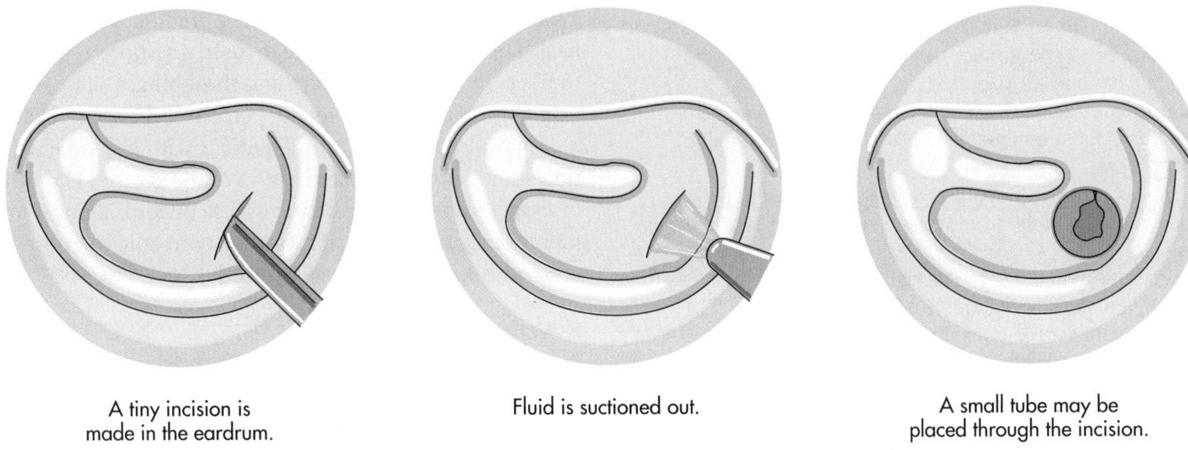

Figure 60-6 Myringotomy and transtympanic tube placement to prevent chronic serous otitis media.

Surgical Management. Surgical intervention may be necessary if attempts to control the infection medically are unsuccessful, and the ossicles become necrotic. Repairing the damage of middle ear infection requires a difficult microsurgical procedure. Tympano-ossiculoplasty repairs the necrotic ossicles and creates a new eardrum. The surgical procedure is still being refined, and a variety of middle ear prostheses are available (Figure 60-7). The surgical procedure is often performed in an ambulatory surgery center with the patient under local anesthesia and sedation. Tympano-ossiculoplasty is not always successful, but it does restore sound transmission for some patients (see Guidelines for Safe Practice box).

Diet. Diet does not play a role in the management of otitis media, but patients may modify their diet in response to symptoms. Increasing the daily intake of fluids is generally recommended in the presence of fever.

Activity. No particular activity restrictions are included in the management of middle ear infections. Patients who are experiencing significant ear pain and fever may be more comfortable resting and avoiding activity.

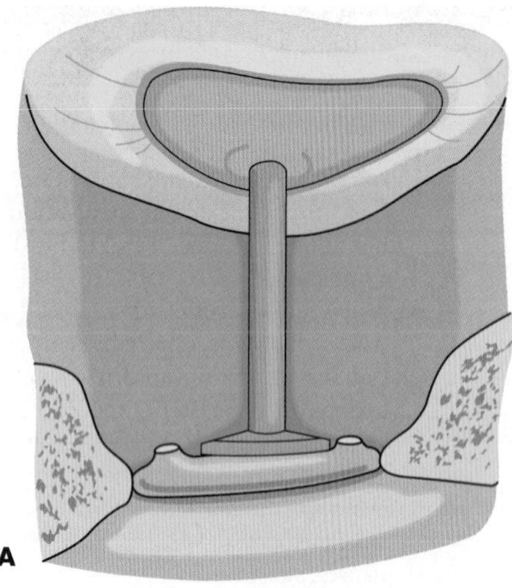

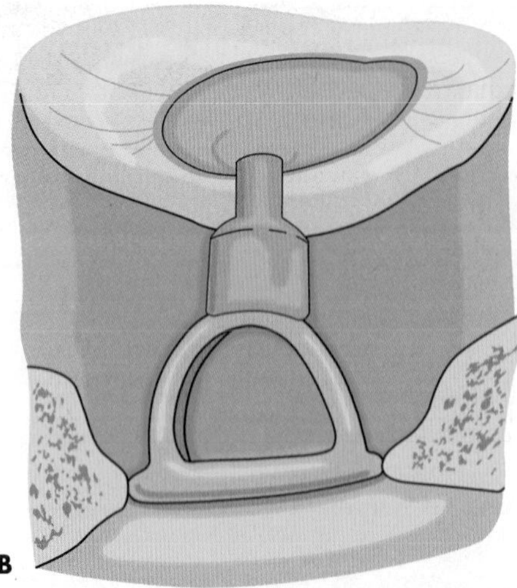

Figure 60-7 Middle ear prostheses. **A,** Schuring ossicle columnella prosthesis for total ossicular replacement surgery. **B,** Schuring ossicle cup prosthesis for incus replacement surgery.

Guidelines for Safe Practice

Ear Surgery

Most patients undergoing ear surgery have extremely short hospitalizations. Thus patient teaching is a major focus of nursing care. The patient must understand what to expect after discharge and how to promote healing during the recovery period.

The nurse explains to the patient that:

- Decreased hearing is expected initially from the presence of swelling and packing in the ear.
- Cracking or popping noises are commonly heard in the affected ear and are expected.
- Minor earache and discomfort in the cheek and jaw are common, but should be managed effectively with mild analgesics.
- Dizziness or lightheadedness may also be present initially, and caution must be used when getting out of bed and walking.
- Bleeding and drainage are negligible so a cotton ball frequently provides an adequate dressing.

Following surgery, the nurse instructs the patient to:

- Sneeze, cough, or blow nose with the mouth open as needed for the first week after surgery.
- Blow the nose gently as needed, one side at a time.
- Avoid vigorous activity until approved by the surgeon.
- Change cotton ball dressing as prescribed.
- Report any drainage other than a slight amount of bleeding to the surgeon.
- Keep ear dry for 6 weeks after surgery.
  - Do not shampoo the hair without a barrier.
  - Protect the ear when necessary with two pieces of cotton (outer piece saturated with petrolatum).
- Avoid loud noisy environments.
- Balance ear pressure as needed by holding nose, closing mouth, and swallowing.
- Avoid air travel until cleared by the surgeon.
- AVOID HEAVY LIFTING, STRAINING, OR VIGOROUS ACTIVITY FOR 3 WEEKS.

Referrals. Referrals are not necessary for patients with acute otitis media that responds promptly to treatment with antibiotics. Patients with chronic otitis media may be referred to a surgeon for correction of complications or to an audiologist if extensive hearing loss occurs.

NURSING MANAGEMENT

ASSESSMENT

When assessing the patient with a middle ear infection, the health history should include focused questions related to pain in the ear that is often severe and throbbing, a sense of fullness or pressure in the ear, and any perceived change in hearing.

Physical assessment of the patient with a middle ear infection should focus on examination of the ear for (1) drainage—bloody, serous, or purulent; (2) inflamed, bulging tympanic membrane; and (3) perforation of tympanic membrane. The patient should also be assessed for fever.

NURSING DIAGNOSES

Nursing diagnoses are determined from analysis of patient data. Nursing diagnoses for the patient with a middle ear infection may include but are not limited to:

Diagnostic Title	Possible Etiologic Factors
1. Acute pain	Infection, buildup of fluid in ear spaces, swelling, trauma
2. Deficient knowledge: treatment of otitis, self-care after surgery	Lack of exposure to information and skills

EXPECTED PATIENT OUTCOMES

Expected patient outcomes for the person with a middle ear infection may include but are not limited to:

1. Will state that pain is decreased to a manageable level
2. Will describe required self-care accurately

INTERVENTIONS

1. Relieving Pain

Patients with otitis media are rarely admitted to an acute care setting and need to be instructed about self-care. The nurse instructs the patient about the use of all medications (see Table 60-3) and the importance of taking the antibiotic exactly as prescribed for the full course of the prescription. Analgesics may be necessary to successfully control the ear pain until the antibiotic begins to reduce the severity of the inflammation. The nurse encourages the patient to use these medications for comfort and to remain at rest until the antibiotic has demonstrated effectiveness. Reduced physical activity does appear to be helpful in controlling pain.

2. Patient/Family Education

The nurse instructs the patient to avoid getting water in the ear during treatment. This includes showering and shampooing as well as swimming. Commercial ear plugs or other barriers may be used as temporary protection during shampooing. If an ear wash is prescribed, the nurse teaches the patient and a designated family caregiver how to perform this treatment safely at home.

EVALUATION

To evaluate the effectiveness of nursing interventions, compare patient behaviors with those stated in the expected patient outcomes. Achievement of outcomes is successful if the patient with middle ear infection:

- **1a.** States that no pain is present in the affected ear.
- **1b.** Is free of drainage, redness, edema, and itching in the ear canal.
- **2a.** Explains and demonstrates prescribed treatments.
- **2b.** Identifies symptoms that need to be reported promptly to a health care provider (otorrhea, decrease in hearing, and return of pain).

GERONTOLOGIC CONSIDERATIONS

Middle ear infection can occur at any point in the life span, but is not a common problem in older adults. When it does occur, management is the same as for any other patient. However, early infection may go undiagnosed unless pain is severe because older adults frequently experience itching in the ear or blockage with cerumen.

SPECIAL ENVIRONMENTS FOR CARE

Critical Care

Patients being treated for middle ear infection would never be expected to need critical care management. Otitis media is a community-based infection that the patient can manage effectively at home. Even surgical intervention is at most a 1- to 2-day hospitalization, which would not be expected to need critical care intervention unless catastrophic complications develop.

Community-Based Care

Because middle ear infection is a community-based problem, the entire discussion is appropriate to this setting. Patients need written as well as oral instruction and may require temporary home visiting if no one is available to assist the patient with treatments such as ear washes.

COMPLICATIONS

The primary complications of middle ear infection are perforation of the eardrum and conductive hearing loss. The hearing loss usually resolves with effective treatment of the infection, but may be permanent if chronic disease is present. Acute perforations also tend to heal spontaneously and without residual problems, but complex situations may require surgical closure of the perforation.

Cholesteatoma may result from chronic otitis media. In this condition epithelium from the external ear canal enters and extends into the middle ear, usually through a tympanic membrane perforation. The skin forms a saclike growth that traps debris and puts increasing pressure on the structures of the middle ear. The chronic infection causes cholesterol granules to be deposited within the sac, which gives the growth its name. Surgical excision may become necessary if pressure is causing damage or necrosis to the delicate ear structures. Limited procedures are generally attempted to preserve hearing, but either an open or closed mastoidectomy may be performed.

PROBLEMS OF THE INNER EAR

Sensorineural hearing loss is the most common inner ear disorder and may occur in conjunction with an identified ear problem or in isolation. The hearing loss is usually incomplete but is frequently progressive. Loss of discrimination (understanding of words) is a characteristic feature of sensorineural hearing loss. The inner ear is so delicate that it does not lend itself to surgical correction or repair. Hearing loss is discussed at the beginning of the chapter.

Acoustic Neuroma

Etiology/Epidemiology

Benign and malignant tumors can involve the inner ear by extension through the temporal bone, but acoustic neuroma is by far the most common lesion affecting the inner ear. An acoustic neuroma is a benign tumor of the eighth cranial nerve. It is a slow-growing lesion that can occur at any age and usually occurs unilaterally. The tumor typically grows at the point where cranial nerve VIII enters the internal auditory canal, the temporal bone, and may extend into the brainstem. The tumor is more common in women and tends to occur in persons between 30 and 60 years old.

Pathophysiology

Acoustic neuromas arise from the neurilemmal sheath (sheath of Schwann) along the vestibular branch of the acoustic nerve and spread to the cochlear branch. Early diagnosis is important because the tumor can grow and compress the facial nerve and arteries within the ear canal and can also extend intracranially at which point, the chance of preserving hearing and facial nerve function is reduced. In rare cases, the pressure of the tumor can become life-threatening. Symptoms include tinnitus, vertigo, and a progressive unilateral loss of ability to hear high-pitched sounds. Disorders of the facial nerve may emerge if the tumor is compressing this structure as well.

Collaborative Care Management

Acoustic neuromas are treated surgically, usually by a neurosurgeon. Computed tomography scans can show tumors greater than 2 cm, but the patient's hearing is usually already compromised by the time the tumor is this large. Technical challenges of the surgical procedure include preservation of both hearing and facial nerve function. Many patients experience some degree of residual hearing loss after treatment.

MENIERE'S DISEASE

Etiology/Epidemiology

Meniere's disease or syndrome, also called idiopathic endolymphatic hydrops, is an uncommon form of vertigo of unknown etiology.[1] A virus is believed to play a role in etiology, but this relationship has not been proven. The disease occurs when the normal fluid and electrolyte balance of the inner ear is disrupted. Diagnosis is based on the presence of a classic triad of symptoms plus a prodromal symptom of fullness or pressure in the involved ear. The classic triad consists of episodic true vertigo, sensorineural hearing loss, and tinnitus.

The prevalence of Meniere's disease in the United States is approximately 40 persons per 100,000. Men and women are affected about equally. Peak onset occurs is the fourth decade and the disease is usually diagnosed in persons younger than 60 years.[5] The disease usually begins unilaterally but may progress to both ears in 10% to 78% of patients. Family history is significant. Symptoms may be exacerbated during the menstrual cycle in women who experience significant premenstrual fluid retention.

Pathophysiology

The underlying pathologic changes of Meniere's disease include overproduction and defective absorption of endolymph, which increases the volume and pressure within the membranous labyrinth until distention results in rupture and mixing of the endolymph and perilymph fluids. The two fluids have significantly different compositions, and the mixture disrupts the fluid and electrolyte balance within the labyrinth. Classic Meniere's disease attacks last from 2 to 3 weeks, approximately the time required to close the rupture and restore the fluid balance. Symptoms range from mild to incapacitating and include vertigo, tinnitus, and fluctuating sensorineural hearing loss from degeneration of the hair cells. Prodromal symptoms include tinnitus, ear fullness, and hearing loss. Ninety-five percent of patients experience vertigo associated with nausea, vomiting, and ataxia.

Meniere's disease is relatively uncommon, but the symptom of dizziness or vertigo is second only to headache as the most common chronic symptom reported by patients in the United States. Vertigo, or spinning, is the medical term for dizziness, but dizziness is described in such varied terms that it is almost impossible to accurately define the symptom. Spinning, or vertigo, may be the most common form of dizziness. Other "feelings" include lightheadedness, giddiness, imbalance, veering in one direction while walking, unsteadiness, or a vague feeling of uncertainty during changes in body position. Questions that can be used to explore vertigo are presented in Box 60-1. Initially symptoms of Meniere's disease last less than 2 hours, although altered balance may last up to 2 days. As the disease progresses symptoms last hours to days, and the episodes occur with less warning and are more disabling. Because the balance system can compensate, dizziness is usually not present consistently but is episodic. Early in the course of the disease the patient is asymptomatic between episodes, but as the disease progresses, recovery between attacks is incomplete and permanent tinnitus, moderate to severe hearing loss, and chronic unsteadiness may result.

Collaborative Care Management

The diagnosis of Meniere's disease is established after eliminating other causes of the patient's symptoms. Because there is no known cure, management of the disease is focused on control of symptoms. A variety of medications may be used in the attempt to control disabling symptoms. Antiemetics and anticholinergics may be administered during an acute attack to decrease autonomic nervous system activity. Diuretics and vasodilators are helpful to some patients in restoring the proper fluid balance in the inner ear. Other patients may respond to drugs that reduce vestibular impulses and sedatives. Treatment protocols have used more than 50 different medications. Usually a combination of agents can be found that adequately control the patient's symptoms.

Patients with severe vertigo sometimes profit from vestibular rehabilitation, which teaches labyrinthine compensatory exercises combined with physical therapy. Balance exercises decrease dizziness by helping the brain to compensate for the damaged balance system. Movements that trigger dizziness are repeated rather than avoided. Avoiding dizziness is more comfortable for the patient but does not help the balance system regain its function and compensate for losses.

If the patient's symptoms cannot be satisfactorily controlled with medical interventions, a variety of surgical procedures may be performed. Endolymphatic sac procedures involve decompression and various forms of shunts. These procedures are designed to reduce the fluid pressure within the labyrinth and control vertigo. A destructive procedure in which the membranous labyrinth is removed either subtotally or totally through the oval window or through the mastoid bone is called a labyrinthectomy.

Vestibular nerve surgery destroys the vestibular nerve in the affected ear while attempting to preserve hearing. With any surgery on the vestibular system, there is a risk of causing hearing loss and creating chronic vertigo.

Patient/Family Education. Diet therapy is frequently quite helpful in controlling the symptoms associated with Meniere's disease. The nurse encourages the patient to follow a low-salt diet and avoid excess use of caffeine, sugar, monosodium glutamate, and alcohol. The intake of food and fluid is distributed over the course of the day. Some patients are able to achieve significant symptom improvement from diet modification alone.

Patients need clear instructions about how to manage an acute attack of vertigo. The nurse instructs the patient to immediately lie down on a firm surface if possible, loosen the clothing, and close the eyes until the acute vertigo stops. Driving and operating machinery should not be attempted during attacks. Between attacks the patient can resume normal activities but should avoid swimming under water, which may cause a loss of orientation.

Loss of balance places the person with vertigo at high risk for falls. The nurse assists the patient to explore ways to increase the safety of the home environment. The nurse reminds the patient of the importance of sitting or lying down at the onset of dizziness to reduce the risk of falls. The nurse advises the patient to avoid ladders, work on roofs or trees, or climbing in high places until the vertigo is controlled. Balance therapy can be extremely helpful in supporting the balance network in the brain, and the nurse reinforces the importance of daily practice with these exercises. Careful adherence to the medication regimen is also discussed.

Because the brain must integrate data from the vestibular, visual, and proprioceptive systems to maintain balance, other disorders can also result in vertigo and balance disturbances. Other vestibular disorders are summarized in Table 60-4. A Nursing Care Plan for a patient with Meniere's disease follows.

TABLE 60-4 Vestibular Disorders

Disorder	Definition	Cause (Most Common)	Vertigo	Tinnitus	Hearing Loss
Vestibular neuronitis	Infection of the vestibular nerve with sudden onset	Virus	First attack most severe, subsequent attacks less severe		
Labyrinthitis	Infection of the labyrinth of the inner ear	Virus, bacteria	Severe vertigo diminishing with time	May or may not be present	Permanent sensorineural loss
Benign paroxysmal positional vertigo	Degenerative debris free-floating in the endolymph	Idiopathic (many theories)	Positional vertigo with quick head movements or position change		
Presbyastasis (presbyvertigo)	Balance disorder of aging	Degenerative changes of the vestibule	Imbalance when standing/walking, leading to falls and injuries		

Nursing Care Plan — *Patient With Meniere's Disease*

DATA Mrs. B. is a 59-year-old schoolteacher. During the past 6 months she has had three attacks of vertigo, which she describes as "whirling in space" and incapacitating. In addition, she has suffered fluctuating hearing and noise (tinnitus) in her left ear, nausea and vomiting, and a sense of fullness or pressure in the left ear. She is anxious and concerned about the possibility of a brain tumor.

Mrs. B. was seen in consultation by an otologist, who examined her and ordered an audiogram, tympanometry, electronystagmography, and auditory brainstem response. Subsequently, Mrs. B. was diagnosed with Meniere's disease. Her treatment regimen includes a sodium-restricted diet (allowing 1500 mg of sodium); hydrochorothiazide (HCTZ), 50 mg orally per day; labyrinthine compensatory exercises; and niacin, 100 mg orally three times a day, to control her attacks of vertigo.

NURSING DIAGNOSIS **Anxiety related to fear and intermittent incapacitating attacks of vertigo**
GOALS/OUTCOMES Will report a reduction in anxiety following use of coping strategies

NOC Suggested Outcomes
- Anxiety Control (1402)
- Coping (1302)
- Knowledge: Disease Process (1803)

NIC Suggested Interventions
- Anxiety Reduction (5820)
- Coping Enhancement (5230)
- Teaching: Disease Process (5602)

Nursing Interventions/Rationales
- Acknowledge patient's anxiety. *To validate the patient's feelings and demonstrate empathy for her concerns.*
- Explore with patient her concerns and fears about her decreased hearing and effects of dizziness. *To determine the level of anxiety the patient is experiencing and assist with planning interventions to address her fears and concerns.*
- Teach patient about her disease and correct misunderstandings about her medical diagnosis. *Anxiety is often caused by lack of or inaccurate information. Teaching the patient and correcting misunderstandings often decrease feelings of apprehension.*

Nursing Care Plan Patient With Meniere's Disease—cont'd

- Determine which coping strategies have helped the patient deal with anxiety in the past. *Coping strategies that have been successful in the past are likely to be successful again.*
- Encourage realistic hopes about outcome of disease process. *Prepares the patient for possible outcomes and reduces anxiety.*
- Refer patient to support services as needed. *To provide access to additional support persons who have experience in dealing with patients with the same or similar problems.*

Evaluation Parameters

1. Accurately verbalizes signs of anxiety
2. Uses anxiety-lowering strategies
3. Explains cause of vertigo
4. Demonstrates use of positive coping strategies

NURSING DIAGNOSIS **Deficient knowledge (disease process, symptom control) related to lack of previous experience with disease process**

GOALS/OUTCOMES Patient verbalizes understanding of disease process and methods to control symptoms

NOC Suggested Outcomes

- Knowledge: Disease Process (1803)
- Knowledge: Medications (1808)
- Safety Behavior: Fall Prevention (1909)

NIC Suggested Interventions

- Teaching: Disease Process (5602)
- Teaching: Prescribed Medications 5616)
- Fall Prevention (6490)

Nursing Interventions/Rationales

- Teach patient about the disorder, therapy, and need for medical follow-up care. *To increase understanding of the disease and its treatment so the patient can assume self-care with confidence.*
- Help patient identify actions that may precipitate vertigo. *Understanding factors that precipitate dizziness may help lessen their occurrence.*
- Teach patient methods of preventing dizziness. *To decrease the frequency of vertigo attacks.*
- Encourage patient to move slowly and not turn her head suddenly when experiencing dizziness. *To decrease dizziness and prevent falls and injury.*
- Encourage patient to use background noise when tinnitus is distressing. *Background noise is distracting and masks the effects of tinnitus.*
- Teach patient to use measures to enhance communication. *If hearing loss is present, the patient will need to learn effective measures for ensuring communication.*
- Teach patient the need for maintaining fluid intake >2500 ml/day. *Dehydration may occur from vomiting and use of diuretics.*
- Reinforce the need for taking prescribed medications. *Adherence to the prescribed medication schedule may reduce the occurrence of vertigo.*
- Identify home environmental factors that place the patient at increased risk for falls. *To prevent injury from modifiable factors such as scatter rugs and lack of handrails in the bathtub.*

Evaluation Parameters

1. Describes disease process accurately
2. Uses methods to control symptoms
3. Accurately describes methods to protect personal safety

NURSING DIAGNOSIS **Ineffective individual coping related to chronic dizziness**

GOALS/OUTCOMES Will identify and use coping strategies

NOC Suggested Outcomes

- Coping (1302)

NIC Suggested Interventions

- Coping Enhancement (5230)
- Emotional Support (5270)

Nursing Care Plan — *Patient With Meniere's Disease—cont'd*

Nursing Interventions/Rationales

- Make decisions regarding safety of patient if or when she is unable to do so. *To prevent injury when the patient is unable to make decisions because of overwhelming stress.*
- Assist patient with identification of coping strategies that have been successful in the past. *Coping strategies that have been successful in the past are likely to be successful in new situations.*
- Avoid overloading the patient with information. *People who are not coping well do not have the capacity to comprehend large amounts of information.*
- Assist patient with identification of personal strengths. *Patients who are not coping well may not be able to recognize their personal or family strengths. Focusing on strengths may help the patient use those strengths.*
- Teach and encourage use of relaxation techniques when feeling particularly overwhelmed. *Provides diversion, which may facilitate coping.*
- Teach the patient ways to protect herself from injury when experiencing dizziness. *Knowledge of how to protect herself may increase her self-confidence and help her cope better with the situation.*

Evaluation Parameters

1. Identifies past effective coping strategies
2. Uses coping strategies to decrease stress and anxiety
3. Voices ability to cope with effects of disease process
4. Voices ability to manage chronic condition successfully

Critical Thinking Questions

1. Describe how you think you might feel if you were told that you had a significant and permanent hearing loss.
2. Compare and contrast the pathophysiology, clinical manifestations, and assessment parameters for conductive and sensorineural hearing loss.
3. What measures or precautions could you suggest to the patient who has vertigo?
4. How are upper respiratory infections and otitis media related?

References

1. Bennett JC, Plumb F: *Cecil textbook of medicine,* ed 21, Philadelphia, 2000, WB Saunders.
2. Brackmann DE, Shelton C, Arriaga MA: *Otologic surgery,* ed 2, Philadelphia, 2001, WB Saunders.
3. Collins JG: Prevalence of selected chronic conditions: United States 1990-1992: National Center for Health Statistics, *Vital Health Statistics* 10(194):1, 1997.
4. Griest SE, Bishop PM: Tinnitus as an early indicator of permanent hearing loss, *AAOHN J* 46(7):325, 1998.
5. Guntinas O: Acute vestibular syndrome, *N Engl J Med* 339(10):151, 1999.
6. LaRosa S: Primary care management of otitis externa, *Nurse Pract* 23(6):131, 1998.
7. National Institute for Occupational Safety and Health (NIOSH) Fact Sheet: *Work related hearing loss,* Washington, DC, 1999, USDHHS.
8. Panhorst B: Noise exposures, *AAOHN* 46(1):4, 1998.
9. Stewart MG, Coker NJ: Outcomes and quality of life in conductive hearing loss, *Otolaryngol Head Neck Surg* 123(5):87-88, 2000.
10. US Department of Health and Human Services: *Healthy people 2010: understanding and improving health,* Washington, DC, 2000, USDHHS.

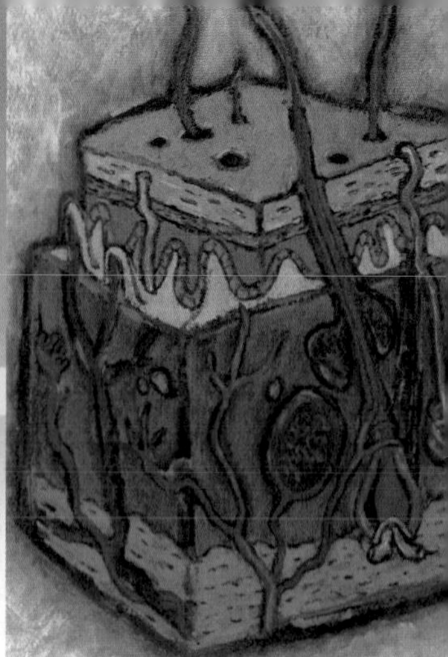

61 Assessment of the Skin

Marianne C. Tawa

Objectives

After studying this chapter, the learner should be able to:

1. Correlate the structures of the skin with their functions.
2. Define guidelines and parameters for assessment of the skin and accessory structures.
3. Identify specific changes in the skin associated with physiologic aging.
4. Describe primary and secondary skin lesions, lesion arrangement, and configuration.

The skin is the largest organ of the body, accounting for approximately 15% of the total body weight. It is exposed to the external environment and provides the first line of defense of the body; yet at the same time it is affected by changes in the internal environment. Thus assessment of the skin and its associated appendages hair, nails, and glands provides insight into how individuals are affected by and cope with both external and internal environments. Information gathered in this assessment provides the basis for identification of actual or potential nursing problems related to the skin, infection, fluid and electrolyte imbalances, nutritional imbalances, or inadequate oxygenation of tissues. Baseline observations facilitate early and accurate identification of changes that may occur.

ANATOMY AND PHYSIOLOGY

Structure of the Skin

The skin is composed of three major layers: the epidermis, the dermis, and the subcutaneous tissue (Figure 61-1). The epidermis is the outermost structure of the skin. It possesses the unique ability to regenerate itself by forming new cells on an ongoing basis. The primary cell of the epidermis is the keratinocyte or squamous cell. Keratinocytes produce keratin, which is a resilient, insoluble, fibrous protein. The epidermis consists of five histologically distinct layers, each of which is named for the stage of reproductive activity of the keratinocyte that occurs within it. The innermost basal cell layer, also known as the stratum basale, basement membrane, or stratum germinativum gives rise to new cells through mitosis. After cell division has taken place in the basal cell layer, one basal cell from each cell division remains behind while the other migrates upward. The migrating cell passes through the intermediate layers of the stratum spinosum, stratum granulosum, and stratum lucidum, further flattening and differentiating along the way. Twenty-eight days later on average, the mature keratinocyte reaches the stratum corneum or horny cell outermost layer of the epidermis. The horny cell layer is predominately composed of keratin, which is responsible for the vital barrier function of skin.

Another critical but less commonly found cell in the epidermis is the melanocyte. Melanocytes are dendritic pigment producing cells derived from the neural crest during embryologic development. They form pigment granules called melanosomes, which contain melanin and provide color to skin, eyes, and hair. Melanocytes also play a role in protection from ultraviolet light. Langerhan cells, derived from bone marrow, are also found in the epidermis and serve an immunologic function related to antigen presentation.

The second layer of skin, called the *dermis* or *cutis*, is located beneath the epidermis and is demarcated by the basement membrane. At 1 to 4 mm the dermis is significantly thicker than the epidermis and provides structural support as well as mass to the skin. The dermis consists of connective tissue components including collagen, elastin, and reticulum fibers as well as water, ground substance, sensory and postganglionic nerves, blood vessels, and lymphatics. The dermis surrounds and supplies nutrition and electrolytes to the skin appendages such as sweat glands, sebaceous glands, and hair follicles.

The third layer of skin is the subcutaneous tissue, which consists of fat cells or lipocytes separated by fibrous walls composed of collagen and blood vessels. This fatty tissue layer conducts heat only one fourth as rapidly as does other tissues and thus serves as the heat insulator of the body. Subcutaneous tissue also provides a cushioning effect, is a storage site for caloric reserve, and anchors the other two layers to supportive structures (e.g., muscle, tendon, bone). The density of subcutaneous tissue varies from location to location in the body. For example, the waist and hips typically possess ample subcutaneous tissue, whereas the eyelids and nipples lack it. Distribution of subcutaneous tissue is regulated by sex hormones, genetics, age, and eating habits.

Eccrine sweat glands are present everywhere on the body surface except for the ear canal, penis, labial tissue, lips, and

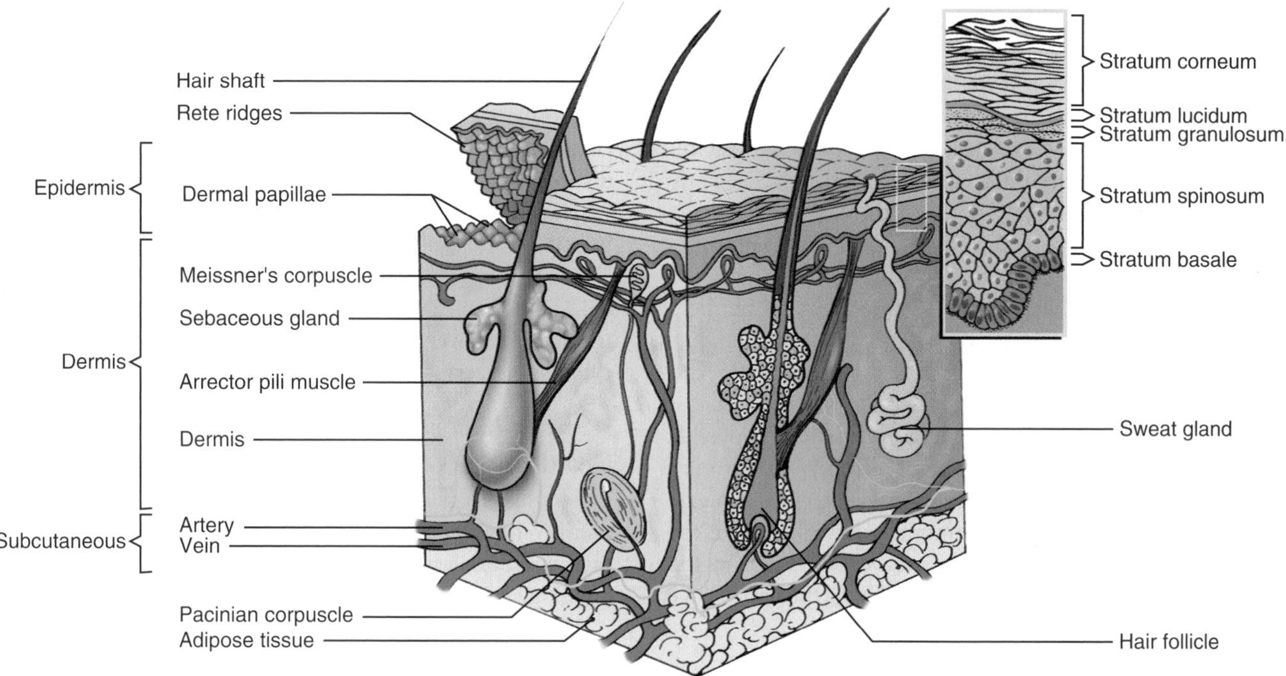

Figure 61-1 Anatomy of the skin.

nail beds. The heaviest concentration of eccrine glands is found on the palms of the hands and soles of the feet, head, trunk, and extremities. Eccrine sweat is an odorless, colorless, hypotonic solution, which is directly secreted to the surface of the skin. Eccrine glands participate in the heat-regulating mechanisms of the body and their activity is under the control of the sympathetic nervous system. Thermal, mental, and gustatory stimuli promote eccrine gland secretion.

Apocrine glands are located mainly in the axilla, umbilical area, breast, genitals, external ear canal, and eye lid. Apocrine glands under the direction of epinephrine and norepinephrine produce a milky, odorless, sterile secretion. At the skin surface level, the fluid comes in contact with bacteria present on the hair follicle or skin and results in body odor. These glands have no identifiable biologic function.

Sebaceous glands are found on all areas of the body except for the top and bottom surfaces of the hands and feet. Sebaceous glands are most often associated with hair follicles. The greatest density of these glands occurs on the scalp, face, chest, and back. Sebaceous glands under the influence of androgenic hormones produce sebum. This is a lipid-containing substance, which may play a role in lubrication and synthesis of vitamin D in the skin.

Functions of the Skin

Protection

The outermost layer of the epidermis, the stratum corneum, is a relatively impermeable layer of tightly packed flat cells that protects the underlying tissue from the outer environment. A small number of nonpathogenic bacteria reside in this horny layer of skin. Lack of moisture in this layer keeps the microorganism number low, as growth is impeded. Bacteria attempting to penetrate hair follicles are deterred by the sebum. Fat-soluble substances such as moisturizing lotions can penetrate the skin by passively diffusing through the hair follicles and sebaceous glands.

Intact skin is the first line of defense against bacterial and foreign-substance invasion, slight physical trauma, heat, or ultraviolet rays. When the skin is exposed to environmental factors such as pressure, friction, and internal shearing forces, the epidermis is compressed to the depth of the supporting structures (i.e., bone). With prolonged exposure the capillary bed within the dermis and the larger vessels within the subcutaneous tissue become occluded, causing ischemia of the tissues in the area. If the ischemia is not reversed by removing the source of pressure, cellular death is imminent and the skin's defensive line is jeopardized.

Scraping or stripping the surface of the skin (e.g., by the removal of tape or the use of razors without shaving cream) can weaken the epidermis. Once the barrier has weakened, permeability to bacteria, drugs, and other foreign substances is increased. Percutaneous absorption of medications through the skin can be enhanced when the skin surface is disrupted or denuded. Epidermis that becomes extremely dry may fissure and crack more readily. Moist skin surface areas can become macerated, thus providing a medium for bacterial overgrowth.

Mucous membranes, although continuous with the stratum corneum, are somewhat protected from the external environment. Fluids and other substances such as certain drugs can be absorbed through the mucous membranes.

Heat Regulation

Body temperature is controlled by radiation of heat from the surface of the skin, conduction of heat from skin to other objects or air, removal of heat by air currents on the skin (convection), and evaporation of water from skin surfaces. Insensible water evaporation from the skin and lungs occurs at a rate of 600 to 1000 ml/day. On a hot day the only way the body can lose heat is by evaporation, and anything that restricts evaporation under these conditions will increase body temperature. The blood vessels of the skin help control body temperature by constricting in cold environments to promote conservation of heat and dilating in warm environments to promote loss of heat by radiation. These mechanisms help maintain a constant internal body temperature.

Sensory Perception

The skin contains receptor endings of nerves responsible for sensing pain, touch, heat, and cold. Through the stimulation of these nerve endings, a person is able to communicate with the immediate external environment. Distribution of the sensory endings is generalized; however, certain areas of the body have more than other areas. For example, the hands have a higher concentration than the forearms.

Excretion

Water lost through the skin is a factor in maintaining water balance in the body. Salt as well as water is lost through excessive sweating. A person can become acclimatized to a continually hot environment, however, and the amount of salt lost decreases over time.

Vitamin D Production

Synthesis of vitamin D takes place in the skin by the effect of sunlight (ultraviolet rays). Vitamin D is necessary in the metabolism of calcium and phosphorus.

Decorative

The skin, hair, and nails individually and collectively contribute to one's body image, which can be aesthetically pleasing or displeasing. Because the skin and its appendages are the parts of the body most readily visible to the outside world, they play an important role in the impression made by a person on others. Individuals with skin disorders both acute and chronic can develop marked alterations in self- esteem and confidence.

PHYSIOLOGIC CHANGES WITH AGING

Many skin changes occur as a person ages. Observable changes result primarily from loss of subcutaneous tissue, degeneration of collagen and elastic fibers, loss of melanocytes, increased capillary fragility, decreased secretion of sweat glands, hormonal changes, and overexposure to environmental elements.

The skin loses its elasticity and becomes loose and wrinkled. Exposed areas may be thickened, but in general the skin becomes thinner, drier, and more fragile. There are fewer hair follicles and as a result absorbtion of fat-soluble substances is decreased. Benign growths such as, seborrheic keratoses, solar lentigines (brown spots), and vascular hyperplasias such as cherry angiomas and senile purpura (red to purple ecchymotic spots) develop in middle to elder years. Changes in the color, texture, and quantity of hair is another age associated finding in older adults. Nails may become thickened, brittle and discolored with advancing age.

Age-related changes also place elders at risk for skin problems. Elders are more likely to have one or more chronic diseases and to be taking medications that can produce skin disorders. Dry skin changes set the stage for pruritus (itching) with frequent scratching that can disrupt the epidermis. Skin infections such as candidiasis caused by yeast organisms and impetigo caused by the gram-positive organisms group A beta-hemolytic *Streptococcus* or *Staphylococcus aureus,* may then result. Lower extremity venous insufficiency in elders can cause stasis dermatitis.

ASSESSMENT

Health History

Patient history is an important component of the skin assessment. When patients report the presence of a rash, change in pigmentation, lesions, or new skin symptoms such as itching, burning, or pain, the following information must be obtained.

- Usual skin condition: appearance, color, moisture, texture, and integrity
- Onset of the problem: initial location—when changes were first noted; skin appearance at onset; other associated symptoms such as pain or itching
- Changes since onset: change in location, change in size or appearance; onset of new associated symptoms such as pain or itching
- Possible causes: exposure to known contact allergens such as poison ivy, rubber, nickel, or fragrance. If cause is unknown, ask about:
  - Exposure to potential sensitizing substances, such as metals, chemicals, detergents, solvents, or plant life
  - Use of new pharmacologic agents either prescription or over the counter
  - Work that may cause contact with potential skin irritants or require hands to be constantly in water
  - Participation in recreational activities (e.g., painting, camping, or gardening) that may involve exposure to sensitizing substances
  - Exposure to ultraviolet light (sun) producing exaggerated sunburn, photosensitivity
  - Change in climate
  - Increase in stress level
- Alleviating factors: clinician-prescribed or self-prescribed. Note how and when used.
- Psychologic reaction to skin changes, including the ability to work, recreate, or interact on a social or intimate level

Because the history assists not only in assessing the patient's health status but also in identifying needs for health information and instruction, assessing for good health practices relating to dermatologic system function is essential (see Patient Teaching box).

Physical Examination

Methods of Assessment

Direct inspection with a good light is the basic method of skin assessment. Palpation is used in addition, to identify tem-

Patient Teaching
Maintenance of Healthy Skin

To maintain healthy skin, adults should:
- Prevent drying and irritation of the skin
- Avoid overbathing.
- Use tepid water and pH neutral soaps that are less drying.
- Lather gently and pat dry.
- Apply an emollient cream or lotion immediately after bathing
- Drink plenty of water.
- Eat a well-balanced diet.
- Get an adequate amount of sleep.
- Exercise regularly.

Perform self-skin assessment monthly. Report any new growths or changes in preexisting lesions such as moles to their health care provider.

Older adults and others with an impaired immune response should report early signs of skin infection to their health care provider because of the risks of delayed healing and spread.

perature, areas of tenderness, and the density and induration of lesions. A systematic head-to-toe skin assessment can be conducted while the related health history is obtained. When the history identifies potential or existing problems, involved areas of the skin are reassessed as needed. Remember that data obtained from physical assessment of the skin not only relates to dermatologic problems but also provides an indication of overall health status. Detailed principles of effective skin assessment are presented in the Guidelines for Safe Practice box.

Guidelines for Safe Practice
Skin Assessment Techniques

1. Be prepared: Adequate lighting is crucial to examination of the skin. Natural lighting is preferred. If the lighting is inadequate, lesions may be missed or described inaccurately. If the room temperature is not well controlled, vasoconstriction or vasodilation can occur leading to false impressions.
2. Be systematic: If only some parts of the skin are inspected, an important observation may be missed.
3. Be thorough: Look at all areas carefully. If the person is lying down, be sure to examine the back, especially the sacral area. Expose areas of tissue hidden by skin folds. For example lift breasts and separate gluteal folds. Maintain patient privacy as you progress sequentially through the examination. Make certain to examine the mucous membranes of the oral cavity.
4. Be specific: When lesions are identified, describe them in terms of shape, size using the metric system, location, color, and other characteristics.
5. Compare right side with left side. When observing changes in skin color or tissue shape, always compare one side of the body with the other to differentiate structural from pathologic changes, as well as symmetry of manifestation.
6. Record the data: Unrecorded data are lost data. Baseline observations indicating normality or abnormality are needed for comparison with subsequent findings. Changes need to be recorded to determine progress toward achieving desired outcomes.
7. Use appropriate technique: Palpation is used during physical assessment of the skin. Lesions are palpated for density, induration, and tenderness. Standard Precautions (see Chapter 10) need to be observed during palpation, and the examiner must determine whether it is appropriate to use gloves.

Components of the General Skin Assessment

Objective data to be collected when examining the skin for general health status include skin color and pigmentation, temperature, moisture, elasticity, mobility and turgor, texture, thickness, odor, hygiene, and presence of lesions.

Color. The normal components of skin color are brown, yellow, red, and blue. Brown coloration or pigmentation is due to the presence of melanin in the skin. Melanin formation requires the amino acid tyrosine, the enzyme tyrosinase, and molecular oxygen. Variations in pigmentation occur in different parts of the body. An increase in pigmentation occurs on the exposed skin surfaces of the head, neck, arms, and hands. Conversely, a decreased pigmentation is observed on the nonexposed skin surfaces of the genitalia, palms, and soles. Hyperpigmentation, or an overall increase in the brown component of skin color, occurs normally in some persons as a genetic factor (dark skin). The skin of darkly pigmented persons does not contain more melanocytes, but the melanocytes are larger and produce more melanin. Pigmented skin offers more protection from ultraviolet radiation; hence dark skin reacts less to sunlight and skin cancer incidence is reduced. Because of the greater amount of melanin in dark skin, however, alterations in pigmentation occur more frequently in African-Americans than in other races. Fair complexioned individuals can acquire increased pigmentation from the effects of sun exposure (tanning). Because melanin is formed in the basal cell layer and gradually migrates to the surface where it is cast off, acquired pigmentation from sun exposure (tan) fades. Hyperpigmentation also may occur with radiation therapy as a result of activation of tyrosinase. Hyperpigmentation induced in this manner fades slowly and may be long-lasting. In addition, certain endocrine diseases, pregnancy, oral contraceptive use, and nutritional and metabolic disorders can produce hyperpigmentary skin changes. Hyperpigmentation may follow an inflammatory process in the skin as seen with eczema, acne vulgaris, drug eruptions, and skin infections. Cutaneous neoplastic processes such as T-cell lymphoma of the skin may produce hyperpigmented patches and plaques. Hydroquinone (bleach) with salicylic acid or with retinoic acid interferes with tyrosinase activity.

Hypopigmentation occurs normally in some persons as a genetic factor (light skin). Albinos have a congenital inability to produce melanin. Severe trauma can destroy melanin-producing cells and result in hypopigmentation (scar tissue). Some healthy persons develop a condition called vitiligo, in which there is a failure of melanin formation. Sharply demarcated, white (amelanotic) patches typically distributed over the face, joints, hands, and legs are the hallmarks of this skin disorder. Vitiligo is thought to be an autoimmune disease in which vitiligo antibodies are produced to melanocytes. Other causes for acquired hypopigmentation include the aftermath of an inflammatory process such as atopic dermatitis or psoriasis, infections such as tinea versicolor, and certain neoplastic skin processes.

The red component of skin color comes from the blood supplied to the skin. The rate of blood flow through the skin is highly variable because of its function in heat control. The blood vessels are innervated by the sympathetic nervous system; thus vasoconstriction occurs with the neuroendocrine response to stressors. With vasoconstriction, smaller amounts of blood pass through the vessels, producing decreased redness; a dark skin becomes dull and gray and a light skin whiter (pallor). Vasodilation increases the amount of oxygenated blood flow, and the skin acquires a reddish color (erythema). Vascular flush areas of the body are the "butterfly" band from cheek to cheek across the nose, neck, upper portion of the chest, flexor surfaces of the extremities, and genital areas.

Changes in blood composition also affect skin color. Excess deoxygenated hemoglobin gives a bluish tint (cyanosis) to the skin and mucous membranes, whereas an excess of bile pigment results in a yellowish tint to the skin and sclerae of the eyes.

Changes in skin color are best observed in areas with the least amount of pigmentation and that are free of the masking effects of tanning or cosmetics. Thus the lips, mucous membranes of the mouth, earlobes, nail beds, conjunctivae, sclerae, and the palms of the hands and the soles of the feet are the preferred areas. The lips in particular show rapid color changes. Inaccurate assessment of skin color may be attributed to factors such as poor lighting, extremes in room temperature, the presence of edema, poor hygiene, or positioning. See Table 61-1 for examples of skin color changes

Assessment of dark-skinned individuals is more difficult than assessment of light-complexioned individuals because color changes are less obvious. Other supportive data are often needed to assist in reaching a conclusion. For example, when the skin is inflamed, the erythema (redness) may not be clearly visible. Thus the involved area must be palpated to check for warmth and edema.[7] Strategies for the accurate assessment of dark skin are presented in the Guidelines for Safe Practice box.

Skin color changes will be seen best in areas of lesser pigmentation, which include the lips, areas around the mouth, mucous membranes, conjunctivae, earlobes, nail beds, palms, and soles. The sclerae of many dark-skinned persons contain fatty deposits with carotene, giving the sclerae a yellowish tinge.[4] In these persons, jaundice will have to be determined by other signs, such as bile in the urine or feces.

Loss of redness provided by the blood produces grayish or dull tones rather than pallor. This sign may be difficult to observe by the untrained eye. Grayish or dull tones can be visualized best in the lips, mucous membranes, conjunctivae, and nail beds. Cyanosis also gives the skin a grayish or dull tone because of loss of redness. Areas of lesser pigmentation, including the earlobes, palms, and soles, are assessed for signs of cyanosis.

Temperature. Skin temperature is regulated by both vasoconstriction and vasodilation. If an excess amount of heat is being produced within the body, such as with fever or exercise, or if heat from the external environment increases, the sym-

TABLE 61-1 Skin Color Changes

Physiology	Causative Conditions
Redness (Erythema)	
Vasodilation: more rapid blood flow, more oxygenated blood giving a reddish hue	Blushing, heat, inflammation, fever, alcohol ingestion, extreme cold (below 15° C), hot flushes, polycythemia
Whiteness (Pallor)	
Vasoconstriction: slower blood flow, less blood in capillaries	Cold, fear, shock
Partially obstructed blood flow: less blood in capillaries	Vasospasm, thrombus, narrowed vessels, arterial insufficiency
Fluid between blood vessels and skin surface	Edema
Decreased oxygenation of blood from decreased hemoglobin	Anemia
Loss of melanin	Vitiligo
Bluish (Cyanosis)	
Deoxygenated hemoglobin seen in earlobes, lips, mucous membranes of mouth, nail beds	Heart or lung disease, inadequate respiration, peripheral blood vessel obstruction, venous disease, cold, anxiety
Yellow (Jaundice)	
Increased bile pigment in blood eventually distributed to skin and mucous membranes and to sclera of eye	Liver disease, obstruction of bile ducts, chronic uremia, rapid hemolysis
Brown	
Increased melanin deposits: normal in brown-black races	Aging, sunburn; anterior pituitary, adrenal cortex, or liver disease
Dullness	
Vasoconstriction in dark skin	Cold, fear, shock
Partially obstructed blood flow in dark skin	Vasospasm, thrombus, narrowed vessels, arterial insufficiency
Fluid between blood vessels and skin surface in dark skin	Edema

pathetic centers in the hypothalamus are inhibited and vasodilation occurs. An increase in the amount of blood flow creates a sensation of warmth on the skin. This also occurs with hyperthyroidism. A local inflammation of the skin or underlying tissue also produces vasodilation; this is part of the inflammatory response. Cold skin is caused by vasoconstriction as a result of sympathetic stimulation. Diseases such as hypothyroidism also can contribute to skin coolness. To assess the temperature of the skin use the backs of the fingers, which are more sensitive than the fingertips.

Moisture. Skin is assessed as being dry, moist, or oily. Dry skin is frequently seen in the elderly person because of decreased activity of the sebaceous glands. Dry skin and mucous membranes also are seen in persons who are dehydrated as water moves from the cells into the intravascular compartments. Persons with hypothyroidism have thick, dry, leathery skin.

Guidelines for Safe Practice

Assessment of Dark Skin

1. Check skin color in areas of least pigmentation: sclerae, conjunctivae, buccal mucosa, tongue, lips, nail beds, palms, and soles.
2. Palpate as well as inspect, especially if inflammation or edema is suspected.
3. Correlate findings with the patient's history.
4. Remember that pallor in brown-skinned patients may present as a yellowish brown tinge to the skin and in black-skinned patients as "ashen-gray" because of the absence of underlying red tones in the skin.
5. Check for cyanosis by inspecting the nail beds, lips, palpebral conjunctiva, earlobes, palms, and soles. Compare to baseline color whenever possible.
6. Observe for jaundice in that portion of the sclera that is observable when the eye is open. Since fatty deposits containing carotene, which give the sclerae a yellow appearance, are common in dark-skinned individuals, also observe the posterior portion of the hard palate. Do this in bright daylight for best discrimination of color.
7. Assess for edema by observing for areas of the skin that appear lighter in color, as edema reduces the intensity of color because of the increased distance between the external epithelium and the pigmented layers. Palpate for a "tight" feeling to the skin.
8. Observe for petechiae over areas of lighter pigmentation such as the abdomen, gluteal areas, the volar aspect of the forearm, in the palpebral conjunctiva and in the buccal mucosa.
9. Differentiate petechiae and ecchymoses from erythema by exerting pressure over the affected area and observing for color change. Erythema will blanch but petechiae and ecchymoses remain unchanged.
10. Assess rashes by palpating for changes in skin texture.
11. Remember the oral mucosa, including the gums, borders of the tongue, and lining of the cheeks, of dark-skinned individuals may have a normal freckling of pigmentation. Also the gingivae normally may have either a blotch or evenly distributed dark blue color.

Moist skin is caused by the presence of water or sweat on the surface. Overheating produces sweating. Persons with hyperthyroidism have moist, smooth skin. Some persons have more effective sweat mechanisms than others. Stressors, shock, or any situation that stimulates the sympathetic nervous system will cause increased fluid loss through the sweat glands (diaphoresis). Inasmuch as vasoconstriction occurs simultaneously with stimulation of the sympathetic nervous system, the skin is cold and wet (clammy).

Oily skin is frequently encountered at puberty. Excess sebum formation by the sebaceous glands may lead to blocking of the follicular orifices, resulting acne lesions and sebaceous cysts.

Elasticity, Mobility, and Turgor. The skin is highly elastic and moves freely over most areas. It loses its mobility when it becomes stretched; this occurs with edema, when the interstitial spaces become filled with fluid. Skin becomes rigid in the person with scleroderma, a collagen disease, as a result of collagenous fibrosis of the tissue. Turgor is tissue tension and is measured by the speed of the skin's return to a normal position of fullness after it has been stretched. Decreased skin turgor is a normal assessment finding in elderly persons. In others, decreased turgor indicates dehydration of the tissue or extreme weight loss. To assess elasticity and turgor, a portion of skin over the sternum is picked up (elasticity) and the speed of return to normal is assessed (turgor). To assess hydration status of an elderly patient, the nurse should examine the mucous membranes. Skin that has decreased turgor will remain for a few seconds in a fold ("tenting") before returning slowly to normal (Figure 61-2).

Texture. The skin is normally soft and smooth with some roughened areas over exposed areas such as the elbows. The skin of older adults may be rough and lack underlying tissue substance (atrophy). Hypertrophic scarring, also known as keloid formation, is another example of a textural change in the skin.

Thickness. Normal skin is uniformly thin over most of the body except over the palms and soles. A callus, or painless overgrowth of epidermis, may develop over these areas as a result of pressure or friction. Thickened skin over pressure sites like elbows and soles occurs with aging.

Odor. Clean skin is usually free of odor except for areas that contain the apocrine sweat glands. Odor occurs because of bacterial composition of protein matter. Some draining skin lesions may produce an odor.

ACCESSORY STRUCTURES

Hair

Hair growth, pattern, and distribution are indicators of the person's general state of health.[3] Excessive hair growth (hypertrichosis) usually is related to heredity or hormonal changes. Hair loss (alopecia) occurs normally with age, especially in some men. Abnormal hair loss may be caused by hormonal imbalance (androgen excess), thyroid disease, general ill health, infections of the scalp, chronic liver disease, stressors, or drugs (e.g., chemotherapeutic agents/hormones). Hair loss on the dorsum of the toes may indicate decreased arterial circulation. The hair shaft is an inert structure, and changes occur over time as a

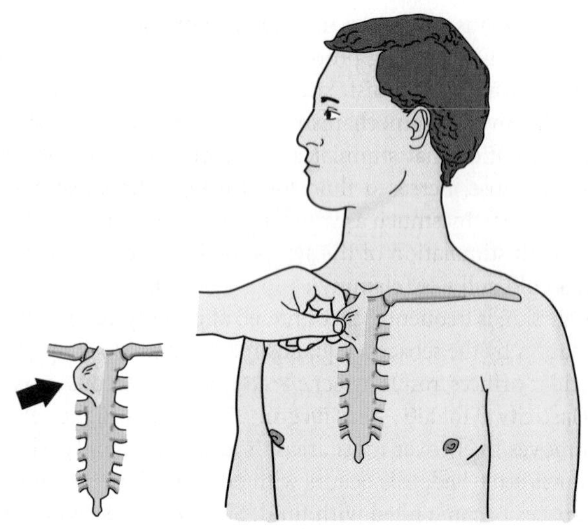

Figure 61-2 Examination of skin turgor. Tenting of the skin over the sternum occurs with decreased skin turgor.

result of hormonal activity and the availability of nutrients to the bulb at the base of the hair root.

When assessing hair, color, amount, pattern, distribution, as well as cleanliness of scalp and facial hair should be noted. If the patient is wearing a wig or other hairpiece, this should be removed temporarily for inspection of any remaining hair and the scalp. Because it is easy to miss lesions on the scalp, ask the patient to assist by indicating areas of itching, pain, or roughness.

Hair should also be assessed for signs of infestation with the crab-louse (pediculosis). Nits are the eggs of the lice and are found embedded on hair strands. They are observed as small, glistening, grayish specks along the hair shaft close to the scalp. Hair of dark-skinned individuals should be assessed for traumatic alopecia. This type of hair loss results from hair care practices such as tight hair curlers, cornrow braiding, hot combing, or the use of picks because black hair shafts are highly susceptible to breakage. Wetting or softening the hair before combing may help prevent trauma to it.

Nails

The appearance of the nails changes with age and states of illness. Changes in nail plate texture may indicate metabolic disease, nutritional imbalances including vitamin deficiency, or digestive disturbance. Pale nail beds and poor capillary return (slow return to normal color after the nail is pinched) may indicate hypoxia or anemia. Capillary refill is normally less than 3 seconds. Clubbing of the nails refers to the elimination of the small concave portion at the base of the nail by soft tissue growth. Normally the angle between the nail base and the fingernail is approximately 160 degrees. Early clubbing is present when the angle increases to 180 degrees or more. The mechanism of clubbing is not understood, but occurs with certain diseases associated with chronic hypoxia (see Chapter 19).

The epithelial lining of the nail bed is usually inert. The nail is affixed to the nail bed, and both move outward as the nail grows. The epithelial lining of the nail bed can lose its inert quality in the presence of inflammatory processes such as with psoriasis, chronic hand eczema, or fungal nail plate infections. When this occurs, the nail bed keratinizes and horny masses collect under the nail, resulting in deformity of the nail and possible separation from the nail bed.[6]

Paronychia, an infection of the tissue surrounding the nail, is characterized by red, shiny skin and painful swelling. The infection can be due to trauma or underlying skin diseases. The usual infecting organisms are staphylococcus, yeast, and molds. If the nail is lost, it usually will grow back unless the nail bed has been injured.

SKIN LESIONS

When individual lesions or skin rashes are observed, they should be described in terms of type, color, size, shape, configuration and arrangement, distribution, and texture. Primary lesions are visual and/or palpable changes in the structure of the skin unchanged by time or environment. Secondary skin lesions are those due to environmental influences or natural evolution, such as scratching, rubbing, infection, or therapy.

Type

Use of proper descriptive terminology (Table 61-2) by the nurse is essential to clear, accurate communication about skin lesions. For example, use of the term vesicle provides a clear picture of a lesion that is clear, fluid-filled, and smaller than 1 cm. Figure 61-3 illustrates the most common types of lesions.

Color

Color of lesions varies from pale, brown, red, to normal background pigmentation. Color helps to identify whether the lesion may be secondary to an inflammatory process, infection, sun exposure, or heredity. For example, café-au-lait spots (French for coffee with milk) are congenital pale tan macules.[1]

Size

The metric system is used for measurement. If a metric ruler is not available, the size of a lesion can be estimated by measuring a portion of one's finger to use as a gauge.

Shape and Demarcation

Shape describes the contour of a lesion. Examples include round, oval, polygonal (many sided), and asymmetric. Demarcation refers to the sharpness of the edge of the lesion, that is, whether it is discrete or diffuse.

Texture

The lesion is described as being rough or smooth, dry or moist, and on the surface or deeply penetrating into the tissue. Alterations in texture may occur as a result of scarring. Keloids are firm, raised, shiny hypertrophic scars that grow beyond the wound, often with clawlike projections. Although keloids are seen in all races, they are much more prevalent in the African-American population.[5] Highly susceptible areas for keloid growth include the sternum, mandible, ear, and neck.

TABLE 61-2 Types of Skin Lesions

Observed Skin Changes	Differentiation	Term	Example
Change in Color or Texture			
Spot	Circumscribed; flat; color change	Macule	Freckle
Discoloration (reddish purple)	Bleeding beneath the surface; injury to tissue	Contusion	Bruise
Soft whitening	Caused by repeated wetting of skin	Maceration	Between toes after soaking
Flake	Dry cells of surface	Scale	Dandruff; psoriasis
Roughness from dried fluid	Dry exudate over lesions	Crust ("scab")	Eczema, impetigo
Roughness from cells	Leathery thickening of outer skin layer	Lichenification	Callus on foot
Change in Shape			
Fluid-filled lesions	Less than 1 cm; clear fluid	Vesicle	Blister; chickenpox
	Greater than 1 cm; clear fluid	Bulla	Large blister, pemphigus
	Small, thick yellowish fluid (pus)	Pustule	Acne
Solid mass, cellular growth	Less than 1 cm	Papule	Small mole; raised rash
	1 to 2 cm	Nodule	Enlarged lymph node
	Greater than 2 cm	Tumor	Benign or malignant tumor
	Excess connective tissue over scar	Keloid	Overgrown scar
Swelling of tissue	Generalized swelling; fluid between cells	Edema	Inflammation; swelling of feet
	Circumscribed surface edema; transient; some itching	Wheal ("hive")	Allergic reaction
Breaks in Skin Surfaces			
Oozing, scraped surface	Loss of superficial structure of skin	Abrasion	"Floor burn"; scrape
Scooped-out depression	Loss of deeper layers of skin	Ulcer	Pressure or stasis ulcer
Superficial linear skin breaks	Scratch marks, frequently by fingernails	Excoriations	Scratching
Linear cracks or cleft	Slit or splitting of skin layers	Fissure	Athlete's foot
Jagged cut	Tearing of skin surface	Laceration	Accidental cut by blunt object
Linear cut, edges approximated	Cutting by sharp instrument	Incision	Knife cut
Vascular Lesions			
Small, flat, round, purplish, red spot	Intradermal or submucous hemorrhage	Petechia	Bleeding tendency, decreased platelets; vitamin C deficiency
Spider-like, red, small	Dilation of capillaries, arterioles, or venules	Telangiectasis	Liver disease, vitamin B deficiency
Discoloration, reddish purple	Escape of blood into tissue	Ecchymosis	Trauma to blood vessels

Blanching Test

Some vascular lesions blanch when direct pressure is applied and then swiftly return to their original color once the pressure is alleviated. Skin lesions without a vascular component remain unchanged with pressure. The blanching test can be performed with a glass slide or a handheld magnifying lens.

Configuration

Configuration refers to the arrangement or pattern of lesions in relation to other lesions.[1] Skin lesions can occur discretely or in groupings. These groupings may be arranged as linear, following a line; annular, ringlike; confluent, merging together; or serpiginous, serpentlike. Disseminated refers to multiple scattered lesions diffusely distributed over the body (Figure 61-4).

Distribution

Distribution takes into consideration both the arrangement of lesions over an area of skin as well as the pattern. Terms used to describe distribution include discrete (isolated), localized, regional, and generalized. Symmetric, exposed, intertriginous (skin fold), dermatonal (following spinal nerves path), and random are examples of patterns seen with common skin disorders such as eczema, yeast infections, and herpes zoster (shingles).

See Table 61-3 for normal skin assessment findings in adults and variations in older adults.

Assessment measures and variations in normal findings relevant to the care of older adults are presented in the Gerontologic Assessment box. Also identified are disorders common in older adults, which may be responsible for abnormal assessment findings.

Macule—flat; nonpalpable; circumscribed; less than 1 cm in diameter; brown, red, purple, white, or tan
Examples: Freckles; flat moles; rubella; rubeola

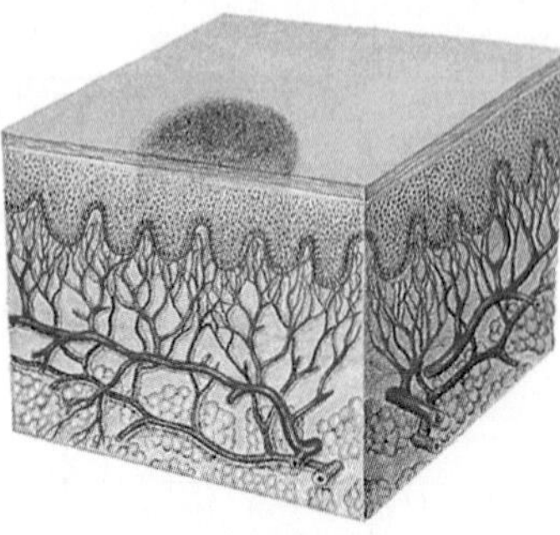

Papule—elevated; palpable; firm; circumscribed; less than 1 cm in diameter; brown, red, pink, tan, or bluish red
Examples: Warts; drug-related eruptions; pigmented nevi

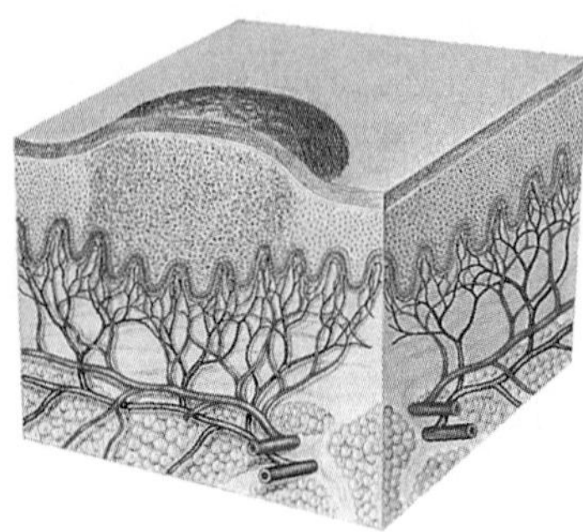

Plaque—elevated; flat topped; firm; rough; superficial papule greater than 1 cm in diameter; may be coalesced papules
Examples: Psoriasis; seborrheic and actinic keratoses

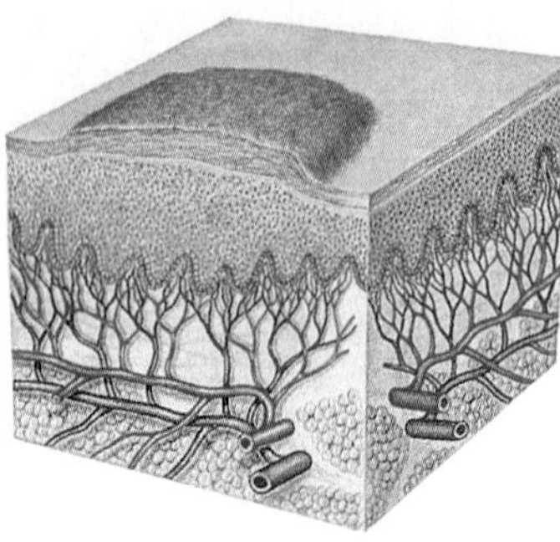

Wheal—elevated; irregular-shaped area of cutaneous edema; solid, transient, changing; variable diameter; pale pink with lighter center
Examples: Urticaria; insect bites

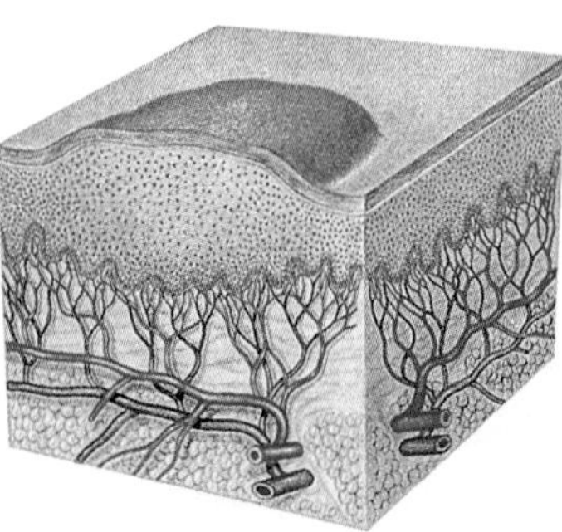

Nodule—elevated; firm; circumscribed; palpable; deeper in dermis than papule; 1 to 2 cm in diameter
Examples: Erythema nodosum; lipomas

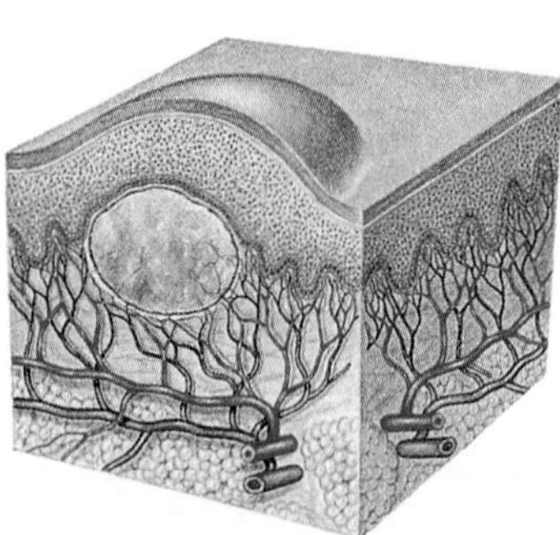

Crust—dried serum, blood, or purulent exudate; slightly elevated; size varies; brown, red, black, tan, or straw
Examples: Scab on abrasion; eczema

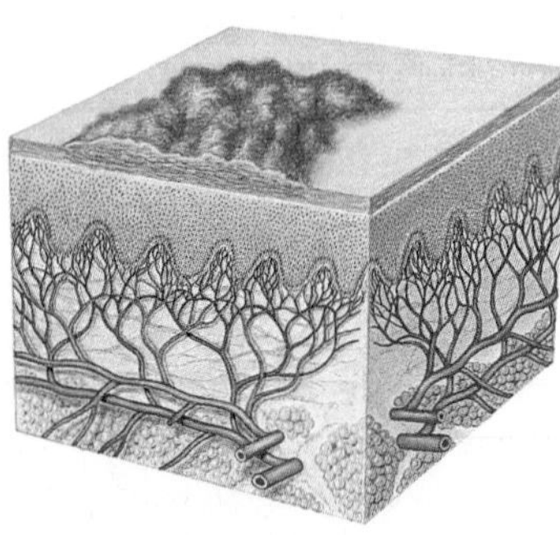

Scale—heaped-up keratinized cells; flaky exfoliation; irregular; thick or thin; dry or oily; varied size; silver, white, or tan
Examples: Psoriasis, exfoliative dermatitis

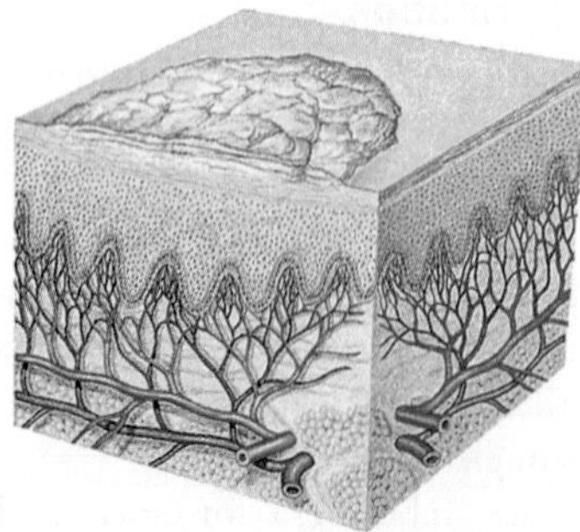

Figure 61-3 Common skin lesions.

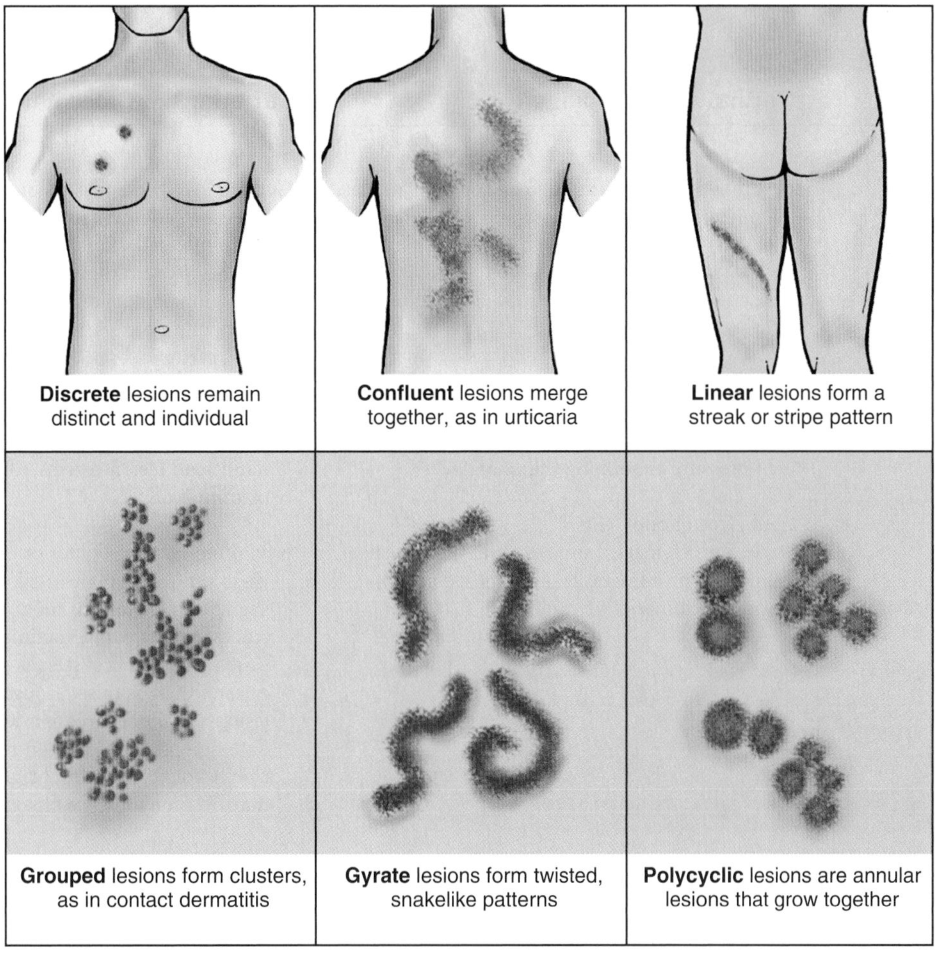

Figure 61-4 Examples of arrangements or configurations of lesions.

TABLE 61-3 Normal Skin Findings in Adults and Variations in Older Adults

Assessment Parameter	Normal Adult Findings	Variations in Older Adults
Skin		
Color tone	Deep to light brown in African-Americans; whitish pink to ruddy with olive or yellow overtones in Caucasians	Skin of Caucasian persons tends to look paler and more opaque
Pigmentation uniformity	Sun-darkened areas; areas of lighter pigmentation in dark-skinned persons (palms, lips, nail beds); labile pigmentation areas associated with use of hormones or pregnancy; callused areas appear yellow; crinkled skin areas darker (knees and elbows); dark-skinned (Mediterranean origin) persons may have lips with bluish hue; vascular flush areas (cheeks, neck, upper chest, or genital area) may appear red, especially with excitement or anxiety; skin color masked through use of cosmetics or tanning agents	More freckles; uneven tanning; pigment deposits; hypopigmented patches
Surface temperature	Cool to warm	
Moisture	Minimum perspiration or oiliness felt; dampness in skin folds; increased perspiration associated with warm environment of activity; wet palms, scalp, forehead, and axilla associated with anxiety	Increased dryness, especially of extremities; decreased perspiration; changes may be hard for patient to accept

Adapted from Thompson JM, et al: *Mosby's manual of clinical nursing,* ed 2, St Louis, 1989, Mosby; modified from Borners A, Thompson J: *Clinical manual of health assessment,* St Louis, 1984, Mosby.

Continued

TABLE 61-3 Normal Skin Findings in Adults and Variations in Older Adults—cont'd

Assessment Parameter	Normal Adult Findings	Variations in Older Adults
Skin–cont'd		
Elasticity, mobility Turgor	Skin moves easily when lifted and returns to place immediately when released	General loss of elasticity; skin moves easily when lifted but does not return to place immediately when released; skin appears lax; increased wrinkle pattern more marked in sun-exposed areas, in fair skin, and in expressive areas of face; pendulous parts sag or droop (under chin, earlobes, breasts, and scrotum)
Texture	Smooth, even, soft; some roughness on exposed areas (elbows and soles of feet)	Flaking and scaling associated with dry skin, especially on lower extremities
Thickness	Wide body variation; increased thickness in areas of pressure or rubbing (hand and feet)	Thinner skin, especially over dorsal surface of hands and feet, forearms, lower legs, and bony prominences
Hygiene	Clean, free of odor	
Lesions	Striae (stretch marks) usually silver or pinkish; freckles (prominent in sun-exposed areas); some birthmarks	Nevi often become lighter or disappear, seborrheic keratoses (pigmented, raised, warty, slightly greasy lesions most often found on truck or face); senile (actinic) keratoses on exposed surfaces, first seen as small reddened areas and then as raised, rough, yellow-to-brown lesions; senile sebaceous adenomas (yellowish flattened papules with central depressions); cherry adenomas (tiny, bright, ruby red, round; may become brown with age)
Nails		
Configuration	Nail edges smooth and rounded; nail base angle 160 degrees; nail surface flat or slightly curved	Toenails may be thickened and distorted with increased linear grooves/ridges
Consistency	Smooth, hard surface; uniform thickness	Fingernails may be more brittle or may peel Accentuated longitudinal lines
Color	Variations of pink; pigment deposits in nail beds of dark-skinned individuals	Toenails may lose translucence and luster and may become yellow
Adherence to nail bed	Nail base feels firm when palpated	
Hair		
Surface characteristics	Scalp smooth; hair shiny; vellus hair short, fine, inconspicuous, and unpigmented; terminal hair coarser, thicker, more conspicuous, and usually pigmented	Sebaceous hyperplasia may extend into scalp
Distribution and configuration	"Normal" varies with individual; hair present on scalp, lower face, nares, ears, axillae, anterior chest around nipples, arms, legs, back, buttocks; female pubic configuration forms inverted triangle; hairline may extend up linea alba; male pubic configuration is upright triangle with hair extending up linea alba to umbilicus	Increased facial hair (especially in women); bristly quality; men may have coarse hair in ears, nose, and eyebrows; decreased scalp hair, symmetric balding in men (most often frontal or occipital); decreased pubic and axillary hair
Texture	Scalp hair may be fine or coarse; fine vellus hair over body; coarse terminal hair pubic and axillary areas	Facial hair coarse; body hair fine
Color	Wide variation from pale to black; color may be masked or changed with rinses or dyes	Graying; whitening; hairs that do not lose pigment often become darker
Quantity	"Normal" varies with individuals; gradual symmetric balding of scalp hair in some men	General disease of body and scalp hair

Gerontologic Assessment

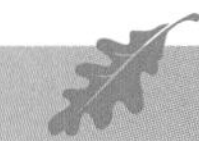

Assess color, pigmentation uniformity, temperature, moisture, texture, thickness and turgor, elasticity and mobility of the skin.
- Normal age-related changes occur in all of these assessment components and are summarized in Table 61-3.
- Inspect skin for intactness, infections, and lesions.
- The thin, dry skin characteristic of the older adult predisposes to skin breakdown. Once breakdown occurs, there is increased risk of infection because of the decreased immune response of the older adult. A number of skin lesions, both benign and malignant, occur with significantly increasing frequency among older adults.

Assess risk of medication-related photosensitivity. Obtain a complete list of medications used, including over-the-counter preparations and review for preparations that can cause an enhanced response to sunlight.
- Many medications taken by older adults can cause hypersensitivity. Among are thiazide diuretics, tetracyclines, sulfa drugs, and certain psychotropics.

COMMON DISORDERS IN ELDERS

Dry Skin Changes—*Xerosis*
Stasis dermatitis of the lower extremities
Benign skin tumors—*Cherry angiomas, spider veins, skin tags ,and seborrheic keratoses*
Skin cancer—*Basal cell carcinoma, squamous cell carcinoma, and melanoma*
Drug reactions
Herpes zoster
Rosacea
Seborrheic dermatitis

DIAGNOSTIC TESTS

Most skin disorders are diagnosed by careful physical assessment. However, diagnostic tests may be used when further information is required to confirm a diagnosis.

Laboratory Tests

Tzanck Prep Test

Skin disorders that produce vesicles or blisters can be further differentiated by performing a Tzanck prep. Wright's or Giemsa stain is used to perform the prep. The vesicle is unroofed with a cotton swab or blade and the base of the vesicle is scraped to obtain cells for examination.[2] Herpes virus will reveal giant multinucleated cells under the microscope.[5] Other skin disorders that can produce vesicles such as poison ivy (allergic contact dermatitis) will not reveal giant cells with the Tzanck prep.

Potassium Hydroxide (KOH) Prep Test

If a fungal infection is suspected, a potassium hydroxide (KOH) prep will assist in the identification of fungal forms. Dry scale is scraped from the lesion onto a slide using a No. 15 blade, glass slide, or coverslip. One or two drops of 20% KOH are placed onto the slide and gently heated. Examination under the microscope reveals hyphae and spores.

Culture

Gram stain and culture and sensitivity of weeping or pustular lesions can be performed to rule in or out bacterial sources for infection. Streptococci and staphylococci are the most common organisms responsible for producing skin infections. Wound cultures can easily be obtained using a cotton swab/culture media and swabbing the exudates from the lesion surface.

Special Tests

Skin Biopsy

Samples of skin lesions may be obtained for examination of the cells of the epidermis, dermis, and subcutaneous tissue. Biopsies can be performed by shave technique (does not require sutures), punch, using a circular-sharp cutting instrument (sutures optional), and excisional biopsy where a full-thickness specimen is often removed for diagnosing skin cancers (requires sutures). The skin is anesthetized before performing a skin biopsy with an intradermal injection of xylocaine. Bleeding can be managed with sutures, electrodessication, or topical hemostatic agents.[2]

Patch Testing

Patch testing is used to both identify and document the causative agent in allergic contact dermatitis and is sometimes helpful in screening when a secondary change takes place on a preexisting rash. Standard concentration samples of suspected allergens are applied to the skin. Minute quantities of the products are placed under an occlusive dressing on the forearms or upper portion of the back. The patches are removed 48 hours after application, and the sites are assessed for swelling or vesicle formation. Because delayed reactions are possible, sites should be reevaluated in 72 hours up to 1 week.

Wood's Lamp

A handheld ultraviolet A Wood's lamp may be used to assist in the diagnoses of certain fungal infections affecting the scalp and body. Certain species of fungi will fluoresce bright blue, green, or gold colors when illuminated by the lamp.

References

1. Anderson DN, lexicographer: *Mosby's medical, nursing, and allied health dictionary,* ed 6, St Louis, 2002, Mosby.
2. Dermatology Nurses's Association: *Dermatology nursing essentials: a core curriculum,* Pittman, NJ, 1998, Anthony J. Janetti.
3. Dermatology Nurse's Association: *Dermatology nursing basics—core proceeding book from annual convention,* Linden, NJ, 2001, Anthony J Janetti.
4. Fitzpatrick TB et al: *Color atlas and synopsis of clinical dermatology,* New York, 2000, McGraw-Hill Professional Publishing.
5. Habif T: *Skin disease: diagnosis and treatment,* ed 3, St Louis, 2001, Mosby.
6. Irwin MJ: Assessing color changes for dark-skinned patients, *Adv Clin Care* 6(6):8, 1991.
7. Leasia MS, Monahan FD: *A practical guide to health assessment,* ed 2, Philadelphia, 2001, WB Saunders.

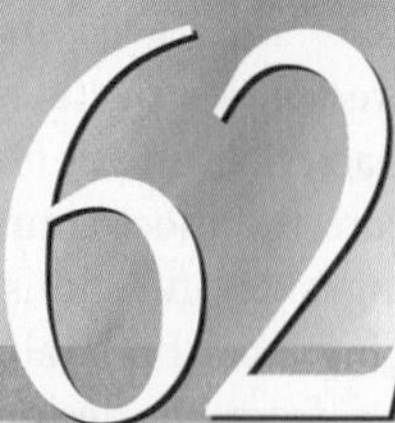

62 Problems of the Skin

Marianne C. Tawa, Sharon Aronovitch

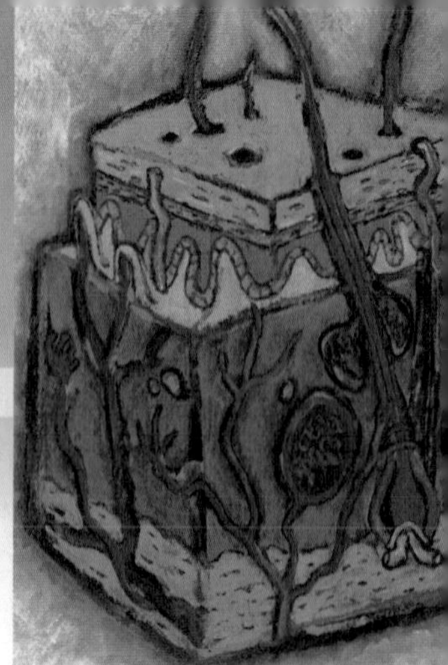

Objectives

After studying this chapter, the learner should be able to:

1. Describe general nursing interventions for patients with dermatologic disorders.
2. Relate the psychologic effects of dermatologic problems.
3. Explain the pathogenesis, physical examination features, and therapeutic interventions for fungal, viral, and bacterial infections of the skin.
4. Describe collaborative care management strategies for patients with follicular disorders.
5. Discuss preventive measures and interventions for eczematous dermatitis and psoriasis.
6. Identify skin manifestations that may result from systemic disease.
7. List skin cancer risk factors and identifying features for premalignant versus malignant lesions.
8. Correlate preventive and early intervention measures for pressure ulcers.
9. Develop an individualized nursing care plan for the patient with a pressure ulcer.

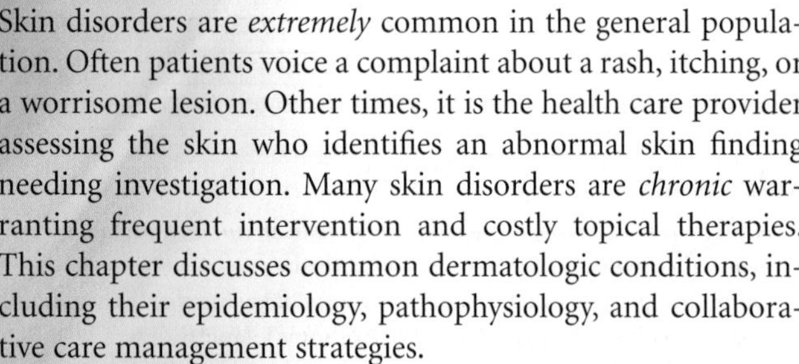

Skin disorders are *extremely* common in the general population. Often patients voice a complaint about a rash, itching, or a worrisome lesion. Other times, it is the health care provider assessing the skin who identifies an abnormal skin finding needing investigation. Many skin disorders are *chronic* warranting frequent intervention and costly topical therapies. This chapter discusses common dermatologic conditions, including their epidemiology, pathophysiology, and collaborative care management strategies.

INFESTATIONS

PEDICULOSIS

Etiology/Epidemiology

Pediculosis (lice infestation) is often found among populations who live in overcrowded dwellings with inadequate hygiene facilities. It is also common in children, many of whom acquire head lice in their day care and classroom environments. Pediculi (lice) are most often found among people who live in overcrowded dwellings with inadequate hygiene facilities.

Pathophysiology

Diagnosis is made by inspection of the appropriate body part. A magnifying glass may be helpful for visualizing the nits attached to the hair shaft. Patients may experience symptoms of itching, particularly at night. Other symptoms include hivelike papules and plaques distributed randomly on the trunk and extremities. Frequent scratching of the scalp may set the stage for skin breakdown, secondary bacterial infections, and enlarged cervical lymph nodes.

Three types of lice infest humans: the head louse, the body louse, and the pubic louse. Lice obtain their nutrition by sucking blood from the skin. The head louse *(Pediculus humanus capitis)* attaches itself to the hair shaft and lays about eight eggs a day. The eggs are firmly attached to the hair or threads of clothing and hatch in 1 week. Head lice may be viewed with a hand lens or flashlight and appear as grayish, glistening oval bodies.[9] The head louse is usually confined to the scalp and beard.

Transmission of head lice occurs through direct person to person contact and also through use of other infected persons' hats, brushes, or combs.

The body louse *(Pediculus humanus corporis)* resides chiefly in the seams of clothing around the neck, waist, and thighs. The bite causes minute hemorrhagic points and severe itching. Transmission is by direct body-to-body contact or by shared clothing and linens.

The pubic louse *(Phthirus pubis)* differs slightly from the head and body louse. It resembles a tiny crab, having clawlike pincers that attach firmly to the pubic hair. Nits are visible in the pubic hair. *P. pubis* is transmitted by sexual contact, bed clothing, towels, and occasionally toilet seats.

Collaborative Care Management

Diagnosis is made through inspection of the appropriate body part. A magnifying glass may be helpful for visualizing the nits attached to the hair shaft. Patients with pediculosis experience itch, particularly at night, and can have hivelike papules and plaques distributed randomly on the trunk and extremities. Frequent scratching of the scalp or other areas may result in skin breakdown, secondary bacterial infections, and enlarged cervical lymph nodes.

Treatment of pediculosis consists of topical application of a pediculicide such as 1% permethrin (Nix or Elimite lotion). Pyrethrins (RID) and the pediculicide gamma benzene hexachloride (1% lindane, Kwell shampoo) are used as second- and third-line treatment options. When pyrethrin products or lindane is used, a second application in 7 to 10 days may be necessary. Directions for both application and duration of treatment time differ according to the product and body location. Pediculicides are not used on eyebrows or eyelashes because of potential eye irritation or sensitization. If eyelashes are infested, nits are removed and petrolatum jelly is applied to smother the lice.

Patient/Family Education. Patients are instructed on the proper application of the pediculicide. Lindane is contraindicated in pregnant and lactating women, as well as newborns. The focus of nursing care is to identify infected persons and educate them about the etiology of pediculosis and prevention of its spread.

Contacts should be evaluated for infestation and treated if necessary. Persons with head lice should be instructed to soak combs, brushes, and hair utensils in hot water. Clothing and bedding should be laundered in the hot water cycle.

SCABIES

Etiology/Epidemiology

Scabies is caused by the female mite *(Sarcoptes scabiei)*. Scabies infestations occur in all age-groups, races, social, and economic classes. Residential communities, shelters, college dormitories, and other crowded living environments are conducive to mite transmission.[11] Close skin-to-skin contact is the typical transmission route, although the mite can live for 2 days on clothing or bedding.

Pathophysiology

The female itch mite penetrates the stratum corneum and burrows into the skin. Within several hours of skin penetration, the itch mite lays a large number of eggs and deposits fecal pellets. The larvae mature in 10 to 14 days and move to the skin surface, where the females are impregnated; the cycle then repeats itself. The incubation period varies, but often a long period elapses before symptoms are noted. Delayed hypersensitivity is thought to be a major factor in the lapse between infestation and symptoms. The incubation period in persons with no previous exposure is 4 to 6 weeks.

The classic symptom for scabies infestation is intense itching—particularly at night time. It is thought to be secondary to an immune response to the mite. Initial skin assessment may reveal the presence of threadlike linear or serpiginous shaped gray-brown burrows, which are less than 1 mm wide. Later papules, hivelike plaques, and nodules may be noted on physical examination. Lesions tend to be concentrated in the web spaces of the fingers, around the wrists, axillae, breasts, waist, thighs, lower buttocks, and genitalia (Figures 62-1 and 62-2). The head and neck are rarely involved. Secondary infections with excoriations and pustules may result from repeated scratching.

Collaborative Care Management

Diagnosis is based on identifying the itch mite under the microscope. The mite is removed from the end of a burrow with a pointed scalpel blade, or the entire burrow is sliced off, placed on a slide with glycerol or mineral oil, and examined under a microscope. If the burrows are not yet visible, mineral oil may be applied to the skin to aid in identification of the burrows.

The goals of therapy are elimination of the itch mite and treatment of complications. To eliminate the mite, the patient

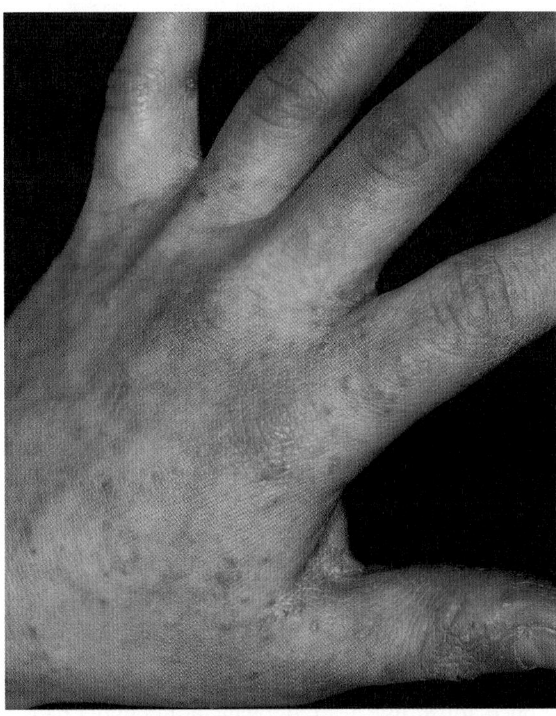

Figure 62-1 Scabies. Tiny vesicles and papules in the finger webs and back of the hand.

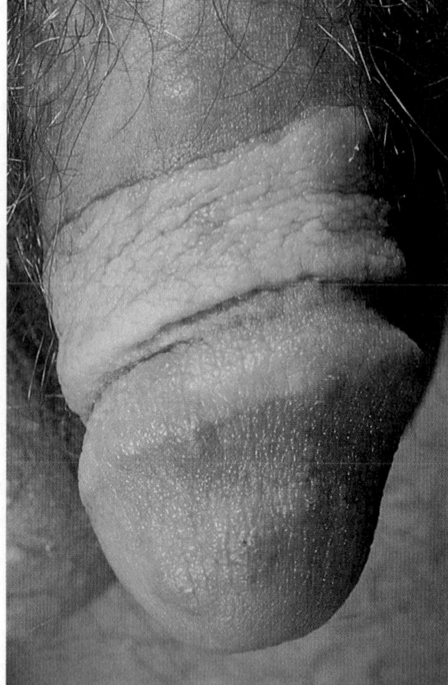

A

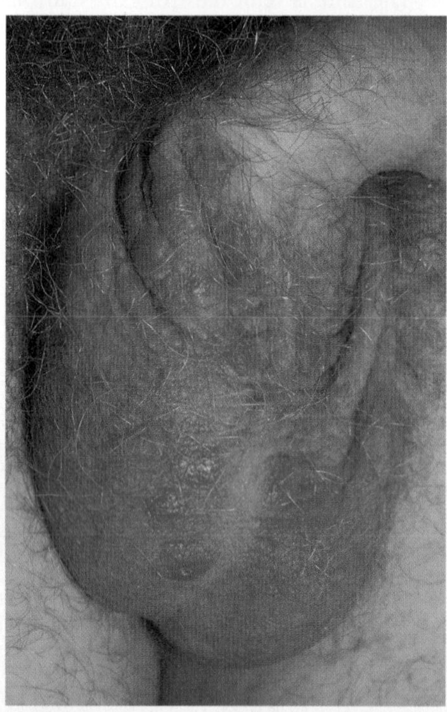

B

Figure 62-2 **A,** Eroded papules on the glans is a highly characteristic sign of scabies. **B,** An established infestation of the penis and scrotum. Large papules may remain after appropriate therapy and sometimes require treatment with intralesional steroids.

and close contacts are treated with either permethrin (Elimite 5% cream) or gamma benzene hexachloride (lindane, Kwell), which are used as follows:

Permethrin (Elimite 5% cream)

Applied at bedtime head to toe including under nails.

Showered off in 8 hours.

Treatment is repeated in 14 days if symptoms persist.

Gamma benzene hexachloride (lindane, Kwell)

Applied at bedtime in a thin layer over the entire body from neck down.

Washed off in 8 to 12 hours.

Treatment repeated in 1week only if living mite identified.

For postscabitic itching and dermatitis, low-potency topical corticosteroids are applied bid for 1 to 2 weeks. Secondary infections are treated with topical or systemic antibiotics.

Patient/Family Education. As with pediculosis, patient education is the primary intervention. Scabies is easily transmitted between individuals and larger groups. Close contacts need to be identified and treated for infestation even in the absence of symptoms. Some patients experience shame and guilt when they learn the diagnosis; a nonjudgmental attitude with explanations of methods of control may help these patients cope with their feelings.

Teaching for the patient with scabies includes:

- All family members/close physical contacts should be treated simultaneously, whether or not symptoms are present.
- Detailed directions for application of the prescribed scabicide should be given.
- Underclothing and linens should be washed in hot water on the day of treatment and dried in the dryer or ironed after dry; clothing and bedding that cannot be laundered need to be placed in plastic bags for several weeks to avoid reinfestation.

Symptoms of itching may persist for up to 2 weeks after treatment.

FUNGAL INFECTIONS

Fungi are larger and more complex than bacteria. They may be unicellular, such as yeasts, or multicellular, such as molds. Many types are pathogenic to humans, causing common skin disorders such as tinea corporis *(ring worm)* or more serious systemic diseases such as blastomycosis. Certain types of fungi produce minor symptoms, whereas others produce significant inflammatory or hypersensitivity reactions.

CANDIDIASIS

Etiology/Epidemiology

Candida albicans, a yeastlike fungus, normally inhabits the gastrointestinal tract, mouth, and vagina, but not usually the skin. Candidiasis (moniliasis), the inflammatory infection caused by the organism's overgrowth on the skin, is caused by the toxins that are released. Some predisposing factors permitting overgrowth of *C. albicans* are pregnancy, oral contraceptives, inhaled corticosteroids, poor nutrition, antibiotic therapy, diabetes mellitus and other endocrine diseases, and immunosuppressed states. Yeast thrives in warm, moist environments, such as the perineum, oral cavity, and intertriginous skin folds of the breast and groin.

Pathophysiology

Overgrowth of *C. albicans* causes the clinical infection candidiasis. Candidiasis involving the mucosa of the mouth is called thrush. The lesions appear as white milk curdlike plaques on the buccal mucosa and may extend down the esophagus. Oral candidiasis can be painful, with symptoms of burning and dysphagia. Vaginal candidiasis produces local mucosal inflammation and thick, white vaginal discharge. Skin infection with the candida organism favors the occlusive body folds of the breasts, groin, and intergluteal region. Moist, macerated patches with vesicles and pustules can produce pruritus and burning. A classic clinical sign of candidiasis is the presence of satellite lesions at the periphery of the general inflammation (Figures 62-3 and 62-4).

Collaborative Care Management

Diagnosis of candidiasis is made by history, clinical features, and microscopic examination.

Treatment is aimed at eliminating predisposing factors. Other measures include keeping the skin dry to avoid maceration and wearing loose, absorbent clothing. Powders may lessen skin fold rubbing. Nystatin (Mycostatin), clotrimazole (Lotrimin, Mycelex), ciclopirox (Loprox), ketoconazole (Nizoral), itraconazole (Sporanox), and fluconazole (Diflucan) are all effective against yeast organism.

Patient/Family Education. The primary focus of patient teaching is prevention. The need to eliminate warm/moist environments that support the growth of the organisms is explained. The importance of thorough drying after bathing is stressed. A second focus is early detection. Patients are taught to carefully assess mucous membranes and skin folds. Immunosuppressed patients may be on an oral antifungal medication long term. Medication teaching is critical with an emphasis on method of administration, side effect profile, and compliance.

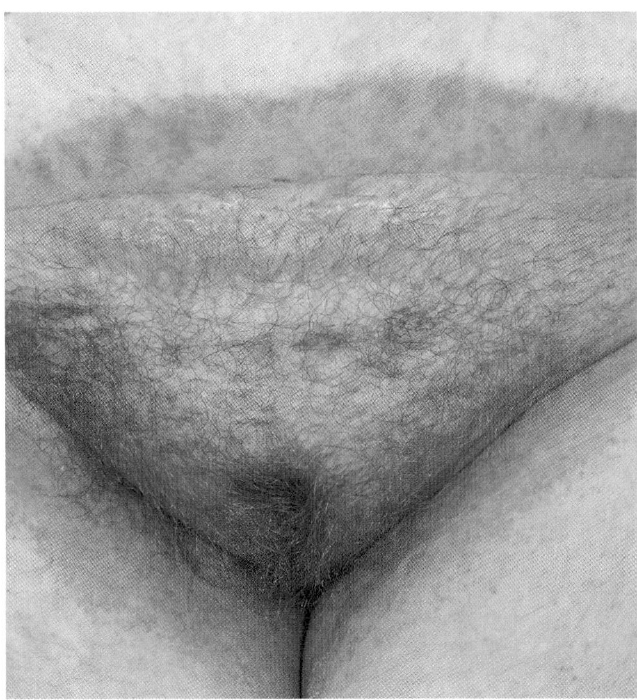

Figure 62-3 Candidal intertrigo. The overhanging abdominal fold and groin area are infected in this obese patient.

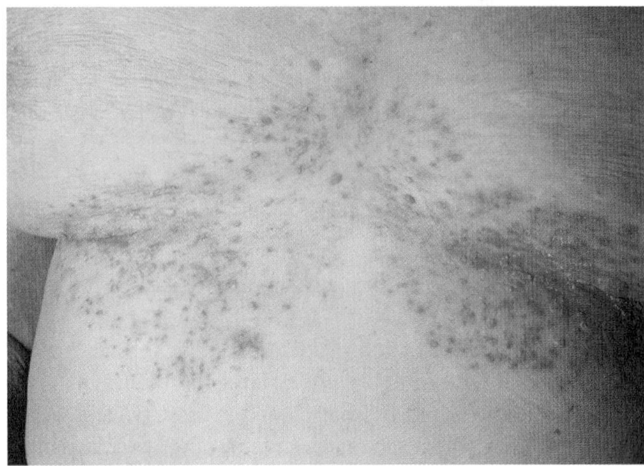

Figure 62-4 Candidiasis under the breast. There are several moist, red papules with a fringe of white scale.

DERMATOPHYTE/TINEA INFECTIONS

Dermatophyte infections occur on nonviable keratinized skin, hair, and nails. Tineas represent a distinct class of fungi both botanically and pathologically. Acquisition is from soil, animal, or human contacts. The incidence of infection is low because of host cellular immunity. The usual fungi causing infection are microsporum, trichophyton, and epidermophyton. Diagnosis of a dermatophyte infection is made by clinical history and physical examination along with microscopy. The variants are named for the location of the rash: tinea capitis, tinea corporis, tinea cruris, tinea pedis, and tinea unguium.

Tinea Capitis

Etiology/Epidemiology

Tinea capitis (scalp) infection is transmitted readily person to person, especially in crowded conditions. Minor scalp trauma facilitates implantation of the spores. Tinea capitis has a worldwide distribution, primarily among prepubertal children.

Pathophysiology

The characteristic rash is round, erythematous, scaly, with pustules appearing at the edge of the lesion (Figure 62-5, *A*). Hair loss *(black dot alopecia)* occurs, with the hair shaft broken off at the base of the scalp. Hair loss is temporary, as the lesions usually heal without scarring. Tinea capitis is usually noninflammatory, but a purulent, boggy progression into *kerion* may develop. In certain situations infected hairs placed under a Wood's light will fluoresce a blue-green color.

Collaborative Care Management

Griseofulvin (Grisactin, Fulvicin, Gris-PEG), an antifungal antibiotic, remains quite effective in the treatment of tinea capitis. High-fat meals aid in the absorption of this drug. There are many drug-drug interactions associated with this medication; thus it is not favored in adults. Another oral antifungal agent choice is itraconazole (Sporanox). This triazole antifungal agent is broad spectrum, but also has many drug

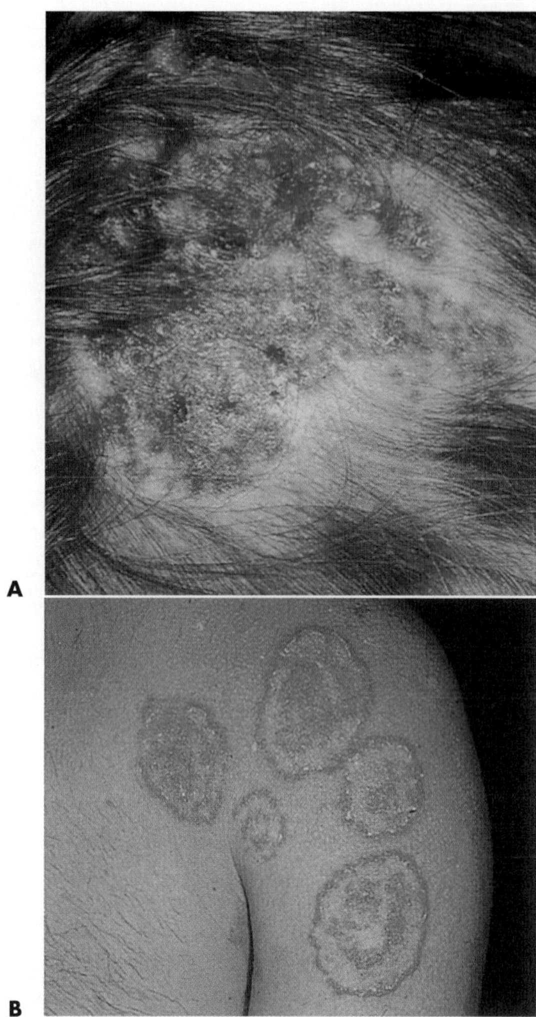

Figure 62-5 A, Tinea capitis. B, Tinea corporis.

interactions. Topical antifungal agents offer assistance only when infection is mild.

Patient/Family Education. Patient teaching focuses on assisting the patient/family to understand the treatment regimen. The scalp should be shampooed at least twice a week. Cutting the hair short facilitates shampooing but may cause psychologic trauma for some children; therefore the hair is best left at an acceptable length.

Tinea Corporis and Tinea Cruris

Etiology/Epidemiology

Tinea corporis (colloquially called *ringworm*) is a common pediatric infection, but can occur in adults, particularly those residing with infected persons. Dermatophytes favor hot and humid climates. Tinea cruris, commonly referred to as *jock itch,* occurs most commonly in men, especially those who wear occlusive athletic wear, or participate in cycling.

Pathophysiology

Tinea corporis typically occurs on the nonhairy exposed parts of the body with ring-shaped plaques, erythematous scaling border, and central clearing. (Figure 62-5, *B*). Lesions of tinea cruris occur in the warm, moist, intertriginous areas of the groin. The lesions are bilateral and extend outward from the groin along the inner thigh. The color ranges from brown to red, scaling is absent, and pruritus is usually present.

Collaborative Care Management

Mild infections are treated with topical antifungals.

Patient/Family Education. Because the dermatophytes thrive in moist, warm environments, patients are instructed to keep the affected areas clean and dry; use a bland dusting powder to promote dryness, and wear loose underclothing.

Tinea Pedis

Etiology/Epidemiology

The most common dermatophyte infection is tinea pedis, or *athlete's foot.* Tinea pedis is rarely seen in children or women but is widespread among young men, especially those wearing sneakers/athletic shoes in hot environments. Walking barefoot in gymnasiums or around swimming pools does not necessarily lead to a tinea infection; conversely, however, susceptible persons will acquire it regardless of their activities.

Pathophysiology

The most common form of tinea pedis is the intertriginous form. The fungal involvement usually begins in the toe webs, especially in the fourth interspace, and may extend to the undersurface of the toes or onto the plantar surface. The person may be asymptomatic or may experience itching and burning in the affected area. The nail plate may become discolored, thickened, or distorted *(onychomycosis).* Tinea pedis is often confused with other foot eruptions, such as eczematous dermatitis/contact dermatitis, or psoriasis.

Collaborative Care Management

Therapy for tinea pedis is topical with antifungal agents. Twice daily application of the medication for at least 1 month is critical, as relapse is quite common. When thick, chronic, scaling plaques are evident, keratolytic agents such as lactic or glycolic acid moisturizers can be helpful in decreasing scale accumulation. If the eruption become acutely inflamed with vesicles and bullae, soaks with Domeboro solution (aluminum acetate) followed by application of the topical antifungal may be used. Systemic antifungal agents are used when the infection proves to be nonresponsive to topical therapy. Nail plate infections generally require systemic antifungal agents, as the densely packed keratin of the nail does not permit adequate absorption of topical agents.

Patient/Family Education. Patients with tinea infections are taught meticulous foot and nail care. They are also advised to wear socks made of an absorbent material, such as cotton, and to change them more than once a day to keep the feet dry. Wearing sandals or going barefoot may also be suggested as ways to control moistness of the feet and toes.

BACTERIAL INFECTIONS

Skin infections may result from loss of skin integrity or from altered host resistance. Minute perforations in the stratum

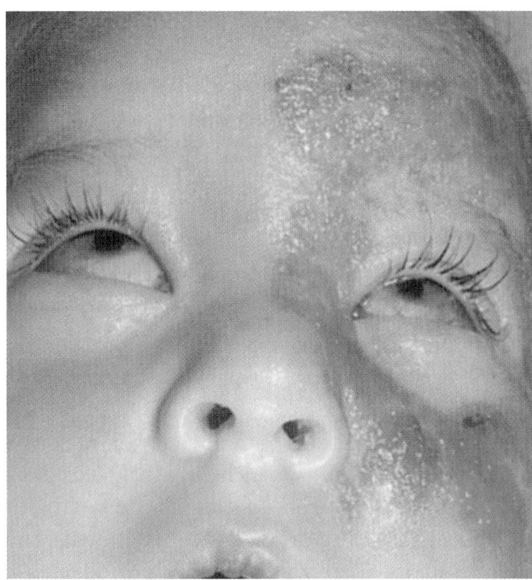

Figure 62-6 Impetigo. Note characteristic crusting.

corneum layer of the epidermis permit entry of microorganisms. Most bacteria that normally inhabit the skin are nonpathogenic. Pathogenic bacteria such as *Staphylococcus aureus* and *Streptococcus pyogenes* can penetrate the outer skin layer, causing the superficial skin infections impetigo and folliculitis.

IMPETIGO

Etiology/Epidemiology

Impetigo is a common, contagious, superficial skin infection caused by beta-hemolytic streptococci or *S. aureus.* Presence of the staphyloccocal organism in the nares predisposes certain patients to impetigo. Although impetigo may occur in any age-group, children are most often affected. Impetigo occurs more commonly in the summer or early fall. The exposed surfaces of the face, arms, and legs are the most common locations for infection. Factors that promote development of impetigo include tropical climates, poor hygiene, poor nutrition, and compromised health. There are few symptoms associated with this infection.

Pathophysiology

Streptococcal impetigo begins as a small, thin-walled vesicle that ruptures easily and leaves a weeping denuded spot. It becomes pustular and dries to form a honey-colored crust that appears stuck on the skin (Figure 62-6). The process, which is superficial, may extend below the crust. Staphylococcal impetigo is characterized by smaller vesicles that enlarge into bullae, rupture, and form shallow erosions. If untreated, impetigo may last for several weeks with new lesions forming.

Collaborative Care Management

Treatment consists of maintaining rigorous topical hygiene. Antimicrobial soaps and washes may be used to decrease the bacterial environment. Crusts must be removed and the lesions washed gently two or three times a day to prevent further crust formation. Warm soaks or saline compresses may be necessary to soften crusts that adhere firmly. Topical antibiotics for the selected organism are applied two to three times a day for approximately 10 days. Systemic antibiotics may be prescribed if the infection is extensive or the patient is at risk.

Patient/Family Education. Teaching focuses on the contagious potential of the disease and methods to prevent the spread of infection. Good hand washing technique for patient and family members is reinforced. Patients are directed to use personal towels and linens and to launder them after the first day of treatment.

FOLLICULITIS

Etiology/Epidemiology

Folliculitis is inflammation of the hair follicle caused by infection, chemical irritation, or physical trauma. *S. aureus* is the most common gram-positive bacteria causing infection.

Gram-negative bacteria such as pseudomonas can infect patients who are receiving antibiotics long term or those who use hot tubs. The infection may be caused by drainage from other infected lesions. Predisposing factors include chronic illness, mechanical irritation from shaving or clothing, hot tub use, or infection in close contacts. Pseudofolliculitis, seen commonly in the military and in African-American males, occurs in the beard region. Sharp cut hair emerge from the follicle, curve, and reenter the skin, causing a chronic low-grade irritation.

Pathophysiology

Bacterial infections of the hair follicle may be superficial in the epidermis around the hair follicle or deep in the tissue surrounding both the lower and upper portions of the hair follicle. Deep folliculitis produces a more severe inflammatory response. Sycosis barbae, *barber's itch,* is a deep folliculitis of the beard. Hordeolum (stye) is a deep folliculitis of the eyelashes (see Chapter 58). Typically there is swelling of the surrounding eyelid and crusting along its edge.

Collaborative Care Management

Treatment of superficial folliculitis includes aggressive hygiene with antimicrobial cleansers and soaps. In addition, topical antibiotics such as mupirocin or neosporin may be applied two to three times a day. Warm compresses may be used to encourage resolution of deep folliculitis.

Patient/Family Education. Nursing management focuses on teaching patients about the prescribed therapy and avoidance of predisposing factors.

FURUNCLES AND CARBUNCLES

Etiology/Epidemiology

Furuncles (boils) are a deep folliculitis that originates either from a superficial folliculitis or as a deep nodule around the hair follicle. Furunculosis is the appearance of several furuncles. An infection that involves several surrounding hair follicles is termed a carbuncle. The causative organism is usually staphylococcus, but occasionally furuncles can be caused by other gram-positive and gram-negative bacteria. Both furuncles and carbuncles develop with obesity, poor nutritional states, debilitation, and poorly controlled diabetes mellitus.

Pathophysiology

Local swelling, erythema, and tenderness are the presenting symptoms. Within 3 to 5 days the lesion becomes elevated or "points up," the surrounding skin becomes shiny, and the center or "core" turns yellow. Carbuncles have several cores. The furuncle (boil) will rupture spontaneously, or may require surgical incision and drainage. With drainage, the pain is immediately alleviated. The drainage progresses from yellow purulent material to serosanguineous discharge. Drainage usually subsides within a few hours to a few days; the redness and swelling subside gradually. Furuncles/carbuncles are commonly seen on the face, neck, breasts, axillae, buttocks, thighs, perineum, and groin.

Collaborative Care Management

Warm compresses are used to aid in bringing the boil to a head. As the boil drains, care must be taken to keep the infected discharge off the surrounding skin. Systemic antibiotics may be prescribed based on the results of wound culture and sensitivity or Gram stain. Incision and drainage of the boil may be required. Strict adherence to Standard Precautions is essential in the care of persons with boils or carbuncles. Furuncles and carbuncles tend to recur in susceptible individuals.

Patient/Family Education. Patient teaching focuses on preventing the spread of the infection. Patients are cautioned to keep their hands away from the discharge to prevent spread of infection.

ERYSIPELAS

Etiology/Epidemiology

Erysipelas is a form of localized cellulitis usually caused by a hemolytic streptococcus and *S. aureus* (Figure 62-7). Older adults with poor host resistance are at risk for this infection. Erysipelas may develop after a puncture wound, ulcer, or chronic dermatitis.

Pathophysiology

Before the development of systemic antibiotics, erysipelas was a serious infection. It is characterized by localized inflammation and swelling of the skin and subcutaneous tissues. Typical sites of infection are the face, scalp, hands, and genitalia. A sharp, erythematous line demarcates infected skin from normal skin. The infected area is warm to palpation. The infection spreads via the lymphatic system and bloodstream.

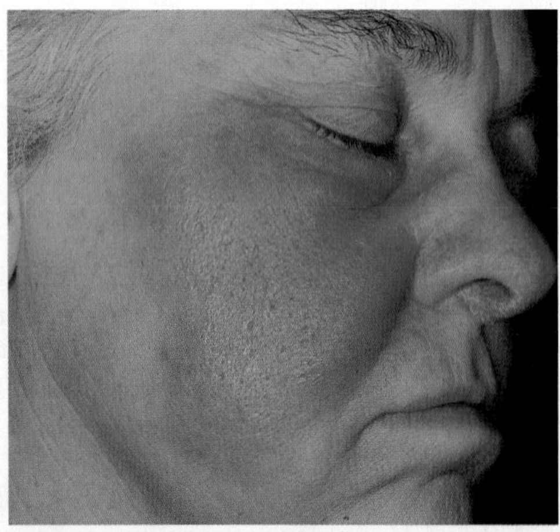

Figure 62-7 Cellulitis. Acute phase with intense erythema.

Collaborative Care Management

Gram stain, culture, and sensitivity determine the appropriate antibiotic treatment. Local lesions are immobilized and elevated to decrease local edema. Domeboro soaks are used to decrease discomfort and dry up bullous lesions. Moist heat may also be used. If abscess formation occurs, incision and drainage may be indicated.

Patient/Family Education. Patient education focuses on treatment recommendations, which may include soaks, elevation, and administration of antibiotics. It is imperative that the patient understand the importance of completing the course of prescribed antibiotic therapy.

VIRAL INFECTIONS

WARTS

Etiology/Epidemiology

Warts are benign epidermal tumors caused by the human papilloma virus (HPV). There are approximately 65 subtypes of the virus causing infection on skin and mucosal surfaces. The incidence of HPV is high in the general population, with children and young adults more commonly affected.

Pathophysiology

Warts are benign skin growths that grow in a variety of shapes. Transmission of the virus is by skin-to-skin contact. The common wart is a small, circumscribed, painless, hyperkeratotic papule usually seen on the extremities, especially the hands. Filiform warts are slender fingerlike projections occurring mostly on the face and neck. Plantar warts grow inward from the pressure on the soles of the feet and may be painful. They are differentiated from calluses by the disruption of normal plantar skin lines on the soles of the feet. Warts that develop in the anogenital region (condyloma acuminata) are grayish with a cauliflower-like appearance and may burn or itch. Anogenital warts are acquired by sexual activity or rarely by autoinnoculation. Certain subtypes of HPV possess cancer-transforming potential.

Collaborative Care Management

There are several treatments for warts, most of which are destructive modalities. Warts often spontaneously resolve without intervention. Treatment for both common and plantar warts include keratolytic acids (salycylic and lactic acids), cryosurgery with liquid nitrogen, electrosurgery, laser surgery, and surgical excision, rarely. Anogenital (condyloma acuminatum) HPV infections are treated with multiple modalities including caustic acids, podophyllum resin, imiquimod cream (topical immune response agent), as well as cryotherapy and laser surgery.

Patient/Family Education. Patient teaching focuses on the viral etiology of HPV, mode of transmission, and implications of treatment. Patients may seek resources for *alternative* therapies, which include hypnosis and biofeedback. Sexually transmitted disease prevention should be strongly emphasized in all patients with genital tract disease. In addition, the need for examination of sexual partners should be stressed.

HERPES SIMPLEX

One of the most common viruses found in humans is the herpes simplex virus (HSV), which occurs as two similar yet serologically different strains, type 1 and type 2. Type 1 virus is found primarily on the face or in the mouth and is colloquially referred to as fever blisters or cold sores. It is also occasionally found in the eyes (keratitis). Type 2 is associated with genital tract infection transmitted by sexual contact. Transmission of HSV is primarily skin to skin or skin to mucosa. The incubation period may be anywhere from 2 to 20 days. Details of HSV infection are found in Chapters 32 and 56.

HERPES ZOSTER

Etiology/Epidemiology

Herpes zoster, or shingles, is caused by the same virus (varicella-zoster) that causes varicella (chickenpox). Varicella is believed to be the primary infection in a nonimmune host, whereas herpes zoster is thought to be the response in a partially immune host. Herpes zoster occurs more commonly in older adults, because of the natural decline in cellular immunity seen with normal aging. Although herpes zoster is far less communicable than chickenpox, persons who have not had chickenpox may develop herpes zoster after exposure to the vesicular lesions of persons with it. For this reason, susceptible persons should not care for patients with herpes zoster. Herpes zoster occurs more frequently in persons with HIV disease, lymphatic cancers, and post organ/marrow transplantation. In rare circumstances it may recur.

Pathophysiology

In herpes zoster clusters of vesicular lesions are arranged in a linear fashion. They follow the course of the peripheral sensory nerves and hence the lesions never cross the midline of the body (Figure 62-8). They often are unilateral but nerve groups on both sides of the body can be involved. Two thirds of persons with herpes zoster develop lesions over thoracic dermatomes, and the remainder show involvement of the trigeminal nerve with lesions on the face, eye, and scalp. The rash develops first as macules but progresses rapidly to vesicles and/or bullae. The fluid becomes turbid, and crusts develop and drop off in about 10 days.

Malaise, fever, itching, and pain over the involved area may precede the rash. If vesicles develop within 1 to 2 days after the initial pain symptoms, the lesions usually clear in 2 to 3 weeks; but if the vesicles develop over a period of 1 week, a prolonged course can be expected.

Discomfort from pain and itching is the major problem with herpes zoster. The pain may vary from a light burning sensation to a deep visceral-type pain, and it may be intermittent or constant. It usually persists for up to 4 weeks. In about 10% of patients, a pain syndrome called postherpetic neuralgia develops.

Collaborative Care Management

For some patients no pharmacologic treatment is prescribed for herpes zoster. If the infection is identified early (within 48 to 72 hours of first lesions), or in high risk individuals, antiviral therapy is helpful. Acyclovir (Zovirax) accelerates healing and reduces acute pain. It is given orally in high doses (800 mg five times a day for 1 week). In severe infections acyclovir may be given intravenously. Because acyclovir can precipitate in renal tubules, drinking fluids should be encouraged. Although acyclovir does not prevent postherpetic neuralgia, it may reduce its severity. Famciclovir, similar to acyclovir, is used for uncomplicated cases of acute herpes zoster in patients who are immunocompromised. As with acyclovir, famciclovir has been shown to reduce the duration of postherpetic neuralgia.

Analgesics may be required for pain management. Aspirin, with or without codeine, is often effective; meperidine (Demerol) may be needed for severe pain. Nonsteroidal antiinflammatory drugs (NSAIDs) are usually ineffective. Local discomfort may be relieved by topical antipruritic agents such as, Sarna, Prax, PrameGel, or oatmeal colloid preparations. Domeboro soaks (aluminum acetate) applied as a cool compress may provide local relief and quicken drying of the vesicles. Loose clothing helps minimize contact with the affected area. Patients should avoid exposure to highly susceptible persons (those who have not had chickenpox or are immunosuppressed).

Postherpetic neuralgia usually lasts less than 1 year but may persist for many years. The pain is always present with superimposed sharp pain episodes. Because the pain results from nervous system damage, it does not respond well to usual pain therapies. Multidisciplinary approaches to pain management are often required. Local application of capsaicin cream may provide some pain relief. Tricyclic antidepressants are commonly prescribed. Transcutaneous electrical nerve stimulation may be tried initially, although it usually is not effective on a long-term basis. Narcotics are avoided because of the persistence of the pain and potential for addiction. Because the pain can become an all-consuming part of the patient's

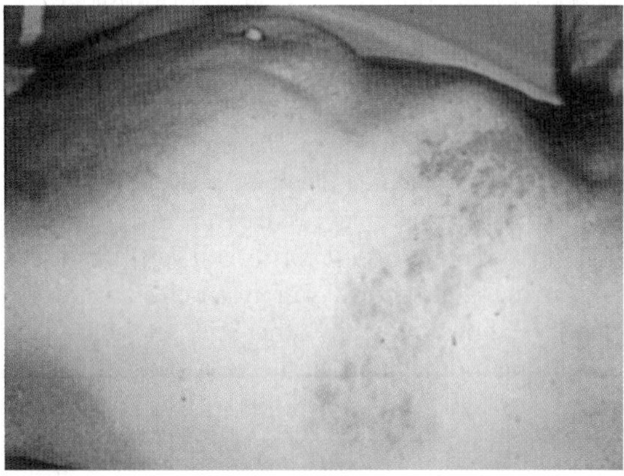

Figure 62-8 Herpes zoster.

life, ongoing evaluation of the impact on the patient functionally and socially and ongoing supportive counseling are helpful.

Patient/Family Education. Patient and family education to prevent spread of infection is important. Patients should be educated regarding the course of the disease and possible complications. Patients and family should receive information regarding treatments and medications. Nursing care focuses on helping patients deal with the postherpetic neuralgia. (For a complete discussion of chronic pain, see Chapter 12.)

ACNE

ACNE VULGARIS

Etiology/Epidemiology

Acne vulgaris, a common skin disease, is seen in 80% of adolescents, but it may also occur in adults. It affects approximately 70 million persons annually in the United States. Acne is multifactorial. Acne pathology is thought to be related to free fatty acids, endocrine effects, stressors, heredity, and infection. Diet has been essentially ruled out as a causative factor, but none of the other factors have been demonstrated conclusively. Acne occurs at puberty, when the sebaceous glands are stimulated by androgens and is often found to be common within families. Acne is more quiescent in summer months.

Pathophysiology

At puberty, sebaceous glands undergo enlargement from androgen stimulation. Sebum is released, passed through the follicular canal, and combined with sebaceous gland cell fragments, epidermal cells (keratin), and bacteria. At this time, triglycerides in the sebum are hydrolyzed to glycerol and free fatty acids. The sebum and debris may become plugged in the hair follicle to form an open comedo (blackhead) if it is at the surface or a closed comedo (whitehead) if it is below the surface (Figure 62-9). The dark color of the blackhead is melanin, not dirt, and results from passage of melanin from the adjoining epidermal cells.

Inflammatory lesions apparently develop from the escape of sebum into the dermis, which then serves as an irritant, causing an inflammatory reaction. Free fatty acids may also be an irritant in the follicle itself. Acne occurs mostly on the face and neck, upper chest, and back, although the upper arms, buttocks, and thighs may also be involved. Comedones are the first visible signs, and the skin is characteristically oily. The inflammatory lesions include papules, pustules, nodules, and cysts. Superficial lesions may resolve in 5 to 10 days without scarring, but large lesions last for several weeks and often result in scarring. The typical scar resembles an old volcano (ice-pick scar); however, many other sizes and shapes may result, depending on the depth and extent of the inflammatory lesions.

The extent of the lesions varies greatly. Some persons have only a few small lesions. Many adolescents have several lesions that peak at ages 16 to 18 years of age and then slowly resolve.

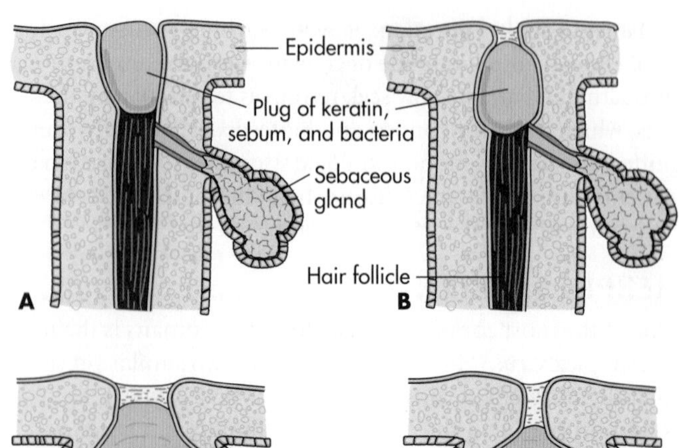

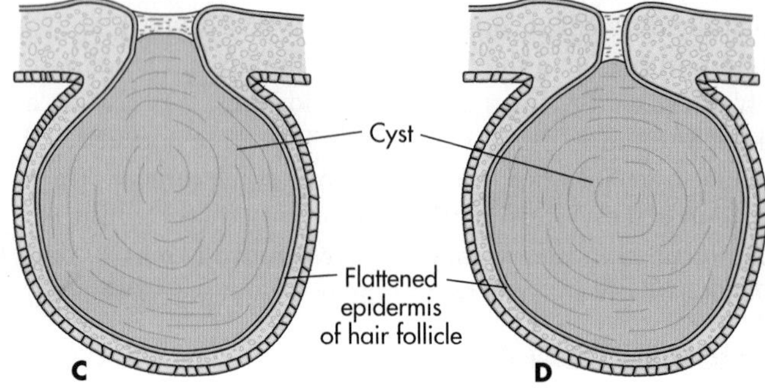

Figure 62-9 Formation of lesions in acne vulgaris. **A,** Open comedo (blackhead), early stage. **B,** Closed comedo (whitehead), early stage. **C,** Cyst formation in open comedo, advanced stage. **D,** Cyst formation in closed comedo, advanced stage.

A small percentage of the population develops severe nodular-cystic acne.

Collaborative Care Management

Treatment of acne consists of topical, systemic, intralesional, and surgical approaches.

Topical agents commonly prescribed are benzoyl peroxides, retinoids and retinoid-like drugs (tretinoin, adapalene, tazarotene, azelaic acid), and antibiotics (clindamycin, erythromycin, sulfa based). Systemic antibiotic therapy with tetracyclines, erythromycin, or trimethoprin-sulfamethoxazole is indicated for inflammatory acne lesions. Isoretinoic acid (Accutane), a vitamin A acid analog, is an alternate type of systemic therapy. Side effects of isoretinoic acid include dry lips, conjunctiva and skin, hair loss, muscle aches, photosensitivity, mood disturbance, elevated lipids, and birth defects. Low progestin-containing oral contraceptive agents may offer benefit to certain female patients. Intralesional corticosteroid therapy is used for the cysts of severe acne, whereas dermabrasion and laser resurfacing procedures can be used to revise scars. Chemical peels with alphahydroxy and/or more penetrating acids (trichloroacetic acid) may be used as an adjuvant therapy with both topical/oral medications or as postacne therapy.

Counseling and teaching are the major nursing strategies. Acne can be a significant life stressor, particularly in the adolescent years. Behavioral responses to the altered body image produced by acne flares may be anger, hostility, shyness, depression, and withdrawal. Psychologic counseling may be necessary in select situations.

Patient Teaching
The Patient With Acne

PREVENTIVE MEASURES

Keep hands and hair away from the face.
Avoid masks, straps, and cradling of the face.
Shampoo hair daily.
Avoid exposure to oils and greases.
Eat a well-balanced diet and avoid any foods that appear to cause skin flare-ups.

GENERAL SKIN CARE

Wash face two to three times a day with mild cleansers. Do not overwash.
Use over-the-counter (OTC) salicylic, sulfa, or benzyl peroxide agents under the direction of health care provider.
Avoid vigorous rubbing of the skin.
Use only H_2O-based cosmetics.
Never leave cosmetics on face overnight.

DRUG THERAPY

Follow the prescribed therapy; it may take up to 8 weeks to realize benefit from both topical and systemic therapy.
Expect skin desquamation, especially with topical tretinoin.
Avoid using multiple OTC agents while on medical therapy.
Remove cosmetics before applying topical medications.
Avoid exposure to direct sunlight if using topical tretinoin or taking drugs such as tetracyclines and sulfa antibiotics (photosensitivity).
Pregnancy prevention is mandatory for Accutane therapy (possibility of birth defects).

Patient/Family Education. Dispelling acne myths is a critical nursing intervention (foods such as chocolate, pizza, soda, and french fries do *not* cause acne) because understanding the nature of acne helps the person understand the necessary care. Teaching is directed toward general health care of the skin and guidelines for therapy (see the Patient Teaching box).

The lesions in acne develop when the pilosebaceous follicles become plugged; therefore activities that contribute to occlusion of the follicles are to be avoided. Hair and hands should be kept away from the face. Loose clothing prevents pressure over the follicles, and tight collars should not be worn. The skin should be kept clean. Greasy, oil-based cosmetics may be occlusive and plug up the follicles. Medication teaching, including drug interactions, pregnancy prevention, and side-effect profiles, should be reviewed in detail with the patient and family. Daily sun protection is advised with most agents to avoid photosensitivity reactions.

ACNE ROSACEA

Etiology/Epidemiology

Acne rosacea is a follicular eruption of the skin with both a vascular and acne component. It affects 30- to 50-year-olds, women more than men, but men tend to have more severe manifestations. The cause is unknown. Many theories abound, but none have been proven. Fair complexioned individuals are more inclined to manifest symptoms of acne rosacea. A familial predisposition to acne rosacea is also seen.

Pathophysiology

Acne rosacea begins with erythema over the central face, cheeks, and nose. Flushing and blushing are classic symptom associated with this finding. Papules, pustules, cysts, and enlargement of superficial blood vessels (telangectasias) ensue. Years of acne rosacea can lead to an irregular, bulbous thickening of the skin of the distal part of the nose (rhinophyma), with a red-purple discoloration and dilated follicles.[10]

Collaborative Care Management

Rosacea responds slowly to treatment and relapses are common. In moderate to severe cases, topical/oral antibiotics or isotretinoin may be used. Telangectasias and rhinophyma can be modified with laser surgery. Elimination of rosacea triggers is crucial to managing the disease. Anything that induces flushing such as heat, cold, wind, sunlight, alcohol, and spicy foods can exacerbate symptoms. Daily sun protection is strongly recommended.

Patient/Family Education. Patients and family should be educated on the disease and the therapy selected. Identification of rosacea triggers and their avoidance should be stressed. Use of mild cleansers and avoidance of alcohol-based products and fragrances may reduce symptoms.

ECZEMATOUS DERMATITIS

Eczema is characterized by superficial inflammation of the skin. The terms eczema and dermatitis are often used interchangeably. There are approximately 20 forms of eczema, each of which is triggered by certain flare factors such as dryness, change in environment or temperature, infection, and stress. Dermatitis is often classified arbitrarily according to specific features, such as cause, pattern, and age. Some common types of dermatitis are described in Table 62-1 and are discussed in more detail in the succeeding text. Regardless of the cause, the lesions in any dermatitis follow a characteristic pattern. Initially, erythema and local edema are followed by vesicle formation with oozing and then crusting and scaling. If the dermatitis persists, there will be evidence of excoriation from scratching and thickening of the skin, and the color becomes more brownish. Secondary infection may result.

CONTACT DERMATITIS

Etiology/Epidemiology

Contact dermatitis is caused by exposure to substances in the environment. (Table 62-2). Contact dermatitis occurs in both irritant and allergic forms. Irritant contact dermatitis is a nonallergic reaction occurring in any person on contact with a sufficient concentration of an irritant.[12] It occurs four times more commonly than allergic contact dermatitis. Mechanical irritation may result from wool or glass fibers. Chemical irritants include acids, alkalies, solvents, detergents, and oils commonly found in cleaning compounds, insecticides, and industrial compounds. Biologic irritants include urine, feces, and toxins from insects or aquatic plants. Persons engaged in wet work such as food handlers, health care workers, and childcare providers are more prone to irritant contact dermatitis.

TABLE 62-1 Types of Dermatitis

Type	Cause	Characteristics
Contact (Figure 62-10)	External agents	Site and pattern of lesions depend on exposure pattern (e.g., linear, angular) Itching a major symptom
Atopic	Hypersensitivity reaction, hereditary	Itching a major symptom Lesions caused by scratching
Lichen simplex chronicus	Stasis, irritants, psychologic factors	Itching a major symptom Lesions caused by scratching
Seborrheic (Figure 62-11)	Pitysporum orbiculare overgrowth likely with genetic and environmental influences	Erythematous, scaly (e.g., dandruff)
Nummular	Unknown	Coin-shaped lesions Severe itching
Stasis	Altered circulation	Erythema, edema Lesions may develop from trauma Itching may be severe

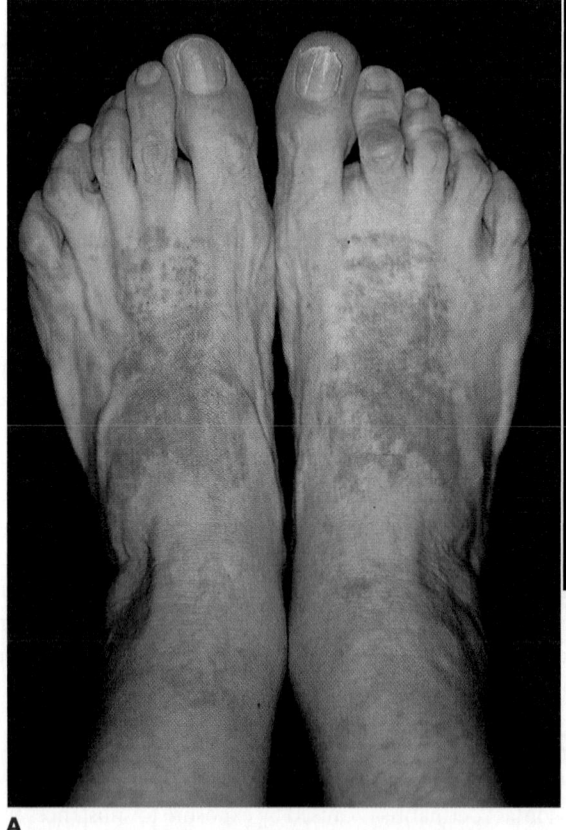

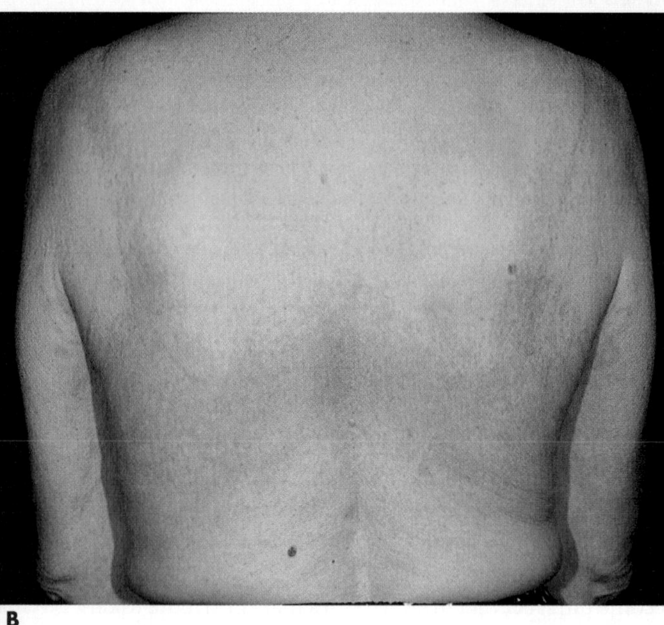

Figure 62-10 **A,** Shoe contact dermatitis. Sharply defined plaques formed under a shoe lining impregnated with rubber cement. **B,** Allergic contact dermatitis to spandex rubber in a bra.

Allergic contact dermatitis is a cell-mediated type IV delayed hypersensitivity immune reaction from contact with a specific antigen (Figure 62-10, *B*). Many compounds can cause sensitization under specified conditions. Typical antigens include poison ivy, synthetics, industrial chemicals, drugs (e.g., sulfanilamide or penicillin), and metals (especially nickel and chromate). Once the skin has been sensitized, further contact with the sensitizing substance will produce an eczematous reaction. The sensitizing allergen may reach the site by direct contact; by indirect contact, such as transmission by animals, from one part of the body to the other by the hands, or on clothing; or by the air, as in smoke. Investigation of possible exposures including medications, products (e.g., household cleaning, cosmetics, hobbies), occupational environment, and recreational activities may provide insight into possible etiologies for the contact event.

Pathophysiology

The characteristic lesions of contact dermatitis appear sooner in an irritant contact than in the allergic type; however,

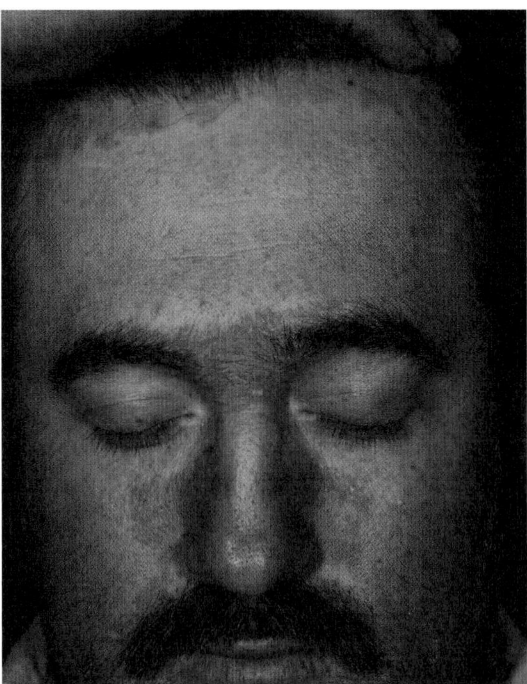

Figure 62-11 Seborrheic dermatitis in an adult with extensive involvement in all of the characteristic sites.

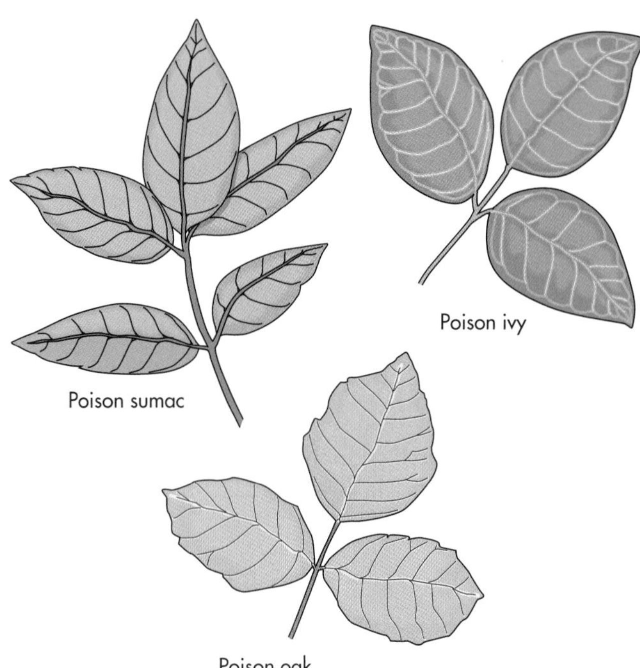

Figure 62-12 Typical leaves of poison sumac, poison ivy, and poison oak.

TABLE 62-2 Common Causes of Allergic/Irritant Contact Dermatitis

Area	Cause
Face/scalp/ears	Cosmetics, hair care products, jewelry, cleansers, sunscreen, contact lens solution, metals (especially nickel), glasses
Neck	Perfumes, clothing (especially wool)
Trunk, axillae	Deodorants, clothing, perfumes, laundry products
Arms/hands	Poison ivy, oak, and sumac; jewelry; nickel, etc., in watchbands
	Detergents and other cleansers, gloves
Legs/feet	Medication for "athlete's foot," shoes

the onset and appearance vary, depending on the type and concentration of the irritant. The rash develops on the exposed areas, particularly the more sensitive areas, such as the dorsal rather than the palmar surface of the hands. When contact dermatitis is suspected but the agent is unknown, patch testing may be carried out,[16] or the environment may be manipulated to exclude suspected agents.

Collaborative Care Management

Weeping vesicular lesions are treated with Domeboro soaks (aluminum acetate) applied one to two times a day. Crusts and scales are not removed but are allowed to drop off naturally as the skin heals. Topical corticosteroids (mid to potent range) are applied twice a day to affected areas for approximately 2 weeks. Face, genital, and skin fold sites warrant weaker steroid formulations such as hydrocortisone 0.5% to 1%. Oral corticosteroids may be prescribed for generalized rash manifestations or significant hand and face involvement. Rarely oral antibiotics are used when secondary infection ensues. Itching may be eased by oral antihistamines, topical antipruritic agents, or colloidal oatmeal baths and lotions.

Patient/Family Education. The primary focus of patient teaching is prevention. Contact dermatitis may be prevented by avoiding the irritating or sensitizing substance whenever possible. Patients and family members should be educated to recognize the leaves of *Rhus* plants—poison ivy, oak, and sumac (Figure 62-12). Persons walking in areas where poison ivy grows need to protect the skin by wearing appropriate clothing. If contact with poison ivy is suspected, symptoms may be averted by immediately rinsing the skin for 15 minutes with running water to remove the resin before skin penetration occurs. Remove clothing carefully to avoid skin contact.

The person who develops a sensitivity to material encountered in the living or working environment may need to consider a permanent change of environment if other measures are unsuccessful. Gloves may be used if the person is handling irritant or allergenic substances. Persons sensitive to detergents may need to wash their clothes and bathe with a mild soap product.

ATOPIC DERMATITIS

Etiology/Epidemiology

Atopic dermatitis is a common inflammatory skin condition linked to a larger group of atopic diseases including asthma and hayfever. Approximately 40% to 50% of persons with atopic dermatitis develop manifestations of asthma and/or hay fever. Upwards of 50% to 60% of patients with atopic dermatitis come from families with one or more atopic diseases. Atopic dermatitis is chronic and relapsing with several factors contributing to flares. Controlling environmental influences such as climatic changes and humidity levels can prove challenging for both patient and caregiver alike. Exacerbating factors include sudden changes in temperature or humidity; exercise; psychologic stress; fibers such as wool, fur, or nylon; detergents; and perfumes. Atopic dermatitis is most common in children. Up to 75% of children with atopic dermatitis develop symptoms by 6 months of age. It usually disappears or becomes less severe between the ages of 2 and 3 years but can recur in late childhood or adolescence. Resolution of symptoms is seen by age 30 in a large number of adults.

The major symptom of atopic dermatitis is intense pruritus.[14] Chronic rubbing and scratching produces eczematous skin findings, followed by skin thickening *(lichenification)* and alteration in pigmentation (hypopigmentation or hyperpigmentation).

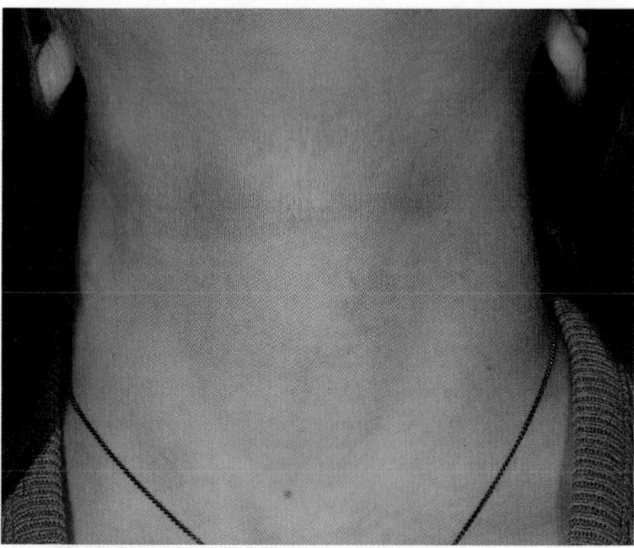

Figure 62-13 Atopic dermatitis. Classic appearance of erythema and diffuse scaling about the neck.

Pathophysiology

The protective barrier function of the skin is diminished greatly in the atopic population. Lipid content changes in the epidermis permit water loss from the cells resulting in dry skin. Persons with atopic dermatitis are highly sensitive with a lowered threshold to pruritus. Even minor stimuli can produce intense episodes of itching. Increased levels of IgE and shifts in helper T-cell lymphocytes in the skin are the characteristic immunologic-mediated abnormalities seen in atopic dermatitis. There is a marked tendency toward vasoconstriction of superficial blood vessels, and the skin blanches readily. Cold and low humidity are poorly tolerated because of drying effects. Heat and high humidity are also poorly tolerated because vasodilation increases the inflammatory reaction, thus aggravating the dermatitis and causing increased itching and discomfort. The initial clinical presentation for atopic dermatitis is rough, dry skin that may appear as early as the first month of life. Infants may develop moist, oozing, crusting lesions on the scalp and face, with spread to the trunk and extensor aspects of the arms and legs. Later, the lesions become localized to the flexures of the neck (Figure 62-13), wrists, antecubital and popliteal fossae, eyelids, and behind the ears. The erythema is dusky, and excoriations may become secondarily infected. By the late twenties or early thirties the lesions usually disappear, but they may recur at a later date as chronic hand or foot eczema.

The compromised barrier function of the skin in atopic dermatitis places individuals at increased risk for acquiring viral, fungal, and bacterial infections of the skin.

Collaborative Care Management

There is no cure for atopic dermatitis, but symptoms can be controlled. Hydrating the skin is the cornerstone of therapy. Applying an occlusive moisturizing agent three to four times a day (preferably emollients in a *water-in-oil* base) works to reestablish a well-hydrated stratum corneum. Topical corticosteroid therapy is the principal pharmacologic agent used in the management of atopic dermatitis. Weaker potency corticosteroids are selected for the pediatric population, with ointment vehicles proving to be more hydrating. More potent topical corticosteroids should be reserved for adults, with education regarding method of application, duration of use, and potential side effects. Topical corticosteroids may be used in concert with wet wraps, which can enhance drug absorption and play a role in decreasing pruritus. Systemic corticosteroids may be given for a limited period to those with severe atopic eczema.

Systemic therapy with sedating antihistamines at night (when itching is more intense) can be helpful. Treatment of secondary bacterial skin infections with appropriate antibiotics may be warranted. In some instances, patients may benefit from phototherapy with ultraviolet (UV) B or UV A + psoralen (PUVA). Tacrolimus ointment (Protopic) is a new topical immunosuppressive drug used in the management of atopic dermatitis. Clinical trials and current practice demonstrate efficacy, with few systemic side effects.

Patient/Family Education. Patient education is the major focus of care. Successful management of atopic dermatitis is achieved through patient, family, and health care provider collaboration. Provision of comprehensive written skin care instructions and demonstration of techniques for application of topical drugs are critical nursing measures. Addressing the social-emotional concerns of patients with atopic dermatitis is another challenging area for intervention. Chronic manifestations of this skin disease can set the stage for social isolation, poor self-esteem, anxiety, and sleep disturbance (see Patient Teaching box).

LICHEN SIMPLEX CHRONICUS

Lichen simplex chronicus (LSC) is a localized, well-circumscribed, eczematous eruption caused by repeated rubbing and scratching. It tends to occur in areas that can be easily reached, such as the wrists, ankles, and back of the scalp. Stress factors are thought to be involved. Once itching is initiated by an insect bite, rash, or nonspecific irritant, the *itch-scratch* cycle

Patient Teaching
The Patient With Atopic Dermatitis

1. Use only gentle cleansers and soaplike products.
2. Take a relaxing warm bath for 15 to 20 minutes; gently pat away excess H_2O and immediately apply a moisturizer. Reapply moisturizers throughout the day when skin is dry.
3. Wet wraps may be used in place of soaking; wraps permit evaporation, which cools the skin, thus decreasing pruritus.
4. Apply corticosteroids in a thin layer and rub in well; do not use fluorinated corticosteroid on the face.
5. Avoid wool, fur, or rough fibers against the skin; they act as irritants and cause itching.
6. Avoid overheating that increases sweating, leading to itching. Wear loose, light clothing in hot weather. Air conditioning promotes comfort.
7. Avoid sunburn—wear a sunscreen with a minimum of SPF No. 15.
8. Avoid excessive cold that dries the skin.
9. Wash all new garments before wearing to remove potentially irritating chemicals.
10. Consult health care provider if eczema worsens.

ensues. Scratching becomes habitual. The skin becomes excoriated, and thickened geometric-appearing plaques result. Itching is often worse at night. Potent topical corticosteroids applied to the involved sites are the treatment of choice for LSC. Occlusive dressings with plastic wrap or tape (Cordran tape) applied for 3 to 7 days may enhance the steroid effects.

SEBORRHEIC DERMATITIS

Seborrheic dermatitis is an eczematous eruption that typically occurs on the hairy areas of the scalp, eyebrows, face, central chest, and sometimes genital skin folds. Inflammatory changes around the sebaceous gland and hair follicle produce the characteristic symptoms of redness and greasy scales. The cause is unknown, but overgrowth of yeast organisms on the skin is strongly postulated. Family history of the skin disease may be found. Seborrheic dermatitis is chronic, with symptoms often worse in the winter months. Mild to moderate seborrheic dermatitis of the scalp is treated with tar, selenium, zinc, or ketoconazole shampoo preparations. These products exert an antimicrobial effect on the microbial flora found at the hair follicle unit. More significant scalp involvement may require topical corticosteroids to flatten thick scaly plaques. Facial sites are treated with low potency topical steroids and/or topical antifungal agents.

NUMMULAR DERMATITIS

Nummular dermatitis is a chronic condition of uncertain cause occurring most commonly in middle-age or older men. The lesions of nummular dermatitis are typically 4 to 10 cm, erythematous, and coin shaped. The rash has a predilection for the dorsal aspects of the hands, extensor surfaces of the lower extremities, and buttocks. Itching may be severe. A background of dry skin can promote flare-ups of eczematous dermatitis. Treatment consists of hydrating the skin with moisturizing lotions, topical corticosteroid agents, and tar products.

STASIS DERMATITIS

Stasis dermatitis is a common eczematous eruption of the lower extremities occurring in older persons. It is usually preceded by varicosities and poor circulation. With the reduction in venous return from the legs, substances normally carried away by the circulation remain in the tissues causing irritation. The skin is often brawny colored with associated edema. Itching may or may not occur. Scratching may produce breaks in the epidermis, which can become secondarily infected. The most important treatment for stasis dermatitis is prevention by careful attention to the treatment of peripheral vascular conditions and prevention of constriction of the circulation to the extremities (see Chapter 25). Treating lower extremity edema with elevation, compression stocking, and Unna boots where applicable will ultimately decrease the dermatitis skin changes. Topical corticosteroids will improve the eczematous changes. Domeboro soaks may be useful when weeping lesions are present.

SKIN REACTIONS FROM SYSTEMIC FACTORS

DRUG HYPERSENSITIVITY REACTIONS

Etiology/Epidemiology

Drug hypersensitivity reactions can be caused by almost any drug. The rash occurs as a result of gradual accumulation of the drug or because of antibodies that develop in response to a component of the medication. Skin manifestations from drugs may have a nonallergic or an allergic basis. Commonly seen skin reactions include maculopapular lesions, purpura, vesicles, bullae, ulcers, and urticaria (Table 62-3). The reactions can appear at any time, but the onset is usually sudden.

Pathophysiology

Type I anaphylactic (urticaria, angioedema), type II cytotoxic (cellular injury), type III immune complex (serum sickness), or type IV cell-mediated (allergic contact dermatitis, allergic photosensitivity) hypersensitivity reactions may occur. Some drugs may have combined reactions; for example, penicillin may produce both type I and type III reactions. Allergic contact dermatitis is commonly seen with drugs used topically. The rash is often bright red, semiconfluent, macular and papular, generalized, and bilateral. Hypersensitivity occurs early when previous sensitization has taken place.

Photosensitivity may occur with certain drugs and may take one of two forms: phototoxicity or photoallergy (Table 62-4). Phototoxicity may occur in any person taking a photosensitive drug and results from the reaction of the drug (chemical) with radiant energy, particularly UV light. Broad-spectrum sunscreens, which cover the spectrum of UV A (e.g., zinc oxide, titanium dioxide, or parasol 1789), may reduce potential photosensitivity reactions. Photoallergic reactions are cell-mediated (type IV) hypersensitivity reactions; therefore

TABLE 62-3 Skin Reactions to Common Medications

Reaction	Medication
Erythematous rash (maculopapular)	Antibiotics, sulfonamides, thiazide diuretics, barbiturates, phenylbutazone
Purpura (ecchymosis, petechiae)	Thiazides, sulfonamides, barbiturates, anticoagulants
Mucocutaneous lesions (vesicles, bullae, ulcers)	Sulfonamides, penicillins, barbiturates, phenylbutazone
Urticaria	Penicillins, streptomycin, tetracycline, insulin, aspirin, dyes, adrenocorticotropic hormone, antiserum

TABLE 62-4 Drug Photosensitivity

Reaction	Symptoms	Drugs
Phototoxicity	Resembles sunburn (erythema, edema, vesicles)	Coal tar derivatives Psoralens Tetracycline Nalidixic acid Sulfanilamide Declomycin Chlorpromazine Certain dyes
Photoallergy	Resembles eczema (exudative papules and vesicles, urticaria, lichenification)	Diuretics (thiazides) Phenothiazines Oral hypoglycemics Griseofulvin Nonsteroidal antiinflammatory agents Retinoids

they affect only a small group of persons after several sensitizing exposures of drug and sunlight.

Collaborative Care Management

Treatment of drug hypersensitivity reactions consists of stopping the drug and treating the symptoms with cool, moist compresses; antihistamines (for pruritus); and topical and systemic corticosteroids. Photosensitivity can be prevented by avoiding direct sunlight on the skin when taking a drug with photosensitivity effects and/or using broad-spectrum sunscreens that cover the spectrum of UV A. Photo-protective clothing may also be helpful in this setting.

Patient/Family Education. The primary goal of patient education is prevention by making sure patients know the drug(s) to which they are allergic. The patient or family member should know the specific drug name and type of reaction. A Medic-Alert bracelet may be beneficial. Allergy information should be documented on the patient's record. Nursing care also focuses on helping the patient comply with treatment.

EXFOLIATIVE DERMATITIS

Etiology/Epidemiology

Exfoliative dermatitis is a rare, generalized dermatitis. In most cases the cause is unknown, but the disease may be associated with other types of dermatitis or with a lymphoma, or it may be the result of a drug reaction.

Pathophysiology

The onset of exfoliative dermatitis may be rapid or insidious and consists of an elevated temperature and a generalized erythema, followed by extensive scaling (exfoliation). Pruritus may be present, and the lesions often become infected. Loss of large amounts of water and protein from the skin leads to hypoproteinemia, weight loss, and difficulty with temperature control. Heart failure may occur in elderly patients. Death may result from overwhelming infection or circulatory collapse.

Collaborative Care Management

Therapy consists of maintaining fluid balance and preventing infection. Methods used to prevent infection in patients with burns are applicable (see Chapter 63). All drugs are discontinued as potential causative factors, although antibiotics may be started after culture and sensitivity tests of infected lesions. Oral corticosteroids are given for severe cases. Daily baths followed by application of petrolatum to the skin promote comfort.

Patient/Family Education. Patient teaching focuses on the course of the disease, rationales for treatment, and the management of signs and symptoms and use of comfort measures.

ERYTHEMA MULTIFORME

Etiology/Epidemiology

Erythema multiforme (EM) is a common, self-limiting inflammation of the skin and mucous membranes in genetically susceptible persons. Episodes of the disease may be single, recurrent, or, rarely, continuous. Although it is usually mild, EM may progress to a toxic epidermal necrolysis type of illness. Erythema multiforme is classified as major or minor. The major type is also described as the severe bullous form or Stevens-Johnson syndrome. Both forms are thought to be a cell-mediated immune response to relevant antigens. The responsible agent usually can be identified. Medications that can trigger erythema multiforme include phenytoin, carbamazepine, sulfonamides, NSAIDs, allopurinol, and certain antibiotics (particularly cephalosporins). Drugs, not infection, are thought to be responsible for the severe bullous form of the disorder.

Infections that cause EM include mycoplasmal pneumonia, chickenpox, hepatitis B, infectious mononucleosis, and herpes simplex, which is the most common. More unusual causes of EM include systemic lupus erythematosus, lymphoma, leukemia, radiation therapy, pregnancy, and reactions to vaccinations, particularly hepatitis B.

Pathophysiology

Erythema multiforme may affect the skin and mucous membranes or solely the skin. Episodes of the disease usually

TABLE 62-5 Skin Reactions of Some Communicable Diseases

Disease	Cause	Incubation Period (Days)	Place of Rash Origin	Skin Lesions
Measles (rubeola)	Rubeola virus	11 (8-14)	Face	Pink macular-papular rash; lesions coalesce
German measles; 3-day measles (rubella)	Rubella virus	14-21	Face	Pink macular-papular rash; lesions usually discrete; may coalesce
Scarlet fever (scarlatina)	Hemolytic streptococcus	1-3	Neck, chest	Bright red (scarlet) macules (pinpoint)
Chickenpox (varicella)	Varicella-zoster virus	14-21	Back, chest	Macule, papule, vesicle, crust; lesions at different stages
Smallpox	Variola virus	12 (7-21)	Face	Macule, papule, vesicle, crust; lesions all at same stage
Typhoid fever	*Salmonella typhosa*	14 (7-21)	Abdomen	Macular rash

last for 1 to 3 weeks. Characteristic lesions of EM are flat topped, sharply marginated, dusky red papules and targetoid (bulls eye–like) lesions. The rash has an affinity for the backs of the hands, palms and soles, and extensor limbs. With the major variant of EM (bullous variety), the rash occurs on the dorsa of the hands, palms, knees, feet, and elbows. The oral cavity may be affected by blisters progressing to erosion of the entire oral mucosa and lips. Conjunctivitis may occur, progressing to corneal opacity. If the genital mucosa become involved, adhesions may result as a long-term complication. The skin findings may be preceded by fever, chest pain, and arthralgia. Severe cases may be confused with toxic epidermal necrolysis. If the triggering agent is herpes simplex, EM usually occurs 7 to 10 days after the onset of the herpes infection.

Collaborative Care Management

A single episode of EM may not require treatment. Any suspected triggering agent is discontinued and symptoms treated. Topical corticosteroids may help to reduce local inflammation, itching, and burning. Systemic corticosteroids administered early may alleviate the pain-related symptoms. Sedating antihistamines such as hydroxyzine may be of some use. Persons with ocular and oral-mucosal involvement, or the severe bullous type (Stevens-Johnson syndrome) warrant close supervision and supportive hospitalization. Individuals with extensive blistering should be treated as burn patients (see Chapter 63).

Intravenous or enteral feeding may be indicated for persons with extensive oral involvement. Protective dressings should be applied to prevent secondary infection. Caution must used when choosing the appropriate antibiotic therapy because Stevens-Johnson syndrome is triggered by drugs. Systemic steroids are indicated for the treatment of patients with severe cases of EM. Steroids are effective in reducing fever and aiding symptomatic relief but do not significantly affect morbidity or mortality rate. Skin lesions may take weeks to heal, and systemic steroids may delay the healing process. The risk/benefit ratio should be considered, particularly in older patients, before prescribing systemic steroids. Oral antiviral agents such as acyclovir may help with herpes-associated recurrent EM reactions. Azathioprine is an option for suppressing attacks in severe disease.

Patient/Family Education. The patient with any type of EM needs support and education throughout diagnosis and treatment. Initially other disorders causing blistering must be considered, and the patient will require support during this time. Education is needed regarding the medications prescribed, including administration, dosing, and side effects. Nursing care is supportive and includes baths, soaks, oral care, and dressings. Thorough explanations should accompany treatments. Patients and family require teaching regarding the course of the disease, complications, possible triggers, and recurrences. The relationship between herpes simplex and episodes of erythema multiforme should be explained.

INFECTIOUS DISEASES

Communicable diseases, such as measles, chickenpox, and scarlet fever produce skin reactions (Table 62-5). Nodes and hemorrhagic spots in the skin also accompany severe acute rheumatic fever.

PAPULOSQUAMOUS DISEASES

Papulosquamous diseases are characterized by papular, scaly lesions. Common disorders in this category of dermatoses are psoriasis and pityriasis rosea.

PSORIASIS

Etiology/Epidemiology

Psoriasis is a chronic disease of epidermal proliferation characterized by exacerbations and remissions. Scaling, erythema, and pruritus are the hallmark symptoms of this disorder. It is thought to be genetically linked. Psoriasis is associated with certain human leukocyte antigens. The immune system plays a key role in this disease, as it responds to systemic immunosuppressive agents. There are no specific precipitating factors for the majority of persons; however, some people may develop exacerbations after climatic changes, stressors, trauma, infections, or drugs. Approximately 20% of the population is affected by psoriasis with equal distribution in both genders. There is a higher incidence of psoriasis among Caucasians and a lower incidence among the Japanese, Native Americans, and people of West-African origin. Psoriasis occurs in all ages but is less common among children and older persons. Approximately one third of cases of psoriasis occur in persons younger than 20 years of age.

Pathophysiology

The rapid production and turnover of skin cells at the epidermal layer creates the scaling papules and plaques of psoriasis. The turnover time for normal skin is 28 days. Once the basal cell divides, the keratinocyte takes approximately 14 days to flatten and differentiate as it progresses upward, ultimately reaching the stratum corneum layer. It takes an additional 14 days for this cell to be sloughed off. In psoriasis, cellular turnover takes place at an accelerated rate of 3 to 4 days.

The papules and plaques of psoriasis are raised, erythematous, sharply circumscribed, with a silvery-white scale (Figure 62-14). Removal of the scale usually results in a characteristic pinpoint bleeding called the Auspitz phenomenon. In darker-skinned persons, the plaques may appear purple. Psoriatic lesions can occur anywhere on the body, but are more commonly found on the scalp, elbows, knees, and sacral-lumbar areas. Beefy red lesions may be observed in an acute flare-up. Nail changes occur in 10% to 50% of patients with psoriasis. Characteristic nail changes are pitting, yellowish discoloration, oil drop or salmon patches, leukonychia (whitening of the nail), splinter hemorrhage, and onycholysis (separation of the nail from the nail bed).

The common forms of psoriasis are psoriasis vulgaris, guttate psoriasis, pustular psoriasis, and erythrodermic psoriasis. In psoriasis vulgaris the plaques are symmetric, large and small, with silvery white scale adherent. An outbreak of guttate psoriasis may follow streptococcal pharyngitis or viral upper respiratory infection. Palmoplantar psoriasis occurs on the volar surfaces of the hands and feet and can be quite debilitating for some individuals. In generalized pustular psoriasis ,patients have a history of a plaque-type psoriasis, later developing pustules on an erythematous base, eventually forming pools of pustules. Other symptoms include fever, chills, arthralgia, hypocalcemia, and leukocytosis. Flare-ups of the disease may be triggered by discontinuing use of systemic steroids for a plaque-type of psoriasis. Erythrodermic psoriasis, as the name implies, produces a red coloration of the skin with a desquamative scale over most of the body. Inflammatory vasodilatory mechanisms are responsible for problems in temperature regulation, hypoalbuminemia, pedal edema, and high-output cardiac failure.

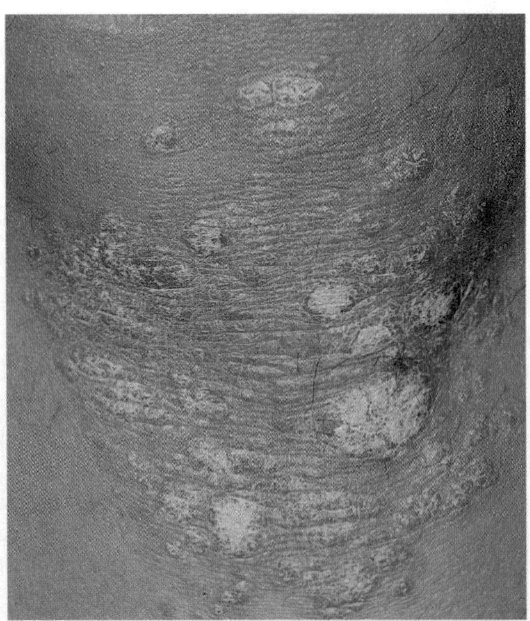

Figure 62-14 Psoriasis. Note silvery scaling.

An accompanying arthritis (psoriatic arthritis) occurs in approximately 3% to 4% of the population with or without skin disease findings. Presentation of the arthritis varies; it may manifest as an asymmetric oligoarthropathy, it may affect mainly the distal interphalangeal joints, or it may cause a severely debilitating type of joint disease.

Collaborative Care Management

For localized manifestations of psoriasis (large and small plaque type) application of topical corticosteroids for a defined period of time may be used. Potential for steroid-induced side effects occurs with prolonged use of these agents. Coal tar products (soaks, gels, creams, and shampoos) may play a role in decreasing pruritus while diminishing epidermal cell turnover.

Calcipotriene (Dovonex), a vitamin D_3 derivative, can be effective in inhibiting the proliferation of keratinocytes. Calcipotriene may be used in concert with topical steroid therapy. The use of calcipotriene is not indicated for the treatment of widespread psoriasis because of the risk for systemic absorption with elevated calcium levels.

UV light inhibits DNA synthesis, thus slowing the rapid skin cell growth. Ultraviolet light is divided into 3 wavelengths: UVC (long), UVB (middle), and UVA (short). UVC is not used in skin therapeutics. The combination of tar and UVB light, known as the Goeckerman regimen, is a widely used form of therapy for patients with psoriasis.

Photo chemotherapy (psoralen with UVA light [PUVA]) is used for diffuse disease, thicker plaques, or when other therapies have not been effective. Psoralens are taken 1 to 2 hours before exposure to the UV light; dose is based on body weight. Methotrexate, the systemic retinoid; Soriatane, a vitamin A derivative; and cyclosporine, an immunosuppressive agent are used in advanced disease.[13] These drugs require regular laboratory monitoring of complete blood count, liver function, and lipids.

Patient/Family Education. Most patients with psoriasis are treated on an ambulatory basis. One approach to therapy has been the establishment of psoriasis day care centers where patients visit daily for a designated time period to receive aggressive topical therapy, light treatment, and education pertaining to self-care. Patients with psoriasis may require intervention to cope with feelings surrounding perceived altered body image.

The disease is not curable and may wax and wane continuously. Lesions may regress with treatment, only to recur in the same area again. Teaching for individuals who have psoriasis is summarized in the Guidelines for Safe Practice box.

PITYRIASIS ROSEA

Etiology/Epidemiology

Pityriasis rosea is a common, benign, self-limiting dermatosis of unknown etiology.[12] A viral source has been postulated, but never proven. Common, with worldwide distribution, the disease affects all races and occurs most commonly in women, adolescents, and young adults. Seventy-five percent of cases occur in persons 10 to 35 years old. The incidence is higher in the early spring and autumn months.

Pathophysiology

The initial symptom is usually a 2- to 10-cm solitary oval lesion (herald patch) with a thin, scaly border and yellowish center, appearing most often on the trunk, proximal arms, and legs. The herald patch usually precedes other lesions by 1 to 30 days. A generalized eruption of multiple pink branlike scaly patches follows the herald patch. The distribution of lesions is often in long axes running parallel to each other and on the trunk, which creates a "Christmas tree"–like appearance. The eruption is self-limiting, lasting approximately 6 to 8 weeks. Recurrences of pityriasis rosea are extremely rare.

Treatment measures are few, because most patients do not experience symptoms. Topical corticosteroids and antipruritic agents may be used if itching is present. Emollients are needed as the lesions dry up. Low-dose UV B phototherapy may be beneficial when the rash is diffuse or itching is significant. Exposure to natural sunlight (to the point of minimal erythema) will also speed disappearance of the lesions and relieve itching. The patient should be cautioned against sunburn.

Guidelines for Safe Practice

The Patient With Psoriasis

Teaching should include information on the etiology and chronicity of psoriasis, as well as the following instructions:

- Reduce episodes of psoriasis flare-ups by avoiding skin trauma (injuries, sunburn, infections), extremes of temperature, and stress.
- Shampoo hair frequently to remove scales. If scalp has plaques, use tar, zinc, or selenium shampoos (e.g., T gel, DHS Zinc, Head and Shoulders) for 10 minutes before rinsing. Presoften thick plaques with mineral oil the night before a morning shampoo; use a fine-toothed comb to remove loose scales.
- Avoid self-medication, particularly when receiving prescribed therapy.
- Apply topical medications in a thin layer.
- Monitor for side effects of medications.
- Seek medical follow-up care during periods of exacerbation.

Patient/Family Education. Nursing care is essentially symptomatic and includes assisting with and teaching about application of topical corticosteroids, baths, and emollients. Educating patients on the limited course of pityriasis rosea is another supportive measure.

BULLOUS DISEASES (BLISTERING DISORDERS)

PEMPHIGUS VULGARIS

Etiology/Epidemiology

Pemphigus vulgaris (PV) is an acute or chronic, serious, blistering disorder of the skin and mucous membranes. The cause of PV is thought to be autoimmune. Rare, but worldwide, PV occurs primarily in persons between 40 and 60 years old, with equal incidence in men and women and a higher incidence among Jewish persons.

Pathophysiology

PV is characterized by large bullae that appear all over the body and on the mucous membranes. Tissue injury results from circulating autoantibodies that bind to the structural proteins within the epidermis. Blister formation occurs above the stratum basalis. Healing is commonly associated with the development of postinflammatory hyperpigmentation, rather than scarring. The lesions break and are followed by crusts and scarring. The disease is characterized by acantholysis (cells slip past one another and fluid accumulates between them). By placing the thumb firmly on the skin and exerting lateral sliding pressure, the upper epidermis can be dislodged, resulting in erosion or blister (Nikolsky's sign). A Tzanck test can identify acantholytic cells. Secondary bacterial infections of the crust can lead to sepsis. Patients can succumb to PV if treatment is delayed.

Collaborative Care Management

Hospitalization is usually required for rigorous skin care and monitoring of drug effects. The treatment of choice for severe PV is high-dose systemic corticosteroids. The dose is gradually reduced as skin improvement is noted. Immunosuppressive agents such as methotrexate, cyclophosphamide, and azathioprine may be added to reduce the corticosteroid dose requirements.

Nursing care of the person with severe PV can be a challenge. Stryker frames may be used to help the person change position painlessly and to prevent weight bearing on raw surfaces. Air mattress or flotation systems may be used to reduce surface pressure on skin and promote comfort. Domeboro solution, potassium permanganate, and oatmeal products with oil delivered as baths or compresses to oozing lesions help control odor and remove crusts. Infection is a major concern because of the immunosuppressive effects of drug therapy. Topical antibiotics are helpful for reducing the bacterial flora on the skin. Special mouth care is required for mouth lesions, and bland diets are more easily tolerated.

Patient/Family Education. Emotional support and encouragement of both patient and family are extremely important. Patients may fear rejection because of their appearance, and they need evidence of continued family and staff interest and attention. The risk for disturbed body image and social isolation is high.

Patients should be encouraged to adhere to a balanced diet to promote further wound healing. General skin care measures should be reinforced. Medication instruction regarding the mechanism of action, side effects, and drug-drug interactions should be reviewed with both patient and family. Eliciting a return demonstration on application of topical agents and dressings by the patient and/or family member is another important nursing intervention.

TUMORS OF THE SKIN

Skin cell growths may develop from the epidermis, sebaceous or sweat glands, melanocytes, and mesodermal tissue (e.g., connective or vascular tissue).

KERATOSIS (BENIGN LESION)

The term keratosis refers to any cornification or growth of the horny layer of the skin. Examples of keratoses include corns and calluses, warts, and seborrheic and actinic (solar) keratosis (Table 62-6).

PREMALIGNANT LESIONS

Skin lesions that may evolve into a malignant state include actinic keratosis, keratoacanthoma, leukoplakia, Bowen's disease, and atypical nevi or moles. The term premalignant does not imply that all of the lesions will become malignant but that the tendency to become malignant exists (Table 62-7).

MALIGNANT LESIONS

Malignant skin lesions include squamous cell carcinoma, basal cell carcinoma, and malignant melanoma (Table 62-8).

Etiology

Malignant melanoma is a tumor of the melanocytes, occurring on both sun-exposed and nonexposed skin surfaces. Malignant melanoma often develops from a preexisting pigmented mole or nevi, although it may arise from healthy skin. Precursor lesions to melanoma are atypical or dysplastic nevi, congenital nevi, and lentigo maligna. There is a genetic predisposition to melanoma; 10% of persons with melanoma have a first-degree relative with the disease.[1]

Epidemiology

Malignant melanoma is increasing more rapidly than any other malignancy.[17] It is the most common cancer. Alarmingly, the death rate is also increasing and is second only to lung cancer. Currently, 1 in 70 persons will develop malignant melanoma. This increase may be due in part to increased sun exposure, thinning of the ozone layer, and other uncontrollable factors. Persons at increased risk include those with a previous melanoma, multiple atypical nevi (atypical mole syndrome), fair-complexioned individuals, (especially those with light hair and light eyes), and persons with a history of childhood blistering sunburns. The mean age of diagnosis is 40 years.

TABLE 62-6 Keratoses: Etiology, Appearance, and Treatment

Type of Lesion	Etiology	Appearance	Treatment
Corns	Pressure, ill-fitting shoes	Center core that thickens inwardly, pain with pressure, usually occur on toes	Felt pad with center hole to relieve pressure, properly fitting shoes; corn will recur if pressure not relieved
Callus	Constant pressure on plantar surface of foot; can also occur on palmar surface of hands	Thickening of horny layer of skin	Relief of pressure, regular massage with softening lotion or creams
Seborrheic keratoses (Figure 62-15, *A*)	Normal aging process, rarely develop into malignancy; must distinguish from actinic keratoses, which have malignancy potential	Large, darkened, greasy warts usually on trunk, less often on scalp, face, and proximal extremities; sudden increase in number and size may indicate a gastrointestinal malignancy	No treatment except for cosmetic reasons or constant irritation; may be removed by curettage, electrodesiccation, or liquid nitrogen
Dermatosis papulosa nigra	Seborrheic keratoses in African-Americans	Small, pedunculated, heavily pigmented	Same as for seborrheic keratoses
Actinic keratoses (Figure 62-15, *B*) (senile, solar)	Chronic exposure to solar irradiation; occur on exposed areas of skin; light-skinned persons most vulnerable Approximately 25% evolve to squamous cell carcinoma (evidenced by a rapid increase in size of lesion)	Round or irregular, red-brown to gray in color with dry, scaly appearance Surrounding skin usually dry and wrinkled from overexposure to sun	Protective clothing, sunscreens; removal by curettage, liquid nitrogen therapy, dermabrasion, electrodesiccation, large lesions by excision; multiple lesions may be treated with topical application of 1%-5% 5-fluorouracil cream

Pathophysiology

Major classifications of melanoma include melanoma in situ, superficial spreading melanoma, lentigo maligna melanoma, nodular melanoma, and acral-lentiginous melanoma. The most common is the superficial spreading type, which accounts for 70% of all melanomas.

Nodular melanoma carries the worst prognosis. Survival rates for primary localized melanomas after excision are 90% to 98%. The survival rate for other stages ranges from 5% to 80%. Staging is based on tumor size, affected lymph nodes, and metastases. The tumor arises from melanocytes. Responsible for the biosynthesis and transport of melanin, these cells

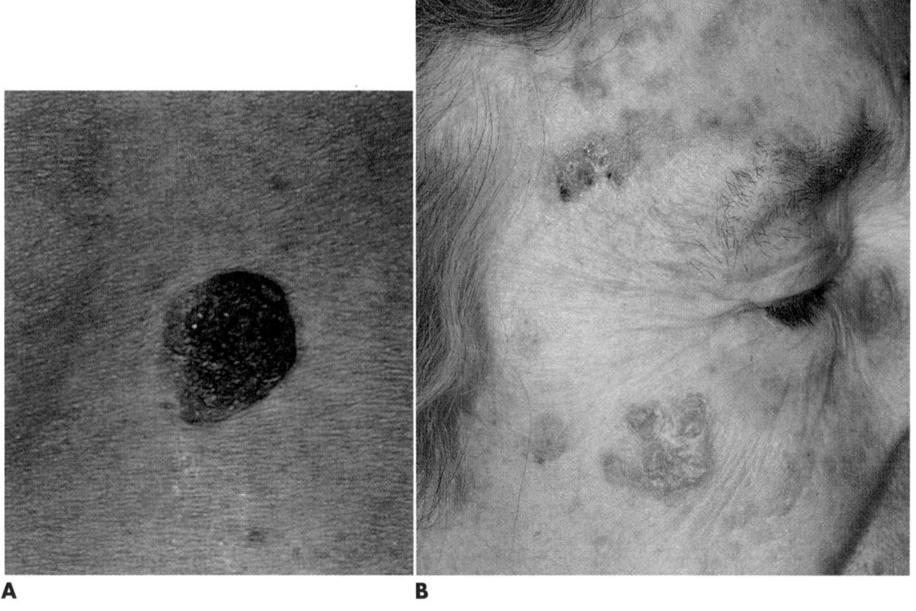

Figure 62-15 **A,** Seborrheic keratosis. **B,** Actinic (senile) keratosis.

TABLE 62-7 Premalignant Lesions: Etiology, Appearance, and Treatment

Lesion	Etiology	Appearance	Treatment
Leukoplakia	Unknown causes and external irritants such as poor-fitting dentures, cheek biting, and pipe and cigarette smoking; chronic maceration, friction, and senile atrophy may lead to vaginal leukoplakia	Mucous membranes develop thickened, white patches of keratinized cells, which may eventually lead to squamous cell carcinoma Erythroplakia (red or red and white patches) of the mouth has a higher malignancy potential than leukoplakia	Prevention by removal of causative factors; inspection of mouth, mucous membranes; dental care for rough teeth, proper-fitting dentures; large lesions are usually surgically excised, and a biopsy is performed; benign lesions may be removed by electrodesiccation Surgical excision, cryotherapy, curettage and electrodesiccation, carbon dioxide laser therapy, 5-fluorouracil cream or solution
Bowen's disease	Chemical carcinogens; occurs on older, light-skinned men; also called squamous cell carcinoma in situ Persons affected are at higher risk of developing other malignancies	Widely distributed, sharply demarcated brown plaques, although a single lesion may exist	
Pigmented nevi (moles)	Most are harmless, but others may be dysplastic, precancerous, or cancerous Changes in a mole that require immediate attention: Development of a ring of new pigment around the base Development of uneven pigmentation Sudden growth Loss of hair Bleeding	Present on most persons, regardless of skin color; may be flat, raised, prominent, or hairy; color ranges from tan to black Atypical (dysplastic) moles usually occur on the upper back in males and on the legs in females (refer to malignant melanoma section for further discussion)	Biopsy and excision of suspicious lesions; to help remember the characteristics of malignant moles, the American Cancer Society has developed the mnemonic *ABCD:* *Asymmetry* of borders *Border* irregularity *Color* blue-black or variegated *Diameter* 0.6 mm

TABLE 62-8 Nonmelanoma Skin Cancers: Etiology, Appearance, and Treatment

Lesion	Etiology	Appearance	Treatment
Squamous cell carcinoma (Figure 62-16)	Unknown; may arise from actinic keratoses, Bowen's disease, or leukoplakia	If precursor was premalignant lesion, the lesion will be indurated and surrounded by an inflammatory base. New lesions appear as a firm keratotic nodule with an indurated base. Lip or ear lesions may metastasize to regional lymph nodes. Lesions on hair-bearing areas rarely metastasize.	Prevention and early detection. Removal by surgical excision or Mohs' micrographic surgery (surgery in which the lesion is removed in successive thin horizontal layers along a grid pattern until the undersurface and borders of the removed tissue is free of malignant cells), curettage with electrodesiccation, irradiation, or chemosurgery (for treatment of tumors without well-defined borders). A dressing is applied with a fixative paste such as zinc chloride; removal of the dressing removes malignant tissue. Reapplication is usually necessary.
Basal cell carcinoma	Unknown; most common malignant tumor affecting light-skinned persons over age 40; primarily occurs over hairy areas that contain pilosebaceous follicles	Translucent appearance, color from flesh to pale pink with a few telangiectatic vessels across the surface. Rarely metastatic if treated.	If untreated, tumors become locally invasive with severe tissue destruction, infection, and hemorrhage. If untreated, metastasizes to bone, lung, and brain. Treatment depends on site and extent of tumor: surgical excision or Mohs' micrographic surgery, curettage with electrodesiccation, irradiation, and chemosurgery.

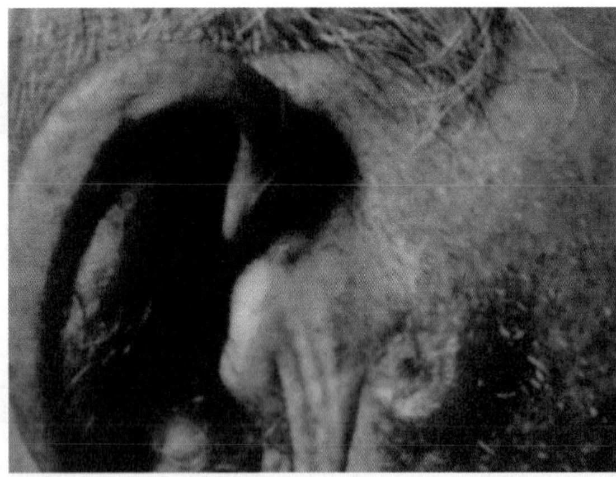

Figure 62-16 Squamous cell carcinoma in infra temporal area, one of the most common sites for this tumor.

are most commonly found in the basal layer of the epidermis and eye, but are also found in the meninges, alimentary and respiratory tracts, and lymph nodes. Contained in each melanocyte is a melanosome, an organelle that synthesizes the pigment. In melanoma, the melanosome is abnormal or absent. Atypical melanocytes proliferate along the basal layer of the epidermis; when the melanocytes invade the dermis, the lesion is considered malignant. There is a radial growth phase in each type of melanoma; the length of time of this phase varies. Melanoma is staged, as are other cancers, depending on the depth of tumor at the time of excision and presence of lymph node and solid organ metastases.

Tumors occur most commonly on the head, neck, and lower extremities. The lesions vary considerably in appearance, some with deep pigmentation, irregular scalloped borders, and surrounding erythema or halo. Others may possess variegated pigmentation (yellow, blue, black, gray) or absence of color altogether (Figure 62-17). Late changes include bleeding and ulceration. The incidence of metastasis from malignant melanoma is high and depends on the depth of invasion. Metastasis typically occurs first to the regional lymph nodes and then by hematogenous spread to the lungs, liver, brain, and other areas.

Collaborative Care Management

Diagnostic Tests. As in all malignancies, confirmation of diagnosis is by biopsy. Excisional skin biopsies with sufficient margins to determine the depth of invasion and provide staging information are performed on suspicious pigmented lesions. Electrodessication, curettage, shaving, and cryotherapy are contraindicated in mole evaluations, as they do not provide sufficient tissue to rule in or rule out malignant melanoma.

Surgical Management. Surgical intervention in malignant melanoma by far offers the best potential for cure. Once the diagnosis of malignant melanoma is made by skin biopsy, a wide surgical excision is performed. Removing an appropriate margin of tissue surrounding the lesion decreases the chance of local recurrence. Surgical margins for primary cutaneous melanoma are determined by the thickness of the lesion. Patients with intermediate-thickness melanoma (>1 mm deep) may elect to undergo sentinel lymph node mapping. A negative sentinel lymph node is highly predictive that the remainder of

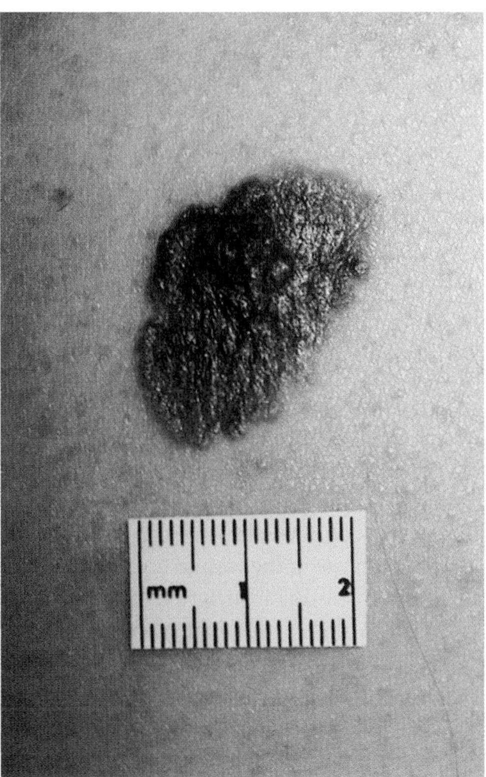

Figure 62-17 Malignant melanoma. Note asymmetry of borders, size >6 mm, and color.

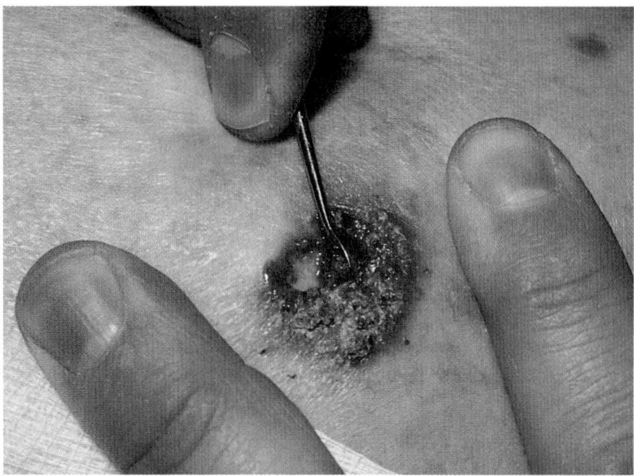

Figure 62-18 Curettage of inflamed seborrheic keratosis.

the nodal basin will also be negative. If the sentinel lymph node is positive, a completion lymphadenectomy is usually recommended to determine the number of positive lymph nodes. Therapeutic lymph node dissection is indicated for persons with clinically enlarged regional nodes after cytologic confirmation of metastatic disease. Regional lymphadenectomy may be indicated for palliative purposes as well.

Medical Management. Metastatic malignant melanoma is resistant to currently available systemic chemotherapeutic agents. The drug used most successfully is dacarbazine (DTIC), with an overall response rate of 10% to 28%, depending on disease site. Indicated as treatment for surgically unresectable advanced metastatic melanoma, DTIC can be administered on an outpatient basis. Other chemotherapeutic agents are sometimes used in the clinical trial setting. Isolated limb perfusion and infusion therapy can provide maximal chemotherapeutic effect in an involved limb. Hyperthermia, in addition to vascular perfusion of chemotherapy through an isolated region, allows high concentrations of chemotherapeutic agents to be administered to the extremity with minimal systemic toxicity.

High-dose interferon has recently been shown to result in a small but significant improvement in both disease-free and overall survival rates. Interferon treatment is both costly and potentially toxic. Lower-dose interferon therapy results in less toxicity but does not result in a survival benefit. Other biologic response modifiers, such as recombinant interleukin-2 and monoclonal antibodies, are options for select individuals in the clinical trial setting. Immunotherapy with tumor vaccines to stimulate the host's system to react to the melanoma is the subject of many clinical trials at this time. Local radiation is sometimes used to offer local control at a site of a deeper melanoma.

Ambulatory Dermatologic Surgical Procedures. The following sections discuss dermatologic surgical procedures performed by clinicians in an ambulatory setting:

Dermatologic Surgery. Treatment of skin lesions by dermatology providers often includes removal of skin lesions. Superficial skin lesions involving only the epidermis can be removed easily by various means; deep lesions involving the dermis, such as some cancers, are removed with full-thickness skin excision.

Shave Biopsy/Excision. Superficial lesions rising above the plane of the skin surface can be removed by shaving technique. A No. 15 scalpel blade is typically used. The entire lesion may be removed for diagnosis. Hemostasis is obtained with pressure, Drysol or Monsel's solution, or Gelfoam.

Curettage. Curettage is the scraping or scooping out of a superficial lesion with a curette, a spoon-shaped, sharp-edged instrument. A local anesthetic is usually injected around the lesion before curettage (Figure 62-18). Hemostasis is accomplished with a chemical styptic such as ferric chloride or Monsel's solution, with gelatin foam, or by electrocoagulation. Lesions removed by curettage include seborrheic keratosis, actinic keratosis, basal cell carcinomas, and warts.

Punch Biopsy. Punch biopsies are used to provide tissue for histologic evaluation (e.g., suspected skin cancers, unusual dermatoses), as well as to remove small, benign lesions. After the patient receives a local anesthetic, a punch is used to remove deep lesions up to 10 mm in diameter. The tissue is then sent for biopsy. Punch biopsies may be closed with sutures. Secondary intention wound healing is sometimes selected by the clinician. In this situation hemostasis can be obtained with gelatin foam packing.

Cryosurgery. Tissue can be destroyed by rapid freezing with substances such as liquid oxygen, carbon dioxide snow or gas, liquid nitrogen, dichlorodifluoromethane (Freon), or nitrous oxide. Carbon dioxide snow and liquid nitrogen are most commonly used. The rapid freezing causes formation of intracellular ice, which destroys the cell membranes and produces cell dehydration. Cryosurgery is commonly used for removing skin tumors (benign and malignant) and warts.

Although the procedure usually is not painful, a tingling pain occurs when the freezing substance is applied and may be uncomfortable for some persons, particularly if multiple lesions are treated.

Tissue necrosis may not be evident until 24 hours after cryosurgery. A clear or hemorrhagic bulla forms during the first day, but inflammatory reactions and bleeding are usually absent. A serous exudate occurs during the first week, followed by eschar or crust formation. The crust drops off in 3 to 4 weeks as the underlying tissue heals. Hypopigmentation may occur because melanocytes are highly vulnerable to freezing.

Electrosurgery. Electric current may be used in dermatologic surgery to remove tissue and to control bleeding. Electrodesiccation is the drying of tissue by means of a monopolar current through the needle electrode. Electrofulguration is a form of electrodesiccation in which the needle electrode is held close to, rather than inserted into, the tissue, thus spraying the area with sparks. Bipolar current is used for electrocoagulation, which coagulates the tissue, curtailing capillary bleeding, and for electrosection, which cuts the tissue. Delayed bleeding may occur, especially from electrocoagulation, and may alarm the unprepared patient. The bleeding can be easily controlled by direct pressure. After most uses of electrosurgery, the wound is left exposed for air drying. Dressings may be used if the area is subject to frequent trauma or rubbing or if oozing is present. The wound may be wiped with 70% alcohol to hasten drying. A hemostatic nonocclusive dressing may be made by covering the wound with Gelfoam powder and tape.

Diet. No special diet is prescribed for persons undergoing dermatologic surgery. However, the patient should be encouraged to have a nutritionally balanced diet both before and after surgery to enhance healing of tissues.

NURSING MANAGEMENT OF PATIENT UNDERGOING DERMATOLOGIC SURGERY

PREOPERATIVE CARE

Regardless of the type and extent of the surgery, the patient and family need preoperative teaching. This may be done in a variety of settings, depending on the type of procedure planned. Teaching should include specifics regarding the location and extent of incision, any postoperative activity limitations, and any special postoperative care needs. Information should be included regarding the anesthetic options available. See Chapter 16 for further discussion of preoperative preparation of the patient.

POSTOPERATIVE CARE

After surgery, the patient requires care and monitoring as described in Chapter 18. If a malignant lesion was removed, the patient may be instructed to seek follow-up care at closer intervals. If metastasis occurs, the nursing care focuses on helping the patient understand the treatment and its side effects. The patient is confronted with many physical problems, as well as psychoemotional problems such as fear of cancer, loss of health, and fear of dying.

After superficial skin surgery the patient is instructed not to remove the crust (scab), which acts as a protection (healing occurs under the crust). The crust should be kept as dry as possible; if it gets wet, it should be patted dry. Alcohol may be applied and allowed to evaporate. Makeup may be used over the crust. The crust may be left uncovered or may be covered with an adhesive bandage. Signs of redness, edema, or pain should be reported to the health care provider.[7]

After deep skin surgery, the wound is usually bandaged and the patient is given specific instructions for care by the clinician. Aspirin and other drugs that alter blood coagulation should be avoided for 7 days before and after surgery to decrease the potential for postoperative bleeding.[7]

The patient and family require an explanation about the treatments that may be performed postoperatively or prescribed for home care. They also require teaching regarding the care of healthy skin and steps to prevent further damage to the skin as discussed next.

Avoiding Causative Agents

The first step in preventing dermatologic conditions is avoiding the causative agent, which may be a specific antigen, a contact irritant, a microorganism, trauma, direct sunlight, or an insect. Instructing the person to avoid a known causative agent is preventive medicine; however, it may not be that simple. Many dermatologic diseases have no known cause or are hereditary. Unfortunately, once the mechanism of the disease is known, it is not always possible to remove the triggering factors. Occasionally, symptoms may persist long after the agent is removed. Therefore major responsibilities of the nurse include education of the patient about measures that promote rest, methods that decrease emotional stress, the need for good nutrition, and the need to closely observe sites to determine changes in skin conditions.

Cleansing

Bathing is an essential element of skin care. The frequency of skin cleansing is individualized according to need and patient preference. The outer layer of skin cells and perspiration are acidic, and their presence inhibits the life and growth of harmful bacteria; however, a normal flora of bacteria grow in acidity and act as the skin's protection. Strong soaps that are alkaline in reaction may neutralize this protective acid condition of the skin. They may also remove the oily secretion of the sebaceous glands, which lubricates the outer skin layers and contributes to their health. Removal of excess oil and scale or debris is sometimes necessary to facilitate the absorption of medication, promote healing, and enhance the appearance of the skin. For example, in psoriasis removal of scale by mechanical means and slowing of skin metabolism are prime objectives.

Normal skin should be washed with pH-neutral, soaplike agents to remove excess oils and excretions and to prevent odor. Care must be taken not to cause drying or irritation. After showering the skin can be patted dry, and lotion applied to prevent drying. Maintaining a proper degree of hydration in the skin prevents dryness and itching, which may lead to scratching, excoriation, and further trauma. Hydrating the stratum corneum, or outer layer of skin, may be accomplished by soaking in a tub of water for 20 to 30 minutes and then immediately applying a lubricating lotion or cream. This application of a cream prevents the rapid loss of water from the skin surface.

Sunlight

Sunlight, particularly UV light, is damaging to the skin. Ultraviolet light is termed actinic, meaning photochemically active radiation. UVA light contributes to aging and carcinogenesis of the skin. The UVB light spectrum leads to burning and activation of melanin, which produces tanning. Chronic tanning will later produce the undesirable skin changes of wrinkling, pigmentary disturbances (e.g., brown spots), and leatherlike textural changes. Tanning parlors should be avoided, as they use both the damaging UVB and/or UVA light spectrums to produce tans, which carry the same harmful skin cancer risks as natural sunlight.

The way to protect against UV rays is to block the rays. The rays may be blocked by opaque clothing, umbrellas, wide brimmed hats, or other screening aids; by avoiding sun exposure between 10 AM and 3 PM; or by selected sunscreens. The optimal sunscreens have a sun protection factor (SPF) of 15 or greater.[16] Sunscreens can be easily removed by swimming or sweating, thus reapplications are necessary. Sun screen labels indicate whether or not a product is *water resistant* or *water proof.* Eyes should be protected with UV-protective sunglasses. UV light has stronger effects at high altitudes (where there is less atmosphere to absorb the rays) and at the equator (where the sun is closer to the earth); therefore additional protection is required in these locations. Persons with dermatoses that are exacerbated by UV light or those who have an illness that is photo-exacerbated should avoid sunlight if possible or generously apply broad-spectrum (UVA-UVB) sunscreens. Rashes caused by photosensitivity resulting from certain medications appear abruptly and are widespread, symmetric, and bright red. Classes of medications that enhance photosensitivity include certain tetracyclines, sulfa drugs, antihypertensives, diuretics, oral hypoglycemics, psychotropic drugs, and NSAIDs.

Nutrition

Balanced nutrition plays an important role in maintaining intact, healthy skin. Essential nutrients involved in this endeavor include protein, vitamin C, iron, and zinc.[8] Some dermatologic disorders may be directly associated with dietary intake. Excessive dryness of the skin and thickening of the stratum corneum at the hair follicle openings may be caused by nutritional deficiencies. Elevated blood lipid levels caused by hyperlipoproteinemia may take the form of xanthomas on the skin surface. Persons experiencing hypersensitivity reactions may be placed on restrictive diets to exclude intake of known causative agents or as a diagnostic tool to identify causative agents. Food labels should be read carefully to determine whether the product or food additive contains the agent the hypersensitive person is to avoid. Patients and family members should be educated on the specific dietary restrictions inherent to their treatment plan.

Observation of Changes

Care of normal skin includes regular observation of pigmented skin areas, moles or nevi, as well as other newly acquired skin growths. Any change in size, color, or general appearance should be reported to a health care provider.

Dangers of Self-Treatment

People should be urged to seek attention from a health care provider when skin conditions develop. Although skin diseases rarely cause death, they may be reflections of serious systemic illness and can account for much discomfort and for serious interruption of work and other activities. Many persons are inclined to rely on the advice of friends, local pharmacists, or home remedies. Each individual's skin reacts differently to treatment, and the skin that is already irritated or inflamed may respond violently to inexpert treatment. Medications prescribed previously for an unrelated skin disorder may produce an unfavorable response in a new skin problem. Medications without expiration dates should be discarded. The person may be spared much discomfort and expense by consulting a specialist when symptoms first develop and before a mild skin condition becomes a serious problem.

Psychologic Care

A certain degree of "beauty orientation" exists in Western culture. Television and print media advertisements use beautiful models to attract the consumer. Beauty is culturally defined. Cosmetics to enhance good looks are extensively used by women as well as men. Therefore skin diseases or physical defects that detract from "good looks" can produce altered perspectives on self-image.

A person's emotional reaction to a skin disorder or deformity must not be underestimated. Pride in oneself and the ability to think well of and regard oneself favorably in comparison with others are essential to the development and maintenance of a well-integrated personality. Every person who has a defect or is physically challenged, particularly if the defect is conspicuous to others, suffers from some threat to emotional security. The extent of the emotional reaction and the amount of maladjustment that follows depend on the individual's personality and ability to cope with emotional insults. Physical insults, whether they be induced by skin disease or trauma, almost invariably lead to disruptive life experiences. The child who has severe atopic dermatitis, especially involving the face, may be ridiculed at school; the adolescent girl who has pitted acne scars may be self-conscious and avoid social situations; and the young man with a posttraumatic scar on his face may be refused a sales job. Under any of these circumstances, the individual may withdraw from a society that is unkind. The defect may be used to justify failure, avoid responsibility, or justify striking out against an unkind society.

Skin diseases that produce marked alterations in the visible body surfaces can alter the person's body image. Societal onlookers may recoil when viewing persons with severe skin diseases. They may fear potential threats of contagiousness, although most often this is unwarranted. Nurses and other health care providers should possess insight into their own possible responses to viewing severe skin problems, before delivering care. Patients with skin disorders should be provided with an open, accepting, nurturing health care environment.

BOX 62-1 Common Causes of Pruritus

Dry skin
Skin irritants: plastic or glass fibers, wool, plant products, insects
Drug reactions
Psychogenic reactions
Infectious diseases
Infestation: hookworm
Systemic diseases: obstructive biliary disease, uremia, diabetes mellitus
Neoplasia: Hodgkin's disease, leukemia, lymphoma

Relief of Pruritus (Itching)

Pruritus, or itching, is a cutaneous symptom that provokes the desire to scratch. It is caused by repetitive low-frequency stimulation of C fibers. These C fibers are similar to, but different from, the C fibers that transmit pain stimuli. Itching can be produced by mechanical stimulation of the skin or by chemical mediators. Itching primarily occurs in the skin, certain mucous membranes, and eyes. The areas most sensitive to itching are the nostrils, mucocutaneous junctions, external ear canals, and perineum.

Pruritus can be caused by any irritating substance that disrupts the integrity of the stratum corneum layer of the skin, or can result from certain systemic diseases (Box 62-1). One of the most common causes of pruritus is dry skin. Dry skin can accompany certain skin disorders such as atopic dermatitis, occur as a result of overbathing with drying soaps, or happen as a normal manifestation of aging. Physiologic factors that can intensify itching include vasodilation, tissue anoxia, and circulatory stasis. Whatever the etiology, pruritus ranges from a simple annoyance to a severe, distressing, exhausting problem.

Pruritus leads to the motor response of scratching. Persons with intense itching can severely excoriate the skin by digging deeply into the skin with their fingernails. Persons with generalized pruritus may be observed to be in constant motion-twisting, rubbing, and scratching repeatedly.

A major step in treating patients with pruritus is to attempt to remove the itch stimuli and break the itch-scratch cycle. Cold causes vasoconstriction and will provide some relief. Hydration in a tepid bath followed by the application of an emollient lotion is helpful. Cornstarch or colloidal oatmeal preparations may be added to the bath. Topical corticosteroids decrease the inflammatory effects and play a role in decreasing pruritus symptoms.[5] Topical antipruritic agents such as Sarna lotion and pramoxine hydrochloride applied two to three times a day can decrease the itch-scratch cycle. Oral antihistamines, both sedating and nonsedating agents, may offer some benefit.

The awareness of pruritus may be more acute during the night because of a decrease in diverting stimuli. Cool, light, nonrestrictive bed clothing may help allay itching. Hot, dry environments are not conducive to managing itch symptoms. Attempts should be made to humidify the living quarters with use of humidifiers and moist heat systems.

Temperature Control

Maintenance of optimal body temperature can be an issue for persons with dermatologic problems. Patients with generalized flush (erythroderma) or extensive atopic or exfoliative dermatitis may be losing body heat at an abnormally increased rate. Ambient room temperature should be maintained at 32.2° C (90° F) or greater, so as to ensure patient comfort. Care must be taken to avoid chilling, particularly after bathing when compresses or dressings are applied.

Therapeutic Baths and Soaks

Baths or soaks are recommended to relieve pruritus, remove exudates, hydrate dry skin, dehydrate weeping, moist skin, or to provide antimicrobial actions (Table 62-9). Too frequent bathing or soaking can lead to dry skin. The application of emollient lotions or creams immediately after bathing or soaking will enhance the hydrating effects of the product.

Tub baths may be administered to cleanse the skin before therapeutic topical therapy, to relieve generalized pruritus, or to provide direct therapy (e.g., Domeboro or tar baths). During cleansing baths special attention is given to intertriginous areas, where creams and topical medications may collect. Older adults should be provided with a safe environment for bathing to avoid falls. Lifts may be required with the hospitalized patient. If a lift is not available, sitting on a chair under a gentle shower is the next best alternative to a cleansing bath (see Guidelines for Safe Practice box, p. 1971, top).

Wet dressing intervention provides cooling, drying, antipruritic, or debriding effects. Plain tap water or physiologic saline may be used, or medications may be added. An astringent effect may be obtained through the use of Burow's solution (Domeboro, Buro-Sol, Bluboro), 1:20 or 1:40 dilution. Potassium permanganate ($KMnO_4$) has antimicrobial and drying effects. All tablet crystals must be thoroughly dissolved to prevent chemical burning of the skin. Potassium permanganate should not be used on the face. Silver nitrate ($AgNO_3$), 0.5%, is an antimicrobial agent that is often used in the treatment of burns. Both $KMnO_3$ and $AgNO_3$ can stain skin and cloth (see Guidelines for Safe Practice box, p. 1971, bottom).

TABLE 62-9 Preparations Commonly Used for Baths or Soaks

Substance	Effect	Suggested Actions
Colloids: oatmeal, cornstarch, soybean powder	Antipruritic, drying	Tub surfaces become very slippery; support person to prevent falls.
Potassium permanganate $KMnO_4$	Antifungal, drying, deodorizing	Strain pulverized tablet through cheesecloth to prevent irritation; stains surfaces and linens.
Burow's solution (aluminum acetate)	Antibacterial, drying	Commonly used for soaks.
Sulfur bath suspension	Antibacterial	Rinse body with tepid water after bath to remove residual sulfur particles.
Tar preparations: Balnetar, Zetar, Alma-Tar, Polytar	Antipruritic, moisturizing	Do not use soap with tar baths.
Bath oils: Alpha-Keri, Jeri-Bath, Domol	Antipruritic, moisturizing	Tub surfaces may become slippery.

Guidelines for Safe Practice

Baths and Soaks

1. The water temperature should be of comfort to patient (usually 32° to 38° C, or 90° to 100° F).
2. Medication should be completely dissolved while tub is filling.
3. The soak should last 20 to 30 minutes.
4. To prevent falls when oils or colloids are added to the water, patients are assisted in and out of the water.
5. A rubber mat is used to prevent slipping.
6. The skin is patted, not rubbed, dry to avoid skin irritation.
7. Creams or ointments are applied immediately after the bath to retain skin moisture.
8. After a medicated bath, the tub is cleaned as follows:
   a. Pour 1 cup of bleach into used tub water.
   b. Let bleach stand in water for 5 minutes.
   c. Wipe sides and bottom of tub.
   d. Drain and clean tub as usual.

Guidelines for Safe Practice

Applying Wet Dressings

1. Prepare solution to be applied at room temperature. Sterility is not required.
2. Soak dressing thoroughly in solution.
3. Protect bed or clothing with towels, bath blanket, flannel squares, etc.
4. Wring out dressings–they should be wet but not dripping.
5. Apply dressings in smooth layers (two to four layers) to involved areas. Wrap fingers and toes separately, and wrap joints so that they can bend.
6. Remove, soak, and reapply dressings before they dry (that is, every 3 to 5 minutes).
7. Continue treatment for 20 to 30 minutes.
8. Pat skin dry.

Medications

Medications are delivered to patients with skin disorders via topical, intralesional, or systemic routes. Topical therapy is preferable, as it has the potential for decreased systemic side effects. The disadvantages of topical therapy are the time requirements for applications, volumes needed, and potential aesthetic concerns. Dermatologic topical medications are delivered to the target organ (skin) via several *vehicle* systems. A vehicle is the substance in which the medication is placed for application to the skin. Creams, ointments, lotions, gels, solutions, and powders are the usual *vehicle* systems used to deliver topical medication. The degree of inflammation observed in a rash will influence the choice of vehicle selected to treat it. Patient instruction on method of application will enhance the treatment regimen. (Table 62-10). The nurse should be aware of the pharmacologic actions of the topical medication prescribed, as well as the actions of the vehicle system.

The Dermatologic Formulary lists the broad categories of agents used in management of skin disorders along with examples of select products.

Topical Corticosteroids

Glucocorticosteroids are the most potent antiinflammatory substances available. They possess the unique ability to inhibit cell division. In dermatologic care, corticosteroids are used to treat a variety of skin disorders because of their antiinflammatory, antiproliferative, and antipruritic properties. Topical corticosteroids differ in their antiinflammatory effects, ranging from low to very high potency. Hydrocortisone is of low potency. Some corticosteroids, such as triamcinolone acetonide (Aristocort, Kenalog), vary in potency depending on the dose. Topical steroids in an ointment vehicle are usually more potent and have a greater lubricating effect than cream vehicles of the same agent. Fluorinated corticosteroids are of stronger potency and thus have a greater potential for causing the local side effects of skin atrophy, purpura, striae, rosacea, and folliculitis. Fluorinated corticosteroids should not be used on the face, skin folds, or genital sites. Hypothalamic-pituitary-adrenal axis suppression is a rare occurrence with topical corticosteroid therapy. It can happen, however, in the setting of a super potent agent applied to large surface area for an extended period of time. Occlusive dressings enhance the effects of topical corticosteroids. Occlusion can offer benefit for (1) dermatoses of palms and soles, (2) thick psoriatic plaques, (3) localized plaques of lichen simplex chronicus, and (4) extensive, severe, steroid-responsive dermatitis. The affected area should be occluded only when directed by the health care provider. Plastic wrap is good for occluding small areas. Plastic (nonlatex)

TABLE 62-10 Factors Influencing Vehicle Selection and Patient Instructional Tips

Factor	Vehicle
Degree of Inflammatory Process	
Acute Inflammation	Wet dressings
Marked erythema, edema, blistering, tenderness, pruritus, oozing, crusting	Powders Solutions Lotions
Subacute Inflammation	Lotions Aerosols Creams
Oozing and crusting subsided Erythema and edema less acute but still present	Gels
Chronic Inflammation	Gels
Limited erythema, scaling, fissures Pruritus	Ointments
Location of Skin Condition	
Scalp—lotions, gels, solutions Intertriginous areas—lotions, powders, creams	
Activity of Medication in Given Vehicle	
Chemical formulation of active ingredient versus vehicle	

Application	Instructional Tips
Creams	Indicated for hair-bearing areas, moist lesions, and intertriginous folds. Apply in direction of hair growth evenly and sparingly.
Ointments	Indicated for dry and fissured skin surfaces. Hydrating skin prior to application may improve effectiveness. Avoid moist/occlusive surfaces >> potential for irritation and maceration.
Lotions	Indicated for large surface areas, intertriginous folds, hair-bearing areas and oozing sites. Shake well prior to application.
Powders	Indicated for intertriginous folds and other sites where moisture trapping occurs. Apply with puff or shaker. Remove starch or cellulose containing powders before re-application.
Solution/Spray/Aerosol	Indicated for hair-bearing areas or large surface areas. Spray aerosol 6 inches from skin in bursts.
Gels	Indicated for hair-bearing surfaces and facial sites—may be dehydrating. Irritation can be minimized by applying to dry skin.

From Dermatology Nurses Association: *Dermatology nursing essentials: a core curriculum,* Linden, NJ, 1998, Anthony J. Janetti.

gloves may be used on hands and plastic bags on feet. Plastic garment bags or large trash bags may be used for the trunk, with holes cut for head and arms. Plastic suits (sauna suits) are available for total body occlusion. Lesions are usually occluded at night for an 8-hour period. The patient should be monitored for potential complications, including candida infections, sweat retention, and folliculitis.

Application of Topical Medications

Gloves are worn for protection when applying topical medications. Powders should be sprinkled into the gloved hand and then applied to the skin to avoid aerosolization of the agent. Powders should be used sparingly to prevent caking. Cornstarch is not suggested because it encourages growth of yeast organisms. Lotions with a water or alcohol base are applied by patting gently. Lotions with an oily base are applied thinly and evenly with the palm of the gloved hand. Ointments are applied with gloved hand and tend to spread with greater ease than creams. If a dressing is to be applied, the ointment may be spread on the dressing with a tongue blade before application to the skin. Some topical medications, such as coal tar products, are removed before other topical treatments are imposed.

Home Care

The vast majority of patients with dermatologic disorders do not require inpatient hospitalization. Patient teaching is critical to successful self-care management in the outpatient population. Key teaching points are described in the Guidelines for Safe Practice box. Clear, concise written instructions tailored to the specific language and age requirements of the patient is optimal. Many dermatology organizations and related pharmaceutical companies provide free patient education literature on skin disorders, skin cancer prevention, and use of dermatologic topical products.

Dressing procedures are sometimes costly and complex. These patients will benefit from a home health referral to assist with teaching, as well as community financial resources.

Guidelines for Safe Practice

Teaching the Patient With a Dermatologic Disorder

1. Nature of the disorder (cause, preventive measures, acuity or chronicity, symptoms requiring medical follow-up care)
2. Treatment modalities to be carried out at home (soaks, baths, medicated dressings)
3. Special precautions to be observed during treatment, such as the following:
   a. Avoid nonporous coverings over dressings, unless ordered
   b. Completely dissolve tablets or crystals in baths or soaks
   c. Avoid excessive rubbing of medication over lesions
   d. Apply thin layers of lotions or powders
4. Prescribed medication regimens: route of administration, vehicle to be used, dose, frequency, duration of topical application, side effects, where supplies can be obtained
5. Ways to promote socialization with others when disfiguring dermatologic lesions are present

PRESSURE ULCERS

Etiology

Pressure ulcers are defined by the National Pressure Ulcer Advisory Panel (NPUAP) as lesions caused by unrelieved pressure against soft tissue, usually over bony prominences. For many years, pressure ulcers were incorrectly termed bed sores or decubitus ulcers. The Latin definition of the term decubitus implies lying flat, and decubitus therefore was correctly changed to pressure after it was ascertained that one could develop a pressure ulcer while in any body position, on any body location, and from any source of pressure (internal secondary to bone or body weight, as well as external). Risk factors for pressure ulcers are associated with both intrinsic and extrinsic factors. Extrinsic factors include moisture, shear, friction, and pressure, which can also be internal pressure. Intrinsic risk factors relate to characteristics of the patient's skin structure that are determined by factors such as the amount of collagen, age, nutritional status, and use of steroids; presence of spinal cord injury or other alterations in mobility and perception; and degree of perfusion. Factors affecting perfusion of the skin include blood pressure, extracorporeal circulation, serum protein, albumin and prealbumin levels, hemoglobin and hematocrit levels, smoking, vascular disease, administration of vasoactive medication, and either a pronounced increase or decrease in body temperature.

Epidemiology

Pressure ulcers are nonselective. They can occur in any age-group, ethnic population, or socioeconomic group. Attempts have been made to estimate the financial burden of the pressure ulcer problem; however, research has been limited and inconsistent. Some studies estimate that $11.5 billion is expended annually on products for pressure ulcer management. Attempts to estimate the cost of an individual pressure ulcer also have been unsuccessful. Conservative estimates of the cost of treatment for one stage I or stage II pressure ulcer range from $125 to $200 with treatment of one stage II or IV pressure ulcer to be between $14,000 and $23,000.[4]

The NPUAP reviewed more than 800 available manuscripts in an attempt to define the scope of the problem and has concluded that the incidence and prevalence of pressure ulcers in various health care settings are high enough to warrant concern. Clinical Practice Guidelines,[6] nationally accepted standards of care, were established and reviewed for validity based on that manuscript review.

The estimated prevalence of pressure ulcers is approximately 12% in skilled care facilities[18] and 10.8% in acute care facilities,[3] of which 8.5% are intraoperatively acquired.[2] Home care agencies report that 29% of their patients have a pressure ulcer[15] with a much greater incidence in certain high-risk populations, such as patients with a spinal cord injury. An estimated one in five patients die each year from complications of pressure ulcers.

Pathophysiology

Unrelieved pressure causes cellular necrosis as a result of vascular insufficiency. The pathophysiology of pressure ulcers is outlined in Table 62-11. Box 62-2 presents the stages of pressure ulcers.

Collaborative Care Management

Pressure ulcers have been identified as primarily a nursing problem, but they require collaboration with the entire health care team for effective resolution. Management includes interventions designed to control chronic disease symptomatology that affects healthy integument, such as medication regulation to keep glucose levels within normal limits and measures to promote optimal tissue perfusion and oxygenation. The correct product for treatment of pressure ulcers must be ordered. Products chosen inappropriately for wound management can cause more tissue damage or delay healing. A discussion of common treatment modalities used in the management of pressure ulcers follows.

Diagnostic Tests. No specific laboratory tests assist with diagnosis of pressure ulcers. Related laboratory examinations pertinent to risk factors should be used as a predictor of potential alteration in skin integrity. Open, draining ulcers may require culture and sensitivity to identify pathogens and determine appropriate antibiotics.

Medications. There are no particular medications for pressure ulcers. Antibiotics are used if an infection is present. Vitamins, minerals, and essential and nonessential amino acids are prescribed to facilitate improvement in the patient's nutritional status.

Treatment. More than 2000 products exist as purported treatment measures for pressure ulcers. Representative product categories are discussed in Table 62-12.

Surgical Management. Some patients with wounds qualify for surgical intervention. Surgeons perform myocutaneous flaps and skin grafts of various levels, depending on the patient's physical condition, compliance level, and type of wound.

TABLE 62-11 Normal Function, Pathophysiology, and Clinical Manifestations of Pressure Ulcers

Normal Function	Pathophysiology	Clinical Manifestations
Microvasculature: capillaries supply tissue needs of oxygenated blood and nutrients	Pressure applied to soft tissue compresses capillaries, distorting structure and occluding blood flow	Ischemia at first, followed by reactive hyperemia
Sympathetic response	Compensation by increased shunting of capillary circulation to area under pressure; capillaries increase permeability and leak fluid into tissues	Tissue edema and inflammation
Capillary walls lined with endothelial cells; platelets flow smoothly through microvessels	Endothelial cells disrupted, platelets aggregate, and thrombi form in capillaries and lead to cellular death	Erythema that may or may not resolve once pressure source is removed
Intact skin as the body's protective mechanism	Cellular death leads to tissue necrosis	Pressure ulcer with visible tissue damage, described by stages (see Box 62-2)

BOX 62-2 Stages of Pressure Ulcers

Stage 1

An observable pressure-related alteration of intact skin whose indicators as compared to the adjacent or opposite area on the body may include changes in one or more of the following:

- Skin temperature (warmth or coolness)
- Tissue consistency (firm or boggy feel)
- Sensation (pain, itching).

The ulcer appears as a defined area of persistent redness in lightly pigmented skin, whereas in darker skin tones, the ulcer may appear with persistent red, blue, or purple hues.

Stage 2

Partial-thickness skin loss involving epidermis, dermis, or both. The ulcer is superficial and presents clinically as an abrasion, blister, or shallow crater.

Stage 3

Full-thickness skin loss involving damage to, or necrosis of, subcutaneous tissue that may extend down to, but not through, underlying fascia. The ulcer presents clinically as a deep crater with or without undermining of adjacent tissue.

Stage 4

Full-thickness skin loss with extensive destruction, tissue necrosis, or damage to muscle, bone, or supporting structures (e.g., tendon, joint capsule). Undermining and sinus tracts also may be associated with stage 4 pressure ulcers.

NOTE: If eschar (dead leathery tissue) is present, pressure ulcers cannot be accurately staged.

These surgical interventions are discussed in Chapter 64. See the Research box for a discussion of intraoperative control of hypothermia and the correlation between core body temperature and the development of pressure ulcers.

Diet. Patients with wounds require additional protein (1.5 to 2 g/kg/day) and calorie intake to assist with tissue regeneration on a cellular level. A well-balanced diet is sufficient to maintain healthy skin; however, most patients with identified risk factors are not eating a well-balanced diet. Protein supplementation in balanced amounts is helpful. Only a medical nutritionist, a physician with a subspecialty practice in nutritional management, or a registered dietitian can accurately determine a balance of demand and replacement that will be therapeutic for the patient. Research also suggests that supplemental vitamins A and C; the minerals zinc, copper, and manganese; and amino acids (glutamine, arginine, and cysteine) plus a multiple vitamin help stimulate wound healing on a cellular level.

Activity. As discussed earlier, the more independently active the patient is, the lower the risk of pressure ulcer formation and the greater the chances of wound healing. The key factor related to wound healing is the removal of the causative agent(s). Regardless of the treatment prescribed for wound care, if the patient or the nurse does not relieve the pressure, wound healing will not occur.

Referrals. Many disciplines have become involved with wound-healing modalities. There are now many professional associations associated with wound care that exist for the podiatrist, registered nurse, physical therapist, registered dietitian, and scientists involved in the advancement of wound care. At present nurses and physicians receive minimal education about either the products and/or principles of wound healing. A nursing specialty has evolved over the last 30 years called wound, ostomy, and continence nursing (previously known as enterostomal therapy or ET nursing). Wound, ostomy, continence (WOC) nurses are nationally recognized as leaders in the wound care arena and are an active part of the NPUAP. If an institution does not have a WOC nurse on staff, the Wound, Ostomy and Continence Nurses Society in California can provide a referral to the closest practitioner. This organization can be contacted by calling 800-826-0268, or through the Internet at www.wocn.org.

TABLE 62-12 Products Used to Treat Pressure Ulcers

Category	Example
Exudate Absorption	
Copolymer starch dressings	Absorption dressing Duoderm granules
Calcium alginates (absorb exudate, as well as release calcium on a cellular level—stimulates angiogenesis)	Kaltostat Sorbsan Algosteril
Debridement	
Enzymatic	Accuzyme Santyl Panafil Biozyme C
Wet-to-dry dressings*	100% cotton gauze in many forms (4 × 4, kerlex)
Wound Protection, Insulation, and Mild Absorption	
Hydrocolloids (waxy pectin adhesive dressings that provide an optimal wound environment)	Duoderm Restore Tegasorb Ultec
Transparent dressings (thin, adhesive dressings that support the microenvironment for cellular regeneration)	Tegaderm Bioclusive OpSite Blister film Polyskin
Polyurethane foam dressings (nonadhesive; some assist with odor control)	Allevyn Lyofoam EpiLock Carrasyn
Hydrogel dressings (gel in a tube or a nonadherent sheet; have a topical soothing effect; varied in thickness)	Elasto-Gel Vigilon Second Skin

NOTE: Research suggests that wounds heal most effectively in a moist, natural environment, with a clean, debris- and necrotic-free wound area. Dressings and interventions are all designed with these principles in mind. Several have other added benefits that are discussed separately within each category.

*Solutions used vary according to preference of physician; most common solution is normal saline.

Research

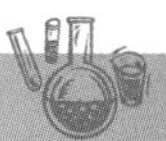

Reference: Scott EM: Effects of warming therapy on pressure ulcers: a randomized trial, *AORN J* 73:921-927, 929-933, 936-938, 2001.

Pressure ulcers are a serious and expensive health care problem. In the acute care setting up to 25% of pressure ulcers occur during a surgical procedure. The patients at greatest risk for developing a pressure ulcers are those individuals having operations related to reconstructive surgery of existing pressure ulcers, or vascular, cardiac, or orthopedic procedures.

All patients receiving general anesthesia are at risk for developing hypothermia (less than 96.8° F). Hypothermia typically occurs in older patients and those with large surface areas of the body exposed, an opened peritoneal cavity, or receiving large amounts of unwarmed irrigation fluid. Hypothermia has been associated with deviations in serum potassium, postoperative instability, myocardial ischemia within the first 24 hours after surgery, increased mortality, increased arterial blood pressure, cardiovascular complications, protein metabolism, and decreased subcutaneous oxygen tension resulting from vasoconstriction.

The purpose of this study was to test the hypothesis that intraoperative control of hypothermia would reduce the development of pressure ulcers.

A prospective, randomized clinical trial was conducted. The methods of care tested were the use of forced-air warming therapy with the simultaneous warming of intravenous fluids compared to the standard therapy of automatic regulation of ambient temperature, minimal patient exposure during preparation time, and use of warmed blankets for immediate postoperative care. Results of the study, although not statistically significant, showed that the development of pressure ulcers was decreased by nearly 50% in patients who received warming therapy. This study supports the hypothesis that there is a correlation between core body temperature and the development of pressure ulcers.

NURSING MANAGEMENT OF PATIENT WITH PRESSURE ULCER

A holistic approach to nursing management of the patient with a pressure ulcer contains four components: (1) controlling the contributing factors by reduction or elimination, (2) supporting the host, (3) optimizing the microenvironment based on principles of wound healing, and (4) providing education for patients and caregivers.

ASSESSMENT

Most pressure ulcers can be prevented if the nurse is diligent about assessment and appropriate interventions. Not all interventions are within the scope of nursing practice; therefore a multidisciplinary leadership approach as recommended by the NPUAP is important. Prevention can be accomplished only when the nurse has identified those patients at high risk for development of pressure ulcer. Many "assessment tools" are available. Currently only two tools are cited in the Clinical Practice Guidelines[2] as valid and research based; these are the Norton and Braden scales. Most institutions incorporate information from one or both of these tools while developing their own tool.

Assessment tools consider both extrinsic and intrinsic factors that contribute to alterations in skin integrity. The Norton scale (Figure 62-19), which was developed for use in a geriatric population, examines the patient's general health and mental status and levels of mobility, activity, and continence. Simple to use, this tool leaves much room for nursing judgment within the specific areas. These areas are scored from 1 to 4, and a total is calculated. The lower the total number of points, the greater the risk the patient has for skin breakdown. The Braden scale is more specific, providing explanations for each score the patient is given (Figure 62-20, p. 1978). This tool was based on the original work of the Norton Scale. The areas scored in this tool include the patient's levels of sensory

Norton Scale

A Physical condition	B Mental state	C Activity	D Mobility	E Incontinence	Total Score
4 Good	4 Alert	4 Ambulant	4 Full	4 Not	______
3 Fair	3 Apathetic	3 Walks with help	3 Slightly limited	3 Occasional	
2 Poor	2 Confused	2 Chairbound	2 Very limited	2 Usually urine	
1 Bad	1 Stupor	1 Bedrest	1 Immobile	1 Double incontinence	

Norton Plus Scale
(For determining high risk for pressure sores)

Check ONLY if YES	YES
Diagnosis of diabetes	____
Diagnosis of hypertension	____
Hematocrit (M) <41%	____
(F) <36%	____
Hemoglobin (M) <14 g/dl	____
(F) <12 g/dl	____
Albumin level <3.3 g/dl	____
Febrile >99.6°F	____
5 or more medications	____
Changes in mental status to confused, lethargic within 24 hours	____
TOTAL Number of Checkmarks	
Norton Scale Score	____
Minus total from above	____
Norton Plus Score	____

Figure 62-19 Norton Scale and Norton Plus Scale.

perception, mobility, nutrition, and activity, as well as the presence or absence of moisture, friction, and shear. Once again, a number is assigned for each parameter, the total is calculated, and the lower the score, the greater the risk factor.

A skin risk assessment tool should be completed at the time of a patient's admission to a facility and thereafter on either a weekly basis or when there has been a change in the patient's condition, such as surgery. Some institutions have established protocols to complete successive skin risk assessment at intervals longer than every week if the patient is residing in a long-term care facility.

Once a wound has developed, the nurse is responsible for periodic assessments to determine whether the plan of care continues to be effective. Institutional policies differ on the frequency of assessments, so the term *periodic* has been adopted by the NPUAP to offer general guidelines while allowing flexibility for individual care settings.

A staging classification system as detailed in Box 62-2 is helpful for the nurse in determining the appropriate interventions for a particular wound based on the depth of the tissue involved; however, it is not an all-inclusive tool. A wound covered with necrotic tissue (eschar) cannot be staged because the depth of tissue damage cannot be ascertained. To appropriately evaluate and document pressure ulcers, the nurse also must assess the size, color, presence of exudates, odor (if present), and presence of slough or necrotic tissue.

Size

Sizing the wound determines the size and occasionally the type of dressing(s) required. The nurse should measure size of the wound by its length, width, and depth at the deepest point. The depth of the wound is measured by inserting a sterile applicator and comparing depth with measurements on a wound-measuring guide. Other general parameters to assess include presence of undermining or sinus tracts in the wound, condition of the surrounding skin, and the presence of foreign bodies in wound (e.g., sutures, orthopedic hardware).

A more accurate wound assessment can be obtained by taking a photograph of the wound. The photograph should be labeled to identify the patient and date and should indicate where the length, width, and depth were measured for future accuracy in measurements. An irregularly shaped wound should be traced if a photograph cannot be obtained. Medicare requires accurate sizing of the wound for reimbursement of home care dressing supplies.

Color

The color of wounds provides information about vascular supply, infection, healthy versus necrotic tissue, and nutritional status. "Healthy" full-thickness wounds have a beefy-red, granular appearance. If the wound bed is pale, this may be a reflection of a low hemoglobin level. Necrotic tissue is white, yellow, gray, or black. Certain infections also change the color of a wound bed. *Pseudomonas* species can produce greenish drainage on the wound bed.

Exudate

Wound drainage should be assessed for amount, color, consistency, and odor. Infected wounds generally produce large amounts of odorous drainage. Documentation should be as objective and descriptive as possible. Terms such as small, moderate, and large are subjective and should be avoided.

NURSING DIAGNOSES

Nursing diagnoses are determined from analysis of patient data. Nursing diagnoses for the patient with a pressure ulcer may include but are not limited to:

Diagnostic Title	Possible Etiologic Factors
1. Impaired skin integrity and/or risk for impaired skin integrity	Nutritional deficit; prolonged immobility; advanced age; decreased hemoglobin, serum albumin, and prealbumin levels
2. Deficient knowledge	Lack of knowledge regarding treatment regimen and follow-up care, and adequate nutrition

EXPECTED PATIENT OUTCOMES

Expected patient outcomes for the patient with or at risk for a pressure ulcer may include but are not limited to:

1a. Will be discharged with intact skin or with a healing wound that is free of infection

1b. Will be free of observable pressure-related alterations of intact skin

2. Will demonstrate with caregiver, if appropriate, ability to implement a program of continuing therapeutic and/or preventive care, including measures to reduce or relieve pressure on the skin, manage incontinence/moisture, and maintain adequate nutrition

INTERVENTIONS

1. Promoting/Maintaining Skin Integrity

Interventions in the management of a patient with a pressure ulcer include activities in the areas of prevention, protection, rehabilitation, and education (see Nursing Care Plan). The nurse needs to keep in mind that many of these same interventions can be used in a nursing care plan for the prevention of impaired skin integrity.

Prevention focuses on either reducing or relieving pressure to bony prominences. One way to achieve this goal is by instituting a schedule of turning the patient at least every 2 hours. The use of pressure relieving and/or reduction surfaces for the bed and/or chair should also be incorporated into the patient's plan of care; however, in many institutions this represents an additional cost.

The skin is inspected at regular intervals for signs of early irritation and/or breakdown. Moisturization of the skin is important to maintain its soft, elastic state. Massaging moisturizer or lotion over bony prominences should be avoided, as this action may cause the rupture of blood vessels and possible injury to friable tissue. Incontinence of stool and urine should be controlled (i.e., diapers) or diverted (i.e., Foley catheter, fecal incontinence pouch) to keep excess moisture and irritants away from the skin. A moisture barrier, preferably one with either dimethicone or petrolatum, should be applied per the manufacturer's directions or as needed in between incontinence episodes once the patient has been cleaned of body waste.

Reduction or elimination of shear and friction is accomplished using a lift sheet when moving the patient in bed or out of bed. The head of the bed should be no higher 30 degrees to avoid shear by the patient sliding to the foot of the bed.

A summary of preventive interventions can be found in the Guidelines for Safe Practice box.

Protection of the skin and wound environment includes the use of aseptic technique and Standard Precautions for the prevention of infection. The patient is monitored for clinical signs and symptoms of infection every shift and these are reported as appropriate.

Rehabilitation to the patient's highest level of optimal functioning is an important goal in both the treatment and/or prevention of pressure ulcers. The patient should be involved in planning his or her activity schedule as much as possible. Gradually increasing the patient's activity level assists with restoration to an optimal level of functioning.

As the patient's expenditure of energy increases with activity, nutritional intake needs to be adjusted to meet this need. Optimal nutrition is best provided to the patient by obtaining a consult with either a registered dietitian or medical nutritionist. Many patients require specialized diets to maintain a high caloric intake in order to meet the demands of healing a wound, as well as maintaining life. Nurses should, however, be cognizant of the nutritional requirements related to supplementation of vitamins, minerals, and amino acids that facilitate the healing process.

2. Patient Education

Patient and family education is an integral part of the patient's plan of care. The patient and caregiver must be taught about the need for continued interventions to prevent recurrence. This includes instruction on dressing and intervention techniques. Many of the preventive measures described in the Guidelines for Safe Practice box can be taught to the patient and his or her family.

EVALUATION

To evaluate the effectiveness of nursing interventions, compare patient behaviors with those stated in the expected patient outcomes. Nursing care is successful if the patient with a pressure ulcer:

1a. (1) Has intact skin, or a decrease or no increase in pressure ulcer size.

(2) Demonstrates active wound healing, as evidenced by a clean, granular wound bed, minimal serosanguineous drainage, and no signs of infection (pain, tenderness, fever, induration, surrounding erythema, increased drainage).

1b. Has intact skin free of pressure-related changes such as abnormal warmth or coolness, firm or boggy tissue consistency, pain or itching, persistent redness in lightly pigmented skin or in darker skin, persistent red, blue, or purple hues.

Patient's name		**Evaluator's name**
Sensory perception Ability to respond meaningfully to pressure-related discomfort	**1. Completely limited:** Unresponsive (does not moan, flinch, or grasp) to painful stimuli, due to diminished level of consciousness or sedation, **OR** limited ability to feel pain over most of body surface.	**2. Very limited:** Responds only to painful stimuli. Cannot communicate discomfort except by moaning or restlessness, **OR** has a sensory impairment that limits the ability to feel pain or discomfort over ½ of body.
Moisture Degree to which skin is exposed to moisture	**1. Constantly moist:** Skin is kept moist almost constantly by perspiration, urine, etc. Dampness is detected every time patient is moved or turned.	**2. Moist:** Skin is often but not always moist; linen must be changed at least once a shift.
Activity Degree of physical activity	**1. Bedfast:** Confined to bed.	**2. Chairfast:** Ability to walk severely limited or nonexistent. Cannot bear own weight and/or must be assisted into chair or wheelchair.
Mobility Ability to change and control body position	**1. Completely immobile:** Does not make even slight changes in body or extremity position without assistance.	**2. Very limited:** Makes occasional slight changes in body or extremity position but unable to make frequent or significant changes independently.
Nutrition Usual food intake pattern	**1. Very poor:** Never eats a complete meal. Rarely eats more than ⅓ of any food offered. Eats 2 servings or less of protein (meat or dairy products) per day. Takes fluids poorly. Does not take a liquid dietary supplement, **OR** is NPO and/or maintained on clear liquids or IV for more than 5 days.	**2. Probably inadequate:** Rarely eats a complete meal and generally eats only about ½ of any food offered. Protein intake includes only 3 servings of meat or dairy products per day. Occasionally will take a dietary supplement, **OR** receives less than optimum amount of liquid diet or tube feeding.
Friction and shear	**1. Problem:** Requires moderate to maximum assistance in moving. Complete lifting without sliding against sheets is impossible. Frequently slides down in bed or chair, requiring frequent repositioning with maximum assistance. Spasticity, contractures, or agitation leads to almost constant friction.	**2. Potential problem:** Moves feebly or requires minimum assitance. During a move, skin probably slides to some extent against sheets, chair, restraints, or other devices. Maintains relatively good position in chair or bed most of the time but occasionally slides down.

Figure 62-20 Braden Scale for predicting pressure ulcer risk.

2. Demonstrates with caregiver, if appropriate, ability to implement a program of continuing therapeutic and/or preventive care, including measures to reduce or relieve pressure on the skin, manage incontinence/moisture, and maintain adequate nutrition.

GERONTOLOGIC CONSIDERATIONS

Many of the changes in the skin associated with aging predispose the older adult to the development of pressure ulcers. Thinning of the epidermis makes the skin more prone to injury. Adhesion of the epidermis to the dermis is decreased and accompanied by a decrease in skin elasticity, allowing the skin to be easily stretched and deformed. The skin is a less effective barrier against infection, bruising, and water loss. In addition, thermal regulation and the ability to perceive touch and pain are decreased. Excessive pressure may not be well perceived in the older adult and coexisting neurologic deficits may compound the problem.

With the application of shearing forces, the epidermal-dermal attachment may weaken and allow the skin layers to separate. A blister forms and eventually ruptures, leaving a flap of skin with uneven edges, called a skin tear. Persons who require assistance with moving in bed or transfers are at risk for the development of skin tears caused by shearing forces. Frequent bathing with an alkaline soap can dry older adults' skin by altering the natural acidic mantle of the epidermis. The use of emollient soaps and moisturizers is recommended by moisturizing the skin either during or after bathing.

		Dates of assessment				
3. Slightly limited: Responds to verbal commands but cannot always communicate discomfort or need to be turned, **OR** has some sensory impairment that limits ability to feel pain or discomfort in 1 or 2 extremities.	**4. No impairment:** Responds to verbal commands. Has no sensory deficit which would limit ability to feel or voice pain or discomfort.					
3. Occasionally moist: Skin is occasionally moist, requiring an extra linen change approximately once a day.	**4. Rarely moist:** Skin is usually dry; linen requires changing only at routine intervals.					
3. Walks occasionally: Walks occasionally during day but for very short distances, with or without assistance. Spends majority of each shift in bed or chair.	**4. Walks frequently:** Walks outside the room at least twice a day and inside room at least once every 2 hours during waking hours.					
3. Slightly limited: Makes frequent though slight changes in body or extremity position independently.	**4. No limitations:** Makes major and frequent changes in position without assistance.					
3. Adequate: Eats over ½ of most meals. Eats a total of 4 servings of protein (meat, diary products) each day. Occasionally will refuse a meal, but will usually take a supplement if offered, **OR** is on a tube feeding or TPN regimen, which probably meets most of nutritional needs.	**4. Excellent:** Eats most of every meal. Never refuses a meal. Usually eats a total of 4 or more servings of meat and dairy products. Occasionally eats between meals. Does not require supplementation.					
3. No apparent problem: Moves in bed and in chair independently and has sufficient muscle strength to lift up completely during move. Maintains good position in bed or chair at all times.						
		Total score				

Figure 62-20, cont'd

Because of these numerous predisposing factors, older adults are at greater risk for pressure ulcers. Predisposing factors include (1) anemia, (2) poor nutrition, (3) decreased albumin, (4) decreased mobility, (5) thinning of skin and loss of the subcutaneous cushion, (6) drug therapy such as glucocorticoids and NSAIDs, (7) incontinence, and (8) comorbid conditions (e.g., hypertension, coronary artery disease, diabetes) or use of sedatives that interfere with sensory perception, natural shifting of body position, or turning in bed.

Pressure ulcers can develop not only in those confined to bed but also in those confined to a sitting position. The ulcers occur whenever pressure is allowed to be maintained. Ulcers can occur on the head, shoulders, or lower back if a recumbent position is maintained. In the side-lying position the patient can develop a pressure ulcer on the hips, ankles, and the pinna of the ear. Sitting promotes ulcers on the buttocks. The underside of the scrotum can be injured with shearing and pressure.

Measures to prevent and treat pressure ulcers are the same for the older adult as for any person. The only difference is that tissue, because of the predisposing factors, is damaged more quickly, so more frequent position changes and inspections need to be implemented. Many hospitalized older adults require dietary measures to improve nutrition to prevent pressure ulcers. Also, many older adults require use of pressure relieving and/or reducing surfaces (e.g., specialty mattresses or beds) and padding for chairs, if immobilization is required.

Nursing Care Plan — Patient With a Pressure Ulcer

DATA Mrs. M. is a 79-year-old widow. She has a history of hypertension, congestive heart failure (CHF), obesity, and degenerative joint disease. She is right-hand dominant. Mrs. M. lives alone in her own home; an adult daughter lives nearby. Mrs. M. actively attends social activities at a local senior center.

This morning she was admitted to the hospital for a left cerebrovascular accident (CVA), or brain attack. Nursing assessment findings include:

- Alert and oriented times 3 but appears depressed
- Dysphagia
- Incontinent of urine and stool
- Right-sided hemiparesis
- +2 pitting edema of the lower extremities
- Bruise on the sacrum from a previous fall
- Generalized dry skin
- Height, 65 inches; weight, 180 pounds
- Braden scale = 12
- Vital signs: temperature, 36.9° C; pulse, 92; respirations, 18; blood pressure, 142/88

Mrs. M.'s prescribed medications include:

- Lisinopril 10 mg bid
- Furosemide 40 mg qd
- Digoxin 0.125 mg qd
- Heparin 5000 U q12h SQ
- Ibuprofen (Motrin) 800 mg tid

Collaborative management is focused on preventing any further neurologic events or deficits, promoting nutrition, preventing aspiration, controlling hypertension, preventing increased CHF, promoting mobility and independence, preventing injury, and psychologic support. A skin tear is present on the sacrum and is a stage II pressure ulcer. Mrs. M. is transferred to a subacute division for physical and occupational therapy. The heparin has been discontinued, and the patient is on a mechanical soft diet and transfers with the assistance of one person.

NURSING DIAGNOSIS **Impaired skin integrity related to immobility and mechanical forces**
GOALS/OUTCOMES Will achieve progressive healing of pressure ulcer

NOC Suggested Outcomes

- Tissue Integrity: Skin and Mucous Membranes (1101)
- Wound Healing: Secondary Intention (1103)
- Immobility Consequences: Physiologic (0204)

NIC Suggested Interventions

- Pressure Management (3500)
- Pressure Ulcer Care (3520)
- Pressure Ulcer Prevention (3540)

Nursing Interventions/Rationales

- Assess skin every shift and as needed. *Frequent assessment allows for early recognition of skin changes, effectiveness of treatment, and preventive measures.*
- Assess areas of redness for ability to blanch. *Areas of nonblanchable erythema indicate increased pressure, which can easily progress to ulceration.*
- Document Braden scale weekly. *The Braden scale is a reliable tool for predicting pressure ulcer risk. The patient's initial score of 12 places her at risk for pressure ulcer development.*
- Assess and record changes in wound and surrounding tissue with each dressing change. Document size and depth. *To monitor progress of healing and detect any complications or infection.*
- Use appropriate barrier dressings and topical agents on sacral wound. *The physician or skin care specialist nurse determines protocols. Proper medication and treatment are essential for wound healing.*
- Turn patient every 2 hours and post the turning schedule. *Rotation of body position promotes adequate blood flow and avoids prolonged pressure on any one part.*
- Pad bony prominences. *Padding reduces pressure on skin over bony prominences, which are susceptible to breakdown as a result of tissue necrosis.*
- Elevate heels off of mattress. *The heels are susceptible to breakdown, and elevation avoids pressure.*
- Avoid massaging reddened areas. *Massage of areas under pressure may lead to further tissue injury.*
- Use emollient soap, moisturize skin after bathing, and keep perianal area clean and dry. *To prevent drying of the skin and prevent heel ulcer formation. Contamination of the perianal area with feces or urine may speed skin breakdown and cause infection.*
- Provide bowel and bladder training; avoid use of diapers and plastic pads. *Continence of urine and stool decreases the patient's risk of skin ulcer development. Increased moisture and decreased ventilation increase the risk of pressure ulcer development.*
- Avoid shearing forces (e.g., use of turning sheet or pull sheet). *To prevent injury or further tissue breakdown.*
- Keep sheets clean and dry; avoid wrinkling. *Moisture increases risk of breakdown, and wrinkled areas may cause increased pressure.*
- Use Egg Crate mattress on bed and seat cushion on wheelchair. *Provides padding, decreases pressure.*

Nursing Care Plan *Patient With a Pressure Ulcer—cont'd*

- Perform passive range of motion on affected extremities and promote active range of motion on unaffected extremities. *Promotes circulation and prevents complications associated with immobility.*
- Teach patient and daughter techniques for maintaining mobility/range of motion and promote ambulation and a regular exercise program. *Patient and family involvement in the treatment program increases success in attaining goals. An exercise program enhances circulation, promotes general health, decreases stress, and aids in weight control.*
- Encourage maximal participation in activities of daily living (ADLs). *Allows the patient some sense of control and independence. The patient is right handed and has right-sided hemiparesis, so she may need additional assistance with ADLs.*
- Employ safety precautions and fall prevention measures. *To prevent further injury to skin or other tissues.*
- Encourage elevation of legs when sitting. *To promote venous return and reduce the formation of edema (the patient has a history of CHF, edema).*
- Assess patient's need for analgesia before dressing changes. *To increase the patient's ability to tolerate dressing changes, which can be painful.*

Evaluation Parameters

1. Evidence of pressure ulcer healing
2. Decreased size of pressure ulcer
3. Absence of complications
4. Participates in prevention and treatment programs

NURSING DIAGNOSIS **Imbalanced nutrition: more than body requirements related to inadequate dietary control or lack of resources**

GOALS/OUTCOMES Will achieve weight within 5 pounds of ideal

Nursing Interventions/Rationales

- Assess patient's caloric needs, and promote nutritionally adequate diet and fluid intake while restricting excess calories. *To promote tissue healing without promoting obesity. Fluid intake of less than 800 ml/day increases the risk of pressure ulcer development.*
- Monitor serum albumin, protein, and complete blood count (CBC) results. *To assess the patient's protein stores, which are necessary for tissue healing. An albumin level lower than 3.0 is a risk factor for development of pressure ulcers. Protein needs are increased to maintain a positive nitrogen balance and aid in healing. CBC results may indicate infection or anemia.*
- Encourage patient and family to become involved in setting goals for dietary changes, documenting food intake, and meal planning. *There is greater probability that changes will be made when the patient is involved in planning those changes. Patients know their own likes and dislikes, financial resources, and ability to make dietary changes. Participation allows the patient greater control over her situation.*
- Help patient identify an acceptable weight loss schedule. *Permanent weight loss is generally gradual weight loss based on sound dietary principles. Fad diets should be avoided. The patient's agreement with the weight loss plan ensures greater probability of compliance.*

Evaluation Parameters

1. Loses weight gradually after making dietary modifications
2. Albumin and total protein remain within normal limits
3. Ingests adequate protein to promote healing

SPECIAL ENVIRONMENTS FOR CARE

Home Care Management

Many persons at high risk for pressure ulcers are sent home with these same risk factors. Thus the family or other caregiver must know all the interventions, including proper positioning techniques, use of protective devices, and proper nutrition.

If a pressure ulcer has developed, the caregiver may have to continue treatment measures initiated in the health care facility after discharge to the home. The caregiver must know how to do the treatment, the frequency of the treatment, safety precautions for self, how to dispose of used dressings, and what type of inspection to implement with each treatment. The caregiver must also know what changes need to be reported to the health care provider (i.e., home care nurse, primary care physician) immediately.

Most patients sent home with pressure ulcers should have a referral to a home health care agency. The home care nurse

Guidelines for Safe Practice

Interventions To Prevent Pressure Ulcers

INCONTINENCE

- Cleanse skin after each episode of incontinence. Check incontinent patients frequently.
- Assess causative factors of incontinence.
- Contain urine and feces in absorbent products that control moisture and exposure to skin; plastic-lined products can contribute to the problem. If appropriate, manage incontinence with a Foley catheter or fecal incontinence pouch.
- Minimize moisture next to skin from any source.

NUTRITIONAL DEFICITS

- Collaborate with dietitian to assess for optimal nutritional support.
- Assess for symptoms of nutritional compromise (decreased appetite and subsequently less oral intake; serum albumin level of less than 3-3.5 g/dl or a serum prealbumin level of less than 20 mg/dl; Hgb level of less than 10 g/dl; signs and symptoms of dehydration, including thirst, poor skin turgor, and dry mucous membranes; elevated hematocrit and serum sodium levels).

SKIN CARE AND EARLY TREATMENT MEASURES

- Inspect skin at regular intervals, at least daily, frequency determined by institutional policy (e.g., every shift instead of daily) and patient degree of risk. A head-to-toe inspection should be conducted, with attention to intertriginous areas and bony prominences.
- Bathing schedule should be developed according to patient preference, institutional policy, and general skin condition. Use a mild cleansing agent, and avoid water temperature extremes.
- Assess environmental factors, such as temperature and humidity, for contribution to skin condition.
- Lubricate skin with emollient lotions or moisturizers. Avoid lotion with scents or high alcohol contents.
- Avoid massage.

ALTERATIONS IN MOBILITY/ACTIVITY

- Reposition patient at least every 2 hours.
- Use position pillows or foam wedges to separate skin areas in contact with each other or to assist with maintaining positions. Use cautiously because these devices can become an additional source of pressure if not properly placed.
- Heels should be elevated off of bed surfaces with supportive pillows. Heel protectors help reduce friction.
- Avoid positioning directly onto trochanter. Place patient more appropriately into 30 degree side-lying position.
- Elevating the head of the bed centers all body weight directly over the pelvic triangle. It is best to keep the degree of elevation to 30 degrees, if possible.
- To reduce friction and shear, use lifting devices to raise patient in bed, rather than dragging patient across the surface of the bed.
- A pressure reduction of relief device should be used for all patients at risk of pressure ulcer formation.
- Patients in wheelchairs and other chairs should be taught to shift weight and have pressure-reducing surfaces on which to sit.

can help the caregiver establish routines at home, obtain supplies most economically, and store supplies appropriately. The home care nurse can assist the caregiver in gaining confidence while performing treatments. Additionally, the home care nurse can ensure that the patient's nutritional needs are met and an appropriate frequency and technique for change in position are maintained.

Most persons at home with pressure ulcers have many other physiologic or psychosocial needs. The home care nurse can help the caregiver develop routines to meet these other needs and also obtain assistance to provide some respite.

COMPLICATIONS

Most complications associated with pressure ulcers are the sequelae of infection. In addition, if the patient has undergone surgical intervention, the complications associated with anesthesia and surgery are potential problems (see Research box and Chapter 20 for a discussion of postoperative care and complications). If the pressure ulcer becomes infected, the infection may spread to the bloodstream, and sepsis may result. Osteomyelitis is another potential complication, requiring long-term intravenous antibiotics and possible surgical intervention. In a patient with alterations in mobility, extensive pressure ulcers may result in further immobility. For example,

Research

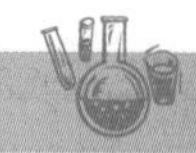

Reference: Shah JL: Postoperative pressure sores after epidural anaesthesia, *Br Med J* 321(7266): 941-942, 2000.

Epidural anesthesia offers the patient undergoing major surgery fewer side effects. However, the side effects known to be associated with epidural anesthesia include a dural puncture wound, motor block with resulting temporary paralysis, and hypotension. It is well documented that young and fit patients do not develop pressure ulcers as a result of epidural anesthesia.

This study reports three cases of young, healthy women between 33 and 52 years of age requiring either a hysterectomy or vulvectomy for cancer. One patient noticed blisters on her heels on the second postoperative day, another on the fourth postoperative day. The third patient did not complain of heel discomfort while hospitalized, but returned to clinic for a 3-week follow-up appointment with heel ulcers. The commonality between these three cases is the administration of epidural anesthesia with resultant paralysis for up to 2 postoperative days, systolic blood pressure of 95 mm Hg or less during the surgical procedure, and an operative time of at least 2.5 hours.

Results of this small case study support previously documented studies that have demonstrated that length of operative procedure greater than 2 hours, hypotensive state during surgery, and immobility are contributing factors to the development of pressure ulcers.

a person with spinal cord injury with a pressure ulcer on the buttocks or sacral area may have to spend an extended period of time lying prone, with all pressure off the affected area. In such instances, the patient is not allowed to sit in his or her wheelchair.

If contamination of the pressure ulcer with bowel contents is a problem, some surgeons perform a temporary colostomy to prevent potential contamination of the wound. The colostomy is reversible after healing has occurred.

To prevent infection the nurse must carefully monitor the wound for size, including depth, type of drainage, and presence or absence of granulation tissue. The patient must be monitored for signs and symptoms of systemic infection.

Psychologic support for both the patient and family is important because of the length of time required for treatment and healing. Depression and social isolation, particularly in the older patient, may be a sequelae of treatment for pressure ulcers.

Critical Thinking Questions

1. Discuss two risk factors for malignant melanoma and further describe strategies for prevention of the disease.
2. Describe three important patient teaching interventions for self-care management of severe atopic dermatitis.
3. What nursing interventions would be appropriate for a patient experiencing a disturbed body image as a result of a dermatologic condition or an extensive pressure?
4. What are the risk factors for pressure ulcers?
5. What nursing approaches would you prescribe for an obese 60-year-old patient with diabetes mellitus who has neuropathy and is wheelchair-bound?

References

1. Arndt KA: *Manual of dermatologic therapeutics,* ed 5, Boston, 1995, Little Brown.
2. Aronovitch SA: Intraoperatively acquired pressure ulcer prevalence: a national study, *J Wound Ostomy Continence Nurs* 26(3):130, 1999.
3. Barczak CA et al: Fourth national pressure ulcer prevalence survey, *Adv Wound Care* 10(4):18, 1997.
4. Beckrich K, Aronovitch SA: Hospital-acquired pressure ulcers: a comparison of costs in medical vs. surgical patients, *Nurs Econ* 17(5):263, 1999.
5. Bueller HA, Bernhard JD: Review of pruritus therapy, *Dermatol Nurs* 10(2):101-107, 1998.
6. Clinical Practice Guidelines: *Pressure ulcers in adults: prediction and prevention,* Washington, DC, 1992, USDHHS.
7. Dermatology Nurses Association: *Dermatology nursing essentials: a core curriculum,* Linden, NJ, 1998, Anthony J Janetti.
8. Dermatology Nurses Association: *Dermatology nursing basics course,* Linden, NJ, 2001, Anthony J Janetti.
9. Fitzgerald T: *Nursing health assessment,* Philadelphia, 1994, Springhouse.
10. Fitzpatrick TB et al: *Color atlas and synopsis of clinical dermatology,* New York, 1997, McGraw-Hill.
11. Gioshes SE: Scabies: case presentation, *Dermatol Nurs* 9(4):58, 1997.
12. Habif T: *Clinical dermatology— a color guide to diagnosis and therapy,* ed 3, St Louis, 1997, Mosby.
13. McClelland PB: New treatment options for psoriasis, *Dermatol Nurs* 9(5):295-304, 1997.
14. Nicol NH: Managing atopic dermatitis in children and adults, *Nurse Pract* 25(4):58-59, 63-64, 69-70, April 2000.
15. Oot-Giromini BA: Pressure ulcer prevalence, incidence and associated risk factors, *Decubitus* 6(5):24-32, 1993.
16. Robins P: Sun Sense: *A complete guide to prevention. early detection, and treatment of skin cancer,* New York, 1996, The Skin Cancer Foundation.
17. Ruszkowski A et al: Patch testing basics: patient selection, application techniques, and guidelines for interpretation, *Nurse Pract* (suppl) February, 1995 pp. i-vi.
18. Spector D, Fortinsky RH: Pressure ulcer prevention in an Ohio nursing home, *J Aging Health* 10(1):62-68, 1998.

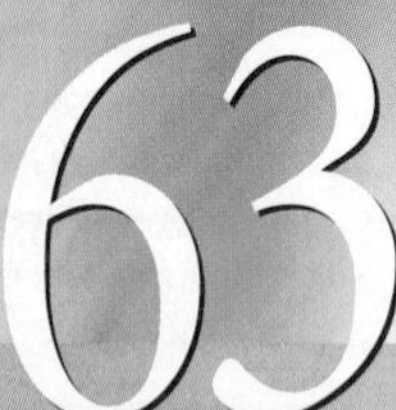

Burns

Diane E. Fritsch, Lynne C. Yurko

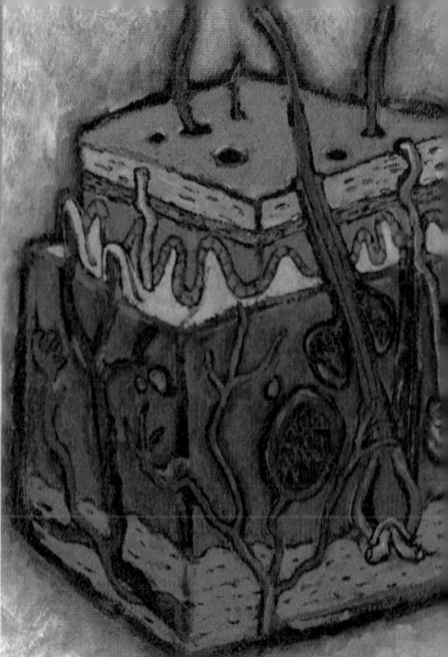

Objectives

After studying this chapter, the learner should be able to:

1. Describe the assessment of the burn patient, including the extent, location, and etiology of the burn.
2. Differentiate among the three phases of a major burn.
3. Describe emergency care for a major burn.
4. Compare interventions for replacing body fluids, preventing infection, promoting nutrition and mobility, and providing emotional support during the three phases of burn care.
5. Identify appropriate wound care for partial-thickness and full-thickness burns.
6. Identify learning needs of the patient with burns.
7. Discuss preventive measures for populations at risk for burn injury.

Etiology

The skin is the largest human organ. A burn injury occurs as a result of destruction of the skin from direct or indirect thermal forces. Burns are caused by flame, scalding with steam or hot fluids, direct contact with hot surfaces, chemicals, electrical current, and radiation. Burn injuries are in many respects the worst of all tragedies an individual can experience. A major burn is accompanied by an overwhelming insult to the patient physically and psychologically and may be catastrophic in terms of cost and suffering to the family involved.

Epidemiology

Approximately 1 million people suffer a thermal injury each year in the United States. Although the annual number of burn injuries has decreased by 50% since the 1960s, 45,000 persons are admitted to hospitals and more than 4500 persons die as a result of burn injury each year.[3] Injury is often a result of the victim's own action. This is particularly true for older adults, whose burns often are caused by the ignition of clothing when cooking or smoking. Scald injuries are the most frequent type of injury, but flame injury is more serious. The direct cost of treating a burn injury can be high. Average hospital costs for patients injured by flame range from $36,000 to $117,000.[25] Costs are higher for large burns, and indirect costs related to lost wages and property loss contribute to the extensive cost of a burn injury.

Pathophysiology

The depth of a burn is dependent on the temperature of the burning agent and the length of time during which it is in contact with the skin. Early tissue damage may occur at temperatures of 104° F (40° C). Irreversible damage to the dermis occurs at temperatures of 158° F (70° C).[25] Burn injuries are described as superficial (first-degree burns), superficial or deep partial thickness (second-degree burns), or full thickness (third-degree burns) according to the degree of destruction of the epidermal and dermal layers of the skin (Figure 63-1).

Superficial, or first-degree, burns involve only the epidermal layer of the skin. Sunburns are commonly first-degree burns. Also, areas of first-degree burns may surround deeper burns. Partial-thickness or dermal (second-degree) burns are characterized by destruction of the epidermis and varying depths of the dermis. These burns are likely to be painful because nerve endings have been injured and exposed, but they have the ability to heal because part of the epithelial cells is not destroyed. The presence of blisters often indicates a more superficial partial-thickness injury. Blisters may increase in size as a result of continuous exudation and collection of tissue fluid. During the healing phase of a partial-thickness burn, dryness and itching are common and are caused by increased vascularization of sebaceous glands, reduction of secretions, and decreased perspiration.

Full-thickness (third-degree) burns include destruction of the epidermis and the entire dermis, as well as possible damage to the subcutaneous layer, muscle, and bone. Nerve endings are destroyed, resulting in a painless wound. Eschar, a leathery covering composed of denatured protein, may form as a result of surface dehydration. Black networks of coagulated capillaries may be seen. Full-thickness burns require skin grafting because the destroyed tissue is unable to epithelialize. Often a deep partial-thickness burn may convert to a full-thickness burn because of infection, trauma, or decreased blood supply.

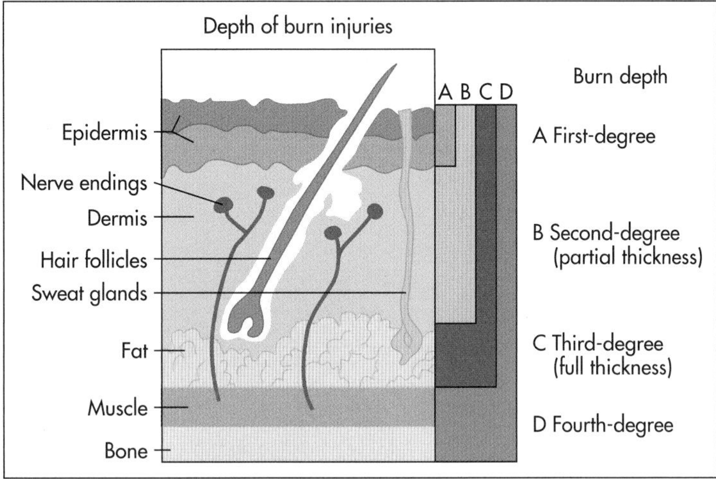

Figure 63-1 Levels of skin involved in burn injury.

As a result of burns, normal skin structure and function are impaired. The protective barrier function of the skin is diminished; sweat and sebaceous glands are destroyed; the number of functioning sensory receptors is decreased; body fluids escape; and there is a lack of temperature control. The severity of these impairments depends on the extent of the burn and the depth of the damage.

Local Tissue Response. Damage to the skin from a thermal injury results in immediate tissue changes. These changes are known as the zones of injury.[14] If the heat damage is severe enough, a zone of coagulation is formed. In this area the protein has been coagulated and the damage is irreversible. Surrounding this area is the zone of stasis, in which the blood vessels are damaged, resulting in decreased perfusion. The cells in this area are still viable but because of poor blood flow and tissue edema are at risk for death over the next few hours or days. Tissue in the zone of stasis is at risk for further necrosis because of other factors such as dehydration and infection. Thorough wound care, hydration, and prevention of infection are essential in limiting further destruction of this area. At the outer edge of the burn is the zone of hyperemia, or inflammation. Here blood flow is increased because of vasodilation from the release of vasoactive substances. This increased blood flow brings leukocytes and nutrients necessary to promote wound healing.

Systemic Response to Burn Injury. Virtually every organ system is affected by a major burn injury. Systemic changes known as burn shock develop with a burn of greater than 25% of the total body surface area (TBSA).[18] Burn shock is both a hypovolemic and a cellular shock. It results from the release of cellular mediators and vasoactive substances, such as histamine, serotonin, prostaglandins, and interleukin-1, from the damaged tissue. These substances induce a systemic inflammatory response (see Chapter 11) in which immediately following a brief period of vasoconstriction, increased vascular permeability, resulting in significant hypovolemia and edema, occurs. This phase begins at injury, peaks in 12 to 24 hours, and lasts for 48 to 72 hours.

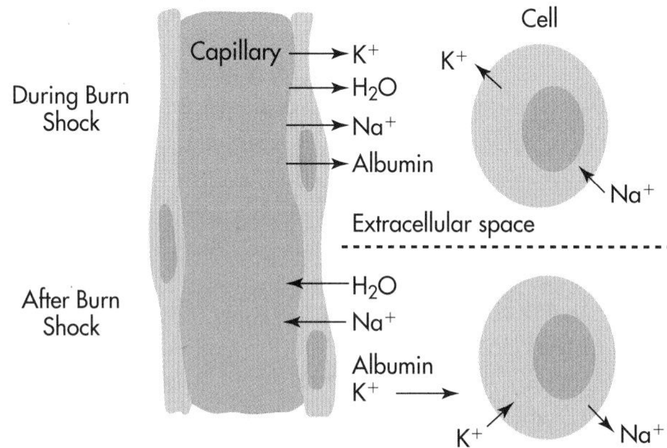

Figure 63-2 Fluid and electrolyte shifts associated with burn shock.

During the burn shock phase, intravascular fluid is lost through evaporation from the wound and also through edema formation. Vasodilation and increased capillary permeability result in the movement of fluid, electrolytes, and protein from the intravascular space to the interstitial space. Fluid movement is caused by both oncotic and osmotic forces. Serum protein moves out of the intravascular compartment into the interstitial spaces as a result of the increased capillary permeability. Fluid moves with the protein as a result of a change in oncotic forces (Figure 63-2). When capillary permeability is reestablished, this protein is unable to move back into the intravascular space. The lymphatic system becomes overloaded and is unable to recirculate the protein, and significant hypoproteinemia ensues. The sodium level within the damaged tissue rises, further moving water from the intravascular space, increasing wound edema and hypovolemia. Significant local and systemic edema occurs. Edema may be severe in highly vascular areas such as the face. Patients with large-surface-area burns experience edema throughout the body that can impair peripheral circulation by compressing circulatory vessels in an extremity. Figure 63-3 illustrates the fluid shifts that occur during burn shock.

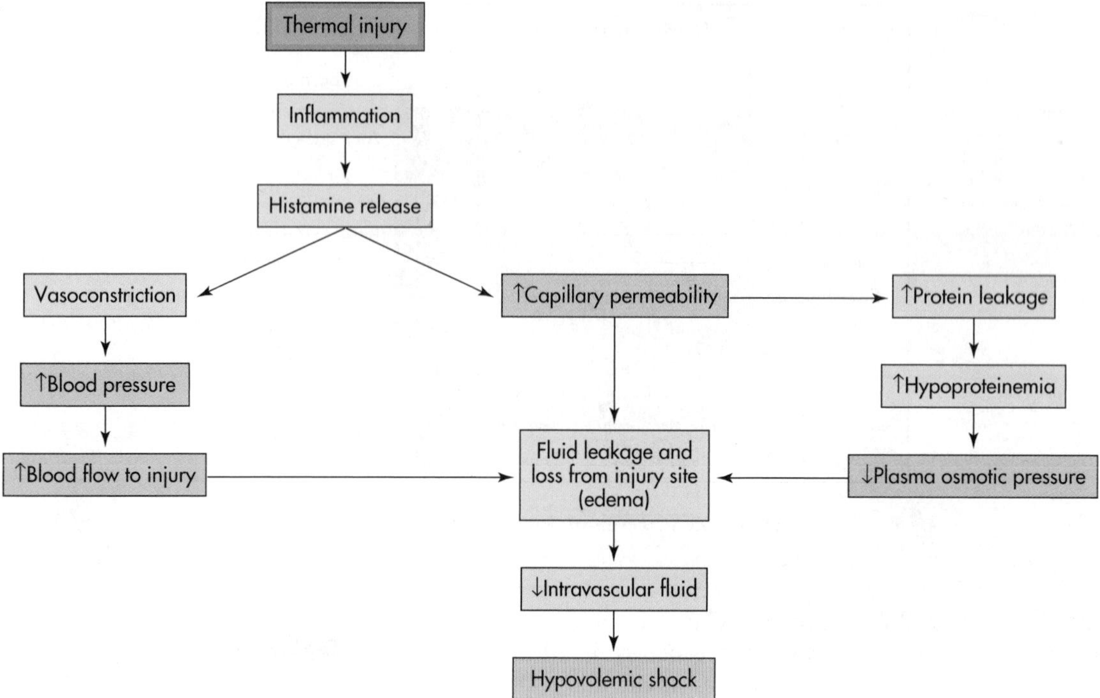

Figure 63-3 Flow diagram of fluid shifts resulting in hypovolemic shock.

Immediately after a burn injury, cardiac output is decreased because of the release of catecholamines (e.g., epinephrine and norepinephrine), vasopressin (antidiuretic hormone), and antiogensin II, which causes an intense but brief vasoconstriction and increased systemic vascular resistance and increased cardiac workload.[17] The blood pressure may be elevated, and the patient is tachycardic. This physiologic response assists in the initial attempt to conserve fluid, but its increased capillary force also promotes burn edema. Cardiac function continues to be depressed even after adequate fluid resuscitation, pointing to the myocardial depressant effects of inflammatory mediators, such as tumor necrosis factor, that are released from the burn wound.[13,15] Figure 63-4 presents an overview of the pathophysiologic changes seen with a severe burn.

Pulmonary function may be affected even in the absence of an inhalation injury. Increased work of breathing occurs as a result of edema formation and from an increased pulmonary vascular resistance that develops from the release of mediators such as serotonin.[30] In addition, the patient may be at risk for airway obstruction from oropharyngeal swelling that increases once fluid resuscitation begins.[32]

The kidneys, liver, and intestines are also affected during a major burn. Decreased blood flow to the kidneys as a result of hypovolemia, vasoconstriction, and a significant release of antidiuretic hormone places the patient at risk for renal failure. Patients at greatest risk for renal failure have had a delay in their initial fluid resuscitation or develop sepsis.[7] Hepatic perfusion is also compromised, contributing to liver ischemia.[28] Finally, the decreased bowel perfusion makes the patient prone to a paralytic ileus. Breakdown of the small intestine may occur, causing bacteria to move or translocate across the intestinal wall into the blood vessels, promoting the development of sepsis.

The last significant effect of a burn injury is the compromise of the immune system. The break in skin integrity destroys the body's first line of defense. A complex change in the body's immune system results in bone marrow depression, causing immunosupression and a shorter lifespan of red blood cells. Damaged tissue triggers the release of the inflammatory cytokine cascade. The release of these cytokines (tumor necrosing factor and interleukins) impairs the function of lymphocytes, macrophages, and neutrophils, increasing the risk of infection.[21] The nutritional deficit that occurs also decreases the burn patient's ability to fight infection. For the patient with a major burn injury, infection and resulting sepsis and multisystem organ dysfunction have serious consequences.

After the period of burn shock, the patient remains acutely ill. This period is characterized by hypermetabolism and impaired nutrition. A negative nitrogen balance begins at the onset of the burn and is the result of tissue destruction, protein loss, and the stress response. It continues throughout the acute phase and is secondary to continued loss of protein from the wound, resulting from tissue catabolism due to immobility and an increased metabolic rate. Special attention to the nutritional needs of the patient is an integral part of the comprehensive care during this time. The patient is vulnerable to significant weight loss as a result of fluid evaporation from the wound and loss of solid body mass secondary to increased metabolism.

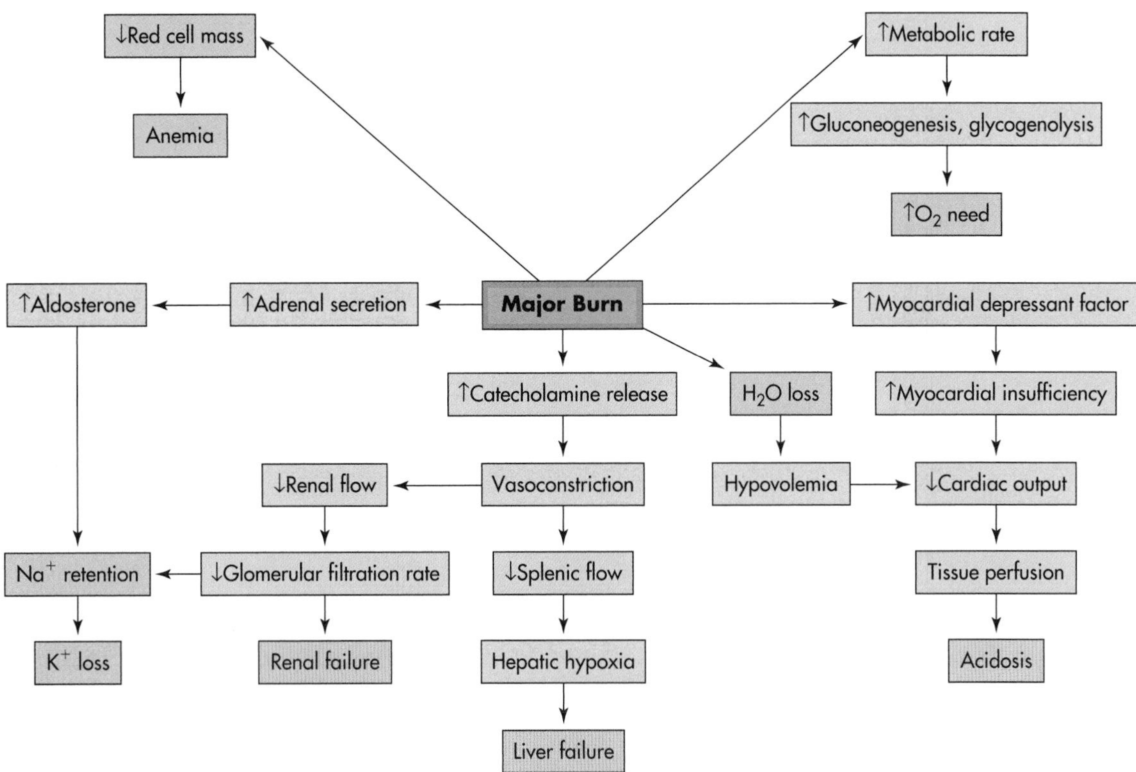

Figure 63-4 Overview of pathophysiology of a major burn.

Complications of the gastrointestinal system occur commonly after thermal injury. Gastric and duodenal ulceration has been reported in severely burned patients. Bleeding is the major clinical problem for patients with these lesions. Treatment is aimed at prevention and is best accomplished by antacids, H_2 blockers, and enteral feedings. Cholecystitis, pancreatitis, and hepatic dysfunction may also be seen as a result of tissue ischemia from hypoperfusion.

PHASES OF TREATMENT

Management of a person with a burn injury is extensive and costly. Discharge planning begins on admission using a multidisciplinary approach (see Clinical Pathway) to ensure that quality and cost-effective care is provided.

Three phases of treatment can be identified in the care of the severely burned patient: the emergent, acute, and rehabilitation phases. The emergent phase refers to the first 24 to 48 hours after a burn. During this time the patient is admitted, the severity of the injury is determined, first aid and wound care are given, and burn shock is treated. The acute phase of treatment begins at the end of the emergent phase and lasts until all of the full-thickness wounds are covered with skin grafts or partial-thickness wounds are healed. The physical healing time is determined by the patient's medical condition, nutritional status, and ability to heal. A 40% injury requires approximately 40 days to heal. The rehabilitation phase focuses on the patient's return to a useful place in society. Two areas of concern during this phase are (1) the restoration of function over joint surfaces that were scarred and (2) emotional assistance for the patient and family. The rehabilitation of the patient actually begins during early hospitalization and is addressed throughout the hospital stay. After the initial discharge, the patient may require emotional assistance and counseling, and many readmissions may be necessary for reconstructive procedures. Emotional and social healing depends on each patient's ability to cope with a new body image and society's acceptance of the change in the patient's physical appearance.

Emergent Phase

Collaborative Care Management

The goals of management during the emergent phase, the first 24 to 48 hours after a burn, are to (1) secure the airway, (2) support circulation by fluid replacement, (3) keep the patient comfortable with analgesics, (4) prevent infection through careful wound care, (5) maintain body temperature, and (6) provide emotional support.

Prehospital Care and First Aid. At the scene of a burn injury, the first priority is to remove the victim from the hazardous environment and stop the burning process, since the length of exposure to the causative agent is directly related to the severity of the injury. The method by which this is accomplished varies with the type of burn (see Guidelines for Safe Practice box).

Scald injury is the most common burn injury and may affect a widespread area. Scald injury is related to the temperature of the liquid and length of exposure. Thus initial care consists of cooling the skin with cool water.

clinical pathway — *Extensive Burns Without (Prior to) Surgery and After Surgery (Post Op Day 6)*

DRG: ____________ ACTUAL LOS: ____________
EXPECTED LOS: ____________ DISCHARGE DATE: ____________ (page 1 of 2)
ADMIT DATE: ____________

ATTENDING PHYSICIAN: ____________________

CONSULTS:
SOCIAL WORK OT/PT CHILD LIFE PHARMACY
NUTRITION CARE MANAGEMENT PASTORAL CARE
(Initial when complete in shaded box)

Authors:
R. Fratianne, M.D.
C. Brandt, M.D.
Lynne Yurko, R.N.
Burn Team

Metro Health Medical Center
Cleveland, Ohio

	(EMERGENT PHASE)		(ACUTE PHASE Day 3)		(REHABILITATION PHASE 1 Week Prior to Discharge)
ELEMENTS	**DAY 1**	**DAY 2**		**DISCHARGE**	**OUTCOMES**
Diagnostic Testing	Chem 7&11 → EKG Cultures (Wound) Tox Screen Sickle Cell CBC/Diff Platelets PT/PTT Type & screen Pre-albumin q Mon & Thur 24 hr. Urine q Sun & Wed UA Chest X-Ray Refer to DVT Protocol Testing for premorbid condition ABG with Respiratory Symptoms →	daily → CBC → Chest X-Ray Repeat abnormal Lab findings Evaluation for Chest X-ray	Reassess Lab needs according to results daily Cultures (wound) → q Mon & Wed → SW assessment (within 5 working days) ABGs with ventilator or O2 therapy changes	Reassess Lab needs according to results daily	1. Patient will maintain a balanced metabolic state. 2. Patient with/without acute respiratory insult will maintain optimal airway/ pulmonary function.
Medications/ IV Therapy	Vitamins Minerals Stool Softener (when on bedrest) Fluid/colloid resus. **Peds: 2-4cc/kg/% TBSA Burned plus 1/2 maintenance: Monitor Urine Output for .5-1 cc/hr **Adult: 4cc/kg/% TBSA Burned (Monitor Urine output 30-50 cc/hr) IV Catheter sites rethread day 3 and changed day 6 Routine IV Protocols: Adult and Peds. Pain Management/Assessment — Pain Scale Daily H_2 Blockers Tetanus Proph. Immunization status/Peds		Antibiotics per culture or wound assessment → IV: fluids or IIP →		1. Patient maintains optimal cardiac and circulatory status. 2. Patient will attain a self-identified acceptable level of pain relief. 3. Absence of clinical signs of IV infiltration, site infection, line occlussion or thrombophlebitis.
Treatments	Wound care protocol → Routine care protocol until discharge Isolation Weight	assists with wound care → Weight / Weight	performs wound care → Weight daily / Weight / Weight	until discharge Weight daily	1. Patient will remain free from wound infection/wound related sepsis. 2. Burns heal without complications.

Treatments (cont'd)	Grid pediatric < 12 yrs. Splinting → Positioning → Evaluate for pressure relief (Low air loss bed) P/T & O/T ROM			Reassess — Reassess — ADL When appropriate	Plan Discharge Needs Plan Discharge Needs	3. Unburned skin integrity will be maintained. 4. Patient will maintain or attain optimal level of function. 5. Patient will have daily periods of rest/sleep.
Nutrition	Tube Feeding per Protocol Nutrition Screen →	Nasojejunal Tube placement in 24 hours		Advance Diet According to needs		Patient will maintain or achieve optimal nutrition status.
Activity	May be bedrest or up to chair with activity as tolerated P/T & O/T ROM Exercise Child Life planning →			Increase activity to ambulating independently Gym Program —	Independent with exercise program	Patient will maintain/attain an optimal level of functioning.
Assessment and Monitoring	Standard Medical H+P I+O → Standard Nursing Assessment on admit and q8 hours S.W. Consultation for patient and family → Photo Permit Signed Photos on admit and weekly → Pastoral Care Assessment within 3 days Cardiac Monitor/Pulse Ox —			Assess I&O monitoring needs DC Monitors when non-critical		1. Patient will maintain a balanced metabolic state. (For age and stage of recovery) 2. Stable Cardiac Rhythm 3. Identify needed spiritual/religion support. 4. Identify patient's faith group/religion denomination to determine spiritual response.
Patient/Family Education	Emergent Care Teaching → Orient to: 1. Unit 2. Burn Injury 3. Infection Control Initiate Learning Pathway → Patients/Families told clergy can be contacted Pastoral Care consultation for patient & family.		Evaluate Home and resources available for discharge Educate Pt./Family on Burn Recovery Process → Follow through to home care Gym Program introduced Educate Nutritional Requirements	Acute Care Teaching →	Rehab Teaching	1. Patient/Caregiver response/interactions are appropriate for phase of injury. 2. Patient/caregiver will participate in the total management of care. 3. Patient/caregiver response & intervention demonstrates adaptation to injury.
Discharge Planning	Diet Visitor Booklet Education Pack		Videos Discharge Class Diet Adult Support Group	OT/PT recommendations (for Discharge)	Wound Care Instruction Complete Outpatient Plans complete Follow-up Appointments Made OT/PT teaching complete Diet Instructions complete as appropriate.	1. Patient/Caregiver will verbalize/demonstrate an understanding of post-hospital care and follow-up requirements. 2. Patient reenters society at preburn status/or makes adjustments. 3. Appropriate sacramental/religious rites will be offered.

IIP, intermittent infusion plug.

Guidelines for Safe Practice

Prehospital Care of Major Burns

1. Remove victim from source of burn.
2. Douse with water and remove nonadherent smoldering clothing to stop the burning process.
3. If chemical burn, carefully remove clothing and flush wound with large amounts of water.
4. If electrical burn and victim is still in contact with electrical source, do not touch victim. Remove electrical source with a dry, nonconductive object.
5. Establish patent airway and assess for inhalation injury. Give oxygen if available.
6. Check peripheral pulses to assess circulatory status.
7. Assess and initiate treatment for injuries requiring immediate attention.
8. Remove tight-fitting jewelry or clothing.
9. Cover burn with a moist sterile or clean cover.
10. Cover victim with a warm, dry cover to prevent heat loss.
11. Transport victim to the nearest medical facility.

Flame and flash injuries, the second most common types of burn injury, are commonly associated with an inhalation injury if the burn occurred in a closed space. These injuries may occur from house fires (caused by smoking in bed or children playing with matches) or ignited gasoline or propane. The amount and duration of the flame determine the depth of the injury, which often consists of combined partial- and full-thickness burns. In the case of fire, flames should be extinguished, flammable or hot material removed from the victim, and the victim and rescuer removed from the unventilated or hazardous surroundings. If clothing is on fire, the victim's first reaction is to run, which only fans the flames. In this case the best intervention is to stop the person; wrap him or her in a blanket, coat, sheet, or towel; and roll him or her on the ground to exclude oxygen and thereby put out the fire. The rule is "stop, drop, and roll." Similarly, for people who are confined to a wheelchair or limited in their movement as a result of a disability, a blanket or rug should be used to smother a fire and the victim should drop to the ground and roll to smother all flames if possible. The victim should never stand, because this will cause the flames and smoke to engulf the facial area, possibly igniting the hair and causing an inhalation injury. Any water source can be used to extinguish flames, cool the burn, or dilute the chemical unless the victim is still in contact with an electrical source. Once all flame is extinguished, clothing (except clothing that adheres to the burned area), jewelry, and debris are carefully removed. Any clothing removed should be saved for possible analysis of flammability.

Contact burns occur from direct contact with a hot substance, such as hot metal, stoves, hot tar, or irons. The area of burn is usually confined to the area where the substance came into contact with the skin.

Chemical burns are usually the result of accidents in homes or industry but may be the result of a deliberate assault on an individual. Household chemical burns may be caused by drain cleaners, disinfectants, or other chemicals used in the home. Industrial chemicals such as strong acids (hydrochloric), alkali, and organic compounds such as phenol and petroleum products (gasoline) are common causes of chemical burns. Thousands of chemicals are in use today, and exposure to them may cause thermal injury. The severity of the injury is related to the chemical involved, its concentration, the length of exposure, and the immediate treatment. Treatment should include irrigation of the area with copious amounts of water or saline.[31] Serious burns to the eyes may occur whenever a chemical splashes onto the face. Treatment includes careful irrigation of the eye with water. Adequacy of the irrigation is determined by testing a sample of the irrigated fluid with litmus paper to test for the presence of acid or alkali. Ingestion of noxious chemicals may burn the upper gastrointestinal tract. These burns are difficult to treat and often cause complications.

Electrical burns pose a special hazard to the victim because the TBSA of the burn is not always apparent and is often internal. Dysrhythmias and neurologic dysfunction are common.[31] Extreme care must be taken when removing the victim from the electrical source to prevent a similar injury to the rescuer.

Once burning is stopped, a primary survey of the patient's condition is made. Airway, breathing, and circulation are assessed. Then the patient's clothing is removed, and a brief neurologic examination is performed. Next a secondary assessment is completed if the patient has no life-endangering injuries. During the secondary assessment a more thorough head-to-toe assessment is made and a history is obtained. The history includes the mechanism of injury; medical history, including allergies; and medications the patient is taking. It is during this secondary assessment that the burn wound is evaluated and treated, because life-threatening conditions are always cared for before the burn wound.[2]

Burn wounds are covered with dressings dampened with normal saline or water, which eases the pain, reduces edema, and prevents evaporation of body water. The patient's entire body is wrapped in a dry cover to prevent heat loss. Ice should never be used, because sudden vasoconstriction causes severe shifting of body fluids and may increase the depth of injury. Although sterile dressings are preferred, clean dressings may be used because all dressings will be removed when the patient arrives at the medical facility. Oils, salves, and ointments should never be used on burns before evaluation at the hospital.

Standard Precautions should be followed whenever there is a possibility of exposure to blood or other body fluids. This includes the wearing of a gown, gloves, a mask, and eye protection. Initial care of the person with a major burn in the emergency department is summarized in the Guidelines for Safe Practice box.

Pain Relief. In the prehospital period, pain from extensive burns is best controlled by gentle and minimal handling and by application of dressings to exclude air from the burned surfaces. The degree of pain is usually inversely proportional to the depth of the burn injury. As mentioned earlier, full-thickness burns are usually painless because nerve endings have been destroyed.

Guidelines for Safe Practice

Initial Treatment of Major Burns in the Emergency Department

1. Establish airway.
2. Initiate fluid therapy by intravenous (IV) catheters.
3. Insert indwelling catheter for hourly urine measurement.
4. Insert nasogastric tube to remove stomach contents and prevent gastric distention.
5. Manage pain by IV narcotics in small, frequent doses.
6. Assess circulation distal to circumferential burns.
7. Provide tetanus prophylaxis.

Transporting the Burn Victim. Burns are often more severe than they first appear to be; therefore even patients with burns that appear to be superficial should be seen by a physician. The hospital or burn center should be notified before a burn victim is transported so that they have time to prepare for the patient's arrival.

Transfer of the patient should not be delayed because of difficulty in establishing an intravenous (IV) line. The American Burn Association teaches that an IV line is not necessary if the patient is less than 60 minutes from the hospital. When an IV line is established, the recommended solution is lactated Ringer's solution infused at 500 ml/hr for an adult and 250 ml/hr for a child age 5 years or older. No IV lines are recommended for children younger than age 5.[1]

For obviously small burns fluids may be given by mouth with caution. With large burns nothing should be given by mouth because fluids decrease peristalsis. Also, patients with large burns, or those who have inhaled smoke, may vomit and thus are at risk for aspiration.

Patients with major burns should be transported to a regional burn center. Currently 139 hospitals in the United States have burn care centers. These burn units are located throughout the country, and most are found in major medical centers in urban areas. Canada has 17 burn care centers.[8] To optimize burn care, the American Burn Association has created a national standard for voluntary review of burn centers according to a systematic approach to burn care. The verification is granted for a 3-year period by the American Burn Association and the American College of Surgeons.[3] Because of potential management problems, the American Burn Association recommends transfer of patients to a burn center on the basis of burn size, depth, mechanism, and comorbid factors[2] (Box 63-1).

Emergency Department Management. Rapid and efficient care is essential in the emergency department management of the victim with a major burn (see Guidelines for Safe Practice box). If any respiratory distress is present, an airway is established. Prophylactic intubation may be initiated if any heat or smoke has been inhaled, or if the head, neck, or face is involved. Inhalation injuries are best managed with controlled ventilation because swelling of the upper airway can progress to obstruction (Figure 63-5). Endotracheal intubation is preferred over a tracheostomy. Edema of the respiratory passages commonly subsides within a few days after the initial injury; therefore surgery of the airway should be avoided. Depending on the severity of symptoms, emergency treatment may include oxygen, suctioning, and postural drainage.

After an airway has been established, circulatory support is addressed. Fluid is best replaced through two large-caliber peripheral IV catheters. Placement of these catheters is preferred through an unburned site to prevent the introduction of infection. An indwelling urinary catheter is inserted to adequately monitor urine output. Hourly urine output measurements are used as a guide to the adequacy of fluid (plasma volume) replacement.

Patients with burns of more than 20% of the TBSA are more prone to nausea, vomiting, and an ileus.[2] Oral fluids are not recommended, since they create a threat of vomiting and aspiration. A nasogastric tube is inserted and attached to suction to prevent gastric distention.

BOX 63-1 Burn Center Referral Criteria

- Partial-thickness burns greater than 10% of the total body surface area
- Burns that involve the face, hands, feet, genitalia, perineum, or major joints
- Third-degree burns in any group
- Electrical burns, including lightning injury
- Chemical burns
- Inhalation injury
- Burn injury in patients with preexisting medical disorders that could complicate management, prolong recovery, or affect mortality
- Any patient with burns and concomitant trauma (such as fractures) in which the burn injury poses the greatest risk of morbidity or mortality
- Burned children in hospitals without qualified personnel or equipment for the care of children
- Burn injury in patients who will require special social, emotional, and/or long-term rehabilitative intervention

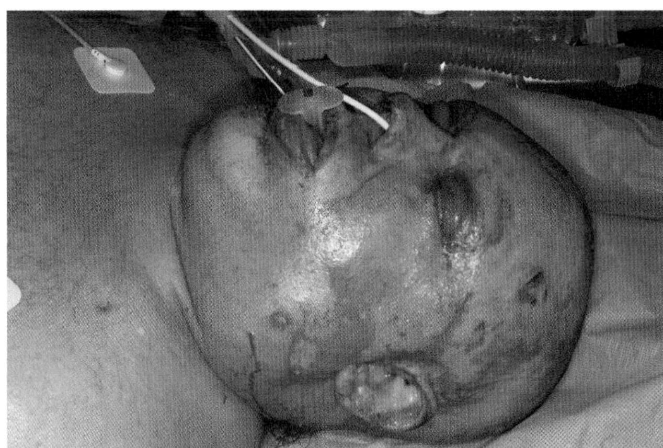

Figure 63-5 Deep partial-thickness face burn from molten steel, resulting in facial swelling requiring intubation for airway control.

Medications. Morphine sulfate is the drug of choice for pain relief and is given intravenously in small increments (2 to 4 mg). A morphine drip can be used and titrated to the patient's pain. No medication of any kind should be given intramuscularly or subcutaneously, because it may pool and be absorbed later when cardiac output and blood pressure improve. Large doses of sedatives and analgesics are avoided because of the danger of respiratory depression and the potential for masking other symptoms.

Tetanus prophylaxis is given in the emergency department. Tetanus toxoid is administered if the patient has been previously immunized but has not received tetanus toxoid in the preceding 5 years. If information about prior tetanus immunization is not known, a dose of human tetanus–immune globulin hormone is administered and an active tetanus immunization program is begun.[2]

Treatments. Replacing fluids and electrolytes (fluid resuscitation) is an essential part of the treatment of burn victims and is instituted as soon as the severity of the burn and the patient's condition are known (Box 63-2). Ideally, fluid therapy is started within an hour after a severe burn to prevent the onset of hypovolemic shock.

Fluids administered during the first 48 hours are given to maintain circulating blood volume. Additional fluids and electrolytes are added to replace losses from vomiting or from nasogastric drainage. Two types of fluids are considered when calculating the needs of the patient: crystalloids and colloids.

Crystalloids may be isotonic or hypertonic. Isotonic solutions, such as lactated Ringer's solution or physiologic (0.9%) sodium chloride, do not generate a difference in osmotic pressure between the intravascular and interstitial spaces. Thus large amounts of fluids are required to restore and maintain the intravascular volume. Hypertonic salt solutions have a milliosmolar content of 400 to 600 (280 to 300 mosm is isotonic), thus creating an osmotic pull of fluid from the interstitial space back to the depleted intravascular space. The use of hypertonic solutions decreases the amount of fluid a patient needs during resuscitation,[32] which helps decrease burn tissue edema and minimizes cardiopulmonary complications (pulmonary edema and congestive heart failure).

The consensus formula for fluid resuscitation is based on the Parkland formula.[2] With the use of this formula, the patient's fluid requirements for the first 24 hours following injury are estimated. For adults the formula is:

2 to 4 ml of lactated Ringer's solution ×
Body weight (in kg) × Percent burn

BOX 63-2 Indications for Fluid Resuscitation

Burns greater than 20% of the total body surface area (TBSA) in adults
Burns greater than 10% of the TBSA in children
Patient older than 65 years of age or younger than 2 years of age
Patient with preexisting disease that would reduce normal compensatory responses to minor hypovolemia (i.e., cardiac or pulmonary disease or diabetes)

Because blood volume falls most rapidly and edema increases most significantly in the first 8 hours, IV replacement is accomplished at a rapid rate. One half of the total amount calculated is given in the first 8 hours after the injury. The time is calculated from the time of injury, not from the time emergency care was initiated. In the second 8-hour period one fourth of the total amount of calculated lactated Ringer's solution is given, and in the third 8-hour period the remaining one fourth is given. For example, if a patient weighing 75 kg has a 70% TBSA burn, the fluid requirements are:

- 4 ml lactated Ringer's solution × 75 kg × 70% = 21,000 ml needed over the first 24 hours.
- One half is needed in the first 8 hours: $\frac{1}{2}$ × 21,000 = 10,500 ml in 8 hours, or 1312 ml/hr.
- One fourth is needed in each of the next two 8-hour periods: $\frac{1}{4}$ × 21,000 = 5250 ml in 8 hours, or 656 ml/hr.

Colloids may also be used as part of the fluid replacement protocol.[12] The use of colloids is avoided in the first 12 hours after a burn because of the capillary permeability caused by the burn injury. This capillary permeability begins to close at 12 hours, and after this time patients may receive colloids such as fresh-frozen plasma, albumin, or dextran. These colloids supply volume but also generate oncotic pressure, which helps pull fluid back into the intravascular space. Fresh-frozen plasma is also beneficial in restoring lost clotting factors. Red blood cells are used only if the patient has had a significant loss or destruction of red blood cells.

During the second 24 hours after a burn, one half to two thirds of the initial 24-hour volume is generally required. During this second 24-hour period, colloid solutions are also used to replace intravascular volume once capillary permeability significantly decreases.

After the first 48 to 72 hours the patient may begin to mobilize fluid as edema reabsorption occurs. The urine output increases dramatically and may not be a reliable guide to fluid needs. Hence fluid needs are assessed by measuring serum and urine electrolyte levels. Fluid replacement, using 5% dextrose–containing fluids, is based on patient assessment. If dehydration occurs from diuresis, fluid replacement therapy is continued until blood volume is stabilized. Potassium may be added to the IV fluid because of potassium losses in the urine. The patient is monitored closely for signs of water intoxication or pulmonary edema.

NURSING MANAGEMENT OF PATIENT DURING EMERGENT PHASE

ASSESSMENT

Many factors are considered in determining the severity of a burn injury. These include the size and depth of the burn, the cause of injury, and the patient's preinjury health status.

Health History

Knowledge of circumstances surrounding the burn injury is extremely valuable in the management of a burn victim. Identifying the mechanism of injury is of prime importance because the nature of the agent has a direct effect on prognosis and treatment. This information can be obtained from either the burn victim or witnesses to the event. Data should include:

How the burn injury occurred

When the burn injury occurred

Duration of contact with the burning agent

Location where the burn injury occurred (enclosed area suggests possibility of smoke inhalation and/or carbon monoxide poisoning)

Whether or not there was an associated explosion (suggests possibility of other injuries)

Determining the patient's age and medical history is also necessary, since these factors may modify treatment. Patients over age 60 and those under age 2 have a higher mortality rate than a young adult with the same percentage of burn. Preexisting endocrine, pulmonary, cardiovascular, or renal disease or a history of drug abuse decreases a victim's ability to cope with severe burns. A prior illness, such as diabetes or renal failure, may become acute during the postburn phase. The physiologic stress seen with the burn may exacerbate a latent disease process or worsen an already active process and thus increase mortality. Diabetes and chronic obstructive pulmonary disease may be aggravated, or patients with arteriosclerotic heart disease may develop a myocardial infarction.

Because most burn patients require topical and systemic therapy with a number of drugs, allergies and drug sensitivities must also be determined and documented.

Physical Examination

As part of the determination of the severity of the burn injury, the size and depth of the burn are assessed. For adults the "rule of nines" is used to determine the size of the burn. The percentage of the TBSA burned is estimated with the use of charts that depict anterior and posterior drawings of the body. In adults the body is divided into areas equal to multiples of 9% (Figure 63-6). In clinical practice the burned area is shaded in on the drawings, and the amount of body surface burned is calculated from the shaded areas. Calculations are modified for infants and children younger than 10 years of age because of their relatively larger head and smaller body (consult a pediatric textbook for these figures). The depth of the burn injury is evaluated on the basis of appearance, color, and sensation (Table 63-1). The burn is classified as superficial (first degree), superficial partial thickness (Figure 63-7) or deep partial thickness (second degree) (Figure 63-8), or full thickness (Figure 63-9). A laser Doppler is being used more often to evaluate the blood flow in the injured tissue to assist in definitive diagnosis of the depth of injury.[26]

Body Part Involved

The body part involved is an important factor in evaluating the severity of a burn. The part of the body burned must be considered when the severity of the burn is estimated; a 3% burn of the anterior surface of the thigh is not as serious as a 3% burn to the neck, face, or perineal area. Injuries that involve cosmetic and functional areas of the body require a long period of recovery because of both physical and emotional reactions to

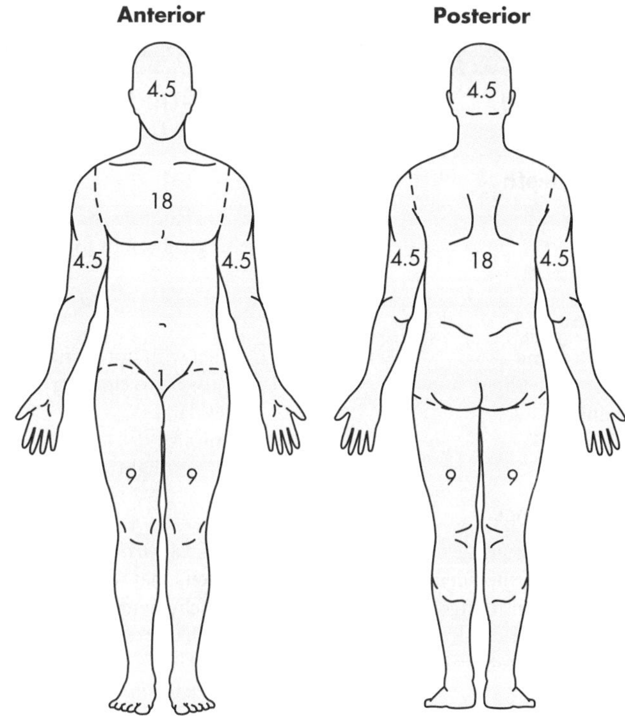

Figure 63-6 Rule of nines.

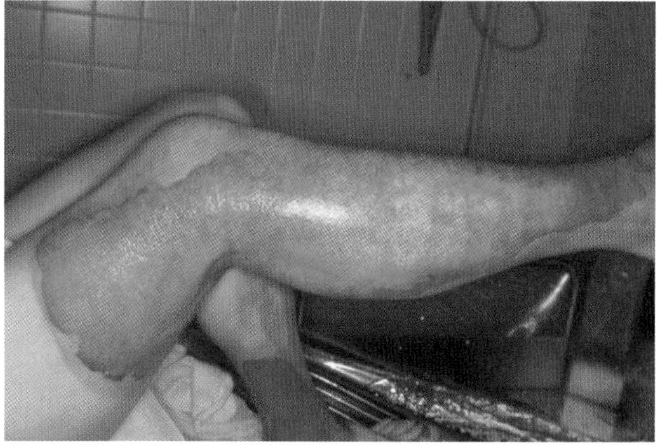

Figure 63-7 Superficial partial-thickness burn to leg.

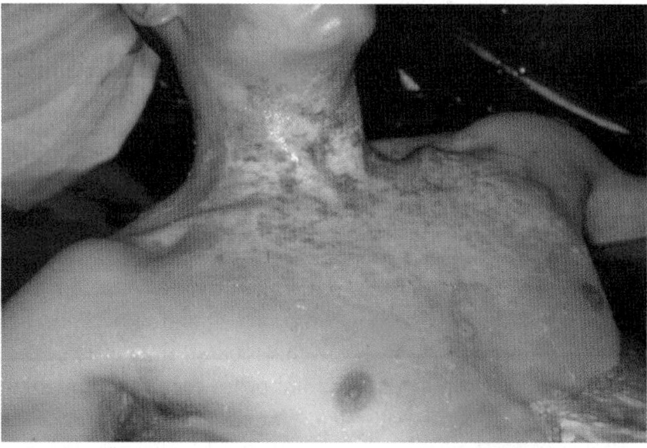

Figure 63-8 Deep partial-thickness burn to chest and neck.

TABLE 63-1 Characteristics of the Depth of Burn Injury

Superficial (First-Degree) Burn	Partial-Thickness (Second-Degree) Burn	Full-Thickness (Third-Degree) Burn
Skin Depth		
Epidermis	Entire epidermis, partial dermis Sweat glands, hair follicles intact	Epidermis, dermis Extends to subcutaneous tissue, possibly muscle and bone
Cause		
Flash flame Ultraviolet light Sunburn	Contact with hot liquids or solids Flash flame to clothing Direct flames Chemicals Ultraviolet light	Contact with hot liquids or solids Flame Chemicals Electrical contact
Appearance		
Dry, no blisters Minimal or no edema Blanches with fingertip pressure, and color returns when pressure removed.	*Superficial partial injury* Blisters that will increase in size Blanches with fingertip pressure and color returns when pressure returns Moist *Deep partial injury* Blisters present are slower to increase in size Blanching decreased, prolonged Less moisture	Dry with leathery eschar Charred vessels visible under eschar Blisters rare, but thin-walled blisters that do not increase in size may be present No blanching with pressure
Color		
Increased redness	*Superficial partial injury* Pink *Deep partial injury* Pale, mottled with dull, white, tan, cherry red areas	White, charred, dark tan, black, dark red
Sensation		
Painful	Very painful	No pain Deep throbbing Nerve endings dead
Healing Time		
2-5 days with peeling No scarring May discolor	*Superficial partial injury* 5-21 days, no grafting *Deep partial injury* 21-35 days without complications May convert to full-thickness burn and require grafting	No healing potential Requires excision and grafting

the burn injury. Burns of the face, hands, and feet require extensive, meticulous care and extensive physical and occupational therapy. Burns of the head, neck, and chest may also involve injury to the respiratory tract and result in severe respiratory distress. Burns of the perineum are difficult to manage because of the potential for contamination and infection. The circumferential, or encircling, burn of a limb, the neck, or the chest has serious consequences. This type of burn causes constrictive contraction of the skin and produces a tourniquet effect that may impair breathing and/or circulation.

The factors determining the severity of burns are summarized in Box 63-3.

NURSING DIAGNOSES

Nursing diagnoses are determined from analysis of patient data. Nursing diagnoses for the person with burns during the emergent phase may include but are not limited to:

Diagnostic Title	Possible Etiologic Factors
1. Ineffective airway clearance	Tracheobronchial edema, obstruction, secretions
2a. Deficient fluid volume (burn shock)	Abnormal fluid loss: movement of fluid from intravascular to interstitial space; evaporation

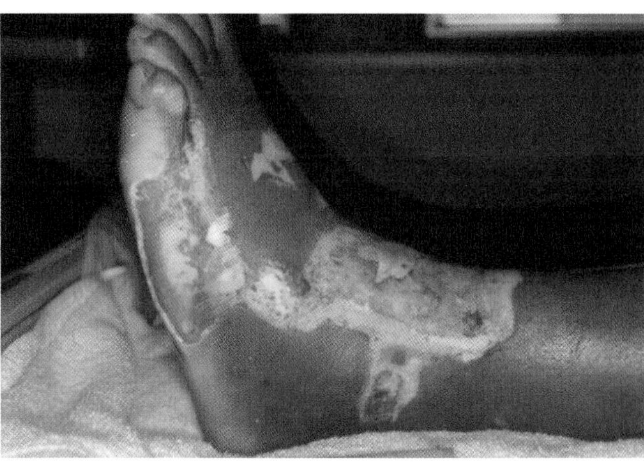

Figure 63-9 Full-thickness burn to anterior ankle.

BOX 63-3 Factors Determining Severity of Burns

Size of burn
Depth of burn
Age of victim
Body part involved
Mechanism of injury
History of cardiac, pulmonary, renal, or hepatic disease
Injuries sustained at time of burn

3.	Hypothermia	Impaired temperature regulatory mechanisms; wound exposure to environment
4.	Risk for infection	Break in skin integrity
5.	Impaired skin integrity	Burn injury, impaired perfusion
6.	Acute pain	Trauma, exposure of nerve endings
7.	Anxiety	Threat of death, situational crisis

EXPECTED PATIENT OUTCOMES

Expected patient outcomes for the burn-injured patient during the emergent phase include but are not limited to:

1. Will maintain a patent airway, adequate oxygenation, and ventilation
2. Will maintain euvolemia
3. Will not have a drop in body temperature to less than 98.6° F (37° C)
4. Will remain free of infection
5. Will have no further tissue loss
6. Will achieve an acceptable level of pain relief
7. Will verbalize concerns and will not appear to be anxious

INTERVENTIONS

1. Maintaining a Patent Airway

Persons who are burned on the face and neck or those who have inhaled flame, steam, or smoke are observed closely for signs of laryngeal edema and airway obstruction. Data indicating potential or existing inhalation injury are outlined in Box 63-4.

BOX 63-4 Factors Determining Inhalation Injury and/or Potential Airway Obstruction

Burns to face and neck
Singed hairs, nasal hair, beard, eyelids or eyelashes
Intraoral charcoal, especially on teeth and gums
Brassy cough
Hoarseness
Copious sputum production
Carbonaceous sputum
Burn injury that has occurred in a closed space
Smell of smoke on victim's clothes or on victim
Respiratory distress

BOX 63-5 Signs of Adequate Fluid Resuscitation

Clear sensorium
Pulse: <120 beats/min
Urine output: 30 to 50 ml/hr (adult)
Systolic blood pressure: 100 mm Hg
Central venous pressure: 5 to 10 mm Hg
Pulmonary capillary wedge pressure: 5 to 15 mm Hg
Blood pH normal range: 7.35 to 7.45 and base deficit ≥6

Adequate ventilation and oxygenation may be possible with the victim breathing room air; however, when any inhalation injury has occurred, it is best to give oxygen. When smoke is inhaled, carbon monoxide binds with hemoglobin, displacing oxygen. High carboxyhemoglobin levels impair tissue oxygenation, resulting in tissue asphyxia. Providing the victim with 100% oxygen by mask reverses this condition. If the victim is in respiratory distress or has a suspected inhalation injury, endotracheal intubation may be necessary.[2]

2. Maintaining Fluid Volume

During fluid resuscitation, adequate volume is assessed by monitoring mental status, vital signs, peripheral perfusion, body weight, and urine output. A 15% to 20% weight gain in the first 72 hours of resuscitation is anticipated. Significant laboratory measurements include serum and urine electrolytes, serum and urine osmolality, and hematocrit values. Hourly urine output is commonly used as a gauge for adequate fluid replacement. Fluid should be titrated to ensure an output of 0.5 ml/kg/hr, or 30 to 50 ml/hr. The most common reasons for a urine output below 30 ml/hr, which is indicative of insufficient fluid replacement, are that the calculated fluid replacement is behind schedule and/or the patient's fluid requirements are greater than predicted. The urine is observed for color and analyzed for the presence of blood. The physician is notified if hematuria is present.

Other clinical criteria that indicate adequate resuscitation are pulse rate of 120 beats/min or less, central venous pressure in the low to normal range, pulmonary artery end-diastolic pressure in the low to normal range, and mental lucidity (Box 63-5).

Acidosis indicates that fluids have not been given in sufficient quantities to maximize tissue perfusion. Anaerobic metabolism ensues when the metabolic tissue requirements are not met during resuscitation. Recent studies have indicated that the presence of a base deficit, particularly less than −6, is a good indicator of the patient being inadequately fluid resuscitated.[16]

When edema resorption begins after the first 48 to 72 hours, serum and urine electrolyte levels, not urine output, are used to guide fluid needs, and the patient is monitored closely for signs of water intoxication or pulmonary edema.

Patients may complain of moderate to severe thirst during this period. Aggressive oral hygiene may alleviate patient discomfort. If oral fluids are permitted, accurate recording of ingested fluids is important. Unlimited oral intake and failure to measure it may provide too much fluid in the circulating blood, resulting in water intoxication.

3. Maintaining Body Temperature

The loss of skin greatly decreases the severely burned patient's ability to regulate body temperature. The environment must be heat controlled and kept warmer than usual. Room temperature is maintained at 80° to 85° F (26.7° to 29.4° C) with a humidity of 40% to 50%. Drafts must be eliminated. Fluid warmers, heat lamps, and warming blankets are used during burn shock. Prolonged exposure to air is avoided. Exposed areas of the body are covered with sterile sheets and blankets to decrease the loss of body heat through the open wounds while other areas of the burn are being cleansed.

4, 5. Providing Initial Wound Care

Care of the burn wound can be delayed until all first aid measures have been initiated. Wound care should be carried out carefully and with as little discomfort to the patient as possible. One of the most important factors to be considered in wound care is that the patient has lost the ability to withstand infection in the area where the skin is damaged or destroyed. The goals of initial wound care are:

- Cleanse the wound to eliminate or decrease the dead tissue and debris that serve as the media for bacterial growth.
- Prevent further destruction of viable skin.
- Provide for patient comfort.

During the admission procedure the burn wound and the entire body are washed to remove dirt and debris, as well as loose dead tissue on the burned areas. Detergents or antiseptic preparations are effective cleansing agents. Gentle cleansing with gauze is effective in removing dead tissue without causing further tissue damage.

All hair in and around the burn wound is shaved and wiped off the skin because hair attracts and shelters bacteria. Singed hair is clipped short to avoid bacterial contamination of the wound.

Firm, intact blisters may remain undisturbed because they are a natural protective and pain-free dressing. If the blisters are broken and the epidermis is separated, loose tissue must be debrided.

After the wound is cleaned and before a dressing is applied, cultures of the wound are obtained. Baseline cultures provide information about organisms present in the wound at the time of admission. Prophylactic antibiotics are usually not indicated.

Photographs are taken on admission and at intervals during the patient's hospitalization. These pictures provide a record of the appearance of the burn wound on admission, before the application of topical therapy, and during the healing process.

The constricting effect of nonviable tissue (eschar) from a full-thickness injury to the chest, neck, or extremities is an early complication. Edema forming rapidly under the constricting eschar produces a tourniquet effect that causes occlusion of venous and arterial circulation and may result in ischemic necrosis, especially in unburned areas distal to the constrictive eschar. Frequent monitoring of distal pulses is part of an ongoing assessment to ensure uninterrupted vascular flow to all extremities. Extremities should be monitored for signs and symptoms of circulatory compromise, including diminished peripheral pulses, decreased capillary refill, paleness or cyanosis, decreased temperature, and increased pain or paresthesia. It may be necessary to monitor circulation every 15 minutes.

Circumferential burns of the neck and chest can lead to constriction of chest wall expansion and airway compromise, resulting in respiratory distress. Monitoring chest excursion, respiratory rate, and ventilator settings, if the person is intubated, for high pressures and low tidal volume is part of the respiratory assessment.

Treatment of the constricting effects of the eschar is an escharotomy, which is performed on the burn unit. An escharotomy is a linear surgical incision through the burn eschar that releases the constriction caused by the full-thickness injury (Figure 63-10). Patients have limited pain during an escharotomy because the nerve endings have been damaged by the burn.

6. Providing Comfort

The patient is kept as comfortable as possible by gentle handling of the burn areas and by keeping the wounds covered so that air does not reach them. Small doses of morphine are given intravenously.

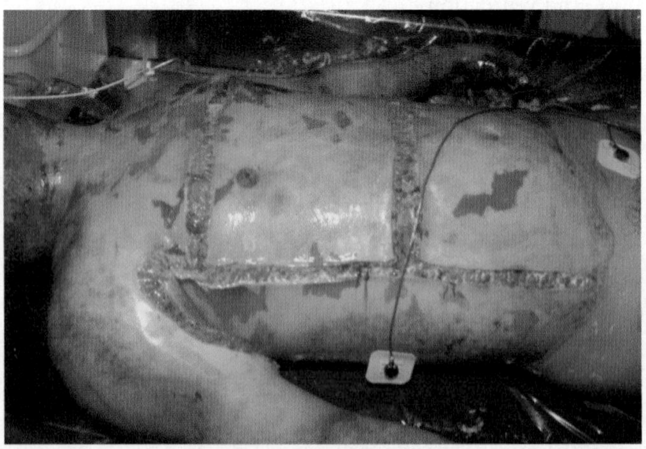

Figure 63-10 Escharotomies to full-thickness chest burns.

7. Providing Emotional Support

Patients with significant burn injury receive a profound insult to their body and self-image. They are aware that they may not survive, which causes fear and helplessness. The shock and pain of the accident, the chaos and rush to the hospital, and the unknown surroundings and people all intensify the emotional stress.

The nurse spends the most time with the patient and has a considerable influence on the patient's psychologic adjustment. Interventions that can be used to reassure the patient and alleviate anxiety include:

- Identify self to the patient.
- Orient the patient to the surroundings.
- Describe the basis for physical symptoms (skin loss, pain, and cold).
- Explain the equipment and procedures to be used in treatment.

Patient/Family Education

Health Promotion/Prevention. Nurses can help prevent accidental burns by participating in health education programs that stress fire prevention and the consequences of fires, such as burns, deformities, and death. Nurses can also promote legislation that would control hazardous practices and make working and living environments safer. Community health nurses are in an unusually advantageous position to recognize unsafe practices in the home and to help families develop safe habits of living. Nurses can raise the awareness of patients and the community to the burn problem through education and burn awareness campaigns (Figure 63-11).

Prevention programs can be developed to highlight seasonal activities that result in burn injuries (Box 63-6). Approximately 80% of all accidental burns occur in the home and are caused primarily by ignorance, carelessness, and the curiosity of children. More than 35% of all fire and burn injuries involve children playing with matches and cigarette lighters. Prevention focuses on teaching parents and others caring for children to keep matches and cigarette lighters out of the reach of children.

Smoke detectors are present in 13 out of 14 homes. Half of home fires and three fifths of fire-related deaths occur in homes without smoke detectors. About one third of homes with smoke detectors have fire-related deaths because the smoke detector does not work. Working smoke detectors awaken people to the fire and allow them time to escape to safety.[22] Prevention includes teaching:

1. All homes should have working smoke detectors on each level of the home and in the hallway outside of the bedrooms.
2. Batteries should be tested periodically and changed twice yearly—in the spring and the fall. In states and countries with time changes between standard and daylight saving time, battery changes can be timed to coordinate with these time changes. Batteries should never be removed for the reason that they go off during cooking, since it is easy to forget to replace them.
3. In most cities in the United States, the fire department will install smoke detectors free of charge to older adults and others unable to do so for themselves. Fire departments in many communities have free smoke detectors for those unable to afford them. People who use home oxygen therapy should not smoke or be around flames.

Fire Sales are No Bargain
A working smoke detector
is the best buy of your life

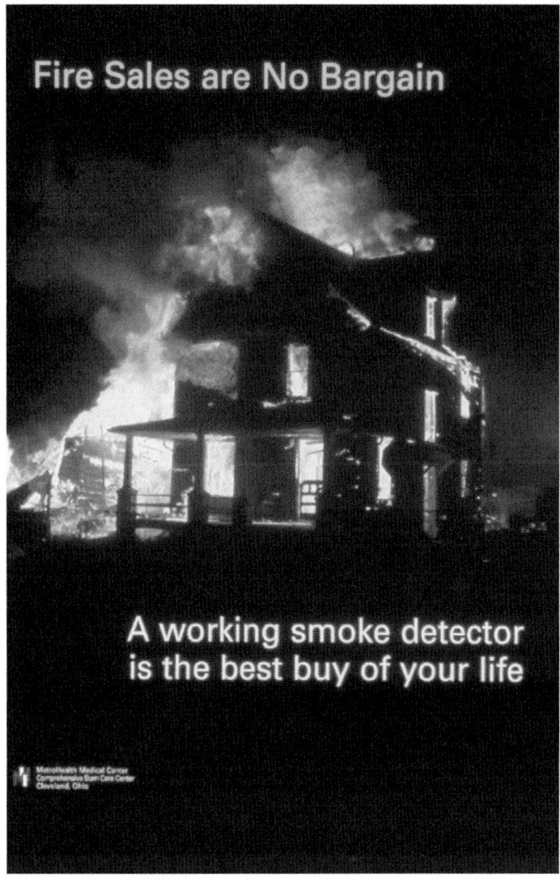

Figure 63-11 Sample burn prevention poster.

BOX 63-6 Seasonal Causes of Burn Injuries

Season	Causes
Spring	Barbecuing, charcoal Burning leaves, yard cleanup Overheated radiators Gasoline (lawnmowers, engines)
Summer	Sun exposure Fireworks Beach activity Sun-heated surfaces (tar, asphalt, sand)
Fall	Hot liquids Yard cleanup Candles Halloween activities
Winter	Holiday activities Fireplaces Hot liquids Woodburning stoves/space heaters Electrical wires

The oxygen should be at least 10 feet from an open flame (e.g., cigarettes, lighters, pilot lights, candles). The high risk of burn injury can be reduced with patient and family education.[6]

Burn injuries to adults are most often related to accidents while they are cooking, using microwave ovens, or smoking or otherwise using matches. Burns commonly occur when a person is distracted while cooking or falls asleep while smoking. Prevention centers on teaching persons of all ages to be especially careful of scald burns when using microwave ovens. Scald burns occur when the power of the microwave is underestimated, and all users need to be educated about the safe use of these ovens. Smokers need to be reminded to never smoke in bed, to be particularly careful about falling asleep while smoking and sitting in overstuffed furniture, and to be sure that cigarettes are completely extinguished, especially before going to bed.

Although sunburn may not be thought of as a burn, even a relatively mild burn over a large portion of the body can cause changes in fluid distribution and dehydration. Camp nurses should keep this in mind when they present educational programs for camp counselors and campers. Emphasis is on the proper use of sunscreen products, the need to use a sunscreen with at least a skin protector factor (SPF) of 15, and the need to limit the time spent in the sun.

Each year there is an increased demand for careful inspection and regulation of places housing the ill and infirm. The elderly are often housed in old and nonfireproof structures from which they may not be able to escape if a fire occurs. Nurses can be involved to exert necessary pressure to ensure that adequate measures are taken to bring structures up to the fire code and to ensure that there is a fire evacuation plan. Basic fire prevention programs in all health care facilities should include one mock evacuation drill annually.

Another facet of fire prevention programs focuses on places where large numbers of persons congregate, such as schools, theaters, and sports arenas. Laws regulating public buildings require hinged doors that swing outward, draperies and decorations that are fireproof, and stairways with special fire doors in new apartment buildings and hotels. Smoke detectors and sprinkler systems are required in new buildings and residential health care facilities.

In fire prevention programs, emphasis should be placed on the special needs of the disabled. They are at higher risk for burn injury because of their inability to rapidly evacuate from unsafe situations (Box 63-7).

The government's role in fire prevention centers around laws designed to protect the public. For example, rigid enforcement of laws requiring that industrial products be labeled when they are known to be flammable and that new products be tested carefully for their flammable qualities before being placed on the market is further evidence of government efforts to protect the public from accident by fire. Industry can be made safer by constant vigilance of management in cooperation with fire safety officers and health care professionals to identify hazards and implement a safety program. All chemicals should be labeled, and antidotes should be identified and available. A core group of every workforce should be versed in emergency treatment of all types of burns for the protection of every employee.

The Surgeon General's report on goals to be achieved by 2010 include an increase in functioning residential smoke alarms and a reduction in residential fire deaths. These goals are particularly focused at high-risk groups: American Indian/Alaska natives and African-Americans.[29] The goals for all groups are summarized in the Healthy People 2010 box.

BOX 63-7 Safety Measures to Be Observed by the Disabled

- Develop a fire escape plan. Keep exit routes free of clutter and have two escape routes. Do not include windows with bars in the escape routes. All windows with bars should have a quick-release feature for easy removal.
- Keep a whistle by the bed to alert rescuers where you are or to warn others of fire. The fire department will place a sticker in your bedroom window to assist firefighters in locating you should a fire occur.
- Keep eyeglasses, dentures, keys, a flashlight, and a telephone near your bedside in case of an emergency.
- People using oxygen should not smoke or be near fire with oxygen in use.
- Smokers should use large, deep ashtrays and never smoke in bed.
- Set the hot water heater thermostat at 120° F (48.9° C) or less, with installation of valves in the bathrooms that regulate water temperature.
- Turn handles of pans to the back of the stove when cooking. Do not wear clothing with loose sleeves when cooking. Double-check that the stove is off after cooking.

Healthy People 2010

Goals per 100,000 People for Reduction in Residential Fire Deaths and Presence of Functioning Smoke Alarms

The Surgeon General's goals for 2010 related to burn injury are focused on decreasing residential fire deaths through the presence of a functioning smoke alarm on every floor.

GOAL 1: REDUCE THE INCIDENCE OF RESIDENTIAL FIRES

1998 baseline: 1.2 per 100,000 people
2010 target: 0.2 per 100,000 people

GOAL 2: INCREASE TOTAL POPULATION LIVING IN RESIDENCES WITH FUNCTIONING SMOKE ALARMS ON EVERY FLOOR

1998 baseline: 88%
2010 target: 100%

The highest identified risk groups are African-Americans, American Indians or Alaska Natives, and Hispanic or Latino populations. 1998 baseline data reflect higher rates of residential fires and a lower presence of smoke alarms among these groups.

From US Department of Health and Human Services: *Healthy People 2010: understanding and improving health,* Washington, DC, 2000, USDHHS.

EVALUATION

To evaluate the effectiveness of nursing interventions, compare patient behaviors with those stated in the expected patient outcomes. Achievement of patient outcomes is successful if the patient:

1. Maintains a patent airway, adequate oxygenation, and ventilation.
1a. Is free of stridor and adventitious breath sounds.
1b. Has Po_2 >80 mm Hg and Pco_2 <45 mm Hg.
1c. Has carboxyhemoglobin level <10%.
2. Overcomes fluid deficit and is free of signs of fluid excess.
2a. Has urine output of 30 to 50 ml/hr (0.5 ml/kg) in adults or 1 to 2 ml/kg/hr in children.
2b. Has electrolytes within normal limits.
2c. Has normal sensorium.
2d. Has systolic blood pressure >100 mm Hg.
2e. Has heart rate <120 beats/min.
2f. Has pH between 7.35 and 7.45 and base excess ≥6.
2g. Has limited tissue edema.
2h. Has minimal fluid weight gain.
2i. Exhibits no signs of pulmonary edema.
3. Maintains a body temperature between 98.6° and 101.3° F (37° and 38.5° C).
4. Shows no evidence of wound infection.
4a. Wound appears clean.
4b. Has temperature <101.3° F (38.5° C).
4c. Routine wound cultures are obtained on admission and are scheduled for every 3 days.
4d. There is documentation of Standard Precautions or protective gowns, sterile gloves, hats, and masks being worn when caring for the open burn wound.
5. Burn wound shows no evidence of further tissue loss.
6. Is free of unmanageable pain.
6a. Sleeps between treatments.
6b. Does not have elevated vital signs.
6c. Appears relaxed and indicates pain is reduced after receiving morphine.
7. Does not appear to be anxious.
7a. Listens to explanations from staff.
7b. Begins to verbalize concerns about the accident and asks questions about the future.

SPECIAL ENVIRONMENTS FOR CARE

Critical Care Management

Patients who suffer burn injuries require specialized care, which is best obtained in a burn unit. A multidisciplinary team, including surgeons, nurses, physical and occupational therapists, social workers, microbiologists, clergy, child life workers, psychologists, volunteers, and other disciplines, is involved in the approach to care. Nurses working in the burn unit need to provide critical care for patients of all age-groups. They must understand wound care, infection control, and rehabilitation requirements of burn patients. Nurses also need to understand the different types of dressings, including Biobrane porcine, and artificial skin, such as Integra, AlloDerm, and cultured epithelium.

Acute Phase

The acute phase of treatment begins at the end of the emergent phase and lasts until the burn wound is healed. The length of this period varies. If the burn is a partial-thickness injury, the acute phase extends for 7 to 21 days; if the burn is a full-thickness injury over a large percentage of the body requiring surgery for skin grafting, the acute phase may last for months.

During the acute phase the two main foci of management are (1) treatment of the burn wound and (2) avoidance, detection, and treatment of complications. The most common complications are infection (septicemia and pneumonia), renal disease, and heart failure.

Collaborative Care Management

Diagnostic Tests. Laboratory testing during the acute phase focuses on monitoring the patient's fluid and electrolyte balance. Chemistry profiles may be obtained once or twice daily during the patient's critical phase while fluid resuscitation is in progress. Complete blood counts are monitored to assess the patient's white blood cell count and hemoglobin and hematocrit values. Wound cultures are obtained once or twice weekly to track the bacterial colonization of the wounds. Ongoing surveillance of wound cultures is essential for early treatment of infection. Evaluation of nutritional status is monitored through prealbumin levels and urine urea nitrogen. Patients who are intubated or have inhalation injuries require periodic chest x-ray studies. In addition, bronchoscopy is performed on patients with inhalation injuries to assess the degree of injury to the lungs.

Medications. Analgesia is essential for pain control. The most commonly used agents are opioids such as morphine sulfate, fentanyl, and codeine. Patients with major burns may require agents to prevent stress ulcers (e.g., ranitidine, cimetidine, or sucralfate). Systemic antimicrobial agents are used only when evidence of infection is present. Topical antimicrobial agents are applied to the burn wounds on the basis of the depth of injury and wound culture results. Anabolic steroids, such as oxandrolone, have had positive effects during the recovery phase of a major burn. They are used to attenuate the catabolic state, restore lean body mass, and promote wound healing.[9] Current research is focused on the benefits of administration during the acute phase of injury. In addition, many burn patients have preexisting illnesses and require ongoing medication management of their current health problems.

Treatments. For the burn patient, wound care is a major treatment. Depending on the depth and location of the wound, dressing changes are performed once, twice, or three times daily (see Promoting Skin Integrity, p. 2003).

Skin Grafts. Skin grafts are applied to cover the burn wound and speed healing, to control contractures, and to shorten convalescence. Successful grafting reduces the patient's vulnerability to infection and prevents the loss of body heat and water vapor from the open wound. Grafting may be performed for cosmetic or functional purposes during the rehabilitation phase. Most skin grafts are applied between days 3 and 21 after the initial injury, depending on the depth and extent of the burn and the condition of the burn wound base.

A variety of grafts obtained from various sources are used to treat burn wounds (Table 63-2). Grafts may provide permanent or temporary coverage. An autograft is a graft of skin obtained from the patient's own body and is a permanent graft. A homograft, or cryopreserved cadaveric allograft, is a graft of skin obtained from a cadaver 6 to 24 hours after death. It can be used as fresh donor skin (stored in the refrigerator) or frozen donor skin obtained from a tissue bank. A heterograft (xenograft) is a graft of skin obtained from another species, such as a pig. Homografts, heterografts, synthetic substitutes, and biosynthetic dressings (Biobrane) are intended to provide temporary coverage while the burn wound heals. As the wound heals, these temporary coverings are gradually rejected and are easily removed from the newly healed skin. Temporary grafts reduce water, electrolyte, and protein losses at the burn surface; reduce wound pain; and allow the patient freedom of movement. Temporary grafts act like human skin and may be used until the patient is ready for an autograft. Often autografting is delayed as a result of complications such as infection, pneumonia, or the critical status of the patient.

Dermal replacements or synthetic substitutes for skin are currently being developed and used in burn units throughout the United States. Integra, AlloDerm, and cultured epithelium are new products currently available. All of these products are expensive. The product alone may cost $20,000 or more per patient. Cost-effectiveness is being evaluated, with costs and patient outcomes being compared. The ultimate skin substitute would include the following properties: it would be inexpensive, nonantigenic, flexible, and durable; it would also prevent fluid loss, serve as a barrier to infection, adjust to the wound surface, grow with a child, not cause hypertrophic scarring, store easily with a long shelf-life, and be applied in one operation. There currently is not a perfect skin substitute.[27]

Before the graft is placed on the wound, the surgical procedure of tangential excision and/or facial excision is performed in which the necrotic tissue or eschar is removed down to viable tissue or fascia. It is then covered with an autograft or skin substitute. The procedure is best performed between the second and fifth burn day. This technique is used to cover a full-thickness burn injury. Advantages of tangential excision and grafting are outlined in Box 63-8.

Split-thickness skin grafts, full-thickness skin grafts, and primary closure are surgical techniques used to cover the burn wounds (Figure 63-12). Split-thickness skin grafts include the upper layers of skin (epidermis) and part of the middle layer (dermis) but are not taken so deep as to prevent regeneration of the skin at the site from which they are taken (donor site). The grafts are removed with a dermatome blade from almost any unburned part of the body. The sizes of these grafts are determined by the sites available and the area to be covered. Grafts may be used as sheets or are meshed. Meshing of the graft involves taking the sheet of skin after it is removed from the donor and feeding it into a meshing instrument that perforates the sheet with tiny slits. The meshing of the graft makes it more expandable so that it can be stretched to cover wider areas of the body surface (Figure 63-13). Sheet grafts are applied directly to the burn wound without meshing. They result in better functional and cosmetic outcomes and are used on the face, neck, hands, or around joints.

Full-thickness grafts are composed of layers of skin down to the subcutaneous tissue. They are used if there is a well-defined area of full-thickness burn, give a better cosmetic appearance than split-thickness grafts when healed, and are used early in wound management. Areas that benefit from full-thickness grafts are the hands, neck, and face. Full-thickness grafts can also be used in rehabilitation stages to restore body function and to release skin contractures.

Primary closure is another method of burn wound closure. It is used to close small burns by pulling the skin together and suturing the burn area together or by closing the area with local skin flaps.

Graft sites require skilled nursing management. Autografts are secured in surgery with staples, dressings, and splints. Special precautions are taken to prevent sliding, slipping, or movement of the graft. The grafted area may be covered with a large, occlusive, bulky dressing to hold new skin securely in place. Splints applied in the operating room help provide immobilization and maintain the position of the grafted areas.

BOX 63-8 Advantages of Tangential Excision and Grafting

- Decreases hospitalization
- Prevents potential conversion of burn to full thickness by removing necrotic tissue before infection occurs
- Diminishes anxiety and lessens trauma to multiple graftings
- Allows early grafting and early restoration of function
- Reduces scar formation because of use of full-thickness graft

TABLE 63-2 Types of Grafts

Graft	Source	Coverage
Autograft	Patient's own nonburned skin removed and applied to burn	Permanent
Cultured skin	Patient's skin removed in small squares and grown in laboratory conditions into large pieces of skin	Permanent
Integra (artificial skin)	Two-layer man-made membrane used to replace dermis and covered with autograft, forming functional dermis and epidemis	Permanent
AlloDerm	Man-made collagen matrix used to provide dermal layer covered with autograft	Permanent

The dressing remains intact for 48 to 72 hours. Sheet grafts and full-thickness grafts are examined every 24 hours because drainage or blood can accumulate under the graft. This fluid can be removed by aspiration with a needle, rolling the fluid with a cotton tip, or cutting a small slit in the graft to drain the fluid. The graft dressings are removed slowly and carefully so that the graft is not disturbed.

The donor site represents a wound similar to that of a partial-thickness injury. Care of the donor site is as important as care of the graft itself, because donor sites that fail to heal result in an enlargement of the patient's open wound surface. Donor sites may be treated by a variety of methods. One method is covering the exposed surface with Xeroform and leaving it exposed to the air. Exposing the donor site to a heat lamp also promotes healing because, as the drainage from the wound dries, it serves as a protective covering. The site usually heals within 2 weeks. Other methods include the use of OpSite or Biobrane on the donor site. The area is kept wrapped and checked daily for drainage and healing.

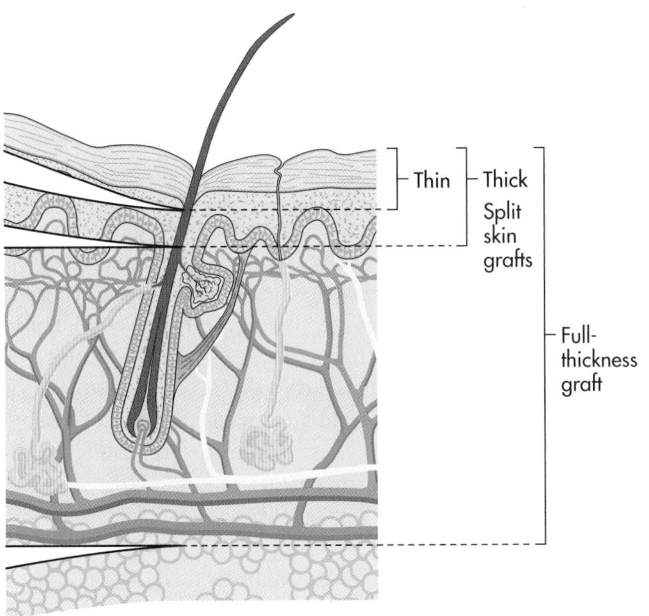

Figure 63-12 Levels of skin involved in thin and thick split-skin grafts and full-thickness grafts.

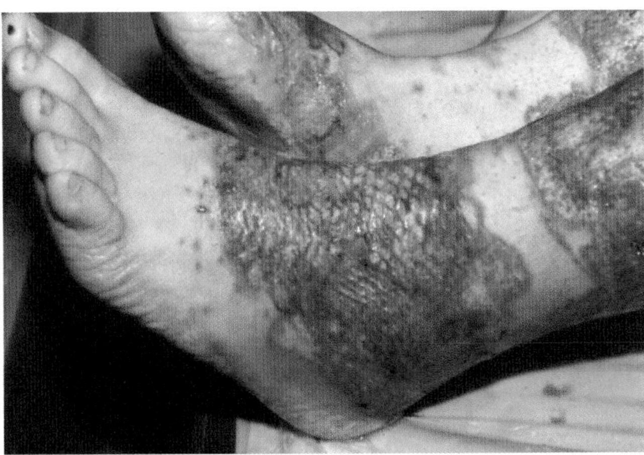

Figure 63-13 Mesh graft to foot.

Many patients complain of severe pain in the donor site, and the nurse should not hesitate to give medications for pain. The pain should subside in 24 to 48 hours as the wound dries. The wound is inspected daily for any signs of infection (erythema, purulent drainage, or foul odor). If infection develops, antibiotics may be administered, and the wound may be treated with wet dressings.

Diet. Metabolism can be increased by two or three times normal after moderate to severe burns because of stress, fluid loss, hypercatabolism, and immobility.[24] Shivering and elevated levels of catecholamines, cortisol, and glucagon present after thermal injury increase oxygen consumption and heat production and deplete liver and muscle glycogen and fat deposits, resulting in negative nitrogen balance and weight loss. Protein is broken down to provide amino acids for use in gluconeogenesis rather than being used to build new tissue. Thus wound healing is prolonged, and the patient's susceptibility to infection increased.

A burn patient remains catabolic until caloric intake exceeds caloric expenditure. This catabolic state may last for days or months, depending on the severity of the burn. The patient's energy and protein requirements equal those needed for normal homeostasis plus those required to offset the catabolic state and repair the burn injury.

Nuritional Assessment. Maintenance of a nutritional support program is critical to survival and is initiated on admission. The goals of the nutritional support program are to establish oral intake as soon as possible and to maintain sufficient caloric and protein intake to restore tissue loss. A team approach provides comprehensive input and integrates the efforts of the patient, physician, nurse, pharmacist, dietitian, and occupational and physical therapists.

A nutritional assessment is made during the first days of the burn injury and includes anthropometric measurements (to determine actual weight compared with ideal weight), indirect calorimetry, and laboratory studies (electrolytes, liver function tests, and urine). The admission assessment provides a baseline against which progress can be evaluated. Twenty-four-hour urine specimens and urea nitrogen findings may be obtained two or three times a week to evaluate the patient's nitrogen balance. Transferrin or prealbumin levels provide sensitive indicators of visceral protein status.[19] Urinary nitrogen and serum albumin levels can be affected by insensible protein loss and hydration status. Albumin's half-life of 20 days makes day-to-day evaluation of albumin difficult to interpret. On the other hand, prealbumin, which has a short half-life of 20 to 25 hours, provides a sensitive indicator of nutritional status and the patient's response to feeding.

Nutritional requirements for the burn patient are highly variable, depending on the extent and depth of injury and the patient's age, gender, preburn nutritional status, and preexisting diseases. Total caloric needs may be as high as 3500 to 5000 calories per day. Calories are provided to the patient as 20% protein, 50% carbohydrate, and 30% fat. Dietitians in burn centers most commonly use the Curreri formula and variations of the Harris-Benedict equation. These formulas are used as a guide to begin nutritional support.

Protein is essential to replace nitrogen lost through the wound and in urine and to promote tissue repair and healing. Protein needs in the adult increase from a normal of 0.8 g/kg of body weight to 1.5 to 3 g/kg. Protein calories must be dedicated to the wound and not used for energy needs. This is accomplished by providing the patient with sufficient carbohydrate and fat for energy use.

Approximately 5 mg/kg/min of glucose is provided. Excessive carbohydrate administration is avoided to prevent increased carbon dioxide production and hyperglycemia. In addition to calories, fat provides fat-soluble vitamins and essential fatty acids. Calories provided by fat are limited to 30% because of the adverse effect that high fat levels have on the immune system.[11]

Vitamin and mineral supplements are essential for optimal wound healing. Vitamins C and A, zinc, and iron are provided at doses higher than the recommended daily allowances. Vitamins A and C have roles as cellular antioxidants and are required for collagen synthesis. Patients may receive as much as 1000 mg of vitamin C and 5000 to 10,000 IU of vitamin A per day. Zinc levels decrease because of increased nitrogen excretion in the urine during the acute phase. Zinc is essential for wound healing and has a key role in immune function. Patients receive supplementation of up to 220 mg/day.[19] Iron may be supplied to treat anemia caused from blood loss after skin grafting.

Feeding Methods. Enteral feeding (oral or tube feeding) is the preferred method for the burn patient. A paralytic ileus or gastric dilation is commonly seen in the severely burned patient as a result of shock, stress, or sepsis. This may limit the patient's ability to tolerate gastric feedings for the first few weeks. Commonly, small-bore feeding tubes are inserted into the duodenum or endoscopically into the jejunum so that feedings may be initiated within the first 24 hours of injury. Early feeding decreases hypermetabolism, improves nitrogen balance, minimizes bacterial translocation from the gut secondary to muscle atrophy, and decreases diarrhea and hospital length of stay.[24] Total parenteral nutrition is generally reserved for patients who are unable to tolerate enteral feeding.

Oral feeding is encouraged whenever possible. However, it is difficult for the patient to consume the number of calories needed from food alone because of pain and decreased gastric motility. Therefore a combination of food by mouth with supplements, such as milk shakes or Ensure, and tube feedings may be necessary to meet the patient's nutritional requirements.

Activity. Physical and occupational therapy is necessary for the burn patient and begin on admission. Collaboration between nurses and the therapists is essential. The patient is encouraged to move about and to ambulate as much as possible. Patients with major burns or those who require mechanical ventilation may only tolerate bed rest and range-of-motion exercises. As soon as hemodynamic and pulmonary stability is achieved, the patient may sit in a chair and then ambulate. The patient is encouraged to assist with self-care as much as possible.

Referrals. Referrals to other services are determined by the needs of the patient. For example, patients with other conditions such as diabetes may require consultation from an expert to assist in managing the diabetes during the acute phase of their burn. Consultation with a psychiatrist may be indicated for patients whose burns were self-inflicted or for those who are having difficulty adjusting to their postburn appearance.

NURSING MANAGEMENT OF PATIENT DURING ACUTE PHASE

ASSESSMENT

During the acute phase, burn patients are often frightened and anxious about their injury and the associated treatments. These responses can be compounded by the intensive care unit environment.

Burn patients experience both physical and psychologic pain. Physical pain is usually focused on specific activities such as wound cleansing and debridement, dressing changes, and physical therapy. The nurse must assess the patient's reaction to pain and intervene appropriately.

Physical Examination

A thorough head-to-toe assessment of the burn patient is performed every 8 hours. This includes checking mental status, vital signs, breath sounds, bowel sounds, dietary intake, motor ability, intake and output, weight pattern, and circulation. It also includes observation of burn wounds, grafts, and any donor site. Purulent drainage, abnormal color, foul odor, redness or swelling in surrounding normal skin, or the presence of healing should be noted. Changes in these parameters from shift to shift or from day to day make further assessment necessary.

NURSING DIAGNOSES

Nursing diagnoses are determined from analysis of patient data. Possible nursing diagnoses for the person with burns during the acute phase may include but are not limited to:

Diagnostic Title	Possible Etiologic Factors
1. Impaired skin integrity	Burn injury, nutritional deficit
2. Risk for infection	Break in skin integrity, impaired immune response
3. Imbalanced nutrition: less than body requirements	Increased metabolic needs, protein losses through wounds, decreased appetite
4. Acute pain	Exposed nerve endings, immobility
5. Deficient fluid volume	Increased fluid loss via evaporation through the burn wound
6. Impaired physical mobility	Splinting after a graft procedure, activity intolerance, depression, decreased strength and endurance
7. Anxiety	Changes in health status/role functioning; situational crisis
8. Ineffective individual coping	Situational crisis, personal vulnerability, ineffective support systems

9. Compromised family coping	Inadequate or incorrect information, temporary family disorganization, role changes
10. Disturbed body image	Loss/change of body parts, function
11. Self-care deficit	Intolerance to activity, pain, musculoskeletal impairment
12. Hypothermia	Exposure of wounds to environment

EXPECTED PATIENT OUTCOMES

Expected patient outcomes for the burn-injured patient during the acute phase include but are not limited to:

1. Will have a clean, healing wound
2. Will be free of pathogenic organisms and signs and symptoms of infection
3. Will have a positive nitrogen balance and wound healing
4. Will report a decreasing and acceptable level of pain
5. Will exhibit signs of adequate fluid balance
6. Will maintain full range of motion
7. Will exhibit reduced anxiety
8. Will exhibit functional coping mechanisms
9. Family will exhibit functional coping mechanisms
10. Will begin to develop a realistic body image
11. Will demonstrate increased ability to perform self-care activities
12. Will have a body temperature between 98.6° and 101.3° F (37° and 38.5° C)

INTERVENTIONS

1. Promoting Skin Integrity

Healing of the burn wound is an essential component of care of the patient. Expert assessment skills are required to monitor the wound during healing and to detect any signs of infection. Wound care may be needed one to three times daily. Wound cleansing, debridement, and dressing application are accomplished during these treatments. The patient is adequately medicated before the procedure. Strict barrier precautions are maintained. Caregivers wear gowns, masks, eye protection, and gloves. The goals of wound care include:

- Prevention of infection
- Removal of devitalized tissue
- Prevention of further destruction of healthy tissue
- Minimalization of pain

Hydrotherapy

Hydrotherapy using a shower, tub, or spray table facilitates the removal of topical medications and loosens debris, sloughing eschar, and exudate. Wound care in a tub permits immersion of the patient into water or antimicrobial solutions. Soaking helps in the removal of topical agents and eschar and helps facilitate range of motion. Generally, tub therapy is limited to 30-minute intervals to prevent heat loss. Tub therapy is avoided in critically ill patients and those with a wound infection, since the infection may be transmitted to other areas of the body through the tub water.

A spray table may be used for patients who are poorly mobile or have wound infections, or during their more critical phase. This method of hydrotherapy allows the patient to be recumbent, and water is provided through the use of temperature-controlled hoses. For patients who are mobile, a regular shower can be used. This method helps the patient resume activities of daily living (ADLs).

Wound Cleansing and Debridement

Thorough cleansing and debridement of the wound is an important part of wound healing. After removal of the gauze dressings, the wound is cleansed with a mild soap or noncytotoxic wound-cleansing agent. Nonadherent exudates or debris is removed. In deeper wounds in which eschar, or devitalized tissue, is present, debridement may be required. Debridement may be surgical, enzymatic, or mechanical. Surgical debridement involves cutting the dead tissue away and is performed in the operating room with the patient under anesthesia. Enzymatic debridement involves the use of a topical enzyme that promotes separation of the eschar from the wound bed. During mechanical debridement, manual removal of eschar using gauze sponges, tweezers, scissors, or other instruments is performed. Because this is a painful procedure for patients, they must be adequately medicated. During this cleansing procedure the wound is carefully assessed for signs of healing or infection.

Methods of Wound Treatment

Different methods of treating the burned area may be used depending on the location of the burn, its size and depth, inpatient versus outpatient care, and the patient's response to therapy. Wounds can be managed by an open or closed method. If an open method is used, a topical agent or wound covering is placed on the wound and is left exposed to the air. More superficial burns of the face may be managed in this manner. A topical agent, such as bacitracin, is applied to the face after cleansing. An open method allows for the wound to be visualized more readily and assists in range of motion because of the absence of constricting dressings. Disadvantages include heat loss and easy accidental removal of the topical agent during patient activity. If a closed method of wound care is used, the topical agent or wound covering is placed on the wound and the wound is covered with a gauze wrap. This method promotes adherence of the topical agent to the wound and limits fluid loss and wound drying.

A number of agents are available for use in managing burn wounds (Table 63-3). Topical agents are creams that are applied directly to the wound. Petroleum-based topical antimicrobial agents, such as bacitracin, provide a barrier protection to the wound and are used for more superficial burns. Other agents, such as silver sulfadiazine and mafenide acetate, are used for full-thickness and deep dermal burns. The cream penetrates through the eschar, treating wound infection and helping the eschar to separate, and the antimicrobial action helps prevent or treat infection. If eschar is present, an enzyme may be applied topically to promote separation of the dead tissue.

TABLE 63-3 Topical Medications and Wound Coverings Used in Burn Therapy

Agent	Indication	Description	Intervention
Topical Agents			
Petrolum-based antimicrobial ointments (e.g., Bacitracin, Neosporin)	Partial-thickness burns	Petroleum-based ointment provides a barrier protection to wound Mild antimicrobial activity Poor penetration of eschar	Cleanse wound thoroughly between applications to prevent caking. Maintain adequate layer to prevent wound drying.
Silver sulfadiazine (Silvadene)	Deep partial- to full-thickness burns Wound infection	Broad-spectrum cream with activity against gram-negative, gram-positive, and *Candida* organisms Penetrates eschar to inhibit bacterial growth at dermis-eschar interface Inhibits epithelial tissue development May cause skin rash May cause transient decrease in white blood cell count for 24-48 hours after application Contraindicated in sulfa allergies	Apply ¼-inch layer directly to wound or impregnated into gauze dressing two or three times daily (painless and somewhat soothing). Repeated application may cause slimy, grayish appearance. Discontinue when eschar is no longer present.
Mafenide acetate (Sulfamylon)	Deep partial- to full-thickness burns Wound infection	Bacteriostatic against gram-negative and gram-positive organisms 11.1% water-soluble cream: Penetrates thick eschar and cartilage Inhibits epithelial tissue development 5% solution: Antimicrobial solution that may be used for prevention and treatment of wound infection	Plan for pain management as it may result in pain on application. Apply cream in ¼-inch layer directed to wound or impregnate into gauze dressing two or three times daily. Monitor for metabolic acidosis, particularly when applied to 40% of total body surface area or greater (inhibits carbonic anhydrase activity). Monitor for allergic rash. Discontinue when eschar is no longer present.
Silver nitrate (5% solution)	Deep partial- to full-thickness burns Wound Infection	Bacteriostatic against gram-positive and gram-negative bacteria Poorly penetrates eschar Application colors tissue black, making wound assessment more difficult	Plan for pain management because application causes pain. Apply carefully as it can stain clothing and linen.
Enzymes			
Collagenase (Santyl)	Deep partial- to full-thickness wounds Wound Infection	Collagen-specific enzyme digests collagen in necrotic tissue Does not harm healthy tissue No antimicrobial properties Active in pH range of 6-8	Apply to areas where eschar exits one or two times daily; cover wound with barrier dressing. Monitor for eschar separation and discontinue when eschar is removed.
Papain urea debriding ointment (Accuzyme)	Deep partial- to full-thickness wounds	Water-insoluble, nonspecific cysteine-protease breaks down nonviable tissue Does not harm healthy tissue No antimicrobial properties Active in pH range of 3-12	Apply to areas where eschar exists one or two times daily with gauze dressing. Monitor for eschar separation and discontinue when eschar is removed. Plan for pain management because application may cause pain.

TABLE 63-3 Topical Medications and Wound Coverings Used in Burn Therapy—cont'd

Agent	Indication	Description	Intervention
Synthetic Wound Coverings			
Acticoat	Partial- and full-thickness burns and donor sites	Polyethylene mesh coated with ionic silver with a rayon/polyester core Broad-spectrum antimicrobial action Maintains moist wound environment Covering may be left in place for several days	Monitor for exudates and infection.
Xeroform	Partial-thickness burns and donor sites	Petrolatum-based fine-mesh gauze impregnated with 3% bismuth tribromophenate Mild antimicrobial properties Provides protective barrier dressing that allows for epithelial tissue development	Apply to clean partial-thickness wounds. Monitor for and maintain adherence to wound; change daily if nonadherent. Monitor for signs of infection.
Scarlet Red	Partial-thickness burns and donor sites	Fine-mesh gauze impregnated with lanolin, olive oil, petrolatum, and red dye Promotes epithelial tissue development and protects wound No antimicrobial properties	Apply to clean partial-thickness wounds. Monitor for and maintain adherence to wound; change daily if nonadherent. Monitor for signs of infection.
Mepitel	Partial-thickness burns and donor sites	Pliable, nonadherent dressing consisting of fine-mesh netting coated with silicone Mild antimicrobial properties Provides protective barrier dressing that allows for epithelial tissue development Pores in dressing allow for dissipation of exudates	Apply to clean, partial-thickness wound or donor site.
Film dressings (e.g., OpSite)	Partial-thickness burns and donor Sites	Semipermeable barrier dressing Dressing allows for wound visualization	
Biosynthetic Wound Coverings			
Biobrane	Partial-thickness burns and donor sites	Semisynthetic wound covering composed of nylon, Silastic, and porcine collagen membrane that binds with wound fibrin, forming a skin substitute, allowing for healing Pores in membrane allow dissipation of exudates No antimicrobial properties An advantage to this is that pain is decreased as a result of fewer dressing changes	Apply to a clean, partial-thickness wound immediately after injury or as a covering for donor sites. Keep in place until wound is healed.
TransCyte	Partial-thickness wounds	Polymer membrane and neonatal human fibroblast cells cultured under aseptic conditions in vitro on a porcine-coated nylon mesh Secretes human dermal collagen, matrix proteins, and growth factors to promote wound healing Pain is decreased as a result of fewer dressing changes	Apply to a clean partial-thickness wound within 24 hours after injury or wound excision. Keep in place until wound is healed.

Continued

TABLE 63-3 Topical Medications and Wound Coverings Used in Burn Therapy—cont'd

Agent	Indication	Description	Intervention
Biosynthetic Wound Coverings–cont'd			
Calcium alginate	Partial-thickness wounds	Dressing composed of nonwoven fabric pad composed of calcium alginate from brown seaweed Calcium alginate ions exchanged with sodium ions on the wound to form a protective, fibrous gel Provides protective barrier, promoting healing and exudate absorption	Remove calcium alginate dressing for wound care, monitoring for wound healing and infection.
Biologic			
Cadaver allograft	Partial-thickness or excised wounds	Human donor skin providing a temporary wound covering prevents water, electrolyte, and protein losses from wound Allograft remains adherent until rejection occurs or is surgically removed May be used as a bridge to final grafting Carries risks of disease transmission	Monitor for adherence and infection.
Pigskin (heterograft, xenograft)	Partial-thickness or excised wounds	Skin from another species (e.g., pigskin) used as a temporary wound covering to protect wound, preventing water, electrolyte, and protein losses May be used as a bridge between full-thickness wound excision and final grafting	Monitor for adherence and infection. Change every 2-3 days, depending on adherence.

Temporary wound coverings may be used on the burn wound. These coverings protect the wound, promote healing, and have varying degrees of antimicrobial action. They may be synthetic, biosynthetic, or biologic. The choice of these agents is based on the depth of the wound and the presence or absence of infection. These coverings may be left in place for 1 day or until the wound heals.

2. Preventing Infection

The burn patient is at tremendous risk for infection. Measures to prevent infection begin at the time the patient is admitted to the hospital and continue until healing is complete. Sources of infection may be endogenous or exogenous. Bacteria that survive in the hair follicles and glands are a source of endogenous infection. In addition, after burn injury, bacteria that normally live in the intestinal tract migrate or translocate across the intestinal wall and spread to the general circulation by way of the lymphatic system. Local and systemic infections (septicemia) are the most common complications of burns and are the major cause of death, particularly in burns covering more than 25% of the body.

Organisms commonly causing burn wound infection include *Pseudomonas aeruginosa, Acinetobacter* organisms, enterococci, and *Staphylococcus aureus.* These organisms are normally found on the skin or in the intestine and become a source of infection. Treatment of antimicrobial-resistant organisms, such as methicillin-resistant *S. aureus* and vancomycin-resistant enterococci, is an increasingly difficult problem in burn centers.

Fungal infections have an increased incidence in burn patients because of the use of broad-spectrum antibiotics. *Candida albicans,* which normally is found in the gastrointestinal tract, accounts for the majority of fungal infections. Cultures of the patient's wound may be taken on admission and at biweekly intervals to determine the presence of bacteria and their sensitivity to antibiotics.

Infection is commonly the cause of deterioration in the condition of a burn patient. Signs of infection include erythema and edema at the wound edges, increasing pain, odor, drainage, and decreasing function. The wound may show changes in color from red to violet, dark brown, or black. Tissue necrosis may occur (Figure 63-14).

Signs of sepsis in the burn patient are:

- Change in sensorium
- Fever
- Tachypnea
- Tachycardia
- Paralytic ileus (decreased tolerance of feedings)

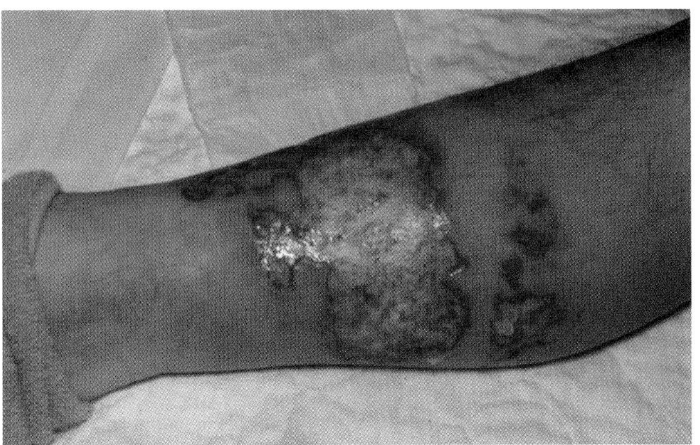

Figure 63-14 Leg burn with cellulitic wound infection.

- Abdominal distention
- Oliguria

To prevent the introduction of exogenous organisms into the wound, strict adherence to Standard Precautions is essential. Persons with upper respiratory tract infections should not be permitted near the patient. Thorough wound cleansing is necessary to remove the debris that acts as a media for bacterial growth. Placing the severely burned patient in a special burn unit can decrease the possibility of infection because the unit environment is specifically equipped for infection control. If the patient is cared for in a general hospital unit, a private room is essential, and all equipment needed by the patient remains in the room.

3. Providing Nutrition

Planning, collaboration, and ingenuity are required to ensure that the patient receives adequate nutritional support. An oral diet is encouraged whenever possible. The patient's food preferences are determined, and the family is encouraged to bring favorite foods from home. Care is coordinated so that mealtimes are relaxed and not associated with other procedures, such as wound care. A social situation can be created by having burn patients eat together or with family members. Pain medication is provided so that the patient is comfortable. Coordination with occupational therapy staff is essential if the patient needs assistive devices to hold utensils and cups.

Patients unable to consume sufficient calories orally require tube feedings. Continuous feedings are provided when requirements are high. As the patient begins to eat orally, tube feedings may be provided overnight, allowing the patient to eat during the day. Calorie counts are essential to monitor the patient's progress.

Monitoring the patient's nutritional status is an ongoing process. Weight loss and gain are monitored daily during the critical phase and biweekly as the wounds heal. Initially, weight gain occurs because of fluid retention. As diuresis occurs, the patient's weight decreases as a result of fluid loss. Significant weight loss reflects protein loss and loss of fat reserves and muscle mass. Prealbumin, urine urea nitrogen balance, and cholesterol levels are obtained.

Guidelines for Safe Practice

Minimizing Pain During Dressing Changes

1. Provide analgesic medications before dressing change.
2. Provide clear explanation to gain patient's cooperation.
3. Handle burned areas gently.
4. Use sterile technique (infection causes increased pain).
5. Encourage patient to participate in treatment whenever possible.
6. Use distraction (e.g., radio or conversation) and relaxation techniques when appropriate.

The patient's tolerance of feeding is monitored by evaluating bowel function. Diarrhea may be a problem for patients receiving antibiotics or tube feedings. Commonly, burn patients have difficulties with constipation as a result of administration of opioids and decreased activity. Stool softeners, laxatives, and increased fluid intake may be provided.

4. Promoting Comfort

Pain management is a component of the Patient Bill of Rights and is a major part of the burn patient's care. Uncontrolled pain affects all aspects of recovery, including tolerance of wound care, ability to eat, mobility, wound healing, and psychologic adjustment. Acute pain is most successfully managed with narcotics. The methods and routes of administration are carefully evaluated on an individual basis. Attention is paid to pain management needs during dressing changes and other daily activities. During dressing changes, parenteral narcotics are given to achieve rapid onset of action. The use of agents such as ketamine, fentanyl, and self-administered nitrous oxide may be beneficial for some patients. The Guidelines for Safe Practice box outlines nursing interventions during dressing change.

Planning for patient comfort from pain, itching, or general discomfort includes a plan for procedural, background, and breakthrough pain. The nursing plan of care and assessment includes pain assessment with vital signs. An around-the-clock approach to pain management is essential for the burn patient. Undermedication may occur if the patient fears becoming addicted and fails to report pain or if the nurse fails to adequately evaluate the degree of pain. The use of a numeric analog scale in which the patient rates the pain helps determine whether the pain is being adequately controlled. Providing medication at frequent intervals helps maintain ongoing comfort. Time-released opioids and patient-controlled analgesia are also viable options.

Physiologic pain may be induced or aggravated by loneliness and depression. The patient's complaint of pain may be an indication of unmet emotional needs that can be addressed with the use of presence, touch, music therapy, or diversional activities. Anxiety about anticipated procedures and sleep deprivation may increase the amount of pain experienced by the patient. Patients experiencing posttraumatic stress disorder (PTSD) report higher levels of pain.[5] Interventions may include the use of antianxiety medication and nonpharmacologic methods such as music therapy, meditation, or relaxation exercises (see Research box).

5. Maintaining Fluid Balance

To assess for fluid volume deficit, the patient is weighed daily on the same scale, in the same amount of clothing, at the same time daily. A careful record is kept of the weights. Electrolytes are monitored by frequent blood chemistry analyses. Fluids are offered on a regular basis, and a careful record is kept of all intake and output.

Patients are taught the importance of maintaining fluid and electrolyte balance after discharge and the need to notify their health care provider immediately if they experience weight loss accompanied by headache, lightheadedness, fatigue, decreased urine output, irritability, or rapid pulse, which are signs of fluid deficit, or an increase in fatigue, abdominal distention, anorexia, vomiting, constipation, muscle cramps, paresthesia, or confusion, which are signs of electrolyte imbalance. They are also taught to eat a well-balanced diet with sufficient fluid intake.

6. Promoting Range of Motion

As the patient's wounds heal and pain is controlled, the patient is encouraged to do range-of-motion exercises on a regular schedule. The nurse provides assistance and support as needed, with the goal being that the patient will be able to perform them independently. The patient and family are taught the importance of range-of-motion exercises in preventing or minimizing contractures. Physical and occupational therapists are involved in helping the patient improve range of motion.

7. Relieving Anxiety

A burn injury is a sudden, unexpected event. Its impact on psychologic well-being is enormous, and promoting mental health is a major component of the burn patient's care. The psychologic responses in the emergent phase are related to the threat to survival. During the acute phase a variety of behaviors may be seen. (See Table 63-4 for a summary of psychologic responses.) As the patient becomes aware of the extent of the injury and begins to evaluate its implications for his or her life, many problems may occur that affect the ability of both the patient and the family to cope with the situation.

Nurses play a major role in maintaining and restoring the patient's mental health. Pain plays a significant role in the patient's level of anxiety and is commonly identified by patients as the worst part of their hospital stay. Controlling pain assists in decreasing anxiety.

Ongoing education is imperative to assist the patient in understanding the care given and to make realistic plans for the future. It is important for the patient to maintain a sense of hope for the future so that he or she can resume a normal life. Without hope, the patient has less ability to cope, a sense of failure, and less-gratifying interpersonal relationships.

Emotional recovery from a burn injury is slower than physical recovery. Symptoms of psychologic distress are present in a large number of patients up to 1 year after a burn injury. These symptoms include intrusive and distressing memories of the burn injury and avoidances of thoughts and feelings related to the burn.[10] In addition, patients may have increased irritability, anxiety, and sleep disturbances[23] (see Table 63-4).

Those individuals who adjust well after a burn injury have characteristics in common. Those who had positive experiences before the injury are better able to deal with the consequences of a burn injury. In addition, they have family and other social supports available to them. They can engage others in their care and are able to revise their self-image in a realistic and positive manner.

Burn-injured persons are also at risk for the development of PTSD. In this condition symptoms occur after a psychologically traumatic event that would be considered outside the range of normal human experience.[4] Symptoms of PTSD include:

- Reexperiencing the trauma in dreams or intrusive recollections
- A numbed response to the environment, such as decreased interest or detachment
- An exaggerated startle response
- Sleep disturbance
- Guilt about having survived the event, especially if others did not
- Avoidance of activities that arouse recollections of the event

The size and severity of the burn and the degree of disfigurement do not consistently predict the patient who will de-

Research

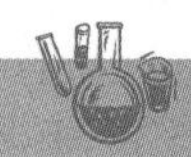

Reference: Weinberg K et al: Pain and anxiety with burn dressing changes: patient self report, *J Burn Care Rehabil* 21:157-161, 2000.

The ability of nurses to adequately manage the patient's pain and anxiety during wound care is a critical part of each patient's care. The presence of anxiety can confound the patient's pain experience and may make pain control more difficult. The purpose of this study was to describe the relationship between self-reported pain and anxiety, time, and dressing changes during the first 5 days in a burn unit. A convenience sample of 24 adult burn-injured patients who had burns covering less than 50% of the total body surface area was used. A visual analog pain thermometer scale of 0 to 10 and a visual analog anxiety scale of 0 to 10 were used to elicit the patient's self-report of pain and anxiety. Patients were asked to rate their pain and anxiety immediately before, immediately after, and ½ hour after the burn dressing change. The results indicated that pain and anxiety scores peaked at day 4, and that the presence of pain correlated with anxiety. The patients' anxiety scores were highest before the procedure and lowest ½ hour after the dressing change. Although the anxiety score decreased after the dressing change, the pain score remained high. The authors concluded that anxiety levels decreased because the patient realized that wound care was complete until the next day. The fact that the pain score remained high despite decreasing anxiety scores indicated that the patients were able to differentiate between pain and anxiety. Interventions should be directed at pain and anxiety based on the patient's self-report.

velop PTSD. Patients are more likely to develop PTSD if there is an actual or perceived lack of social support, the presence of a maladaptive coping style, and high emotional distress. Patients may be nonsymptomatic during hospitalization but develop PTSD after discharge.[5] Therefore ongoing psychologic evaluation and intervention is necessary during hospitalization and during the months that follow.

8, 9. Promoting Effective Coping of the Patient and Family

The nurse should explore with the patient how he or she coped with stressful events in the past. It is important to remember that some patients were raised to be stoic when in pain or distress. Other patients were encouraged to express their feelings openly. Nurses should support the patient's coping style unless the patient indicates that he or she would be interested in exploring new methods of coping.

Relaxation exercises, meditation, and music therapy may be useful in helping the patient cope with pain and other stressors. In some situations hypnosis may be used with the goal of having the patient develop the ability to induce self-hypnosis during dressing changes and other stressful events.

Patients are usually helped to cope if they are kept fully informed about what is planned for their care and what will be expected of them during various treatments. Coping with unexpected events can be very upsetting, especially when patients have had to give up most of their independence.

Families, like patients, cope best when they are kept fully informed and have a realistic understanding of what lies ahead for the patient. The family can be deeply disrupted by a serious burn to a family member. Initially the family is concerned about the patient's survival and needs careful explanations of what is being done for the patient and why. The explanations may need to be repeated more than once because family members may be too distressed to comprehend what they are being told.

Social workers are helpful in exploring the family's concerns about role disruptions, plans for child care, financial

TABLE 63-4 Psychologic Reactions to Severe Burns

Definition	Behavior Exhibited	Nursing Approach
Conservation, Withdrawal		
Decreased interaction with environment as an immediate response to serious injury Occurs immediately after injury and may last for first 1-2 weeks Protective value to self (may be mistaken for depression)	Decreased interaction with environment, staff, family Often keeps eyes closed, sleeps, remains immobile	Avoid forcing patient to deal with situation. Provide supportive environment. Provide ongoing information on status and care.
Denial		
Protective, unconscious defense mechanism Helps relieve anxiety caused by threat to life, limb, self	Denies extent of injury, loss of limb, loss of others in accident May acknowledge the loss but not the impact	Support patient. Avoid forcing patient to deal with fears. Answer questions honestly. Provide information in small doses over time.
Regression		
Patient returns to earlier ways of coping with stress May exhibit childlike behaviors	Assertive, demanding, temper tantrums Tearful, clings to dependent relationships	Avoid attacking and responding negatively to behavior exhibited. Acknowledge patient's difficulty in coping. Encourage and reward positive behaviors and independence.
Anger and Hostility		
Angry, agitated behavior in response to a perceived wrong, loss of control Grieving response	Angry, agitated, hostile to staff and family	Encourage verbalization of frustration. Avoid responding directly to anger. Provide choices and control. Assist patient in searching for meaning to injury.
Depression		
Extent of injury becomes distorted and impacts patient's sense of worthiness and self-esteem	Degrading comments about self Sleep disturbances, decreased appetite, generalized slowing, poor motivation	Acknowledge the loss. Focus patient on realistic expectations.
Anxiety		
Fear and threat to self as a result of injury	Restlessness, agitation, difficulty in following instructions, poor memory, easily startled	Support patient. Acknowledge fears. Provide information in small, frequent doses.

concerns, and the family members' own feelings of distress. Often family members require considerable support from health care professionals to work through their own feelings before they can be supportive to the patient. The burn team members meet to decide who will provide what support to the family.

Family members can best provide realistic support to the patient when they have accurate knowledge about what the patient will experience at each step in the recovery process. They also need information about community resources available to them and the patient.

10. Promoting a Positive Body Image and Self-Concept

A burn wound, especially a large one, presents a serious challenge to the patient's self-concept. As the patient's condition improves, he or she may express a desire to view the burned area. The burn team assesses the readiness of the patient to view the burned area and decides which members of the burn team will be present when the viewing occurs. If the patient desires, a family member or another support person may be present.

The patient is encouraged to express how he or she feels about the changed appearance. Individual counseling may be necessary for some patients as they integrate the change in their appearance into their self-concept. Other patients benefit from being referred to a patient support group where they can meet other patients in various stages of recovery. The group may be led by a nurse, social worker, psychologist, or other health care professional experienced in working with burn patients. Knowledge about the patient's coping style can help determine whether individual or group therapy or both will be recommended to the patient.

11. Encouraging Self-Care Activities

The patient is encouraged to participate as much as possible in his or her own care. Independence in ADLs is supported. Some patients require more encouragement than others in assisting with tasks such as wound care. It is important that the patient be involved in developing a daily plan of care, including meal selection, time of treatments, rest periods, therapy, and socialization.

12. Preventing Hypothermia

Room temperature is maintained at 80° to 85° F (26.7° to 29.4° C) with a 40% to 50% humidity. Care is taken to limit wound exposure time during dressing changes.

EVALUATION

To evaluate the effectiveness of nursing interventions, compare patient behaviors with those stated in the expected patient outcomes. Achievement of patient outcomes is successful if the patient:

1. Has skin integrity reestablished.
1a. Shows wound healing.
1b. Shows no hypertrophic scarring.
1c. Is able to perform skin care.
2. Is free of wound or systemic infection.
2a. Shows no pathogenic organisms from wound culture.
2b. Has no signs of systemic infection (i.e., fever, tachypnea, tachycardia, paralytic ileus, or oliguria).
3. Has optimal nutritional status.
3a. Has protein and caloric intake adequate to meet calculated needs.
3b. Has positive nitrogen balance, indicated by normal prealbumin and albumin levels.
3c. Maintains preburn weight.
3d. Has no diarrhea or constipation.
4. Manifests adequate pain control.
4a. Rates pain control as acceptable.
4b. Has no physical signs of pain (e.g., tachycardia, diaphoresis, splinting of body parts, or protective movement).
4c. States is able to sleep.
4d. Is able to perform self-care.
5. Has adequate fluid balance.
5a. Has stable weights.
5b. Has blood levels of sodium and potassium within normal limits.
5c. Has balanced intake and output.
5d. Has good skin turgor.
6. Exhibits full range of motion.
6a. Moves arms and legs through range of motion several times daily.
6b. Performs ADLs with no or minimal assistance.
7. Exhibits reduced anxiety.
7a. Appears relaxed and calm.
7b. Has normal vital signs.
7c. Listens quietly to explanations from staff and asks appropriate questions about the future.
8. Demonstrates effective coping.
8a. Uses relaxation and meditation techniques during dressing changes and other stressful events.
8b. Verbalizes realistic appraisal of life situation.
8c. Discusses resources available to assist with changes in lifestyle.
9. Family or significant other(s) demonstrates effective coping.
9a. Is realistically supportive of patient.
9b. Uses counseling and other services in adjusting to changes in family.
10. Develops a realistic body image and self-concept.
10a. Is able to look at and touch burned areas.
10b. Verbalizes feelings about change in appearance and grieving for former self.
10c. Verbalizes ways appearance could be improved (e.g., makeup).
11. Understands the treatment regimen.
11a. Is able to explain daily routine after discharge.
11b. Discusses resources available after discharge.
11c. States name of person to call in case of an emergency.
11d. States date and time of follow-up visit.
11e. Performs self-care with minimal assistance.
11f. Feeds self.

11g. Dresses self.
11h. Maintains hygiene and grooming.
11i. Changes dressing with assistance of significant other.
12. Maintains normothermia.
12a. Understands importance of avoiding chilling.
12b. Takes temperature daily.

GERONTOLOGIC CONSIDERATIONS

Gerontologic considerations are summarized in Box 63-9.

Rehabilitation Phase

Rehabilitation begins at the time of admission. However, rehabilitation as the third stage of treatment begins when the patient's burn is reduced to less than 20% of the TBSA and the patient is capable of assuming some self-care activity. The principles of management are to return the patient to a productive place in society and to accomplish functional and cosmetic reconstruction. Rehabilitation does not end when the patient is discharged. It may take from 2 to 5 years after discharge for the patient to reach a maximal level of emotional and physical adjustment.

Collaborative Care Management

Diagnostic Tests. Specific diagnostic testing during the rehabilitation phase depends on the patient's condition and progress toward goals. Overall, limited testing is required. Evaluation of nutritional status (prealbumin and urine urea nitrogen measurements) and monitoring for the presence of infection (complete blood counts and wound and/or blood cultures) may be necessary.

Medications. The number of medications prescribed decreases as the patient progresses through the rehabilitation phase. As wounds heal, less analgesia is required, and antimicrobial agents are prescribed only for documented infections.

Treatments. As burn wounds continue to heal, only minimal wound care is necessary. This may be performed by the patient in an outpatient clinic or in the home. When reconstructive procedures are performed, more extensive wound care is necessary.

Surgical Management. Initial skin grafting is completed during the acute phase. However, the patient may require reconstructive surgery to improve function and plastic surgery to re-form ears, noses, or eyelids during the rehabilitation phase. Scar tissue and contractures commonly occur 1 to 2 years after the burn and may require additional skin grafting.

Diet. Nutritional requirements continue to decrease, and vitamin supplements are no longer necessary. A well-balanced diet with adequate fluid intake is encouraged.

Activity. Optimal function is the goal of rehabilitation. Physical and occupational therapy is provided in inpatient rehabilitation settings, in outpatient settings, or in the home.

BOX 63-9 Gerontologic Considerations in Burn Care

Epidemiology

The incidence of burn injury in the home is disproportionately higher than for younger adults.
One third of all those who die in residential fires are older adults.
Older adults are at a higher risk for burn injury because of:
- Thinner skin, which is less resistant to heat
- Decreased mobility and reaction time
- Visual and hearing impairments that decrease the ability to evaluate danger
- Living in older homes, which may have faulty wiring, poor heating systems, or no smoke detectors

Flame injury is the most common type of burn injury.
Inhalation injury occurs more often in older adults than in younger persons because of their inability to escape the fire.

Aging Changes That Affect Recovery From Burn Injury

Overall mortality is higher than in younger adults.
Reserve capacity of organ systems is diminished.

Cardiovascular System

Cardiac response to burn shock is impaired because of:
- Lower cardiac output
- Coronary atherosclerosis
- Decreased baroreceptor response to volume changes

All of these put older adults at risk for cardiac failure.

Pulmonary System

Decreased elasticity of the thoracic cage and decreased number and efficiency of alveoli make older adults more prone to hypoxia, hypoventilation, and atelectasis.

Immunologic System

Older adults have diminished host resistance and impaired cell-mediated and humoral immunity.
Older adults are more prone to infection and sepsis and have decreased ability to combat infection.

Wound Healing

Diminished inflammatory response
Increased healing time
Decreased tolerance of wound excision and grafting

Management Considerations

Carefully assess cardiac status during burn resuscitation.
Monitor response to fluid volume administration (hypotension).
Monitor breath sounds for the onset of pulmonary edema.
May require the use of a pulmonary artery catheter to adequately evaluate urine output.
Monitor for early signs of respiratory failure.
Mobilize patient as soon as possible.
Provide pulmonary hygiene.
Prevent infection.
Monitor for early signs of complications, such as mental status changes, ileus, wound drainage, and temperature changes (especially hypothermia).
Promote nutritional intake.
Provide thorough wound care.

Referrals. In promoting the patient's return to full function, referrals may be made to agencies that can facilitate reintegration into society. Patients requiring a change in vocation are referred to a vocational counselor, and those who continue to have difficulty adjusting to their injuries are referred for psychologic care.

NURSING MANAGEMENT OF PATIENT DURING REHABILITATION PHASE

ASSESSMENT

The patient must be helped to maintain range of joint motion to prevent scars from healing in positions that will result in deformity. Complaints of pain and pressure should not be overlooked, because damage may occur from an improperly applied splint or poor positioning. It is important that patients understand why ambulation or motion is necessary even though it may be painful.

The emotional impact of a severe burn is enormous. The psychologic scars last forever and affect the victim and family for the rest of their lives. The extent to which the family unit adapts affects how the patient reacts to his or her new body image, as well as his or her feelings of self-worth.

The hospital environment and hospital personnel influence the adaptation process. In the immediate postburn period the nurse is primarily concerned with physiologic survival of the patient. At the same time, the nurse must be able to identify psychologic problems and coping mechanisms of the patient and family.

The nurse is responsible for assessing the patient's responses to positioning, splinting, and exercise and the ability of the patient and family to perform daily wound care after discharge. Correct positioning must be maintained to avoid the development of contractures. The splinted limb is assessed for adequate circulation, cyanosis, and temperature and the presence of pulses. Exercise, ADLs, and ambulation must be continuously assessed for patient tolerance, both physically and emotionally. Complete and comprehensive instructions of wound and dressing care followed by return demonstration are necessary before discharge.

NURSING DIAGNOSES

Nursing diagnoses are determined from analysis of patient data during the rehabilitation phase. Nursing diagnoses for the person with burns may include but are not limited to:

Diagnostic Title	Possible Etiologic Factors
1. Impaired physical mobility	Pain, decreased strength and endurance, contractures
2. Self-care deficit	Intolerance to activity; musculoskeletal impairment
3. Disturbed body image	Loss/change of body parts and/or function
4. Risk for impaired skin integrity	Nutritional deficit, fragile new tissue
5. Chronic pain	Joint, tissue contractures
6. Ineffective individual coping	Situational crisis, ineffective support systems
7. Compromised family coping	Inadequate or incorrect information; temporary family disorganization, role changes
8. Deficient knowledge	Unfamiliarity with burn injury

EXPECTED PATIENT OUTCOMES

Expected patient outcomes for the burn-injured patient during the rehabilitation phase include but are not limited to:

1. Will achieve full range of motion and physical activity consistent with desired levels
2. Will perform ADLs
3. Will develop a realistic image of self and make alterations needed in daily activities
4. Will have intact, healed tissue
5. Will report decreased pain
6. Will demonstrate effective coping mechanisms and develop a realistic plan for the future
7. Family will demonstrate effective coping mechanisms
8. Will verbalize understanding of treatments and demonstrate wound care and exercises

INTERVENTIONS

1. Promoting Mobility

As the survival rate of patients with larger and deeper burns increases, so does the challenge to maintain optimal functioning and cosmetic results. The percentage of patients with joint limitations increases in accordance with the degree and extent of their burns. Although these patients may be critically ill, their rehabilitation needs must be addressed immediately. A comprehensive program of positioning, splinting, exercise, ambulation, and ADLs must begin on the first or second day after the burn and be carried through until after discharge. Any delays in initiating treatment will be detrimental to the patient's ultimate functional outcome. Contractures are among the most serious long-term complications of burns today. They result from muscle and joint stiffening, skin grafting, and prolonged bed rest. Although occupational and physical therapists are primarily responsible for addressing the patient's rehabilitation needs during all phases of the patient's recovery, the nurse is responsible for ensuring that all their recommendations are followed.

Therapeutic Positioning

Therapeutic positioning—placing body parts in antideformity positions—is vital to the prevention of burn contractures. The patient must be repositioned in bed (side-lying, supine, or prone position) frequently and regularly around the clock. Correct positioning varies, depending on the area of the body burned (Table 63-5). Maintaining appropriate positioning helps maintain extremities and joints in the position of normal function and decrease contractures. Beds with pressure-reducing capability or low air loss may be necessary to limit skin pressure.

TABLE 63-5 Therapeutic Positioning for the Burn

Area Burned	Description of Position
Neck	No pillow Towel roll under cervical spine Neck splint
Shoulder	90-degree abduction, neutral rotation Elbow splint may be used to aid in maintaining position
Axilla	Abduction with 10- to 15-degree forward flexion and external rotation Support abducted arm with suspension from intravenous (IV) pole or bedside table Axilla splint
Elbow	Extension Support extended arm on bedside table, foam trough Elbow splint
Hand	Hand splint
Dorsal surface	Flexion
Palmar surface	Hyperextension
Hip	Extension with neutral rotation Supine with lower extremity extended Prone position (if medically appropriate) Trochanter roll Foam wedge along lateral aspect of thigh Knee or long leg splint
Knee	Extension Prone position (if medically appropriate) Patient out of bed with lower extremities extended and elevated Knee splint
Ankle	Dorsiflexion Padded footboard with heels free of pressure Ankle splint

Prolonged rest in a semi-Fowler's position or with the pillow pushing the head forward must be avoided, even though many patients like this position because it enables them to see about the room better. The bed can often be turned so that the patient can look about without having to assume positions that may lead to the formation of contractures. The bedside table may be changed from one side of the bed to the other at intervals to stimulate other body positions.

Splints

Splints prevent or correct contractures and immobilize joints after grafting. They are custom-made devices that are often molded directly on the patient to ensure optimal conformity (Figure 63-15). It is the responsibility of the nurse to apply the splint properly and according to an established schedule. An improperly applied splint can promote contractures and lead to additional complications. The nurse assesses the splinted limb for adequate circulation, cyanosis, temperature, and the presence of pulses. Complaints of pain and pressure should be assessed because damage may occur with an improperly applied splint. Some physicians prefer to use the open method of treatment and use frequent exercise instead of splinting to prevent contractures.

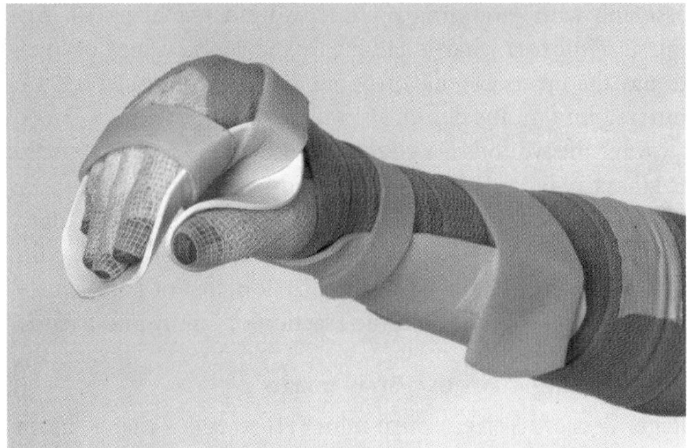

Figure 63-15 Hand splint to maintain functional position.

Exercises and Ambulation

Exercises for prevention and correction of contractures are begun as soon as the patient is stable. Active exercises are preferred, although exercises performed with active assistance and the use of gentle pressure may be more realistic. Supervision by a physical or occupational therapist is desirable. Exercises may be performed more easily in water and may be done concurrently with dressing changes if the patient is able to tolerate the activity. Continuous passive pressure motion devices may be used to prevent contractures of affected joints. When burns are completely covered (by healing or by graft), exercises may be performed in an occupational therapy or physical therapy department, where the patient may benefit from a change in environment.

Ambulation decreases the risk of thromboemboli and renal calculi, promotes optimal ventilation, helps maintain range of motion and strength in the lower extremities, orients the patient to the environment, and provides a sense of functional independence. Patients who have large burns have less ability to tolerate activity and require a progressive approach to mobilization. Initially the patient may need to be transferred with maximal assistance onto a stretcher chair and progress to a sitting position. Gradually the patient may progress to a standing pivot transfer into a nearby chair and eventually ambulate with minimal assistance. Before getting out of bed, an elastic bandage support must be applied to the lower extremities to prevent venous stasis, edema, and orthostatic hypotension.

2. Promoting Self-Care

One of the ultimate goals in the rehabilitation of the burn patient is to maintain or restore the patient's independence in performing ADLs. The occupational therapist aids in this process by selecting activities appropriate to the patient's medical, physical, and mental status. Activities that the nurse can encourage are self-feeding, telephoning, reading mail, and assisting with grooming or burn wound management. The nurse reinforces what is taught by the physical and occupational therapists so that progress can be continued on the nursing unit, in the clinic, or in the home.

After the wounds are healed, the long recuperative process begins, accompanied by the realization of endless implications for the future. Burns on the face make adjustment particularly difficult. Different kinds of fears include fear of death, pain, disfigurement, prolonged hospitalization, loss of job security, disruption of lifestyle, and the reaction of family and friends.

3. Promoting a Positive Body Image

Regardless of its size, a burn injury represents a change in the individual's perception of self. As the burn heals, the patient must deal with a new appearance. The patient must have the opportunity to talk about concerns or fears. Some patients may be unable to discuss these with their family or significant others. The nurse must be prepared to listen actively and help the patient accept changes in appearance. The patient must be allowed to grieve for the loss of the former self. However, the patient should be encouraged to focus on the positive aspects of self.

To the adolescent, the thought of being different or conspicuous may be unbearable. If possible, the patient should see facial burns only after being prepared for the experience. The patient will need support and understanding to cope with his or her image in the mirror. The patient will exhibit readiness by asking to look in the mirror. Interaction with other burn patients who are further along in the healing process may help the patient believe that recovery is possible. In some cases the recovery is very good, and although differences in skin pigmentation remain, the redness that accompanies healed burn wounds often fades considerably within a few months. Pigmentation problems are more acute for persons with brown or black skin. Their healed skin may be a different shade, freckled, or whitish. Commercial makeup products that help blend skin tones are available.

4. Promoting Skin Integrity

Preventing Scarring

Whenever a wound of connective tissue heals, hypertrophic scarring will occur unless the skin adheres to the underlying structure. Hypertrophic scarring results from the overgrowth and overproduction of tissue. This occurs especially in areas of stress and movement, such as the hands, legs, and chest (Figure 63-16). The thickened, rigid scar that results may later cause contractures. The application of controlled, constant pressure to the surface of an immature scar will reduce the scar and leave a smooth, pliable tissue. If this pressure is applied to new, healthy tissue, hypertrophic scarring will be decreased. The pressure garment, a specially designed elastic woven material, provides tridimensional control. The custom-made garment is fitted to each patient individually. Until the garment is completed, bandages can be used for a pressure dressing.

Even though pressure garments help decrease the formation of thick, disfiguring scars, patient acceptance is a problem. The garments are uncomfortable and make the patient warm, especially during hot weather. They must be tight enough to produce the 24 mm Hg of pressure required to exceed capillary pressure to be effective in reducing edema and scar formation. The patient must wear the garment 23 hours a day for 6 months to a year.

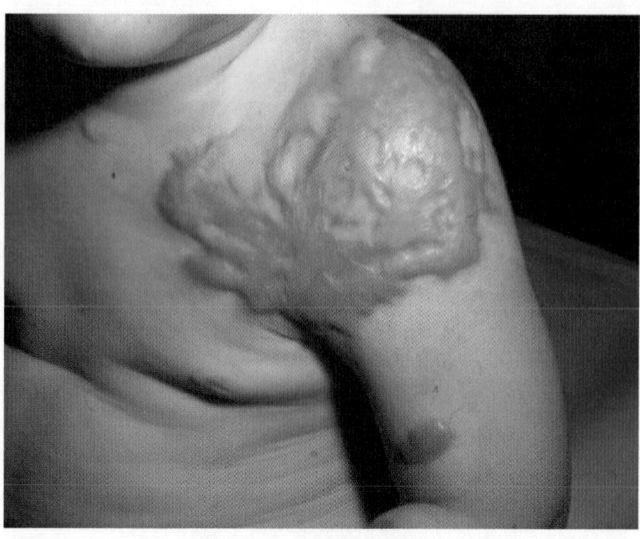

Figure 63-16 Severe hypertropic scarring.

A plan for exercise and splinting must be established before discharge. To prevent scar contractures, daily therapy sessions may be necessary for several weeks or months. The occupational therapist can develop aids to help with the ADLs.

5. Promoting Comfort

Although less severe, pain remains a problem during the rehabilitation phase. Small areas of skin may remain open and continue to require dressing changes. In addition, newly healed skin is sensitive. Physical and occupational therapy and increasing activity may result in discomfort. Interventions are focused on administration of analgesics, diversional activities, relaxation techniques, and providing information about what the patient can expect. Daily hydrotherapy helps the patient to relax tense muscles.

6, 7. Facilitating Individual and Family Coping

After discharge, the patient continues to adjust to temporary or permanent function loss, cosmetic disfigurement, and the reactions of others. The ability to manage depends on coping mechanisms before the burn, the severity and site of the burn, and the reaction of others. The patient's adaptation to these changes can be evaluated during outpatient visits when the burn team and appropriate personnel are available.[20]

Follow-up care may not take place at the institution where the patient was hospitalized. The burn team members may need to contact their counterparts in the community to plan follow-up care. If possible, a member of the follow-up team should visit the patient in the hospital before discharge.

Job retraining may be necessary if the burn injury caused loss of joint function or other physical limitations that prevent

Guidelines for Safe Practice

Teaching the Patient With a Burn

1. Patient/significant other verbalizes understanding of:
   a. Pathophysiology of the burn process
   b. Depth and percentage of the injury
   c. Functions of the skin
   d. Need for fluid replacement
2. Knowledge of the healing process
   a. Nutritional requirements
   b. Infection control measures
   c. Rationale for wound management
      (1) Hydrotherapy and debridement
      (2) Topical agents
      (3) Grafting
   d. Scar formation
      (1) Stages of development
      (2) Use of elastic bandage or pressure garments
      (3) Use of cosmetics and prosthetics
   e. Purpose of occupational and physical therapy toward improved mobility
      (1) Level of activity
      (2) Prescribed exercises
3. Pain management
   a. Relationship of pain to depth of injury
   b. Pain control options
      (1) Analgesics
      (2) Diversional activities
      (3) Meditation
      (4) Relaxation exercises
4. Discharge needs
   a. Skin care for healed areas
      (1) Protection from sun
      (2) Avoidance of chemical irritants
      (3) Increased sensitivity
      (4) Blister formation
   b. Skin care for open areas
      (1) Prescribed dressing
      (2) Application
      (3) Abnormal conditions
5. Application and care of pressure garments
6. Home care needs
   a. Care of clothing
   b. Cleanliness of the dressing change area (i.e., shower/bathtub)
   c. Adaptation of the home environment (i.e., handicap rails in bathtub or shower area)
7. Nutritional needs
   a. Basic four food groups
   b. Relationship of dietary intake to the healing process
8. Emotional readjustment
   a. To new body image
   b. Emotional reactions that may develop at home
      (1) Nightmares/flashbacks
      (2) Grief
      (3) Isolation
      (4) Depression
9. Dealing with reactions of others
10. Options for increasing social activity

the patient from returning to former employment. The local office of the State Labor and Industry Board can assign a vocational counselor to help the patient return to the workforce. Even if retraining cannot begin for several months, the contact with the vocational counselor and anticipation of retraining may help the patient look beyond immediate problems and think about the future.

8. Facilitating Learning

Discharge Teaching

Before discharge, burn patients and their families have a great need for education so that they can take increasing responsibility for their own care. Discharge teaching involves the entire burn team, who work together to prepare the patient and family for discharge.

Early discharge planning accomplishes two goals. First, it helps solve problems early. For example, if the patient's house burned and needs to be repaired, the family may need to relocate. This could be done before discharge, thus preventing the added stress of moving after discharge. Second, early discharge planning emphasizes the future. If discharge is discussed, the patient and his or her family may realize more quickly that recovery and return to home are possible.

Complete and comprehensive instructions followed by return demonstration contribute to learning the necessary skills to be independent in self-care activities after discharge. Patients with a major burn should not be discharged from the hospital until they can care for themselves physically, with assistance if necessary, and are prepared to meet the stresses involved in returning to their former living patterns. Teaching priorities are summarized in the Guidelines for Safe Practice box.

A major goal in discharge teaching is to prevent excessive scar formation by exercising, splinting, and applying pressure dressings. If these methods are not effective, reconstructive surgery may be necessary. A patient recovering from a major burn may need 12 to 18 months to achieve complete wound healing.

Instructions should include how to care for the healed graft and nongrafted areas. Signs and symptoms of complications, including areas that may blister and break down, and signs of infection are also addressed.

An example of written discharge instructions is provided in the Guidelines for Safe Practice box, and a Nursing Care Plan is found on pp. 2016 to 2018. Written instructions should include the name and phone number of a physician or nurse whom the patient may call with questions or problems concerning follow-up care. A referral may be made to a home health agency that may be of assistance in dressing the patient's wounds at home.

Nursing Care Plan — Patient With a Burn

DATA Mr. W. is a 63-year-old retired man with a history of adult-onset diabetes, diabetic neuropathy, peripheral vascular disease, and hypertension. The evening before admission to the hospital, Mr. W. filled his bathtub at home to soak his feet. Without checking the water temperature with his hands, he placed his feet and legs in the tub to soak for approximately 20 minutes. Because of decreased sensation in his feet and legs, he was unaware of the hot water temperature. On removing his feet from the tub, he noticed that his legs were bright red. The next morning his skin was still bright red and had blisters and weeping. After evaluation in the emergency department, he was admitted to the burn center.

Mr. W.'s wounds were cleansed with water and mild soap. Nonadherent skin was removed, an initial wound culture was obtained, and photos were taken. The wounds are dark red with poor capillary refill and assessed to be a 10% total body surface area, deep partial-thickness burn, circumferential from the toes to midcalf bilaterally.

Nursing assessment reveals:

- Mr. W. controls his diabetes by watching what he eats and taking an oral hypoglycemic agent. He does not monitor his blood glucose level routinely.
- Mr. W. lives alone in a two-story home. His daughter lives in the same city.
- Peripheral pulses are present on Doppler examination only.
- Mr. W. has diminished sensation in his lower extremities but identifies a burning, throbbing pain.
- Mr. W.'s blood pressure is 148/90, and his blood glucose level is 204 mg/dl.

NURSING DIAGNOSIS **Impaired skin integrity related to thermal injury**
GOALS/OUTCOMES Burn wounds will heal without complications

NOC Suggested Outcomes

- Tissue Integrity: Skin and Mucous Membranes (1101)
- Wound Healing: Secondary Intention (1103)

NIC Suggested Interventions

- Skin Care: Topical Treatments (3584)
- Skin Surveillance (3590)
- Wound Care (3660)

Nursing Interventions/Rationales

- Assess wounds with each dressing change for evidence of healing or infection. *Early detection of wound infection is essential to prevent deterioration of the wound and development of systemic infection.*
- Perform wound care (hydrotherapy and debridement) as prescribed using strict asepsis. *Meticulous wound care is essential to remove nonviable tissue, protect viable tissue, prevent infection, and promote healing.*
- Apply topical ointments/creams as prescribed. *Topical wound agents may change daily, depending on the condition of the wound. They promote healing and prevent infection.*
- Administer vitamins and minerals (vitamin A, ascorbic acid, and zinc) as ordered. *To promote wound healing. These agents are required for wound healing.*
- Monitor blood glucose levels before meals and at bedtime. *Poorly controlled diabetes mellitus impairs wound healing and promotes infection. Burn injury affects diabetes control because of the stress of the illness and hypermetabolism (for major burns).*
- Limit patient ambulation. Maintain leg elevation when in chair or bed. *To prevent edema from leg dependency. Increased edema at the burn site results in decreased tissue perfusion.*

Evaluation Parameters

1. Unburned skin remains intact
2. Absence of burn complications

NURSING DIAGNOSIS **Risk for infection related to loss of skin integrity and diabetes mellitus**
GOALS/OUTCOMES Will remain free of wound infection

NOC Suggested Outcomes

- Immune Status (0702)
- Risk Control (1902)
- Tissue Integrity: Skin and Mucous Membranes (1101)

NIC Suggested Interventions

- Skin Surveillance (2590)
- Infection Protection (6550)
- Wound Care (3660)

Nursing Interventions/Rationales

- Assess wounds during each dressing change for signs of localized infection. *Infection may be reflected by erythema at the wound edges; a pale, mottled, dry appearance of the wound; and purulent, foul-smelling drainage. The presence of wound infection will affect the type of topical agent selected.*
- Monitor for signs and symptoms of systemic infection (temperature elevation, altered sensorium, and elevated white blood cell [WBC] count). *Early detection of infection will allow for the appropriate selection of systemic or topical antimicrobial agents.*

Nursing Care Plan — Patient With a Burn—cont'd

- Obtain a wound sample for culture twice weekly, as ordered. *Tracking bacterial colonization of the wound allows for early detection of pathogens so that treatment can be initiated.*
- Maintain aseptic wound technique and thorough cleansing of equipment and hydrotherapy tubs/tables. *Prevents cross-contamination of bacteria between patients that may cause infection.*

Evaluation Parameters

1. Evidence of wound healing
2. Absence of purulent drainage, increased redness
3. Absence of fever, elevated WBC count
4. Accurately lists signs and symptoms of infection

NURSING DIAGNOSIS **Acute pain related to tissue injury**
GOALS/OUTCOMES Will achieve pain-free status

NOC Suggested Outcomes

- Pain Level (2102)
- Pain Control (1605)

NIC Suggested Interventions

- Pain Management (1400)
- Analgesic Administration (2210)
- Progressive Muscle Relaxation (1460)

Nursing Interventions/Rationales

- Assess pain level using a pain rating scale of 1 to 10 at least every 4 hours, during wound care, and during physical therapy. *Determining the patient's perception of pain assists with selection of an appropriate analgesic agent and dose.*
- Administer analgesia around the clock. *Burn pain is constant. Better pain control can be achieved when pain medication is administered on a scheduled basis.*
- Provide analgesia before hydrotherapy and wound care. *Pain will increase during wound care and physical therapy. Pain control allows for more active participation by the patient.*
- Maintain elevation of legs while in bed or chair. *Dependent leg positions increase pain because of venous pooling and the formation of edema.*
- Encourage use of nonpharmacologic methods of pain control (imagery, distraction, relaxation). *Nonpharmacologic methods increase pain control when used in conjunction with pharmacologic agents.*

Evaluation Parameters

1. Reports pain reduced or controlled
2. No facial grimace or expressions of pain
3. Demonstrates use of nonpharmacologic methods of pain control
4. Reports satisfaction with pain control measures

NURSING DIAGNOSIS **Risk for ineffective therapeutic regimen management related to lack of knowledge of burn process, treatment regimen, signs and symptoms of complications, and burn injury prevention**
GOALS/OUTCOMES Will develop and follow a plan for maintaining therapeutic regimen

NOC Suggested Outcomes

- Knowledge: Treatment Regimen (1813)
- Participation: Health Care Decisions (1606)
- Adherence Behavior (1600)

NIC Suggested Interventions

- Learning Facilitation (5520)
- Teaching: Prescribed Procedure/Treatment (5618)
- Self-Modification Assistance (4470)

Nursing Interventions/Rationales

- Assess patient's physical and cognitive ability to perform wound care. *The patient's ability to perform wound care will help determine discharge needs (i.e., home health care versus performing by self).*
- Instruct patient to apply lotion to affected skin areas two or three times each day. *Lotion helps maintain moisture of newly healed tissue and prevents tissue breakdown. Newly healed skin is prone to itching, flaking, and dryness.*
- Encourage patient to wear socks and well-fitted shoes. *Tight shoes predispose healed areas of the feet to tissue breakdown. This is especially important for patients with diabetes who have decreased sensation in their feet.*

Continued

Nursing Care Plan — Patient With a Burn–cont'd

- Avoid exposure of healed wounds to chemicals or extremes in temperature. *Tissue is fragile initially and will easily be reinjured.*
- Provide patient with a bath thermometer to assess the temperature of water before bathing. *Decreased sensation of the feet from diabetic neuropathy limits the patient's ability to determine the water temperature. The water temperature should be 100° to 105° F (37.8° to 40.5° C).*
- Instruct patient to turn the temperature of his home hot water tank down to 54.4° C (130° F). *A water temperature of 150° F (65.5° C) (a common hot water tank setting) will result in full-thickness burns in approximately 1 second. It takes 30 seconds for a full-thickness burn to occur at 130° F (54.4° C), decreasing the possibility of future injury.*

Stress importance of maintaining blood glucose levels within normal range. *Poorly controlled diabetes mellitus contributes to diabetic neuropathy and infection and impairs healing.*

Refer patient to community resources as appropriate. *The patient may need assistance with controlling diabetes or changing lifestyle habits to prevent future injuries.*

Evaluation Parameters

1. Verbalizes understanding of wound care needs
2. Performs wound care accurately
3. Identifies skin care for healed areas
4. Identifies actions that predispose to burn injury
5. Verbalizes need to control blood glucose levels within normal range

EVALUATION

To evaluate the effectiveness of nursing interventions, compare patient behaviors with those stated in the expected patient outcomes. Achievement of patient outcomes is successful if the patient:

1. Has full range of motion and mobility.
1a. Demonstrates exercise program for the prevention and control of contractures.
2. Is able to perform ADLs.
2a. Cares for own burn scars and applies dressings as necessary.
2b. Performs daily routine without assistance.
3. Has a realistic body image.
3a. Speaks openly about change in appearance.
3b. Participates in activities with nonburned persons.
3c. Presents self positively.
4. Maintains skin integrity.
4a. Identifies techniques to prevent breakdown of healed areas (e.g., protection from sun, exposure to harsh chemicals, use of lubricating lotions, and proper use of pressure garments).
5. Controls pain.
5a. Rates pain control as acceptable.
5b. States is able to sleep.
5c. Is able to perform daily routines without increasing pain.
6. Exhibits positive coping behaviors.
6a. Identifies alterations in personal situation and identifies strategies to improve it.
6b. Develops positive self-concept.
6c. Reintegrates into the community.
7. Family exhibits positive coping behaviors.
7a. Family identifies alterations in patient's and family's situation and identifies strategies to improve it.
8. Understands the treatment regimen.
8a. Is able to explain daily routine and the reasons for it.
8b. Discusses hospital and community resources available for assistance.
8c. States date and time of next medical follow-up.
8d. States name of health care provider to call in an emergency.

COMMUNITY-BASED CARE

Patient support services need to be available through rehabilitative and outpatient services. With patients being discharged earlier, education about their care requirements and wound care is generally completed after discharge. Treatment plans and teaching for all patients start at the onset of injury and continue throughout their course of healing whether they are in the hospital or are being treated in an outpatient setting. All team members are available, and resources are provided to patients and families at the different levels of healing. Support groups are available to assist patients with resocialization and coping with their burn injury for many years after their discharge.

COMPLICATIONS

Complications may occur during any phase in burn management. The most common complications are wound infections, contractures, and psychologic problems, with some persons developing PTSD. Each of these conditions has been discussed within the chapter.

Guidelines for Safe Practice

Discharge Instructions for the Patient With a Burn

We on the burn team are happy to see that you are able to go home. To ensure the speediest possible recovery, it is important that you be able to care for yourself and recognize problems that may interfere with your complete recovery.

If any of the following occur, please call the hospital and ask for the Burn Clinic. The nurse will be able to assist you.

1. Healed area breaking open (Cover with a clean dressing.)
2. Formation of blisters
3. Signs of infection
   a. Fever, temperature higher than 100.4° F (38° C)
   b. Redness, pain, swelling, hardness, or warmth in or around the wound or any other part of the body
   c. Increased or foul-smelling drainage from the wound
4. Problems with your elastic bandages or Jobst garment, such as improper fit, formation of blisters, or opening of the healed area underneath

Your first clinic appointment will be on ______.

BATHING

Bathing or showering daily in your usual manner cleans the wounds, especially the ones that are still open.

1. Check the water and be sure to adjust the temperature to a warm and comfortable level. Your skin is more sensitive to extra heat or cold and can be easily injured.
2. Wash gently with a clean, soft washcloth, using a mild detergent soap such as Dial or Ivory. Be careful not to rub too hard so as not to disturb the grafted areas. Avoid harsh or deodorant soaps.
3. Rinse skin thoroughly after washing.
4. Dry thoroughly.
5. Apply specific dressing as instructed.

CARE FOR BURN WOUND

These are your guidelines for the care of your burn wound. During this time, look at the involved areas and note any changes that need to be reported.

1. Wash hands.
2. Remove dressing and dispose of in a paper bag or wrap in newspaper.
3. Wash hands.
4. Wash open area with a clean soft washcloth and Dial or Ivory soap and water. Use a clean towel and washcloth with each dressing change.
5. Rinse skin well with plain water.
6. Wash hands.
7. Apply dressing as described below.
8. Wear gloves. Wash basin or bathtub with a disinfectant such as Lysol.
9. Wash hands.

CARE OF CLOTHING

When you are discharged, you may find that healed burn areas are sensitive to harsh detergents, fabric softeners, and clothing dyes. If you are sensitive, we suggest the following:

1. Launder new clothing before use, by machine or by hand, with a detergent free of additives.
2. Rinse clothes twice.
3. Do not use fabric softeners.
4. If you have open burns or a healed area that opens, wash all clothes separately from those of other family members.
5. Scarlet Red ointment will permanently stain clothing.
6. If dyes used in clothing cause irritation, wear white articles.
7. Wear loose-fitting clothing.

ELASTIC BANDAGES

You have been taught to put on your own elastic bandages while in the hospital, but if you do have a problem with this, please notify the Burn Clinic. It is also important that you know how to care for them and understand problems that occur.

1. If they are too loose, they will be ineffective and must be rewrapped.
2. If they are too tight, they will cause discomfort, numbness, tingling, and puffiness and must be rewrapped.
3. They must be worn for a long period of time, probably 6 to 12 months, to be effective, so please do not stop wearing them until your doctor tells you.
4. To care for your elastic bandages:
   a. Hand wash with a mild detergent in cold water.
   b. Towel dry.
   c. Lay flat to dry.

PRESSURE GARMENT

You have been taught to put on your pressure garment while in the hospital, but if you have a problem with this, please notify the Burn Clinic. It is also important that you know how to care for it and understand problems that can occur.

1. If it is too loose, it will be ineffective and you will require a new garment.
2. If it is too tight, it will cause discomfort, numbness, and tingling. Do not wear it if this occurs, but notify the Burn Clinic as soon as possible.
3. To care for your pressure garment:
   a. Hand wash with a mild detergent in cold water.
   b. Towel dry.
   c. Lay flat to dry.

DIET

A well-balanced diet is important as your burn wound continues to heal. Be sure to include meat, milk products, breads and cereals, and fruits and vegetables in your diet.

YOUR EMOTIONS

It is not uncommon to feel blue or let down after you go home. The Burn Support Group meets every Thursday to help you.

Courtesy Comprehensive Burn Center, MetroHealth Medical Center, Cleveland, Ohio.

Critical Thinking Questions

1. Two 30-year-old men are brought to the emergency department after burns from a house fire. One man has a partial-thickness burn, and the other has a full-thickness burn. What subjective data would help differentiate these two types of burns?
2. Incorporating general principles of psychologic care, develop one nursing approach for each of the following patient responses to a severe burn: withdrawal, regression, anger/hostility, and depression.
3. Describe the burn prevention teaching for a 60-year-old man with chronic obstructive pulmonary disease and diabetes being discharged home while receiving oxygen therapy.
4. Discuss the differences in priorities of care during the emergent and rehabilitation phases of burn injury.

References

1. American Burn Association: *Advanced burn life support course: prehospital manual,* Chicago, 1994, ABA.
2. American Burn Association: *Advanced burn life support course: provider's manual,* Chicago, 2001, ABA.
3. American College of Surgeons: Resources for optimal care of patients with burn injury. In *Resources for optimal care of the injured patient 1999,* Chicago, 1998, ACS.
4. American Psychiatric Association: *Diagnostic and statistical manual of mental disorders: DSM-IV-TR,* ed 4, Washington, DC, 2000, APA.
5. Baur KM, Hardy PE, Van Dorsten B: Posttraumatic stress disorder in burn populations: a critical review of the literature, *J Burn Care Rehabil* 19:230-240, 1998.
6. Chang TT, Lipinski CA, Sherman HF: A hazard of home oxygen therapy, *J Burn Care Rehabil* 22:71-74, 2001.
7. Chrysopoulo MT et al: Acute renal dysfunction in severely burned adults, *J Trauma* 46:141-144, 1999.
8. Committee on the Organization and Delivery of Burn Care: *Burn care resources in North America 1999-2000,* Chicago, 1999, American Burn Association.
9. Demling RH, DeSanti L: Oxandrolone, an anabolic steroid, significantly increases weight gain in the recovery phase after major burns, *J Trauma* 43:47-51, 1997.
10. Ehde DM et al: Post-traumatic stress symptoms and distress 1 year after burn injury, *J Burn Care Rehabil* 21:105-111, 2000.
11. Gamiel Z, DeBiasse MA, Demling RH: Essential microminerals and their response to burn injury, *J Burn Care Rehabil* 17:264-272, 1996.
12. Gordon M, Goodwin CW: Initial assessment, management, and stabilization, *Nurs Clin North Am* 32(2):237-249, 1997.
13. Huang YS et al: Pathogenesis of early cardiac myocyte damage after severe burns. *J Trauma* 46:428-432, 1999.
14. Jackson DM: The diagnosis of the depth of burning, *Br J Surg* 40:588-596, 1953.
15. Kao CC, Garner WL: Acute burns, *Plast Reconstr Surg* 101:2482-2492, 2000.
16. Kaups KL, Davis JW, Dominic WJ: Base deficit as an indicator of resuscitation needs in patients with burn injuries, *J Burn Care Rehabil* 19:346-348, 1998.
17. Kramer GC, Nguyen TT: Pathophysiology of burn shock and burn edema. In Herndon DN, editor: *Total burn care,* London, 1996, WB Saunders.
18. Lund T: Edema generation following thermal injury: an update, *J Burn Care Rehabil* 20:445-452, 1999.
19. Mayes T, Gottschlich MM, Warden GD: Clinical nutritional protocols for continuous quality improvements in the outcomes of patients with burns, *J Burn Care Rehabil* 18:365-368, 1997.
20. Mertens, DM, Jenkins ME, Warden GD: Outpatient burn management, *Nurs Clin North Am* 32(2):343-364, 1997.
21. Munster AM: The immunological response and strategies for intervention. In Herndon DN, editor: *Total burn care,* London, 1996, WB Saunders.
22. National Fire Prevention Association: *Information about smoke alarms, 2001,* website: http://nfpa.org.
23. Patterson DR et al: Describing and predicting distress and satisfaction with life for burn survivors, *J Burn Care Rehabil* 21:490-498, 2000.
24. Ramzy PI, Barret JP, Herndon DN: Thermal injury, *Crit Care Clin* 15:333-352, 1999.
25. Rutan RL: Physiologic response to cutaneous burn injury. In Carrougher GJ, editor: *Burn care and therapy,* St Louis, 1998, Mosby.
26. Schiller WR et al: Laser Doppler evaluation of burned hands predicts need for surgical grafting, *J Trauma* 43:35-39, 1997.
27. Sheridan RL, Tompkins RG: Skin substitutes in burns, *Burns* 25:97-103, 1999.
28. Tadros T, Traber DL, Herndon DN: Hepatic blood flow and oxygen consumption after burn and sepsis, *J Trauma* 49:101-108, 2000.
29. US Department of Health and Human Services: *Healthy People 2010: understanding and improving health,* Washington, DC, 2000, USDHHS.
30. Warden GD: Fluid resuscitation and early management. In Herndon DN, editor: *Total burn care,* London, 1996, WB Saunders.
31. Winifree J, Barillo DJ: Nonthermal injuries, *Nurs Clin North Am* 32(2):275-296, 1997.
32. Yowler CJ, Fratianne RJ: Current status of burn resuscitation, *Clin Plast Surg* 27:1-10, 2000.

Selected Bibliography

CHAPTER 1: MEDICAL-SURGICAL NURSING TODAY

Nursing Shortage

American Association of Colleges of Nursing: *Faculty shortages intensify nation's nursing deficit,* Washington DC, 1999, AACN.

American Association of Colleges of Nursing: *1999-2000 enrollment and graduations in baccalaureate and graduate programs in nursing,* Washington DC, 2000, AACN.

American Association of Colleges of Nursing: *The baccalaureate degree in nursing as minimal preparation for professional practice,* Washington DC, 2000, AACN.

American Hospital Association: The hospital workforce shortage: immediate and future, *TrendWatch* 3(2):2, 2001.

Minnick A: The RN workforce in 2005: retirement and the baby boomers, Paper presented at the November meeting of the American Academy of Nursing, Alexandria, Va, 1999.

Nevidjon B, Erickson, JI: The nursing shortage: solutions for the short and long term, *Online J Issues Nurs* 6(1):manuscript 4, 2001.

Peterson CA: Nursing shortage: not a simple problem—no easy answers, *Online J Issues Nurs* 6(1):manuscript 1, 2001.

Prescott P: The enigmatic nursing workforce, *J Nurs Adm* 2:59, 2000.

Taft S: The nursing shortage, *Online J Issues Nurs* 6(1):overview, 2001.

William M Mercer: *Attracting and retaining registered nurses—survey results,* Chicago, 1999, Author.

CHAPTER 2: COMPLEMENTARY AND ALTERNATIVE THERAPIES

General

Fadiman A: *The spirit catches you and you fall down,* New York, 1997, Farrar, Straus, Giroux.

Freeman LW, Lawlis GF: *Complementary and alternative medicine: a research-based approach,* St Louis, 2001, Mosby.

Guzzetta CE: *Essential readings in holistic nursing,* Gaithersburg, Md, 1998, Aspen Publishing Inc.

Hutchinson CP: Healing touch: an energetic approach, *Am J Nurs* 99(4):43, 1999.

Klotz LK et al: Impact of complementary healing modalities on quality of life and treatment adherence for a family with breast cancer: a case study approach, *Int J Hum Caring* 3:7, 1999.

Snyder M, Lindquist R: *Complementary/alternative therapies in nursing,* New York, 1998, Spring Publishing.

Spencer J, Jacobs J: *Complementary/alternative medicine: an evidence-based approach,* St Louis, 1998, Mosby.

Biologically Based Treatments

Barrett B et al: Assessing the risks and benefits of herbal medicine: an overview of scientific research, *Alternative Ther* 5:40, 1999.

Blumenthal M et al: *The German Commission E Monographs: therapeutic monographs on medicinal plants for human use,* Austin, Tx, 1998, American Botanical Council.

Buckle J: Use of aromatherapy as a complementary treatment for chronic pain, *Alternative Ther* 5:42, 1999.

Gruenwald J et al, editors: *PDR for herbal medicine,* Montvale, NJ, 1998, Medical Economics Company.

Murphy J: Preoperative considerations with herbal medicine, *AORN J* 69:173, 1999.

PDR for herbal medicine, ed 2, Montvale, NJ, 2000, Medical Economics.

PDR for nonprescription drugs and dietary supplements, ed 20, Montvale, NJ, 1999, Medical Economics.

Peirce A: *The American Pharmaceutical Association guide to natural medicine,* New York, 1999, William Morrow.

Waddell DL et al: Three herbs you should get to know, *Am J Nurs* 101(4):48, 2001.

Wilt TJ et al: Saw palmetto extracts for treatment of benign prostatic hyperplasia: a systematic review, *JAMA* 280:1604, 1998.

CAT Journals

Alternative Therapies in Health and Medicine
InnoVision Communication, a division of the American Association of Critical Care Nurses
101 Columbia
Aliso Viejo, Ca 92656

Alternative Medicine Review: A Journal of Clinical Therapeutics
Thorne Research, Inc.
PO Box 3200
Sandpoint, Idaho 83864
208-263-1337
Fax 208-265-2488

HerbalGram
American Botanical Council
PO Box 144345
Austin, Tx 78714-4345
512-926-4900
Fax 512-926-2345
www.herbalgram.org

Integrative Medicine: Integrating Complementary and alternative medicine
Elsevier Science Ltd.
PO Box 800
Oxford OX5 1DX, United Kingdom

CHAPTER 3: PROMOTING HEALTHY LIFESTYLES

Health Promotion and Prevention

Andersen RE: Healthy people 2010 steps in the right direction, *PhysicianSports Med* 28(10):7, 2000.

Burggraf V, Barry RJ: Healthy People 2010: protecting the health of older individuals, *J Gerontol Nurs* 16, 2000.

Jaret P: Healthy people 2010: helping people change, *Hippocrates* 14(1):25, 2000.

Kavanaugh T et al: Risk profile and health awareness in male offspring of parents with premature coronary health disease, *J Cardiopulmon Rehabil* 20(3):172, 2000.

Sheahan SL: Documentation of health risks and health promotion counseling by emergency department nurse practitioners and physicians, *J Nurs Scholarship* 32(3):245, 2000.

Wieck KL: Health promotion for inner-city minority elders, *J Community Health Nurs* 17(3):131, 2000.

Nutrition and Weight Management

Author: Sibutramine in patients with hypertension, *Nurses Drug Alert* 24(10):76, 2000.

Beamer BA: Exercise to prevent and treat diabetes mellitus, *Physician Sports Med* 28(10):85, 2000.

Berkowitz VJ, Rock CL: A view on high-protein, low-carb diets. High-protein, low-carbohydrate diets: do they work? *J Am Diet Assoc* 100(11):1300, 2000.

Lenaghan NA: The nurse's role in smoking cessation, *Med Surg Nurs* 9(6):298, 2000.

Terry P: What should we do about excess weight? *J Am Diet Assoc* 100(11):1303, 2000.

Winkleby MA et al: Ethnic and socioeconomic differences in cardiovascular disease risk factors: findings for women from the Third National Health and Nutrition Examination Survey, 1988-1994, *JAMA* 280(4):356, 1998.

Exercise

Chen J, Miller WJ: Health effects of physical exercise, *Health Rep* 10(3):35, 1999.

Crespo CJ: Encouraging physical activity in minorities eliminating disparities by 2010, *Physician Sports Med* 28(10):36, 2000.

Fontaine KR: Physical activity improves mental health, *Physician Sports Med* 28(10):83, 2000.

McKinney R, Andersen RE: Exercise benefits patients with osteoarthritis, *Physician Sports Med* 28(10):71, 2000.

Sherwood NE, Jeffery RW: Behavioral determinants of exercise: implications for physical activity interventions, *Annu Rev Nutr* 20:21, 2000.

Regimen Adherence

Hays BJ et al: Public health nursing data building the knowledge base for high-risk prenatal clients, *MCN Am J Matern Child Nurs* 25(3):151, 2000.

Kaiser KL et al: Patterns of health resource utilization, costs and intensity of need for primary care clients receiving public health nursing case management, *Nurs Case Manage* 4(2):53, 1999.

Nisbeth O et al: Effectiveness of counseling over 1 year on changes in lifestyle and coronary heart disease risk factors, *Patient Educ Counseling* 40:121, 2000.

Svedlund M, Axelsson I: Acute myocardial infarction in middle-aged women: narrations from the patients and partners during rehabilitation, *Intensive Crit Care Nurs* 16(4):256, 2000.

Thomson P: A review of behavioral change theories in patient compliance to exercise-based rehabilitation following acute myocardial infarction, *Coron Health Care* 3(1):18, 1999.

Tobin B: Getting back to normal: women's recovery after a myocardial infarction, *Can J Cardiovasc Nurs* 11(2):11, 2000.

Smoking Cessation

Gauen S: Ways to help patients quit smoking, *Am J Health Syst Pharm* 56(5):425, 1999.

Martinelli AM: Testing a model of avoiding environmental tobacco smoke in young adults, *J Nurs Scholarship* 31(3):237, 1999.

Sarna L: Higher priority on tobacco control. Nursing knowledge for the 21st century: opportunities and challenges, *J Nurs Scholarship* 32(4):332, 2000.

White J: Wellness Wednesdays: health promotion and service learning on campus, *J Nurs Educ* 38(2):69 1999.

CHAPTER 4: NURSING CARE OF OLDER ADULTS

General

Chang SO: The conceptual structure of physical touch in caring, *J Adv Nurs* 33(6):820, 2001.

Ebersole P: Leaders in geriatric nursing: Kathleen Cole Buckwalter, *Geriatr Nurs* 22(2):92, 2001.

Smyth C et al: Creating order out of chaos: models of GNP practice with hospitalized older adults, *Clin Excellence Nurse Pract* 5(2):88, 2001.

Stiles T, Lucyk B: Surfing the gray wave, *RN* 13(2):8, 2001.

Trenethick MJ: Thriving, not just surviving: the importance of social support among the older, *J Psychosocial Nurs* 35(9):27, 1997.

Wynkle ML: Gerontological nursing research: challenges for the new millennium, *J Gerontol Nurs* 27(4):7, 2001.

Zigmond et al: Circumstances at HIV diagnosis and progression of disease in older HIV-infected Americans, *Am J Public Health* 91(7):1117, 2001.

Assessment

Ennis BW et al: Diagnosing malnutrition in the older, *Nurse Pract* 26(3):52, 2001.

Heath H, White I: Sexuality and older people: an introduction to nursing assessment, *Nurs Older People* 13(4):29, 2001.

Katsma DL, Souza CH: Older pain assessment and pain management knowledge of long-term care nurses, *Pain Manage Nurs* 1(3):88, 2000.

Klaas D: Testing two elements of spirituality in depressed and non-depressed older adults, *Int J Psychiatr Nurs Res* 4(2):452, 1998.

Maher S: Assessing age-related sleep disorders, *Nurs Older People* 13(3):27, 2001.

Miller J et al: The assessment of acute confusion as part of nursing care, *Appl Nurs Res* 10(3):131, 1997.

Spencer G: The role of exercising in successful ageing, *Prof Nurse* 15(2):105, 1999.

Traynor V, Dewing J: RCN news: assessing admirals, *Nurs Older People* 13(3):30, 2001.

Watson R: Assessing the musculoskeletal system in older people, *Nurs Older People* 13(5):29, 2001.

Watson R: Assessing the gastrointestinal (GI) tract in older people: the lower GI tract, *Nurs Older People* 13(1):27, 2001.

Willis T, Ford P: Assessing older people—contemporary issues for nursing, *Nurs Older People* 12(9):16, 2000.

CHAPTER 5: CHRONIC ILLNESS

General

Allonzo AA: The experience of chronic illness and post-traumatic stress disorder: the consequence cumulative adversity, *Soc Sci Med* 50:1475, 2000.

Barker DJP: A new model for the origins of chronic disease, *Med Health Philosophy* 31, 2001.

Fried LP et al: Association of comorbidity with disability in older women: the women's health and study, *J Clin Epidemiol* 52:27, 1999.
Nesbitt BJ, Heidrich SM: Sense of coherence and illness appraisal in older women's quality of life, *Nurs Health* 23(1):25, 2000.
Stroupe KT et al: Does chronic illness affect the adequacy of health insurance coverage? *J Health Polit Policy Law* 25:309, 2000.
Thorne SE: The science of meaning in chronic illness, *Int J Nurs Stud* 36:397, 1999.
Thorne SE et al: Attitudes toward patient expertise in chronic illness, *Int J Nurs Stud* 37:303,2000.

Ethnicity and Health

Silverman M et al: Self care for chronic illness: older African-Americans and Whites, *J Cross-Cultural Gerontology* 14:169,1999.

CHAPTER 6: LOSS, GRIEF, DYING, AND END-OF-LIFE CARE

General

Coyle N, Layman-Goldstein M: Pain assessment and management in palliative care. In Matzo MI, Sherman DW, editors: *Palliative care nursing: quality care to the end of life,* New York, 2001, Springer.
Edmonds P et al: Is the presence of dyspnea a risk factor for morbidity in cancer patients? *J Pain Symptom Manage* 19(1):15, 2000.
Ellershaw J et al: Care of the dying: setting standards for symptom control in the last 48 hours of life, *J Pain Symptom Manage* 21(1):12, 2001.
Furman J: Preventing chronic grief, *Nursing 2002,* 32(2):56, 2002.
Given BA et al: Family support in advanced cancer, *CA Cancer J Clin* 51 (4):213, 2001.
Hermann CP. Spiritual needs of dying patients: a qualitative study, *Oncol Nurs Forum* 28(1):67, 2001.
Hickman SE et al: Family reports of dying patients' distress: the adaptation of a research tool to assess global symptom distress in the last week of life, *J Pain Symptom Manage* 22(1):565, 2001.
Panke JT: Difficulties in managing pain at the end of life, *Am J Nurs* 102(7):26, 2002.
Smith-Stoner M: How to build your "hope" skills, *Nursing 99* 29(9):49, 1999.
Teno JM et al: Validation of Toolkit After-Death Bereaved Family Member Interview, *J Pain Symptom Manage* Sept22(3):752-758, 2001.
Volker DL: Oncology nurses' experiences with requests for assisted dying from terminally ill patients with cancer, *Oncol Nurs Forum* 28(1):39, 2001.
Wildiers H, Menten J: Death rattle: prevalence, prevention and treatment, *J Pain Symptom Manage* 23(4):310, 2002.

Communication

Becker R: Teaching communication with the dying across cultural boundaries, *Br J Nurs* 8(14):938, 1999.
Linkewich B et al: Communicating at life's end, *Can Nurse* 95(5):41, 1999.
Stanley KJ: Silence is not golden: conversations with the dying, *Clin J Oncol Nurs* 4(1):34, 2000.

The Dying Experience

Costello J: Nursing older dying patients: findings from an ethnographic study of death and dying in elderly care wards, *J Adv Nurs* 35(1):59, 2001.
Dendaas NR: Prognostication in advance cancer: nurses' perceptions of the dying process, *Oncol Nurs Forum* 29(3):493, 2002.
Fox A: Dying at home: supporting patient choices, *Nurs Times* 95(5):50, 1999.
McGrath P: Caregivers' insights on the dying trajectory in hematology oncology, *Cancer Nurs* 24(5):413, 2001.
Middlewood S et al: Dying in hospital: medical failure or natural outcome? *J Pain Symptom Manage* 22(6):1035, 2001.
Rooda LA et al: Nurses' attitudes toward death and caring for dying patients, *Oncol Nurs Forum* 26(10):1683, 1999.
Tarzian AJ: Caring for dying patients who have air hunger, *J Nurs Scholarship* 32(2):137, 2000.
Tolle SW et al: Family reports of barriers to optimal care of the dying, *Nurs Res* 49(6):310, 2000.
Yang MH, McIlfatrick S: Intensive care nurses' experiences of caring for dying patients: a phenomenological study, *Int J Palliat Nurs* 7(9):435, 2001.
Yedidia MJ, MacGregor B: Confronting the prospect of dying: reports of terminally ill patients, *J Pain Symptom Manage* 22(4):807, 2001.

End of Life

Campbell ML: End of life care in the ICU: current practice and future hopes, *Crit Care Nurs Clin North Am* 14(2):197, ix, 2002.
Fins JJ et al: End-of-life decision-making in the hospital: current practice and future prospects, *J Pain Symptom Manage* 17(1):6, 1999.
Norton SA, Talerico KA: Facilitating end-of-life decision-making: strategies for communicating and assessing, *J Gerontol Nurs* 26(9):6, 2000.
Pierce SF: Improving end-of-life care: gathering suggestions from family members, *Nurs Forum* 34(2):5, 1999.
Steinhauser KE et al: Preparing for the end of life: preferences of patients, families, physicians, and other care providers, *J Pain Symptom Manage* 22(3):727, 2001.
Zuckerman C, Wollner D: End of life care and decision making: how far we have come, how far we have to go: review, *Hosp J* 14(3-4):85, 1999.

Ethical and Legal Issues

Ladd RE, Pasquerella L, Smith S: What to do when the end is near: ethical issues in home health care nursing, *Public Health Nurs* 17(2):103, 2000.

Grief and Bereavement

Furman J: Preventing chronic grief, *Nursing 2002* 32(2):56, 2002.
Krohn B: When death is near: helping families cope, *Geriatr Nurs* 19(5):276, 1998.

Quality of Life

Annells M, Koch T: "The real stuff": implications for nursing of assessing and measuring a terminally ill person's quality of life, *J Clin Nurs* 10(6):806, 2001.

Palliative and Hospice Care

Coyle N, Layman-Goldstein M: Pain assessment and management in palliative care. In Matzo MI, Sherman DW, editors: *Palliative care nursing: quality care to the end of life,* New York, 2001, Springer.
Kulbe J: Stressors and coping measures of hospice nurses, *Home Health Nurse* 19(11):707, 2001.
McGrath P et al: "What should I say?": qualitative findings on dilemmas in palliative care nursing, *Hosp J* 14(2):17, 1999.
Moody LE et al: Assessing readiness for death in hospice elders and older adults, *Hosp J* 15(2):49, 2001.
Owens MR et al: A pilot program to evaluate pain assessment skills of hospice nurses, *Am J Hosp Palliat Care* 17(1):44, 2000.
Ronaldson S, Devery K: The experience of transition to palliative care services: perspectives of patients and nurses, *Int J Palliat Nurs* 7(4):171, 2001.

CHAPTER 7: EMERGENCY CARE

General

Arslanian-Engoren C: Gender and age bias in triage decisions, *J Emerg Nurs* 26(2):117, 2000.

Bell K: Identification and documentation of bite marks, *J Emerg Nurs* 26(6):628, 2000.

Blank FS, Keyes M: Thrombolytic therapy for patients with acute stroke in the ED, *J Emerg Nurs* 26(1):24, 2000.

Cheung DS, Kharasch M: Evaluation of the patient with closed head trauma: an evidence based approach, *Emerg Med Clin North Am* 17(1):9, 2001.

Killerman A, Heron S: Firearms and family violence, *Emerg Med Clin North Am* 17(3):699, 1999

Ledrey LE, Fuagmo D: SANE: advocate, forensic technician, nurse? *J Emerg Nurs* 27(1):91, 2001.

Linden J: Sexual assault, *Emerg Clin* 17(3):685, 1999.

Pasqualone GA, Fitzgerald SM: Munchausen by proxy syndrome: the forensic challenge of recognition, diagnosis and reporting, *Crit Care Nurs Q* 22(1):52, 1999.

Wright V, Akers, A: The community awareness rape education (CARE) program for high school students, *J Emerg Nurs* 26(2):182, 2000.

Yam M: Seen but not heard: battered women's perceptions of the ED experience, *J Emerg Nurs* 26(5):464, 2000.

CHAPTER 8: CRITICAL CARE

General

Ahrens T: Role of technology in achieving clinical and cost impact in acute and critical care, *Crit Care Nurs Clin North Am* 11:1, 1999.

Alspach JG: *Core curriculum for critical care nursing,* ed 5, Philadelphia, 1998, WB Saunders.

Dyson M: Intensive care unit psychosis, the therapeutic nurse-patient relationship and the influence of the intensive care setting: analyses of interrelating factors, *J Clin Nurs* 8:284, 1999.

Hurlock-Chorostecki C: Holistic care in the critical care setting: application of a concept through Watson's and Orem's theories of nursing, *CACCN* 10:20, 1999.

Llenore E, Ogle KR: Nurse-patient communication in the intensive care unit: a review of the literature *Aust Crit Care* 12:142, 1999.

Lynn-McHale DJ, Carlson KK: *AACN Procedure manual for critical care,* ed 4, Philadelphia, 2001, WB Saunders.

Maddox M et al: Psychosocial recovery following ICU: experiences and influences upon discharge to the community *Intensive Crit Care Nurs* 17:6, 2001.

Pastores SM, Halpern NA: Striving to get new technology into the critical care environment: strategies and a checklist to improve your chances of success, *J Crit Illness* 15:351, 2000.

Redeker NS: Sleep in acute care settings: an integrative review, *J Nurs Scholarship* 32:31, 2000.

CHAPTER 9: COMMUNITY-BASED CARE

Community-Based Nursing

Feensta C: Community based and community focused: nursing education in community health, *Public Health Nurs* 17(3):155, 2000.

Iliffe S, Drennan V: Primary care for older people: learning the lessons of history, *Community Pract* 73(5):602, 2000.

Jarrett NJ et al: Terminally ill patients' and lay-carers' perceptions and experiences of community-based services, *J Adv Nurs* 29(2):476, 1999.

McElmurry BJ, Keeny GB: Primary health care, *Annu Rev Nurs Res* 17:241, 1999.

Schmidt SM et al: Epidemiologic determination of community-based nursing case management for stroke, *J Nurs Adm* 29(6):40, 1999.

Van-Ort S, Townsend J: Community-based nursing education and nursing accreditation by the Commission on Collegiate Nursing Education, *J Prof Nurs* 16(6):330, 2000.

Home Care

Anderson AA et al: Unplanned hospital readmissions: a home care perspective, *Nurs Res* 48(6):299, 1999.

Hall D: Change, continuity and function of the community health visitor, *Community Pract* 73(12):870, 2000.

Hays BJ et al: Quantifying client need for care in the community: a strategy for managed care, *Public Health Nurs* 16(4):246, 1999.

Madigan EA, Fortinsky RH: Alternative measures of resource consumption in home care episodes, *Public Health Nurs* 16(3):198, 1999.

Murray TA: Using role theory concepts to understand transitions from hospital-based nursing practice to home care nursing, *J Contin Educ Nurs* 29(3):105, 1998.

Rice R: Home visit safety, *Geriatric Nursing* 19(4):241, 1998.

Rice R: Infection control in the home: 1998 update, *Geriatric Nursing* 19(5):297, 1998.

Case Management

Aubry T et al: Family-focused case management: a case study of an innovative demonstration program, *Can J Community Mental Health* 19(1):63, 2000.

Boosfeld B, O'Toole M: Technology-dependent children: transition from hospital to home, *Paediatr Nurs* 12(6):20, 2000.

Doerge JB: Creating an outcomes framework, *Outcomes Manage Nurse Pract* 4(1):28, 2000.

Finch L: Long-term rehab. Going home, *Rehabil Manage* 13(7):70, 2000.

Hays BJ et al: Quantifying client need for care in the community: a strategy for managed care, *Public Health Nurs* 16(4):246, 1999.

Smith R: Long-term rehab. Making sense of the magnitude of options, *Rehabil Manage* 13(7):66, 2000.

Walsh J: Recognizing and managing boundary issues in case management, *Care Manage* 2(2):79, 2000.

Young MG: Recognizing the signs of elder abuse, *Patient Care* 34(20):56, 2000.

Patient Teaching

Alexander E: Crossing barriers to diabetes education, *Pract Nurse* 20(6):332, 2000.

Author: If patients ask..., *RN* 64(1):8, 2001.

Author: Confidentiality. Patient teaching: easy as ABC? *Nursing* 30(9):80, 2000.

Ehiri BI: Improving patient compliance among hypertensive patients: a reflection on the role of patient education, *Int J Health Promot Educ* 38(3):104, 2000.

Jones KR et al: Establishing a comprehensive database for home parenteral nutrition: six years of data, *Nutr Clin Pract* 15(6):279, 2000.

Rycroft-Malone J et al: Nursing and medication education, *Nursing* 14(50):35, 2000.

Shawyer GW, Cox RH: Need for physician referral of low-income, chronic disease patients to community nutrition education programs, *J Nutr Elderly* 20(1):17, 2000.

Documentation

Bjorvell C et al: Development of an audit instrument for nursing care plans in the patient record, *Qual Health Care* 9(1):6, 2000.

Currell R et al: Nursing record systems: effects on nursing practice and health car outcome, *Cochrane Library* 1:19, 2001.

Glover D: Communicating with colleagues: documentation, *Nurs Times* 96(31):47, 2000.

Johnson T: Functional health pattern assessment on-line: lessons learned, *Comput Nurs* 18(5):248, 2000.

McEvoy M: Development of a new approach to palliative care documentation, *Int J Palliative Nurs* 6(6):288, 2000.

Nahm R, Poston I: Measurement of the effects of an integrated, point-of-care computer system on quality of nursing documentation and patient satisfaction, *Comput Nurs* 18(5):220, 2000.

CHAPTER 10: LONG-TERM CARE

Internet Sites

American College of Health Care Administrators, www.achca.org.
American Health Care Association, www.ahca.org.
American Medical Director Association, www.amda.com.
American Society of Consulting Pharmacy, www.ascp.com.
Health Care Financing Administration, www.hcfa.gov.
Medicare, www.medicare.gov.
National Association of Director of Nursing Administration in Long Term Care, www.nadona.org.
National Citizen's Coalition for Nursing Home Reform, www.nccnhr.org/.

Nursing Issues

Author: Long-term care nurses ignored, *Nurs Times* 97(8):8, 2001.
Doyle C: Reflections: practice profile. Applying sound principles of medication use for older people, *Nurs Older People* 12(9):37, 2000.
Gray J: Brave change of heart...long-term care, *Nurs Stand* 15(20):3, 2001.
Saba VK et al: Challenges for data management in long-term care. In *Essentials of computers for nurses: informatics for the new millennium,* New York, 2001, McGraw-Hill.
Trossman S: Yes, there is a staffing crisis in long-term care, *Am Nurse* 33(3):1, 2001.
Willis T, Ford P: Assessing older people—contemporary issues for nursing, *Nurs Older People* 12(9):16, 2000.

Resident Care

Caro FG et al: Performance-based home care for the elderly: the quality of circumstances protocol, *Home Health Care Serv* 18(4):1, 2000.
Dabelko HI, Balaswamy S: Use of adult day services and home health care services by older adults: a comparative analysis, *Home Health Care Serv* 18(3):65, 2000.
Ennis BW et al: Diagnosing malnutrition in the elderly, *Nurse Pract* 26(3):52, 2001.
Katsma DL, Souza CH: Elderly pain assessment and pain management knowledge of long-term care nurses, *Pain Manage Nurs* 1(3):88, 2000.
Thomas S, MacMahon D: Health care and older people: setting the scene, *Community Nurs* 15(2):8, 2001.

Administrative Issues

Author: Stats and facts. Nursing staff shortages in long-term care facilities, *Manage Care Interface* 13(11):46, 2000.
Goforth L: Paying the piper: the crisis in chronic care, *Home Health Care Serv* 18(3):1, 2000.
Riggs CJ, Rantz MJ: A model of staff support to improve retention in long-term care, *Nurs Admin Q* 25(2):43, 2001.
Ross MM et al: End-of-life care fore seniors: the development of a national guide, *J Palliative Care* 16(4):47, 2000.
Ryden MB et al: Value-added outcomes: the use of advanced practice nurses in long-term care facilities, *Gerontologist* 40(6):654, 2000.

CHAPTER 11: INFLAMMATION AND INFECTION

General

Bentley DW et al: Practice guidelines for evaluation of fever and infection in long-term care facilities, *J Am Geriatr Soc* 49:2, 2001.
Burger ET: Preparing adult patients for international travel, *Nurse Pract* 26:5, 2001.
Corwin EJ: Understanding cytokines, *Biol Res Nurs* 2:1, 2000.
Cunha BA: Effective antibiotic-resistance control strategies, *Lancet* 357:9265, 2001.
Feudtner C, Marcuse EK: Ethics and immunization policy: promoting dialogue to sustain consensus, *Pediatrics* 107:5, 2001.
Jones RN: Resistance patterns among nosocomial pathogens, *Chest* 119:2, 2001.
Loeb M: Antibiotic use in long-term care facilities: many unanswered questions, *Infect Control Hosp Epidemiol* 21:10, 2000.
Stephenson J: Researchers describe latest strategies to combat antibiotic-resistant microbes, *JAMA* 285:18, 2001.
Ward D: Implementing evidence-based practice in infection control, *Br J Nurs* 9:5, 2000.
Watzl B: Review on nutrition and immunity in man, *Am J Clin Nutr* 73:6, 2001.

CHAPTER 12: PAIN

General

Madjar I: *Giving comfort and conflicting pain,* Edmonton, Alberta, 1998, Qual Institute Press.
Miaskowski C: *Cancer pain management,* ed 2, Boston, 1999, L Jones & Bartlett Publishers.
Snyder M, Lindquist R: *Complementary/alternative therapies in nursing,* ed 3, New York, 1998, Springer Publishing.
Wall PD, Melzack R: *The textbook of pain,* ed 4, Edinburgh, 1999, Churchill Livingstone.

CHAPTER 13: FLUID, ELECTROLYTE, AND ACID-BASE IMBALANCE

Fluid and Electrolyte Imbalance

General

Cummings B et al: *A.D.A.M.® interactive physiology CD: Fluid, electrolyte, and acid/base balance,* 1999, website: Benjamin/Cummings Publishing and adam.com®.
Metheny NM: *Fluid and electrolyte balance nursing considerations,* ed 4, Philadelphia, 2000, JB Lippincott.
Springhouse Corporation Staff: *Fluids and electrolytes made incredibly easy,* ed 2, Springhouse, Pa, 2001, Springhouse.

Fluid Imbalance

Metheny N: Focusing on the dangers of D_5W, *Nursing 97* 27(10):55, 1997.
Klotz, RS: The effects of intravenous solution on fluid and electrolyte balance, *J IV Nurs* 21(1):20, 1998.

Electrolyte Imbalance

Castialione V, Kearney K: Hyperkalemia, *Am J Nurs* 100:55, 2000.
DeJong MJ: Hyponatremia, *Am J Nurs* 98(12):36, 1998.
Fabious DB: How to recognize electrolyte imbalances on an ECG, *Nursing 98* 28:32hn1, 1998.
Rose BD: *Clinical physiology of acid-base and electrolyte disorders,* ed 5, New York, 2000, McGraw-Hill.

Nursing Management

Hall JC: Choosing nutrition support: how and when to initiate, *Nurs Case Management* 4(5):212, 1999.
Mentes JC: Hydration management protocol, *J Gerontological Nurs* 26(10):6, 2000.
Powers FA: Your elderly needs I.V. therapy...Can you keep her safe? *Nursing 99* 29:54, 1999.

Acid-Base Balance

General

Heitz UE, Horne MM: *Pocket guide to fluid, electrolyte and acid-base balance,* ed 4, St Louis, 2000, Mosby.

Keyes JL: *Fluid, electrolyte, and acid-base regulation,* 1999, Universe.com, Inc.

Rose BD et al: *Clinical physiology of acid-base and electrolyte disorders,* New York, 2000, McGraw-Hill.

Thomson WS, Adams JF, editors: *Clinical acid-base balance,* London, 1997, Oxford University Press.

CHAPTER 14: SHOCK

Etiology

Cardiogenic shock complicating acute myocardial infarction: results of the SHOCK Trial Registry, *J Am Coll Cardiol* 36(3) (Suppl A):1063, 2000.

Harvnak M, Boujoukos A: Hypotension, *AACN Clin Issues Adv Pract Acute Crit Care* 8(3):303, 1997.

Noskin GA, Phair JP: Approach to the patient with bactermia and sepsis. In Kelly WN, editor: *Textbook of internal medicine,* ed 3, Philadelphia, 1997, Lippincott-Raven.

Physiology

Asuncion MM, Koushik VS: Shock state and the elderly, *Clin Geriatr* 8(8):40, 45, 2000.

Collins T: Understanding shock, *Nurs-Stand* 14(49):35, 2000.

Malone AM: Hemodynamic monitoring: basic principles and clinical application, *Support Line* 23(1):17, 2001.

Pathophysiology

Baxter F: Septic shock, *Can J Anaesth* 44(1):59, 1997.

Jumar A et al: Myocardial dysfunction in septic shock, *Crit Care Clin* 16(2):251, 2000.

Shoemaker WC: Shock states: pathophysiology, monitoring, outcome prediction and therapy. In

Shoemaker WC et al, editors: *Textbook of critical care,* ed 3, Philadelphia, 1995, WB Saunders.

Terr AL: Anaphylaxis and urticaria. In Stites DP et al, editors: *Medical immunology,* ed 9, Stamford, Conn, 1997, Appleton & Lange.

Clinical Manifestations

Diebel LN et al: Effect of acute hemodilution on intestinal perfusion and intramucosal pH after shock, *J Trauma Injury Infect Crit Care* 49(5):800, 2000.

Marik PE: The clinical features of severe community-acquired pneumonia presenting as septic shock, *J Crit Care* 15(3):85, 2000.

Stoll EH: Clinical focus: sepsis and septic shock, *Clin J Oncol Nurs* 5(2):71, 2001.

Werfel P: Avoid assessment traps, *J Emerg Med Services* 25(8):20, 2000.

Management

Chu SH, Hsu RB: Current status of artificial heats and ventricular assist devices, *J Formos Med Assoc* 99(2):79, 2000.

Criss E: Trauma management in the new millennium: patient care 2000, *J Emerg Med Serv* 12: 34, 38, 1999.

Cunha B, Gill V: Antimicrobial therapy in sepsis. In Fein A, editor: *Sepsis and multiorgan failure,* Baltimore, 1997, Williams & Wilkins.

Cuzzocrea S et al: Antioxidant therapy: a new pharmacological approach in shock, inflammation, and ischemia/reperfusion injury, *Pharmacol Rev* 53(1):135, 2001.

Jindal N et al: Pharmacologic issues in the management of septic shock, *Crit Care Clin* 16(2):233, 2000.

Jordan KS: Fluid resuscitation in acutely injured patients, *J Intravenous Nurs* 23(2):81, 2000.

Liepert DJ, Rosenthal MH: Management of cardiogenic, hypovolemic and hyperdynamic shock, *Curr Rev Perianesthesia Nurs* 22(9):103, 2000.

Menon V et al: Lack of progress in cardiogenic shock: lesions from the GUSTO trials, *Eur Heart J* 21(23):1928, 2000.

Mower et al: How to respond to shock, *Dimensions Crit Care Nurs* 20(2):22, 2001.

Voelckel WG et al: Vasopressin improves survival after cardiac arrest in hypovolemic shock, *Anesth Analg* 91(3):627, 2000.

CHAPTER 15: CANCER

General

American Cancer Society: *Cancer prevention and early detection: facts and figures 2001,* Atlanta, 2001, The Society.

Calzone KA: Genetic predisposition testing: clinical implications for oncology nurses, *Oncol Nurs Forum* 24:712, 1997.

Swan DK, Ford B: Chemoprevention of cancer: review of the literature, *Oncol Nurs Forum* 24:719, 1997.

Tranin A: Genetics and breast cancer risk, *Contemporary Issues in Breast Cancer,* 2001, website: http://www.ons.org.

Yarbo CH et al: *Cancer symptom management,* ed 2, Boston, 1999, Jones and Bartlett.

Surgery

Tucci RA, Bartels KL: Ovarian cancer surgery: a clinical pathway, *Clin J Oncol Nurs* 2:65, 1998.

Zack E: Sentinel lymph node biopsy in breast cancer: scientific rationale and patient care, *Oncol Nurs Forum* 28:997, 2001.

Radiation Therapy

Abel LJ et al: Nursing management of patients receiving brachytherapy for early stage prostate cancer, *Clin J Oncol Nurs* 3:7, 1999.

Gosselin TK, Waring JS: Nursing management of patients receiving brachytherapy for gynecologic malignancies, *Clin J Oncol Nurs* 5:59, 2001.

Chemotherapy

Gralla RJ et al: Recommendations for the use of antiemetics: evidence-based, clinical practice guidelines, *J Clin Oncol* 17:2971, 1999.

Kosier MB, Minkler P: Nursing management of patients with an implanted Ommaya reservoir, *Clin J Oncol Nurs* 2:63, 1999.

Labovich TM: Transfusion therapy: nursing implications, *Clin J Oncol Nurs* 1:61, 1997.

Myers J: Hypersensitivity reaction to paclitaxel: nursing interventions, *Clin J Oncol Nurs* 4:61, 2000.

National Cancer Institute/Cancer Therapy Evaluation Program (CTEP): Common Toxicity Criteria, 1999, website: http://ncictephelp@ctep.nci.nih.gov.

Oncology Nursing Society: *Cancer chemotherapy guidelines and recommendations for practice,* ed 2, Pittsburgh, 1999, Oncology Nursing Press.

Wickham RS et al: Taste changes experienced by patients receiving chemotherapy, *Oncol Nurs Forum* 26:697, 1999

Biotherapy

Kiley KE, Gale DM: Nursing management of patients with malignant melanoma receiving adjuvant alpha interferon-2b, *Clin J Oncol Nurs* 2:11, 1998.

Complementary and Alternative Therapy

Decker GM, Myers J: Commonly used herbs: implications for clinical practice, *Clin J Oncol Nurs* 5 (Suppl): 2001.

CHAPTER 16: PREOPERATIVE NURSING

Assessment

Shortall SP, Perkins LA: Interpreting the ins and out of pulmonary function tests, *Nursing 99,* 29(12):41, 1999.

Wiens A: Preoperative anxiety in women, *AORN J* 68:74, 1998.

Antibiotic Therapy

Glaser V: Emerging infections: new pathogens and changing resistance patterns, *Patient Care Nurse Practitioner* 3(4):24, 2000.

Glover TL: How drug-resistant microorganisms affect nursing, *Orthopaedic Nurs* 19(2):19, 2000.

Jacobson AF: Research for practice controlling VRE, *Am J Nurs* 99(6):68, 1999.

Kupecz D: Linezolid: a new class of antibiotic, *Nurse Pract* 25(11):62, 2000.

Reece SM: The emerging threat of antimicrobial resistance: strategies for change, *Nurse Pract* 24(11):70, 1999.

Young MG: New developments in antibiotics, *Patient Care Nurse Practitioner* 3(8):25, 2000.

Complementary and Alternative Therapy

D'Epiro NW: Homeopathy: can like cure like? *Patient Care Nurse Practitioner* 2(12):7, 1999.

Karch AM, Karch FE: The herb garden, *Am J Nurs* 99(6):12, 1999.

Miller J, Ingram L: Perioperative nursing and animal-assisted therapy, *AORN J* 72(3):477, 2000.

Waddell DL et al: Three herbs you should get to know, *Am J Nurs* 101(4):48, 2001.

Youngkin EQ, Thomas DJ: Vitamins: common supplements and therapy, *Nurse Pract* 24(11):50, 1999.

Informed Consent

Dunn D: Exploring the gray areas of informed consent, *Nursing 99* 29(7):41, 1999.

Elderly

Adams W et al: Alcohol problems in the elderly, *Patient Care Nurse Pract* 3(10):68, 2000.

Bailes B: Hypothyroidism in elderly patients, *AORN J* 69(5):1026, 1999.

Ennis BW et al: Diagnosing malnutrition in the elderly, *Nurse Pract* 26(3):52, 2001.

Kee CCC, Miller V: Perioperative care of the older adult with auditory and visual changes, *AORN J* 70(6):1012, 1999.

Sheahan SL: Medication used and misuse by the elderly, *Adv Nurse Pract* 8(12):41, 2000.

Patient Education

Coslow BF, Eddy ME: Effects of preoperative ambulatory gynecological education: clinical outcomes and patient satisfaction, *J Perianesthesia Nurs* 13(1):4, 1998.

Dunn D: Preoperative assessment criteria and patient teaching for ambulatory surgery patients, *J Perianesthesia Nurs* 13(5):274, 1998.

Krenzischek DA et al: Evaluation of ASPAN's preoperative patient teaching videos on general, regional, and minimum alveolar concentration/conscious sedation anesthesia, *J Perianesthesia Nurs* 16(3):174, 2001.

Sleep Apnea

Gupta RM et al: Postoperative complications in patients with obstructive sleep apnea syndrome undergoing hip or knee replacement: a case-control study, *Mayo Clin Proc* 76:897, 2001.

CHAPTER 17: INTRAOPERATIVE NURSING

General

Fossum S et al: A comparison study on the effects of prewarming patients in the outpatient surgery setting, *J Perianesthesia Nurs* 16(3):187, 2001.

Kleinbeck SVM, McKennet M: Challenges of measuring intraoperative patient outcomes, *AORN J* 72(5):91, 2000.

Phippen ML, Wells MP: *Patient care during operative and invasive procedures,* Philadelphia, 2000, WB Saunders.

Anesthesia

Hemmings HC, Hopkins PM: *Foundations of anesthesia basic and clinical sciences,* St Louis, 2000, Mosby.

Kreger C: Getting to the root of pain spinal anesthesia and analgesia, *Nursing 2001* June:31, 2001.

Miller D: Taking the sting out of local anesthesia, *Patient Care Nurse Pract* March:49, 2000.

Bloodless Surgery

Grogan A: Bringing bloodless surgery into the mainstream, *Nursing 99* 29(11):58, 1999.

Ozawa S et al: A practical approach to achieving bloodless surgery, *AORN J* 74(1):34, 2001.

Employee Safety

Perry J: The bloodborne pathogens standard, 2001: what's changed? *Nurs Manage* 32(6):25, 2001.

Stringer B et al: Quantifying and reducing the risk of bloodborne pathogen exposure, *AORN J* 73(6):1135, 2001.

Talikwa L: Clearing the air of surgical smoke, *Managing Infect Control* 1(1):58, 2001.

Infection Control

Crosby CT, Mares AK: Skin antisepsis: the basics, *Managing Infect Control* 1(1):38, 2001.

Steelman VM: Prion diseases: an evidenced-based protocol for infection control, *AORN J* 69(5):946, 1999.

Latex Allergy

Baena de Nires Kioes NHM, Mendes Lopes RA: Latex allergy in health care personnel, *AORN J* 72(1):42, 2000.

Dyck RJ: Historical development of latex allergy, *AORN J* 72(1):27, 2000.

Floyd PT: Latex allergy update, *J Perianesthesia Nurs* 15(1):26, 2000.

Hudson ME: Dental surgery in pediatric patients with spina bifida and latex allergy, *AORN J* 74(1):57, 2001.

Patient Positioning

Meltzer B: A guide to patient positioning, *Outpatient Surgery Magazine* 11(4):48, 2001.

Sterilization

Frieze M: Sterilization solutions for the new millennium, *Managing Infect Control* June:18-20, 2001.

May T: Keeping up with sterilization system technology, *Managing Infection Control* May:62-64, 2001.

Mayworm D: Four options for low-temperature sterilization, *Outpatient Surgery Magazine* 11(4):73, 2001.

Mayworm D: What you need to know about eto, *Outpatient Surgery Magazine* 11(3):67, 2001.

Spry C: Low-temperature sterilization, *Infection Control Today* 5(5):14, 2001.

Wound Closure

King ME, Kinney AY: A sticky solution to wound repair, how to apply a topical liquid that mends simple lacerations, *Nursing 2001* 31(3):52, 2001.

Shearer DC, Blunt E: The latest choice in wound closure, when and how to use dermabond, *Adv Nurse Practitioners* 8(5):85, 2000.

CHAPTER 18: POSTOPERATIVE NURSING

General

Baltimore JJ: Postlaryngospasm pulmonary edema in adults, *AORN J* 70(3):468, 1999.

Brenner ZR: Preventing postoperative complications, what's old, what's new, what's tried-and-true, *Nursing 99* 29(10):34, 1999.

Knoerl DV et al: Evaluation of orthostatic blood pressure testing as discharge criterion from PACU after spinal anesthesia, *J Peranesthesia Nurs* 16(1):11, 2001.

Saar LM: Use of a modified postanesthesia recovery score in phase II perianesthesia period of ambulatory surgery patients, *J Perianesthesia Nurs* 16(2):82, 2001.

Anticoagulation Therapy

Gibbar-Clements et al: The challenge of warfarin therapy, *Am J Nurs* 1000(3):38, 2000.

Nadeau C et al: The challenges of oral anticoagulation, *Patient Care Nurse Practitioner* 3(12):12, 2000.

Stillwell SB: When you suspect epidural hematoma, *Am J Nurs* 100(9):68, 2000.

Complementary and Alternative Therapy

Buckle J: Aromatherapy in perianesthesia nursing, *J Perianesthesia Nurs* 14(6):336, 1999.

VanKooten M: Non-pharmacologic pain management for postoperative coronary artery bypass graft surgery patients, *J Nurs Scholarship* 31(2):157, 1999.

Pain

Barnes S: Pain management: what do patients need to know and when do they need to know it? *J Perianesthesia Nurs* 16(2):107, 2001.

Kozuh JL: NSAIDs and antihypertensives: an unhappy union, *Am J Nurs* 100(6):40, 2000.

McCaffery M, Ferrell BR: Opioids and pain management, what do nurse know? *Nursing 99* 29(3):48, 1999.

Meltzer B: 5 oral pain meds: an in-depth look at 5 popular prescription pain-killers, *Outpatient Surgery Magazine* 11(5):52, 2001.

Pasero C: Oral patient-controlled analgesia, it can work the hospital, *Am J Nurs* 100(3):24, 2000.

Platt A, Reed B: Meet new pain standards with new technology, *Nurs Manage* 23(3):40, 2001.

Preemptive Analgesia

Goodwin SA: A review of preemptive analgesia, *J Perianesthesia Nurs* 13(2):109, 1998.

Gottschalk A: New concepts in acute pain therapy: preemptive analgesia, *Am Fam Physician* 63(10):1979, 2001.

Kissin I: Preemptive analgesia, *Anesthesiology* 93(4):1138, 2000.

Rhiner M, Kedziera P: Managing breakthrough pain: a new approach, *Am J Nurs Suppl* March:3-12, 1999.

Siwek J: Preemptive analgesia: decreasing pain before it starts, *Am Fam Physician* 63(10):1924, 2001.

CHAPTER 19: ASSESSMENT OF THE RESPIRATORY SYSTEM

General

Horne C, Derrico, D: Mastering ABGs, *Am J Nurs* 99:8, 1999.

Hueston WJ et al: Does acute bronchitis really exist? A reconceptualization of acute viral respiratory infections, *J Fam Pract* 49:5, 2000.

Smith-Sims K: Hospital-acquired pneumonia, *Am J Nurs* 101:1, 2001.

Tierney LM et al: *Current medical diagnosis and treatment,* ed 37, Stamford, Conn, 1998, Appleton & Lange.

Wilson S, Giddens J: *Health assessment for nursing practice,* ed 2, St Louis, 2001, Mosby.

Wong F: A new approach to ABG interpretation, *Am J Nurs* 99:8, 1999.

CHAPTER 20: UPPER AIRWAY PROBLEMS

General

Bethel M, Rose J: Sinus and bronchial treatment, *Aromatic News* Fall:9, 2000.

Coleman EA: Emergency: anthrax, *Am J Nurs* 101(12):48, 2001.

Hatcher T: The proverbial herb, *Am J Nurs* 101(2):36, 2001.

Henderson CW: Women affected differently than men, *Women's Health Weekly* September 9: 12, 2000.

Jacobs MR, Weinberg W: Disease management. Evidence-based guidelines for treatment of bacterial respiratory tract infections in the era of antibiotic resistance, *Manage Care Interface* 14(4):68, 2001.

Kearney K: Emergency: epiglottitis, *Am J Nurs* 101(8):37, 2001.

West B, Jones NS: Endoscopy-negative, computed tomography-negative facial pain in a nasal clinic, *Laryngoscope* 111(4):581, 2001.

Wilmoth D et al: Pulmonary care. Caring for adults with cystic fibrosis, *Crit Care Nurse* 21(3):34, 2001.

Sinusitis

Anon J: Guidelines for managing otitis media and sinusitis, *Manage Care Interface* Suppl A:11, 2001.

Dixson RK: The why and how of endoscopic surgery, *Semin Perioperative Nurs* 9(4):163, 2000.

Doty RL, Mishra A: Olfaction and its nasal obstruction, rhinitis and rhinosinusitis, *Laryngoscope* 111(3):409, 2001.

Klein L: Sinusitis: when to treat and how, *RN* 64(1):42, 2001.

Meletis CD: Natural approaches to sinusitis relief, *Alternative Complementary Ther* 6(2):69, 2000.

Phillips CD: Screening sinus CT and paranasal imaging, *Appl Radiol* 30(5):9, 2001.

Trotto NE: A prudent prescription for acute sinusitis, *Patient Care* 35(7):54, 2001.

Allergies

Gasbarro R: Identifying and managing patients with asthma and allergy, *Drug Topics* 145(7):68, 2001.

Lucas BD: Common test for cat allergies not always needed, *Patient Care* 33(12):12, 1999.

Montanaro A, Tilles SA: Update in allergy and immunology, *Ann Intern Med* 134(4):291, 2001.

Voelker R: NGF implicated in allergy, *JAMA* 283(24):3189, 2000.

Cancer

Armstrong WB, Meyskens FL: Chemoprevention of head and neck cancer, *Otolaryngol Head Neck Surg* 122(5):728, 2000.

Gleich LL: Gene therapy for head and neck cancer, *Laryngoscope* 110(5):708, 2000.

John LD: Quality of life in patients receiving radiation for non-small cell lung cancer, *Oncol Nurs Forum* 28(5):807, 2001.

Lennie TA et al: Educational needs and altered eating habits following a total laryngectomy, *Oncol Nurs Forum* 28(4):667, 2001.

Schaefer KS: Periomedicine. Oral care for the patient with head and neck cancer, *Access* 15(5):56, 2001.

CHAPTER 21: LOWER AIRWAY PROBLEMS

General

Abraham IL et al: Profiling care and benchmarking best practice in care of hospitalized elderly: the Geriatric Institutional Assessment Profile: *Nurs Clin North Am* 34:1, 1999.

Ahrens T, Tucker K: Pulse oximetry, *Crit Care Clin North Am* 11:1, 1999.

Corrin, B: *Pathology of the lung,* Philadelphia, 2000, Churchill Livingstone.

Doenges ME, Moorhouse MF: *Nurse's pocket guide: diagnoses, interventions and rationales,* Philadelphia, 1998, FA Davis.

Keegan L: The environment as a healing tool, *Nurs Clin North Am* 36:1, 2001.

Rakel RE, Bope ET, editors: *Conn's current therapy,* Philadelphia, 2001, WB Saunders.

Shoulders-Odom B: Using an algorithm to interpret arterial blood gases, *Dimensions Crit Care* 19:1, 2000.

Tate J, Tasota FJ: Using pulse oximetry, *Nursing* 30:9, 2000.

Witek TJ: The fate of inhaled drugs: the pharmacokinetics and pharmacodynamics of drugs administered by aerosol, *Respir Care* 45:7, 2000.

Zielinski J: Long-term oxygen therapy in conditions other than chronic obstructive pulmonary disease, *Respir Care* 45:2, 2000.

Acute Lung Injury and Acute Respiratory Distress Syndrome

Ball C: Use of the prone position in the management of acute respiratory distress syndrome, *Intensive Crit Care Nurs* 15:4, 1999.

Brower RG, Fessler HE: Mechanical ventilation in acute lung injury and acute respiratory distress syndrome, *Clin Chest Med* 21:3, 2000.

Cawley MJ et al: Mechanical ventilation and pharmacologic strategies for acute respiratory distress syndrome, *Pharmacotherapy* 18:1, 1998.

Gillette MA, Hess DR: Ventilator-induced lung injury and the evolution of lung-protective strategies in acute respiratory distress syndrome, *Respir Care* 46:2, 2001.

Petty TL: In the cards was ARDS: how we discovered the acute respiratory distress syndrome, *Am J Respir Crit Care Med* 163:3, 2001.

Phillips JK: Management of patients with acute respiratory distress syndrome, *Crit Care Clin North Am* 11:2, 1999.

Asthma

Autio L, Rosenow D: Effectively managing asthma in young and middle adulthood, *Nurs Pract* 24:1, 1999.

Burns SM, Lawson C: Pharmacological and ventilatory management of acute asthma Exacerbations, *Crit Care Nurse* 19:4, 1999.

Horuichi T, Castro M: The pathobiologic implications for treatment. Old and new strategies in the treatment of chronic asthma, *Clin Chest Med* 21:2, 2000.

Huss K, Huss RW: Genetics of asthma and allergies, *Nurs Clin North Am* 35:3, 2000.

Janson S et al: Use of biological markers of airway inflammation to detect the efficacy of nurse-delivered asthma education, *Heart Lung* 30:1, 2001.

Lindberg M et al: Asthma nurse practice: a resource-effective approach in asthma management, *Respir Med* 93:8, 1999.

Miracle V, Winston M: Take the wind out of asthma, *Nursing* 30:8, 2000.

Owen CL: New directions in asthma management, *Am J Nurs* 99:3, 1999.

COPD

Baker S, Flynn MB: New hope for patients with emphysema: lung reduction surgery, *Heart Lung* 28:6, 1999.

Calverley PM: COPD: early detection and intervention, *Chest* 117(Suppl 2):5, 2000.

Enright PL, Crapo RO: Controversies in the use of spirometry for early recognition and diagnosis of COPD in cigarette smokers, *Clin Chest Med* 21:4, 2000.

Farrero E et al: Impact of a hospital-based home care program on the management of COPD patients receiving long-term oxygen therapy, *Chest* 119:2, 2001.

Frey JI: Gender differences in coping styles and coping effectiveness in chronic obstructive pulmonary disease groups, *Heart Lung* 29:5, 2000.

Petty TL: Definitions, causes, course, and prognosis of chronic obstructive pulmonary disease, *Respir Care Clin North Am* 4:3, 1998.

Cystic Fibrosis

Bolyard DR: Sexuality and cystic fibrosis, *Am J Matern Child Nurs* 26:1, 2001.

Goetsche LL: Lung transplantation in patients with CF, *Am J Nurs* 101:7, 2001.

Hodson ME: Treatment of cystic fibrosis in the adult, *Respiration* 67:6, 2000.

Lanuza DM et al: Research on the quality of life of lung transplant candidates and recipients: an integrative review, *Heart Lung* 29:3, 2000.

LiPuma JJ: Burkholderia cepacia: management issues and new insights, *Clin Chest Med* 19:3, 1998.

Maurer JR et al: International guidelines for the selection of lung transplant candidates. The International Society for Heart and Lung Transplantation, the American Thoracic Society, the American Society of Transplant Physicians, the European Respiratory Society, *Heart Lung* 27:4, 1998.

Ochoa LL, Richardson GW: The current status of lung transplantation: a nursing perspective, *AACN Clinical Issues* 10:2, 1999.

Dyspnea

Ambrose MS: Chronic dyspnea, *Nursing* 98:4, 1998.

Knebel AR et al: Dyspnea management in alpha-1 antitrypsin deficiency: effect of oxygen administration, *Nurs Res* 49:6, 2000.

Manning HL: Dyspnea treatment, *Respir Care* 54:11, 2000.

McBride S et al: The therapeutic use of music for dyspnea and anxiety in patients with COPD who live at home, *J Holistic Nursing* 17:3, 1999.

Truesdell S: Helping patients with COPD manage episodes of acute shortness of breath, *Med Surg Nurs* 9:4, 2000.

Lung Cancer

Adjei AA: Primary lung cancer. In Rake RE, Bope ET, editors: *Conn's current therapy 2001,* Philadelphia, 2001, WB Saunders.

Giarelli E et al: A standardized nursing intervention protocol for patients with cancer redefines the relationship among patients, caretakers, and nurses, *Am J Nurs* 100:12, 2000.

Petty TL: Screening strategies for early detection of lung cancer: the time is now, *JAMA* 284:15, 2000.

Tarzian AJ: Caring for dying patients who have air hunger, *J Nurs Scholarship* 32:2, 2000.

Mechanical Ventilation

Burns SM: Making weaning easier. Pathways and protocols that work, *Crit Care Nurs Clin North Am* 11:4, 1999.

Burns SM, Dempsey E: Long-term ventilator management strategies: experiences of two hospitals, *AACN Clinical Issues* 11:3, 2000.

Burns SM et al: Design, testing, and results of an outcome-managed approach to patients requiring prolonged mechanical ventilation, *Am J Crit Care* 7:1, 1998.

Chatburn RL, Primiano FP: A new system for understanding modes of mechanical ventilation, *Respir Care* 46:6, 2001.

Mathews PJ, Mathews LM: Reducing the risks of ventilator-associated infections, *Dimensions Crit Care* 19:1, 2000.

Powers J, Bennett SJ: Measurement of dyspnea in patients treated with mechanical Ventilation, *Am J Crit Care* 8:4, 1999.

Seneff MG et al: The impact of long-term acute-care facilities on the outcome and cost of care for patients undergoing prolonged mechanical ventilation, *Crit Care Med* 28:2, 2000.

Tasota FJ, Dobbin K: Weaning your patient from mechanical ventilation, *Nursing* 30:10, 2000.

Tobin MJ: Advances in mechanical ventilation, *N Engl J Med* 344:26, 2001.

Wilmoth D: New strategies for mechanical ventilation. Lung protective ventilation, *Crit Care Clin North Am* 11:4, 1999.

Pneumonia

Baine WB, Yu W, Summe JP: Epidemiologic trends in the hospitalization of elderly Medicare patients for pneumonia, 1991-1998, *Am J Public Health* 91:7, 2001.

Bartlett JG et al: Community-acquired pneumonia in adults: guidelines for management. The Infectious Diseases Society of America, *Clin Infect Dis* 26:4, 1998.

Ellstrom KE: Breathing easier in the intensive care unit: pneumonia, *Crit Care Nurs Clin North Am* 11:4, 1999.

Goldman M et al: Fungal pneumonias: the endemic mycoses, *Clin Chest Med* 20:3, 1999.

Harris JR et al: Risk factors for nosocomial pneumonia in critically ill trauma patients. *AACN Clinical Issues* 11:2, 2000.

Ibrahim EH et al: Experience with a clinical guideline for the treatment of ventilator-associated pneumonia, *Crit Care Med* 29:6, 2001.

Lieberman D, Lieberman D: Community-acquired pneumonia in the elderly: a practical guide to treatment, *Drugs Aging* 17:2, 2000.

Muder RR: Management of nursing home-acquired pneumonia: unresolved issues and priorities for future investigation, *J Am Geriatr Soc* 48:1, 2000.

Murphy M et al: A multihospital effort to reduce inpatient lengths of stay for pneumonia, *J Nurs Care Q* 13:5, 1999.

Pulmonary Embolism

Berman AR: Pulmonary embolism in the elderly, *Clin Geriatr Med* 17:1, 2001.

Christie F: Pulmonary embolism, *Am J Nurs* 98:11, 1998.

Hartmann IJ et al: Diagnosing acute pulmonary embolism: effect of chronic obstructive

pulmonary disease on the performance of D-dimer testing, ventilation/perfusion scintigraphy, spiral computed tomographic angiography, and conventional angiography, *Am J Respir Crit Care Med* 162:6, 2000.

Koutkia P, Wachtel TJ: Pulmonary embolism presenting as syncope: case report and review of the literature, *Heart Lung* 28:5, 1999.

Lewis AM: Respiratory emergency, *Nursing* 29:8, 1999.

Reidel M: Acute pulmonary embolism 1: pathophysiology, clinical presentation, and diagnosis, *Heart* 85:2, 2001.

Respiratory Failure

Behrendt CE: Acute respiratory failure in the United States: incidence and 31-day survival, *Chest* 118:4, 2000.

Borum ML et al: The effect of nutritional supplementation on survival in seriously ill hospitalized adults: an evaluation of the SUPPORT (Study to Understand Prognoses and Preferences for Outcomes and Risks of Treatments) data, *J Am Geriatr Soc* 48:5, 2000.

Bryan CL, Homma A: Acute respiratory failure. In Rakel RE, Bope ET, editors: *Conn's current therapy 2001,* Philadelphia, 2001, WB Saunders.

McCord M: Respiratory failure: after the intensive care unit, *Crit Care Clin North Am* 11:4, 1999.

Sarcoidosis

Gibson GJ: Sarcoidosis: old and new treatments, *Thorax* 56:5, 2001.

Smoking Cessation

Fiore MC: Treating tobacco use and dependence: an introduction to the US Public Health Service Clinical Practice Guideline, *Respir Care* 45:10, 2000.

Froelicher ES, Christopherson DJ: Women's initiative for nonsmoking (WINS): design and methods, *Heart Lung* 29:6, 2000.

Halpern MT et al: Smoking cessation in hospitalized patients, *Respir Care* 45:3, 2000.

Ruppert RA: The last smoke: your patients can quit smoking for life, *Am J Nurs* 99:11, 1999.

Tanoe LT: Cigarette smoking and women's respiratory health, *Clin Chest Med* 21:1, 2000.

Ward T: Using psychological insights to help people quit smoking, *J Adv Nurs* 34:6, 2001.

Warren CW et al: Tobacco use by youth: a surveillance report from the Global Youth Tobacco Survey project, *Bull WHO* 78:7, 2000.

Tuberculosis

Anderson P: TB caccines: progress and problems, *Trends Immunol* 22:3, 2001.

Jack W: The public economics of tuberculosis control, *Health Policy* 57:2, 2001.

Packham S: Tuberculosis in the elderly, *Gerontology* 47:4, 2001.

Pomerantz BJ: Pulmonary resection for multi-drug resistant tuberculosis, *J Throac Cardiovasc Surg* 212:3, 2001.

Raynor D: Reducing the spread of tuberculosis in the homeless population, *Br Nurs J* 9:13, 2000.

Reves R: Tuberculosis and other myobacterial diseases. In Rake RE, Bope ET, editors: *Conn's current therapy 2001,* Philadelphia, 2001, WB Saunders.

Small PM, Fujiwara PI: Management of tuberculosis in the United States, *N Engl J Med* 345:3, 2001.

Snell JJ: Current management of tuberculosis, *Expert Opin Pharmacother* 1:1, 1999.

Stone CL: Building academic and practical knowledge in nursing through TB skin testing certification in a BSN curriculum, *Public Health Nurs* 18:3, 2001.

Van Wormer LM: Tuberculosis: the latest, *CRNA* 11:1, 2000.

CHAPTER 22: ASSESSMENT OF THE CARDIOVASCULAR SYSTEM

General

Ebell MH: Evaluation of the patient with suspected deep vein thrombosis, *J Fam Pract* 50(2):167, 2001.

Greene P: Recognizing young people at risk for sudden cardiac death in preparticipation sports physicals, *J Am Acad Nurs Pract* 12(1):11, 2000.

Heikkila J et al: Gender differences in fears related to coronary arteriography, *Heart Lung* 28(1):20, 1999.

Kennedy MS, Zolot JS: Predicting organ damage in hypertensive patients, *Am J Nurs* 101(2):20, 2001.

Lloyd-Jones DM et al: Differential impact of systolic and diastolic blood pressure level on JNC-VI staging, *Hypertension* 34:381, 1999.

Schakenbach L: Myoglobin can detect heart muscle damage in two hours, *RN* 63(12):101, 2000.

Shi L et al: Validating the adult primary care assessment tool, *J Fam Pract* 50(2):161, 2001.

Tobin LJ: Evaluating mild to moderate hypertension, *Nurse Pract* 24(5):22, 1999.

Tyrell A: Abdominal aortic aneurysm: diagnosis, treatment, and implications for advanced practice nursing, *J Am Acad Nurse Pract* 11(9):397, 1999.

Zecchin RP et al: Is nurse-supervised exercise stress testing safe practice? *Heart Lung* 28(3):175, 1999.

CHAPTER 23: CORONARY ARTERY DISEASE AND DYSRHYTHMIAS

Coronary Artery Disease—Stable Angina and Acute Coronary Syndrome

Alligood KA, Iltz JL: Update on antithrombotic use and mechanism of action, *Prog Cardiovasc Nurs* 16:81, 2001.

AHA/ACC Conference Proceedings: Measuring and improving quality of care: a report from the American Heart Association/American College of Cardiology First Scientific Forum on Assessment of Healthcare Quality in cardiovascular disease and stroke, *Circulation* 101:1483, 2000.

Bridges EJ, Woods SL: Cardiovascular chronobiology: do you know what time it is? *Prog Cardiovasc Nurs* 16:65, 2001.

Drew BJ, Krucoff MW: Consensus statement for practice: multilead ST-segment monitoring in patients with acute coronary syndromes: a consensus statement for healthcare professionals, *Am J Crit Care* 8(6):372, 1999.

Gibbons RJ et al: ACC/AHA/ACP-ASIM pocket guidelines for management of patients with chronic stable angina: a report of the American College of Cardiology/American Heart Association Task Force on Practice Guidelines, 2000.

Gibbons RJ et al: ACC/AHA/ACP-ASIM guidelines for the management of patients with chronic stable angina: executive summary and recommendations: a report of the American College of Cardiology/American Heart Association Task Force on Practice Guidelines (Committee on Management of Patients with Chronic Stable Angina), *Circulation* 99:2829, 1999.

Jairath N: Implications of gender differences on coronary artery disease risk reduction in women, *AACN Clinical Issues* 12(1):17, 2001.

Roettig ML, Tanabe P: Emergency management of acute coronary syndromes, *J Emerg Nurs* 26(6 Suppl):S1, 2000.

Ryan TJ et al: ACC/AHA pocket guidelines for the management of patients with acute myocardial infarction: a report of the American College of Cardiology/American Heart Association Task Force on Practice Guidelines, April 2000.

Steinke EE: Sexual counseling after myocardial infarction, *Am J Nurs* 100(12):38, 2000.

Percutaneous Coronary Interventions

Morris NB: Brachytherapy: savior or tease, *Crit Care Nurs Clin North Am* 11(3):333, 1999.

Nickolaus MJ et al: Advances in interventional cardiology: beyond the balloon, *Nurs Clin North Am* 35(4):897, 2000.

Reynolds S et al: Head of bed elevation, early walking, and patient comfort after percutaneous transluminal angioplasty, *Dimensions Crit Care Nurs* 20(3):44, 2001.

Thorbs N et al: Coronary rotational atherectomy: a nursing perspective, *Crit Care Nurse* 20(2):77, 2000.

Dysrhythmias

Boyle J, Rost MK: Present status of cardiac pacing: a nursing perspective, *Crit Care Nurs Q* 23(1):1, 2000.

Falk RH: Medical progress: atrial fibrillation, *N Engl J Med* 344(14):1067, 2001.

Fenton JM: The clinician's approach to evaluating patients with dysrhythmias, *AACN Clinical Issues* 12(1):72, 2001.

Gilbert CJ: Common supraventricular tachycardias: mechanisms and management, *AACN Clinical Issues* {au: journal name ok?} 12(1):100, 167, 2001.

Paul S: ECGs and pacemakers: understanding advanced concepts in atrioventricular block, *Crit Care Nurse* 21(1):56, 2001.

Teplitz L: Treating tachyarrhythmias with radiofrequency catheter ablation, *Dimensions Crit Care Nurs* 19(3):28, 2000.

Tresch DD: Evaluation and management of cardiac arrhythmias in the elderly, *Med Clin North Am* 85(2):527, 2001.

White E: Patients with implantable cardioverter defibrillators: transition to home, *J Cardiovasc Nurs* 14(3):42, 2000.

Diet and Heart Disease

Goldberg IJ et al: Wine and your heart: a science advisory for healthcare professionals from the Nutrition Committee, Council on Epidemiology and Prevention, and Council on Cardiovascular Nursing of The American Heart Association, *Circulation* 103:472, 2001.

Krauss RM et al: AHA Scientific Statement: AHA Dietary guidelines revision 2000: a statement for healthcare professionals from the Nutrition Committee of the American Heart Association, *Circulation* 102:2284, 2000.

Kris-Etheron {au: initial?} et al: Summary of the scientific conference on dietary fatty acids and cardiovascular health: conference summary from the Nutrition Committee of the American Heart Association, *Circulation* 103(7):1034, 2001.

Lichtenstein AH et al: Stanol/sterol ester-containing foods and blood cholesterol levels: a statement for healthcare professionals from the Nutrition Committee of the Council on Nutrition, Physical Activity, and Metabolism of the American Heart Association, *Circulation* 103(8):1177, 2001.

Logan P, Clarke S: Nutritional and medical therapy for dyslipidemia in patients with cardiovascular disease, *AACN Clinical Issues* 12(1):40, 2001.

Pradka LR: Lipids and their role in coronary heart disease, *Nurs Clin North Am* 35(4):981, 2000.

CHAPTER 24: HEART FAILURE, VALVULAR PROBLEMS, AND INFLAMMATORY PROBLEMS OF THE HEART

Heart Failure

Albert N: Implementation strategies to manage heart failure outcomes, *AACN Clinical Issues* 11(3):396, 2000.

Beattie S: Heart failure with preserved LV function: pathophysiology, clinical presentation, treatment, and nursing implications, *J Cardiovasc Nurs* 14(4):24, 2000.

DeWald T et al: Current trends in the management of heart failure, *Nurs Clin North Am* 35(4):855, 2000.

Grady KL et al: American Heart Association statement: team management of patients with heart failure, *Circulation* 102(19):2443, 2000.

Halm MA, Penque S: Heart failure in women, *Prog Cardiovasc Nurs* 15:121, 2000.

MacCallum EM: The role of beta-blockers in the management of patients with heart failure, *Dimensions Crit Care Nurs* 20(1):24, 2001.

MacKlin M: Managing heart failure: a case study approach, *Crit Care Nurse* 21(2):2001.

Mendzef SD: Neurohormonal factors in heart failure, *Nurs Clin North Am* 35(4):841, 2000.

Obias-Manno D: Unconventional applications in pacemaker therapy, *AACN Clinical Issues* 12(1):127, 170, 2001.

Richardson L: Women and heart failure, *Heart Lung* 30(2):87, 2001.

Inflammatory Heart Disease

Bayer AS et al: Diagnosis and management of infective endocarditis and its complications, *Circulation* 98(25):2936, 1998.

Colletti C: Emergency! Pericarditis, *Am J Nurs* 99(10):35, 1999.
Lewandowski DM: Myocarditis, *Am J Nurs* 99(8):44, 1999.
Miracle VA: Put the brakes on pericarditis, *Nursing* 31(4):44, 2001.
Pawsat DE, Lee JY: Inflammatory disorders of the heart: pericarditis, myocarditis, and endocarditis, *Selected Topics in Emergency Cardiac Care* 16(3):665, 1998.
Sparacino PS: Cardiac infections: medical and surgical therapies, *J Cardiovasc Nurs* 13(2):49, 1999.

Cardiomyopathy

Corish C, Miracle V: Peripartum cardiomyopathy: educate women with PPCM about grave health risks of future pregnancies, *Am J Nurs* 101(Suppl):25, 2001.
Gargiulo J: Hypertrophic cardiomyopathy: preventing tragic endings, *Am J Nurs* 100(8):24JJ, {au: page no. ok?} 2000.

Coronary Artery Bypass Surgery

Allen JK: Changes in cholesterol levels in women after coronary artery bypass surgery, *Heart Lung* 28:270, 1999.
Banks TA: Radial artery harvesting, *Am J Nurs* 100:21, 2000.
Bourassa MG et al: Quality of life after coronary revascularization in the United States and Canada, *Am J Cardiol* 85:548, 2000.
Deliargyris EN et al: Preoperative factors predisposing to early postoperative atrial fibrillation after isolated coronary artery bypass grafting, *Am J Cardiol* 85:763, 2000.
King KK et al: Concerns and risk factor modification in women during the year after coronary artery surgery, *Nurs Res* 49:167, 2000.
Lindsay GM et al: Coronary artery disease patients' perceptions of their health and expectation of benefit following coronary artery bypass grafting, *J Adv Nurs* 32:1412, 2000.
Redecker NS, Wykpisz E: Effects of age on activity patterns after coronary artery bypass surgery, *Heart Lung* 28:5, 1999.
Reger TB, Vargas G: The return of the radial artery in CABG, *Am J Nurs* 99(9):26, 1999.
Van Kooten ME: Non-pharmacologic pain management for postoperative coronary artery bypass graft surgery patients, *J Nurs Scholarship* 31:157, 1999.
Wilson DE, Tracy MF: CABG and the elderly, *Am J Nurs* 100:24AA-TT, 2000.

Valvular Heart Disease and Surgery

Baptisti MM: Aortic valve replacement, *RN* 64:58, 2001.
Livorsi-Moore J et al: Port access, *Am J Nurs* 99:52, 1999.
Mehta NJ et al: Stenotrophomonas maltophilia endocarditis of prosthetic aortic valve: report of a case and review of the literature, *Heart Lung* 29:351, 2000.

Heart Surgery—General Considerations

Beattie S: A portrait of post-op a-fib, *RN* 63:26, 2000.
Brown MM: Implementation strategy: one-stop recovery for cardiac surgical patients, *AACN Clinical Issues* 11:412, 2000.
Chuk PK: Vital signs and nurses' choices of titrated dosages of intravenous morphine for relieving pain following cardiac surgery, *J Adv Nurs* 30:858, 1999.
Davies N: Patients' and carers' perception of factors influencing recovery after cardiac surgery, *J Adv Nurs* 32:318, 326, 2000.
Heckman R: Ultrasound use in cardiothoracic surgery, *AORN J* 73:142, 144, 155, 159, 164, 2001.
Innerarity S: Hypomagnesemia in acute and chronic illness, *Crit Care Nurs Q* 23:1, 2000.
King KM: Gender and short term recovery from cardiac surgery, *Nurs Res* 49:29, 2000.
Odell M: The patient's thoughts and feelings about their transfer from intensive care to the general ward, *J Adv Nurs* 31:322, 2000.
Prince SE, Cunha BA: Postpericardiotomy syndrome, *Heart Lung* 26:165, 1997.
Stewart M et al: Group support for couples coping with a cardiac condition, *J Adv Nurs* 33:190, 2001.

CHAPTER 25: VASCULAR PROBLEMS

Hypertension

Ambler SK, Brown RD: Genetic determinants of blood pressure regulation, *J Cardiovasc Nurs* 13(4):59, 1999.
Bushnell KL, Smith LA: Hypertension clinical outcomes in a nurse practitioner managed care setting, *Semin Nurs Manage* 6(3):155, 1998.
Chase S: Hypertensive crisis, *RN* 63(6):62, 2000.
Karch A, Karch F: When a blood pressure isn't routine, *Am J Nurs* 100(3):23, 2000.
Kozuh J: NSAIDs and antihypertensives: an unhappy union, *Am J Nurs* 100(6):40, 2000.
McPaul K: New hypertension guidelines, *AAOHN J* 47(3):114, 1999.
Miracle VA: Act fast during a hypertensive crisis, *Nursing* 31(9):50, 2001.
Skolnik N et al: Combination antihypertensive drugs: recommendations for use, *Am Fam Physician* 61(10):3049, 2000.
Tobin LJ: Evaluating mild to moderate hypertension, *Nurse Pract* 24(5):22, 25, 29, 1999.
Wang, C, Abbott LJ: Development of a community based diabetes and hypertension preventive program, *Public Health Nurs* 15(6):406, 1998.

Peripheral Arterial Disease

Adams S: Evaluation and conservative management of chronic lower extremity arterial disease, *Clinical Excellence for Nurse Practitioners* 3(2):88, 1999.
Braun C et al: Components of an optimal exercise program for the treatment of patients with claudication, *J Vasc Nurs*17(2):32, 1999.
Fahey V: *Vascular nursing,* ed 3, Philadelphia, 1999, WB Saunders.
Sloan H, Wills EM: Ankle-brachial index: calculating your patient's vascular risk, *Nursing* 99(10):58, 1999.
Sparks RD: The answer is Buerger's disease, and the question is, *West J Med* 168(4):286, 1998.

Venous Disease

Anderson L: Ischemic venous thrombosis. Its hidden agenda, *J Vasc Nurs* 17(1):1, 1999.
Breen P: DVT: what every nurse should know, *RN* 63(4):58, 2000.
Hess CT: Putting the squeeze on venous ulcers, *Nursing* 31(9):58, 2001.
Johnson M: Treatment and prevention of varicose veins, *J Vasc Nurs* 15(3):65, 1997.
Nunnelee J: Low molecular weight heparin, *J Vasc Nurs* 15(2):94, 1997.
Rudolph D: Pathophysiology and management of venous ulcers, *J Wound Ostomy Continence Nursing* 25(5):248, 1998.

CHAPTER 26: ASSESSMENT OF THE HEMATOLOGIC SYSTEM

General

Banaldi-Junkins CA et al: Hematopoiesis and cytokines: relevance to cancer and aging, *Hematol Oncol Clin North Am* 14:45, 2000.
Caen JP et al: Regulation of megakaryocytopoiesis, *Haemostasis* 29:27, 1999.
Hevehan DL et al: Physiologically significant effects of pH and oxygen tension on granulopoiesis, *Exp Hematol* 28:267, 2000.
Kaushansky K: Thrombopoietin and hematopoietic stem cell development, *Ann NY Acad Sci* 872:314, 1999.
Keen ML: Hemoglobin and hematocrit: an analysis of clinical accuracy, *ANNA J* 25:83, 1998.

Lahaye L, Biddle C: AANA Journal course: update for nurse anesthetists—the ruddy globule: the erythrocyte—its biology, chemistry, and functional variations, *AANA J* 68:463, 2000.

Maloy BJ: Hematopoiesis, stem cells, and transplantation, *J Intravenous Nurs* 23:298, 2000.

Oertel LB: Monitoring warfarin therapy, *Nursing 99* 29:41, 1999.

Stohlawetz PJ et al: Effects of erythropoietin on platelet reactivity and thrombopoiesis in humans, *Blood* 95:2983, 2000.

Weatherall, DJ, Provan, AB: Red cells 1: inherited anemias, *Lancet* 355:1169, 2000.

Wendling F: Thrombopoietin: its role from early hematopoiesis to platelet production, *Haematologica* 84:158, 1999.

Wilson CI et al: The peripheral blood smear in patients with sickle cell trait: a morphologic observation, *Lab Med* 31:445, 2000.

CHAPTER 27: HEMATOLOGIC PROBLEMS

Anemia

Nayak LH et al: Appropriateness of iron therapy in elderly long-term care residents, *Ann Long-term Care* 7(1):2, 1999.

Provan D, Wetherall D: Red cells II: acquired anemias and polycythemia, *Lancet* 355(9211):1260, 2000.

Ryan C: We made the perfect decision... nurse Lisa Nash...made medical history by genetically selecting her baby, *Nurs Times* 96(43):10, 2000.

Hemoglobinopathy

Clark C: Donation from HLA-Identical sibling donor good for thalassemic patient, *Transplant Weekly* March 1, 1999.

Mentzer WC, Kan YW: Prospects for research in hematologic disorders: sickle cell disease and thalassemia, *JAMA* 285(5):640, 2001.

Leukemia

McGarth P: Its horrendous—but really, what can you do? Preliminary findings on financial impact of relocation for specialized treatment, *Aust Health Rev* 23(3):94, 2000.

Medoff E: Oncology today: leukemia, *RN* 63(9):43, 2000.

Zevrack B: Quality of life of long-term survivors of leukemia and lymphoma, *J Psychosoc Oncol* 18(4):39, 2000.

Lymphoma

Grant WB: Ecological study of dietary and smoking links to lymphoma, *Altern Med Rev* 5(6):563, 2000.

Stremick K, Gallagher E: Malignant lymphomas: Hodgkin's disease and non-Hodgkin's lymphoma, *Am J Nurs* April supplement:18, 52, 2000.

Stem Cell Transplant

Baker F et al: Reintegration after bone marrow transplantation, *Cancer Pract* 7(4):190, 1999.

MMWR: Guidelines for preventing opportunistic infections among hematopoietic stem cell transplant recipients, *MMWR* (49[RR-10]): 1-95, 97-125, CE 1-7, 2000.

Smith ME et al: Issues and care of the post bone marrow transplant patient, *Home Health Care Consultant* 6(7):2, 1999.

CHAPTER 28: ASSESSMENT OF THE ENDOCRINE SYSTEM

General

DeGroot L, Jameson JL, editors: *Endocrinology,* ed 4, Philadelphia, 2001, WB Saunders.

Nusynowitz ML: Thyroid imaging. *Lippincott's Prim Care Pract* 3(6):546; quiz 556, 1999.

Watson R: Assessing endocrine system function in older people, *Nurs Older People* 12(9):27, 2000.

CHAPTER 29: PITUITARY, THYROID, PARATHYROID, AND ADRENAL GLAND PROBLEMS

General

Burgess JR et al: Osteoporosis in multiple endocrine neoplasia type 1: severity, clinical significance, relationship to primary hyperparathyroidism, and response to parathyroidectomy, *Arch Surg* 134(10):1119, 1999.

Chou FF et al: General weakness as an indication for parathyroid surgery in patients with secondary hyperparathyroidism, *Arch Surg* 134(10):1108, 1999.

DeGroot L, Jameson JL, editors: *Endocrinology,* ed 4, Philadelphia, 2001. WB Saunders.

Dorn LD, Cerrone P: Cognitive function in patients with Cushing syndrome: a longitudinal Perspective, *Clin Nurs Res* 9(4):420, 2000.

Luken KK: Clinical manifestations and management of Addison's disease, *Am Acad Nurse Pract* 11(4):151, 1999.

Shen WT et al: Laparoscopic vs open adrenalectomy for the treatment of primary Hyperaldosteronism, *Arch Surg* 134(6):628, 1999; discussion 631.

Subramaniam R et al: Retroperitoneoscopic excision of phaeochromocytoma: haemodynamic events, complications and outcome, *Anaesth Intensive Care* 28(1):49, 2000.

Terpstra TL, Terpstra TL: Syndrome of inappropriate antidiuretic hormone secretion: recognition and management, *Medsurg Nurs* 9(2):61, 2000; quiz 69. Review. PMID: 11033692 [PubMed indexed for MEDLINE]

Acromegaly

Coskeran P: Management and treatment of patients with acromegaly, *Nurs Times* Mar 95(13):50, 1999.

Sachse D: Acromegaly, *Am J Nurs* 101(11):69, 73, 77, 2001.

Adrenal Gland

Carson PP: Emergency: adrenal crisis, *Am J Nurs* 100(7):49, 2000.

Williams M: Disorders of the adrenal gland, *Semin Perioperative Nurs* 7(3):179, 1998.

Hypothyroidism

Bailes BK: Hypothyroidism in elderly patients, *AORN J* 69(5):1026, 1999.

Elliott B: Diagnosing and treating hypothyroidism, *Nurse Pract* 25(3):92, 99, 2000.

Nayback AM: Hyponatremia as a consequence of acute adrenal insufficiency and hypothyroidism, *J Emerg Nurs* 26(2):130, 2000.

Shelton BK: Hypothyroidism in cancer patients. *Nurse Pract Forum* 9(3):185, 1998.

Thyroid

Czenis AL: Thyroid disease in the elderly, *Adv Nurse Pract* 1999 7(9):38; quiz 45, 1999.

Stajduhar KI et al: Thyroid cancer: patients' experiences of receiving iodine-131 therapy, *Oncol Nurs Forum* 27(8):1213, 2000.

Walpert N: The highs and lows of autoimmune thyroid disease, *Nursing 98* 28(12):58, 1998.

Thyrotoxicosis

Dahlen R: Managing patients with acute thyrotoxicosis, *Crit Care Nurse* 22(1):62, 2002.

Lincoln NB et al: Patient education in thyrotoxicosis, *Patient Educ Couns* 40(2):143, 2000.

CHAPTER 30: DIABETES MELLITUS AND HYPOGLYCEMIA

General

Aiello JH: Preventing diabetic nephropathy: the role of primary care, *Nurse Pract* 23(2):12, 1998.

Bartol T: Putting a patient with diabetes in the driver's seat, *Nursing 2002* 32(2):53, 2002.

Baumann LC et al: Clinical outcomes for low-income adults with hypertension and diabetes, *Nurs Res* 51(3):191, 2002.

Cameron BL: Making diabetes management routine, *Am J Nurs* 102(2):26, 2002.

Fain JA: Lowering the boom on hyperglycemia, *Nursing 2001* 31(8):48, 2001.

Flood L, Constance A: Diabetes and exercise safety, *Am J Nurs* 102(6):47, 2002.

Konick-McMahan J: Riding out a diabetic emergency, *Nursing 99* 29(9):34, 1999.

Peters J et al: Diabetes care delivery in the community, *Prof Nurse* 16(1):844, 2000.

Tkaks NC: Hypoglycemia unawareness, *Am J Nurs* 102(2):34,

CHAPTER 31: ASSESSMENT OF THE GASTROINTESTINAL SYSTEM

General

Blazys D: Use of lavage in treating overdose, *J Emerg Med* 26(4):343, 2000.

Carlson E: Irritable bowel syndrome, *Nurse Pract* 23(1):82, 86, 1998.

Centers for Disease Control and Prevention: Outbreaks of *Escherichia coli* O157:H7 infections among children associated with farm visits-Pennsylvania and Washington, *JAMA* 285(18):2320, 2001, website: http://www.cdc.gov/health/diseases.htm.

King V: Is test-and-eradicate or prompt endoscopy more effective for treatment of dyspepsia in *Helicobacter pylori*-positive patients? *J Fam Pract* 49(11):1048, 2000.

Pisarra VH: Recognizing the various presentations of appendicitis, *Nures Pract* 24(8):42, 44, 49, 52, 1999.

Wilson SF, Giddens JF: *Health assessment for nursing practice,* ed 2, St Louis, 2001, Mosby.

CHAPTER 32: MOUTH AND ESOPHAGUS PROBLEMS

General

Galvan TJ: Dysphagia: going down and staying down, *Am J Nurs* 101(1):37, 2001.

McHale JM et al: Expert nursing knowledge in the care of patients at risk of impaired swallowing, *J Nurs Scholarship* 30(2):137, 1998.

Prisco MK: Evaluating neck masses, *Nurse Pract* 25(4):30, 2000.

Quinn KL, Reedy A: Esophageal cancer: therapeutic approaches and nursing care, *Semin Oncol Nursing* 15(1):17, 1999.

Shugars DC, Patton LL: Detecting, diagnosing and preventing oral cancer, *Nurse Pract* 22(6):105, 1997.

Spiess A, Kahrilas P: Treating achalasia, *JAMA* 280(7):638, 1998.

Gastroesophageal Reflux Disease

Ault DL, Schmidt D: Diagnosis and management of gastroesophageal reflux, *Nurse Pract* 23(6):81, 88, 1998.

Bunting T: Putting the lid on gastroesophageal reflux, *Nursing* 31(6):46, 2001.

Castell DO: A practical approach to heartburn, *Hosp Pract* 34(12):89, 1999.

DeVault K et al: Updated guidelines for the diagnosis and treatment of gastroesophageal reflux disease, *Am J Gastroenterol* 94(6):1434, 1999.

Goldsmith C: Gastroesophageal reflux disease, *Am J Nurs* 98(9):44, 1998.

Middlemiss C: Gastroesophageal reflux disease: a common condition in the elderly, *Nurse Pract* 22(11):51, 1997.

Resto MA: Gastroesophageal reflux disease, *Am J Nurs* 100(9):24D, 2000.

Scott M, Gelhot A: Gastroesophageal reflux disease: diagnosis and management, *Am Fam Physician* 59(5):1161, 1999.

CHAPTER 33: STOMACH AND DUODENUM PROBLEMS

Peptic Ulcer Disease

Aronson B: Update on peptic ulcer drugs, *Am J Nurs* 98(1):41, 1998.

Centers for Disease Control and Prevention, Division of Bacterial and Mycotic Diseases, *Helicobacter pylori* and peptic ulcer disease, 2001, website: http://www.cdc.gov/ulcer/md.htm.

Heslin JM: Peptic ulcer disease, *Nursing* 27(1):34, 1997.

Saunders CS: *H. pylori* infection: simplifying management, *Patient Care* 33(23):118, 1999.

Schuster J: Misoprostol and diarrhea, *Nursing* 28(4):68, 1998

GI Bleeding

Hines SE: Current management of upper GI tract bleeding, *Patient Care* 34(2):20, 2000.

Kamen BJ: Combating upper GI bleeding, *Nursing* 29(7):32hn1, 1999.

Laskowski-Jones L: Managing hemorrhage, *Nursing* 27(9):36, 1997.

Gastric Cancer

Graham DY: *Helicobacter pylori* infection is the primary cause of gastric cancer, *J Gastroenterol* 35(suppl 12):90, 2000.

Kodama M, Kodama T: In search of the cause of gastric cancer, *In Vivo* 14(1):125, 2000.

La Vecchia C, Franceschi S: Nutrition and gastric cancer, *Can J Gastroenterol* 14(Suppl D):51D, 2000.

O'Connor K: Gastric cancer, *Semin Oncol Nurs* 15(1):26, 1999.

Onishi K, Miaskowski C: Mechanisms and management of gastric cancer, *Cancer Nurs* 19(3):187, 1998.

Roukos DH: Current status and future perspectives in gastric cancer management, *Cancer Treat Rev* 26(4):243, 2000.

Nutrition/Malnutrition

Cammon SAR, Hackshaw HS: Are we starving our patients? *Am J Nurs* 100(5):43, 2000.

Dudek SG: Malnutrition in hospitals: who's assessing what patients eat? *Am J Nurs* 100(4):36, 2000.

Springhouse Corporation Staff: Evaluating nutritional disorders, *Nursing* 30(11):22, 2000.

Enteral and Parenteral Nutrition

Bliss DZ, Lehmann S: Tube feeding: administration tips, *RN* 62(8):2931, 1999.

Bliss DZ, Lehmann S: Tube feeding: immune boosting formulas, *RN* 62(8):26, 1999.

Bowers S: All about tubes, *Nursing* 30(12):41, 2000.

Bowers S: Nutrition support for malnourished acutely ill adults, *Medsurg Nurs* 8(3):145, 1999.

Cheever KH: Early enteral feeding of patients with multiple trauma, *Crit Care Nurse* 19(6):40, 1999.

Fellows LS et al: Evidence-based practice for enteral feedings: aspiration prevention strategies, bedside detection, and practice change, *MEDSURG Nursing* 9(1):27, 2000.

Kohn-Keeth C: How to keep feeding tubes flowing freely, *Nursing* 30(3):58, 2000.

Loan T et al: Debunking six myths about enteral feeding, *Nursing* 28(8):43, 1998.
Metheny NA et al: pH, color and feeding tubes, *RN* 61(1):25, 1998.
O'Brien B et al: G-tube site care: a practical guide, *RN* 62(2):52, 1999.

CHAPTER 34: INTESTINAL PROBLEMS

General

Aronson BS: Ruptured diverticulum, *Nursing* 28(9):33, 1998.
Breitfeller JM: Peritonitis, *Am J Nurs* 99(4):33, 1999.
Kamen BJ: Battling lower GI bleeding, *Nursing* 29(8):32hn1, 1999.
Lewis AM: Gastrointestinal emergency, *Nursing* 29(4):52, 1999.
Pisarra VH: Recognizing the various presentations of appendicitis, *Nurse Pract* 24(8):42, 44, 49, 52, 1999.

Foodborne Illness

Cerrato PL: When food is the culprit, *RN* 62(6):52, 1999.
Juckett G: Prevention and treatment of traveler's diarrhea, *Am Fam Physician* 60:119, 1999.
Mackenzie DL: When *E. coli* turns deadly, *RN* 62(7):28, 1999.
Newland J: Traveler's diarrhea, *Am J Nurs* 97(4):161, 1997.

Irritable Bowel Syndrome

Carlson E: Irritable bowel syndrome, *Nurse Pract* 23(1):82, 1998.
Heitkemper M, Jarrett M: Irritable bowel syndrome, *Am J Nurs* 101(1):26, 2001.
Springhouse: Living with irritable bowel syndrome, *Nursing* 29(9):38, 1999.

Inflammatory Bowel Disease

Botomoan V et al: Management of inflammatory bowel disease, *Am Fam Physician* 57(1):57, 71, 1998.
Cerrato PL: Omega-3 fatty acids: nothing fishy here, *RN* 62(8):59, 1999.
Klonowski E, Masoodi J: The patient with Crohn's disease, *RN* 62(3):32, 1999.
Martin FL: Ulcerative colitis, *Am J Nurs* 97(8):38, 1997.
Rayhorn N: Understanding inflammatory bowel disease, *Nursing* 29(12):57, 1999.
Read TE, Kodner IJ: Colorectal cancer: risk factors and recommendations for early detection, *Am Fam Physician* 59(11):3083, 2001.

Bowel Cancer

Cavalieri J, Franklin B: Hereditary nonpolyposis colon cancer, *Am J Nurs* 98(10):42, 1998.
Dammel T: Fecal occult blood testing, *Nursing* 27(7):44, 1997.
Held J: Caring for a patient with colon cancer, *Nursing* 27(4):34, 1997.
Griffith S, Kane K: What is the most cost effective screening regimen for colon cancer? *J Fam Pract* 50(1):13, 2001.
Pontieri-Lewis V: Colorectal cancer: prevention and screening, *Medsurg Nurs* 9(1):9, 2000.
Saddler D, Ellis C: Colorectal cancer, *Semin Oncol Nurs* 15(1):58, 1998.

Bowel Surgery

Dunn D: Common questions about ileoanal reservoirs, *Am J Nurs* 97(11):67, 1997.
Young M: Caring for patients with coloanal reservoirs for rectal cancer, *Medsurg Nurs* 9(4):193, 2000.

Ostomy Care

Ball EM: A teaching guide for a continent ileostomy, *RN* 63(12):35, 2000.
Bradley M, Pupiales M: Essential elements of ostomy care, *Am J Nurs* 97(7):38, 1997.
Bryant D, Fleischer I: Changing an ostomy appliance, *Nursing* 30(11):51, 2000.
Thompson J: A practical ostomy guide, *RN* 63(11):61, 2000.

CHAPTER 35: GALLBLADDER AND EXOCRINE PANCREATIC PROBLEMS

Cholecystitis

Farrar JA: Acute cholecystitis, *Am J Nurs* 101(1):35, 2001.
Leitzmann MF et al: A prospective study of coffee consumption and the risk of symptomatic gallstone disease in men, *JAMA* 281:2106, 1999.
Leitzmann MF et al: The relation of physical exercise to risk for symptomatic gallstone disease in men, *Ann Intern Med* 128:417, 1998.
Stabile BE: Laparoscopic cholecystectomy-associated bile duct injuries, *West J Med* 168(1):40, 1998.

Pancreatitis

Evans JD et al: Outcome of surgery for chronic pancreatitis, *Br J Surg* 84(5):624, 1997.
Haber PS, Pirola RC, Wilson JS: Clinical update: management of acute pancreatitis, *J Gastroenterol Hepatol* 12(3):189, 1997.
McLave SA, Ritchie CS: Artificial nutrition in pancreatic disease: what lessons have we learned from the literature? *Clin Nutr* 19(1):1, 2000.
Meissner JE: Caring for patients with pancreatitis, *Nursing* 27(10):50, 1997.
Pasero CL: Assessing and treating the pain of pancreatitis, *Am J Nurs* 98(11):1415, 1998.
Varona B et al: Food intake of patients with chronic pancreatitis after onset of the disease, *Am J Clin Nutr* 65(3):851, 1997.

CHAPTER 36: ASSESSMENT OF THE HEPATIC SYSTEM

General

Author: Antiviral briefs, *AIDS Patient Care STDs* 14(3):169, 2000.
Cabot S: A healthy liver and weight loss, *Positive Health* 37:33, 1999.
Chin NT et al: Seroprevalence of viral hepatitis in older nursing home population, *J Am Geriatr Soc* 47(9):1110, 1999.
Dieterich, DT: Chronic hepatitis C: update on diagnosis and treatment, *Consultant* 40(9):1590, 2000.
Ellet, MLC: Hepatitis C, E, F G, and non-AG, *Gastroenterol Nurs* 23(2):67, 2000.
Hatcher T: The proverbial herb, *Am J Nurs* 101(2):36, 2001.
Weisiger RA, Lyman EB: *Sleisinger and Fordtran's gastrointestinal and liver disease,* Philadelphia, 1999, WB Saunders.

CHAPTER 37: HEPATIC PROBLEMS

General

Carillo EH et al: Evolution in the treatment of complex blunt liver injuries, *Curr Probl Surg* 38:1, 2001.
Fetrow CW, Avila JR: *Professionals handbook of complementary and alternative medicines,* Springhouse, Pa, 1999, Springhouse.
Knudson MM, Maull KI: Nonoperative management of solid organ injuries, *Surg Clin North Am* 79:1357, 1999.
Schiff ER et al, editors: *Schiff's diseases of the liver,* ed 8, vol 1, Philadelphia, 1998, Lippincott-Raven.
Udobi KF et al: Role of ultrasonography in penetrating abdominal trauma, *J Trauma Injury Infect Crit Care* 50:475, 2001.
Wolfe M: *Therapy of digestive disorders,* Philadelphia, 2000, WB Saunders.

Hepatitis

Benson L et al: Advances in the treatment of hepatitis C: combination therapy with interferon alfa-2b and ribivirin, *J Am Acad Nurse Pract* 12(9):364, 2000.

Chene BL, Decker AP: Battling hepatitis C, *RN* 64(4):54, 2001.

Dougherty AS, Dreher HM: Hepatitis C: Current treatment for an emerging epidemic, *Medsurg Nurs* 10(1):9, 2001.

Haiduven DJ: Planning a hepatitis C postexposure management program for health care workers: issues and challenges, *AAOHN J* 48(8):370, 2000.

Jefferson T et al: Vaccines for preventing hepatitis B in health care workers, *Cochrane Library* issue 2:16, 2001.

Seeff LB: Natural history of hepatitis C, *Am J Med* 107:102, 1999.

Biliary/Liver Cirrhosis

Author: Complementary healthcare practices, *Gastroenterol Nurs* 24(1):38, 2001.

Helton WS et al: Tranjugular intrahepatic portasystemic shunt vs surgical shunt in good-risk cirrhotic patients, *Arch Surg* 136:17, 2001.

Molmenti EP et al: Hepatobiliary malignancies, *Surg Clin North Am* 79:43, 1999.

Nazarian GK et al: Refractory ascites: midterm results of treatment with a transjugular intrahepatic protosystem shunt, *Radiology* 205:173, 1997.

Liver Failure

Adam SJ: Palliative care for patients with a failed liver transplant, *Intensive Crit Care Nurs* 16(6):396, 2000.

Lee W, Williams R: *Acute liver failure,* Cambridge, 1997, Cambridge University Press.

Radovich PA: Use of transjugular intrahepatic portosystemic shunt in liver disease, *J Vasc Nurs* 18(3):83, 2000.

Trotto NE: Meeting the challenge of alcoholic liver disease, *Patient Care* 34(11):112, 2000.

CHAPTER 38: ASSESSMENT OF THE RENAL SYSTEM

General

Cook L: The value of lab values, *Am J Nurs* 99(5):66, 71, 73, 1999.

Rahman M et al: A comparison of standardized versus "usual" blood pressure measurements in hemodialysis patients, *Am J Kidney Dis* 39(6):1226, 2002.

CHAPTER 39: KIDNEY AND URINARY TRACT PROBLEMS

General

Astor BC et al: Association of kidney function with anemia: the Third National Health and Nutrition Examination Survey (1988-1994), *Arch Intern Med* 162(12):1401, 2002.

Callahan MB et al: A model for patient participation in quality of life measurement to improve rehabilitation outcomes, *Nephrol News Issues* 13(1):33, 1999.

CHAPTER 40: KIDNEY FAILURE

General

Caress AL et al: A descriptive study of meaning of illness in chronic renal disease, *J Adv Nurs* 33(6):716, 2001.

Dialysis

Dimkovic N, Oreopoulos DG: Chronic peritoneal dialysis in the elderly, *Semin Dial* 15(2):94, 2002.

Gregory N: Assessing the impact of concomitant therapies on anemia in dialysis patients.

Case study of the anemic patient, *Nephrol Nurs J* 27(3):320; quiz 324, 2000.

Karahan OI et al: Continuous ambulatory peritoneal dialysis, *Acta Radiol* 43(2):170, 2002.

Klang B et al: Predialysis education helps patients choose dialysis modality and increases disease-specific knowledge, *J Adv Nurs* 29(4):869, 1999.

Kutner NG, Jassal SV: Quality of life and rehabilitation of elderly dialysis patients, *Semin Dial* 15(2):107, 2002.

Vlaminck H et al: The dialysis diet and fluid non-adherence questionnaire: validity testing of a self-report instrument for clinical practice, *J Clin Nurs* 10(5):707, 2001.

Wolfson M: Nutrition in elderly dialysis patients, review, *Semin Dial* 15(2):113, 2000.

End-Stage Renal Disease

Hagren B et al: The haemodialysis machine as a lifeline: experiences of suffering from end-stage renal disease, *J Adv Nurs* 34(2):196, 2001.

Harris TT et al: Subjective burden in young and older African-American caregivers of patients

with end-stage renal disease awaiting transplant, *Nephrol Nurs J* 27(4):383, 355; discussion 392, 405, 2000.

Krishnan M et al: Epidemiology and demographic aspects of treated end-stage renal disease in the elderly, *Semin Dial* 15(2):79, 2000.

Roth C, Culp K: Renal osteodystrophy in older adults with end-stage renal disease, *J Gerontol Nurs* 27(7):46; quiz 54, 2001.

White Y, Grenyer BF: The biopsychosocial impact of end-stage renal disease: the experience of dialysis patients and their partners, *J Adv Nurs* 30(6):1312, 1999.

Hemodialysis

Curtin RB et al: Hemodialysis patients' noncompliance with oral medications, *ANNA J* 26(3):307; discussion 317, 1999.

Oka M, Chaboyer W: Dietary behaviors and sources of support in hemodialysis patients, *Clin Nurs Res* 8(4):302; discussion 314, 1999.

Thomas-Hawkins C: Symptom distress and day-to-day changes in functional status in chronic hemodialysis patients, *Nephrol Nurs J* 27(4):369; discussion 380, 428, 2000.

Welch JL, Davis J: Self-care strategies to reduce fluid intake and control thirst in hemodialysis Patients, *Nephrol Nurs J* 27(4):393, 2000.

Kidney Transplantation

Rao VK: Kidney transplantation in older patients: benefits and risks, *Drugs Aging* 19(2):79, 2002.

Wainwright SP et al: Psychosocial recovery from adult kidney transplantation: a literature review: review, *J Clin Nurs* 8(3):233, 1999.

Renal Failure

Lindqvist R et al: Perceived consequences of being a renal failure patient, *Nephrol Nurs J* 27(3):291; discussion 298, 2000.

McCann K, Boore JR: Fatigue in persons with renal failure who require maintenance haemodialysis, *J Adv Nurs* 32(5):1132, 2000.

Neild GH: Multi-organ renal failure in the elderly, *Int Urol Nephrol* 32(4):559, 2001.

Van de Noortgate N et al: The dialytic management of acute renal failure in the elderly: review, *Semin Dial* 15(2):127, 2002.

Wade-Elliott R: Caring for the elderly with renal failure: gastrointestinal changes, *ANNA J* 26(6):563, 596; quiz 570, 1999.

CHAPTER 41: ASSESSMENT OF THE NERVOUS SYSTEM

General

Brohi K, Wilson-MacDonald J: Evaluation of unstable cervical spine injury: a 6-year experience, *J Trauma Injury Infect Crit Care* 49(1):76, 2000.

Ignatavicius D: Resolving the delirium dilemma, *Nursing 99* 29(10):41, 1999.

Ishikawa K et al: Characteristics of infection and leukocyte count in severely head-injured patients treated with mild hypothermia, *J Trauma Injury Infect Crit Care* 49(5):912, 2000.

Jean WC et al: Gunshot wound to the head resulting in a vertebral artery pseudoaneurysm at the base of the skull, *J Trauma Injury Infect Crit Care* 50(1):126, 2001.

Leake NB: Looks can be deceiving: the behind-the-scenes battle of fibromyalgia, *Adv Nurse Practitioners* 9(6):41, 42, 44, 45, 51, 52, 56, 2001.

Marx JA, Biros MH: Who is at low risk after head or neck trauma, *N Engl J Med* 343:138, 2000.

Mayer DM et al: Speaking the language of pain, *Am J Nurs* 101(2):44, 2001.

Muller D: Brainstem conundrum: the Chiari I malformation, *J Am Acad Nurse Pract* 13(4):154, 2001.

Wijdicks EF: Current concepts: the diagnosis of brain death, *N Engl J Med* 344(16):1215, 2001.

Zimmerman PG: Development of a Glasgow Coma Scale teaching video, *J Emerg Nurs* 26(5):421, 2000.

CHAPTER 42: TRAUMATIC AND NEOPLASTIC PROBLEMS OF THE BRAIN

Seizures

Hilton G: Seizure disorders in adults: evaluation and management of new onset seizures, *Nurse Pract* 22(9):42, 1997.

Lewis AM: Neurologic emergency, *Nusing* 29(10):54, 1999.

Long L, Reeves A: The practical aspects of epilepsy: critical components of comprehensive patient care, *J Neurosci Nurs* 29(4):249, 1997.

McNew CD et al: How to help your patient with epilepsy, *Nursing* 27(9):57, 1997.

Shafer PO: Epilepsy and seizures—advances in seizure assessment, treatment and self management, *Nurs Clin North Am* 34(3):743, 1999.

Snively C et al: Vagal nerve stimulator as a treatment for intractable epilepsy, *J Neurosci Nurs* 30(5):286, 1998.

Headache

Anonymous: Headaches: treatments vary with the type, *Mayo Clin Health Lett* 19(9):1, 2001.

Blumenthal HJ, Rapoport AM: The clinical spectrum of migraine, *Med Clin North Am* 85(4):897, 2001.

Mannix LK: Epidemiology and impact of primary headache disorders, *Med Clin North Am* 85(4):887, 2001.

Mathews NT: Serotonin 1D(5-HT) agonists and other agents in acute migraine, *Neurol Clin* 15(1):61, 1997.

Moloney MF et al: Caring for the woman with migraine headaches, *Nurse Pract* 25(2):17, 2000.

Brain Tumors

Berweiler U et al: Reservoir systems for intraventricular chemotherapy, *J Neurooncol* 38:141, 1998.

Doolittle N et al: Blood brain barrier disruption for the treatment of malignant brain tumors. The national program, *J Neurosci Nurs* 30(2):81, 1998.

Increased Intracranial Pressure

Alvarez del Castillo M: Monitoring neurologic patients in intensive care, *Curr Opin Crit Care* 7(2):49, 2001.

Hilton G: Cerebral oxygenation in the traumatically brain-injured patient: are ICP and CPP enough? *J Neurosci Nurs* 32(5):278, 2000.

Kajs-Wylie M: Antihypertensive therapy for the neurological patient: a nursing challenge, *J Neurosci Nurs* 31(3):142, 1999.

Stewart-Amidei C: Neurologic monitoring in the ICU, *Crit Care Nurs Q* 21(3):47, 1998.

Central Nervous System Infection

King D: Central nervous system infection, *Nurs Clin North Am* 34(3):761, 1999.

Head Trauma

Davella D et al: Guidelines for the treatment of adults with severe head trauma—criteria for surgical treatment, *J Neurosurg Sci* 44(1):19, 2000.

Marion ND, Speigel TP: Changes in the management of severe traumatic brain injury: 1991-1997, *Crit Care Med* 28(1):16, 2000.

McCarthy G, Quin G: Future inpatient management of patients with minor head injuries, *Emerg Med J* 17(2):153, 2000.

McNair ND: Traumatic brain injury, *Nurs Clin North Am* 34(3):637, 1999.

Meagher RJ, Narayan RK: The triage and acute management of severe head injury, *Clin Neurosurg* 46:127, 2000.

Procaccio F et al: Guidelines for the treatment of adults with severe head trauma: criteria for medical treatment, *J Neurosurg Sci* 44(1):11, 2000.

Segatore M: Corticosteroid and traumatic brain injury: status at the end of the decade of the brain, *J Neurosci Nurs* 31(4):239, 1999.

Sullivan J: Positioning of patients with severe traumatic brain injury: research based practice, *J Neurosci Nurs* 32(4):204, 2000.

Wilberger JE: Contemporary treatment paradigms in head injury, *Clin Neurosurg* 46:143, 2000.

CHAPTER 43: VASCULAR AND DEGENERATIVE PROBLEMS OF THE BRAIN

Cerebral Vascular Disease

Fedorov EM: Helping patients with dysphagia, *Am J Nurs* 101:24GG, 2001.

Hafsteinsdottir TB, Brypdonck M: Being a stroke patient: a review of the literature, *J Adv Nurs* 26(3):580, 1997.

Hock HH: Brain attack, *Nurs Clin North Am* 34(3):689, 1999.

Treib J et al: Treatment of stroke on an intensive stroke unit: a novel concept, *Intensive Care Med* 26:1598, 2000.

Multiple Sclerosis

National Multiple Sclerosis Society: www.nmss.org.

Noseworthy JH et al: Medical progress: multiple sclerosis, *N Engl J Med* 343(13):938, 2000.

Ross AP: Neurologic degenerative disorders, *Nurs Clin North Am* 34(3):725, 1999.

Parkinson's Disease

Barker S et al: Parkinson's disease: a holistic approach, *Am J Nurs* 98(11):48A, 1998.

Conley CC, Kirchner JT: Medical and surgical treatment of Parkinson's disease: strategies to slow symptom progression and improve quality of life, *Postgrad Med* 106(2):41, 1999.

Herndon CM et al: Parkinson's disease revisited, *J Neurosci Nurs* 32(4):216, 2000.

Jacopini G: The experience of disease: psychosocial aspects of movement disorders, *J Neurosci Nurs* 32(5):263, 2000.
Parkinson's Disease Foundation: www.parkinsons-foundation.org.
Ross AP: Neurologic degenerative disorders, *Nurs Clin North Am* 34(3):725, 1999.
Young R: Update on Parkinson's disease, *Am Fam Physician* 59(8):2155, 1999.

Myasthenia Gravis

Cunning S: When the dx is myasthenia gravis, *RN* 63(4):26, 2000.
Hopkins LC: Clinical features of myasthenia gravis, *Neurol Clin* 12(2):243, 1994.
Grohar-Murray ME: Self-care actions to manage fatigue among myasthenia gravis patients, *J Neurosci Nurs* 30(3):191, 1998.
Kokontis L, Gutmann L: Current treatment of neuromuscular diseases, *Arch Neurol* 57(7):939, 2000.
Myasthenia Gravis Foundation of America: www.myasthenia.org.
Ross AP: Neurologic degenerative disorders, *Nurs Clin North Am* 34(3):725, 1999.

Amyotrophic Lateral Sclerosis

Carter GT et al: Expanding the role of hospice care in amyotrophic lateral sclerosis, *Am J Hospital Palliative Care* 16(6):707, 1999.
National ALS Association: www.alsa.org.
Nowotny ML: Reflections: my journey with amyotrophic lateral sclerosis, *J Neurosci Nurs* 30(1):68, 1998.
Ross AP: Neurologic degenerative disorders, *Nurs Clin North Am* 34(3):725, 1999.
Walling AD: Amyotrophic lateral sclerosis, *Am Fam Physician* 59(6):1489, 1999.

Guillain-Barré Syndrome

Kokontis L, Gutmann L: Current treatment of neuromuscular diseases, *Arch Neurol* 57(7):939, 2000.
Sulton LL: A multidisciplinary care approach to Guillain-Barre syndrome, *Dimen Crit Care Nurs* 20(1):16, 2001.
Worsham T: Easing the course of Guillain-Barre syndrome, *RN* 63(3):46, 2000.

CHAPTER 44: SPINAL CORD AND PERIPHERAL NERVE PROBLEMS

Spinal Cord Injury

Black T: Moving into the millennium with new SCI standards, *Spinal Cord Injury Nurs* 17(2):69, 2000.
Blair ME: Assistive technology: what and how for persons with spinal cord injury, *Spinal Cord Injury Nurs* 17(3):110, 2000.
Burke DA et al: Incidence rates and populations at risk for spinal cord injury: a regional study, *Spinal Cord* 39:274, 2001.
Chonin AT et al: Providing rehab care? *Am J Nurs* 100(7):78, 2000.
Lathbury K: The road ahead: managing a spinal cord injury, *Case Manager* 11(3):55, 2000.
Lucke KT: Pulmonary management following acute SCI, *J Neurosci Nurs* 30(2):91, 2000.
Mitcho K, Yanko JR: Acute care management of spinal cord injuries, *Crit Care Nurs Q* 22(2):61, 1999.
Predergast V, Sullivan C: Acute spinal cord injury: nursing considerations for the first 72 hours, *Crit Care Nurs Clin North Am* 12(4):499, 2000.
Senior K: Spinal cord repair: are we getting closer? *Lancet* 355(9212):1340, 2000.
Wald A: Help and hope for patients with spinal cord injury, *Nurs Spectrum* 11A(15):8, 1999.

Cranial Nerve Disorders

Costa M: Trigeminal neuralgia, *Am J Nurs* 98(6):42, 1998.
Domanico S: Bell's palsy: a case study, *Internet J Adv Nurs Pract* 12(1):1, 1998.
Jackson EM et al: Trigeminal neuralgia: a diagnostic challenge, *Am J Emerg Med* 17(6):1, 1999.
Kumar GK et al: When is facial pain trigeminal neuralgia? *Postgrad Med* 104(4):149, 155, 199, 1998.
Love RMK: Bell's palsy isn't fatal, but patients need special attention, *RN* 62(2):12, 1999.
Mosiman W: Taking the sting out of trigeminal neuralgia, *Nursing* 31(3):86, 2001.
Noone J, Longe S: Bell's palsy in the primary care setting: a case study, *Clin Excellence Nurse Pract* 2(4):206, 1998.

CHAPTER 45: ASSESSMENT OF THE MUSCULOSKELETAL SYSTEM

General

Corbett JV: Laboratory tests and diagnostic procedures in orthopaedic nursing practice, *Nurs Clin North Am* 33(4):685, 1998.
Heibler K: Mobility health assessment, *Orthopaedic Nurs* 17(4):30, 1998.
Maher AB et al, editors: *Orthopaedic nursing,* ed 3, Philadelphia, 2002, WB Saunders.
Mangini M: Physical examination of the musculoskeletal system, *Nurs Clin North Am* 33(4):685, 1998.
O'Hanlon-Nichols {au: initial?}: A review of the adult musculoskeletal system, *Am J Nurs* 98(6):48, 1998.
Seidel HM et al: *Mosby's guide to physical examination,* ed 4, St Louis, 1999, Mosby.
Unger J, Selfridge-Thomas J: The preparticipation evaluation. In *Nursing contact hours for nurse practitioners,* Atlanta, 2001, American Health Consultants.

CHAPTER 46: TRAUMA TO THE MUSCULOSKELETAL SYSTEM

General

Barnett R et al: A patient-oriented approach to the management of musculoskeletal injuries, *Therapeutic Bull: Suppl Clinician News* 6(2): 2002.
Goldstein TS: *Geriatric orthopaedics: rehabilitative management of common problems,* ed 2, Gaithersberg, Md, 1999, Aspen.
Maher AB et al, editors: *Orthopaedic nursing,* ed 3, Philadelphia, 2002, WB Saunders.
Parsons LC et al: Orthopaedic trauma: managing secondary medical problems, *Crit Care Nurs Clin North Am* 13(3):433, 2001.

Fractures

Byrne T: Orthopaedic essentials: the setup and care of a patient in Buck's traction, *Orthopaedic Nurs* 18(2):79, 1999.
Davis P, Barr L: Principles of traction, *J Orthop Nurs* 3(4):222, 1999.
Feldt KS, Oh HL: Pain and hip fracture outcomes for older adults, *Orthopaedic Nurs* 19(8):35, 2000.
Pifer G: Casting and splinting: prevention of complications, *Top Emerg Med* 22(3):48, 2000.
Sims M, Whiting J: Pin-site care, *Nurs Times* 96(48):46, 2000.

Complications of Fractures

D'Heere MS et al: Fat embolism syndrome, *J Trauma Nurs* 6(3):73, 1999.
Tumbarello C: Acute extremity compartment syndrome, *J Trauma Nurs* 7(2):30, 2000.

CHAPTER 47: DEGERATIVE DISORDERS

General

Evans CZH, Robbins PD: Gene therapy in orthopaedics, *Orthopaedic Nurs* 19(1):16, 2000.
Slowikowski RD, Flaherty SA: Epidural analgesia for postoperative orthopaedic pain, *Orthopaedic Nurs* 19(1):23, 2000.
Turkowski B: Preventing DVT in orthopaedic patients, *Orthopaedic Nurs* 19(3):93, 2000.

Complementary and Alternative Therapies

Carmack BJ: Companion animals: social support for orthopaedic clients, *Nurs Clin North Am* 33(4):701, 1998.
Herdtner S: Using therapeutic touch in nursing practice, *Orthopaedic Nurs* 19(5):77, 2000.
Stupay S, Siversten L: Herbal and nutritional supplement use in the elderly, *Nurse Pract* 25(9):56, 2000.

Rheumatoid Arthritis

Berard A et al: Patterns of drug use in rheumatoid arthritis, *J Rheumatol* 27(7):1648, 2000.
Genovese MC, Davis JS: Decision making in medicine. Current management of rheumatoid arthritis, *Hosp Pract* 36(2):21, 29, 35, 2001.
Infante R, Lahita RG: Rheumatoid arthritis: new disease modifying and anti-inflammatory drugs, *Geriatrics* 55(3):30, 35, 39, 2000.
Leine-Kilpi H et al: Nursing study of the significance of rheumatoid arthritis as perceived by patients using the concept of empowerment, *J Orthop Nurs* 3(3):138, 1999.
MacLean CH et al: Quality of care for patients with rheumatoid arthritis, *JAMA* 284(8):984, 2000.
Oh TM et al: Rehabilitation of orthopaedic and rheumatologic disorders: connective tissue diseases, *Arch Phys Med Rehabil* 81(3)(suppl 1):S60, 78, 101, 2000.

Degenerative Joint Disease

American College of Rheumatology Subcommittee on Osteoarthritis: Recommendations for the medical management of osteoarthritis of the hip and knee, *Arthritis Rheum* 43(9):1905, 2000.
Brander VA et al: Rehabilitation of orthopaedic and rheumatologic disorders: degenerative joint disease, *Arch Phys Med Rehabil* 81(3)(Suppl 1):S 67, 78, 101, 2000.
Burmeister A: The use of glucosamine and chondroitin sulfate in the treatment of osteoarthritis, *Physician Assistant* 24(11):46,49,52, 2000.
Leslie M: Knee osteoarthritis management therapies, *Pain Management Nurs* 20:51, 2001.
Moon LB, Backer J: Relationships among self-efficacy, outcome expectancy, and postoperative behaviors in total joint replacement patients, *Orthopaedic Nurs* 19(2):77, 2000.
Schlesinger N: Osteoarthritis: pathology, epidemiology, and risk factors, *Physical Med Rehabil: State of the Art Rev* 15(1):1, 2001.
Seemann S: Interdisciplinary approach to a total knee replacement program, *Nurs Clin North Am* 35(2):405, 2000.
Sharkey NA et al: The role of exercise in the prevention and treatment of osteoporosis and osteoarthritis, *Nurs Clin North Am* 35(1):209, 2000.
Showalter A et al: Patients' and their spouses' needs after total joint arthroplasty: a pilot study, *Orthopaedic Nurg* 19(1):49,62, 2000.
Watson MC et al: Nonaspirin, non-steroidal anti-inflammatory drugs for osteoarthritis of the knee, *Cochrane Library,* Oxford, Issue 2, 2001.

Gout

Hill J: Gout: its causes, symptoms, and treatment, *Nurs Times* 95(47):48, 1999.
Tucker F: Acute gouty arthritis: diagnosis and treatment, *Physician Assistant* 23(11):32, 1999.

Autoimmune Connective Tissue Diseases

Barwick ARW: Understanding lupus, *Nurs Standard* 14(46):47, 53, 2000.
Brown AC: Lupus erythematosus and nutrition: a review of the literature, *J Ren Nutr* 10(4):170, 2000.
Petri M: Approach to the management of systemic lupus erythematosus, *J Clin Outcomes Management* 7(8):56, 2000.
Sontheimer RD, Kovalchik P: Cutaneous manifestations of rheumatic diseases: lupus erythematosus, dermatomyositis, scleroderma, *Dermatol Nurs* 10(2):81, 1998.

Metabolic Bone Diseases

Eck JC et al: Vertebroplasty: a new treatment strategy for osteoporotic compression fractures, *Am J Orthop* 21(3):1234, 2002.
Ioannidis G et al: Quality of life in osteoporosis, *Nurs Clin North Am* 36(3):481, 2001.
Lewis T et al: Caring for the patient with Paget's disease of the bone, *Nurse Pract* 24(7):50, 53, 57, 1999.
Lucasey B: Corticosteroid-induced osteoporosis, *Nurs Clin North Am* 36(3):455, 2001.
McClung B, McClung M: Pharmacologic therapy for the treatment and prevention of osteoporosis, *Nurs Clin North Am* 36(3):433, 2001.
Meiner SE: An expanding landscape: osteoporosis treatment options today, *Adv Nurse Pract* 7(7):27, 80, 1999.

Low Back Pain

Mazanec D: Diagnosis and management of low back pain in older adults, *Clin Geriatr* 8(13):63, 2000.

Disorders Affecting the Muscles

Kagen LJ: How to evaluate the patient who has muscle disease, *J Musculoskeletal Med* 17(7):407, 2000.
Krivickas LS, Carlson NL: Myopathies, *Physical Med Rehabil: State of the Art Rev* 13(2):307, 1999.

CHAPTER 48: ASSESSMENT OF THE IMMUNE SYSTEM

General

Deasy J: How the immune system responds to infection, *J Am Acad Physician Assistants* 10(5):73, 1997.
Lahita RG: Gender and the immune system, *J Gender Specific Med* 3(7):19, 2000.
National Cancer Institute (NCI), 2001: Internet document: *Understanding the immune system,* website: http://rex.nci.nih.gov/behindthenews/uis/uisframe.htm.
Ploegh HL: Immune and other responses to viral infections, *Nutr Rev* 58:51, 2000.
Risi GF, Tomascak V: Prevention of infection in the immunocompromised host, *Am J Infect Control* 26(6):594.{au: year?}
Sobel JD: Pathogenesis of urinary tract infection: role of host defenses, *Infect Dis Clin North Am* 11(3):531, 1997.
Sun LZ et al: The American cornflower: a prophylactic role involving nonspecific immunity, *J Alternative Complementary Med* 5(5):437, 1999.
Yoshikawa TT: State of infectious diseases health care in older persons, *Clin Geriatr* 7(5):55, 1999.

CHAPTER 49: IMMUNOLOGIC PROBLEMS

General

Rohde T et al: Glutamine, exercise, and the immune system—is there a link? *Exerc Immunol Rev* 4:49, 1998.

Chronic Fatigue Syndrome

Dimitrov MG: Neuropsychological assessment of chronic fatigue syndrome, *J Chronic Fatigue Syndrome* 3(4):31, 1997.

Goldstein JA: The pathophysiology of chronic fatigue syndrome and related neurosomatic disorders, *J Chronic Fatigue Syndrome* 6(2):83, 2000.

Uslan D: Perspectives on CFS and impairment: proposed guidelines for disability determination, *J Chronic Fatigue Syndrome* 3(4):75, 1997.

Werbach MR: Chronic fatigue syndrome: how far have we come? *J Nutr Environmental Med* 10(3):181, 2000.

Latex Allergy

Buhr V: Screening patients for latex allergies, *J Am Acad Nurse Pract* 12(9):380, 2000.

Criss E: Latex allergies: a growing concern for both EMS providers and patients, *J Emerg Med Serv* 25(10):42, 2000.

Davis BR: Perioperative care of patients with latex allergy. *AORN J* 72(1):47, 2000.

Drake C: Online connections. Internet resources about latex allergy, *AORN J* 72(1):107, 2000.

Dyck RJ: Historical development of latex allergy, *AORN J* 72(1):27, 2000.

Fetter MS: Nursing's hazards to health, *Medsurg Nurs* 12(3):197, 2000.

Lopes MH, Lopes RA: Latex allergy in health care personnel, *AORN J* 72(1):42, 2000.

Suleyman F: Addressing the problem of latex glove allergy, *Community Nurse* 6(3):26, 2000.

Hypersensitivity Reactions

Howatson-Jones IL: Adverse reactions to contrast media, *Professional Nurse* 15(12):771, 2000.

Schonwald S: Methylprednisolone anaphylaxis, *Am J Emerg Med* 17(6):583, 1999.

Shuster J: Adverse drug reaction: amphotericin B reaction, *Nursing 2000* 30(11):89, 2000.

Snooks H et al: Care of patients with anaphylactic shock, *Prehospital Immediate Care* 4(1):51, 2000.

Transfusions

Glover G, Powell F: Blood transfusions, *Emerg Nurse* 4(4):10, 1997.

Raife TJ: Adverse effects of transfusions caused by leukocytes, *J Intravenous Nurs* 20(5):238, 1997.

CHAPTER 50: HIV INFECTIONS AND AIDS

General

Abbaticola MM: A team approach to the treatment of AIDS wasting, *J Assoc Nurse AIDS Care* 10(1):45, 2000.

Corti ME et al: Disseminated histoplasmosis and AIDS: clinical aspects and diagnostic methods for early detection, *AIDS Patient Care Standards* 14(3):149, 2000.

Cosby C et al: Hematological complications and quality of life in hospitalized AIDS patients, *AIDS Patient Care Standards* 14(5):269, 2000.

Fisher LR et al: AIDS, anemia, and an abnormal platelet count, *Hosp Pract* 34(10):39, 1999.

Frich LM, Borgbjerg FM: Pain and pain treatment in AIDS patients: a longitudinal study, *J Pain Symptom Manage* 19(5):339, 2000.

Hirschhorn L: Women and HIV: closing the treatment gap, *Patient Care* 33(6):187, 1999.

Jones KM: Human immunodeficiency virus disease: managing respiratory complications through the life span, *Crit Care Nurs Clin North Am* 11(4):455, 1999.

Keithley JK et al: HIV/AIDS and nutrition implications for disease management, *Nurs Case Manage* 5(2):52, 2000.

Lambotte O et al: Nosocomial bacteremia in HIV patients: the role of peripheral venous catheters, *Infect Control Hosp Epidemiol* 21(5):330, 2000.

Ungvarski PJ, Trzcianowska H: Neurocognitive disorders seen in HIV disease, *Issues in Mental Health Nurs* 21(1):51, 2000.

CHAPTER 51: ORGAN TRANSPLANTATION

General

Alcoser PW, Burchett S: Bone marrow transplantation: immune system suppression and reconstitution, *Am J Nurs* 99(6):1999.

Augustine SM: Heart transplantation: long term management related to immunosuppression, complications, and psychosocial adjustments, *Crit Care Nurs Clin North Am* 12(1):69, 2000.

Becker C, Petlin A: Heart transplantation, *Am J Nurs* (May Suppl):8, 1999.

Bush WW: Overview of transplantation immunology and the pharmacotherapy of adult solid organ transplant recipients: focus on immunosuppression, *AACN Clin Issues Adv Practice Acute Critical Care* 10(2):253, 1999.

Denton MD et al: Immunosuppression strategies in transplantation, *Lancet* 353(9158):26, 1999.

Glaser V: Bone marrow transplantation for cancer: exploring the options, *Patient Care 2000* 34(5):74, 2000.

Good EW: Caring for patients with donor organs, *Nursing 2000* 30(6):34, 2000.

Johnson E et al: Preventing fungal infections in immunocompromised patients, *Br J Nurs* 9(17):1154, 2000.

Penko ME, Tirbaso D: An overview of liver transplantation, *AACN Clin Issues Adv Practice Acute Critical Care* 10(2):176, 2000.

Poole P, Greer E: Immunosuppression in transplantation: a new millennium in care, *Crit Care Nurs Clin North Am* 12(3):315, 2000.

CHAPTER 52: ASSESSMENT OF THE REPRODUCTIVE SYSTEM

General

American College of Obstetricians and Gynecologists: *Adult manifestations of childhood sexual abuse,* ACOG Educational Bulletin No 259, Washington, DC, 2000, American College of Obstetricians and Gynecologists.

American College of Obstetricians and Gynecologists: *Primary and preventive care: periodic assessments,* ACOG Committee Opinion, No 246, Washington, DC, 2000, American College of Obstetricians and Gynecologists.

DeMasters J: HRT: a clinician's guide to understanding the dilemma, *AWHONN Lifelines* 4:27, 2000.

Furniss K: Tomatoes, Pap smears, and tea? Adopting behaviors that may prevent reproductive cancers and improve health, *J Obstet Gynecol Neonatal Nurs* 29:641, 2000.

North American Menopause Society: *Menopause core curriculum study guide,* 2001, website: http://www.menopause.org/proedu/studyguide.html.

North American Menopause Society: A decision tree for the use of estrogen replacement therapy or hormone replacement therapy in postmenopausal women: consensus opinion of the North American Menopause Society, *Menopause* 7:76, 2000.

North American Menopause Society: Clinical challenges of perimenopause: consensus opinion of the North American Menopause Society, *Menopause* 7:5, 2000.

North American Menopause Society: The role of calcium in peri- and postmenopausal women: consensus opinion of the North American Menopause Society, *Menopause* 8:84, 2001.

North American Menopause Society: The role of isoflavones in menopausal health: consensus opinion of the North American Menopause Society, *Menopause* 7:215, 2000.

Shepherd J et al: Interventions for the encouraging of sexual lifestyles and behaviors intended to prevent cervical cancer (Cochrane Review). In *The Cochrane Library,* 1, Oxford, 2001, Update Software.

CHAPTER 53: WOMEN WITH REPRODUCTIVE PROBLEMS

General

American College of Obstetricians and Gynecologists: *Adult manifestations of childhood sexual abuse,* ACOG Educational Bulletin No. 259, Washington, DC, 2000, ACOG.

American College of Obstetricians and Gynecologists: *Surgical alternatives to hysterectomy in the management of leiomyomas,* ACOG Practice Bulletin No. 16, Washington, DC, 2000, ACOG.

Wyatt K et al: Premenstrual syndrome, *Clin Evidence* 4:1121, 2000.

CHAPTER 54: PROBLEMS OF THE BREAST

General

Baron R: Sensory alterations after breast cancer surgery, *Clin J Oncol Nurs* 2(1):17, 1998.

Gross RE: Current issues in the surgical treatment of early stage breast cancer, *Clin J Oncol Nurs* 2(2):55, 1998.

Gross RE et al: A flowsheet for documenting independent nursing visits after breast cancer, *Oncol Nurs Forum* 26(4):775, 1999.

Harris RL: Consistency of patient information: is this happening? *Cancer Nurs* 20(4):274, 1997.

Lauri S, Sainio C: Developing the nursing care of breast cancer patients: an action research approach, *J Clin Nurs* 7:424, 1998.

Leddy SK: Incentives and barriers to exercise in women with a history of breast cancer, *Oncol Nurs Forum* 24(5):885, 1997.

Rees CE, Bath PA: Meeting the information needs of adult daughters of women with early breast cancer, *Cancer Nurs* 23(1):71, 2000.

Seegers BL et al: Self care and breast cancer recovery, *Cancer Pract* 6(6):339, 1998.

Skrutkowska M, Weijer C: Do patients with breast cancer participating in clinical trials receive better nursing care? *Oncol Nurs Forum* 24(8):1411, 1997.

Sladek ML et al: A critical pathway for patients undergoing one-day breast cancer surgery, *Clin J Oncol Nurs* 3(3):99, 1999.

Adjuvant Therapy

Craddock RB et al: An intervention to increase use and effectiveness of self-care measures for breast cancer chemotherapy patients, *Cancer Nurs* 22(4):312, 1999.

Hebert-Croteau N et al: Compliance with consensus recommendations for the treatment of early stage breast carcinoma in women, *Cancer* 85(5):1104, 1999.

Johnson JE et al: The effects of nursing care guided by self-regulation theory on coping with radiation therapy, *Oncol Nurs Forum* 24(6):1041, 1997.

Knobf MT: Natural menopause and ovarian toxicity associated with breast cancer therapy, *Oncol Nurs Forum* 25(9):1519, 1998.

Longman AJ et al: Pattern of association over time of side effects burden, self-help, and self-care in women with breast cancer, *Oncol Nurs Forum* 24(9):1555, 1997.

Mock V et al: Effects of exercise on fatigue, physical functioning, and emotional distress during radiation therapy for breast cancer, *Oncol Nurs Forum* 24(6):991, 1997.

Schwartz AL: Daily fatigue patterns and effect of exercise in women with breast cancer, *Cancer Pract* 8(1):16, 2000.

Wengström Y et al: Effects of a nursing intervention on subjective distress, side effects and quality of life of breast cancer patients receiving curative radiation therapy, *Acta Oncol* 38(6):763, 1999.

Whenery-Tedder M: A positive approach to chemotherapy, *Nurs Times* 93(23):2, 1997.

Wickham RS et al: Taste changes experienced by patients receiving chemotherapy, *Oncol Nurs Forum* 26(4):697, 1999.

Genetics

Amlung S et al: Genetic predisposition to breast and ovarian cancer: a case study, *AACN Clin Issues* 9(4):555, 1998.

Baron RH, Borgen PI: Genetic susceptibility for breast cancer: testing and primary prevention options, *Oncol Nurs Forum* 24(3):461, 1997.

Bove CM et al: Presymptomatic and predisposition genetic testing: ethical and social considerations, *Semin Oncol Nurs* 13(2):135, 1997.

Biesecker BB: Psychological issues in cancer genetics, *Semin Oncol Nurs* 13(2):120, 1997.

Cain S: Breast cancer genetics and the role of tamoxifen in prevention, *J Am Acad Nurse Pract* 12(1):21, 2000.

Hoffman W, Schlag PM: BRCA1 and BRCA2- breast cancer susceptibility genes, *J Cancer Res Clin Oncol* 126:487, 2000.

Jenkins J: Educational issues related to cancer genetics, *Semin Oncol Nurs* 13(2):141, 1997.

Kash KK et al: Psychosocial aspects of cancer genetics: women at high risk for breast and ovarian cancer, *Semin Surg Oncol* 18:333, 2000.

Steinberg KK: Risks associated with genetic testing: health insurance discrimination or simply business as usual, *JAMA* 55(4):241, 2000.

Williams JK: Principles of genetics and cancer, *Semin Oncol Nurs* 13(2):68, 1997.

Lymphedema

Carter BJ: Women's experiences of lymphedema, *Oncol Nurs Forum* 24(5):875, 1997.

Földi E: The treatment of lymphedema, *Cancer* 83:2833, 1998.

Meek AG: Breast radiotherapy and lymphedema, *Cancer* 83:2788, 1998.

Mortimer PS: The pathophysiology of lymphedema, *Cancer* 83:2798, 1998.

Passik SD, McDonald MV: Psychosocial aspects of upper extremity lymphedema in women treated for breast carcinoma, *Cancer* 83:2817, 1998.

Pressman PI: Surgical treatment and lymphedema, *Cancer* 83:2782, 1998.

Rinehart-Ayers ME: Conservative approaches to lymphedema treatment, *Cancer* 83:2828, 1998.

Rockson SG: Precipitating factors in lymphedema: myths and realities, *Cancer* 83:2814, 1998.

Thiadens SR: Current status of education and treatment resources for lymphedema, *Cancer* 83:2864, 1998.

Prevention/Screening

Deane KA: The role of the breast clinic nurse, *AORN J* 66(2):304, 1997.

Gulitz E et al: Missed screening opportunities among older women, *Cancer Pract* 6(5):289, 1998.

Holm CJ et al: Health beliefs, health locus of control, and women's mammography behavior, *Cancer Nurs* 22(2):149, 1999.

Leslie NS, Roche BG: The effectiveness of the breast self-examination shield, *Oncol Nurs Forum* 24(10):1759, 1997.

Northouse LL et al: Coping with a breast biopsy: how healthcare professionals can help women and their husbands, *Oncol Nurs Forum* 24(3):473, 1997.

Poole K, Lyne PA: The 'cues' to diagnosis: describing the monitoring activities of women undergoing diagnostic investigations for breast disease, *J Adv Nurs* 31(4):752, 2000.

Rimer BK, Bluman LG: The psychosocial consequences of mammography, *J Natl Cancer Inst Monogr* 22:131, 1997.

Psychoemotional Issues

Carroll S: Breast cancer part 3: psychosocial care, *Prof Nurse* 13(12):877, 1998.

Hoskins CN: Breast cancer treatment-related patterns in side-effects, psychological distress, and perceived health status, *Oncol Nurs Forum* 24(9):1575, 1997.

Lehto RH, Cimprich B: Anxiety and directed attention in women awaiting breast cancer surgery, *Oncol Nurs Forum* 26(4):767, 1999.

Survivors of breast cancer: illness uncertainty, positive reappraisal, and emotional distress, *Oncol Nurs Forum* 25(3):555, 1998.

Pelusi J: The lived experience of surviving breast cancer, *Oncol Nurs Forum* 24(8):1343, 1997.

Pozo-Kaderman C et al: The psychosocial aspects of breast cancer, *Nurse Pract Forum* 10(3):165, 1999.

Rendle K: Survivorship and breast cancer: the psychosocial issues, *J Clin Nurs* 6:403, 1997.

Samarel N et al: Women's perceptions of group support and adaptation to breast cancer, *J Adv Nurs* 28(6):1259, 1998.

Sandgren AK et al: Telephone therapy for patients with breast cancer, *Oncol Nurs Forum* 27(4):683, 2000.

Wyatt GK, Friedman LL: Physical and psychosocial outcomes of midlife and older women following surgery and adjuvant therapy for breast cancer, *Oncol Nurs Forum* 25(4):761, 1998.

Quality of Life

Ashing-Giwa K et al: Quality of life of African-American and white long-term breast carcinoma survivors, *Cancer* 85(2):418, 1999.

Bloom JR et al: Intrusiveness of illness and quality of life in young women with breast cancer, *Psychoooncology* 7:89, 1998.

Bull AA: Quality of life in women with recurrent breast cancer, *Breast Cancer Res Treat* 54:47, 1999.

Dorval M et al: Long term quality of life after breast cancer: comparison of 8-year survivors with population controls, *J Clin Oncol* 16(2):487, 1998.

Dorval M et al: Type of mastectomy and quality of life for long term breast carcinoma survivors, *Cancer* 83(10):2130, 1998.

Ferrell BR et al: Quality of life in breast cancer part I: physical and social well-being, *Cancer Nurs* 20(6):398, 1997.

Ferrell BR et al: Quality of life in breast cancer part II: psychological and spiritual well-being, *Cancer Nurs* 21(1):1, 1998.

Ferrell BR et al: Quality of life in breast cancer survivors: implications for developing support services, *Oncol Nurs Forum* 25(5):887, 1998.

Lee CO: Quality of life and breast cancer survivors: psychosocial and treatment issues, *Cancer Pract* 5(5):309, 1997.

Longman AJ et al: Side-effects burden, psychological adjustment, and life quality in women with breast cancer: pattern of association over time, *Oncol Nurs Forum* 26(5):909, 1999.

Sexuality and Body Image

Bruner DW: Assessing women's sexuality after cancer therapy: checking assumptions with the focus group technique, *Cancer Nurs* 21(6):438, 1998.

Ganz PA et al: Life after breast cancer: understanding women's health-related quality of life and sexual functioning, *J Clin Oncol* 16(2):501, 1998.

McPhail G: Menopause as an issue for women with breast cancer, *Cancer Nurs* 22(2):164, 1999.

Price B: Explorations in body image care: Peplau and practice knowledge, *J Psychiatr Ment Health Nurs* 5:179, 1998.

The Elderly

Bailes JS: Health care economics of cancer in the elderly, *Cancer* 80(7):1348, 1997.

Ganz PA: Interaction between the physician and the older patient, *Cancer* 80(7):1323, 1997.

Kantor DE, Houldin A: Breast cancer in older women: treatment, psychosocial effects, interventions, and outcomes, *J Gerontol Nurs* 25:19, 1999.

Krupat E et al: Patient assertiveness and physician decision-making among older breast cancer patients *Soc Sci Med* 49:449, 1999.

Savage SA, Clarke VA: Older women's illness representations of cancer: a qualitative study, *Health Educ Res* 13(4):529, 1998.

Schain W: Psychosocial issues and life-cycle concerns of women with breast cancer, *Cancer Prev Control* 1:122, 1997.

Smith-Bindman R et al: Is screening mammography effective in elderly women? *Am J Med* 108:112, 2000.

Wenzel LB et al: Age-related differences in the quality of life of breast carcinoma patients after treatment, *Cancer* 86(9):1768, 1999.

Wyatt GK et al: Complementary therapy use among older cancer patients, *Cancer Pract* 7(3):136, 1999.

CHAPTER 55: MEN WITH REPRODUCTIVE PROBLEMS

General

Castellsagué X et al: Male circumcision, penile human papillomavirus infection, and cervical cancer in female partners, *N Engl J Med* 346:1105, 2002.

Gann PH et al: Strategies combining total and percent free prostate specific antigen for detecting prostate cancer: a prospective evaluation, *J Urol* 167:2427, 2002.

Hernández-Díaz S: Iatrogenic legacy from diethylstilbestrol exposure, *Lancet* 359:1081, 2002.

CHAPTER 56: SEXUALLY TRANSMITTED DISEASES

General

Brackbill RM et al: Where do people go for treatment of sexually transmitted diseases? *Fam Plann Perspect* 31(1):10, 1999.

DiClemente RJ et al: Condom carrying is not associated with condom use and lower prevalence of sexually transmitted diseases among minority adolescent females, *Sex Transm Dis* 28(8):444, 2001.

Lahoti S et al: Screening and treatment of sexually transmitted diseases. Part 1: chlamydia, gonorrhea, and bacterial vaginosis, *J Pediatr Health Care* 14(1):34, 2000.

Miller HG et al: Correlates of sexually transmitted bacterial infections among U.S. women in 1995, *Fam Plann Perspect* 31(1):4, 23, 1999.

Orr DP et al: Subsequent sexually transmitted infection in urban adolescents and young adults, *Arch Pediatr Adolesc Med* 155(8):947, 2001.

Parks DK et al: Screening and treatment of sexually transmitted diseases. Part 2: trichomonas, human papillomavirus infection, and genital herpes simplex virus, *J Pediatr Health Care* 14(3):130, 2000.

Patel K: Sexually transmitted diseases in adolescents: focus on gonorrhea, chlamydia, and trichomoniasis—issues and treatment guidelines, *J Pediatr Health Care* 12(4):211, 1998.

Shrier LA et al: Randomized controlled trial of a safer sex intervention for high risk adolescent girls, *Arch Pediatr Adolesc Med* 155:73, 2001.

Smith MU, DiClemente RJ: STAND: a peer educator training curriculum for sexual risk reduction in the rural South, *Prev Med* 30:441, 2000.

Gonorrhea

Cecil JA et al: Features of *Chlamydia trachomatis* and *Neisseria gonorrhoeae* infection in male army recruits, *J Infect Dis* 184(9):216, 2001.

Evans B et al: Rates of gonorrhea and chlamydia in black ethnic groups, *Sex Transm Infect* 77(5):390, 2001.

Low DE: The new oral cephalosporins in community-acquired infection, *Clin Microb Infect* 6(Suppl 3):64, 2000.

Sheff B: *Neisseria gonorrhoeae, Nursing* 30(7):76, 2000.

Wiest DR et al: Empiric treatment of gonorrhea and chlamydia in the ED, *Am J Emerg Med* 19(4):274, 2001.

Herpes Genitalis

Chandrasekar PH: Identification and treatment of herpes lesions, *Adv Wound Care* 2(5):254, 1999.

Kelley LS: Evaluating change in quality of life from the perspective of the person: advanced practice nursing and Parse's goal of nursing, *Holistic Nurs Practice* 13(4):61, 1999.

Swanson JM et al: Effects of psycho-educational interventions on sexual health risks and psycho-social adaptation in young adults with genital herpes, *J Adv Nurs* 29(4):840, 1999.

Human Papillomavirus

Boyer LE et al: Hispanic women's perceptions regarding cervical cancer screening, *J Obstet Gynecol Neonatal Nurs* 30(2):240, 2001.

Mancuso P: Dermatologic manifestations of infectious diseases in pregnancy, *J Perinatal Neonatal Nurs* 14(1):17, 2000.

Mashburn J: Evolution of the evidence-based Papanicolaou smear, *J Midwifery Womens Health* 46(3):181, 2001.

Bacterial Vaginosis

Belkengren R, Sapala S: Pediatric management problems: bacterial vaginosis (BV), *Pediatric Nurs* 25(2):200, 1999.

Trichomonas

Schmid G et al: Prevalence of metronidazole-resistant trichomonas vaginalis in a gynecology clinic, *J Reprod Med* 46(6):545, 2001.

CHAPTER 57: ASSESSMENT OF THE VISUAL SYSTEM

General

Fitzpatrick M: Ophthalmologists eye: new examination tool, *JAMA* 286(13):1576, 2001.

Gupta D: An O.D.'s primer on ultrasound, *Rev Optometry* 138(10):41, 2001.

Nichols L: Oopen your eyes to dilation regimens, Part 1, *Rev Ophthalmol* 8(6):100, 2001.

Pandit RJ et al: Effectiveness of testing visual fields by confrontation, *Lancet* 358(9290):1339, 2001.

CHAPTER 58: PROBLEMS OF THE EYE

General

Gallemore RP, Boyer DS: Retinal detachment: the best treatment is prevention, *Rev Ophthalmol* 8(4):121, 2001.

Hamilton DR et al: Watch for steroid-induced glaucoma after LASIK, *Rev Ophthalmol* 9(6):143, 2002.

Murdoch I: Glaucoma: latest developments in diagnosis and treatment, *Pulse* 62(23):51, 2002.

Weintraub JM et al: Postmenopausal hormone use and lens opocities, *Ophthalamic Epidemiol* 9(3)179: 2002.

CHAPTER 59: ASSESSMENT OF THE AUDITORY SYSTEM

General

Alper C et al: *Decision-making in ear, nose, and throat disorders,* Philadelphia, 2001, WB Saunders.

Gates G: *Current therapy in otolaryngology: head and neck surgery,* ed 6, St Louis, 1998, Mosby.

CHAPTER 60: PROBLEMS OF THE EAR

General

Ayache D et al: Perilymphatic pressure measurement in Meniere's disease, *Ann Otol Rhinol Laryngol* 3(7):643, 2002.

Brookler KH: Caloric test results in a patient with Meniere's syndrome, *Ear Nose Throat J* 81(2):84, 2002.

Grossan M: Safe, effective techniques for cerumen removal, *Geriatrics* 55(1):80, 2000.

Marcincuk MC, Roland PS: Geriatric hearing loss: understanding the causes and providing appropriate treatment, *Geriatrics* 57(4):44, 2002.

Meyer SE, Megerson CA: Patients perceived outcomes after stapedectomy for otosclerosis, *Ear Nose Throat J* 79(11):846, 2000.

Ott MC, Lundy LB: Tympanic membrane perforation in adults, *Postgrad Med* 110(5):81, 2001.

Russell F, Mulholland K: Prevention of otitis media by vaccination, *Drugs* 62(10):1441, 2002.

Sadovsky R: Temperature of saline solution for ear irrigation, *A Fam Physician* January 2000, website: http://www.aafp.org/afp/20000101/tips/20.html.

CHAPTER 61: ASSESSMENT OF THE SKIN

General

Bickley LS: *Bates's guide to physical examination and history taking,* ed 7, Philadelphia, 1999, JB Lippincott.

Physiology of the Skin

Dermatology Nurses's Association: *Dermatology nursing essentials: a core curriculum,* Pitman, NJ, 1998, Anthony J Janetti.

Lesion Description and Identification

Dermatology Nurse's Association: *Dermatology nursing basics: core proceeding book from anuual convention,* New Jersey, 2001, Anthony J. Janetti Co.

Fitzpatrick TB et al: *Color atlas and synopsis of clinical dermatology,* ed 4, New York, 2000, McGraw-Hill Professional Publishing

Habif T: *Clinical dermatology: a color guide to diagnosis and therapy,* ed 3, St Louis, 1997, Mosby.

Odon RB et al: *Andrews' diseases of the skin: clinical dermatology,* ed 9, Philadelphia, 2000, WB Saunders.

CHAPTER 62: PROBLEMS OF THE SKIN

General

Kamines MS et al: *Atlas of cosmetic surgery,* Philadelphia, 2002, WB Saunders.

Jacknin J: *Smart medicine for the skin: a comprehensive guide to understanding conventional and alternative therapies to heal common skin problems,* Avery, New York, 2001.

McGovern TW et al: Cutaneous manifestations of biological warfare and related threat agents, *Arch Dermatol* 133(3):311, 1999.

Nguyen P et al: Aggressive squamous cell carcinomas in persons infected with the human immunodeficiency virus, *Arch Dermatol* 138(6):758, 2002.

CHAPTER 63: BURNS

General

Barret JP, Herndon DN: *Color atlas of burn care,* London, 2001, WB Saunders.

Carrougher GJ, editor: *Burn care and therapy,* St Louis, 1998, Mosby.

Cortiella J, Marvin JA: Management of the pediatric burn patient, *Nurs Clin North Am* 32(2):311, 1997.

Herndon DN, editor: *Total burn care,* London, 1996, WB Saunders.

Kagan RJ, Smith SC: Evaluation and treatment of thermal injuries, *Dermatol Nurs* 12(5):334, 338, 347, 2000.

Moore FD: Then and now: treatment volume, wound coverage, lung injury, and antibiotics: a capsule history of burn treatment at mid-century, *Burns* 25:733, 1999.

Nelson LA, Thompson DD: Burn injury, *Plast Surg Nurs* 18(3):159, 176, 184, 1998.

Roberts AH: Burn prevention: where now? *Burns* 26:419, 2000.

Pathophysiology

Ahrns KS, Harkins DR: Initial resuscitation after burn injury: therapies, strategies, and controversies, *AACN Clin Issues* 10(1):46, 1999.

Gibran NS, Heimbach DM: Current status of burn wound pathophysiology, *Clin Plastic Surg* 27:11, 2000.

Luterman A: Burns and metabolism, *J Am Coll Surg* 190:104, 2000.

Ramzy PI et al: Thermal injury, *Crit Care Clin* 15:333, 1999.

Ryan CM et al: Objective estimates of the probability of death from burn injuries, *N Engl J Med* 338:362, 1998.

Saffle JR: Predicting outcomes of burns, *N Engl J Med* 338:387, 1998.

Wysocki AB: Skin anatomy, physiology, and pathophysiology, *Nurs Clin North Am* 34(4):777, 1999.

Phases of Treatment

American Burn Association: *Advanced burn life support,* Chicago, 2001, American Burn Association.

Demling RH, DeSanti L: Management of partial thickness facial burns (comparison of topical antibiotics and bio-engineered skin substitutes), *Burns* 25:256, 1999.

Flynn MB: Identifying and treating inhalation injuries in fire victims, *DCCN* 18(4):18, 1999.

Hansbrough JF, Franco ES: Skin replacements, *Clin Plastic Surg* 25:407, 1998.

Neely AN, Holder IA: Antimicrobial resistance, *Burns* 25:17, 1999.

Richard R: Assessment and diagnosis of burn wounds, *Adv Wound Care* 12(9):468, 1999.

Rose DD, Jordan EB: Perioperative management of burn patients, *AORN J* 69(6):1211, 1213, 1215, 1999.

Sheridan RL: Evaluating and managing burn wounds, *Dermatol Nurs* 12(1):17, 21, 30, 2000.

Still JM, Law EJ: Primary excision of the burn wound, *Clin Plastic Surg* 27:23, 2000.

Wielbelhaus P, Hansen SL: What you should know about managing burn emergencies, *Nursing* 31(1):36, 2001.

Illustration Credits

Chapter 1 1-2 From National Sample Survey of Registered Nurses, Washington, DC, 2000, HRSA, Bureau of Health Professions, Division of Nursing; 1-2 From U.S. Bureau of the Census, 2001; 1-3, 1-4 From American Association of Colleges of Nursing: *2000-2001 Enrollment and graduations in baccalaureate and graduate programs in nursing,* Washington, DC, 2001, AACN.

Chapter 3 3-1 From U.S. Department of Agriculture, Washington, DC; 3-2 Redrawn from Pender NJ: *Health promotion in nursing practice,* ed 2, East Norwalk, Conn, 1987, Appleton & Lange; 3-3 Source: NHLBI Obesity Education Initiative, NIH, www.nhlbi.nih.gov.

Chapter 4 4-1 Redrawn from Ebersole P, Hess P: *Toward healthy aging: human needs and nursing response,* ed 5, St Louis, 1998, Mosby.

Chapter 5 5-4 From Paterson BL: The shifting perspectives model of chronic illness, *J Nurs Scholarsh,* First Quarter, 2001.

Chapter 6 6-1 Modified from Aguilera DC: *Crisis intervention: theory and methodology,* ed 7, St Louis, 1994, Mosby.

Chapter 7 7-1 Courtesy University of Virginia Medical Center, Charlottesville, Va.

Chapter 8 8-1 Redrawn from *Waiting room survival guide,* ed 2, Washington, DC, 1993, Foundation for Critical Care; 8-2 Redrawn from Jackle M., Halligan, M: *Cardiovascular problems: a critical care nursing focus,* Bowie, Md, 2001, Robert J. Brady. In Sole ML et al: *Introduction to critical care nursing,* ed 3, Philadelphia, 2001, WB Saunders.

Chapter 9 9-1 From Monahan FD, Neighbors M: *Medical-surgical nursing: foundations for clinical practice,* ed 2, Philadelphia, 1998, WB Saunders.

Chapter 10 10-1 Source: Hobbs FB, Damon BL: *65+ in the United States,* U.S. Bureau of the Census, Current Population Reports, Special Studies, pp 23-190, April 1996; 10-3, 10-4 From HCFA33-OSCAR Form 671: F9, current surveys as of September 2000; 10-6, 10-7 From *Long-term care facility resident assessment instrument (RAI) user manual,* HCFA, October 1995.

Chapter 12 12-6 Redrawn from Watt-Watson JH, Donovan MI: *Pain management: nursing prospective,* St Louis, 1992, Mosby; 12-7 Adapted from McCaffery M, Beebe A: *Pain: clinical manual for nursing practice,* St Louis, 1989, Mosby.

Chapter 13 13-11 From Monahan FD, Neighbors M: *Medical-surgical nursing: foundations for clinical practice,* ed 2, Philadelphia, 1998, WB Saunders.

Chapter 14 14-1, 14-2, 14-3, 14-4 From Monahan FD, Neighbors M: *Medical-surgical nursing: foundations for clinical practice,* ed 2, Philadelphia, 1998, WB Saunders; 14-5 Courtesy The Jobst Institute, Toledo, Ohio.

Chapter 15 15-1 From Szarka C et al: *Curr Probl Cancer* 15:6, 1994; 15-4, 15-9 From Lewis SM et al: *Medical-surgical nursing: assessment and management of clinical problems,* ed 5, St Louis, 2000, Mosby; 15-15 From Monahan FD, Neighbors M: *Medical-surgical nursing: foundations for clinical practice,* ed 2, Philadelphia, 1998, WB Saunders; 15-16, 15-17 Redrawn from LaRocca JC, Otto SE: *Pocket guide to intravenous therapy,* ed 3, St Louis, 1997, Mosby; 15-18 From World Health Organization: *Cancer pain relief,* ed 2, Geneva, 1996, WHO.

Chapter 16 16-1, 16-2, 16-3 Courtesy University Hospitals of Cleveland, Cleveland, Ohio.

Chapter 17 17-8, 17-9 From Elkin MK et al: *Nursing interventions and clinical skills,* ed 2, St Louis, 2000, Mosby.

Chapter 18 18-1 Redrawn from Litwack K: *Post Anesthesia care nursing,* ed 2, St Louis, 1995, Mosby; 18-3 Courtesy MetroHealth System, Cleveland, Ohio; 18-4B Redrawn from Canobbio MM: *Cardiovascular disorders,* St Louis, 1990, Mosby; 18-6A Redrawn from Morison M: *A colour guide to the nursing management of wounds,* London, 1992, Mosby-Wolfe.

Chapter 19 19-2, 19-6 From Beare PG, Myers JL: *Adult health nursing,* ed 3, St Louis, 1998, Mosby; 19-5 From Lewis SM et al: *Medical-surgical nursing: assessment and management of clinical problems,* ed 5, St Louis, 2000, Mosby; 19-8 Redrawn from Price SA, Wilson LM: *Pathophysiology: clinical concepts of disease processes,* ed 5, St Louis, 1997, Mosby; 19-12 Modified from Talbot L, Meyers-Marquardt M: *Pocket guide to critical care assessment,* ed 3, St Louis, 1997, Mosby; 19-16 Redrawn from Seidel HM et al: *Mosby's guide to physical examination,* ed 4, St Louis, 1999, Mosby; 19-17 Redrawn from Stillwell S, Randall E: *Pocket guide to cardiovascular care,* ed 2, St Louis, 1994, Mosby; 19-18, 19-22 From Monahan FD, Neighbors M: *Medical-surgical nursing: foundations for clinical practice,* ed 2, Philadelphia, 1998, WB Saunders; 19-19 From Talbot L, Meyers-Marquardt M: *Pocket guide to critical care assessment,* ed 3, St Louis, 1997, Mosby; 19-21 Redrawn from Spearman CB et al: *Egan's fundamentals of respiratory therapy,* ed 5, St Louis, 1990, Mosby.

Chapter 20 20-1, 20-2, 20-4, 20-5, 20-7, 20-8, 20-11, 20-15, 20-16, 20-17, 20-18, 20-20 Redrawn from Schuller DE, Schleuning AJ: *Otolaryngology: head and neck surgery,* ed 8, St Louis, 1994, Mosby; 20-10 From Gruber RP, Peck GC: *Rhinoplasty: state of the art,* St Louis, 1993, Mosby; 20-12 From Monahan FD, Neighbors, M: *Medical-surgical nursing: foundations for clinical practice,* ed 2, Philadelphia, 1998, WB Saunders; 20-13 From Beare PG, Myers JL: *Adult health nursing,* ed 3, St Louis, 1998, Mosby; 20-24 From Lewis SM et al: *Medical-surgical nursing: assessment and management of clinical problems,* ed 5, St Louis, 2000, Mosby; 20-25 Redrawn from Kaplow R, Bookbinder M: *Heart Lung* 23(1):59, 1994.

Chapter 21 21-1 From Lewis SM et al: *Medical-surgical nursing: assessment and management of clinical problems,* ed 5, St Louis, 2000, Mosby; 21-2, 21-3 From Potter PA, Perry AG: *Fundamentals of nursing: concepts, process, and practice,* ed 5, St Louis, 2001, Mosby; 21-4 From Des Jardins T, Burton GG: *Clinical manifestations and assessment of respiratory disease,* ed 3, St Louis, 1995, Mosby; 21-5

From Monahan FD, Neighbors M: *Medical-surgical nursing: foundations for clinical practice,* ed 2, Philadelphia, 1998, WB Saunders; 21-12, 21-13, 21-14, 21-15, 21-17, 21-20 From McCance KL, Huether SE: *Pathophysiology: the biologic basis for disease in adults and children,* ed 4, St Louis, 2002, Mosby; 21-24 Courtesy DePaul Health Center, St Louis; 21-25 From Sorrentino SA: *Mosby's assisting with patient care,* St Louis, 1999, Mosby; 21-26 Courtesy Ballard Medical Products, Draper, Utah.

Chapter 22 22-5 Redrawn from Thompson JM, Wilson SF: *Health assessment for nursing practice,* St Louis, 1996, Mosby; 22-8, 22-24, 22-25, 22-26 Redrawn from Conover MS: *Understanding electrocardiography: arrhythmias and the 12-lead ECG,* ed 6, St Louis, 1992, Mosby; 22-12, 22-13 From Thibodeau GA, Patton KT: *Anatomy and physiology,* ed 5, St Louis, 2003, Mosby; 22-18, 22-19, 22-20, 22-22 Redrawn from Kinney MR et al: *Comprehensive cardiac care,* ed 7, St Louis, 1991, Mosby; 22-29 Redrawn from Daily EK, Schroeder JS: *Techniques in bedside hemodynamic monitoring,* ed 5, St Louis, 1994, Mosby.

Chapter 23 23-2 From Huether SE, McCance: *Understanding pathophysiology,* ed 2, St Louis, 2000, Mosby.

Chapter 24 24-3 Redrawn from Konstam M et al: *Heart failure: evaluation and care of patients with left ventricular systolic dysfunction.* Clinical Practice Guideline No. 11. AHCPR Publication No. 94-0612. Rockville, MD: Agency for Health Care Policy and Research, Public Health Service, U.S. Department of Health and Human Services, June 1994; 24-4 Redrawn from Kissane IM: *Anderson's pathology,* ed 9, St Louis, 1990, Mosby; 24-5, 24-11, 24-12 From Monahan FD, Neighbors M: *Medical-surgical nursing: foundations for clinical practice,* ed 2, Philadelphia, 1998, WB Saunders; 24-6, 24-7, 24-8, 24-9, 24-10, 24-13, 24-16 From Beare PG, Myers JL: *Adult health nursing,* ed 3, St Louis, 1998, Mosby; 24-14C Courtesy St Jude Medical, Inc, St Paul, Minn.

Chapter 25 25-3, 25-9, 25-10, 25-14 From Lewis SM et al: *Medical-surgical nursing: assessment and management of clinical problems,* ed 5, St Louis, 2000, Mosby; 25-4 Courtesy LoGerfo FW, Boston, Mass; 25-5 From Black J et al: *Medical-surgical nursing: clinical management for positive outcomes,* ed 6, Philadelphia, 2001, WB Saunders; 25-6, 25-12 From Kamal A, Brockelhurst IC: *Color atlas of geriatric medicine,* ed 2, St Louis, 1991, Mosby; 25-7 Courtesy Otto Bock Health Care, Minneapolis, Minn; 25-13 Courtesy Kendall Company, Mansfield, Mass; 25-15 From Lofgren KA: Varicose veins. In Haimovici H, editor: *Vascular surgery: principles and techniques,* Oxford, 1976, Blackwell Science, Ltd; 25-16 From Belch JJF et al: *Color atlas of peripheral vascular diseases,* ed 2, 1996, Mosby-Wolfe.

Chapter 26 26-1 From McCance KL, Huether SE: *Pathophysiology: the biologic basis for disease in adults and children,* ed 4, St Louis, 2002, Mosby; 26-2 From Monahan FD, Neighbors, M: *Medical-surgical nursing: foundations for clinical practice,* ed 2, Philadelphia, 1998, WB Saunders; 26-3 From Pagana KD, Pagana TJ: *Mosby's manual of diagnostic and laboratory tests,* ed 2, St Louis, 2002, Mosby.

Chapter 27 27-5 From Porth CM: *Pathophysiology: concepts of altered health status,* ed 6, Philadelphia, 1998, JB Lippincott.

Chapter 28 28-3, 28-4, 28-10 Redrawn from McCance KL, Huether SE: *Pathophysiology: the biologic basis for disease in adults and children,* ed 4, St Louis, 2002, Mosby; 28-5, 28-6 Redrawn from Thibodeau GA, Patton KT: *Anatomy and physiology,* ed 5, St Louis, 2003.

Chapter 29 29-1 From Mendeloff AI, Smith DE, editors: Acromegaly, diabetes, hypermetabolism, proteinuria, and heart failure. Clin Pathol Conference, *Am J Med* 20:133, 1956; 29-2 From Shapiro LM, Buchalter MB: *Color atlas of hypertension,* London, 1992, Wolfe; 29-5 Courtesy Dr Jeffrey Hurwitz. From Bingham BJ et al: *Atlas of clinical otolaryngology,* St Louis, 1992, Mosby; 29-6 From Bergman LV and Associates, Cold Spring, NY; 29-7 From Hall R, Evered DC: *Color atlas of endocrinology,* ed 2, St Louis, 1990, Mosby; 29-9 From Lewis SM et al: *Medical-surgical nursing: assessment and management of clinical problems,* ed 5, St Louis, 2000, Mosby.

Chapter 30 30-1 Data from National Institute of Diabetes and Digestive and Kidney Diseases, National Information Clearinghouse, National Institutes of Health: Diabetes Statistics, NIH Publication No. 96-3926, 1995; 30-9 From U.S. Department of Agriculture, Washington, DC; 30-11, 30-12 From Lewis SM et al: *Medical-surgical nursing: assessment and management of clinical problems,* ed 5, St Louis, 2000, Mosby.

Chapter 31 31-3, 31-4 From Thibodeau GA, Patton KT: *Anatomy and physiology,* ed 5, St Louis, 2003; 31-5, 31-11 From Monahan FD, Neighbors M: *Medical-surgical nursing: foundations for clinical practice,* ed 2, Philadelphia, 1998, WB Saunders; 31-12 Courtesy Olympus America, Inc., Mehlville, NY.

Chapter 32 32-1, 32-4 From Lewis SM et al: *Medical-surgical nursing: assessment and management of clinical problems,* ed 5, St Louis, 2000, Mosby; 32-2 From Callen JP et al: *Color atlas of dermatology,* Philadelphia, 1993, WB Saunders; 32-5 From Zuidema GD: *Shackelford's surgery of the alimentary tract,* ed 4, vol 1, Philadelphia, 1996, WB Saunders.

Chapter 33 33-10 From Beare PG, Myers JL: *Adult health nursing,* ed 3, St Louis, 1998, Mosby.

Chapter 34 34-3, 34-4, 34-19, 34-21 From Wilcox CM: *Atlas of clinical gastrointestinal endoscopy,* Philadelphia, 1995, WB Saunders; 34-23 From de los Ríos Magriña E. *Atlas of therapeutic proctology,* Philadelphia, 1984, WB Saunders.

Chapter 35 35-3 After Siegel JH et al: Mechanical lithotripsy of common duct stones. *Gastrointest Endosc* 36(4):353, 1990. Copyright American Society of Gastrointestinal Endoscopy.

Chapter 36 36-1, 36-2 From Thibodeau GA, Patton KT: *Anatomy and physiology,* ed 5, St Louis, 2003, Mosby; 36-3 From Copstead LC, Banasik JL: *Pathophysiology: biological and behavioral perspectives,* ed 2, Philadelphia, 2000, WB Saunders; 36-4 Redrawn from McCance KL, Huether SE: *Pathophysiology: the biologic basis for disease in adults and children,* ed 4, St Louis, 2002, Mosby.

Chapter 37 37-1 Redrawn from McCance KL, Huether SE: *Pathophysiology: the biologic basis for disease in adults and children,* ed 4, St Louis, 2002, Mosby; 37-2 Courtesy Invacare Corporation, Elyria, Ohio; 37-4B From Lewis SM et al: *Medical-surgical nursing: assessment and management of clinical problems,* ed 5, St Louis, 2000, Mosby; 37-5, 37-6, 37-7, 37-8B, C From Beare PG, Myers JL: *Adult health nursing,* ed 3, St Louis, 1998, Mosby; 37-8A From Townsend CM et al: *Sabiston textbook of surgery; the biological basis of modern surgical practice,* ed 16, Philadelphia, 2001, WB Saunders.

Chapter 38 38-4 From Thibodeau GA, Patton KT: *Anatomy and physiology,* ed 5, St Louis, 2003; 38-5 Redrawn from Thibodeau GA, Patton KT: *Anatomy and physiology,* ed 5, St Louis, 2003.

Chapter 39 39-2 From Brundage DJ: *Renal disorders,* St Louis, 1992, Mosby; 39-3 From American Medical Association: JAMA patient page: urinary tract infections, *JAMA* 283(12):1646, 2000; 39-4 From Kissane JM: *Anderson's pathology,* ed 9, St Louis, 1990, Mosby; 39-8, 39-15 From Weiss RM et al: *Comprehensive urology,* London, 2001, Mosby International Limited.

Chapter 40 40-1 Redrawn from McCance KL, Huether SE: *Pathophysiology: the biologic basis for disease in adults and children,* ed 4, St Louis, 2002, Mosby; 40-2 From Smith T: *Renal nursing,* London, 1997, Bailliere-Tindall; 40-6 From Lewis SM et al: *Medical-surgical* *nursing: assessment and management of clinical problems,* ed 5, St Louis, 2000, Mosby.

Chapter 41 41-1, 41-5, 41-13, 41-14, 41-26 From Monahan FD, Neighbors M: *Medical-surgical nursing: foundations for clinical practice,* ed 2, Philadelphia, 1998, WB Saunders; 41-2, 41-3, 41-4, 41-9, 41-10, 41-12 From Thibodeau GA, Patton KT: *Anatomy and physiology,* ed 5, St Louis, 2003; 41-11 From Beare PG, Myers JL: *Adult health nursing,* ed 3, St Louis, 1998, Mosby; 41-16 Courtesy Scott Bodell.

Chapter 42 42-2, 42-10, 42-11, 42-13, 42-16 From Monahan FD, Neighbors M: *Medical-surgical nursing: foundations for clinical practice,* ed 2, Philadelphia, 1998, WB Saunders; 42-7, 42-8, 42-12 Redrawn from Barker E: *Neuroscience nursing,* St Louis, 1994, Mosby.

Chapter 43 43-5 43-10B, 43-11 From Lewis SM et al: *Medical-surgical nursing: assessment and management of clinical problems,* ed 5, St Louis, 2000, Mosby; 43-7, 43-10A Redrawn from *Recovering from a stroke,* Dallas, 1994, American Heart Association; 43-9 Redrawn from *The one-handed way,* Dallas, 1994, American Heart Association; 43-14 Redrawn from Rudy E: *Advanced neurologic and neurosurgical nursing,* St Louis, 1984, Mosby; 43-16 From Perkin GD et al: *Atlas of clinical neurology,* ed 2, London, 1993, Gower Medical Publishing.

Chapter 44 44-9 From Murphy M: Traumatic spinal cord injury: an acute care rehabilitation perspective, *Crit Care Nurs Q* 22(2):51, 1999; 44-12 Courtesy Zimmer, Inc., Warsaw, Ind; 44-14 Courtesy Acromed Corporation; Cleveland, Ohio; 44-15 Courtesy Kinetic Concepts, San Antonio, Tex; 44-17 Courtesy Sammons Preston, A Bissell Healthcare Company, Bolingbrook, Ill; 44-21 Redrawn from Chipps E et al: *Neurologic disorders,* St Louis, 1992, Mosby.

Chapter 45 45-1, 45-4, 45-9, 45-11, 45-12 Redrawn from Thompson JM et al: *Mosby's clinical nursing,* ed 5, St Louis, 2002, Mosby; 45-2, 45-3, 45-8 From Thibodeau GA, Patton KT: *Anatomy and physiology,* ed 5, St Louis, 2003, Mosby; 45-6, 45-7 From McCance KL, Huether SE: *Pathophysiology: the biologic basis for disease in adults and children,* ed 4, St Louis, 2002, Mosby; 45-13 From Thompson JM et al: *Mosby's clinical nursing,* ed 5, St Louis, 2002, Mosby; 45-14, 45-19, 45-21, 45-22, 45-25, 45-29 From Seidel HM et al: *Mosby's guide to physical examination,* ed 4, St Louis, 1999, Mosby; 45-30 From Gregory B: *Perioperative nursing series: orthopaedic surgery,* St Louis, 1994, Mosby.

Chapter 46 46-1, 46-21 Courtesy Rocky Shepheard, New London, Ohio; 46-2, 46-3 From Lewis SM et al: *Medical-surgical nursing: assessment and management of clinical problems,* ed 5, St Louis, 2000, Mosby; 46-8 Courtesy Acromed Corporation, Cleveland, Ohio; 46-10 Courtesy Smith & Nephew, Memphis, Tenn; 46-13 Courtesy Zimmer, Inc, Warsaw, Ind; 46-16 Courtesy Stryker Instruments, Kalamazoo, Mich.

Chapter 47 47-1, 47-28, 47-29, 47-45 From McCance KL, Huether SE: *Pathophysiology: the biologic basis for disease in adults and children,* ed 4, St Louis, 2002, Mosby; 47-2, 47-14, 47-30, 47-31, 47-41, 47-42, 47-43 From Kamal A, Brockelhurst JC: *Color atlas of geriatric medicine,* ed 2, St Louis, 1991, Mosby; 47-3 From Sorrentino SA: *Assisting with patient care,* St Louis, 1999, Mosby; 47-4, 47-7, 47-8 47-9, 47-10, 47-11 Courtesy Sammons Preston, A Bissell Healthcare Corporation, Bolingbrook, Ill; 47-12 From Habif TP: *Clinical dermatology,* ed 3, St Louis, 1996, Mosby; 47-13 From Doherty M: *Color atlas and text of osteoarthritis,* London, 1994, Wolfe; 47-18, 47-21 Courtesy Zimmer, Inc., Warsaw, Ind; 47-19 Courtesy Dupuy Orthopaedics, Inc, Warsaw, Ind; 47-22 Courtesy OrthoLogic Corp, Phoenix, Ariz; 47-23, 47-24 From Gregory BA: *Perioperative nursing series: orthopaedic surgery,* St Louis, 1994, Mosby; 47-25 From Dieppe P et al: *Arthritis and rheumatism in practice,* London, 1991, Gower; 47-26 Redrawn from Mourad L: *Orthopedic disorders,* St Louis, 1991, Mosby; 47-27 From Lewis SM et al: *Medical-surgical nursing: assessment and management of clinical problems,* ed 5, St Louis, 2000, Mosby; 47-32 Redrawn from the National Osteoporosis Foundation: *Osteoporosis Report* 13(1):8, Spring 1997, Washington, DC; 47-34 From Beare PG, Myers JL: *Adult health nursing,* ed 3, St Louis, 1998, Mosby; 47-46, 47-47 From Damjanov I, Linder, J: *Anderson's pathology,* ed 10, St Louis, 1996, Mosby; 47-48, 47-49 From American Academy of Orthopaedic Surgeons: *Instructional Course Lectures,* vol 33, St Louis, 1984, Mosby.

Chapter 48 48-1 From Lewis SM et al: *Medical-surgical nursing: assessment and management of clinical problems,* ed 5, St Louis, 2000, Mosby; 48-7, 48-8, 48-11 From Monahan FD, Neighbors M: *Medical-surgical nursing: foundations for clinical practice,* ed 2, Philadelphia, 1998, WB Saunders.

Chapter 49 49-3, 49-7, 49-8 Redrawn from McCance KL, Huether SE: *Pathophysiology: the biologic basis for disease in adults and children,* ed 4, St Louis, 2002, Mosby; 49-4 From McCance KL, Huether SE: *Pathophysiology: the biologic basis for disease in adults and children,* ed 4, St Louis, 2002, Mosby; 49-5 From Monahan FD, Neighbors M: *Medical-surgical nursing: foundations for clinical practice,* ed 2, Philadelphia, 1998, WB Saunders.

Chapter 50 50-1, 50-2 From Centers for Disease Control and Prevention: *Current status of the HIV/AIDS epidemic in the U.S.,* HIV/AIDS Surveillance Report, 2000, CDC; 50-3 From Centers for Disease Control and Prevention: *Proportion of AIDS cases, by race/ethnicity and year of report, 1985-1999, United States,* 2000, CDC; 50-4, 50-7 From Monahan FD, Neighbors M: *Medical-surgical nursing: foundations for clinical practice,* ed 2, Philadelphia, 1998, WB Saunders; 50-8 From Callen JP et al: *Color atlas of dermatology,* Philadelphia, 1993, WB Saunders.

Chapter 51 51-1 Redrawn from Chabelewski FL: Donation and transplantation, *Nursing Curriculum,* 1996; 51-3, 51-4, 51-5, 51-6, 51-7 Redrawn from Smith SL: *Tissue and organ transplantation: implications for professional nursing practice,* St Louis, 1990, Mosby.

Chapter 52 52-1, 52-2, 52-3, 52-5, 52-12 From Lowdermilk DL et al: *Maternity & women's health care,* ed 7, St Louis, 2000, Mosby; 52-4, 52-9, 52-13, 52-14, 52-16, 52-17, 52-18 From Monahan FD, Neighbors M: *Medical-surgical nursing: foundations for clinical practice,* ed 2, Philadelphia, 1998, WB Saunders; 52-6, 52-7, 52-8, 52-11 From Seidel HM et al: *Mosby's guide to physical examination,* ed 4, St Louis, 1999, Mosby; 52-10, 52-20 Redrawn from Gillenwater JY et al: *Adult and pediatric urology,* ed 3, St Louis, 1996, Mosby.

Chapter 53 53-1 From Lewis SM et al: *Medical-surgical nursing: assessment and management of clinical problems,* ed 5, St Louis, 2000, Mosby; 53-2, 53-3, 53-5 From Monahan FD, Neighbors M: *Medical-surgical nursing: foundations for clinical practice,* ed 2, Philadelphia, 1998, WB Saunders; 53-4 Redrawn from Wong DL et al: *Maternal child nursing care,* ed 2, St Louis, 2002, Mosby; 53-13 From Beare PG, yers JL: *Adult health nursing,* ed 3, St Louis, 1998, Mosby; 53-14 From Seidel HM et al: *Mosby's guide to physical examination,* ed 4, St Louis, 1999, Mosby; 53-15 Redrawn from Herbst A et al: *Comprehensive gynecology,* ed 2, St Louis, 1992, Mosby.

Chapter 54 54-1 Data from Centers for Disease Control and Prevention: *U.S. mortality public use data tapes 1960-1997, U.S. Mortality Volumes 1930-1959,* National Center for Health Statistics, 2000, CDC; 54-2 Data from American Cancer Society: *NCI Surveillance, Epidemiology, and End Results Program,* Atlanta, 1999, ACS; 54-3, 54-4 From Seidel HM et al: *Mosby's guide to physical examination,* ed 4, St Louis, 1999, Mosby; 54-6 From Powell DE,

Stelling CB: *The diagnosis and detection of breast disease,* St Louis, 1994, Mosby; 54-10 Courtesy Active, Inc., Kalamazoo, Mich; 54-11 Redrawn from *Reach to recovery exercises after breast surgery,* No 4669-PS, Atlanta, 1996, American Cancer Society.

Chapter 55 55-1, 55-2, 55-4 From Seidel HM et al: *Mosby's guide to physical examination,* ed 4, St Louis, 1999, Mosby; 55-8 From Lowdermilk DL et al: *Maternity & women's health care,* ed 7, St Louis, 2000, Mosby; 55-10 From Beare PG, Myers JL: *Adult health nursing,* ed 3, St Louis, 1998, Mosby.

Chapter 56 56-1, 56-2, 56-3, 56-4, 56-5, 56-6 From Centers for Disease Control and Prevention: *Tracking the hidden epidemics: trends in STDs in the United States,* 2000, CDC.

Chapter 57 57-2, 57-3 Redrawn from Stein HA et al: *Ophthalmic terminology: speller and vocabulary builder,* ed 3, St Louis, 1992, Mosby; 57-4, 57-8 Redrawn from Newell FW: *Ophthalmology: principles and concepts,* ed 8, St Louis, 1996, Mosby; 57-6 From Elkin MK et al: *Nursing interventions and clinical skills,* ed 2, St Louis, 2000, Mosby; 57-7, 57-11 From Thompson JM, Wilson SF: *Health assessment for nursing practice,* St Louis, 1996, Mosby; 57-12 From Seidel HM et al: *Mosby's guide to physical examination,* ed 4, St Louis, 1999, Mosby; 57-13 From Ragling EM, Roper-Hall MJ: *Eye injuries,* London, 1986, Gower Medical Publishing; 57-15 From Lewis SM et al: *Medical-surgical nursing: assessment and management of clinical problems,* ed 5, St Louis, 2000, Mosby.

Chapter 58 58-3 Redrawn from Stein HA et al: *The ophthalmic assistant: fundamentals in clinical practice,* St Louis, 1988, Mosby; 58-4 Courtesy Department of Ophthalmology and Visual Sciences, University of Iowa Health Care, Iowa City, Iowa; 58-9 From Sorrentino SA: *Mosby's textbook for nursing assistants,* ed 5, St Louis, 2000, Mosby.

Chapter 59 59-1, 59-2, 59-3, 59-7, 59-8 From Seidel HM et al: *Mosby's guide to physical examination,* ed 4, St Louis, 1999, Mosby; 59-5, 59-6 From Sigler BA, Schuring LT: *Ear, nose, and throat disorders,* St Louis, 1994, Mosby.

Chapter 60 60-2 Courtesy CLG Photographics, St Louis; 60-5, 60-6 Redrawn from Sigler BA, Schuring LT: *Ear, nose, and throat disorders,* St Louis, 1994, Mosby.

Chapter 61 61-1, 61-4 From Monahan FD, Neighbors M: *Medical-surgical nursing: foundations for clinical practice,* ed 2, Philadelphia, 1998, WB Saunders; 61-3 From Seidel HM et al: *Mosby's guide to physical examination,* ed 4, St Louis, 1999, Mosby.

Chapter 62 62-1, 62-2, 62-3, 62-4, 62-5, 62-7, 62-10, 62-11, 62-13, 62-14, 62-15, 62-18 From Habif TP: *Clinical dermatology,* ed 3, St Louis, 1996, Mosby; 62-6 Courtesy Antoinette Hood, MD, Department of Dermatology, University of Indiana School of Medicine, Indianapolis, Ind; 62-8 Courtesy Wellcome Foundation, Ltd; 62-16 Courtesy Gary Monheit, MD, University of Alabama at Birmingham School of Medicine, Birmingham; 62-17 From Mackie RM: *Skin cancer,* ed 2, St Louis, 1996, Mosby; 62-19 From Norton D et al: *An investigation of geriatric nursing problems in hospital,* Edinburgh, 1975, Churchill-Livingstone; 62-20 Copyright Braden B, Bergstrom N, 1988.

Chapter 63 63-11 Courtesy Comprehensive Burn Care Center, MetroHealth Medical Center, Cleveland, Ohio.

Index

E

Q

R

S

T

V

X

Y

Z

Guidelines

Patient Teaching

Nursing Care Plan